TROPICAL INFECTIOUS DISEASES

Commissioning Editor: *Sue Hodgson*
Development Editor: *Sharon Nash*
Editorial Assistant: *Kirsten Lowson*
Project Manager: *Frances Affleck*
Design: *Stewart Larking*
Illustration Manager: *Merlyn Harvey*
Illustrator: *Robert Britton*
Marketing Manager(s) (UK/USA): *Richard Jones/Helena Mutak*

THIRD EDITION

TROPICAL INFECTIOUS DISEASES

Principles, Pathogens and Practice

RICHARD L. GUERRANT MD
Thomas H. Hunter Professor of International Medicine
Director, Center for Global Health, Division of Infectious Diseases and International Health
University of Virginia School of Medicine
Charlottesville, VA, USA

DAVID H. WALKER MD
Carmage and Martha Walls Distinguished University Chair in Tropical Diseases
Director, Center for Biodefense and Emerging Infectious Diseases
Professor and Chair, Department of Pathology
University of Texas Medical Branch
Galveston, TX, USA

PETER F. WELLER MD FACP FIDSA
Professor of Medicine, Harvard Medical School
Professor, Immunology and Infectious Diseases Department, Harvard School of Public Health
Chief, Infectious Disease Division
Vice Chair of Research, Department of Medicine, Beth Israel Deaconess Medical Center
Boston, MA, USA

For additional online content visit
www.expertconsult.com
Expert CONSULT

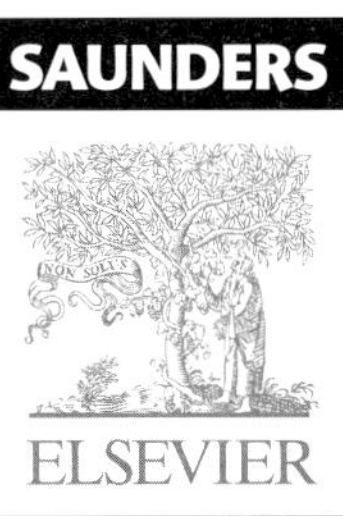

Edinburgh, London, New York, Oxford, Philadelphia, St Louis, Sydney, Toronto

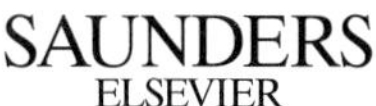

SAUNDERS is an imprint of Elsevier Inc.

First edition 1999
Second edition 2006

Notices

Knowledge and best practice in this field are constantly changing. As new research and experience broaden our understanding, changes in research methods, professional practices, or medical treatment may become necessary. Practitioners and researchers must always rely on their own experience and knowledge in evaluating and using any information, methods, compounds, or experiments described herein. In using such information or methods they should be mindful of their own safety and the safety of others, including parties for whom they have a professional responsibility.

With respect to any drug or pharmaceutical products identified, readers are advised to check the most current information provided (i) on procedures featured or (ii) by the manufacturer of each product to be administered, to verify the recommended dose or formula, the method and duration of administration, and contraindications. It is the responsibility of practitioners, relying on their own experience and knowledge of their patients, to make diagnoses, to determine dosages and the best treatment for each individual patient, and to take all appropriate safety precautions.

To the fullest extent of the law, neither the Publisher nor the authors, contributors, or editors assume any liability for any injury and/or damage to persons or property as a matter of products liability, negligence or otherwise, or from any use or operation of any methods, products, instructions, or ideas contained in the material herein.

Saunders

British Library Cataloguing in Publication Data

Tropical infectious diseases: principles, pathogens and practice. – 3rd ed.
1. Tropical medicine.
I. Guerrant, Richard L. II. Walker, David H., 1943-
III. Weller, Peter F.
616.9′883-dc22

ISBN-13: 9780702039355

A catalogue record for this book is available from the British Library

Library of Congress Cataloging in Publication Data
A catalog record for this book is available from the Library of Congress

The publisher's policy is to use **paper manufactured from sustainable forests**

Printed in China

Last digit is the print number: 9 8 7 6 5 4 3 2 1

CONTENTS

Foreword x
Preface xii
List of Contributors xiii

SECTION I: Principles and General Considerations

1 Principles of Parasitism: Host–Parasite Interactions 1
Juan P. Olano, Peter F. Weller, Richard L. Guerrant, David H. Walker

2 The Perfect Storm: Climate, Ecosystems and Infectious Diseases 8
Fernando J. Torres-Vélez, Corrie Brown

3 Epidemiology and Biostatistics 11
Edward T. Ryan, Megan Murray

4 Social and Cultural Factors in Tropical Medicine: Reframing Our Understanding of Disease 17
Rebecca Dillingham, David A. Walton, Paul E. Farmer

5 Nutrition and Micronutrients in Tropical Infectious Diseases 23
Margaret Kosek, Robert E. Black

6 Host Genetics and Susceptibility to Infection 32
Graham S. Cooke, Michael Levin, Robert J. Wilkinson, Geoffrey Pasvol

7 Disease Eradication and Control 40
David L. Heymann

8 Vector Biology 45
José M.C. Ribeiro, Jesus G. Valenzuela

9 Immunology, Host Defense, Immunodeficiencies, and Vaccines 52
Lisa A. Spencer, Anne Nicholson-Weller

10 Vaccines in the Tropics 63
Alan D.T. Barrett

11 Tropical Infectious Diseases and Malignancy 71
Catherine de Martel, Silvia Franceschi, Julie Parsonnet

12 Chemotherapy of Parasitic Diseases 76
Richard D. Pearson, Peter F. Weller, Richard L. Guerrant

13 Chemotherapy of Bacterial, Fungal, and Viral Diseases 95
Thomas L. Holland, Nathan M. Thielman, Richard D. Pearson

14 Global Surveillance for Emerging Infectious Diseases 105
Ray R. Arthur, James W. LeDuc, James M. Hughes

SECTION II: Pathogens

Part A: Bacterial and Mycobacterial Infections

15 Enteric *Escherichia coli* Infections 110
Theodore S. Steiner, Nathan M. Thielman, Richard L. Guerrant

16 Typhoid and Paratyphoid (Enteric) Fever 121
Myron M. Levine, Milagritos D. Tapia, Anita K.M. Zaidi

17 Nontyphoidal Salmonellosis 128
Christopher C. Moore, Patrick Banura, David A. Pegues, Samuel I. Miller

18 Shigellosis 137
Gerald T. Keusch, Mohammed A. Salam, Dennis J. Kopecko

19 *Campylobacter* Infections 145
Ban Mishu Allos, Albert J. Lastovica

20 Cholera Infections 150
Myron M. Levine, Debasish Saha, A.S.G. Faruque, Samba O. Sow

21 "Noncholera" *Vibrio* Infections 157
J. Glenn Morris, Jr, G. Balakrish Nair

22 Enteric *Clostridium* Infections 162
Cirle A. Warren

23 *Helicobacter pylori* Infections 167
Barry J. Marshall, Robert H. Gilman

24 Meningococcal Disease 174
Alexandre Leite de Souza, Diederik van de Beek, W. Michael Scheld

25 Gonococcal and Other Neisserial Infections 184
Joseph A. Duncan, Lillian B. Brown, Peter A. Leone

26 *Haemophilus ducreyi* Infections 191
Allan R. Ronald

27 *Haemophilus influenzae* 193
Mark C. Steinhoff, Thomas Cherian, Elizabeth P. Schlaudecker

28 Donovanosis 196
Nigel O'Farrell

29 Pneumococcal Infections 199
Keith P. Klugman, Charles Feldman

30 Group A Streptococcal and Staphylococcal Infections 203
Dennis L. Stevens, Amy E. Bryant

31 Pertussis 212
Joshua C. Eby, Erik L. Hewlett

32 Legionellosis 215
Thomas J. Marrie, Paul S. Hoffman

33 Melioidosis 219
Sharon J. Peacock, David A.B. Dance

34 Diphtheria 223
Anna Kabanova, Rino Rappuoli

35 Tuberculosis and Atypical Mycobacterial Infections 228
Edward C. Jones-Lopez, Jerrold J. Ellner

36 *Mycobacterium ulcerans* Infection (Buruli Ulcer) 248
Wayne M. Meyers, Douglas S. Walsh, Françoise Portaels

37 Leprosy 253
Douglas S. Walsh, Wayne M. Meyers

38 Anthrax 261
G. Raghurama Rao, David H. Walker

39 Bartonelloses 265
Christoph Dehio, Ciro Maguiña, David H. Walker

40 Brucellosis 271
Eduardo Gotuzzo, Georgios Pappas

41 Plague 276
Paul S. Mead

42 Tetanus 284
Barnett R. Nathan, Thomas P. Bleck

Part B: Spirochetal Infections

43 Treponemal Infections 289
Joseph D. Tucker, Arlene C. Seña, P. Frederick Sparling, Xiang-Sheng Chen, Myron S. Cohen

44 Relapsing Fever and Other *Borrelia* Diseases 295
Alan G. Barbour

45 Leptospirosis 303
Wun-Ju Shieh, Charles Edwards, Paul N. Levett, Sherif R. Zaki

Part C: Chlamydial Infections

46 Trachoma 308
Chandler R. Dawson, Julius Schachter

47 *Chlamydia trachomatis* Infections of the Genital Tract (Including Lymphogranuloma Venereum) 314
David Mabey, Rosanna W. Peeling

48 Psittacosis 320
Thomas J. Marrie

Part D: Rickettsial and Ehrlichial Infections

49 Spotted Fever Group Rickettsioses 323
Daniel J. Sexton, David H. Walker

50 Typhus Group Rickettsioses 329
David H. Walker, Didier Raoult

51 Scrub Typhus 334
Ik-Sang Kim, David H. Walker

52 Ehrlichioses and Anaplasmosis 339
J. Stephen Dumler

53 Q Fever 344
Thomas J. Marrie

Part E: Viral Infections

54 Measles 347
Jon K. Andrus, Ciro A. De Quadros, Carlos Castillo-Solorzano

55 Hendra and Nipah Viral Infections 352
Thomas G. Ksiazek, K.B. Chua, Paul A. Rota, Pierre E. Rollin

56 Human Herpesvirus Infections 355
S. David Hudnall, Lawrence R. Stanberry, Paul D. Griffiths

57 Smallpox and Related Orthopoxviral Infections 369
Peter B. Jahrling

58 Respiratory Viral Infections 378
José Luiz Proença-Módena, Gustavo Olszanski Acrani, Cynthia B. Snider, Eurico Arruda

59 Severe Acute Respiratory Syndrome (SARS) 392
Mei-Shang Ho

60 Enterovirus Infections, Including Poliomyelitis 398
Mark A. Pallansch

61 Rotavirus Infections 406
Juana Angel, Manuel A. Franco, Harry B. Greenberg

62 Calicivirus Infections 411
Gagandeep Kang, Mary K. Estes, Robert L. Atmar

63 Astroviruses, Enteric Adenoviruses, and Other Gastroenteritis Viral Infections 416
Roger I. Glass, Joseph S. Bresee

64 Enteric Viral Hepatitis A and E 420
Shahid Jameel, Rakesh Aggarwal

65 Viral Hepatitis C 427
Miriam J. Alter

66 Hepatitis B and Deltavirus Infections 433
Ding-Shinn Chen, Pei-Jer Chen

67 Overview of Viral Hemorrhagic Fevers 441
C.J. Peters, Sherif R. Zaki

68 Arenavirus Infections 449
Delia A. Enría, James N. Mills, Dan Bausch, Wun-Ju Shieh, C.J. Peters

69 Rift Valley Fever 462
C.J. Peters, Shinji Makino, J.C. Morrill

70 Crimean-Congo Hemorrhagic Fever 466
Onder Ergonul, Michael R. Holbrook

71 Hantavirus Infections 470
Charles F. Fulhorst, Frederick T. Koster, Delia A. Enría, C.J. Peters

72 Sandfly Fever, Oropouche Fever, and Other Bunyavirus Infections 481
Robert B. Tesh, Pedro F.C. Vasconcelos

73 Filovirus Infections 483
Victoria Wahl-Jensen, C.J. Peters, Peter B. Jahrling, Heinz Feldmann, Jens H. Kuhn

74 Yellow Fever 492
J. Erin Staples, Thomas P. Monath

75 Dengue and Dengue Hemorrhagic Fever 504
Eng Eong Ooi, Duane J. Gubler

76 Japanese Encephalitis, West Nile, and Other Flavivirus Infections 511
Robert B. Tesh, Tom Solomon

77 Tick-borne Encephalitis and Omsk Hemorrhagic Fever 515
Christian W. Mandl, Michael R. Holbrook

78 Alphavirus Infections 519
Scott C. Weaver, David W. Smith

79 Rabies 525
Thomas P. Bleck

80 Human Papillomavirus Infections 532
William Bonnez, Gerhard Lindeque

Part F: Retroviral Infections

81 Human Retroviral Infections in the Tropics 541
Steven J. Reynolds, Pascal O. Bessong, Thomas C. Quinn

Part G: Fungal Infections

82 Dermatophytosis 559
Michael B. Smith, Michael R. McGinnis

83 Mycetoma 565
Ahmed Hassan Fahal

84 Chromoblastomycosis and Phaeohyphomycosis 569
Tadahiko Matsumoto, Chester R. Cooper, Paul J. Szaniszlo

85 Histoplasmosis, Blastomycosis, Coccidioidomycosis, and Cryptococcosis 573
Gregory M. Anstead, Tihana Bicanic, Eduardo Arathoon, John R. Graybill

86 Paracoccidioidomycosis 582
Ricardo Negroni, Gregory M. Anstead, John R. Graybill

87 Penicilliosis Marneffei 586
Khuanchai Supparatpinyo, Gregory M. Anstead, John R. Graybill

88 Mucocutaneous and Deeply Invasive Candidiasis 589
Shmuel Shoham, Marcio Nucci, Thomas J. Walsh

89 Mucormycosis 597
Thomas J. Walsh, Emmanuel Roilides, John H. Rex, Michael R. McGinnis

90 Entomophthoramycosis, Lobomycosis, Rhinosporidiosis, and Sporotrichosis 603
Duane R. Hospenthal

91 Pneumocystosis 608
Peter D. Walzer, A. George Smulian, Robert F. Miller

Part H: Protozoan Infections

92 Enteric Amebiasis 614
Kristine M. Peterson, Upinder Singh, William A. Petri, Jr

93 Intestinal Flagellate and Ciliate Infections 623
David R. Hill, Theodore E. Nash

94 Cryptosporidiosis 633
Aldo A.M. Lima, Amidou Samie, Richard L. Guerrant

95 *Cyclospora*, *Isospora*, and *Sarcocystis* Infections 641
Ynés R. Ortega, Jean W. Pape

96 Malaria 646
Stephen L. Hoffman, Carlos C. (Kent) Campbell, Nicholas J. White

97 Babesiosis 676
Sam R. Telford III, Peter F. Weller, James H. Maguire

98 African Trypanosomiasis (Sleeping Sickness) 682
Jacques Pépin, John E. Donelson

99 American Trypanosomiasis (Chagas Disease) 689
Louis V. Kirchhoff

100 Leishmaniasis 696
Selma M.B. Jeronimo, Anastacio de Queiroz Sousa, Richard D. Pearson

101 Pathogenic and Opportunistic Free-Living Amebae: *Acanthamoeba* spp., *Balamuthia mandrillaris*, *Naegleria fowleri*, and *Sappinia pedata* 707
Govinda S. Visvesvara, Sharon L. Roy, James H. Maguire

102 Microsporidiosis 714
Louis M. Weiss, David A. Schwartz

103 Toxoplasmosis 722
Joseph D. Schwartzman, James H. Maguire

Part I: Nematode Infections

104 Lymphatic Filariasis 729
Thomas B. Nutman, James W. Kazura

105 Loiasis and *Mansonella* Infections 735
Amy D. Klion, Thomas B. Nutman

106 Onchocerciasis 741
Achim M. Hoerauf

107 Zoonotic Filariasis 750
Mark L. Eberhard

108 Dracunculiasis 759
Ernesto Ruiz-Tiben, Donald R. Hopkins

109 Toxocariasis and Larva Migrans Syndromes 763
James S. McCarthy, Thomas A. Moore

110 Trichinellosis 768
Fabrizio Bruschi, K. Darwin Murrell

111 Angiostrongyliasis 774
John H. Cross†, Kao-Pin Hwang

112 Other Tissue Nematode Infections 778
Yezid Gutierrez

113 Enterobiasis 788
Thomas A. Moore, James S. McCarthy

114 Trichuriasis 791
Nilanthi R. de Silva, Edward S. Cooper

115 Ascariasis 794
David J. Diemert

116 Hookworm Infections 799
Peter J. Hotez

117 Strongyloidiasis 805
Afzal A. Siddiqui, Robert M. Genta, Ismael Maguilnik, Steven L. Berk

Part J: Cestode Infections

118 Introduction to Tapeworm Infections 813
Herbert B. Tanowitz, Murray Wittner, A. Clinton White, Jr

119 Cysticercosis 815
Hector H. Garcia, Christina M. Coyle, A. Clinton White, Jr

120 Echinococcosis 824
Peter M. Schantz, Peter Kern, Enrico Brunetti

121 *Taenia* and Other Tapeworm Infections 839
Murray Wittner, A. Clinton White, Jr, Herbert B. Tanowitz

Part K: Trematode Infections

122 Schistosomiasis 848
Charles H. King

123 Liver, Lung, and Intestinal Fluke Infections 854
Siddhartha Mahanty, J. Dick Maclean†, John H. Cross†

Part L: Ectoparasitic Infections

124 Arthropods, Tongue Worms, Leeches, and Arthropod-borne Diseases 868
Jerome Goddard

SECTION III: Practice: Approach to the Patient in the Tropics

125 Distinguishing Tropical Infectious Diseases from Bioterrorism 879
Juan P. Olano, C.J. Peters, David H. Walker

126 Health Advice for International Travel 887
Jay S. Keystone, Robert Steffen, Phyllis E. Kozarsky

127 Migrant, Immigrant, and Refugee Health 902
Luis S. Ortega, Rachel B. Eidex, Martin S. Cetron

128 Infectious Diseases in Modern Military Forces 910
Alan J. Magill, Bonnie L. Smoak, Truman W. Sharp

129 Gastrointestinal Symptoms 916
Luis M. Valdez, Eduardo Gotuzzo, Nathan M. Thielman, Herbert L. DuPont

130 Fever and Systemic Symptoms 925
Mary E. Wilson, Andrea K. Boggild

131 Eosinophilia 939
Mary E. Wilson, Peter F. Weller

132 Cutaneous Lesions 950
Steven D. Mawhorter, David L. Longworth

133 Hepatobiliary Disease 975
Mohammad S. Khuroo, Mehnaaz S. Khuroo

134 Approach to the Patient in the Tropics with Pulmonary Disease 982
Gregory J. Martin

135 Ocular Disease 991
Edward T. Ryan, Marlene Durand

136 Neurologic Disease 1017
Tom Solomon, Mustapha A. Danesi, Frank J. Bia, Thomas P. Bleck

137 Approach to the Patient in the Tropics with Anemia 1024
Saad H. Abdalla, Geoffrey Pasvol

138 Sexually Transmitted and Urinary Tract Infections 1033
Arlene C. Seña, Allan R. Ronald, Kimberley K. Fox, Myron S. Cohen

139 Approach to the Patient with HIV and Coinfecting Tropical Infectious Diseases 1046
Christopher L. Karp, Siddhartha Mahanty

140 Delusional Parasitosis 1066
Kathryn N. Suh, Jay S. Keystone

141 Tropical Infectious Disease Concerns in Pregnancy 1072
Raul E. Isturiz, Eduardo Gotuzzo

Index 1082

FOREWORD

CRISIS IN THE MAINTENANCE OF GLOBAL HEALTH

This third edition of the now classic *Tropical Infectious Diseases: Principles, Pathogens and Practices* emerges at a time of crisis in the struggle to maintain global health. Present challenges include the serious consequences of uncontrolled growth in human population; climatic extremes that create humanitarian disasters, and international spread of new, virulent, and treatment-resistant pathogens; and failures and derelictions by politicians and international organizations in the quest for a fairer distribution of resources. Some of these problems were identified in my Forewords to the first (1999) and second (2006) editions of this marvellous book but, since then, they have intensified, unabated.

AN INCREASING ROLE FOR THE SPECIALITY OF TROPICAL MEDICINE

The speciality of Tropical Medicine (with Tropical Infectious Diseases as its largest component) is an unusually broad discipline. It encompasses sciences as diverse as economics, anthropology, zoology, agriculture, epidemiology, and molecular biology, equipping it to meet many of the challenges to maintaining global health. The increasing role and relevance of this approach is argued persuasively by each succeeding chapter of this book, which has been scrupulously edited by the successful team of Dick Guerrant, David Walker and Peter Weller. The third edition is resplendent in full color, a great advantage for the memorable display of clinical images, life cycles, and tables. The standardized distribution maps are a particular delight – making the lack of them for important pathogens, such as Borrelioses (with multiple agents and incomplete data as noted in Chapter 44) and Parastrongyliasis (with a broadening global range as noted in Chapter 111), all the more frustrating! – but users should beware of unwarranted certainty that a disease does not occur outside the prescribed area (e.g., malaria in Great Exuma, Bahamas occurring in travelers to March 2008). Some second-edition maps have been corrected (e.g., in Chapter 43, pinta is restored to southern Mexico and yaws to Java). The convenience and compactness of compression into a single volume is at the expense of relegating the plentiful and welcome references to a website, a cost- and space-saving inconvenience for readers of the hard copy. It is gratifying that the proportion of international authors has been increased with each new edition and that some exciting new chapters have been added. However, Karr's apothegm "plus ça change, plus c'est la même chose" is highly apposite. What is so reassuring about the invigoratingly new and fresh presentation of this third edition of *Tropical Infectious Diseases* is that it continues to reemphasize, with supporting arguments and evidence, the fundamental tenets of our specialty. The following are but three examples.

POVERTY, HUMAN DISASTERS, AND TROPICAL DISEASE (CHAPTERS 2, 7)

The link between poverty, tropical developing countries, and (often classic tropical) infectious diseases is undeniable. It is partly explained by underlying deficiencies in nutrition (Chapter 5), sanitation, and safe food and water supplies, but the role of climate and vulnerability to natural disasters has become increasingly obvious in recent earthquake, flood, and famine tragedies (Chapter 2). Nobel economics laureate Amartya Sen has emphasized the political devisiveness of human disasters, both within and between nations, a principle well illustrated by the January 2010 Haitian earthquake.[1] The climate change debate continues and, in mid 2010, critical diversions of the jet stream in the upper atmosphere are likely to have caused both the devastating floods in Pakistan and north-eastern China and the heat wave in Russia. In the aftermath of natural disasters, infectious diseases become the leading cause of death. For example, in the Bengal famine of 1943–6, 80% of the 2–3 million excess deaths were attributable to endemic infections, principally malaria, other fevers and diarrhoeal diseases.[1] In the response to such cataclysmic events, the experience, skills and multidisciplinary approach of Tropical Medicine professionals can be of decisive importance (Chapters 2, 7).

EMERGING PATTERNS OF TROPICAL DISEASES (CHAPTER 14)

Since the publication of the second edition, the attention of WHO and national public health bodies has been largely preoccupied or distracted by the threat of an H1N1 influenza pandemic. The redistribution of massive funding towards this contingency has had serious repercussions for control of other major diseases, especially the neglected tropical infectious diseases. The wisdom and propriety of WHO's interpretation of the epidemiology and handling of this emergency is now the subject of intense enquiry.[2,3] In the meantime, other less publicized viral pandemics have swept across tropical regions. Chikungunya (Chapter 78) appeared in western Indian Ocean islands in early 2005 causing 100,000s of cases during which the A226V mutation was selected, allowing transmission by *Aedes albopictus* mosquitoes and increased virulence, and followed by spread to India (1.42 million reported cases), elsewhere in South Asia, Africa, and in rural Emilia-Romagna in Italy where autochthonous transmission was established for a while in 2007.[4]

Human encroachment on the natural environment with consequent ecologic disturbance and degradation has been associated with the emergence of lethal pathogens including filoviruses (Chapter 73), arenaviruses (Chapter 68), henipaviruses/paramyxoviruses (Chapter 55), rhabdoviruses (Chapter 79), and coronaviruses (Chapter 58). Growing evidence implicates distinctive mammalian vectors, many of which are bats whose importance for human health is becoming apparent.[5]

GLOBALIZATION OF TROPICAL PATHOGENS WITH THEIR RESISTANCE TO THERAPEUTIC AGENTS (CHAPTERS 12, 13, 15, 35, 96, 122)

The geographic dimension, so integral to Tropical Medicine, is well illustrated by the global threat now posed by Gram-negative Enterobacteriaceae with resistance to carbapenem conferred by the

^{bla}NDM-1 (New Delhi metallo-beta-lactamase) gene. A collaborative study between UK, India, and Pakistan has revealed that many patients in UK harbouring NDM-1 organisms had travel, hospital, or other links with India and Pakistan.[6] NDM-1 importations from the Indian subcontinent have also been reported in other European countries, North America, and Australia. Multiply antibiotic-resistant *Acinetobacter baumannii-calcoaceticus* complex bacteria were imported in military and civilian casualties from field hospitals in Iraq to USA and UK where they pose an increasing risk to immunocompromised or severely ill patients in intensive care units.[7] Another example would be the spread of extensively and totally resistant *Mycobacterium tuberculosis*.[8] The breakthrough achieved in the treatment of multiply-resistant *Plasmodium falciparum* malaria (Chapter 96) is currently threatened by emergence of artemisinin resistance. Artesunate-resistant *P. falciparum* was first confirmed in Pailin on the Cambodia–Thailand border in 2008[9] but is now suspected in other border areas of countries along the Mekong River (Cambodia, China (Yunnan Province), the Lao People's Democratic Republic, Myanmar, Thailand, and Vietnam) although its presence in South America and African countries is unconfirmed.[10] Another wonder drug, praziquantel, which revolutionized the treatment of schistosomiasis (Chapter 122) may also be losing its efficacy against *S. mansoni* in Senegal, Egypt[11] and Uganda.

Much is happening in the world of tropical infectious diseases but both continuity and change in this fascinating field are brilliantly reflected in Guerrant, Walker, and Weller's book, which I strongly recommend as a comprehensive, critical, up-to-date, and beautifully presented review.

David A. Warrell
University of Oxford, UK
August 2010

REFERENCES

1. Sen A. Human Disasters. In Warrell DA, Cox TM, Firth JD, eds. *Oxford Textbook of Medicine*. 3rd ed. Oxford: Oxford University Press; 2010: 119.
2. British Medical Journal Correspondence: Laurell AC, Herrera JR. What happened in Mexico? BMJ. 2010;340:c3465. Zarocostas J. WHO swine flu review committee promises to probe links with drug industry. BMJ. 2010;341:c3648.
3. Lancet Infectious Diseases. Leading Edge. WHO failing in duty of transparency. *Lancet Infectious Diseases*. 2010;10:505.
4. Townson H, Nathan MB. Resurgence of chikungunya. *Trans R Soc Trop Med Hyg*. 2008 Apr;102(4):308.
5. Wong S, Lau S, Woo P, Yuen KY. Bats as a continuing source of emerging infections in humans. *Rev Med Virol*. 2007 Mar-Apr;17(2):67.
6. Kumarasamy KK, et al. Emergence of a new antibiotic resistance mechanism in India, Pakistan, and the UK: a molecular, biological, and epidemiological study. *Lancet Infect Dis*. 2010 Aug 10. [Epub ahead of print]
7. Scott P, et al. An outbreak of multidrug-resistant *Acinetobacter baumannii-calcoaceticus* complex infection in the US military health care system associated with military operations in Iraq. *Clin Infect Dis*. 2007 Jun 15;44(12):1577.
8. Gandhi NR et al. Multidrug-resistant and extensively drug-resistant tuberculosis: a threat to global control of tuberculosis. *Lancet*. 2010 May 22;375(9728):1830.
9. Dondorp AM et al. Artemisinin resistance: current status and scenarios for containment. *Nat Rev Microbiol*. 2010 Apr;8(4):272.
10. WHO. Prevention and treatment of artemisinin-resistant falciparum malaria: update for international travellers. *Wkly Epidemiol Rec*. 2010 May 21;85(21):195.
11. Doenhoff MJ, Cioli D, Utzinger J. Praziquantel: mechanisms of action, resistance and new derivatives for schistosomiasis. *Curr Opin Infect Dis*. 2008;21:659.

PREFACE

In our rapidly changing world, both tropical infectious diseases and, contemporaneously, the third edition of *Tropical Infectious Diseases: Principles, Pathogens and Practice* have evolved substantially since the first and second editions of the book in 1999 and 2006. New agents and new threats from terrorism, increasing antimicrobial resistance, and climate and ecologic changes have created some "perfect storms," as noted in a new Chapter 2 by Torres-Velez and Brown. Other entirely new chapters by new authors include those on Vaccines, SARS, separate Hepatitis A–E chapters, Crimean-Congo hemorrhagic fever, Tick-borne Encephalitis and Omsk Hemorrhagic Fever, Human Papillomavirus, and mucormycosis. In addition, the number of authors has increased from 231 to 271, with the number of international contributors nearly doubling from 54 to 102, representing 38 (including 15 new) countries around the world.

As well as the new, topically pertinent chapters, all chapters from the previous edition have been thoroughly revised and updated, and this third edition also benefits from new, full color presentations of illustrative, clinical and scientific material throughout. Life cycle diagrams that follow the original format of human involvement in the top half and environmental stages in the bottom half, with clinically pertinent boxes annotating the human disease manifestations of infection during the pathogens' development in humans, are also presented in full color. Further life cycle diagrams have been included to illustrate additional microbial pathogens. The book has been condensed into a more handy single volume, while still retaining our philosophy and mission of providing useful, authoritative, scholarly, and contemporary knowledge. Consistent with our interests in providing a fully referenced text that is evidence-based and founded in current published knowledge, all chapters are fully referenced; the references are easily accessible, together with their abstracts, via on-line links.

What has *not* changed is our steadfast commitment to comprehensive excellence that combines cutting edge molecular and pathophysiologic science and epidemiology with practical clinical and field experience and is reflected throughout by our outstanding authors. Our authors are the best in their fields, and we are privileged to benefit from their perspectives on the most relevant science, medicine and epidemiology of tropical infectious diseases. To them we owe a huge debt of gratitude.

Finally, we thank our superbly capable and organized Development Editor, Sharon Nash. Likewise, we thank Mary Ann Winecoff, Rachel Stella, Doris Baker, and Sherrill Hebert, our Publishing Director, Sue Hodgson, and our Project Manager, Frances Affleck, whose labors have made this completely new, full color volume possible. We also acknowledge our spouses, Nancy, Margie, and Anne, who have again supported us as we have endeavored with our authors to produce an extensively updated third edition of *Tropical Infectious Diseases: Principles, Pathogens and Practice*.

Richard L. Guerrant, MD
David H. Walker, MD
Peter F. Weller, MD

CONTRIBUTORS

Saad H. Abdalla, MD
Honorary Clinical Senior Lecturer, Department of Medicine, Imperial College London, London, UK
Chapter 137

Gustavo Olszanski Acrani, PhD
Research Fellow, Department of Cell Biology and Virology Research Center, University of São Paulo School of Medicine, Ribeirão Preto, SP, Brazil
Chapter 58

Rakesh Aggarwal, MD DM
Professor, Department of Gastroenterology, Sanjay Gandhi Postgraduate Institute of Medical Sciences, Lucknow, India
Chapter 64

Ban Mishu Allos, MD
Assistant Professor of Medicine and Preventive Medicine, Vanderbilt University School of Medicine, Nashville, TN, USA
Chapter 19

Miriam J. Alter, PhD
Robert E. Shope Professor in Infectious Disease Epidemiology, Director, Infectious Disease Epidemiology Program, Institute for Human Infections and Immunity, Professor, Department of Internal Medicine, University of Texas Medical Branch, Galveston, TX, USA
Chapter 65

Jon K. Andrus, MD
Deputy Director, Pan American Health Organization, Washington, DC, USA
Chapter 54

Juana Angel, MD PhD
Professor, Instituto de Genética Humana, Facultad de Medicina, Pontificia Universidad Javeriana, Bogotá, Colombia
Chapter 61

Gregory M. Anstead, MD PhD
Associate Professor, Department of Medicine, Division of Infectious Diseases, University of Texas Health Sciences Center, Director, Immunosuppression and Infectious Diseases Clinics, South Texas Veterans Healthcare System, San Antonio, TX, USA
Chapters 85, 86, and 87

Eduardo Arathoon, MD
Director Médico, Clínica Familiar Luis Ángel García, Asociación de Salud Integral, Guatemala City, Guatemala
Chapter 85

Eurico Arruda, MD PhD
Professor of Microbiology, Department of Cell Biology and Virology Research Center, University of São Paulo School of Medicine, Ribeirão Preto, SP, Brazil
Chapter 58

Ray R. Arthur, PhD
Director, Global Disease Detection Operations Center, Division of Global Disease Detection and Emergency Response, Center for Global Health, Centers for Disease Control and Prevention, Atlanta, GA, USA
Chapter 14

Robert L. Atmar, MD
Professor, Departments of Medicine and Molecular Virology and Microbiology, Baylor College of Medicine, Houston, TX, USA
Chapter 62

Patrick Banura, MBChB MPH
Head of Department, Department of Community Health, Masaka Regional Referral Hospital, Masaka, Uganda
Chapter 17

Alan G. Barbour, MD
Professor, Microbiology & Molecular Genetics and Medicine, School of Medicine, University of California-Irvine, Director, Pacific-Southwest Regional Center of Excellence for Biodefense and Emerging Infections, Irvine, CA, USA
Chapter 44

Alan D.T. Barrett, PhD
John D. Stobo MD Distinguished Chair in Vaccinology, Director, Sealy Center for Vaccine Development, Professor, Department of Pathology, University of Texas Medical Branch, Galveston, TX, USA
Chapter 10

Dan Bausch, MD MPH&TM
Associate Professor, Department of Tropical Medicine, Tulane School of Public Health and Tropical Medicine, Associate Professor, Department of Medicine, Section of Infectious Diseases, Tulane University Medical Center, New Orleans, LA, USA
Chapter 68

Steven L. Berk, MD
Professor and Dean, School of Medicine, Texas Tech University Health Science Center, Lubbock, TX, USA
Chapter 117

Pascal O. Bessong, MSc PhD
Head, Department of Microbiology, Principal Investigator, AIDS Virus Research Laboratory, University of Venda, Thohoyandou, South Africa
Chapter 81

Frank J. Bia, MD MPH
Professor (Emeritus) Internal Medicine, Yale School of Medicine, Medical Director, AmeriCares, Stamford, CT, USA
Chapter 136

Tihana Bicanic, MD
Research Fellow and Honorary Consultant in Infections Disease, Department of Infectious Diseases, St George's University of London, London, UK
Chapter 85

Robert E. Black, MD MPH
Edgar Berman Professor and Chair, Department of International Health, Johns Hopkins Bloomberg School of Public Health, Baltimore, MD, USA
Chapter 5

Thomas P. Bleck, MD FCCM
Professor of Neurological Sciences, Neurosurgery, Medicine, and Anesthesiology, and Assistant Dean, Rush Medical College, Associate Chief Medical Officer (Critical Care), Rush University Medical Center, Chicago, IL, USA
Chapters 42, 79, and 136

Andrea K. Boggild, MSc MD FRCPC
Staff Physician, Tropical Disease Unit, Division of Infectious Diseases, Department of Medicine, University Health Network-Toronto General Hospital, Toronto, ON, Canada
Chapter 130

William Bonnez, MD
Associate Professor of Medicine, Infectious Diseases Division, University of Rochester School of Medicine, Rochester, NY, USA
Chapter 80

Joseph S. Bresee, MD
Chief, Epidemiology and Prevention Branch, Influenza Division, Centers for Disease Control and Prevention, Atlanta, GA, USA
Chapter 63

Corrie Brown, DVM PhD
Josiah Meigs Distinguished Professor, Department of Veterinary Pathology, College of Veterinary Medicine, University of Georgia, Athens, GA, USA
Chapter 2

Lillian B. Brown, MPH PhD
Research Associate Department of Epidemiology, University of North Carolina – Chapel Hill School of Medicine, Gillings School of Global Public Health, Chapel Hill, NC, USA
Chapter 25

Enrico Brunetti, MD
Assistant Professor of Infectious Diseases, University of Pavia, Staff Physician, Division of Infectious and Tropical Diseases, IRCCS S. Matteo Hospital Foundation, Pavia, Italy
Chapter 120

Fabrizio Bruschi, MD
Professor of Parasitology, Department of Experimental Pathology, MBIE, Università di Pisa, Scuola Medica, Pisa, Italy
Chapter 110

Amy E. Bryant, PhD
Research Scientist, Infectious Disease Section, Veterans Affairs Medical Center, Boise, ID; Affiliate Assistant Professor, Department of Medicine, University of Washington, Seattle, WA, USA
Chapter 30

Carlos C. (Kent) Campbell, MD MPH
Director, Malaria Control Program, PATH, Seattle, WA, USA
Chapter 96

Carlos Castillo-Solorzano, MD MPH
Regional Advisor on Vaccines and Immunization, Pan American Health Organization, Washington, DC, USA
Chapter 54

Martin S. Cetron, MD
Director, Division of Global Migration and Quarantine, NCEZID, CDC, National Center for Emerging and Zoonotic Infectious Diseases, Atlanta, GA, USA
Chapter 127

Ding-Shinn Chen, MD
Distinguished Chair Professor, Division of Gastroenterology and Hepatology, Department of Internal Medicine, National Taiwan University College of Medicine, Staff Physician, Hepatitis Research Center, National Taiwan University Hospital, Taipei, Taiwan
Chapter 66

Pei-Jer Chen, MD PhD
Professor, Division of Gastroenterology and Hepatology, Department of Internal Medicine, National Taiwan University College of Medicine, Staff Physician, Hepatitis Research Center, National Taiwan University Hospital, Taipei, Taiwan
Chapter 66

Xiang-Sheng Chen, MD PhD
Professor and Vice-Director, National Center for STD Control, Nanjing, China
Chapter 43

Thomas Cherian, MD
Coordinator, Expanded Programme on Immunization, Department of Immunization, Vaccines and Biologicals, World Health Organization, Geneva, Switzerland
Chapter 27

K.B. Chua, MBBS MMed MD PhD FRCPE FRCPath
Consultant Virologist, National Public Health Laboratory, Ministry of Health Malaysia, Selangor, Malaysia
Chapter 55

Myron S. Cohen, MD
J. Herbert Bate Distinguished Professor, Medicine, Microbiology and Immunology and Public Health, Chief, Division of Infectious Diseases, Director, Institute of Global Health and Infectious Diseases, The University of North Carolina at Chapel Hill, Chapel Hill, NC, USA
Chapters 43 and 138

Graham S. Cooke
Senior Lecturer Infectious Diseases, Imperial College London, UK Honorary Associate Professor, University of KwaZulu Natal, South Africa
Chapter 6

Chester R. Cooper, Jr, PhD
Professor of Biological Sciences, Department of Biological Sciences, Youngstown State University, Youngstown, OH, USA
Chapter 84

Edward S. Cooper, MBBS FRCP
Clinical Consultant, Partnership for Child Development, Department of Infectious Disease Epidemiology, Imperial College, London, UK
Chapter 114

Christina M. Coyle, MD MS
Professor of Clinical Medicine, Albert Einstein College of Medicine, Director of the Tropical Medicine Clinic, Bronx Municipal Hospital, Jacobi Medical Center, Bronx, NY, USA
Chapter 119

John H. Cross[†], PhD
Professor, Tropical Public Health, Department of Preventive Medicine and Biometrics, Uniformed Services University of the Health Sciences, Bethesda, MD, USA
Chapters 111 and 123

David A.B. Dance, MB ChB MSc FRCPath
Regional Microbiologist (South West), Health Protection Agency, Plymouth, Devon, UK
Chapter 33

[†]deceased

Mustapha A. Danesi, MB FRCPI FMCP FWACP
Professor, Department of Medicine, College of Medicine, University of Lagos, Consultant Physician and Neurologist, Clinical Department of Medicine, Lagos University Teaching Hospital, Lagos, Lagos State, Nigeria
Chapter 136

Chandler R. Dawson, MD
Professor Emeritus of Ophthalmology, Francis I. Proctor Foundation, University of California, San Francisco, San Francisco, CA, USA
Chapter 46

Catherine de Martel, MD PhD
Fellow, International Agency for Research on Cancer, Lyon, France
Chapter 11

Ciro A. De Quadros, MD
Executive Vice-President, Albert B. Sabin Vaccine Institute, Washington, DC, USA
Chapter 54

Anastacio de Queiroz Sousa, MD
Associate Professor of Medicine, Department of Clinical Medicine, School of Medicine, Federal University of Ceara, Director, Hospital São Jose for Infectious Diseases, Fortaleza, Ceara, Brazil
Chapter 100

Nilanthi R. de Silva, MBBS MSc MD
Professor of Parasitology, Faculty of Medicine, University of Kelaniya, Kelaniya, Ragama, Sri Lanka
Chapter 114

Alexandre Leite de Souza, MD
Infectious Diseases Specialist, Department of Medical Sciences, University of São Paulo School of Medicine (FM USP), São Paulo, Brazil
Chapter 24

Christoph Dehio, PhD
Professor of Molecular Microbiology, Biozentrum of the University of Basel, Basel, Switzerland
Chapter 39

David J. Diemert, MD FRCP(C)
Assistant Professor, Department of Microbiology, Immunology and Tropical Medicine, The George Washington University School of Medicine, Director of Clinical Trials, Sabin Vaccine Institute, Washington, DC, USA
Chapter 115

Rebecca Dillingham, MD MPH
Center for Global Health, Assistant Professor of Medicine, Division of Infectious Disease and International Health, University of Virginia Health System, Charlottesville, VA, USA
Chapter 4

John E. Donelson, PhD
Professor of Biochemistry, Carver College of Medicine, University of Iowa, Iowa City, Iowa, USA
Chapter 98

J. Stephen Dumler, MD
Professor, Associate Director of Clinical Microbiology, Director of Parasitology Laboratory, Division of Medical Microbiology, Department of Pathology, The Johns Hopkins University School of Medicine, The Johns Hopkins Hospital; Department of Molecular Microbiology and Immunology, The Johns Hopkins University Bloomberg School of Public Health, Baltimore, MD, USA
Chapter 52

Joseph A. Duncan, MD PhD
Assistant Professor of Medicine and Pharmacology, University of North Carolina School of Medicine, Department of Medicine, Division of Infectious Diseases, Chapel Hill, NC, USA
Chapter 25

Herbert L. DuPont, MD
Chief of Internal Medicine, St. Luke's Episcopal Hospital, Director, Center for Infectious Diseases, The University of Texas School of Public Health, Vice Chairman, Department of Medicine, Baylor College of Medicine, Houston, TX, USA
Chapter 129

Marlene L. Durand, MD
Assistant Professor of Medicine, Harvard Medical School, Director, Infectious Disease Service, Massachusetts Eye and Ear Infirmary, Physician, Massachusetts General Hospital, Boston, MA, USA
Chapter 135

Mark L. Eberhard, PhD
Director, Division of Parasitic Diseases, Centers for Disease Control and Prevention, Atlanta, GA, USA
Chapter 107

Joshua C. Eby, MD
Assistant Professor, Division of Infectious Diseases and International Health, Department of Medicine, University of Virginia School of Medicine, Charlottesville, VA, USA
Chapter 31

Charles Edwards, MB BS FRCPC FACP
Department Head, Department of Medicine, Queen Elizabeth Hospital, St Michael, Barbados
Chapter 45

Rachel B. Eidex, PhD
Chief, Refugee Health Program for Africa, Division of Global Migration and Quarantine, Centers for Disease Control and Prevention,
Nairobi, Kenya
Chapter 127

Jerrold J. Ellner, MD
Professor of Medicine, Boston University School of Medicine, Chief, Section of Infectious Diseases, Boston Medical Center, Boston, MA, USA
Chapter 35

Delia A. Enría, MD MPH
Director, Instituto Nacional de Enfermedades Virales Humanas, Pergamino, Argentina
Chapters 68 and 71

Onder Ergonul, MD MPH
Professor of Infectious Diseases, Marmara University, School of Medicine, Istanbul, Turkey
Chapter 70

Mary K. Estes, MD
Professor, Departments of Molecular Virology and Microbiology and Medicine, Baylor College of Medicine, Houston, TX, USA
Chapter 62

Ahmed Hassan Fahal, MBBS FRCS MD MS
Professor of Surgery, Mycetoma Research Centre, University of Khartoum, Khartoum, Sudan
Chapter 83

Paul E. Farmer, MD PhD
Maude and Lillian Presley Professor of Social Medicine, Chair, Department of Global Health and Social Medicine, Harvard Medical School, Chief, Division of Global Health Equity, Brigham and Women's Hospital, Co-founder, Partners in Health, Boston, MA
Chapter 4

A.S.G. Faruque, MBBS MPH
Scientist, International Centre for Diarrhoeal Disease Research, Bangladesh (ICDDR,B), Dhaka, Bangladesh
Chapter 20

Charles Feldman, MB BCh DSc PhD
Professor of Pulmonology and Chief Physician, Charlotte Maxeke Johannesburg Academic Hospital and University of the Witwatersrand, Division of Pulmonology, Department of Internal Medicine, Faculty of Health Sciences, University of the Witwatersrand Medical School, Johannesburg, South Africa
Chapter 29

Heinz Feldmann, MD
Chief, Laboratory of Virology, Division of Intramural Research, NIAID, NIH, Rocky Mountain Laboratories, Hamilton, MT, USA
Chapter 73

Kimberley K. Fox, MD MPH
Medical Epidemiologist, Centers for Disease Control and Prevention, Atlanta, GA, USA
Chapter 138

Silvia Franceschi, MD
Head, Section of Infections, International Agency for Research on Cancer, Lyon, France
Chapter 11

Manuel A. Franco, MD PhD
Professor, Instituto de Genética Humana, Facultad de Medicina, Pontificia Universidad Javeriana, Bogotá, Colombia
Chapter 61

Charles F. Fulhorst, DVM DrPH
Professor, University of Texas Medical Branch at Galveston, Department of Pathology, Galveston, TX, USA
Chapter 71

Hector H. Garcia, MD PhD
Professor, Department of Microbiology, School of Sciences, Director, Center for Global Health, Universidad Peruana Cayetano Heredia, Lima, Peru
Chapter 119

Robert M. Genta, MD
Chief for Academic Affairs, Caris Life Sciences, Irving, Texas, Clinical Professor of Pathology and Medicine (Gastroenterology), University of Texas Southwestern Medical Center at Dallas, Staff Pathologist, Dallas Veterans Affairs Medical Center, Dallas, TX, USA
Chapter 117

Robert H. Gilman, MD DTM&H
Professor, International Health, Director, Institute of Tropical Medicine and Public Health, Johns Hopkins Bloomberg School of Public Health, Baltimore, MD, USA
Chapter 23

Roger I. Glass, MD PhD
Director, Fogarty International Center, National Institutes of Health, Bethesda, MD, USA
Chapter 63

Jerome Goddard, PhD
Associate Extension Professor of Medical and Veterinary Entomology, Mississippi State University, Department of Entomology and Plant Pathology, Mississippi State University, MS, USA
Chapter 124

Eduardo Gotuzzo, MD FACP FIDSA
Director, Instituto de Medicina Tropical "Alexander von Humboldt," Universidad Peruana Cayetano Heredia, Head, Departamento de Enfermedades Infecciosas Tropicales y Dermatológicas, Hospital Nacional Cayetano Heredia, Lima, Peru
Chapters 40, 129, and 141

John R. Graybill, MD
Professor of Medicine (Emeritus), Department of Medicine, Division of Infectious Diseases, University of Texas Health Science Center, San Antonio, TX, USA
Chapters 85, 86, and 87

Harry B. Greenberg, MD
Senior Associate Dean for Research, Joseph D. Grant Professor of Medicine and Microbiology and Immunology, Stanford University School of Medicine, Stanford, CA, USA
Chapter 61

Paul D. Griffiths, MBBS MD DSc FRCPath
Professor of Virology, University College London Medical School, Centre for Virology, UCL Medical School, London, UK
Chapter 56

Duane J. Gubler, ScD FAAAS FIDSA
Professor and Director, Program on Emerging Infectious Diseases, Duke-NUS Graduate Medical School, Singapore, Asia-Pacific Institute of Tropical Medicine and Infectious Diseases, University of Hawaii, Honolulu, Hawaii, USA
Chapter 75

Richard L. Guerrant, MD
Thomas H. Hunter Professor of International Medicine, Director, Center for Global Health, Division of Infectious Diseases and International Health, University of Virginia School of Medicine, Charlottesville, VA, USA
Chapters 1, 12, 15, and 94

Yezid Gutierrez, MD PhD
Retired, Formerly Adjunct, Laboratory Medicine, Cleveland Clinic, Cleveland, OH, USA
Chapter 112

Erik L. Hewlett, MD
Professor of Medicine, Division of Infectious Diseases and International Health, Department of Medicine, University of Virginia School of Medicine, Charlottesville, VA, USA
Chapter 31

David L. Heymann, MD
Professor, Infectious Disease Epidemiology, London School of Hygiene and Tropical Medicine, Head and Senior Fellow, Chatham House Centre on Global Health Security, London, UK
Chapter 7

David R. Hill, MD DTM&H FRCP FFTM
Honorary Professor, London School of Hygiene and Tropical Medicine, Director, National Travel Health Network and Centre, University College London Hospitals, NHS Foundation Trust, London, UK
Chapter 93

Mei-Shang Ho, MD MPH
Fellow, Institute of Biomedical Sciences, Academia Sinica, Taipei, Taiwan
Chapter 59

Achim M. Hoerauf, MD
Professor of Microbiology and Parasitology, Director and Chair, Institute of Medical Microbiology, Immunology and Parasitology, University of Bonn Medical Center, Bonn, Germany
Chapter 106

Paul S. Hoffman, PhD
Professor of Medicine and Microbiology, Division of Infectious Diseases and International Health, University of Virginia School of Medicine, Charlottesville, VA, USA
Chapter 32

Stephen L. Hoffman, MD DTMH DSc(Hon)
Chief Executive and Scientific Officer, Sanaria Inc., Rockville, MD, USA
Chapter 96

Michael R. Holbrook, PhD
Senior Scientist, Battelle Memorial Institute, National Institutes for Health-Integrated Research Facility, Ft. Detrick, MD, USA; Adjunct Associate Professor, Department of Pathology, and Department of Microbiology and Immunology, The University of Texas Medical Branch, Galveston, TX, USA
Chapters 70 and 77

Thomas L. Holland, MD
Fellow, Infectious Diseases, Duke University Medical Center, Durham, NC, USA
Chapter 13

Donald R. Hopkins, MD MPH
Vice President, Health Programs, The Carter Center, Atlanta, GA, USA
Chapter 108

Duane R. Hospenthal, MD PhD FACP FIDSA
Chief, Infectious Disease Service, Brooke Army Medical Center, Fort Sam Houston, Texas, Professor of Medicine, Edward Hébert School of Medicine, Uniformed Services University of Health Sciences, Bethesda, MD, USA
Chapter 90

Peter J. Hotez, MD PhD
Distinguished Research Professor and Chair, Department of Microbiology Immunology and Tropical Medicine, George Washington University, School of Medicine and Public Health, Washington, DC, USA
Chapter 116

S. David Hudnall, MD
Professor of Pathology and Laboratory Medicine, Director of Hematopathology, Yale University School of Medicine, New Haven, CT, USA
Chapter 56

James M. Hughes, MD
Professor, Division of Infectious Diseases, Department of Medicine, School of Medicine, Professor, Hubert Department of Global Health, Rollins School of Public Health, Emory University, Atlanta, GA, USA
Chapter 14

Kao-Pin Hwang, MD
Department of Pediatrics, Chang Gung Memorial Hospital, Kaohsiung, Taiwan
Chapter 111

Raul E. Isturiz, MD FACP
Senior Consultant, Centro Medico de Caracas, Department of Internal Medicine, Infectious Diseases Section, Caracas, Venezuela
Chapter 141

Peter B. Jahrling, PhD
Director, NIAID Integrated Research Facility, Fort Detrick, Frederick, MD, USA
Chapters 57 and 73

Shahid Jameel, PhD
Senior Scientist and Group Leader, Virology, International Centre for Genetic Engineering and Biotechnology (ICGEB), New Delhi, India
Chapter 64

Selma M.B. Jeronimo, MD
Professor, Department of Biochemistry, Bioscience Center, Universidade Federal do Rio Grande do Norte, Natal, Brazil
Chapter 100

Edward C. Jones-Lopez, MD MS
Assistant Professor of Medicine, Section of Infectious Diseases, Boston University School of Medicine and Boston Medical Center, Boston, MA, USA
Chapter 35

Anna Kabanova, MD
PhD student, Novartis Vaccines and Diagnostics, Siena, Italy
Chapter 34

Gagandeep Kang, MD FRCPath PhD
Professor, Department of Gastrointestinal Sciences, Christian Medical College, Tamil Nadu, India
Chapter 62

Christopher L. Karp, MD
Gunnar Esiason/Cincinnati Bell Chair, Director, Division of Molecular Immunology, Professor of Pediatrics, Cincinnati Children's Hospital Research Foundation, University of Cincinnati College of Medicine, Cincinnati, OH, USA
Chapter 139

James W. Kazura, MD
Professor of International Health and Medicine, Director, Center for Global Health and Diseases, Case Western Reserve University School of Medicine, Cleveland, OH, USA
Chapter 104

Peter Kern, MD DTM&H FIDSA
Professor of Infectious Diseases, Head, Division of Infectious Diseases, Comprehensive Infectious Diseases Center, Ulm University Hospital and Medical Center, Ulm, Germany
Chapter 120

Gerald T. Keusch, MD
Professor of International Health and of Medicine, Associate Director, National Emerging Infectious Diseases Laboratories, Director, Collaborative Core, Special Assistant to the President for Global Health, Boston University, Boston, MA, USA
Chapter 18

Jay S. Keystone, MD MSc (CTM) FRCPC
Professor of Medicine, Tropical Disease Unit, Toronto General Hospital, Toronto, ON, Canada
Chapters 126 and 140

Mehnaaz S. Khuroo, MBBS MD
Consultant Pathologist, Jawahir Lal Nehru Memorial Hospital, Rainawari, Srinagar, Kashmir, J&K, India
Chapter 133

Mohammad S. Khuroo, MD DM FRCP (Edin) FACP MACP Emeritus
Director, Digestive Diseases Centre, Dr Khuroo's Medical Clinic, Srinagar, Kashmir, J&K, India
Chapter 133

Ik-Sang Kim, MD PhD
Professor, Department of Microbiology and Immunology, Seoul National University College of Medicine, Seoul, Korea
Chapter 51

Charles H. King, MD
Professor of International Health, Center for Global Health and Diseases, Case Western Reserve University School of Medicine, Cleveland, OH, USA
Chapter 122

Louis V. Kirchhoff, MD MPH
Professor, Division of Infectious Diseases, Department of Internal Medicine, Department of Epidemiology, University of Iowa, Staff Physician, Department of Veterans Affairs Medical Center, Iowa City, IA, USA
Chapter 99

Amy D. Klion, MD
Head, Eosinophil Pathology Unit, Laboratory of Parasitic Diseases, National Institute of Allergy and Infectious Diseases, Bethesda, MD, USA
Chapter 105

Keith P. Klugman, MD PhD
William H. Foege Professor of Global Health, Hubert Department of Global Health, Rollins School of Public Health; Professor of Epidemiology and Infectious Diseases, Emory University, Atlanta, GA, USA, Co-Director of Respiratory and Meningeal Pathogens Research Unit, Medical Research Council and University of the Witwatersrand, Johannesburg, South Africa
Chapter 29

Dennis J. Kopecko, PhD
Senior Research Scientist and Chief, Laboratory of Enteric and Sexually Transmitted Diseases, US Food and Drug Administration, Center for Biologics Evaluation and Research, Bethesda, MD, USA
Chapter 18

Margaret Kosek, MD
Assistant Scientist, Department of International Health, Johns Hopkins Bloomberg School of Public Health, Baltimore, MD, USA
Chapter 5

Frederick T. Koster, MD
Assistant Scientist, Respiratory Immunology and Asthma Program, Lovelace Respiratory Research Institute, Albuquerque, NM, USA
Chapter 71

Phyllis E. Kozarsky, MD
Professor of Medicine, Emory University School of Medicine, Atlanta, GA, Expert Consultant, Division of Global Migration and Quarantine, CDC, Atlanta, GA, USA
Chapter 126

Thomas G. Ksiazek, DVM PhD
Professor, Galveston National Laboratory, Department of Pathology, University of Texas Medical Branch, Galveston, TX, USA
Chapter 55

Jens H. Kuhn, MD PhD MS
Managing Consultant/Lead Virologist, Integrated Research Facility, Division of Clinical Research/NIAID/NIH, Fort Detrick, Frederick, MD, USA
Chapter 73

Albert J. Lastovica, PhD
Extraordinary Professor of Food Microbiology, Department of Biotechnology, Faculty of Natural Sciences, University of the Western Cape, Bellville, South Africa
Chapter 19

James W. LeDuc, PhD
Professor, Microbiology and Immunology, Robert E. Shope MD and John S. Dunn Distinguished Chair in Global Health, Director, Galveston National Laboratory, University of Texas Medical Branch, Galveston, TX, USA
Chapter 14

Peter A. Leone, MD
Professor of Medicine, University of North Carolina, Medical Director, HIV/STD Prevention and Care, North Carolina Department of Health and Human Services Communicable Diseases Branch, University of North Carolina, Chapel Hill, NC, USA
Chapter 25

Paul N. Levett, PhD ABMM FCCM
Assistant Clinical Director, Provincial Laboratory, Saskatchewan Health, Regina, Saskatchewan, Canada
Chapter 45

Michael Levin, FMed Sci FRCPCh
Professor of Paediatrics and International Child Health, Department of Paediatrics, Division of Medicine, Imperial College, London, UK
Chapter 6

Myron M. Levine, MD DTPH
Simon and Bessie Grollman Distinguished Professor and Director, University of Maryland School of Medicine, Center for Vaccine Development, Baltimore, MD, USA
Chapters 16 and 20

Aldo A.M. Lima, MD PhD
Professor and Director, INCT Institute of Biomedicine and Center for Global Health, Department of Physiology and Pharmacology, School of Medicine, Federal University of Ceará, Fortaleza, Brazil
Chapter 94

Gerhard Lindeque, MD FCOG(SA) FRCOG
Professor of Obstetrics and Gynaecology, University of Pretoria, Pretoria, South Africa
Chapter 80

David L. Longworth, MD
Chair, Medical Institute, Cleveland Clinic, Cleveland, OH, USA
Chapter 132

David Mabey, DM FRCP
Professor of Communicable Diseases, London School of Hygiene and Tropical Medicine, London, UK
Chapter 47

J. Dick Maclean†, MD FRCPC MRCP(UK) DCMT(Lond)
Formerly Professor of Medicine and Director, McGill Centre for Tropical Diseases, McGill University, Senior Physician, Division of Tropical Diseases, Department of Medicine, Montreal General Hospital, Montreal, Quebec, Canada
Chapter 123

Alan J. Magill, MD FACP FIDSA – COL/MC
Director, Division of Experimental Therapeutics, Walter Reed Army Institute of Research, Silver Spring, MD, USA
Chapter 128

Ismael Maguilnik, MD
Professor of Internal Medicine, Gastroenterology, Federal University of Rio Grande do Sul, Brazil, Head of Endoscopy, Department of Clinical Hospital, Federal University of Rio Grande do Sul, Brazil
Chapter 117

†deceased

Ciro Maguiña, MD
Director, Adjunto del IMT-AVH-UPCH, Departamento de Medicina, Universidad Peruana Cayetano Heredia, Médico Infectólogo Tropicalista, Departamento de Medicina Tropical, Hospital Nacional Cayetano Heredia, Lima, Peru
Chapter 39

James H. Maguire, MD MPH
Professor of Medicine, Brigham and Women's Hospital, Boston, MA, USA
Chapters 97, 101, and 103

Siddhartha Mahanty, MBBS MPH
Staff Clinician, Laboratory of Parasitic Diseases, National Institute of Allergy and Infectious Diseases, National Institutes of Health, Bethesda, MD, USA
Chapters 123 and 139

Shinji Makino, DVM PhD
Edgar and Mary Frances Monteith Distinguished Professorship in Viral Genetics, Professor, Department of Microbiology and Immunology, The University of Texas Medical Branch, Galveston, TX, USA
Chapter 69

Christian W. Mandl, MD PhD
Associate Professor of Virology, Department of Virology, Medical University of Vienna, Vienna, Austria, Vice President, Novartis Vaccines and Diagnostics, Cambridge, MA, USA
Chapter 77

Thomas J. Marrie, MD
Dean, Faculty of Medicine, Dalhousie University, Halifax, Nova Scotia, Canada
Chapters 32, 48, and 53

Barry J. Marshall, AC FRACP FAA FRS
Clinical Professor of Microbiology, The University of Western Australia, Faculty of Life and Physical Sciences, School of Biomedical Biomolecular and Chemical Sciences, Discipline of Microbiology and Immunology, Crawley, WA, Australia
Chapter 23

Gregory J. Martin, MD
Captain, Medical Corps, US Navy, National Naval Medical Center, Associate Professor of Medicine and Preventive Medicine, Uniformed Services University, Bethesda, MD, USA
Chapter 134

Tadahiko Matsumoto, MD DMSc
Assistant Director of Clinical Medicine and Consultant Dermatologist, Yamada Institute of Health and Medicine, Tokyo, Japan, Clinical Professor, Department of Dermatology, Juntendo University, Tokyo, Japan, Clinical Professor, Department of Dermatology, Kurume University, Kurume, Japan
Chapter 84

Steven D. Mawhorter, MD DTM&H
Staff Physician and Director, International Traveler's Health Clinic, Department of Infectious Diseases, Cleveland Clinic, Associate Professor of Medicine, Cleveland Clinic Lerner College of Medicine of Case Western Reserve University, Cleveland, OH, USA
Chapter 132

James S. McCarthy, MD
Professor of Medicine and Senior Consultant in Infectious Diseases, Royal Brisbane and Women's Hospital, Queensland Institute of Medical Research, University of Queensland, Brisbane, Australia
Chapters 109 and 113

Michael R. McGinnis, PhD
Fungus Testing Lab, Department of Pathology, University of Texas Health Science Center at San Antonio, Professor Emeritus, Department of Pathology, University of Texas Medical Branch, Galveston, TX, USA
Chapters 82 and 89

Paul S. Mead, MD MPH
Chief, Epidemiology and Surveillance Activity, Bacterial Diseases Branch, Division of Vector-borne Infectious Diseases, Centers for Disease Control and Prevention, Fort Collins, CO, USA
Chapter 41

Wayne M. Meyers, MD PhD DSc
Visiting Scientist, Department of Environmental and Infectious Disease Sciences, Armed Forces Institute of Pathology, Washington, DC, USA
Chapters 36 and 37

Robert F. Miller, MB BS FRCP
Reader in Clinical Infection, University College London, London, UK
Chapter 91

Samuel I. Miller, MD
Professor of Medicine, Microbiology, Genome Sciences, Adjunct Professor of Immunology, University of Washington School of Medicine, Seattle, WA, USA
Chapter 17

James N. Mills, PhD
Chief, Medical Ecology Unit, Division of Viral and Rickettsial Diseases, National Center for Infectious Diseases, Centers for Disease Control and Prevention, Atlanta, GA, USA
Chapter 68

Thomas P. Monath, MD
Partner, Kleiner Perkins Caufield and Byers, Harvard, MA, USA
Chapter 74

Christopher C. Moore, MD
Assistant Professor, Division of Infectious Diseases and International Health, Department of Medicine, University of Virginia, Charlottesville, VA, USA
Chapter 17

Thomas A. Moore, MD FACP
Clinical Professor, Department of Medicine, University of Kansas School of Medicine, Wichita, KS, USA
Chapters 109 and 113

J.C. Morrill, DVM PhD
Visiting Professor, Department of Microbiology and Immunology, University of Texas Medical Branch, Galveston, TX, USA
Chapter 69

J. Glenn Morris, Jr, MD MPH&TM
Director, Emerging Pathogens Institute, Professor of Medicine (Infectious Diseases), College of Medicine, Adjunct Professor, College of Public Health and Health Professions, University of Florida, Gainesville, FL, USA
Chapter 21

Megan Murray, MD
Associate Professor of Epidemiology, Department of Epidemiology, Harvard School of Public Health, Boston, MA, USA
Chapter 3

K. Darwin Murrell
Adjunct Professor, USUHS School of Medicine, Department of Preventive Medicine and Biometrics, Bethesda, MD, USA, Honorary Professor, Faculty of Life Science, University of Copenhagen, Denmark
Chapter 110

G. Balakrish Nair, PhD
Director, National Institute of Cholera and Enteric Diseases, Beliaghata, Kolkata, India
Chapter 21

Theodore E. Nash, MD
Head, Gastrointestinal Parasites Section, Laboratory of Parasitic Diseases, National Institutes of Allergy and Infectious Diseases, National Institutes of Health, Bethesda, MD, USA
Chapter 93

Barnett R. Nathan, MD
Assistant Professor, Department of Neurology, University of Virginia, Charlottesville, VA, USA
Chapter 42

Ricardo Negroni, MD
Honorary Professor of Microbiology and Parasitology, University of Buenos Aires School of Medicine, Consultant, Francisco Javier Muñiz Hospital, Buenos Aires, Argentina
Chapter 86

Anne Nicholson-Weller, MD
Professor of Medicine, Harvard Medical School, Divisions of Allergy/Inflammation and Infectious Diseases, Department of Medicine, Beth Israel Deaconess Medical Center, Boston, MA, USA
Chapter 9

Marcio Nucci, MD
Associate Professor, Department of Internal Medicine, Chief, Mycology Laboratory, University Hospital, Universidade Federal do Rio de Janeiro, Rio de Janeiro, Brazil
Chapter 88

Thomas B. Nutman, MD
Head, Helminth Immunology Section and Head, Clinical Parasitology Unit, Laboratory of Parasitic Diseases, National Institute of Allergy and Infectious Diseases, Bethesda, MD, USA
Chapters 104 and 105

Nigel O'Farrell, MD FRCP
Consultant Physician, Ealing Hospital, London, UK
Chapter 28

Juan P. Olano, MD
Associate Professor, Department of Pathology, Director, Residency Training Program, Member, Center for Biodefense and Emerging Infectious Diseases, University of Texas Medical Branch, Galveston, TX, USA
Chapters 1 and 125

Eng Eong Ooi, BMBS PhD
Associate Professor, Program in Emerging Infectious Diseases, Duke-NUS Graduate Medical School, Singapore
Chapter 75

Luis S. Ortega, MD
Chief, Asia Regional Program, Division of Global Migration and Quarantine, National Center for Emerging and Zoonotic Infectious Diseases, Centers for Disease Control and Prevention, Atlanta, GA, USA
Chapter 127

Ynés R. Ortega, PhD MPH
Associate Professor, Center for Food Safety, University of Georgia, Griffin, GA, USA
Chapter 95

Mark A. Pallansch, PhD
Chief, Polio and Picornavirus Laboratory Branch, Centers for Disease Control and Prevention, Atlanta, GA, USA
Chapter 60

Jean W. Pape, MD
Professor of Medicine, Center for Global Health, Division of Infectious Diseases, Department of Medicine, Weill Medical College of Cornell University, New York, NY, USA, Director, Les Centres GHESKIO, Port-au-Prince, Haiti
Chapter 95

Georgios Pappas, MD
Physician, Institute of Continuing Medical Education of Ioannina, Ioannina, Greece
Chapter 40

Julie Parsonnet, MD
George DeForest Barnett Professor of Medicine and Professor of Health Research and Policy, Stanford University School of Medicine, Stanford, CA, USA
Chapter 11

Geoffrey Pasvol, MA MB ChB DPhil FRCP FRCPE
Professor, Wellcome Centre for Clinical Tropical Medicine, Imperial College London, Wright Fleming Institute, London, UK
Chapters 6 and 137

Sharon J. Peacock, BM BA MSc FRCP FRCPath PhD
Professor of Clinical Microbiology, Department of Medicine, University of Cambridge, Addenbrooke's Hospital, Cambridge, UK
Chapter 33

Richard D. Pearson, MD
Professor of Medicine and Pathology, Division of Infectious Diseases and International Health, University of Virginia School of Medicine, Charlottesville, VA, USA
Chapters 12, 13, and 100

Rosanna W. Peeling, PhD
Professor and Chair of Diagnostic Research, London School of Hygiene and Tropical Medicine, London, UK
Chapter 47

David A. Pegues, MD
Professor of Medicine, Division of Infectious Diseases, David Geffen School of Medicine, Los Angeles, CA, USA
Chapter 17

Jacques Pépin, MD FRCPC MSc
Professor of Infectious Diseases, University of Sherbrooke, Sherbrooke, Quebec, Canada
Chapter 98

C.J. Peters, MD
Professor of Pathology and Microbiology and Immunology, Center for Biodefense and Emerging Infectious Diseases, WHO Collaborating Center for Tropical Diseases, University of Texas Medical Branch, Galveston, TX, USA
Chapters 67, 68, 69, 71, 73, and 125

Kristine M. Peterson, MD MPH
Assistant Professor, Division of Infectious Diseases, University of Virginia Health System, Charlottesville, VA, USA
Chapter 92

William A. Petri, Jr, MD PhD
Professor and Chief, Wade Hampton Frost Professor, Division of Infectious Diseases, University of Virginia Health Sciences Center, Charlottesville, VA, USA
Chapter 92

Françoise Portaels, PhD
Professor and Head, Unit of Mycobacteriology, Department of Microbiology, Institute of Tropical Medicine, Antwerp, Belgium
Chapter 36

José Luiz Proença-Módena, PhD
Research Fellow, Department of Cell Biology and Virology Research Center, University of São Paulo School of Medicine, Ribeirão Preto, SP, Brazil
Chapter 58

Thomas C. Quinn, MD MSc
Professor of Medicine, International Health, Epidemiology, and Molecular Microbiology and Immunology, Division of Infectious Diseases, The John Hopkins Medical Institutions, Baltimore, MD, USA
Chapter 81

G. Raghurama Rao, MD
Former Professor and Head of Department of Dermatology, Andhra Medical College, Andhra Pradesh, India
Chapter 38

Didier Raoult, MD PhD
Professor, Unité des Rickettsies, Faculté de Médecine, Marseille, France
Chapter 50

Rino Rappuoli, PhD
Global Head of Vaccine Research, Novartis Vaccines and Diagnostics, Siena, Italy
Chapter 34

John H. Rex, MD
Vice President Clinical Infection, AstraZeneca Pharmaceuticals; Adjunct Professor of Medicine, University of Texas Medical School, Houston, TX, USA
Chapter 89

Steven J. Reynolds, MD MPH FRCPC DTM&H
Senior Clinician, National Institute of Allergy and Infectious Diseases, National Institutes of Health, Washington, DC, USA
Chapter 81

José M.C. Ribeiro, MD PhD
Chief, Vector Biology Section, Laboratory of Malaria and Vector Research, NIAID, National Institutes of Health, Rockville, MD, USA
Chapter 8

Emmanuel Roilides, MD PhD
Professor of Pediatrics, Third Department of Pediatrics, Aristotle University, Hippokration Hospital, Thessaloniki, Greece
Chapter 89

Pierre E. Rollin, MD
Deputy Branch Chief, Special Pathogens Branch, Centers for Disease Control and Prevention, Atlanta, GA, USA
Chapter 55

Allan R. Ronald, MD FRCPC MACP
Distinguished Professor Emeritus, University of Manitoba, Winnipeg, Manitoba, Canada
Chapters 26 and 138

Paul A. Rota, PhD
Lead Scientist, Measles Team, Measles, Mumps, Rubella and Herpesviruses Laboratory Branch, Centers for Disease Control and Prevention, Atlanta, GA, USA
Chapter 55

Sharon L. Roy, MD MPH
Medical Epidemiologist, Waterborne Disease Prevention Branch, Division of Foodborne, Waterborne, and Environmental Diseases, Centers for Disease Control and Prevention, Atlanta, GA, USA
Chapter 101

Ernesto Ruiz-Tiben, PhD
Director, Dracunculiasis Eradication, The Carter Center, Atlanta, GA, USA
Chapter 108

Edward T. Ryan, MD
Associate Professor of Medicine, Harvard Medical School; Associate Professor of Immunology and Infectious Diseases, Harvard School of Public Health; Director, Tropical and Geographic Medicine, Massachusetts General Hospital, Boston, MA, USA
Chapters 3 and 135

Debasish Saha, MBBS MS
Clinical Epidemiologist, Bacterial Diseases Programme, Medical Research Council (UK) Laboratories, Banjul, The Gambia, West Africa
Chapter 20

Mohammed A. Salam, MD
Director, Clinical Sciences Division, International Centre for Diarrhoeal Disease Research, Bangladesh (ICDDR,B), Dhaka, Bangladesh
Chapter 18

Amidou Samie, BSc MSC PhD
Senior Lecturer, Department of Microbiology, University of Venda, Thohoyandou, South Africa
Chapter 94

Julius Schachter, PhD
Professor Emeritus of Laboratory Medicine, Chlamydia Laboratory, University of California, San Francisco, San Francisco, CA, USA
Chapter 46

Peter M. Schantz, MD VMD PhD
Epidemiologist and Senior Service Fellow, Division of Parasitic Diseases/NCZVED/CCID, National Center for Infectious Diseases, Centers for Disease Control and Prevention, Atlanta, GA, USA
Chapter 120

W. Michael Scheld, MD
Professor of Medicine, Division of Infectious Diseases and International Health, Department of Medicine, University of Virginia School of Medicine, Charlottesville, VA, USA
Chapter 24

Elizabeth P. Schlaudecker, MD
Pediatric Infectious Diseases Fellow, Division of Infectious Diseases, Cincinnati Children's Hospital Medical Center, Cincinnati, OH, USA
Chapter 27

David A. Schwartz, MD MSHyg FCAP
Associate Clinical Professor of Pathology, Department of Pathology, Vanderbilt University School of Medicine, Nashville, TN, USA
Chapter 102

Joseph D. Schwartzman, MD
Professor of Pathology, Department of Pathology, Dartmouth Medical School, Lebanon, NH, USA
Chapter 103

Arlene C. Seña, MD MPH
Clinical Associate Professor, Division of Infectious Diseases, University of North Carolina at Chapel Hill, Chapel Hill, NC, Medical Director, Durham County Health Department, Durham, NC, USA
Chapters 43 and 138

Daniel J. Sexton, MD FACP FIDSA
Professor, Department of Medicine, Division of Infectious Diseases, Duke University Medical Center, Durham, NC, USA
Chapter 49

Truman W. Sharp, MD MPH (Capt, MCUSN)
Commanding Officer, US Naval Medical Research, Unit No. 3, Cairo, Egypt
Chapter 128

Wun-Ju Shieh, MD MPH PhD
Pathologist, Infectious Diseases Pathology Branch, Division of High-Consequence Pathogens & Pathology, Centers for Disease Control and Prevention, Atlanta, GA, USA
Chapters 45 and 68

Shmuel Shoham, MD
Scientific Director, MedStar Clinical Research Center, Washington Hospital Center, Assistant Professor of Medicine, Georgetown University School of Medicine, Washington, DC, USA
Chapter 88

Afzal A. Siddiqui, PhD
Professor, Microbiology and Immunology, Internal Medicine, Pathology, School of Medicine, Texas Tech University Health Sciences Center, Lubbock, TX, USA
Chapter 117

Upinder Singh, MD
Associate Professor, Chief, Division of Infectious Diseases and Geographic Medicine, Stanford University School of Medicine, Stanford, CA, USA
Chapter 92

David W. Smith, BMedSc MBBS FRCPA FACTM
Clinical Professor, School of Biomedical, Biomolecular and Chemical Sciences and School of Pathology and Laboratory Medicine, University of Western Australia, Nedlands, Western Australia, Australia
Chapter 78

Michael B. Smith, MD MS
Terminology Manager, Clinical Informatics, SNOMED Terminology Solutions, College of American Pathologists, Northfield, IL, USA
Chapter 82

Bonnie L. Smoak, MD PhD MPH (Col, MCUSA)
Associate Professor, Department of Preventive Medicine and Biometrics, Uniformed Services University of the Health Sciences, Bethesda, MD, Director, Division of Preventive Medicine, Walter Reed Army Institute of Research, Silver Spring, MD, USA
Chapter 128

A. George Smulian, MD
Chief, Infectious Disease Section, Cincinnati VA Medical Center, Associate Professor of Medicine, University of Cincinnati, Cincinnati, OH, USA
Chapter 91

Cynthia B. Snider, MD MPH
Infectious Diseases Fellow, University of Virginia, Charlottesville, VA, USA
Chapter 58

Tom Solomon, BA BM BCh FRCP DCH DTMH PhD
Chair of Neurological Science, Head of Brain Infections Group and Director of Institute of Infection and Global Health, University of Liverpool, Liverpool, UK
Chapters 76 and 136

Samba O. Sow, MD MS
Associate Professor of Medicine, General Director, Center for Vaccine Development-Mali (CVD-MALI), ex-Institut Marchoux, Ministry of Health, Bamako, Mali
Chapter 20

P. Frederick Sparling, MD
Professor of Medicine and Microbiology and Immunology, University of North Carolina School of Medicine, Chapel Hill, NC, USA
Chapter 43

Lisa A. Spencer, PhD
Assistant Professor of Medicine, Harvard Medical School, Division of Allergy/Inflammation, Department of Medicine, Beth Israel Deaconess Medical Center, Boston, MA, USA
Chapter 9

Lawrence R. Stanberry, MD PhD FAAP
Reuben S. Carpentier Professor and Chairman, Department of Pediatrics, College of Physicians and Surgeons, Columbia University, New York, NY, USA
Chapter 56

J. Erin Staples, MD PhD
Medical Epidemiologist, Arboviral Diseases Branch, Division of Vector-borne Infectious Diseases, Centers for Disease Control and Prevention, Fort Collins, CO, USA
Chapter 74

Robert Steffen, MD Hon FFTM/ACTM
Emeritus Professor of Travel Medicine, University of Zurich Center of Travel Medicine, WHO Collaborating Centre for Travellers' Health, Zurich, Switzerland
Chapter 126

Theodore S. Steiner, MD
Associate Professor of Medicine, University of British Columbia, Vancouver, Canada
Chapter 15

Mark C. Steinhoff, MD
Director, Global Health Center, Professor of Pediatrics, Division of Infectious Diseases, Cincinnati Children's Hospital Medical Center, University of Cincinnati College of Medicine, Cincinnati, OH, USA
Chapter 27

Dennis L. Stevens, PhD MD
Chief, Infectious Disease Section, Veterans Affairs Medical Center, Boise, ID, Professor, Department of Medicine, University of Washington School of Medicine, Seattle, WA, USA
Chapter 30

Kathryn N. Suh, MD FRCPC
Associate Professor of Medicine, Division of Infectious Diseases, The Ottawa Hospital, Ottawa, ON, Canada
Chapter 140

Khuanchai Supparatpinyo, MD
Professor of Infectious Disease, Department of Medicine, Faculty of Medicine, Chiang Mai University, Chiang Mai, Thailand
Chapter 87

Paul J. Szaniszlo, PhD
Professor Emeritus, The University of Texas at Austin, Section of Molecular Genetics and Microbiology, Austin, TX, USA
Chapter 84

Milagritos D. Tapia, MD
Assistant Professor, University of Maryland School of Medicine, Center for Vaccine Development, Baltimore, MD, USA
Chapter 16

Herbert B. Tanowitz, MD
Professor of Pathology and Medicine, Director of the Diagnostic Parasitology Laboratory, Jacobi Medical Center, Albert Einstein College of Medicine, Bronx, NY, USA
Chapters 118 and 121

Sam R. Telford III, ScD
Associate Professor, Tufts University, Cummings School of Veterinary Medicine, North Grafton, MA, USA
Chapter 97

Robert B. Tesh, MD
Professor of Pathology and Microbiology and Immunology, Center for Biodefense and Emerging Infectious Diseases, University of Texas Medical Branch, Galveston, TX, USA
Chapters 72 and 76

Nathan M. Thielman, MD MPH
Associate Professor of Medicine, Director, Duke Global Health Residency Program, Division of Infectious Diseases and International Health, Duke Global Health Institute, Duke University, Durham, NC, USA
Chapters 13, 15, and 129

Fernando J. Torres-Vélez, DVM PhD
Veterinary Pathologist, Infectious Disease Pathogenesis Section, Comparative Medicine Branch (CMB), National Institute of Allergy and Infectious Diseases (NIAID), National Institutes of Health (NIH), Bethesda, MD, USA
Chapter 2

Joseph D. Tucker, MD MA
Instructor in Medicine, Harvard Medical School, Assistant in Medicine, Massachusetts General Hospital, Boston, MA, USA
Chapter 43

Luis M. Valdez, MD
Associate Professor of Medicine, Universidad Peruana Cayetano Heredia, Internal Medicine-Infectious Diseases Specialist, British American Hospital, Lima, Peru
Chapter 129

Jesus G. Valenzuela, PhD
Chief, Vector Molecular Biology Section, Laboratory of Malaria and Vector Research, NIAID, National Institutes of Health, Rockville, MD, USA
Chapter 8

Diederik van de Beek, MD PhD
Neurologist, Department of Neurology, Center of Infection and Immunity Amsterdam (CINIMA), Academic Medical Center University of Amsterdam, Amsterdam, The Netherlands
Chapter 24

Pedro F.C. Vasconcelos, MD PhD
Chief, Department of Arbovirology and Hemorrhagic Fevers, Director, WHO Collaborating Center for Research, Diagnostic Reference and Training on Arbovirus, Director, National Institute for Viral Hemorrhagic Fevers, Instituto Evandro Chagas/SVS/MS, Ananindeua, Brazil, Professor of Pathology, Pará State University, Belém, Brazil
Chapter 72

Govinda S. Visvesvara, PhD
Research Microbiologist, Division of Foodborne, Waterborne, and Environmental Diseases, Centers for Disease Control and Prevention, Atlanta, GA, USA
Chapter 101

Victoria Wahl-Jensen, MS PhD
Managing Consultant/Virologist, Integrated Research Facility, Division of Clinical Research/NIAID/NIH, Fort Detrick, Frederick, MD, USA
Chapter 73

David H. Walker, MD
Carmage and Martha Walls Distinguished University Chair in Tropical Diseases, Director, Center for Biodefense and Emerging Infectious Diseases, Professor and Chair, Department of Pathology, University of Texas Medical Branch, Galveston, TX, USA
Chapters 1, 38, 39, 49, 50, 51, and 125

Douglas S. Walsh, MD FAAD
Chief, Department of Immunology and Medicine, United States Army Medical Component, Armed Forces Research Institute of Medical Sciences (AFRIMS), Bangkok, Thailand
Chapters 36 and 37

Thomas J. Walsh, MD FACP FAAM FIDSA
Professor of Medicine, Director, Transplantation – Oncology, Infectious Diseases Program, Weill Cornell Medical College, New York, Presbyterian Hospital, New York City, New York, USA
Chapters 88 and 89

David A. Walton, MD
Instructor in Medicine, Department of Internal Medicine, Brigham and Women's Hospital, Boston, MA, USA
Chapter 4

Peter D. Walzer, MD MSc
Associate Chief of Staff for Research, Cincinnati VA Medical Center, Professor of Medicine, University of Cincinnati, Cincinnati, OH, USA
Chapter 91

Cirle A. Warren, MD
Assistant Professor, Center for Global Health, Division of Infectious Disease and International Health, Charlottesville, VA, USA
Chapter 22

Scott C. Weaver, PhD
Professor, Department of Pathology, Scientific Director, Galveston National Laboratory, Director, Institute for Human Infections and Immunity, University of Texas Medical Branch at Galveston, Galveston, TX, USA
Chapter 78

Louis M. Weiss, MD MPH
Professor of Pathology, Division of Parasitology and Tropical Medicine, Professor of Medicine, Division of Infectious Diseases, Albert Einstein College of Medicine, Bronx, NY, USA
Chapter 102

Peter F. Weller, MD FACP FIDSA
Professor of Medicine, Harvard Medical School, Professor, Immunology and Infectious Diseases Department, Harvard School of Public Health, Chief, Infectious Disease Division, Vice Chair of Research, Department of Medicine, Beth Israel Deaconess Medical Center, Boston, MA, USA
Chapters 1, 12, 97, and 131

A. Clinton White, Jr, MD FACP FIDSA
Paul R. Stalnaker MD Distinguished Professor, Director, Infectious Disease Division, Department of Internal Medicine, University of Texas Medical Branch, Galveston, TX, USA
Chapters 118, 119, and 121

Nicholas J. White, OBE DSc MD FRCP FMedSci FRS
Professor of Tropical Medicine, Mahidol University and Oxford University, Faculty of Tropical Medicine, Mahidol University, Bangkok, Thailand
Chapter 96

Robert J. Wilkinson, MA PhD BM BCh DTM&H FRCP
Wellcome Trust Senior Fellow, MRC Programme Leader, Imperial College London, MRC National Institute for Medical Research, University of Cape Town, Cape Town, South Africa
Chapter 6

Mary E. Wilson, MD FACP FIDSA
Associate Professor of Global Health and Population, Harvard School of Public Health, Boston, MA, USA
Chapters 130 and 131

Murray Wittner, MD PhD
Professor Emeritus, Director, International Health and Travel Medicine Clinic, Montefiore Medical Center, Bronx, NY, USA
Chapters 118 and 121

Anita K.M. Zaidi, MBBS SM FAAP
A. Sultan Jamal Professor of Pediatrics and Child Health, Department of Pediatrics and Child Health, Aga Khan University, Karachi, Pakistan
Chapter 16

Sherif R. Zaki, MD
Chief, Infectious Disease Pathology, Centers for Disease Control and Prevention, Atlanta, GA, USA
Chapters 45 and 67

Access the complete reference list online at http://www.expertconsult.com

CHAPTER 1

Principles of Parasitism: Host–Parasite Interactions

Juan P. Olano • Peter F. Weller • Richard L. Guerrant • David H. Walker

INTRODUCTION

The relationship between two living organisms can be classified as parasitic, symbiotic, or commensal.[1-3] This same classification scheme can be used to describe relationships between microorganisms and more complex living organisms that act as hosts. The term *parasite* is used here in its broad sense to mean a microorganism interacting with another organism (either vertebrate or invertebrate) in the same ecologic niche.

The following definitions are used in this chapter:

Parasitism: Association between two different organisms wherein one benefits at the expense of the other. All infectious agents causing illness belong to this category.

Commensalism: Association between two organisms in which one derives benefit from the other without causing it any harm. This intermediate category is not uniformly accepted. Often, upon detailed analysis, the relationship turns out to be either parasitic or symbiotic.[2]

Symbiosis or *mutualism*: Both organisms benefit from the relationship. The type of relationship also depends on host factors. For example, bacteria normally inhabiting the bowel live in an apparent commensal or (by inhibiting potential pathogens) symbiotic relationship with humans. However, in cases of cirrhosis with consequent hepatic insufficiency, bacteria can become a dangerous source of ammonia that leads to hepatic encephalopathy. A commensal relationship can be transformed into a potentially harmful one.

MICROBIAL FACTORS

Principles of Microbial Evolution and Classification

The Earth is approximately 4.5 to 5 billion years old. There is good fossil evidence of microbial life approximately 3.5 billion years ago. Microbial life (stromatolites) was mostly photosynthetic, unicellular, and anaerobic.[1,4] Eukaryotes, bacteria, and archaea evolved from a still hypothetical universal common ancestor.[5-7] Eukaryotes then evolved into protozoans, metazoans, plants, and animals, as we know them today. Moreover, there is strong evidence that primitive eukaryotic cells established relationships with bacterial organisms that later evolved into cytoplasmic organelles, such as chloroplasts in plants and mitochondria in animals.[8]

To put things into perspective, approximately five-sixths of the history of life on Earth has been exclusively microbial. Human beings appeared on the planet only 2 million years ago as very late newcomers to the biosphere. Life was initially anaerobic, but with the appearance of photosynthetic organisms and chloroplasts, oxygen was released into the atmosphere for the first time.[9] Radiation in the upper atmosphere created the ozone layer from molecular oxygen, which then shielded the Earth's surface from dangerous radiation. Nucleic acids were therefore protected from harmful mutations. Organisms had to evolve to survive in the presence of oxygen. A few of the ancient anaerobes were able to survive in the highly oxidant atmosphere, and they represent the anaerobes as we know them today.

The phylogeny of living organisms is based on molecular approaches, particularly analysis of ribosomal RNA.[5,6,10] Because of the antiquity of the protein synthesis machinery, these molecules are excellent evolutionary clocks. For prokaryotes, the 16S subunit of ribosomes is the most useful for classification purposes.

Viruses deserve special comment because of their molecular simplicity and at the same time their importance as human pathogens and as possible agents of hereditary changes and cancer.[11,12] A virus is a genetic element with either DNA or RNA coated by protein of viral origin and sometimes enveloped by lipid material of host origin. Some viruses have enzymes that are necessary for their replication. The only criterion that these organisms fulfill to be considered living organisms is that of reproduction. They are inert particles when outside of the host cell, and once they have access into a cell they become active and the cell is subverted to produce more viral particles. Sometimes the cell dies in the process, and sometimes the relationship is stable. Viral hosts include bacteria, protozoa, animals, and plants.

The classification of viruses is based on different criteria than the ones used for other organisms. The major criteria are type of nucleic acid, presence or absence of an envelope, manner of replication, and morphologic characteristics.[12,13]

Simpler forms of self-replicating organisms include virusoids and viroids.[14,15] The former are satellite RNAs that are found encapsidated in the proteins encoded by their helper virus (e.g., hepatitis caused by the hepatitis D virus delta agent in conjunction with hepatitis B virus). The viroids are mostly plant pathogens that consist of single-stranded circular RNA molecules.

The concept of "infectious agent" was revolutionized by the discovery of proteinaceous infectious agents known as prions. These proteins are responsible for neurodegenerative diseases in animals and humans. The protein particles lack nucleic acids but still are able to reproduce and trigger conformational changes in host proteins, leading to cell death.[16,17]

In contrast, protozoa are nucleated, single-cell organisms that, depending on the species, replicate by means as simple as binary fission (e.g., *Trichomonas*) or as complex as involving multiple sexual and asexual stages in both animal and invertebrate hosts (e.g., plasmodia). Protozoa include amebae (e.g., *Entamoeba histolytica*), flagellates (e.g., *Giardia lamblia*), ciliates (e.g., *Balantidium coli*), and sporozoa (e.g., *Cryptosporidium*). Even more complex are helminths, which are multicellular metazoan organisms with highly developed internal organs, including alimentary and reproductive tracts. The helminths include nematodes (roundworms), cestodes (tapeworms), and trematodes (flukes). Many helminths have complex life cycles with multiple developmental stages both in the animal host and in intermediate invertebrate or vertebrate hosts. Because of their size, helminths, the macroparasites, are solely extracellular pathogens; because of their prolonged life cycles and generation times, their capacity for genetic alteration is diminished compared to smaller, simpler microbes (the microparasites).

Development of Microbial Virulence

Evolution of Virulence

The traditional view assumes that natural selection would favor evolution toward a benign coexistence between host and parasite.[18,19] A modern view of evolution of virulence focuses on the tradeoff between the benefits that pathogens accrue through increased exploitation of hosts and the costs that result from any effects of disease that reduce transmission to susceptible hosts.[19,20] From this point of view, virulence could be the evolved as well as the primitive stage of the association between host and parasite, depending on the development of enhanced rather than reduced transmission.

According to Levin[19] and Levin and Svanborg-Eden,[20] there are three alternative models to explain evolution of a microparasite's virulence: direct selection, coincidental evolution, and short-sighted within-host selection. The direct selection model states that there is a direct relationship between the parasite's virulence and its rate of infectious transmission. The best documented and often cited example is that of the dramatic changes in virulence that the myxoma virus underwent after being released into the wild in Australia to "control" the population of wild rabbits. In the beginning, rabbit mortality and viral transmission rates were high. As the population of rabbits was decimated, the virulence of the virus decreased and its rate of transmission actually increased. This outcome is explained by the longer survival and duration of the period of shedding of the virus. At the same time, more resistant rabbits increased in number due to the selection process.[21]

According to the coincidental evolution model, the factors responsible for the virulence of a microparasite evolved for some purpose other than to provide the parasite with some advantage within a host or for its transmission to other hosts. Clostridial toxins are good examples in this category. There is no beneficial reason to kill a human host who became infected by *Clostridium tetani* spores from soil in order for the parasite to survive. They are mostly soil bacteria and do not need humans for their survival.[19]

Short-sighted within-host evolution posits that the parasites responsible for the morbidity and mortality of the host are selected for as a consequence of within-host evolution since that produces a local advantage for their survival within the host. The host dies and the rate of transmission would decrease. This is an example of evolutionary myopia in which the long-term consequences of killing a host would not matter to the parasite.[22,23] Natural selection is a local phenomenon that happens at a given time and place and goes perfectly with this model. Bacteria such as *Neisseria meningitidis* that normally live attached to human pharyngeal epithelial cells sometimes invade the central nervous system (CNS) and kill the host. Their replication in the CNS is favored since competition is low and defenses are not as abundant as in the tonsillar areas.[19]

It follows from the previous paragraphs that evolutionary theories addressing virulence have predicted that virulence of microbes evolves in response to changes in conditions or tradeoffs. One of the most commonly considered "tradeoffs" is between the benefit of a high within-host microbial density (allowing efficient transmission to the next host) and the cost of a reduced longevity of the infection in the host due to high parasite density that tends to kill the host.

Other approaches have been proposed such as the role of how pathogenic mechanisms affect virulence evolution. According to this model, pathogenic mechanisms that manipulate host immunity or escape from the host immune response (longer survival in the host) dominate as causes of virulence compared to mechanisms that incrementally alter transmission (higher microbial density and increased mortality).[24,25] Furthermore, natural selection would act more strongly on mutations influencing clearance than on mutations influencing transmission.[26]

Another cited model to explain dynamics of virulence evolution is the so-called "source–sink" model in which evolution of bacterial pathogens is evaluated from ecological points of view that microbes switch from permanent (source) and transient (sink) habitats.[27]

The generation times of mammalian hosts are much longer than those of microorganisms. Therefore, genetic mutations in these hosts, on which natural selection acts, take longer to become part of a large population. Nevertheless, there is evidence that specific microorganisms can exert selective pressure on the gene pool of human hosts. The evidence is strongest for the potentially lethal infections caused by falciparum malaria. In regions of the world where falciparum malaria is endemic, including Africa, there is a high prevalence of genetic mutations that alter hemoglobin structure or synthesis, decreasing or abolishing falciparum malaria parasites' survival.[28] The selective pressure of malaria on human gene expression is not confined solely to affecting erythrocytes but also likely involves the immune system, cytokines, and other systems.[29]

Other Modes of Altering Virulence and Pathogenicity

Although the selective pressures of evolution generally exert changes over a multitude of centuries, there are other mechanisms that may more rapidly alter microbial pathogenicity, virulence, and drug susceptibility. The expression of mutated genes in microorganisms is heightened when there are greater numbers of organisms and their generation times are brief. Hence, altered gene expression in helminths will be slow to be expressed, whereas in microparasites genetic alterations will be likely to develop. For mycobacterial infections, large numbers of bacilli that persist for a long time facilitate the genetic emergence of drug resistance to a single agent, and this likelihood underlies the principle of using more than a single drug to treat tuberculosis. Even more rapidly dividing microparasites can develop genetic alterations, and this is especially true when the fidelity of genetic replication is poor. This is prominent in human immunodeficiency virus type 1 (HIV-1), whose reverse transcriptase lacks a 3′ exonuclease proofreading activity.[30] Alterations in cell tropism, pathogenicity, and drug sensitivity are frequent in HIV-1 infections. Again, several antiviral agents must be employed concomitantly to circumvent the highly frequent mutations that alter drug susceptibility in HIV-1 strains.

In addition to their own genetic material, many classes of microparasites either contain or are capable of acquiring transferable genetic elements in the form of plasmids, transposons, or bacteriophages. These transferable genetic elements also provide a means for the spread of resistance to antibacterial drugs, an increasing problem in all regions of the world.[31]

Causes of Acute or Chronic Infections in Individuals

One obvious impact of an infectious disease is on the individual infected. Hence, in any region of the world independent of other infectious diseases or malnutrition, the acute infection will cause morbidity and potential mortality in the infected human host. Among otherwise healthy people, the immediate impact of the infection is the symptomatic acute illness. For some infections that have prolonged courses, their impact may also continue over many years. Chronic infections include most of those caused by helminthic parasites, which characteristically live for years; persisting mycobacterial infections; and retroviral infections (HIV-1, HIV-2, and human T-cell lymphotropic virus type 1). Finally, the sequelae of some infections can include the development of neoplasms. Examples include hepatocellular carcinomas associated with chronic hepatitis B and C viral infections, bladder tumors with urinary schistosomiasis, cholangiocarcinomas with biliary fluke infections, and gastric adenocarcinomas and lymphomas associated with *Helicobacter pylori* infections.

Causes of Widespread Infections in Populations

Infectious diseases may affect not only individuals but also large groups of people or entire populations due to epidemic or highly endemic transmission. Throughout human history, a few microorganisms have been responsible for great epidemics and massive numbers of dead or crippled people as a result of infections spreading locally or throughout the world.[32–35] Typhus has been associated almost always with situations that involve overcrowding, famine, war, natural disasters, and poverty. The outcomes of several European wars were affected by the morbidity and mortality inflicted by typhus or other diseases on the military. Typhus epidemics were common during the world wars of the twentieth century and in the concentration camps where the ecological conditions were ideal for such a disease to spread.[30] Today, typhus and other rickettsioses are still public health problems in some countries, but overall the disease was brought under control after its life cycle was described and antibiotics, insecticides, and public health measures became available.[34]

Bubonic plague, caused by *Yersinia pestis*, is another disease that has shaped history, especially in Europe during the Middle Ages.[35] Millions of people were affected by pandemics that spread throughout the continent. Tuberculosis, smallpox, and measles had a tremendous effect on the native populations of the Americas after Columbus's voyages to the New World. It has been estimated that 90% of the population in Mexico was killed by these pathogens, which were novel to the native residents.

Acquired immunodeficiency syndrome (AIDS) represents the modern pandemic that will continue to affect human history for at least decades. Other examples are cholera and influenza, which are capable of causing pandemics.[36]

In addition to widespread diseases caused by epidemic spread of infections, some infectious diseases, because of their highly endemic prevalence in populations, continue to affect large segments of the world's population. These include enteric and respiratory infections, measles, malaria, tuberculosis and schistosomiasis. Furthermore, even the staggering mortality and morbidity of these tropical infectious diseases do not control populations but are associated with population overgrowth. This is true not only across the different countries of the world but also throughout the history of developed countries. Thus, the impact of these infections is not solely on the individual but, because of their highly endemic or epidemic occurrence, on populations. This has consequences on economic, political, and social functioning of entire societies.[37]

Polyparasitism and Effects on Nutrition and Growth

In an otherwise healthy and fully nourished person, a new infection is likely to be the only active infection in that person. In contrast, in regions where enteric and other infections are highly prevalent because of inadequate sanitation and poor socioeconomic conditions, adults and especially children may harbor several infections or be subject to repeated episodes of new enteric pathogens. Thus, the polyparasitism of multiple concurrent or recurrent infections adds a new dimension to the impact of acute infections, not often encountered in developed countries.

Moreover, the subclinical impact of a number of tropical infectious diseases is beginning to become apparent. Increasing data suggest that even "asymptomatic" giardial,[38] cryptosporidial,[39] and enteroaggregative *Escherichia coli*[40] infections may be very important in predisposing to malnutrition, thus reflecting a clinically important impact, even in the absence of overt clinical disease such as diarrhea. Likewise, chronic intestinal helminth infections also have a major impact on nutrition in those with already marginal nutrition. Anthelminthic therapy in these children, who lack symptomatic infections, has led to increases in growth, exercise tolerance, and scholastic performance.[41,42]

MICROBIAL INTERACTIONS WITH HUMAN HOSTS

Just as microorganisms have evolved over centuries or longer, mammalian hosts have evolved to contain and limit the deleterious consequences of infections with diverse microbes. The human immune system is composed of multiple elements, including those of innate immunity and those of adaptive immunity. Many of the elements of innate immunity are more primitive and found in invertebrate organisms, whereas the adaptive immune responses have evolved further in vertebrate hosts. Microorganisms that successfully infect human hosts must, at least in the short term, overcome elements of the host immune system, which then may react further to attempt to control these infections.

The study of microbial pathogenesis has been revolutionized with the advent of comparative genomics and the multitude of genomic tools that have become available in the last two decades or so. The first bacterium whose genome was fully sequenced was that of a laboratory strain of *Haemophilus influenzae* in 1995, followed by *Mycoplasma genitalium* the same year. Since then over 250 bacterial genome sequences have become available. Discovery of virulence genes has therefore expanded rapidly and has benefited from other strategies such as powerful computational methods, genetic signatures, analysis of physical linkage to accessory genetic elements, and biochemical and genetic approaches that depend on comprehensive genome sequence information.[43] Furthermore, proteomics-based methods have also been used in combination with genome-sequence analysis to define new virulence factors.[43] For obligate intracellular pathogens, whose genetic manipulation is far more difficult than for other microbes, the use of genomic and post-genomic tools (genomic-microarray methods and proteomics) has been virtually the only path to discovery of virulence factors. In general, these tools have advanced the understanding of virulence factors in pathogenic microorganisms exponentially.

Microorganisms that infect humans are exogenous to the host and must colonize or penetrate epithelial barriers to gain access to the host. Except for infections acquired during the intrauterine period, infectious agents must bridge host epithelial surfaces, the keratinized epithelium of the skin, or the mucosal epithelium of the respiratory, gastrointestinal, or genitourinary tracts. Ultimately, there are four types of microbial localization in the host (***Fig. 1.1***). Some microbes will enter intracellular sites either within the cytoplasm or within vesicular or vacuolar compartments in cells. Other microbes remain extracellular, either at epithelial surfaces or within the host in the blood, lymph, or tissues.

Interactions at Epithelial Barrier Surfaces

The barrier functions occurring at epithelial surfaces are part of the innate host defenses and are important in determining the outcome of interactions of potential pathogens with the host. Interactions at epithelial barriers involved in defense against external microbes include not only the physical properties of the epithelial surfaces but also the overlying mucous phase, the ciliated or other propulsive activities facilitating microbe clearance, and the normal microbial flora.

Normal Flora

Vertebrate warm-blooded organisms, such as humans, are an ideal site for the survival of many microbes and provide a rich source of organic material and a constant temperature and pH. Microbes coexist with us in and on our bodies, especially on epithelial surfaces where there is contact with the outside world, such as the bowel, upper respiratory tract,

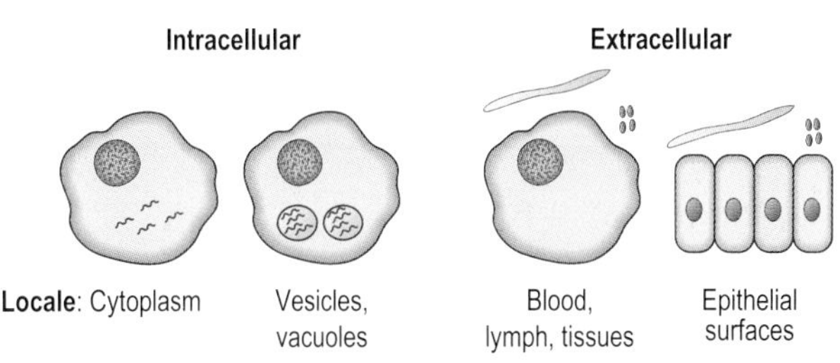

Figure 1.1 Microbial localization.

mouth, skin, and distal portions of the genitourinary tract.[1,2,43] Most of these microorganisms are highly adapted to live with us and do not cause any harm. The presence of the same type of microorganisms at a particular site in the absence of disease is called colonization. Normal colonizing microbial flora help to limit access by potentially pathogenic microorganisms. One condition predisposing to infection is the alteration of the normal epithelial flora, as occurs with antibiotic therapy, since this may allow for the proliferation of pathogenic organisms normally held in balance by the endogenous normal microbial flora. Examples include *Candida* vaginitis or the development of pseudomembranous colitis due to toxigenic *Clostridium difficile*, which may complicate antibiotic therapy.

Adhesion to the Epithelium

Microorganisms maintain themselves in or on their host by adhesion to cells or the extracellular matrix. Adhesins are encoded by chromosomal genes, plasmids, or phages.[44] They are usually divided into fimbrial and afimbrial adhesins.[45] Fimbrial adhesins are present in organisms such as *Neisseria gonorrhoeae* and are in part responsible for the attachment to genitourinary tract epithelium, preventing the bacteria from being washed out by the urine stream.[46,47] An example of an afimbrial adhesin is the filamentous hemagglutinin of *Bordetella pertussis*, which is responsible for the attachment of *B. pertussis* to epithelial cells in the respiratory tract.[48] Adhesins attach to receptors in the host. These receptors include proteins, glycolipids, and carbohydrates exposed on the surface of cells or in the extracellular matrix.[44] Integrins are one class of proteins present on eukaryotic cell surfaces that can serve as bacterial receptors.[44] *Helicobacter pylori* binds to Lewis blood group antigen present in the gastric epithelium.[49] *Neisseria* has a ligand that binds to CD66 molecules on epithelial cells.

Some pathogens have even more evolved interactions with the host and activate signal transduction mechanisms in the host cell, which in turn upregulate other molecules that aid in the adhesion process.[2,44] Certain strains of enteropathogenic *E. coli* possess type III secretion or contact-mediated systems.[50] In such cases, the secretion and synthesis of virulence factors is modulated by contact with host surfaces. The systems are complex (more than 20 genes are involved) and have not been elucidated completely at the molecular level.[51,52]

Penetration of the Epithelial Barriers

Some microbes do not have the means to penetrate skin barriers and are only able to gain access through bites produced by arthropods (e.g., rickettsiae, arboviruses, plasmodia, and filariae).[53,54] In such cases, microbes may be introduced by direct inoculation (e.g., rickettsiae, arboviruses, and plasmodia) or may gain access by migrating through the puncture site (filariae). Other microbes (e.g., skin bacteria and fungi) depend on mechanical disruption of the skin (e.g., due to burns, trauma, or intravenous catheters) to invade deeper structures.[55] Still others invade when defenses on mucosal surfaces are lowered due to combined local or generalized immunosuppression and altered mucosal integrity (mucositis) due to chemotherapy or malnutrition (e.g., *Candida* spp. and anaerobic and other enteric bacteria in the bowel). Some microbes do not invade tissues at all and affect the host locally and systemically by liberating toxins at the site of colonization (e.g., diphtheria exotoxin).[44]

For enteric pathogens, some, including poliovirus, *Salmonella enterica* serovar Typhimurium, *Salmonella enterica* serovar Typhi, *Campylobacter jejuni*, *Yersinia enterocolitica*, and *Yersinia pseudotuberculosis*, gain access to the host across the intestinal epithelium by utilizing uptake in specialized epithelial M cells.[56] Internalization of some microorganisms is also achieved through other mechanisms, such as sequential "zipper-like" encircling of the organisms triggered by bacterial ligands and cellular receptors, as occurs in infections caused by *Listeria monocytogenes*.[44] The trigger mechanism of the bacteria induces massive rearrangements of cytoskeletal proteins such as actin, which results in membrane ruffles, as occur with shigellosis and salmonellosis.[44]

In the genitourinary tract, invasion of some agents (e.g., HIV-1) is facilitated by mucosal erosions caused by other infectious agents.[57]

Spread from the Portal of Entry

Once the organisms gain access to the body after overcoming the first lines of defense, they either spread to other sites of the body or reproduce locally and often invade surrounding tissues. Local spread is facilitated by a number of factors, including collagenases, hyaluronidases, fibrinolysis, and other enzymes. They are produced by a wide range of organisms, and the role of these enzymes in invasion is, in some cases, controversial.[2]

Lymphatic spread occurs in most cases once the organisms gain access to subepithelial tissues or serosal surfaces. Lymphatic vessels are distributed in most tissues of the body, with few exceptions such as the brain. Lymph is carried by lymphatic vessels to regional lymph nodes, where it circulates through the node and eventually returns to the systemic circulation through the thoracic duct and the great lymphatic vein. One to three liters of lymph is returned to the systemic circulation every day. Most pathogens are filtered in lymph nodes before reaching the systemic circulation, but some actually reproduce either in the endothelium of lymphatic vessels (e.g., *Mycobacterium leprae*)[2,58] or in tissue macrophages present in the lymph nodes (e.g., *Brucella* spp.) or lymphocytes (HIV and herpesviruses, including Epstein–Barr virus).[59] Some organisms reach the systemic circulation after overwhelming the defenses in the lymph nodes (e.g., *Bacillus anthracis* and *Y. pestis*).

Microorganisms carried in the blood are transported either extracellularly (e.g., most of those causing bacteremia) or intracellularly. Intracellular pathogens are carried by red blood cells (e.g., *Plasmodium, Babesia,* Colorado tick fever virus, and *Bartonella*), monocytes (e.g., measles virus, cytomegalovirus, and *Toxoplasma*), or neutrophils (e.g., *Anaplasma phagocytophilum*, *Ehrlichia ewingii*, and some pyogenic bacteria).[2,60]

Once in the blood, by initial lymphatic or hematogenous spread, the microorganisms have access to virtually any site in the body. However, some pathogens exhibit tropism for certain tissues. This tropism depends on multiple factors, including the anatomy of the microcirculation in a given tissue (fenestrated capillaries versus continuous endothelial lining), receptors present on certain endothelial cells, and the presence of mononuclear phagocytic cells in organs such as bone marrow, liver, and spleen.[2] Other less common routes of spread include peripheral nerves (e.g., rabies and varicella zoster virus), cerebrospinal fluid (after the organisms traverse the blood–brain barrier), and serosal cavities.

Localization in the Host

Microbes that have gained access to the host at or through epithelial barriers then, depending on the properties and size of the pathogens, have the capacity either to seek intracellular sites or remain extracellular (see *Fig. 1.1*). Mechanisms of host immune responses to the microorganisms vary depending on their sites of localization.

Intracellular Localization

Specific microorganisms use highly developed processes to gain access to and survive within host cells. The microorganisms may reside either in the cytoplasm or within vesicular or vacuolar compartments of targeted cells.

Targeting and penetration of cells is governed by the interactions of microbial surface proteins that may engage host cell molecules that function as receptors for the microbial ligands. The entry of malarial parasites into erythrocytes is a good example, and the nature of the erythrocyte receptors used by different malarial parasite species governs which red blood cells are infected. *Plasmodium vivax* binds to the Duffy blood group antigens present on some people's red blood cell membranes. The expression of the Duffy blood group antigen is genetically determined, and this antigen is present mostly in whites and Asians and largely absent in blacks of sub-Saharan African ancestry.[61–64] This genetic absence of a receptor on red blood cells required for vivax malaria's survival explains why vivax malaria is rare in regions of Africa. *Plasmodium vivax* also exhibits a characteristic restriction in the age of erythrocytes it infects. Only young red blood cells and reticulocytes are susceptible to infection, even though the Duffy blood group antigen is present on red blood cells of all ages. The basis for this restriction to younger red blood cells also rests with receptor-mediated limitations. *Plasmodium vivax* parasites contain reticulocyte-binding proteins, which recognize and bind to reticulocyte-specific antigens on the red blood cell surface.[65,66] Thus, host cell receptor–microbial ligand interactions have an impact on the geographic range of infections based on host genetic differences in requisite receptor expression and on the specific cells that a microbe may enter.

Another example of the intricacies of microbe–receptor interactions has been recognized with HIV-1. Although CD4 is the primary cellular receptor for HIV entry, binding to CD4 alone is not sufficient for entry of HIV-1 into cells. Cellular coreceptors that are members of the chemokine receptor family of seven-transmembrane G protein-coupled molecules are also important. T-cell tropic strains use the CXCR-4 chemokine receptor, and macrophage tropic HIV-1 strains use the CCR-3 and CCR-5 chemokine receptors as coreceptors in concert with CD4. The differences among strains of HIV-1 in their capacities to bind to different chemokine receptor–coreceptors may help explain differences in cell tropism and pathogenicity, the lack of infectability of nonprimate cells, and, for those with genetically altered coreceptors, the apparent resistance to HIV-1 infection of some individuals.[67–70]

Typical of those etiologic agents that have an intracellular localization are viruses. The entry of these agents into cells is increasingly recognized to be dependent on their interactions with specific host cell proteins that act as their "receptors." For instance, host cell molecules that function as viral receptors include multiple isoforms of membrane cofactor protein (CD46), a complement regulatory protein, for measles; the integrin, intracellular adhesion molecule-1 (ICAM-1), for rhinovirus; erythrocyte P antigen for parvovirus B19; and the C3d complement receptor (CR2) for Epstein–Barr virus.[71–74]

Microbes that exist principally within the cytoplasm are sequestered from many immune response mechanisms active on extracellular pathogens, including antibody and phagocytic cells. Viral intracellular proteins will be processed and displayed with class I major histocompatibility complex (MHC) proteins, which enable CD8 cytotoxic T cells to recognize and kill the virally infected cell.

Other microbes are internalized within phagocytic cells, especially macrophages. Once internalized in host cells, organisms such as *Salmonella*, *Mycobacterium*, *Chlamydia*, and *Legionella* use an extraordinary assortment of mechanisms to prevent their phagocytic vacuole from fusing with the host cells' acidifying lysosomes.[75–77] For some parasites, the intracellular environment is an important determinant of parasitism. For example, *Leishmania* and *Coxiella* (unlike other pathogens) benefit from the acidic environment of the macrophage phagolysosome. *Leishmania* use the proton gradient across the lysosome to drive the energy-dependent uptake of two important substrates: glucose and proline.[78] Thus, *Leishmania* amastigotes actually survive in the macrophage phagolysosome because they benefit from its proton gradient and because they avoid activating the processes that normally kill ingested microorganisms. Leishmanial lipophosphoglycan inhibits the action of β-galactosidase, chelates calcium, inhibits protein kinase C and the oxidative burst, and may scavenge toxic oxygen metabolites.[79]

Conversely, other intracellular pathogens such as *Toxoplasma gondii* survive within the macrophage by using an alternative pathway of entry that avoids fusion of the parasitophorous vacuole with lysosomes.[76,80] In contrast, dead or antibody-coated *T. gondii* enter via the Fc receptor and are routed to a different intracellular compartment, which fuses with the lysosome, and are then killed in the phagolysosome.[76,80,81]

Other organisms, such as *Shigella*, *Listeria*, and *Rickettsia*, breach their vacuolar membrane to multiply freely in the cytoplasm and may also usurp host cellular actin to propel their further spread to neighboring cells, continuing to exploit their intracellular sanctuary.[82–84]

Immune responses against microbes within macrophages rely heavily on class II MHC-mediated presentation of host antigenic peptides to T-helper 1 (Th1) types of CD4$^+$ T cells, which then augment the microbicidal activities of the macrophages.

Extracellular Localization

Some types of microbes that remain extracellular typically reside at epithelial surfaces, including bacteria such as *N. gonorrhoeae*, *H. pylori*, *Vibrio cholerae*, and *E. coli*, and helminths such as adult *Ascaris lumbricoides*, hookworms, and *Trichuris trichiura*. Mucosal immune responses, including IgA and leukocytes, participate in host immune reactions to these pathogens.

Other microbes that survive extracellularly are present within the blood, lymph, or tissues of the host, and these organisms include fungi, viruses, bacteria, protozoa, and notably the helminths. Multicellular helminths, due to their large size, remain forever extracellular and may be found in the blood (e.g., microfilariae), lymph (adult lymphatic filarial worms), tissues (migrating larvae and adult stages of some helminths), and cerebrospinal fluid. Host defense against extracellular pathogens uses antibodies, complement, phagocytic cells, and, for helminths, IgE, eosinophils, and mast cells.[85]

Tissue Damage

There are multiple mechanisms by which microbes inflict damage on host tissues.

Direct Damage or Alteration of Host Cell Function

Host cells can be killed directly by the infectious agent, as in some viral or bacterial infections that are highly cytopathic (e.g., yellow fever virus in hepatocytes and *Salmonella* in macrophages).[86,87] Some microorganisms multiply intracellularly until the cell bursts and dies (e.g., *Rickettsia prowazekii*).[34] Some bacteria, viruses, and other parasites, such as *Shigella*, HIV-1, and *Listeria*, can induce apoptosis of host cells.[59,88,89] Apoptosis is triggered by different mechanisms, such as activation of the interleukin-converting enzyme pathway.[90,91] This form of programmed cell death is probably more widespread as a mechanism of cell death in infectious diseases than previously thought.

Damage is sometimes caused by toxins secreted by bacterial cells (exotoxins). In this case, bacteria can either invade host tissues or colonize mucosal sites and then release toxins at the mucosal site that are absorbed systemically and cause distant damage.[92] Exotoxins can act through different pathways that damage the components of the cell membranes such as phospholipids[88,93] or affect signaling pathways (e.g., *V. cholerae*).[44,94] Other exotoxins, such as streptolysins and listeriolysins, alter membrane permeability. Still others, such as exfoliatin (e.g., *Staphylococcus aureus*) and elastase (e.g., *Pseudomonas* spp.), are capable of degrading extracellular elements.[2] Some toxins are translocated to the intracellular environment, where they affect multiple enzymatic systems. These toxins are classified according to their enzymatic activity, such as adenosine diphosphate (ADP) ribosyl transferase (e.g., diphtheria toxin, *P. aeruginosa* exotoxin A, and pertussis toxin), depurinase (e.g., *Shiga* toxin), adenylate cyclase (e.g., pertussis hemolysin and anthrax edema factor), and zinc protease (e.g., tetanus).[94] The end result ranges from blockade of protein synthesis and cell death or blockade of exocytosis (especially CNS neurotransmitters at the synaptic cleft)[95,96] to increases of cyclic adenosine monophosphate (AMP) or cyclic guanosine monophosphate (GMP) and changes in cell permeability.[94] Still other organisms, such as *C. difficile*, produce toxins that change basic cell signaling transducers such as Rho to alter cell function or affect their spread. Finally, organisms can interact with host cell or microbial transcriptional regulation of genes (such as iron-binding proteins for uropathogenic *E. coli*[92,97]) or cytokine release (such as *H. pylori* or enteroaggregative *E. coli*[40,98–100]) to enhance their survival or elicit pathogenic responses. The evolutionary advantages to a microbe of its remarkable array of traits that we call "virulence" hold many of the clues to their control, if we can but truly understand them.

Endotoxins are a subset of lipopolysaccharides present in the outer membrane of Gram-negative bacteria that can trigger a wide variety of responses in the host, including massive cytokine release leading to hypotension and shock.[101,102] These deleterious effects occur with high-grade invasion of the blood by Gram-negative bacteria, including enteric Gram-negative bacteremias and meningococcemia.

Indirect Damage

Damage to the host may also develop as a consequence of immune reactions to the infectious agents. One scheme for classifying immunopathologic responses divides the reactions into four types based on the elements of the immune response involved.[103]

Type I reactions involve elements of strong Th2 responses that lead to increased IgE, eosinophilia, and eosinophil and mast cell activation. Adverse reactions of this type include the development of urticaria (with several helminthic parasites), the occurrence of potentially life-threatening anaphylactic shock in IgE-mediated mast cell degranulation (e.g., triggered by systemic release of antigens from echinococcal cysts[104]), and exuberant eosinophilic infiltration of tissues due to migrating helminth larvae (e.g., Löffler's pneumonia with the pulmonary migration of *Ascaris* larvae).

Type II reactions are also dependent on elements of Th2 cell responses that lead to increased IgM and then IgG antibodies directed toward the infectious agents. These antibodies, if cross-reactive with host antigens, may lead to complement-mediated cytotoxicity or antibody-dependent cell-mediated cytotoxicity by natural killer cells, which have Fc receptors. An example of this type of immunopathologic response is the uncommon hemolytic anemia associated with *Mycoplasma pneumoniae* infection that is mediated by complement-induced hemolysis triggered by IgM (cold agglutinin) antibodies against erythrocyte I antigen.

Type III reactions are caused by the deposition of immune complexes. When neither antibody nor antigen is present in excess of the other, the complexing of antibodies with soluble antigen results in the formation of immune complexes that may cause disease. This may develop acutely as antibody titers rise in the presence of microbial antigens, causing the syndrome of serum sickness. In addition, when soluble antigen is persistently abundant, sustained formation of immune complexes develops, leading to chronic immune complex-mediated tissue damage (especially glomerulonephritis), as found in subacute bacterial endocarditis, chronic hepatitis B antigenemia, and chronic *Plasmodium malariae* infections.[105]

Type IV reactions include adverse reactions mediated by macrophages and cytotoxic T cells. Examples are damage caused by granulomas in leprosy, tuberculosis, tertiary syphilis, and fungal infections. Likewise, granulomas developing around schistosomal eggs, depending on their location, may cause ureteral obstruction or hepatic presinusoidal lesions. Other deleterious inflammatory reactions in this category are mediated by parasite-elicited host cytokines, such as the hepatic fibrosis elicited by schistosomal eggs.

IMMUNE INTERACTIONS

Immune Evasion

The human immune system has evolved in concert with microbes and is very sophisticated, especially with regard to host defenses against microbes, but the system is not perfect. Interactions of the immune system with microbes are an ongoing affair. Microbes have a high mutation rate compared to human beings. Microbes have evolved a diversity of mechanisms that can enable microorganisms to subvert immediate immunologically mediated elimination (***Table 1.1***). Persistence within the host is necessary for the propagation of some parasites.

There are multiple mechanisms by which microbes can persist in the body and evade the immune system. Tolerance is defined as specific reduction in the response of the immune system to a given antigen.[106,107] In the case of transplacental infection, the fetus develops a certain degree of tolerance to antigens to which it is exposed. The immune system of fetuses is rather incompletely developed *in utero*, and microorganisms survive easily. Cytomegalovirus infects the fetus transplacentally and produces extensive damage to multiple tissues. After delivery, infants continue shedding virions for weeks to months because they are unable to destroy the virus. Other mechanisms include the production of superantigens that stimulate a large population of T cells, which then become deleted if the encounter occurs during early development. Exposure to massive amounts of antigen in the circulation can also lead to tolerance.[2,103] Immunosuppression is a well-demonstrated phenomenon that occurs during certain infections caused by viruses, bacteria, protozoa, and helminths. These infections usually involve the lymphoid tissues and macrophages and hamper the immune response.

Table 1.1 Mechanisms of Immune Evasion Used by Pathogenic Microbes

Type of Immune Response	Immune Evasion Mechanisms
Innate immunity	Block natural killer cells
	Recognition avoidance
	Complement inactivation or blockage
	Avoidance of phagocytosis by macrophages and polymorphonuclear neutrophils
	Manipulation of cell surface
Early induced response	Modulation of inflammatory response
	Interference with signaling pathways
	Interference with RNAi
	Antimicrobial peptide degradation
	Modulation of endosomal trafficking
	Modulation of cytoskeleton
Adaptive immunity	Induce apoptosis
	Interfere with receptors and signaling
	Modulation of antigen presentation and processing
	Modulation of cell maturation
	Superantigens
Protective immunity	Antigenic variation
	Phase shift
	Escape mutants

Intracellular pathogens that are able to spread from cell to cell without exposure to the extracellular compartment can avoid exposure to some elements of the immune system. In other cases, pathogens reside in sites relatively inaccessible to the immune system, such as glandular luminal spaces or kidney tubules. In many infections, antibodies are produced but do not effect microbial killing. Sometimes, antibody avidity is low, the epitopes against which the antibody is directed are not critical to the microorganism's survival, or the mechanism of immune elimination is not antibody dependent.[2]

Other microorganisms have developed means of counteracting specific elements of immune responses, such as production of an IgA-degrading enzyme, IgAase, by certain strains of *N. gonorrhoeae*.[108] Some strains of amebae also produce proteases that destroy complement.[2] Reactivation of infections in old age due to waning immunity has been well demonstrated in cases of tuberculosis and varicella zoster virus, allowing transmission to new hosts.

One well-studied mechanism of immune evasion is the capability of changing the antigenic structure by genetic mutation or by programmed sequential expression of genes encoding different surface antigens.[109] Antigenic drift and recombination between influenzaviruses affecting humans and animals are well documented. *Borrelia recurrentis* and *Trypanosoma gambiense* are also capable of changing their surface antigens after antibodies control the initial bloodstream infection.[110,111] The new antigens are not recognized by the antibodies, allowing relapse of the infection. Parasites in which sexual reproduction is possible benefit enormously.[112] Genetic variability introduced by crossing over during meiotic divisions is much greater than the variability introduced by asexual reproduction. As many as four crossovers on a single pair of chromosomes have been demonstrated in *P. falciparum*.[113]

Microparasites also have multiple mechanisms by which they can evade the initial line of defense provided by phagocytes. These strategies include killing of the phagocyte (e.g., *Streptococcus pyogenes* and *Entamoeba histolytica*), inhibition of chemotaxis (e.g., *Clostridium perfringens*), decreased internalization of microbes by phagocytic cells (e.g., *T. gondii*), inhibition of opsonins (e.g., *Treponema pallidum*), inhibition of phagolysosome fusion (e.g., *M. leprae* and *Mycobacterium tuberculosis*), and escape from the phagosome into the cytoplasm (e.g., *Rickettsia* spp., *Trypanosoma cruzi*, and *Listeria*).[2,44,75,92] With cell-to-cell spread, microorganisms may be minimally exposed to complement, antibodies, or phagocytes in the extracellular or intravascular spaces.[77,78] Rickettsial infections spread from cell to cell throughout the infected foci in the endothelial layer of the microvasculature.[82,83,94]

Macroparasites, the helminths, have evolved diverse mechanisms that enable them to survive *in vivo*.[85] Characteristically, helminths live for months to years in infected hosts within the lumen of the bowel, within tissues, or in the blood or lymphatic vessels. Many helminths are in intimate and recurring contact with all elements of the immune system. As a consequence of their size, helminthic worms do not use intracellular mechanisms to evade immune responses but have evolved a number of capabilities that permit their survival. For instance, interference with antigen processing has been well documented in animal models and patients infected with the filarial nematodes *Brugia malayi* and *Onchocerca volvulus*. These helminths produce a family of proteins called the cystatins that are capable of inhibiting proteases responsible for antigen degradation and subsequent presentation through MHC class II pathways in antigen-presenting cells. These proteins are also capable of modulating T-cell proliferation and elicit upregulation of interleukin-10 (IL-10) expression. Other modulators include helminthic derivatives of arachidonic acid such as lipoxin A4, which is capable of blocking production of IL-12 in dendritic cells. Helminthic prostaglandins can also inhibit IL-12 production by dendritic cells. Since helminths have very complex genomes (~21 000 protein-encoding genes in some of them), they are capable of producing a large variety of proteins. Some of them are cytokines and related proteins also capable of modulating the host immune response to their advantage. For example, *B. malayi* has been shown to express transforming growth factor (TGF)-β-like proteins capable of binding TGF-β human receptors. Other cytokines include macrophage-migration inhibition factors produced by several nematodes including *B. malayi*. Blockade of effector mechanisms has also been demonstrated in some helminth infections, including proteases that target effector molecules such as eotaxin. Neutrophil proteases can also be inhibited by serpins.

EMERGING INFECTIOUS DISEASES

The concept of emerging infectious diseases is not new but has been the focus of attention due to the resurgence of old infectious diseases that were thought to be controlled and the recognition of new pathogens as humans increase their interaction with the biosphere. By definition, an emerging infectious disease is one that has newly appeared in the population or has existed but is rapidly increasing in incidence or geographic range.[114] Others define emerging infections as "new emerging or drug resistant infections whose incidence in humans has increased within the last two decades, or whose incidence threatens to increase in the near future." Emerging infections are classified by some as newly emerging, re-emerging/resurging, and deliberately emerging. Since 1967, after a widely publicized statement from the US Surgeon General declaring victory in the war against infectious diseases, more than 85 new pathogens have been described. These include viruses, bacteria, protozoans, and helminths. These pathogens can cause a wide diversity of syndromes including acute respiratory infections (influenza A H1N5, H1N1, SARS-CoV, Sin Nombre virus, human metapneumovirus), systemic diseases caused by viral hemorrhagic fever viruses (Lassa, Ebola, dengue), encephalitic syndromes (Nipah virus, West Nile virus), arthropod-borne agents (*Borrelia burgdorferi*, *Rickettsia* spp., *Ehrlichia* spp., *Anaplasma*), enteric pathogens (*Cryptosporidium*, microsporidia), chronic viral diseases (HIV-1 and 2, human T-cell lymphotropic virus types 1–3, human herpesviruses 6–8), hepatotropic viruses (hepatitis C and E), and other infectious agents.

The factors involved in the emergence or reemergence of infectious diseases are complex and include ecological changes (deforestation, reforestation, flooding, and climatic changes), changes in human demographics and behavior (sexual, cultural, and war), increased international travel, technological advances (organ transplantation and antibiotics), microbial evolution with the appearance of antibiotic-resistant or antigenically distinct strains, and deficiencies in surveillance and public health policy.[113,115–117] The classic triad of microbe, host, and environment is again exemplified.

TROPICAL INFECTIOUS DISEASES

Globally, as assessed in terms of disability-adjusted life years (DALYs), which measure morbidity and mortality,[118] infectious diseases in 1990 accounted for 36.4% of total DALYs. Infectious disease DALYs were considerably in excess of those attributable to cancer (5.9%), heart disease (3.1%), cerebrovascular disease (3.2%), or chronic lung disease (3.5%).[119]

However, these calculations admittedly miss the disproportionate impact of tropical infectious diseases on the still rapidly increasing populations living in impoverished, tropical areas, and they grossly underestimate the major developmental impact of common childhood enteric, helminthic, and other infections.[38,120–122] For those caring for individual patients with infectious diseases, appropriate diagnosis and treatment are important considerations for the individual. Even more important is the consideration of approaches that will lead to diminished acquisition of infectious diseases. For some infectious agents, immunization holds promise, as witnessed by the successful global eradication of smallpox and the potential eradication of poliomyelitis. Greater progress in the control of infectious diseases, however, rests with improvements related to socioeconomic conditions of the population at risk. In developed countries, tuberculosis was diminished well before the introduction of the first antimicrobial agents active against *M. tuberculosis*, and the reduction was attributable to improved socioeconomic conditions. For the major infectious diseases of the tropics, improvements in sanitation, living conditions, and general public health will be critical in helping control the impact of the diverse infectious agents that currently contribute to human morbidity and mortality. The impact of these infections is related not only to their effect on the health of the infected individual but also to their contribution to the morbidity associated with malnutrition and to their larger societal impact as an impediment to the full development of the political, economic, and social potential of entire populations.

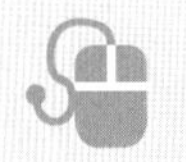
Access the complete reference list online at
http://www.expertconsult.com

CHAPTER 2

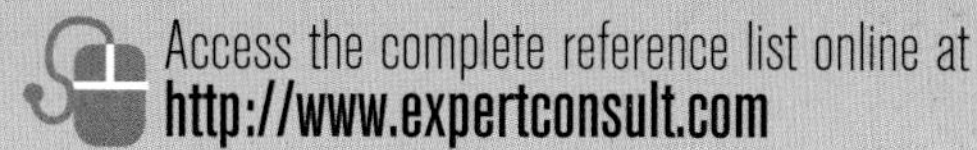
Access the complete reference list online at
http://www.expertconsult.com

The Perfect Storm: Climate, Ecosystems and Infectious Diseases

Fernando J. Torres-Vélez • Corrie Brown

The studies of emerging diseases and environmental changes are linked together in a manner reminiscent of the old adage about the forest and the trees. Each new disease that occurs is studied in significant depth, that is, with an intense focus, as on a single tree. However, it is often the overall environmental changes, or the proverbial forest, that is the greatest influence on the actual emergence of that disease. In recent decades the world has experienced a plethora of new and reemerging pathogens – human immunodeficiency virus, Hantavirus, Nipah virus (NiV), severe acute respiratory syndrome, Rift Valley fever, and bluetongue among others. A common denominator in the appearance of these diseases has been some modification of the environment, intensification or regional variations of normal atmospheric phenomena such as El Niño-Southern Oscillation (ENSO), as well as more specifically human-induced environmental changes.[1] Some of these anthropogenic factors are habitat encroachment by the growing human population, putting humans in closer contact with animals harboring pathogens previously unknown to infect people. Other instances involve impacts that humans have been having on the environment for decades, brewing today's global climate changes. Over the last decade, the scientific investigations into climate change have expanded logarithmically and now comprehensive and elegant multidisciplinary studies are beginning to illuminate potential disease problems due to climate change.

Climate is usually defined in a specific area as the "average weather," the mean and variation of atmospheric components such as temperature, precipitation, and wind, over time, traditionally 30 years. The overall global climate is powered by a fraction of the total solar radiation reaching the planet. Approximately one-third of all the incoming solar energy never makes it to the Earth's surface but rather is reflected back to space by atmospheric components. Of the remaining two-thirds absorbed by the Earth, an equal amount must be radiated back to space, to prevent an ever-increasing surface temperature. Clouds and gases, such as water vapor and carbon dioxide (CO_2), absorb much of the thermal radiation emitted by land and oceans, retransmitting it to Earth in a desirable greenhouse effect. This natural greenhouse effect allows for temperatures that are compatible with life processes as we know them. Water vapor and CO_2 are the most important greenhouse gases and significant increases in either can cause an enhanced greenhouse effect which has an overall effect of climate warming. Oceans and plants serve as natural CO_2 buffers by absorbing a great deal of what is generated. However, human activity is offsetting this natural system by burning fossil fuels and clearing forests.[2]

In addition to the anthropogenic contribution to global warming, external factors such as volcanic eruptions can have a major impact on the global climate. This was clearly illustrated in 1991 after Philippine's Mount Pinatubo's eruption when a global cooling and drying of the atmosphere was recorded.[3] Also there are poorly understood, coupled air–sea climatic events, such as ENSO, which can alter the climate of vast geographical areas for extended periods of times. During the ENSO, there is a reversal of surface air pressures between the eastern and western tropical Pacific, bringing a weakening and often reversal of trade winds. This allows for warmer water from the western Pacific to flow toward the east and build up off the coast of South America. The change in trade winds brings rain to the dry eastern Pacific, leaving extensive drought in the western Pacific. Volcanic eruptions or ENSO can be influenced by or combined with anthropogenic-induced global warming to augment further climate changes or contribute to adverse climatic events.[4–7]

A global authority on climate change was established by the United Nations Environment Programme and the World Meteorological Organization in 1989 in the form of the Intergovernmental Panel on Climate Change (IPCC). The IPCC is composed of scientists from around the world who review and assess scientific and technical data relevant to the understanding of climate change. They are charged with providing the world with a clear scientific view on the current state of climate change and its potential environmental and socioeconomic consequences. This panel has concluded that the observed climate changes cannot be explained by just natural factors. There is agreement that disease incidence and distribution are likely to change, although the manner in which this will happen is complex and difficult to specify.[2]

Below are three examples of infectious diseases that have emerged as a result of some of the climatic changes described above. The first, bluetongue, and its spread into northern Europe may be the only clear example of disease spread directly related to global warming. The second, Rift Valley fever, has reemerged several times in Eastern Africa in recent years, largely as a result of expanded ENSO impacts. The third, NiV, emerged in Malaysia due to a combination of direct anthropogenic effects and socioeconomic pressures, combined with ENSO effects.

BLUETONGUE

Bluetongue virus extension into northern Europe is undoubtedly the best example of a livestock disease expanding its range based on climate change, although the intensive outbreaks experienced in the last 2 years demonstrate the multiplicity of factors that play a role.

Bluetongue is an arthropod-borne disease, capable of infecting all ruminants, but with most severe clinical disease in sheep, in which there is severe depression, lameness, and often facial and tongue swelling, and abortion in pregnant animals. In cattle there is usually minimal clinical disease, but these animals can remain viremic for months, and so serve as the main reservoir of infection.[8] Bluetongue virus (BTV) is a segmented dsRNA virus in the Orbivirus genome, family *Reoviridae*. The disease is endemic in much of Africa and over large segments of the Americas, with distribution coinciding with the range of *Culicoides* spp., the responsible insect vector. The main Asian-African vector is *Culicoides imicola*. The disease has occurred in North Africa and the Middle East, making sporadic incursions into southern Europe, as *Culicoides* are easily transported on wind. The "envelope" or range of usual *C. imicola* distribution includes the southernmost parts of Europe, which are the regions that have been sporadically affected by bluetongue over the last few decades. Farther north in Europe, there are other *Culicoides* species known as the Palearctic species, *C. pulicaris* and *C. obsoletus*. Although both had been proven to be capable of transmitting bluetongue experimentally, they were not functioning in the natural epidemiology of infection prior to 2008.

Over the last several years, there have been documented increases in nighttime and winter temperatures and also changes in moisture conditions.[9] Warming trends in Europe created an environment for enhanced replication and survival of all of these *Culicoides* species, and, in some cases, shortened cold periods allowed for the vectors to persist throughout the winter. The range of *C. imicola* has expanded in recent years with the expansion shown to be coincident with warming.[10] The warming not only improved and expanded the populations of *Culicoides*, but also enabled enhanced viral replication within the vector.

Several strains of BTV have made incursions into Europe since the late 1990s. One of these, BTV-8, came from Africa and moved through Italy and up into Germany and the United Kingdom, affecting areas that had never before experienced bluetongue disease. It is hypothesized that the enhanced *C. imicola* population in southern Europe helped to fuel an outbreak. With expanding populations of *C. imicola* and the Palearctic species, there was more extensive overlap of these different species. A "handover" event occurred probably multiple times, in which the new host species picked up the virus from the endemic host. Once the virus was established within the Palearctic species, it was able to move to more northerly climes.[11] The increased temperatures in these more northerly areas, especially the shortened winter period, ensured that the Palearctic species would survive through the season during which BTV would have otherwise been expected to die back. As a result, there was sustained transmission of the disease in new areas.

This extension of BTV into northern Europe resulted in disease in many countries that had never before experienced the disease. More than 3000 outbreaks of bluetongue were reported to the World Organization for Animal Health in 2008 from northern European countries, and hundreds of thousands of ruminants died or were euthanized to prevent spread.[12]

RIFT VALLEY FEVER

Rift Valley fever virus is a segmented, enveloped, single-stranded RNA virus in the genus *Phlebovirus*, family *Bunyaviridae*. It has a wide variety of hosts but severe disease is seen most commonly in ruminants, especially sheep and goats, where it can present as an "abortion storm," death of neonates, and hepatic disease. It is also zoonotic and in humans presents as a febrile, flu-like illness, with some experiencing severe liver pathology or vascular complications. Mortality in humans ranges from 1% to 5% but in some outbreaks has been much higher.[13,14]

The virus is transmitted transovarially in mosquitoes and, under dry climatic conditions, can survive in *Aedes* mosquito eggs for years and maybe decades. With excessive rainfall, the mosquito eggs will hatch, and carry virus to susceptible ruminants, which experience a high viremia. Then *Culex* mosquitoes serve to transport the infection from animal to animal and, occasionally, animal to human.

The disease was first described around Lake Naivasha, in the Kenyan portion of Africa's Rift Valley, in 1930, and remained confined to the larger geographic zone of the Rift Valley for more than 40 years, with sporadic outbreaks occurring, usually associated with heavy rainfall.[15]

However, since 1977, Rift Valley fever has been recorded outside this zone on multiple occasions, all of which are associated with increases in flooding allowing for extensive mosquito replication. In 1977, Rift Valley fever surfaced in Egypt, and there was an extensive outbreak involving thousands of human and animal cases. Building of the Aswan dam in the years prior to this outbreak was probably an important factor as this hydrological project permitted controlled flooding of agricultural lands and subsequent enhanced mosquito habitats.[16] Then, in 1987, there was another outbreak, this time across the continent to West Africa, in Mauritania. In this case, Rift Valley fever occurred subsequent to completion of the Diama dam on the Senegal river, another project that created increased standing water for mosquito amplification.[17] In both of these cases, Egypt and Mauritania, there were human-induced changes to the environment, in the form of dam-building which created more standing water and therefore greater habitat possibilities for vectors of disease.

In 1997, there was a large outbreak in the Horn of Africa, beginning in northern Kenya and eventually moving to affect five different countries in the region, with large losses of domestic ruminants and extensive human infection.[18] This outbreak was attributed to excessive rainfall, which was brought about by the ENSO effect.[19] Then again in 2006–2007 there was another less extensive outbreak in the Horn of Africa, also attributed to heavy rainfall due to ENSO. However, by the time of this outbreak, climatic prediction models had been developed, and so sufficient warnings of a potential outbreak were distributed 2–6 weeks before the outbreak, dampening the overall impact because of preparedness and mitigation efforts, involving prompt suspicion and documentation of the diagnosis with aborted or ill animals and selected use of the available vaccine, isolation, and mosquito precautions and control.[20]

NIPAH

NiV is a newly described virus belonging in the *Henipavirus* genus of the *Paramyxoviridae* family. It emerged in Malaysia in the late 1990s in both humans and swine. In pigs, the disease occurred primarily as a respiratory ailment, with severe coughing, and was initially called "barking pig syndrome." The virus replicated in the respiratory tract of pigs and presumably was disseminated by aerosol to humans who developed a multisystemic disease, with predominant encephalitis and high case-fatality rate. During the course of the outbreak, there were 105 human deaths, almost all of which were closely associated with pig rearing or slaughter. To control the disease approximately one million pigs were slaughtered. The disease has reappeared, on a much smaller scale, in small clusters in humans in India and Bangladesh, but without any associated swine disease.[21–24]

Early molecular characterization of NiV revealed its relatedness to Hendra virus (HeV), another novel *Paramyxovirus* previously discovered in Australia only a few years before.[25,26] As HeV was shown to have a reservoir in pteropid bats (large fruit bats called flying foxes), these animals were studied for a possible role in NiV epidemiology. Approximately 3 years after the initial outbreak in Malaysia, NiV was isolated from the urine of these bats as well as from partially eaten fruits consumed by the animals.[27] Subsequent detection of NiV antibodies and RNA in bats' saliva and urine in Thailand, Cambodia, and India further strengthened the hypothesis that flying foxes of the genus *Pteropus* were the natural reservoir.[28–30]

With subsequent outbreaks taking place without pigs as the intermediate host, the ecologic and epidemiologic picture of NiV became more intricate and complex than originally thought. What was the role of pigs during its first emergence? What factors promoted infection of pigs during the first emergence?

During the 1990s, swine production in Malaysia moved to a more intensive system with high turnover of piglets. In addition, most farms were often combining fruit production with the use of pig waste as fertilizer, resulting in many trees overhanging pigpens. Extensive slash and burn practices in the region and an extended dry season brought up by the ENSO promoted changes in migration patterns of the *Pteropus* bats to areas of plentiful food availability, the pig/fruit farms.[31] It is believed that the combination of these production techniques, land use, and climate changes provided the ideal conditions for NiV's emergence in swine, from which it was aerosolized easily to humans. A unique set of factors brought two species with historically distinct ecological niches into close contact. Furthermore, the intense production practices allowed for a subtle introduction, circulation, and establishment of the virus into a new amplifying host, the pig. Retrospective serologic studies indicate that the first human cases in Malaysia predated the 1997 outbreak, indicating that the virus may have been circulating at low levels prior to the known emergence. The intensive management (high turnover of piglets) likely allowed a small amount of virus in select pigs to be widely circulated through transport and extensive sales associated with the rapidly developing intensive swine industry. As more animals became infected, there was increased possibility for transmission to people, and an outbreak occurred in the human population.[32] Recent outbreaks in India and Bangladesh have been attributed to direct contact with the bat's body fluids.[24,33]

CONCLUSION

As we continue contributing to global climate changes, modifying and encroaching into new habitats, there will undoubtedly be new instances of disease emergence and modifications of existing epidemiologic patterns.

To pinpoint emerging problems at their source and help to prevent their spread, it will be critical that health professionals become aware of the potential for novel or unexpected infections and to work more closely with veterinary, agricultural, and climate experts to understand better and control these emerging and expanding global health threats.

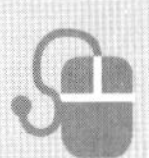

Access the complete reference list online at **http://www.expertconsult.com**

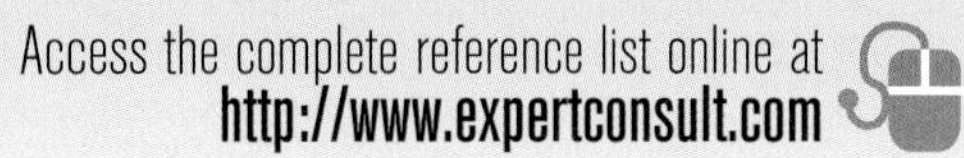
Access the complete reference list online at
http://www.expertconsult.com

CHAPTER 3

Epidemiology and Biostatistics

Edward T. Ryan • Megan Murray

Epidemiology is the science of investigating the occurrence, causes, and prevention of disease in human populations. Epidemiologic tools may be used to estimate disease frequency, uncover or confirm associations between risk factors and disease occurrence, and define the impact of preventive and curative measures to combat disease. As one of the primary disciplines of the field of public health, epidemiology is of great importance to human health worldwide, especially in the developing world. A fundamental understanding of epidemiologic principles – including basic terminology; study design and hypothesis testing; and data collection, analysis, and interpretation – is, therefore, necessary to the understanding of biomedical sciences.

OVERVIEW AND TERMINOLOGY

Measures of Disease Frequency

Prevalence is a measure of the total number of existing cases of a disease or condition in a specific population at a particular time. Prevalence is usually expressed as a fraction or percentage of a population, but it can also be given as the number of cases per 1000, 10 000, or 100 000 people. In contrast to prevalence, which enumerates *all* cases of a disease, *incidence* is a measure of the number of *new* cases of disease occurring over a specified period. Incidence is, therefore, expressed as the number of cases that occurred in a population of a given size per a unit time. Thus, if a cohort of 1000 individuals is followed for 1 year and 100 of these individuals develop a specific disease, the incidence rate of that disease would be 0.1, or 100 per 1000 per year.

Measures of Effect

In addition to measuring frequency of occurrence of a disease, epidemiologic studies measure the strength of an association between a specific risk factor and the incidence of a disease or medical condition, or between a specific intervention or treatment and the prevention or resolution of a disease. For instance, the effect of a risk factor on disease frequency can be estimated by comparing the incidence of disease in a group that has been exposed to a specific risk factor to the incidence of disease in a group that has not been exposed.

Infectious Disease Terms

There are a number of definitions specific to the epidemiologic study of infectious diseases. A disease that occurs regularly in a population is said to be *endemic*. When a disease occurs at a frequency higher than is expected, it is said to be *epidemic*. A localized epidemic may be referred to as an *outbreak*. Diseases in animals are said to be *enzootic* or *epizootic*. After infection, there often follows a period of *latency*, defined as the duration of time from infection to onset of infectiousness. The period of time immediately following infection may also be an *incubation* period, defined as the time from infection to development of symptomatic disease. If the incubation period is longer than the latent period for a specific disease, individuals may infect others prior to the onset of recognizable illness. An *attack rate* refers to the proportion of a population that develops an infectious disease over a given period. The term *secondary attack rate* refers to the proportion of *exposed* individuals who become ill. The secondary attack rate is often measured among the household members of a known index case, since it is relatively easy to count the number of exposed individuals and follow them over time.

The *basic reproductive number*, often expressed as R_0, is defined as the expected number of secondary infectious cases generated by an average infectious case in a population in which everyone is susceptible. This quantity determines the potential for an infectious agent to start an outbreak, the extent of transmission in the absence of control measures, and the ability of control measures to reduce spread. R_0 can be expressed as a product of the number of contacts each infectious individual has per unit time (k), the probability of transmission per contact between an infectious case and a susceptible person (b), and the mean duration of infectiousness, D:

$$R_0 = bkD$$

Although it is a highly simplified summary of a pathogen's epidemic potential, R_0 may be used to predict outcome following an introduction of an infection into a population. If R_0 is greater than 1, the number of people infected will grow and an epidemic will take place; if R_0 is less than 1, the disease will die out.

In real epidemics, it is useful to replace the *basic reproductive number* with the *effective reproductive number*, denoted R, which is defined as the *actual* average number of secondary cases infected by a primary case. R is usually less than R_0, since it reflects both the impact of control measures instituted over time and the depletion of a susceptible population as previously infected individuals acquire immunity. *Herd immunity* results when a vaccine not only protects a vaccinated individual from contracting an infection but also prevents that individual from spreading the infection to others.

STUDY DESIGN

Understanding scientific–medical studies requires knowledge of a number of fundamental epidemiologic and statistical concepts, the first of which concerns study design. Studies may be designed to measure disease frequency (incidence and prevalence) or to measure an effect (e.g., how effective is drug A compared with drug B in the treatment of individuals with a certain medical condition). A classic type of study that measures disease frequency is a *surveillance study*, which tracks the frequency of a disease in a population over time. It is effectively a reporting system. It may be *active*, in which case people with disease are actively sought, or *passive* where cases are reported that present to medical attention. It may be hospital- or clinic-based or community-based. It may report specific well-defined diseases or, if diagnostic capabilities are limited, it may report syndromes (e.g., the syndrome of ulcerative genital disease as opposed to genital herpes, chancroid, or syphilis, specifically). Surveillance systems are a fundamental tool in public health because they provide critical information on disease burden and changes in disease frequency over time that may alert public health authorities to epidemic disease.

Studies that *measure an effect* may measure the effectiveness of a new drug or vaccine; alternatively, they measure the effect of a possible risk factor on disease frequency (e.g., the effect that smoking has on the risk of developing lung cancer). The optimal study for measuring effect is a *clinical trial*. Randomized clinical trials are prospective studies in which individuals are randomized to one of at least two study arms and followed for the outcome of interest over time. The major advantage of this type of study is that the random nature of group assignment ensures that people in one group will not differ systematically from people in another group in some way that would influence outcome. Another way to say this is that the purpose of randomization is to eliminate potential confounding factors (whether suspected or not suspected) that are associated with both exposure and outcome.

If the random assignment is completely unknown to both the study participants and researchers, it is called a *double-blind randomized trial*. If one of the study arms receives a treatment or intervention and the other receives a placebo, the trial is called a *placebo-controlled trial*. Since it is unethical to offer one group a placebo if there is available a treatment of known benefit, many trials compare the efficacy of a new intervention to that of a standard therapy; these trials are called *equivalence studies*. An example of a randomized double-blind equivalence study would be one that compares the efficacy of two drugs, drug A and drug B, for the treatment of shigellosis. To ensure that both participants and researchers are blinded to the intervention, the drug preparations should look and taste the same, be administered on the same dosing schedule, and given by the same route. Follow-up of the two groups should be identical.

It is often impossible to conduct a clinical trial, especially when the exposure of interest is not an intervention or a treatment but some kind of environmental or genetic factor. In this case, a *cohort study* can be conducted to estimate association between risk factor and outcome. In a cohort study, groups of individuals with different exposure histories are identified and followed over time. As an example, imagine that we want to study the relationship between smoking and lung cancer. We could identify individuals who smoke and those who do not and follow them over time to see if the incidence of lung cancer between the two cohorts is different. This type of study has several possible shortcomings, one of which is that it may take years or decades for an individual to develop a disease or outcome after initial exposure. Another problem inherent in this type of study is the fact that the two cohorts of exposed and unexposed people may differ in ways other than just the basis of the exposure of interest (a *confounding influence*). For example, a confounding influence in our study may be the effect of alcohol consumption on the development of lung cancer (for instance, if individuals who drink heavily were more likely to smoke than those who do not drink heavily).

An alternative study design is a *case-control study*. In this type of study, exposures of people who experience an outcome of interest are compared to exposures of those who have not had such an outcome. This type of study is especially useful for a rare disease or when there is a prolonged period of time between exposure and outcome. Continuing our example of examining the relationship of smoking and lung cancer, in a case-control study, we would identify individuals who have developed lung cancer and a group of "controls" who have not developed lung cancer. We could then ascertain the smoking histories of individuals in the study and try to determine whether they were consistently different between cases and controls. Since case-control studies often involve retrospective collection of exposure data obtained after a subject knows his or her diagnosis, there is a potential for *recall bias*. Another potential problem in case-control studies involves the selection of controls. Ideally, cases should be chosen from the population that gave rise to cases and should be selected without regard to exposure status. Case-control and cohort studies are also referred to as *observational studies*, since there is no intervention.

HYPOTHESIS TESTING

When designing a study, researchers should first *state the hypothesis* that they want to test. For example, "we hypothesize that drug A is effective in treating salmonellosis." The hypothesis should be stated before data are collected. A common pitfall of studies is to first collect data and *then* to analyze data for comparisons that reach statistical significance. Such a fishing expedition may uncover real differences, but may also uncover differences related to chance alone.

A placebo-controlled double-blind randomized trial would be the best way to test our hypothesis that our new drug A is "effective" in treating individuals with salmonella gastroenteritis. When designing this study, researchers should first select relevant and measurable endpoints that will distinguish whether individuals who get the drug "do better." Primary endpoints may be days of diarrhea; days of fever; duration of bacterial shedding of salmonella organisms in stool; and/or the presence or absence of infectious complications, bacteremia, or death. These outcomes should be as clinically relevant and precise as possible; that is, definitions of what constitutes diarrhea and fever should be established before the study is undertaken, the same amount of stool and blood should be collected and processed from all study enrollees to ensure equality of assessment, and data should be recorded and reported as accurately and completely as possible.

After the hypothesis is stated, the researchers should next formulate the *null hypothesis*. In this step, the investigators should assume that no true difference exists between the two study groups (those who get drug A and those who get the placebo). A decision should then be made as to what constitutes a statistically significant result. *Statistical significance* is usually conveyed through a statistic known as the *P value*; results are often considered significant if the *P* value is less than a cutoff value (or "alpha level") of 5%. The *P* value refers to the probability that one would observe a result equal to or more extreme than the study result under the null hypothesis. One way to interpret this is to say that if a difference is shown between the two groups, there is a 95% chance that the difference is true (or a less than 5% chance that the difference is due to chance alone).

The *alpha level* is a cutoff value for a *P* value for a hypothesis test that is often set, somewhat arbitrarily, at 0.05. A *type I error* occurs when the null hypothesis is incorrectly rejected when it is in fact true, that is, when there is no difference between drug A and a placebo. A test with an alpha level of 0.05 should lead to type I errors no more than 5% of the time. Unlike the *P* value that varies with the data, alpha levels are chosen in advance and indicate the specific *P* value that will be considered significant. A *type II* (or *beta*) *error* occurs when the null hypothesis is not rejected even when there is truly a difference between the two arms of the study, that is, between drug A and the placebo. Type II errors may occur when a study is not large enough to detect a difference, or when individuals are not followed for an adequate amount of time for differences between groups to become apparent. Most well-designed studies aim for a type II error rate between 10% and 20%. The *power* of a study refers to the probability that the null hypothesis is rejected when it is false, and it is thus given the expression

$$\text{Power} = 1 - \text{Probability of a type II error}$$

Therefore, most studies aim for 80–90% power (i.e., an 80–90% chance that if the null hypothesis is not rejected it is correct). It is this power calculation that determines the number of individuals who need to be enrolled in a study.

Only after the hypothesis has been stated and a study appropriately designed and adequately powered should data be collected and stored. Once this is completed, data analysis may begin. In this step, investigators determine the estimated effect of the intervention or exposure, and the probability that the observed difference between the two study groups would occur if no true difference exists in the larger population.

Data Expression and Analysis

Data may be expressed in many ways. When an exposure or outcome is expressed in terms of a continuous variable such as age or weight, the differences between groups may be expressed by comparing *mean* or *median* values for the two groups. Both these statistics are measures of central tendency, meaning that they describe the middle, or average, value of the data. The mean is the *arithmetic* average, which is simply obtained by summing the observations and dividing the sum by the number of observations. For instance, if we measure the days of diarrhea following administration of drug A to patients with salmonellosis, we may find that one patient had diarrhea for 2 days, another for 3 days, another for 4 days, another for 5 days, and another for 20 days. The mean would be a summation divided by the number evaluated (2 + 3 + 4 + 5 + 20 (equals 34) divided by 5 = 6.8). The *median* is the value that divides the data in half; 50% of the observations have values lower than the median, and 50% have values greater than the median. The median is also referred to as the 50th centile. Using the median rather than the mean lessens the impact of outliers, since the actual values of extreme data points do not affect the median. Another way of reducing the effect of extreme outlier observations is to use the *geometric mean*, which is often used with data measured on a logarithmic scale. The geometric mean is calculated by multiplying the observed values and taking the *n*th root, where *n* is the number of observations. For the preceding example, this would be given by

$$\sqrt[5]{(2)(3)(4)(5)(20)} = 4.7$$

The term *standard deviation* measures the spread of the individual observations around the mean. It is given by the formula

$$s = \sqrt{\sum \frac{X - \bar{X}}{n-1}}$$

where X represents the value of each individual observation, $\bar{X}$ represents the mean, and n represents the number of observations. The *standard error of the mean* indicates the degree of uncertainty in calculating estimate from a sample. A standard error may be calculated from the standard deviation by dividing the standard deviation by a square root of *n* (with *n* representing the number of values measured).

Range refers to the interval from the minimum to the maximum value in a set of quantitative measurements. For instance, the arithmetic mean in our example would be 6.8, the geometric mean would be 4.7, the median would be 4, and the range would be 2 through 20.

Data that are *normal* or *normally distributed* are symmetrically distributed around a mean. A classic example of normally distributed data is a bell-shaped curve (e.g., a population-based IQ evaluation; ***Fig. 3.1***).

Characteristics that we might want to study may be measured in a variety of ways. Observed data may be *dichotomous*, *categorical*, or *continuous*. If data can take only one of two values, they are defined as *dichotomous*. Returning to our smoking and lung cancer example, we could describe smoking in terms of the dichotomous variables "ever" or "never" smoked.

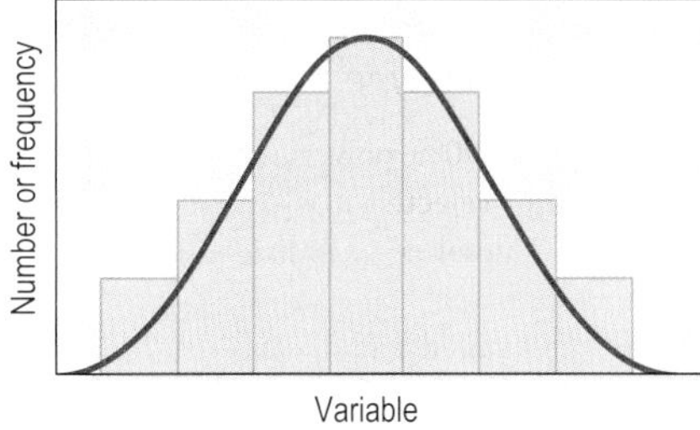

Figure 3.1 Normal distribution.

Categorical observations have values that fit into categories. For example, we might characterize race or ethnicity using a categorical variable. Some data categories describe ascending levels of intensity or severity. For example, we could describe smoking history as "none," "light," "moderate," and "heavy." When categorical data are ordered in this way, they are *ordinal*. Finally, data may be measured on a *continuous* scale. Again, referring to our smoking example, we could measure smoking in terms of the number of cigarettes consumed. At analysis, continuous data may be transformed into categorical data (but not vice versa).

Once we have summarized our data into the groups we are comparing, we need to decide whether the data differ between groups. If data are dichotomous, we may compare proportions, for example, the proportion of "ever" smokers who develop lung cancer to "never" smokers who develop lung cancer. For instance, imagine in our study that 5 smokers develop lung cancer out of a cohort of 100, while only 1 of 100 nonsmokers develops lung cancer. These data could be presented in a table of observed frequencies as follows:

	Lung Cancer	No Lung Cancer	Total
Ever smoked	5	95	100
Never smoked	1	99	100
	6	194	200

Under the null hypothesis, we assume that there is no difference in the incidence of lung cancer among smokers and nonsmokers. Given that 6 cases of lung cancer occurred among the 200 people we followed, we can come up with a table of "expected" frequencies under the null hypothesis.

	Lung Cancer	No Lung Cancer	Total
Ever smoked	3	97	100
Never smoked	3	97	100
	6	194	200

We can use the *chi-square test* statistic to ask how likely it would be that we obtained the observed frequencies if the null hypothesis were true. The chi-square statistic is given by the formula

$$\chi^2 = \sum_{\text{ALL CELLS}} \frac{(O-E)^2}{E}$$

where *O* is observed frequency and *E* is expected frequency. If the chi-square test is small, this suggests that there is no difference between the groups; if it is large, we assume that a difference exists.

Other statistical tests are available to analyze data. The choice of optimal test depends on a number of variables, including data type and number of groups. For instance, for continuous data that are normally distributed, we could compare the means of two groups using the *t test* for comparing means. When data are not normally distributed, other tests would be required; these usually are based on "order statistics" and include such nonparametric methods as the *Mann–Whitney U test*, the *Kruskal–Wallis* test and the *Wilcoxon matched rank test*, among others. The *ANOVA* (analysis of variance) test may be used to compare more than two groups that are normally distributed. The Mann–Whitney U test is used for evaluating two groups that are not normally distributed, and the Kruskal–Wallis test may be used for evaluating more than two groups that are not normally distributed.

Analysis of data may disclose "associations." For instance, returning to our example of smoking and lung cancer, we may find that smoking and lung cancer are statistically associated. Although variables that are found to be associated with an outcome are often called *risk factors*, a statistical association does not imply a cause and effect relationship between that variable and outcome. The *relative risk* is the probability of an outcome if a risk factor/association is present divided by the probability of the outcome if the risk factor/association is absent. For instance, in our example of the cohort study of smokers and nonsmokers, we imagined a study in which we have followed 100 individuals who smoke and 100 individuals who never smoked. We saw that 5 of the 100 smokers developed cancer (probability 0.05), but that only 1 of 100 nonsmokers developed lung cancer (probability 0.01). The relative risk is, therefore, 0.05 divided by 0.01, or 5. A relative risk of 5 implies that individuals who smoke are five times more likely to develop lung cancer than individuals who do not smoke.

In case-control studies, it is the researcher who determines how many study and control participants are evaluated, and so a true disease frequency in the population as a whole cannot be established. In this case, we cannot estimate the relative risk, since we do not actually know the risk of disease in the unexposed population. An approximation of the relative risk for case-control studies is the *odds ratio*. To understand the difference between a risk and an odds ratio, think of the probability (or risk) of throwing a six-sided die in a game of chance and having the die land with six black dots facing up (1 in 6 chance). The odds of throwing a six on the other hand will be the number of times the die will land with six black dots showing divided by the number of times six dots will not be uppermost (1 to 5). An odds ratio is, therefore, the odds of developing an outcome if an association is present, divided by the odds of an outcome if the association is absent. Both the relative risk and the odds ratio are easy to calculate from a 2 × 2 table.

	Lung Cancer	No Lung Cancer	Total
Ever smoked	*A*	*B*	*A* + *B*
Never smoked	*C*	*D*	*C* + *D*
	A + *C*	*B* + *D*	*A* + *B* + *C* + *D*

$$\text{RR} = \frac{A/(A+B)}{C/(C+D)}$$

$$\text{OR} = \frac{[A/(A+C)]/[C/(A+C)]}{[B/(B+D)]/[D/(B+D)]} = \frac{A/C}{B/D} = \frac{AD}{BC}$$

Confidence intervals are a way of combining information about the strength of an association with information about the effects of chance in obtaining the observed results. A 95% confidence interval (CI) is most commonly used. An association is usually reported as an odds ratio (OR) or relative risk (RR) with a 95% CI.

The final stage of analyzing a study is extrapolation. We may extrapolate to an individual or to a group. For instance, based on a relative risk or odds ratio of 5 for smoking and lung cancer, we could conclude that if an individual smoked, he or she may be five times more likely to develop lung cancer than if he or she did not smoke. We may also speak of an *attributable risk percent*. The advantage of this concept is that it allows us to think of a portion of the risk of developing a disease that may be eliminated among those who do not have the risk factor. Attributable risk percentage may be thought of as

$$(\text{RR} - 1/\text{RR}) \times 100\%$$

For instance, in our study, we found that smoking was associated with a relative risk of 5 of developing lung cancer. This may not seem like an overly large risk of developing lung cancer; however, the attributable risk percent is 5 − 1/5 = 80%. This suggests that 80% of lung cancer in our study population could have been prevented if our study participants had never smoked.

UNDERSTANDING DIAGNOSTIC LABORATORY TESTS

In many instances, laboratory tests are part of a case definition (e.g., detection of serum antibodies against human immunodeficiency virus (HIV) in a study involving individuals infected with HIV). It should be recalled that a test is often a surrogate marker to distinguish a disease-free group from a diseased group. Assuming a normal distribution in both groups of whatever marker we are measuring (e.g., a serum antibody level), we can imagine that the disease-free and diseased groups do not overlap at all with regard to the specific blood test of interest (***Fig. 3.2A***). Often, however, the two groups do overlap, and some individuals in the diseased group will have tests with lower values than some of the individuals in the disease-free group (***Fig. 3.2B***).

In establishing the utility of a test, therefore, we must first establish the reference interval for disease-free individuals. *Sensitivity* and *specificity* of a test are then measured compared with a "gold standard." *Sensitivity* measures the probability that those with a disease will have a positive test when individuals with the disease are identified by the gold standard. *Specificity* measures the probability that those who do not have the disease will test negative by the test being evaluated. There usually is a tradeoff between the sensitivity and specificity of a specific test. For example, if we choose X as the cutoff value for a positive test on ***Figure 3.2B*** of overlapping curves, we will achieve 100% sensitivity – but at the cost of misclassifying many negative cases as positive ones, that is, reducing specificity. Conversely, we could maximize specificity by moving our cutoff value for a positive test rightward to the Y position, but in so doing, we would compromise our ability to identify a true case of disease.

For example, imagine that we are evaluating a new test to diagnose schistosomiasis, and imagine that we will compare this test to a gold standard in a village with a population of 1000 individuals of whom 500 actually have schistosomiasis by our gold standard. Imagine that our new test correctly identifies 400 infected individuals but incorrectly identifies 100 truly infected individuals as not having schistosomiasis when in fact they are infected (*false negative*). Also imagine that our new test incorrectly labels 50 individuals as having schistosomiasis who do not (*false positive*).

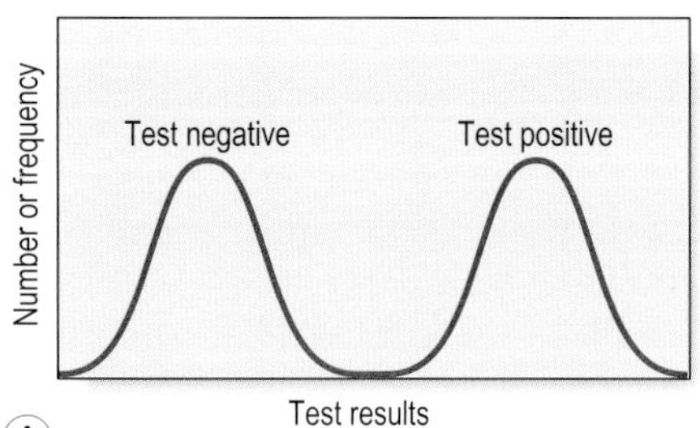

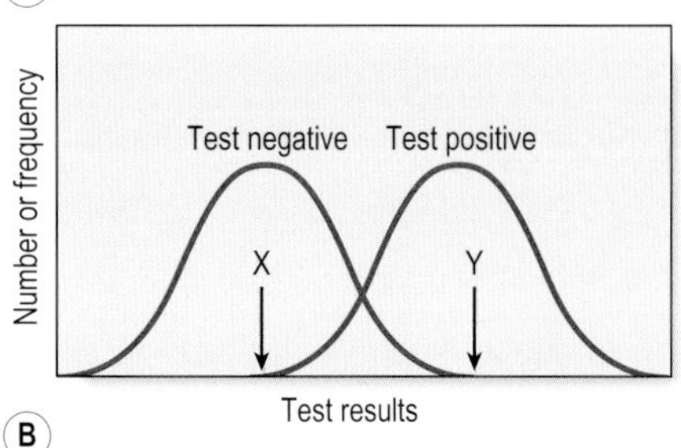

Figure 3.2 **(A)** Normal distribution in which two groups do not overlap. **(B)** Two groups that overlap.

Test	Gold Standard Disease	Gold Standard Disease-Free
Positive	400 (*a*)	50 (*b*)
Negative	100 (*c*)	450 (*d*)
	500	500

Sensitivity and specificity are calculated as:

$$\text{Sensitivity} = \frac{a}{a+c} = \frac{400}{500} = 0.80 \text{ or } 80\%$$

$$\text{Specificity} = \frac{d}{b+d} = \frac{450}{500} = 0.90 \text{ or } 90\%$$

Our test will, therefore, have a sensitivity of 80% and a specificity of 90%. The actual utility of this test, however, will rest not only on its sensitivity and specificity but also on the prevalence of the disease in question in our population of interest. In our preceding example, there was a 50% prevalence of schistosomiasis (500 infected individuals who lived in a population of 1000). If we assume that the "true" prevalence of schistosomiasis in a different village is 20%, at a population level, the average individual in that village will have a 20% chance of having the disease before the test is performed (in reality, certain individuals will be at higher or lower risk of having schistosomiasis on the basis of age, sex, and other factors). Assuming that we are evaluating 1000 individuals (with 20% of them having the disease), and assuming that we are using our new test with a sensitivity of 80%, we would assume that 160 of the 200 individuals with the disease will be correctly identified by the test:

Test	Gold Standard Disease	Gold Standard Disease-Free
Positive	160	80 false positives
Negative	40 false negatives	720
	200	800

The remaining 20% of these individuals will be incorrectly labeled as negative ($n = 40$; false negatives). Specificity equals 90%; therefore, 90% of those who are disease-free will be correctly labeled as negative (90% of 800; 720 true negatives). The remaining 10% of individuals who are disease-free will be incorrectly labeled as positive (10% of 800; 80 false positives).

Now let us imagine that we are applying our same test in a different village (Village Y) in which schistosomiasis is much more prevalent and 75% of the population has the disease:

Test	Gold Standard Disease	Gold Standard Disease-Free
Positive	600	25 false positives
Negative	150 false negatives	225
	750	250

Finally, let us imagine that we use our test in a third village (Village Z), in which schistosomiasis is much rarer and the true probability of disease is only 2% (only 2% of the population is infected). Then our table would look like this:

Test	Gold Standard Disease	Gold Standard Disease-Free
Positive	16	98 false positives
Negative	4 false negatives	882
	20	980

Now, let us analyze the predictive value of positive and negative test results in each of these villages. The *positive predictive value* refers to the probability that one who tests positive truly has the disease, while the *negative predictive value* refers to the probability that one who tests negative actually does not have the disease. The crucial point to understand is that the predictive value depends not only on the sensitivity and specificity of the test itself but also on the disease prevalence in the population being evaluated.

Test	Gold Standard Disease	Gold Standard Disease-Free	
Positive	*a* = number of individuals diseased and positive	*b* = number of individuals disease-free and positive	*a* + *b* = total number of test positives
Negative	*c* = number of individuals diseased and negative	*d* = number of individuals disease-free and negative	*c* + *d* = total number of test negatives

The following formulae are used for calculating the predictive value of a positive test and the predictive value of a negative test:

$$\text{Predictive value of a positive test} = \frac{a}{a+b}$$ [Proportion of individuals with a positive test who actually have the disease]

$$\text{Predictive value of a negative test} = \frac{d}{c+d}$$ [Proportion of individuals with a negative test who actually do not have the disease]

Using the preceding calculated numbers, and assuming a 2% pretest probability of disease (as in Village Z):

$$\text{Predictive value of a positive test} = \frac{a}{a+b} = \frac{16}{16+98} = 14\%$$

$$\text{Predictive value of a negative test} = \frac{d}{c+d} = \frac{882}{4+882} = 99.5\%$$

Similarly, if we assume a 75% pretest probability as in Village Y:

$$\text{Predictive value of a positive test} = \frac{a}{a+b} = \frac{600}{600+25} = 96\%$$

$$\text{Predictive value of a negative test} = \frac{d}{c+d} = \frac{225}{150+225} = 60\%$$

Therefore, using exactly the same test, with exactly the same sensitivity and specificity, we can generate the following table of positive and negative predictive values of our test in villages with different prevalences of the disease in question:

	Pretest Probability		
	2% (Village Z)	20% (Village X)	75% (Village Y)
Predictive value of a positive test	14%	66.7%	96%
Predictive value of a negative test	99.5%	94.7%	60%

This means that there is an 86% chance that a positive test obtained in Village Z with a 2% pretest probability of disease is falsely positive. Similarly, there is a 40% chance that a negative result is in fact falsely negative in Village Y with a pretest probability of disease of 75%. This is despite the fact that we are using the same test with the same sensitivity and specificity in each village. It is, therefore, crucial to understand that the interpretation of laboratory tests (whether in a study or in clinical practice) should be understood in context.

ACKNOWLEDGMENTS

We are grateful to Margaret Bikowski and Sam Riley for assistance with figures. This work was supported in part by a grant from the US Centers for Disease Control and Prevention, U19CI000514 (ETR).

Access the complete reference list online at
http://www.expertconsult.com

Access the complete reference list online at
http://www.expertconsult.com

CHAPTER 4

Social and Cultural Factors in Tropical Medicine: Reframing Our Understanding of Disease

Rebecca Dillingham • David A. Walton • Paul E. Farmer

BARRIERS TO CARE AND THE PERSISTENT PATHOGENS: A BIOSOCIAL APPROACH

By the close of the twentieth century, the world's ranking infectious pathogens – from well-known malaria and filariasis to the more recently described human immunodeficiency virus (HIV) – could be controlled by the tools of modern medicine and public health. And yet, none of these diseases, or other important "tropical diseases," has been brought to heel. None of them, even those without a nonhuman host, have been eradicated. Some epidemic diseases continue to expand. Still others mutate to become drug-resistant pathogens for which there are no clear therapies. Vaccines, in the event they exist, are not always delivered effectively in the settings in which they are most needed. The cumulative burden of these diseases remains unchanged, and in some cases is growing; this burden weighs most heavily on the world's poorest billion inhabitants.

This chapter examines this central irony of twenty-first century medicine: the persistence of morbidity and mortality due to infectious diseases years after effective vaccines, cures, suppressive treatments, and preventive strategies have been discovered. The forces inhibiting the successful application of existing scientific knowledge are not primarily biological or cultural; they are, rather, economic and structural barriers to change. Using what may be called a *biosocial model,* this chapter will describe these barriers to health and will highlight several approaches to overcome them.

Because modern epidemics are almost invariably rooted in social conditions, some long-standing and others changing rapidly, inquiry that does not draw on the social sciences is unlikely to offer a comprehensive or accurate understanding of these plagues. The mechanisms by which social forces shape epidemics are not readily revealed by single methodologies, but rather by interdisciplinary research that links qualitative and quantitative methods. A biosocial model calls into question the very term *tropical diseases*, since in the past many of the pathogens discussed in this textbook caused significant mortality far from the tropics. The dozen or so diseases grouped under this rubric have little in common in terms of pathogenesis, chronicity of infection, modes of transmission (some are vector-borne, others are not), or efficacy of existing control and treatment strategies. But whether we consider what are often termed the "neglected diseases" (African trypanosomiasis, dengue, leishmaniasis, schistosomiasis, Chagas' disease, lymphatic filariasis, and onchocerciasis) or the largest infectious killers (diarrheal and respiratory diseases, human immunodeficiency virus (HIV), tuberculosis (TB), and malaria), there are important similarities to consider. All of these diseases afflict the poor disproportionately and are linked to social conditions. For each disease, there exist important deliverables: new and improved diagnostics and therapeutics that could affect the distribution and outcomes of these epidemics. In each instance, new discoveries could substantially decrease the morbidity and mortality associated with these persistent pathogens, but social and economic barriers hamper effective control strategies.

The mechanisms by which social forces delay health progress are in large measure those leading to the propagation of new epidemics such as HIV. We begin this review with a case study of HIV and TB in rural Haiti, since many of the barriers to care are best seen by closely examining individual illness trajectories and since TB is often the leading cause of death among patients living with HIV disease in resource-poor settings. The case study is followed by a review of structural barriers to effective HIV prevention and care. Next, a brief description of the challenges of implementing insecticide-treated bednets (ITNs) and artemisinin-based combination therapies (ACTs) illustrates how poverty, the primary social barrier, limits effective implementation of proven prevention and treatment strategies. Finally, we will explore the implications of this review for effective control of these and other leading infectious killers.

AIDS AND TUBERCULOSIS IN HAITI: JOSEPH'S STORY

On the afternoon of March 17, 2003, four men appeared at the public clinic in Lascahobas, Haiti, each carrying a leg of a makeshift stretcher. (The Lascahobas health clinic in central Haiti is a partnership between the nonprofit organization Partners In Health/Zanmi Lasante and the Haitian Ministry of Health. When it began providing voluntary counseling and testing and treatment for HIV in late 2002, Lascahobas became rural Haiti's second full-service HIV clinic.) On the stretcher lay a young man, Joseph, eyes closed and seemingly unaware of the 5-mile journey he had just taken on the shoulders of his neighbors. When they reached the clinic after the 4-hour trip, they placed him on an exam table. The physician tried to interview him, but Joseph was already moribund. His brother recounted the dying man's story.

Joseph, 26, had been sick for months. His illness had started with intermittent fevers, followed by coughing, weight loss, weakness, and diarrhea. His family, too poor to take him to a hospital, brought Joseph to a traditional healer. Joseph would later explain: "My father sold nearly all that he had – our crops, our land, and our livestock – to pay the healer, but I kept getting worse. My family barely had enough to eat, but they sold everything to try to save me."

Joseph was bedridden 2 months later. He became increasingly emaciated and soon lost all interest in food. As he later recalled, "My mother, who was caring for me, was taking care of skin and bones."

Faced with what they saw as Joseph's imminent death, his family purchased a coffin. Several days later, a community health worker employed by the Lascahobas clinic visited their house. The health worker was trained to recognize the signs and symptoms of TB and HIV and immediately suspected that the barely responsive Joseph might have one or both of these diseases. Hearing that their son might have one last chance for survival, Joseph's parents pleaded with their neighbors to help carry Joseph to the clinic since he was too sick to travel on a donkey and too poor to afford a ride in a vehicle.

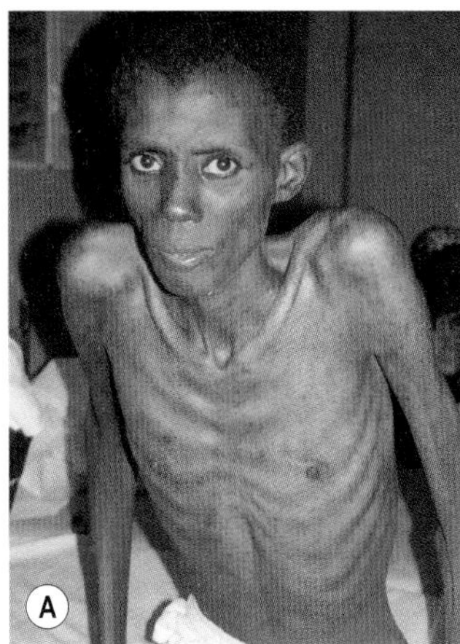

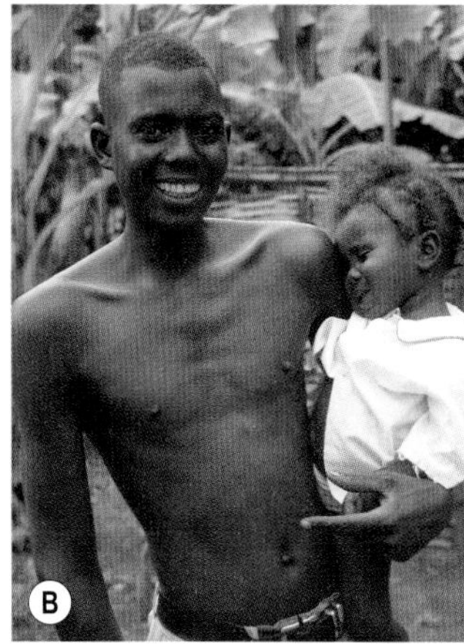

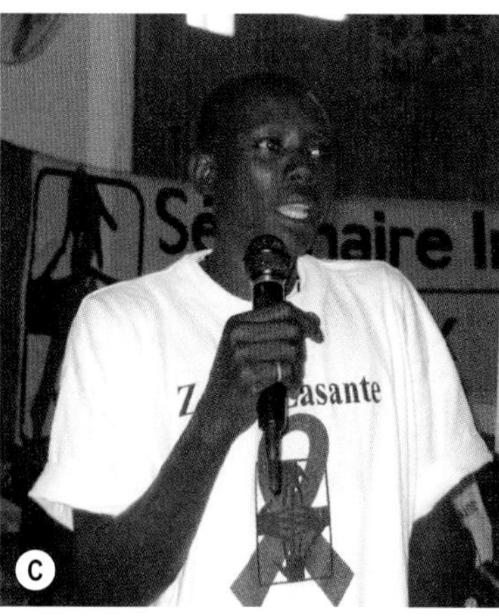

Figure 4.1 The "Lazarus effect": effective, accessible treatment for HIV and TB brought Joseph back from the brink of death. His experience, and that of hundreds of thousands of other impoverished patients in rural Haiti now receiving free medical care through a public–private partnership, is renewing his community's faith in the health sector and restoring hope to the destitute sick everywhere. **(A)** March 2003: Joseph, before treatment. **(B)** September 2003: Joseph after treatment for HIV and TB, with his healthy niece. **(C)** August 2004: Joseph speaks at a health and human rights conference.

At the clinic, Joseph was diagnosed, as per the community health worker's suspicions, with advanced HIV and disseminated TB (*Fig. 4.1A*). He was hospitalized and given antiretrovirals and antituberculous medications. Like his family, however, Joseph had lost faith in the possibility of recovery. He remembers telling his physician early in the course of his treatment, "I'm dead already, and these medications can't save me."

Despite his doubts, Joseph dutifully took his medications each day, and he slowly began to improve. Several weeks later, he was able to walk. His fevers subsided and his appetite returned. After discharge, he received directly observed therapy (DOT) for both HIV and TB from a neighbor serving as an *accompagnateur*. (For a more detailed discussion of community-based approaches to HIV treatment and care, see Farmer et al.[1]) After 4 months of therapy, Joseph had gained 30 pounds (*Fig. 4.1B*).

Now, Joseph is employed as an HIV outreach worker, often speaking in front of large audiences about his experience (*Fig. 4.1C*). "When I was sick ... I couldn't farm the land, I couldn't get up to use the latrine; I couldn't even walk. Now I can do any sort of work. I can walk to the clinic just like anyone else. I care as much about my medications as I do about myself. There may be other illnesses that can break you, but AIDS isn't one of them. If you take these pills, this disease doesn't have to break you."

STRUCTURAL BARRIERS TO EFFECTIVE HIV AND TUBERCULOSIS CONTROL

By the end of 2008, 4 million people in resource-limited settings had initiated antiretroviral therapy (ART), a 10-fold increase in 5 years. Despite this impressive scale-up of the provision of ART, Joseph's experience is typical in many ways and instructive in most. In December 2008, only 44% of those who needed ART were receiving it. The rate of coverage among infected children was even lower.[2] In addition, budgetary decisions by donor countries, including the United States, limit the expansion of ART programs, making rationing of the life-saving therapy increasingly common in some countries in Africa.[3]

Joseph's story is similar to that of tens of millions worldwide suffering from HIV and TB. He lives in great poverty; he sought care unsuccessfully until he simply gave up. His family did what they could to save his life, selling off meager assets and receiving contradictory advice from neighbors and from traditional healers in a country in which trained medical personnel are rare and most care is fee-for-service. Joseph's experience is exceptional in that he lived in an area of Haiti in which treatment for both HIV and TB had recently come to be considered a public good and made available to poor patients who could not afford user fees.[4] Treatment for these two chronic infectious diseases is supervised not by physicians or nurses – who do play a role in the diagnosis of illness – but by community health workers who are also one's neighbors.[5] In the following sections, we review these topics in greater detail by examining an emerging literature that explores socioeconomic barriers to effective care for HIV and tuberculosis.

The "Brain Drain"

One significant and often-invoked barrier to effective care in resource-poor settings is the lack of medical personnel. In what has been termed the "brain drain," large numbers of physicians and nurses are leaving their home countries in order to pursue opportunities abroad, leaving behind health systems that are understaffed and ill-equipped to deal with the epidemic diseases that ravage local populations. A recent survey reports that one-fifth of African physicians and one-tenth of African nurses work abroad; some countries have lost as many as 70% of their health care professionals.[6] The World Health Organization (WHO) estimates that there is a global deficit of 2.4 million doctors, nurses, and midwives, with the greatest number needed in sub-Saharan Africa.[7] This deficit of health care workers, while appalling, conceals further inequalities in health care staffing within countries. Rural–urban disparities in health care personnel mirror disparities of both wealth and health. Fewer than 55% of all people in the world live in urban areas, but over 75% of physicians and more than 60% of nurses are concentrated there.[7] In addition to inter- and intranational transfer of personnel, HIV itself is contributing to personnel shortages across Africa. Although data on the prevalence of HIV among health professionals are scarce, the available numbers suggest substantial and adverse impacts on an already overburdened health sector. The situation in Malawi is instructive, where a ranking cause of loss of health care workers is premature death, often from AIDS.[8] The shortage of medical personnel in the areas hardest hit by HIV has profound implications for prevention and treatment efforts in these regions. The cycle of health sector impoverishment, brain drain, and consequent lack of personnel to fill positions, when they are available, conspires against ambitious programs to bring antiretroviral drugs to those living with both HIV and poverty. Furthermore, the education of medical trainees is jeopardized as the ranks of the health and academic communities continue to shrink due to migration or disease.

A proper biosocial analysis of the brain drain reminds us that health personnel flight – almost always from poor to less poor regions – is not simply a question of desire for more equitable remuneration. Epidemiologic trends and access to the tools of the trade are also relevant, as are working conditions more generally. In many of the settings now losing skilled health personnel, the advent of HIV has led to a sharp rise in tuberculosis incidence; other opportunistic infections have also become, in the eyes of providers, insuperable challenges. Together, these forces have conspired to render the provision of proper care impossible, as the comments of a Kenyan medical resident suggest: "Regarding HIV/AIDS, it is impossible to go home and forget about it. Even the simplest opportunistic infections we have no drugs for. Even if we do, there is only enough for a short course. It is impossible to forget about it ... Just because of the numbers, I am afraid of going to the floors. It is a nightmare thinking of going to see the patients. You are afraid of the risk of infection, diarrhea, urine, vomit, blood ... It is frightening to think about returning."[9]

When providing care for the sick becomes a nightmare for those at the beginning of clinical training, physician "burn-out" soon follows among those who carry on in settings of impoverishment. In the public-sector institutions put in place to care for the poorest, the confluence of epidemic disease, lack of resources with which to respond, and user fees has led to widespread burn-out among health workers. Raviola and colleagues offer an important biosocial study linking epidemiology, the experience of providers, and an understanding of the political economy of the Kenyan health care system: "I don't see a future for the medical profession here," concluded a resident at Kenyatta National Hospital in Nairobi. "Why? It is expensive. You have to invest a lot. There is no government support. People can't afford care here."[9]

The WHO focused its 2006 report, "Working together for health," on the issue of developing an equitable distribution of health care workers. The report highlights strategies to build stronger health care systems within which workers can actually provide care, to improve educational opportunities throughout health care workers' careers, and to provide adequate, reliable compensation.[7] While countries are still developing their national plans based on this report, an example of a successful program in Ghana, a country that lost 68% of its medical school graduates between 1993 and 2000, demonstrates how an emphasis on the development of in-country training and support of young physicians can persuade them to stay. In 2002, Ghana's parliament allocated US$3 million to develop postgraduate training programs for physicians, the "Ghana College of Physicians and Surgeons."[10] The "Safe Motherhood Initiative" in obstetrics and gynecology, one of the new specialty training programs, had retained 37 of 38 of its trainees at the time of their report.[11]

Structural Adjustment and Access to Care

The large-scale socioeconomic forces at work in the differential distribution of sickness and health often stem from decisions made far from hospital wards or even national capitals. Many African countries in fact registered improvements in health systems and indices in the years following independence. Kenya, for example, saw infant mortality decline by more than 58% between 1963 and the early 1990s.[12] However, the economic crises of the 1970s and 1980s left many of these postcolonial nations mired in mounting debts to offshore creditors. African governments needed loans to pay interest on the outstanding debts and to meet basic social spending needs. The World Bank and the International Monetary Fund became the principal creditors in this arena, and these institutions soon found themselves the chief sources of funding for health and development projects in poor countries. Loans came with strict requirements such as the imposition of sweeping economic "reforms" in favor of a "free market" system designed to stimulate the economy and fix perceived imbalances in trade and government budgets. These economic austerity measures – termed "structural adjustment programs" – had profound and often deleterious effects on the health of many countries, as mandatory reductions of government budgets led to sharp declines in funding for the health sector. In Nigeria, for example, per capita expenditure on health care fell by more than 70% between 1980 and 1987.[13] Some have argued that structural adjustment programs in fact increased risks for HIV infection in Africa.[14]

Cuts in health care spending led to the closing of public health posts, clinics, and hospitals in many parts of sub-Saharan Africa. Even basic services – from first-aid to prenatal care – were slashed from the operating budgets of many Ministries of Health. Between 1990 and 1992, 14 African countries – all mired in structural adjustment programs – saw at least a 10% decline in the level of polio vaccination. Botswana topped the list with a 24% reduction in polio vaccine coverage during this time.[15]

The collateral damage of economic austerity programs in sub-Saharan Africa also directly affected health care professionals. Thousands of doctors and nurses across the continent lost their jobs as a result of budget restructuring. Many emigrated overseas, and funds for health care worker education disappeared, threatening the future supply of trained professionals.[16] For example, in late 2003, an estimated 4000 Kenyan nurses were unemployed secondary to economic policies that restricted recruitment of health workers into the public sector.[17] The damage done by structural adjustment remains, but encouraging changes have occurred. The advent of substantial and sustained funding from large charitable foundations and donor countries to address the health problems of the poor has changed the discussion from *whether* to develop and support the systems needed to provide access to care to *how* to provide it.[18]

User Fees

Another legacy of economic austerity programs is the widespread institution of "user fees" for health services that were formerly free of charge, with the intent of generating revenue for the health sector. Instead of revitalizing the health sector, however, user fees often sharply reduce the ability of the poor to access medical care.[19]

For example, UNICEF and the WHO introduced the Bamako Initiative in 1987, with the approval of the Health Ministries of the WHO African Region, to try to improve access to primary care by creating a structure to generate revenue for clinics. The initiative includes the provision of generic essential drugs by donor agencies or national governments to district and village health management committees. These drugs are then sold to the public at a profit, which is then, theoretically, used to buy back the initial stock of drugs and to improve the quality of health centers. Despite widespread support from decision makers and a great deal of positive press, several studies have reported a decline in attendance rates for health services as a result of the user charges stipulated by the Bamako Initiative.[20,21] A longitudinal study conducted in the Democratic Republic of the Congo revealed a 40% decrease in health service utilization between 1987 and 1991 after the adoption of the Bamako Initiative.[22]

Other studies also document deleterious effects of user fees. Despite exemptions for children and the indigent, Mbugua and colleagues found that attendance at rural Kenyan government health facilities plummeted by 41% after user fees were introduced, and rebounded after fees were abolished.[23] In a cross-sectional study of 37 countries in sub-Saharan Africa, even the money-minded World Bank concluded that user fees decreased utilization of health services.[24] Another study revealed that the number of men reporting to sexually transmitted disease (STD) public clinics in Kenya fell by 40% after user charges were introduced in 1989; the authors concluded that the introduction of user fees in STD clinics likely increased the number of untreated STDs in the population.[25] This association has clear implications for HIV treatment and prevention efforts, as HIV is a sexually transmitted disease in much of the world.

While user fees remain a topic of debate among some donors, many countries have developed strategies to eliminate them.[26] Uganda eliminated user fees in 2001 with a subsequent increase in utilization of services and without any decline in measured or perceived quality of service.[27] Other countries, like Rwanda and Cambodia, have implemented programs to provide government-subsidized health care to the poor through health insurance and a health equity fund respectively.[26,28] In Haiti, a careful analysis by Médecins du Monde demonstrated that the elimination of user fees in clinics that the organization co-manages with the Haitian Ministry of Health resulted in a dramatic increase in clinic usage with a coincident reduction in cost per unit of care delivered. The authors of the report make a strong argument and provide important empiric evidence of the benefits of both augmenting the "supply-side" of the health care equation with new clinics and personnel *as well as* the "demand-side" by eliminating the often insurmountable barrier of user fees.[29]

Economic Costs and Adherence to HIV Therapy

As HIV treatment programs in resource-poor settings undergo expansion, advocates and pundits alike agree that medication adherence is paramount to the success of these initiatives. Requiring patients to pay for ART is an enormous barrier to adherence. Data from individual programs have shown that adherence is significantly reduced at sites in which patients are forced to pay even nominal fees for their medications.[30,31]

In addition, dramatic clinical consequences, beyond poor adherence, result from charging the poor for ART. Ivers et al report in a meta-analysis of clinical cohorts from resource-limited settings that providing free medications contributes most to increasing the proportion of patients with a suppressed viral load, a critical parameter for HIV-infected patients.[32] Similarly, the Antiretroviral Therapy in Lower-Income Countries (ART-LINC) collaboration documents results from 23 clinical cohorts in Africa, Asia, and South America. In analyses from this group, the risk of death for patients in fee-for-service programs was nearly five-fold higher than in programs that provided medications at no cost (HR: 4.64; 95% CI: 1.11–19.41).[33,34]

These studies suggest that charging for ART excludes the poor from access to care, increases the likelihood that acquired resistance will develop through inadequate therapy, and leads to unnecessary loss of life. As Mukherjee has noted, "a human rights-based – rather than market-based – approach is the only realistic strategy for an epidemic that is concentrated in the poor and marginalized communities who have neither access to health care nor the ability to pay for treatment."[35]

Unfortunately, the direct costs of ART are not the only financial burdens faced by HIV-infected individuals and their families. The economic toll of HIV before the patient is even diagnosed leads to further impoverishment and delays in seeking and receiving effective care. Lessons from the long-entrenched TB epidemic are instructive. In Bangladesh, where all TB services and medications are provided free of charge, the average total loss of income before proper diagnosis and treatment was estimated to be US$245, or nearly 4 months of a family's yearly income.[36] In Thailand, even after diagnosis at a government hospital, 80% of patients incurred significant costs for travel and food during hospital visits. In the same study, up to 15% of patients were forced to sell household assets and use bank loans to cope with illness-related expenses.[37]

These data on the deleterious effects of direct and indirect costs of therapy have obvious implications for the successful provision of lifelong HIV treatment. Fortunately, some programs have addressed the problem of hidden costs. One such example, the HIV Equity Initiative, the program in which Joseph was treated, covers indirect costs with a package of benefits that includes a monthly transportation stipend and emergency transportation coverage at a cost of US$60 per patient per year. In partnership with the World Food Programme, the HIV Equity Initiative also provides nutritional support to those in need, at a cost of approximately US$450 per family per year.[38] Ensuring access to food combats another critical threat to adherence to ART: hunger.[39,40]

Civil Conflict and Natural Disaster

The noxious synergy of civil strife and poverty has a well-documented negative impact on the health of the poor. Conflict contributes to the deterioration of existing public health infrastructure in addition to creating conditions that decrease access to clean water and shelter, which can in turn lead to increased incidence of infectious pathogens. In an editorial on the violence that engulfed Haiti in 2004, Farmer laments the near-total collapse of the health sector.[41] As easy targets for violence, as well as often being overwhelmed by the consequences of violence, hospitals are increasingly prone to acute staff shortages, stockouts of medications and supplies, and even closure.[42] More lasting effects also follow conflict due to exacerbation of the "brain drain." A study of the migration of African health professionals documented the loss of more than 40% of the physicians between 1990 and 2000 from the war-ravaged countries of Angola, Congo-Brazzaville, Guinea-Bissau, Liberia, Mozambique, Rwanda, and Sierra Leone.[6]

The direct impact of conflict on HIV and TB epidemics has also been documented. In Sierra Leone, 23% of tuberculosis clinics closed between 1990 and 1994 secondary to violence and war.[43] The Rwandan genocide in 1994 is believed to have contributed to the expansion of the HIV epidemic to rural areas of that country.[44] The civil war in Guinea-Bissau in 1998–1999 is linked to a doubling of the HIV-1 seroprevalence in that country.[45]

At the time of this writing, just weeks after a 7.0 earthquake devastated Haiti's capital city, it is also impossible to ignore the effects of natural disasters on the health sector. Like human-generated violence, events such as earthquakes, tsunamis, and hurricanes tend to reinforce preexisting social inequalities and strain health systems. In addition to leaving over 200 000 people dead and nearly 300 000 more wounded, the January 12, 2010 earthquake in Haiti collapsed the country's largest nursing school, killing 100–150 students and faculty, including the entire second-year nursing class. Clearly, this heartbreaking loss will have significant long-term repercussions for Haiti's already-strained health sector human resources.

Stigma

The role of stigma as a major barrier to care for HIV patients has been extensively reviewed elsewhere.[46–49] However, recent experiences in resource-poor settings suggest that the introduction of effective HIV treatment and care programs can help destigmatize what was once considered a fatal disease.[49] In communities in rural Haiti, dramatic, visible recoveries after initiation of antiretroviral treatment, dubbed the "Lazarus effect," have led to a sharp decline in HIV-related stigma.[50] While the contours of discrimination vary from country to country, AIDS-related stigma will likely decrease as access to treatment improves and as people come to realize that HIV is a manageable disease.

THE COST OF MALARIA

Malaria's human toll is enormous. Nearly 250 million people suffer from malarial disease each year, and the disease annually kills almost 1 million people, mostly pregnant women and children under 5. The poor disproportionately suffer the consequences of malaria. Fifty-eight percent of malaria mortality occurs in the poorest 20% of the world's population; 90% of malaria mortality is registered in sub-Saharan Africa.[51] The differential magnitude of this burden of mortality is greater than that associated with any other disease.[52] Despite suffering the greatest consequences of malaria, the poor are precisely those least able to access effective prevention and treatment tools.[53]

Rolling Back Malaria

Due in part to differences in vector distribution and climate, resource-rich countries offer few blueprints for malaria control and treatment that are applicable in tropical settings. In 2001, African heads of state endorsed the WHO Roll Back Malaria (RBM) campaign, which prescribes strategies appropriate for sub-Saharan African countries. RBM recommends a three-pronged strategy to reduce malaria-related morbidity and mortality: the use of insecticide-treated bednets (ITNs), combination antimalarial therapy with an artemisinin-containing medication (ACT), and indoor residual spraying. In the first years of this program, uptake of these strategies was disappointing, but beginning in 2004, a growing number of malaria-endemic countries have adopted these principles and implemented programs.[53] This may in part reflect a fivefold increase in international funding for malaria programs between 2003 and 2009 from

US$0.3 billion to US$1.7 billion.[51] A closer look at the differential success in increasing access to ITNs and to ACTs is useful when considering the importance of careful attention to the economic and social complexities revealed through a biosocial lens.

The initially limited success of the scale-up of ITN coverage was indicative of the campaign's inadequate acknowledgment of the economic barriers that preclude the destitute sick from accessing critical preventive technologies. Despite proven efficacy and what are considered "reasonable costs," the 2003 RBM report revealed disappointing levels of ITN coverage. In the 28 African countries surveyed, only 1.3% (range, 0.2–4.9%) of households owned at least one ITN, and less than 2% of children slept under an ITN.[54] The RBM strategy initially emphasized the importance of commercial markets as sources of ITNs for African populations.[55] A precedent supporting this emphasis was the prior existence in countries such as Madagascar and Mali of local markets for untreated bednets. Presumably, therefore, a demand for bednets existed prior to the RBM campaign, as did a distribution system with points of sale.[56] However, this market approach, even with the application of subsidized social marketing strategies, did not result in large increases in coverage in the first years of the RBM campaign.

Several studies attempted to define willingness to pay (WTP) and actual payment for ITNs in African countries in order to understand why market-based strategies were unsuccessful. Policy-makers often utilize WTP to determine appropriate pricing for social marketing projects and to project revenue and demand.[57,58] Guyatt and colleagues provide an important critique of WTP studies from their work in highland Kenya. The 2002 study compared the attitudes of people living in homesteads that had been provided with heavily subsidized ITNs ($n = 190$) to households that had no bednets and had not been targeted by other health care initiatives ($n = 200$). Ninety-seven percent of all households expressed willingness to pay for nets; however, only 4% of those willing to pay offered spontaneously to meet the suggested price of 350 KSh (Kenyan shillings). After being prompted that "nets are expensive," 26% of respondents expressed willingness to pay the full price. This study did not actually offer nets for sale; therefore, the number of nets actually purchased cannot be compared. However, this study did contextualize the hypothetical WTP for ITNs by comparing it to other household costs: the price of an ITN equaled the cost of sending three children to primary school for a year. By contextualizing the nets' relative cost, the authors called into question the likelihood that families in this district, over half of whom fall below the Kenyan poverty line, would actually be able to purchase ITNs despite their "willingness to pay."[59]

Given the barriers to purchasing ITNs, especially among the poorest of the poor, many researchers and development professionals involved in malaria programs called for the free distribution of nets, stressing their importance as a public health measure: "the priority for Africa should be to adopt ITNs as a public good – like childhood vaccines."[60]

A great deal of progress has been made over the past 5 years, and observational studies of large, community-based programs to distribute no-cost ITNs confirm their ability to dramatically increase coverage by ITNs as well as the feasibility of combining distribution with other existing public health services such as vaccination campaigns and antenatal care clinics.[61–63] The 2009 RBM report reflects the success of the change in policy: the WHO estimates that at the end of 2008, 31% of households owned ITNs, compared to 17% in 2006 and <2% in 2003.[51] This rapid increase suggests that participating countries could potentially reach the RBM goal of 100% coverage by 2015.

The use of ACTs to treat malaria is critical for effective treatment of individuals and for the prevention of the evolution of drug-resistant parasites. While the goal of 100% appropriate treatment is as yet unrealized, the WHO reports steady progress with a fivefold increase in the percentage of children with fever treated with an ACT in Africa from 2006 to 2008 (from 3% to 16%). Further progress on this strategy is hampered by limited supplies of ACTs and the high cost of therapy, which may in part explain why 37 countries still permit the use of artemisinin-based monotherapy. Rapid action is needed, as resistance to artemisinins has already emerged on the Cambodia–Thailand border.[51]

Emulating the strategy pioneered to increase access to medications for drug-resistant TB may be helpful for ACTs as well, and a global subsidy fund has already been created to purchase therapeutics for countries that need them.[64,65] In addition, careful attention to the features of programs that successfully ensure appropriate diagnosis and treatment of malaria – such as the employment of community health workers and the use of blister packs – will provide important guidance in the struggle to bring proven prevention and treatment techniques to the poorest, especially in rural settings.[65]

HARNESSING SCIENCE TO CONTROL EPIDEMIC DISEASE: A BIOSOCIAL CHALLENGE

All of what are now often considered tropical diseases – AIDS, African trypanosomiasis, dengue, leishmaniasis, malaria, schistosomiasis, TB, Chagas' disease, lymphatic filariasis, and onchocerciasis – are more notable for their differences than for their similarities. Some are caused by viral pathogens; others by parasites or bacteria. Some are vector-borne; others have no known nonhuman hosts. Some of these infections are vaccine-preventable; for others, reliable prevention methods are still under development. While their efficacy varies widely, prevention and/or treatment options are available for each of these diseases. Why, then, do these infections remain ranking causes of death and debility in the twenty-first century?

In truth, the so-called "tropical" diseases are more linked to social and economic class than to latitude. Although new basic knowledge, especially if generated by "use-inspired basic research,"[66] will lead to improved diagnostic and therapeutic tools, and even as the pace of discovery increases due to our emerging understanding of the genomic structure of the pathogens and vectors in question, it is increasingly clear that social and economic barriers constitute formidable obstacles to the effective and equitable deployment of technologies new and old. As Farmer and Becerra wrote,

> *The phenomena that concern us – epidemic and endemic disease – are not solely biological; neither are they purely social. Yet conventional studies typically rely on disciplinary approaches and fail to reveal the full complexity of these epidemics. Only by embracing a transdisciplinary, biosocial approach can we hope to describe fully these "tropical" epidemics, and intervene successfully. For example, when yet another hydroelectric dam alters rates of schistosomiasis or filariasis, we must also study the "behavior" of policymakers at development agencies if we are to understand the distribution and outcome of schistosomiasis and filariasis. When recurrent drug stockouts characterize a tuberculosis control program, the "knowledge, attitudes, beliefs and practices" of patients may have only limited relevance to the emergence of drug resistance, whereas fluctuating drug prices, tariffs, and poor drug quality might prove determinant. When poor bloodscreening practices mean rising rates of American trypanosomiasis, it is an anthropology of blood banking and bloodbankers, rather than scrutiny of patients' notions, that is called for.*[67]

In seeking to understand the distribution and outcomes of infectious diseases in a broader social context, it is clear that a rising tide of social inequality is making it increasingly difficult to bring research to the bedside (in fact, many do not sleep in beds, but on mats or worse). This rising outcome gap may well prove the biggest challenge facing epidemic disease control in the coming decades. That is, as we develop new tools – vaccines and other preventives, diagnostics, and drugs – our failure to distribute them equitably means that the poor will do worse than ever. This has been seen starkly with regard to TB, malaria, HIV, and other epidemics: although the diseases occur in many settings, virtually all deaths are registered among the poor. From an equity perspective, the situation has gotten worse since new tools were developed.

Each of the settings in which these deaths occur is beset by socioeconomic barriers to care, and these barriers vary from site to site. In some places, health care reform has weakened the public delivery systems. In others, such systems are absent or beyond the reach of the majority. But not all the news is bad. Structural obstacles can be surmounted, as we saw in considering community-based care for AIDS in rural Haiti, based on previous successful efforts to treat tuberculosis in the same setting.[68] Promising developments also have occurred in the prevention and treatment of malaria in many countries in Africa and Asia, and in reducing maternal mortality in Asia, Latin America and the Caribbean, northern Africa, and Oceania.[69]

We conclude that a great deal more research is required if we are to have better diagnostics; more powerful, less toxic drugs; new control strategies; and effective vaccines for tropical diseases. However, without a complementary analysis of social factors like those described in this chapter, the long-term deployment of old and new interventions to combat "tropical disease" will risk failure. In some cases, failure will simply maintain the alarmingly unequal topography of health care outcomes around the globe, even for "easily treatable" diseases. However, as we have learned from the ravages of multidrug-resistant TB and malaria, failure is an unacceptable option: any efforts that result in failure exacerbate inequalities rather than diminish them, creating infections that are increasingly difficult to treat. Relinquishing our responsibility to treat these diseases in poor people is not an option; rather, we must seek to understand social as well as molecular mechanisms of treatment failure. The social mechanisms may stem from problems with policy-making and implementation, but they will result in the development of resistance to drugs and insecticides, continued unacceptable rates of morbidity and mortality, and the persistence of pathogens that should be controlled thanks to the science of tropical medicine.

ACKNOWLEDGMENT

The authors wish to acknowledge Alice Yang and Zoe Agoos for their invaluable contributions to the conceptualization, research, and revision of this chapter.

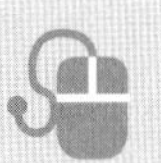

Access the complete reference list online at **http://www.expertconsult.com**

Access the complete reference list online at
http://www.expertconsult.com

CHAPTER 5

Nutrition and Micronutrients in Tropical Infectious Diseases

Margaret Kosek • Robert E. Black

INTRODUCTION

In addition to the toll in morbidity and mortality due to tropical infectious diseases, many infectious diseases common to all regions of the world last longer, are more clinically severe, and are more likely to have a fatal outcome in impoverished regions in the tropics because of the complex interactions between infection, protein-calorie malnutrition, and micronutrient deficiencies. The intent of this chapter is to provide an insight into these interactions through a review of the supporting evidence linking the nutritional and micronutrient status of the host, the patency of the immune system, and the course and outcome of infections of global importance. Although these interactions generally are accompanied and exacerbated by poverty, political instability, and the lack of access to adequate health care, the interaction between nutrition and infection has an immediate direct adverse effect on health.

Despite modest improvements in indices over the last 15 years, protein energy malnutrition (PEM) and micronutrient deficiencies remain highly prevalent in low- and middle-income countries.[1,2] In the year 2005 the World Health Organization (WHO) estimated that 20.2% of children under the age of 5 were underweight (weight for age $Z < -2$), 32.0% were stunted (height for age $Z < -2$) and 3.5% were severely wasted (weight for height $Z < -3$; standard definition of severe acute malnourishment) using the newly derived WHO standards of 2005.[3] Of the micronutrients with a demonstrated importance in determining the severity of infectious diseases it is estimated that clinical vitamin A deficiency (xerophthalmia) affects 5.17 million preschool children, while subclinical vitamin A deficiency affects another 190 million.[4] Iron deficiency and consequent anemia are detected in a high proportion of children and adults in developing countries.[5] Zinc deficiency is considered to be common in developing countries and recent estimates based on stunting and the adequacy of zinc in the available food supply suggest that nearly all low- or middle-income countries have a moderate to high risk of zinc deficiency.[6] It is clear that in developing areas the interaction of malnutrition and infectious disease becomes a key determinant in health outcomes and an important factor in the transmission and ecology of infectious diseases.

NUTRITION–INFECTION INTERACTIONS: PRINCIPLES

A guiding principle in the relationship between nutrition and infection has been the belief that dietary inadequacy both predisposes to infection and worsens outcome. This long-held principle suggests that nutritional interventions should play a critical role in thwarting the impact of infections. Growth faltering in infancy, a good marker of nutritional deprivation,[7] is strongly associated with an increased incidence, duration, and severity of infectious diseases as revealed in numerous prospective studies carried out in areas with a high prevalence of malnutrition.[8–12] Prospective birth cohort studies in diverse regions of the globe reveal that breastfed children have strikingly similar growth patterns in the absence of economic and hygiene environments that restrict growth.[13,14] However, the majority of the world's children live in conditions that begin to develop shortfalls in anthropometric indicators at 3 months of life, with acceleration of growth faltering when weaning foods are introduced, and the incidence of both diarrhea and respiratory illness increases in the second half of infancy (***Fig. 5.1***). Cutaneous anergy was noted to be present in malnourished patients, which led to the hypothesis that malnourished individuals suffered disproportionately from infectious diseases because of immune deficits.

These relationships led to attempts to minimize the impact of infectious diseases in children in the developing world through food or nutrient supplements early in life prior to or during the period when anthropometric indicators deviate from standards in well-nourished populations. Multiple planned interventions in the 1970s and 1980s sought to demonstrate that the provision of more protein or limiting amino acids to the diet[15,16] and then more energy[17] (when the protein supplements failed to obtain the desired response) would reduce morbidity due to infectious diseases. However, prior to the dramatic success of supplementation with vitamin A in the 1990s, interventions to curb the burden of infectious disease through nutritional supplementation were not clear successes. A recent review of 10 studies measuring the impact of complementary feeding interventions on morbidity found the effects to be both inconsistent and modest.[18]

Early studies had also noted that kwashiorkor, the most severe form of PEM, was often preceded by an infection such as acute diarrheal disease,[19] measles,[20] or chickenpox.[21] The evidence for the effect of a cycle of enteric infections and malnutrition is particularly well documented. There is good evidence that even asymptomatic gastrointestinal infections lead to growth faltering[22,23] and high burdens of overt diarrhea are a major contributor to stunting.[24] Measured observations of children during infectious disease episodes show that such episodes cause anorexia, nutrient malabsorption, micronutrient wasting, and growth deficits.[25–30] Diverse infections often occur at a rate that continually delays the ability of a child to achieve adequate catch-up in nutritional status or linear growth and the child enters a cycle of repeated infections and worsening nutritional status.

These observations taken together lead to the current thinking of the relationship between nutritional status and infection as bidirectional. Not only could PEM or micronutrient deficiencies worsen infectious disease morbidity, infections could in turn lead to deterioration in nutritional and micronutrient status (***Fig. 5.2***). To maximally diminish the burden of infectious disease in malnourished populations, disease control measures must be instituted in parallel with appropriately targeted nutritional interventions.

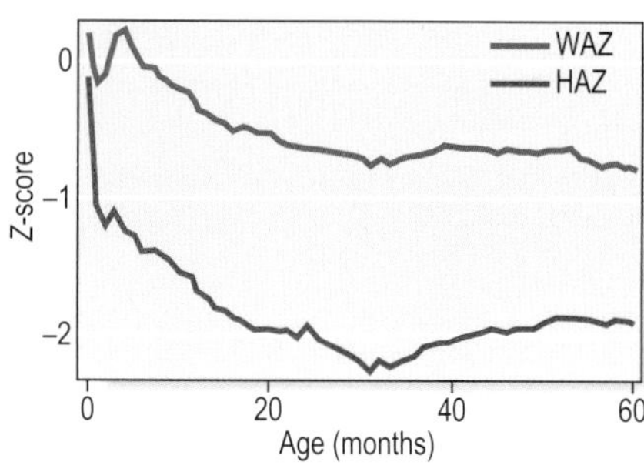

Figure 5.1 Mean weight (WAZ) and height for age (HAZ) measures of a cohort of children in rural Peru demonstrating progressive downward deviation from international standards typical for children living in impoverished settings.

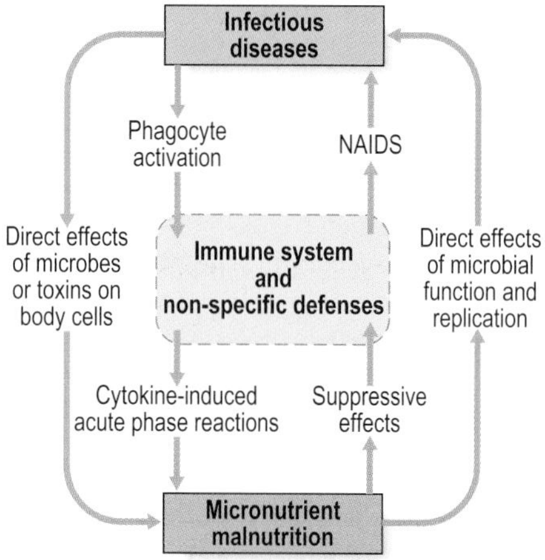

Figure 5.2 A schematic representation of the interactions between infectious diseases and malnutrition. NAIDS, nutritionally acquired immune dysfunction.

EFFECTS OF MALNUTRITION ON INFECTION (BOX 5.1)

Protein Energy

The degree to which the above interactions occur and the extent of their actual impact gained clarity when several prospective community-based studies accurately characterized the relationship between anthropometrics and child mortality rates in the early 1990s.[31,32] These estimates have recently been improved to delineate estimates based on underweight (low weight for age), stunting (low height for age), or wasting (low weight for height) status and by the use of updated nutritional data based on improved growth standards.[33] The expansion of estimates from basing predictors exclusively on underweight status (weight for age) is helpful as it can be applied in more varied epidemiologic contexts. The effect of undernutrition on anthropometric indicators varies in different epidemiologic contexts – stunting and wasting are highly correlated in Asia but poorly correlated in Latin America and Africa, and having a predictive model in which the three major indices can be used for imputation is a significant advance.[34] There is a steep progressive increase in the odds of mortality that is directly related to the degree of undernutrition (***Table 5.1***). A severely underweight child has 9.7 times the odds of dying as a child who is not underweight. Similar trends are seen in wasting and stunting. Diarrhea is consistently the cause of death that is most altered by nutritional status of the host, although strong relationships also exist for pneumonia and measles. The observed association of altered nutritional status on malarial outcome is lesser in magnitude and inconsistent among studies. It is worth noting that, as most malnourished children are mildly to moderately undernourished as measured by anthropometrics, the

Box 5.1 General Effects of Malnutrition on the Immune System

Protein Energy Malnutrition
- Decreased mucosal integrity
- Impeded macrophage migration
- Diminished T-lymphocyte help in immune responses dependent on mature CD4 cells (cell-mediated immunity)
- Delayed kinetics and deficient antibody responses to certain antigens, particularly polysaccharide
- Depressed amounts of mucosal secretory IgA and specific secretory IgA antibodies in response to mucosal infections
- *In vivo* consumption of complement, depressed plasma levels of most complement components and activities affecting both alternate and classic pathways of complement activation
- Deficient serum opsonic activity
- Favors type 2 response

Vitamin A Deficiency
- Decreased mucosal integrity
- Altered cytokine expression leads to type 1 immune responses

Zinc Deficiency
- Decreased macrophage chemotaxis
- Decreased neutrophil activity
- Decreased T-cell response to antigen stimulation
- Favors type 2 responses
- Diminished opsinin activity

Iron Deficiency
- Decreased neutrophil chemotaxis and bacteriocidal effects

greatest number of deaths modulated by the effect of nutrition on infectious disease outcome occur in children belonging to these categories. The new estimates now assign 2.2 million deaths and 21% of disability-adjusted life-years (DALYs) in children under the age of 5 years to the combined effects of severe wasting, stunting, and intrauterine growth restriction.[33]

Micronutrients

Micronutrients may have direct effects on the progression of an infection. The availability of key micronutrients in tissues or fluids can influence the growth and replication of infectious agents. For example, iron is required for the propagation of malaria and *Salmonella*; vitamin B_{12} is required for *Diphyllobothrium latum*. More frequently, micronutrients mediate their effect on the morbidity from infectious disease by modulating the immune system. A particular micronutrient deficiency rarely occurs in an isolated manner but rather overlaps with other micronutrient deficiencies and PEM (for symptoms of specific nutrient deficiencies, recommended replacement dosages, and recommended daily intakes, see ***Table 5.2*** available online). Nevertheless, large prospective field trials have demonstrated the benefits derived from dietary supplements with vitamin A and zinc, which have been shown to reduce the incidence, severity, and duration of various infectious diseases. Micronutrients with a role in protein synthesis (e.g., thiamine, riboflavin, pantothenic acid, and essential amino acids) are all needed for the production of antibodies. The nonessential amino acids arginine and glutamine appear to provide important benefits for antigen-specific immunity and improved mucosal integrity,[35] and essential polyunsaturated fatty acids are needed to produce prostaglandins, lipoxins, and thromboxanes. This review will be limited to vitamin A, zinc, iron, and selenium as data in these areas are more complete.

Vitamin A

Vitamin A modifies the severity of infectious diseases, with profound effects on childhood mortality.[36,37] Childhood xerophthalmia, the most reliable indicator of vitamin A deficiency, is linked to a higher risk of morbidity and mortality. Severe untreated xerophthalmia (with corneal involvement) has a high risk of concomitant morbidity, malnutrition, and mortality, with case-fatality rates for severe infections ranging from 5% to over 50%.[38] Milder, noncorneal xerophthalmia, while not blinding,

Table 5.1 Odds Ratio of Death by All Causes and by Common Etiologies in Children Under 5 as a Result of Deficits in Principal Anthropometric Indicators

	Severe (< −3)	Moderate (< −2)	Mild (−2 to < −1)	Greater than −1
Weight for Age (WAZ)				
All cause	9.7 (5.2–17.9)	2.5 (1.8–3.6)	1.8 (1.2–2.7)	1.0
Diarrhea	9.5 (5.5–16.5)	3.4 (2.7–4.4)	2.1 (1.6–2.7)	1.0
Pneumonia	6.4 (3.9–10.4)	1.3 (0.9–2.0)	1.2 (0.7–1.9)	1.0
Malaria	1.6 (1.0–2.7)	1.2 (0.5–3.5)	0.8 (0.2–3.2)	1.0
Measles	6.4 (4.6–9.1)	2.3 (1.7–3.2)	1.3 (1.1–1.5)	1.0
Height for Age (HAZ)				
All cause	4.1 (2.6–6.4)	1.6 (1.3–2.2)	1.2 (0.9–1.5)	1.0
Diarrhea	4.6 (2.7–8.1)	1.6 (1.1–2.5)	1.2 (0.9–1.7)	1.0
Pneumonia	3.2 (1.5–6.7)	1.3 (0.9–2.1)	1.0 (0.6–1.6)	1.0
Malaria	2.1 (0.9–4.9)	1.0 (0.8–3.6)	0.7 (0.5–0.9)	1.0
Measles	2.8 (1.4–5.8)	1.7 (0.8–3.6)	0.7 (0.5–0.9)	1.0
Weight for Height (WHZ)				
All cause	9.4 (5.3–16.8)	3.0 (2.0–4.5)	1.5 (1.2–1.9)	1.0
Diarrhea	6.3 (2.7–14.7)	2.9 (1.8–4.5)	1.2 (0.7–1.9)	1.0
Pneumonia	8.7 (4.8–15.6)	4.2 (3.2–4.5)	1.6 (1.1–2.4)	1.0
Malaria	2.3 (1.6–3.2)	3.0 (1.0–8.9)	0.9 (0.3–2.6)	1.0
Measles	6.0 (4.3–8.3)	3.7 (2.5–5.5)	1.8 (0.9–3.6)	1.0

95% confidence intervals are displayed.
(Adapted from Black RE, Allen LH, Bhutta ZA, et al. Maternal and child undernutrition: global and regional exposures and health consequences. Lancet. 2008;371:243–260.)

also increases the risk of morbidity and death. Preschool Indonesian children with night blindness (XN), Bitot's spots (X1B), or both conditions (representing "mild xerophthalmia") were three, six, and nine times more likely to die, respectively, within 3 months of diagnosis than their nonxerophalmic peers.[36] The association was strong and consistent across age, illness, and anthropometric data, suggesting a causal role of vitamin A deficiency in child mortality. Excess mortality also extended to siblings of xerophthalmic children.[39] Xerophthalmic "clusters" occur within households and communities.[40]

Intervention trials indicate that vitamin A supplementation modifies the severity, more than the incidence, of certain infectious diseases, as is the general trend with other forms of malnutrition. This effect is most apparent from its impact on all-cause mortality among preschool children. The initial trial conducted in Indonesia found that 1–6-year-old children receiving 60 000 μg retinol equivalents of vitamin A every 6 months died at a 34% lower rate than children in villages not receiving supplements.[41] Subsequently five trials showed significant reductions in the mortality of children 6 or more months of age, ranging from 19% in Ghana to 54% in southern India,[38] while two trials failed to show an impact on mortality. A meta-analysis of these trials revealed a mortality reduction of 23% in all countries with the use of vitamin A in children over the age of 6 months.[38] The effect of vitamin A supplementation given earlier than 6 months of age remains controversial, because three trials in Asia have shown reductions in mortality in early infancy,[42–44] but two trials in Africa have found no benefit.[45,46] Two trials of neonatal vitamin A supplementation are planned for Africa and one for India. Current estimates are that half a billion doses of vitamin A are distributed yearly and this results in the prevention of 350 000 deaths in children annually.[47]

One of the clearest synergistic relationships between a micronutrient and infection is that of vitamin A and measles. Vitamin A treatment during measles can profoundly decrease the morbidity, the incidence of secondary complications, and mortality. Although the degree of reduction has varied in trials using different doses, a recent meta-analysis found that results of randomized controlled trials giving two doses of 200 000 IU vitamin A revealed an overall reduction in all-cause mortality of 67%.[48,49] Furthermore, there was a 47% reduction in the incidence of croup and a 77% reduction in pneumonia-specific mortality and the duration of diarrheal episodes was significantly shortened in the supplemented groups. The measured impact of the effect of vitamin A for the primary prevention and treatment of diarrhea and respiratory tract infections yields conflicting findings. Several studies have noted a decrease in the duration and severity of diarrheal disease in children receiving vitamin A as primary prophylaxis.[50,51] Other trials have failed to do so, but recent work evaluating the risk of vitamin A supplementation on different diarrhea etiologies reveals differing effects, which may offer an explanation for these divergent findings.[52,53] In a meta-analysis of eight double-blind randomized controlled trials of vitamin A prophylaxis, no effect on diarrheal disease incidence was found and a mild negative effect (relative risk (RR) 1.07, 95% confidence interval (CI) 1.02–1.12) was noted on the incidence of respiratory disease.[54] Additionally, vitamin A given as adjunctive therapy in children hospitalized with pneumonia was associated with a decreased oxygen saturation and increased respiratory distress in Peru[55] and there was a nonsignificant trend towards higher mortality in vitamin A-supplemented children hospitalized with pneumonia in Tanzania.[56]

Children with xerophthalmia or severe malnutrition or any child with measles should be treated according to guidelines from the WHO: 200 000 IU of vitamin A orally on presentation, 200 000 IU the following day, and another 200 000 IU 2–4 weeks following the infection to reestablish liver stores. Children under the age of 1 year should receive half-doses. The use of vitamin A as routine adjunctive therapy for respiratory infections and diarrhea is not indicated.

Zinc

The classical syndrome of severe zinc deficiency is seen in acrodermatitis enteropathica, a rare genetic disorder characterized by dermatitis, linear growth deficits, anorexia, irritability, and chronic diarrhea. However, even milder degrees of zinc deficiency are associated with an increased risk of infectious diseases. Despite the lack of a reliable and widely used indicator of zinc status on which to base estimates of prevalence of this condition, the clinical trials of supplementation showing significant and large impacts on common child diseases in diverse geographic zones and populations indicate that zinc deficiency is a common condition in children in developing regions.[57] The use of zinc supplementation for the primary prevention of diarrheal disease is supported by trials in diverse areas of the world. A meta-analysis informed by 15 studies has shown a decrease in the incidence of acute diarrhea of 14% and persistent diarrhea of 25%.[58]

A recent meta-analysis of 14 trials of zinc as an adjunctive treatment for acute diarrhea suggests that zinc decreases the duration of acute diarrheal episodes by 0.5 days ($P = 0.002$).[59–73] The strength of effect is significantly greater in persistent diarrhea where zinc therapy decreases the probability of persistence of diarrhea on a given day by 21% compared with the control group (RR 0.79; 95% CI 0.65–0.96).[59,74–77] Effectiveness trials have shown that populations receiving adjunctive zinc therapy for diarrhea have lower subsequent rates of diarrheal diseases, hospitalizations for diarrhea, and hospitalization for pneumonia.[78,79] There is a WHO UNICEF recommendation that zinc supplements should be used in the treatment of acute diarrhea along with oral rehydration therapy; this may be done at the modest cost of $0.20 for a course of treatment[80,81] and implementation is accelerating in many countries.[82]

Twelve studies evaluating the effect of zinc supplementation on respiratory illness were included in a recent meta-analysis that showed a modest effect of a 8% decrease in incidence (95% CI 0.85–0.99).[58] The utility of zinc in preventing more severe respiratory illness, defined as either pneumonia or acute lower respiratory tract infection, has been estimated to be decreased by 20–35%.[83]

Findings from three studies on the utility of zinc supplementation for the primary prevention of falciparum malaria are more conflicting. In the Gambia[84] and Papua New Guinea[85] small studies revealed reductions in health center attendance attributable to falciparum malaria by 30% and 38% respectively, although only the later study reached statistical significance. In Burkina Faso a larger study found no difference in the incidence of falciparum malaria diagnosed by active household surveillance in zinc-supplemented children.[86] A multicenter trial in Ecuador, Ghana, Tanzania, Uganda, and Zambia revealed no difference in time to reduction of fever or anemia in children receiving zinc as an adjunctive therapy for falciparum malaria.[87]

More recently, zinc given in addition to standard nutritional therapy was associated with lower incidences of morbidity for diarrhea and all-cause mortality in children with severe PEM.[88] Given the large attenuating effects on the two principal causes of mortality in children, diarrhea and pneumonia, it is not surprising that two large studies in different epidemiologic contexts showed trends towards a decrease in mortality of 7% (95% CI 6–19%) in Tanzania and 8% (95% CI 0.83–1.31) in Nepal, although neither trial's findings was statistically significant.[89,90] However, in these trials there was a statistically significant 18% reduction in zinc-supplemented children who were at least 12 months of age. It is abundantly clear that zinc, through diminishing the severity of the most prevalent causes of morbidity and mortality of children in the developing regions, has an important and as yet unrealized potential to improve global child health. As supplementation may be needed at least weekly, the application of this intervention will not be as easy as providing high-dose vitamin A every 6 months. Alternative approaches for primary prevention include fortifying basic foodstuffs or the promotion of the use of animal-based protein, which is a good source of zinc.[91,92]

Iron

Iron deficiency, with related anemia, is the most commonly identified micronutrient deficiency globally.[93] Dietary intakes in tropical zones are generally marginal and often confounded by blood loss associated with menstruation and/or infection with hookworm or schistosomes. Anemia may either be a symptom of nutritional deficiency or a response to active infection. Both iron-deficiency anemia and the anemia induced by infection lower serum iron levels and therefore may alter the outcome of infections. The assessment of relationships is complicated by several factors. The first is the definition of anemia and the failure of many investigators to distinguish between iron-deficiency anemia, anemia resulting from infection, and the hereditary hemoglobinopathies.[94] For investigational settings the best evidence for the measure of iron status of an individual is the soluble transferrin receptor:log ferritin[95] or plasma zinc protoporphyrin:heme ratio,[96] but these measures are rarely available in limited resource settings where the highest prevalence of iron deficiency occurs. ***Table 5.3*** provides a guide for the evaluation of common laboratory tests used to differentiate causes of anemia.

Table 5.3 Iron-Deficiency Anemia Versus the Anemia of Infection[a]

Variable	Iron-Deficiency Anemia	Anemia of Infection
Red blood cell count	Depressed	Depressed
Hemoglobin	Depressed	Depressed
Hematocrit	Depressed	Depressed
Plasma iron	Depressed	Depressed
Plasma transferrin	*Markedly elevated*	*Normal or depressed*
Transferrin saturation	Markedly reduced	Reduced
Plasma ferritin	*Reduced*	*Normal or increased*
Tissue iron stores	*Markedly reduced*	*Normal or increased*
Zinc protoporphyrin	*Elevated*	*Normal*
Soluble transferrin receptor	*Elevated*	*Normal*
Iron therapy	*Corrects the anemia*	*Fails to correct the anemia*

[a]Key differences are in italics.

Studies of iron supplementation have led to possible examples of nutrition–infection antagonisms. Review of trials indicated that provision of iron supplements results in an increased density of malaria parasites in the blood and possibly clinical malaria.[97] More alarming was a clinical trial in preschool children in Zanzibar that was halted due to a 12% (95% CI 2–23) increase in mortality and 11% (95% CI 1–23%) increase in hospitalizations in children receiving iron and folic acid. A subanalysis in a group of children who received more extensive malaria therapy showed that iron-deficient children were at risk of severe morbidity and benefited from iron supplementation, but iron-replete children still had an adverse effect.[98–100] A similar trial in Nepal where malaria is not endemic showed no adverse effects (nor any benefit regarding mortality) associated with iron supplementation.[101] Currently, the recommendation for universal iron supplementation in preschoolers is limited to nonmalarious areas. Universal iron supplementation should not be undertaken in malarious regions; however, the treatment of individuals with iron deficiency is still indicated and should be accompanied by effective malaria therapy. Improved screening to identify iron-deficient children correctly should target interventions to avoid adverse outcomes in malarious areas.[96]

Evidence for nutritional antagonism is not restricted to *Plasmodium* species. Viral infections such as hepatitis C and human immunodeficiency virus (HIV) and bacterial infections such as *Vibrio vulnificus* are more severe in iron-overloaded individuals.[102,103] A meta-analysis of iron supplementation trials found that iron-supplemented children have more diarrhea.[104] An enteric pathogen that appears to have a complex and possibly antagonistic relation with iron is salmonella. Experimental infection studies in rats have demonstrated that severe iron deficiency enhances resistance to infection and that mild deficiency enhances susceptibility.[105,106] This may explain disparate findings from often-cited observational studies that salmonella infections in Guam were often associated with iron-supplemented formula.[107] Iron supplementation has not been shown conclusively to affect the risk of lower respiratory infections.[104] Despite the importance of adequate iron status in the development of children and the productivity of adults, iron supplementation has risks as well as benefits in regard to infectious diseases.[108]

Selenium

One of the most novel recent observations regarding the interaction between a host and an infectious agent has come from investigations into the origin and pathogenesis of Keshan's disease, an epidemic cardiomyopathy in China.[109] Epidemiologic investigations revealed that only populations living in areas with selenium-deficient soils developed the disease.[110] Subsequently blood and tissue samples from cases revealed coxsackieviruses.[111] Laboratory mice fed on selenium-sufficient diets could be infected with a strain of coxsackievirus B4 and develop only mild limited cardiomyopathy while selenium-deficient animals developed a severe cardiomyopathy upon infection with the same coxsackievirus B4 strain.[112] It was subsequently noted that coxsackieviruses that did not normally exhibit cardiotoxicity in selenium-sufficient animals became cardiotoxic following passage through selenium-deficient animals. Viral sequencing of the virus after passage through selenium-deficient animals confirmed genotypic changes while strains passed exclusively through selenium-replete animals had no genotypic changes.[113] This appears to be an example of a novel type of interaction between host and infectious agent in which the infectious agent increases in virulence because of a specific deficit in a host's nutritional status. A recent trial demonstrated a reduction in the incidence of diarrhea in selenium-supplemented pregnant Tanzanian women,[114] but high selenium levels (≥114 μg/L) in the same setting were also associated with increased HIV-1 RNA levels, suggesting that micronutrient status may increase the risk of HIV transmission.[115] This transmission risk should be clarified before developing supplementation guidelines for selenium in this population.

INFECTION-RELATED METABOLIC ALTERATIONS COMPROMISE HOST NUTRITIONAL STATUS (BOX 5.2)

Infectious diseases may produce primary direct losses of body nutrients or secondary losses mediated through the inflammatory cytokine response and catabolic effects. Loss of iron due to hookworm and schistosomes and macronutrients from geohelminths illustrate the consequences of infectious agents. Direct losses may also result from toxins produced by the pathogen, such as toxigenic stains of enteropathogens that result in sizable losses of electrolytes, water, and bicarbonate. Despite these important examples of direct effects, indirect effects account for the majority of the impact of pathogens on the host's nutritional status. There is an innate link between the immune and endocrine systems, and the metabolic changes associated with even mild infections can have an important effect on the nutritional status of the host. The inflammatory response induces constitutional symptoms, alteration in the metabolism of proteins and carbohydrates, and redistribution of minerals between physiologic compartments.

Constitutional Symptoms

Constitutional symptoms of infection are fever, anorexia, malaise, headache, and myalgia; the first two have clear effects on the nutritional status of the host. The hallmark sign of infection, fever, is induced by the release of interleukin-1 (IL-1), IL-6, and tumor necrosis factor-α (TNF-α) which act at the level of the hypothalamus to alter the temperature set point. This host response is felt to be a favorable adaptive response, but it comes at a substantial metabolic cost. For the augmentation of body temperature by 1°C, the basal metabolic rate increases by 12–23%.[116] Therefore, for a strong febrile response of 40°C, the basal metabolic rate increases 30–60% over baseline needs.

Fever is generally accompanied by anorexia. Although the reason for this host response is not clear, its effects can be important. In a well-controlled study in Bangladesh, 41 children between 6 and 35 months of age with diarrhea and an age-matched control group were studied. It was found that children hospitalized with acute watery diarrhea, despite an educational intervention and "coaching," consumed only 47–58% of the total calories consumed by the healthy control group.[117] Breastfeeding abrogated the changes to a large extent, but not completely.[118] A recent study in Peru suggests that peptide YY is a key mediator of anorexia during acute diarrheal infections.[117]

Box 5.2 Effects of Infection on Host's Nutritional Status

Decreased intake (anorexia)	Increased basal metabolic rate
Protein catabolism and negative nitrogen balance	Increased gluconeogenesis
Depletion of carbohydrate stores	Decreased absorption (symptomatic and asymptomatic gastrointestinal infections)
Altered fat metabolism	Micronutrient sequestration (Fe, Zn)
Pseudodiabetic state: hyperinsulinemia, increased insulin resistance, raised glucagons and glucocorticoid levels	Nutrient wasting (Zn loss in diarrhea, protein and vitamin A loss in shigellosis)

Alterations in Protein Metabolism

Protein catabolism occurs in even subclinical infections.[119,120] Cytokine release triggers skeletal muscle proteolysis via increased levels of corticosteroids by the ubiquitin proteasome pathway.[121,122] Liberated amino acids are taken up in part by the liver where IL-6-mediated transcriptional regulation leads to the enhancement of transcription and translation of essential acute-phase proteins such as C-reactive protein, complement, serum amyloid, and α-antitrypsin while down-regulating synthesis of exported proteins such as albumin and transferrin.[123,124] Despite active proteolysis of muscle, serum amino acids levels are lower than at steady state because of rapid uptake by the liver and immune cells.[125]

Not all amino acids released by proteolysis are recycled; branched amino acids, for example, are used for energy and the released nitrogen is excreted in the urine. Some amino acids, such as phenylalanine, are not recyclable and are also excreted in the urine. The loss of protein, especially during serious infections, is not trivial. It is estimated that, in moderate infections, the average daily protein loss is 0.6 g/kg/day, the recommended daily intake for adults. Losses in dysentery are somewhat higher, 0.9 g/kg/day, and in severe infections, including typhoid fever, daily protein loss approached 1.2 g/kg/day.[126] While proteolysis may serve in the short term as a source of amino acids for new protein synthesis, the continuous consumption of proteins must, at a given point, have adverse consequences for the host.

Alterations in Carbohydrate Metabolism

The inflammatory response induces a metabolic state characterized by increased gluconeogenesis secondary to cytokine upregulation of the rate-limiting enzyme phosphoenolpyruvate carboxykinase[127] even when exogenous carbohydrate intake is adequate. Serum levels of insulin, glucagon, and corticosteroids are all increased. The metabolic result is a syndrome of hyperinsulinemia, insulin resistance,[128] depressed glycogenesis and fat catabolism,[129] and enhanced peripheral glucose uptake and utilization.

Alterations in Mineral Metabolism

The divalent cations iron and zinc are highly protein-bound. During the inflammatory response, significant shifts in the distribution of these minerals occur. Iron and zinc are sequestered by the cytokine-induced synthesis of their binding proteins, ferritin and metallothionein. Sequestration of the minerals is in direct proportion to the severity of the infection; zinc levels can fall to half normal levels and iron can become almost undetectable.[130]

GASTROINTESTINAL INFECTIONS

Gastrointestinal infections have a particularly strong role in inducing a compromise in host nutritional status. Malabsorption in gastrointestinal illness may result from the epithelial destruction by the pathogen or alternately the immune response to the pathogen. Even common diarrheal illnesses can have a profound impact on nutrient absorption. In symptomatic rotavirus infection, the most common cause of acute severe diarrheal illness worldwide, there is a 42% decrease in the absorption of nitrogen and fat, a 48% decrement in the absorption of carbohydrates, and a 55% decrease in the total energy absorption.[131] These indices for malabsorption are slightly more severe in both enterotoxigenic *Escherichia coli* infections and in shigellosis.[28,131] In shigellosis,[132] protein loss is sizable and important and vitamin A is wasted.[30] Giardiasis and ascariasis lead to the malabsorption of vitamin A.[27] Large losses of zinc occur in diarrhea.[133]

EFFECTS OF MALNUTRITION ON HOST IMMUNE FUNCTION

Innate Immunity: Physical Barriers

The primary physical barrier to infection, the integument, is affected by a wide variety of nutrient deficiencies. Skin lesions are one of the cardinal signs of kwashiorkor. PEM, or even more milder forms of nutritional depletion, can be correlated with decreased gastrointestinal mucosal integrity as measured by the lactulose:mannitol ratio, and this in turn is correlated with growth deficits.[134,135] Similarly, vitamin A deficiency has been found to have a similar effect on gut integrity by the same test.[136] Striking histological changes are noted in the epithelia of vitamin A-deprived animals characterized as metaplastic hyperkeratosis that are rapidly reversible upon vitamin A repletion.[137,138] While severe zinc deficiency results in characteristic skin lesions,[139] mild to moderate zinc deficiencies also compromise the integrity of the gastrointestinal and respiratory epithelia.[140,141] Indeed, specific nutrient deficiencies are often manifest by epithelial lesions: dermatosis and mucosal atrophy are noted in pellagra; dermatosis and dermatitis, cheilosis and angular stomatitis are manifest in pyridoxine deficiency; and subcutaneous atrophy and tissue fragility are seen in scurvy. The nonessential amino acid glutamine also appears to have a role in the maintenance of intestinal epithelial integrity.[35]

Innate Immunity: Phagocytic Cells

Neutrophils and macrophages are the first-line generalized response to invading organisms. There is some dispute about diminished neutrophil chemotaxis and adhesion in PEM,[142–144] but there does appear to be a diminished bactericidal killing despite a normal generation of oxidative metabolites.[143,145] Additionally, serum opsinin activity is notably depressed in patients with PEM[146] and this is likely to diminish further the microbicidal functions of neutrophils. Zinc facilitates neutrophil activity directly[147–149] and indirectly through the stimulation of opsonic activity.[149]

Macrophages play a dual role in host defense. Once activated by lymphokine signals, macrophages may act directly as a microbicidal effector against intracellular pathogens, including viruses, certain bacteria, and fungi, as well as protozoa. In addition to these direct functions, macrophages are the key antigen-presenting cells for T-lymphocyte proliferative responses and cytokine production. Although it is clear that malnourished hosts are at an increased risk of infection due to intracellular pathogens, it is difficult to separate the direct effects on macrophage phagocytosis and microbial function from the indirect effects due to impaired antigen presentation and reduced T-cell responses that are necessary to stimulate normal macrophage activation. Despite this, it has been noted in murine models that macrophages from protein-restricted animals are abnormally sensitive to apoptotic stimuli.[150] In children with PEM, a markedly delayed and diminished macrophage migration was noted using the Rebuck window technique.[144] In addition, in murine models, diminished adhesion, activation, and delayed phagocytosis were demonstrated.[151,152]

Macrophages appear to have decreased antigen-presenting capacity and possibly a diminished capacity for normal coordinated signaling with T cells. A study of activated macrophages from protein-restricted and protein-sufficient diets revealed that the phagocytosis of *Candida albicans* and the generation of superoxide in response to phorbol myristate acetate were significantly diminished in the low-protein diet group using cells from both unprimed and bacille Calmette-Guérin (BCG)-primed animals, suggesting direct effects of malnutrition on the macrophage.[153] Furthermore, a marked decrease in macrophage production of nitric oxide and prostaglandin E_2 was observed, which would be expected to enhance lymphocyte proliferation by diminishing the negative regulatory signals for these cells. Whether this macrophage defect resulted from decreased secretion of interferon-γ (IFN-γ) by the responding T cells or decreased response of macrophages to IFN-γ signaling is not clear.

There is evidence for both altered intracellular signaling following endotoxin stimulation[154] and altered cytokine responses under multiple experimental conditions in PEM. In one study of cytokine response, the plasma levels of IL-6 and the p55 and p75 soluble receptors for TNF-α were elevated in children with PEM, especially in the presence of severe PEM with edema, independent of the presence of clinical infection.[155] In contrast, another study with Turkish children without apparent infection found decreased IL-1 levels compared with control subjects, but IL-1 increased during infection in a manner similar to that of the controls.[156] These findings are consistent with prior data in humans showing that *in vitro* production of IL-1 by lipopolysaccharide-stimulated peripheral blood monocytes was depressed in severe PEM compared with controls.[157,158]

In humans with acrodermatitis enteropathica the monocyte chemotactic response is suppressed and can be normalized by the addition of zinc *in vitro*.[141,159] In a murine model zinc deficiency was found to affect adversely monocyte uptake and killing of *Trypanosoma cruzi* in a dose-dependent manner,[160] and zinc-deficient mice exhibited macrophage-mediated depression of T-cell proliferation that could be corrected *in vitro* by the addition of zinc.[161] The extent to which these events occur in common infections in humans remains unclear.

Adaptive Immunity

Protein Energy Malnutrition

PEM profoundly affects the adaptive immune response through diverse mechanisms. Abundant data show that T cells are especially affected, particularly T-helper cells, and these deficits are largely mediated through defects in the T-cell maturation process. However, important alterations in B-cell function, immunoglobulins, and complement are also present. Understanding the effects of PEM is further complicated because study populations almost certainly suffered micronutrient deficiencies at a time when they were not readily identified and the accurate attribution of immune deficits to one aspect of undernutrition is not possible.

Over the past 150 years, a number of studies have documented a major impact of malnutrition on lymphocytes, long before the concepts of T and B lymphocytes were proposed and methods were developed to identify them. For example, anatomical and histopathologic examination of the thymus, spleen, and lymph nodes in persons dying of malnutrition revealed involution of the thymus and depletion of populations of lymphocytes from the peripheral lymphoid organs, now known to be predominantly populated with T lymphocytes. However, the number of circulating lymphocytes was only mildly diminished or often normal. Later, when it was possible to distinguish T cells from B cells, it was noted that there was a decrease in the number of mature functioning T lymphocytes, an unchanged number of B cells, and an increase in the number of cells which expressed neither T- or B-cell markers (null cells).[162,163] However, the degree of malnutrition as assessed by anthropometry did not correlate with the percentage of mature and immature T lymphocytes in circulation, and there was considerable individual variation.[163] More recent studies using monoclonal antibodies to identify lymphocyte subpopulations in Bolivian infants with severe PEM and thymic involution (greater than 90% decrease in thymic size by ultrasonography) showed a statistically significant decrease in the percentage of mature CD4+ cells, an increase in the percentage of CD1a+ precursor cells and CD8+ Tc and Ts cells, and no change in the percentage of CD21+ B cells in the malnourished, as compared with normally nourished, controls.[164] All these findings support a significant deficit affecting the T-cell maturation process in individuals with PEM.

The mechanisms that mediate the deficit in T-cell maturation are not clear. The thymic epithelium produces a variety of zinc-binding peptides, such as thymosin and thymulin, which have been shown to drive maturation of T lymphocytes *in vitro*. Lymphocytes from Bolivian children with protein energy malnutrition incubated with thymulin *in vitro* showed an increased percentage of CD4+ cells at the expense of CD1a+ precursors, with no observed change in the percentage of CD21+ B lymphocytes.[164] Studies from lymphocytes of Guatemalan children undergoing incubation with thymosin 5 show consistent findings.[165] These findings taken together strongly suggest that the thymic microenvironment is altered *in vivo* and that this alteration causes severe abnormalities in T-cell number and function, especially in the maturation of CD4+ cell lines.

Th lymphocytes also differentiate along two functionally polarized lines, Th1 and Th2, under a diverse range of influences including the cytokine milieu, the nature of the protein ligand, cortisol, norepenephrine, and microbial burden.[166] Th0 cells are stimulated to differentiate into Th1 cells under the influence of IL-12 and produce IL-2, IFN-γ, and TNF-β. IFN-γ stimulates antigen presentation through the up-regulation of both major histocompatibility class I and class II molecules on a wide variety of cell types. IL-12, among other things, blocks the differentiation of Th0 cells into Th2 cells. The response mediated by Th1 cells, a type 1 response, is characterized by a strong cell-mediated immune response and phagocytic activity and a relatively weaker humoral response. On the other hand Th2 cells differentiate under the influence of IL-4 and secrete IL-4, IL-5, IL-10, and IL-13. IL-4, IL-10, and IL-13 stimulate B-cell development, antibody production, and immunoglobulin class switching. Furthermore, IL-4 inhibits the differentiation of T0 cells into T1 cells. The response mediated by Th2 cells, type 2 immunity, is characterized by a strong humoral response. The tendency of one response (type 1 or type 2) to limit the other results is a polarization of the immune response.

The extent to which PEM alters Th polarization is not well studied. However, in one study of Turkish children with PEM, IL-6 was noted to be significantly elevated whereas TNF-β levels were not different from the control group, leading the authors to conclude that PEM favored a type 2 response.[167] Findings from a murine model support this hypothesis.[168] Delayed-type hypersensitivity skin response is a measure of cell-mediated immunity, which is dependent on Th1 cell activity. Defects in skin test reactivity to recall antigens such as tuberculin and *Candida albicans* are prevalent in individuals with PEM. This is not a new observation: during the mid-1960s, prior to the discovery of the T- and B-lymphocyte lineages and T-cell subpopulations, diminished prevalence and size of the tuberculin reaction were observed in African children with PEM compared to better nourished children from the same environment, and the tuberculin response to BCG vaccine was blunted.[169,170] Because tuberculosis has long been associated with malnutrition, the adverse effects of PEM on cell-mediated immunity responses, the principal host defense against *Mycobacterium tuberculosis*, may be an important determinant of outcome. In fact, one study has shown that peripheral blood monocytes from malnourished tuberculosis patients produced no more IFN-γ when stimulated *in vitro* than controls, suggesting that defective IFN-γ responses by Th1 cells in malnutrition contribute to the susceptibility of malnourished hosts to tuberculosis.[171]

The percentage of B lymphocytes in the circulation remains in the normal range in PEM patients, consistent with the preservation of the cellularity of B-lymphocyte-rich regions of the peripheral lymphoid organs. These cells are functional, and PEM patients usually have elevated serum levels of immunoglobulin G (IgG), IgM, and IgA, especially in the presence of infections. However, normal immunoglobulin levels do not mean that antibody production is normal as well. The key determinant is likely to be the amount and quality of specific antibody present and the ability of B cells to produce antibodies in response to new antigens.

There are limited data on the production of specific antibodies in PEM patients, mostly from studies using the response to vaccines as the experimental model. The majority of these have involved the use of the T-lymphocyte-dependent protein tetanus toxoid and typhoid vaccine, which contains both T-dependent protein antigens, the flagellar H antigens of *Salmonella typhi*, and T-independent somatic O antigens. Because of the large body of evidence to show that Th cells are diminished in PEM and the additional information that the immune response seems to be type 2 primed in PEM, the expectation is that PEM will inhibit the response to tetanus toxoid and flagellar H antigens and not significantly affect the response to the O polysaccharide. However, PEM patients appear to respond well to tetanus[172] and to flagellar antigens but not to polysaccharide antigens,[173,174] suggesting that at least some T-dependent responses occur normally, but that there is a defect in the response to carbohydrate antigens.[175] Other vaccines have been tested, with variable results, sometimes,[176–178] but not always[179,180] showing a compromised antibody response. In a study of household contacts of adult cholera patients in Bangladesh, children 1–8 years of age were given two oral doses of cholera toxin B subunit, the nontoxic portion of cholera toxin, or placebo within 24 hours of the hospitalization of the index adult patient. Although one-third of the children became infected with cholera (half symptomatic with diarrhea), malnourished children (weight for age <70% of the standard) did not differ from well-nourished children in the concentrations of salivary total immunoglobulin A, initial serum antitoxin, or vibriocidal antibodies or in their serologic response to colonization, disease, or the toxin B subunit.[181]

Although total IgG levels are normal or elevated in PEM, antipolysaccharide antibodies are commonly of the IgG_2 or IgG_4 subclass. Thus, in response to respiratory infections with encapsulated organisms such as *Streptococcus pneumoniae* or *Haemophilus influenzae* type b (Hib), IgG_2 and IgG_4 antibodies are either made locally in the lung or are transported into pulmonary secretions.[182] It is possible that the susceptibility of children with PEM to bacterial-encapsulated respiratory pathogens is due to defects in the production of optimal IgG subclass antibodies, but the question has not been fully addressed. On the other hand, trials of the Hib conjugate vaccine in the Gambia effectively eliminated Hib disease, including in children with mild to moderate malnutrition.[183]

Can we make sense of the different vaccine challenges used to elicit antibody responses and the variable results obtained? Perhaps this may be simply a matter of kinetics. In PEM patients have generally tested the antibody response at the end of 4 weeks or longer following booster doses, and the early response, detectable within days of immunization, has not been examined. However, in real infections (in contrast to immunization), the kinetics of the immune response is likely to be crucial to adequate host defenses. Therefore, normal percent seroconversion or even levels of antibody weeks after the original vaccine dose, or even later following a booster dose, do not predict whether or not the early responses were also normal. In one study of the response to measles vaccine a delay in specific immune response, measured on days 21 and 42 postimmunization, was noted in children with PEM.[184] The late response may represent a catch-up synthesis of antibody in PEM, sufficient to induce protection against a subsequent infection, but if the early response is delayed or of diminished magnitude in response to the actual infectious agent then the severity of the infection is likely to be greater.

The secretory immune system has also been assessed in individuals with PEM and consistently found to be deficient.[185] For example, a study of the response to measles and oral polio vaccines revealed diminished sIgA levels in saliva and specific IgA antibody responses following immunization of these patients.[186]

When measured in PEM patients, all components of serum complement except C4 have been observed to be significantly reduced, especially C3 and factor B.[187] As a result both the classical and the alternate pathways are affected, although *in vitro* assays of complement-dependent hemolysis indicate that the compromise to the antibody-independent and early-acting alternate pathway is more severe.[188–190] The high degree of activation of complement and elevated level of circulating complement–antibody complexes and the paradoxical fall seen in C3 levels in children with PEM and a concurrent infection[186] all suggest that complement activity is at least in part explained by a consumptive process, probably amplified by deficits in synthesis of complement components.[188]

Vitamin A

Despite the large amount of data demonstrating a clear benefit of vitamin A on child survival there is a paucity of data on the mechanisms by which vitamin A deficiency alters immune function. Vitamin A-deficient children have a decreased CD4/CD8 and cell ratio that can be normalized with vitamin A.[191] However, the strongest effects of vitamin A deficiency on adaptive immunity are regulated through the induction of a cytokine profile that favors a type 1 over a type 2 response[192–194] that can inhibit antibody responses, especially to polysaccharide antigens.[195] Vitamin A has an important role in the differentiation and homing of regulatory T cells,[196,197] and there is evidence of modulation of antigen presentation and secretory immunoglobulin production at the level of the gut.[197,198] In animal models high levels of vitamin A augment the type 2 response, even when stimulated by a type 1 antigen such as influenza A.[199] Possible adverse effects of vitamin A on immune responses were suspected when a defect was noted in the seroconversion rate of 6-month-old children given vitamin A at the time of measles immunization. As a practical way to give vitamin A was through the delivery structure provided by immunization, this early finding raised concern; however, a group of subsequent studies that measured the immunologic response to measles,[200] oral polio[201] and diphtheria, pertussis, and tetanus[202] vaccines failed to show any adverse event of concurrent vitamin A administration on the antibody response to any of the antigens in these vaccines.

Zinc

Zinc deficiency has diverse effects on adaptive immunity. The most profound deficits induced by zinc deficiency involve T-cell-mediated immune responses, especially type 1 responses. Zinc-deficient mice have reduced numbers of T cells, reduced proliferative responses to both mitogens and specific antigens, decreased IL-2 production and decreased antibody levels to a T-dependent antigen but not a T-independent antigen.[203] All of these changes were reversible with zinc supplementation.[157,203,204] These results are consistent with findings in children with PEM in whom nutritional rehabilitation failed to correct thymic gland involution (measured by chest radiographs) until 2 mg/kg/day of zinc was added to their diet. In malnourished children with diminished delayed-type hypersensitivity (DTH) skin test results, zinc has been demonstrated to augment DTH responsiveness.[205,206] More recently, lymphocyte proliferative responses were greater in children with shigellosis receiving adjunctive zinc therapy than in controls.[207]

Zinc deficiency inhibits thymulin activity and thereby limits both intrathymic and extrathymic T-cell differentiation.[208] Zinc deficiency also limits peripheral T-cell activation and division through diminished IL-2 production,[209] and by decreasing the activity of NF-κB[210] and down-regulating the interaction between IL-2 and IL-2 receptors the responsiveness of T cells to IL-2 is reduced.[211] In addition to decreased IL-2, production of IFN-γ and TNF-α, cytokines critical for a normal type 1 response, is compromised[209] while the production of the type 2 cytokines IL-4, IL-5, IL-6, and IL-10 remains intact,[209,212] leading to a distinct polarization in T-cell response.

Animal studies also support some degree of impairment of B cells due to zinc deficiency, although the effects seem less than that seen in T cells. Pre-B cells and immature B cells, but not mature B cells, are reduced in number during zinc deficiency secondary to glucocorticoid-mediated apoptosis.[213] The patency of the humoral response in zinc deficiency appears to be highly dependent on the antigen. In a murine model induced zinc deficiency had no detectable effect on the IgM response following immunization with a pneumococcal polysaccharide vaccine,[214] whereas in the same murine model with a T-cell-dependent pneumococcal surface protein A vaccine, the IgG response was significantly decreased at both 14 and 28 days. In animals who underwent subsequent pneumococcal challenge, zinc-deficient animals exhibited heavier colonization and were more likely to become septicemic and die than controls.[215] In humans zinc deficiency augments the risk for the development of symptomatic disease in carriers of pneumococcus.[216] In children zinc was shown to augment the antibody response to serotype 9V, but not other serotypes in children receiving the heptavalent vaccine.[217] Recent studies of the immunologic response to the oral killed whole cell plus cholera toxin B subunit cholera vaccine revealed an increased serum vibriocidal response and a decreased cholera toxin response in zinc-supplemented individuals.[218–221] In one of these studies fecal anticholera toxin was increased.[218] Vibriocidal antibodies are directed against a lipopolysaccharide antigen and should be a T-independent response while cholera toxin is a protein and should induce a T-dependent humoral response.

CLINICAL POINTERS

Generally, professionals in public health have accepted the large body of evidence linking malnutrition and infection and act to implement appropriate interventions. Clinicians, however, routinely fail to recognize malnutrition, particularly milder forms, or to institute and monitor adequate nutritional therapy in patients with concurrent infections. Even mild to moderate malnutrition can be an important determinant in the outcome of an infectious disease. Patient management will be optimized only when clinicians incorporate appropriate nutritional therapy and counseling into clinical practice. Conversely, cytokine-induced losses of muscle mass and body nutrients occur during infections, even in previously well-nourished individuals who receive prompt and effective therapy. These losses can be fully reversed by convalescent feedings and micronutrient supplementation. Despite adequate replacement diets it generally takes 2–3 times as long to replete an individual as it took to deplete them[22] and the period of nutritional convalescence will depend on both the chronicity and the severity of the infection. In general it is recommended that children should receive 30% more calories and 100% more protein to allow for catch-up growth during convalescence. Plentiful early and frequent feedings are especially important for infants and children in order to reinitiate an anabolic state and prevent a cycle of intensified progressive malnutrition often associated with frequent or recurring infections.

Individuals with severe wasting (weight-for-height Z-score < -3) greatly benefit from management accorded by structured protocols. Implementation of WHO standardized management protocols has greatly improved outcome measures and decreased case-fatality rate following protocol institution.[222,223] A meta-analysis of nine studies estimated that the facility-based WHO protocol reduced mortality from acute malnutrition by 55% as compared with conventional treatments.[222,224–228] Because malnourished patients suffer atrophy of the intestinal mucosa, along with diminished production of hydrochloric acid and digestive enzymes, refeeding may be clinically difficult. Adequate amounts of potassium, phosphate, magnesium, zinc, and other vitamins must be replaced judiciously and energy requirements and intake measured and adjusted carefully during therapy.[222,229] Weight gain must be accurately measured, recorded, and diligently monitored to assess the adequacy of response to therapy. Infections are common and need to be identified and treated early. Although this intensive inpatient treatment approach is highly effective, it must be noted that in settings of limited political stability and skilled motivated staff, the implementation of these protocols is compromised significantly and coverage is in many instances unacceptably low.[225,230] There is growing evidence that ready-to-use therapeutic food in Malawi, Ethiopia, Sudan, and the Niger used largely on an outpatient basis may obtain mortality rates as low as 4–5%, an important finding that will facilitate the expansion of treatment programs in areas with limited health infrastructure.[231–233] Notably ongoing studies document very low default rates as well as mortality rates.[234]

Because important forms of malnutrition cause lymphoid atrophy, quick estimation of tonsillar size in a malnourished child provides instantaneous clinical information about the potential functional competence of the immune system. Tonsils virtually disappear during severe malnutrition.

Vitamin A deficiency is widespread in developing countries, and a careful eye examination is a mandatory part of patient evaluation. Both corneal xerophthalmia (xerosis, ulceration, necrosis) and mild xerophthalmia are authentic clinical indicators that the patient faces an increased risk of morbidity and mortality, as well as blindness. Prompt treatment with vitamin A is essential. Because vitamin A deficiency generally occurs in clusters, the presence of xerophthalmia in an index patient should raise the suspicion that family members and possibly the community as a whole share the deficiency. Vitamin A prophylaxis and dietary counseling should reach out beyond the index patient. As vitamin A deficiency increases mortality and the severity of infections before evidence of xerophthalmia, children in most developing countries should receive vitamin A at regular intervals. High-dose vitamin A administration is a mandatory part of treatment for all children with measles. Although beyond the scope of this chapter, biofortification of the food supply through improvement of the quality of foods rather than supplementation of individuals with vitamin A and other micronutrients is critical if we are to address the nutritional needs of the 9 billion people who will populate this planet by 2050.

While adequate iron intake is necessary to prevent iron-deficiency anemia, caution needs to be exercised in regard to infectious diseases. It is recommended that iron supplements be withheld until initial management of severe malnutrition, which may be accompanied by serious infections. Children who present with infectious diseases and anemia should not be started on iron supplements until the infection is treated. The possible increase in some infections such as malaria and diarrhea with routine iron supplementation needs to be considered along with the possible benefits in deciding if this should be done in various settings.

Preschool children with diarrhea should receive zinc (10 mg/day for 10–14 days; half this in children <6 months) along with oral rehydration therapy, including increased fluids and continued feeding. Routine zinc supplementation, either daily or weekly, should be considered in populations where children have poor-quality diets and a high prevalence of stunting.

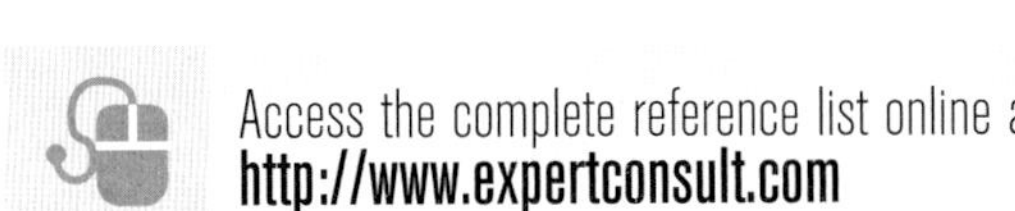

Access the complete reference list online at
http://www.expertconsult.com

CHAPTER 6

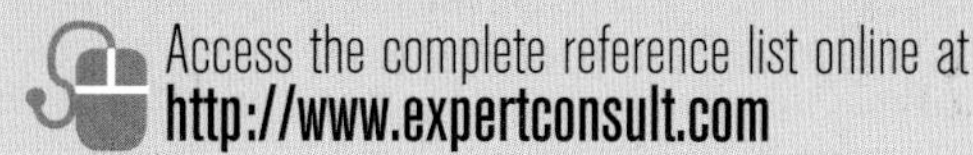
Access the complete reference list online at
http://www.expertconsult.com

Host Genetics and Susceptibility to Infection

Graham S. Cooke • Michael Levin • Robert J. Wilkinson • Geoffrey Pasvol

By 1950, the concept that the genetic diversity within the host may influence the outcome of infection became apparent, and malaria served as a prototype. All but a few infectious diseases are characterized by variation in both disease pattern and severity, even in epidemic circumstances, indicating that host response has an important influence on the outcome of disease. A classic study highlighted the importance of host genetic makeup in our susceptibility to infection.[1] The cause-specific risk of dying in adopted children was compared, depending on whether their biologic (genetically related) or adoptive (environmentally related) parent died prematurely before the age of 50 years. The results were striking. The death of a biologic parent resulted in an increased relative risk of dying in the adoptee of 5.8 for infectious diseases, more than for cardiovascular disease (4.5) and much more than for cancers (1.2). The advent of molecular biology and major advances in our understanding of the structure and function of the immune system have provided tools for the more precise dissection of genetic factors that influence the outcome of infection for the immune response through generations of natural selection.

GENERAL CONCEPTS

There are a number of genetic features and general concepts that apply to any consideration of the genetic basis of resistance (or susceptibility) to infectious disease:

1. The traits involved are complex. It is often impossible to find a genetic marker that shows complete co-segregation with a complex trait. The reasons are well reviewed:[2]
   a. Incomplete penetrance and phenocopy: A mutant gene product may have a major influence, but its effect may be compensated for by other mechanisms. Alternatively, a given mutant may give rise to a phenotype that can also arise in the absence of that mutant (phenocopy).
   b. Genetic heterogeneity: Mutations in any one of several genes (e.g., in a biochemical or immunological pathway) may give rise to the same phenotype. An example is given by deficiencies of the interacting complement factors C3, I, or H, which may predispose to infection with encapsulated bacteria.
   c. Polygenic inheritance: Some traits may require the simultaneous presence of variation in multiple genes. This is the case for most infectious diseases.
   d. A high frequency of a disease-associated allele makes the attribution of risk and linkage analysis more difficult. For example, a number of studies have examined the relationship between human leukocyte antigen (HLA)-DR2 and tuberculosis. The universal problem has been the high general frequency of this allele in the populations under study. Since the HLA-DR2 allele is present in approximately 40% of people in southern India, and in 60% of patients with tuberculosis,[3] a major effect may be missed as a consequence of the difficulty in attributing risk.
2. The protection conferred may only be relative. The possession of red blood cells negative for the Duffy antigen, and the resistance it provides against vivax malaria, is one of the few examples in humans of absolute genetic protection against an infection,[4] although recently a few exceptions to this have been documented in a few individuals.[5] In most other circumstances protection is relative. Although people with the sickle cell trait have up to 90% protection against malaria, they can undoubtedly become infected and die of falciparum malaria. Glucose-6-phosphate dehydrogenase (G6PD) deficiency may provide between 50% and 60% protection, whereas people with α-thalassemia may have as small a margin of protection as 5%.[6] Thus, "protection" is rarely absolute and should only be discussed at the population, rather than the individual, level.
3. The heterozygous rather than homozygous state may confer overall protection. This is the classic concept of "hybrid vigor." A "double dose" of a protective gene may not be additive in the protection it provides and could even be deleterious. An example of this phenomenon occurs in sickle cell carriers (AS) who have a reduced risk of dying of falciparum malaria: patients with sickle cell disease (SS) were thought to be at increased risk of death in the face of malaria. To complicate matters, this may however not be the case: in Kenya, SS patients were recently found to be at reduced risk from malaria, but this does not exclude the likelihood of SS patients dying from sickle cell disease itself or something else, e.g., severe sepsis.[7]
4. Protection may be highly specific. Protection offered by a genetic trait may be specific on a number of counts. First, protection may exist not only for a disease, for example, malaria, but also for malaria caused by a specific species of parasite. Thus, sickle cell trait carriers are protected against falciparum malaria but not against nonfalciparum *Plasmodium* species (i.e., *P. vivax, P. ovale,* and *P. malariae*). Second, protection may be specific for a particular clinical or pathologic form of the disease. An example of this is the class I major histocompatibility complex (MHC) antigen B53, which is associated with protection against both cerebral malaria and severe malarial anemia, whereas the class II haplotype, DRB1*1302, is only protective against anemia.[8] Alternatively, protection may apply to only a particular age group: for example, sickle cell trait carriers living in an endemic area for malaria are mainly protected between the ages of approximately 6 months and 5 years, at the time when passively acquired, antibody-mediated protection from the mother has waned and the individual has not as yet developed actively acquired immunity. Sickle cell trait may hasten the development of acquired immunity.
5. Where an apparently deleterious allele persists in a population, there is likely to be selective pressure in favor of that persistence,

perhaps mediated by protection against an infectious disease. For example, homozygosity for a rare polymorphism at position −308 in the tumor necrosis factor (TNF) promoter region confers a 7.7 times increased risk of dying of cerebral malaria (i.e., increased susceptibility). The persistence of the rare allele in the population at a frequency of 16% implies that it confers protection against another, as yet unidentified, infection or disease.[9]

ELEMENTS OF THE IMMUNE SYSTEM

Nonimmune Mechanisms

Molecular genetics has made extraordinary advances in the understanding of the genetic basis and potential treatment of a large number of inherited conditions, some of which may confer protection against conditions prevalent in the tropics. Beyond malaria, one such condition is cystic fibrosis caused by a mutation in the chloride transporter cystic fibrosis transmembrane conductance regulator gene (CFTR) on chromosome 7.[10] The mutant CFTR with phenylalanine at position 508 resists the entry of both *Pseudomonas* and *Salmonella typhi* into epithelial cells.[11,12] Clinically, this gives rise to differing consequences: *Pseudomonas* is not internalized and thereby multiplies to high numbers in abnormally viscid secretions that cannot be cleared. There is an association between genotypes in CFTR and susceptibility to typhoid fever.[13]

Innate Immunity

Excepting the unique example of innate protection by red blood cell variants in malaria, the innate system consists of three major elements: serum factors, phagocytic cells, and natural killer cells. Complement is a proteolytic cascade system consisting of at least 24 serum proteins and 11 membrane-bound proteins. The majority of the complement components are present in the plasma as inactive precursors. Triggering of the complement cascade results in opsonization or lysis of infecting organisms. Chemotactic molecules such as C5a are generated and immune complexes are solubilized. Activation can occur via the binding of antigen-bound immunoglobulin (Ig) G or IgM to the first complement C1 (classical pathway). The alternative, antibody-independent pathway involves the activation of C4 and C2 by a plasma serine protease in complex with mannose-binding lectin (MBL), which in turn is bound to suitable carbohydrate ligands present on the surface of bacteria or viruses. The genes for many of the complement components have been identified and the effect of deficiency is listed in ***Table 6.1***. Phagocytes, in the form of dendritic cells, also process and present antigens from microorganisms to lymphocytes. Major interest in how phagocytes recognize pathogens was stimulated by the discovery of the Toll-like receptors (TLRs), whose differential engagement by pathogens can induce overlapping yet distinct patterns of gene expression that contribute to an inflammatory response.[14] In addition, antigen-presenting cells (APCs) employ other pattern recognition receptors, including complement receptor 3 (CR3), scavenger receptors, the mannose receptor, and various other C-type lectins such as DC-SIGN. Polymorphic variation within these receptors contributes to susceptibility to infection.[15,16]

Acquired Immunity

The predominant effector and regulatory cell in the acquired response is the lymphocyte. B lymphocytes produce antibody that attaches to foreign organisms, facilitating their destruction by a number of mechanisms. Their response is regulated by regulatory T cells, mainly $CD4^+$. In addition, cytotoxic T cells, mainly $CD8^+$, can be effector cells that kill infected cells. All T lymphocytes recognize foreign antigen presented by an APC via MHC class I and II molecules. One of the features of the genes of the MHC region is the high degree of polymorphism. The class I genes encode the antigen-presenting molecules HLA-A, -B, and -C and the class II region genes HLA-DR, -DQ, and -DP. Both regions are located on the short arm of chromosome 6. In between the class I and II regions is the class III region, which encodes a number of genes also involved in the immune response, such as the genes for the complement factors C2 and C4 and factor B and that for the cytokine TNF. There is evidence to support the hypothesis that natural selection acts to maintain MHC polymorphism for several reasons. First, unusual allelic frequency distributions occur at MHC loci. Second, the patterns of nucleotide substitution show an enhanced rate of nonsynonymous (amino acid-altering) substitution in the codons encoding the peptide-binding region of the molecules. Third, polymorphisms at certain MHC loci are very long-lasting. Fourth, introns at MHC loci are homogenized by recombination and subsequent genetic drift.[17] There is a considerable body of evidence to support the idea that infectious diseases are a force maintaining MHC diversity.[18]

Cytokines

Cytokines, produced by many immune cells, act as soluble effector and regulatory molecules. A very large number of molecules have been described and the literature abounds with studies of association between elevation or depression of a given cytokine and disease. The fact that most cytokine genes are polymorphic has resulted in a large number of studies relating such polymorphism to susceptibility or resistance to various infections (see ***Table 6.4***). In fact, there is considerable redundancy within the cytokine network, with circuits of cytokines acting in tandem to regulate inflammatory processes, and so studies of single cytokines can be poorly informative. Variation with cytokine genes is clearly of most interest when polymorphism is shown to have potential functional correlates, as is the case for the molecules of the MHC.

TECHNIQUES OF GENETIC DISSECTION

Most human genetic studies referred to here can be categorized as linkage analysis or association studies, and on occasions both are employed to pin down genetic influences on disease.

Single pedigree analysis of human traits has been used with great success in infectious diseases (see below), for example in the study of disseminated mycobacterial infection.[19]

A genome-wide widely used method in recent years compares the observed and expected distributions of the number of alleles shared between affected siblings ("affected sib pair analysis"). Studies in infectious diseases, including leprosy, tuberculosis, and hepatitis, have yielded important results outlined below that have led to novel insights into disease pathogenesis and potential therapy.

The great strength of affected sib pair analysis is its ability to screen the human genome for novel disease loci, separated from any prior biological hypothesis. Its great weakness is the ability to power studies sufficiently to detect small genetic effects from single loci. With the realization that many genetic effects, particuarly in infectious diseases, are small, association studies of greater power are once again returning to favor.

Association Studies

The commonest design for case-control studies involves the comparison of one group (disease-affected) with another (usually a healthy population control). An early example of a genetic case-control study is that of Allison,[20] who determined that normal (AA) controls were more likely to have parasitemia with *P. falciparum* than people with sickle cell trait (AS). There are weaknesses in case-control studies, some of which relate to the general concepts outlined above. However, in recent years the enormous investment in genomic data sets has led to a description of over 1.42 million single nucleotide polymorphisms (SNPs) which exist in the human genome.[21] Dramatic advances in the ability to type SNPs and the collection of ever larger study populations has led to a renaissance in case-control studies which can explore genetic associations across the genome (genome-wide association studies (GWAs)). The results of these studies are beginning to be published for infectious diseases,[22,23] and offer

Table 6.1 Inherited Conditions Predisposing to Infectious Diseases and Their Genetic Basis

Syndrome	Clinical Features	Defect	Genetic Basis	References
Chronic granulomatous disease	Presents in the first years of life with severe recurrent bacterial and fungal infections	Failure of intracellular O_2 production	X-linked or autosomal recessive with defects in NADPH oxidase subunits	115
X-linked immunodeficiency syndromes	Chronic sinopulmonary infections, chronic diarrhea, and hepatitis			
X-linked agammaglobulinemia	As above	Agammaglobulinemia	Mostly due to mutation in Bruton's tyrosine kinase gene	116
Common variable immunodeficiency	As above		Multiple	117
Hyper-IgM syndrome	As above	Lack of IgG, IgA, and IgE	Mutation in CD154 (CD40 ligand)	118
Wiskott–Aldrich syndrome	Eczema, thrombocytopenia, recurrent infections, autoimmune disorders, IgA nephropathy	Mutations in the Wiskott–Aldrich protein, a regulator of platelet and lymphocyte function		119
Severe combined immunodeficiency	Severe and persistent infection from early life	Decreased T cells and abnormal thymic differentiation	Mutations in IL-2Rγ, Jak3, IL-7Rα, RAG1, TAG2, Artemis, CD3δ, adenosime deaminase, and CD45	120
C1	Systemic lupus erythematosus-like illness and increased susceptibility to infection	Lack of expression of C1q, C1r, or C1s		99
C3	Increased susceptibility to encapsulated bacteria			99
Factors I and H	As above	Both are cofactors for C3; deficiency therefore gives rise to the same susceptibility		99
C4	Bacterial meningitis	Failure of C4B expression		99
Properdin	Meningococcal disease	X-linked		99
C5–C9	Meningococcal disease			99
Mannose-binding lectins (MBLs)	Unusual and recurrent infection; carriage of hepatitis B	Mutation in codon 52 or 54 of exon 1 of the MBL gene		121

yet further new insights into disease pathogenesis. There is current debate[24,25] as to whether future studies should focus on ever larger population studies or more detailed genetic analysis as high-throughput sequencing, rather than SNP typing, becomes possible. Given the persisting need for new insights into the control of so many infectious diseases, both approaches are likely to have merit.

INHERITED CONDITIONS PREDISPOSING TO INFECTIOUS DISEASE

A number of well-characterized genetic defects that predispose to infection have been characterized at the molecular level (see *Table 6.1*). In general, these predispose to severe sepsis and the mutations responsible are so deleterious that they do not persist in populations at other than a minute frequency. Major advances in our understanding of immunity to common intracellular pathogens has derived from the analysis of small numbers of patients (often children) with severe recurrent atypical mycobacterial or *Salmonella* infections, who have mutations in the interleukin (IL)-12- and interferon (IFN)-γ-driven type 1 cytokine pathway (*Table 6.2*). This knowledge has prompted the search for less deleterious variants in these genes that may predispose to intracellular pathogens.[26,27]

STUDIES ON THE GENETIC INFLUENCE OF INFECTIOUS DISEASE IN HUMANS

Table 6.3 shows some HLA associations with infectious disease in humans. *Table 6.4* shows additional illustrative non-MHC and class III MHC genes with allelic variants that have been associated with infectious disease. Associations for selected diseases are discussed in more detail in the following sections.

Malaria

Genetic resistance to malarial infection has, of all infections, been best characterized, largely because polymorphisms of the red blood cell membrane and the red blood cell's contents are easily recognized by relatively simple laboratory methods, such as blood group typing, enzyme assays, and hemoglobin electrophoresis (*Table 6.5*).[4,28] In 1949, J. B. S. Haldane introduced the concept of "balanced polymorphism," whereby carriers of a recessive trait, for example, thalassemia, may be at a selective advantage of surviving severe falciparum malaria compared to both normal people and those with severe thalassemia.[29] This "malaria hypothesis" predicted that the frequency of thalassemia carriers would increase until offset by the resultant increase in the number of severely affected people in the population who would die prematurely, thus achieving a state of balanced polymorphism. α-Thalassemia is usually caused by the deletion of one of the linked pair of α-globin genes. The normal genotype is αα/αα; heterozygotes (αα/α–) are clinically normal, and homozygotes (α–/α–) have a mild anemia. There is good evidence that thalassemia is maintained in Melanesia as a consequence of natural selection by, and protection from, malaria.[6] This may be a result of altered plasmodial surface antigen expression in thalassemic cells.[30]

It was thus somewhat surprising that in Espiritu Santo (one of the islands of Vanuatu), the incidence of both the less severe vivax and falciparum malaria in homozygous thalassemic children aged 0–4 years was approximately twice as high as in αα/αα children.[31] The incidence of the rarely severe vivax malaria was particularly high in thalassemia

Table 6.2 Novel Genetic Immunodeficiency Syndromes that Predispose to Intracellular Infection

Molecule	Phenotype	Mutation	References
IFN-γ receptor I	Severe atypical mycobacterial infection	Point mutation at nucleotide 395 that introduces a stop codon	19
IFN-γ receptor II	*Mycobacterium fortuitum* and *M. avium* infection	Homozygous dinucleotide deletion at nucleotides 278 and 279, resulting in a premature stop codon	122
IL-12p40	BCG and *Salmonella enteritidis* infection	Point mutation at nucleotide position 2116	123
IL-12β1 receptor subunit	Severe mycobacterial and salmonella infections	A variety of missense and deletion mutations	124, 125
Stat-1	Disseminated BCG or *M. avium* infection	Point mutation at nucleotide position 2116	126

IFN, interferon; IL, interleukin; BCG, bacille Calmette-Guérin.

Table 6.3 Summary of Reported Associations between Major Histocompatibility Complex Alleles and Infectious Diseases

Disease	Effect	Allele(s)	Population	References
Protection				
HIV	Reduced progression	DQB1*0302, DRB1*0401	US, hemophiliacs	127
	Diminution in maternally transmitted virus	DRB1*1501 DRB1*1300	Whites, US Black and Hispanic, US	128
	Resistance to infection	A*0205	US, MSM	39
Hepatitis B	Transient infection	DRB1*1302	Multiple	92–94
Dengue shock syndrome	Reduced severity	B13	Thailand	129
Hepatitis C	Reduced severity	DR5	Multiple	130–132
Tuberculosis	Protective	A1 supertype	India	133
Typhoid	Protective	TNFA*2 [308].DRBI*0301 haplotype	Vietnam	134
Falciparum malaria	Reduced severity of cerebral disease and of anemia	B53	Gambia	8
	Reduced anemia	DRB1*1302-DQB1*0501	Gambia	8
Leishmaniasis	Mucosal disease	DR2		135
Filariasis	Reduced elephantiasis	DR3	Indonesia	77
Onchocerciasis	Localized disease	DQB1*0500	West Africa	78
Increased Susceptibility				
Dengue shock syndrome	Increased severity	A2	Thailand	129
HIV	More rapid CD4 decline	DQB1*0501–DRB1*0101	US, hemophiliacs	127
	Increased progression to AIDS	DQB1*0603–DRB1*1300, DQB1*0301, DRB1*1400	US, hemophiliacs	127
	More rapid CD4 decline	A1-B8-DR3	US, Scotland	37, 38
Tuberculosis	Increased severity of pulmonary disease	DR2	Multiple	48, 50, 53, 136
	Susceptibility and severity	A3 supertype	India	133
Typhoid	Increased susceptibility	TNFα*1 [-308].DRB1*04 extended haplotype	Vietnam	134
Leprosy	Tuberculoid disease	DRB1*1502	India	80, 81
	Lepromatous disease	DRB1*1501	India	80, 81
Lyme disease	Chronic course	DR2, DR4	US	137,138
	All forms	A2, C3	Germany	139
Schistosomiasis	Hepatosplenomegaly	B5, B44, DQB1*0201	Multiple	73–75, 140
Filariasis	Elephantiasis	B27, DQ5		77

HIV, human immunodeficiency virus; AIDS, acquired immunodeficiency syndrome; MSM, men who have sex with men.

homozygotes younger than 30 months old. The authors postulated that infection by vivax malaria at this age, perhaps because thalassemia is characterized by a mild increase in the number of immature red blood cells (reticulocytes), which are the preferred red blood cell habitat of *P. vivax*, may result in cross-reactive immunity to the lethal effects of *P. falciparum*. Another possibility is that the *P. falciparum* strains present on the island studied may be less virulent, because severe falciparum malaria on this island is much less frequent than elsewhere in the world.[31]

In another case-control study, the protection of both G6PD-deficient hemizygotes (males) and heterozygote females against falciparum malaria, in both West and East Africa, was demonstrated, appearing to resolve an age-old debate on the importance of this genotype in the face of severe falciparum malaria.[32] However, a more recent study was not able to confirm protection in heterozygous females.[33]

Protection against two life-threatening manifestations of malaria, cerebral disease and anemia, is associated in The Gambia with the class I antigen HLA-B53. Protection against anemia only was conferred by the class II extended haplotype DRB1*1302-DQB1*0501.[8] Because HLA-B53 is rare in populations not exposed to malaria, it was proposed that the frequency in The Gambian population studied was due to natural

Table 6.4 Non-Major Histocompatibility Complex (MHC) and Class III MHC Genes with Allele-Specific Associations with Infection

Gene	Allele	Effect	References
Cytokines and Chemokines			
Tumor necrosis factor (TNF)-α	TNFA*2[-308]	Increased severity of falciparum malaria, meningococcal disease, and mucocutaneous leishmaniasis	9, 109, 141, 142
Interleukin-1 (IL-1) complex	IL-1Ra A2-ve/IL-1β+3953) A1 +ve	Increased DTH and pleural tuberculosis	143
IL-8	Haplotype 2	Increased susceptibility to respiratory syncytial virus infection	144
IL-8	−251 IL-8 promoter	Increased inflammation and susceptibility to travelers' diarrhea	145
IL-10	ATA haplotype	Spontaneous clearance or more rapid fibrosis	146, 147
RANTES	In1.1C allele	Accelerated progression of HIV	148
SDF-1	3′ A/3′ A	Delayed or accelerated progression of HIV	44, 149
Interferon-γ	+874 SNP	Increased susceptibility to tuberculosis	27
Receptors			
CCR2	64I allele	Slower progression of HIV	43
CXP5	32-bp deletion	Slower progression of HIV	41–43
	CCR5P1 haplotype	Rapid progression of HIV	44
IL-12 receptor β1	R214-T365-R378 allele (2)	Increased susceptibility to tuberculosis	26
Vitamin D receptor	VDR tt and ff genotypes	Resistance to tuberculosis and hepatitis B	61, 62
TLR4	Multiple	Increased susceptibility to meningococcal disease	105
TLR5	392 stop codon	Increased susceptibility to legionnaires' disease	150
Various			
SLC11A1	Various	Susceptibility to tuberculosis	175–177
Haptoglobin	2-2	Increased severity of pulmonary tuberculosis	136, 151, 152
Mannan-binding lectin (MBL)	Codon 52, 54, and 57 variants	Increased risk of meningococcal disease and pneumococcal disease; decreased risk of tuberculous meningitis	100, 153

HIV, human immunodeficiency virus; DTH, delayed-type hypersensitivity.

Table 6.5 Red Cell Variants Believed to Provide Protection Against Malaria

Variant	Distribution	Postulated Mechanism	References
Hemoglobinopathies			
Hb S	Sub-Saharan Africa, Indian subcontinent	Premature removal of infected cells, reduced multiplication, induced sickling, reduced cytoadherence	154, 155
Hb C	West Africa	Impairment of merozoite release	156
Hb E	Southeast Asia	Increased phagocytosis	157
Hb F	Global	Sensitivity to oxidant stress	158
α-Thalassemia	Global in malaria endemic areas	Increased IgG binding, sensitivity to oxidant stress	6, 30
β-Thalassemia	Mediterranean, Southeast Asia, West Africa	Increased IgG binding, sensitivity to oxidant stress	159
Red Cell Enzymes			
Glucose-6-phosphate dehydrogenase deficiency	Worldwide	Sensitivity to oxidant stress	32
Pyridoxal kinase	Sporadic	Unknown	160
Red Cell Membrane			
Melanesian (band III) ovalocytosis	Melanesia	Reduced invasion	161
Duffy antigen negativity	West Africa mainly; also East Africa	*Plasmodium vivax* only, failure of invasion	162
Blood group O	Worldwide	Poor rosette formation	163
Glycophorin B deficiency	West Africa	Decreased invasion	164

selection. Because red blood cells do not express class I molecules, the site of cytotoxicity is presumably the infected liver cell. Cytotoxic cells do contribute to antimalarial immunity and it was possible to show that a nonamer peptide eluted from the HLA-B53 molecule was able to induce such responses in people exposed to malaria.[34]

The cytokine TNF is encoded by a gene within the MHC class III region on the short arm of chromosome 6 and transcription is under the control of a promoter that lies 5′ to the structural gene. TNF, especially when produced in excess, is implicated in the pathogenesis of a number of severe infections, including Gram-negative sepsis, tuberculosis, human immunodeficiency virus (HIV) infection, and malaria. Homozygosity for a polymorphism in the promoter region, involving a guanine-for-adenine substitution at position −308 relative to the start codon, is associated with a 7.7 times increased risk of death from cerebral malaria.[9] The functional significance of this polymorphism, however, is controversial. Recently, a number of non-MHC and class III MHC genes with allele-specific

Table 6.6 Examples of Non-Major Histocompatibility Complex (MHC) and Class III MHC Genes with Allele-Specific Associations with Malaria

Gene	Variant	Effect	Population	References
Protection				
CR-1	CR1-deficient	Severe disease	Papua New Guinea	165
Fc-γ receptor IIa (CD32)	R131 allele, rather than the RR131 genotype	Severe disease	Children in The Gambia	166
CD36 gene	Heterozygosity for a nonsense mutation	Severe disease	Kenyan children	167
Intercellular adhesion molecule-1 (ICAM)	ICAM-1Kilifi (change from Lys to Met in the loop that interacts with parasitized red blood cells)	Severe disease	Children in Gabon	168
CD40 ligand (CD40L)	Males hemizygous for the CD40 L-726C (not significant in females)	Severe disease	The Gambia	169
Nitric oxide synthase 2 gene (NOS2)	NOS2 (Lambarene) (NOS2-G954C)	Severe and mild disease	Gabon	170
Increased Susceptibility				
TNF-α	TNFA*2 [–308].	Increased severity of cerebral malaria	Children in The Gambia	9
TNF-α	TNF-238 A	Increased risk of severe malarial anemia	Children in The Gambia	142
TNF (promoter region)	OCT-1-binding genotype	Increased susceptibility to cerebral malaria	Children in The Gambia	171
Fc-γ receptor IIa (CD32)	HH131 genotype	Severe disease	Children in The Gambia	166
Inducible nitric oxide synthase promoter	Longer forms of CCTTT microsatellite repeat	Severe disease	Adults in Thailand	172
Haptoglobin	Hp1-1	Severe disease	Children in Ghana	173
No Effect				
Complement receptor 1 (CD35)	Gene underlying the Knops antitheticals antigens S11/S12 and McC(a)/McC(b)	No association	Children in The Gambia	174

associations with malaria have been described and more examples of these will no doubt follow (*Table 6.6*). Some of these genetic variants have shown protection against severe disease and others increased susceptibility that may vary, for instance, with the malarial disease phenotype or the population studied, and they would fail to recognize an advantage in the face of some other as yet unidentified selection pressure.

Clearly many genes regulate the susceptibility to malaria and its consequences. Whilst sickle hemoglobin is regarded as important and as a paradigm in genetic resistance to malaria, it must be remembered that, on its own, it may form only a small proportion (perhaps as low as 2%) in the total variability of the incidence of malaria.[35] Moreover the protective effects of sickle hemoglobin might be reduced rather than enhanced by the presence of another so-called protective genetic variant in the population such as α+-thalassemia.[36]

Human Immunodeficiency Virus

There is variability in the natural history of HIV infection. Three categories of infected people have attracted attention: (1) those who progress rapidly; (2) long-term nonprogressers (LTNP); and (3) people who are very likely to have been exposed but who do not seroconvert. Initial interest centered on the MHC with reports that rapid progression is associated with the HLA-A1-B8-DR3 extended haplotype.[37,38] It has been reported that the HLA A*0205 is associated with resistance against infection,[39] an observation that fits with a number of reports that ascribe protection against HIV infection to antiviral $CD8^+$ T cells.[40] The phenomenon of heavily exposed but persistently uninfected people also came to prominence when the coreceptors for HIV infection were described in the mid-1990s. For T-tropic viruses the coreceptor is CXCR-4, and CCR-5 is the coreceptor for M-tropic viral strains. A defective CCR-5 allele, which contains a 32-base pair deletion, prevents expression of CCR-5 at the cell surface. Homozygotes for this mutation are resistant to HIV infection, and infected heterozygotes have slower disease progression, a finding that has been widely reproduced.[41–43]

Attendant on the discovery of CXCR-4 and CCR5 as the coreceptors for HIV, a large number of studies have also examined genetic variants in both the chemokine ligands and receptors on susceptibility and the progression of HIV. Thus, a multisite haplotype of the CCR5 regulatory region containing a promoter allele, CCR5P1, that increases CCR5 expression is associated with rapid progression to acquired immunodeficiency syndrome (AIDS), particularly in the early years after infection.[44] HIV-1-infected individuals carrying the CCR2-64I allele progressed to AIDS 2–4 years later than individuals homozygous for the common allele.[43] Varying findings, however, have been made with respect to the ligands. For example, it has been shown that the In1.1C allele associated with a down-regulation of RANTES (CCL5) expression associates with rapid progression in an African-American cohort. However, in a study of Ugandans with relatively late disease,[45] the In1.1C allele was associated with protection from death, emphasizing how the same polymorphism can associate with profoundly different effects in different populations and different epidemiological settings.

More recently, GWAs have investigated HIV disease progression, but also the phenotypes of viral load set point (plasma HIV RNA level) and HIV DNA level. The most striking findings have confirmed the strength of association with polymorphism within the HLA region, particularly the HCP5 gene.[22,46] Although few non-HLA loci have been identified, there are some[47] that could open avenues for further work.

Tuberculosis

Research on genetic susceptibility to tuberculosis presents typical and some exceptional difficulties with respect to phenotyping. Because most tuberculosis infection in adults is latent, the phenotyping of control subjects for association studies also presents difficulties, particularly in the setting of HIV infection. Should controls be tuberculin skin test-positive and thus likely to be infected and assumed resistant, or should they be negative? Few, if any, studies have addressed this issue in detail and most case-control studies to date have compared individuals with disease to those without disease (regardless of exposure). Associations between HLA and pulmonary disease have been described frequently and HLA-DR2 has consistently been reported.[48–51] The two largest studies that typed class I alleles failed to detect any association.[52,53] Beyond the MHC, the relationship between the human SLC11A1 gene and tuberculosis has already been discussed. In general, the association with polymorphism in the SLC11A1 gene, like many in tuberculosis, has been hard to replicate. More robust appears to be the association between polymorphism in the IFN-γ pathway and disease. The finding that polymorphism in the IFN-γ gene is associated with tuberculosis[27] has been replicated elsewhere[54,55] and polymorphism within the receptor IFNGR1 has also been implicated.[54] Further insight into immune protection has come from studies on DC-SIGN,[56,57] MCP-1,[58] SP100,[59] and NOD2.[60]

An example of where candidate gene work has potentially advanced the field is the study of vitamin D receptor status. Homozygotes for a noncoding polymorphism at codon 352 (genotype tt) of the vitamin D receptor gene were significantly under-represented among Gambians with tuberculosis, an association that was supported by analysis of a separate population of Asians in west London.[61,62] The study from London made an attempt to analyze gene–environment interaction by concurrent determination of serum vitamin D levels. Acquired deficiency of vitamin D was far more powerfully associated with tuberculosis than genetic variation in its receptor. Both studies are biologically plausible because 1,25-dihydroxyvitamin D_3 decreases the intramacrophage growth of *Mycobacterium tuberculosis*.[63] These findings have led to further work currently evaluating vitamin D supplementation in the treatment of tuberculosis.[64]

Genome-wide scans on affected sibling pairs have detected moderate linkage of tuberculosis to different chromosomal regions. In Africa, linkage was found to chromosomes 15q, Xq, and 20q13[65] with the linkage on chromosome 20 replicated[66] and in Brazil to chromosome 17q11.2.[67,68] Chromosome 17q11.2 has some interesting candidates, including a number of chemokine genes and the inducible nitric oxide synthase gene (NOS_2). The link with chromosome Xq is also interesting because a male excess of tuberculosis is reported in many populations, and one gene, CD40 ligand, has been associated with disease.[69] Fine mapping has the potential to refine these linkages and, within the region of linkage on chromosome 20, the replication of association with MC3R polymorphism and disease offers a new avenue of biological exploration in tuberculosis. This hitherto unexplored target in tuberculosis has been the subject of work in other inflammatory diseases and provides a good example of how hypothesis-free work can open up new areas of research. Overall, the lack of a clear major genetic susceptibility locus for tuberculosis is consistent with the possibility that most of the genetic component of susceptibility to tuberculosis is dispersed among many loci. Results of ongoing GWAs are therefore awaited with interest and are likely to provide important insights into the biology of this persistent disease.

Helminthic Infections

An exhaustive review of human genetic susceptibility to helminth infection has been published.[70] Two features of helminth infections have attracted genetic study. The first is that, within populations, helminths tend to be overdistributed (i.e., a few people harbor high parasite burdens). Notwithstanding the environmental, behavioral, and parasitic factors that contribute to this feature, there is evidence that the intensity of helminth infection is partially under genetic control. The second feature is that sequelae, particularly of invasive helminth infection, arise because of immunopathology. Thus, fibrosis in schistosomiasis or the dichotomy between microfilaremia or hypersensitivity in filarial infection may have genetic correlates. In particular, a great deal of attention has been paid to the possibility that variants of genes that predispose to atopy protect against helminths.

Two whole genome-based linkage analyses have productively related the intensity of helminth infection to specific chromosomal regions. In a landmark study of a quantitative trait, microsatellite mapping of 11 informative families in Brazil indicated that the control of intensity of *Schistosoma mansoni* infection mapped to a single region of chromosome 5, most closely to the colony-stimulating factor receptor 1 gene (CSF1R) but also to a region containing the genes for the important type 2 cytokines IL-4, -5, and -13.[71] Also, the intensity of *Ascaris* infection was linked to genes on chromosomes 1 and 13, with the most plausible candidate being the B-lymphocyte stimulator protein (BlyS).[72]

Hepatosplenic schistosomiasis is believed to be largely due to the immune response to egg antigens, and there have been a number of studies on the role of HLA. Studies from Egypt and a single study from South America have consistently related HLA-B5 to hepatosplenomegaly in *S. mansoni* infection.[73,74] Studies of *S. japonicum* infection tend to be small, yielding multiple HLA associations, although in the largest of these HLA-B44 was a risk factor for the development of hepatosplenic disease.[75] In a more recent molecular analysis restricted to class II alleles, it was reported that hepatosplenic disease is associated with DQB1*0201.[76]

Lymphatic filariasis caused by *Wuchereria bancrofti* and *Brugia malayi* is characterized by a spectrum of manifestations from asymptomatic microfilaremia to deforming elephantiasis. Tissue damage in elephantiasis is suspected to be immune-mediated. In a study of patients with filariasis, the frequency of HLA-B27 and -DQ5 was increased and that of HLA-DR3 decreased in patients with elephantiasis compared to other patients older than age 45.[77] DQB1*0501 has also been associated with patients with localized, as opposed to generalized, onchocerciasis.[78]

Other Diseases

Leprosy

The polar spectrum of clinical leprosy offers an opportunity to investigate the effect of genetic factors on disease expression, but most effort has been directed toward determining susceptibility. An early application of transmission disequilibrium testing suggested linkage of susceptibility to the MHC locus on chromosome 6.[79] At least five studies have indicated an association between leprosy and HLA-DR2, which is strongest for tuberculoid disease. In two studies from India it appears that tuberculoid leprosy associates with DRB1*1502 and lepromatous disease with DRB1*1501.[80,81] However, others concluded that susceptibility to leprosy *per se* is probably not controlled by HLA-linked genes.[82] Variability in results might be explained by the observation that non-HLA genes within the MHC are associated with disease susceptibility.[83]

Three whole-genome scans for leprosy susceptibility in different populations have been reported with different results. The first to be published was a study of the genomes of 224 families from south India, containing 245 independent affected sib pairs, mainly with paucibacillary leprosy. A major susceptibility locus was identified on chromosome 10p13[84] with another on the short arm of chromosome 20.[85] The linkage within chromosome 10 might well be attributable to DC-SIGN polymorphism, also associated with tuberculous disease.[56] Work in Vietnam later reported a major locus of diseases susceptiblity within 6q25.2-q27 (away from the MHC),[86] specifically to 17 markers located in a block of approximately 80 kilobases overlapping the 5 centimorgan regulatory region shared by the Parkinson's disease gene PARK2 and the coregulated gene PACRG.[87] The same study reproduced the association in a large case-control analysis in Brazil. The Vietnamese study also found weaker evidence of linkage to 6p21.3 (including the MHC loci).[86] Further work has established that this linkage is probably due to polymorphism of the lymphotoxin-α which reduces gene expression and increases susceptibility to leprosy, particularly in those under 25 years of age.[88]

Hepatitis B

A considerable number of studies have been conducted on susceptibility to hepatitis B virus (HBV) infection and on susceptibility to develop hepatocellular carcinoma. Early attention focused on understanding why some individuals cleared HBV infection whilst in others infection persisted. Mutations in codons 52, 54, or 57 in exon 1 of the MBL gene reduce serum MBL levels and may be associated with an opsonic defect. An early analysis showed that a mutation in codon 52 is more common in white, but not Asian, patients with chronic HBV infection,[89] but subsequent studies did not associate MBL mutations with hepatitis B.[90,91] An early study also associated HLA-DRB1*1302 with transient HBV infection in Gambian adults and children.[92] This association has been inconsistently replicated in other populations, although a significant protective effect of HLA-A*03 was reported for Caucasians[93,94] and more recently HLA-A*02 amongst Japanese.[95]

The recent availability of a range of potent antivirals to reduce disease progression in HBV has reduced interest in genetics of disease progression. However, a genome-wide screen of siblings with persistent HBV infection identified the class II receptor gene cluster as a major locus determining HBV persistence, consistent with the known benefits of IFN-α treatment in some patients.[96] Similarly, the widely available hepatitis B vaccine is very effective, but there is interest in understanding genetic factors associated with vaccine responsiveness. A recent study from The Gambia found CD11a polymorphism to be associated with peak anti-HBs levels, a surrogate for long-term durability of vaccine responses.[97]

Meningococcal Disease

Most individuals acquiring new strains of meningococci, despite lacking specific antibody for several weeks, do not develop invasive disease following nasopharyngeal acquisition of new strains of meningococci.[98] This suggests that innate immune mechanisms are often effective in containing the organism. Host molecules relevant to innate immunity to meningococci include plasma proteins such as complement, MBL, and C-reactive protein, as well as the extensive range of pattern recognition receptors on cell surfaces, such as the TLRs, CD14, and mannose receptors.

Deficiency in terminal components of the complement pathway and properdin with recurrent meningococcal disease are well recognized[99] and are shown in ***Table 6.1***. Individuals possessing functional variants in the gene for MBL that led to reduced plasma concentrations of the protein have increased susceptibility to meningococcal disease.[100]

Factor H is an important regulator of the alternate pathway of complement activation. A functional polymorphism in the promoter of the factor H gene is associated with increased levels of the protein, and leads to susceptibility to group C meningococcal infection. As this polymorphism is common in Caucasian populations, its effect on disease susceptibility within the population is large.[101] The finding that defects in all three pathways of complement activation (classical, MBL, and alternate) lead to meningococcal disease suggests that this is a critical pathway for containment of the infection.

The host innate immune response to invading microorganisms is triggered following recognition of common structural motifs present on bacteria and viruses through a range of pattern recognition receptors.[102] Endotoxin (lipopolysaccharide (LPS)) is able to trigger innate immune responses following recognition by a number of host proteins and surface receptors, including the family of TLR4 and the CD14 molecule.[102,103] The importance of TLRs in containing Gram-negative organisms was first identified in mice with mutations in the LPS locus. LPS receptor-deficient mice (homologous to TLR-4 deficiency in humans) are unable to respond to bacterial endotoxin and show enhanced susceptibility to infection with *Salmonella*, *Neisseria*, *Escherichia coli*, and other Gram-negative organisms.[104] An excess of rare TLR-4 coding changes was found in patients with meningococcal disease compared to controls utilizing complete sequencing of the TLR-4 gene ($P = 2 \times 10^{-6}$; odds ratio 27).[105] This study suggests a critical role for endotoxin sensing in containment of meningococcal disease. TLR-4 is only one of a large number of proteins involved in the detection of endotoxin and other bacterial structures; these include other TLR receptors, CD14, and the accessory proteins, including MYD88, MD2, as well as the downstream regulators of cellular activation.[106] Some or all of these may contribute to the recognition of Gram-negative organisms and the activation of defensive host inflammatory responses.

An extensive body of evidence suggests that patients with fulminant and fatal meningococcal disease have an excessive and uncontrolled inflammatory response often under genetic control, with activation involving both cellular and noncellular inflammatory pathways.[107,108] Following the initial report that heterozygosity for the −308 promoter polymorphism in the TNF gene was associated with an increased (2.5 times) risk of death in meningococcal disease,[109] an association between outcome of meningococcal disease and other polymorphisms in the IL-10 and IL-1 pathway was reported.[110,111] Purpura fulminans is the most dramatic complication of meningococcal sepsis, leading to peripheral gangrene and often requiring amputation of limbs and digits. Predisposition to purpura fulminans may also have a genetic basis. A functional polymorphism in the plasminogen activator inhibitor gene is associated with meningococcal outcome.[112] The same applies to the factor V Leiden gene.[113] Patients possessing the 4G allele within the PAI-1 promoter gene produce higher levels of plasminogen activator inhibitor but are at increased risk of death, confirmed in a much larger subsequent study.[114] These genetic differences in the key regulators of the antithrombotic and thrombolytic pathways likely explain the occurrence of purpura fulminans associated with meningococcal disease.

CLINICAL RELEVANCE

For most practitioners of tropical medicine, the association of disease with genetic polymorphisms may appear attractive intellectually but of very little clinical relevance. We are only on the fringe of discovery of genetic factors influencing host resistance or susceptibility to infection and the explosion in genetic technology is likely to yield many more novel findings in years to come. For families identified with inherited genetic defects there are clear benefits for their management and important insights into disease protection.

How will the dissection of more complex disease lead to clinical benefit, particularly in the tropics? Genotyping is now a routine tool when choosing antiretroviral combinations for HIV patients in a developed-world setting. Such clincial application is unlikely to be realistic in the forseeable future when resources are scarce, but a knowledge of the population prevalence of alleles predisposing to drug toxicity can inform choices about the best treatment.

The emergence of clinical genotyping to predict the development or outcome of disease has been slow for many complex diseases, and infections are no exception. In the tropics such applications are equally fanciful. The greatest contribution of host genetics is likely to be in informing better biological prevention and treatment methods. Examples of this are described above but the translation of discovery to practice is slow and uncertain. We are only just beginning to see how the science of genetics can benefit those populations that need progress most.

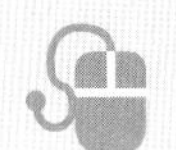

Access the complete reference list online at
http://www.expertconsult.com

CHAPTER 7

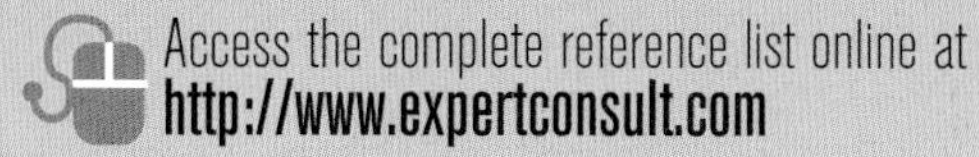
Access the complete reference list online at
http://www.expertconsult.com

Disease Eradication and Control

David L. Heymann

INTRODUCTION

Since the global certification of smallpox eradication in 1980 there has been widespread interest in infectious disease eradication as a public health goal, despite doubts that had developed with failures in the eradication of hookworm and yellow fever in the early 1900s, yaws in the 1940s, and malaria in the 1950s. Each of these previous efforts to eradicate was associated with optimism when they were begun because of newly obtained scientific knowledge or potential interventions, and from their failure valuable lessons were learned.

The hookworm eradication strategy was based on mass screening of stools of children for evidence of hookworm infection, their treatment with newly identified curative drugs, and the construction of sanitary facilities.[1,2] Among the lessons learned from this effort was the importance of sustained political will to provide for such basic public health services as sanitation – and the need for sustainable supplies of drugs and other public health goods as the basis for successful public health programs.

The strategy for yellow fever eradication targeted destruction of the breeding sites of the mosquito vector *Aedes aegypti*, based on the newly understood epidemiology of yellow fever transmission and that lowering mosquito densities decreased yellow fever virus transmission.[3] When it was discovered in the 1930s that the yellow fever virus had a natural reservoir among jungle mammals as well, and that the transmission force in Africa differed from that in Latin America where the strategy had been developed, it was understood that eradication could not be accomplished using the available technologies and resources.[4]

The strategy for the eradication of yaws was aimed at reducing the prevalence of the infectious agent through mass screening to identify persons with the characteristic lesions of yaws, and treatment with penicillin in hopes that prevalence could be decreased low enough to inhibit and finally interrupt transmission.[5] When it was realized that mild and subclinical/latent infection also occurred, and that this permitted continued transmission, it was clearly understood that the eradication strategy would require enhanced screening with a yet to be developed field diagnostic test, and additional costs.

Finally, the malaria eradication strategy relied on the use of residual spraying of the interior walls of dwellings where mosquitoes settled after biting, with the newly developed insecticide DDT. Mosquitoes would thus be killed and transmission decreased. The malaria eradication strategy also included clinical case detection and treatment with currently existing antimalarial drugs.[6] During the course of eradication efforts the mosquito vector developed resistance to DDT, and the malaria parasite developed resistance to antimalarials. The ability to cope with these two issues using existing technologies limited the ability to alter the eradication strategy to compensate, and the eradication program was discontinued.

These lessons, combined with the lessons from the successful effort to eradicate smallpox, have increased understanding of the biological and epidemiological characteristics of infectious agents that could be candidates for eradication.

IDENTIFYING CANDIDATE INFECTIOUS AGENTS FOR ERADICATION

The concept of eradication is an important public health goal because eradication results in decreased human suffering and death, and anticipated cost savings once eradication has been achieved. The estimated mortality of smallpox in 1967 compared to the mortality of AIDS, tuberculosis, and malaria as recently estimated by the World Health Organization and UNAIDS clearly demonstrates the power of eradication in decreasing infectious disease mortality (***Fig. 7.1***).

During the past 30 years efforts have been made to apply the lessons from various eradication programs in order to more clearly understand the biological and epidemiological characteristics of an infectious agent that determine the feasibility of its eradication, to more precisely define the public health terms used to describe eradication, and to use these characteristics and public health terms to systematically assess the feasibility of eradication of known infectious agents.

Biological and Epidemiological Characteristics of Infectious Agents That Determine the Feasibility of Eradication

The feasibility of eradicating smallpox had been clearly demonstrated in the first half of the twentieth century by routine vaccination programs in many industrialized and developing countries that reached the level of herd immunity necessary to interrupt transmission of the variola virus, the causative agent of smallpox. The World Health Assembly passed a resolution to eradicate smallpox worldwide in 1967, and in those countries that still had endemic smallpox, routine vaccination programs were at first supplemented by mass vaccination campaigns in order to rapidly develop herd immunity. As smallpox epidemiology became better understood through investigation of outbreaks that occurred as part of the eradication program, the strategy evolved from one of mass vaccination to search and containment: active identification of cases and their contacts through searches for persons with clinical signs of smallpox, and ring vaccination of households neighboring the household of those who had clinical signs, and vaccination of their household and other close contacts.[7]

The program successfully interrupted transmission of smallpox in all remaining endemic countries, and in 1980, after a rigorous certification process which included surveys for clinical disease and residual facial scarring associated with smallpox, the World Health Organization declared smallpox eradicated from the world. After this declaration all countries were asked to destroy any smallpox virus specimens remaining in laboratories, or to provide them to one of two WHO Collaborating Centers for storage under maximum biosecurity conditions.

A number of endemic countries had been reluctant to participate in smallpox eradication despite the World Health Assembly resolution, and

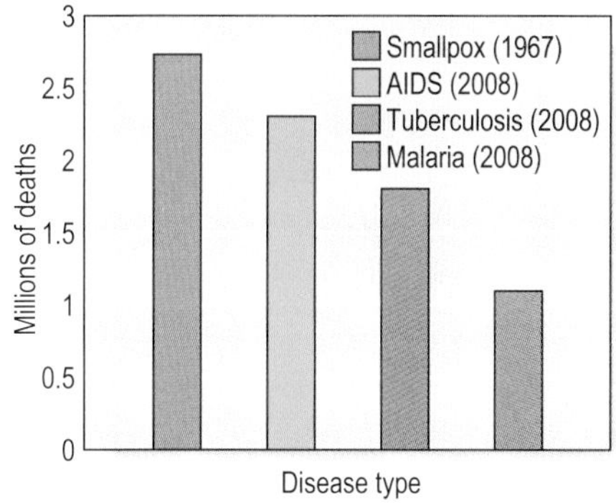

Figure 7.1 Estimated smallpox mortality, 1967, and recent mortality estimated from AIDS, tuberculosis, and malaria: the power of eradication in decreasing infectious disease mortality. (Source: World Health Organization).

others were torn by civil war, and eradication activities could be conducted only during brief intervals. Eradication was accomplished, however, by ensuring continued government commitment and international coordination that provided technical expertise and external finances to these and other endemic countries.

Through retrospective analysis, the success of eradication has been attributed to the following biological and epidemiological characteristics of smallpox by public health experts throughout the world, including D.A. Henderson who led the successful smallpox eradication effort:[8]

Burden of Disease Variola major, the predominant form of smallpox, had a case-fatality rate of 20–30% in unvaccinated persons, with an estimated mortality of over 2.7 million in 1967, the year that smallpox eradication was begun. It was clearly understood to be a serious threat by governments in both industrialized and developing countries, comparable to mortality of the three major infectious diseases today for which there are no vaccines: AIDS, tuberculosis and malaria (***Fig. 7.1***).

Environmental Persistence There were no animal reservoirs and no insect vectors involved anywhere in the transmission cycle of smallpox. Humans were the only reservoir, and the variola virus could not amplify independently in the environment. Interrupting transmission in humans was therefore the only necessary target to accomplish eradication.

Transmission Potential The secondary attack rate of smallpox was estimated to be approximately 30% in nonimmunized populations, resulting in transmission from each infected person to two to five additional close and unvaccinated contacts. With this relatively low secondary attack rate it was possible to contain the spread of infection by vaccinating potential contacts and to trace the origin of infection to detect other possible outbreaks.

Clinical Expression Every person infected with the variola virus developed a characteristic rash that was readily identifiable by health workers and the general population, and transmission occurred only during the time the rash was present. Approximately three-fourths of those who had variola major were left with lifelong residual pockmarks on the face, and clinical signs and residual scarring could easily be used to identify the geographic area of transmission so that search and containment could be targeted. These two characteristics also facilitated certification of eradication once transmission had been interrupted.

Susceptibility to Reinfection Infection with the variola virus caused solid immunity to reinfection, and those who recovered from disease ceased to carry the variola virus. Vaccination with smallpox vaccine provided solid immunity in an estimated 95% or more of vaccinated persons and, if given within 4 days of infection, was thought to attenuate the course of disease in those already infected.

Box 7.1 Generally Accepted Biological and Epidemiological Criteria for Assessing Feasibility of Eradication of an Infectious Agent

Burden of disease	Susceptibility to reinfection
Environmental persistence	Long-term effectiveness of intervention
Transmission potential	
Clinical expression	

Long-Term Effectiveness of Interventions Smallpox vaccine was inexpensive, lyophilized and thermostable for 30 days or more at temperatures of 37°C, providing complete protection from one dose for up to 20 years in those who were successfully vaccinated.

The lessons learned from smallpox eradication have led to six generally accepted biological and epidemiological criteria for assessing the feasibility of eradication of an infectious agent (***Box 7.1***).

These biological and epidemiological criteria – along with other considerations based on political will and available or potential financing – were variously used in the late twentieth century by governments, political leaders, and public health experts to make the decision to eradicate two additional infectious agents – the wild poliovirus and *Dracunculus medinensis*. These decisions, now embedded in World Health Assembly resolutions, have led to the establishment of the two global eradication initiatives that are currently under way (see later in the chapter).

Public Health Terms to Describe Eradication

Though many of the biological and epidemiological criteria in ***Box 7.1*** had been used in the decision-making process to eradicate wild poliovirus and *Dracunculus medinensis*, questions remained as to whether a more precise assessment of the feasibility of eradication was possible. In 1997, a group of public health experts was therefore assembled in a Dahlem (Germany) workshop for an interdisciplinary exchange of ideas on disease eradication. The workshop formally reviewed all present and past efforts to eradicate infectious diseases, with a goal of developing additional criteria to strengthen the assessment of eradication feasiblity.[9] The workshop concluded that additional criteria would provide a more valid assessment, and that these included differences between the level of reduction that could potentially be achieved for infection and disease; the need for long term sustainability once these reductions had been achieved; and the extent of the geographic area where disease was present.

A definition for eradication, and four other public health terms, were proposed by the workshop in hopes that they would provide a context that would facilitate the assessment of the feasibility of eradication. A few years after the Dahlem workshop, after the deliberate use of anthrax spores to cause harm, fear of bioterrorism added an additional consideration to the feasibility of eradication in many countries where bioterrorism was perceived as a threat.[10] Added to this perceived threat was the fact that the entire genomes of many different infectious agents had been published and understood, and that infectious agents that had been eradicated from nature could potentially be reintroduced if successfully synthesized *de novo*.

Table 7.1 attempts to provide a summary of the public health definition of eradication, and of the other terms determined to strengthen the assessment of infectious agents for eradication, as proposed from the Dahlem workshop. In addition, a further dimension has been added to this summary table that incorporates the perceived fears related to bioterrorism.

ASSESSMENT OF THE FEASIBILITY OF ERADICATION OF KNOWN INFECTIOUS AGENTS

Ten or so years before the Dahlem workshop, resolutions had been passed by the World Health Assembly to eradicate the wild poliovirus and *Dracunculus medinensis* using many of the biological and epidemiological

Table 7.1 Definitions of Public Health Terms Related to Eradication of Infectious Agents Based on Dahlem Workshop on the Eradication of Infectious Diseases and Considerations Related to Bioterrorism

Public Health Term	Reduction in Disease	Reduction in Infection	Geographic Area	Sustainability
Control	Reduction of morbidity and mortality to a locally accepted level		Wherever disease exists and control efforts are made	Continued intervention required to maintain reduction
Elimination of disease	Reduction of incidence to zero		Wherever disease exists and elimination efforts are made	Continued intervention required to maintain reduction
Elimination of infection		Reduction of infected humans to zero	Wherever infection exists in humans and elimination efforts are made	Continued intervention required to prevent reestablishment
Eradication		Permanent reduction of infected humans to zero	Worldwide	Intervention measures no longer required unless risk of accidental or deliberate reintroduction of infectious agent
Extinction		Infectious agent no longer exists in humans, nature or laboratory	Worldwide	Intervention measures no longer required unless risk of deliberate reintroduction of *de novo* synthesized infectious agent

Table 7.2 Biological and Epidemiological Feasibility of Eradication of Wild Poliovirus and *Dracunculus medinensis* Using General Criteria

Criterion	Wild Poliovirus	*Dracunculus medinensis*
Burden of disease	High in 125 countries prior to beginning eradication (1000 children paralyzed per day)	High in areas of poverty in certain geographic areas of the Middle East, South Asia and Africa with severe morbidity
Environmental persistence	Unable to persist in environment/no reservoir other than humans/no amplifying vector	Unable to persist in environment/no reservoir other than humans/no vertical transmission in amplifying vector
Transmission potential	High attack rate (virtually all children by age 5) and virus can be physically carried in gut of those who are immune, for times estimated as long as 1 month	High in villages in endemic regions where sanitation is poor
Clinical expression	Incomplete (up to 500 or more asymptomatic infections for each child with paralysis)	Infection leads to visible clinical signs
Susceptibility to reinfection	Reinfection does not occur once immunity obtained to all three virus types	Reinfection thought to occur
Long-term effectiveness of intervention	Solid immunity after vaccination but requires cold chain for vaccine transport	Clean water prevents infection

criteria now summarized in ***Box 7.1***.[11,12] ***Table 7.2*** shows retrospectively, and for comparative purposes, a feasibility assessment of wild poliovirus and *Dracunculus medinensis* based on the biological and epidemiological criteria for the feasibility of eradication outlined in ***Box 7.1***.

There are clearly differences in the biological and epidemiological characteristics of the wild poliovirus and the smallpox virus, especially as regards transmission potential and clinical expression. The biological and epidemiological characteristics of *Dracunculus medinensis*, however, are more similar to those of the variola virus. Neither of these infectious agents persists in the environment, both cause a high burden of disability-causing disease, and both have effective and relatively inexpensive interventions – factors that appear to have been important in the decision to eradicate. High levels of political will associated with better controlling of both these infections in countries and internationally, and present and projected financial resources available internationally, have led these programs to the brink of success.

Polio Eradication

A World Health Assembly resolution to eradicate polio was passed in 1988 at a time when polio was endemic in 125 countries, and an estimated 1000 children were being paralyzed each day from one of three polioviruses (type 1, 2 or 3).[9] Polio is passed from person to person through fecal/oral contact, mainly by ingesting unclean water in areas where sanitation is substandard (see Chapter 60). The strategy for polio eradication is based on developing herd immunity to all three virus types that will protect individuals from infection, and at the same time decrease incidence to lower levels so that eventually transmission cannot be sustained. The strategy consists of continuation and strengthening of routine immunization programs that include polio vaccination, vaccination campaigns, usually during the low season of polio transmission, to increase herd immunity, and surveillance to assure that all possible cases of polio are reported, completely investigated, and confirmed/genetically sequenced in a network of quality-controlled public health laboratories.

Vaccination campaigns are either scheduled as national immunization days, or as supplemental vaccination campaigns – sometimes called mopping up campaigns – in areas where transmission is identified by surveillance. All campaigns target children under 5 years of age, and supplemental campaigns often consist of door-to-door vaccination in addition to vaccination at fixed sites on specified days.

Great progress has been made in polio eradication since 1988. By 1999, transmission of endemic type 2 poliovirus had been interrupted worldwide, and by 2008 all but four of the original 125 countries had interrupted transmission of all three types of wild poliovirus. The four countries that remained polio endemic for polio types 1 and 3 virus were Afghanistan, India, Nigeria, and Pakistan.

Virus exportation, mainly of type 1 poliovirus, has occurred from two of these countries – India and Nigeria. Origins of the exported viruses have been confirmed by surveillance, and exportation has been a persistent risk to eradication efforts. During 2008, for example, 13 countries were reinfected. In many of these countries poliovirus again began to circulate, requiring increased financial resources to conduct vaccination campaigns. The problem of exportation has been heightened by rumors of deliberately contaminated polio vaccine that ignited a controversy in Kano State, northern Nigeria, in mid-2003 and led to the immediate and official suspension of immunization activities.[13] Such rumors – the substance of which varies from the contamination of polio vaccine with HIV at the time of manufacture to the deliberate addition of hormones to permanently sterilize young girls – have plagued the poliomyelitis eradication efforts since their beginning, and led to decreased vaccination coverage and herd immunity.

Other causes of decreased vaccination coverage in the remaining endemic countries include civil disturbance and inability to physically reach children to provide vaccine, and less than optimal seroconversion to the oral polio vaccine in certain areas of India where transmission force is extremely intense due to dense populations and substandard sanitation.[14] Despite these obstacles, the world is now close to eradicating polio, with just over 1600 children with polio-associated paralysis having been found through surveillance in 2009, but efforts by countries to interrupt the last chains of transmission must be strengthened, and problems that interfere with vaccinating children resolved.

Once transmission of all three types of wild poliovirus has been interrupted worldwide and certified through continued surveillance, an additional strategy will be required. Because of the risk of live attenuated polio vaccine to revert to its virulent form, countries that are now using oral poliovirus vaccine to eradicate polio must stop its use in order to eliminate the risks of paralytic poliomyelitis from vaccine-associated paralytic polio and circulating vaccine-derived and Sabin poliovirus.[15] Finally, wild polioviruses in laboratories around the world must be destroyed after certification of eradication, or consolidated in designated laboratories under secure conditions to minimize the risk of reintroduction. Inactivated polio vaccine production, from wild poliovirus stocks, must also be placed under biosecure conditions in order to minimize the risk of accidental release and reintroduction of virus. Some countries are also contemplating whether wild poliovirus – either natural or biosynthesized – could pose a risk to eradication, and in these same countries continued vaccination strategies are being considered for the post-eradication era.

Dracunculiasis Eradication

Dracunculiasis is caused by the parasitic worm *Dracunculus medinensis* and is characterized by the gradual emergence of a female worm from an ulcer, usually in the leg (see Chapter 108). When a person with dracunculiasis immerses the infected part in cold water, the worm releases thousands of larvae that are ingested by a small cyclopoid crustacean that inhabits the water. When a person drinks water containing the infective cyclops, the cyclops are killed but the infective larvae are liberated and penetrate the wall of the intestine; mature worms then migrate through subcutaneous tissues to the leg where they continue to mature and from where females deposit their larvae when in contact with water.

Intensive control efforts for dracunculiasis began in 1982, and early success led to a World Health Assembly resolution in 1991 to eradicate the disease.[12] The eradication strategy is to interrupt transmission to humans by preventing ingestion of the minute cyclopoid crustacean containing the larval parasites. Several methods are used: providing safe water supplies with new wells, destruction of the crustacean in water by the use of the insecticide temephos, and health education to promote filtration or boiling of water before ingestion. Infected persons are identified through surveys and reports, are treated by removal of the adult worm and wound care, and counseled not to enter the water and thus contaminate it.

Foci of infection of dracunculiasis in the Middle East and South Asia have been eliminated using this strategy, and infection is thought to be currently limited to Sudan, Ghana, Mali, Nigeria, and Niger. By 2003, the incidence of dracunculiasis worldwide had decreased from an estimated 3.5 million infections in 20 countries in 1986, to just over 9500 reported infections in 5 countries in 2007.[12] The majority of infections are in Sudan, where continuing civil disturbance has caused a problem in operations, and Ghana. Continued active surveillance and mapping of infected villages, followed by implementation of the eradication strategy, are required in order to complete eradication.

Comparison of Polio and Dracunculiasis Eradication Programs

Polio and dracunculiasis eradication activities to date have greatly decreased the burden of morbidity, as expressed by disability, caused by these two infections. Three WHO regions have now been certified as polio free, despite the differences in biological and epidemiological characteristics of the wild polio and smallpox viruses, especially as regards transmission potential and clinical expression that have required intensive surveillance to identify children with paralytic polio, and numerous costly vaccination campaigns to stop transmission from those who are asymptomatically infected. But the risk of imported wild poliovirus and the development of vaccine derived circulating polioviruses continues to exist in these regions. Dracunculiasis eradication has likewise been certified in many countries, is much less costly and is sustainable over the long term, possibly reflecting its closer similarity in biological and epidemiological characteristics to the variola virus.

Of great importance is that both infectious agents cause a high burden of disease that has generated political will to eradicate, and that neither persists in the environment nor has a reservoir other than humans, and both have inexpensive and effective interventions, characteristics that have clearly been shown to be among the most important factors that led to the success of the smallpox eradication program.

As for smallpox eradication, availability of resources has been crucial in the accomplishments that have been made in both eradication programs to date. In fact, it is the availability of resources, and the continued political will of endemic countries and the international community, that appear in part to have compensated for the biological and epidemiological characteristics that would have otherwise been thought to lead to failure. To date it is estimated that polio eradication has cost in excess of 5 billion US dollars, while the cost of dracunculiasis eradication, which benefits from a highly sustainable and simple technology, has been estimated at 90 million US dollars during the first 10 years of intensive operations. Ensuring continued political commitment and funding are challenges for both programs, and will be among the keys to success.

Assessment of the Feasibility of Eradication of Other Known Infectious Agents

Biological and epidemiological criteria have been used to assess the feasibility of eradication of the poliovirus and *Dracunculus medinensis*. The five public health terms defined by the Dahlem workshop (***Table 7.2***) are also useful when deciding the feasibility of eradication of other infectious agents, and for identifying other public health strategies for infectious agents that do not appear to be eradicable. These terms have generally been simplified operationally to two major terms: eradication and elimination as a public health problem.[16]

With these two terms currently in use – eradication and elimination as a public health problem – no further infectious agents have been clearly identified for eradication by the World Health Assembly at present, though several diseases have been targeted for elimination as public health problems. They include onchocerciasis, leprosy, and lymphatic filariasis, and intensified control programs, using consensus control strategies, are currently under way.[17–21] A measles elimination target has likewise been set, and there is currently discussion as to whether the elimination target should be changed to one of eradication. Other diseases that are being or have been considered for elimination as public health problems include urban rabies, hepatitis B, and congenital syphilis.

Eradication is a worthy and important public health goal. Based on the synthesis of international understanding and recommendations presented in this chapter, it is clear that biological and epidemiological characteristics of an infectious agent are important in determining whether eradication is feasible, followed by an assessment of political will and available or potentially available finances.

Assessment of the feasibility of eradication can be further strengthened, and other control options identified, by examining the potential level of reduction in prevalence or incidence of the infectious agent possible, the geographic extent of the disease caused by the agent, and the long-term need for sustainability of control activities to maintain the reductions gained. In some instances where eradication of an infectious agent is not considered feasible by this assessment, targeting reduction in incidence or prevalence of an infectious disease in order to eliminate it as a public health problem, while understanding the need to sustain the intervention after the reduction target has been attained, has provided the impetus needed to increase political will and financing for better control of those infectious diseases that at present cannot be eradicated.

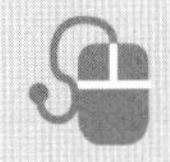

Access the complete reference list online at
http://www.expertconsult.com

Access the complete reference list online at
http://www.expertconsult.com

CHAPTER 8

Vector Biology

José M.C. Ribeiro • Jesus G. Valenzuela

INTRODUCTION

Many parasites, from viruses to nematodes, are transmitted to humans by arthropod vectors. As noted in several chapters of this book, these invertebrates are important in transmitting some of the most devastating human diseases. Because parts of the life cycle of such parasites are dependent on the life cycle of the vector itself, understanding the epidemiology and transmission dynamics of such diseases necessarily includes understanding the factors affecting the life cycle of their vectors.

Ticks are specialized mites related to spiders and thus arachnids (having eight legs in the adult stage). Insects are hexapods. Because of the many similarities in their life cycle and transmission of pathogens to humans and other vertebrates, medical entomologists lump ticks and insects as arthropod vectors in medical entomology textbooks.

Although in a few cases pathogens are transmitted mechanically from one host to another by vectors in their attempt to feed, the general rule is for the pathogen to develop an intricate life cycle within the vector host. This life cycle may take from several days to months (as with some tick-borne pathogens). The time taken for the parasite to complete the life cycle within its vector is called the *extrinsic incubation period*, which is the time in the vertebrate from infection to the first appearance of symptoms. Some pathogens develop exclusively within the digestive tract of the vector, such as *Trypanosoma cruzi* or *Leishmania* spp., whereas others develop within several compartments of the vector. Thus, *Plasmodium*, *Theileria*, and *Babesia*, as well as most arboviruses, will eventually locate themselves within the vector salivary glands after crossing the gut, disseminating into the hemolymph, and finally invading the salivary glands. Filarial worms, depending on the species, develop in different vector organs (muscle, coelomic fat body, or malpighian tubules) and exit by puncturing through the vector's mouthparts while the vector attempts to feed.

VECTOR LIFE CYCLE STRATEGIES

Most bloodsucking arthropods are oviparous, with the exception of some Diptera (including the tsetse) which are ovoviviparous (the egg hatches within the uterus and the larva feeds on secretions produced by milk glands). Two basically different growth strategies are observed: those having complete metamorphosis (*holometabolous*; ***Fig. 8.1***) and those having incomplete metamorphosis (*hemimetabolous*; ***Fig. 8.2***). Holometabolous insects follow the model of the butterfly, the caterpillar being very different from the adult animal. Hemimetabolous development follows the cockroach model, the immature animal being similar to the adult. In all cases the immature animal feeds after coming out of the egg, and molts to a larger stage, shedding its old cuticle in a process called ecdysis. The newly emerged insect has a soft cuticle, ingests air or water, and enlarges itself before the cuticle hardens again. This feeding and molting process occurs from two to five times before the arthropod molts to an adult. Before molting to the adult, the general appearance of the insect or tick is similar (only larger) to the newly hatched form. The last molt in hemimetabolous animals transforms the arthropod into an adult having sexually mature reproductive organs and fully developed wings (in species having wings they are found only in the adult stage). In holometabolous insects (all ticks are hemimetabolous), the last immature molt leads to a pupa, where metamorphosis to the adult stage occurs. All immature stages of holometabolous insects are called *larvae*, whereas all immature stages of hemimetabolous insects are called *nymphs*. In hard ticks (Ixodidae), there are two immature stages: the first is called a larva and the second a nymph.

Nymphs and adults of hemimetabolous insects and ticks thus have the same general appearance (varying in size), usually sharing the same habitat and feeding on the same types of food. However, larvae and adults of holometabolous insects are very different, have different habitats, and have different feeding habits. Immature and adult ticks, as well as nymphs and adult kissing bugs (triatomids) and bed bugs, all feed solely on blood, while larvae and adults of mosquitoes and sandflies feed on very different things, with only the adult female insect feeding on blood. Thus control of holometabolous insects involves two completely different strategies: those aimed at the immature and those aimed at the adult stages of the vector.

LIFE SPAN, REPRODUCTIVE CAPACITY, AND VECTOR ABUNDANCE

Insects and ticks also vary greatly in their life span and reproductive capacity. Mosquitoes, for example, can complete a life cycle within 1–2 weeks, while some ticks take several years and even more than a decade if food is scarce. Additionally, a single female may produce only a few offspring (such as the tsetse), several hundred (mosquitoes), or thousands (ixodid ticks). Of course, most offspring of such insects never become adults, as only one female needs to achieve maturity to replace the preceding one and keep the vector population size constant. However, changes in the environment that make it possible for a larger number of larvae and nymphs to become adults can create explosive increases in vector abundance, and thus create epidemic conditions. In the case of mosquitoes, an unusually good rainy season may produce several generations resulting in a large number of adults. Ticks, with their longer life cycles, have populations that can fluctuate on a yearly basis, as can be the case with winter weather fluctuations in New England affecting the density of the deer tick, the vector of Lyme disease. Vector abundance normally exhibits a large variance both temporally and spatially, and this is reflected in the time and spatial dynamics of vector-borne diseases.

The life span of a vector relative to the time taken for the parasite to complete its invertebrate life cycle is also very important for understanding the dynamics of vector-borne diseases. For example, most malaria parasites take at least 1 week to complete their life cycle in the adult

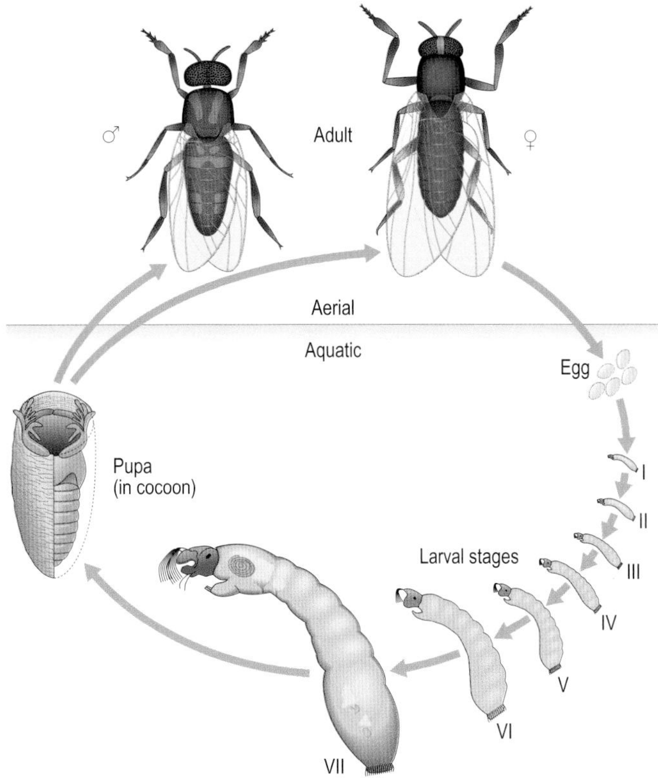

Figure 8.1 Life history of a holometabolous insect, represented by the life cycle of a black fly, *Simulium damnosum*. Note the very different aspects of immature and adult insects that share different habitats. (Modified from Beaty BJ, Marquardt WC. The Biology of Disease Vectors. Fort Collins: University Press of Colorado; 1996.)

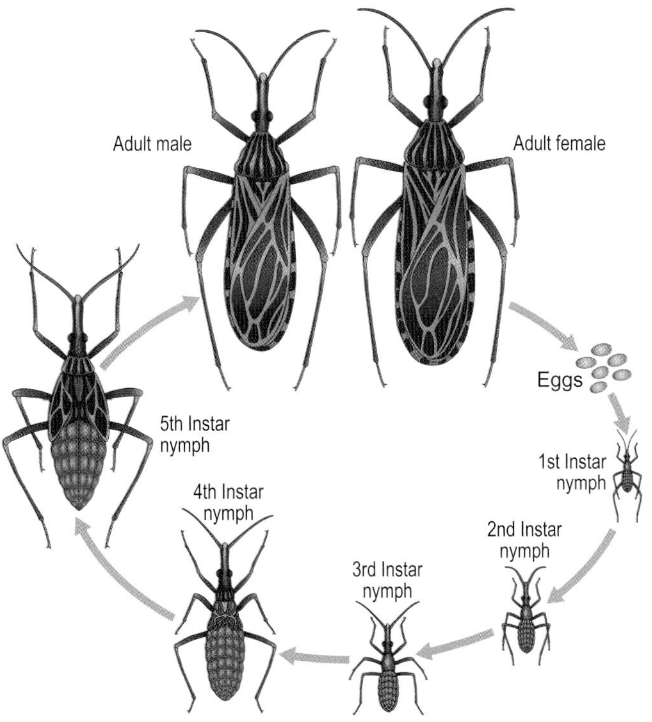

Figure 8.2 Life history of a hemimetabolous insect, represented by the life cycle of a triatomine bug, *Rhodnius prolixus*. Note the similar appearance of all instars, which also share the same source of food. (Modified from Beaty BJ, Marquardt WC. The Biology of Disease Vectors. Fort Collins: University Press of Colorado; 1996.)

female mosquito, but most mosquitoes die of old age in less than a week. Thus, the longevity of the adult female mosquito is a very important variable determining how many secondary cases a single case of malaria can generate given a certain number of mosquitoes available per person. On the other hand, ticks can outlive most of their rodent hosts, and this can be very important in the perpetuation of viral diseases of short duration (e.g., diseases that either kill the host or to which the host becomes immune) in a small-sized rodent population.

HOST SPECIFICITY

There are two basic strategies followed by those animals that feed on vertebrate blood: a hunting strategy, where the insect actively searches for its prey (most bloodsucking arthropods are micropredators, not parasites), and an ambush strategy, where the insect or tick positions itself to maximize contact with its host or prey. The tsetse, horse fly, and mosquito are good hunters, whereas most ticks and fleas maximize ambush.

To locate their hosts, vectors use visual cues, temperature gradients (including infrared "vision"), and olfaction. For example, some tsetse species are attracted by anything larger than a dog that moves at a certain speed (including a car), are even more attracted if the object smells like cattle urine, and are really excited over a warm surface. Carbon dioxide and water vapor are common attractants to many ticks and hematophagous insects. The smell of human feet (made possible by the same genus of bacteria that ferments Limburger cheese) was shown to be attractant to *Anopheles gambiae*, a highly anthropophilic mosquito.

Host specificity is a very important concept for understanding the dynamics of vector-borne diseases, as they have a squared value in the equations of transmission dynamics. For example, a mosquito needs to feed once on a person with malaria to acquire the *Plasmodium* parasite and feed again on another person several days later to deliver the parasite. If only 50% of the population of a particular mosquito species feed on humans, and only 50% of the mosquitoes feeding on the sick person acquire gametocytes (the parasite stage infectious for the mosquito), then only 50% of this 50%, or only 25% of the entire population, would then transmit the parasite to humans. *An. gambiae* mosquitoes feed almost exclusively on humans (greater than 98%), even when other sources of blood (e.g., cattle) are available, and this is one of the reasons this mosquito is such a good malaria vector. On the other hand, some vectors are relatively nonspecific, and they may become good bridge vectors for transferring zoonotic pathogens, such as *Ixodes scapularis* transmitting *Borrelia burgdorferi* from the white-footed mouse to humans.

VECTOR COMPETENCE

Vector-borne parasites can be very selective in the host species in which they complete development. For example, human malaria can be transmitted only by mosquitoes of the genus *Anopheles*. This may be due to many biologic reasons varying from the time the mosquito peritrophic matrix is formed (a chitinous dialysis membrane-like structure that forms around the blood meal inside the mosquito gut that may serve as a barrier to the invading parasites), to the mosquito's ability to mount a melanotic reaction to the developing oocyst, and to the sporozoite's ability to find the mosquito salivary gland and survive the mosquito's hemolymph defense system. Other mosquitoes can develop heavy sporozoite infections of the salivary glands, even when feeding on lightly parasitemic hosts. This biologic ability of a vector to serve (or not) in the parasite's life cycle to its infective stage is called *vector competence*. It is actually expressed as the fraction of a particular vector population or species that can transmit the parasite after taking an infectious blood meal. In many cases the term *vector potential* is used synonymously with vector competence, mainly in a context where a potential vector species from a certain geographic area is being investigated for its ability to carry a parasite from another geographic area. For example, a medical entomologist from California may check whether local *Culex* mosquitoes are able to complete the life cycle of a virus found in Japan. The results of such tests of vector competence may indicate the potential for that particular Japanese viral disease to appear in California.

VECTORIAL CAPACITY

Even when determining that a particular arthropod species is competent for the parasite to complete its life cycle, this does not mean that such a vector will be important in maintaining disease transmission in the real world. For example, in the laboratory one may force a mosquito or tick to take a meal from a host it will never find or prefer to feed on in its habitat. Or the life span of the vector may be so short, compared to the extrinsic incubation period, that most of the vectors are dead before transmission occurs. Or the abundance of the vector may be so low that it will not sustain transmission of the pathogen in real-life conditions. To understand the role of a particular vector in the transmission of a particular pathogen, the concept of *vectorial capacity* was developed by Macdonald.[1] Vectorial capacity includes not only the concepts of vector competence but also those of vector abundance, host specificity, vector longevity, and the time taken for the parasite to develop its life cycle within the vector (extrinsic incubation period). Vectorial capacity has a precise numerical meaning which represents the number of infective bites generated by a single case of a particular vector-borne disease, on a per day basis. This concept was developed by workers in the field of malariology and may be adapted to understand several other vector-borne diseases where vector survival is on the same order of magnitude as the extrinsic incubation period (this includes most mosquito-, sandfly-, black fly-, and flea-borne diseases).

In formal numerical terms the Macdonald vectorial capacity equation can be expressed as:

$$VC = m \cdot a^2 \cdot b \cdot p^n / -\ln p$$

where

VC = vectorial capacity (number of mosquito infective bites generated by a single parasitemic patient)

m = number of mosquitoes available per person

a = human biting rate

b = vector competence

p = probability of the vector surviving 1 day

n = extrinsic incubation period.

This equation can be understood in a very straightforward way by following each term and its relationship to the transmission dynamics of the parasite in the invertebrate host. It is quite obvious that the number of secondary disease cases of a mosquito-borne disease would be proportional to the number of vectors available per person (***Fig. 8.3***); that is, the more mosquitoes, the more chance of one case generating another case of malaria. The number of mosquitoes, however, has to be qualified regarding their host specificity, as described above. If only 10% of the mosquitoes feed on a person, only a maximum of 1% could potentially deliver the parasite back to human hosts, because in order to transmit the disease they would have to feed again on people, assuming that on the second blood-feeding the mosquitoes have the same chance of feeding on either a human host or another host (this is a nontested assumption of the MacDonald model!). Vectorial competence would further interfere with the ultimate number of infective bites, as not all vectors may develop the parasite to its infective stage (and that was why "a maximum of 1%" was written above). The term p^n expresses the number of mosquitoes surviving the length of time associated with the intrinsic incubation period. When collected from the wild, mosquito mortality follows roughly an exponential decay curve, and thus the number of mosquitoes surviving n days would be exactly p^n. For example, if a mosquito has a 90% probability of surviving 1 day, then the number of mosquitoes that would survive 10 days would be 0.9^{10} or 34.9% of the initial mosquito population (see ***Fig. 8.3***). Thus, at the end of the extrinsic incubation period, only a fraction of the vectors would be delivering the pathogen. However, even considering the number of mosquitoes that survive n days, these mosquitoes would not survive forever, and would continue to die. Because most infected

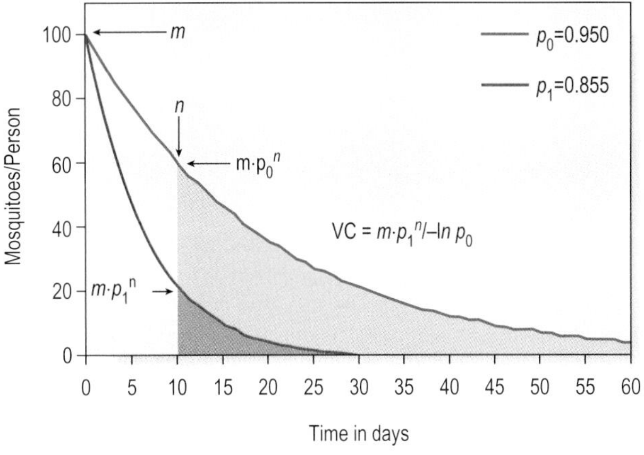

Figure 8.3 Graphical representation of two different sets of equal numbers of mosquitoes (100) biting a person infected with malaria at day 0. One set (p_0) has a daily survival rate of 0.95 whereas the other set (p_1) has a rate of 0.855. The human biting rate and vector competence are equal to 1 in both mosquito sets. Note that the two sets of mosquitoes die at different rates and continue to bite people without transmitting disease until n (extrinsic incubation period) days have elapsed. After this time interval, mosquitoes have infected salivary glands and surviving insects will produce infective bites. The total number of infective bites will be proportional to the number of mosquitoes surviving n days multiplied by their life expectancy in days. The result is equal to the vectorial capacity (VC) and is numerically equal to the marked areas under the curve. Note that a 10% change in the survival rate leads to a ninefold change in the vectorial capacity.

mosquitoes do not have their mortality rate significantly changed due to infection with the parasite, we can assume that the daily survival rate of such mosquitoes is still p. To calculate the number of infective bites delivered for the remainder of the life of the mosquitoes, one would have to integrate the area under the survival curve for those mosquitoes. We know from calculus that to calculate the area under an exponential with a rate p, the solution is $1/-\ln p$. Thus the area under the mosquito survivorship curve from day n (the extrinsic incubation period) until all mosquitoes are dead represents the vectorial capacity of a particular vector–pathogen association.

The above considerations are very helpful in understanding the interrelationships of the several variables affecting the transmission dynamics of many vector-borne diseases. For example, it becomes clear that the main parameter affecting vectorial capacity is the term p^n, which has an exponential value. Indeed some of the best mosquito vectors are long-lived when compared with other species. The human biting rate is a quadratic term, whereas mosquito abundance m and vector competence b are linear terms. Indeed many poorly anthropophilic vectors such as *An. albimanus* or *An. culicifascies* will only transmit human malaria when they are extremely abundant (and thus the m term compensates for the low value of a^2). Similarly, *Aedes aegypti* is a poor vector for urban yellow fever in Nigeria (the virus strain was of sylvatic origin), having poor vectorial competence b, but when conditions favor extremely abundant mosquito numbers, epidemics have occurred.[2]

The equation above with its parameters is an extreme simplification of what occurs in real life, but useful insights are obtained even when appreciating its limitations. Many of the terms are considered constants, but in real life they may be functions of other parameters. For example, the extrinsic incubation period changes with temperature; this is an important variable with most malarial and viral pathogens. Increased temperature may reduce incubation time significantly, increasing the vectorial capacity in larger proportion due to the exponential behavior of p^n. Similarly, increased humidity may significantly increase daily survival of mosquitoes (that otherwise may easily die of dehydration), also affecting vectorial capacity in an exponential fashion. The human biting rate of a particular vector species may also change with the repertoire of hosts in a given location. For example, many mosquitoes will prefer cattle or horses for a blood meal, but when "progress" arrives and horses and cattle disappear, the same species may start to bite humans preferentially and create a condition for human disease transmission.[3]

BASIC REPRODUCTIVE RATE

To convert the vectorial capacity equation into the basic reproductive rate (R_0) of the particular disease, one has to include the terms that represent the life cycle of the parasite in the human host. These are represented by the number of days that the infection lasts in the vertebrate host, expressed by the disease recovery rate r (measured as the probability per day of reverting to the nonparasitemic state), and by the probability c that the new secondary host will acquire the infection once bitten by the vector. We thus have

$$R_0 = \mathrm{VC} \cdot c/r$$

It is interesting to note the regulatory effect of vertebrate host immunity on R_0. The more time that a person stays sick (and thus the smaller the recovery rate r), the more mosquitoes are infected and the larger the disease R_0. However, in hyperendemic situations people acquire some immunity and the recovery rate is much faster (larger); also, the chance of getting infected by an infective bite (c) is smaller due to immunity. Both terms thus conspire to bring down R_0 in hyperendemic conditions. Conversely, this is why it is difficult to accomplish sustained control of malaria in hyperendemic conditions: as herd immunity goes down, the disease reproductive rate fights back. In the process of controlling the disease (and thereby reducing immunity), the scenario may change from one of "calm" or "quiet" endemicity to one of severe epidemics. Accordingly, if the current effort of indoor residual spraying in Africa is not sustained, epidemics affecting both young children and adults will certainly happen a few years after vector control suspension.

VECTOR LONGEVITY

The equations above are useful for understanding the dynamics of vector-borne diseases when the vector is relatively short-lived with reference to the extrinsic incubation period of the particular pathogen. Other scenarios for transmission can happen where vector longevity, for example, is not an important issue. Ticks are often more long-lived than their vertebrate hosts, as is the case with most rodents. Population size is an important determinant of the perpetuation of many infectious diseases that leads to lifelong immunity. For example, it is postulated that a human population settlement of at least 200 000 people is necessary to produce enough nonimmune children to sustain measles. One can, however, envision a small population of rodents (fewer than 1000) and their ticks sustaining a virus that produces lifelong immunity by the "ping-pong" effect of the virus being shuttled from the vertebrate to invertebrate hosts on an annual basis. For example, let us imagine a rodent population in sub-Saharan Africa that typically breeds in the annual rainy season, and their ticks, which also feed on an annual cycle. During the rainy season, both larvae and nymphs feed on the rodents simultaneously for a period of 2 months. Infected nymphs can transmit the virus to nonimmune rodents, and a few days later these rodents transmit the pathogen to larvae, which will feed again only in the next year (after molting to nymphs), when young, nonimmune rodents are available. A disease of short duration, without relapses, conferring lifelong immunity can thus perpetuate itself even within a host population of small size. The same reasoning applies in the absence of vectors if the pathogen can live long enough in the environment to reinfect young mice, as is the case with the North American hantavirus. Because rodents have a relatively short life span, they need a relatively small population size to keep diseases in an enzootic state for a pathogen. On the other hand, rodents can achieve very large population sizes, which makes the situation still worse. This may be one of the explanations for the continuous emergence of pathogens associated with rodent hosts; i.e., rapidly generating rodents can maintain cycles of pathogens even when they induce lifelong immunity.

TRANSOVARIAL TRANSMISSION

Some vector-borne pathogens can be transovarially transmitted from the adult female to its offspring. Some mosquitoes can have a small or substantial portion of their eggs containing viruses which will continue their development in the mosquito larvae up to the adult stage. In this case, the first bite of the adult female may inoculate the pathogen into the vertebrate host. Transovarial transmission is often referred to as *vertical* transmission of a pathogen, to differentiate it from *horizontal* transmission, when one vector acquires a pathogen from a vertebrate host. *Sexual* transmission of mosquito-borne viruses was also demonstrated in some rare cases, where male (non-blood-feeding) mosquitoes that were infected by the transovarial route could transfer the virus to females via copulation; this also occurs with African swine fever virus in argasid ticks.

In some cases transovarial transmission of a pathogen is an essential feature of the pathogen life cycle. For example, cattle babesiosis *(Babesia bovis)* is transmitted by the cattle tick *(Rhipicephalus microplus)*, which is a single-host tick. *Rhipicephalus* larvae attach to a host, staying with the same animal for life, until the adult female tick takes a large blood meal, drops off, lays thousands of eggs, and dies. There is no way of continuation of the *Babesia* life cycle without transovarial transmission of the protozoa from mother to young larvae.

Transovarial transmission may be an important route for the perpetuation of other pathogens that are also transmitted horizontally. For example, a mosquito-borne virus causing epizootics or epidemics might lead to increased herd immunity of the vertebrate hosts that prevents further spread of the virus within the vertebrate population. The virus could perpetuate in nature during the interepidemic period by vertical transmission, until the herd immunity goes down again and a new invasion of the vertebrate population by the pathogen can occur. Even if vertical transmission is relatively inefficient (e.g., if only 10% or less of the offspring become infective), the large number of horizontally infected vectors during epidemic times could lead to a few vertically infected individuals after several mosquito generations, enough to initiate a new epidemic after herd immunity decreases. This is again a case of the ping-pong transmission described above for tick-borne pathogen scenarios, but due to the much shorter life of mosquitoes, vertical transmission allows for the pathogen to hide within vectors until vertebrate herd immunity goes down.

MODES OF VECTOR-BORNE DISEASE TRANSMISSION

In most cases vectors are not born with parasites they transmit, but rather they get infected while blood-feeding. Once they have reached the vector's gut, parasites either continue to live there, such as *Leishmania* and *Trypanosoma*, or they cross the insect midgut epithelium into their vector's hemocoel, an open cavity between the digestive system and the cuticle, filled by hemolymph, the insect's blood, and other insect organs. Once in the hemolymph, parasites such as *Plasmodium* and several arboviruses will accumulate in their vectors' salivary glands. When vectors salivate into their hosts' skin in their attempt to obtain a blood meal, parasites are thus inoculated. Mosquito-borne parasitic worms can invade the thoracic muscles, fat body, or malpighian tubules of their vectors where they develop into infectious stage 3 larvae, whereupon they leave the nursing organ and go back into the hemolymph. These worms are too big to invade the salivary glands, but while the vector is feeding, triggered by the sudden temperature increase, they puncture the vector cuticle, actively moving into the vertebrate skin where they attempt to penetrate the tissue through the feeding wound. In many cases the worm dehydrates before it can achieve its goal, and this is one of the reasons why filarial transmissions such as that of *Wuchereria* are found only in humid places. Gut-dwelling parasites can be transmitted either when they are regurgitated into the vertebrate host, such as *Leishmania* and flea-borne plague, or when they are delivered in the vector feces, such as occurs with American trypanosomes. Defecation while feeding is relatively common with vectors because of the relatively huge blood meal, which compresses the insect rectum, and also because of the very fast water transport from the midgut to the hemolymph and from there to the rectum via the malpighian tubules, the kidney equivalent in arthropods. Interestingly, desert-dwelling triatomines are not good vectors, because they conserve water so well that they end up not defecating on their hosts. However, rodent reservoirs may acquire the disease while eating the triatomines.

Role of Vector Saliva in Parasite Transmission

Most vector-borne parasites invade their vertebrate hosts in sites were the vector has injected saliva. In the case of saliva-borne pathogens such as malaria, it is important to stress that sporozoites are not delivered into the vertebrate host circulation, as most diagrams show, but rather are released inside the host skin, from where they actively move into the blood circulation, in the case of human malaria. When mosquitoes reach a blood vessel, they suck the blood so fast that all sporozoites end up in the mosquito gut and are lost. *Leishmania* organisms, although not delivered via vector saliva, are delivered in the same wound where salivation occurs, thus the inoculation is coincident with a site exposed to their vector's saliva. Blood-feeders' saliva contains an array of pharmacologically active components that assist them to obtain a blood meal. This salivary cocktail includes potent anticoagulants, antiplatelet substances, vasodilators and immunomodulators, allowing blood-feeders to disarm the vertebrate's hemostatic and inflammatory system to their advantage. This pharmacologically modulated site may result in a better environment for pathogen establishment; in fact, *Leishmania major* parasites when co-injected into mice with sandfly saliva result in greater infection as compared to animals inoculated with parasites alone. The same phenomenon has been observed in transmission of viruses by ticks and in transmission of viruses by mosquitoes.

Vertebrate immune responses generated to the bites of arthropod vectors can influence vector feeding and/or the efficiency of pathogen transmission. In the case of ticks, repeated feeding in non-natural hosts results in immune responses that lead to tick rejection. However, immune-mediated tick rejection does not occur, or is milder, when ticks feed on natural hosts. On the other hand, in the case of *Phlebotomus* sand flies, repeated feeding in mice results in delayed-type hypersensitivity that allows sandflies to probe and feed faster in these animals. These immune responses, however, have a deleterious effect on some pathogens transmitted by vectors. Immune responses to *Ixodes scapularis* in natural and non-natural hosts result in protection against *Borrelia burgdorferi* infection. Similarly, immune responses to sandflies results in protection against *Leishmania major* infection, and a strong correlation exists between individuals generating immune responses to the sandfly *Lutzomyia longipalpis* and being protected against *Leishmania chagasi* infection. Therefore, in some vector-borne diseases, pre-exposure to vector saliva may result in immune responses capable of preventing parasite transmission We should emphasize that probably not all immune responses to vector bites are protective against all vector-borne pathogens, as not all individuals respond identically to insect bites. This will probably depend on the biology of the pathogen in its vertebrate host. In the case of human malaria, for example, sporozoites tend to leave the bite site within minutes in their journey to the hepatocyte, thus not being exposed for very long to immune effects of a sensitized skin. However, presentation of circumsporozoite antigen, which remains in the sporozoite trails, will be done in the context of anti-saliva immunity. Therefore, the role of saliva in parasite transmission seems to be a two-edged sword phenomenon. On the one hand, salivary secretions have a positive impact on pathogen or parasite establishment in vertebrate hosts not previously exposed to salivary components. This enhancement effect may be due to the potent bioactive, anti-inflammatory and immunosuppressive properties of the vector's saliva. On the other hand, salivary secretions have a detrimental effect on transmission of pathogens and parasites in a vertebrate host previously exposed to vector salivary components. This may be due to neutralization of the salivary bioactive components or to indirect killing of the pathogen generated by cellular immune responses to salivary proteins. Vector salivary secretions are therefore an important component in the transmission of pathogens or parasites and for this reason are being targeted as an alternative approach to control vector-borne diseases.

VECTOR IDIOSYNCRASIES

Following are summaries of the life cycle aspects of the most important vectors.

The order Diptera includes all flies, those insects containing only one pair of wings in the adult stage, and a pair of halters, which are atrophied wings. They are all holometabolous, having usually four larval stages or instars, one instar of a nonfeeding pupa, and finally the adult male and female. In some species of mosquitoes and many sandflies, larvae can withstand prolonged periods without food in diapause during the dry or cold season.

Mosquitoes

All larval instar stages of mosquitoes are aquatic. *Aedes* eggs are laid singly at the edge of the water; these embryonate and stay dormant until they are covered by water again. *Culex* eggs are laid together in a raft on the surface of the water, while *Anopheles* eggs are laid singly on the water surface or on mud, both hatching after a few days. The female mosquito, depending on the species, may choose either small containers or large bodies of water to lay her eggs. Also, the quality of the water chosen for oviposition will vary with the mosquito species. Usually *Aedes* and *Anopheles* mosquitoes will choose relatively clear water, and the larvae will not withstand too much suspended organic matter or scum, whereas *Culex* mosquitoes will thrive in such environments. Thus urban *Culex pipiens* will develop in great numbers in pit latrines, while *Aedes (Stegomyia)* spp. may thrive in small containers containing drinking or rain water. Developmental time from egg to adult may take from 5 days to 3 weeks, depending on the species, temperature, and larval food supply. Only the adult female mosquito feeds on blood, which is used for egg development; usually more than 100 eggs per blood meal are produced. Both male and female mosquitoes take sugar-rich meals, which energize flight. Mosquitoes are vectors of many arboviral diseases such as dengue and yellow fever (transmitted by *Aedes* mosquitoes), malaria (only anopheline mosquitoes transmit human malaria), bancroftian filariasis (mainly by *Culex*, but also *Anopheles* mosquitoes), and brugian filariasis *(Aedes)*.

Sandflies

These insects belong to the family Psychodidae, which also contains the sewer flies. Sandflies are vectors of arboviral, bacterial (*Bartonella*), and protozoal (*Leishmania*) human diseases. Immature sandflies are terrestrial, the larvae usually inhabiting mature, organically rich soil that has a composition similar to potting compost. Most vectors belong either to the New World genus *Lutzomyia* or to the Old World genus *Phlebotomus*. They may live within human dwellings, but are more commonly associated with peridomestic organic trash, rodent or other vertebrate nests, or forest soil. The immature life cycle of many important vector species is not known precisely. The time from egg to adult can be 45 days or longer depending on temperature. Some species have only one cycle per year, the third instar being the overwintering stage. Only adult female flies feed on blood, and both adults also feed on sugary solutions produced by aphids, fruits, or flower nectar. Adults do not fly well and show a typically "hopping" flight, close to the wall or another substrate.

Black Flies

Black fly larvae are all aquatic and need moving water to feed. Most species attach to a substrate within a fast-moving plume of water, where they open their feeding fans to catch nutrients in the form of particulate organic matter. *Simulium neavei* is an important vector of onchocerciasis in central Africa and occurs in lakes where it is attached to the gills of crabs. The flow of water on the gills is sufficient for oxygen exchange in an otherwise calm body of water. Developmental time from egg to adult varies with temperature and species from 2 to nearly 4 months. Adults are good fliers and may disperse with the wind for many miles from their breeding site. Similarly to mosquitoes and sandflies, only the adult female feeds on blood.

Horse Flies and Deer Flies (Tabanids)

These large flies are vectors of *Loa loa* filariasis in West Africa and can also mechanically transmit equine infectious anemia virus to horses. Whether they can also transmit other viruses by mechanical transmission is as yet unknown. Carnivorous larvae emerge from eggs deposited in moist grass and soil, where they feed on other insects, such as grubs. Male horse flies feed on vegetable material and do not bite. Females feed by making relatively large and painful cuts in the skin. The flies feed from the hematomas that accumulate in such lesions. They are usually not very efficient feeders, feeding several times per day, often flying from one host directly to another.

Tsetse

The tsetse (the word *tsetse* means fly destructive to cattle, thus the name tsetse fly is redundant) is an ovoviviparous vector of African trypanosomiasis. The female fly has a uterus wherein an individual egg hatches, the resulting larva feeding on secretions provided by milk glands. About every 10–15 days, the female fly deposits a large third instar, a larva that burrows into the ground and immediately pupates giving rise a few weeks later (3–4 weeks or longer) to another adult fly. Both male and female flies feed exclusively on blood. An adult female fly can at most produce six to eight such offspring, half of which are males. Tsetses thus have low reproductive capacity, and their population can be relatively easily controlled by trapping adult flies with ox urine-baited traps. Indeed, capture of 75% of the adult population can reduce the R_0 of the fly population to lower than unity and thus to local extinction. An equivalent effort for mosquitoes would require trapping of more than 95% of the adult population because of their larger reproductive capacity. Different species of tsetse can show different host specificities (from crocodiles to wart hogs and humans), as well as different habitat requirements (dry savanna, or riverine environments). Accordingly, each particular African trypanosomiasis scenario will be linked to the particularities of the bionomics and life cycle of the particular trypanosome vector.

Fleas (Siphonaptera)

These holometabolous organisms are always associated with the nest of their hosts, and thus a close relationship usually exists between a flea species and its host. This may explain why there are about 200 genera of fleas, while all remaining bloodsucking arthropods make up another 240 genera. Fleas are vectors of rickettsial (murine typhus) and bacterial (*Yersinia* plague organisms) pathogens. Also, fleas infected with *Yersinia pestis* develop a "blocked" gut, causing them to move from host to host and spread the bacterial pathogen. When the flea's natural zoonotic hosts start to die from disease, the hungry fleas may attack other host species, bridging the pathogen from an epizootic or enzootic to an epidemic cycle. Similarly, fleas that are left in empty burrows may attack anything that looks like food after a period of starvation. Both male and female fleas feed exclusively on blood. Females lay their eggs in the host's nest, the larvae feeding on a mix of organic material comprising skin keratin remains mixed with dried host blood which is squirted from the anus of the adult flea while it feeds. Thus small blood spots found in the bed linen of humans are an indication of flea-feeding activity.

Lice (Anoplura)

These are wingless hemimetabolous insects that live their entire lives associated either with human hair (*Pediculus humanus capitata*) or with the human body, where they stay attached to human clothes (*Pediculus humanus corporis*). When laid, eggs are attached to hairs or clothes. All instars feed exclusively on blood. The insects are sensitive to a decrease in temperature, so the body lice will survive only in conditions where clothes cannot be washed and changed regularly, as is the case following social turmoil and in homeless populations. Only *P. humanus corporis* is incriminated as a vector of louse-borne typhus and louse-borne relapsing fever. The insecticide DDT was actually discovered during World War II in a program to find novel pediculicides. The Allies were anticipating huge mortality from louse-borne typhus after the invasion of Italy.

Kissing Bugs (Hemiptera)

Hemiptera is the insect order with the common name of bugs (as flies represent the Diptera). The family Reduviidae has predacious, plant-feeding and blood-feeding insects. All are hemimetabolous, developing through five nymphal instars. The subfamily Triatominae comprises about 125 species in 15 genera, all having exclusively blood-feeding habits. Nymphs and adults live associated with nests, burrows, or habitations of their hosts. Kissing bugs can be very selective for their hosts; some are associated exclusively with birds, others with bats, and so on. Kissing bugs are vectors of *Trypanosoma cruzi*, the causative agent of Chagas' disease. This disease has a zoonotic cycle, as well as an endemic cycle. Thus, vectors maintaining the zoonotic cycle are associated with wildlife or domesticated animals, and vectors associated with human disease are found in the domestic environment. Other species may be found within the peridomestic environment, particularly in chicken pens, stables, woodpiles that harbor rodents, and so forth. Some species of the genera *Triatoma*, *Panstrongylus*, and *Rhodnius* became highly adapted to the human environment. Nymphs and adults take large meals of blood (5–10 times their own weight in blood) in 10–30 minutes. They usually attack their victims while the host is sleeping, biting the face, thus the name kissing bug, or *barbeiros* (barbers) in Portuguese, or *vinchuca* or *chincha* in Spanish. The large meal triggers a diuresis in the bugs, which then defecate while still feeding, carrying *T. cruzi* to their vertebrate host. The life cycle from egg to adult may take less than 6 months to 2 years depending on the species. *Rhodnius* may go from egg to adult in 6 months, having only five meals of blood, each blood meal taking less than 15 minutes. Adult females copulate once and are fertilized for life, laying their eggs in the same places in which they hide. Both male and females feed on blood, and may do so several times during adult life. Most domestic species are associated with poor housing construction (mud and stick) that creates small holes and cracks in the walls (most *Triatoma* and *Panstrongylus*), or with dirt floors (*Triatoma dimidiata*), or with thatched roofs (most *Rhodnius*). Accordingly, endemic Chagas' disease is highly correlated with poverty in rural areas of Central and South America.

Control of kissing bugs is relatively simple compared to that of other vector-borne diseases and great progress has been made in the past 50 years in reducing domestic Chagas' disease transmission in South America. As zoonotic cycles continue to exist, Chagas' disease may disappear for a time in some areas only to reemerge later as favorable conditions reappear and a bridge from the sylvatic to the human disease cycle takes place. Accordingly, research emphasis on bugs is shifting from domestic species to those that are peridomestic and may serve as bridge vectors.

Bed Bugs (Hemiptera)

Bed bugs belong to the family Cimicidae and, similarly to the triatomines, are exclusively blood-feeders and associate themselves with the nests of their hosts, thus their name. Unlike triatomines, though, the adult stage has no wings. Of the 91 reported species, 2 are of importance to humans, namely *Cimex lectularius,* found in subtropical and temperate zones, and *C. hemipterus*, found in tropical/equatorial areas. These insects are not incriminated as vectors of any human disease, although they can be infected in the laboratory with protozoa and viruses. More importantly, they can accumulate in large numbers in human dwellings and cause severe dermatitis due to hypersensitivity reactions, mostly in the form of urticarial papules. The bugs hide themselves well in mattresses and in wall crevices, biting at night; their victims accordingly may not be aware that they are sleeping in the company of a thriving bed bug population, and may show up in the physician's office without a clue as to their dermatitis. When DDT started to be used, bed bugs virtually disappeared from urban environments, but lately they have made a comeback including in Europe and the United States.

Ticks (Acari)

For medical entomologic purposes, we can consider ticks as coming in two varieties: hard (family Ixodidae) and soft (family Argasidae). All feed exclusively on blood, but can also produce a hygroscopic saliva that captures moisture from the air. Thus, these arthropods can survive long periods of time without desiccating. Indeed, some soft ticks can withstand years without a blood meal and without dehydrating. There is, however, a limit to the degree of air humidity at which the saliva can draw water from the atmosphere, and this in great part limits the range of different tick species, on both a macro- and a microgeographic scale.

Hard Ticks (Ixodidae)

Hard ticks have two immature stages, a six-legged larval stage and an eight-legged nymphal stage; the adults also have eight legs. Ticks are vectors of many arboviral, rickettsial, microbial, and even filarial organisms (the last not of human importance). Ticks can take huge meals compared to their size, and stay attached to feed on their hosts for several days to weeks. Adult females take a single blood meal, drop off the host, and produce many hundreds to thousands of eggs before dying. Typically, larval ticks take microliter or submicroliter meals, nymphs will take several microliters, and an adult will take hundreds of microliters to over 1 mL of blood. Hard ticks can be classified as being one-, two-, or three-host species. For example, the cattle tick *R. microplus* is a one-host tick. Thus larvae coming from eggs deposited in the field ambush a cow, and stay with the same animal for life. Two-host ticks will attach to a host as a larva, continue with the host after the nymphal molt, and detach from the vertebrate after the nymphal meal. They molt to adults in the environment, and then search for another host. This strategy allows the tick to use one set of hosts (usually smaller animals) for the immature stages, and another set (usually larger animals) for the adult stages. Many three-host tick species will feed on birds or rodents in their immature stages and on deer or other larger mammals as adults. There are also three-host species associated with small vertebrates, but in this case the adult female takes smaller meals and lays a smaller number of eggs. Note that transmission of pathogens is potentially larger in three-host tick species, and that transovarial transmission is an important component to be considered.

Soft Ticks (Argasidae)

Soft ticks have a variable number of immature stages or instars depending on the species and availability of blood. Unlike hard ticks, which stay attached to their hosts for several days, soft ticks usually take meals lasting from a few minutes to 1 hour. Some tick species, such as *Ornithodoros coriaceus*, may produce large and painful hematomas in their hosts. Soft ticks are usually associated with nests or burrows of their hosts, or the places where host animals rest. They are vectors of arboviral and microbial diseases, such as the relapsing fever borreliosis.

Trombiculid Mites

These mites are not ticks, but, like ticks, are also acari. They can transmit rickettsial pathogens, like *Orientia tsutsugamushi* (scrub typhus). Only the six-legged larvae of these mites feed on tissue fluid, nymphs and adults being predacious on other arthropods. Transovarial transmission of the pathogen is thus required for maintenance of disease foci.

VECTOR CONTROL

One can either kill vectors, or avoid contact with them by various means, to prevent vector-borne diseases. In the case of holometabolous insects, control will differ if one is committing larvicide or adulticide, because these stages have different ecological settings. Some examples of vector control follow below.

Malaria is transmitted by several anopheline mosquito species that have different breeding site preferences, different adult resting preferences, and different degrees of anthropophilic behavior. In the case of *An. gambiae*-transmitted malaria, the mosquito breeds in small pools of clear and recently collected water, open to the sun at least for part of the day. Most of these are associated with human activities, such as tire tracks, irrigation seepages, cattle hoof prints, and so on. Larval control may be difficult because of the scattered nature and small size of the sites. On the other hand, *An. funestus* breeds in permanent water bodies, avoiding predators by hiding in the emerging vegetation. Cleaning the edges of ponds or introduction of some fish species can give some control to *An. funestus* breeding. Both *An. gambiae* and *An. funestus* are anthropophilic, resting inside human dwellings, making this behavior amenable to the use of indoor insecticide spraying to kill the adult mosquitoes.

Dengue is transmitted by *Ae. aegypti* and *Ae. albopictus* mosquitoes. These mosquitoes lay eggs just above the water line within small containers with clean water. The eggs embryonate and sustain desiccation for many months. When the container is again flooded, the larvae hatch and are the first insects to exploit the new environment. *Ae. aegypti* prefers containers closely associated with humans, whereas *Ae. albopictus* will breed peridomestically. Sanitation around human habitation, as well as habit changes (such as emptying water in flower pots), can accomplish a lot to avoid mosquito breeding. Indoor spraying for *Ae. aegypti* is also effective, but less so for the more exophilic biter *Ae. albopictus*.

Bancroftian filariasis is transmitted by many species of mosquitoes, but the main vector worldwide is *Culex pipiens quinquefasciatus*. This mosquito can survive, and thrive, in highly organic polluted waters that would kill by suffocation any *Aedes* or anopheline larvae. *Culex* larvae have a strong and long siphon tube that allows them to break through the scum of such breeding sites. Indeed, pit latrines and sewers can lead to breeding of enormous numbers of *Culex* mosquitoes. Sanitation measures as well as larvicides can be of use to control filariasis.

Control of hemimetabolous Chagas' disease-transmitting bugs is done with indoor residual spraying, which kills all stages of the vector. Chagas' disease control has been very successful in South America where vector transmission was reduced following indoor spraying, together with economic and population changes.

Repellents are substances that prevent landing, or probing and feeding by vectors. A good repellent has to be volatile, which makes it last a shorter time, and thus frequent applications may be needed for effective control. Some repellents may have toxicity to children and should be used with care.

Physical means of prevention include house screening and bednets for nighttime-biting vectors. Bednets are increased in efficacy by having them impregnated with pyrethroid insecticides. Large-scale trials of impregnated bednets for malaria control are being completed, and followed up by distribution of such nets to affected populations.

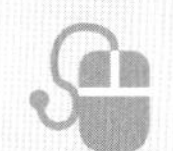

Access the complete reference list online at
http://www.expertconsult.com

CHAPTER 9

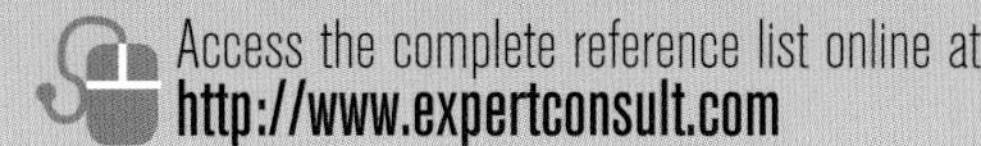
Access the complete reference list online at
http://www.expertconsult.com

Immunology, Host Defense, Immunodeficiencies, and Vaccines

Lisa A. Spencer • Anne Nicholson-Weller

INTRODUCTION

This chapter (1) introduces basic concepts of innate and adaptive immunity; (2) examines how immune responses are regulated and directed to antimicrobial immunity; and (3) considers deficiencies of the immune system that predispose to infections. Fuller discussions of these topics are available in cited references and immunology texts.[1–4] While we outline how the immune system should work, it is important to consider that all successful pathogens have evolved strategies to avoid some key element(s) of immunity. These strategies are discussed as the virulence factors in the chapters about specific pathogens.

Box 9.1 lists abbreviations used extensively in this chapter.

Conceptually, the immune system can be considered in two parts: innate and adaptive immunity. The phylogenetically older innate system is the only immune system of invertebrates. Innate immunity is critical in identifying microbes as "nonself" and in discriminating between benign and dangerous pathogens. In vertebrates the innate system is retained and beginning at the level of cartilaginous fish, an additional adaptive immune system functions. The adaptive immune system introduces a higher level of specificity and efficiency to immune effector functions and introduces the potential for immunologic memory, protecting hosts from second exposures to the same pathogenic organisms. Adaptive immunity relies on innate immunity to determine whether or not a pathogen is harmful, and to prevent unnecessary immune-mediated tissue damage. Therefore, while we conceptually divide the immune response into innate and adaptive components, in reality both arms participate in an intricate, coordinated response; instructing and honing one another throughout immune responses to optimize antimicrobial defense while minimizing collateral tissue damage. Differences between the innate and adaptive immune systems are summarized in ***Table 9.1***.

INNATE IMMUNITY

Innate immune mechanisms are inherited, invariant, and highly conserved throughout the evolution of nonfungal eukaryotes. The innate system combines physical attributes, soluble mediators, and cellular components to accomplish two essential functions: (1) formation of a rapid, first line of defense against pathogens; and (2) integration of pathogen and environmental cues to instruct the initiation of an appropriate ensuing adaptive immune response.

Innate immune barriers, including skin and other epithelial surfaces, physically block pathogen entry. Mucosal fluid layers of the respiratory, gastrointestinal, and genitourinary tracts contain soluble antimicrobial factors and function both as physical barriers and a medium for washing microbes away through peristaltic motion in the gut or the activity of ciliated epithelium in the airways. In addition to serving as physical barriers, epithelial layers of various body cavities have additional roles. Importantly, nonpathogenic "friendly" flora colonize host surfaces, making it more difficult for pathogens to colonize. A notable complication of antibiotic therapy is the decimation of antibiotic-sensitive normal flora throughout the host, which gives potential pathogens an advantage.

Innate immune cells situated at epithelial barriers (e.g., epithelial cells, tissue-specific macrophages, and Paneth cells) sense microbes and respond by secreting antimicrobial molecules and cellular chemoattractants. Other innate immune barrier cellular constituents function to: (1) kill infected cells; (2) phagocytose and kill microbes; (3) release soluble factors that bind microbes (e.g., natural antibody) or enhance antimicrobial capacities of neighboring cells (e.g., cytokines); and/or (4) extract information about pathogens and infection to initiate and instruct appropriate adaptive immune responses. Components of innate immunity are summarized in ***Table 9.2***. Foundational to the efficient functioning of both soluble mediators and cellular constituents of innate immunity is the capacity to recognize pathogens as foreign, a process elegantly achieved through use of pattern recognition molecules (PRMs).

Pattern Recognition Molecules

Fluid phase molecules and cell-associated receptors can recognize pathogens and trigger innate immune responses. These "sensors" of innate immunity, pathogen recognition molecules (PRMs), recognize vital, conserved molecular patterns that evolved in viruses, bacteria, parasites, and fungi. These molecular motifs, not shared by metazoans and higher animals, are called pathogen-associated molecular patterns (PAMPs).[5] Phylogenetically distinct glycomes (the full complement of sugars associated with an organism) between organisms provide an especially rich source of PAMPs. Some common microbial PAMPs are noted along with host molecules that recognize them in ***Table 9.3***.

Host Fluid Phase PRMs

Some fluid phase PAMP sensors are directly microbicidal (e.g., defensins and cathelicidins); others opsonize or tag microbes and their products to enhance the uptake or recognition of pathogens by cells of the innate and adaptive immune systems (e.g., complement and natural antibody). The complement system has three pathways for recognizing PAMPs: (1) the lectin pathway, which uses mannan-binding lectin and ficolins as sensors;[6] (2) the classical pathway, which may be activated by direct C1q binding, or indirectly when "natural" IgM antibodies bind PAMPs and subsequently recruit C1q; and (3) the alternative pathway that is activated by PAMPs that lack sialic acid. Both the classical and alternative pathways can continuously and slowly activate C3, and the same is likely true for the lectin pathway.[7,8] Both fluid phase and membrane-bound inhibitors keep complement pathways in check until a PAMP is recognized, then the scale is tipped toward activation, which under most conditions is kept localized and transient.[9] Factor H binds sialic acids of host cells and prevents the alternative complement pathway from assembling. Many microbial PAMPs lack sialic acid and without factor H binding the alternative

Box 9.1 Some Abbreviations Used in this Chapter

APC, antigen-presenting cell; BCR, B-cell receptor; CTL, cytotoxic T lymphocyte; DAMP, damage-associated molecular pattern; CR, complement receptor; DC, dendritic cell; Ig, immunoglobulin; IFN, interferon; MHC, major histocompatibility complex; PAMP, pathogen-associated molecular pattern; PRM, pattern recognition molecule; TCR, T-cell receptor; Th, T helper; TLR, Toll-like receptor.

Table 9.1 Complementary Attributes of the Innate and Adaptive Immune Systems

Attribute	Innate Immunity	Adaptive Immunity
Location of genes	Germline	Germline with significant rearrangements/ mutations occurring in peripheral lymphoid tissues during life
Time of onset	From conception	During life, but only after exposure to specific immunogen
Discrimination of foreignness	Good	Poor
Specificity	Low	High
Capacity to contain invading pathogens	Low	High

Table 9.2 Components of Innate Immunity

Barriers	Soluble	Cellular Mediators
Epithelial surfaces	Fluid phase PRMs (see Table 9.3A)	Phagocytes (monocytes, macrophages, neutrophils)
Mucous layers	Antimicrobial peptides	Natural killer (NK) cells
Flushing motions	Cytokines	B-1 cells
Normal microbial flora		Eosinophils, basophils, and mast cells

pathway is activated on the microbial surface. All three complement pathways activate serine esterases that cleave and activate C3 yielding C3a, a soluble anaphylotoxin, and C3b, which has transient reactivity to form covalent thioester or amide bonds with nearby sugars or amino groups, respectively. C3 activation is significantly amplified compared with other steps in the complement sequence, in part because C3 is present in plasma in higher molar concentrations and the C3 cleaving enzyme of the alternative pathway can be recruited to amplify the activation of the lectin and classical pathways. C5 binds to C3b docked adjacent to C3-cleaving enzymes and once cleaved the resultant C5b condenses with C6, C7, C8, and C9 to form the nonselective C5b–9 channel, while C5a is released in the fluid phase. The C5b–9 complex is often referred to as the "membrane attack complex," but this is a misnomer. While excessive C5b–9 activity is associated with pathology, under normal circumstances C5b–9 has hormone-like activity in that it provides a Ca^{2+} influx and activates G-coupled protein(s) in autologous cells, which can lead to a spectrum of nonlytic cellular responses.[10] In terms of host defense, human deficiencies of C5, C6, C7, or C8 and to a lesser extent C9 are associated with a predisposition to *Neisseria meningitidis* meningitis and disseminated *N. gonorrhoeae* (see Chapters 25 and 26), indicating critical roles for C5b–9 in host resistance to *Neisseria* species.[11]

Complement proteins that potentially remain bound to the PAMP, mannan binding lectin, C1q, C4b, and C3b, are all opsonic and use the same receptor, namely complement receptor 1 (CD35),[12–14] which is expressed on erythrocytes and phagocytes, as well as some other cells.[15] On erythrocytes, complement receptor 1 (CR1) ligates complement-opsonized particles (microbes and immune complexes); and during passage through the liver and spleen, the particles are removed by resident phagocytes; and erythrocytes return to circulation: a process known as immune adherence-mediated clearance. C3b, the major complement opsonin, in part because of its molar abundance, facilitates phagocytosis by neutrophils and monocytes. The importance of opsonization by immunoglobulin (Ig) and C3b for the subsequent phagocytosis and killing by neutrophils is underscored by the fact that if any of these factors is missing there is a marked susceptibility to extracellular pathogens, including *Streptococcus pneumoniae* and other streptococcal species. C3b can be further processed by the serine protease factor I to iC3b and then C3dg using as cofactors CR1 or H for the first step, and CR1 for the second step. Regulated processing of C3b generates C3 ligands that engage different receptors, each with distinctive cellular expression. iC3b ligates CR3 (CD11b/CD18), which is expressed on neutrophils and macrophages predominantly; and C3dg ligates CR2 (CD21), which is expressed on B cells and dendritic cells predominantly.

Fluid phase fragments of activation of C4, C3, and C5, namely C4a, C3a, and C5a, known as anaphylatoxins, reinforce the inflammatory response. In addition, the widespread expression of receptors (R) for C3a and C5a suggests that these anaphylatoxins are more broadly involved. Indeed, C3a acting in the absence of a specific receptor potentiates chemokine CXCL12 stimulation of bone marrow B cells, which demonstrates a role for complement in the maturation of B cells.[16] A list of soluble PAMP sensors is included in ***Table 9.3A***.

Cell-Associated PRMs

Ligation of cell-associated PRMs (***Table 9.3B***) promotes phagocytosis of microbes and microbial products and activates immune cell functions. Cell-associated PRMs are expressed on cell surfaces and within intracellular compartments, facilitating exposure to their cognate pathogenic ligands. One example is cell surface-expressed complement receptors, which bind complement-tagged molecules, facilitating phagocytosis and further activation of innate immune cells. Other examples are Toll-like receptors (TLRs), transmembrane receptors expressed on immune cells, as well as on the endothelium, epithelium, and fibroblasts, that recognize a spectrum of PAMPs, and include surface-expressed TLR 1, 2, 4, 5, and 6, and intracellular TLR 3, 7, 8, and 9. Signaling through TLRs activates immune cells, and provides specific information on the type of pathogen encountered (***Fig. 9.1***). The ability of individual TLRs to recruit different adaptor proteins and the heterodimerization of TLRs provides for a multitude of potential signaling outcomes.

In addition to extracellularly expressed PRMs, intracellular compartments also express PAMP sensors. Transmembrane TLRs expressed within endosomal compartments bind PAMPs associated with phagocytosed material within phagosomes, and elicit signaling cascades that activate immune cells (***Fig. 9.1***). Cellular processes, such as autophagy, are in place to encourage the delivery of intracellular PAMPs to TLR-expressing endosomal compartments.[17]

Moreover, innate immune cells express numerous cytosolic PRMs, including nucleotide-binding oligodimerization domain containing (Nod)-like receptors (NLR) (e.g., Nod1 and Nod2) and retinoic acid-inducible gene I-like receptor (RIG-1) family members that activate proinflammatory signaling cascades and antimicrobial pathways in response to recognition of cytosolic PAMPs, including viral and bacterial nucleotides.[18] These PRMs are especially important in recognizing bacteria that have escaped or evaded endolysosomal compartments. A subset of NLRs (i.e., Ipaf and Cryopyrin) respond to cytosolic PAMPs through induction of inflammasomes, multimeric protein complexes controlling caspase 1 activation and downstream secretion of caspase-1-dependent proinflammatory cytokines (i.e., interleukin (IL)-1β, IL-18).[19]

Notably, some inflammasomes are activated in response to cellular effects of microbial infection (i.e., potassium efflux), as opposed to

Table 9.3 Innate Immunity: Pathways for the Detection of Foreign Particles

A. Fluid Phase PRMs

Pattern Recognition Molecule (PRM)	Foreign PAMP Recognized	Recruits Complement?
Mannan-binding lectin (MBL)	Polymannose carbohydrates	Yes
Natural IgM antibody	Bacterial carbohydrates	Yes
Alternative complement pathway	Nonsialylated carbohydrates	Yes
Direct C1q binding	Negatively charged surfaces, complexes of anions–cations	Yes
Surfactant protein A (SPA)	Phospholipids	No
Surfactant protein D (SPD)	Phospholipids	No
Defensins	Broadly recognize bacteria, enveloped and nonenveloped viruses and fungi	No
Cathelicidins	Broadly recognize bacteria, enveloped viruses and fungi	No

B. Cell-associated PRMs

Pattern Recognition Molecule (PRM)	Foreign PAMP or DAMP Recognized
Cell surface:	
Killer inhibitory receptors (KIRs)	Viral-associated deficient MHC I expression on host cells
Mannose-binding receptor (CD206)	Polymannose carbohydrates
TLR1	Triacylated bacterial lipoproteins
TLR2	Diacylated and triacylated bacterial lipoproteins
TLR4	Lipopolysaccharide (LPS)
TLR5	Flagellin
TLR6	Bacterial lipoproteins
Complement receptors: CR1, CR2, CR3	Polymannose carbohydrates, negatively charged surfaces, complexes of anions–cations, necrotic cells, and PAMPs recognized by IgM or IgG, which activate complement
Dectin-1	β-Glucan, fungal cell wall components
Intracellular – endosomal:	
TLR3	dsRNA
TLR7	ssRNA
TLR8	Ligand unknown
TLR9	Unmethylated CpG DNA
Intracellular – cytosolic:	
RIG-I	Cytosolic, short dsRNA or 3′-triphosphate ssRNA
MDA5	Cytosolic, dsRNA
ISD sensor	Cytosolic DNA
Nod1	Peptidoglycan (PGN) molecules containing an unusual amino acid unique to PGN from most Gram-negative bacteria (i.e., *Shigella flexneri, Escherichia coli, Pseudomonas aeruginosa, Helicobacter pylori*), and only specific Gram-positive bacteria
Nod2	Muramyl dipeptide (MDP), a conserved structure in most types of PGN, therefore a more general sensor of bacteria; newly recognized as a viral sensor
Ipaf	Intracellular flagellin (important for response to *Salmonella enterica* serovar Typhimurium and *Legionella pneumonophila*)
Cryopyrin	Bacterial RNA and monosodium urate or calcium pyrophosphate dehydrate crystals released by damaged cells
NALP3	Potassium efflux, bacterial secretion systems

direct interaction with microbial PAMPs. Signs of cellular stress are commonly referred to as "alarmins," or DAMPs, for **d**amage-**a**ssociated **m**olecular **p**atterns. Integration of signals achieved through simultaneous recognition of PAMPs and DAMPs provides a means by which innate immune cells can assess through PRMs not only the type of pathogen encountered, but also the degree of pathogenicity. This is especially important for innate immune cells specialized in presentation of microbial antigens to the adaptive system (i.e., dendritic cells). In these cells, effects of PRM activation include upregulation of specific costimulatory molecules (i.e., CD80, CD86, CD40; molecules providing costimulatory signals to T-helper cells), and induction of immunomodulatory cytokine secretion and molecule expression (i.e., Notch ligands; molecules providing a polarizing signal to antigen-specific T-helper cells) (***Fig. 9.1***). The sum total of these specific signals will determine the subset of T-helper cells generated, and thereby the type of adaptive response elicited.

Cellular Constituents of Innate Immunity

Cellular constituents of innate immunity are listed in ***Table 9.2***. Natural killer (NK) cells are a family of innate immune leukocytes that are directly cytotoxic to some tumor and virus-infected cells. NK cells express a cohort of activation receptors with a ligand repertoire that is still ill defined but includes viral hemagglutinins and markers of cell stress, including stress-induced expression of the major histocompatibility complex (MHC) I-like MICA and MICB molecules. Signaling through NK cell activation receptors leads to transient recruitment and phosphorylation of adaptor molecules containing ITAM (immunoreceptor tyrosine-based activation motif) domains and initiates intracellular signaling cascades resulting in release of perforin and cytolytic enzymes from NK cells. Perforin creates pores in target cells, which are then destroyed by cytolytic enzymes. In addition to activation receptors, NK cells express

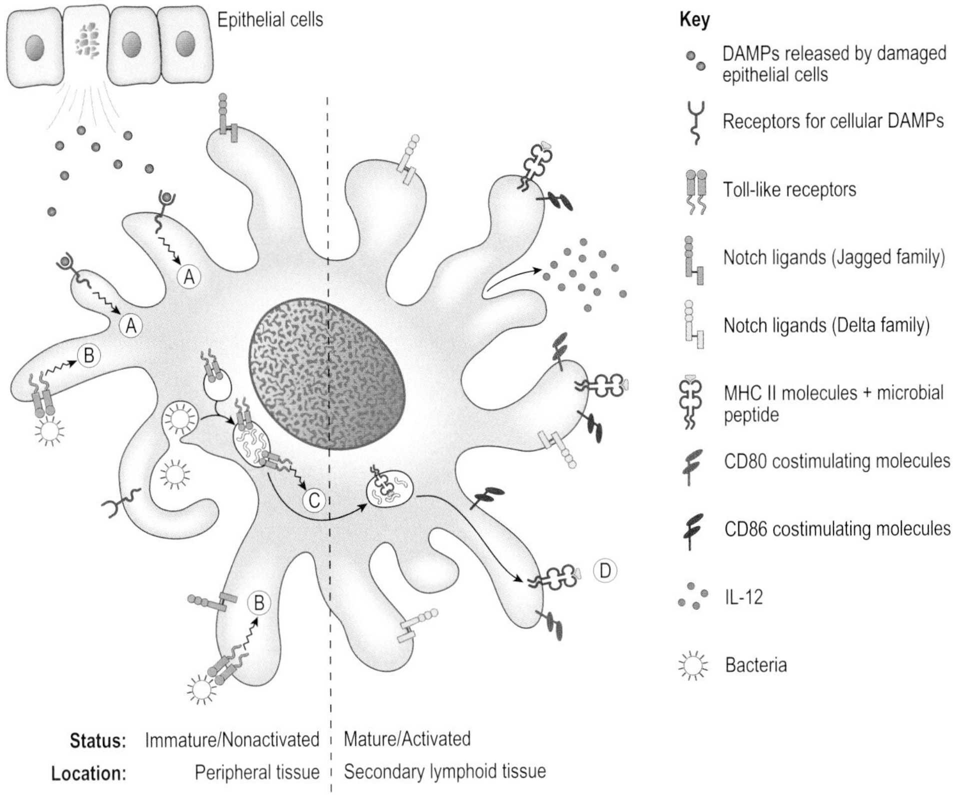

Figure 9.1 Activation of antigen presenting cells (APCs). Activation of cellular pattern recognition molecules by damage-associated molecular patterns (DAMPs) released from damaged tissue cells (A) and pathogen-associated molecular pattern (PAMPs) associated with intact (B) or phagocytosed (C) microbes, leads to expression of ingested microbial peptides associated with MHC II (D), upregulation of costimulatory molecules (e.g., CD80, CD86), modulation of immunomodulatory molecules (e.g., Notch ligands), and secretion of immunomodulatory cytokines (e.g., interleukin (IL)-12).

a highly diverse range of inhibitory receptors. The cytoplasmic tails of inhibitory receptors contain ITIM (immunoreceptor tyrosine-based inhibitory motif) domains that, upon activation, recruit phosphatases that interact with and dephosphorylate the adaptor molecules associated with activating receptors, counteracting activation signals and maintaining the NK cell's inhibitory state. The best known of the NK cell inhibitory receptors (CD94:NKG2A heterodimers and members of the KIR (killer cell immunoglobulin-like receptor) family of receptors) recognize various distinct alleles of MHC I, a set of molecules expressed by all nucleated cells. Therefore, normal expression of MHC I by target cells delivers a tonic inhibitory signal to the NK cell, thereby preventing NK cell-mediated killing of a healthy cell. Many virus-infected or transformed cells have diminished class I expression, which is a pathogen-directed strategy to avoid the adaptive immune system. These abnormal host cells are targets for NK cells. NK cells also express CD16, an Fcγ receptor recognizing an invariate region of IgG. Ligation of NK cell-expressed CD16 provides a strong activation signal, and cells coated with IgG are targeted for destruction by NK cells in a process termed antibody-dependent cell-mediated cytotoxicity (ADCC). In addition to cytotoxic functions, NK cells rapidly secrete cytokines, specifically interferon (IFN)-γ, capable of promoting antiviral immunity and modulating adaptive immunity.

Phagocytic cells include neutrophils, monocytes, and dendritic cells (DCs). Neutrophils, the most numerous white blood cell type in circulation, are critical first responders to sites of infection, as evidenced by the high prevalence of serious infections in patients with genetically determined neutrophil dysfunction or neutropenia.[20] Under the appropriate stimulus, monocytes can migrate into tissues and become macrophages. Macrophages are important in clearing cellular debris, but become more effective in host defense once "educated" through cytokine signals provided by adaptive immunity. Most often phagocytes (both neutrophils and macrophages) depend on the complement system for recognizing the "foreignness" of the particle, by recognizing and binding the complement tag using CR1 (CD35), CR3 (CD11b/CD18), and C3Ig as receptors. However, monocytes and macrophages can recognize the PAMPs, polymannose and polyglucan, directly by two receptors. The mannose receptor (CD206) (not to be confused with serum mannan-binding lectin) is a C-type lectin,[21,22] and there are two glucan receptors, Dectin-1 and the lectin-binding site of CD11b/CD18.[23] Once digested, phagocytosed material passes through the endocytic pathway in phagosomes and is "digested" within phagolysosomes, compartments formed when phagosomes fuse with lytic enzyme-containing lysosomes. Importantly, the process of phagocytosis not only functions in eliminating pathogens and cell debris, but is also a critical means by which the local microenvironment is sampled by innate immune cells. Phagocytes (especially macrophages and DCs) extract information concerning the nature of the pathogen and extent of infection through integration of signals generated by the phagocytosed material through cell-expressed PRMs and environmental cues. These signals are crucial to improving the antimicrobial activities of innate immune cells and in the development of an appropriate adaptive immune response, in large part by provoking specific cytokine secretion by macrophages and DCs, and by upregulating costimulatory and immunomodulatory molecules on DCs (*Fig. 9.1*).

Mast cells, basophils, and eosinophils, like neutrophils, are distinct in their content of numerous intracellular granules. Unlike neutrophils, basophils and eosinophils are found in very low numbers in the blood (eosinophils represent 1–5% of circulating white blood cells, and basophils <1%), and mast cells are primarily tissue-dwelling. Traditionally mast cells, basophils, and eosinophils had been considered solely for their terminal effector functions. For example, allergen-specific IgE antibodies bind to IgE receptors on mast cells within tissues, and upon secondary exposure to the same allergen, mast cell-bound IgE antibodies are crosslinked by allergen, leading to release of pre-formed, granule-derived chemical mediators (including histamine) from mast cells, resulting in local or systemic anaphylaxis. Likewise, deposition of eosinophil-derived cationic proteins (i.e., major basic protein (MBP), eosinophil cationic protein (ECP), and eosinophil peroxidase (EPO)) can kill helminth parasites *in vitro*, and mediate tissue damage in allergic inflammation, fueling the supposition that eosinophils function as end-stage effector cells in allergy and helminth parasitic infections. However, more recent studies have begun to reveal additional roles for mast cells, basophils, and eosinophils in the earlier stages of disease processes, and highlight non-redundant contributions of these granulocytes in the initiation and modulation of an ensuing adaptive response, as reviewed in references 24–27.

B-1 lymphocytes residing predominantly in the peritoneal, pleural, and pericardial cavities release IgM antibodies referred to as "natural antibodies" in light of their secretion apparently without a need for specific antigenic activation. Like conventional B cells (also known as B-2 lymphocytes), B-1 lymphocytes are derived from bone marrow stem cells. However, unlike their B-2 counterparts, B-1 cells are self-renewing and do not undergo all the differentiation steps of conventional B cells, resulting in a limited repertoire of rearranged immunoglobulin genes. The resultant limited repertoire of antibody specificity provided by B-1 cells led to their categorization as innate immune, as opposed to adaptive immune, cells and is consistent with the fact that B-1 immunoresponsiveness has been selected over generations of a species to respond to common, invariant immunologic epitopes of pathogens. B-1 lymphocyte-derived natural IgM is an important fluid phase PRM that provides a first line of defense against microbial infections prior to the generation of subsequent isotypes (i.e., IgG, IgE, etc.) of antibody.

Dendritic cells (DCs) link innate immunity with adaptive immunity. They act as sentinels throughout the body, picking up antigen and presenting it to cells of the adaptive immune system. Importantly, along with the pathogen, DCs extract information from the tissue environment itself, largely through expression of PRMs, to determine the extent of infection, and utilize this information to inform the adaptive system. DCs are the most important antigen-presenting cell (APC).

There are several subsets of DCs, including: Langherhans DCs found in epidermal layers of skin; interstitial DCs found in most other organs (except the brain); monocyte-derived DCs arising from monocytes migrated into tissues; and plasmacytoid DCs, derived from plasmacytoid DC precursors. Additional designations can be assigned to further divide DC subsets, a topic of ongoing studies. Regardless of origin or phenotype, DCs function to pick up antigen and present it to T lymphocytes. Immature Langerhans and interstitial DCs lie dormant within tissues, extending their long dendrites through epithelial junctions to sample both tissue and luminal environments, until "awakened" by pathogens or evidence of tissue damage through activation of DC-expressed PRMs. While immature, DCs take up antigen efficiently by phagocytosis, receptor-mediated endocytosis, and pinocytosis. In the presence of a microbial infection, the combination of pathogen- and tissue-derived signals activates DCs, inhibiting their capacity for further phagocytic uptake, and inducing the specific expression of soluble (i.e., cytokines) and surface-expressed molecules (i.e., costimulatory receptors) that relay information on the type and severity of infection to antigen-specific interacting T cells (***Fig. 9.1***). Mature DCs migrate to lymph nodes, where they display processed pieces of the antigen within surface-expressed MHC class II (MHC II) molecules and interact directly with T cells of the adaptive immune system to initiate adaptive responses. Thus, DCs are considered a critical bridge between innate and adaptive responses.

A unique subset of DCs, termed follicular DCs (FDCs), appear to develop within B-cell follicles of lymph nodes. These cells are not phagocytic and do not express MHC II. Rather, FDCs express high levels of complement receptors (CR1, CR2, and CR4) and Fc receptors, allowing FDCs to efficiently capture antibody–antigen complexes. FDCs serve as an antigenic reservoir within the lymph nodes important for the maturation and diversification of B cells.

Cytokines are the soluble mediators that are used to spread the danger signals of innate and adaptive immunity. Chemokines, interleukins, and interferons are part of this expansive family. We limit our discussion of cytokines to interferons (IFNs), so named because they "interfere" with viral replication. Type 1 IFNs consist of a family of IFN-α and a single IFN-β that are released in response to ligation of RIG-1 and/or TLRs 3, 7, 8, and 9. Type 1 IFN signaling through its receptor results in activation of the family of "IFN responsive genes" that limit viral infection by eliminating viral components from cells, inducing apoptosis of infected cells, and preventing the infection of new cells. Plasmacytoid DCs are a major source of IFN-α and are likely responsible for directing an antiviral adaptive Th1 response. Tumor necrosis factor (TNF)-α signaling synergizes with the antiviral activity of type1 IFNs.[28] IFN-γ is the only type 2 IFN, and while it is secreted by all activated immune cells, T cells and NK cells are the major sources. One of its prime functions is to upregulate expression of MHC class I for antigen processing and presentation. Humans genetically deficient in type 1 IFNs are susceptible to herpes simplex encephalitis, while those with deficiencies in the IFN-γ signaling pathway are susceptible to infections with atypical mycobacteria, intracellular organisms that do not infect normal hosts.[29]

Requisite to accomplishing the goals of innate immunity, the specific recruitment of cells and mediators to the site of infection is initiated through release of soluble factors from affected tissue cells, and involves a complex interplay between surface molecules expressed by the vascular endothelium and circulating leukocytes, coordinated by soluble chemoattractants. Emigration of cells from the blood circulation into tissues (diapedesis) is well described in basic immunology texts,[1–4] as are inflammatory cascades resulting in the robust recruitment of neutrophils and other specific immune cells into infected sites. Once in tissues, leukocytes will crawl to the infection. Only at that localized site will the innate immune mediators cause the resident cells to upregulate surface intercellular adhesion molecule 1 (ICAM-1), which can be made by all nucleated cells, and engages the β2 integrins of the arriving leukocytes, causing their further activation.[30]

Synthesis

The innate immune system has a limited number of responses, all of which are encoded in the germline. The main objectives of innate immune responses are to prevent entry of pathogens, kill or tag pathogens that have circumvented physical protective barriers, "sense" the type and severity of the infectious threat and use this information to instruct the adaptive immune system. These feats are largely accomplished by soluble and cell-associated molecules recognizing conserved motifs common to whole classes of pathogens and evidences of cell and tissue damage. This concept of microbial infection-associated "danger signals" serving to dictate immune activation derives from theories originally set forth by Charles Janeway,[31] and developed and espoused by Polly Matzinger and Ephraim Fuchs.[32] Ironically, as vaccines are engineered to be less toxic, the purified vaccine antigen(s) often escape detection by the innate immune system and therefore fail to elicit the danger signals necessary to stimulate a robust adaptive immune response.

ADAPTIVE IMMUNITY

Unlike the immediate mobilization of innate immunity, antigen-specific adaptive immunity requires time, generally on the order of 7–10 days, to fully develop. However, in contrast to the invariant collection of PRMs available to the innate immune system, the adaptive system can generate an almost unlimited array of antigen-specific receptors because of ongoing gene rearrangement in lymphocytes, driven by antigenic exposures of individuals. In addition, the adaptive immune system is capable of immunologic memory, providing for very rapid, antigen-specific immunity against subsequent exposure to the same pathogen. The goal of vaccines is to harness this aspect of adaptive immunity.

Components of the Adaptive Immune System

Lymphoid Organs

The lymphoid system is conceptually divided into a central and a peripheral system. The central system generates the lymphocytes (B and T cells) from stem cells in the bone marrow and provides for further differentiation of B cells in the bone marrow and T cells in the thymus. The peripheral lymphoid system (including tonsils, peripheral lymph nodes, spleen, and the mucosal lymphoid tissues) is where the lymphocytes encounter antigens and initiate adaptive immune responses. Antigen entering the body from tissues is carried by the lymph and filtered and concentrated within lymph nodes, while antigens in the blood are filtered and concentrated by the spleen. Processed antigen is also carried to lymphoid tissue by antigen-presenting cells (APCs), such as DCs. In most lymph nodes and the spleen, lymphocytes are concentrated in the white pulp. T cells are found in the central region and B cells are found in the germinal centers, toward the periphery of the organ or node.[1-4]

Cell Types of the Adaptive Immune Response

Cells of the adaptive immune system include T and B lymphocytes. In contrast to the broad-spectrum pattern recognition receptors of innate immune cells, lymphocytes express highly specific cell surface receptors, recognizing antigenic epitopes that are potentially unique to a single pathogen. Upon encountering their cognate antigenic epitope, lymphocytes proliferate rapidly and their progeny differentiate into effector cells and memory cells. Effector B cells become plasma cells, and secrete copious amounts of a soluble form of their cell surface antigen receptor in the form of antibodies. Effector T cells may be directly cytotoxic to target cells ($CD8^+$ T cells) or provide "help" to other cell types, effectively regulating the type of immune response generated ($CD4^+$ T cells). Memory cells (both B and T) maintain an antigenic record of the infectious agent, and are responsible for the very rapid generation of antigen-specific immunity in response to reinfection by the same microbe.

Lymphocyte Development and Activation

Development of B Lymphocytes and the Humoral Response

During B-cell maturation in the bone marrow, the heavy and light chain immunoglobulin genes are rearranged, allowing for a large repertoire of possible antigenic specificities among B-cell receptors (BCRs) in the B-cell pool. However, in a single B cell, once a successful rearrangement is achieved, further rearrangement is blocked. Therefore, all immunoglobulin (or antibody) molecules expressed on or secreted by a single B cell share the same antigenic specificity. The heavy and light immunoglobulin chains include variable and constant regions. Variable regions provide antigenic specificity. The heavy chain constant region (μ, γ, α, δ, or ε) utilized during gene rearrangement determines the isotype of the expressed BCR, and mature B cells generally emerge from the bone marrow expressing μ heavy chains (IgM). B cells that do not encounter an antigen recognized by their membrane Ig experience a relatively short life span. However, crosslinking of BCRs by cognate antigen delivers an activation signal leading to proliferation and generation of effector and memory B cells. This division is termed clonal proliferation to reflect the fact that each daughter cell expresses identical BCRs. Activated B cells localize in the germinal centers of lymph nodes where further mutations of the immunoglobulin heavy and light chain genes occur, and selection mediated by interactions with antigen-laden follicular DCs leads to B cells capable of secreting high-affinity antibodies.[1-4]

Costimulation of Effector B Cell Responses Involves Innate Immunity and T-Helper Cells

Although antigenic crosslinking of surface immunoglobulin provides B cells with a primary stimulatory signal, in most cases B cells require a second signal, provided by activated $CD4^+$ T cells, to undergo full activation and clonal proliferation. Generation of these activated $CD4^+$ T cells requires PRM-generated costimulatory signals from innate immune cells (see later in the chapter). These B–T-cell interactions occur within secondary lymphoid tissue, in a zone at the periphery of germinal centers.

Complement can effect another type of costimulation, triggered by innate immunity directly. If antigen is first recognized as foreign and tagged with complement component C3b, which is processed to C3dg, the threshold amount of antigen needed to evoke a B-cell response is lowered by a factor of 10 000.[33] One reason C3dg-tagged antigen is efficient is that the CD21/CD19 signaling complex is costimulated with the BCR. CD21 is the receptor for C3dg and may facilitate uptake of antigen, while CD19 gives a positive signal to B cells.

As the immune response progresses, the efficacy of humoral immunity is further enhanced with concurrent genetic rearrangements of the heavy chain constant region, changing the isotype of the BCR while maintaining the strict antigen specificity encoded by the variable regions. These rearrangements are influenced by cytokines secreted by activated $CD4^+$ T cells. As heavy chain constant regions are rearranged, gene segments upstream of the new region are excised; B-cell transitions to new isotypes (i.e., from IgM to IgG) are thus unidirectional. Once secreted the specific biological properties of the five isotypes of human immunoglobulins depend primarily on the cellular expression pattern and signaling pathways utilized by the specific Fc receptors (FcRs) engaged by the various isotypes (***Table 9.4***). FcRs are broadly expressed on both innate and adaptive immune cells. As the adaptive immune system is engaged, its products, including antigen-specific antibodies, work together with the innate immune system to direct and enhance an antimicrobial response. For example, IgE bound to an allergen will crosslink FcεRs on mast cells and induce degranulation; while IgG bound to a virus-infected cell will crosslink FcγRs on NK cells and stimulate the NK cells to kill the infected cell through ADCC. The roles of the FcγRs in directing innate and adaptive immune responses have been recently reviewed.[34]

Development of T Lymphocytes and Cell-Mediated Immunity

T-cell precursors generated in the bone marrow migrate to the thymus where T-cell receptor (TCR) gene rearrangement takes place and positive and negative selection occur. Variable (V), joining (J), diversity (D), and constant (C) region genes come together to form αβ or γδ TCRs. TCR diversity is even greater than that for BCRs owing to the large number of J and D region genes. Following a successful TCR rearrangement, cells undergo "positive selection" to ensure that only those T cells which react with self-MHC can mature, followed by a process of "negative selection," during which time most T cells that recognize "self-peptides" are eliminated.[1-4]

When mature T cells exit the thymus the majority express a functional TCR in association with either CD4 or CD8 molecules on their cell surfaces. Upon appropriate antigenic stimulation, CD8-expressing T cells will become cytotoxic effector cells, with the capacity to destroy infected or malignant cells, while CD4-expressing T cells will become "helper" effector cells with the capacity to regulate the type and intensity of the immune response.

Unlike B cells, which directly recognize antigenic epitopes expressed on pathogens or their products, T cells recognize antigenic epitopes of peptides generated through proteolytic processing by innate immune accessory cells, and displayed on the innate immune cell surface within a specialized groove of an MHC molecule (detailed below).

Costimulation of Effector T-Cell Responses

As with B-cell activation, interaction with cognate antigen is not sufficient to fully activate T cells. Rather, control of $CD4^+$ "helper" T-cell activation is in part regulated by a number of T cell-expressed accessory molecules, called "costimulatory" molecules (e.g., CD28, CD40L), that must be engaged by an APC in order for the T cell to respond.[35] Reciprocal APC ligands, which are induced by exposure to PAMPs, are CD80 and CD86

Table 9.4 Physical, Chemical, and Biologic Properties of Human Immunoglobulins

Property	IgM	IgG	IgA	IgD	IgE
Molecular weight	970	160	170–340	184	188
Serum concentration (mg/dL)	45–150	800–1500	90–325	0–8	<0.025
Light chains	κ or λ	κ or λ	κ or λ	κ or λ	κ or λ
Heavy chains (subgroups)	μ	γ1, γ2, γ3, or γ4	α1 or α2	δ	ε
J chain	Yes	No	In dimeric form	No	No
Time of synthesis[a]	First	Later			
Half-life in serum (days)	5	23	6	3	2.5
Localization	Serum	Serum, amniotic fluid, tissues	Serum, secretions, tears, colostrum, saliva, gastrointestinal and genitourinary tracts	Serum	Serum, tissues
Complement activation					
Classical pathway	++++	++	0	0	0
Alternative pathway	+	+	+	+	+
Opsonic activity	++	++++	0		
Lytic activity[b]	++++	++	0		
Inhibition of bacterial adherence	+	+	+++		
Viral neutralization	++	++	++		
Reaginic activity	0	Only IgG_4	0	0	++++
Binds Fcγ receptors on phagocytes, promoting phagocytosis	0	++++	0	0	0
Binds Fcε receptors on mast cells, inducing degranulation	0	0	0	0	++++
Binds Fcα and transferrin (Tfn) receptors	0	0	++++	0	0

[a]Because IgM antibody is produced early in infection and usually does not persist after months, IgM antibody can be an indicator of recent infection. Further, IgM antibody does not cross the placenta (in contrast to IgG), so IgM antibodies against a pathogen in a neonate are indicative of intrauterine or postnatal infection of the child and are independent of maternal antibodies.

[b]Only through activation of complement.

(for CD28) and CD40 (for CD40L).[36] One important outcome of costimulatory interactions is the activation of integrins, providing stable adhesion between T cells and APCs, thereby enhancing the possibility of stimulating an immune response.[37] Of note, costimulatory signals between APCs and T cells are commonly referred to as "signal 2" (peptide–MHC II interaction with the TCR is considered "signal 1"). In a later section we will describe a "third signal" transmitted between APCs and $CD4^+$ T cells that dictates which type of T-helper (Th) effector cell is generated (see *Fig. 9.1*).

Activation of $CD8^+$ cytotoxic T cells also includes checks and balances; APCs displaying peptide within the context of MHC I to $CD8^+$ T cells must first be "licensed" through PRM activation on an APC and/or an activated T-helper cell. Thus, the ability of the innate immune system to appropriately recognize pathogens and upregulate costimulatory molecules on APCs provides an important control over the immune system: interaction between a peripheral lymphocyte that binds antigen presented by an APC that lacks costimulatory molecules leads to functional paralysis of the lymphocyte, or tolerance.[37]

MHC and Antigen Presentation to T Cells: A Closer Look

MHC, also designated HLA for "human leukocyte antigen," is translated from a region of highly polymorphic genes.[1–4] The MHC has two types of gene products: class I and class II. Both classes of MHC contain a "groove" in which processed peptide binds.[38]

MHC I Presentation of Intracellular Proteins to $CD8^+$ T Cells

Some of the proteins synthesized endogenously by the host cell's ribosomes, as is the case for viral proteins, are normally degraded in the constitutive proteosome, an organelle designed to break down denatured or nonessential proteins to peptides. Some of these peptides are transported into the endoplasmic reticulum (ER) by the TAPs (transporters of antigen presentation), where peptides usually of 8–9 amino acids in length are loaded into the groove of nascently synthesized class I molecules. The MHC class I–peptide complex is then transported through the Golgi complex and expressed on the cell surface (*Fig. 9.2*).[39] In the case of an intracellular infection, "immunoproteosomes" are induced by IFN-γ and replace some of the constitutive proteosomes. The two types of proteosomes have distinctive proteolytic specificities and thereby enhance the repertoire of available peptides for presentation to T cells.[40] Therefore, MHC I–peptide complexes essentially function as "flags" on the surface of cells, revealing a sampling of their intracellular contents. Nonself peptides (foreign, e.g., viral and malignancy-associated peptides) complexed with MHC I will be recognized by activated cytotoxic T lymphocytes (CTLs), which can then lyse the virus-infected or abnormal cell (*Fig. 9.3*). Because, potentially, any nucleated cell could be infected with a virus, all cells in the body, except erythrocytes, express class I MHC and are thereby scrutinized by CTLs for evidence of a foreign peptide. Activated CTLs are capable of eliminating infected cells by several mechanisms, including the release of granule-derived cytotoxins (perforin, granzyme) and the engagement of T cell-expressed Fas ligand to target cell-expressed Fas to elicit apoptosis (programmed cell death) of the target cell. CTLs also release cytokines that contribute to host defense. For instance, these cells release IFN-γ, which inhibits viral replication and activates macrophages for intracellular killing and antigen presentation (type 1 macrophages). A virulence strategy employed by some viruses (e.g., herpesviruses) is to downregulate host MHC I expression to avoid destruction by CTLs. (Importantly, as discussed above, NK cells are effective at eliminating host cells with lowered surface MHC I expression.) Host peptides are also presented by class I MHC, but are generally not recognized, since most self-recognizing T cells are eliminated in the thymus and never circulate. Those T cells reacting with host peptides with low affinity are normally removed in the periphery.

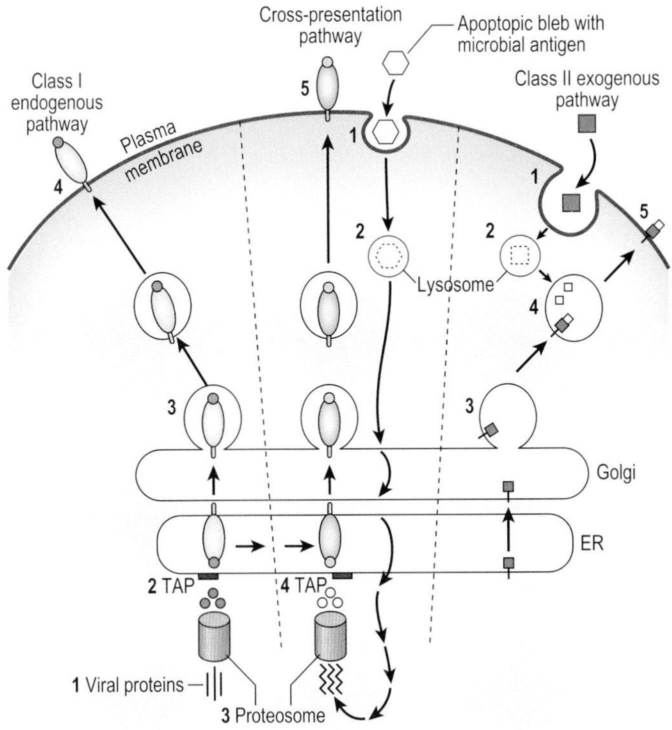

Figure 9.2 The pathways for processing antigens for presentation with major histocompatibility complex (MHC) molecules. Intracellular antigens (*left*), such as those derived from viruses, are degraded in the proteosome (1); complexed with TAP (transporter associated with antigen processing) (2); and exported from the Golgi as an MHC class I antigen–peptide complex (3), which are then expressed on the outer plasma membrane (4). Extracellular antigens (*right*) are phagocytosed or endocytosed (1), and degraded in lysosomes (2). Class II MHC molecules are synthesized and leave the Golgi in vesicles (3) that fuse with late endosomes containing antigenic peptides allowing the peptides to complex with MHC class II proteins (4), and the peptide-MHC class II complexes move to the plasma membrane (5). Cross-presentation (*center*) occurs when exogenous antigens, usually in a complex with apoptotic debris, are internalized by phagocytosis or endocytosis (1), and move through a lysosomal compartment (2) to the proteosome (3). Thereafter, the degraded peptides are bound to TAP (4) for movement into the endoplasmic reticulum (ER) and Golgi for complexing with MHC class I proteins for transport and expression at the plasma membrane (5).

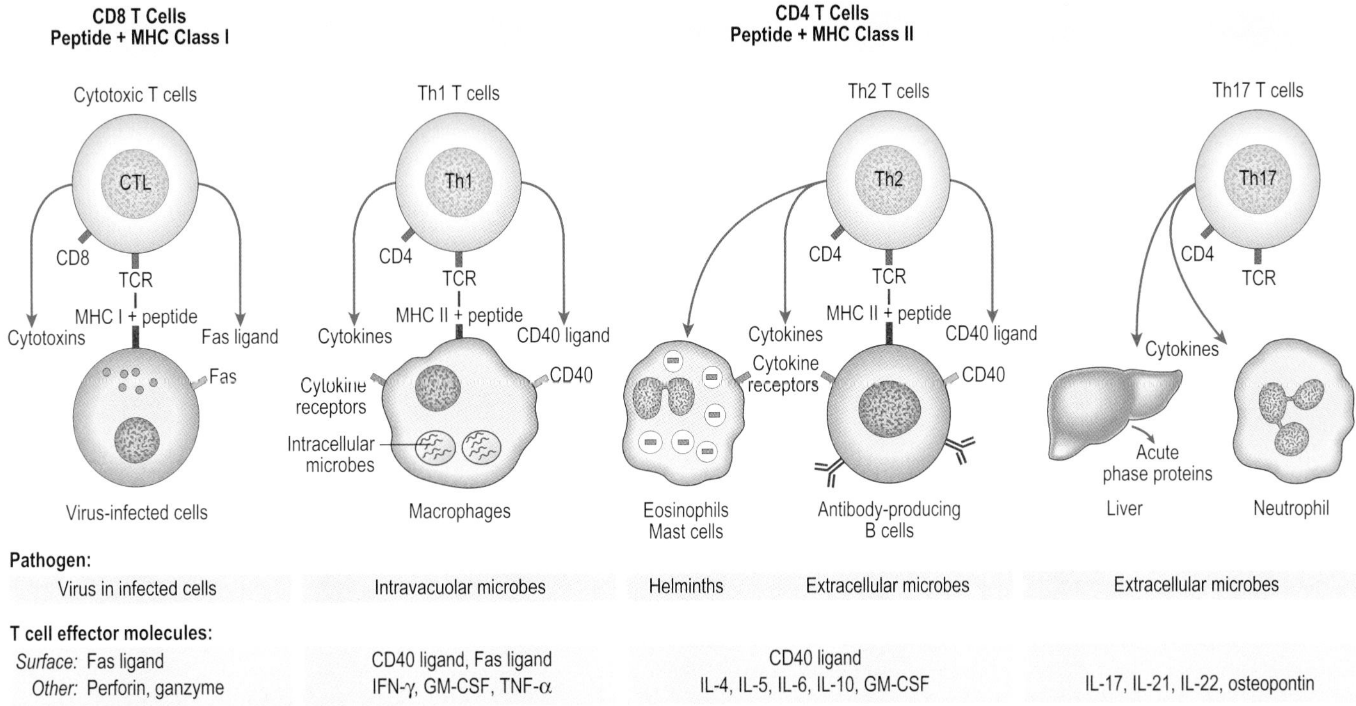

	CD8 T Cells	Th1 T cells	Th2 T cells		Th17 T cells
Pathogen:	Virus in infected cells	Intravacuolar microbes	Helminths	Extracellular microbes	Extracellular microbes
T cell effector molecules:					
Surface:	Fas ligand	CD40 ligand, Fas ligand	CD40 ligand		
Other:	Perforin, ganzyme	IFN-γ, GM-CSF, TNF-α	IL-4, IL-5, IL-6, IL-10, GM-CSF		IL-17, IL-21, IL-22, osteopontin

Figure 9.3 Responses of T-lymphocyte subsets to infectious agents. CD8$^+$ T cells respond to antigens from intracellular pathogens, such as viruses, presented with class I major histocompatibility complex (MHC) molecules. These cytolytic CD8$^+$ T cells lyse infected target cells by release of toxic proteins (perforin, granzyme) and by induction of apoptosis (programmed cell death) by engagement of Fas. CD4$^+$ T cells can be directed to develop into T-helper 1 (Th1) cells that stimulate macrophage killing of intracellular pathogens (cell-mediated immunity); T-helper 2 (Th2) cells that produce antibody or enhance eosinophil- and mast cell-mediated responses to helminthic parasites; proinflammatory T-helper 17 (Th17) cells that exert cytopathic effects on tissues and are implicated in autoimmunity; or T-regulatory cells (T_{reg}) (*not shown*) that prevent excessive tissue damage by dampening T-cell activities. GM-CSF, granulocyte-macrophage colony-stimulating factor; IFN-γ, interferon-γ; IL-4, etc., interleukins; TNF-α, tumor necrosis factor-α.

MHC II Presentation of Extracellular Proteins to Helper T Cells

A different pathway of antigen presentation is followed for molecules synthesized outside the cell, such as those from the extracellular pathogen *S. pneumoniae*. In this case, APCs, which are primarily DCs, monocytes, macrophages, and B lymphocytes, sample the extracellular milieu. This sampling might take the form of phagocytosis of particles, such as bacteria or apoptotic or necrotic cell debris, by monocytes or macrophages, or endocytosis and pinocytosis of soluble samples by any of the APCs. PRMs within phagocytic and endosomal intracellular compartments of the APCs sense PAMPs in the internalized samples, leading to cellular activation and upregulation of costimulatory molecules and MHC II expression. The larger antigens are proteolytically degraded, and the derived peptides are loaded onto MHC II molecules within endocytic vesicles and are expressed on the surface of the APC (***Fig. 9.2***).[41] $CD4^+$ helper T cells recognize antigens bound to class II MHC. Generation and selection of antigen-specific effector helper T cells are requisite for costimulation of antibody and CTL responses and rely upon the broad sampling of microbes and apoptotic or necrotic host cells from the extracellular milieu (***Fig. 9.3***). A key virulence strategy for some bacteria is to interfere with host cell expression of microbial peptide-loaded MHC II molecules, either through resisting phagocytic engulfment (e.g., encapsulated bacteria such as *S. pneumoniae* and *N. meningitidis*), escaping phagosomes (e.g., *Shigella flexneri*), or by decreasing MHC II surface expression (e.g., *Salmonella*).

CD1 and Cross-Presentation

Two addenda to the classic distinction of class I and class II pathways of antigen presentation are necessary. First, lipid and glycolipid antigens (i.e., those derived from *Mycobacterium* species), are presented by CD1 proteins on NK-T cells. Distinguishing features of the CD1 proteins are that they have limited diversity and their cytoplasmic tails target them to distinct endosomal compartments for the potential loading of lipids from different intracellular pathogens.[42] The second addendum to the class I/class II paradigm is the concept of "cross presentation." Cross presentation occurs when an antigen made outside the APC is internalized by endocytosis or phagocytosis, and instead of complexing with class II MHC, it is routed to a compartment containing class I MHC (see ***Fig. 9.2***).[43,44] At least one pathway involves proteosome digestion and complexing of the peptide with class I in the ER in the usual manner. Antigenic material, either from apoptotic infected cells or complexed with heat shock proteins from stressed or necrotic cells, is favored for cross presentation.[45,46]

MHC Diversity

In humans, the MHC, or HLA, genes are located on chromosome 6. There are three major polymorphic genes for class I (A, B, and C).[1–4] Because these genes are codominant, a cell will commonly express six different MHC class I molecules (three from each parent). The class II polymorphic genes are DR, DP, and DQ, all composed of α and β chains. Many individuals also have a gene for an extra DR β chain, either of which can combine with the DR α chain. Thus, class II MHC heterozygous individuals can express eight different polymorphic alleles (four from each parent). The reason an individual needs so many possible MHC proteins is to be able to generate a diverse array of grooves in the MHC molecules, such that there would be a groove to fit at least some antigens from each potential pathogen. Although this strategy works most of the time, there are some MHC types that have been linked to susceptibility to certain pathogens (see ***Table 6.3***), or to an increased frequency of certain immunologic diseases, such as ankylosing spondylitis and reactive arthritis.[47–49] The reason the human species maintains such a large and diverse MHC repertoire likely relates to the selection advantage of being able to react to numerous and diverse pathogens. Although an evolving pathogen might find a susceptible MHC-"deficient" type in a few individuals, others in the population will have different and functional MHC types and therefore will not be susceptible to the altered pathogen.

Responses of the Adaptive Immune System

Anergy and Tolerance

Anergy is a state of global immunologic unresponsiveness, which can be remedied by removal or addition of one or more factors.[1–4] For instance, an abundance of IL-10 leads to downregulation of costimulatory molecules on APCs such that they are unable to activate T cells to respond in the presence of specific antigen. Removal of IL-10 from the system leads to restoration of responsiveness.

Tolerance is different from a state of anergy and occurs when the immune system is unable to respond to a specific antigen.[1–4] There are multiple steps in the immune response that are susceptible to tolerance, providing a safeguard to prevent the immune system from reacting against itself. Immature B cells that react with multivalent self-antigens are destroyed by programmed cell death, or apoptosis, a process referred to as "clonal deletion." Immature B cells that react with soluble self-antigens are rendered inactive by the downregulation of their surface IgM and their signaling potential. Finally, when CD4 T cells bind an APC expressing antigen-MHC but no costimulatory molecules, these T cells will be rendered tolerant. Tolerance can be induced experimentally in animals and has been shown to be partially dependent on the form and the route of administration of the antigen. High doses of antigen, orally administered antigen, or repetitive doses of low concentrations of antigen may all lead to tolerance. Successful vaccine strategies must avoid inducing tolerance.

Maturation of Productive Antimicrobial Immune Responses

Immune Regulation by T-Helper Cells

As described above, activated T-helper cells provide critical costimulatory signals to adaptive immunity (i.e., for the generation of effector B cells and licensing of CTLs), and also promote immunity through stimulating the activities of innate immune cells (i.e., "educating" macrophages to kill their intracellular microbes). The majority of these functions are accomplished through the secretion of specific cytokines. Thus, a key aspect governing the generation of any appropriate immune response is the development of activated T-helper cell subsets secreting the appropriate cytokines. Through studies of disease processes in mice and humans, data have emerged highlighting several distinct subsets of effector helper T cells, based upon the specific pattern of cytokines secreted. Of note, it is likely that additional subsets or further classifications within subsets will continue to be identified as more sophisticated analyses of microbial infections are performed. Moreover, the feasibility of plasticity between discrete subsets throughout an immune response remains to be fully resolved. Nonetheless, we can describe the maturation of effective immune responses as Th1, Th2, Th17, or T regulatory through describing the cytokine profile of the respective T-helper cell subset(s) generated.

Polarization of naïve T cells into the distinct effector cell subsets appears to be dictated by a series of "third signals" transmitted between the APC and the cognate antigen-specific T cell. As with costimulatory factors, DC sensing of PAMPs through DC-expressed PRMs is critical in modulating surface-expressed polarizing molecules (i.e., Notch ligands) and the secretion of soluble immunomodulatory cytokines (i.e., IL-4, IL-12) (***Fig. 9.1***). For example, DCs expressing surface Jagged 1 Notch ligands and secreting IL-4 will instruct Th2 differentiation in antigen-specific naïve $CD4^+$ T cells; DCs stimulated to upregulate Delta Notch ligands and secrete IL-12 will promote polarization to a Th1 phenotype; and Delta 4-expressing DCs, in the presence of cytokines such as IL-6 and TGF-β promote Th17 polarization.[50,51] Because the type of immature DC defines its repertoire of PAMP receptors,[52] the DC subset may be a factor in the propensity for induction of Th1, Th2, Th17, or T_{reg} phenotypes. The tissue microenvironment, with its distinctive exposure to foreign antigens and array of innate immune cells, also influences the ability of resident immature DCs to polarize T-helper cells. T-helper cell subsets and their associated immune responses are described below.

Th1 Responses: Cell-Mediated Immunity and Delayed Type Hypersensitivity

During infections with intracellular pathogens, signals from Th1 lymphocytes enable full activation of CTLs. For some intracellular pathogens that live within vesicles or vacuoles, such as mycobacteria, neither antibody nor CTLs have access to the pathogens. Rather, macrophages harboring these pathogens must be activated by antigen-specific Th1 lymphocytes to kill the pathogens.[53] Antigen-committed Th1 cells recognize their cognate microbial peptide complexed with MHC class II on the surface of an infected macrophage, and secrete macrophage-activating cytokines, including IFN-γ, TNF-α, and granulocyte-monocyte colony-stimulating factor (GM-CSF). CD40 ligand on the Th1 lymphocyte engages CD40 on macrophages and also contributes to macrophage activation (***Fig. 9.3***). The "classically" activated macrophage uses upregulated nitric oxide and oxygen radicals to aid in killing pathogens in phagolysosomes.[54] A less productive form of Th1 immunity is known as delayed type hypersensitivity. Contact dermatitis, such as sensitivity to poison ivy, is a common form of delayed type hypersensitivity.

Th2 Responses: Antibody Production and Immediate Hypersensitivity

Th2 responses participate in host defense against extracellular pathogens in two ways. First, through Th2-expressed CD40L signaling of B cell-expressed CD40, and through secretion of Th2 cytokines, including IL-4 and IL-6, Th2 cells activate B cells to produce antibodies and undergo isotype switching, whereby immunoglobulin synthesis matures from IgM to include other classes of immunoglobulins. Antibodies function to directly neutralize some pathogens and toxins, to opsonize pathogens facilitating their phagocytosis by cells such as neutrophils and macrophages, and to activate complement for enhanced opsonization or lysis of some bacteria. Antibody may also enhance NK cell functions by means of antibody-dependent cellular cytotoxicity (ADCC). The varying functions of the specific antibody isotypes are summarized in ***Table 9.4***.

A second role of Th2 cells is to "alternatively" activate macrophages to produce Th2 cytokines instead of Th1 cytokines. The end result is that the macrophage becomes more efficient at presenting peptides from extracellular microbes, and secretes extracellular matrix components, such as fibronectin. This process is important for tissue repair processes, and in the formation of granulomas surrounding some extracellular parasites or their products (i.e., schistosome eggs). Epithelioid cells and granulomatous fibrosis are the histologic hallmarks of alternatively activated macrophages.[54]

Activation of the Th2 pathway can lead to immediate hypersensitivity, an IgE-dependent form of allergy. The reaction is initiated when IgE antibodies that are bound via their Fc region to the IgE receptors bind their specific antigens ("allergens"). Crosslinking of the IgE receptors (expressed principally on mast cells) stimulates the activation and release of mediators from these cells, which may cause localized urticaria, or systemic anaphylaxis. IL-4 from Th2 lymphocytes strongly promotes the synthesis of IgE; the Th2 cytokines IL-5 and GM-CSF stimulate eosinophil differentiation and activation; and IL-4 acts on mast cells. IgE, eosinophils, and mast cells are involved in host defense against the extracellular helminthic parasites. On the other hand, a dysregulated Th2 response leads to chronic inflammation, asthma being a prime example.[55]

Th17 Responses: Inflammation and Autoimmunity

Th17 is a more recently identified T-helper cell subset that mediates tissue damage through secretion of highly proinflammatory cytokines. Th17 cells are characterized by their secretion of IL-17A, IL-17F, IL-21, IL-22, and osteopontin. IL-17 is a strongly proinflammatory cytokine that stimulates the release of acute phase proteins, enhances granulopoiesis, and promotes neutrophil recruitment; IL-21 promotes the growth and maturation of NK cells and B cells; and IL-22 stimulates acute phase protein release and synergizes with IL-17 to enhance secretion of antimicrobial peptides. The Th17-driven proinflammatory response is particularly effective in host defense against extracellular microbes, e.g., *S. pneumoniae*, fungi and some protozoa. On the other hand, owing to their proclivity toward inflammation, Th17 cells are increasingly implicated in graft rejection, allergic pulmonary inflammatory diseases and autoimmune diseases (e.g., rheumatoid arthritis and psoriasis).

Regulatory T Cells

In both mice and humans there are subsets of T cells, that when depleted or genetically deficient, predispose to autoimmunity and/or uncontrolled inflammation. Study of these "regulatory" T cells (T_{reg}) remains a rapidly evolving field, and is the subject of numerous recent reviews.[56–58] Natural T_{reg} cells (nT_{reg}) are generated in the thymus and likely limit autoimmune responses, while inducible T_{reg} cells (iT_{reg}) are generated in the periphery, potentially a means of downregulating inflammation. A major transcription factor associated with $CD4^+$ T_{reg} cells is FoxP3 (although a subset of $FoxP3^-$ regulatory T cells is induced in the periphery). In humans, genetic deficiency of Foxp3 is associated with IPEX (immune dysregulation, polyendocrinopathy, enteropathy, and X-linked syndrome).[59,60] In addition, $CD8^+$ T_{reg} cells have been described (reviewed in Smith and Kumar).[61]

IMMUNOPATHOLOGY

Autoimmunity

Tolerance to self-antigens occurs at multiple steps beginning early in development and continues for the life of the organism. Autoimmunity occurs when there is a breaking of tolerance to self-antigens, which likely occurs as the result of both an environmental insult and a genetical predisposition. Environmental insults may be an infection or tissue damage; and genetic predispositions include any of the following: (1) primary immunodeficiencies that are associated with abnormal control of pathogens;[62] (2) defective clearance of apoptotic debris as in deficiencies of early complement components;[63,64] (3) gain of function mutations leading to increased expression of an immune activator, for example the B-cell activator CR2;[65] (4) loss of function mutations for an immune regulator, for example the inhibitory FcR, FcγRIIB;[34] (5) certain MHC alleles that predispose to autoimmune disease, such as the association of the class I MHC B27 allele with ankylosing spondylitis. This might be the result of the physical characteristics of the MHC groove as a determinant of what peptides can be presented, or tight linkage to an as yet undiscovered susceptibility gene.

Other Forms of Immunopathology

Immune responses to infections may contribute to pathologic changes in non-autoimmune ways. When the host is unable to eliminate microbial or parasitic antigens, such as occurs in subacute bacterial endocarditis and chronic *Plasmodium malariae* infections, the host's antibodies will complex with shed microbial antigens to form immune complexes. Normally immune complexes are tagged with complement, bound to erythrocyte CR1 and delivered by erythrocytes to phagocytes of the liver and spleen for removal. An excess of immune complexes can overwhelm this normally anti-inflammatory process, leading to tissue inflammation due to the activation of cells by their FcγRs. This may develop acutely or chronically as antibody titers rise, causing the syndrome of serum sickness.

The recruitment and activation of phagocytes in response to infections also may contribute to tissue damage owing to the exuberant local release of leukocyte granule proteins and generation of oxidants. Thus, the pyogenic response of neutrophils to bacterial infections can be partially deleterious, as with the chronic neurologic sequelae following bacterial meningitis.[66] Likewise, eosinophil activation in response to helminthic infections and allergic diseases, such as asthma, can damage host cells.[55] Finally, the inability to silence activated immune cells by either apoptosis due to mutations in the Fas–Fas ligand signaling pathway, or by lysis due to perforin mutations that disable CTLs and NK cells leads to autoimmune lymphoproliferative syndrome (ALPS) and hemophagocytic lymphohistiocytosis (HLH), respectively.[67,68]

IMMUNODEFICIENCIES AND INFECTION

Genetic deficiencies (see Chapter 6, ***Tables 6.1–6.6*** and reference 67), as well as acquired defects in the immune system may be associated with susceptibility to infections, and the pattern of infection – affected tissue and specific pathogen(s) – gives insight as to the defect. Many of the classic neonatal phenotypes of severe immunodeficiency states have now been recognized with a more moderate phenotype in adults. Thus, an appreciation of immunodeficient states is relevant for any age. The new onset of infection in a previously healthy host can herald the presence of an underlying acquired disease such as HIV infection or a hematologic malignancy, which are important to rule out. When it is relevant to consider a genetically determined immunodeficient state depends on the family history, age of the patient, chronicity and pattern of infections. There are no easy rules, but there are some recurrent themes, such as severe periodontal disease when neutrophils are defective; the similar susceptibility of patients to encapsulated Gram-positive organisms when individuals are deficient in IgG, neutrophils, or complement C3; and the association of some "signature" organisms, such as *Aspergillus* spp. and *Burkholderia cepacia* with chronic granulomatous disease. Common variable immunodeficiency presents at any age and usually is heralded by recurrent pyogenic respiratory infections, which is characteristic of IgG deficiency. However, a subset of these patients present with autoimmune phenomena that cloud the ultimate diagnosis.[69,70]

VACCINES

Vaccines have had an enormous positive impact on public health and remain one of the most cost-effective means of preventing infectious diseases (see Chapter 10). The efficacy of most vaccines rely on an IgG response that is strong and ideally recruits memory lymphocytes. Early vaccines relied on killed or attenuated pathogens as immunogens, but the toxicity of the former and the chance for reverting to virulent forms of the latter have encouraged the design of recombinant subunit immunogens for use in vaccines. However, "clean" immunogens are not recognized by pattern recognition receptors and without an innate response to prime adaptive immunity no protective immunity ensues. To circumvent this problem adjuvants are mixed with the immunogen, and the role of the adjuvant is to stimulate an innate response and cause the upregulation of costimulatory molecules on the APC and the T cell. "Alum" (aluminum hydroxide) is the most common adjuvant in use, although its mode of action remains controversial.[71]

Antibodies directed against capsular carbohydrates were known to be protective against *S. pneumoniae*, *Haemophilus influenzae*, and *N. meningitidis*, but making vaccines presented a special problem since purified carbohydrate does not usually elicit T-cell help and as a consequence the immune response is weak and short-lived. To circumvent this problem the purified carbohydrate is coupled to protein so that the antigen-presenting B cells will present both the peptides and the carbohydrate and be able to receive help from T cells responsive to the peptides.[72] The modified inactive diphtheria toxin CRM197 is commonly used as the "carrier protein." Using a protein that has been included in another vaccine, namely the DTP (diphtheria-tetanus-pertussis), ensures that there will be ample numbers of T-helper cells to provide help to the B cells presenting the carbohydrate antigen. To make use of the role TLRs have in innate immunity, some new vaccines are being developed that have the immunogen coupled to TLR ligands. Going forward, fresh insights from immunologic research will continue to inform the development and effective use of vaccines.

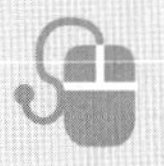

Access the complete reference list online at **http://www.expertconsult.com**

Access the complete reference list online at
http://www.expertconsult.com

CHAPTER 10

Vaccines in the Tropics

Alan D.T. Barrett

INTRODUCTION

The impact of vaccination on the health of the world's peoples is hard to exaggerate. With the exception of safe water, no other modality, not even antibiotics, has had such a major effect on mortality reduction and population growth (Stanley Plotkin, vaccinologist, 1999).

As elegantly stated by Stanley Plotkin, vaccination is probably the most effective public health intervention of all time. This is especially true in developing countries, where poverty limits those who can afford health care. Given the large quantity of research undertaken on vaccine development over a long period time (centuries), it is somewhat surprising that only a total of 31 vaccines are in use today. This is in part due to the long and complex road to the development of a vaccine. There are expectations not only that a vaccine will give long-term protective immunity from the infectious disease but also that it will be 100% safe, such that any side-effects due to immunization are unacceptable. Given these expectations, at the present time the process of vaccine development from discovery to licensure takes 18–20 years, and consequently is very expensive at approximately US$ 500 million. In this chapter the routine immunization schedules and travelers' vaccines will be outlined, and how vaccines are implemented in the tropics is followed by a description of the vaccine development pathway and a discussion of vaccines in development.

ROUTINE IMMUNIZATIONS

As in developed countries, there are routine immunizations given to children and adults in poor countries. The World Health Organization (WHO) has recommendations for vaccines for all age groups: childhood, adolescent, and adult immunizations (***Tables 10.1 and 10.2***). This information is frequently updated as new vaccines become available, and detailed information on all vaccines is available.[1] Many of the vaccines recommended by the WHO are the same as those used in developed countries, such as the United States,[2] but there are some differences. For example, the WHO recommends BCG vaccine (bacillus Calmette-Guérin is a live attenuated vaccine against tuberculosis) for all children after birth and the live attenuated poliomyelitis vaccine for all children, but does not recommend the live attenuated chickenpox (varicella) vaccine, whereas the United States does not recommend BCG vaccine, utilizes the inactivated poliomyelitis vaccine, and has incorporated the varicella vaccine into the routine childhood immunization schedule.

It should be emphasized that the WHO provides recommendations as not all vaccines will be required in all regions of the world. As indicated in ***Tables 10.1 and 10.2***, there are a number of vaccines that are required only in certain areas of the world where the diseases are found; many of these vaccines are used for travelers who visit these areas from other parts of the world (see below). Examples would be yellow fever where the disease is found in tropical South America and sub-Saharan Africa but not Asia, whereas Japanese encephalitis is found in Asia but not Africa or South America. The objective is to aid decision-making of the most advantageous immunization schedules for health care providers in each region/country to prevent vaccine-preventable diseases and maintain lifelong immunity. In this situation health care providers include not only those who are responsible for administering the vaccine but also national decision-makers, immunization managers, regulatory authorities, and Ministers of Health. This process is not only important for public health officials but also it helps vaccine producers evaluate potential markets.

VACCINES FOR TRAVELERS

In the 21st century air travel makes it possible to reach any destination in the world within 24 hours. The WHO estimates that at any one time more than 500 000 persons are in aircraft. Travel vaccine portfolios are an important component for most vaccine producers, and travel medicine clinics are equally important as sites to provide the appropriate vaccines for travelers (see Chapter 126). The emphasis is on appropriate vaccines as it is important that individuals only receive vaccines for which there is demonstrable risk of the traveler being exposed to the natural disease. For example, individuals visiting Peru would want to receive yellow fever vaccine if they were visiting the jungle areas of Peru but would not want to receive the vaccine if they were visiting Lima, the capital of Peru, as this city is on the coast where the mosquito vectors that transmit the virus are not found. Similarly, intracountry travelers need to be considered for vaccination when they travel to different regions of a country. Public health agencies such as the United States Centers for Disease Control and Prevention have a website that is continually updated on recommendations of vaccines for travelers to different regions of the world.[3]

ECONOMICS OF VACCINE DEVELOPMENT

Given the cost to develop a vaccine, economic evaluation and viability are very important criteria and are based on who will pay for the vaccine and how much they are willing to pay. However, in reality, this decision-making process is more complicated as the number of people who might benefit from the vaccine, the population that is targeted for immunization, and the severity of the disease that will be prevented by immunization are all important points that need to be considered. Consequently, estimates of market need are then influenced by the quantity of vaccine that is needed, the shelf-life of the vaccine, and a predicted vaccine purchase price.

Until recent times, it has been considered that there are more individuals in a developing country who would benefit from a vaccine than in a developed country, but there may be fewer financial resources

Table 10.1 Recommended Routine Immunization – Summary of World Health Organization Position Papers

Antigen	Children	Adolescents	Adults
Recommendations for All			
BCG	1 dose		
DTP	3 doses Booster (DTP) 1–6 years of age	Booster (Td)	Booster (Td) in early adulthood or pregnancy
Haemophilus influenzae type b	3 doses, with DTP		
Hepatitis B	3–4 doses, with DTP	3 doses (for high-risk groups if not previously immunized)	
HPV		3 doses (girls)	
Pneumococcal (conjugate)	3 doses, with DTP		
Polio (oral polio vaccine)	3 doses, with DTP		
Rotavirus	Rotarix vaccine: 2 doses with DTP RotaTeq vaccines: 3 doses with DTP		
Measles	2 doses		
Recommendations for Certain Regions			
Japanese encephalitis	Live attenuated vaccine: 1 dose Booster after 1 year Mouse brain-derived vaccine: 2 doses Booster after 1 year, then every 3 years	Mouse brain-derived vaccine Booster every 3 years up to 10–15 years of age	
Yellow fever	1 dose, with measles		
Recommendations for Some High-Risk Populations			
Typhoid	Vi vaccine: 1 dose; Ty21a vaccine: 3–4 doses Booster dose 3–7 years after primary series		
Cholera	Dukoral (WC-rBs): 3 doses ≥ 2–5 years, booster every 6 months; 2 doses adults/children > 6 years, booster every 2nd year Shanchol & mORCVAX: 2 doses ≥ 1 year, booster dose after 2 years		
Meningococcal (polysaccharide)	1 dose		
Hepatitis A	2 doses		
Rabies	3 doses		
Recommendations for Immunization Programs with Certain Characteristics			
Mumps	2 doses, with measles		
Rubella	1 dose	1 dose (alternative strategy adolescent girls and child bearing age women)	
Influenza (inactivated)	First vaccine use: 2 doses Revaccinate annually: 1 dose only	1 dose from 9 years of age Revaccinate annually	

BCG, bacillus Calmette-Guérin; DTP, diphtheria, tetanus, pertussis; Td, tetanus, diphtheria; HPV, human papillomavirus.
(Adapted from http://www.who.int/immunization/policy/Immunization_routine_table1.pdf. Updated 9 June 2010.)

available to purchase the vaccine such that the market need may be perceived as insufficient to support the vaccine development. However, improvements in transportation have made it possible to travel rapidly to anywhere in the world and now infectious diseases are considered a world problem rather than a problem of individual countries. This opens doors for vaccine producers to have larger markets than previously thought, but this is matched by the need to work with multiple national regulatory authorities (NRAs).

PRIVATE-PUBLIC PARTNERSHIPS

Prevention of infectious diseases by immunization is advantageous due to both public health reasons and economics, and is thought to save at least 3 million lives each year. It is estimated that an additional US$1 billion per year in immunizations would save 10 million more lives over the next decade.[4] Until recently, market forces alone were insufficient to meet the health care priorities of resource-poor populations. However, the last 15 years have seen a marked change in vaccine development for diseases found in developing countries due to large-scale involvement of entities such as the WHO, Bill and Melinda Gates Foundation, Global Alliance for Vaccines and Immunization (GAVI), and the Program for Appropriate Technology in Health (PATH).

Global Alliance for Vaccines and Immunization

GAVI[5] is a private–public partnership of United Nations Children's Fund (UNICEF), Bill and Melinda Gates Foundation, WHO, and World Bank that started in 2000. The program is targeted at developing countries, and only those that are the poorest. In 2009, there were 72 GAVI-eligible countries, which include approximately half of the world's population; however, each country is assessed for each aspect of the program, and not all countries are eligible for all parts of the program.

The first phase was a 5-year plan (2000–2005) aimed at extending and improving the quality of immunization programs by two approaches: supplying new and underused vaccines and strengthening vaccine delivery systems. The former focused on *Haemophilus influenzae* type b (Hib), hepatitis B, and yellow fever vaccines, and the latter focused on implementation of disposable autodisable syringes to prevent reuse of syringes and associated equipment that have the potential to cause infections. The 5-year plan provided grants for supply of vaccines, with the expectation that countries would increase their national contribution, leading to subsequent financial sustainability.

The second phase is a 10-year plan (2006–2015) that is increasing the range of vaccines included in the program (pneumococcus and rotavirus),

Table 10.2 Recommended Routine Immunizations for Children

Antigen		Age at First Dose	Doses in Primary Series	Interval between Doses			Booster Dose
				First to Second	Second to Third	Third to Fourth	
Recommendations for All Children							
BCG		As soon as possible after birth	1				
DTP		6 weeks (min.)	3	4 weeks (min.)	4 weeks (min.)		1–6 years of age
Haemophilus influenzae type b		6 weeks (min.) with DTP1, 24 months (max.)	3	4 weeks (min.) with DTP2	4 weeks (min.) with DTP3		
Hepatitis B	Option 1	As soon as possible after birth (<24 hours)	3	4 weeks (min.) with DTP1	4 weeks (min.) with DTP3		
	Option 2	As soon as possible after birth (<24 hours)	4	4 weeks (min.) with DTP1	4 weeks (min.) with DTP2	4 weeks (min.) with DTP3	
HPV		Quadrivalent 9–13 years of age Bivalent 10–13 years of age	3	Quadrivalent – 2 months (min. 4 weeks) Bivalent – 1 month (max. 2.5 months)	Quadrivalent: 4 months (min. 12 weeks) Bivalent – 5 months		
Pneumococcal (conjugate)		6 weeks (min.) with DTP1	3	4 weeks (min.) with DTP2	4 weeks (min.) with DTP3		
Polio (oral polio vaccine)		6 weeks (min.)	3	4 weeks (min.) with DTP2	4 weeks (min.) with DTP3		
Rotavirus	Rotarix	6 weeks (min.) with DTP1, 15 weeks (max.)	2	4 weeks (min.) with DTP2 no later than 32 weeks of age			
	RotaTeq	6 weeks (min.) with DTP1, 15 weeks	3	4 weeks (min.) – 10 weeks with DTP2	4 weeks (min.) with DTP3 no later than 32 weeks of age		
Measles		9–15 months (6 months min.)	2	4 weeks (min.)			
Recommendations for Children Residing in Certain Regions							
Japanese encephalitis	Mouse brain-derived	1 year	2	4 weeks (min.)			After 1 year and every 3 years up to 10–15 years of age
	Live attenuated	9–12 months	1				After 1 year
Yellow fever		9–12 months with measles	1				
Recommendations for Children in Some High-Risk Populations							
Typhoid	Vi PS	2 years (min.)	1				Every 3 years
	Ty21a	Capsules 5 years (min.)	3 or 4	1 day	1 day	1 day	Every 3–7 years
Cholera		2 years (min.)	2	7 days (min.)			
Meningococcal (polysaccharide)		2 years (min.)	1				
Hepatitis A		1 year (min.)	2	6–18 months			
Rabies		As required	3	6 days	14 days		Every 5 years
Recommendations for Children Receiving Vaccinations from Immunization Programs with Certain Characteristics							
Mumps		12–18 months with measles	2	1 month (min.) to school entry			
Rubella		9–15 months with measles	1				
Influenza (inactivated)		6 months (min.)	2	1 month			

BCG, bacillus Calmette-Guérin; DTP, diphtheria, tetanus, pertussis; Td, tetanus, diphtheria; HPV, human papillomavirus. (Adapted from http://www.who.int/immunization/policy/Immunization_routine_table2.pdf. Updated 9 June 2010.)

but has found that financial sustainability is a significant problem. GAVI has an accelerated development and implementation plan program for pneumococcal and rotaviral vaccines that aims to shorten the period between vaccines being proven safe and effective for use and their introduction in developing countries. In addition, the Hib initiative has been expanded into a pentavalent vaccine program where one immunization incorporates vaccines for five diseases (Hib, diphtheria, tetanus, pertussis, and hepatitis B). A vaccine investment strategy has been developed where the WHO provided a list of 18 diseases in 2007 to be considered for investment. From this list GAVI has selected four diseases for consideration of financial support (cervical cancer, Japanese encephalitis, rubella, and typhoid).

Access of developing countries to vaccines is a key component of GAVI, and this is being achieved via two financial initiatives. Advance market commitments (AMCs) are designed to stimulate the development and manufacture of vaccines specifically for developing countries. The pilot AMC is for a new vaccine to target pneumococcal disease (due to *Streptococcus pneumoniae*) with the aim of supporting up to 60 of the world's poorest countries to introduce pneumococcal vaccine by 2015. The second initiative is the International Finance Facility for Immunization that borrows on capital markets against donor countries' pledges and raises funds through bonds. This novel financial mechanism aims to provide US$4 billion in funds between 2006 and 2015.

Program for Appropriate Technology in Health

PATH[6] originated in the 1970s and has expanded extensively in the last 30 years and considers itself "a catalyst for global health." It focuses on a number of areas to improve public health, including advancing technologies, strengthening systems, and encouraging healthy behaviors, and works in over 70 countries. One of the foci of PATH is vaccine development with projects on technologies to improve the safety, effectiveness, and efficiency of vaccine delivery in countries that are disproportionately affected by vaccine-preventable infectious diseases.

Supporting the design, development, scale-up, production, commercialization, and distribution of technologies solely through the public sector is clearly beyond available resources and not economically viable within the countries that need the vaccines. Thus, public–private collaborations are indispensable for investment in suitable technologies to further vaccine development in developing countries. PATH has developed and refined many approaches for identifying and advancing vaccine-related technologies, and works collaboratively in partnerships with vaccine and technology companies, public and private sector partners, research institutes, universities, other nongovernmental organizations, research consortia, and international agencies to further vaccine development. All of the above are key to advancing candidate vaccines to usage in the community and improving public health. Projects have included maintaining the cold chain and issues that impact vaccine delivery and effectiveness at point of use, such as bench and field testing, technology transfer, scale-up, licensing, and market and product introduction for a number of vaccines, including *Shigella*, enterotoxigenic *Escherichia coli*, rotavirus, Japanese encephalitis, pneumococcal disease, seasonal and pandemic influenza, and cervical cancer.

World Health Organization

The WHO has a number of programs that are focused on vaccines. Most are in the "Immunization, Vaccines, and Biologicals" program,[7] whose mission is a "world in which all people at risk are protected against vaccine-preventable disease" and provides recommendations on policy, guidelines, and information on vaccines. Within WHO, the Strategic Advisory Group of Experts on Immunization was established in 1999 to be the principal advisory group for vaccines and immunization that makes the key recommendations on immunizations (including global policy, strategies, technology, research and development, vaccine delivery, and relationships to other health interventions) and reviews and endorses all immunization-related materials prior to publication. The Weekly Epidemiological Record[8] is used to publish all WHO recommendations on immunizations, in French and English, with additional translations available in Arabic, Chinese, Russian, and Spanish. Currently, the WHO provides immunization policy recommendations on most components of vaccine implementation (***Box** 10.1*), and 24 vaccine-preventable diseases (***Box** 10.2*),[9] and position papers are frequently updated.

Box 10.1 Components of Vaccine Implementation

- Program management
- Procurement
- Vaccine quality
- Cold-chain regimen and equipment
- Vaccine handling
- Open-vial policy
- Establishing recommendations for vaccine use: universal and targeted vaccination
- Vaccine administration
- Contraindications
- Adverse events following immunization (AEFI) (also termed serious adverse events)
- Outbreak control
- Postlicensure assessment of safety and efficacy (population studies)
- Waste management
- Immunization coverage
- Vaccine-preven disease surveillance
- Research
- Community outreach and education – health professionals and public
- Cost-effectiveness

(Modified from www.who.int/immunization/policy/en/index.html.)

Box 10.2 Catalog of Available Immunization Policy Recommendations

- Bacillus Calmette-Guérin (BCG)
- Cholera
- Diphtheria
- Diphtheria, tetanus, and pertussis (DTP)
- Hepatitis A
- Hepatitis B
- *Haemophilus influenzae* type b (Hib)
- Human immunodeficiency virus (HIV)
- Influenza
- Japanese encephalitis
- Measles
- Meningococcal disease
- Measles, mumps, and rubella (MMR)
- Mumps
- Pertussis
- Pneumococcal disease
- Polio
- Rabies
- Rotavirus
- Rubella
- Tetanus
- Typhoid
- Varicella
- Yellow fever

Global Immunization Vision and Strategy (GIVS)

GIVS was recently established by WHO and UNICEF as a global 10-year program (2006–2015) to enhance immunizations.[10] The objectives are to immunize more people against more diseases, introduce newly available vaccines and technologies, manage immunization programs with respect to global relationships (i.e., implementation will depend on the specific needs of a country/region), and integrate immunizations with other health interventions. The overall goal is to reduce vaccine-preventable disease mortality and morbidity by two-thirds by 2015 compared to 2000.[11] In its first few years this program has significantly increased routine immunization coverage, but the challenge will be to sustain immunization coverage in future years.

United Nations Prequalified Vaccines

A very important issue for implementation of a vaccine is "prequalification." This refers to a service provided by the WHO to the United

Nations for designating a vaccine from a particular producer as having suitable quality assurance (e.g., safety, efficacy, potency, thermostability) to be purchased by United Nations agencies. This process is very important as a particular vaccine may be manufactured by multiple producers in different countries, and a prequalification designation informs Ministries of Health and NRAs that a particular vaccine from a producer meets standards required for immunization. In addition, prequalified vaccines have a price negotiated between the producer and United Nations. This is advantageous for both producers (as they have a defined market) and countries (as they will know the price of the vaccine and whether or not they can afford to incorporate the vaccine in their immunization program).

As one would expect, not all vaccines manufactured by all producers are prequalified. At present 24 of the 55 worldwide vaccine producers have one or more prequalified vaccine products. Currently, WHO has prioritized the following 12 vaccines for prequalification in 2009–2010: (1) bivalent oral polio vaccine; (2) dengue vaccine; (3) diphtheria-tetanus-pertussis-hepatitis B-*Haemophilus influenzae* type b pentavalent vaccine; (4) inactivated poliovirus vaccine; (5) seasonal influenza vaccine; (6) measles and measles-containing combination vaccines; (7) meningococcus type A-containing conjugate vaccines; (8) monovalent polio vaccines; (9) pneumococcal vaccines; (10) rotavirus vaccine; (11) tetanus-diphtheria vaccine (for adults); and (12) yellow fever vaccine. Note that a dengue vaccine has not been licensed yet but is being included now as the process of prequalification has many steps. This list is updated annually.

VACCINE SAFETY

Significant efforts have been made in the last 20 years by regulatory authorities and manufacturers to improve and ensure the safety of vaccines. Nonetheless, technologic advances and increasing knowledge about vaccines have led to investigations focused on the safety of current vaccines, which has an ever-increasingly important role on public confidence in immunization. While great efforts have been made in producing vaccines, they have little use if the target population will not have confidence to receive the vaccine. As a consequence, it is essential that concerns regarding vaccine-related adverse events are rapidly and effectively addressed in order to maintain confidence in a vaccine, and ultimately maintain immunization coverage and reduce disease incidence. Adverse events are defined as any undesirable experience associated with the use of a medical product in a patient. In particular, serious adverse events are the major concern. These are defined by the US Food and Drug Administration as adverse events involving death, life-threatening condition, hospitalization (initial or prolonged), disability, or congenital anomaly, or requiring intervention to prevent permanent impairment or damage. It was in this background that the WHO established the Global Advisory Committee on Vaccine Safety (GACVS) in 1999 to respond promptly, efficiently, and with scientific thoroughness to vaccine safety issues of potential global importance. The GACVS meets twice a year and publishes its discussions/recommendations in the WHO Weekly Epidemiological Record.

In 1999, the Brighton Collaboration[12] was established. at a meeting in Brighton, UK, and was subsequently officially inaugurated in fall 2000. The Collaboration consists of volunteers from developed and developing countries with expertise in patient care and public health and members of scientific, pharmaceutical, regulatory, and professional organizations who are experts in the field of immunization safety and in corresponding medical specialties. The Collaboration aims to facilitate the development, evaluation, and dissemination of high-quality information about the safety of human vaccines.[13]

VACCINE DEVELOPMENT PATHWAY

Given that we have vaccines to control relatively few infectious diseases and the huge successes of current vaccines in controlling infectious diseases, there is an urgent need to develop more vaccines, but the process is not straightforward. The vaccine development pathway involves four distinct phases: (1) basic science/discovery; (2) preclinical development; (3) clinical research; and (4) postlicensure activities.

Basic Science/Discovery

Basic science discoveries are fundamental to the development of new vaccines. It is significant that many of the vaccines that are used today are due to discoveries made in universities (e.g., poliomyelitis, measles, and yellow fever) that were subsequently exploited by industry to produce the vaccine. Nearly all the current live attenuated vaccines were generated empirically before the advent of NRAs, and it is unlikely that many of the current vaccines we take for granted (e.g., smallpox, yellow fever, and BCG) would be approved in the modern era. Where it was not possible to generate live attenuated vaccines, the logical alternative was to take the wild-type organism and chemically inactivate it, and use it as a killed vaccine. While this process has been important in the development of vaccines against some important infectious diseases, killed vaccines suffer from the limitation that booster immunizations are required to maintain a protective immune response. The development of "genetic engineering" techniques revolutionized vaccine development, and the first recombinant subunit vaccine was the hepatitis B vaccine where the surface antigen (HBsAg) was expressed in yeast. Subsequently, many candidate vaccines have been developed or are in development using genetic engineering techniques, and these are described in detail for specific pathogens in the relevant chapters of this book.

The major objective of the discovery/basic science phase is to identify candidate antigen(s), i.e., the gene(s) (and protein(s) encoded) that induce an immune response (i.e., an antigen that is immunogenic is defined as an immunogen). Characterization of the candidate immunogens demonstrates the ability of the immunogen to stimulate a protective immune response in a small animal model. Clearly, development of a small-animal model that resembles the disease seen in humans is very important. The immunogen needs to be presented optimally to the immune system, and this may involve the development of a platform technology (e.g., vaccinia) to deliver the immunogen and/or adjuvants to enhance the immune response.

Preclinical Development

There is a considerable lag period between a discovery and its commercial exploitation. Following a successful basic science/discovery phase, a candidate vaccine moves to the preclinical development phase. Once the initial discovery has been made there is a need to carry out comprehensive characterization of the candidate vaccine before clinical research can be undertaken. This is somewhat easier for killed and subunit products than live vaccines where the attenuated phenotype has to be carefully documented and the potential of reversion thoroughly investigated. Once completed, generation of the prototype vaccine is a critical step in the development pathway. This step not only demonstrates the technical feasibility of producing the candidate vaccine but will start the process for meeting the regulatory requirements that will later be obligatory by NRAs for ultimate licensure.

Before entering clinical trials, candidate vaccines are tested to evaluate safety, immunogenicity, and, when possible, efficacy in animal models. Nonclinical safety assessment includes tests to determine the direct toxicity of the candidate vaccine and other components of the formulation, the lack of contaminants, impurities, and adventitious agents, and the potential of the vaccine directly or indirectly to trigger other preexisting conditions.[14] In general, vaccine toxicology is assessed in single-dose and repeat-dose studies in two mammalian species, typically one rodent and one nonrodent (often a nonhuman primate). The vaccine is usually given by the route of administration planned for clinical use and tested at the maximum proposed human dose. The repeat-dose studies typically include one dose more than anticipated for use in humans. The repeat-dose studies are aimed at determining a dose where no adverse effect is observed. The toxicology assessments generally include mortality, clinical signs, food consumption, body weight, temperature, clinical chemistry, hematology, gross pathology, and histopathology. Depending on the constituents of the candidate vaccine, other specific tests may be required, such as potential of a live viral vaccine to establish a persistent infection, a DNA vaccine to integrate into the host genome, or additional genetic and reproductive toxicology studies for vaccines that will potentially be administered to pregnant women.[15] Recent years have seen the development of new vaccine platforms, novel adjuvant systems, and unique delivery systems, and it is very likely that expanded safety testing will be required that is appropriate for the constituents and technology.[16] As one would expect, the more detailed the studies, the longer it takes for a vaccine to reach licensure, and this explains in part the ever-increasing timeline for the vaccine development pathway.

Preclinical immunogenicity studies focus on the importance of understanding the protective immune response. They involve investigations of the ability of the candidate vaccine to induce humoral and/or cellular immune responses, and the innate immune response, in relevant animal models. In an ideal situation, a vaccine immunogen will stimulate both neutralizing antibodies and a cell-mediated immune response that will stimulate long-term memory $CD8^+$ and $CD4^+$ T cells. With preclinical immunogenicity studies the aim is to demonstrate a protective immune response in an animal model that can be translated to a protective immune response in humans, both qualitatively and quantitatively. We often know a lot about the immune response induced by vaccine immunogens in common small-animal models, such as mice, but this is currently not matched by our knowledge in humans, and in some situations the mouse immune response is not representative of that seen in humans. However, recent years have seen a substantial move from obtaining data in small-animal models to equivalent studies in higher animals and humans.[17] Although these studies are very important in early preclinical development of a vaccine candidate, most are not undertaken under good laboratory practices or a comparable quality system and therefore have limited use for preclinical development towards licensure. Ultimately, the studies on the protective immune response will lead to the development of correlate(s) of protection. While the immune response is complex and many different parameters are measured, a correlate of protection has to be assessable by uniform assays. Candidate vaccines that reach studies in (nonhuman or human) primates are often referred to as being in "advanced development."

Clinical Research

The prelicensure evaluation of vaccines in humans proceeds in a stepwise manner through an increasingly complex series of clinical trials. The first studies, referred to as phase I trials, are safety and immunogenicity studies performed in a small number of closely monitored healthy volunteers, normally young adults. These are generally short-term studies that may examine a range of vaccine dosages. The study design may be uncontrolled open-label or more often are randomized, double-blind, placebo-controlled. Inclusion of a placebo group is important in assessing adverse events that may occur during the trial. As stated above, there is an expectation that all vaccines will be 100% safe with no adverse events associated with immunization. Phase I clinical trials follow a similar approach for nearly all vaccines. Phase II studies involve larger numbers of healthy volunteers, possibly volunteers at risk for the target disease. The design may examine optimum dosage and dosing regimen and focus on safety and immunogenicity, and some efficacy data may be collected. These larger sample sizes provide greater power to detect less common adverse events. Phase II trials are randomized, blinded, and placebo-controlled. Phase III trials may enroll hundreds to thousands of individuals depending on the prevalence of the target disease. Generally thousands of volunteers are included in phase III trials in order to assess for rare adverse events. The phase III trials must be randomized, double-blinded, and placebo-controlled. For tropical diseases, the ability to undertake efficacy studies depends on the prevalence of the disease and the capacity to have strong epidemiologic data on incidence in areas where clinical trials will be undertaken. For some diseases, such as diarrheal diseases, this is relatively straightforward, while for other diseases, such as Ebola hemorrhagic fever, this is more difficult as the disease does not occur reproducibly over periods of time, the geographic location varies, and the relative numbers of cases are small.

Following successful completion of the clinical trials program, the next step in the vaccine development pathway is submission of a biologics license application (BLA) or the equivalent to the NRA.[18] This includes product labeling, which should permit health care providers to understand the vaccine's proper use, its potential risks and benefits, information to be conveyed to patients and parents, and how to deliver the vaccine safely. Because the safety of a vaccine may not be apparent until it is used widely in the population, approval of the new product may be contingent upon undertaking postmarketing studies, also referred to as phase IV studies. It should be noted that, in the United States, phase III clinical studies to provide data on safety in a statistically significant population size need to be completed before the application for a BLA, whereas, in Europe, phase III studies may be undertaken after the vaccine has been approved as postmarketing safety studies.

NATIONAL REGULATORY AUTHORITIES

NRAs and national control laboratories (NCLs) play a critical role in the vaccine development process as these entities will ultimately set the conditions for regulation, licensure, surveillance, and control of a vaccine in each country. The NRA ensures that the quality, manufacturing, storage, distribution, dispensing, efficacy, and safety of a vaccine are all appropriate for a particular vaccine product. The emphasis is often on consistency such that every lot of vaccine meets the same standards. The NCLs provide vaccine reference preparations, including antigen and antibody standards and other materials, for ensuring consistency in vaccines. These standards normally have defined biological activity expressed in international units so that vaccines manufactured by different producers in different countries can be compared and standardized. The NRAs and NCLs are critical as currently 55 countries have vaccine manufacturers, and there are at least 76 NRAs. The challenge for NRAs is to keep up with the continuing improvements in science and technology associated with the entire process of vaccine development.

With advances in vaccine development comes increased complexity, and this has resulted in the steady increase in requirements for each vaccine before licensure is approved. This is readily seen in the United States with the Food and Drug Administration and in Europe with the European Medicines Agency, but is also true of all NRAs. Due to the expanding global nature of the vaccine industry, multiple NRAs and rules present increasing challenges to the development and implementation of new vaccines. To address this growing problem, regulatory agencies and manufacturers in the United States, Europe, and Japan established the International Conference on Harmonization.[19] This is complemented by the WHO, which has the Global Training Network on Vaccine Quality that was established in 1996 with the aim of improving vaccine quality practices. In addition, the WHO Expert Committee on Biological Standardization consults and provides consensus views on important regulatory issues and provides guidance documents for use by NRAs and industry. These are published as Technical Report Series.[20] Another important consideration is that vaccines for tropical diseases require clinical trials to be undertaken in countries where the diseases are found while the vaccine may be manufactured in a different country. Thus, each NRA has a critical role in vaccine development. With this in mind, the Developing Countries Vaccine Regulators Network has been established to share the experiences of multiple countries and facilitate licensure of vaccines.

VACCINE DEVELOPMENT – PRIORITY DISEASES

In addition to information on currently available vaccines, the WHO plays a very active role in vaccine development with respect to the future

Table 10.3 Diseases for Vaccine Research and Development

Bacterial diseases	- Buruli ulcer *(Mycobacterium ulcerans)* - **Diphtheria** - Group A *Streptococcus*-associated diseases - Group B *Streptococcus*-associated diseases - ***Neisseria meningitidis*** meningitis (groups **A**, B, **C, Y, W-135**) - **Pertussis** - *Staphylococcus aureus*-associated diseases - Gastric cancer (*Helicobacter pylori*) - **Tetanus** - Trachoma
Enteric diseases	- Norovirus-associated diarrhea - *Campylobacter* diarrhea - **Cholera** - Enterotoxigenic *Escherichia coli* (ETEC) diarrhea - **Rotavirus** diarrhea - Shigellosis - **Typhoid** fever
Hepatitis	- **Hepatitis A** - **Hepatitis B** - Hepatitis C - Hepatitis E
Parasitic diseases	- Amebiasis - Hookworm disease - Leishmaniasis - Malaria (pre-erythrocyte, blood, and sexual stages) - Schistosomiasis
Respiratory diseases	- ***Haemophilus influenzae B*** pneumonia and invasive disease - **Influenza** - **Measles** - **Mumps** - Parainfluenza-associated pneumonia (PIV-3) - **Pertussis** - Respiratory syncytial virus (RSV) pneumonia - Severe acute respiratory syndrome (SARS) - ***Streptococcus pneumoniae*** pneumonia and invasive disease - **Tuberculosis**
Sexually transmitted diseases	- Cervical cancer (**human papillomavirus**) - *Chlamydia trachomatis*-associated genital diseases - Gonorrhea - Herpes simplex type 2 genital ulcers - HIV/AIDS
Vector-borne viral diseases	- Dengue - **Japanese encephalitis** - **Tick-borne encephalitis** - West Nile virus-associated disease - **Yellow fever**
Cancer-related diseases	- Cervical cancer (**human papillomavirus**) (see sexually transmitted diseases, above) - Gastric cancer (*Helicobacter pylori*) - Liver cancer (**hepatitis B**) - Liver cancer (hepatitis C) - Nasopharyngeal cancer (Epstein–Barr virus)
Zoonotic diseases	- Anthrax - Crimean-Congo hemorrhagic fever - Ebola hemorrhagic fever - Hepatitis E diarrhea - Lassa fever - Leishmaniasis - Leptospirosis - Lyme disease - Marburg hemorrhagic fever - Plague - **Rabies** - Rift Valley fever - Tularemia
Other viral diseases	- **Mumps** - **Poliomyelitis** - **Rubella** - **Smallpox**

HIV/AIDS, human immunodeficiency virus/acquired immunodeficiency syndrome.
Diseases in **bold** have vaccines commercially available.
Experimental vaccines are available for diseases shown in *italic* as investigational new drugs (INDs).
(Modified from www.who.int/vaccine_research/diseases/portfolio/en/index.html.)

implementation of vaccines in advanced development. The WHO has identified 68 diseases where vaccines can reduce the morbidity and/or mortality (***Table** 10.3*). This is a large list and includes diseases where no commercial vaccines exist and vaccines that are already available but are not utilized to maximum effect in poor countries. The WHO has vaccine position papers on 21 of these diseases and agents (tuberculosis, cholera, diphtheria, Hib, hepatitis A, human papillomavirus, influenza, Japanese encephalitis, measles, meningococcal disease, mumps, pertussis, pneumococcus, polio, rabies, rotavirus, rubella, tetanus, typhoid, varicella, and yellow fever).

There are 24 diseases for which vaccine development is a priority, either as improved vaccines or as new vaccines (*Box 10.3*). For some of these diseases we already have vaccines (e.g., rabies and Japanese encephalitis), but the current vaccines are not affordable or cannot be manufactured at the large numbers of doses required for mass immunization campaigns. For other diseases, there are no vaccines currently available

Box 10.3 Priority Areas for Research and Development of New Vaccines

Diarrheal diseases	Malaria
Acute respiratory infections	Measles
Caliciviruses	Meningococcal vaccines
Campylobacter	Parainfluenza
Cholera	*Streptococcus pneumoniae*
Dengue	Rabies
Enterotoxigenic *Escherichia coli* (ETEC)	Rotavirus
Haemophilus influenzae	Respiratory syncytial virus (RSV)
Human immunodeficiency virus (HIV)	Severe acute respiratory syndrome (SARS)
Human papillomavirus	*Shigella*
Influenza	Tuberculosis
Japanese encephalitis	Typhoid

(e.g., respiratory syncytial virus), or there are vaccine candidates available that need further clinical development (e.g., malaria).

THE FUTURE

A combination of scientific, technologic, and economic advances in the last 30 years is leading to a very optimistic future for vaccines for tropical diseases. However, these are mostly based on candidate vaccines that are already in at least advanced-stage preclinical development. Major challenges remain for a number of infectious diseases where our understanding of an immunogen that induces protective immunity is very limited or the agent has evolved mechanisms of overcoming the host immune response. Many of these diseases are found in tropical countries, and new advances are needed in discovery/basic science to generate appropriate immunogens for development as candidate vaccines.

Access the complete reference list online at
http://www.expertconsult.com

Access the complete reference list online at http://www.expertconsult.com

CHAPTER 11

Tropical Infectious Diseases and Malignancy

Catherine de Martel • Silvia Franceschi • Julie Parsonnet

INTRODUCTION

Until a few decades ago, cancer was considered a disease of the industrialized world. This common wisdom stemmed from the belief that the modern lifestyle – with its cigarettes, highly refined diet, and exposure to environmental pollutants – was the preeminent cause of cancer, and that malignancy was the price paid for development. Indeed, annual age-standardized cancer mortality rates in industrialized nations regularly range above 100 per 100 000 population for females and 150 per 100 000 for males. In minority groups, mortality rates exceeding 300 have been reported.[1,2] In contrast, cancer incidence and mortality rates are lower in developing countries. For example, Sri Lanka reports mortality rates of 69.6 for males and 63.2 for females.[1]

Yet, although the proportion of all deaths due to cancer in industrialized nations still far exceeds that in developing tropical nations, it is incorrect to conclude that cancer is not an important concern in developing countries. In fact, developing countries already bear the brunt of the world's cancer. Of the estimated 10.9 million new cases of cancer diagnosed worldwide in 2002, 5.8 million (53.7%) occurred in the developing world. Moreover, the mortality and incidence of cancer in the developing world is grossly underestimated.[1] In most developing countries, cause of death statistics do not exist, and cancer registry coverage, although improving, is sparse and of poor quality. For instance, cancer registries currently encompass around 10% of the African population, compared to 99% of the North American population.[3,4] Cancer diagnoses, when registered, are often based on incomplete information, as diagnostic capabilities are limited and postmortem examinations are rare. Thus, the number, types, and distribution of cancer cases are not known with any reasonable degree of certainty. Vast inaccuracies in the estimates of the population that constitutes the denominator of incidence (or mortality) rates further blur the picture. Yet, despite these deficiencies in data, it is clear that among the elderly, cancer is a leading cause of death in the developing world as well as in the industrialized West.

With the registry information that is available, certain trends are apparent. The demographic and epidemiologic transitions that accompany economic development have led to a gradually increasing median age and a growing proportion of older individuals. At present, approximately 9% of the population of developing countries is over the age of 60; this figure is expected to rise to 20% by 2050.[5] This trend, together with growing tobacco use, urbanization, industrialization, and disposable income, foretells a rapid increase in chronic disease, including cancers, in all but the very poorest countries. Globally, cancer mortality is expected to approximately double by 2020; in the developing world, however, rates are expected to rise fivefold.[6] Nevertheless, it should not be assumed that populations of developing countries are homogeneous with respect to their cancer pattern. For a long time, investigators have recognized extreme differences in cancer prevalence between or even among populations. For example, in a study of bladder cancer in Durban, South Africa, 95% of the tumors in white Africans and 30% in black Africans were transitional cell carcinoma, whereas 53% of the black patients, but only 2% of the white Africans, had squamous cell carcinoma. Ova of *Schistosoma haematobium* were seen in microscopic sections of the bladder tumors in 85% of the patients with squamous cell carcinoma, but in only 10% of the patients with transitional cell carcinoma.[7] Such studies can be extremely useful in unraveling the etiology and epidemiology of cancer among populations by pinpointing differences in risk factors.

As an increasing proportion of the world's cancer burden falls on developing countries, the demand will grow for costly and sophisticated resources for diagnosis and treatment of malignancies. Low- and middle-income countries combined, representing 84% of the world's population, accounted for only 12% of global health spending in the year 2002.[8] The inevitable increase in cancer incidence in tropical countries in future decades will provide a powerful economic incentive to focus on prevention to any extent possible. The questions are: what should we prevent and how do we prevent it?

INFECTION AS A PREVENTABLE CAUSE OF CANCER

Acute infectious diseases, notably diarrheal diseases, malaria, human immunodeficiency virus (HIV), and tuberculosis, are universally recognized as the major cause of premature mortality in developing countries, particularly among infants and children. Ironically, it is now evident that, among adults, many cancers are also caused by infectious diseases. That infection might lead to malignancy is still often greeted with surprise and skepticism by individuals in developed countries, and betrays ignorance about cancers that afflict developing countries. Worldwide, infection is among the most important causes of cancer. Experts from the International Agency of Research on Cancer (IARC) estimated conservatively that 18% of all malignancies, 26% in developing countries, and as many as 36% in Africa were attributable to infectious agents in 2002.[9] The culpable agents are mainly *Helicobacter pylori*, human papillomavirus (HPV), and hepatitis B and C viruses (HBV and HCV), causing gastric, cervix uteri, and liver cancers, respectively. In terms of overall mortality age-adjusted numbers, cancers of the stomach for men and cervix uteri for women rank second and third worldwide, whereas liver cancer ranks third and sixth for men and women, respectively.[1] Thus, although cancer may be widely perceived as a consequence of industrial and environmental pollutants, in reality, infection with certain widespread pathogens is second only to smoking as a cause of death from malignancy (***Fig. 11.1***). In addition, certain parasites such as *Clonorchis sinensis*, *Opisthorchis viverrini*, or *Schistosoma haematobium* and viruses such as human T-cell leukemia virus type 1 (HTLV-1) are significant causes of cancer in restricted geographic areas.[10–12] Epstein–Barr virus (EBV) is unique in its ability to cause a broad range of cancers, including cancers of the nasopharynx, a large proportion of Hodgkin's and Burkitt's lymphoma, and a non-negligible fraction of

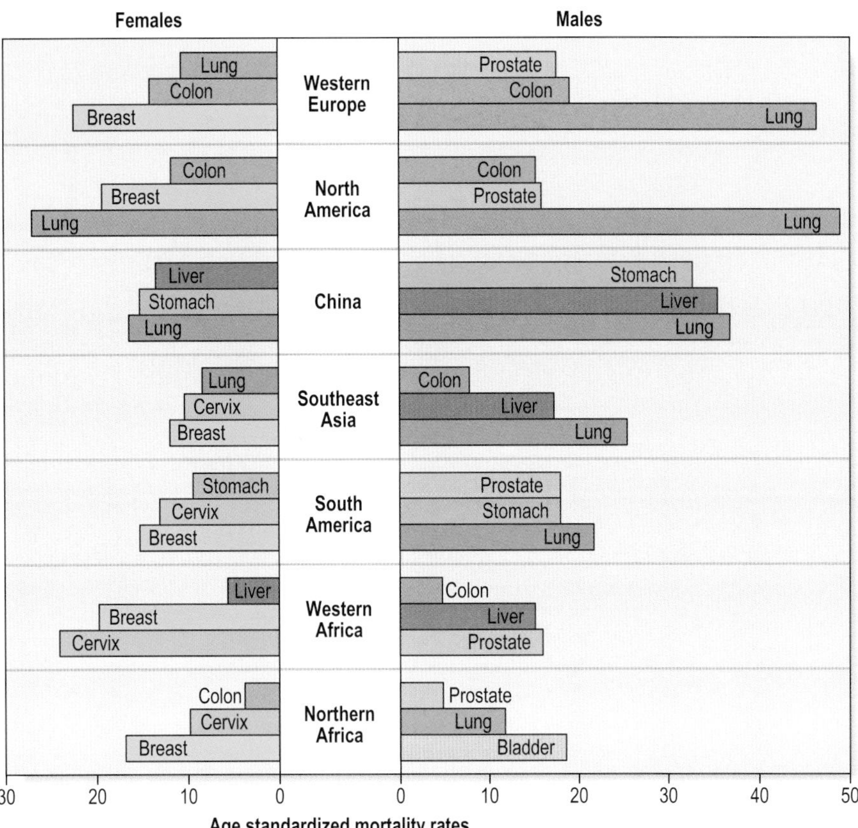

Figure 11.1 Estimates of the three leading causes of cancer death, by region. (Adapted from Ferlay J, Bray F, Pisani P, Parkin DM. GLOBOCAN 2002: Cancer Incidence, Mortality and Prevalence Worldwide, Version 2.0. IARC Cancer Base No. 5. Lyon: IARC Press; 2004.)

stomach cancer and non-Hodgkin's lymphoma (NHL) other than Burkitt's lymphoma.[9,13]

The impact of pathogen-induced malignancy is particularly pronounced in countries in the transition from low-to-medium-resource to high-resource economies. Adults in these populations who were infected with carcinogenic microbes such as HBV or *H. pylori* in childhood are experiencing a rapid increase in life expectancy. Since each year of chronic infection adds to the cumulative cancer risk, the number of cancer cases related to infection early in life would be expected to parallel the overall increase in longevity. The AIDS epidemic has also deeply affected the distribution of cancers worldwide by increasing the occurrence of cancers known or suspected to be of infectious origin.[14] Risk for Kaposi's sarcoma (KS) and NHL is multiplied 100-fold in immunosuppressed patients. In Africa, and especially in sub-Saharan Africa where the AIDS epidemic is raging, KS is the most common cancer in males and one of the most common in females.[4] To a lesser extent, Hodgkin's lymphoma and cancers of the cervix uteri and anus are also fostered by HIV-related immunosuppression.[15–17] Although antiretroviral therapy, where it is available, has diminished the incidence of some cancers associated with severe immunosuppression (i.e., KS, brain or immunoblastic NHL), antiretroviral therapy has not yet shown a beneficial effect on other cancers (i.e., cervix uteri).[17]

In many respects, the predominance of infection-related cancer can be looked upon as good news. Infectious diseases are often preventable or treatable. Consequently, knowledge of specific infectious causes and the epidemiology of the pathogens involved provides a blueprint for control of those particular malignancies. The feasibility of control is demonstrated by the dramatic decline in infection-related malignancy in industrialized nations. Gastric cancer, for example, was among the leading causes of cancer death in the United States as recently as 1945, but now is far less common. The decline of cancer at this site occurred without the benefit of vaccines or specific interventions. General improvements in socioeconomic status, sanitation, and hygiene appear to be responsible for a substantial reduction in many infection-related malignancies, as they are for many acute infectious diseases in industrialized nations.

It is important to note, however, that chronic infections are not the only important class of carcinogenic exposure in developing countries. Throughout the world, the threat from cigarette smoking cannot be overstressed. Lung cancer alone accounts for 12.4% of all new malignancies diagnosed worldwide.[1] Where cigarettes may have been too expensive for the average person to purchase two or three decades ago, the epidemic is still less pronounced. But as socioeconomic conditions improve, corresponding increases in cigarette smoking augur poorly for the future.[18] In China, for instance, the increase in tobacco smoking and tobacco-related death parallels that seen in the United States, with a 40-year offset.[19] This rise may translate into several hundred million deaths from tobacco-related diseases in 2030.

Alcohol consumption is also strongly associated with cancer risk, notably of the upper aero-digestive tract and liver sites, as illustrated recently in a population-based study in Russia.[20] Also important is the relative absence of fresh fruits and vegetables from the diets of poorer countries. Exposure to dietary carcinogens such as mycotoxins (e.g., aflatoxin), nitrates, and salt also magnifies cancer risk. Thus, although cancers related to infection may be quite common in developing countries, attention must be paid to other factors that can also be addressed by public health interventions.

INFECTIONS THAT CAUSE CANCER

Many infectious agents have been posited to cause cancer. The IARC reviews epidemiologic and basic science information on suspected cancer-causing agents on a regular basis. It then classifies these agents as definite, probable, possible, not classifiable, or unlikely causes of cancer (group 1, 2A, 2B, 3, and 4, respectively). To date, international experts have carried out extensive evaluations of liver flukes, schistosomes, *H. pylori*,

Organism	IARC Classification[a]	Tumor Sites with Sufficient Evidence for Carcinogenicity in Humans	Attributable Fraction[b]
Viruses			
Hepatitis B virus	Group 1	Hepatocellular carcinoma	54%
Hepatitis C virus	Group 1	Hepatocellular carcinoma	31%
		Non-Hodgkin's lymphoma	NS
Alpha papillomaviruses (HPV) types			Cervical cancer: 100% for all viruses
HPV16	Group 1	Cervical, anogenital cancers	
HPV18, 31, 33, 35, 39, 45, 51, 52, 56, 58, 59	Group 1	Cervical cancers	
HPV68	Group 2A	Cervical cancers	
HPV26, 53, 66, 67, 70, 73, 82, 30, 34, 69, 85, 97	Group 2B	Cervical cancers	
HPV6, 11	Group 3	Cervical cancers	
Beta papillomaviruses types			
HPV5, 8	Group 2B	Skin cancers	NS
Human T-cell leukemia virus type 1 (HTLV-1)	Group 1	Adult T-cell leukemia and lymphoma	1%
Epstein–Barr virus	Group 1	Burkitt's lymphoma	81%
		Other non-Hodgkin's lymphoma	NS
		Hodgkin's disease	46%
		Nasopharyngeal carcinoma	98%
Human herpesvirus 8 (HHV-8)	Group 1	Kaposi's sarcoma	100%
Human immunodeficiency virus 1 (HIV-1) (indirect action through immunosuppression)	Group 1	Kaposi's sarcoma	100%
		Non-Hodgkin's lymphoma	NS
		Hodgkin's disease	NS
		Cervical, anal cancers	NS
		Conjunctival cancers	NS
Human immunodeficiency virus 2 (HIV-2)	Group 2A	Immunodeficiency related cancers	
Bacteria			
Helicobacter pylori	Group 1	Non-cardia gastric carcinoma	74–78%
		Gastric lymphoma	74–79%
Other *Helicobacter* spp.	NS	Cholangiocarcinoma, biliary tract	NS
Campylobacter jejuni	NS	Immunoproliferative small intestinal disease	NS
Mycobacterium ulcerans	NS	Squamous cell carcinoma (skin)	NS
Salmonella enterica serovar Typhi	NS	Cholangiocarcinoma	NS
Chronic or recurrent urinary tract infections	NS	Bladder cancer	NS
Chronic osteomyelitis or wound infections	NS	Squamous cell carcinoma	NS
Parasites			
Opisthorchis viverrini	Group 1	Cholangiocarcinoma	NS
Clonorchis sinensis	Group 1	Cholangiocarcinoma	NS
Schistosoma haematobium	Group 1	Bladder cancer	4%
Schistosoma japonicum	Group 2B	Hepatocellular and rectal cancers	NS

Table 11.1 Infectious Agents Purported to Cause Malignancy

[a]From "Overall Evaluations of Carcinogenicity to Humans" as evaluated in IARC Monographs Volumes 1–100; Bouvard V, Baan R, Straif K, et al. A review of human carcinogens – Part B: biological agents. Lancet Oncol 2009;10(4):321–322.
[b]From Parkin DM. The global health burden of infection-associated cancers in the year 2002. Int J Cancer 2006;118(12):3030–3044.
NS, not specified.

HBV, HCV, human herpesvirus 8 (HHV-8), HPV, HTLV, HIV, and EBV (*Table 11.1*).[21] Other infectious agents that have not yet been evaluated by the IARC, but are suspected to cause cancer, are listed in *Table 11.1*. Because the great majority of these pathogens are reviewed elsewhere in this book, we will not discuss their biological or epidemiological characteristics or clinical manifestations. Instead, we focus here on the general features and control of the infection-induced malignancies.

All types of oncogenic agents enhance cell proliferation. The mechanisms by which this occurs can be quite variable, however, ranging from induction by viral oncogenes of cell growth factors to stimulation of growth by inflammatory intermediaries. A simplified scheme of infection-related oncogenesis can be used to categorize the malignancies into one of two types: either tumors caused by the integration of oncogenic DNA into the host cell, or those induced by chronic inflammation. Agents with oncogenes directly immortalize cells, while inflammatory carcinogenic agents do not. Immunosuppression may be important for development of malignancies related to oncogene integration. This is not thought to be always the case for inflammation-related malignancy. Transplant recipients and HIV-infected people, for instance, show neither an excess nor a lack of stomach cancer.[14] Finally, cancers related to infection appear to occur only after a long incubation period, with the remarkable exception of a few viruses and cancers, e.g., the short incubation period between EBV infection and the development of Burkitt's lymphoma in young children in sub-Saharan Africa, and the rapid onset of KS and NHL after organ transplantation.[14]

The importance of chronic inflammation in inducing cancer was first exemplified by two diseases not uncommon to the tropics: chronic, draining osteomyelitis and Buruli ulcers (caused by *Mycobacterium ulcerans*) (see Chapter 36). These chronic, inflammatory conditions, if left untreated, cause aggressive squamous cell carcinomas.[22] In each instance, carcinogenesis appears to depend not on specific oncogenic genes or gene products produced by the infectious agent, but rather on the organism's ability to persist despite the host's efforts to combat its presence. Inflammation is thought to induce cancer by stimulating production of reactive oxygen and nitrogen species that damage DNA, proteins, and membranes. Proliferation is a pro-mutagenic effect, permitting more cells to be susceptible to DNA damage and mutation. It also fosters selective growth of mutant clones.[23–27] We now recognize that many infections, including *H. pylori*, *S. haematobium*, *O. viverrini*, and HBV, are at least in part linked to cancer by their ability to foster an inflammatory response. In support of this, phenotypes of *H. pylori* that cause more inflammation are more closely related to malignancy.[28,29] Treatment of *S. haematobium* leads to marked decreases in inflammatory cells within the bladder, and associated declines in chromosomal damage.[30]

Mechanisms for lymphomagenesis are different from those for epithelial tumors. In the context of chronic inflammation, B-cell migration and proliferation are driven by T cells stimulated by a locally persistent antigen, such as *H. pylori* in the stomach.[31] This chronic lymphoid stimulation can eventually lead to B-cell mucosa-associated lymphoid tissue (MALT) lymphomas as first described in the stomach and since then at several cancer sites (e.g., in the small intestine with *Campylobacter jejuni*, or in the ocular adnexa with *Chlamydia psittaci*).[32–34]

Some oncogenic viruses, such as HPV and EBV, may lead more directly to cancer by integration of viral oncogenes or oncogene promoters into nuclear DNA. Resultant viral oncoproteins interact with and inactivate host tumor suppressor proteins such as p53, uncoupling normal growth control processes and leading to cellular transformation.[35,36] Oncogenic viruses can also induce production of cell growth factors, stimulating the host cell's reproduction, and accordingly their own. Other viruses, such as HIV, are not direct carcinogens but, by limiting the host's immune response, foster carcinogenic effects of relatively quiescent infectious agents. For example, HIV-related cellular immunodeficiency fosters carcinogenesis by EBV and HHV-8, viruses that are seldom carcinogenic in immunocompetent hosts, but frequently cause NHL and KS in immunosuppressed people.[14]

The etiology of infection-induced cancer is made more complex by the multifactorial causes of certain tumors on the one hand, and multiple outcomes following certain infections on the other. The importance of a specific agent in causing malignancy (its "attributable risk") depends on its prevalence (***Fig. 11.2***).[37] For example, in high-incidence areas of hepatitis, primary hepatocellular carcinoma (HCC) is commonly associated with chronic infection with HBV or HCV. In general, HBV is the main virus found in HCC cases in Asian, African, and Latin American countries, whereas HCV predominates in Japan, Pakistan, Mongolia, and Egypt.[38] In areas where hepatitis viruses are less prevalent, they will be a less common factor in HCC. In Sweden, for example, Widell and colleagues tested 95 sera from 299 HCC patients for serological or immunological signs of such infection.[39] They found only 5% HBV infection and 17% HCV infection, but almost 80% of the cases were seronegative for both viruses. Thus, chronic viral hepatitis appeared to play a minor role in induction of HCC in Sweden, where alcohol-related cirrhosis is a much more common risk factor.

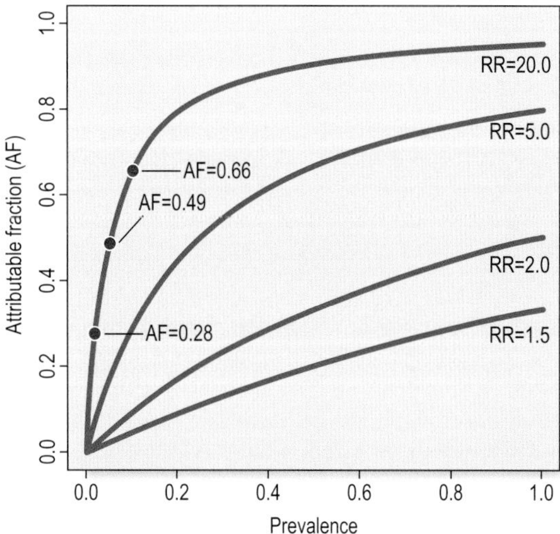

Figure 11.2 The fraction of disease attributable to a given risk factor (i.e., infection) is a function of the prevalence and the relative risk (RR) of exposure to this risk factor. Underestimation of the prevalence and/or RR can lead to the underestimation of the corresponding attributable fraction (AF). This is especially true for infections with low prevalence rates and strong associations with cancer, for example hepatitis C virus. (From de Martel C, Franceschi S. Infections and cancer: established associations and new hypotheses. Crit Rev Oncol Hematol 2009;70(3):183–194.)

Like any other cause of cancer, infections may be important, even necessary, but not sufficient for the induction of cancer. Just as most smokers do not get lung cancer, most infections with potentially carcinogenic pathogens do not proceed to a malignancy. For example, the large and diverse group of HPVs is implicated in causation of a variety of proliferative conditions, some of which (warts, epithelial cysts, intraepithelial neoplasias, anogenital, orolaryngeal and oropharyngeal papillomas, keratoacanthomas, and other types of hyperkeratoses) are relatively benign.[40] Virtually all cancers of the cervix uteri and more than 50% of other anogenital cancers may be attributed to certain high-risk HPV types that may act as solitary carcinogens or in concert with cofactors.[9] The progression of HPV-associated squamous epithelial lesions to cervical cancer is enhanced by smoking, use of hormonal contraception, or certain concurrent sexually transmitted agents, such as herpes simplex virus or chlamydia, and is clearly associated with HIV-induced immunosuppression.[41–43] Similarly, heavy exposure to aflatoxin B1 is widely considered to be a cocarcinogen with HBV; although either is capable of inducing HCC, the combination appears to behave synergistically in regions where both agents are endemic.[44] Although 90% of the world's population is thought to be infected with EBV, the two tumors classically linked to EBV occur in limited geographic areas. Burkitt's lymphoma is found in hyperendemic malarial areas of Africa and New Guinea, and nasopharyngeal carcinoma in parts of Southeast Asia, northern Africa and among the Inuit population, suggesting the presence of genetic susceptibility or other geographic cofactors.[45,46]

PREVENTION OF INFECTION-RELATED MALIGNANCIES

Each carcinogenic pathogen has unique features that may facilitate or frustrate efforts to control or prevent the associated cancers. Yet, of the many oncogenic infections, only for EBV infection is primary prevention impossible to attain by available public health measures.

Prevention at the primary level – that is, by blocking an initial infection – may be accomplished in the case of HBV by immunization of infants with a recombinant DNA or plasma-derived vaccine. The HBV vaccine has already proved effective in protecting inoculated children against chronic carriage and HCC.[47,48] In Taiwan, an intensive vaccination program in newborns began in 1984. The incidence of HCC in children 6–9 years of age declined from 0.51 per 100 000 children for those born before the program to 0.15 for those born after, a reduction by a factor of four.[49] Since 1991, the HBV vaccine is recommended as part of the WHO's Expanded Programme on Immunizations. It is currently given as part of routine childhood immunizations in 164 countries with a global coverage rising from 15% in 1996 to around 60% in 2006. The other tremendous accomplishment in primary prevention concerns cancer of the cervix uteri. A vaccine against the two main oncogenic HPV types (16 and 18, which account for at least 70% of cervical cancers) is now available, with efficacy trials showing a protection of more than 95% among HPV-uninfected young women.[50] Other efforts are under way to develop vaccines against infectious agents, including HCV and *H. pylori*.[51,52] Unfortunately, vaccine development often constitutes high-risk financial research for pharmaceutical companies. In helminthology, in particular, a dearth of research activity renders the prospect of successful vaccines remote.

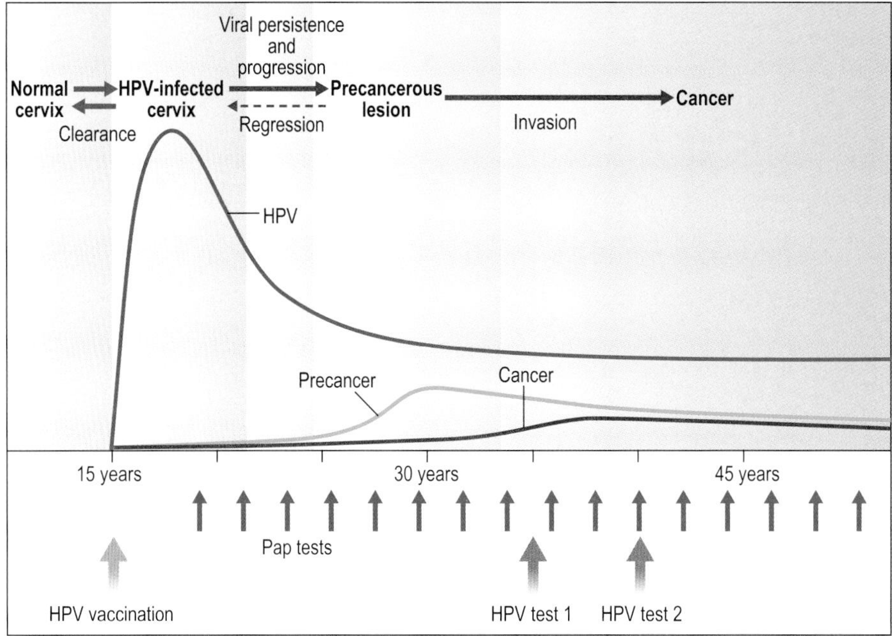

Figure 11.3 The natural history of human papillomavirus (HPV) infection and cervical cancer. The peak prevalence of transient infections with carcinogenic types of HPV (blue line) occurs among women during their teens and twenties, after the initiation of sexual activity. The peak prevalence of cervical precancerous conditions occurs approximately 10 years later (green line) and the peak prevalence of invasive cancers at 40–50 years of age (red line). (The peaks of the curves are not drawn to scale.) The conventional model of cervical cancer prevention is based on repeated rounds of cytologic examination, including Papanicolaou smears, and colposcopy (small blue arrows). Alternative strategies include HPV vaccination of adolescents (large beige arrow), one or two rounds of HPV screening at the peak ages of treatable precancerous conditions and early cancer (large reddish-brown arrows), or both. (Schiffman M, Castle PE. The promise of global cervical-cancer prevention. N Engl J Med 2005;353(20):2101–2104)

If a vaccine is available, it has to be proved cost-effective to be widely implemented. Rupnow and colleagues evaluated whether a *H. pylori* vaccine could be a cost-effective strategy for gastric cancer prevention in the United States, where US$50 000 is considered a reasonable amount to pay for 1 year of life. Despite the low incidence of gastric cancer in the US population, a vaccine administered to infants would be cost-effective, with a time horizon beyond 40 years.[53] In industrialized nations such as Japan, where gastric cancer rates are higher, it is likely that a national vaccination program would be even more warranted. However, it is probable that very few developing countries will be able to afford such vaccine without substantial financial help.

In the absence of vaccines, primary prevention depends largely on global public health measures and education. Prevention programs for schistosomiasis include education of the public in proper disposal of excreta to avoid contact with contaminated water. Infection with the oriental liver flukes *O. viverrini* and *C. sinensis* (see Chapter 123) can be prevented by refraining from eating raw or partially fermented freshwater fish. Educational campaigns in endemic areas of northeastern Thailand and elsewhere, however, have had only limited success in dislodging long-ingrained traditional dietary practices. *H. pylori* infection appears to diminish in conjunction with improved household sanitation and hygiene. The spread of sexually transmitted and bloodborne infections can be greatly reduced by "safe sex" and "safe injection" practices, together with systematic testing of blood supplies, and drug rehabilitation programs. Campaigns against overuse of injected medications could also be extremely useful in developing countries where there is a popular belief that injections are preferable to oral medication.

Secondary prevention, intended to impede the development of an existing infection to an advanced stage, is the rationale behind screening programs such as the Papanicolaou smear for signs of premalignant changes that may lead to cervical cancer. This cancer prevention strategy has proved an extraordinarily cost-effective method of health promotion. Where the Papanicolaou smear is widely employed, cervical cancer deaths have plummeted. Moreover, since certain types of HPV have been identified as a necessary cause of cervical cancer, a combination of primary prevention through vaccination and secondary preventive screening for carcinogenic HPV in older women will likely eliminate cervical cancer as a major threat to women[54,55] (*Fig. 11.3*). Some preliminary studies also suggest that therapeutic vaccines may have a role to play in regression of cervical lesions related to HPV in humans.[56–59] Other secondary prevention strategies include case finding, and treatment of infections that cause cancers (i.e., trematode, or *H. pylori*). Although there is no curative treatment for HIV, tremendous progress has been made in recent years in delivering antiretroviral treatment, even in some low-resource areas. Control of HIV has proved an effective way to limit immunosuppression-related malignancies. New perspectives for HCV treatment (see Chapter 65), for instance using small-molecule inhibitors, have shown promise in clinical trials that could translate into cancer prevention within a few years.[60]

The epidemiology of carcinogenic pathogens is closely related to the social and economic characteristics of the human populations that harbor them. As these characteristics evolve, disease prevalence will also change even without biomedical intervention. For example, the disappearance of *H. pylori* from industrialized Western countries occurred without any specific intervention, indeed, without even the knowledge that the organism existed. Just as the rainforest flora transform following subtle human disturbances, we can expect our own resident human flora to evolve with changes in behavior, social structure, sanitation, and environmental context. As old organisms wane and new organisms emerge, we can anticipate further changes in the epidemiology of infection-induced malignancies.

Access the complete reference list online at **http://www.expertconsult.com**

CHAPTER 12

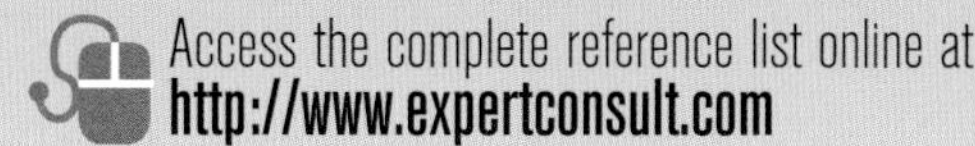
Access the complete reference list online at
http://www.expertconsult.com

Chemotherapy of Parasitic Diseases

Richard D. Pearson • Peter F. Weller • Richard L. Guerrant

INTRODUCTION

Many drugs are used in treating parasitic diseases, which is not surprising given the genetic diversity and varying life cycles of parasites. Treatment of helminth infections is summarized in sections on intestinal and systemic nematodes, trematodes, and cestodes. Therapy of protozoan infections follows and is divided into the treatment of malaria, luminal parasites, the kinetoplastida, and other systemic protozoan infections. More complete discussions of the pharmacology and mechanisms of action of the antiparasitic drugs can be found elsewhere.[1] Substantial additional information about indications, dosing, and toxicity is available in the pathogen-specific chapters and in the *Medical Letter on Drugs and Therapeutics*, Drugs for parasitic infections (www.medicalletter.org),[2] as summarized in the tables in this chapter.

TREATMENT OF INTESTINAL NEMATODES

The benzimidazoles, albendazole and mebendazole, have broad spectra of activities against intestinal nematodes, including *Ascaris lumbricoides,* the hookworms *Ancylostoma duodenale* and *Necator americanus, Trichuris trichiura, Enterobius vermicularis,* and others (***Table 12.1***). Pyrantel pamoate is active against the hookworms, *A. lumbricoides, E. vermicularis*, and some other intestinal nematodes, but it is not effective against *T. trichiura*. The benzimidazoles and pyrantel pamoate have replaced a number of older anthelminthics such as piperazine, which were more toxic or less effective. Resistance to the benzimidazoles, observed in veterinary pathogens, has not yet emerged as a problem among nematodes that infect humans. Ivermectin is the recommended treatment of *Strongyloides stercoralis.* Albendazole is an alternative. In immunocompromised persons or those with disseminated strongyloidiasis, prolonged or combined therapy with both drugs is often used. Thiabendazole, previously the drug of choice for strongyloidiasis, has substantial untoward effects and is no longer available in the United States. Either albendazole or ivermectin can be used for treating cutaneous larva migrans.

Albendazole, because of its broad spectrum of activity and favorable pharmacokinetics, is the drug of choice for many helminthic infections.[2,3] It has activity against the common soil-transmitted nematodes. A single dose is curative in approximately 90% of *A. lumbricoides* infections, 75% of hookworm infections, and 30% of *T. trichiura* infections.[4] In persons who are not cured, worm burdens are substantially reduced. Mass treatment programs employing a single dose of albendazole 400 mg have improved the nutritional status and fitness of children infected with *A. lumbricoides*, hookworms, and/or *T. trichiura*.[5] Albendazole should be given daily for 3 days in those with heavy *T. trichiura* infections. Reinfection is common in highly endemic settings, and retreatment at intervals of several months is recommended. Albendazole is effective in treating cutaneous larva migrans.[6] It is used at higher dosage and for longer duration for echinococcal infections,[7,8] neurocysticercosis,[9] and trichinellosis. Albendazole is also used for the treatment of intestinal microsporidiosis due to *Encephalitozoon (Septata) intestinalis* and ocular and disseminated microsporidia infections, but not all microsporidia are susceptible.[10]

Albendazole binds to tubulin in susceptible parasites, inhibits microtubule assembly, decreases glucose absorption, and inhibits fumarate reductase in helminths. It does not inhibit glucose metabolism in humans. Albendazole is poorly water-soluble, but it is well absorbed when administered with a fatty meal. There is rapid first-pass metabolism in the liver to albendazole sulfoxide, which has excellent anthelminthic activity. The serum half-life of albendazole sulfoxide is 8–9 hours, and the concentration in cerebrospinal fluid (CSF) is approximately 40% of that in serum. Concurrent administration of dexamethasone, often administered to patients being treated for neurocysticercosis, increases serum levels by approximately 50%.[11] Concentrations of albendazole sulfoxide in echinococcal cysts are approximately 25% of those in serum. Elimination of albendazole sulfoxide and other metabolites is primarily through the kidney.

Albendazole is usually well tolerated when given as a single dose for the treatment of soil-transmitted intestinal nematode infections, although some patients develop gastrointestinal (GI) discomfort or experience migration of adult *A. lumbricoides* from the nose or mouth or in the stool. Albendazole is embryotoxic in animals and contraindicated during pregnancy. High-dose, prolonged therapy for echinococcal disease or other indications is occasionally complicated by alopecia, bone marrow suppression, or hepatocellular injury.

Mebendazole, administered twice daily for 3 days, was widely used for the treatment of *Ascaris lumbricoides,* the hookworms *Ancylostoma duodenale* and *Necator americanus, Trichuris trichiura,* and *Enterobius vermicularis* prior to the introduction of albendazole.[12] A single dose of mebendazole 500 mg has been used in mass treatment programs for soil-transmitted helminths. Mebendazole also kills the adult and has some activity against invasive larvae of *Trichinella spiralis*.[13] Like albendazole, mebendazole selectively binds to helminthic tubulin, blocks its assembly into microtubules, and inhibits glucose uptake, leading to depletion of glycogen stores and ultimately parasite death. Glucose metabolism is not affected in humans.

Mebendazole is only slightly soluble in water and is relatively poorly absorbed from the GI tract,[12] which limits its effectiveness against tissue-dwelling helminths. The serum half-life of absorbed drug is 2.5–5.5 hours. Mebendazole is metabolized in the liver and excreted in the urine. Mebendazole is relatively well tolerated in the doses used to treat intestinal nematodes. Transient abdominal pain and diarrhea occur in small numbers of recipients. Prolonged, high-dose therapy used in the treatment of echinococcal liver cysts has been associated with alopecia, hepatocellular injury, and bone marrow suppression. Mebendazole is contraindicated during pregnancy.

Thiabendazole has a broad spectrum of anthelminthic activity, but because of its toxicity, its use has been limited to strongyloidiasis. Nausea, vomiting, diarrhea, dizziness, tinnitus, and other neurological side effects,

Table 12.1 Treatment of Nematode (Roundworm) Infections

Infection	Drug	Adult Dosage	Pediatric Dosage
***Ancylostoma caninum* Infection (Eosinophilic Enterocolitis)**			
Drug of choice	Albendazole[a]	400 mg once	400 mg once
	or mebendazole	100 mg bid × 3 days	100 mg bid × 3 days
	or pyrantel pamoate[a]	11 mg/kg (max. 1 g) × 3 days	11 mg/kg (max. 1 g) × 3 days
	or endoscopic removal		
***Ancylostoma duodenale*, see Hookworm Infection**			
Angiostrongyliasis (*Angiostrongylus cantonensis, A. costaricensis*)[b]			
Anisakiasis (*Anisakis* spp.)			
Treatment of choice	Surgical or endoscopic removal[c]		
Ascariasis (*Ascaris lumbricoides*, Roundworm)			
Drug of choice[e]	Albendazole[a]	400 mg once	400 mg once
	or mebendazole	100 mg bid × 3 days or 500 mg once	100 mg bid × 3 days or 500 mg once
	or ivermectin[a,d]	150–200 μg/kg once	150–200 μg/kg once
Capillariasis (*Capillaria philippinensis*)			
Drug of choice	Mebendazole[a]	200 mg bid × 20 days	200 mg bid × 20 days
Alternative	Albendazole[a]	400 mg daily × 10 days	400 mg daily × 10 days
Cutaneous Larva Migrans (Creeping Eruption, Dog and Cat Hookworm)			
Drug of choice	Albendazole[a]	400 mg daily × 3 days	400 mg daily × 3 days
	or ivermectin[a,d]	200 μg/kg daily × 1–2 days	200 μg/kg daily × 1–2 days
***Dracunculus medinensis* (Guinea Worm) Infection**			
Drug of choice	See footnote[e]		
***Enterobius vermicularis* (Pinworm) Infection**			
Drug of choice[f]	Mebendazole	100 mg once; repeat in 2 weeks	100 mg once; repeat in 2 weeks
	or pyrantel pamoate	11 mg/kg base once (max. 1 g); repeat in 2 weeks	11 mg/kg base once (max. 1 g); repeat in 2 weeks
	or albendazole[a]	400 mg once; repeat in 2 weeks	400 mg once; repeat in 2 weeks
Filariasis[g]			
• ***Wuchereria bancrofti, Brugia malayi, B. timori***			
Drug of choice[h]	Diethylcarbamazine[i,j]	6 mg/kg/day in 3 doses × 12 days	6 mg/kg/day in 3 doses × 12 days

[a]An approved drug but considered investigational for this condition by the Food and Drug Administration.

[b]*A. cantonensis* causes predominantly neurotropic disease. *A. costaricensis* causes gastrointestinal disease. Most patients infected with either species have a self-limited course and recover completely. Analgesics, corticosteroids, and careful removal of cerebrospinal fluid at frequent intervals can relieve symptoms from increased intracranial pressure (Lo Re V III and Gluckman SL. Am J Med. 2003;114:217). Treatment of *A. cantonensis* is controversial and varies across endemic areas. No anthelminthic drug is proven to be effective and some patients have worsened with therapy (Slom TJ, et al. N Engl J Med. 2002;346:668). Mebendazole and a corticosteroid, however, appear to shorten the course of infection (Tsai H-C, et al. Am J Med. 2001;111:109; Chotmongkol V, et al. Am J Trop Med Hyg. 2006;74:1122). Albendazole has also relieved symptoms of angiostrongyliasis (Chen XG, et al. Emerg Infect Dis. 2005;11:1645).

[c]Repiso Ortega A, et al. Gastroenterol Hepatol. 2003;26:341. Successful treatment of anisakiasis with albendazole 400 mg PO bid × 3–5 days has been reported, but the diagnosis was presumptive (Moore DA, et al. Lancet. 2002;360:54; Pacios E, et al. Clin Infect Dis. 2005;41:1825).

[d]Safety of ivermectin in young children (<15 kg) and pregnant women remains to be established. Ivermectin should be taken on an empty stomach with water.

[e]No drug is curative against *Dracunculus*. A program for monitoring local sources of drinking water to eliminate transmission has dramatically decreased the number of cases worldwide (Barry M. N Engl J Med. 2007;356:2561). The treatment of choice is slow extraction of the worm combined with wound care and pain management (Greenaway C. CMAJ. 2004;170:495).

[f]Since family members are usually infected, treatment of the entire household is recommended.

[g]Antihistamines or corticosteroids may be required to decrease allergic reactions to components of disintegrating microfilariae that result from treatment, especially in infection caused by *Loa loa*. Endosymbiotic *Wolbachia* bacteria may have a role in filarial development and host response, and may represent a potential target for therapy. Addition of doxycycline 100 or 200 mg/day × 6–8 weeks in lymphatic filariases and onchocerciasis has resulted in substantial loss of *Wolbachia* and decrease in both micro- and macrofilariae (Taylor MJ, et al. Lancet. 2005;365:2116; Debrah AY, et al. PloS Pathog. 2006;e92:0829); but use of tetracyclines is contraindicated in pregnancy and in children <8 years old.

[h]Most symptoms are caused by adult worm. A single-dose combination of albendazole (400 mg) with either ivermectin (200 μg/kg) or diethylcarbamazine (6 mg/kg is effective for reduction or suppression of *W. bancrofti* microfilaria, but the albendazole/ivermectin combination does not kill all the adult worms (Addiss D, et al. Cochrane Database Syst Rev. CD003753; 2004).

[i]For patients with microfilaria in the blood, *Medical Letter* consultants start with a lower dosage and scale up. d1: 50 mg; d2: 50 mg tid; d3: 100 mg tid; d4–14: 6 mg/kg in 3 doses (for *Loa Loa* d4–14: 9 mg/kg in 3 doses). Multidose regimens have been shown to provide more rapid reduction in microfilaria than single-dose diethylcarbamazine, but microfilaria levels are similar 6–12 months after treatment (Andrade LD, et al. Trans R Soc Trop Med Hyg. 1995;89:319; Simonsen PE, et al. Am J Trop Med Hyg. 1995;53:267). A single dose of 6 mg/kg is used in endemic areas for mass treatment (Figueredo-Silva J, et al. Trans R Soc Trop Med Hyg. 1996;90:192; Noroes J, et al. Trans R Soc Trop Med Hyg. 1997;91:78).

[j]Diethylcarbamazine should not be used for treatment of *Onchocerca volvulus* due to the risk of increased ocular side-effects including blindness associated with rapid killing of the worms. It should be used cautiously in geographic regions where *O. volvulus* coexists with other filariae. Diethylcarbamazine is contraindicated during pregnancy. See also footnote[o].

Table 12.1 Treatment of Nematode (Roundworm) Infections—cont'd

Infection	Drug	Adult Dosage	Pediatric Dosage
• ***Loa loa***			
Drug of choice[k]	Diethylcarbamazine[i,j]	6 mg/kg/day in 3 doses × 12 days	6 mg/kg/day in 3 doses × 12 days
• ***Mansonella ozzardi***			
Drug of choice[e]	See footnote[l]		
• ***M. perstans***			
Drug of choice[e]	Albendazole[a]	400 mg bid × 10 days	400 mg bid × 10 days
	or mebendazole[a]	100 mg bid × 30 days	100 mg bid × 30 days
• ***M. streptocerca***			
Drug of choice[m]	Diethylcarbamazine	6 mg/kg/day × 12 days[j]	6 mg/kg/day × 12 days[j]
	Ivermectin[a]	150 μg/kg once	150 μg/kg once
• **Tropical Pulmonary Eosinophilia (TPE)[n]**			
Drug of choice	Diethylcarbamazine	6 mg/kg/day in 3 doses × 12–21 days	6 mg/kg/day in 3 doses × 12–21 days
• ***Onchocerca volvulus* (River Blindness)**			
Drug of choice	Ivermectin[o]	150 μg/kg once, repeated every 6–12 months until asymptomatic	150 μg/kg once, repeated every 6–12 months until asymptomatic
Gnathostomiasis (*Gnathostoma spinigerum*)			
Treatment of choice[q]	Albendazole[a]	400 mg bid × 21 days	400 mg bid × 21 days
	or ivermectin[a]	200 μg/kg/day × 2 days	200 μg/kg/day × 2 days
	± surgical removal		
Gongylonemiasis (*Gongylonema* sp.)[p]			
Treatment of choice	Surgical removal		
	or albendazole[a]	400 mg × 3 days	400 mg × 3 days
Hookworm Infection (*Ancylostoma duodenale, Necator americanus*)			
Drug of choice	Albendazole[a]	400 mg once	400 mg once
	or mebendazole	100 mg bid × 3 days or 500 mg once	100 mg bid × 3 days or 500 mg once
	or pyrantel pamoate[a]	11 mg/kg (max. 1 g) × 3 days	11 mg/kg (max. 1 g) × 3 days
Moniliformis moniliformis			
Drug of choice	Pyrantel pamoate[a]	11 mg/kg once, repeat twice, 2 weeks apart	11 mg/kg once, repeat twice, 2 weeks apart
Oesophagostomum bifurcum			
Drug of choice	See footnote[q]		
Strongyloidiasis (*Strongyloides stercoralis*)			
Drug of choice[r]	Ivermectin	200 μg/kg/day × 2 days	200 μg/kg/day × 2 days
Alternative	Albendazole[a]	400 mg bid × 7 days	400 mg bid × 7 days

[k]In heavy infections with *Loa loa*, rapid killing of microfilarie can provoke encephalopathy. Apheresis has been reported to be effective in lowering microfilarial counts in patients heavily infected with *Loa loa* (Ottesen EA. Infect Dis Clin North Am. 1993;7:619). Albendazole may be useful for treatment of loiasis when diethylcarbamazine is ineffective or cannot be used, but repeated courses may be necessary (Klion AD, et al. Clin Infect Dis. 1999;29:680; Tabi TE, et al. Am J Trop Med Hyg. 2004;71:211). Ivermectin has also been used to reduce microfilaremia, but albendazole is preferred because of its slower onset of action and lower risk of precipitating encephalopathy (Klion AD, et al. J Infect Dis. 1993;168:202; Kombila M, et al. Am J Trop Med Hyg. 1998;58:458). Diethylcarbamazine, 300 mg PO once/week, has been recommended for prevention of loiasis (Nutman TB, et al. N Engl J Med. 1988;319:752).

[l]Diethylcarbamazine has no effect. A single dose of ivermectin 200 μg/kg reduces microfilaria densities and provides both short- and long-term reductions in *M. ozzardi* microfilaremia (Gonzalez AA, et al. W Indian Med J. 1999;48:231).

[m]Diethylcarbamazine is potentially curative due to activity against both adult worms and microfilariae. Ivermectin is active only against microfilariae.

[n]Boggild AK, et al. Clin Infect Dis. 2004;39:1123. Relapses occur and can be treated with a repeated course of diethylcarbamazine.

[o]Diethylcarbamazine should not be used for treatment of this disease because rapid killing of the worms can lead to blindness. Periodic treatment with ivermectin (every 3–12 months), 150 μg/kg PO, can prevent blindness due to ocular onchocerciasis (Udall DN. Clin Infect Dis. 2007;44:53). Skin reactions after ivermectin treatment are often reported in persons with high microfilarial skin densities. Ivermectin has been inadvertently given to pregnant women during mass treatment programs; the rates of congenital abnormalities were similar in treated and untreated women. Because of the high risk of blindness from onchocerciasis, the use of ivermectin after the first trimester is considered acceptable according to the World Health Organization. Doxycycline (100 mg/day for 6 weeks), followed by a single 150 μg/kg dose of ivermectin, resulted in up to 19 months of amicrofilaridermia and 100% elimination of *Wolbachia* species (Hoerauf A, et al. Lancet. 2001;357:1415).

[p]Wilson ME, et al. Clin Infect Dis. 2001;32:1378; Molavi G, et al. J Helminth. 2006;80:425.

[q]Albendazole or pyrantel pamoate may be effective (Ziem JB, et al. Ann Trop Med Parasitol. 2004;98:385).

[r]In immunocompromised patients or disseminated disease, it may be necessary to prolong or repeat therapy, or to use other agents. Veterinary parenteral and enema formulations of ivermectin have been used in severely ill patients with hyperinfection who were unable to take or reliably absorb oral medications (Orem J, et al. Clin Infect Dis. 2003;27:152; Tarr PE. Am J Trop Med Hyg. 2003;68:453; Marty FM, et al. Clin Infect Dis. 2005;41:e5). In disseminated strongyloidiasis, combination therapy with albendazole and ivermectin has been suggested (Lim S, et al. CMAJ. 2004;171:479).

Table 12.1 Treatment of Nematode (Roundworm) Infections—cont'd

Infection	Drug	Adult Dosage	Pediatric Dosage
Trichinellosis (*Trichinella spiralis*)			
Drug of choice	Steroids for severe symptoms *plus*		
	Albendazole[a]	400 mg bid × 8–14 days	400 mg bid × 8–14 days
Alternative	Mebendazole[a]	200–400 mg tid × 3 days, then 400–500 mg tid × 10 days	200–400 mg tid × 3 days, then 400–500 mg tid × 10 days
***Trichostrongylus* Infection**			
Drug of choice	Pyrantel pamoate[a]	11 mg/kg base once (max. 1 g)	11 mg/kg once (max. 1 g)
Alternative	Mebendazole[a]	100 mg bid × 3 days	100 mg bid × 3 days
	or albendazole[a]	400 mg once	400 mg once
Trichuriasis (*Trichuris trichiura*, Whipworm)			
Drug of choice	Mebendazole	100 mg bid × 3 days or 500 mg once	100 mg bid × 3 days or 500 mg once
Alternative	Albendazole[a]	400 mg × 3 days	400 mg × 3 days
	or ivermectin[a]	200 µg/kg/day × 3 days	200 µg/kg/day × 3 days
Visceral Larva Migrans (Toxocariasis)[s]			
Drug of choice	Albendazole[a]	400 mg bid × 5 days	400 mg bid × 5 days
	or mebendazole[a]	100–200 mg bid × 5 days	100–200 mg bid × 5 days

[s]Optimum duration of therapy is unknown; some consultants would treat for 20 days. For severe symptoms or eye involvement, corticosteroids can be used in addition (Despommier D. Clin Micro Rev. 2003;16:205).

(Derived from the *Medical Letter on Drugs and Therapeutics*, Drugs for parasitic infections, www.medicalletter.org, October 2008. Recommendations that differ from those of the Medical Letter are marked with an asterisk.)

as well as elevated liver enzymes, are common. It is contraindicated during pregnancy. Topically applied thiabendazole is well tolerated and effective in the treatment of cutaneous larva migrans.[14]

Pyrantel pamoate,[15] a depolarizing neuromuscular blocking agent, is active against *E. vermicularis*, the hookworms, and *A. lumbricoides*. It is poorly absorbed after oral administration and generally well tolerated. Some recipients experience transient GI side effects or, less commonly, headache, drowsiness, insomnia, dizziness, or hypersensitivity reactions. It is not recommended for use during pregnancy. Muscles of susceptible nematodes undergo depolarization and an increase in spike discharge frequency that leads to a short period of calcium-dependent stimulation resulting in irreversible paralysis. The worms are subsequently expelled in the feces. Pyrantel also inhibits helminth acetylcholinesterases. Piperazine, which paralyzes worms by causing hyperpolarization, and pyrantel are mutually antagonistic and should not be administered together.

Ivermectin, a macrocyclic lactone produced by *Streptomyces avermitilis*, has a broad spectrum of activity against helminths and arthropods. It is the preferred treatment of strongyloidiasis,[2,16,17] onchocerciasis, and cutaneous larva migrans. However, failures can occur in persons with strongyloidiasis, leading to the use of multiple doses or combination therapy with albendazole, particularly in immunocompromised patients with disseminated disease.[2] Ivermectin has activity against *Ascaris lumbricoides* and *Trichuris trichiura*, but not hookworms. It has activity against blood-sucking arthropods and can be used in the treatment of scabies and lice. Ivermectin, well absorbed after oral administration, is highly protein-bound, has a serum half-life of 12 hours, and accumulates in adipose tissue and in the liver. It is subject to enterohepatic recirculation and eliminated in the stool. Ivermectin activates the opening of gated-chloride channels in susceptible helminths and arthropods, resulting in an influx of chloride ions and paralysis of the pharyngeal pumping mechanism of helminths. It is generally well tolerated in persons treated for strongyloidiasis or scabies, but it can elicit pruritus, dizziness, and other symptoms in those with filarial diseases in response to dying parasites.

TREATMENT OF SYSTEMIC NEMATODES

Diethylcarbamazine is the drug of choice for several filarial infections, including *Wuchereria bancrofti*, *Brugia malayi*, *B. timori*, *Mansonella streptocerca*, and *Loa loa*, and for tropical pulmonary eosinophilia.[2,18] It has been used in combination with albendazole in single-dose, mass treatment programs[19] and even added to salt to control infection among residents in *W. bancrofti*-endemic areas. Diethylcarbamazine damages or kills adult worms of these species. While it is not directly toxic to microfilariae, it promotes their killing by the host's immune responses. Diethylcarbamazine can be used prophylactically to prevent *L. loa* infections in endemic areas. *Mansonella perstans* is sensitive to albendazole or mebendazole, but not diethylcarbamazine (see ***Table 12.1***). Of note, diethylcarbamazine kills microfilariae of *Onchocerca volvulus*, but it is not used for the treatment of onchocerciasis because the rapid release of parasite antigens along with lipopolysaccharide and other substances from *Wolbachia*, the endosymbionts that they harbor, can elicit severe systemic and ocular inflammatory reactions.[20] Ivermectin, which is associated with much less severe reactions, is the drug of choice. *Wolbachia* are also a potential target for treatment. Long-term administration of doxycycline, which is active against them, results in a substantial reduction in micro- and macrofilariae.[20]

Diethylcarbamazine, a piperazine derivative, is well absorbed orally and has a half-life of 8 hours. The parent drug and its metabolites are excreted through the kidney. Side effects include those due to the drug and those that result from the release of parasite antigens and *Wolbachia* lipopolysaccharide. They include nausea, vomiting, anorexia, headache, malaise, weakness, and arthralgias. In patients with *W. bancrofti* or *B. malayi* infection, localized swelling or nodules may develop along lymphatics during treatment, or there may be transient lymphedema or hydrocele formation. Diethylcarbamazine is no longer used in patients with onchocerciasis because it can elicit the Mazzotti reaction, which is characterized by hypotension, pruritus, fever, tachycardia, wheezing, chorioretinitis, and uveitis secondary to the release of microfilarial antigens and *Wolbachia* lipopolysaccharide. Life-threatening encephalopathy has been reported in patients with heavy *L. loa* infections who received the drug.

Ivermectin is the drug of choice for the treatment of onchocerciasis,[21,22] killing microfilariae in the skin and eye. It does not kill adult *O. volvulus*, but it decreases production of microfilariae. Retreatment is usually necessary at 6–12-month intervals. Ivermectin has activity against microfilaria of *W. bancrofti*, *B. malayi*, and *L. loa*, but it does not kill the adult worms and is not used in the treatment of these infections.

TREATMENT OF CESTODES AND TREMATODES

Among the platyhelminths, praziquantel[23,24] is the drug of choice for the treatment of all adult cestodes (tapeworms) in the human intestinal tract (*Table 12.2*). Niclosamide is active against human tapeworms as well, but prolonged therapy is necessary for *Hymenolepis nana*, the dwarf tapeworm, which is capable of autoinfection. Nitazoxanide, discussed later as an antiprotozoal drug, is an alternative for *H. nana*, and has activity against *Taenia saginata* and potentially other tapeworms. Both albendazole and praziquantel[25,26] can kill cysticerci of *T. solium* in the central nervous system (CNS) of humans. Albendazole is preferred for neurocysticercosis due to its favorable pharmacokinetics. Corticosteroids are typically administered concomitantly with anthelminthic drugs to reduce the inflammatory response elicited by released cysticercal antigens and the concomitant increase in intracranial pressure. The concurrent use of corticosteroids increases the serum level of albendazole and decreases that of praziquantel. Albendazole is also used for echinococcal diseases. Prolonged albendazole therapy cures approximately one-third of patients with *Echinococcus granulosus* cysts, and it is given prior to and during percutaneous drainage procedures or surgery to prevent seeding of the peritoneum. It is also used for the suppression of inoperable *E. granulosus* and *E. multilocularis* infections.

Praziquantel is the drug of choice for the treatment of *Schistosoma* species and most other trematodes (flukes) that infect humans (*Table 12.3*).[23,24] The principal exception is *Fasciola hepatica*, which responds to the veterinary fasciolide, triclabendazole, and to a lesser extent bithionol.[27,28] The adverse effects of these anthelminthic drugs are summarized in *Box 12.1*.

Praziquantel is rapidly taken up by susceptible platyhelminths. Studies of the tapeworm *Hymenolepis diminuta* indicate that it causes blebs in the neck of the tapeworm and the release of calcium from endogenous stores, which results in paralysis and expulsion of the worm from the GI tract.[29] In the case of schistosomes, praziquantel damages the tegument, resulting in intense vacuolation and increased permeability to calcium.[30] Adult schistosomes are paralyzed and translocated to the liver through the portal circulation. Sequestered antigens are exposed on the parasite's surface allowing for the binding of antibodies and phagocytes and immune destruction.

Praziquantel is well absorbed after oral administration. There is extensive first-pass metabolism, and the metabolites, which are inactive, are excreted in the urine. Praziquantel is approximately 80% protein-bound; the serum half-life is 4–6 hours. The concentration in the CSF is approximately 15–20% of that in plasma.[31] The concurrent administration of corticosteroids, which is often done in patients undergoing treatment for

Table 12.2 Treatment of Cestode (Tapeworm) Infections

Infection	Drug	Adult Dosage	Pediatric Dosage
Adult (Intestinal Stage)			
Diphyllobothrium latum (Fish), *Taenia saginata* (Beef), *T. solium* (Pork), *Dipylidium caninum* (Dog)			
Drug of choice	Praziquantel[a]	5–10 mg/kg once	5–10 mg/kg once
Alternative	Niclosamide	2 g once	50 mg/kg once
Hymenolepsis nana (Dwarf Tapeworm)			
Drug of choice	Praziquantel[a]	25 mg/kg once	25 mg/kg once
Alternative	Nitazoxanide[a,b]	500 mg once or bid × 3 days[c]	1–3 years: 100 mg bid × 3 days[c] 4–11 years: 200 mg bid × 3 days[c]
Larval (Tissue Stage)			
Echinococcus granulosus (Hydatid Cyst)			
Drug of choice[d]	Albendazole[a]	400 mg bid × 1–6 months	15 mg/kg/day (max. 800 mg) × 1–6 months
E. multilocularis			
Treatment of choice	See footnote[e]		
Taenia solium (Cysticercosis)			
Treatment of choice	See footnote[f]		
Alternative	Albendazole[a]	400 mg bid × 8–30 days; can be repeated as necessary	15 mg/kg/day (max. 800 mg) in 2 doses × 8–30 days; can be repeated as necessary
	or praziquantel[a]	100 mg/kg/day in 3 doses × 1 day, then 50 mg/kg/day in 3 doses for 29 days	100 mg/kg/day in 3 doses × 1 day, then 50 mg/kg/day in 3 doses × 29 days

[a]An approved drug but considered investigational for this condition by the Food and Drug Administration (FDA).

[b]Nitazoxanide may be effective against a variety of protozoan and helminth infections (Bobak DA. Curr Infect Dis Rep. 2006;8:91; Diaz E, et al. Am J Trop Med Hyg. 2003;68:384). Nitazoxanide is available in 500-mg tablets and an oral suspension; it should be taken with food.

[c]Juan JO, et al. Trans R Soc Trop Med Hyg. 2002;96:193; Chero JC, et al. Trans R Soc Trop Med Hyg. 2007;101:203; Diaz E, et al. Am J Trop Med Hyg. 2003;68:384).

[d]Patients may benefit from surgical resection or percutaneous drainage of cysts. Praziquantel is useful preoperatively or in case of spillage of cyst contents during surgery. Percutaneous aspiration–injection–reaspiration (PAIR) with ultrasound guidance plus albendazole therapy has been effective for management of hepatic hydatid cyst disease (Smego RA Jr, et al. Clin Infect Dis. 2003;37:1073; Nepalia S, et al. J Assoc Physicians India. 2006;54:458; Zerem E, Jusufovic R. Surg Endosc. 2006;20:1543).

[e]Surgical excision is the only reliable means of cure. Reports have suggested that in nonresectable cases use of albendazole (400 mg bid) can stabilize and sometimes cure infection (Craig P. Curr Opin Infect Dis. 2003;16:437; Lidove O, et al. Am J Med. 2005;118:195).

[f]Initial therapy for patients with inflamed parenchymal cysticerosis should focus on symptomatic treatment with antiseizure medication (Yancey LS, et al. Curr Infect Dis Rep. 2005;7:39; del Brutto AH, et al. Ann Intern Med. 2006;145:43). Patients with live parenchymal cysts who have seizures should be treated with albendazole together with steroids (dexamethasone 6 mg or 40–60 mg prednisone 40–60 mg daily) and an antiseizure medication (Garcia HH, et al. N Engl J Med. 2004;350:249). Patients with subarachnoid cysts or giant cysts in the fissures should be treated for at least 30 days (Proaño JV, et al. N Engl J Med. 2001;345:879). Surgical intervention (especially neuroendoscopic removal) or cerebrospinal fluid diversion followed by albendazole and steroids is indicated for obstructive hydocephalus. Arachnoiditis, vasculitis, or cerebral edema is treated with prednisone 60 mg/day or dexamethasone 4–6 mg/day together with albendazole or praziquantel (White AC, Jr. Annu Rev Med. 2000;51:187). Any cysticercoidal drug may cause irreparable damage when used to treat ocular or spinal cysts, even when corticosteroids are used. An ophthalmic exam should always precede treatment to rule out intraocular cysts.

(Derived from the *Medical Letter on Drugs and Therapeutics*, Drugs for parasitic infections, www.medicalletter.org, October 2008.)

Table 12.3 Treatment of Trematode (Fluke) Infections

Infection	Drug	Adult Dosage	Pediatric Dosage
Fluke, Hermaphroditic, Infection			
Clonorchis sinensis (Chinese Liver Fluke)			
Drug of choice	Praziquantel[a]	75 mg/kg/day in 3 doses × 2 days	75 mg/kg/day in 3 doses × 2 days
	or albendazole[a]	10 mg/kg × 7 days	10 mg/kg × 7 days
Fasciola hepatica (Sheep Liver Fluke)			
Drug of choice[b]	Triclabendazole	10 mg/kg once or twice[c]	10 mg/kg once or twice[c]
Alternative	Bithionol	30–50 mg/kg on alternate days × 10–15 doses	30–50 mg/kg on alternate days × 10–15 doses
	or Nitazoxanide[a]	500 mg bid × 7 days	1–3 years: 100 mg q 12h × 7 days 4–11 years: 200 mg q 12h × 7 days >12 years: 500 mg q 12h × 7 days
Fasciolopsis buski, Heterophyes heterophyes, Metagonimus yokogawai (Intestinal Flukes)			
Drug of choice	Praziquantel[a]	75 mg/kg/day in 3 doses × 1 day	75 mg/kg/day in 3 doses × 1 day
Metorchis conjunctus (North American Liver Fluke)[e]			
Drug of choice	Praziquantel[a]	75 mg/kg/day in 3 doses × 1 day	75 mg/kg/day in 3 doses × 1 day
Nanophyetus salmincola			
Drug of choice	Praziquantel[a]	60 mg/kg/day in 3 doses × 1 day	60 mg/kg/day in 3 doses × 1 day
Opisthorchis viverrini (Southeast Asian Liver Fluke)			
Drug of choice	Praziquantel[a]	75 mg/kg/day in 3 doses × 2 days	75 mg/kg/day in 3 doses × 2 days
Paragonimus westeramani (Lung Fluke)			
Drug of choice	Praziquantel[a]	75 mg/kg/day in 3 doses × 2 days	75 mg/kg/day in 3 doses × 2 days
Alternative[d]	Bithionol	30–50 mg/kg on alternate days × 10–15 doses	30–50 mg/kg on alternate days × 10–15 doses
Schistosomiasis (Bilharziasis)			
Schistosoma haematobium			
Drug of choice	Praziquantel	40 mg/kg/day in 2 doses × 1 day	40 mg/kg/day in 2 doses × 1 day
S. japonicum			
Drug of choice	Praziquantel	60 mg/kg/day in 3 doses × 1 day	60 mg/kg/day in 3 doses × 1 day
S. mansoni			
Drug of choice	Praziquantel	40 mg/kg/day in 2 doses × 1 day	40 mg/kg/day in 2 doses × 1 day
Alternative	Oxamniquine[e]	15 mg/kg once[f]	20 mg/kg/day in 2 doses × 1 day[f]
S. mekongi			
Drug of choice	Praziquantel	60 mg/kg/day in 3 doses × 1 day	60 mg/kg/day in 3 doses × 1 day

[a]An approved drug but considered investigational for this condition by the Food and Drug Administration.

[b]Unlike infections with other flukes, *Fasciola hepatica* infections may not respond to praziquantel. Triclabendazole (Egaten, Novartis) may be safe and effective but data are limited (Askoy DY, et al. Clin Microbiol Infect. 2005;11:859). It is available from Victoria Pharmacy, Zurich, Switzerland (www.pharmaworld.com; 41-1-211-24-32) and should be given with food for better absorption. Nitazoxanide also appears to have efficacy in treating fascioliasis in adults and children (Favennec L, et al. Aliment Pharmocol Ther. 2003;17:265; Rossignol JF, et al. Trans R Soc Trop Med Hyg. 1998;92:103; Kabil SM, et al. Curr Ther Res. 2000;61:339).

[c]Keiser J, et al. Expert Opin Invest Drugs. 2005;14:1513.

[d]Triclabendazole may be effective in a dosage of 5 mg/kg once/day × 3 days or 10 mg/kg bid × 1 day (Calvopiña M, et al. Trans R Soc Trop Med Hyg. 1998;92:566). See also footnote[b].

[e]Oxamniquine, which is not available in the United States, is generally not as effective as praziquantel. It has been useful, however, in some areas in which praziquantel is less effective (Ferrari ML, et al. Bull WHO. 2003;81:190; Harder A. Parasitol Res. 2002;88:395). Oxamniquine is contraindicated in pregnancy. It should be taken after food.

[f]In East Africa, the dose should be increased to 30 mg/kg, and in Egypt and South Africa to 30 mg/kg/day × 2 days. Some experts recommend 40–60 mg/kg over 2–3 days in all Africa (Shekhar KC. Drugs. 1991;42:379).

(Derived from the *Medical Letter on Drugs and Therapeutics*, Drugs for parasitic infections, www.medicalletter.org, October 2008.)

neurocysticercosis, reduces the CSF concentration of praziquantel and may decrease its efficacy.

Praziquantel is frequently associated with mild, transient side effects, including headaches, lassitude, dizziness, nausea, vomiting, and abdominal discomfort, but these are seldom severe enough to interrupt therapy. Apparent untoward reactions due to the release of parasite antigens have been reported in patients treated for schistosomiasis and pulmonary paragonimiasis. Increased intracranial pressure resulting from the release of cysticercal antigens is a potentially life-threatening event in patients receiving praziquantel for neurocysticercosis, and corticosteroids are usually administered concurrently.[32,33] Praziquantel is contraindicated in people with cysticerci in the eye or spinal cord because of the deleterious consequences of local inflammatory reactions. The concurrent administration of cimetidine, ketoconazole, or miconazole can inhibit the metabolism of praziquantel and increase serum levels.

Niclosamide is active against adult tapeworms in the GI tract.[34] It is very poorly absorbed, which limits its spectrum of activity to intestinal organisms. It is thought to uncouple oxidative phosphorylation in the mitochondria of adult cestodes and may also interfere with anaerobic metabolism. As the adult tapeworm dies, there is destruction of the

Box 12.1 Adverse Effects of Anthelminthic Drugs

Drugs Used for Nematode Infections

Albendazole (Albenza – GlaxoSmithKline)

Occasional: abdominal pain; migration of *Ascaris* through mouth and nose; reversible alopecia; increased serum transaminase activity
Rare: leukopenia; rash; renal toxicity

Diethylcarbamazine citrate USP[a] (Hetrazan)

Frequent: severe allergic or febrile reactions in patients with microfilariae in the blood or skin; gastrointestinal disturbances
Rare: encephalopathy (with treatment of heavy *Loa loa* infection)

Ivermectin (Stromectol – Merck)

Occasional: Mazzotti-type reaction seen in onchocerciasis, including fever, pruritus, tender lymph nodes, headache, joint and bone pain
Rare: hypotension

Mebendazole (Vermox – McNeil)

Occasional: diarrhea, abdominal pain, migration of *Ascaris* through mouth and nose
Rare: leukopenia, agranulocytosis, hypospermia

Pyrantel pamoate (Antiminth – Pfizer)[b]

Occasional: gastrointestinal disturbances, headache, dizziness, rash, fever

Drugs Used for Cestode and Trematode Infections

Albendazole (Albenza – GlaxoSmithKline) – See Above

Bithionol[a] (Bitin – Tanabe, Japan)

Frequent: photosensitivity reactions, vomiting, diarrhea, abdominal pain, urticaria
Rare: leukoplakia, toxic hepatitis

Oxamniquine (Vansil – Pfizer)[b]

Occasional: headache, fever, dizziness, somnolence, nausea, diarrhea, rash, insomnia, hepatic enzyme changes, electrocardiogram changes, electroencephalogram changes, orange-red discoloration of urine
Rare: seizures, neuropsychiatric disturbances

Praziquantel (Biltricide – Bayer)

Frequent: abdominal pain, diarrhea, malaise, headache, dizziness
Occasional: sedation, fever, sweating, nausea, eosinophilia, fatigue
Rare: pruritus, rash, edema, hiccups

[a]*Available from the CDC Drug Service, Centers for Disease Control and Prevention, Atlanta, GA 30333; telephone (404) 639-3670; evenings, weekends, and holidays (404) 639-2888.*
[b]*Not available in the United States.*

Box 12.2 Adverse Effects of Antimalarial Drugs

Artemether with Lumefantrine

(Coartem – Novartis)

Occasional: headache, dizziness, anorexia and weakness. Lumefantrine inhibits CYP206 and can thereby reduce the metabolism of other drugs that prolong the Q-T interval
Rare: hypersensitivity reactions, including urticaria, angioedema, and bullous eruption. Possible neuropathic effects

Artesunate

(Intravenous from Centers for Disease Control, Walter Reed Army Institute of Research)

Occasional: bradycardia, dizziness, nausea and vomiting
Rare: hypersensitivity reactions, seizure, cerebellar dysfunction (ataxia, gait, slurred speech)

Atovaquone

(Mepron – GlaxoSmithKline, Malarone (with proguanil) – GlaxoSmithKline)

Occasional: abdominal pain, nausea, vomiting, diarrhea, headache

Chloroquine HCl and Chloroquine Phosphate

(Aralen – Sanofi, and Others)

Occasional: pruritus, vomiting, headache, confusion, depigmentation of hair, skin eruptions, corneal opacity, weight loss, partial alopecia, extraocular muscle palsies, exacerbation of psoriasis, eczema, and other exfoliative dermatoses, myalgias, photophobia
Rare: irreversible retinal injury (especially when total dosage exceeds 100 g, discoloration of nails and mucous membranes, nerve-type deafness, peripheral neuropathy and myopathy, heart block, blood dyscrasias, hematemesis

Mefloquine

(Lariam – Roche)

Frequent: vertigo, lightheadedness, nausea, other gastrointestinal disturbances, nightmares, visual disturbances, headache, insomnia
Occasional: confusion, psychological disturbance
Rare: psychosis, hypotension, convulsions, coma, paresthesias

Primaquine Phosphate USP

Frequent: hemolytic anemia in glucose-6-phosphate dehydrogenase deficiency
Occasional: neutropenia, gastrointestinal disturbances, methemoglobinemia
Rare: central nervous system symptoms, hypertension, arrhythmias

Proguanil

(Paludrine – Wyeth-Ayerst, AstraZeneca), or with atovaquone (Malarone – GlaxoSmithKline)

Occasional: oral ulceration, hair loss, rash, scaling of palms and soles, urticaria
Rare: hematuria (with large doses), vomiting, abdominal pain, diarrhea (with large doses), thrombocytopenia

Quinine Dihydrochloride and Sulfate

(Many Manufacturers)

Frequent: cinchonism (tinnitus, headache, nausea, abdominal pain, visual disturbance)
Occasional: deafness, hemolytic anemia, other blood dyscrasias, photosensitivity reactions, hypoglycemia, arrhythmias, hypotension, drug fever
Rare: blindness, sudden death if injected too rapidly

scolex and proximal portion with expulsion of the remainder of the worm in the feces.

Niclosamide is usually well tolerated, but it can cause mild GI or systemic symptoms and, rarely, a rash. It kills adult *T. solium*, but the disintegration of the worm and the release of viable ova into the intestinal lumen raise the theoretical possibility of autoinfection. For this reason, many physicians prefer praziquantel for intestinal *T. solium* infection. When niclosamide is used, it is often followed by a purge to expedite removal of the worm. In the case of *Hymenolepis nana*, 5–7 days of niclosamide are needed to cure infection, whereas a single dose of praziquantel is effective, and it is consequently recommended.

Oxamniquine is an alternative to praziquantel for the treatment of *Schistosoma mansoni* infections.[35] Although the precise mechanism of its action is uncertain, it produces marked alterations in the tegument of adult schistosomes, but it does so over a period of days, in contrast to praziquantel, which acts in hours. Higher doses of oxamniquine are recommended for treatment in some areas of Egypt and equatorial Africa. Oxamniquine is well absorbed orally and has a half-life of 1.0–2.5 hours. The parent drug and its metabolites are cleared through the kidney and can produce an orange or red discoloration of the urine. Potential side effects include dizziness, drowsiness, skin rash, and GI disturbances, including abdominal pain, diarrhea, nausea, vomiting, and loss of appetite. Seizures occur rarely. Oxamniquine is contraindicated in people with epilepsy and during pregnancy.

TREATMENT OF SYSTEMIC PROTOZOAL INFECTIONS: MALARIA, BABESIOSIS, AND TOXOPLASMOSIS

Malaria

The prophylaxis (see ***Tables 96.5 and 126.3 and Box 12.2***) and treatment of malaria (***Table 96.4 and Boxes 12.2, 96.3, and 96.4***) are of great importance in the tropics. In endemic areas measures should be taken to minimize transmission by anopheline mosquito bites. They include room screens, insecticide impregnated bed nets, long-sleeve clothing and pants, the application of insect repellents with diethylmetatolumide (DEET) or alternatives to exposed skin, and the use of permethrin on clothing. But even with these measures, chemoprophylaxis is necessary.[36–38] The Centers for Disease Control and Prevention (CDC) provide recommendations for the prevention and treatment of malaria by country.[36]

Chloroquine is the drug of choice for prophylaxis in areas with chloroquine-sensitive *Plasmodium falciparum,* and chloroquine-sensitive *P. vivax, P. ovale, P. malariae,* and *P. knowlesi*.[2,36–38] Chloroquine resistance has not been reported in the latter three species. Primaquine is used to prevent later relapses of *P. vivax* and *P. ovale* due to persistent hypnozoites in the liver.

P. falciparum and, to a lesser extent, *P. vivax,* are notable among protozoa for their propensity to develop resistance to chemotherapeutic agents. Chloroquine resistance is widespread among *P. falciparum*. Only in Central America west of the Panama canal, Haiti and adjacent areas of the Dominican Republic, and some areas of the Middle East can *P. falciparum* isolates be considered chloroquine-sensitive. Chloroquine-resistant *P. vivax* is prevalent in Indonesia and to a limited degree in some other areas.[39] Doxycycline, the fixed combination of atovaquone–proguanil (Malarone), or mefloquine is used for chemoprophylaxis in areas where chloroquine-resistant *P. falciparum* or *P. vivax* are endemic.[2,36–38] The untoward effects of mefloquine, particularly the neuropsychiatric toxicity, have been a source of substantial concern and limit its use.[40] Provided that the recipient has normal glucose-6-phosphate dehydrogenase (G6PD) levels, daily primaquine is another option for prophylaxis in special circumstances.

Chloroquine remains the treatment of choice in areas with sensitive *Plasmodium* species. There are several options for the treatment of chloroquine-resistant falciparum malaria. Quinine sulfate with tetracycline has been the mainstay of treatment for years. They have been replaced in many areas of the world by artemisinin derivates administered in combination with a second antimalarial drug to prevent relapse and emergence of drug resistance. The fixed drug combination, artemether–lumefantrine (Coartem), has been widely used and is licensed in the United States. The fixed drug combination, atovaquone–proguanil (Malarone), can also be used in uncomplicated cases. Mefloquine is another option, but toxicity is common at the dosage used for treatment. Resistance to mefloquine and quinine has become common in rural areas of Thailand and elsewhere in Southeast Asia, and resistance to artemisinins has been reported as well in recent years. In persons unable to take oral medications in the United States, intravenous quinidine gluconate or artesunate, which is available through the CDC, are options. Intravenous quinine dihydrochloride is available in some areas of the world, but not the United States, as are a number of artemisinin derivates.

Chloroquine, a 4-aminoquinoline, remains the drug of choice for the prophylaxis and treatment of chloroquine-sensitive *P. vivax, P. ovale, P. malariae,* and *P. falciparum* malaria. Its mechanism of action has been extensively studied. It is concentrated in the hemoglobin-containing digestive vesicles of asexual intraerythrocytic parasites. Chloroquine inhibits the parasite's heme polymerase that incorporates ferriprotoporphyrin IX, which is potentially toxic to the parasite, into insoluble, nontoxic, crystalline hemozoin.[41] Chloroquine-resistant strains of *P. falciparum* actively transport chloroquine out of the intraparasitic compartment. Although this can be blocked by calcium channel inhibitors *in vitro*, chloroquine resistance has not been effectively reversed in humans. Hydroxychloroquine (Plaquenil) is also effective for prophylaxis against chloroquine-sensitive *Plasmodium* species.

Chloroquine has a bitter taste, but it is well absorbed from the GI tract. The half-life, which varies, averages 4 days, permitting once-weekly administration for prophylaxis. Approximately half of the parent drug is excreted unchanged in the urine and the remainder is metabolized in the liver. Chloroquine is generally well tolerated when used at the doses recommended for the prophylaxis and treatment of malaria. Side effects include headache, nausea, vomiting, blurred vision, dizziness, and fatigue. Some Africans and African-Americans experience pruritus, which responds to antihistamines. Rare side effects include depigmentation of hair, exacerbation of psoriasis, blood dyscrasias, seizures, neuropsychiatric effects, and reactions in people with porphyria. Retinal damage has occurred in people receiving chloroquine at high doses for the treatment of rheumatologic disorders, but it has not been documented as a problem in people taking it weekly over many years for malaria prophylaxis.[42] Chloroquine has been used for chemoprophylaxis during pregnancy.

Children are more sensitive than adults to the toxic effects of chloroquine, and cardiopulmonary collapse and death have occurred following accidental overdoses and in adults attempting suicide. As little as 1 g of chloroquine can be fatal in children unless treatment is initiated with mechanical respiration, diazepam to control seizures, and blood pressure support.[43] An intravenous preparation of chloroquine is available outside the United States, but it must be given slowly and with great caution because of its propensity to produce respiratory depression, heart block, hypotension, cardiovascular collapse, and seizures.

Primaquine, an 8-aminoquinoline, is the only drug currently available that can eradicate hypnozoites of *P. vivax* and *P. ovale* in the liver. It is administered to people with *P. vivax* and *P. ovale* infection to prevent relapses. The identification of relatively resistant strains of *P. vivax* in the Southwest Pacific, Southeast Asia, South America, and East Africa[44–46] led to an increase in the dosage recommended.[2] Primaquine can also be used in special circumstances for prophylaxis against chloroquine-resistant *P. falciparum* and other forms of malaria, but recipients must be tested to ensure that they do not have G6PD deficiency.[47] Primaquine plus clindamycin is an alternative to trimethoprim-sulfamethoxazole for the prophylaxis and treatment of *Pneumocystis jirovecii* in persons who cannot tolerate sulfonamides.

Primaquine is well absorbed orally and rapidly converted to carboxyprimaquine, which has a half-life of approximately 7 days. The precise mechanism of action is unknown, but it is thought to interfere with mitochondrial function and possibly the transport of vesicles in the parasite. Primaquine is generally well tolerated, although some recipients experience abdominal cramps, epigastic distress, and nausea. The major concern is hemolysis in people with G6PD deficiency.[48] The G6PD status of the recipient should be determined before it is administered. Altered dosage schedules can be used in Africans with more limited G6PD deficiency. Rarely, primaquine causes neutropenia, methemoglobinemia, leukopenia, or granulocytopenia. Primaquine is contraindicated during pregnancy and in breast-feeding mothers because life-threatening hemolysis may occur in the fetus or baby if they are G6PD-deficient. Travelers should be warned not to give the drug to fellow travelers who have not been screened for G6PD deficiency.

Quinine sulfate, a cinchona alkaloid, is the oldest of the antimalarials.[49] With the exception of quinine-resistant *P. falciparum* strains in Thailand and adjacent areas of Southeast Asia, quinine is effective against all five *Plasmodium* species, including chloroquine-resistant *P. falciparum*. The mechanism of its action is unknown, but quinine is thought to act at the level of the parasites' hemoglobin-containing digestive vesicle and may interfere with ferriprotoporphyrin IX metabolism. Quinine has a very bitter taste. It is rapidly absorbed after oral administration and has a half-life of 16–18 hours in people with malaria. It is metabolized in the liver, and the native drug and its metabolites are excreted in the urine. Quinine has the poorest therapeutic-to-toxicity ratio of any antimalarial drug. The side effects, known collectively as cinchonism, include tinnitus, decreased hearing, headache, nausea, vomiting, dysphoria, and visual disturbances. They are dose-related and reversible. Quinine has also been associated with severe hypoglycemia in people with heavy *P. falciparum* infections due to the utilization of glucose by the parasites and release of insulin from the pancreas.[50] Hypoglycemia can be prevented or treated by the administration of intravenous glucose. Rare complications with quinine include massive hemolysis in patients with heavy *P. falciparum* infections resulting in hemoglobinuria and renal failure (black water fever), cutaneous hypersensitivity reactions, agranulocytosis, and hepatitis. Quinine can cause respiratory paralysis in people with myasthenia gravis. It stimulates uterine contractions and can produce abortions, but it has saved the lives of many pregnant women with *P. falciparum* malaria.

Quinidine gluconate, the stereoisomer of quinine, is used for the intravenous treatment of patients with acute malaria who cannot take quinine by mouth.[51,52] Quinidine gluconate is well known for its role in the treatment of ventricular ectopy. Once widely used in coronary care units in the United States, it has been replaced by newer cardiac medications and is no longer stocked in many hospitals. Its side effects include prolongation of the Q-T interval, arrhythmias, and hypotension, particularly if it is infused too rapidly. People receiving intravenous quinidine should be monitored in an intensive care setting and changed to the oral quinine as soon as they can take medications by mouth. Where it is available, intravenous quinine dihydrochloride can be used if quinidine is not available. It, too, can produce myocardial depression, peripheral vascular collapse, respiratory depression, and death. Patients must be monitored closely during its infusion. Intravenous therapy with either drug should be terminated as soon as the patient is able to take oral drugs. Intravenous artesunate is a more rapidly acting and safer alternative when parenteral therapy is needed.

Mefloquine, a quinoline methanol compound derived from quinine, has been used for the prophylaxis and treatment of chloroquine-resistant *P. falciparum* malaria.[53] It is active against all five *Plasmodium* species, including those that are resistant to chloroquine, but mefloquine-resistant strains of *P. falciparum* are common in rural areas of Thailand and adjacent countries, and they have been reported from some other regions of the world. Mefloquine is available for oral administration only and is slowly and incompletely absorbed. It is 99% protein-bound and has a variable half-life ranging from 6 to 23 days, with a mean of approximately 14 days. It is metabolized and excreted slowly through the bile and feces. Mefloquine appears to interfere with the food vacuoles of the intraerythrocytic asexual stage of the parasite.

Considerable attention has been paid to the untoward effects of mefloquine, and its use for prophylaxis has steadily decreased in favor of doxycycline and atovaquone–proguanil, better-tolerated alternatives. Transient nausea, dizziness, vivid dreams, fatigue, and lassitude occur in a subset of recipients, but it is the potential for less common neuropsychiatric reactions, including anxiety, depression, acute psychosis, and seizures, that limits its use. Mefloquine is contraindicated in people with a history of epilepsy or psychiatric problems. It can depress atrial–ventricular conduction and should not be used by patients with cardiac conduction defects. Mefloquine may be used in people taking beta-blockers if they have no underlying arrhythmias. Mefloquine also has antibacterial activity, and it can inactivate the live oral typhoid vaccine (*Salmonella typhi* Ty21a) if administered concurrently. Rare side effects include exfoliative erythroderma, agranulocytosis, and paresthesias. Mefloquine is not approved by the Food and Drug Administration for use during pregnancy or in children who weigh less than 15 kg, but it has been used in situations in which the potential benefits are judged to outweigh the risks.[54]

Halofantrine, a 9-phenanthrenemethanol, has activity against the asexual, intraerythrocytic stages of chloroquine-sensitive and chloroquine-resistant strains of *P. falciparum, P. vivax, P. ovale*, and *P. malariae*. Although not available in the United States, it has been used in Africa. Halofantrine is variably absorbed after oral administration; higher levels are obtained if the drug is taken with a fatty meal. The half-life of the native drug is 1 or 2 days and that of its active metabolite is 3–5 days. It is excreted primarily in the feces. Halofantrine produces prolongation of the Q-T interval and has been associated with sudden death.[55] It should be avoided unless no alternative is available.

Doxycycline taken daily provides effective prophylaxis against all *Plasmodium* species. Either tetracycline or doxycycline is typically administered with quinine in the treatment of acute chloroquine-resistant malaria. The tetracyclines do not act quickly enough to be used alone for treatment. Doxycycline is well absorbed after oral administration. It is generally well tolerated, but GI symptoms may occur. Doxycycline can also cause severe "pill" esophagitis if it does not pass through to the stomach. Consequently, it should be taken with a full glass of water and the recipient should remain upright for at least an hour after ingestion. Other potential untoward effects include photosensitivity dermatitis, *Candida albicans* vaginitis, and antibiotic-associated colitis. Finally, tetracyclines should not be used in children younger than 8 years of age because of the potential for dental staining, or in pregnant women.

Pyrimethamine alone or with sulfonamides was used in the prevention and treatment of malaria, but resistance is now widespread, and they are seldom indicated. The two agents inhibit sequential steps in the folic acid metabolic pathway. Sulfonamides reduce the activity of dihydropteroate synthetase and reduce the binding of *p*-aminobenzoic acid to it. Pyrimethamine preferentially inhibits dihydrofolate reductase in susceptible parasites. Fansidar[56] is a fixed combination of pyrimethamine (25 mg) and sulfadoxine (500 mg), a long-acting sulfonamide with a half-life of 5–9 days. Fansidar has been associated with life-threatening cutaneous hypersensitivity reactions in people allergic to sulfonamides, is no longer available in many countries, and is not recommended for malaria chemoprophylaxis.

The fixed combination of atovaquone–proguanil (Malarone; adult tablets contain atovaquone 250 mg and proguanil 100 mg) has assumed an increasingly important role in the prevention and treatment of uncomplicated *P. falciparum* infections.[57,58] Malarone is better tolerated than mefloquine or doxycycline for prophylaxis, but more expensive. Atovaquone also is an alternative for the treatment of *Pneumocystis jirovecii*.[59]

Atovaquone is a highly lipophilic compound with low aqueous solubility. Administration with food enhances its absorption twofold. Plasma concentrations do not increase proportionately with dose. Atovaquone is highly protein-bound, with a half-life exceeding 60 hours. There is extensive enterohepatic cycling, and it is eventually excreted unchanged in the feces. Atovaquone selectively inhibits electron transport at the level of the cytochrome bc_1 complex, which results in collapse of the parasite's mitochondrial membrane potential. It also affects pyrimidine biosynthesis, which is obligatorily coupled to electron transport in *Plasmodium* through ubiquinone/ubiquinol. Resistance develops rapidly when atovaquone is used alone to treat malaria. It is generally well tolerated but can cause GI side effects, including nausea, vomiting, and diarrhea, as well as skin rash and pruritus.

Proguanil is slowly absorbed after oral administration. The serum level falls to zero within 24 hours, so it must be taken daily for prophylaxis. Its triazine metabolite, cycloguanil, inhibits dihydrofolate reductase in susceptible *Plasmodium*. Resistance is well documented among *Plasmodium* species when the drug is used alone. Proguanil acts synergistically with atovaquone to collapse mitochondrial membrane potential in *Plasmodium*. It is generally well tolerated. At higher doses it can cause nausea, vomiting, abdominal pain, and diarrhea. Hematological effects occur rarely.

The combination of atovaquone–proguanil (Malarone) is administered daily for prophylaxis. It is begun 1–2 days before exposure. It needs to be continued for only 7 days after exposure, unlike chloroquine, doxycycline and mefloquine, that must be continued for 4 weeks. It does not kill hypnozoites of *P. vivax* or *P. ovale*. Atovaquone–proguanil is generally well tolerated, but abdominal pain, nausea, vomiting, diarrhea, headache, pruritus, and rash may occur. The GI side effects are more common with the higher treatment doses. Asymptomatic, transient elevations of liver enzymes have also been observed with treatment doses. The combination is contraindicated during pregnancy.

Artemisinin derivatives, which include artesunate, artemether, and arteether, are sesquiterpene lactones derived from the Chinese herbal medication quinghaosu, which comes from the wormwood plant, *Artemisin annua*.[60–62] They are endoperoxide-containing compounds. In the presence of intraparasitic iron, they are thought to be converted into free radicals and other intermediates that alkylate specific malarial proteins and act rapidly to kill intraerythrocytic parasites. They should be administered with a second antimalarial drug to prevent relapses and the development of resistance to single-agent therapy. The artemisinins are widely used around the world for the treatment of acute chloroquine-resistant *P. falciparum* and other forms of malaria.[60,61] The route of administration varies; some are administered orally, whereas others are available intravenously, intramuscularly, or by suppository. The fixed combination of artemether–lumefantrine (Coartem) is used worldwide and has been approved in the United States for the treatment of acute, uncomplicated, chloroquine-resistant malaria.[61] Intravenous artesunate is available from the CDC under an investigational new drug for the treatment of chloroquine-resistant *P. falciparum* infections in persons who cannot take oral medications and for whom intravenous quinidine is not available or tolerated.[62]

Artemeter, other artemisinins, and lumefantrine are blood schizontocides. They are rapidly cleared from the circulation. The short half-life of the artemisinin derivatives precludes their use for malaria prophylaxis. Adverse effects are infrequent and typically mild with the artemisinins. They include headache, dizziness, anorexia, and weakness in adults. Rare hypersensitivity reactions, including urticaria, angioedema, and bullous eruptions, have been noted in postmarketing surveillance. Lumefantrine inhibits CYP206 and can thereby reduce the metabolism of drugs that prolong the Q-T interval, so attention must be given to its potential drug–drug interactions. Neuropathic effects have been reported in dogs given chronic, high-dose artemisinin therapy.

Toxoplasmosis, Babesiosis, and *Pneumocystis* Pneumonia

Like *Plasmodium* species, *Toxoplasma gondii* and *Babesia* species are important pathogens of the phylum Apicomplexa. The medications used to treat them and their untoward effects are summarized in ***Table 12.4 and Box 12.3***. They include several of the antimalarial drugs discussed previously and the antibiotics clindamycin, azithromycin, and spiramycin that act at the ribosomal level. Pyrimethamine and sulfadiazine are recommended for the treatment of toxoplasmosis. Clindamycin is an alternative to sulfadiazine for people with sulfonamide allergies. The macrolide, spiramycin, is recommended for the treatment of toxoplasmosis during pregnancy. Atovaquone plus azithromycin is the best-tolerated regimen for the treatment of babesiosis. Clindamycin and quinine are also effective but have more side effects. Trimethoprim-sulfamethoxazole is the drug of choice for the treatment and prevention of *Pneumocystis jirovecii* infection, as summarized in ***Table 12.4***. Alternatives for treatment include primaquine plus clindamycin, trimethoprim plus dapsone (a sulfone widely used in the treatment of leprosy), pentamidine, or atovaquone. Alternatives for prophylaxis include dapsone alone, dapsone plus pyrimethamine, pentamidine aerosol and atovaquone.

Box 12.3 Adverse Effects of Drugs Used to Treat Other Protozoa

Atovaquone

(Mepron – GlaxoSmithKline)

Frequent: rash, nausea
Occasional: nausea, vomiting, diarrhea, rash
Rare: renal papillary necrosis, severe hypoalbuminemia, epidermal necrolysis, optic atrophy, agranulocytosis, neonatal hyperbilirubinemia after use in pregnancy

Dapsone

(Jacobus)

Frequent: rash, transient headache, gastrointestinal irritation, anorexia, infectious mononucleosis-like syndrome
Occasional: cyanosis due to methemoglobinemia and sulfhemoglobinemia, other blood dyscrasias, including hemolytic anemia, nephrotic syndrome, liver damage, peripheral neuropathy, hypersensitivity reactions, increased risk of lepra reactions, insomnia, irritability, uncoordinated speech, agitation, acute psychosis

Pyrimethamine USP

(Daraprim – GlaxoSmithKline)

Occasional: blood dyscrasias, folic acid deficiency
Rare: rash, vomiting, convulsions, shock, possibly pulmonary eosinophilia, fatal cutaneous reactions with pyrimethamine-sulfadoxine (Fansidar)

Spiramycin

(Rovamycine – Aventis)

Occasional: gastrointestinal disturbances
Rare: allergic reactions

TREATMENT OF INTESTINAL AND VAGINAL PROTOZOA

Several major luminal pathogens, *Entamoeba histolytica, Giardia lamblia*, and *Trichomonas vaginalis*, which live under anaerobic conditions in the intestine or vagina, are susceptible to metronidazole or tinidazole.[63,64] Of the two, tinidazole is better tolerated. The recommended treatment of these and other intestinal protozoan infections and the associated untoward effects are summarized in ***Table 12.5 and Box 12.4***, respectively. Nitazoxanide, which is available in oral formulation, is approved for the treatment of giardiasis and cryptosporidiosis. It is the only drug reported to be effective for *Cryptosporidium* infections in immunocompetent persons. Relapses occur in those with acquired immunodeficiency syndrome (AIDS). Trimethoprim-sulfamethoxazole, which inhibits successive steps in the folic acid pathway, is effective for the treatment of *Cystoisospora belli* and *Cyclospora cayetanensis*. Ciprofloxacin, a fluoroquinolone that inhibits topoisomerase II, is an alternative. Albendazole is used to treat intestinal microsporidiosis due to *Encephalitozoon (Septata) intestinalis* and ocular and disseminated disease caused by susceptible microsporidia species.

Metronidazole, a nitroimidazole that is active only under anaerobic conditions, is used in the treatment of *E. histolytica, G. lamblia*, and *T. vaginalis* as well as for anaerobic bacterial infections. It is activated by reduction of its 5-nitro group through a sequence of intermediate steps involving microbial electron transport proteins of low redox potential. It is concentrated in anaerobic organisms and serves as an electron sink. Metronidazole is rapidly absorbed after oral administration and has a half-life of 8 hours. More than half of each dose is metabolized in the liver. The metabolites and remaining parent drug are excreted in the urine. Nausea, vomiting, diarrhea, and a metallic taste are often associated with metronidazole use and may lead to discontinuation of the drug. These side effects are less common with the lower doses (250 mg three times a day) recommended for the treatment of giardiasis than with the higher doses used for

Box 12.4 Adverse Effects of Drugs Used in the Treatment of Luminal Protozoal Infections

Diloxanide Furoate[a]

(Furamide - Boots)

Frequent: flatulence
Occasional: nausea, vomiting, diarrhea
Rare: diplopia, dizziness, urticaria, pruritus

Iodoquinol

(Yodoxin – Glenwood, Others)

Occasional: rash, acne, slight enlargement of the thyroid gland, nausea, diarrhea, cramps, and pruritus
Rare: optic neuritis, optic atrophy, loss of vision, peripheral neuropathy after prolonged use in high dosage (for months), iodine sensitivity

Metronidazole

(Flagyl – Searle, Others)

Frequent: nausea, headache, metallic taste, anorexia
Occasional: vomiting, diarrhea, insomnia, weakness, stomatitis, vertigo, tinnitus, paresthesias, rash, dry mouth, dark urine, urethral burning, disulfiram-like reaction with alcohol, candidiasis
Rare: seizures, encephalopathy, pseudomembranous colitis, ataxia, leukopenia, peripheral neuropathy, pancreatitis

Nitazoxanide

(Alinia – Romark)

Occasional: gastrointestinal side-effects

Paromomycin (Aminosidine)

(Humatin – Monarch)

Frequent: gastrointestinal disturbances with oral use
Occasional: vestibular nerve damage (mainly auditory) and renal damage when aminosidine is given IV, vertigo, pancreatitis

Tinidazole

(Tindamax – Presutti))

Occasional: metallic taste, nausea, vomiting, rash

Albendazole (see Box 12.1)

[a]*Not available in the United States.*

Table 12.4 Treatment of Other Protozoal Diseases and Pneumocystis

Infection	Drug	Adult Dosage	Pediatric Dosage
***Acanthamoeba* Keratitis**			
Drug of choice	See footnote[a]		
Amebic Meningoencephalitis, Primary and Granulomatous			
• ***Naegleria***			
Drug of choice	Amphotericin B[b,c]	1.5 mg/kg/day in 2 doses × 3 days, then 1 mg/kg/day × 6 days plus 1.5 mg/day intrathecally × 2 days, then 1 mg/day every other day × 8 days	1.5 mg/kg/day in 2 doses × 3 days, then 1 mg/kg/day × 6 days plus 1.5 mg/day intrathecally × 2 days, then 1 mg/day every other day × 8 days
• ***Acanthamoeba***			
Drug of choice	See footnote[d]		
• ***Balamuthia mandrillaris***			
Drug of choice	See footnote[e]		
• ***Sappinia diploidea***			
Drug of choice	See footnote[f]		
Microsporidiosis			
• **Ocular (*Encephalitozoon hellem, E. cuniculi, Vittaforma corneae (Nosema corneum)*)**			
Drug of choice	Albendazole[b,g]	400 mg bid	
	plus fumagillin[h]		
• **Intestinal (*E. [Septata] intestinalis* and *E. bieneusi*)**			
Drug of choice	Fumagillin[i]	20 mg tid × 14 days	
• ***E. intestinalis***			
Drug of choice	Albendazole[b,g]	400 mg bid × 21 days	

[a]Topical 0.02% chlorhexidine and polyhexamethylene biguanide (PHMB, 0.02%), either alone or in combination, have been used successfully in a large number of patients. Treatment with either chlorhexidine or PHMB is often combined with propamidine isethionate (Brolene) or hexamidine (Desmodine). None of these drugs is commercially available or approved for use in the United States, but they can be obtained from compounding pharmacies. Leiter's Park Avenue Pharmacy, San Jose, CA (800-292-6773; www.leiterrx.com) is a compounding pharmacy that specializes in ophthalmic drugs. Propamidine is available over the counter in the United Kingdom and Australia. Hexamidine is available in France. The combination of chlorhexidine, natamycin (pimaricin), and debridement also has been successful (Kitagawa K, et al. Jpn J Ophthalmol. 2003;47:616). Debridement is most useful during the stage of corneal epithelial infection. Most cysts are resistant to neomycin; its use is no longer recommended. Azole antifungal drugs (ketoconazole, itraconazole) have been used as oral or topical adjuncts (Shuster FL, Visvesvara GS. Drug Resist Update. 2004;7:41). Use of corticosteroids is controversial (Hammersmith K. Curr Opin Ophthalmol. 2006;17:327; Awwad ST, et al. Eye Contact Lens. 2007;33:1).

[b]Not approved by the Food and Drug Administration for this indication.

[c]However, a *Naegleria fowleri* infection was treated successfully in a 9-year-old girl with combination of amphotericin B and miconazole both intravenous and intrathecal, plus oral rifampin (Seidel JS, et al. N Engl J Med. 1982;306:348). Amphotericin B and miconazole appear to have a synergistic effect, but *Medical Letter* consultants believe the rifampin probably had no additional effect (Visvesvara GS, et al. FEMS Immunol Med Microbiol. 2007;50:1). Parenteral miconazole is no longer available in the United States. Azithromycin has been used successfully in combination therapy to treat *Balamuthia* infection, but was changed to clarithromycin because of toxicity concerns and for better penetration into the cerebrospinal fluid. *In vitro*, azithromycin is more active than clarithromycin against *Naegleria*, so may be a better choice combined with amphotericin B for the treatment of *Naegleria* (Deetz TR, et al. Clin Infect Dis. 2003;37:1304; Schuster FL, Visvesvara GS. Drug Resistance Updates. 2004;7:41). Combinations of amphotericin B, ornidazole and rifampin (Jain R, et al. Neurol Indian. 2002;50:470) and amphotericin B, fluconazole and rifampin have been used (Vargas-Zepeda J, et al. Arch Med Res. 2005;36:83). Case reports of other successful therapy have been published (Schuster FL, Visvesvaria GS. Int J Parasitol. 2004;34:1001).

[d]Several patients with granulomatous amebic encephalitis (GAE) have been successfully treated with combinations of pentamidine, sulfadiazine, flucytosine, and either fluconazole or itraconazole (Visvesvara GS, et al. FEMS Immunol Med Microbiol. 2007;50:1, epub Apr 11). GAE in a patient with acquired immunodeficiency syndrome (AIDS) was treated successfully with sulfadiazine, pyrimethamine, and fluconazole combined with surgical resection of the central nervous system lesion (Seijo Martinez M, et al. J Clin Microbiol. 2000;38:3892). Chronic *Acanthamoeba* meningitis was successfully treated in 2 children with a combination of oral trimethoprim/sulfamethoxazole, rifampin, and ketoconazole (Singhal T, et al. Pediatr Infect Dis J. 2000;20:623). Disseminated cutaneous infection in an immunocompromised patient was treated successfully with IV pentamidine, topical chlorhexidine, and 2% ketoconazole cream, followed by oral itraconazole (Slater CA, et al. N Engl J Med. 1994;331:85) and with voriconazole and amphotericin B lipid complex (Walia R, et al. Transplant Infect Dis. 2007;9:51). Other reports of successful therapy have been described (Schuster FL, Visvesvara GS. Drug Resistance Updates. 2004;7:41). Susceptibility testing of *Acanthamoeba* isolates has shown differences in drug sensitivity between species and even among strains of a single species; antimicrobial susceptibility testing is advisable (Schuster FL, Visvesvara GS. Int J Parasitol. 2004;34:1001).

[e]*B. mandrillaris* is a free-living ameba that causes subacute to fatal GAE and cutaneous disease. Two cases of *Balamuthia* encephalitis have been successfully treated with flucytosine, pentamidine, fluconazole and sulfadiazine, plus either azithromycin or clarithromycin (phenothiazines were also used) combined with surgical resection of the central nervous system lesion (Deetz TR, et al. Clin Infect Dis. 2003;37:1304). Another case was successfully treated following open biopsy with pentamidine, fluconazole, sulfadiazine and clarithromycin (Jung S, et al. Arch Pathol Lab Med. 2004;128:466).

[f]A free-living ameba once thought not to be pathogenic to humans. *S. diploidea* has been successfully treated with azithromycin, pentamidine, itraconazole, and flucytosine combined with surgical resection of the central nervous system lesion (Gelman BB, et al. J Neuropathol Exp Neurol. 2003;62:990).

[g]Albendazole must be taken with food; a fatty meal increases oral bioavailability.

[h]Chan CM, et al. Ophthalmology. 2003;110:1420. Ocular lesions due to *E. hellem* in patients infected with human immunodeficiency virus (HIV) have responded to fumagillin eyedrops prepared from Fumidil-B (bicyclohexyl ammonium fumagillin) used to control a microsporidial disease of honey bees (Garvey MJ, et al. Ann Pharmacother. 1995;29:872), available from Leiter's Park Avenue Pharmacy (see footnote *a*). For lesions due to *V. corneae*, topical therapy is generally not effective and keratoplasty may be required (Davis RM, et al. Ophthalmology. 1990;97:953).

[i]Oral fumagillin (Flisint – Sanofi-Aventis, France) has been effective in treating *E. bieneusi* (Molina JM, et al. N Engl J Med. 2002;346:1963), but has been associated with thrombocytopenia and neutropenia. Highly active antiretroviral therapy (HAART) may lead to microbiologic and clinical response in HIV-infected patients with microsporidial diarrhea. Octreotide (Sandostatin) has provided symptomatic relief in some patients with large-volume diarrhea.

Table 12.4 Treatment of Other Protozoal Diseases and Pneumocystis—cont'd

Infection	Drug	Adult Dosage	Pediatric Dosage
• **Disseminated (*E. hellem, E. cuniculi, E. intestinalis, Pleistophora* sp., *Trachipleistophora* sp., and *Brachiola vesicularum*)**			
Drug of choice	Albendazole[b,g]	400 mg bid	
***Pneumocystis jirovecii* (Formerly *carinii*) Pneumonia (PCP)[j]**			
Drug of choice	Trimethoprim (TMP)/ sulfamethoxazole (SMX)	TMP 15 mg/SMX 75 mg/kg/day, PO or IV in 3 or 4 doses × 21 days	TMP 15 mg/SMX 75 mg/kg/day, PO or IV in 3 or 4 doses × 21 days
Alternatives	Primaquine[b,k]	30 mg base daily × 21 days	0.3 mg/kg base daily × 21 days
	plus clindamycin[b,l]	600 mg IV q6h × 21 days, or 300–450 mg PO q6h × 21 days	15–25 mg/kg IV q6h × 21 days, or 10 mg/kg PO q6h × 21 days
	or trimethoprim[b]	5 mg/kg tid × 21 days	5 mg/kg tid × 21 days
	plus dapsone[b]	100 mg daily × 21 days	2 mg/kg tid × 21 days
	or pentamidine	3–4 mg/kg IV daily × 21 days	3–4 mg/kg IV daily × 21 days
	or atovaquone	750 mg bid × 21 days	1–3 months: 30 mg/kg/day × 21 days 4–24 months: 45 mg/kg/day × 21 days >24 months: 30 mg/day PO × 21 days
Primary and Secondary Prophylaxis[m]			
Drug of choice	Trimethoprim/ sulfamethoxazole	1 tablet (single- or double-strength) daily or 1 double-strength tablet 3 days/week	TMP 150 mg/SMX 750 mg/m^2/day in 2 doses 3 days/week
Alternative	Dapsone[b]	50 mg bid, or 100 mg daily	2 mg/kg/day (max. 100 mg) or 4 mg/kg (max. 200 mg) each week
	or dapsone[b]	50 mg daily or 200 mg each weeks	
	plus pyrimethamine[n]	50 mg or 75 mg each weeks	
	or pentamidine	300 mg aerosol inhaled monthly via Respirgard II nebulizer	≥5 years: 300 mg inhaled monthly via Respirgard II nebulizer
	or atovaquone[b,o]	1500 mg daily	1–3 months: 30 mg/kg/day 4–24 months: 45 mg/kg/day >24 months: 30 mg/kg/day
Toxoplasmosis (*Toxoplasma gondii*)[p]			
Drug of choice	Pyrimethamine[p]	25–100 mg/day × 3–4 weeks	2 mg/kg/day × 2 days, then 1 mg/kg/day (max. 25 mg/day) × 4 weeks[q]
	plus Sulfadiazine[r]	1–1.5 g qid × 3–4 weeks	100–200 mg/kg/day × 3–4 weeks

[j]*Pneumocystis* has been reclassified as a fungus. In severe disease with room air PO_2 ≤70 mmHg or Aa (alveolar – arterial) gradient ≥35 mmHg, prednisone should also be used (Gagnon S, et al. N Engl J Med. 1990;323:1444; Caumes E, et al. Clin Infect Dis. 1994;18:319).

[k]Primaquine phosphate can cause hemolytic anemia, especially in patients whose red cells are deficient in glucose-6-phosphate dehydrogenase (G6PD). This deficiency is most common in African, Asian, and Mediterranean peoples. Patients should be screened for G6PD deficiency before treatment. Primaquine should not be used during pregnancy. It should be taken with food to minimize the nausea and abdominal pain. Primaquine-tolerant *P. vivax* can be found globally. Relapses of primaquine-resistant strains may be retreated with 30 mg (base) × 28 days.

[l]Oral clindamycin should be taken with a full glass of water to minimize esophageal ulceration.

[m]Primary/secondary prophylaxis in patients with HIV can be discontinued after CD4 count increases to >200 × 10^6/L for >3 months.

[n]Plus leucovorin 25 mg with each dose of pyrimethamine. Pyrimethamine should be taken with food to minimize gastrointestinal adverse effects.

[o]Atovaquone is available in an oral suspension that should be taken with a meal to increase absorption.

[p]To treat central nervous system toxoplasmosis in HIV-infected patients, some clinicians have used pyrimethamine 50–100 mg/day (after a loading dose of 200 mg) with sulfadiazine and, when sulfonamide sensitivity developed, have given clindamycin 1.8–2.4 g/day in divided doses instead of the sulfonamides. Treatment is usually given for at least 4–6 weeks. Atovaquone (1500 mg bid) plus pyrimethamine (200 mg loading dose, followed by 75 mg/day) for 6 weeks appears to be an effective alternative in sulfa-intolerant patients (Chirgwin K, et al. Clin Infect Dis. 2002;34:1243). Atovaquone must be taken with a meal to enhance absorption. Treatment is followed by chronic suppression with lower dosage regimens of the same drugs. For primary prophylaxis in HIV patients with <100 × 10^6/L CD4 cells, either trimethoprim-sulfamethoxazole, pyrimethamine with dapsone, or atovaquone with or without pyrimethamine can be used. Primary or secondary prophylaxis may be discontinued when the CD4 count increases to >200 × 10^6/L for >3 months (MMWR Morb Mortal Wkly Rep. 2004;53(RR15):1). In ocular toxoplasmosis with macular involvement, corticosteroids are recommended in addition to antiparasitic therapy for an anti-inflammatory effect. In one randomized single-blind study, trimethoprim-sulfamethoxazole was reported to be as effective as pyrimethamine/sulfadiazine for treatment of ocular toxoplasmosis (Soheilian M, et al. Ophthalmology. 2005;112;1876). Women who develop toxoplasmosis during the first trimester of pregnancy should be treated with spiramycin (3–4 mg/day). After the first trimester, if there is no documented transmission to the fetus, spiramycin can be continued until term. If transmission has occurred *in utero*, therapy with pyrimethamine and sulfadiazine should be started (Montoya JG, Liesenfeld O. Lancet. 2004;363:1965). Pyrimethamine is a potential teratogen and should be used only after the first trimester.

[q]Congenitally infected newborns should be treated with pyrimethamine every 2 or 3 days and a sulfonamide daily for about 1 year (Remington JS, Desmonts G. In: Remington JS, Klein JO, eds. Infectious Disease of the Fetus and Newborn Infant, 6th ed. Philadelphia: Saunders; 2006:1038).

[r]Sulfadiazine should be taken on an empty stomach with adequate water.

(Derived from the *Medical Letter on Drugs and Therapeutics*, Drugs for parasitic infections, www.medicalletter.org, October 2008.)

Table 12.5 Treatment of Luminal Protozoa

Infection	Drug	Adult Dosage	Pediatric Dosage
Amebiasis (*Entamoeba histolytica*)			
• Asymptomatic			
Drug of choice	Iodoquinol[a]	650 mg tid × 20 days	30–40 mg/kg/day (max. 2 g) in 3 doses × 20 days
	or paromomycin[b]	25–35 mg/kg/day in 3 doses × 7 days	25–35 mg/kg/day in 3 doses × 7 days
Alternative	Diloxanide furoate[c]	500 mg tid × 10 days	20 mg/kg/day in 3 doses × 10 days
• Mild to Moderate Intestinal Disease			
Drug of choice[d]	Metronidazole	500–750 mg tid × 7–10 days	35–50 mg/kg/day in 3 doses × 7–10 days
	or tinidazole[e]	2 g once daily × 3 days	≥3 years: 50 mg/kg/day (max. 2 g) in 1 dose × 3 days
	followed by either		
	Iodoquinol[a]	650 mg tid × 20 days	30–40 mg/kg/day (max. 2 g) in 3 doses × 20 days
	or paromomycin[b]	25–35 mg/kg/day in 3 doses × 7 days	25–35 mg/kg/day in 3 doses × 7 days
• Severe Intestinal and Extraintestinal Disease			
Drug of choice	Metronidazole	750 mg tid × 7–10 days	35–50 mg/kg/day in 3 doses × 7–10 days
	or tinidazole[e] *followed by either* iodoquinol *or* paromomycin as described for mild to moderate intestinal disease above	2 g once daily × 5 days	≥3 years: 50 mg/kg/day (max. 2 g) × 3 days
Balantidiasis (*Balantidium coli*)			
Drug of choice	Tetracycline[f,g]	500 mg qid × 10 days	40 mg/kg/day (max. 2 g) in 4 doses × 10 days
Alternatives	Metronidazole[f]	750 mg tid × 5 days	35–50 mg/kg/day in 3 doses × 5 days
	or iodoquinol[f]	650 mg tid × 20 days	30–40 mg/kg/day (max. 2 g) in 3 doses × 20 days
***Blastocystis hominis* Infection**			
Drug of choice	See footnote[h]		
Cryptosporidiosis (*Cryptosporidium*)			
• Non-HIV-Infected			
Drug of choice	Nitazoxanide[d]	500 mg bid × 3 days[f]	1–3 years: 100 mg bid × 3 days 4–11 years: 200 mg bid × 3 days ≥12 years: 500 mg bid × 3 days
• HIV-Infected			
Drug of choice	See footnote[i]		

HIV, human immunodeficiency virus.

[a]Iodoquinol should be taken after meals.

[b]Paromomycin should be taken with a meal.

[c]Not available commercially. It may be obtained through compounding pharmacies such as Panorama Compounding Pharmacy, 6744 Balboa Blvd, Van Nuys, CA 91406 (800-247-9767) or Medical Center Pharmacy, New Haven, CT (203-688-6816). Other compounding pharmacies may be found through the National Association of Compounding Pharmacies (800-687-7850) or the Professional Compounding Centers of America (800-331-2498, www.pccarx.com).

[d]Nitazoxanide may be effective against a variety of protozoan and helminth infections (Bobak DA. Curr Infect Dis Rep. 2006;8:91; Diaz E, et al. Am J Trop Med Hyg. 2003;68:384). It was effective against mild to moderate amebiasis, 500 mg bid × 3 days, in a recent study (Rossignol JF, et al. Trans R Soc Trop Med Hyg. 2007;101:1025). It is approved by the Food and Drug Administration (FDA) only for treatment of diarrhea caused by *Giardia* or *Cryptosporidium* (Med Lett Drugs Ther. 2003;45:29). Nitazoxanide is available in 500-mg tablets and an oral suspension; it should be taken with food.

[e]A nitroimidazole similar to metronidazole, tinidazole appears to be as effective and better tolerated than metronidazole (Med Lett Drugs Ther. 2004;46:70). It should be taken with food to minimize gastrointestinal adverse effects. For children and patients unable to take tablets, a pharmacist can crush the tablets and mix them with cherry syrup (Humco, and others). The syrup suspension is good for 7 days at room temperature and must be shaken before use (Fung HB, Doan TL. Clin Ther. 2005;27:1859). Ornidazole, a similar drug, is also used outside the United States.

[f]Not FDA-approved for this indication.

[g]Use of tetracyclines is contraindicated in pregnancy and in children <8 years old. Tetracycline should be taken 1 hour before or 2 hours after meals and/or dairy products.

[h]Clinical significance of these organisms is controversial; metronidazole 750 mg tid × 10 days, iodoquinol 650 mg tid × 20 days, or trimethoprim-sulfamethoxazole 1 double-strength tablet bid × 7 days have been reported to be effective (Stenzel DJ, Borenam PFL. Clin Microbiol Rev. 1996;9:563; Ok UZ, et al. Am J Gastroenterol. 1999;94:3245). Metronidazole resistance may be common in some areas (Haresh K, et al. Trop Med Int Health. 1999;4:274). Nitazoxanide has been effective in clearing organism and improving symptoms (Diaz E, et al. Am J Trop Med Hyg. 2003;68:384; Rossignol JF. Clin Gastroenterol Hepatol. 2005;18:703).

[i]No drug has proven efficacy against cryptosporidiosis in advanced acquired immunodeficiency syndrome (AIDS) (Abubakar I, et al. Cochrane Database Syst Rev. 2007;1:CD004932). Treatment with highly active antiretroviral therapy (HAART) is the mainstay of therapy. Nitazoxinide (Rossignol JF. Aliment Pharmacol Ther. 2006;24:807), paromomycin (Maggi P, et al. Clin Infect Dis. 2000;33:1609), or a combination of paromomycin and azithromycin (Smith NH, et al. J Infect Dis. 1998;178:900) may be tried to decrease diarrhea and recalcitrant malabsorption of antimicrobial drugs, which can occur with chronic cryptosporidiosis.

Table 12.5 Treatment of Luminal Protozoa—cont'd

Infection	Drug	Adult Dosage	Pediatric Dosage
Cystoisosporiasis (*Cystoisospora belli*; formerly *Isospora belli*)			
Drug of choice[m]	Trimethoprim (TMP)/ sulfamethoxazole[f] (SMX)	TMP 160 mg/SMX 800 mg (1 double-strength tablet) bid × 10 days	TMP 5 mg/kg/day, SMX 25 mg/kg/day bid × 10 days
Cyclosporiasis (*Cyclospora cayetanensis*)			
Drug of choice[j]	Trimethoprim/sulfamethoxazole[f]	TMP 160 mg/SMX 800 mg (1 double-strength tablet) bid × 7–10 days	TMP 5 mg/kg/day, SMX 25 mg/kg/day bid × 7–10 days
***Dientamoeba fragilis* Infection[k]**			
Drug of choice	Iodoquinol	650 mg tid × 20 days	30–40 mg/kg/day (max. 2 g) in 3 doses × 20 days
	or paromomycin[f]	25–35 mg/kg/day in 3 doses × 7 days	25–35 mg/kg/day in 3 doses × 7 days
	or tetracycline[e–g]	500 mg qid × 10 days	40 mg/kg/day (max. 2 g) in 4 doses × 10 days
	or metronidazole[f]	500–750 mg tid × 10 days	35–50 mg/kg/day in 3 doses × 10 days
Giardiasis (*Giardia duodenalis*)			
Drug of choice	Metronidazole[e]	250 mg tid × 5–7 days	15 mg/kg/day in 3 doses × 5–7 days
	Tinidazole[e]	2 g once	50 mg/kg once (max. 2 g)
	Nitazoxanide[d]	500 mg bid × 3 days	1–3 years: 100 mg q12h × 3 days 4–11 years: 200 mg q12h × 3 days ≥12 years 500 mg q12h × 3 days
Alternatives[l]	Paromomycin[f,m]	25–35 mg/kg/day in 3 doses × 5–10 days	25–35 mg/kg/day in 3 doses × 5–10 days
	Furazolidone	100 mg qid × 7–10 days	6 mg/kg/day in 4 doses × 7–10 days
	Quinacrine[n]	100 mg tid × 5–10 days	2 mg/kg tid × 5–10 days (max. 300 mg/day)
Microsporidiosis, Intestinal			
• *E. bieneusi*			
Drug of choice	Fumagillin[o]	20 mg/day tid × 14 days	
• *E. (Septata) intestinalis*			
Drug of choice	Albendazole[p]	400 mg bid × 21 days	
Trichomoniasis (*Trichomonas vaginalis*)			
Drug of choice[p]	Metronidazole	2 g once *or* 500 mg bid × 7 days	15 mg/kg/day in 3 doses × 7 days
	or tinidazole[d]	2 g once	50 mg/kg once (max. 2 g)

[j]Usually a self-limited illness in immunocompetent patients. Immunosuppressed patients may need higher doses, longer duration (TMP/SMX qid × 10 days, followed by bid × 3 weeks) and long-term maintenance. In sulfonamide-sensitive patients, pyrimethamine 50–75 mg daily in divided does (plus leucovorin 10–25 mg/day) has been effective.

[k]Norberg A, et al. Clin Microbiol Infect. 2003;9:65; Vandenberg O, et al. Int J Infect Dis. 2006;10:255.

[l]Another alternative is albendazole 400 mg/day × 5 days in adults and 10 mg/kg/day × 5 days in children (Yereli K, et al. Clin Microbiol Infect. 2004;10:527; Karabay O, et al. World J Gastroenterol. 2004;10:1215). Combination treatment with standard dose of metronidazole and quinacrine × 3 weeks has been effective for a small number of refractory infections (Nash TE, et al. Clin Infect Dis. 2001;33:22). In one study, nitazoxanide was used successfully in high doses to treat a case of *Giardia* resistant to metronidazole and albendazole (Abboud P, et al. Clin Infect Dis. 2001;32;1792).

[m]Poorly absorbed; may be useful for treatment of giardiasis in pregnancy.

[n]Quinacrine should be taken with liquids or after a meal.

[o]Oral fumagillin (Flisint: Sanofi-Aventis, France) has been effective in treating *E. bieneusi* (Molina J-M, et al. N Engl J Med. 2002;346:1963) but has been associated with thrombocytopenia and neutropenia. HAART may lead to microbiologic and clinical response in HIV-infected patients with microsporidial diarrhea. Octreotide (Sandostatin) has provided symptomatic relief in some patients with large-volume diarrhea.

[p]Albendazole must be taken with food; a fatty meal increases oral bioavailability.

(Derived from the *Medical Letter on Drugs and Therapeutics*, Drugs for parasitic infections, www.medicalletter.org, October 2008.)

amebiasis (750 mg three times a day). Other side effects include headache, dizziness, vertigo, and numbness. Potentially severe disulfiram-like reactions occur in patients who ingest alcohol while taking metronidazole.

Tinidazole, another 5-nitroimidazole, has a similar mechanism of action and spectrum of activity. It has been widely used throughout the world for the treatment of giardiasis, intestinal amebiasis, and trichomoniasis. In comparison to metronidazole, it has a longer half-life, a shorter and less complicated dosing regimen, and fewer side effects.

Since neither metronidazole nor tinidazole reliably eradicates cysts of *E. histolytica*, a luminal agent is used with them in people with amebiasis. The luminal agents include paromomycin, diloxanide furoate, and iodoquinol. Any of these agents can be used alone in people with asymptomatic cyst excretion.

Paromomycin (aminosidine), an aminoglycoside poorly absorbed from the GI tract, reaches high concentrations in the intestine and is effective against *E. histolytica* cysts.[65,66] It is generally well tolerated, although nausea, vomiting, abdominal pain, or diarrhea may occur. Any absorbed paromomycin is excreted by the kidney and, like other aminoglycosides, is potentially ototoxic and nephrotoxic in people with renal failure.

Diloxanide furoate is also poorly absorbed and well tolerated. It is effective in killing *E. histolytica* cysts.[67] Mild GI side effects may occur.

Iodoquinol, a halogenated oxyquinoline, is another alternative. It, too, is poorly absorbed. Side effects include headache, diarrhea, nausea, vomiting, and abdominal pain. Less common are fever, itching, and seizures. Encephalopathy has also been reported.[68] Iodoquinol can cause iodine dermatitis, and its high iodine content can interfere with the results of thyroid function tests for months after therapy.

Nitazoxanide, a 5-nitrothiazole-salicylamide derivative, has a broad spectrum of activity against protozoa and helminths.[69–72] It is licensed in the United States for the treatment of giardiasis and cryptosporidiosis in immunocompetent children. It is also active against *Hymenolepis nana*, other helminths, bacteria, including *Clostridium difficile,* and even some viruses. It is formulated in tablet and liquid forms. It is well absorbed orally and hydrolyzed to its active metabolite, tizoxanide, which undergoes conjugation to tizoxanide glucuronide. The parent compound is not detectable in serum. The maximum concentrations of the metabolites are observed in 1–4 hours. They are both excreted in urine and bile. Tizoxanide is highly protein-bound. Although the mechanism of action is uncertain, tizoxanide is thought to inhibit pyruvate:ferredoxin oxidoreductase enzyme-dependent electron transport reactions essential to the metabolism of anaerobic organisms. Nitazoanide is well tolerated. Abdominal pain, diarrhea, headache, and nausea have been associated with its use, but their frequencies have not been greater than in controls receiving a placebo.

Trimethoprim-sulfamethoxazole is the drug of choice for the treatment of enterocolitis due to *Cystoisospora belli* and *Cyclospora cayetanensis*,[2] inhibiting two sequential steps in the folic acid pathway. Trimethoprim-sulfamethoxazole is generally well tolerated, but it can cause GI symptoms as well as rash, fever, and other hypersensitivity responses in people with sulfonamide allergies. In addition, the combination is associated with frequent side effects in people with AIDS, including rash, fever, and neutropenia.[73]

TREATMENT OF CHAGAS' DISEASE, AFRICAN TRYPANOSOMIASIS, AND LEISHMANIASIS

Trypanosoma cruzi, the etiology of Chagas' disease, and *T. brucei gambiense* and *T. brucei rhodesiense*, the causes of human African trypanosomiasis (sleeping sickness), pose difficult therapeutic challenges. The drugs used to treat *T. cruzi,* nifurtimox and benznidazole, are variably effective and have substantial side effects (***Table 12.6 and Box 12.5***). Treatment is indicated for acute Chagas' disease, recent infections, and indeterminant infections in children, young adults, and possibly older adults.[74] Once cardiac or GI findings of chronic Chagas' disease appear, antiparasitic treatment is no longer indicated. An increasing number of cases of Chagas' disease are being diagnosed in the United States and Canada as a result of immigration and the screening of blood donors.[74] Pentamidine and suramin are used for the treatment of the hemolymphatic stage of *T. brucei gambiense* and *T. brucei rhodesiense* infections, respectively.[75] Melarsoprol is used for CNS involvement. All three drugs are associated with substantial toxicity. The development of eflornithine for the treatment of *T. brucei gambiense* was a substantial advance, but the quantity of drug needed for treatment and the cost have curtailed its use in endemic areas.

Nifurtimox, a nitrofuran, has been used for the treatment of Chagas' disease in the United States.[74,76,77] It is available from the CDC. Nifurtimox lowers mortality in acute Chagas' disease due to myocarditis and meningoencephalitis and shortens the duration of symptoms. It is administered daily for a period of 90–120 days. Side effects occur in more than half of those treated and include anorexia, vomiting, abdominal pain, weight loss, sleep disorders, paresthesias, weakness, and polyneuritis. These untoward effects are usually reversible when the drug is stopped, but they often pose a therapeutic dilemma given the long duration of treatment. Seizures, rash, and neutropenia occur rarely.

Benznidazole, a nitroimidazole, has been widely used for the treatment of acute Chagas' disease in Latin America and for children and young adults with indeterminate *T. cruzi* infections.[74,77–79] It is administered for 30–90 days. It is frequently associated with skin reactions,

Box 12.5 Adverse Effects of Drugs Used to Treat Kinetoplastids

Benznidazole[a]
(Rochagan – Roche)
Frequent: allergic rash, dose-dependent polyneuropathy, gastrointestinal disturbances, psychic disturbances

Eflornithine[a]
(Difluoromethylornithine – Sanofi)
Frequent: anemia, leukopenia
Occasional: diarrhea, thrombocytopenia, seizures
Rare: hearing loss

Melarsoprol
(Mel-B – Specia)
Frequent: myocardial damage, albuminuria, hypertension, colic, Herxheimer-type reaction, encephalopathy, vomiting, peripheral neuropathy
Rare: shock

Miltefosine
(Impavido – Zentaris)
Frequent: nausea; vomiting; diarrhea; "motion sickness"; elevations in liver enzymes, blood urea nitrogen, and creatinine

Nifurtimox
(Lampit – Bayer)
Frequent: anorexia, vomiting, weight loss, loss of memory, sleep disorders, tremor, paresthesias, weakness, polyneuritis
Rare: convulsions, fever, pulmonary infiltrates and pleural effusion

Pentamidine Isethionate
(Pentam 300, NebuPent – Fujisawa)
Frequent: hypotension, hypoglycemia (may be followed by diabetes mellitus), vomiting, blood dyscrasias, renal damage, pain at injection site, gastrointestinal disturbances
Occasional: may aggravate diabetes, shock, hypocalcemia, liver damage, cardiotoxicity, delirium, rash
Rare: Herxheimer-type reaction, anaphylaxis, acute pancreatitis, hyperkalemia, ventricular arrhythmias

Pentavalent Antimonials: Meglumine Antimonate[a]
(Glucantime – Aventis)

Sodium Stibogluconate
(Pentostam – GlaxoSmithKline)
Frequent: muscle and joint pain, fatigue, nausea, transaminase elevations, T-wave flattening or inversion, amylase elevation, pancreatitis
Occasional: weakness, abdominal pain, liver damage, bradycardia, leukopenia, thrombocytopenia, rash, vomiting
Rare: diarrhea, pruritus, myocardial damage, hemolytic anemia, renal damage, shock, sudden death

Suramin Sodium
(Germain – Bayer)
Frequent: vomiting, pruritus, urticaria, paresthesias, hyperesthesia of hands and feet, photophobia, peripheral neuropathy
Occasional: kidney damage, blood dyscrasias, shock, optic atrophy

[a]*Not available in the United States.*

dose-dependent polyneuropathy, GI symptoms, bone marrow suppression, and psychiatric side effects.

Suramin, a toxic drug, is used for the treatment of the hemolymphatic stage of *T. brucei rhodesiense*.[80,81] It is administered intravenously. Suramin is frequently associated with nausea, vomiting, urticarial eruptions, paresthesias, hyperesthesias, and peripheral neuropathy. Less frequent side effects are renal damage, blood dyscrasias, loss of consciousness, and shock.

Pentamidine isethionate, a diamidine, is used for the treatment of the hemolymphatic stage of *T. brucei gambiense*.[82,83] It is an alternative drug for the treatment of leishmaniasis, but toxicity has limited its use. It has also been used for *Pneumocystis* pneumonia in those who cannot tolerate trimethoprim-sulfamethoxazole.[84] Aerosolized pentamidine can be used for prophylaxis against *P. jirovecii* in persons with AIDS, but it does not prevent infection in organs other than the lungs, and there are problems associated with its administration and the venting of exhaled material.

Pentamidine is usually administered intravenously. Intramuscular injections are associated with inflammation and sterile abscesses at the site

Table 12.6 Treatment of the Kinetoplastids: *Leishmania* and Trypanosomes

Infection	Drug	Adult Dosage	Pediatric Dosage
Leishmania			
Visceral[a,b]			
Drug of choice	Liposomal amphotericin B[c]	3 mg/kg/day IV days 1–5 and 14 and 21[d]	3 mg/kg/day IV days 1–5 and 14 and 21[d]
	or sodium stibogluconate	20 mg Sb[v]/kg/day IV or IM × 28 days	20 mg Sb[v]/kg/day IV or IM × 28 days
	or miltefosine[e]	2.5 mg/kg/day (max. 150 mg/day) × 28 days	2.5 mg/kg/day (max. 150 mg/day) × 28 days
Alternative[f]	Meglumine antimonate	20 mg Sb[v]/kg/day IV or IM × 28 days	20 mg Sb[v]/kg/day IV or IM × 28 days
	or amphotericin B[f]	1 mg/kg IV × 15–20 days or every second day for up to 8 weeks	1 mg/kg IV × 15–20 days or every second day for up to 8 weeks
	or paromomycin sulfate[f–h]	15 mg/kg/day IM × 21 days	15 mg/kg/day IM × 21 days
Cutaneous[a,i]			
Drug of choice	Sodium stibogluconate	20 mg Sb[v]/kg/day IV or IM × 20 days	20 mg Sb[v]/kg/day IV or IM × 20 days
	or meglumine antimonate	20 mg Sb[v]/kg/day IV or IM × 20 days	20 mg Sb[v]/kg/day IV or IM × 20 days
	or miltefosine[e]	2.5 mg/kg/day (max. 150 mg/day) × 28 days	2.5 mg/kg/day (max. 150 mg/day) × 28 days
Alternative[j]	Paromomycin[f–h]	Topically bid × 10–20 days	Topically bid × 10–20 days
	or pentamidine[f]	2–3 mg/kg IV or IM daily or every second day × 4–7 doses[k]	2–3 mg/kg IV or IM daily or every second day × 4–7 doses[k]
Mucosal[a,l]			
Drug of choice	Sodium stibogluconate	20 mg Sb[v]/kg/day IV or IM × 28 days	20 mg Sb[v]/kg/day IV or IM × 28 days
	or meglumine antimonate	20 mg Sb[v]/kg/day IV or IM × 28 days	20 mg Sb[v]/kg/day IV or IM × 28 days
	or amphotericin B[f]	0.5–1 mg/kg IV daily or every second day for up to 8 weeks	0.5–1 mg/kg IV daily or every second day for up to 8 weeks
	or miltefosine[f]	2.5 mg/kg/day (max. 150 mg/day) × 28 days	2.5 mg/kg/day (max. 150 mg/day) × 28 days

Sb[v] refers to the amount of pentavalent antimony administered.

[a]To maximize effectiveness and minimize toxicity, the choice of drug, dosage, and duration of therapy should be individualized based on the region of disease acquisition, a likely infecting species, and host factors such as immune status (Herwaldt BL. Lancet. 1999;354:1191). Some of the listed drugs and regimens are effective only against certain *Leishmania* species/strains and only in certain areas of the world (Arevalo J, et al. Clin Infect Dis. 2007;195:1846). *Medical Letter* consultants recommend consultation with physicians experienced in management of this disease.

[b]Visceral infection is most commonly due to the Old World species *L. donovani* (kala-azar) and *L. infantum* and the New World species *L. infantum chagasi*, which is thought to be the same species as *L. infantum*.

[c]Liposomal amphotericin B (AmBisome) is the only lipid formulation of amphotericin B that is approved by the Food and Drug Administration (FDA) for treatment of visceral leishmaniasis, largely based on clinical trials in patients infected with *L. infantum* (Meyerhoff A. Clin Infect Dis. 1999;28:42). Two other amphotericin B lipid formulations, amphotericin B lipid complex (Abelcet) and amphotericin B cholesteryl sulfate (Amphotec), have been used, but are considered investigational for this condition and may not be as effective (Bern C, et al. Clin Infect Dis. 2006;43:917).

[d]The FDA-approved dosage regimen for immunocompromised patients (e.g., infected with human immunodeficiency virus) is 4 mg/kg/day IV on days 1–5, 10, 17, 24, 31, and 38. The relapse rate is high; maintenance therapy (secondary prevention) may be indicated, but there is no consensus as to dosage or duration.

[e]Effective for both antimony-sensitive and -resistant *L. donovani* (Indian); miltefosine (Impavido) is manufactured in 10- or 50-mg capsules by Zentaris (Frankfurt, Germany: info@zentaris.com) and is available through consultation with the Centers for Disease Control and Prevention. The drug is contraindicated in pregnancy; a negative pregnancy test before drug initiation and effective contraception during and for 2 months after treatment are recommended (Murray H, et al. Lancet. 2005;366:1561). In a placebo-controlled trial in patients ≥12 years old, oral miltefosine 2.5 mg/kg/day × 28 days was also effective for treatment of cutaneous leishmaniasis due to *L. (V.) panamensis* in Colombia, but not *L. (V.) braziliensis* or *L. mexicana* in Guatemala (Soto J, et al. Clin Infect Dis. 2004;38:1266). "Motion sickness," nausea, headache, and increased creatinine are the most frequent adverse effects (Soto J, Soto P. Expert Rev Anti Infect Ther. 2006;4:177).

[f]Not FDA-approved for this indication.

[g]Paromomycin IM has been effective against *Leishmania* in India; it has not yet been tested in South America or the Mediterranean and there are insufficient data to support its use in pregnancy (Sundar S, et al. N Engl J Med. 2007;356:2371). Topical paromomycin should be used only in geographic regions where cutaneous leishmaniasis species have low potential for mucosal spread. A formulation of 15% paromomycin/12% methylbenzethonium chloride (Leshcutan) in soft white paraffin for topical use has been reported to be partially effective against cutaneous leishmaniasis due to *L. major* in Israel and *L. mexicana* and *L. (V.) braziliensis* in Guatemala, where mucosal spread is very rare (Arana BA, et al. Am J Trop Med Hyg. 2001;65:466). The methylbenzethonium is irritating to the skin; lesions may worsen before they improve.

[h]Cutaneous infection is most commonly due to the Old World species *L. major* and *L. tropica* and the New World species *L. mexicana, L. (Viannia) braziliensis*, and others.

[i]Although azole drugs (fluconazole, ketoconazole, itraconazole) have been used to treat cutaneous disease, they are not reliably effective and have no efficacy against mucosal disease (Magill AJ. Infect Dis Clin North Am. 2005;19:241). For treatment of *L. major* cutaneous lesions, a study in Saudi Arabia found that oral fluconazole, 200 mg once daily × 6 weeks appeared to speed healing (Alrajhi AA, et al. N Engl J Med. 2002;346:891). Thermotherapy may be an option for cutaneous *L. tropica* infection (Reithinger R, et al. Clin Infect Dis. 2005;40:1148). A device that generates focused and controlled heating of the skin has been approved by the FDA for this indication (ThermoMed – ThermoSurgery Technologies Inc, Phoenix AZ, 602-264-7300, www.thermosurgery.com).

[j]Topical paromomycin should be used only in geographic regions where cutaneous leishmaniasis species have low potential for mucosal spread. A formulation of 15% paromomycin/12% methylbenzethonium chloride (Leshcutan) in soft white paraffin for topical use has been reported to be partially effective in some patients against cutaneous leishmaniasis due to *L. major* in Israel and against *L. mexicana* and *L. (V.) braziliensis* in Guatemala, where mucosal spread is very rare (Arana BA, et al. Am J Trop Med Hyg. 2001;65:466). The methylbenzethonium is irritating to the skin; lesions may worsen before they improve.

[k]At this dosage pentamidine has been effective in Colombia predominantly against *L. (V.) panamensis* (Soto-Mancipe J, et al. Clin Infect Dis. 1993;16:417; Soto J, et al. Am J Trop Med Hyg. 1994;50:107). Activity against other species is not well established.

[l]Mucosal infection is most commonly due to the New World species *L. (V.) braziliensis, L. (V.) panamensis*, or *L. (V.) guyanensis*.

Table 12.6 Treatment of the Kinetoplastids: *Leishmania* and Trypanosomes—cont'd

Infection	Drug	Adult Dosage	Pediatric Dosage
Trypanosomiasis[m]			
T. cruzi **(American Trypanosomiasis, Chagas' Disease)**			
Drug of choice	Nifurtimox	8–10 mg/kg/day in 3–4 doses × 90–120 days	1–10 years: 15–20 mg/kg/day in 4 doses × 90–120 days 11–16 years: 12.5–15 mg/kg/day in 4 doses × 90–120 days
	or benznidazole[n]	5–7 mg/kg/day in 2 divided doses × 30–90 days	≤12 years: 10 mg/kg/day in 2 doses × 30–90 days >12 years: 5–7 mg/kg/day in 2 doses × 30–90 days
T. brucei gambiense **(West African Trypanosomiasis, Sleeping Sickness)**			
• Hemolymphatic Stage			
Drug of choice[o]	Pentamidine[f]	4 mg/kg/day IM × 7 days	4 mg/kg/day IM ×7 days
Alternative	Suramin	100–200 mg (test dose) IV, then 1 g IV on days 1, 3, 7, 14, and 21	Test dose then 20 mg/kg IV, then on days 1, 3, 7, 14, and 21
• Late Disease with CNS Involvement			
Drug of choice	Eflornithine[p]	400 mg/kg/day IV in 4 doses × 14 days	400 mg/kg/day IV in 4 doses × 14 days
	or melarsoprol[q]	2.2 mg/kg/day IV × 10 days	2.2 mg/kg/day IV × 10 days
T. b. rhodesiense **(East African Trypanosomiasis, Sleeping Sickness)**			
• Hemolymphatic Stage			
Drug of choice	Suramin	100–200 mg (test dose) IV, then 1 g IV on days 1, 3, 7,14, and 21	Test dose then 20 mg/kg IV on days 1, 3, 7, 14, and 21
• Late Disease with CNS Involvement			
Drug of choice	Melarsoprol[q]	2–3.6 mg/kg/day IV × 3 days; after 7 days 3.6 mg/kg/day × 3 days; repeat again after 7 days	2–3.6 mg/kg/day IV × 3 days; after 7 days 3.6 mg/kg/day × 3 days; repeat again after 7 days

[m]Barrett MP, et al. Lancet. 2003;362:1469. Treatment of chronic or indeterminate Chagas' disease with benznidazole has been associated with reduced progression and increased negative seroconversion (Viotti R, et al. Ann Intern Med. 2006;144:724).

[n]Benznidazole should be taken with meals to minimize gastrointestinal adverse effects. It is contraindicated during pregnancy.

[o]Pentamidine and suramin have equal efficacy, but pentamidine is better tolerated.

[p]Eflornithine is highly effective in *T. b. gambiense* but not in *T. b. rhodesiense* infections. In one study of treatment of central nervous system disease due to *T. b. gambiense*, there were fewer serious complications with eflornithine than with melarsoprol (Chappuis F, et al. Clin Infect Dis. 2005;41:748). Eflornithine is available in limited supply only from the World Health Organization. It is contraindicated during pregnancy.

[q]Schmid E, et al. J Infect Dis. 2005;191:1922. Corticosteroids have been used to prevent arsenical encephalopathy (Pepin J, et al. Trans R Soc Trop Med Hyg. 1995;89:92). Up to 20% of patients with *T. b. gambiense* fail to respond to melarsoprol (Barrett MP. Lancet. 1999;353:1113). In one study, a combination of low-dose melarsoprol (1.2 mg/kg/day IV) and nifurtimox (7.5 mg/kg PO bid) × 10 days was more effective than standard-dose melarsoprol alone (Bisser S, et al. J Infect Dis. 2007;195:322).

(Derived from the *Medical Letter on Drugs and Therapeutics*, Drugs for parasitic infections, www.medicalletter.org, October 2008.)

of inoculation. It is not absorbed orally. The mechanism of action is not known, but it may interact with the parasite's DNA. Side effects are common and include GI complaints, dizziness, tachycardia, flushing, and hypotension if the drug is infused too rapidly. Renal function is impaired transiently in as many as one-fourth of recipients. A major concern is hypoglycemia that results from the release of insulin from damaged pancreatic beta cells. Patients with higher pentamidine levels appear to be at greater risk. Fatalities have been reported during and after therapy. The development of insulin-dependent diabetes mellitus is a potential long-term outcome.

Melarsoprol, a trivalent arsenical, is administered intravenously for the treatment of African trypanosomiasis with CNS involvement.[80,81] Fever, abdominal pain, vomiting, arthralgias, myocardial toxicity, hypertension, albuminuria, and peripheral neuropathy are common.[80,81] More importantly, approximately 6% of recipients develop allergic encephalitis, which is characterized by headache, dizziness, mental dullness, confusion, ataxia, obtundation, and seizures; overall, 4% of patients die as a consequence.[85,86] Cardiovascular collapse is a rare complication.

Eflornithine (difluoromethylornithine) is effective against the hemolymphatic and CNS stages of *T. b. gambiense* infection.[87–89] It is an enzyme-activated, irreversible inhibitor of ornithine decarboxylase, an important enzyme in the polyamine pathway. It does not have activity against *T. b. rhodesiense*. Eflornithine can be administered orally or intravenously. The ratio of the level in CSF to serum ranges from 0.09 to 0.45; the ratio is highest in patients who have the most severe CNS involvement. Most of the drug is excreted in the urine. In contrast to the other drugs used to treat African trypanosomiasis, eflornithine is relatively well tolerated. Flatulence, nausea, vomiting, and diarrhea can occur, but they are transient. Some recipients develop reversible anemia, thrombocytopenia, or neutropenia. Diplopia, dizziness, or hypersensitivity reactions occur rarely.

The treatment of leishmaniasis is complicated. It depends on the clinical syndrome, likelihood of parasite resistance, and cost and availability of drugs. Amphotericin B is broadly active against *Leishmania* species. When formulated in liposomes, it is targeted to macrophages, the site of leishmanial infection. Liposomal amphotericin B is the drug of choice for visceral leishmaniasis. It is the only drug approved for that indication in the United States. Sodium stibogluconate and meglumine antimoniate, pentavalent antimony-containing compounds, were once the mainstay of treatment. They continue to be used for visceral leishmaniasis in Latin America, but resistance now precludes their use in India and some other areas.[90–92] Miltefosine, the only orally administered antileishmanial agent, is currently available for the treatment of visceral leishmaniasis in India; but resistance has been reported. More recently, parenterally administered paromomycin has been reported to be effective in studies in India.

Treatment of cutaneous leishmaniasis is indicated in persons with large and cosmetically important skin lesions and those infected with *Leishmania* species associated with mucosal disease in the Americas. Pentavalent antimonials are widely used for both cutaneous and mucosal leishmaniasis. Alternatives include liposomal amphotericin B, miltefosine, imidazole antifungals including fluconazole, itraconazole and ketoconazole, amphotericin B deoxycholate, local injection of pentavalent antimony into the lesion, and topical paromomycin. Other therapeutic modalities, including immunotherapy, cryotherapy, and thermotherapy, have been reported to be effective, but data are insufficient to recommend their general use.

Amphotericin B deoxycholate, well known as an antifungal agent, is a highly active antileishmanial drug.[93,94] Its use is limited by the requirement for prolonged parenteral administration and its toxicity. Amphotericin B binds to ergosterol and other sterols and is thought to damage the cytoplasmic membrane of *Leishmania* much as it does the membranes of susceptible fungi. Untoward effects, including fever, chills, malaise, nausea, anorexia, weight loss, and vomiting, accompany administration. Both acute and chronic nephrotoxicity and resulting electrolyte abnormalities are common.

Liposomal amphotericin B (AmBisome) is the treatment of choice for visceral leishmaniasis in the United States and other industrialized areas.[95,96] Delivery of drug to the reticuloendothelial system by liposomes is theoretically attractive since *Leishmania* reside in mononuclear phagocytes. In addition, liposomal amphotericin B is much better tolerated than amphotericin B deoxycholate and the treatment course is shorter. Other lipid-associated amphotericin B preparations appear to be effective, but they have been less extensively studied and are not approved by the Food and Drug Administration.

Stibogluconate is available in the United Kingdom and through the CDC in the United States, whereas meglumine antimoniate is used in French-speaking areas and in Latin America. Although the bioavailability can vary among lots, sodium stibogluconate and meglumine antimoniate appear to be of comparable efficacy and toxic when administered on the basis of their pentavalent antimony content. They are administered intravenously or intramuscularly for systemic therapy. Intralesional injections have been used for cutaneous leishmaniasis in some areas of the world.

Stibogluconate and meglumine antimoniate are administered at a dose of 20 mg of pentavalent antimony (Sb^{V}) per kilogram body weight per day for 20–28 days depending on the clinical syndrome and infecting *Leishmania* species. Their mechanism of action is uncertain. Although most patients are able to complete a full course of therapy, side effects are common and increase with age. They include nausea, vomiting, abdominal pain, anorexia, myalgias, arthralgias, headache, and malaise. Chemical pancreatitis is observed in many patients, and severe pancreatitis occurs in some. It is particularly common in people with renal failure. Nonspecific ST-T-wave changes are common. Less frequent side effects are elevated liver enzymes, bradycardia, leukopenia, thrombocytopenia, and anemia. Renal toxicity, myocardial damage, and shock are rare. Sudden death, possibly from arrhythmia, has been reported in people receiving more than the recommended dose.

Miltefosine (hexadecylphosphocholine) is the only orally administered drug with activity against *Leishmania* species.[97–99] It is currently available for the treatment of visceral leishmaniasis in India, where resistance to pentavalent antimony is common in *L. donovani*. Miltefosine has also been used successfully in the treatment of New World cutaneous leishmaniasis.[98,99] Although the precise mechanism of action is uncertain, it probably affects cell signaling pathways by inhibiting phosphokinase C and protein kinase C and also interferes with the synthesis of glycosylphosphatidylinositol membrane anchors, which are important in *Leishmania* and related kinetoplastids. Miltefosine is relatively well tolerated, but nausea, vomiting, and a sense of "motion sickness" may occur in up to one-third of recipients, particularly at high doses. Elevations of hepatic transaminases, blood urea nitrogen, and creatinine have been noted but usually resolve with continuation of the drug. The side effects seldom result in premature termination of therapy in patients treated for visceral leishmaniasis. Unfortunately, miltefosine resistance has been documented in *L. donovani*.[100] Further studies are needed to define its role in the treatment of visceral leishmaniasis in areas of the world other than India and in the treatment of cutaneous and mucosal leishmaniasis.

Table 12.7 Treatment of Ectoparasites

Infection	Drug	Adult Dosage	Pediatric Dosage
Lice (*Pediculus humanus, P. capitis, Phthirus pubis*)[a]			
Drug of choice	0.5% Malathion[b]	Topically	Topically
	or 1% permethrin[c]	Topically	Topically
Alternatives	Pyrethrins with piperonyl butoxide[c]	Topically	Topically
	or ivermectin[d–f]	200 µg/kg × 3, days 1, 2, and 10	≥15 kg: 200 µg/kg PO
Scabies (*Sarcoptes scabiei*)			
Drug of choice	5% Permethrin	Topically	Topically
Alternatives[g,h,i]	Ivermectin[d,e]	200 µg/kg once[g]	200 µg/kg once[g]
	or 10% crotamiton	Topically once daily × 2 days	Topically once daily × 2 days

[a]Pediculocides should not be used for infestations of eyelashes. Such infestations are treated with petrolatum ointment applied 2–4 times per day × 8–10 days. Oral trimethoprim (TMP)/sulfamethoxazole (SMX) has also been used (Meinking TL. Curr Probl Dermatol. 1996;24:157). For pubic lice, treat with 5% permethrin or ivermectin as for scabies. TMP/SMX has also been effective together with permethrin for head lice (Hipolito RB, et al. Pediatrics. 2001;107:E30).

[b]Malathion is both ovicidal and pediculocidal; two applications at least 7 days apart are generally necessary to kill all lice and nits.

[c]Permethrin and pyrethrin are pediculocidal; retreatment in 7–10 days is needed to eradicate the infestation. Some lice are resistant to pyrethrins and permethrin (Meinking TL, et al. Arch Dermatol. 2002;138:220).

[d]Not approved by the Food and Drug Administration (FDA) for this indication.

[e]Safety of ivermectin in young children (<15 kg) and pregnant women remains to be established. Ivermectin should be taken on an empty stomach with water.

[f]Ivermectin is pediculocidal, but more than one dose is generally necessary to eradicate the infestation (Jones KN, English JC III. Clin Infect Dis. 2003;36:1355). The number of doses and interval between doses have not been established, but in one study of body lice, three doses administered at 7-day intervals were effective (Fouault C, et al. J Infect Dis. 2006;193:474).

[g]Treatment may need to be repeated in 10–14 days. A second ivermectin dose taken 2 weeks later increases the cure rate to 95%, which is equivalent to that of 5% permethrin (Usha V, et al. J Am Acad Dermatol. 2000;42:236; Chosidow O. N Engl J Med. 2006;354:1718; Heukelbach J, Feldmeier H. Lancet. 2006;367:1767).

[h]Lindane (gamma-benzene hexachloride; Kwell) should be reserved for treatment of patients who fail to respond to other drugs. The FDA has recommended it not be used for immunocompromised patients, young children, the elderly, pregnant and breast-feeding women, and patients weighing <50 kg.

[i]Ivermectin, either alone or in combination with a topical scabicide, is the drug of choice for crusted scabies in immunocompromised patients (del Giudice P. Curr Opin Infect Dis. 2004;15:123).

(Derived from the *Medical Letter on Drugs and Therapeutics*, Drugs for parasitic infections, www.medicalletter.org, October 2008.)

Box 12.6 Adverse Effects of Drugs Used in the Treatment of Ectoparasites

Crotamiton
(Eurax – Westwood–Squibb)
Occasional: rash, conjunctivitis

Malathion
(Ovide – Medicis)
Occasional: local irritation

Permethrin
(Nix – GlaxoSmithKline; Elimite – Allergan)

Pyrethrins and Piperonyl Butoxide
(RID – Pfizer, Others)
Occasional: allergic reactions

The aminoglycoside, paromomycin, administered intravenously has also been used successfully in the treatment of pentavalent antimony-resistant *L. donovani* in India. While other parenterally administered aminoglycosides are associated with nephrotoxicity, ototoxicity, or vestibular toxicity, paromomycin has reportedly been well tolerated. It has also been used topically with methylbenzethonium chloride in soft white paraffin for the treatment of cutaneous leishmaniasis caused by *L. major* and other *Leishmania* species.[101]

The imidazole antifungals, ketoconazole,[102] itraconazole,[103] and fluconazole,[104] inhibit ergosterol biosynthesis and vary in their activity against different *Leishmania* species. Failures occur, even with sensitive *Leishmania* species, and their use has been primarily in persons with cutaneous disease.

TREATMENT OF ECTOPARASITIC DISEASES

The major ectoparasites of humans, lice and scabies, can be treated with topical malathion, permethrin, or alternative drugs, or oral ivermectin (***Table 12.7 and Box 12.6***).

Access the complete reference list online at
http://www.expertconsult.com

Access the complete reference list online at http://www.expertconsult.com

CHAPTER 13

Chemotherapy of Bacterial, Fungal, and Viral Diseases

Thomas L. Holland • Nathan M. Thielman • Richard D. Pearson

INTRODUCTION

This chapter provides an overview of major antibacterial, antimycobacterial, antifungal, and antiviral agents but does not include comprehensive information about the pharmacology, indications, dosing, or toxicities of all the chemotherapeutic agents used in the treatment of tropical infectious diseases. The treatment of specific infections is more thoroughly addressed in Section II, Pathogens. Additionally, drugs used against opportunistic infections and potentially serious drug interactions in human immunodeficiency syndrome (HIV)-infected patients are summarized. More complete discussions are found in pharmacology textbooks, and substantial additional information about indications, dosing, and toxicities may be found in *The Medical Letter on Drugs and Therapeutics*.

ANTIBACTERIAL DRUGS

Antibiotics, their pharmacology and indications, form the topic of entire textbooks. The increasingly worrisome emergence of resistance among bacteria has nearly outstripped even the impressive burgeoning of new antibiotics, and effective therapy often requires isolation of the pathogen and sensitivity testing to specific antimicrobial agents. Furthermore, infections in immunocompromised hosts or in "privileged sites," such as cerebrospinal fluid (CSF) or endocarditic vegetations, often require bactericidal agents or synergistic antibiotic combinations. Treatment of common infections such as pneumonia, meningitis, and sepsis is fraught with increasing difficulty because of resistant organisms. For example, *Streptococcus pneumoniae* is increasingly resistant to penicillin and sometimes to cephalosporins and macrolides. *Listeria monocytogenes*, an important cause of meningitis, is resistant to even third-generation cephalosporins. Ampicillin is recommended for its treatment. Macrolides are indicated for "atypical" pneumonia caused by *Mycoplasma pneumoniae*, *Chlamydia pneumoniae*, or *Legionella pneumoniae*. In addition to Gram-negative bacilli, staphylococci, particularly methicillin-resistant *Staphylococcus aureus*, and *Candida* have emerged as important causes of nosocomial infection. Adverse effects of antibiotics are also common, ranging from hypersensitivity reactions, including rash, fever, and anaphylaxis, most often seen with sulfonamides and β-lactam antibiotics, to nephrotoxicity, especially with aminoglycosides. Antibiotic-associated colitis or superinfections can occur with most antibiotics but are especially common with those whose broad spectrum alters the normal oropharyngeal, bowel, and other flora. This section focuses on selective principles of antibiotic therapy within the major classes of antibacterial drugs and lists the infections for which these agents are generally the drug of choice or a primary alternative. These are summarized in ***Table 13.1***.

Shown in ***Figure 13.1*** are the various mechanisms by which antibacterial agents exert either bactericidal or bacteriostatic activity against different microorganisms. The major bacterial cell wall inhibitors are β-lactam agents (such as penicillins, cephalosporins, and carbapenems) and vancomycin. Penicillins differ in their absorption, protein-binding characteristics, metabolism, and renal excretion, but in general all are well distributed throughout the body. In the presence of inflammation, CSF concentrations rise to around 5% of those in plasma. Adjustments in dosages of penicillin are generally not necessary until renal clearance decreases below 30 mL/minute. Penicillin G and penicillin V are active against most non-β-lactamase-producing Gram-positive and Gram-negative cocci. Ampicillin and amoxicillin exhibit broader Gram-negative coverage than penicillin does, but increasing resistance among *Haemophilus influenzae*, *Shigella*, and *Salmonella* has been seen in recent years. Penicillinase-resistant penicillins (e.g., methicillin, nafcillin, dicloxacillin) inhibit staphylococci and streptococci. The carboxypenicillins (carbenicillin and ticarcillin) have extended activity against *Pseudomonas aeruginosa* and other Gram-negative bacilli. Because they are readily destroyed by β-lactamases, these agents are useful primarily when combined with a β-lactamase inhibitor. Ureidopenicillins (e.g., piperacillin, mezlocillin, and azlocillin) also exhibit extended activity against Gram-negative organisms (including *Pseudomonas*), while retaining activity against streptococci. The combination of piperacillin with the β-lactamase inhibitor tazobactam renders this ureidopenicillin more effective against β-lactamase-producing bacteria.

Cephalosporins are classified into generations based on their spectrum of antimicrobial activity. In general, first-generation cephalosporins have good activity against Gram-positive organisms and moderate activity against Gram-negative bacilli such as *Escherichia coli*. Some second generation cephalosporins, such as cefotaxime, have enhanced activity against *Haemophilus* and Gram-negative bacilli, but less activity than first-generation cephalosporins against staphylococci. Third-generation cephalosporins, in general, have less activity against staphylococci and more activity against streptococci, Enterobacteriaceae, *Neisseria*, and *Haemophilus* spp. Notably, ceftazidime and cefoperazone have less activity against streptococci but improved activity against *P. aeruginosa*. Third-generation cephalosporins, like penicillins, are widely distributed into body compartments. Cefotaxime and ceftriaxone enter the CSF and are widely used to treat meningitis. Ceftizoxime (and cefepime) also can be used to treat meningitis. Most cephalosporins are eliminated by renal mechanisms. Cefoperazone and ceftriaxone are primarily excreted by the biliary route. Fourth-generation cephalosporins, including cefepime, have activity against both Gram-positive cocci (comparable to that of cefotaxime or ceftriaxone) and excellent activity against *P. aeruginosa* (comparable to that of ceftazidime).

Penicillins are generally well tolerated. The most important life-threatening side effect is a type I hypersensitivity reaction, which occurs in up to 0.05% of treatment courses. A morbilliform skin eruption occurs in 3–5% of patients. Occasionally, penicillin can cause seizures when given in high doses, particularly in patients with concomitant renal failure. The incidence of anaphylaxis with cephalosporins is even less than that seen with penicillins. It is estimated that fewer than 5% of those who

Table 13.1 Selected Antibacterial Drugs

Drug	Infections for Which Drug is a Top Choice or a Primary Alternative	Some Important Infections *not* Treated by Drug
Bacterial Cell Wall Inhibitors		
β-Lactams • Penicillins	*Streptococcus*[a] *Enterococcus*[a] (with aminoglycoside) *Staphylococcus*[a] (if sensitive) *Neisseria meningitidis* *Bacillus anthracis* *Clostridium perfringens, Clostridium tetani* Anaerobes (oropharyngeal) *Pasteurella multocida* *Spirillum minus* *Streptobacillus moniliformis* *Actinomyces* *Leptospira* *Treponema pallidum, Treponema pertenue* *Capnocytophaga canimorsus* (DF-2) (+ aminoglycoside)	Gram-negatives β-Lactamase-producing *Staphylococcus aureus* *Legionella*
• Aminopenicillins: Ampicillin, amoxicillin	*Enterococcus* (with aminoglycoside) *Listeria monocytogenes* (± gentamicin) *Proteus mirabilis*[a] *Eikenella corrodens*[a]	*Legionella* β-Lactamase-producing Gram-negatives *Staphylococcus aureus* *Haemophilus influenzae*
+ β-Lactamase inhibitor: Amoxicillin + clavulanate Ampicillin + sulbactam	β-Lactamase-producing *H. influenzae* *S. aureus* *Escherichia coli* *Klebsiella pneumoniae* *Moraxella (Branhamella) catarrhalis* Anaerobes	*Legionella* *Acinetobacter* *Pseudomonas* *Citrobacter* *Enterobacter* *Serratia*
• Penicillinase-resistant penicillins: Cloxacillin, dicloxacillin, nafcillin, oxacillin, flucloxacillin	*Staphylococcus*[a] (penicillinase +)	MRSA *Enterococcus*
• Carboxy- and ureidopenicillins + β-lactamase inhibitor: Ticarcillin + clavulanate Piperacillin + tazobactam	*Pseudomonas aeruginosa*[a] (+ aminoglycoside) *Enterobacter* *Escherichia coli* *Klebsiella pneumoniae* *Proteus* spp. *Providencia stuartii* *Acinetobacter* *Bacteroides* Some polymicrobial infections (e.g., diabetic foot ulcer)	Some enterococci *Legionella* *Campylobacter jejeuni* *Listeria*
• Cephalosporins:		All cephalosporins: Enterococci MRSA *Listeria* *Legionella*
First generation (cephalothin and others)	Methicillin-susceptible *Staphylococcus aureus*, streptococci (penicillin-susceptible), *E. coli*, *Klebsiella*,[a] *Proteus* (indole +)	
Second generation (cefuroxime and others)	*Providencia*,[a] *Moraxella (Branhamella) catarrhalis*	
Third generation: cefotaxime, ceftriaxone	*Neisseria gonorrhoeae*[a] (or cefixime or cefpodoxime) *Haemophilus ducreyi*, *Salmonella*, *Borrelia burgdorferi* meningitis, *Campylobacter fetus*	
Ceftazidime	*Pseudomonas aeruginosa*[a] *Burkholderia (Pseudomonas) pseudomallei*[a] (melioidosis)	
Fourth generation: cefepime	*Pseudomonas aeruginosa*, *Enterobacter*, *Klebsiella pneumoniae*	
• Monobactam: Aztreonam	Gram-negatives	All Gram-positives
• Carbapenems: Imipenem, meropenem, doripenem	*Campylobacter fetus* *Enterobacter*[a] (with aminoglycoside) *Acinetobacter*[a] *Citrobacter freundii* *Serratia*	MRSA *Pseudomonas capacia* *Xanthomonas (Stenotrophonomas) maltophilia* *Enterococcus faecium* *Corynebacterium* JK group *Legionella*

Table 13.1 Selected Antibacterial Drugs—cont'd

Drug	Infections for Which Drug is a Top Choice or a Primary Alternative	Some Important Infections *not* Treated by Drug
Vancomycin	MRSA Penicillin-resistant pneumococci (with ceftriaxone or cefotaxime) *Bacillus cereus, Bacillus subtilis* *Corynebacterium* JK group	All Gram-negatives
Plasma Membrane Active Agent		
Daptomycin[b]	*Enterococcus* *Staphylococcus aureus* MRSA	All Gram-negatives Anaerobes
Inhibitors of Bacterial Ribosomal Actions		
Macrolides Erythromycin	*Corynebacterium diphtheriae* (with antitoxin) Streptococci (in penicillin- and cephalosporin-allergic patients) *Campylobacter jejeuni,*[a] *Bartonella* *Bartonella henselae, B. quintana* (or ciprofloxacin for *B. henselae*) *Bordetella pertussis* *Haemophilus ducreyi* (or ceftriaxone or azithromycin) *Legionella* *Chlamydia trachomatis* (inclusion conjunctivitis, pneumonia) *Mycoplasma pneumoniae* (alt. tetracycline) *Ureaplasma urealyticum*	Most Gram-negatives
Clarithromycin[c]	*Helicobacter pylori*[a] (or tetracycline + metronidazole + bismuth	
Azithromycin	*C. trachomatis* (trachoma, urethritis, cervicitis)	
Aminoglycosides		
Streptomycin Gentamicin	*Yersinia pestis* (plague); *Francisella tularensis* (in combination with ampicillin for *Enterococcus, Listeria* or with tetracycline for *Brucella, Pseudomonas mallei*)	Monotherapy for any organism[e]
Tobramycin, amikacin	(in combination with ureidopenicillins for *P. aeruginosa*)	
Tetracyclines[d]	*Brucella*[a] (+ aminoglycoside)	Most hospital-acquired bacteria
Tigecycline	*Enterococcus* including VRE; MRSA; complicated intra-abdominal infections *Calymmatobacterium granulomatis, Vibrio*[a] (alt. cefotaxime for *Vibrio vulnificus*), *Chlamydia psittaci, Chlamydia pneumoniae* (TWAR), *Chlamydia trachomatis* (urethritis, cervicitis, LGV) *Rickettsia, Ehrlichia, Borrelia recurrentis, Borrelia burgdorferi*	*P. aeruginosa, Proteus, Providencia*
Clindamycin	Anaerobes, toxic streptococci, staphylococci (preferred by some)	All Gram-negatives
Chloramphenicol	*Bacteroides*[a] (oropharyngeal strains; or penicillin)	Enterococci MRSA
Linezolid	*Enterococcus* MRSA Highly penicillin-resistant *Streptococcus pneumoniae*	Gram-negatives Anaerobes
Quinupristin/dalfopristin (Synercid)	Vancomycin-resistant *Enterococcus faecium*	*Enterococcus faecalis* Gram-negatives Anaerobes
DNA Gyrase Inhibitors		
Fluoroquinolones[f]		
All	Most enteric Gram-negative bacilli,[a] including *Salmonella*[a] (Typhi and others), *Shigella,*[a] *Vibrio cholerae, Campylobacter jejeuni*	
Ciprofloxacin	Plus: *Bartonella henselae* (cat-scratch bacillus), *Neisseria gonorrhoeae, Haemophilus ducreyi, Pseudomonas aeruginosa*	Anaerobes, streptococci
Ofloxacin	Plus: *Neisseria gonorrhoeae, Chlamydia trachomatis*	Anaerobes, streptococci
Levofloxacin, gatifloxacin, moxifloxacin	Plus: β-lactam-resistant *S. pneumoniae* *Pseudomonas aeruginosa* (ciprofloxacin, levofloxacin)	Some anaerobes

Table 13.1 Selected Antibacterial Drugs—cont'd

Drug	Infections for Which Drug is a Top Choice or a Primary Alternative	Some Important Infections *not* Treated by Drug
Bacterial Folate Antagonists		
Sulfonamides Trimethoprim-sulfamethoxazole	*Moraxella (Branhamella) catarrhalis* *Yersinia enterocolitica*[a] *Aeromonas* *Burkholderia cepacia*[a] *Stenotrophomonas maltophilia*[a] *Nocardia*	*Campylobacter jejuni* Enterococci Anaerobes Most *Pseudomonas* species
Other		
Metronidazole	*Clostridium difficile* *Bacteroides*[a] (gastrointestinal strains) Bacterial vaginosis	Aerobic bacteria

[a]Confirm sensitivity as resistance is increasing (e.g., *Streptococcus pneumoniae* requiring cefotaxime, ceftriaxone, or, for high-level resistance, vancomycin plus rifampin or levofloxacin, gatifloxacin, or moxifloxacin).
[b]FDA-approved for complicated skin and skin structure infections.
[c]Clarithromycin is not recommended for use in pregnancy or in patients receiving terfenadine therapy who have preexisting cardiac abnormalities.
[d]Tetracyclines are generally not recommended for pregnant women or for children less than 8 years of age.
[e]Aminoglycosides are useful only in combination therapy.
[f]Fluoroquinolones are generally not recommended for children or pregnant women.
MRSA, methicillin-resistant *Staphylococcus aureus*; LGV, lymphogranuloma venereum; VRE, vancomycin-resistant enterococci.
See Choice of antibacterial agents. Treatment Guidelines from The Medical Letter 2007;57:33–50, for doses, toxicities, and alternatives.

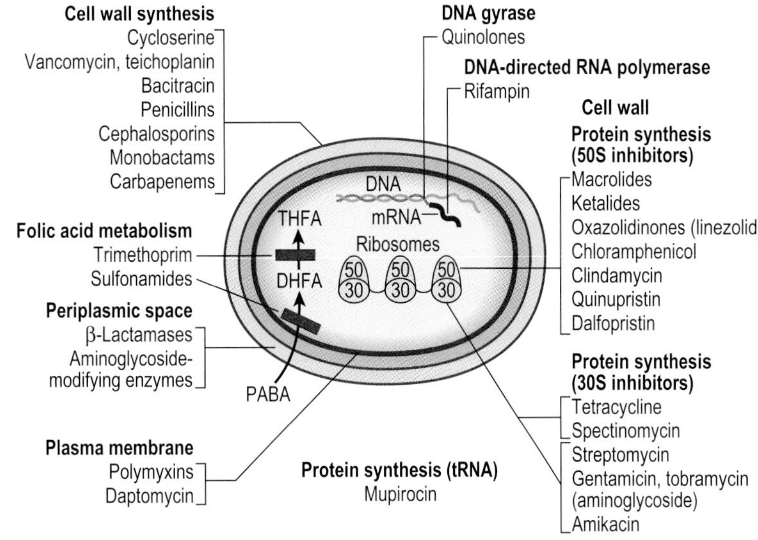

Figure 13.1 Antimicrobial sites of bactericidal or bacteriostatic action on microorganisms. The five general mechanisms are (1) inhibition of synthesis of the cell wall, (2) damage to the outer membrane, (3) modification of nucleic acid and DNA synthesis, (4) modification of protein synthesis (at ribosomes), and (5) modification of energy metabolism within the cytoplasm (at folate cycle). DHFA, dihydrofolate; PABA, para-aminobenzoic acid; THFA, tetrahydrofolate. (Adapted from Brody TE, Larner J, Minneman K, et al. Human Pharmacology: Molecular to Clinical, 3rd ed. St Louis: Mosby-Year Book, 1998.)

have anaphylactic reactions to penicillin are at risk for such a reaction with a cephalosporin.

The carbapenems – imipenem, meropenem, ertapenem, and doripenem – all administered intravenously, are β-lactam antibiotics that are relatively resistant to β-lactamases. Because imipenem is hydrolyzed by a renal dihydropeptidase, it is combined with a renal dehydropeptidase inhibitor, cilastatin. Imipenem and meropenem reach therapeutic concentrations in CSF in patients with meningitis; however, imipenem may cause seizures in patients with underlying brain injury or impaired renal clearance. Clinical experience suggests that carefully adjusting imipenem dosing according to renal function or the use of meropenem may help decrease the risk of seizures. Imipenem, meropenem, and doripenem have excellent activity against Gram-positive and Gram-negative aerobes and anaerobes. Ertapenem, on the other hand, has minimal activity against *P. aeruginosa* or *Acinetobacter*. It offers the advantage of once daily dosing for infections caused by susceptible organisms.

Vancomycin, a glycopeptide cell wall inhibitor unrelated to β-lactams, is not absorbed orally and is primarily used intravenously. It is eliminated by glomerular filtration and is not removed by intermittent hemodialysis or peritoneal dialysis. Dosage should be adjusted in patients with impaired creatinine clearance. Vancomycin is useful for Gram-positive (but not for Gram-negative) bacteria, particularly methicillin-resistant *S. aureus* and methicillin-resistant coagulase-negative staphylococci. Oral vancomycin effectively treats *Clostridium difficile*-associated diarrhea, and is the preferred therapy (over metronidazole) for severe disease. Vancomycin occasionally causes "red-man syndrome," a histamine-mediated phenomenon characterized by erythema, especially around the head and neck, sometimes with hypotension. Vancomycin also can be ototoxic, particularly at higher plasma concentrations or when given in combination with aminoglycosides.

Some new agents with activity targeting Gram-positive bacteria have become available in recent years. Daptomycin is a cyclic lipopeptide that binds to and depolarizes bacterial plasma membranes, resulting in cell death. It offers the advantage of once daily dosing and is a reasonable alternative to vancomycin for complicated skin and skin structure infections as well as for *S. aureus* bacteremia. Linezolid, an oxazolidinone that inhibits protein synthesis at the bacterial ribosome, has clinically useful activity against both *Enterococcus faecium* and *E. faecalis*, including many vancomycin-resistant enterococci and methicillin-resistant staphylococci. It has the advantage of being dosed orally, but its long-term use has been limited primarily by concerns for treatment-associated thrombocytopenia. Quinupristin/dalfopristin, a combination of streptogramins, also inhibits bacterial protein synthesis. It is active against methicillin-resistant *S. aureus* (MRSA) and *E. faecium*, including vancomycin-resistant strains (VRE), but not against *E. faecalis*. Disadvantages of quinupristin/dalfopristin include the requirement for infusion via a central venous catheter and frequent dose-limiting myalgias. Tigecycline is a glycylcycline structurally similar to the tetracyclines that has broad activity against Gram-positives including MRSA and VRE. It also has activity against a broad array of Gram-negative organisms, but notably not against *P. aeruginosa*.

The macrolide antibiotics include erythromycin, clarithromycin, azithromycin, and dirithromycin. Erythromycin has broad Gram-positive activity (including *S. pneumoniae*, *Streptococcus pyogenes*, and *Corynebacterium diphtheriae*) and inhibits *Bordetella pertussis*, legionellae, mycoplasmas, and chlamydiae. Erythromycin is distributed throughout the body but does not achieve adequate concentrations to treat meningitis. The most common adverse effects of erythromycin are gastrointestinal. Transient hearing loss can be seen, especially at high doses. Clarithromycin is associated with fewer gastrointestinal side effects. Its spectrum of activity includes that of erythromycin plus activity against atypical mycobacteria and some *H. influenzae*. It is two to four times more active than erythromycin against staphylococci and streptococci. Azithromycin is better absorbed and better tolerated than erythromycin; it has an extremely long half-life and can be given once daily for 5 days. It is two to four times less active than erythromycin against staphylococci and streptococci, but it is more active against *H. influenzae*. A single 1 g dose is effective for genital chlamydial infections. Erythromycin and clarithromycin should never be coadministered with terfenadine or astemizole because of potential cardiac toxicity (such as torsades de pointes). Telithromycin is the first of a new class of antibiotics, ketalides, which are structurally similar to macrolides but demonstrate enhanced activity against multidrug-resistant *S. pneumoniae*. Telithromycin is approved for mild to moderately severe community-acquired pneumonia.

Aminoglycosides are not absorbed orally but are given primarily by either intravenous or intramuscular injection. The antimicrobial spectrum of activity of aminoglycosides is limited to aerobic and facultative Gram-negative bacilli. Nephrotoxicity occurs in 5–25% of patients and ototoxicity (vestibular or auditory) in 0.5–3.0% of patients. Renal toxicity is usually reversible, whereas ototoxicity often is not. Toxicity can typically be avoided by careful monitoring of blood levels and serial measurements of serum creatinine.

Tetracyclines are broad-spectrum agents that may be administered either orally or intravenously. They are typically well absorbed (best absorbed in the fasting state because tetracyclines chelate with divalent metals), widely distributed in body fluids, and renally excreted. Tetracyclines are the drug of choice for Rocky Mountain spotted fever, ehrlichiosis, and chlamydial infections; *Borrelia burgdorferi*, mycoplasmas, *Vibrio cholerae*, *Brucella* spp., and *Pseudomonas pseudomallei* are usually susceptible. Increasing resistance renders them less useful against many other bacterial strains. Tetracyclines may cause discoloration of teeth and bones in children less than 8 years of age and may cause photosensitivity in any patient.

Chloramphenicol (another inhibitor of bacterial ribosomal activity) is active against a broad range of aerobic and anaerobic Gram-positive and Gram-negative bacteria, chlamydiae, rickettsiae, and *Mycoplasma* spp. It is well absorbed from the gastrointestinal tract and can be given intravenously. Chloramphenicol is widely distributed throughout the body and, because of its lipid solubility, achieves high concentrations in brain tissue and CSF. The dose should be reduced in patients with hyperbilirubinemia. Chloramphenicol may cause reversible bone marrow suppression in adults receiving 4 g or more per day and causes aplastic anemia in 1 in 24 000 to 1 in 40 000 recipients. It has also been associated with optic neuritis and with gray baby syndrome in premature infants.

Clindamycin is well absorbed orally and can be given by intramuscular or intravenous dosing as well. Clindamycin penetrates most body compartments except brain tissue and CSF. Concentrations are inadequate to treat meningitis or other brain infections except toxoplasmosis. The half-life of clindamycin is prolonged in severe liver disease. It is active against most Gram-positive cocci (except enterococci) and many anaerobes. Clindamycin causes diarrhea in up to 20% of patients and pseudomembranous colitis in 3–5% of patients. It is rarely associated with hepatotoxicity and allergic reactions such as rash.

The quinolones constitute another class of antibacterials, DNA gyrase inhibitors, which inhibit DNA synthesis in bacterial but not mammalian cells. They are well absorbed orally and distributed widely. Absorption of several quinolones is impaired in the presence of magnesium, aluminum, calcium, zinc, and iron. Because the newer fluoroquinolones such as levofloxacin, gatifloxacin, and moxifloxacin have good activity against increasingly penicillin-resistant pneumococci, they are often considered for treatment of community-acquired pneumonia. Quinolones are effective against most Enterobacteriaceae, *Haemophilus* spp., Gram-negative cocci, legionellae, mycoplasmas, and chlamydiae. Moxifloxacin also has activity against anaerobes. These agents are not the therapy of choice for infections with staphylococci and penicillin-susceptible streptococci. Although generally well tolerated, all quinolones can cause gastrointestinal upset and central nervous system (CNS) side effects, the latter occurring more commonly in the elderly. Because quinolones cause arthropathy in immature animals, they are not recommended for use in children or pregnant women. Quinolones decrease the clearance of theophylline.

Folic acid synthesis is inhibited by both trimethoprim and sulfonamides. The combination trimethoprim-sulfamethoxazole provides a potent sequential inhibition of folic acid synthesis and is useful in treating *Staph. aureus*, *Strep. pyogenes*, *Strep. pneumoniae*, *E. coli*, *Proteus mirabilis*, *Shigella* spp., *Salmonella* spp., *Pseudomonas cepacia*, *Burkholderia pseudomallei*, *Yersinia enterocolitica*, and *Neisseria gonorrhoeae*. It is also useful in treating several fungal/protozoal infections, including *Pneumocystis jirovecii*, *Isospora belli*, and *Cyclospora cayetanensis*. Hypersensitivity reactions, Stevens–Johnson syndrome, and hematologic toxicities are some of the more common or serious complications of therapy with sulfamethoxazole.

ANTIMYCOBACTERIAL DRUGS

The agents used for mycobacterial infections and their toxicities are summarized in ***Table 13.2***. Susceptible strains of *Mycobacterium tuberculosis* are treated with isoniazid and rifampin with or without pyrazinamide, for 6–9 months. Where significant resistance (i.e., >4% to isoniazid) is possible, a four-drug regimen with isoniazid, rifampin, pyrazinamide, and either ethambutol or streptomycin is used until the sensitivities are known. In cases of multiple drug resistance, additional agents are required to achieve a minimum of three or more drugs to which the organism is susceptible. In addition, clarithromycin or azithromycin, ethambutol, and rifabutin are used in treatment of *Mycobacterium avium-intracellulare* complex infections in persons with acquired immunodeficiency syndrome (AIDS).

ANTIFUNGAL DRUGS

The therapeutic armamentarium against fungi is expanding (***Table 13.3***). For many years, amphotericin B was the only drug available for the treatment of most systemic fungal infections. Its untoward effects and requirement for parenteral administration are problematic (***Table 13.4***). Lipid-associated and liposomal amphotericin preparations, which may be less toxic, are now available. In the United States, these agents are approved for treatment of aspergillosis, candidiasis, and cryptococcosis in patients who are refractory to, or intolerant of, conventional amphotericin B therapy, or as empiric therapy in febrile neutropenia. The introduction of the azoles – ketoconazole, fluconazole, itraconazole, voriconazole, and posaconazole – which are less toxic than amphotericin B and can be administered orally, constituted major advances. The echinocandins caspofungin, micafungin, and anidulafungin have excellent clinical activity against *Candida* spp. and a favorable safety profile, and can also be utilized as second-line agents for *Aspergillus* spp.

Table 13.2 Antimycobacterial Drugs

Drugs	Main Adverse Effects
Primary Agents Against *Mycobacterium tuberculosis*[a]	
Isoniazid (PO or IM, 5 mg/kg/day; 10–20 mg/kg/day for children; max. 300 mg/day for adults and children)	Hepatic toxicity, peripheral neuropathy
Rifampin (PO or IV, 10–20 mg/kg/day to 600 mg/day)	Hepatic toxicity, flu-like syndrome
Pyrazinamide (PO, 15–30 mg/kg/day to 1.5–2.5 g/day)	Hepatic toxicity, arthralgias, hyperuricemia
Ethambutol (Myambutol PO, 15–25 mg/kg/day)	Optic neuritis
Streptomycin (IM, 15 mg/kg/day; 20–30 mg/kg/day for children)	Vestibular toxicity, renal damage
Alternative Antimycobacterial Drugs	
Capreomycin (Capastar IM, 15 mg/kg/day; 15–30 mg/kg/day for children; max. 1 g)	Auditory and vestibular toxicity, renal damage
Kanamycin (Kantrex et al IM or IV, 15 mg/kg/day; 15–30 mg/kg/day for children; max. 1 g)	Auditory and renal toxicity
Amikacin (Amikin IM or IV, 15 mg/kg/day; 15–30 mg/kg/day for children)	
Cycloserine (Seromycin PO 250–500 mg bid; 10–20 mg/kg/day; max. 1 g)	Psychiatric symptoms, seizures
Ethionamide (Trecator-SC, PO 250–500 mg bid; 15–20 mg/kg/day; max. 1 g)	Gastrointestinal disturbances, hepatic toxicity
Ciprofloxacin (Cipro PO, 250–750 mg bid for adults only)	
Moxifloxacin (Avelox PO, 400 mg/day for adults only)	
Gatifloxacin (Tequin PO, 400 mg/day for adults only)	
Ofloxacin (Floxin PO 600–800 mg/day for adults only)	
Para-aminosalicylic acid (PAS; Teebacin PO, 4–6 g bid; 75 mg/kg bid for children; max. 12 g)	Gastrointestinal disturbances
Clofazimine (Lamprene PO 100–200 mg; 1 mg/kg in children)	Gastrointestinal disturbances; ichthyosis; pigmentation of cornea, retina, skin
Additional Agents Particularly Useful for MAC[b]	
Clarithromycin PO, 500 mg bid	Rifabutin and AZT levels
Azithromycin PO, 500 mg qd (500 mg 3 times a week when used as a component of MAC treatment regimen)	
Clarithromycin 500 mg bid or azithromycin 1200 mg qwk or 300 mg qd (for MAC prophylaxis)	
Rifabutin PO 300–450 mg qd	

[a]See Drugs for tuberculosis. Med Lett Drugs Ther 2007;55:15–22, for details regarding indications, doses, and toxicities.
[b]See Table 13.7 for additional details.
AZT, zidovudine; MAC, *Mycobacterium avium-intracellulare* complex.
IM, intramuscularly; IV, intravenously; PO, by mouth; bid, twice a day; qd, every day; qwk, every week.

Table 13.3 Systemic Antifungal Drugs

Antifungal Agent	Diseases for Which This Is the Drug of Choice or a Primary Alternative	Antifungal Agent	Diseases for Which This Is the Drug of Choice or a Primary Alternative
Amphotericin B[a] (0.5–1.5 mg/kg IV)	Aspergillosis Blastomycosis Candidiasis (deep) (± flucytosine) Coccidioidomycosis (± flucytosine) Cryptococcosis Histoplasmosis Mucormycosis Paracoccidioidomycosis Sporotrichosis (systemic)	*Oral azoles*[b] Fluconazole (100–200 mg/day PO)	Candidiasis[c] (oropharyngeal, esophageal, vaginal) Coccidioidomycosis (requires 400–800 mg/day PO) Cryptococcosis (200 mg/day PO, for suppression)
Itraconazole (200 mg daily or bid PO)	Blastomycosis Histoplasmosis Pseudallescheriasis Paracoccidioidomycosis Sporotrichosis (cutaneous, itraconazole or saturated solution of potassium iodide) Chromomycosis (*Fonsecaea pedrosi* and others)	Ketoconazole (400–800 mg/day PO)	Pseudallescheriasis (ketoconazole or miconazole) *Madurella mycetomatis*[d] Blastomycosis Alternative for candidiasis (oropharyngeal, esophageal) Coccidioidomycosis Histoplasmosis Paracoccidioidomycosis

Table 13.3 Systemic Antifungal Drugs—cont'd

Antifungal Agent	Diseases for Which This Is the Drug of Choice or a Primary Alternative	Antifungal Agent	Diseases for Which This Is the Drug of Choice or a Primary Alternative
Voriconazole (6 mg/kg IV q12h for 1 day, then 4 mg/kg IV q12h, then 200 mg bid PO)	Invasive aspergillosis Refractory infection with *Scedosporium apoispermum* or *Fusarium* spp. Esophageal candidiasis	Echinocandins Caspofungin (70 mg IV for 1 day, then 50 mg IV daily) Anidulafungin (200 mg IV ×1, then 100 mg IV q24h) Micafungin (100 mg IV q24h except esophageal candidiasis (150 mg IV q24h))	Invasive candidiasis Invasive aspergillosis
Posaconazole (200 mg PO q6h or 400 mg PO q12h)	Aspergillosis Candidiasis Zygomycoses		

[a]Amphotericin B is given IV over about a 2- to 4-hour interval once a day or in double doses every other day. The duration of therapy with the drug usually ranges from 4 to 12 weeks. To decrease the severity of the initial reaction to the drug, if the patient is not dangerously ill, some clinicians begin with a 1 mg test dose, followed in 2–4 hours, if no severe reaction occurs, by a full therapeutic dose. Pretreatment with acetaminophen (Tylenol and others), aspirin, or hydrocortisone 25 mg IV can decrease the severity of the reactions. Treatment with meperidine (Demerol and others) 25 mg IV can shorten the duration of fever and chills.

[b]The optimal duration of treatment with the oral azole drugs is unclear. Depending on the disease, these drugs are continued for weeks or months or, particularly in AIDS patients, indefinitely. With ketoconazole and itraconazole, AIDS patients may have lower serum concentrations.

[c]For patients with oropharyngeal disease, clotrimazole troches five times daily or nystatin solution (100000 units/mL) 5 mL qid may be effective and are relatively inexpensive. For patients with fluconazole-resistant esophageal disease, an echinocandin or amphotericin B 0.3 mg/kg IV can be used. *Candida krusei* infections are usually resistant to fluconazole. *Candida glabrata* infections are often resistant. Bladder irrigation with 50 mg/L of amphotericin B in sterile water has been used to treat *Candida* cystitis.

[d]Actinomycetoma (with *Actinomadura madurae, Nocardia* and others) requires streptomycin + sulfamethoxazole-trimethoprim or dapsone.

IM, intramuscularly; IV, intravenously; PO, by mouth; q12h, every 12 hours.

See also Antifungal drugs. Treatment guidelines. Med Lett. 2008;65:1–8.

Table 13.4 Toxicities of the Antifunga Drugs

Drug	Toxicity
Amphotericin B	Systemic: fever, chills, headache, hypotension, tachycardia
	Gastrointestinal: nausea and vomiting
	Nephrotoxicity (may be decreased by sodium loading): hypomagnesemia, hypokalemia, renal tubular acidosis
	Hematologic: anemia, thrombocytopenia, mild leukopenia
Flucytosine	Bone marrow depression (increased with renal impairment if dosage adjustments are not made)
Itraconazole	Gastrointestinal: nausea, abdominal pain
	Drug interactions: increases levels of terfenadine and cisapride, which can be fatal; rhabdomyolysis if used concurrently with cyclosporine, lovastatin, simvastatin; absorption dependent on gastric acidity, decreased by H_2 blockers and antacids; others
Ketoconazole	Gastrointestinal intolerance, mild hepatotoxicity
	Others: rash, itching, dizziness, gynecomastia
	Endocrine: gynecomastia, altered libido, decreased potency, menstrual irregularity
	Drug interactions: increases levels of terfenadine and cisapride, which can be fatal; others
Fluconazole	Allergic: rash, Stevens–Johnson syndrome (rare), anaphylaxis (rare)
	Others: serious hepatotoxicity (rare)
	Drug interactions: increases levels of terfenadine and cisapride, which can be fatal; others
Voriconazole	Similar to other azoles except that approximately 30% have transient visual disturbances following dosing
Posaconazole	Generally well tolerated, similar side effect profile to fluconazole
Caspofungin	Generally well tolerated; pruritus and headache are most common
Micafungin	Generally well tolerated, similar to caspofungin
Anidulafungin	Generally well tolerated, similar to caspofungin

ANTIVIRAL DRUGS AND THE TREATMENT OF OPPORTUNISTIC INFECTIONS IN PATIENTS WITH AIDS

The treatment of HIV infection is changing rapidly, and favored regimens combine nucleosides and protease inhibitors (PIs) or non-nucleoside reverse transcriptase inhibitors (NNRTIs). New classes including integrase inhibitors and entry and fusion inhibitors have recently become available. The major antiviral agents and their indications and major toxicities are shown in *Tables 13.5 and 13.6*. Potentially serious drug interactions can occur, especially when protease inhibitors, which can affect the cytochrome P-450 enzyme system in the liver, are used concurrently with antimycobacterial, antifungal, or other agents. The approaches to treatment of opportunistic infections in patients with HIV infection are summarized in *Table 13.7*. Updated treatment recommendations from the US Department of Health and Human Services are frequently posted at http://www.aidsinfo.nih.gov (accessed 4/26/10) and include detailed tables of drug interactions and toxicities.

Table 13.5 Antiviral Drugs (Other than Antiretroviral Agents)[a]

Antiviral (with Representative Adult Dose)	Virus or Disease for Which This Is a First-line Drug	Toxicity
Acyclovir (Zovirax and others) (IV or PO to 800 mg 5 times a day for 5–10 days)	HSV, VSV	Gastrointestinal disturbances, crystalline nephropathy, headache, rash
Valacyclovir (Valtrex), prodrug of acyclovir (up to PO 1 g tid)	HSV, VZV	Similar to acyclovir; prolonged high doses may cause TTP/HUS
Famciclovir (Famvir), prodrug of penciclovir (PO 500 mg bid/tid)	HSV, localized VZV	Headache, nausea, diarrhea
Amantadine (Symmetrel) or rimantadine (Flumadine) (PO 200 mg/day × 5 days)	Influenza A	CNS anxiety, insomnia, confusion (usually minor, less with rimantadine)
Ganciclovir (Cytovene) (IV 5 mg/kg once or twice per day)	CMV retinitis, pneumonia, others	Neutropenia, thrombocytopenia
Foscarnet (Foscavir) (IV 40–60 mg/kg q8h)	For resistant CMV, HSV, VZV	Renal dysfunction, hypocalcemia
Cidofovir (Vistide) (IV 5 mg/kg q2wk)	CMV retinitis (chronic suppression)	Nephrotoxicity, neutropenia, metabolic acidosis, uveitis, ocular hypotony
Interferon-alfa (Roferon-A, Intron-A, Alferon N) (SC or IM 3–10 million units 3 times a week for 4–6 months) or pegylated interferon-alfa 2b (PEG-Intron) (1 μg/kg once a week SC for 48 weeks)	Chronic hepatitis B, C,[b] D	Flu-like symptoms, marrow suppression
Ribavirin (Virazole) (aerosol for 12–18 h/day for 3–7 days, or IV)	RSV, Lassa fever, Sabia virus, CCHF, some hantavirus infections	Teratogenic, embryotoxic, hemolytic anemia
Ribavirin (Rebetrol, Rebetron) (1000–1200 mg/day PO)	Hepatitis C[b]	
Trifluridine (Viroptic) (topical, 1 drop 1% q2h for 10 days)	Ocular and mucocutaneous HSV	Generally well tolerated; occasionally may cause burning and stinging of the cornea
Vidarabine (Vira-A)	(HSV, VZV before acyclovir)	
Lamivudine (Epivir HBV) (100 mg PO once a day for 1–3 years)	Hepatitis B	Generally well tolerated; rare headache, nausea, dizziness
Fomiversen (Vitravene) (330 μg intravitreally q2wk × 2 doses, then monthly)	CMV retinitis	Iritis, vitritis, increased intraocular pressure and vision changes
Valganciclovir (Valcyte) (prodrug of ganciclovir) (900 mg PO bid for 21 days followed by 900 mg once daily)	CMV retinitis, others	Similar to ganciclovir
Ganciclovir intraocular implant (Vitrasert) (4.5 mg intraocularly every 5–8 months)	CMV retinitis	Late retinal detachment
Oseltamivir (Tamiflu) (75 mg PO bid for 5 days for treatment; 75 mg PO once daily for prevention)	Influenza A or B treatment (within 36 hours) and prevention	Nausea and vomiting
Zanamivir (Relenza) (10 mg bid for 5 days by inhaler)	Influenza A or B treatment (within 2 days)	Nasal and throat discomfort, bronchospasm
Penciclovir (Denavir) (1% cream applied q2h while awake for 4 days)	Orolabial HSV	
Adefovir (Hepsera) (10 mg PO daily)	Chronic hepatitis B	Asthenia

[a]See Drugs for non-HIV viral infections. Med Lett Drugs Ther. 2007;59;59–70, for full information about dosing, indications, and toxicities.
[b]For hepatitis C infections, interferon and ribavirin are coadministered.
HSV, herpes simplex virus; VZV, varicella-zoster virus; TTP, thrombotic thrombocytopenic purpura; HUS, hemolytic-uremic syndrome; CMV, cytomegalovirus; RSV, respiratory syncytial virus; CCHF, Crimean-Congo hemorrhagic fever; CNS, central nervous system.
IM, intramuscularly; IV, intravenously; PO, by mouth; SC, subcutaneously; bid, twice a day; tid, three times a day; q8h, every 8 hours; q2wk, every 2 weeks.

Table 13.6 Antiretroviral Drugs (with Usual Doses and Main Adverse Effects)

Antiretroviral	Main Adverse Effects
Reverse Transcriptase (RT) Inhibitors	
Nucleoside and Nucleotide Analogs	
Zidovudine (AZT, Retrovir) PO 200 mg tid or 300 mg bid	Anemia, neutropenia, nausea and vomiting, hemolytic anemia, malaise, myopathy, confusion, hepatitis
Didanosine (dideoxyinosine, ddI, Videx) PO 125–200 mg bid; Videx EC, PO 400 mg daily	Neuropathy, pancreatitis, gastrointestinal upset, decreased absorption with itraconazole
Zalcitabine (dideoxycytidine, ddC, Hivid) PO 0.75 mg tid	Neuropathy, rash, stomatitis, esophageal ulceration, pancreatitis, fever
Stavudine (d4T, Zerit) PO 40 mg bid (30 mg bid if <60 kg)	Neuropathy, transaminitis, rarely pancreatitis, lipoatrophy
Lamivudine (3TC, Epivir) PO 150 mg bid or PO 300 mg daily	Gastrointestinal upset, rare pancreatitis
Tenofovir disoproxil fumarate (Viread) 300 mg PO bid	Asthenia, headache, renal insufficiency
Abacavir (Ziagen) 300 mg PO daily	Hypersensitivity reaction (can be fatal)
Emtricitabine (FTC, Emtriva) 200 mg PO daily	Headache, nausea, skin hyperpigmentation
Non-nucleoside RT Inhibitors	
Efavirenz (Sustiva) 600 mg PO daily	Rash, vivid dreams, dizziness, insomnia, impaired concentration
Nevirapine (Viramune) PO 200 mg bid	Rash
Delavirdine (Rescriptor) PO 400 mg tid	Rash
Etravirine (Intelence) PO 200 mg bid	Rash
Protease Inhibitors	
Saquinavir (Invirase PO 600 mg tid; Fortovase PO 1200 mg tid)	Diarrhea; nausea; abdominal pain; poor bioavailability, especially with Invirase. Decreased levels with rifampin, rifabutin; antihistamine toxicity
Ritonavir (Norvir) PO 600 mg q12h	Diarrhea; nausea and vomiting; paresthesias; transaminitis; asthenia; levels reduced by rifampin, rifabutin, dexamethasone; other drug toxicities
Indinavir (Crixivan) PO 800 mg q8h	Renal stones, hyperbilirubinemia, gastric hypoacidity (decreased ddI absorption), other drug toxicities
Nelfinavir (Viracept) PO 750 mg tid with food or PO 1250 mg bid with food	Diarrhea, asthenia, nausea, abdominal pain, headache, rash
Atazanavir (Reyataz) 400 mg daily	Indirect hyperbilirubinemia, prolonged PR interval, hyperglycemia, fat maldistribution
Fosamprenavir (Lexiva) 1400 mg PO bid	Diarrhea, nausea, vomiting, fat maldistribution, skin rash, hyperglycemia, lipid abnormalities
Darunavir (Prezista) 600 mg PO bid for treatment-experienced patients; 400 mg PO bid for treatment-naïve patients	Gastrointestinal intolerance, headache
Tipranivir (Aptivus) 500 mg PO bid	Transaminitis, elevated triglycerides and cholesterol
Fusion Inhibitors	
Enfuvirtide (Fuzeon, T-20) 90 mg SC bid	Local injection site reactions, increased rate of bacterial pneumonia, hypersensitivity reaction
Maraviroc (Selzentry) 300 mg PO bid or with most protease inhibitors 150 mg PO bid	Diarrhea, nausea, headaches, fatigue
Integrase Inhibitors	
Raltegravir (Isentress) 400 mg PO bid	Nausea, diarrhea, headache, transaminitis

PO, by mouth; SC, subcutaneously; bid, twice a day; tid, three times a day; q12h, every 12 hours.

See Drugs for HIV infection. Med Lett Drugs Ther. 2009;78:11–22, and US Department of Health & Human Services: Guidelines for the Use of Antiretroviral Agents in HIV-1 Infected Adults & Adolescent. Available at www.aidsinfo.nih.gov.

Table 13.7 Drugs Used Against Selected Opportunistic Infections

Infection/Drug	Usual Prophylactic or Suppressive Doses
Pneumocystis Pneumonia (PCP)	
Trimethoprim (TMP)-sulfamethoxazole (SMX) PO or IV 15–20 mg TMP and 75–100 mg SMX/kg/day administered q6h or q8h for 3 weeks	PO 1 double-strength (DS) tab qd or PO 1 single-strength tab qd
Pentamidine isethionate IV 3–4 mg/kg/day for 3 weeks	300 mg inhaled monthly via Respigard II nebulizer
Dapsone (+ trimethoprim 5 mg/kg tid PO for 3 weeks) PO 100 mg/day for 3 weeks	PO 100 mg/day or PO 50 mg bid
Atovaquone PO 750 mg bid for 3 weeks	PO 1500 mg qd
Clindamycin (300–450 mg PO q6h or 600–900 mg IV q6h for 3 weeks) and primaquine (15–30 mg base PO qd for 3 weeks)	–
Prednisone, in addition to TMP/SMX, if patient acutely ill, PO_2 <70 mmHg (40 mg bid for 5 days, then 40 mg qd for 5 days, then 20 mg qd for 11 days)	–
Toxoplasmosis	
Pyrimethamine 200 mg PO ×1, then 50–75 mg PO qd and sulfadiazine PO 1.0–1.5 g q6h plus leucovorin 10–25 mg PO qd, or pyrimethamine + clindamycin	Pyrimethamine PO 25–50 mg qd and sulfadiazine 0.5–1.0 g q6h for suppression; to prevent first episode, TMP-SMX PO 1 DS tab qd
Cryptosporidiosis	
Aminosidine (paromomycin) PO 500–750 mg qid	–
Nitazoxanide PO 0.5–1.0 g bid for 14 days	–
Mucosal Candidiasis	
Nystatin PO 0.5–1.0 mU 3–5 times a day or clotrimazole 10 mg 5 times a day	–
Fluconazole PO 100–200 mg qd	–
Itraconazole oral solution 200 mg PO qd	–
Cryptococcosis	
Amphotericin B deoxycholate 0.7 mg/kg/day + flucytosine 25 mg/kg PO qid for at least 2 weeks, then fluconazole 400 mg PO for 8 weeks	Fluconazole 200 mg PO qd for suppression
Herpes Simplex Virus (HSV) or Varicella-Zoster Virus (VZV) Infections	
Acyclovir 200–800 mg PO 5 times a day or 10 mg/kg IV q8h for 1–2 weeks for VZV	For suppression: 400 mg PO bid
Foscarnet 40 mg/kg IV q8h	40 mg/kg IV qd
Cytomegalovirus (CMV) Infections	
Ganciclovir IV 5 mg/kg q12h	For suppression: IV 5–6 mg/kg qd or 5 times a week or PO 1 g tid
Intraocular ganciclovir implant + valganciclovir 900 mg PO bid with food for 14–21 days, then valganciclovir 900 mg/day	PO 1 g tid
Foscarnet IV 60–90 mg/kg q8–12h	IV 90–120 mg/kg qd
Cidofovir 5 mg/kg/week IV for 2 weeks (beware of nephrotoxicity; probenicid and hydration required)	5 mg/kg every other week (beware of nephrotoxicity; probenicid and hydration required)
***Mycobacterium avium* Complex (MAC)**	
Clarithromycin PO 500 mg bid or Azithromycin PO (500 mg/day, or some use 500 mg 3 times a week) + Ethambutol 15 mg/kg/day + Rifabutin 300 mg PO qd (dose may need to be adjusted for drug interactions)	For primary prophylaxis: Azithromycin 1200 mg/week PO or Clarithromycin 500 mg PO bid
Syphilis	
Penicillin IM 2.4 million units benzathine weekly for 1–3 weeks or doxycycline 100 mg PO bid for 2–4 weeks or IV 12–24 million units/day for 2 weeks or IM 2.4 million units procaine qd for 10 days with 500 mg probenecid PO bid (one of the latter 2 regimens needed for neurosyphilis)	

IV, intravenously; PO, by mouth; bid, twice a day; tid, three times a day; qid, four times a day; qd, every day; q6h, every 6 hours.

(Adapted from Bartlett JG, Gallant JE. The 2004 Abbreviated Guide to Medical Management of HIV Infection; and MMWR 58(RR-4), 2009, available at aidsinfo.nih.gov. (Accessed 9/10/2009).

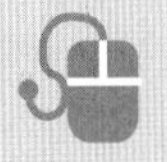

Access the complete reference list online at
http://www.expertconsult.com

Access the complete reference list online at http://www.expertconsult.com

CHAPTER 14

Global Surveillance for Emerging Infectious Diseases

Ray R. Arthur • James W. LeDuc • James M. Hughes

INTRODUCTION

Despite advances in science, technology, and medicine that have improved disease prevention and management, endemic and emerging infectious diseases continue to pose threats to domestic and global health. Established diseases such as malaria, tuberculosis (TB), and human immunodeficiency virus (HIV) infection still proliferate, fueled in part by antimicrobial resistance.[1] The increasing speed and volume of international travel, migration, and trade create new opportunities for microbial spread, and the prospect of a deliberate release of pathogenic microbes underscores the importance of preparedness to address the unexpected.[2,3] The examples of severe acute respiratory syndrome (SARS), a previously unknown disease that spread rapidly around the world in 2003, and pandemic H1N1 influenza in 2009 (***Fig. 14.1***), illustrate the vulnerability of the global community to new microbial threats and highlight the need for increased vigilance and strengthened response capacity.[4,5]

Concerns about global health security led World Health Organization (WHO) Member States to formulate and adopt the revised International Health Regulations (IHR) in 2005.[6] The new requirement for IHR State Parties to develop and maintain defined core capacities for national surveillance and response highlights the importance placed on early recognition of disease events so that measures can be promptly taken to control the threat at its source before the disease can spread to other countries. Furthermore, countries that can provide assistance must help countries that lack available resources. Effective global surveillance requires that each country have a strong national surveillance system.

Recent domestic challenges have included the introduction of West Nile encephalitis[7,8] and monkeypox[9] into the United States; the anthrax episodes of fall 2001;[10] multistate outbreaks involving contaminated food products[11,12] and pandemic H1N1 influenza.[13] Internationally, public health officials have faced the emergence of Nipah virus[14] and SARS,[15] the intensified global spread of dengue,[16,17] Ebola and Marburg outbreaks of unprecedented magnitude,[18,19] the direct avian-to-human transmission of H5N1 influenza,[20,21] and the spread of chikungunya virus from Africa to islands in the Indian Ocean, Asia, and Europe.[22] The 2009 H1N1 influenza pandemic originated in Mexico, but the virus was identified first from cases in the United States.[13] Each of these examples illustrates the global implications of local problems, the role of strong health intelligence networks in addressing emerging infections, and the importance of data on the background rate of diseases in recognizing unusual disease events.[23]

PUBLIC HEALTH SURVEILLANCE

Public health surveillance is the continuous analysis, interpretation, and feedback of systematically collected information used to inform public health decision making.[24] Timely community health information in the hands of trained experts is the foundation for recognition of threats to health. To intervene successfully, disease surveillance systems need to provide a continuous, accurate, and near real-time overview of a population's health. Surveillance systems must be sensitive in terms of their ability to detect outbreaks and other changes in community health status over time, and they must be flexible in adapting novel diagnostic technology to changing health intelligence needs. Given the increasing pace of international travel and globalization and the threat of intentional outbreaks, surveillance activities need to extend beyond the monitoring of disease burden to include the capacity to quickly recognize unusual, unexpected, or unexplained disease patterns. Because many emerging infectious agents are zoonotic,[25] it is also important to integrate veterinary disease reporting networks into systems that monitor diseases of humans, as emphasized by the One Health Initiative.[26]

Astute clinicians and microbiologists are essential for early detection of threats. In the United States, surveillance for notifiable diseases is conducted by state and local health departments, which receive reports from physicians, nurses, and laboratorians who are often the first to observe and report unusual illnesses or syndromes. States voluntarily report nationally notifiable diseases to the Centers for Disease Control and Prevention (CDC) through a standards-based system for collecting and sharing electronic disease reports from health care providers within local health jurisdictions to state and federal public health authorities. In addition to these parameter-based systems, clinicians and state epidemiologists can also contact CDC directly to report disease events if urgent notification is appropriate or if the event is unusual.

Starting in 1994, CDC launched a two-phase initiative to strengthen domestic capacity to respond to the dual threats of endemic and emerging infections. The publication of two strategy documents[27,28] led to the launching of new surveillance initiatives, including the Emerging Infections Program (EIP), a national network for population-based surveillance and research.[29] Several provider-based sentinel surveillance networks were established in collaboration with emergency department physicians, infectious disease clinicians, and travel medicine specialists to provide early warning of events that might be missed by public health surveillance. Additional enhancements to the surveillance effort include development of the National Molecular Subtyping Network for Foodborne Disease Surveillance (PulseNet) as an early warning system for foodborne diseases, the Gonococcal Isolate Surveillance Project (GISP) to monitor antimicrobial resistance in *Neisseria gonorrhoeae*, strengthened surveillance for emerging diseases (e.g., West Nile encephalitis, seasonal and pandemic influenza), and surveillance for outbreaks that might be due to acts of bioterrorism.

CDC also works in partnership with WHO, ministries of health, foundations, development agencies, and other federal agencies to promote national, regional, and international disease surveillance. Recognition of the global nature of the emergence and spread of infectious diseases stimulated the development of a strategy focused on CDC's efforts to enhance global capacity for disease surveillance and outbreak response[30] focusing on six priority areas for protecting domestic and global health, among which are global initiatives for disease control, international

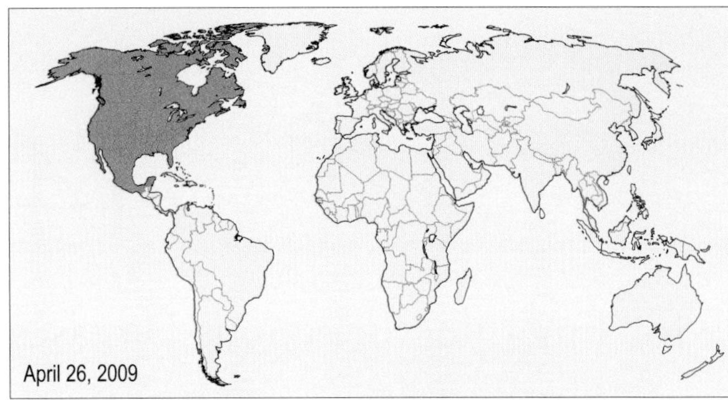

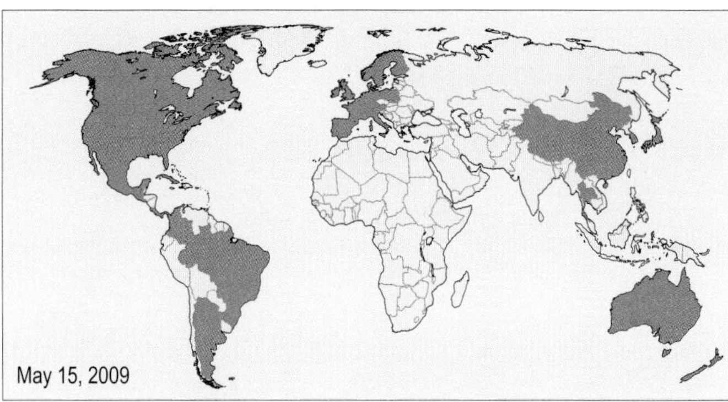

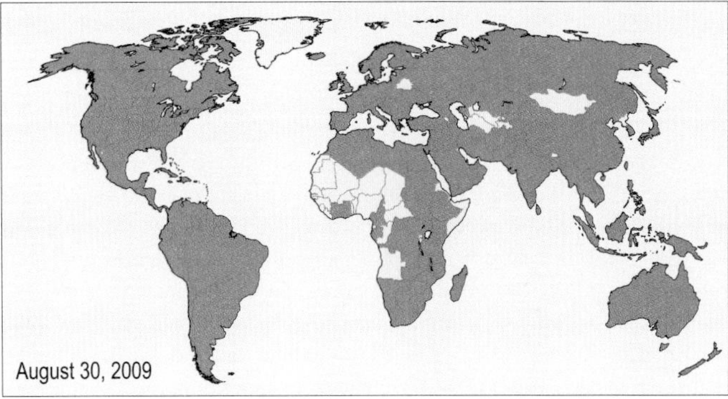

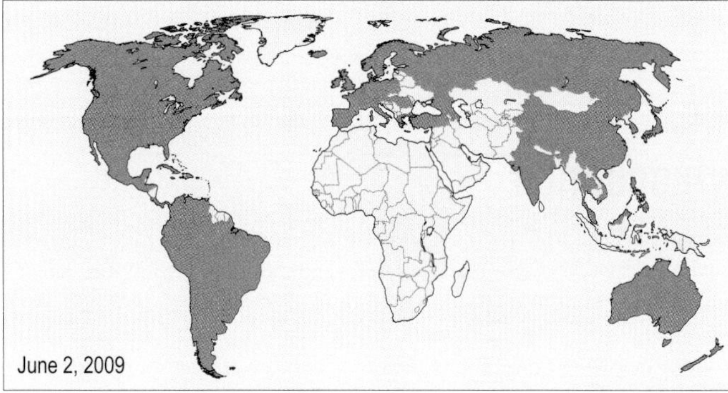

Figure 14.1 Countries with laboratory-confirmed pandemic H1N1 influenza infections – April 26, 2009 to August 30, 2009. (Source: WHO and ministries of health.)

outbreak assistance, and a global approach to disease surveillance. CDC's international activities include creation of the Global Disease Detection program (see below), US–Mexico Border Infectious Disease Surveillance (BIDS) system, development of GeoSentinel, and provision of technical assistance to regional disease surveillance networks in Africa, Asia, Latin America, and the circumpolar regions of Canada and Europe, as well as to WHO's disease-specific global networks.

WHO manages global disease surveillance and response through a composite of partnerships and networks for gathering, verifying, and analyzing international disease intelligence, mainly to support global and regional efforts to eradicate certain diseases, such as poliomyelitis, and to protect the global community against diseases with pandemic potential. The oldest of these networks is the global influenza surveillance network, which was established more than 50 years ago and has served as the prototype for the design and implementation of other systems (see below).[31]

To respond to the increasing number of emerging and rapidly spreading infectious diseases, WHO has developed a global "network of networks" that links local, regional, national, and international networks of laboratories and medical centers into a mega-surveillance network for early warning and response.[32] Formal partners include ministries of health, WHO Collaborating Centers, WHO country and regional offices, and international military groups such as the Global Emerging Infections System of the US Department of Defense.[33]

Event-based outbreak reports are also received from non-governmental organizations, relief workers, private clinics, individual scientists, and public health practitioners and, more recently, from internet-based scanning of media reports. The Public Health Agency of Canada's Global Public Health Intelligence Network (GPHIN), an electronic tool used by WHO since 1997, has demonstrated the value of using internet news sites for reports of outbreaks and unusual disease events. Similar media-scanning systems have been recently developed in other countries.[34] Project Argus at Georgetown University complements the internet-scanning technology with 30–40 analysts who have native language skills and local knowledge to provide context to the reports. The human-based Program for Monitoring Emerging Diseases (ProMED) was established in 1994. Over 40 000 subscribed members in over 160 countries submit reports of disease events.[35] National and multinational public health institutions have established specialized units, modeled on WHO's Alert and Response Operations, for monitoring and verifying event-based reports, coming particularly from countries with weak surveillance and reporting systems. CDC, the European Centre for Disease Prevention and Control, and the French Institute for Public Health Surveillance are a few notable examples.

Global surveillance networks all operate within the framework of the International Health Regulations (IHR), which outline WHO's authority and Member States' obligations to develop surveillance capabilities, report and prevent the spread of disease threats. The revised IHR (2005) entered into force in 2007. Countries were required to complete an assessment of their core surveillance and response capacities within 2 years and then have 3 years to implement the required measures for compliance. The revised IHR are much broader in scope than the preceding regulations. The IHR define a Public Health Emergency of International Concern (PHEIC) as any extraordinary public health event (all hazards) that constitutes a public health risk to other countries through international spread, and potentially requires a coordinated international response. State parties to the IHR are required to notify WHO about events that may constitute a PHEIC, which includes mandatory reporting of four diseases (smallpox, SARS, wild-type poliovirus infections, and novel subtypes of influenza) and an assessment of all other threats using a prescribed algorithm. WHO makes the final assessment of whether an event is a PHEIC. Of the many events reported by countries to WHO since IHR implementation in June 2007, pandemic H1N1 influenza was the first PHEIC declared by the WHO Director General in May 2009.

Whereas the IHR provide the legal framework for global control of infectious diseases, WHO's Global Outbreak Alert and Response Network (GOARN) is the operational arm, i.e., the mechanism by which WHO's partners respond to outbreaks of international importance.[32] GOARN activities are described below.

EXAMPLES OF SPECIALIZED SURVEILLANCE AND RESPONSE NETWORKS

Global Disease Detection Program

CDC's Global Disease Detection (GDD) program, established in 2004, develops and strengthens global capacity to rapidly detect, accurately identify, and promptly contain emerging infectious disease and bioterrorist threats that occur internationally.[36] The central focus of the GDD program are eight Regional Centers in China, Egypt, Guatemala, India, Kazakhstan, Kenya, South Africa and Thailand that build national and regional surveillance and response capacity in support of WHO and IHR (2005) implementation. The Atlanta-based GDD Operations Center is a centralized unit that creates an environment for joining CDC program expertise and disease intelligence from a vast array of sources, and supports CDC response operations when international assistance is requested.

Global Influenza Surveillance Network

Established in 1952, this global network of more than 120 institutions in 99 countries monitors influenza activity and collects the viral isolates that determine the composition of the following year's influenza vaccines[37,38] (*Fig. 14.2*). The isolates are characterized by WHO Collaborating Centers in the United Kingdom, Japan, Australia, and the United States. In addition to guiding the annual composition of recommended vaccines, the network operates as an early warning system for the emergence of influenza variants and novel strains that could signal the emergence of an influenza pandemic.

Global Laboratory Network for Poliomyelitis Eradication

International disease eradication strategies include a strong surveillance component. To support the Global Polio Eradication Initiative, WHO established the Global Laboratory Network for Poliomyelitis Eradication,[39] which uses molecular techniques to determine whether wild-type polio is circulating in areas undergoing eradication efforts. Genomic sequencing capabilities and collaboration among network laboratories have allowed the tracking of virus strains within and among countries and the identification of the origin of viruses imported into polio-free countries.[40]

Global Foodborne Infections Network (formerly known as WHO Global Salm-Surv)

Started in 2000, WHO's Global Salm-Surv is a global network of laboratories and individuals involved in isolation, identification, and antimicrobial resistance testing of *Salmonella* and surveillance of salmonellosis.[41] The scope of the network has recently broadened to include other pathogens and has been renamed the Global Foodborne Infections Network (GFN). The goal is to enhance the capacity and quality of foodborne and enteric pathogen surveillance, serotyping, and antimicrobial resistance testing throughout the world. GFN includes an electronic discussion group; international training courses for microbiologists and epidemiologists working in human health, veterinary and food sciences; external quality assurance testing; and focused research projects on topics such as surveillance enhancement and burden of illness. Member institutions enter their top 15 *Salmonella* serotypes yearly in a web-based country databank that can be searched for serotype frequency nationally, regionally, or globally.

PulseNet International

PulseNet International is a worldwide network of regional and national laboratory networks that utilizes standardized genotyping methods to enhance surveillance and provide early warning of food- and waterborne disease outbreaks, emerging pathogens, and acts of bioterrorism.[42] PulseNet promotes laboratory investigations of foodborne outbreaks through culture confirmation, and laboratories participating in the network use standard laboratory molecular subtyping protocols for all major bacterial pathogens transmitted via food and water and for *Yersinia pestis*. Disease case clusters originating from common source outbreaks, which may otherwise not be detected, are identified by sharing and comparing pulse-gel electrophoresis patterns (PFGE) patterns between participating laboratories.

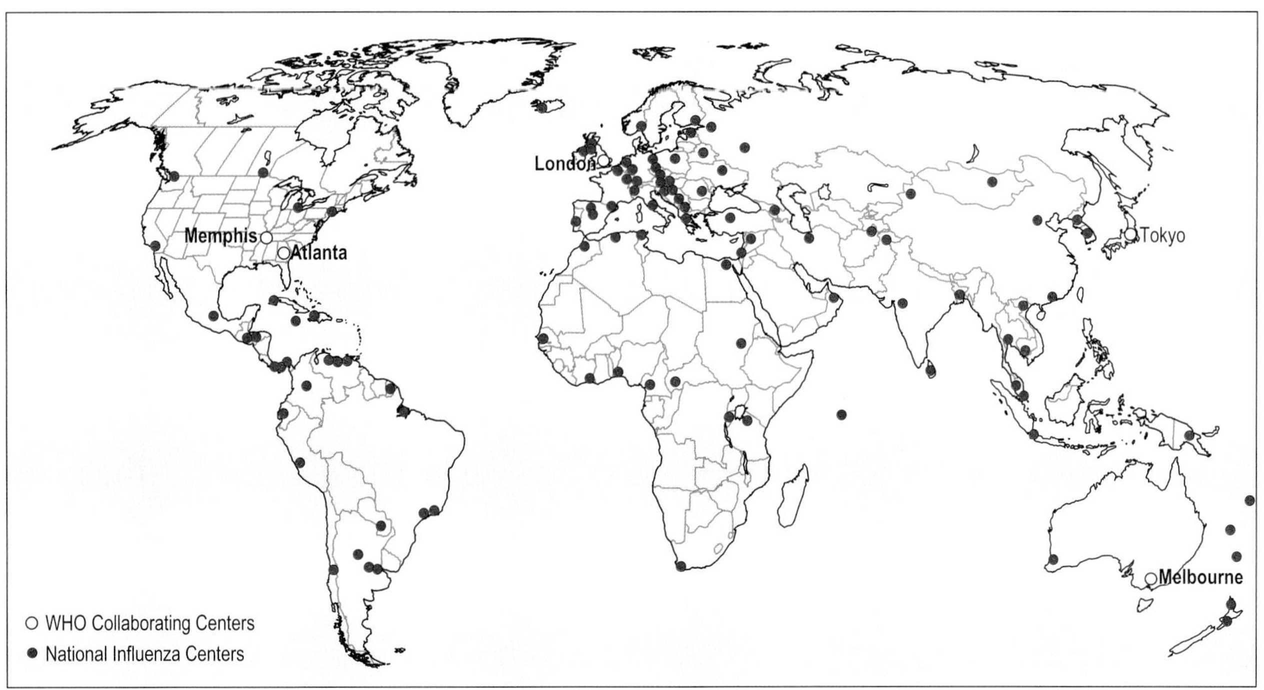

Figure 14.2 WHO Global Influenza Surveillance Network of five Collaborating Centers and 128 national influenza centers in 99 countries – September 24, 2009.

Drug Resistance Surveillance Projects

Surveillance of antimicrobial resistance is fundamental for understanding trends, developing treatment guidelines, and assessing the effectiveness of interventions. In 1994, WHO, the International Union against Tuberculosis and Lung Disease (IUATLD), and other partners launched the Global Project on Anti-Tuberculosis Drug Resistance Surveillance in response to growing concern about drug resistance and its impact on TB control. The purpose of this network of reference laboratories is to measure the prevalence of anti-TB drug resistance (single-drug resistant, multidrug-resistant, and extensively drug-resistant TB) in several countries using standard methods and to study the correlation between the level of drug resistance and treatment policies in those countries.[43] Monitoring antimalaria drug resistance has demonstrated increasing resistance that requires revision of treatment guidelines (see *Fig. 96.4*). Recently, artemisinin resistance has been recognized in Cambodia.[44]

Global Outbreak Alert and Response Network

The Global Outbreak Alert and Response Network (GOARN) was launched in 2000 as a mechanism for combating international disease outbreaks, ensuring the rapid deployment of appropriate technical assistance to affected areas, and contributing to long-term epidemic preparedness and capacity building. GOARN electronically links more than 120 partner institutions and surveillance networks, which together possess the expertise, skills, and resources for rapid outbreak detection, verification, and response.[32] The coordinated response to the large Ebola hemorrhagic fever outbreak in Uganda in 2000 demonstrated the merit of the principles on which the network is based and functions.[18] The importance of GOARN was also evident in 2003, when WHO coordinated the unprecedented global response to SARS. Through GOARN, WHO assembled the international public health, clinical, and research communities to rapidly identify and characterize the causative agent and to contain the spread of this new infectious agent, providing a new standard for future responses to global microbial threats.[4]

THE CRITICAL ROLE OF THE LABORATORY

Microbiology laboratories play a critical role in surveillance for emerging infectious diseases and bioterrorism threats by identifying the microbial cause of disease syndromes, detecting and reporting new or unusual pathogens, and assessing antimicrobial resistance.[45,46] To carry out this role, laboratories require well-equipped, safe, and secure facilities, adequate human and financial resources, access to needed reagents, and robust quality control.

Accurate etiologic diagnosis is dependent on standardization of and scrupulous attention to a series of essential procedures. These include the collection and transport of appropriate clinical specimens, careful handling, accurate and complete labeling, and access to relevant clinical information to guide the testing process. Laboratorians also benefit from knowledge of the local epidemiologic situation. The chain of events is completed when the laboratory provides results to the medical staff to guide clinical management of the patient and to epidemiologists for cluster and trend analysis, monitoring, and response. Specimen collection requires an understanding of the samples needed (e.g., whole blood, serum, cerebrospinal fluid); proper containers for safe transport outside the clinical facility; labeling with information on the source and the time of collection relative to clinical status; proper packaging for shipping; and compliance with regulations for transport. The laboratory to which the specimens are being sent should be notified in advance to facilitate assistance with customs clearance and transport.

The critical needs of the laboratory center around three basic resources: equipment and supplies to safely conduct the required tests, reagents to test for the pathogens of interest, and trained staff to perform the testing. High-quality diagnostic reagents with positive and negative controls are critical, especially for viral diseases or locally unfamiliar diseases. For some agents, such as influenza, dengue, and hantaviruses, commercially available diagnostic kits can be used in settings with minimal laboratory facilities.

Proper biosafety containment and strict adherence to biosafety procedures are critical, as was demonstrated by the recurrence of SARS-CoV infections in Singapore, Taiwan, and China in late 2003/early 2004 due to lapses in laboratory containment.[47–49] Most organisms are classified in one of four biosafety levels (BSL), depending on the seriousness of the disease, their transmissibility, and the availability of effective treatment or vaccines.[50] BSL 3 and 4 are required for handling the most dangerous pathogens and require highly specialized facilities and potentially expensive physical plant requirements.

Field laboratories can be key to the rapid containment of outbreaks of emerging infectious diseases. This was shown in the 2000–2001 outbreak of Ebola hemorrhagic fever in Uganda, when testing at a field laboratory was linked with additional testing at CDC and other reference centers.[18,51]

Pathology laboratories and pathologists have also been critical to identifying the causal agents, describing the pathogenetic processes,[52] and guiding the early phases of the epidemiologic investigations of several recently described diseases, including hantavirus pulmonary syndrome,[53] new variant Creutzfeldt–Jakob disease,[54] SARS,[55] and Lujo virus, a newly recognized hemorrhagic fever-associated arenavirus in southern Africa.[56] Clinicopathologic studies have also helped in understanding diseases such as West Nile virus encephalomyelitis.[57] Immunologic and molecular methods, including immunohistochemistry, *in situ* hybridization, and polymerase chain reaction, have revolutionized the diagnosis and understanding of emerging infectious diseases, showing the importance of pathologists and medical examiners in surveillance.[52]

COMMUNICATIONS

Finally, rapid reliable exchange and dissemination of information on disease incidence and distribution in real time are critical and depend on formal and informal networks. The 2003 global SARS epidemic showed how laboratory scientists, clinicians, and public health experts, aided by electronic communications, rapidly generated the scientific basis for public health action. A "virtual" international network of laboratories, linked by a secure website and daily teleconferences, identified the causative agent and rapidly developed diagnostic tests.

Recently developed and enhanced technologies have helped create web-based public health tools for disease reporting and emergency communications. The US CDC communicates breaking surveillance information to public health officials through two electronic networks: the Epidemic Information Exchange (Epi-X), a secure mechanism for sharing health surveillance information on outbreaks and other unusual events, and the Health Alert Network (HAN), which links local, state, and federal health agencies and provides an electronic platform for emergency alerts and long distance training. Similarly the Early Warning and Response System tracks communicable diseases in Europe.[58] Globally, WHO shares information through Disease Outbreak News on the WHO website, and the *Weekly Epidemiological Record*.

It is also key (and a required core capacity in the IHR) to communicate about risk. Outbreaks of novel or reemerging infectious disease involve scientific uncertainties and high levels of public concern that health officials will be challenged to address. Since the 2001 anthrax attacks and the 2003 global SARS outbreaks, CDC and WHO have been actively involved in efforts to incorporate risk communication into public health practice, as demonstrated during the H1N1 influenza pandemic.

CONCLUSIONS

Future challenges posed by infectious agents are difficult to predict but certainly include the emergence of additional zoonotic agents that cross the species barrier to humans; the emergence of new bacterial strains that are more virulent or resistant to antibiotics; the possible deliberate release of pathogenic microbes by terrorists; the emergence of novel influenza viruses; the likelihood of increased spread of arbovirus infections, particularly dengue, West Nile and chikungunya and yellow fever viruses; and further outbreaks of cholera and foodborne diseases. The best defense against these mobile and resilient pathogens is timely and reliable infectious disease intelligence obtained through global public health surveillance.[32] The international community has made important strides in developing networks for detecting and reporting infectious disease events and enhancing capacity for clinical and laboratory surveillance. Continued commitment and support are needed to optimize these mechanisms to improve the timely detection of unusual disease events, strengthen the ability to share disease intelligence, and inform prevention and containment efforts.

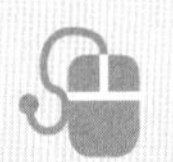

Access the complete reference list online at
http://www.expertconsult.com

CHAPTER 15

Access the complete reference list online at http://www.expertconsult.com

Enteric *Escherichia coli* Infections

Theodore S. Steiner • Nathan M. Thielman • Richard L. Guerrant

INTRODUCTION

Diarrheal illnesses constitute one of the leading infectious causes of death and disability worldwide. It is estimated that 1.9–2.5 million children die annually from diarrheal illnesses, the vast majority in Africa, Asia, and Latin America.[1–4] In a World Bank index of overall disease burden, disability-adjusted life years (DALYs) lost, diarrheal illnesses accounted for 7.3% of the total DALYs lost worldwide in 1990, nearly twice that due to sexually transmitted diseases, including acquired immunodeficiency syndrome (AIDS), and three times that due to malaria.[5] Furthermore, the World Bank DALY calculation for diarrhea counts predominantly its mortality, largely ignoring its even more staggering impact on morbidity and malnutrition.[6,7] Of the varied bacterial pathogens known to cause diarrhea worldwide, enterovirulent *Escherichia coli* collectively constitutes one of the most common, if not the most common, cause of diarrheal illness in tropical regions, particularly where sanitation facilities are limited.[8–10]

E. coli is the major aerobic organism of the normal intestinal flora, with around 10^{7-8} colony-forming units per gram of stool. Although the majority of isolates remain nonpathogenic gut commensals, diverse sets of virulence determinants confer this versatile species with virtually the entire range of pathogenic mechanisms by which bacteria cause diarrhea. Depending on how one deconstructs the complex range of diarrheagenic virulence traits in *E. coli,* anywhere between 5 and 10 different categories can easily be defined. This chapter emphasizes the five major types for which pathogenicity in outbreaks or volunteer studies has been established: enterotoxigenic *E. coli* (ETEC), enteropathogenic *E. coli* (EPEC), enteroaggregative *E. coli* (EAEC), enterohemorrhagic *E. coli* (EHEC), and enteroinvasive *E. coli* (EIEC). Also reviewed is diffusely adherent *E. coli* (DAEC), which has been variably associated with diarrhea in epidemiologic studies, yet possesses defined pathogenic traits that support its role as a true diarrheal pathogen.

THE AGENT

E. coli is a short, nonspore-forming, often fimbriate Gram-negative bacillus which grows readily on simple culture media or synthetic media with as little as glycerol or glucose as its only nutrient. With the exception of many enteroinvasive strains, most *E. coli* organisms are first identified as lactose-fermenting Gram-negative rods on routine culture medium. Other biochemical characteristics include indole production, lack of citrate fermentation, positive methyl red test, and negative urease and Voges–Proskauer reactions. *E. coli* is further characterized by a relatively complex serotyping scheme involving 173 O (lipopolysaccharide), 80 K (capsular), and 56 H (flagellar) antigens, all of which can be subdivided into partial antigens. Although the final number of *E. coli* serotypes is enormously high, 50 000–100 000 or more, the number of pathogenic serotypes in gastrointestinal infections is fairly limited (***Table 15.1***). The current serotyping scheme establishes O and H antigens based on bacterial agglutination; the K antigen is determined by gel immunoprecipitation or phage typing.[11] Each of the major categories of diarrheagenic *E. coli* falls into a relatively, but not absolutely, restricted set of these O:H serotypes which has proved useful in understanding both the pathogenesis and epidemiology of enteric *E. coli* infections.

EPIDEMIOLOGY

Despite the worldwide ubiquity of *E. coli,* most enteric *E. coli* infections are seen in the developing world where sanitation facilities are limited (***Fig. 15.1***). In community-based studies in Bangladesh and Brazil, ETEC alone accounted for up to 15–20% of cases of diarrhea,[8,12] and, overall, ETEC is regarded as the leading identified cause of traveler's diarrhea,[13,14] having been isolated in over half of the cases investigated in some studies.[15,16] Risk factors for ETEC in travelers include the length of stay, lack of adherence to food precautions, and a particular polymorphism haplotype in the gene for interleukin-10 (IL-10).[17]

Young children in the tropics are particularly prone to ETEC infections, with the peak incidence between 6 and 18 months of age.[18] In one prospective longitudinal study, ETEC was identified as the cause of diarrhea as many as two to three times per year per infant,[19] although in other studies the rates have been as low as 39/1000 patient-years.[18] Finally, ETEC can cause foodborne outbreaks in developed areas.[20] Like most enteropathogens, ETEC infection is acquired by ingesting contaminated food or water, and infants are at particular risk at weaning. The infective dose of ETEC is relatively high in the normal host, ranging from 10^6 to 10^{10} colony-forming units.[21,22]

EPEC was the first group of *E. coli* shown to cause diarrhea. In the 1940s epidemiologic investigations implicated EPEC isolates in outbreaks of community-acquired and nosocomial infantile diarrhea in Great Britain.[23] In these initial reports, mortality rates exceeded 50% in some cases.[23] Although EPEC is no longer considered a common cause of diarrhea in most developed nations, sporadic cases and outbreaks have been reported in Great Britain, Finland, and the United States.[24–27] Numerous studies in tropical or developing areas have demonstrated a convincing association of EPEC in infants with diarrhea,[28–33] and in some studies EPEC was identified as the commonest bacterial cause of diarrhea in the youngest children.[33–35] Recent hospitalization has been identified as an important risk factor for EPEC diarrhea in children in São Paulo, Brazil.[28] Older studies have suggested bottle-feeding as a risk factor for EPEC diarrhea,[23,36] and more recent series have demonstrated that breastfeeding is protective.[28,35] Recently, evidence has emerged for the existence of "atypical EPEC," isolates that lack the EPEC adherence factor (EAF) plasmid (see below) but maintain attaching and effacing ability; these appear to be a heterogeneous group of bacteria, whose role in clinical disease is still being investigated (reviewed in reference 37).

Table 15.1 Serogroups Associated with Enterovirulent *Escherichia coli*

Category	Predominant O Serogroups
Enterotoxigenic (ETEC)	LT: 1, 6, 7, 8, 9, 128
	LT + ST: 11, 15, 20, 25, 27, 60, 63, 75, 78, 80, 85, 88, 89, 99, 101, 109, 114, 139, 153
	ST: 12, 78, 115, 148, 149, 153, 159, 166, 167
Enterohemorrhagic (EHEC)	157, 26, 103, 111, 113, + some 50 others
Enteroinvasive (EIEC)	11, 28, 29, 112, 115, 124, 136, 143, 144, 147, 152, 164, 167, 173
Enteropathogenic (EPEC)	18, 26, 44, 55, 86, 111, 114, 119, 125, 126, 127, 128, 142, 145, 157, 158
Enteroaggregative (EAEC)	3, 15, 44, 51, 77, 78, 86, 91, 92, 111, 113, 126, 141, 146
Diffusely adherent (DAEC)	75, 15, 126

LT, heat-labile toxin; ST, heat-stable toxin.

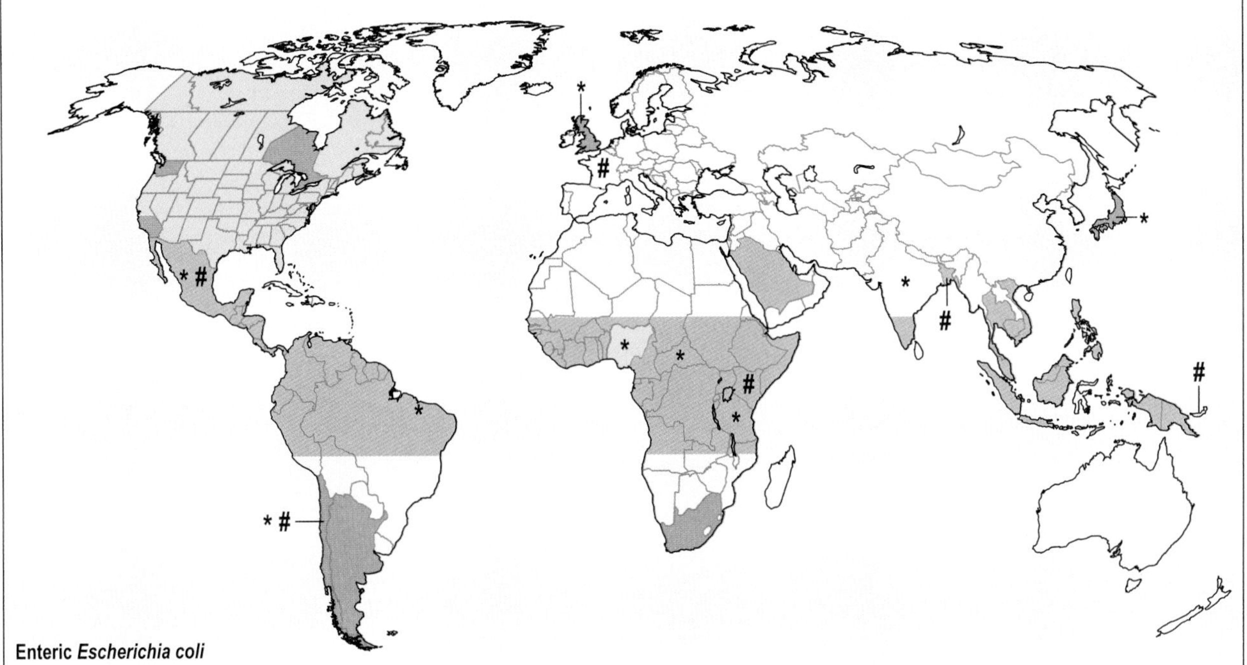

Figure 15.1 Enteric *Escherichia coli* distribution. *Note:* A number of epidemiologic studies have linked enteroaggregative *E. coli* (*) or diffusely adherent *E. coli* (#) with either acute or persistent diarrhea.

EAEC, classically identified by its ability to adhere to HEp-2 cells and glass slides in a "stacked-brick" pattern, is implicated as a significant cause of persistent diarrhea (greater than 14 days) in developing regions.[29,37–40] This endemic pediatric diarrhea was initially felt to be the predominant disease caused by EAEC, but more recent studies have demonstrated that EAEC is nearly as common as ETEC as a cause of adult travelers' diarrhea and also causes outbreak and episodic infections in developed countries.[41–48] In fact, one prospective study in the United States found that EAEC was the leading bacterial cause of acute diarrhea, ahead of *Salmonella* or *Campylobacter*.[49] EAEC has also frequently been identified as a cause of chronic diarrhea in patients with AIDS.[50–53] A recent meta-analysis confirmed a statistically significant association of EAEC carriage with diarrhea in these settings.[54] EAEC is also found more frequently in patients with irritable bowel syndrome than controls, although its role in the pathogenesis of this disorder remains speculative.[55]

Diffusely adherent *E. coli,* so named because of its HEp-2 pattern of adherence, has been variably associated with diarrhea in a number of epidemiologic studies.[32,56–60] In the largest of these, Levine et al.[56] examined 1081 samples from children with diarrhea and matched controls in Chile. An association between DAEC and diarrhea increased with age, reaching a plateau at a relative risk of 2.1 at 48–60 months of age. The increasing list of epidemiologic studies that examine the importance of DAEC in pediatric diarrhea is exhaustive; the reader is referred to several excellent reviews for a comprehensive summary.[61–63]

Although infection with *E. coli* O157:H7 and other EHEC is primarily recognized in developed countries, this pathogen also occasionally plagues the developing world. The majority of outbreaks worldwide are reported in the United States, Canada, the United Kingdom, and Japan, where foods originating from or contaminated by bovine sources are typically implicated.[64–67] EHEC has also been isolated in a number of tropical or developing areas, including Chile, Argentina, India, South Africa, and Swaziland.[58,68–71] Like most of the other enterovirulent *E. coli,* sporadic cases of *E. coli* O157:H7 peak during the warm weather months.[72]

EIEC, which taxonomically is more closely related to *Shigella* than to other *E. coli,* probably accounts for only 1–2% of endemic diarrheal episodes.[73] EIEC infections can be readily transmitted via contaminated food, and the largest outbreak (226 persons affected) in the United States was attributed to contamination of imported Camembert cheese with EIEC serogroup O124.[74]

THE DISEASE

Dictated by diverse sets of virulence determinants, the clinical manifestations of the different types of enterovirulent *E. coli* vary from cholera-like watery secretion with ETEC to dysentery indistinguishable from shigellosis with EIEC. The clinical characteristics of various enteric *E. coli* infections are summarized in ***Table 15.2***.

ETEC characteristically causes an acute watery diarrhea within 8–72 hours after ingestion, which ranges from a mild self-limited illness to dehydrating cholera-like purging.[21,22] Typically, stools are watery and without evidence of inflammation. Fever is usually low-grade or absent. Beyond the diarrhea, ETEC infections in infants and children interrupt normal feeding patterns and lead to diminished long-term linear growth.[8,19]

EPEC infections can be devastating to the neonate. Classically, mortality rates of 25–70% have been reported in outbreaks, where clinical illness is typically characterized by vomiting, low-grade fever, and profuse watery diarrhea. In subjects with experimental EPEC infection, fecal lactoferrin levels are significantly elevated, demonstrating the inflammatory nature of this disease.[75] EPEC may persist, as evidenced in a US daycare center outbreak in which infants' symptoms lasted for a mean of 18 days.[24]

EAEC is prominently linked with persistent diarrhea in children. Fever and grossly bloody stools are rarely associated with clinical infection,[29,39] but fecal lactoferrin levels are often elevated in children with EAEC infections whether they have diarrhea or not, these children having significant growth shortfalls, suggesting that EAEC causes malnutrition and intestinal inflammation, with or without diarrhea.[76] It is notable that in some epidemiologic studies EAEC has not been associated with diarrhea[57,77,78] and that different strains have variably caused diarrhea in human volunteer studies.[79,80] The variable association of EAEC with diarrhea is likely due to heterogeneous expression of virulence determinants, but host factors may also be relevant. For example, travelers with a particular genotype in the IL-8 promoter are more likely to develop symptomatic diarrhea with EAEC infection.[81] The importance of this and other naturally occurring genetic polymorphisms in EAEC infection in other settings remains to be known.

Little is known about the clinical characteristics of DAEC enteric infections, which have been inconsistently associated with diarrhea (except in older children 18–60 months of age). One study found a particular association of DAEC with vomiting.[82] However, its pathogenicity is clouded by two studies involving 51 volunteers challenged with three different DAEC strains.[79,83] Only one individual developed diarrhea. As with EAEC, not all DAEC isolates (as defined by HEp-2 adherence) possess the necessary virulence traits to cause disease. For example, in one case-control study, only DAEC isolates that expressed the *afa* locus were statistically associated with diarrhea.[84]

E. coli O157:H7 and other EHEC cause diarrhea, hemorrhagic colitis, hemolytic–uremic syndrome (HUS), thrombotic thrombocytopenic purpura, and sometimes death. Although infection with *E. coli* O157:H7 typically begins as nonbloody diarrhea, in most cases that come to medical attention the diarrhea becomes bloody by the second or third day of illness. Fevers are seen in fewer than one-third of patients and vomiting in about half. Fecal leukocytes or lactoferrin are typically seen in less than 40% of patients with symptomatic EHEC infection. Uncomplicated

Table 15.2 Clinical Features of Enteric *Escherichia coli* Infections

Type of *E. coli*	Epidemiology/Setting	Incubation Period	Diarrhea	Additional Features	Sequelae
ETEC	Young children > adults in developing world/ travelers to tropics	10–72 hours	Acute watery	Nausea, abdominal cramping; ± low-grade fevers	Interrupted feeding patterns → diminished linear growth
EPEC	Infants in developing world	As short as 9–12 hours	Acute → persistent watery	Positive fecal lactoferrin, vomiting, fever, dehydration	Mortality rates up to 25–70% reported
EAEC	Children in developing world	20–48 hours	Persistent	Fever in 12%; grossly bloody stools in up to 1/3 of patients	May interfere with normal growth patterns
	Travelers to tropics	Unknown	Acute; occasionally persistent	More likely than ETEC to have positive fecal lactoferrin	Occasional persistence
	Patients with AIDS	Unknown	Persistent		Chronic diarrhea
	Endemic diarrhea in developed countries	Unknown	Acute, self-limited	No characteristic or defining features compared to other bacterial pathogens	Usually none
EHEC	All ages Primarily in United States, Canada, Europe, cone of South America	12–60 hours	Acute bloody diarrhea (progressing to hemorrhagic colitis in 38–61%); occasionally nonbloody diarrhea	Fecal leukocytes or lactoferrin in 30–40%; fevers in 0–32%; abdominal pain; moderate leukocytosis	Progression to HUS/TTP in 2–8%; rarely death; complications greatest at extremes of age; long-term renal damage may occur following HUS
EIEC	All ages Primarily in developing regions; occasional outbreaks in industrialized countries	As short as 10–18 hours	Acute watery diarrhea followed by dysentery	Fecal leukocytes or lactoferrin elevated; gross purulence, blood, mucus may be seen in stool; severe abdominal cramps	Hypoglycemia, especially if malnourished
DAEC	Pathogenicity most established in children aged 24–60 months	Unknown	Acute in three studies; persistent in one; not associated with diarrhea in multiple studies	Nausea/vomiting prominent in one study	Unknown

ETEC, enterotoxigenic *Escherichia coli;* EPEC, enteropathogenic *E. coli*; EAEC, enteroaggregative *E. coli*; EHEC, enterohemorrhagic *E. coli*; EIEC, enteroinvasive *E. coli;* DAEC, diffusely adherent *E. coli*; AIDS, acquired immunodeficiency syndrome; HUS, hemolytic–uremic syndrome; TTP, thrombotic thrombocytopenic purpura.

infections typically resolve in about 1 week. Infection with *E. coli* O157:H7 has been confused with a number of other gastrointestinal disorders such as appendicitis, inflammatory bowel disease, and ischemic colitis.[72,85] Local complications may include bowel perforation, toxic megacolon, and stricture.[64,85,86]

The most devastating sequela of EHEC infection, HUS (a constellation of microangiopathic hemolytic anemia, thrombocytopenia, and acute renal failure), occurs most frequently in children between 1 and 4 years of age and in the elderly.[87] The overall rate of HUS in sporadic cases of bloody diarrhea with *E. coli* O157:H7 is between 5% and 10%.[64] A number of studies point to preexisting EHEC infection in 75–95% of children presenting with HUS.[88–91] It is often difficult to document microbiologic evidence of EHEC infection at the onset of HUS symptoms, as persons with HUS typically seek medical attention around 6–12 days after the onset of diarrhea, when the EHEC stool counts are decreasing.[92] Among survivors of HUS, chronic renal disease may develop, as noted in ongoing follow-up from a large waterborne outbreak of EHEC in Walkerton, Ontario. There is also a recent report of an association between HUS and subsequent development of type 1 diabetes mellitus.[93,94] Reported host risk factors for the development of HUS in patients with EHEC diarrhea include the extremes of age,[95] leukocytosis,[96] diminished P1 antigen expression on red blood cells,[97] the use of antimotility agents, and possibly prior antimicrobial therapy (see below).[98]

As with shigellosis, EIEC infection typically causes watery diarrhea followed by dysenteric stools with mucus, fecal leukocytes, and scant blood. Fever, severe abdominal cramps, and malaise are common.

PATHOGENESIS AND IMMUNITY

Summarized in ***Table 15.3*** are the major known virulence determinants for enterovirulent *E. coli,* including their genetic traits, mechanisms of action, and relevant experimental models. Also noted are other enteric bacteria expressing similar virulence determinants, illustrating that the diverse range of virulence traits demonstrated in *E. coli* infections is representative of those present in the majority of bacterial enteropathogens. While not dealt with elsewhere in this book, organisms such as *Aeromonas, Plesiomonas, Klebsiella, Citrobacter, Enterobacter,* and *Yersinia* may produce enterotoxins, as noted in ***Table 15.3***, and may be important enteric pathogens, more often in cooler, temperate climates.

Enterotoxigenic *E. coli*

In order for ETEC to be fully pathogenic the organism must both colonize the small intestine and elaborate one or more enterotoxins. After ingestion in contaminated food or water, ETEC with fimbrial colonization factor antigens (CFAs) attach and multiply *in situ*, thereby overcoming the peristaltic defense mechanism in the proximal small intestine. CFA-I, CFA-II, CFA-IV, and others are distinguished from the type 1 pili, common to almost all *E. coli,* by their ability to agglutinate erythrocytes in the presence of D-mannose. While the receptors for CFAs are not fully known, the Lewis (a) blood group antigen is likely involved in CFA-I attachment, and children carrying this gene are at increased risk for infection with CFA-I-expressing ETEC.[99] Although most ETEC isolates are associated with at least one of the classic CFA types, other additional attachment factors (such as PCFO159, PCFO166, E8775, CS 7, and CS 17), yet to be fully characterized, may also participate in small-intestine colonization.[100–102]

ETEC is defined primarily by the heat-labile (LT) and heat-stable (ST) toxins it elaborates. Of the four known enterotoxins (LT-I, LT-II, STa, and STb) produced by ETEC, LT-I and STa are best established as important secretagogues in humans, and pathogenic strains typically elaborate one or both of these toxins. The LT-I family of toxins are high-molecular-weight proteins (84–86 kDa) remarkably similar to cholera toxin in structure and function. The deduced amino acid sequences of the single enzymatically active (A) subunit and the five binding (B) subunits of LT-I demonstrate approximately 80% homology with that of cholera toxin, and its secretory effect is blocked by antisera to cholera toxin.[103] Given this degree of structural similarity with cholera toxin, it is not surprising that the mechanism of action of LT enterotoxin is nearly identical to that of cholera toxin (***Fig. 15.2***). After binding to a GM_1 ganglioside receptor (or to a 130–140-kDa glycoprotein receptor 20–30 times more prevalent in intestinal brush border than the binding site for cholera toxin)[104] like cholera toxin, LT activates adenylate cyclase via NAD-dependent adenosine diphosphate (ADP) ribosylation of Gs_α. The resultant increase in intracellular cyclic adenosine monophosphate (cAMP) ultimately stimulates chloride secretion and inhibits sodium absorption, leading to the voluminous watery stools characteristic of this infection. LT-induced signaling via cAMP also alters host membrane structure to increase bacterial adherence[105,106] and decreases expression of antimicrobial peptides from epithelial cells.[107] Finally, LT itself can bind to and activate Toll-like receptor 1/2 heterodimers, which may help explain its strong immunogenicity.[108]

The ST toxin family, which bears significant homology with the endogenous intestinal peptide guanylin, also causes fluid and electrolyte secretion.[109] The major ST toxin responsible for diarrhea in humans, STa, is an 18–19-amino-acid enterotoxin with no subunit structure, which contains three disulfide bonds important for biologic activity. As shown in ***Figure 15.3***, STa binds to an extracellular domain of guanylate cyclase, resulting in increased intracellular levels of cyclic guanosine monophosphate (cGMP), which ultimately leads to decreased absorption of sodium and increased chloride secretion.

In addition to *Vibrio cholerae*, occasional other bacteria, including *Klebsiella, Enterobacter, Morganella, Aeromonas, Plesiomonas, Campylobacter,* and *Salmonella* species, have been shown to elaborate LT-like toxins.[8,110–116] An STa-like peptide toxin, EAST-1, is produced by many EAEC and EHEC isolates and causes fluid secretion in a cGMP-dependent manner.[117,118] The gene for East-1 (*astA*) is statistically associated with diarrhea in EAEC infections.[54]

Enteropathogenic *E. coli*

Unlike in ETEC, secretory exotoxin elaboration does not play a role in the pathogenesis of EPEC. The basic pathogenic feature of these organisms is the attaching and effacing lesion, which is characterized by degeneration of the microvillus brush border, with cupping and pedestal formation of the plasma membrane at sites of bacterial attachment, noted histologically[119] (***Fig. 15.4***). ***Figure 15.5*** depicts the four-stage model of EPEC pathogenesis, proposed by Lockman and Kaper,[120] as well as the mechanism of its invasive capacity. Early adherence is mediated by the bundle-forming pilus, which is primarily encoded by the *bfpA* gene. Following binding to cell surface carbohydrates, the bundle-forming pili retract, bringing the bacteria into intimate contact with the host cell. These adherent bacteria then express a type III secretion system (TTSS) "needle complex" that penetrates the host cell membrane and injects bacterial proteins, including the translocated intimin receptor (Tir). After injection, Tir is tyrosine-phosphorylated, leading to recruitment of cytoskeletal elements that form a tall pedestal upon which the bacterium sits. The *eae* gene product, intimin, sits in the bacterial cell wall and binds directly to Tir, helping to anchor the bacterium to the pedestal. A number of additional proteins secreted by the TTSS have been identified, some of which reside along with the TTSS structural proteins in the chromosomal pathogenicity island known as the LEE (locus of enterocyte effacement), which was clearly identified as a virulence trait in EPEC strains in human volunteer studies.[121] Additional non-LEE TTSS effectors have also been characterized, adding additional complexity to the question of how EPEC causes diarrhea.[122,123] Several of these effectors appear to modulate host signaling and are required for full pathogenicity in closely associated animal pathogens (*Citrobacter rodentium*, rabbit enteropathgenic *E. coli*). Some known TTSS effectors of EPEC and other pathogenic proteins are listed in ***Table 15.3***.

Although EPEC organisms do not cause keratoconjunctivitis in guinea pigs, a property classically associated with invasive *Shigella* and EIEC,

Table 15.3 Pathogenic Mechanisms of Enterovirulent *Escherichia coli*

Category[a]	Virulence Determinant	Genetic Locus	Mechanism	Experimental Model	Enteric Bacteria Expressing Similar Virulence Determinants
ETEC[b]	CFA-I–IV	Plasmid	Colonization	MRHA	
	LT I and II	LT-I (plasmid) LT-II (chromosome)	Adenylate cyclase → secretion	18-hour rabbit ileal loops and CHO/Y1 cells	LT-like toxins: *Vibrio cholerae*, *Klebsiella*, *Enterobacter*, *Aeromonas hydrophila*, *Plesiomonas shigelloides*, *Campylobacter*, *Salmonella*
	ST-I (ST_a)	Plasmid	Guanylate cyclase → secretion	4–6-hour rabbit ileal loops and suckling mice	ST-like toxins: *Yersinia enterocolitica*, *Citrobacter freundii*, non-O1 vibrios, EAEC
	ST-II (ST_b)	Plasmid	Cyclic nucleotide-independent HCO_3^- secretion	Piglet loop	
EHEC[b]	SLT-I and II SLT-IIvh and IIvp	Phage	Toxins bind to Gb3 receptor, glycosidase cleaves adenosine-4324 in 28S rRNA of 60S ribosomal subunits to halt protein synthesis	HeLa cell cytotoxicity	SLTs: non-EHEC STEC; Shiga toxin: *Shigella dysenteriae* type 1
	Intimin	Locus of enterocyte effactment (LEE) (chromosomal pathogenicity island)	Intimate adherence to Tir (see below), leading to pedestal formation	Fluorescence actin staining (FAS), pedestal formation	EPEC, *Citrobacter rodentium*, REPEC
	Type III secretion system (TTSS)	LEE	Intimate attachment via Tir injected into cell membrane; actin rearrangement, pedestal formation		EPEC shares many similar genes, although pedestals are qualitatively different; TTSS found in many plant and animal pathogens (e.g., REPEC, *Citrobacter rodentium*, *Salmonella*, *Yersinia*)
	TTSS effectors: Tir	LEE	Binding to intimin, recruitment of actin condensation		
	EspA	LEE	Part of needle complex		
	EspB, D	LEE	Form pores in host cell membrane for effector delivery		
	EspF	LEE	Causes host cell apoptosis		
	EspG, H	LEE	Possibly mediates invasion		
	Map	LEE	Mitochondrial damage		
	NleA	Non-LEE PAI	COPII protein complex; disrupts intracellular protein trafficking[c]		
	Cif (cycle-inhibiting factor)	Non-LEE prophage	Cell cycle arrest by stabilization of cyclin-dependent kinase inhibitors, actin stress fiber formation[d,e]	Cytopathic effects on culture cells	Homologs in *Yersinia pseudotuberculosis*, other nonenteric pathogens
	Other TTSS effectors	Genomic prophage sites	At least 39 translocated proteins identified;[f] most functions unknown	Secretion assays and bioinformatic analyses	Homologs in plant pathogens, *Shigella*
	Accessory toxins: ToxB EspP Ehx (RTX toxin) StcE	pO157 plasmid	Implicated in adhesion, cytotoxicity, tissue edema	Various	Homologs in many pathogenic bacteria
	Flagellin	*fliC* (chromosome)	Motility; IL-8 release via TLR5 activation	Motility and cytokine release	*Salmonella*, EAEC, EPEC
EIEC[b]	IpaA, B, C IpgD (invasion and adhesin proteins)	Plasmid	Cell invasion and spread	Sereny test	Invasion plasmid: *Shigella* spp.
	IscA	Plasmid	Actin nucleation, leading to intracellular spread	Actin microfilament formation and cytoplasmic motility	*Shigella* spp.

Table 15.3 Pathogenic Mechanisms of Enterovirulent *Escherichia coli*—cont'd

Category[a]	Virulence Determinant	Genetic Locus	Mechanism	Experimental Model	Enteric Bacteria Expressing Similar Virulence Determinants
	SepA	Plasmid	Serine protease autotransporter		Various
EPEC[b]	Bundle-forming pilus	60-MDa EAF plasmid (bfpA)	Localized adherence (LA)	LA to Hep-2 cells	
	Intimin/Tir	Chromosomal LEE	Tir injected into host cell becomes tyrosine-phosphorylated and binds intimin on bacterial surface	FAS, pedestal formation	EHEC, *Citrobacter rodentium*, REPEC
	TTSS	LEE, additional PAIs	Similar effectors as in EHEC, above		
	Flagellin	*fliC* (chromosome)	Motility; IL-8 release via TLR5 activation	Motility and cytokine release	*Salmonella*, EAEC, EHEC
EAEC[b]	Aggregative adherence fimbriae (AAF)	60-MDa AA plasmid: *aggA* (AAF/I), *aafA* (AAF/II), *agg3A* (AAF/III), *hdaA* (novel type)	Aggregative adherence (AA), biofilm formation	HEp-2 or HeLa cell AA; biofilm formation in liquid media	
	AggR	Plasmid	Master regulator of virulence genes	PCR or gene probe	
	EAST1	*astA* (AA plasmid)	Guanylate cyclase → secretion	Rabbit ileal loops and Ussing chambers	Found in many EHEC, other *E. coli*
	Dispersin	*aap* (AA plasmid)	Regulates deaggregation during colonization		
	Pet	Plasmid	Cleavage of fodrin, leading to cytoskeletal damage	Ussing chamber; cytotoxicity	Other SPATE family members
	Pic	*pic/set* locus on chromosome	Mucinase; allows growth on mucin		
	ShET-1	*pic/set* locus on chromosome	Possible enterotoxin	Ussing chamber	*Shigella*
	Flagellin	*fliC* (chromosomal)	IL-8 release via TLR5 activation	Motility, cytokine release	*Salmonella*, EPEC, EHEC
	Type VI secretion system	*aai* cluster and a second chromosomal PAI	Unknown function of small, secreted effectors		*Aeromonas*, *Salmonella*, *Vibrio cholerae*
DAEC	Fimbrial adhesin (F1845)	Chromosome	Binding to CD55 (decay accelerating factor) leading to unique cytopathology	Diffuse adherence (DA) to HEp-2 cells	Uropathogenic *E. coli*
	Afimbrial adhesin (AIDA-I)	Plasmid	DA	DA to HEp-2 cells	
	Sat	Chromosome	SPATE family toxin		Other SPATE members

ETEC, enterotoxigenic *Escherichia coli*; CFA, colonization factor antigen; MRHA, mannose-resistant hemagglutination; LT, heat-labile toxin; ST, heat-stable toxin; EAEC, enteroaggregative *E. coli*; EHEC, enterohemorrhagic *E. coli*; SLT, Shiga-like toxin; STEC, Shiga toxin-producing *E. coli*; EPEC, enteropathogenic *E. coli*; REPEC, rabbit enteropathogenic *E. coli*; IL, interleukin; LEE, locus of enterocyte effacement; PAI, pathogenicity island; EIEC, enteroinvasive *E. coli*; PCR, polymerase chain reaction; SPATE, serine protease autotransporter of Enterobacteriaceae; DAEC, diffusely adherent *E. coli*.

[a]See **Table 15.1**.

[b]Pathogenicity in humans established in outbreaks or volunteer studies.

[c]Cell Host Microbe. 2007;2(3):160–71.

[d]PLoS ONE. 2009;4(3):e4855.

[e]Cell Microbiol. 2008;10(12):2496–508.

[f]PNAS. 2006;103(40):14931–14946.

invasion has been observed in clinical specimens, *in vivo* experimental models, and a variety of epithelial cell types *in vitro*.[124–129] Exactly how any of these epithelial cell changes lead to diarrhea has not been fully worked out. Incubation of EPEC with polarized epithelial monolayers results in decreased transepithelial resistance and both TLR5-dependent and -independent secretion of IL-8,[115] possibly reflecting an increase in permeability and inflammation that could contribute to diarrhea.[116] In addition, the loss of microvilli likely leads to malabsorption.[130]

The role of immune responses in EPEC infection is uncertain. The distinctively different age-specific attack rates may be explained by the development of immunity following colonization or infection with EPEC. Certain TTSS effector proteins, especially intimin and Tir, are highly immunogenic in mice,[131] and antibodies against intimin are found in adults living in endemic areas, which could explain the relative lack of EPEC and EHEC infections in adults in these locations.[132] Alternatively, the loss of age-specific receptors may account for the dramatic drop in EPEC infection in patients older than 6 months of age.[133] Several lines of evidence suggest that breast milk may provide passive immunity against EPEC infection. In addition to the association of EPEC infection with bottle-feeding, secretory IgA to the EAF and oligosaccharide fractions of human colostrum and breast milk have been shown to inhibit localized adhesion of EPEC to HEp-2 cells.[134,135]

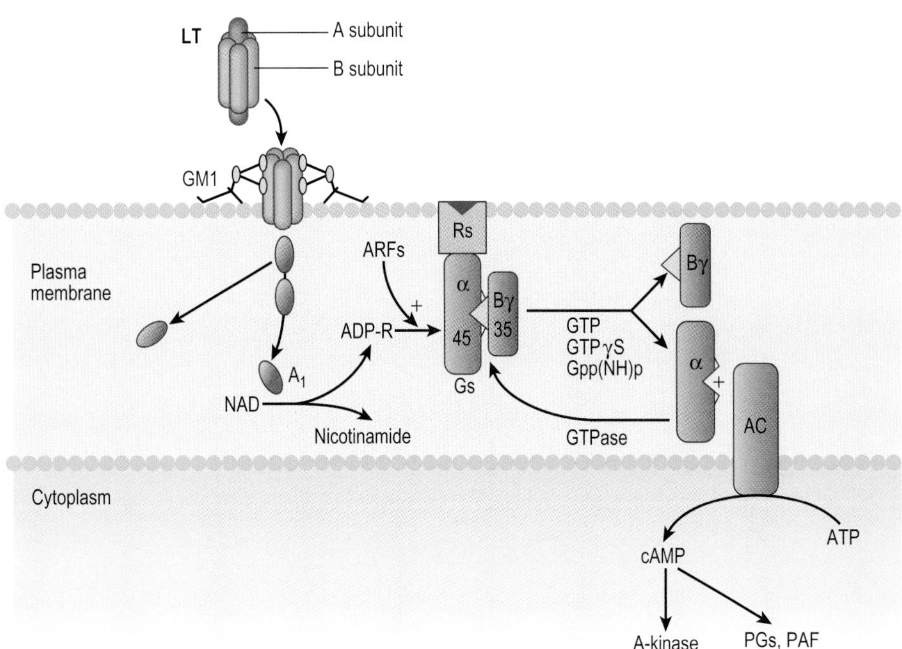

Figure 15.2 Heat-labile toxin (LT), a homolog of cholera toxin, binds to a monosialoganglioside receptor (GM1) via its B subunits, and the A_1 subunit is released from B_5 and A_2 by cleavage of a disulfide bond. This enzymatically active peptide catalyzes the dissolution of NAD to nicotinamide and, in the presence of adenosine diphosphate (ADP) ribosylation factors (ARFs), ADP ribosylates Gs_{α}, which then dissociates from the βγ subunit to activate adenylate cyclase (AC). Cyclic adenosine monophosphate (cAMP) formation, catalyzed by adenylate cyclase, stimulates water and electrolyte secretion by intestinal epithelial cells via protein kinase A, prostaglandin (PG) synthesis, and possibly platelet-activating factor (PAF). ATP, adenosine triphosphate; GTP, guanosine triphosphate.

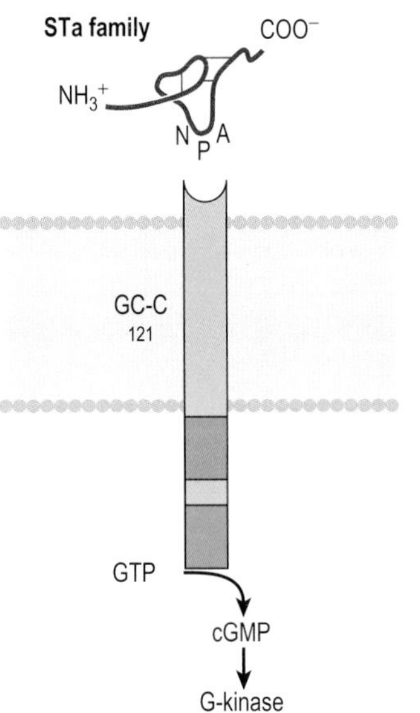

Figure 15.3 Heat-stable enterotoxin (ST), an 18–19-amino acid peptide, binds to an extracellular domain of guanylate cyclase (GC-C) to increase cyclic guanosine monophosphate (cGMP), which activates G kinase, ultimately leading to altered sodium and chloride transport via phosphorylation of membrane proteins. GTP, guanosine triphosphate.

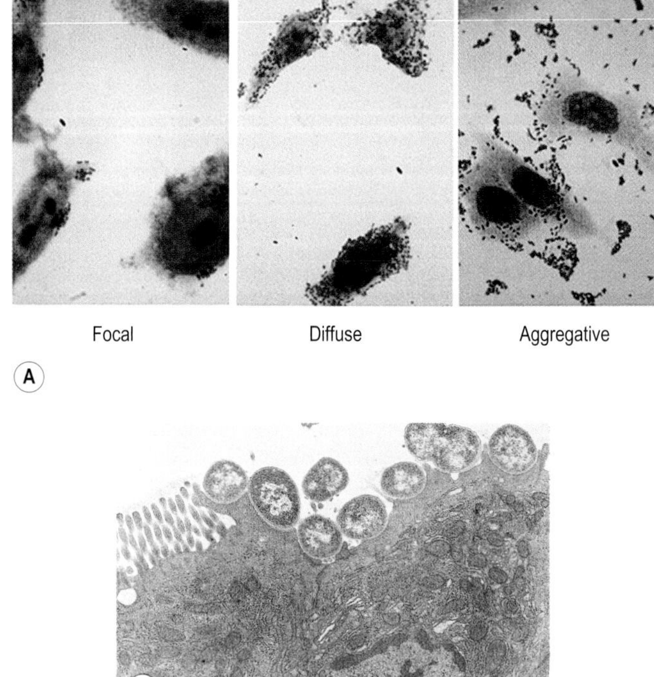

Figure 15.4 **(A)** Three types of HEp-2 cell attachment: locally adherent enteropathogenic *Escherichia coli* (EPEC, left), diffusely adherent *E. coli* (DAEC, center), and enteroaggregative *E. coli* (right). **(B)** EPEC attachment and effacement on human enterocytes in a patient with diarrhea. (Reproduced from Rothbaum R, McAdams AJ, Giannella R, et al. A clinicopathologic study of enterocyte-adherent *Escherichia coli*: a cause of protracted diarrhea in infants. Gastroenterology. 1982;83:441.)

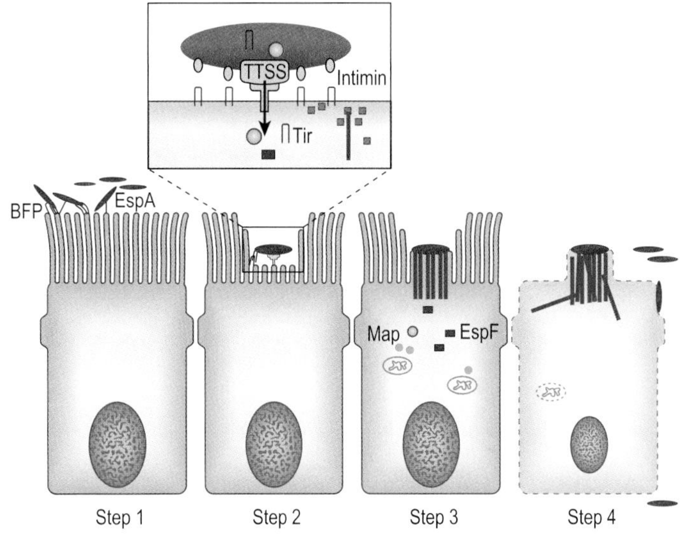

Figure 15.5 Four-stage model of enteropathogenic *Escherichia coli* (and enterohemorrhagic *E. coli*) pathogenesis. Step 1: Bacteria contact the epithelial surface and adhere loosely via bundle-forming pili (BFP) and EspA projections. Step 2: Intimate attachment begins as bacteria inject Tir and other effectors via the type 3 secretion system (TTSS). Tir inserts into the host cell membrane and binds intimin on the bacterial surface. Meanwhile, host proteins are recruited to the cytoplasmic tail of Tir and begin cytoskeletal rearrangements. Step 3: Actin recruited to the contact point with the bacteria forms an elongated pedestal. TTSS effectors alter host cell physiology. Shown are Map, which damages mitochondria, and EspF, which causes apoptosis. Step 4: Pedestal formation and cell damage continue, leading to loss of membrane and mucosal barrier integrity. In addition, invasion of bacteria can occur at this stage.

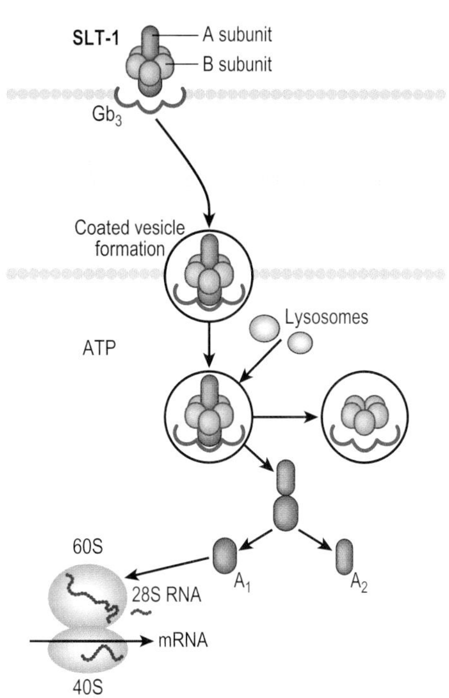

Figure 15.6 Shiga-like toxins (SLTs) I and II produced by enterohemorrhagic *Escherichia coli* bind to globotriaosyl ceramide (Gb_3) via B subunits and undergo receptor-mediated endocytosis. The A subunit, after release into the cytoplasm, is proteolytically degraded to A_1 and A_2 fragments. The former binds to the 60S ribosome and cleaves an adenine residue at position 4324 in 28S ribosomal RNA, thereby halting protein synthesis and causing cell death. ATP, adenosine triphosphate.

Enterohemorrhagic *E. coli*

At least two virulence traits, attaching and effacing ability and Shiga-like toxin (SLT) elaboration, confer pathogenicity to EHEC organisms. Like EPEC, EHEC causes filamentous actin accumulation at the site of attachment in association with "cup and pedestal" formation.[136] As in EPEC, this is achieved through the actions of genes on a chromosomal pathogenicity island analogous to the LEE. However, there are some differences between EPEC and EHEC pedestals: notably, EHEC Tir does not require tyrosine phosphorylation in order to initiate pedestal formation.[137]

What distinguishes EPEC from EHEC more obviously are the SLTs of EHEC. These toxins, which are structurally and functionally similar to the Shiga toxin from *Shigella dysenteriae* I, are also referred to as verotoxins, reflecting their cytotoxicity for Vero cells. Thus, EHEC has been variably referred to in the literature as STEC and VTEC. Current convention is to label as EHEC only those organisms that have both attaching and effacing ability and express one or both SLTs.[138] Non-EHEC STEC, which lack attaching and effacing ability, are frequently identified, although their pathogenic potential is variable.[139,140] At least two immunologically distinct SLTs, both with one A and five B subunits, have been described. The 70-kDa SLT-I is virtually identical to Shiga toxin and is neutralizable by antiserum against Shiga toxin. The smaller 60-kDa SLT-II is neutralized by neither antibodies to Shiga toxin nor SLT-I.[141,142]

Although SLTs alone are capable of stimulating bloody fluid accumulation and mucosal injury in multiple animal models,[143,144] SLT production does not appear to be requisite for developing diarrhea in EHEC infections.[145] In severe disease, particularly when bloody diarrhea is present, it is thought that SLTs gain systemic access and that they play a central role in the development of HUS. It is proposed that SLTs, which inhibit protein synthesis in a number of cell lines *in vitro*, do so in endothelial cells (as shown in ***Fig. 15.6***), ultimately causing them to detach and expose platelets to the subendothelium, thus initiating coagulation.[146] The receptor for the SLT B subunit, globotriaosylceramide or Gb3, is highly expressed in several of the target organs of EHEC/HUS, including the colon, kidneys, and brain.[147–150] In addition, in rabbits SLT-I has been shown to induce a thrombotic microvascular angiopathy similar to that seen in humans with HUS.[143] Epidemiologic data suggest that SLT-II may be more important than SLT-I for progression of *E. coli* O157:H7 infection to HUS.[66,151,152]

The role of antibodies in protecting against EHEC infection or its complications remains unknown. Although the epidemiologic observation of increased rates of infection and complications in young children and the elderly may suggest a role for immunity in preventing infection, reports of recurrent hemorrhagic colitis and HUS associated with recurrent *E. coli* O157:H7 infections argue against a key role for protective immunity.[64,153,154]

Enteroaggregative *E. coli*

Data from several volunteer studies demonstrate marked variability in EAEC pathogenicity in adults.[79,80] This is likely because this category of *E. coli*, defined primarily by a phenotypic assay (stacked-brick HEp-2 cell adherence), includes subsets of *E. coli* with varied (or no) virulence traits. However, phylogenetic analysis suggests that there are three distinct subfamilies of EAEC with common traits, indicating that EAEC is not as heterogeneous a class of bacteria as was once thought. Moreover, there is clinical evidence that strains with a "typical" adherence pattern and strains that express the transcriptional regulator *aggR* and genes in its regulon are more likely to cause diarrhea and intestinal bleeding and inflammation than atypical strains.[46,155–159]

There are a number of identified virulence traits in EAEC. The characteristic HEp-2 adherence is mediated by flexible bundle-forming fimbrial structures, aggregative adherence fimbriae (AAF), of which at least three distinct types exist. Other potential EAEC adhesins include heat-resistant agglutinin 1 (Hra1),[160] a galactose-inhibitable lectin,[161,162] a pilin called HdaA,[163] and type IV pili.[164] Expression of these adherence fimbriae is strongly associated with the ability of EAEC to form biofilms in liquid media;[165] consequently, biofilm formation can serve as a reasonably sensitive, rapid test for EAEC (see below).

The AAF are encoded by two separate gene clusters on the 60-MDa AA plasmid.[135,136] Also encoded on the plasmid is Pet, a member of the serine protease autotransporter toxin family. Pet cleaves host cytoskeletal proteins and may be responsible for many of the cytotoxic effects of EAEC *in vitro*. An additional plasmid protein, dispersin, is expressed during EAEC infection, and serves to release AAF attachments to allow for bacterial dispersion.[166] Many EAEC isolates also encode a plasmid-borne enterotoxin, designated EAST-1, which bears significant homology with the enterotoxin domains of ST and guanylin.[118] Most of the plasmid and chromosomal pathogenicity genes in EAEC are controlled by the plasmid-encoded transcriptional regulator, AggR, and this gene is frequently associated with the presence of other virulence genes and with diarrhea in colonized patients.[167]

In addition to the plasmid virulence traits noted above, EAEC strain 042 (the prototype pathogenic in volunteers) expresses several chromosomal virulence traits. One of these proteins, Pic, is a mucinase that likely contributes to the distinctive intestinal adherence of EAEC.[168,169] The opposite strand from Pic in the same location encodes a protein, ShET-1, that was first identified as an enterotoxin in *Shigella flexneri*.[170] EAEC 042 also expresses a highly inflammatory flagellin, which causes IL-8 release from epithelial cells *in vitro* via Toll-like receptor 5 and appears to be responsible for most of the inflammatory response to EAEC.[171,172] Finally, the EAEC chromosome harbors at least two pathogenicity islands encoding type VI secretion systems, which export small molecules; the roles of the type VI effectors remain largely unknown, but appear to be involved in biofilm formation.[173]

Diffusely Adherent *E. coli*

Less is known about DAEC pathogenesis than about other *E. coli* pathotypes. The diffusely adherent phenotype can be mediated by either fimbrial (F1845) or afimbrial (AIDA-1) adhesins.[174,175] These adhesins are homologous to Afa/Dr adhesins found on many uropathogenic *E. coli* (UPEC), and bind to decay-accelerating factor (CD55), leading to clustering of this protein in the cell membrane and unique ultrastructural changes.[176–179] Toxic effects include loss of tight junction integrity[180] and basolateral cytokine release.[181] In addition, a SPATE-family toxin called Sat was identified in DAEC and found to be strongly associated with urinary tract infections and diarrhea but not asymptomatic colonization in one study population.[182] The similarity between Afa/Dr DAEC and UPEC strains has raised the suggestion that they share a common ancestry and pathogenesis (reviewed in references 183 and 184).

Enteroinvasive *E. coli*

Like *Shigella,* EIEC penetrates and multiplies within colonic epithelial cells, eventually causing cell death and the exuberant host inflammation responsible for much of the dysenteric clinical syndrome. A large 140-MDa plasmid that has extensive homology with the invasion plasmid of *Shigella* species mediates these virulence properties.[185] The invasion plasmid encodes a TTSS that injects effectors IpaA, B, and C, and IpgD, which recruit epithelial cell signaling to create cytoskeletal rearrangements that permit entry of the bacterium (reviewed in reference 138). An additional plasmid-encoded protein, IcsA, localizes to one pole of the bacterial outer membrane where it binds N-WASP, leading to actin condensation. This polar actin condensation pushes the bacterium through the cytoplasm and ultimately into adjacent cells, leading to horizontal spread through the epithelium.[186,187] Other virulence traits expressed by some EIEC isolates include plasmid-encoded enterotoxins, which may explain the watery diarrhea often seen in early stages of EIEC infection.[188,189] EIEC can also trigger inflammation in intestinal epithelial cells by activating the intracellular host peptidoglycan receptor Nod1.[190]

DIAGNOSIS

Because of the ubiquity of *E. coli* in fecal material, definitive diagnosis of enteric infections with enterovirulent *E. coli* often involves sophisticated techniques to detect the virulence traits themselves, many of which are beyond the scope of most clinical diagnostic laboratories. Of the enterovirulent *E. coli,* EHEC is most easily identified because of the dominant prevalence of serotype O157:H7. Because *E. coli* O157:H7, unlike most *E. coli,* does not ferment sorbitol, sorbitol-MacConkey agar is used as a screening medium. Presumptive diagnosis of *E. coli* O157:H7 infection can be made when sorbitol-negative (clear) *E. coli* isolates are shown to agglutinate in the presence of *E. coli* O157 antiserum.[191] However, non-O157 EHEC isolates, which can cause human disease, will be missed by this method. Newer immunologic techniques that detect SLT-I and SLT-II in stool are therefore in widespread use. Screening for EHEC by one of these methods is recommended for all bloody stool samples received in diagnostic laboratories.[192,193]

The enteroadherent *E. coli* types (EPEC, EAEC, and DAEC) are classically identified by the HEp-2 cell adherence assay in which HEp-2 cells are incubated with *E. coli* isolates, washed, stained, and then examined microscopically for adherence patterns. EPEC attaches in focal aggregates (local adherence), EAEC adheres to both HEp-2 cells and glass in a stacked-brick pattern, and, as suggested by the name, DAEC adheres in a diffuse pattern to cells (but not glass). Although a number of technical variations in the HEp-2 cell adherence assay have been described, it appears that the so-called CVD (Center for Vaccine Development, University of Maryland) method or a modification of the UTH (University of Texas, Houston) method to include a 2–4-hour postwash incubation is best able to distinguish all three patterns.[194,195] A simpler version using prefixed HEp-2 cells was shown to be 92% sensitive for detection of EAEC.[196]

Molecular testing for known virulence genes is also widely used to detect EPEC, EAEC, and DAEC. Multiplex and real-time polymerase chain reaction (PCR) protocols are available in specialized laboratories and have shown variable sensitivity and specificity compared to the HEp-2 assay. However, they have the advantage of identifying specific pathogenicity genes, which is advancing scientific understanding of these organisms. Some isolates that show typical HEp-2 adherence patterns may in fact not be pathogenic if they lack an appropriate complement of other virulence traits (e.g., atypical EPEC); this could explain some of the difficulties historically in establishing pathogenicity of EAEC and DAEC in clinical studies. Conversely, there may be *E. coli* that fail to demonstrate HEp-2 adherence yet possess enough other pathogenic traits to act as significant pathogens. Ongoing work may make these molecular tests more widely available for clinical practice.[197]

In addition to molecular and adherence testing, EAEC may also be sensitively identified by a simple quantitative or qualitative assay for biofilm formation when grown in rich media in the absence of cells, although the specificity appears lower than with HEp-2 cells.[198] Biofilms are a reasonable marker for the presence of a necessary complement of other pathogenicity factors, particularly AggR, known to be associated with diarrhea;[199,200] in one study, biofilm was 89% sensitive for the presence of *astA* and *aggR* genes by PCR.[201]

ETEC is distinguished by establishing the presence of characteristic enterotoxins or the genes that encode them. LT or ST can be identified using tissue culture techniques (such as the Chinese hamster ovary cell elongation assay for LT)[202] or cGMP elevations in T84 cells for ST.[109] Less cumbersome techniques include several commercially available immunoassays.[203,204] Genetic techniques using DNA probes or PCR have also been used.[205–209]

Classically, EIEC was identified using the animal model of invasion, such as the Sérény test in which invasion is demonstrated in the conjunctiva of guinea pigs.[210] More recently, molecular techniques using DNA probes and PCR have shown promise as highly sensitive and specific alternatives to the more classic diagnostic methods.[211,212]

TREATMENT AND PROGNOSIS

Rehydration

As with all diarrheal diseases, replacement of lost fluid and electrolytes is the cornerstone of therapy. This is best accomplished with the reduced osmolarity formulation (see ***Table 129.4***). The formulation is based on the physiologic observation that intestinal absorption of sodium is coupled to that of glucose, and that addition of glucose to sodium-containing solutions drives sodium absorption even in the face of ongoing intestinal secretion. Other carbohydrates (rice or maize starch, for example) are as effective as glucose in volume repletion and have the advantage of reducing the amount of diarrhea as well, as shown in several clinical trials.[213–215] Simple and inexpensive, oral rehydration therapy has been credited with saving up to 1 million lives per year.[216] Oral rehydration is preferred over intravenous therapy for several reasons: it is more physiologic (with an intact thirst mechanism, overhydration is avoided), less expensive, less painful, safer (no risk of intravenous catheter infections), and much easier to administer in developing countries.

Successful use of oral rehydration therapy begins with a careful assessment of the patient's hydration status. Guidelines for assessing dehydration in children are listed in ***Table 129.3***. In addition, assessment of capillary refill time,[217] urine output, and urine specific gravity may be useful measures of dehydration and response to rehydration therapy.[218] Oral rehydration is recommended for those with mild to moderate dehydration. When severe dehydration (10% or more of body weight) is present, intravenous therapy with normal saline or Ringer's lactate is recommended, and serum electrolytes should be measured and corrected if oral therapy cannot be given first. As soon as dehydration has been corrected, age-appropriate refeeding can further reduce stool output, decrease the duration of diarrhea, and improve nutritional values.[219,220]

Antimicrobial Therapy

In placebo-controlled trials published in the early 1980s, tetracycline, trimethoprim-sulfamethoxazole, and trimethoprim alone were all shown to decrease the duration of diarrhea in either naturally acquired ETEC infection or in volunteers experimentally infected with the organism.[221,222] Since then, a number of studies of *E. coli* isolates in developing countries have reported increased resistance to multiple antimicrobials, including ampicillin and trimethoprim-sulfamethoxazole.[223–228] Fortunately, the majority of *E. coli* isolates remain sensitive to fluoroquinolones,[225–227,229] and multiple studies have demonstrated the efficacy of these agents in the treatment of travelers' diarrhea, including the subgroups infected with ETEC and EAEC.[45,229–233] Abbreviated courses of quinolone therapy for 3 days[229,233] or even single dose[230] have documented efficacy in patients with travelers' diarrhea. Ciprofloxacin was also effective in curing EAEC diarrhea in a small group of HIV-infected patients.[51] Unfortunately, ciprofloxacin resistance is emerging in multidrug-resistant *E. coli* isolates from travelers treated with ciprofloxacin.[233] Effective therapy for EAEC-associated travelers' diarrhea using the nonabsorbable antibiotic rifaximin has also been demonstrated in a small clinical trial.[234] Single-dose azithromycin, which has the advantage of activity against fluoroquinolone-resistant *Campylobacter* as well as *E. coli*, is as effective as ciprofloxacin in treating travelers' diarrhea and stands as another alternative.[235] Specific therapy for DAEC has not been studied.

Several reports suggest the efficacy of antibiotics in managing EPEC infections,[119,236,237] although the only controlled trial specifically addressing EPEC infections was with 49 Ethiopian children in whom serotype O111:B4 predominated.[237] In this series, complete resolution of diarrhea was seen within 3 days in 73% of cases receiving trimethoprim-sulfamethoxazole (and in 76% in those receiving mecillinam) versus 7% in controls, and bacteriologic cure was confirmed in 53% of those receiving antibiotics versus none in the control group. In addition to rehydration therapy and antibiotics, parenteral nutrition supplementation may be helpful in the severely malnourished patient with EPEC infection.[119] In multiple regions worldwide, antimicrobial resistance among EPEC isolates is emerging;[238–240] if feasible, antimicrobial selection should be guided by susceptibility testing.

The role of antimicrobial treatment in EHEC disease remains uncertain. Although most *E. coli* O157:H7 is susceptible *in vitro* to antibiotics such as ampicillin, carbenicillin, gentamicin, cephalothin, chloramphenicol, quinolones, trimethoprim, and trimethoprim-sulfamethoxazole,[64,241–243] exposure of the organism to sublethal concentrations of trimethoprim-sulfamethoxazole, ciprofloxacin, and tetracycline has been reported to increase SLT release.[244] Of note, ciprofloxacin also stimulates increased release of endotoxin from *E. coli*,[245,246] which can result in significant cytokine release from whole blood and human peripheral blood monocytes.[247,248] There is limited clinical evidence that antibiotics may be harmful in EHEC infection, including a prospective but nonrandomized study,[249] suggesting an association between antibiotic use and progression to HUS. Among retrospective studies from several outbreaks, antibiotics did not appear to influence the duration of symptoms.[64,250] In one retrospective case series of 20 patients with *E. coli* O157:H7 infection, treatment with trimethoprim-sufamethoxazole was significantly associated with the development of HUS.[96] However, other studies report an association of appropriate antimicrobial therapy for more than 24 hours with lack of progression to HUS.[98] In the only prospective randomized therapeutic trial in EHEC diarrhea, the duration of symptoms was not significantly reduced by trimethoprim-sulfamethoxazole, although treatment was begun relatively late in the illness.[251] In addition, the above-mentioned prospective study found a trend toward the development of HUS in the group not receiving antibiotics, although this did not reach statistical significance. A meta-analysis of nine studies (six retrospective and three prospective) did not show a higher risk of HUS following antibiotic administration.[252] The choice of antibiotic is likely to be important: one recent study using gnotobiotic piglets found that ciprofloxacin led to fatal HUS, while azithromycin prevented it.[253] Until further clinical trials are done, no definitive recommendations for antibiotic treatment of EHEC can be given.

Bacillary dysentery associated with EIEC typically responds to appropriate antimicrobials targeting shigellosis. As with *Shigella* species, antibiotic susceptibility patterns vary geographically, and antimicrobials such as ampicillin and trimethoprim-sulfamethoxazole may not be effective against EIEC. Resistance to third-generation cephalosporins and quinolones, including nalidixic acid, is less common.[254,255]

Other Therapies

Bismuth Subsalicylate

In addition to oral rehydration therapy and specific antimicrobial therapy, a number of other agents may help to treat enteric *E. coli* infections. Bismuth subsalicylate has been used ever since the early 1900s as an antidiarrheal agent, and several studies have validated its efficacy in treating diarrhea caused chiefly by enterovirulent *E. coli*.[256] Its efficacy in preventing and treating ETEC infections has been shown in volunteers fed ETEC, as well as in field trials.[257–259] In addition, in a randomized placebo-controlled trial in which the most commonly isolated potential pathogen was *E. coli* with EPEC serotypes, bismuth subsalicylate effected a significant reduction in duration of diarrhea, duration of hospitalization, and stool output in infants and young children with acute watery diarrhea.[259] Nonetheless, antidiarrheal drugs including bismuth subsalicylate are generally not recommended in treating infants with acute diarrhea caused by any pathogen.[218]

Antimotility Agents

Loperamide shortens the time to the last unformed stool in travelers' diarrhea, and may offer some modest benefit in patients infected with ETEC during the first 24 hours of combination therapy with ciprofloxacin;

however, antimotility agents may mask fluid losses and should not be used in children.[260–262] The safety of antimotility agents in EIEC infections is uncertain. Murphy et al.[263] reported no adverse effects in 42 adult patients with dysentery who received loperamide in combination with ciprofloxacin, and, compared with 46 receiving ciprofloxacin alone, this regimen resulted in fewer unformed stools and a shorter duration of diarrhea. Nonetheless, the modest symptomatic improvement seen with antimotility agents in this disease must be weighed against reports of adverse outcomes associated with their use in inflammatory diarrheal illnesses.[264,265] Given reports associating antimotility agents with the development of HUS,[98,266,267] and increased risk of central nervous system manifestations in HUS[268] in EHEC infections, they should clearly be avoided in patients suspected of having hemorrhagic colitis.

Probiotics

There has been significant enthusiasm for the use of live bacterial preparations as "natural" remedies for gastrointestinal illness. While live-culture yogurt has antibacterial activity *in vitro*,[269] it had no significant clinical effect in rabbit EPEC infection in one study.[270] Yogurt was shown to be no more effective than milk in treating acute diarrhea in malnourished children.[271] Newer probiotic preparations containing defined organisms have shown more promise. One such organism, *Lactobacillus* GG, shortens the duration of acute diarrhea in children with rotavirus infection but not bacterial diarrhea.[272–274] In one trial prophylactic administration of *Lactobacillus* GG to undernourished children in Peru did decrease the incidence of diarrheal episodes (5.21 episodes/child/year versus 6.02 for placebo; $P<0.05$).[275] *Lactobacillus* GG was also shown to prevent travelers' diarrhea in two randomized, blinded, placebo-controlled studies, although the effect was limited to travelers to particular areas (Turkey, North Africa).[276,277] Another probiotic, the yeast *Saccharomyces boulardii*, was shown to reduce the duration of diarrhea when given along with oral rehydration solution to children in Myanmar.[278] Despite these promising early studies, the cost-effectiveness of probiotics is not known, and hence there is not yet sufficient evidence to support the routine use of any probiotic preparation in the prevention or treatment of *E. coli* enteric infection.

PREVENTION AND CONTROL

As with the vast majority of pathogens causing diarrheal illness, proper sanitation and hygiene aimed at diminishing the risk of fecal–oral transmission are important for the prevention of enteric *E. coli* infections. Culturally sensitive education on the use of soap and handwashing after defecation and before eating or preparing foods and improvements in the disposal of human waste are the simplest and, perhaps overall, the most effective means of preventing disease caused by most enteric *E. coli*.[279–283] Numerous studies have demonstrated the protective benefits of breastfeeding in preventing diarrheal diseases, including those associated with ETEC and EPEC.[27,284,285] Not only does breastfeeding diminish the risk of fecal–oral exposure from exposure to weaning foods, but breast milk likely affords immunologic protection[286] and may contribute oligosaccharides and other substances which interfere with attachment of *E. coli* to intestinal epithelium.[134,135] Programs that address deficiencies in micronutrients such as vitamin A and zinc have also been shown to improve the severity of diarrhea in developing regions.[287–289] Moreover, a recent study in Bangladesh found that being significantly underweight was a significant risk factor for infection with ETEC as well as *Cryptosporidium* and *Entamoeba histolytica,* highlighting the vicious cycle of diarrheal infection and malnutrition.[290]

Those traveling to the tropics should be advised to eat only those foods that are thoroughly cooked and served piping hot, or fresh fruits that can be peeled. Isolation of diarrheagenic *E. coli* from food handlers,[291] ice,[250] and domestic cats,[292] highlights the ease of acquisition and the need for adherence to these principles.

A live, attenuated whole-cell cholera/choleratoxin B subunit vaccine (Dukoral) is available for travelers and provides short-lived, partial protection against cholera and LT-producing ETEC.[293] A recent study found that, even with the observed 42.6% effectiveness at preventing travelers' diarrhea, the vaccine was still cost-effective.[294] A new transcutaneous patch vaccine using LT significantly reduced the incidence of moderate to severe diarrhea in travelers in a recent phase II trial[295] and may become an alternative in the future.

In general, antibiotic chemoprophylaxis for travelers' diarrhea, although often effective, is not recommended. People who are at high risk of complications from travelers' diarrhea, such as those with diabetes, inflammatory bowel disease, advanced AIDS, or those on immunosuppressive drugs, should be warned that agents such as *Cryptosporidium* are not prevented by antibiotics and may cause far worse disease than ETEC or EAEC. Moreover, the increasing antibiotic resistance of certain pathogens (e.g., *Campylobacter* in Thailand) makes chemoprophylaxis less attractive.

Given the striking association of EHEC infection with bovine sources in developed countries, preventive efforts previously focused primarily on inspection of food products and new microbiologic quality standards.[296] While recent studies suggest that the grain-based diet of industrialized farms encourages colonization with acid-tolerant EHEC strains that may be better adapted to infecting humans, the economic and social implications of changing agricultural practice on this basis have not been measured.[297] Nevertheless, stricter governmental and industrial standards in the handling of food animals may help prevent widespread point source outbreaks. An additional promising tool is a vaccine based on EPEC/EHEC secreted effectors, which reduces EHEC colonization in cattle.[298–300] Widespread use of such vaccines, along with changes in agriculture practice, offers promise in reducing human EHEC infections.

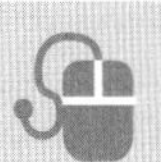

Access the complete reference list online at
http://www.expertconsult.com

Access the complete reference list online at http://www.expertconsult.com

CHAPTER 16

Typhoid and Paratyphoid (Enteric) Fever

Myron M. Levine • Milagritos D. Tapia • Anita K.M. Zaidi

INTRODUCTION

The enteric fevers, including typhoid fever caused by *Salmonella enterica* serovar Typhi (*Salmonella* Typhi) and paratyphoid fever due to *Salmonella* Paratyphi A or *Salmonella* Paratyphi B (or rarely, *Salmonella* Paratyphi C), represent acute generalized infections of the reticuloendothelial system, intestinal lymphoid tissue, and gallbladder. These communicable diseases are restricted to human hosts and human chronic carriers serve as the reservoir of infection. Clinical manifestations of acute infection vary depending on the host, pathogen strain, inoculum size, and vehicle of transmission. Severe clinical illness in the older child or adult is characterized by persisting high fever, abdominal discomfort, malaise, and headache. Before the advent of antibiotics, the disease evolved over several weeks, culminating in a case fatality rate of ~10–20%.[1,2] The protracted, debilitating nature of this febrile illness in untreated (or improperly treated) patients is accompanied by mental cloudiness or stupor. Historically in endemic areas, typhoid comprised ~80% of enteric fever.[3] However, *Salmonella* Paratyphi A has been gaining prominence as a cause of enteric fever in Asia[4,5] and among travelers.[6]

THE AGENT

Salmonella Typhi, *Salmonella* Paratyphi A, and *Salmonella* Paratyphi B are serovars within the genus *Salmonella* of the family Enterobacteriaceae. These Gram-negative, motile bacilli do not ferment lactose.

Taxonomy

Only two species are currently recognized within the genus *Salmonella*, *Salmonella enterica* and *S. bongori*, and only the former is important with respect to human disease. There are six subspecies of *S. enterica*, of which subspecies I, *S. enterica* subspecies *enterica*, contains all the important pathogens that cause human disease. *S. enterica* subspecies *enterica* is further subdivided into >2500 serovars (i.e., distinct serotypes) based on specific somatic O antigens, capsular polysaccharide Vi antigen, and flagellar H antigens expressed by the organism. The antigenic serotyping scheme (Kauffman–White scheme) defines a serovar by its O polysaccharide antigens (and also whether capsular polysaccharide Vi is expressed) and its H flagellar antigens. The serogroup of a *Salmonella* is defined by its O antigens, while serovar is defined by the full antigenic structure that includes the flagellar antigens and whether Vi is expressed. O antigens are part of the lipopolysaccharide (LPS) of the bacterial outer membrane. The lipid A (endotoxin) portion of LPS is a glucosamine-based phospholipid that makes up the outer monolayer of the bacterial outer membrane. Attached to lipid A is a core polysaccharide that is essentially identical in all the important *Salmonella* serovars that cause human disease, particularly invasive disease. The most external surface component attached to the core polysaccharide is an O polysaccharide that consists of terminal O repeat units linked one to another. This is exposed to the environment in *Salmonella* Paratyphi A and B, whereas in *Salmonella* Typhi the capsular Vi (for "virulence") polysaccharide (homopolymer of *N*-acetylgalacturonic acid)[7] covers the O polysaccharide.

The terminal O polysaccharide of *Salmonella* varies in structure depending on the sugars comprising the core unit and their linkages one to another. *Salmonella* Paratyphi A falls into serogroup A, *Salmonella* Paratyphi B into serogroup B, and *Salmonella* Typhi into serogroup D. The O repeat units of *Salmonella* serogroups A, B and D share a common trisaccharide backbone that consists of repeats of mannose, rhamnose, and galactose.[8] Attached to the backbone is another dideoxyhexose sugar that is α-1,3-linked to the mannose residue.[8] If the α-1,3-linked dideoxyhexose sugar is abequose, the resultant structure constitutes immunodominant antigen "4" that defines O serogroup B; if the sugar is paratose, the structure creates immunodominant antigen "2" that defines serogroup A; if the sugar is tyvelose, immunodominant antigen "9" is created that defines O serogroup D.

Some *Salmonella* express two different antigenic forms of flagella, called phase 1 and phase 2. *Salmonella* Typhi and Paratyphi A express only phase 1 flagellar antigens, H:a and H:d, respectively, while *Salmonella* Paratyphi B expresses both phase 1 flagella H:b and phase 2 flagella H:1,2. Bacteriologic confirmation of *Salmonella* Typhi, *Salmonella* Paratyphi A, and *Salmonella* Paratyphi B can be made by agglutination with typing sera or by multiplex polymerase chain reaction (PCR).[9]

Whereas other pathogenic Enterobacteriaceae such as *Shigella* and non-typhoidal *Salmonella* stably carry R factor plasmids encoding antibiotic resistance, until about 1990 this was the exception with typhoid bacilli. The first antibiotic used to treat typhoid fever, chloramphenicol, reported in 1948,[10] was immensely useful for a quarter century thereafter (and remains useful where strains of *Salmonella* Typhi remain susceptible). However, rather suddenly, large-scale epidemics of chloramphenicol-resistant typhoid fever ensued, first in Mexico (1972)[11,12] and then in Southeast Asia (1974).[13] After ~2 years in Mexico, the resistant strain disappeared and was replaced by chloramphenicol-sensitive strains. In 1979 and 1980, chloramphenicol-resistant typhoid appeared in Lima, Peru[14] but these resistant strains also disappeared after a few years and were replaced by chloramphenicol-sensitive *Salmonella* Typhi. In these instances the antibiotic-resistance genes were encoded on plasmids of incompatibility group HI1.[11,14] Beginning in the late 1980s, *Salmonella* Typhi strains resistant to chloramphenicol, amoxicillin, and trimethoprim-sulfamethoxazole disseminated widely throughout Asia.[15–17] Alternative effective antibiotics included oral ciprofloxacin and parenteral ceftriaxone; however, the widespread use of ciprofloxacin and other fluoroquinolones, often in inadequate dosages and duration, encouraged the emergence of fluoroquinolone-resistant strains.[18]

Genomics

The full sequences of the genome of two isolates of *Salmonella* Typhi have been reported including modern multiresistant strain CT18 from Vietnam and venerable strain Ty2, isolated in Russia in about 1915. The genome of the former has 4 809 037 base pairs (bp) and 4599 open reading frames (ORFs),[19] while Ty2 has 4 791 961 bp and 4399 ORFs.[20] There is 98% genomic homology between CT18 and Ty2. A striking revelation was that these genomes have undergone degradation (compared to *Salmonella* Typhimurium); each genome shows >200 pseudogenes, 195 of which are identical. There are also segments of genome present in Typhimurium that are not evident in Typhi. Since more than a dozen of the pseudogenes encode fimbrial attachment factors, loss of these likely explains the narrow human host specificity of Typhi compared to Typhimurium.

Salmonella Typhi also exhibits 10 *Salmonella* pathogenicity islands including ones involved in cell invasion (SPI1), intracellular survival (SPI2) and Vi biosynthesis (SPI7). There is >80% sequence homology with *Salmonella* Typhimurium.

Salmonella Paratyphi A has a 4 585 229 bp genome with 4263 ORFs and considerable homology with *Salmonella* Typhi.[21] Paratyphi A also manifests genomic degradation, with 173 pseudogenes (28 identical to Typhi).[21] *Salmonella* Paratyphi A followed a distinct evolutionary path to evolve into a pathogen exhibiting a similar pathogenesis and host specificity as Typhi.

EPIDEMIOLOGY

Incidence and Geographic Distribution

Typhoid and paratyphoid fevers are associated with poor sanitation and untreated water supplies. Thus, they are endemic in many areas of the developing world, while their transmission is rare in industrialized countries. Typhoid persists as a public health problem in South and Southeast Asia, the Middle East, northeast Africa, sub-Sahara Africa, Central America, parts of the Caribbean and a few regions in South America. In many developing countries with endemic disease, notification data underestimate the burden, due to incomplete reporting and lack of means for bacteriologic confirmation. In contrast, the true magnitude of the typhoid fever problem in some developing countries may be inflated because the clinical picture is easily confused with other febrile infections and laboratory infrastructure for bacteriologic confirmation is usually absent.[3,22] It has been estimated that each year ~21.6 million cases of typhoid fever and 216 510 deaths occur, along with 5.4 million cases of paratyphoid fever.[3]

Population-based surveillance efforts have attempted to quantify the incidence of enteric fever in selected populations by systematically collecting blood cultures from febrile patients.[4,23–26] These efforts have yielded insights on the incidence of typhoid and paratyphoid fever in different populations, age groups, and geographic areas where the incidence of enteric fever was already believed to be moderate or high. Some efforts were based on passive surveillance that required the patients to seek care at established health care facilities, where blood cultures were obtained.[4,23,24] In other efforts, active surveillance was undertaken by visiting households at least weekly to detect persons with fever,[25,26] who then had blood cultures collected. Several household surveillance projects were undertaken in Asian urban slums in Delhi[25] and Dhaka.[26]

Coincident with the pandemic of multiple antibiotic-resistant typhoid fever in South Asia that began in 1989, the risk of developing typhoid fever among US travelers increased to $105/10^5$ for travelers from Asia,[27–29] and to $76/10^5$ for travelers from Africa, similar to annual incidence rates of typhoid in areas of moderate endemicity, yet for travelers exposure usually lasts less than 1 month.[28]

From 1999 to 2006, 1439 of 1830 (79%) US typhoid cases were associated with foreign travel.[29] Travel to three Asian countries (India, Pakistan, and Bangladesh) accounted for 67% of the travel-associated cases; most of these (65%) were visiting family or friends, whereas only 9% were tourists and 3% were on business-related travel.[29]

Seasonality

Endemic typhoid often exhibits seasonality but the peak season varies. In temperate and subtropical areas of developing and transitional countries where typhoid remains endemic, most cases occur during summer. Cases among US travelers increase in the US summer, coinciding with peak travel. In Chile, Ecuador, and Peru, when typhoid was highly endemic, there was a clear peak in summer,[30] while in northern Nigeria[31,32] typhoid peaks during the dry season.

Reservoirs of Infection

Chronic gallbladder carriers constitute the long-term reservoir of *Salmonella* Typhi and *Salmonella* Paratyphi A and B.[33,34] In endemic areas, particularly during "typhoid season," persons with subclinical and clinical infection who are short-term excreters also constitute a reservoir from which the infection can be transmitted. In areas where urinary tract *Schistosoma haematobium* or *S. mansoni* infections are co-endemic with typhoid, chronic urinary bladder carriers of *Salmonella* Typhi may exist.[35]

Modes of Transmission

Typhoid and paratyphoid infection is almost always acquired by ingestion of food or water vehicles contaminated by human excreta that contain *Salmonella* Typhi or *Salmonella* Paratyphi A or B. Typhoid fever is uncommon in modern industrialized countries where populations have access to treated water supplies and sanitation that removes human waste. Among populations in less developed countries that lack such amenities, typhoid fever is often endemic and, from the public health perspective, typically constitutes the most important enteric disease problem of school-age children.[36]

Typhoid fever was endemic in Europe and North and South America in the late nineteenth and early twentieth centuries. A single intervention, the treatment of water supplies by chlorination or sand filtration, broke the cycle of endemicity and diminished the incidence of typhoid, even though the prevalence of chronic carriers in the populations remained high for decades thereafter.[37,38]

Enteric fever may be transmitted by the fecal-oral route via a "short cycle" or a "long cycle." The short cycle is typified by an individual carrier who contaminates food vehicles that are consumed in proximity by family members, or by participants at a communal gathering (e.g., a wedding), or by a carrier handling food in a restaurant.[39] Examples of short-cycle sporadic cases and outbreaks include families served by the infamous cook, "Typhoid Mary,"[40] and restaurant outbreaks in Texas,[41] Maryland,[39] and New York.[42] Most outbreaks in the United States are related to short-cycle transmission.[39,42,43] Examples of long-cycle transmission include contamination of water supplies by sewage,[44] contamination of widely distributed piped municipal water supplies,[44,45] and dissemination of typhoid bacilli via processed contaminated foods transported over long distances.[46]

When outbreaks occasionally occur in industrialized countries, a careful epidemiologic investigation usually incriminates the food or water vehicle responsible and identifies a chronic carrier culpable for the contamination,[39,47,48] or sometimes in sporadic, non-travel-associated cases a chronic carrier, such as an elderly family member.[29,49]

Because clinical microbiologists have increased exposure to *Salmonella* Typhi, they also constitute a high-risk group.[50,51] Transmission of *Salmonella* Typhi within clinical microbiology laboratories may occur by inadvertent aerosol generation. Rarely, direct person-to-person transmission of typhoid through anolingual sexual practices has been reported.[52,53]

Molecular Epidemiology

Useful molecular epidemiologic tools for comparing isolates include pulsed field gel electrophoresis[54–57] and comparison of single nucleotide polymorphisms (SNPs).[58,59]

THE DISEASE

Clinical Spectrum

Typhoid fever and paratyphoid fever exhibit a spectrum of clinical severity. At the population level, paratyphoid generates fewer complications. However, in the individual patient it is not possible on clinical grounds to differentiate whether the enteric fever is caused by *Salmonella* Typhi or *Salmonella* Paratyphi.[60,61] Classic full-blown cases begin with malaise, anorexia, myalgia, fever that increases in stepwise fashion to reach 39–40°C, abdominal discomfort, and headaches.[2,62,63] Without appropriate antimicrobial therapy, fever remains at this level for at least 10–14 days (and sometimes for weeks, if the patient survives). In response to appropriate antibiotics, the fever diminishes, also in stepwise fashion, over several days. During the period of sustained fever, approximately 20% of white patients manifest an exanthem ("rose spots") consisting of subtle, salmon-colored macules, 2–4 mm in size, which blanch with pressure. Rose spots are usually seen on the chest, abdomen, and back; *Salmonella* Typhi can be cultured from rose spots.[64] Constipation is not uncommon in older children and adults, whereas diarrhea may occur in young children with typhoid fever. A bronchitic cough is common in the early stage of illness.

The peripheral leukocyte count in typhoid fever is often <4500/mm^3, which helps in the differential diagnosis. Thrombocytopenia is also common, with platelets <80 000/mm^3. Liver dysfunction, as detected by mildly elevated serum transaminase values, is observed in most patients.

A particularly severe form of typhoid fever is occasionally encountered in which cerebral dysfunction, including obtundation, delirium or coma, and shock are present, requiring corticosteroid therapy with appropriate antimicrobial therapy to avoid a case-fatality rate that can exceed 20%.[65]

Although infants may manifest severe clinical forms of typhoid fever, bacteremic *Salmonella* Typhi infection in children younger than 2 years of age is often remarkably mild and is not recognized clinically as enteric fever but rather as a nondescript febrile syndrome.[66,67]

Relapse

Relapses were observed in about 8% of patients with typhoid fever in the preantibiotic era. The rate in patients treated with the first (chloramphenicol) and second (ampicillin, amoxicillin, and trimethoprim-sulfamethoxazole) generation of antibiotics used for therapy of typhoid ranged from 10% to 35%. The organisms that initiate relapse appear to come from within the reticuloendothelial system. Typhoid bacilli can be recovered from liver biopsies during relapse and from bone marrow many months after the patient has fully recovered from symptoms. Relapses typically occur about 3 weeks after the last febrile day or 2 weeks after cessation of antibiotics and are clinically milder and shorter than the initial illness and respond promptly to appropriate antibiotics. After treatment of acute typhoid fever with oral fluoroquinolones or azithromycin or after parenteral ceftriaxone, relapse is distinctly uncommon.

Intestinal Perforation and Hemorrhage

Two of the most feared complications of typhoid fever, intestinal perforation and hemorrhage, occur in ~0.5–1.0% of cases, particularly those who have been ill for several weeks without proper antibiotic therapy. These complications are consequent to the lesions in gut-associated lymphoid tissue that are so prominent in the gross pathology of *Salmonella* Typhi infection.

Other Complications

Typhoid can affect any human organ system and result in complications.[2] Uncommon complications include typhoid hepatitis, empyema, osteomyelitis, and psychosis.[1,2] More rarely, septic arthritis, meningitis, myocarditis, and empyema of the gallbladder can occur.

Chronic Carriers

Approximately 1–5% of patients with enteric fever, depending on age and sex, become chronic gallbladder carriers of the organism (defined as excretion of the pathogen for more than 12 months after acute infection).[68,69] More rarely, chronic renal carriers occur.

PATHOGENESIS AND IMMUNITY

Pathogenesis

Salmonella Typhi and *Salmonella* Paratyphi A and B are invasive bacteria that efficiently traverse from the lumen across the human intestinal mucosa, eventually to reach the reticuloendothelial system, where, after an 8–14 day incubation, they launch a systemic illness. *Salmonella* Typhi and *Salmonella* Paratyphi A and B are highly host-adapted pathogens, with humans comprising the only natural host and reservoir of infection. Insights into the pathogenesis of typhoid fever comes from four sources: clinicopathological observations in humans,[1,70] volunteer studies,[1,71] studies of a chimpanzee model,[72] and analogies drawn from *Salmonella* Typhimurium and *Salmonella* Enteritidis "mouse typhoid" models.[73]

Susceptible human hosts ingest the pathogen in contaminated food or water. The inoculum size and the vehicle in which it is ingested greatly influence the attack rate for typhoid fever and the incubation period, a relationship documented in volunteer studies in the 1960s.[71] Doses of 10^9 and 10^8 pathogenic *Salmonella* Typhi ingested by volunteers in 45 mL of skim milk induced clinical illness in 98% and 89% of individuals, respectively; doses of 10^5 caused typhoid fever in 28% of volunteers, whereas none of 14 subjects who ingested 10^3 organisms developed clinical illness.[71]

While gastric acid in the fasting normochlorhydric stomach inactivates many typhoid bacilli that are ingested, some foods effectively buffer the acid barrier. After passing through the pylorus and reaching the small intestine, the bacilli rapidly penetrate the mucosa to reach the lamina propria. *Salmonella* Typhi targets M (microfold) cells overlying Peyer's patches and other gut-associated lymphoid tissue,[74] and are then ingested by dendritic cells and macrophages underlying the M cells. However, the bacilli may also invade enterocytes and enter endocytic vacuoles that transit the cells to be released into the lamina propria, without destroying the enterocyte;[75] *Salmonella* may also pass paracellularly between enterocytes.[76] SPI1 encodes the genes for mucosal invasion.

Upon reaching the lamina propria in the nonimmune host, typhoid bacilli elicit an influx of macrophages and dendritic cells that ingest the organisms but are generally unable to kill them. Some bacilli apparently remain within macrophages of the small-intestinal lymphoid tissue. Other typhoid bacilli are drained into mesenteric lymph nodes where further multiplication and ingestion by macrophages take place. SPI2 includes the genes that allow survival in the intracellular environment of mononuclear professional phagocytes. Eventually, there is a release of tumor necrosis factor-α, interleukin (IL)-2, IL-6, and other cytokines by the macrophages (and perhaps by enterocytes).

Postmortem studies have documented the inflammatory responses that occur in the distal ileum in the Peyer's patches and other organized lymphoid aggregations. It is from these lesions in the distal ileum and ascending colon that hemorrhage can occur later in the disease course. Gross bleeding comes from eroded vessels in or near the Peyer's patches. Perforations of the bowel wall occur in the same sections of the gut as the hemorrhages (***Fig. 16.1***).

Shortly after invasion of the intestinal mucosa, a primary bacteremia takes place in which *Salmonella* Typhi is filtered from the circulation by fixed phagocytes of the reticuloendothelial system. The main route by which typhoid bacilli reach the bloodstream in this early stage is by lymph drainage from mesenteric nodes entering the thoracic duct and thence the general circulation. Conceivably, ingestion of a massive inoculum followed by widespread invasion of the intestinal mucosa could result in direct bloodstream invasion. Having gained its intracellular haven

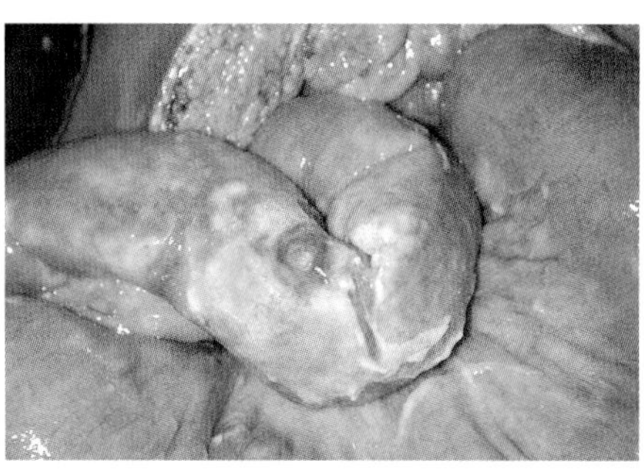

Figure 16.1 Ileal ulcer and perforation due to *Salmonella* Typhi invasive disease in an adult male patient. (Courtesy of Hasnain Zafar, MBBS, FCPS, Aga Khan University, Karachi, Pakistan.)

throughout the organs of the reticuloendothelial system, the pathogen resides therein during the incubation period (usually 8–14 days) until the onset of clinical enteric fever. Clinical illness is accompanied by a fairly sustained, albeit low level (1–10 organisms/mL), "secondary" bacteremia. During bacteremia, the Vi antigen protects the bacteria from the lytic effects of O antibody (if present) and complement.[77] *Salmonella* Typhi strains lacking Vi are rare[78] and somewhat less virulent than Vi-expressing strains.[71]

The bacteremia of typhoid fever persists for several weeks if antibiotic therapy is not given. The symptoms and signs of typhoid fever are not due to circulating endotoxin. Most patients have no serum endotoxin detected by the limulus assay,[79] except patients who present with severe clinical disease and septic shock syndrome, in whom circulating endotoxin can be demonstrated.[65]

During the primary bacteremia typhoid bacilli also reach the gallbladder, an organ for which *Salmonella* Typhi has a remarkable predilection.[72,80] *Salmonella* Typhi can be readily cultured from bile or from bile-stained duodenal fluid in patients with acute typhoid fever.[81–83] In approximately 2–5% of patients, the gallbladder infection becomes chronic.[68] The propensity to become a chronic carrier is greater in females and increases with age at the time of acute *Salmonella* Typhi infection, thereby resembling the epidemiology of gallbladder disease.[68,84] The infection becomes chronic in individuals who have preexistent gallbladder pathology at the time of acute *Salmonella* Typhi infection. Carriers shed as many as 10^9 organisms/g feces,[85] but these organisms travel the length of their gastrointestinal tract without penetrating or causing disease.

Host Factors

Since *Salmonella* Typhi and *Salmonella* Paratyphi are primarily intracellular pathogens, genetic factors are believed to influence not only host susceptibility and the severity of clinical disease but also the generation of cell-mediated immune responses that modulate recovery from clinical infection. In Vietnam and Indonesia, human HLA types have been identified that purportedly affect susceptibility to clinical illness and propensity towards severe disease.[86–88]

Immune Response to Wild-Type Infection

Following acute *Salmonella* Typhi infection, serum antibodies to somatic O and flagellar H antibodies appear, whereas most patients with acute typhoid fever apparently do not manifest rises in serum anti-Vi antibody.[89,90] In contrast, serum Vi antibody is highly elevated in chronic gallbladder carriers.[89,90] Intestinal secretory IgA antibody responses to *Salmonella* Typhi can also be detected.

Measurement of cell-mediated immunity (CMI) in patients with wild-type infection has been limited in the modern era. However, measurement of CMI responses in subjects vaccinated with attenuated strains administered as oral vaccines has generated extensive evidence demonstrating the appearance of classic MHC I-restricted cytotoxic T cells and T cells that secrete cytokines upon exposure to *Salmonella* Typhi antigens.[91]

DIAGNOSIS

Clinical Bacteriology to Isolate the Organism

Confirmation of the diagnosis of enteric fever requires recovery of *Salmonella* Typhi or *Salmonella* Paratyphi from a suitable clinical specimen. Multiple blood cultures should be obtained from patients in whom the diagnosis is suspected clinically. The isolation rate of *Salmonella* Typhi or *Salmonella* Paratyphi from blood cultures depends on many factors, including the volume of blood cultured, the ratio of volume of blood to volume of culture broth (ideally, the ratio should be ≥1 : 8), inclusion of anti-complementary substances in the broth (e.g., sodium polyanethol sulfonate or bile), and whether the patient has already received antibiotics to which the *Salmonella* Typhi is sensitive. If three 5 mL blood cultures are obtained, *Salmonella* Typhi can be recovered from the blood in approximately 65–70% of untreated suspect cases.

The current "gold standard" of bacteriologic confirmation of typhoid fever is the bone marrow culture, which is positive in 85–95% of cases, even when the patient has received antibiotics.[64,81,82,92] The use of duodenal string devices to obtain bile-stained duodenal fluid for culture is also quite useful.[81] The combination of a duodenal string and two blood cultures generally provides a sensitivity of bacteriologic confirmation equal to that achieved with bone marrow cultures, but without the invasiveness of the latter.[81] The bacteriologic culture of skin snips from rose spots also provides a high yield.[64] Stool cultures are generally positive in only 45–65% of cases (somewhat higher in children).

Salmonella Typhi does not ferment lactose; it produces hydrogen sulfide, but does not produce gas. As a consequence, suspicious colonies are evident on usual lactose-containing media as lactose-negative colonies. The biochemical pattern in triple sugar iron agar is rather characteristic, manifested by an acid butt without gas, an alkaline slant, and obvious H_2S production. Fresh isolates typically agglutinate with Vi but not group D antiserum. However, if the bacteria are boiled to remove the Vi capsule, a reaction with group D antiserum is then readily seen. The Vi antigen is an important epidemiologic aid, since its susceptibility to lysis by bacteriophages allows for the classification of 80 definite and stable varieties of typhoid bacilli. This can help identify the source and spread of a specific strain.[93]

Antigen Detection

Over the years many attempts have been made to develop tests that detect *Salmonella* Typhi antigens in blood, urine, or body fluids, thereby providing a rapid diagnostic test for typhoid fever. With few exceptions, these tests have been disappointing and have failed to warrant the enthusiasm of initial reports. Most assays are based on the detection of the O or Vi antigens of *Salmonella* Typhi in blood or urine using coagglutination, ELISA, or countercurrent immunoelectrophoresis.

Nucleic Acid-Based Detection

PCR methods have attempted to amplify *Salmonella* Typhi genes from blood.[94–96] However, even these sensitive assays must grapple with the fact that the level of bacteremia in typhoid is low (~1–10 organisms/mL of blood) and so they have yielded variable results. More importantly, heretofore, these methods have been amenable only to research laboratories and are not presently amenable for use in laboratories in developing countries. Significant hurdles will have to be overcome to adapt them to become practical tests for clinical care even in industrialized country settings to diagnose enteric fever in travelers.

Serodiagnosis by Detecting Antibodies

Serodiagnosis of typhoid fever was described in 1896 by Widal and Sicard,[97] who reported that the serum from patients with typhoid fever agglutinated typhoid bacilli. Variations of the Widal test are still used today in many developing countries to measure agglutinins in serum from patients with suspected enteric fever. The test is more accurate when performed with antigen in tubes rather than on slides. By careful choice of antigen, both O and H antibodies can be selectively measured. Using *Salmonella* Typhi strain O901 (which lacks flagellar and Vi antigens), *Salmonella* Typhi O antibody can be selectively measured. A strain such as *Salmonella* Virginia, which possesses the identical phase 1 flagellar antigen H:d as *Salmonella* Typhi but shares no O somatic antigens with serovar Typhi, can be used to measure H agglutinins.[98] Most patients with typhoid fever have elevated levels of O and H antibody at the time of onset of clinical illness.[98] Although the prevalence of H antibodies in adults living in endemic areas is generally too elevated for the test to be useful in that age group,[98,99] it can be useful as a diagnostic test in children <10 years of age in endemic areas and in persons of any age from non-endemic areas.[98] One study from Indonesia supported the use of the slide test for O agglutinins of *Salmonella* Typhi, even for adults in that endemic area.[100]

Two tests, TyphiDot and TUBEX, that detect antibodies to purified *Salmonella* Typhi antigens are in use in some endemic areas.[101–104] In some venues results have been promising,[101–104] although neither test is completely satisfactory.

TREATMENT AND PROGNOSIS

Antimicrobials

The report by Woodward et al[10] in 1948 that chloramphenicol could successfully treat typhoid fever ushered in a new era during which this oral antibiotic served to control typhoid mortality globally, as the case fatality dropped from ~15% to <1%. However, the emergence of resistance to chloramphenicol in the 1970s, and then sequentially to other antimicrobials commonly used to treat enteric fever (amoxicillin and trimethoprim-sulfamethoxazole initially, and later ciprofloxacin) has severely limited therapeutic options in endemic settings with high rates of drug-resistant typhoid.[11,15,17,18,54,56,105–110] The subsequent emergence of multiresistant *Salmonella* Paratyphi A strains has further complicated the treatment of enteric fever.[105,106] Appropriate therapy for enteric fever is no longer straightforward and requires consideration of severity of illness and local susceptibility patterns (***Table 16.1***). The management of typhoid and paratyphoid acquired in South and Southeast Asia is particularly challenging because of high disease burden, dearth of clinical microbiology facilities to make a definitive diagnosis and provide antimicrobial susceptibility, and widespread prevalence of multidrug resistance including strains with decreased susceptibility to fluoroquinolones.[105–110] Moreover, resistant typhoid and paratyphoid are now a global problem.[6,29,111] Over one-third of typhoid infections in the United States recently reported to the Centers for Disease Control and Prevention exhibited reduced susceptibility to fluoroquinolones, with most resistant infections associated with travel to South Asian countries.[29]

Drug-susceptible uncomplicated typhoid and paratyphoid can effectively be managed in outpatient settings with chloramphenicol, amoxicillin, ciprofloxacin, or ofloxacin (***Table 16.1***). Although as effective as chloramphenicol, ciprofloxacin has the advantage of more convenient dosing and lower clinical relapse rates.[106,112]

There are no well-established guidelines for the treatment of uncomplicated typhoid in drug-resistant areas. WHO recommends cefixime as an alternative[113] and this has been used extensively and successfully in the management of typhoid in South Asia. However, reports of high failure rates observed in Nepal and Vietnam despite *in vitro* susceptibility are concerning.[114,115]

Oral azithromycin has emerged as another therapeutic option and is increasingly used as first-line therapy in areas of high multidrug resistant

Table 16.1 Antimicrobial Therapy of Typhoid and Paratyphoid Fever

Disease Severity	Antimicrobial Drug Susceptibility	Antimicrobial Agent	Route	Duration	Pediatric Dose	Adult dose
Uncomplicated typhoid fever[a]	Empiric therapy in areas of low MDR[c] and NARST[d] or known susceptible strain	Ciprofloxacin *or* ofloxacin	PO	7–10 days	10 mg/kg bid	500 mg bid
		Chloramphenicol	PO	14 days	15–20 mg/kg qid	500 mg qid
		Amoxicillin	PO	14 days	25–33 mg/kg tid	25–33 mg/kg tid
		Trimethoprim-sulfamethoxazole	PO	14 days	4–5 mg/kg bid[g]	160 mg bid
	Empiric therapy in areas with high MDR[c] and NARST[d] or known resistant strain	Azithromycin	PO	7 days	15–20 mg/kg OD	1 g loading, then 500 mg OD
		Cefixime	PO	14 days	15–20 mg/kg OD	15–20 mg OD
		Gatifloxacin[f]	PO	7 days	10 mg/kg OD	10 mg/kg OD
						Maximum dose 400 mg
Severe or complicated typhoid fever[b]	Strain known to be fully susceptible to FQs[e]	Ciprofloxacin *or* ofloxacin	IV	10–14 days	10 mg/kg bid	500 mg bid
	FQ resistant or decreased susceptibility[e] (NARST)[d] or unknown	Ceftriaxone	IV	10–14 days	75 mg/kg OD	2–4 g OD
		Cefotaxime	IV	10–14 days	50 mg/kg tid	500 mg to 1 g tid

[a]Uncomplicated typhoid fever – patient does not have signs of systemic toxicity and can tolerate oral therapy.

[b]Severe typhoid – patient appears toxic or obtunded or has prolonged fever, and/or evidence of organ system dysfunction.

[c]MDR – multidrug resistance to certain first-line agents – chloramphenicol, trimethoprim-sulfamethoxazole, amoxicillin.

[d]NARST – Nalidixic acid resistant *Salmonella* Typhi. Nalidixic acid resistance correlates with decreased susceptibility to fluoroquinolones and is associated with clinical failure on fluoroquinolone therapy.

[e]FQ – Fluoroquinolones. *Salmonella* Typhi strains with decreased susceptibility to FQs have minimum inhibitory concentrations (MIC) of 0.125 μg/mL or higher. FQ resistant strains have MIC values of 4 μg/mL or higher.

[f]Gatifloxacin is a newer generation fluoroquinolone that is effective in NARST typhoid. Gatifloxacin is no longer available in the United States or Canada as an oral formulation because of concerns with dysglycemia among elderly patients, but it is still available in some Asian countries.

[g]Dosage is based on the trimethoprim component.

PO, by mouth, IV, intravenously; bid, twice a day; tid, three times a day; qid, four times a day; OD, once a day.

and nalidixic acid-resistant (a marker for decreased susceptibility to fluoroquinolones) typhoid.[116] A newer fluoroquinolone, gatifloxacin, has shown good clinical outcomes in nalidixic-resistant strains.[110,114]

Severe or complicated typhoid should be managed, if possible, in hospital with parenteral antibiotics (preferably intravenous ceftriaxone) and careful monitoring to ensure good clinical outcomes (***Table 16.1***). Switching to an oral agent to which the strain is (or is presumed) susceptible can occur once the patient is afebrile.

Corticosteroids for Severe Clinical Illness

Prompt administration of high-dose dexamethasone reduces case fatality in patients with severe typhoid fever without increasing the occurrence of complications, carriers, or relapse among survivors.[65,117] After starting antibiotics, a loading dose of 3 mg/kg of dexamethasone should be administered by slow intravenous infusion over 30 minutes, followed by 1 mg/kg given at the same rate every 6 hours for eight additional doses; the total duration of corticosteroid therapy is 48 hours. Patients with normal mentation and circulatory status do not require corticosteroids, while those with borderline mental or circulatory status should be monitored intensively every 15 minutes. If the patient's condition deteriorates, they should receive dexamethasone (or an equivalent corticosteroid) immediately because a delay in initiating therapy increases mortality.

PREVENTION AND CONTROL

Safe Water and Food

Since enteric fever pathogens are typically acquired via the ingestion of contaminated water or food, enteric precautions should be taken when living or traveling in endemic areas. Only treated (boiled or otherwise treated) water should be consumed and foods that may be fecally contaminated (e.g., uncooked salad vegetables) should be avoided.

Typhoid and Paratyphoid Vaccines

Ty21a Live Oral Vaccine

Ty21a, an attenuated strain of *Salmonella* Typhi that is safe and protective as a live oral vaccine, was developed in the early 1970s by chemical mutagenesis of pathogenic strain Ty2.[118] Characteristic mutations in this strain include an inactivation of the *galE* gene that encodes an enzyme involved in LPS synthesis and the inability to express Vi polysaccharide, along with approximately two dozen additional mutations.

Ty21a proved to be remarkably well tolerated in placebo-controlled clinical trials.[36] Multiple double-blind, placebo-controlled studies that utilized active surveillance methods to assess the reactogenicity of Ty21a in adults and children showed that adverse reactions were not observed significantly more often in the vaccine recipients than in the placebo group for any symptom or sign. In large-scale field trials with Ty21a, involving approximately 465 000 schoolchildren in Chile and 32 000 in Egypt, and approximately 20 000 subjects from 3 years of age to adults in Indonesia, passive surveillance failed to identify vaccine-attributable adverse reactions or other safety issues.[119–124]

Controlled efficacy field trials of Ty21a emphasize that the formulation of the vaccine, the number of doses administered, and the spacing of the doses markedly influence the level of protection that can be achieved.[120–123,125,126] Two formulations, including enteric-coated capsules and a "liquid" formulation in which lyophilized vaccine is reconstituted along with buffer powder into a vaccine cocktail, are licensed; however, in recent years only the enteric coated capsule formulation has been manufactured. Based on a field trial in Chile that demonstrated that three doses of Ty21a in enteric-coated capsules given on an every other day schedule conferred 67% efficacy over 3 years of follow-up and 62% protection over 7 years of follow-up,[120,127] this formulation and schedule are used throughout the world – except for the United States and Canada, which recommend a four-dose regimen. This was based on results of a large-scale, randomized comparative trial carried out in Santiago, Chile where recipients of four doses of Ty21a in enteric-coated capsules (every other day schedule) experienced a significantly lower incidence of typhoid than those allocated to receive two or three doses.[126] Ty21a confers significant cross-protection against *Salmonella* Paratyphi B[123] but not against *Salmonella* Paratyphi A.[123]

In the mid-1980s, a "liquid suspension" formulation of Ty21a that was amenable to large-scale manufacture was prepared with two packets, one with the lyophilized vaccine and the other with buffer,[122] to be mixed in a cup containing 100 mL of water for ingestion. Randomized placebo-controlled field trials carried out in Santiago, Chile[122] and Plaju, Indonesia[123] showed the liquid formulation of Ty21a to be better (significantly so in the Santiago trial) than the enteric coated capsule formulation[122,123] and to protect young children as well as older children.

Vi Polysaccharide Parenteral Vaccine

In the 1970s and early 1980s, methods were developed to purify Vi capsular polysaccharide so that it was 99.8% free of contaminating LPS and was not denatured.[77,128–131] This was an important breakthrough because as little as 5% impurity with LPS can result in systemic adverse reactions in a few percent of recipients.[129] In contrast, when Vi vaccine is highly purified, it is well tolerated and febrile reactions are observed in only 1–2% of subjects. In clinical trials, well-tolerated 25 μg and 50 μg single parenteral doses of purified Vi stimulated rises of serum Vi antibodies in the vast majority of vaccinated adults and school-age children.[129–131] Administration of subsequent parenteral doses did not achieve boosts in antibody;[132] thus, the Vi polysaccharide functions like a T-cell-independent antigen. Passive surveillance carried out during field trials showed the Vi vaccine to be as well tolerated as the licensed (meningococcal and pneumococcal) polysaccharide vaccines that served as the control preparations in these trials.[130,131]

Two randomized, controlled, double-blind field trials were carried out in Nepal and South Africa to assess the efficacy of a single 25 μg dose of nondenatured purified Vi vaccine. Over 17 months of surveillance in Nepal, the vaccine conferred 72% vaccine efficacy.[131] In South Africa, the vaccine provided 64% protection over 21 months of follow-up[130] and 55% protection over 3 years.[133] The Nepal trial included all ages from preschool to adulthood, whereas the South African trial was performed in schoolchildren. A third controlled field trial was carried out in subjects 3–50 years of age in Guangxi, China and evaluated the protective efficacy of a single 30 μg dose of a Vi polysaccharide vaccine manufactured in China.[134] The vaccine conferred 69% efficacy (95% CI = 28%, 87%) over 19 months of follow-up.

Vi vaccine provides protection after just a single dose. On the other hand, Vi antibody responses cannot be boosted and the efficacy does not appear to persist beyond 3 years. Concern over the relatively short-lived duration of protection of Vi has heightened following an epidemiologic investigation of an outbreak of typhoid fever that occurred among Vi-vaccinated French soldiers deployed to Ivory Coast.[135] Prior to the outbreak, the standard operating procedure had been to immunize French soldiers with Vi vaccine every 5 years. The outbreak investigation revealed that receipt of Vi more than 3 years earlier was associated with a significantly increased risk of developing typhoid fever during the outbreak.[135]

Supporting the epidemiologic observations of Vi efficacy enduring only 2–3 years is a report that monitored the duration of serum Vi antibodies for 3 years after a single inoculation of adults in a non-endemic area. The percentage of subjects with a putative protective level (1.0 μg/mL) of Vi antibody fell from 87% at 1 month post-immunization to 46% after 2 years and to only 35% at 3 years post-immunization.

In a cluster randomized effectiveness trial, Vi conferred indirect protection on non-vaccinated subjects.[136] ***Table 16.2*** summarizes salient characteristics of Ty21a and Vi vaccines.

New Generation Typhoid Vaccines

New engineered strains of *Salmonella* Typhi that contain precise attenuating mutations have been shown in phase I and II clinical trials to be well

Table 16.2 Salient Characteristics of Live Oral Ty21a and Parenteral Vi Polysaccharide Typhoid Vaccines

Parameter of Comparison	Ty21a	Vi
Route of administration	Oral	Parenteral
No. of doses	3 (4 in United States and Canada)	1
Well tolerated	Yes	Yes
Efficacy	~65%	~65%
Duration of efficacy	7 years	Up to 3 years
Herd immunity	Yes	Yes
Serum IgG anti-Vi	No	Yes
Boostable immune responses	Yes	No
Cell-mediated immunity (including cytotoxic lymphocytes)	Yes	No
Amenable for infant immunization	No[a]	No[b]
Protects against Vi-negative strains	Presumably	No
Protects against *Salmonella* Paratyphi	*Salmonella* Paratyphi B only	No[c]
Recommended for pregnant women	No	Yes
Large-scale school-based vaccination	Yes	Yes
Effective in endemic population	Yes	Yes
Effective in travelers	Yes	Yes

[a]Enteric coated capsules cannot be administered to infants.
[b]Vi polysaccharide is a T-independent antigen that is poorly immunogenic in infants.
[c]*Salmonella* Paratyphi A and B do not express Vi.

tolerated and immunogenic after ingestion of a single oral dose. Attractive live oral vaccine candidates include strains M01ZH09,[137–139] Ty800,[140] CVD 908-*htrA*,[141,142] and CVD 909.[143,144]

Vi polysaccharide has been conjugated to carrier proteins such as recombinant exotoxin A of *Pseudomonas aeruginosa* to increase its immunogenicity by conferring T-cell-dependent properties upon the antigen, including the induction of immunologic memory. In adults and children in endemic areas, booster doses of Vi conjugate vaccine clearly increase the titers of antibody over those elicited by a priming dose.[145–147] A randomized, controlled field trial of Vi conjugate in children immunized at ages 2–4 years in Vietnam's Mekong Delta demonstrated 91.5% (CI, 77.1–96.6%) vaccine efficacy over 27 months of active surveillance[146] and 82% efficacy during an additional 19 months of follow-up that utilized a passive surveillance system.[147]

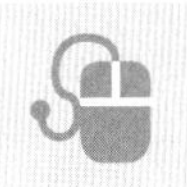

Access the complete reference list online at **http://www.expertconsult.com**

CHAPTER 17

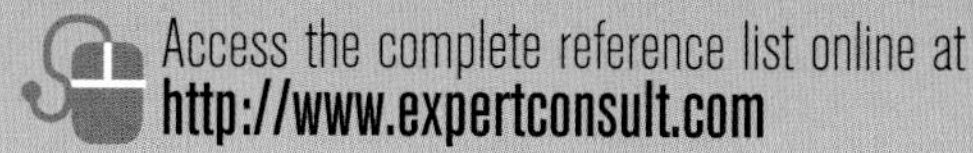
Access the complete reference list online at
http://www.expertconsult.com

Nontyphoidal Salmonellosis

Christopher C. Moore • Patrick Banura • David A. Pegues • Samuel I. Miller

INTRODUCTION

Nontyphoidal *Salmonella* species have been isolated from most animals, including domestic and wild mammals, reptiles, and birds, and are a major source of foodborne disease throughout the developed and developing world.[1] *Salmonella* is readily transmitted to humans by contaminated food or poor sanitation. Although infection most often results in self-limited acute gastroenteritis, nontyphoidal *Salmonella* is one of the leading causes of bacteremia in sub-Saharan Africa.[2] The widespread distribution of *Salmonella* in the environment, its increasing prevalence in the global food chain, and its virulence and adaptability have an enormous medical, public health, and economic impact worldwide.

THE AGENT

Salmonella is a genus of the family of Enterobacteriaceae; they are 2–3 × 0.4–0.6 μm Gram-negative nonspore-forming facultatively anaerobic bacilli.[3] The genome sequences of *typhimurium* strain LT2 consists of 4 857432 base pairs and 5599 coding sequences, including 204 pseudogenes,[4] remarkably similar to that of other Enterobacteriaceae, but with 8% of genes unique to subtype 1 *Salmonella* that may be involved in adaptation to warm-blooded hosts.

The genus *Salmonella* has two species: *S. choleraesuis*, with six subspecies (I, II, IIIa, IIIb, IV, and VI), and *S. bongor*, which formerly was subspecies V.[5] *S. choleraesuis* subspecies I contains almost all the serotypes pathogenic for humans. Because *S. choleraesuis* refers to both a species and a serotype, the species designation *S. enterica* has been recommended and widely adopted. According to the current *Salmonella* nomenclature system, the full taxonomic designation *S. enterica* subspecies *enterica* serotype *typhimurium* can be shortened to *S.* serotype *typhimurium* or *S. typhimurium*.

Members of the seven *Salmonella* subspecies can be grouped into one of more than 2400 serotypes (serovars) according to somatic O, surface Vi, and flagellar H antigens and habitats.[6] *S. enterica* subspecies *enterica* (I with 1454 serotypes) is found in warm-blooded animals while subspecies *salmae* (II with 489 serotypes), *arizonae* (III with 84 serotypes), *diarizonae* (IIIb with 324 serotypes), *houtenai* (IV with 70 serotypes), *indica* (IV with 12 serotypes), and *S. bongori* (V with 20 subtypes) are found in cold-blooded animals and the environment (total = 2463 serotypes). All subspecies have occurred in humans.[6] For simplicity, most *Salmonella* serotypes are named for the city in which they were defined, and the serotype is often used as the species designation.[5] Although serotyping of all surface antigens can be used for formal identification, most laboratories perform a few simple agglutination reactions that define specific O-antigen serogroups, designated as groups A, B, C_1, C_2, D, and E *Salmonella*.[7]

EPIDEMIOLOGY

Incidence

In many countries the incidence of human *Salmonella* infections has increased markedly, although good population-based surveillance data are mostly lacking. In the United States, the incidence rate of nontyphoidal *Salmonella* infection has doubled in the last two decades, with an estimated 1.4 million cases occurring annually.[8,9] In 2006, the estimated incidence rate of salmonellosis (13.6 per 100000 population) was highest among 11 potentially foodborne diseases under active surveillance and varied little by geographic region (***Fig. 17.1***).[10] In 2006, *S. typhimurium*, *S. enteritidis*, and *S. newport* were the three most common serotypes, together accounting for greater than 40% of all laboratory-confirmed cases of human salmonellosis.[11]

Nontyphoidal *Salmonella* causes a small but significant proportion of diarrhea among travelers[12] and among young children in developing countries.[13] However the true incidence rate of nontyphoidal *Salmonella* infection in resource-limited settings is unknown due to lack of laboratory infrastructure.[14,15] The incidence of salmonellosis is highest during the rainy season in tropical climates and during May to October in temperate climates in the northern hemisphere, coinciding with the peak in foodborne outbreaks (***Fig. 17.2***).[16]

Reservoirs and Transmission to Humans

In humans, nontyphoidal *Salmonella* infections are most often associated with food products and are the most frequently identified agent of foodborne disease outbreaks (***Fig. 17.3***).[17] Food of animal origin, including meat, poultry, eggs, and dairy products, can become contaminated with *Salmonella*.[17] For example, 43% of beef carcasses in Senegal were positive for *Salmonella* in the slaughterhouse while at the same time 87% of beef sampled in retailers was *Salmonella*-positive.[18,19] Eating uncooked or inadequately cooked foods cross-contaminated with these products may lead to human infection. In the developed world, nontyphoidal salmonellosis is most often associated with consumption of poultry and eggs,[17,20] but many food vehicles have been implicated in transmission to humans.[17,21] Although foodborne outbreaks predominate, waterborne outbreaks of salmonellosis have also been reported.[22] Salmonellosis associated with exotic pets is a resurgent public health problem, with an estimated 3–5% of all cases of salmonellosis in humans associated with exposure to exotic pets, especially reptiles.[21] Transmission between humans is less frequent but can occur.

Antimicrobial Resistance

Antimicrobial resistance among human nontyphoidal *Salmonella* isolates is increasing worldwide and is likely due, in part, to the widespread use of antimicrobial agents for the empirical treatment of febrile syndromes and as growth promoters in animal production.[23–25] High rates of resistance (>50–100%) to chloramphenicol, trimethoprim-sulfamethoxazole, and ampicillin have been reported from Africa, Asia, and South America. In Malawi resistance to these three antibiotics increased among *S. enteritidis* isolates to >90% in 1999 followed by a gradual decline in resistance during 2001–2004. In contrast, >90% of *S. typhimurium* isolates were resistant to ampicillin and trimethoprim-sulfamethoxazole throughout the period studied, but additional resistance to chloramphenicol was rapidly acquired among *S. typhimurium* during 2001–2002, suggesting acquistion of a plasmid conveying a multidrug-resistant phenotype. Resistance to multiple antibiotics by *S. typhimurium* or *S. enteritidis* paralleled their incidence of bacteremia. Strains remained susceptible to ciprofloxacin and third-generation cephalosporins (***Figs 17.4 and 17.5***).[16] In South Africa, by 2002, *Salmonella isangi* expanded to account for 20% of nontyphoidal *Salmonella* and was found to contain an extended-spectrum β-lactamase.[26] Increasing minimal inhibition concentrations (MICs) of ciprofloxacin against nontyphoidal *Salmonella* have also recently been reported in Kenya, Nigeria, and Senegal.[27–29] Multidrug-resistant nontyphoidal *Salmonella* has emerged in developed countries, including the United States (***Table 17.1 and Fig. 17.3***).[30] Resistant *Salmonella* isolates are associated with recent treatment with an antimicrobial agent, systemic infections, hospitalization, and death.[31,32]

Of particular concern is the worldwide emergence of a distinct strain of multidrug-resistant *S. typhimurium*, characterized as definitive phage type 104 (DT104), that is resistant to at least five antimicrobials – ampicillin, chloramphenicol, streptomycin, sulfonamides, and tetracyclines.[33] The DT104 strain has broad host reservoirs and is difficult to control in domestic livestock, leading to its widespread clonal dissemination among food animals, especially cattle, and humans in Europe, the United States, Canada, and the Middle and Far East.[33–36] Although not known to be more virulent than susceptible *S. typhimurium* strains, infection with DT104 may be associated with greater morbidity and mortality, possibly reflecting inadequate empirical antimicrobial therapy.[37]

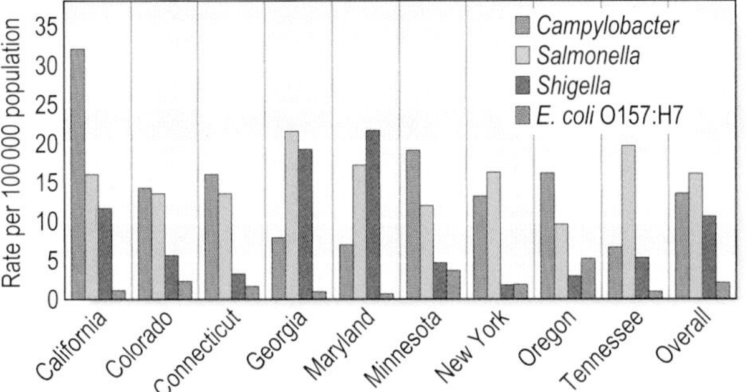

Figure 17.1 Incidence rate per 100 000 population of laboratory-confirmed *Salmonella*, *Campylobacter*, *Shigella*, and *Escherichia coli* O157:H7 infections by selected sites in the United States, Foodborne Diseases Active Surveillance Network, 2002. (Reproduced from Centers for Disease Control and Prevention. Preliminary FoodNet Data on the Incidence of Foodborne Illnesses – Selected Sites, United States, 2002. MMWR. 2003;52:340–343.)

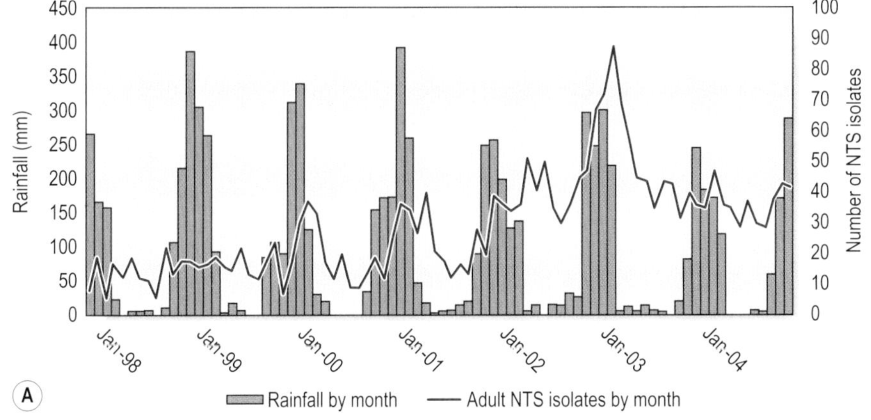

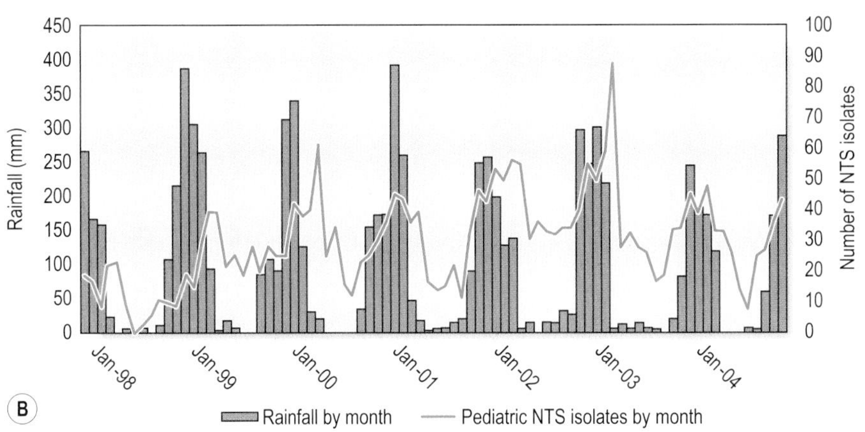

Figure 17.2 The relationship between seasonal rainfall and the incidence of nontyphoidal salmonellae (NTS) bacteremia among **(A)** adults and **(B)** children, by month, 1998–2004. (Reprinted with permission from Gordon MA, Graham SM, Walsh AL, et al. Epidemics of invasive *Salmonella enterica* serovar *enteritidis* and *S. enterica* serovar *typhimurium* infection associated with multidrug resistance among adults and children in Malawi. Clin Infect Dis. 2008;46:963–969.)

Outbreaks and sporadic cases of nontyphoidal *Salmonella* resistant to third-generation cephalosporins have been reported in both developed and developing countries.[38] Resistance to third-generation cephalosporins is conferred by conjugative plasmid-encoded β-lactamases from functional groups 1 (AmpC) and 2 (TEM).[38,39] Recent surveys in the United States found that 5.1% of *Salmonella* isolates from cattle and pigs and 1.6% of isolates from humans were ceftriaxone-resistant (MIC $\geq$ 16 μg/mL).[30] Fluoroquinolone-resistant *Salmonella* strains have emerged among humans

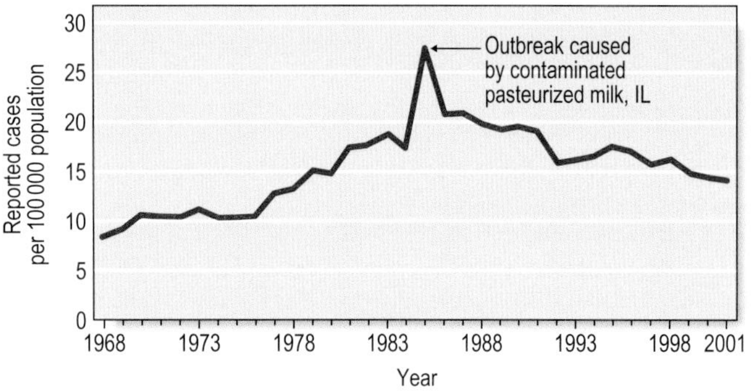

Figure 17.3 Incidence rate per 100 000 population of nontyphoidal salmonellosis by year, United States, 1968–2001. (Reproduced from Centers for Disease Control and Prevention. Summary of Notifiable Diseases, United States, 2001. MMWR. 2003;50:96.)

Table 17.1 Antimicrobial Resistance of *Salmonella* Isolates, United States, 2000

	Salmonella typhi **(*n* = 177)**	***Salmonella*** **non-*typhi*** **(*n* = 1378)**
	n **(% Resistant)**	***n*** **(% Resistant)**
Amikacin	2 (1.1)	0 (0)
Amoxicillin–clavulanic acid	0 (0)	54 (4)
Ampicillin	16 (9)	219 (16)
Cefoxitin	3 (1.7)	43 (3)
Ceftriaxone	0 (0)	18 (1.3)
Cephalothin	2 (1.1)	54 (4)
Chloramphenicol	19 (11)	138 (10)
Ciprofloxacin	0 (0)	5 (0.4)
Gentamicin	1 (0.6)	37 (3)
Nalidixic acid	41 (23)	34 (2)
Streptomycin	18 (11)	223 (16)
Sulfamethoxazole	21 (12)	235 (17)
Tetracycline	19 (11)	256 (19)
Trimethoprim	16 (9)	29 (2) sulfamethoxazole

(Adapted from Centers for Disease Control and Prevention. NARMS 2000 Annual Report. Available online at http://www.cdc.gov/narms/annuals.htm.)

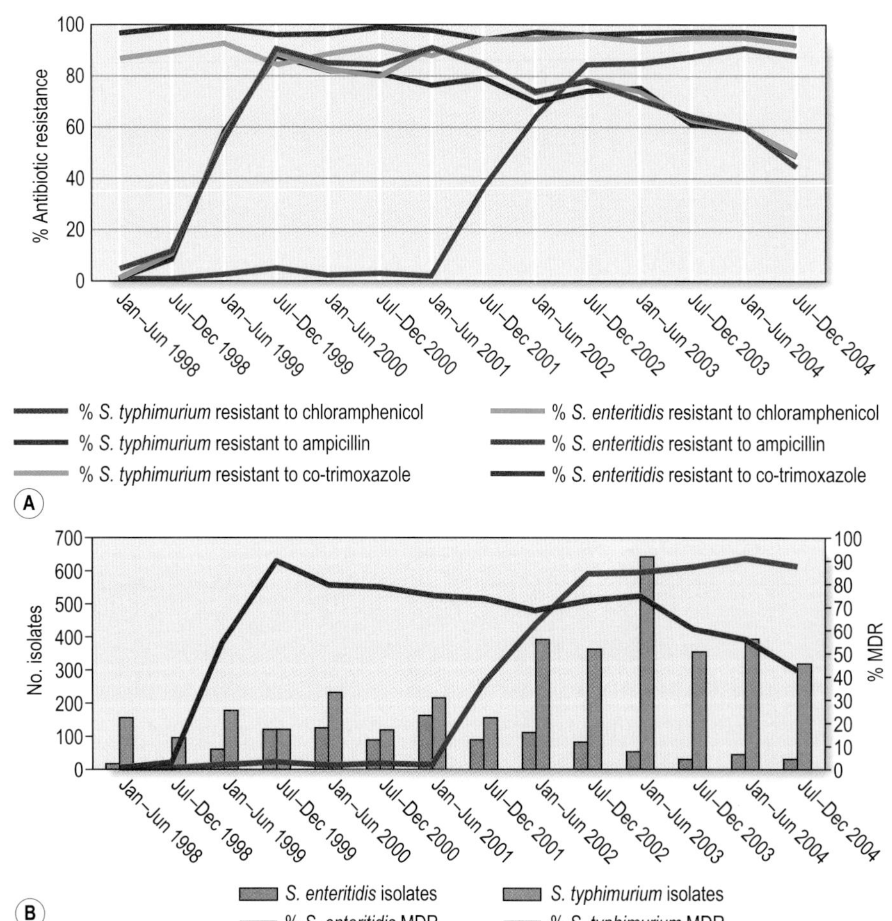

Figure 17.4 (A) The emergence of resistance to chloramphenicol, ampicillin, and trimethoprim-sulfamethoxazole among *Salmonella enterica* serovar *enteritidis* and *S. enterica* serovar *typhimurium* isolated from adults and children, 1998–2004. **(B)** The relationship between emergence of multidrug resistance (MDR) and the incidence of nontyphoidal salmonella (NTS) bacteremia caused by *Salmonella enterica* serovar *enteritidis* and *S. enterica* serovar *typhimurium* among adults and children, 1998–2004. (Reprinted with permission from Gordon MA, Graham SM, Walsh AL, et al. Epidemics of invasive *Salmonella enterica* serovar *enteritidis* and *S. enterica* serovar *typhimurium* infection associated with multidrug resistance among adults and children in Malawi. Clin Infect Dis. 2008;46:963–969).

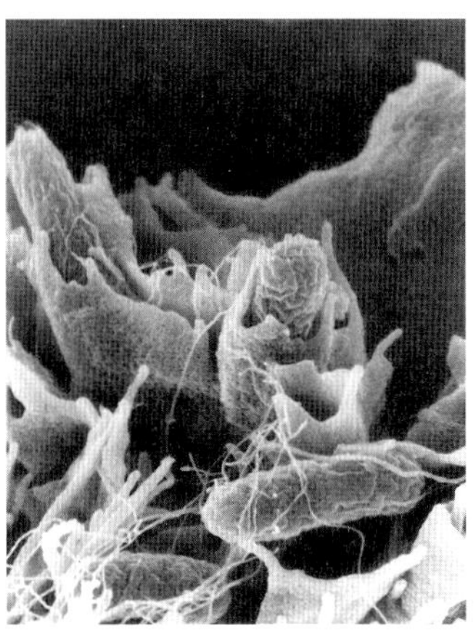

Figure 17.5 Scanning electron micrograph showing *Salmonella typhimurium* entering a Hep-2 cell through bacteria-mediated endocytosis. Membrane ruffles extend from the cell surface, enclosing and internalizing adherent bacteria. (Reprinted with permission from Ohl ME, Miller SI. *Salmonella*: a model for bacterial pathogenesis. Annu Rev Med. 2001;52:259–274. ©2001 Annual Reviews. www.annualreviews.org.)

and animals, and resistance is due to mutations of the intracellular targets DNA gyrase (gyrA or gyrB) or topoisomerase IV, or to overproduction of efflux pumps.[40–42] Emergence of fluoroquinolone resistance among human *Salmonella* isolates is clearly linked with the use of fluoroquinolones as growth promoters in food animals.[24,43]

International Spread of Salmonellosis

Changes in food consumption and the rapid growth of international trade in agricultural food products have facilitated the dissemination of new *Salmonella* serotypes associated with fresh fruits and vegetables.[44] Human or animal feces may contaminate the surface of fruits and vegetables and may not be removed by washing. Recent foodborne sources of outbreaks of salmonellosis associated with fresh produce include cantaloupe, tomatoes, unpasteurized orange juice, cilantro, and raw seed sprouts. Soaking seeds in sodium hypochlorite can reduce, but not eliminate, the risk of sprout-associated illness, and thus immunocompromised persons should not eat sprouts.[45] Outbreaks associated with manufactured food products include icecream (United States, *S. enteritidis*), pasteurized milk (United States, *S. typhimurium*), powdered milk products and infant formula (Canada and United States, *S. tennessee*), unpasteurized goats milk cheese (France, *S. paratyphi*), processed foods containing peanuts, including peanut butter, frozen dinners, and ready-to-eat snacks. The highest concentrations of fecal organisms in drinking water sources in Africa occur at the onset of the wet season and this may be associated with increased risk of waterborne nontyphoidal salmonellosis.[16,46]

THE DISEASE

Clinical Manifestations

Gastroenteritis

Infection with nontyphoidal *Salmonella* most often results in self-limited acute gastroenteritis that is indistinguishable from that due to many other enteric bacterial pathogens. Within 6–48 hours of ingestion of contaminated food or water, nausea, vomiting, and diarrhea occur.[47] In most cases, stools are loose, of moderate volume, and without blood. Stools may be watery and of large volume ("cholera-like") or of small volume associated with tenesmus, pus, or blood ("dysentery-like").[45] Fevers (38–39°C), abdominal cramping, nausea, vomiting, and chills are frequently reported. A comparison of community-acquired nontyphoidal *Salmonella* gastroenteritis versus bacteremia in Kenya revealed that a higher proportion of children with gastroenteritis reported with symptoms of diarrhea and vomiting compared to children who had bacteremia, indicating that nontyphoidal bacteremia without gastroenteritis may be an emerging disease in Africa.[48] Headache, myalgias, and other systemic symptoms can also occur. Microscopic examination of stools shows neutrophils and, less frequently, red blood cells. Infrequently, *Salmonella* can cause a syndrome of pseudoappendicitis or can mimic the intestinal changes of inflammatory bowel disease.[47] Toxic megacolon is a rare but potentially life-threatening complication.[49]

Diarrhea is usually self-limited, typically lasting for 3–7 days.[47] Diarrhea that persists for more than 10 days should suggest another diagnosis. If fever is present, it usually resolves within 48–72 hours. Occasionally, patients require hospitalization for dehydration, and death occurs infrequently. In the United States, nontyphoidal *Salmonella* infections result in an estimated 2.2 hospitalizations per 1 million population and 582 deaths per year.[9] More deaths occur among the elderly, especially those residing in long-term care facilities, and among immunocompromised patients.[20,50–52]

After resolution of gastroenteritis, the mean duration of carriage of nontyphoidal *Salmonella* in the stool is 4–5 weeks and varies by *Salmonella* serotype.[53] Antimicrobial therapy may increase the duration of carriage.[53] In addition, a higher proportion of neonates have prolonged carriage; in one study, 50% of neonates were still excreting *Salmonella* at 6 months.[54] However, the delayed clearance of infection in neonates does not result in permanent carriage; almost all chronic carriers are adults.[53,54]

Bacteremia

Nontyphoidal *Salmonella* is now being recognized as a leading cause of bacteremia in sub-Saharan Africa.[2,55] This may be due in part to an association between nontyphoidal *Salmonella* bacteremia and malaria, malnutrition, human immunodeficiency virus (HIV) infection and possibly schistosomiasis. In a study from Mozambique, the incidence of childhood bacteremia was 425 cases per 100 000 person-years with nontyphoidal *Salmonella* bacteremia, accounting for 120 cases per 100 000 person years. However, the true incidence of bacteremia is likely to be much higher in resource-limited settings because the incidence of bacteremia among children who die before reaching the district hospital is frequently unable to be determined and because of limited laboratory facilities to make the diagnosis.[2,14,56]

Classically, *S. choleraesuis* and *S. dublin* produce sustained bacteremia with fever, but any *Salmonella* serotype can cause bacteremia.[47] Fever and splenomegaly are predictive of *Salmonella* bacteremia; they occurred in 95% and 38% of adult patients in Malawi.[55,57] Similar findings have also been noted in Kenya.[58] Nontyphoidal *Salmonella* bacteremia occurs without or remote to gastrointestinal symptoms in both adults and children.[55,58] While only 1–4% of immunocompetent individuals with *Salmonella* gastroenteritis have positive blood cultures,[53] infants and children less than 3 years old, the elderly, and the immunocompromised, including those with acquired immunodeficiency syndrome (AIDS), may develop recurrent *Salmonella* bacteremia despite antimicrobial therapy.[50,59–63] *Salmonella* has a propensity for infection of vascular sites, and high-grade or persistent bacteremia suggests an endovascular infection.[64] Endovascular infection occurs in 10–25% of persons over 50 years of age, usually involves the aorta, and most commonly results from seeding atherosclerotic plaques or aneurysms.[65,66] Mortality rates range from 14% to 60% and are lower with prompt diagnosis and combined medical and surgical therapy.[67,68]

Salmonellosis and HIV Infection

In studies among HIV-infected persons in Africa, *Salmonella* species are one of the most frequent causes of bacteremia, are often multidrug-resistant, and are associated with high mortality (24–80%) and recurrence rates (43%).[55,69] HIV-infected individuals have a 20–100-fold increased risk of salmonellosis compared with the general population.[50] Of 2517 children with nontyphoidal *Salmonella* bacteremia in Malawi during 1998–2004, 19–35% were HIV-infected; 85% were <3 years old. Of 2439 Malawian adults with nontyphoidal *Salmonella* bacteremia,

95–98% were HIV-infected.[16] *Salmonella* is more likely to cause severe invasive disease (fulminant diarrhea, enterocolitis, rectal ulceration, recurrent bacteremia, focal infections, meningitis, and death) in persons with AIDS compared with infection in immunocompetent persons or asymptomatic HIV infection.[70,71]

Recurrent nontyphoidal *Salmonella* bacteremia is an AIDS-defining illness resulting from incomplete clearance of the primary infection because of impaired cell-mediated immunity. Without maintenance antimicrobial therapy, up to 45% of individuals with HIV infection will have recurrent bacteremia.[70] In resource-rich settings, among those with HIV, the incidence of recurrent nontyphoidal *Salmonella* bacteremia has declined, likely because of the direct bactericidal activity of antiretrovirals on *Salmonella* species, the impact of highly active antiretroviral therapy on immune reconstitution, and the use of trimethoprim-sulfamethoxazole for the prevention of *Pneumocystis* pneumonia.[70,72,73]

Localized Infections

Localized infections develop in approximately 5–10% of persons with *Salmonella* bacteremia, and the presentation may be delayed.[74] Extraintestinal complications of salmonellosis and their management are summarized in ***Table 17.2***.

Chronic Carrier State

The chronic carrier state is defined as the persistence of *Salmonella* in stool or urine for periods longer than 1 year. From 0.2% to 0.6% of patients with nontyphoidal salmonellosis develop chronic carriage,[75] a lower frequency than that observed in *S. typhi* infection.[66,76,77] The frequency of chronic carriage is higher in women, in persons with biliary abnormalities or concurrent bladder infection with *Schistosoma haematobium*, and in infants.[62,78] Asymptomatic carriers of nontyphoidal *Salmonella* have also been described in Africa.[79,80]

PATHOGENESIS AND IMMUNITY

Interactions with Gastrointestinal Tract and Induction of Enteritis

As few as 10^3 bacteria may produce nontyphoidal gastroenteritis and the ingested dose is an important determinant of incubation period and disease severity.[81] Gastric acidity represents the initial barrier to *Salmonella* colonization.[82] Infants have relative gastric achlorhydria, compared to adults, which may contribute to their risk of nontyphoidal *Salmonella* disease. Salmonellae express multiple fimbriae that contribute to tight adherence to intestinal epithelial cells in culture and are required for colonization in animal models.[83]

Salmonellae invade intestinal epithelial cells by bacteria-mediated endocytosis (***Fig. 17.4***).[84,85] Shortly after bacteria adhere to the apical epithelial surface, profound cytoskeletal rearrangements occur in the host cell, disrupting the normal epithelial brush border and inducing formation of membrane ruffles that reach out and enclose adherent bacteria in large vesicles. Following bacterial internalization, a fraction of *Salmonella*-containing vesicles transcytose to the basolateral membrane, and the apical epithelial brush border reconstitutes.

Salmonellae encode a type III secretion system (TTSS) within pathogenicity island 1 (the SPI-1 TTSS) that is required for bacteria-mediated endocytosis and intestinal epithelial invasion. Type III secretion systems subvert host cell function through the translocation of virulence proteins directly from the bacterial cytoplasm into the host cell. Two SPI-1 translocated proteins, SipC and SipA, promote *Salmonella* invasion through direct interactions with the actin cytoskeleton. SipC inserts into the host cell plasma membrane and nucleates actin polymerization at the site of *Salmonella* attachment.[86,87] SipA enhances actin polymerization through stabilization of actin filaments and reduction of the critical concentration for polymerization.[86–88] Additional SPI-1 translocated proteins contribute to invasion by targeting members of the Rho family of monomeric GTP-binding proteins (G proteins). Rho family proteins regulate the structure and dynamics of the actin cytoskeleton and are required for formation of the membrane ruffles that mediate *Salmonella* internalization.[89] The SPI-1 translocated proteins SopE and SopE2 act as GDP/GTP exchange factors and induce membrane ruffling following microinjection into epithelial cells.[90,91] SopB is an additional SPI-1 translocated protein that acts as an inositol polyphosphatase within the host cell.[92] This activity indirectly stimulates Rho GTPases and promotes membrane ruffling.[93] SipA and SipC act in concert with downstream cellular effectors of activated Rho GTPases to initiate and spatially direct the actin rearrangements that lead to *Salmonella* internalization.[87]

Salmonella serotypes clinically associated with gastroenteritis induce a secretory response in intestinal epithelium and initiate recruitment and transmigration of neutrophils into the intestinal lumen.[94] The SPI-1 TTSS is also required for these responses. Stimulation of Rho GTPase signaling by SopE and SopE2 also leads to activation of MAP kinase pathways and synthesis of proinflammatory cytokines.[91,95,96] Simultaneously, a SipA N-terminal region triggers apical secretion of the potent neutrophil chemoattractant hepoxillin A3.[97]

Salmonellae also utilize the SPI-1 TTSS to deliver proteins that down-regulate the host inflammatory response associated with *Salmonella* invasion. The SptP protein inactivates Rho GTPase signaling by acting as a GTPase-activating protein (Rho GAP).[98] By reversing MAPK and MAPKK activation, both Spt P GAP and tyrosine phosphatase activities directly oppose the activity of SopE and SopE2 and reduce membrane ruffling and proinflammatory signaling. The plasmid-mediated effector SpvC also directly inhibits Erk, Jnk, and p38 MAPKs through its phosphothreonine lyase activity.[99,100] In addition, the SspH1 and AvrA proteins inhibit NF-κB activation and related host cell cytokine synthesis.[101,102]

Table 17.2 Extraintestinal Infectious Complications of Salmonellosis

Site	Incidence	Risk Factors	Manifestations	Complications	Mortality	Diagnosis	Treatment
Endocarditis[66,168]	0.2–0.4%	Preexisting valvular heart disease	Valvular vegetation, infected mural thrombus	Valve perforation, relapse (20–25%), pericarditis	~70%	Blood culture, echocardiography	Early valve surgery + 6 weeks Pceph 3, Pamp, P/PO fluoroquinolone
Arteritis[68,169,170]	Rare	Atherosclerosis, aortic aneurysm, endocarditis, prosthetic graft, myelodysplasia	Prolonged fever, pain in back, chest, or abdomen	Mycotic aneursym, aneurysm rupture, aortoenteric fistula, vertebral osteomyelitis	14–60%	Blood culture, CT or nuclear scan	Early surgical bypass + 6 weeks Pceph 3, Pamp, P/PO fluoroquinolone

Table 17.2 Extraintestinal Infectious Complications of Salmonellosis—cont'd

Site	Incidence	Risk Factors	Manifestations	Complications	Mortality	Diagnosis	Treatment
Central nervous system[171–173]	0.1–0.9%	Infants (especially neonates)	Meningitis, ventriculitis, brain abscess, subdural empyema, encephalopathy	Seizures, mental retardation, hydrocephalus, brain infarction, relapse	~20–60%	CSF culture, CT or MRI scan	≥3 weeks Pceph 3, Pamp, carbapenem
Pulmonary[66,74]	Rare	Lung malignancy, structural lung disease, sickle cell anemia	Pneumonia	Lung abscess, empyema, bronchopleural fistula	~25–60%	Respiratory culture, chest radiograph	≥2 weeks P/POabx
Bone[174,175]	<1%	Sickle cell anemia, male gender, connective tissue disease, immunosuppression	Femur, tibia, humerus, lumbar vertebrae	Relapse, chronic osteomyelitis	Very low	Bone radiograph	≥4 weeks Pceph 3, Pamp, P/PO fluoroquinolone + surgery for sequestra
Joint: reactive[176,177]	0.6%	HLA-B27, antibiotic therapy	≥3 joints involved (especially knee, ankle, wrist, and sacroiliac)	Prolonged symptoms (mean duration 5.5 months)	Negligible	Joint fluid examination and culture	Nonsteroidal anti-inflammatory agent
Joint: septic[178]	0.1–0.2%	Osteoarthritis, connective tissue disease, sickle cell disease, prosthetic joint	Knee, hip, shoulder	Joint destruction osteomyelitis	Very low	Joint fluid examination and culture	Repeated needle aspiration + ≥4 weeks P/POabx
Muscle/soft tissue[179]	Rare	Local trauma, male gender, diabetes, HIV infection	Abscess, pyomyositis	Osteomyelitis, endovascular infection, frequent relapse	~33%	Ultrasonography, aspiration	Drainage + ≥2 weeks Pabx
Hepatobiliary[180]	Rare	Cholelithiasis, cirrhosis, amebic abscess, echinococcal cyst, hepatocellular carcinoma	Hepatomegaly, cholecystitis, hepatic abscess	Rupture with secondary peritonitis, subphrenic abscess, spontaneous bacterial peritonitic	~10%	Ultrasonography, aspiration	Drainage + ≥2 weeks Pabx
Splenic	Rare	Sickle cell anemia, splenic cyst, splenic hematoma	Splenomegaly	Left-sided empyema, subphrenic abscess, rupture with secondary peritonitis	<10%	Ultrasonography, aspiration	≥2 weeks Pabx, ± percutaneous drainage or splenectomy
Urinary[61,181]	0.6%	Urolithiasis, malignancy, renal transplantation	Cystitis, pyelonephritis	Renal abscess, interstitial nephritis, relapse	~20%	Urine culture, ultrasonography	Removal of structural abnormality + 1–2 weeks Pabx + ≥6 weeks PO fluoroquinolone or TMP-SMX
Genital[66]	Rare	Pregnancy, renal transplantation	Ovarian abscess, testicular abscess, prostatis, epididymitis	Abscess	Very low	Ultrasonography, aspiration	Drainage of collection + 1–2 weeks Pabx + ≥6 weeks PO fluoroquinolone or TMP-SMX
Soft tissue[182]	<1%	Local trauma immunosuppression	Pustular dermatitis, subcutaneous abscess, wound infection	Septic thrombophlebitis, endophthalmitis	~15%	Drainage culture	≥2 weeks Pabx + drainage of collection

Pceph 3, parenteral third-generation cephalosporin; Pamp, parenteral ampicillin; P/PO FQ, parenteral or oral fluoroquinolone; CT, computed tomography; CSF, cerebrospinal fluid; MRI, magnetic resonance imaging; P/PO, parenteral or oral antimicrobial (e.g., quinolone, ampicillin, TMP-SMX, chloramphenicol or third-generation cephalosporin); HLA, human leukocyte antigen; HIV, human immunodeficiency virus; TMP-SMX, trimethoprim-sulfamethoxazole; P/POabx, parenteral or oral antibiotics.

Interactions with Macrophages and Systemic Infection

Salmonellae are facultative intracellular pathogens, and bacterial replication within macrophages is essential for the production of systemic disease.

The PhoP/PhoQ two-component regulatory system senses the intracellular environment and induces transcription of more than 40 *Salmonella* genes required for survival within macrophages.[103] Activation of the PhoP/PhoQ regulon leads to widespread modifications in the protein and lipopolysaccharide components of the bacterial inner and outer membranes.[104,105] These surface modifications confer resistance to antimicrobial factors within the phagosome, including antimicrobial peptides. PhoP/PhoQ-regulated lipopolysaccharide modifications alter the charge density and fluidity of the outer membrane, discouraging antimicrobial peptide insertion in the membrane.[105,106] In addition, PhoP/PhoQ-regulated modifications in lipid A structure produce a lipopolysaccharide molecule with significantly less proinflammatory signaling activity.[105]

Salmonellae express enzymes that inactivate microbicidal reactive oxygen and nitrogen species produced within the macrophage. Resistance to nitric oxide (NO) results in part from bacterial synthesis of homocysteine, an NO antagonist.[107] *Salmonella* mutants unable to synthesize homocysteine are hypersensitive to NO and are less virulent. In addition, salmonellae produce at least one superoxide dismutase that inactivates reactive oxygen species.[108] A second *Salmonella* type III secretion system is encoded in *Salmonella* pathogenicity island 2 (SPI-2); it translocates proteins across the membrane of the *Salmonella*-containing vacuole (SCV) into the macrophage cytosol and is necessary for the survival of *Salmonella* in the macrophage.[109] SPI-2 translocated proteins appear to prevent the maturation of the SCV into a mature phagolysosome, thus creating an intracellular compartment favorable for bacterial replication. Several SPI-2 translocated proteins localize to the surface of the SCV and may alter its fusion with other membranous compartments within the macrophage.[110–114] SPI-2-mediated modifications in the SCV lead to exclusion of the NADPH oxidase and inducible NO synthase from the vacuolar membrane, allowing the bacterium to evade the reactive oxygen and nitrogen species produced by these enzymes.[115,116]

SpvB is a *Salmonella* virulence protein that is secreted into the macrophage cytoplasm, thus promoting disassembly of actin networks around the vacuole.[109,117] SpvB promotes bacterial dissemination beyond the intestine in animals and bacteremia in humans.[118] Other bacterial factors, including incompletely characterized cytotoxin genes and genes required for synthesis of essential nutrients and iron acquisition, also are important in systemic pathogenesis.[119–121]

Host Response and Immunity

The innate immune system senses invasive *Salmonella* infections using Toll-like receptors (TLR) that recognize conserved elements of bacterial structure, including recognition of lipopolysaccharide by TLR4, bacterial lipoproteins by TLR2, and flagellin by TLR5.[122] Activation of these receptors on phagocytes and epithelia leads to synthesis of cytokines that orchestrate the acute inflammatory response and instruct the subsequent antigen-specific immune response. Mice lacking a functional TLR4 response are highly susceptible to *Salmonella* infection.[123] The initial control of *S. typhimurium* replication in host tissue requires recruitment and activation of macrophages.[124] Macrophage activation and efficient killing of *Salmonella* are associated with production of interferon-γ (IFN-γ), interleukin-12 (IL-12), and tumor necrosis factor-1 (TNF-α).[125–127] Humans with mutations in the IFN-γ and IL-12 receptor genes develop severe infections with nontyphoidal *Salmonella* serotypes.[128,129]

HIV infection is strongly associated with invasive salmonellosis, and defects in macrophage phagocytosis and oxidative burst have been described in HIV-infected individuals.[130–133] In an *ex vivo* study using human alveolar macrophages from HIV-infected patients from Malawi there was an increased secretion of TNF-α, IL-10, and IL-12 in response to *S. typhimurium* challenge, regardless of IFN-γ priming. This cytokine dysregulation showed a relationship with peripheral CD4 cell count, with marked decline at values less than 250 cells/μL. Therefore, dysregulation of proinflammatory cytokine release, including IL-12 by macrophages during *Salmonella* infection may underlie the susceptibility to severe salmonellosis in patients with HIV infection. The defect was not reversed by IFN-γ and may represent a proinflammatory effect of HIV infection upon the macrophage or the alveolar milieu.[134]

Final clearance of infection and immunity to rechallenge requires a Th1-type CD4 T-cell response and production of specific antibodies by B cells.[126,135,136] Sera from healthy Malawian children aged more than 16 months contained anti-*Salmonella* antibody and successfully killed *S. typhimurium*. However, sera from most healthy children less than 16 months, those most likely to suffer *Salmonella* bacteremia, lacked *Salmonella*-specific antibody and sera lacking antibody did not kill *S. typhimurium* despite normal complement function. Addition of *Salmonella*-specific antibody enabled killing of *S. typhimurium*.[4] The importance of cellular immunity in controlling *Salmonella* infection in humans is demonstrated by the extreme susceptibility of individuals with HIV infection, lymphoproliferative diseases, or immune suppression following transplantation.[50,60,61,70,137]

DIAGNOSIS

Isolation and Identification

Freshly passed stool is preferred for the isolation of *Salmonella*. Stool is plated directly onto agar plates. Low-selective media, such as MacConkey agar and deoxycholate agar, and intermediate-selective media, such as *Salmonella-Shigella*, xylose-lysine-deoxycholate, or Hektoen agar, are widely used to screen for both *Salmonella* and *Shigella* species. New selective chromogenic media, such as CHROMagar and COMPASS agar, are more specific than other selective media, reduce the need for confirmatory testing and time to identification, and increasingly are used for the primary isolation and presumptive identification of *Salmonella* from clinical stool specimens.[138] Combining chromogenic agar with xylose-lysine-deoxycholate agar may improve sensitivity.[139] Tetrathionate- and selenite-based enrichment broths are often used to facilitate the recovery of low numbers of organisms.[138] Highly *Salmonella*-selective media, such as selenite with brilliant green, may help identify suspected carriers. Bismuth sulfite agar, with an indicator of hydrogen sulfite production and which does not contain lactose, can be used for the detection of the 1% of *Salmonella* strains (including most *Salmonella* serogroup C strains) that ferment lactose.[140]

After primary isolation, possible *Salmonella* isolates can be tested in commercial identification systems or inoculated into screening media such as triple sugar iron and lysine iron agar. Rapid IgM antibody-based serologic tests have been developed and may supplement stool culture for the diagnosis of acute *Salmonella* infection.[141] Isolates with typical biochemical profiles for *Salmonella* should be serogrouped with commercially available polyvalent antisera or sent to a reference or public health laboratory for complete serogrouping. Polymerase chain reaction (PCR) methods for diagnosis are rapidly emerging and may reach practical ease for diagnosis in some settings.[142]

Molecular Typing

Subtyping methods are frequently used for epidemiologic purposes to differentiate strains of common *Salmonella* serotypes. Phenotyping methods may be useful for characterizing outbreak-associated strains and sporadic multidrug-resistant isolates, and include bacteriophage typing, plasmid profile analysis, antimicrobial susceptibility, and biotyping. More discriminative genotyping techniques, including ribotyping, pulsed-field gel electrophoresis, insertion sequences analysis, PCR-based fingerprinting, and multilocus sequence typing, have been used in epidemiologic studies to differentiate strains within a given serotype.[142] Genomic DNA analysis using microarrays may complement the other genotyping methods.[143] However, lack of standardization and time requirement limit the widespread use of these genotyping techniques.

TREATMENT AND PROGNOSIS

Gastroenteritis

Nontyphoidal *Salmonella* gastroenteritis is usually a self-limited disease, and therapy should primarily be directed to the replacement of fluid and electrolyte losses. In a large meta-analysis, antimicrobial therapy for uncomplicated nontyphoidal *Salmonella* gastroenteritis, including short-course or single-dose regimens with oral fluoroquinolones, amoxicillin, or trimethoprim-sulfamethoxazole, did not significantly decrease the length of illness, including duration of fever or diarrhea, and was associated with an increased risk of relapse, positive culture after 3 weeks, and adverse drug reactions.[144] In fact, some early reports suggested that children treated with ampicillin or amoxicillin were more likely to have both prolonged excretion and clinical relapse compared to those who were given placebo.[145] Fluoroquinolone therapy may rapidly convert the results of stool cultures to negative immediately after therapy but this is of uncertain clinical benefit, and there is no difference in long-term clearance of *Salmonella* compared to placebo-treated control patients.[146] Therefore, antimicrobials should not be used routinely to treat uncomplicated nontyphoidal *Salmonella* gastroenteritis or to reduce convalescent stool excretion.

Although fewer than 5% of all patients with *Salmonella* gastroenteritis develop bacteremia, certain individuals are at increased risk for invasive infection and may benefit from preemptive antimicrobial therapy. Antimicrobial therapy should be considered for neonates, persons older than 50 years, and those with immunosuppression or cardiac valvular or endovascular abnormalities, including prosthetic vascular grafts. Treatment consists of an oral or intravenous antimicrobial administered for 48–72 hours or until the patient becomes afebrile. Longer treatment may result in a higher rate of chronic carriage and relapse. For susceptible organisms, treatment with an oral fluoroquinolone, trimethoprim-sulfamethoxazole, or amoxicillin is adequate. Although fluoroquinolones are not recommended for administration to children less than 10 years of age, they may have a role in treating severe nontyphoidal salmonellosis in this age group.[147,148] A trial in Turkey also demonstrated that intravenous immunoglobulin (500 mg/kg on days 1, 2, 3, and 8) in combination with cefoperazone when administered to preterm neonates with *S. typhimurium* infection reduced the mortality, complications, and duration.[149]

Bacteremia

Current World Health Organization (WHO) guidelines for empiric therapy of childhood sepsis recommend penicillin and chloramphenicol or ampicillin and gentamicin as initial treatment, but increasing resistance and limited penetration of gentamicin into cells limit their effectiveness.[16,150] The WHO recommends a third-generation cephalosporin in areas where resistance to other agents is known to be common. Therefore empirical therapy for life-threatening bacteremia or focal infection should include a third-generation cephalosporin and a fluoroquinolone until susceptibilities are known.[150]

If bacteremia is high-grade (i.e., >50% of three or more blood cultures is positive), one should search for endovascular abnormalities by echocardiogram or other imaging techniques, such as computed tomography or indium-labeled white blood cell scan. Low-grade bacteremia not involving vascular structures should be treated with intravenous antimicrobial therapy for 7–14 days. Six weeks of intravenous therapy with a β-lactam antibiotic, such as ampicillin or ceftriaxone, is recommended to treat documented or suspected endovascular infection. Intravenous ciprofloxacin followed by prolonged oral therapy may be an option, but published clinical experience is limited.[67] Chloramphenicol should not be used to treat endovascular infection because of high failure rates.[64,151] Early surgical resection of infected aneurysms or other infected endovascular sites is recommended.[67,68] Patients with infected prosthetic vascular grafts that could not be resected have been maintained successfully on chronic suppressive oral therapy.[152] When there is failure to respond to appropriate antimicrobial therapy, in the right setting, a search for schistosomiasis coinfection as well as for focal disease should be initiated.[62]

Recurrent *Salmonella* Bacteremia in Individuals with AIDS

In persons with AIDS and a first episode of *Salmonella* bacteremia, 1–2 weeks of intravenous antimicrobial therapy followed by 4 weeks of oral fluoroquinolone therapy (e.g., ciprofloxacin 500–750 mg twice daily) should be administered to attempt eradication of the organism and to decrease the risk of recurrent bacteremia.[153] Long-term secondary prophylaxis or suppressive therapy with an oral fluoroquinolone or trimethoprim-sulfamethoxazole should follow the initial 6-week primary therapy in patients with a CD4 cell count < 200 cells/mm^3 or those who relapse.[153,154] Fluoroquinolones and zidovudine have a synergistic antibacterial effect against *Salmonella*; administration of both drugs may dramatically decrease the risk of recurrent infection.[155] Trimethoprim-sulfamethoxazole may also help prevent other opportunistic infections, including *Pneumocystis* pneumonia.

Chronic Carrier State

Chronic carriage of nontyphoidal *Salmonella* is managed similarly to typhoid carriage. Amoxicillin (3 g for adults or 100 mg/kg for children divided three times a day for 3 months), trimethoprim-sulfamethoxazole (one double-strength tablet twice a day for 3 months), or ciprofloxacin (750 mg twice daily for 4 weeks) is effective in eradication of chronic carriage associated with susceptible strains, with cure rates of more than 80%.[156,157] Amoxicillin and fluoroquinolones are concentrated in bile and fluoroquinolones have superior intracellular penetration. Shorter courses in endemic areas may lead to resistant infections.[158] If anatomic abnormalities, such as biliary or kidney stones, are present, surgery combined with antimicrobial therapy may be required for eradication.[75]

PREVENTION AND CONTROL

The prevention and control of salmonellosis require both an understanding of the complex cycles of transmission and ongoing surveillance to characterize trends in *Salmonella* occurrence and to identify outbreaks. Control of foodborne salmonellosis requires barriers to the introduction and multiplication of *Salmonella* from the farm to the table.[159] In resource-limited settings, protection of source water, increased access to centrally treated safe water, strategies such as the use of narrow-mouthed, spigoted containers for water storage, and treatment of water at home by chlorination, solar disinfection, filtration, flocculation, or a combination of maneuvers may reduce the risk of infection with *Salmonella* and other diarrheal infections.[160–162]

Recognition of foodborne outbreaks requires that clinicians have a high index of suspicion, order the appropriate laboratory test, and promptly report positive culture results to local public health departments. Vaccination of feed animals, limiting the use of antimicrobials as growth promoters, and improved food safety practices should further reduce the burden of foodborne salmonellosis. The use of algorithms and rapid molecular subtyping have improved the ability to detect clusters and outbreaks of salmonellosis.[163] Establishment of cooperative international surveillance systems has facilitated rapid data exchange for the prevention of human salmonellosis associated with widely distributed agricultural and manufactured foods.[164,165]

Outbreaks occur when commercial kitchens serve *Salmonella*-contaminated foods that have been insufficiently cooked or mishandled.[51] It is reasonable to allow food handlers to return to work with careful personal hygiene after diarrhea is resolved. Two consecutive negative stool samples should only be required for food handlers whose work involves touching unwrapped foods that are consumed raw or served without further cooking. Routine surveillance of food handlers for asymptomatic stool carriage of *Salmonella* is not recommended.

To limit the risk of nosocomial transmission to patients and health care workers, patients excreting *Salmonella* should be managed with standard precautions, including the use of barrier precautions, such as gloves, when performing direct patient care or handling soiled articles. Control of *Salmonella* outbreaks in long-term care facilities or neonatal care areas may be difficult because of poor compliance with isolation precautions and the increased susceptibility of these patients.[166] Although *Salmonella* infection in newborns, the elderly, or immunocompromised can be severe, the risk of transmission of *Salmonella* from health care workers to patients appears to be low.[167] Once health care workers are asymptomatic and passing formed stool, they should be allowed to return to work if standard precautions are observed. However, local and state regulations may require work exclusion for health care workers with salmonellosis until two or more stool cultures obtained at least 24 hours apart are negative.

Access the complete reference list online at
http://www.expertconsult.com

Access the complete reference list online at
http://www.expertconsult.com

CHAPTER 18

Shigellosis

Gerald T. Keusch • Mohammed A. Salam • Dennis J. Kopecko

INTRODUCTION

Shigellosis is an infection of the large bowel caused by one of the many serotypes of the genus *Shigella*. While it is a disease typically associated with poverty, poor hygiene, and crowded living conditions in developing countries, as well as an important contributor to childhood malnutrition where such conditions prevail, it also remains a frequent cause of diarrhea in developed countries.[1] It has been difficult to reliably determine the burden of shigellosis because etiological data are infrequently collected from representative populations around the world. In addition, the organism is fragile and may not survive long enough to be identified in clinical samples when they are obtained.[2] Studies in rural Peru have demonstrated that active surveillance increases yield by 20-fold compared to passive methods.[3] Previous retrospective analysis of published data estimated the annual global burden at >200 million infections and 1.1 million deaths, 99% in the developing world.[4] In such settings, *Shigella* species cause as many as 5–15% of all diarrhea cases and most episodes of bloody diarrhea or dysentery in infants and children seeking care in clinics or hospitals. In Bangladesh, the isolation rate in rural Matlab is approximately twice that of urban Dhaka. While these mortality figures are likely an overestimate, *Shigella* are responsible for a significant portion of the residual 1–1.5 million non-rotavirus diarrhea deaths annually, even in settings where dehydration is effectively treated early with oral rehydration therapy (ORT).

In contrast, in developed countries shigellosis typically presents as mild to moderate watery diarrhea, indistinguishable from other etiologies. These patients are not investigated microbiologically, and thus go unreported. The number of laboratory confirmed *Shigella* isolates reported to the US Centers for Disease Control and Prevention (CDC), around 10 000–15 000, fluctuates year by year. The isolation rate appears to be slowly trending downward from an average of 6.4/100 000 per year between 1968 and 1988 to 5.6/100 000 per year between 1989 and 2002.[5] It reached an all-time low of 3.5/100 000 in 2006, the latest year reported;[6] this is several hundred-fold lower than the incidence in developing countries. Seventy-five to 80% of infections in infants and young children are due primarily to *S. sonnei*, and are commonly acquired at day-care centers. The true incidence of shigellosis in the United States is estimated by CDC as around 444 000 cases/year.[7]

For reasons not well understood, there is a recent trend to less severe disease in some developing regions of the world.[8] This may be related to reduced transmission of and mortality due to the most virulent serotype, *S. dysenteriae* type 1, which occurs almost exclusively in developing countries. Systematic surveillance in both rural and urban Bangladesh documents its virtual disappearance since outbreaks in 1984 and 1994. Previous large-scale epidemics due to *S. dysenteriae* type 1, especially during humanitarian emergencies, have been associated with high attack rates (6–39%) and case-fatality rates (1.5–9%).[9] Whether the current trends will be sustained is not yet clear. Improved hygiene, sanitation, nutrition, and access to health services in many developing countries are encouraging developments; however, *Shigella* epidemiology has always been unpredictable and full of surprises.

THE AGENT

Shigella was identified by Kiyoshi Shiga just over a century ago during a severe outbreak of bloody diarrhea in Japan,[10] and ultimately named in his honor. They are Gram-negative highly host-adapted bacilli within the family Enterobacteriaceae, infecting only humans and some nonhuman primates.[11] *Shigella* cannot be differentiated from *Escherichia coli* by DNA relatedness, and were they discovered today would be classified within the genus *Escherichia*.[12] It remains a separate genus because of the distinctive clinical illnesses *Shigella* cause. Unlike most *E. coli* and *Salmonella*, *Shigella* do not possess flagella and are nonmotile. There are biochemical differences between *Shigella* and other Enterobacteriaceae, but aside from the inability to ferment lactose, these are of little importance for diagnosis or, apparently, for virulence.

Shiga's original isolate is now known as *S. dysenteriae* type 1. At least 14 additional *S. dysenteriae* serotypes have been described, some associated with clinical disease and outbreaks.[13,14] There are three additional species, *flexneri* (14 serotypes/subtypes), *boydii* (20 serotypes), and *sonnei* (1 serotype, multiple phage/colicin types).[1] Although *S. dysenteriae* can be distinguished from other *Shigella* by its inability to ferment mannitol, in practice all species are identified initially by their inability to utilize lactose or produce hydrogen sulfide, and then are distinguished serologically.

EPIDEMIOLOGY

Shigella are present wherever humans are. Direct person-to-person spread is the major route of transmission, facilitated by the very low inoculum required for infection. In experimental human studies just 10–100 *S. dysenteriae* type 1 cause infection and clinical disease in 10–20% of nonimmune subjects.[15] This is one reason why *Shigella* is so readily transmitted within clinical microbiology laboratories.[16] Large numbers of organisms are excreted in stool; post-infection carriage in stool is self-limited, although occasional chronic carriers are reported. Further transmission is fecal-oral, typically due to contamination of the hands with infected feces. Failure to wash hands after defecation often leads to transfer of organisms directly or via an intermediate object (fomite) to the mouth of a susceptible individual. *Shigella* may also contaminate food or water directly or indirectly from feces, resulting in common-source outbreaks. Flies attracted to human feces can also transfer *Shigella* to food or water, and, especially where open defecation is practiced, the use of traps to reduce the fly population can diminish the incidence of shigellosis.[17] *Shigella* can also be sexually transmitted via anal-oral contact. In the United States, men (76%) and *S. flexneri* (52.6%) predominate, although the proportion of *S. sonnei* (46.1%) has been increasing.[18] Because significant environmental or animal reservoirs do not exist, shigellosis

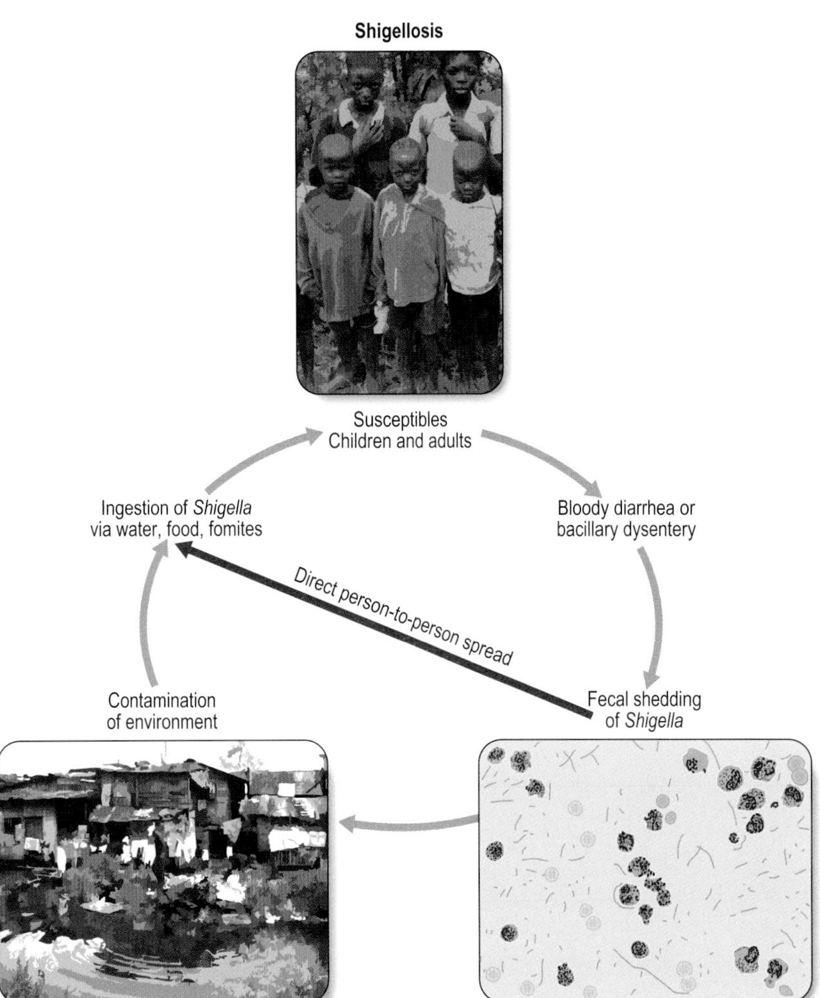

Figure 18.1 Life cycle/pathogenesis of *Shigella* species in urban and rural populations. *Shigella* are highly adapted to humans, and do not have a reservoir outside of the human intestine. The cycle is therefore from the stool of an infected individual to the mouth of a susceptible individual, generally referred to as fecal-oral transmission. Because the inoculum necessary to transmit infection is so small, the common pathway is direct person-to-person contact; however, stool can directly contaminate food or water or be transferred by flies, or organisms can be transmitted through anal-oral sex or through inanimate objects handled by individuals whose hands have been in contact with infected material.

can theoretically be controlled by effective environmental sanitation and personal hygiene. However, chlorinated drinking water and environmental sanitation have not yet eliminated shigellosis from the United States. The life cycle for *Shigella* infection is illustrated in ***Figure 18.1***.

Incidence is highest in children 1–5 years of age, presumably because good personal hygiene is much more difficult to achieve in the young and they have not yet acquired specific immunity. In many disease-endemic countries shigellosis peaks during the hot dry season, when water for handwashing and household hygiene is in short supply. Outbreaks also occur in the rainy season, presumably because feces are washed from the environment into drinking water sources. In the United States, *S. sonnei* infection peaks in late summer and early fall. Shigellosis is very common in day-care centers, where susceptible infants and toddlers cluster. Poor sanitation on native American reservations has, for many years, resulted in especially high rates of shigellosis and infant mortality; federal programs to construct sanitary facilities and improve access to clean water have reduced this disparity.[5]

S. dysenteriae type 1 was the dominant species when originally discovered in 1896, but was replaced by *S. flexneri* after World War I and virtually disappeared. Following World War II, *S. sonnei* gradually became the principal isolate in industrialized countries while *S. flexneri*, particularly serotypes 2a, 2b and 3a, has persisted in developing countries (***Fig. 18.2***).[19] There are a few exceptions, such as Thailand, where *S. sonnei* has also replaced *S. flexneri* as the most common isolate.[20] It has been suggested that contamination of water in some developing countries with *Pleisiomonas shigelloides*, which expresses the same O antigen as *S. sonnei*, induces a cross-reactive O-antigen-specific immunity to *S. sonnei*.[21] The fourth species, *S. boydii*, is present primarily in the Indian subcontinent and has always been uncommon elsewhere. Specific *Shigella* clones can rapidly move around the world, evidenced by food-associated outbreaks of an identical *S. sonnei* in Denmark and Australia, associated with baby corn imported from Thailand.[22] *S. dysenteriae* type 1, the only species known to cause epidemics, reemerged during 1969–1972 in Mexico and Central America, affecting children and adults alike, with high mortality rates.[1] Similar outbreaks in South Asia and Africa followed; in the past decade, however, incidence has sharply diminished.

Shigella has evolved relatively recently from ancestral *E. coli* serotypes,[12] and its major virulence properties, encoded on a plasmid, have not yet stabilized genetically by integration into the chromosome. The continuing detection of new *Shigella* serotypes in South Asia suggests that the genus is still evolving, which may be partly responsible for the changing epidemiology of shigellosis.

PATHOGENESIS AND IMMUNITY

Shigella cause a superficial invasive colitis involving the epithelium and lamina propria, in contrast to noninvasive enterotoxigenic pathogens such

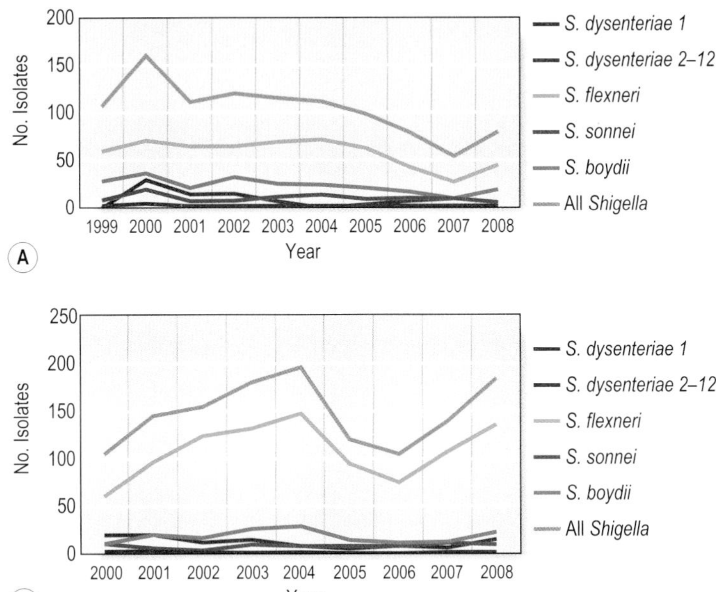

Figure 18.2 Isolation of *Shigella* species in a systematic 2% microbiological sampling of fecal specimens at ICDDR,B Hospital in Dhaka **(A)** and from all patients presenting to the rural ICDDR,B Matlab Hospital **(B)**. *S. flexneri* accounts for approximately 75% of all isolates in both settings. In contrast (not shown), the vast majority of isolates in developed countries are *S. sonnei*. (Source: ICDDR, B.)

as *Vibrio cholerae* or systemic invaders such as *Salmonella enterica* serovar Typhi.[25] When excreted in stool *Shigella* are noninvasive but resistant to low pH, due to activation of a glutamate-dependent acid-resistance system transcriptionally upregulated during the stationary growth phase.[23] This property allows the organisms to tolerate exposure to a pH below 2.5 for several hours and facilitates their survival through the stomach. *Shigella* genes for cell invasion are activated in the small bowel, in advance of reaching the preferred target, the terminal ileum and colon. The combination of acid resistance and efficient host cell invasion contributes to the low inoculum needed for infection and disease. Invasion of the intestinal epithelium proceeds through a complex and intricate mechanism, mediated by both microbial and host proteins.[24,25] Intimate biochemical "cross-talk" signals between *Shigella* and various host cell types activate specific bacterial and host genes necessary for disease pathogenesis, particularly a bacterial type 3 secretion system (TTSS) and invasion mediators, which trigger essential host cell responses, cytoskeletal rearrangements, and release of inflammatory cytokines.[26,27]

Our understanding of microbial invasion and the ensuing host-mediated pathogenesis of disease has undergone dramatic advancement in recent decades. The pathologic consequences of *Shigella* are now thought to be due largely to a microbially induced exaggerated host inflammatory response resulting in intestinal mucosal damage. The mucus-covered gut epithelium is a major defense barrier against most enteric microbes, and is endowed with intracellular and extracellular receptors to recognize microbial invasion and activate the innate immune system. Indeed, nonmotile *Shigella* cannot penetrate mucus-covered intestinal cells. Instead, using its unique molecular mechanisms, *Shigella* initially traverse the mucosa through non-mucin-covered specialized antigen-processing microfold (M) cells, without disrupting them.[28] They encounter the underlying lymphoid follicles within the mucosa, are ingested by resident macrophages and lyse the phagosomal vacuole and enter the cytoplasm where they multiply. The consequence is apoptotic death of the infected macrophage[29] and release of intracellular stores of the inflammatory cytokines interleukin-1β (IL-1β) and IL-18.[25,30] Invasive pathogens like *Shigella* also bind host Toll-like receptors (TLRs) on the basolateral epithelial cell membrane, upregulating proinflammatory cytokine genes and increasing secretion of IL-8 and tumor necrosis factor-α (TNF-α). Invasion of colonic cells *in vitro* is associated with upregulation of IL-1, IL-4, IL-6, IL-8, TNF-α, and gamma interferon (IFN-γ).[31] This has been confirmed *in vivo* using rectal biopsy samples from acutely ill or convalescing shigellosis patients.[32] Severe illness is associated with markedly increased IL-1β, IL-6, TNF-α, and IFN-γ expression. IL-1β and IL-8 both induce migration and activation of polymorphonuclear neutrophils (PMNs), leading to recruitment of PMNs and their transmigration between epithelial cells into the gut lumen.[33]

Shigella lipopolysaccharide (LPS) is another critical signal for PMN adherence and migration. LPS translocated from the luminal to the basal side of intestinal epithelial cells during *Shigella* invasion interacts with circulating host LPS-binding protein and is recognized by the PMN ligand, CD14. This leads to upregulation and activation of the PMN adherence ligand CD11b/CD18, required for transepithelial PMN migration.[34] Migration of PMNs between intestinal epithelial cells disrupts the integrity of interepithelial cell tight junctions and allows *Shigella* in the lumen to gain entry to the submucosa and the basolateral epithelial surface where they trigger TLRs and amplify the production of proinflammatory cytokines.

Invasion of the colonic mucosa is divisible into three stages: primary translocation of *Shigella* across M cells and infection of follicular macrophages, secondary release from dead macrophages of bacteria that now invade the basolateral surface of adjacent epithelial cells, and tertiary amplification of epithelial cell invasion following disruption of the tight junction (***Fig. 18.3***). All three are essential to disease pathogenesis. In a rabbit model, blocking IL-1 by pretreatment with IL-1 receptor antagonist, or inhibiting neutrophil chemotaxis and migration by antibody to PMN CD18, prevents progression of infection and clinical disease.[35] Attraction and activation of PMNs triggers degranulation and damage of surrounding tissue,[36] even though organisms are efficiently killed by a mechanism that does not require oxygen.[37] *Shigella* pathogenesis is a double-edged sword, engaging innate immune responses that are both defensive (PMN-mediated killing) and offensive (destabilization of epithelial cohesion and mucosal damage) in nature. The imbalance of the response to *Shigella*, to some degree, mimics the excessive immunologic response of inflammatory bowel diseases.

Invasion of intestinal M cells and epithelial cells depends on the TTSS, a microbial needle-like secretion apparatus that injects effector proteins, invasion plasmid antigens (Ipas), through the host cell membrane into the cytoplasm[24] (Fig. 18.3) . IpaA modulates the activities of Cdc42, Rac, and Rho, small GTPases that control actin polymerization and cytoskeletal alterations.[39] This leads to the internalization of *Shigella* within a host-membrane bound endosome (***Fig. 18.4***). Subsequent lysis of the endosomal membrane is due to IpaB and IpaC, releasing organisms into the cytoplasm. Mutations that inhibit endosomal lysis also block bacterial

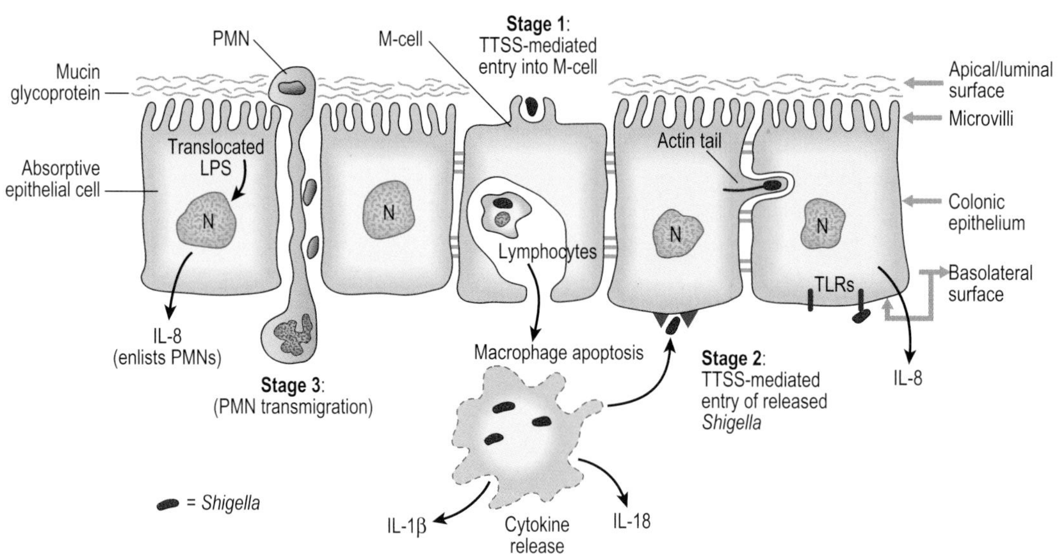

Figure 18.3 Stages of *Shigella* pathogenesis. The colonic mucosal epithelial cells are coated with mucin glycoprotein at the apical surface. Specialized microfold (M) cells, not covered by mucin, overlay lymphoid follicles filled with macrophages, dendritic cells, and lymphocytes, to sample entering antigens/pathogens and present them to the immune system for a response. *Shigella* entry into the mucosa involves three discrete stages. In stage 1, ingested *Shigella* utilize their type 3 secretion system (TTSS) needle to trigger invasion across the apical surface of M cells. This entry process involves a reorganization of actin filaments which results in the entry of *Shigella* into the cytoplasm. The bacteria pass through the M cells where they encounter and are engulfed by macrophages. The consequence is macrophage apoptosis, resulting in the release of IL-1β, IL-18, and viable organisms. In stage 2, the released *Shigella* interact with Toll-like receptors (TLRs), upregulating the production of IL-8, which is further enhanced by *Shigella* lipopolysaccharide (LPS) translocated during infection. *Shigella*, released from dead macrophages, invade the basolateral surface of absorptive epithelial cells utilizing their TTSS, quickly lyse the endosomal vacuole and reach the cytoplasm where they can multiply, triggering more inflammation. Intracellular *Shigella* also nucleate an actin tail at one pole of the rod-shaped bacterium. This constantly growing tail of contractile proteins serves as a "motor" pushing the bacteria to the plasma membrane and into the adjacent cell, now surrounded by a double membrane. When these bacteria escape into the cytoplasm the process repeats as infection proceeds laterally without exiting the epithelial cells. The third stage of invasion involves IL-8 mediated enlistment of polymorphonuclear neutrophils (PMNs) and their paracellular migration between adjacent epithelial cells, breaching the normally tight intercellular junctions. This allows bacteria in the gut lumen to pass between host cells to the basolateral space where they interact with TLRs and further upregulate inflammation. *Shigella* are effectively killed by PMNs; however, this causes more tissue damage due to the ensuing degranulation. Disease pathogenesis is due to the death and sloughing of small patches of colonic epithelial cells creating focal microulcerations, with leakage of underlying blood/lymphatic vessels in the lamina propria and the loss of serum protein. N, nucleus.

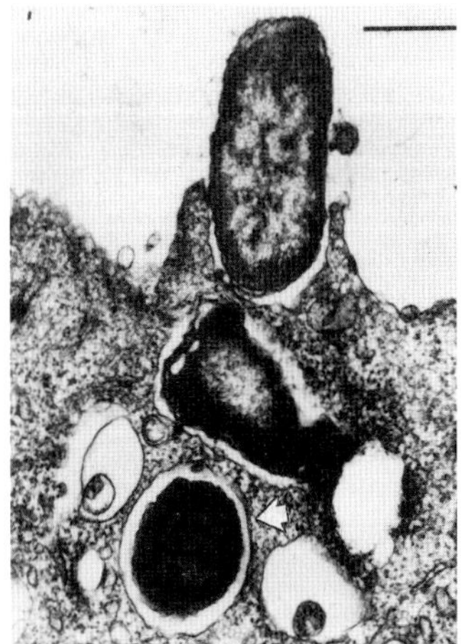

Figure 18.4 Invasion of cultured HeLa cell monolayers by *Shigella flexneri*. The bacterial cell at the top of the figure has initiated the reorganization of epithelial cell cytoskeleton, and the actin-based movement of the host cell membrane to form a phagocytic vacuole is evident. The two pseudopods of host cell origin will fuse at the top, engulfing the bacterium within a membrane-bounded endosome, as shown at the lower portion of the cell (white arrowhead).

multiplication and are avirulent. Multiplying organisms express IcsA, an adenosine triphosphatase, energizing the polymerization of actin filaments at one end of the bacterium, forming an actin tail and propelling the organisms forward.[40] IcsA-negative strains cannot generate an actin tail or move intracellularly, and are greatly reduced in virulence.[41] The actin polymerization effect is often referred to as the "actin motor." It can drive *Shigella* to the plasma membrane, creating membrane-bound protrusions at the host cell intermediate junction (***Fig. 18.5***), leading to invasion of the adjacent host cells within a double-membrane endosome.[42] When this vesicle is lysed, organisms released into the cytoplasm continue the process. Invasion requires host cell E-cadherin, a calcium-dependent cell adhesion molecule localized to intermediate junctions below the tight junction.[43] The clinical correlate of cell-to-cell invasion, bacterial multiplication, and necrosis and sloughing of infected epithelial cells, is focal microulcerations, occurring primarily in the terminal ileum and colon, with the greatest intensity in the distal colon and rectum.

Shigellosis persists longer in children than in adults, perhaps reflecting immunologic immaturity in young children. Clearance of infection likely involves a combination of normal intestinal cell turnover, microbial death due to innate defenses (e.g., PMNs), down-modulation of inflammation, and the development of specific local immunity. Strong epidemiologic evidence indicates that immunity to *Shigella* is serotype-specific and based on LPS O antigens, although its precise nature, whether mucosal IgA, serum IgG, or some cellular immune mechanism, is not known.

Shiga toxin (Stx)-producing *S. dysenteriae* type 1 is epidemiologically linked to the development of hemolytic-uremic syndrome (HUS). The importance of Stx is supported by the ability of serotypes of *E. coli*

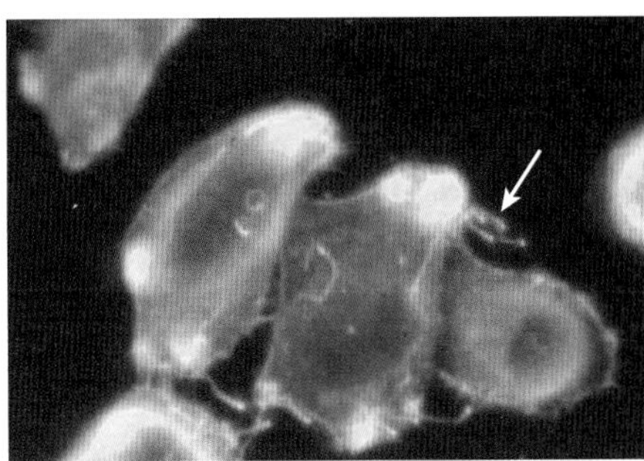

Figure 18.5 Intracellular movement of *Shigella flexneri* within HeLa cells stained with fluorescein-labeled phalloidin, which specifically binds to polymerized actin. The actin tails, labeled by the dye, appear as bright streaks within the cytoplasm, and as they are created the organism is propelled forward by the force of actin contraction, the "actin motor." Organisms that reach the plasma membrane protrude beyond the plane of the cell (arrow), a display termed fireworks, and can be seen approaching the plasma membrane of adjacent cells.

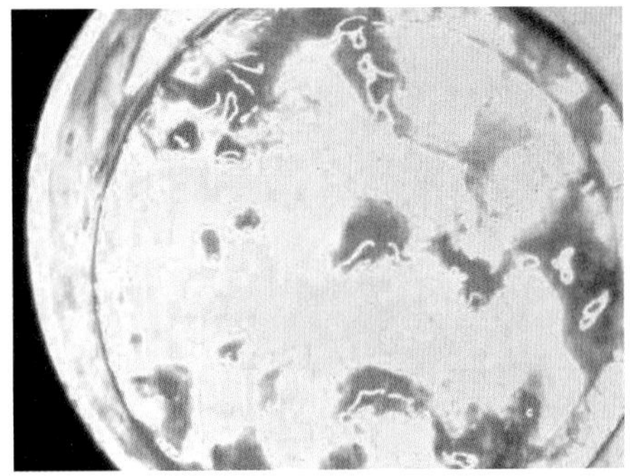

Figure 18.6 Typical dysenteric stool is a small-volume mix of blood and pus. Such stools may be passed 30 or more times per day, often with increased pain (tenesmus).

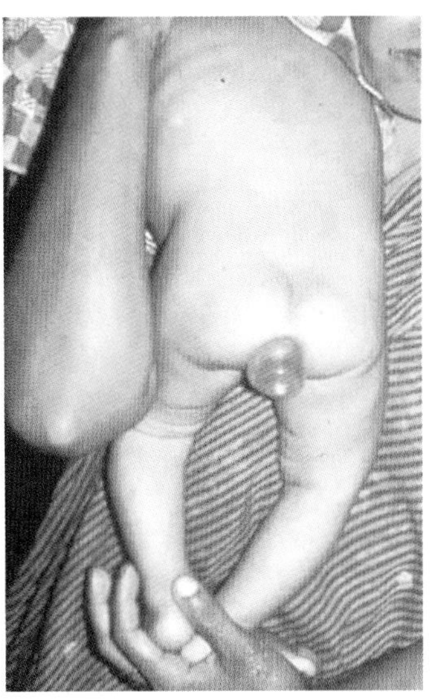

Figure 18.7 Bangladeshi child with rectal prolapse, a consequence of intense proctitis due to invading *Shigella* and the resulting inflammatory response.

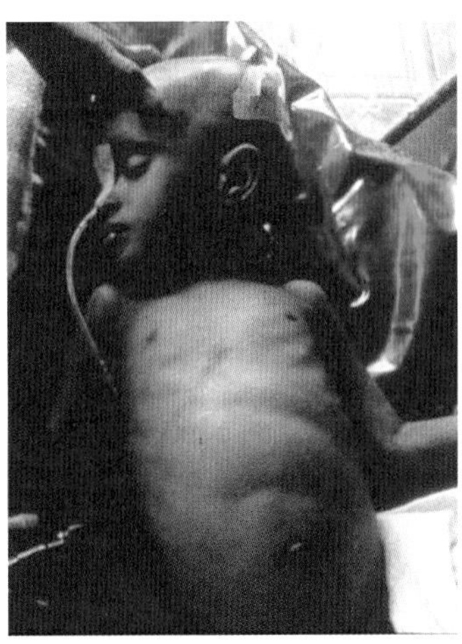

Figure 18.8 Bangladeshi child with toxic megacolon caused by *Shigella dysenteriae* type 1 infection. The dilated loops of bowel are clearly discernible beneath the abdominal wall.

(such as O157:H7) that produce structurally and biochemically similar toxins (Stx1 and Stx2) to cause HUS.[44] Shiga toxins are known to bind glycolipid receptors on endothelial cells, essential in the pathogenesis of HUS.[45]

THE DISEASE

Clinical Manifestations and Complications

Shigellosis typically begins with malaise and fever, 24–72 hours after ingestion of the organism. This is followed by diarrhea, usually watery at the outset, but containing many leukocytes when examined microscopically. Diarrhea may become bloody or progress to dysentery, a syndrome characterized by the triad of small volume, grossly bloody, mucopurulent stools (***Fig. 18.6***), abdominal cramping, and tenesmus, a painful straining with the urge to pass stool. Shigellosis is often referred to as bacillary dysentery to distinguish it from amebic dysentery due to the protozoan *Entamoeba histolytica*.

These manifestations result from inflammation, intense proctocolitis, and ulcerations of the colonic mucosa. Dysentery is not an invariable consequence of *Shigella*, and is in large part determined by the virulence of the infecting strain, the infectious dose, and the susceptibility of the individual. Most patients with *S. sonnei* infections never develop grossly bloody diarrhea or dysentery, whereas most patients with *S. dysenteriae* type 1 infection do. Host factors, some undoubtedly genetic, others related to nutritional status or other co-morbidities such as HIV/AIDS, also determine severity in individuals.[46,47]

Shigella dysentery is associated with profound anorexia.[48] Because the stomach and small bowel are not directly involved in shigellosis, neither vomiting nor severe dehydration is prominent, although mild-moderate dehydration occurs due to stool water losses, increased insensible water loss from fever, and reduced food and fluid intake. The intensity of the proctitis can be so severe that rectal prolapse occurs, especially in young children with *S. dysenteriae* type 1 or *S. flexneri* infection[49] (***Fig. 18.7***). Functional intestinal obstruction and toxic megacolon (***Fig. 18.8***) may develop with severe inflammation, most commonly with *S. dysenteriae* type 1 infections.[50] Although infection with *Shigella* usually does not progress beyond the lamina propria, colonic or distal ileal perforation can occur, most typically in neonates or malnourished children.[51] Bacteremia due to the infecting *Shigella* itself or another luminal organism, especially in malnourished or immunocompromised patients, is a complication in 5–10% of patients in Bangladesh.[52] Bacteremic infection in the United States is extremely uncommon, and >99% of isolates reported to CDC are from feces.[5]

Shigellosis is associated with a number of systemic complications. Patients may present with a generalized motor seizure, especially young children with high fever and *S. flexneri* or *S. dysenteriae* type 1 infection.[53] More than one seizure is rare; however, patients can become obtunded or even comatose, usually in association with metabolic aberrations such as severe hypoglycemia or hyponatremia.[54] Hypoglycemia, due to lack of food intake and an inadequate gluconeogenic response, may be profound (plasma glucose <1 mmol/L). Hyponatremia is associated with dysentery, and is due to sodium loss in the stool plus secretion of antidiuretic hormone in amounts inappropriate for the serum sodium concentration, possibly triggered by hypoalbuminemia and decreased intravascular oncotic pressure in patients with severe dysentery. In Bangladesh serum sodium concentrations less than 125 mmol/L are present in approximately 50% of all patients with severe *S. dysenteriae* type 1 and 25% of those with *S. flexneri* infection.

The most dramatic systemic complication of shigellosis is HUS, characterized by microangiopathic hemolytic anemia, thrombocytopenia, and oliguric renal failure. HUS occurs exclusively in *S. dysenteriae* type 1 infection[55] and is usually first noted 1–5 days after dysentery develops, often as intestinal manifestations are subsiding. Renal failure and hemolytic anemia can be severe; thrombocytopenia is usually less marked, with platelet counts in the range of 25 000–100 000/mm^3 and no bleeding manifestations other than in the gut. HUS may be incomplete, with any manifestation occurring in isolation.[56] Shigellosis has a profound effect on nutrition, and wherever shigellosis is hyperendemic it is a major contributor to the high prevalence of malnutrition in children. First, energy requirements are increased due to high fevers.[57] Second, inflammatory cytokines released in the host response[58] cause muscle protein catabolism, altered priorities for acute phase protein synthesis, and anorexia with decreased food intake. Third, these patients lose considerable amounts of protein due to transudation of serum across the damaged gut mucosa.[59] These changes persist long into convalescence. In developing countries, severe *Shigella* infections due to *S. dysenteriae* type 1 and *S. flexneri* almost double the subsequent rate of persistent (greater than 14 days) diarrhea and acute malnutrition, and increase mortality by 10-fold in such patients.[60]

Shigella (and other invasive enteric bacteria such as nontyphoidal *Salmonella*, *Campylobacter*, and *Yersinia*) can initiate reactive (sterile) arthritis, sometimes accompanied by tendinitis, conjunctivitis, uveitis, urethritis, or erythema nodusum.[61] This clinical constellation, previously termed Reiter's syndrome, is an autoimmune process occurring 2–3 weeks post infection. It is highly associated with the HLA-B27 haplotype, and in these individuals arthritis can be acute or chronic, and can result in severe joint damage.

DIAGNOSIS

Although all O-antigens of *Shigella* can now be detected by DNA microarray methods,[62] in practice specific diagnosis still depends on stool culture. This is best done directly from fresh stool samples, which increases yield compared to rectal swabs.[1] If culture cannot be done rapidly (best at the bedside) stool should be inoculated to transport media such as buffered glycerol-saline or Cary–Blair medium. Use of a moderately selective medium for Gram-negative organisms, such as MacConkey or deoxycholate citrate agar (DCA), and a more highly selective medium such as xylose-lysine-deoxycholate (XLD), Hektoen enteric (HE), or *Salmonella-Shigella* (SS) agar, optimizes yields. *Shigella,* as well as *Salmonella*, does not change the color of the pH indicator in these media because they cannot ferment lactose. Lactose-negative colonies can be identified and subcultured to triple sugar iron (TSI) agar or Kligler iron agar (KIA). On these media *Shigella* produce an alkaline slant, confirming lactose negativity, and an acid butt due to anaerobic fermentation of glucose, are nonmotile and do not produce hydrogen sulfide or gas. Putative isolates fulfilling these criteria can be serologically confirmed, speciated and serotyped with specific antisera.[1] It has been suggested that *S. dysenteriae* type 1 could be rapidly identified by testing for catalase activity, since it is catalase negative, compared to other *Shigella* and most Enterobacteriaceae which are catalase positive.[63]

In many areas of the tropics, microbiology is not readily available and diagnosis is based on clinical and simple laboratory features. While some practitioners in endemic areas still believe that dysentery is commonly amebic in etiology, there is ample evidence that patients with dysentery are far more likely to be infected with *Shigella* than with *E. histolytica.*[64]

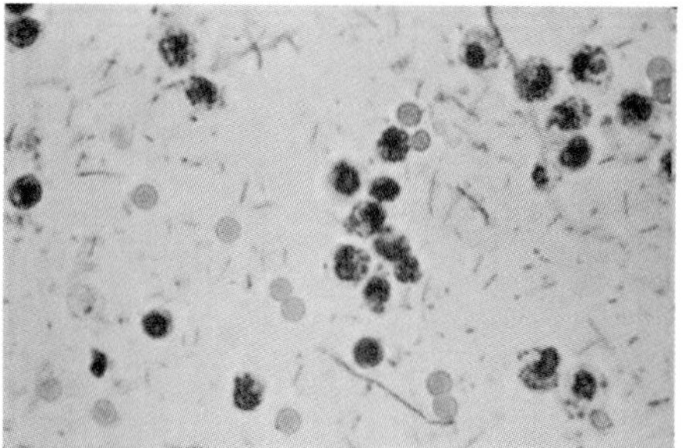

Figure 18.9 Fecal smear of shigellosis.

Clinical and laboratory features in amebic and bacillary dysentery differ sharply. Shigellosis is suggested by a short pre-hospitalization illness, high fever, and the presence of abundant fecal leukocytes, greater than 50 neutrophils per high-power field (***Fig. 18.9***).[65] Amebiasis is more often chronic, and leukocytes are few or absent in the stool because the parasite lyses PMNs. Mere presence of amebic cysts in stool is not diagnostic, as the vast majority are nonpathogenic strains of *E. dispar.* Virulent *E. histolytica* are suggested by identification of motile trophozoites containing ingested erythrocytes in fresh stool preparations.[66] More specific diagnosis is possible with ELISA or PCR, and sharply reduces the false positives with microscopy alone. In the absence of confirmed amebiasis, patients with frank dysentery should be presumed to have shigellosis and treated empirically for this infection. In developing countries the diagnosis of clinical dysentery can often be established by community health workers who either observe the characteristic stool or obtain a history of bloody stools from the mother, who are reliable historians in reporting bloody diarrhea.[67]

Rapid methods have been developed to diagnose shigellosis, including fluorescent antibody staining for *S. dysenteriae* type 1, which has high sensitivity (92%) and specificity (93%),[68] immunomagnetic isolation of bacteria followed by PCR[69] or monoclonal antibody[70] confirmation, and isotope- or enzyme-labeled DNA probes for virulence markers specific for *Shigella*, although some of the latter are also present in the rare *Shigella*-like enteroinvasive *E. coli.*[71,72] A rapid simple dipstick method has been devised for *S. flexneri* 2a, the most common serotype in developing countries.[73] Although these may become commercially available, cost will remain a major deterrent to their use in resource-limited settings. The only reliable rapid commercially available method in routine use is an enzyme immunoassay for Shiga toxin in stool. A positive test is indicative of *S. dysenteriae* type 1 or an Stx-producing *E. coli* serotype, such as O157. This test is used primarily in developed countries for rapid diagnosis of Stx-producing *E. coli.*[74,75] Serologic testing for O-antigen antibody is useful for epidemiologic studies of shigellosis but not for diagnosis of acute disease, especially in endemic areas where the majority of the population may be seropositive from prior infections.[76]

TREATMENT AND PROGNOSIS

Except for mild-moderate watery diarrhea due to *S. sonnei* in well-nourished individuals, for which antibiotics are not warranted, antimicrobial therapy is the cornerstone of treatment for shigellosis. In the absence of effective antimicrobial therapy, mortality from bloody diarrhea or dysentery due to *Shigella* is appreciable; *S. dysenteriae* type 1 and *S. flexneri* in developing countries have been associated with mortality rates in excess of 10%, particularly in the young and the elderly.[77] In this setting, even *S. sonnei* can be lethal, especially among individuals sick enough to seek hospital care. Effective antimicrobial therapy given within 72 hours of symptoms not only brings prompt clinical resolution but also reduces the likelihood of HUS.[78] All persons who have dysentery and presumed *Shigella* infection should therefore be treated with an appropriate antimicrobial agent when first seen; the results of culture and susceptibility testing, if available, can then be used subsequently to modify treatment when necessary.

To be useful in resource-poor settings, an antimicrobial agent should be safe for use in children under 5 years, proven clinically effective in controlled trials, administered orally, and affordable.[79] Because of the ever rising prevalence of multidrug-resistant strains, selection of an appropriate agent has become increasingly difficult.[80] Older oral drugs, such as chloramphenicol and tetracycline, and trimethoprim-sulfamethoxazole and ampicillin, until recently the drugs of choice for shigellosis, are no longer first-line choices because of drug resistance (***Fig. 18.10***).[81] Some agents effective *in vitro*, such as oral extended-spectrum cephalosporins (e.g., cefixime), are ineffective *in vivo*.[82] Older nonabsorbable agents, such as furazolidone, are ineffective, despite advertising claims to the contrary. A newer nonabsorbable agent, rifamixin, has been shown to be effective when given prophylactically to prevent illness in human challenge experiments with *S. flexneri*. If safe and useful for established infection and substantiated in field trials, rifamixin may become another option for multidrug-resistant infections.[83]

Unfortunately, current options for treating *Shigella* infections in developing countries are limited and recommendations are subject to change as drug resistance develops (***Table 18.1***). Nalidixic acid, previously useful against multiresistant strains, is no longer reliable because of increasing resistance.[84] Newer fluoroquinolones, such as ciprofloxacin, the macrolide azithromycin, and the β-lactam pivamdinocillin, remain effective,[85,86] although emerging resistance to ciprofloxacin and azithromycin is of concern.[87,88] Short course (3-day) ciprofloxacin is proven effective, and reduces the cost of treatment.[89] The parenteral agent ceftriaxone is also effective, even when given for just 2 days.[90] The major constraints currently are cost and the need for parenteral administration, which precludes its use at the community level. It is a good initial option for individuals with severe illness treated in health care facilities wherever multidrug resistance is common. Unfortunately, ceftriaxone resistance is also beginning to emerge.[91] Depending on the drug, a course of treatment in Bangladesh can cost the equivalent of 1 day to 3 weeks' earnings for the poorest, those with an income less than US$1 per day.

If empiric antimicrobial treatment for severe shigellosis does not result in clinical improvement within 48 hours, infection with a drug-resistant strain or another organism should be considered, and therapy modified. It is essential to know local drug resistance patterns to devise an empirical strategy for first- and second-line drugs. This necessitates a surveillance system and adequate laboratory capacity, neither of which may be available in developing countries.

Because patients with shigellosis are rarely severely dehydrated, intravenous rehydration is not necessary. There are no contraindications to

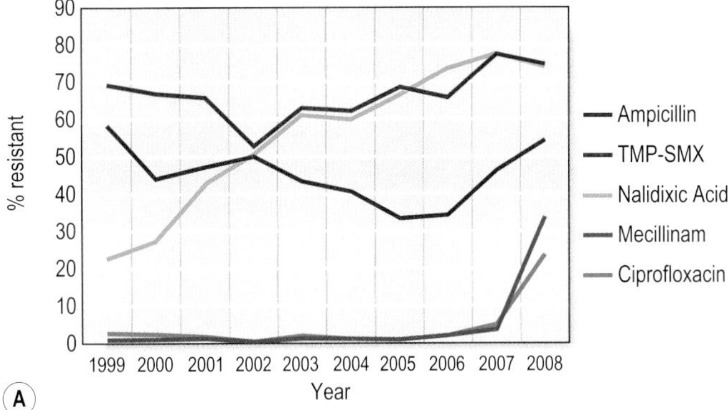

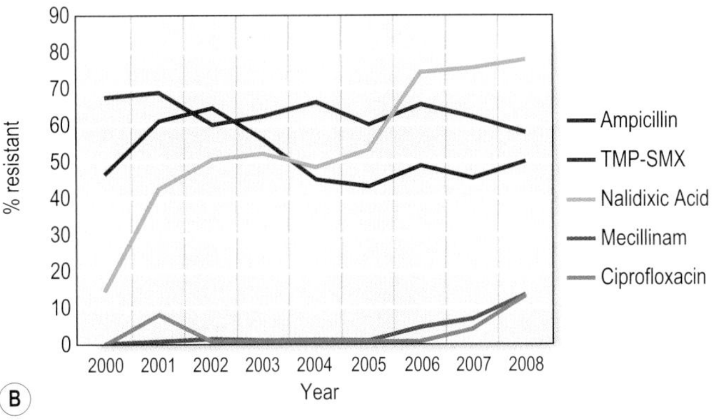

Figure 18.10 Antimicrobial sensitivity of strains isolated in Dhaka (urban) and Matlab (rural) Bangladesh. These isolates were obtained through a 2% systematic surveillance of patients seen at the ICDDR,B Hospital in Dhaka, Bangladesh **(A)** and from the culture of all patients seen at the Matlab Hospital **(B)**. Over the past decade, more than 70% of strains have become resistant to nalidixic acid, more than 60% to trimethoprim-sulfamethoxazole, and 30–60% of strains to ampicillin. Of concern is the recent emergence of resistance to mecillinam and ciprofloxacin. (Source: ICDDR, B.)

Table 18.1 Current Antimicrobial Agents for Treatment of Shigellosis in Tropical Countries

Agent	Adult Dose	Pediatric Dose[a]	Frequency	Duration	Total Treatment Cost in Dhaka[b] (Pediatric/Adult)
Pivamdinocillin[c]	400 mg	20 mg/kg	4 times daily	5 days	US$3.50/7.00
Ciprofloxacin	500 mg	10 mg/kg	Twice daily	3 days[d]	US$1.30/1.30
Azithromycin	500 mg on day 1, 250 mg/day thereafter	10 mg/kg on day 1, 5 mg/kg thereafter	Once daily	5 days	US$2.50/1.75[e]
Ceftriaxone	2 g	100 mg/kg	Once daily	5 days	US$11–14/18–22
Trimethoprim and Sulfamethoxazole	160 mg / 800 mg	4 mg/kg / 20 mg/kg	Twice daily	5 days	Most *S. dysenteriae* type 1 and *S. flexneri* strains are resistant. May still be useful for *S. sonnei* if drug resistance is limited
Ampicillin	500 mg	25 mg/kg	4 times daily	5 days	Most *S. dysenteriae* type 1 and *S. flexneri* strains are resistant. May still be useful for *S. sonnei* if drug resistance is limited

[a]Maximum pediatric dose is the adult dose.
[b]Calculated on the basis of packaged drugs in Dhaka, and for a 10 kg child.
[c]Not available in many countries, including the United States.
[d]Prolonged use in children is contraindicated because of risk of arthritis. This is not an issue for treatment of acute shigellosis.
[e]Because of the packaging of pediatric formulation of azithromycin, it costs more to purchase a pediatric course of treatment than a full course for an adult.

ORT, and it is useful to manage mild-moderate dehydration that may occur. Severe hyponatremia, a serious complication, can be treated with either intravenous normal saline or a bolus of 3% NaCl; close clinical monitoring is required. Increasing serum sodium concentration by 6–8 mmol/L in 24 hours is considered safe.[92] Patients with shigellosis should be fed to the extent they are willing to eat (breast milk or solid foods, depending on age) to prevent hypoglycemia and malnutrition. Anorexia responds to effective antimicrobial therapy.[93] Restoration of nutritional status is most rapidly achieved if sufficient calories and high-quality protein are provided during convalescence; however, it takes considerably longer to replenish nutrient stores than it does to create the deficit during infection. Parents of a child recovering from shigellosis must be encouraged to feed their child more than normal during convalescence until satisfactory weight gain has occurred. This may be difficult in settings of poverty and food insecurity.

Treatment of complications is largely supportive. Patients with seizures do not need anticonvulsant therapy, since more than one seizure is uncommon. HUS may require transfusion and peritoneal dialysis; however, mortality from *S. dysenteriae*-associated HUS remains higher than observed in HUS due to other etiologies,[94,95] perhaps because the disease is more severe, the host is more malnourished, or because facilities for managing this complication are limited where *S. dysenteriae* type 1 outbreaks occur. Toxic megacolon due to transmural colitis and microvascular thrombosis is an ominous complication, with mortality rates as high as 50%. Colectomy can be lifesaving but often not feasible in developing countries, because complex postoperative support is unavailable and subsequent long-term care for a child with a colectomy is difficult to ensure. Conservative management with antibiotics, fluids, nasogastric suction, and limited surgical intervention if intestinal perforation occurs – with or without megacolon – may be the better strategy.[96,97] Rectal prolapse resolves on its own as the inflammation wanes; in the interim, the prolapsed tissues should be kept moist and protected against injury. Suspected bacteremia should be treated with parenteral, broad-spectrum antibiotics.

PREVENTION AND CONTROL

Because of the low inoculum and person-to-person transmission, the primary method of preventing shigellosis remains good personal hygiene,[98,99] although access to potable water and sanitary disposal of feces is often lacking where the disease is most prevalent. Caretakers of children should be encouraged to wash their hands after contact with stool or soiled clothes, and always before preparing food. Handwashing with soap is preferred, but if unavailable then traditional practices using sand or ash, or even with water alone, are better than not washing at all. In addition to resistance to change of established behaviors, the lack of water in or near the household is a major handicap. Where open defecation is practiced, simple fly control can reduce the prevalence of *Shigella* infection.[100]

While immunization could have significant impact, it has proved difficult to develop safe and effective *Shigella* vaccines, in part because the mechanisms of protective immunity remain unclear and because there are many antigenically distinct serotypes involved.[101] Pioneering early vaccine studies demonstrated that protective immunity against shigellosis is serotype-specific.[102] Experimental human shigellosis models support this concept, as prior infection is highly protective against reinfection with the same species and serotype.[103,104] Because traditional parenteral killed vaccines have been ineffective,[105] attention has shifted to alternative approaches, including oral immunization with live attenuated *Shigella*[106] or *Salmonella* Typhi expressing *Shigella* O-antigens,[107] isolated *Shigella* cell surface components,[108] or parenteral O-polysaccharide-protein conjugates.[109] A limited multivalent vaccine of the most common serotypes would be very useful. To date, no acceptably safe and sufficiently effective vaccine has been developed; too often the most immunogenic vaccines have been the most reactogenic, while other vaccine approaches with acceptable reactogenicity have not been very immunogenic. The lack of a good animal model of shigellosis has also limited *Shigella* vaccine development. Finally, despite the lack of success thus far, the search for common protective component(s) for a serotype-independent vaccine should not be abandoned.

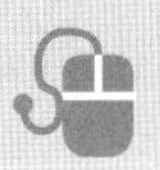

Access the complete reference list online at
http://www.expertconsult.com

Access the complete reference list online at http://www.expertconsult.com

CHAPTER 19

Campylobacter Infections

Ban Mishu Allos • Albert J. Lastovica

INTRODUCTION

Campylobacters are bacteria that often produce an acute gastrointestinal illness. Infections with these organisms occur in every part of the world, including arctic, temperate, and tropical climates.[1] In developing countries, especially those in tropical areas, they are hyperendemic and important causes of morbidity and possibly mortality in young children. *Campylobacter* infections also are an important cause of diarrhea in persons residing in developed countries who travel to developing countries in the tropics.[2,3]

THE AGENT

Campylobacter species are microaerophilic, comma-shaped, Gram-negative rods that were first recognized as causes of infectious abortion in animals in the early twentieth century[4] and later were determined also to cause infectious abortion in women.[5] Over the next decades, the organisms were reported to cause bacteremia, meningitis, endocarditis, and abscesses in immunocompromised patients.[6,7] A group of related organisms also were isolated from the blood of patients with diarrhea.[8] During the last three decades of the twentieth century, campylobacters were recognized as one of the most common bacterial causes of diarrhea worldwide.

Although the organisms were first called *Vibrio*, they were assigned to a new genus, *Campylobacter*, in 1973;[9] this scheme was later modified so that the opportunistic organism was called *Campylobacter fetus*, and the related vibrios were called *C. jejuni* and *C. coli*.[10] In 2000, the complete genome of *C. jejuni* was sequenced.[11]

Currently the whole genome sequences for eight *Campylobacter* species have been determined.[12] The use of filtration with antibiotic-free culture systems[13] and other newer techniques[14,15] have led to the recognition that many other "atypical" species of *Campylobacter* and closely related genera also may produce human disease[16] (***Table 19.1***). Such species include *C. fetus*, *C. concisus*, *C. curvus*, *C. lari*, *C. insulaenigrae*,[17] *C. jejuni* subsp. *doylei*, *C. rectus*, *C. sputorum*, *C. upsaliensis*, *Helicobacter cinaedi*, *Helicobacter fennelliae*, *Arcobacter butzleri*, *Arcobacter cryaerophila*, and *C. hyointestinalis*. New pathogenic species of *Campylobacter* are being identified with some regularity.

In tropical countries such as South Africa, such "atypical" campylobacters comprise more than 50% of the *Campylobacter* species isolated.[18–20] In contrast, in the United States and other developed nations, *C. jejuni* accounts for greater than 95% of *Campylobacter* species isolated.[21] Other studies of *Campylobacter*, in Thailand,[22] Hong Kong,[23] and the Central African Republic,[24] show a higher incidence of *C. coli* relative to that seen in industrialized nations. However, since methods designed to optimize detection of *C. jejuni* might not support growth of other species, the contribution of these organisms to the burden of human disease may be underestimated. An efficient isolation and identification protocol for all species of *Campylobacter* and the related genera *Helicobacter* and *Arcobacter* has been developed.[20]

Campylobacters grow best at the body temperatures of warm-blooded animals. Optimal growth for *C. jejuni* is at 42°C at which campylobacters will survive only a few days, but at 4°C they can persist for weeks in substances such as water, feces, urine, or milk.[25] Similarly, the organism may flourish and grow in an alkaline environment but will not last 5 minutes at pH less than 2.3.[25]

EPIDEMIOLOGY

The epidemiology of *Campylobacter* infections is markedly different in tropical developing countries than in the developed world (***Table 19.2***). Infections are hyperendemic among young children. In tropical countries such as Bangladesh, South Africa, The Gambia, Zaire, India, Australia, Indonesia, and China, the rate of isolation of *Campylobacter* is greatest in infants and declines with age.[26] Although national surveillance programs for campylobacteriosis do not exist in developing countries, estimates from laboratory-based surveillance suggest that the incidence of this infection among children less than 5 years of age may be more than 100 times higher than the rate among children in developed nations.[27] Campylobacters frequently can be isolated from asymptomatic children and adults in developing countries.[28] In contrast, in developed countries, infection is almost always recognized in association with illness, recognized asymptomatic infections are uncommon, and young children are not at greatest risk.

In the developing nations mentioned previously, breastfed children are usually protected, but a high rate of infection with concomitant watery diarrhea is observed after they are weaned.[29] In addition to early weaning, close proximity to animals and lack of toilets are important risk factors for the development of early-childhood diarrheal illnesses in general, and those caused by *Campylobacter* in particular.[27,30] The apparent absence of multiple infections within a household[31] suggests that person-to-person transmission is not an important mode of spread, even in developing countries. Infections in adults and older children usually are asymptomatic and durations of excretion are short, suggesting that acquired immunity is protective. The importance of acquired protective immunity is further supported by studies in developing countries showing that rising serum antibodies to *Campylobacter* are associated with a lower rate of infection.[32,33]

Outbreaks of *Campylobacter* infection, which occur regularly in developed countries, do not occur in developing countries because of this high level of immunity. Campylobacters are ubiquitous in the environment in tropical climates and infections occur year-round. The late summer and early fall peak in the incidence of *Campylobacter* infections observed in temperate climates is not seen in tropical countries.[26,28,34]

Table 19.1 Clinical and Epidemiologic Features Associated with "Atypical" Campylobacters and Related Organisms

Species	Clinical Presentation	Epidemiological Data
C. coli	Fever, diarrhea, abdominal pain	Clinically and epidemiologically similar to *C. jejuni*
C. fetus	Bacteremia, sepsis, meningitis, vascular infection, abortion	Found in healthy sheep and cattle; may cause spontaneous abortion and infertility
C. hyointestinalis	Watery or bloody diarrhea, vomiting, abdominal pain	Causes proliferative enteritis in swine
C. insulaenigrae	Enteritis, bacteremia	Isolated from healthy seals and a porpoise
C. jejuni subsp. *doylei*	Diarrhea, bacteremia	Increasing evidence as a human pathogen
C. lari	Abdominal pain, diarrhea	Seagulls colonized; transmitted to humans via contaminated water
C. sputorum	Pulmonary, axillary, groin and perianal abscesses	Has been isolated from dairy cows
C. upsaliensis	Watery diarrhea, low-grade fever, abdominal pain, bacteremia, occasionally abortion, abscesses	Found in dogs, cats; may have autumn seasonality in tropical countries
H_2-requiring campylobacters[a]	Periodontitis, diarrhea, rarely bacteremia	Role as a human pathogen not established
Helicobacter cinaedi, H. fennelliae	Chronic mild diarrhea, proctitis, abdominal cramps, bacteremia	Increased in homosexual men and in children in developing countries; may cause bacteremia in HIV+ hosts
H. pullorum	Rare human pathogen, occasionally associated with diarrhea, rarely bacteremia	Isolated from asymptomatic hens and from hens with hepatitis
H. rappini	Gastroenteritis; a few reports document bacteremia	Animal reservoir not known
Arcobacter butzleri	Fever, diarrhea, abdominal pain, nausea, rarely bacteremia	Enzootic in human primates
Arcobacter cryaerophilia	Diarrhea, rarely bacteremia	Isolated from mussels in brackish water

[a]Includes *C. retus*, *C. curvus*, and *C. concisus*.

Table 19.2 Clinical and Epidemiologic Characteristics of Campylobacter Infections in Developed Versus Tropical Developing Countries

Characteristic	Developed Countries	Developing Countries
Peak age group affected	15–29 years	<2 years
Endemicity of infection	Endemic	Hyperendemic
Occurrence of outbreaks	Common	Rare
Seasonality	Summer and fall peaks	Year-round
Predominant mode of transmission	Food-borne	Uncertain
Clinical expression	Inflammatory	Noninflammatory
Asymptomatic infection	Uncommon	Usual
Nature of diarrhea	Inflammatory[a]	Watery
Abdominal cramps	Common	Rare
Bacterial load in stools of infected persons	High	Low
Presence of immunity in typical adult	No	Yes

[a]Stools frequently contain gross or occult blood, and leukocytes.

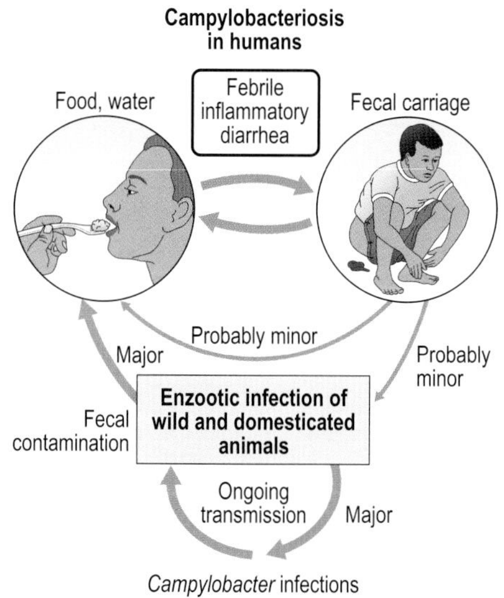

Figure 19.1 *Campylobacter* infections life cycle.

Although rotavirus, enterotoxigenic *Escherichia coli*, and *Shigella* infections are more common than *Campylobacter* as causes of diarrhea in tropical countries,[30,35,36] campylobacters are among the most common bacterial cause of community-acquired diarrhea in developed countries.[37–39] However, even in developing countries, *Campylobacter* infections are increasing and in some areas surpassing *Shigella* and *E. coli* as causes of diarrhea.[40] Furthermore, the prevalence of *Campylobacter* infections is higher in tropical climates than in cooler ones. Even among healthy, asymptomatic children in countries such as Bangladesh, South Africa, The Gambia, and Central African Republic, *Campylobacter* may be isolated from 10% to 40% of children from a single culture.[28,31,41–43] *Campylobacter* infection is one of the most common causes of diarrhea among travelers to developing countries[44] and in Thailand is the most common cause.[33,45]

Most human infections with *Campylobacter* in developing countries occur because of consumption of or exposure to animals or their products (***Fig. 19.1***). Campylobacters live as commensals in the gastrointestinal tract of a variety of animals, especially avian species. Not surprisingly, campylobacters are frequently isolated from poultry and other animals in developing countries,[46–51] but the extent of the contribution of this source to human illness has not been determined.[52] Interestingly, even in developed nations, the incidence of infection in rural areas is higher, similar to patterns observed in developing nations.[53] In Africa, campylobacters also have been isolated from surface domestic water sources used for human consumption[54] and from dairy products.[55] The main vehicles of human infection in developed countries are water, milk, raw meat, and most importantly, poultry. Person-to-person transmission of *Campylobacter* is infrequent in both developed and developing countries.

THE DISEASE

In developing countries, the clinical consequences of infection with *Campylobacter* differ from those seen in the developed world. When children in tropical settings develop diarrhea as a result of *Campylobacter* infection, it frequently is watery and there usually is little or no evidence of an inflammatory process.[56] Although symptomatic infection is most likely to occur during the first few months and years of life, asymptomatic infections outnumber symptomatic ones by 2 to 1, even among children less than 5 years of age.[57] Infection among children in tropical countries is quite common; more than two infections per year are likely during the first 5 years of life.[31,57] Among young children in Bangladesh, the estimated rate is eight *Campylobacter* infections per year.[28]

In developed areas, *Campylobacter* infections usually produce an acute gastrointestinal illness that is indistinguishable from illness caused by other "inflammatory" enteric bacteria such as *Salmonella* and *Shigella*. Illness usually begins abruptly with abdominal cramps and diarrhea. Children in developing countries who develop symptomatic *Campylobacter* infection also typically experience loose stools with mucus, along with fever and vomiting.[58] However, although half of *Campylobacter*-infected patients presenting for medical attention in developed countries have bloody diarrhea,[37] in tropical climates the diarrhea usually does not contain blood. Less than one-third of *Campylobacter*-infected children in Thailand have bloody stools; most have mucoid stools that are neither watery nor bloody; about one-third have watery diarrhea.[22,58] *Campylobacter* infections among persons living in tropical areas also are less likely to produce abdominal cramps.[28] The illness usually resolves within 1 to 2 weeks; about 20% of patients will have relapsing symptoms lasting several weeks. Although *Campylobacter* infections occur frequently in HIV-infected persons residing in developed countries,[59] a similar phenomenon is not always observed in developing nations.[60–62]

Complications of *Campylobacter* infections are rare and usually the result of local invasion. Massive gastrointestinal hemorrhage may occur. Other complications include cholecystitis, pancreatitis, obstructive hepatitis, and splenic rupture.[63–66] Neonatal sepsis and death can occur if the mother is infected during the third trimester.[67] Extraintestinal complications of *Campylobacter* infections are rare[68] but are more common in malnourished children. Such complications include bacteremia, meningitis, and purulent arthritis. *C. jejuni*, *C. upsaliensis*, and other *Campylobacter* species have been associated with pediatric bacteremia.[20] Infection may lead to fulminant sepsis and death. The postinfection complication, Guillain–Barré syndrome (GBS), occurs at an estimated rate of 1 per 2000 infections.[69] A particularly severe form of GBS, acute motor axonal neuropathy, occurs in seasonal epidemics among children in rural China and also may be associated with preceding *C. jejuni* infection.[70] Reactive arthritis also may occur after *Campylobacter* infection and is most common in persons who carry the HLA-B27 phenotype.[71–73] *C. jejuni* was recently implicated as a cause of immunoproliferative small intestine disease (a form of lymphoma) in a 45-year-old woman in Cameroon.[74]

In patients in developed countries, the pathologic lesion of *Campylobacter* enteritis is infiltration of the lamina propria with acute and chronic inflammatory cells and destruction of epithelial glands with crypt abscess formation.[75] The site of tissue injury is usually the jejunum, ileum, and colon.[75,76] This nonspecific colitis may be indistinguishable from ulcerative colitis or Crohn's disease; hence the importance of diagnosing this treatable infection before immunosuppressive therapy is given for inflammatory bowel disease. The pathology of *Campylobacter* enteritis among patients in tropical and developing countries has not been well described but, based on the clinical presentation, is presumably milder.

PATHOGENESIS AND IMMUNITY

Three factors important in the ability of *Campylobacter* to produce illness include the dose of organisms reaching the small intestine, the host's immunity to the organism, and the virulence of the particular strain. Infection leads to multiplication of the organism in the intestine. The number of bacterial cells required to cause illness is unknown, but a high dose is likely needed to infect 50% of subjects.[77] In general, the higher the inoculum, the shorter the incubation period (usually 1 day to 1 week) and the higher the attack rate.

In developed countries, *Campylobacter*-infected persons shed between 10^6 and 10^9 colony-forming units per gram of stool.[25] However, the intestinal bacterial load is lower among similarly infected persons in developing nations.[32] Furthermore, in developing areas, the duration and number of organisms excreted are highest in infants and decline with age, also consistent with increasing acquisition of immunity.[58]

Characteristics of campylobacters that enable them to adhere to and invade intestinal cells include the presence of flagella, high molecular-weight plasmids, superficial adhesins, fimbriae, and chemotactic factors.[77–85] Campylobacters must be flagellated to colonize, invade, and cause disease.[86] *In vivo* studies have demonstrated that flagella synthesis genes are needed for maximal *C. jejuni* invasiveness.[87,88] Although the bacteria do not possess fimbriae per se, fimbriae-like filaments enable the organisms to attach to epithelial cells.[89] Additionally, several *C. jejuni* surface proteins (e.g., PEB1, CadF) appear to function in attachment and subsequent colonization and invasion.[89] Invasion of epithelial cells by *C. jejuni* results in cellular injury and, ultimately, in diarrhea. The mechanism of invasion is complex and not completely understood.[90]

Despite early reports to the contrary,[91] the low level of enterotoxin production that occasionally has been observed *in vitro* does not appear to be important in the pathogenesis of *Campylobacter* infections.[85,92] Enterotoxin production cannot be demonstrated *in vivo*, and infected patients do not form antibodies against enterotoxin.[93] All *C. jejuni* isolates possess a gene that codes for cytolethal distending toxin; however, not all isolates produce this toxin, and its role in causing disease is not established.[94] Some have suggested the toxin may play a role in pathogenesis by inducing death of macrophages, thus suppressing innate immunity.[95,96] Specific immunity to *Campylobacter* may be acquired and plays a crucial role in curtailing disease severity. In developing countries where these infections are hyperendemic, infection and illness rates decline with age, again suggesting the acquisition of immunity. Volunteer studies also have shown that short-term specific immunity to *Campylobacter* occurs.[77,97] Humoral immunity appears to play an important role in containing *Campylobacter* infection. After infection, serum antibodies (IgA, IgG, and IgM) peak in 2–4 weeks, then rapidly decline.[98] The importance of humoral immunity is further supported by studies showing that in hypogammaglobulinemic patients, *Campylobacter* infections are severe, prolonged, and difficult to eradicate.[99] Children in tropical settings develop steadily rising serum IgA antibodies to *Campylobacter*. Once these high levels are achieved, IgG levels, which also rise through early childhood, begin to decline.[58,100,101] These data suggest that frequent exposure to *Campylobacter* leads to the development of solid "gut immunity," which precludes sensitization of IgG-producing cells. Such gut immunity correlates well with the declining incidence of infection with age, the lower proportion of infections that are symptomatic, and the reduced bacterial level and duration of excretion.[58] Recent studies showed that campylobacters induced maturation and cytokine production in dendritic cells, indicating that these bacteria elicit innate immune responses.[102]

Persons with human immunodeficiency virus (HIV) infection have more frequent, persistent, severe, and extraintestinal *Campylobacter* infections than the general population in developed nations.[103,104] Although these observations could suggest that cellular immunity also plays an important role in protection against *Campylobacter*, many such patients have defects in humoral responses as well.

Serum killing of *Campylobacter* species occurs via complement-mediated bactericidal activity.[105] This could explain why bacteremia due to *Campylobacter* species is uncommon except in immunodeficient persons, or is due to the serum-resistant *C. fetus*.[105] Serum-resistant campylobacters have been isolated from the cerebrospinal fluid of patients with meningitis.[106]

DIAGNOSIS

In developing countries, the simplest and most inexpensive method for diagnosis of *Campylobacter* infection is direct examination of stools after Gram or Wright staining. Stools also can be directly examined for the presence of white blood cells or lactoferrin and erythrocytes, which are nonspecific findings associated with inflammatory agents but which also suggest the presence of a bacterial enteric pathogen, such as *Campylobacter*.

The gold standard for detection of *Campylobacter* infection is culture of the organism from stool, blood, or other site of infection. Because *Campylobacter* infection cannot be differentiated from infections due to other bacterial enteric pathogens on clinical grounds, isolation of the organism using a selective technique is the only way to make the diagnosis with certainty. Cephalothin-containing selective media will suppress most fecal flora while permitting the growth of most *C. jejuni* strains. However, some *Campylobacter* species (and even a few *C. jejuni* strains) are cephalothin-susceptible, and must be isolated on less selective media or on antibiotic-free media after filtration of the stool sample.[20] In tropical countries, many patients may have mixed infections with *Campylobacter* and other enteric pathogens.[22,58] In addition, several species of *Campylobacter* and related species may be co-isolated from the same clinical sample.[20] Therefore, the precise contribution of *Campylobacter* infection to these children's illnesses may be difficult to assess.

Campylobacter infection also may be mistaken for inflammatory bowel disease. *Campylobacter* enterocolitis may produce crypt abscesses (which are frequent in ulcerative colitis) and granulomas (which are common in Crohn's disease).[75,76,107] Persons suspected of having inflammatory bowel disease should have cultures for several different *Campylobacter* species performed as part of their diagnostic workup.

Serologic testing occasionally may be useful for detecting recent *Campylobacter* infection.[105,108] However, this technique is unlikely to be helpful in tropical developing countries where infection is hyperendemic and background infection rates are high. Polymerase chain reaction (PCR) to detect *Campylobacter* in stools is beginning to be used in some clinical laboratories in developed nations.[109,110] However, the clinical significance of a positive PCR assay in a patient in a developing country might be difficult to interpret and the costs associated with such testing preclude wide usage.

TREATMENT AND PROGNOSIS

Antimicrobial treatment of *Campylobacter* infections, if initiated early in the illness, reduces the duration of bacterial excretion in stools.[111,112] However, most patients with *Campylobacter* enteritis, and certainly those with asymptomatic or mild infection, do not need antimicrobial therapy. Even patients whose symptoms lead them to seek medical care may not require measures other than encouragement to keep well hydrated. Occasionally, intravenous fluids are needed, especially in the very young and very old. In developing countries, oral hydration solutions are the best method of maintaining fluid and electrolyte balance, unless volume depletion is severe. The prognosis for most patients with *Campylobacter* infection is favorable; symptoms usually resolve within 1 week without antimicrobial therapy.

Antibiotics should be given to *Campylobacter*-infected patients in certain high-risk groups or clinical circumstances. Because *Campylobacter* infection may have deleterious effects on the fetus, pregnant women should receive prompt therapy.[67] Similarly, HIV-infected or other immunocompromised patients should receive antibiotics. With the expanding HIV epidemic in developing countries, extraintestinal infection will be increasingly common. Immunocompetent persons with fever greater than 38.3°C (101°F), bloody stools, symptoms lasting more than 1 week, or worsening symptoms also may benefit from antimicrobial therapy.

Campylobacters are susceptible to a wide variety of antimicrobial agents, including macrolides, quinolones, nitrofurans, and aminoglycosides. Care should be taken before prescribing tetracycline because more than 20% of campylobacters are resistant.[113,114] Susceptibility to ampicillin, metronidazole, and trimethoprim-sulfamethoxazole is variable. There is almost universal resistance of *Campylobacter* to cephalosporins, penicillin, vancomycin, and rifampin.

Erythromycin remains the treatment of choice for most patients with infections due to *Campylobacter*. Erythromycin has low toxicity, has a relatively narrow spectrum of activity, and is inexpensive. Because erythromycin stearate is incompletely absorbed, it can exert a local effect throughout the bowel, in addition to its systemic effects. In most developed countries, the rate of erythromycin resistance among *Campylobacter* species has remained under 10%.[115–117] Higher rates of resistance have been reported from developing countries, such as Thailand,[35] but resistance remains low in other countries, such as India and Kenya.[118,119] The rate of erythromycin resistance is substantially higher among *C. coli* strains.[114,120–122] The newer macrolides, azithromycin and clarithromycin, have excellent activity against *Campylobacter*.[123–126] Although they achieve higher concentrations in tissue, they provide little clinical advantage over erythromycin and are considerably more expensive. Strains resistant to erythromycin also will be resistant to these newer macrolides. The activity of clindamycin against *C. jejuni* is equivalent to that of erythromycin.

At one time, it appeared that quinolones, such as ciprofloxacin, had emerged as the treatment of choice for bacterial diarrhea in general and for *Campylobacter* enteritis in particular.[127] Unfortunately, rapidly emerging resistance of campylobacters to quinolones in tropical regions and in other parts of the world has limited their effectiveness.[112,128,129] Widespread use of fluoroquinolones in poultry has led to the transfer of antibiotic-resistant strains to humans.[130,131] Nalidixic acid resistance commonly but not invariably crosses with resistance to ciprofloxacin.[114] Resistance to this agent has paralleled the increasing resistance to fluoroquinolones.

In special circumstances when therapy is required, and when a patient is intolerant of many agents or when a strain has an unusual antibiotic resistance pattern, alternative agents such as chloramphenicol may be used; nearly all campylobacters are susceptible to chloramphenicol.[114,132] This agent is especially useful in tropical developing countries because of its low cost. For persons with bacteremia and other extraintestinal suppurative infections, gentamicin and imipenem are active against campylobacters and the rate of resistance to these agents is less than 1%. Gentamicin is ineffective against *Campylobacter* in the gut; therefore, oral therapy with an effective, absorbable drug also must be given.

PREVENTION AND CONTROL

Campylobacters are so ubiquitous in the environment of most tropical developing nations that there is no possibility of reducing the reservoirs of infection. Rather, prevention must focus on interrupting the path of transmission to humans from animals, animal products, or environmental sources contaminated by animals or humans. Poultry, livestock, pets, and wild animals are the major reservoirs. Therefore, as for many bacterial enteric pathogens, a basic tenet of prevention is adequate hand washing; this is especially important in tropical areas for people who handle animals and food within a household. Especially important is the awareness of the necessity for proper cooking and storage of foods of animal origin.

The safe disposal of sewage and the protection and purification of water supplies also are fundamental to control of most diseases due to enteric pathogens, including *Campylobacter*. Programs to improve water safety in developing countries may impact the number of infections.[133] Excreta from sheep, cattle, and wild and domestic birds should not be allowed to contaminate a community's water supplies. Chlorination reliably inactivates *Campylobacter*.[134]

Control of *Campylobacter* infections in developing countries will likely be difficult unless an effective vaccine is developed. Because of the diversity of serotypes of *C. jejuni*, the possibility of vaccination for prevention of infection must be based on group antigens. Since *Campylobacter* infection of humans is "accidental" given that humans are not required for completion of their life cycle, the natural acquisition of immunity in developing countries and the identification of group antigens suggest that vaccination will be feasible. There is no proven benefit of antibiotic prophylaxis to prevent *Campylobacter* infection in travelers to tropical and subtropical environments.

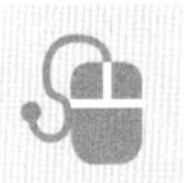

Access the complete reference list online at
http://www.expertconsult.com

CHAPTER 20

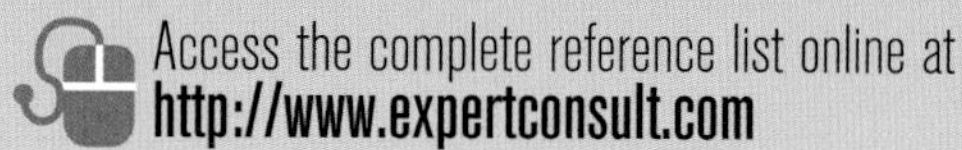
Access the complete reference list online at
http://www.expertconsult.com

Cholera Infections

Myron M. Levine • Debasish Saha • A.S.G. Faruque • Samba O. Sow

INTRODUCTION

Cholera is a diarrheal illness caused by *Vibrio cholerae* O1 (and less often by serogroup O139), which in its severe form, cholera gravis, can rapidly and fatally dehydrate adults as well as children. Besides its clinical severity in the individual patient, cholera is one of the few bacterial diseases that is capable of true pandemic spread. Since 1961, when the seventh pandemic caused by *V. cholerae* O1 biotype El Tor began on the island of Sulawesi, El Tor cholera has progressively extended to involve all the inhabited continents. Since cholera is spread by contaminated water and food vehicles, its transmission is facilitated wherever populations are not served by treated water supplies and sanitation.

Several events in the last decade of the twentieth century and the first decade of the twenty-first century exemplify the epidemiologic and clinical importance of cholera and demonstrate why it commands special attention:

1. The return of cholera to Latin America in 1991, after a century of absence, and its rapid dissemination, leading to more than 1 million cases by 1994;[1]
2. The explosive outbreak of El Tor cholera in Rwandan refugees in Goma, Zaire, resulting in ~70 000 cases and 12 000 deaths in July 1994;[2,3]
3. The appearance in 1992–1993 of epidemic cholera in the Indian subcontinent caused, for the first time, by a *V. cholerae* serogroup other than O1, so-called O139 Bengal;[4,5]
4. An enormous epidemic of cholera in Zimbabwe in 2008–2009 (estimated at >92 000, with >4000 deaths) that exposed glaring deteriorations in that country's water and sanitation infrastructure and inability of its health care delivery system to respond effectively to an epidemic.[6,7]

THE AGENT

Medical historians debate whether cholera existed in ancient populations in the Indian subcontinent and the Middle East, but since 1817 at least seven distinct pandemics of cholera have occurred. The first six pandemics originated in the Ganges delta, from where they spread across several continents.

During the third and fourth pandemics, John Snow made hallmark descriptions of the epidemiology of cholera in London, suggesting that it was a contagion and incriminating its spread via sewage-contaminated municipal water,[8] insights made several decades before Robert Koch isolated the causative bacterium in Egypt in 1883, during the fifth pandemic.[9]

In the 1950s, S.N. De in India demonstrated that cell-free supernatants of *V. cholerae* caused fluid accumulation in isolated loops of rabbit intestine, thereby implying the existence of an enterotoxin.[10] In the late 1960s, cholera enterotoxin (CT) was purified to homogeneity and shown to be composed of two different types of subunits noncovalently linked.[11] Also in the late 1960s, oral glucose/electrolyte solutions were shown to be effective in rehydrating patients with mild and moderate cholera, a clinical breakthrough that eventually revolutionized the therapy of diarrheal dehydration of all etiologies.[12]

V. cholerae, a motile Gram-negative facultative anaerobe with a unipolar flagellum, prefers alkaline (pH 6–10), brackish (elevated sodium) environments. This chitinase-producing species comprises part of the autochthonous flora of brackish water environments, where it is closely associated with zooplankton and other fauna having chitinous exoskeletons.[13] *V. cholerae* is a well-defined species based on biochemical tests and DNA homology studies,[14] but one that is not homogeneous with regard to the potential to cause epidemic human disease. Taxonomists currently recognize more than 200 serogroups of *V. cholerae*. Within the species, an important discrimination exists among strains with respect to the production of cholera enterotoxin, O serogroup, and the potential for epidemic spread. Prior to 1992, only enterotoxigenic *V. cholerae* within the O1 serogroup were recognized as the etiologic agents of endemic and epidemic cholera. Within the O1 serogroup, there exist two main serotypes, Inaba and Ogawa, and two biotypes, classical and El Tor.[14] Whereas either biotype can cause the spectrum of clinical manifestations from asymptomatic infection to cholera gravis, the ratio of mild to severe cases is higher for the El Tor biotype. Characteristics that differentiate the El Tor biotype include a resistance to polymyxin B, ability to agglutinate chicken erythrocytes, and a susceptibility to specific typing phages. El Tor tends to be much hardier than classical biotype and survives better in the environment and in the human intestine. Even as *V. cholerae* El Tor progressively spread to involve multiple continents, classical biotype *V. cholerae* persisted in the Ganges delta, along with El Tor, throughout much of the first two decades of the pandemic. Despite the disappearance of classical biotype vibrios in the 1990s as a cause of endemic or epidemic cholera, the genetic legacy of classical biotype persists as early in the twenty-first century in Mozambique and India El Tor variant strains came to be recognized that carry phages encoding classical cholera toxin.[15]

V. cholerae O1 strains can shift between Inaba and Ogawa, with the change more often going from Ogawa to Inaba. DNA sequence analysis of genes (rfb) encoding the O1 antigen reveals that the sequences for Inaba and Ogawa antigens are almost identical and that some serotype shifts are the consequence of minor alterations in the sequence of rfbT.[16,17]

Beginning in late 1992, large-scale epidemics of typical clinical cholera caused by a serogroup other than O1 were reported in India and Bangladesh,[4,5] marking the first time that epidemic disease was attributed to another serogroup. Molecular analysis of the causative agent, O139 Bengal, reveals that it possesses the identical virulence attributes and other characteristics as *V. cholerae* El Tor (e.g., sequences encoding El Tor cholera toxin and toxin coregulated pili, resistance to polymyxin).[14] It appears that the epidemic O139 strain was derived by a deletion event in the genes that encode O1 of an El Tor strain followed by the acquisition of a large fragment of new DNA encoding O139. During 1993, O139 spread to Thailand, Burma, Pakistan, and China, and importations were also reported in the United States and United Kingdom. At the time, it was feared that these epidemiologic events might be the harbingers of an eighth cholera pandemic with O139 as the etiologic agent. However, in 1995 and 1996 the incidence of O139 diminished in the Indian subcontinent and this serogroup disappeared from several countries that it had invaded in the previous 2 years. Since O139 disease has become endemic in Bengal, health authorities for the past decade have maintained surveillance to see whether O139 disease resurges and spreads to other continents in pandemic form.

Other O1 and O139 strains do not produce CT, do not cause cholera, and are not involved in epidemics. *V. cholerae* strains of serogroups other than O1 or O139 are associated with diarrhea or other clinical syndromes such as bacteremia; however, these other serogroups do not cause explosive epidemics or have pandemic potential.

EPIDEMIOLOGY

Incidence and Geographic Distribution

Because of its pandemic nature, cholera ebbs and flows across vast geographic distances over time. The Ganges delta is the ancestral home of cholera, where it has persisted in interpandemic periods as "Asiatic cholera." As the seventh pandemic of El Tor cholera progressively spread from its origin in the early 1960s on the island of Sulawesi in Indonesia, it has become endemic in many areas where it first appeared in epidemic form. Thus, cholera is now endemic in the Philippines, Southeast Asia and in multiple countries in sub-Saharan Africa (***Fig. 20.1***). During the early 1990s it was endemic for several years in Peru, Ecuador, and some other Latin American countries.

Typically, when cholera newly invades an immunologically naive population, the highest incidence is observed in young adult males. As the disease becomes increasingly endemic, the incidence increases in women and children; eventually, the peak incidence is found in young children.

Seasonality

In most endemic areas, cholera exhibits a seasonal pattern.[18] The disease typically appears simultaneously in multiple geographically separate foci. This pattern has also been seen as cholera invades new territory. For example, in 1991 when the cholera invasion of South America began with an explosive and extensive epidemic in Peru, large outbreaks appeared almost simultaneously in three distinct cities spanning a 900-km stretch along the Pacific coast.[18]

Recent data suggest that the explosive rise of cases early in many epidemics may be explained in part by hyperinfective vibrios released into water sources lacking vibriophages, while curtailment of the epidemic may correlate with an increase in lytic phages in the water.[19,20]

Reservoirs of Infection

Since humans are the only known host of cholera and chronic carriers are extremely rare, it was previously assumed that in endemic areas mild and asymptomatic infections serve as the reservoir to maintain the disease until the next cholera season when conditions would once again favor enhanced transmission. However, the appearance of a single case of cholera in Texas in 1973 in a fisherman, caused by an unusual highly hemolytic El Tor Inaba strain,[21] followed 5 years later by an outbreak of approximately two dozen cases of the identical strain in which poorly cooked seafood was incriminated as the vehicle,[22] led to the identification of an environmental focus of infection in the Gulf of Mexico. This El Tor Inaba strain was found in the brackish waters of Gulf estuaries, where it was associated with shrimp and other crustacea eaten as local seafood. Identification of a similar environmental focus of free-living enterotoxigenic *V. cholerae* O1 El Tor in Queensland, Australia, further supports the contention that brackish water environmental niches can serve as the reservoir of *V. cholerae* O1.[23]

Colwell[13] reports that *V. cholerae* can enter a "viable but nonculturable" state that allows them to survive harsh environmental conditions by means of a kind of bacterial hibernation. More recently this has been referred to as an "active but not culturable" state.[19] When the toxigenic *V. cholerae* eventually encounter favorable conditions of temperature,

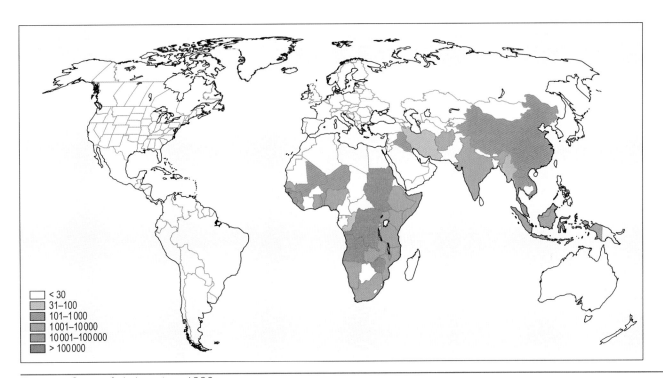

Figure 20.1 Cases of cholera since 1990.

salinity, and pH, they can rejuvenate, regaining the potential to metabolize and grow.[13] These may also be the conditions under which zooplankton blooms occur.

Modes of Transmission *(Fig. 20.2)*

Most of our knowledge about the vehicles of transmission of cholera stems from case-control investigations, which have demonstrated waterborne as well as foodborne transmission.[24,25] When El Tor cholera struck Latin America in explosive fashion in 1991, faulty municipal water and sewage systems, contaminated surface waters, and unsafe domestic water storage methods resulted in extensive waterborne cholera transmission.[26,27] Beverages prepared with contaminated water and sold by street vendors, ice, and even commercial bottled water have been incriminated.[28]

V. cholerae O1 may gain access to food in a primary manner, as by the natural association of vibrios with the chitinous exoskeletons of shrimp, crabs, and oysters in certain estuarine environments,[13,22,29] or food may be secondarily contaminated during preparation or handling.[30] The most commonly implicated food vehicle worldwide has been raw or undercooked seafood, including mussels, shrimps, oysters, cockles, clams, fish, salt fish, and ceviche (uncooked fish or shellfish marinated in lemon or lime juice).

Cooked grains, beans, and rice with sauces have also been repeatedly incriminated in cholera transmission. A small inoculum of enterotoxigenic *V. cholerae* introduced by an infected food handler into one of these types of food and stored without refrigeration can increase by several logs within 8–12 hours. In several instances, cholera has been transmitted by vegetables or fruit irrigated with raw sewage or doused with sewage to freshen them.[31]

During outbreaks or seasonal epidemics, cholera may spread via multiple modes of transmission, depending on local customs, climate, and other factors.[32] Finally, if pathogenic *V. cholerae* O1 and O139 persist in environmental reservoirs, then transmission across long distances can occur via the ballast water of large ships, as they intake ballast water in one port and discharge it prior to entering another port thousands of miles away.[33]

Person-to-person contact spread of cholera virtually never occurs; transmission occurs typically via large inocula in food or water vehicles and a large inoculum is required for cholera to manifest clinically.[34]

New findings suggest that for a few hours after being shed, toxigenic *V. cholerae* remain in a hypertransmissible state.[19,20,35] Thus, in a crowded

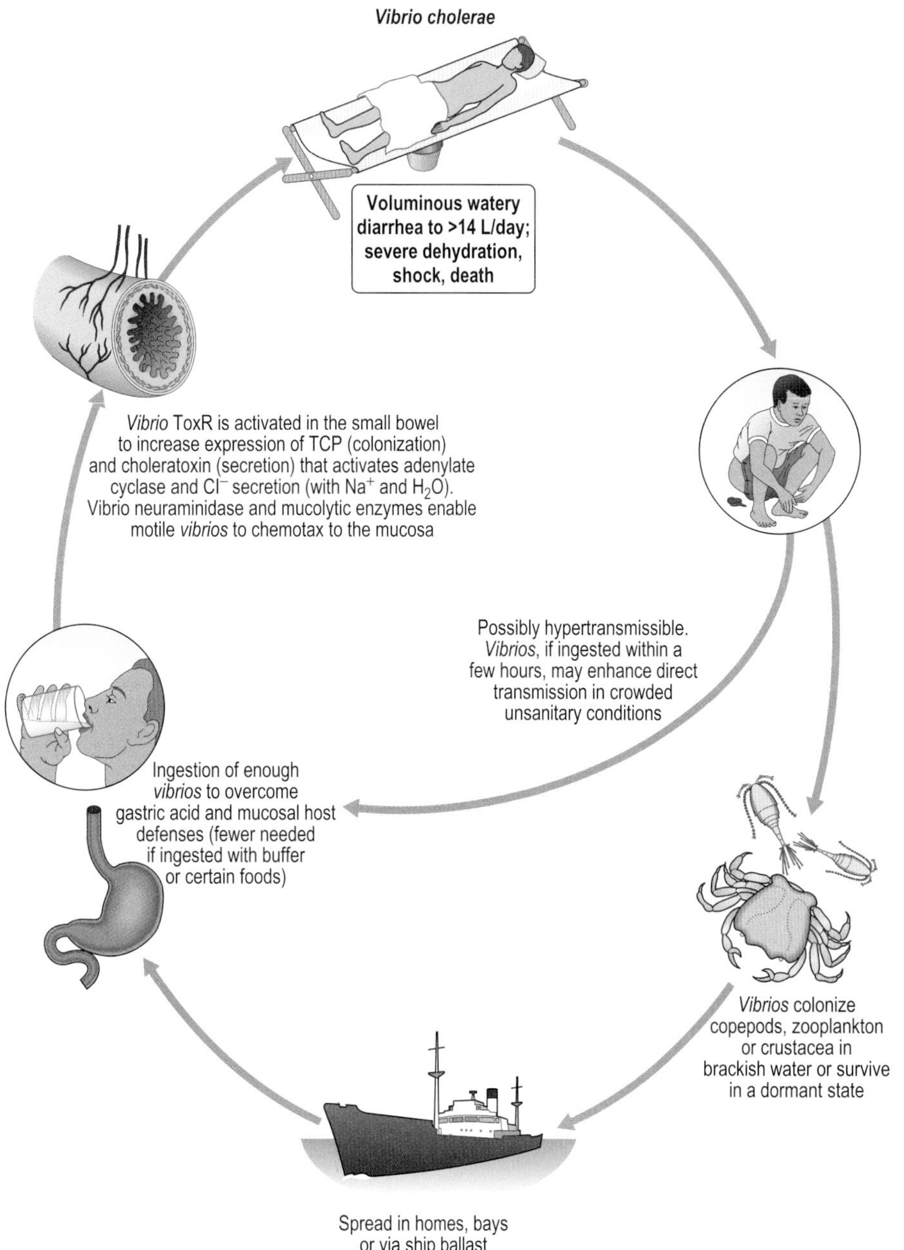
Vibrio cholerae
Voluminous watery diarrhea to >14 L/day; severe dehydration, shock, death
Vibrio ToxR is activated in the small bowel to increase expression of TCP (colonization) and choleratoxin (secretion) that activates adenylate cyclase and Cl^- secretion (with Na^+ and H_2O). Vibrio neuraminidase and mucolytic enzymes enable motile vibrios to chemotax to the mucosa
Possibly hypertransmissible. Vibrios, if ingested within a few hours, may enhance direct transmission in crowded unsanitary conditions
Ingestion of enough vibrios to overcome gastric acid and mucosal host defenses (fewer needed if ingested with buffer or certain foods)
Vibrios colonize copepods, zooplankton or crustacea in brackish water or survive in a dormant state
Spread in homes, bays or via ship ballast

Figure 20.2 *Vibrio cholerae* life cycle. TCP, toxin coregulated pili.

setting where other susceptible human hosts and facile modes of transmission exist, the infectious dose may be unusually low and spread from an acute case may be explosive.[19]

International Surveillance and Disease Notification

Cholera was the disease for which modern public health surveillance and reporting was first organized and bears the code 001 in the international classification of diseases. Along with plague and yellow fever, by international convention, cholera is a notifiable disease. In 1994, 94 countries, the largest number ever, reported cholera to the World Health Organization (WHO), signifying the cumulative effect of epidemics in Africa, Asia, and Latin America. Nevertheless, for reasons involving trade, fear of food embargos, and effects on tourism, many countries delay reporting cholera cases to the WHO or do not report at all. For example, from international health statistics in the late 1980s, Bangladesh appears to have had little or no cholera. Yet at the same time as those "official" statistics were generated, large-scale field trials were carried out to evaluate cholera vaccines in which hundreds of confirmed cases were documented.[36] In 2005, 52 countries reported cholera cases.

Host Risk Factors

Known host factors that greatly increase the risk of developing cholera gravis include blood group O,[37] hypochlorhydria,[38,39] and a lack of background immunity.[40] In both endemic and epidemic situations, persons of blood group O are clearly at much greater risk of developing cholera gravis than persons of other blood groups.[37,41] When cholera invades a new, immunologically naive population, persons with hypochlorhydria (e.g., with partial gastrectomy) have often been the index case.[42] In endemic areas the highest incidence of cholera usually is seen in children 1–4 years of age. The age-specific incidence falls thereafter and the prevalence and geometric mean titer of serum vibriocidal antibody rise, as increasing immunity is acquired.[43] However, there is one interesting exception to this pattern: women of child-bearing age exhibit a high incidence.[18]

Molecular Epidemiology

Molecular biologic techniques have been applied to analyze *V. cholerae* O1 and O139 strains in order to determine relationships and to deduce the origin or derivation of strains. The techniques include Southern blotting of restricted chromosomal DNA with specific probes, examination of restriction fragment length polymorphism (ribotyping), pulsed-field gel electrophoresis, multilocus enzyme electrophoresis (electropherotyping), comparison of DNA sequences, polymerase chain reaction (PCR) methods, and full or partial genome sequencing.[44–48] Application of these molecular subtyping methods has revealed that there are four major clonal groups of *V. cholerae* O1 El Tor strains worldwide: (1) seventh pandemic; (2) US Gulf coast; (3) Australia; and (4) Latin America. The US Gulf coast and Australian strains, each representing an environmental reservoir, are closely related. The seventh pandemic and Latin American strains are also similar. It has also been shown that the O139 epidemic strains of 1992–1994 are closely related (indeed, virtually identical) to strains of the El Tor seventh pandemic clone.

THE DISEASE

The incubation period is usually 18–40 hours but can be as short as 12 hours or as long as 72 hours, depending on the inoculum ingested and the susceptibility of the host. The first symptoms are queasiness, nausea, and abdominal gurgling, followed by the onset of diarrhea. In severe cholera, the stools rapidly become like voluminous rice water with a fishy smell (up to 1.0–1.25 L/h in teenagers and adults) and are high in electrolyte content. Vomiting is common during the first 6–12 hours of illness but usually disappears as voluminous purging continues.[49]

Table 20.1 Electrolyte Content of Cholera Stools in Older Versus Younger Children

	Adult or Older Child (mEq/L)	Young Child (mEq/L)
Na^+	135	100
Cl^-	100	90
K^+	15	30
HCO_3^-	40	30

The electrolyte composition of cholera stools depends on the age of the patient and the purge rate. At peak purge, the isotonic "rice water" stools of adults and older children have high Na^+ (circa 135 mEq/L) and bicarbonate (circa 45 mEq/L) concentrations, as shown in ***Table 20.1***. In young children, the Na^+ concentration typically does not exceed 100 mEq/L at peak purge.

As fluid and electrolyte deficits rapidly increase, signs of moderate and then severe dehydration appear. The patient has dry mucous membranes, an increased thready pulse rate, hypotension, sunken eyes, decreased skin turgor, decreased urine output, and thirst. Severely dehydrated patients have altered mental status, Kussmaul breathing, lethargy, stupor, and cold clammy skin. Cramping of peripheral skeletal muscles and of abdominal muscles consequent to acute potassium and calcium losses may cause extreme discomfort.

Complications

Hypovolemic shock, hyponatremia, hypokalemia, metabolic acidosis, and occasional hypocalcemia due to acute and huge loss of water and electrolytes are the major complications of cholera.[50] If timely intervention is not initiated these all can lead to death. Severe hypoglycemia from inadequate gluconeogenesis and exhaustion of glycogen stores is an uncommon complication seen in pediatric patients who manifest acute convulsions and even coma if serum glucose concentrations fall below 1 mmol/L.[51] In patients with severe dehydration and a marked decrease in renal perfusion, acute renal failure can occur. Very rarely, pulmonary edema can ensue if large volumes of intravenous fluids without bicarbonate are rapidly infused in a patient with severe acidosis, but inadequate fluid replacement is much more common. Rarely, septicemia due to *V. cholerae* has also been reported.

PATHOGENESIS AND IMMUNITY

Pathogenesis

There are few infections in which the molecular pathogenesis has been as well elucidated as cholera. One can think of *V. cholerae* O1 and O139 as complex and elegant living delivery systems for cholera toxin, which is responsible for the severe purging characteristic of cholera gravis. Studies in volunteers have shown that the ingestion of as little as 5 μg of purified cholera enterotoxin induces a clinical syndrome that closely resembles the severe purging of cholera gravis.[52] Nevertheless, subsequent volunteer studies with *V. cholerae* O1 vaccine candidate strains harboring deletions in genes encoding the enzymatically active (A) subunit, both A and B (binding) subunits of cholera toxin, or the entire cholera toxin virulence cassette (which encodes two other toxins and a minor fimbrial colonization factor) showed that some strains retained the ability to cause mild diarrhea and other gastrointestinal symptoms,[53] possibly via a mechanism that involves intestinal inflammation.[54,55] Moreover, whereas ingestion of purified cholera toxin alone may induce a syndrome of severe purging, the fully pathogenic vibrios that cause cholera in nature must carry multiple virulence factors that result in a stepwise progression ultimately resulting in severe diarrhea.

Following ingestion, pathogenic *V. cholerae* O1 or O139 must survive the formidable gastric acid barrier and pass through the pylorus to reach the proximal small intestine, the critical site of host–parasite interaction. Ingestion, without buffer, of 10^6 viable pathogenic *V. cholerae* by fasting North American volunteers resulted in neither infection nor diarrhea because the vibrios were destroyed by gastric acid.[34] In contrast, if 10^6 vibrios were administered with sodium bicarbonate buffer or food, cholera developed in approximately 90% of the volunteers.[34] Indeed, when administered with buffer, as few as 10^3 *V. cholerae* O1 El Tor caused diarrhea in approximately 67% of volunteers, although the stool volume was less than in subjects who ingested higher doses of vibrios.[34]

Once in the small intestine, the vibrios are believed to sense their environment by means of ToxR, a protein that is the product of a master regulatory gene, toxR.[56] Activation of toxR leads to expression of cholera toxin and toxin coregulated pili (TCP), the most important intestinal colonization factor,[57,58] as well as to the indirect activation (via toxT) of approximately 17 other genes involved with bacterial adaptation to survival in the human intestine. As neuraminidase and other vibrio enzymes break down the mucus barrier on the surface of the intestine, motility plays a critical role as the unipolar flagellum propels the organisms toward the enterocyte surface, attracted by chemotactins.

TCP constitutes the major intestinal colonization factor for *V. cholerae* O1 and O139.[57,58] The TCP of El Tor and O139 are genetically and antigenically identical but differ somewhat from TCP of classical biotype. The genes for TCP biogenesis are found within a 40-kb vibrio pathogenicity island. A mutant strain of *V. cholerae* O1, unable to express TCP, was unable to colonize the intestine of volunteers or to stimulate good vibriocidal antibody responses.[59] Surprisingly, although TCP must be expressed in order to elicit vibriocidal antibodies, specific antibody responses to TCP itself are not observed.[60]

The observation that early vaccine strains deleted of *ctxA* nevertheless were able to cause mild diarrhea, abdominal cramps, nausea, occasional vomiting, and low-grade fever[61] led to a search for possible accessory enterotoxins elaborated by *V. cholerae*. Two new toxins, zonula occludens toxin (Zot)[62] and accessory cholera enterotoxin (Ace),[63] encoded by genes located in the cholera toxin virulence cassette, were described. Subsequently, it was found that the *ctx* virulence cassette is actually the genome of a lysogenic filamentous bacteriophage (designated CTX-phi) and that Zot and Ace also play roles in phage morphogenesis.[64] CTX-phi comprises two regions, core and RS2.[64] The former encodes cholera toxin and several proteins, including Ace, that participate in phage packaging and secretion. Genes within the RS2 region encode products required for replication (*rstA*), integration (*rstB*), and regulation of CTX-phi (*rstR*).[64] Notably, the attachment factor for the toxin-encoding phage is TCP.

Immune Response

Following *V. cholerae* O1 infection, robust serum vibriocidal antibody responses and rises in immunoglobulin G (IgG) cholera antitoxin are observed.[65,66] Approximately 90% of complement-dependent vibriocidal antibodies are directed toward the O antigen, with the remaining 10–15% of antibodies being against protein antigens. In immunologically primed individuals, strong SIgA intestinal antibody responses follow cholera infection. However, significant rises in SIgA anti-lipopolysaccharide (LPS) and antitoxin are surprisingly sparse in nonprimed individuals. The detection of gut-derived, trafficking IgA antibody-secreting cells that make specific antibody to LPS and CT antigens is a good measure of priming of the intestinal immune system.[67]

Whereas infection-derived immunity to cholera is believed to be mediated by intestinal mucosal SIgA antibodies, curiously, serum vibriocidal antibodies are the best correlate of protection.[40,68] These serum antibodies are presumed to be a proxy for the stimulation of intestinal antibodies. Serum anti-B subunit responses are more prominent in pediatric cholera patients, while serum antibody responses to LPS and TCP are more prominent in adults.[69]

Whereas high titers of specific vibriocidal antibodies appear after *V. cholerae* O1 infection, vibriocidal responses following O139 infection are weak and rather nonspecific.[70] A correlate of protection for O139 cholera has not yet been identified.

DIAGNOSIS

V. cholerae O1 or O139 infection is diagnosed by isolation of the organism in stool culture, followed by agglutination with O-specific antisera.[14,25] Speciation of O1 is performed with Inaba and Ogawa typing antisera. Confirmation of the enterotoxigenicity of isolates is usually performed in reference laboratories by means of PCR or DNA probes that detect cholera toxin genes or by immunoassays or bioassays that detect toxin.

Dark-field microscopy can provide a rapid presumptive diagnosis when used in conjunction with specific antisera. The motility of vibrios is seen to become immobilized in the presence of specific antibody. Various immunoassays that detect vibrio antigen have been used as rapid diagnostic tests.[71–73] A commercial colorimetric immunoassay directed against O1 and O139 antigens (Cholera and Bengal SMART, direct fluorescent assay, New Horizons Diagnostics Corp.) greatly facilitates presumptive diagnosis.[71,72] PCR techniques can detect *V. cholerae* O1 and O139 in clinical specimens and in food even when viable vibrios are no longer present.[14]

TREATMENT AND PROGNOSIS

The three pillars to treating patients with cholera are: (1) aggressive rehydration therapy; (2) administration of antibiotics; and (3) treatment of complications. Aggressive rehydration by oral and intravenous routes to repair fluid and electrolyte deficits and to replace the prodigious ongoing diarrheal losses is the cornerstone of therapy of cholera.[74] Appropriate antimicrobials are an important adjunct to fluid therapy, as they diminish the volume and duration of purging and rapidly curtail the excretion of vibrios, thereby diminishing the chance of secondary transmission. Finally, as rehydration therapy has become increasingly effective, patients surviving from hypovolemic shock and severe dehydration manifest certain complications, such as hypoglycemia, that must be recognized and promptly treated. If these fundamental guidelines are followed properly, case fatality, even during explosive epidemics in developing countries, can be kept below 1%.[74,75] On the other hand, failure to comply with these basic proven clinical rules can result in unacceptably high case fatality.[3,6]

Fluid Therapy

Fluid therapy is divided into two phases: (1) rapid replacement of water and electrolyte deficits, known as rehydration phase; and (2) maintenance phase to infuse fluids to replace ongoing losses. Fluid and electrolyte deficits should be replenished as rapidly as possible (within 2–4 hours of initiation). Patients suffering from severe dehydration with or without overt shock usually lose 10% of their body weight and must be rapidly rehydrated with intravenous fluids. The time recommended for rehydration in adult and pediatric populations is 3 and 6 hours respectively. In adults 30% of the total required fluid is administered in the first half an hour, while in children it is 1 hour. Patients with cholera gravis generally require several liters of intravenous fluids to stabilize them to the point where oral rehydration can begin. In adults with cholera gravis, 8–12 liters of intravenous fluids may be required before oral hydration alone can keep up with losses. Cholera patients with mild or moderate dehydration and moderate purge rates (<500 mL/h) can usually be managed with oral rehydration alone.

Intravenous Rehydration

The optimal intravenous solutions for treating cholera have a polyelectrolyte composition similar to that of the cholera stool. The most extensively used intravenous rehydration fluid worldwide for treatment of cholera is Ringer's lactate, because it is so widely available commercially. Ringer's lactate contains Na^+ 130 mEq/L, K^+ 4 mEq/L, Ca^{2+} 3 mEq/L, Cl^- 111 mEq/L, and lactate (precursor of HCO_3^+) 29 mEq/L. Because the concentration of K^+ in Ringer's lactate is too low, supplemental K^+ must be administered either by adding a sterile KCl (or similar potassium salt) solution to the Ringer's solution to increase the concentration of K^+ to 15–20 mEq/L, or by initiating oral rehydration. In some endemic countries such as Bangladesh, a balanced polyelectrolyte solution such as "Dhaka Solution" is used for intravenous rehydration. It contains Na^+ 133 mmol/L, K^+ 13 mmol/L, Cl^- 98 mmol/L and acetate equivalent to 48 mmol/L of bicarbonate.[76]

Aggressive rehydration with adequate volumes of fluid and appropriate electrolytes leads to rapid clinical improvement in the patient (e.g., stronger pulse, elevation of blood pressure, increase in skin turgor, and improved state of consciousness), which is also reflected in simple laboratory assays (e.g., fall in hematocrit and in plasma specific gravity). Once renal perfusion is reestablished in the severely dehydrated patient, normal homeostatic mechanisms begin to combat acidosis and regulate serum electrolyte concentrations.

The volume of all diarrheal losses and vomitus must be measured in the patient with cholera. Once the patient has had replacement of his or her deficit and is in the stage of maintenance therapy, fluid management is generally based on 4-hour periods. The total fluid losses during the previous 4-hour period constitute the volume of fluids that will be administered to the patient during the next 4 hours. As diarrheal losses begin to diminish, the 4-hourly replacement requirements will decrease accordingly.

Oral Rehydration

Oral rehydration therapy was developed in the 1960s based on the discovery that glucose-mediated cotransport of sodium and water across the mucosal surface of the small intestine epithelium remains intact during cholera infection despite the effect of cholera toxin.[77] If the diarrhea is copious, large volumes of oral rehydration fluids must be ingested to keep up with ongoing losses.

The oral rehydration solution (ORS) currently recommended by WHO for treatment of cholera is composed of Na^+ 90 mEq/L, Cl^- 80 mEq/L, K^+ 20 mEq/L, citrate$^-$ 30 mEq/L, and glucose 111 mmol/L. Packets containing sufficient salts and glucose to prepare 1 liter of rehydration solution are widely available in developing countries. Each packet contains 3.5 g NaCl, 2.9 g sodium citrate, 1.5 g KCl, and 20 g glucose. In some areas of the world cereal-based oral rehydration solutions (that provide multiple, actively transported substrates) have become popular for the treatment of cholera,[78] although in some controlled trials no advantage was shown over glucose-based oral rehydration solutions.[79] Reduced-osmolarity rehydration solutions (Na^+ 75 mEq/L, Cl^- 65 mEq/L, K^+ 20 mEq/L, citrate$^-$ 30 mEq/L, and glucose 75 mmol/L) are controversial for treatment of cholera[80] because, although the rate and volume of purging are reduced versus standard ORS, some patients develop hyponatremia (albeit usually asymptomatic and of moderate degree).

The regimen for calculating the amount of ORS to be administered to replace ongoing losses differs by age. Since the Na^+ concentration in cholera stools is approximately 135 mEq/L in adults, one-and-a-half volumes of oral rehydration solution containing 90 mEq/L must be given for every volume of rice water diarrheal stool passed in order to replace Na^+ losses. In contrast, in young children in whom the Na^+ concentration of cholera stools is only approximately 100 mEq/L, ongoing losses can be replaced on the basis of a 1 : 1 ratio of ORS to volume of diarrheal stool. There is a practical limit to the volume of ORS that can be consumed on an hourly basis; in older adults and teenagers, the upper limit is approximately 750 mL/h.

Occasionally, there may be difficulty in promptly introducing an intravenous line in a cholera patient with severe dehydration. In such patients, the patient's head and upper torso should be elevated and a nasogastric tube should be inserted to initiate rehydration with ORS until venous access can be obtained.

Antimicrobial Therapy

Appropriate antibiotics decrease the duration of diarrhea, total diarrheal stool volume, and duration of excretion of *V. cholerae*, and therefore serve as an important adjunct to rehydration therapy. Antibiotic treatment should be based on local sensitivity as resistance to widely used agents is common (***Table 20.2***). Tetracycline or its derivative doxycycline were used extensively but resistance has become widespread. The recommended pediatric dosage is 50 mg/kg/day in four divided doses for 3–5 days, whereas the regimen for teenagers and adults is 500 mg four times daily for 3–5 days. Doxycycline has the advantage of being administered once daily in a dose of 4–6 mg/kg for children or 300 mg for teenagers and adults for 3–5 days. However, teeth staining with prolonged courses in children and contraindications in pregnancy and increasing resistance limit tetracycline use.

Alternative antimicrobial regimens that are usually effective include (5-day courses of therapy): erythromycin (pediatric dosage is 40 mg/kg/day in four divided doses; adult dosage is 250 mg four times daily); trimethoprim-sulfamethoxazole (pediatric dosage is 8 mg/kg/day trimethoprim and 40 mg/kg/day sulfamethoxazole in two divided doses; adult dosage is 160 mg trimethoprim and 800 mg sulfamethoxazole twice daily); furazolidone (pediatric dosage is 5 mg/kg/day in four divided doses; adult dosage is 100 mg every 6 hours); ampicillin (pediatric dosage is 50 mg/kg/day in four divided doses; adult dosage is 500 mg every 6 hours). Ciprofloxacin 250 mg once daily for 3 days is also a useful regimen,[81] while experience with single-dose ciprofloxacin has been inconsistent.[82,83] Single-dose azithromycin (1 g in adults) has been shown to be effective in treating cholera in both adults and children. In one randomized, controlled clinical trial, a single dose of azithromycin

Table 20.2 Antibiotics Available for the Treatment of Cholera

Antibiotics	Adult Dose	Pediatric Dose	Comments
Tetracycline or doxycycline	500 mg 6-hourly for 3 days 300 mg single dose		Recommended for adults but reports of resistance; not recommended for use in children and pregnant women
Erythromycin or azithromycin	250 mg 6-hourly for 3 days 1 g single dose	40 mg/kg/day 6-hourly for 5 days 20 mg/kg body weight single dose	Recommended and widely used
Ciprofloxacin	500 mg once daily for 1–3 days	20 mg/kg body weight as single dose	Recommended and has advantage of single dose
Trimethoprim-sulfamethoxazole	160 mg trimethoprim and 800 mg sulfamethoxazole 12-hourly for 3 days	8 mg/kg/day trimethoprim and 40 mg/kg/day sulfamethoxazole 12-hourly for 3 days	Reports of growing resistance
Ampicillin	500 mg 6-hourly ×3 days	50 mg/kg/day 6-hourly ×3 days	Reports of increasing resistance and not widely used
Furazolidone	5 mg/kg/day 6-hourly ×3–7 days	100 mg 6-hourly ×3–7 days	Reports of high resistance and not widely used

(20 mg/kg, maximum dose 1 g) was as effective as 3 days of erythromycin therapy (12.5 mg/kg every 6 hours).[84] Trimethoprim-sulfamethoxazole use should be avoided in areas where O139 is known to be prevalent, since *V. cholerae* O139 is typically resistant to this antimicrobial.[85] During epidemics in developing countries, single-day or single-dose antibiotic therapy (such as 1 g of ciprofloxacin or 300 mg of doxycycline for adults or 1 g of azithromycin) may be necessary in resource-constrained settings,[86,87] particularly if antibiotics are in short supply. However, the concern with single-dose therapy is that this may accelerate the emergence of resistance.

PREVENTION AND CONTROL

Wherever human populations live under conditions of underdevelopment, characterized by a lack of treated water supplies and sanitation to remove human fecal waste, the transmission of all enteric infections, including cholera, is favored. When an epidemic of cholera occurs, the first priority is to diminish case fatality by providing rehydration facilities, arranging rapid transport of patients to those facilities, and educating the population to seek treatment promptly when diarrhea begins. Prompt initiation of surveillance to identify the major foci of disease is critical in order to prioritize where scarce treatment and transport resources must be allocated. Mass-media health messages are useful to educate the population on the symptoms of cholera, advise where to seek treatment, starting home-based management with ORS until the patient can be transferred to the nearest health center, and publicize what water sources or foods should be avoided and what practices should be discontinued or encouraged. In many instances, control of the epidemic can be achieved by incriminating the most important vehicles of transmission through epidemiologic case-control studies and then taking appropriate measures to eliminate consumption of the incriminated vehicle or to discontinue certain high-risk behaviors.

Safe Water and Food

The threat of epidemic cholera often leads to emergency orders to boil all drinking water, advice that in many situations is impractical, expensive, and environmentally untenable. Rather, chemical disinfection with sodium or calcium hypochlorite is a preferred alternative because it can be implemented at all levels from municipal or community reservoirs through distribution systems to household storage containers.[88] Hypochlorite-treated water retains residual free chlorine, so that if *V. cholerae* are introduced after treatment they cannot readily survive. It has been proposed that in endemic areas such as the Ganges river delta where cholera is endemic and is often associated with consumption of brackish surface waters containing zooplankton to which toxigenic *V. cholerae* and O139 are adherent, filtering the surface water through multiple layers of sari cloth may be a protective practice.[89]

Defecation in the open air should be discouraged and emergency pit latrines should be built. Disinfectants such as cresol or lime should be used to disinfect stools and vomitus. Hand-washing with soap after defecation and before taking food can reduce the transmission substantially.

Simple modifications in food preparation practices markedly reduce the risk of cholera during epidemics. For example, the use of lemons, limes, and yogurt can acidify foods so that *V. cholerae* do not survive.[90]

Chemoprophylaxis

In endemic areas or epidemic areas where secondary transmission within households is shown to be a frequent event, a short (3-day) course of tetracycline (or another cited antibiotic) administered to household contacts can diminish transmission within households.[91] However, such use of antibiotics must be strictly controlled because indiscriminate use in the community can rapidly lead to antibiotic resistance. This was the situation in Guayaquil, Ecuador, in 1991, following the introduction of cholera into that community. An attempt at mass chemoprophylaxis rapidly led to the appearance of *V. cholerae* O1 strains that had acquired resistance to tetracycline as well as several other antibiotics.[92]

Cholera Vaccines

There are currently three licensed cholera vaccines, two of which are widely available. These include the B subunit/killed whole-cell oral vaccine (BS/WCV)[93,94] and a mix of killed whole-cell O1 and O139 vibrios. The other licensed vaccine, live oral *V. cholerae* O1 strain CVD 103-HgR,[95,96] is not presently being manufactured, although manufacture might begin again in the future. The BS/WCV is marketed under the trade name Dukoral (SBL, Stockholm, Sweden). The bivalent killed whole-cell oral vaccine, Shanchol, is marketed by Shanta Biotech, Hyderabad, India. Neither of these nonliving oral cholera vaccines is presently licensed in the USA. The oral vaccines have distinct advantages over the old parenteral vaccine. They are easy to administer and are more potent in stimulating local intestinal immune responses.

An advantage of the BS/WCV is its complete safety, even in immunocompromised subjects. A drawback to the BS/WCV is the need for two to three doses to confer protection. The nonliving vaccine elicits only modest serum vibriocidal responses but strong antitoxin responses. If time and circumstances allow preemptive immunization, the BS/WCV can be successfully delivered despite the need for two spaced doses.[97] Two randomized, controlled field trials assessed the efficacy of a two-dose regimen of the commercial formulation of the BS/WCV. Two doses of BS/WCV conferred 86% protection upon young adult Peruvian military personnel over approximately 5 months of follow-up.[93] A two-dose regimen did not confer significant protection upon Peruvian civilians (children and adults) during a year of follow-up.[94] However, administration of a third dose conferred greater than 60% protection during a second year of follow-up.[94]

The safety, immunogenicity, and efficacy of the prototype killed whole-cell bivalent (O1 and O139) vaccine was established in a cluster randomized, placebo-controlled, double-blind field trial in Kolkata, India, where, over 2 years of follow-up, a two-dose regimen conferred 67% protection against culture-confirmed cholera.[98]

CVD 103-HgR, the licensed live oral cholera vaccine that is not presently manufactured, showed several practical advantages over the killed vaccines, the main being its immunogenicity and efficacy following ingestion of a single dose, with protection already evident within 8 days.[99] A single-dose regimen of CVD 103-HgR did not confer long-term protection against El Tor cholera in an endemic area but cholera incidence plummeted after initiation of the trial.[100] When CVD 103-HgR was used by the WHO in control of an epidemic of cholera in Micronesia (a situation where time and logistical constraints made it untenable to administer other than a single-dose vaccine), the single-dose live cholera vaccine exhibited 79% efficacy under field conditions.[101]

Travelers

When cholera invaded Latin America in 1991, travel-associated cases of cholera increased markedly, in particular among US travelers. Besides cholera in travelers, persons were infected in the United States when contaminated foods (e.g., seafood) were illegally brought into the United States by travelers and from foodborne outbreaks related to air travel.[102]

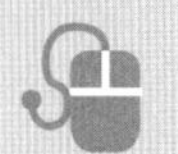

Access the complete reference list online at http://www.expertconsult.com

Access the complete reference list online at http://www.expertconsult.com

CHAPTER 21

"Noncholera" *Vibrio* Infections

J. Glenn Morris, Jr • G. Balakrish Nair

INTRODUCTION AND THE AGENT

In the early days of work with *Vibrio cholerae,* strains that did not agglutinate with serum from cholera patients were designated as "nonagglutinating," "non-O1" or "noncholera" vibrios.[1,2] They were initially thought to be nonpathogenic, until the 1950s when human disease outbreaks due to these "noncholera" strains began to be identified and investigated. Within the species *V. cholerae* over 200 O groups have now been identified. Strains in O-group 1 were regarded as the sole cause of epidemic cholera until 1992, when *V. cholerae* strains subsequently classified as O-group 139 (syn. Bengal) first appeared and spread in epidemic form across the Indian subcontinent.[3,4] However, serogroup is not a consistent marker for pathogenicity, as there are environmental *V. cholerae* O1 and O139 strains that do not carry the genes for standard virulence factors such as cholera toxin,[5,6] while strains in other serogroups (such as O37) have been found to be closely related genetically to epidemic O1 strains and have caused outbreaks of cholera-like illness.[7] Toxigenic strains of *V. cholerae* serogroup O141 and O75 have been associated with sporadic cholera-like diarrhea in the United States[8,9]; localized outbreaks of diarrheal illness have been caused by O10 and O12 strains in 1994 in Peru,[10] O6 and O14 strains in Khmer refugee camps in Thailand,[11] and O10 strains in India[12] (see map, ***Fig. 21.1***). In general, however, non-O1/O139 *V. cholerae* strains have been associated with mild, sporadic illness, or with asymptomatic colonization.[13]

In addition to the initially observed diversity within the species *V. cholerae* itself, many "noncholera" strains were subsequently found to be so distinct from *V. cholerae* as to constitute separate species. Fujino and coworkers first isolated what we now know as *V. parahaemolyticus* from clinical samples and from shirasu (dried sardines) associated with an outbreak of gastroenteritis that occurred in Osaka in 1950.[14] A new *V. parahaemolyticus* clonal group that appeared to have increased virulence (as reflected by increased hospital admissions) emerged in the mid-1990s within serogroup O3:K6.[15] Members of this clonal group, as defined by multilocus sequence typing (MLST) and other molecular markers, have now been identified in 22 different serogroups.[15] These strains have been associated with a pandemic of *V. parahaemolyticus* gastroenteritis that has spread to virtually all parts of the world, including the United States.[16–18]

Aside from *V. cholerae* and *V. parahaemolyticus*, nine other *Vibrio* species that can infect humans (or that have been isolated from humans) are now recognized. *V. fluvialis,*[19] *V. furnissii,*[20] *V. hollisae* (recently moved to a new genus, *Grimontia*)[21] and *V. mimicus*[22] have been associated primarily with diarrheal disease. *V. alginolyticus* and *V. damsela*[20] generally cause wound infections. *V. vulnificus*, initially described in 1979 as a "lactose-positive marine *Vibrio*," is recognized as an important cause of septicemia in alcoholics and immunosuppressed hosts; cases have been reported primarily from Korea, Taiwan, and the Gulf Coast region of the United States.[23–25] A newly described biogroup of *V. vulnificus*, biogroup 3, has been implicated in serious wound infections associated with exposure to live tilapia in Israel.[26] Descriptions of infections with *V. cincinnatiensis*, *V. carchariae*, and *V. metschnikovii* have been restricted to case reports, and the significance of their isolation from humans remains to be determined. ***Table 21.1*** lists the *Vibrio* species associated with human illness, together with data on numbers of reported cases and deaths in the United States for 2007.[27] Numerous other *Vibrio* species (currently totaling 92; http://www.bacterio.cict.fr/uw/vibrio.html) inhabit a variety of marine niches, but are not known to be pathogenic to humans.

EPIDEMIOLOGY

Incidence

In the United States, *V. parahaemolyticus* is the most common noncholera *Vibrio* species isolated from patients, followed by *V. alginolyticus*, *V. vulnificus*, and the "nonepidemic" or non-O1/O139 strains of *V. cholerae* (***Table 21.1***). At a global level, *V. parahaemolyticus* is again the most commonly isolated noncholera vibrio: it has been implicated as the cause of one-fourth of foodborne disease cases in Japan,[28] and was the most common etiology for foodborne disease outbreaks between 1994 and 2005 in coastal provinces of China.[17] After decreasing in the early 1990s, the reported incidence of *V. parahaemolyticus* more than doubled between 1996 and 1998, with the appearance of a new clonal group of pandemic *V. parahaemolyticus* strains within serotype O3:K6 and associated serovariants O4:K68, O1:K25, and O1:KUT.[29,30] This specific clone of *V. parahaemolyticus* and its serovariants has spread into Asia, the Americas, Africa, and Europe (***Fig. 21.2***), although recent reports suggest that the pandemic has peaked, with a decline in incidence now being observed.

Non-O1/O139 (nonepidemic) *V. cholerae* has been isolated from 2–3% of patients with diarrheal illness in tropical areas (including travelers).[13] As with other *Vibrio* species, isolation rates are higher in coastal areas: an isolation rate of 16.4% was reported from Cancún, Mexico,[31] as compared with no isolations in a study in Mexico City.[32] In Calcutta, a cholera-endemic area, the isolation rate for nonepidemic strains of *V. cholerae* among patients hospitalized with diarrhea has been reported to vary between 2.7% and 4.9%, with no temporal clustering of any particular serogroup and no pronounced seasonality.[33]

Carriage

Long-term human carriage of *Vibrio* species is unusual; chronic carriers do not appear to play a role in the epidemiology of the disease. However, short-term carriage or asymptomatic infections may be relatively common. From a cohort of 479 physicians attending a meeting in New Orleans who agreed to submit stool samples, 51 stool samples were positive for noncholera vibrios (*V. parahaemolyticus*, nonepidemic *V. cholerae*, *V. vulnificus*, *V. fluvialis*, and *V. mimicus*), of which 36 were from asymptomatic individuals.[34] In a large study in Iran in 1971, 1.6% of pilgrims

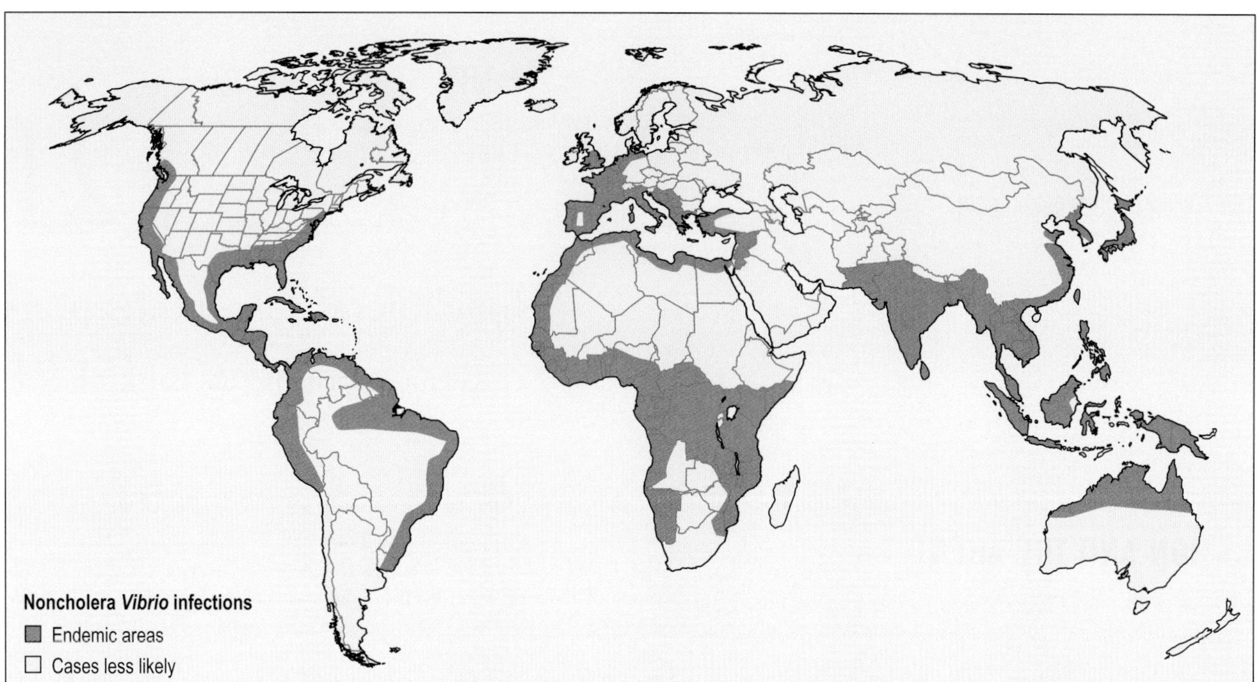

Figure 21.1 Noncholera *Vibrio* infections.

Table 21.1 *Vibrio* species Implicated as Causes of Human Disease and Number of Deaths Associated with Infection with these Species

	Clinical Presentation			
Species	**Gastroenteritis**	**Wound Infections**	**Septicemia**	**No. of Cases (No. of Deaths)[a]**
V. cholerae				
Epidemic (CTX+ O1, O139)	++	(+)	–	9 (0)[b]
Nonepidemic[c]	++	+	+	49 (3)
V. mimicus	++	+	–	10 (0)
V. parahaemolyticus	++	+	(+)	232 (0)
V. fluvialis	++	+	+	19 (1)
V. furnissii	++	–	–	0 (0)
Grimontia hollisae[d]	++	+	(+)	6 (0)
V. vulnificus	+	++	++	95 (30)[e]
V. angiolyticus	–	++	–	100 (0)
V. damsela	–	++	–	2 (0)
V. cincinnatiensis	–	–	(+)	0 (0)
V. carchariae	–	(+)	–	0 (0)
V. metschnikovii	(+)	–	(+)	1 (0)

[a]Data reflect *Vibrio* infections reported to the Centers for Disease Control and Prevention during 2007. Data are from the 35 states that reported cases; for many of these states, reporting of *Vibrio* infections is not routine, and consequently numbers may not reflect the true number of cases. 2007 data from http://www.cdc.gov/nationalsurveillance/PDFs/CSTEVibrio2007.pdf.

[b]Data include 4 cases associated with foreign travel, and one case associated with imported food.

[c]Data include 5 non-toxigenic *V. cholerae* O1.

[d]Formerly identified as *Vibrio hollisae*.

[e]The 30 reported deaths are from a group of 83 cases for which data on death were available.

++, Most common clinical presentation; +, neither rare nor most common clinical presentation; (+), rare clinical presentation; –, a clinical presentation that is not seen.

(Modified from Morris JG Jr. Cholera and other types of vibrioses: a story of human pandemics and oysters on the half shell. Clin Infect Dis 2003;37:272–280.)

returning from Mecca were estimated to be carriers of noncholera *V. cholerae* (compared with 0.015% of persons leaving for Mecca).[35] In Calcutta, 15.3% of family contacts of *V. parahaemolyticus* diarrhea cases were found to be carrying the organism, with excretion continuing for up to 5 days.[36] Carriage of *Vibrio* species by wild and domestic animals is also well described: nonepidemic *V. cholerae* has been isolated from dogs in Calcutta[37]; from cows, goats, dogs, and chickens in India[38]; from ducks in Denmark;[39] from seagulls in England; and from horses, lambs, and bison in Colorado.[40]

Transmission

As shown in the "life cycle" (***Fig. 21.3***), the marine or estuarine environment serves as the primary reservoir for these organisms. In

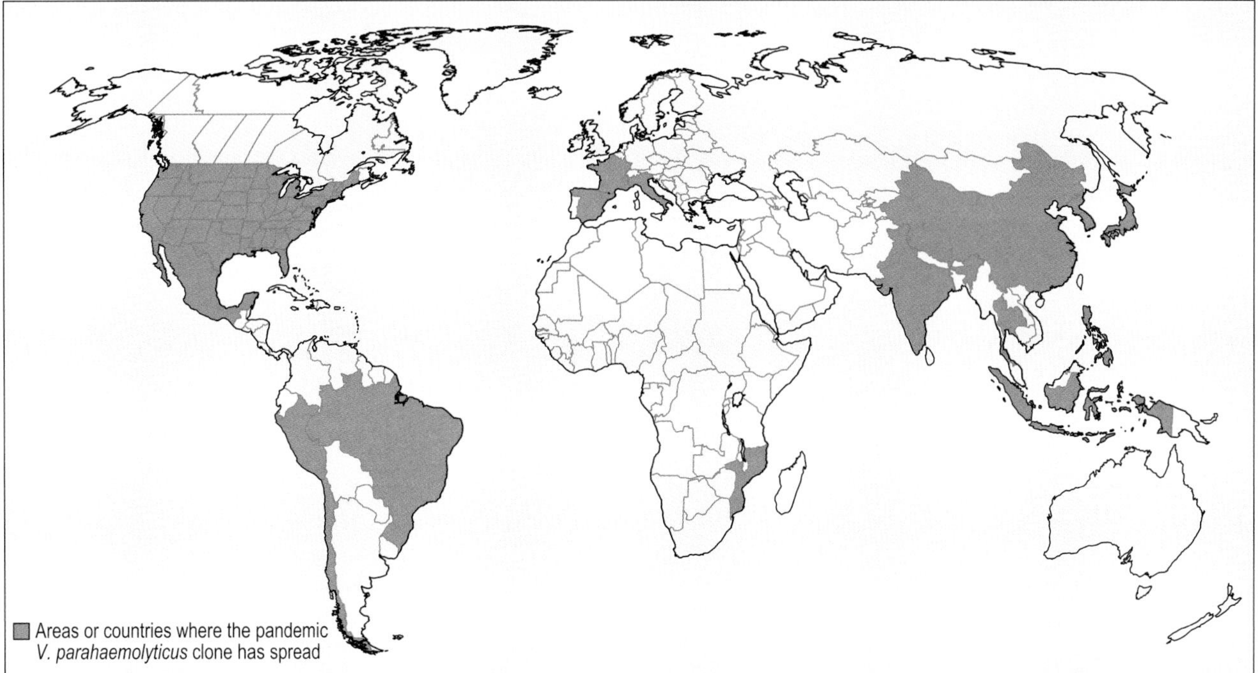

Figure 21.2 Dissemination of the new pandemic *V. parahaemolyticus* clone.

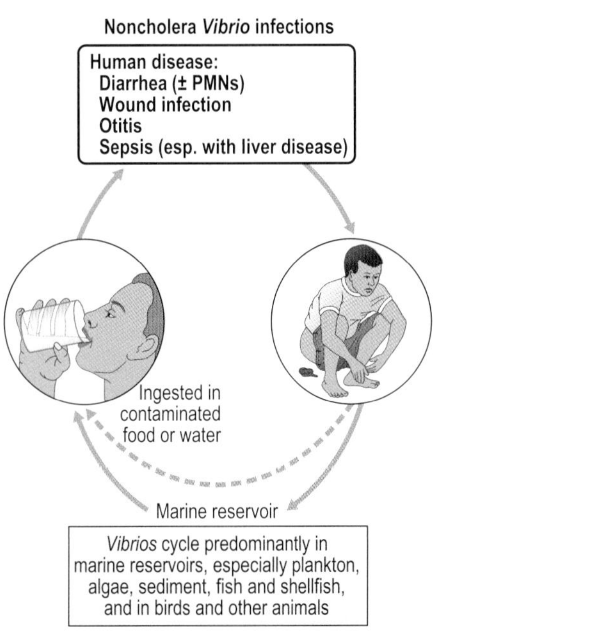

Figure 21.3 Noncholera *Vibrio* transmission. PMNs, polymorphonuclear neutrophils.

temperate regions, virtually all cases can be linked back to raw or undercooked seafood.[41] US non-O1/O139 *V. cholerae* and *V. vulnificus* cases are often associated with raw oyster consumption,[42,43] and there were major US *V. parahaemolyticus* outbreaks linked with oysters in 1997 (Washington State) and 1998 (Texas, New York, Connecticut, and Washington State).[44] The pattern is less clear in poverty settings, possibly because of the increased risk of fecal contamination of food and water sources, or cross-contamination of foods by seafood vehicles.[31]

Ecology/Distribution/Seasonality

Vibrios are ubiquitous in the marine environments, estuaries, and freshwater throughout the world. While most are halophilic (i.e., require salt for growth), *V. cholerae* can grow in freshwater, and has been isolated from freshwater lakes.[45] In temperate climates, counts of vibrio bacteria vary seasonally: in the summer (when water temperatures exceed 20°C), vibrios can easily be isolated from water, suspended particulate matter, plankton, algae, sediment, fish, and shellfish; during the winter months, they decline markedly in number and are found primarily in sediments.[14,46] Among other possible natural reservoirs, egg masses of the nonbiting midge *Chironomus* spp. (Diptera)[47] and unicellular free-living protozoa such as *Acanthamoeba* species[48] have recently been shown to harbor *V. cholerae*. Vibrio counts are independent of the level of fecal coliforms; these are naturally occurring, free-living organisms that can be present in "pristine" waters that are free of fecal contamination.

Vibrios can be concentrated in oysters, with numbers of *V. parahaemolyticus* and *V. vulnificus* 100 times higher than the surrounding water.[46] Non-O1 *V. cholerae* have been isolated from 14% of randomly selected oyster shell stock,[49] and virtually all summer-harvested oysters along the US Gulf Coast and Chesapeake Bay carry *V. vulnificus* and/or *V. parahaemolyticus*, with counts that can exceed 10^4/g.[44,46,50] *V. cholerae* and *V. vulnificus* can shift to a "viable but nonculturable" form, which may permit them to survive for extended periods in the environment under adverse conditions.[51–53] *V. cholerae* (and possibly other species) also have the ability to acquire a "rugose" morphology, associated with the production of a surface polysaccharide that promotes cell aggregation and protective biofilm-like masses of cells[54] that extend their environmental survival and transmission.

Human illnesses due to vibrios are seen in coastal areas around the world (see ***Fig. 21.1***). In Japan, where consumption of seafood (including raw and undercooked seafood) is common, *V. parahaemolyticus* accounts for a large proportion of foodborne illness. *V. vulnificus* has emerged as a significant health problem in Korea and Taiwan, linked again with consumption of raw or undercooked seafood.[24,55] In temperate areas illness tends to follow a seasonal pattern.[41,56] Increasing water temperatures in coastal areas in the United States (possibly related to global climate change) may serve as a cofactor in an increasing incidence of *V. parahaemolyticus* in the United States.[57] In the Rias of Galicia, Spain, salinity was the primary factor that appeared to govern the temporal and spatial distribution of *V. parahaemolyticus*, whereas seawater temperature had a secondary effect and only modulated the abundance in periods and areas of reduced salinities.[58] Seasonality is less apparent in tropical areas.

Host Factors

In cases of vibrio gastroenteritis, sex, race, or blood group have not shown any consistent correlation with disease. The median age of persons with vibrio gastroenteritis varies with geographic location. In Cancún, Mexico, for example, children less than 1 year of age were at highest risk of infection with nonepidemic *V. cholerae*,[31] whereas in Bangladesh and Thailand cases tended to occur in older children and adults. In a survey of 14 sporadic nonepidemic *V. cholerae* infections in the United States,[42] the median patient age was 45, which may reflect the older age of the population that consumes raw oysters. Factors that decrease gastric acidity may increase the risk of infection.

Host factors play a much more important role in the epidemiology of sepsis due to *Vibrio* species. Virtually all patients with sepsis due to *V. vulnificus* and nonepidemic *V. cholerae* have an underlying chronic medical illness,[23–25,41,43,59,60] with persons with underlying liver disease, including alcoholic cirrhosis or hemochromatosis, appearing to be at highest risk. Based on the number of cases reported to the Florida Health Department between 1981 and 1992, the annual rate of illness from *V. vulnificus* infection in adults with self-reported liver disease in Florida who ate raw oysters was 7.2 per 100000 adults, 80 times the rate for adults without known liver disease who ate raw oysters (0.09 cases per 100000 population).[43] The risk of sepsis due to *V. parahaemolyticus* also appears to be increased by the presence of underlying chronic illness, although the association does not appear to be as strong as that seen with *V. cholerae* and *V. vulnificus*. Risk may also be increased in patients with decreased gastric acidity.

THE DISEASE

Primary clinical presentations vary by species and may include gastroenteritis, wound and ear infections, and septicemia. Vibrio gastroenteritis typically involves diarrhea, abdominal pain, and sometimes nausea and vomiting. Reported sporadic noncholera *V. cholerae* illnesses are relatively severe. Among 14 sporadic cases in the United States,[42] the median duration of illness was 6.4 days. All had diarrhea, 71% had fever, but only 21% had nausea and vomiting. One-fourth had bloody diarrhea. In volunteers[61] and outbreaks[62,63] duration of illness has generally been in the range 12–24 hours, with incubation periods of 10–24 hours (range, 5.5–96 hours).[61] *V. parahaemolyticus* produces a similar spectrum of gastrointestinal illness with diarrhea (98%), abdominal cramps (89%), nausea (76%), vomiting (55%), and fever (52%).[64] In both the United States and Japan, illness tends to be mild, with a median duration (in US foodborne outbreaks) of 2.4 days.[64] Bloody stools were noted in 29% of *V. parahaemolyticus* cases reported to the Centers for Disease Control and Prevention.[64] More severe illness with dysentery may occur;[65,66] hypotension and shock occurred in three of five *V. parahaemolyticus* cases in one outbreak in Great Britain, and there were 20 deaths among the 272 patients involved in the Japanese outbreak where *V. parahaemolyticus* was first identified.[14] The incubation period for *V. parahaemolyticus* is usually 12–24 hours.

Vibrio species have been isolated from seawater-exposed wounds[13,41] and have been implicated as a cause of otitis and, rarely, pneumonia associated with near-drowning episodes.[13] While infection can occur in normal hosts, complications, including sepsis, are more likely in persons who are immunocompromised or have chronic underlying illnesses.[41]

Septicemia, due primarily to encapsulated strains of *V. vulnificus* and *V. cholerae*, occurs almost exclusively in persons who have underlying liver disease, are alcoholic, diabetic, or are in some way immunocompromised.[23–25,59,60] One-third of patients with *V. vulnificus* septicemia present in shock.[23–25] Thrombocytopenia is common, and there is often evidence of disseminated intravascular coagulation; gastrointestinal bleeding is not infrequent. The mortality rate is greater than 50%, with mortality exceeding 90% among patients who become hypotensive within the first 24 hours of hospitalization. Three-fourths of patients with *V. vulnificus* septicemia have characteristic bullous skin lesions;[23–25,67] identification of these skin lesions in the appropriate epidemiologic setting should prompt aggressive, specific therapy for this pathogen. While there are fewer data on patients with *V. cholerae* septicemia, the clinical presentation is comparable to that seen with *V. vulnificus* (although skin lesions are not as prominent); the mortality rate in a recent case series from Taiwan was 47%, with a rate in excess of 60% noted in an older US series.[59,60]

PATHOGENESIS AND IMMUNITY

Nonepidemic *V. cholerae* strains likely cause gastroenteritis through a number of different mechanisms, analogous to the multiplicity of mechanisms described for diarrheagenic *Escherichia coli*. Some non-O1/O139 *V. cholerae* strains carry the genes for and produce cholera toxin (CT).[7,52] CT-producing strains were isolated from 29% of cases of sporadic non-O1 *V. cholerae* gastroenteritis in Bangladesh; patients infected with these strains had more severe and prolonged diarrhea, with greater weight loss.[68] However, CT production is relatively uncommon among clinical isolates of nonepidemic serotypes of *V. cholerae*.[13,69]

A subgroup of *V. cholerae* strains produces a heat-stable enterotoxin (designated NAG-ST)[70] that closely resembles the heat-stable enterotoxin of enterotoxigenic *E. coli*. Volunteer and epidemiologic studies suggest that these strains cause diarrhea in humans.[11,61] Other possible virulence factors include the colonization factor TCPA, toxins within the RTX toxin gene family,[71] the hemolysin HLYA, pathogenicity islands identified in epidemic *V. cholerae* O1 strains (VSP-1, VSP-2), and type three secretion systems (TTSS).[72,73] However, there are not strong data linking any one factor with illness. In studies in volunteers,[61] two out of three nonepidemic *V. cholerae* strains tested did not cause human disease, suggesting that many, if not most, of the strains outside of known pathogenic subgroups are nonpathogenic commensals.

The pathogenicity of *V. parahaemolyticus* isolates has traditionally been correlated with the production of the thermostable direct hemolysin (Vp-TDH), which is responsible for the beta hemolysis (the Kanagawa phenomenon) seen when 96% of clinical isolates (but only 1% of environmental isolates) are plated on Wagatsuma agar.[14,74,75] Kanagawa hemolysis correlates with the presence of an 80 kb pathogenicity island on chromosome II, including two *tdh* genes and a set of genes for the TTSS.[76] Volunteer studies also demonstrated the importance of Vp-TDH: Kanagawa-positive strains produced diarrhea whereas doses of up to 10^9 Kanagawa-negative strains failed to do so in 15 volunteers.[77] Furthermore, studies with isogenic mutants have shown that deletion of the Vp-TDH gene results in loss of enterotoxic activity in laboratory models (Ussing chamber and rabbit ileal loop assays).[78]

A second group of hemolysins, Vp-TDH-related hemolysins, or Vp-TRH, can be found in certain clinical isolates, especially those that are Kanagawa-negative.[79–81] These hemolysins are genetically related to Vp-TDH (sharing about 70% sequence homology) but are more diverse (less than 2.8% divergence among most Vp-TDH versus 16% between two subgroups of Vp-TRH). Studies of *V. parahaemolyticus* from the west coast of the United States and from Thailand have linked clinical illness with isolation of urease-positive, Kanagawa-negative strains from stool cultures.[82,83] These strains have been shown almost always to carry the *tdh* gene.[84] *V. parahaemolyticus* has been shown to have at least two sets of genes encoding TTSS, which share genetic lineages with similar systems found in nonepidemic *V. cholerae*.[85] TTSS1 is a Ysc-plus-Psc system present on the large chromosome, and appears to be intrinsic to the species based on G+C content. TTSS2 is detected only in Kanagawa-positive strains, is not similar to any particular TTSS of other bacteria, and is located on the small chromosome.[15] Recent studies have identified yet another novel TTSS system, similar to TTSS2, this time in a *trh*-positive strain.[85] Infection with *V. parahaemolyticus* results in B-cell responses and an acute inflammatory response that is self-limiting.[86] Within hours of infection, *V. parahaemolyticus* utilizes its TTSS to cause induction of autophagy, cell rounding and then cell lysis that eventually results in the proinflammatory death of an infected host cell.[87] A four-way

BLAST analysis of the genome sequences of different *V. parahaemolyticus* strains has shown that the new highly virulent clone arose from a prepandemic O3:K6 isolate that acquired at least seven novel regions, which included both a TTSS and a T6SS.[88] However, precise factors which account for the increased virulence attributed to "pandemic" strains remain elusive.[15]

Encapsulation appears to be a key virulence factor for strains that cause septicemia.[89,90] *V. vulnificus* strains produce a polysaccharide capsule. Most nonepidemic strains of *V. cholerae* also produce a capsule, with the degree of encapsulation correlating significantly with the risk of sepsis.[91] *V. cholerae* O1 strains (i.e., epidemic cholera strains) are not encapsulated and have not been associated with septicemia. Interestingly, *V. cholerae* O139 Bengal strains are encapsulated[92] and do appear to be able to cause septicemia in susceptible hosts. Encapsulation provides vibrios with protection against serum bactericidal activity and allows bacteria to resist opsonization and phagocytosis. Antibodies directed against the capsular polysaccharide are protective in animal models.[93]

In rep-PCR analyses, *V. vulnificus* strains from clinical sources tend to cluster together, suggesting that these strains carry gene sequences (including virulence factors) not present in environmental strains.[94] Work on virulence factors in *V. vulnificus* includes those associated with iron acquisition, cytotoxicity, motility, and expression of proteins involved in attachment and adhesion; however, other than encapsulation, there are no specific factors that have been clearly linked with increased risk of sepsis.[95]

DIAGNOSIS

Although some *Vibrio* species will grow on media routinely used for isolating stool pathogens, selective thiosulfate, citrate, bile salts, and sucrose medium (TCBS agar) is the standard. Except for a few strains of *Grimontia hollisae*, all pathogenic vibrios will grow on this medium, producing colonies that are yellow (sucrose fermenters such as *V. cholerae*) or blue-green (nonsucrose fermenters such as *V. parahaemolyticus*). Isolates from wounds and blood will also grow on any standard culture medium, including blood agar.

Confirmation of the genus and species employs standard biochemical panels. As many vibrios are halophilic, the addition of 1% NaCl to growth media is often necessary to prevent false-negative reactions. When examining environmental samples, especially water samples, concentration procedures or selective enrichment broths may be needed.

Serotyping is available for *V. cholerae* through the National Institute of Health, Tokyo, and may prove useful in analysis of outbreak-related strains. PCR and probe-based methods for identification of critical genes in many of these species are increasingly available on an experimental basis.[96–98] Both MLST and pulsed-field gel electrophoresis[99] and recently variable number of tandem repeats analyses[100,101] have been used to type *Vibro* species.

TREATMENT AND PROGNOSIS

Treatment

As in any diarrheal disease, volume repletion is the most important element of therapy in patients with vibrio gastroenteritis. Antimicrobial therapy in cholera has been shown to reduce the duration of diarrhea and the excretion of vibrios. While there are no controlled trials of therapy in vibrio gastroenteritis, the use of antimicrobial therapy in more severe cases is reasonable. Although tetracycline and ciprofloxacin have been drugs of choice, resistance is increasing,[102] and single-dose azithromycin (which has been effective in the treatment of severe cholera in adults) may be a reasonable alternative.

Wound infections require débridement and antimicrobial therapy; again, tetracycline, ciprofloxacin, or azithromycin appear to be reasonable choices. For patients with septicemia, prompt, effective antimicrobial therapy is critical,[23] as is supportive care (ideally in an intensive care unit setting). Although no controlled trials are available, a combination of minocycline (100 mg every 12 hours orally) and cefotaxime (2.0 g every 8 hours intravenously) or a "newer" fluoroquinolone has been recommended for treatment of sepsis caused by *V. vulnificus*,[103,104] and are reasonable for sepsis caused by other *Vibrio* species.

Hyperimmune serum against the *V. vulnificus* capsular polysaccharide does protect against death in animal models, even when administered after onset of symptoms.[93] However, both *V. vulnificus* and nonepidemic *V. cholerae* have a large number of different capsule types, and preliminary data suggest that antisera directed against one capsular type is not cross-protective; the resultant need for a multivalent product makes it more difficult to produce a useful therapeutic immunoglobulin.

Prognosis

The prognosis in vibrio gastroenteritis is excellent, with virtually all patients showing a complete recovery within a matter of days. Surprisingly high rates of mortality have been reported in some *V. parahaemolyticus* outbreaks, perhaps related to cardiac arrhythmias.

The prognosis for patients with *V. cholerae* or *V. vulnificus* septicemia is much more guarded. Mortality rates among these patients exceed 50%, with survivors often having long-term disability related to multiorgan system failure and the consequences of prolonged hospitalization in an intensive care unit.

PREVENTION AND CONTROL

Given the ubiquitousness of this organism in nature, total prevention is unlikely so long as people eat raw or undercooked seafood. Risks can be reduced by adhering to proper food-handling techniques, including techniques to minimize cross-contamination within kitchens and prevent growth of bacteria in food vehicles. Provision of safe supplies of food and water (i.e., with minimal fecal contamination) is essential, particularly in developing countries. No vaccines are currently available for these pathogens; vaccination would also be of uncertain utility, given the relative infrequency (and generally self-limited nature) of most of these infections.

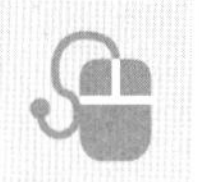

Access the complete reference list online at
http://www.expertconsult.com

CHAPTER 22

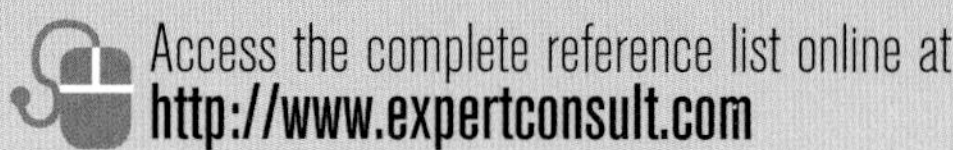
Access the complete reference list online at
http://www.expertconsult.com

Enteric *Clostridium* Infections

Cirle A. Warren

INTRODUCTION

Clostridial species are obligate anaerobic, Gram-positive, spore-forming bacilli. They are found in soil, sewage, marine sediments, intestinal tracts of human and other animals and decaying animal and plant products.[1] Of more than 150 known species of *Clostridium*, about 20 are associated with human or animal disease.[1,2] Four clostridia, *C. difficile*, *C. perfringens*, *C. botulinum*, and *C. septicum*, are associated with human disease involving the gastrointestinal tract as either the source or site of infection.

THE AGENT

The two major features that are important in clostridial disease transmission and pathogenesis are sporulation and toxin production, respectively. Most clostridia sporulate under conditions suboptimal for growth. Both vegetative bacteria and spores find their way to the environment, food, and feeds and eventually gain entry into the human gastrointestinal tract. *C. difficile* spores contaminate the hospital environment and can be transmitted from patient to patient through the hands of health care providers.[3] Because *C. difficile* spores resist desiccation and routine environmental decontamination, they may survive on hard surfaces for months.[4] *C. perfringens* can grow between 15 and 50°C and generation time is 20 minutes at 33–49°C.[5] Spores germinate and vegetative cells multiply during slow cooling or inadequate heating of food. Toxin production occurs after ingestion during sporulation in the small intestines. *C. botulinum* grows and produces toxin in anaerobic conditions with pH <4.5, low salt and sugar content, and temperature of 4–121°C.[6] Toxigenic clostridia secrete biologically active proteins (toxins) that are responsible for most of the observed effects in *in vitro* and *in vivo* studies and human disease.[1,6–8]

CLOSTRIDIUM DIFFICILE INFECTION

EPIDEMIOLOGY

Since it was first described as the cause of antibiotic-associated diarrhea and pseudomembranous colitis in 1978,[9] *C. difficile* has been recognized as the most common known cause of hospital-acquired infection in resource-sufficient countries.[10,11] *C. difficile* has been isolated from either diarrheal or non-diarrheal stools, from either hospitalized individuals or those coming from the community across all age groups in Asia, Africa, and South America.[12–15] Very recently, there was a heightened concern about the emergence of strains causing international outbreaks and severe disease. In 2000, the incidence rates of *C. difficile* infection (CDI) and fulminant *C. difficile* colitis were noted to have increased in a university hospital in Pittsburgh, Pennsylvania.[16] A retrospective study of the first 2 years of the outbreak showed an increase in nosocomial CDI from 2.7 to 6.8 cases per 1000 discharges with associated increases in deaths and colectomies.[17] Since then, several other locations in the United States,[18,19] Canada,[20,21] and Europe[22,23] reported a similar trend. The rising rates and severity of CDI were attributed to strains characterized as group BI by restriction endonuclease analysis (REA), as North American pulse-field type NAP1 by pulse-field gel electrophoresis (PFGE), as ribotype 027 (BI/NAP1/027), and as toxinotype III.[18] These strains have initially been described to have an 18 bp deletion at the negative regulator gene *tcdC*, causing 16-fold and 23-fold increases in toxin A (TcdA) and toxin B (TcdB), respectively.[24] Subsequent studies revealed a single bp deletion at position 117 of the open reading frame which renders the *tcdC* non-functional.[25,26] The presence of binary toxin (CdtA, CdtB) has also been identified with these strains although the clinical significance of this feature has yet to be proven.[27] Historically, BI strains were fluoroquinolone and clindamycin sensitive while other historic strains causing outbreaks were clindamycin resistant.[18] However, the newly emerged BI/NAP1/027 isolates have also acquired fluoroquinolone resistance, in addition to clindamycin resistance.[18] This strain was linked not only to the widespread nosocomial outbreaks but also to a rise in community-associated disease, infections in younger populations including children and pregnant women, and cases with no previous exposure to antibiotics.[28–31] More recently, other strains such as polymerase chain reaction PCR ribotypes 001 and 078 were reported in certain outbreaks and severe cases of CDI in Europe.[32–34]

Data on the relative importance of the above emerging *C. difficile* strains in areas other than North America and Europe, especially in resource-limited settings, are scant. Although the incidence of CDI seems to be increasing in other parts of the globe as well, genotyping data are usually not available.[35] Since the late 1990s, there have also been outbreaks of CDI from TcdA-negative/TcdB-positive (A−/B+) strains occurring in Canada,[36,37] the Netherlands,[38] and Japan.[39] More recently, increasing incidence of A−/B+ strains were also noted in Ireland (95% of isolates),[40] Korea (21.4% of isolates),[41] and Argentina (86.4% of isolates).[42] Molecular typing of recovered isolates reveal that these strains were of toxinotype VIII and PCR ribotype 017. In isolates subjected to antibiotic susceptibility testing, resistance to macrolide, lincosamide, and streptogramin (MLS) (isolates also carried the *ermB* gene that encodes MLS resistance) and to fluoroquinolone was also noted. In another study, clonal worldwide spread of these strains has been suggested based on characterization of isolates coming from the United States, Canada, United Kingdom, Poland, Netherlands, France, and Japan.[43] The disease caused by A−/B+ strains has the same spectrum as that caused by A+/B+ strains, ranging from asymptomatic carriage to fulminant colitis. However, various authors have documented increased severity of disease and an increased association with pseudomembranous colitis.[44,45]

Human Carriage, Animal Infection and the Environment

C. difficile, including toxigenic strains, can be isolated in 2–3% of healthy adults.[46] Among hospitalized adult patients, colonization rates increased to 20–40%.[46,47] In the absence of an outbreak, up to 20% of residents of long-term care facilities had been reported to be colonized and as many as 70% may acquire the organism within 2 weeks of antibiotic therapy.[48] A significant proportion of residents already harbor the organism on admission and an additional 10–20% may get colonized during their stay.[48,49] Infants and children are known reservoirs of *C. difficile* with the highest carriage rates reported among neonates (up to 70%), decreasing to 6% at age 2 and down to adult rates in older children.[50] Traditionally, infants and children are at low risk of CDI although sporadic cases of severe disease have been reported.[50] The advent of BI/NAP1/027 may have changed the epidemiology of the disease in children. Pediatric patients without recent exposure to health care facility and/or antibiotics have been reported to have acquired severe colitis.[29,51]

Typical of the ubiquitous nature of clostridia, *C. difficile* has also been isolated from soil, water, animal feces, and food items.[52–56] Interestingly, even retail meats, cooked and uncooked, and ready-to-eat salads have been shown to harbor the organism.[52,54,57] The isolates that came from these retail foods are of the emerging strains discussed above, suggesting that food may be a potential source for virulent *C. difficile*. In addition to the hospital and long-term care facilities, the bacterium has also been isolated in a few studies in day care centers and veterinary facilities.[55,58,59] CDI has been known to occur in horses, dogs, and ratites.[60,61] More recently, infection was also noted in neonatal piglets and calves.[61,62] In a study looking at the genetic relationship of toxinotype V strains from human and animal specimens, a high degree of similarity was seen in some of the isolates.[63] Indeed, ribotypes 027, 017, and 078 from recent human isolates can all be isolated from either calves, horses, or pigs.[60] Whether animal reservoirs and transmission via foods are the possible sources of *C. difficile*, especially for community-acquired infections, remains to be proven.

THE DISEASE

Individuals infected with *C. difficile* present with a wide of range of presentations from asymptomatic colonization to fulminant disease. Severe pseudomembranous colitis may be complicated by toxic megacolon, perforation, severe sepsis, septic shock, or death. Diarrhea is usually reported but may be absent in the presence of severe colonic dysmotility (ileus) causing "toxic megacolon".[64] Stool is characteristically inflammatory, with or without gross or occult bleeding. Endoscopic, radiologic, and histopathologic findings are reviewed under "diagnosis" below.

Risk Factors

The three main risk factors for the development of CDI are antibiotic exposure, old age, and hospitalization. All antibiotics have been associated with subsequent infection but the most frequently implicated in outbreaks and sporadic diseases are clindamycin then penicillins (since 1970s), cephalosporins (since 1980s), and lately, fluoroquinolones (since 2000).[65,66] With the advancement in metagenomics technology and burgeoning interest in the microbial communities in humans,[67] the role of antibiotics in perturbing the intestinal microbiota and subsequent development of CDI is gradually being elucidated. It has long been noted that the indigenous intestinal flora protects against colonization by and overgrowth of *C. difficile* and other enteric pathogens,[68,69] A recent study involving human volunteers has shown that antibiotic (ciprofloxacin) administration decreases the diversity of the gut microbiota, the magnitude and duration of which varies between individuals.[70] Although recovery of the taxonomic composition of the intestinal communities occurred 4 weeks after the end of treatment, several taxa failed to recover even after 6 months. Microbial diversity has also been observed to be decreased in a patient with antibiotic-associated diarrhea.[71] Discontinuation of antibiotic was followed by resolution of diarrhea and reversal of the changes in the fecal microbial flora. Findings from murine studies suggest that antibiotics not only reduce species diversity of intestinal microbiota and promote growth of *C. difficile* but may also induce toxin production, trigger a "supershedder state," and enhance spore-mediated transmission of infection.[72,73]

The high incidence, recurrence, and mortality rates of CDI in individuals of advanced age have been attributed to the inability of the waning immune system to mount an antibody response against *C. difficile* toxin A.[74,75] With the advent of the NAP1/BI/027 outbreaks, the vulnerability of elderly people to fulminant colitis and complications of CDI infection became more visible. From 1999 to 2006, the age-adjusted death rate for CDI increased by at least 30% per year in the entire US population (http://www.cdc.gov/nchs/data/nvsr/nvsr57/nvsr57_14.pdf). Approximately 90% of deaths occurred in persons aged ≥65 years. Elderly patients with CDI usually come from long-term health care facilities, have comorbid conditions, suffer from complications such as gastrointestinal bleeding or dehydration, are admitted to the intensive care unit, need colectomy, and are more likely to die compared with the younger patients.[76,77] Hospitalization is a major risk factor as this is usually the site of initial encounter with the *C. difficile* spores transmitted from the contaminated environment to the patient through the hands of health care workers.[78] In this environment, susceptible patients (including the elderly and the immunocompromised) are also frequently exposed to multiple antibiotics for various clinical indications.

PATHOGENESIS AND IMMUNITY

The main virulence factors that are known to cause clinical disease in CDI are the two large toxins TcdA (308 kDa) and TcdB (270 kDa). Both toxins are glucosyltransferases which inactivate Rho, Rac, and Cdc42, resulting in actin condensation and subsequent cytoskeletal changes, apoptosis, and cell death of target cells.[8] TcdA and TcdB are encoded by *tcdA* and *tcdB*, respectively. The two toxin genes are located in a 19.6 kb pathogenicity locus (PaLoc). *tcdC*, a gene that lies downstream of *tcdA*, functions as a negative regulator of toxin production. The hyperproduction of toxins in the NAP1/BI/O27 strains has been attributed to the deletions in *tcdC* resulting in the loss of its regulatory activity.[18,25,79] The toxins have three major domains: C-terminal or C-repetitive domain (receptor-binding), translocation domain (cysteine protease), and N-terminal (enzymatic) domain.[8,80] Both toxins enter the cell through receptor-mediated endocytosis. The N-terminal domain cleaves from the whole toxin via a cysteine protease activity and is translocated into the cytosol.[81,82] The glucosyltransferase activity is then carried out by the N-terminal domain. In addition to changes in the cytoskeletal organization, disruption of epithelial tight junctions and induction of apoptosis, Tcds also induce an intense inflammatory response characterized by infiltration of inflammatory cells, especially neutrophils, activation of submucosal neurons, secretion of cytokines, chemokines and arachidonic acid metabolites, and production of substance P and reactive oxygen intermediates.[8,83] Recent reports described the involvement of intracellular kinases and transcription factors in the induction of prostaglandin and chemokine syntheses.[84,85] The direct link between glucosylation of the small GTPases and induction of the inflammatory cascade is yet to be elucidated.

DIAGNOSIS

The gold standard for laboratory diagnosis had been the cytotoxin assay. Because of the unavailability of tissue culture facility in most hospitals, the most commonly used diagnostic method was enzyme immunoassay. Systematic review of the commercially available toxin detection (enzyme immunoassay) tests revealed unacceptably low sensitivity of some of the assays and the overall low positive predictive value of the method (<50% in some kits).[86] Molecular techniques to detect gene encoding for TcdB are increasingly being used for their rapid turnaround time and improved sensitivity rates.[87] However, because of the increased possibility of getting

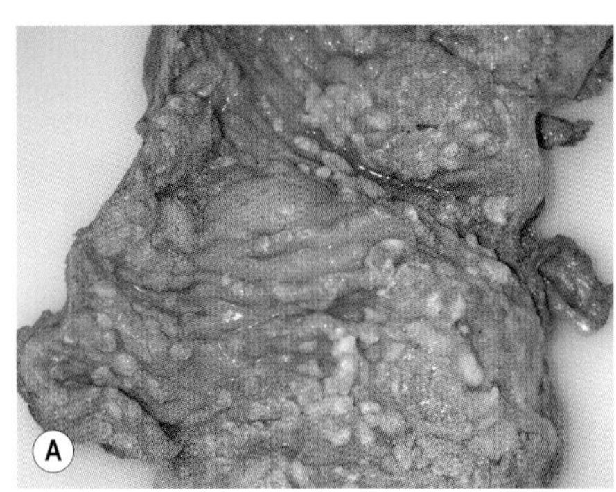

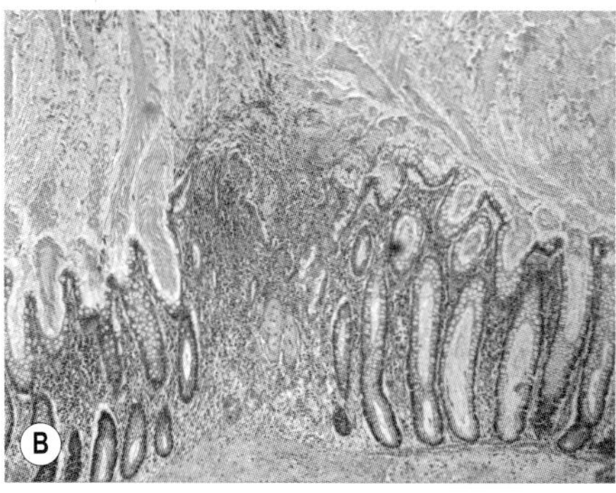

Figure 22.1 **(A)** Gross pathology: Punctate and geographic areas of pseudomembranes (*fibrin*, necrotic mucosal cells and leukocytes) with intervening normal *colonic* mucosa. **(B)** Histology: A focal *raised* area of necrotic colonic mucosa ("volcanic eruption") overlain by a thick exudate of fibrin and degenerating mucosal and inflammatory cells. (Courtesy of Drs Randy Robinson and Cirle Warren.)

false positive results, some investigators recommend two-step (or more) diagnostic algorithms.[88–90]

Radiologic procedures such as abdominal X-rays or CT scan may be helpful in diagnosis but are especially valuable in assessing for complications of pseudomembranous colitis such as toxic megacolon and perforation.[91,92] The characteristic "pseudomembranes" in severe disease are usually visualized during either endoscopy (proctosigmoidoscopy or colonoscopy, if performed) or in gross specimens taken from patients requiring colectomy (***Fig. 22.1A***). Histologic studies usually reveal a "volcano eruption"-like appearance of the necrotic intestinal epithelium infiltrated by acute inflammatory cells (mostly neutrophils) and overlain by thick fibrinous exudate with degenerating epithelial and inflammatory cells (***Fig. 22.1B***).

TREATMENT AND PROGNOSIS

First-Line Treatment For years, metronidazole has been the preferred first-line therapy for CDI because of its equivalent efficacy with vancomycin at a more affordable cost. However, a recent randomized controlled trial showed that vancomycin is more effective than metronidazole for severe disease (cure rates of 97% and 76%, respectively).[93] In this study, vancomycin was given at 125 g orally four times a day for 10 days. Severe disease was described as either the presence of pseudomembranous colitis or admission to the intensive care unit; or two of the following: age >60 years, temperature of 38.3°C, albumin level <2.5 mg/dL, or white blood cell count >15 000 cells/mm^3. For mild disease, metronidazole at 250 mg four times a day resulted in a cure rate of 90% compared with 98% in those given vancomycin ($P = 0.36$).

Alternative Agents Nitazoxanide, an antimicrobial agent that interferes with anaerobic metabolism of bacteria and protozoa, has been reported to be as effective as vancomycin in a small randomized, double-blind study. The sustained response rate from nitazoxanide (500 mg two times a day for 10 days) was 89%.[94] Rifaximin, a semisynthetic derivative of rifamycin, is a non-absorbed antibiotic that has activity against *C. difficile*. Initial studies suggest its efficacy for recurrent CDI but development of microbial resistance has been noted.[95,96] Other antimicrobial agents undergoing phase III clinical trials include ramoplanin, a new lipoglycodepsipeptide, and difimicin (OPT-80 and PAR-101), a minimally-absorbed microcycle.[97,98] Tolevamer, an anionic polymer that binds TcdA and TcdB, has been shown to be inferior to metronidazole and vancomycin for primary CDI but the relapse rate was significantly less.[99,100] Studies on the role of active vaccination in treatment are under way.

Fulminant Colitis In cases of seriously ill patients, vancomycin given by mouth or by retention enema and intravenous metronidazole are usually administered.[101,102] Although evidence for its efficacy is anecdotal, intravenous immunoglobulin (IVIG) has been used by others for severe disease as well. Surgical intervention is usually indicated for toxic megacolon and perforation but must also be considered early on for unresponsiveness to medical therapy.[103,104]

Recurrent Disease Recurrence of CDI occurs in up to 30% of patients treated with antibiotics.[102] The initial recurrence is usually treated with a repeat course of either metronidazole or vancomycin.[105] For the second episode, most experts recommend tapered followed by pulsed dosing of oral vancomycin.[106,107] From the third recurrence onwards, different management strategies have been tried but the evidence for their efficacy mostly comes from anecdotal reports or small studies. These strategies include vancomycin plus probiotics,[108] vancomycin followed by rifaximin,[96] nitazoxanide,[109] probiotics,[110] toxin-binding resins, IVIG,[109] fecal bacteriotherapy,[111] and chronic low-dose vancomycin suppressive therapy.

PREVENTION AND CONTROL

The hospital continues to be the major source of *C. difficile* spores. To reduce the incidence of CDI, infection control measures targeting the environment, personal hygiene, and barrier methods must be in place.[112] Disinfection with a 1 : 10 dilution of concentrated sodium hypochlorite (i.e., bleach) is effective in reducing environmental contamination.[113] Other commonly used hospital cleaning agents may not only be non-sporicidal but may even induce sporulation. The use of gloves is proven to be effective in reducing transmission of *C. difficile* during care of patients with CDI.[114] Alcohol-based hand sanitizers are not effective in killing *C. difficile* spores and thus should not be used alone in decontaminating the hands. Proper hand washing technique with use of soap and water is important. Patients with symptomatic CDI should be promptly identified and isolated.

Exposure to antibiotics is a major risk factor in the development of CDI. Antibiotic restriction, in combination with other infection control measures, has been shown to reduce institutional rates of CDI.[115,116]

C. PERFRINGENS FOOD POISONING AND OTHER DIARRHEAL DISEASES

EPIDEMIOLOGY

C. perfringens is the second most common cause of reported foodborne disease outbreaks and outbreak-associated illnesses in the United States.[117] From 2001 to 2005, the Centers for Disease Control and Prevention (CDC) reported a mean of 51 outbreaks (2077 cases) per year where *C. perfringens* was either the confirmed or suspected etiology. Inadequate food (usually animal meats) storage and reheating are the associated risk factors and outbreaks occur mostly in restaurants, institutions, and social gatherings.[5]

THE AGENT, PATHOGENESIS, IMMUNITY, AND THE DISEASE

C. perfringens type A food poisoning is due to the production of the enterotoxin CPE, which is generated in the small bowel during sporulation of the ingested vegetative cells (at least 10^7).[118,119] CPE binds to enterocytes and increases membrane permeability and Ca^{2+}-dependent cell death.[7] Villous shortening and epithelial desquamation are evident in histology. Abdominal pain, nausea, and diarrhea occur 6–24 hours after intake of contaminated food.[5,119] Symptoms are self-limiting and last for 24 hours only. Mortality is extremely rare but lately a few patients have been reported to develop severe, even fatal, enterocolitis resembling necrotizing enteritis.[120,121]

C. perfringens type C food poisoning (or necrotizing enteritis, enteritis necroticans, or "pigbel" or "Darmbrand") is a syndrome of acute abdominal pain, bloody diarrhea, and segmental necrotic inflammation of the small intestines 5–6 hours to a few days after ingestion of contaminated food. The disease was mainly seen in communities where protein deprivation, meat-feasting (e.g., pig-feasting in Papua New Guinea), staple diets containing trypsin inhibitors (e.g., sweet potatoes) and intestinal parasitism (especially ascariasis) coexist.[5,122] More recently, case reports of enteritis necroticans in diabetic patients from the developed world have emerged.[123,124] β-Toxin, produced by vegetative cells, is the predominant toxin thought to be involved in the pathophysiology of the disease.[5,125] Current evidence suggests that β-toxin is pore-forming and causes membrane permeability that leads to cell death.[7] Endothelial cells have recently been suggested to be the main target of the toxin, which causes vascular necrosis, hemorrhage, and tissue necrosis.[126,127]

C. perfringens is also being increasingly recognized as a cause of antibiotic-associated diarrhea. In a prospective study of 4659 patients with clinical suspicion of antibiotic-associated diarrhea (AAD), the prevalences of *C. difficile* cytotoxin, *C. perfringens* enterotoxin, and *Staphylococcus aureus* enterotoxins were 12.7%, 3.3%, and 0.2%, respectively.[128] Age greater than 70 years was a common risk factor for all pathogens but female gender and use of antacid were more associated with *C. perfringens* infection than with the others. History of exposure to specific antibiotic classes was not observed to be a risk factor. Low prevalence rates of *C. perfringens* AAD were also seen in other reports.[129,130] DNA fingerprinting and pulse-field electrophoresis (PFGE) studies indicated that nosocomial transmission, indeed, also occurs.[128,131,132]

DIAGNOSIS

Identification of foodborne *C. perfringens* infection requires appropriate epidemiologic and clinical settings as the organism and its toxins may be detected in the environment or food and stool of healthy individuals.[5,133,134] Reverse passive latex agglutination and enzyme-linked immunosorbent assay can demonstrate enterotoxin and PCR assay can detect the gene encoding for the toxins.[5,131,135] PFGE can identify the presence of the responsible strain in the environmental samples or the patients in sporadic disease, foodborne outbreaks, or nosocomial infection.

TREATMENT AND PREVENTION

Proper food handling, storage, and heating is the mainstay in preventing food poisoning. *C. perfringens* type A illness is usually self-limiting and thus does not require antibiotics. Fluid and electrolyte resuscitation is the first line of treatment. In cases of severe necrotizing enterocolitis, antimicrobial treatment with or without surgical intervention may be necessary. In general, clostridial species (except *C. difficile*) are very sensitive to penicillin G.[136] However, broad-spectrum antimicrobial regimens may be needed in complicated cases, for example perforation, secondary peritonitis, or abscess formation. Indications for surgery include persistent toxicity, persistent intestinal obstruction, suspected perforation, and severe bleeding.[2] *C. perfringens* type C disease in endemic communities has been shown to be preventable using a β-toxoid vaccine.[137,138]

FOODBORNE AND INTESTINAL BOTULISM SYNDROMES

EPIDEMIOLOGY

Ingestion of home-canned and home-fermented food is the traditional risk factor for foodborne botulism caused by *C. botulinum*.[139–142] Ingestion of raw muktuk (skin and pink blubber layer) from beached whale has been linked to botulism.[143] More recent outbreaks also involved commercially produced food items. In 2006, an international (United States and Canada) outbreak of severe botulism was attributed to a carrot juice produced by one manufacturer.[144] In 2007 an outbreak in Texas and Indiana was linked to a commercially canned chili sauce and subsequent recall of the implicated brand and other meat products produced at the canning factory.[145]

THE AGENT, PATHOGENESIS, IMMUNITY, AND THE DISEASE

The gastrointestinal tract is one of the portals of entry for botulinum toxin. The toxin is absorbed primarily in the duodenum and jejunum and systemically distributed to the peripheral cholinergic synapses, where it binds to presynaptic receptors and inhibits release of acetylcholine.[146] Human botulism is usually caused by toxin types A, B, E, or F. Three clinical syndromes of botulism related to the gut are recognized: foodborne botulism, infant botulism, and adult intestinal botulism.[6] Foodborne botulism is caused by ingestion of food contaminated by botulinum toxin. Typically, foodborne illness is defined by the toxin-induced neuroparalytic symptoms after a history of intake of contaminated food. Gastrointestinal symptoms are more commonly seen in cases of toxin types B and E illness than other toxin types.[6,147] Diarrhea, nausea, constipation, and abdominal cramps are reported to occur in botulism.[148] Gastrointestinal symptoms are variably associated with or followed by neurologic symptoms such as cranial nerve palsies and descending flaccid paralysis. The neurologic symptoms are ascribed to the botulinum (neuro)toxins and their cleavage of synaptobrevin II to prevent vesicular docking and release of acetylcholine to prevent peripheral cholingeric synaptic transmission. The etiology of enteric symptoms is unknown. Animal experimentation has not produced gastrointestinal symptoms with administration of any of the toxin types used.[6]

Infant botulism is caused by toxins formed by colonizing *C. botulinum* in the gastrointestinal tract of babies <1 year old. Constipation, poor feeding, and lethargy may be the initial presentation, which may progress to cranial neuropathies and respiratory weakness.[149] Consumption of honey has been associated with infant botulism in 15% of cases.[150] *C. butyricum* and *C. barati* have also been implicated in some cases.[151] Adult intestinal botulism is a rare disease caused by botulinum-producing *Clostridium* spp. colonizing the intestinal tract of adults who usually have anatomical or functional bowel disorders or who have been exposed to antimicrobial agents.[152,153]

DIAGNOSIS

The definitive diagnosis of foodborne botulism entails a history of ingestion of suspect food and detection of botulinum toxin in the food source or in either sera (early), gastric content, or stool (late) of a patient with neuroparalytic symptoms.[154] Suspected cases in the United States should be immediately discussed with the state epidemiologist and the CDC. The standard test is the mouse bioassay performed in a few public health laboratories. A less sensitive alternative test is enzyme-linked immunosorbent assay. Currently, a rapid mass spectrometry-based assay to detect and identify the neurotoxins is being developed.[155,156]

TREATMENT AND PREVENTION

Patients suspected to have botulism should be placed in intensive care for frequent monitoring and ventilatory support, if needed. Botulinum antitoxin is the only specific treatment for botulism. This can be obtained in consultation with the CDC. For foodborne botulism, wound botulism, and botulism of unknown cause in the United States, contact the state department or the CDC Director's Emergency Operations Center

(770–488–7100). For infant botulism, contact the California Department of Health Services, Infant Botulism Treatment and Prevention Program (510–540–2646).[6] Prevention requires diligence with heating well above boiling (hence pressure cooking) before canning.

CLOSTRIDIUM SEPTICUM

C. septicum is a known cause of gas gangrene involving infected war wounds and is also implicated in some cases of neutropenic enterocolitis.[1] Atraumatic or spontaneous *C. septicum* infections have more consistently been associated with malignancy, especially intestinal adenocarcinoma in adults.[157–159] Myonecrosis and bacteremia are common presentations. A recent review of 47 cases of *C. septicum* infection in children has identified 22 (47%) cases of myonecrosis.[160] Malignancy was found in 49%, cyclic or congenital neutropenia in 21%, hemolytic-uremic syndrome in 11%, structural bowel ischemia in 4% and local extremity trauma in 6%. The development of the disease is mainly attributed to *C. septicum* α-toxin, a pore-forming cytolytic protein that causes rapid cell death.[161,162] Antibiotics with or without surgical intervention are the mainstay of treatment.

SUMMARY

Clostridial species causing human disease gain access to the gastrointestinal tract through exposure to contaminated environment or food, causing asymptomatic colonization of the gastrointestinal tract or symptomatic infection of either healthy or immunocompromised hosts. In colonized individuals, symptoms may develop later during conditions that increase the host vulnerability (e.g., antibiotics, other intestinal diseases, age). Symptomatic disease ranges from mild to life-threatening presentations and management depends on the specific species and illness involved. Optimal prevention and control of sporadic cases and outbreaks entails an understanding of the transmission of the organism, the intestinal milieu, and pathogen–host interactions.

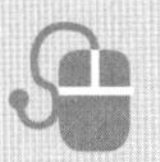

Access the complete reference list online at **http://www.expertconsult.com**

Access the complete reference list online at
http://www.expertconsult.com

CHAPTER 23

Helicobacter pylori Infections

Barry J. Marshall • Robert H. Gilman

INTRODUCTION

Helicobacter pylori colonizes the mucus layer of the human stomach and causes inflammation termed *active chronic gastritis*.[1] *H. pylori* can easily be identified using simple techniques available in all microbiology laboratories. It infects more than half of the population, is more common in tropical countries, and can cause peptic ulceration or gastric cancer. In the tropics it may be associated with reduced gastric acid,[2] increased diarrhea, and malnutrition.[3] *H. pylori* can be diagnosed by direct examination of gastric mucosal biopsy tissue obtained at endoscopy, or via gastric mucus obtained using a string capsule, or noninvasively using serology, a urea breath test, or a fecal antigen test. Cure of the infection is possible in most patients with a 2-week treatment using combinations of antimicrobial agents and acid-lowering drugs.[4] In areas with poor sanitation, reinfection is common.[5–7] Thus there is interest in preventing new infections by developing an oral vaccine, without success to date.

THE AGENT

H. pylori is the type strain of a new genus of spiral-shaped bacteria, *Helicobacter*. Their morphology and sheathed flagella may facilitate motility in the mucus layer of the gastrointestinal tract. *H. pylori* is microaerophilic, but not anaerobic, found in the mucus layer of the gut, between the anaerobic lumen and the oxygenated mucosa.

H. pylori is a Gram-negative spiral, 3.5 μm long × 0.6 μm thick, with 1.5 wavelengths and four to seven sheathed flagella at one end of the organism (***Fig. 23.1***). In tissues *H. pylori* appears spiral and lies close to the gastric epithelial cells and in the mucus glands. Squashed or smeared fresh gastric biopsy specimens may be stained by Gram stain or examined by phase contrast microscopy.[8,9] In histologic sections *H. pylori* stains well with Giemsa, toluidine blue, or silver stains. Hematoxylin and eosin (H&E) stain does not adequately demonstrate *H. pylori*.

In culture, *H. pylori* appears longer and spiral forms are less obvious, with comma shapes and U-shapes (unseparated dividing organisms) being seen.[10]

H. pylori is a highly genetically diverse organism, which in part probably allows it to develop in a host's micro-niches after transmission, as well as making it relatively immune resistant. Also this wide variation means that accurate genotyping can identify a unique organism in nearly every individual host.

Culture

H. pylori grows in reduced O_2 at 37°C as generated by a commercial *Campylobacter* kit in a gas jar or a 10% CO_2 incubator in 4–6 days on fresh (preferably) chocolate or blood agar. The generated "*Campylobacter*" atmospheres are also available as premixed cylinders that can be used to fill a sealable plastic bag with a moist paper towel inside. If nothing else is available, a candle jar with moist paper towels in the bottom will provide an adequate atmosphere, and even gas-generating methods such as the "steel wool and Alka Seltzer"[11] can be used.

Selective Media

Although *H. pylori* can be isolated easily from gastric biopsy samples onto nonselective media, 20% of patients have bacterial contamination of the biopsy, and overgrowth of commensal flora will make isolation of *H. pylori* difficult. To maximize the isolation rate, a selective medium can be made by adding vancomycin, trimethoprim, and amphotericin to the culture medium.[12] Ready-made selective media for *H. pylori* culture are available,[13] or *Campylobacter* isolation media such as Skirrow's medium may also be used.[14]

Identification

On blood or chocolate agar, transparent or pale-yellow 1–2 mm "water spray" colonies appear after 3–6 days. They are strongly positive for catalase, oxidase, and rapid urease (with a pink color observed within 5 minutes of applying a colony to Christensen's urea agar). The organism also grows in broth such as shaking tubes of *Brucella* broth[15] or in gas-permeable shaking bags[16] in a CO_2 incubator, or in fermenters.[17]

Pitfalls

When subculturing *H. pylori*, one should always examine the Gram's stain morphology of *H. pylori* as well as perform the biochemical identification tests described earlier. Contaminating organisms may appear similar to the naked eye and are often urease, oxidase, or catalase positive.

EPIDEMIOLOGY

H. pylori infects more than 70% of persons in most developing countries and about 30% of persons in developed countries. In societies that have recently emerged to affluence (such as Japan), *H. pylori* is still quite common and infects most persons over the age of 40 years. As standard of living, education and hygiene improved in the twentieth century, most countries noted a dramatic fall in *H. pylori* prevalence, especially in children.

H. pylori is acquired in childhood, probably by the fecal-oral route; it has been isolated from the feces of children in The Gambia[18] and polymerase chain reaction (PCR) techniques have shown the organism in water from Peru.[5] In developing countries, children may be infected at the rate of 15% per annum so that most of the population is infected by adulthood.[19] The initial infection with *H. pylori* may be lost spontaneously but then reacquired from the environment, before the child maintains a stable permanent gastric infection, amidst intrafamilial spread via

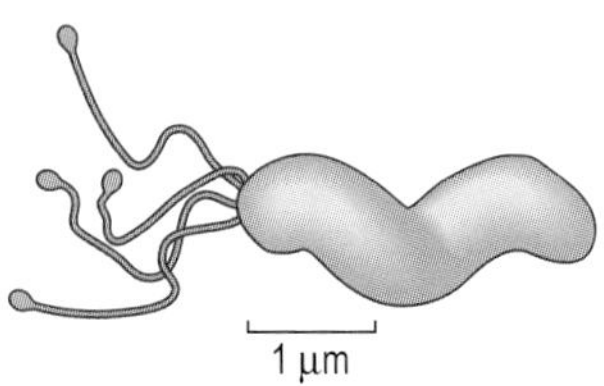

Figure 23.1 *Helicobacter pylori* (3.5 ×0.6 μm) has a smooth wall and four to seven sheathed flagella arising from only one end of the cell. These features distinguish it from *Campylobacter* spp., which have rough cell walls and a single, thinner, unsheathed flagellum at each end of the cell. Other *Helicobacter* spp. have distinguishing features such as many flagella and axial filaments (*H. felis* from cats) or flagella sprouting from the sides of the organism (*H. mustelae* from ferrets). Mature organisms appear as spiral forms with 1.5 wavelengths.

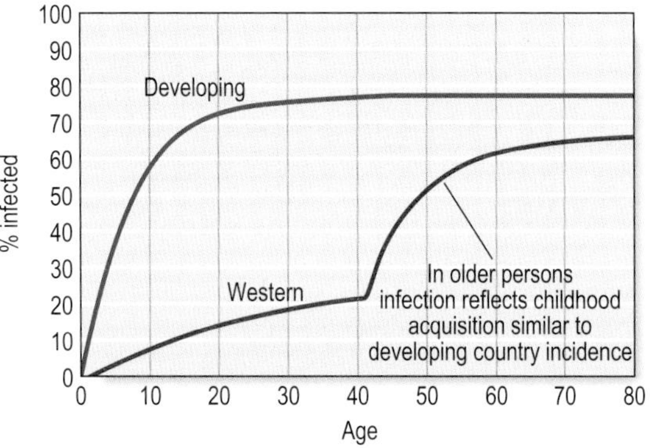

Figure 23.2 The prevalence of *Helicobacter pylori* in developing and Western countries. In developed countries, *H. pylori* is decreasing in prevalence so that most of the infections are in those over the age of 50 years who likely acquired the infection during childhood. The infection in young persons is only seen in immigrants from high-risk countries.

stools or even aerosols of vomitus,[20,21] with young children amplifying infections.[22]

H. pylori DNA is sometimes present in dental plaque,[23] but live organisms are rarely culturable from the oral cavity. Organisms might occasionally be carried to the mouth in gastric reflux, but probably do not reside there, and are rarely transmitted directly (67 infants born to infected mothers had only one new *H. pylori* infection by breath test during a 12-month period).[24] The rate of reinfection after treatment in developed countries is low but in developing countries up to 30% of a treated adult population will be reinfected within a 30-month period; most of these recurrences are due to new infections (by DNA analysis of the strains), suggesting common fecal-oral spread (***Fig. 23.2***). Genotyping has demonstrated that in developed countries transmission is often mother to child whereas in developing countries infection is more often from sources outside of the family.[25]

PATHOGENESIS AND IMMUNITY

Acute Infection

Upon ingestion, the urease enzyme of *H. pylori* enables it to survive in acid by generating ammonia and bicarbonate from urea present in the gastric juice.[26] Vague epigastric discomfort and even vomiting may commence 72 hours after ingestion of the organism. Gastric acid secretion may initially increase. Symptoms usually settle after several days as the bacterium induces achlorhydria,[20,27,28] perhaps via the action of a bacterial toxin,[29] ammonia, or the presence of cytokines, especially interleukin-1β (IL-1β).[30]

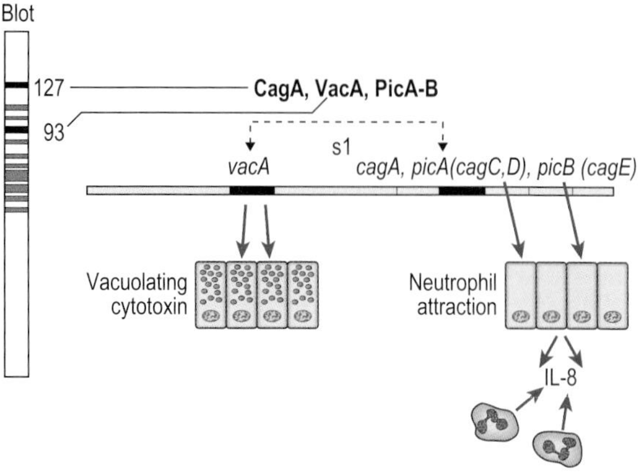

Figure 23.3 Relationships of cytotoxin genes and proteins. The left side diagrams a representative immunoblot pattern of a patient with a duodenal ulcer and *Helicobacter pylori* infection. The 127 kDa band is the cytotoxin-associated gene A (*cagA*) product. The *cagA* pathogenicity island has a higher guanine + cytosine content than the rest of the *H. pylori* genome. This suggests that the *cagA* gene group has long ago been imported from a different genus. The *vacA* (vacuolating toxin A) gene has two main subunits (s and m), and these can each be in two subtypes (s1, s2, and m1, m2). When s2 is present, the cytotoxic potential of the organism is very weak and is not usually associated with peptic ulcer, and the *cagA* island is usually absent.

In the tropics, achlorhydria has long been associated with malnutrition and susceptibility to enteric infections such as *Vibrio cholerae* and enterotoxigenic *Escherichia coli* infections.[31,32,33]

The achlorhydria of acute *H. pylori* is "chemically induced" and is reversible, unlike that seen after many years of the chronic *H. pylori* infection, where atrophy of gastric mucosa causes acid secretion to be irreversibly diminished.[34] The gastric atrophy and attendant achlorhydria and decreased excretion of vitamin C may also contribute to iron deficiency anemia seen in subjects with *H. pylori*.

Attachment

H. pylori's several attachment mechanisms enable it to selectively colonize gastric mucosa but not intestinal mucosa. *H. pylori* adheres to Lewis B antigen,[35] phosphatidylethanolamine,[36] and ganglioside GM_3,[37] all of which are present on the gastric mucus epithelial cells. In addition, *H. pylori* synthesizes Lewis X antigen, which may be a mechanism of "molecular mimicry" to make the organism similar to the host tissue, thus attenuating the immune response.[38] Once attached, *H. pylori* induces IL-8 production, which attracts neutrophils.[39] Deep colonization in the acid-secreting mucosa may also induce IL-1 secretion by inflammatory cells that inhibits acid secretion.

Cytotoxins

The most notable *H. pylori* cytotoxin is CagA, one component of some 30 genes in the *cagA* pathogenicity island, which encodes a "type IV" secretion system. A hollow pilus-like structure injects the CagA toxin protein into the epithelial cell. CagA toxin emulates two growth factors causing the epithelial cell to adopt a less structured, more mobile, primitive form, thus disrupting epithelial integrity and allowing nutrients to leak out to the *H. pylori*. In developed countries, CagA is present in only 60% of strains, whereas in most tropical or developing countries over 90% of strains are CagA-positive.

Linked to CagA is VacA toxin, a membrane pore causing leaky intracellular organelles and the appearance of "vacuoles" in the cells. The two *vacA* subunits "s" and "m" can each exist in two forms, s1 or s2, and m1 or m2; only s1 (with m1 or m2) is associated with active cytotoxin (***Fig. 23.3***).[40] Other toxins are BabA (blood-group antigen binding toxin A)[41] and DupA (duodenal ulcer promoting gene). Toxin-producing strains (CagA, VacA, BabA) are associated with duodenal ulcer or with gastric cancer and upregulate mucosal inflammation. Interleukin polymorphisms in the patient, such as IL-1β and its receptor, modulate inflammatory responses to virulent strains to increase cancer risk by 5–50-fold.[42–44]

H. pylori also activates both IL-10 and IL-17, which increase T_{reg} cells and downgrade host immunity, thereby contributing to *H. pylori's* propensity for lifelong infection.

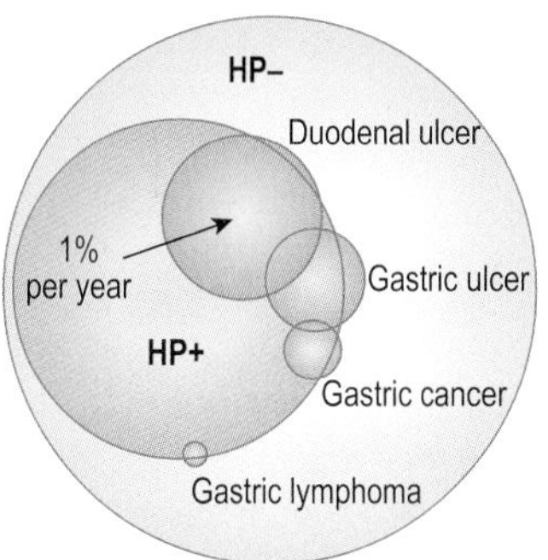

Figure 23.4 Disease associations with *Helicobacter pylori* (HP). The large circle represents a typical population in a developed country where 60% of persons are *not* infected with *H. pylori*. The darker circle represents the 40% of persons who *are* infected with *H. pylori*. Even so, nearly all the duodenal ulcers and gastric ulcers occur in the *H. pylori*-positive group. Each year, 1% of infected patients undergo transition from asymptomatic gastritis to symptomatic peptic ulcer. Note that most gastric adenocarcinomas and gastric mucosa-associated lymphoid tissue (B-cell) lymphomas also occur in the *H. pylori*-positive persons. Controversy reigns as to the role of *H. pylori* in persons with dyspepsia but in whom ulcers are not found: should *H. pylori* be treated in these persons, or ignored?

THE DISEASE

Asymptomatic Infection

All people with *H. pylori* infection have histologic gastritis, but this lesion is usually asymptomatic. Thus, the acute infection may be a short-lived vomiting illness in young children, but the bacterium is never cleared. The asymptomatic chronic infection has been linked to slight growth impairment in children,[45,46] and iron deficiency is certainly associated, but many reported disease associations might be socioeconomic. Pediatric and non-gastric disorders associated with "asymptomatic" *H. pylori* have been reviewed elsewhere.[47] The natural history of lifelong gastritis is explained in detail below.

Active Chronic Gastritis

Active chronic gastritis with polymorphonuclear and mononuclear cells (lymphocytes and plasma cells) in the gastric mucosa is associated with nearly all *H. pylori* infections.[44] Neutrophilic invasion of the necks of mucous glands may occur when gastritis is severe.[48–51] In the antrum of the stomach, *H. pylori* is most numerous on the surface of the epithelium (beneath the mucus layer) but it also lives in the mucus-secreting glands. In the body of the stomach (corpus), almost all of the organisms are found on the surface. Inflammation occurs near the bacteria. Thus in the corpus, the appearance is that of a "superficial gastritis," whereas in the antrum, the inflammation is deeper. In either place the lesion can be associated with lymphoid follicles.[52]

In long-standing chronic active superficial gastritis, the superficial inflammation includes a predominance of polymorphonuclear neutrophils, with chronic lymphocytic inflammation surrounding destroyed remnants of gastric deep glands. As this deep inflammation extends, the deep glands become scattered, shallow islands separated by chronic inflammation called chronic atrophic gastritis. Another way deep glands are replaced is through intestinal metaplasia. Metaplastic epithelium may be due to the ingress and proliferation of bone-marrow-derived stem cells. Although not inherently premalignant, these proliferating stem cells are susceptible to DNA damage from ingested gastric carcinogens, or endogenous carcinogens generated from the abnormal flora of the hypochlorhydric stomach. The possible link between inflammation, stem cells and cancer has been proposed by Houghton.[53] The degree of deep glands lost through either inflammation or intestinal metaplasia determines how extensive is the chronic atrophic gastritis.[54] Chronic atrophic gastritis is a precancerous lesion probably due to the effects of long-term hypochlorhydria and the resultant presence of abnormal gastric flora. In general, inflammation, both superficial and deep, is more severe in the antrum, less in the corpus, and least in the cardia.[55] In both the antrum and the corpus, the preceding lesions may be associated with lymphoid follicles, which are rarely seen in the gastric mucosa except after *H. pylori* infection.[56]

H. pylori attachment damages the cytoskeleton of the epithelial cells so that they bulge out rather than maintain a flat luminal surface. Under periodic acid–Schiff staining, the apical mucus content is reduced and cells are shorter, termed the destructive mucin lesion of the covering gastric epithelium.[51,57]

Over the lifetime of the infected person, inflammation may destroy the glandular elements (atrophy) and intestinal cells often replace gastric mucus-secreting epithelium (intestinal metaplasia). The resulting atrophic gastritis is the final "burned out" phase of *H. pylori* infection, usually seen in older persons. In tropical countries, however, where *H. pylori* may have been present from a very early age, atrophic gastritis may be seen in young adults and is believed to be a major risk factor for gastric cancer.[58]

Duodenal and Gastric Ulcer

The most obvious disease associated with *H. pylori* is peptic ulceration (***Fig. 23.4***). More than 90% of duodenal ulcers are associated with toxin-producing *H. pylori*.[59] When a patient with a duodenal ulcer does not have *H. pylori* infection, etiologic factors such as Zollinger–Ellison syndrome or nonsteroidal anti-inflammatory drug (NSAID) use are likely.[60]

In gastric ulcer, two causes prevail, and many patients will have both. Most gastric ulcers have *H. pylori* with chronic gastritis. The stomach is also directly exposed to ingested agents such as an NSAID and is more likely than the duodenum to ulcerate in response to these agents. About 50% of gastric ulcers in the United States are caused by NSAIDs rather than *H. pylori*.[50]

In tropical countries where NSAIDs are less widely used and *H. pylori* is very common, most gastric ulcers are caused by *H. pylori*.[61] Perhaps because of this, gastric ulcers are more likely to be malignant and require endoscopy and biopsy for histologic examination.

Duodenal ulcer likely starts with *H. pylori* colonization mainly in the antrum, leading to high acid secretion but a defective mucosal barrier. Inflammation in the antrum impairs the growth of D cells (which make somatostatin) and thus decreases their inhibitory effects on the gastrin-producing G cells. This results in higher gastrin production, which may in turn, over the lifetime of the patient, cause a hyperplasia of the acid-secreting mucosa. Gastric mucus cells normally present in the duodenal bulb become colonized with *H. pylori*, seeded from the infection present in the antrum. Neutrophil invasion of the duodenal epithelium (duodenitis) increases susceptibility to ulceration. Inflammation is more severe when the *H. pylori* secretes CagA, thus associating the cytotoxin with duodenal ulcer.[62,63]

All persons with peptic ulcer should be tested for *H. pylori* and treated with antimicrobial agents if positive.[4,64] Ulcer recurrence is less than 10% when *H. pylori* is eradicated, whereas more than 90% of ulcers recur when the bacterium persists.[65] Thus, most patients are cured of their ulcer disease with effective antibiotic treatment.[66]

Gastric Cancer

Adenocarcinoma

Worldwide, gastric cancer is the second most common cancer, the high prevalence areas being Brazil, Colombia, Korea, China, and Japan. *H. pylori* infection affects more than half the population.[66] The incidence of gastric cancer has declined in the United States since 1930. It was the most common cancer, but now it ranks about ninth.[67]

H. pylori confers an approximately sixfold risk of gastric cancer, accounting for about half of all gastric cancers.[66] Thus, in most tropical countries where *H. pylori* is prevalent, gastric cancer is also common. In India, Bangladesh, the Middle East, southern China, and some African countries, however, *H. pylori* is prevalent but gastric cancer is not. This paradox suggests that genetic, dietary, and other unknown environmental factors are also important in the etiology of adenocarcinoma.[67,68]

The proposed chain of events in gastric carcinoma starts with a very early (age 1–5 years) infection with *H. pylori* so that the corpus mucosa is damaged during childhood. In this setting, ulcers are unlikely but a large area of the stomach is involved in the process. Bone marrow stem cells occasionally migrate into the gastric mucosa where they proliferate and produce intestinal metaplasia. Damaged areas coalesce into chronic atrophic gastritis and acid secretion diminishes, eventually allowing other organisms to colonize the stomach.[69–71] In this setting, nitrates can be changed to nitrites and then to nitrosamines, which are carcinogenic. In the presence of ammonia, inflammation itself can cause nitrosamines to form in the mucosa. Inflammation is more severe when the *H. pylori* secretes toxin, thus associating several cytotoxins with gastric cancer. The presence of proliferating stem cells in an environment containing carcinogens leads to gastric cancer risk.

The Ulcer–Cancer Controversy

It has been well demonstrated that CagA toxin-positive strains of *H. pylori* are associated with both duodenal ulcer (a high-acid state) and stomach cancer (a low-acid state). Paradoxically, patients who have duodenal ulcer are protected from developing stomach cancer. This implies that acid protects from the carcinogenic effects of *H. pylori*. Even in Japan, where stomach cancer is common, it is quite rare for a person with duodenal ulcer to develop the malignancy.[72]

One proposed explanation for this is the age of acquisition of the infection. In a tropical country where *H. pylori* is acquired in early childhood and nutrition may be poor, the infection causes severe damage to the acid-secreting area of the stomach.[58] Poor nutrition probably also assists this tendency to develop an asymptomatic low-acid state.[73]

Factors related to gastric cancer associated with *H. pylori* infection include hypochlorhydria, virulence of the infecting strain, genetic factors of the host, micronutrients in the diet, and geographic location of the patient.[3] If *H. pylori* is acquired in late childhood or in the adult years, the infection tends to affect mainly the antrum of the stomach, leaving the acid-secreting part of the stomach (the corpus) intact to cause duodenal ulcer disease.

It is also likely that carcinogenic potential of *H. pylori* is related to the type of CagA toxin. Its potency (and, ultimately, the severity of the related inflammation), is proportional to the number and avidity of phosphorylation sites it has. In European strains the phosphorylation sites can be absent, single or may have up to four copies. In many East Asian strains, however, one of the copies is optimized for a potent pharmacologic effect.[74,75] However, since disease is also modulated by dietary and other environmental factors, a particular CagA toxin type is not necessarily associated with a high cancer risk in every ethnic group.

Lymphoma

H. pylori eradication therapy should be the initial step in the treatment of proven or suspected gastric lymphoma. Up to 90% of mucosa-associated lymphoid tissue (MALT) lymphomas are associated with *H. pylori*.[76] These indolent B-cell lymphomas are sometimes driven by continuing *H. pylori* antigenic stimulus and regress when *H. pylori* infection is treated.[77,78] MALT lymphoma is cured in 70% of patients in whom *H. pylori* is eradicated.[79]

DIAGNOSIS

The diagnosis of *H. pylori* may be by invasive or noninvasive methods, or both, as shown in ***Table 23.1***. Endoscopic biopsy of gastric mucosa is the usual invasive method, although minimally invasive methods can include blind biopsy, nasogastric aspiration, or the gastric string test.[80] Noninvasive tests are primarily serologic tests that detect IgG antibody to *H. pylori*, urea breath tests (UBT) to detect gastric urease, and fecal antigen tests.

Table 23.1 Accuracy of Diagnostic Tests for *Helicobacter pylori* Infection in 268 Patients Undergoing Esophagogastroduodenoscopy

Tests	Sensitivity (%)	Specificity (%)	Positive Predictive Value (%)	Negative Predictive Value (%)
Invasive				
Biopsy: chronic inflammation[a]	100	66.3	84.4	100
Biopsy: acute inflammation[b]	86.7	93.7	96.2	79.5
Biopsy: Warthin–Starry silver stain[c]	93.1	99.0	99.4	88.7
CLOtest®[d]	89.6	100	100	84.1
Noninvasive				
^{13}C-urea breath test[e]	90.2	95.8	97.5	84.3
Fecal antigen test[f]	94.1	91.8	93.4	92.6
Serum IgG[g]	91.3	91.6	95.2	85.3
Serum IgA	71.1	85.3	89.8	61.8

[a]Chronic inflammation present in gastric antral biopsies.
[b]Acute inflammation present in gastric antral biopsies.
[c]Warthin–Starry stain of gastric antral biopsy.
[d]Rapid urease test conducted on gastric antral biopsy with results ascertained at 24 hours.
[e]^{13}C-urea breath test 60 minutes after administration of 150 mg ^{13}C-labeled urea.
[f]Data from Vaira D, Malfertheiner P, Megraud F, et al. Diagnosis of *Helicobacter pylori* infection with a new non-invasive antigen-based assay. HpSA European study group. Lancet. 1999;354(9172):30–33.
[g]Serum antibodies to *H. pylori*.
(Data from Cutler AF, Havstad S, Ma CK, et al. Accuracy of invasive and noninvasive tests to diagnose *Helicobacter pylori* infection. Gastroenterology. 1995;109:136.)

Invasive Tests

Histology

For histologic study from intact mucosa, mucosal biopsy specimens are taken away from any visible lesion, to allow distinction of active chronic gastritis from changes due to acute ulcer healing. Biopsies for *H. pylori* should be in addition to biopsies taken to exclude malignancy. Optimally at least five biopsies should be taken for the appropriate histologic diagnosis. Whenever possible biopsies should be down to the muscularis mucosae so that a better reading of chronic gastritis can be made. The biopsies should be taken two from the antrum, within 2–3 cm from the pylorus (one from the distal lesser curve and the other from the distal greater curve), two from the corpus, one from the mid-corpus, and another from the lesser curve angular notch.[80] In addition to routine H&E sections, the specimens should be stained with Giemsa or a silver stain such as Warthin–Starry or Genta stain.[81]

Culture

For culture biopsies may be moistened with a single drop of saline for prompt transport to the laboratory in a sterile tube. In some studies, organisms have remained viable in snap frozen biopsies.[82]

Blind gastric mucosal biopsies, gastric aspirates, and gastric string tests are less sensitive. Biopsy material, gastric mucus, and gastric juice can also be examined with polymerase chain reaction (PCR) or immunologic methods, but at present these are not reproducible in different laboratories and have no particular advantage over culture or histology. Stool immunoassay or PCR may also be used to detect *H. pylori* especially in children where, although less sensitive than biopsy, it is highly specific and is highly acceptable to parents and patient. Real-time PCR of stool for *H. pylori* has also be used to define clarithromycin resistance, giving same day results without the need of culture.[83]

Urease Test

H. pylori's urease allows its rapid detection in gastric biopsy material. The biopsy is placed in a medium containing urea and a pH indicator. Urease converts urea to ammonia and the pH rises with a subsequent color change.[84] *H. pylori* urease produces a positive reaction in a few minutes, a result that is so specific for *H. pylori* that other diagnostic material is often unnecessary and may be discarded to save expense.[85]

Noninvasive Tests

Infection is almost always accompanied by a rise in specific IgG antibody to *H. pylori*. IgM is present during the acute infection but is not well studied because acute infections are rarely documented. IgA is present in 80% of persons with *H. pylori*, but the absence of IgA does not exclude infection. Thus, in most cases, IgG is the best predictor of *H. pylori* infection (***Fig. 23.5***), and is available in ELISA kits, with a sensitivity and specificity approaching 95%. However, IgG may remain positive up to 2 years after successful treatment.[86] Thus the urea breath test is a better test for cure. However, if carefully validated, serology can help predict bacterial eradication. A 10% drop in ELISA absorbance at 1 year predicted *H. pylori* eradication in 84% of Mexican treated patients.[87] IgG can even be detected in urine and gingival secretions.

A fecal antigen test for *H. pylori* is less sensitive than the urea breath test at detecting *H. pylori* after treatment, but fecal tests are ideal when the UBT is unavailable, and in very young children.

UBT rely on the breakdown of isotope-labeled urea by urease (from *H. pylori*) in the stomach (***Fig. 23.6***). The ^{14}C UBT only takes 10 minutes and requires a single breath sample. The ^{13}C test takes 40 minutes and requires a baseline plus a 20–30 minute test sample. Both tests are highly accurate and the choice of which to use depends on availability and cost. Although the ^{14}C UBT uses a trace of radioactive carbon, the dose is very small – equal to less than 24 hours of background exposure, so it is not excluded from use in women or children.[88]

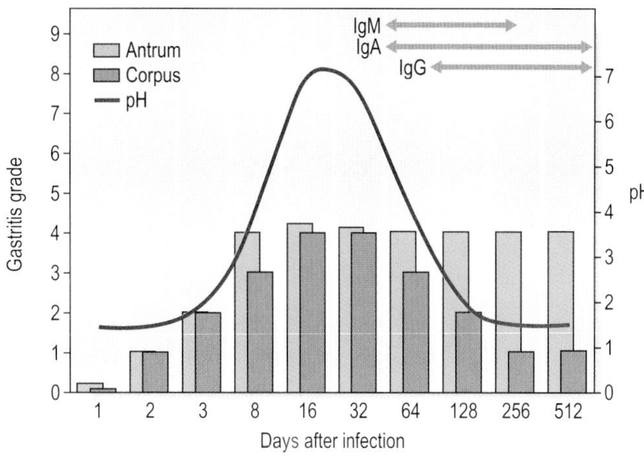

Figure 23.5 The natural history of *Helicobacter pylori* infection. The horizontal axis shows the time scale in days over 18 months. The left vertical axis is gastritis grade as represented in the columns showing antral and corpus mucosa inflammation graded 0–4. The right vertical axis shows the pH of gastric juice on a scale of 0–7. Note that corpus mucosa inflammation subsides after 3 months, whereas antral inflammation remains. As the corpus mucosa returns to near normal, acid secretion revives and gastric pH falls to normal acidic levels. Variable early responses are seen in IgA and IgM. IgG is present after the fourth week and remains as the most stable antibody response in nearly all infected persons.

Diagnostic Criteria for Research Studies

Table 23.1 gives comparative data on the accuracy of diagnostic tests.[89,90] Although histology is accurate, an experienced pathologist is required, and is aided by the updated Houston–Sydney classification. However, altered muscle bundles can still give a false impression of atrophy.

Concordance between two different methods such as histology and culture, urease test and culture, histology and serology, or urease test and serology help prove the diagnosis.

Although complicated by frequent reinfection in developing areas, two negative tests (UBT or fecal antigen) will suffice, the first at 4 weeks post therapy and the second at 6–8 weeks post therapy.

TREATMENT AND PROGNOSIS

Eradication treatment is recommended for patients with peptic ulcer disease and the rare patient with gastric lymphoma.

In the tropics, regimens containing metronidazole are much less effective, and furazolidone is an alternative in a 10-day regimen that includes bismuth and amoxicillin. Rapid recurrence after successful eradication is well documented in Peru, Bangladesh, and Turkey.[6] Reinfection is most likely caused by fecal contamination of water or food.

Experience suggests that:

- *In vitro* sensitivity to an antibiotic does not predict *in vivo* efficacy. Therefore, use tested antibiotic combinations that are proven to work.
- Acid appears to protect *H. pylori* from antibiotics; therefore, the most successful treatments include strong acid suppression with proton pump inhibitors.
- Eradication usually requires 7–14 days of treatment (longer does not increase cures but does increase side effects).
- *H. pylori* does not typically develop resistance to amoxicillin, bismuth, tetracycline, and furazolidone. Therefore they may be reused, and sensitivity testing for them is not required.

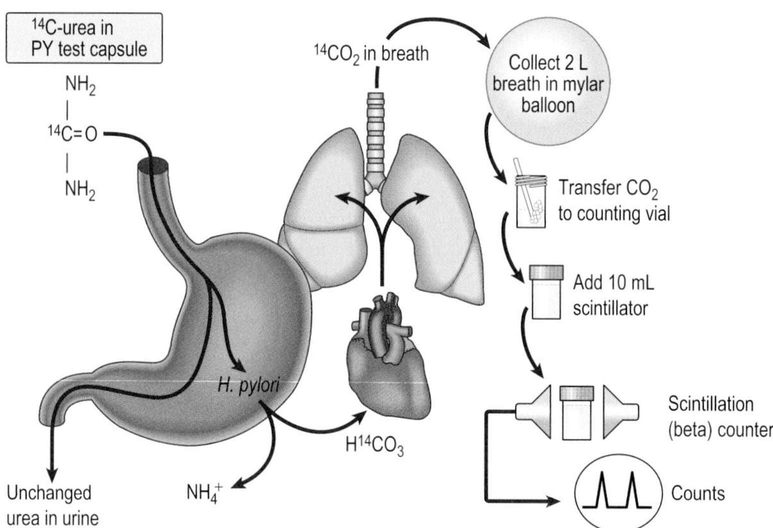

Figure 23.6 The urea breath test. Urea labeled with an isotope of carbon (a capsule of ^{14}C-urea in this illustration) is swallowed by the fasted patient. Ten to 15 minutes later, a breath sample is collected into a balloon, processed as shown, and then counted in a scintillation counter. $^{14}CO_2$ can be detected in the breath of a patient infected with *Helicobacter pylori*. When *H. pylori* is not present, the urea remains intact and there is no $^{14}CO_2$ in the breath. Unchanged ^{14}C-urea is excreted in the urine. Since more than 90% of the isotope is excreted within 3 days, radiation exposure is exceedingly small, about the same as natural background in 24 hours (0.3 mrem). In the ^{13}C-urea breath test, the patient first swallows a high-fat meal or drink, which serves to delay gastric emptying. Ten minutes later, a baseline breath sample is collected and a solution of isotope is swallowed. Diagnostic breath samples are collected 20–40 minutes later. Breath samples are analyzed in an isotope ratio mass spectrometer.

Table 23.2 Treatment Options for *Helicobacter pylori*[a]

Group	Description	Duration
A[b]	Bismuth	
	• Bismuth subsalicylate (Pepto Bismol) 525 mg (2 tablets) qid	14 days
	• Bismuth subcitrate (DeNol) 120 mg (1 tablet) qid	14 days
B	Penicillin	
	• Amoxicillin IG bid	7 or 10 or 14 days
C	Macrolide	
	• Clarithromycin 500 mg bid[c]	7 or 10 or 14 days
	• Josamycin 1000 mg bid	7 days
D	Nitroimidazole	
	• Metronidazole 500 mg	7 or 10 or 14 days bid or tid[c]
	• Tinidazole 1000 mg daily	7 or 10 or 14 days
E	Tetracycline	
	• Tetracycline 500 mg qid	14 days
F	Quinolone	7 or 10 or 14 days
	• Ofloxacin 500 mg bid	7–14 days
	• Levofloxacin 250 mg bid	7–14 days
	• Ciprofloxacin 500 mg bid	14 days
G	Nitrofurans	
	• Furazolidone 200 mg bid[c]	7 or 10 or 14 days
H	Ansamycin	
	• Rifabutin 150 mg bid	14 days
I	Proton pump inhibitors (use double a normal dose)	
	• Omeprazole 40 mg tid (has been superseded by esomeprazole in most countries)	
	• Esomeprazole 40 mg tid	
	• Lansoprazole 30 mg tid	
	• Pantoprazole 40 mg tid	
	• Rabeprazole 20 mg tid	

[a]Treatment priorities are normally: IBC → IBD → IBEG. For penicillin allergy choose ICD or IAED IFH.
[b]When Pepto Bismol is not available, substitute DeNol 1 tablet qid.
[c]Side effects are likely as doses of clarithromycin, metronidazole, and furazolidone increase.
bid, twice a day; tid, three times a day; qid, four times a day.

Box 23.1 Treatments in Common Usage

Esomeprazole 20 mg bid, clarithromycin 500 mg bid, and amoxicillin 1 g bid (7–10 days)	Rabeprazole 20 mg bid, amoxicillin 1 g bid, levofloxacin 250 mg bid (10 days)
Esomeprazole 20 mg bid, clarithromycin 250 mg bid, and metronidazole 400 mg bid (7 days)	Omeprazole 20 mg bid, amoxicillin 1 g bid, furazolidone 200 mg bid, and bismuth subsalicylate (De-Nol) 240 mg (2 tabs) bid (14 days)
Bismuth (subsalicylate or citrate) 1 tablet qid,[a] tetracycline 500 mg qid, metronidazole 250 mg qid (1–1.5 g daily) (10–14 days)	

[a]Addition of a proton pump inhibitor probably enhances the cure rate.
bid, twice a day; qid, four times a day.

- *H. pylori* quickly becomes resistant to the following drugs: metronidazole (and other "idazoles"), clarithromycin (and other "macrolides"), and rifabutin. ***Box 23.1*** outlines doses used in therapy, while ***Table 23.2*** gives treatment options.

Treatment of resistant *Helicobacter* infections and newer treatment combinations, such as "sequential therapy," have been recently reviewed.[91]

PREVENTION AND CONTROL

In developing countries, *H. pylori* recurrence after successful treatment occurs at rates 10–20 times higher than in developed countries. In addition, bacterial counts of *H. pylori* in gastric biopsies taken in recurrence are similar to those in biopsies taken prior to treatment. The high reinfection rate and lack of change in the *H. pylori* bacterial counts suggest there is little natural immunity after infection.

Given the rapid recurrence of *H. pylori* infection in impoverished tropical areas, goals for control of infection must include improved sanitation. Although eradication of *H. pylori* to prevent cancer may be unrealistic at present, prevention of gastric ulcer and duodenal ulcer recurrence for periods of a year or two may be helpful even where recurrence is high. Ethnic and cultural factors are also important; in Malaysia, prevalence rates among the Malays ranged from 12% to 29%, while among the Chinese they ranged from 27% to 58%, and for Indians between 49% and 52%.[92]

The ability of treatment to reverse precancerous lesions is unclear. Treatment may reverse dysplasia but not intestinal metaplasia. Patients treated for *H. pylori* who had gastric atrophy were at increased risk for developing gastric cancer. In patients with severe intestinal metaplasia associated with atypical changes or dysplasia, it is probably worthwhile to eradicate *H. pylori*. In patients with gastric lymphoma, eradication is mandatory because tumor regression occurs when *H. pylori* infection is treated. There is no evidence to date, however, that eradicating *H. pylori* in patients with gastric cancer will affect the course except to prevent further new cancers.

Reinfection with *H. pylori* makes vaccine use highly attractive yet it also suggests that finding an effective vaccine may be difficult. Vaccines need to work in children to prevent early infection in order to protect against ulcer disease and gastric cancer. Since natural immunity to reinfection is weak, a more immunogenic vaccine might help prevent recurrence of *H. pylori* infection after effective antimicrobial therapy.

H. pylori infection is one of the most common infections in the tropics, significantly associated with peptic ulcer disease, gastric cancer, and possibly with other enteric infections. New diagnostic, therapeutic, and preventive measures will undoubtedly determine the evolving approaches to better controlling the consequences of *H. pylori* infections worldwide.

Access the complete reference list online at
http://www.expertconsult.com

CHAPTER 24

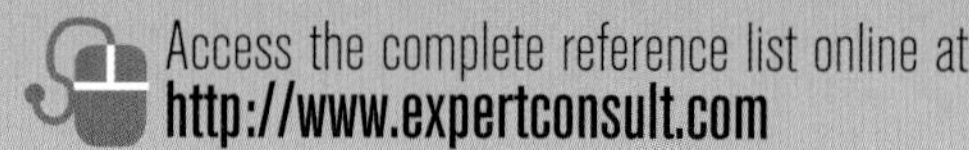
Access the complete reference list online at
http://www.expertconsult.com

Meningococcal Disease

Alexandre Leite de Souza • Diederik van de Beek • W. Michael Scheld

INTRODUCTION

Meningococcal disease is caused by *Neisseria meningitidis*. Vieusseux described meningococcal sepsis in 1805. Two centuries later, advances have been made in public health measures, effective vaccines, antimicrobial therapy, diagnostic procedures (such as real-time polymerase chain reaction, PCR), and (potentially) anti-inflammatory drugs.[1–3] Supportive care can maintain homeostasis by monitoring hemodynamic status, administering vasoactive agents, and providing respiratory and renal support. However, meningococcal disease continues to pose serious problems worldwide, influenced by geography, season, climate, meningococcal phenotype, host genetic polymorphisms, and population demographics.[4–8] Although focal outbreaks and epidemics occur in more developed areas, the incidence varies widely, and in the so-called meningitis belt of sub-Saharan Africa, hyperendemic and epidemic meningococcal disease frequently occurs.[4] Meningococcal infections continue to pose an important public health threat in the tropics because mortality is high, serious neurologic and other sequelae occur, and vaccine strategies are currently suboptimal.

History

Meningococcal disease was first reported in the city of Geneva by Vieusseux in 1805. He hypothesized that meningococcal infection, rather than being transmitted through direct person-to-person contact, was spread by "bad air": "*Le mal parut tenir à une constitution particulière de l'air, et non à une contagion se communiquant de proche en proche.*" ("The malady appears to possess a constitution that favors transmission through the air, rather than that of a contagion that is communicated by close personal contact.").[1] Across the Atlantic, the first reported cases of this "singular and very mortal disease" occurred in Medfield, Massachusetts, where nine persons afflicted with this illness died between March 8 and March 31 of the following year (1806). The patients were treated with Fowler's mineral solution (arsenite of potash) and wine. Danielson and Mann recorded these first observations of meningococcal infection and its empiric therapeutic approach in the United States in 1806 and many of the early descriptions were collated in a treatise by Elisha North of Connecticut in 1811.[9]

Anton Weichselbaum of Vienna first isolated meningococci in 1887. The organisms were obtained from the cerebrospinal fluid (CSF) of six patients with meningitis and were initially named *Diplococcus intracellularis meningitidis*. The lumbar puncture was introduced by Quincke in 1891 and major CSF alterations associated with meningitis were recognized by the turn of the century.[10]

The first truly significant therapeutic modality for any form of meningitis was developed by Simon Flexner in 1913 and consisted of systemic and intrathecal administration of antimeningococcal antisera raised in horses. Although toxic, antisera therapy reduced the mortality of meningococcal meningitis from approximately 80% to 30% during World War I and for decades thereafter. The first successful account of therapy of meningococcal meningitis with an antimicrobial agent was published in 1937;[11] nine patients survived after receiving subcutaneous and intraspinal injections of sulfanilamide and the sole death occurred despite eradication of the organism from CSF. Although sulfonamide resistance among meningococci was common by the mid-1960s and led to the abandonment of this class of agents for the treatment and prophylaxis of meningococcal disease, this event spurred interest in the development of immunoprophylaxis, leading to several safe and effective meningococcal vaccines. In Brazil, the first confirmed case of meningococcal infection was reported in 1906 by Godinho in the city of São Paulo at the Emílio Ribas Institute of Infectology, although much time would pass before the disease became generally recognized.[1]

THE AGENT

Neisseria species are non-spore-forming, oxidase-positive, nonmotile, Gram-negative cocci (measuring approximately 0.8 μm by 0.6 μm) that usually appear as biscuit- or kidney-shaped diplococci on smears of infected fluids. Since other organisms may appear similar morphologically, identification rests on biochemical and immunologic techniques. Sugar fermentation reactions are usually sufficient for speciation within the genus *Neisseria*.[12] Meningococci characteristically ferment glucose and maltose to acid. The organisms grow rapidly on blood, chocolate, gonococcal, or enriched Mueller–Hinton agar in a moist 3–10% CO_2 environment at 35–37°C. A modified Thayer–Martin medium is employed for meningococcal isolation from contaminated sites, as in detection of the carrier state. The organism is rather fastidious, susceptible to drying and chilling, so all specimens should be inoculated promptly.

The ultrastructural characteristics of meningococci are complex. Surface components include capsular polysaccharide, fimbriae or pili, lipooligosaccharides (LOS), and outer membrane proteins (OMPs); several of these structures are important virulence determinants.[1,10,12] Major classification schemes of meningococci divide organisms into serogroups based on structural differences among capsular polysaccharides and agglutination reactions with specific antisera. Invasive isolates are uniformly encapsulated, whereas carrier strains are often unencapsulated (nongroupable). The serogroups have very important epidemiologic and prevention-related implications. Thirteen serogroups are currently recognized and designated A, B, C, D, E, H, I, K, L, X, Y, Z, and W-135.[10,12] Most meningococcal disease is caused by organisms in serogroups A, B, C, and Y, although the proportion of cases caused by serogroup W-135 is increasing in some areas.[10]

Further classification of meningococci within serogroups into serotypes is based largely on the analysis of OMP profiles in the cell envelope.[10,12] Variations in protein porB are currently classified into serotypes 1 through 21. This classification scheme is useful in epidemiologic studies and as a basis for the preparation of subtype vaccines. Further classification into subserotypes is based on variations in protein porA.[13]

Subserotypes P1.1 through P1.16 are currently recognized. Variations in LOS are utilized for subdivision into immunotypes (L1 through L12).[14] Techniques for subclassification of meningococci are generally available only in research or reference laboratories but are extremely useful in epidemiologic studies. In addition to classification by serogroup, serotype, subserotype, and LOS immunotype, many reports have focused on multilocus enzyme electrophoresis.[15,16] This latter technique led to the realization that epidemics caused on a worldwide basis by a strain of serogroup A meningococci are derived from a single clone.

The standard for epidemiologic research has become multilocus sequence typing (MLST).[16] MLST analysis determines genetic variation in seven housekeeping genes of the meningococcus and has shown that most cases of disease are caused by a few clonal complexes of related sequence types, the hypervirulent lineages.

There are various genes in the meningococcal genome that are potential virulence factors in the human host.[17–19] One of the most promising advances regarding meningococcal pathogenesis was the discovery of the complete genome sequences of the serogroup A[20] and B[21] organisms.[17] Meningococci spontaneously produce a wide range of genetic variations due to the hyperdynamic nature of the meningococcal genome.[22] For the meningococci to adapt to the changing environments and to evade the host immune defenses, concomitant genome diversification and genome preservation are required.[22] In the cellular environment within a human host, meningococci can indeed uptake DNA by retracting type IV pili, which are long projections that surround the bacterial cell surface, and introducing DNA into the meningococcal cell through the outer and inner membranes.[22] In addition, the ability of meningococci to exchange the genes responsible for the biosynthesis of their capsules, including the switch from serogroup C to B or vice versa, has been recognized.[17,23] These factors have critical implications for understanding meningococcal pathogenesis, for developing vaccine prevention strategies based on capsular polysaccharide, and for epidemiologic investigations, and suggest a strategy by which meningococci escape vaccine-induced or natural protective immunity.[23]

EPIDEMIOLOGY

Transmission and Carriage

The World Heath Organization estimates that at least 500 000 new cases of meningococcal infection occur every year, resulting in more than 50 000 deaths.[1] The bacterial pathogen *N. meningitidis* is an obligate commensal of the human nasopharyngeal mucosa. Typically, this microorganism spreads from person to person by airborne droplets or via direct physical contact, such as kissing.[1] Meningococci are found in the airways of 10% of the healthy population, and the rate of colonization might exceed 50%, especially in individuals with viral respiratory tract illness.[1,24] Meningococcal colonization may result in an asymptomatic carrier state (which is most common) or endemic, hyperendemic (i.e., in the meningitis belt between epidemics at approximately 10–50 cases per 100 000 per year), or epidemic disease.[10] Meningococci persist asymptomatically in the nasopharynx for periods ranging from several weeks to months to as long as 1–2 years.[25] Sporadic cases of disease occur at the much lower annual rates of 1–5 per 100 000.[1,7] During this colonization phase, protective antibodies to the strain are usually induced.[26]

Although, as noted previously, at least 13 capsular serogroups of meningococci have been described, most human disease is caused by serogroups A, B, C, Y, and W-135, and these strains cause nearly all outbreaks of disease. This section describes recent epidemiologic trends for the major serogroups.

Serogroup A

Serogroup A organisms are the most common cause of large epidemics.[4,17,27] These outbreaks may lead to incidence rates as high as 300–1000 cases per 10^5 population.[28] For example, the annual incidence reached 370 cases per 100 000 population in the greater São Paulo area in 1974, with 31 000 cases reported per year.[28] Attack rates are highest in children and young adults and some investigators have reported that, compared with the age distribution of disease in endemic cases, higher proportions of the disease occur in older children during epidemics. In some areas of the world, serogroup A meningococcal epidemics recur in a periodic pattern.[4,27] The African meningitis belt (***Fig. 24.1***), stretching from Ethiopia in the east to The Gambia in the west, frequently experiences epidemic disease and in some countries epidemics occur every 8–12 years. ***Figure 24.2*** shows the incidence of disease and outbreak history in a typical meningitis belt country, Niger, for a 70-year period. This area of sub-Saharan Africa is dry with an average yearly rainfall of 300 mm and with winter seasons that feature warm, dry, and dusty winds (the harmattan).[29] Outbreaks typically begin with the onset of the dry season in January and end abruptly with the coming of the rains in May or June.[4,27] Although conjectural, the distinct seasonality is striking and may be related to the drying effect on mucous membranes, seasonal transmission of respiratory viruses, or other factors.[4,27]

In a study of serogroup A meningococcal strains from epidemic waves from the 1950s through the early 1980s,[30] individual epidemics and most

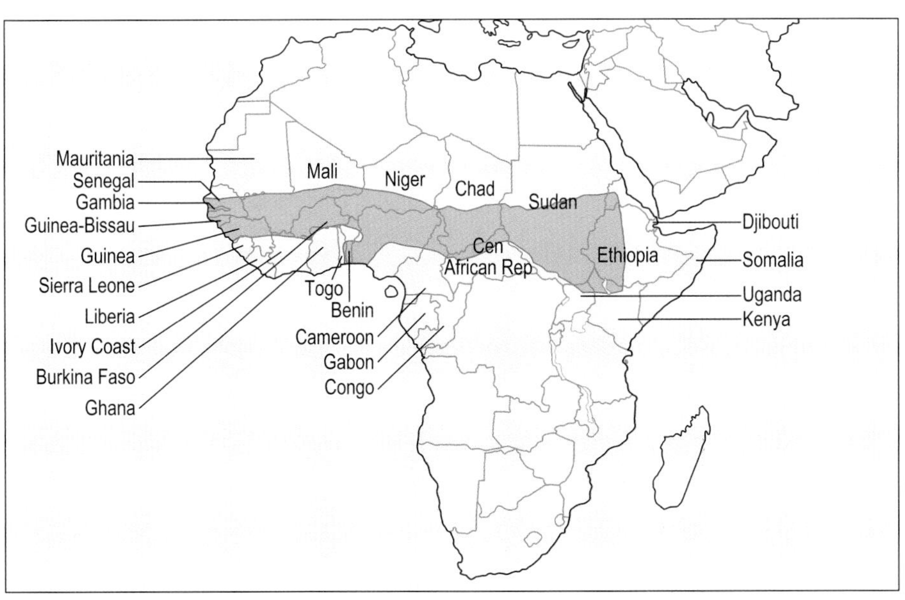

Figure 24.1 The sub-Saharan Africa "meningitis belt."

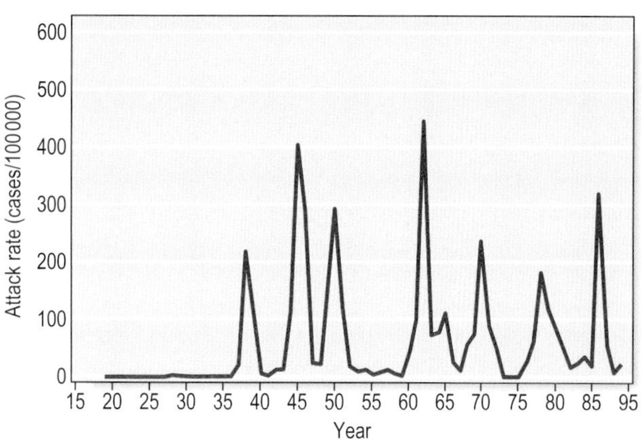

Figure 24.2 The epidemiology of meningitis in Niger. a country located in the "meningitis belt," from 1919 through 1989. (From Riedo FX, Plikaytis BD, Broome CV. Epidemiology and prevention of meningococcal disease. Pediatr Infect Dis J 1995;14:643.)

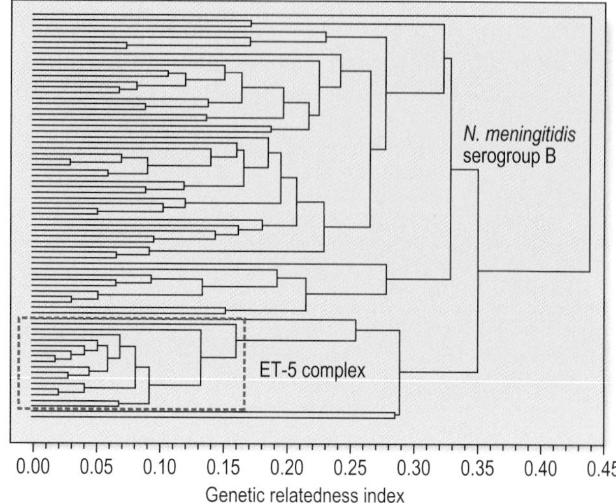

Figure 24.3 Multilocus enzyme electrophoresis dendrogram of serogroup B meningococci showing the location of the enzyme type 5 (ET-5) complex.

waves of epidemics lasting several years were due to single strains. Molecular epidemiology showed that a serogroup ST-5 clone predominated and was responsible for epidemics in the meningitis belt countries until 1999.[27] However, starting in 1995, a new, closely related ST-7 clone emerged, which has spread throughout the meningitis belt and is responsible for the major epidemic waves.

Major epidemics in the meningitis belt are heralded by a "shift to the right" toward older age groups (i.e., adolescents instead of 5- to 9-year-old children), a predictive feature of explosive epidemics.[10,14] It is possible that introduction of new strains into populations that have not previously (or at least recently) been exposed to them leads to higher attack rates in older children compared to endemic or hyperendemic disease.[28] This could occur without assuming the new organisms have any inherent increased invasiveness or transmission potential. Introduction of newer strains with different antigenic determinants into the population places older children and young adults at risk since they have never "seen" this strain and may not be immunologically protected as they were from previously circulating strains.[28]

In 1996, the biggest wave of meningococcal meningitis outbreaks ever recorded hit West Africa.[4,27] An estimated 250 000 cases and 25 000 deaths occurred in Niger, Nigeria, Burkina Faso, Chad, and other countries and paralyzed medical care systems locally. The outbreak stopped with the spring rains as usual but continued into the next winter season.[4,27] The strain isolated was from the III-1 clone, which has caused a series of outbreaks in Africa since 1988, according to the Centers for Disease Control and Prevention (CDC).

Serogroup B

Group B organisms, ST-32 and ST-41/44 complexes, have recently emerged as important pathogens in northern Europe, Cuba, Chile, US Pacific Northwest, and New Zealand, causing serious local outbreaks peaking in the 10- to 20-year-old age group. The continued high prevalence of serogroup B meningococcal disease has important implications because of the current lack of a widely available vaccine effective against this serogroup. In the early 1990s, increasing rates of meningococcal disease in the general population and focal outbreaks were documented in Oregon.[31] The overall rate of disease, which had been in the range of 1–2 cases per 100 000 population, similar to that in the United States in general, rose steadily to approximately 5 cases per 100 000. The age distribution in the cases also rose, consistent with epidemic disease caused by the other serogroups, but data soon showed that most of the cases were caused by serogroup B. Further subtyping data identified an enzyme type strain previously seen only very rarely in the United States, designated ET-301. This strain caused 80% of all serogroup B disease in Oregon and was closely related to other strains identified by Caugant and colleagues as the ET-5 complex (*Fig. 24.3*) that was later identified as complex ST-32.[32,33] Strains from this group have caused increased rates of disease, usually with overall incidence rates between 5 and 15 cases per 100 000 population per year in Norway, the Netherlands, Cuba, and throughout much of Latin America in the 1980s and early 1990s. In contrast to serogroup A and C outbreaks, which even in the absence of large-scale immunization programs usually run their course over a period of 2–3 years in a given area, serogroup B ET-5 outbreaks tend to cause prolonged elevations of disease rates in the same areas, persisting for up to a decade.[34]

Serogroup C

Large-scale outbreaks due to serogroup C have occurred frequently in the tropics. For example, the attack rate was 517 cases per 100 000 inhabitants during a serogroup C epidemic in Burkina Faso.[10,14] In July 1971, a dramatic epidemic of sulfonamide-resistant serogroup C meningococcal infection emerged in São Paulo. Interestingly, a particular phenomenon occurred in the period from 1972 to 1974, when there was an overlapping of two epidemic waves in São Paulo, one caused by serogroup C and another, larger epidemic caused by serogroup A.[1] Initially, 91% of all meningococcal infection was caused by *N. meningitidis* serogroup C strains, while in 1974, 90% of the strains were serogroup A. Indeed, it was one of the most widespread meningococcal epidemics in history. In 1975, mass vaccination of millions of Brazilians over several days with vaccine A plus C put an end to this epidemic, which was responsible for thousands of deaths.

In most developed countries, meningococcal disease, usually caused by serogroup B, C, or Y meningococci, has slowly decreased in incidence (*Fig. 24.4*). However, in the late 1980s and early 1990s, disturbing small outbreaks and an increased incidence of serogroup C disease were identified in a number of countries, particularly Canada.[35,36] The outbreaks usually involved between 5 and 20 children or young adults in small geographic areas and the fatality rate (10–15%) and burden of serious sequelae caused increasing alarm. Most of the recent Canadian outbreaks and cases were caused by one specific serogroup C strain, designated enzyme type (ET)-15, which was identified as MLST sequence type 11.[37] This type increased in Canadian strain collections from 5% of all invasive isolates in 1985 to over 65% by 1990 and resulted in a large-scale immunization program. The ET-15 strain and four other closely related clonal strains were also implicated in a marked increase in outbreaks of serogroup C meningococcal disease in the United States, where it remains among the most prevalent causes of meningococcal meningitis (*Table 24.1*). Multiple outbreaks of serogroup C meningococcal disease occurred

Serogroup	Percentage of Isolates
C	32
B	24
Y	31
W-135	6
A	<1

Table 24.1 *Neisseria meningitides* Serogroups Responsible for Invasive Disease: United States, 1995

(Adapted from Broome CV, Wenger JD, Schuchat A, et al. Changing epidemiology of bacterial meningitis in the United States. Presented at the 36th Interscience Conference on Antimicrobial Agents and Chemotherapy, New Orleans, LA, September 1996, abstract S64.)

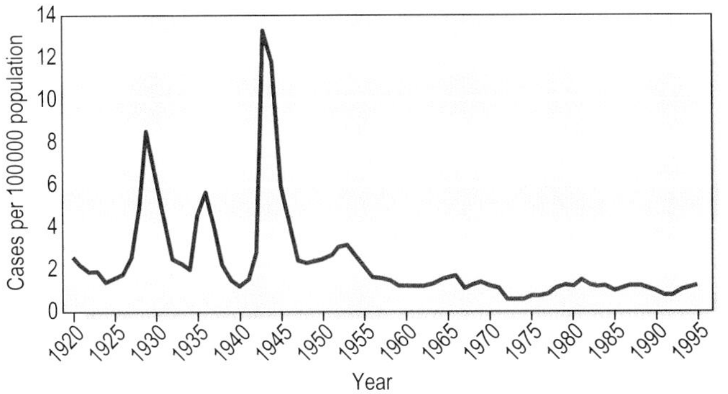

Figure 24.4 The incidence of reported meningococcal disease in the United States by year, 1920–1995.

and mass immunization campaigns were conducted in more than 10 separate sites between 1990 and 1993.[35]

In the developed world, invasive infections due to *Neisseria meningitidis* serogroup C have increased over the past decade.[38] Routine immunization with the meningococcal serogroup C protein-polysaccharide conjugate vaccines has been undertaken in several countries with reductions in the disease burden of bacterial meningitis. Concerns that routine vaccination may result in an increase in meningococcal disease due to non-C serogroups have not been realized.

Serogroup W-135

Serogroup W-135 strains (ST-11 complexes) caused worldwide outbreaks in 2000–2002 associated with the Hajj pilgrimage, and in part of the meningitis belt countries. During the outbreak of meningococcal disease coinciding with the Hajj pilgrimage in March 2000, the attack rate of W-135 disease was 25 cases per 100000 pilgrims.[39] All outbreak-associated isolates of serogroup W-135 were members of a single clone of the hypervirulent ET-37/ST-11 complex, which occurred as the result of expansion of a clone that had been in circulation since 1970.[40] It has been estimated that a majority of the 12000 meningitis cases in Burkina Faso in 2002 were of the W-135/ST-11 complex.[41]

Serogroup Y

Serogroup Y disease has emerged in the United States. In 1989–1991 this serogroup was responsible for 2% of meningococcal infections, but the incidence has risen gradually since 1995. Today, around one-third of cases in the United States are caused by this serotype.[42]

THE DISEASE

At the dawn of the twentieth century, Herrick noted that: "For a satisfactory understanding of the complications of epidemic cerebrospinal meningitis a proper knowledge of the fundamental nature of disease is necessary," and that "the result of the study of epidemic cerebrospinal meningitis has been the establishment of the disease as primarily a bloodstream invasion from the initial focus in the upper air-passages with usual but not constant localization in various susceptible parts of the body."[43] The clinical manifestations of meningococcal disease vary from transient fever and bacteremia to fulminant disease with death within hours of the onset of symptoms.[44] Meningitis and septic shock caused by *N. meningitidis* infection have mortality rates of 4–15% and 40%, respectively.[44,45]

Table 24.2 Symptoms and Signs of Bacterial Meningitis

Symptom or Sign	Percentage
Headache	≥90
Fever	≥90
Meningismus	≥85
Alteration in consciousness	≥80
Petechiae/purpura	≈50
Vomiting	≈30
Seizures	≈30
Focal neurologic findings	≈25
Myalgias	≈20
Ocular palsies	≈10
Hemiparesis	<5
Papilledema	<1

Wolfe and Birbara[46] described four major clinical syndromes, but variations of these scenarios occur and the patients may progress from one to another syndrome.

1. **Bacteremia without sepsis.** In the setting of an upper respiratory illness or viral exanthem, blood cultures are drawn which are reported as positive for *N. meningitidis*, often after discharge. Occult bacteremia with recovery in the absence of antimicrobial therapy is rare, but serum concentrations of bacteria in children are often low, from 22 to 325 organisms per milliliter of blood.[47]
2. **Meningococcemia without meningitis.** The patient is clinically septic with signs of malaise, weakness, headache, and hypotension developing shortly after admission or before in the presence or absence of skin rash and leukocytosis.
3. **Meningitis with or without meningococcemia.** Headache, fever, and meningeal signs predominate with a cloudy CSF. The state of the sensorium varies from fully alert to deeply obtunded. The deep tendon and superficial reflexes are unaltered and there are no pathologic reflexes.
4. **Meningoencephalitis.** Profound obtundation with meningeal signs and a cloudy CSF are characteristic. Furthermore, the deep tendon reflexes and superficial reflexes are either absent or, rarely, hyperactive and pathologic reflexes are frequently present.

It is worth noting that the wide range of clinical expressions requires a high index of suspicion for meningococcal disease, especially in an endemic situation with sporadic cases. The symptoms and signs of bacterial meningitis are listed in ***Table 24.2***. Meningococcal meningitis differs somewhat from other forms of bacterial meningitis with headache, confusion, and stiff neck in less than half of the patients.[48] In infants and small children, fever and vomiting are often the only early clue to central nervous system (CNS) involvement, and these patients are frequently brought to the hospital only after an insidious impairment in consciousness or convulsions occur.[12] Evidence of meningeal irritation is common, except in the very young and very old. Focal neurologic signs and seizures have been less common in meningococcal meningitis when compared to pneumococcal meningitis or disease due to *Haemophilus influenzae*.[49] Cerebral infarction occurs in 15–20% of adults with bacterial meningitis, typically in patients with pneumococcal meningitis,[50,51] but stroke caused by *N. meningitidis* may affect adults and children alike, and has been linked

Box 24.1 Differential Diagnosis of Fever, Altered Sensorium, and Petechial Rash

Meningococcal disease	Septic shock
Rickettsial infections (e.g., Rocky Mountain spotted fever)	Viral meningitis
Staphylococcus aureus endocarditis	Viral hemorrhagic fevers
Streptococcus pneumonia, Haemophilus influenza (especially with splenectomy)	"Noninfectious": thrombotic, thrombocytopenic purpura (TTP), hemolytic-uremic syndrome (HUS), vasculitis, and heatstroke[64]

to serogroups B, C, and Y.[45,52] In addition, *N. meningitidis* has been implicated in various neurological complications: tetraplegia (spinal cord infarction); cranial nerve dysfunction (principally of the sixth, seventh or eighth cranial nerves); subdural empyema; hydrocephalus; seizure disorders; spinal cord dysfunction (myelitis); visual impairment; brain abscesses; brainstem infarction and late effects, such as cognitive impairment.[45,51–55] A complex web of cells and molecules has been implicated in meningococcal pathogenesis.[1,2,44,45,56–59] The pathogenesis of stroke in a patient with meningococcal meningitis is believed to involve multiple molecular/cellular mechanisms and pathogenic pathways, including upregulation of cytokines and, subsequently, downregulation of coagulation inhibitors and endothelial injury and coagulopathy and ischemia dysfunction.[45,52,56,59] Reactive oxygen species and reactive nitrogen intermediates have also been identified as critical mediators of the pathogenesis of bacterial meningitis.[2,57] A systemic inflammatory response also increases the risk of stroke and myocardial infarction.[60]

Meningococcal sepsis is the prototype of septic shock, requiring aggressive intensive care.[1] The clinical features of meningococcal septic shock emerge when perfusion of the vital organs (brain or heart) is maintained at the expense of perfusion of organs such as kidney, skin, and gut.[61] Shock results from a combination of hypovolemia caused by capillary leak syndrome, myocardial dysfunction, altered vasomotor tone, and impaired cellular metabolism.[61] Impaired consciousness and petechial skin lesions, when present, arise relatively late in the course of the infection.[62,63] Lesions analogous to petechial skin lesions can be seen in various conditions: sepsis caused by *Streptococcus pneumoniae*, Group A streptococci, *Staphylococcus aureus*, or *H. influenzae*; infections caused by rickettsiae or viruses; and illnesses such as heatstroke (***Box 24.1***).[1,64] Severe muscle tenderness of the lower extremities is one of the earliest clinical signs of neisserial sepsis and can be critical to early recognition and diagnosis.[62,65]

Although the differential diagnosis is wide (***Box 24.1***), the presence of petechiae and fever with an altered sensorium is a medical emergency. The petechial eruption is characterized by discrete lesions 1–2 mm in diameter, most frequently on the trunk and lower extremities, rapidly progressing to more extensive ecchymotic lesions (***Figs 24.5, 24.6, and 24.7***). Petechiae correlate with thrombocytopenia and coagulopathy, particularly disseminated intravascular coagulation (DIC). Response of petechiae early in the disease to therapeutic modalities is an important prognostic variable that can be assessed at the bedside by proper attention to the number of lesions and progression within a defined area of the skin.[4,9]

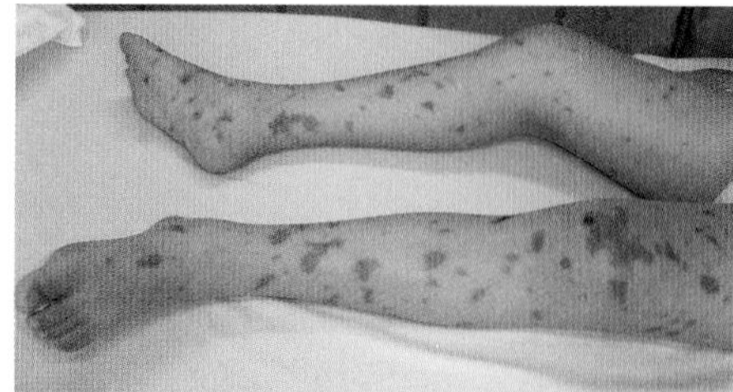

Figure 24.5 Petechial lesions on the lower limbs in a patient with meningococcal infection.

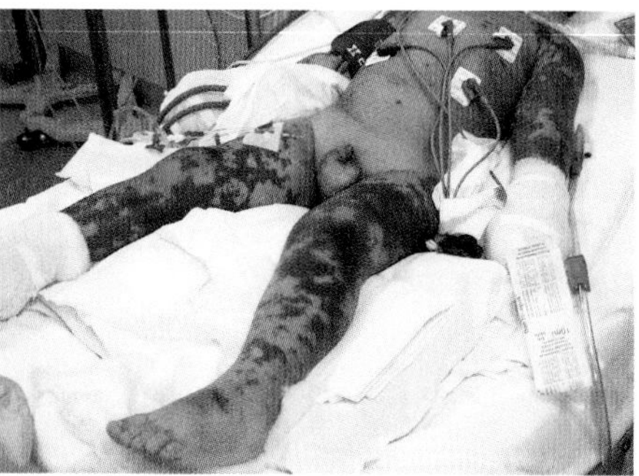

Figure 24.6 Striking petechial and purpuric rash in a patient with meningococcal septic shock.

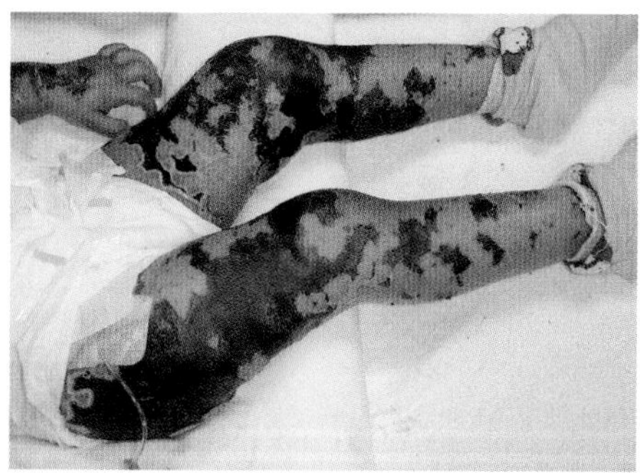

Figure 24.7 Meningococcal purpura fulminans can progress to profound tissue necrosis of the lower limbs, leading to drastic physical sequelae such as skin scars and amputations, which have a significant impact on quality of life.

Meningococcal Pericarditis

Pericardial effusion, with or without cardiac tamponade, is a well-documented complication of meningococcal disease and is seen in 6–16% of cases of septic pericarditis.[66] In addition, pericardial involvement has been described in 3–19% of patients with meningococcal infection and may affect children and adults alike.[66,67] Recently, meningococcal pericarditis has been classified on the basis of clinical and pathobiological criteria: primary, disseminated, and immunoreactive pericarditis. *Primary* meningococcal pericarditis is defined by the isolation of *N. meningitidis* in the pericardial fluid or blood cultures, without meningitis, meningococcal sepsis or other foci of meningococcal infection. In *disseminated* meningococcal disease with pericarditis, there is direct invasion of the pericardium, resulting in a septic pericarditis and the onset of symptoms is usually within the first week of meningococcal sepsis. Primary pericarditis and disseminated meningococcal disease with pericarditis often require treatment with steroidal or nonsteroidal anti-inflammatory drugs and pericardiocentesis in those patients in whom the progressive accumulation of pericardial fluid leads to tamponade, in addition to antibiotics. *Immunoreactive* meningococcal pericarditis is a late complication of meningococcal disease, occurring 6–16 days after the initiation of treatment and is probably an immunopathologic process. No bacteria are detectable in the pericardial fluid. Improvement with anti-inflammatory treatment, either salicylates or corticosteroids, is common. These three types of neisserial pericarditis are typically associated with serogroup C, B, and W-135, occurring at much higher rates in W-135 infection than in serogroup B or C infection.[66,68] Meningococcal pericarditis may be associated with higher pericardial fluid cytokine concentrations than those found in blood, favoring local production.[67] Meningococcal cells can be seen within pericardial fluid but the molecular mechanisms by which these microorganisms interact with the pericardial barrier, as well as the chain of events involved in septic meningococcal pericarditis remain unknown.[68,69]

Meningococcal Peritonitis

In patients with meningococcal infection, atypical presentations such as complications involving abdominal organs, which may present as an acute abdomen, have also been well documented, e.g., peritonitis, splenic rupture, cholecystitis, pelvic inflammatory disease, mesenteric adenitis, ileitis, and pericarditis.[70] Peritonitis caused by *N. meningitidis* is rare but affects adults and children alike and has been linked to serogroups B, C, W135, and Z.[70] We recommend immunological and molecular techniques for the diagnostic evaluation and clarification of meningococcal septic phenomena, especially after the administration of antibiotics.[66,67,70]

Myocardial Dysfunction

Myocardial involvement is widely recognized as playing a central role in the pathophysiology of meningococcal sepsis and can be a critical factor for patient outcomes.[1] The incidence of myocardial depression in meningococcal septic shock is higher than in other types of sepsis.[71] Histopathological evidence of meningococcal myocarditis was seen in 78% of 200 fatal cases of meningococcal infection (85% of adults and 57% of children).[72]

Myocardial dysfunction during neisserial sepsis can cause lung edema, as well as vascular collapse, leading to impaired tissue perfusion and multiple organ failure. Life-threatening cardiac dysfunction occurs 7–10 days after bacterial invasion. Unexpected severe lung edema may emerge at days 3–7 when peripheral edema is mobilized, especially during bradyarrhythmias.[71] Furthermore, fatal cases can unexpectedly arise from asystole caused by inflammation of the conduction system.[1] Heart failure can be recognized at the early stage of the illness by a fixed tachycardia that does not respond to fluid loading. Typically, echocardiographic study displays a dilated, hardly contracting myocardium with an increased left-ventricle end-diastolic diameter, a reduced shortening fraction (<0.30), and a decreased left ventricular ejection fraction (left-ventricle end-diastolic diameter <50%).[71]

Myocardial cell dysfunction emerges as a result of multiple pathophysiologic events that are associated with meningococcal sepsis, including profound electrolyte, acid–base, and metabolic imbalances such as: hypoxemia, acidemia, hypokalemia, hypocalcemia, hypophosphatemia, hypomagnesemia, hypoglycemia, and disturbed fatty acid metabolism.[1,61] Five of 22 patients with meningococcal sepsis showed signs of myocardial ischemia characterized by increased levels of troponin I.[1] Myocardial contractility usually improves with volume resuscitation and correction of electrolyte and acid–base disturbances. However, critically ill patients with ongoing septic shock despite adequate volume resuscitation may need inotropic support to improve myocardial function. Key supportive measures to maintain homeostasis include fluid resuscitation, electrolyte replacement, monitoring of central venous oxygen saturation, cardiovascular support, and mechanical ventilation as necessary.

The precise nature of the myocardial depressant factors has not been fully deciphered.[73] Pathan et al reported that interleukin-6 (IL-6) induced a dose-dependent myocardial depression, and that tumor necrosis factor alpha (TNF-α) had no significant effect on myocyte contractility.[73] The biological effect of IL-6 is mediated by the IL-6 receptor, composed of an 80 kDa ligand binding subunit and a 130 kDa signal transducing element.[71] Myocardial cells that do not possess the 80 kDa ligand binding subunit may use soluble IL-6R to mediate IL-6 signals.[71] Despite the drastic myocardial dysfunction during the inflammatory phase of meningococcal infection, patients who survive regain normal myocardial function.[61]

Respiratory Tract Infections

Although nasopharyngeal colonization with meningococci renders sputum cultures imprecise in the diagnosis, meningococcal pneumonia occurs in conjunction with meningococcemia or meningitis in 8–15% of cases.[74,75] *N. meningitidis* also can be a primary respiratory pathogen.[68] Primary meningococcal pneumonia, once considered rare, is now recognized as the most common form of meningococcal disease in military recruits and has been reported in 4.5% of all cases of bacterial pneumonia in a general hospital population.[75] However, the clinical presentations of meningococcal infections other than meningitis or meningococcal sepsis may lead to erroneous diagnosis.[68]

A recent clinical study demonstrated that meningococcal pneumonia was most frequently diagnosed in patients aged >70 years (20 of 33 patients), and 54.5% of the strains belonged to serogroup W135, although these strains had heterogeneous phenotypes.[68] Meningococcal pneumonia was identified on the basis of classical symptoms and signs (fever, dyspnea, cough, and radiologic findings) associated with the isolation of *N. meningitidis* from blood.[68] A review of 58 patients with meningococcal pneumonia over a 25-year period documented a shift in antimicrobial therapy from predominantly penicillin to cephalosporins; overall fatality was 8.6%.[76] The serogroups responsible were as follows: Y, 44%; B, 18%; W-135, 16%; and C, 14%.

N. meningitidis and Atypical Sites

In recent decades, there have been remarkable changes in the epidemiological behavior of *N. meningitidis*, and the human nasopharynx is no longer the only recognized primary site of the initial stage of meningococcal infection.[1] The pathogen has been found in the mucous membranes of the endocervix, anus, urethra, and conjunctiva.[77–79] The ability of meningococci to colonize mucous membranes other than the nasopharynx is critically linked to direct inoculation of *N. meningitidis* into the mucus from an exogenous source, via orogenital sex or vertical transmission.[77,80] Colonization is a key step in the sequence of events leading to neisserial infection. In general, meningococcal infection occurs within 10 days after colonization. However, there have been cases of neisserial infection following prolonged carriage of a pathogenic strain.

Chronic Meningococcemia

Chronic meningococcemia is defined as bacteremia caused by *N. meningitidis* lasting more than 1 week and presenting without meningeal signs.[81] This intriguing syndrome is characterized by fever, rash, and arthritis. Cutaneous manifestations seen in up to 50% of the cases include purpuric papules, nodules, and urticarial eruptions.[81] The syndrome is similar to that observed with chronic gonococcemia for which it is often mistaken. Rompalo et al contrasted the isolation of gonococci with that of meningococci from blood or synovial fluid cultures from 1970 to 1972 (15:1) to similar studies from 1980 through 1983 (9:5).[82] *N. meningitidis* infection may rarely present as chronic meningitis or encephalopathy.[83]

Meningococcemia in the Setting of Complement Deficiency

Complement or properdin deficiency predisposes persons to the occurrence of meningococcal disease (see Chapter 9).[84–86] Interestingly, the degree of severity of meningococcal infection is often less and case-fatality rates are low when terminal complement components are affected. In all other respects, the clinical course is similar to that outlined previously.

PATHOGENESIS AND IMMUNITY

Meningococcal disease is exclusive to humans. The meningococcal carrier state is fundamental to the development of invasive disease.[10,12,14,25,28] Approximately 6% of the population develops nasopharyngeal colonization with *N. meningitidis* yearly. Nasopharyngeal carriage rates vary markedly with age and the population under study but are approximately 5–15%, rising from 0.5% in children 3–48 months old to approximately 20–40% in young adults. Carriage persists for weeks to months and occasionally years and largely accounts for the increased risk of disease in household contacts of an index case. Although uncharacterized host and environmental factors, including prior viral upper respiratory tract infection, contribute to containment of infection or invasion, host immunity also plays an important role. Those persons recently colonized with meningococci appear to be at greatest risk of invasive disease.[25]

The age-specific incidence of meningococcal infection is inversely proportional to the presence of serum bactericidal antibodies against serogroups A, B, and C. More than 50% of infants possess bactericidal antibody at the time of birth as a result of transplacental transfer. Immunoglobulin G (IgG) antibody to serogroup B polysaccharide, however, is lacking in neonates. This contributes to the occurrence of serogroup B meningococcal disease in this age group, and since serogroup B meningococcal capsular antigen is identical to the capsular polysaccharides of *Escherichia coli* K1 and certain types of serogroup B streptococci, these organisms are also major causes of neonatal sepsis and meningitis.[87] The inverse link between occurrence of invasive disease and bactericidal antibody was first documented during an outbreak of serogroup C meningococcal meningitis among US Army recruits in 1968.[88]

Several risk factors for meningococcal disease have been identified, but the cause of differences in susceptibility and outcome between individuals and populations remains unknown.[5] In the 1980s, studies of adopted children and twins revealed that genetics are major determinants of susceptibility to infectious diseases. New genetic research techniques have also identified host genetic polymorphisms that influence severity and outcome in meningococcal disease. Recently, several other studies further suggested that genetics play a role in susceptibility of meningococcal disease. However, despite intensive research efforts, no polymorphism has been definitively shown to affect susceptibility to meningococcal and pneumococcal disease. The polymorphisms or haplotypes in IL-1 receptor antagonist, surfactant protein A2, carcinoembryonic antigen cell adhesion molecules 3 and 6, and complement factor H found with meningococcal disease were based on insufficient sample sizes.[5,7]

Although recovery from invasive meningococcal disease generally confers lifelong immunity against the homologous serogroup, this is not the major immunizing process. Nasopharyngeal colonization, particularly with serogroup B, C, or Y, may elicit the development of bactericidal activity, primarily directed against the colonizing strain but also active against heterologous organisms within 5–12 days of acquisition.[10] Nasopharyngeal colonization with nongroupable meningococci or *Neisseria lactamica*, virtually nonpathogenic organisms, may confer protective immunity against other meningococci with invasive potential. The carriage rates of pathogenic meningococci are far too low in children to account for antibody formation and the importance of other cross-reacting organisms, outside the genus *Neisseria*, have also been proposed. Paradoxically, an exuberant IgA response to meningococci may actually enhance the development of systemic disease.

In addition to bactericidal antibody, an intact complement system is also a component of the host's defenses against invasive meningococcal disease (see Chapter 9).[44,84–86] Recurrent or chronic neisserial infections have been associated with rare isolated deficiencies of late complement components (C5, C6, C7, or C8, and perhaps C9).[44,84–86] Screening for complement defects is useful in families with recurrent or chronic neisserial infections and perhaps for individuals after only one episode of invasive meningococcal disease.[86] Complement deficiency also appears to predispose to meningitis caused by nongroupable meningococci and *Neisseria*-related bacteria (i.e., *Moraxella* or *Acinetobacter* species).[89] Depletion of early complement components (C1, C3, or C4) because of an underlying disorder such as nephrotic syndrome, hepatic failure, the presence of C3 nephritic factor, or multiple myeloma may predispose to the first episode of invasive meningococcal disease.[10] Properdin dysfunction, with normal concentrations, also predisposes to invasive meningococcal disease; this defect is reversible with vaccination.[90] Asplenic states also increase the risk of serious infections by encapsulated organisms, especially *Haemophilus influenzae* or *Streptococcus pneumoniae*, but also meningococci. Although all of the preceding factors (particularly recent colonization with a pathogenic strain in a nonimmune host) undoubtedly contribute to the pathogenesis of overt meningococcal disease, the precise determinants contributing to the clinical illness (as opposed to the usual outcome of asymptomatic carriage) are poorly defined. Even during epidemics, only 1 in 1000–5000 colonized patients develops disease.[10,14] Various predisposing factors have been proposed to explain this discrepancy, including crowding, low socioeconomic status, poor general health, a preceding upper viral respiratory tract infection, and alcoholism. Simultaneous outbreaks of meningococcal and influenza infections have been described in institutional and community settings.[91] The role of viral infections in the enhancement of meningococcal dissemination is unproven and the precise factors that contribute to the development of overt clinical illness are at present poorly understood.[91,92]

Box 24.2 Putative Meningococcal Virulence Factors

Capsular polysaccharide	Outer membrane proteins
Pili	Outer membrane vesicles or blebs
IgA protease	
Lipopolysaccharide (endotoxin)	Metabolic pathways (e.g., iron)

The time from nasopharyngeal acquisition to bloodstream invasion is short, usually 10 days or less. The incubation period may also be quite short, since "secondary" cases commonly occur within 1–4 days of the index case.[10,12] Once the organism is bloodborne, more than 90% of meningococcal disease is manifested as meningitis and/or meningococcemia. As noted previously, the clonal nature, even among clones of closely related organisms, suggests the complex interplay among virulence characteristics[10] (***Box 24.2***).

As noted previously, all isolates from invasive infections are encapsulated (i.e., serogroup-positive), but 20% to more than 50% of isolates from carriers are unencapsulated (nontypable). The capsular polysaccharide appears to be essential to virulence, probably because of its antiphagocytic properties which allow the organism to escape host-phagocytic clearance mechanisms within the CSF or bloodstream. Pili are protein surface appendages composed of identical pilin repeated subunits and include the major adhesions Opa and Opc.[93] Pili are important mediators of meningococcal adhesion to human nonciliated columnar nasopharyngeal epithelial cells, an important early step in the development of the carrier state.[1,94] Extracellular proteases that cleave the IgA1 heavy chain in the hinge region are elaborated by pathogenic *Neisseria* species (i.e., meningococci and gonococci). Besides pili at least seven other adhesins have been described. Carcinoembryonic antigen cell adhesion molecules (CEACAMs) are cell-surface molecules in nasopharyngeal epithelium and neutrophils that interact with opacity-associated adhesin proteins of the meningococcus.[95]

Meningococcal lipopolysaccharide (LPS) resembles *H. influenzae* LPS by a lack of the O-antigenic polysaccharide side chain found in enteric bacteria despite a smooth phenotype and proven virulence and is more properly referred to as a lipooligosaccharide (LOS). This endotoxin is a major component of the outer membrane of the meningococcus and is crucial in the pathogenesis of sepsis and meningitis.[96] It is now well established that LPS is sensed by mammalian cells through Toll-like receptor 4 (TLR4), in combination with coreceptors MD-2 and CD14.[97] Activation of this complex leads to recruitment of the adapters MyD88, Mal, TRIF, and TRAM to the cytoplasmic domain of TLR4.[98] These adapters initiate signal transduction pathways that lead to induction of innate immunity. These pathways are classified in a so-called "MyD88-dependent" pathway involving MyD88 and Mal, and a "MyD88-independent" pathway involving TRIF and TRAM. Hallmarks of MyD88-dependent and MyD88-independent signaling are induction of proinflammatory cytokines and type I interferon, respectively. While the response to LPS can be beneficial to the host by containing a beginning infection, it can also be detrimental when excessive stimulation occurs through growth of large numbers of bacteria in the bloodstream as happens during sepsis. The host responds to bacterial endotoxin with proinflammatory gene expression and activation of coagulation pathways. A recent study showed that a substantial proportion of meningococcal clinical isolates may have LPS with underacylated lipid A due to mutations in the lpxL1 gene.[99] The resulting low-activity LPS may have an important role in virulence by aiding the bacteria to evade the innate immune system.

Although the specific role for outer membrane proteins (OMPs) in meningococcal virulence is unclear, these organisms release substantial amounts of cell surface material in the form of outer membrane vesicles or blebs containing OMPs and LPS during growth *in vitro* and *in vivo* in the absence of cell lysis, a process exacerbated by antimicrobial agents. These outer membrane vesicles or blebs represent relevant vehicles for CNS tissue damage during meningococcal infection.[100] Finally, tissue invasion may also be facilitated by the ability of meningococci to obtain iron from transferrin, hemoglobin, and lactoferrin. Animals subjected to iron overload are more susceptible to fatal meningococcal infection.

DIAGNOSIS

Patients with a petechial or purpuric eruption, fever, and altered sensorium represent a medical emergency; the differential diagnosis is listed in ***Box 24.1***. Between 50% and 75% of children with meningococcemia have a purpuric or petechial rash, principally on the trunk and lower extremities (***Figs 24.5, 24.6, and 24.7***). Petechiae are found in the skin, mucous membranes, and conjunctivae but not in the nail beds. Petechial rashes should be promptly examined microscopically in the initial evaluation of a patient with suspected meningococcemia after aspiration or making a "touch preparation" on a glass slide[1,63]; approximately 70% of these preparations will reveal the organisms, usually within vacuolated neutrophils if meningococcemia is present (***Fig. 24.8***). In approximately 20–25% of patients with meningococcemia, the organisms may be visualized on the peripheral blood smear, especially in a buffy coat preparation (***Fig. 24.9***). Although the sensitivity is low, this simple test can be quite valuable in the initial approach.

The gold standard for the definitive diagnosis of invasive meningococcal disease remains culture of the organism from a normally sterile body fluid; the CSF and blood are the most common sites of positive cultures by the preceding techniques.[10] It is worth noting that CSF cultures are often positive in the presence of suspected meningococcemia, even in the absence of clinical signs of overt meningitis.[101] Meningococci are often cultured from CSF specimens that appear virtually normal by cytologic and chemical analyses in the early phases of illness. The mean concentration of meningococci in CSF specimens is approximately 10^5 colony-forming units (CFU) per milliliter with a wide range from approximately 10^2 CFU/mL to greater than 10^7 CFU/mL.[102,103]

The diagnosis of meningococcal meningitis requires examination of the CSF.[3] As discussed previously, culture remains the gold standard and CSF Gram stains in the presence of meningococcal meningitis have an overall sensitivity of approximately 70% in untreated patients. Other CSF values are highly variable. In an analysis of 58 patients with meningococcal meningitis,[48] the median leukocyte count was approximately 1200/mm^3, with a range of less than 10/mm^3 to more than 65 000/mm^3. Polymorphonuclear leukocytes predominate overwhelmingly in untreated patients. CSF protein concentrations range from 25 mg/100 mL to more than 800 mg/100 mL, with a median value of approximately 150 mg/100 mL, while 75% of CSF specimens reveal glucose concentrations below 40 mg/100 mL. All of these values may be altered significantly by prior antimicrobial treatment.[12,48]

Detection of meningococcal antigen in CSF by various techniques, including counterimmunoelectrophoresis, latex agglutination, and cold agglutination, have demonstrated variable sensitivity and specificity despite the capability of detecting 0.5 μg or less of meningococcal antigen under standardized test conditions.[3,12] False negative results are common.[104] Meningococcal antigen may be detected in urine by these techniques despite negative CSF specimens. These tests should only be considered in Gram-negative cases.

Recently, the polymerase chain reaction (PCR) has been applied to the diagnosis of invasive meningococcal disease.[3] For example, Ni and colleagues examined 54 CSF samples with appropriate controls by PCR in a blinded fashion.[105] The sensitivity and specificity of PCR for the diagnosis of meningococcal meningitis were both 91%. PCR may be most appropriate in Gram-negative cases, especially in patients receiving prior antimicrobial therapy, but requires special techniques and is expensive. Multiplex PCR has proven effective in the diagnosis of meningococcal disease, especially in the setting of prior antimicrobial administration.[106,107] The technique can be used to rapidly type strains of critical value in an evolving epidemic.[33] A more broad-based PCR technique utilizing 16S RNA may differentiate bacterial from viral meningitis, even in partially treated or Gram-negative cases, but is not specific for meningococcal disease and not widely available.[108] Nevertheless, in selected cases, PCR is a valuable adjunct for the diagnosis of meningococcal infections where resources are available.[3] In most tropical regions, especially during an epidemic, suspected meningococcal meningitis is treated empirically without attempt at specific microbiologic confirmation. Finally, the differential diagnosis of petechial skin lesions with fever in the tropics includes many etiologies (e.g., viral hemorrhagic fevers, rickettsial infections, etc.) rarely encountered in temperate climates.

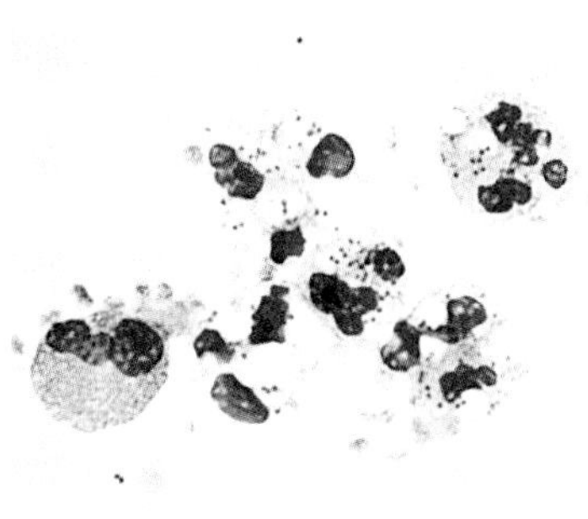

Figure 24.8 "Touch prep" (impression preparation) of a petechial lesion in a case of meningococcemia, depicting the organisms and polymorphonuclear leukocytes (Giemsa stain).

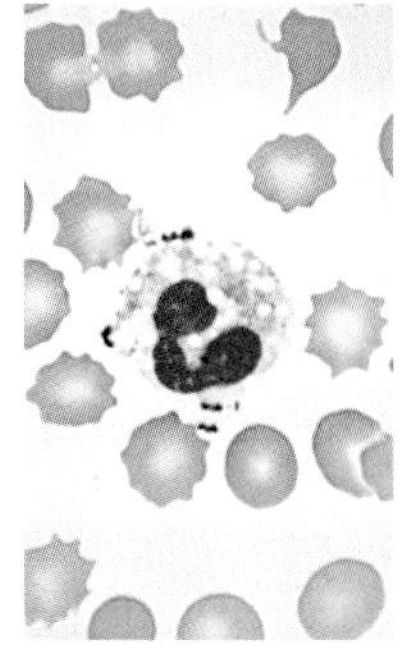

Figure 24.9 Buffy coat preparation of a peripheral blood smear in meningococcemia, displaying leukocyte-associated meningococci (Wright stain).

TREATMENT AND PROGNOSIS

Antimicrobial and Adjunctive Therapies

For penicillin-susceptible strains of *N. meningitidis*, penicillin G 300 000 units/kg per day intravenously (IV), in divided doses every 4 hours, or ampicillin 400 mg/kg per day, in divided doses every 4 hours, are the preferred antibiotics for the treatment of invasive meningococcal disease.[3,10,12] A 5-day course of therapy is adequate for most cases of uncomplicated meningococcal meningitis. Meningococcal resistance to penicillin has been reported.[109] β-Lactamase-producing isolates are still very rare, but penicillin-resistant strains that do not produce β-lactamase appear to have a reduced affinity for penicillin-binding proteins (e.g., PBP-2 and PBP-3) and have been reported from Spain, the United Kingdom, and other countries.[110,111] In Spain, the number of relatively penicillin-resistant meningococcal isolates reached 20% in 1989.[110] However, in the United States in 1991, only 3 of 100 isolates submitted to the CDC had minimum inhibitory concentrations (MICs) of penicillin of 0.125 μg/mL.[112] Because of the low frequency of resistance in some areas, routine sensitivity testing of meningococcal isolates is not indicated; nevertheless, surveillance for resistance should continue. Meningitis due to relatively penicillin-resistant meningococci (MICs in the range of 0.1–0.8 μg/mL) has been managed successfully with currently recommended doses of penicillin or a third-generation cephalosporin (e.g., cefotaxime, ceftriaxone).[3] Ceftriaxone (100 mg/kg per day IV in two divided doses) or cefotaxime (200 mg/kg per day IV in three divided doses) is effective. Chloramphenicol is an effective substitute in the penicillin-allergic patient at a dosage of 100 mg/kg per day up to a maximum of 4 g per day total dose in four divided doses, as chloramphenicol-resistant meningococci, although reported, remain rare.[10,12] Chloramphenicol is often the preferred agent in resource-limited settings and is often administered in an oily vehicle by the intramuscular (IM) route to sustain chloramphenicol concentrations in blood over prolonged periods of time.[10]

Although various adjunctive therapies have been reported to improve outcome in patients with bacterial meningitis, treatment of meningococcal meningitis with steroids has been debated in the literature for years.[57] Evidence from recent studies supports the use of adjunctive steroids for all cases of community-acquired bacterial meningitis, regardless of whether the causative pathogen has been identified.[113] Current practice guidelines and expert opinion recommend that dexamethasone (10 mg) should be administered intravenously every 6 hours for 4 days in adult patients who have suspected bacterial meningitis.[113] In most childhood studies, a 4-day regimen of dexamethasone (0.4 or 0.6 mg/kg per day) divided into four daily doses was used.[113] In addition, glycerol (a hyperosmolar agent and an osmotic diuretic) is another instrument that has been assessed as a novel adjunctive tool in the treatment of bacterial meningitis.[57] A recent multicenter trial was undertaken in six Latin American countries where 654 infants and children (2 months to 16 years) with bacterial meningitis were randomly assigned to one of four treatment arms: oral glycerol (1.5 g/kg every 6 hours for 48 hours), intravenous dexamethasone (0.15 mg/kg every 6 hours for 48 hours), oral glycerol plus intravenous dexamethasone, and placebo.[114] Patients who received glycerol, or glycerol and dexamethasone had fewer severe neurologic sequelae than those who received placebo. Five properties of glycerol make its widespread use possible and desirable: it can be taken orally, is inexpensive, is easily available, has no special storage requirements, and is safe.[114] Notably, glycerol is also a scavenger of free oxygen radicals, and this action may further alleviate meningeal inflammation.[114] Further studies regarding the effects of glycerol therapy for bacterial meningitis are warranted before this adjunctive tool can be routinely recommended.

In the management of meningococcal disease, the emphasis must still be placed on early diagnosis and prompt initiation of antibiotic therapy, which continue to be the cornerstones of the successful management of this dramatic illness, reducing morbidity and mortality rates.[1] In fact, the combination of three clinical studies has shown a statistically significant case-fatality reduction from 11.5% (41/358) to 4.7% (6/127) in patients given antibiotics before hospital admission.[115–117] Meningococci in CSF are killed within 3–4 hours after intravenous treatment with an adequate dose of antibiotic, and concentrations of endotoxin in plasma fall by 50% within 2 hours.[1] Meningococcal infection may progress rapidly, even after the appropriate treatment has commenced.[61] Therefore, patients should be closely monitored for early signs of severe sepsis or shock.

Supportive Care

In the early twentieth century, the prognosis of meningococcal infection was dramatically changed by the introduction of meningococcal antiserum and antimicrobial therapy.[1] However, despite significant improvements in supportive care, as well as treatments involving modulation of the inflammatory and coagulation cascades, the mortality rate has changed little in recent years. Studies of modulation of the host inflammatory cascade have produced controversial results, demonstrating that the intricacies of the pathogenesis of meningococcal disease continue to preclude predicting the benefit of any given intervention.[1,61]

Monitoring of systolic blood pressure in children may be insufficient to detect the development of meningococcal septic shock.[1,61] Children are able to compensate for loss of up to 40% of their circulating volume without developing hypotension, and may therefore have a normal blood pressure until shock is advanced.[61] Despite septic shock, preservation of brain perfusion is usually present, and the apparent alert status of the children can mislead physicians to underestimate the true degree of cardiovascular derangements. The possibility of meningococcal septic shock must be suspected when a patient presents with urinary output <0.5 mL/kg for at least 1 hour; capillary refilling time ≥3 seconds; cold extremities; or tachycardia.[1]

Virtually all patients show some evidence of coagulopathy during meningococcal sepsis, and coagulation status can be assessed by observing the size and number of skin lesions, together with platelet counts and measurement of prothrombin and activated partial thromboplastin times.[1,63] Strategies designed to treat hemostatic imbalances, such as blood and plasma exchange, which improve disseminated intravascular coagulation (and perhaps remove cytokines), appear to be safe and to reduce mortality.[115] In fact, in two series reported in 1992 (each with 13 patients), mortality decreased from 78% and 60% (historical control patients) to 24% and 8%, respectively, in patients treated with blood and plasma exchange.[115]

Management of meningococcal sepsis and homeostasis often requires early and aggressive correction of hypovolemia and electrolyte disorders; administration of vasoactive drugs; the establishment of central venous access in order to perform fluid resuscitation and to assess cardiovascular function (by measuring central venous oxygen saturation); assessment and constant monitoring of platelet counts plus hemoglobin levels; treatment of coagulopathy (transfusion of fresh-frozen plasma plus vitamin K administration); as well as early mechanical ventilation and renal replacement therapy as necessary.[1] Interestingly, improvement in limb perfusion was achieved after hyperbaric oxygenation in 12 (86%) of 14 patients with purpura fulminans caused by different pathogens.[115] The treatment of meningococcal sepsis can be extremely complex. Therefore, treatment ideally should be given in a facility capable of administering critical medical care. Such capacity is defined as follows: having dialysis and mechanical ventilation equipment available; having physicians and nurses that are skilled in intensive care medicine; and having orthopedic, vascular, and plastic surgeons that take a multidisciplinary approach to treating patients with ischemic tissue damage.[1] Obviously, such facilities may not be available in many resource-constrained environments.

PREVENTION AND CONTROL

Chemoprophylaxis

Several agents reliably eradicate the carrier state, although for a varying duration of time.[118] Rifampicin, ceftriaxone, azithromycin, and quinolones all have activity against meningococci in the nasopharynx.[98] Minocycline eradicates the carrier state rapidly and eradication persists for up to 6–10 weeks after treatment.[12,119] Unfortunately, vertiginous reactions limit the usefulness of this agent. Rifampin is also highly effective but can result in the emergence of rifampin-resistant meningococci in approximately 10–27% of patients receiving this agent.[120] Ciprofloxacin, ofloxacin, and azithromycin have been shown in controlled studies to eradicate nasopharyngeal carriage following a single dose for up to 1 month in a high proportion (95% or more) of subjects.[121–123] Currently, rifampin is the recommended therapy for meningococcal prophylaxis at a dosage of 600 mg every 12 hours in adults and 10 mg/kg every 12 hours in children (both for 2 days),[12] although ceftriaxone and quinolones are highly effective, and the one dose strategy ensures compliance.

The group at greatest risk of secondary cases of meningococcal disease includes household contacts of the index case and these persons should receive chemoprophylaxis. Similar high-risk situations occur in closed populations, including college dormitories, military barracks, nursery schools, day care centers, and chronic care hospitals.[124] The use of chemoprophylactic agents in these groups should be individualized based on the intensity of exposure. Health care personnel rarely require chemoprophylaxis except when intimate contact (such as mouth-to-mouth resuscitation) with the index patient is performed.[125]

Immunoprophylaxis

Shortly after the recognition of sulfonamide-resistant meningococci, and the obvious implications for prevention of secondary cases through chemoprophylaxis, efforts to develop immunogenic vaccines against the major meningococcal serogroups intensified. Following the example provided by the *H. influenzae* type b conjugate vaccines, preparations of serogroup A, C, or W-135 polysaccharide chemically conjugated to proteins have been evaluated in clinical trials.[126–129] The experience with serogroup C conjugate vaccine in the United Kingdom is illuminating. Although rates vary widely in Europe, the annual incidence of meningococcal disease in the United Kingdom is higher than in the United States (approximately 3–5 cases/100 000 population/year vs. 1.0–1.5 cases/100 000 population/year). In 1997, the serotype distribution in the United Kingdom was as follows: B, 54%; C, 38%; other, 8%; and most deaths due to serogroup C occurred in children less than 2 years of age and in adolescents 15–20 years old. Licensed serogroup C vaccines have conjugated the polysaccharide to CRM-197 mutant diphtheria toxin or tetanus toxoid.[130] There was an approximately 90% reduction in serogroup C disease in the vaccinated group,[131] while no change in serogroup B disease occurred in the United Kingdom overall. In addition, carriage was reduced (although low)[132] and invasive disease declined approximately 67% in the unvaccinated older population.[133]

In the United States, a quadrivalent meningococcal polysaccharide vaccine conjugated to diphtheria toxoid (MCV4) was approved in 2005.[134] The vaccine consists of cell surface polysaccharides from serogroups A, C, Y, and W-135 covalently linked to diphtheria toxoid. The conjugated vaccine evokes a powerful immune response by stimulating a T-cell-dependent immune response, leading to both a strong primary response and a strong anamnestic response at reexposure.[135] The conjugate vaccines also lead to a reduction in nasal carriage, thereby decreasing transmission through herd immunity. In the United States, the immunogenicity of MCV4 in younger children was assessed in a randomized, double-blind, controlled trial in 1398 healthy children.[136] In 2- to 10-year-old children, MCV4 had a safety profile similar to that of PSV-4 (quadrivalent polysaccharide vaccine) and elicited significantly higher and more persistent serum bactericidal antibody responses against meningococcal serogroups A, C, Y, and W-135 than did the licensed polysaccharide vaccine.[136]

The Advisory Committee on Immunization Practices (ACIP) recommends routine vaccination with one dose of MCV4 in those aged 11–18 years at the earliest opportunity.[137] In addition, ACIP recommends routine vaccination for persons aged 19–55 years who are at increased risk for meningococcal disease: college freshmen living in dormitories, microbiologists routinely exposed to isolates of *N. meningitidis*, military recruits, travelers to or residents of countries in which meningococcal infection is hyperendemic or epidemic, persons with terminal complement component deficiencies, and persons with anatomic or functional asplenia. In 2008, the Food and Drug Administration (FDA) approved expanding the use of MCV4 to include children 2–10 years old who are at increased risk for meningococcal infection.[138] These children include travelers to or residents of countries in which meningococcal disease is hyperendemic or epidemic, children who have terminal complement component deficiencies, and children who have anatomic or functional asplenia.

The current WHO strategy for control of meningitis epidemics in the African meningitis belt stresses mass vaccination with meningococcal polysaccharide vaccines to halt the outbreak and sound case management to curb the lethality of the disease.[139] Current internationally marketed polysaccharide meningococcal vaccines are A/C, A/C/W135, or A/C/Y/W135 multivalent products.[139] However, polysaccharide vaccines are not able to prime immunological memory and are poorly immunogenic in infants and young children. The dramatic burden caused by group A meningococci in Africa could be potentially prevented and eliminated by the use of an effective Men A conjugate vaccine. However, no group A conjugate vaccines have yet been licensed for use in Africa.[4,139] The lack of progress in developing a meningococcal A conjugate vaccine for Africa led to the creation of the Meningitis Vaccine Project (MVP) in 2001 as a partnership between the WHO and PATH with funding from the Bill & Melinda Gates Foundation.[4,139] MVP aims to eliminate meningococcal epidemics as a public health problem in sub-Saharan Africa through the development, manufacture, testing, and introduction of conjugate meningococcal vaccines.[4,139]

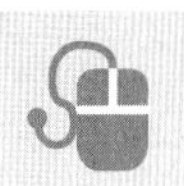

Access the complete reference list online at
http://www.expertconsult.com

CHAPTER 25

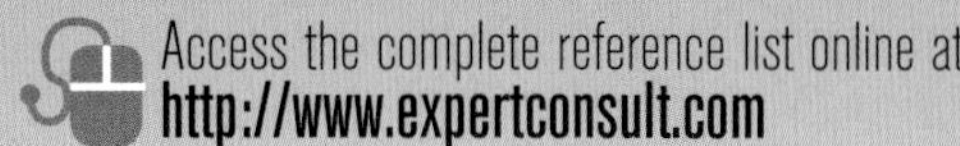
Access the complete reference list online at
http://www.expertconsult.com

Gonococcal and Other Neisserial Infections

Joseph A. Duncan • Lillian B. Brown • Peter A. Leone

INTRODUCTION AND THE AGENT

The sexually transmitted disease commonly known as gonorrhea is caused by the bacterium *Neisseria gonorrhoeae*. *N. gonorrhoeae* is a Gram-negative diplococcus that is aerobic, nonmotile, and nonspore-forming. It belongs to the family Neisseriaceae, which contains the genera *Neisseria, Moraxella, Eikenella, Simonsiella, Alysiella, Kingella*, and *Acinetobacter*.[1] The genus *Neisseria* is composed of 10 species, all of human origin, despite which two of these species are pathogenic to humans: *N. gonorrhoeae* and *N. meningitidis*.[2] The latter is an etiologic agent of a common form of bacterial meningitis. *N. gonorrhoeae* is the cause of urethritis, cervicitis, pelvic inflammatory disease (PID), and associated infections and is distantly related to *Neisserialactamica*, which can occasionally be a human pathogen. All *Neisseria* species are oxidase-positive, but only *N. gonorrhoeae* typically invades the upper reproductive tract; 20% of women with gonococcal cervicitis develop PID.[3] Gonorrhea is occasionally invasive, and 0.3–3.0% of mucosal infections progress to disseminated gonococcal infection (DGI).[4] Perhaps the most important impact of gonorrhea is facilitation of acquisition of human immunodeficiency virus (HIV)[5,6] and shedding of HIV in semen.[7]

EPIDEMIOLOGY

Although the overall incidence of gonorrhea has declined since 1975, it remains the second most commonly reported communicable disease in the United States. The case rate of US gonococcal infection decreased from 371.5 per 100 000 population in 1986 to 116.2 per 100 000 in 2003.[8] The 2003 rate was the lowest ever reported for the United States; however, the rate of reported gonorrhea has since reached a plateau and remained relatively stable (119 per 100 000 in 2007).[9] Rates of gonorrhea remain high regionally – in the southeast; among some ethnic groups – African-Americans and Hispanics; and among certain behavioral risk groups – men who have sex with men (MSM) and adolescents.[9] The highest incidence of gonorrhea occurs in adolescents and young adults, and the prevalence increased between 2005 and 2007 among 15–24-year-olds, especially among 15–19-year-old females (647.9 per 100 000 population) and 20–24-year-old males,[9] possibly reflecting their greater number of partners, higher likelihood of unprotected intercourse, and choice of partners, who themselves have a higher incidence of disease.[10,11] The prevalence rate for African-Americans was approximately 2%, which was 36 and 14 times greater than Caucasian men and women, respectively.[11]

The global incidence of gonorrhea remains high, with an estimated 62 million new cases each year.[12,13] Overall rates for the disease remain low in most of Europe but are high in populations of immigrants and low socioeconomic status, and importation from other countries accounts for 14–25% of cases of gonorrhea diagnosed in Europe.[14–16] Although accurate information is limited and infection is often underdiagnosed or under-reported, gonorrhea rates are highest in the developing world, especially sub-Saharan Africa, South and Southeast Asia, the Caribbean, and Latin America. In developed countries, prevalence is also highest in the most marginalized individuals socially and economically, with lower socioeconomic factors, ethnic minority status, and younger age being major correlates of risk.

Poverty increases risk for gonorrhea;[9,17] impoverished groups often have limited access to health care, are reluctant to seek prompt treatment, may engage in drug or substance abuse, and often populate concentrated areas with high disease rates. In 2007, African-Americans accounted for 70% of total reported cases of gonorrhea in the United States.[9] The rate of gonorrhea for African-Americans was 19 times higher than among whites in 2007 (662.9 cases per 100 000 versus 34.2). The infection rate of gonorrhea among American Indian/Alaskan natives (107.1) and among Hispanics (69.2) was 3 and 2 times higher, respectively, than the rate among non-Hispanic white Americans.[9,17]

Transmission

Gonorrhea may be the sexually transmitted disease (STD) most efficiently spread from person to person. Transmission following a single episode of vaginal intercourse is approximately 70–80% from male to female and 20–30% from female to male.[18,19] Transmission through either receptive or insertive rectal intercourse may be less efficient than by vaginal intercourse. Oral-to-genital transmission is probably the least common and least efficient means of transmission. Although specific rates are not available, it has been reported that transmission is greater through fellatio than cunnilingus. In MSM, oral–genital contact may account for up to 50% of all urethral infections. As with other STDs, gonorrhea prevalence and transmission can be partially explained by applying the concept of "core group" transmitters. By definition, members of the core group are individuals who are more likely to become infected and more likely to transmit the disease to others. As a result of their high level of sexual activity and frequency of partner change, these individuals have the greatest influence in sustaining the epidemic of gonorrhea.[20]

THE DISEASE

The clinical manifestations of gonorrhea are numerous and vary from local asymptomatic disease to dissemination. The initial site of infection, the infecting strain of gonorrhea, host immunity, and other coinfections all influence the spectrum of clinical disease.

Gonococcal Infection in Men

In men, gonococcal urethritis is the most common manifestation of infection. Following inoculation of the anterior male urethra, *N. gonorrhoeae* attaches to and infects columnar epithelial cells. The incubation period may range from 24 hours to 14 days, but 75% of men develop symptoms (dysuria and discharge) within 4 days of infection.[21,22] Dysuria usually precedes the development of purulent discharge by approximately 24 hours. Although 90% of newly acquired infections are symptomatic, about 50% of all infections in the community have few to no symptoms.[23] If left untreated, gonococcal urethritis usually resolves over the course of several weeks, with the majority of cases becoming asymptomatic within 6 months.[24]

Since the widespread availability of effective antimicrobial therapy in the 1940s, local complications in men have become rare. However, *N. gonorrhoeae* causes about 10% of acute epididymitis. Other complications include acute or chronic prostatitis, orchitis, seminal vesiculitis, posterior urethritis, and infection of Tyson's and Cowper's glands.[25]

Sexual practices determine the site of infection. In homosexual males, the rectum is the only site of gonococcal infection in 40% of reported cases. Rectal infection occurs through direct inoculation by receptive anal intercourse and often results in symptomatic disease,[26,27] ranging from mild pruritus and painless rectal discharge to severe rectal pain and bloody, mucopurulent discharge. Diagnosis is best made by anoscopy and culture, since external inspection may reveal few signs of infection. Without treatment the patient can become a chronic, asymptomatic carrier. Pharyngeal infection occurs in up to 25% of homosexual men and 7% of heterosexual men who engage in oral–genital contact with an infected partner. Over 90% of pharyngeal infections are asymptomatic but can produce an exudative pharyngitis or tonsillitis. The pharynx is the only site of infection in 5% of patients with gonococcal infection. Pharyngeal infection clears spontaneously in nearly all cases within 12 weeks of infection.[28–30]

Gonococcal Infection in Women

The clinical presentation of gonorrhea in women is varied, and about 50% of women with endocervical infection are asymptomatic. Although the columnar epithelial cells of the endocervix are the initial site of infection, up to 30% of women with untreated infection develop upper reproductive tract infection or PID.[31] In the presence of endocervical infection, infection usually also involves the urethra.

The incubation period for gonorrhea is longer in women than in men but is usually less than 10 days. The clinical presentation is highly variable and includes vaginal discharge secondary to mucopurulent cervicitis, abnormal menstrual bleeding, and anorectal discomfort.[26,31] Dysuria is also a common symptom of gonococcal infection in women. It is often mistaken for acute bacterial cystitis and should be suspected in young, sexually active women with pyuria in the absence of bacteria. Women who present with dysuria should have a pelvic examination as well as examination of the urethra for inflammatory exudate, and visualization of the cervix for signs of endocervical involvement and specimen collection.

PATHOGENESIS AND IMMUNITY

N. gonorrhoeae is a strict human pathogen and is highly adapted to survival in and dissemination from the human urogenital tract. The host environment for gonococcus varies depending on the sex of the host (male and female genital tracts are quite different at the anatomical and cellular level) and stage of infection (resting mucosa, inflamed mucosa, and nonmucosal human tissue each present different challenges to the organism).[32] *N. gonorrhoeae* utilizes numerous surface and secreted factors to facilitate infection of its human host. These factors are involved in: (1) attachment; (2) local proliferation; (3) penetration or invasion; and (4) survival or avoidance of host defense mechanisms. Because of the variation in host environment, many, if not all, of these factors involve cell surface components that may be subject to phase or antigenic variations. Phase variation refers to the ability of the organism to turn the expression of a gene on or off, while antigenic variation refers to the ability of the organism to change the physical structure of the molecule, including proteins, lipids, and saccharides.

Lipooligosaccharide

Lipooligosaccharide (LOS), the lipid A-containing structure in the outer membranes of Neisseriae (including the gonococcus), has a relative paucity of glycosylation when compared to lipopolysaccharide of enteric Gram-negative species. LOS variation has been implicated in antigenic variation and escape from immunologic surveillance, resistance to complement and other host antimicrobial factors, and bacterial adherence to host substrate.[1–4,33–36] Variations in gonococcal LOS are largely due to phase-variable expression of genes involved in LOS biosynthesis, those in the *lgtABCDE* operon and *lgtG*, which determine core oligosaccharide structure and *lst*, which determines LOS sialylation.[5–7,37–39] Sialylation of LOS facilitates binding of complement regulatory molecule, factor H, inducing high levels of complement resistance.[8,40] Gonococcal LOS sialylation also helps it resist killing by polymorphonuclear leukocytes. Gonococci lacking the *lst* gene have reduced virulence in murine models of gonorrhea, and LOS from gonococci isolates from human urethral exudate is highly sialylated, suggesting that LOS sialylation is important in pathogenesis.[9,10,41,42] Phosphoethanolamine decoration of the oligosaccharide and lipid A moiety is an additional structural modification of gonococcal LOS that is mediated by the *lpt3*, *lpt6*, and *lptA* genes, respectively.[11–13,43–45] Structural changes in LOS are mediated by phase-variable expression of many of these biosynthetic genes.[5,37] The interaction of gonococcal LOS with the human asialoglycoprotein receptor (ASGP-R) allows entry into primary human urethral epithelial cells.[46] Gonococcal LOS is also known to interact with Toll-like receptor-4, dendritic cell-SIGN (CD209), and the inflammasome to activate inflammatory signaling in host immune cells.[13–15,45,47,48] The potency of immune signaling activation has been correlated in some cases to variations in LOS structure.[13,16,45,49] The role of variability in LOS-induced inflammatory signaling remains to be determined.

Type IV Pilus

Type IV pili often facilitate bacterial DNA uptake from the environment, mediate twitching motility, and effect attachment to host cells.[50] The main structural protein, pilin, is encoded by the *pilE* gene. The gonococcal genome also contains multiple, silent incomplete variant copies of pilin-encoding genes, *pilS*.[51] Antigenic variation occurs with translocation of DNA from a *pilS* locus into a homologous region of the expressed *pilE* locus. The resulting alterations in the structure of the pili are thought to allow evasion of host adaptive immune response. If the *pilS*-derived sequence blocks transcription or expression of functional pilin, phase variation occurs. Analysis of gonococcus isolated from human challenge studies has demonstrated that *pilE* antigenic variation occurs early in human infection.[52,53] Nonpiliated gonococcal colony variants isolated *in vitro* demonstrate reduced infectivity in human challenge studies, suggesting the pilus is important to infection of the male genital tract.[54,55] Unfortunately, studies demonstrating that gonococcal strains lacking *pilE* or other pilus structural proteins are less infectious than isogenic wild-type strains in human challenge studies or mouse models of disease have not been reported to date. CD46, or membrane cofactor protein, and the human complement regulator C4B-binding protein have both been identified as putative host epithelial cell receptors for the gonococcal pilus.[17,18,56,57] The pilus is thought to be decorated with the pilC proteins PilC1 and PilC2, whose expression is also controlled by phase variation. PilC is critical for binding of piliated gonococci to human epithelial cells.[58] PilC appears to bind to a yet-to-be-identified receptor on epithelial cells rather than CD46 or complement regulator C4B-binding protein.[19,59] Pilus-mediated binding is known to induce host cell signaling including activation of host protein kinases and mobilization of calcium ion flux, presumably through activation of cytoskeleton-mediated mechanosensation. This signaling leads to cytoskeletal rearrangements and induction of antiapoptotic gene expression in host cells. The role of these host cellular responses in the pathogenesis of gonococcal infections is an active area of research.

Porin

N. gonorrhoeae expresses a single porin protein from the *porB* locus. PorB is highly abundant, representing about 50% of all gonococcal outer-membrane protein. Unlike many other gonococcal outer-membrane proteins, PorB amino acid sequences are relatively conserved between strains.[20,21,60,61] Gonococcal PorB falls largely into two immunologically defined serotypes (P1A and P1B). Interestingly, gonococci of the P1A serotype are more frequently associated with disseminated gonococcal diseases, whereas P1B-expressing gonococcal strains are more commonly isolated from cases of urethritis and cervicitis. DGI is frequently associated with asymptomatic infection of mucosal surfaces, rather than symptomatic gonorrhea with robust local inflammation.[22,62] The mechanism by which gonococcal porin may facilitate these different forms of infection is not clearly defined. However, gonococci expressing P1A invade host cells more rapidly than those expressing P1B. Expression of certain P1A genes is also associated with increased resistance to complement-induced killing.[23,63] Gonococcal porin can also induce activation of at least two signaling pathways in host cells: (1) host cell apoptosis and (2) inflammatory signaling through the Toll-like receptor-2 pathway.[24,25,64,65] Through mechanisms that have not been elucidated, gonococcal PorB has been found to incorporate into mammalian cell membranes. Insertion of PorB in mammalian cells results in formation of functional ion channels and activates cell death in epithelial-, monocyte-, and lymphocyte-derived cells.[24,64] Gonococcal PorB contains a region of homology with the mitochondrial voltage-dependent ion channel, which results in its targeting mitochondria in epithelial cells and is required for the induction of apoptosis.[26,27,66,67]

Opacity Proteins

Opa proteins are a family of 11 or 12 related proteins that increase the colonial opacity of gonorrhea when viewed under a dissecting microscope.[53] Opa proteins undergo frequent phase and antigenic variation, with up to four or five different Opa genes being simultaneously expressed with a change in frequency of about 0.001 per cell per generation.[68]

Opa antigenic variation is regulated by translational frame shifting, which is due to a high-frequency, spontaneous variation in the number of CTCTT oligonucleotide repeats in the signal-encoding sequence of the Opa region.[69] Each Opa contains two hypervariable regions (HV-1 and HV-2), which are surface-exposed and promote the intimate attachment of gonococci to the host cell.[70,71] New Opa gene alleles can arise in a strain predominantly from recombination of alleles within a single strain or from acquisition and recombination of other gonococcal strains.[28,72] When gonococci that express no Opa proteins (all Opa gene expression phase shifted off) are used in experimental infection in the urethra of male volunteers, the recovered bacteria all express at least one Opa protein.[29,73] Similar findings with regard to Opa expression have been noted in a murine model of vaginal gonorrhea.[30,74] These data suggest Opa protein expression is required early in urethral infection and that phase shifting of Opa expression occurs during human infection.[75,76] Opa proteins can mediate both bacterial adherence and endocytosis by eukaryotic cells.[77] Antibodies directed against these regions decrease cell adherence, but no cross-reacting Opa antibodies have been found to block adherence.

Several studies suggest that only a few Opa types may be able to mediate cellular attachment or induce endocytosis.[77] Opa binds to host heparin sulfate proteoglycans and to protein surface receptors known as carcinoembryonic antigen-like cell adhesion molecules (CEACAMs, formerly referred to as CD66 antigens).[78,79] The phase-shifting expression of various Opa proteins may provide gonococci with the ability to bind to various host cell types depending on the specific Opa proteins expressed by the bacteria and the differential expression of CEACAM family members by different host cell types.[80] CEACAM engagement on professional phagocytic cells results in the activation of host cell Src tyrosine kinases, Hck and Fgr, which is then followed by Rac activation. Rac activation, in turn, triggers cytoskeletal rearrangement and internalization of the gonococcus.[81] In addition to triggering signaling events responsible for phagocytosis of the gonococcus, activation of CEACAM-1 on host lymphocytes by binding of Opa52 leads to activation of the immunoreceptor tyrosine-based inhibitory motif. This signaling pathway results in reduced antibody production and induces cell death in B lymphocytes.[31,32,82,83] Opa52-mediated activaiton of CEACAM-1 may therefore represent a mechanism by which the gonococcus inhibits adaptive immune response to infection by the bacteria.

Although Opa expression seems to be an important factor in the initiation of gonococcal infection, gonococcal isolates from the upper genital tract of women are less likely to express Opa than isolates from the lower genital tract.[84] Increasing the number of Opa variants that a host has developed antibodies against does not increase susceptibility to the acquisition of gonococcal infection but does reduce the risk for developing salpingitis.[85]

Reduction Modifiable Protein

Unlike the antigenic variability associated with gonococcal surface structures, reduction modifiable protein (Rmp) has relative antigenic stability within the species and the genus *Neisseria*.[86–89] Rmp is physically associated with Por on the outer membrane of gonococci and is highly immunogenic for noncomplement-fixing antibodies. Host antibodies directed against Rmp bind to the Por–Rmp complex and prevent deposition of complement-fixing anti-Por antibodies.[90] Once bound, antibodies to Rmp increase the deposition of C3 and C9 and redirect terminal complement complex to nonlytic sites.[91–93] The presence of anti-Rmp antibodies also correlates with an increased risk of gonococcal mucosal infection.[94] Rmp is closely related to the outer-membrane protein 3 (OmpA) of *Escherichia coli* and the class 4 protein of meningococcus.[92] It is possible that Rmp antibodies are acquired in the absence of gonococcal infection by colonization of the intestinal tract by *E. coli* or by nasopharyngeal colonization with meningococcus. In essence, gonococci can use the host immune response against other organisms as its way of preventing an effective response to itself.

IgA Protease

N. gonorrhoeae and many other mucosal pathogens secrete an exoenzyme known as immunoglobulin A1 (IgA_1) protease.[33,95] Gonococcal IgA_1 protease protects the bacteria from host immune responses by cleaving the hinge region of IgA, which is the primary secreted antibody active at mucosal surfaces. Further studies have demonstrated that IgA_1 protease has additional host substrates that are likely to play a role in the pathogenesis of gonorrhea. IgA_1 protease also cleaves the lysosomal-associated membrane protein-1 (LAMP-1) which appears to reduce the ability of lysosome/endosome to mediate killing of the gonococcus and to facilitate transcytosis of the gonococcus across polarized epithelial cells.[34,35,96,97] IgA protease also induces production of proinflammatory and immunomodulatory cytokines from human monocytic cells.[36,37,98,99] Thus IgA protease of *N. gonorrhoeae* likely helps establish infection through effects on epithelial cells and controlling host immune responses to infection. However, IgA protease-deficient gonococci caused human experimental male uthrethritis; thus this protein is not essential to establish human male infection.[38,100] Its role in female infection remains unclear.

Future work in this field that focuses on pathogen-derived factors involved in the initiation and maintainance of infection and on the host molecules that mediate the host response to *N. gonorrhoeae* is essential to identify vaccination strategies aimed at reducing the burden of gonococcal-associated diseases.[101]

DIAGNOSIS

Cervical or urethral exudate should be examined by Gram stain and by culture. Mucopurulent cervicitis is defined by the presence of a yellow-green discoloration on a swab after insertion into the endocervix. In the absence of infection, the swab would remain white or be coated by a clear mucoid discharge. Culture or other diagnostic tests should be used to differentiate gonococcal cervicitis from other causes of cervical inflammation, such as chlamydia and herpes simplex. The endocervical Gram stain sensitivity is only 50% and must demonstrate intracellular Gram-negative diplococci to discriminate between *N. gonorrhoeae* and other *Neisseria* and Gram-negative species that normally inhabit the vagina and cervix.[102] Whenever possible, it is essential to confirm the diagnosis of gonococcal infection through either culture or direct or amplified genetic probes.

Other local sites of infection in women include gonococcal proctitis, which is found in 35–50% of women with cervicitis and is usually asymptomatic. It can be the only site of infection in 5% of women.[51,103] If symptoms are present, they are similar to those shown by men. Although sore throat and pharyngitis in the STD clinic are often associated with a history of fellatio, gonorrhea or other sexually transmitted infections are not usually isolated.[103,104] Most pharyngeal infections are asymptomatic and clear spontaneously. Pharyngeal gonorrhea is found in 10–20% of women with endocervical infection,[104] is associated with an apparent increased risk of dissemination, and has been associated with sexual transmission.[104,105]

Local infection of the endocervix extends to the uterus, fallopian tubes, or adjacent structures in about 15% of women.[106–108] Factors contributing to upper tract infections include menstruation, use of an intrauterine device, a history of douching, adolescent age, or previous history of PID. Clinical signs and symptoms of upper tract infection involve some or all of a constellation including lower abdominal pain, dyspareunia, abnormal menstrual bleeding, adnexal and cervical motion tenderness, fever, and other complaints consistent with an intraabdominal infection. Endocervical Gram stain may be helpful and yield a presumptive diagnosis by the presence of intracellular Gram-negative diplococci, but it is negative in 40–60% of women with PID.[102] Therefore, the diagnosis of PID is usually made on clinical grounds and cannot be distinguished from nongonococcal PID. None of the clinical signs and symptoms has both high sensitivity or specificity for PID. Use of three clinical variables – a high erythrocyte sedimentation rate, fever, and adnexal tenderness – correctly classified only 65% of laparoscopically diagnosed PID.[109] Because of the lack of a diagnostic clinical sign or symptom, the differential diagnosis remains broad and includes ectopic pregnancy, urinary tract infection, pyelonephritis, appendicitis, proctocolitis, and endometriosis.

Early diagnosis and treatment are essential to prevent the complications of PID. Infertility is strongly associated with a history of PID and occurs with increasing frequency in 11% of women who have had one episode, in 23% with two episodes, and in 75% with three or more episodes of PID. Other sequelae include chronic pelvic pain and ectopic pregnancy.[102,110]

Other urogenital complications from gonorrhea in women include perihepatitis (Fitz-Hugh–Curtis syndrome), which presents as acute right or bilateral upper-quadrant tenderness, frequently with signs and symptoms of PID.[111] Infection of Bartholin's gland duct presents with local erythema and pus at the posterior third of the labia majora.

Infection with gonorrhea during pregnancy is similar in clinical presentation to that in nonpregnant women. However, in women with gonococcal infection, there are higher rates of spontaneous abortion, premature rupture of membranes, acute chorioamnionitis, postpartum endometriosis, and premature delivery.[112,113] Asymptomatic women may transmit infection throughout the pregnancy and postpartum period. In particular peripartum transmission to the newborn may result in infection of the conjunctiva, rectum, or respiratory tract.[114,115] Gonococcal ophthalmia can be prevented by routine screening for endocervical infection during pregnancy and by the prophylactic use of 1% silver nitrate, erythromycin, or tetracycline ophthalmic solution.[93] These agents may not be available in developing countries. A single application of povidone-iodine 2.5% is an inexpensive alternative with a broad spectrum of activity against chlamydia, gonococcus, HIV, and herpes simplex.[116,117] Given the high rates of tetracycline-resistant *N. gonorrhoeae* (TRNG), tetracycline may no longer be adequate as prophylactic therapy.[4]

Disseminated Disease

DGI is relatively rare, occurring in 0.5–3.0% of untreated mucosal infections.[4] Most DGI occurs in persons with asymptomatic mucosal infection. This may be partially due to infection by a distinct clone that typically causes minimally symptomatic mucosal infection but is prone to systemic dissemination. This clone exhibits the arginine, hypoxanthine, and uracil (AHU) auxotype, PorIA serovar, and serum-resistant phenotype. Host factors are also important with women, accounting for about 70% of disseminated disease and bacteremia, often beginning during menses. Patients with terminal complement component deficiency are particularly susceptible to systemic infection with the gonococcus and meningococcus.[109]

The clinical manifestations of DGI are a result of gonococcal bacteremia, although patients typically lack the classic signs of bacteremia, that is, high fever, leukocytosis, or systemic toxicity.[4] The most common presentation of DGI is polyarthritis. Gonococcal arthritis can, however, present as monarticular arthritis, the most common cause of acute arthritis in young adults. An important clinical finding that helps differentiate gonococcal arthritis from other infectious causes is tenosynovitis, which often occurs over the involved joint and is sometimes accompanied by erythema.[110] Skin lesions, which typically occur throughout this period, appear as sparse, pustular lesions with surrounding erythema on the distal extremities. Lesions are present in 50–75% of patients but number fewer than 30 in most cases.[111,112]

Purulent arthritis is a later manifestation of the arthritis-dermatitis syndrome associated with DGI and occurs in approximately 30–40% of patients with DGI. Synovial fluid cultures are usually sterile but are more frequently positive in patients with synovial fluid leukocyte counts greater than 40 000/μL.[113] Blood and skin lesion cultures are usually also sterile, with the overall yield of blood cultures being less than 30% but decreasing with the duration of clinical illness.[114] This may be due to the intermittent, low level of bacteremia, the extraordinary nutritional requirements of the gonorrhea strains most likely to disseminate, and the role of immunocomplex deposition as a cause of local inflammation.

Other manifestations of DGI include mild pericarditis, endocarditis, and meningitis (each of which is seen in fewer than 3% of patients with DGI).[113–115]

To confirm the diagnosis of DGI, tests for gonococcal infection should be obtained from all mucosal sites. In more than 80% of patients, gonococci can be isolated from genital, rectal, or pharyngeal sites. In cases in which tests are negative from all mucosal sites, isolation of *N. gonorrhoeae* from sexual partners may be the only means to confirm diagnosis.

Culture

The gold standard for detection of *N. gonorrhoeae* used to be the culture. Nucleic acid amplification tests (NAATs) are now the standard. The main benefits of culture are lower cost, high specificity, and the ability to do additional studies, such as antimicrobial susceptibility testing. The disadvantages of culture can be substantial in developing countries because of the stringent storage and transport requirements of culture media, the fastidious growth requirements of *N. gonorrhoeae*, and the delay in obtaining results. Test performance, available technology, cost, and prevalence of gonorrhea must be taken into account when selecting diagnostic tests to be used for identifying gonococcal infection. Ideally, the test should be highly sensitive, specific, rapid, and inexpensive.[116]

The yield of gonococcal culture largely depends on the anatomic site of the culture and the use of selective or nonselective media. Selective media contain several antibodies to prevent the overgrowth of genitourinary, enteric, and oral flora. Modified Thayer-Martin (MTM) is probably the most widely used selective medium, with an overall sensitivity of 80–95% for isolation of *N. gonorrhoeae*. Other selective media include NYC (New York City), Martin-Lewis (ML), and GC-Lect. There are significant differences among these media. MTM lacks serum and inhibits the growth of 3–10% of *N. gonorrhoeae* strains because of its high concentration of vancomycin (3 µg/mL) relative to other media. Additionally, it is difficult to predict when vancomycin-sensitive strains may be present, because of geographic variation in prevalence. Vancomycin-sensitive strains are more likely to be found in heterosexuals, whites, and asymptomatic carriers. Moreover, growth of vancomycin-sensitive strains largely depends on the size of the inoculum; smaller inocula are more likely to be inhibited. GC-Lect medium has some advantage over MTM for the isolation of vancomycin-sensitive strains owing to its lower concentration of vancomycin (2 µg/mL) and the presence of supplemental nutrients. NYC medium is serum-enriched and also has a vancomycin concentration of 2 µg/mL. NYC medium is translucent and therefore facilitates both the selection of oxidase-positive colonies and viewing under a stereomicroscope. Production variability and increased cost render NYC less useful than MTM.

To prevent the overgrowth of gonococcal colonies with normal flora, it is best to use selective media in sites with a higher concentration of easily cultured bacteria, such as the rectum, pharynx, and endocervix. Nonselective media can be used for urethral specimens from men with symptomatic urethritis because of the high concentration of gonococci relative to that of other genital flora.

In women, it is rare to detect infection in other mucosal sites without first finding it in the cervix. For women who have undergone a hysterectomy, urethral testing is indicated. Consideration of tests obtained from the accessory gland ducts, pharynx, and rectum is based on clinical presentation, site of sexual contact, and cost.

Gram Stain

Low cost and rapidity of diagnosis make Gram stain of clinical specimens an important test for the evaluation of gonorrhea in the clinical setting. Gram stain is considered positive if neutrophils with intracellular Gram-negative diplococci are observed. It is considered negative in the absence of Gram-negative diplococci, and equivocal following observation of extracellular Gram-negative or morphologically atypical-appearing organisms.[116,117] Because it is not possible to distinguish *N. meningitidis* from *N. gonorrhoeae* by Gram stain, it is sometimes necessary to confirm the diagnosis through culture. Other nonpathogenic *Neisseria* species are usually not present as intracellular organisms.

The sensitivity and specificity of the Gram stain smear vary, depending on the site of infection and the presence or absence of symptoms. For symptomatic urethritis in men, the high sensitivity and specificity, 95% and 98%, respectively, suffice for diagnosis.[117–120] In asymptomatic males, the sensitivity is significantly lower and requires a culture to rule out gonococcal infection. Lower sensitivity (40–60%) is also seen in Gram stains of endocervical samples from symptomatic women, although it retains a high specificity in these cases. Owing to high specificity, it is possible to make a presumptive diagnosis on the basis of a positive smear. The high intraobserver variability in preparing and reading endocervical Gram stains renders unreliable the reading of a negative Gram stain.[116,119] Although sometimes useful, the Gram-stained smear of the rectum, pharynx, and other sites should be used only in conjunction with cultures or other diagnostic tests to confirm diagnosis.

Nucleic Acid Amplification Tests

NAAT methodology involves amplification of specific *N. gonorrhoeae* DNA or RNA sequences by polymerase chain reaction (PCR), strand displacement assay (SDA), or transcription-mediated assay (TMA). Ligase chain reaction is no longer commercially available. NAATs have reported sensitivities and specificities from urethral and endocervical specimens that are comparable to culture.[121,122] The advantages of these tests over culture are the rapidity of results and the high sensitivity compared with culture. The latter has allowed testing for *N. gonorrhoeae* by NAATs to be applied to urine specimens, urethral, vaginal, rectal, and pharyngeal swabs.[123,124] Urine-based testing or, in the case of females, a self-collected vaginal swab permits screening of populations outside the traditional clinic setting and identification of the asymptomatic carrier of *N. gonorrhoeae* without invasive testing.

NAAT tests are currently not approved by the US Food and Drug Administration for use in the rectum, pharynx, and conjunctiva; however, some public and private laboratories have established performance specifications for their NAAT with rectal and pharyngeal swab specimens, thereby allowing results to be used for patient management. Laboratories that establish performance specifications for the use of NAATs with nongenital specimens must ensure that specificity is not compromised by cross-reaction with nongonococcal *Neisseria* species. The sensitivity of NAATs for the detection of *N. gonorrhoeae* in genital and nongenital anatomic sites is superior to culture but varies by NAAT type.[125]

The high sensitivity of NAATs has a trade-off in that specificity is not 100%. There can be false-positive results when screening is performed in low-prevalence populations.[126] Caution must be given to use of NAATs in screening asymptomatic populations. Even with reported high specificity, there is reason to be concerned that a poor positive predictive value with vaginal swabs may occur with PCR; this is less of an issue for TMA and SDA.[127] In the future, commercially available NAATs may identify resistance genes. Correlation of genetic markers of resistance to clinical isolates will still need to be made prior to widespread use of this technology as part of resistance monitoring.

TREATMENT AND PROGNOSIS

Antimicrobial Resistance

Control of gonococcal disease has depended heavily on the use of highly effective and preferably single-dose antibiotic therapy.[128] As early as the 1950s, however, reduced susceptibility to penicillin was reported.[129] Unfortunately, antimicrobial resistance has continued to evolve and spread since that time. Antibiotic resistance remains disproportionately represented in less developed nations and in socially marginalized groups. The reasons for the development of resistance are complex but can be attributed to four major factors: (1) poor compliance with prescribed therapy; (2) inadequate dosing of antibiotics; (3) circumstances causing low or inadequate antibiotic serum levels; and (4) conditions favoring the selection of resistance mutations (such as the widespread use of antimicrobial agents in the general population).

Antibiotic resistance occurs through two main mechanisms: chromosomal and plasmid-mediated resistance. Chromosomal resistance is encoded at several different loci and usually occurs as a stepwise, incremental resistance pattern. The single exception to stepwise chromosomal resistance is spectinomycin, to which high-level resistance occurs after a single alteration to the ribosomal target.[130,131] Plasmid resistance usually occurs as a one-step change to high-level resistance and rapidly spreads through a population.

Therapeutic regimens should be based on the knowledge of the *in vitro* sensitivity of prevalent gonococci in the immediate region. A strong argument can be made that regional susceptibility patterns are more important than strain susceptibility in a given individual.[132] This is especially important because most treatment occurs prior to obtaining the antimicrobial susceptibilities on a particular gonococcal isolate. Increasing minimum inhibitory concentrations (MICs) to antimicrobial therapy partially explains the rise in treatment failure, which further highlights the importance of monitoring resistance patterns in order to select treatment regimens accurately. In turn, this can further the discovery of new resistance patterns as they develop. Ideally, this monitoring should be a continuous surveillance program. Owing to financial constraints, point prevalence studies at repeated intervals can be performed to follow temporal changes in susceptibility patterns.

The specific incidence of antibiotic resistance is geographically variable, but effective treatment is a common challenge in several countries. In the United States, the Far East, and western and central Africa,[133] treatment with penicillin and tetracycline is unreliable owing to the appearance in gonococci of plasmids that produce β-lactamase, resulting in penicillinase-producing *N. gonorrhoeae* (PPNG); of plasmids that mediate high-level TRNG; and emergence over many decades of chromosomally mediated penicillin- and tetracycline-resistant *N. gonorrhoeae* (CMRNG).[133–135] PPNG strains are characterized by the production of β-lactamase and have MICs for penicillin greater than or equal to 16 μg/mL. CMRNG strains are characterized by the lack of β-lactamase production and have penicillin MICs less than 8 μg/mL. A strain can have plasmid-mediated resistance to both penicillin and tetracycline (PPNG-TRNG). Chromosomal-resistant strains usually have MICs less than or equal to 2 μg/mL for tetracycline, penicillin, or cefoxitin. In general, chromosomal resistance occurs through alterations in antimicrobial-binding proteins or through decreased net permeability of the gonococcal outer membrane.[129,136]

In reaction to widespread penicillin and tetracycline resistance, the Centers for Disease Control and Prevention (CDC) in 1987 ceased to recommend the first-line use of these agents for treatment of gonorrhea. It then began advocating the use of third-generation cephalosporins and selected fluoroquinolones.[137,138] Quinolone-resistant *N. gonorrhoeae* strains are now widely disseminated throughout the United States and the world. As of April 2007, quinolones are no longer recommended in the United States for the treatment of gonorrhea and associated conditions such as PID. Consequently, only one class of antimicrobials, the cephalosporins, is still recommended and available for the treatment of gonorrhea in the United States. The CDC website (http://www.cdc.gov/std/gisp) can provide the most current information.

Fortunately, ceftriaxone continues to be effective with no reported resistance. Cefixime had been the only oral cephalosporin recommended by the CDC for the treatment of uncomplicated gonococcal infection. Cefpodoxime has, in the past, been used as a replacement for cefixime.[139] There is concern, however, regarding the potential emergence of strains resistant to the use of a 200-mg dose of cefpodoxime and a similar concern of emerging resistance to cefixime. The clinical data for cefpodoxime are sparse, at best, with limited clinical data reported in the literature. Although it appears that cefpodoxime therapy at 200 mg and 400 mg may be equivalent, a 400-mg dose should be used for treatment.[140] Monitoring for the emergence of resistance or evidence of clinical treatment failure is recommended for areas where cefpodoxime or cefixime is used as first-line treatment for uncomplicated gonococcal infection.

The concern over potential cefixime resistance stems from the application of a therapeutic index, defined by the ratio of peak serum concentration to MIC. The recommended therapeutic index is a ratio greater than 3 to 4 : 1, as determined by the use of penicillin G for the treatment of gonococcal urethritis.[141] Antimicrobial agents with a therapeutic index greater than 4 are highly effective in curing gonorrhea. Relative to other therapies, cefixime demonstrates a low peak serum level. The recommended dose of cefixime, 400 mg PO, produces a peak serum level of 4 μg/mL, while 500 mg of ceftriaxone IM produces peak serum concentrations of 42–45 μg/mL. This concentration is more than 1000 times greater than the MIC for *N. gonorrhoeae*.[142,143]

Fluoroquinolone resistance (QNRG) is widespread and has been noted in the Far East, Australia, Africa, Europe, and (most recently) the United States.[144] Fluoroquinolone resistance is chromosomally mediated and affects all members of this class of drug. Widespread increases in QNRG have been noted in MSM throughout the United States. This prompted the CDC initially to issue behavior-specific recommendations on treatment of gonorrhea but, because prevalence of QNRG is high among those with gonococcal infection, fluoroquinolones are no longer recommended for the treatment of gonococcal infection.

Antimicrobial Therapy

Ideally, antimicrobial therapy for gonorrhea should be safe, inexpensive, and achieve rapid serum and tissue levels at least three to four times greater than the MIC of the infecting gonococcal strain. Treatment regimens for uncomplicated gonorrhea should cure at least 95% of infections by a single dose of therapy. The continued evolution of gonococcal resistance has led to significant changes to the 2002 recommendations. The ideal therapeutic index (ratio of peak serum concentration to MIC of 3–4 : 1) is achieved with the recommended regimens of cefixime or ceftriaxone. Ceftriaxone, cefixime, and ciprofloxacin all clear *N. gonorrhoeae* in less than 24 hours from the urethral mucosa and semen of men.[145] Because of the rapid clearance of infection and the high potency of the recommended treatment regimens, test of cure is not indicated following treatment for uncomplicated gonorrhea with current cephalosporin regimens. The high rate of coinfection with chlamydia in most geographic areas – 15–20% among men and 30–50% among women – necessitates empirical treatment of chlamydia infection with all gonorrhea treatment regimens.[146,147] Current recommendations in the United States call for ceftriaxone 250 mg IM with cefixime 400 mg PO as an alternative therapy, plus treatment for possible coinfection with *C. trachomatis* with either single-dose azithromycin 1.0 g PO, or with doxycycline 100 mg PO two times per day for 7 days.[147,148] Consideration should be given to using a regimen containing ceftriaxone or azithromycin where syphilis prevalence remains high.[149]

Alternative regimens for those unable to take cephalosporins include spectinomycin 2 g IM, kanamycin 2 g IM, or gentamicin 240 mg IM.[150–152] Because of the low risk of cross-reactions between penicillin and cephalosporins with single-dose therapy, cephalosporins may be used in patients with penicillin allergies, unless there is a history of an immediate IgE-mediated hypersensitivity reaction.

Pharyngeal gonococcal infection may be treated with ceftriaxone 250 mg IM. An alternative regimen for those unable to be treated with cephalosporins is ciprofloxacin 500 mg or ofloxacin 400 mg PO. Local prevalence of quinolone-resistant gonorrhea must be kept in mind with test of cure for areas where prevalence is ≥5% or is unknown.[150] When considering alternative regimens, it is important to note that spectinomycin is ineffective against pharyngeal infection.[151] Its use in the United States has been limited to pregnant women who are unable to take cephalosporins.

Gonorrhea in pregnancy is best treated with ceftriaxone 250 mg IM, plus a regimen active against *C. trachomatis* with erythromycin base 500 mg PO, four times a day for 7 days, or amoxicillin 500 mg PO three times a day for 7 days, or azithromycin 1.0 g PO.[150,151] Pregnant women for whom cephalosporins are contraindicated may be treated with spectinomycin 2 g IM once. Pregnant women should have rectal and endocervical cultures for *N. gonorrhoeae* obtained 3–7 days following therapy as a test of cure.

DGI requires hospitalization for observation of response to therapy and to insure compliance. The recommended initial regimen for DGI is ceftriaxone 1 g IM or IV every 24 hours.[150,151] If patients are allergic to cephalosporins, therapy should include spectinomycin 2 g IM every 12 hours.[150] Resolution of symptoms usually occurs within 24–48 hours of initiation of therapy. In patients with a prompt clinical response to therapy and whose compliance is likely, therapy can be completed on an outpatient basis, with an oral regimen of cefixime 400 mg twice per day or cefpodoxime 400 mg twice per day, or (if QRNG is not a consideration) ciprofloxacin 500 mg twice per day or ofloxacin 400 mg twice per day to complete 7–10 days of total antibiotic therapy.[150]

Meningitis and endocarditis require high-dose intravenous therapy with a highly active agent that achieves adequate tissue levels in the site of infection, such as ceftriaxone 1–2 g IV every 12 hours. The duration of therapy should be a minimum of 10–14 days for gonococcal meningitis and a minimum of 4 weeks for gonococcal endocarditis.[150]

PID requires prompt treatment to reduce the incidence of chronic infection, chronic pelvic pain, and infertility. Women must be evaluated to distinguish PID from appendicitis and ectopic pregnancy. Severely ill women – those with high fever, severe pain, or inability to tolerate oral fluids – should be treated in the hospital until they are afebrile and have clinically improved. Outpatient therapy is best limited to nonpregnant, compliant women with mild-to-moderate disease. Follow-up examination is performed within 48–72 hours to monitor for clinical improvement in signs and symptoms. The two main therapeutic options appear in ***Table 25.1***.

Table 25.1 Therapy for Pelvic Inflammatory Disease in Women

Outpatient Therapy	Inpatient Therapy[a]
Option A	**Option A**
Ceftriaxone 250 mg IM	Cefoxitin 2.0 g IV every 6 hours
or	*or*
Cefoxitin 2.0 g IM with probenecid 1.0 g PO	Cefotetan 2.0 g IV every 12 hours
plus	*plus*
Doxycycline 100 mg PO, twice per day for 14 days	Doxycycline 100 mg IV every 12 hours
Option B	**Option B**
Ofloxacin 400 mg PO, twice per day for 14 days	Clindamycin 900 mg IV every 8 hours
plus	*plus*
Metronidazole 500 mg PO, twice per day for 14 days	Gentamicin loading dose IV or IM (2 mg/kg of body weight), followed by a maintenance dose (1.5 mg/kg) every 8 hours

[a]Intravenous (IV) therapy should be continued for a minimum of 48 hours after clinical improvement and, once the patient is switched to oral therapy, completed with doxycycline 100 mg orally (PO) twice per day for a total of 14 days of antimicrobial therapy.[9]
IM, intramuscular.

PREVENTION AND CONTROL

Despite widely available effective therapy, the persistence of gonorrhea at epidemic levels demonstrates the failure of current control programs. Persistence of STDs in a community can be described by the equation:[153]

$$R_o = BcD$$

Where R_o (the reproductive rate) is greater than 1, the disease will increase in prevalence in the community. The reproductive rate is dependent on the efficiency of transmission (B), the rate of sexual partner change (c), and the duration of infectiveness (D). Attempts to reduce the reproductive rate can be directed at interventions that may alter these factors.

Barrier methods remain one of the most effective means of reducing the transmission of gonorrhea.[154] For men, this includes the use of latex or polyurethane condoms. The current version of the female polyurethane condom has been demonstrated to reduce the transmission of trichomoniasis, but studies evaluating its effectiveness in reducing the transmission of gonorrhea have not been published.[155] The major drawbacks to all barrier methods are noncompliance and unacceptability. The female condom presents identical problems. These issues are further complicated by male resistance to the use of the female condom.

Methods which allow more autonomy in initiation by females include the use of vaginal microbicidal agents. When used intravaginally, the currently available agent, nonoxynol-9, reduces the risk of gonorrhea by 10–70%.[156] Since nonoxynol-9 is a detergent that can disrupt the lipid bilayers of cell membranes, it can cause mucosal irritation and ulcers and thus increase the risk of HIV transmission. As a result, nonoxynol-9 as means of gonorrhea prevention is no longer recommended.

Vaccines offer the hope of reducing the efficiency of transmission. Crude killed, whole-cell vaccines have been tried in humans and primates, but they are likely to be more toxic than subunit vaccines and offered no protection in human trials.[157] To date, subunit vaccines directed against Pil and Por have not prevented infection in human volunteers.[158,159] Future vaccines may target PilC, TbpB (an immunogenic component of the transferrin receptor), or FrpB (a partially conserved outer-membrane iron-repressed protein).[60] DNA vaccines offer a highly promising approach to effective immunogenic response but have yet to be studied for a gonococcal vaccine. A study using a DNA vaccine for priming an antibody response to PorB resulted in a high titer and long-lasting antibody response in an animal model.[160]

Until the availability of an effective vaccine, behavioral intervention remains a crucial strategy for reducing the spread of gonorrhea. Behavioral intervention aims to increase condom use/acceptability and both to delay sexual debut and reduce the rate of partner change. Transmission of gonorrhea is further influenced by factors that affect health care utilization. The essential components of an effective control program are providing increased access to health care, providing the opportunity for treatment at the earliest presentation of symptoms, identifying high-risk groups for targeted interventions, screening high-risk asymptomatic patients for infection, identifying and treating sexual partners of patients with gonorrhea, and rescreening those identified with infection 3–4 months after treatment.[150]

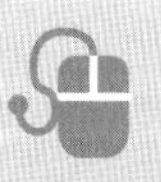

Access the complete reference list online at
http://www.expertconsult.com

Access the complete reference list online at http://www.expertconsult.com

CHAPTER 26

Haemophilus ducreyi Infections

Allan R. Ronald

INTRODUCTION

Haemophilus ducreyi has been a leading cause (along with syphilis and herpes simplex virus) of genital ulcers. Most prevalent in tropical developing areas, it predisposes to increased HIV acquisition and should be an important target of sexually transmitted disease (STD) control programs.

THE AGENT

The organism *H. ducreyi* is no longer classified taxonomically by 16S rRNA within the *Haemophilus* genus but rather is included within the *Actinobacillus* cluster. The organisms stain faintly negative with Gram stain and are arranged in "school of fish" or "railway tracks" patterns. *H. ducreyi* grows best on media supplemented with vitamins, vancomycin to inhibit growth of Gram-positive organisms, and charcoal to absorb toxic substances.[1] *H. ducreyi* has a capsule, pili, and several virulence factors.[2]

EPIDEMIOLOGY

H. ducreyi is spread through sex. The organism has no known reservoir other than persons with ulcers. The annual global incidence of chancroid has been reduced dramatically since 1990 and is now probably below 500 000. Historically more than 99% of cases occurred in developing countries, particularly eastern and southern Africa, India and Southeast Asia. In 2007 chancroid still accounted for 12% of genital ulcer disease (GUD) in Malawi and about 1% of GUD in Botswana and South Africa.[3,4] However, during the past 8 years, no chancroid has been reported elsewhere with the exception of a few cases from the South Pacific islands. Following exposure, uncircumcised men are three times more susceptible to infection. Among female sex workers in Nairobi, Kenya during the 1980s as many as 10% had *H. ducreyi* infection.[5] The organism is readily transmitted heterosexually during unprotected intercourse with a risk of infection that exceeds 50%.[5] GUD enhances the probability of HIV transmission. *H ducreyi* ulceration recruits lymphocytes and macrophages to the mucosal surface and provides ready entry for HIV from the genital secretions of the sexual partner.[5] HIV-infected persons who acquire *H. ducreyi* excrete HIV in the ulcer and expose subsequent sexual partners to increased risk of infection. The contribution of chancroid to the HIV epidemic may have been as much as one-third of the total incidence in some regions.[6]

THE DISEASE

Chancroid is characterized by single or multiple shaggy undermining ulcers on the genitalia. *H. ducreyi* does not cause systemic, invasive infection. The ulcers are usually painful, often quite superficial, and in about 40% of patients, associated with inguinal lymphadenitis. If untreated, the adenitis proceeds to bubo formation and may drain spontaneously, creating an inguinal abscess. In men, about half the ulcers occur on the prepuce and the rest on the glans, in the urethra, on the penile shaft, and on the scrotum and adjacent skin. Kissing lesions are common. In women the lesions occur commonly at the vestibular entrance, particularly on the posterior fourchette. However, numerous lesions are frequently widely present on the inner aspects of the labia majora and on the labia minora. Despite the apparent classic features of chancroid, numerous studies have shown that clinical etiologic identification and differentiation from syphilis, genital herpes, and granuloma inguinale is not possible.[7] As a result, syndromic management to include chancroid is essential for all patients with genital ulcer disease (GUD) if chancroid is endemic in the region. Recently *H. ducreyi* has been cultured from chronic cutaneous ulcers in children in the South Pacific islands.[8]

PATHOGENESIS AND IMMUNITY

H. ducreyi has cytotoxic and hemolytic proteins that are important determinants of virulence in both animal models and in human volunteer studies.[2] The host response is predominantly mononuclear with a preponderance of activated T lymphocytes and macrophages.

DIAGNOSIS

H. ducreyi can be transported in supplemented thioglycollate transport media and kept for up to 24 hours at 4°C.[1] However, ideally the culture should be plated immediately onto specially prepared chocolate media.[1] Growth is optimal at 32°C in a CO_2 environment with 100% humidity. A candle jar with a moistened paper towel provides a satisfactory environment. Growth often is not apparent before 48 hours. The opaque yellow-gray colony can usually be moved intact across the agar surface. Polymerase chain reaction (PCR) technology has been adapted to identify *H. ducreyi* from genital ulcer specimens and can be combined with PCR primers and probes for *Treponema pallidum* and herpes simplex virus.

TREATMENT AND PROGNOSIS

Chancroid is effectively treated with the macrolides and the fluoroquinolones. Most strains are resistant to ampicillin, tetracycline, and sulfonamides. Erythromycin, prescribed for 7 days in a dose of 500 mg three times a day or ciprofloxacin, prescribed as a single daily dose of 500 mg for 3 days, have cure rates in excess of 95%.[9] Inguinal buboes should be incised or aspirated if they become fluctuant.

PREVENTION AND CONTROL

Chancroid elimination requires implementation of conventional STD control initiatives. Primary prevention strategies include promotion of safer sex, widespread use of condoms, and partner referral with empiric treatment of contacts.[10] If chancroid is known to be present in a region, early diagnosis and appropriate syndromic treatment at the first point of contact with the health system can usually prevent wide dissemination. Routine examination of sex workers with empirical treatment of GUD rapidly reduces the reservoir of this pathogen. These STD control measures are very effective, even in resource-limited societies.[10] *H. ducreyi* has currently been eliminated from large regions where it was once the commonest STD and probably facilitated millions of HIV transmissions. However, reintroductions can occur as long as some countries have endemic disease, and until global eradication is achieved continuing surveillance and a capacity for outbreak response is essential.

Access the complete reference list online at
http://www.expertconsult.com

Access the complete reference list online at http://www.expertconsult.com

CHAPTER 27

Haemophilus influenzae

Mark C. Steinhoff • Thomas Cherian • Elizabeth P. Schlaudecker

INTRODUCTION

Haemophilus influenzae is among the most common causes of bacterial meningitis and other invasive infections in infants and young children throughout the world. Historically in the developing world, it has not been recognized as a vaccine-preventable cause of serious morbidity, long-term disability, and death. The availability of an effective vaccine against *H. influenzae* type b (Hib), which can virtually eliminate Hib disease, underscores the importance of determining the burden of vaccine-preventable illness caused by Hib. It also deserves recognition as a tropical illness in view of its global swathe of illness and death.[1,2]

THE AGENT

F. Pfeiffer in 1889 first described the "influenza bacillus" in Germany during an influenza epidemic, mistakenly reporting it as the cause of influenza. The genus *Haemophilus* ("blood-loving" in Greek) was formally named in 1920, to mark its requirement for blood substances in artificial media.

H. influenzae is a small, fastidious Gram-negative bacterium that requires hemin (X factor) and nicotinamide adenine dinucleotide (NAD, or V factor) for growth on artificial media. NAD is not available in routine blood agar, which accounts for its apparent absence in laboratories that do not use chocolate agar (made by heating blood so that red blood cells lyse and release V factor), or supplemented media such as Fildes or Leventhal agar. Some strains of the organism elaborate a polysaccharide capsule that permits classification into six distinct capsular serotypes (a through f). The capsular subtype b (Hib) causes over 90% of all invasive infections. Other strains do not elaborate a capsule and hence cannot be typed on the basis of the capsule; they are collectively referred to as non-typable *H. influenzae* (NTHi). In addition, *H. influenzae* can be biochemically typed into six biotypes (I through VI). The biotypes and the capsular serotypes are distinct typing methods, not correlated with each other. The entire Hib chromosome was sequenced in 1995, the first free-living organism to be DNA-sequenced.

EPIDEMIOLOGY

H. influenzae is part of the normal human nasopharyngeal flora and spreads by the airborne or direct contact routes from person to person. Nonencapsulated strains are frequently found in the upper respiratory tract. Among encapsulated strains, invasive type b is carried by 7–15% of children in high-risk populations, such as Alaskan natives and some African populations.[3] The rates of carriage of invasive type b organisms vary significantly with age and socioeconomic factors but are markedly decreased in vaccinated populations. The Hib serotype causes most invasive disease, including bacteremia, meningitis, epiglottitis, pneumonia and empyema, septic arthritis, and cellulitis. In North America and Europe, the peak incidence of invasive Hib disease is from 6 to 12 months of age; in West Africa and India, the peak incidence is from 6 to 8 months.[4,5]

Reported incidence rates of Hib disease vary widely, but in the absence of vaccination, the estimated global incidence of invasive Hib disease and pneumonia is 1342 cases per 100 000 children less than 5 years of age.[1,6] The incidence rate ranges from 544 cases per 100 000 in the Americas to 1822 cases per 100 000 in Southeast Asia. Among Eskimo and Native American children under 5 years of age, rates of Hib meningitis of up to 254 per 100 000 have occurred.[6] In India, the minimal Hib meningitis incidence is estimated to be 32 per 100 000 in infants less than 12 months of age, with an annual incidence of 7.1 per 100 000 in children less than 5 years of age.[7] Throughout the world, Southeast Asia has the largest numbers of cases and deaths attributed to Hib, followed by Africa, the western Pacific, and the eastern Mediterranean.[1] In the year 2000, the total number of deaths attributed to Hib disease was estimated to be 371 000, of which 50% occured in six countries: India, Nigeria, Ethiopia, DR Congo, China, and Afghanistan.[1,6]

THE DISEASE

Unencapsulated *H. influenzae* strains may cause sinusitis, otitis media, and bronchitis and may also cause pneumonia in children in developing countries or in adults with immune defects. Hib strains cause meningitis, bacteremia, pneumonia, epiglottitis, septic arthritis, pericarditis, and occult febrile bacteremia, as well as placentitis and peripartum septicemia in mothers (***Table 27.1***). A small proportion of invasive disease is caused by other capsular types, notably, a and f.

About half of all reported invasive infections caused by Hib are meningitis, and before the introduction of Hib vaccine, Hib accounted for the majority of childhood bacterial meningitis cases worldwide, outside the meningococcal belt of Africa.[1,6] The clinical characteristics of Hib meningitis are similar among children of developing or developed countries, although the case-fatality rates may reach 40% in the former.[1] Complications included subdural effusions, and central nervous system sequelae occur in 3–47% of survivors of Hib meningitis, with deafness being a common finding.[8,9] Hib epiglottitis was common in older children in North America and Europe but is rarely reported in developing countries.[5] Hib pneumonia is said to be infrequent in developed countries. However, in developing countries, data on Hib pneumonia are mixed; lung tap and Hib vaccine studies indicate that Hib may cause 4–30% of severe pneumonias in hospitalized patients.[10,11]

PATHOGENESIS AND IMMUNITY

Carriage of Hib in the nasopharynx is mediated by pili, which facilitate attachment to epithelial cells, and an immunoglobulin (Ig) A_1 protease protects the organism from mucosal antibodies. Carriage increases

Table 27.1 Worldwide Spectrum of All Classical (Nonbacteremic Pneumonia Excluded) *Haemophilus influenzae* Type B (Hib) Diseases, Taken from Data for 3931 Patients in 21 Studies from Various Parts of the World

Hib Diseases	Percentage
Meningitis	52
Pneumonia	12
Epiglottitis	10
Septicemia	8
Cellulitis	5
Osteoarticular	4
Others	3
Multifocal	6

(Modified from Peltola H. Worldwide *Haemophilus influenzae* type b disease at the beginning of the 21st century: global analysis of the disease burden 25 years after the use of the polysaccharide vaccine and a decade after the advent of conjugates. Clin Microbiol Rev. 2000;13:302–317.)

following infection with influenza or other viruses. Most carried strains are nonencapsulated. Following carriage, encapsulated strains may invade the bloodstream and infect secondary sites, whereas nonencapsulated strains mainly cause disease by contiguous spread.

Type b strains have a pentose polysaccharide capsule composed of repeating units of phosphoribosyl phosphate (PRP), which is a critical virulence factor. The other serotypes have hexose polysaccharide capsules and are far less frequent in invasive disease. It has been known since the 1930s era of serotherapy that IgG antibody directed against the capsular polysaccharide can be used for therapy and is protective in an animal model. Specific anti-PRP antibody mediates opsonophagocytosis and is correlated with protection. The age-specific incidence of disease in human infants is inversely correlated with the proportion of infants with protective levels of serum anti-PRP antibody.

DIAGNOSIS

H. influenzae is diagnosed by microbiologic isolation of the organism from a sterile site such as cerebrospinal fluid (CSF), blood, lung aspirate, joint, or bone. The characteristic small, flat, colorless colonies are seen on subculture on chocolate agar. Hib excretes capsular polysaccharide, which can be found by antigen detection techniques such as latex agglutination in the blood, CSF, and urine. Other polysaccharide detection methods include coagglutination, countercurrent immunoelectrophoresis, and enzyme immunoassay. The sensitivity of urine antigen tests is variable, and false positives may occur in colonized children or those who have recently received Hib vaccine. The advent of polymerase chain reaction (PCR) techniques has introduced a new Hib detection technique. In the setting of meningitis epidemics or previously treated children, PCR techniques have increased the ability to detect Hib rapidly.[12]

TREATMENT AND PROGNOSIS

Ampicillin or chloramphenicol has been the treatment of choice for all forms of invasive *H. influenzae* disease, but resistance to ampicillin emerged during the 1970s and to chloramphenicol in the 1990s and has reduced their usefulness in many regions.[5] Third-generation cephalosporins should be used for initial treatment depending on local susceptibility patterns. Cefotaxime 200 mg/kg/day in four doses or ceftriaxone 100 mg/kg once daily are regimens of first choice. Treatment for meningitis and sepsis syndromes should be continued for 7–10 days. Osteomyelitis requires a longer course of therapy, usually 2 weeks of parenteral therapy followed by 2–4 weeks of an oral regimen.

Controlled trials in children with Hib meningitis have shown that dexamethasone 0.15 mg/kg every 6 hours, given for 2–4 days with a third-generation cephalosporin, reduces the occurrence of hearing loss, probably by modifying the inflammatory response.[13] More recent studies suggest that dexamethasone is not an effective adjuvant therapy in developing countries.[14,15] This difference in effectiveness may be related to the higher proportion of more serious cases, typically admitted later in the disease course, frequently seen in hospitals in developing regions.

PREVENTION AND CONTROL

The virtual elimination of invasive Hib disease in many regions by immunization is an outstanding success story of modern public health (***Fig. 27.1***). Polysaccharide PRP vaccines were effective in older children but were immunologically ineffective in infants at greatest risk. Conjugation of the polysaccharide to proteins stimulates a T-cell-dependent antibody response in infants, with immunologic priming. Four different Hib PRP–protein conjugate vaccines effective in infants are now available, including two combination vaccines. In 2009, Hiberix, another Hib conjugate vaccine, was licensed in the United States for booster dosing only. The World Health Organization (WHO) supports the use of a pentavalent vaccine immunizing against diphtheria, tetanus, pertussis, hepatitis B, and Hib. The vaccines have similar efficacy but differ in immunologic details.

Hib meningitis virtually disappeared a few years after the introduction of protein-conjugated Hib PRP vaccines for infants in 1991 in the United States. This status was achieved even though the level of immunization among infants was lower than 80% in many urban regions, suggesting that reduction of carriage in vaccines had a herd effect that resulted in protection of unvaccinated infants.[16] The experience of rapid reduction or disappearance of Hib meningitis within 1–2 years of introduction of routine immunization was replicated in Europe,[17] South America,[18] West Africa,[19,20] Uganda,[21] and India.[7,22] Hib vaccination is clearly efficacious as well as cost-effective.[23]

Current US practice is to administer three doses of oligosaccharide–CRM conjugate Hib vaccine (HbOC) or PRP-T vaccine at 2, 4, and 6 months of age or two doses of PRP-OMP at 2 and 4 months, with a booster at 5–18 months. Because of the success of universal infant immunization in developed countries, and the reports of high efficacy of Hib conjugate vaccine in the prevention of invasive disease, the WHO recommends that conjugate Hib vaccines should be included in all routine infant immunization programs.[6,24] The WHO frequently updates recommendations for vaccination. Hib vaccines combined with diphtheria–tetanus–pertussis (DTP) or hepatitis B vaccines are in use in the United States, and combination pentavalent vaccines with Hib, DTP, and inactivated polio vaccine (IPV) are available elsewhere. A new pneumococcal vaccine (PCV-10) with *H. influenzae* protein D as a carrier has shown efficacy against otitis media caused by NTHi. Emerging data on immune responses to protein D in this vaccine suggest that this may provide added protection against disease caused by unencapsulated strains.[25]

Passive immunization with monthly injections of human IgG can prevent Hib disease, although this is not feasible in developing regions. Preventive treatment of unvaccinated household infant contacts with rifampicin is recommended in North America to reduce the 1–4% secondary attack rate in household and daycare contacts.

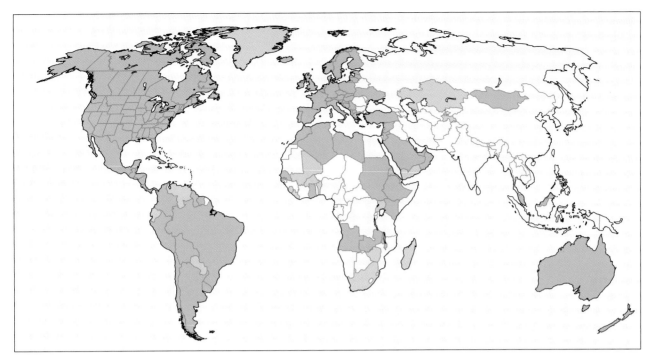

136 countries introduced infant immunization schedule

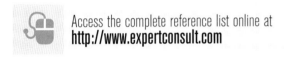

- Hib$^3 \geq 80\%$ (102 countries or 53%)
- Hib$^3 < 80\%$ (26 countries or 13%)
- Hib vaccine introduced but no coverage data reported (8 countries or 4%)
- Hib^3 vaccine not introduced (57 countries or 30%)

Figure 27.1 Countries having introduced *Haemophilus influenzae* type b (Hib) vaccine and infant Hib coverage, 2008. (Reproduced from World Health Organization. http://www.who.int/immunization_monitoring/diseases/Hib/en/index.html.)

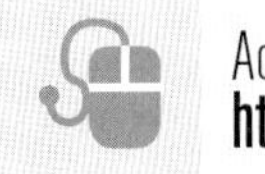

Access the complete reference list online at
http://www.expertconsult.com

CHAPTER 28

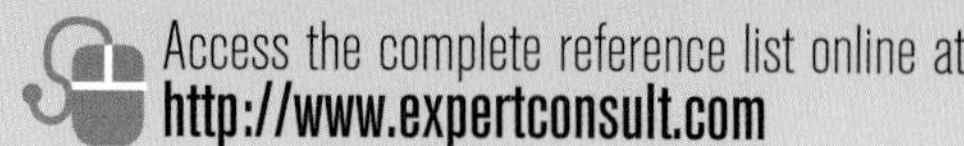
Access the complete reference list online at
http://www.expertconsult.com

Donovanosis

Nigel O'Farrell

INTRODUCTION

Donovanosis is a cause of genital ulceration found in a few diverse tropical countries. The condition has been known under many names, including serpiginous ulceration of the groin, ulcerating granuloma of the pudenda, granuloma genitoinguinale, infective granuloma, granuloma inguinale tropicum, chronic venereal sores, granuloma venereum, and more commonly, granuloma inguinale. This variation in terminology has led to many cases of donovanosis being mistaken for lymphogranuloma venereum, a condition caused by *Chlamydia trachomatis* serovars L1–L3.

Donovanosis was first described by McLeod, Professor of Surgery in Calcutta, in 1882[1] and the causative organism was recognized by Donovan in Madras in 1905.[2] Until recently the organism has been classified as *Calymmatobacterium granulomatis*, a Gram-negative bacillus. However, based on evidence of a phylogenetic similarity of 99% with *Klebsiella pneumoniae* and *K. rhinoscleromatis*, a proposal has been put forward that the organism be reclassified as *K. granulomatis* comb. nov.[3] Lesser phylogenetic similarities with *Klebsiella* species have also been reported and further confirmatory studies are needed to determine whether *C. granulomatis* is indeed a unique species.[4]

THE AGENT

Classical Donovan bodies measure 1.5 × 0.7 μm and are usually found in macrophages and epithelial cells of the stratum malpighii. Characteristically there is a large mononuclear cell 25–90 μm in diameter with intracytoplasmic cysts filled with deeply stained Donovan bodies.[5] Initial attempts to culture the causative organism were unconvincing until 1943 when Anderson reported its isolation on the yolk sac of chick embryos and proposed a new genus, *Donovania*, and species, *granulomatis*.[6,7] Electron microscopy studies typically show organisms with Gram-negative morphology and a large capsule but no flagella. Filiform vesicular protrusions may be seen on a corrugated cell wall.[8]

EPIDEMIOLOGY

Donovanosis has an unusual geographic distribution. Currently, it is found in Papua New Guinea, South Africa – KwaZulu-Natal and Eastern Transvaal, parts of India and Brazil, and in aboriginal communities in Australia. Sporadic cases are occasionally reported elsewhere in southern Africa, the West Indies, and South America. The largest epidemic recorded was in Papua New Guinea where 10 000 cases were reported in a population of 15 000 between 1922 and 1952.[9]

Following the move to syndromic reporting of sexually transmitted infections (STIs) in many developing countries, routine reporting of donovanosis has diminished considerably even in endemic areas. Prior to this change, a significant epidemic emerged in Durban where 3153 cases were reported from the main STI clinic in 1997.[10] Donovanosis also accounted for 11% and 16% of genital ulcers in men and women respectively in an earlier Durban study.[11,12] However, by 2004 the prevalence of donovanosis in Durban had decreased significantly.[13] In Papua New Guinea, the incidence of donovanosis is now decreasing but the condition was the second most common cause of genital ulceration in five health centers in 1989–1990.[14] In Pondicherry, south India, donovanosis accounted for 14% of genital ulcer cases in an STI clinic between 1993 and 1997.[15] In the Northern Territory region of Australia, reported cases decreased to less than 10 per year by 2002 from an estimated 300 cases in 1998 following the introduction of an eradication program.[16]

Donovanosis is generally regarded as an STI albeit one with low infectivity. The case for sexual transmission is supported by the following: a history of sexual exposure before the appearance of lesions, increased incidence in most sexually active age groups, anal lesions in homosexual men practicing receptive anal intercourse, genital infection predominant, frequent concomitant STIs, and outbreaks linked to sex work. Although infection with donovanosis in sexual partners of index cases is not invariable, epidemiological treatment is advised, as lesions may not always be immediately obvious.

THE DISEASE

The incubation period is uncertain. Experimental lesions have been induced in humans 50 days after inoculation and this duration is probably a reasonable estimate.[17] The condition usually starts as a firm papule or subcutaneous nodule that subsequently ulcerates. Four types of lesions are reported: (1) ulcerogranulomatous – the commonest type – beefy-red, nontender, fleshy ulcers that bleed readily to the touch; (2) hypertrophic or verrucous type – usually with a raised irregular edge, sometimes dry; (3) necrotic – offensive smelling ulcer causing tissue destruction; (4) sclerotic or cicatricial lesion with fibrous and scar tissue.

The genital area is affected in 90% of cases and the inguinal region in 10% (***Fig. 28.1***). The usual sites of infection are, in men, coronal sulcus (***Fig. 28.2***), prepuce, frenum, and in women, the labia minora and fourchette. Cervical lesions are uncommon but may mimic carcinoma. Extragenital lesions occur in 6% of cases and are usually associated with genital disease. Sites of infection include lip, gums, cheek, palate, pharynx, neck, nose, larynx, and chest.[18] Lymph gland enlargement is uncommon. Disseminated donovanosis is rare but secondary spread to liver and bone may occur and is often associated with pregnancy and cervical lesions. Extragenital lesions may be difficult to differentiate from rhinoscleroma caused by *Klebsiella rhinoscleromatis.* Carcinoma is a serious but rare complication.

As a cause of genital ulceration that bleeds readily, it is not surprising that donovanosis is a risk factor for human immunodeficiency virus (HIV) infection. In Durban the proportion of men diagnosed with donovanosis and HIV increased significantly as the duration of lesions increased,

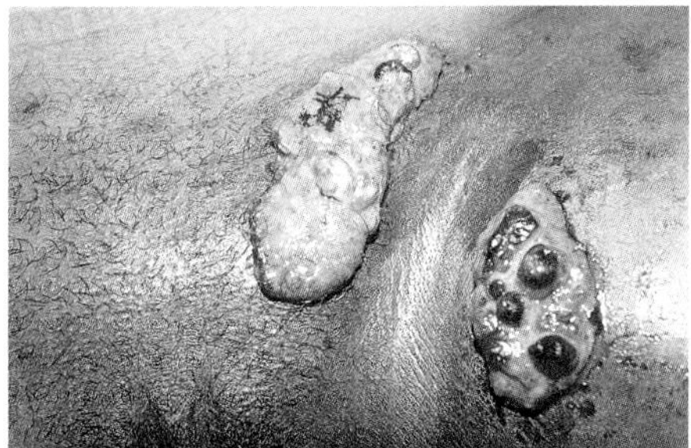

Figure 28.1 Inguinal lesions of donovanosis.

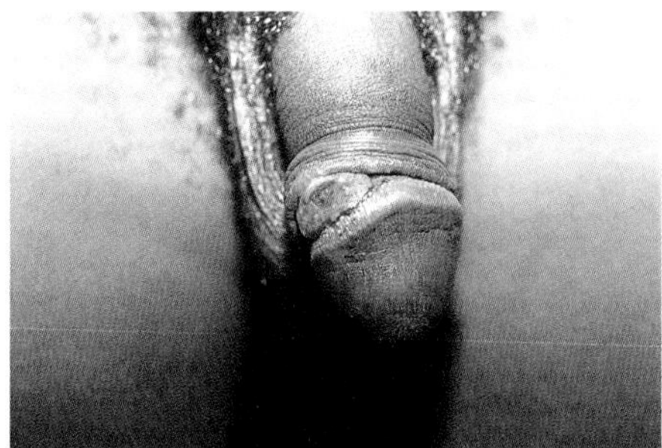

Figure 28.2 Typical penile donovanosis lesions.

suggesting that HIV was acquired through sexual intercourse despite ulceration.[19]

DIAGNOSIS

In endemic areas a clinical diagnosis of genital donovanosis by experienced observers has a reasonably high positive predictive value.[20] If possible, confirmation of the diagnosis should be made before antibiotics are given so that definitive treatment can be given. The diagnosis is made by identifying intracellular Donovan bodies, sometimes capsulated, within large mononuclear cells in smears obtained either from tissue smears or biopsy samples (*Fig. 28.3*).

Tissue smears can be performed cheaply and quickly in busy clinics. However, to achieve the maximum positive yield, specimens must be prepared carefully. Debris should be removed from the ulcer by gently rolling a cotton-tipped swab across the lesion to minimize bleeding. Another swab should then be both rolled firmly across the ulcer to collect material and then across a glass slide so that material is spread evenly. The slide is air-dried and stained by a rapid Giemsa method using eosin and thiazine solutions.[21] If multiple swabs are taken to detect other pathogens and donovanosis is suspected clinically, the tissue smear should be taken first so that an adequate amount of material can be collected.

In clinics where patients are likely to return, a crushed tissue smear using a slow overnight Giemsa method is preferable.[22] Pieces of tissue obtained by using a forceps and scalpel from the advancing surface of the ulcer are crushed between two slides and then stained.[23] If time and resources allow, biopsy specimens may offer a greater chance of confirming the diagnosis. The best stains to use are either Giemsa or silver. Histologic changes of donovanosis show epithelial proliferation with a heavy inflammatory infiltrate of plasma cells, neutrophils, and few lymphocytes. Biopsy is invariably required to confirm the diagnosis for necrotic and sclerotic ulcers and sometimes for hypertrophic lesions.

Culture of the causative organism has recently been the subject of a resurgence of interest. After a gap of 35 years, culture was reported from two centers in 1997 – in Durban using a monocyte co-culture system[24] and in Darwin with a modified chlamydia culture system using human epithelial cell lines.[25]

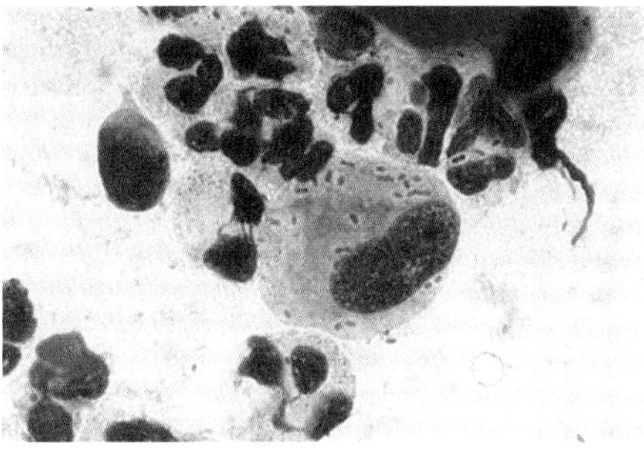

Figure 28.3 Tissue smear stained by rapid Giemsa (RapiDiff) technique showing numerous Donovan bodies in a monocyte.

Polymerase chain reaction (PCR) methods have also been developed for donovanosis.[4,26] In Darwin, amplification of *Klebsiella*-like sequences was achieved using primers targeting the *phoE* gene. A diagnostic PCR was developed using the observation that two unique base changes in the *phoE* gene eliminate Hae111 restriction sites, enabling clear differentiation from closely related species of *Klebsiella*.[26,27] A colorimetric PCR test has since been developed for use in diagnostic laboratories,[28] as has a genital ulcer multiplex PCR that includes *C. granulomatis*.[29]

Serologic testing with an indirect immunofluorescence method using tissue sections from known donovanosis cases has been undertaken but the sensitivity of this method is low for early lesions.[30] Other diagnostic methods, now superseded, include antigen detection, complement fixation, and skin tests.

In communities where donovanosis is prevalent, practitioners should have a high index of suspicion and be able to make a reasonably accurate clinical diagnosis in most cases. However, other causes of genital ulceration – primary syphilis, condylomata lata of secondary syphilis, chancroid and large HIV-associated herpes ulcers – should also be considered. Amebiasis and carcinoma may mimic necrotic donovanosis. Dual infection with one or more of the classical causes of genital ulcers should always be considered, particularly if there is a delay in seeking medical attention. In developed countries, a history of travel to and sex in an endemic country may point to a diagnosis of donovanosis.[31]

TREATMENT AND PROGNOSIS

WHO guidelines recommend azithromycin 1 gram followed by 500 mg daily.[32] In Australia, either azithromycin 1 gram weekly for 4–6 weeks or 500 mg once daily for 1 week were both effective.[33] The US Centers for Disease Control and Protection (CDC) recommend azithromycin 1 gram weekly for at least 3 weeks or until all lesions have healed.[34] Other antibiotics should probably be given for 3 weeks or until all lesions are healed and include: co-trimoxazole 160–800 mg twice daily, ciprofloxacin 750 mg twice daily, doxycycline 100 mg twice daily. Gentamicin 1 mg/kg three times daily intramuscularly or intravenously can be given if there is no response in the first few days with other regimens. Ceftriaxone, norfloxacin, and trovofloxacin have also proved effective. Surgery may have to be undertaken for intractable lesions that cause gross tissue destruction.

The introduction of syndromic STI management has significant implications for the management of donovanosis. Traditional syndromic algorithms for genital ulcers have advised treating for syphilis and chancroid, although more recently herpes management has also been included. Optimal treatment for donovanosis differs from chancroid and areas with significant prevalences of donovanosis should therefore have their own local algorithms that will ensure adequate treatment for possible cases. A good example of this local approach is in Australia where azithromycin is the drug of choice when donovanosis is suspected amongst aboriginals.[33] In the past azithromycin has often been excluded from treatment protocols because of cost but its price has decreased considerably and it should now be the universal first choice treatment for donovanosis.

A neglected aspect in the management of donovanosis is the psychological distress that some patients, particularly those with long-standing disease, are subjected to. The importance of case management for donovanosis is therefore still very important. Many patients present with long-standing disease and have sought health care previously elsewhere. In these cases confirmation of the diagnosis should be sought so that specific treatment can be given for donovanosis. Patients should be seen in a confidential setting and informed that they have an unusual condition that will respond to antibiotics over time. Poor genital hygiene may be a predisposing factor[18] and the need to wash behind the foreskin in men with subpreputial lesions should be mentioned. The report that azithromycin for one week is effective is particularly important for the management of patients who have to travel long distances.

It is unclear whether HIV alters the response of donovanosis ulcers to treatment. In Durban the clinical response to treatment was unaltered in HIV-positive pregnant women[35] but in India ulcers took slightly longer to heal in HIV-positive individuals than in those who were HIV-negative.[36] Although there are no data about azithromycin for donovanosis in HIV-positive subjects, it would be surprising if it were not shown to be effective.

PREVENTION AND CONTROL

The fact that significant numbers of donovanosis cases are found in only a few geographical locations makes the condition particularly suitable for targeted initiatives for disease control. In Papua New Guinea the large epidemic was controlled by annual examination, registration of the population, compulsory treatment, and assistance from the police in detaining patients reluctant to cooperate with the authorities.[9] Also in Papua New Guinea, in Goilala District, where 3.4% of the local population were infected with donovanosis, successful control measures included house-to-house visits with on-site medical examinations.[37] When antibiotics first became available in the United States, donovanosis elimination programs were initiated by some states. More recently a donovanosis eradication program targeting aboriginal and Torres Strait Islander populations in Australia commenced in 1996.[38] This intervention has reduced the numbers of cases significantly and owes much to strong political commitment supported with resources to heighten awareness of donovanosis at the primary health care level.

Female sex workers have been implicated as source contacts of index cases in the United States[39] and Papua New Guinea,[40] and usually have detectable lesions if infected. Clearly health care providers working with sex workers in donovanosis endemic areas should be targeted to increase awareness of donovanosis.

Control of genital ulcers is one strategy that could be important in limiting the spread of HIV.[41] It is therefore noteworthy that the numbers of cases of HIV attributable to heterosexual sex is still very low in Northern Territory, Australia, where a sustained program to eliminate donovanosis has now been in place for some years.[42] Global eradication of donovanosis remains a distinct possibility but will require significant inputs from those in endemic areas if it is to be accepted onto the WHO disease eradication agenda.[43]

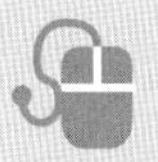

Access the complete reference list online at
http://www.expertconsult.com

Access the complete reference list online at http://www.expertconsult.com

CHAPTER 29

Pneumococcal Infections

Keith P. Klugman • Charles Feldman

INTRODUCTION

Acute respiratory infections are the leading cause of infectious disease mortality[1] and a large fraction of that mortality is attributable to the pneumococcus *Streptococcus pneumoniae*[2] (***Fig. 29.1***). Until 1965, acute respiratory infections caused 25% of all deaths in children younger than 5 years old in European countries with low adult life expectancy (<45 years) compared to 4% of childhood deaths in countries with longer adult life expectancy (>70 years).[3] During the 1980s, acute respiratory infections were thought to cause a mean of 18.8% of mortality in children younger than 5 years old in developing countries.[3] More recent evidence from a clinical trial conducted in rural Gambia in the 2000s suggests this to be an underestimate, as protection (probably incomplete) against just 9 of 91 pneumococcal serotypes reduced all-cause mortality in infants by 16%.[4] The percentage of infant mortality attributable to pneumonia increases as the infant mortality rate increases.[5] Most fatal pneumonia in children is caused by *S. pneumoniae* with a diminishing fraction due to *Haemophilus influenzae* type B as immunization against that pathogen is rolled out in developing countries.[6] The pneumococcus is also the most important cause of pneumonia in adults.[7,8] It is also a leading bacterial pathogen in the cause of meningitis throughout the world, including tropical countries.[9] It is estimated that about three of every four children in the world will have had at least one episode of acute otitis media by the age of 3 years and the pneumococcus is the leading bacterial pathogen responsible for between 25% and 50% of cases of acute otitis media.[10] The pneumococcus is an important cause of sinusitis[11] and can also rarely cause other infections such as peritonitis (associated with infections of the reproductive organs[12] or with nephrotic syndrome),[13] endocarditis, septic arthritis, osteomyelitis, epidural and brain abscesses, as well as soft tissue infections.[14]

THE AGENT

The pneumococcus is a Gram-positive coccus that is usually identified on the basis of optochin susceptibility and bile solubility. It can also be identified by its reaction with specific antisera. There are currently 93 pneumococcal serotypes described.[15,16]

Although the first observation of the organism now known as *S. pneumoniae* was made by Klebs in 1875,[17] the significance of this observation eluded him[18] and the discovery of the organism is often credited to Pasteur[19] and Sternberg,[20] who in 1881 passaged the organism from human saliva in rabbits and noticed that it caused a fatal septicemia in the animals. After much debate, it was recognized in 1883 to be a cause of lobar pneumonia by Friedländer.[21]

Fifty years later, driven by a desire to understand the lethal events in pneumococcal pneumonia, Griffith[22] and Alloway[23] demonstrated that the capsular polysaccharide was the essence of virulence of pneumococci, and capsular production could be naturally transferred as a heritable trait by an exogenous chemical substance, the transforming principle. In 1944, Avery, MacLeod, and McCarty[24] showed that the transforming principle was DNA. Over the next 50 years, the study of pneumococcal infection produced the first nonprotein vaccine,[25] suggested mechanisms for the action of penicillin and antibiotic tolerance,[26] and uncovered the complex structure and inflammatory properties of Gram-positive peptidoglycan.[27,28] Historically, the pneumococcus has thus provided a rich resource for the discovery of important tenets in medicine.[29]

PATHOGENESIS AND IMMUNITY

With the use of genome sequencing[30,31] and new genetic strategies amenable to mutation of Gram-positive bacteria,[32–37] many new virulence determinants of the pneumococcus and their regulatory mechanisms have been identified (***Fig. 29.2***). It is becoming increasingly clear that the microorganism possesses a myriad of putative virulence factors and that the mechanisms of pathogenesis are highly complex and multifactorial.[38] Many of the virulence factors have overlapping activities and functions, such that factors considered essential for lung infection may also play an important role in nasopharyngeal colonization.[32,33]

Targeting Pneumococci to Several Niches in the Host

Successful colonization of the upper respiratory tract by *S. pneumoniae* is an essential first step in the pathogenesis of pneumococcal infections.[38] Pneumococci bind to nasopharyngeal cells by several cell surface proteins, such as the choline-binding proteins, that act as "adhesins."[39,40] One of the major adhesins of the pneumococcus has been identified as PspC (previously known as CbpA).[41–45]

The factors that are responsible for transition from colonization to invasive disease have not been fully elucidated.[38] Progression to overt disease is more frequent upon acquisition of a new serotype[46] or following a viral respiratory tract infection, particularly influenza.[47] Upon gaining access to the lung, pneumococci adhere to and invade cytokine-activated lung and endothelial cells by binding to the platelet-activating factor (PAF) receptor on the cells. Pneumococci bound to the PAF receptor are internalized and migrate across eukaryotic cells in a vacuole, suggesting this as a route of entry for invasive disease.[48]

Invasion and host tissue damage is the result of the coordinated activity of several virulence determinants. The microorganism undergoes spontaneous phase variation marked by a switch from an opaque to a transparent colony morphotype.[49,50] While the former are adapted to nasopharyngeal colonization, displaying less capsule and more "adhesin," the latter have more capsule, which is strongly antiphagocytic, and are better suited to survival in the bloodstream.[42,50]

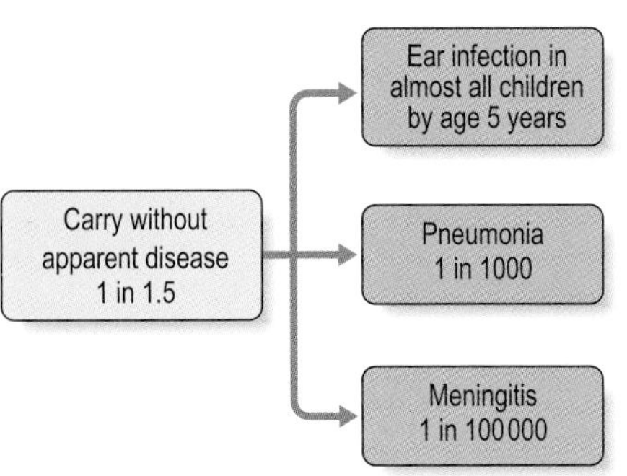

Figure 29.1 Prevalence of pneumococcal infection in children.

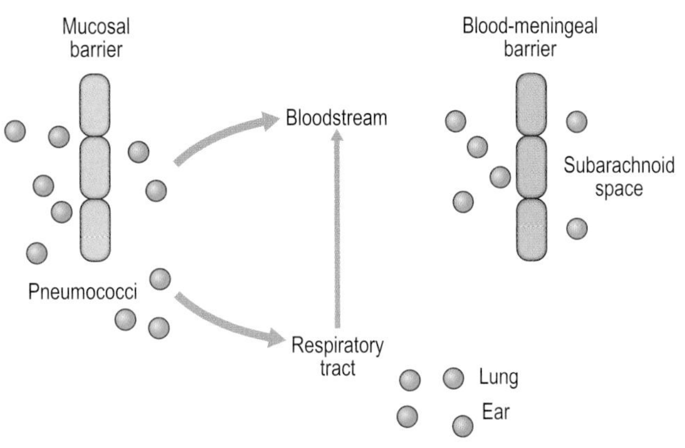

Figure 29.2 Pathogenesis of pneumococcal infection.

Invasion and host tissue damage is also potentiated by the production of a number of toxins by the pneumococcus including pneumolysin, hydrogen peroxide, hyaluronidase, neuraminidase, and various others.[40,42,51,52] Once in the bloodstream, progression to pneumococcal meningitis usually occurs in conjunction with a high-grade septicemia. Invasion of the subarachnoid space may relate to the ability of the pneumococci to bind to and traverse cerebral vascular endothelial cells by binding to the PAF receptor using cell wall choline and CbpA.[53] Pneumococcal toxins, such as pneumolysin, also appear to contribute to the pathogenesis of meningitis.[54]

Inflammation in Response to Pneumococcal Cell Wall

The cell wall, which is responsible for initiating inflammation, is composed of interlinked disaccharide peptides that form a network.[27] This backbone is decorated with a polyribitol teichoic acid which is unusual in that it contains phosphorylcholine.[55] The phosphorylcholine and the chemical composition of the cell wall building blocks are critical to the inflammatory activity of the cell wall.[28]

All the signs and symptoms of pneumococcal pneumonia, otitis media, and meningitis can be produced by instilling purified, protein-free pneumococcal cell wall into the appropriate organ.[28,56] The greater the release of cell wall during infection, the greater the inflammatory response and the more acute the course of disease.[57] Cell wall interacts with all elements of the acute inflammatory response. Components of the cell wall bind to CD14,[58] LPS binding protein,[58] and other soluble carrier proteins that then present the cell wall to Toll-like receptor (TLR) 2.[39,59–61] Intracellular cell wall is recognized by NOD2.[62,63] These interactions activate transcription of acute phase response genes through NF-κB.[51] This results in the production of cytokines (particularly interleukin-1 and tumor necrosis factor) and chemokines (such as PAF), as well as the initiation of procoagulant activity.

Inflammation in Response to Pneumococcal Toxins

Various enzymes and several toxins contribute to the pathogenesis of invasive pneumococcal disease.[42,64] One of the best studied factors is pneumolysin, a 53 kDa, cytolytic, thiol-activated protein toxin, produced by almost all clinically relevant pneumococci. The toxin has multiple effects on both the hosts' cellular and humoral immune systems.[42,64–66] Pneumolysin has been reported to interact with TLR4, which contributes to innate and adaptive immunity to the pneumococcus and triggers the production not only of interleukin-8, but also of various other proinflammatory cytokines.[67] Furthermore, recombinant pneumolysin on its own is able to induce the salient histologic features of pneumococcal infection in the rat lung *in vivo*.[68] Some secreted proteins and cell wall components are directly cytotoxic in that they kill eukaryotic cells. This toxicity can arise either by necrosis or by apoptosis.[69] Pneumolysin and hydrogen peroxide and probably cell wall itself have been shown to induce apoptosis of epithelial, endothelial, neuronal, and immune cells.[70–73]

Pneumococcal Clearance

Clearance of pneumococci involves recruitment of leukocytes in a β_2 integrin-dependent fashion and subsequent phagocytosis. Depending on the chemistry of the capsule, phagocytosis can be avid or fail completely. The most virulent serotypes in mice are 3, 4, and 6,[73] while a variety of serotypes including 3 and 19F have been implicated in increased mortality in humans.[74] Type-specific anticapsular antibody is the critical element in protective immunity. Phagocytosis is also promoted by the strong ability of cell wall to fix complement and the ability of the acute phase reactant, C-reactive protein, to bind to the phosphorylcholine of the pneumococcal teichoic acid.[75,76]

EPIDEMIOLOGY

Important risk factors for pneumococcal infections in adults are smoking and chronic obstructive pulmonary disease, other underlying systemic diseases such as liver failure, renal failure, alcoholism, sickle cell disease, lymphoma, and leukemia, and primary immunodeficiencies, including IgG subclass deficiencies. Invasive pneumococcal disease is common, however, in crowded communities as disparate as the crowded huts of rural villages in Papua New Guinea,[77] remote villages in Alaska in winter,[78] and the jails of modern urban America.[79] The disease is more common in winter, probably due to increased carriage[80] and increased antecedent viral infections at that time of the year.

The emergence of human immunodeficiency virus (HIV) infection as a specific risk factor for invasive pneumococcal disease was first described when an excess of pneumococcal pneumonias was found among patients with acquired immunodeficiency syndrome (AIDS) in 1984.[81] The incidence of pneumococcal bacteremia in AIDS patients was subsequently shown to be about 100 times greater than that in patients without AIDS.[82] In some African countries HIV is now the dominant risk factor for invasive pneumococcal disease in adults[83,84] and children.[85] Risk factors for invasive pneumococcal disease in HIV-infected persons include a CD4 count of <200 cells/μL, a previous history of pneumonia, and a serum albumin value below 3 g/dL.[86] HIV-infected patients with pneumonia have an increased incidence of bacteremia and, in particular, recurrent bacteremias.[11,87] Although it is commonly reported that HIV-infected patients usually respond well to standard antibiotic therapy,[11,87] a recent study comparing HIV-infected and HIV-uninfected cases with bacteremic pneumococcal pneumonia indicated that when the cases are stratified according to age and severity of illness, HIV-infected cases have a poorer prognosis, which correlates with the degree of immunocompromise as indicated by the CD4 cell count.[88] There are data[89] to suggest that pediatric serotypes/groups are more common in HIV-infected persons,[83,90] particularly women.[83] Highly active antiretroviral therapy (HAART) decreases the burden of pneumococcal disease but residual risk remains elevated, particularly in those individuals that continue to smoke.[91–93]

Antibiotic Resistance

Penicillin resistance of the pneumococcus was first described by Hansman and coworkers among strains isolated from Papua New Guinea in 1967.[94] Until the 1980s the focus of resistance was Papua New Guinea, South Africa, and Spain;[95] while the incidence of resistance in most developed countries remained low, very few data were available from developing countries. The 1990s witnessed a dramatic increase in resistance worldwide (***Fig. 29.3***) including Southeast Asia.[96] Studies in Pakistan,[97] South Africa,[98,99] and elsewhere documented a similar rate of resistance in isolates obtained from nasopharyngeal swabs from children attending outpatient clinics, or on admission to hospital, compared with isolates from blood and cerebrospinal fluid (CSF). This allowed the possibility of determining the incidence of resistance in small field trials that focus on nasopharyngeal carriage. Such studies have been reported from many countries including the Central African Republic,[100] Zambia,[101] and Malawi.[102] Although a direct association between the total use of antibiotics in a given country and antibiotic resistance has not been documented in developing countries, this association has been documented for the pneumococcus in Europe.[103] Antimicrobial agents are freely available in most developing countries but there are some poor countries with populations not exposed to antibiotics and these populations may harbor pneumococci with very low levels of resistance. Such a situation has been documented in Lesotho[104] and in Nepal.[105] Macrolide resistance is increasingly common in pneumococci but may be expected to be more common in developed countries where these more expensive drugs are widely used. In developing communities mass treatment with azithromycin for trachoma may increase the isolation of macrolide-resistant pneumococci, particularly if these strains are preexistent in the community.[105,106] Among the oral agents, resistance to trimethoprim-sulfamethoxazole is of particular concern because of its widespread use in treatment of pneumonia, as prophylaxis in HIV-infected patients in developing countries, and its ability to select multiresistant strains.[102] Fansidar therapy for malaria has been shown to select trimethoprim-sulfamethoxazole resistance in pneumococci isolated from the nasopharynx of exposed children in Malawi.[107]

DIAGNOSIS

Pneumococcal infections are diagnosed primarily by culture of the organism from appropriate clinical samples such as CSF, blood, pleural fluid, or purulent sputum. Confirmation of a pneumococcal cause of otitis media requires tympanocentesis. Although not routinely used diagnostically, lung puncture is required to establish the true cause of pneumonia. Other approaches to diagnosis include the detection of pneumococcal DNA antigen especially in CSF. Real-time polymerase chain reaction (PCR) has shown a correlation between increasing amounts of pneumococcal DNA in CSF and mortality.[89] PCR is now the modality of choice to detect pneumococcal empyema and a number of novel approaches including Binax and Luminex based detection of antigen in CSF and urine are under investigation.[108–110]

TREATMENT AND PROGNOSIS

Meningitis

The mainstay of treatment of pneumococcal meningitis in many developing countries has been intravenous penicillin or ampicillin, usually given in combination with chloramphenicol. This combination is no longer reliably effective as failure occurs even with intermediately penicillin-resistant strains which are now widespread globally.[111,112] The cephalosporins, cefotaxime or ceftriaxone, are now generic and the preferred agents for the management of pneumococcal meningitis. The emergence of cephalosporin resistance in pneumococci in the United States,[113] together with evidence of increased CSF bactericidal activity against these strains after the addition of vancomycin,[114] suggests that vancomycin may be added empirically to these cephalosporins for management of pneumococcal meningitis. The decision to use combination therapy will depend on the prevalence of strains with minimum inhibitory concentrations of cefotaxime or ceftriaxone greater than 2 μg/mL. In most developing countries such strains are currently rare.[115] Dexamethasone is widely given in developed countries as adjunctive therapy for the management of both adult and pediatric pneumococcal meningitis,[116,117] but data from randomized trials in Malawi do not suggest such a benefit in that setting.[115,118]

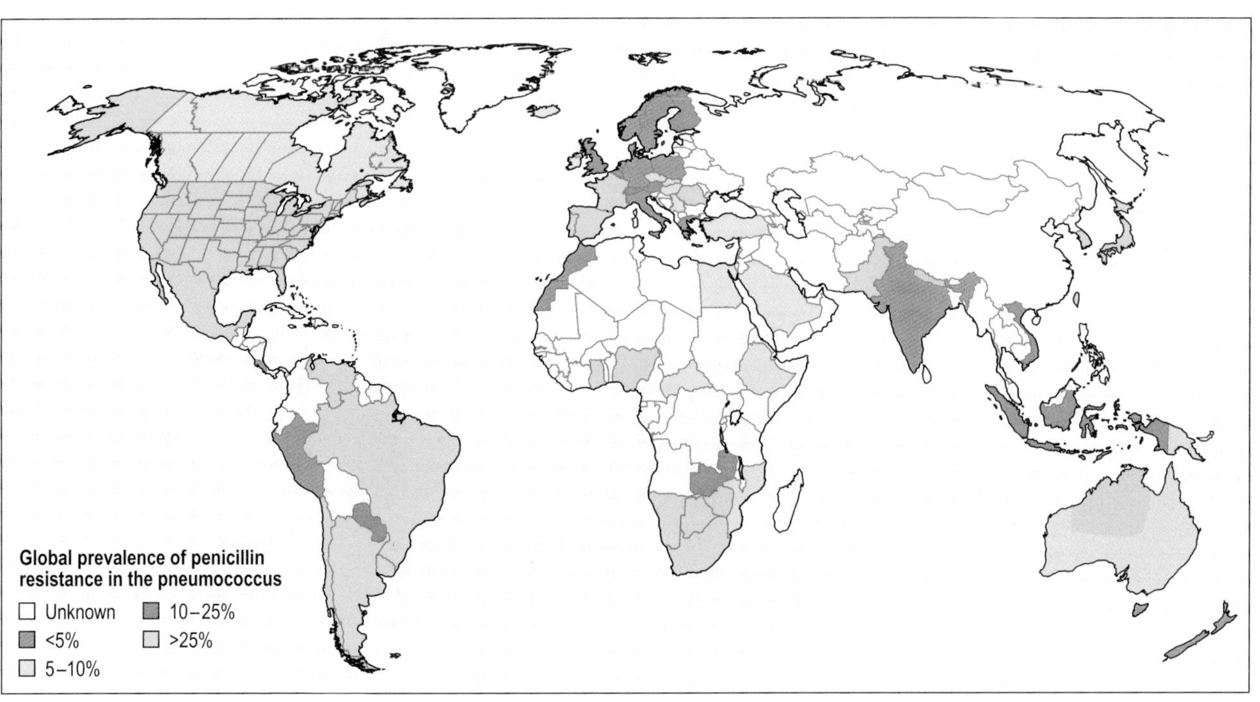

Figure 29.3 Global prevalence of penicillin resistance in the treatment of pneumococcal meningitis.

Pneumonia

The treatment of choice for mild–moderate pneumonia is oral amoxicillin. Pneumococcal resistance to β-lactams does not appear to influence the outcome of pneumonia treated with these agents[119] and in pediatric patients oral amoxicillin has been shown to be more effective than co-trimoxazole, and equivalent to inpatient parenteral ampicillin, in the outpatient management of sicker cases with pneumococcal pneumonia.[120,121] Intravenous management with penicillin or ampicillin is appropriate treatment for severe infections treated as inpatients and the breakpoint for resistance to penicillin in the treatment of non-meningeal infections has been raised from 2 μg/mL to 8 μg/mL.[122] In penicillin-allergic patients new fluoroquinolones that are highly active against pneumococci are probably the drugs of choice,[123] although their cost may be prohibitive in developing countries. Very severe pneumonias may be treated with combination therapy using a β-lactam and a macrolide based on several observational studies[124,125] but prospective randomized trials of combination therapy have not been performed to date.

Otitis Media

In terms of the penetration of drugs into the middle ear, the spectrum of activity of different agents against pneumococci, and retained activity against resistant strains, high-dose amoxicillin is the most appropriate oral agent for the management of otitis media.[126]

PREVENTION AND CONTROL

The currently approved adult vaccine consists of the capsular polysaccharides from 23 of the most common serotypes.[127] While the vaccine has been widely advocated for the prevention of invasive pneumococcal disease in developed countries, the vaccine does not appear to protect against pneumonia in the high-risk groups to whom it is given,[128] and although it may be useful in reducing invasive disease in HIV patients on HAART,[129] it may enhance disease in HIV-infected persons who are not on antiretroviral therapy.[130] The basis for the ineffectiveness appears to be its inability to elicit a T-cell-dependent immune response. This can be overcome by conjugating a protein to the polysaccharide, a process successfully used to introduce a seven-valent pneumococcal vaccine into the United States in 2000.[131] Seven- and nine-valent pneumococcal conjugate vaccines are highly effective in preventing sepsis and meningitis in children due to vaccine serotypes,[132,133] even in HIV-infected children;[133] they reduce radiographically proven pneumonococcal pneumonia by 25% in fully immunized children[133] and induce herd immunity in the population.[131] Vaccine introduction in the United States initially reduced the fraction of antibiotic-resistant strains[134] and also reduced pneumococcal meningitis.[135] Although the vaccine reduces pneumococcal otitis, its overall efficacy against otitis is reduced by serotype replacement.[136] The emergence of replacement serotypes such as 19A[137] and 6C[138] is of concern and has led to the development of a 13-valent formulation. Nonetheless the seven-valent vaccine is recommended as a priority by WHO for introduction into the immunization schedule of countries where mortality exceeds 50/1000 live births or where more than 50 000 children die annually.[139] Conjugate pneumococcal vaccine has recently been shown to protect against vaccine type disease when given to HIV infected adults,[140] but its use in adults remains investigational. A protein-based vaccine is being sought to extend protection to capsular types not in the conjugate vaccine formulation.

Antibiotic prophylaxis has been attempted in communities such as Papua New Guinea with high rates of disease,[141] but because of the emergence of resistance it is reserved for patients at particularly high risk, for example children with sickle cell disease.[142] These patients require pneumococcal vaccine and are a priority group to receive conjugate pneumococcal vaccine.[143] There are innovative funding mechanisms such as the Advance Market Commitment[144] which should help to overcome the barrier of cost and accelerate introduction of conjugate vaccine into developing countries. Conjugate vaccination of adults is currently subject to clinical trials.

ACKNOWLEDGMENTS

The authors would like to acknowledge the contribution of Elaine Tuomanen, MD, St Jude's Children's Research Hospital, Memphis, TN, for her contribution to this chapter in the 2nd edition of this book.

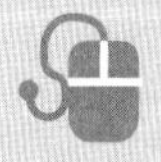

Access the complete reference list online at
http://www.expertconsult.com

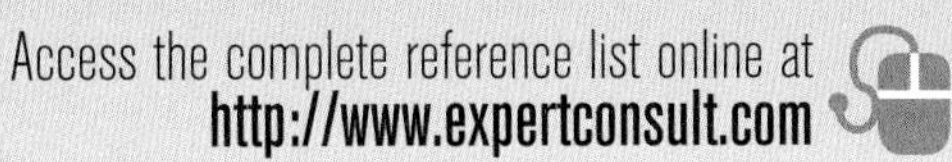
Access the complete reference list online at
http://www.expertconsult.com

CHAPTER 30

Group A Streptococcal and Staphylococcal Infections

Dennis L. Stevens • Amy E. Bryant

INTRODUCTION

Streptococcus pyogenes (group A streptococcus; GAS) is unique among human pathogens in its ability to cause a wide variety of clinical infections and postinfectious sequelae.[1] Further, in its coevolution with humans, GAS has developed a myriad of molecular strategies to circumvent important host defense mechanisms.[2] Thus, in pathogenesis of both acute GAS infections and the well-known postinfectious sequelae, it is the unique host/pathogen interaction that accounts for the diverse disease spectrum and the resultant morbidity and mortality. This chapter emphasizes these host–microbe relationships to explain the unique epidemiologic and pathogenic features of *S. pyogenes* and, in the next section, *Staphylococcus aureus*.

STREPTOCOCCAL INFECTIONS

THE AGENT

S. pyogenes is a Gram-positive, catalase-negative coccus that divides in a single plane, thus forming chains of bacteria. Lancefield[3] developed a classification scheme based on the acid-extractable polysaccharide and, to date, groups of streptococci from A to O have been defined by such typing. Commercially available rapid latex agglutination tests have simplified strain typing. Although the bacitracin susceptibility test has proved very reliable as a presumptive marker for GAS, both false negative and false positive results are problematic. GAS may be grown aerobically or anaerobically and, in general, growth is enhanced in the presence of 10% carbon dioxide.

EPIDEMIOLOGY

The epidemiology of GAS infections is a dynamic process geographically and temporally. The declining prevalence and severity of both rheumatic fever (RF) and scarlet fever in the twentieth century in developed countries may have been related to improved socioeconomic conditions, timely antibiotic treatment of streptococcal pharyngitis, and secondary prophylaxis for RF.[4] However, these declines are more likely due to cyclic variation in the virulence of the organism. The recent outbreaks of pharyngitis, acute RF, and the newly recognized streptococcal toxic shock syndrome (Strep TSS) support this concept.

Historically, RF was common in the northern United States, though currently it is rare in developed countries but remains problematic in developing nations, especially those in tropical environments.[4] Impetigo is also more common in tropical areas, though elevation above sea level is also a factor that increases the prevalence of disease.[1] It is likely, though unproven, that skin carriage is higher in tropical areas than temperate climates, though the inverse is true for throat carriage. Recently, invasive GAS infections, such as Strep TSS and necrotizing fasciitis, have been described with increased frequency in North America and Europe[5–16] and subsequently throughout tropical areas as well. The diversity of infectious diseases caused by GAS is illustrated in ***Box 30.1***.

THE DISEASE

GAS, perhaps more than any other pathogen, has the ability to cause diverse infections. The clinical characteristics of each of these are described in the following sections.

Pharyngitis and the Asymptomatic Carrier

The natural reservoirs of *S. pyogenes* are human skin and mucous membranes, and nearly 5% of all people, regardless of age, are pharyngeal carriers. Carriage reaches rates of 15–50% in school-age children (~5–15 years of age) in temperate climates during epidemics of GAS pharyngitis where transmission occurs via aerosolized droplets. The cardinal manifestations include sore throat, submandibular and anterior cervical adenopathy, fever of greater than 38°C, and pharyngeal erythema with exudates. Acute pharyngitis is sufficient to induce antibody against streptococcal M protein, streptolysin O (SLO), DNase, and hyaluronidase, and, if present, pyrogenic exotoxins. GAS pharyngitis may progress to scarlet fever, bacteremia, suppurative head and neck infections, Strep TSS, carrier state, RF, or poststreptococcal glomerulonephritis depending on the interaction between specific streptococcal virulence factors and the various immunologic defense molecules of the human host.

During GAS epidemics, particularly where RF or poststreptococcal glomerulonephritis is prevalent, treatment of asymptomatic carriers may be necessary, and programs that use monthly injections of benzathine penicillin effectively reduce the incidence of GAS pharyngitis and RF.

Scarlet Fever

Recent outbreaks of scarlet fever in the United States and Great Britain have been associated with strains of GAS that produce pyrogenic exotoxin C.[17] The cases have been notably mild and the illness has been referred to as "pharyngitis with rash." Scarlet fever has not always been a mild disease; around 1900, mortality rates of 25% were common on both sides of the Atlantic.

Scarlet fever has been divided into the following types: mild, moderate, toxic, and septic. Thus, benign scarlet fever may be either mild or moderate, and the fatal or malignant form may be either septic or toxic. Historically, the toxic cases invariably began with a severe sore throat, marked fever, delirium, skin rash, and painful cervical lymph nodes. In severe toxic cases, fulminating fevers of 107°F, pulse rates of 130–160 beats per minute, severe headache, delirium, convulsions, little if any skin rash, and death within 24 hours were the usual findings. These cases

Box 30.1 Streptococcal Infections and Sequelae

Cellulitis	Pharyngitis
Erysipelas	Pneumonia
Impetigo	Poststreptococcal glomerulonephritis
Mastoiditis	Rheumatic fever
Myonecrosis	Sinusitis
Necrotizing fasciitis	Streptococcal toxic shock syndrome
Otitis media	
Peritonsillar abscess	

occurred before the advent of antibiotics, antipyretics, and anticonvulsants, and deaths were the result of uncontrolled seizures and hyperpyrexia. The term "septic scarlet fever" refers to the form characterized by local invasion of the soft tissues of the neck and complications such as upper airway obstruction, otitis media with perforation, profuse mucopurulent drainage from the nose, bronchopneumonia, and death. Note that necrotizing fasciitis and myositis were not previously observed in association with scarlet fever.

Soft Tissue Infections

Erysipelas

Erysipelas is caused exclusively by *S. pyogenes* and is characterized by the abrupt onset of fiery-red swelling of the face or extremities.[18] Distinctive features are well-defined margins, particularly along the nasolabial fold; a scarlet or salmon-red color; rapid progression; and intense pain. Flaccid bullae filled with clear fluid may develop during the second to third day of illness, yet extension to deeper soft tissues, bacteremia, and shock occur only rarely. Surgical débridement is rarely required and treatment with penicillin is very effective. Swelling may progress despite treatment, though fever, pain, and intense redness diminish usually within 24–48 hours. Desquamation of the involved skin occurs 5–10 days into the illness and scarring of the skin does not occur. Infants and elderly adults are most commonly afflicted. Erysipelas has become less severe since the early 1900s even before antibiotic treatment became available.

Streptococcal Pyoderma (Impetigo Contagiosa)

The thick, crusted skin lesions of streptococcal pyoderma frequently have a golden-brown color resembling dried serum.[18] Children between 2 and 5 years of age are most commonly infected. Epidemics occur throughout the year in tropical areas or during the summer months in more temperate climates and are usually associated with poor hygiene. Initially, colonization of the unbroken skin occurs either exogenously from patients with impetiginous lesions or endogenously by contamination of the skin with oropharyngeal organisms. Development of impetiginous lesions requires 10–14 days and is initiated by minor trauma such as an abrasion or insect bite, which facilitates intradermal inoculation. Patients with impetigo should receive penicillin, particularly when numerous sites of the skin are involved, though treatment does not prevent poststreptococcal glomerulonephritis. Topical treatment with an agent effective against Gram-positive bacteria, such as bacitracin or mupirocin, is also effective. About 50% of cases of impetigo currently are caused by *Staphylococcus aureus* including methicillin-resistant *S. aureus* (MRSA).

Cellulitis

GAS may invade the epidermis and subcutaneous tissues, resulting in local swelling, erythema, and pain.[18] The skin becomes indurated and, in contrast to erysipelas, is a pinkish color. Patients with lymphedema secondary to lymphoma, filariasis, or surgical node dissection (mastectomy, carcinoma of the prostate, etc.) are predisposed to development of GAS cellulitis, as are those with chronic venous stasis and superficial dermatophyte infection of the toes. Saphenous vein donor site cellulitis may be due to group A, C, or G streptococci. Cellulitis associated with a primary focus (e.g., an abscess or boil) is more likely caused by *S. aureus*. Aspiration of the leading-edge and punch biopsy yield a causative organism in 15% and 40% of cases, respectively. Patients respond quickly to penicillin, though in some cases where staphylococcus is of concern, nafcillin or oxacillin may be a better choice, or one may need cover for MRSA infection (discussed later in this chapter). If bluish or violet discoloration develops or if bullae become apparent, a deeper infection such as necrotizing fasciitis or myositis should be considered (see section below on necrotizing fasciitis). Particularly when such patients demonstrate systemic toxicity, a serum creatine phosphokinase level should be obtained and, if elevated, prompt surgical inspection and débridement should be performed.

Lymphangitis

Cutaneous infection with bright red streaks ascending proximally is most commonly associated with GAS, though groups C and G have also been implicated. Prompt antibiotic treatment is mandatory because bacteremia and systemic toxicity develop rapidly once infected lymphatic fluid reaches the thoracic ducts.

Necrotizing Fasciitis

Necrotizing fasciitis, originally called streptococcal gangrene, is a deep-seated infection of the subcutaneous tissue that results in progressive destruction of fascia and fat but may spare the skin itself,[18] though in nearly 50% of cases, all layers of the skin as well as subcutaneous tissue and underlying muscle are destroyed. Within the first 24 hours, swelling, heat, erythema, and tenderness develop and rapidly spread proximally and distally from the original focus. During the next 24 hours, the erythema darkens, changing from red to purple to blue, forming blisters and bullae that contain clear, yellow fluid.[19] The purple areas become frankly gangrenous and extensive necrosis of the subcutaneous tissue ensues. Patients become increasingly toxic and develop shock and multiorgan failure. In the past, aggressive fasciotomy and débridement and application of Dakin's solution topically achieved mortality rates as low as 20%, even before antibiotics were available. The increased severity of necrotizing fasciitis that has occurred among recent cases of Strep TSS relative to shock, multiorgan failure, and mortality could be due to the increased virulence of GAS itself.

Myositis and Myonecrosis

Historically, streptococcal myositis has been an extremely uncommon GAS infection, and only 21 cases were documented from 1900 to 1985.[20] Recently, an increased prevalence of GAS myositis has been reported in the United States, Norway, and Sweden.[5,6,21] While GAS infection of the skin can penetrate to deeper structures, primary myositis and myonecrosis have been described precisely at sites of antecedent non-penetrating trauma such as a muscle strain or deep hematoma.[5] In these cryptic "no-portal" types of GAS infections, hematogenous translocation of GAS from the oropharynx to the injured site likely occurs, though most patients do not report symptomatic pharyngitis or tonsillitis. In an experimental model, Bryant and colleagues have recently shown that interaction of circulating GAS with surface-expressed vimentin on damaged muscle cells mediates development of these cryptic infections at sites of muscle injury.[22] Severe pain at the site of infection may be the only initial presenting symptom and later in the course, swelling and erythema, violaceous bullae, skin sloughing and extreme toxicity develop. Muscle compartmental syndromes may develop rapidly. In most cases a single muscle group is involved; however, because patients frequently have bacteremia, there may be other sites of myositis or abscess. Distinguishing streptococcal myositis from spontaneous gas gangrene caused by *Clostridium perfringens* or *C. septicum* may be difficult, although the presence of crepitus or gas in the tissue would favor a diagnosis of clostridial infection. Myositis is easily distinguished from necrotizing fasciitis anatomically by means of surgical exploration or incisional biopsy, though clinical features of both conditions overlap and 30–40% of patients may have both. Though soft tissue radiography, computed tomography (CT), and magnetic resonance imaging (MRI) may be useful in localizing the site of infection, these generally show only edema or soft tissue swelling and do not distinguish myonecrosis or myositis from soft tissue damage due to blunt trauma. Increasing quantities of muscle enzymes in the serum may provide a useful clinical clue of deep infection. In published reports, the case-fatality rate of necrotizing fasciitis is between 20% and 50%, whereas that of GAS myositis is between 80% and 100%. Aggressive surgical débridement is of extreme importance because of the poor efficacy of penicillin described in human cases as well as in experimental streptococcal models of myositis (see Treatment section).

Streptococcal Toxic Shock Syndrome

In the mid-1980s, reports of invasive GAS infections associated with bacteremia, deep soft tissue infection, shock, and multiorgan failure began to appear in the medical literature from North America and Europe.[5,21] Though all ages may be affected, the greatest increases have occurred among previously healthy persons from 15 to 50 years of age. Mortality rates of 30–70% have been described in patients with Strep TSS, in spite of aggressive modern treatment measures. The Strep TSS is defined as any GAS infection associated with the sudden onset of shock and organ dysfunction.

Acquisition of Group A Streptococcus and Predisposing Factors

The most common GAS infections resulting in Strep TSS are soft tissue infections (necrotizing fasciitis, myonecrosis), pneumonia, postpartum sepsis, septic joint, peritonitis, and empyema. For soft tissue infection, the portals of entry are surgical site, chickenpox, insect bites, slivers, burns, and minor abrasions. The portal of entry of streptococci could not be ascertained in 45% of cases but many infections occurred precisely at sites of minor, nonpenetrating trauma (e.g., muscle strain, ankle sprain, subcutaneous hematoma, etc; see prior section). Early on, the only symptoms may be fever and severe pain. In adults, a viral-like prodrome suggestive of influenza precedes the onset of Strep TSS by several days. The use of nonsteroidal anti-inflammatory drugs (NSAIDs) to treat pain or suppress fever may mask the presenting symptoms or predispose the patient to more severe disease.[22]

Symptoms

Pain is a common initial symptom of Strep TSS, is abrupt in onset and severe, and may not be associated with tenderness or physical findings early in the course of infection. The pain most commonly involves an extremity, but may also mimic peritonitis, pelvic inflammatory disease, deep vein thrombophlebitis, acute myocardial infarction, or pericarditis.

Physical Findings

Fever is the most common presenting sign, although on admission to the hospital 10% of patients in one report had profound hypothermia secondary to shock. Confusion may be present in over half of the patients and, in some, it progresses to coma or combativeness. In our report,[5] 80% of patients had tachycardia and 55% had systolic blood pressure of less than 110 mmHg on admission. Although 45% of patients had normal blood pressure (systolic pressure >110 mmHg) on admission, in all of these patients hypotension developed within the subsequent 4 hours. Soft tissue infection evolved to necrotizing fasciitis or myositis in 70% of patients, and in these cases surgical débridement, fasciotomy, or amputation was required. An ominous sign was the progression of soft tissue swelling to formation of vesicles and then bullae, which took on a violaceous or bluish coloration. Among patients with no soft tissue infection on admission, a variety of clinical presentations were observed; these included endophthalmitis, myositis, perihepatitis, peritonitis, myocarditis, and overwhelming sepsis. Patients who experience shock and multiorgan failure without clinical evidence of local infection have a worse prognosis because definitive diagnosis and surgical débridement may be delayed.

Laboratory Test Results

Evidence of renal involvement was apparent at the time of admission by the presence of hemoglobinuria and elevated serum creatinine level. The serum albumin level was moderately low (3.3 g/dL) on admission and dropped further (2.3 g/dL) by 48 hours. Hypocalcemia, including ionized hypocalcemia, was detectable early in the hospital course. The serum creatine phosphokinase (CPK) level is a useful test to detect deeper soft tissue infections, such as necrotizing fasciitis or myositis.

The initial laboratory studies demonstrated only mild leukocytosis, but a dramatic left shift (43% of white blood cells were band forms, metamyelocytes, and myelocytes). The mean platelet count was normal on admission but dropped to approximately 120 000 cells/mm^3 within 48 hours, frequently in the absence of criteria for disseminated intravascular coagulopathy (DIC).

Bacteriologic Cultures

GAS was isolated from blood in 60% of cases, and from deep tissue specimens in 95%.

Clinical Course

Shock was apparent early in the course and management was complicated by profound capillary leak.[5] Adult respiratory distress syndrome (ARDS) occurred frequently (55%) and complicated fluid resuscitation. Renal dysfunction preceded hypotension in many patients and progressed or persisted for 48–72 hours despite treatment. In all patients who survived, serum creatinine levels returned to normal within 4–6 weeks. Overall 30–70% of patients have died despite aggressive treatment, including administration of intravenous fluids, colloid, pressors, mechanical ventilation, and surgical intervention, including fasciotomy, débridement, exploratory laparotomy, intraocular aspiration, amputation, and hysterectomy.

Characteristics of Clinical Isolates of Group A Streptococci

M protein types 1, 3, 12, and 28 of GAS have been the most common isolates from patients with shock and multiorgan failure. These strains have also been isolated with increasing frequency from patients with pharyngitis, erysipelas, and asymptomatic carriers. M protein types 1 and 3 producing pyrogenic exotoxins A or B, or both, have been found most commonly in isolates from patients with severe infection in Norway, Sweden, Great Britain, and the United States.[5,10,11]

Postinfectious Sequelae

Rheumatic Fever

The prevalence of acute RF (ARF) in the Western world decreased dramatically after World War II (0.5–1.88 cases per 100 000 school-age children per year).[23] In contrast, in India and Sri Lanka the prevalence of ARF has remained 140 per 100 000 for children between 5 and 19 years of age. Socioeconomic factors seem to be important because the highest rates in all countries have been among the impoverished in large cities. Although improved living conditions and the development of penicillin have had important roles in reducing the prevalence of ARF in the United States, the decreases actually began before antibiotics were available. In recent years there has been a resurgence of ARF among US military recruits and in the civilian population among predominantly white middle-class children.[24] A particularly frightening aspect of these recent civilian cases has been the low incidence of symptomatic pharyngitis (24–78%). Thus, our modern primary prevention strategy (diagnosis of acute GAS pharyngitis with penicillin treatment within 10 days) would not have prevented ARF in these cases.[25]

Variations in the expression of virulence factors of "rheumatogenic strains" of *S. pyogenes* may best explain these fluctuations in ARF. M protein types isolated from RF patients (i.e., types 1, 3, 5, 6, 14, 18,

19, and 24)[4] have a common antigenic domain that is immunologically cross-reactive with human heart tissue. Understanding this molecular mimicry holds great promise for the elucidation of the immune mechanisms resulting in clinical ARF. One other marker for rheumatogenicity is the mucoid appearance of fresh pharyngeal isolates from patients with ARF. In recent times in the United States, such strains have been of type 18.

Although certain M protein types are strongly associated with ARF, such strains may cause other GAS infections as well. For example, types 1 and 3 have also been associated with poststreptococcal glomerulonephritis and Strep TSS. Further, epidemics of pharyngitis caused by these rheumatogenic strains are not invariably associated with epidemics of RF.

That host factors determine the clinical outcome of GAS infection is suggested by the observation that persons with certain human leukocyte antigen (HLA) class II antigens are predisposed to development of ARF. Further, Stollerman[23] suggests that a gradual acquisition of susceptibility to ARF by schoolchildren occurs after repeated infections. This is supported by the observations of Ayoub and associates, who state that ARF is uncommon in children less than 2 years old and that antibody response to streptococcal antigens is exaggerated in children with ARF compared with those with GAS pharyngitis alone.[26] In addition, Zabriskie and colleagues[27] have shown that patients with ARF demonstrate increased expression of the B-cell alloantigen D8/17 in comparison with unaffected family members, including identical twins. That some strains of GAS can cause ARF in any person is suggested by the observation that the attack rate of ARF can vary from 388 cases per 100 000, as seen in soldiers in World War II, to 1 per 100 000 today. Such fluctuations among relatively homogeneous populations separated in time suggest changes in the relative rheumatogenicity of GAS and not unique host factors.

The clinical manifestations of ARF are multiple and, because each is not specific for ARF, several criteria must be met to establish a definitive diagnosis.[4] Simply put, two major manifestations or one major and two minor manifestations plus, in either case, evidence of an antecedent GAS infection are required for definitive diagnosis. The major manifestations and the frequency with which they occur during first attacks of ARF are as follows: arthritis (75%), carditis (40–50%), chorea (15%), and subcutaneous nodules (<10%). The minor manifestations are fever, arthralgia, heart block, the presence of acute phase reactants in the blood (C-reactive protein, leukocytosis, and elevated erythrocyte sedimentation rate), and prior history of ARF or rheumatic heart disease. Carditis, when present, occurs during the first 3 weeks of illness and may involve the pericardium, myocardium, and endocardium. Patients with pericarditis may have chest pain or pericardial effusion, whereas those with myocarditis may have intractable heart failure. Manifestations of acute endocarditis include the development of new murmurs of mitral regurgitation or aortic regurgitation, the latter being sometimes associated with a low-pitched apical mid-diastolic flow murmur (Carey Coombs murmur). Murmurs of mitral stenosis and aortic stenosis are not detected acutely during first attacks of ARF but are chronic manifestations of rheumatic heart disease. Migratory arthritis involves several joints, most frequently the knees, ankles, elbows, and wrists, in more than 50% of patients.

Each involved joint has evidence of inflammation that characteristically resolves within 2–3 weeks with no progression to chronic arthritis or articular damage. Subcutaneous nodules occur several weeks into the course of ARF and are found over bony surfaces or tendons. They last only 1–2 weeks and have, in some cases, been associated with severe carditis. Erythema marginatum is an evanescent, nonpainful, erythematous eruption occurring on the trunk or proximal extremities. Individual lesions can develop and disappear within minutes, but the process may wax and wane over several weeks or months. Sydenham's chorea often occurs later in the course than other manifestations of ARF and is characterized by rapid nonpurposeful choreiform movements of the face, hands, and feet. Attacks usually disappear during sleep but may persist for 2–4 months.

Poststreptococcal Glomerulonephritis

Acute glomerulonephritis (AGN) can follow either pharyngeal or skin infection and is associated with GAS strains possessing M protein types 12 and 49, respectively.[1] During epidemics of skin or pharyngeal infection produced by a nephritogenic strain, attack rates of 10–15% have been documented with latent periods of 10 days after pharyngitis and 3 weeks after pyoderma. Nonspecific symptoms include lethargy, malaise, headache, anorexia, and dull back pain. The classic signs of AGN are all related to fluid overload and are manifested initially by edema, both dependent and periorbital. Hypertension develops in most patients and is usually mild. Severe cases may be characterized by ascites, pleural effusion, encephalopathy, and pulmonary edema, though evidence of heart failure per se is lacking. Evidence of glomerular damage by renal biopsy has been documented in nearly 50% of contacts of siblings with AGN, suggesting that, as in ARF, subclinical disease is not uncommon after infection with certain strains of GAS. Unlike ARF, but similar to scarlet fever, glomerulonephritis occurs most commonly in children between 2 and 6 years of age. Like ARF and scarlet fever, AGN may affect several members of the same family. Recurrences or secondary attacks occur only rarely and there is little to suggest that AGN progresses to chronic renal failure.

The differential diagnosis of poststreptococcal AGN must include Henoch–Schönlein disease, polyarteritis nodosa, idiopathic nephrotic syndrome, leptospirosis, hemolytic-uremic syndrome (*Escherichia coli* O157:H7), and malignant hypertension. The diagnosis is simpler if there has been a recent history of symptomatic GAS pharyngitis, impetigo, or scarlet fever. Elevated or rising antibody titers to streptococcal antigens such as ASO, anti-DNase A or B, or antihyaluronidase are helpful, though ASO titers may be low in patients with pyoderma. A careful urinalysis to document proteinuria and hematuria should be performed, but it is mandatory to demonstrate red blood cell casts because the latter is the hallmark of glomerular injury. The blood urea nitrogen and creatinine values are elevated and, if nephrotic syndrome is present, the serum cholesterol level may be elevated and serum albumin concentration low. Twenty-four-hour excretion of protein is usually less than 3 g and total hemolytic complement and C3 levels are markedly reduced. The potential role of streptococcal infections in predisposing to other syndromes such as pediatric autoimmune neuropsychiatric disorder associated with streptococcal infection (PANDAS) remains unclear.[28]

PATHOGENESIS AND IMMUNITY

S. pyogenes causes multiple and distinct clinical syndromes and has developed unique ways to circumvent host defense mechanisms. Adherence of GAS to the mucosal epithelium is crucial to the pathogenesis of pharyngitis and RF and it occurs via the complex interaction of fibronectin-binding protein, lipoteichoic acid, peptidoglycan, and M protein with cell surface structures including fibronectin. Penetration of epithelial cells is important in invasive diseases such as bacteremia, though the mechanisms by which GAS reaches the deeper tissue are not fully understood. Studies by Hanski and Caparon[29] suggest that carbon dioxide and oxygen may alter expression of M protein and fibronectin-binding protein. Once within the tissues, GAS evades the host's inflammatory defenses by destroying or inactivating complement-derived chemoattractants (e.g., via C5a peptidase),[30] dysregulating endogenous complement inhibitory factors (such as factor H),[31] and by binding or inactivating immunoglobulin (via M and M-like proteins). M protein, in the absence of M-type-specific antibody, protects GAS from phagocytosis and secreted streptolysin O (SLO) in high concentration destroys approaching phagocytes. Distally, lower concentrations of SLO stimulate polymorphonuclear neutrophil (PMN) adhesion to endothelial cells, effectively preventing continued granulocyte migration.

Cytokines, in particular tumor necrosis factor (TNF) and interleukin-1 (IL-1), are produced by immune cells in response to many different GAS factors, including peptidoglycan, SLO, and streptococcal pyrogenic exotoxin B (SPEB). These cytokines mediate the development of fever, shock, and multiorgan failure associated with Strep TSS, but are also responsible for the fever and rash associated with scarlet fever. In addition, the pyrogenic exotoxins and some M protein fragments are superantigens, meaning they bind simultaneously to the MHC class II of the antigen-presenting cell (APC) and to certain V_β regions of the T-cell receptor in the absence of classical antigen processing. This causes activation of both cell types, resulting in proinflammatory cytokine production by APCs as well as clonal proliferation of T lymphocytes with massive production of the lymphokines interferon-γ (IFN-γ), IL-2, and TNF-β. Together, the monokines and lymphokines mediate hypotension and stimulate leukostasis, resulting in shock, microvascular injury, multiorgan failure, and, if excessive, death.

Another prominent feature of severe GAS infections is rapid tissue destruction. Recent studies in animals demonstrated that SLO dose dependently induces intravascular aggregates of platelets and neutrophils in sufficient quantities to effectively curtail vascular blood flow to the site of toxin injection. This process may contribute to the rapid tissue destruction observed in human cases of necrotizing fasciitis and myonecrosis.

Bacterial Cell Structure and Extracellular Products

Capsule

Some strains of GAS possess luxuriant capsules of hyaluronic acid, resulting in large mucoid colonies on blood agar. In recent times this mucoid phenotype has been associated with M protein types 1, 3, and 18 strains isolated from patients during epidemics of streptococcal pharyngitis and secondary RF.[4] Strains that are highly mucoid adhere to and invade epithelial cells less well than nonmucoid strains. However, a keratinocyte receptor (CD44) has been shown to bind to hyaluronic acid capsule. Once a barrier has been breached, the capsule may provide protection from phagocytosis and in general these mucoid strains are more virulent if injected subcutaneously.[32]

M Proteins

M protein is a coiled α-helical surface protein consisting of four distinct regions (A–D). Region A near the N-terminal is highly variable, and antibodies to this region confer type-specific protection, likely due to enhanced opsonization.[31] Within the more conserved B–D regions lies an area that binds one of the complement regulatory proteins (factor H). The net effect is to stearically inhibit antibody binding and complement-derived opsonin deposition, thus effectively camouflaging the organism against immune surveillance. Lastly, a proline-glycine-rich region intercalates the protein into the bacterial cell wall, and a hydrophobic region acts as a membrane anchor. In the absence of type-specific antibody, M protein inhibits the phagocytosis of *S. pyogenes* by PMNs, and fragments of M protein can act as superantigens.[33]

Over 150 different M types of GAS are recognized by either serologic typing (antibody recognition) or by sequencing of the *emm* gene itself. The regulation of M-protein synthesis is not firmly established but *emm* appears to be part of a virulence (*vir*) operon that includes an upstream control sequence and other virulence factor genes.[30] Observations by Lancefield[3] suggest that the quantity of M protein produced decreases with passage on artificial media and conversely increases rapidly with passage through mice. During untreated pharyngitis, the quantity of M protein produced by an infecting strain progressively decreases during convalescence.

Cell Wall

The cell wall is composed of a peptidoglycan backbone embedded with lipoteichoic acid (LTA). Besides their structural functions, both peptidoglycan and LTA have important interactions with the host immune system (see later discussion).

Cytoplasmic Membrane

Little is known about the cytoplasmic membrane, though it clearly serves as an effective barrier to the external milieu. It is also the site of cell wall synthesis which is orchestrated by five different penicillin-binding proteins (PBPs). Cell-wall degradation and synthesis during chain elongation is a dynamic process whose control is a reflection of the metabolic status of the organism. All PBPs are expressed during log-phase growth of GAS, and it is at this stage that penicillin's effects are greatest.[34] As organisms reach the stationary phase of growth, PBP prodution is curtailed and, in the absence of its targets, penicillin's efficacy is reduced.

Streptolysin O

SLO belongs to a family of pore-forming, oxygen-labile, thiol-activated cholesterol-dependent cytolysins (CDCs) and causes the broad zone of beta hemolysis surrounding colonies of GAS on blood agar plates. Exogenous cholesterol inhibits hemolysis both *in vitro* and in situations where serum cholesterol is high (e.g., nephrotic syndrome); thus, elevated antistreptolysin (ASO) titers occur because either cholesterol or anti-ASO antibody "neutralizes" SLO. Several CDCs, including SLO, have been cloned and sequenced and striking homology exists among them in a 13- to 15-amino acid region near the conserved cysteine residue.[35] The significance of SLO in pathogenesis is discussed later in this chapter.

Deoxyribonucleases A, B, C, and D

Expression of deoxyribonucleases (DNases) *in vivo* elicits production of anti-DNase antibody during and after infection. Antibodies to DNase A and DNase B have proved useful in the serologic diagnosis of pharyngeal and skin infections.[1,18] The importance of these enzymes in the pathogenesis of GAS infections has not been proved.

Hyaluronidase

Hyaluronidase hydrolyzes the hyaluronic acid in deeper tissues and may facilitate the spread of GAS along fascial planes. Anti-hyaluronidase titers rise following GAS infections, especially those involving the skin.

Pyrogenic Exotoxins A, B, C, MF, and SSA

The pyrogenic exotoxins A, B, C, MF, and SSA, also called scarlatina toxins and erythrogenic toxins, induce lymphocyte blastogenesis, potentiate endotoxin-induced shock,[36] induce fever, suppress antibody synthesis, and act as superantigens.[37,38]

The gene for streptococcal pyrogenic exotoxin A (*speA*) is transmitted by bacteriophage,[39] and stable toxin production depends on lysogenic conversion in a manner analogous to that for diphtheria toxin production by *Corynebacterium diphtheriae*. Factors controlling SPEA production are not fully understood, though the quantity of SPEA produced can vary dramatically from decade to decade.[40] Historically, SPEA-producing strains have been associated with severe cases of scarlet fever and, more recently, with Strep TSS.[5]

Although all GAS possess the gene for SPEB (*speB*), the quantity of toxin produced varies greatly and its regulation is highly complex. Several different roles in pathogenesis have been postulated for SPEB, mostly based on its *in vitro* proteolytic and superantigenic activities. SPEB cleaves pre-IL-1β to release biologically active IL-1β, activates matrix metalloproteases that disrupt endothelial integrity and induce apoptosis, and cleaves fibronectin, vitronectin, immunoglobulin, and serum properdin such that bacterial survival and dissemination may be facilitated. SPEB also cleaves the terminal portion of M protein, rendering the organism more susceptible to phagocytosis by normal serum but protecting it from opsonization by M-type-specific antibody. SPEB, like other superantigens, induces production of both monokines and lymphokines that mediate fever, shock, and tissue injury. However, proteolytic cleavage of some superantigens by SPEB reduces their proliferative and immunomodulatory activities. Despite this panoply of activities, SPEB's role in pathogenesis remains to be established with certainty. For instance, some studies have shown that insertional inactivation of *speB* decreases mouse lethality[41] while others using a similar approach failed to demonstrate a role for *speB* in virulence.[42] This discrepancy remains to be resolved.

Pyrogenic exotoxin C (SPEC), like SPEA, is bacteriophage-mediated and its expression is likewise highly variable. Hallas[17] demonstrated that mild cases of scarlet fever in England have been associated with strains of GAS producing SPEC.

Streptococcal superantigen (SSA) was described in an M type 3 GAS strain isolated from a patient with Strep TSS.[43] SSA resembles the other pyrogenic toxins, though its distribution and its role in pathogenesis have not been defined.

Mitogenic factor (MF) has all the features of other pyrogenic exotoxins, is a potent inducer of cytokines and lymphokines, and has been found in most strains of GAS examined.[44,45]

Many other GAS superantigens have been described, though their roles in pathogenesis remain unknown.[46]

Protein F

Protein F is a fibronectin-binding protein that contributes to the adherence of GAS to epithelial surfaces.[46] Production of protein F is inversely related to carbon dioxide concentrations in the milieu.[29]

C5a Peptidase and Interleukin-8 Cleaving Enzyme

IL-8 cleaving enzyme is a cell envelope protease that cleaves the chemoattractant IL-8.[47] Similarly, C5a peptidase, an enzyme produced by most strains of GAS, cleaves the complement activation factor C5a[30] – itself a potent chemoattractant. These virulence factors, alone or in combination, may thus thwart the migration of phagocytes to the site of infection.

TREATMENT AND PROGNOSIS

Emergence of Erythromycin Resistance

The first erythromycin-resistant strain of GAS was isolated in Great Britain in 1959 and, by 1975, resistant strains had also been isolated in the United States, Canada, and Japan. Although the prevalence of erythromycin resistance among GAS strains has remained low (3.6–4.0%) in most Western countries, in Japan resistance increased from 8.5% to 72% between 1971 and 1974. Similarly, erythromycin resistance had been a rare finding in Sweden; however, in 1984, an epidemic of pharyngitis (294 cases) caused by erythromycin-resistant GAS was reported. Marked increases in erythromycin resistance have also been documented in Finland, Australia, and Spain, and recently, Pittsburgh.

Sulfonamide Resistance

Sulfonamide resistance currently is reported in fewer than 1% of GAS isolates.

Therapeutic Failure of Penicillin

The major problem in the treatment of severe GAS infections with penicillin is a lack of *in vivo* efficacy, despite impressive *in vitro* susceptibility. Penicillin failure in pharyngitis, tonsillitis, or mixed infections has been attributed to inactivation of penicillin *in situ* by β-lactamases produced by co-colonizing organisms such as *Bacteroides fragilis* or *Staphylococcus aureus*. Active selection of such β-lactamase-producing organisms following treatment with penicillin is well documented and leads to bacteriologic failure in 40–80% of patients. In support of the role of β-lactamase in bacteriologic failures, Smith and Kaplan described cure rates of 90% in such failures if the second treatment consisted of amoxicillin plus clavulanate compared with only a 29% cure with a second regimen of penicillin.[48] In addition, antibiotics that are unaffected by β-lactamase activity (e.g., amoxicillin with clavulanate, erythromycin, or clindamycin) have a greater efficacy than penicillin in patients with recurrent GAS tonsillitis. In penicillin-allergic patients with acute GAS pharyngitis, erythromycin, cephalosporins, and clindamycin are reasonable alternatives, and all have had greater bacteriologic efficacy than penicillin in clinical trials.

Genotypic penicillin tolerance could also explain penicillin's lack of efficacy in tonsillitis or pharyngitis. Tolerant strains demonstrate a slower rate of growth, a slower rate of bacterial killing by penicillin, and an absence of β-lactam-induced cell lysis. Penicillin-tolerant GAS strains have been isolated from 11 of 18 cases of penicillin treatment failures of acute tonsillitis compared with 0 of 15 from successfully treated patients. Penicillin-tolerant strains have also caused epidemics of pharyngitis.

Penicillin also has reduced efficacy in the treatment of severe streptococcal infections in humans (i.e., streptococcal bacteremia, pneumonia, myositis, and Strep TSS) and laboratory animals. In a murine model of myonecrosis, penicillin was effective only if given early or if small numbers of GAS were used to initiate infection. With larger inocula, or if treatment was delayed, penicillin was no more effective than placebo. Thus, penicillin's efficacy declined as the infection became more severe, due to reduced expression of the PBPs by stationary phase organisms.[34] In contrast, clindamycin had excellent efficacy even if treatment was delayed up to 16 hours due to its ability to suppress bacterial virulence factor production, its longer postantibiotic effect, its indifference to the inoculum size and bacterial stage of growth, and its ability to attenuate TNF synthesis.

STAPHYLOCOCCAL INFECTIONS

In tropical climates, the most common *S. aureus* infection is pyomyositis, though impetigo, cellulitis, carbuncles, and furuncles are also very common. In cities where intravenous drug abuse is prevalent, endocarditis and bacteremia have also been described. *S. epidermidis* is also an important cause of intravascular, central nervous system shunt, and prosthetic joint infections. Similarly, *S. saprophyticus* and *S. intermedius* cause urinary tract and dog bite infections, respectively, in Western cultures and likely cause similar problems in tropical countries as well.

THE AGENT

Staphylococci are Gram-positive cocci that divide in two planes, thus yielding the classic clusters of cocci. *S. aureus* colonies cause beta hemolysis on sheep blood agar plates and appear as large moist colonies that may develop a golden hue with prolonged growth or when incubated at room temperature for a few hours.

EPIDEMIOLOGY

The normal reservoir of *S. aureus* and *S. epidermidis* is human skin. In addition, the nasal passage may harbor *S. aureus* and may provide an inoculum source for those with recurrent furunculosis. *S. aureus* causes infection in healthy persons as well as compromised patients and is distributed among all people worldwide. Clinical settings with specific staphylococcal infections are listed in ***Box 30.2***.

THE DISEASES

Folliculitis, Carbuncles, and Abscesses

Abscesses can develop from skin organisms introduced into the deeper tissue, from seeding of the skin from hematogenous sources such as bacteremia associated with endocarditis, or contiguously from infectious foci in the lung or gastrointestinal tract. In the former case, hair follicles serve as a portal of entry for a number of bacterial species, though *S. aureus* is the most common cause of localized folliculitis. Recurrent folliculitis is most common in black males in association with shaving (folliculitis barbae). Folliculitis can progress to small subcutaneous abscesses

Box 30.2 Staphylococcal Infections

Bacteremia	Pneumonia
Cavernous sinus thrombosis	Septic arthritis
Cellulitis	Staphylococcal scalded skin syndrome
Endocarditis	Staphylococcal toxic shock syndrome
Furunculosis	Suppurative thrombophlebitis
Impetigo	Surgical incision site infection
Myositis	
Necrotizing fasciitis	
Osteomyelitis	

(furuncles), which either resolve with antibiotic treatment alone or progress to form very large, exquisitely painful carbuncles that require surgical drainage as well as antibiotics. Certain individuals seem predisposed to develop recurrent *S. aureus* infections (recurrent furunculosis) and most have underlying factors such as poor hygiene, nasal carriage of staphylococcus, or neurodermatitis. Though it is suggested that diabetic patients are prone to such infections, there are few data to support this concept. In contrast, patients with Job's syndrome classically have recurrent *S. aureus* infections. In addition, these patients have eosinophilia and high levels of immunoglobulin E (IgE) antibody in serum.

Treatment of recurrent furunculosis may require surgical incision and drainage as well as anti-staphylococcal antibiotics such as nafcillin parenterally or dicloxacillin orally for methicillin-sensitive *S. aureus* (MSSA; see later section on MRSA). A recent randomized trial compared antibiotics (trimethoprim/sulfamethaxazole) with placebo in pediatric patients with MRSA skin abscesses and found no difference in outcome, though those treated with antibiotics had fewer new lesions.[49] Prevention is difficult, but some success has been realized with intranasal bacitracin or mupirocin ointment and hexachlorophene (pHisoHex) baths (in adults). Prophylactic antibiotics should be used only in severe cases.

Sebaceous glands empty into hair follicles and the ducts, if blocked (sebaceous cyst), may resemble a staphylococcal abscess or may become secondarily infected. Chronic folliculitis is uncommon except in acne vulgaris where normal flora, for example, *Propionibacterium acnes*, may play a role. Hidradenitis suppurativa occurs in either acute or chronic forms and can lead to recurrent axillary or pudendal abscesses.

Impetigo

Impetigo contagiosa is caused by *S. pyogenes*, and bullous impetigo by *S. aureus*. Both skin lesions may have an early bullous stage but then appear as thick crusts with a golden-brown color. It is important to distinguish impetigo contagiosa because of its potential relationship to poststreptococcal glomerulonephritis.

Pyomyositis

Pyomyositis is usually due to *S. aureus*, is common in tropical areas but rare in temperate climates, and typically there is no known portal of entry. The most common presenting features are muscle pain (100%) and fever (81%).[50] Blood cultures are positive in 14.3% of cases, complications include bronchopneumonia (23.1%) and empyema (19.2%), and mortality is low (7.7%). In one series there was an association with tuberculosis of the dorsal-lumbar spine.[50] Recently a dramatic increase in pyomyositis has been described in children in the United States caused by both MSSA and MRSA strains.[51] No contiguous portal of entry was observed; however, most developed infection at the exact site of a recent muscle strain or a minor non-penetrating injury (e.g., bruise). Infection remains localized and shock does not occur, unless strains produce toxic shock syndrome toxin-1 (TSST-1) or certain enterotoxins. In contrast, primary myositis caused by *S. pyogenes* is generally associated with severe systemic toxicity, including Strep TSS.

Empyema

S. aureus is the most common cause of empyema in the pediatric age group in tropical areas and has the highest prevalence in the hottest most humid months.[52] Predisposing conditions include prior pustular skin lesions, measles, chickenpox, and blunt trauma to the chest. Only 4% of strains have been MRSA, but this could increase dramatically in the future. In one report, chest tube drainage was effective in 78% of cases; however, the remaining patients required decortication.[52]

Endocarditis

S. aureus is an important cause of acute endocarditis worldwide. Intravenous drug abuse is the most common risk factor and in 50% of cases involves the right side of the heart. Still, fulminant staphylococcal bacteremia with endocarditis can occur in patients with no risk factors. The major complications regardless of cause are acute destruction of the aortic valve with sudden-onset pulmonary edema. In such cases, it may be necessary to replace the aortic valve immediately to prevent the development of left ventricular dilatation and subsequent myocardiopathy. Patients with right-sided endocarditis are less prone to cardiovascular collapse but may develop multiple staphylococcal abscesses of the lung. Regardless of the location of the vegetations, some patients develop metastatic abscesses of the liver, spleen, bones, and kidney. (See also later discussion of MRSA.)

Staphylococcal Toxic Shock Syndrome

Epidemiology

Toxic shock syndrome associated with *S. aureus* infections was originally referred to as TSS,[53] though in this chapter it is designated Staph TSS to distinguish it from the toxic shock syndrome caused by group A streptococcus (Strep TSS). The vast majority of Staph TSS cases occur in white females aged 15–19 years.[54–59] The incidence of Staph TSS was highest in 1980 (2.4–16/100 000 population),[57,58,60–63] with northern California having the lowest[63] and Colorado[62] having the highest infection rates. Numerous epidemiologic studies established that the illness was associated with the female menstrual cycle and that vaginal *S. aureus* colonization and infection played a significant role.[54–62] TSST-1 was isolated from *S. aureus*[64,65] and found to be produced by >90% of menstrual Staph TSS strains.[66]

Since its peak in 1980, a marked and persistent decline in Staph TSS has ensued and many possible explanations exist. First, there may have been enhanced reporting of cases in 1980 owing to extensive media coverage. Second, this decline could be related to education of the patients at risk, loss of virulence of the microbe, or acquisition of immunity to the putative toxins by a significant segment of the population. Lastly, some suggest that the reduced prevalence was due to removal of Rely tampons. Clearly, this latter notion does not fully explain the decline because menstrual cases of Staph TSS continue to occur. For further discussions about the epidemiologic studies implicating tampons, and the Rely brand in particular, the reader is referred to the literature.[54–57,67,68]

Nonmenstrual cases of Staph TSS were described among both sexes, regardless of age, and were associated with surgical procedures such as rhinoplasty with Teflon stents or nasal packing.[69] Nonmenstrual cases have also been associated with a variety of primary *S. aureus* infections, including cutaneous infection, postsurgical or postpartum infection, focal tissue infection, and pneumonia with or without antecedent influenza infection.[70] In contrast to menstrual Staph TSS, TSST-1 has been detected in only half of strains isolated from patients with nonmenstrual Staph TSS.[66,69] Staphylococcal enterotoxin B (SEB) and, to a lesser extent, enterotoxins A (SEA) and C (SEC) have been found in the remaining strains.[71–74] In addition, case reports suggest that strains that produce TSST-1 together with SEC may be more likely to cause fatalities,[72,73] but luckily both toxins are rarely found together in the same strain.[74]

Clinical Presentation

A prodromal period of 2–3 days precedes the physical manifestations of Staph TSS and consists of malaise, myalgia, and chills.[75] Fever begins soon thereafter, followed by symptoms of lightheadedness, modest confusion, and lethargy. The majority of patients develop diarrhea early in the course. Symptoms of hypovolemia, due in part to capillary leak and diarrhea, then predominate and include hyperventilation, palpitations, and dizziness on standing. Confusion, a prominent feature of Staph TSS, may affect some patients' ability to recognize the seriousness of their illness, resulting in delayed treatment.

When patients are first examined, fever, tachycardia, tachypnea, and hypotension are usually present. A transient, erythematous rash has been observed in over 50% of patients and may be either diffuse or patchy in distribution.[75] Many patients have marked peripheral vasodilation associated with high cardiac output and thus erythematous skin may represent maximal capillary dilation due to toxins or endogenous mediators. The capillary leak mentioned previously may not be apparent until fluid resuscitation has been undertaken. Desquamation of skin, particularly at sites of a previous erythematous rash, occurs between 7 and 14 days.[75]

Pathogenesis and Immunity

TSST-1 and staphylococcal enterotoxins are the major virulence factors associated with cases of Staph TSS. The genetic determinants for TSST-1 and SEB are variably expressed from a mobile genetic element, likely a transposon.[76] Some environmental conditions that enhance TSST-1 production include neutral pH, iron, trace elements such as magnesium and calcium, and oxygen.[68] Extrapolation of these findings to the association of menstrual Staph TSS with tampon use has been difficult if not controversial. Some suggest that tampons could (1) increase vaginal partial oxygen pressure during placement, and (2) supply surfactants and magnesium – either of which could result in enhanced toxin production.[70]

TSST-1 and staphylococcal enterotoxins stimulate T-cell proliferation (blastogenesis) via the superantigen mechanism,[77] which requires viable T lymphocytes bearing a specific V_β repertoire, and either an antigen-presenting cell (APC) or a fragment of the MHC class II receptor.[78] Other accessory molecules (e.g., CD4, ICAM-1, CD11a, CD28, CD2) may also participate [79,80] Superantigen-driven immune cell activation generates vast quantities of the lymphokines IL-2, IFN-γ, and TNF-β[77,81,82] as well as the monokines TNF-α, IL-1, and IL-6,[37,81] though their production dynamics are quite different. Specifically, during the first 24 hours, monokines predominate. By 48 hours, TNF-β and other lymphokines are detectable, and by 72 hours, equal quantities of TNF-α and TNF-β can be measured.[81]

Mechanisms controlling superantigen-driven cytokine production are poorly understood, but both counterregulatory cytokines and accelerated programmed cell death (apoptosis)[72] are likely involved. For instance, in a mouse model of SEB-induced shock, V_β-selective clonal expansion occurred 24–48 hours after administration of SEB.[83,84] On day 3, clonally expanded cells were apoptotically depleted, resulting in anergy.[83,84] This expansion–deletion sequence occurred predictably *in vivo* when high concentrations of superantigen were used but also occurred with low dosages.[85] Further, Miethke and coworkers[86] demonstrated that shortly after sublethal SEB challenge, mice became resistant to an otherwise lethal dose of SEB plus D-galactosamine.[86] Lymphocytes harvested from these animals lost the ability to release TNF-β and IL-2.[86] Though the authors hypothesized release of corticosteroids suppressed subsequent T-cell responsiveness, counterregulatory cytokines likely play a more important role. For example, IL-10, a regulatory lymphokine, inhibited TSST-1-induced synthesis of TNF-β and IFN-γ production by 68% and 86%, respectively,[87] leading the authors to suggest that administration of IL-10 might be a rational treatment for superantigen-induced disease.[87] Experimental studies showing that IL-10 protected animals from lethal SEB challenge support this hypothesis.[88]

TREATMENT AND PROGNOSIS

Patients with Staph TSS will be profoundly hypotensive, tachycardic, and febrile, and may have evidence of coagulopathy. The general supportive measures described for Strep TSS apply to Staph TSS as well. Clearly, in menstrual cases, early removal of the tampon and irrigation of the vaginal vault are important. Similarly, in nonmenstrual cases, surgical débridement, drainage, and removal of stents and packing are vital.[89]

Antibiotic treatment based on *in vitro* susceptibility would suggest that nafcillin, first- or second-generation cephalosporins, vancomycin, clindamycin, erythromycin, and fluoroquinolones would be reasonable choices. A variety of these antibiotics have been used in the past 15 years, and the mortality rate for Staph TSS remains at about 3% for menstrual cases and is two- to threefold higher for nonmenstrual cases.[68]

As with Strep TSS, shock and organ failure in patients with Staph TSS are clearly the consequence of bacterial toxin-mediated effects on the immune system. Thus, antibiotics that suppress protein (toxin) synthesis might be more efficacious than cell wall-active antibiotics. Indeed, clindamycin,[90–92] erythromycin,[92] rifampin,[92] and fluoroquinolones[92] each significantly suppressed TSST-1. In contrast, five different β-lactam antibiotics, including nafcillin and cephalosporins, increased TSST-1 in culture supernatants.[92] Recently, Stevens et al demonstrated that nafcillin enhanced the production of TSST-1, α-hemolysin and the Panton–Valentine leukotoxin in both MSSA and MRSA by increasing the quantity and duration of mRNA expression.[93] In contrast, linezolid and clindamycin inhibited toxin production.[93] Unfortunately, there has been no controlled clinical trial comparing different antibiotics; however, these experimental results suggest that antibiotic susceptibility alone may not necessarily predict success.

The potential use of immunoglobulin to treat Staph TSS has a sound basis. First, patients who develop Staph TSS have low to absent antibody titers against TSST-1 or enterotoxins or both.[68] Second, the general population in both the United States and Europe has significant antibody titers against these toxins and titers increase with age.[68] Finally, data from experimental animal studies demonstrate that neutralizing antibody against TSST-1 is therapeutic.[94,95] There have been no prospective studies done in humans.

The usefulness of corticosteroids in shock has been studied for many years. Corticosteroid therapy is not currently considered to be an effective treatment in the United States, though some centers in Europe currently use this treatment. Todd[89] advocates corticosteroids for patients with "severe Staph TSS unresponsive to initial antibiotic therapy."

Cellulitis

Because of the diverse causes of cellulitis, empirical choices of antibiotic therapy depend greatly on the clinical factors described previously. Once cultures and sensitivities are available, choices are much easier and more specific. The physician must first decide if the patient's illness is severe enough to require parenteral treatment. For presumed streptococcal or staphylococcal cellulitis, nafcillin, cephalothin, cefuroxime, vancomycin, or erythromycin are good choices. Cefazolin and ceftriaxone have less activity against *S. aureus* than cephalothin, though clinical trials have shown a high degree of efficacy. Ceftriaxone may be a useful choice for outpatient treatment because of once-per-day dosing. Similarly, teicoplanin, like vancomycin, has excellent activity against *S. pyogenes* and both *S. aureus* and *S. epidermidis* and may be given once per day by intravenous or intramuscular injection. For patients being treated with oral drugs, dicloxacillin, cefuroxime axetil, cefpodoxime, or erythromycin (or clarithromycin or azithromycin) are effective treatments. For known group A, B, C, or G streptococcal infections, penicillin or erythromycin should be used orally or parenterally. In serious group A streptococcal infections, clindamycin is superior to penicillin. This is probably because in this type of infection, wherein large numbers of bacteria are present, streptococci are in a stationary phase of growth and do not express a full complement of PBPs. In contrast, clindamycin is not affected by inoculum size or stage of growth. In addition, clindamycin suppresses production of extracellular toxins by both *S. aureus* and *S. pyogenes*.

Methicillin-Resistant *S. aureus* Infections

During the past 15 years, the prevalence of MRSA has steadily increased in all communities worldwide. Until 2002, MRSA was strictly associated with hospital-associated (HA) infections and the greatest risk factors were prior hospitalization, surgical procedures, and recent antibiotic exposure, particularly fluoroquinolones, β-lactam antibiotics, and vancomycin. Currently, a dramatic increase in community-associated (CA) MRSA infections has been reported. These are most commonly associated with soft tissue infections, though pneumonia, toxic shock syndrome, and necrotizing soft tissue infections have been described.[96,97]

Like MSSA, MRSA strains cause cellulitis, furunculosis, carbuncles, and impetigo. In addition, MRSA causes soft tissue abscesses associated with localized skin necrosis and ulceration ("spider bites"). Necrotizing fasciitis associated with patients with hepatitis C and diabetes has been reported in adults in Los Angeles[97] and pyomyositis has been reported from children in Chicago and Houston (see previous section on pyomyositis). Unlike necrotizing fasciitis caused by GAS, patients with MRSA-associated necrotizing fasciitis rarely develop shock, organ failure or extensive necrosis of tissue.

Hemorrhagic/necrotizing pneumonitis caused by MRSA strains harboring the genes for the Panton–Valentine leukocidin is associated with high mortality (60%) and rapid progression in previously healthy young adults.[98] Risk factors include influenza virus infection, prior MRSA colonization, or contact with a family member with previous MRSA infection. Hemoptysis and a rapid decline in neutrophil count were important clinical clues. That this entity is not well recognized by physicians is suggested by the fact that 80% of patients with hemorrhagic necrotizing pneumonitis were treated initially with ceftriaxone.

Vancomycin has been the drug of choice, though it is slowly bactericidal and does not penetrate tissues, particularly the lung, very well. The widespread use of vancomycin parallels a clear increase in resistance in MRSA (reviewed in reference 99). First, "MIC creep" in MRSA has been widely reported in the United States. Second, frank resistance to vancomycin (MICs >32 μg/mL) has occurred, largely in dialysis patients. Third, intermediate vancomycin resistance (defined as MICs of 2–4 μg/mL) appears related to thick-walled MRSA strains with increased binding sites for vancomycin. Fourth, vancomycin heteroresistance has been demonstrated using larger inocula for susceptibility testing in which a subpopulation (1–10%) is constitutively resistant to vancomycin, is not picked up by conventional antimicrobial susceptibility testing, and is associated with vancomycin failures. A macro-E-test is being to developed to provide clinicians with important information that could predict failure.

Several new agents exist and several more are in the pipeline. Linezolid has been shown to be an effective agent for skin and soft tissue infections, bacteremia, and pneumonia caused by MRSA.[100] Daptomycin, which is rapidly bactericidal, has also been approved for MRSA skin and skin structure infections, bacteremia, and right-sided endocarditis.[101] Linezolid may also be more effective than vancomycin for MRSA pneumonia due to better tissue penetration,[102] and a clinical trial comparing these agents is currently underway. Daptomycin should not be used for pneumonia because it was shown to be less effective than ceftriaxone for community-acquired pneumococcal pneumonia. This is partly due to poor tissue penetration and direct binding of daptomycin to lung surfactant. Tigecycline, a minocycline derivative, has been approved for skin and skin structure infections and also intra-abdominal infections.[103]

Unfortunately, HA MRSA strains are also resistant to many other antibiotics. CA MRSA strains are less likely to be resistant to trimethoprim-sulfamethoxazole and tetracyclines, but inducible clindamycin resistance has emerged as a potential problem in 20–30% of strains. These dynamic changes in the susceptibility of *S. aureus* cause great difficulty in recommending specific treatments for both HA and CA MRSA. The clinician must factor in the prevalence of MRSA in his or her environment, the seriousness of the infection, and the site and type of infection when selecting empiric antibiotics. It is more important than ever to obtain cultures and rely on sensitivities to guide subsequent treatment.

PREVENTION AND CONTROL

Prevention and control of streptococcal and staphylococcal infections and their sequelae are best accomplished by careful personal hygiene and prompt treatment of early infections. Extensive regimens to eradicate carriage may have a role in selected cases of recurring infections.

Access the complete reference list online at
http://www.expertconsult.com

CHAPTER 31

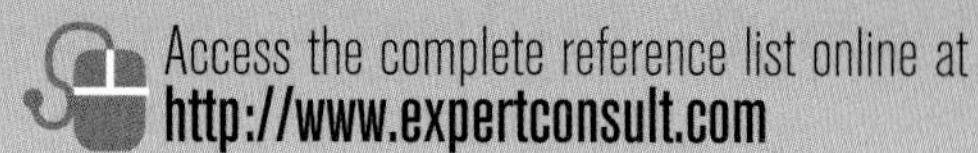
Access the complete reference list online at
http://www.expertconsult.com

Pertussis

Joshua C. Eby • Erik L. Hewlett

INTRODUCTION

Pertussis, or whooping cough, remains a significant cause of morbidity and mortality worldwide. Despite the availability of effective vaccines, an estimated 17 million cases and 300 000 deaths occur annually.[1] The highest incidence is in developing countries, where malnutrition and limited supportive care contribute to a high (4%) case-fatality rate in infants.[2,3] Even in countries where pertussis vaccination is widely available, there has been a resurgence of pertussis disease with the greatest increase among adolescents and adults.[4–10]

THE AGENT

Pertussis is caused by coccobacillary organisms from the genus *Bordetella*. *B. pertussis* and *B. parapertussis* are responsible for whooping cough in humans, although *B. parapertussis* does not produce pertussis toxin, a major virulence factor of *B. pertussis*.[11,12] *B. pertussis* is believed to be the predominant cause of pertussis morbidity and mortality and is the focus of World Health Organization (WHO) pertussis surveillance.[1] Other *Bordetella* species, including *B. bronchiseptica*, *B. avium*, *B. hinzii*, *B. holmesii*, and *B. trematum*, are primarily animal pathogens, which have been reported to infect humans, often via transmission from animals.[13–18]

EPIDEMIOLOGY

Pertussis has a worldwide distribution, but there is lack of active surveillance in many countries and a paucity of data from some regions of the world. Pertussis persists in communities as an endemic disease, with 3–5-year epidemic cycles superimposed. Outbreaks occur in settings in which pertussis transmission is most likely to occur, such as crowded working and living environments and communities with low vaccination rates.[19] Although incidences of pertussis in unimmunized populations have been reported to reach 6000 per 100 000 child-years <15 years of age and 18 000 per 100 000 child-years <5 years of age,[3] widespread pertussis vaccination elicits declines to <20 per 100 000 person-years.[1,10,20] In some countries with high vaccination rates, a decrease in incidence has been followed by a subsequent rise in incidence, with rates as high as 300–500 cases per 100 000 person-years.[5,7,21] This increase in incidence may reflect an epidemiologic shift to older age groups and infants being affected. Prior to the use of whole-cell pertussis vaccine, many infants had passive immunity from maternal antibodies delivered transplacentally and possibly in breast milk (***Fig. 31.1***).[22–24] As a result, pertussis was primarily an illness of young children (aged 2–10 years), who acquired limited natural immunity from their primary infection and were boosted throughout their lives by exposures to infected individuals. In the setting of widespread pediatric immunization, maternal pertussis antibodies are lacking and infants are often born unprotected. Even though immunization is often initiated in the first 2 months of life, protective immunity is generally not obtained until the third dose. Immunity from vaccination wanes over a 10–12-year period following the dose at age 6 years (***Fig. 31.1***).[4,8–10,25] Affected adolescents and adults are capable of transmitting pertussis to each other and to infants, and most infant cases of pertussis can be traced to exposure to an adolescent or adult contact.[26–28]

THE DISEASE

Pertussis infection is transmitted via aerosol droplet, during close exposure to a person with active infection. After an asymptomatic incubation period ranging from 1 to 3 weeks, the classical syndrome of whooping cough begins, with the catarrhal phase, during which symptoms include rhinorrhea, watery eyes, dry cough, mild conjunctival injection and low-grade fever. This phase of about one week cannot be distinguished clinically from other upper respiratory tract infections. As the illness progresses to the paroxysmal phase, infected individuals may develop the characteristic paroxysmal cough, a series of short expiratory bursts, followed by an inspiratory gasp that produces the typical whoop. Paroxysms and whooping are relatively uncommon in infants, who may have apneic episodes as their only symptom. The paroxysmal cough can be associated with additional symptoms, such as post-tussive emesis, cyanosis, facial flushing, and syncope, and laboratory finding of leukocytosis with lymphocyte predominance.[29–31] Adults and adolescents may be asymptomatic or exhibit nonclassical symptoms and signs.[27,31,32]

During the prolonged (weeks to months) paroxysmal phase, there can be significant morbidity and mortality, especially under conditions in which malnutrition and dehydration occur. The principal complications include pneumonia (caused by *B. pertussis* or other pathogens), conjunctival hemorrhages and central nervous system (CNS) dysfunction. CNS abnormalities can present as encephalopathy or seizures in infants, young children, and even adults.[9,29,33] Paroxysms decrease in frequency and intensity during the convalescent phase, which can last several months. During this time, infection with unrelated respiratory pathogens or any irritating stimulus can precipitate recurrence of the paroxysmal cough.

PATHOGENESIS AND IMMUNITY

B. pertussis produces a number of virulence factors that interact in an orchestrated sequence of events to produce the clinical disease of pertussis. Despite knowledge of the mechanisms of action of many of these factors at the cellular and molecular level, their exact target tissues and pathophysiology remain a matter of speculation. A current working model for the pathogenesis of pertussis involves adhesins, toxins, and other virulence factors.[34,35] The adherence factors – filamentous hemagglutinin (FHA), pertactin (PRN), and fimbriae (FIM) – appear to be involved in the attachment of *B. pertussis* to ciliated respiratory epithelia, but no single factor is absolutely essential to establishment of infection and several of these have been shown to have other effects, such as the

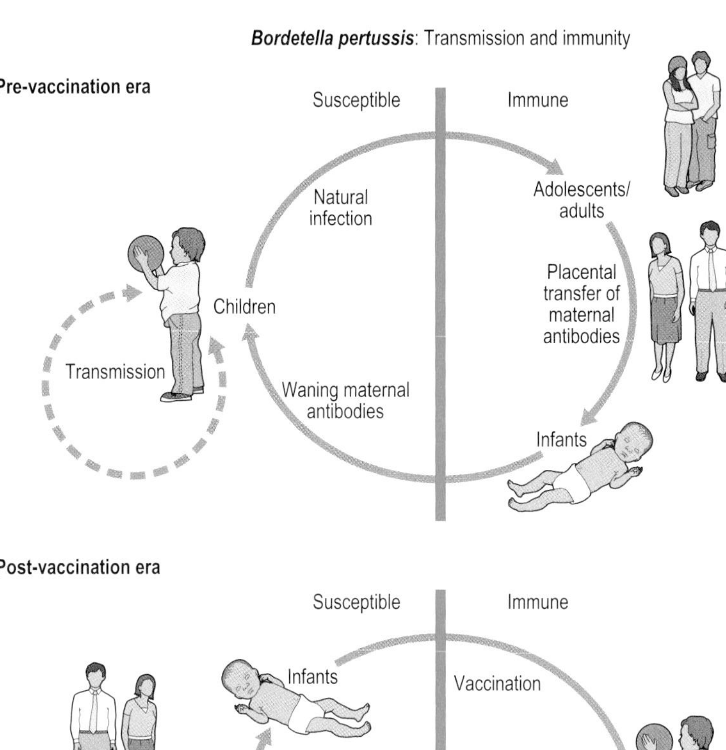

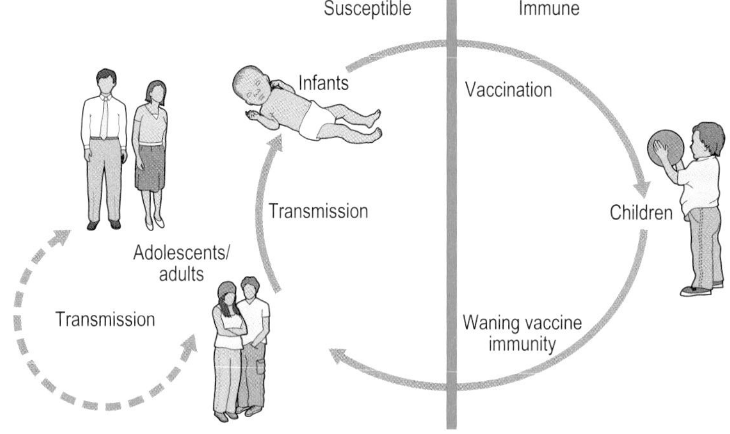

Figure 31.1 *Bordella pertussis*: transmission and immunity.

immunomodulation produced by FHA.[36] The release of tracheal cytotoxin (TCT), a breakdown product of the bacterial peptidoglycan, causes ciliostasis and death of the tracheal ciliated epithelial cells. Adenylate cyclase toxin (ACT) produces an accumulation of cyclic adenosine monophosphate (cAMP) intracellularly, which impairs the function of leukocytes and may affect other cell types. Other pathogenic factors produced by *B. pertussis* (dermonecrotic toxin, tracheal colonization factor, and an autotransporter/serum resistance factor, BrkA) have also been described.

The best-known and most extensively studied product of *B. pertussis* is pertussis toxin (PT), which induces lymphocytosis, enhances insulin secretion, inhibits intracellular signal transduction, and impairs the function of phagocytes. PT is not expressed by *B. parapertussis* or other *Bordetella* species and is not necessary for causing a coughing syndrome, but appears to be the primary determinant of severe disease and sequelae. Strains not expressing PT have, however, been isolated from patients in France.[37] PT is the only virulence factor that disseminates systemically, but the target tissues through which PT elicits its pathogenic effects and specific symptoms remain to be elucidated.[38]

DIAGNOSIS

Historically, the diagnosis of pertussis infection has been limited by a lack of a sensitive and specific diagnostic method that is also practical for widespread use. Isolation of the *B. pertussis* organism by culture is very specific, but has low sensitivity, even in experienced laboratories. Serologic detection of antibodies to components of pertussis has been used in epidemiologic studies and vaccine efficacy trials. There is not, however, a standardized methodology for pertussis serology, and case definitions based on serologic criteria vary amongst published studies.[7,8,31,39,40] Although the Centers for Disease Control and Prevention (CDC) does not recommend serology as a method for diagnosis, the WHO includes paired serological assay in its case definition of pertussis. For diagnosis by a one-time serologic test, the Massachusetts Department of Public Health has utilized a cutoff of >20 μg/mL for anti-PT IgG measured by enzyme-linked immunosorbent assay, and has reported a 63% sensitivity using culture and/or direct fluorescence antibody staining as the gold standard.[41]

Polymerase chain reaction (PCR) assays for *B. pertussis* are highly sensitive and specific and are increasingly available for routine diagnosis in clinical settings.[29,42] Because PCR does not require a viable organism, the diagnosis of pertussis infection can sometimes be made in patients who have already received treatment with antibiotics or who present for care later in the course of illness.[43] Recent advancements in PCR allow discrimination between *B. pertussis* and *B. parapertussis.*[44–46] Despite these advantages, PCR is more costly and less widely available and flaws in PCR technique and/or interpretation have led to misidentification of cough illnesses in the United States as pertussis outbreaks.[47] Finally, although a very infrequent problem, PCR cannot detect antibiotic resistance that has been reported in strains of *B. pertussis*.

According to the 1997 CDC recommendations, a case of pertussis is defined clinically as "a cough illness lasting at least 2 weeks with one of the following: paroxysms of coughing, inspiratory 'whoop,' or post-tussive vomiting, without other apparent cause (as reported by a health professional)." A patient with pertussis is classified as a *definite case* if the clinical case definition is met, in conjunction with supporting laboratory (culture or PCR) or epidemiologic (direct linkage to a definite case) evidence. A *probable case* meets the clinical criteria, but without laboratory confirmation.[48]

TREATMENT

Infants with pertussis disease are at the greatest risk for complications and neurologic sequelae and, for this reason, supportive therapy is critical. These patients often require hospitalization for close monitoring, frequent nasotracheal suctioning, supplemental oxygen, and parenteral hydration and nutrition, in addition to treatment with antibiotics. Although some antibiotics have been shown to eliminate *B. pertussis* from the respiratory tract, thereby reducing transmission, their efficacy in reducing the severity and duration of disease is dependent on early initiation of therapy. Macrolide and azalide antibiotics (erythromycin, clarithromycin, and azithromycin) are recommended for treatment of pertussis[49] in ages ≥1 month old. Azithromycin is recommended for children <1 month old. Though microbiologic cure of pertussis is difficult to assess, azithromycin and clarithromycin appear as effective as erythromycin and better tolerated.[50–52] For adults, azithromycin is administered as 500 mg orally once, followed by 250 mg on days 2–5. Dosing for children is 10 mg/kg orally daily for 5 days for children <6 months, or 10 mg/kg orally once, followed by 5 mg/kg on days 2–5 for children ≥6 months. Clarithromycin is dosed as 15 mg/kg daily (maximum 1 g/day) orally in two divided doses for 7 days. Erythromycin (particularly the estolate ester) is recommended at a daily dose of 40–50 mg/kg orally (maximum 2 g/day) divided into four doses, for a full 14-day course to prevent bacteriologic relapse. When a macrolide is not available or cannot be tolerated, trimethoprim-sulfamethoxazole can be used in children ≥2 months old, but there are few published reports validating its use in pertussis treatment.[53] Adjunctive therapy with corticosteroids[54] or β_2-adrenergic agonists[55,56] has been suggested to be of some symptomatic benefit in severely affected individuals, but their efficacies in this setting have not been documented and require further study.

PREVENTION AND CONTROL

In the pre-vaccine era, immunity to pertussis infection was acquired and maintained through clinical disease, followed by repetitive exposure to *B. pertussis* as it circulated in the community. It was soon recognized that acquisition of antibodies to the organism correlates with resistance to infection.[57] In the 1950s, a killed, whole-cell pertussis vaccine, combined with diphtheria and tetanus toxoids and aluminum-containing adjuvants (DTwP vaccine), was developed and used widely. Although this vaccine achieves an efficacy of greater than 80% if properly prepared, there has been significant variability in the vaccine product made by different manufacturers, resulting in lower efficacy with some products.[58] In addition, the use of the whole-cell vaccine, in some countries, has been limited by its associated reactogenicity, which includes pain, swelling, fever, anorexia, and vomiting.[59,60] In younger children and infants, there were reports of encephalopathy and neurologic sequelae temporally associated with DTwP but no conclusive evidence that DTwP causes CNS damage.[59,61,62]

Because of concern over the safety of DTwP in the 1970s and 1980s, several acellular pertussis (aP) vaccines were developed using PT and one or more of the following components: PRN, FHA, or FIM. These vaccines have similar efficacy and decreased reactogenicity compared with whole-cell vaccines and they are now licensed and available in combination with diphtheria and tetanus toxoids (DTaP) in most developed countries. The complexity of producing purified vaccine components entails a production cost that is, however, unreasonable for most developing countries.

WHO continues to recommend use of whole-cell pertussis vaccine in some parts of the world, because of its lower cost of production and its greater availability, especially in countries that manufacture their own vaccine. In countries where the reactogenicity of the whole-cell vaccine caused decreased acceptance of pertussis immunization, WHO recommends use of the acellular vaccine.[1]

Countries that instituted routine pertussis immunization in the 1950s observed a drop in pertussis incidence, followed many years later by a resurgence in cases with a greater proportion in adolescents and adults.[1,4,5,7,8,10,29] The duration of protection from whole-cell vaccines is 10–12 years[29] but is yet to be determined for aP vaccines. It has been observed that some *B. pertussis* strains isolated from previously vaccinated individuals have genetic variations in the virulence factors corresponding to vaccine components, suggesting possible adaptation of the organism to the acellular vaccines.[37,63,64] Whether evolution of *B. pertussis*, in countries with high vaccination rates, is related to the rise in incidence remains to be determined.

Countries that implement more widespread pertussis immunization strategies will likely see a similar epidemiologic shift in disease from young children to adolescents and adults. For example, following the initiation of infant pertussis immunization in Senegal, there was a decline in incidence in every age group (including a 79% reduction in the 6–23-month age group). During a subsequent 8-year period, the median age of individuals experiencing pertussis rose from 4.1 to 6.2 years of age, and cases in children less than 5 years old dropped from 60% to 38%.[3]

Clinical trials of the newer acellular pertussis vaccines have demonstrated safety, immunogenicity,[29,65,66] and efficacy[21] in adolescents and adults. In 1998, France was the first country to recommend a booster dose of acellular pertussis vaccine for adolescents. Since then, vaccination of adolescents and adults with acellular pertussis vaccine has been endorsed in multiple European countries, Canada, Australia, Japan, and, more recently, the United States.[10,25,27,48] An adolescent booster dose supports humoral and cell-mediated immunity for several years[67] and, in Canada, adolescent booster doses of acellular pertussis vaccine have resulted in a decrease in pertussis incidence across all age groups.[68]

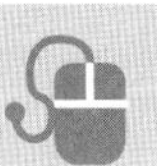

Access the complete reference list online at
http://www.expertconsult.com

Access the complete reference list online at
http://www.expertconsult.com

CHAPTER 32

Legionellosis

Thomas J. Marrie • Paul S. Hoffman

INTRODUCTION

From July 21 to 24, 1976, the 58th Annual Convention of the American Legion was held at a hotel in Philadelphia. One hundred and eighty-two of the attendees at the convention developed pneumonia.[1] One hundred and forty-seven (81%) were hospitalized and 29 (16%) died. This outbreak of pneumonia, of apparent unknown cause, triggered an exhaustive epidemiologic and microbiologic investigation by the Centers for Disease Control and Prevention (CDC) culminating in the isolation of a new microorganism, *Legionella pneumophila*, approximately 6 months later.[2]

It soon became apparent from analysis of stored serum samples that this organism had caused disease prior to 1976, and prospective studies showed that the spectrum of illness ranged from a nonpneumonic, mild, self-limited febrile illness (Pontiac fever)[3] to a pneumonic illness that varied from mild to severe. The latter was often accompanied by multisystem disease.[1,4] The pneumonic form of the illness following infection with *Legionella* is referred to as legionnaires' disease (LD).

THE AGENT

There are more than 30 species in the family Legionellaceae.[5] *Legionella pneumophila* serogroup 1 accounts for most of the cases of LD. Legionellaceae are Gram-negative, aerobic, non-spore-forming bacilli that measure 0.3–0.9 μm wide by 2–20 μm long. These organisms require special media for growth. Charcoal yeast extract agar buffered to pH 6.9 and containing α-ketoglutarate along with cefamandole, polymyxin B, and anisomycin to prevent growth of other microorganisms is the primary medium used for isolation of these organisms. Addition of α-ketoglutaric acid to the medium promotes growth of *Legionella* likely by stimulation of oxygen-scavenging enzymes.

These organisms are visualized poorly, if at all, by Gram stain. In tissue, silver impregnation stains such as the Dieterle or Warthin–Starry method allow visualization of the organism.

EPIDEMIOLOGY

Once the microorganism had been isolated, it was characterized and diagnostic reagents became available. In 1981, 5 years after the initial outbreak, England and colleagues[6] reported on the first 1000 cases of sporadic LD in the United States. The authors noted that most cases occurred during June to October – 71% of patients were male, and 88% were white. During the 2 weeks before onset of this illness, 37% had traveled overnight, 29% had visited a hospital, and 5% had been hospitalized 2 days before onset of illness. Twenty-three percent lived within sight of a construction or excavation site, and 32% had been exposed to a construction or excavation.

As we have learned more about the epidemiology of this disease, these were all seminal observations. With these original observations in mind, it is instructive to examine the report of Marston and associates,[7] which analyzed *Legionella* surveillance data on 3254 patients reported to the CDC from 1980 through 1989. Disease rates did not vary by year but were higher in the northern states and during the summer. The mean age of patients with LD was 52.7 years compared with 34.7 years for the US population. In contrast to earlier reports, people with LD were now more likely to be black. They were also more likely to be smokers and have diabetes, cancer, acquired immunodeficiency syndrome (AIDS), or end-stage renal disease. Indeed, the observed number of cases among patients with AIDS was 42-fold higher than expected. Risk factors for mortality in the study of Marston and coworkers were older age, male sex, nosocomial acquisition of disease, immunosuppression, end-stage renal disease, and cancer. Twenty-three percent of the cases were nosocomially acquired.

Soon after the description of LD, it was evident that cases could occur sporadically or in clusters. Furthermore, these cases could be community or nosocomially acquired. As with most infectious diseases, outbreaks provided an opportunity to learn about the mechanisms of transmission of LD. In most instances, *Legionella* is transmitted to humans by inhalation of aerosols containing the bacteria. Outbreaks have been associated with exposure to a variety of aerosol-producing devices, including showers,[8,9] a grocery store mist machine,[10] cooling towers,[11–16] whirlpool spas,[17,18] decorative fountains, and evaporative condensers.[19,20] It is also likely that aspiration of contaminated potable water by immunosuppressed patients is a mechanism whereby *Legionella* is acquired.[21–23]

Legionella pneumophila multiplies in potable water that contains amebae but not in filtered amebae-free water.[24] Amebae are natural hosts for legionellae.[25]

Legionellosis is believed to occur worldwide, but data are limited or nonexistent for many countries. It is likely that legionellosis is very uncommon in areas without water heaters and complex water distribution systems. However, even in these areas, aspiration of contaminated natural water, such as following boating accidents, can result in LD. LD has been found throughout North America, Europe, the United Kingdom, Argentina, Brazil, Singapore, Thailand, and Australia (***Fig. 32.1***). LD has been reported from South Africa,[26] China,[27] and Zambia.[28] A few cases of LD have been reported in India. The major problem is that serologic tests and culture for legionellae are not available in most tropical countries. Indeed, Harris and Beeching[29] state that the Western approach to the management of pneumonia "with hospitalization and administration of antibiotics to cover typical and 'atypical' [e.g., *Legionella*] organisms is not appropriate for much of the tropics." However, in areas where studies have been carried out, *Legionella* and LD have been found. This situation is exemplified by data from Singapore. There were 144 cases of LD from 1991 to 1995, and there was widespread contamination of water (33% of 2774 cooling towers and 18.8% of 16 outdoor fountains) by *Legionella* in that country.[30]

In a study of community-acquired pneumonia (CAP) requiring admission to hospital, conducted at 15 centers throughout Canada, the

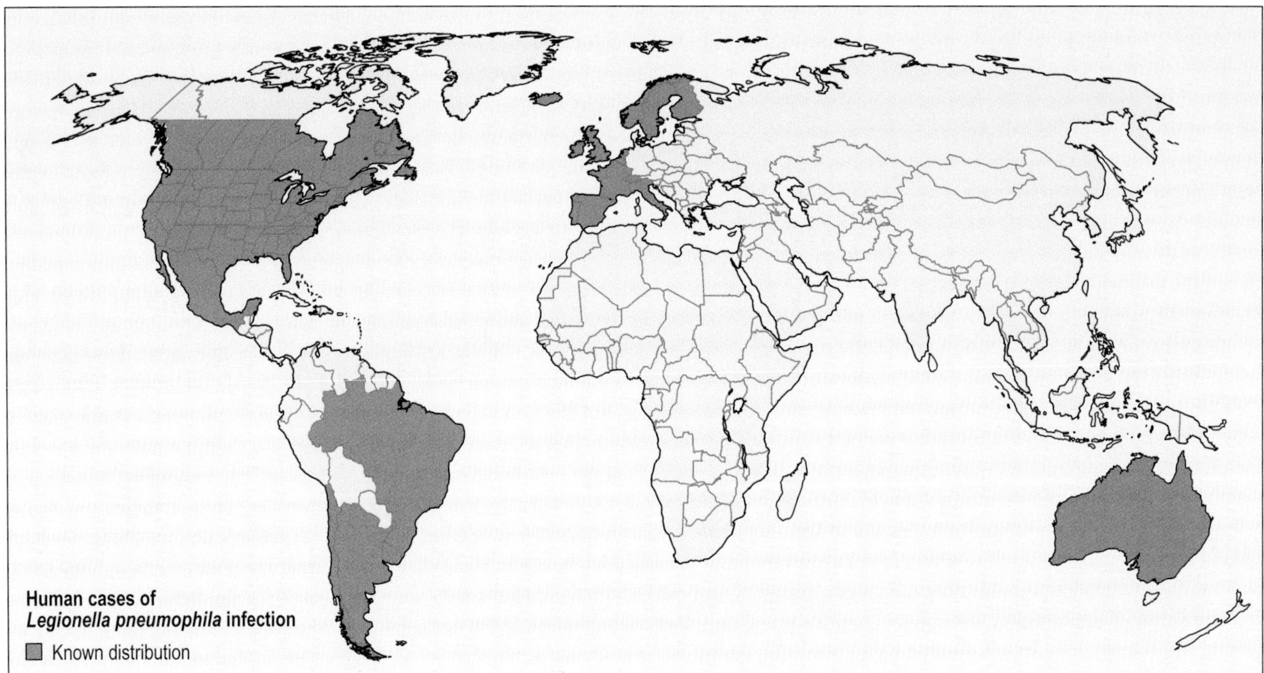

Figure 32.1 Human cases of *Legionella pneumophila* infection have also been reported from Singapore, Thailand, South Africa, China, Zambia, India, and the Caribbean.

investigators found that 3.2% of the 850 patients had LD.[31] When only those who had urine tested for *Legionella* antigen were considered, patients from the Halifax site (7/163 versus 11/660) had a higher rate of LD.[31] The number of reported cases of legionellosis in the United States increased by 70% from 1310 cases in 2002 to 2223 in 2003.[32] The eastern United States showed most of the increases in age-adjusted incidence rates after 2002.[32] Investigators from the CDC noted an association between increased rainfall in the Mid-Atlantic states and the increasing rate of LD.[33] Indeed, a 1 cm increase in rainfall was associated with a 2.6% increase in LD.[33]

LD can also be a travel-related illness. In a study in Europe, Joseph identified 113 outbreaks of LD that were really travel-associated clusters involving 315 persons.[34] Travel within Europe accounted for 88% of the cases. The remainder were associated with travel to the Americas, Caribbean, Far East, Africa, and Middle East[34]. In these instances, the source is usually contaminated water aerosols, although the location may be beautiful such as a spa pool on a cruise ship,[35] or water fountains at a Dutch flower show.[36] LD can be acquired quite a distance from a contaminated source such as a cooling tower or an air scrubber, where the exhaust can be carried by prevailing winds. Cases have been documented at 3 km,[13] 6–7 km,[37] and 10 km[38] from such sources. In fact, the investigation of an outbreak of LD is often challenging, requiring a multidisciplinary team, and represents some of the most exciting of epidemiological investigations.

Table 32.1 Comparison of Selected Features of Nosocomial Legionnaires' Disease from Three Reports[a]

Feature	Korvick and Yu[40]	Kirby et al[4]	Marrie et al[41]
No. studied	65	20	55
Male:female ratio	62:3	14:6	33:22
Mean age (years)	59.2	52.3	58.6
No. died	16 (24.6)	14 (70)	35 (63.3)
Immunosuppressed	27 (41.5)	18 (90)	40 (73)
Malignancy	19 (29)	7 (35)	16 (29)
Assisted ventilation	NS	NS	33 (60)
Cough	60 (92)	14 (70)	37 (67)
Chills	50 (77)	6 (30)	37 (67)
Diarrhea	30 (47)	3 (15)	12 (22)
Dyspnea	23 (36)	7 (35)	35 (64)
Chest pain	21 (33)	11 (55)	8 (15)
Hemoptysis	22 (34)	6 (30)	1 (2)
Legionella isolate	5 (8)	NS	40(70)

[a]Numbers in parentheses refer to percentage.
NS, not stated.

THE DISEASE

Legionellosis consists of two diseases: Pontiac fever and LD. The former is a self-limited febrile illness. The incubation period is 24–48 hours. There is a 90% or greater attack rate among those exposed, and recovery occurs in approximately 1 week. Malaise, myalgia, fever, chills, headache, and nonproductive cough are common symptoms. There is no pneumonia.[39]

LD is a pneumonic illness with a wide spectrum of severity and frequency of extrapulmonary manifestations. Initially, patients with LD have a nonproductive cough, but later in the course of the illness it can be productive. Occasionally, hemoptysis occurs, and the clinical picture may mimic pulmonary embolus.

Rales and signs of consolidation are evident on examination. There may be relative bradycardia. Some patients have watery diarrhea and headache; confusion and lethargy dominate the clinical picture in others. The pneumonia may continue to progress despite appropriate treatment, and respiratory failure may ensue. In severe LD, clinical improvement is not seen for 4 or 5 days after appropriate antibiotic therapy has been instituted.

Disseminated intravascular coagulation, thrombocytopenia, rhabdomyolysis, glomerulonephritis, pyelonephritis, pericarditis, and pancreatitis may complicate the clinical course. Hyponatremia and hypophosphatemia are common. ***Table 32.1*** summarizes selected features of nosocomial LD as reported from three different institutions.[4,40,41]

The radiographic manifestations of LD consist of alveolar opacities that may be segmental or lobar and unilateral or bilateral. Pleural effusions

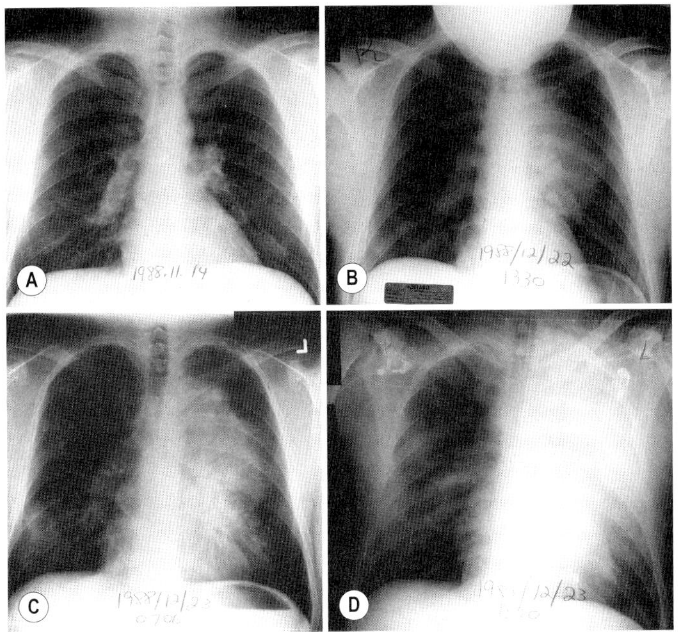

Figure 32.2 **(A–D)** Serial chest radiographs of a 42-year-old man with chronic lymphocytic leukemia who was admitted December 22, 1988, with legionnaires' disease. The rapid progression of the pneumonia is evident. The radiograph dated November 14, 1988 **(A)** was taken when he was well.

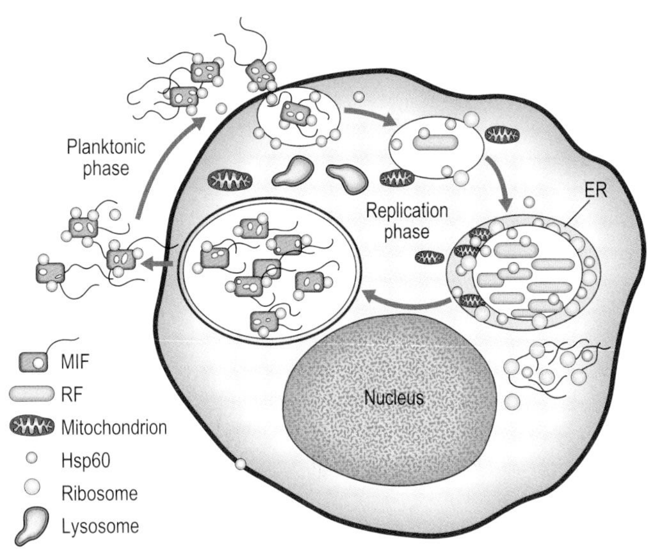

Figure 32.3 *Legionella pneumophila* developmental cycle. *Legionella pneumophila* enters natural hosts and macrophages by phagocytosis. The bacteria are invasive of nonphagocytic cell lines. Depicted are the mature intracellular forms (MIFs) entering a host cell and contained within an endosomal membrane. Displayed on the surface of MIFs that stain red by the Gimenez stain is Hsp60, a surface-associated protein that promotes attachment and invasion. The endosome does not fuse with lysosomes and recruits vesicles, mitochondria, and ribosomes. The *Legionella*-laden endosome becomes surrounded by the endoplasmic reticulum (ER), producing a replication-proficient environment. During this period, MIFs germinate into vegetative replicative forms (RF) and no longer stain red with Gimenez stain. The bacteria initiate rounds of replication, and late in infection the RFs differentiate into the nonreplicating MIFs. Following destruction of the host cell, MIFs are released into the environment. MIFs are initially motile, but they lose motility after 24 hours and further differentiate into a planktonic cyst that can remain infectious for extended periods while between hosts.

occur. Progression of the opacities is common (***Fig. 32.2***). Indeed, in severe LD, progression of the pneumonia continues for 4 or 5 days after institution of appropriate antibiotic therapy. Examination of pulmonary tissue infected by *Legionella* reveals a fibrinopurulent lobar pneumonia or bronchopneumonia.[42] Polymorphonuclear leukocytes, predominantly neutrophils, and macrophages are found within the alveoli. Leukocytoclasis is a common feature. A mixed interstitial inflammatory pattern may accompany the airspace inflammation. Thrombosis of small vessels, septic vasculitis, and alveolar wall necrosis can occur.

PATHOGENESIS AND IMMUNITY

The legionellae are intracellular parasites of protozoa in natural environments, and humans become infected by inhalation of aerosols containing bacteria or amebae laden with the organisms.[43] In the lung, legionellae are phagocytosed by alveolar macrophages, in which they abrogate phagosome–lysosome fusion and replicate in an endosome surrounded by the endoplasmic reticulum.[44] It is generally believed that *Legionella* plies a common infection strategy in both natural hosts and human macrophages,[45] as depicted in ***Figure 32.3***. In this regard, the legionellae are naturally invasive of host cells and rely on a type IV secretion system to deliver effector proteins into their hosts that both alter cell signal transduction pathways and initiate remodeling of the endosome. Once intracellular, the bacteria-laden endosome recruits small vesicles, mitochondria, and ribosomes and within 4–6 hours becomes enveloped by the endoplasmic reticulum, establishing the replicative endosome.[44] Bacterial growth begins at this time and continues in macrophages for ~24 hours, at which time the macrophage disintegrates, and the bacteria are released. Macrophage death results from apoptosis and is mediated by the caspase system and several adaptor molecules.[46] The released bacteria are often phagocytosed by other macrophages, dendritic cells, and epithelial cells, thus perpetuating the infection.

A new developmental form of *L. pneumophila* has been identified and characterized in natural hosts and in nonphagocytic HeLa cell cultures that resembles a cyst or spore.[47,48] It is noteworthy that in a murine model of LD, inoculation of *L. pneumophila*-infected *Hartmannella vermiformis* resulted in an eightfold increase in intrapulmonary *L. pneumophila*.[49] These observations are consistent with reports that *L. pneumophila* harvested from amebae are more infectious upon reinfection than are *in vitro*-grown bacteria. Mature intracellular forms (MIFs) are also approximately 100-fold more infectious than *in vitro*-grown bacteria. Since airborne amebae are found in water aerosols,[8] they may serve as a reservoir or transmission vehicle for delivery of highly infectious MIFs to humans.

Virulence of *Legionella* is considered multifactoral and complex since the bacteria must not only establish the replicative endosome but also acquire all nutrients from the host cell, including amino acids, organic acids, iron, and other micronutrients.[50,60] Avirulent mutants do not replicate in macrophages and are defective in expression of transmission traits that include sensitivity to sodium chloride, osmotic resistance, motility, and surface location of heat shock protein 60 (Hsp60).[52–54] Immunity against *L. pneumophila* requires development of a cellular immune response.[61] Antibodies are not effective against *L. pneumophila* because opsonized bacteria are more efficiently phagocytosed. Interactions of *Legionella* with murine macrophages and dendritic cells also induce an array of cytokines and chemokines. An interleukin-1β (IL-1β) response is produced upon binding of the bacteria to macrophages.[62] Interestingly, IL-12 and interferon-γ (IFN-γ) are commonly detected in serum of infected patients or in animal models, but in macrophage culture *Legionella* specifically represses IL-12 production by macrophages.[63] It is believed that most of the IL-12 is produced by dendritic cells.[64] Among the cytokines detected in murine models or in human infection are IL-1α, IL-1β, IL-4, IL-6, IL-12, and IL-18.

The lack of viable markets for vaccines against *Legionella* has limited research initiatives in this area. In one study, vaccination of guinea pigs with the purified major outer membrane protein OmpS protected guinea pigs against an LD_{100} lethal challenge, whereas immunization with purified Hsp60 provided little protection.[65] Production of IFN-γ has a protective effect by promoting activation of macrophages. Activated macrophages limit the intracellular replication of *Legionella* by decreasing the expression of transferrin receptors and limiting the availability of iron to the bacteria.[66]

Legionella pneumophila serves as a model system for the study of innate immunity because, as a resident in aquatic protozoa, it has not evolved mechanisms to evade the human immune system. Toll-like receptors TLR2, TLR4, TLR5, and TLR9 are activated during infection with *L. pneumophila*.[67] Ironically, human infection represents a dead end or failure in the life cycle of *Legionella* and provides an explanation for why immunocompromised people are so susceptible to infection.[45] Thus, whatever *Legionella* can do to interfere with the host immune system appears to occur by chance and not by the design of evolution.

DIAGNOSIS

A high index of suspicion is necessary in diagnosing sporadic cases of LD. Outbreaks of pneumonia usually trigger a workup for *Legionella*, so these are easier to diagnose.

Isolation of the organism from respiratory secretions is the definitive diagnostic method. Detection of *Legionella* antigen in urine by enzyme-linked immunosorbent assay is approximately 80% sensitive and more than 95% specific.[68,69] This test is readily available for *L. pneumophila* serogroup 1. Diagnostic kits are also available for detection of antigens of *L. pneumophila* 1 to 6. *Legionella* antigen is excreted in the urine for days to weeks (rarely up to 1 year) after the onset of pneumonia.

Demonstration of a fourfold rise in antibody titer between acute and convalescent serum samples using an indirect immunofluorescence whole-cell assay can also be used to diagnose LD. Up to 12 weeks may be required to demonstrate a fourfold rise in antibody, so serology is not useful for the acute management of this disease. A single or static titer of 1 : 256 or greater is no longer considered satisfactory for the diagnosis of LD.[70] Polymerase chain reaction (PCR) applied to respiratory secretions, pulmonary tissue, or pleural fluid is currently undergoing evaluation as a diagnostic method.[71,72] In particular, PCR of material obtained by throat swab is an attractive approach, but the sensitivity and specificity of such a strategy have yet to be defined.

TREATMENT AND PROGNOSIS

Quinolones are the drugs of first choice. Azithromycin is also effective in the treatment of LD.[73] Doxycycline is also active against *L. pneumophila* and has been used to treat LD. Erythromycin used to be considered the drug of choice. It is given in a dose of 1 g intravenously every 6 hours. At this dosage, reversible ototoxicity may occur.[74] Rifampin (300 mg twice daily) orally is given until clinical improvement occurs, at which time it can be discontinued. Relapses occur with treatment of less than 21 days' duration.

Data from a prospective, non-randomized study indicate that levofloxacin (and presumably other quinolones) are superior to macrolides for the treatment of severe LD.[75] In this study carried out in Murcia, Spain, 3.4% of the patients receiving levofloxacin had complications compared with 27.2% of those receiving macrolides; the levofloxacin patients had a shorter length of stay – 5.5 versus 11.3 days. Addition of rifampin to levofloxacin provided no additional benefit. Azithromycin appears to be the best macrolide for the treatment of LD.[73]

Early administration of antibiotics (within 8 hours of admission to hospital) to patients with severe LD has been associated with better outcomes.[76]

PREVENTION AND CONTROL

When cases of nosocomial LD are diagnosed, the potable water distribution system of the hospital should be cultured for *Legionella*. If *Legionella* is found, heating the water to 160°F (70°C) for several days and then flushing hot water throughout all the outlets can result in temporary reduction of the concentration of *Legionella* in the water. Hyperchlorination or the addition of copper and silver ions to the water supply can also control contamination of the potable water and result in cessation of outbreaks of nosocomial LD. If Legionellaceae cannot be eradicated from the water supply, all organ transplant recipients and all those who are receiving corticosteroids should not drink the water and should not shower in the water. In addition, on-site or nearby cooling towers should have the coolant water cultured for *Legionella*.

Outbreaks of LD on board cruise ships and at flower shows emphasize the importance of surveillance for this infection and control of *Legionella* in a variety of water distribution systems.[77]

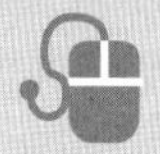

Access the complete reference list online at
http://www.expertconsult.com

Access the complete reference list online at
http://www.expertconsult.com

CHAPTER 33

Melioidosis

Sharon J. Peacock • David A.B. Dance

INTRODUCTION

Melioidosis is an infection caused by the Gram-negative bacillus *Burkholderia pseudomallei*. This disease has emerged over the past 25 years as an important cause of morbidity and mortality in Southeast Asia and northern Australia, and is also endemic in other tropical regions. *B. pseudomallei* has been classified as a "Category B" agent by the US Centers for Disease Control and Prevention.[1]

THE AGENT

Melioidosis was first recognized as a fatal "glanders-like" illness in Burma in 1911 by Alfred Whitmore.[2] The genetic similarity of the causative organism to that of glanders, *B. mallei*, has since been confirmed by multilocus sequence typing and whole genome sequencing.[3–5] Animal and human infections with Whitmore's bacillus were later recognized by Stanton and Fletcher in the Federated Malay States.[6] They considered the disease to be a zoonosis and coined the term melioidosis. Workers in French Indochina subsequently showed that the organism was really an environmental saprophyte.[7] *B. pseudomallei* was previously classified in various genera (e.g., *Malleomyces*, *Pfeifferella*, *Actinobacillus*, *Bacillus*, *Pseudomonas*) but, along with other members of ribosomal RNA (rRNA) homology group II of the genus *Pseudomonas* (e.g., *P. cepacia*), it was assigned to the new genus, *Burkholderia*, by Yabuuchi in 1992.[8]

EPIDEMIOLOGY

Geographic Distribution

The main areas of melioidosis endemicity are Southeast Asia and northern Australia. An estimated 2000–5000 cases occur each year in Thailand,[9] while up to 50 cases are diagnosed annually in both Singapore and Australia. In recent years the known distribution of areas endemic for melioidosis has expanded to include Cambodia, Laos, Vietnam, Indonesia, southern China, the Indian subcontinent, Hong Kong, and Taiwan.[10,11] Sporadic cases have been reported from the Pacific islands, central Africa, Central and South America, and the Caribbean.[10,11] The disease is probably underdiagnosed in many of these regions, because relatively sophisticated laboratory facilities are necessary to confirm the diagnosis. Reports of cases in Iran and an epizootic that occurred in France during the 1970s[12] suggest that infection may be transmitted in nontropical regions.

Reservoirs and Transmission

B. pseudomallei is readily isolated from soil and surface water in endemic areas.[13,14] Humans and a wide range of animals are thought usually to become infected by inoculation or contamination of wounds or mucosae with soil or surface water, although a specific exposural incident is only identified in 6–25% of cases.[15,16] Infections occurred in a disproportionate number of helicopter crewmen during the Vietnam War, possibly through inhalation of aerosols generated by the rotors.[17] Two recent outbreaks in Australia have been traced to potable water supplies, although the mode of transmission was uncertain.[18,19] There is no evidence that insect vectors play a role in transmission. Melioidosis occurs in a wide range of animal species (including rodents, primates, sheep and goats, pigs, cattle, horses, deer, dogs and cats, dolphins, koalas, kangaroos, camels, crocodiles, and birds). Transmission from animals to humans has rarely been reported,[20] and person-to-person spread is also extremely uncommon.[21] Iatrogenic infection from contaminated injections and laboratory-acquired infections have also been reported occasionally, resulting in the classification of *B. pseudomallei* as a Hazard Group 3 pathogen.

Descriptive Epidemiology

Melioidosis predominantly affects people in regular contact with soil and water. In northeast Thailand, melioidosis accounts for 18% of community-acquired septicemias,[22] and in the Northern Territory of Australia it is the commonest cause of fatal community-acquired sepsis.[16] The annual incidence of human melioidosis in Ubon Ratchathani province in northeast Thailand in 2006 was 21.3 per 100 000 population (unpublished data, D. Limmathurotsakul and S. Peacock), which is comparable to figures reported from northern Australia and Papua New Guinea (19.6 and 20.0 per 100 000 population per year, respectively).[23,24] All age groups can develop melioidosis, but incidence peaks between the ages of 40 and 60 years. The male : female ratio is 3 : 2 in Thailand but is higher in Australia and Singapore, probably because of differences in exposure to soil during rice farming. Melioidosis is markedly seasonal in most settings (an exception being Singapore),[25] with approximately 75% of cases presenting during the rainy season and the highest incidence occurring during especially heavy monsoons.[16] Most cases of melioidosis appear to be recently acquired.[26] Risk factors for melioidosis include the presence of diabetes mellitus, chronic renal failure, immunosuppressive treatments including steroids, thalassemia, chronic liver disease, chronic lung disease (including cystic fibrosis), and kava consumption, one or more of which are found in 60–80% of cases.[15,16,27,28] The association with diabetes mellitus is particularly strong and may increase the relative risk of infection by up to 100-fold.[15] There is no evidence that human immunodeficiency virus infection predisposes to melioidosis.[29]

THE DISEASE

The clinical spectrum of *B. pseudomallei* infection is extremely broad, and none of the clinical classifications of melioidosis is entirely satisfactory. Infections may be acute or chronic and localized or disseminated, but one form of the disease may progress to another and individual patients are often difficult to categorize. Several reviews have summarized the clinical manifestations of melioidosis.[2,6,10,16,17,22,30]

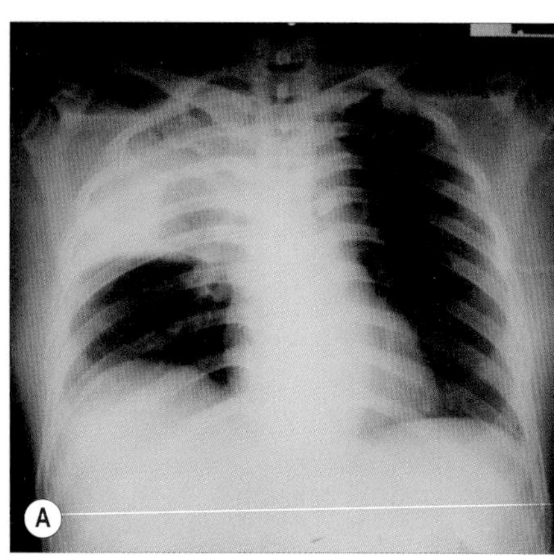

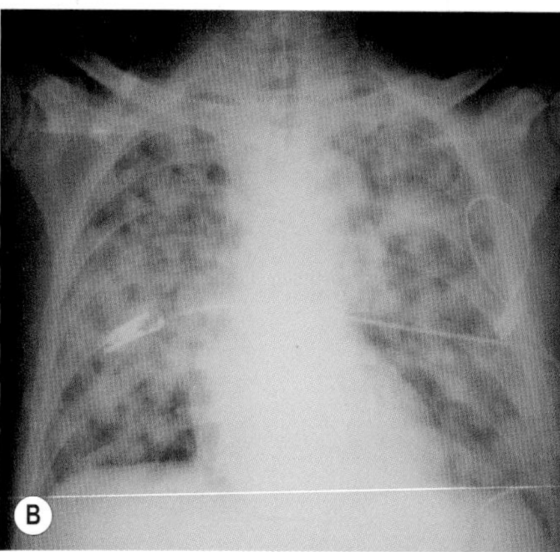

Figure 33.1 Chest radiographs of two patients with melioidosis. **(A)** Right upper lobe consolidation in a patient with bacteremia, pneumonia, pyelonephritis, and subcutaneous abscesses. **(B)** Widespread bilateral shadowing in a patient with bacteremia, pneumonia, and multiple abscesses in the liver and spleen. (From Dance DAB. Melioidosis. In: Cook G, Zumla A, eds. Manson's Tropical Diseases, 22nd ed. London: WB Saunders; 2009.)

Mild and Subclinical Infections

In endemic areas such as northeast Thailand, 80% of children have antibodies to *B. pseudomallei* by the time they are 4 years old.[31] Seroconversion provides evidence of exposure to *B. pseudomallei*, but the clinical consequences are usually asymptomatic or sufficiently trivial not to reach medical attention.

Latent Infections

Long periods of latency have been observed between exposure to *B. pseudomallei* and the onset of clinical features of infection, the maximum recorded being 62 years.[32] The development of infection after prolonged latency usually occurs at times of intercurrent stress (e.g., other acute infections, burns or trauma, malignancies, diabetes mellitus), when cellular immunity is likely to be suppressed. The sites and mechanisms of persistence are unknown, although clinically silent, chronic, localized foci of melioidosis in the lung, liver, or spleen have been reported in animals. The proportion of seropositive patients who harbor latent infection is unknown.

Septicemic Melioidosis

Approximately 50–60% of cases of culture-positive melioidosis have positive blood cultures.[15,16] Most of these present clinically as community-acquired sepsis syndrome, with a short history (median, 6 days; range, 1 day to 2 months) of high fever and rigors, although some have a less acute, typhoidal illness with a swinging fever, often associated with profound weight loss.[22] Patients with multiple, noncontiguous foci of infection, which probably reflect bacteremia at some stage, behave similarly. Only half have evidence of a primary focus of infection, usually in the lung or skin and subcutaneous tissues. Confusion, stupor, jaundice, and diarrhea may also be prominent features. Initial investigations usually reveal anemia, a neutrophil leukocytosis, coagulopathy, and evidence of renal and hepatic impairment. Such patients often deteriorate rapidly, developing widespread metastatic abscesses, particularly in the lungs, liver, and spleen, and metabolic acidosis with Kussmaul's breathing. Once septic shock has supervened, the untreated mortality approaches 95%, with many patients dying within 48 hours of hospital admission. Other poor prognostic features include absence of fever, leukopenia, azotemia, and abnormal liver function tests.[22] A high level of bacteremia (>50 CFU/mL) is associated with a fatal outcome.[33]

If the patient survives this acute phase, the manifestations of the multiple septic foci that result from bacteremic dissemination become prominent. Any site or tissue may be involved, but the most common foci are the lungs, liver, spleen, prostate, and skin and soft tissues. An abnormal chest radiograph is found in 60–80% of patients, the most common pattern being widespread shadowing[34] (*Fig. 33.1*). Multiple liver and splenic abscesses are also common (*Fig. 33.2*). Cutaneous pustules or subcutaneous abscesses occur in 10–20% of cases.[22] Secondary lesions may occur in any other tissue or organ (e.g., kidneys, bones and joints, brain). "Neurological melioidosis," characterized by peripheral motor weakness, brainstem encephalitis, aseptic meningitis, and respiratory failure, is now thought to reflect direct invasion of the central nervous system rather than being toxin-mediated.[16,35]

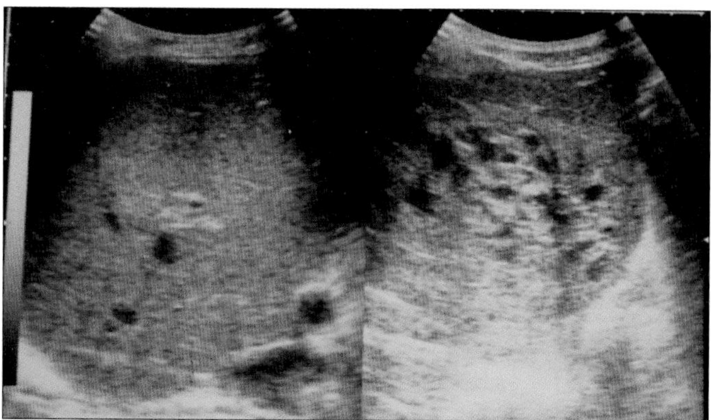

Figure 33.2 Abdominal ultrasound showing multiple liver abscesses in a patient with septicemic melioidosis ("Swiss cheese liver"). A similar picture may be seen in the spleen.

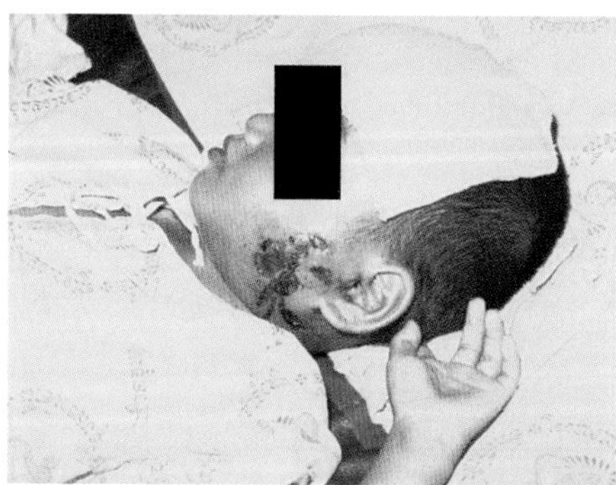

Figure 33.3 Child with suppurative parotitis. In this case the overlying skin is involved, and there is facial nerve palsy.

Localized Melioidosis

Localized melioidosis in the lung can be confused with tuberculosis, with cavitating pneumonia accompanied by profound weight loss.[36] Relative sparing of the apices and the infrequency of hilar adenopathy may help to distinguish the two.[34] There is a predilection for the upper lobes, although any lung zone may be affected. Complications include pneumothorax, empyema, and purulent pericarditis, and ultimately progression to septicemia. Acute suppurative parotitis (*Fig. 33.3*) is a characteristic manifestation of melioidosis in Thai children, accounting for approximately one-third of pediatric cases,[37] but has rarely been reported elsewhere. This strong age–site association probably reflects ascending infection after oral contamination with muddy water. Most cases are unilateral and result in parotid abscesses that require surgical drainage, although they may rupture spontaneously into the auditory canal. Facial nerve palsy and septicemia are rare complications. Other sites include cutaneous and subcutaneous abscesses, lymphadenitis, osteomyelitis and septic arthritis, liver or splenic abscesses, cystitis, pyelonephritis, prostatic abscesses, epididymo-orchitis, keratitis, and brain abscesses.

Pathology

Although *B. pseudomallei* is a pyogenic organism, the pathological features of lesions of melioidosis may vary from an acute, necrotizing inflammation with abscess formation to a chronic granulomatous inflammation, depending on the duration of the infection, and sometimes a mixed picture is seen.[38] It is difficult to make a specific histopathologic diagnosis, but features that may be helpful include the presence of intracellular "globi" of Gram-negative bacilli combined with giant cells against a background of acute necrotizing inflammation.[39]

PATHOGENESIS AND IMMUNITY

Bacterial Virulence Factors

The organism possesses several potential virulence determinants and strains of the organism undoubtedly vary in virulence.[40] Lipopolysaccharide (LPS) is presumably important during septicemia, although the biologic effects of *B. pseudomallei* LPS differ from those of enterobacterial LPS.[41] Polysaccharide capsule is required for virulence in experimental animal models.[42,43] Capsule expression is induced in the presence of serum and appears to interfere with deposition of complement factor C3b on the bacterial cell surface.[43] Other putative virulence determinants include a heat-labile, lethal exotoxin with a molecular weight of approximately 31 kDa,[44] various other toxins and enzymes (e.g., hemolysin, lecithinase, lipase, and proteases),[45] a siderophore (malleobactin),[46] flagella,[47] type IV pili,[48] and a type III secretion system.[49] Six type VI secretion systems have been noted in the *B. pseudomallei* genome,[50] although the investigation of their role in disease pathogenesis has not yet been published. Quorum sensing, a cell-density dependent communication system involved in coordination of gene regulation via *N*-acyl-homoserine lactones, has been described for *B. pseudomallei*, disruption of which leads to reduced bacterial virulence in an animal model.[51] *B. pseudomallei* is able to survive intracellularly,[52] which probably contributes to the recalcitrant nature of melioidosis, its potential for long periods of latency, and its tendency to relapse.[53] Spread between cells occurs via a process involving actin rearrangement into a comet tail appearance within membrane protrusions.[54] A type III secretion system (TTSS3) that shares homology with the *inv/spa/prg* TTSS of *Salmonella enterica* serovar Typhimurium and the *ipa/mxi/spa* TTSS cluster of *Shigella flexneri* appears to play a central role in this process.[49,55]

Host Defense

The innate and adaptive immune response to *B. pseudomallei* has been reviewed in detail elsewhere.[56,57] Evidence from studies in experimental animals suggests that antibodies to exotoxin, LPS, flagellin, flagellin–LPS conjugates, and capsular polysaccharides may all have some protective effect. In human infections, the level of antibody to lipopolysaccharide but not capsular polysaccharide was significantly higher in patients who survived melioidosis than in those who died.[58] Production of interferon-γ appears to be particularly important in protection in some mouse models.[59] The fact that C57BL/6 mice are considerably more resistant to infection by *B. pseudomallei* than BALB/c mice also suggests a role for cellular immunity in host defense.[60] On the other hand, an overaggressive host response may actually contribute to pathogenesis, and raised levels of several proinflammatory cytokines have been found to be associated with a poor outcome in human melioidosis.[61–63]

DIAGNOSIS

Melioidosis is difficult to diagnose on clinical grounds alone, so where possible laboratory confirmation by detection of *B. pseudomallei* should be sought. This requires relatively sophisticated facilities, which are not available in many endemic areas. Because of the potential for latency, the diagnosis should be considered in any patient who has ever visited an endemic area who presents with septicemia or abscesses, particularly if there is evidence of an underlying disease such as diabetes mellitus.

Microscopy and Culture

The organism should be sought in blood, pus, throat swab, sputum, urine, or any other specimen appropriate to the clinical presentation. Microscopy of a Gram-stained smear may reveal bipolar or unevenly staining Gram-negative rods, but this has a low specificity and sensitivity. Direct immunofluorescent microscopy may be helpful in endemic areas, but is not widely available.[64] Isolation and identification of *B. pseudomallei* is diagnostic, since asymptomatic carriage has never been reported. The organism grows readily on most laboratory media, although it may take 48 hours or more to develop characteristic colonial morphology. The sensitivity of culture may be increased by the use of selective media.[65] Culture of a throat swab alone using these selective techniques has an overall sensitivity of 36% for the diagnosis of melioidosis (79% in sputum-positive patients), which is particularly useful in children or others who cannot produce sputum.[66] Identification of cultures may be conducted using conventional biochemical tests, commercial kits, or latex agglutination tests, but may be delayed or incorrect because many microbiologists are not familiar with the characteristics of the organism. Consequently, if melioidosis is suspected, the laboratory should always be warned to ensure that appropriate techniques and containment measures are employed.

Detection of Antigens and Nucleic Acids

Several rapid diagnostic techniques for the detection of *B. pseudomallei* antigens have been developed, but most of these currently have suboptimal sensitivity when used directly on clinical samples and/or are not widely available.[67,68] A conventional polymerase chain reaction (PCR) assay targeting the 16S rRNA gene for the detection of *B. pseudomallei* in clinical specimens was reported to have a high diagnostic sensitivity but lacked specificity.[69] Several real-time PCR assays have been developed,[70–74] and two of these have undergone clinical evaluation for the detection of *B. pseudomallei* in clinical specimens.[73,74] One assay had a diagnostic sensitivity of 91%,[73] but the second had a much lower sensitivity of 61%[74]; the reasons for this disparity are unclear. The diagnostic sensitivity of PCR is highest for pus samples but is low for blood.[73,74] Loop-mediated isothermal amplification (LAMP) has been developed for the detection of *B. pseudomallei*, which on clinical evaluation was shown to have a diagnostic sensitivity of 44%.[75] At the present time, molecular diagnostics are not sufficiently sensitive to replace culture for the diagnosis of melioidosis.

Detection of Antibodies

The serodiagnostic test most widely used in endemic areas is an indirect hemagglutination (IHA) test, which detects antibodies to a mixture of crude heat-stable antigens.[76] The test is poorly standardized, and there is considerable interlaboratory variation between the titers regarded as positive. The IHA and other currently available serologic tests are not useful in regions where melioidosis is endemic because the healthy indigenous population is often seropositive.[31] Serologic testing may have a greater diagnostic utility in persons who do not normally reside in regions endemic for melioidosis, including returning travelers and laboratory workers following accidental laboratory exposure to *B. pseudomallei*.[77] Different IHA titers have been used to infer a positive result, but a single raised titer (>1 :40) in someone from a non-endemic area, or a rising titer, is suggestive of exposure to *B. pseudomallei*. A negative serologic test does not rule out exposure or infection since some patients with culture-proven melioidosis do not have detectable antibodies.[78]

TREATMENT AND PROGNOSIS

Supportive Treatment

Patients with septicemic melioidosis usually require aggressive supportive treatment and should ideally be managed in an intensive care unit. Particular attention should be paid to correction of volume depletion and septic shock, respiratory and renal failure, and hyperglycemia or ketoacidosis. Abscesses should be drained whenever possible.

Specific Treatment

B. pseudomallei is intrinsically resistant to many antibiotics, including aminoglycosides and early β-lactams. Until the mid-1980s, various empirical combination regimens were used to treat melioidosis, usually including a tetracycline, chloramphenicol, and co-trimoxazole. Several more recent studies, which have been well summarized elsewhere,[10,30,79] have provided a sound evidence base for the treatment of severe melioidosis. Treatment comprises two phases: an acute phase, the aim of which is to reduce mortality, and an eradication phase, the aim of which is to reduce the risk of relapse. The mortality of acute severe melioidosis has been substantially reduced by the use of ceftazidime, imipenem, or cefoperazone-sulbactam.[80–85]

A striking reduction in mortality from 95% to 10% in patients with melioidosis shock associated with the use of meropenem plus co-trimoxazole with adjunctive granulocyte colony-stimulating factor (G-CSF) was reported from the Royal Darwin Hospital, northern Australia in 2004.[86] A subsequent randomized, placebo-controlled trial of G-CSF in ceftazidime-treated patients with severe sepsis caused by suspected melioidosis conducted in northeast Thailand did not show a mortality benefit associated with G-CSF therapy.[87]

Ceftazidime 50 mg/kg per dose (up to 2 g) every 6–8 hours, or meropenem 25 mg/kg per dose (up to 1 g) every 8 hours is currently the treatment of choice for melioidosis and should be given for a minimum of 10–14 days, and longer (4–8 weeks) for deep-seated infection according to the clinical response. Trial data do not support the addition of trimethoprim-sulfamethoxazole (TMP-SMX) during this initial phase, although some clinicians elect on grounds of drug penetration to add TMP-SMX 8/40 mg/kg (up to 320/1600 mg) every 12 hours for treatment of patients with neurologic, prostatic, bone, or joint melioidosis. Amoxicillin-clavulanate therapy is an alternative but is associated with a higher failure rate,[88] and ceftriaxone and cefotaxime should not be used.[89]

Following parenteral treatment, prolonged oral antibiotics are needed to prevent relapse, which occurs in up to 23% of patients,[26,53] and is more common in patients with more severe disease. This can be reduced to less than 10% if antibiotics are given for a total of 20 weeks.[90] The current treatment recommendation for oral eradication therapy is TMP-SMX plus doxycycline.[91] TMP-SMX is given every 12 hours using a dose based on weight (2 × 160–800 mg (960 mg) tablets if more than 60 kg; 3 × 80–400 (480 mg) tablets if 40–60 kg; and 1 × 160–800 mg (960 mg) or 2 × 80–400 (480 mg) tablets if adult less than 40 kg). Dosing of doxycycline is 2.5 mg/kg per dose up to 100 mg orally every 12 hours. A clinical trial being conducted in Thailand to determine the equivalence of TMP-SMX with or without doxycycline is nearing completion. Amoxicillin-clavulanate therapy is preferable for oral eradication treatment in children and in pregnant or lactating women, but is associated with a higher rate of relapse compared with TMP-SMX plus doxycycline.[90,92] Consensus guidelines have been developed for dosing of amoxicillin-clavulanate in melioidosis, which in the oral eradication phase should be used at a dose of 20/5 mg/kg three times a day with a maximum dose of 1500/375 mg three times a day for patients >60 kg, and a lower maximum dose for patients <60 kg of 1000/250 mg three times per day.[93] The fluoroquinolones, with or without azithromycin, and doxycycline alone are all associated with unacceptable relapse rates.[92,94–96] In patients with mild localized disease, the preceding oral regimens may be used, although the optimal agents and duration of treatment remain to be defined.

Outcome and Follow-up

Even with optimal treatment, the mortality from acute severe melioidosis is high (30–47%). In patients who survive, there is often chronic morbidity resulting from both the disease itself and the underlying conditions. Patients require long-term follow-up to detect relapse. Susceptibility tests should be carried out on isolates obtained during or after treatment, since resistance may emerge in 5–10% of cases.[97]

PREVENTION AND CONTROL

B. pseudomallei is ubiquitous in the environment in endemic areas, so it is difficult for those whose occupations involve soil and water contact to avoid exposure. Common sense would suggest that those particularly at risk (e.g., diabetic patients) should avoid regular contact with contaminated environments or use hand and foot protection, although the effectiveness of this has not been evaluated. Elimination of the organism from soil using disinfectants was attempted in the French outbreak,[12] but is probably futile. There is no *B. pseudomallei* vaccine licensed for human use, although experimental vaccines are under development and have been used in animals.[98] The organism should be handled in containment level 3 facilities in the laboratory. Patients should ideally be nursed in standard isolation, although person-to-person spread is very rare.

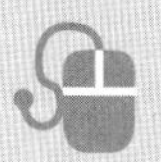

Access the complete reference list online at
http://www.expertconsult.com

Access the complete reference list online at http://www.expertconsult.com

CHAPTER 34

Diphtheria

Anna Kabanova • Rino Rappuoli

INTRODUCTION

Diphtheria is caused by infection with the Gram-positive bacillus *Corynebacterium diphtheriae* which carries a lysogenic bacteriophage containing the gene coding for diphtheria toxin. Toxinogenic strains produce a powerful exotoxin that is responsible for the most severe manifestations of the disease. Thanks to successful vaccination with a nontoxic form of diphtheria toxin, today diphtheria is a rare disease and most physicians have never seen one case. Recent outbreaks in Russia indicate that, in the absence of effective vaccination, the disease can come back quickly.

Prior to the introduction of effective childhood vaccination programs, diphtheria was a major cause of childhood mortality. In 1884, Löffler reported isolation of the organism from patients with diphtheria and demonstration of its pathogenicity in animals.[1] He hypothesized that a potent poison was formed at the site of the local lesion because the organism was usually found only in the site of inoculation in the respiratory tract. In 1888, Roux and Yersin[2] reported that sterile filtrates from cultures of the diphtheria bacillus were lethal to guinea pigs, with development of lesions identical to those found in animals infected with the organism. This was followed by the demonstration of immunity in animals that had received iodine-treated toxin, and the passive transfer of this immunity to other animals by Von Behring in 1890.[3] In 1894, Roux and Martin used equine antitoxin for treatment of children, with a dramatic reduction in mortality.[4] The first vaccines were mixtures of toxin and antitoxin; these were replaced by diphtheria toxoid in the 1920s.

The organism is usually transmitted by direct person-to-person contact. Both symptomatic persons with diphtheria and asymptomatic carriers can transmit the organism, although symptomatic persons are thought to be more highly infectious than carriers. Transmission by fomites may occur, and milk-borne outbreaks have been reported (***Fig. 34.1***).

THE AGENT

Corynebacteria are taxonomically related to the mycobacteria and *Nocardia*. *C. diphtheriae* is a pleomorphic, nonmotile, Gram-positive bacillus. A selective medium containing tellurite is essential for primary isolation. Four biotypes – gravis, mitis, intermedius, and belfanti – can be distinguished based on colonial morphology on tellurite blood agar and biochemically.[5]

Although other virulence factors exist, the most significant virulence factor is diphtheria toxin, a 58-kDa protein produced by strains carrying β-corynebacteriophage. The phage encodes the toxin, and nontoxigenic strains can be converted to toxin production by this phage.[6] Lysogenic *C. diphtheriae* strains produce diphtheria toxin only when the medium is depleted of iron. The chromosome of *C. diphtheriae* contains two specific recombination sites, and allows the stable integration of two copies of corynephage DNA in the bacterial genome. Because each phage carries one copy of the *tox* gene, double lysogens produce twice the toxin produced by monolysogens. As discussed later, this feature has been very important for obtaining strains hyperproducing CRM197, a nontoxic form of diphtheria toxin, that has been proposed as a new vaccine candidate.[7,8]

Rarely, other *Corynebacterium* species (*C. pseudotuberculosis* and *C. ulcerans*) can produce toxin. Sequence analysis of 16S ribosomal RNA has demonstrated that these species are closely related to *C. diphtheriae*.[9]

EPIDEMIOLOGY

Due to the high mortality rate and frequency of infections, diphtheria was one of the first infectious diseases for which mass vaccination was implemented. Prompted by outbreaks after World War II, the World Health Organization (WHO) introduced routine immunization of infants and young children in industrialized countries. This immunization led to dramatic reductions in diphtheria cases and, remarkably, even eliminated the circulation of toxigenic *C. diphtheriae* among individuals.[10] In developing countries, diphtheria toxoid was included in the Expanded Programme on Immunization beginning in the 1970s. Vaccination coverage of infants with three doses of diphtheria toxoid in developing countries rose from 5% in 1974 to 79% by 1992.[11] Between 70 000 and 90 000 cases of diphtheria were reported each year during the 1970s to WHO; by the 1990s, this had decreased to 22 000–27 000 cases each year, representing a decrease worldwide of about 70% over a 20-year period. The reduction in reported cases of diphtheria globally during this period was largely due to reductions in reported cases of diphtheria in developing countries.[12] Global vaccination coverage of infants rose from 75% in 1990 to 91% in 2007.[13]

The consequence of the successful diphtheria vaccination was a decreased attention to vaccination and to the disease itself. However, immunity against diphtheria in the adult population has decreased, and large segments of adults in many industrialized countries have been reported to have antibody titers below the protective level of 0.01 IU/mL and, consequently, to be susceptible to diphtheria.[6,11] Outbreaks of diphtheria in immunized populations started to occur when toxinogenic strains, imported from the countries in which diphtheria was still endemic, were introduced in an adult population that did not receive boosters of diphtheria toxoid after the basic vaccination in childhood. The number of diphtheria cases has strikingly increased from the mid-1980s in several countries in Eastern Europe. Furthermore, a massive epidemic of diphtheria in the Russian Federation in the mid-1990s caused approximately 125 000 cases and 4000 deaths.[14] Molecular typing has demonstrated that the outbreak was associated with the emergence of an epidemic clone of *C. diphtheriae* biotype gravis in Russia, although other strains circulated concurrently.[15] In response to the epidemic, vaccine coverage of both children and adults has increased in most countries of the former Soviet Union, and the incidence of disease has been dramatically reduced. Although clinical diphtheria is now rare in most developed countries,

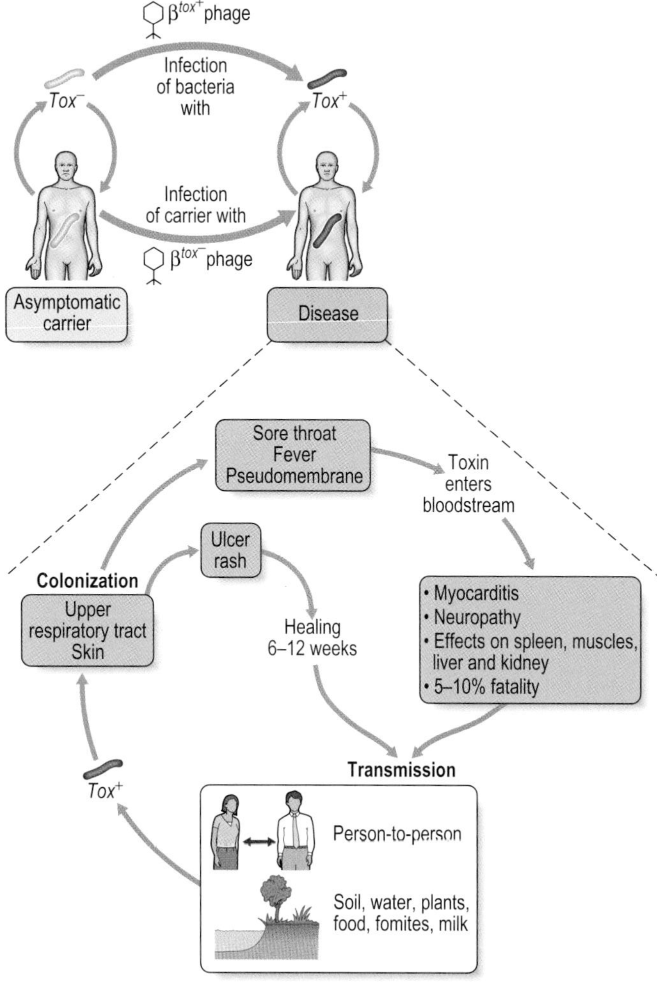

Figure 34.1 Life cycle of *Corynebacterium diphtheriae*.

circulation of *C. diphtheriae* may persist in selected populations within those countries.[16]

Diphtheria epidemics among adolescents and young adults have also been reported in a number of countries such as Jordan, Lesotho, Algeria, China, Ecuador, and Afghanistan.[16,17] The common features of these epidemics are that they occurred following a period of high immunization coverage among young children and that cases of diphtheria were predominantly reported among adolescents and young adults, populations not covered by the immunization program.[11] The current epidemiological situation matches the incidence rates of disease with the infant vaccination coverage level (***Fig. 34.2***). The main countries of Southeast Asia still report vaccination coverage below 90% and this coincided with more than 6000 cases in India, Indonesia, and Nepal in 2008.[13]

In temperate climates, epidemics of respiratory diphtheria are seen in susceptible populations, with a seasonal increase in the fall and winter. Mortality rates of 5–10% are typically reported. In endemic areas of tropical climates and subtropical climates, cutaneous infection is thought typically to occur repeatedly in childhood, conferring immunity. Because toxin is poorly absorbed from cutaneous sites, severe manifestations of diphtheria toxin are infrequent.[16]

Group A *Streptococcus* is frequently isolated from cases of both respiratory and cutaneous diphtheria. It is unknown if one infection predisposes to the other, or if they are frequently co-isolated, because both infections may be associated with similar risk factors.

THE DISEASE

Following an incubation period of 2–5 days, the illness begins with malaise, sore throat, anorexia, and low-grade fever. The hallmark of respiratory diphtheria is the pseudomembrane (***Fig. 34.3***), which may be seen in the posterior oropharynx, and may extend into the larynx or trachea or upward into the nose. The pseudomembrane is composed of fibrin, cellular debris, and bacteria and may be white, gray, or black, and is typically firmly adherent, resulting in bleeding if forcibly removed. Soft-tissue swelling of the neck results in the so-called bull-necked appearance. In vaccinated persons, the membrane may be follicular and nonconfluent.

The most serious complications of diphtheria are respiratory obstruction, if the membrane is extensive, and complications due to distant

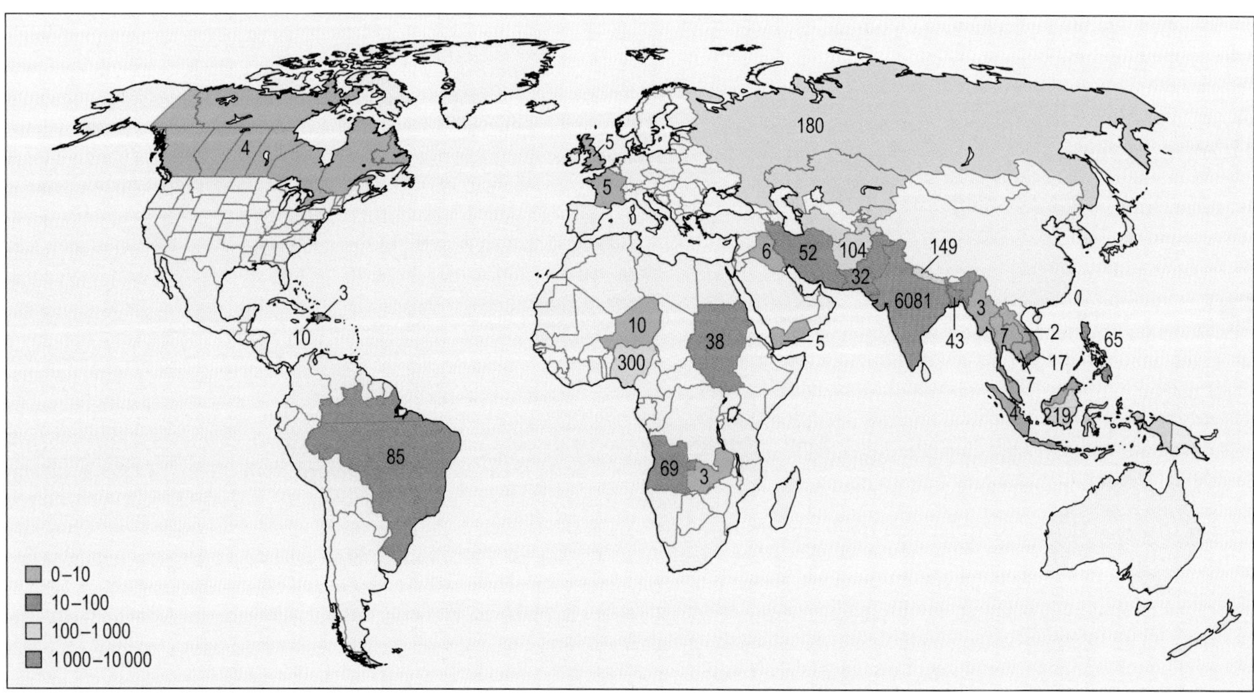

Figure 34.2 Diphtheria incidence according to World Health Organization statistics, years 2007–2008.

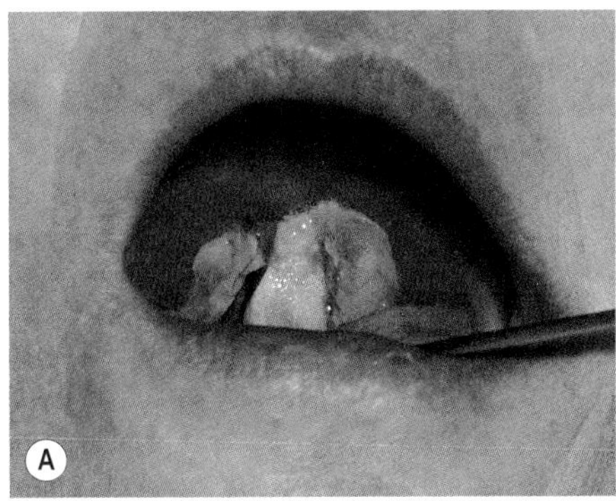

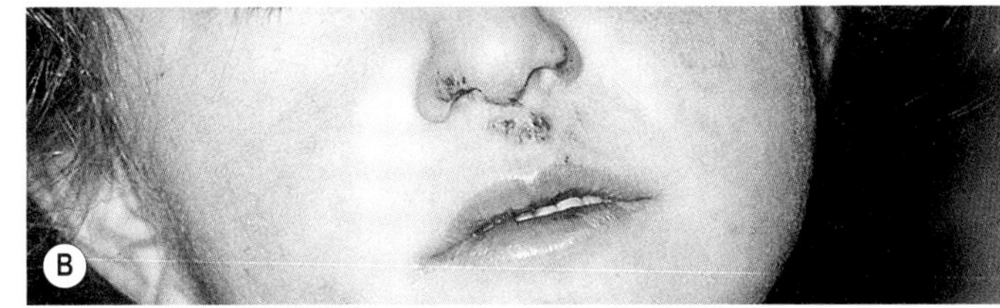

Figure 34.3 (A) Pseudomembrane in a patient with respiratory diphtheria. (Courtesy of Dr Peter Strebel, Centers for Disease Control and Prevention, Atlanta, GA.) **(B)** Cutaneous diphtheria in a child with nasal diphtheria. (Courtesy of Dr Linda Quick, Centers for Disease Control and Prevention, Atlanta, GA.)

effects of the toxin, most commonly myocarditis or neuropathy.[18] Myocarditis typically occurs 7–14 days after onset of disease. The most common electrocardiographic complications are flattening and inversion of T waves, ST-segment changes, and conduction abnormalities, including complete heart block. The prognosis appears to be worse in cases of diphtheria myocarditis with conduction disturbances or ventricular ectopy.[19] Permanent cardiac damage due to diphtheria myocarditis is rare, but recovery may be prolonged. Pathologically, scattered foci of hyaline and granular degeneration are seen early in the course, followed by fibrosis.

Neuropathy may be seen either early or late in the course of illness. Palatal neuropathy and other cranial nerve palsies are often seen early in the course – as early as the first week of illness – while ocular palsies, diaphragmatic paralysis, and paralysis of limbs are generally seen later in the course of illness. Electrophysiologic studies demonstrate slowing of conduction, prolongation of distal motor latency, and, in severe cases, conduction block. Diaphragmatic paralysis may necessitate ventilatory support. If the patient survives, ultimately complete recovery is expected. Pathologic changes include segmental demyelination of nerve fibers within sensory ganglia and demyelination of adjacent peripheral nerves and anterior and posterior roots.

Other complications include renal failure, thrombocytopenia, and coagulation abnormalities. Disseminated intravascular coagulation may occur in severe cases.

Cutaneous diphtheria may occur as a secondary infection following impetigo, other skin infections, or injury. Primary diphtheria typically begins as a vesicle or pustule that progresses to a punched-out ulcer, most commonly seen on the extremities. Lesions may be single or multiple. The ulcer initially is painful and covered with a dark pseudomembrane, but later becomes anesthetic. Healing usually occurs spontaneously over 6–12 weeks, but the course may be more prolonged.[20] Complications due to systemic absorption of diphtheria toxin may be seen, but are uncommon. Cutaneous diphtheria is more common in tropical and subtropical areas than in temperate areas.

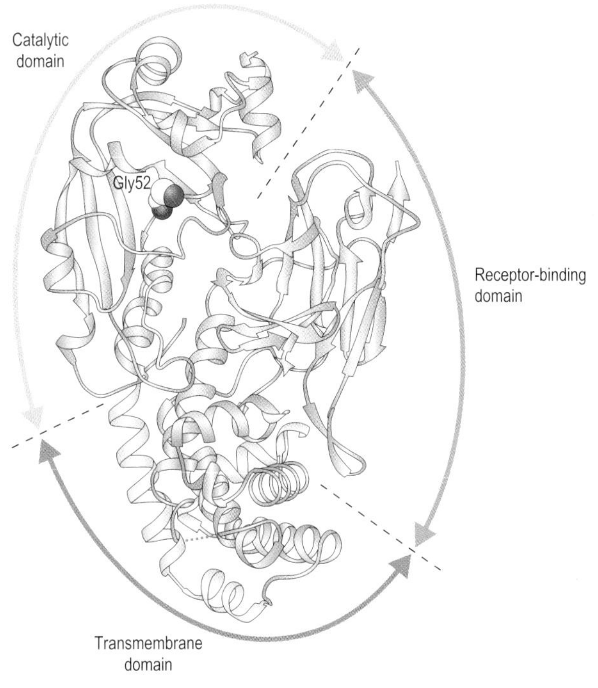

Figure 34.4 Three-dimensional structure of the functional domains of diphtheria toxin. High-lighted amino acid glycine in position 52 is substituted with glutamine in the CRM197 variant. (Redrawn from Broker M, Dull PM, Rappuoli R, et al. Chemistry of a new investigational quadrivalent meningococcal conjugate vaccine that is immunogenic at all ages. Vaccine. 2009;27:5574–5580.)

Diphtheria Toxin: Pathogenicity and Application for Vaccine Development

Diphtheria toxin is a 58.350-Da protein comprising 535 amino acid residues. It is synthesized as a single polypeptide, but in its active form is proteolyzed to two polypeptide chains linked by a disulfide bond. The C-terminal B fragment (345 residues) contains the transmembrane and receptor-binding domains, and the N-terminal A fragment (190 residues) contains the catalytic domain (***Fig. 34.4***).[21] On the cell surface, diphtheria toxin binds to heparin-binding epidermal growth factor precursor, and the toxin–receptor complex undergoes receptor-mediated endocytosis. The A fragment is then translocated across the endocytic membrane into the cytosol. Once in the cytosol, the catalytic domain catalyzes the transfer of adenosine diphosphate (ADP) ribose from nicotinamide adenine dinucleotide (NAD) to elongation factor-2, halting protein synthesis and resulting in cell death.[22] Although diphtheria toxin is the major virulence factor in *C. diphtheriae,* other virulence factors exist. Nontoxigenic *C. diphtheriae* strains can cause typical respiratory diphtheria with pseudomembrane, although toxin-related complications such as myocarditis and neuropathy are not seen. Invasive disease due to nontoxigenic strains of *C. diphtheriae* is well documented.[23]

In 1920s, the introduction by Ramon and Glenny of an effective method to inactivate toxins fully by formaldehyde treatment permitted the introduction of the diphtheria toxoid as a vaccine component of common use.[24,25] Briefly, the crude supernatant of the hypertoxigenic *C. diphtheriae* strain PW8 grown in a fermenter is treated with 0.75% formaldehyde or glutaraldehyde, and kept at 37°C for 4–6 weeks to allow complete detoxification of diphtheria toxin.[6] Formaldehyde treatment induces cross-linkage between an ε-amino group of lysine and another amino acid-reactive group, leading to the intermolecular and intramolecular protein cross-linking. Under these circumstances, the antigen purity is never higher than 60–70% due to covalent coupling of contaminant small peptides to the toxin molecules. To avoid this problem, alternatively, diphtheria toxin can be first purified (85–95%). While removing the toxicity, the treatment also changes the epitopes of the molecule with a potential reduction of the immunogenicity and protective efficacy of the toxoid.

To avoid the issue, a number of mutants that had lost toxicity were generated in the 1970s. These proteins were called cross-reacting material (CRM), since they were immunologically related to diphtheria toxin. Of the different diphtheria toxin mutants obtained by nitrosoguanidine or by site-directed mutagenesis, CRM197 is the most popular (***Fig. 34.4***). This mutant is completely devoid of enzymatic activity due to the single amino acid substitution (Gly52→Glu mutation) and can be easily obtained with a purity above 95%. The isolation of a strain of *C. diphtheriae* (C7) containing two phages stably integrated into the chromosome permitted optimization of the system for CRM197 production.[8] The stability and immunogenicity of CRM197 were additionally increased when the molecule was subjected to a very mild treatment with formaldehyde; in other terms it required only 1/100 of the formalin needed for inactivation of the wild-type antigens.[7]

Consequently, CRM197 effectively elicited neutralizing immunity during clinical trials.[26] It has not been able to replace diphtheria toxoid in the vaccine against diphtheria. However, its high purity and well-proven safety made this molecule the ideal carrier for polysaccharide conjugate vaccines. Today CRM197 is the carrier for licensed conjugate vaccines against *Haemophilus influenzae*, pneumococcus, and meningococcus, and is used to vaccinate most children globally.[27–29]

DIAGNOSIS, TREATMENT, AND PROGNOSIS

The diagnosis of diphtheria is often made initially on clinical grounds. Because of the importance of early treatment with diphtheria antitoxin, clinicians should not wait for laboratory confirmation to initiate treatment.

The diagnosis is confirmed by isolation of *C. diphtheriae* from the site of infection by growing it on the tellurite-containing selective medium. For evaluation of patients with suspected respiratory diphtheria, both nasopharyngeal and throat swabs should be obtained. For suspected cases of diphtheria infection of nonrespiratory sites, the lesion swab is taken. Once isolated, the organism should be characterized by biotype and evaluated for production of toxin. The standard method of toxigenicity testing is the Elek immunoprecipitation test. A polymerase chain reaction (PCR) assay for the *tox* and *dtxR* genes has been developed. PCR may be performed directly on clinical specimens, providing a rapid confirmatory test.[30]

The differential diagnosis of respiratory diphtheria includes bacterial and viral pharyngitis, infectious mononucleosis, Vincent's angina, acute epiglottitis, and peritonsillar abscess.

The mainstay of treatment of diphtheria is diphtheria antitoxin. Because diphtheria antitoxin does not neutralize intracellular diphtheria toxin, it is essential that it be given as early in the course of illness as possible; prognosis clearly worsens the later in the course of illness that antitoxin is administered. Available preparations of diphtheria antitoxin are of equine origin and may produce immediate or delayed reactions. A history of prior horse serum exposure or allergy should be obtained and hypersensitivity test performed.[31] If the patient is sensitive to horse serum, the indications for use of diphtheria antitoxin should be reevaluated. If antitoxin is indicated, the patient should be desensitized; standard protocols for desensitization are published.[32]

If there is no history of hypersensitivity to equine serum and the sensitivity test is negative, the total recommended dose of antitoxin should be given without delay. The dose is determined by the site and extent of local disease and the severity and duration of illness. For anterior nasal diphtheria, 10 000–20 000 units of diphtheria antitoxin is recommended, with increasing doses for the tonsillar form (15 000–25 000 units), pharyngeal or laryngeal diphtheria of 48 hours' or less duration (20 000–40 000 units), nasopharyngeal disease (40 000–60 000 units), and extensive disease of greater than 3 days' duration or with brawny swelling of the neck (80 000–120 000 units).[33] The preferred route of administration is intravenous, because peak antitoxin levels may not be reached for several days following intramuscular administration. The patient should be carefully monitored during administration of antitoxin and the infusion stopped if there are signs of shock. During the testing or infusion of diphtheria antitoxin, a 1:100–1:1000 solution of epinephrine should be available and ready for emergency use if needed.

Toxin-mediated complications are uncommon in cutaneous diphtheria, but have occurred. Use of antitoxin may be indicated in patients with extended, multiple pseudomembranous lesions.[20]

Although antimicrobial agents are of secondary importance in the treatment of diphtheria, they will hasten clearing of the organism and may result in less risk of transmission of diphtheria to others. Agents of choice are penicillin or erythromycin, which are highly active against *C. diphtheriae.* Until the patient can swallow easily, parenteral administration is recommended, with dosages of intramuscular procaine penicillin G (25 000–50 000 units/kg/day for children and 1.2 million units/day for adults in two divided doses) or parenteral erythromycin (40–50 mg/kg/day with a maximum dosage of 2 g/day). Once the patient can swallow easily, oral erythromycin in four divided doses or oral penicillin 125–250 mg four times a day can be substituted to complete the 14-day course of therapy.[16] In mild cases, oral therapy may be used for the complete course of treatment. Erythromycin resistance has been reported in areas where erythromycin has been used widely for treatment of cutaneous diphtheria; likewise, tetracycline and rifampin resistance have also been reported.[34]

Without antitoxin treatment, respiratory diphtheria is frequently fatal, with case-fatality rates of 30–50% reported. With the introduction of diphtheria antitoxin for treatment of diphtheria, mortality has decreased to 5–10% in most series. In diphtheria, receipt of antitoxin within the first 2–3 days of illness is clearly associated with reduced mortality. Disease in vaccinated persons is usually mild.

PREVENTION AND CONTROL

Once a case is recognized, the following measures are recommended to limit further spread. Strict isolation should be maintained until elimination of the organism is demonstrated by negative cultures of two samples obtained at least 24 hours apart after completion of antimicrobial therapy. Close contacts should be identified and evaluated for signs and symptoms of diphtheria. As soon as nasopharyngeal and pharyngeal swabs are obtained for culture, antimicrobial prophylaxis should be administered regardless of prior vaccination status. Recommended regimens include a single dose of intramuscular benzathine penicillin G (600 000 units for children less than 6 years of age and 1.2 million units for persons older than 6 years of age) or a 7–10-day course of oral erythromycin (40 mg/kg/day for children and 1 g/day for adults). Although there is some evidence that erythromycin may be more effective at eradication of the carrier state than penicillin, a single dose of benzathine penicillin administered intramuscularly may be preferred if compliance is in doubt. Persons who continue to harbor the organism after treatment with either agent should receive an additional 10-day course of erythromycin and follow-up cultures should be obtained. Vaccination status of contacts should be assessed and, if indicated, vaccine administered. Surveillance of close contacts should be maintained for at least 7 days, but hospitalization in the absence of clinical illness is not indicated.[35] Reporting of cases of diphtheria to public health authorities is required by law in many countries.

Vaccination of infants with diphtheria toxoid in combination with tetanus toxoid and whole-cell pertussis vaccines (DTP) in many countries of the world has resulted in dramatic reductions in diphtheria incidence globally. Today 117 countries (61% globally) achieved over 90% vaccination coverage of infants with three doses of diphtheria toxoid.[13] Successful pediatric vaccination programs against diphtheria have resulted in high levels of immunity in this age group; however frequent booster vaccinations are required to maintain herd immunity in the adult population.[11,36]

In developing countries, the highest priority for diphtheria prevention and control is to reach a high coverage rate for the primary series of three doses of DTP in infants. In endemic areas, infant immunization will protect young children from diphtheria, although it will not prevent continued circulation of the organism, and immunity of older children and adults will be maintained by reexposure.[8]

Diphtheria toxoid is administered to children less than 7 years of age with tetanus toxoid and acellular pertussis vaccine (DTaP); DTaP may also be combined with other vaccines in combination vaccines that decrease the number of injections that need to be administered simultaneously.[37,38] US immunization authorities recommend that children receive DTaP at 2, 4, and 6 months of age, with booster doses at 15–18 months and 4–6 years. Adult formulation tetanus and diphtheria toxoids (Td) are recommended every 10 years, beginning at age 11–12 years. Travelers to diphtheria-endemic areas are at risk of contracting diphtheria and should be age-appropriately immunized prior to travel.[39] With the increasing number of doses of diphtheria toxin that are now recommended, reactogenicity is likely to increase. Although further purification of extraneous proteins residing in the toxoid may help to ameliorate this problem, optimal future diphtheria vaccines should provide protection of longer duration, with fewer injections. Genetically detoxified pertussis and diphtheria toxoids are thought to provide a safer DTaP vaccine that contains lower amounts of proteins and that induces equal or higher levels of specific antibodies.[6]

While the present vaccine made by diphtheria toxoid is quite satisfactory, future developments may be the substitution of DTaP components with new recombinant antigens, the development of new administration modes and vaccine combination with modern adjuvants. In developing countries, where vaccination is not yet fully practiced and the disease is still responsible for a remarkable percentage of deaths, development of a single-dose vaccination may solve the logistic difficulty of delivering multiple doses necessary to give protection.

Access the complete reference list online at
http://www.expertconsult.com

CHAPTER 35

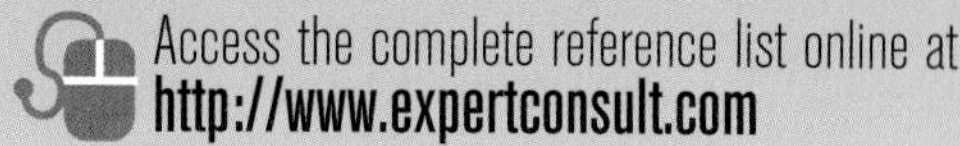
Access the complete reference list online at
http://www.expertconsult.com

Tuberculosis and Atypical Mycobacterial Infections

Edward C. Jones-Lopez • Jerrold J. Ellner

INTRODUCTION

Tuberculosis (TB) is a chronic necrotizing granulomatous disease caused by the acid-fast bacillus *Mycobacterium tuberculosis* or the closely related species *M. bovis* and *M. africanum*. It is spread primarily by inhalation of aerosolized infectious droplet nuclei from patients with active pulmonary TB. The lungs are the main portal of entry. The most common manifestation of TB in humans is pulmonary disease, but nearly all organ systems can be involved. The most frequent sites of extrapulmonary disease are the lymph nodes, pleura, and bones and joints. Although TB occurs worldwide, more than 95% of cases and 98% of deaths occur in developing countries. Miliary and meningeal TB in children and TB occurring in human immunodeficiency virus (HIV)-coinfected people are important causes of death in areas of high prevalence. The emergence of multidrug-resistant (MDR) and extensively drug-resistant (XDR) TB poses a threat to global health. Advances in diagnostics, therapies and vaccines may provide the necessary new tools to impact effectively on TB control. *M. bovis* is still a significant cause of human disease in developing countries.

THE AGENT

M. tuberculosis is a slender nonmotile bacillus approximately 2–4 μm in length. It is an obligate aerobic organism and grows best in tissues with high ambient oxygen tensions, such as the apices of the lung or the renal cortex. The cell wall consists of a waxy coat containing mycolic acid and other complex lipopolysaccharides. This unique cell wall gives members of the genus *Mycobacterium* their characteristic acid-fast staining property and is increasingly associated with its propensity to evade the immune system and strain-specific virulence.[1] After staining with carbol fuchsin, mycobacteria are not decolorized by washing with acid alcohol. Mycobacteria take up other stains, such as Gram's stain, poorly. *M. tuberculosis* typically appears as a slender solid or beaded organism, and virulent strains are often aggregated in clumps in culture. The complete genome of a virulent laboratory strain of *M. tuberculosis* H37Rv was the first to be sequenced,[2] leading to new knowledge about the pathogenesis and virulence of TB and promising to accelerate the identification of new targets for diagnostic testing, treatment, and vaccine development. The sequencing of multiple strains of *M. tuberculosis* and speciation by the study of single nucleotide polymorphisms (SNPs) has allowed grouping into six major SNP-cluster groups and five subgroups[3] and subtypes. Heterogeneity of the organism may explain differences in immunopathogenesis and clinical manifestations of TB.

M. africanum can be reliably distinguished from *M. tuberculosis* only by biochemical testing. The clinical features, drug susceptibility, and outcomes of *M. africanum* disease are similar to those of *M. tuberculosis*. The bovine tubercle bacillus, *M. bovis*, shares greater than 95% DNA homology with *M. tuberculosis* and causes disease in humans, cattle, deer, badgers, and other animals. Speciation can be performed only by specialized laboratories. Most strains are niacin positive, do not reduce nitrate, and are resistant to pyrazinamide.

TB is predominantly spread by droplet nuclei that are generated during coughing and sneezing by people with active pulmonary TB. Direct transmission by heavily infected body secretions from fistulas and skin lesions occurs infrequently. Cutaneous TB from direct inoculation occurs rarely in pathologists ("prosecutor's wart") and laboratory workers. Fomites (eating utensils, clothing, and bedding) play no role in TB transmission among humans. Large-droplet nuclei rapidly settle out of air currents or are removed by the mucociliary ladder in the upper airway and present little danger. Bacteria in small droplets are rapidly killed by drying and exposure to ultraviolet light. Tubercle bacilli in droplet nuclei measuring 1–5 mm in diameter remain suspended in air for long periods, where they can be inhaled and reach the distal airspaces to establish a primary focus of infection. The number of bacilli needed to produce infection is low; infection in humans may occur when as few as one to five bacilli impact in a terminal alveolus.

The risk of infection is related to the duration and severity of exposure to infectious droplet nuclei. The length of exposure must generally be prolonged; brief casual exposures usually do not result in infection.[4] On the other hand, even protracted and intense exposure of household contacts only leads to transmission of infection in about 50% of exposed persons.[5] The density of infectious droplet nuclei in the air in proximity to an active TB case is related to the smear status of the index case (bacillary density), cough frequency and cough strength, the presence of cavitary lung disease, and the number of air exchanges (ventilation) in the area. Because up to 1000–10 000 acid-fast bacilli (AFB) per milliliter of sputum must be present for a positive AFB smear,[6] smear-positive people are the most important sources of transmission of TB in the community. Recent studies suggest that even strongly smear positive cases differ in their ability to generate aerosols containing viable organisms (K. Fennelly and E. Jones López, unpublished observations). Different studies have indicated that 30–60% of people heavily exposed to smear-positive individuals with pulmonary TB become infected. For programmatic purposes, AFB smear-negative patients usually are considered to be noninfectious. In fact, they may account for up to 17% of new cases.[7] Crowded housing also leads to increased transmission of TB due to repeated and prolonged exposure and decreased air exchanges. Most transmission of TB occurs in household contacts – that is, people living in the same residence with an infectious smear-positive case. Intimate contact such as sharing a bed with a patient with TB poses the greatest risk. Outbreaks of TB have occurred in settings where HIV-infected people congregate such as residential shelters, prisons, and hospitals.[8]

EPIDEMIOLOGY

TB is a major global health problem. Up to one-third of the world's population is believed to be infected with *M. tuberculosis*, based on tuberculin skin test (TST) surveys. The World Health Organization (WHO) estimates that 9.27 million new TB cases occurred in 2007, and TB is the second leading cause of death due to an identified infectious pathogen worldwide, exceeded only by HIV/AIDS.[9–11] Fifty-five percent of cases occurred in Asia and 31% in Africa. India contributes 2 million cases and China over 1 million cases; 1.37 million or 15% occurred in the HIV-infected, 79% of which were in Africa. There were 1.3 million deaths in HIV-uninfected and 456 000 deaths in HIV-infected people (the latter representing 33% of all HIV-infected deaths). Up to 7% of all deaths and 26% of preventable deaths in developing countries are due to TB.[12,13] There were approximately 0.5 million cases of MDR TB and 55 countries reported at least one case of XDR TB. TB predominantly affects young adults in their most productive years of life and has substantial impact on economic development. It is also increasingly an urban problem. Two-thirds of the world's population will live in cities by 2025; many will live in crowded, substandard housing with poor ventilation in large cities in developing countries in Asia and Africa.

Tuberculosis and Human Immunodeficiency Virus Interactions

HIV infection currently is the greatest risk factor known for the progression of latent *M. tuberculosis* infection to active TB (reactivation or postprimary TB) and for the rapid progression of new infection (primary TB). Thirty to 40% of all new TB cases in many African countries occur in HIV-coinfected people, with rates as high as 60–70% in some eastern and southern African nations.[10] Increasing rates of HIV coinfection in countries such as Botswana have led to rapid increases in the incidence of TB despite the introduction of more effective TB treatment strategies using the directly observed therapy, short course strategy.[14] Globally, approximately 15% of all new TB cases – more than double the percentage in 1990 – occur in HIV-infected people.[2,9,10]

The lifetime cumulative risk of developing active TB in HIV-infected people is markedly higher than the 5–10% lifetime risk in TST-positive HIV-uninfected people.[15,16] The increased risk begins within the first year after HIV infection and is sustained for at least the first 4–5 years after HIV infection; the relative risk of TB is 2.9 despite the absence of overt immunosuppression.[17] The rapid increase in risk following HIV infection is associated with an early depletion of *M. tuberculosis*-specific T-helper 1 (Th1) cells in peripheral blood,[18] most likely a consequence of the massive loss of CD4 T cells from gut-associated lymphoid tissue that occurs immediately after HIV infection.[19] The reported risk of developing active TB in TST-positive HIV-infected people is 8% per year.[13–16] Increasing TB cases among HIV-infected people also pose a threat to public health because TB can be spread to both HIV-infected and HIV-noninfected people in the community. Some suggest that little transmission occurs from HIV-infected people because of a relatively short period of infectiousness prior to diagnosis and treatment or demise.[20,21] Other factors that may play a role in reduced transmission from HIV-infected people is the greater proportion with pulmonary TB that are sputum smear negative and the fall in AFB density with CD4 count in smear positives.[22] However, because transmission may ultimately depend on several factors such as environmental conditions, bacillary load, cough strength and frequency, and the rheology of secretions (K. Fennelly and E. Jones-López, unpublished observations), there is conflicting evidence about whether HIV-infected patients are equally infectious as HIV-uninfected TB patients.[23]

The clinical manifestations of TB in HIV-coinfected people are highly dependent on which infection occurs first and the degree of immunosuppression. In developing countries with a high prevalence of TB, many people become infected with *M. tuberculosis* during childhood and early adolescence. Most will not develop active TB after primary infection but will enter a prolonged period of clinical latency. People with latent TB infection who later become coinfected with HIV have a subsequent 5–8% annual risk of developing reactivation TB, resulting in a 40–70% cumulative lifetime risk of TB disease. The risk depends on the severity of HIV-related immunosuppression and the activity of the latent focus. TB developing early after HIV infection when CD4 counts are high presents predominantly as pulmonary disease with typical clinical and radiographic manifestations. With advanced HIV-related immunosuppression, the presentation becomes more atypical (lower lobe non-cavitating infiltrates and intrathoracic adenopathy) with an increase in extrapulmonary disease.

People who are infected with HIV and who then later become infected with *M. tuberculosis* frequently develop rapidly progressive primary TB. This is typical in countries of low TB prevalence and in outbreak settings. Active sputum smear-positive TB developed within 4 months in 37% of HIV-infected people exposed to two TB patients in a group home for HIV-infected people in San Francisco.[24] In a nosocomial TB outbreak in Italy, 8 of 18 (44%) HIV-infected patients exposed to a single sputum smear-negative TB patient developed active TB within 60 days of diagnosis of the index case.[25] In areas with a high prevalence of TB, HIV-infected people successfully treated for TB also are at increased risk to develop recurrent TB due to reinfection. In a prospective study of South African mine workers, 62% of relapses in HIV-infected adults were due to reinfection compared to 6% in HIV-noninfected individuals.[26] Secondary preventive therapy with isoniazid was 55% effective in reducing TB recurrence in this high transmission setting.[27]

Despite good clinical and microbiologic responses to TB chemotherapy,[28–32] the development of active TB in HIV-infected people appears to be associated with shortened survival,[32,33] possibly due to immune activation and consequent increased HIV replication.[34,35] The case-fatality rate of TB in HIV is approximately 33%. TB is now the leading cause of death in HIV-infected people globally, especially in sub-Saharan Africa, where it has been found at postmortem examination in 40–54% of HIV-infected adults.[36,37] Globally, 26% of all deaths due to TB in 2007 occurred in HIV-infected people.[38] Increased access to antiretroviral therapy (ART) has had a profound impact on dual infection. The incidence of TB is decreased by more than 80%.[39,40] The protective effect was greatest in symptomatic patients and those with advanced immunodeficiency.

Tuberculin Skin Test

TST is widely used in epidemiologic surveys to assess the prevalence and estimate the annual rate of TB infection and in clinical practice to assess whether a person has been infected with *M. tuberculosis* and has latent TB infection (LTBI). Skin testing should be performed by intradermal injection (Mantoux method) of 5 tuberculin units of purified protein derivative of tuberculin (PPD) per 0.1 mL, usually into the skin of the volar surface of the forearm. Correctly placed injections produce an immediate raised wheal. The test should be read as the number of millimeters of palpable induration present after 48–72 hours.

The operating characteristics of the test are dependent on the population tested, the amount of nonspecific cross-reactions (generally small reactions) due to prior BCG vaccination or infection with environmental mycobacteria, and the cut point used. Most people with reactions greater than 10 mm are infected with *M. tuberculosis*. A cut point of 5 mm is recommended when testing HIV-infected people, although this recommendation has been recently contested.[41] A positive TST indicates only prior infection with *M. tuberculosis* and not active disease. Up to one-fourth of newly diagnosed patients with active pulmonary TB have negative tuberculin reactions.

False-negative PPD tests can be caused by protein-calorie malnutrition, other diseases such as sarcoidosis and HIV infection, intercurrent viral infections, and immunosuppressive drugs such as corticosteroids. When present, the size of a previously positive TST reaction may wane over time, but remain susceptible to TST-induced boosting. Repeated testing of such a patient may result in the perception of new TST conversion suggesting recent infection. Two-step tuberculin tests in which PPD testing is repeated on people with a negative initial PPD skin test 1–5 weeks later can be used to identify this booster phenomenon. If the second PPD test is reactive, the positive test should be ascribed to boosting rather than to recent infection.

Positive TST skin reactions due to BCG vaccination wane with time. Routine neonatal BCG vaccination has little impact on the size of the TST reaction in adults; however, it may be a confounding factor in people revaccinated at school age or adolescence.[42,43] Recent knowledge about the important role of T lymphocytes and interferon-γ (IFN-γ) in tuberculosis has led to the development of *in vitro* diagnostic tests known as interferon-γ release assays (IGRA) to detect tuberculous infection. The two commercially available IGRA tests (QuantiFERON-TB, Cellestis, Australia, and T-SPOT.*TB*, Oxford Immunotec, UK) are both based on antigen-specific stimulation of IFN-γ release from mononuclear cells in a peripheral blood sample. The use of mycobacterial antigens including early secreted antigen-6 (ESAT-6), culture filtrate protein-10 (CFP-10), and TB 7.7 that are found in *M. tuberculosis*, but not in BCG or most other nontuberculous mycobacteria, enhances the specificity of these new tests. These assays offer the advantages that they can be done in a single visit, there is little interobserver variability, and there are no boosted responses. Over the past 3–5 years, IGRAs have gained widespread use in clinical settings and are increasingly used interchangeably with the TST to evaluate for *M. tuberculosis* infection. However, IGRAs have several important limitations:[44] (1) they have not been sufficiently validated in large prospective studies for reliability over time (stability); (2), as with the TST, IGRAs do not reliably distinguish LTBI from active TB disease; (3) a growing number of studies, particularly among HIV-infected subjects and household contacts of infectious TB cases, show discordance between IGRA and TST results in individuals likely to be *M. tuberculosis* infected; (4) their performance in programmatic conditions in high TB prevalence countries[45] is not well validated. The high cost of newer tests limits their use to TB programs in high-income settings, where the intended goal is to eradicate *M. tuberculosis* infection with these targeted LTBI treatment programs.[46]

Neither TST nor IGRAs indicate the time since *M. tuberculosis* infection occurred (recent TST converters are at higher risk of disease progression); nor can they discern the viability of the infecting strain.

THE DISEASE

Risk Factors for Progression from Infection to Active Tuberculosis

Most people infected by *M. tuberculosis* do not develop active TB following their initial infection (primary TB); infection is typically marked only by the development of a positive TST or IGRA test result, with only 5–10% of HIV-uninfected people developing active TB during their lifetime.[15] The risk is greatest in the first 2 years following infection and then declines. The risk of developing primary TB is associated with more intense exposure and is higher for people infected through contact with an index sputum smear-positive TB case.[4] The age at the time of TB infection is also important; those infected in infancy, adolescence, or old age are more likely to develop active TB.

The risk of developing progressive primary or reactivation TB is increased in immunocompromised people; the degree of risk varies with the underlying disease-impairing host defenses. The risk of developing TB among HIV-infected people was 79-fold greater than in HIV-noninfected people in one study[47] and may be up to 170-fold higher in patients with acquired immunodeficiency syndrome (AIDS).[48] People with silicosis, end-stage renal disease, certain malignancies such as head and neck cancers, lymphomas, poorly controlled diabetes mellitus, chronic malnutrition, rapid weight loss, chronic treatment with corticosteroids and other immunosuppressive drugs such as tumor necrosis factor-α (TNF-α) inhibitors, and those who smoke tobacco are also at increased risk of developing TB, although the relative risk is much less than that of HIV-infected people. The duration and dose of corticosteroid use associated with an increased risk of TB are unknown; however, treatment for less than 3 or 4 weeks with doses of 15 mg of prednisone or less daily probably causes little increased risk.

Primary Tuberculosis

TB infection is usually acquired by the inhalation of droplet nuclei containing viable tubercle bacilli that are phagocytosed by alveolar macrophages to establish a primary nidus of infection. In the nonimmune host, the bacilli multiply intracellularly, kill the cell, and then spread to the draining hilar lymph nodes or to the bloodstream via the thoracic duct. Most primary infections are asymptomatic, but some people develop fever, nonproductive cough, dyspnea, and, occasionally, erythema nodosum. Symptoms are more common in children than in adults. Crepitations from alveolar consolidation and focal wheezes due to bronchial compression by enlarged intrathoracic lymph nodes may be present. Lesions demonstrable on chest film include small patchy alveolar infiltrates in the middle and lower lung fields, often with unilateral hilar adenopathy. Bronchial compression by enlarged nodes may produce upper or middle lobe collapse. Small transient pleural effusions occur in 10% of patients.

The vast majority of immunocompetent people develop an effective immune response against *M. tuberculosis* and contain their primary infection, leaving only small calcified parenchymal scars (Ghon complex), usually in the middle and lower lung fields. If the corresponding draining hilar lymph node is visible, the radiographic lesion is termed a Ranke complex (***Fig. 35.1A***). Small scars due to arrested lesions from seeding of tubercle bacilli to the apical regions of the lung at the time of primary infection are known as Simon's foci (***Fig. 35.1B***). In many people, however, residua of the primary focus are undetectable on subsequent chest radiographs.

Following primary infection, immunocompetent people develop specific acquired resistance to reinfection. Although incompletely understood, the protective immune mechanisms appear to include T-lymphocyte-dependent activation of macrophages to destroy tubercle bacilli. Specific acquired resistance is long-lasting, possibly due to repeated primary but clinically latent foci of infection. Conditions such as HIV infection associated with immunosuppression may lead to lowered resistance to exogenous reinfection.[26] Reinfection is most likely to contribute substantially to new cases of TB in areas of high prevalence and transmission.

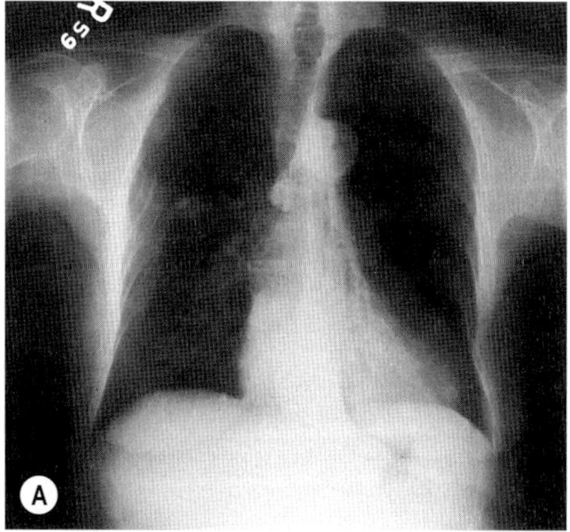

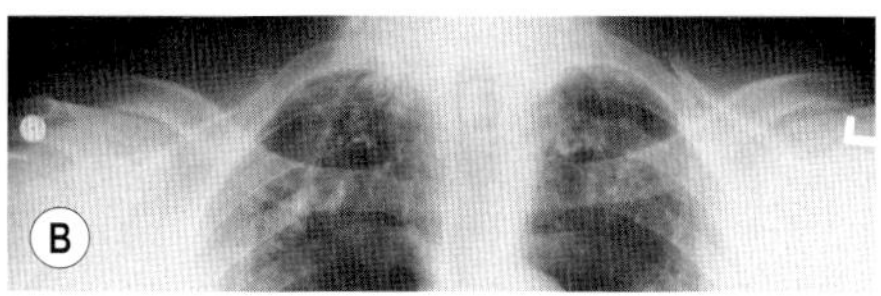

Figure 35.1 Remote arrested tuberculosis. **(A)** Calcified right mid-lung field lesion (Ghon focus) with calcified hilar lymph nodes. The combination of a Ghon focus and a draining lymph node is known as a Ranke complex. Note left lower lobe bronchiectasis secondary to remote tuberculosis. **(B)** Calcified apical tuberculous foci (Simon's foci).

Progressive Primary Tuberculosis

People who fail to develop specific acquired immune responses following primary TB infection may develop progressive primary TB. This form of disease is most common in young children, the immunocompromised, and the elderly. Miliary or meningeal disease may result after widespread hematogenous dissemination of tubercle bacilli. The clinical presentation is frequently cryptic with nonspecific symptoms such as malaise and fatigue or fever of unknown origin.[49] Progressive primary disease in young adults presents with fever, productive cough, night sweats, weight loss, and upper lobe cavitary lesions, which can be reliably distinguished from reactivation TB only when recent PPD skin test conversion has been documented.[50] The period of clinical latency in those that progress to active TB may be measured in days or weeks (mainly in children and people with advanced HIV disease) or as long as several months. In a study in Uganda, the duration of the latent period between exposure, infection, evidence of early disease and the onset of symptoms among household contacts of an infectious TB case was as long as 22 months.[51]

Reactivation (Postprimary Tuberculosis)

Although acquired immune responses are crucial to mycobacterial killing and the prevention of progressive pulmonary or disseminated disease after primary infection, they do not totally eradicate all viable tubercle bacilli. Low numbers of dormant, slowly metabolizing organisms persist in small, walled-off fibrocaseous lesions in the lung and other organs seeded during the initial bacillemia. These foci may "break down" years to decades later in the presence of waning immunity to produce active local or disseminated disease.

The lungs are the most common site of reactivation TB. Chronic cough productive of purulent sputum of greater than 2 or 3 weeks' duration, night sweats, weight loss, and anorexia are the most frequent complaints. From 40% to 60% of patients are afebrile at presentation. The onset of symptoms usually is insidious. Approximately one-fifth of patients with reactivation TB have no chest symptoms and the diagnosis is detected on a routine chest radiograph.[52]

Hemoptysis may occur and varies from blood-streaked sputum due to endobronchial lesions to massive, sometimes fatal, hemoptysis in patients with far-advanced cavitary disease. Large subpleural lesions may cause adjacent pleural inflammation and pleuritic chest pain. TB is characterized by brisk local inflammation and thrombosis of small pulmonary vessels contiguous to active lesions resulting in the loss of perfusion to poorly ventilated, diseased lung areas. This may explain the relatively low frequency of dyspnea in active TB until the disease is very extensive. Rarely, large lesions or cavities rupture into the pleural space producing a pneumothorax and chest pain and sudden dyspnea.

Signs of consolidation, coarse or fine crepitations and bronchial breath sounds, are present on auscultation over affected lung zones. In some instances, crepitations may be heard only after the patient has been instructed to take several deep breaths, cough vigorously, and take further deep breaths ("post-tussive rales"). Low-pitched amphoric breath sounds (named for their resemblance to the sound produced by blowing across the opening of a wide-mouthed jug) may be heard over large cavities. Dullness to percussion and decreased tactile and vocal fremitus at the lung bases indicate the presence of concomitant pleural effusion or thickening.

The chest radiographic findings in reactivation TB are varied.[52,53] In many cases, they are more extensive than suggested by physical examination of the thorax. Lesions are characteristically localized to the apical and posterior segments of the upper lobes (***Fig. 35.2***) and the superior (dorsal) segment of the lower lobes, although other areas may be involved less frequently. The reasons underlying the predilection for reactivation TB to occur in the lung apices are not known with certainty but have been conjectured to be due to higher ambient oxygen tensions favoring mycobacterial growth or to decreased lymphatic clearance from these areas. Intrathoracic lymphadenopathy is uncommon in reactivation TB. The radiographic lesions are usually asymmetrical and begin as areas of consolidation with focal infiltrates. Local inflammation and host responses lead to caseation and pulmonary necrosis. If these areas liquefy and rupture into a bronchus, cavities result. Early cavities are thin-walled and have surrounding infiltrates, and only approximately 10% have visible air–fluid levels.

Caseous necrosis and cavitation are critical events in the natural history of TB because local conditions in the cavity are conducive to rapid bacillary growth. TB can then be spread to other areas of the lung by spillage of caseous material from cavities into the airways with subsequent bronchial and aerogenous spread. The upper airways may become involved, resulting in tuberculous laryngitis and otitis media. Infectious sputum may be swallowed, leading to tuberculous enteritis or peritonitis.

Parenchymal lesions heal by fibrosis, leaving round or linear scars. Small cavities may be obliterated by fibrosis and contraction; however, large thick-walled cavities often persist. Such lesions, even when sterilized by effective anti-TB chemotherapy, may later become colonized by *Aspergillus* or other, atypical mycobacteria. Erosion and rupture of small nonthrombosed pulmonary arteries in the walls of chronic tuberculous cavities (Rasmussen's aneurysm) can produce massive life-threatening hemoptysis. Late hemoptysis may also be due to fungal infection of residual cavities (mycetoma), bronchiectasis, or erosion of old calcified nodes into a central bronchus, and it does not necessarily imply that active TB disease is present.

Reactivation TB also presents with lower-lobe disease ranging from dense, poorly resolving lobar or segmental infiltrates to atelectasis or large mass lesions or cavities.[54,55] The last-named are often mistaken for lung cancers or putrid lung abscesses. Lower-lobe TB may be more common in diabetic patients and immunosuppressed hosts. The diagnosis often is delayed because of failure to consider TB, especially when such patients fail to respond to empirical treatment for pyogenic pneumonia

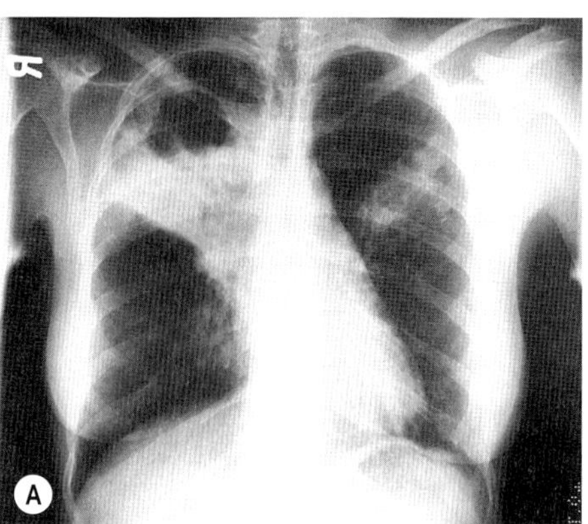

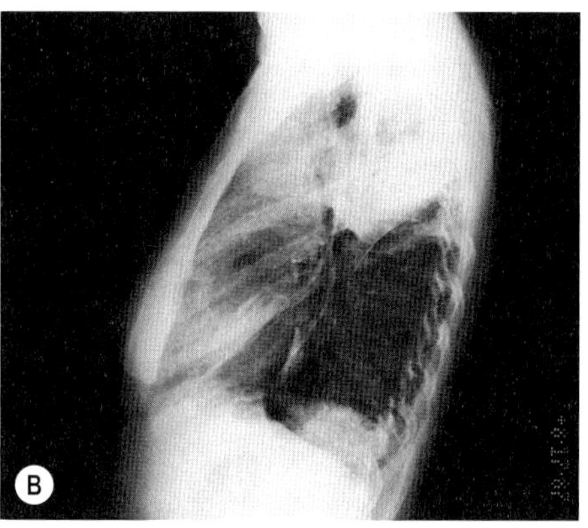

Figure 35.2 Posteroanterior **(A)** and left lateral **(B)** chest X-rays showing typical reactivation (postprimary) tuberculosis in the adult. Bilateral upper lobe fibrocavitary disease affects predominantly the apical and posterior segments of the right upper lobe.

or mixed aerobic–anaerobic lung abscess. Rarely, patients with reactivation TB present with normal chest X-rays and positive acid-fast bacilli (AFB) smears and cultures resulting from endobronchial lesions or old tuberculous nodes that have eroded and are discharging into the bronchial tree.

For detailed information, the reader is referred to several excellent reviews of the radiographic manifestations of TB in normal and immunocompromised hosts.[53,56–58]

Pediatric Tuberculosis

Children usually acquire tuberculous infection from close contact with an infectious, typically sputum smear-positive, adult. Most infections are contracted from someone living in the same household. The younger the child, the more likely it is that he or she has been infected by a household member. Malaise, fever, failure to thrive, and erythema nodosum may occur with progressive primary disease. Contrary to the usual presentation in adults with productive cough and chest pain, cough is an infrequent presenting complaint in children with TB except for those with endobronchial disease. Because pulmonary necrosis and cavitation are less frequent in children, the bacillary burden is usually lower; therefore, children are less likely to be sputum AFB smear positive and a source of transmission to others. Clinical symptoms, radiographic signs, and sputum positivity in children's cases begin to resemble adult cases of TB at approximately 15 years of age.

The diagnosis of TB in children is problematic.[59–61] Children often do not produce sputum for examination. Gastric lavage can be performed to obtain swallowed sputum, but the process is time-consuming and uncomfortable for young children and has a low sensitivity of approximately 50%. In most instances, a presumptive diagnosis is made and anti-TB treatment is initiated based on the constellation of a positive TST reaction in a child with compatible chest film findings and exposure to a known infectious case or residence in a high-prevalence area. This conservative approach is warranted because children are at high risk of progressive TB and miliary and meningeal disease.

Pulmonary Tuberculosis in Immunocompromised Patients

Patients who are mildly immunocompromised may present with typical reactivation TB with cough, sputum production, malaise, and weight loss and a radiographic picture of apical fibrocavitary disease.

Severely immunocompromised patients are at high risk of developing progressive primary TB if recently infected and for reactivation of latent TB infection. These patients may present with disseminated disease or overwhelming pneumonia and adult respiratory distress syndrome. The spectrum of chest radiographic lesions ranges from abnormalities comparable to those in primary TB to diffuse pulmonary infiltrates, often without cavitation, and miliary disease.[56] The absence of cavitation and the presence of diffuse or lower lung field location of the infiltrates often results in delayed diagnosis and treatment and likely contributes to the high mortality of TB in immunocompromised patients.

Tuberculosis in People with Human Immunodeficiency Virus Infection

M. tuberculosis is a highly virulent human pathogen and produces disease throughout the course of HIV infection. During the early stages of HIV infection when host defenses are less impaired, TB usually presents with clinical and radiographic features consistent with typical reactivation-type fibrocavitary disease.[62,63]

As HIV infection progresses, the clinical and radiographic presentation of TB becomes more atypical. With progressive immunosuppression, if once positive, the TST may revert to negative. TB in severely immunosuppressed HIV-infected people is characterized by an increase in disseminated and extrapulmonary forms of disease. In one representative study of patients with advanced AIDS and TB, 38% of patients had pulmonary TB only, 30% had extrapulmonary disease only, and 32% had both pulmonary and extrapulmonary disease.[29] Widespread TB was present in 54% of adult patients dying with AIDS in an autopsy series from Côte d'Ivoire and was thought to be the primary cause of death in 32%,[37] but it was much less common (2%) in HIV-infected children dying at the same institution.[64]

Pulmonary disease is present in 65–93% of HIV-infected patients with TB.[28,29,65–70] Chest films often show lower lung zone or diffuse infiltrates, mediastinal or hilar lymphadenopathy, pleural involvement, and a lower frequency of cavitary disease (***Fig. 35.3***). Around 5–8% of HIV-infected people with proven pulmonary TB have a normal chest radiograph.[71,72] Unlike TB in HIV-noninfected patients, where positive blood cultures occur in fewer than 5% of patients, mycobacterial blood cultures are positive in 26–42% of patients with AIDS and TB,[73–75] including one-third of patients with occult disseminated disease.

The yield of sputum microscopy for the diagnosis of TB also may be lower in HIV-infected people, making diagnosis more difficult in programs where microscopy is the only available diagnostic test. Studies from developing and industrialized countries suggest that HIV-infected TB patients have smaller numbers of bacilli in the sputum and a lower frequency of positive sputum AFB smears (45–67%) than HIV-noninfected

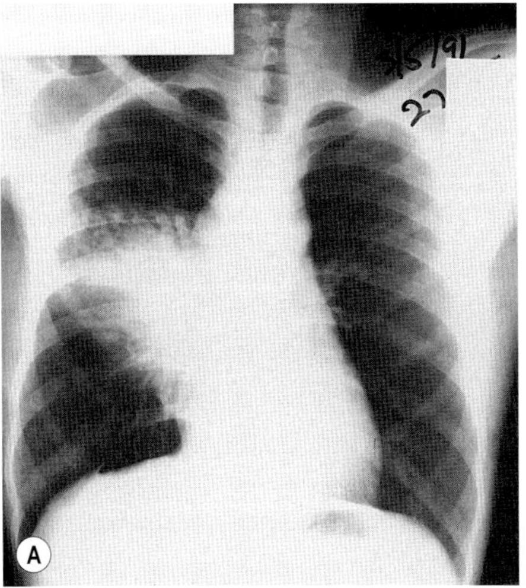

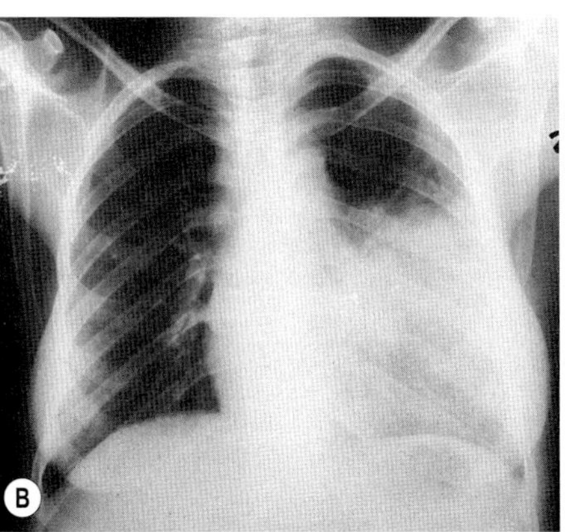

Figure 35.3 Atypical presentations of pulmonary tuberculosis in HIV-infected adults. **(A)** Right mid-lung field infiltrate with ipsilateral hilar adenopathy and absence of cavitation resembling primary tuberculosis. **(B)** Dense mid and lower lung field infiltrates.

people.[76–80] Sputum cultures are positive in 62–93% of cases, comparable to HIV-noninfected patients.[29,78,81] The increased number of smear-negative cases probably reflects the contribution of noncavitary cases.

The histopathologic findings in the lungs of HIV-infected patients with active TB are characterized by higher bacillary burdens and poorly organized local inflammation compared with HIV-noninfected TB patients. Greater numbers of AFB and more poorly formed granulomas are present in patients with more severe degrees of immunosuppression and lower CD4 lymphocyte counts.[82] In fact the pathology may be dominated by foamy epithelioid cells/macrophages which are loaded with intracellular organisms. Despite the higher tissue burdens of tubercle bacilli in HIV-infected TB patients, epidemiologic studies from both developing and industrialized countries have shown that HIV-infected patients are comparably or less infectious than HIV-noninfected patients.[83–88] Whereas the traditional explanations refer to decreased cavitary lung disease, etc., we recently have found that decreased cough strength is a factor as well (K. Fennelly, unpublished observations).

Tuberculosis during Treatment with TNF Inhibitors

Another special case of interest is the development of TB as a complication of treatment with TNF inhibitors. The first reports indicated an increase risk of TB in patients treated for rheumatoid arthritis with infliximab, the TB occurring a median of 16 weeks after starting therapy.[89] Extrapulmonary TB was 3 times more frequent and disseminated TB 12 times. Subsequent studies suggested that this was a complication of all forms of anti-TNF therapy but somewhat more common and occurring earlier when antibody blocked the surface as well as soluble TNF as contrasted to receptor blockade, which does not affect cell surface antibody.[90] These observations indicate the ongoing importance of TNF in maintaining granuloma integrity as well as latency of TB. They mandate attempts to diagnose and treat latent TB infection in individuals about to start treatment with this class of agents.

Extrapulmonary Tuberculosis

Tuberculosis can affect nearly all organ systems. Most cases of extrapulmonary disease represent reactivation TB due to the breakdown of previously dormant foci established during the primary infection. A few forms of extrapulmonary disease, such as tuberculous pleurisy and phlyctenular conjunctivitis, represent hypersensitivity reactions to mycobacterial proteins and occur following primary infection. Approximately 20% of HIV-noninfected patients with TB have extrapulmonary disease.

In developing countries with a high prevalence of TB infection, extrapulmonary TB frequently occurs in children and young adults. This is in contrast to industrialized nations, where extrapulmonary TB is more frequent in the elderly, presumably due to reactivation of TB in the setting of declining immunity related to aging. The frequency of disseminated TB and some forms of extrapulmonary TB, such as tuberculous meningitis (TBM), is clearly increased among HIV-infected people.

Several points about extrapulmonary tuberculosis require emphasis. Diagnosis is frequently more difficult than that for pulmonary disease. Miliary, meningeal, and abdominal TB frequently present with nonlocalizing systemic symptoms, such as fever and failure to thrive. Cutaneous anergy to TST occurs in 35–50% of patients with these forms of TB. One-fourth to one-third of people with HIV infection with extrapulmonary TB lack clinical and radiographic evidence of active or remote pulmonary TB. Therefore, normal chest films and a negative TST cannot be used definitively to exclude the diagnosis of TB. In a recent study from Taiwan, the diagnostic performance of IGRAs in extrapulmonary TB varied according to the site of disease; in 138 patients with definite and probable TB, the sensitivity of T-SPOT.*TB* ranged from 100% for TBM, tuberculous pericarditis, and intestinal TB, to 95% for lymphadenitis, to 43% for tuberculous peritonitis.[91] Common forms of extrapulmonary TB are discussed in the following sections.

Tuberculous Pleurisy

Tuberculosis can involve the pleural space by direct extension, hematogenous seeding, or, most frequently, extension or rupture of a subpleural caseous focus into the pleural space. Tuberculous pleurisy with effusion usually develops 3–6 months after primary infection.[92] Around 5–20% of HIV-noninfected adults have pleural effusions at the time of diagnosis with intrathoracic TB, and TB is the most common cause of pleural effusions in many developing countries.[93,94]

Relatively few bacilli are present in the pleural space so that the pleuritis has been attributed to an *in situ* delayed-type hypersensitivity (DTH) response to mycobacterial proteins. Exudative pleural effusions have been induced experimentally in tuberculin-sensitized guinea pigs by injecting tuberculin into the pleural space.[95] PPD-specific T lymphocytes are present in the pleural fluid in greater numbers than in the peripheral blood in patients with TB pleurisy.[96] These lymphocytes are predominantly T-helper cells. The marked local inflammation is mediated by the release of high levels of several cytokines, including IFN-γ, interleukin (IL-2), and TNF-α, by activated PPD-specific T lymphocytes and macrophages.[97–101]

Tuberculous pleurisy typically presents with the abrupt onset of fever, cough, and pleuritic chest pain, but it may have a more chronic course with fever, weight loss, and malaise. In one study, two-thirds of patients had symptoms for less than 1 month and one-third were ill for less than 1 week.[102] Chest films show a small to moderate-sized pleural effusion with visible parenchymal disease in one-third to one-half of cases. When unilateral, the effusions are more frequently right-sided (57%).[82] Approximately 10% have bilateral effusions.[103,104] Initial PPD skin tests are negative in one-third of cases but become reactive in nearly all patients if retested 6–8 weeks later.[103] Tuberculin anergy may seem paradoxical given the vigorous DTH response in the pleural space. Mononuclear suppressor cells have been detected in the circulation, but not the pleural fluid, of PPD anergic patients with tuberculous pleurisy.[105,106]

The pleural effusion is usually an exudate containing greater than 50% lymphocytes. Neutrophils may predominate in the first few weeks after the development of the effusion. Owing to the chronic pleural inflammation, it is unusual to find more than 5% mesothelial cells.[107] Low pleural fluid glucose is present in only approximately 20% of cases[103] but is an important diagnostic clue when present because the differential diagnosis of low pleural fluid glucose (<60 mg/dL) is limited, with few exceptions, to four conditions: malignancy, empyema, rheumatoid arthritis, and TB. Other ancillary tests useful in the diagnosis of tuberculous pleurisy include measurement of pleural fluid adenosine deaminase and IFN-γ.[108]

Patients with suspected tuberculous pleurisy should undergo PPD skin testing and examination of the sputum and pleural fluid. Many patients with minimal parenchymal disease will have negative sputum smears due to the low bacillary burden. Sputum and gastric aspirate AFB smears are positive in less than one-third of patients.[103] AFB smears of pleural fluid also have a low diagnostic yield and mycobacterial cultures are positive in less than 25%.[103,109] Closed pleural biopsy with the Abrams or Cope needle is a very useful diagnostic technique. The presence of granulomas in pleural tissue, even in the absence of AFB or caseation, is highly suggestive of TB. A single pleural biopsy will demonstrate granulomas in approximately 60% of cases.[110] If multiple biopsy specimens are examined, the diagnostic yield increases to approximately 90%. Portions of the biopsy material should be submitted for histologic evaluation and special stains and other portions should be cultured. AFBs are seen in tissue sections in 5–18% of patients.[109,110] Using the combination of pleural biopsy histology and cultures, 85–95% of cases can be diagnosed.[109,110] Pleural biopsy cultures may still be positive up to several weeks after patients have been started on empirical anti-TB chemotherapy.

Pleural TB is frequent in HIV-infected patients, and pleural involvement has been reported in 28–38% of HIV-infected patients with TB.[74,93] The size of the effusions is similar to that of HIV-noninfected patients, although the duration of symptoms may be longer.[111] The diagnostic yield on pleural biopsy is also similar to that of HIV-negative patients; however, pleural fluid cultures are significantly more likely to be positive in

HIV-positive patients (75% versus 24%).[111] Inoculation of liquid as well as solid culture media enhances diagnosis.

In HIV-noninfected persons, tuberculous pleurisy is generally a self-limited condition with spontaneous resolution of the effusion even without specific anti-TB treatment; 41–65% of these patients will later develop active TB, the majority within the first 3 years after the episode of pleurisy.[112,113] Tuberculous pleurisy responds extremely well to modern chemotherapy regimens. Isoniazid and rifampicin (called rifampin in the United States) given daily for 9 months, or daily for 1 month followed by twice-weekly treatment for 5 or 8 months, cures more than 98% of patients.[114,115] Six-month short-course regimens including pyrazinamide are also highly effective. If the clinical suspicion for TB is high and pleural biopsy is unavailable or the biopsy histology and special stains are negative, another reasonable option is empirical treatment with specific anti-TB chemotherapy with repeat PPD skin testing and reevaluation in 4–6 weeks. Repeated thoracocenteses are unnecessary. Intrapleural corticosteroids are of little value. A tapering course of adjunctive oral corticosteroids (prednisolone, 0.75 mg/kg per day) given during the first 2 or 3 months of anti-TB treatment was shown in one placebo-controlled study to increase the rate of resolution of symptoms and pleural fluid resorption but did not alter the extent of residual pleural thickening.[116] Corticosteroids probably are of marginal benefit in patients with small effusions and mild symptoms.

Large necrotic tuberculous foci or cavities occasionally rupture into the pleural space to produce a true tuberculous empyema. The pleural fluid is thick and cloudy with a high density of bacilli. An etiologic diagnosis usually can be established quickly by simple microscopy and culture of the pleural fluid. Tuberculous empyemas are usually associated with far-advanced cavitary disease. Treatment is difficult, may need to be prolonged, and should be given in conjunction with a chest consultant.[117] Drainage or decortication is often required. Secondary complications include extension through the chest wall, producing chest wall abscesses and draining fistulas.

Miliary Tuberculosis

The term miliary tuberculosis is used to describe disseminated TB resulting from hematogenous spread associated with characteristic lesions on chest radiography. Miliary lesions are diffuse 1 or 2 mm rounded opacities scattered throughout all lung fields and are named for their resemblance to millet seeds. Early lesions may be indistinct and easily missed (***Fig. 35.4A***). Advanced lesions may coalesce and appear as larger rounded lesions that occasionally cavitate (***Fig. 35.4B***). In developing countries with a high prevalence of TB, most cases occur following primary infection. In industrialized countries, the majority of cases arise from breakdown and hematogenous seeding from old latent foci in the lung or other organs. Pathologically, the pulmonary lesions consist of aggregates of macrophages and lymphocytes in granulomas with or without caseous necrosis. In severely immunocompromised patients, such as patients with advanced AIDS, little tissue inflammation may be present and many bacilli may be visible.

Systemic symptoms predominate in patients with miliary TB despite the numerous pulmonary lesions. The chest is generally clear to auscultation. A minority have lymphadenopathy or hepatosplenomegaly. Choroidal tubercles, which are raised white-yellow plaques visible in the choroid on fundoscopic examination, are pathognomonic but occur in fewer than 15% of cases. Fever, weight loss, and failure to thrive are frequent, and miliary TB may be a cause of fever of unknown origin in the elderly.[49] Hematologic abnormalities ranging from leukopenia to leukemoid reactions occur in 10% of cases.[118] Patients may present with headache, confusion, personality change, and focal neurologic deficits due to concomitant central nervous system (CNS) involvement with TBM.

The diagnosis of miliary TB is usually straightforward when typical radiographic lesions are present. The initial chest X-ray may, however, be negative. In such cases, a computed tomography (CT) scan my reveal miliary infiltrates. The PPD skin test is positive in only 52–72% of cases.[119–122] Patients with neurologic symptoms and signs should undergo lumbar puncture and cerebrospinal fluid (CSF) examination. Hyponatremia may be a clue to the syndrome of inappropriate secretion of antidiuretic hormone due to CNS disease. The diagnostic yields of sputum AFB smears and culture, urine and gastric aspirate culture, and tissue biopsies in patients with miliary TB are listed in ***Table 35.1***. Routine mycobacterial cultures may take 3 or more weeks to become positive. In urgent situations, when available, fiberoptic bronchoscopy with transbronchial lung biopsy has a diagnostic yield of 75–100%.[120,126,127] When classic necrotizing granulomas are present, a presumptive diagnosis can be reached quickly. Treatment with the standard short-course regimens described later is recommended for cases of miliary TB.

Tuberculous Meningitis

TB involves the CNS in three ways. Tuberculomas are parenchymal mass lesions that produce focal symptoms by acting as space-occupying lesions. Tuberculous spondylitis (***Fig. 35.5***) can result in spinal cord compression or radiculopathy. The most frequent form of CNS TB is TBM. This is the most life-threatening form of extrapulmonary TB and was uniformly fatal before the advent of antituberculous chemotherapy. It is still a leading cause of death and chronic disability in infants and children with TB.[128]

Unlike areas of the developing world with a high prevalence of TB where the infant or child develops TBM in the setting of progressive primary infection or miliary disease, in more developed nations TBM is more frequently seen in adults and the elderly in association with reactivation TB. The HIV pandemic has also been associated with increased case rates of CNS TB. TBM occurs five times more frequently in HIV-infected people than in those who are HIV seronegative.[129] Around 5–10% of HIV-infected patients with TB have CNS involvement, predominantly as

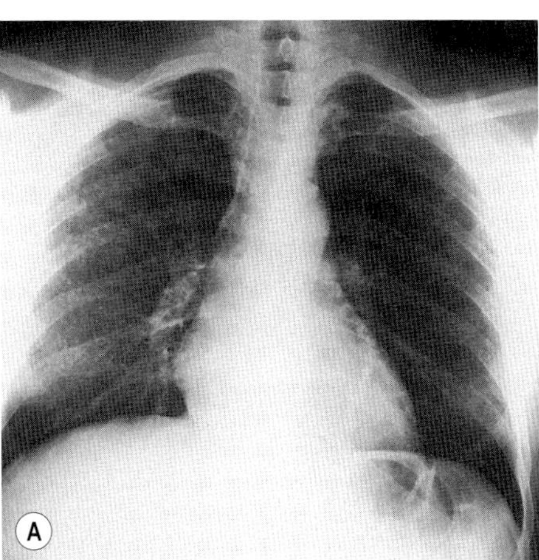

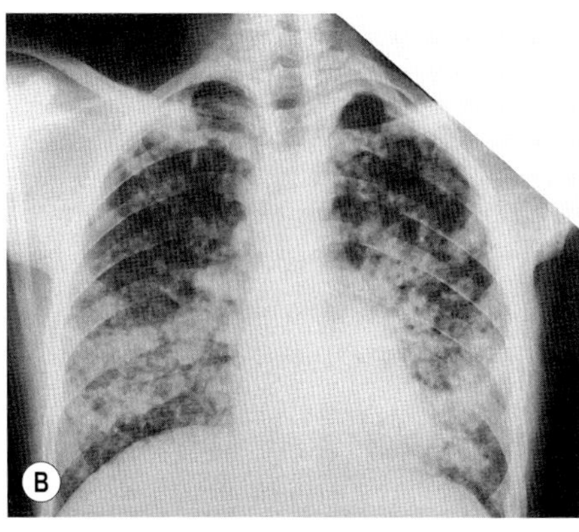

Figure 35.4 **(A)** Early miliary tuberculosis. Diffuse 1 or 2 mm rounded opacities involve all lung fields. **(B)** Coalescence of smaller lesions in advanced miliary disease.

Series	Sputum AFB Smears	Sputum Culture	Gastric Aspirate Culture	Urine Culture	Bone Marrow Biopsy and Culture	Liver Biopsy	Lymph Node Biopsy
Berger and Samortin[123]	–	50	–	–	80	100	100
Munt[121]	33	63	–	14	33	67	62
Gelb et al[122]	–	55	–	23	100	82	60
Grieco and Chmel[124]	–	–	–	–	–	60	80
Bobrowitz[125]	18	66	–	–	–	–	–
Maartens et al[120]	33	62	75	33	86	100	100
Kim et al[126]	33	76	100	59	45	59	–

Table 35.1 Yield of Diagnostic Studies in Miliary Tuberculosis (Percentage with Positive Histology or Culture)

AFB, acid-fast bacilli.

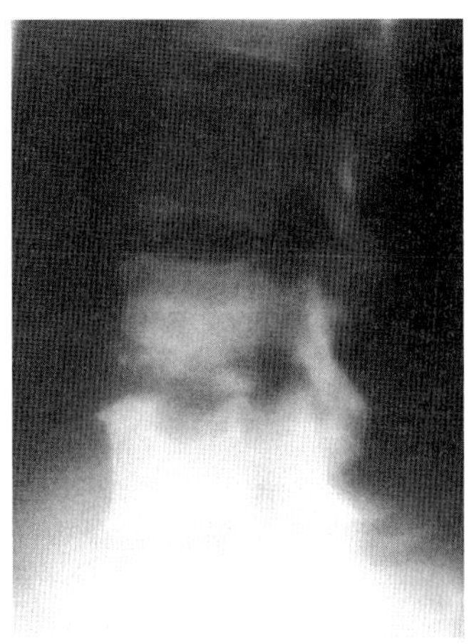

Figure 35.5 Tuberculous spondylitis. Lytic lesion involving the anterior and inferior aspect of the L3 vertebra and the posterior and superior aspects of the L4 vertebra with early sparing of the disk space.

meningitis.[29,129–131] Further, TBM may develop during treatment of TB as a form of TB-IRIS (see section below on immune reconstitution inflammatory syndrome (IRIS) and unmasking TB). TBM resembles many other forms of chronic meningitis. It occurs without other evidence of extracranial TB in a significant minority of cases, further increasing difficulties in diagnosis.

TBM usually results from the rupture of a subependymal tuberculous focus into the CSF provoking a brisk local inflammatory and immunologic response.[132,133] The severe inflammatory responses in the subarachnoid space cause most of the symptoms and ultimate morbidity of TBM. Pathologic lesions include: (1) a thick gelatinous basilar exudate capable of entrapping cranial nerves and blood vessels and blocking normal CSF resorptive pathways; (2) a severe arteriolitis and perivasculitis with subsequent endarteritis and thrombosis of nutrient vessels to the brain parenchyma, resulting in ischemia and infarction; and (3) severe comorbidity due to debility and secondary infection.

Adults may develop TBM in the setting of progressive primary disease or miliary TB similar to children. However, they may also develop it due to late meningeal seeding and subependymal tubercle formation from bacilli spread systemically from the breakdown of small cryptic smoldering or previously dormant renal and osseous foci.[132] Most cases have other clinical or radiographic stigmas of TB in other extracranial sites, but a few have no other apparent evidence of TB outside of the CNS.

Common clinical manifestations at the time of presentation for medical attention include headache, fever, irritability, and, in children, episodes of protracted vomiting. Fever is present in 47–100% of cases,[134,135] and meningismus is present in 57–90% of cases;[136,137] decreased level of consciousness, papilledema, and cranial nerve palsies (most commonly of the sixth cranial nerve, followed by palsies of the third, fourth, and seventh cranial nerves) are seen less frequently. The clinical presentation of TBM is similar in HIV-positive and -negative people.[129,138] A definitive study was performed in two tertiary referral hospitals in Ho Chi Minh City in Vietnam and compared 96 HIV-infected to 432 HIV-infected patients with TBM.[139] HIV-associated TBM was similar in terms of neurologic manifestations although other extrapulmonary involvement, in particular lymph node involvement, was more common (32.5% versus 18.5%), CSF cultures were more likely to be positive (41.7% versus 29.6%) and all-cause mortality at 6 months was increased 2.9-fold. This cohort was not treated with ART, which can be expected to modify the outcome.

In adults, the presentation of TBM is similar to many other forms of chronic meningitis, with fever, meningismus, headache, and an abnormal level of consciousness.[125] The combination of leptomeningeal signs, especially new or evolving cranial nerve palsies, a chest film picture consistent with TB, and a CSF profile of hypoglycorrhachia with lymphocytic pleocytosis should suggest the diagnosis. The differential diagnosis is vastly different in the setting of HIV infection in which cryptococcal meningitis and other opportunistic infections are increased in frequency.

The duration of symptoms prior to hospital admission varies from a few days to 6 months. Initial TSTs were positive in 31–61% of adult[140,141] and 50–96% of pediatric cases.[128,142] Sputum smears and cultures or gastric aspirate cultures were positive in 14–51% of cases.[136,143] The chest radiograph is helpful diagnostically: 44–88% of all adult and pediatric patients have radiographic abnormalities compatible with pulmonary TB.[137,144] Approximately 20% will have a miliary pattern. Bone marrow biopsy and liver biopsy are other good sites for diagnostic sampling in miliary disease. CT and nuclear magnetic resonance imaging (MRI) of the head, where available, are useful in detecting concomitant tuberculomas and complications such as hydrocephalus. Hyponatremia is present in 37–73% of patients[145,146] due to the syndrome of inappropriate antidiuretic hormone secretion.[147] Owing to the increased incidence of TBM in HIV-infected people, patients should be offered HIV testing.

The usual CSF findings consist of hypoglycorrhachia (CSF glucose <40 mg/dL) in 32–88% of patients,[145,148] elevated protein levels, and a lymphocytic pleocytosis with 100–500 cells/mL.[149] This pattern of abnormalities is generally the same across all age groups. The fluid is usually clear or ground glass in appearance. Markedly elevated protein levels (>500 mg/dL) and xanthochromic fluid may occasionally be seen in severe cases complicated by hydrocephalus with spinal subarachnoid block. An early predominance of polymorphonuclear leukocytes occurs in 6–45% of cases but there is a rapid shift to lymphocytic pleocytosis.[135,136]

The CSF glucose characteristically declines as the disease progresses. A rising CSF protein may signal the development of obstruction to CSF recirculation due to worsening basilar or spinal arachnoiditis. With appropriate treatment, the CSF findings normalize in the following order: glucose, CSF protein, and CSF cell counts.[143] CSF abnormalities may take up to 3–6 months to resolve completely.[150]

The yield from direct AFB smears of CSF ranges from 0% to 87%.[137,146] CSF mycobacterial cultures are positive in 40–83%.[137,151] Examination of fluid from the last tube collected at lumbar puncture, larger volumes of CSF (5–20 mL), or staining the clot (pellicle), if one forms, may increase the yield of direct AFB smears. Newer techniques, including measurement of CSF adenosine deaminase, antibodies against mycobacterial proteins, polymerase chain reaction (PCR) analysis, and assays to detect mycobacterial antigens, have been developed but have not entered widespread use due to limited sensitivity and specificity.[152–154]

A high level of clinical suspicion, however, is necessary to diagnose many cases of TBM. Only one-fourth to one-third of patients will have a history of exposure to a known case of TB, although such information should be sought. The chest X-ray, if consistent with TB, provides an important diagnostic clue. Acid-fast smears and cultures of secretions and tissues from other organs may provide important supportive evidence. Sputum examination should be performed in patients with pulmonary involvement. Cultures of gastric aspirates may be useful alternatives in children. The yields of sputum and gastric aspirate smears and cultures range from 14% to 51%.[136,143]

Lumbar puncture and examination of the CSF form the cornerstones of diagnosis in TBM. The differential diagnosis of subacute or chronic lymphocytic meningitis, with or without hypoglycorrhachia, is broad and includes fungal meningitis, "aseptic" viral meningitis, parasitic infestations of the CNS, acute syphilitic meningitis, brain abscesses, subdural hematomas, carcinomatous meningitis, and other rarer diseases.[155] The most important differential diagnostic concern in immunocompromised patients is cryptococcal meningitis. The immediate diagnostic value of the lumbar puncture lies in the rapid exclusion of bacterial meningitis and subarachnoid hemorrhage and the demonstration of cell counts and chemistries consistent with TBM. Multiple lumbar punctures (up to three to four taps of 10–20 mL of CSF) are indicated if the diagnosis remains in doubt as the yield from cultures and smears increases with serial taps[137] and the evolution of CSF chemistries and cell counts (development of lymphocytic pleocytosis and progressive fall in glucose) can be followed.

A diagnostic algorithm has been proposed and validated for HIV-uninfected patients to distinguish TBM from bacterial meningitis.[156] It relies on five dichotomized clinical variables (age <36, duration of illness >6 days, WBC count <15 000, CSF cell count <900, and CSF neutrophils <75%).

Most of the first-line anti-TB drugs achieve good levels in the CSF. In the presence of meningeal inflammation, isoniazid achieves levels in the CSF comparable to those in the blood.[157] Rifampicin levels are 20–50% of those in the peripheral blood.[158] Ethambutol, pyrazinamide, and ethionamide all penetrate the CNS relatively well. The notable exceptions are the aminoglycosides that penetrate even inflamed meninges poorly.

Modern short-course chemotherapy regimens (described later) including isoniazid, rifampicin, pyrazinamide, and ethambutol achieve good cure rates.[159] Most authorities treat TBM for at least 1 year. A randomized controlled trial has defined the efficacy of adjunctive dexamethasone therapy for TBM.[160] Patients with TBM were allocated to receive treatment with dexamethasone intravenously for 2 weeks beginning with a dose of 0.4 mg/kg per day, followed by a tapering regimen of oral corticosteroids for 4 weeks. The corticosteroid-treated group showed improved survival (relative risk of death, 0.69) but there was no effect on severe neurologic residua in the survivors. Treatment effects were similar across subgroups stratified by disease severity and HIV infection. Corticosteroids may achieve these salutary effects by blunting severe local inflammation with vasculitis and entrapment of small cerebral blood vessels and cranial nerves. In fact serial MRI scans showed that treatment with dexamethasone halved the development of infarction (27% versus 58%), may have accelerated clearing of hydrocephalus but did not affect the development of tuberculomas in 24%.[161]

Elevated intracranial pressure (ICP) and hydrocephalus are common in TBM, especially in children. Ventriculoatrial or ventriculoperitoneal shunting procedures may be required for neurologic deterioration despite appropriate antituberculous chemotherapy and ICP-reducing measures, progressively increasing ICP, and the presence of severe hydrocephalus on imaging studies. The overall prognosis is determined by the severity of neurologic involvement at the time of presentation and the duration of illness.[128,134,137,148,162,163] Comatose patients have the highest mortality and the greatest risk of permanent neurologic sequelae.

Tuberculous lymphadenitis, bone and joint, renal, genital, pericardial, abdominal, and other rare forms of turberculosis are detailed in the online section of this chapter.

Immune Reconstitution Inflammatory Syndrome and Unmasking Tuberculosis

Treatment of HIV-associated TB with ART may result in paradoxical worsening of known TB (TB-IRIS) or new clinical findings in previously inapparent TB (unmasking TB).[164] TB-IRIS occurs when TB treatment precedes ART and unmasking TB when ART precedes the diagnosis of TB. There is intense interest in determining the pathogenesis of TB-IRIS. TB-IRIS is more likely to occur when the CD4 count is low, viral load high, and interval between treatment of TB and beginning ART short. The frequency of TB-IRIS varies between 8% and 43%, and whereas the case definition usually stipulates onset within 3 months of starting ART, in fact the median time of onset is 14 days. In a recent single site report from Kampala Uganda, TB-IRIS occurred in 29% of HIV-infected patients a median of 5 weeks after initiation of ART.[165] The manifestations are quite varied and often mimic progression of TB. For this reason it is important to exclude drug resistance of the isolate, nonadherence to treatment on the part of the patient, and alternative opportunistic infections. The clinical manifestations usually are reversible but become more serious if there is respiratory failure or neurologic involvement. In Uganda, only 7% of early deaths after initiation of ART could be ascribed to TB-IRIS.[166] A recent study from South Africa characterized neurologic manifestations of TB-IRIS.[167] Neuro-IRIS accounted for 12% of all TB-IRIS, occurred a median of 14 days after initiating ART, and was characterized by TBM, tuberculoma, or both, or radiculomyelopathy. One-fourth had neuro-TB that was exacerbated following ART; 91% of patients were treated with corticosteroids, 13% died, and 17% were lost to follow-up.

It is difficult to separate the entity of "unmasking TB" from missed diagnosis at the time ART is started and not surprisingly the adequacy of screening is an important determinant of the frequency of apparent unmasking. Unfortunately, the limited implementation of treatment of latent TB infection may be a contributor to unmasking TB and some such cases are potentially avoidable. The overall frequency varies with the incidence of TB in the population ranging from 1.3 per 100 patients in European and North American cohorts to 23% in a community-based South African cohort. In the Ugandan cohort 5.9% developed TB in the first 6 months and 2.7% thereafter with a median of 5 weeks. In a high incidence setting it is likely that some late unmasking cases represent progression of primary or reinfection TB. Unmasking TB tends to be relatively typical in presentation.

PATHOGENESIS AND IMMUNITY

The interaction between *M. tuberculosis* and the host is influenced by the genetics of both. It is assumed that certain humans express enhanced levels of innate resistance accounting for lack of infection despite certain exposure, for example in household contacts. The innate local host defenses that prevent establishment of infection manifest by TST conversion in exposed people are not understood. Strains of *M. tuberculosis* also differ in their virulence and their induction of host cytokines that may modify the granulomatous tissue reaction as well as the TST. After inhalation, droplet nuclei containing small numbers of viable tubercle bacilli are deposited in the terminal airspaces. The initial site of exposure/infection is most often in the lower or middle lobes due to the higher ventilation of these lung regions. The potential interaction of ingested bacilli with antibody is a potentially important area of limited investigation. In the lung, tubercle bacilli are phagocytosed by alveolar macrophages and dendritic cells. Tubercle bacilli also have the capacity to invade alveolar type 2 epithelial cells. This results in expression of the antimicrobial peptide human beta defensin-2.[168] The initial interactions also involve Toll-like receptors (TLRs) on the phagocyte surface that are ligated by the lipoglycan lipoarabinomannan, trehalose dimycolate, and other bacterial cell wall constituents. Phagocytosis, invasion, and ligation of TLRs result in the production of chemokines that attract blood monocytes and lymphocytes to form an inflammatory focus.

About one-half of intensely exposed household contacts fail to manifest *M. tuberculosis* infection presumably due to innate resistance. Recent advances in understanding innate immunity have demonstrated T-cell and IFN-γ independent pathways that may allow direct killing of *M. tuberculosis* by macrophages without dissemination of tubercle bacilli or development of adaptive immunity.

In the immunologically naïve host lacking sufficient innate resistance, the bacilli have the capacity to multiply intracellularly, ultimately leading to necrotic cell death with release of more bacilli into the alveolar space. T cells drawn to the inflammatory focus do not have immunologic memory. Certain T-cell populations (e.g., γδ T cells and natural killer cells) may, however, activate alveolar macrophage and monocyte killing of the bacteria to provide some local control of the infection.

When innate immunity fails to contain *M. tuberculosis*, subsequent events are determined by whether the host is immunocompetent and whether the immune system is mature. Bacilli released by lysed cells spread from the alveolar spaces to the regional lymph nodes and then hematogenously throughout the body. In the absence of a competent immune response, infection progresses to disease (primary progressive TB). Tissue inflammation and damage are minimal. The clinical presentation may be atypical with predominance of lower lobe disease, noncavitary opacities, and extrapulmonary manifestations. Some adults present with typical upper lobe cavitary lung disease. Immunodeficient hosts, infants, and children may, however, develop miliary disease and TB meningitis.

More than 95% of infected humans control the primary infection and have no clinical symptoms. In them, the initial interactions between the bacillus and host cells lead to induction of specific acquired immunity against *M. tuberculosis*. This immunity controls the primary infection and maintains foci of persistent organisms as clinically latent. The balance of cytokines and receptors expressed by antigen-presenting cells determines whether T-cell differentiation occurs along the Th1 pathway generally associated with protective immunity or the Th2 pathway in which antibody formation dominates. Th1 cells produce IFN-γ and IL-2, enhance macrophage microbicidal activity, and augment DTH. Th2 cells produce predominantly deactivating cytokines, including IL-4, IL-5, IL-6, and IL-10, and favor B-cell growth and antibody production.

M. tuberculosis infection thus results in the differentiation of naïve T cells into effector T cells that expand to great numbers in the host. CD4 T cells differentiate into Th1 and Th2 cells, whereas CD8 T cells differentiate into cytotoxic T cells. Together, the effector CD4 and CD8 T-cell compartments of the adaptive immune response put forth a coordinated effort to clear the infection. As infection clears, the effector T cells undergo extensive apoptosis and T-cell numbers return to homeostasis in the host. Importantly, during this time period, a small number of antigen-specific T cells survive either as short-lived T effector memory or as long-lived central memory T cells.[169]

CD4 T lymphocytes play an important role in immune defenses against TB. Depletion of CD4 cells in mice results in uncontrolled BCG infection,[170] whereas adoptive transfer of CD4 cells from sensitized animals confers protection against TB.[171] The risk of developing pulmonary TB and severe forms of extrapulmonary disease correlates with declining CD4 lymphocyte counts in HIV-infected people.[172,173] The tremendously increased risk of reactivation of a clinically latent TB infection in HIV-infected people (and in the setting of treatment with TNF inhibitors) redefines the concept of latency. Clearly, active immune surveillance involving CD4 lymphocytes is essential for controlling bacterial replication at these sites. In addition to CD4 cells, CD8 cells contribute to protective immunity.[174,175] The role of γδ T cells, CD4–CD8–, and natural killer cells to acquired immunity is unclear. Evidence has emerged supporting a role for antibody in protection, requiring a rethinking of basic concepts of immunity and pathogenesis.[176,177]

The development of effective specific acquired immunity responses occurs concomitantly with the development of specific DTH responses demonstrated by a reactive tuberculin skin test, which can usually be detected 4–6 weeks after initial TB infection.

In people who develop protective immune responses, the initial focus of infection usually heals by fibrosis or after undergoing caseation and calcification. Regional lymph nodes also heal over several months. Small numbers of viable tubercle bacilli may survive in these foci for decades in a dormant state. Breakdown of these foci in the setting of waning immunity due to aging, immunosuppressive medications, HIV infection, or other medical illnesses as discussed previously can result in reactivation of the previously well-contained infection, leading to clinically apparent disease.

Protective immune responses against TB developed after primary infection usually protect against subsequent exogenous reinfection with other strains of *M. tuberculosis*. Studies using restriction fragment length polymorphism DNA fingerprinting, however, indicate that exogenous reinfection and progressive TB disease may contribute substantially to TB morbidity in densely crowded slums in high-burden countries[178] and in immunocompromised groups such as alcoholics residing in public shelters[179] and HIV-infected patients in large urban areas.[180,181] Reinfection TB has also been documented to occur in HIV-infected people in Africa[26] and may be most important in crowded urban areas of developing countries and in closed environments, principally mines, where high rates of TB disease and transmission occur.

During the period of clinical latency, effective host defenses against the development of active TB are characterized by strong Th1-like patterns presumably reprimed at local sites of bacterial replication. IL-12 appears to be the critical cytokine in the development of protective immunity and IFN-γ in its expression. Genetic defects in the expression of these cytokines or their receptors lead to predisposition to disseminated mycobacterial infections. TNF-α is critical to maintaining granuloma integrity.

When the immune host is exposed to mycobacterial antigens as occurs in reactivation TB, a brisk *in situ* DTH response occurs and may contribute to tissue damage. This is the case in pleural TB and TB peritonitis, pericarditis, and meningitis. When the balance between mycobacterial replication and host immunity shifts, usually because of immunosuppression, reactivation TB ensues. At the pulmonary focus there is a vigorous inflammatory response with unregulated expression of cytokines. The immune response no longer controls bacterial replication, contributing instead to tissue damage.

Systemically, patients with progressive TB show a Th2 pattern with depression of DTH, *in vitro* blastogenesis, and production of IL-2 and IFN-γ. Their circulating T cells express IL-4, and serum immunoglobulin G levels to *M. tuberculosis* proteins are increased. The inflammatory response leads to programmed cell death or apoptosis and development of cavities. There is overproduction of the immunosuppressive cytokines TGF-β and IL-10, which depress IFN-γ expression.[182] As patients are treated, the suppression by these cytokines diminishes, unmasking a protracted primary defect in T-cell function. This acquired immunosuppression may be a factor in bacterial persistence and the requirement for lengthy courses of chemotherapy as well as the increased risk of reinfection seen in treated TB patients.

With the sequencing of the genome of *M. tuberculosis* it is possible to explore the role of differences in virulence of the organism in pathogenesis. For example, certain strains, such as CDC1551, appear to induce more cytokine production, larger granulomas, and more DTH.[183] The relative role of host and bacterial genetics as opposed to acquired comorbidities in influencing the progression of infection and disease is an area of active research.

Drug Resistance

Soon after the introduction of streptomycin for the treatment of TB, treatment failures due to drug resistance were noted when patients were treated with single agents. Drug resistance develops from random chromosomal mutations, which occur spontaneously at low rates in wild-type strains of *M. tuberculosis*. The rate of natural resistance varies for specific agents: 1 in 0.5×10^4 bacilli for ethambutol, 1 in 3.5×10^6 for isoniazid, 1 in 3.8×10^6 for streptomycin, and 1 in 3.1×10^8 for rifampicin. Combination chemotherapy was introduced in the 1950s to overcome acquired drug resistance by ensuring that sufficient numbers of drugs were given such that all organisms present in a patient were susceptible to one or more of the drugs used. Solid caseous foci contain approximately 10^2 to 10^4 bacilli, whereas cavitary lesions contain approximately 10^7 to 10^9 bacilli.[184] The probability of a single tubercle bacillus being resistant to more than one drug is the product of the probabilities of resistance to each drug. A cavitary lesion before treatment may already contain 10 to 1000 organisms resistant to a single drug, but it is unlikely that such a lesion contains bacilli resistant to two or more drugs; for example, 1 in $10^6 \times$ 1 in 10^6 means that only 1 in 10^{12} bacilli would be expected to be resistant to both drugs.

Monotherapy, inappropriate treatment regimens, or the addition of a single drug to the regimen of patients failing treatment select for the outgrowth (clinical resistance) of populations of mutant resistant organisms and the development of MDR TB. The presence of MDR limits options for successful treatment and cure of the patient and may lead to the spread of drug-resistant TB to others in the community.

The term *primary drug resistance* refers to the presence of resistance to one or more antituberculous medications in a patient who has never been treated for TB. Primary drug resistance rates are a reflection of natural drug resistance and the successful application of TB treatment by the TB control program in the community. *Acquired drug resistance* refers to drug resistance in patients with a prior history of TB treatment. Acquired drug resistance is often due to poor compliance, poor absorption or bioavailability of drugs, and the addition of single agents to the regimens of patients who are already failing treatment (***Box 35.1***). Poorly organized TB treatment programs can lead to the rapid development of drug resistance in both developing and industrialized countries. Once initial resistance has developed, acquisition of resistance to additional drugs is more likely (a phenomenon known as amplification of resistance); the use of standardized treatment regimens may lead to amplification of drug resistance in certain settings.[185]

The term *multidrug-resistant (MDR) TB* refers to *M. tuberculosis* isolates resistant to at least isoniazid and rifampicin. The development of rifampicin resistance is a crucial event because overall success rates with four-drug short-course initial and retreatment regimens in patients with isoniazid or streptomycin resistance are only slightly less than those with fully drug-susceptible organisms,[186] whereas treatment outcomes in the presence of both isoniazid and rifampicin resistance are poor. Multiple drug resistance necessitates the use of more toxic, more expensive, and less effective second- and third-line agents for TB treatment. Many developing countries cannot afford these second- and third-line agents.

A multinational laboratory survey[187] and a hospital-based outbreak of fatal disease[188] in South Africa established XDR TB as a major new public health concern. XDR TB is defined as caused by an organism that is MDR with additional resistance to a fluoroquinolone plus one of the injectables (amikacin, kanamycin, capreomycin). Globally, approximately 5–10% of MDR isolates fulfill these criteria for XDR TB. In an outbreak among HIV-infected patients in KwaZulu-Natal, 52 of 53 patients died after a median of 16 weeks of hospitalization. With recognition of the outbreak, improved diagnosis and management reduced the case-fatality rate from 98% to 84%.[189] The best outcome data come from Peru where a comprehensive interdisciplinary management team, and regimens that were individualized based on drug susceptibility testing resulted in 60.4% cure rates and 22.9% case-fatality rate,[190] an outcome similar to MDR TB.

Box 35.1 Factors Associated with Acquired Drug Resistance

Incomplete or intermittent therapy	Patient noncompliance
Physician error	Inappropriate isoniazid preventive therapy (failure to exclude active tuberculosis)
Inadequate initial treatment regimen	

Current estimates are that 500 000 cases of MDR TB occur annually with 110 000 deaths.[9] Twenty-seven countries account for 85% of the estimated cases, with most cases found in India, China, the Russian Federation, and South Africa. The prevalence of drug-resistant and MDR TB is higher in previously treated individuals.[191] Even in countries thought to have low burdens of MDR TB, retreatment cases are at substantial risk. For example, in retreatment cases at a referral hospital in Kampala, Uganda, 12.7% were MDR TB.[192] Taking a careful history regarding prior TB treatment and exposure to individuals with known drug-resistant TB is the most important way to identify patients at risk for having drug-resistant TB.

DIAGNOSIS

Routine methods for the diagnosis of TB are based on demonstration of the organism on smears and cultures obtained from infected secretions or tissues from affected organs. Newer methods involve the detection of specific *M. tuberculosis* antigens or antibodies to mycobacterial proteins and the identification of specific *M. tuberculosis* DNA in clinical specimens.

Standard procedures begin with microscopic examination of smears made from potentially infected secretions and tissues and culture of these materials on a variety of media. Hot and cold carbol fuchsin (Ziehl–Neelsen and Kinyoun) methods are the most widely used. The number of AFB that must be present in a sample for a positive AFB smear has been estimated to be 10^3–$10^4/\mu L$,[6,193] but good laboratories with experienced microscopists who spend adequate time examining slides likely have a lower threshold for detection. The use of fluorochrome stains such as auramine–rhodamine allows more rapid screening of sputum smears with a sensitivity comparable to those of the Ziehl–Neelsen or Kinyoun methods. The rate of sputum smear positivity is dependent on the bacillary load, which is in turn dependent on the extent of disease and the presence of cavitary lesions. Pretreatment smears are negative in 22–61% of new pulmonary TB cases and are more common in patients with minimal and noncavitary disease,[194–197] which occurs more frequently in patients with HIV coinfection.

Clinical specimens can be cultured on a variety of media. The most popular are opaque egg-based Löwenstein–Jensen and clear oleic acid–albumin agar-based Middlebrook media. Löwenstein–Jensen medium is inexpensive but small early colonies can be detected earlier on transparent agar-based media. Cultures should be examined weekly until positive or for 8 weeks. Organisms from positive cultures are then speciated using morphologic and biochemical techniques to identify them as *M. tuberculosis* or atypical mycobacteria. Using conventional egg- or agar-based media, 4–8 weeks are required for cultures to become positive, especially for paucibacillary and smear-negative samples. The long culture period is due to the long dividing times of mycobacteria (12–18 hours), which means that 3 or more weeks are required for growth from a single cell to a visible colony on solid media. Drug susceptibility testing by conventional techniques requires an additional 2–4 weeks.

Sputum specimens can be collected at the time of examination, in the early morning, and as overnight pooled collections. Early morning specimens are preferred because in these samples the tracheobronchial secretions have collected in the airways overnight and have a higher yield and a lower contamination rate. Multiple specimens should be examined. The diagnostic yield increases with up to five specimens but most of the enhanced yield is achieved with the first two or three samples.[198] Increased sputum production can also be induced by the inhalation of normal or hypertonic (3%) saline aerosols in adults unable to spontaneously produce sputum. The resulting secretions are thinner than spontaneously expectorated sputum and the laboratory must be made aware that the sample is an induced specimen to prevent it from being discarded as unsatisfactory. In children and young adults unable to produce sputum, gastric aspiration can be performed, preferably in the early morning before the patient rises, to sample respiratory secretions that have been swallowed and pooled in the stomach. Mycobacteria die quickly in acidic stomach contents, and gastric aspirates should be processed promptly or neutralized with buffer. The sensitivity of AFB smears of gastric aspirates is only 23–30%; however, positive smears are highly reliable for the diagnosis of TB.[199,200]

Where available, bronchoscopy is useful for diagnosis in cases in which sputum specimens are repeatedly negative and other samples are unavailable and an empirical trial of treatment is inadvisable. Samples can be obtained by washing, brushing, bronchoalveolar lavage, and transbronchial lung biopsy. Specimens obtained at bronchoscopy are rarely the only positive specimens in patients with TB when final culture results are available.[201–203] The principal value of bronchoscopy, therefore, is in allowing the diagnosis to be established quickly in seriously ill or immunocompromised patients (including patients with AIDS) by demonstrating necrotizing granulomas or AFB in histologic sections of tissue.[121,201–203] Transbronchial biopsy with the fiberoptic bronchoscope may be particularly valuable for the rapid evaluation of suspected cases of miliary disease.[120,127,205]

Newer methods have been developed to increase diagnostic sensitivity and to shorten the time needed to diagnose TB and perform drug susceptibility testing.[206,207] Systems based on automated or semi-automated detection of growth in enriched liquid media can detect growth more rapidly than detection of visible colonies on solid media. Radiometric culture methods such as the BACTEC 460 system rely on the detection of radioactive ^{14}C released from a labeled palmitic acid substrate in liquid media by metabolically active mycobacteria and significantly shorten the time until detection of a positive culture (BACTEC 460 system is currently being discontinued). The newer nonradiometric mycobacterial growth indicator tube (BACTEC MGIT 960) system is based on oxygen quenching in the presence of replicating mycobacteria and is now the preferred automated culture system. Using appropriate decontamination methods and culture media, it is possible to directly inoculate susceptibility testing media from clinical specimens, eliminating the lengthy primary culture step.

Traditional systems for speciating mycobacteria have relied on biochemical parameters, colonial morphology and rate of growth, and gas or liquid chromatography. Rapid methods using DNA probes have been developed that bind specifically to mycobacterial RNA from a single species; binding is detected photometrically. Probes are commercially available for *M. tuberculosis* complex (includes *M. tuberculosis* and *M. bovis*), *M. avium* complex, *M. avium*, *M. intracellulare*, *M. kansasii*, and *M. gordonae*. These tests require only a few hours to perform.

Several nucleic acid amplification assays have been developed for mycobacterial diagnosis based on PCR, strand displacement or transcription-mediated amplification, reporter phage, and ligase chain reaction methods. In general, these tests have performed well on smear-positive respiratory specimens (sensitivity, 82–100%; specificity, 93–100%) but less so on smear-negative specimens (sensitivity, 51–88%; specificity, 97–100%).[206] The Centers for Disease Control and Prevention recommend that nucleic acid amplification testing be performed on at least one respiratory specimen from a patient with signs and symptoms of pulmonary TB for whom a diagnosis of TB is being considered but has not yet been established.[208] Molecular amplification tests are expensive and require significant infrastructure and staff training for reliable performance.

Conventional drug susceptibility testing against first-line anti-TB drugs can be performed using the critical concentration or indirect proportion methods on solid media but requires 2 or 3 weeks to perform after a positive culture is obtained.[209,210] The time to obtain results is reduced using enriched liquid culture systems such as the BACTEC 460 or MGIT 960 systems. Resistance to rifampicin is due in the great majority of cases to mutations in a short sequence of the *rpoB* gene of the bacterial RNA polymerase, and rapid PCR-based methods have been developed to assess whether resistance to rifampicin is present, a reliable marker for MDR TB.[185] Resistance to other key drugs is due to a variety of mechanisms and mutations, and rapid genotypic testing for resistance is less reliable at this time.

TREATMENT

Modern TB treatment is based on the use of potent short-course, multiple-drug regimens that sterilize the sputum rapidly. TB treatment is divided into two phases – the initial intensive phase lasting 1 or 2 months that kills the rapidly dividing, rapidly metabolizing organisms, followed by a 4–7-month continuation phase that kills the remaining slowly metabolizing organisms. The most useful first-line drugs for TB treatment include isoniazid, rifampicin, ethambutol, pyrazinamide, and streptomycin. Adult and pediatric dosages are summarized in ***Table 35.2***. Combination therapy with these agents forms the foundation of current TB chemotherapy.

First-Line Drugs

Streptomycin

Streptomycin was introduced for the treatment of tuberculosis in 1948 soon after its discovery. It must be given parenterally and penetrates most

Table 35.2 Dosages of First-Line Antituberculosis Drugs Used in Adults and Children[a]

Drug	Daily Dose	Twice Weekly Dose	Thrice Weekly Dose
Isoniazid	5 mg/kg PO (10–15 mg/kg in children); maximum 300 mg/day	15 mg/kg PO (20–30 mg/kg in children); maximum 900 mg/dose	15 mg/kg PO (20–30 mg/kg in children); maximum 900 mg/dose
Rifampicin	10 mg/kg PO (10–20 mg/kg in children); maximum 600 mg/day	10 mg/kg PO (10–20 mg/kg in children); maximum 600 mg/day	10 mg/kg PO (10–20 mg/kg in children); maximum 600 mg/day
Pyrazinamide	Weight 40–55 kg = 1000 mg; 56–75 kg = 1500 mg; above 76 kg = 2000 mg PO (15–30 mg/kg in children); maximum 2 g/day	Weight 40–55 kg = 2000 mg; 56–75 kg = 3000 mg; above 76 kg = 4000 mg PO (50–70 mg/kg in children); maximum 4 g/dose	Weight 40–55 kg = 1500 mg; 56–75 kg = 2500 mg; above 76 kg = 3000 mg PO (50–70 mg/kg in children); maximum 3 g/dose
Ethambutol[b]	Weight 40–55 kg = 800 mg; 56–75 kg = 1200 mg; above 76 kg = 1600 mg PO (15–25 mg/kg in children)	Weight 40–55 kg = 2000 mg; 56–75 kg = 2800 mg; above 76 kg = 4000 mg PO (50 mg/kg in children)	Weight 40–55 kg = 1200 mg; 56–75 kg = 2000 mg; above 76 kg = 2400 mg PO (25–30 mg/kg in children)
Streptomycin	15 mg/kg IM (20–40 mg/kg in children); maximum 1 g/day	25–30 mg/kg IM (adults and children); maximum 1.5 g/dose	25–30 mg/kg IM (adults and children); maximum 1.5 g/dose

[a]Children younger than 12 years old.

[b]Ethambutol is not recommended for treatment in children younger than 12 years old who cannot be reliably monitored for ophthalmologic toxicity but should be considered in cases of drug-resistant tuberculosis.

IM, intramuscularly; PO, orally.

body spaces and tissues, including inflamed meninges. The initial use of streptomycin monotherapy for cavitary TB in the 1940s was quickly followed by the observation that following initial remarkable improvement, after 3 months of treatment up to 80% of patients treated with streptomycin had streptomycin-resistant bacilli.[211] When combined in various regimens with subsequent agents, such as isoniazid, *p*-aminosalicylic acid, and ethambutol, streptomycin proved highly useful in TB treatment. Streptomycin is a first-line bactericidal agent with a minimum inhibitory concentration (MIC) against *M. tuberculosis* of 8 μg/mL. Streptomycin is usually given by intramuscular (IM) injection at a dose of 15 mg/kg per day (up to 1 g per day) for the first 1 or 2 months of treatment. The drug is renally excreted and the dose should be decreased in patients with underlying renal insufficiency. Major side effects include ototoxicity (vestibular more than hearing loss) and nephrotoxicity and are related to the cumulative dose.

Isoniazid

Isoniazid (isonicotinic acid hydrazide) was introduced for the treatment of tuberculosis in 1952. Isoniazid is a mycobactericidal drug with an MIC against *M. tuberculosis* of 0.05–0.2 μg/mL. It is well absorbed when administered orally (PO) with good tissue and CNS penetration. It can also be administered parenterally by IM injection. Usual doses are 5 mg/kg per day up to 300 mg per day in adults. Higher doses can be given when intermittent dosing is used (twice- or three-times-weekly administration); however, these should not exceed 900 mg/dose because of the increased risk of neurotoxicity, specifically seizures.

The frequency of adverse reactions to isoniazid in HIV-uninfected patients is approximately 5%.[212] The most common adverse reactions are rash, fever, peripheral neuropathy, and jaundice. Rarer adverse events include neutropenia, thrombocytopenia, seizures, encephalopathy, antinuclear antibody-positive small-vessel vasculitis, dyspepsia, red blood cell aplasia, optic neuritis, methemoglobinemia, urinary retention, and pellagra. Severe and rarely fatal hepatitis may occur during isoniazid preventive therapy. Elevations of serum aminotransferases occur in 10–20% of all subjects receiving isoniazid preventive therapy.[213] These increases, developing during the initial weeks of therapy, are generally asymptomatic and frequently resolve despite continuation of the drug. People who consume ethanol (alcohol; especially on a daily basis), those with preexisting liver disease, and pregnant and postpartum black and Hispanic women are at increased risk of hepatotoxicity.[214,215] Hepatotoxicity is usually reversible if the medication is stopped when initial symptoms of hepatotoxicity, including nausea, anorexia, malaise, and dull upper abdominal discomfort, occur. Health care workers and patients need to be aware of these symptoms and the importance of stopping isoniazid treatment and seeking medical attention if they occur.

Isoniazid therapy is also associated with the development of a dose-dependent peripheral sensorimotor neuropathy via interactions with pyridoxine and pyridoxal-5-phosphate metabolism. Peripheral neuropathy develops in only 1–2% of well-nourished patients receiving 3–5 mg/kg per day of isoniazid, but it is more frequent in malnourished people, pregnant women, and patients with diabetes mellitus, chronic renal failure, and alcoholism. Isoniazid peripheral neuropathy can be prevented or reversed in nearly all cases by supplemental oral pyridoxine 25–50 mg per day. Where available, pyridoxine supplementation should be given to all patients receiving isoniazid.

Rifampicin

Rifampicin is a first-line bactericidal agent that inhibits DNA-dependent RNA polymerase, leading to the death of the bacilli. Rifampicin is well absorbed with good penetration of inflamed meninges. The MIC against *M. tuberculosis* is approximately 0.5 μg/mL. The usual dose is 10 mg/kg per day (up to 600 mg per day). Rifampicin is a potent hepatic enzyme inducer and has many clinically significant drug interactions affecting the dosing of other medications, such as warfarin sodium (Coumadin), theophylline, and HIV protease inhibitors, nevirapine and several other frequently used medications. Rifampicin increases the metabolism of estrogens and can result in decreased efficacy of hormonal contraceptive and breakthrough bleeding. The principal side effects are gastrointestinal intolerance, skin rashes, cholestatic jaundice, and hepatitis. A flulike syndrome characterized by malaise, fever, chills, headache, and myalgias can occur and is more frequent with intermittent dosing. Hemolytic anemia and thrombocytopenia are rare complications but require permanent discontinuation of the drug. Body secretions, including urine, sweat, and tears, appear orange or orange-red during rifampicin treatment. Rifampicin is the single most effective antituberculous drug currently available and constitutes the backbone of short-course (6 months) modern treatment regimens; resistance to rifampicin requires treatment to be extended to 9 or 12 months.

Ethambutol

Ethambutol is primarily a mycobacteriostatic agent given to prevent the emergence of drug resistance to other first-line drugs. It has low CSF penetration. The MIC is 1–5 μg/mL. Usual dosages are 15–25 mg/kg per day. The drug is renally excreted and the dosage should be reduced in patients with renal insufficiency. The most important side effect of ethambutol is retrobulbar neuritis, which presents as blurred vision or decreased peripheral and color vision. The frequency of ocular toxicity is lower at the 15 mg/kg per day dose that is recommended when ethambutol is continued after the intensive phase of therapy. Patients receiving ethambutol should be instructed about symptoms of ocular toxicity. Simple visual acuity and color vision screening at follow-up clinic visits may help detect this complication early. Ethambutol should not be prescribed for young children who cannot report visual symptoms reliably. Ocular toxicity is reversible in most cases after discontinuation of the drug.

Pyrazinamide

Pyrazinamide is an important first-line bactericidal agent first used in TB treatment in the 1950s. Early concerns about hepatotoxicity relegated it to a minor role until the 1970s, when a series of important clinical trials conducted by the British Medical Research Council clearly established its important role in rapid sterilization of tuberculous lesions with resultant shortening of the duration of chemotherapy from 9–12 months to 6 months. Pyrazinamide is highly active in the acidic intracellular environment against organisms in macrophages. It has good tissue penetration, including the CSF. Usual doses are 15–30 mg/kg per day, up to 2 g per day. The most frequent side effects are gastrointestinal intolerance, hepatotoxicity, arthralgias, asymptomatic hyperuricemia due to blockade of urate excretion, and, rarely, acute gouty arthritis. Pyrazinamide does not appear to further increase the risk of hepatotoxicity when used in combination with isoniazid and rifampicin.[216] Minor arthralgias occur frequently and can usually be treated with salicylates or nonsteroidal inflammatory agents such as indomethacin while continuing the drug. The major value of pyrazinamide is its early sterilizing activity against intracellular organisms during the initial intensive phase of treatment.[217]

Second-Line Antituberculosis Drugs

Several other agents are available for the treatment of known or suspected drug-resistant TB cases, which is 5–10 times more frequent in patients previously treated for TB (i.e., retreatment TB).[218] As a whole, these drugs are more toxic, less well tolerated, and less effective for TB treatment. Their use is indicated only for drug-resistant TB and as substitute agents when first-line drugs cannot be tolerated by the patient. Treatment involving second-line drugs also must be given for long durations of 18–24 months. Several of these agents must be given parenterally. Many are not readily available in developing countries due to their expense. When possible, the treatment of MDR TB and XDR TB is best suited to referral centers with specialized laboratories, trained personnel, and access to surgical facilities (surgical resection of large, necrotic lung cavitary lesions and other procedures are frequently indicated).[219]

Box 35.2 Important Principles in Treatment of Tuberculosis

Use combination chemotherapy with at least two drugs to which the patient's organism can reasonably be expected to be susceptible	Adequate doses of bioavailable drugs must be given consistently for an adequate duration of time for cure to be achieved
Never add a single drug to a failing regimen	Both the patient and the physician share responsibility for successful treatment
The principal role of bacteriostatic drugs is to prevent emergence of resistant organisms during combination chemotherapy	

Initial Tuberculosis Treatment Regimens

Many national and international organizations have published excellent comprehensive guidelines for TB treatment that are very valuable for clinicians.[220–224] This section discusses general principles of treatment (***Box 35.2***) and some suggested highly effective short-course regimens. The use of such regimens is feasible and highly cost-effective under program conditions.[225,226] Although the availability of regular supplies of high-quality drugs and the prescribing of adequate regimens in adequate doses for adequate durations are essential, it is important to stress the critical roles of the health care team, patient adherence to treatment, social factors, and political commitment in achieving good outcomes in TB control.

Four drugs should be prescribed initially unless local drug-resistance rates to first-line anti-TB drugs are known to be low (<2%).[220] Treatment with rifampicin, isoniazid, and pyrazinamide is critical to the success of 6-month short-course regimens. Rifampicin and isoniazid should be given for the entire duration of 6-month regimens for optimal efficacy. Pyrazinamide is necessary only during the first 2 months of treatment of drug-susceptible TB. Where available, the use of fixed-dose combination tablets decreases the number of pills to be taken, lessens the risk that patients may take only some of their drugs, and is strongly recommended by WHO.[222]

Patient compliance is a crucial factor in treatment failure and the development of acquired drug resistance. Whenever possible, TB treatment should be administered as directly observed therapy (DOT), where a health care worker or lay supervisor observes the patient swallow each dose of medication. DOT has been shown to be a highly effective (and cost-effective) strategy for TB treatment in both industrialized and developing countries.[225,227]

The following 6-month regimens have been shown to be highly effective in initial TB treatment:[217,228,229]

1. Two months of daily isoniazid, rifampicin, ethambutol, and pyrazinamide followed by 4 months of isoniazid and rifampicin administered two or three times weekly.
2. Two weeks of daily isoniazid, rifampicin, ethambutol, and pyrazinamide followed by 6 weeks of twice-weekly isoniazid, rifampicin, ethambutol, and pyrazinamide followed by 4 months of twice-weekly isoniazid and rifampicin.
3. Six months of three-times-weekly isoniazid, rifampicin, and pyrazinamide.

If drug susceptibility testing is performed and the isolate is fully drug susceptible, ethambutol may be discontinued. If the patient cannot tolerate pyrazinamide, excellent results may be achieved in patients with fully susceptible TB with 9 months of isoniazid and rifampicin. Six months of treatment with the previous regimens is generally adequate for patients with pulmonary TB who have satisfactory clinical and bacteriologic responses to treatment. Based on data suggesting that patients with initial cavitary disease who do not convert their sputum cultures to negative after 2 months of treatment are at high risk for relapse, some authorities now recommend extending treatment for an additional 3 months with isoniazid and rifampicin for such patients.[220,224]

In developing countries with limited supplies of rifampicin, 2 months of daily ethambutol, isoniazid, rifampicin, and pyrazinamide followed by 6 months of daily isoniazid and ethambutol[222] or 6 months of isoniazid and thiacetazone[223] is widely used, although relapse rates are higher than with regimens containing rifampicin during the entire course of treatment.[230] Longer treatment regimens without a potent rifampicin and pyrazinamide-containing intensive phase, such as 2 months of daily isoniazid, thiacetazone, and streptomycin followed by 10 months of isoniazid and thiacetazone, can also be utilized but are associated with lower cure rates and high rates of cutaneous drug reactions in areas with a high prevalence of HIV coinfection.[231–234]

Patients should be instructed to cover their mouth and nose with a handkerchief or tissue when coughing. Masks and an initial period of respiratory isolation are desirable for hospitalized patients with smear-positive disease, where available. These measures can be discontinued when the number of bacilli visible on sputum smears and cough frequency decrease. Short-course chemotherapy regimens rapidly sterilize the sputum. Sputum smears may take longer to clear than sputum cultures, especially when rifampicin-containing regimens are used. Sputum smear-positive, culture-negative status was observed during the first 4–20 weeks of treatment in 20% of patients in one large series.[196] This phenomenon presumably is due to the visualization of nonviable organisms on sputum smears. Adequate respiratory isolation facilities are not available in many hospitals, however, and the primary emphasis in infection control should be on maintaining a high clinical suspicion for TB and the rapid diagnosis and treatment of infectious sputum smear-positive individuals. Although smear-positive patients are thought to be most infectious, there may be significant variability in infectiousness regardless of smear results.[235–238]

Routine monitoring of hepatic function tests is not recommended. Proper patient education about TB, the need for full completion of treatment, and common side effects is important. In addition to DOT visits, patients should routinely be seen in the clinic on a monthly basis to review progress. At a minimum, the sputum should be examined monthly until conversion, at the end of treatment, and whenever clinical symptoms warrant. Around 77–90% of patients treated with rifampicin-containing short-course regimens should be culture negative (more than 75% smear negative) after completing 2 months of treatment, and essentially all should be culture negative after 3 months.[225,239–242] Reduction in cough frequency, resolution of fever and chest pain, and weight gain are the most important clinical signs of response to treatment. Defervescence occurred within 2 weeks in 64–93% of patients with pulmonary TB treated with rifampicin-containing regimens.[243,244] Serial chest radiography should not routinely be used to monitor response to treatment. One fourth to one-third of patients with good clinical and microbiologic responses to treatment have worsening of radiographic lesions during the initial months of treatment. Chest films should be taken when the clinical course is complicated by new hemoptysis, poor response to treatment, or other significant changes in the patient's condition. In cases of poor response to treatment, if the chest film has not improved after 3 months of treatment, noncompliance, malabsorption of anti-TB drugs, drug-resistant TB, an incorrect initial diagnosis, or other concomitant chest disease should be considered. An end-of-treatment film may be helpful as a future baseline for comparison.

Patients should be instructed to return to the clinic promptly for medical attention when symptoms of drug toxicity occur. Early signs of hepatotoxicity (nausea, malaise, anorexia, and upper abdominal discomfort) should be emphasized. Minor drug reactions may be managed symptomatically with continuation of anti-TB treatment. Moderate or severe suspected drug reactions should be treated by discontinuation of TB treatment, appropriate medical management, and serial observation of the patient until the reaction subsides. At the discretion of the treating clinician, stepwise reinstitution of the anti-TB drugs at full dosage beginning with the least likely offending drug may be considered on a case-by-case basis, or alternative drugs may be substituted. The use of desensitization schedules with escalating doses of drugs such as isoniazid is not recommended. The reintroduction process should not be prolonged to avoid long periods of monotherapy. The implicated drug should be discontinued if the reaction occurs during rechallenge and the regimen modified appropriately by the addition of new replacement drugs. Most adverse drug reactions to anti-TB drugs are reversible upon discontinuation of the offending medication.

There are several promising developments in the treatment of TB.[245] Rifapentine, a long-acting rifamycin, has been shown to be effective when administered once weekly during the continuation phase of treatment in HIV-noninfected patients.[246] Newer fluoroquinolones, including levofloxacin, gatifloxacin, and moxifloxacin, are highly active against *M. tuberculosis* and may allow shortening of treatment to less than 6 months. In a trial from India, 4- and 5-month regimens including an initial intensive phase containing ofloxacin, isoniazid, rifampicin, and pyrazinamide were highly successful in patients with smear-positive tuberculosis, resulting in relapse rates of less than 4%.[247] New compounds including PA-824, a nitroimidazole active against slowly dividing organisms, and more recently OPC-67683, are in early testing.[248] Other drugs at different stages in the discovery pipeline are TMC-207 (diarylquinoline), SQ-109 (ethylenediamine) and PNU-100480, a new oxazolidinone with potent anti-TB activity, in addition to the early bactericidal activity shown by linezolid.[249] In a recent study, the addition of TMC-207 to a standard regimen for the treatment of MDR TB decreased the time to sterilization of sputum and increased the proportion of patients that converted their sputum.[250]

Special Situations

Pediatric Tuberculosis

Microbiologic confirmation of the diagnosis of TB is difficult in young children and the decision to treat is often based on known close contact with an infectious smear-positive case, compatible clinical symptoms and radiographic findings, and lack of response to empirical treatment with broad-spectrum antibiotics targeted against common bacterial pathogens. Regimens used in children are comparable to those in adults with appropriate dose modifications[220] (see ***Table 35.2***). Local formularies should be consulted about available preparations of anti-TB drugs for children. Ethambutol should be avoided in infants and young children who cannot report symptoms of ophthalmologic toxicity. Radiographic and clinical response should be monitored, with improvement expected over 2 or 3 months. Intrathoracic lymphadenopathy may take up to 2 years to fully resolve in children, and the persistence of lymphadenopathy is not, in itself, an indication for prolonged therapy.

Pregnancy and Lactation

TB treatment regimens used in pregnant and lactating women are similar to regimens used in nonpregnant women.[220,251,252] Few data are available on the potential teratogenicity of pyrazinamide and some programs avoid its use in pregnancy. Isoniazid and rifampicin have good long-term safety records in pregnant and lactating women, and daily treatment with isoniazid and rifampicin for 9 months is highly effective in drug-susceptible TB. Treatment of drug-resistant TB during pregnancy is complex, and such patients should be evaluated by a specialist. Successful treatment of MDR TB during pregnancy has been reported.[253]

The risk of isoniazid hepatotoxicity may be increased during pregnancy and the early postpartum period. Aminoglycosides should be avoided during pregnancy due to the risk of irreversible ototoxicity in the fetus. Pregnant women are more susceptible to development of isoniazid-associated peripheral neuropathy and should receive pyridoxine 25–50 mg per day while on TB treatment. Breastfeeding is safe while on TB chemotherapy.[254]

Extrapulmonary TB

Extrapulmonary TB is associated with lower bacillary burdens than pulmonary disease; therefore, extrapulmonary disease can generally be treated with standard short-course regimens that are effective for pulmonary disease.[228,255] Owing to the serious implications of relapsed disease at sites of potentially limited drug penetration, most clinicians treat miliary, meningeal, and skeletal TB for 12 or more months. Adjunctive surgical débridement and stabilization of bone and joint tuberculosis should be considered in addition to chemotherapy on a case-by-case basis. There is evidence from controlled clinical trials that short courses of corticosteroids (1 mg/kg per day prednisone or the equivalent rapidly tapered over 4–6 weeks) may be useful in cases of TBM, pericarditis, and severe serofibrinous pleurisy. Corticosteroids have also been used in cases of extensive pulmonary TB with severe clinical toxicity or acute respiratory failure. Corticosteroids can be given safely in conjunction with anti-TB chemotherapy.

Tuberculosis Treatment in Human Immunodeficiency Virus-Coinfected Patients

The treatment of choice for pulmonary TB in HIV-infected patients is short-course combination chemotherapy with regimens including isoniazid, rifampicin, ethambutol, and pyrazinamide that are effective in more than 95% of patients with drug-susceptible TB when administered for a full course of treatment.[28,29,31,32,81] A meta-analysis indicates that rifampicin should be continued for at least 3 months.[256] Due to increased relapse rates (in some instances with acquired rifampicin resistance) in HIV-infected patients treated with twice-weekly therapy, daily treatment during the intensive phase and at least thrice-weekly treatment during the continuation phase are highly recommended.[257,258] In contrast, regimens that do not include rifampicin as a principal component are associated with an increased incidence of severe cutaneous hypersensitivity reactions, lower rates of sputum conversion, higher treatment failure and relapse rates, and increased mortality compared with rifampicin-containing regimens in HIV-infected patients.[231,234,259]

Compliance is critical to good outcomes in the treatment of TB in HIV-infected people. DOT may be especially valuable in this setting.[260] Ambulatory treatment is fully satisfactory for the majority of patients with uncomplicated disease.

When treated with appropriate regimens, clinical and microbiologic responses to treatment are comparable to responses in HIV-noninfected patients. An extended duration of anti-TB chemotherapy is not routinely indicated in HIV-infected patients;[31] however, the microbiologic response to therapy should be closely monitored with serial sputum examinations. Treatment should be prolonged if the response to treatment is slow or otherwise unsatisfactory.[220] It is of note that virologic response to ART is unaffected by anti-TB therapy.[261]

Rarely, patients being started on anti-TB chemotherapy develop transient worsening of fever, lymphadenitis, cerebral tuberculomas, pulmonary infiltrates, pleural effusions, or other signs and symptoms of TB – so-called paradoxical reactions. Paradoxical reactions occur in HIV-uninfected people but appear to be more frequent in HIV-infected patients and in some studies have occurred more frequently in patients being started on ART and anti-TB treatment at the same time.[262] Paradoxical reactions usually occur within the first 2 months of ART, often during the initial 2–3 weeks of treatment, and may be more frequent in patients with low CD4 counts. The cause of paradoxical reactions is unclear; however, they may be due to reconstitution of host immune responses and heightened inflammatory responses after beginning anti-TB and possibly ART.[263] In fact, there is an associated increase in expression of mycobacterial reactive IFN-γ-producing Th1 cells.[264] Clinical deterioration should be ascribed to paradoxical reactions only after careful evaluation for treatment failure, malabsorption, noncompliance, drug toxicity, or another concomitant opportunistic infection. Mild paradoxical reactions are usually self-limited and may be treated symptomatically. Some authorities recommend a short course of several weeks of prednisone or methylprednisolone beginning at 1 mg/kg per day for patients with severe paradoxical reactions.[220]

Two studies of HIV-infected South African and Haitian adults assessing whether secondary prophylaxis with isoniazid after initial treatment could prevent recurrent TB showed a 55–82% decrease in recurrent disease in patients receiving isoniazid.[265,266] Patients with advanced HIV infection benefited the most, leading some authorities to recommend expansion of preventive therapy guidelines to include secondary isoniazid prophylaxis in patients with advanced HIV/AIDS living in areas with a high prevalence of TB. The timing of initiating ART and the antiretroviral drugs and regimens used in treating HIV-infected patients with TB who are not currently on ART is an evolving area of clinical practice. There are three clinical trials in progress that address this issue so that a clear answer should be forthcoming. A recent study indicated that integrated as compared to sequential management of TB-HIV was associated with a 56% improved survival.[267] Rifampicin is a potent hepatic microsomal enzyme inducer and alters the metabolism of many drugs. ART with protease inhibitors and non-nucleoside reverse transcriptase inhibitors has significant drug interaction during rifampicin therapy, resulting in low serum concentrations of the antiretroviral drugs and high rifampicin levels. In severely immunosuppressed patients (CD4 count <200/μL) deaths due to HIV-related complications may occur early during TB treatment. Therefore, many authorities recommend beginning concomitant ART early. Rifabutin has fewer drug interactions and, where available, can be used as an alternative to rifampicin. Other options include using ART regimens including efavirenz and avoiding nevirapine[268] and protease inhibitors initially. In fact the study by Boulle et al indicated that the virologic outcome is poorer when nevirapine is used in TB-HIV, whereas this is not the case with efavirenz. Recommendations and guidelines are rapidly changing and the clinician should consult with a specialist skilled in the treatment of both TB and HIV/AIDS for assistance.

Drug-Resistant Tuberculosis

From a tuberculosis control program standpoint, drug-resistant *M. tuberculosis* isolates are as infectious and virulent as drug-susceptible strains.[269,270] The clinical presentation of drug-resistant TB is similar to that of drug-susceptible TB; however, drug-resistant TB is difficult to treat and associated with worse outcomes.

Whereas initial isoniazid or streptomycin monoresistance has only minimal impact on the outcome of 6 months of treatment with rifampicin-containing short-course regimens,[186] the presence of rifampicin resistance or resistance to both isoniazid and rifampicin (MDR TB) is serious. Prolonged treatment with more toxic and expensive agents is required. Although initial studies reporting clinical outcomes among MDR TB patients were discouraging, recent work shows improving trends, with as many as 80% of patients responding to treatment.[271] With appropriate consultation and supervision, community-based therapy for MDR TB has been successful in some settings.[272] Patients have improved outcomes when their treatment regimen contains a minimum of three drugs to which their isolate is susceptible,[273] but it is generally recommended to build a regimen with at least four effective drugs.[274] A single agent should never be added to a failing regimen.

Cases of drug-resistant TB should be managed by specialized units and consultants whenever possible because treatment requires a good laboratory and access to more expensive and toxic drugs. Retreatment of treatment failures, relapses, and cases of suspected drug-resistant TB should be carefully monitored and administered as DOT. Under program conditions, failures and relapses of TB after an initial course of short-course chemotherapy are rarely multiple drug-resistant. Routine drug susceptibility testing of initial pretreatment isolates, although optimal, is not absolutely necessary. Patients with acquired drug resistance to isoniazid or isoniazid and streptomycin can still be cured by retreatment regimens such as the standard 8-month IUATLD (International Union Against Tuberculosis and Lung Disease) retreatment regimens consisting of 2 months of streptomycin, ethambutol, isoniazid, rifampicin, and pyrazinamide, followed by 1 month of ethambutol, isoniazid, rifampicin, and pyrazinamide, and concluding with 5 months of daily or three-times-weekly isoniazid, ethambutol, and rifampicin.[223] Drug susceptibility testing should be performed in patients with treatment failure or relapse, especially after unsuccessful retreatment.

The most important management principle in treating patients with resistance to one or more drugs is the administration of at least two new drugs to which the patient's isolate is susceptible. Initial isoniazid mono-resistance can be treated with the retreatment regimens described previously; with a 9-month regimen of rifampicin, ethambutol, and pyrazinamide for 2 months followed by rifampicin and ethambutol for 7 months;[275] or with 6 months of rifampicin, ethambutol, and pyrazinamide.[220] Patients whose isolates are resistant to rifampicin alone may be treated with isoniazid and ethambutol for 18 months or isoniazid, pyrazinamide, and streptomycin for 9 months.[276]

Treatment for MDR TB (resistant to at least isoniazid and rifampicin) involves prolonged therapy and the use of drugs with substantial side effects. Patients with suspected MDR TB should be managed in consultation with a specialist experienced in the management of MDR TB. General principles of management include the initial use of five drugs that are likely to be active, including an injectable one, until sputum cultures are negative, then continuing with three drugs. The most efficacious (bactericidal) drugs available should be used in adequate and tolerable doses for an adequate duration. If the patient is failing standard short-course treatment with isoniazid, rifampicin, pyrazinamide, and ethambutol and MDR TB is suspected, one approach is to add a fluoroquinolone such as ofloxacin or levofloxacin, an injectable drug such as kanamycin or amikacin, and possibly ethionamide. Authorities recommend continuing treatment for at least 12–15 months after sputum culture conversion. In the setting of localized disease, continued sputum positivity, massive hemoptysis, or inability to tolerate medical treatment, surgical resection of diseased lung tissue may play an adjunctive role in the treatment of MDR TB.[277,278] Detailed information about the treatment of drug-resistant TB can be obtained from several excellent sources.[223,279–282] The optimal management of XDR TB is not yet known. A backbone regimen containing capreomycin, cycloserine, and *p*-aminosalicylic acid was effective in Peru.[190] The high activity of a new anti-TB compound TMC207 against MDR TB may presage an important role in XDR TB management.[283] Similarly, the finding that the combination of meropenem plus amoxicillin-clavulanate is highly active *in vitro* against XDR TB isolates may indicate another therapeutic avenue to pursue.[284]

PREVENTION AND CONTROL

Tuberculosis Control

There are three principal strategies for the prevention and control of TB. Primary preventive measures include BCG vaccination and interruption of transmission, case finding, and treatment. Preventive therapy – the administration of drugs given after a person has become infected by *M. tuberculosis* to prevent the development of active TB – is an approach targeted at secondary prevention of new cases.

Owing to their higher bacillary burden, sputum smear-positive people with active TB (50% of all TB cases) are the principal source of TB transmission in the community. The highest priority in TB control programs and the fundamental approach advocated by IUATLD and WHO is the rapid identification and treatment of new cases of sputum smear-positive pulmonary TB detected through passive case finding. Because these infectious cases transmit TB to others, treatment of smear-positive cases benefits the affected individual and the community. When fully implemented, efficient case finding and effective treatment of smear-positive TB cases can quickly reduce mortality due to TB and the incidence of the disease in high-prevalence areas.

Bacille Calmette–Guérin Vaccination

Bacille Calmette-Guérin (BCG) is a living attenuated strain of *M. bovis* derived by serial passage in culture by Calmette and Guérin between 1908 and 1918. It is the basis of several inexpensive, safe vaccines widely used for the prevention of TB. BCG is a component of the United Nations Expanded Program on Immunization and is the world's most widely used vaccine. It is usually given as a single intradermal injection soon after birth.

Results of 21 large clinical trials of various BCG vaccines have yielded conflicting data about the efficacy of BCG in the prevention of TB.

Protective efficacy ranged from 10% to 81% in these studies.[285] Meta-analyses of these studies suggest that BCG vaccines are approximately 50% protective against the development of TB.[286] In some tropical countries, such as Malawi, BCG vaccine protects against leprosy but not TB. The protective efficacy of BCG vaccines against TB was decreased or absent in trials done in countries closer to the equator, possibly due to the higher frequency of naturally occurring infection with nontuberculous mycobacteria in these areas, which may be cross-protective against TB. Several different strains of BCG are used in making BCG vaccines. Genomic studies comparing various BCG strains have identified deletions, duplications, and single nucleotide polymorphisms that may also account for some of the difference in protection among various BCG vaccines.[287] In contrast to data showing variable prevention of pulmonary TB, there is more solid evidence that BCG is approximately 85% effective in preventing miliary and meningeal TB, the two most life-threatening forms of TB, in childhood.[288] The protective efficacy and duration of protection of BCG vaccination in immunocompromised people, such as those infected with HIV, are unclear.

Complications of BCG vaccination are infrequent and consist mainly of local lymphadenopathy or lymphadenitis; disseminated disease is rare. The rate of complications may be slightly higher in HIV-infected people but is still very low,[289] and WHO recommends that BCG vaccination be administered to infants early in life, even when the mother is known or suspected of being HIV infected. BCG vaccination should be withheld only from people with symptomatic HIV infection.[290]

Vaccines against TB that are under development include DNA vaccines, protein and peptide vaccines with new adjuvants, recombinant BCG and other live vectors expressing immunodominant mycobacterial antigens, naturally or rationally attenuated strains of mycobacteria, and nonpeptide vaccines.[291] Several candidate vaccines are entering human testing.

Treatment of Latent TB Infection

Treatment of LTBI, formerly termed TB-preventive therapy, has two principal benefits – an individual health benefit through prevention of TB and an important benefit to the community wherein decreased transmission of new *M. tuberculosis* infections will lead to an eventual lowering of case rates in the entire population. Interest in the use of isoniazid to prevent TB disease in people with previous *M. tuberculosis* infection began in the late 1950s. In HIV-noninfected people, 6–12 months of isoniazid preventive therapy was clearly shown to provide long-term health benefits. Isoniazid decreases the occurrence of TB by approximately 65% (range, 25–92%);[292] protection lasts up to 19 years and may be lifelong.[293]

Effectiveness is strongly correlated with the duration of preventive therapy and patient compliance. Maximal benefit in HIV-noninfected people was observed with 6–12 months of isoniazid preventive therapy, with no further advantage resulting from treatment exceeding 1 year.[294] In a large study from eastern Europe, the protective efficacy of isoniazid preventive therapy in patients with fibrotic residual lesions on chest radiography was only slightly reduced with 6 months of treatment, from 75% to 65%, compared with 12 months of therapy, whereas side effects were more frequent with the longer regimen.[295] Efficacy increases with compliance and was as high as 90% in highly compliant patients in some clinical trials; however, even patients with intermittent compliance over a sustained course of therapy benefit substantially from isoniazid preventive therapy.[16] Based on the previous data, 9 months of treatment with isoniazid is now the recommended regimen for treatment of latent TB infection for children and most adults. Three months of treatment with isoniazid and rifampicin has also been shown to be effective for the prevention of TB.[296–298]

The principal safety consideration regarding isoniazid preventive therapy is isoniazid-related hepatotoxicity. In a placebo-controlled trial of 6–12 months of isoniazid preventive therapy, the overall incidence of hepatotoxicity was 0.5%.[299] The incidence of hepatotoxicity increased with age, from 0.3% in people 20–34 years old to 1.2% in patients 35–49 years old, and with increased length of therapy. Ethanol consumption (especially on a daily basis), preexisting liver disease, possibly pregnancy, and the postpartum period[214,215] are also associated with hepatotoxicity.

Data from seven controlled clinical trials have shown that preventive therapy is also effective in PPD-positive (PPD ≥5 mm) HIV-infected people.[300] Six to 12 months of isoniazid, 3 months of isoniazid plus rifampicin, and 2 or 3 months of rifampicin and pyrazinamide provide approximately 56–60% short-term protection against TB. The combination of rifampicin and pyrazinamide is no longer recommended for treatment of latent TB infection because of an increased rate of severe hepatotoxicity and fulminant hepatic failure.[299] PPD-negative and anergic individuals have not been shown to benefit from preventive therapy against TB.[296,302,303]

The duration of the protective effect of TB preventive therapy in HIV-infected people is unknown.[304] Data from Zambia and Uganda suggest that benefits extend for 1–3 years[305,306] and may be longer after treatment with rifampicin-containing regimens.[305]

Increased access to ART certainly impacts on the need for preventive therapy. The effect of ART on TB incidence is greatest at CD4 counts below 200 and in the presence of symptoms (WHO stage 3 or 4).[39] However, at the low CD4 strata there was substantial residual risk of TB despite ART, indicating a role for preventive therapy in this group. Further ART reduced TB incidence in the CD4 200–350 strata, indicating that preventive therapy should be considered if there is no access to ART for this group. A recent study indicates that ART reduced the hazard rate for TB by 64% whereas the reduction was 89% when ART followed preventive therapy.[307] The overriding issue is, however, limited implementation of preventive therapy in HIV-infected people.

Decisions to prescribe isoniazid preventive therapy should balance the risks of developing active TB and the risk of isoniazid toxicity. HIV-infected people, close household contacts of smear-positive TB patients, and recent TST converters are among those at highest risk of developing active TB. Other groups of people with positive PPD skin tests for whom TB preventive therapy should be considered are listed in ***Box 35.3***. Active TB must be excluded prior to beginning preventive therapy.

The daily dosage of isoniazid for preventive therapy is 5 mg/kg (10 mg/kg in children) up to a maximum dose of 300 mg. Isoniazid can also be given twice weekly at a dose of 15 mg/kg up to a maximum dose of 900 mg when supervised preventive therapy is warranted, although the protective efficacy of intermittent regimens has not been studied. Pyridoxine 25–50 mg per day should be administered to prevent isoniazid-associated peripheral neuropathy. Routine biochemical monitoring of serum transaminases in patients receiving isoniazid preventive therapy is of limited value in people younger than 35 years of age but should be considered in older people, drinkers, and those with underlying liver disease. When serum liver function tests are monitored, discontinuation of isoniazid should be considered if the levels exceed three to five times the upper limit of normal. All people receiving isoniazid preventive therapy should be instructed to seek medical attention if symptoms of

Box 35.3 Tuberculin Skin Test-Positive Patients for Whom Tuberculosis Preventive Therapy Should Be Considered

- HIV-infected patients and people at high risk for HIV such as intravenous drug users
- Close contacts of new infectious TB cases (especially sputum smear-positive cases)
- Recent purified protein derivative skin test converters
- People with underlying medical conditions placing them at high risk of developing TB (poorly controlled diabetes mellitus, prolonged corticosteroid therapy, leukemia, Hodgkin's disease, head and neck cancer, end-stage renal disease, conditions associated with rapid weight loss, and chronic protein-calorie malnutrition)
- Recent immigrants from countries with a high prevalence of TB
- Institutionalized people (prisons, nursing homes, etc.)

hepatotoxicity, such as malaise, dark urine, nausea, and abdominal pain, develop and should be seen at the clinic at least monthly.

Only limited experience is available with drugs other than isoniazid for preventive therapy in patients who have been exposed to known or suspected cases of drug-resistant TB or where isoniazid was not tolerated. Treatment with 4 months of daily rifampicin[298] has been used in instances in which the index TB case is resistant to isoniazid or in which the patient could not tolerate isoniazid. Six months of ethambutol plus pyrazinamide or pyrazinamide plus ofloxacin have been used as preventive therapy in high-risk patients who were infected after exposure to cases of MDR TB, although side effects, mainly gastrointestinal intolerance, have been frequent with the latter regimen.

ATYPICAL MYCOBACTERIA

Several species of mycobacteria other than *M. tuberculosis* have been implicated as important human pathogens in the past three decades. Although the number of cases of disease due to these organisms is much less than those due to *M. tuberculosis* in developing countries, atypical mycobacteria are responsible for many serious infections in immunocompromised people in the United States and Europe, including disseminated *M. avium* complex (MAC) disease in patients with advanced AIDS. Several species cause chronic pulmonary disease and lymphadenitis, the most common clinical manifestations of disease in HIV-noninfected people (*Table 35.3*).

Table 35.3 Common Disease Syndromes Associated with Atypical Mycobacterial Species in Humans

Syndrome	Species
Chronic pulmonary disease	*M. avium-intracellulare* (MAC) complex
	M. kansasii
	M. abscessus
	M. xenopi
	M. fortuitum complex
	M. simiae
	M. malmoense
	M. szulgai
Skin and soft tissue	*M. marinum* (swimming pool infections or fish tank granulomas)
	M. fortuitum complex
	M. chelonae
	M. abscessus
	M. ulcerans (Buruli ulcer)
	M. haemophilum
Skeletal infections	*M. fortuitum* complex
	MAC complex
	M. kansasii
	M. marinum
	M. terrae
Lymphadenitis	MAC complex
	M. scrofulaceum
	M. fortuitum complex
	M. malmoense
	M. kansasii
	M. haemophilum
	M. genavense
Disseminated disease	MAC complex
	M. kansasii
	M. scrofulaceum
	M. fortuitum complex
	M. chelonae
	M. haemophilum

Disease due to representative species will be discussed. The reader is referred to the excellent comprehensive reviews by Wolinsky,[308] Pitchenik and Fertel,[309] and Wallace[310] for further information.

There are several important distinctions between human disease due to nontuberculous mycobacteria and TB. Atypical mycobacteria are less virulent human pathogens and tend to produce disease in immunocompromised people or people with underlying structural lung disease. Pulmonary disease, lymphadenitis, and disseminated disease are the most common clinical manifestations of disease due to atypical mycobacteria. Nontuberculous mycobacteria are environmental organisms and many species can be isolated from soil, water, dust, milk, and birds or animals in temperate climates. There is little evidence of human-to-human transmission of these organisms, and patients with atypical mycobacterial disease are generally not considered infectious to others. Lastly, many of these organisms can colonize humans without producing invasive disease.

Nontuberculous mycobacteria are usually classified based on the rapidity of growth on solid media and the production of pigment when incubated in light (photochromogens) or darkness (scotochromogens; Runyon classification). Photochromogens (group I) include *M. kansasii*, *M. marinum*, and *M. simiae*; scotochromogens (group II) include *M. scrofulaceum*, *M. szulgai*, *M. xenopi*, *M. gordonae*, and *M. flavescens*; nonchromogens (group III) include *M. avium-intracellulare*, *M. ulcerans*, *M. gastri*, *M. terrae*, *M. triviale*, and *M. malmoense*; and rapid growers (group IV) include *M. fortuitum*, *M. abscessus*, *M. chelonae*, and *M. smegmatis*. Nontuberculous mycobacteria cannot be reliably distinguished from *M. tuberculosis* by AFB smear microscopy and positive smears should be presumed to indicate active TB until proven otherwise. Speciation is difficult and time-consuming and was previously done only by reference laboratories using colonial morphology, pigment production, and biochemical testing methods. Recently, several species- or species group-specific DNA probes have become available (GenProbe) that allow rapid differentiation of *M. tuberculosis*, *M. kansasii*, MAC, and the common laboratory waterborne contaminant *M. gordonae*.

Lymphadenitis

Nontuberculous mycobacteria are a common cause of pediatric cervical lymphadenitis. Most children present with unilateral submandibular and high anterior cervical lymph node enlargement.[311] Most are afebrile, appear healthy, and no immunologic abnormalities can be detected. The pathogenesis is unclear but may be related to oropharyngeal trauma from teething and the fact that young children commonly put objects in their mouths. MAC is now the most frequently recovered species, replacing *M. scrofulaceum* and *M. fortuitum*.[311] Many children with nontuberculous lymphadenitis have positive TST tests. Tuberculin skin tests may be useful in suggesting an underlying mycobacterial cause of the enlarged nodes but are not helpful in distinguishing cases due to *M. tuberculosis* and other nontuberculous mycobacteria. The chest X-ray is usually normal in children with lymphadenitis due to nontuberculous mycobacteria. A tuberculous cause is more likely when associated pulmonary stigmas are present and the supraclavicular and posterior cervical nodes are affected.

The treatment of choice is surgical – total excision of the affected nodes. Incision and drainage and simple biopsy are not recommended because they frequently result in the formation of chronically draining fistulas and sinus tracts requiring difficult cleanup surgery. Antibiotic treatment has not previously been shown to be useful; however, experience with regimens that contain newer agents, such as clarithromycin and fluoroquinolones, has been limited and these drugs may play a role in the future treatment of this condition.

Skin and Soft Tissue Infections

M. marinum causes chronic papular lesions and cellulitis when inoculated into the skin traumatized in association with exposure to fresh or saltwater marine environments, including fish tanks. Tenosynovitis can occur if deeper structures are injured, and rarely a sporotrichoid picture with nodules developing proximal to the site of the initial lesion may occur. The diagnosis is made by history, a consistent appearance of the lesion, and biopsy and culture. *M. marinum* grows best at low temperatures, and culture at 28–30°C (rather than 37°C) is required for optimal isolation. *M. haemophilum* and *M. fortuitum* also produce nodular skin lesions, usually in severely immunocompromised people. Deep chronic lower-extremity skin ulcers are produced by *M. ulcerans* in tropical Africa (Buruli ulcer) and Australia. *M. ulcerans* produces a potent family of toxins, the mycolactones, which are responsible for the severe, protracted local tissue destruction.[312] *M. kansasii*, *M. fortuitum*, *M. chelonae*, and MAC can also produce skeletal disease, frequently involving the hand, which resembles TB but usually requires surgical treatment.

Chronic Pulmonary Disease

MAC, *M. kansasii*, *M. malmoense*, *M. fortuitum*, *M. xenopi*, and *M. chelonae* are the most common nontuberculous mycobacteria causing chronic respiratory disease. Concomitant chronic obstructive pulmonary disease (COPD), pneumoconioses (especially silicosis), chronic bronchiectasis, head and neck and lung cancers, and alcoholism are recognized risk factors for disease due to nontuberculous mycobacteria. Fast-growing species such as *M. fortuitum* and *M. chelonae* sometimes produce chronic pneumonia in patients with rheumatoid lung disease, achalasia, cystic fibrosis, and underlying lipoid pneumonia. Nontuberculous mycobacteria may also colonize the lower airway without producing invasive disease, especially in the presence of other chronic structural lung diseases. Therefore, care must be taken to distinguish between colonization and invasive disease. Bronchoscopes and respiratory therapy equipment can become contaminated with waterborne nontuberculous mycobacteria if not properly decontaminated between uses. Diagnostic criteria established by the American Thoracic Society for the diagnosis of nontuberculous mycobacteria as etiologic pathogens in patients with compatible clinical and radiographic findings require persistently positive AFB smears and isolation of the organism by moderately heavy growth in culture from two or more sputum or bronchoscopic specimens and the exclusion of other possible causes such as TB or other endemic mycoses such as histoplasmosis or cryptococcosis.[313] Despite retrospective series claiming subtle differences between the chest radiographic findings in pulmonary diseases due to nontuberculous mycobacteria and *M. tuberculosis*, in day-to-day clinical practice the radiographic findings in these two conditions are indistinguishable. Apical fibrocavitary disease with scarring, contraction, and volume loss are the most common findings.

Disease Due to *M. avium-intracellulare* Complex

The MAC is a group of slowly growing mycobacteria that cause cervical lymphadenitis and chronic, slowly progressive necrotizing pneumonia in HIV-noninfected children and adults, respectively, and disseminated disease in patients with AIDS.

Chronic Pulmonary Disease

Clinical series from the pre-HIV era emphasized the role of MAC as a cause of chronic necrotizing apical pneumonia similar to TB in elderly men with COPD, bronchiectasis, remote TB, or lung cancer.[314] The underlying lung disease was believed to predispose to colonization with MAC, which then resulted in a chronic, slowly progressive, necrotizing pneumonia in a small number of individuals. Patients presented with chronic productive cough, weight loss, fever, and night sweats with fibrocavitary infiltrates on chest film.

In industrialized countries such as the United States, the prevalence of chronic pulmonary disease due to MAC appears to be increasing[315] for unclear reasons, and the spectrum of disease has widened recently. MAC disease has been described as presenting as slowly progressive middle lung field noncavitating nodular infiltrates and persistent cough without fever or weight loss in middle-aged, nonsmoking women with no prior history of respiratory disease.[316,317] Fibrocavitary lesions are much less common in these patients. Chest CT scans demonstrated nodular interstitial disease and bronchiectasis in these patients, which was believed to be due to the nontuberculous mycobacterial disease. Many of these patients succumbed to slowly progressive respiratory failure.

Treatment of pulmonary MAC disease requires prolonged multiple-drug chemotherapy. The organism is highly resistant to many drugs used to treat TB. Recurrence after treatment is frequent. The course of the disease and long-term outcome vary significantly among patients; however, substantial morbidity is common and some patients die of slowly progressive respiratory failure and cor pulmonale. In HIV-noninfected people, cavitary lung disease due to MAC is often indolent, and in some patients noncavitary disease improves or resolves without treatment. In people with concomitant lung diseases such as bronchiectasis or COPD, treatment of the underlying condition with smoking cessation, bronchodilators, and antibiotics should be optimized. MAC is resistant *in vitro* to many antibiotics. When treatment is necessary, multiple drugs should be used and, when possible, isolates should be submitted to a reference laboratory for susceptibility testing. The azalide and macrolide antibiotics, azithromycin and clarithromycin, are highly active against MAC. One suggested initial regimen is clarithromycin or azithromycin, rifampicin, ethambutol, and amikacin or streptomycin for 2 or 3 months followed by clarithromycin or azithromycin, rifampicin, and ethambutol for a total of 24 months.[318] Treatment of pulmonary MAC disease must be prolonged. Side effects are frequent, and early consultation with a unit experienced in the management of these patients is advised whenever possible.

Disseminated Disease in Human Immunodeficiency Virus-Infected Patients

Although TB is the most common serious mycobacterial disease affecting HIV-infected people worldwide, disseminated MAC infection is a common late opportunistic infection among HIV-infected people in the United States and Europe. The incidence of disseminated MAC disease has decreased greatly due to the advent of highly active ART and effective chemoprophylaxis. Disseminated MAC disease has been infrequently reported in HIV-infected patients from developing countries in Africa,[319,320] despite the fact that the organism is present in great numbers in the soil and water.[321] Disseminated MAC infection in patients with AIDS usually presents with fever, chronic diarrhea, night sweats, anorexia, hepatosplenomegaly, abdominal lymphadenopathy, fatigue, and weight loss.[322] Severe anemia and elevated serum alkaline phosphatase are often present. In contrast to HIV-noninfected patients, significant pulmonary disease due to MAC is uncommon in patients with AIDS.

Disseminated MAC infection occurs late in the course of HIV infection and contributes significantly to morbidity and mortality.[323,324] The median peripheral blood CD4 lymphocyte count at the time of diagnosis in several studies was less than 50/µL, and disseminated MAC infection has been reported only rarely in patients with CD4 counts greater than 100/µL. The pathogenesis of disseminated MAC infection in AIDS is unclear. The frequent isolation of MAC from the sputum or stool of patients with AIDS before the diagnosis of disseminated MAC disease suggests that primary infection via inhalation or ingestion of the organism usually precedes disseminated disease.

The diagnosis of disseminated MAC infection in AIDS is usually straightforward. Blood cultures are positive in more than 90% of cases; bone marrow, liver, and lymph node biopsies also have very high diagnostic yields. Although MAC has significant *in vitro* resistance to many antimycobacterial drugs, treatment with newer drug regimens has led to improvement in symptoms, clearing of mycobacteremia, and increased survival. The new macrolides and azalides, clarithromycin and azithromycin, are highly active against MAC. Combination therapy with clarithromycin 500 mg twice daily or azithromycin 600 mg once daily plus ethambutol 15 mg/kg per day is highly effective. The addition of an aminoglycoside[325] or rifabutin[326] adds little to the effectiveness of treatment with a macrolide plus ethambutol. Rifabutin has significant interactions with many antiretroviral drugs. Chemoprophylaxis against disseminated MAC infection is now recommended by many authorities for HIV-infected people whose CD4 lymphocyte counts are less than 50/μL.[327] Azithromycin 1200 mg once weekly and clarithromycin 500 mg twice daily are the most widely used regimens and decrease the incidence of disseminated MAC infection by approximately 60%.[328,329] Rifabutin can be used alternatively for preventive therapy in people who are intolerant of macrolides but is less effective. Data from several clinical trials have shown that chemoprophylaxis against MAC can be safely discontinued in patients who have a sustained increase in their CD4 count to greater than 100/μL for more than 3 months after beginning ART.[330]

Disease Due to *M. kansasii*

M. kansasii causes chronic pulmonary disease similar to reactivation TB and disseminated disease in patients with advanced AIDS. Disease due to this pathogen occurs sporadically throughout the world but is most common in the central and southwestern United States and in England and Wales. In HIV-noninfected patients with pulmonary disease, treatment with isoniazid, rifampicin, and ethambutol for 18–24 months or until sputum cultures have been negative for 12 months is recommended.[313] *M. kansasii* usually responds well to treatment. The duration of therapy required in patients with AIDS is unknown.

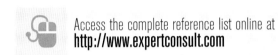

Treatment

Treatment of disease due to nontuberculous mycobacteria is long and difficult. Few clinical trials have been done to guide therapy. Atypical mycobacteria are usually resistant to most anti-TB drugs, although several other classes of chemotherapeutic drugs have activity against some species. The value of drug susceptibility testing in guiding treatment is controversial, and reliable testing is available only through a few specialized laboratories. Susceptibility testing is best established in the treatment of *M. kansasii* disease and for assessing susceptibility to macrolides and azalides for MAC infection.

The effectiveness of drug therapy is highly variable, even with combination therapy. Thorough surgical débridement is important in localized disease. *M. marinum* infections limited to superficial tissue can be treated with doxycycline, trimethoprim-sulfamethoxazole, or ciprofloxacin. Deeper or extensive infections require treatment with combination therapy with rifampicin, ethambutol, and possibly streptomycin. Sulfonamides, cefoxitin, amikacin, ciprofloxacin, and imipenem are active against *M. fortuitum*. Infections due to *M. scrofulaceum* should be treated with the same regimens used for MAC infections.[331] Treatment of MAC and *M. kansasii* infections was described earlier. The reader is encouraged to consult the published guidelines of the American and British Thoracic Societies for detailed information about the treatment of specific mycobacterial infections.[313,332]

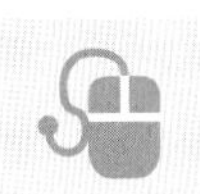

Access the complete reference list online at
http://www.expertconsult.com

CHAPTER 36

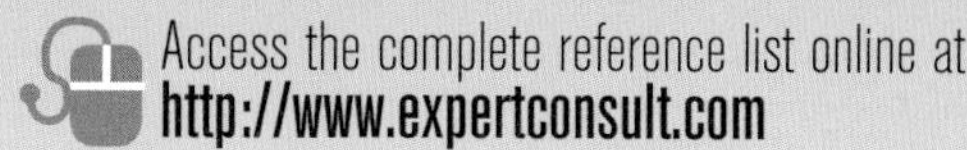
Access the complete reference list online at
http://www.expertconsult.com

Mycobacterium ulcerans Infection (Buruli Ulcer)

Wayne M. Meyers • Douglas S. Walsh • Françoise Portaels

INTRODUCTION

Buruli ulcer (BU), caused by *Mycobacterium ulcerans,* is an indolent necrotizing infection of the skin, subcutaneous tissue, and bone. Synonyms for BU are Bairnsdale or Searles' ulcer in Australia, and Kumusi ulcer in Papua New Guinea. Dodge and Lunn named the disease in 1962 after the geographic site of the first large epidemic investigated, in Buruli County, Uganda, now Nakasongola District.[1] Cook described the disease in 1897 in Uganda.[2] Because BU appears in forms other than ulcers, many investigators prefer the term *M. ulcerans* disease. BU is the third most common mycobacterial infection of humans, after tuberculosis and leprosy. The World Health Organization (WHO) in 1998 recognized BU as a re-emerging infection, most pronounced in West Africa, where the disease is a major public health problem because of frequent disabling and stigmatizing complications.[3,4]

THE AGENT

MacCallum and colleagues were the first to isolate *M. ulcerans* in culture in 1948 from a patient in Australia.[5] Portaels et al first reported isolation of the organism from the environment in 2008.[6] The organism is an acid-fast bacillus (AFB) that grows optimally at 30–32°C on mycobacteriologic media such as Löwenstein–Jensen medium and is a slow-grower.[7] *M. ulcerans* is microaerophilic, exquisitely sensitive to ultraviolet radiation, and sensitive to temperatures of 37°C or higher, properties consistent with the concept that, in nature, this organism is related to wetland environments; however, the ultimate source of the organism remains obscure.[8] *M. ulcerans* and *Mycobacterium marinum* share many common properties, including similar environmental relationships, optimal growth temperatures, identical mycosides, and molecular biologic properties.[9]

The necrotizing and immunosuppressive toxin elaborated by *M. ulcerans* is a polyketide known as mycolactone.[10–13] A cluster of genes in a plasmid of *M. ulcerans* encodes polyketide synthases and polyketide-modifying enzymes that produce mycolactone.[14] Variations of the 16S rRNA gene sequences of *M. ulcerans* are related to geographic origin and divide the species broadly into African, American, Asian, and Australian strains.[15] Insertion sequences, apparently specific for *M. ulcerans*, are used to identify the organism by polymerase chain reaction (PCR).[16]

EPIDEMIOLOGY

With few exceptions, BU is focally endemic in rural wetlands of tropical countries, especially in terrain that has seasonal flooding. A few individuals acquire the disease outside of tropical latitudes: southern Australia, China, and Japan. Reported incidence rates currently are highest in West Africa (Benin, Côte d'Ivoire, Ghana, Liberia, Nigeria, and Togo). Other endemic countries include Angola, Burkina Faso, Cameroon, Democratic Republic of the Congo, Equatorial Guinea, French Guiana, Gabon, Guinea, Indonesia, Kenya, Malaysia, Papua New Guinea, Peru, Republic of the Congo, Sudan, Suriname, and Uganda (***Fig. 36.1***).[17] Recent reemergence of BU is most often attributed to environmental changes: deforestation, topographic human-made alterations (dams, irrigation systems), and increasing numbers of people doing manual basic agriculture in wetlands.[18] Highest frequencies of BU (approximately 75%) are in children 15 years of age and younger, and in the elderly. For all ages, sexes are affected equally and no racial predisposition is known.[19] Most lesions are on the limbs, with highest frequencies on the lower extremities. Anecdotal observations on genetically related siblings in families of multiple parentage suggest inherited predisposition factors, but none has been identified.

Increasing evidence links the etiologic agent to flora and fauna of stagnant or slow-flowing water.[20] In Australia, speculation is increasing that BU may be a zoonosis transmitted by mosquitoes from possums.[21] *M. ulcerans* was first identified in 1999 in aquatic insects and other water-dwelling animals by molecular biologic methods.[22] There are no reports of transmission from patients to contacts. In Australia, koalas and possums acquire BU in nature.[23] Rats, mice, cows, armadillos, and other animals are susceptible experimentally.[24] Mode of transmission is an active area of inquiry.

With the initial discovery of *M. ulcerans* in water bugs (*Naucoris* spp. and Belostomatidae spp.) in Benin, West Africa, insects have been implicated as reservoirs of transmission.[7] Passage of *M. ulcerans* to mice by the bite of infected water bugs has been reported, suggesting that these insects may play a role in natural transmission.[25] However, many lesions in humans arise at sites of antecedent trauma, rendering it likely that the skin at the site was superficially contaminated by *M. ulcerans*, which was inoculated into the skin or subcutaneous tissue by the trauma.[26] Reported trauma has been as severe as gunshot or land mine wounds or as slight as a hypodermic injection. BU has developed at the site of a human bite and a snakebite.[27,28] Contamination of the skin may result from direct exposure to stagnant water, aerosols, insect bite, insect saliva or feces, or from fomites.

There are multiple reports of imported BU in nonendemic countries, for example, Canada, France, Germany, and the United States.[29–33]

THE DISEASE

From assumed trauma-induced disease, initial lesions appear in the skin from 2 weeks to 3 years later, or even longer.[26] Mean incubation periods are estimated to be 2–3 months in most reports. Anecdotal evidence of markedly prolonged onset of disease after leaving an endemic area suggests that latent infection is possible.

Connor and Lunn in 1966 were the first to describe the clinicopathology of a large number of patients, in Uganda.[34] *M. ulcerans* disease presents in a spectrum of forms. A proposed schema for the classification of these forms and their natural history is presented in ***Figure 36.2***. After infection, the disease may remain localized or may disseminate directly, bypassing the nodular stage.

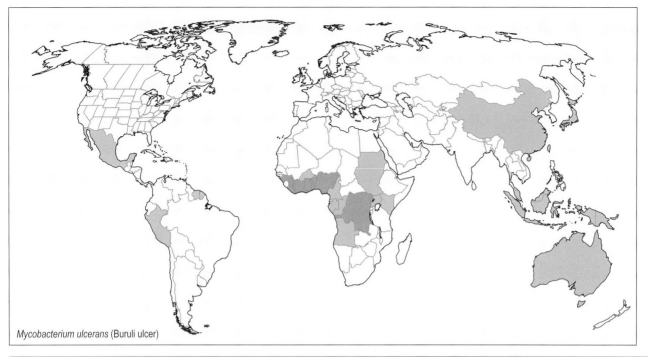

Figure 36.1 World distribution of Buruli ulcer. Red represents countries with a higher number of cases, and yellow a lower number of cases.

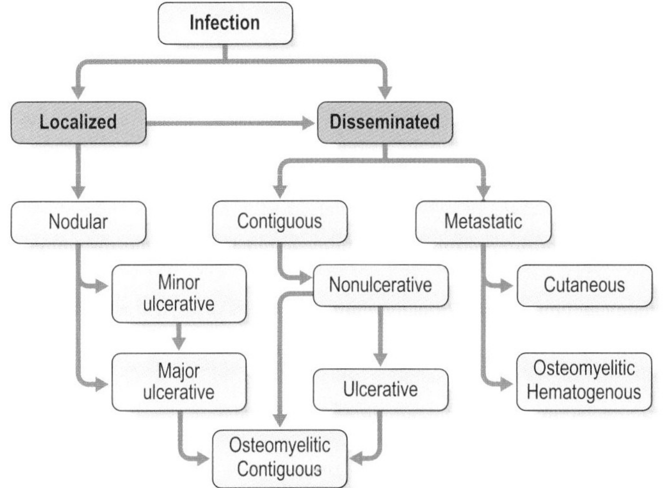

Figure 36.2 Proposed classification of clinical forms of active *M. ulcerans* disease.

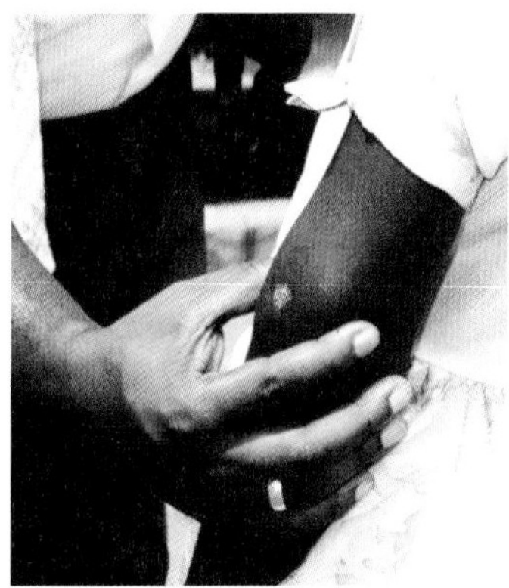

Figure 36.3 Nodular form of Buruli ulcer with incipient ulceration in a child in Ghana.

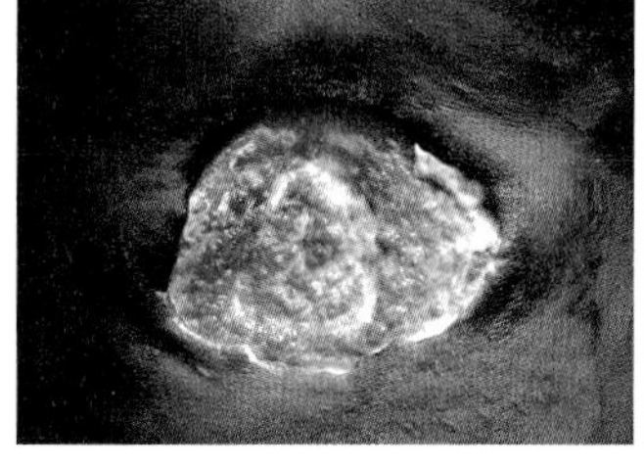

Figure 36.4 Major ulcerative form of Buruli ulcer in an Angolan man covering entire epigastrium. Note the central slough and undermined and indurated borders.

Localized Disease

Nodule

This form develops as a single, firm, movable, nonpainful nodule (2–4 cm in diameter) in the subcutaneous tissue and lower dermis (***Fig. 36.3***).[35,36] Microscopically, there is contiguous coagulation necrosis of the lower dermis and panniculus and sometimes the fascia. In the center of the lesion there are clusters of AFB. Significantly, the necrosis extends far beyond the AFB. Some nodules contain mineralized foci and vasculitis. There are remarkably few inflammatory cells.

Nodulo-ulcerative Forms

Minor Ulcer

This small ulcer (1–2 cm in diameter) develops at the site of a nodule, has a slightly undermined edge, a necrotic center, and is sharply demarcated. The ulcer tends to self-heal early without complications. Microscopically, minor ulcers have narrow, undermined edges. The central necrotic slough is sharply defined and contains numerous AFB. This slough and AFB are extruded through the ulceration defect, and scarring ensues.

Major Ulcer

This form also arises by ulceration of the epidermis over a nodule (***Fig. 36.4***). When fully developed, the ulcer has well-demarcated, undermined edges surrounded by induration. The ulcer base contains a whitish necrotic slough resembling cotton wool. Major ulcers may be large,

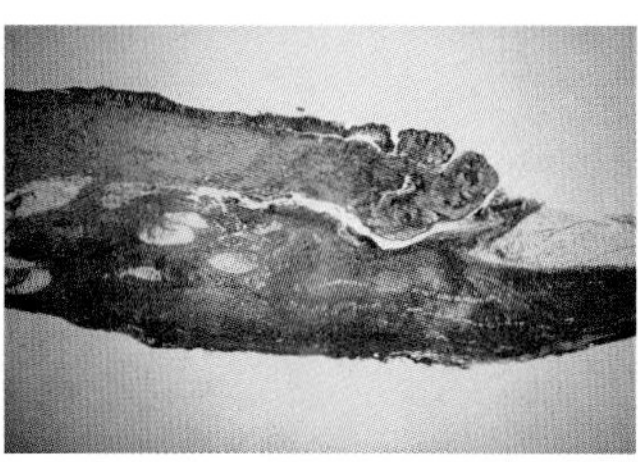

Figure 36.5 Movat-stained section of edge of ulcer from lesion in Figure 36.4 (×2.5). There is re-epithelialization of the undermined flap, with contiguous coagulation necrosis of the subcutaneous tissue.

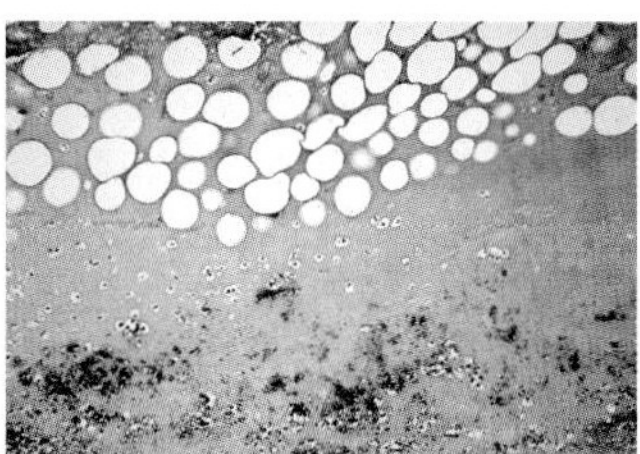

Figure 36.6 Subcutaneous tissue of a major ulcer. There are islands of dead fat cells (ghosts) and massive numbers of acid-fast bacilli in an area of coagulation necrosis. Ziehl–Neelsen stain, ×25.

destroying wide areas of skin and structures such as eyes and genitalia. Healing often produces cicatricial contractures, which can be disabling when located over articulations. Contiguous osteitis sometimes develops subjacent to the ulcer, destroying bone. Metastatic disease may spread from such lesions, but not as frequently as in directly disseminated disease. In Australia, the initial lesion occasionally presents as a painless pustule less than 1 cm in diameter and may progress to a major ulcer.[37] Microscopically, there is an ulcer with undermined re-epithelializing edges. Adjacent epidermis is often hyperplastic. In the ulcer base and surrounding tissue there is contiguous coagulation necrosis down to and including the fascia (*Fig. 36.5*). In the panniculus the fat cells are swollen and dead, but their ghost outlines are retained. The interlobular septa are necrotic and thickened. Vasculitis is common. Clusters of AFB are usually plentiful and mostly extracellular (*Fig. 36.6*).

Disseminated Disease

Plaque

Plaques are elevated, indurated lesions with irregular but delineated borders. Lesions are more than 2 cm in diameter and can be 15 cm or more in largest dimension. Skin is reddened or discolored. Plaques may arise from nodules but usually there is no evidence for a nodule. In late stages, plaques may break down and develop into one or more ragged ulcers. The appearance of these ulcers differs strikingly from the sharply defined, symmetrical ulcers that develop from localized disease. Microscopically, there is contiguous coagulation necrosis of the panniculus, extending into the dermis and fascia. AFB are confined largely to the panniculus and fascia. Vasculitis and mineralization are common.

Edematous Form

Edematous lesions are characterized by diffuse, non-painful, firm, nonpitting thickening of the skin, with margins that are frequently imperceptible. Often there are color changes of the skin. Lesions range from small (5 cm in diameter) to massive, sometimes involving an entire extremity or most of the trunk. There usually is no evidence for a nodule.[38] Microscopically, there is massive contiguous coagulation necrosis similar to that seen in other forms. AFB are most plentiful in the deep panniculus and fascia. Some specimens suggest that the AFB tend to proliferate just above the fascial plane. Necrosis extends far beyond the AFB.

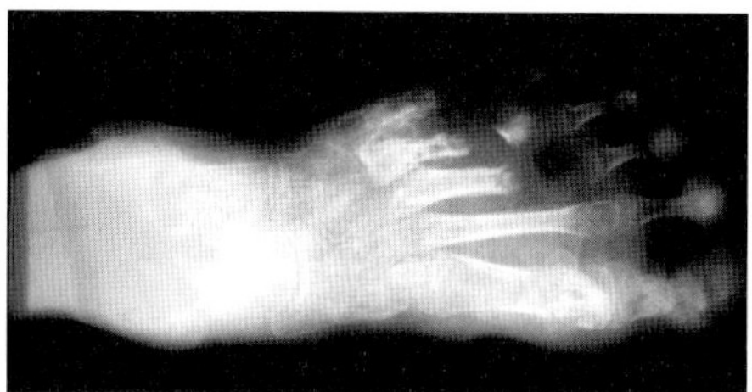

Figure 36.7 Radiograph shows contiguous osteomyelitis of the phalanges and metatarsal bones directly under a major ulcer of *M. ulcerans* disease on the dorsum of the foot.

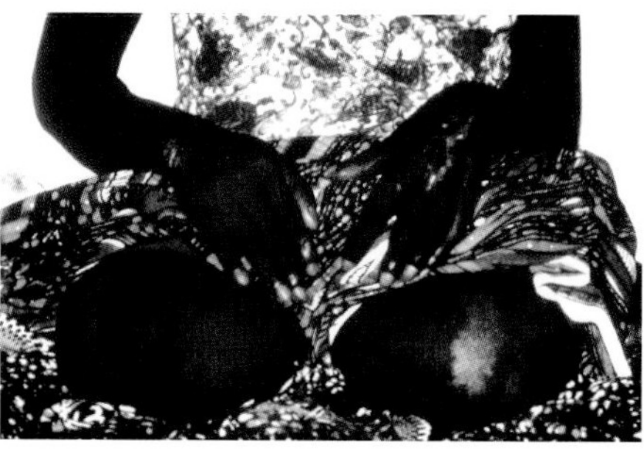

Figure 36.8 Amputations resulting from metastatic spread to bone of lower extremities. There is also spread to both wrists in this 13-year-old girl in Benin.

Metastatic Disease

Potentially, *M. ulcerans* may enter the lymphatic system or bloodstream from any form of BU; however, it is probably more frequent in disseminated disease. Although clinical lymphadenopathy is not common in BU disease, local and regional lymph nodes reveal invasion by *M. ulcerans* of the afferent lymphatic vessels and cortical sinuses, often with extension into the medullary areas with necrosis. Targets for metastatic spread seem to be limited to skin and bone. Osteomyelitis, either contiguous (*Fig. 36.7*) or metastatic, is observed in 10–15% of BU patients.[39,40] Hematogenous spread appears to involve the epiphyseal/metaphyseal level initially in long bones, but the bones of the hands and feet are likewise affected.[32] Sometimes the soft tissue surrounding a bone is so severely damaged that the bone becomes infarcted. Severe deformity and amputations are common sequelae of bone involvement (*Fig. 36.8*). Microscopically, there is coagulation necrosis of the bone marrow and destruction of all osseous tissues.

PATHOGENESIS AND IMMUNITY

The pathogenesis of *M. ulcerans* infection is related closely to at least two known properties of the etiologic agent: optimal growth at 30–32°C and elaboration of a potent toxin.[35] Temperature requirement favors initial onset of lesions in skin. The toxin destroys tissue, providing a nutrient medium for bacillary proliferation and isolating the organism from immunocompetent cells. *In vitro*, the toxin is also directly immunosuppressive to both B and T cells.[11] Variations in clinical and histopathologic presentations of BU suggest that some individuals have highly effective innate resistance, some develop resistance early and others late, and a few seem to be totally anergic.[41]

Cutaneous responses to "burulin" (a purified sonicate of *M. ulcerans*) reveal that BU infections stimulate a specific cell-mediated immune response in patients as healing begins.[42] This correlates well with the histopathologic appearance of delayed-type hypersensitivity granulomas in older lesions as they begin to heal. The immunosuppression of T cells, and the immunologically isolated status of BU lesions resulting from the local necrosis limit the sensitization of immunocompetent cells in early and advancing stages of the disease.[11] The ultimate effect is T-cell anergy, which prevents the development of the Th1 cellular response. Eventually there is sufficient immunostimulation by antigens of *M. ulcerans* to promote proliferation of peripheral blood mononuclear cells and production of interferon-γ to facilitate a Th1-type granulomatous response.[43-46] Sera from patients contain antibodies against soluble *M. ulcerans* antigens; however, their importance in pathogenesis and diagnosis is unknown.

Data on coinfection of BU and HIV are insufficient to establish increased susceptibility of patients with HIV/AIDS to BU. Anecdotal observations suggest that BU disease is more aggressive in HIV-infected patients.[47]

DIAGNOSIS

Experienced observers can usually make the diagnosis clinically.[48] In ulcerated lesions, Ziehl–Neelsen stains of exudates from the undermined edge often reveal clusters of AFB, predominantly extracellular. The same material, after decontamination, may be used for culture on Löwenstein–Jensen media. Incubation temperature must be 30–32°C. Transport media may be employed if stains and cultures cannot be performed locally. Molecular diagnostic analysis of exudates, biopsy specimens, or fine-needle aspirates using PCR techniques is useful for the identification of *M. ulcerans*.[9,16,49,50]

Specimens for histopathologic analysis should be obtained from the undermined edge of the ulcer and include all levels, including fascia. In nonulcerative disease (plaque or edematous), specimens should be taken from the presumed center of the lesion. Ellipses of tissue are better than punch biopsy specimens. The differential diagnosis is extensive. In the collection of specimens studied at the Armed Forces Institute of Pathology (AFIP), where the primary clinical diagnosis was BU, the authors have noted numerous other infectious and noninfectious inflammatory diseases and neoplasms as primary histologic diagnoses.

TREATMENT AND PROGNOSIS

A number of therapeutic drug trials are in progress and gaining wide acceptance; however, excisional surgery remains popular (***Figs 36.9 and 36.10***).

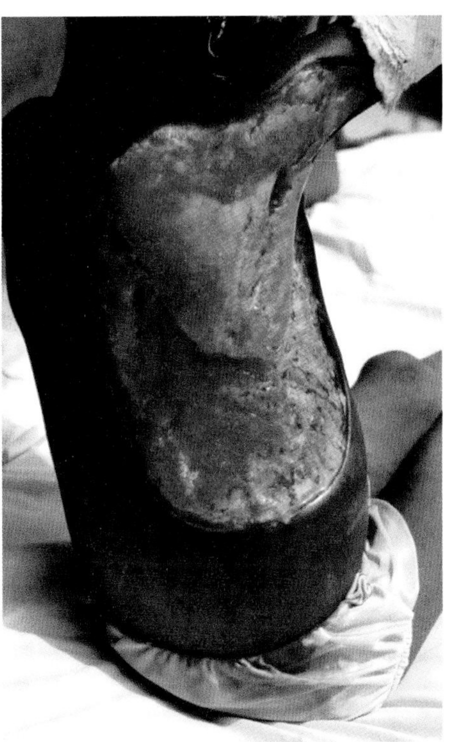

Figure 36.9 Excised edematous lesion in a 9-year-old girl in Togo. Pockets of active disease are recurring in the borders.

Papules, nonulcerated nodules and small ulcers are widely excised and usually closed primarily. Plaques and edematous disease are excised widely down to or through the fascia if necrotic. Any involved muscle should be excised. Determining the limits of lateral extension of disease is often difficult, and is an active area of research.[38,51] Experienced surgeons may be able to determine these limits by palpation, but exploratory incisions and blunt dissections are useful to establish the limits of excision. Marginal recurrences are frequent and must be further excised. Split-skin autografting is usually performed after sufficient granulation tissue has developed.

Postoperative care, especially physiotherapy, is essential for the prevention of contractures (***Fig. 36.11***). The skin graft must cover the lesion completely to minimize actinic damage. Bone lesions should be managed by specialists.[52] Heat therapy without surgical excision is successful for appropriate lesions but must be applied assiduously, keeping the base of ulcers at 40°C by fully controlled heating jackets or other devices.[53,54]

Current WHO recommendation for antibiotic therapy is an 8-week course of daily oral rifampin (10 mg/kg) and streptomycin (15 mg/kg) by intramuscular injection.[55] Early and limited lesions can be effectively treated with this combination of antibiotics without surgery.[56,57] Surgery

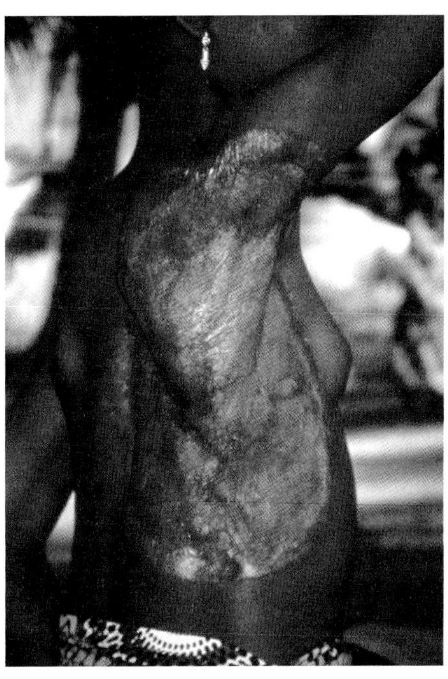

Figure 36.10 Patient in Figure 36.9 seen 5 years after complete excision and autologous split-skin grafting.

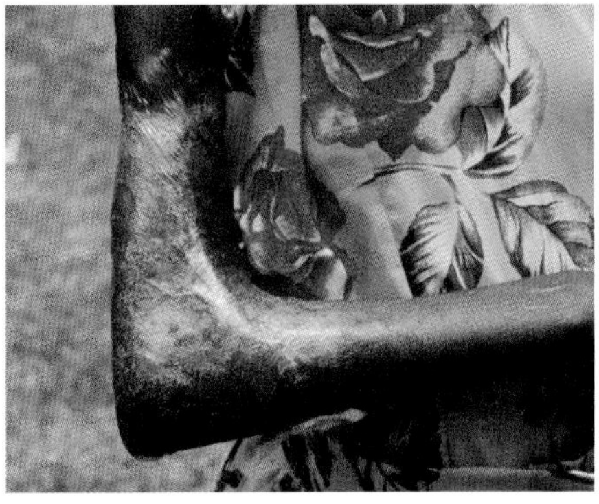

Figure 36.11 Frozen elbow from contracture scarring of a large, healed Buruli ulcer in a Ghanaian girl.

may still be needed for some large ulcers; however, the need and the best timing for surgery requires clarification.[58]

Prognosis is unpredictable. Surgically managed early small lesions have an excellent prognosis. However, any lesion may recur locally or spread metastatically after initial therapy, threatening significant tissue loss, and increasing the danger of cosmetic and disabling deformities and amputations. Secondary septicemia, tetanus, and gas gangrene sometimes are fatal. Without initial appropriate treatment, patients are likely to become severely disabled, increasing the stigma of the disease. Disabled patients are prone to develop psychosocial problems and may become a socioeconomic burden to the community and the health care delivery system.[4,59]

PREVENTION AND CONTROL

In tropical rural settings where BU is endemic, protection against contamination of the skin is virtually impossible. Protected water sources in villages reduce exposure to *M. ulcerans*, but in most endemic countries, providing wells is not a priority. Thus, environmentally oriented plans for control of BU have seldom been successful, leaving vaccination programs the only viable alternative.

Neonatal BCG vaccination protects against BU, but only for 6–12 months, although it may protect against osteomyelitis in BU-infected patients.[40,60] Subunit vaccines based on virulence factors or antigens of *M. ulcerans* are being studied.[61]

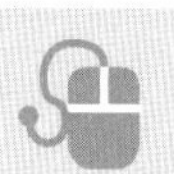

Access the complete reference list online at
http://www.expertconsult.com

Access the complete reference list online at http://www.expertconsult.com

CHAPTER 37

Leprosy

Douglas S. Walsh • Wayne M. Meyers

INTRODUCTION

Leprosy is a chronic infection caused by *Mycobacterium leprae*, affecting mainly the cooler body areas: skin, upper respiratory passages, anterior segments of eyes, superficial segments of peripheral nerves, and testes. The traditional, pervasive, social stigma attached to leprosy may be traced to the disfigurement, deformity, mutilations, and blindness related to damaged tissues. In cultures influenced by Judeo-Christian orthodoxy, the ostracism leprosy patients suffer is frequently severe and, in part, attributable to what is called leprosy in the Old Testament.[1] The Hebrew word *tsara'ath* was translated *lepra* in the Septuagint, the first Greek version of the Old Testament (third century BC). Subsequent Latin and English translations of the Bible used *lepra* and *leprosy*, respectively. The original Hebrew word denoted a group of diseases, none of which had recognizable clinical features of leprosy, and referred generally to ceremonial uncleanness.[2] Cultures never influenced by Judaic laws, however, frequently had similar attitudes toward leprosy – for example, the Chinese as early as the eighth century BC.[3] To reduce stigma, the International Leprosy Association in 1948 abandoned the word "leper" for "leprosy patient."[4] Today, the term "Hansen's disease" is a frequent synonym for leprosy.[5] Prevention of disability and conservation of cosmetic integrity are of great importance to preserve productivity and social acceptance.

THE AGENT

M. leprae, measuring 0.5 μm × 4.0–7.0 μm, is an acid-fast bacillus (AFB) in the order Actinomycetales and family Mycobacteriaceae. The Ziehl–Neelsen method stains *M. leprae* in smears, but in tissue sections the Fite–Faraco method is optimal. Acid-fastness is related to mycolic acid in the cell wall.[6] Staining properties of *M. leprae* in skin smears or biopsy specimens are important in the rapid assessment of the therapeutic efficacy of antileprotics. Viable organisms stain solidly, and as they degenerate, stain irregularly, then become granular, and eventually nonacid-fast. Persistence of bacillary carcasses in tissues or in smears can be visualized by silver staining techniques.[7] In patients with multibacillary (disseminated) leprosy, carcasses may remain in macrophages for several years after the leprosy bacilli have lost acid-fastness.

In 1873, in Norway, Hansen proposed that the bacillary bodies he saw in unstained tissue fluids from lepromatous nodules were the cause of leprosy. This was the first described mycobacterium and, notably, the first bacterial pathogen associated with chronic human disease. Although *M. leprae* is considered an obligate intracellular parasite, investigators occasionally report *in vitro* cultivation in cell-free media. All such claims remain unsubstantiated.[8]

As *M. leprae* is not cultivable, identification of candidate organisms as *M. leprae* depends on ancillary criteria, as follows: (1) fails to grow on routine mycobacteriologic media; (2) infects the foot pads of mice in a manner consistent with that of *M. leprae*;[9] (3) acid-fastness is abolished by exposure to pyridine;[10] (4) invades nerves of hosts; (5) suspensions of killed bacilli produce a characteristic "lepromin" reaction pattern when injected into the skin of leprosy patients, with each of the various clinical forms;[11] (6) produces phenolic glycolipid-1 (PGL-1), a presumed species-specific antigen;[12] and (7) displays species-specific DNA sequences.[13]

Cell walls of *M. leprae* contain arabinogalactan, mycolates, peptidoglycan, and protein.[14] Constituents of the cell wall appear to play a significant role in the *M. leprae*–host cell interaction, both in protecting the parasite and in stimulating immune responses.[15,16] The *M. leprae* genome contains 3 268 203 base pairs with a G + C content of 57.8%. Only 1604 or 49.5% of the genes encode proteins, compared with 3959 or 90.8% for *Mycobacterium tuberculosis*. This represents a massive deficit of metabolic capabilities for *M. leprae* that probably explains why it has not been cultivated *in vitro*.[17]

The assumed gene decay of *M. leprae* may contribute to the long multiplication time of 13 days for *M. leprae* in the foot pads of immunologically intact mice, and to the normally long incubation period of human leprosy, estimated at 3–5 years. In less resistant hosts, such as nude mice, generation times may be as short as 26 hours,[18] approaching that of 18 hours for *M. tuberculosis*. This may help explain the short incubation periods in some highly susceptible infants under 1 year of age.[19]

Preferential localization of lesions of leprosy to cooler body surfaces, selective growth in foot pads of normal mice, and the marked susceptibility of armadillos (body temperature 32–35°C) suggest that the optimal growth temperature for *M. leprae* is below 37°C.[20,21]

EPIDEMIOLOGY

Leprosy and its transmission do not require a tropical environment. Historically, the disease has afflicted people in nearly every part of the world, including countries traversed by the Arctic Circle, but its geographic origins are only now being unraveled.[22] Today the higher prevalence rates in the tropics are best attributable to socioeconomic factors (***Fig. 37.1***). In 1995 the World Health Organization (WHO) estimated there were 1.8 million people in the world with active leprosy, a marked reduction over earlier decades (12–15 million).[23] In 2008, the WHO reported about 250 000 new leprosy cases, and estimated prevalence had dropped to 213 000.[24] However, incidence likely remains much higher, with reductions reflecting fewer case finding efforts. Moreover, a considerable portion of reduced prevalence may be artificial, attributable to redefinition of a case of leprosy, as only individuals under chemotherapy for leprosy are counted as cases. Prevalence rates vary: Southeast Asia has 75% (India alone, 65%), Africa 12%, and the Americas 8% (***Fig. 37.1***). In the United States there are an estimated 6500 people with a history of leprosy; about 150 new cases are reported annually, most in immigrants.[25]

Infected humans are the most common source of leprosy, and the most common mode of transmission of leprosy is believed to be nasorespiratory.[26] Secretions from the nasal mucosa of untreated lepromatous

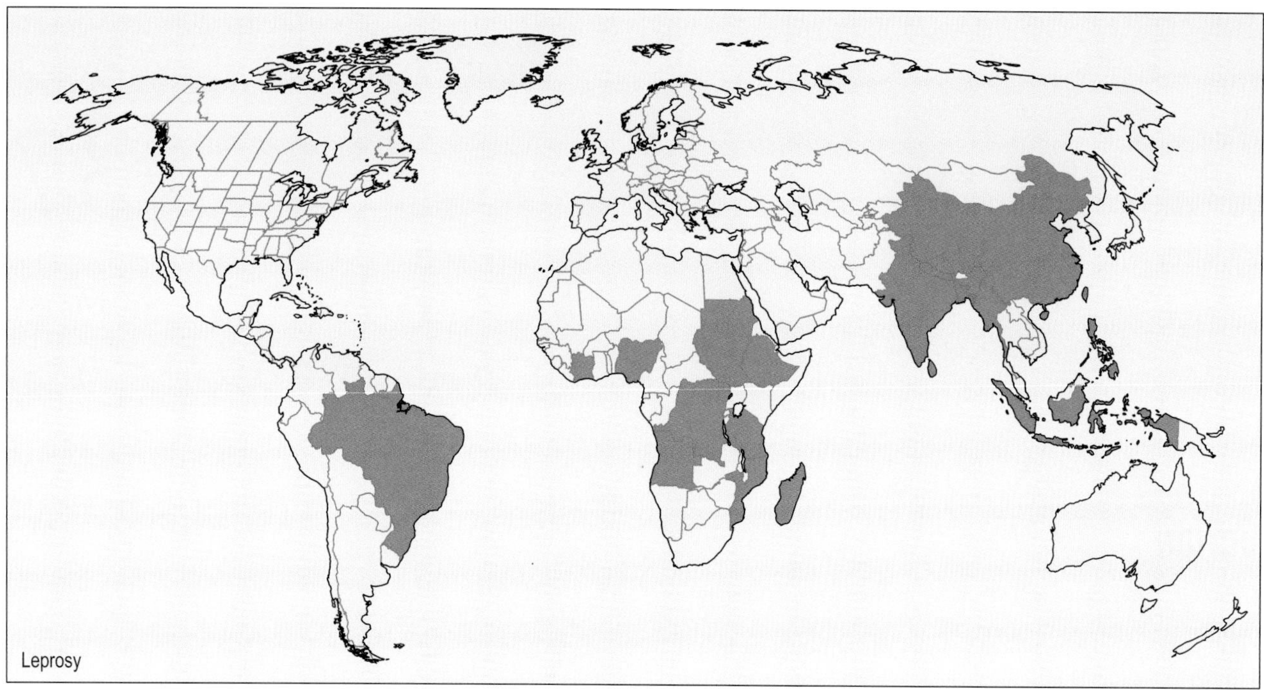

Figure 37.1 Leprosy is present in nearly every country. The countries highlighted on the map contributed 94% of all leprosy cases reported in 2007. (Adapted from World Health Organization, SEA-GLP-2009.3.)

patients contain many viable leprosy bacilli.[27] However, direct skin-to-skin contact or fomites may play a role.[28] *M. leprae,* after drying in the shade, in India, remain viable for up to 5 months, and in wet soil for 46 days.[29] Thus, the leprosy bacilli could be carried in aerosols to the nasal mucosa, perhaps binding to fibronectin and then to fibronectin receptors on mucosal cells.[30]

Transmission through mother's milk or transplacental infection is plausible. Breast tissue and mother's milk of multibacillary patients may contain large numbers of *M. leprae,* putting their nursing infants at risk.[31] There is increasing evidence for transplacental transmission of leprosy. Cord blood contains *M. leprae*-specific IgA and IgM antibodies, and titers of these antibodies rise in some infants of lepromatous mothers over 3–24 months after birth.[32,33] Leprosy in infants under 1 year of age is well known. In one series of 49 infants, the youngest diagnosed was 2 months old; only about half of the mothers had clinical leprosy.[19] This suggests transient subclinical *M. leprae* bacteremia during gestation.

Nonhuman reservoirs of leprosy are well known. Naturally acquired leprosy in armadillos was first detected in Louisiana in 1974 and, focally, up to 60% of armadillos are infected.[34–36] Similarly, indigenous leprosy has been detected in chimpanzees and monkeys in West Africa, and elsewhere.[37–39] Humans may acquire leprosy from wild, naturally infected armadillos.[40–43]

In most endemic areas, only 5–10% of infected persons develop progressive clinical disease. Children may constitute 20–30% of cases.[44,45] In adults, the male to female ratio is 2–3 : 1, but in children, 1 : 1. Specific immunologic parameters in Ethiopia suggest that occupational contacts (e.g., health care workers) have the highest sensitization rates to *M. leprae* (58%), followed by household contacts (47%), and non-contacts in endemic areas (29%).[46]

Lower prevalence rates of leprosy correlate directly with adequate housing and higher living standards. This is perhaps the best explanation for the disappearance of leprosy from northern Europe beginning just after the Middle Ages, and explains the tendency for leprosy to prevail today in poorer areas, primarily the tropics. Other public health factors common to the tropics may influence the prevalence of leprosy. For example, there is a marked frequency of intestinal nematode infections in lepromatous leprosy in Brazil, and probably in most tropical climates. Diniz attributes this association to a modulation of host immune response by parasites, downregulating Th1 and upregulating Th2 responses.[47]

The genetic epidemiology of leprosy is slowly being unraveled. In a survey in India, if one twin had leprosy, the odds of leprosy in a monozygotic twin were 89%, versus 17% for a dizygotic twin.[48] Newer data indicate susceptibility loci on chromosomes 6 (HLA-DR) and 10, and polymorphisms in interleukin (IL)-10, tumor necrosis factor-α (TNF-α), and Toll-like receptor genes may influence leprosy development, form of disease, and risk of reactions.[49–52]

PATHOGENESIS AND IMMUNITY

Bacteremia is common in multibacillary leprosy, and found in up to 15% of paucibacillary patients.[32,53] Invasion and multiplication of *M. leprae* in dermal lymphatic and vascular endothelial cells probably plays a major role in the hematogenous spread of the bacillus.[54] Scollard showed that *M. leprae* invades peripheral nerves via blood (and possibly lymphatic) vessels of the perineurium, gaining access to the endoneurial compartment.[55] Colonization of endothelial cells by *M. leprae* may cause ischemia of nerves, contributing to peripheral neuritis. The Schwann cell of peripheral nerves is the classic target for *M. leprae.*[56] Rambukkana has shown that laminin-2 in the basal lamina of the Schwann cell–axon unit binds to *M. leprae*, and ultimately that the α-dystroglycan receptor of the Schwann cells binds with laminin-2.[57] This is a postulated mechanism of infection of Schwann cells.

Immunopathogenesis

Leprosy is a paradigm for observing the range of clinical and pathologic interactions between variable host responses and a bacterium with relatively stable virulence. The immune response determines a patient's position in the spectrum of disease (***Table 37.1***), reflecting the popular Ridley–Jopling classification.[58] For the major disease forms, tuberculoid is characterized by one or several small, well-demarcated lesions, borderline shows a modest number of medium-sized lesions, and lepromatous presents with widespread, poorly defined lesions.

The immunologic capability of an individual, including patients, vis-à-vis *M. leprae*, is assessed by the intradermal inoculation of 0.1 mL of *lepromin*, a suspension of heat-killed *M. leprae* (1.6×10^8 organisms/mL), obtained today from experimentally infected armadillos.[11] The response

Group	Clinical Features	Histologic Features	Lepromin Reaction	Bacillary Density
Indeterminate (I)	Vaguely defined, hypopigmented or erythematous macule	Often indistinguishable from "mild nonspecific dermatitis" Lymphocytes and histiocytes around skin appendages and nerves	Weakly positive or negative	Negative or scanty
Tuberculoid (TT)	One or few anesthetic macules or plaques Borders well defined Peripheral nerve involvement common	Epithelioid-lymphocyte granulomas, with or without giant cells, in skin and nerves No subepidermal clear zone AFB in nerves, but rare	Strongly positive	Rare
Borderline-tuberculoid (BT)	Lesions similar to TT, more numerous Borders less distinct than TT Satellite lesions may form around larger lesions Peripheral nerve involvement common	Granulomas similar to TT Nerves infiltrated AFB frequently found in nerves	Positive	Scanty
Borderline (BB)	More lesions than BT Borders less distinct than BT Satellite lesions common Peripheral nerve involvement common	Epithelioid cells and histiocytic infiltrations focalized by lymphocytes Nerves show increased cellularity AFB readily found in nerves	Negative or weakly positive	Negative
Borderline-lepromatous (BL)	Lesions similar to BB, more numerous Some nerve damage	Histiocytic infiltrations show tendency to evolve toward epithelioid and foamy cells Lymphocytes present Nerves have less cellular infiltration AFB plentiful in nerves	Negative	Heavy
Lepromatous (LL)	Multiple, non-anesthetic, macular or papular, symmetrically distributed lesions No neural lesions until late Late complications of madarosis, leonine facies, testicular damage	Foamy histiocytes contain numerous AFB Few lymphocytes Subepidermal clear zone (Grenz) Numerous AFB in nerves and perineurium without significant intraneural cellular infiltration	Negative	Very heavy

Table 37.1 Criteria for Classification of Leprosy

AFB, acid fast bacilli.

is evaluated by measuring the diameter of induration at the injection site 3–4 weeks postinoculation (Mitsuda reaction).[59] Because high percentages of all normal populations react,[60] this skin test is never diagnostic but is useful for classification of disease: TT and BT patients are strongly positive (greater than 5 mm); LL, weakly or nonreactive (0–2 mm); and BL and BB have intermediate reactions (3–5 mm) (see ***Table 37.1***).

Modified lepromin tests using a high concentration of leprosy bacilli show that lepromatous patients cannot clear *M. leprae* from the reaction site, whereas tuberculoid patients destroy the bacilli efficiently.[61] Thus, survival and multiplication of *M. leprae* in macrophages determine the form of leprosy: if macrophages destroy *M. leprae* rapidly, minimal or no lesions develop, but if macrophages do not control multiplication of *M. leprae,* disseminated disease follows.

The level of cell-mediated immunity (CMI) to *M. leprae* determines the progression of disease, but precise mechanisms are unclear. In lepromatous patients there may be anergy to a variety of antigens,[62] but most strikingly to *M. leprae*.[63] In advanced lepromatous disease, total circulating T lymphocytes may be decreased, but T-cell subset ratio variations are inconsistent.[64] However, T lymphocyte–macrophage interactions in lepromatous patients are disrupted, perhaps by T-suppressor cell activity, with deficient production of interferon-γ (IFN-γ) and IL-2 and less macrophage activation.[65,66] This deficiency can be overcome, evidenced by injection of recombinant IL-2 and IFN-γ into lepromatous lesions causing influx of $CD4^+$ T cells, activating macrophages, and reducing bacillary load.[67–69] IFN-γ and IL-2 may have some therapeutic effect, but generate TNF-α, typically associated with deleterious reactions.[70]

In tuberculoid lesions, the CD4/CD8 T-cell ratio is 2 : 1, with a Th1-like profile characterized by mRNA transcripts for proinflammatory cytokines IL-2, IFN-γ, and IL-12 that induce strong CMI.[71–73] In lepromatous lesions, the CD4/CD8 ratio is 1 : 2, with a Th2-like profile characterized by mRNA transcripts for anti-inflammatory cytokines IL-4 and IL-10 which are associated with weak CMI, but strong humoral responses.[71] These findings support the paradigm that robust CMI limits disease, and that humoral immunity has little effect, largely determining the type of leprosy (see ***Table 37.1***).

Factors determining generation of a Th1 or Th2 response during infection with *M. leprae* are not fully understood. In addition to genetic predisposition (see Epidemiology section), one important factor may be innate responses, when *M. leprae* is first encountered. Toll-like receptors on innate immune cells may recognize mycobacterial lipoproteins, generating cytokines that mediate specific responses in a Th1 or Th2 direction.[74–76]

Clinical Leprosy

The Ridley–Jopling system (see ***Table 37.1***), derived from clinical and histopathologic criteria, is often used to classify leprosy forms. In contrast, the WHO classification for field workers is based on the bacterial burden in tissues: paucibacillary (PB), patients with skin smears negative for AFB, or five or fewer cutaneous lesions; and multibacillary (MB), patients with skin smears positive for AFB, or more than five lesions.[77] Some versions of the WHO classification exclude skin smears, but using lesion numbers alone is prone to error.

Indeterminate leprosy (I) is usually the earliest lesion, and presents as poorly defined macules, mildly hypopigmented in dark skin and slightly erythematous in lighter skin (***Fig. 37.2***). Texture, amount of hair, sensation, and sweating in the lesion are, at most, only slightly changed. Histopathologically, there are a few lymphocytes around neurovascular bundles (***Fig. 37.3***). These changes are nonspecific unless AFB are found in nerves, arrectores pilorum muscles, or in the subepidermal area (***Fig. 37.4***).[78] Diagnosis of indeterminate lesions often requires close cooperation between the histopathologist and clinician. Lesions may

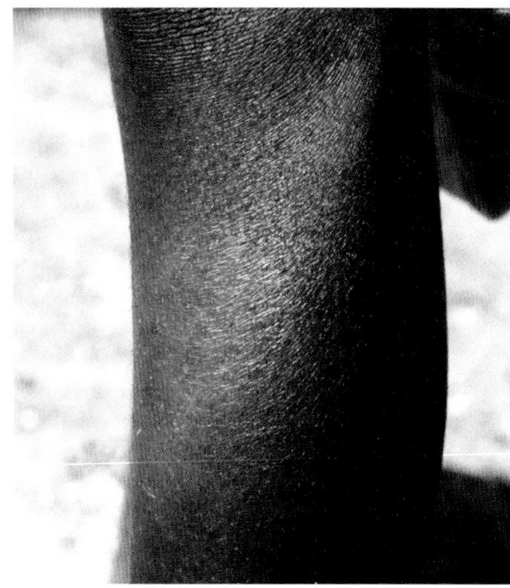

Figure 37.2 Hypopigmented macule of indeterminate leprosy on the calf of an Indian child.

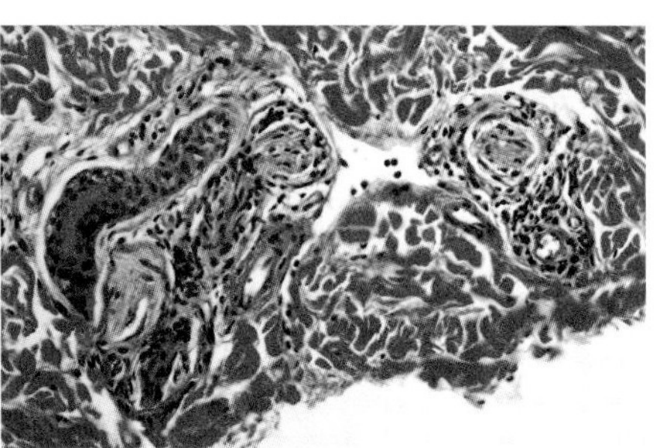

Figure 37.3 Indeterminate leprosy showing mild infiltrations of lymphocytes and histiocytes in the lower dermis, along neurovascular channels (hematoxylin and eosin).

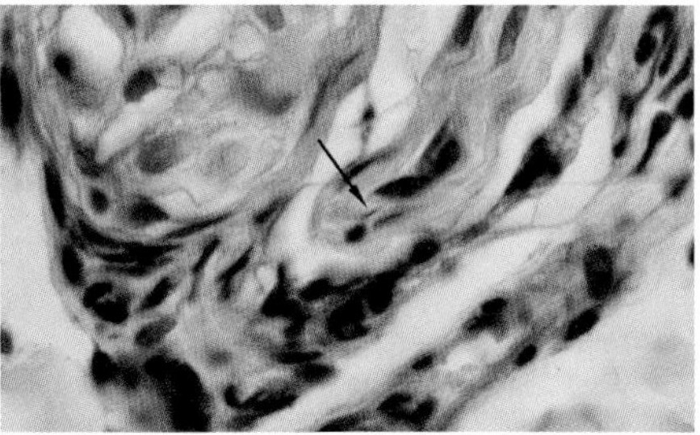

Figure 37.4 Nerve in subcutaneous tissue from specimen in Figure 37.3 showing a few lymphocytes around the intact nerve and a few acid-fast bacilli (arrow) (Fite–Faraco).

self-heal, remain unchanged for long periods, or progress to other forms of leprosy.

Tuberculoid leprosy (TT) patients have a single or few lesions, which may be macular or infiltrated. Borders are well defined and often finely papulated (***Fig. 37.5***). Sensation and sweating in lesions are impaired, and hair is frequently absent. Cutaneous nerves and peripheral nerve trunks are often enlarged in the region of lesions (***Fig. 37.6***). Sections of skin show epithelioid cell granulomas that invade nerves and often the epidermis (***Fig. 37.7***). AFB are rare and are found most consistently in nerves, papillary dermis, or arrectores pilorum muscles.

Borderline leprosy is divided into three major subgroups: borderline-tuberculoid (BT) midborderline (BB), and borderline-lepromatous (BL). This area of the spectrum is unstable, especially BB. BT lesions resemble those of TT but often are more numerous, with less distinct margins. In

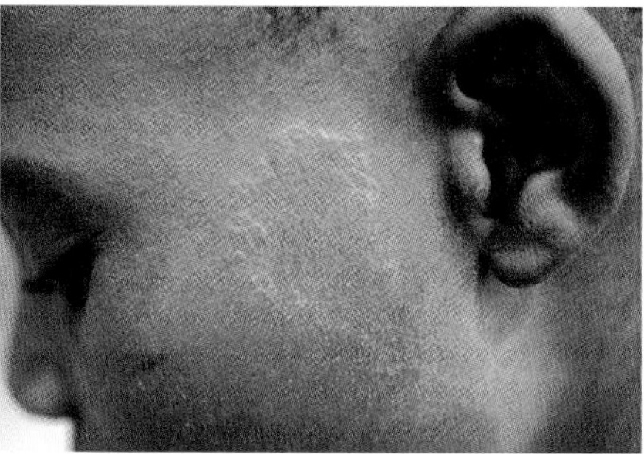

Figure 37.5 Tuberculoid leprosy in a 12-year-old Congolese boy. This was the only lesion, and it had a well-defined papulated border with central healing.

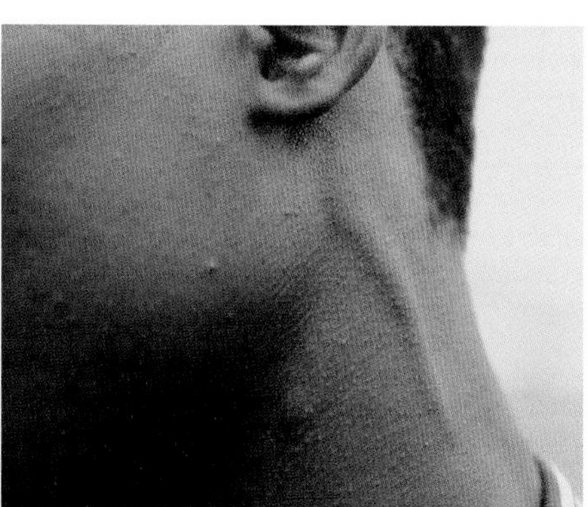

Figure 37.6 A large macule of tuberculoid leprosy in a Congolese boy near the angle of the mandible is barely visible, but accompanied by a thickened great auricular nerve.

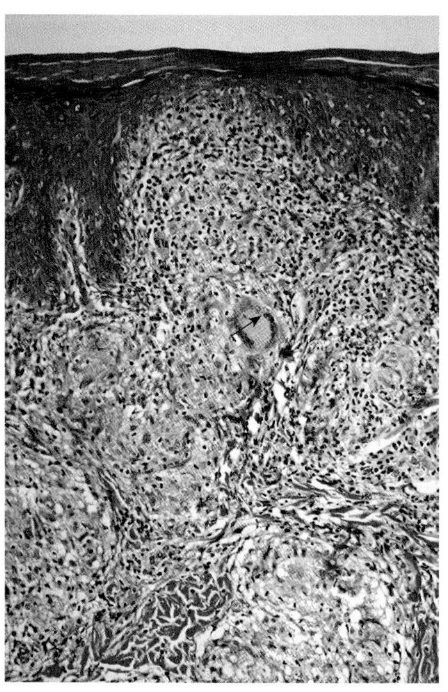

Figure 37.7 Tuberculoid leprosy with dense granulomatous infiltration in the upper and middle dermis. The granulomas are composed of epithelioid cells, Langhans giant cells (arrow), and lymphocytes, and are invading the epidermis (hematoxylin and eosin).

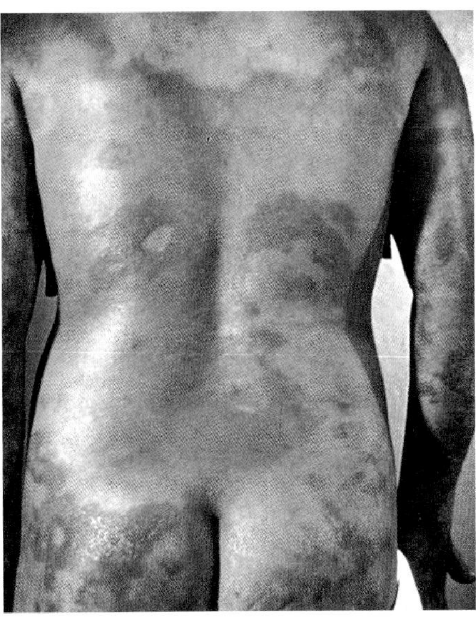

Figure 37.8 Borderline lepromatous leprosy in a Filipino. There are many plaques, some with defined borders and others vague. There is some characteristic "central clearing" within some plaques. The erythematous lesions suggest that the patient is undergoing a reversal reaction (type 1).

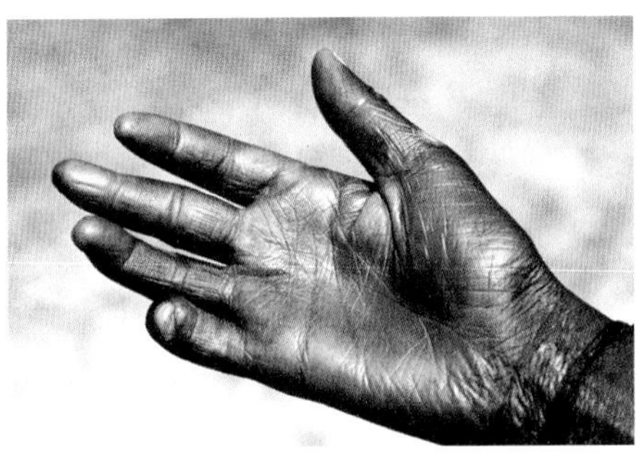

Figure 37.9 Hand of Indian adolescent girl with borderline leprosy showing neuropathic changes: damage and scarring of skin from insensitivity, atrophy of intrinsic muscles of hand, and clawing of fourth and fifth digits (ulnar nerve paralysis). There was also anhidrosis from autonomic nerve damage.

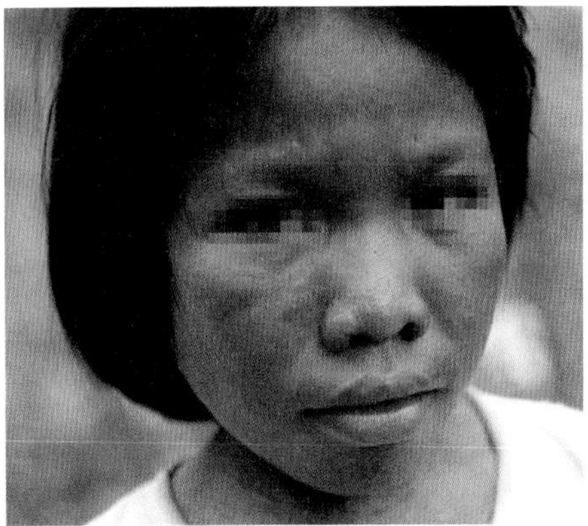

Figure 37.10 Advanced lepromatous leprosy in an adolescent Filipino girl. Skin of face is diffusely thickened, especially the alae nasi. Eyebrows are thinned.

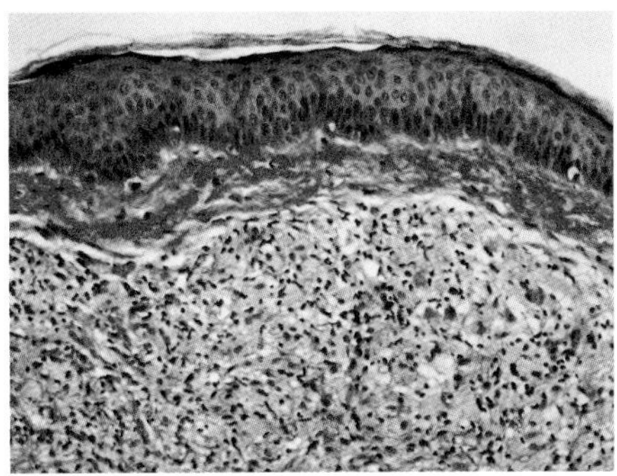

Figure 37.11 Advanced polar lepromatous leprosy showing replacement of dermis by foamy histiocytes (lepra cells), and a thin subepidermal clear zone (hematoxylin and eosin).

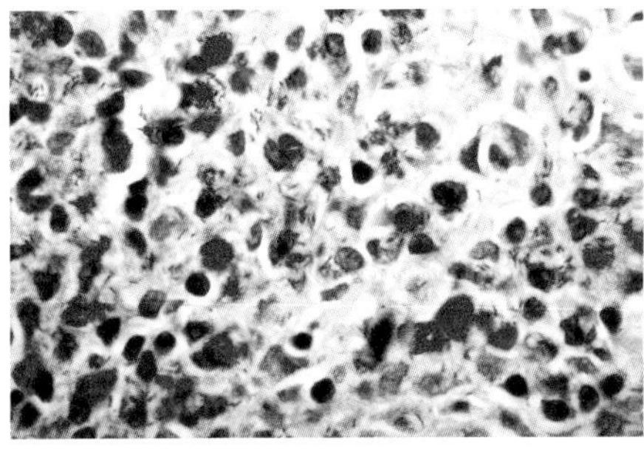

Figure 37.12 Higher magnification of same specimen shows clumps of *Mycobacterium leprae* in histiocytes (Fite–Faraco).

BL there are widespread plaques, often with distinctive central clearing, and nodules (***Fig. 37.8***). Histopathologically, BT shows well-formed granulomas with few AFB, whereas BL is nearly anergic with many AFB in histiocytes and nerves. Damage to cutaneous and peripheral nerves develops early and is often severe and widespread (***Fig. 37.9***). Reversal reactions (type 1) are common with resulting neuropathic changes, especially in the hands, feet, and face.

Lepromatous leprosy (LL) infiltrates nearly the entire skin, with cellular exudates heaviest in the cooler areas, such as the ears, the central face, and the extensor surfaces of the thighs and forearms (***Fig. 37.10***). Physical examination may easily miss the subtle macules of early LL. Damage to nerves develops slowly but relentlessly. There is insensitivity of hands and feet, and loss of some body hair (e.g., eyebrows) at later stages. Other areas involved are the upper respiratory tract from the nasal mucosa to the larynx, the eye, lymph nodes, and testes. Sterility and gynecomastia may follow leprous orchitis. Histopathologically, macrophages densely infiltrate the dermis but leave a subepidermal clear zone (***Fig. 37.11***). Nerves are rather well preserved until late. AFB abound in nerves, macrophages, blood vessel walls, and arrectores pilorum muscles, with many AFB in clumps and globi (***Fig. 37.12***).

Occasionally in LL, especially in relapses, elevated firm nodules appear in the skin, referred to as histoid leprosy.[78] Histologically, the macrophages resemble fibrocytes arranged in whorls, as in dermatofibromas, and contain numerous AFB.

In patients of Latin American ancestry, particularly Mexicans, there is a highly anergic form of LL called Lucio leprosy. Infiltration of skin is so diffuse that the diagnosis is often missed. In advanced stages, Lucio's phenomenon may develop, characterized by obstructive vasculitis causing dermal infarcts and ulcers, often involving massive areas of the skin. Recently, *M. leprae*, as the cause of Lucio leprosy, has been questioned.[79]

Occasionally pure neural leprosy affects peripheral nerves in the absence of cutaneous lesions. Biopsy specimens of nerves may show any form of leprosy, but most are borderline disease. Patients present with one or more painful enlarged peripheral nerve(s) accompanied by sensory loss, paresis, or muscular wasting.

Reactions

The course of leprosy is often punctuated by acute reactional episodes. Reactions are divided into two categories: type 1 or reversal reactions (*Fig. 37.13*), and type 2, or erythema nodosum leprosum (ENL) (*Fig. 37.14*).

Reversal reactions are most frequent in borderline leprosy and represent an episodic upgrading of cell-mediated immunity. Existing cutaneous lesions become swollen and erythematous. Neuritis is common and is responsible for much of the sensory loss and deformities of borderline leprosy. By repeated reversal reactions, borderline lesions may gradually upgrade toward tuberculoid disease. Today, with defined short-term therapeutic regimens for treatment, caretakers are confronted with differentiating relapsing leprosy from upgrading reversal reactions. Criteria for *relapse* include increased number of lesions, skin smear positive for AFB (BB and BL patients), tissue reaction inconsistent with reversal reaction, and favorable response to antileprosy therapy; for *reversal reaction* criteria include exacerbation at sites of previous lesions, skin smear negative for AFB, tissue reaction suggesting reversal reaction, and rapid response to anti-inflammatory therapy (e.g., steroids).[80] Lepromin-positive patients with IgM antibodies to PGL-1 are at greatest risk of reversal reactions, suggesting participation of both humoral and cell-mediated components.[81]

Sensitized T lymphocytes proliferate in reversal reactions, releasing cytokines that attract and activate macrophages.[82] Tissue reaction shows edema, increased numbers of lymphocytes, epithelioid cells, and giant cells. This is the only instance where hyperergic lesions of leprosy may show necrosis in granulomas and dermal nerves. Increased TNF-α may provoke this necrosis.[70]

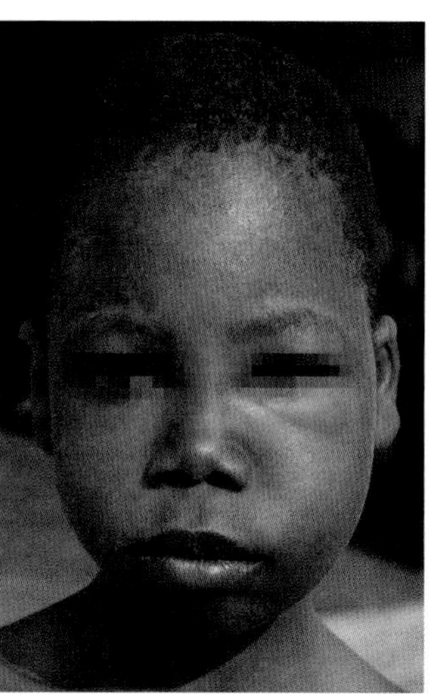

Figure 37.13 Reversal reaction (type 1) in an 8-year-old Congolese boy with borderline-tuberculoid leprosy. The left side of his face is swollen, and mild palsy is present from damage to the facial nerve. The reaction responded rapidly to steroid therapy.

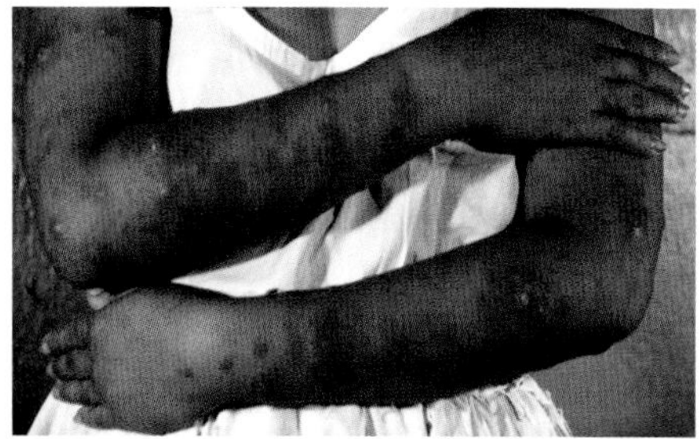

Figure 37.14 Erythema nodosum leprosum in a Filipino adolescent girl with lepromatous leprosy. Papules on upper extremities are erythematous and tender.

ENL develops in approximately 50% of all lepromatous patients. Clinically, there is rapid onset of tender subcutaneous nodules, often accompanied by fever, synovitis, and iridocyclitis. These lesions resemble the Arthus phenomenon and probably are related to immune complexes that form locally by the release of antigens of *M. leprae* that combine with circulating antibody, probably modulating T-lymphocyte populations *in situ*. T-helper cells within lesions increase, and TNF-α is produced.[83,84] Histopathologically, neutrophils usually infiltrate the lesion, often accompanied by vasculitis and ulceration. Elevation of serum amyloid A and C-reactive protein may help establish the diagnosis in atypical lesions.[85] Secondary amyloidosis in LL is seen most frequently in patients with chronic ENL.

DIAGNOSIS

History of contact or residence in endemic areas raises suspicion of leprosy in a patient with chronic lesions of the skin. The cardinal signs of leprosy are hypoesthetic lesions of the skin, enlarged peripheral nerves, and AFB in skin smears. In the absence of another clear diagnosis, any one of these observations suggests leprosy. Delay in diagnosis is often prolonged following the first visit to a physician for leprosy-related symptoms; in the United States this period averages 1 to 1½ years. Such delay may result in irreversible sequelae.

Experienced observers can often make the diagnosis clinically. However, histopathologic evaluation is strongly recommended for confirmation of diagnosis and classification.

Physical Examination

The entire skin surface should be examined. Vague changes are best seen in direct sunlight. Peripheral nerves are palpated for enlargement and tenderness. Cutaneous nerves in or near lesions may be enlarged. Unexplained damage to hands or feet, or any muscle weakness (e.g., clawhand or footdrop) or sensory deficit strongly suggests peripheral neuropathy. Lepromatous patients may have a chronic stuffy nose.

Sensory changes in lesions are tested for light touch with a few fibers of cotton or calibrated nylon bristles, and for heat–cold discrimination by warm and cool water in test tubes. Sensory changes are the most important criterion for clinical diagnosis; thus repeated testing is recommended in doubtful situations.

Laboratory Findings

Skin smears are obtained from multiple sites (usually six to eight) and should include the edge of macules or plaques, nodules, both earlobes, and the nasal mucosa. Skin smears are made by squeezing a fold of skin between thumb and forefinger, and making a short shallow slit in the skin with a razor blade or scalpel. The instrument is then turned 90° to the slit and the sides of the slit scraped. The fluid thus obtained is spread on a slide over a circle approximately 1 cm in diameter, heat-fixed, and stained by the Ziehl–Neelsen method. Smears must be performed and microscopically evaluated by experienced personnel to avoid misinterpretation.[86]

Serologic tests for the *M. leprae*-specific PGL-1 antigen and antibodies to PGL-1 are available.[87,88] Specificity is high, and most lepromatous patients are positive. Paucibacillary patients, however, are frequently nonreactive. Lepromatous patients have PGL-1 antigen in serum and urine.[89,90] Polymerase chain reaction (PCR) assays are able to detect small numbers of *M. leprae* in tissue sections, skin, and nasal smears.[13] Because of potential contamination in laboratories in endemic areas, PCR data must be interpreted carefully and correlated clinicopathologically.[13,91] Sera from lepromatous patients may give false positive reactions for syphilis in cardiolipin-based assays.

Histopathology

Biopsy specimens should be taken from the edges of lesions and should include the entire thickness of the skin and subcutaneous tissue.

Occasionally, damaged nerves may appear only in the subcutaneous tissue. Punch biopsy specimens are most convenient, but should be as large as is cosmetically acceptable for the site chosen. The specimen should be fixed in 10% buffered formalin for routine evaluation. If molecular studies are anticipated, the specimen must be preserved in 70% ethyl alcohol.[92] To demonstrate *M. leprae* optimally in tissue sections, the Fite–Faraco method is essential.[93] A diagnosis of leprosy is made only when the evidence is convincing; "consistent with leprosy" must be avoided in histopathologic evaluations.

Differential Diagnosis

A limited list of differential diagnoses is given here:

1. **Changes in pigmentation.** Superficial mycoses, scars, birthmarks, postinflammatory changes, and cutaneous filariasis (onchocerciasis and streptocerciasis).
2. **Infiltrated lesions.** Leishmaniasis, lymphoma, granuloma annulare, granuloma multiforme (Mkar disease), lupus erythematosus, psoriasis, pityriasis rosea, sarcoidosis, and neurofibromatosis.
3. **Peripheral neuropathies.** Syringomyelia, lead toxicity, diabetes mellitus, primary amyloidosis, and familial hypertrophic neuropathy.

TREATMENT AND PROGNOSIS

Because of known drug-resistant strains of *M. leprae*, especially to dapsone and rifampin, monotherapy is avoided.[94] The type of antibacterial multidrug therapeutic (MDT) regimen employed is usually based on the WHO simplified classification of PB or MB, and follows the WHO recommended combination of drugs,[95–97] as follows:

1. **Single lesion regimen.** Some clinicians treat single skin lesions with a single dose combination of rifampin 600 mg, ofloxacin 400 mg, and minocycline 100 mg. In the authors' view, there are insufficient long-term follow-up data on efficacy to recommend the general use of this therapeutic approach. Such patients should be treated at least by the PB regimen.
2. **Paucibacillary regimen.** Rifampin (600 mg), given once monthly under supervision, plus dapsone (100 mg/day), for 6 months. Treatment is then discontinued.
3. **Multibacillary regimen.** Rifampin (600 mg) and clofazimine (300 mg), given once monthly under supervision, plus dapsone (100 mg/day) and clofazimine (50 mg/day) for at least 12 months; however, some authorities recommend continuation of treatment for 24 months.[51] Clofazimine darkens the skin, especially lesions, and is stigmatizing in some communities.[98] If this is unacceptable, prothionamide, ethionamide or minocycline may be substituted. Pediatric doses of the WHO MDT regimens are given in *Table 37.2*.

In the United States, the National Hansen's Disease Program (NHDP) recommends the following regimens[99]:

1. **PB disease:** dapsone (100 mg) and rifampin (600 mg), both daily, for 12 months.
2. **MB disease:** dapsone (100 mg), rifampin (600 mg), and clofazimine (50 mg), all daily, for 24 months. If the patient is on corticosteroids, the rifampin (600 mg) is given monthly.

Table 37.2 Dosage of Multiple-Drug Therapy for Children with Leprosy

Weight (kg)	Percentage of Adult Dose
<15	25
15–30	50
31–45	75
>45	100

(From Jopling WH. Handbook of Leprosy. London, William Heinemann, 1984.)

MDT regimens are intended to address increasing prevalence of drug-resistant *M. leprae*, as well as residual dormant *M. leprae* not killed by MDT, often called "persisters," in patients who otherwise respond well clinically. Persisters begin multiplying after antileprosy treatment is discontinued, and may be responsible for some relapses, even after full MDT courses.[100]

Relapse rates following MDT are viewed as acceptably low by most authorities, ranging from 0% to 10% in most studies; the higher rates are generally associated with higher pre-MDT bacterial burdens.[101,102] In some locations, relapses are highest in PB patients, suggesting incorrect classification. Indeed, clinicians using the WHO system often misclassify MB patients and place them in the PB category, leading to undertreatment. Although the results of WHO MDT appear excellent, long-term follow-up remains essential.[103] *M. leprae* resistance to components in the WHO MDT regimen, especially dapsone and rifampin, is well established, and the role of persisters is not fully resolved.[104] As such, MDT regimens should be given regular reappraisal, with a focus on drugs, dosage, duration, and long-term follow-up.

Several other potent antileprosy drugs and combinations are under evaluation and may eventually be included in multidrug regimens. These include the fluoroquinolones pefloxacin, ofloxacin and moxifloxacin, the macrolide clarithromycin, and the tetracycline minocycline.[105–108] Rifampin, ofloxacin, and minocycline (ROM), given together at monthly intervals 12–24 times, is an alternative MDT regimen.[109]

Efficacy of chemotherapy in lepromatous patients can be assessed by clinical progress and the staining property of *M. leprae* in skin smears or biopsy specimens. The response of tuberculoid and borderline patients is best measured by the clinical response and histopathologic evaluation. Viability of *M. leprae* from patients can be determined by mouse foot pad inoculation, or by a variety of faster metabolic assays.[110]

Care of insensitive hands and feet and correction of physical disabilities are essential in the comprehensive treatment of affected patients. This is an extensive topic, and the reader is directed to appropriate texts on the subject.[111–113]

Therapy for Reactions

Reactions in leprosy are considered a *medical emergency*. Appropriate treatment should be instituted immediately, and the patient followed closely.

1. **Reversal reaction.** If the reaction is accompanied by peripheral neuritis, the affected part is immobilized by a splint and analgesics and corticosteroids given orally. Up to 80 mg of prednisone daily is given initially and tapered off over 2–3 months to a minimally effective level as long as neuritis persists. If long-term prednisone therapy is required, an alternate-day regimen may be attempted. Although supported by some, the usefulness of clofazimine as an adjunct to corticosteroids in reversal reactions has not been established.[114] Antileprosy therapy is continued during treatment for reactions.
2. **Erythema nodosum leprosum (ENL).** Because all MDT regimens for MB leprosy contain clofazimine, which has significant anti-inflammatory activity, severe ENL is encountered less frequently today. In milder forms of ENL, therapy may require only mild analgesics. Severe ENL requires more aggressive therapy, especially when there is iritis, neuritis, cutaneous ulceration, or orchitis.

Thalidomide is the most active drug for ENL, initially given at 100 mg three to four times daily.[115] The dose is then tapered to the minimum effective level. Thalidomide is prescribed only for men and nonfertile females. Some clinicians will administer the drug only to inpatients under direct supervision. Efficacy of thalidomide may depend in part on the inhibition of TNF-α production, but other cytokines may be affected. If thalidomide cannot be used, prednisone is given, as for reversal reactions. Clofazimine may also be increased to 300 mg/day, but an effect usually takes 4–6 weeks.[116] It is unclear if TNF-α antagonists (e.g., infliximab), generally used for autoimmune disorders, will affect leprosy.[117]

Iridocyclitis is a serious complication: local corticosteroids must be added to systemic anti-inflammatory treatment, and ophthalmologic consultation obtained.

PREVENTION AND CONTROL

There are no recommendations for prevention of infection in endemic areas. Chemoprophylaxis of close contacts using rifampin may be useful, perhaps for a short period, but is probably not appropriate for large populations.[118,119]

Current control programs are based on the principles that: (1) the number of contagious patients is reduced by chemotherapy, and (2) the surveillance of contacts will detect early leprosy. Execution of these principles requires intensive programs in education of the public and training of medical personnel to diagnose leprosy and deliver treatment. A rapid low-cost test for PGL-1 detection offers promise for the identification of contacts of leprosy patients at risk and could be incorporated into control programs.[120] Skin tests specific for leprosy would represent a marked advance in early diagnosis, and are under study.[121] Studies to identify proteins for use in rapid diagnostic tests for leprosy (serological) are ongoing.[122] If such tests are established, given that many exposed individuals do not develop disease, the ethical management of positive reactors without clinical findings must be resolved.

Effective vaccination offers the best approach for eliminating leprosy in humans.[123] Initial evaluation in Venezuela of a WHO vaccine composed of heat-killed *M. leprae* plus bacille Calmette-Guérin (BCG) did not confer protection against leprosy.[124] A single BCG vaccination gives varying levels of protection in different geographic areas. In Malawi, repeated BCG vaccinations gave an overall protection rate of 50% against leprosy, with 95% protection in children under 15 years old, suggesting one feasible option.[125,126] Other trials of vaccines based on cultivable mycobacteria (*Mycobacterium w* and the ICRC bacillus) are in progress in India.[127] The development of vaccines based on subunit mycobacterial antigens is being pursued.[51]

Unlike the association of tuberculosis and human immunodeficiency virus (HIV), HIV infection may not be a significant risk factor for leprosy in most populations.[128,129] However, in some populations in Africa, HIV infection had an overall 2.2 relative risk for leprosy, and up to 23% of multibacillary infections were HIV seropositive.[130] Moreover, recent observations of leprosy presenting as part of the HIV immune reconstitution inflammatory syndrome (IRIS) emphasizes that HIV–leprosy interactions are not yet fully understood.[131]

There is cautious optimism that rigorous application of the WHO's MDT regimens will interrupt transmission of leprosy, and diminish incidence. The WHO goal is to "eliminate" leprosy as a public health problem, defined as a prevalence of ≤1 active leprosy patient per 10 000 population, in all countries. As of 2007, "elimination" had been achieved in all but three countries, Brazil, Nepal, and Timor-Leste, although notably high rates remained in several other countries, especially India (***Fig. 37.1***). Focus is now on programs giving special attention to these and other high endemic areas. To maintain patient confidence and provide complete care, it should be mandatory that all such programs include resources for follow-up and management of the physical disabilities and social stigma of patients who have completed fixed-duration therapeutic regimens.[51,132] This requires integration of leprosy control operations into the general health care programs of endemic countries, a formidable task.

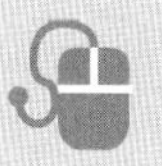

Access the complete reference list online at
http://www.expertconsult.com

Access the complete reference list online at http://www.expertconsult.com

CHAPTER 38

Anthrax

G. Raghurama Rao • David H. Walker

INTRODUCTION

Anthrax is primarily a zoonotic disease of herbivorous animals, caused by *Bacillus anthracis*, a large (1 × 3–10 μm), Gram-positive, aerobic spore-forming bacillus (***Fig. 38.1***). Humans acquire the natural disease as an occupational hazard or by accidental contact with infected animals and their by-products. The disease is one of the oldest recorded infections of humans and animals. It was the first human disease for which a specific pathogen was established by Robert Koch, in 1876. A live attenuated animal vaccine was developed and tested by Louis Pasteur in 1881.[1–3]

THE AGENT

B. anthracis is part of the *B. cereus* group. Except for *B. anthracis*, all members of this group are resistant to penicillin because they produce chromosomally encoded β-lactamases.[4] Recently, β-lactamase producing strains of *B. anthracis* have also been reported.[5,6] *B. anthracis* has a 5.3 Mb genome encoding 5508 proteins.[7] Seven *gerA* family sensors recognize small molecules such as nutrients and ions leading to germination of the spores.[8] Virulence of *B. anthracis* is attributed to the production of two factors, a γ-linked poly-D-glutamic acid capsule and a three-component protein exotoxin termed anthrax toxin complex. Two plasmids, pX01 and pX02, encode the toxins and capsule synthesis genes, the synthesis of which is controlled by *atxA* and *acpA* regulator genes.[9] Sporulation involves not only synthesis of the spore coats but also loading with components needed during early germination.[8] The very limited genetic diversity of *B. anthracis* suggests that it has spread as a clone throughout the world.

EPIDEMIOLOGY

Naturally occurring anthrax remains a public health problem in agricultural regions throughout the world, especially in South and Central America, the Caribbean, southern and eastern Europe, Africa, Asia, and the Middle East, where livestock are not vaccinated because of poor veterinary services (***Fig. 38.2***).[1–3,10] Frequent outbreaks of animal and human anthrax continue to occur in Africa[11,12] and southern India.[13–17] *B. anthracis* is a potential agent of biological warfare. One of the largest epidemics of inhalational anthrax occurred in the city of Sverdlovsk, Russia in 1979 due to accidental release of anthrax spores from a military biological weapons facility.[18] Anthrax is virtually eliminated from the United States, but in 2001 an outbreak of 22 cases of anthrax was reported to be due to bioterrorism.[2]

Transmission

B. anthracis spores can remain viable and infective in the soil for many years, even decades. They are a potential source of infection for grazing livestock, but they generally do not represent a direct infection risk for humans.[1] Domestic and wild herbivores, including sheep, goats, cattle, water buffalo, antelopes, elephants, giraffe, and zebras, are highly susceptible to fatal infection.[19–21] During periods of drought when grasses are scarce and short, herbivores ingest spore-contaminated soil along with the short vegetation. In other settings, it has been proposed that rainfall carries spores to low areas. Infected animals shed the bacilli during terminal hemorrhage from all natural orifices and contaminate the surrounding soil. On exposure to air, the vegetative forms sporulate, and these spores are resistant to many disinfectants and adverse environmental conditions. Opening the carcass, whether for butchering meat, harvesting the hide, or necropsy, increases the quantity of spores in the environment. Predators and carrion birds accomplish not only this result but also can transport anthrax organisms to distant places. Thus, the cycle of deposition of spores in the soil and their consumption by herbivores continues.

Humans become incidentally infected when contacting spores on dead animals or their meat, hides, hair or wool. The most common form of the disease, cutaneous anthrax, occurs when spores enter skin damaged by a cut or abrasion in persons involved in butchering or skinning an infected animal.[1–3,10,16,17] Inhalation of spores causes illness mainly in manufacturing settings, including the domestic weaving of contaminated wool, and in laboratory workers.[1–3,10,22–24] Ingestion of raw or undercooked meat may cause a severe enteric disease that has been described mainly in tropical Africa and Asia.[1,25–27] There is circumstantial evidence that biting flies transmit anthrax not only to humans but also among animals.[5,11,12,28] Direct person-to-person transmission of anthrax is extremely rare.[1] Therefore isolation of infected cases is not required.

THE DISEASE

Human Anthrax

The four clinical forms of human anthrax – cutaneous, oropharyngeal, gastrointestinal, and inhalational – are determined by the portal of entry of *B. anthracis*. More than 90% of cases are cutaneous, and even if untreated 80% or more of these infections remain localized. A high proportion of patients with inhalational, oropharyngeal and gastrointestinal forms and 20% of patients with the cutaneous form develop systemic bacteremia and if not treated promptly succumb to fatal effects of the anthrax toxins.[1–3]

Cutaneous Anthrax

Cutaneous anthrax occurs mainly on exposed parts of the body, usually the hands, fingers, face, or neck.[1–3,14–17] Single lesions are common, but multiple lesions can also occur. The spores are introduced through a skin lesion (cut or abrasion) or by means of a fly bite. After an incubation period of 1–7 days (usually 2 or 3 days), a painless, often pruritic papule resembling an insect bite develops at the site of inoculation over a period of 24–48 hours. The papule enlarges and becomes vesicular with clear or serosanguineous fluid containing numerous bacilli. The vesicle enlarges and satellite vesicles may develop. Striking, non-pitting gelatinous edema surrounds the lesion. Fever, malaise, and regional lymphadenopathy are often associated features. Subsequently, the vesicle becomes hemorrhagic, cloudy and ruptures towards the end of the first week and undergoes necrosis, forming an ulcer. A black eschar of 1–5 cm forms over the ulcer (anthrax is derived from word *anthrakitis*, the Greek word for coal, in reference to the color of the lesion). The characteristic painless ulcer with black eschar and surrounding edema is the hallmark of cutaneous anthrax (***Fig. 38.3***) and serves to differentiate it from a wide range of infectious and noninfectious conditions such as furuncles, impetigo, erysipelas, cellulitis, milker's nodule, orf, glanders, plague, syphilitic chancre, ulceroglandular tularemia, rickettsial diseases, leishmaniasis, and arachnid bites. Over the next 2–3 weeks, the eschar detaches and falls off, and healing occurs without leaving a permanent scar. Resolution of the ulcer is not hastened by antibiotic treatment. A small proportion of untreated cases develop massive edema of the face, eyelids, head, and neck (***Fig. 38.4***), sites interfering with respiration, and causing toxic shock due to septicemia, or meningitis. Secondary infection of the ulcer is uncommon but would be indicated by the recurrence of fever with lymphangitis, local pain, and purulent discharge. The skin lesion usually manifests edema involving most prominently the upper dermis with formation of a subepidermal bulla that is sloughed, leaving an ulcer. The fully formed eschar comprises coagulation necrosis of the skin with anthrax bacilli, vasculitis, edema, hemorrhage, and leukocytic exudates extending deep into the subcutaneous fat but not the skeletal muscle.[29,30]

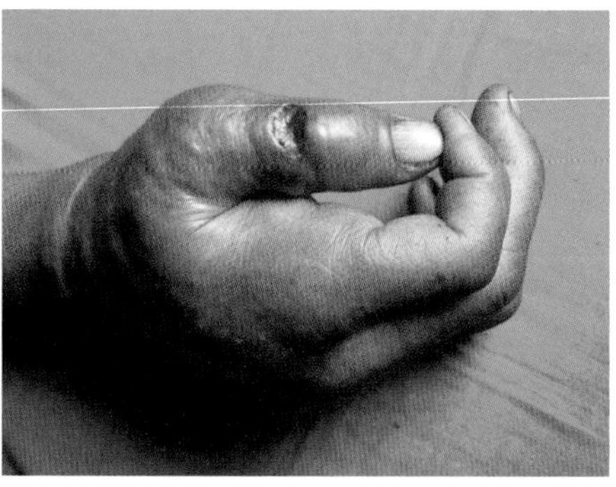

Figure 38.3 A characteristic ulcer with black eschar and edema.

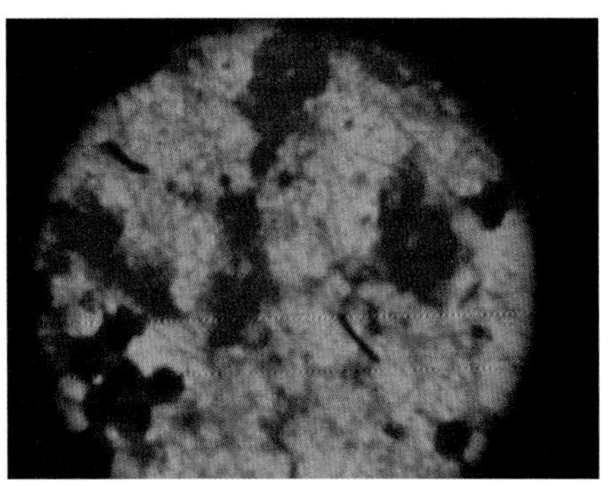

Figure 38.1 Photomicrograph of Gram-positive *Bacillus anthracis* in the soft tissue of cutaneous anthrax.

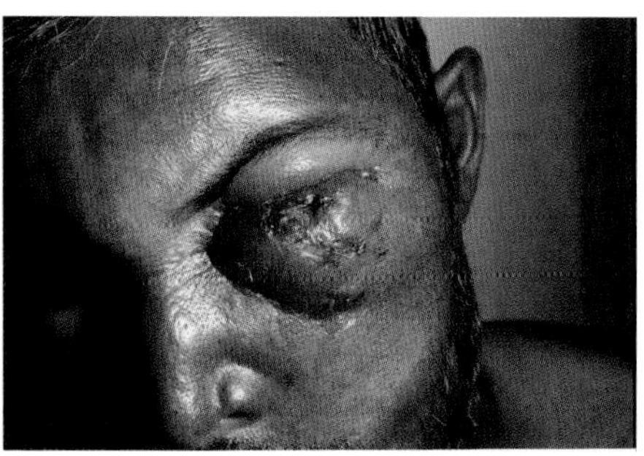

Figure 38.4 Massive gelatinous edema of the eye with ulcer.

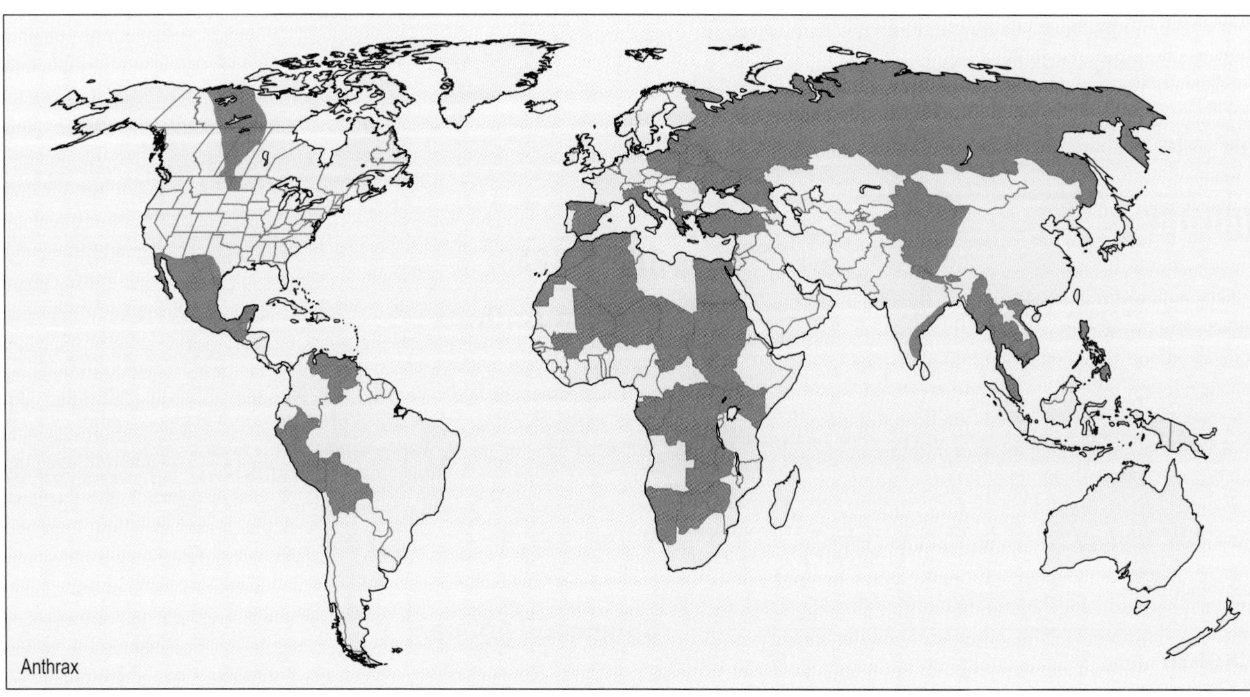

Figure 38.2 Global distribution of anthrax.

Oropharyngeal and Gastrointestinal Anthrax

Oropharyngeal Anthrax

Oropharyngeal anthrax is the result of deposition of spores in the oropharynx, which causes typical anthrax-like nodules or ulcers on the tonsils, pharynx, or hard palate. The symptoms include fever, severe throat pain, dysphonia, dysphagia, and airway compromise due to lymphadenitis.[1,2,31,32] The oral lesions undergo necrosis and ulceration, and often develop a white to gray pseudomembrane in the second week. In the differential diagnosis, diphtheria, complicated tonsillitis, streptococcal pharyngitis, Vincent's angina, Ludwig's angina, and parapharyngeal abscess should be considered.

Gastrointestinal Anthrax

The symptoms of gastrointestinal anthrax appear 2–5 days after ingestion of raw and undercooked meat containing spores.[1,2] The mortality rates have been estimated at 4–50%.[25–27]

The lesions may occur anywhere in the gastrointestinal tract during septicemic anthrax including the esophagus, stomach, duodenum, jejunum, and ileum, but following ingestion the lesion involves the terminal ileum and cecum.[33] The characteristic lesion is a single, superficial ulcer with extensive surrounding edema. The lesion may bleed, and hemorrhage may be massive and fatal in some cases.[34] Massive hemorrhagic enlargement of mesenteric lymph nodes and extensive ulceration can result in intestinal obstruction, bleeding, perforation, and ascites.[25–27] The early symptoms are nonspecific and include nausea, vomiting, anorexia, asthenia, mild diarrhea, and fever. Early diagnosis is difficult, resulting in mortality greater than 50%. The differential diagnosis includes food poisoning (in the early stages), dysentery (amebic or bacterial), gastroenteritis (bacterial or viral), and acute abdomen due to other reasons.

Inhalational Anthrax

Extremely rare and fatal unless treated early in the course, inhalational anthrax occurs as an industrial disease associated with contaminated wool, hair, other animal products (woolsorter's disease) and also with bioterrorist acts.[1,2,22–24] It results from inhalation of *B. anthracis* spores smaller than 5 µm. The spores germinate, replicate in mediastinal lymph nodes and secrete toxins.[35,36] The incubation period ranges from 1 to 7 days, but may be as long as 60 days.[2] The initial symptoms may resemble influenza, including productive cough, myalgia, fatigue, and fever. After several days, the symptoms may progress to severe dyspnea, cyanosis and shock. Chest radiographs show pleural effusions and mediastinal widening due to lymphadenopathy. Meningitis, often hemorrhagic, occurs in up to half of patients with inhalational anthrax. The course of illness averages 4 days with death occurring after 24 hours of hospitalization. The mortality is 100% in untreated cases. The differential diagnosis includes influenza, mycoplasmal pneumonia, legionnaires' disease, psittacosis, and fungal and viral pneumonias.

Other Rare Forms of Anthrax

Anthrax Meningitis

Anthrax meningoencephalitis is considered to be a rare and serious complication of any of the three forms of anthrax due to hematogenous spread of the bacilli to the central nervous system.[1–3,10–14] Cases have also been reported without any identifiable primary portal of entry.[37,38] It resembles meningitis due to other causes although it is frequently hemorrhagic. The case fatality is nearly 100%. The diagnosis is confirmed by demonstration of Gram-positive capsulated organisms in cerebrospinal fluid.

Anthrax Sepsis

Sepsis develops after the lymphohematogenous spread of *B. anthracis* from the primary lesion (cutaneous, gastrointestinal, or pulmonary). Clinical features are high fever, toxemia, and shock, with death following in a short time. Definitive diagnosis is made by the isolation of *B. anthracis* from the primary lesion and from blood cultures.[1–3,10–14]

PATHOGENESIS AND IMMUNITY

Clinical manifestations of anthrax occur when spores gain access to the body and germinate within macrophages or dendritic cells.[1] Phagocytosis plays an important role in the dissemination of *B. anthracis*.[1] After germination, *B. anthracis* secretes three plasmid-encoded proteins: protective antigen, lethal factor, and edema factor, which act in combination as toxins.[1,2,39] Protective antigen (PA), an 83 kDa protein, binds by its C-terminus preferentially to a cell surface receptor, capillary morphogenesis protein 2, is cleaved by a host protease (furin) to yield a 63 kDa polypeptide, and with a coreceptor (low-density lipoprotein receptor-related protein) assembles into a heptameric β-barrel prepore that is capable of binding lethal factor (LF) and/or edema factor (EF). In association with a lipid raft, the prepore enters the cell by receptor-mediated endocytosis via a clathrin-coated pit. Acidification of the endosome results in insertion of the 14-strand PA β-barrel pore and proton-driven transport of LF and EF into the cytoplasm.[40–44] EF, an 89 kDa protein, is a calmodulin-dependent adenylate cyclase that increases the intracellular cyclic adenosine monophosphate, resulting in the interstitial edema occurring around the eschar.[45,46] LF is a zinc metalloprotease[47] with activity that digests mitogen-activated protein kinases 3 and 6,[48] and thereby disrupts signal transduction pathways in eukaryotic cells. For some years, the primary cell type affected in anthrax pathogenesis has been regarded as the macrophage, but recently evidence that favors dendritic cells has accumulated.[1]

A key pathologic lesion apparently explaining the lethal hemorrhagic meningitis and hematogenous hemorrhagic pneumonia of disseminated anthrax is vasculitis.[1,36] The induction of apoptosis in endothelial cells by lethal toxin may play a role in the vascular lesions.[1] Pathogenicity of *B. anthracis* requires the presence of the plasmid-encoded, highly negatively charged antiphagocytic, poly-D-glutamic acid capsule.[1]

DIAGNOSIS

The diagnosis of anthrax depends on recognition of a cutaneous or oropharyngeal lesion, typical signs and symptoms, and history of exposure or potential exposure to an infected animal or its products. Laboratory confirmation is by examination of Gram-stained smears of vesicular fluid, skin or oropharyngeal ulcer base, ascites, or pleural or cerebrospinal fluid, culture, immunohistochemical identification of *B. anthracis*, serological studies, and polymerase chain reaction (PCR). On Gram stain, the bacilli are Gram-positive and occur singly or in short chains, with the organisms being surrounded by a capsule. The ends of the bacilli are truncated or often concave and somewhat swollen so that a chain of bacilli presents a "bamboo stick' appearance. On methylene blue stain the bacterial cell is blue whereas the surrounding capsule is pink (M'Fadyean reaction).[1,4] The specimens are cultured on sheep blood agar aerobically at 35–37°C. After 15–24 hours of incubation, characteristic grayish white, non-motile, non-hemolytic and Gram-positive colonies with ground-glass appearance are observed.[1,4] Specific identification is achieved by γ-phage lysis or by staining with monoclonal antibodies to the capsule and cell wall antigens. Skin biopsies are not mandatory for the confirmation of diagnosis, but they are useful for immunohistochemistry and PCR studies. More recently, enzyme-linked immunosorbent assay and electrophoretic immunotransblot techniques have been found to be more sensitive and specific in detecting the antibodies against PA, LF, EF, and capsule than other reported immunoassays.[1,49] PCR methods are available for confirming the presence of virulence factor (capsule and toxin) genes. Primers to protective antigen (*pag*), lethal factor gene (*lef*), *capB* and *capC* genes and S-layer genes are effective.[1,16,17,50] PCR is a useful tool to confirm anthrax, particularly if the culture is negative because of prior antibiotic treatment.

TREATMENT AND PROGNOSIS

Penicillin G is still the drug of choice in the therapy of naturally occurring anthrax though the organism is susceptible to a wide range of broad-spectrum antibiotics. Ciprofloxacin and doxycycline have become primary treatment alternatives in recent years. In mild uncomplicated cases of cutaneous anthrax, the treatment usually recommended is intramuscular procaine penicillin 500–600 mg (800 000 to 1 million units) every 12–24 hours for 3–7 days. Oral penicillin V (500 mg every 6 hours) or amoxicillin (500 mg every 8 hours) for 3–7 days are alternatives. For children also, penicillin is the antibiotic of choice, and in general half-adult doses are given to children younger than 10 years.[1] Cutaneous lesions usually become sterile within the first 24 hours after commencement of therapy, and the accompanying edema usually subsides within 24–48 hours, but antibiotic therapy will not alter the clinical effects of the toxin. In life-threatening systemic cases, high-dose intravenous penicillin (4 million units every 4–6 hours) or ciprofloxacin (400 mg every 12 hours) may be combined with an antibiotic, which also has good penetration into the central nervous system.[1] Clarithromycin, clindamycin, vancomycin, or rifampicin is suggested as supplementary antibiotics for inhalational anthrax and streptomycin for gastrointestinal anthrax; vancomycin or rifampicin are suggested for anthrax meningitis. The duration of treatment is 10–14 days. In the event of bioterrorism, multidrug regimens are recommended.[2,51,52] Ciprofloxacin and doxycycline are generally contraindicated for children and pregnant women but can be used in life-threatening emergencies. Though systemic corticosteroid treatment is controversial, it may be used in severe cases along with intensive supportive care, in addition to antibiotic therapy. Surgical interventions generally are not beneficial.

PREVENTION AND CONTROL

Prevention of human anthrax depends on prevention of animal anthrax by effective animal vaccination programs. This has largely been achieved in Europe and the United States. A live, unencapsulated, avirulent *B. anthracis* strain 34F2 (Sterne) vaccine is in use the world over. The protection by a single dose is said to last about one year; therefore, annual boosters are recommended for livestock in endemic areas. Control measures include quarantine of animals on farms where cases have been confirmed, vaccination of all livestock on the farm and adjacent areas, and treatment of animals with antibiotics. Antibiotics should not be given 10 days before or after vaccination to avoid killing the live attenuated bacterial vaccine. The dead animals should not be opened and should be disposed of by incineration or rendering. Deep burial of infected carcasses with slaked lime, a less favored option,[1] disinfection of the premises with 5% formaldehyde, and soil decontamination measures should be initiated as soon as possible, once the outbreak is identified.[1]

Anthrax is a notifiable disease. Humans are protected by public awareness programs regarding the dangers of contact with infected animals or their meat and products. Vaccines[1,53] have been developed for humans; a live spore vaccine similar to Sterne veterinary vaccine has been used effectively in the former USSR. An improved anthrax vaccine adsorbed on aluminum hydroxide (AVA) is the only FDA-approved one in the United States. It is prepared from a cell-free culture filtrate of a toxigenic, non-encapsulated strain of *B. anthracis*. The filtrate contains all the toxin components (LF, EF, and PA) and does not contain dead or live bacteria. This vaccine is recommended in high-risk populations such as laboratory workers and certain military personnel. The vaccination schedule of AVA consists of three subcutaneous injections at 0, 2, and 4 weeks and 6, 12, and 18 months with yearly boosters. Post-exposure prophylaxis against *B. anthracis* with ciprofloxacin is recommended following aerosol exposure to *B. anthracis* spores in a laboratory setting or bioterrorist incident.[2,51]

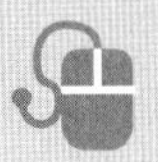

Access the complete reference list online at
http://www.expertconsult.com

Access the complete reference list online at http://www.expertconsult.com

CHAPTER 39

Bartonelloses

Christoph Dehio • Ciro Maguiña • David H. Walker

INTRODUCTION

The genus *Bartonella* of the α2-Proteobacteria comprises 26 species. All bartonellae are arthropod-borne pathogens that cause long-lasting intraerythrocytic infections in their specific mammalian reservoir host(s), including the two human-specific pathogens *B. bacilliformis* and *B. quintana*. Incidental human infection by at least seven species adapted to various animal reservoirs does not lead to intraerythrocytic bacteremia, but these zoonotic infections can cause a broad range of clinical manifestations.[1] The great majority of cases of human bartonellosis are caused by only three species: the two human-specific pathogens and the cat-adapted zoonotic pathogen *B. henselae*. *B. bacilliformis* is the etiologic agent of a sandfly-transmitted febrile hemolytic anemia (Oroya fever) and chronic cutaneous angiomatosis (verruga peruana) endemic to Andean tropical Peru, Ecuador, and Colombia. *B. quintana*, the causative agent of trench fever during World Wars I and II, currently affects the louse-infested poor.[2] *B. henselae* is the primary cause of cat-scratch disease.[3] In immunocompromised persons, particularly those infected with human immunodeficiency virus (HIV), *B. henselae* and *B. quintana* cause opportunistic infections frequently manifested as cutaneous bacillary angiomatosis resembling verruga peruana.[4] *B. henselae* and *B. quintana*, as well as *B. alsatica*, *B. elizabethae*, *B. koehlerae*, *B. vinsonii* subsp. *arupensis* and subsp. *berkhoffii* are etiologic agents of infective endocarditis.[5–12] *B. rochalimae* has been reported to cause bacteremia with fever, and *B. grahamii* to cause neuroretinitis (***Table 39.1***).[13–15] All other species of the genus *Bartonella* cause persistent asymptomatic infections of their respective mammalian reservoir(s), but have not yet been associated with human disease.[1,8,16–22]

The acute hemolytic form of *B. bacilliformis* infection occurred catastrophically during the construction of Peru's Central Railway from Lima to Oroya, from which the designation Oroya fever is derived.[23–25] At least 7000 workers died between 1869 and 1873 as the railroad construction passed from 1000 to 3000 meters above sea level, roughly along the Rimac River valley, where the sandfly vector abounds. The connection between Oroya fever and verruga peruana was vividly and dramatically demonstrated in 1885 by a Peruvian medical student, Daniel Carrión, who, seeking to prove that the cutaneous disease was infectious, had himself inoculated experimentally with material from a patient's skin lesion.[23–27] Only as death from severe febrile disease and anemia approached did he realize that the verruga had contained the etiologic agent of Oroya fever. Both manifestations of the infection are now known as Carrión's disease.

In 1961 Vinson and Fuller[28] reported the isolation of *B. quintana* after prolonged cultivation on blood agar; subsequent infection of human volunteers with this isolate fulfilled Koch's postulates.[29]

Visualization of bacteria in silver-stained lesions of cat-scratch disease in 1983 and the discovery in 1990 that the sequence of a polymerase chain reaction (PCR) product of the 16S ribosomal DNA (rDNA) from bacillary angiomatosis lesions was the same as that from a novel species, *B. henselae*, isolated from the blood of immunocompromised patients, were important milestones in the elucidation of the medical importance of this organism.[30–34] Subsequently, cat-scratch disease patients were shown to develop antibodies to *B. henselae* and to be infected with this bacterium.[35]

THE AGENT

B. bacilliformis is an aerobic, facultative intracellular 1–3 μm pleomorphic bacillus with a poorly staining Gram-negative cell wall and 2–16 unipolar flagella conferring a high degree of motility.[36] *B. henselae* does not contain flagella but exhibits a characteristic twitching movement. It expresses on the cell surface the trimeric autotransporter adhesin (TAA) BadA, which forms major surface appendages.[37,38] *B. quintana* also expresses TAA, the variably-expressed outer membrane proteins VompA to VompD.[39] *B. henselae* and *B. quintana* are metabolically rather inert in that they test negative for glucose oxidation, indole production, nitrate reduction, and catalase, oxidase, and urease activity.

Bartonellae require hemin, with *B. quintana* having the highest hemin requirement for growth among bacteria.[40] *B. quintana* has five heme receptors that are all expressed and are predicted to be β-barrel outer membrane proteins with eight transmembrane domains and four extracellular loops. The *ialA* invasion gene of *B. bacilliformis* is a dinucleoside polyphosphate hydrolase more similar to eukaryotic plant diadenosine tetraphosphate hydrolases than to the bacterial enzymes.[41] It likely removes the toxic substrate that accumulates during invasion and oxidative stress generated by host defenses with useful adenosine triphosphate as a byproduct of its catabolism.

Growth of bartonellae is slow, requires 5% CO_2, hemin, and an optimal temperature of 35°C for *B. quintana* and *B. henselae* and 28°C for *B. bacilliformis*.

EPIDEMIOLOGY

The reservoir host of *B. bacilliformis* is the human, who may remain persistently bacteremic for months after recovery.[42–45] A wildlife reservoir was postulated, since isolated cases have occurred in persons exposed to vectors for a single night in deserted areas.[46] However, no confirmed isolations of *B. bacilliformis* have been obtained from fauna in the endemic areas. The classically accepted vector in Peru is the female hematophagous sandfly, *Lutzomyia verrucarum*, which is found in narrow river valleys between 500 and 3200 meters above sea level (***Fig. 39.1***). More recently, cases have occurred in high rainforest regions.[47] South American bartonellosis also occurs in Colombia and Ecuador, where *L. verrucarum* is absent (***Fig. 39.2***).[48] The most likely vector in Colombia is the highly anthropophilic *L. columbiana*, but at present the disease is apparently seldom documented in Colombia.[43] The probable vectors in Ecuador, where cases occur in low-lying coastal areas as well as the Andes, are unknown. Although sandflies are incompletely studied in South America, more than

Table 39.1 Etiology and Transmission of Human Bartonelloses

Species	Disease	Reservoir Host	Arthropod Vector
B. bacilliformis	Oroya fever (acute)	Human	*Lutzomyia verrucarum* (sandfly)
	Verruga peruana (chronic)		
B. quintana	Trench fever	Human	*Pediculus humanus corporis* (human body louse)
	Bacillary angiomatosis		
	Endocarditis		
B. henselae	Cat-scratch disease	Cat	*Ctenocephalides felis* (cat flea)
	Bacillary angiomatosis		
	Endocarditis		
B. alsatica	Endocarditis	Rabbit	Not known
	Lymphadenitis		
B. clizabethae	Endocarditis	Rat	Not known
B. koehlerae	Endocarditis	Cat	Not known
B. grahamii	Neuroretinitis	Mouse	*Ctenophthalmus nobilis nobilis* (rodent flea)
B. rochalimae	Bacteremia with fever	Fox	*Pulex simulans* (false human flea)
B. vinsonii subsp. *arupensis*	Endocarditis	Mouse	Not known
	Bacteremia with fever		
B. vinsonii subsp. *berkhoffii*	Endocarditis	Dog/coyote	Not known

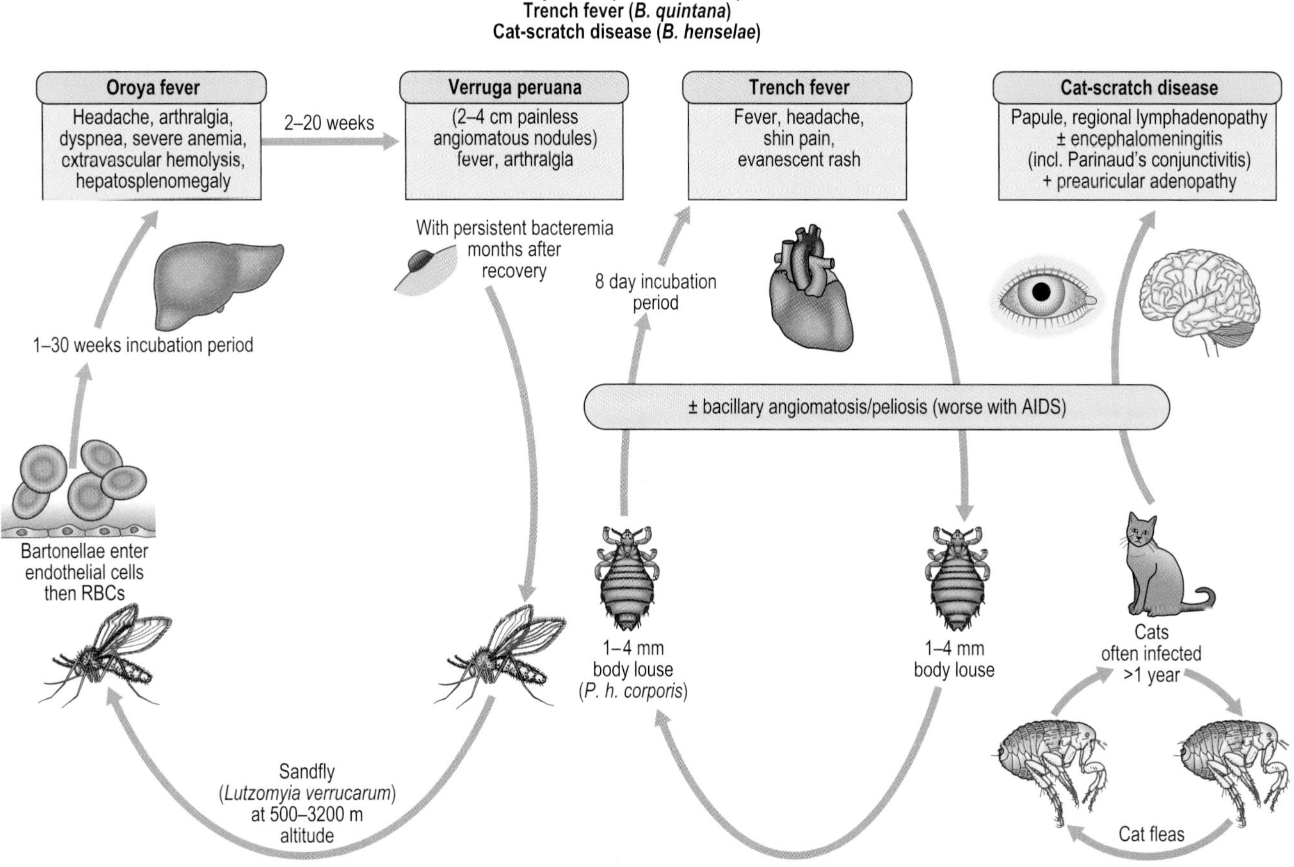

Figure 39.1 Infection cycle of the three major human pathogenic *Bartonella* species: Carrión's disease (*B. bacilliformis*); trench fever (*B. quintana*); cat-scratch disease (*B. henselae*).

500 different species have been described with two-thirds of them in the Americas, more than 60 in Ecuador, and approximately 120 in Peru.[49,50] Serologic studies suggest that in endemic areas more than 60% of the population has been infected.[51] In such populations 0.5–10% are bacteremic at any given time.[43,45,52] A prospective population-based study in an endemic site identified a high incidence (12.7 infections/100 person-years) that was greatest in children less than 5 years of age and declined with age.[52] The affected pediatric population commonly belongs to a low income population. Higher incidence was associated with the increased humidity, temperature, and sandfly population during El Niño-influenced weather. As expected with a human reservoir and transmission by indoor sandfly bites in the evening and night, 70% of cases

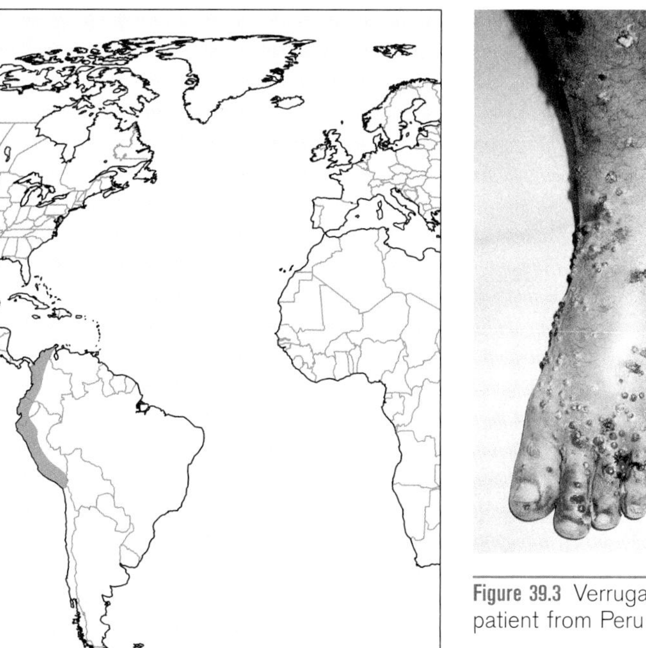

Figure 39.2 Global distribution of *B. bacilliformis.*

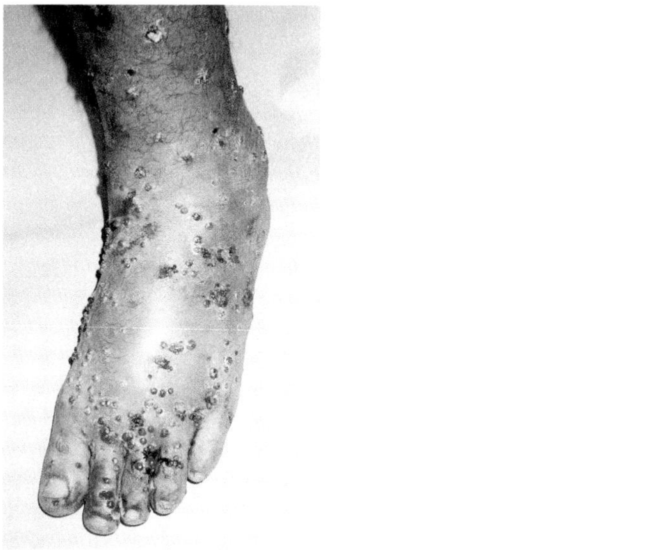

Figure 39.3 Verruga peruana skin lesions on the foot and leg of a patient from Peru infected with *B. bacilliformis.*

clustered in 18% of households. Mothers in endemic areas expect the verruga to occur in their children and are concerned if, after a certain febrile illness that they consider to be bartonellosis, the children do not develop the skin lesions, fearing more severe complications and death. Epidemics occur when immunologically naive persons are exposed to the infection because of population migration or introduction of infected sandflies.[25,42]

The human louse, *Pediculus humanus corporis*, was recognized as the human-to-human vector of epidemic trench fever in the European theaters of World Wars I and II (***Fig. 39.1***). *B. quintana* infections have also occurred in North Africa, Ethiopia, Japan, China, Mexico, and Bolivia and more recently in the United States and France among immunocompromised patients, particularly those with HIV infection, as well as among homeless persons who abuse alcohol.[28,53–58] After immunocompetent persons recover from untreated *B. quintana* infection, asymptomatic intraerythrocytic bacteremia may continue for months.[59] It is likely that *B. quintana* is a prevalent but as yet poorly recognized agent of human infections in the tropics.[60]

The reservoir of *B. henselae* is the domestic cat throughout the world, particularly in warm, humid climates where *Ctenocephalides felis* cat fleas thrive.[61,62] A substantial proportion of domestic cats are infected, and bacteremia is prolonged, lasting months to more than a year.[61,63] Cat fleas transmit *B. henselae* between cats and possibly by contaminating cat scratch or bite wounds with flea feces (***Fig. 39.1***).[64,65] The bacteria remain infectious in flea feces for prolonged periods. There are two genotypes of *B. henselae* that have variable prevalences in different geographic regions with imperfect concordance between the distributions of human and cat genotypes.[66,67] Cat-scratch disease and other manifestations of *B. henselae* infection occur throughout the tropics.

Bartonella endocarditis, most frequently caused by *B. quintana* or *B. henselae*, is not related to the immune status of the host but rather to the risk factors for infection.[68] Case reports of endocarditis caused by *B. alsatica*, *B. elizabethae*, *B. koehlerae* or *B. vinsonii* subsp. *arupensis* and spp. *berkhoffii*, of neuroretinitis caused by *B. grahamii*, and of bacteremia with fever caused by *B. rochalimae* and *B. vinsonii* subsp. *arupensis* are difficult to link with the natural reservoir–vector cycles.[5,8–13,69] Conversely high seroprevalence of antibodies to rat-associated *B. elizabethae* among urban intravenous drug abusers has not been correlated with clinical manifestations.[70]

THE DISEASE

The incubation period of Carrión's disease is considered to be 21 days (from Carrión's experimental infection) with a range of 1–30 weeks and a mean of 2 months. The two clinical forms of the disease – Oroya fever and verruga peruana – may occur sequentially, sometimes with an intervening clinically silent period, or either form may occur alone.[24,25,42–44,71,72] The usual gradual onset of systemic symptoms of malaise, somnolence, anorexia, myalgia, headache, pain in the back and extremities, chills, and fever accompany erythrocyte parasitization levels as high as 100% (***Fig. 39.1***). The mononuclear phagocytic system removes and destroys a major portion of the infected red blood cells after 2–4 weeks, resulting in severe anemia with erythrocyte counts in some cases below $10^6/\mu L$, accompanied by hepatosplenomegaly, generalized lymphadenopathy, jaundice, dyspnea, and mental status changes.[43,73,74] The facultative intracellular bartonellae invade endothelial cells, particularly in skin and lymph nodes. Patients with severe infection develop pericardial effusion, myocarditis, coma, convulsions, delirium, acute respiratory distress, anasarca, acute renal failure, and multiple organ failure.[75,76] Infection during pregnancy may result in transplacental infection, abortion, fetal death, and maternal death. The duration of Oroya fever is between 1 and 6 weeks with variation from mild to fatal with a mortality rate of approximately 40% in the preantibiotic era, 8% in current hospital settings, 88% in a recent outbreak in a remote rural area, and 0.7% in a contemporary population-based study.[42,73] Death frequently occurs owing to infection-induced immunodeficiency and consequent opportunistic infections that intervene in 30% of cases caused by bacteria (e.g., salmonellae, staphylococci, or *Mycobacterium tuberculosis*), protozoa (e.g., *Toxoplasma* or amebae), fungi (e.g., *Histoplasma* or *Pneumocystis*), and viruses (e.g., herpesvirus or hepatitis B virus).[27] Salmonellosis was formerly the most frequent fatal complication in hospitalized patients.[77] Inversion of the T-lymphocyte helper and suppressor subset ratio and development of skin test anergy reflect transient immunosuppression underlying the appearance of opportunistic infections.[78,79]

Two to 20 weeks after recovery from Oroya fever or without any preceding illness, arthralgia, fever, and a series of crops of verrucae appear as painless erythematous 0.2 to 4 cm papules, sessile or subdermal nodules, or large angioma-like cutaneous lesions (***Fig. 39.3***). The lesions are prone to bleed and occur particularly on the head and extremities; sometimes they also occur on the nasal, conjunctival, and oral mucosa, but they have never been described in internal organs – this tropism may reflect the temperature optimum of 28°C for growth of *B. bacilliformis.*

These lesions consist of proliferations of vascular endothelial cells and dermal dendrocytes with interspersed macrophages, lymphocytes, and plasma cells.[79–81] In verrucae, bartonellae are observed extracellularly.[79,81] Individual verrucae dry up and slough in a few weeks, leaving no scars. Crops of verrucae can occur for months or exceptionally for years.[82,83] In an endemic area, 11% of infections were acute hemolytic Oroya fever; 37% of the infected population had verruga peruana preceded by symptoms of Oroya fever, 31.5% developed verruga peruana without preceding acute hemolytic illness, and 20.5% were asymptomatic. Overall only 7% of this medically underserved population was hospitalized, and none died.[52] In an outbreak in a nonendemic area where the disease had not previously occurred, 77.5% of the population developed antibodies against *B. bacilliformis*, 13.8% had symptoms (fever, headache, and bone and joint pain) of Oroya fever, and verruga peruana occurred in 17.6% with only 4.8% of the population manifesting the biphasic course.[84]

Trench fever or acute *B. quintana* infection has a variable incubation period that averages 8 days.[29,53,58] The clinical course varies from mild and afebrile to moderately severe with a long clinical course and numerous relapses. Some patients suffer a single febrile episode of 4–5 days often accompanied by malaise, headache, pain that is particularly severe in the shins, and an evanescent rash that is visible mainly in lightly pigmented skin. Other patients have continuous fever for up to 6 weeks or a course with three to eight periodic febrile episodes of about 5 days' duration from which the name *B. quintana* is derived. Contemporary *B. quintana* infection of homeless alcoholic persons typically manifests only as fever unless associated with *Bartonella* endocarditis.[54,56,57] Yet among homeless French persons, 14% are bacteremic, 80% of whom are afebrile. Prolonged *B. quintana* bacteremia can persist for 300 to 443 days after onset. In Europe, chronic lymphadenopathy has been associated with granulomatous *B. quintana* infection of the lymph nodes.[85]

The clinical manifestations of *B. henselae* infection include cat-scratch disease, unilateral follicular conjunctivitis, neuroretinitis, retinochoroiditis, encephalitis, meningitis, encephalopathy, persistent or relapsing febrile bacteremia, hepatosplenic lesions, infective endocarditis, osteomyelitis, atypical pneumonia, erythema nodosum, bacillary angiomatosis, bacillary peliosis, and inflammatory or vasoproliferative lesions in virtually any organ (***Fig. 39.1***).[3,4,30–32,34,61,66,86–96] Cat-scratch disease typically manifests as a papule at the site of inoculation of organisms by cat scratch or bite and by regional lymphadenopathy with or without fever in 25–60% of patients 3–12 days after injury and 1–2 weeks before onset of constitutional symptoms. *B. henselae* stimulates an inflammatory reaction in immunocompetent hosts that manifests most often as regional (epitrochlear, axillary, and/or cervical) lymphadenopathy that resolves in a median of 7 weeks and undergoes suppuration in 15%. Peruvian studies have detected antibodies to *B. henselae* and *B. clarridgeiae*.[97,98] The formation of mature granulomas leads to the elimination of the organisms. In immunocompromised patients, especially those with AIDS, *B. henselae* and *B. quintana* infections stimulate the proliferation and migration of endothelial cells, resulting in cutaneous bacillary angiomatosis and in some patients similar vascular proliferations in the spleen and liver (bacillary peliosis), lymph node, lung, bone, gastrointestinal tract, brain, mouth, nose, and anus.[99] The lesions resemble verruga peruana with lobular proliferations of endothelial cells.[100] They also contain neutrophils, leukocytoclastic debris, and extracellular amorphous granular material that is revealed by Warthin–Starry silver staining to be microcolonies of bartonellae. Although *B. henselae* and *B. quintana* are facultative intracellular bacteria, intracellular bartonellae are not characteristic of *B. henselae* and *B. quintana* bacillary angiomatosis.[37] In some patients, the disseminated lesions are neither angioma-like nor granulomatous but rather a mixture of nonspecific inflammation and fibrosis.

Bartonella endocarditis affects mainly middle-aged patients who present with fever (83%), often develop emboli (43%) from the large vegetations that involve the aortic valve more often than the mitral valve, and occasionally suffer renal failure owing to mesangioproliferative glomerulonephritis.[68] *B. henselae* most often affects previously damaged valves, and *B. quintana*, previously normal valves. Chronic myocarditis has been reported in association with evidence for *Bartonella* infections.[101,102]

PATHOGENESIS AND IMMUNITY

In Oroya fever, the facultatively intracellular *B. bacilliformis* is introduced into the vasculature by the bite of a sandfly and is taken up by endothelial cells of capillaries, sinusoidal lining cells, and red blood cells (***Fig. 39.1***).[103–105] Bartonellae induce invaginations in the erythrocyte cell membrane by an uncharacterized molecule – deformin – and entry into the red blood cell is mediated by proteins encoded by the two-gene invasion locus *ialA*/*ialB* and motility provided by flagella.[36,106–110] Entry of *B. bacilliformis* into endothelial cells is dependent on Rho-GTPase, which is activated by the bacteria.[111] *B. quintana* circulate inside 0.001–0.005% of human erythrocytes, sequestered from immune attack.[59] Although *in vitro* cultivation of *B. quintana* in human red blood cells shortens the cells' life span, anemia does not occur, in marked contrast with extravascular hemolysis in Oroya fever.[59,112] Entry of human erythrocytes by *B. quintana* (as well as cat erythrocytes by *B. henselae*) is probably dependent on the type IV secretion system Trw, which is essential for the invasion of erythrocytes by *Bartonella tribocorum* in an experimental rat infection model.[113] The Trw system is absent from the ancestral species *B. bacilliformis*, while flagella are absent from the more recently evolved and closely related species *B. quintana*, *B. henselae*, and *B. tribocorum*, suggesting that the Trw system has functionally replaced flagella in the process of erythrocyte invasion.[114,115] A distinct type IV secretion system, VirB/VirD4, that is present in *B. quintana*, *B. henselae*, and *B. tribocorum* (but not in *B. bacilliformis*) plays a prominent role in the infection of endothelial cells and possibly nucleated cells.[116–118] The VirB/VirD4 system injects several bacterial effector proteins (Bep = ***B**artonella* **e**ffector **p**rotein) that subvert multiple cellular functions in favor of the pathogen, for example to trigger bacterial uptake via cytoskeletal rearrangement or to inhibit host cell apoptosis.[116,119–122]

The pathogenesis of enhanced angiogenesis in *Bartonella*-associated verruga peruana, bacillary angiomatosis, and peliosis may involve the adhesin BadA, endothelial mitogenic factors (e.g., GroEL) secreted by the bacteria, paracrine and autocrine angiogenic effects of vascular endothelial growth factor from macrophages and overlying epidermis, interleukin (IL)-1β from macrophages and IL-8 and angiopoietin 2 from endothelial cells, inhibition of endothelial apoptosis by an unidentified bacterial component, and possibly decreased levels of antiangiogenic IL-12 and interferon (IFN)-γ in immunocompromised persons.[38,123–126] Moreover, in *B. henselae* and *B. quintana* infections, vascular proliferation and apoptosis is modulated by the activity of VirB/VirD4-translocated Bep effector proteins.[121,122,126]

Host defenses against bartonellae involve strong cell-mediated immunity associated with delayed-type sensitivity and Th1-type cytokines (IFN-γ and IL-12). Homeless persons with chronic *B. quintana* bacteremia lack specific antibodies and have lower production of tumor necrosis factor-α, IL-1β, and IL-6 by peripheral blood mononuclear cells and greater production of immunosuppressive IL-10 after *B. quintana* stimulation, which may underlie the failure of the immune system to clear the infection.[127] Antibodies clear bartonellae when they are released from infected erythrocytes.[128]

DIAGNOSIS

Oroya fever, with an early clinical differential diagnosis including typhoid fever, malaria, brucellosis, hepatitis, tuberculosis, leptospirosis, sepsis, sylvatic yellow fever, typhus, paracoccidioidomycosis, histoplasmosis, hematologic malignancy, and hemolytic or aplastic anemia, can be diagnosed by detection of *B. bacilliformis* within erythrocytes in stained blood smears (***Fig. 39.4***). Caution is recommended, however, because of the frequency of artifacts.[43,72] Epidemiologic data are essential. The bacteria can be cultivated from blood in 71–83% of cases by incubating for up to 6 weeks at 28°C on Columbia agar supplemented with 5% defibrinated blood or other blood- or hemin-supplemented media, with detection of colonies after an average of 18 days. Diagnosis can also be achieved by PCR even on blood spotted onto a card and can be differentiated from

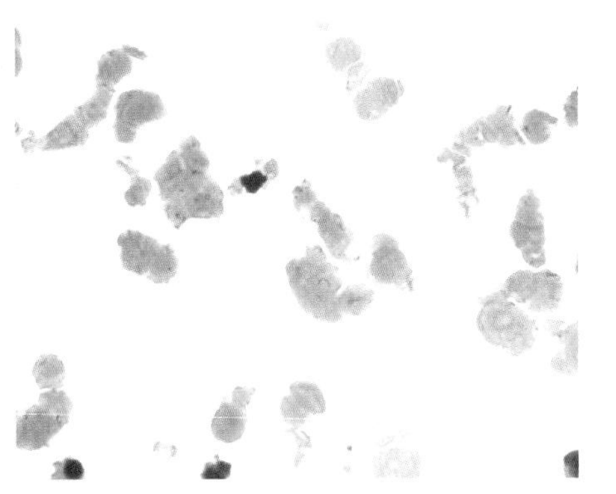

Figure 39.4 Peripheral blood smear of a Peruvian patient with Oroya fever. A high proportion of erythrocytes contain *B. bacilliformis*.

other bartonellae.[52,129–131] Serologic diagnosis of *B. bacilliformis* infection can be established by enzyme immunoassay, IgM or IgG indirect immunofluorescence, indirect hemagglutination, and immunoblot detection of a 17 or 18 kDa antigen.[51,84] The diagnosis of verruga peruana, for which the clinical differential diagnosis includes hemangiomas, pyogenic granuloma, bacillary angiomatosis, Kaposi's sarcoma, chickenpox, molluscum contagiosum, and malignant melanoma, can be confirmed by histopathology.[79,83,132] Culture of *B. bacilliformis* from the skin lesions is difficult because of frequent contamination and its slow growth.

The diagnosis of cat-scratch disease can be established by immunofluorescence antibody (IFA) test, enzyme immunoassay serology, culture, or PCR of lymph node aspirate or biopsy.[35,88] IFA serology provides best results with low passage bacterial antigen cocultivated with cells. Agar-grown antigens yield lower titers, and endpoint titers vary with different commercial products. Thus, a fourfold rise in titer or seroconversion is more convincing than a single high titer. Enzyme immunoassay serology for cat-scratch disease detects IgM antibodies in 53% of sera during the first 3 months, reverting to negative thereafter. IgG antibodies are detected in 92% although initially negative in 28% followed by seroconversion. IgG antibodies remain detectable in only 25% of patients after 1 year.[98] There is considerable serologic cross-reactivity between *B. quintana* and *B. henselae*. Bacteremia with *B. quintana* or *B. henselae* can be diagnosed by saponin or EDTA freeze–thaw lysis of erythrocytes to release intracellular bartonellae, followed by centrifugation and incubation at 35°C in a humid 5% CO_2 atmosphere on chocolate or Columbia blood agar for more than a month, for colonial growth to be visible.[67,133] Organisms are identified by twitching motility in wet mounts, immunofluorescent staining with specific antibodies, and molecular methods. In a recent large series of cases of cat-scratch disease, *B. henselae* DNA was detected by PCR in 31% of lymph node biopsies and 55% of lymph node aspirates, and *B. henselae* was isolated from 27% of lymph node biopsies and 11% of lymph node aspirates after a median of 21 days.[67] The most cost-effective diagnosis of cat-scratch disease relies on the combination of clinical manifestations and serology. The etiologic diagnosis of bacillary angiomatosis and *Bartonella* endocarditis can be established on resected tissues by a combination of histopathology and immunohistology, PCR, or culture.[54,100,134] *Bartonella* antibodies are usually absent in immunocompromised patients with bacillary angiomatosis. *Bartonella* endocarditis is diagnosed more effectively by real-time PCR than by culture, and an IFA titer of at least 800 is strongly supportive of the diagnosis.[67,135] The species of *Bartonella* endocarditis can be determined by cross-absorption immunoblotting.[136]

TREATMENT AND PROGNOSIS

Oroya fever was treated traditionally with chloramphenicol (50 mg/kg daily up to 3 g/day) and after defervescence with half the dose for 10 days because of chloramphenicol's activity against salmonellosis, a classically described life-threatening secondary infection.[73,137] In recent years, therapeutic failure with chloramphenicol due to overwhelming infections (e.g., *Pseudomonas* sp., *Enterobacter* sp., *Acinetobacter* sp.) has changed the drug of choice to ciprofloxacin in children and adults. The dosage of ciprofloxacin for the acute phase is 500 mg twice a day orally for 10 days. The dosage for children younger than 15 years is 250 mg twice a day orally for 10 days.[138] Mutations of *gyrA* in organisms grown in the presence of ciprofloxacin suggest the potential development of resistance.[139] Transfusions of packed red blood cells may be needed to treat the severe anemia in approximately 10% of patients. It must be remembered that throughout the disease the bone marrow is hyperactive, liberating immature erythrocyte precursors. Once the infection is under control, recovery from anemia is surprisingly prompt. For severe cerebral complications (coma, convulsions due to cerebral hypoxia, and edema), short courses of dexamethasone have been employed.[137] The verrucae can be treated with oral rifampin (10 mg/kg daily for 14–21 days), which is more effective and convenient than the formerly used streptomycin. Alternative drugs are oral erythromycin, ciprofloxacin, and azithromycin.[83,138,140,141]

The signs of uncomplicated cat-scratch disease are mainly the manifestations of an effective immune response, and antibiotic treatment has little or no effect on the course of disease although azithromycin may hasten the resolution of lymphadenopathy.[142] *In vitro* susceptibility tests for *B. quintana* and *B. henselae* correlate poorly with clinical experience. Many antimicrobial agents are bacteriostatic, but aminoglycosides such as gentamicin are bactericidal against *B. henselae*.[140,143] Ocular bartonellosis is treated with doxycycline (100 mg every 12 hours) because of superior ocular penetration with a 2- to 4-week course in immunocompetent patients and 4 months or longer in immunocompromised patients.[87] In practice, bacillary angiomatosis is treated with oral doxycycline (100 mg twice a day) or oral erythromycin (0.5–1.0 g four times a day) for 2–3 months and longer if resolution is incomplete or relapse occurs. Oral tetracycline, minocycline, chloramphenicol, clarithromycin, and azithromycin have also been used successfully. In a series of 101 patients with *Bartonella* endocarditis, among whom 12 died and two suffered relapses, full recovery was more likely if the patient was treated with an aminoglycoside, and survival was more likely if the patient was treated for a minimum of 14 days with an aminoglycoside.[68] Endocarditis and, in many cases, bacteremia and visceral bacillary angiomatosis or peliosis are treated intravenously. *Bartonella* endocarditis requires cardiac valve replacement in 76% of cases usually for hemodynamic reasons. The intraerythrocytic niche of *B. quintana* presents a therapeutic challenge. Testing of antimicrobial agents against intraerythrocytic *B. quintana* reveals that doxycycline, fluoroquinolones, and β-lactams are not bactericidal, gentamicin and rifampin are bactericidal at 4 μg/mL, but the peak intraerythrocytic concentration of gentamicin (0.26 μg/mL) occurs after 24 hours and is not bactericidal.[112] Most likely gentamicin kills *B. quintana* only after its release from red blood cells. Chronic *B. quintana* bacteremia in homeless persons is effectively cleared by treatment with gentamicin (3 mg/kg in one intravenous dose daily) for 14 days followed by oral doxycycline (200 mg/day) for 28 days.[144]

PREVENTION AND CONTROL

Control efforts for *B. bacilliformis* infections are directed mainly against adult sandflies. Peridomestic exposure to *Lutzomyia* is reduced by spraying houses, nearby animal shelters, and other structures with residual insecticides and by the use of fine-mesh screens. Area control of sylvan sandflies is not currently achievable, and resistance to insecticides is at least a potential concern. Individual protection using insect repellants and fine-mesh bednets is feasible and in endemic areas should focus on infants and children. An effective measure for workers in endemic areas is to leave the dangerous areas before dusk and set up camp elsewhere; in the Andes, a relatively short distance may mean a difference of several hundred meters in elevation.

Reduction in *B. henselae* transmission can be achieved via elimination of cat fleas and avoidance of traumatic injury by cats. Prophylaxis for *Mycobacterium avium* complex infections or other reasons with macrolides seems to protect also against *Bartonella* infections in HIV-infected persons.[145]

Control of trench fever depends on killing human body lice with insecticides and improved socioeconomic conditions that make it possible to kill lice as clothes are washed routinely in hot, soapy water. Intensive treatment of human infections would reduce the reservoir of *B. quintana*.

Reduction of infection in the known reservoirs of bartonelloses, for example humans (*B. bacilliformis* and *B. quintana*) and cats (*B. henselae*), could be theoretically be accomplished by vaccination. It is also conceivable that an agent for which there is no non-human reservoir, such as *B. bacilliformis* and *B. quintana*, might eventually be eradicated.

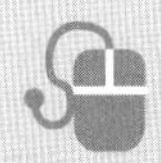

Access the complete reference list online at
http://www.expertconsult.com

Access the complete reference list online at http://www.expertconsult.com

CHAPTER 40

Brucellosis

Eduardo Gotuzzo • Georgios Pappas

INTRODUCTION

In 1887, Sir David Bruce described "a disease of long duration with fever, profuse perspiration, splenomegaly, frequent relapses, rheumatoid or neuralgic pain, swelling of the joints and orchitis" seen in his patients in Malta, and he isolated the pathogen from the spleen of his autopsy studies.[1] Brucellosis still poses important problems in animals and humans in some regions of the world.[2–4]

THE AGENT

Brucella is a slow-growing, aerobic, catalase-positive, nonmotile Gram-negative coccobacillus in the Alphaproteobacteria (α_2 group) with *Bartonella (Rochalimaea) henselae* and *Agrobacterium tumefaciens*.[5,6] As shown in ***Table 40.1 and Figure 40.1***, the species are largely host-specific: *B. melitensis* (the cause of Malta fever) has sheep and goats as reservoir, *B. abortus* (the cause of Bang's disease) causes abortions in cattle, *B. suis* is derived from aborting swine, while *B. canis* can be isolated from aborting beagle dogs. Two other organisms considered nonpathogenic to humans (*B. ovis* and *B. neotomae*) have been isolated from sheep and wood rats, respectively.[7,8] In recent years, novel *Brucella* species have been isolated from marine mammals and are provisionally called *B. ceti* (isolated from marine mammals such as whales, dolphins, porpoises), and *B. pinnipedialis*, (isolated from seals and walruses).[9] These species have been shown to be pathogenic for humans.[10] Another novel *Brucella* species, *B. microti*, has been isolated from red foxes in Central Europe, although human disease has not been documented until now.[11]

EPIDEMIOLOGY

Brucellosis is largely an occupational disease of developing countries or poor rural regions of the developed world.[12] In addition to the classical endemic regions in the Middle East,[13,14] the Mediterranean, and Latin America,[13,15–19] the disease has recently emerged, sometimes amidst geopolitical unrest in central Asia (including Kyrgyzstan, Kazakhstan, Turkmenistan), the Balkan Peninsula (Albania, Bosnia-Herzegovina, and Bulgaria), and even Mongolia.[20] Typically in northern Greece the disease is constantly reintroduced through the northern borders, similar to that seen in Texas and California from neighboring Mexico.[21] Increasing cases have also recently been reported in South Korea, which had been brucellosis-free.[22] The disease is also importated through international travel or specific patterns of migration; as in Germany, where most cases are observed in Turkish-origin immigrants who travel during the summer to their hyperendemic homeland and return infected or carrying infected dairy products.[23]

In endemic regions, the principal pathogen implicated is *B. melitensis*; males and females are equally infected, and 20–25% of cases are children. Infections are typically acquired through the consumption of dairy products, especially nonpasteurized goat's cheese and untreated milk.[24,25] Some outbreaks, including those in family groups, have been reported from common sources, often from contaminated edible products.[26–32] *B. melitensis* may symptomatically infect up to 50% of family members.[25,33] A Saudi Arabian study evaluated household members of patients with acute brucellosis through serological screening: two members or more tested positive in 42% of the families. The risk factor in these families was raw milk ingestion.[34]

The lowest attack rates are in young children, probably related to food habits rather than to immunity. Evidence does not support human to-human transmission, except in rare cases of infection via bone marrow transplantation,[35] blood transfusion, and a possible case of transmission to a sexual partner via the organism in semen.[36] Women develop more severe brucellosis[25,36,37] with more articular involvement[33] and more severe thrombocytopenia[38] with *B. melitensis* infections.

In travelers to endemic areas, the use of antacids and H_2-receptor inhibitors has been considered a risk factor, in addition to the consumption of "typical" local food prepared with unpasteurized cheese or milk.[39,40]

B. abortus is the second commonest species infecting humans, and is typically an occupational disease in abattoir workers,[9] butchers, veterinarians, and farmers, usually affecting adult men (and occasionally family members), who become infected through the skin and conjunctiva.[10,11] *B. suis* is an enzootic disease in swine, while *B. canis* has infected only a few dog breeders.[41,42]

Brucella remains the commonest laboratory-acquired infection, as two recent studies, one from the United States and one from Spain, have demonstrated.[43,44]

THE DISEASE

It is useful to stratify the different clinical presentations of brucellosis due to *B. melitensis*.[45] However, it is less helpful in the evaluation of patients with *B. abortus* or *B. suis* infections, because chronic or recurring forms are infrequent.

Acute Form (Classical Febrile Brucellosis)

In acute *B. melitensis* infections, patients typically present with evening fever (38°C (100°F) or greater), with profuse or patchy sweating, malaise, headache, and weight loss (3–10 kg in 1–2 weeks). Half of these patients have arthralgias and one-third have arthritis, often with myalgias and back pain. Mild anemia, leukopenia, and hepatic involvement are frequent,[46–50] but psychiatric and urologic complications are rare. Constipation is common in endemic brucellosis; however, patients may present with diarrhea and fever, especially travelers from developed countries.

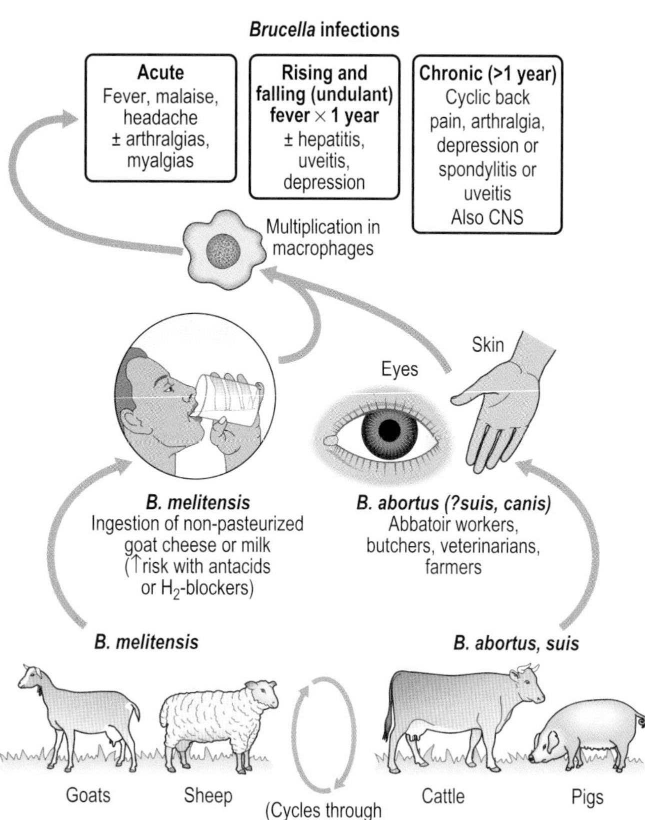

Figure 40.1 Brucellosis life cycle.

Table 40.1 Brucellosis: Epidemiologic and Clinical Differences

	Brucella abortus	*Brucella melitensis*
Principal reservoir	Cattle	Goats
Transmission	Worker's disease: veterinarians, farmers, butchers	Consumption of unpasteurized goat cheese
Age	Adults 20–45 years	All ages, 25% children
Sex	>95% male	50% female
Geographic location	United States	Arabian countries; Latin America: Peru, Mexico, Argentina; Mediterranean countries: Spain, Italy, France, Greece, Portugal
Pathogenicity	Low	High
Subclinical-to-clinical case ratio	8:1	<1:1
Clinical pattern	Mild disease; no chronic form; mortality <0.1%	More severe form, frequent relapses: chronic form 1–5%; mortality 1%
Outbreaks	Rare	Frequent in the United States with imported dairy products
Family cases	Rare	Occasional

Relapsing or Undulant Form (Malta Fever)

This is the "classical pattern" described by Bruce[1] and is observed after 2 months with the disease. In the preantibiotic era, 75% of patients developed this form, with rare cases persisting beyond 1 year. This form represents 25–30% of cases in endemic areas and usually reflects incomplete treatment, failure of standard treatment, or lack of a proper initial diagnosis and therapy. Hepatic involvement and arthritis are common, as is a mild depressive mood, and occasionally uveitis and orchiepididymitis in young males.[51] This form may also present as a fever of unknown origin.[52]

Chronic Brucellosis

Two patterns of chronic brucellosis (lasting more than 1 year) may be seen. The first is a cyclic course with back pain, arthralgias, sweating, and depressive mood. This pattern is very similar to the chronic fatigue syndrome and occurs more frequently in women, especially women older than 40 years of age. The second chronic form is localized brucellosis: spondylitis or uveitis (or episcleritis) without fever or systemic symptoms. This form is frequent in adults (representing 5–10% of cases in endemic areas), affects both sexes equally, but is rare in children. In addition to the preceding clinical forms, the following sections detail complications (often localized) that may be seen (listed in order of decreasing frequency).

Arthritis

Several forms of arthritis are listed in ***Table 40.2***.

Peripheral arthritis is the most common presentation, affecting young adults and children; most cases involve monoarticular arthritis in the knee or hip.[45,53] However, some patients have polyarthritis and other rheumatoid-like syndromes. Peripheral arthritis likely involves two pathogenic mechanisms: (1) Reactive arthritis is associated with poly- or pauciarticular involvement, where *Brucella* is not isolated from the joint. This form is associated with high circulating immune complex levels,[54] has a good prognosis, and often remits spontaneously.[14,55–57] (2) Alternatively, infectious monoarticular arthritis can occur, in which the organism can be isolated from synovial fluid when the proper culture medium is used. The prognosis depends on appropriate antibiotic treatment. Low levels of lactate in synovial fluids have been reported to be associated with the isolation of *Brucella* from the joint.[58] Even biopsy of the synovial fluid does not distinguish between reactive and infectious arthritis (both are exudative and inflammatory); only the clinical pattern and the appropriate culture can define which process is involved. More unusual forms include sternoclavicular arthritis[59,60] and extra-articular rheumatism (tendinitis, bursitis, and fibrositis) seen in approximately 10% of adult women.

Sacroiliitis is the second most frequent articular lesion.[61,62] It is usually unilateral, more frequent in young adults, seen in both sexes, and often associated with pain on movement (Lasègue's sign). The bone scan is helpful in diagnosis.

Spondylitis occurs in 5–10% of patients with brucellar arthritis.[45,53,63] A Hungarian study noted the association of human leukocyte antigen (HLA)-B27 with brucellar spondyloarthritis;[64] however, this association is less impressive in our Peruvian familial studies of brucellar arthritis.[65–67] Narrowing of the disk space (diskitis) is the earliest sign; however, the presence of lytic and blastic lesions and the erosion of the anterosuperior

Table 40.2 Arthritis in Brucellosis Related to Age and Clinical Form

Brucellosis Clinical Form	Brucellar Arthritis	Peripheral Arthritis	Sacroiliitis	Spondylitis	Age
Acute	20–35%	Frequent	Frequent	Rare	Children, young adults
Subacute	25–40%	Common	Frequent	Common	Young adults, children
Chronic	40–60%	Rare	Rare	Frequent	Mainly >40 years

Table 40.3 Differential Diagnosis of Tuberculous Versus Brucellar Spondylitis

	Tuberculosis Spondylitis	Brucellar Spondylitis
Age	Young adults (20–40 years)	>40 years old
Sex	More common in males	Slightly more frequent in females
Main localization	Dorsal	Lumbar
Two or more vertebrae	<10%	20–30%
Paravertebral abscess	Very common	10–20%
Radiography	Lytic lesion (rare, blastic)	Lytic and blastic lesion
Sequelae (gibbus or humpback deformity)	Common	Rare

part of the vertebral body ("parrot beak") are the most characteristic presentations.[68–70] This form is rare in children; most patients are older than 40 years of age. Important differential diagnostic considerations are other infectious spondylitis such as tuberculous (*Table 40.3*) and *Staphylococcus aureus* spondylitis. *S. aureus* spondylitis is painful and presents with fever, a symptom less commonly seen with tuberculous spondylitis and occasionally in brucellar spondylitis, given that it is a late complication. The pain of brucellar spondylitis is exacerbated by lying down, which distinguishes it from ostearthropathic pain, which improves with rest.[71] In addition, brucellar spondylitis, with its diskitis and reduction of the intervertebral space, must be distinguished from neoplastic metastases that affect vertebral bodies.

Hepatitis

Although the presence of hepatomegaly is frequent (50–70%) and increased alkaline phosphatase is common, clinical hepatitis is less frequent and is detected in approximately 3–6% of adults. Granulomatous hepatitis appears to be common with *B. melitensis* infections in Latin America and Greece, and may occur in association with the development of a cell-mediated immune response.[49,50,72] Hepatitis may be severe with bone and hematologic changes.[11,73–76]

Hematologic Involvement

Mild anemia and leukopenia with lymphocytosis are common in uncomplicated brucellosis.[77–79] Lymphopenia may correlate with severity.[79] Bone marrow aspiration frequently shows iron deficiency (up to 35%, even in males); iron deficiency has been associated with more aggressive courses in animals,[48] a finding that could explain the greater severity of brucellosis with greater iron deficiency and thrombocytopenia in women than in men.[33,37,38] Severe thrombocytopenia may require steroid therapy, and in some patients with persistent thrombocytopenia after 2 months of treatment and proven bacteriologic cure, splenectomy may be necessary.[38,80] Rare complications of brucellosis include Evans's syndrome,[78,79] with pancytopenia and cytophagocytosis,[81–84] which can be confused with malignant histiocytosis. Pancytopenia is caused by granulomas in bone marrow.[47] Severe thrombocytopenia may cause fatal central nervous system (CNS) hemorrhage.

Genitourinary Complications

Brucellosis is a common cause of orchiepididymitis in endemic areas. Although typically responding to classical treatment, in isolated cases disease progression to abscess and necrosis may necessitate orchiectomy.[85] Differential diagnosis from space-occupying lesions is of paramount importance in the context of brucellar involvement.

Neurologic Involvement

Neurobrucellosis is reported in 1–5% of adults, but is a rare complication in children.[86–89] It usually involves meningitis or encephalitis. The cerebrospinal fluid (CSF) is similar to that in other chronic meningitides with increased lymphocytes and protein; CSF cultures are positive in 10–20% of cases.[90] The clinical pattern is characterized by fever, headache, neck rigidity, and altered consciousness. In contrast to tuberculous meningitis, the cranial nerves are usually not involved in neurobrucellosis. Guillain–Barré syndrome can be seen in young adults with acute brucellosis; brain abscesses are rare.[91–95] The CNS may also be involved in *Brucella* endocarditis or from bleeding in severe thrombocytopenia; both are associated with a poor prognosis.

Other Complications

One of the risk factors for travelers from developed countries to endemic areas is the use of antacids or H_2-receptor antagonists. In these patients, gastrointestinal symptoms are frequent, mainly subacute diarrhea (although among residents of endemic areas, constipation is more common).[39,96]

Brucella endocarditis can occur in a previously normal aortic valve (50–70% of *Brucella* endocarditis), and it remains the leading cause of death in brucellosis.[86,87] When the patient recovers, the valve often becomes calcified. Despite some reported success with medical treatment alone, most experts recommend valve replacement and 2–3 months of antibiotic therapy.[97–99]

In chronic brucellosis (with *B. melitensis*), psychiatric disorders are common. These include "brucellar neurasthenia," chronic fatigue, amnesia, and depression.[100,101] In the preantibiotic era, suicide was one of the causes of death.[102,103] Symptoms often persist after the infection is cured; antidepressant or other symptomatic therapy may be required for 3–6 months.

Eye Involvement

Eye involvement is an unusual complication that may occur in subacute or chronic forms of brucellosis. Anterior or posterior uveitis is the most common ocular manifestation of *Brucella* infection.[104,105] Panuveitis often results in loss of vision.[106–110] Other ocular lesions include papilledema, optic neuritis, and episcleritis.[108,109,111–113] In patients without proper treatment, secondary glaucoma, cataracts, retinal detachment, and phthisis bulbi have been reported.[104–107]

Brucellosis in Children and Pregnancy

Brucellosis produces mild to moderate disease in children, but the chronic form is rare. Relapses in children are usually due to incomplete treatment. Hepatitis and arthritis are often seen in children. The arthritis is usually peripheral, but hip or knee arthritis may be seen.[13,16,114–116]

Brucellosis during pregnancy is associated with poor fetal prognosis with a high rate of abortion, miscarriage, prematurity, and fetal death.[18,86,117] The incidence of spontaneous abortion in Saudi Arabia in the first and second trimesters was 43%, whereas the incidence of intrauterine fetal death in the third trimester was 2%.[118] Prompt treatment with co-trimoxazole, co-trimoxazole/rifampin, or rifampin for 6 weeks plus an aminoglycoside greatly improved the fetal prognosis.[118,119] A few cases of congenital brucellosis have been reported, but early diagnosis and proper treatment should prevent most congenital infection.

Brucellosis in Immunocompromised Patients

Some reports, but not others,[120] have described more frequent relapse in human immunodeficiency virus patients.[121,122] In endemic areas, caution should be applied to patients receiving immunocompromising medications for other reasons (either as chemotherapy for cancer or as biological agents for chronic autoimmune diseases), since brucellosis may emerge, or reemerge after many years in cases of chronic latency, and complicate the clinical picture, particularly in patients with autoimmune arthritis.[110,123]

PATHOGENESIS AND IMMUNITY

B. melitensis is more acid- and serum-resistant and is likely acquired frequently via oral ingestion. The 2–3-week incubation period likely involves invasion, perhaps analogous to typhoid fever, with multiplication in macrophages since the organism is able to survive intracellularly. Its smooth lipopolysaccharide (LPS) appears to be responsible for the resistance of *Brucella* to serum, but its immunogenicity is greatly inferior to that of the LPS of other Gram-negative pathogens.[124] *Brucella* infections are likely acquired via small or subclinical skin abrasions, conjunctival inoculation, or perhaps less commonly via the respiratory route. The tendency of *B. abortus* to localize in placental tissue in cattle may well relate to the enrichment of placental tissue with erythritol, which may stimulate the growth of this organism.[125]

Unlike *B. melitensis* and *B. suis,* which tend to cause abscesses in experimental animals, *B. abortus* tends to cause granuloma formation in mice.[126] Immune responses, initially immunoglobulin M (IgM) then proceeding to IgG, clearly do not provide full protective immunity, since relapsing disease can occur. The role of cell-mediated immunity is suggested by the formation of granulomas and likely determines the characteristic recovery from and partial resistance to subsequent reinfection. Th1 and cytotoxic T-cell immunity appears to be important in host defenses against the pathogen.[127]

DIAGNOSIS

Since the protean clinical and routine laboratory manifestations are not specific to brucellosis, a thorough history of occupation, travel, and consumption of unpasteurized milk or milk products is key to making the diagnosis (***Figs 40.2 and 40.3***). Although it requires biosafety level 3 precautions, the isolation of *Brucella* provides a definitive diagnosis. The best procedure is bone marrow culture,[128,129] with a yield of 92% (versus 70% with two blood cultures; $P<0.001$) and with faster growth (4.32 days versus 6.65 days; $P<0.01$). The best medium, Ruiz-Castañeda,[130] was modified by Gotuzzo et al.[128] through the addition of sodium polyethylene sulfonate and cysteine. With the new DuPont isolator and Bactec techniques, the isolation is improved.[131,132] Bone marrow culture is especially important in difficult clinical cases with epidemiologic suspicion of brucellosis, and when serologic tests are negative (as seen in relapsing uveitis,[107] unexplained fever, or with hematologic abnormalities).[3] However, the diagnosis of brucellosis is often made by serology;[130,133] in a large series in the United States, only 17% of cases had bacteriologic isolation.[134] The rose Bengal test remains an inexpensive, sensitive, and specific test; however, it is not useful in follow-up of patients or in diagnosing relapses.[15,125,135,136] 2-Mercaptoethanol is used to detect IgG antibody.[136,137] However, well-standardized *Brucella* antigen (usually from the smooth, cross-reacting *B. abortus* strain, which may miss rough *B. canis* infections) and dilution to exclude false-negative prozone effects are key to the diagnosis. Antigens often used in "febrile agglutinins" are frequently nonspecific with cross-reactions from cholera, tularemia, or *Yersinia* infections.

Polymerase chain reaction (PCR) methods using ribosomal RNA have been developed.[138] Real-time PCR can further evaluate the bacterial load, which can remain positive, even years after clinical cure with antibiotic therapy.[139,140] These findings may have major implications for the pathophysiology of the disease and the nature of chronic brucellosis.[141]

Brucella as a Bioterrorism Agent

Brucella is listed as a potential agent for a biologic attack by the Centers for Disease Control and Prevention, being the first biological weapon developed in the 1950s.[142] *Brucella* spp. aerosols are easy to prepare and disseminate. Even 10–100 bacteria can produce human disease, and it poses substantial risk for laboratory-acquired infection.[143–145] In the laboratory, attack rates can be as high as 30–100% depending on the inoculum size and the worker's position. *Brucella* needs to be handled with the biosafety guidelines of a level 3 organism.[146–148] A strategy of antibiotic

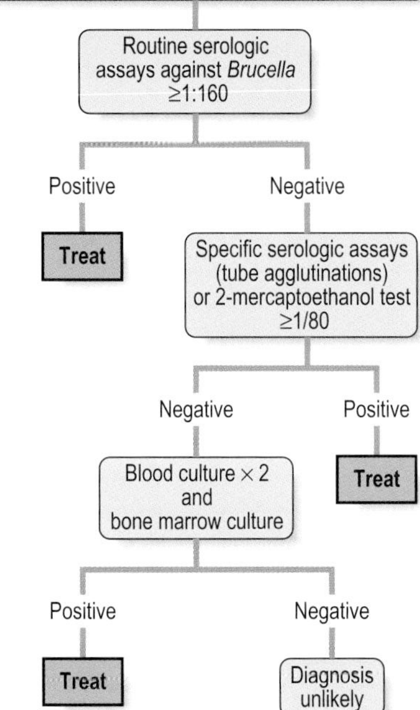
Subacute brucellosis
Suspected because of:
(a) a previous diagnosis of brucellosis with incomplete treatment or
(b) an appropriate epidemiologic background, including:
1. Travel to Latin America, the Mediterranean, or Arab countries
2. Consumption of unpasteurized cheese
3. Laboratory employment (bacteriology division)
4. Veterinarian or farm worker
Routine serologic assays against Brucella ≥1:160
Positive
Negative
Treat
Specific serologic assays (tube agglutinations) or 2-mercaptoethanol test ≥1/80
Negative
Positive
Blood culture × 2 and bone marrow culture
Treat
Positive
Negative
Treat
Diagnosis unlikely

Figure 40.2 Algorithm for the diagnosis and treatment of subacute brucellosis.

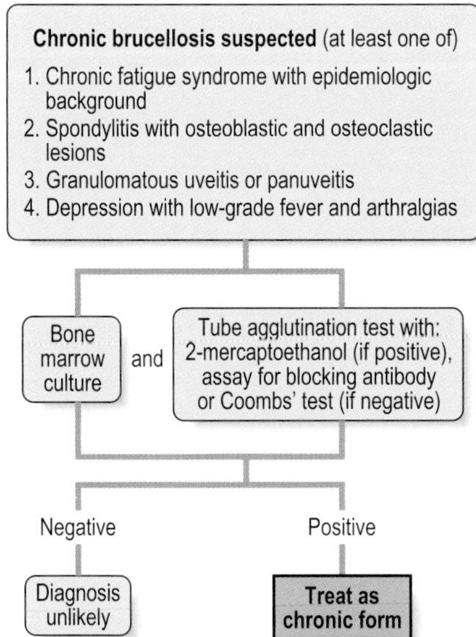
Chronic brucellosis suspected (at least one of)
1. Chronic fatigue syndrome with epidemiologic background
2. Spondylitis with osteoblastic and osteoclastic lesions
3. Granulomatous uveitis or panuveitis
4. Depression with low-grade fever and arthralgias
Bone marrow culture
and
Tube agglutination test with: 2-mercaptoethanol (if positive), assay for blocking antibody or Coombs' test (if negative)
Negative
Positive
Diagnosis unlikely
Treat as chronic form

Figure 40.3 Algorithm for the diagnosis and treatment of chronic brucellosis.

prophylaxis combined with serologic follow-up of exposed workers is provided in a report from Quebec after a large exposure of workers to *B. melitensis*.[149] A model to evaluate the economic impact and potential medical care in a brucellosis postattack intervention was reviewed with emphasis on pulmonary aerosol use.[150]

TREATMENT AND PROGNOSIS

Although several antibiotics have *in vitro* activity against *Brucella,* effective agents must be active intracellularly (particularly in an acidic environment where *Brucella* reside), produce a rapid decrease in fever, reduce or treat complications, and have a low rate of relapse. Because of the high rate of relapse with monotherapy, two antibiotics are typically recommended.[91,151–154] Tetracyclines, and particularly doxycycline, constitute the mainstay of therapy, possessing excellent intracellular activity. However, patients should avoid sun exposure because doxycycline occasionally causes photosensitivity.[155] Doxycycline for 6 weeks combined with either streptomycin (15 mg/kg daily for 2–3 weeks) or rifampin (600–900 mg once daily for 6 weeks) has been recommended. Although the rifampin-containing combination is inferior, clinicians and patients often prefer its convenience. However, rifampin may increase the clearance of doxycycline and reduce the doxycycline half-life in serum (mainly in rapid acetylators),[156] and meta-analyses have shown more relapses with rifampin plus doxycycline than with streptomycin and doxycycline.[41,157–159] The combination of doxycycline with gentamicin should be considered the first alternative regimen, although the optimal duration of gentamicin administration is debated. Evidence against the use of co-trimoxazole in two-antibiotic regimens, and of the potential for fluoroquinolone-containing regimens alone, has been noted. The duration of treatment should be extended for spondylitis: a meta-analysis showed that treating for 3 months improved outcomes.[160] In children, the relapse rate is low after 4 weeks of treatment.[13,16] In pregnant women and children younger than 7 years of age, tetracyclines are contraindicated. Some studies have described the use of rifampicin in combination with aminoglycoside (or co-trimoxazole).[13,16,18,86,161]

PREVENTION AND CONTROL

Because brucellosis is a zoonosis, the best control measure is prevention, with pasteurization of dairy products and use of gloves and masks by veterinarians and farmers. In the laboratory, careful adherence to safety guidelines and precautions is imperative.[161] As a zoonosis in domestic animals, brucellosis is prevented by serologic testing and elimination of infected cattle and by routine pasteurization of milk. In addition, immunization of calves with a *B. abortus* strain 19 vaccine and of goats with a *B. melitensis* strain rev-1 vaccine is helpful. Some have used a live attenuated *Brucella* vaccine in persons at high risk, but this is not widely available. Improved animal husbandry and use of animal control measures and milk pasteurization have substantially reduced brucellosis in many areas.

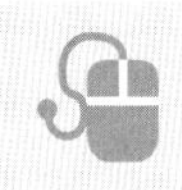

Access the complete reference list online at
http://www.expertconsult.com

CHAPTER 41

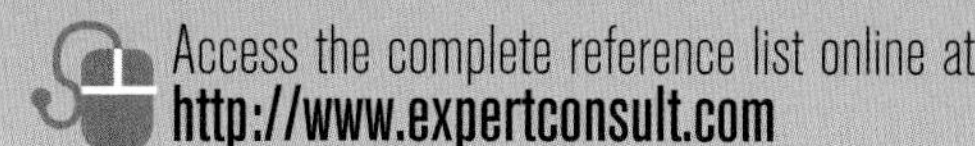
Access the complete reference list online at
http://www.expertconsult.com

Plague

Paul S. Mead

INTRODUCTION

Plague is an uncommon but life-threatening zoonosis caused by the Gram-negative bacillus *Yersinia pestis*. Humans acquire infection through the bite of infected rodent fleas, by handling or ingesting infected animal tissues, or by inhaling contagious airborne particles. Most human infections occur in rural areas of the developing world, where sanitation is poor and humans live in close association with rodent reservoirs. The principal clinical forms of plague are bubonic, septicemic, and pneumonic. Bubonic and septicemic plague account for approximately 80% and 15% of primary cases, respectively. Pneumonic plague can occur as a primary infection but more often develops as a complication of bubonic or septicemic plague. All forms of plague can be cured if diagnosed and treated promptly; however, even short delays can lead to overwhelming endotoxemia, organ failure, and death.

Plague has caused three major pandemics over the past 1500 years. The "Justinian" pandemic began in the mid sixth century AD and killed an estimated 40 million persons while spreading from central Africa to the Mediterranean, Europe, and Asia Minor. The second pandemic began in the fourteenth century in Central Asia and traveled along caravan routes to reach the Near and Middle East. Entering Messina by ship in 1347, the "Black Death" spread swiftly through Europe and the British Isles. Although some historians contend that this rapid advance suggests an alternative etiology,[1] recent evidence from archeological and transmission studies strongly supports the role of *Y. pestis* as the cause of the Black Death.[2-4] Medieval plague persisted in Europe for several centuries and is thought to have killed a quarter or more of some affected populations.

The last global surge of plague, the third or so-called modern pandemic, arose in the latter half of the nineteenth century in Yunnan Province, China. It struck Hong Kong and from there spread by rat-infested steamships to port cities throughout the world, including several in the United States.[5-7] It was in Hong Kong that Alexandre Yersin established the etiology of plague by isolating the plague bacillus from enlarged lymph nodes of plague victims in 1894.[8] Four years later in Bombay, Paul-Louis Simond identified the plague bacillus in the tissues of dead rats; he subsequently proposed that rat fleas transmitted the bacillus from rat to rat, and from rats to humans. Within 30 years of its appearance, the third plague pandemic resulted in 26 million human cases and more than 12 million deaths, most of them in India.[5]

After 1900, the global spread of plague was limited by regulations that controlled rats in ports and imposed inspection and rat-proofing of ships. *Y. pestis* did, however, become newly established among urban and rural rodent populations in many previously unaffected areas of the Americas, Europe, Africa, and Asia, resulting in scattered zoonotic foci that still exist throughout the world.[9,10] In San Francisco, between 1900 and 1908, major outbreaks of rat-borne plague killed more than 200 persons. By 1908, plague was epizootic among ground squirrels in counties surrounding the city,[7] and in subsequent years spread to wild rodent populations throughout California and other states in the western third of the country. The last outbreak of urban plague and of person-to-person pneumonic transmission in the United States occurred in Los Angeles in 1924–1925. By the middle of the twentieth century, cities in the United States and elsewhere had enforced higher sanitary standards and building codes, effective insecticides and rodenticides had become widely available, and several classes of antibiotics had been shown to be efficacious in treating plague. Most human plague since then has been sporadic and rural in distribution. Outbreaks have been relatively slow to develop and readily controlled by a combination of surveillance, early diagnosis and treatment, and flea and rat suppression.[11] The major exceptions to this generalization were the large rat-borne plague epidemics that occurred from 1962 to 1975 in war-torn Vietnam and in the 1990s in Madagascar.[12,13]

Plague can be prevented through steps to reduce risks of exposure, and outbreaks can be readily halted using standard public health measures. Cases should be reported immediately to local health authorities so that appropriate investigative and control measures can be implemented promptly. Routine reporting of plague cases is not required under World Health Organization (WHO) international health regulations; however, individual cases and outbreaks must still be reported if, as in the case of pneumonic plague, they potentially constitute an international concern.[14] Concern has been raised over plague as a potential weapon of terrorism, and *Y. pestis* has been classified as a Category A select agent subject to federal laws governing its management and transport. Medical and public health response plans have been developed to counter the threat of an intentional release.[15]

THE AGENT

Y. pestis is a nonmotile, nonsporulating, Gram-negative coccobacillus in the family Enterobacteriaceae.[6,16] It is microaerophilic, nonfastidious, oxidase- and urease-negative, non-lactose-fermenting, and biochemically unreactive. *Y. pestis* grows slowly but well on a wide variety of common media (e.g., brain-heart infusion broth, sheep blood agar, chocolate agar, and MacConkey agar). Growth occurs across a wide range of temperatures (4–40°C) and pH (5.0–9.6), but is optimal at 28°C and pH 7.4. In the environment, *Y. pestis* is rapidly killed by temperatures above 40°C and by desiccation. Incubation at 37°C for 24 hours on agar yields pinpoint, transparent colonies that are easily overlooked, especially if there is contamination of the culture by other bacteria. At 48 hours, colonies are typically gray, 1–2 mm in diameter, and have an irregular "hammered metal" appearance when viewed under magnification. In broth, *Y. pestis* grows in flocculent clumps, typically attached to the sides of the tube in downwardly projecting stalactite forms that leave a clear broth. With polychromatic stains such as Wayson, Wright, or Giemsa, plague bacilli from clinical specimens demonstrate a characteristic bipolar appearance resembling closed safety pins (***Fig. 41.1***). Although not truly encapsulated, *Y. pestis* produces an envelope that contains the unique fraction 1 (F1) glycoprotein surface antigen. Diagnostic specimens can be safely handled under Biosafety Level 2 (BSL-2) procedures, but manipulation of isolates requires BSL-3 measures to adequately protect laboratory workers.[16]

Genomic studies suggest that the plague bacillus evolved from *Y. pseudotuberculosis* as recently as 1500 to 20 000 years ago.[17–19] This transition from enteric to flea-borne pathogen was made possible by the acquisition of several virulence factors that allow survival in rodents, humans, and fleas.[6,20–22] Most of these virulence factors are encoded on three plasmids, of approximate sizes 9.5, 70, and 110 kb. The 9.5 kb plasmid (pPCP1) encodes a bacteriocin (pesticin) that promotes iron uptake and a temperature-dependent plasminogen activator (Pla). At ambient temperatures, the plasminogen activator protease facilitates the formation of a bolus of blood and aggregated bacteria in the flea midgut, which blocks the flea's proventriculus and leads to regurgitation of infective material when the "blocked" flea attempts to feed. The 70 kb plasmid (pCD1 or pLcr) encodes gene products active in low calcium environments. These products include *Yersinia* outer surface proteins (Yops) and soluble V antigen, thought to be essential to *Y. pestis* survival in macrophages. The Yop virulon includes a type III secretory system that injects Yop effector proteins into the cytosol of eukaryotic cells. These factors downregulate the immune response of macrophages, epithelial and endothelial cells, and induce apoptosis by blocking signaling pathways.[23] The 110 kDa plasmid

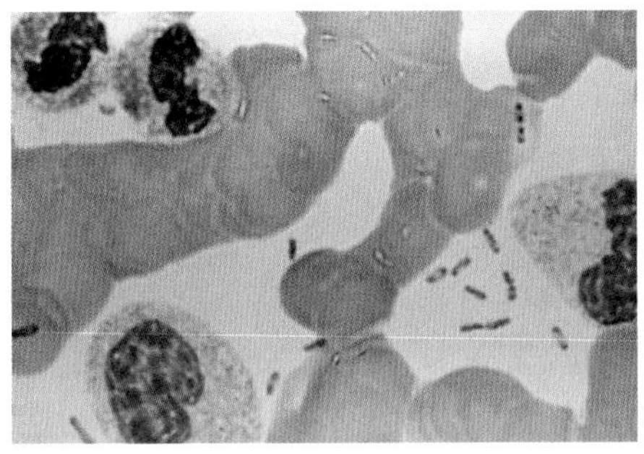

Figure 41.1 Peripheral blood smear from a patient with plague septicemia, showing characteristic bipolar-staining *Y. pestis* (Wright stain, oil immersion).

(pFra or pMT1) contains genes for the F1 envelope glycoprotein antigen and a murine exotoxin. F1 antigen is produced only by organisms growing at 30°C or greater. *Y. pestis* strains expressing F1 antigen are able to resist phagocytosis in the absence of opsonizing antibodies. The murine toxin (Ymt) is highly toxic to mice and rats, but is not known to be toxic in humans. In the flea midgut, Ymt plays a critical role in protecting *Y. pestis* from a cytotoxic digestion product of blood plasma.

Chromosomally encoded virulence factors include a lipopolysaccharide endotoxin and a pigment factor, the hemin storage locus (*hms*) that regulates the absorption of exogenous iron. When *Y. pestis* is grown on media with Congo red, a heme-analog dye, iron absorption is indicated by pigment production. Strains that do not produce pigment have diminished virulence in mammals and are unable to induce blocking in the flea gut. Hemin storage locus products expressed in the low temperature (28°C or less) environment of the flea assist in forming blockage of the flea gut necessary for efficient transmission.[21,22] An additional chromosomally encoded product, the pH 6 antigen (Psa), inhibits phagocytosis of *Y. pestis* in mammals.

Y. pestis isolates have been classified into three biotypes based on their ability to ferment glycerol and reduce nitrate: Antiqua, Medievalis, and Orientalis. Relict populations of the Antiqua biotype are found in Africa, southeastern Russia, and central Asia; the Medievalis biotype is found around the Caspian Sea; and the Orientalis biotype occurs in Asia and the Western hemisphere. Although these phenotypes have been thought to reflect strains associated with the first, second, and third pandemics, respectively,[24] studies using multiple molecular techniques suggest that *Y. pestis* isolates represent up to eight genetically distinct populations that do not correlate entirely with biovar.[17] Limited archeological evidence suggests that all three pandemics were caused by strains of the Orientalis phenotype.[25]

EPIDEMIOLOGY

Plague foci are distributed throughout the world (***Fig. 41.2***) and involve a diverse array of host and vector species[10,26–29] (***Box 41.1***). Transmission among rodents and fleas is often described in terms of enzootic and epizootic cycles (***Fig. 41.3***).[10,27,28] Enzootic cycles help sustain the organism over time and involve relatively resistant rodent species living in remote,

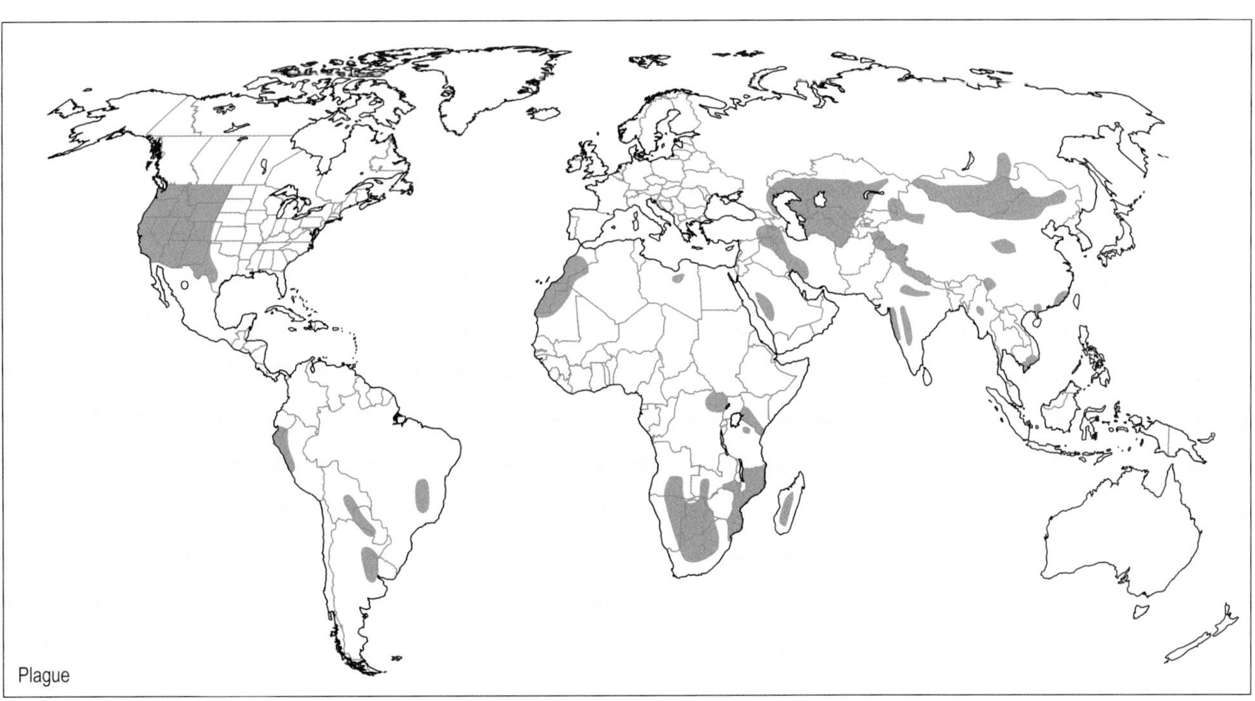

Figure 41.2 Global distribution of known plague foci.

Box 41.1 Plague Foci

North American Plague Foci

Wild rodent plague has been reported west of the 100th meridian in 17 contiguous western states and in some areas of adjacent Canada and Mexico.[9,30] The major plague sites are the southwestern focus, comprising mainly semi-arid grassland plateaus, foothills, and forested uplands of northeastern Arizona, most of New Mexico, southern Utah, and southern Colorado; the Pacific Coast focus, comprising mostly valley grassland, foothills, and the montane habitat of California and southern Oregon; the Great Basin focus, encompassing parts of Utah, Nevada, and southern Idaho; and the Rocky Mountain and northern focus, comprising mostly northern Colorado, Wyoming, and Montana.[9,29] The principal rodent hosts in the southwestern focus are various burrowing ground squirrels (*Spermophilus* spp.), prairie dogs (primarily *Cynomys gunnisoni*), wood rats (*Neotoma* spp.), antelope ground squirrels (*Ammospermophilus* spp.), deer mice (*Peromyscus maniculatus*), and related species. The major rodent hosts in the various niches of the Pacific Coast focus include *Spermophilus* spp., especially the California ground squirrel (*S. beecheyi*), the golden-mantled ground squirrel (*S. lateralis*), chipmunks (various *Tamias* spp.), deer mice and other *Peromyscus* spp., and voles (*Microtus* spp.). Other important hosts in the United States include various small ground squirrels (*S. elegans*, *S. beldingi*, and *S. townsendi*) in the Rocky Mountain and Great Basin regions, and the black-tailed prairie dog (*Cynomys ludovicianus*) in the Great Plains region. Epizootics of plague have recently occurred in urban tree squirrel (*Sciurus niger*) populations in cities along the eastern foothills of the Colorado Rocky Mountains, but pose a small risk to humans because these squirrels are parasitized by nonanthropophagic fleas. Since 1950, a few cities in the United States have rarely been found to have *Y. pestis*-infected rats (e.g., Tacoma, San Francisco, Los Angeles, Dallas). However, no widespread epizootics or human plague cases have resulted, possibly because the rats have been infested with only small numbers of fleas or with flea species that are inefficient vectors of *Y. pestis*. The principal fleas transmitting plague among wild rodent epizootic hosts in the United States include various ground squirrel fleas (*Oropsylla montana* (*Diamanus montanus*), *Hoplopsyllus anomalus, Thrassis* spp., *Opisocrostis* spp., *Oropsylla idahoensis*), prairie dog fleas (*Opisocrostis* spp.), wood rat fleas (*Orchopeas* spp.), and chipmunk fleas (*Eumolpianus eumolpi*).[9,29] *O. montana* is the most important vector of *Y. pestis* to persons in the United States because it is a competent host that readily feeds on a wide range of rodents, and on other mammals, including humans.

South American Plague Foci

In South America, active enzootic plague foci exist in Brazil, Bolivia, Peru, and Ecuador, and have been described previously in Paraguay, Argentina, and Venezuela. *Y. pestis* infection in these foci has been variously found in commensal rats (*Rattus* spp.), cotton rats (*Sigmodon* spp.), rice rats (*Oryzomys* spp.), field mice (*Akodon* spp.), cane mice (*Zygodontomys* spp.), wild cavies, and domesticated guinea pigs (*Cavia* and *Galea* spp.).[5,28] Domestic guinea pigs are reared in homes for food in the Andean region and are considered a potential commensal risk of infection to humans; human plague outbreaks in the Andean region, including a recent extensive bubonic plague epidemic in northern Peru and a mixed bubonic/pneumonic plague outbreak in Ecuador, have been suspected to be associated in the domestic environment with infected guinea pigs as well as *R. rattus*. A previously active plague area in northeastern Brazil has been quiescent over the past 20 years. The various fleas that serve as principal vectors in South American foci are *X. cheopis* on *Rattus* spp. and *Polygenis* and *Pleochaetis* spp. on wild rodents. *Pulex irritans,* the human flea (which also parasitizes domesticated guinea pigs), has been implicated as a potential transmitter of plague to humans in some Andean outbreaks.

African Plague Foci

Widely scattered active plague foci exist in East and southern Africa, including Democratic Republic of the Congo (previously Zaire), Uganda, Kenya, Tanzania, Zambia, Zimbabwe, Mozambique, Botswana, South Africa, Namibia, and Angola, and on the Indian Ocean island of Madagascar.[5,10,28,31] Less active foci exist in some northern African states (e.g., Libya, Algeria). The principal wild rodent hosts in Africa include gerbils (*Tatera* and *Desmodillus* spp.), swamp rats (*Otomys* spp.), various grass mice (*Arvicanthis* spp.), multimammate rats (*Mastomys* spp.), and commensal rats (*Rattus* spp.). One scenario describes plague in grassland gerbil populations spreading to multimammate rats in agricultural fields, and then to commensal rats in villages, resulting in human plague outbreaks. The principal flea vectors of wild rodent hosts are *Xenopsylla* and *Dinopsyllus* spp., while *X. cheopis* and *X. braziliensis* are the principal flea species involved in transmission among commensal rats and to humans.

Asian Plague Foci

The most important Eurasian plague hosts are gerbils (various *Meriones* spp.) in Iran, Kurdistan, Transcaucasia, other areas around the Caspian Sea, and the plains of southeastern Russia and Kazakhstan; marmots (*Marmota* spp.) in Central Asia, including mountainous Khazakstan, northeastern China, Mongolia, Manchuria, and in Transbaikalia; and ground squirrels (*Spermophilus* spp.) in Mongolia, northern-central China, the central Asian plains and steppes, and some areas around the Caspian Sea.[5,10,28] The primary flea vectors on gerbils are *Xenopsylla* and *Nosopsyllus* spp.; on marmots, various *Oropsylla*, *Rhadinopsylla*, and *Citellophilus* spp.; and on ground squirrels, *Citellophilus* and *Neopsylla* spp.

In India, the gerbil, *Tatera indica*, has been described as the principal wild rodent maintenance host.[5,10,28] Although it lives principally in open grassland sites in its natural state, it does invade agricultural fields and village peripheries. Other maintenance hosts include *Mellardia meltada*, various field mice, and palm squirrels (*Funambulus* spp.). The important commensal rat species are *Bandicota bengalensis*, *B. indica*, *R. rattus*, and *R. norvegicus*. Investigations in Maharashtra in western-central India suggest that *Y. pestis* may spread from reservoir gerbil populations in open grasslands to peridomestic *R. rattus* populations through intermediary populations of bandicoot rats (*B. bengalensis*). The primary vectors of plague in India are *X. cheopis* and *X. astia*.

The principal rodent hosts in Myanmar, Vietnam, and Indonesia are *R. rattus* subsp. *diardii* and the Polynesian rat (*R. exulans*).[5,10,28] *R. rattus* subsp. *flavipectus* is an important host in southern China. *R. norvegicus* and the bandicoot *B. indicus* have been described as important hosts in Vietnam. The shrew, *Suncus murinus*, has been described as a possibly important host of plague in Vietnam and Indonesia. *X. cheopis* is the principal vector of plague in southern China, Myanmar, Vietnam, and Indonesia; *X. astia* (a less efficient vector) is also found on rats in Myanmar and Vietnam. *Stivalius cognatus*, a rat flea, is considered to be an important secondary vector of plague in Indonesia.

sparsely populated areas. In enzootic cycles, infection spreads slowly, mortality among rodent populations is unremakable, and the risk of human infection is generally low. In contrast, epizootic cycles are characterized by rapid transmission among highly susceptible rodent hosts, resulting in mass die-offs of rodent populations and accelerated dispersal of infected fleas. Epizootics among rodent populations living in close proximity to humans pose an increased risk of human infection. Of particular concern are epizootics involving the commensal black and Norwegian rats (*Rattus rattus* and *R. norvegicus*) and their highly efficient rat flea vectors (*Xenopsylla cheopis* and *X. braziliensis*).[5,10,11] These species are adapted to live intimately with humans and historically are thought to have played an important role in pandemic spread of plague.

Humans are incidental hosts who become infected through the bite of infected rodent fleas, by handling or ingesting infected animal tissues, or

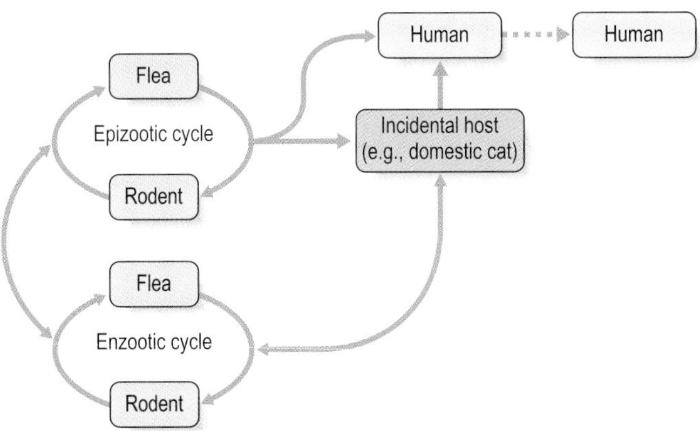

Figure 41.3 Plague transmission cycles demonstrating hosts and principal routes. *Y. pestis* usually cycles between rodents and fleas in enzootic (maintenance) or epizootic (amplifying) cycles. Infection may be transmitted to humans or other incidental mammalian hosts through flea bites or through direct contact with or consumption of infected animal tissues. Pet dogs and cats may further promote transmission by bringing infective rodent fleas into the home environment. Plague pneumonia can be transmitted from one person to another or from cats to humans through infective respiratory droplets.

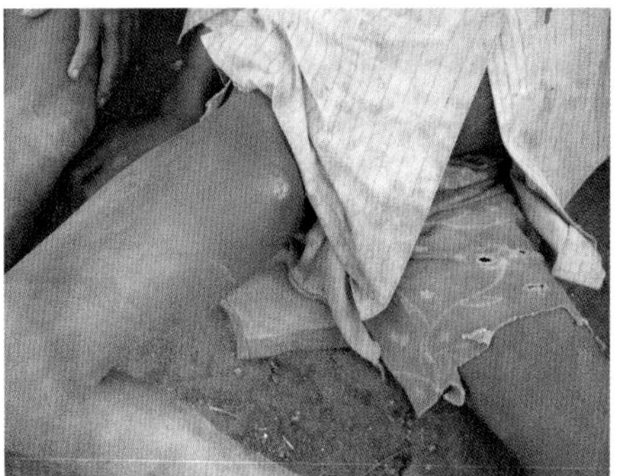

Figure 41.4 Right inguinal bubo with surrounding edema.

by inhaling contagious airborne particles. The risk of human infection varies with environmental circumstances and human behaviors. Low socioeconomic status is an important risk factor because infestation by rats and their fleas is associated with poor housing and unsanitary conditions. In addition, humans may be exposed through contact with other, incidentally infected domestic and wild mammals. Cats are highly susceptible to plague and can transmit infection to humans through respiratory secretions, resulting in primary pneumonic plague.[32,33] Dogs are relatively resistant to illness but may still play a role in human infection by transporting rodent fleas into the domestic environment.[34] For example, a recent study in New Mexico found that plague patients were significantly more likely than controls to have allowed dogs to sleep on their bed at night.[35] Hunters may become infected through direct inoculation while skinning or otherwise handling carcasses of infected rodents, rabbits and hares, domestic and wild felids, and coyotes.[10,32,36] This is a particular risk among marmot hunters in Mongolia and northeastern China.[37] Direct inoculation is associated with an increased risk of septicemia and a high fatality rate. Ungulates, including antelope, deer, camels, dromedaries, and goats, are also susceptible to plague; handling and ingesting undercooked meat of these animals has been responsible for limited human plague outbreaks in northern Africa, the Middle East, and Central Asia.[38] Once infected, humans with pneumonic plague pose a risk for person-to-person transmission, a risk that is enhanced in the cramped living quarters of nomadic hunters and impoverished populations.

Routine reporting of plague cases to the WHO was discontinued after 2003. During the 15-year period from 1989 to 2003, a total of 38 359 human cases (approximately 2500 cases a year) and 2845 deaths (7%) were reported to the WHO by 25 countries.[39] Nearly 80% of cases were reported from Africa, 15% from Asia, and the remainder from the Americas. Countries reporting more than 1000 cases include Madagascar, Tanzania, Democratic Republic of the Congo, Vietnam, Mozambique, Namibia, and Peru. A recent report of human plague in Algeria, 50 years after the last occurrence, underscores the potential for reemergence.[39] In Madagascar, outbreaks have occurred in coastal urban as well as rural highland areas.[13,40] In the tropics, plague incidence usually peaks in the cooler, moist months of the year. Following the extraordinary epidemics of pneumonic plague involving tens of thousands of cases in Manchuria in the period 1910–1926, pneumonic plague outbreaks around the world have occurred only sporadically, usually involving three or fewer generations of cases, and typically affecting family members, close friends, and care providers of pneumonic plague patients. The 1994 outbreak of reported pneumonic plague in Surat, India, probably involved fewer than 100 cases.[41] Small clusters of cases of pneumonic plague have more recently been reported from China, Ecuador, Madagascar, and northern India.

In the United States, 447 plague cases (~9 cases per year) and 65 deaths (15%) were reported during 1960–2008[42] (Centers for Disease Control and Prevention (CDC), unpublished data). Although plague in animals occurs in 17 of the contiguous western states, more than 80% of human cases are reported from the southwestern states of New Mexico, Arizona, and Colorado, and approximately 10% from California.[32,43] In the United States, flea-borne plague is highly seasonal, occurring most often between May and October; winter plague cases are uncommon and usually associated with hunting. More than half of plague exposures in the United States are thought to occur in the general area of patients' homes.[36] This is particularly true in the southwest, where homes in rural and semi-rural areas are often situated near habitats of highly plague-susceptible animals, such as prairie dogs, rock squirrels, and woodrats.[10] In the Sierra Nevada mountains of California and Nevada, epizootic plague in chipmunks and ground squirrels is a risk to visitors to public parks. Hikers, campers, and hunters throughout the western United States have a small but definite risk of exposure, especially in the warmer months of the year.

THE DISEASE

Plague takes several clinical forms depending in part on the route of exposure.[5,15,44,45] The most common primary form is bubonic plague, which accounts for 80–85% of cases in the United States. An additional 15% of patients present with septicemic plague, and 1–3% with pneumonic or other forms of plague.[15] The usual incubation period for all forms is 2–7 days, but can be as short as 1 day for patients with primary pneumonic plague.

Bubonic Plague

Bubonic plague typically begins with fever (38–40°C), headache, chills, myalgias, arthralgias, and a feeling of weakness.[44] Simultaneously or shortly thereafter, the patient notices tenderness and pain in regional lymph nodes proximal to the site of inoculation of the plague bacillus. The femoral and inguinal groups of nodes are most commonly involved, followed by the axillary and cervical nodes. Upper body sites may be relatively more involved in children than adults. The enlarging bubo(es) becomes progressively swollen, painful, and tender, and the patient typically guards against palpation and limits movement. The surrounding tissue often becomes edematous, and the overlying skin may be erythematous, warm, and tense, and may desquamate (*Fig. 41.4*). Inspection of the skin surrounding or distal to the bubo sometimes reveals the site of a flea bite marked by a small papule, pustule, scab, or ulcer. Larger pustular lesions (furuncles or carbuncles), ulcers, and eschars may rarely occur and can be confused with those caused by tularemia or anthrax. Treated in the uncomplicated state with an appropriate antibiotic, bubonic plague usually responds quickly, with disappearance of fever and resolution of other systemic manifestations over 2–5 days. Buboes often remain enlarged and tender for a week or more after treatment has begun and can occasionally become fluctuant. Without effective antimicrobial treatment, bubonic plague may progress to an increasingly toxic state of fever, tachycardia, lethargy, agitation and, occasionally, convulsions and delirium. Plague patients typically have white blood cell counts of 12 000–25 000/μL, with a predominance of immature polymorphonuclear leukocytes. Leukemoid reactions showing white blood cell counts as high as 50 000/μL or more can occur.[45] Mild forms of bubonic plague, called pestis minor, have been described in South America and elsewhere; in these cases, the patients are ambulatory, only mildly febrile, and have subacute buboes. Differential diagnostic possibilities for bubonic plague include streptococcal or staphylococcal adenitis, tularemia, cat-scratch disease, mycobacterial infection, acute filarial lymphadenitis, chancroid and other sexually transmitted diseases that cause regional lymphadenitis, and strangulated inguinal hernia. The bubo of plague is usually distinguishable from lymphadenitis of most other causes by its rapid onset, extreme tenderness, accompanying signs of toxemia, and usual absence of cellulitis or obvious ascending lymphangitis.

Septicemic Plague

Septicemic plague is a sudden, nonspecific febrile illness that occurs in the absence of apparent regional lymphadenitis.[46–48] It is characterized by rapidly progressive, overwhelming endotoxemia and dissemination of infection, and the diagnosis of plague is often not suspected until preliminary blood culture results are reported by the laboratory. Patients may have gastrointestinal symptoms such as nausea, vomiting, diarrhea, and abdominal pain, making a correct clinical diagnosis even more challenging.[49] If not treated early with appropriate antibiotics and aggressive supportive care, septicemic plague is usually fulminating and fatal. In the United States from 1960 to 2008, 20 of 72 primary septicemic plague cases were fatal, yielding a case-fatality rate of 28%. Differential diagnostic possibilities include any other overwhelming systemic infection, including Gram-negative sepsis with other agents, meningococcemia, and bacterial endocarditis. Some patients develop adult respiratory distress syndrome (ARDS), which can lead to confusion with other conditions such as hantavirus pulmonary syndrome and severe acute respiratory syndrome (SARS).

Pneumonic Plague

Pneumonic plague occurs in two forms, primary and secondary, both of which are potentially contagious and frequently fatal.[5,50] Primary plague results from direct inhalation of plague bacteria into the lungs. Onset is sudden with chills, high fever, headache, body pains, weakness, dizziness, and chest discomfort. Cough, sputum production, increasing chest pain, tachypnea, and dyspnea typically predominate on the second day of illness and may be accompanied by hemoptysis, increasing respiratory distress, cardiopulmonary insufficiency, cyanosis, and circulatory collapse. Principally an alveolar process, primary pneumonic plague is characterized by sputum that is initially watery or mucoid, and quickly becomes blood-tinged or frankly bloody. Chest signs in primary plague pneumonia may indicate localized pulmonary involvement in the early stage, with rapidly developing segmental consolidation before bronchopneumonia spreads to other segments and lobes of the same and opposite lung. Liquefaction necrosis and cavitation may develop at sites of consolidation and may leave significant residual scarring.

Secondary pneumonic plague arises through hematogenous spread from a bubo or other untreated source. It manifests first as an interstitial pneumonitis in which sputum production is scant, and the sputum is more likely to be inspissated and tenacious in character than the sputum found in primary pneumonic plague. In the United States from 1960 to 2008, 55 cases of secondary plague pneumonia and 11 cases of primary plague pneumonia were reported to the CDC, with no known secondary transmission to contacts and an overall case-fatality rate of 42% (CDC, unpublished data, 2009). Observers of pneumonic plague in the early twentieth century remarked on minimal auscultatory findings, the appearance of toxemia, and the frequency of sudden death, as compared to patients with other bacterial pneumonias.[50] Differential diagnostic possibilities include other bacterial pneumonias such as mycoplasma pneumonia, legionnaires' disease, staphylococcal or streptococcal pneumonia, tularemia pneumonia, and Q fever. Severe viral pneumonia, including hantavirus pulmonary syndrome and SARS, could be confused with plague.

Because respiratory spread of *Y. pestis* occurs by infective droplets, only persons with close respiratory exposure have a high risk of infection. Primary plague pneumonia is considered more contagious than secondary pneumonia because it is more likely to produce copious watery sputum, and the patient may be mobile and expose a wider circle of individuals in the early stage of contagiousness.

Meningeal Plague

Meningitis is an unusual manifestation of plague, occurring in 18 (4%) of 447 cases reported to CDC during 1960–2008 (CDC, unpublished data, 2009). Most cases were late complications of bubonic plague, and 14 patients (78%) survived. Although meningitis may be a part of the initial presentation of plague, its onset is often delayed and may be the result of insufficient antibiotic treatment of the primary illness.[51] Chronic, relapsing meningeal plague over periods of weeks and even months was described in the preantibiotic era. Plague meningitis presents as typical bacterial meningitis, with fever, headache, altered mental status, meningismus, and a polymorphonuclear leukocytic pleocytosis.

Pharyngeal Plague

Plague pharyngitis is an unusual condition and presents with fever, sore throat, and cervical lymphadenitis. In its early stages, it may be clinically indistinguishable from more common causes of pharyngitis. Cervical or submandibular buboes usually develop secondary to the pharyngeal involvement. Cases arise following respiratory droplet exposure, or from the ingestion of undercooked meat.[5,38] Pharyngeal plague may give rise to secondary plague pneumonia. Care providers working in plague-endemic areas should be alert to the possibility of plague in the differential diagnosis of acute bacterial pharyngitis. Pharyngeal colonization with *Y. pestis* sometimes occurs without symptoms among contacts of persons with pneumonic plague. Epidemiological observations do not suggest that persons with pharyngeal carriage present a contagious threat to others.

PATHOGENESIS AND IMMUNITY

Y. pestis inoculated through the skin or mucous membranes is carried via lymphatics to regional lymph nodes. This early stage of infection may be facilitated by macrophages which engulf but do not kill the pathogen, providing it with both transportation to the lymph node and a protected, intracellular niche in which to acclimatize to the mammalian host.[23] Growing intracellularly at 37°C, the bacteria begin expressing F1 envelope antigen, a key factor in their ability to resist subsequent phagocytosis by polymorphonuclear lymphocytes.[6,23] Within the lymph node, *Y. pestis* initiates an intense inflammatory reaction, creating a bubo. Initially the affected lymph nodes are edematous, congested, and have minimal inflammatory infiltrates and vascular injury. However, microscopic examination of fully developed buboes reveals infiltration by polymorphonuclear leukocytes, hemorrhagic necrosis with destruction of normal architecture, and dense concentrations of extracellular bacilli.[52] Affected nodes may be surrounded by a serosanguineous effusion, and when several adjacent lymph nodes are involved, a boggy, edematous mass can result. Spontaneous bubo rupture and suppurative drainage may occur.

Bacteremia is common in plague and can result in seeding of other organs. In addition, untreated bacteremia can reach high levels, leading to excessive release of proinflammatory mediators, such as tumor necrosis factor-α and other cytokines. The resulting systemic inflammatory response may lead to hypotension, disseminated intravascular coagulation, acute renal failure, ARDS, and irreversible shock.[44] Affected tissues contain inflamed microvasculature occluded by fibrin thrombi, resulting in necrosis and hemorrhage. Blockage of vessels in acral sites can lead to gangrene of fingertips, toes, ears, and nose.[52] These cutaneous signs may be the origin of the term "Black Death." Patients who recover from plague typically have elevated antibodies to various antigens, including the diagnostically useful F1 antigen.

Pneumonic plague can result from inhalation of infective respiratory droplets from a person or animal with respiratory plague or secondary to hematogenous spread in a patient with bubonic or septicemic plague. It can result also from inhalation of *Y. pestis* in a laboratory accident.[53] Primary plague pneumonia generally begins as a lobular process and then extends by confluence, becoming lobar and then multilobar. Typically, plague organisms are most numerous in the alveoli. Secondary plague pneumonia begins more diffusely as an interstitial process, with organisms initially most numerous in the interstitial spaces. In untreated cases of both primary and secondary plague pneumonia, the usual findings are diffuse pulmonary hemorrhage, necrosis, and scant neutrophilic leukocyte infiltration.[50]

DIAGNOSIS

A high index of clinical suspicion, a careful clinical and epidemiologic history, and a thorough physical examination are required to make a timely diagnosis of plague. A delayed or missed diagnosis of plague is associated with a high case-fatality rate, and infected travelers who seek medical care after they have left endemic areas (peripatetic plague cases) are especially at risk.[43,54] When plague is suspected, close communication is essential between clinicians and the diagnostic laboratory, and between the diagnostic laboratory and a qualified reference laboratory. Laboratory tests for plague are highly reliable when conducted by persons experienced in working with *Y. pestis*, but such expertise is usually limited to specialized reference laboratories. Because of recent concerns with possible bioterrorism, a network of participating laboratories across the United States has been developed with the ability to make rapid and confirmatory diagnoses. All state public health laboratories now have this capability and can, if necessary, forward materials to the CDC for rapid advanced procedures.[55]

When plague is suspected, specimens should be obtained promptly for microbiologic studies, chest radiographs taken, and effective antimicrobial therapy initiated empirically. Appropriate diagnostic specimens for smears and culture include blood in all patients, lymph node aspirates in those with suspected buboes, sputum samples or tracheobronchial aspirates in those with suspected pneumonic plague, and cerebrospinal fluid in those with meningeal signs. A portion of each specimen should be inoculated onto suitable media (e.g., brain-heart infusion broth, sheep blood agar, chocolate agar, or MacConkey agar). Smears of each specimen should be stained with Wayson or Giemsa stain, and with Gram stain, and examined using light microscopy. If possible, the specimens should also be examined using direct fluorescent antibody (FA) testing.[16] An acute phase serum specimen should be collected for *Y. pestis* antibody testing, followed by a convalescent phase specimen collected 3–4 weeks later. For diagnosis in fatal cases, autopsy tissues should be collected for culture, FA testing, and histological processing, including buboes, samples of solid organs (especially liver, spleen, and lung), and bone marrow. For culture, specimens should be sent to the laboratory either fresh or frozen on dry ice and not in preservatives or fixatives. Cary–Blair or a similar holding medium can be used to transport *Y. pestis*-infected tissues.

Laboratory confirmation of plague is best achieved through the isolation of *Y. pestis* from body fluids or tissues. When the patient's condition allows, several blood cultures taken over a 45-minute period before treatment may increase the chances of successful isolation. *Y. pestis* strains are readily distinguished from other Gram-negative bacteria by polychromatic and immunofluorescence staining properties, characteristics of growth on microbiologic media, biochemical profiles, and confirmatory lysis by the *Y. pestis*-specific bacteriophage.[16] Automated systems may misidentify *Y. pestis* as other species. Laboratory mice and hamsters are susceptible to *Y. pestis* and are used in specialized laboratories to make isolations from contaminated materials and for virulence testing.

In the absence of a positive culture, plague can be confirmed by demonstrating a fourfold or greater change in serum antibodies to *Y. pestis* F1 antigen by passive hemagglutination (PHA) testing or by detecting a serum antibody titer of 128 or greater in a single serum sample from a patient with a compatible illness who has not received plague vaccine. The specificity of a positive PHA test is confirmed by F1 antigen hemagglutination inhibition (HI) testing. A small percentage of plague patients will develop diagnostic antibody levels within 5 days after illness onset, most seroconvert within 1–2 weeks, a few seroconvert more than 3 weeks after onset, and <5% fail to seroconvert.[56] Early specific antibiotic treatment may delay seroconversion by several weeks. Following conversion, serologic titers diminish gradually over months to years. Enzyme-linked immunosorbent assays (ELISAs) for detecting IgM and IgG antibodies to *Y. pestis* are useful in identifying antibodies in early infection and in differentiating them from antibodies developed in response to previous vaccination. Recently, antigen capture ELISA procedures, polymerase chain reaction assays, and handheld immunodiagnostic antigen detection tests for rapid, early diagnosis have been developed and are being evaluated. The handheld devices allow diagnostic testing of clinical materials at the bedside, even under primitive conditions.[57]

TREATMENT AND PROGNOSIS

Untreated, plague is fatal in over 50% of bubonic cases and in nearly all cases of septicemic or pneumonic plague. The overall plague case-fatality rate in the United States in the past 50 years has been approximately 15%.[15] Fatalities are almost always due to delays in seeking treatment, misdiagnosis, and delayed or incorrect treatment. Rapid diagnosis and appropriate antimicrobial therapy are essential. The case-fatality rate is very high for pneumonic plague patients who begin treatment more than 18–24 hours after the onset of pulmonary symptoms.

Effective antibiotic therapy should be given immediately after obtaining diagnostic specimens. Streptomycin has been considered the drug of choice since its introduction in the 1940s, and prompt administration can reduce mortality in bubonic plague to 5% or less. Streptomycin should be administered intramuscularly in two divided doses daily, in a dosage for adults of 30 mg/kg of body weight per day for 7 days, or for at least 3 days after remission of fever and other symptoms. Most patients improve rapidly and become afebrile after about 3 days of therapy.[44] Streptomycin is ototoxic and nephrotoxic, although the risk of severe vestibular damage and hearing loss is considered to be small in the short courses required for treating plague. Streptomycin should be used cautiously in pregnant women, in older patients, and in patients with hearing difficulty.

Streptomycin is not always readily available, and gentamicin has been proposed as an acceptable alternative based on *in vitro* susceptibility studies, animal models, and case series.[15,48,58–61] Retrospective analysis of 50 patients in New Mexico suggests that gentamicin, or a combination of gentamicin and doxycycline, is at least as efficacious as streptomycin.[62] A randomized trial of 65 patients in Tanzania found that 94% of those treated with gentamicin recovered.[63] Studies of patients with other diseases indicate that gentamicin is less ototoxic but more nephrotoxic than streptomycin. Renal toxicity associated with gentamicin is usually mild and reversible, and the drug is generally considered safer than streptomycin for use in pregnant women and children. For these and other considerations, gentamicin has been recommended as an alternative in first-line treatment of plague in the event of a bioterrorist attack and is included in the US strategic national stockpile.[15]

For patients with contraindications to the use of aminoglycosides, tetracycline and chloramphenicol are effective alternatives. Doxycycline has become the tetracycline of choice because of its ease of administration, rapid and efficient absorption after ingestion, and its superior ability to achieve and maintain peak serum concentrations following oral administration. Doxycycline treatment should be initiated with a loading dose, either intravenously or orally depending on the severity of illness. In adults, a loading dose of 200 mg every 12 hours on the first day rapidly achieves a peak serum concentration of approximately 8 μg/mL, and is followed by a daily dosage of 100 mg every 12 hours.[61,64] Tetracycline is administered to adults in an initial loading dose of 2 g, followed by a usual dose of 2 g/day in four divided doses. Doxycycline or tetracycline can also be used to complete a course of treatment begun with an aminoglycoside. When used as principal treatment, a tetracycline should be given for 7–10 days, or for at least 3 days after fever and other symptoms have subsided.[15]

For conditions in which high tissue penetration is important, such as plague meningitis, pleuritis, or myocarditis, chloramphenicol is considered the drug of choice.[15,58] It may be used separately or in combination with an aminoglycoside. A loading dose of 25–30 mg/kg of body weight is given, followed by 50–60 mg/kg of body weight per day in four divided doses. As indicated by clinical response, chloramphenicol dosage may be reduced to a daily dose of 25–30 mg/kg to lessen the magnitude of reversible bone marrow suppression. The irreversible marrow aplasia associated with chloramphenicol is so rare (estimated to occur in 1 in 40 000 patients) that its consideration should not deter its use in patients who are seriously ill with plague infection.

Ciprofloxacin, a fluoroquinolone, has shown promise *in vitro* and in laboratory animal studies,[65–67] but case series demonstrating its utility in human plague have not been reported. Penicillins, cephalosporins, and macrolides have poor efficacy and should not be used. Trimethoprim-sulfamethoxazole has been used successfully to treat bubonic plague, but is not considered a first-line choice and is not recommended for treating severe forms of the disease. In general, antimicrobial treatment should be continued for 7–10 days or for at least 3 days after the patient has become afebrile. Patients begun on intravenous antibiotics may be switched to oral regimens as indicated by clinical response. Improvement is usually evident 2–3 days from the start of treatment, even though lessening fever may continue for several more days.

Consequences of delayed treatment of plague include disseminated intravascular coagulation, ARDS, and other complications of bacterial sepsis and endotoxemia. Patients with these disorders require intensive monitoring and close physiologic support. Buboes may require surgical drainage if they threaten to rupture. Abscessed lymph nodes rarely can be a cause of recurrent fever in patients who have otherwise had satisfactory recovery; the cause may be occult when intrathoracic or intra-abdominal nodes are involved. Viable *Y. pestis* organisms have occasionally been isolated from buboes 1–2 weeks into convalescence.

Natural resistance to recommended antimicrobials is exceedingly rare. Most resistant strains have shown only partial resistance to a single agent and have not been associated with treatment failures. In 1995, two clinical isolates with plasmid-mediated drug resistance were recovered in Madagascar, one with high-level resistance to streptomycin, the second resistant to multiple drugs including streptomycin, chloramphenicol, ampicillin, tetracycline, and sulfonamides.[58] Both patients recovered despite being treated per protocol with streptomycin and trimethoprim-sulfamethoxazole. The plasmids conferring resistance in these two strains are believed to have arisen independently, possibly through horizontal gene transfer in the flea midgut.[58] In the absence of antimicrobial pressure on wild rodent populations, it is questionable whether such resistance would be expected to propagate in nature. To date these remain the only such natural isolates identified among thousands tested worldwide. Antimicrobial resistance is not known to have emerged during treatment of plague in humans, and relapses following recommended courses of treatment are virtually unknown.

PREVENTION AND CONTROL

Surveillance, environmental management, and personal protective measures are the cornerstones of prevention and control.[11,68,69] Surveillance includes environmental monitoring to determine sites of plague activity, inspection of rodent habitats for signs of epizootics, collecting and testing of fleas from abandoned burrows, trapping and testing of live rodents and their fleas for *Y. pestis* infection, and testing of animals found sick or dead from suspected plague. In some circumstances, carnivore seropositivity is used as an indicator of rodent plague activity in an area. Dogs and wild canines readily seroconvert following exposure but retain elevated antibody levels for less than a year, making them useful sentinels of recent plague activity in an area.

Personal protective measures include avoidance of areas with known epizootic plague (these may be posted by government authorities); avoidance of sick or dead animals; use of repellents, insecticides, and protective clothing when there is a potential for exposure to rodent fleas; and use of gloves when handling animal carcasses. The practice of letting domestic dogs and cats sleep on the same bed as humans should be discouraged in endemic areas.

Postexposure prophylaxis for 7 days with doxycycline or other tetracycline, chloramphenicol, or ciprofloxacin is recommended for persons who have had a known close exposure to a pneumonic plague patient in the prior 7 days. Oral doxycycline or ciprofloxacin has been recommended for postexposure prophylaxis in the event of a terrorist attack with *Y. pestis*.[15] Pre-exposure prophylaxis may occasionally be recommended for persons who are unable to avoid visiting or residing in an area where a plague outbreak is in progress or who are screening or caring for plague patients in unusual circumstances, such as an outbreak. To reduce the risk of airborne droplet spread, plague patients should have a chest radiograph to rule out pulmonary involvement. Patients with suspected pneumonic plague should be managed in isolation under respiratory droplet precautions until the patient has responded clinically and sputum cultures are negative (sputum typically is sterile within 24–48 hours of beginning treatment). Persons caring for sick animals (especially cats) in plague-endemic areas should take precautions to avoid contamination with infectious exudates or expelled respiratory secretions.[33]

Sources of rodent food (garbage, feed for livestock and pets) and shelter (brushpiles, junk heaps, woodpiles) should be eliminated in domestic, peridomestic, and working environments, and buildings and food stores should be rodent-proofed. Controlling fleas with insecticides is a principal public health measure in situations where epizootic plague activity places humans at high risk. This includes insecticidal dusting and spraying of rodent burrows, rodent runs, and other sites where rodents and their fleas are found. In known plague foci, pet owners should consider using flea control products to protect their pets and potentially reduce their risk of exposure. The decision to control plague by killing rodents should be left to public health authorities and should only be carried out in conjunction with effective flea control. Killing rodents has no lasting benefit without environmental sanitation.

In the event of a plague epidemic, measures should rapidly be taken to control spread, as described in international regulations and guidelines for plague control.[11,68] These measures include delineation of infected areas, rapid detection and treatment of cases and exposed contacts, isolation and monitoring of suspected human plague cases and case contacts, and control of fleas and rodents in plague-infected areas, in port facilities, and on ships and other conveyances as indicated.

A formalin-killed vaccine was available for many years for use by persons who worked with *Y. pestis* in the laboratory or were otherwise at high risk of exposure. However, it is no longer available for use in the United States. Concern for bioterrorism has stimulated renewed efforts to develop safe, rapidly acting, and efficacious vaccines using advanced molecular approaches.[68] At present, the most promising candidates are recombinant subunit vaccines that express F1 and V antigens of *Y. pestis* and appear to protect animals against infective aerosol exposures.[70–72] Other approaches under investigation include passive immunization with aerosolized monoclonal antibodies[73] and vaccines based on attenuated *Y. pseudotuberculosis*.[74,75]

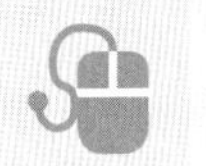

Access the complete reference list online at **http://www.expertconsult.com**

ACKNOWLEDGMENT

The contributions of David Dennis, MD to this chapter in previous editions are gratefully acknowledged.

CHAPTER 42

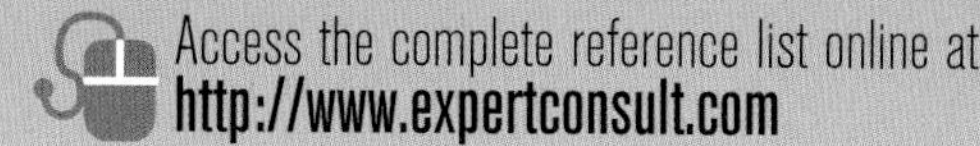
Access the complete reference list online at
http://www.expertconsult.com

Tetanus

Barnett R. Nathan • Thomas P. Bleck

INTRODUCTION

Tetanus remains a significant health concern throughout the world. Though falling in developed countries, tetanus, particularly neonatal tetanus (with up to 90% mortality), continues to be a significant cause of morbidity and mortality in tropical and developing regions.[1–5] Muscle relaxants and ventilatory support have made the treatment of acute tetanus possible, though critical intensive care may not be available in developing areas. An effective vaccine *is* clearly effective in reducing mortality, particularly from neonatal tetanus.[6]

The characteristic muscle rigidity and trismus of tetanus was described in ancient Egypt and Greece.[7,8] In the eighteenth century, tetanus was thought to be a result of nerve injury or even epilepsy.[9] In the nineteenth century, Sir William Gowers accurately noted that: "Tetanus is a disease of the nervous system characterized by persistent tonic spasm, with violent brief exacerbations. The spasm almost always commences in the muscles of the neck and jaw, causing closure of the jaws (trismus, lockjaw), and involves muscles of the trunk more than those of the limbs. It is always acute in onset, and a very large proportion of those who are attacked die."[10] Nicolaier reported a strychnine-like toxin from anaerobic soil bacteria in 1884,[11] and 6 years later Behring and Kitasato demonstrated that immunization with an inactivated extract of this bacterium prevented tetanus.[12]

In the eighteenth century neonatal tetanus was known as the "7-day disease" or "9-day fits"[13,14] because it usually presents about 1–2 weeks postpartum. In 1887, Beumer determined that the umbilicus was the portal of entry for neonatal tetanus.[15]

THE AGENT

Clostridium tetani is a slender, obligate anaerobic bacillus measuring 0.5–1.7 μm by 2.1–18.1 μm.[16] Although classified as a Gram-positive organism, it may stain variably, especially in tissue or older cultures.[17] Most strains are slightly motile, and have abundant peritrichous flagella during growth.[18] The mature organism loses its flagella and forms a spherical terminal spore,[19] thus looking like a squash racket (***Fig. 42.1***).[20] The spores resist extremes of temperature and moisture, are stable at atmospheric oxygen tension, can survive indefinitely and are viable after exposure to ethanol, phenol, or formalin. Spores are killed by 100°C for 4 hours, autoclaving at 121°C and 103 kPa (15 psi) for 15 minutes, or with iodine, glutaraldehyde, or hydrogen peroxide.

Spores can be isolated from animal feces and are ubiquitous in the environment, including soil and even carpets. Hence any breach in skin defenses such as wounds, burns, animal bites, human bites,[21] and even insect bites may result in inoculation of the spores.[22] About 80% of tetanus cases in the United States result from acute injuries (punctures and lacerations); 20% result from more chronic wounds.[23] Wounds occur indoors or outdoors (29% versus 21%),[24] and 7–21% of tetanus cases are cryptogenic.[24]

C. tetani grows best at 37°C on a variety of media (including blood agar) as long as oxygen is excluded. Standard anaerobic transport and isolation are important in culturing the organism. However, diagnostic and therapeutic decisions should not be made based on the culture, since cultures are frequently negative in patients with clinical tetanus, and routine bacteriologic studies do not indicate whether a strain of *C. tetani* carries the toxin plasmid.

EPIDEMIOLOGY

About 1 million cases of tetanus occur annually worldwide (or about 18 per 100 000 population per year),[1] but reported cases of tetanus are significantly lower than this estimate (***Fig. 42.2***). In tropical and developing countries tetanus continues to be a significant problem, even though neonatal cases have decreased. Neonatal tetanus accounts for approximately half of the total number of cases worldwide and has up to a 90% mortality rate.[4,5] Eighty percent of worldwide neonatal tetanus cases occur in Bangladesh, China, Ethiopia, India, Indonesia, Kenya, Nepal, Nigeria, Pakistan, Somalia, Sudan, Uganda, Vietnam, and Zaire.[25] Approximately 120 000 deaths occur annually in Africa due to neonatal tetanus, which accounts for 10–30% of infant deaths in many countries.[26] A recent study from a tertiary care hospital in Nigeria reported a 42.9% case-fatality rate.[27]

Since the 1980s it is estimated that the number of deaths from neonatal tetanus has been reduced by 75% through vaccination before or during pregnancy and with clean delivery and cord care practices.[25] Effective neonatal intensive care, including mechanical ventilation, can markedly improve survival.[28] Vaccinating expectant mothers protects her long term and her newborn during the first few weeks of life. The World Health Organization had hoped to eliminate maternal and neonatal tetanus by 2005,[29] but war and inadequate resources have delayed this achievement.

THE DISEASE

Tetanus is classified into four clinical subtypes: generalized, localized, cephalic, and neonatal. These four clinical subtypes represent the site of toxin action, either predominantly at the neuromuscular junction or at more central inhibitory systems. Incubation time (the time from spore inoculation to first symptoms) for all clinical types seems to vary depending on the ultimate severity of the disease, with more severe disease developing more quickly (8.3 ± 4.7 days) and mild disease taking longer (11 ± 6.7 days).[30] The length of the incubation period also varies with the distance of the inoculation site from the central nervous system (CNS), so that injuries to the lower extremities have longer incubation periods than those occurring at more proximal sites.

Generalized tetanus is the most commonly recognized form of the disease. Trismus, or lockjaw, is the most common presenting sign. It is caused by rigidity of the masseter muscles, which in turn prevents the opening of the mouth, and its severity can be gauged by measuring the distance between the upper and lower teeth with the mouth maximally opened. Trismus results in the classic and characteristic risus sardonicus (*Fig. 42.3*), a facial expression which consists of lateral extension of the corners of the mouth, raised eyelids, and wrinkling of the forehead. These facial features may at times be subtle and may require comparisons with old photographs or confirmation of a change by the patient's family or friends.

Involvement of other muscle groups can then follow the onset of trismus: first the neck, then the thorax and abdomen, and finally the extremities. Tetanic spasms or generalized spasms resemble opisthotonos, decerebrate posturing, or even seizures, and are elicited by both external (noises, drafts of air, touching the patient) or internal (full bladder, coughing) stimuli. The tetanic spasms last for a few seconds to minutes and occur at irregular intervals. These spasms are extremely painful, and full consciousness is retained; this helps differentiate them from seizures or decerebrate posturing. Tetanospasmin is epileptogenic in experimental models, but true epileptic seizures in tetanus are rare. Respiratory compromise is the most serious early problem in generalized tetanus. Spasm of the glottis may occur and results in death via asphyxiation. The diaphragm and abdominal musculature are also frequently affected and this can result in apnea. This effect may be either central or directly at the neuromuscular junction (NMJ),[31] causing paralysis of these muscles. Deep tendon reflexes are usually hyperactive. After several days of illness, autonomic dysfunction, usually a hypersympathetic state, is noted in patients with severe tetanus. Autonomic dysfunction is now the leading cause of death in tetanus patients.[32] It is characterized by labile hypertension and tachycardia, arrhythmias, peripheral vascular constriction, diaphoresis, pyrexia, increased carbon dioxide output, increased urinary catecholamine excretion, and sometimes hypotension. The disease may continue to progress for 10–14 days, reflecting the time it takes for the toxin to be transported to the CNS. Recovery then begins, usually taking about 4 weeks. Without antitoxin, the disease persists for as long as the toxin is produced. Because toxins are produced in insufficient quantities to stimulate an immune response, patients who survive tetanus have little natural immunity and recurrent tetanus is well documented.[33,34]

Localized tetanus is characterized by fixed rigidity of the muscles at or near the site of injury. This may be mild, may persist for months, and usually resolves spontaneously. The muscle may be painful, and deep tendon reflexes may be brisk. The toxin may affect the NMJ, causing weakness, as well as rigidity. Partial immunity to the toxin may be responsible for preventing further hematogenous spread and generalized tetanus,[35] but unless treated, localized tetanus frequently evolves to the generalized form.

Cephalic tetanus occurs with injuries to the head or at times is associated with *C. tetani* infections of the middle ear.[36] Patients have weakness of the facial musculature, and facial paresis is common.[37] Dysphagia[38] and extraocular muscle[39] involvement also have been reported. The incubation period is usually 1–2 days. This is an unusual

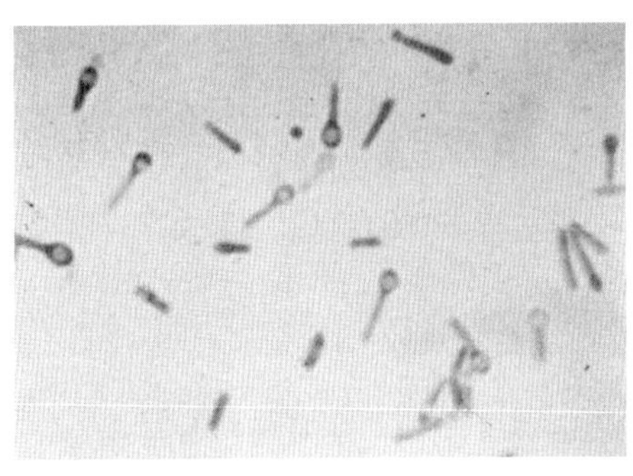

Figure 42.1 Gram stain of a culture of *Clostridium tetani*. (Original magnification: ×1000.) (From Bleck T, Brauner JS: Tetanus. In: Scheld WM, Whitley RJ, Durack DT, eds. Infections of the Central Nervous System, 2nd ed. New York: Raven Press; 1996. Courtesy of P.C. Schrechenberger and A. Kuritza.)

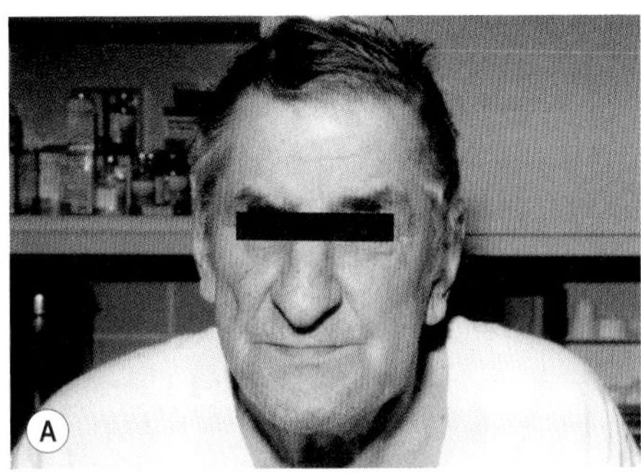

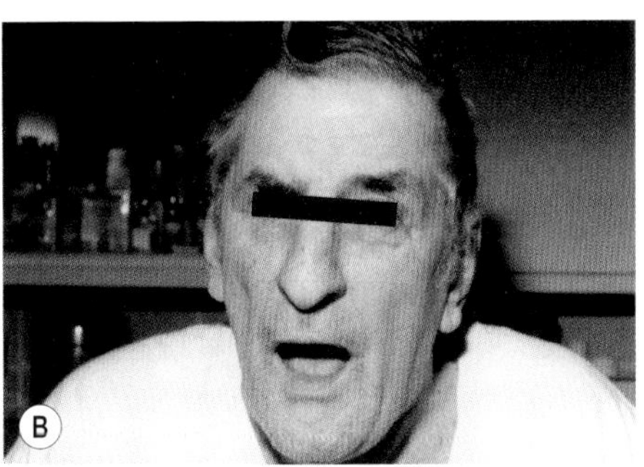

Figure 42.3 **(A)** Risus sardonicus. Note the straightened upper lip at rest. **(B)** Trismus. The patient was instructed to open his mouth as fully as possible. (From Bleck T, Brauner JS: Tetanus. In: Scheld WM, Whitley RJ, Durack DT, eds. Infections of the Central Nervous System, 2nd ed. New York: Raven Press; 1996.)

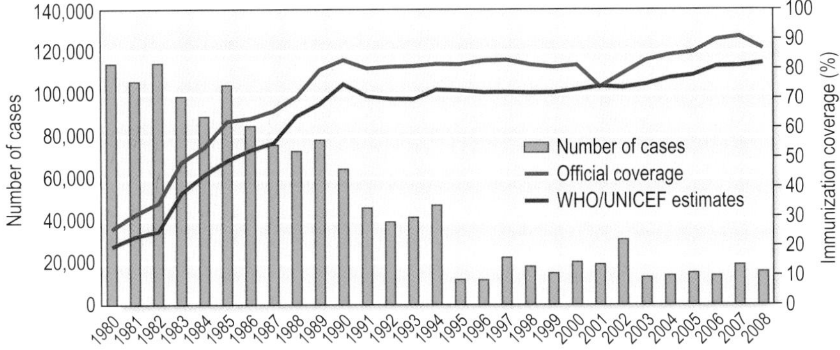

Figure 42.2 Total tetanus global annual reported cases and DTP3 coverage, 1980–2008. (From WHO Vaccine-Preventable Diseases: Monitoring System 2009 Global Summary. WHO/IVB/2009. Copyright World Health Organization 2009.)

form of tetanus, and it too can evolve to the generalized form if left untreated.

Neonatal tetanus is a generalized form of the disease and is far more common in developing countries than in the developed world. It is the leading cause of neonatal mortality in many parts of the world, and of the diseases that can be vaccinated against it is second only to measles as a cause of childhood death.[40] It usually follows an infection of the umbilical stump, often because of improper wound care. In addition, a lack of maternal immunity to tetanus, which, if present, would be passively transferred to the neonate, is necessary for the development of this disease. Four factors seem to play a role in developing neonatal tetanus: (1) the length of the stump (a shorter stump appears to increase the risk), (2) the care with which the cord is ligated, (3) the cleanliness of the instruments and dressings, and (4) the cleanliness of the environment.[41] The incubation period is from 1 to 10 days postpartum, and the mortality rate is up to 90%, with the largest numbers of deaths in the first week of the disease. The infants usually are weak, irritable, and unable to suck. Tetanic spasms occur later, and the opisthotonic posturing must be differentiated from neonatal seizures or other metabolic or congenital abnormalities that cause posturing in this age group. The hypersympathetic state described previously also is common and is frequently the cause of death. Developmental retardation is common in those who survive.[42]

PATHOGENESIS AND IMMUNITY

The spores of *C. tetani* germinate and the bacteria proliferate when the redox potential of the tissue is low. Once the bacteria are growing, two exotoxins are produced: tetanospasmin and tetanolysin. The clinical significance of tetanolysin is unclear. It may aid in the damage of viable tissue near the wound site, lowering the redox potential and allowing for continued growth of anaerobes, perhaps by disrupting membrane channels.[43,44] There also is evidence that tetanolysin can cause electrocardiographic abnormalities and disseminated intravascular coagulation when given systemically in experimental animals.[45]

Tetanospasmin, or "tetanus toxin," is believed to cause all the typical clinical manifestations of tetanus. It is synthesized as a single 151 kDa (1315-amino acid) chain.[46,47] This molecule is then cleaved by a bacterial protease into a heavy chain and a light chain, connected by a disulfide bridge,[48] which is necessary for toxin activity.[49] Papain cleaves the heavy chain at lysine 865, leaving a 50 kDa chain. This is termed the *C fragment*;[50] an N-terminal light chain, still linked by the disulfide bridge, is variously called the *B fragment* or the *A-B fragment*. These chains are thought to affect different phases of toxin binding, cell entry, and toxicity. The DNA for this polypeptide resides on a single plasmid;[51] strains of *C. tetani* that do not have this plasmid have no toxigenic properties. Tetanospasmin inhibits neurotransmitter release at the presynaptic terminal,[52] and this accounts for the clinical presentation of tetanus. The toxin first binds and then passes through the presynaptic membrane,[53] perhaps through uncoated vesicles[54,55] or through pores in phospholipid and ganglioside vesicles.[56] The toxin enters the cytoplasm via an acidic vacuole (similarly to diphtheria toxin). Other toxins, such as cholera, must enter via the Golgi apparatus before membrane translocation.[57] Once in the cytoplasm of the presynaptic terminal, tetanospasmin cleaves the protein (synaptobrevin) that "docks" the neurotransmitter vesicle to the membrane, ultimately for fusion and then release.[58] Thus, because synaptobrevin is cleaved, the vesicle is unable to fuse with the membrane and the neurotransmitter cannot be released.

Tetanospasmin travels via retrograde transport back to the cell body and can then cross several orders of synaptically connected neurons. This process allows the toxin to move from the NMJ of alpha motor neurons to the spinal cord and ultimately to the brain, and helps explain its effects on the NMJ, autonomic function, and the CNS. The heavy chain of the toxin is necessary for the retrograde transport of the toxin to the cell body.[59] Tetanospasmin is also spread hematogenously but must still enter the CNS via neurons and retrograde transport. Any toxin that has not entered a neuron is potentially accessible to antitoxin antibody, but toxin that is intraneuronal or intra-axonal is not, and this helps explain the delay in improvement for several days after initiation of treatment.

Once transported to the spinal cord, tetanospasmin affects the inhibitory neurons. These neurons use either glycine or γ-aminobutyric acid (GABA) and normally inhibit the alpha motor neurons. Without this inhibition, the motor neuron increases its firing rate, ultimately causing rigidity of the muscle innervated by this neuron. Without this inhibition, the normal relaxation of antagonist muscles is impaired, and the characteristic tetanic spasm occurs, in response to movement or stimulation. The toxin is transported into the brainstem,[60] but the clinical relevance of this is unclear.

Tetanospasmin disinhibits sympathetic reflexes at the spinal cord level, implying that hyperadrenergic findings do not depend on the hypothalamus or brainstem;[61] however, the development of the syndrome of inappropriate antidiuretic hormone secretion may support hypothalamic involvement.[62] Patients with tetanus occasionally develop bradycardia and hypotension,[63] as well as disruption of gastric motility,[64] indicating that parasympathetic function is also disrupted.

The effects of tetanospasmin at the NMJ have been established for more than 40 years.[65] More recent studies show a presynaptic defect in the release of acetylcholine (similar to botulism) demonstrated by single-fiber electromyography (EMG).[66] NMJ recovery presumably depends on sprouting new synapses, but the original junctions eventually recover, after which the new ones are pruned. Although frequently overlooked, there may be significant weakness in tetanus, and the tetanospasmin effect on the NMJ is likely the reason.

DIAGNOSIS AND DIFFERENTIAL DIAGNOSIS

The diagnosis of tetanus is primarily clinical. Trismus, muscle rigidity, stimulus-induced tetany, and a history of a wound or injury within the previous 3 weeks is highly suggestive of generalized tetanus. Likewise, a newborn with a poor suck and increased muscle rigidity and spasms, in the setting of poor umbilical hygiene and a mother with no immunization history, likely has neonatal tetanus. EMG may demonstrate findings consistent with increased excitability of the motor neurons as well as NMJ blockade, although this is not specific for tetanus. *C. tetani* is rarely cultured from the wound, and in any case a positive culture does not prove the presence of the disease. Blood and serum studies are usually normal or non-specific, and cerebrospinal fluid (CSF) is usually normal. For the most part, laboratory studies help evaluate for other entities in the differential diagnosis.

Symptoms caused by strychnine, a direct antagonist at the glycine receptor, mimic tetanus. Abdominal muscle rigidity between spasms is more common in tetanus than strychnine toxicity, and trismus frequently occurs later with strychnine. A history of strychnine intoxication may be elicited, and the toxin may be found in the serum, urine, or gastric contents. Dystonic reactions to dopamine antagonists may be confused with tetanus; however, torticollis and oculogyric crisis can be seen in the former but never with tetanus. A brief trial of an anticholinergic agent, such as benztropine or diphenhydramine, which usually relieves dystonic reactions, can further differentiate dystonia from tetanus. Tetany produced by hypocalcemia or alkalosis is usually accompanied by Chvostek's sign (spasm of the facial muscles elicited by tapping on the facial nerve in the region of the parotid gland) and Trousseau's phenomenon (tapping the palm and eliciting palmar spasm). Tetany from these metabolic causes usually involves the extremities rather than the axial musculature, and trismus is much less common. Associated serologic studies confirm the diagnosis. Generalized seizures may be confused with tetanus, but the former, by definition, involve a loss of consciousness. Both, however, respond to benzodiazepines. Conversion reaction or "pseudotetanus" is a disorder in which the patient's movements resemble tetanus. Patients with psychiatric disease can at times be distracted, their movements or postures inconsistent, and there may be a history suggestive of secondary gain. Finally, while the nuchal rigidity of meningitis may resemble the neck stiffness of tetanus, the CSF in tetanus is invariably normal.

TREATMENT

A patient with generalized tetanus or neonatal tetanus requires the facilities and the expertise of an intensive care unit (ICU) to survive. A review of 335 consecutive tetanus patients revealed that survival drastically improved after the development of ICUs (with mortality decreasing from 44% to 15%) and that the major improvement came from prevention of death due to respiratory failure.[67] The mainstays of treatment include (1) neutralizing existing toxin before it enters the nervous system, (2) inhibiting further production of tetanus toxin, (3) muscle relaxation and sedation, (4) management of autonomic instability, and (5) ventilatory, nutritional, and general ICU support. A time-based protocol that the authors have found effective in generalized tetanus is shown in ***Box 42.1***.

Treatment of generalized tetanus should begin with administration of human tetanus immunoglobulin (HTIG). Blake and colleagues[68] demonstrated that a single dose of 500 IU is as effective as the standard dose of 3000–5000 IU. The smaller amount can be given as a single dose; this is important as each intramuscular (IM) injection is a potential stimulus for a tetanic spasm. Equine antitetanus serum may be more readily available, particularly in developing regions, but it has a much higher incidence of adverse reactions. It is dosed at 10 000 to 1 million units intramuscularly (IM). Once the tetanus toxin has entered the motor neuron, it is no longer possible to neutralize it with the antibody. Intrathecal administration of HTIG is possible (although not approved by the US Food and Drug Administration (FDA)) and some authors report that it may be advantageous;[69] however, other studies have failed to demonstrate a benefit.[70] Débriding the portal of entry does not change the course of the disease, although it may help prevent secondary infection. Antibiotic treatment should be initiated at the outset. Metronidazole is superior to penicillin with significantly less progression of the disease, shorter hospitalization, and improved survival.[71] Penicillin, a GABA antagonist, may have a negative effect.[72] Furthermore, the infection may persist despite the administration of penicillin.[73] The dose of metronidazole is 500 mg intravenously (IV) every 6 hours for 7–10 days.

Muscle relaxation is best accomplished with benzodiazepines or baclofen. Diazepam, lorazepam, and midazolam are all effective. With all three agents, very large doses are required to control tetanic spasms; doses in excess of 500 mg per 24 hours of diazepam, 200 mg per 24 hours of lorazepam, and 0.1–0.3 mg/kg per hour of midazolam may be required. Intrathecal administration of baclofen also is effective.[74,75] If GABA receptor agonists, such as benzodiazepines or baclofen, are unsuccessful in controlling the muscle spasms, then neuromuscular blockade is necessary. Vecuronium (6–8 mg per hour) or pancuronium bromide as a bolus of 0.1 mg/kg, then infusion of 0.3–0.6 mg/kg per minute, can be used. Vecuronium is preferred, since it is less likely to cause autonomic instability. A recent case report demonstrated the *in*effectiveness of

Box 42.1 Management Protocol for Generalized Tetanus

I. Diagnosis and Stabilization: First Hour after Presentation

A. Assess airway and ventilation. If necessary, prepare for endotracheal intubation and neuromuscular junction blockade (e.g., vecuronium 0.1 mg/kg).

B. Obtain samples for antitoxin level, strychnine and dopamine antagonist assays, electrolytes, blood urea nitrogen, creatinine, creatine kinase, and urinary myoglobin determination. If meningitis is part of the patient's differential diagnosis, perform a lumbar puncture.

C. Determine the portal of entry, incubation period, period of onset, and immunization history.

D. Administer benztropine 1–2 mg intravenously (IV) or diphenhydramine 50 mg IV to aid in excluding a dystonic reaction (see text for caveat).

E. Administer a benzodiazepine IV (diazepam in 5 mg increments, or lorazepam in 2 mg increments) to control spasms and decrease rigidity. Initially, employ a dose adequate to produce sedation and minimize reflex spasms. If this dose compromises the airway or ventilation, intubate using a short-acting neuromuscular blocking agent prior to transferring the patient to a quiet, darkened area of the intensive care unit.

II. Early Management Phase: First 24 Hours

A. Administer human tetanus immunoglobulin (HTIG), 500 units intramuscularly (IM).

B. At a different site, administer IM an absorbed tetanus toxoid such as tetanus-diphtheria vaccine 0.5 mL or diphtheria-tetanus-pertussis vaccine 0.5 mL, as appropriate for age. Adsorbed tetanus toxoid without diphtheria toxoid is available for patients with a history of reaction to diphtheria toxoid; otherwise, the correct combination for the patient's age should be employed.

C. If intrathecal administration of antitoxin is being considered, it should be administered at this point.

D. Begin metronidazole 500 mg IV every 6 hours for 7–10 days.

E. Perform a tracheostomy after placement of an endotracheal tube and under neuromuscular junction blockade if spasms produce any degree of airway compromise, or if dysphagia or difficulty managing secretions occurs.

F. Débride the wound if this is indicated for its own management (this has no apparent effect on the course of tetanus).

G. Place a soft, small-bore nasal feeding tube or a central venous hyperalimentation catheter.

H. Administer benzodiazepines as needed to control spasms and produce sedation. If adequate control is not achieved, institute long-term neuromuscular junction blockade (e.g., with a vecuronium infusion or intermittent pancuronium injections). Continue benzodiazepines for sedation with electroencephalographic monitoring to ensure somnolence.

I. Initiate physical therapy for pulmonary toilet and passive range-of-motion exercises as soon as the patient has been stabilized pharmacologically. Additional sedation should be given before each treatment, and again during the treatment if the therapy provokes spasms.

III. Intermediate Management Phase: Next 2–3 Weeks

A. Treat sympathetic hyperactivity with IV labetalol 0.25–1.0 mg/min or morphine 0.5 1.0 mg/kg per hour. Consider epidural blockade with local anesthetics. Avoid diuretics for blood pressure control, because volume depletion will worsen autonomic instability.

B. If hypotension is present, place a pulmonary artery catheter and an arterial line, and administer fluids, dopamine, or norepinephrine.

C. Sustained bradycardia usually requires a pacemaker. Atropine or isoproterenol may be useful during pacemaker placement. External pacing should be avoided unless the patient is under neuromuscular junction blockade.

D. Begin prophylactic heparin to prevent pulmonary embolism.

E. Use a flotation bed, if possible, to prevent skin breakdown and peroneal nerve palsies. Otherwise, ensure frequent turning and employ antirotation boots.

F. Maintain benzodiazepines until neuromuscular junction blockade, if employed, is no longer necessary, and the severity of spasms has diminished substantially. Taper the dose over 14–21 days.

G. Begin rehabilitation planning.

IV. Convalescent Stage: 2–6 Weeks

A. When spasms are no longer present, begin physical therapy. Many patients require supportive psychotherapy.

B. Before discharge, administer another dose of the appropriate tetanus toxoid combination.

C. Schedule a third dose of toxoid to be given 4 weeks after the second.

(Adapted from Bleck T, Brauner JS. Tetanus. In: Scheld WM, Whitley RJ, Durack DT, eds. Infections of the Central Nervous System, 2nd ed. New York: Raven Press; 1996.)

rocuronium in controlling tetany and spasms.[76] Of course, when paralytic agents are used, the patient must be intubated and ventilated with positive pressure. More likely, the patient will need to be intubated on presentation; this is done so as to protect the airway, which may occlude during tetanic spasms. Control of autonomic instability can be achieved with a variety of agents. Intravenous labetalol, a combined α- and β-blocker, is the treatment of choice. Esmolol, clonidine, and morphine sulfate are also effective. Magnesium sulfate infusions can help with many aspects of the disease.[77] For bradycardia and hypotension, a temporary pacemaker may be necessary for the former, while fluid boluses and sympathomimetics (e.g., norepinephrine) may be required for the latter. The nutritional requirements of tetanus patients may be extraordinary, but once they are sedated and their spasms and autonomic activity suppressed, their nutritional requirements are similar to those of other critically ill patients. Gastric emptying may be impaired, and therefore, central venous nutrition may be necessary.

There is no standard regimen for the treatment of neonatal tetanus; however, it is treated much like generalized tetanus. Tetanus antitoxin should be administered to neutralize the tetanospasmin that has not yet entered neurons. Human antitetanus immunoglobulin is preferred with a single dose of 3000–5000 units IM, but as noted previously a smaller dose may also be effective (although not specifically tested in children). Equine antitoxin is more widely used because of its availability, but serum sickness or allergic reactions are a significant concern. A single dose of 5000 units of equine antiserum is appropriate. A recent study in neonatal tetanus failed to show any advantage for intrathecal antitoxin.[71] Although débridement of the wound or infected umbilical stump may be surgically indicated, there is no evidence that débridement itself helps prevent progression of the disease. Eradication of the organism can be accomplished with penicillin 100 000 units/kg per day, although penicillin, being a GABA antagonist, can theoretically act synergistically with tetanospasmin and worsen spasms. Metronidazole may be a better choice. Sedation and muscle relaxation of the neonate can be accomplished with a variety of agents including, for acute control of spasms, paraldehyde 0.3 mL/kg IM or diazepam 1–2 mg/kg IM or IV; and for chronic sedation, phenobarbital 5 mg/kg every 6 hours, or diazepam 1–2 mg/kg every 6 hours. Chronic ICU support must also be maintained as described previously for generalized tetanus.

PREVENTION AND CONTROL

Active immunization with tetanus toxoid is one of the most effective preventive measures in medicine. Preventing one case of tetanus saves enough health-care expense to immunize several thousand people.[78] Active immunization with three IM injections of alum-adsorbed tetanus toxoid (10 lyophilized units, 0.5 mL) provides almost complete immunity for 5 years. Routine immunization in the infant begins at 6 weeks to 2 months of age with two other immunizations at 1- to 2-month intervals. A fourth vaccination should be given 1 year after the third, and a fifth at 4–6 years of age. Children under 7 years of age should receive the combined diphtheria-tetanus-pertussis (DTP) vaccine, while the tetanus-diphtheria (Td) vaccine is recommended for those older than 7. Several studies demonstrate that the pertussis component of the vaccine can be given in acellular rather than cellular form with fewer side effects and better efficacy in preventing pertussis.[79] This DTP vaccine has been approved by the FDA.[80] The complete series must be given to ensure adequate antibody titers. Routine boosters should be administered every 10 years.

In the developing world, neonatal tetanus remains a significant problem owing to large numbers of unimmunized women of childbearing age. A single dose of tetanus toxoid administered to unimmunized pregnant women in their third trimester provides protective antibody titers to both the mothers and their babies.[81] Both human immunodeficiency virus-infected adults and infants also have the ability to develop protective tetanus antibody titers.[82,83]

Immunization after an injury that might cause tetanus (contaminated wound, puncture, burn, frostbite, avulsion, and crush injury) should be performed if no tetanus booster has been given within the previous 5 years. An injured patient should be boosted with the adsorbed Td vaccine if none has been administered within the last 10 years. If a prior immunization history is unavailable, then a series of three monthly Td injections should be performed. HTIG should also be administered (250–500 IU) to a patient with no clear previous vaccination history, particularly if the wound is likely to cause tetanus. Most authors agree that both HTIG and tetanus toxoid can be given simultaneously, as long as different sites are used. ***Tables 42.1 and 42.2*** represent the current recommendations of the American College of Emergency Physicians for immunization after injury in children less than 7 years of age and in older children and adults.[84]

On the horizon are other methods of immunization. Sustained-release tetanus toxoid may be available in the future, allowing for a vaccination schedule with fewer doses.[85] Oral immunization has been demonstrated in mice by genetically engineering a mutant live *Salmonella* Typhi strain to carry a fragment of the tetanospasmin gene (fragment C),[86] and oral or nasal administration of liposome-incorporated tetanus toxoid may be possible.[87]

Table 42.1 Guide to Tetanus Prophylaxis in Wound Management in Children under 7 Years Old

Patient's History of Adsorbed Tetanus Toxoid	Clean Minor Wounds		All Other Wounds	
	DPT (or Td)	HTIG	DPT (or Td)	HTIG
Less than three doses or unknown	Yes[a]	No	Yes[a]	Yes
Three or more doses	No[b]	No	No[c]	No

[a]The primary immunization series should be completed.
[b]Yes, if the routine immunization schedule has lapsed (to make up for missed doses).
[c]Yes, if the routine immunization schedule has lapsed, or if more than 5 years since the last dose of tetanus toxoid.
DPT, diphtheria-pertussis-tetanus vaccine; HTIG, human tetanus immunoglobulin; Td, tetanus-diphtheria vaccine.
(Adapted from Tetanus immunization for adults and children in the ED. Information paper. ACEP Online August 1996; available at: http// www.acep.org/policy/PM000604.htm.)

Table 42.2 Guide to Tetanus Prophylaxis in Wound Management in Children Older Than 7 Years of Age and Adults

Patient's History of Adsorbed Tetanus Toxoid	Clean Minor Wounds		All Other Wounds	
	Td	HTIG	Td	HTIG
Less than three doses or unknown	Yes	No	Yes	Yes
Three or more doses	No[a]	No	No[b]	No

[a]Yes, if more than 10 years since last dose.
[b]Yes, if more than 5 years since last dose.
HTIG, human tetanus immunoglobulin; Td, tetanus-diphtheria toxoids adsorbed (for use in adults and children over 7 years of age).
(Adapted from Tetanus immunization for adults and children in the ED. Information paper. ACEP Online August 1996; available at: http:// www.acep.org/policy/PM000604.htm.)

Access the complete reference list online at **http://www.expertconsult.com**

Access the complete reference list online at http://www.expertconsult.com

CHAPTER 43

Treponemal Infections

Joseph D. Tucker • Arlene C. Seña • P. Frederick Sparling
Xiang-Sheng Chen • Myron S. Cohen

INTRODUCTION

Despite the availability of simple and inexpensive treatment options for those with treponemal infections, this ancient group of diseases remains a modern plague of global importance. Venereal syphilis (*Treponema pallidum* subsp. *pallidum*) has a particularly important position in the field of global health not only because it has an impact on pregnancy outcomes and increases human immunodeficiency virus (HIV) transmission, but also because it can be difficult to diagnose. While the advent of penicillin (PCN) was an important landmark in the fight against syphilis, the "great imitator" (so called because of its myriad clinical manifestations) has made a resurgence in the past decade, accelerated by incomplete case-finding in resource-limited areas with a heavy disease burden and persistent risky sexual behaviors among high-risk individuals. This chapter focuses on key epidemiologic, diagnostic, and clinical aspects of *T. pallidum* subsp. *pallidum* infection, then briefly introduces yaws (*T. pallidum* subsp. *pertenue*), pinta (*T. carateum*), and endemic syphilis (*T. pallidum* subsp. *endemicum*).

THE AGENT

All four pathogenic treponemes belong to the Spirochaetaceae family of bacteria, named for their spherical shape when examined under darkfield microscope. Human pathogenic treponemes measure 6–15 μm in length and 0.2 μm in diameter, enveloped by a cytoplasmic membrane and a loosely associated outer membrane. Between these two membranes are a peptidoglycan scaffolding and several endoflagella, responsible for the characteristic corkscrew motility of the organism. However, none of the four treponemes that cause human disease (*T. pallidum* subsp. *pallidum*, *pertenue*, and *endemicum*, and *T. carateum*) can be distinguished based on microscopy or serological findings. Genetic analyses permit differentiation of treponemal subspecies and individual *T. pallidum* subsp. *pallidum* subtypes based on variability in *tpr* and other genes.[1] *T. pallidum* can only survive for hours to days outside the mammalian host. None of the four pathogenic treponemes can be cultured *in vitro*, complicating efforts to create a vaccine and understand better the unique pathophysiology of treponemal infections.

HISTORY

Few diseases have the richly described lore of venereal syphilis infection. Steeped in stigma and moral implications, the disease was referred to as the "French disease" in Italy and the "Italian disease" in France. A heavy burden of syphilis among foreign sailors purchasing sex at port contributed to the notion that this was a disease of the "other," and syphilis-associated stigma persists to today. Conventional accounts of the history of syphilis often start with a Naples outbreak in 1495, the year following Christopher Columbus's return to the Old World. However, whether Christopher Columbus and his crew brought syphilis back from the New World or whether syphilis predated Columbus remains a matter of contention. Molecular epidemiological analyses of Old World and New World skeletons have been used to help shed light on the issue, supporting that Columbus and his men brought syphilis from the New World.

In 1905 Schauddin and Hoffmann discovered the bacteria causing syphilis. In the same year, the term "treponeme" was coined, derived from the Greek roots meaning "to turn" and "thread." The subsequent development of the Wasserman test allowed for a more systematic analysis of the clinical manifestations of syphilis infection independent of other sexually transmitted infections.

EPIDEMIOLOGY

T. pallidum subsp. *pallidum* infections are acquired chiefly through unprotected sex, although there are reports of other transmission routes that include placental (congenital syphilis), blood transfusion, kissing, giving premasticated food to babies, and direct inoculation (***Fig. 43.1***). Syphilis eradication has been the goal for decades in many regions with a low prevalence, but sustained syphilis eradication campaigns have proved elusive. Based on public health campaigns focused on eliminating prostitution, screening high-risk individuals, and treating syphilis infections, primary syphilis was nearly eliminated from China during the 1960s. Sexual syphilis transmission rates during primary and secondary infection approximate 0.5 per act of unprotected intercourse with substantial variation based on immune status, timing, and clinical manifestations.[2] After inoculation, an incubation of 3–90 days ensues at which point the primary chancre of syphilis appears. Transmission is primarily from patients with either primary or secondary lesions, especially chancres, mucous patches, and condyloma lata. Syphilis may be transplacentally transmitted for about 8 years after the initial infection; only rarely are cases of congenital syphilis acquired through the birth canal.

Syphilis is an important sexually transmitted infection in many regions of the world. Within the United States, the number of new syphilis cases reached a nadir in 1998, at which point the US Centers for Disease Control and Prevention launched a nationwide syphilis elimination effort in the United States. However, the spread of syphilis among men who have sex with men (MSM) stymied this effort. Syphilis incidence in the United States displays substantial variation based on ethnicity and location, with a disproportionate burden of new US syphilis cases among African-Americans in the south.

Beyond high-income nations of the world, syphilis remains a major public health problem in many low-income nations. Unfortunately, many such low-income regions with a substantial burden of syphilis also have

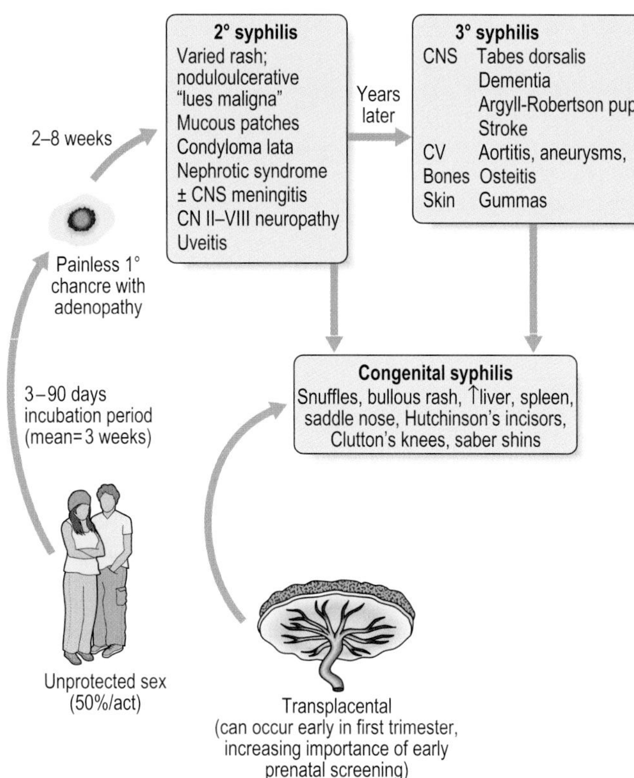

Figure 43.1 Life cycle of treponemal infections.

generalized HIV epidemics (***Table 43.1***). The World Health Organization (WHO) estimated that there are over 10 million syphilis cases each year among those aged 15–49 years.[3] Syphilis is an important etiology of genital ulcer disease in Asia and Africa. China and many parts of Asia have substantial syphilis epidemics, fueled by massive social changes in the last 20 years.[4] In 2008, syphilis overtook tuberculosis as the most commonly reported infection in Shanghai, increasing the importance of syphilis prevention and treatment programs. Unlike the increasing homosexual HIV epidemics in urban middle- and high-income nations among MSM, syphilis is more commonly a heterosexually transmitted infection in low-income nations. However, syphilis spread among MSM in low-income areas is growing alongside increases in the absolute size of MSM populations in these areas. Vertical syphilis transmission is also a major public health concern in many low-income nations where antenatal screening systems are often suboptimal.

THE DISEASE

Sexually transmitted syphilis infection causes a wide spectrum of clinical manifestations which led Sir William Osler to remark, "Know syphilis and the whole of medicine is open unto you." The classic description of a painless genital ulcer belies the innumerable clinical manifestations of syphilis infection. Early syphilis infection refers to the first year after infection and is further subdivided into primary syphilis, secondary syphilis, and early latent syphilis based on clinical presentation. Following the initial symptoms, untreated patients with syphilis will have spontaneous resolution of symptoms and enter the latent phase of infection. The majority of relapses occur in the first year, and this period is called early latent syphilis. Late latent syphilis cases (>1 year of disease) are less

Table 43.1 Global Burden of Syphilis Infection by Region, Estimated for 2005

Region	Male Cases	Female Cases	Total Cases
North and South America	1.2 million	1.2 million	2.4 million
Africa (excluding North Africa)	1.9 million	1.5 million	3.4 million
North Africa and Middle East	300 000	300 000	600 000
Europe	200 000	200 000	400 000
Southeast Asia (includes India, not China)	1.5 million	1.5 million	3 million
Western Pacific region (includes China)	500 000	500 000	1 million
Total	5.6 million	5.0 million	10.6 million

(Source: World Health Organization, as presented at the 2009 International Society for Sexually Transmitted Diseases Research Conference in London.)

infectious, but there can be *in utero* transmission in pregnant women during this stage.

The classically described primary lesion of syphilis, the chancre, is a painless well-circumscribed ulcer on any surface of the body at the initial point of contact, typically accompanied by unilateral or bilateral lymphadenopathy. Atypical dermatological manifestations of the primary chancre or the absence of any other skin findings are common in primary syphilis, demanding a low threshold for diagnostic testing. Among those with HIV infection, cutaneous manifestations may include a greater number of lesions, but there are relatively few differences in clinical manifestations.[5] Accompanying firm, nonpainful inguinal lymphadenopathy is found in many patients with primary syphilis, but is more generalized in secondary syphilis. Dissemination of infection often occurs in primary infections, but systemic signs and symptoms typically develop a few weeks after the primary stage.

Primary lesions of syphilis spontaneously resolve in 3–6 weeks, but may persist in approximately 10% of patients.[6] Secondary syphilis can result in a number of clinical manifestations, including dermatological manifestations (including noduloulcerative lesions, called lues maligna), genital lesions, as well as gastrointestinal, renal, constitutional, and central nervous system (CNS) manifestations. Macular, maculopapular, papular, and pustular rashes are consistent with the disseminated stage of secondary syphilis infection. The first lesions may be quite pale and are found on the trunk. A squamous, flaking appearance over the rash should suggest syphilis when seen. Hyperpigmentation is common in the lesions. A predilection of the rash for the palms and soles is a useful diagnostic clue in some cases of secondary syphilis. Mucous patches, painless white/gray lesions on the top of the tongue or other mucosal surfaces, and condyloma lata, white/gray plaques in the perineum or intertriginous areas, can both be present in secondary syphilis. Secondary-stage *T. pallidum* infections can trigger a nephrotic syndrome or glomerulonephritis in the kidney or an elevated serum alkaline phosphatase and mildly elevated total bilirubin, suggesting hepatocellular inflammation in the liver.

Approximately 40% of syphilis patients have some CNS symptoms, ranging from mild headache to frank meningitis. Treponemal invasion of the CNS may occur at any point in syphilis infection, ranging from early syphilis to late latent syphilis. Cerebrospinal fluid (CSF) analyses from patients with neurosyphilis may reveal increased total protein and a pleocytosis. Neurological manifestations of secondary syphilis include isolated cranial neuropathies (especially II–VIII), Erb's paralysis, amyotrophic meningomyelitis, uveitis, and tinnitus, among others.

Late or tertiary syphilis is an insidious disease process that can affect any organ years after the initial infection, but focusing on the CNS, cardiovascular system, bones, and skin. The clinical manifestations of late neurosyphilis include tabes dorsalis (dorsal column degeneration resulting in altered sensation), dementia, Argyll Robertson pupils, seizures, and otitis. Cardiovascular lesions associated with late syphilis encompass aortitis, and ascending thoracic aneurysms. Gummas are granulomatous lesions that can occur in virtually any organ, but are now rare. HIV infection may increase the risk of gummas.

As syphilis makes a resurgence in many regions of the world, recognizing the clinical manifestations of congenital syphilis remains important. Early syphilis infection in the mother carries the greatest risk of transmission to the fetus, but any stage of syphilis has the potential for *in utero* syphilis transmission. Early clinical signs of congenital syphilis include rhinitis (snuffles), an often vesicular or bullous rash, anemia, hepatosplenomegaly, jaundice, and neurological symptoms. Children born with syphilis may have clinical manifestations such as saddle-nose deformity, protruding mandible, high palatal arch, Hutchinson's incisors, Clutton's joints (bilateral painless swelling of the knees), and saber shins. The wide array of clinical manifestations of syphilis underscores the importance of prompt diagnostic testing.

DIAGNOSIS

Syphilis diagnostic algorithms revolve around serological test results, traditionally with the initial use of a sensitive nontreponemal test followed by a specific treponemal test for confirmation (***Fig. 43.2***). However, the development of rapid treponemal syphilis tests and automated newer treponemal detection assays expand opportunities for using the treponemal test as an initial screening tool. None of the serological tests can differentiate *T. pallidum* subsp. *pallidum* from yaws, pinta, or endemic syphilis.

While serologic tests are central to syphilis diagnosis, darkfield microscopy for direct visualization of spirochetes can be a useful adjunct, especially in cases of early infection when primary lesions are present and antitreponemal antibodies cannot be detected by serology. Transudate from moist lesions that have a higher burden of treponemes (condyloma lata, primary chancre, etc.) are more likely to reveal the characteristic corkscrew-shaped organisms under darkfield microscropy (***Fig. 43.3***). The sensitivity of darkfield examination can approach 80%,[7] but a low organism burden, sampling problems, or partial treatment can all lead to false-negative results. Direct fluorescent antibody testing is another direct test and may be available in some laboratories, and can also be useful for identifying *T. pallidum* from primary or secondary lesions, including differentiating pathogenic treponemes in oral or rectal specimens from nonpathogenic treponemes. Polymerase chain reaction from oral ulcer swabs appears to be a sensitive and specific adjunct in syphilis diagnosis (especially early syphilis infections), but the required laboratory facilities and personnel would limit its use in many low-income settings.

Nontreponemal syphilis tests are relatively inexpensive, quantitative, and can be used to track infection status over time. Nontreponemal tests use antigen containing cardiolipin, lecithins, and cholesterol, each of which flocculates when it reacts with immunoglobulin M (IgM) and IgG antibodies produced by a host. The rapid plasma reagin (RPR) and Venereal Disease Research Laboratory (VDRL) tests are the most common nontreponemal tests. The sensitivity of RPR ranges from 77–100% in early infection to 100% in secondary infection alongside a specificity of 98%.[8] A fourfold decrease in RPR or VDRL titer (equivalent to two dilutions) within 6–24 months depending on the stage of infection is the benchmark for adequate response to syphilis treatment, but persistently elevated RPR/VDRL titers can result from a biological false positive test, treatment failure, or reinfection. Biologic false-positive nontreponemal tests may present in a wide variety of clinical settings, including pregnancy, infections (HIV, tuberculosis, leprosy, endocarditis, malaria), chronic inflammatory disorders (lupus, rheumatoid arthritis, antiphospholipid syndrome), intravenous drug users, following viral infections or vaccinations, or in relation to drug or allergic reactions. A prozone phenomenon can occur when the amount of antigen–antibody complexes overwhelms the nontreponemal assay, resulting in a false-negative result, especially in secondary syphilis, HIV coinfection, and pregnancy. Dilutions should be performed in cases where there is a high index of clinical suspicion of syphilis infection.

Treponemal tests which include rapid point-of-care tests and newer enzyme immunoassays (EIAs) for *T. pallidum* have the advantage of high sensitivity and specificity, but cannot distinguish present from treated infections. The traditional treponemal tests detect antitreponemal antibodies and include the fluorescent treponemal antibody absorption (FTA-Abs) and the agglutination tests (*T. pallidum* particle agglutination, the *T. pallidum* heamagglutination, and the microhemagglutination assay (MHA TP)). The rapid treponemal tests use immunochromatographic strips and a lateral flow format to detect IgG, IgA, or IgM directed against syphilis.[8] These rapid tests can be stored at room temperature, do not

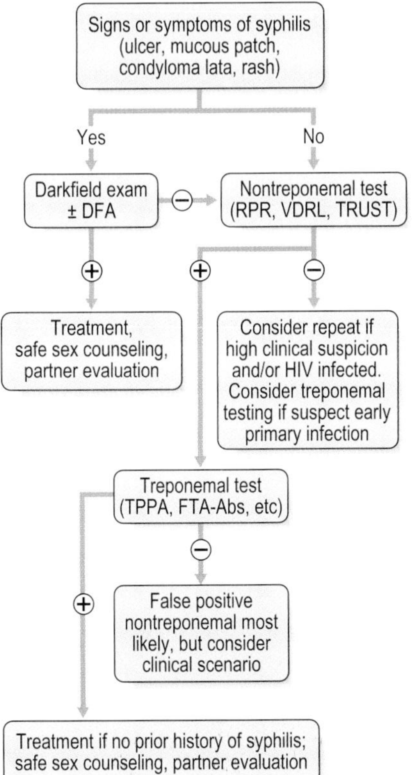

Figure 43.2 Traditional diagnostic algorithm for syphilis screening. DFA, direct fluorescent antibody; RPR, rapid plasma reagin; VDRL, Venereal Disease Research Laboratory; TRUST, toluidine red unheated serum test; TPPA, *T. pallidum* particle agglutination; FTA-Abs, fluorescent treponemal antibody absorption; HIV, human immunodeficiency virus.

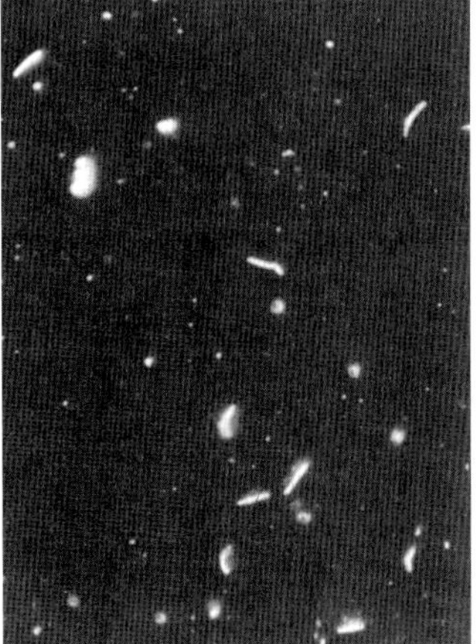

Figure 43.3 Darkfield microscopy examination of the corkscrew-shaped spirochete. (Reproduced from Mandel G, Bennett J, Dolin R (eds) Principles and Practice of Infectious Diseases, 7th ed. Philadelphia, PA: Elsevier, 2010.)

require equipment, and can use whole blood from fingerpricks. The EIAs for *T. pallidum* use either wild-type *T. pallidum* or recombinant antigens to coat a microtiter plate of wells that react with antitreponemal antibodies. Early EIAs were targeted toward antitreponemal IgG, but newer assays are available that can detect IgM as well, increasing their utility in diagnosing congenital syphilis or primary syphilis.

The sensitivity of most treponemal tests ranges from 70% to 100% with a specificity ranging from 97% to 99%.[8] Unlike nontreponemal tests, the treponemal tests are not quantitative and generally remain positive even after treatment. These tests are also plagued by biologic false-positive results, more commonly found in intravenous drug users, patients with infections (including leprosy, Lyme, leptospirosis), and inflammatory conditions (lupus). Although treponemal tests have traditionally been the confirmatory test of choice for syphilis, the advent of inexpensive rapid treponemal tests in low-income regions and automated EIAs in large-scale laboratories may alter traditional diagnostic algorithms. When used as screening tests, positive rapid tests or EIAs should be followed by nontreponemal tests for confirmation and to determine titers that can be monitored after treatment.[9] When a positive rapid test or EIA is accompanied by a negative RPR, a thorough patient history is important to rule out prior treated syphilis or early syphilis. If resources allow, a second treponemal test is recommended for further evaluation of patients without a prior history of syphilis who are positive on treponemal screening and negative by "confirmatory" nontreponemal testing.

Neurological tests for syphilis infection include CSF VDRL and various forms of treponemal testing from CSF specimens. Whereas the CSF VDRL offers a high specificity in identifying patients with neurosyphilis, the treponemal tests (CSF-FTA unabsorbed, CSF-Abs, CSF MHA-TPHA, CSF MHA-TP) generally provide higher sensitivity and result in better negative predictive values. Among patients who are suspected of having congenital syphilis, the most effective diagnostic tests are Western blots for *T. pallidum* specific IgM and immunofluorescent antigen detection from either nasopharyngeal or umbilical specimens.

TREATMENT AND PROGNOSIS

Benzathine penicillin (PCN) G is the treatment of choice for syphilis among adults who do not have neurological involvement. There have been no cases of *T. pallidum* resistant to PCN, although treatment failures can occur. Quantitative VDRL/RPR tests should become nonreactive 1–5 years following treatment, with the duration of time dependent on the syphilis stage, severity of illness, and HIV status. Early syphilis infections (primary, secondary, early latent) in adults may be treated with 2.4 million units of benzathine PCN intramuscularly administered as a single dose. This provides adequate drug levels for approximately 2–3 weeks and is a reasonable treatment course in immunocompetent individuals. Despite the lack of clinical evidence to guide this treatment decision, many providers will treat early syphilis in HIV-infected patients with more than a single dose of PCN in an effort to prevent or treat early CNS invasion. Late latent syphilis cases and syphilis of unknown duration require a longer course of 2.4 million units of benzathine PCN weekly for a total of three injections. Persons with neurosyphilis require aqueous crystalline PCN 3.0–4.0 million units intravenously every 4 hours for 10–14 days or ceftriaxone 1 g daily intramuscularly or intravenously for 14 days.

Syphilis patients allergic to PCN have other potential treatment regimens, including doxycyline, tetracycline, and possibly azithromycin. The treatment duration of doxycyline for early syphilis in adults is 14–15 days, while late latent syphilis cases and syphilis of unknown duration require 28 days of treatment. Azithromycin 2.0 g as a single dose has been demonstrated to have equivalent efficacy as benzathine PCN for early syphilis in a study from Tanzania,[10] and also has activity against gonorrhea and chlamydia. However, the identification of a point mutation conferring resistance to azithromycin has been reported in isolates from the United States, Ireland,[11] Canada, and China, making this a suboptimal alternative for syphilis treatment.[11]

All pregnant women with syphilis should receive PCN and pregnant women who are allergic to PCN should be desensitized. Ceftriaxone treatment failures of syphilis in pregnancy have been reported, making ceftriaxone a poor antibiotic choice. Doxycycline and tetracycline are not viable treatment options because of the possibility of adverse effects on the mother or the fetus. Cases of congenital syphilis should be treated with aqueous crystalline PCN G at 100 000–150 000 U/kg intravenously in two or three divided doses for at least 10 days or procaine PCN G 50 000 U/kg/day intramuscularly daily for at least 10 days. PCN should be given to all neonates born to mothers with syphilis except when there is adequate documentation of serologically effective syphilis treatment.

Following initiation of syphilis therapy, patients may experience a Jarisch–Herxheimer reaction, a transient immunologic reaction due to release of antigenic substances from the spirochetes upon treatment. This typically occurs 1–2 hours after antibiotics, and consists of fever, chills, myalgias, headache, hyperventilation, flushing, and mild hypotension. The Jarisch–Herxheimer reaction can be seen predominantly after treatment for primary or secondary syphilis, and may persist for 12–24 hours. Supportive therapy with antipyretic or anti-inflammatory agents is recommended.

PREVENTION AND CONTROL

While clinicians need to know the essential clinical, diagnostic, and therapeutic parameters related to *T. pallidum*, there are several key public health issues related to syphilis that are worthy of further discussion. *T. pallidum's* synergistic relationship with HIV infection, high transmission rate, and impact on pregnancy outcomes make it a key sexually transmitted infection to control.

Syphilis infection increases the risk of both acquiring and transmitting HIV infection, and the shared sexual risk behaviors make coinfection more common. HIV testing is therefore recommended for all patients diagnosed with syphilis. The mechanism of synergy between syphilis and other ulcerative sexually transmitted infections and HIV is likely related to decreased physical skin barriers and ulcer recruitment of monocytes that express increased CCR5. Unfortunately, as discussed before, patients with HIV and syphilis may have false-positive or false-negative syphilis serologies, making definitive diagnosis difficult. HIV-infected patients may have earlier and more extensive CNS involvement during syphilis infection, increasing the importance of a complete neurological examination and CSF diagnostics in cases where there is suspicion of neurosyphilis.

Partner notification plays an important public health role in syphilis control efforts, and empiric treatment should be provided to all sex partners exposed during the infectious period of the index case. All individuals with newly diagnosed or reported early syphilis infection should be offered partner services in concert with local public health officials.[12]

Syphilis has a wide range of deleterious outcomes in the context of pregnancy. Animal models suggest that *T. pallidum* invades the fetal compartment at 9–10 weeks of pregnancy, increasing the importance of early prenatal testing. Syphilis during pregnancy can cause miscarriage, stillbirth, hydrops fetalis, growth restriction, premature delivery, and perinatal death. Research from 1001 pregnancies in the preantibiotic era found that 17% resulted in abortion, 22% led to prenatal death, and 21% of cases resulted in congenital syphilis.[13] Screening for syphilis routinely in women attending prenatal clinics is therefore critical to prevent complications during pregnancy and congenital infections.

ENDEMIC TREPONEMATOSES

Although less common than *T. pallidum* subsp. *pallidum* infections, the endemic treponematoses are important – yaws (*T. pallidum* subsp. *pertenue*), endemic syphilis (*T. pallidum* subsp. *endemicum*), and pinta or bejel (*T. carateum*). There are no serological tests that can distinguish syphilis from the endemic treponematoses. While there are some similar clinical characteristics, none of the endemic treponematoses have any impact on pregnancy outcomes or are thought to affect HIV transmission.

The four treponemal bacteria are alike insofar as none can be cultured *in vitro*. They are spread chiefly by direct contact, with the addition of fomite transmission in endemic syphilis. Each of the three endemic treponemes has a specific geographic distribution, generally within the 30th parallels in the northern and southern hemispheres (***Fig. 43.4***). Yaws has the largest geographic distribution, affecting rural rainforest regions where high humidity and poor hygiene likely enhance person-to-person transmission. Pinta is also more common in rainforest regions, but is only found in the Americas and the Caribbean islands. Endemic syphilis is principally found in the dry and arid climate of North Africa and the Arabian peninsula. Yaws and endemic syphilis both disproportionately affect children, while pinta occurs more frequently in individuals aged 14–30 years old.

Similar to venereal syphilis, endemic treponematoses have a diversity of clinical manifestations. The typical early lesion is a raised papule at the site of inoculation, followed by regional lymphadenopathy. In pinta, long-term infections are characterized by multiple small scaly papules that expand and form psoriasiform plaques called pintids. Yaws and endemic syphilis have late infections manifested by cutaneous lesions and potentially involvement of bones and joints (***Fig. 43.5***). None of the endemic treponematoses has cardiovascular or neurological sequelae.

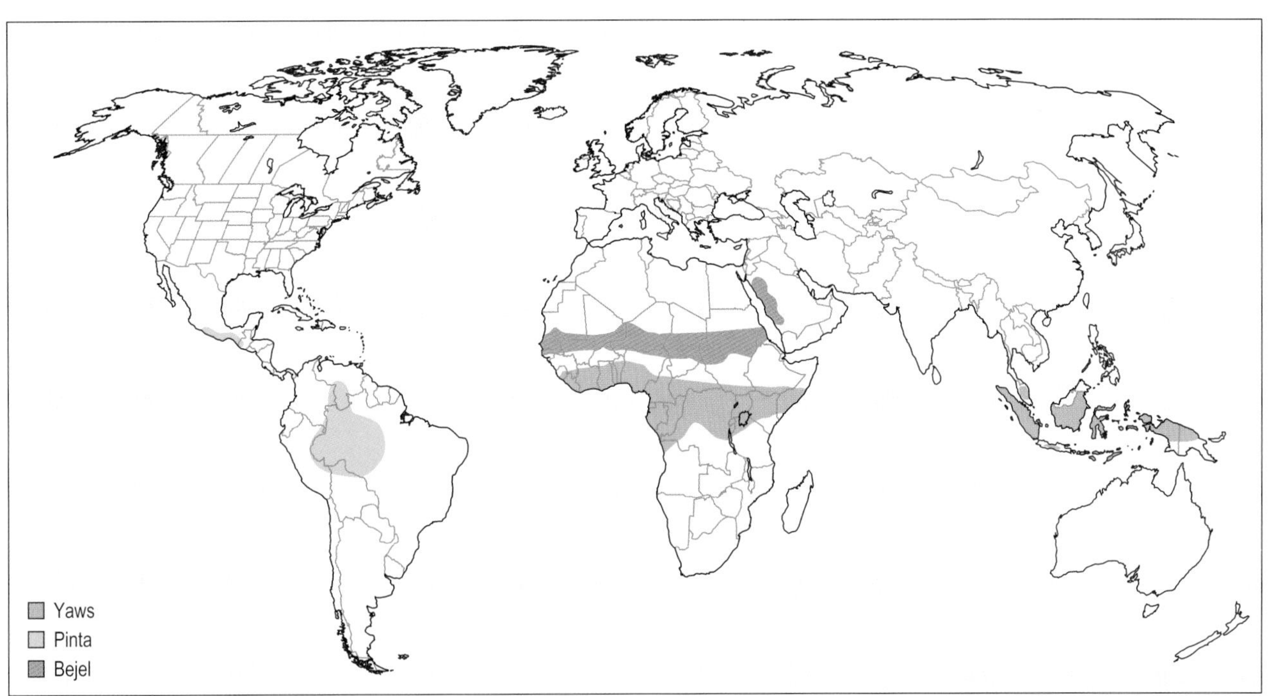

Figure 43.4 Geographic distribution of endemic treponematoses.

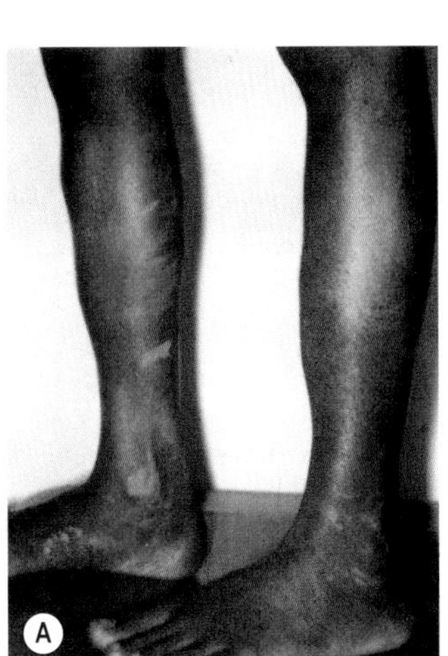

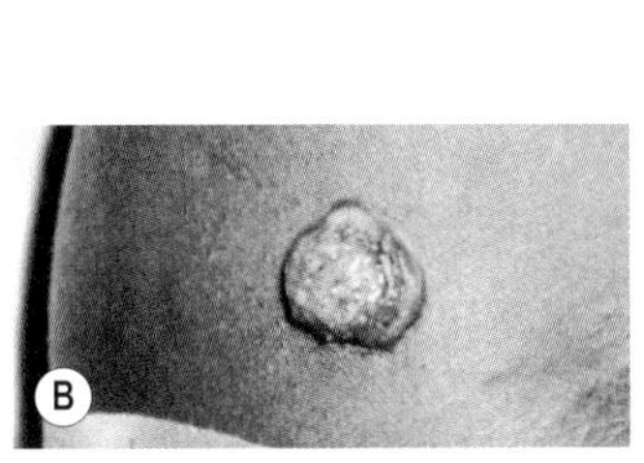

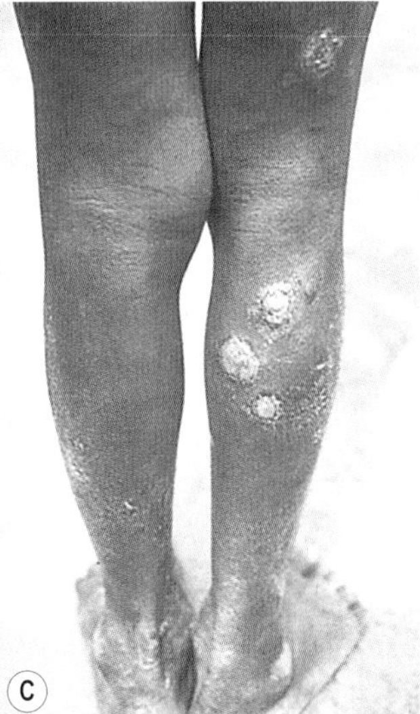

Figure 43.5 (A) Early ulcer from a patient with cutaneous yaws. (Reproduced from Perine PL, Hopkins DR, Niemel PLA et al. Handbook of Endemic Treponematoses. Geneva: World Health Organization, 1984.) **(B)** Initial, solitary yaws papilloma (frambesioma) on the upper thigh. (Reproduced from Perine PL, Hopkins DR, Niemel PLA, et al. Handbook of Endemic Treponematoses: Yaws, Endemic Syphilis, and Pinta. Geneva: World Health Organization, 1984.) **(C)** Bony deformity of the tibiae due to yaws osteoperiostitis. (Reproduced from Perine PL, Hopkins DR, Niemol PLA, et al. Handbook of Endemic Treponematoses: Yaws, Endemic Syphilis, and Pinta. Geneva: World Health Organization: 1984.)

Since most endemic treponematoses are diagnosed in regions with limited laboratory capacity, clinical diagnosis is quite common. The diagnosis can be confirmed using the same treponemal and nontreponemal serologies used in the diagnosis of venereal syphilis infection. Once a patient has a confirmed diagnosis, PCN is the treatment of choice for endemic treponematoses. The WHO recommends treating endemic treponemes with benzathine PCN G 600 000 units for those under 10 years of age, and 1.2 million units for those older than 10 years. All close contacts should receive treatment to prevent the spread of infection.

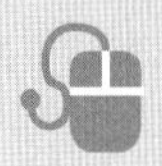

Access the complete reference list online at
http://www.expertconsult.com

Access the complete reference list online at http://www.expertconsult.com

CHAPTER 44

Relapsing Fever and Other *Borrelia* Diseases

Alan G. Barbour

INTRODUCTION

Physicians have recognized relapsing fever as a clinical entity since the time of Hippocrates. There are few if any other diseases that are characterized by two or more episodes of high fever separated by week-long periods of well-being.[1,2] During the fevers there are high densities of bacteria in the blood. Relapsing fever occurs in two major forms: louse-borne and tick-borne. The ticks that transmit relapsing fever are soft-bodied (argasid) ticks. Isolated cases and epidemics have occurred in equatorial regions, temperate zones, and the sub-arctic in all hemispheres. Louse-borne relapsing fever has had, like plague and typhus, periods of huge impact on human health.[3]

The recognition of Lyme borreliosis (or Lyme disease) as a clinical entity is more recent.[4,5] The clinical manifestations of Lyme borreliosis are diverse and may mimic other infectious and noninfectious disorders. In contrast to relapsing fever, bacteria are sparse in the blood. Lyme borreliosis is transmitted by hard-bodied or ixodid ticks. Whereas relapsing fever exists on most continents, Lyme borreliosis has been documented to date only in the Nearctic (North America) and the Palearctic (Europe and temperate Asia) ecological regions.[1]

THE AGENTS

The agents of relapsing fever and Lyme borreliosis are spirochetes, which are spiral or wavy filamentous bacteria with these characteristics: (a) two cell membranes with a periplasmic space between, and (b) flagella that are inserted at each end and traverse the length of the cell in the periplasmic space.[6] Members of the genus *Borrelia* are host-associated microorganisms and not free-living (***Table 44.1***). Viable borrelias are extracellular in their reservoir and vector hosts. Outside their hosts *Borrelia* spp. are susceptible to drying, hypotonic or hypertonic solutions, detergents, and temperatures above 41°C. The cells have widths of approximately 0.2 µm and lengths of 10–30 µm; they can be visualized by dark field or phase contrast microscopy but not standard light microscopy without special stains. They are microaerophilic microorganisms and grow in a complex medium that contains, among other ingredients, serum, glucose, albumin, peptides, vitamins, a thickening agent such as gelatin, and *N*-acetylglucosamine, the building block for an arthropod's chitin exoskeleton.[7,8]

Although borrelias do not have lipopolysaccharides with the characteristics of endotoxins, they do have abundant outer membrane lipoproteins that are potent B-cell mitogens and stimulators of inflammatory cytokines, such as tumor necrosis factor.[9] The lipoproteins are anchored at their N-terminal ends by fatty acids embedded in the fluid membrane of the spirochetes. *Borrelia* species also have abundant glycolipids that may elicit an immune response during infection.[10]

The genome of *Borrelia* spp. comprises a linear chromosome and several linear and circular plasmids. The G + C contents are about 30%. There are three major clades of *Borrelia* species: (1) the relapsing fever group (***Table 44.1***), (2) the Lyme borreliosis group, which includes the most common agents of Lyme borreliosis – *B. burgdorferi*, *B. afzelii*, and *B. garinii* – as well as several related species not associated with human disease, and (3) the hard tick-borne species *B. lonestari*, *B. theileri*, and *B. miyamotoi* of uncertain medical significance.[11]

EPIDEMIOLOGY

Ecology and Epidemiology of Tick-Borne Relapsing Fever

Except for *B. recurrentis*, the sole louse-borne agent, *Borrelia* species are transmitted by argasid ticks of the genus *Ornithodoros* and, less commonly, the genus *Carios*.[12] *Ornithodoros* ticks have two or more nymphal stages between larval and adult stages; ***Figure 44.1*** shows several sizes of *O. turicata*. Most species of argasid ticks feed on a single or a very limited number of hosts. *Ornithodoros* ticks are noted for their longevity, up to 15–20 years, and their ability to survive without a blood meal for several years. Transovarial transmission by their vectors is common among tick-borne *Borrelia* species, thus providing for survival when vertebrate hosts are absent or sparse. Reservoirs of the relapsing fever *Borrelia* species include a variety of mammals, most commonly rodents (***Fig. 44.2***), but may include birds as well. The natural reservoir for the tick-borne species *B. duttonii* appears to be humans.

Ornithodoros ticks feed for less than 30 minutes and usually at night. Most people are not aware of their bite. A sign of an *Ornithodoros* tick bite may be a small papule with a central eschar that appears within a few days of exposure. The spirochetes are present in the salivary gland at the onset of feeding, and the pathogens enter the host with the saliva soon after the tick begins to feed. The risk of relapsing fever after a single bite of an infected tick is 50% or higher.

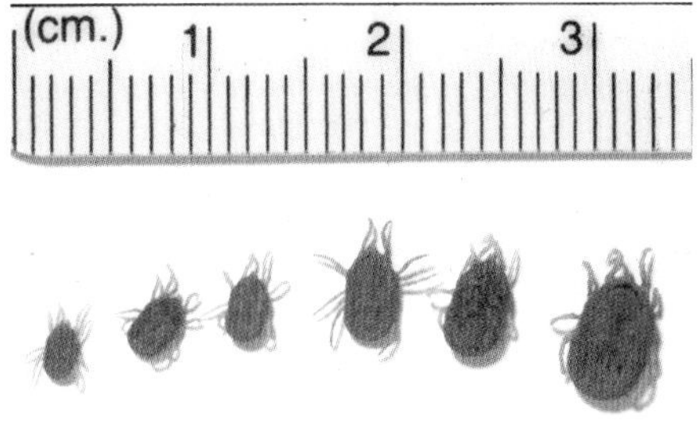

Figure 44.1 Nymphal and adult *Ornithodoros turicata* ticks collected from a cave in which several people acquired tick-borne relapsing fever.

Table 44.1 Common *Borrelia* Species that Cause Diseases of Humans

Species	Disease[a]	Ecological Region	Arthropod Vectors	Primary Reservoir[b]
Borrelia afzelii	LB	Palearctic	*Ixodes ricinus, I. persulcatus*	Mammals
B. burgdorferi	LB	Nearctic/Paleartic	*I. scapularis, I. pacificus/I. ricinus*	Mammals
B. crocidurae	TBRF	Palearctic	*Ornithodoros erraticus*	Mammals
B. duttonii	TBRF	Afro-tropical	*O. moubata*	Humans
B. garinii	LB	Palearctic	*I. ricinus, I. persulcatus*	Birds
B. hermsii	TBRF	Nearctic	*O. hermsi*	Mammals
B. hispanica	TBRF	Palearctic	*O. marocanus*	Mammals
B. latyschewii	TBRF	Palearctic	*O. tartakovskyi*	Mammals
B. mazzottii	TBRF	Nearctic	*O. talaje*	Mammals
B. parkeri	TBRF	Nearctic	*O. parkeri*	Mammals
B. persica	TBRF	Palearctic	*O. tholozani*	Mammals
B. recurrentis	LBRF	Global[c]	*Pediculus humanus*	Humans
B. turicatae	TBRF	Nearctic	*O. turicata*	Mammals
B. venezuelensis	TBRF	Neotropical	*O. rudis*	Mammals

[a]LB, Lyme borreliosis; TBRF, tick-borne relapsing fever; LBRF, louse-borne relapsing fever.
[b]Primary reservoir for maintenance of species in nature.
[c]*B. recurrentis* probably originated in Palearctic or Afro-tropical regions.

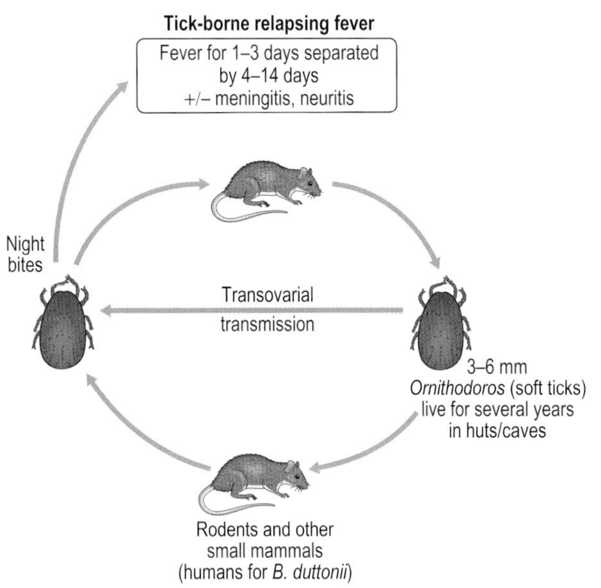

Figure 44.2 Life cycle of tick-borne relapsing fever.

Tick-borne relapsing fever occurs in the Palearctic, Nearctic, Afro tropical, and Neotropical ecological regions (***Table 44.1***). Human infections have not been well-documented in the Indo-Malayan, Australasia, or Oceania ecological regions. Reports of relapsing fever from areas with rainforests or monsoon forests are probably attributable to louse-borne infection or the importation of infected ticks with livestock. With the speed and frequency of international travel, persons with relapsing fever may initially seek care in their home countries.[13]

In the United States and Canada, most cases of autochthonous relapsing fever are due to *B. hermsii* and *B. turicatae*.[14,15] Although vectors and reservoirs for these species are widely distributed in the western and central United States, human disease incidence is highly focal. Among 450 cases of relapsing fever identified in the United States over 14 years, 13 counties accounted for half of the cases.[16] *O. hermsi*, the vector of *B. hermsii*, is found in forested mountains at elevations ranging from 1000 to 2700 meters, depending on the latitude, throughout the western United States and British Columbia. Common hosts for *O. hermsi* are chipmunks and squirrels. Most cases of *B. hermsii* infection can be traced to sleeping in or near cabins and rustic houses that have rodents nesting in the roof, under eaves, in walls, under porches, or in wood piles.

O. turicata, the vector of *B. turicatae*, is found in desert, semi-desert and scrub landscapes of the southwestern and south-central United States, as well as drier areas of central Mexico and an isolated focus in Florida,[1,2,12] *O. turicata* ticks reside in rodent burrows or in caves and overhanging rock ledges that shelter large animals. In Mexico *O. turicata* has also been found in human habitats, especially those with pigsties. Humans become infected with *B. turicatae* by entry into caves, crawling under houses, or sleeping in structures with walls infested with *O. turicata*. *B. parkeri* is closely related to *B. turicatae*, but human infections are rare, probably because humans seldom encounter the tick vector, *O. parkeri*. *O. talaje*, the vector of *B. mazzottii*, overlaps the distribution of *O. turicata* in the southwestern United States and extends as far as south as Guatemala. Tick-borne relapsing fever has been reported in Panama, where the natural hosts include monkeys, opossums, and armadillos. The vector in Panama as well as Venezuela and Colombia is *O. rudis*, and the agent is *B. venezuelensis*.

Tick-borne relapsing fever remains a common infection of rural villages in parts of sub-Saharan Africa.[17–19] Many cases are associated with human habitats with thatched roofs or mud walls or floors. While most cases in sub-Saharan Africa are attributable to either *B. duttonii* or *B. crocidurae*, a new species has been observed in Tanzania.[20,21] Human infections from *B. persica*, *B. latyschewii*, and *B. hispanica* also continue to occur in Central Asia, Iran, North Africa, and the Middle East. The range of *B. persica* extends from the Mediterranean area and the Middle East to Central Asia.[1,22] *B. persica*'s vector, *O. tholozani*, lives in houses and buildings, as well as burrows and caves.[23] In Central Asia and the Caucasus region, *B. latychevi* is a less likely agent of relapsing fever, because its vector ticks rarely inhabit human dwellings. In the past, the range of *B. hispanica* included the Iberian peninsula as well as Greece, Cyprus, and North Africa. Endemic relapsing fever has been reported again in Spain, but it is caused by a *Borrelia* sp. that may be distinct from *B. hispanica*.[24,25]

Ecology and Epidemiology of Louse-Borne Relapsing Fever

The vector is the body louse (***Fig. 44.3***), *Pediculus humanus corporis*, which only feeds on humans in nature. *B. recurrentis* appears to be a louse-adapted variant of the tick-borne species *B. duttonii*.[26] Nonhuman primates can be experimentally infected with *B. recurrentis*, but humans are the critical reservoirs for maintenance of the pathogen in nature. After entering the midgut of the feeding louse, *B. recurrentis* move to the hemolymph where they may persist for the approximately 3-week life span of the louse. They do not migrate to the salivary glands or appear in the feces. Humans

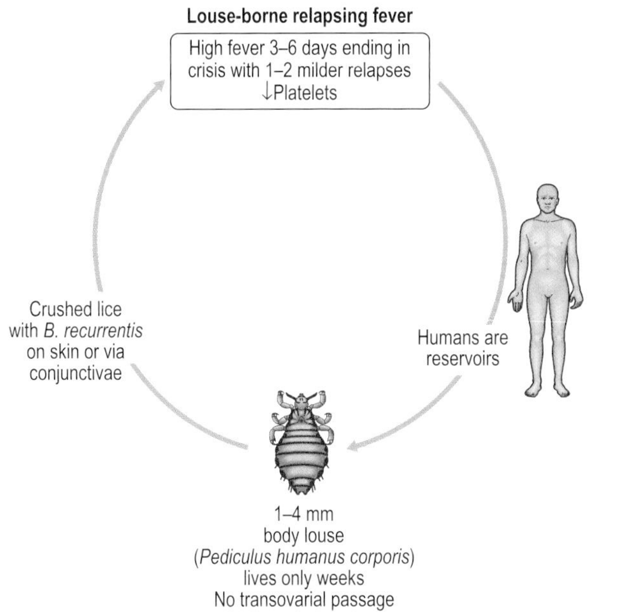

Figure 44.3 Life cycle of louse-borne relapsing fever.

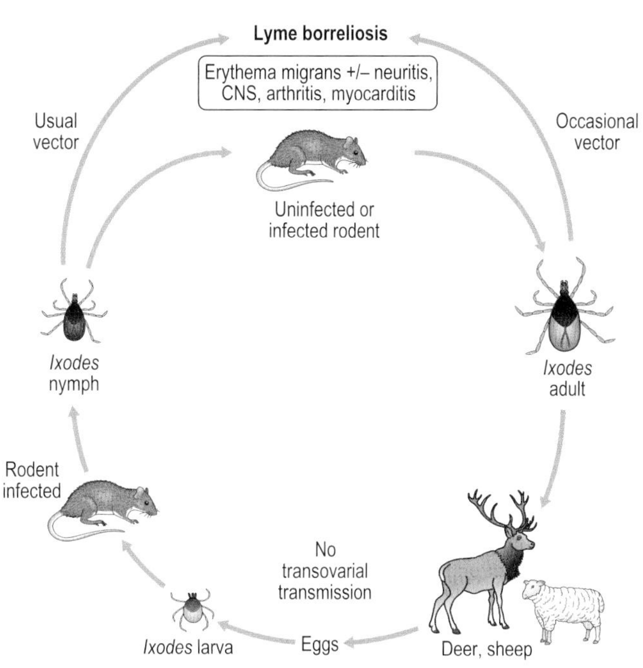

Figure 44.4 Life cycle of Lyme borreliosis.

become infected with *B. recurrentis* when they crush an infected louse with fingers or teeth. The organism is introduced at the bite site, the skin of the crushing fingers, the conjunctivae when people rub their eyes, or through the mucous membranes of the mouth.

B. recurrentis infection still occurs in the Horn of Africa, particularly in the highlands of Ethiopia, where it has been endemic for decades.[3,27–29] Transmission is highest during the rainy season when the poor gather together in shelter, and infected lice move from one person to another. As reflected by such colloquial names as "famine fever" and "vagabond fever," factors that predispose to louse-borne relapsing fever epidemics include famine, war, and refugees. Precipitating conditions for outbreaks are crowding, limited changes of clothing, and lack of access to washing. Millions of cases of louse-borne relapsing fever occurred around the disrupted times of the two world wars of the twentieth century.

Ecology and Epidemiology of Lyme Borreliosis

The vectors of Lyme borreliosis agents are species of the *Ixodes* genus (*Fig. 44.4*) of hard ticks in temperate regions of the northern hemisphere: *I. scapularis* in the eastern United States, *I. pacificus* in the western United States, *I. ricinus* in Europe, and *I. persulcatus* across Russia to northern Asia.[1,12] *B. burgdorferi* is the sole agent in North America. This species also occurs in Europe, but most cases in Europe, Russia, and northern Asia are caused by *B. afzelii* or *B. garinii*. Transovarial transmission of the pathogen by *Ixodes* spp. ticks is rare or nonexistent. Ticks usually acquire the infection when they feed as larvae or nymphs on small mammals or birds. After the molt, nymphs or adults feed on other mammals and birds, thus perpetuating the *Borrelia* spp. in nature. The usual hosts for the adult ticks are large mammals, such as deer or sheep. Humans most commonly become infected through the bite of nymphs, which are small enough to go unnoticed. Unlike argasid ticks, which feed for only short periods of time and transmit the spirochetes from the start of feeding, ixodid ticks feed for several days before dropping off. *B. burgdorferi* and other Lyme borreliosis species must migrate from the midgut to the salivary glands over 1–2 days before they begin to enter the host.

Lyme borreliosis is the most common vector-borne disease in the United States, primarily in the northeastern and north-central regions, and throughout much of Europe.[30] The risk is highly focal, though, and depends on the characteristics of the environment and the degree of exposure to infected nymphs. A canopied forest with an undergrowth of grass and low shrubs is a typical landscape. Humans come in contact with ticks through recreational and work activities in this environment and also around their homes, which may abut forests and wood-stands. Unlike some *Ornithodoros* species, the *Ixodes* ticks that transmit Lyme borreliosis do not reside in dwellings.

Table 44.2 Clinical and Laboratory Features of Tick-Borne Relapsing Fever (RF), Louse-Borne RF, and Lyme Borreliosis

Characteristic	Tick-Borne RF	Louse-Borne RF	Lyme Borreliosis
Fever ≥39°C	Common	Common	Rare
Duration without treatment	Days–weeks	Days	Weeks–years
Fever relapses	Multiple	Few	None
Local skin rash	No	No	Common
Neurologic involvement	Common	Rare	Common
Joint involvement	No	No	Common
Spirochetes on blood smear	Yes	Yes	No
Antibiotic therapy	Several doses	Single or few doses	Several doses
Jarisch–Herxheimer reaction	Moderate	Moderate–severe	Mild or none

THE DISEASE

Table 44.2 summarizes the common and distinguishing features of tick-borne relapsing fever, louse-borne relapsing fever, and Lyme borreliosis. The hallmark of relapsing fever is the sudden onset of two or more episodes of fever spaced by afebrile periods. The temperature may reach 43°C and is usually above 39°C. In the louse-borne form the first episode of unremitting fever lasts 3–6 days and is typically followed by a single milder episode. During tick-borne relapsing fever there are multiple febrile periods of 1–3 days each. *Figure 44.5* shows the temperature pattern of two cases of tick-borne relapsing fever. In both forms of relapsing fever the intervals between fevers are generally from 4 to 14 days. The first fever episode ends by crisis, which is characterized by rigors, hyperpyrexia, and elevations of pulse and blood pressure over about

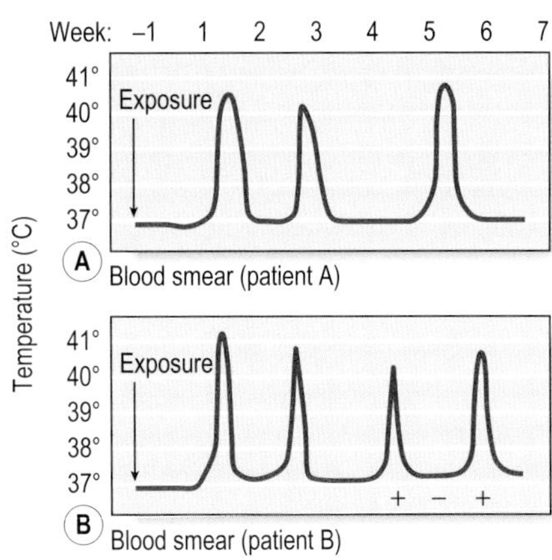

Figure 44.5 (A and B) Temperature curves in two cases of tick-borne relapsing fever. The exposure to ticks occurred 1 week before onset of first fever. Wright-stained blood smears of the patient in **B** were examined and were assessed as positive (+) or negative (–) with respect to the presence of spirochetes (see Fig. 44.7).

15–30 minutes. This phase is followed by a few to several hours of profuse diaphoresis, falling temperature, and hypotension. Deaths from untreated relapsing fever are most common during the crisis and its immediate aftermath.

Accompanying the first and subsequent fevers may be headache, neck stiffness, arthralgia, and myalgia. The patient may complain of dizziness and have an unsteady gait. On examination the patient may be delirious, apathetic, or stuporous. Most patients with relapsing fever have splenomegaly, which may present as abdominal or left shoulder pain. More than half of patients with louse-borne relapsing fever and about 10% of patients with tick-borne relapsing fever have enlarged liver, and clinical or laboratory evidence of hepatitis. Cholestasis is not prominent.

In louse-borne relapsing fever, epistaxis, skin petechiae and/or ecchymoses are common. They probably are attributable to thrombocytopenia, impaired production of clotting factors by the liver, and/or blockage of small vessels by aggregates of spirochetes. Platelet counts may fall below 50 000/μL. In both forms of relapsing fever leukocyte counts are usually in the normal range or only slightly elevated; there may be leukopenia during the crisis.

Although louse-borne relapsing fever patients often present with a clouded sensorium, this is probably attributable to microemboli and proinflammatory cytokines rather than spirochete invasion of the brain.[31] Direct neurologic involvement is more common in tick-borne relapsing fever. Meningitis or meningoencephalitis are consequences of this invasion. There may be residual hemiplegia or aphasia. Cranial neuritis, most commonly of the seventh or eighth cranial nerves, typically first appears during the second or third febrile period of tick-borne relapsing fever. The presentation is unilateral or bilateral Bell's palsy or deafness. Other neurologic manifestations during tick-borne relapsing fever are radiculopathy and myelitis. Iridocyclitis or panophthalmitis may leave the patient visually impaired.

Myocarditis appears to be common in louse-borne and tick-borne relapsing fever and may be the proximate cause of death in some fatal cases.[32] The most common evidence of myocarditis are gallops on cardiac auscultation and a prolonged QT_c interval. Some patients have cardiomegaly and pulmonary edema. Acute respiratory distress syndrome may occur in the absence of evidence of myocarditis.[33] Relapsing fever during pregnancy frequently leads to abortion or stillbirth in experimental infections and human cases. There may be transplacental transmission of the infection or a newborn may be infected at birth.[34–37] Congenital malformations as a consequence of relapsing fever have not been reported.

During early infection with *B. burgdorferi*, *B. afzelii*, or *B. garinii*, the most frequent skin manifestation is erythema migrans, an erythematous patch or target-like skin lesion of 2 cm or more diameter at the site of the tick bite.[38] After dissemination of the microorganisms, erythema migrans lesions may appear in numerous locations. Temperatures of 39°C or higher are uncommon during Lyme borreliosis. Other manifestations of the early disseminated stage are polyarthralgias, radiculopathy, cranial nerve palsies, meningoencephalitis, and myocarditis.[4,5,39] The greatest morbidity with Lyme borreliosis occurs in patients with late or chronic infections, i.e., those lasting months to years. In these patients there may be chronic pauciarticular arthritis, debilitating dysfunction of the central and/or peripheral nervous system, or a persistent inflammatory skin disorder, acrodermatitis chronica atrophicans.

PATHOGENESIS

A *Borrelia* infection of humans almost always begins with contact with a tick or louse bearing the spirochetes. Rarely the disease is acquired through (1) accidental inoculation of infected blood, (2) contact of blood with abraded or lacerated skin, mucous membranes, or the conjunctiva, or (3) transplacental or perinatal transmission from mother to fetus.[34,35] Transmission to humans by aerosol, fomites, human saliva, urine, feces, or sexual contact has not been documented.

A single spirochete is sufficient to initiate relapsing fever.[6] Having gained access to the blood, the organisms multiply there at a rate of one cell division every 6–12 hours until they number 10^5 to 10^8/mL blood. The incubation period between exposure and the first fever is between 3 and 12 days. From the blood the spirochetes may invade the central nervous system (CNS), eye, liver, and other organs. Aggregations of *Borrelia* with erythrocytes or platelets produce microemboli.[40,41] Live and dead spirochetes may accumulate in large numbers in the spleen and liver as the microemboli, immune complexes, and other aggregates are filtered out of the blood.

Recurrence of fever after the initial immune response is the result of the recovery of the spirochete population in the blood. Early microbiologists recognized that the new crop of *Borrelia* were antigenically distinct from the original infecting organism.[42] Populations that predominate during each relapse are assigned different serotype names. For example, a rat infected with serotype A had serotypes B and C in the blood during the first relapse and second relapse, respectively. There is a rough order to the appearance of serotypes during infection, but it is not absolutely fixed. Characteristically, antiserum to serotype A could passively protect mice from infection with serotype A but not serotypes B or C. Similarly, antisera against serotypes C or B were effective against the homologous serotype but not against others.

The varying antigens that determine serotype identity are a set of outer membrane lipoproteins called variable membrane proteins.[43] These proteins are of two sizes: variable small proteins (Vsp) of about 20 kDa and variable large proteins (Vlp) of about 40 kDa.[44] A single strain of *B. hermsii* may be capable of producing thirty to forty different variable major proteins, about equally divided in number between Vsps and Vlps. There can be as little as 30% identity in amino acid sequences between two different variable major proteins of the same strain of a relapsing fever *Borrelia* sp., which accounts for the lack of cross-reactivity between antisera.[45,46]

There is a complete or near-complete gene for each Vsp or Vlp protein.[47] In any single cell only one of the genes is expressed, usually at a site near the end of a linear plasmid. The thirty or forty other *vsp* and *vlp* genes in the genome are silent in their storage locations on other plasmids. The expression site, in distinction to the silent sites, has a promoter in front of the *vsp* or *vlp* gene. A different *vsp* or *vlp* gene spontaneously replaces the one at the expression site at an estimated frequency of 10^{-4} to 10^{-3} per cell generation.[46] The newly appearing serotype is still in low numbers at the time the immune system responds to the first serotype with an outpouring of antibodies, and thus escapes as the original infecting serotype is cleared from the blood.

There are two ways in which a gene at the expression site is replaced by another.[48] The most common mechanism is a nonreciprocal, unidirectional recombination between two linear plasmids. A simplified

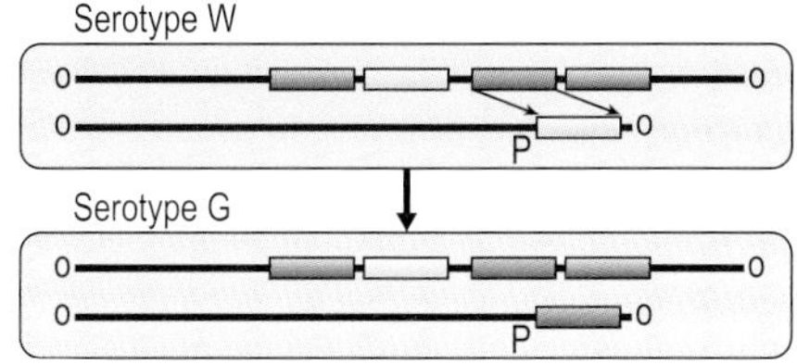

Figure 44.6 Schematic representation of molecular events in an antigenic switch from serotype W (yellow) or serotype G (orange) in relapsing fever *Borrelia* spp. In this switch, there is an intermolecular gene conversion in which the donor sequence is a silent *vmp* gene in a tandem array of silent genes, which are denoted by yellow, blue, or orange or pink boxes, on a linear plasmid. The target sequence is an extra copy of the yellow *vmp* gene that is next to the telomere (O) of another linear plasmid and downstream from a promoter (P). The *vmp* gene at the silent location is unchanged in the recombination.

representation of such a switch in these genes is shown in ***Figure 44.6***. The boundaries for the recombination are blocks of sequence identity between silent and expression sites around and flanking the 5′ and 3′ ends of the expressed and silent genes.[47] The loose programming of the appearance of serotypes is determined by the combination of (1) the degree of sequence identity between the 5′ ends of silent and expressed genes and (2) the distance between the end of the silent gene and the next recombination block to the 3′ direction.[49]

The second mechanism by which a new variable major protein gene is expressed is intramolecular rather than the intermolecular recombination between two plasmids. For the second mechanism to occur, there must be untranscribed gene downstream from the expressed gene and in the same orientation.[50] A deletion between short direct repeats at the 5′ ends of each of the two genes effectively excises the sitting gene. The one behind moves up with deletion to take its place next to the promoter.

Variable membrane proteins also have a role in tissue localization during infection. Within a given species, certain serotypes can invade the brain, while other serotypes, identical but for the variable membrane protein, cannot.[51] Some species of *Borrelia*, such as *B. duttonii* in Africa and *B. turicatae* in North America, are particularly neurotropic.[31]

The presentation of Lyme borreliosis is categorized as early localized, early disseminated, and late disease, according to the duration and extent of the infection.[5] It begins locally as a rash about 1–2 weeks after a tick has attached for >24 hours. In the skin the spirochetes move centrifugally, thus enlarging the diameter of the lesion over several days to weeks. In some patients the borrelias also circulate in the blood during acute infection but at a density that is undetectable by light microscopy of blood. If fever occurs, it is mild. During the bacteremia, the infection disseminates to other organs and tissues, commonly the joints, heart, and nerves and brain. Late manifestations of Lyme borreliosis are the result of persistence of spirochetes and the provocation of inflammation in the tissues and organs, mainly the brain, nerves, skin, heart, and large joints, rather than reappearance of spirochetes in the blood.

IMMUNITY

In animals infected with relapsing fever *Borrelia* spp., IgM antibodies alone are sufficient to limit or eliminate infection from the blood.[52,53] Experimental animals with deficient T-cell function, such as nude mice, clear spirochetes from the blood as effectively as their immunocompetent counterparts.[54] Because specific antibodies, even Fab monomers, to outer membrane proteins can kill borrelias in the absence of complement or phagocytes,[53,55] deficiencies in the latter immune effectors may not hinder clearance of borrelias from the blood. Host defense deficiencies that do increase severity of relapsing fever are asplenia and impaired B-cell function. During infection animals and human patients have antibodies to a number of different components of spirochetes, but only those directed against the Vsp and Vlp appear to be effective in controlling infection.[46,52]

The immune response often is not successful in clearing borrelias from the brain, cerebrospinal fluid (CSF), or eye.[31]

Infection with *B. burgdorferi* or related species is more severe in mice with profound immune deficiencies, but the infection is not fatal. For immunocompetent mice, tissue pathology and spirochete burden is determined by genetic factors of both the host and the pathogen.[56] Experimental animals are passively protected against infection by immune sera or monoclonal antibodies alone. Immunity is usually strain-specific. While cell-mediated immunity to *B. burgdorferi* appears not to play a necessary or even sufficient role in an effective immune response to infection or vaccination, T-cell responses to a pathogen or host antigen may be responsible for a form of reactive arthritis of one or a few large joints that a minority of untreated patients in North America experience.[57]

PATHOLOGY

In fatal cases of relapsing fever gross findings include widespread petechiae, enlarged spleen and liver, and an edematous, congested brain.[3,31,58] The most common histologic findings in fatal cases are swelling of endothelial cells, microvascular leakage, perivascular mononuclear cell infiltrates, microabscesses, and hemorrhages. Fatal cases of louse-borne relapsing fever frequently have myocarditis with histiocytic infiltrates and microhemorrhages. The spleen and liver, but seldom the kidneys or adrenals, often have focal areas of necrosis. Although bleeding is a common complication of louse-borne relapsing fever, evidence of intravascular coagulation is not prominent.

The spirochetes can be detected in tissue sections with silver stains or by immunofluorescence. Borrelias move through or between endothelial cells as they leave the blood for tissues, but they do not appear to proliferate in these or phagocytic cells. The spirochetes are usually found in perivascular locations, sometimes as tangles of bacteria. In autopsy cases and experimentally infected animals, spirochetes are commonly found in the spleen, liver, brain, eye, and kidney. In the brain the spirochetes are around the meninges.[31,59] The severity of relapsing fever generally correlates directly with the numbers of spirochetes in the blood.[60]

Fatalities from Lyme borreliosis itself are extremely rare. The usual pathologic specimen is a skin biopsy, which if taken from the leading edge of the expanding skin rash, can reveal spirochetes by silver stain or immunofluorescence.[38] Biopsies of synovial tissue of patients with frank arthritis reveal acute and chronic inflammation with proliferative synovium.[57] The presence of spirochetes in joint tissue can be demonstrated by polymerase chain reaction (PCR) but almost never by microscopy.

DIAGNOSIS

Recurrent fevers at intervals of a few to several days suggest the diagnosis of relapsing fever. If these are accompanied by the crisis phenomenon, hepatomegaly or splenomegaly, cranial neuritis in the case of tick-borne relapsing fever, or jaundice and petechiae in the case of louse-borne relapsing fever, and an epidemiologic history of exposure to body lice or soft-bodied ticks, then relapsing fever is highly likely. Relapsing fever may be confused with rickettsioses, malaria, typhoid, brucellosis, Colorado tick fever, dengue, leptospirosis, rat-bite fever, or meningococcemia, depending on the epidemiologic circumstances. Coinfection with malaria parasites may occur with either tick- or louse-borne relapsing fever.[61,62] Patients with louse-borne relapsing fever may have epidemic typhus as well.

In early localized Lyme borreliosis there is usually, but not always, erythema migrans, and mild fever. In early disseminated Lyme borreliosis, polyarthralgia, multiple erythma migrans lesions, symptoms and signs of meningeal irritation, radiculopathy, seventh or other cranial nerve palsy, and heart block may occur singly or in different combinations. Late Lyme arthritis may resemble pauciarticular rheumatoid arthritis, juvenile rheumatoid arthritis, or reactive arthritis. The diagnosis of "chronic Lyme disease" has been applied by some practitioners to long-standing disorders with nonspecific symptoms, such as malaise, poor

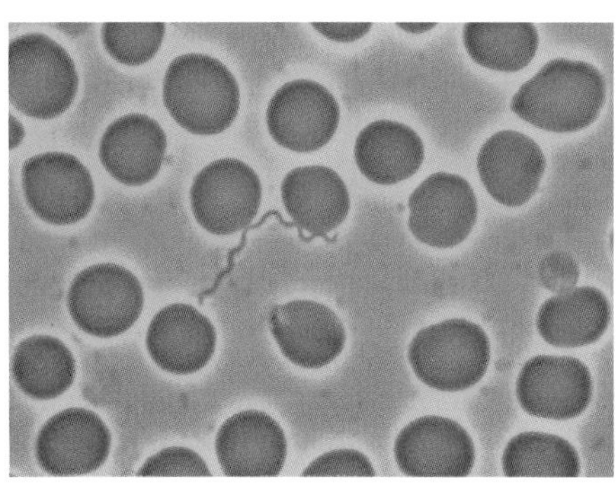

Figure 44.7 A single *Borrelia hermsii* spirochete in a Wright-stained thin blood smear of a case of tick-borne relapsing fever.

concentration, myalgias, and easy fatigability. When empirical antibiotic therapy fails in these cases, there is little or no evidence that these symptoms are attributable to active infection with a *Borrelia* species.[63,64] The few geographic areas where transmission of both Lyme borreliosis and relapsing fever occur are far western North America and some areas bordering the Mediterranean.

If the diagnosis of relapsing fever is suspected, a smear or wet-mount of blood that is obtained during a febrile period should be prepared. Once the temperature is declining or has returned to normal range in absence of antipyretics, visual detection of spirochetes in unconcentrated blood is unlikely. Giemsa or Wright stain of a methanol-fixed thin smear reveals the spirochetes if their density in the blood is greater than 10^5/mL (***Fig. 44.7***). In health facilities with automated blood smear analysis, a manual examination of the blood smear should be requested. With a thick smear, concentrations of 10^4 or more organisms per milliliter of blood can be detected. The smear is treated with acridine orange or fluorescein-labeled anti-*Borrelia* antibody and then examined under ultraviolet light.[46,65] After low-speed centrifugation of anticoagulated blood followed by high-speed centrifugation of the resultant plasma provides a pellet for staining and microscopic examination, as few as 10 spirochetes/mL may be detected.[66]

Phase contrast or dark field microscopy reveals motile spirochetes in blood diluted ~1:1 in phosphate-buffered saline under a coverslip and examined at approximately ×400 magnification. Coiling and bending movements of the spirochetes as they swim among the erythrocytes are tell-tale signs. Centrifugation of the anticoagulated blood in a capillary tube and examination of the buffy coat increases the sensitivity of microscopy to 10^3 spirochetes/mL.[67] When relapsing fever is suspected, inoculation of blood or CSF into young mice, rats, or Syrian hamsters may reveal a *Borrelia* sp. Infection of the mouse can be enhanced by the severe combined immunodeficiency phenotype or splenectomy.[46,51,68] Blood of the inoculated mice is examined daily for presence of the spirochetes for 1 week.

In vitro cultivation is an alternative for recovery of the organism from the blood, but it is not widely available. Kelly's medium and its derivative, Barbour–Stoenner–Kelly medium, support the growth of most *Borrelia* spp.[69,70] Selection against contaminants is achieved by supplementation of the medium with rifampin, phosphomycin, an aminoglycoside, and/or amphotericin B. Tubes of medium are inoculated with several drops of blood or other specimen and incubated at 34–37°C in tightly capped tubes for up to 2 weeks. More rapid than culture for direct detection is PCR, which is increasing in use for diagnosis.[17,71,72] PCR of DNA extracts of the blood or from culture medium provides a means for identification of the species of *Borrelia* on the basis of DNA sequences.[73]

Serologic assays are seldom used for relapsing fever. Enyzme-linked immunosorbent assays (ELISA) and immunofluorescence assays based on whole cell antigen are available at some reference laboratories, but they are not standardized. An immunoassay using a recombinant form of GlpQ protein, which is found in relapsing fever *Borrelia* spp. but not in the Lyme disease *Borrelia* spp., demonstrates higher specificity than whole cell assays in studies of both tick-borne and louse-borne relapsing fever.[15,74]

In contrast to relapsing fever, laboratory confirmation of the diagnosis of Lyme borreliosis usually rests on measurement of antibodies to a Lyme borreliosis *Borrelia* sp. and not direct recovery or detection of the agent itself. Serologic testing is widely available, and the options are the following: (1) a whole cell-based ELISA followed by confirmatory immunoblot for those samples with positive or borderline reactions, and (2) a subunit ELISA based on a conserved region of Vls proteins of *B. burgdorferi* or a combination of recombinant antigens.[75,76]

Analysis of the CSF is indicated in cases of suspected relapsing fever or Lyme borreliosis when there are signs of meningitis or meningoencephalitis.[31,39] Documentation of mononuclear pleocytosis and/or mildly to moderately elevated protein concentration in the CSF provides justification for use of intravenous antibiotic therapy of tick-borne relapsing fever and Lyme borreliosis (see below). CSF analysis under these conditions also rules out most other nonviral infectious causes of meningitis.

TREATMENT AND PROGNOSIS

Paul Ehrlich and colleagues successfully used organic arsenicals to treat patients with relapsing fever, but since the advent of antibiotics beta-lactam and tetracycline compounds have been the drugs of choice for *Borrelia* infections. Minimum inhibitory concentrations of penicillin and tetracycline for *Borrelia* spp. are less than 0.1 μg/mL.[6,69,77] Relapsing fever *Borrelia* spp. are also susceptible to macrolides, chloramphenicol, coumermycins, and vancomycin, but there is less experience with these antibiotics. Borrelias are not susceptible to rifampin, metronidazole, and sulfa drugs and are relatively resistant to most quinolones and aminoglycosides. There is no evidence that *Borrelia* spp. have acquired resistance to any antibiotics. For relapsing fever, within 4–8 hours of the first dose of an effective antibiotic most patients will no longer have detectable spirochetes in the blood.

Single doses of 100 mg of doxycycline, 500 mg of tetracycline, or 500 mg of erythromycin stearate or ethyl succinate are effective oral antibiotics for adults with louse-borne relapsing fever.[78–80] For all children the oral dose of erythromycin is 12.5 mg/kg up to 500 mg. For children older than 8 years the oral dose of doxycycline is 2 mg/kg up to 100 mg, and the oral dose of tetracycline is 12.5 mg/kg up to 500 mg. An alternative single dose oral treatment is chloramphenicol at 500 mg for adults and 12.5–25 mg/kg up to 500 mg for children.[81] The overall recurrence rate after therapy is less than 5%. Tetracyclines appear to have better efficacy and are preferred over erythromycin, except for pregnant and nursing women and for children under 9 years old. When the patient cannot take tetracycline by mouth, the intravenous dose is 250 or 500 mg for adults. Parenteral treatment with intramuscular penicillin G procaine is 600 000–800 000 units for adults and 400 000 units for children.

Tick-borne relapsing fever cases occur sporadically or in limited outbreaks. Accumulated anecdotal experience suggests that the recurrence rate is 20% or more after single dose treatments.[15,58,82] From their residence in the brain, spirochetes can reinvade the blood once antibiotic levels have declined below minimum inhibitory concentrations.[83] The preferred treatment for non-pregnant, non-lactating patients aged 9 years or older is tetracycline 500 mg or 12.5 mg/kg, orally every 6 hours for 10 days, or doxycycline 100 mg or 4 mg/kg, twice daily for 10 days. When tetracyclines are contraindicated, the alternative is erythromycin 500 mg or 12.5 mg/kg, orally every 6 hours for 10 days. Beta-lactam antibiotics are administered parenterally rather than orally and are drugs of choice, if central nervous system involvement is suspected, and there are no contraindications. There are no published trials of treatment of relapsing fever with CNS involvement, but the protocol for therapy of Lyme borreliosis with this complication (see below) would likely be effective.

In general the treatment of Lyme borreliosis is similar to the treatment of tick-borne relapsing fever, except that tetracycline and beta-lactam antibiotics are usually favored over macrolide antibiotics.[39,84,85] For early localized or early disseminated disease the recommended oral antibiotic treatment for non-pregnant, non-lactating patients aged 9 years or older is doxycycline, 100 mg maximum or 4 mg/kg twice daily, amoxicillin, 500 mg maximum or 16.7 mg/kg three times daily, or cefuroxime axetil, 500 mg maximum or 15 mg/kg twice daily, for 14–21 days. Children younger than 9 years and pregnant or lactating women are treated with amoxicillin or cefuroxime axetil. For disseminated early disease when CNS involvement is suspected or when patients are hospitalized with atrioventricular heart block and/or myopericarditis, parenteral antibiotics are administered: penicillin G 3–4 million units maximum or 33 000–67 000 units/kg every 4 hours, ceftriaxone 2 g maximum or 50–75 mg/kg, once a day or in two divided doses, or cefotaxime 2 g maximum or 50–67 mg/kg every 6 or 8 hours for 10–14 days. Late Lyme borreliosis with arthritis and without clinical evidence of neurologic involvement can be treated with oral antibiotics as described for early disease but for 28 days. For late neurologic disease parenteral therapy is administered for 2–4 weeks.

Jarisch–Herxheimer Reaction

Relapsing fever is one of the few infections for which antibiotic therapy poses a significant risk of death or further morbidity, for reasons other than anaphylaxis or overdosage. Within a few hours of the first dose of an antibiotic, 80–90% of patients with louse-borne relapsing fever and 30–40% of patients with tick-borne relapsing fever experience a worsening of symptoms.[86,87] In a minority of patients the reaction is life-threatening or fatal. A mild Jarisch–Herxheimer reaction (J-HR) occurs during the first day or two after start of antibiotics for some patients with early localized or disseminated Lyme borreliosis.

J-HR is essentially the same as the "crisis" that shortly follows the appearance of neutralizing antibodies in the blood. In both situations the borrelias are lysed and their contents are released into the circulation. Within 1–2 hours the patient experiences intense rigors and becomes restless and apprehensive. The temperature elevates 1–2°C, and the pulse rate and blood pressure rise. This is followed over the next few hours by profuse sweating, exhaustion, a decline in temperature, fall in blood pressure, and leukopenia. In an animal model of the J-HR, the same changes in temperature and white blood cell count occur after treatment of infected mice with antibiotics or infusion of ruptured spirochetes.

The abundant lipoproteins of the spirochetes likely act on the Toll-like 2 receptors of macrophages and other cells.[9,50] This ligand–receptor binding induces the release of inflammatory cytokines.[88,89] Levels of tumor necrosis factor (TNF), interleukin (IL)-6, and IL-8 rise several-fold over pretreatment levels during the J-HR in patients treated for louse-borne relapsing fever.[90] The anti-inflammatory cytokine IL-10 rises to high levels in response and partially mitigates deleterious proinflammatory effects.[91]

Therapy with penicillin in comparison to tetracyclines has a somewhat lower risk of producing a severe J-HR,[80] but this may be at the cost of a delay in illness resolution and possibly a higher disease recurrence risk.[80,92] Administration of corticosteroids, pentoxifylline, antipyretics, or naloxone have been of limited or no benefit in reducing morbidity or mortality from J-HR. Infusion of antibodies to human TNF prior to administration of penicillin reduced the severity of J-HR in a clinical trial,[93] but this treatment is expensive.

Anticipation of the reaction and provision of monitoring or constant nursing attention will permit resuscitative measures, such as volume expansion and digoxin, to be started.[29] Placement of an intravenous line with infusion of saline before administering the antibiotic is recommended. The pathophysiology of J-HR includes dilatation of the vasculature and low systemic resistance, increased tissue demands for oxygen from fever and inflammation, and myocardial dysfunction. If each of these aspects is addressed, as for example by increasing the blood volume, providing an inotropic agent, and reduction of core body temperature by tepid water sponge baths or acetaminophen, the chances of recovery from a severe J-HR or from a severe crisis are improved.

PROGNOSIS

Untreated louse-borne relapsing fever and tick-borne relapsing fever historically have had mortality rates of 10–70% and 4–10%, respectively. With timely treatment with appropriate antibiotics, the death rates are reduced to 2–5% for the louse-borne form and to less than 2% for tick-borne relapsing fever. Malnourished individuals, infants, and pregnant women are at a higher risk of more severe disease.[28] Prognosis is poorer if the patient is stuporous or comatose on admission or if there is diffuse bleeding, myocarditis, poor hepatic function, bronchopneumonia, or coinfection with typhus, typhoid, or malaria. The mortality rate from J-HR in louse-borne relapsing fever is approximately 5%. Some patients have survived the crisis or J-HR, only to die suddenly later that day or next, perhaps from an arrhythmia.

Mortality from Lyme borreliosis is rare. There have been no recorded fatalities from J-HR with Lyme borreliosis. Some patients with chronic pauciarticular arthritis do not substantially benefit in the short term from one or two courses of antibiotic therapy, but many eventually show improvement.

PREVENTION AND CONTROL

Louse-borne relapsing fever can be prevented by avoiding infestation or contact with human body lice. Although humans are reservoirs of the infection, there is no direct human-to-human transmission, with the exception of transplacental or perinatal transmission or contact with blood. The body louse lives in clothing and only attaches to the body when feeding. Reduction of crowding, improved personal hygiene, and better access to washing facilities greatly decrease the potential for louse-borne diseases. More specific and immediate measures for de-lousing patients and household or shelter contacts are bathing, shaving of the scalp, and application of one of the following: 1% lindane shampoo (Kwell) or powder; 0.5% permethrin powder; 1% permethrin soap, lotion, or shampoo; 10% DDT powder; 5% carbaryl powder; or 1% malathion powder.[58,94] The insecticides can be mixed with talcum powder. Infested clothes and bedding materials should be washed in water at a temperature of at least 60°C with either soap or 7% (w/v) DDT. If possible, the clothing and bedding should then be ironed.

Log cabins and similar wood structures in forested areas with enzootic transmission are a particular risk for tick-borne relapsing fever when rodents nest in roofs, walls, and woodpiles, under eaves and porches, and in burrows under the house. In other natural environments ticks may be in caves or natural shelters where animals sleep and nest. In inhabited areas the ticks may be in thatched roofs, mud walls, and crawl spaces under houses. In more agrarian environments, domestic animals, such as pigs, goats, and sheep, may be reservoirs for infection of humans, if the livestock are adjacent to the living quarters, and the ticks have access to the human household as well as the livestock. Sleeping on floors of buildings with suspected infestation should be avoided. Beds are preferably metal and at a distance from walls. Insecticide-impregnated mosquito nets around the bed may be useful. For entry into infested caves, DEET can be applied to the exposed skin, and permethrin can be sprayed on clothing. Efforts should be made to make the structure rodent-proof.[95,96] Interiors of buildings infested with *Ornithodoros* ticks can be sprayed or fumigated with 0.5% diazinon, 0.5% malathion, or 0.5% lindane.

When *Ornithodoros* tick bites occur, such as during exploration of a cave or vacation in a cabin located in an area endemic with tick-borne relapsing fever, prophylactic doxycycline (200 mg orally the first day and then 100 mg a day for 4 days), or as an alternative, tetracycline (500 mg orally four times daily for 3 days), will reduce the risk of infection if taken within 2 days of the exposure by nonpregnant individuals 9 years of age or greater.[97] This regimen may also prevent illness after accidental inoculation with infected blood or culture medium in the laboratory, hospital, or clinic. At present there is not a vaccine for either louse-borne relapsing fever or tick-borne relapsing fever.

Prevention of Lyme borreliosis depends on avoidance of tick bites in endemic areas through (1) personal protection measures, such as application of repellents, appropriate clothing, and inspection for ticks after exposures, (2) community and residential acaricides and landscape management, (3) reduction in the numbers or competencies of reservoir and vector hosts, and (4) prophylactic antibiotics for higher-risk tick bites.[5,98] A vaccine against Lyme borreliosis was approved for commercial use in the United States, but it is no longer on the market or available.

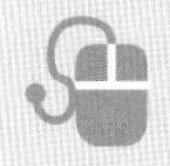

Access the complete reference list online at
http://www.expertconsult.com

Access the complete reference list online at http://www.expertconsult.com

CHAPTER 45

Leptospirosis

Wun-Ju Shieh • Charles Edwards • Paul N. Levett • Sherif R. Zaki

INTRODUCTION

Leptospirosis is a zoonotic disease caused by pathogenic spirochetes of the genus *Leptospira*. In 1907, Stimson described the microorganism in renal tubules of a patient who died of so-called yellow fever.[1] The spirochete was first isolated in Japan by Inada and coworkers in 1915,[2] nearly 30 years after Weil described the clinical disease in 1886.[3] Its relatively recent discovery belies the long history of leptospirosis, which was probably known much earlier in China and Japan by names such as "rice harvest jaundice" and "autumn fever."[4,5]

THE AGENT

Leptospires (from the Greek *leptos*, fine, and *speira*, a coil) are thin, finely coiled, filamentous spirochetes measuring 6–20 × 0.1 μm, with characteristic curved or hooked ends. The genus *Leptospira* contains both pathogenic and nonpathogenic strains. Traditionally, pathogenic leptospires have been included in the species *L. interrogans*, which contains at least 250 antigenically distinct variants known as serovars.[6,7] The genus *Leptospira* was reclassified, based on DNA relatedness,[8–10] into 16 species, including at least seven pathogenic species: *L. interrogans, L. borgpeterseni, L. inadai, L. noguchii, L. santarosai, L. weillii,* and *L. kirschneri*. Identification of *Leptospira* isolates is important because different serovars cause different clinical diseases and have different host specificities.

EPIDEMIOLOGY

Leptospirosis is an infectious disease of worldwide distribution (***Fig. 45.1***). Because it is most prevalent in areas where diagnostic capabilities are limited, and because its clinical presentation varies, few reliable data on its global incidence are available. Nevertheless, this disease has been described as the most common zoonosis affecting many species of wild and domestic animals, such as rodents, livestock, wild mammals, dogs, and cats.[6] Human infection can occur either through direct contact with infected animals or, much more commonly, through indirect contact with water or soil contaminated by the urine of infected animals.[11] Person-to-person transmission is extremely rare since the human is a dead-end host for leptospiral dissemination.[5] In contrast, leptospires can survive for long periods in the renal tubules of infected animals without causing illness. Most human infections occur in young adult men and children and result from occupational or environmental exposure.[11] Epidemiologic studies indicate that infection is commonly associated with certain occupations, such as farmer, sewage worker, veterinarian, and animal handler. Leptospirosis can also be transmitted during recreational activities, such as hiking, picnicking, swimming, and canoeing.[12–15]

Leptospires can survive in untreated water for months or years, but they cannot survive desiccation or salt water.[11] Only sporadic cases of leptospirosis occur in arid climates and deserts. In comparison, the disease is endemic in tropical and temperate areas, areas with heavy precipitation, and areas with high levels of subsurface water. Hence, China, Southeast Asia, Africa, and South and Central America have immense areas where the disease is endemic. Leptospirosis occurs sporadically in these areas, with a peak seasonal incidence in summer; large epidemics have been reported after periods of unusually heavy rainfall and monsoons.

THE DISEASE

The incubation period of leptospirosis ranges from 2 to 26 days (usually 7–12). In general, it can be divided into two distinct clinical syndromes: 90% of patients present with a mild anicteric febrile illness, and 10% are severely ill with jaundice and other manifestations (Weil's syndrome). Both anicteric and icteric leptospirosis may follow a biphasic course. In the first or septicemic phase, patients usually present with an abrupt onset of fever, chills, headache, myalgias, skin rashes, nausea, vomiting, conjunctival suffusion, and prostration. The fever may be high and remittent, reaching a peak of 40°C before defervescence. Conjunctival suffusion (***Fig. 45.2***) is characteristic and usually appears on the third or fourth day. Myalgias usually involve the muscles in the calf, abdomen, and paraspinal region and can be severe. When present in the neck, myalgias may cause nuchal rigidity reminiscent of meningitis. In the abdomen, myalgia may mimic acute abdomen, leading to confusion with surgical intraabdominal emergencies.[15–17] The cutaneous manifestations in mild leptospirosis include transient urticarial, macular or maculopapular, erythematous, or purpuric rash.[18] The first phase lasts 3–9 days, followed by 2 or 3 days of defervescence, after which the second or "immune" phase develops. The second phase is characterized by leptospiruria and correlates with the appearance of immunoglobulin M (IgM) antibodies in the serum. Fever and earlier constitutional symptoms recur in some patients, and signs of meningitis, such as headaches, photophobia, and nuchal rigidity, may develop. Central nervous system involvement in leptospirosis most commonly occurs as aseptic meningitis.[19–21] Complications such as optic neuritis, uveitis,[22,23] iridocyclitis,[24] chorioretinitis,[25] and peripheral neuropathy occur more frequently in the immune phase[26] (***Fig. 45.3***). Prolonged or recurrent uveitis was demonstrated in 2% of patients with onset several months after symptoms of clinical leptospirosis.[27]

In icteric leptospirosis, persistent high fever and jaundice may obscure the two phases.[26] The severe form of leptospirosis is usually associated with hepatic dysfunction, renal insufficiency, hemorrhage, myocarditis,[28,29] and a high mortality. Hemorrhage can occur as petechiae, purpura, conjunctival hemorrhage, gastrointestinal hemorrhage, and pulmonary hemorrhage. Severe pulmonary hemorrhage has been described in China,[30] Korea,[31] and since 1996 in Nicaragua,[32,33] where patients died of pulmonary hemorrhage with no significant renal dysfunction or jaundice (***Fig. 45.4***). Other less common manifestations of leptospirosis are generalized lymphadenopathy,[32,34] pharyngitis, acalculous cholecystitis,[17,35] and adult respiratory distress syndrome.[36]

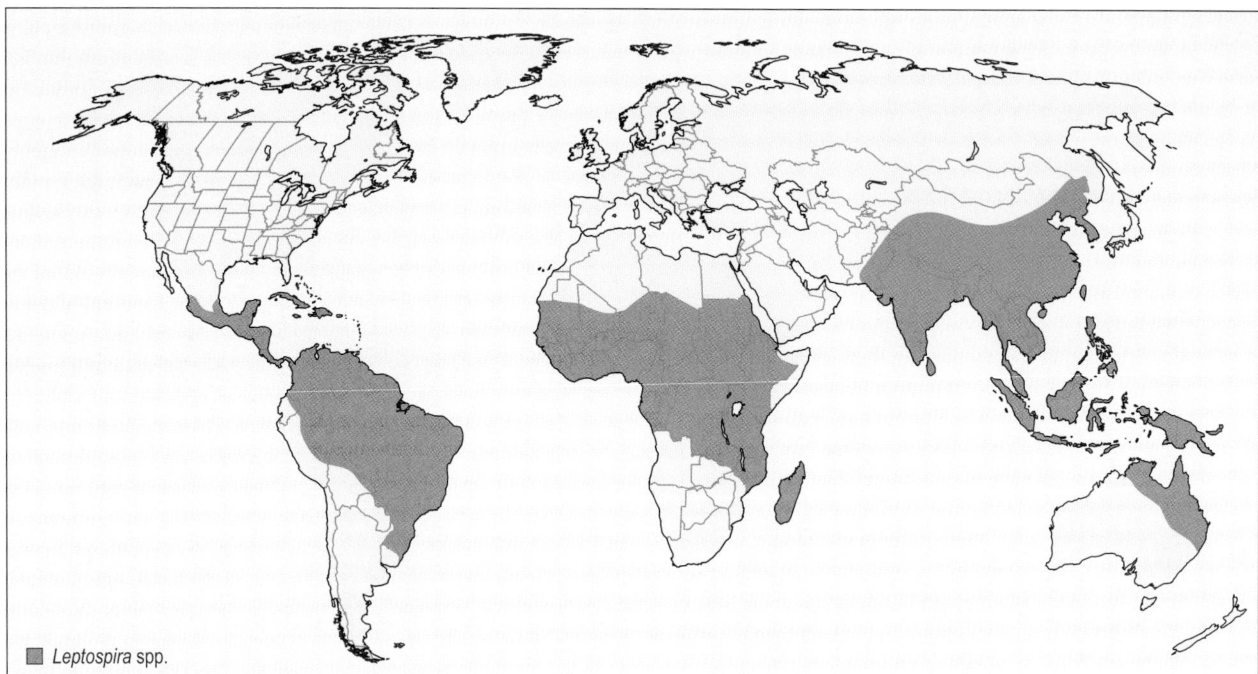

Figure 45.1 Geographic distribution of leptospirosis.

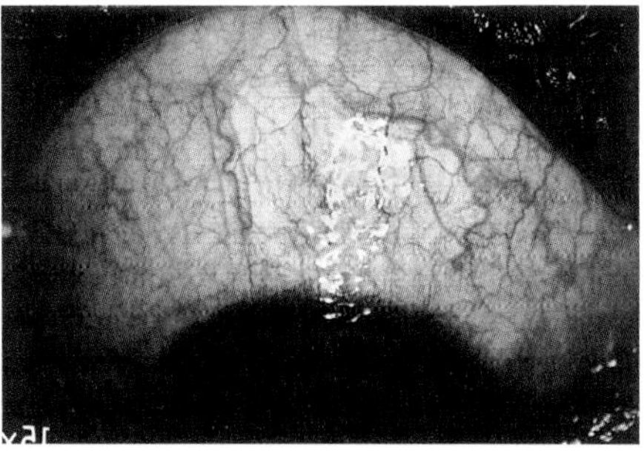

Figure 45.2 Jaundice and conjunctival suffusion in severe leptospirosis.

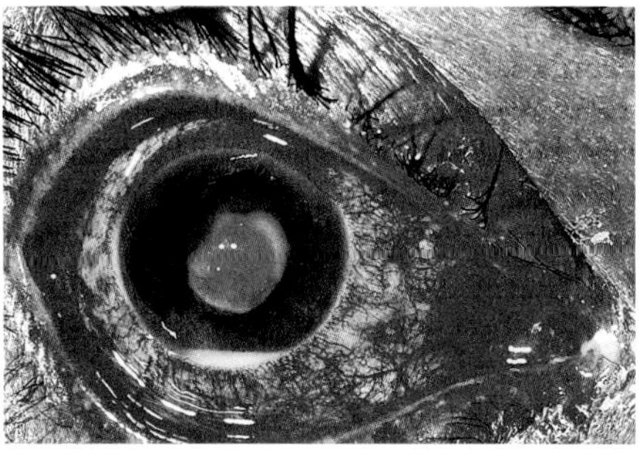

Figure 45.3 Hypopyon uveitis with posterior synechiae. (Courtesy of Dr S. R. Rathinam, Aravind Eye Hospital, Madurai, India.)

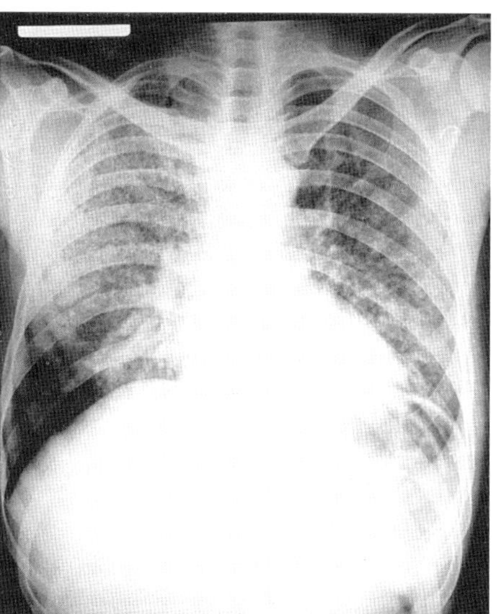

Figure 45.4 Bilateral pulmonary infiltrates as seen in chest radiograph of a patient who died of massive pulmonary hemorrhage.

Most of the routine laboratory tests show nonspecific findings. The white blood cell count can be low, normal, or elevated, but it is usually associated with a left shift. Mild anemia and thrombocytopenia are common; hemolytic anemia and disseminated intravascular coagulation have been described in severe cases.[37] Thrombocytopenia is observed in more than 50% of patients and is significantly associated with renal failure.[38,39] Liver, renal, and central nervous system involvement may be present in any combination. Liver involvement may be mild or severe, with bilirubin levels reaching 60–80 mg/dL in extreme cases.[40] Hepatomegaly occurs more often in icteric disease but is observed in as many as 15% of anicteric cases. Serum alkaline phosphatase, lactate dehydrogenase, aspartate aminotransferase, and alanine aminotransferase may all be elevated.[41] Usually, the levels are two or three times greater than the upper limits of normal and infrequently reach the higher ranges typical of acute viral hepatitis. Hyperamylasemia occurs frequently in severe disease, but pancreatitis is rare. Proteinuria, pyuria, hematuria, and hyaline or granular casts are common findings on urinalysis, even in the absence of renal dysfunction.[42] Renal function impairment is primarily a result of tubular damage; however, hypovolemia may play a critical role in the subsequent development of renal insufficiency.[43,44] In the cerebrospinal fluid (CSF), neutrophils usually predominate in the early course of meningitis but are surpassed by lymphocytes after the seventh day. The CSF protein level may be normal or elevated up to 300 mg/dL, while the glucose concentration is normal. Although abnormal CSF findings are reported in as many as 80% of leptospirosis cases, only half of the patients have neurologic symptoms.

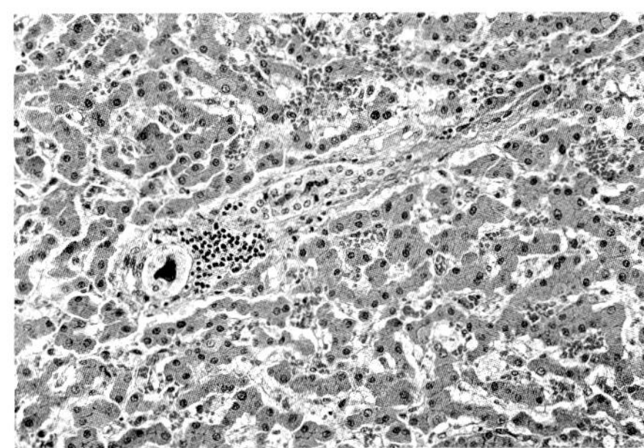

Figure 45.5 Low-power magnification of liver that shows a portal area infiltrated with a moderate number of lymphocytes. Note prominent portal ductal and canalicular bile plugs, sinusoidal dilation, and hypertrophic Kupffer cells containing phagocytosed erythrocytes. (Hematoxylin and eosin; original magnification ×50.)

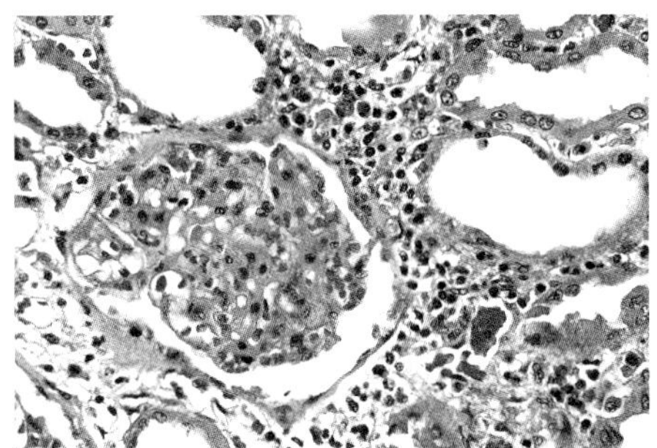

Figure 45.6 Photomicrograph of kidney showing tubular dilation and an interstitial mononuclear infiltrate. Note swelling and focal denudation of tubular epithelial lining cells. (Hematoxylin and eosin; original magnification ×100.)

Various electrocardiographic and chest radiographic abnormalities are common in patients with leptospirosis.[45,46] Arrhythmia or significant cardiac irritability was documented in 35% of patients who were subjected to continuous cardiac monitoring for 24 hours.[26] The significant arrhythmias were atrial fibrillation, flutter, and tachycardia. Premature ventricular contractions are common and can progress to ventricular fibrillation. Echocardiograms on 88 patients in one study revealed pericarditis and small pericardial effusions in 6% of patients.[26] The chest radiographic abnormalities can include pulmonary edema, diffuse pneumonitis, nonsegmental or basal linear opacities, and pleural effusions.[47,48]

The prognosis of leptospirosis depends on the severity of the disease and associated complications. Anicteric leptospirosis usually has a good prognosis, but fatal pulmonary hemorrhage and myocarditis have been reported in anicteric cases.[32,33] The case-fatality rate for Weil's syndrome is 15–40% and is higher for patients older than age 60 years.[49]

In fatal cases, various degrees of jaundice are usually present.[41] Generalized petechiae or ecchymosis in the skin and most internal organs also occur commonly. Microscopically, there is systemic vasculitis with endothelial injury. The damaged endothelial cells usually show different degrees of swelling, necrosis, and denudation. The main histopathologic changes are usually observed in the liver, kidney, heart, and lungs.[32,41,50–52] Hepatic lesions include mild degenerative changes in hepatocytes, prominent hypertrophy and hyperplasia of Kupffer cells, erythrophagocytosis, and cholestasis[53] (***Fig. 45.5***). Focal necrosis with occasional acidophilic bodies may occur, but there is no particular zonal distribution of the necrosis. Mild to moderate mononuclear cell infiltrates are present in portal tracts. In the kidney, the main histopathologic feature is diffuse tubulointerstitial inflammation characterized by a cellular infiltrate, including lymphocytes, plasma cells, macrophages, and polymorphonuclear leukocytes (***Fig. 45.6***). Tubular necrosis is also a common finding. Glomeruli show mild hyperplasia of mesangial cells and occasional infiltration with inflammatory cells.[54] Grossly, the lungs are heavy and severely congested, with focal areas of hemorrhage. Microscopically, the lungs are congested with foci of intra-alveolar hemorrhage[32] (***Fig. 45.7***). In some cases, pulmonary lesions include diffuse alveolar damage and variable degrees of airspace disorganization.

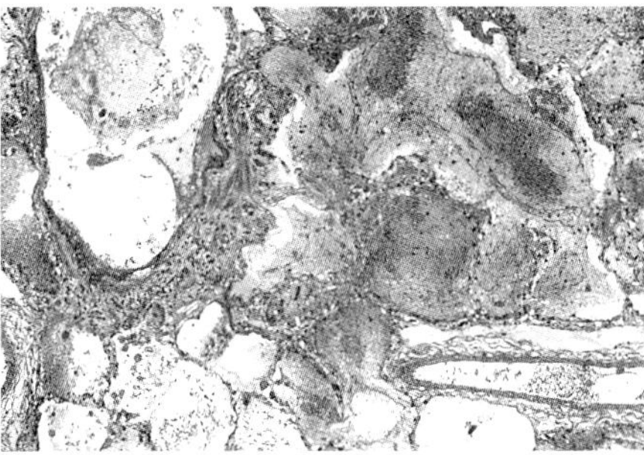

Figure 45.7 Lung in a fatal case with massive pulmonary hemorrhage. Extensive hemorrhage and fibrin are seen within the alveoli. Note mild interstitial inflammatory response and sloughing of bronchial epithelium. (Hematoxylin and eosin; original magnification ×25.)

PATHOGENESIS AND IMMUNITY

The leptospires can penetrate abraded skin or intact mucous membranes, after which they enter the circulation and rapidly disseminate to various tissues.[7] Penetration and invasion of tissues are presumably accomplished through a burrowing motion produced by a pair of axial filaments and release of hyaluronidase.[55] The dissemination and proliferation of the spirochetes in various tissues result in a systemic illness with a broad spectrum of clinical manifestations, including fever, headache, chills, myalgia, abdominal pain, and conjunctival suffusion; more severe manifestations include renal failure, jaundice, meningitis, hypotension, hemorrhage, and hemorrhagic pneumonitis (***Fig. 45.8***).

The pathogenesis of leptospirosis is not fully understood (see Fig. 45.8); there is a marked disparity between the profound clinical illness and the paucity of histologic lesions. In the septicemic (first) phase of human infections and experimental animal models, vascular injury is seen in various organs.[43,56–60] Spirochetes can be found in the walls of capillaries and medium- and large-sized vessels[32] (***Fig. 45.9***). The exact mechanism of vascular damage is not clear. A direct toxic effect of the leptospires has been proposed to cause the vascular injury, but no bacterial endotoxin has been demonstrated. In the immune (second) phase of illness, the host immune response, including immune complex deposition, may play a role in endothelial injury.[28,38]

Recent advances in genomics and proteomics are leading to a better understanding of leptospiral virulence mechanisms.[61]

DIAGNOSIS

The differential diagnosis of leptospirosis depends on the epidemiology of acute febrile illnesses in the particular area. A high index of suspicion is needed in endemic areas, and leptospirosis must be considered when a patient presents with acute onset of fever, headache, and myalgia. However, in locations where dengue fever or malaria is also present, the differentiation may be very difficult because of the similar clinical manifestations. Laboratory confirmation is crucial, especially when these diseases are occurring simultaneously during the rainy season. Other conditions to be considered in the differential diagnosis include influenza, meningitis or encephalitis, viral hepatitis, rickettsioses, typhoid fever, Kawasaki syndrome, septicemia, toxoplasmosis, brucellosis, yellow fever, hantavirus infection, and legionnaires' disease. When the patient presents with jaundice during or after an acute febrile illness, leptospirosis must be differentiated from other causes of jaundice. The high level of bilirubin in Weil's disease with mild to modest elevation of transaminases assists in the differentiation from viral hepatitis, which usually has a much

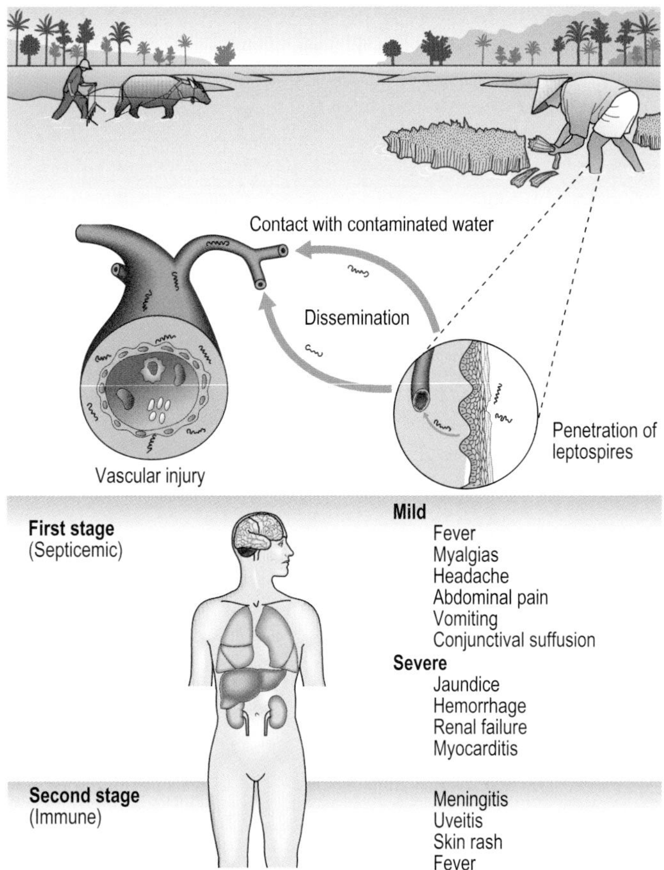

Figure 45.8 Pathogenesis and clinical characteristics of leptospirosis. (Courtesy of Nadia Zaki.)

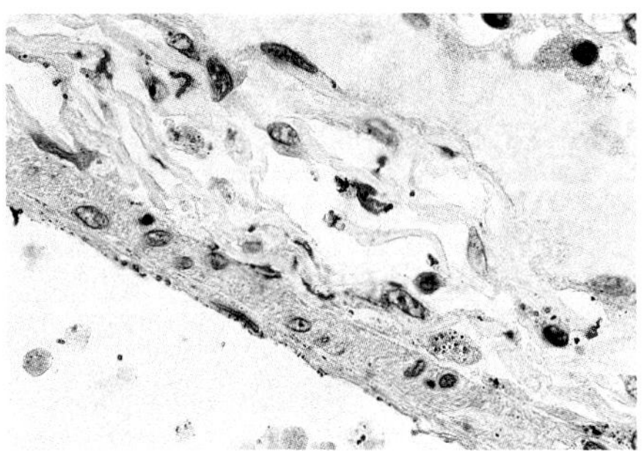

Figure 45.9 High-power magnification of a medium-size pulmonary vessel showing intact and granular forms of leptospires. Note mononuclear cells within the vessel wall and focal denudation of endothelial cells. (Immunoalkaline phosphatase staining; original magnification ×25.)

higher level of transaminases for any given level of bilirubin. A high serum creatine phosphokinase concentration or thrombocytopenia would also favor a diagnosis of leptospirosis. A good history should help to differentiate patients with alcoholic hepatitis.

The definitive diagnosis of leptospirosis depends on laboratory findings. The presence of leptospires may be confirmed by direct detection of the organisms or indirectly by serologic methods. Direct methods include microscopy, antigen detection, DNA detection, and culture. Microscopic methods include examination of tissue samples by dark-field, histological staining, and immunohistochemical (IHC) staining methods. Visualization of leptospires by dark-field microscopic examination of body fluids such as blood, urine, CSF, or dialysate fluid is insensitive and lacks specificity.[62] Approximately 10^4 leptospires/mL are necessary for one cell per field to be visible by dark-field microscopy.[63]

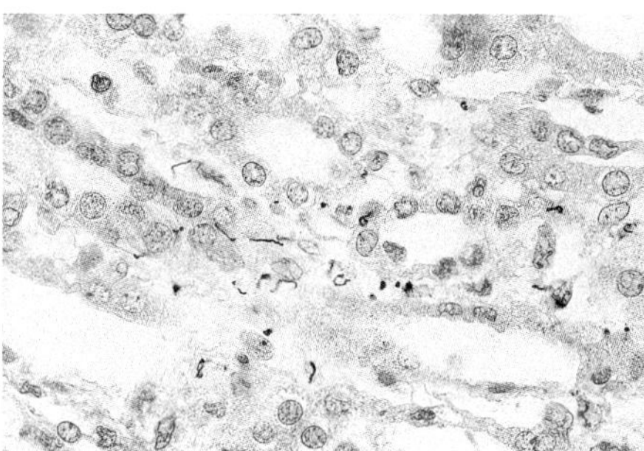

Figure 45.10 Immunostaining of leptospires in kidney. Note intact forms with typical terminal hooks and granular forms of the bacterium. (Immunoalkaline phosphatase staining; original magnification ×158.)

The Dieterle, Steiner, and Warthin–Starry silver impregnation stains can demonstrate leptospires in tissues and body fluids; these silver stains also need special expertise in interpretation since confusion with nerve fibers, cell membrane fragments, and fibrin filaments can occur. IHC staining techniques using immunoalkaline phosphatase[17,32,64] or immunoperoxidase[65] staining methods can readily demonstrate leptospiral antigens and intact leptospira in various tissues (***Fig. 45.10***). Examination of postmortem human tissues, such as kidney, liver, lymph node, and lung, by the immunoalkaline phosphatase method has proved to be a valuable tool in the investigation of leptospirosis outbreaks.[32]

Isolation of leptospires requires special media,[66,67] and unless there is a high index of suspicion cultures are rarely performed while the patient is bacteremic during the acute phase of the illness. Leptospires grow slowly, and cultures may not be positive until several weeks after collection. These factors combine to lower the recovery rate of leptospires and render culture almost invariably unhelpful for individual patient management. However, culture remains valuable for serovar identification of isolates by serologic or molecular methods.[68,69]

Several conventional polymerase chain reaction (PCR) primer pairs have been described for amplification of leptospires,[68] but only two methods have been subjected to extensive clinical evaluation.[70,71] Using these two primer pairs, leptospiral DNA has been amplified from serum,[68,69,71,72] urine,[68,69,73,74] aqueous humor,[75] CSF,[73,76,77] and a number of tissues obtained at autopsy.[78] Sensitive real-time PCR assays have been developed for a number of targets.[79–83] One limitation of PCR is the inability to identify the infecting serovar by sequencing the amplified product.[68]

Because of the difficulties associated with culturing leptospires and the generally low index of clinical suspicion at the time of presentation, the majority of cases of leptospirosis are diagnosed by serology. The reference standard assay is the microscopic agglutination test (MAT), in which live antigens representing different serogroups of leptospires are reacted with serum samples and then examined for agglutination by dark-field microscopy.[84] This test requires significant expertise and resources to perform and interpret, and its use is restricted to a few reference laboratories.

A serologically confirmed case of leptospirosis is defined by a fourfold rise in MAT titer to one or more serovars between acute phase and convalescent serum specimens run in parallel. A titer of at least 1:800 in the presence of compatible symptoms is strong evidence of recent or current infection.[11] Suggestive evidence for recent or current infection includes a single titer of at least 1:200 obtained after the onset of symptoms.[85] Cross-reactions occur between different serogroups, especially in acute-phase samples.[86] Cross-reactivity in acute samples is due to IgM antibodies, which may persist for several years.[87] The MAT is a serogroup-specific assay and cannot be used to interpret reliably the identity of the infecting serovar.[88] Knowledge of the presumptive serogroup may be of epidemiological value in determining potential exposures to animal reservoirs.

Diagnostic application of the MAT is limited by low sensitivity when acute serum samples are tested.[89] Other agglutination assays that detect total immunoglobulins, such as the indirect hemagglutination assay, suffer from similarly low sensitivities on acute specimens but have high sensitivities when acute and convalescent specimens are tested.[86] IgM antibodies are detectable from the fifth day of illness, and commercial IgM detection assays are available in different formats.[86,90–93] Use of these assays as screening tests offers the potential to enhance the diagnostic capacity of many laboratories, especially those in developing countries, where most cases of leptospirosis occur.

TREATMENT AND PROGNOSIS

Death seldom ensues in anicteric leptospirosis, and treatment with antibiotics within the first 4 days of illness will reduce the duration of illness and alleviate the symptoms. Either oral doxycycline 100 mg twice daily for 7 days or penicillin 2.4–3.6 million units/day in divided doses for 7 days is effective in shortening the clinical course.[94,95] An *in vitro* study has suggested that cefotaxime has better minimum inhibitory concentration levels than penicillin and may serve as an alternative choice. Jarisch–Herxheimer-type reactions can occur after initiation of antibiotic treatment.[96] Unless there is a high index of suspicion, most cases are not confirmed at an early stage. Treatment therefore has to be early and empirical when the diagnosis is considered in the appropriate setting.

Patients presenting with severe disease are usually jaundiced or have renal insufficiency as part of Weil's disease. They should be treated with meticulous attention to electrolyte balance and rehydration to prevent anuric renal failure. If early signs of renal failure or prerenal azotemia are present, aggressive rehydration over 48–72 hours with intensive monitoring of the outcome may be beneficial.[97] If acute renal failure occurs, peritoneal dialysis, hemodialysis, or continuous venovenous hemofiltration are all effective therapies. The jaundice requires no treatment. Patients should have serial electrocardiograms performed, and if any abnormality is detected, they should be placed under continuous electrocardiographic monitoring. Arrhythmias in patients with myocarditis should be evaluated and appropriate treatment instituted. Aggressive specific therapy for hemorrhage, hypotension, respiratory failure, or change in level of consciousness is warranted. Controversy still exists as to whether antibiotics are of any value in the treatment of Weil's disease. From several clinical studies, it was concluded that penicillin has little effect on the clinical outcome of severe leptospirosis, except for leptospiruria.[96,98,99] In any controversy, patients should be given the benefit of the doubt. Intravenous penicillin or cefotaxime should therefore be given in this group of patients. It was also suggested that all patients with anicteric leptospirosis be treated irrespective of the time in the course of illness. Further studies need to be done with more clearly defined criteria for severe disease and patient exclusion to answer the question as to the efficacy of antibiotics in Weil's disease.

PREVENTION AND CONTROL

Strategies to prevent and control leptospirosis focus mainly on reducing direct contact with infected animals and contaminated water or soil.[11] The risk of contact with infected animals may be reduced by the institution of appropriate sanitation measures among veterinarians, farmers, and others who handle animals. Since rodents are important natural reservoirs for leptospires, reduction of rodent populations can reduce the incidence of human leptospirosis in endemic areas. However, in places with poverty and poor sanitation, reduction of exposure to rodents may be difficult. Prevention of indirect exposure, or exposure to contaminated water or soil, is more difficult, but a common recommendation is to wear rubber boots and protective clothing and, where possible, to avoid exposure to contaminated rivers, streams, still water, and mud.

Prevention programs for domestic animals have long included leptospira vaccines.[100–103] Effective vaccines are available for cattle, swine, and dogs. The vaccine for cattle generally includes *L. interrogans* serovar hardjo; the vaccine for swine usually includes serovars pomona, grippotyphosa, canicola, and icterohaemorrhagiae; and the vaccine for dogs includes *L. interrogans* serovars canicola and icterohaemorrhagiae. Vaccinated dogs are protected against clinical leptospirosis but continue to shed live leptospires. Immunization of humans is not a common practice, but trials of human vaccines to specific serovars have been attempted successfully in mines in Japan and rice fields in Italy and Spain. Vaccine trials are under way in China, Korea, and Cuba. The major problem with vaccination of humans is that immunity is serovar-specific, and it is very difficult to select all the potentially important serovars for the vaccines.[104–106]

To be effective, the vaccine must include the serovar(s) responsible for the majority of infections in the community. In addition, the incidence of disease should be high enough to justify immunization of people considered to be at high risk for leptospirosis.

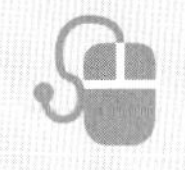

Access the complete reference list online at
http://www.expertconsult.com

CHAPTER 46

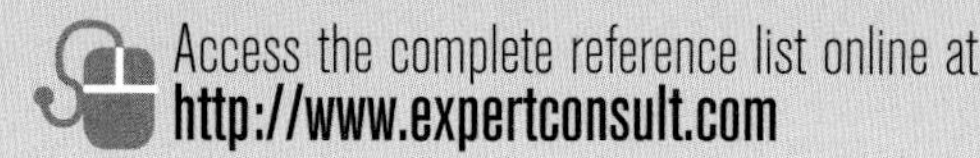
Access the complete reference list online at
http://www.expertconsult.com

Trachoma

Chandler R. Dawson • Julius Schachter

INTRODUCTION

Trachoma is a chronic conjunctivitis that can progress to scarring of the conjunctiva, painful inturned eyelashes, and corneal scarring with blindness. Blinding trachoma is still highly endemic in many developing countries, where 84 million people have active, infectious trachoma, 7.6 million have trachomatous inturned eyelids needing corrective surgery, and 6 million are blind from the disease.[1,2]

The disease was once distributed throughout the world but has disappeared from temperate climates with industrialization and improving socioeconomic and hygienic conditions. Today, most trachoma is found in tropical and subtropical areas. It is endemic in many countries in Africa, was common in the southern Mediterranean and Middle East, and is present in South Asia, some parts of China, Australasia, and South and Central America.[2]

Blinding endemic trachoma of developing countries is caused by infections with *Chlamydia trachomatis* serovars A, B, Ba, or C. Eye infection caused by the sexually transmitted serovars D through K can produce conjunctivitis resembling the early inflammatory phases of endemic trachoma, but without conjunctival scarring and blindness.

A major effort to control blinding trachoma was established by the World Health Organization (WHO) in 1997 as the "Global Elimination of Blinding Trachoma by 2020 (GET 2020)."

THE AGENT

Biologic Characteristics

Chlamydia trachomatis, the causative agent of trachoma, is one of three species within the genus *Chlamydia* that are human pathogens.[3] It also contains serovars that cause genital tract disease and is now identified as the most common sexually transmitted bacterial pathogen (see Chapter 47). *C. psittaci* is almost ubiquitous among avian species and causes the human disease psittacosis, but also includes other strains of mammalian origin (see Chapter 48). *C. pneumoniae* is a human pathogen with a worldwide distribution.[4] It is a major cause of respiratory disease and an etiologic candidate in cardiovascular disease.

Chlamydiae have a complex cell wall (similar to Gram-negative bacteria in composition), both DNA and RNA, prokaryotic ribosomes, and metabolic enzymes that would permit independent existence, except that they lack energy-production mechanisms. Moulder[5] thus termed the chlamydiae "energy parasites" and credited their obligate intracellular parasitism to this trait.

A characteristic of the obligately intracellular chlamydiae is their developmental growth cycle. The extracellular form is the elementary body, and it alone is infectious and responsible for cell-to-cell spread and person-to-person transmission. Following attachment, the elementary body enters the host cell, apparently by receptor-mediated endocytosis. If the particles are viable, or do not have antibody attached, they prevent lysosomal fusion and undergo replication in the phagosome. Within 6–8 hours of ingestion, the elementary body is reorganized into a reticulate body (the only form that replicates). This larger, thin-walled form diverts the host cell's synthetic functions for its own metabolic purpose and proceeds to divide by binary fission. Reticulate bodies are not infectious. After 18–24 hours, reticulate bodies reorganize into elementary bodies and thus become infectious again. Subsequently, the inclusion may disrupt and exit as elementary bodies from the host cell to infect new cells. The full cycle takes about 72–96 hours for the trachoma biovar. These intracytoplasmic collections of elementary bodies constitute the inclusions that may be seen in cytologic smears stained by Giemsa or immunofluorescence methods.

Although all chlamydiae share a genus-specific antigen, there is little DNA homology among *C. trachomatis*, *C. psittaci*, and *C. pneumoniae*.[3] These three species of chlamydiae are distinguished by several features. The elementary body of *C. pneumoniae* is pear-shaped with a large periplasmic space, whereas the elementary bodies of the other two species are round with little or no periplasmic space. The inclusions of *C. trachomatis* accumulate glycogen and thus stain with iodine, whereas the inclusions of *C. psittaci* and *C. pneumoniae* do not. The inclusions of *C. trachomatis* are more compact than those of *C. psittaci* and *C. pneumoniae*. A fourth difference is their response to sulfonamides: *C. trachomatis* is sensitive, but *C. psittaci* and *C. pneumoniae* are not.

C. trachomatis can be further subdivided into two biovars: one that causes lymphogranuloma venereum (LGV) and the other causing trachoma and oculogenital infections. They differ significantly in biologic activity. LGV strains are more invasive and can infect many tissues in addition to epithelial cells (e.g., lymph node invasion, forming the characteristic bubo). This property permits more active cell-to-cell transmission in cell culture and the use of animal inoculation (e.g., mouse) for diagnostic purposes. The oculogenital strains, constituting the trachoma biovar, consist of at least 12 serotypes.[6] They are not readily invasive in cell culture and *in vivo* grow only in columnar and squamocolumnar epithelial cells (conjunctivae, respiratory tract, urethra, cervix, rectal mucosa).

Previously, it had not been possible to identify biologic properties that differentiate the serovars associated with blinding trachoma from those of the trachoma biovar associated with genital tract disease. Recently, however, two sets of genes have been identified that suggest such a differentiation. The polymorphic membrane protein gene designated *pmpH* differs in ways that are consistent with each of these three disease-causing groups of *Chlamydia trachomatis*.[7] This observation suggests distinct evolutionarily divergent patterns for this gene.

More exciting, because of the functional implication, have been the findings relevant to the presence of a tryptophan synthase.[8] This enzyme converts indole into tryptophan. The isolates from trachoma do not have the enzyme, whereas isolates of genital tract origin do (whether they are LGV or oculogenital biovars). Gamma-interferon is an important host response to chlamydial infection and is known to interfere with the completion of the chlamydial developmental cycle. Its action is thought to be due to tryptophan depletion. *In vitro* interferon's inhibitory effect in cell culture can be reversed by adding indole, if the chlamydiae possess a functional tryptophan synthase. This "indole rescue" was only observed with isolates of genital tract origin (mainly serotypes D through K and L1, L2 and L3). This likely represents selection for a survival characteristic of the organism. The authors, Caldwell et al, posit that presence of the enzyme allows for productive infection in the genital tract where normal flora may produce indole, thus allowing the chlamydiae to escape the interferon effect. However, they do suggest that coinfection with *Haemophilus influenzae* could provide the missing tryptophan. Giemsa-stained smears and bacterial cultures from children with blinding trachoma provide ample evidence that *H. influenzae* and other bacterial pathogens are relatively common in trachoma endemic communities.[9] Indeed, it may be these coinfecting bacteria that enhance the intensity of inflammation to potentially blinding levels.[8]

Antigenic Composition and Diversity

Human strains have been classified into more than 18 serovariants (serovars) and 2 biovariants (biovars): the trachoma biovar (serovars A through K and subtype variants) and the LGV biovar (serovars L1 to L3).[8] Infections with the trachoma biovar strains are limited to columnar mucous epithelium resulting in ocular infections, inclusion conjunctivitis, and trachoma, as well as genital tract infections. Serovars A, B, Ba, and C are typically associated with endemic trachoma, whereas all the other serovars have been found in the genital tract (although generally with a preponderance of serovars D and E). Virulence differences have yet to be identified that could account for this distribution of serovars. Even between the biovariants, the molecular basis of virulence differences is unknown.

All chlamydiae share a common lipopolysaccharide (LPS), which is similar in structure but less complex than LPS from Gram-negative bacteria.[10] Significantly, chlamydial LPS is antigenically distinct from that of most other bacteria and in the past was an important target for culture-independent diagnostic assays. Another essential antigenic component is the surface-exposed major outer membrane protein (MOMP).[11] MOMP is antigenically complex and displays both serovar-specific and species-specific antigens shared by strains that cause human infection.[12] The latter antigen was also used for culture-independent detection of *C. trachomatis*. Consequently, diagnostic assays that detect LPS will identify all chlamydial species, whereas assays that detect MOMP will not identify *C. psittaci* or *C. pneumoniae*. Unlike LPS antigens, MOMP antigens are targets of host immunity. This conclusion has been supported by an association of immune protection with serovar specificity and by *in vitro* neutralization of infectivity using anti-MOMP monoclonal antibodies.[13]

EPIDEMIOLOGY

Trachoma has a worldwide distribution (***Fig. 46.1***), and blinding trachoma is still a major public health problem in sub-Saharan Africa; the Middle Eastern crescent; Central, South, and East Asia; and limited areas of the Americas, Australasia, and the Pacific islands.[1,2] Nonblinding trachoma is present in a much larger region of these same areas, which includes most of the drier subtropical and tropical countries. Trachoma was once prevalent and severe in many countries of Europe, North America, and Asia, but it regressed and disappeared with the rising living standards that accompanied industrialization and economic development.

Trachoma rarely occurs under the living conditions in developed countries and in many urban communities of developing countries. In persons with clinically healed trachoma, however, there may be recurrences of active disease, following treatment with topical corticosteroids, with recurrent atopic conjunctivitis, and in old age. This recurrent adult disease does not present a significant public health risk, however.

In communities with blinding trachoma, most children are infected by the age of 1 or 2 years, and active inflammatory trachoma is most prevalent in 2- to 5-year-olds. The prevalence of active disease then declines steadily, although some adults continue to have signs of active disease.[14] Thus children are the chief reservoir of ocular chlamydial infection in communities with endemic trachoma. Blinding lesions (inturned eyelids and corneal scarring) are the outcome of repeated or persistent bouts of severe or moderate-intensity inflammatory disease. These blinding sequelae are generally observed in adults but may occur in childhood as

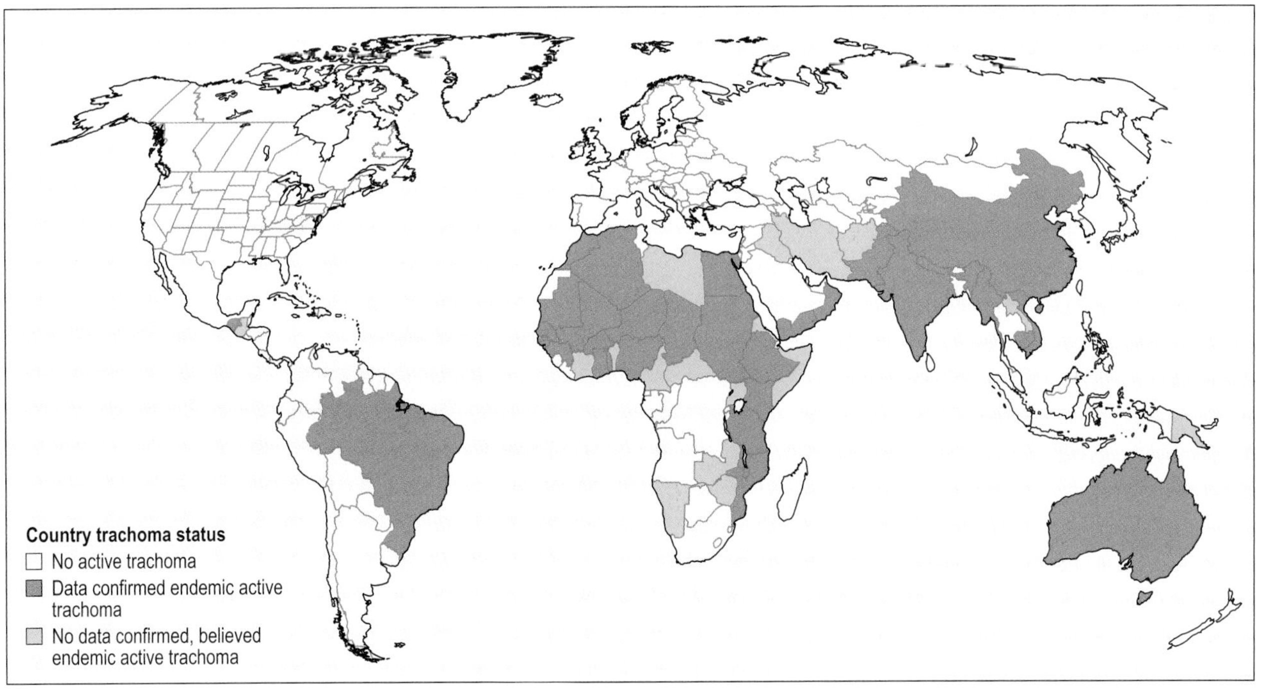

Figure 46.1 Global distribution of trachoma to 2005. (From the World Health Organization (figure at http://gamapserver.who.int/mapLibrary/Files/Maps/global%20active%20may%202006.jpg, accessed March 16, 2010).)

the result of very severe inflammation. Among the environmental features of greatest importance are the presence of young children in the household, crowding, and the unavailability of safe water and household latrines.[15,16] The behavioral risk factors associated with the severity of trachoma are primarily reflected by dirty faces of young children and the lack of latrines in households.

In many endemic areas, the open disposal of human wastes contributes to an increase in the fly population (*Musca sorbens* in Africa and Asia, *M. vetustissima* in Australia, and *Hippletes* sp. in the Americas). The flies cluster on children's eyes, feed on ocular discharges, and can transfer these discharges to the eyes of other children in the same family within 15–30 minutes.[17–19] In the southern Mediterranean and California, seasonal outbreaks of these flies have been associated with epidemics of purulent conjunctivitis, usually caused by *H. influenzae* and other bacterial pathogens.[9] Children with endemic trachoma can also harbor chlamydiae and other bacterial pathogens in the upper respiratory and lower gastrointestinal tracts.[20] Thus, transmission might also occur by aerosol droplet spread and fecal contamination of fomites, as well as by flies.

THE DISEASE

In communities with endemic trachoma, the disease often has inapparent or gradual onset. Initially, trachoma presents as conjunctivitis characterized by the formation of lymphoid follicles in the subconjunctival tissue and inflammatory infiltration (papillary hypertrophy) of the conjunctiva (***Fig. 46.2***). In children under 2 years of age, the papillary reaction with inflammatory thickening of the conjunctiva may be the predominant sign, and follicles may not be prominent. The disease involves the entire conjunctiva, but its effects are most noticeable on the upper tarsus, which has been selected as a diagnostically critical area for examination to determine the degree of trachomatous inflammation and scarring.[21]

As chronic trachoma progresses, it causes scarring of the conjunctiva (***Fig. 46.3***), with fine linear and small stellate scars in milder cases, or broad confluent or synechial scars in severe cases. With severe scarring, there is mechanical distortion of the lids, particularly of the upper tarsus, to produce inturned eyelashes (***Fig. 46.4***). The disease also can destroy the mucus-secreting conjunctival goblet cells and injure the lacrimal glands and tear ducts. Thus, constant corneal abrasion by the inturned eyelashes and deficient tear secretion can lead to corneal ulceration followed by opacification and visual loss. The deep trachomatous scarring in the upper tarsus and fornix may also produce defects in lid closure with exposure of the cornea, which also predisposes to traumatic and infectious damage to the cornea.

During the inflammatory infectious phases, trachoma produces lesions of the cornea ranging from fine punctate defects in the epithelium (epithelial keratitis) to infiltrates of the superficial stromal connective tissue and superficial neovascularization (vascular pannus). A unique characteristic of trachoma is the formation of lymphoid follicles at the conjunctival–corneal junction (limbus), which on resolution leave characteristic depressions at the limbus called Herbert's peripheral pits (see ***Fig. 46.3***).

The degree of conjunctival scarring is directly proportional to the intensity and duration of inflammation.[22] Very severe scarring occurs in children as young as 4 or 5 years of age. Inturned eyelids are uncommon at this age, however, and tend to occur in late adolescence and early adult life, long after the active inflammatory disease has subsided. This late onset of inturned lids in adults may be due to repeated episodes of infection with the development of more scarring and gradual contraction of the lid margin.

The older MacCallan classification of the clinical disease is rarely used now, and there are two related systems recommended by the WHO to describe the clinical findings.[21,23] For this clinical evaluation, signs involving the upper tarsal conjunctiva are used as a convenient index of the disease. These conjunctival signs include lymphoid follicles, diffuse infiltration, papillary hypertrophy, conjunctival scarring, inturned eyelashes, and corneal opacity.

The detailed WHO descriptive system emphasizes grading of the intensity of inflammatory disease on the basis of tarsal follicles and of diffuse inflammation and papillary hypertrophy. Cicatricial signs include conjunctival scarring, inturned eyelashes, and corneal opacity.[21] This detailed description has been useful for clinical research in field studies.

A simplified description was introduced in 1987 by the WHO for use by primary health care workers (***Box 46.1***).[23] This simplified system was developed for use by nonspecialist health workers in developing countries, using a handlight and loupe for examination. A specific series of interventions is linked to the clinical findings.

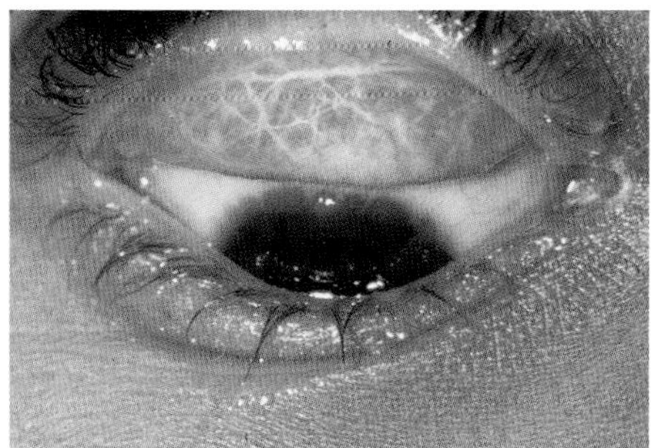

Figure 46.3 Trachoma scarring. The white bands in the everted conjunctiva in a 6-year-old in Tunisia are the scars caused by chronic trachomatous inflammation. The round lesions at the corneal–scleral border are lymphoid follicles and will resolve, leaving a shallow depression (Herbert's pits), a unique sign of trachoma.

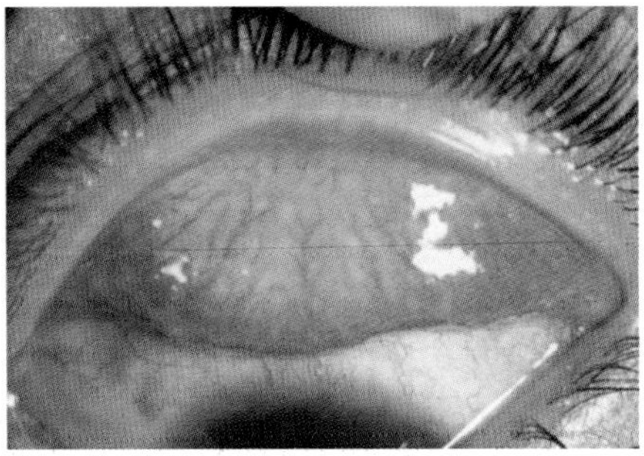

Figure 46.2 Active infectious trachoma in a 7-year-old Tunisian boy. The upper eyelid has been everted to expose the tarsal conjunctiva. The lymphoid follicles (white avascular spots) are diagnostic of infectious trachoma. The large vertical blood vessels are dilated as is the diffuse bed of capillary tufts (papillary hypertrophy).

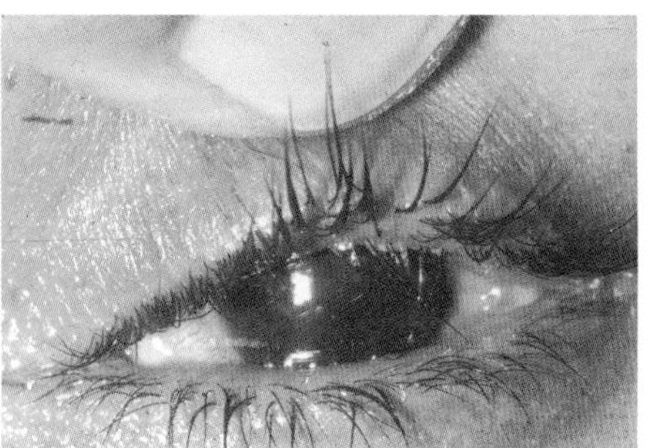

Figure 46.4 Trichiasis caused by trachoma. The inturned eyelids in this 32-year-old Tunisian woman have caused the eyelashes to turn in and abrade the cornea. This constant trauma is painful and eventually induces ulceration and corneal scarring with loss of vision. The surgical correction of inturned eyelids is a cornerstone of the SAFE strategy for trachoma control.

Box 46.1 Simplified Description of Trachoma for Primary Eye Care

Trachoma follicles	Five or more lymphoid follicles on the central area of the upper tarsal conjunctiva
Trachomatous inflammation	Diffuse inflammation of the tarsal conjunctiva that obscures more than half of the normal deep tarsal vessels
Trachomatous scarring	Any characteristic scarring of the tarsal conjunctiva
Trichiasis or entropion	At least one or more deviated lashes touching the eyeball
Corneal opacity	Easily visible corneal opacity or scarring over the pupil

(From Thylefors B, Dawson CR, Jones BR, et al. A simple system for the assessment of trachoma and its complications. Bull WHO. 1987;65:477.)

To identify the presence or absence of trachoma in a community, individual cases must have at least two of the following signs: (1) follicles in the upper tarsal conjunctiva, (2) limbal follicles or their sequelae, Herbert's pits (see ***Fig. 46.3***), (3) typical conjunctival scarring, and (4) vascular pannus more extensive at the superior limbus.[21] Communities with blinding trachoma have a high prevalence of older persons with severe visual loss caused by corneal opacity and a substantial prevalence of potentially disabling trachomatous lesions, specifically inturned eyelashes.[14] These irreversible changes are the long-term outcome of prolonged or recurrent inflammatory disease of moderate or severe intensity. Communities with nonblinding trachoma may have a low incidence of potentially blinding lesions and little if any visual loss from trachoma.

In communities with blinding trachoma, chlamydial infection is always present, but other ocular microbial pathogens appear to contribute significantly to the intensity of trachoma and to lesions that impair vision.

PATHOGENESIS AND IMMUNITY

The host response of the human conjunctiva in trachoma is characterized both clinically and histologically by the presence of lymphoid follicles with germinal centers.[24–26] In the early stages of trachoma, epithelial and subepithelial tissues are infiltrated with lymphocytes and polymorphonuclear leukocytes. Where the conjunctiva is bound down over the tarsal plate, the epithelium is elevated by infiltrating inflammatory cells to form papillae with vascular tufts and folds of epithelium between the elevations.

Early in the disease, collections of lymphocytes appear in the submucosa just beneath the epithelium or deeper within the connective tissue. These early follicles do not have germinal centers and appear to consist mostly of small lymphocytes. As the disease progresses, the collections of lymphocytes develop into lymphoid germinal centers, with an outer layer of small, dense lymphocytes and an inner center of lighter-staining cells with more cytoplasm. Unlike central lymph nodes, these lymphoid follicles are displaced toward the surface. The lymphocytes of the subepithelial follicles appear to be infiltrating the overlying conjunctival epithelium, which is flattened and loosened over the follicle itself, allowing ready access of foreign material into the follicle. Lymphoid follicles in the conjunctiva can also occur deeper in the connective tissue and are not necessarily adjacent to the conjunctival epithelium. Between follicles, the epithelium and submucosal layers are diffusely infiltrated with lymphocytes and some polymorphonuclear cells.

In more advanced stages of trachoma, the follicle itself becomes necrotic, and connective tissue forms in and around the follicles, producing scarring. The formation of Herbert's pits by follicles at the corneoscleral junction (limbus) is evidence that the follicle (during its formation in this confined space) can erode the connective tissue without causing any overt ulceration or connective tissue reaction with scarring.

Macrophages are frequently present in the epithelium and in the follicles themselves. Plasma cells are distributed throughout the conjunctiva. Between the follicles, there is marked lymphocytic infiltration. In addition, the capillaries are dilated, and the whole conjunctival layer is thickened by the cellular infiltration with the formation of papillary villi. As scarring takes place, islands of epithelium between the elevated papillae may become trapped and form epithelial-lined cysts, which fill with desquamated debris to form yellow structures, clinically identified as "post-trachomatous degeneration." Progressive scarring produces inward deformation of the lid margins with inturned eyelashes (trichiasis and entropion), which constantly abrade the cornea to produce corneal scarring and blindness.[24]

DIAGNOSIS

The laboratory methods for identifying *C. trachomatis* in patients with trachoma are essentially the same procedures that have been used to diagnose chlamydial genital tract infections (see Chapter 47). There have been many evaluations of the sensitivity and specificity of these tests for diagnosis of sexually transmitted diseases. It is far more difficult to perform rigorous evaluations in trachoma-endemic areas because of the difficulties in maintaining cold chains and establishing appropriate "gold standards" for comparison. In developing countries, the time-honored Giemsa stain may still be of use in detecting chlamydial inclusions in conjunctival scrapings from some cases of severe active trachoma.[27] Antigen detection methods, such as direct fluorescent antibody (DFA) and enzyme immunoassay (EIA), are also of some use, but they are far less sensitive than the newer nucleic acid amplification tests (NAATs).[28] These are probably the tests of choice for field studies because they do not require maintenance of a cold chain and the specimens can be sent to reference laboratories or be tested locally.

C. trachomatis can be identified in cytologic scrapings or in tissue specimens by recognition of characteristic intracytoplasmic inclusions.[27] Such identification in conjunctival epithelial cells, and less frequently in cervical epithelial cells, constituted the only technique available at the time when trachoma and oculogenital diseases were first recognized at the beginning of the twentieth century, until the organism was isolated in embryonated eggs in 1957 by Tang and associates in Beijing.[29]

The use of cytology in diagnosis was supplanted by cell culture isolation methods and then by modern nonculture diagnostic tests that detect chlamydial antigens or genes. For many years, the most sensitive method for identification of infection of the genital tract was isolation in cell culture. Direct methods of detection of chlamydial DNA (DNA probes) have not been more sensitive than EIA procedures or cell culture. However, the introduction of NAATs in the mid-1990s revolutionized chlamydial diagnostics.[30,31] These tests are highly specific and more sensitive than other diagnostic tests, including culture. The broad-based use of NAATs greatly improved the management of genital infection. Second generation tests have provided incremental improvement in NAAT performance, and at this writing the detection of rRNA seems to be the most sensitive assay for trachoma research.[32]

Isolation

The method of choice for recovery of *C. trachomatis* is cell culture using McCoy, HeLa-229, BHK-21, or L-929 cells. A necessary step in cell cultivation of strains other than LGV is centrifugation of the inoculum onto the cells. In addition, the cells are treated to enhance infection; Gordon and colleagues, who developed the modern cell culture technique, irradiated McCoy cells.[33] Cycloheximide has been substituted for irradiation, and cycloheximide-treated McCoy cells are the most widely used cultivation method at present.[34] Specimen material is inoculated into individual vials with cell sheets on coverslips within them or into wells of microtiter plates that have been implanted with cells. They can be examined at 48–96 hours after inoculation. Intracytoplasmic inclusions are recognized by iodine, Giemsa, or more commonly by fluorescent antibody (FA) staining. Iodine stain only identifies *C. trachomatis* strains. FA stains are more sensitive and can be species-specific (to MOMP) or genus-specific (to LPS).

Antigen and Nucleic Acid Probes

In the 1980s and 1990s, other nonculture diagnostic methods were evaluated and widely used, including DFA, EIA, and DNA probe methods. There are a number of DFA kits commercially available. Although they differ primarily in specificity and in ease of laboratory use, the general principle is the same. A cytologic smear is fixed (at which stage it can be stored), stained with a fluorescein-conjugated monoclonal antibody, and examined by ultraviolet microscopy. Elementary bodies are recognized as small apple-green dots. When the test is performed by experienced persons, the sensitivity can be as high as 90%, but is more often 70–80% when compared to cell culture. The specificity is usually 98% or greater in the hands of experienced microscopists. Thus, it is an excellent screening test for high-risk populations, but less useful in low-prevalence populations.[28,35]

The EIA class of tests is designed for immunochemical detection of dissolved antigenic components. The tests have been designed with the use of plastic to absorb chlamydial LPS or with antigen capture in a sandwich format.[36]

Both DFA and EIA are technologically easier and are less difficult to transport than cell culture specimens. However, they have lower sensitivity and specificity. The DFA has the advantage of a verifiable sample quality, and rapidity (as little as 30 minutes). EIA requires less training and experience because its indicator is more objective; it is automated, and more suitable for batch processing.

Direct nucleic acid probes were commercially available and popular for diagnosis of genital infection, but were less sensitive than culture, although highly specific.[36] They have been replaced by NAATs which are far more sensitive than cell culture and extremely specific.[30,31,37] The newer TMA (rRNA) test is substantially more sensitive in testing clinical specimens from trachoma cases.[32] Chlamydial nucleic acid can be detected in epithelial cell specimens and in male and female urine samples.[38,39]

Although noninvasive sampling (urine) is important for diagnosing sexually transmitted diseases, conjunctival swabs are needed to collect specimens for trachoma. Cell culture is problematic because of the requirement to maintain a cold chain and loss of infectivity that may follow freeze–thaw. While NAATs may be the most sensitive tests, they have the same drawback as other nonculture assays: there is no propagated organism available for further identification (e.g., serologic markers) or testing for antibiotic sensitivity.

Serologic and Immunologic Diagnostic Methods

Although a variety of serologic methods have been used in the past to detect antibodies, the indirect immunofluorescence method, first developed by Bernkopf, has been simplified and standardized in an indirect microimmunofluorescence (MIF) test by Wang and associates.[40] At present, this is the most commonly used test for evaluation of host response to trachoma or to oculogenital agents. For LGV, the complement fixation (CF) test can be used, although the MIF test is more sensitive and specific. The MIF test employs elementary bodies of all known immunotypes, grown in yolk sac or cell culture, as antigens. Antigen dots, in a diluted yolk sac suspension, are placed on a slide in a specific pattern. Serial dilutions of serum, tears, or local secretions are applied, followed by fluorescein-conjugated antihuman immunoglobulin. An obvious advantage of the test is that the conjugate may be prepared against any immunoglobulin class, thus permitting titration of IgG-, IgM-, or IgA-specific antibody. A counterstain is added to the conjugate to permit clearer identification of specific fluorescence in the dots to which antibody-containing serum has been applied. If differentiation of specific immunotypes is sought, the antigens can be evaluated separately. For many purposes, antigen pools can be used.

A CF test is available to measure host response to any chlamydial infection.[41] It is still the most commonly used test for psittacosis and LGV, but it is too insensitive for trachoma or oculogenital infections. Usually, the antigen for the CF is obtained from an LGV strain grown in yolk sac and is prepared by boiling and treatment with phenol.

TREATMENT AND CONTROL

WHO initiated a major effort to control blinding trachoma in 1997 as the "Global Elimination of Blinding Trachoma by 2020 (GET 2020)."[2] A nongovernmental organization, the International Trachoma Initiative (ITI) was established in 2001 to distribute the 135 million doses of azithromycin donated by Pfizer Inc. for trachoma control. The ITI assists ministries of health in affected countries to develop systematic national trachoma control programs.

In trachoma-endemic regions, the goal of trachoma intervention programs is elimination of trachoma as a blinding disease. The new programs are based on four components of the SAFE strategy: **S**urgery to correct inturned eyelids; **A**ntibiotics to eliminate the reservoir of chlamydial infection in the community and to reduce inflammation in individuals; **F**acial cleanliness in young children and the promotion of personal hygiene; **E**nvironmental changes to reduce transmission of trachoma through the elimination of exposed human fecal material and provision of clean water supplies.[42,43]

Surgery

The surgical correction of inturned eyelids (trichiasis) from trachoma is performed with tarsal rotation procedures.[44] Recurrent trichiasis after surgery has been observed regularly; for example, 11% after 1 year in Vietnam.[45] A comparison of surgical cases done by ophthalmologists or by trained eye care workers in Ethiopia showed no difference in the rates of recurrence at 6 months (14.6%) in the two groups.[46] A Cochrane Review[47] of interventions for trachomatous trichiasis found that:

- No trials showed that interventions prevented blindness.
- Bilamellar tarsal rotation of 180° was more effective than unilamellar rotation.
- Community-based surgery compared to health centers increased convenience for patients with no increase in complications.
- Surgery done by trained ophthalmic assistants was as effective as that by ophthalmologists.
- Double sticking plaster (adhesive tape) was more effective than epilation as a temporary measure.
- Oral azithromycin at the time of surgery did not improve outcomes.

A 3- to 4-year follow up of 214 operated cases in The Gambia showed recurrences in 42%, but corneal opacification had improved in 36 of 78 (46%) previously scarred eyes.[48]

For patients blind from trachomatous corneal scarring, corneal transplant surgery has a poor outcome. The reduced flow of tears, loss of mucus from goblet cell destruction, exposure by distorted lids, and inadequate follow-up care all contribute to graft failure in such patients.

Antibiotics

The objectives of antibiotic treatment are to reduce the pool of chlamydial infection in the community and severity of active trachoma, and thus the risk of blindness, in individual cases. Sulfonamides, tetracyclines, erythromycin, other macrolides and azalides, and rifampin are effective against trachoma. Most control programs utilized oral sulfonamides up to the early 1960s, then topical tetracycline ointment to the mid-1990s. Antibiotic treatment in endemic communities (active trachoma in more than 20% of children) was based on the supervised application of topical antibiotic to all persons in a community ("mass therapy").[21] In other settings school children were treated by repeated application of topical antibiotic.

The advent of oral azithromycin has led to a renewed interest in trachoma control because it is effective with one to three doses and can be taken by children as young as 6 months old.[49] The compliance is very high with a single dose, and the drug is well tolerated. The new recommendation for this community treatment is azithromycin, given as a single dose (20 mg/kg body weight for children, or 1 g for adults; height can be used as a surrogate for weight in children).[42] Because Pfizer Inc. has donated oral azithromycin for trachoma control (135 million doses committed), there is no cost of this antibiotic to programs involved in trachoma control, but there are still substantial costs for distributing it to large populations.

Initial case-control studies showed that oral azithromycin was as effective as or better than topical oxytetracycline ointment.[49–51] A subsequent trial of village-wide oral azithromycin (1 dose weekly for 3 weeks) compared to oxytetracycline ointment (1 dose daily for 42 days) in Egypt, Tanzania, and The Gambia showed a substantial reduction of chlamydial infection by both treatments, but only a modest effect on clinically active trachoma.[52] The new goal of antimicrobial treatment is the elimination of chlamydial eye infection and thus of infectious trachoma. Elimination of trachoma in one village in Tanzania was achieved by an initial azithromycin dose (94% compliance) and topical tetracycline to active cases for 18 months.[53] However, most studies have shown that a single mass treatment does not eliminate chlamydial infection and that multiple annual treatment cycles are needed to reduce the infectious load.[54,55] In practice, mass treatment with oral azithromycin is carried out in communities or regions with 10% or more active trachoma in children. One study of treatment in three African countries predicted that mass treatment could be discontinued when infection rates reached 5% in children.[56] In a large scale study in Ethiopia, a single treatment of oral azithromycin for trachoma was associated with reduced mortality in 1- to 9-year-olds.[57]

The evaluation of antibiotic treatment has been based on the clinical diagnosis of active trachoma. After treatment, however, clinical trachoma activity is no longer an adequate surrogate for chlamydial eye infection, because the clinical signs of disease persist after the infection has resolved.[58] To determine the need for further rounds of mass treatment, it will be necessary to test for chlamydial eye infection, preferably by one of the nucleic acid amplification tests. A study in Ethiopia showed that twice yearly community-wide treatment for 3 years reduced clinically active trachoma in 1- to 5-year-olds from about 80% to 20%, but PCR-detected infection rates from 48% to zero.[55]

Face Washing and Hygiene

Personal hygiene intervention is based on studies indicating that young children with dirty faces had a significant risk for active trachoma.[16] In most of these cases "dirty faces" included children with nasal and ocular discharge which is probably caused by infections with other bacteria. Such coinfections could provide the "indole rescue" for the trachoma strains to escape the deficiency of tryptophan as suggested by Caldwell et al.[8] Nevertheless "face washing" has been incorporated into improving the hygiene of young children in trachoma control activities.[59]

Environment

Environmental controls include latrines to reduce fly density and adequate water supplies by building wells or distribution systems.[15–17] These activities are important for community development. Even relatively small changes such as providing screening of latrines for the privacy of women can have a large impact on people's lives. The development of wells and water distribution systems are capital intensive and may not have an immediate effect on infectious trachoma.[60]

The Outlook for Trachoma Elimination

It is roughly a decade since the GET 2020 program was initiated. Tens of millions in trachoma endemic areas have received oral azithromycin. Many thousands have had surgery to correct lid deformity. There have been notable successes where there was sufficient infrastructure to support the control program. For example, multiple annual rounds of azithromycin have effectively eliminated trachoma as a problem in Morocco.[61] Very severe trachoma problems, with large unmet needs for surgical intervention, have become obvious (e.g., Ethiopia). There is a clear need for operational research to answer questions (assessment methods, need for long-term treatment programs, when to stop), and it is clear that some countries cannot afford to implement the program, even with large donations. But, progress is being made.

Access the complete reference list online at
http://www.expertconsult.com

CHAPTER 47

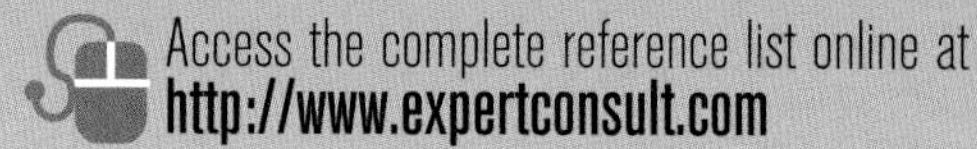
Access the complete reference list online at
http://www.expertconsult.com

Chlamydia trachomatis Infections of the Genital Tract (Including Lymphogranuloma Venereum)

David Mabey • Rosanna W. Peeling

INTRODUCTION

The *Chlamydia* are pathogenic bacteria that are only able to replicate inside eukaryotic host cells. They are unable to synthesize high energy compounds such as adenosine triphosphate, and depend on the host cell to provide them. Their unique developmental cycle distinguishes them from all other bacteria. It involves alternation between a metabolically inert, infectious, spore-like elementary body (EB), which can survive in the extracellular environment, and a metabolically active, replicating reticulate body (RB), which cannot. The chlamydial developmental cycle (***Fig. 47.1***) is completed in about 48 hours *in vitro*. The *Chlamydia* have their own order (Chlamydiales) and family (Chlamydiaceae).

C. trachomatis was first described by Halberstaedter and von Prowazek in 1907, who observed cytoplasmic inclusions in conjunctival scrapings taken from children with trachoma and from monkeys inoculated with ocular material from these children.[1] They named them *Chlamydozoa*, from the Greek words *chlamys* (cloak) and *zoon* (animal), because of the way in which the inclusions were draped around the nucleus. Similar inclusions were soon observed in conjunctival scrapings taken from neonates with conjunctivitis, and from the cervix of their mothers. *C. trachomatis* was first isolated, in mouse brain and subsequently in eggs, from a patient with lymphogranuloma venereum (LGV) in the 1930s.[2] The more fastidious trachoma biovar was not isolated until 1957, in eggs, from a case of trachoma,[3] and in 1959 from the cervix of the mother of an infant with ophthalmia.[4] It was first grown in cell culture in 1965,[5] and this made it possible for the first time to study the epidemiology and clinical features of *C. trachomatis* infection on a large scale.

THE AGENT

Classification

The *Chlamydia* were formerly classified as four species belonging to a single genus, *Chlamydia*: *C. trachomatis*, a human pathogen causing ocular and genital infections; *C. pneumoniae* causing mainly human respiratory disease; *C. psittaci* infecting birds and other animals; and *C. pecorum*, a pathogen of cattle and sheep. A recent taxonomic reclassification, based on ribosomal DNA sequence data, divided the Chlamydiaceae into two genera, *Chlamydia* and *Chlamydophila*.[6] However, this official taxonomy has not been fully adopted by all researchers, some of whom favor a single genus, *Chlamydia,* comprising nine species, namely: *C. trachomatis*, *C. pneumoniae*, *C. psittaci* (birds), *C. abortus* (sheep), *C. felis* (cats), *C. pecorum* (cattle), *C. suis* (pigs), *C. muridarum* (mice), and *C. caviae* (guinea pigs).[7] The first two are primarily human pathogens, while *C. psittaci*, *C. abortus*, and *C. felis* cause zoonotic infections, which are transmitted occasionally to humans from infected animals.

Biology

Chlamydia probably evolved from host-independent, Gram-negative ancestors. The chlamydial envelope possesses bacterial inner and outer membranes. The infectious elementary body is electron-dense, DNA-rich and approximately 300 nm in diameter. The cell wall does not contain peptidoglycan, and its rigidity is maintained by extensive disulfide linking of the major outer membrane protein (MOMP), which makes up some 60% of the outer membrane. The EB binds to the host cell and enters by "parasite-specified" endocytosis. Fusion of the chlamydia-containing endocytic vesicle with lysosomes is inhibited, and the elementary body begins its unique developmental cycle within the eukaryotic cell. MOMP is reduced to a monomeric form and acts as a porin, allowing nutrients to enter the organism from the host cell. After about 8 hours the EB differentiates into the larger (800–1000 nm), noninfectious, metabolically active RB. This divides by binary fission. By 20 hours post-infection, a proportion of RBs has begun to reorganize into a new generation of EBs (***Fig. 47.1***). These reach maturity up to 30 hours after entry into the cell and rapidly accumulate within the endocytic vacuole, which typically contains more than 1000 organisms. They are released by lysis of the host cell between 30 and 48 hours after the start of the cycle.

The species *C. trachomatis* contains two biovars: the more invasive LGV biovar, which can replicate in macrophages, invades lymph nodes and causes a systemic infection, and the more common trachoma biovar, which is largely confined to squamocolumnar epithelial cells of the eye and genital tract. Both contain several serovars, identified by the micro-immunofluorescence test, defined by the presence of serovar-specific epitopes on the MOMP.[8,9] There are three LGV serovars (L1–L3). The trachoma biovar contains serovars A, B, Ba, and C, which cause trachoma and are now largely confined to the developing world, and serovars D–K, which cause genital and oculogenital infections worldwide. The trachoma serovars A, B, Ba, and C, which have a predilection for the eye, differ from serovars D–K in that they are unable to synthesize tryptophan due to disruption of the *trpA* gene.[10]

Genetics

Chlamydia have one of the smallest bacterial genomes, containing around 1 million base pairs. Virtually all strains of *C. trachomatis* also contain a 4.4 MDa plasmid of unknown function. Genomes of *C. trachomatis* serovars A, B, D, and L2 have been sequenced, and show a high level of conservation of gene order and content (>99%).[11,12] A high degree of genetic conservation is also seen across *Chlamydia* species, with *C. trachomatis* and *C. muridarum,* for example, being >95% identical in DNA sequence. The fact that *Chlamydia* replicate within an intracellular vacuole probably explains the high degree of conservation, since it does not allow them to exchange genetic material with other bacteria.

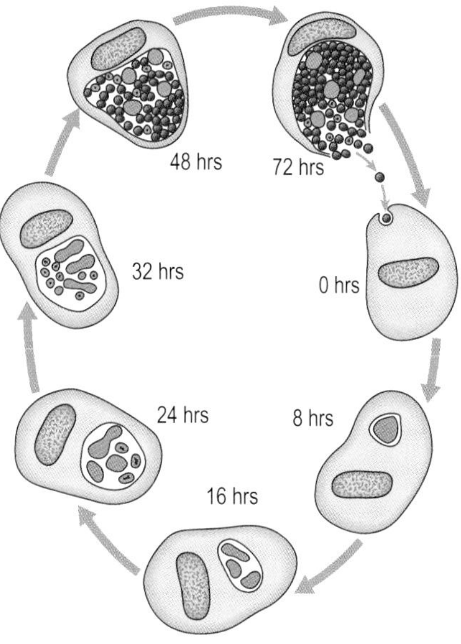

Figure 47.1 The chlamydial developmental cycle.

EPIDEMIOLOGY

C. trachomatis is the most common bacterial sexually transmitted infection (STI). It is common in all sexually active populations, and prevalence is usually highest in the young. In the United Kingdom, the number of reported chlamydial infections trebled between 1996 and 2005.[13] Similar increases were seen in other Western countries including Sweden and Canada over this period.[14] It is not clear to what extent this is due to an increased incidence, or to an increase in the number of people tested using the more sensitive nucleic acid amplification tests, which have been widely used since the late 1990s. The overall incidence of reported chlamydial infection in the United Kingdom in 2005 was 223 per 100 000 total population, with the highest rate (1300/100 000) in females aged 16–19 years. Few countries outside Western Europe and North America have accurate reporting systems for STIs. The World Health Organization has estimated the worldwide incidence of STIs from prevalence data and the estimated duration of infection. This analysis suggests that, in 2005, there were 101 million new cases of genital chlamydial infection.[15]

Molecular Epidemiology

Typing isolates of *C. trachomatis* is potentially of great value. It could help to map sexual networks, and to distinguish between treatment failure and reinfection in clinical trials. If associations could be found between particular strains and particular clinical findings, it could help to identify virulence determinants of *C. trachomatis*, thereby increasing our understanding of the pathogenesis of *C. trachomatis* infection.

The first typing method for *C. trachomatis*, the microimmunofluorescence test, was developed more than 30 years ago.[8] It was based on the ability of polyclonal antisera to distinguish 13 (later increased to 17) serotypes of *C. trachomatis*. Since the early 1990s, many studies have been published in which genital and ocular strains of *C. trachomatis* were genotyped following amplification of the *ompA* gene, which encodes the MOMP, either by sequencing, or by restriction fragment length polymorphism (RFLP) analysis of the amplified product; but *ompA* genotyping has not been sufficiently discriminatory to distinguish between persistent infection, on the one hand, and reinfection with a common genotype, on the other. More recently, a multilocus sequence typing (MLST) method, targeting six variable genes identified through genome sequencing projects, has been used.[16] This method was able to identify 32 genetic variants among 47 Swedish isolates, whereas *ompA* sequencing was only able to identify 12. MLST was used to investigate a new variant of *C. trachomatis* which appeared in Sweden and was missed by commonly used nucleic acid amplification tests due to a deletion in the target plasmid. The new variant was clonal in origin.[17] Future studies using MLST are likely to shed new light on the epidemiology and pathogenesis of *C. trachomatis* infection.

Lymphogranuloma venereum is a rare disease in industrialized countries, but is endemic in parts of Africa, Asia, South America, and the Caribbean. The reported sex ratio is greater than 5 : 1 (male : female), probably because of the easier recognition of disease. The epidemiology of infection is poorly defined because LGV is often indistinguishable clinically from chancroid and other causes of genital ulceration with bubo formation, and it has been difficult to obtain laboratory confirmation. LGV is an uncommon cause of genital ulceration in Africa. Ten percent of patients with buboes presenting to a sexually transmitted disease clinic in Bangkok were found to have LGV, and an epidemic of LGV has been reported among crack cocaine users in the Bahamas.[18,19] In 2003, an outbreak of LGV proctitis due to the L2 serovar was reported among homosexual men in the Netherlands, and in the subsequent three years over 1000 cases were reported in homosexual men across Western Europe, the United Kingdom, North America, and Australia. The majority of affected men have been HIV-positive.[20]

PATHOGENESIS AND IMMUNITY

After an incubation period of 5–10 days, *C. trachomatis* elicits an acute inflammatory response with a purulent exudate. A period of chronic inflammation ensues, with the development of subepithelial follicles, and this leads eventually, in some cases, to fibrosis and scarring. This scarring process is responsible for much of the morbidity associated with *C. trachomatis*, in both the genital tract and the eye. It is particularly likely to occur after repeated infections.[21,22]

It has been difficult to study virulence determinants of *C. trachomatis*, since it has not so far proved possible to manipulate *Chlamydia* genetically. However, the availability of the complete genome sequences of several *C. trachomatis* strains has provided some insights. The serovar D genome contains genes homologous with those coding for virulence factors in other bacteria, including a cytotoxin gene, and genes encoding a type III secretion pathway. A conserved chlamydial protease, proteasome-like activity factor (CPAF), is secreted into the host cell cytoplasm, where it interferes with the assembly and surface expression of HLA molecules and inhibits apoptosis.[11,12,23] A recent study has identified, in a nonhuman primate model, genetic variations in six genes of *C. trachomatis* that appear to be associated with increased virulence.[24]

The epidemiology of *C. trachomatis* infection suggests that a degree of protective immunity follows natural infection. The prevalence and bacterial load of ocular infection is lower in adults than in children in trachoma endemic communities, and the duration of infection is shorter.[25,26] Similarly, genital *C. trachomatis* infection is most prevalent in the youngest sexually active age groups, and the chlamydial isolation rate for men with nongonococcal urethritis is lower in those who have had previous episodes.[27] Trachoma vaccine trials in the 1960s showed that killed whole organism vaccines provided some degree of protection against ocular *C. trachomatis* infection in humans and nonhuman primates.[28] Serovar-specific monoclonal antibodies to MOMP neutralize *C. trachomatis in vitro*, but there are few data to suggest that either IgG or IgA antibody is protective in humans. The intracellular development of *C. trachomatis* is inhibited by interferon-γ (IFN-γ), and there is evidence from animal models and from studies of ocular infection in humans that cell-mediated immune responses mediated by CD4 T lymphocytes are important for the clearance of infection.[28,29]

Unfortunately, vaccine studies in primates also showed that vaccination could provoke more severe disease on subsequent challenge, suggesting that much of the damage caused by *C. trachomatis* infection may be immunopathologic in origin in keeping with the histopathology of *C. trachomatis* infection, in which the lymphoid follicle is the hallmark.

Follicles contain typical germinal centers, consisting predominantly of B lymphocytes, with T cells, mostly CD8 cells, in the parafollicular region. The inflammatory infiltrate between follicles comprises plasma cells, dendritic cells, macrophages, and polymorphonuclear leukocytes, with T and B lymphocytes. Fibrosis occurs at a late stage in trachoma and pelvic inflammatory disease. T lymphocytes outnumber B cells and macrophages. Biopsies from patients with cicatricial trachoma and persisting inflammatory changes show a predominance of CD4 cells, but those from patients in whom inflammation has subsided contain mainly CD8 cells.[30]

A chlamydial heat shock protein (Hsp60), homologous with the GroEL protein of *Escherichia coli,* elicits antibody responses that are associated with the damaging sequelae of *C. trachomatis* infections in both the eye and genital tract.[31,32] *In vitro* studies show that IFN-γ interferes with the chlamydial development cycle, leading to persistent infection with continuing release of Hsp60. It is not known whether the immune response to Hsp60 is itself the cause of immunopathologic damage, or merely a marker of more severe or prolonged infection. Gene expression at the site of infection has been studied to identify molecular pathways to fibrosis following ocular *C. trachomatis* infection in humans. Matrix metalloproteinase 9 (MMP9) appears to play an important role. Case-control studies have identified polymorphisms in several immune response genes (encoding TNF-α, IFN-γ, and IL-10) associated with the development of severe scarring following ocular *C. trachomatis* infection,[33,34] and one study suggested that the polymorphism in the IL-10 gene associated with scarring trachoma led to increased IL-10 secretion at the site of infection.[35]

In recent years research has focused on the development of a subunit vaccine against *C. trachomatis* which provides protection without eliciting immunopathology. Purified preparations of the MOMP were protective in murine models, provided that the native trimeric structure of the protein was maintained.[36] In nonhuman primates, a similar preparation of MOMP reduced peak shedding from the ocular surface, but had no effect on the duration of infection or on ocular disease.[37]

THE DISEASE

The clinical manifestations of genital *C. trachomatis* infection are similar to those of gonorrhea, but are usually less severe, as *C. trachomatis* infection elicits a less intense acute inflammatory response than *Neisseria gonorrhoeae*. Many chlamydial infections are asymptomatic. Long-term sequelae such as infertility are generally caused by fibrosis and scarring following prolonged or repeated infections, and may develop even in those with few or no symptoms. The clinical manifestations of chlamydial infection are summarized in ***Table 47.1***.

Table 47.1 Human Diseases Caused by *Chlamydia*

Species	Serovars	Disease
C. trachomatis	A, B, Ba, C	Trachoma
	D–K	Urethritis, epididymitis
		Cervicitis, pelvic inflammatory disease
		Curtis–Fitz-Hugh syndrome
		Adult and neonatal conjunctivitis
		Neonatal pneumonia
		Reactive arthritis
	L1, L2, L3	Lymphogranuloma venereum
		Proctocolitis
C. psittaci	Many	Pneumonia, endocarditis, abortion
C. pneumoniae	Only one	Community-acquired pneumonia
		Bronchitis

Clinical Manifestations in Men

Urethritis

C. trachomatis is detectable in the urethra of up to 50% of men with symptomatic nongonococcal urethritis. The incubation period is 7–21 days, compared to 2–5 days for gonorrhea. Patients present with a history of dysuria, usually accompanied by a mild-to-moderate mucopurulent urethral discharge. *C. trachomatis* is responsible for a proportion of cases of chronic (persistent/recurrent) non-gonococcal urethritis. Since mixed infections are common, treatment of gonococcal urethritis with an antibiotic ineffective against *C. trachomatis* may result in post-gonococcal urethritis.

Epididymitis

C. trachomatis is responsible for up to 70% of cases of acute epididymitis in young men (35 years of age or younger) in developed countries.[38] Patients present with unilateral scrotal pain, swelling, and tenderness, often accompanied by fever. Most give a history of current or recent urethral discharge, In developing countries, although chlamydiae are important, *Neisseria gonorrhoeae* is the major cause of acute epididymitis. In patients older than 35 years, epididymitis/epididymo-orchitis tends to be caused by urinary tract pathogens. There is no good evidence that chlamydial epididymitis or chlamydial urethral infection leads to male infertility.

Proctitis

Proctitis in men who practice receptive anal intercourse may be due to LGV or non-LGV strains of *C. trachomatis*. The non-LGV strains cause a milder disease, which may be asymptomatic or give rise to rectal pain, bleeding, and mucopurulent anal discharge.

Prostatitis

There is no evidence that *C. trachomatis* causes acute symptomatic prostatitis. Transperineal biopsies from patients with chronic nonbacterial prostatitis show chronic inflammation, but chlamydiae have not been detected by culture or direct immunofluorescence techniques, although polymerase chain reaction (PCR) tests are positive in about 10%. Such largely negative observations, and the failure to detect chlamydial antibody, suggest that *C. trachomatis* is not often implicated directly in the chronic disease.

Clinical Manifestations in Women

Cervicitis

C. trachomatis typically infects the columnar epithelial cells of the endocervix. It does not affect the squamous epithelium of the vagina. *C. trachomatis* is associated with a mucopurulent discharge from the cervix visible on speculum examination, and with hypertrophic cervical ectopy that tends to bleed on contact. Studies in many parts of the world have found that the prevalence of cervical *C. trachomatis* infection is no higher among women who complain of vaginal discharge than among those who do not, suggesting that it is not a cause of symptomatic vaginal discharge.

Urethritis

C. trachomatis has been implicated as a cause of the urethral syndrome, in which women present with dysuria, frequency and sterile pyuria.[39] Clinical signs of urethritis, such as urethral discharge or meatal redness, are not usually found.

Pelvic Inflammatory Disease

C. trachomatis may spread from the endocervix to the endometrium and fallopian tubes, causing pelvic inflammatory disease (PID). This is more likely to occur after trauma to the cervix due, for example, to termination of pregnancy, insertion of an intrauterine contraceptive device, or delivery. Histologic evidence of endometritis can be found in up to 50% of women with mucopurulent cervicitis due to *C. trachomatis*, and is more common in those with a history of abnormal vaginal bleeding. Classical signs of PID may be present (fever, lower abdominal pain and tenderness, and cervical motion tenderness), but chlamydial PID may be subclinical. Spread to the peritoneum may result in perihepatitis (the Curtis–Fitz-Hugh syndrome), sometimes confused with acute cholecystitis in young women, peri-appendicitis and other abdominal complaints. *C. trachomatis* infection has also been associated with postpartum endometritis.[40]

C. trachomatis is the major cause of PID in developed countries. Infertility may be the first indication of asymptomatic tubal disease. It occurs in about 10% of women following a single upper genital tract infection and in possibly half of those after two or three episodes. Infertility may result from endometritis, from blocked or damaged fallopian tubes, or perhaps from abnormalities of ovum transportation caused by damage to the ciliated epithelial surface. Other consequences of salpingitis are chronic pelvic pain and ectopic pregnancy. Following chlamydial PID, the risk of ectopic pregnancy increases seven- to tenfold.

Pregnancy Outcome

There is conflicting evidence on the effect of *C. trachomatis* on pregnancy. Some studies have shown *C. trachomatis* infection to be associated with low birth weight and preterm delivery, but others have failed to confirm this. In general, *C. trachomatis* was diagnosed and treated at a later stage of gestation in those studies that found a correlation between infection and adverse birth outcome than in those that did not.[41–44]

Other Conditions of the Female Genital Tract

C. trachomatis has been weakly associated with bartholinitis and should be considered in the absence of other known pathogens. A significant association between cervical chlamydial infection and cervical squamous cell carcinoma, but not adenocarcinoma, has been established, and it has been suggested that chlamydial infection may enhance the effect of oncogenic papillomaviruses.

Clinical Manifestations Occurring in Both Sexes

Adult Paratrachoma (Inclusion Conjunctivitis) and Otitis Media

Adult chlamydial ophthalmia commonly results from the accidental transfer of infected genital discharge to the eye. It usually presents as a unilateral follicular conjunctivitis, acute or subacute in onset. The features are swollen lids, mucopurulent discharge, papillary hyperplasia, and later follicular hypertrophy and occasionally punctate keratitis. About one-third of patients have otitis media, and complain of blocked ears and hearing loss. The disease is generally benign and self-limiting. Patients and their sexual contacts should be investigated for genital chlamydial infection and managed appropriately.

Reactive Arthritis

Arthritis occurring with or soon after nongonococcal urethritis is termed "sexually acquired reactive arthritis" (SARA). Conjunctivitis and other features characteristic of Reiter's syndrome are seen in about one-third of patients. Evidence of chlamydial infection, by a specific serological response or by the presence of *C. trachomatis* elementary bodies or DNA and antigen in the joints, is found in at least one-third of cases. *C. trachomatis* has also been associated in the same way with "seronegative" arthritis in women. Viable chlamydiae have not been detected in the joints of patients with SARA, which is probably the result of immunopathology. Despite this, early tetracycline therapy has been advocated by some investigators.[45]

Neonatal Infections

Although intrauterine chlamydial infection can occur, the major risk of infection to the infant is from passing through an infected cervix. Conjunctivitis appears in 20–50% of infants exposed to *C. trachomatis* infecting the cervix at birth. A mucopurulent discharge and occasionally pseudomembrane formation occur 1–3 weeks later. It usually resolves without visual impairment.

About half of the infants who have conjunctivitis also develop pneumonia, although a history of recent conjunctivitis and bulging eardrums is present in only half of the cases. Chlamydial pneumonia usually begins between the fourth and eleventh week of life, preceded by upper respiratory symptoms. There is tachypnea, a prominent, staccato cough, but usually no fever, and the illness is protracted. Radiographs show hyperinflation of the lungs with bilateral diffuse, symmetrical, interstitial infiltration and scattered areas of atelectasis.[46] Children infected during infancy are at increased risk of obstructive lung disease and asthma.

Lymphogranuloma Venereum

Lymphogranuloma venereum (LGV) is a systemic, sexually transmitted disease caused by serovars L1, L2, and L3 of *C. trachomatis*.

The clinical course of LGV can be divided into three stages. The primary stage at the site of inoculation; the secondary stage in the regional lymph nodes, and/or the anorectum; and the tertiary stage of late sequelae affecting the genitalia and/or rectum.

In the **primary stage**, after an incubation period of 3–30 days, a small, painless papule, which may ulcerate, occurs at the site of inoculation: usually the prepuce or glans in men; anorectal and rectosigmoid colon sites in homosexual men; the vulva, vaginal wall, or occasionally the cervix in women. Extragenital primary lesions on fingers or tongue are rare. The primary lesion is self-limiting and may pass unnoticed by the patient. Among patients with LGV presenting with buboes in Thailand, more than half had not been aware of an ulcer.[18]

The **secondary stage** occurs some weeks after the primary lesion. It may involve the inguinal lymph nodes, or the anus and rectum. The inguinal form is more common in men than women, since the lymphatic drainage of the upper vagina and cervix is to the retroperitoneal rather than the inguinal lymph nodes. LGV proctitis occurs in those who practice receptive anal intercourse, probably due to direct inoculation.

The cardinal feature of the inguinal form of LGV is painful, usually unilateral, inguinal and/or femoral lymphadenopathy (bubo). Adenopathy above and below the inguinal ligament gives rise to the "groove sign" in 10–20% of cases. Enlarged lymph nodes are usually firm and often accompanied by fever, chills, arthralgia, and headache. Biopsy reveals small discrete areas of necrosis surrounded by proliferating epithelioid and endothelial cells. These areas of necrosis may enlarge to form stellate abscesses, which may coalesce and break down to form discharging sinuses, although this phenomenon occurs in less than a third of patients with inguinal disease. In women, signs include hypertrophic suppurative cervicitis, backache, and adnexal tenderness.

Anorectal involvement is seen predominantly in homosexual men. Clinical features include a purulent anal discharge, anorectal pain and bleeding due to acute hemorrhagic proctitis or proctocolitis. There may be pronounced systemic signs of fever, chills and weight loss. Proctoscopy reveals a granular or ulcerative proctitis from which large numbers of polymorphonuclear leukocytes are seen in rectal smears. CT or MRI scans may show pronounced thickening of the rectal wall, with enlargement of iliac lymph nodes. Enlarged inguinal nodes may also be palpable.

Extragenital infection can cause lymphadenopathy outside the inguinal region. For example, cervical adenopathy due to LGV has been reported after oral sex. A follicular conjunctivitis has also been described following direct inoculation of the eye, which may be accompanied by pre-auricular lymphadenopathy. Other rare manifestations of the secondary stage include acute meningoencephalitis, synovitis, and cardiac involvement.

The **tertiary stage** appears after a latent period of several years, but all late complications are rare today because of the use of broad-spectrum antibiotics. Chronic untreated LGV leads to fibrosis, which may cause lymphatic obstruction and elephantiasis of the genitalia in either sex, or rectal strictures and fistulas. Rarely, it can give rise to the syndrome of esthiomene (Greek: "eating away"), with widespread destruction of the external genitalia.

DIAGNOSIS

The laboratory diagnosis of chlamydial infection depends on detection of the organisms or their antigens or nucleic acid and, to a much lesser extent, on serology. The highest bacterial load is found in the endocervix in women and in the urethra in men. An endocervical swab is therefore needed for the diagnosis of *C. trachomatis* infection by culture or antigen detection assay. However, the greater sensitivity of nucleic acid amplification tests (NAATs) for *C. trachomatis* means that self-administered vaginal swabs and "first-catch" urine specimens give equivalent results to endocervical swabs when using these assays. First-catch urine specimens have replaced intraurethral swabs for the diagnosis of chlamydial urethritis in males when NAATs are employed. Samples to be tested by NAATs can be transported to the laboratory at room temperature, making home-based screening for *C. trachomatis* possible.

Culture

The growth of chlamydiae in cultured cells, rather than in embryonated eggs, more than 40 years ago revolutionized the diagnosis of *C. trachomatis* infection. Centrifugation of specimens onto cycloheximide-treated McCoy or HeLa cell monolayers, followed by incubation and then staining with a fluorescent monoclonal antibody, to detect inclusions, has been used widely for the diagnosis of *C. trachomatis* infection. One blind passage may increase sensitivity. However, cell-culture techniques are no more than 70% sensitive when compared to NAATs, and are labor intensive. Because culture is essentially 100% specific, it still has a role in medicolegal cases.

Direct Immunofluorescence

Detection of elementary bodies using species-specific fluorescent monoclonal antibodies is rapid and, for *C. trachomatis* oculogenital infections, highly sensitive and specific in the hands of skilled observers. However, it is subjective, and not suitable for high throughput testing. It is therefore best used in settings where few specimens are tested, and for confirming positive results obtained with other tests.

Enzyme Immunoassays

Enzyme immunoassays that detect chlamydial antigens, usually the group-specific lipopolysaccharide, were widely used before NAATs became available. However, the lower limit of detection is 1000 organisms or more, and these tests are only about 70% sensitive compared to NAATs, which are now much more widely used.

Nucleic Acid Amplification Tests (NAATs)

By enabling enormous amplification of a nucleic acid sequence specific to the chlamydial species, the PCR assay, the strand displacement assay (SDA), and the transcription-mediated amplification (TMA) technique have overcome problems of poor specificity and particularly of poor sensitivity, since they will detect 10–100 organisms. Commercial assays based on each of these three amplification methods are available and are widely used.[47,48] The first two assays amplify nucleotide sequences of the cryptic plasmid, which is present in multiple copies in each chlamydial elementary body. However, the recently described Swedish variant of *C. trachomatis* harbors a deletion in the plasmid that gives rise to false negative results with these assays.[17] The TMA reaction is directed against rRNA, which is also present in multiple copies. These sensitive assays have replaced culture as the "gold standard" for the diagnosis of *C. trachomatis* infection.

Point of Care Tests

Several point of care tests are available for the diagnosis of *C. trachomatis* infection, but they are less sensitive than NAATs.[49] One such test, in dipstick format, which detects the lipopolysaccharide of *C. trachomatis* and can give a result within 15 minutes of sample collection, has been evaluated by the manufacturer on first-catch urine samples from men and self-collected vaginal swabs from women. In men, it was found to be 83% sensitive (95% confidence interval 74–89%), and 98.5% specific, compared with the Roche Amplicor PCR assay.[50] In women, it was 83% sensitive and 98.9% specific.[51] This test is not yet commercially available, and has not been independently evaluated.

Serological Tests

Serological tests are not generally helpful in diagnosing *C. trachomatis* infection, since they do not distinguish between past and current infection. They may be helpful in the diagnosis of PID, LGV, and in the Curtis–Fitz-Hugh syndrome, since antibody titers tend to be higher in these conditions than in uncomplicated cervical infections. *C. trachomatis* IgM antibody is the gold standard for the diagnosis of chlamydial pneumonia in babies.

TREATMENT AND PROGNOSIS

Chlamydiae are intracellular, and hence insensitive to aminoglycosides and other antibiotics that do not penetrate cells efficiently. Tetracyclines and macrolides are the mainstay of treatment for *C. trachomatis* infections. Ofloxacin is active against *C. trachomatis* at a dose of 300 mg twice daily for 7 days, but is not widely used. Treatment is often started before a microbiological diagnosis can be established, so additional broad-spectrum antibiotics are needed to cover gonococcal and, in the case of PID, anaerobic infections. Treatment of patients' partners is essential to prevent reinfection.

Uncomplicated *C. trachomatis* infections are treated with a single 1 g dose of azithromycin or with doxycycline (100 mg twice daily for 7 days). Chlamydial PID is treated with a 14-day course of doxycycline (100 mg twice daily). Tetracycline resistance has been reported in laboratory isolates of *C. trachomatis*, but clinically significant resistance has not been reported. Doxycycline is contraindicated in pregnancy. Azithromycin as a single 1 g dose, and amoxicillin (500 mg three times daily for 7 days) have both been shown to be safe and effective in pregnant women.[52,53] Ophthalmia neonatorum and neonatal pneumonia due to *C. trachomatis* should be treated with erythromycin syrup by mouth, 50 mg/kg daily divided into four doses, for 14 days.

There has been no adequately powered study comparing antibiotic regimens for LGV. Recommended treatment for both bubonic and anogenital LGV is doxycycline (100 mg twice daily), or erythromycin (500 mg four times daily), for 21 days. Azithromycin has been used successfully in some cases, although a 1 g dose immediately is unlikely to be sufficient, and the optimal regimen is unknown. Fever and bubo pain subside rapidly after antibiotic treatment is started, but buboes may take several weeks to resolve. Large collections of pus should be aspirated, using a lateral approach through normal skin. Rectovaginal fistulas, rectal strictures, and esthiomene require surgical correction with antibiotic coverage.

PREVENTION AND CONTROL

Health education and condom promotion, especially for the youngest sexually active age groups, may help to reduce the incidence of genital *C. trachomatis* infection. Syndromic management of symptomatic infections, and partner notification, may also play a role but, since a high proportion of chlamydial infections are asymptomatic in both sexes, these measures are unlikely to be successful on their own. A screening program for *C. trachomatis* at the primary health care level in the United States has reduced the incidence of upper genital tract infection and its complications in women.[54] Screening programs have been introduced in some European countries, in which young people presenting to health services for any reason are offered a test for *C. trachomatis*; but the public health impact of such opportunistic screening programs remains to be demonstrated.[55]

Access the complete reference list online at
http://www.expertconsult.com

CHAPTER 48

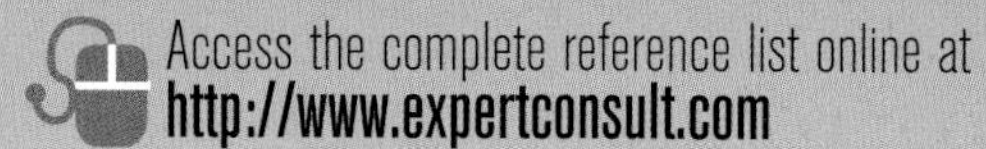
Access the complete reference list online at
http://www.expertconsult.com

Psittacosis

Thomas J. Marrie

INTRODUCTION

Psittacosis was first described by Ritter in 1879.[1] At that time he was investigating a household outbreak of a severe respiratory illness that was associated with contact with sick parrots. In 1892 Morange applied the name *psittacosis* (Greek *psittakos*, parrot) to this illness because of its association with sick parrots. In 1930 the causative agent, *Chlamydia psittaci*, was isolated at about the same time by Bedson in the United Kingdom, Krumwide in the United States, and Lemonthol in Germany.[2]

THE AGENT

Chlamydiae are obligate intracellular prokaryotes with a small genome of approximately 1.2 megabases. Some strains of *C. psittaci* contain a plasmid.[2] The family Chlamydiaceae has two genera: *Chlamydia* with *C. trachomatis*, *C. muridarum*, and *C. suis*; and *Chlamydophila* with *C. abortus*, *C. caviae*, *C. felis*, *C. pecorum*, *C. pneumoniae*, and *C. psittaci*. *Chlamydophila psittaci* has eight serovars, six of which have been isolated from birds (A through F) and two (WC and M56) that have been isolated from mammals. Chlamydiae exhibit morphologic and structural similarities to Gram-negative bacteria. The life cycle is initiated when an elementary body (the extracellular form) attaches to a susceptible epithelial cell. The elementary body then enters the epithelial cell by receptor-mediated endocytosis, where it undergoes reorganization into a much larger replicating form, the reticulate body. The reticulate body divides by binary fission to produce an ever-enlarging inclusion. The morphology of the elementary and reticulate bodies of *C. psittaci* and *C. trachomatis* are similar. *C. psittaci* forms multiple small inclusions in a single infected cell, with each infected elementary body developing its own inclusion. Kaltenboeck and colleagues[3] compared the sequences of the *ompA* gene (which encodes major outer membrane protein) of 10 strains of *C. psittaci*, 11 strains of *C. pecorum*, one *C. pneumoniae* strain, and two *C. trachomatis* strains. Two clusters were present: *C. trachomatis* and another cluster consisting of three major groups of *ompA* alleles: the psittacosis group, *C. pneumoniae*, and the polyarthritis group (ruminant and porcine chlamydial alleles).

EPIDEMIOLOGY

It is likely that all birds are susceptible to infection with *C. psittaci*. Over 150 avian species (57 of the parrot family) representing 10 orders have been documented as hosts for this microorganism. These include members of the parrot family (macaws, cockatoos, parakeets, budgerigars), finches (canaries, bullfinches, goldfinches, sparrows), poultry (hens, ducks, geese, turkeys), and pigeons, pheasants, egrets, gulls, and puffins. Birds transmit the infection to their nestlings, which in turn shed the organism during periods of both illness and health. In bird populations there is a baseline prevalence of 5–8% carriage of *C. psittaci*. This may increase to 100% when the birds are subjected to the stress of shipping, crowding, and breeding. Strains from turkeys and other psittacine birds are most virulent for humans.[2,4] A more recent review found that 467 species belonging to 30 orders of birds had been infected by *C. psittaci*.[5] Most human infections result from avian strains of *C. psittaci*, but other strains from animals are occasionally implicated. The disease has occurred in ranchers following exposure to infected goats, cows, and sheep.[6] Endocarditis has been attributed to avian and non-avian strains, and cats have spread feline pneumonitis to humans and other mammals.[7,8] The organism is resistant to drying and can remain viable for a week at room temperature.

Infected birds excrete *C. psittaci* in feces for several months. Nasal and lacrimal secretions may be infectious.[9] Transmission via eggs has been demonstrated in ducks. In experimental avian infections, the incubation period is 5–10 days. In turkeys, virulent *C. psittaci* strains cause pericarditis, weight loss, air sacculitis, and bronchopneumonia.[9] The mortality rate is low in natural infection.[9] In infected ducks and geese, conjunctivitis, rhinitis, polyserositis, pericarditis, and splenomegaly are common findings.[9] In pigeons, air sacculitis, hepatomegaly, and splenomegaly occur. In psittacine birds, splenomegaly, hepatomegaly, enteritis, sinusitis, and air sacculitis are frequently seen.[9]

Psittacosis is distributed widely (***Fig. 48.1***). In northern latitudes sporadic cases are acquired by contact with imported birds that have not been quarantined and treated with tetracycline prior to sale. Psittacosis in tropical countries is more likely to occur where parrots are caged and kept as household pets; however, there is very little published about psittacosis in the tropics. Psittacosis is an occupational hazard for abattoir workers (turkeys, chickens), farmers or ranchers (ducks, turkeys), laboratory workers (technicians in veterinary research facilities can be involved in outbreaks), pet shop employees (psittacine birds), and veterinarians.[10] In the United States, about 100–250 cases of psittacosis are reported to the Centers for Disease Control and Prevention (CDC) in Atlanta each year.[11] Sporadic psittacosis is often underdiagnosed. In a recent study of 149 patients with pneumonia treated on an ambulatory basis, the author found that two cases (1.3%) were due to *C. psittaci*. Neither case was suspected by the physician to be psittacosis. In a study of 539 patients with community-acquired pneumonia in Canada, 2 patients had pneumonia due to feline strains of *C. psittaci*.[12]

Feral pigeons are common in almost every city in the world. Data from[11] European countries indicate that 19.4–95.6% of pigeons sampled were seropositive for *C. psittaci*.[12] To 2004 there have been 101 case reports of ornithosis in humans where the route of transmission could be traced to contact with feral pigeons.[13] In all likelihood this is a gross underestimate.

Five severe cases of psittacosis associated with duck farms were noted in France between January and March 2006.[14]

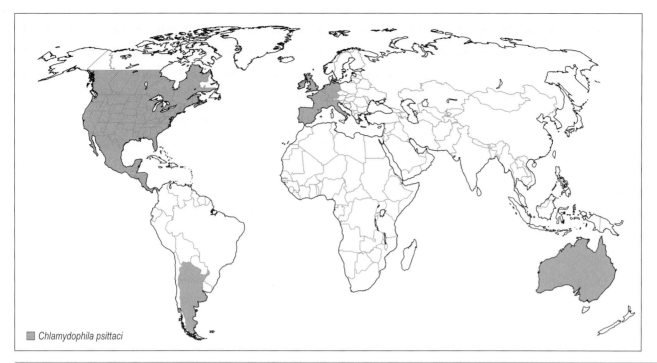

Figure 48.1 *Chlamydophila psittaci* distribution.

THE DISEASE

The clinical spectrum of *C. psittaci* infection is wide, ranging from a subclinical illness to rapidly progressive pneumonia.[2] The incubation period is from 5 to 15 days. Fever, rigors, sweats, and headache are common. Cough occurs in 50–100% of patients, but it usually appears late in the course of illness and usually is nonproductive.[11] The cough, however, may be productive of mucoid sputum, and rarely there is hemoptysis. Some patients, up to 19% in one series, have no respiratory symptoms.[15] There is also a mononucleosis-like form of the illness with fever, pharyngitis, hepatosplenomegaly, and lymphadenopathy. A typhoidal form presents with fever, bradycardia, and malaise. In a series of 135 cases from Australia, there were five modes of presentation: (1) fever with rigors, sweats, and constitutional symptoms but no localizing features, occurring in 41% of the patients; (2) prominent cough and occasionally dyspnea in association with fever in 33%; (3) severe headaches suggestive of meningitis; (4) diarrhea, which occurred in two patients; and (5) pharyngitis, which occurred in 21 patients.[16] An alteration of mental status was noted in 12%.

There are many extrapulmonary manifestations of psittacosis. These include Horder's spots (a pink, blanching maculopapular eruption resembling the rose spots of typhoid fever), acrocyanosis, superficial venous thrombosis, and splinter hemorrhages. Panniculitis, erythema multiforme, and erythema nodosum are cutaneous manifestations.[17] Encephalitis, meningitis, cerebellar involvement, cranial nerve palsies, intracranial hypertension, and transverse myelitis are central nervous system manifestations.[18] Acute renal failure,[19] pancreatitis, and thrombocytopenic purpura have also complicated psittacosis.[20] Other manifestations include reactive arthritis[21] and hemophagocytosis.[22] Endocarditis is a rare extrapulmonary manifestation of psittacosis.

Psittacosis during pregnancy is uncommon, but when it occurs it may be severe. An outbreak of sheep-associated psittacosis in the Faroe Islands in 1938 resulted in infection of 14 pregnant women, 11 of whom died.[23] A number of other cases of sheep-associated psittacosis involving pregnant women have been reported,[7,15] and a case of parakeet-associated psittacosis during pregnancy has been reported.[24] *C. psittaci* appears to have a predilection for the placenta.

Severe respiratory insufficiency due to psittacosis is uncommon, with only 12 reported cases from 1963 to 1993. Ten of these 12 had a history of exposure to birds. Seven had neurologic manifestations, six had gastrointestinal symptoms, and four were in acute renal failure requiring hemodialysis.[25] Eight patients (67%) died, three within 48 hours of admission. While uncommon, fatalities do still occur from this disease.[26]

The white blood cell count is usually normal in psittacosis. Eosinophilia may occur during convalescence. Macfarlane and colleagues[27] compared the radiographic features of 10 patients with *C. psittaci* pneumonia, 49 with legionnaires' disease, 91 with pneumococcal pneumonia, and 46 with mycoplasmal pneumonia. No distinctive pattern was seen for any group. Forty percent of the psittacosis patients had multilobe involvement, and 20% had a pleural effusion. In this series, none of the patients with psittacosis showed radiographic deterioration following admission, as compared with 65% of the patients with legionnaires' disease, 52% of those with bacteremic pneumococcal pneumonia, and 25% with mycoplasma pneumonia. Fifty percent of the patients with psittacosis pneumonia showed clearing of the radiographic opacities by 4 weeks; however, 30% were still unresolved by 12 weeks. In a review of 43 cases of psittacosis, Coutts and colleagues[28] found that 12 (28%) had a normal chest radiograph. Segmental consolidation was most frequent (31%); 21% had lobar consolidation, and 19% had multilobar involvement.

The pleural fluid in psittacosis may have a high adenosine deaminase level.[29] This could result in confusion with tuberculosis, since an adenosine deaminase level of greater than 43 IU/L in pleural fluid is believed to be sensitive and specific for tuberculosis.

PATHOGENESIS AND IMMUNITY

Human infection with *C. psittaci* follows inhalation of contaminated aerosols shed by infected birds. A study at 39 breeding facilities for psittacine birds in Belgium gives further insight into the transmission of *C. psittaci*.[30] Forty-nine (19.2%) of 308 psittaciformes were positive for *C. psittaci* by nested polymerase chain reaction/enzyme immunoassay. Six of 46 (13%) bird owners had *C. psittaci* DNA detected in respiratory secretions – 4 of the 6 were culture positive. All 4 had mild respiratory illness.[30] Antibiotics are used widely in these bird breeding facilities, raising the very real possibility of drug-resistant strains of *C. psittaci* in the future. The mechanism whereby *C. psittaci* is introduced into a flock of birds is poorly understood. Many investigators think that wild birds, which can be infected by the same strains as domestic flocks, play a major role in this process.[31] It is likely that vertical transmission occurs in flocks.[31]

In turkeys *C. psittaci* infects epithelial cells and macrophages in the respiratory tract.[32] This is followed by septicemia and localization of the organisms in epithelial cells and macrophages in various organs.[32] It is still unclear whether humoral or cell-mediated immunity is the most important host defense against *C. psittaci*. The major outer membrane protein (MOMP) has been identified as a protective antigen.[33,34] Plasmid DNA expressing *C. psittaci* serovar A MOMP was used to vaccinate turkeys and was shown to be effective.[35]

DIAGNOSIS

A high index of suspicion is necessary to make the diagnosis of psittacosis. Confirmation is by serologic test – the microimmunofluorescence (MIF) test is more sensitive and species-specific than the complement fixation test (CF). *Chlamydophila psittaci* may also be isolated in tissue culture, but most laboratories do not have the capability of cultivating chlamydiae. An antibody titer of 1 : 64 by the CF test is considered diagnostic. A fourfold rise in titer is also diagnostic. The CF test is family-specific and does not distinguish *C. trachomatis* from *C. pneumoniae* or *C. psittaci* infection. *C. psittaci* DNA can be detected in respiratory secretions using polymerase chain reaction. Wong and associates[36] studied 78 patients in whom a diagnosis of psittacosis was made on the basis of appropriate clinical symptoms following exposure to sick birds. The CF test identified 36 of 78 (46%) as positive, while the MIF test identified 48 of 78 (61%). The investigators used eight strains of *C. psittaci* in the MIF test. Others have noted that the MIF test can be falsely negative.[24] Thus, more than one strain of *C. psittaci* should be used in the MIF test. Wong and coworkers[36] noted four serologic reaction patterns among their 78 patients: (1) positive CF and MIF tests (46%); (2) anticomplementary or negative CF test and positive MIF test (15%); (3) positive serologic response to *C. pneumoniae* (9%); and (4) negative antibody titer using both CF and MIF tests (29%).

TREATMENT AND PROGNOSIS

Treatment is with tetracycline or doxycycline for 10–21 days.[2] Response to treatment is usually prompt. Some patients have severe fatigue that persists for 2–3 months following resolution of the acute illness. A longer course of treatment has been recommended to prevent relapse. Erythromycin is an alternative to treatment with a tetracycline but may be less efficacious in severe cases. There is less than a 1% mortality rate in treated cases.

PREVENTION AND CONTROL

Infected birds should be treated with tetracycline, chlortetracycline, or doxycycline for at least 45 days. Ideally, all imported birds should be treated prophylactically for *C. psittaci*. The CDC have issued recommendations for the control of *C. psittaci* among humans and birds, and these should be used whenever a case of psittacosis is encountered. All cases of psittacosis should be reported to a medical officer of public health for appropriate follow-up and tracing of infected birds.[37]

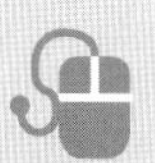

Access the complete reference list online at http://www.expertconsult.com

Access the complete reference list online at
http://www.expertconsult.com

CHAPTER 49

Spotted Fever Group Rickettsioses

Daniel J. Sexton • David H. Walker

INTRODUCTION

During the first decade of the twentieth century, a young American investigator, Howard Ricketts, discovered that ticks were vectors of a then mysterious illness, Rocky Mountain spotted fever (RMSF), that the causative organism circulated in nature between ticks and mammals, and that infected ticks transmitted the causative organism to their progeny.[1,2] Ricketts's discoveries paved the way for later investigators to discover rickettsial diseases occurring in the tropics.

Rickettsia species of the spotted fever group (SFG) cause human diseases in tropical Africa, Asia, Australia, South America, Central America, and Mexico (***Table 49.1***). The recognized geographic range of known rickettsial diseases, such as rickettsialpox, has expanded from urban to suburban and rural areas. African tick bite fever (ATBF), flea-borne spotted fever, Flinders Island spotted fever, *R. parkeri* infection, and Japanese spotted fever are now recognized in new countries. Rickettsial infections are neglected and poorly recognized by physicians in many tropical and subtropical locations. Indeed, medical science has focused insufficient efforts in the diagnosis and antimicrobial treatment of rickettsial infections in subtropical and tropical areas.

THE AGENT

Rickettsiae are small (0.3 × 1.0 μm) Gram-negative obligately intracellular bacteria that reside in various cells of their arthropod hosts and in the cytosol of human endothelial cells.[3] The genus *Rickettsia* is divided into the typhus group and SFG on the basis of antigenic differences in the immunodominant lipopolysaccharides (LPS) and the presence of outer-membrane protein A (OmpA) in SFG rickettsiae.[4] Studies of evolutionary genetic relationships have determined that *R. australis, R. akari,* and *R. felis* comprise the transitional group, a clade between the typhus group and SFG.[5,6] Other clades of presumed nonpathogenic ancestral *Rickettsia* are found in insects, leeches, amebae, and protists.[7]

OmpA, OmpB, and two other cell surface autotransporter proteins, Sca1 and Sca2, are adhesins; OmpB and Sca2 trigger rickettsial entry into cells by induced phagocytosis.[8–13] OmpA contains a series of hydrophilic tandem repeat units that vary in number and order, and OmpB is a 135-kDa S-layer protein, which is the processed form of a 168-kDa precursor.[14–18] Species- and strain-specific epitopes are located on these proteins.[19–21]

Molecular studies of the taxonomy of *Rickettsia* species reveal close genetic relationships that in other genera such as *Orientia* would lump many of these organisms into a smaller number of named species.[22–24] For example, *R. africae* and *R. parkeri* show minimal differences, as do *R. japonica* and *R. heilongjiangiensis*.[25,26] The genetic conservatism of these bacteria may be related to their intracellular location and prolonged survival in arthropod hosts that in turn mitigated immune-selective pressure.

Rickettsiae have undergone remarkable gene reduction. Their genomes are as small as 1.1 Mb. They rely upon the host's cytosolic environment to obtain amino acids, phosphorylated sugars, and adenosine triphosphate by effective rickettsial transport systems. The following SFG and transitional group rickettsiae cause human diseases: *R. rickettsii, R. conorii, R. africae, R. australis, R. sibirica, R. japonica, R. honei, R. parkeri, R. slovaca, R. felis, R. aeschlimannii, R. monacensis, R. massiliae, R. helvetica,* and *R. akari*.[27–45]

EPIDEMIOLOGY

Human infections with SFG and transitional group rickettsiae are transmitted by ticks, fleas (*R. felis*), and mites (*R. akari*) (***Fig. 49.1***). Their distribution is determined by complex relationships involving their particular rickettsial reservoirs (***Fig. 49.2***). Some *Rickettsia* depend completely on transovarian maintenance in their arthropod host; other *Rickettsia* circulate in zoonotic cycles involving an arthropod host and its vertebrate host. In the latter instance the host develops sufficent rickettsemia or co-feeding opportunity to infect another tick or mite serially. Highly pathogenic bacteria such as *R. rickettsii* and *R. conorii* have a deleterious effect on their tick host that results in death of the infected tick lineage after several generations of transovarian passage.[46,47] This harmful interaction correlates with a low prevalence (less than one *R. rickettsii*-infected *Dermacentor* tick or one *R. conorii*-infected *Rhipicephalus* tick per 1000 ticks) even in endemic regions.[48] These rickettsiae rely upon their virulence to maintain horizontal transmission in their vertebrate host and establish new infected tick lines via generation of sufficient concentrations of rickettsiae in the blood to allow feeding ticks to acquire infection.

In contrast, less pathogenic organisms such as *R. africae* are present in up to 80% of their host ticks with which they appear to have a successful long-term nondeleterious relationship.[49] Uninfected ticks may also acquire rickettsial infection by co-feeding; that is, they may ingest rickettsiae that are injected into the skin by an adjacent tick. Whether obtained from blood or infected saliva of another feeding tick, rickettsiae then traverse the tick's gut barrier and hemolymph to invade the tick salivary glands.

Field and experimental studies of zoonotic maintenance of rickettsiae in nature have been performed in Brazil where the incidence and geographic distribution of *R. rickettsii* infection have corresponded to the population of capybaras. These large rodents develop subclincal infection via transmission by *Amblyomma cajennense* ticks, and develop rickettsemia capable of subsequently infecting *A. cajennense* nymphal ticks.[50] *Didelphis aurita* opossums also are susceptible to subclinical infection with *R. rickettsii* and develop intermittent rickettsemia capable of infecting feeding nymphal *A. cajennense* ticks.[51] In experimental settings higher proportions of *R. sanguineus* and *A. aureolatum* than *A. cajennense* acquire *R. rickettsii* from experimentally infected guinea pigs.[52] Naturally infected ticks of all three species are found in Brazil. It can be hypothesized that the

Table 49.1 Epidemiology of Spotted Fever Group Rickettsioses Listed in Order of Decreasing Clinical Severity

Agent	Disease	Geographic Distribution	Maintenance in Nature	Human Transmission
Rickettsia rickettsii	Rocky Mountain spotted fever, Brazilian spotted fever	North, Central, and South America	Transovarial maintenance in *Dermacentor, Rhipicephalus,* and *Amblyomma* ticks; less extensive horizontal transmission from tick to mammal to tick	Tick bite
R. conorii	Boutonneuse fever, Mediterranean spotted fever, Kenya tick typhus, Israeli spotted fever, Indian tick typhus, Astrakhan spotted fever	Mediterranean basin, Africa, Asia	Transovarial maintenance in *Rhipicephalus* ticks	Tick bite
R. sibirica	North Asian tick typhus, lymphangitis-associated rickettsiosis	Russia, China, Mongolia, Pakistan, Kazakhstan, Kyrgyzstan, Tadzhikistan, France, Niger, Mali, South Africa, Portugal	Transovarial maintenance in *Dermacentor, Haemaphysalis,* and *Hyalomma* ticks; horizontal transmission from tick to mammal to tick	Tick bite
R. japonica	Japanese spotted fever	Japan, Korea	Presumably a transovarial tick host	Tick bite
R. australis	Queensland tick typhus	Eastern Australia	Transovarial transmission in *Ixodes* ticks	Tick bite
R. felis	Flea-borne spotted fever	North and South America, Africa, Asia, Europe, presumably worldwide	Transovarial transmission in *Ctenocephalides felis* fleas	Unknown
R. akari	Rickettsialpox	United States, Ukraine, Croatia, Turkey, Mexico, possibly worldwide	Transovarial transmission in *Liponyssoides sanguineus* mites; horizontal transmission from mite to mouse to mite	Mite bite
R. honei	Flinders Island spotted fever	Australia, Thailand	Transovarial transmission in *Aponomma* ticks	Tick bite
R. heilongjiangensis	Far Eastern spotted fever	Eastern Russia, Thailand, China		Tick bite
R. parkeri	Maculataum disease	North and South America	Transovarial maintenance in *Amblyomma* ticks	Tick bite
R. africae	African tick bite fever	Sub-Saharan Africa, Caribbean	Transovarial maintenance in *Amblyomma* ticks	Tick bite
R. slovaca	Tick-borne lymphadenopathy; *Dermacentor*-borne necrosis, eschar, lymphadenopathy	Europe	Transovarial maintenance in *Dermacentor* ticks	Tick bite
R. aeschlimannii, R. massiliae, R. monacensis, R. helvetica, R. amblyommii	Not named	Incompletely defined	Presumably transovarian transmission in ticks	Tick bite

occurrence of temporal and geographic clusters of human cases of *R. rickettsii* in Brazil may have resulted from spillover of sylvatic cycles involving *Amblyomma* ticks, capybaras, and opossums to free-ranging dogs. Infected dogs could in turn infect *R. sanguineus* ticks that progressively infect other dogs, thus creating a large population of *R. rickettsii*-infected peridomestic brown dog ticks that are capable of transmitting spotted fever to humans.[53–55] Such transmission has been described in Mexico and on an Indian reservation in Arizona,[56] and may be partially responsible for the clusters of cases in Brazil.

SFG rickettsiae are transmitted when rickettsiae are inoculated via arthropod saliva into the person's skin after several hours of feeding by ticks or mites. In most endemic locations there is a demarcated seasonal occurrence of rickettsial infections. Climatic factors that affect tick activity and human activities that bring persons in contact with infected ticks have a substantial effect on the epidemiology of these arthropod-borne infections.[57] Tick prevalence and questing behavior while seeking a host for a blood meal are affected by temperature and humidity, which vary from one region to another.

Human SFG and transitional group rickettsioses currently under active investigation in the tropics include pathogens recognized in Africa (*R. africae, R. conorii, R. sibirica* mongolotimonae strain, *R. felis, R. aeschlimannii*), Latin America (*R. rickettsii, R. akari, R. parkeri, R. felis*), Asia (*R. conorii, R. sibirica, R. japonica, R. honei, R. heilongjiangensis, R. felis*), and Australia (*R. australis, R. honei, R. felis*).[24–35,49,58–74] Some of these pathogens are highly associated with a particular arthropod vector (e.g., *R. conorii* with *Rhipicephalus sanguineus* brown dog ticks)[75]; others are found in related ticks (e.g., *Rickettsia africae* with *A. variegatum, A. hebraeum,* and *A. lepidum*); still others are transmitted by unrelated ticks (e.g., *R. rickettsii* by *Dermacentor variabilis, D. andersoni, A. cajennense, A. aureolatum,* and *R. sanguineus*). Ticks that feed on humans only during their adult stage are more frequently detected and reported by patients than when smaller larvae and nymphs transmit infection during an unrecognized tick bite.

R. africae is transmitted by highly aggressive *A. hebraeum* ticks in southern Africa and by *A. variegatum* in sub-Saharan Africa and the West Indies.[76] Outbreaks involving clusters of travelers in rural areas and soldiers in southern Africa[77,78] and endemic cases in Cameroon suggest that *R. africae* causes a high incidence of infections among indigenous persons.[79] It is also the most commonly imported rickettsiosis in travelers.[77]

RMSF is known to occur in the United States, Mexico, Costa Rica, Panama, Colombia, Brazil, and Argentina.[28–30,61,71–74,80–85] The principal vectors of *R. rickettsii* in the tropics are *A. cajennense, A. aureolatum,* and

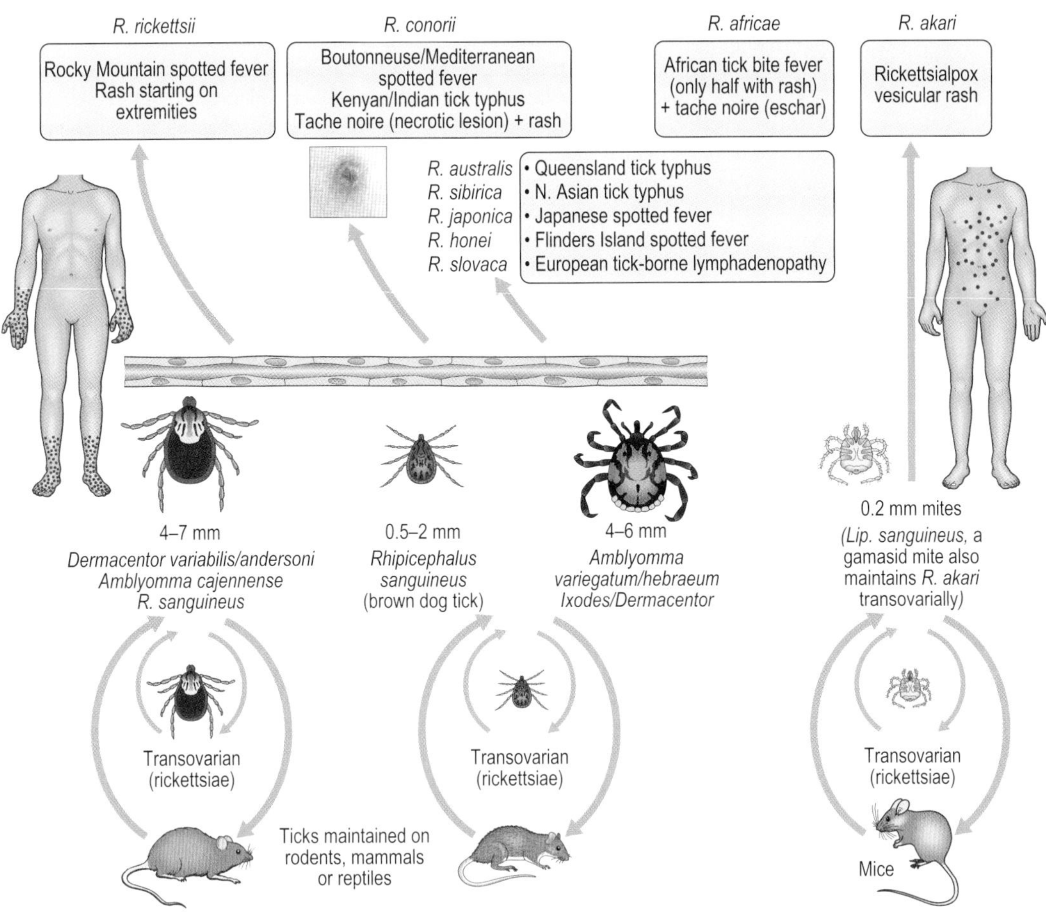

Figure 49.1 Spotted fever rickettsial diseases life cycle.

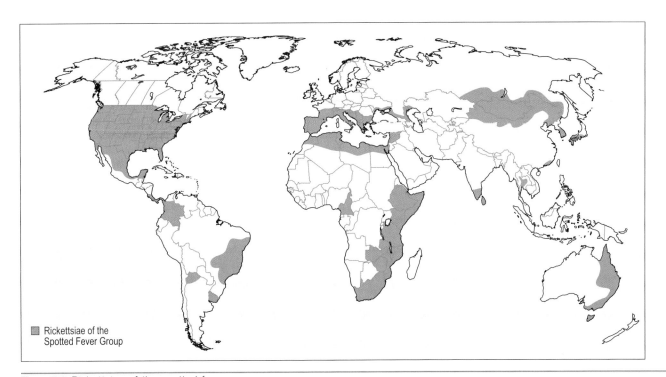

Figure 49.2 Rickettsiae of the spotted fever group.

R. sanguineus. *R. australis* infection occurs along the entire eastern coastal regional of Australia,[86] where the primary vector of *R. australis* is *Ixodes holocyclus* (the scrub tick), the principal human-biting tick in Australia. *I. holocylus* also feeds on a wide array of domestic and wild animals, many of which have been shown to have antibodies against SFG rickettsiae.[86,87] *R. akari*, the cause of rickettsialpox, has been identified in the United States, Ukraine, Croatia, Korea, Mexico, and Turkey.[42,62,88,89]

Misdiagnosis of SFG rickettsial infections is common because the clinical features of rickettsial infections mimic those of many other infectious diseases. Clinical studies of patients with acute febrile illness suspected to be dengue, typhoid, or malaria in whom these diagnoses have been excluded have shown that SFG rickettsioses are prevalent in study sites in Latin America and Africa.[49,79,90] Results of serosurveys of healthy subjects undertaken with the aim of assessing the incidence of undiagnosed infections due to SFG rickettsiae are difficult to interpret because of crossreactivity due to shared antigens such as LPS. Thus previous conclusions that highly virulent organisms, such as *R. rickettsii,* cause a high prevalence of asymptomatic infections are unlikely to be valid. Indeed, most subjects in such studies likely had greater exposure to organisms that appear to cause mild or asymptomatic infection (e.g., *R. amblyommii*).[91–96]

Studies of SFG rickettsioses, diagnosed serologically in Thailand, Laos, Hong Kong, and Sri Lanka, lack confirmation by rickettsial isolation or polymerase chain reaction (PCR) identification of the etiologic species of *Rickettsia*.[97–102] In other studies in Taiwan, the Philippines, Hainan Island, Indonesia, Mexico, Ecuador, Peru, Brazil, and many sub-Saharan African countries, antibodies to undetermined SFG rickettsiae have been found in humans, but their significance is similarly difficult to interpret without simultaneous rickettsial isolation or PCR identification.[102–106]

THE DISEASE

SFG rickettsioses vary in severity. For example, the case-fatality rate in untreated RMSF averages approximately one in four; in contrast, infections due to organisms such as *R. slovaca* and *R. aeschlimannii* produce illnesses that are rarely, if ever, fatal and may remain afebrile (see ***Table 49.1***). Several entities will be described individually because of their severity and occurrence in tropical countries (RMSF and boutonneuse fever), high prevalence (ATBF), or unique clinical presentation (*R. slovaca*-associated tick-borne lymphadenopathy). Other SFG rickettsioses have similar clinical manifestations with nonspecific symptoms at onset and during the course. The proportions of patients with different rickettsial infections with signs such as eschars, rash, presence of maculopapules, vesicles, petechiae, regional lymphadenopathy, lymphangitis, and severe illness are highly variable.

Rocky Mountain Spotted Fever

After an incubation period of 2–14 (average 7) days, RMSF typically begins suddenly with fever, muscle aches, and headache.[107,108] Nausea, vomiting, and abdominal pain are common in the early phases of illness. Occasionally patients with these symptoms also develop abdominal tenderness that leads to misdiagnosis of an acute surgical abdomen that in turns leads to a negative exploratory laparotomy.

There is wide variability in the evolution, distribution, and appearance of skin rash in patients with RMSF. Rash usually appears on days 3–5 after onset of fever, but it may appear earlier or later, or not at all in some patients. Rocky Mountain spotless fever occurs in 10–15% patients.[109] Such cases may end fatally. Rash may be absent or difficult to recognize in African-American patients. Although skin rash is classically described as beginning on the wrists and ankles, before it spreads centripetally, this presentation is frequently not present. Rash may occur on the palms and soles, but this is often detectable only late in the course of illness in many of these patients. Some patients with RMSF have localized rashes on one body region or rashes that appear late in illness manifesting only as a small number of petechial lesions.[109] Skin necrosis or gangrene occurs in a small but important minority of patients, particularly those in whom diagnosis and treatment are delayed.[110,111]

Neurological complications such as meningoencephalitis, coma, and seizures may be life-threatening. Cerebrospinal fluid pleocytosis and/or elevated protein concentration may occur in up to half of the minority of patients who have severe or prominent enough symptoms to undergo lumbar puncture. Focal neurologic deficits, meningismus, ataxia, photophobia, or transient deafness may also occur and lead to diagnostic confusion with other infectious diseases. Pulmonary manifestations, including cough, radiographic alveolar infiltrates, interstitial pneumonia, and pleural effusions, may be present in some cases. Adult respiratory distress syndrome (ARDS) may require mechanical ventilation and supplemental oxygen. In such cases, there is minimal myocardial dysfunction with noncardiogenic pulmonary edema caused by increased vascular permeability associated with intense rickettsial infection of the pulmonary microcirculation. However, the same vasculitic process may involve the heart, resulting in histologic and electrocardiographic changes typical of myocarditis or heart block. Thus, careful assessment of cardiac function is needed to distinguish patients with RMSF complicated by ARDS from those with heart failure due to *Rickettsia*-induced myocarditis. In severe cases, increased vascular permeability results in edema, hypovolemia, decreased glomerular filtration, and prerenal azotemia.[112] In patients with severe hypotensive shock, oliguric acute renal failure may be associated with acute tubular necrosis.[113] Aside from a petechial rash, severe hemorrhagic phenomena seldom occur. Similarly, despite frequent thrombocytopenia, true disseminated intravascular coagulation is rare.[114,115]

Boutonneuse Fever (Mediterranean Spotted Fever)

Boutonneuse fever differs from RMSF in that it has a lower untreated case-fatality rate (4% versus 23%); the presence of a *tache noire* (eschar), a 1-cm focus of vascular rickettsial infection and injury leading to epidermal and dermal necrosis at the site of tick bite inoculation of rickettsiae in 72% of cases; and lower incidence of myalgia, petechiae, stupor, and cough.[116] Illness can be severe in patients with underlying disease such as cardiac failure or diabetes, old age, alcoholism, and glucose-6-phosphate dehydrogenase deficiency.[117–119] Also a recent study in Portugal indicates that the Israeli strain of *R. conori* causes a higher case-fatality rate and more severe clinical course than in those infected with Malish strain.[118]

African Tick Bite Fever

ATBF is a milder illness than boutonneuse fever, and no fatalities have been documented. After an incubation period of 5–7 days, patients with ATBF typically experience the abrupt onset of fever (59–100%), nausea, fatigue, headache (62–83%), myalgia (63–87%), nuchal myalgia (81%), eschars (53–100%), which are typically multiple (21–54%), painful regional lymphadenopathy (40–100%), rash (15–46%) that is either maculopapular (14–26%) or vesicular (0–21%), and aphthous stomatitis (0–11%).[76,120]

Patients from Uruguay, Brazil, and Argentina infected with the closely related SFG rickettsia *R. parkeri* also have illness similar to ATBF, with eschars and painful lymphadenopathy more often than rash.[64,121,122] North American patients infected with *R. parkeri* have eschars, fever, headache, myalgia, maculopapular or vesicular rash, and occasionally tender regional lymphadenopathy.[36]

Tick-borne Lymphadenopathy and Other SFG Rickettsioses

R. slovaca infection occurs in Europe during the cold months when *Dermacentor* ticks attach, usually to the occipital scalp, followed 7–9 days later by the presence of an eschar and painful regional (often cervical) lymphadenopathy. Illness is seldom accompanied by fever or rash.[123,124] The complications of prolonged alopecia at the site of the eschar (24%) and asthenia persisting even after doxycycline treatment suggest the possibility of co-involvement of other factors or agents.

Although other SFG rickettsioses are clinically similar, it should be noted that there is growing recognition of severe cases of Japanese spotted fever, including fatalities and patients with meningoencephalitis, multi-organ failure, and coagulopathy.[125–127] Fatal cases of Queensland tick typhus have also been reported.[128] The recognized incidence of rickettsialpox has risen owing to more attention to evaluation of eschars in the wake of bioterrorist-associated cases of cutaneous anthrax. Human infections with a novel strain of *R. sibirica* have been documented in France, Portugal, and Africa: nearly half of these patients manifest rope-like lymphangitis extending from the eschar toward the regional lymph nodes.[129–131]

PATHOGENESIS AND IMMUNITY

SFG rickettsiae grow and undergo reactivation of virulence in the salivary glands of ticks and mites and then are inoculated into the dermis of the skin during feeding. Presumably rickettsiae initially spread regionally via lymphatic vessels to the regional lymph nodes and later spread hematogenously throughout the body. These obligately intracellular bacteria grow mainly in endothelial cells and to a lesser extent in macrophages. They enter the endothelium by attachment of adhesins, such as OmpB, to a cell membrane protein such as Ku70, and induce cytoskeletal rearrangements in association with protein tyrosine kinase, phosphoinositide-3-kinase, and ubiquitin ligase resulting in clathrin- and caveolin 2-dependent phagocytosis.[8–13,132] Rickettsiae rapidly lyse phagosomal membranes via rickettsial phospholipase D, hemolysin C, and other enzymes, and escape into the cytosol where they replicate by binary fission.[133] SFG rickettsiae stimulate actin-based mobility via their protein RickA, which activates the host's Arp 2/3 complex that triggers nucleation of actin polymerization.[134,135] The actin tail that forms at one pole of the SFG *Rickettsia* propels it through the cytosol and via filopodia to the extracellular space or for cell-to-cell spread.

SFG rickettsiae injure endothelial cells by stimulation of their production of reactive oxygen species that damage cell membranes by lipid peroxidation.[136] The most important pathophysiologic effect of endothelial injury is increased vascular permeability leading to edema.[137–139] Endothelial permeability appears to be caused not only by rickettsia-mediated damage, but also by the effects of interleukin (IL)-1β, tumor necrosis factor (TNF)-α, and interferon (IFN)-γ, such as dissociation of adherens junctions p120-catenin and β-catenin and formation of inter-endothelial cell gaps, as well as cyclooxygenase-2-dependent production of prostaglandin E_2 and prostacyclin.[140,141] SFG rickettsiae manipulate the endothelial cells to serve as an efficient host for their growth by inhibiting apoptosis via activation of NF-κB, leading to inhibition of caspases 3, 8, and 9 and inhibition of release of cytochrome *c* from mitochondria.[142,143]

Immunity to SFG rickettsiae is mediated principally by T lymphocytes. Both CD4 and CD8 T lymphocytes secrete proinflammatory cytokines, especially IFN-γ, which along with TNF-α, IL-1β, and RANTES activate endothelial cells, macrophages, and hepatocytes to kill intracellular rickettsiae via synthesis of nitric oxide and hydrogen peroxide and/or limitation of available tryptophan via its degradation by indoleamine 2,3-dioxygenase.[144,145] Following human infection by *R. africae*, serum levels of the immune mediators IFN-γ, TNF-α, and RANTES are elevated.[146] CD8 lymphocytes provide a critical host defense with perforin-dependent elimination of infected cells by major histocompatibility complex class I-dependent cytotoxic T-lymphocyte activity.[147] Dampening of the infection early in the course by innate immunity includes Toll-like receptor 4-dependent activation of dendritic cells, most likely by rickettsial LPS, leading to NK cell activation with secretion of IFN-γ.[148–152] Antibodies to OmpA and OmpB contribute to control of infection and are effective in preventing reinfection.[153] Severe illness is associated with higher serum levels of TNF p55 and p75 receptors and IL-6.[154] A human IFN-γ single nucleotide polymorphism (SNP) is associated with resistance to boutonneuse fever, and an interaction of IFN-γ and IL-10 SNP genotypes is associated with susceptibility.[155]

DIAGNOSIS

The clinical diagnosis of SFG rickettsiosis is often difficult. This difficulty is underscored by the fact that cases are sometimes only first suspected at autopsy, even in areas where sophisticated medical care and diagnostic testing are available.[156] Fever, headache, and myalgias are nearly universal features of SFG rickettsial infections, but such symptoms are present in many other infectious diseases. Skin rash occurs in most but not all patients with *R. conorii*, *R. australis*, and *R. rickettsii* infection, but occurs in only half of patients with *R. africae* infection. A localized necrotic skin lesion (an eschar or *tache noire*) commonly occurs at the site of rickettsial inoculation by tick bite in patients with infection caused by *R. conorii* (except in Israel), *R. australis, R. japonica, R. africae, R. parkeri, R. slovaca, R. aeschlimannii, R. heilongjiangensis,* and *R. honei*, and by mite bite for *R. akari*. Rarely, such eschars occur in patients with *R. rickettsii* infection as well.[157] It is important to note that skin rash, eschar, and a history of tick bite may be absent or easily overlooked in some patients with SFG rickettsial infections; thus the absence of a rash or history of tick bite should not eliminate the possibility of a rickettsial disease in a febrile patient with other compatible symptoms, signs, and laboratory abnormalities, such as thrombocytopenia, mental status changes, or renal insufficiency. On the other hand, a history of a recent tick bite or tick contact can be of enormous help in diagnosing SFG rickettsioses in a patient with fever and nonspecific symptoms such as myalgias, headache, and gastrointestinal complaints. Similarly, when present, an eschar is often a critical clinical diagnostic sign of SFG rickettsioses, but the presence of an eschar is not in itself diagnostic of SFG rickettsiosis as similar lesions occur in scrub typhus, cutaneous anthrax, tularemia, primary syphilis, and chancroid.

The diagnosis of a SFG rickettsial infection can be established by isolation or molecular detection of the causative organism from blood or tissue and by immunohistochemical methods that visualize SFG rickettsiae in skin biopsy specimens.[158–164] *R. conorii* and *R. africae* have also been detected in circulating endothelial cells using immunomagnetic beads to capture the detached endothelial cells and immunocytologic techniques to demonstrate the rickettsiae.[165] SFG rickettsial infection can be confirmed retrospectively using a variety of serologic methods as antibodies appear late in the course or even late convalescence in ATBF.[166–169] Most of the standard serologic techniques, such as the microimmunofluorescent antibody test, cannot distinguish among infections with the different SFG rickettsial species, and Weil–Felix *Proteus* agglutination assays are both insensitive and nonspecific.[170,171] Molecular technology, such as real-time PCR, and use of biopsies of eschars and skin and even eschar swabs, has improved the laboratory diagnoses of SFG rickettsial infections, but the diagnostic sensitivity remains to be proven early in the course of disease, and adaptation to a point of care and low cost are important for resource-limited settings.[172–178]

Because SFG rickettsial infections often begin with nonspecific symptoms and because subsequent physical and laboratory findings such as a skin rash and thrombocytopenia are easily confused with an array of other diseases prevalent in the tropics, the clinical diagnosis of SFG rickettsial infections must rest on a synthesis of epidemiologic factors such as season of the year, possible exposure to ticks or tick-infested environments, and the clinical findings. It is difficult (and sometimes impossible) initially to distinguish SFG rickettsial infections from dengue, typhoid fever, malaria, drug reaction, and exanthematous viral infections such as measles, rubella, and arboviral and enteroviral disease. Occasionally, severe infection due to *R. rickettsii* or *R. conorii* can mimic meningococcemia, staphylococcal bacteremia, toxic shock syndrome, leptospirosis, viral hemorrhagic fever, or thrombotic thrombocytopenic purpura.

TREATMENT AND PROGNOSIS

Two drugs are the mainstays of treatment of all SFG rickettsial diseases: tetracycline and chloramphenicol. Tetracyclines such as doxycycline are generally the preferred agents, even for young children.[179] Despite the fact that doxycycline is safe and appropriate as initial therapy of children with suspected RMSF (and other SFG rickettsioses), there is evidence that unfounded fears of toxicity may result in a hesitance to use this drug as empiric therapy for RMSF. For example, fewer than 5% of children presenting to a Texas children's hospital with a suspected rickettsiosis actually received doxycycline or chloramphenicol as initial theapy.[180] An analysis of the outcome of 6338 patients with RMSF reported to the Centers for Disease Control and Prevention from 1981 to 1990 suggested that older patients, those treated with chloramphenicol only, patients not receiving a tetracycline as primary therapy, and those with delay in institution of therapy greater than 5 days had higher mortality rates.[181] Chloramphenicol is the preferred agent for pregnant women and for persons with severe illness, in whom it is difficult or impossible to distinguish between a rickettsial infection and meningococcal infection. Josamycin, which is not available in the United States, has also been proposed for pregnant women.[182] Quinolones have been shown to have activity against SFG rickettsiae *in vitro*, and in boutonneuse fever quinolones have been shown to be as effective as doxycycline in reduction in the duration of fever and are apparently superior in the rapidity of amelioration of other symptoms.[183–185] Although azithromycin and clarithromycin have been shown to provide equivalent successful outcome as chloramphenicol in children with mild Mediterranean spotted fever, neither they nor fluoroquinolones can be recommended at the present time for patients with moderate or severe SFG rickettsiosis.[186]

Duration of treatment of SFG rickettsial infections has not been studied systematically in a large cohort of humans. Although treatment regimens using doxycycline to treat Mediterranean spotted fever for time periods as short as 1–2 days have been reported to be as efficacious as 10-day regimens, similar studies have not been undertaken for treatment of other SFG rickettsiae such as *R. rickettsii* and *R. australis*.[187] Additionally, relapse of *R. conorii* infection in children treated with short courses of doxycycline has been reported.[188] In light of these data, most authorities recommend that tetracycline, chloramphenicol, or ciprofloxacin be continued for 7 days or until the patient has been afebrile for at least 48 hours and is improving clinically.

PREVENTION AND CONTROL

The tick vectors of SFG rickettsiae are widespread, and control of tick populations is generally not feasible. A vaccine is not available for any SFG rickettsia. Thus, avoidance of tick bite is the only preventive method available. Tick repellants and protective clothing reduce the risk of tick exposure, but are less acceptable to persons in a warm, humid environment. Regular inspection and removal of ticks from the body prior to inoculation of rickettsiae-infected saliva also reduce the likelihood of infection.

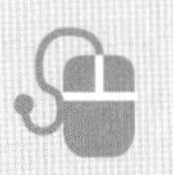

Access the complete reference list online at
http://www.expertconsult.com

Access the complete reference list online at
http://www.expertconsult.com

CHAPTER 50

Typhus Group Rickettsioses

David H. Walker • Didier Raoult

INTRODUCTION

Murine typhus, usually misdiagnosed as another ailment, is among the most prevalent febrile illnesses in the tropics.[1–5] Louse-borne typhus is historically one of the most devastating infections and a continuing cause of morbidity and mortality among isolated, impoverished populations.[6] Rickettsiae are small, obligately intracellular, Gram-negative bacteria that have an arthropod host as at least a portion of their ecologic niche. The typhus group comprises *Rickettsia prowazekii* (epidemic louse-borne typhus, recrudescent typhus, and flying squirrel-associated typhus) and *R. typhi* (murine typhus). Typhus infections were first described by Fracastorius in 1546 based on observations during an Italian epidemic in 1528.[7,8] Half of the deaths among Napoleon's 700 000 soldiers during the Russian campaign of 1812 were likely caused by typhus, just one example of the tremendous effect of typhus on history.[9] Milder forms of typhus described by Brill in 1898 in New York among emigrees from European typhus zones and by Paullin in 1913 in Atlanta were proved during the 1930s to be recrudescent *R. prowazekii* infection and rat flea-transmitted *R. typhi* infection, respectively.[10–15] Antibiotic-resistant *R. prowazekii* strains have been developed, and both *R. prowazekii* and *R. typhi* are aerosol-transmitted biothreats.[16–18]

THE AGENT

Typhus group rickettsiae have a small (1.1×10^6 base pairs) genome, a 135-kDa major, immunodominant S-layer protein arranged tetragonally on the cell wall surface, peptidoglycan, and abundant lipopolysaccharide, and are highly adapted to the intracellular environment rich in amino acids and phosphorylated sugars for which they possess specific mechanisms for transport from host cytoplasm.[19–25]

Typhus rickettsiae both produce adenosine triphosphate (ATP) via the tricarboxylic acid cycle and acquire it using five adenosine diphosphate (ADP)/ATP translocases.[26] The obligately intracellular lifestyle led to marked genome reduction, reflecting loss of genes such as lipid and nucleotide biosynthesis. The single circular genome contains fewer than 900 genes, numerous split genes with internal stop codons, and relics of obsolete genes.

The rickettsial ecologic cycle involves adaptation to arthropod and mammalian hosts in which the availability of nutrients and oxygen and other conditions varies tremendously. Rickettsiae contain unusual split spoT genes, which may be functional in the stringent response – an increase in diguanosine pentaphosphate – by catabolism of the toxic molecules to ATP.[27] Rickettsiae also contain autotransporters and some type IV secretion components but lack others not useful in the intracellular environment.[19,24]

EPIDEMIOLOGY

Typhus group rickettsiae have a louse or flea vector and are transmitted mainly in the insect's feces (***Fig. 50.1***). *R. prowazekii* infects a high proportion of southern flying squirrels (*Glaucomys volans*) in the eastern United States and is transmitted among squirrels by their lice and fleas without deleterious effects to the reservoir or arthropod hosts.[28] Typhus fever appeared in Spain during the late 1400s or early 1500s and was described in Mexico in 1545. Native Americans might have established the louse–human cycle after infection by ectoparasites of flying squirrels in the eastern United States or by *Amblyomma* ticks in Mexico.[29,30] *R. prowazekii* is poorly adapted to human body lice (*Pediculus humanus corporis*) as rickettsial growth in the louse gut epithelium results in highly infectious louse feces and also rupture of the louse's intestine with extravasation of blood turning its body red and death of the louse.[31] Lice do not maintain *R. prowazekii* transovarially.

After recovery from acute infection, *R. prowazekii* persists in many persons as an asymptomatic, latent infection. Years or decades later, presumably owing to waning immunity, rickettsial reactivation causes milder illness with sufficient rickettsemia to infect a portion of feeding body lice. Lice do not tolerate febrile body temperatures and leave patients seeking a new host. These infected lice transmit rickettsiae to nonimmune subjects and ignite an epidemic under conditions of general lousiness. Recrudescent typhus usually occurs within 10 years after acute typhus but may occur more than 30 years afterward. Louse-borne typhus epidemics occurred in Europe during and after World War I, involving 30 million cases and 3 million deaths in Russia alone.[32] In impoverished, cold, mountainous areas such as tropical Andes, Guatemala, Ethiopia, and other African and Asian countries, louse-borne typhus is an endemic disease.[6,33–39] Typhus that disappeared for 25 years prior to the civil war reemerged in Rwanda, Burundi, and Congo, apparently becoming endemic.[34,36] It also reappeared after 30 years in Algeria and Russia, and an autochthonous case occurred in a homeless person in France in 2003.[36–39]

Body lice are strictly adapted to humans and live in clothing rather than on the body, upon which they feed five times a day. Endemic *R. prowazekii* is characterized by localized outbreaks mainly among the young, since most older persons are the immune reservoir of sporadic recrudescent typhus. Travel and lousiness can introduce *R. prowazekii* into other areas, including warm tropical locations where a nonimmune population could suffer an epidemic (***Fig. 50.2***). Lessons from epidemic louse-borne typhus that affected 45 000–100 000 patients during the civil war in Burundi are that many fatalities can smolder in louse-infested populations of prisons and refugee camps for years without an accurate diagnosis and the disorder of war severely impedes effective epidemic control.[34,40,41] Latent *R. prowazekii* infections in populations where body lice are present emphasize the need for vigilance.[42]

R. typhi occurs worldwide, particularly in warm, humid, coastal environments of the tropics and subtropics (***Fig. 50.3***).[1,3–5,43–53] Prevalent in many areas although seldom investigated, murine typhus was identified recently in southern India, Indonesia, Philippines, Ethiopia, Mexico, Taiwan, New Zealand, Laos, Colombia, Brazil, Greece, and Texas.[54–66] Among displaced Khmers at the Thai–Cambodian border, 70% of patients with unexplained fever had murine typhus.[4] In Thailand and Laos, murine typhus is among the most common causes of acute febrile illnesses.

Although there is field and laboratory evidence for seven genera and 11 species of fleas, three species of lice, and three species of mites serving as vectors of *R. typhi*, the epidemiologic and ecologic evidence in most parts of the world points to the oriental rat flea, *Xenopsylla cheopis*, as the major vector and peridomestic *Rattus* species as critical vertebrate hosts. Rickettsiae-laden flea feces are scratched into the pruritic flea bite wound. Some infections are probably caused by flea bite. *R. typhi* might also be transmitted by rubbing infected flea feces into the conjunctiva or by inhalation of aerosols from dried flea feces, in which rickettsiae survive for years.

R. typhi is maintained mainly by horizontal transmission from infected flea to rat to flea. Fleas remain infected for a normal life span and pass the infection transovarially to a small fraction of offspring. Rats are highly susceptible to infection with *R. typhi*, develop sufficient rickettsemia to infect fleas imbibing their blood, and do not usually develop illness. Murine typhus can spread inland along lines of transportation wherever *Rattus*, *X. cheopis*, and *Rickettsia typhi* are carried.[67,68] Although severely reduced incidence was associated with DDT dusting and rat control, murine typhus persists in southern Texas and southern California, where cat fleas, *Ctenocephalides felis*, are apparently the vector, and opossums are possibly the reservoir.[69–71] History of exposure to rat- and rat flea-infested environments or flea bite is seldom recalled. Many patients are food handlers or are exposed to a focus with infected rats and rat fleas at work or home, usually unknowingly.[52,67,72,73]

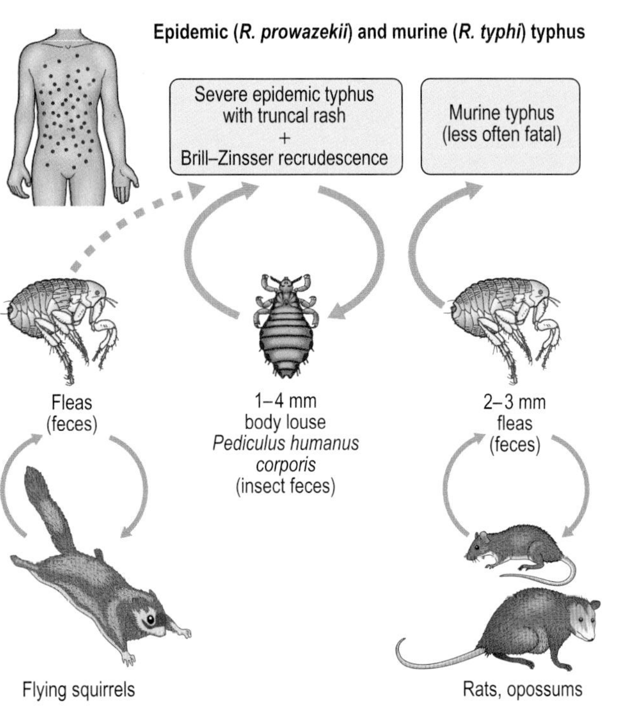

Figure 50.1 Epidemic (*Rickettsia prowazekii*) and murine typhus (*R. typhi*) life cycle.

THE DISEASE

The typhus fevers have clinical similarities with differences in severity according to host factors, the greater virulence of *R. prowazekii,* and antirickettsial treatment.[46,52,72–75] Recrudescent typhus is milder, presumably because of stimulation of anamnestic immunity. Epidemic typhus is a very severe disease that kills previously healthy people, including the early scientific investigators Ricketts and von Prowazek. It is not clear whether flying squirrel-associated typhus is milder because of better nutrition, health, and medical care or whether flying squirrel strains are less virulent.[76–79] Murine typhus is substantially less severe than louse-borne typhus, although 10% of hospitalized patients are admitted to the intensive care unit and 4% die.[72,73,80]

Antibiotic-era patients with epidemic typhus in Ethiopia manifested fever and headache (100%), chills (82%), rash (recognized only in 38% of these patients with pigmented skin), conjunctivitis (53%), muscle tenderness (70%), nausea (32%), vomiting (10%), abdominal pain (30%),

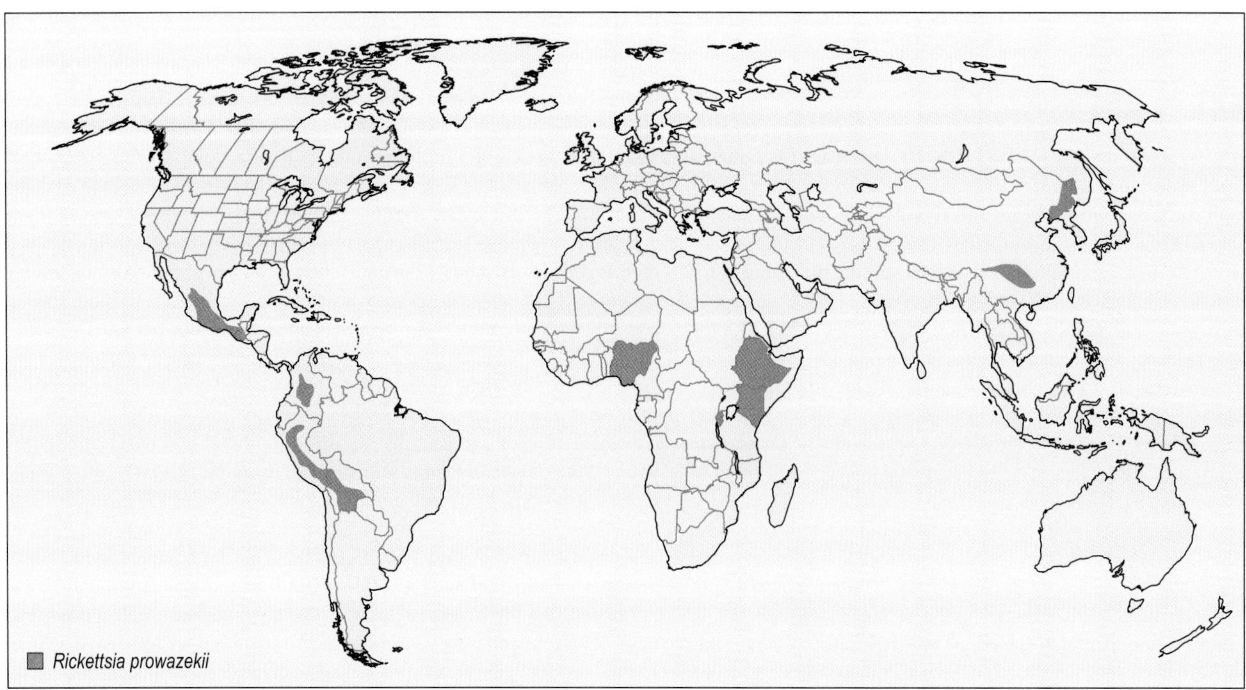

Figure 50.2 Epidemic louse-borne typhus fever.

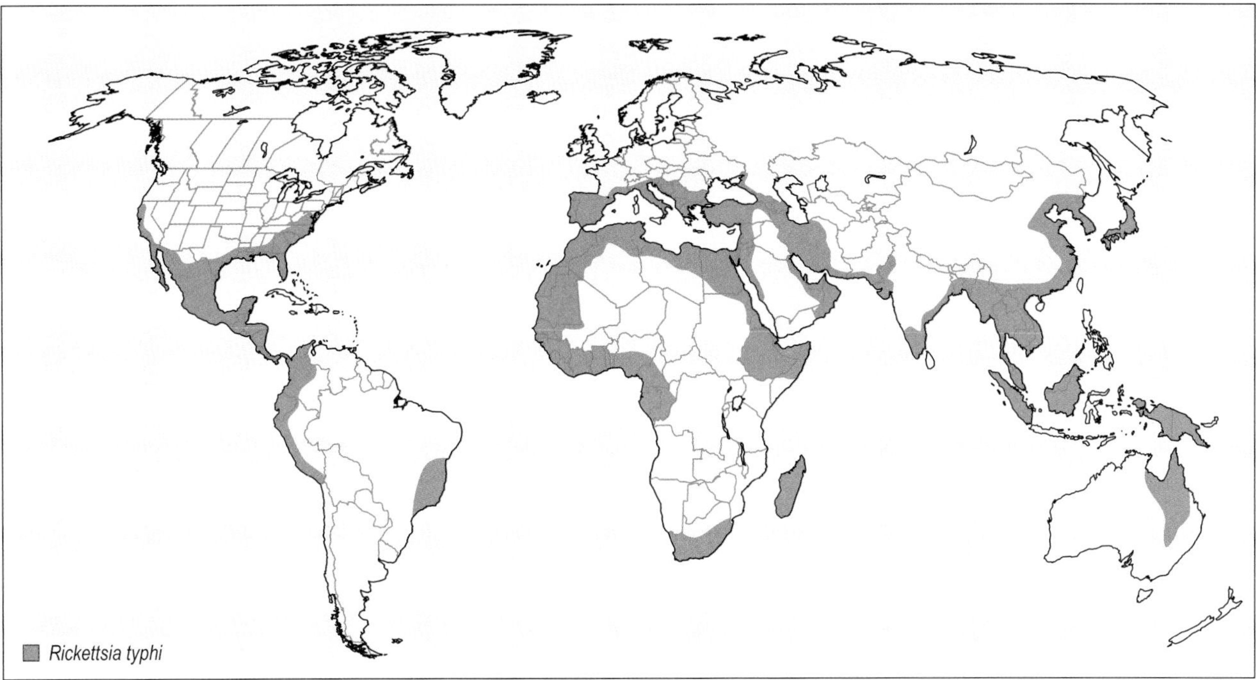

Figure 50.3 *Rickettsia typhi* map.

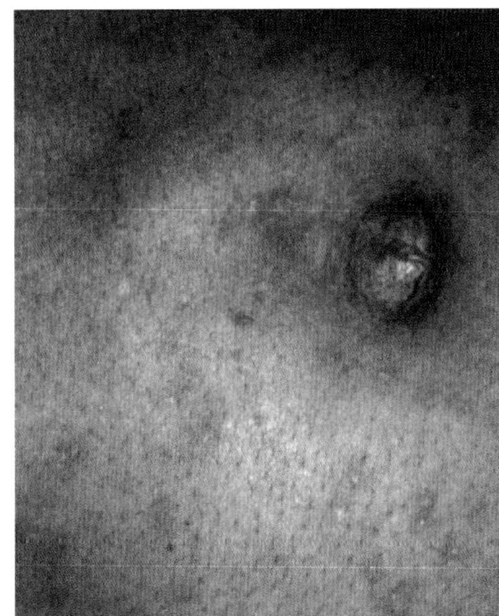

Figure 50.4 Rash of louse-borne typhus in a patient during the epidemic in Burundi.

jaundice (17%), cough (38%), photophobia (33%), and no fatalities.[6] Laboratory evaluation demonstrated mild, normocytic, normochromic anemia (48%); thrombocytopenia (43%); mildly elevated serum aspartate transaminase (63%), alanine transaminase (35%), serum bilirubin (20%), lactate dehydrogenase (82%), creatine kinase (31%), blood urea nitrogen (31%), and creatinine (2%); and mild hypoproteinemia (38%). In the preantibiotic era, the fatality rate of epidemic typhus was usually at least 10% and as high as 60%. The patients in the Burundi epidemic suffered from prominent myalgia, fever, delirium, stupor, confusion, dry cough, conjunctivitis, constipation, as well as coma and gangrene in some severe cases, and a 15% case-fatality rate. Even in darkly pigmented patients, a rash is often visible in the axilla (***Fig. 50.4***).[34,40] Chest roentgenograms frequently reveal interstitial pneumonia. Flying squirrel-associated typhus is characterized by fever (100%), headache (81%), maculopapular rash (66%), confusion (44%), and myalgia (42%).[78] Patients with Brill–Zinsser recrudescent typhus suffer fever, intense headache, myalgia, nausea, dulled sensorium, congested conjunctiva, constipation, and maculopapular rash appearing on the back and abdomen on day 5–7 and spreading rapidly.

Contemporary murine typhus in Thailand, southern Texas, and Greece, after an incubation period of 1–2 weeks, manifests fever (98–100%), headache (42–100%, occurring less frequently in children), chills (64–92%), rash (2–71% varying with skin pigmentation), myalgia (45–71%), nausea (31–59%), vomiting (23–40%), diarrhea (5–26%), abdominal pain (11–31%), jaundice (3–11%), confusion (2–8%), and seizures (2–4%).[4,5,46,52,72] The rash is macular or maculopapular in 78% and petechial in under 10%.[46] Experimental infections documented an incubation period of 8–16 days (mean 11.1 days), a prodrome usually of 2 days' duration, rash in 79% usually after 4 days of illness, and average duration of fever of 12 days.[81] In some patients, the signs, symptoms, and cerebrospinal fluid (CSF) mononuclear cell-predominant pleocytosis and increased protein concentration are similar to viral and leptospiral meningoencephalitis.[82] Central nervous system (CNS) abnormalities may also occur in patients with normal CSF. Chest radiographs reveal infiltrates, atelectasis, pulmonary edema, or pleural effusions in 20% or more of cases.[72] Laboratory evaluation reveals thrombocytopenia (48%); hyponatremia (60%); hypocalcemia (79%); elevated serum urea (27%) and creatinine (21%); hypoalbuminemia (89%); and elevated serum aspartate transaminase (90%), alanine transaminase (73%), alkaline phosphatase (60%), lactate dehydrogenase (87%), and creatine kinase (21%).[72] Severe manifestations include acute renal failure (usually prerenal azotemia), respiratory failure requiring intubation, severe encephalitis, intracerebral hemorrhage, hematemesis, cardiac conduction abnormalities, jaundice, intravascular hemolysis due to glucose-6-phosphate dehydrogenase deficiency or hemoglobinopathy, and exploratory laparotomy for suspected acute surgical abdomen.[46,52,72,82–84] Pediatric murine typhus is frequently mild.[85,86] Hospitalized pediatric cases have fever (100%), rash (80%), headache (77%), abdominal pain (60%), vomiting (43%), cough (40%), thrombocytopenia (60%), hyponatremia (66%), and hypoalbuminemia (46%).[85]

PATHOGENESIS AND IMMUNITY

Typhus rickettsiae attach to the endothelial cell membrane, rapidly stimulate entry by induced phagocytosis, and quickly escape from the phagosome into the cytosol, where they divide every 8–10 hours.[87] Only after the endothelial cell is greatly distended with rickettsiae does it burst, resulting in cell death and release of organisms. Macrophages are a minor target cell. Injury to infected endothelium results in vascular lesions in the skin, brain, and other organs manifesting as rash, encephalitis, and increased vascular permeability, resulting in edema, hypovolemia, hypotension, hypoalbuminemia, azotemia, and hyponatremia.[88–90] Very few infected, injured blood vessels thrombose and cause ischemic necrosis.[88] Virulence of *R. prowazekii* is associated with gene deletion and dependence on the host.[91] Avirulent Madrid E strain, used previously as a vaccine, differs from virulent *R. prowazekii* by a methyltransferase gene mutation leading to absent expression and reduced methylation of OmpB.[92] Rickettsiae have phospholipase activity that plays a role in entry, escape from the phagosome, and cell injury.[93–95] The genomes of *R. prowazekii* and *R. typhi* reveal several candidates for membranolytic function, including hemolysins A and C, phospholipase D, and phospholipase A homologs.[25,93–98] Rickettsial phospholipase D and hemolysin C mediate phagosomal escape by ordinarily vacuole-bound *Salmonella enterica*.[93] However, a *pld* deletion mutant of *R. prowazekii*, although attenuated, retains the ability to escape the phagosome, possibly owing to redundant membranolytic proteins.[94,95,99] An ortholog of an iron-associated superoxide dismutase is predicted to remove reactive oxygen species and favor rickettsial intracellular survival.[25] Rickettsial infection of endothelium and macrophages *in vitro* stimulates secretion of prostaglandin E_2, prostaglandin I_2, leukotriene B_4, and platelet-activating factor, which along with interleukin-1, tumor necrosis factor-α (TNF-α), and other cytokines are hypothesized to contribute to the pathophysiology of typhus not caused directly by rickettsial killing of endothelial cells.[100–102]

Typhus lesions comprise small blood vessels with swollen endothelium and perivascular accumulation of lymphocytes and macrophages.[88] Intradermal rickettsial inoculation results in prompt perivascular infiltration of CD8 and CD4 T lymphocytes in immune humans.[103] Typhus rickettsiae are killed by nitric oxide synthesized by murine endothelial cells and macrophages, activated by interferon-γ (IFN-γ) and TNF-α.[104,105] IFN-γ and CD8 T lymphocytes are critical effectors of immune clearance of *R. typhi* in mice.[106] Cytotoxic T lymphocytes recognize typhus rickettsial antigens on infected cells.[107] Protective immunity appears to be mediated mainly by cellular mechanisms of adaptive immunity, but innate immunity and antibodies likely contribute also.[108] Latent *R. prowazekii* resides in lymph nodes of healthy persons long after recovery from acute typhus fever, but the mechanism of reactivation of *R. prowazekii* is poorly understood.[109]

DIAGNOSIS

The nonspecific flu-like symptoms prior to the appearance of the exanthem, which may never occur, particularly in dark-skinned persons, are nearly impossible to recognize as louse-borne typhus or murine typhus.[4,6,72] Typhus was confounded historically with malaria and typhoid and is frequently misdiagnosed in Africa as these two diseases currently occur in similar settings there.[34,39,40,110] In Southeast Asia murine typhus is commonly confounded with scrub typhus and leptospirosis.[111]

Prominent cough and pulmonary signs suggest pneumonia or bronchitis; neurologic signs with or without CSF abnormalities raise the consideration of viral or bacterial meningoencephalitis; gastrointestinal symptoms and abdominal tenderness suggest viral and bacterial enterocolitis or acute surgical abdomen; elevated hepatic enzymes or jaundice suggest the possibility of viral hepatitis. The differential diagnosis includes typhoid fever; relapsing fever; malaria; leptospirosis; arboviral, enteroviral, filoviral, and arenaviral infections; meningococcemia; measles; secondary syphilis; and toxic shock syndrome. Even where murine typhus infections are well known to the medical community, the initial correct clinical diagnosis is made in only 10% of cases.[72] The Burundi epidemic of typhus, after years of smoldering activity, was recognized only by the investigation of the death of an emergently repatriated Swiss nurse. Murine typhus is among the most prevalent febrile illnesses in the tropics but usually remains misdiagnosed in those seeking medical attention and undiagnosed in those without access to health care. Typhus infections also occur in travelers returning from endemic areas.[110,112,113]

Often the first clue of a typhus group infection is a serologic result, even the least sensitive and least specific of which are not necessarily available in many tropical locations. Although the serologic diagnosis of rickettsial diseases is generally retrospective, the relatively long incubation period and lateness in the course when typhus infection is usually considered allow time for the generation of a detectable antibody response in the first serum sample of some patients.[114] The extensive cross-reactivity among typhus group rickettsiae permits use of either of them as test antigen, but does not allow easy demonstration of which agent stimulated the antibody response. Fewer than half of patients with epidemic typhus have a fourfold higher titer against *R. prowazekii* than against *R. typhi*. Cross-absorption, although capable of specific diagnosis, is laborious, expensive, and seldom undertaken.[115] The standard is the indirect immunofluorescent antibody assay (IFA), which requires an ultraviolet microscope that is seldom available in resource-limited settings.[116] An immunoglobulin G (IgG) titer of 128 or an IgM titer of 32 is considered to be diagnostic. The cutoff titer should be determined by the prevalence and titers of antibodies in local healthy persons. Serodiagnosis can be achieved from blood spotted on to filter paper and mailed to a reference laboratory.[117] The indirect immunoperoxidase antibody assay requires only a light microscope and has equivalent sensitivity and specificity as IFA.[4,5,52] Comparison of a rapid, simple dot enzyme-linked immunosorbent assay (ELISA) with IFA and the historic, but now archaic, Weil–Felix *Proteus* agglutination test demonstrated sensitivity and specificity of the dot ELISA of 89% and 98%, respectively, and of *Proteus* OX-19 agglutination, 72% and 98%, respectively, at a cutoff titer of 320.[114,118] In certain settings, even *Proteus* OX-19 agglutination is a useful tool in recognizing the occurrence of typhus fevers. Whether or not patients with recrudescent typhus produce IgM antibodies to *R. prowazekii* is controversial.[119]

Immunohistologic demonstration of typhus group rickettsiae in a cutaneous biopsy or necropsy tissues establishes the diagnosis of a typhus group infection.[89,120,121] An etiologic diagnosis of a specific *Rickettsia* species infection requires isolation and identification of the obligately intracellular organisms in cell culture (e.g., shell vial centrifugation-enhanced system), or polymerase chain reaction (PCR) amplification of a rickettsial gene and species identification by restriction fragment length polymorphism analysis or sequencing.[59,122–125] While these methods are not routinely available owing to cost and paucity of expertise in rickettsiology, their application on a selective basis establishes the presence and stimulates awareness of the various typhus fevers in a particular region. *R. prowazekii* can be detected by PCR in lice removed from patients even after being sent via mail to a reference laboratory.[126] Ultimately, timely presumptive diagnosis of the individual patient relies on knowledgeable clinical suspicion. Implementation of public health measures to control epidemic typhus or rats and rat fleas depends on a precise diagnosis. A bioterrorism attack of aerosol-transmitted typhus would be very unlikely to be considered diagnostically before the onset of rash, possibly not even then.[17]

TREATMENT AND PROGNOSIS

Patients with typhus infections treated before severe hypotension, acute renal or respiratory failure, or severe CNS disease occurs usually respond dramatically to antirickettsial therapy, particularly doxycycline, with defervescence within 48–72 hours.[46,52,72] Louse-borne typhus fever has been treated successfully in some settings with a single 200-mg oral dose of doxycycline.[34] Single-dose doxycycline treatment has greater than 80% efficacy in murine typhus but is not recommended because relapses may occur.[52] Patients can be treated with oral doxycycline (100 mg twice daily), tetracycline (25–50 mg/kg/day in four divided doses), or chloramphenicol (60–75 mg/kg/day in four divided doses). Patients who are comatose or vomiting are treated intravenously, and doxycycline or chloramphenicol is recommended for patients with renal failure. Pregnant patients should be evaluated individually and treated with either chloramphenicol (early trimester) or doxycycline (late trimester) if necessary. Treatment should, if possible, be continued for 2–3 days after defervescence to avoid relapse. Ciprofloxacin has been associated with treatment failure, but retrospective analysis of Greek patients with murine typhus showed that ciprofloxacin is as effective as chloramphenicol.[127–129]

Clinical experience, the intracellular niche, and presence of β-lactamase and several multidrug transport analogs in the genomes emphasize the natural resistance of *R. prowazekii* and *R. typhi* to most classes of antibiotics.[19,25] The lack of therapeutic response of the 63% of pediatric patients with murine typhus to treatment with a third-generation cephalosporin is a typical situation;[85] in louse-borne typhus, the outcome can be fatal.[128] It is advisable to avoid giving sulfonamide-containing antimicrobials to patients suspected of typhus because these drugs exacerbate the disease. Strains of *R. prowazekii* resistant to chloramphenicol[15] or tetracycline have been selected in the laboratory, and transformation to antimicrobial resistance has been performed by molecular methods.[130] Thus, the specter of a bioterrorism attack with *R. prowazekii* or *R. typhi* resistant to all antibiotics is a threat that has not been addressed. Supportive care, including intensive care nursing, avoidance of pressure sores, dialysis, mechanical ventilation with supplemental oxygen, transfusions, amputation of gangrenous extremities, and antimicrobial treatment of opportunistic pneumonia, may be required in some severely ill patients.

PREVENTION AND CONTROL

Control of epidemic and endemic typhus fevers depends on marked reduction in the vector and, in some cases, the reservoir populations. Murine typhus decreased from more than 5000 cases reported yearly in the southern United States during the 1940s to fewer than 100 annual cases following repeated dusting of rat passageways with DDT, killing rats, and modifying buildings to prevent entry of rats. Epidemics of louse-borne typhus have been curtailed by use of insecticides such as lindane powder for delousing and washing clothes in hot water to kill the lice. Dusting powder containing 1% permethrin applied in doses of 30–50 mg per adult on both the inside and outside of clothing and on bedding can be repeated at 6-week intervals to kill lice. Some louse populations are resistant to some insecticides.[131] The large Burundi epidemic was controlled by immediate treatment of patients with 200 mg doxycycline.[34] Vaccination has been used with apparent success to prevent louse-borne typhus.[131] Killed *R. prowazekii* vaccines required boosters and seemed to reduce the severity of illness in persons whose protection was only partial. A live attenuated strain was used as an effective vaccine under epidemiologic conditions where dose-dependent local and systemic reactions during the 2–3-day period after immunization, mild to moderate symptomatic infection 9–14 days after inoculation in approximately 14% of recipients, and the possibility of reversion to virulence were acceptable.[132]

Currently, there is no licensed vaccine. Development of a highly effective, safe vaccine that would provide protection against all rickettsial infections is a feasible goal.[133] However, the lack of awareness of the true disease burden of these infections by public health agencies and the unlikeliness of commercial profit to be gained from the perceived target populations of the neglected poor in the tropics mitigate against vaccine development.

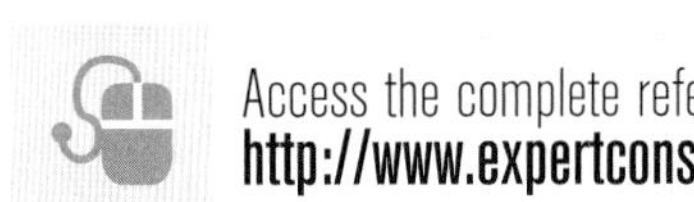

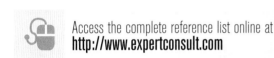

Access the complete reference list online at
http://www.expertconsult.com

CHAPTER 51

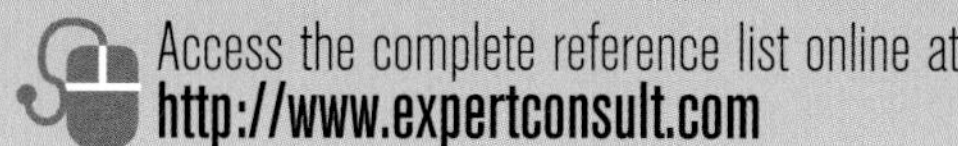
Access the complete reference list online at
http://www.expertconsult.com

Scrub Typhus

Ik-Sang Kim • David H. Walker

INTRODUCTION

Scrub typhus or tsutsugamushi disease is an acute febrile disease prevalent in Eastern Asia, and the western Pacific Ocean. The first record of apparent scrub typhus was described in China in AD 313.[1] The etiologic agent, *Orientia tsutsugamushi* discovered by Nagayo, is transmitted to humans during feeding of infected trombiculid mite larvae (chiggers).[2] Scrub typhus became known to the Western world during World War II when scrub typhus caused tens of thousands of cases in Allied and Japanese troops. Currently, one billion persons in the endemic areas are at risk for scrub typhus, and one million new infections occur annually.[3,4]

EPIDEMIOLOGY

Scrub typhus is confined to the "tsutsugamushi triangle" extending from far eastern Russia in the north, to northern Australia in the south, and to Pakistan and Afghanistan in the west. The endemic area includes Korea, Japan, China, Thailand, Laos, Cambodia, Vietnam, Malaysia, Myanmar, India, Sri Lanka, Nepal, Indonesia, Papua New Guinea, and the intervening Pacific and Indian Ocean islands (***Fig. 51.1***).[5–9] Endemic areas range from typical tropical secondary growth (scrub) vegetation to temperate zones (e.g., Kashmir, Korea, and Mount Fuji) and even the Himalayas above 3000 m elevation.[10–12] The ecologic factors underlying the reemergence of scrub typhus that has been documented recently in India, Sri Lanka, northern China, and the Maldives and Micronesia are not known.[8,13–15]

The agent, *O. tsutsugamushi*, is transmitted to humans by larvae of trombiculid mites (chiggers) during feeding. More than 45 species of trombiculid mites are known to be infected with *O. tsutsugamushi* in nature, but only limited numbers are proven to transmit scrub typhus including *Leptotrombidium pallidum*, *L. akamushi*, *L. scutellare*, *L. deliense*, *L. arenicola*, *L. imphalum*, *L. chiangraiensis*, and *L. pavlovskyi*. *L. pallidum* and *L. scutellare* are the major vectors in Korea and Japan.[16] *L. scutellare* and *L. deliense* transmit the disease in northern and southern China, respectively.[17] *L. deliense* is the major vector in Taiwan, Southeast Asia, India, and Papua New Guinea,[18] and *L. arenicola* is usually found in sandy beaches of Malaysia and Indonesia.[19]

The life cycle of trombiculid mites consists of four stages: eggs, larvae, nymphs, and adults (***Fig. 51.2***).[20] Nymphs and adults feed on eggs of small arthropods underneath the surface of the soil, whereas chiggers come onto the surface and parasitize vertebrate hosts. Chiggers on dead leaves, low vegetation, or soil recognize the presence of vertebrates and move to attach to them. Chiggers incise the host's epidermis with chelicerae and form feeding tubes (stylostomes) by their secretions and host tissues. The duration of feeding varies by mite species, but is usually 1–3 days. More than 6 hours are required for transmission of the infection.[21] Although there are certain endemic landscapes, such as shrubby fringes between fields and forest, banks of rivers, and abandoned rice fields, the chiggers may be found at any location that is suitable for rodent populations. Seasonal occurrence of scrub typhus correlates with the local period of trombiculid mite larval appearance.[22]

Trombiculid mites maintain *O. tsutsugamushi* by transovarian infection.[23] Rodents are key to the population density of the chiggers but are not a reservoir of *O. tsutsugamushi*; only a low proportion of chiggers acquire *O. tsutsugamushi* from infected rodents, and chiggers infected by feeding neither develop a generalized infection nor transmit the organisms transovarially to their offspring.[24] The proportion of *O. tsutsugamushi*-infected mites in a population varies by species and geography ranging from 0% to 10%. Moreover, the distribution of infected mites in an endemic area is not even; there are "mite islands" in which the prevalence of *O. tsutsugamushi*-infected mites is high.[25,26] *O. tsutsugamushi* infections alter the sex ratio in some mite species, with the majority of progeny being female.[27]

Prospective, longitudinal studies in peninsular Malaysia have revealed scrub typhus as the cause of 18.3–23.3% of febrile admissions at two hospitals.[28] In two communities the incidence of *O. tsutsugamushi* infection was 3.2–3.9% per month; the seroprevalence was 48–53%, with an age-dependent increase to greater than 80% above age 44 years.[29,30] Exposure to remote scrub and forested areas of Laos, Vietnam, and Cambodia results in seroconversion at a rate of 484 per 1000 person-years.[30] Laboratory infection via aerosol has been reported.[31]

THE AGENT

O. tsutsugamushi is a small (0.5 × 1.2–3.0 μm), strictly intracellular coccobacillary bacterium. In contrast with *Rickettsia, O. tsutsugamushi* has no or little lipopolysaccharide (LPS) or peptidoglycan and has a thicker outer leaflet of the cell wall than the inner leaflet. The 16S rRNA gene similarity between *O. tsutsugamushi* and *Rickettsia* is 90.2–90.6%.[32]

The major outer membrane proteins of 110, 80, 70, 60, 56, 47, 42, 35, 28, and 22 kDa are distinct from those of other Rickettsiaceae.[33] The 56 kDa transmembrane protein is the most abundant, comprising about 20% of total bacterial protein. Amino acid homology of the protein among the strains varies from 59% to 82%. The protein contains four variable regions located in the hydrophilic regions of the molecule.[34] Direct repeat of short DNA sequences, and frame-shift mutation by deletion or addition of a base resulting in substitution and deletion of several amino acids are frequently present in the variable regions. The remarkable antigenic diversity of and strain-specific immunity to *O. tsutsugamushi* are determined by the 56 kDa protein, which despite vast genetic and antigenic diversity, is genetically stable in a particular strain. The 47 kDa protein of *O. tsutsugamushi,* a homolog of HtrA, is located in the outer membrane. The protein is antigenic and has significant sequence homology to human HtrA. More than 20% of scrub typhus patients' sera cross-react with recombinant human HtrA.[35] The 60 kDa protein, an analog of heat shock protein 60, is located in the cytoplasm. The 22 kDa protein

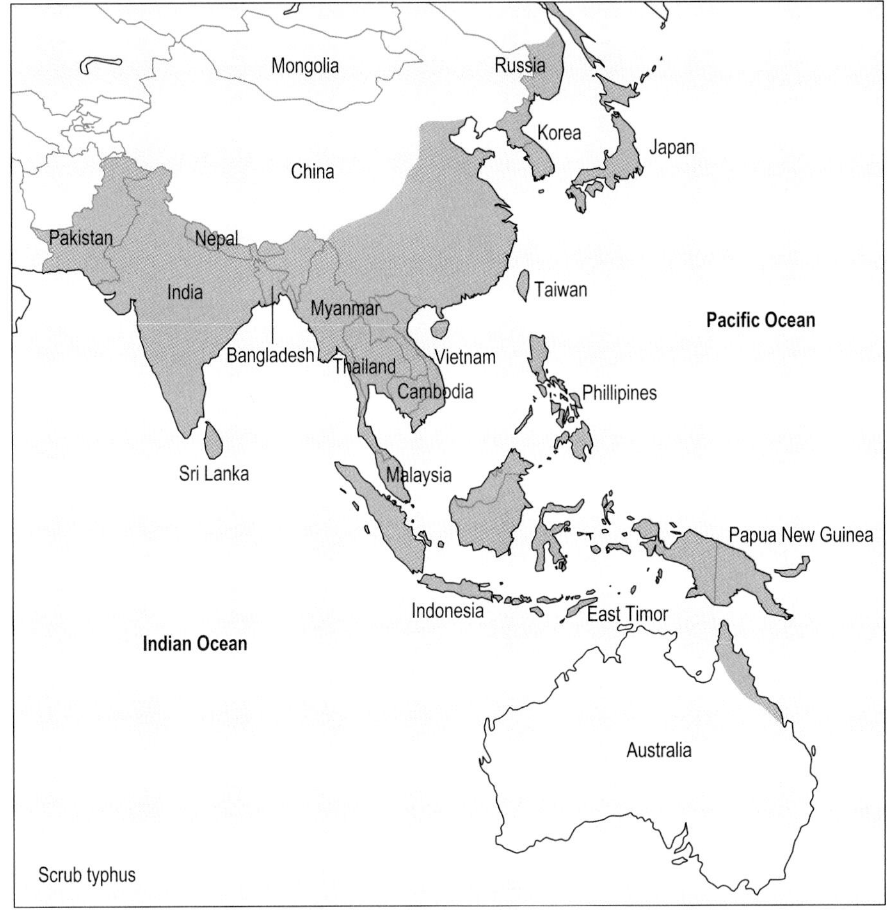

Figure 51.1 Geographic distribution of scrub typhus.

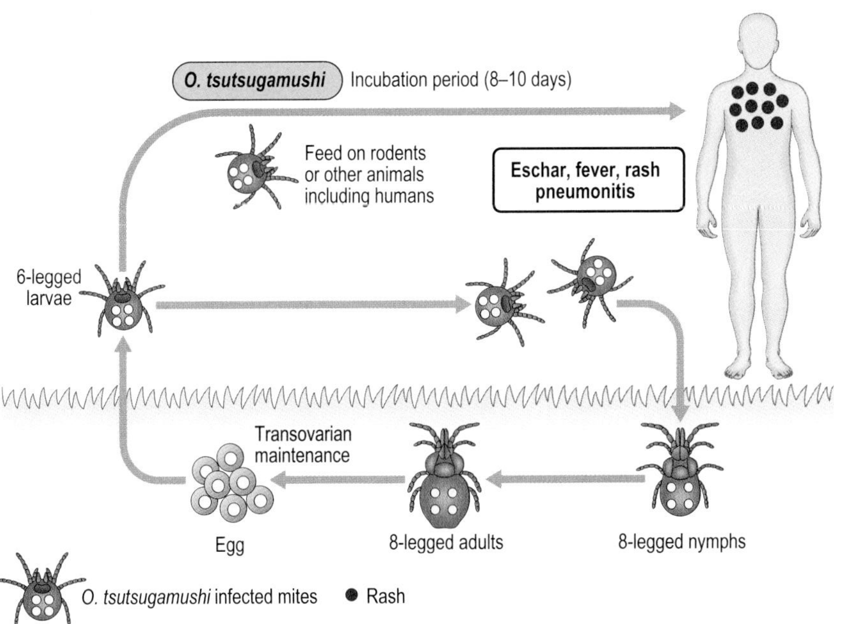

Figure 51.2 Transmission of *O. tsutsugamushi* to the human.

is antigenic, shows sequence variation among strains, and inhibits the protective effects of other immunogens of *O. tsutsugamushi*.[36]

Antigenic heterogeneity of *O. tsutsugamushi* was recognized by cross complement fixation, cross neutralization and cross protection assays. There are more than 70 different strains of *O. tsutsugamushi*. The prototype strains are Karp, Gilliam, and Kato isolated from New Guinea, Myanmar, and Japan, respectively. New strains of *O. tsutsugamushi* distinct from these prototype strains are found in Thailand, Taiwan, Malaysia, Japan, Korea, and China.[37,38] There are geographical differences in the strain distribution. *O. tsutsugamushi* isolates from China, Japan, and Korea are phylogenetically different from the isolates from Southeast Asia including the prototype Gilliam and Karp strains. The divergent evolution may be attributable to vertical transmission in different mite species.[39,40]

The complete genome sequence of *O. tsutsugamushi* reveals a circular chromosome of 2.1 Mbp and G + C content of 30.5%. The *O. tsutsugamushi* genome is unique in that up to 40% of the genome consists of repeated sequences. The repeats are composed of transposases, conjugative type IV secretion system, and reverse transcriptases.[41,42] *O. tsutsugamushi* has an incomplete tricarboxylic acid cycle that lacks functional *gltA* and *acnA* genes. *O. tsutsugamushi* has five genes for ATP/ADP translocases that can exploit host ATP as a source of energy. *O. tsutsugamushi* lacks genes for LPS synthesis, but retains the pathways for peptidoglycan synthesis. *O. tsutsugamushi* has six genes for *Sca* family proteins, which play roles as adhesins and invasins in *Rickettsia*.[43]

THE DISEASE

The clinical symptoms vary depending on the duration of illness, strain of *O. tsutsugamushi*, immune status and other host factors of the patient.[44–47] At the early stage of the disease, the clinical symptoms are fever, rash, eschar, myalgia, and lymphadenopathy, and it is difficult to distinguish scrub typhus clinically from many other febrile diseases. As the disease progresses, serious inflammation and injury, such as interstitial pneumonia, acute respiratory distress syndrome, meningoencephalomyelitis, myocarditis, gastrointestinal bleeding, acute renal failure, hypotensive shock, and disseminated intravascular coagulation (DIC) may occur.[48–50] The incubation period is 5–20 days. The chigger bite is usually painless, and patients seldom notice it. A lesion begins to form 6–10 hours after the bite at the feeding site where a red papule appears and enlarges. The papule is not well demarcated, and a black-brown scab in the center forms the eschar, a focus of cutaneous necrosis resembling a cigarette burn.[51] The eschar is usually well developed by the time fever appears, frequently appearing on the chest, abdomen, back, arm, and leg, and is also found on the scalp, axilla, genitalia, and other sites.[52–54] Thorough physical examination of skin is required for its detection. The detection rate of an eschar varies greatly from 7% to 97%.[55,56]

Almost all scrub typhus patients develop fever and headache. The body temperature rises abruptly to 38–39°C, frequently accompanied by muscle pain and malaise.[57,58] The maculopapular rash appears on the trunk 3–4 days after the onset of fever and spreads to the arms and legs. Rash is reported in low proportions of some case series. Regional lymphadenopathy develops in the drainage of the eschar and is usually present when the eschar appears. Generalized lymphadenopathy develops 2–3 days later. Bacteremia is detected 1–3 days before the onset of fever.[59]

Respiratory symptoms are frequent. About 40% of scrub typhus patients complain of cough at the time of admission.[48] Interstitial pneumonia, pulmonary edema, pleural effusion, cardiomegaly, and/or focal atelectasis are observed by chest radiography in these patients.[60] Congestion of blood vessels in interlobular septa and alveolar walls, hemorrhagic edema, diffuse alveolar damage with hyaline membrane formation, and interstitial pneumonia with mononuclear cell infiltrations are observed at autopsy.[61] The presence of respiratory symptoms is closely associated with severity of illness.[44] Conjunctival injection frequently occurs at the onset of the disease, and subconjunctival hemorrhage often develops 7–10 days later in association with capillary dilatation and increased vascular permeability. There is no discharge.[59,62] Gastrointestinal symptoms including nausea, vomiting, abdominal pain, diarrhea, hematemesis, and melena also occur frequently. Mucosal bleeding, multiple erosions or ulcers, and vascular bleeding are observed by endoscopy in the stomach and duodenum. Gastric lesions are more frequent and severe than the duodenal lesions.[63,64] The central nervous system (CNS) is frequently affected. Headache, nausea, vomiting, transient hearing loss, confusion, neck stiffness, delirium, and mental changes are common. Convulsions and coma may occur.[65] *O. tsutsugamushi* is identified in the cerebrospinal fluid of 24% of the scrub typhus patients with no clinical signs of CNS involvement, suggesting that CNS invasion is common.[66] Acute renal failure develops frequently in severe cases, but may also occur in mild cases.[67] Myocarditis, pericarditis, and relative bradycardia may develop, but congestive heart failure is rare. *O. tsutsugamushi* can be found in the vascular endothelial cells of the myocardium and cardiac myocytes.[68,69] Modest elevations of hepatic aminotransferases are frequent, and some patients develop jaundice. Thrombocytopenia and elevation of C-reactive protein occur often.[50] DIC, rhabdomyolysis, presence of atypical lymphocytes in peripheral blood, and hemophagocytosis in bone marrow have been reported rarely.[70,71] Fetal loss has been reported.[72] A case of transplacental transmission was described, but transplacental transmission could not be confirmed in other cases.[73]

The case-fatality rate in the preantibiotic era ranged from 0% to 30%, possibly with a geographic variation suggestive of differences in virulence. Untreated the average risk of fatality is approximately 7%. Risk factors for severity include increased age and greater bacterial load at the time of admission.[74]

PATHOGENESIS AND IMMUNITY

Infection follows the bite of a trombiculid mite. However, the entire sequence of events that begins with entry via dermis and ultimately results in disseminated infection is not well understood. Larval feeding on vertebrates likely stimulates *O. tsutsugamushi* release from salivary gland cells of mites and transmission to humans mixed with mite saliva.[70] *O. tsutsugamushi* enters cells by induced phagocytosis, but the molecular mechanisms remain largely unknown. The 47 kDa *Orientia* protein binds heparan sulfate, and the 56 kDa protein binds fibronectin. Experimental findings suggest that 47 kDa and 56 kDa proteins and fibronectin play important roles in internalization of *O. tsutsugamushi* into cells. Increased invasion of *O. tsutsugamushi* into cells which overexpress syndecan-4 and inhibition of entry by antibodies to integrin $\alpha5\beta1$ or Arg-Gly-Asp peptide suggest that syndecan-4 and integrin $\alpha5\beta1$ are potential receptors.[75–77] *O. tsutsugamushi* enters by a clathrin-dependent endocytic pathway and escapes from the endosome into the cytosol. Maturation and acidification of the *Orientia*-containing endosome are essential for bacterial exit into the cytosol.[78] *O. tsutsugamushi* in the cytosol moves using microtubules to the microtubule-organizing center near the nucleus where *Orientia* replicates.[79] Organisms that have been released from a cell are usually surrounded by the host plasma membrane. This structure may serve to stabilize the organism during extracellular existence and possibly protect the organism from harmful materials in the saliva of mites and the host immune system.[80]

In the eschar *O. tsutsugamushi* is present predominantly in dendritic cells, which may represent the initial target cell. The mode of *O. tsutsugamushi* dissemination from the eschar to the internal organs is suggested by animal experiments and clinical observations to be lymphogenous to the regional lymph nodes, followed by spread to target organs via the blood. Human dermal microvascular endothelial cells infected with *O. tsutsugamushi in vitro* are activated to express interleukin (IL)-8 and monocyte chemoattractant protein (MCP)-1 just after the infection, and scrub typhus patients have a high serum concentration of soluble endothelial cell-specific adhesion molecule (sE-selectin) in the early stage of the disease.[81,82] These findings suggest that endothelial cells have a central role in the systemic inflammation.

The main target cells of *O. tsutsugamushi* in humans are vascular endothelial cells and macrophages of the reticuloendothelial system, although *Orientia* also infect cardiac myocytes.[83] The basic histopathologic findings in scrub typhus are multiplication of *O. tsutsugamushi* in the endothelial cells lining the small blood vessels, perivasculitis and focal interstitial mononuclear cell infiltrations and accompanying edema. Perivasculitis with mononuclear cell infiltrations may involve the lung, heart, brain, kidneys, gastrointestinal tract, liver, spleen, and lymph node.[83,84]

The mechanism of tissue destruction is unclear. Direct cytotoxicity of *O. tsutsugamushi*, reactive radicals, and cytokines produced by the host immune response are potential pathogenic mechanisms. Primary human endothelial cells infected with *O. tsutsugamushi* develop cytopathic changes.[85] However, only a limited number of *O. tsutsugamushi* are observed in lung and liver lesions of some patients in spite of severe histological changes, suggesting the involvement of immunopathologic mechanisms in tissue injury.[61,86] Increased serum levels of tumor necrosis factor (TNF)-α, interferon (IFN)-γ, and IL-10 as well as upregulation of TNF-α, IFN-γ, IL-1α, IL-1β, IL-6, and IL-10 in peripheral blood mononuclear cells are observed in scrub typhus patients. TNF-α levels in severe cases are higher than in nonsevere cases.[87,88] *O. tsutsugamushi* inhibits apoptosis of infected cells by blocking intracellular calcium release.[89]

Immunity to *O. tsutsugamushi* is strain-specific. Immunity to heterologous strains can develop, but is of only short duration. Volunteers who have recovered from scrub typhus one or two months previously are completely resistant to infection by heterologous strains, but most volunteers who have recovered from scrub typhus one or two years previously are susceptible to heterologous reinfection and suffer similar symptoms and signs as observed in patients with no past history of scrub typhus. Immunity to homologous strains persists for years. The lesion at the inoculation site and the incubation period differ according to the susceptibility of the host. Eschars do not occur in resistant volunteers challenged with *O. tsutsugamushi*.[46]

Experimental studies suggest that protective immunity to scrub typhus is mediated by Th1 cells, as demonstrated by adoptive transfer of antigen-specific, IFN-γ-producing T cells, development of delayed type hypersensitivity, and IFN-γ production by T cells in response to *O. tsutsugamushi* antigen.[90–92] Antibodies to *O. tsutsugamushi* increase the uptake of *O. tsutsugamushi* by neutrophils and macrophages and enhance bacterial clearance from blood. The growth of antibody-coated *O. tsutsugamushi* in activated macrophages is inhibited efficiently.[93] However, passive transfer of hyperimmune sera does not protect mice.[94] These results suggest that humoral immunity facilitates the uptake of *O. tsutsugamushi* by macrophages and that cellular immunity including IFN-γ and cytotoxic T lymphocytes plays a central role in the killing of *O. tsutsugamushi*.

Skin lesions in scrub typhus patients contain more CD8 than CD4 T lymphocytes as well as macrophages, all of which are likely cellular effectors.[95]

DIAGNOSIS

Early diagnosis is important to prevent the progression of scrub typhus to severe generalized disease. The diagnosis can be simple in a patient who has visited an endemic area and presents with a fever, rash, eschar, lymphadenopathy, and acute hearing loss. Unfortunately, this scenario is rarely the case. Clinical suspicion is based on the presence of fever, rash, conjunctival effusions, lymphadenopathy and epidemiological clues in endemic regions, but scrub typhus is often difficult to differentiate from other febrile diseases or drug eruptions and is an often overlooked cause of both pyrexia and pneumonitis of undetermined cause.[44,96–98] Scrub typhus without fever is rare, but some case series report low percentages of patients with eschar and rash, particularly in endemic regions where reinfection is common.[99,100] The presence of an eschar is helpful for the diagnosis, but it does not always develop, and it is difficult to find in some situations. Caution must be taken not to confuse other lesions with eschars. Eschars may occur in the genital region, where they often lose their crust. Thus they can be confused with the ulcers of syphilis, chancroid, or lymphogranuloma venereum.[53] A rash that is hemorrhagic, particularly if associated with leukopenia and thrombocytopenia, suggests dengue rather than scrub typhus.[96] Marked myalgia, liver involvement, and raised serum creatinine levels suggest leptospirosis rather than scrub typhus. However, dual infections with leptospirosis and scrub typhus have been reported.[101] Typhoid fever and malaria are prominent in the differential diagnosis, but plasmodia are generally detectable in blood films from Asian patients with malaria, and enteric fever rarely causes generalized lymphadenopathy or conjunctival suffusion.[102] The laboratory diagnosis is crucial. The Weil–Felix test, the first serological test developed for the diagnosis of scrub typhus, detects cross-reactive antibodies to *Proteus mirabilis* OX-K strain, but the sensitivity is low, and false positive results may occur in leptospirosis, relapsing fever, and *Proteus* urinary tract infection. The indirect immunofluorescent antibody assay (IFA) has high sensitivity and specificity, but specific antibodies to *O. tsutsugamushi* are often absent in the early stage of the disease.[103] IFA and immunoperoxidase assay (IPA) are the serological methods recommended by the World Health Organization and have been considered as the gold standard methods for the serodiagnosis of scrub typhus. The antigen preparation is important in IFA and IPA. Because there are more than 70 strains of *O. tsutsugamushi*, and the antigenicity of strain-specific antigen is usually stronger than species-specific antigens, it is recommended to include local strains of *O. tsutsugamushi* in addition to the prototype strains, Karp, Kato, and Gilliam, in the preparation of IFA slides. An acute stage negative result does not exclude a current infection, and a positive result does not confirm the current infection, especially in endemic areas. Rising IgG antibody titer or IgM titer greater than 1 : 80 has been proposed to have diagnostic significance. However, each laboratory should establish cutoff levels based on the local prevalence and titers of antibodies, with a titer of 1 : 400 being appropriate in some highly endemic regions. A fourfold rise in titer between acute and convalescent samples yields a definitive diagnosis.[104] IFA or IPA requires special equipment and experienced personnel for interpretation of the test. Serologic methods based on the recombinant 56 kDa protein include a passive hemagglutination test, enzyme-linked immunosorbent assay (ELISA), dipstick test, and immunochromatography assay.[105–108] The tests are easy to perform and are adequate for screening a large number of samples, but are less effective than IFA or IPA.[105]

O. tsutsugamushi can be isolated from patients, rodents, and mites by inoculating laboratory mice or cell culture. Isolation of *Orientia* by intraperitoneal mouse inoculation is relatively easy; after 10–14 days, *O. tsutsugamushi* can be observed in peritoneal cavity exudate using Giemsa stain or IFA. If *O. tsutsugamushi* are not observed, blind passage to mice of homogenate of the spleen and liver improves the isolation rate. Patients' buffy coat cells homogenized with a Dounce homogenizer are inoculated onto established cell lines.[109]

O. tsutsugamushi may be detected by polymerase chain reaction (PCR) amplification from cells of blood, eschars, and other tissues. EDTA-treated blood is preferred over heparinized blood. Currently, PCR amplification targeting four different genes, 56 kDa protein gene, 47 kDa protein gene, *groEL*, and 16S rRNA, have been described. There are large differences in sensitivity among these assays. A recent report of loop-mediated isothermal PCR targeting *groEL* offers promise of high sensitivity and specificity, low cost, simplicity, and no need for a thermal cycler or sophisticated reader.[110] PCR amplification based on the 56 kDa protein gene is adequate for genotype or serotype determination, and PCR amplification based on *groEL* is used for the differentiation of *O. tsutsugamushi* from *Rickettsia*.[111,112] Administration of doxycycline and rifampicin reduces the sensitivity of PCR to 10% after 4 days of antibiotic therapy.[113]

The strain of *O. tsutsugamushi* can be determined by cross-complement fixation, cross-neutralization, and cross-protection tests and IFA using strain-specific monoclonal antibodies. Currently, PCR amplification and sequence determination are frequently used for the identification of the strain of *O. tsutsugamushi*.

TREATMENT AND PROGNOSIS, PREVENTION AND CONTROL

Early empirical treatment with antimicrobial agents should be considered. Early antibiotic treatment shortens the disease course, prevents serious complications, and reduces mortality. A day of delay in antibiotic therapy increases the risk of death by 20%.[44] Doxycycline is the drug of choice for the treatment of scrub typhus. Fever usually disappears within 24–60 hours after the beginning of therapy. Tetracycline is as effective as doxycycline, but is more hepatotoxic. Chloramphenicol is an alternative, but is less effective than doxycycline. Azithromycin is as effective as doxycycline with fewer adverse effects.[114,115] Telithromycin, roxithromycin, clarithromycin, and rifampicin have also been used successfully. Parenteral therapy should be given to patients who are vomiting or have severe disease. In areas where parenteral formulations of tetracyclines are unavailable, chloramphenicol is a useful alternative for treatment of severe disease. Time to defervescence in rifampicin-treated patients is shorter than that of doxycycline-treated patients.[116] Quinolones and cephalosporins are not recommended for the treatment of scrub typhus.[72] Antibiotic administration generally alters the clinical course rapidly. Most scrub typhus patients with multiorgan failure are treated with doxycycline, azithromycin, or rifampicin without complications. Scrub typhus that responds poorly to doxycycline and chloramphenicol has been reported in Thailand.[117] Scrub typhus during pregnancy has been treated with azithromycin, chloramphenicol, or rifampin.[73,118]

Doxycycline appears to be an excellent antibiotic for the prevention of scrub typhus among personnel exposed to high risk of infection. Chemoprophylaxis can be considered for travelers and soldiers who visit endemic areas. Weekly doses of 200 mg of doxycycline can prevent *O. tsutsugamushi* infection.[119] Contact with chiggers can be reduced by applying repellent to the tops of boots, socks, and on the lower trousers, wearing long sleeves, by not sitting or lying directly on the ground, and removal of harborage for peridomestic rodents.[120] Unfortunately, these measures are frequently not practiced by those exposed occupationally. Thorough washing and changing clothes after work exposure also reduce risk of infection. No vaccine is available for scrub typhus.

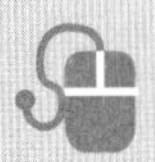

Access the complete reference list online at
http://www.expertconsult.com

Access the complete reference list online at http://www.expertconsult.com

CHAPTER 52

Ehrlichioses and Anaplasmosis

J. Stephen Dumler

INTRODUCTION

As human activities increasingly enter habitats of ticks and their hosts, exposure to previously unrecognized microbes that evolved within mammalian–tick enzootic cycles occurs, and significant new human pathogens emerge. Important examples include obligately intracellular bacteria related to the genus *Rickettsia* that are in the family Anaplasmataceae and the genera *Ehrlichia* and *Anaplasma*.[1–3] *Neorickettsia sennetsu* was identified as a cause of a mononucleosis-like illness in Japan in 1954, and since 1986 at least four new distinct species in the family Anaplasmataceae have been identified as tick-borne human pathogens.[1–6]

THE AGENTS

Anaplasmataceae are classified based on similarities in *rrs* (16S ribosomal RNA genes), *groESL*, *rpoB*, and *gltA*.[3,7,8] *N. sennetsu* infects mostly mononuclear phagocytes, has never been identified in humans outside the Far East, and is likely transmitted by ingestion of trematode-infested fish. *Ehrlichia chaffeensis* infects peripheral blood monocytes and tissue macrophages and is the major cause of human monocytotropic ehrlichiosis (HME).[1,2,6,9,10] *Anaplasma phagocytophilum* infects neutrophils.[3,11,12] *E. ewingii*, another pathogen of neutrophils, is a significant human pathogen, particularly among immunocompromised patients.[5,13] A role for *Wolbachia* spp. infecting filarial nematodes is proposed in complicating human filariasis (see Chapters 101–106).[14] Finally, 30 patients with *E. canis* infection were identified in Venezuela.[15] Given the propensity for some Anaplasmataceae to infect both animals and humans, it is not surprising that some are emerging as significant human diseases in tropical regions.

With the exception of *Wolbachia* spp., each of the Anaplasmataceae pathogenic for humans lives within endosomes in professional phagocytic cells.[16,17] These intracellular bacteria attach to ligands on phagocytic cells, are engulfed, and subvert intracellular endosomal trafficking to allow replication within the vacuole.[18,19] Another common theme is the changing variety of surface immunogenic proteins, which probably contributes to immune evasion in persistently infected reservoir hosts but could allow infection of new niches among alternative hosts such as humans.[20–22] The closely related genera *Ehrlichia* and *Anaplasma* are tick-transmitted, whereas *Neorickettsia* spp. rely on infection of trematodes and their hosts, and *Wolbachia* symbionts of *Brugia*, *Onchocerca*, and other filarial nematodes are passed transovarially.[23–26] Increasing evidence suggests the induction of immunopathologic responses such as overproduction of proinflammatory molecules including tumor necrosis factor-α (TNF-α) as a pathogenetic mechanism.[27–29]

Developments such as the growth of *E. canis* and *E. chaffeensis* in the canine DH82 or human THP-1 macrophage cell lines,[10,30,31] *A. phagocytophilum* in human HL-60 promyelocytic cells,[32] and several species in tick cell cultures[33] allow more comprehensive investigation and improvement of diagnostics. The genome sequences of *E. chaffeensis*, *E. canis*, *E. ruminantium*, *A. phagocytophilum*, *N. sennetsu*, *A. marginale*, *W. pipientis*, and several other *Wolbachia* spp. are completed and should propel research.

HUMAN MONOCYTOTROPIC EHRLICHIOSIS

THE AGENT: *EHRLICHIA CHAFFEENSIS*

E. chaffeensis has a wide ultrastructural variety.[34] In general, two types of cells are observed within vacuoles of host cells: dense-core cells, with a central condensation of ribosomes and DNA fibrils, and reticulate cells, where these components are evenly distributed throughout. Reticulate cells are noninfectious replicating forms, and the *E. chaffeensis* p120 adhesin is differentially expressed on infectious nonreplicating dense-core cells.[35]

E. chaffeensis strains have considerable genomic diversity and variable pathogenicity in severe combined immunodeficiency (SCID) mice, suggesting genetically determined virulence.[36] Protein immunoblots reveal dominant antigens of 200, 120, 66, 55, 44, 29, 28, and 22 kDa.[37,38] Variation in specific epitopes also exists.[39] The immunodominant p28 family of proteins is encoded by at least 22 contiguous paralogs that are independently transcribed and may function as porins.[22,40] The 120-kDa adhesin[35] and another surface-exposed protein, variable-length polymerase chain reaction (PCR) target (VLPT), contain variable numbers of tandem repeats.[41] Components of a type IV secretion mechanism expressed by *E. chaffeensis* assemble at the bacterial membrane and in parasitophorous vacuoles of infected macrophages.[42,43] A 200-kDa ankyrin-containing protein is translocated into infected macrophages and eventually localizes within the nucleus. There it interacts with adenine-rich motifs within Alu-Sx elements, potentially contributing to bacterial regulation of host gene expression.[44]

EPIDEMIOLOGY

HME has clinical and geographic similarities to Rocky Mountain spotted fever (RMSF).[1,2,6,45] Onset is associated with tick exposure and bites, and the major vector is *Amblyomma americanum*, the Lone Star tick (***Fig. 52.1***).[1,2,6,23] Lone Star ticks are found across areas of the south-central and southeastern United States where HME is endemic. All stages of *A. americanum* feed on deer, the major reservoir.[46] Deer experimentally inoculated with *E. chaffeensis* become persistently and subclinically infected.[47] White-tailed deer (*Odocoileus virginianus*) in the southeastern and central United States are often infected or have serologic evidence of infection.[46] White-tailed deer in areas devoid of Lone Star ticks lack evidence of exposure to *E. chaffeensis* until Lone Star ticks spread into those regions.[48] Many canids have serologic evidence of *Ehrlichia* infections, and dogs can be persistently infected subclinically with *E. chaffeensis*.[49–51]

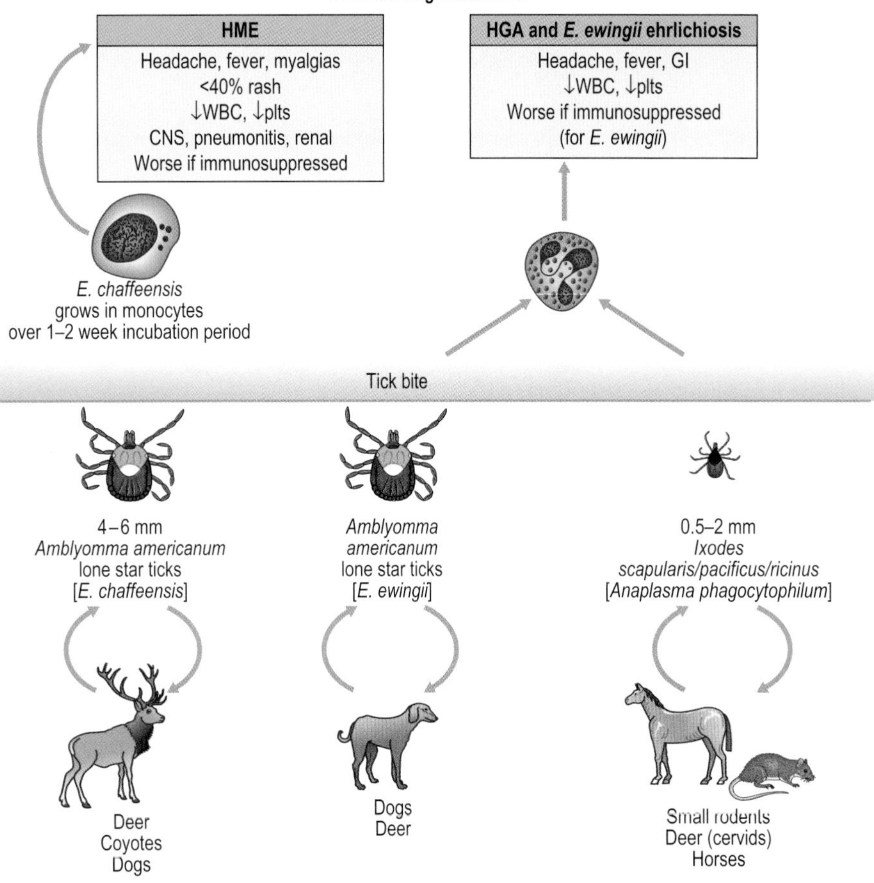

Figure 52.1 Life cycles of human monocytic ehrlichiosis (HME, with *Ehrlichia chaffeensis*) and human granulocytic ehrlichiosis (anaplasmosis) (HGA with *Anaplasma phagocytophilum*) or infection with *E. ewingii*. WBC, white blood cell count; CNS, central nervous system; GI, gastrointestinal.

Prior investigations indicate that human infection occurs at a rate similar to or greater than RMSF. Active, prospective case identification in southeastern Missouri suggests that HME occurs at rates of 2–5 per 100 000 population – 10-fold higher than with passive reporting, and possibly more than an order of magnitude even higher.[1,2,6,52–54] Serologic studies suggest that infection with *E. chaffeensis* or an antigenically related organism also occurs in Europe, Africa, Asia, and Latin America.[4,15,55–59] Asymptomatic seroconversion could confound seroprevalence and diagnostic studies[60]; moreover, mild infection with *E. ewingii* could account for some serologic reactions in tick-exposed populations.[61] Most infections in North America occur from April through September, with a peak in July, when the ticks are active.[1,2,6]

THE DISEASE

Most individuals with HME have an undifferentiated febrile illness 1–4 weeks after tick exposure.[1,2,6,54,62] The mean age is 48 years, although infections occur in children.[63] Most patients reside in rural areas, but rural zip codes and seroprevalence are not correlated.[63] Frequent findings include headache, myalgias, and malaise, while gastrointestinal, respiratory, or central nervous system (CNS) abnormalities or rash is present in fewer than 40% of patients (***Table 52.1***). Laboratory features include leukopenia, thrombocytopenia, and elevations in serum hepatic transaminase concentrations (***Table 52.2***). Severe manifestations include meningoencephalitis, a toxic shock-like syndrome, respiratory insufficiency, acute renal failure, severe hepatitis, myocarditis, and prolonged fever.[28,64–70] The case-fatality rate is 3%, and immunosuppressed persons (e.g., human immunodeficiency virus (HIV)-infected, organ transplant recipients, or corticosteroid-treated) are at risk of overwhelming fatal infection.[13,70–72] Early diagnosis and treatment prevent severe disease.[1,2,6] Pathologic features include perivascular lymphohistiocytic infiltrates without vasculitis, small noncaseating granulomas in bone marrow, and evidence of macrophage activation. Bone marrow is generally hypercellular or normocellular. Hepatocellular apoptosis and, in severe cases, necrosis of liver, spleen, and lymph nodes have been observed.[28,68,72–74] Except in immunocompromised patients, the bacterial load of *E. chaffeensis* is low, underscoring that disease is mediated by host factors.[74]

PATHOGENESIS AND IMMUNITY

Entry of *E. chaffeensis* into macrophages is mediated by p120 and possibly other adhesins to host cell E- and L-selectin, probably at cholesterol-rich membrane lipid rafts or caveolae and glycosylphosphatidylinositol-anchored proteins.[42,75] Binding of a heat-sensitive protein on *E. chaffeensis* initiates host cell phospholipase C and tyrosine kinase activation and mobilizes cytosolic free calcium in association with bacterial entry.[42,76] Entry is receptor-mediated and is impeded by transglutaminase inhibitors, but clathrin binding is not involved. Once internalized, *E. chaffeensis* alters the parasitophorous vacuole, leading to its accumulation of cellular transferrin receptors after activation of iron-responsive protein-1 that inhibits degradation of transferrin mRNA transcripts.[19] This effect leads to iron availability for bacterial growth and to redirection of the parasitophorous vacuole into a receptor salvage pathway that avoids lysosomal fusion. Iron acquisition by *E. chaffeensis* involves ferric (Fe III) iron binding to a ferric-binding protein (Fbp) that shares structural homology and iron-binding capacity with Fbps of other Gram-negative bacteria and is found extracellularly on dense-cored ehrlichiae.[76] Treatment with

Symptom or Sign	Monocytotropic Ehrlichiosis[62,94,180-184] (*n* = 234-422)	Granulocytotropic Anaplasmosis[93,120,123,138,185-192] (*n* = 24-531)
Fever	96% (93–100%)	100% (75–100%)
Myalgia	68% (48–93%)	78% (40–100%)
Headache	72% (67–81%)	89% (61–100%)
Malaise	77% (69–84%)	97% (47–100%)
Nausea	57% (38–68%)	44% (35–53%)
Vomiting	47% (7–59%)	20% (18–34%)
Diarrhea	25% (10–31%)	17% (9–22%)
Cough	28% (24–31%)	20% (0–29%)
Arthralgias	41% (40–43%)	56% (21–100%)
Rash	26% (17–66%)	3% (0–50%)
Stiff neck	21% (13–28%)	22% (0–50%)
Confusion	20% (7–50%)	17% (0–17%)

Table 52.1 Median Percentages of Ehrlichiosis Patients with Specific Symptoms or Signs at Any Time during the Course of Illness (Min.–Max.%)

Laboratory Abnormality	Monocytotropic Ehrlichiosis[54,62,94,180,183] (*n* = 250-308)	Granulocytotropic Anaplasmosis[87,93,105,120,186-190,192] (*n* = 59-344)
Leukopenia	60% (56–74%)	55% (26–77%)
Thrombocytopenia	79% (57–94%)	75% (53–92%)
Anemia	50% (25–57%)	28% (6–50%)
Elevated serum aspartate transaminase	88% (52–100%)	83% (32–100%)
Elevated serum creatinine	24%	15% (0–70%)

Table 52.2 Median Percentages of Ehrlichiosis Patients with Specific Abnormal Laboratory Findings at any Time during the Course of Illness (Min.–Max.%)

desferoxamine diminishes ehrlichial growth, probably because iron is a cofactor in oxidative phosphorylation, a critical metabolic pathway for *Ehrlichia* that cannot utilize glucose or glucose-6-phosphate as energy sources.[19,77] Down-regulation of host RAB5A, SNAP23, and STX16 during infection could underlie altered endosomal trafficking and inhibition of lysosome fusion.[78] The mechanism by which *E. chaffeensis* alters host gene transcription is not clear, although a 200-kDa ankyrin motif-containing protein translocated into the infected cell nucleus binds to DNA in association with altered transcription of *TNF*, *STAT1*, and *CD48*.[44] Similarly, a 47-kDa protein with multiple tandem repeats is secreted and interacts with host proteins involved in cell signaling, transcriptional regulation, and vesicle trafficking.[79]

Infection of macrophages with *E. chaffeensis* results in production of interleukin (IL)-1β, IL-8, and IL-10, but not TNF-α, IL-6, or granulocyte–macrophage colony-stimulating factor (GM-CSF), suggesting a relative lack of proinflammatory signals and potential immunosuppression.[80] Inflammatory chemokines IL-8, monocyte chemotactic protein-1, and macrophage inflammatory protein-1α are produced in response to *E. chaffeensis* p120 and p200 through interactions with pattern recognition receptors. Typical lipopolysaccharide–CD14 interaction does not account for the cytokine responses, since IL-1β induction by *E. chaffeensis* is not inhibited by monoclonal antibodies to CD14 and *E. chaffeensis* lacks lipopolysaccharide biosynthetic pathways. Moreover, *E. chaffeensis* inhibits the expression of mRNA of IL-12, IL-15, and IL-18, cytokines that are key to effective Th1 cellular immunity. Notably, down-regulation of TLR2 and TLR4 genes in *E. chaffeensis*-infected cells results from inhibition of p38 mitogen-activated protein kinase, leading to reduced transcription factor PU.1 activity.[81] Furthermore, ehrlichiae down-regulate the expression of major histocompatibility complex class II on infected cells, a potential mechanism of evading innate and acquired immune responses.[82] Animal models indicate that humoral immunity, particularly to an epitope on P28–19, a strong CD4 Th1 cell IFN-γ response, synergy of IFN-γ and TNF-α, and CD8 cytotoxic T lymphocytes act together to control infection.[29,83–88]

The mechanism by which *E. chaffeensis* damages infected cells is unknown. *In vitro* infection causes cytolysis of infected cells,[10,88–91] some with many morulae, suggesting simple mechanical lysis. The *in vivo* correlate is necrosis associated with abundant *E. chaffeensis* organisms in spleen, liver, and other mononuclear phagocyte-rich tissues of infected immunocompromised patients.[28,72] In contrast, most immunocompetent patients do not develop tissue necrosis, and *E. chaffeensis* are sparse in lesions that include perivascular lymphohistiocytic infiltrates, granulomas, apoptotic hepatocytes, and apoptotic γ/δ T lymphocytes in blood during early convalescence.[28,74,92] These latter pathologic findings in the absence of significant quantities of *E. chaffeensis* suggest the contribution of host responses in the disease process.

DIAGNOSIS

Diagnosis is most often based on serologic studies,[1,2,6,52] which should include both *E. chaffeensis* and *A. phagocytophilum* antigens, since clinical similarity and serologic cross-reactivity occur in many cases.[54,93] Seroconversion, fourfold rise in antibody titer to greater than or equal to 128, or a single serum titer greater than or equal to 256 in a patient with a consistent illness provides evidence of infection.[54] Peripheral blood smears should be examined for ehrlichial morulae (***Fig. 52.2***) in leukocytes, but, except in immunocompromised patients, these are helpful in fewer than 10% of cases.[1,2,6,94] PCR amplification of *E. chaffeensis* DNA from acute-phase blood is between 56% and 95% sensitive, is highly specific, and provides timely information.[54,94,95] *E. chaffeensis* may be cultured from clinical samples in various cell lines, but the method is neither sensitive nor timely.[10,39,54,94]

THE AGENT: *EHRLICHIA EWINGII*

Known as a canine pathogen of neutrophils since the 1960s, *E. ewingii* is a distinct cause of undifferentiated febrile illness following tick bites in

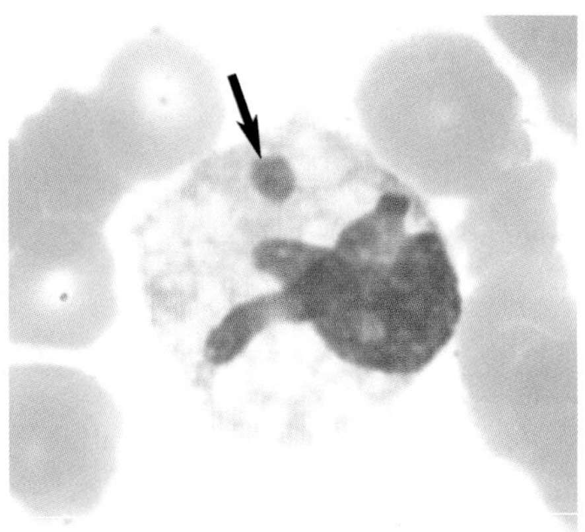

Figure 52.2 Peripheral blood mononuclear cell with intracytoplasmic aggregate (morulae) of *Ehrlichia chaffeensis* (arrow). (Wright stain; original magnification ×1000.)

geographic regions that overlap the distribution of HME and RMSF.[5,13] The bacterium is more closely related to and shares more antigens with *E. chaffeensis* than with *A. phagocytophilum*.[3,13,61] It is likely that some patients with a diagnosis of HME actually have *E. ewingii* because of serologic cross-reactions and since 10% of suspected HME patients in Missouri had *E. ewingii* instead.[5] *E. ewingii* is transmitted by *A. americanum* and possibly *Dermacentor variabilis* ticks (Fig. 52.1).[96,97] Similar to *E. chaffeensis*, white-tailed deer are persistently infected with *E. ewingii* in nature and are likely the most important reservoir, although a role for dogs is also possible.[98,99] Although only a few infected individuals are described, immunocompromised persons, including those with HIV or with organ transplants, are most often infected.[5,13] In general, the illness is similar to HME, but it is milder and with fewer complications and no deaths. As the bacterium has not yet been cultivated *in vitro*, no specific serologic test is available and serodiagnosis cannot be reliably achieved using surrogate *E. chaffeensis* testing. Although infected neutrophils may occasionally be observed in peripheral blood, definitive identification currently depends on detection of *E. ewingii* nucleic acids in clinical samples.[5,100]

HUMAN GRANULOCYTOTROPIC ANAPLASMOSIS

THE AGENT: *ANAPLASMA PHAGOCYTOPHILUM*

A. phagocytophilum contains many protein antigens, and the immunodominant major surface protein-2 (Msp2) 44-kDa proteins (p44) are encoded by 105 paralogous pseudogenes able to recombine into a single expression site.[21,101–104] Recombination by gene conversion or combinatorial mechanisms generates antigenic variants that could promote persistence in the reservoir by immune evasion. In hosts with significant clinical signs, including humans, persistent infection is not documented. Msp2 complexes in *A. phagocytophilum* are also involved in adhesion to fucosylated surface proteins of neutrophils, including platelet selectin glycoprotein ligand-1.[105–107] After binding, the bacteria are internalized within endosomes that do not mature but acquire some bacterial type IV secretion apparatus proteins.[42] A 155-kDa protein AnkA that is secreted by the bacterium is intially phosphorylated by Abl-1, a process that in part determines *A. phagocytophilum* entry into cells.[108,109] Thereafter, AnkA enters into the host cell nucleus, and complexes with host cell chromatin, where it modulates host cell histone structure and transcription of genes critical for pathogen survival.[110–112]

EPIDEMIOLOGY

Human granulocytotropic anaplasmosis (HGA) was first identified in febrile patients who reported tick bites.[11,12,113] *Ixodes persulcatus* complex ticks, including *I. scapularis*, *I. pacificus*, *I. ricinus*, and *I. persulcatus*, are naturally infected, and, except for *I. persulcatus,* each is proven competent for transmission of *A. phagocytophilum* (Fig. 52.1).[24–26,114,115] Small rodents appear to be a major reservoir, but cervids, ruminants, raccoons, and rabbits, among other animals, are infected in nature and may be important reservoirs.[115–119] The lack of transovarial transmission in ticks emphasizes the critical role of the mammal–tick–mammal transmission cycle and *Anaplasma* persistence in mammalian reservoirs.[24] HGA is most frequently recognized in the upper Midwest and northeastern United States and occasionally in northern California, areas that have a high incidence of *Ixodes* tick-related diseases,[12,93,120] including coinfections with Lyme disease and babesiosis.[121–124] Passive case collection reveals incidences as high as 58 and 51 cases per 100 000 population in the upper Midwest and Connecticut, respectively.[93,125,126] A high worldwide seroprevalence rate indicates that HGA probably is widely distributed and significantly underdiagnosed.[127–130] Most cases occur in May–July, when nymphal-stage ticks are active.[93]

On a worldwide basis, a high percentage of *Ixodes* spp. ticks, particularly those in the *I. persulcatus* complex, harbor *A. phagocytophilum*. The highest proportions of infected ticks are *I. scapularis*, in the northeastern and upper midwestern United States, where infection may be found in up to 50% (median 11%).[115,131,132] Up to 7% (median 2%) of *I. pacificus* in California and up to 33% of *I. persulcatus* and *I. ricinus* in Asia and Europe (median 5% and 4%, respectively) are infected.[133–135] Infection also occurs in *Dermacentor* ticks (*D. variabilis* and *D. occidentalis* in California), in Korean *Haemaphysalis longicornis*, and in several *Ixodes* spp. that seldom bite humans (*I. dentatus*, *I. trianguliceps*).[117,134,136,137] Transovarial transmission of *A. phagocytophilum* has not been demonstrated.[24,25]

THE DISEASE

HGA is an undifferentiated febrile illness with headache, myalgias, rigors, and malaise; gastrointestinal, respiratory, and CNS abnormalities occur in a minority of patients[93,120,138] (see ***Table 52.1***). Rash is rare. The median age is between 43 and 60 years, with up to a 2:1 male predominance. Leukopenia (26–77% of patients), thrombocytopenia (53–92%), and elevations in serum hepatic transaminases (32–100%) are often present[93,120,138] (see ***Table 52.2***). The manifestations of severe illness can include prolonged fever, shock, confusion, seizures, pneumonitis, acute renal failure, rhabdomyolysis, acute abdomen, hemorrhage, opportunistic infections, and death;[93,120,139–143] misdiagnosis and late therapy contribute to severe morbidity. CNS infection and cerebrospinal fluid pleocytosis are rare, but complications include seventh cranial nerve palsy, brachial plexopathy, and demyelinating polyneuropathy.[144–146] The case-fatality rate is probably less than 0.5%, but 50% or more of infected patients require hospitalization, even in Europe, where disease is considered to be milder.[93,113] Opportunistic infections, including disseminated candidiasis, herpes esophagitis, cryptococcal pneumonitis, and invasive pulmonary aspergillosis, are major causes of death in patients with and without immunocompromise.[93,139,147]

PATHOGENESIS AND IMMUNITY

The pathogenesis of HGA is not well understood but appears to be related to inadequate control of inflammation triggered by *A. phagocytophilum* infection.[27,147] Limited pathologic examinations of human tissues show macrophage activation, similar to that in *E. chaffeensis* infection, except lacking granulomas.[93,139,147] Neutrophil infection by *A. phagocytophilum* activates chemokine expression, motility, and degranulation but deactivates endothelial cell adhesion and transcytosis, respiratory burst, and apoptosis.[148–153] Such changes allow longer persistence of infected cells in blood that can be ingested by feeding ticks. However, the prolonged activation may contribute to increasing inflammation and bystander cell injury accompanied by reduced ability to control other infections. Infection mediates early responses by interaction with macrophage

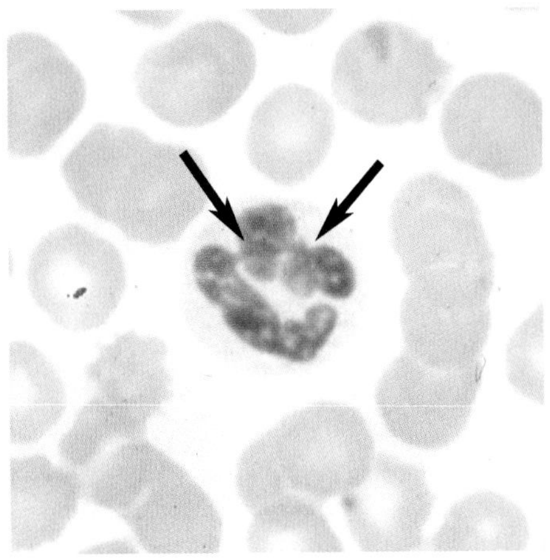

Figure 52.3 Peripheral blood neutrophil with intracytoplasmic aggregate (arrow) of anaplasmae in a patient with human granulocytic anaplasmosis. (Wright stain; original magnification ×1000.)

Toll-like receptor-2 but not Toll-like receptor-4, and inflammasome activation is also likely.[154–156] These interactions also incite production of Th1 proinflammatory cytokines, which are responsible for most inflammatory tissue injury in animal models.[27,157] How *A. phagocytophilum* manipulates the neutrophil is not elucidated, but a role for the type 4 secretion system substrate AnkA, encoded in the bacterial genome, occurs in early bacteria–cell interactions and late with its interaction at the promoters, leading to regulation of critical host defense gene transcription as with *CYBB* (*gp91*^{phox}).[109,112,158]

DIAGNOSIS

Retrospective diagnosis is mostly by serologic tests.[113,159,160] Occasional serologic cross-reactions with *E. chaffeensis* occur, but the homologous titer is usually higher.[32,113] A fourfold increase, seroconversion, or a high single antibody titer (usually ≥640) in a patient with a consistent illness is confirmatory. Careful examination of Giemsa- or Wright-stained peripheral blood smears (***Fig. 52.3***) can be diagnostic in 18–80% of patients during the acute phase.[113] PCR diagnosis is rapid and relatively sensitive, whereas culture is not timely.[113,161]

NEORICKETTSIOSIS

THE AGENT: *NEORICKETTSIA SENNETSU*

Originally recognized as an infectious mononucleosis-like illness in Japan, *N. sennetsu* infections are documented in Malaysia and Laos and might occur in other areas of Asia where raw or undercooked fish is eaten.[162,163] Complex cycles of bacterial infection involve trematodes, the cercariae of which infect snails and aquatic insects.[164] These are in turn ingested by a variety of animals, including fish, mammals, and birds, that may be reservoirs.[165] Fatal infection has never been reported. Diagnosis by serology or culture is available in very few laboratories.

EHRLICHIAL, ANAPLASMAL, AND NEORICKETTSIAL INFECTIONS

TREATMENT

Because severity of HME and HGA can result from therapeutic delays, patients should be treated empirically. Most defervesce within 24–48 hours after doxycycline or tetracycline treatment.[1,2,62,113] Chloramphenicol should not be used, since minimal inhibitory concentrations cannot be effectively achieved *in vivo*.[166–168] The preferred adult regimen is oral doxycycline 100 mg twice daily or tetracycline 250–500 mg every 6 hours. For children, doxycycline 4.4 mg/kg in two divided doses per day or tetracycline 25–50 mg/kg/day in four divided doses is recommended. Therapy is administered for at least 3 days after defervescence, and some physicians treat for 14–21 days. *N. sennetsu* ehrlichiosis also responds to treatment with tetracycline. Some evidence suggests efficacy of rifampin.[166–170] Resistance to fluoroquinolones in *Ehrlichia* is mediated by an amino acid change in GyrA, suggesting the potential for resistance in *A. phagocytophilum* as well, where fluoroquinolones are observed to be at best inhibitory only.[171,172]

PREVENTION AND CONTROL

Simple precautions aimed at reducing tick exposure, including avoiding tick-infested habitats, wearing appropriate barrier clothing, using tick repellents, and removing attached ticks, will lower the risk of disease. Conflicting data exist regarding a "grace period" during which transfer of the infectious agents is delayed immediately after tick attachment for HME and HGA. Some studies suggest a significant reduction in transmission if ticks are removed within 36 hours,[173,174] whereas others show a high transmission rate within 24 hours,[175] suggesting that daily tick removal may not be sufficient to prevent *A. phagocytophilum* transmission.

WOLBACHIA-RELATED COMPLICATIONS OF FILARIASIS

Wolbachia spp. reside in a cytoplamic vacuole and are diversely distributed throughout the world of insects, arthropods, helminths, and crustaceans.[176] These bacteria have diverse effects on their hosts' population dynamics, usually leading to feminization of gender ratios with bacterial survival only in females. Mechanisms that distort gender ratio include cytoplasmic incompatibility between infected and uninfected parents, parthenogenesis, and feminization of genetic males. In addition, endosymbiont bacteria of helminths can influence the survival of larval instars.

The inflammatory complications of lymphatic filariasis and river blindness are part of the pathogenesis of these infections (see Chapters 104–106).[177] These inflammatory processes are associated more often with death of the nematodes, whether naturally or by therapeutic intervention. Much of the subsequent inflammation can be attributed to innate responses of the host toward endosymbiont bacterial components, in part through CD14, Toll-like receptor-4, or other innate immune receptors.[177] Clinical trials to assess the effect of doxycycline treatment in lymphatic filariasis have demonstrated depletion of *Wolbachia* from adult worms and microfilariae, inhibition of embryogenesis, declining microfilariae quantities, and reduced spermatozoa present in female genital tracts.[178,179] Doxycycline eradication of bacterial endosymbionts in filarial nematodes coupled with antifilarial treatment reduces both microfilaremia and adverse reactions in *Brugia malayi* infections.[178]

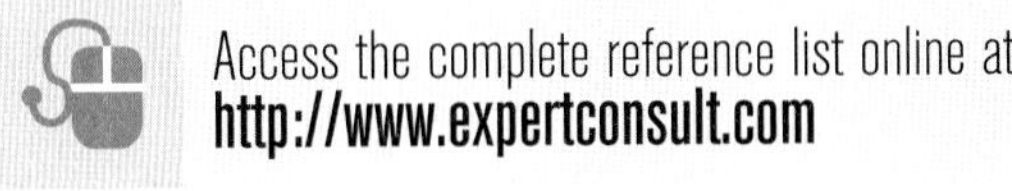

Access the complete reference list online at
http://www.expertconsult.com

CHAPTER 53

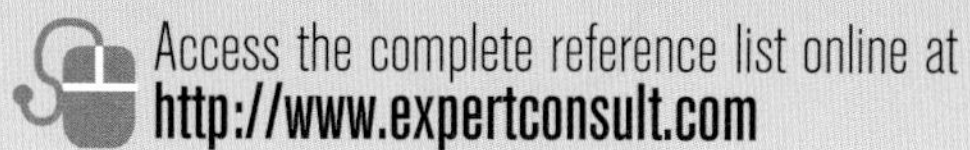
Access the complete reference list online at
http://www.expertconsult.com

Q Fever

Thomas J. Marrie

INTRODUCTION

Q fever is a disease that results from infection with the microorganism *Coxiella burnetii*. It was described by Dr E.H. Derrick in August 1935, at which time he investigated an outbreak of undiagnosed febrile illness among workers at the Canon Hill Abattoir in Brisbane, Australia.[1] Shortly thereafter the organism responsible for this outbreak was isolated and eventually named *Coxiella burnetii* in honor of Dr Herald Rae Cox and Sir Frank Macfarlane Burnet, two scientists who contributed so much to our knowledge of this disease.[2]

THE AGENT

C. burnetii is the sole species of its genus, and on the basis of 16S ribosomal RNA (rRNA) phylogeny it has been placed in the γ subdivision of Proteobacteria, with a specific but distant relationship to *Legionella*. It is an obligate phagolysosomal parasite of eukaryotes and measures 0.3–1.0 μm (***Fig. 53.1***).[3] Recently *C. burnetii* has been grown in a cell-free medium.[4] It forms spores and has survived for 586 days in tick feces at room temperature, for longer than 160 days in water, for 30–40 days in dried cheese made from contaminated milk, and for up to 150 days in soil. In nature and in laboratory animals, it exists in the phase I state. Repeated passage of phase I organisms in embryonated chicken eggs leads to conversion to phase II avirulent forms.[5,6]

The 1 995 275 base pair genome and 37 393 base pair plasmid of *C. burnetii* phase I, Nine Mile strain, have been sequenced.[7] *C. burnetii* is a Centers for Disease Control and Prevention (CDC) category B bioterrorism agent.[8,9] It has been calculated that a concentration of 100 cells/m^3 and an exposure time of 30–60 minutes can deposit more than one cell in the lung.[10]

EPIDEMIOLOGY

Q fever is found worldwide, including tropical countries, with the exception of New Zealand (no data are available about prevalence in Greenland and northernmost North America). In 1955, a review of the geographic distribution of Q fever indicated that it was found in Algeria, Belgian Congo (now Democratic Republic of the Congo), the Cameroons (Cameroon), Egypt, Ubangi Shari (Central African Republic), Kenya, Libya, Madagascar, Rhodesia (now Zimbabwe), and South Africa.[11] More recent studies indicate that Q fever is endemic in Zimbabwe, Tunisia, and northeast Africa.[12–14] Q fever is a zoonosis. There is an extensive wildlife and arthropod (mainly ticks) reservoir of *C. burnetii*.[15] Cattle, sheep, and goats are the animals that usually are the source of transmission of this microorganism to humans.[15] However, cats, dogs, and rabbits are also important in this regard. *C. burnetii* localizes to the uterus and mammary glands in female mammals. During pregnancy, reactivation occurs (although primary infection can occur as well), and the organism multiplies in the placenta, reaching 10^9 guinea pig infective doses per gram of tissue. These organisms are shed into the environment at the time of parturition. Humans become infected after inhaling organisms aerosolized at the time of parturition or later when organisms in dust are stirred up on a windy day. Infected animals can shed *C. burnetii* in milk or feces for months.

A study of 508 US veterinarians attending their annual convention revealed that 22.2% had antibodies to *C. burnetii*.[16] Contamination of water by *C. burnetii* is not uncommon, and such contamination can persist for some time;[17] indeed *C. burnetii* has been shown to survive for >100 days in tap water.[18]

In the United States between 1948 and 1977 a total of 1168 cases were reported to the CDC, a mean of 58.4 cases per year, while from 2000 to 2004 there were 255 cases from 37 states, a mean of 51 cases per year.[19,20]

McQusiton[20] reported that sheep and goats in the United States have a higher seroprevalence for *C. burnetii* than cattle, and she also noted an extensive wildlife reservoir for this organism in the United States.[20] Just over 94% of 316 bulk milk tanks throughout the United States tested at the beginning of 2000 had *C. burnetii* DNA detected.[21]

An outbreak of Q fever associated with a horse-boarding ranch in Colorado in 2005 was due to spread of infection from two herds of goats that had been acquired by the owners.[22] Sawyer and coworkers[23] in 1985 asked laboratories in the United States to submit to them all samples of serum that they had tested for hepatitis and for respiratory infection. Six (0.6%) of the 959 originally submitted for hepatitis testing had acute Q fever, as did 4 (0.6%) in the respiratory cohort. They concluded that Q fever was uncommon in the United States.

Karakousis et al[24] reported a case of chronic Q fever and reviewed all the published cases of chronic Q fever from the United States. They could only find seven such cases from 1976 to 2004, likely a gross underestimate. Q fever peaked in West Germany in 1964 at 450 cases during that year.[25]

Q fever continues to be diagnosed frequently in Australia with a rate of 30 cases per million per year.[26–28] Males are predominantly involved with a male : female ratio of 5.3 : 1.[21] One of the unique risk factors for Q fever in Australia is kangaroo hunting.[29]

Q fever has emerged as a travel-associated illness.[30–33]

THE DISEASE

In most instances, humans become infected with *C. burnetii* following inhalation of contaminated aerosols (***Fig. 53.2***).[34] Certain occupational groups are at high risk of *C. burnetii* infection; these include abattoir workers and veterinarians. Those who live in the vicinity of farms with infected animals are also at high risk of infection. High winds can disperse *C. burnetii*-contaminated dust 10 or more kilometers from these farms.[35,36]

It is likely that ingestion of *C. burnetii*-contaminated milk also causes infection, although the experimental evidence for this in humans is inconclusive. Rarely, infection has occurred via the percutaneous route following crushing of infected ticks between the fingers or as a result of transfusion of contaminated blood. Vertical transmission from mother to

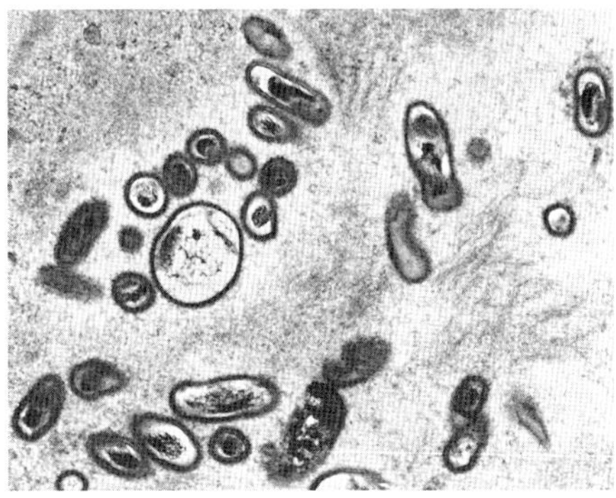

Figure 53.1 Transmission electron micrograph of a cardiac vegetation from a patient with *Coxiella burnetii* endocarditis showing *C. burnetii* cells (×23 335).

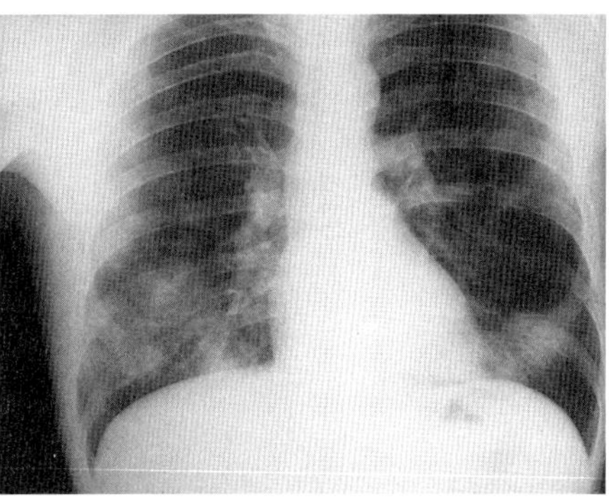

Figure 53.3 Chest radiograph of a young man who developed Q fever pneumonia following exposure to the products of conception of an infected parturient cat. Note the multiple rounded pulmonary opacities.

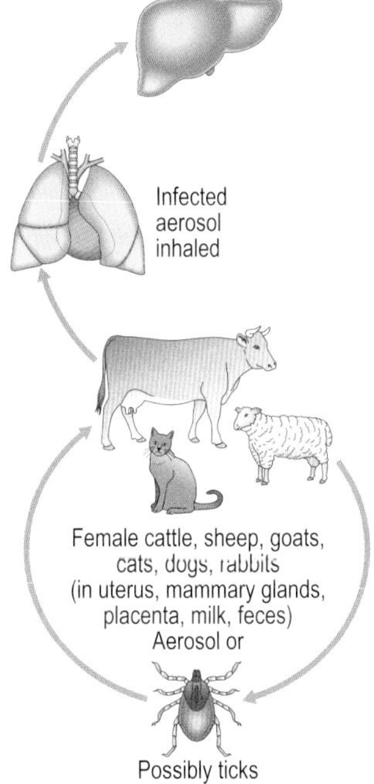

Figure 53.2 Q fever (*Coxiella burnetii*) life cycle.

infant can occur, and person-to-person transmission at the time of autopsy has rarely been reported. Recently, sexual transmission of Q fever has been documented, but this also seems to be very uncommon.

Several outbreaks of *C. burnetii* have occurred in institutions using pregnant sheep for research. These infected pregnant sheep were usually transported along crowded corridors, and a large number of employees in these institutions developed Q fever.

The incubation period for Q fever in humans is about 2 weeks with a range of 2–29 days. A dose–response effect has been demonstrated both experimentally and clinically. *Coxiella burnetii* is one of the most infectious agents known to man, as a single microorganism is capable of initiating infection. The resulting illness in humans can be divided into acute and chronic varieties.

Acute Q Fever

Self-limited Illness

Self-limited illness is the most common manifestation of Q fever. In areas where Q fever is endemic, ≥12% or more of the population have antibodies to *C. burnetii*, and most of these infections are subclinical or undiagnosed. A study from the south of Spain found that 108 of 505 adults (21%) who had fever for more than 1 week and less than 3 weeks had Q fever. All of these patients had normal chest radiographs.

Pneumonia

This illness is more severe than the self-limited febrile illness. The major manifestations are fever; severe headache, often with retro-orbital pain; and cough. Surprisingly, a large number of patients with Q fever pneumonia may not have cough. In our studies in Nova Scotia of 51 patients with radiographically documented Q fever pneumonia, only 14 (27%) had cough.[34] This cough is usually nonproductive. In most instances the pneumonia is of mild to moderate severity and can be treated on an outpatient basis. However, occasionally the pneumonia can be severe and rapidly progressive, resulting in respiratory failure requiring assisted ventilation. Nausea, vomiting, and diarrhea occur in 10–30% of patients with Q fever pneumonia. The most common physical finding is inspiratory crackles. About 5% of Q fever patients with pneumonia have splenomegaly.

The radiographic features of Q fever pneumonia are variable. Subsegmental and segmental pleural-based opacities are common. Multiple rounded opacities are suggestive of this illness, especially the variety that follows exposure to parturient cats (***Fig. 53.3***). Pleural effusions occur in about one-third of patients. Hilar lymphadenopathy may also be present.

Pulmonary tissue has been examined in only a small number of patients with Q fever pneumonia. In these instances the bronchial epithelial lining has been abnormal, and the interstitial space has contained edema along with infiltration by lymphocytes and macrophages. The alveolar spaces are filled with macrophages. We studied one patient with a pseudotumor due to *C. burnetii*. In this instance the lung mass was composed of a mixture of macrophages, multinucleate giant cells, plasma cells, and lymphocytes.

The white blood cell count is usually normal, although one-third of patients have leukocytosis. A slight elevation in hepatic transaminase levels occurs in almost all of these patients.

Hepatitis

There are three presentations of Q fever hepatitis: (1) pyrexia of unknown origin with mild to moderate elevation of hepatic enzymes; (2) a hepatitis-like picture; (3) incidental hepatitis. Liver biopsy reveals distinctive "doughnut" granulomas, that is, a granuloma with a central lipid vacuole and fibrin deposits.

Neurologic Manifestations

Aseptic meningitis or encephalitis complicates up to 1% of cases of Q fever. In some geographic areas the neurologic manifestations of Q fever are much more common than in others. In a study from Plymouth, England, Reilly and coworkers reported a 22% incidence of neurologic manifestations among 103 patients with Q fever.[37] These manifestations included residual weakness, recurrent meningitis, blurred vision, paresthesias, and sensory loss involving the left leg. Other neurologic manifestations of Q fever have included hallucinations, dysphagia, and hemifacial pain suggestive of trigeminal neuralgia. Rarely, behavioral disturbances, cerebellar signs and symptoms, cranial nerve palsies, extrapyramidal disease, Miller Fisher syndrome, and demyelinating polyradiculoneuritis have been reported in Q fever.

Chronic Q Fever

The usual manifestation of chronic Q fever is culture-negative endocarditis. Most of these patients have fever, and nearly all have abnormal native heart valves or prosthetic heart valves. Hepatomegaly or splenomegaly, or both, occur in about half of patients with Q fever endocarditis, and one-third have marked clubbing of the digits. Marked hyperglobulinemia (≥70 g/L) is common and is a useful clue to diagnosis.[38] Microscopic hematuria is usually present. Arterial emboli complicate the clinical course of about one-third of patients with Q fever endocarditis.

In Q fever endocarditis, the vegetation is quite smooth and may form nodules on the valve. Microscopically, there is subacute and chronic inflammatory cell infiltrate, and many large foamy macrophages full of characteristic microorganisms are readily seen by electron microscopy (see ***Fig. 53.1***).

Q Fever in the Immunocompromised Host and During Pregnancy

A recent study of 66 human immunodeficiency virus type 1 (HIV-1) seropositive persons living in Bangui, Central Africa Republic, found that 11 (16.7%) were also seropositive for *C. burnetii*. Two of the seven HIV-infected patients for whom clinical data were available had a history compatible with symptomatic Q fever.[39] Investigators in France found that 10.4% of 500 HIV-positive persons in Marseilles had Q fever antibodies at a titer equal to or greater than 1 : 225 compared with 4.1% of 925 healthy blood donors. They also found that 5 of 63 patients hospitalized with Q fever from 1987 to 1989 in Marseilles were HIV-positive. In France, 20% of patients with chronic Q fever were immunocompromised. These patients had cancer, chronic myeloid leukemia, acquired immunodeficiency syndrome (AIDS), renal transplantation, chronic alcoholism, or were receiving corticosteroid therapy or renal dialysis. Q fever has caused fatal interstitial pneumonia in an 11-year-old boy with the genetic condition chronic granulomatous disease of childhood. Acute Q fever during pregnancy is associated with premature birth (35%) and abortion or neonatal death (43%).

PATHOGENESIS AND IMMUNITY

Increasing knowledge of the pathogenesis of *C. burnetii* infection includes its avoidance of death in macrophages by producing superoxide dismutase, inhibiting cathepsin fusion with the phagosome, and adaptation to the acidic phagolysosome. Chronic Q fever more likely results from differences in the host response than differences in *Coxiella* virulence.[40–51]

DIAGNOSIS

In most countries the diagnosis of Q fever is made by showing a fourfold increase in antibodies between acute and convalescent serum samples using the indirect immunofluorescence test (preferred) or a complement fixation test. The organism can be cultured from a variety of tissues, but this has to be carried out in a biosafety level 3 laboratory. Polymerase chain reaction can be used to amplify *C. burnetii* DNA from a variety of clinical specimens.

TREATMENT AND PROGNOSIS

The prognosis is excellent in acute Q fever, with mortality being extremely rare. Fluoroquinolones and rifampin are the most active agents against *C. burnetii in vitro*. A 10-day course of tetracycline, doxycycline, or a fluoroquinolone will adequately treat acute Q fever. Macrolides have also been used to treat acute Q fever; however, some strains of *C. burnetii* are resistant to macrolides. Q fever pneumonia during pregnancy should be treated with co-trimoxazole for the duration of the pregnancy. In one retrospective study this approach reduced obstetric complications from 81% to 44%. There were no intrauterine fetal deaths in the co-trimoxazole treated group.[52] Those patients with a "chronic Q fever serological profile" should be treated with doxycycline and hydroxychloroquine for 1 year following delivery.[52]

There is one report of recurrent Jarisch–Herxheimer reaction complicating the treatment of Q fever pneumonia.[53]

Patients with cardiac valvular lesions who develop acute Q fever should be followed with serological testing every 3 months, and if the serological profile of chronic Q fever develops, they should be treated with doxycycline and hydroxychloroquine as for Q fever endocarditis. Alternatively preemptive treatment with doxycycline and hydroxychloroquine can be given to these patients for 1 year.[54]

Chronic Q fever should be treated with two antimicrobial agents for at least 3 years.[55] Some authorities recommend lifelong therapy for chronic Q fever. The best regimen is probably doxycycline and hydroxychloroquine. The hydroxychloroquine alkalinizes the phagolysosome rendering doxycycline bactericidal.[56] Hydroxychloroquine is given in a dose of 200 mg three times per day, and the dose is adjusted to maintain a serum concentration between 0.8 and 1.2 μg/mL. It was recently found that doxycycline levels vary among patients and that a serum level of 5 μg/mL should be reached to obtain high success rates.[57] In one case a patient died because the minimum inhibitory concentration of *C. burnetii* to doxycycline was 8 μg/mL.[58] Antibody titers should be determined every 6 months during therapy and every 3 months for the first 2 years after the cessation of therapy. Valve replacement is frequently necessary but should be dictated by the patient's hemodynamic status. Patients are considered cured when the IgG phase I antibody titer is less than 1 : 800 and IgM and IgA antibody titers are less than 1 : 50 by microimmunofluorescence.

PREVENTION AND CONTROL

A formalin-inactivated *C. burnetii* whole-cell vaccine protects against infection and has a 1% rate of induration developing at the inoculation site. The vaccine is available in Australia. The use of only seronegative pregnant sheep in research facilities and control of ectoparasites on livestock are measures that can reduce Q fever infection. It is wise not to accept blood donations from those who reside in an area where there is an outbreak of Q fever and for up to 2 months following cessation of the outbreak.

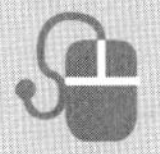

Access the complete reference list online at
http://www.expertconsult.com

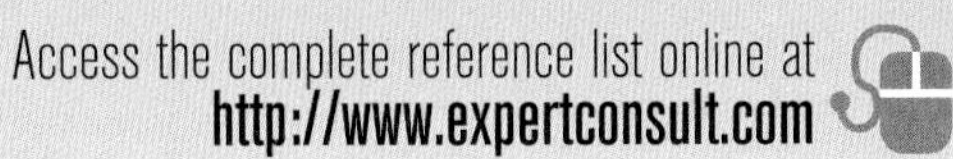
Access the complete reference list online at
http://www.expertconsult.com

CHAPTER 54

Measles

Jon K. Andrus • Ciro A. De Quadros • Carlos Castillo-Solorzano

INTRODUCTION

The origin of the word "measles" likely stems from the Medieval Latin word *miser*, meaning miserable.[1] Historically epidemics of measles have been huge killers of children and have been known to have changed the course of history.[2]

As recently as 1997, more than 36 million measles cases and approximately 1 million measles-related deaths were estimated worldwide. In 1997, measles accounted for more deaths than those caused by all other vaccine-preventable diseases combined.[3] In 2007, as a result of enhanced measles immunization activities, the World Health Organization (WHO) estimated that the numbers of measles deaths globally had declined to approximately 200 000.[4] However, the overwhelming majority of measles deaths still occur among infants and young children living in developing countries.

THE AGENT

Measles virus is an RNA virus of the genus *Morbillivirus* of the *Paramyxoviridae* family.[5] It is the most infectious virus known to man.[6] The virus is antigenically stable, but is quite sensitive to ultraviolet light, heat, and drying. In 1998, the WHO published standardized procedures and protocols for the genetic characterization of wild-type measles viruses and to establish a consistent system for describing genotypes.[7] Genotypes are now grouped into different clades. The ability to effectively monitor accelerated control and elimination programs will be enhanced by continued characterization of viruses isolated from outbreaks around the world.[8,9]

EPIDEMIOLOGY

Measles occurs worldwide. In countries with temperate climates, transmission increases in late winter and early spring. In tropical countries, transmission increases after the rainy season. Prior to measles vaccination, epidemics occurred every 2 or 3 years. The duration of epidemics varied according to population size, crowding, and population immunity. Where measles is endemic, most children are infected by age 10 years. When measles was endemic in the United States, >90% of persons were infected by age 15 years.[10] Countries with higher vaccination coverage levels may have epidemics spaced further apart, approximately every 5–7 years. As the numbers of susceptible individuals increase over time and become large enough to sustain widespread transmission, explosive outbreaks may occur even in countries with high vaccine coverage levels.

The incubation period of measles from the time of exposure to the onset of fever is usually 10 days and an additional 4 days for the onset of rash. Measles is most communicable 1–3 days before the onset of fever and cough. Secondary attack rates among susceptible household contacts are reported to be more than 80%.[11] Outbreaks have been reported in populations in which only 3–7% of the individuals were susceptible.[12–14] There is a marked reduction in communicability of the virus following the appearance of the rash.

THE DISEASE

The disease starts with the onset of fever, malaise, cough, and a runny nose. Conjunctivitis and bronchitis are commonly present. Patients have a harsh, nonproductive cough throughout the febrile period. Cough persists for 1 or 2 weeks in uncomplicated cases. Cough is often the last symptom to disappear. Young children commonly have lymphadenopathy. Older children may also have photophobia and arthralgias.[15]

Within 2–4 days after the onset, other signs begin. A characteristic red maculopapular rash usually begins behind the ears and then on the face, ultimately spreading to the trunk and upper extremities. The rash may not be as striking in dark-skinned children. The rash peaks in 2 or 3 days, usually lasting from 3 to 7 days. After this period, the rash may undergo fine desquamation (***Fig. 54.1***). Malnourished children are more likely to suffer more severe exfoliation.

Infected children in developing countries are more likely to experience complications such as pneumonia, diarrhea, and otitis media.[16] Pneumonia, in particular, causes significant morbidity and mortality.[17] Measles virus may cause pneumonia, but more commonly the pneumonia is a secondary infection with other viral agents or bacteria. Chronic diarrhea in developing countries after acute measles is another complication[18] which adversely contributes to the nutritional status of children.[19]

Malnourished children experience more severe measles.[20] The disease causes malaise and decreased food intake. Metabolic requirements increase because of fever. Parents may inappropriately withhold food during an acute illness. All these factors contribute to undernutrition. Undernutrition of children with measles produces vitamin A deficiency and keratitis, resulting in a higher incidence of childhood blindness in developing countries.[21]

Febrile convulsions are the most common neurologic complication. Less common complications include encephalitis or postinfectious encephalopathy, occurring in approximately 1 in 1000 infected children; and subacute sclerosing panencephalitis (SSPE), a rare chronic, degenerative neurologic disorder associated with the persistent infection of the central nervous system with a defective measles virus.[22] SSPE typically manifests several years after measles infection.

PATHOGENESIS AND IMMUNITY

Measles virus is transmitted from person to person via respiratory droplets or airborne spray to mucous membranes in the upper respiratory tract or the conjunctiva, or by direct contact with nasal or throat secretions of infected persons. Transmission occurs less frequently by articles freshly contaminated with infected nasal and throat secretions. Humans

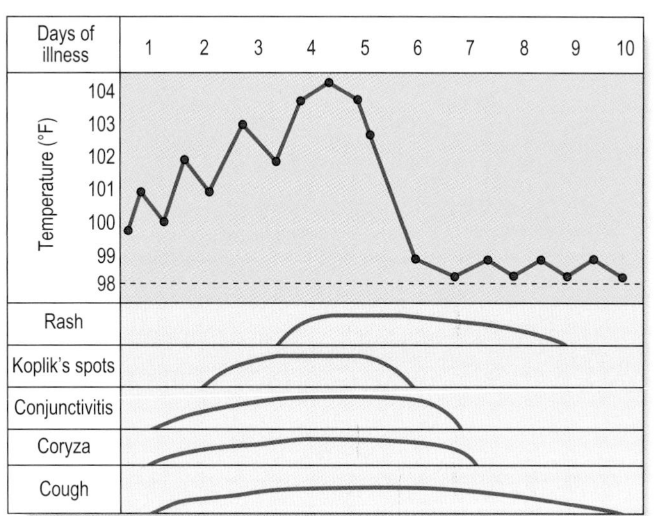

Figure 54.1 Schematic clinical course of a typical case of measles.
(From Krugman S, Katz SL, Gershon A, et al, eds. Infectious Diseases in Children, 9th edn. St Louis, Mosby-Year Book, 1992:224.)

serve as the only reservoir for the virus. Although monkeys in captivity may become infected, measles transmission among monkeys in the wild does not appear to contribute substantially to virus persistence in nature.

Following exposure of a susceptible host to an infected person, measles virus replicates in the respiratory tract. The virus then spreads and multiplies in local lymphatic tissues, subsequently leading to primary viremia.[23] Lymphoid tissue, skin, gastrointestinal tract, lungs, and liver are end-organs that may become infected. Acute measles infection may cause a suppression of the immune system, persisting for several months.[24] This immunosuppression may contribute in part to the increased susceptibility of children with measles to secondary bacterial and viral infections such as pneumonia and gastroenteritis. Children with vitamin A deficiency are at particular risk for such complications and associated mortality.[20]

DIAGNOSIS

Prior to the availability of measles vaccine and rapid scale-up of coverage, measles infection could be diagnosed on clinical grounds with reasonable accuracy. Koplik's spots are pathognomonic, and in endemic countries may be seen on the buccal mucosa in more than 80% of cases if frequent, careful examinations are performed, especially before the rash appears.[25]

In countries with high vaccination coverage, the large number of other childhood exanthematous illnesses makes laboratory testing critical for case confirmation. The differential diagnosis of measles includes rubella, scarlet fever, roseola, dengue fever, early stages of chickenpox, Kawasaki syndrome, toxic shock syndrome, enterovirus and adenovirus infections, rickettsial diseases, and drug hypersensitivity rashes.[15]

For surveillance of measles elimination, virus isolation remains the "gold standard" for the laboratory confirmation of suspected measles cases and for providing opportunities to monitor the molecular epidemiology of viral transmission.[6,26,27] Because of technical challenges, viral isolation is performed only in specialized laboratories. Therefore, more commonly laboratory confirmation of suspect measles cases relies on antibody testing that documents an appropriate immunologic response to measles by the host. Antibody can be detected at rash onset and then peaks approximately 1 month after infection. Immunoglobulin M (IgM) antibody testing is most commonly used in the field, with specimens taken from the host for testing with the first visit to the health system. By 6 weeks after infection IgM antibodies fall below detectable levels, in contrast to immunoglobulin G (IgG), which may be detected for years after infection. The IgM test offers the advantage of determining acute infections with one test. The IgG test is considered positive in the context of a fourfold antibody titer rise of paired acute to convalescent sera. Since the early 1980s, enzyme immunoassays (EIAs) have been made available for both IgM and IgG testing, in contrast to the previously used complement fixation, neutralization, and hemagglutination assays.[28–31]

For measles elimination, the Pan American Health Organization (PAHO) recommends that countries of the Americas use selected commercially available EIA tests with an excellent record of sensitivity and specificity, supported by virus isolation from at least one case in each chain of transmission. This approach has proven essential for sustaining progress achieved in the measles elimination effort of the Americas.

TREATMENT AND PROGNOSIS

For uncomplicated measles, treatment is supportive and includes fluids (such as oral rehydration solution), antipyretics, and nutritional therapy. Antibiotics are needed for secondary bacterial infections, if and when they occur, especially to treat bacterial pneumonia. Vitamin A should be administered to severe cases, especially hospitalized children with acute measles. Vitamin A has been demonstrated to reduce mortality substantially. In communities with increased rates of malnutrition or which have experienced increased measles mortality, WHO recommends that vitamin A be given to all children with acute measles infection.[32] Measles consumes vital nutritional reserves of children, and many require 4–8 weeks to recover their premeasles nutritional status.

In developed countries the case-fatality ratio for measles generally ranges between 0.1 and 1.0 per 1000 cases.[33] In contrast, in developing countries the overall case-fatality ratio may range between 3% and 6%, with the highest rate occurring in infants aged 6–11 months.[34] In high-risk populations, case-fatality ratios as high as 20% or 30% have been reported in infants aged <1 year.[35] Moreover, extremely high measles case-fatality ratios have been reported among infants and children living in extremely stressed conditions, such as refugee camps.[36]

PREVENTION AND CONTROL

The original Edmonston strain measles vaccines approved for use in children in 1963 were attenuated, live, and inactivated vaccines. This strain is now no longer used. The vaccines currently in use may have the more attenuated (**more attenu**ated, hence "Moraten") live measles virus strains. The United States primarily uses the Moraten strain vaccine, while other countries generally use the Schwarz vaccine.[37–39]

By 1982, nearly 20 years after approval in the United States, virtually all developing countries in the world with the support of the Expanded Program on Immunization (EPI) had introduced measles vaccine into their routine childhood vaccination schedules. In those early years coverage was very low. To that end, WHO and UNICEF spearheaded the Universal Childhood Immunization initiative in the 1980s to improve levels of coverage. By 1990, the estimated overall global coverage for children aged <2 years reached approximately 80%.

Immunization with live measles vaccine has been demonstrated to be protective for more than 20 years, and immunity is thought to be lifelong.[40] Due to the interference of maternal antibodies, vaccine effectiveness increases substantially after the first 6–9 months of life, peaking at 95% at 12–15 months of age.[41] The development and persistence of serum antibodies following measles vaccination are lower but parallel to the response following natural measles infection. After infection or vaccination, the infant's antibody responses peak in 6–8 weeks.

Absolute contraindications to measles vaccination are few, but include people with the following characteristics: severe immunosuppression, pregnancy, history of anaphylactic reaction to neomycin, or history of recent receipt of immunoglobulin or other blood products.[42] Vaccine can be administered safely and effectively to children with mild acute illnesses. Priority should be given to vaccinating children who are malnourished. Asymptomatic infection with the human immunodeficiency virus should not be considered a contraindication to measles vaccination.[43]

Generally, 5–15% of infants vaccinated with measles vaccine develop a mild fever.[44] Approximately 5% develop a generalized rash 5–10 days after vaccination that lasts for 1–3 days. This vaccine-associated measles is generally mild and well tolerated.[45] Febrile convulsions occur in approximately 1 in 1000 children following measles vaccination.[46] Severe neurologic events following measles vaccination, such as encephalitis and encephalopathy, are estimated to occur in fewer than 1 in 1 million vaccinees.[47]

Since vaccine use, the interval between epidemics has increased, and the magnitude of outbreaks has decreased markedly.[48,49] Traditionally, the vaccination strategy used to control measles in most developing countries had been to target all children between 9 and 12 months with a single dose of vaccine through the routine childhood vaccination program.[50] Most countries that have achieved and maintained high vaccine coverage with measles vaccine have reported a 90% or more reduction in the measles incidence and measles-related deaths compared to the prevaccine era.[51–54] In a review of cost-effective health measures, the World Bank evaluated measles immunization as being one of the most cost-effective public health interventions currently available.[55]

But even with substantial progress in measles vaccination, in the early 1990s, approximately 40 million cases and 1 million deaths occurred each year. Although measles vaccine coverage has markedly increased, large measles outbreaks have continued to occur in developing countries that have failed to achieve and maintain high levels of vaccination coverage.[56,57] Even in countries with strong systems in place capable of achieving high coverage rates, outbreaks have been reported after the accumulation of susceptible persons over time.[58] Factors that have been implicated in these outbreaks include the failure to achieve and maintain sufficiently high levels of vaccination coverage, the occurrence of primary vaccination failure (the failure to seroconvert following vaccination) in approximately 5–10% of vaccinated children, and the accumulation of susceptible children over time.

The Gambia, a country of approximately 1.7 million people on the Atlantic coast of western Africa, was the first developing country to interrupt measles virus transmission and demonstrate that measles elimination was technically feasible. Annual national measles immunization campaigns were initiated starting in 1967.[59] The campaign strategy included mobile vaccination teams targeting initially children aged 6 months to 6 years for vaccination. Subsequent campaigns targeted young children not previously vaccinated. Measles virus transmission was interrupted within 1 year after the program began, and the country remained free of measles during the period 1968–1970.[60] Soon thereafter, the program was discontinued due to lack of financial support; measles virus was introduced from neighboring countries, and transmission was reestablished.[61,62]

After successfully eradicating polio and noting the measles elimination experience in The Gambia, in 1986, Cuba implemented a national measles vaccination strategy using standard-titer, further attenuated measles vaccine. Health authorities conducted a mass measles vaccination campaign, targeting all children 1–14 years of age, regardless of measles disease history or vaccination status. Over a 6-month period, nearly 2.5 million children were vaccinated, resulting in coverage of approximately 98%. Following the campaign, measles surveillance was strengthened, and the reported number of confirmed measles cases rapidly decreased to record low levels. Between 1989 and 1992, fewer than 20 confirmed measles cases were reported annually. Because of the accumulation of susceptible preschool-age children since the prior campaign, a repeat mass measles vaccination campaign was conducted in November 1993 targeting all children 2–6 years of age, regardless of prior vaccination status or measles disease history. More than 880000 children were vaccinated during this campaign, resulting in a 98% coverage. The last serologically confirmed measles case in Cuba occurred in July 1993.[63]

Given the accumulated field experience suggesting that measles elimination was feasible, in 1994 PAHO embarked on an initiative to interrupt endemic transmission of measles in the Western hemisphere by the year 2000. The strategies adopted to eliminate measles were remarkably similar to those of the successful PAHO polio eradication initiative.[64] As additional experience accumulates, the strategies continue to evolve.[65] In brief, the major aim of the strategy is to rapidly interrupt measles transmission and to maintain the interruption in measles virus circulation by sustaining high population immunity. Surveillance is also critical to detect measles transmission and respond accordingly.

The PAHO measles elimination vaccination strategy has three components.[65] Since children aged 1–14 years traditionally had 90% of the infections, the first component is to conduct a one-time only "catch-up" campaign, targeting all children between the ages of 1 and 14 years for measles vaccination during the low season of transmission, regardless of their previous measles vaccination status. The second component is a "keep-up" vaccination campaign which calls upon routine health services to achieve and maintain the highest coverage possible, but at least 90%. Since the risk of an infant being exposed to circulating measles virus is low, the age of routine measles vaccination can be safely increased from 9 months to 12 months of age, thus providing an increase in measles vaccine effectiveness. Efforts are made to achieve 90% coverage in each successive birth cohort in every district. Despite these first two components, susceptibles accumulate, so "follow-up" campaigns are required on average every 4 years as a second opportunity for measles vaccination. "Follow-up" campaigns target all children aged 1–4 years for measles vaccination during the low season of transmission, regardless of their previous vaccination status. In so doing, the "follow-up" campaigns provide children with a second opportunity for complete protection against measles.[66] Campaigns are conducted when the estimated number of accumulated susceptible preschool-age children approaches the number of infants in an average birth cohort. In practice, PAHO recommends that "follow-up campaigns" be conducted every 4 years.[15]

By the end of 1995, all countries of Latin America and the English-speaking Caribbean had conducted catch-up measles vaccination campaigns. The combined regional 1- to 14-year-old measles vaccination coverage is estimated to be 93%.

After essentially eliminating endemic measles disease (***Fig. 54.2***), in 2001–2002 a huge measles outbreak occurred in Colombia and Venezuela, resulting from an initial measles virus importation into Colombia. The virus genotype was D9, and transmission was interrupted with supplemental immunization campaigns in November 2002. This outbreak most likely represents the last endemic transmission in the region. During this outbreak, Colombia reported 139 and Venezuela 2501 measles cases.

Beginning in 2003, Mexico also experienced an outbreak resulting from importation of measles virus. The virus genotype was H1 and was considered to be an importation because this genotype had never been isolated previously in the Americas. H1 genotype is quite common in the Far East. Because measles population immunity was high, the outbreak remained relatively small and contained. During the outbreak period (April 2003 to July 2004), a total of 108 measles cases were reported. All but 2 cases occurred in two contiguous states and the Federal District of Mexico City. From February 2006 to 2007, Venezuela reported 122 cases. The first patient was probably exposed to measles virus in Spain. The virus genotypes isolated from this outbreak were all B3, the same genotype circulating in Spain at the time.

These last outbreaks in the region highlight the fact that importations are to be expected if endemic transmission is still occurring in other parts of the world.[67] Beginning in 2003, the implementation of strategies to eliminate rubella and rubella congenital syndrome by 2010 greatly contributed to sustaining the measles elimination achievements, despite the continued threat of measles importations.[68] Prior to 2003, PAHO had been recommending that vaccines used in all measles vaccination strategies contain rubella antigen. The aim was to avoid missing the opportunity to control another serious public health threat or to provide support for other essential health services.[69,70] The measles elimination initiative of the Americas unmasked the silent public health problem of congenital rubella syndrome (CRS). Measles surveillance revealed that rubella was a significant public health concern (***Fig. 54.3***), and approximately 20000 CRS cases were occurring annually in the countries of Latin America and the Caribbean. The magnitude of the CRS problem prior to measles elimination was largely unknown.

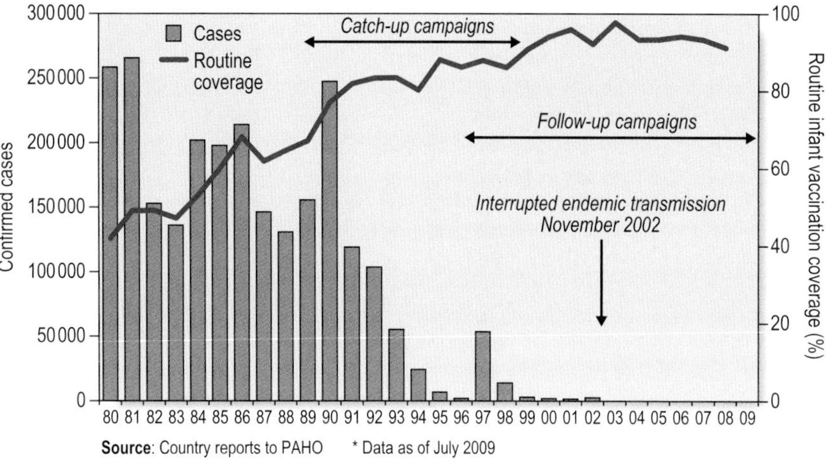

Figure 54.2 Annual reported measles cases in Latin American and Caribbean countries, 1980–2009. (Data from the Pan American Health Organization, Washington, DC.)

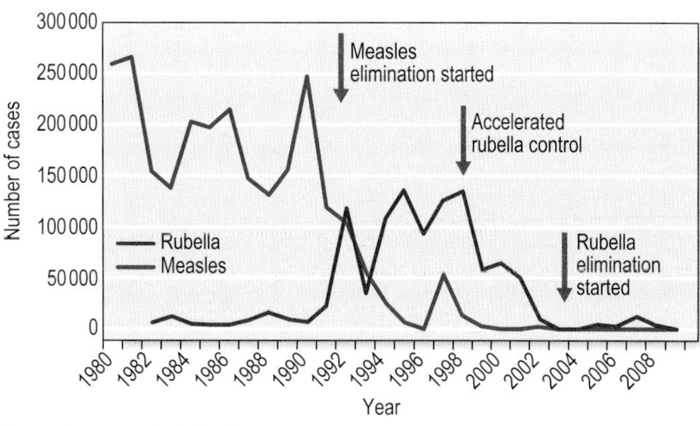

Figure 54.3 Trends in reported measles and rubella cases in the Americas, 1980–2009. (From the Pan American Health Organization Epidemiology Surveillance System, Washington, DC.)

The elimination of rubella and congenital rubella syndrome requires thorough vaccination, rapidly reducing numbers of susceptibles in older populations to prevent the occurrence of congenital rubella syndrome.[68] Therefore, larger, one-time "speed-up" mass rubella campaigns were implemented in all countries, usually targeting both women and men aged <40 years using measles–rubella-containing vaccines. Rigorous analysis of the surveillance and vaccination coverage data determined within each country the lower age targeted for the campaign.

A common feature of all import-related measles outbreaks in countries that have succeeded in stopping endemic transmission is that most cases have either received only one dose of measles-containing vaccine, or have not been vaccinated at all.[71] To support country commitment to maintain their measles elimination status, PAHO has mandated that transmission occurring in a Latin American or Caribbean country as a result of virus importation, which lasts more than a year, should be considered endemic transmission.[72] Such a country would no longer be considered as having eliminated the disease. Critical to maintaining the achievement of measles elimination has been sustaining high-quality surveillance, and maintaining high levels of population immunity with high routine measles coverage and the continued implementation of "follow-up" campaigns with measles–rubella-containing vaccines every 4 years. In so doing, importations once they occur are contained with rapid interruption of transmission much more effectively. As a result of the rubella elimination strategies, the last endemic rubella case reported in the region occurred with date of rash onset on 3 February 2009 in Argentina.[73]

In the United States and other developed countries that have maintained relatively high levels of immunization coverage for several years, two distinct patterns of measles transmission have been observed. Outbreaks have been reported among populations of highly vaccinated school-age children as well as among unvaccinated preschool-age children living in densely populated, poor, urban areas.[74] The outbreaks among vaccinated school-age children have tended to be small and self-limited, whereas those among unvaccinated preschool-age children have frequently been quite large and difficult to control.[75]

In the absence of very high levels of population immunity, efforts to control measles transmission, once an outbreak has started, have proved to be frustrating and often ineffective.[76–78] Due to the very high communicability of measles, many susceptible people are already infected before the outbreak is recognized and control activities implemented. Given the difficulties in controlling measles outbreaks, increased efforts should be made to prevent them. This goal is accomplished by achieving and maintaining very high levels of measles immunity among infants and children.

During the mid-1980s, in order to prevent the occurrence of measles outbreaks among highly vaccinated school-age children, some relatively more developed countries, including Chile, Denmark, Israel, Norway, Sweden, and the United States, instituted a routine two-dose measles vaccination schedule.[79] Moreover, increased efforts have been made to raise measles vaccination coverage among preschool-age children living in impoverished inner-city areas.[80]

Recognizing that measles remained a major killer of children in developing countries, in 2000 WHO and UNICEF began targeting 45 countries in Africa with exceedingly high measles mortality rates.[81] These African countries accounted for >90% of the global measles mortality. The WHO/UNICEF strategy to reduce mortality in Africa was similar to that used by PAHO: rapid reduction of measles susceptibles through measles vaccination and enhanced surveillance to monitor progress.[82] Other core partners supporting this work included the American Red Cross and the US Centers for Disease Control and Prevention. As a result of these efforts, a 74% mortality reduction was achieved from 2000 to 2007. Over the same period, over 11 million deaths from measles were prevented, clearly one of the greatest public health achievements of the last century. The challenge will be to maintain that achievement with the continued threat of importations from other parts of the world.

The challenge for any region embarking on measles elimination will be to maintain high population immunity with excellent immunization coverage and high-quality surveillance, especially to deal with importations. Implementation of measles elimination strategies should uncover the "hidden" disease burden of rubella and congenital rubella syndrome (***Fig. 54.3***). Integrating the elimination of measles with the elimination of rubella will greatly enhance the capacity of countries to sustain progress in the reduction of measles mortality. In addition, countries are encountering new opportunities to expand the benefits of disease control and elimination activities to other aspects of public health, most importantly in improving health care for women and reducing inequities in health care in the poorest countries.[69,70] Adoption of similar strategies in countries worldwide will likely lead to the global eradication of measles early in the twenty-first century.[83-85]

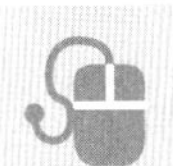

Access the complete reference list online at
http://www.expertconsult.com

CHAPTER 55

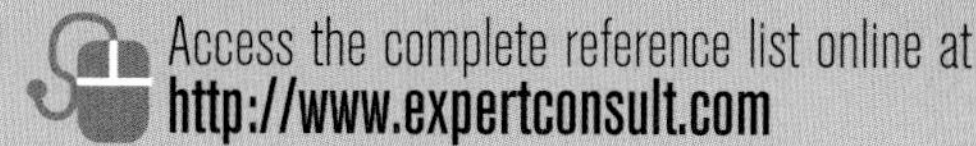
Access the complete reference list online at
http://www.expertconsult.com

Hendra and Nipah Viral Infections

Thomas G. Ksiazek • K.B. Chua • Paul A. Rota • Pierre E. Rollin

INTRODUCTION

Since 1994, when Hendra virus (HeV) was first noted in an outbreak of disease in both race horses and humans in the Brisbane suburb of Hendra, Queensland,[1] the emergence of the henipaviruses continues to be one of the most interesting and intriguing among the zoonotic viruses. Although the Hendra incident was the first noted, it was preceded by an occurrence of disease in horses and humans at Mackay, further north in Queensland.[2,3] Both of these initial incidents involved horses, and the virus was originally called equine morbillivirus; however, field investigations soon revealed that Australian horses were not the likely source of the infection since antibody prevalence was nil in an extensive survey of the equine population.[4,5] Further investigation led to the recognition of flying foxes of the genus *Pteropus* rather than horses as the putative reservoir of the virus in Australia.[6,7] Experimental infections in the laboratory demonstrated that HeV had a wide experimental host range including horses, cats, dogs, rabbits, and laboratory rodents.[8–11]

In the second half of 1998, Malaysia reported an outbreak of encephalitis, initially thought to be caused by Japanese encephalitis virus (JEV). The outbreak had epidemiologic characteristics which were unlike those of the endemic mosquito-borne JEV, and in March 1999 Nipah virus (NiV), a virus that is closely related to HeV, was identified as the etiologic agent of the outbreak.[12,13] Characteristics of this outbreak included exposure to swine as the principal risk factor for infection,[14] with occupations, racial groups, and age groups all associated with this activity. The disease primarily involved the central nervous system with patients progressing to coma and death, particularly if not supported by a ventilator as they entered coma.[15,16] As in Australia, flying foxes of the genus *Pteropus* native to Malaysia were found to be the most likely reservoir of the virus.[17,18] The outbreak was eventually brought to a halt by instituting a system of surveillance and culling swine herds that were contaminated by the virus; there were in excess of 1.1 million swine destroyed and disposed of during the outbreak.[19,20]

In 2001, an outbreak of disease occurred in Siliguri, India, where transmission of the disease included family members and medical staff attending the initial patients. The etiology of the outbreak remained unknown until serum specimens were tested and discovered to have IgM antibodies to NiV. Subsequently, NiV viral RNA was detected by reverse transcriptase polymerase chain reaction (RT-PCR) in the urine of patients, and the viral identity was confirmed by sequencing.[21] Unlike the previous instances in Australia and Malaysia, no intermediate animal host was readily identifiable. Beginning in 2001 Bangladesh has had a number of relatively small outbreaks in an area bordering India to the east.[22–25] These outbreaks are remarkable in that no intermediate domestic animal host has been identified. Epidemiological investigations suggested a number of routes for human infection including direct or indirect contact with fruit bats (*Pteropus giganteus* is the species in this region) in roosting or feeding areas, contamination of food products by the bats, and person-to-person transmission.

Similarly to the emergence of NiV as a human pathogen in Bangladesh, investigation of the ecology of the virus has added additional geographic areas where *Pteropus* spp. or other pteropids have been found to be infected with NiV, HeV or a closely related virus as evidenced by the presence of antibodies, the virus, or virus RNA.[26–36]

THE AGENT

Classification

HeV and NiV are members of a novel genus, *Henipavirus*, within the subfamily *Paramyxovirinae,* family *Paramyxoviridae.*[37] HeV and NiV share 68–92% amino acid identity in their protein coding regions and 40–67% nucleotide homology in the nontranslated regions of their genomes.[38,39]

Genome Structure and Gene Function of HeV and NiV

The single-stranded, negative sense RNA genomes of NiV and HeV have the same gene order, 3′-nucleoprotein (N)–phosphoprotein (P)–matrix protein (M)–fusion protein (F)–attachment protein (G)–RNA dependent RNA polymerase (L)-5′, as the respiroviruses and morbilliviruses. HeV and NiV retain a number of the genetic features found in other paramyxoviruses,[39,40] although the henipaviruses also have several unique characteristics.

The genomes of HeV and NiV are 18 234 and 18 246 nucleotides in length, which, until the characterization of Beilong and J viruses,[41,42] were the largest genomes among the paramyxoviruses with the size due to the large open reading frame for the P gene and the large 3′ nontranslated regions present in several genes.[39,43] The genomes of both HeV and NiV are evenly divisible by six, indicating that the henipaviruses adhere to the rule of six.[44,45] The *cis*-acting[46] sequences that regulate gene expression on the genomes of HeV and NiV including the gene start sites, gene stop sites, RNA editing sites, genomic termini, and intergenic sequences are very closely related to the corresponding sequences within the genomes of respiroviruses and morbilliviruses.[38,39,43,47] The development of minigenome replication assays and reverse genetic systems for NiV[44,48,49] will permit more detailed studies on the genetics and pathogenesis of the henipaviruses.

The P, C, V, and L Proteins of HeV and NiV

The coding strategy for the P gene of the henipaviruses is similar to that of the respiroviruses and morbilliviruses. In each case, a faithful transcript of the P gene codes for the P protein, an essential component of the replication complex, while the transcript encoding the V protein is produced by insertion of non-templated guanosine (G) nucleotides into the mRNA of the P gene to permit access to additional open reading frames.[50]

The V proteins share the same N-terminus as their respective P proteins which, at the editing site, are joined to a unique, C-terminal cysteine-rich open reading frame that is unique to V. The P genes of the henipaviruses also encode C protein, which is produced by ribosomal choice from an overlapping reading frame located near the 5′ terminus of the P gene mRNA.[38,47] The P genes of HeV and NiV also have the capacity to encode a protein that is analogous to the W protein of Sendai virus; W is expressed from an mRNA with a 2 G (guanosine) insertion at the RNA editing site.[51] The P, V, W, and C are present in both infected cells and in sucrose gradient purified virions.[52,53] Studies utilizing eukaryotic plasmid expression systems have shown that P, V, C, and W proteins of NiV, like the analogous proteins of other paramyxoviruses,[54] interfere with the host's innate immune response by inhibiting interferon signaling and induction.[53,55–59] The genes coding for the RNA-dependent RNA polymerase (L protein) of HeV and NiV have a linear domain structure that is conserved in all of the *Mononegavirales*.

The Membrane Glycoproteins of HeV and NiV

The two membrane glycoproteins of HeV and NiV, F and G, are required for cell fusion, and heterotypic mixtures of the G and F proteins of HeV and NiV are also fusion competent.[60,61] The F proteins of the *Paramyxovirinae* are type I membrane glycoproteins that facilitate the viral entry process by mediating fusion of the virion membrane with the plasma membrane of the host cell. F proteins are synthesized as inactive precursors, F_0, that are converted to biologically active subunits, F_1 and F_2, following proteolytic cleavage by a host cell protease.[46]

The attachment proteins of the *Paramyxoviridae* are type II membrane glycoproteins and are responsible for binding to receptors on host cells.[46,62] Unlike many other paramyxoviruses, neither of the henipaviruses has been shown to have erythrocyte binding or neuraminidase activities. The G proteins of the henipaviruses are most closely related to the hemagglutinin neuraminidase (HN) proteins of the respiroviruses.[63] EphrinB2, the membrane-bound ligand for the EphB class of receptor tyrosine kinases, specifically binds to G proteins of henipaviruses and is a functional receptor for HeV and NiV.[64] While EphrinB3 has also been shown to be a functional receptor for both viruses, the binding of NiV to EphrinB3 is much more efficient than the binding of HeV,[65,66] and the G protein of NiV has distinct binding regions for EphrinB2 and EphrinB3.[6] EphrinB3, but not EphrinB2, is expressed in the central nervous system, so the difference in the abilities of HeV and NiV to bind to these cellular receptors is consistent with the neuroinvasiveness of NiV.[65,66]

EPIDEMIOLOGY

The basis for the epidemiology of HeV and NiV, throughout the range of their occurrence, is determined by the reservoirs that maintain them and the means by which the viruses are able to be transferred between the reservoir and the human population. From our perspective, only pteropid fruit bats belonging to the suborder Megachiroptera, family Pteropodidae, have been identified as the natural reservoir hosts of henipaviruses. The four species of pteropid fruit bats (*Pteropus alacto*, *P. poliocephalus*, *P. scapulatus*, *P. conspicillatus*) serve as the reservoir hosts of HeV in Australia.[6,7] The natural reservoir hosts of NiV in Malaysia are *P. vampyrus* and *P. hypomelanus*.[17,67] There are several other pteropid species in the Southeast Asian region which have been found to have evidence of infection with henipaviruses, and these include *P. lylei* in Cambodia and Thailand.[27,29,33] In addition, *P. vampyrus*[28] and *P. hypomelanus* have a wide range in other parts of Southeast Asia and have been found or are likely to have infection with henipaviruses. *P. giganteus*, the *Pteropus* species that is widely distributed throughout South Asia including Bangladesh, parts of Myanmar, Sri Lanka, India, and Pakistan, has serologic evidence of infection.[24,32,68] *P. rufus* as well as two other pteropid species in Madagascar have antibody to NiV, and other genera of pteropid bats in West Africa have antibody or nucleic acid detected by RT-PCR, suggesting the presence of closely related viruses in other hosts and areas.[30,35,36]

Both NiV and HeV are contagious, highly virulent and capable of infecting a wide range of mammalian species in nature and under experimental conditions. Field studies in Malaysia suggest that an interplay of multiple factors could have led to the introduction of the virus from the reservoir bat species to commercial piggeries.[69] The widespread practice of high intensity farming, without the use of sufficient biosecurity practices, certainly facilitated the spread of the virus once it was introduced into the national swine herd. On the infected farms, the disease spread rapidly among pigs owing to direct contact with excretions and secretions such as urine, saliva, and pharyngeal secretions as was confirmed in contact pigs during experimental infections of swine in the laboratory.[70] Other possible means for the mechanical or biological transmission include movement of infected dogs and cats, the repeated use of needles or equipment within farms without sterilization after each use for health interventions, and artificial insemination and sharing of boar semen. The spread of the virus among pig farms within and between states of peninsular Malaysia is due to movement of pigs.[71]

Field investigations demonstrated that farms that did not receive animals from farms with suspected infection remained free from infection, even when these farms were proximate to infected farms.[71] Transmission of NiV to humans could be attributed to close contact with infected pigs.[13,14,72,73] In the Malaysian NiV outbreak human-to-human transmission was rare[74] even though NiV could be isolated from saliva, urine, and nasal and pharyngeal secretions of patients.[75,76] In Bangladesh, unlike the Malaysian outbreak, it appears that virus transmission from bats to humans occurs without involvement of intermediate animal hosts, and human-to-human transmission occurs with some regularity; this may also be the case in India.[21,24,77,78] One observation that may have a bearing on the situation is that very few of the cases in Bangladesh are hospitalized in tertiary care ICU settings, and nursing is, as is traditional in much of the developing world, undertaken by the relatives of the patient, often with no or minimal use of infection control practices. Field investigations indicate that drinking contaminated fresh date palm sap is significantly associated with NiV infection, though eating contaminated fruits could not be excluded.[77] The mode of transmission of HeV virus from pteropid fruit bats to horses is still unclear though the eating of contaminated fruits and/or grass at the roosts or foraging sites of these bats is highly suspected. HeV virus infection in humans is through close contact and care of the infected and sick horses.

Experimental infection and transmission studies of NiV among pigs carried out in the Australian Animal Health Laboratory, Geelong, Australia, established that pigs could be infected by both oral and parenteral inoculation and pigs shed NiV via oronasal routes. Infection was noted to spread quickly to in-contact pigs.[70] Experimental infection of pteropid bats with NiV shows that the infected bats excrete the virus and develop specific antibodies without evidence of illness.[10,79,80] However, the mode of virus transmission and the mechanism of viral persistence in the bat population in the wild are far from clear.

THE DISEASE

In natural infection of humans, pigs, horses, and dogs, the henipaviruses cause systemic infections, though prominent clinical manifestations are confined mainly to the respiratory and central nervous systems.[1,2,12,81]

The virus probably infects its non-natural-reservoir hosts via exposure and contamination of the respiratory mucosa via inhalation of infectious droplets, direct contamination of ocular, oral, or nasal mucosa by self-inoculation or droplet exposure, or through ingestion of contaminated food and liquids. Exposure to contaminated fomites is another possibility in either clinical or natural settings. The tissues lining the oropharynx and respiratory tract with adjoining lymphoid tissue are the major sites of initial viral replication based on histopathological evidence of primary NiV replication in respiratory tract mucosa and lymphoid organs.[15,16]

Following primary viral replication at the entry sites, cell-associated viremia is suggested (similar to measles virus infection). Endothelium, although unlikely to be the primary replication site, serves as the site of secondary virus replication and amplification and also as the means for local spread of infection.[16] The incubation period of NiV infection is estimated to be less than 2 weeks in humans and 7–14 days in pigs based on the affected patients and pigs during the outbreak in peninsular Malaysia. The incubation period of HeV infection is estimated to be 4–18 days in humans and 8–11 days in horses.[2,15,71,82–84]

In NiV infection of humans, the proportion of symptomatic infection is high with only 8–15% of infections resulting in subclinical infection.[15,83–85] The main presenting clinical features at the early stage of acute illness are nonspecific fever, headache, myalgia, and malaise.[15,82,83] More than 50% of the patients subsequently progress to involvement of the central nervous system (CNS) with fever, headache, dizziness, vomiting, and reduced level of consciousness.[15,82,83,85,86] Older patients, especially those having preexisting diabetes mellitus and those with severe brainstem involvement, carry a poorer prognosis.[87] Other poor prognostic factors include the presence of segmental myoclonus (commonly involving diaphragmatic and anterior neck muscles), seizures, and areflexia.

The overall mortality of acute NiV encephalitis is high (approximately 40% in Malaysia and 70% in Bangladesh) because of brainstem involvement.[15] A small number of patients die from complications of acute illness including septicemia, gastrointestinal tract bleeding, renal impairment, hemothorax, pulmonary embolism, and acute atrial fibrillation.[15] In Malaysia, three-quarters of the survivors recovered fully, and a quarter had apparent residual neurological deficits. Approximately 9% of the survivors suffer a second or even a third episode of acute neurological syndrome following initial recovery (relapsed NiV encephalitis), and about 5% who are either asymptomatic or only have mild non-neurological illness initially develop similar acute neurological syndrome at a later date (late-onset NiV encephalitis).[88] Clinical, radiological, and pathological findings suggest that relapsed and late-onset NiV encephalitis is essentially the same disease process but is distinct from acute NiV encephalitis.[88] The mean interval between the first recurrence and the initial infection is about eight and half months. The mortality for relapse or late-onset NiV encephalitis is 18%. This delayed presentation of encephalitis is a feature similar to that seen in a case of fatal meningoencephalitis due to HeV in Mackay, Queensland, Australia; in that instance the patient developed the illness 13 months after the initial infection.[2] Late-onset and relapse encephalitis are attributed to the persistence of infectious NiV in the CNS, although no virus was isolated from the cerebrospinal fluid.[16,88]

In Malaysia, 14% of patients had respiratory involvement and presented with nonproductive cough, and 3 of the 11 affected patients from Singapore had atypical pneumonia with abnormal chest radiographs.[15,89] In Bangladesh, in addition to presentation as acute encephalitis, affected patients also have prominent lung changes and present as acute respiratory distress syndrome, which was not observed among patients in Malaysia. Prominent respiratory involvement affecting Bangladeshi patients may have contributed to human-to-human spread of the disease.[24,78] The absence of accessible tertiary care facilities with respiratory support in Bangladesh and India may also contribute significantly to higher mortality (about 70%) among the affected patients compared to ~40% in the Malaysian outbreak. In Australia, acute HeV infection in humans presents mainly as acute respiratory illness.[1,2] Of the initial two human patients with HeV infection who presented as acute respiratory illness, one died of interstitial pneumonia with respiratory failure and the other had a slow recovery.[1,2] One recent HeV fatality among veterinary practitioners in Australia was marked by more neurological complications.[90]

In pigs, mortality after NiV infection is low, ranging from 5% to less than 15%, but the proportion of animals infected is high, approaching 100%.[71] NiV causes illness in pigs with both CNS and respiratory manifestations, though the clinical patterns of the disease vary according to the age of the pigs. Pigs less than 6 months old usually present with an acute febrile illness with respiratory signs ranging from rapid and labored respiration to a harsh, nonproductive cough and open mouth breathing with severe cough and hemoptysis in severe cases. Neurological signs such as trembling, muscular twitching, spasm and myoclonus, hind-leg weakness with varying degrees of spastic or flaccid paresis and uncoordinated gait may accompany respiratory signs in some affected pigs.[71] In boars and sows, acute febrile illness with labored respiration, increased salivation, and nasal discharge accompany neurological signs such as agitation, head pressing or knocking, mouth clamping, nystagmus, tetanus-like spasm, and seizures. Early abortion may occur in pregnant sows, and sudden death may occur in both boars and sows.[71] HeV causes an acute febrile respiratory and/or neurological illness of short duration in horses which progresses to death within 2–3 days. The main presenting features are fever, rapid and shallow breathing, frothing of saliva and mucous membrane congestion, ataxia, and head pressing.[1,2,91–93]

TREATMENT AND PROGNOSIS

Treatment of patients with HeV or NiV infection is mainly supportive. Ribavirin, a broad-spectrum antiviral agent, was used on an empirical basis in NiV-infected patients during the outbreak in Malaysia.[94] The study employed historical controls, and there was an apparent reduction in mortality. There were no serious side effects encountered in this study. However, tests of ribavirin in experimental animal models have not demonstrated the effectiveness of the drug against lethal NiV infection.[95]

PREVENTION AND CONTROL

A number of experimental vaccines have been developed and found to be effective in protecting laboratory animals against NiV challenge.[96–98] Some of these vaccines may have potential use in livestock, but as is the case for other zoonotic infections, strict biosecurity measures, effective surveillance, and culling of the infected animal population may be the more cost-effective and rapid measure for controlling the spread of disease. It is perhaps more practical to employ a surveillance system that employs sensitive and specific laboratory tests for rapid identification of henipavirus infections for early recognition of their reemergence and then to institute appropriate control.[99] Better understanding of wild animal reservoirs of the henipaviruses and ecological and sociological reasons for emergence into domestic animal and human hosts is warranted.[69] Improved attention to infection control practices in medical facilities and home care settings is certainly worthy of attention in South Asia, where the occurrence of person-to-person transmission has been repeatedly noted in small clusters of cases.[78,100,101] The occurrence of fatal cases in veterinary practitioners in Australia has also emphasized the need for infection control among equine practitioners in areas where an infected reservoir host is known to exist.

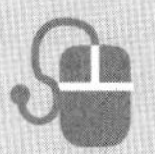

Access the complete reference list online at
http://www.expertconsult.com

Access the complete reference list online at http://www.expertconsult.com

CHAPTER 56

Human Herpesvirus Infections

S. David Hudnall • Lawrence R. Stanberry • Paul D. Griffiths

INTRODUCTION

There are currently nine herpesviruses known to afflict humans – in eight cases, the human is the only known host, while in one case the human rarely plays accidental host to a simian virus. All herpesviruses share certain genetic, structural and biologic characteristics, yet exhibit a bewildering range of clinical disease manifestations (***Table 56.1***).

The human herpesviruses are distributed throughout the world with no significant geographic variation. In many developing areas, including the tropics, children appear to acquire most herpesvirus infections, with the exception of varicella zoster virus (VZV), at an earlier age than in developed countries, presumably due to greater transmissibility and exposure from overcrowding and poor general hygiene. In most cases, primary infection is acquired in early childhood and, with the exception of VZV (varicella), is usually asymptomatic. Symptomatic primary infections with the alphaherpesviruses usually present as mucocutaneous vesicular eruptions – herpes simplex virus (HSV-1) most often localized to the oral region, HSV-2 localized to the genital region, while VZV is most often generalized to cutaneous areas. Primary symptomatic cytomegalovirus (CMV) and Epstein–Barr virus (EBV) infections commonly present in young adults as mononucleosis syndromes with pharyngitis and lymphadenopathy, while human herpesvirus (HHV)-6 infection usually presents with fever and a characteristic macular rash. Little is known of the clinical characteristics of primary HHV-7 and HHV-8 infection. Human infection with cercopithecine virus-1 (CHV-1) usually leads to HSV-like vesicular lesions at the site of inoculation (animal bite) followed rapidly by neurologic symptoms. Those at greatest risk of serious herpesvirus disease include the very young (fetus, newborn) and the immunocompromised (malnourished, persons with acquired immunodeficiency syndrome (AIDS), organ transplant recipients, and cancer patients), who have either immature or deficient immune systems. In these cases, dissemination to visceral organs and the central nervous system (CNS) often leads to a poor outcome.

In most cases following primary infection, herpesviruses persist in the host in a latent state with no recurrence of clinical symptoms. However, a significant number of healthy seropositive persons (20% for EBV) will continue to shed infectious virus intermittently and contribute to the ubiquitous distribution of the herpesviruses. Clinical recurrence in most cases is the result of reactivation of latent infection rather than reinfection. In some cases (e.g., HSV-2), recurrence leads to a clinical illness closely resembling that of the primary presentation but usually of less severity (herpes genitalis), whereas in other cases (e.g., VZV) recurrence leads to a clinical illness which does not resemble the primary presentation and is often of greater clinical severity (herpes zoster). Reactivation may be induced by a variety of stimuli, including sunlight, emotional stress, menses, poor nutritional status, severe illness, trauma, or immunosuppression – all perhaps leading to a transient period of immune suppression.

THE AGENT

All herpesviruses have relatively large and complex double-stranded DNA genomes ranging from 125 kbp to 229 kbp with large (greater than 100 bp) reiterated sequences called terminal repeats at the end(s) of the linear genome. The herpesvirus genome encodes more than 60 genes, including many involved in nucleic acid metabolism and DNA synthesis. The herpes virion is a 120–800 nm particle composed of an estimated 30–35 proteins and consisting of an electron-dense toroidal core containing a linear double-stranded DNA molecule enclosed sequentially by a 100 nm icosadeltahedral nucleocapsid with 162 capsomers, an amorphous tegument layer, and a trilaminar lipid envelope. The envelope is largely derived from host cell nuclear membrane but contains viral glycoproteins important in target cell binding and as targets for neutralizing antibodies. These shared physical properties explain the remarkable ultrastructural similarity of all herpesviruses. After fusion with the target cell, the unenveloped virion migrates to the cell nucleus where the capsid is lost and the linear DNA molecule circularizes in the terminal repeat region(s) to form the closed circular (episomal) form characteristic of the latent cycle. The episomal form replicates during the latent cycle in synchrony with the host genome during S (synthesis) phase through the action of host cell DNA polymerase, while in the lytic cycle replication is driven by viral DNA polymerase. Replication proceeds by a rolling circle mechanism which yields end-to-end concatamers, which are then cleaved at the terminal repeats into monomers. Integration of viral DNA into the host genome does sometimes occur but apparently does not contribute significantly to viral persistence or virus-induced cell transformation.

All herpesviruses exhibit two distinct cycles of infection – the latent and lytic cycles. The latent cycle is characterized by gene expression limited to a few regulatory genes, the products of which are presumably required for maintenance of intranuclear episomal DNA. All viral gene expression is mediated by host cell RNA polymerase II. The latently infected host cell provides a means for virus persistence by remaining viable and serving as a poor target for the host immune system, while retaining the capability of producing infectious virus after switching into the lytic cycle. The lytic cycle is characterized by activation of a large number of viral genes involved in viral DNA replication and virion assembly, most often leading to inhibition of host cell macromolecular synthesis, release of infectious virus, and host cell death. The latent and lytic cycles play complementary roles for the herpesvirus – latency allows for viral persistence while lysis allows for viral spread. However, the factors which govern the balance between the latent and lytic states are poorly understood. Further details of viral replication are available in several excellent texts.[1–5]

The herpesviruses are currently classified on the basis of biologic characteristics by the Herpesvirus Study Group of the International Committee on the Taxonomy of Viruses into three subfamilies – the alpha-, beta-, and gammaherpesviruses. The alphaherpesviruses – HSV,

Table 56.1 Clinical Characteristics of Human Herpesvirus Infection

Virus	Congenital/ Neonatal Infection	Primary Infection	Recurrent Infection	Ocular Disease	Skin Disease	CNS Disease
HSV-1	Rare	Gingivostomatitis, usually in childhood	Herpes labialis	Keratoconjunctivitis, keratitis; most common cause of ulcerative eye infection	Oral mucocutaneous vesicular eruption; intraoral ulcers	Most common sporadic acute viral encephalitis in adults
HSV-2	Congenital infection uncommon; systemic infection in neonate	Herpes genitalis, usually in young adults; a common ulcerative genital infection	Herpes genitalis; usually very mild	Rare	Genital mucocutaneous vesicular eruption	Rare; encephalitis in neonates
VZV	Rare congenital syndrome with skin/autonomic defects; neonatal infection with typical rash	Varicella (chickenpox), usually mild in childhood; adult onset in tropics more severe	Zoster (shingles), usually in older adults	Ophthalmic zoster; rare in varicella	Vesicular eruption; generalized in varicella; dermatomal distribution in zoster	Rarely in elderly with cranial nerve zoster (Ramsay Hunt syndrome)
CMV	Growth and mental retardation (cytomegalic inclusion disease)	Often asymptomatic in childhood; mononucleosis usually in adults	Rare; pneumonia and colitis in immunodeficient	Retinitis in congenital infection	Rare ulcerative perineal eruption in immunodeficient	Encephalitis in congenital infection
EBV	Rare	Often symptomatic in childhood; mononucleosis usually in adolescents/young adults	Burkitt's lymphoma; AIDS lymphoma; post-transplant lymphoma; nasopharyngeal carcinoma	Not reported	Rare maculopapular eruption of trunk and arms	Rare
HHV-6	Rare	Exanthem subitum, in young children	Unknown	Not reported	Maculopapular eruption of trunk and neck	Rare
HHV-7	Rare	? HHV-6-negative exanthem subitum	Unknown	Not reported	? Maculopapular eruption of trunk and neck	Not reported
HHV-8	Not reported	Not reported	Kaposi's sarcoma; primary effusion-based B-cell lymphoma; ? lymphoma; ? Castleman's disease	Not reported	Multifocal macules, plaques, or nodules (Kaposi's sarcoma)	Not reported
CHV-1	Not reported	Vesicular dermatitis at bite site with paresthesia	Not reported	Not reported	Painful vesicular eruption at bite	Severe encephalitis

CHV-1, cercopithecine virus 1; CMV, cytomegalovirus; EBV, Epstein–Barr virus; HHV-6–8, human herpesviruses 6–8; HSV-1, herpes simplex virus type 1; HSV-2, herpes simplex virus type 2; VZV, varicella zoster virus; CNS, central nervous system.

VZV, CHV-1 – have high reproductive rates with rapid spread and lethal lysis of infected cells *in vitro*. Although mucocutaneous epithelia are initially infected, latency is established in the neurons of sensory ganglia. The betaherpesviruses – CMV, HHV-6, and HHV-7 – have low reproductive rates with slow spread and nonlethal cytomegalia of infected cells *in vitro*. Infection may be widespread while latency is likely established in secretory epithelial tissues and leukocytes. The gammaherpesviruses – EBV and HHV-8 – infect lymphocytes, epithelial tissues, and mesenchymal cells, while latency is likely established in B lymphocytes. The gammaherpesviruses are distinct from the other herpesvirus subfamilies in being causally linked to malignant lymphoid, epithelial, and mesenchymal tumors in humans.

The herpesviruses are susceptible to nucleoside analogs such as vidarabine, trifluridine, penciclovir, acyclovir, ganciclovir, famciclovir, and valacyclovir, as well as the viral DNA polymerase inhibitors foscarnet and cidofovir.[6,7] Antiviral drug resistance to both nucleoside analogs and DNA polymerase inhibitors is of concern particularly in the immunocompromised patient.[8] A live, attenuated VZV vaccine (Varivax) is effective in preventing primary varicella (chickenpox) infection, while a higher dose of the same vaccine (Zostavax) is effective in preventing herpes zoster and postherpetic neuralgia. Subunit vaccines against HSV, CMV, and EBV are under development.

HERPES SIMPLEX VIRUSES

THE AGENT

The infectious nature of HSV was first demonstrated by induction of typical dendritic corneal lesions in rabbits from material obtained from human herpes keratitis and herpes labialis lesions.[9] The distinction between the two virus strains, HSV-1 (above-the-belt lesions) and HSV-2 (below-the-belt lesions), was first made in 1968,[10] although it is now recognized that either virus strain can cause comparable primary infection at any anatomic site.[11] HSV virions contain 150 kbp of linear, double-stranded DNA encoding at least 84 proteins.[12] HSV gene expression may be temporally classified into three distinct phases termed alpha (immediate early), beta (early), and gamma (late). Alpha genes are expressed without prior protein synthesis and are largely involved in transcriptional transactivation. Beta genes are dependent upon prior alpha gene expression and encode proteins required for DNA replication. Gamma genes are dependent upon prior DNA replication and encode virion structural proteins. Beta and gamma gene expression is accompanied by inhibition of cellular DNA, RNA, and protein synthesis and by cell death.[13] At least 12 glycoproteins are embedded in the viral envelope; some of these glycoproteins are important in viral infectivity and also as targets of the immune system.[14] The antigenic difference between glycoprotein G (gG) from HSV-1 (gG-1) and HSV-2 (gG-2) is the basis for serologic distinction of the two HSV types.[15] In culture, HSV inhibits host cell macromolecular synthesis and causes rapid cell lysis of a number of cell types.[16,17]

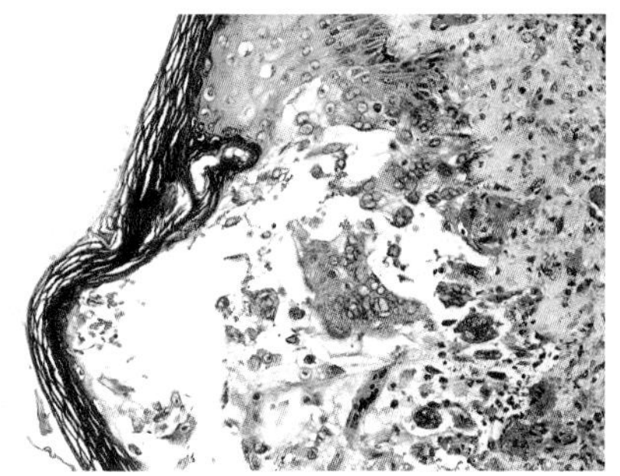

Figure 56.1 Herpes simplex virus type 1 vesicle. (Courtesy of Ravi Sawh, MD, Department of Pathology, UTMB, Galveston, TX.)

EPIDEMIOLOGY

The two strains of the herpes simplex virus, HSV-1 and HSV-2, differ not only in genetic sequence (with approximately 50% sequence homology) but also in biologic and clinical behavior. Both strains are found worldwide with high seroprevalence and no seasonal variation or epidemics. HSV-1 infection is primarily acquired during childhood and adolescence and is more widespread than HSV-2 infection, which is usually acquired during adolescence and early adulthood. HSV-1 seroprevalence exhibits marked geographic variation with relatively low rates (less than 70%) in France, Japan, the United States, and Sweden, and relatively high rates (greater than 95%) in Spain, Italy, Africa, China, and Latin America. Seroprevalence is higher in low socioeconomic groups and in developing regions – by adolescence, up to 80% have anti-HSV-1 antibodies in the developing world, while by the third decade only 60% are seropositive in the developed world.[18] HSV-2 seroprevalence is generally highest in Africa and South America, intermediate in northern Europe and North America, lower in western and southern Europe, and lowest in Asia.[19] Age-specific HSV-2 prevalence is higher in women than men and in populations with higher-risk sexual behaviors. HSV-1 infection is most often acquired through oral transmission following direct contact with either an acutely infected person or a healthy individual who is asymptomatically shedding virus. Primary or initial HSV-1 infection is most often asymptomatic.[20] Asymptomatic oral viral shedding is common in children (20%) while less common (3%) in adults.[21,22] However, unlike varicella, there is no apparent increase in transmission in day-care environments.[23]

THE DISEASE

In infants and children symptomatic primary HSV-1 oral infection follows an incubation period of 2–20 days and is characterized by fever, sore throat, cervical lymphadenopathy, and vesicles in the oral cavity termed gingivostomatitis.[24] In adolescents and adults, symptomatic primary oral HSV-1 (and occasionally HSV-2) infection is most often characterized by a mononucleosis syndrome with pharyngitis, cervical lymphadenopathy, and fever.[25] Acute HSV-1 keratoconjunctivitis causes shallow corneal ulcers that typically have a dendritic appearance and generally heal without corneal scarring. Necrotizing herpetic retinopathies are rare, potentially blinding retinal disorders resulting from ocular infections with HSV-1, HSV-2, VZV, or CMV.[26] Herpetic dermatitis may be seen in athletes (herpes gladiatorum or scrumpox) from person-to-person abrasion, in health care workers on their unprotected fingers (herpetic whitlow), and in patients with eczema in which herpetic superinfection leads to a severe disseminated form termed Kaposi's varicelliform eruption.[27–29] Although rare, HSV-1 encephalitis is the most common cause of acute sporadic viral encephalitis beyond the neonatal period. The early onset of seizures and localizing signs indicating temporal or frontal lobe involvement are characteristic.[30] Disseminated HSV infections outside the neonatal period are rare but can occur in immunocompromised patients and occasionally in pregnancy. Infection in these patients may disseminate by direct extension from the upper oral cavity to involve the trachea and lungs and/or the esophagus and gastrointestinal tract, or dissemination may occur via viremia to involve visceral organs and the central nervous system.[31,32]

Latent HSV-1 in cervical and trigeminal sensory ganglia may reactivate to cause recurrent lesions; it is estimated that 20–40% of primary infections are followed by at least one symptomatic recurrence. The most common recurrent HSV-1 infection is herpes labialis (fever blisters or cold sores).[33,34] Herpes labialis typically presents as small erythematous papules on or about the lips that proceed to a brief vesicular stage before crusting and healing (*Figs 56.1 and 56.2A*). Recurrent HSV-1 infections may also be asymptomatic or take the form of keratoconjunctivitis, keratitis, retinitis, whitlow, cutaneous lesions (gladiatorum), encephalitis, erythema multiforme, duodenal ulcer, or genital herpes, although HSV-1 tends to cause fewer episodes of recurrent genital herpes than does HSV-2.[35] Recurrent keratitis can involve the stroma, and repeated recurrences can produce progressive corneal scarring that can result in blindness.

HSV-2 infection is most often acquired by sexual transmission in adolescents or young adults.[36] It is estimated that 80–90% of HSV-2 infections are asymptomatic, but asymptomatically infected individuals shed virus from genital sites and may transmit virus to sexual partners or newborn infants.[37–41] The most common presentation of HSV-2 infection in adults is herpes genitalis, which is also the most common cause of genital ulcers. The classic presentation of genital herpes is a painful vesicular eruption of the female vulva (*Fig. 56.2B*), vagina, cervix, urethra, and perineum, and of the male glans, preputium, and shaft of the penis. The vesicular lesions typically progress to form shallow painful ulcers, which eventually crust and heal without scarring. Anorectal involvement and cutaneous lesions on the buttocks and thighs are relatively common and may result from anogenital sex or from zosteriform spread of virus from genital to rectal or other adjacent cutaneous sites. Primary infection is often complicated by aseptic meningitis and urinary retention and rarely by transverse myelitis and autonomic dysfunction. Recurrent HSV-2 genital herpes is quite common, and more than 50% of persons with symptomatic primary infection experience recognizable recurrences, typically four to five outbreaks in the first year. HSV-1 is also a common cause of genital herpes.[35,42–44] Recurrent HSV-1 genital herpes is relatively uncommon, and patients having recurrences following a primary infection typically experience only a single outbreak annually. Symptomatic recurrent genital herpes tends to be considerably less severe than the initial outbreak. Subclinical HSV-2 genital infections (asymptomatic shedding) are very common following initial infection in both patients who have experienced symptomatic initial infection and those that are asymptomatically infected.[37–41] HSV shedding, as detected by culture, occurs on about 3% of days for immunocompetent men and women, and more frequently if measured by polymerase chain reaction (PCR) methods or if the individual is HIV-infected.[38,41,45–47]

HSV infection of the fetus or newborn is referred to as neonatal herpes. Most cases occur as a consequence of spread of virus from a mother with genital HSV infection to her infant at the time of delivery, although cases of intrauterine transmission and postpartum acquisition have been documented.[40,48,49] Intrauterine infection early in gestation is a rare cause of intrauterine death and spontaneous abortion.[50] Perinatally acquired neonatal herpes, as with maternal genital herpes, may be due to

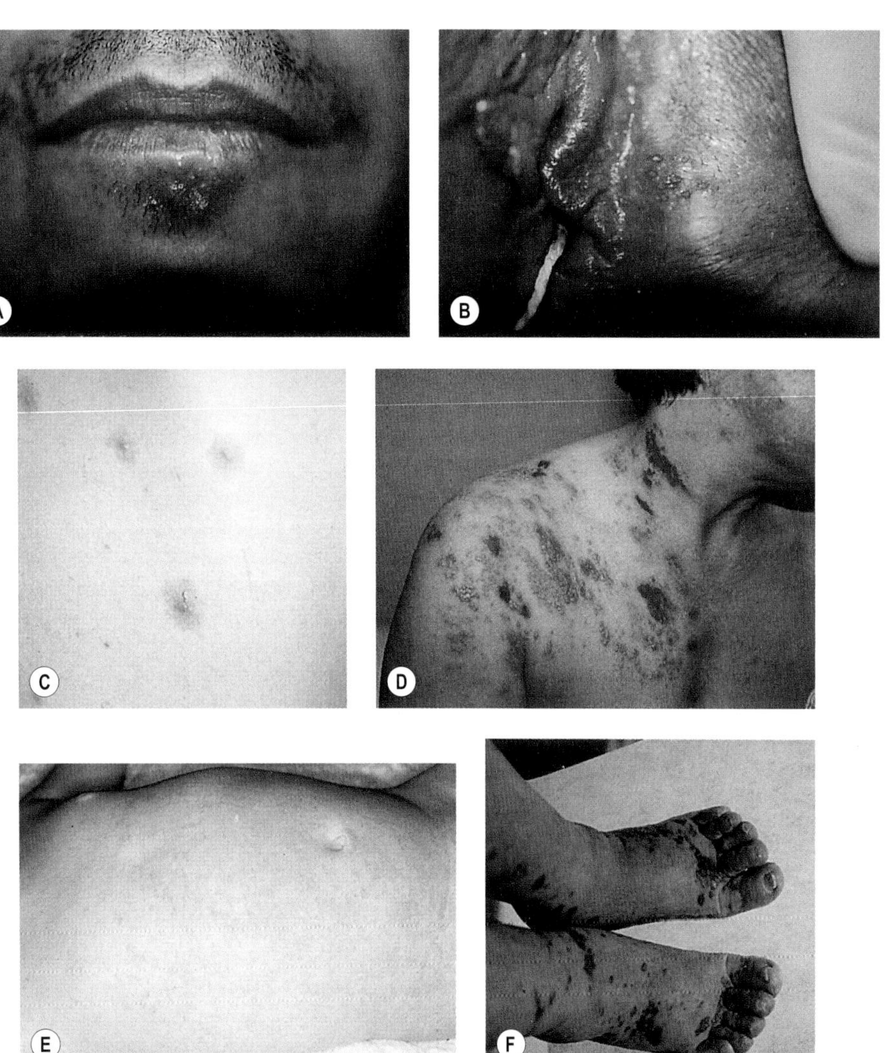

Figure 56.2 Herpetic skin lesions. **(A)** Herpes labialis (primary herpes simplex virus (HSV) type 1. **(B)** Herpes genitalis (primary HSV-2). **(C)** Varicella (primary varicella zoster virus (VZV)). **(D)** Herpes zoster (secondary VZV). **(E)** Exanthem subitum (primary human herpesvirus (HHV) type 6). **(F)** Kaposi's sarcoma (HHV-8). (Courtesy of Stephen Tyring, MD, PhD, University of Texas Medical Branch, Galveston.)

either HSV-1 or HSV-2. The risk of maternal–infant transmission is greatest (approaching 50%) for women experiencing primary genital infection near term, while the risk of transmission for women with a history of genital herpes prior to pregnancy is less than 2%. The difference in risk of transmission probably relates to the presence or absence of HSV-specific maternally derived antibodies that afford the infant some protection against infection and the amount of virus present in the genital tract (high concentrations during the initial infection and several logs less virus during recurrent infections).[51] Most cases of neonatal herpes result from unrecognized or asymptomatic maternal genital herpes.[39,40] Unlike other HSV infections, asymptomatic neonatal herpes probably does not occur. Infection is initiated at a portal of entry: conjunctival sac of the eye, nasopharynx, or a site where the skin is abraded such as occurs with the use of a scalp electrode. Infection that remains localized to the portal of entry results in skin, eye, or mouth (SEM) disease. Without treatment, SEM disease typically progresses to more severe forms of the infection through direct extension to the lungs to produce a necrotizing pneumonitis, via intraneuronal spread to cause CNS disease or through viremic spread to visceral organs resulting in disseminated infection.[51] There is approximately an equal distribution of cases in the SEM, CNS, and disseminated disease categories, but outcome, while generally good for infants with SEM disease, is very poor for infants with disseminated infection with mortality approaching 50% despite antiviral therapy. Infants with CNS disease are likely to survive, but those with HSV-2 infection are very likely to suffer neurologic sequelae.[52]

PATHOGENESIS AND IMMUNITY

In vivo, primary infection begins with replication of virus in epithelial cells, which results in cell death. Virus gains entry to sensory nerve fibers that innervate the portal of entry and move via retrograde axoplasmic transport to the neuron cell body located in sensory ganglia, cervical and trigeminal ganglia in the case of oral infection, and sacral ganglia in the case of genital infection. Once the virus enters the neuronal nuclei, one of two events occurs: either the virus replicates producing progeny virus which moves back to the periphery via anterograde transport where it is released at the nerve ending to infect epithelial cells, or the virus establishes a nonreplicating persistent state referred to as latency.[51,53] In latently infected neurons the virus remains largely quiescent, except for transcription of a small region of the genome that encodes mRNA referred to as the latency-associated transcript (LAT).[54,55] Recurrent HSV infections occur when the latent virus periodically reactivates, resulting in viral production and transport to the periphery where the progeny virus are released from the nerve endings to replicate further in epithelial cells.[53,56] Both the primary and recurrent infections can be symptomatic, characterized by the development of typical herpetic vesicles and ulcers, but more often the recurrent infections are asymptomatic, with virus replication in epithelial cells causing no apparent disease but resulting in virus shedding, which can be transmitted to a susceptible host.[38,57,58] While it is recognized that LAT is involved in the reactivation from latency, the mechanisms responsible for the establishment, maintenance, and reactivation from latency are unknown. Reactivation from the latent state and the development of recurrent infections occur despite the presence of a full range of humoral and cellular immune responses that develop following the primary infection. The development of recurrent infections is facilitated by a variety of immune evasion genes encoded by the virus.[59–63]

DIAGNOSIS

With the possible exception of herpes labialis, the clinical diagnosis of most HSV infections should be confirmed by laboratory testing. While most clinicians feel confident that they can accurately diagnose common HSV infections such as genital herpes, recent studies have shown that the accuracy of clinical diagnoses is poor even for experienced clinicians.[64,65] Four types of laboratory tests are available to help confirm the diagnosis, including viral culture, viral antigen detection, viral nucleic acid detection, and serology. For three of the four laboratory tests (culture, antigen detection, and nucleic acid detection), a lesion must be present in order to obtain the test sample. Serology may be useful in some cases when patients are evaluated after lesions have resolved. The gold standard for HSV diagnosis remains viral isolation by cell culture for cutaneous and ocular infections. Inoculation of fibroblast cell cultures with vesicular or cerebrospinal fluid (CSF) leads to rapid cytopathic change (24–48 hours) indicative of alphaherpesvirus infection (HSV-1, HSV-2, VZV). In general, HSV infection leads more consistently and rapidly to cytopathic change than does VZV. However, clear distinctions among HSV-1, HSV-2, and VZV can be made by the use of direct immunofluorescence using commercially available fluorescence-labeled virus-specific antibodies. Results of positive tests are typically available within 5 days and negative results within 6 days.[66] Detection of HSV antigen by enzyme immunoassay (EIA) is a less sensitive alternative to viral culture and nucleic acid detection, with sensitivities in the range of 65–81% compared to culture and PCR-based methods of viral nucleic acid detection.[67,68] The Tzanck test, the cytologic examination of Wright–Giemsa-stained smears of scrapings from the vesicle base to detect multinucleated giant cells with intranuclear inclusions, should not be used due to its poor sensitivity.[69] Detection of HSV DNA by PCR is not widely available but is the preferred method for examining CSF and is finding increasing use for the diagnosis of mucocutaneous HSV infections. In addition to greater sensitivity, test results may be available within 24–48 hours.[66,68,70–72] Serology may be useful in confirming the clinical diagnosis of a recent illness when lesions are no longer present. Serologic detection of HSV-specific immunoglobulin M (IgM) is generally not useful. The tests are insensitive, and recurrent HSV infection can result in an anamnestic IgM response. For the HSV-seronegative patient, seroconversion by comparison of paired acute and convalescent serum samples is evidence of a recent infection. Increasing titers of virus-specific IgG are not useful in establishing the diagnosis of a recent infection as titers can vary widely in response to recurrent infections. Detection of HSV-2-antibodies in an adolescent or adult is a biomarker for genital herpes. Cases of suspected genital herpes can be confirmed by detection of HSV-2-specific antibodies using type-specific serologic tests that have recently become available commercially. One caveat to remember is that many cases of genital herpes are due to HSV-1, and hence the HSV-2 type-specific serologic tests will not be useful in these cases. Clinicians need to be aware that several FDA-approved HSV antibody tests claim to be type-specific but are remarkably inaccurate. The only type-specific serologic tests with acceptable performance characteristics are those based on differences in the HSV-1 and HSV-2 glycoprotein G.[73,74]

TREATMENT AND PROGNOSIS

Several drugs have proven effective in the treatment of various HSV infections.[75] Intravenous acyclovir is the drug of choice for life-threatening HSV infections and HSV encephalitis. Oral herpes infections in the immunocompetent host have been successfully treated with oral acyclovir and its more bioavailable prodrug, valacyclovir, as well as a related nucleoside analog, famciclovir. Recurrent herpes labialis can also be treated with topical acyclovir and penciclovir and *n*-docosanol, an over-the-counter treatment. A variety of topical preparations have been used in the management of ocular herpes including acyclovir, trifluridine, idoxuridine, and vidarabine. Acyclovir-resistant strains of HSV have been documented in immunocompromised patients but are very rare in patients with an intact immune system.[76] Foscarnet and cidofovir have been successfully used in treatment of acyclovir-resistant HSV disease.[77] However, foscarnet-resistant HSV has been documented in patients with AIDS.[78] Antiviral drugs are useful in the treatment of primary and recurrent HSV infections, and daily suppressive use has proven effective in preventing recurrent oral and genital HSV infections. Latent infection is not altered by treatment with any currently available drug, and when suppressive therapy is discontinued most patients return to a pretreatment recurrence pattern. All life-threatening HSV infections require treatment, and experts feel that all first episode cases of genital herpes should be treated with an oral antiviral drug.

PREVENTION AND CONTROL

Unfortunately, because of the high rate of clinically inapparent infections and healthy carrier states, hygienic measures are not very effective in prevention of HSV infections. However, patients with extensive mucocutaneous disease should be isolated as secretions and contact with lesions may result in transmission. Condom use has been shown to reduce, but not eliminate, the risk of genital HSV transmission.[79,80] A landmark study has shown that suppressive oral valacyclovir therapy (500 mg daily) can also significantly reduce, but not eliminate, the risk of transmission of genital HSV-2 infection among monogamous heterosexual couples.[81] Evidence suggests that cesarean delivery will reduce but not eliminate the risk of maternal–fetal transmission for women with active genital herpes at term.[82] This strategy is not without its consequences since it is estimated that four mothers die from cesarean-related complications for every seven babies prevented from developing fatal neonatal HSV infection.[83] An alternative but as yet unproven strategy is the use of an oral anti-HSV drug by women with a history of genital herpes for the final 4 weeks of gestation. The rationale is to prevent symptomatic recurrences and asymptomatic shedding at term and thereby reduce the risk of maternal–infant transmission. This strategy has been shown to reduce symptomatic and subclinical recurrences in the pregnant woman and to reduce the need for cesarean delivery for active genital herpes. The safety of such therapy in the fetus/newborn and its effectiveness in preventing neonatal herpes have not been established.[84–86] While there have been unsuccessful attempts to develop an effective HSV vaccine for over 60 years,[87] the recent success of an HSV glycoprotein vaccine in protecting women against acquiring genital herpes suggests that the development of a safe and effective HSV vaccine is feasible.[88] Further development of the HSV-2 glycoprotein D vaccine is under way.

VARICELLA ZOSTER VIRUS

THE AGENT

The transmissible agent was demonstrated first in the vesicle fluid of varicella.[89] The connection between varicella and zoster was made by noting varicella among children exposed to family members with zoster.[90] Varicella was induced in susceptible children by inoculation with fluid from zoster lesions.[91] Viruses isolated from varicella and zoster were later shown to be identical biologically, antigenically, and genetically.[92,93] The VZV genome is the smallest of the known human herpesviruses and consists of 125 kb double-stranded DNA with approximately 70 genes.[94] Large portions of the genome are colinear with the HSV-1 genome.[95] The three most abundant viral envelope glycoproteins, gB, gE, and gH, likely are involved in infectivity since they are major targets of neutralizing antibodies. Antigenic similarity between HSV-1 gB and VZV gB leads to serologic cross-reactivity.[96]

EPIDEMIOLOGY

Humans are the only known natural host for VZV, which is associated with two forms of illness – a primary form known as varicella (chickenpox) and a secondary form known as herpes zoster (shingles). VZV is a highly contagious infection spread usually from airborne infectious oral or respiratory secretions or sometimes through direct transfer from skin lesions or via maternal–fetal transmission. Secondary attack rates in susceptible household contacts exceed 85%.[97] In temperate climates, infection rates show a marked seasonal variation, with epidemics in late winter and early spring. In contrast, no seasonal variation is seen in tropical climates. The reasons for this marked difference are not clear, although it has been suggested that heat, humidity, and lack of increased exposure to virus within confined spaces during the winter months may account for some of the difference. In rural India, despite close quarters, unexpectedly low rates of household transmission were documented.[98] In Singapore, varicella has occurred in two very large epidemics separated by 23 years.[99] Although asymptomatic primary infection is rare, serologic studies suggest that subclinical reinfection is common.[100] Rarely, immunocompetent patients may experience second episodes of varicella.[101] Varicella in temperate climates most often presents in preschool and school-age children younger than 10 years of age with the highest incidence in the 3- to 6-year-old group.[102] Despite the prevalence of varicella in childhood, some people in temperate climates do reach adulthood without exposure: a study of military recruits in the United States in the prevaccine era showed that 8% of recruits were seronegative, with a slightly higher seronegative rate in nonwhites and a much higher seronegative rate (20%) in recruits enlisting from outside the United States.[103]

THE DISEASE

Following a 10- to 21-day (typically 14- to 16-day) incubation period, a prodrome of fever, headache, and malaise is followed 24–36 hours later by a diffuse maculopapular rash (***Fig. 56.2C***). In the very young, the prodrome is often unrecognized. The rash is progressive, with successive crops at different stages occurring over a 2- to 7-day period, followed by complete healing within 20 days. The stages of the lesions are successively as follows: macular, papular, vesicular, pustular, and crusting. A hallmark of varicella is the simultaneous presence of lesions at various stages. The rash preferentially involves the trunk, with relative sparing and later involvement of the face and extremities. Oropharyngeal lesions may be seen. In normal, previously healthy children, the disease is generally benign and self-limiting, with the most common complication being secondary bacterial infection of skin lesions. Scarring is another common complication. Neurologic complications include encephalitis and acute cerebellar ataxia.[104] Varicella encephalitis with an incidence of 0.1% typically presents with headaches, seizures, altered thought patterns, and vomiting, with a mortality rate of 5–20% in the pre-antiviral era. Acute cerebellar ataxia is less common (0.025% incidence) than encephalitis and typically presents within 1 week of the rash with ataxia, vomiting, altered speech, vertigo, and/or tremor, with resolution within 2–4 weeks.

In immunodeficient or malnourished children not treated with intravenous acyclovir, the mortality rate ranges from 15% to 18%.[105] These cases are characterized by dissemination, with pneumonia, myocarditis, arthritis, hepatitis, hemorrhage, and encephalopathy (cerebellar ataxia is most common). Superinfection of skin lesions with *Staphylococcus aureus* or *Streptococcus pyogenes* may lead to pyoderma, impetigo, erysipelas, nephritis, gangrene, or sepsis. In the Central American tropics, varicella in young, malnourished children may be complicated by severe diarrhea.

Adults tend to have more severe disease than children, with a 15-fold increase in mortality in untreated subjects. Adult-onset varicella is more often complicated by pneumonitis and encephalitis, with clinically significant pneumonitis in up to 15% of cases. In the prevaccine era, approximately 4% of normal adults in the United States (temperate climate) were VZV seronegative and therefore susceptible to adult-onset varicella.[106] In contrast, in the tropics a much higher percentage of adults is VZV seronegative and therefore susceptible to adult-onset varicella. Persons from tropical areas who relocate to temperate areas are at risk of developing adult-onset varicella, especially if in contact with young children. Maternal varicella in early gestation leads rarely to the congenital varicella syndrome characterized by skin defects, atrophy of extremities, and autonomic nervous system dysfunction.[107,108] Maternal varicella in late gestation may lead to neonatal varicella, with a mortality rate as high as 30% in untreated infants.[109,110]

Recurrent VZV infection is manifest as herpes zoster (shingles), a disease usually seen in adults over 50 years of age. Data suggest racial differences in the risk of developing zoster, with white elderly more at risk than black elderly.[111] Zoster may also occur rarely in childhood. Zoster in immunocompromised patients may be quite protracted and severe. The increased incidence of zoster in the aged as well as in immunocompromised patients is due to decreased anti-VZV cell-mediated immunity.[112,113] There is contradictory evidence that exposure of at-risk seropositive persons to varicella protects against development of zoster, presumably by boosting their cellular immune response.[114] After primary infection, VZV (like HSV) persists in the latent state within nerve ganglia. Nonspecific stimuli such as stress, immunodeficiency, or malignancy have been associated with reactivation of latent virus with involvement of the skin in the nerve distribution supplied by the affected ganglion. Herpes zoster presents after a 3- to 4-day prodrome of fever, malaise, and gastrointestinal disturbance as a painful cutaneous vesicular eruption in a dermatomal distribution (***Fig. 56.2D***). The rash is usually unilateral and along one dermatome only. In severe cases, the eruption may be more generalized and varicelliform. The vesicles heal within 5 days, but postherpetic neuralgia may commence. Postherpetic neuralgia, seen in up to 50% of patients over 50 years old, is defined as constant or intermittent debilitating pain of more than 1 month's duration in the area of the involved dermatome. Infection of the eye, ear, and throat may occur if ophthalmic, trigeminal, or geniculate ganglia are involved. Herpes zoster ophthalmicus is a particularly serious condition, which if untreated may lead to blindness. The Ramsay Hunt syndrome is defined as a triad of involvement of the external auditory meatus, loss of taste in the tongue, and ipsilateral facial palsy. Involvement of the spinal cord may lead to weakness or cranial nerve palsy. The risk of encephalitis is increased in the elderly with cranial nerve involvement and in AIDS patients. Postzoster encephalitis may present in one of three forms: infarcts due to large-vessel vasculitis, multifocal leukoencephalopathy, and ventriculitis.[115]

PATHOGENESIS AND IMMUNITY

VZV replicates in a restricted range of cells *in vitro* resulting in cell death. VZV replicates best in human diploid fibroblasts but also infects primary human keratinocytes.[116] A live attenuated vaccine strain (Oka) is propagated in WI-38 and MRC-5 diploid fibroblast lines. In skin lesions of infected subjects, VZV replication results in high concentrations of cell-free virus in the vesicle fluid; however, in cell culture, the virus remains largely cell associated with little release of infectious virus.[117] Cell-free virus can be obtained by sonication of infected cultures. Infection induces the formation of multinucleated cells with eosinophilic intranuclear inclusions seen both *in vitro* and *in vivo*. Transmission occurs mainly through respiratory spread, and viremia disseminates the virus to mucocutaneous sites, visceral organs, and the peripheral nervous system. Latent infection is established in cranial, dorsal root, and autonomic ganglia.[118–124] The cell specificity of latent virus was previously controversial, but it is now widely agreed that latent VZV resides in neurons.[125] Evidence suggests that at least five viral genes are transcribed during latency, and unlike HSV latency, transcription from the latent VZV genome results in viral protein expression.[126] Like HSV, latent VZV can reactivate, albeit very rarely, to cause recurrent infection (e.g., zoster or shingles). Unlike HSV, reactivation of VZV can result in neuronal injury that causes a prolonged pain syndrome referred to as postherpetic neuralgia.[127]

DIAGNOSIS

The clinical diagnosis of varicella in childhood, now that variola (smallpox) has been eradicated, is not usually difficult. The rash is quite characteristic and only rarely needs to be differentiated from enteroviral exanthem, *S. aureus* infection, drug reactions, contact dermatitis, and disseminated HSV infection. Diagnosis by culture of vesicle fluid is less sensitive than for HSV or CMV and may take 7 days. This method has been supplanted by the more rapid and sensitive shell vial method, which gives results in 1–3 days. Very rapid, sensitive, and specific detection may supplant culture-based systems in the near future as multiplex PCR assays become more widely available.[128] Scrapings of the base of the vesicles reveal multinucleated giant cells with intranuclear inclusions, which cannot reliably be differentiated from HSV. However, immunofluorescence on cultures or scrapings utilizing virus-specific antibodies can differentiate between HSV-1, HSV-2, and VZV. Serologic detection of IgM and a high titer or greater than fourfold rise in IgG anti-VZV antibody may be useful in some cases. Detection of IgM may signify primary infection (chickenpox), while either a high titer or fourfold rise in IgG titer indicates recurrence. However, increased IgM may also be present in recurrence. The clinical diagnosis of herpes zoster in adults is not usually difficult given the characteristic dermatomal pattern of involvement.

TREATMENT AND PROGNOSIS

Although vidarabine and interferon-α have been used in the treatment of severe VZV infection, acyclovir is the drug of choice.[129] Acyclovir is most effective in severe VZV infection if administered intravenously (IV) within 24 hours after the rash develops.[130] Oral acyclovir treatment of otherwise healthy children with chickenpox should be considered, particularly in adolescents and secondary household contacts, although the benefit is modest.[131–134] Due to the detection of acyclovir-resistant strains in patients with AIDS, foscarnet therapy should be considered for severe infection in this setting.[135,136] For herpes zoster, the drugs of choice are famciclovir and valacyclovir. Early treatment of zoster has been shown to shorten the course of cutaneous disease, but the impact of treatment on the duration and severity of postherpetic neuralgia is uncertain.[137] Topical steroids may also be useful in herpetic uveitis and keratitis. Painful zoster may be treated with wet compresses and analgesics containing codeine. Gabapentin, a structural analog of the neurotransmitter γ-aminobutyric acid, is useful in the management of postherpetic neuralgia.[138] Antihistamines may be useful to ameliorate the intense pruritus of varicella in childhood.

PREVENTION AND CONTROL

A live attenuated vaccine (Oka) is licensed in the United States for routine use in healthy, non-immunocompromised susceptible children and adults.[139] The vaccine has been shown to be safe and effective, and its widespread use has resulted in a decline in varicella cases in the United States.[140] The vaccine virus may induce mild varicella and is capable of reactivation with development of herpes zoster.[139] A high dose version of the VZV Oka vaccine (Zostavax) is efficacious in reducing the incidence and burden of illness of zoster and postherpetic neuralgia in older adults.[141,142] The mechanism of action appears to be a boosting of VZV-specific cell-mediated immunity.[143] The boosting appears to be less robust in very elderly patients probably due to immunosenescence.[144] Owing to the high prevalence of the infection in the prevaccine era, its high transmissibility, and the fact that infected persons are contagious 24–48 hours before clinical signs occur, it is difficult to prevent infection by isolation. However, reverse isolation is recommended for hospitalized patients with varicella and for children or immunocompromised adults with herpes zoster. Patients with varicella should be bathed often to prevent staphylococcal and streptococcal superinfection. Immunocompromised children, neonates born to mothers who present with varicella during the week prior to and a few days after birth, and seronegative pregnant females should be treated with varicella zoster immunoglobulin (VZIG) within 96 hours of exposure.[145] VZIG, however, has no effect on the course of herpes zoster or on risk of reactivation.

CYTOMEGALOVIRUS

THE AGENT

Cytomegalovirus (CMV) was first isolated in 1956 by cell culture. The virus was named for the characteristic enlargement of infected fibroblasts noted *in vitro*.[146] CMV grows slowly in cell culture and releases little extracellular virus, features shared with other betaherpesviruses.

EPIDEMIOLOGY

While CMV is ubiquitous, it is not highly transmissible, taking decades for most of a population to become infected.[147,148] In developed countries approximately 60% of adults are CMV seropositive, whereas in developing countries seroprevalence reaches 100%. Multiple studies indicate that disadvantaged groups within populations tend to acquire CMV at an earlier age.[149] Most of these transmissions occur among children in schools and from children to women of childbearing age.[148,150] CMV is frequently acquired perinatally through breastfeeding[151] and infrequently acquired sexually.[152]

THE DISEASE

Most cases of primary CMV infection are asymptomatic. Occasional cases of mononucleosis syndrome or hepatitis occur, and there are rare reports of severe, and even fatal, CMV infections in people with apparently normal immunity. CMV infection in pregnancy is a major medical problem, not for the women themselves but for their fetuses. Approximately 2% of CMV seronegative women seroconvert during pregnancy, and in those cases 32% give birth to infants with congenital CMV infection.[149] In contrast, congenital CMV infection is much less common in infants of women who are CMV seropositive prior to pregnancy (1.4%).[149] However, in communities where CMV seroprevalence is very high (90–100%), approximately twice as many babies with congenital CMV infection are born following recurrent, rather than primary, maternal infection.[149,153] Indeed, it is in parts of the world where virtually 100% of women of childbearing age carry CMV that the incidence of congenital CMV is highest.[149] Overall, congenital CMV infection occurs in 0.7% of newborns, 12.7% of whom have classic symptoms at birth.[153] Approximately 50% of these infants are left with permanent sequelae, particularly sensorineural hearing loss and/or mental retardation.[153] Of the infants who are born without overt symptoms, 13.5% develop permanent disability on follow-up.[153]

In allograft recipients, CMV may induce multiorgan disease, including hepatitis, pneumonitis, gastroenteritis, and retinitis (***Fig. 56.3***). Post-transplant CMV infection may be acquired from the donor organ or be due to reactivation of latent virus in the recipient. The risk of CMV disease is highest in those experiencing primary infection rather than reactivation.[154] CMV is also associated indirectly with graft rejection, fungal infections, and accelerated atherosclerosis in the post-transplant setting.[155] CMV retinitis is a serious condition in AIDS patients with very low CD4 T-cell counts (<100/μL).[156]

PATHOGENESIS AND IMMUNITY

CMV encodes several immunomodulatory genes that interfere with the host immune response.[157] Included among these are genes that downregulate HLA class I expression, block natural killer (NK) cell activating stress signals, and interfere with neutralizing antiviral antibody and complement. The possession of these genes allows CMV to establish "sanctuary sites" within the body from which the virus can reactivate and produce infectious virions.

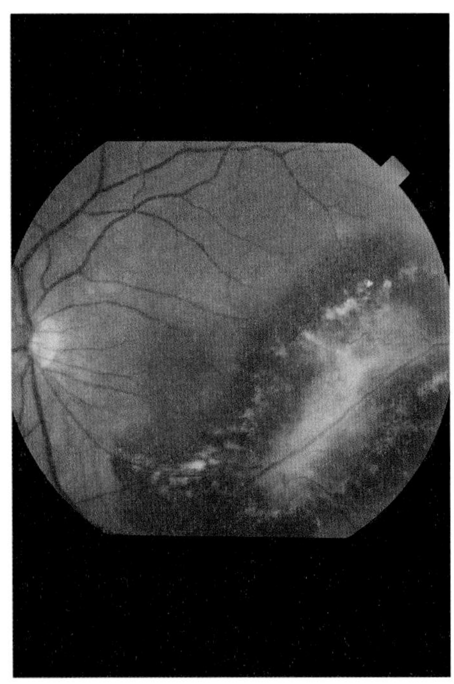

Figure 56.3 The macula of a left eye showing a lesion of active CMV retinitis along the inferior temporal arcade. The CMV retinitis has a white granular appearance of full thickness retinal necrosis and is surrounded by hemorrhage. (slide courtesy Dr. Pauline Wilson).

While these immune evasion strategies are quite effective, CMV is nevertheless highly immunogenic to the host.[158] Indeed, the human immune system commits more resources to controlling CMV than to any other virus, such that CMV-specific T cells accumulate with age and represent the dominant antigen-specific T-cell population in the elderly.[159] Of all CMV antigens, the tegument protein pp65 and the major immediate early antigen are immunodominant.[158]

DIAGNOSIS

Recent CMV infection is demonstrated by detection of CMV IgM antibody, and past infection is demonstrated by detection of CMV IgG antibody by enzyme immunoassay. For detection of recent primary infection in the first trimester of pregnancy, IgM assays are coupled with low avidity IgG assays for diagnosis of asymptomatic primary CMV infection.[160]

In immunocompromised patients, active CMV infection is best detected by quantitative PCR of whole blood. In the post-transplant setting, CMV viral load is carefully monitored, with antiviral treatment initiated when predefined thresholds are reached.[161] Biopsies of affected solid tissues may also be collected for quantitative CMV PCR assay. In contrast to the post-transplant setting, surveillance samples are not collected in AIDS patients since prophylactic anti-CMV therapy has not proven to be beneficial in this patient group.[162]

TREATMENT AND PROGNOSIS

Ganciclovir is the first-line drug used for prevention and treatment of CMV infection in the immunocompromised patient. Administered intravenously, the drug is phosphorylated by the CMV UL97 gene product to its monophosphate form and then by cellular enzymes to its triphosphate form. The triphosphate form is a potent inhibitor of CMV-encoded DNA polymerase.[163] Valganciclovir, the valine ester of ganciclovir, may be used for the treatment or prevention of CMV infection in place of intravenous ganciclovir.[164] Long-term antiviral therapy selects for resistant strains with acquired point mutations or deletions of the UL97 gene.[163] Continued treatment may lead to additional mutational changes in the viral DNA polymerase, producing a highly resistant virus.[163] Foscarnet is used for second-line treatment of CMV infection or disease, especially in patients with documented ganciclovir resistance. It acts as an inhibitor of CMV-encoded DNA polymerase.[163] Acyclovir also has activity against CMV but must be given in high dosage. Maribavir, a newer inhibitor of UL97, which showed promise in a phase II trial,[165] recently failed a phase III trial.

PREVENTION AND CONTROL

Two strategies have evolved for the deployment of antiviral drugs in transplant centers, prophylaxis and preemptive therapy. In prophylaxis, the drug (usually valganciclovir) is given to patients for a defined period of time and then stopped. While CMV is controlled during treatment, frequently a serious rebound infection, often with a resistant strain, may follow cessation of treatment.[166,167] For preemptive therapy, patients are monitored with regular blood samples and treated only if and when significant viremia is detected.[161] Such preemptive therapy is very effective at preventing CMV end-organ disease.[167] The relative advantages of prophylaxis and preemptive therapy have been debated extensively.[166,167] Both are clearly excellent at preventing CMV end-organ disease with a potential advantage for prophylaxis in controlling the indirect effects of CMV but a potential advantage of preemptive therapy in having less late-onset disease with resistant strains.

In AIDS patients, the main objective is to keep the blood CD4 count above 100/μL by manipulation of highly active retroviral therapy (HAART). If this is not possible, then prophylactic valganciclovir can be used to prevent CMV retinitis.[168]

A live attenuated CMV vaccine (Towne strain) developed in the 1980s reduced the severity of CMV end-organ disease but not the incidence of disease or infection.[169] A more modern strategy is to combine only the immunogenic components of CMV with adjuvants. The first randomized controlled trial using this approach reported very positive results.[170] Overall, this vaccine yielded a 50% reduction in the incidence of primary CMV infection.

EPSTEIN-BARR VIRUS

THE AGENT

EBV is a human herpesvirus of the gammaherpesvirus subfamily and genus *Lymphocryptovirus*. Humans are the only known natural host for EBV, although all Old World primate species have closely related lymphocryptoviruses.[171] EBV was first identified as a typical herpesvirus by electron microscopy from a biopsy of endemic African Burkitt's lymphoma.[172] EBV was also shown to cause most cases of infectious mononucleosis.[173] Permanent transformed cell lines harboring EBV can be obtained from infectious mononucleosis blood and from Burkitt's lymphoma tissue.[174] Subsequently, the virus was shown to also be associated with a number of other human diseases, including undifferentiated nasopharyngeal carcinoma (NPC) and other lymphocyte-rich carcinomas, oral hairy leukoplakia in AIDS patients, malignant lymphoma of both B- and T-cell types, and Hodgkin's disease (HD).[175–183] Although *in vitro* only B cells appear to be efficiently infected and transformed, *in vivo* it appears as though the host cell range for EBV is not as restricted – not only B cells but in some cases T cells, epithelial cells, and mesenchymal cells may harbor EBV. EBV gains access to the B lymphocyte through the C3d receptor (CR2, CD21).[184] An EBV strain obtained from a patient with mononucleosis and used to transform marmoset B cells (B95–8) has been cloned and sequenced.[185] EBV DNA contains 172 kb with several sets of repeat elements separated by unique regions containing more than 100 ORFs. Given the importance of the phenomenon of B-cell latency, a great deal of attention has been devoted to the latent genes which encode six nuclear proteins (EBNA1–6), three membrane proteins (LMP1, 2A, 2B), and two highly abundant nonpolyadenylated nuclear RNAs (EBER1, 2). Also,

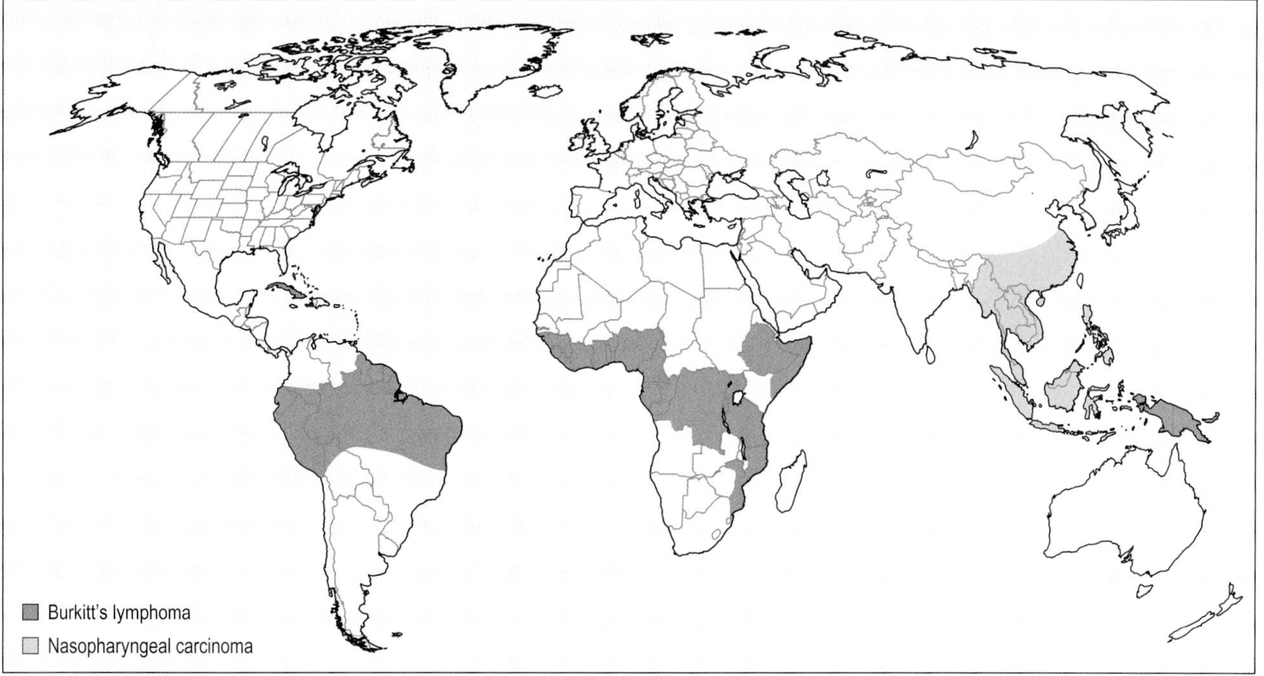

Figure 56.4 Map of the geographic distribution of Epstein–Barr virus-associated Burkitt's lymphoma and nasopharyngeal carcinoma.

there are some EBV genes with homology to human genes, including BHRF1 (bcl2-like), BCRF1 (IL-10-like), and BZLF1 (jun/fos-like).[186–188] It has been suggested that these genes may have been appropriated from the primate genome to provide a survival advantage to EBV-infected cells.[171]

There appear to be two distinct strains of EBV, type 1 (or A type) and type 2 (or B type), which differ in geographic distribution, biologic properties, and genetic sequences.[189,190] The strains differ genetically mostly in the EBNA2, EBNA3, and EBER genes. Type 2 isolates transform B cells *in vitro* with much lower efficiency than type 1 isolates.[191] Although type 2 isolates are more commonly isolated from Asia, Africa, and AIDS patients, they may be recovered not infrequently from the oropharynx of normal persons from the developed world.[189] Although type 1 isolates are more commonly isolated from tumors, no clear difference in pathogenicity of type 1 versus type 2 EBV is established.

EPIDEMIOLOGY

EBV is a human gammaherpesvirus that establishes transient lytic infection of the oropharyngeal mucosal epithelium and chronic latent infection of B lymphocytes. Infection most often occurs following contact with infectious saliva of healthy carriers or patients with infectious mononucleosis. EBV, like the other herpesviruses, has a ubiquitous distribution with an overall adult seroprevalence exceeding 90%. The high rate of seroprevalence is maintained by a large population of healthy carriers – up to 20% of healthy seropositive people in the developed world and 45% of African children excrete virus intermittently in saliva. Unlike CMV, EBV is not recognized as a common congenital or neonatal infection and has not clearly been shown to be transmitted through the genital tract. In the developing world and especially in subequatorial areas of Africa endemic for Burkitt's lymphoma, early childhood infection is the rule and is nearly always asymptomatic. Even in developed countries, many, if not most, primary infections occur in childhood and are subclinical.

THE DISEASE

Primary infection as it occurs in adolescents and young adults classically presents as infectious mononucleosis. Because of the high rate of childhood infection in the tropics, infectious mononucleosis is seldom encountered. Although EBV accounts for the majority of cases of infectious mononucleosis, similar syndromes are caused by CMV, *Toxoplasma*, and viral hepatitis. EBV-associated mononucleosis typically follows an incubation period of 1–2 months and is characterized by several weeks of fever, pharyngitis, malaise, headache, and posterior cervical lymphadenopathy. Laboratory features include atypical lymphocytosis, positive heterophile antibody test (which may be negative in children), positive IgM antiviral capsid antigen (VCA), and elevated IgG anti-VCA. Most of the atypical lymphocytes in peripheral blood express an immunophenotype consistent with activated CD8 cytotoxic T cells, with a smaller increase in NK cells.[192] Other manifestations include mild hepatitis, splenomegaly, encephalitis, polyneuritis, pneumonia, ampicillin-induced rash, and a variety of autoimmune phenomena. In the vast majority of cases, complete spontaneous recovery without recurrence follows. Rarely, however, probably associated with immunodeficiency, either a fatal hemophagocytic syndrome with marrow failure or malignant B-cell lymphoma may intervene. EBV, unlike the other human herpesviruses, with the possible exception of HHV-8, is clearly oncogenic and as such is classically associated with at least three human malignancies – endemic Burkitt's B-cell lymphoma, post-transplant B-cell lymphoma, and NPC (***Fig. 56.4***) – and more loosely associated with other human malignancies – HD, lymphocyte-rich carcinoma, gastric adenocarcinoma,[193,194] smooth muscle tumors,[195,196] some T-cell lymphomas, and other B-cell lymphomas (AIDS-associated, sporadic nonendemic Burkitt's, primary CNS lymphoma).[197] EBV is also associated with Duncan's disease, a fatal infectious mononucleosis-like illness in boys with the rare X-linked lymphoproliferative syndrome.[198] HIV-positive patients and rarely post-transplant patients develop a benign wart-like lesion on the lateral borders of the tongue called oral hairy leukoplakia, which is productively infected with EBV.[179]

PATHOGENESIS AND IMMUNITY

Like the other herpesviruses, EBV may exist in either a latent or a lytic state. However, the predominant mode of B-cell infection appears to lead to latency. Owing to the consistency of patterns of latent EBV gene expression in different cell types, these patterns have been categorized into type I typical of African Burkitt's lymphoma with EBER1/2 and EBNA1 expression, type II in NPC and HD with EBER1/2 and LMP1/2 expression, and type III in latent-transformed B cells with EBER1/2, EBNA1–6, and LMP1/2 expression.[199] As noted previously, at least 10 latent EBV genes are active in EBV-transformed B cells, yet only a few are required for B-cell transformation.[171] Of the latent genes, LMP1 is the only one that has been clearly shown to exhibit transforming function.[200] Although EBV-transformed B cells grow continuously in cell culture, they are normal diploid cells and unable to form tumors in nude mice and are therefore not considered malignant. African Burkitt's lymphoma cells, on the other hand, are not only EBV infected but also have a chromosomal translocation involving the *c-myc* gene on chromosome 8 and one of the immunoglobulin genes on chromosome 2 (κ light chain), 14 (heavy chain), or 22 (λ light chain). These translocations lead to production of excessive amounts of myc protein, a protein important in cell cycle progression.[201,202] The consistent presence of *c-myc* translocations in all cases of Burkitt's lymphoma, whether EBV positive or EBV negative, emphasizes the dominant role of the *c-myc* gene translocation in the genesis of Burkitt's lymphoma. The primacy of *c-myc* activation has also been shown *in vitro* by inducing proliferation of EBV-transformed B cells independent of EBNA2 and LMP1 activity.[203] However, the presence of single-sized fused EBV terminal repeats most consistent with monoclonal virus within tumors has led to the suggestion that EBV is not simply a passenger but is playing an important role in growth of the tumor.[204] The set of latent EBV genes (type II) active in NPC differs from that seen in transformed B cells and includes unusual complementary strand transcripts from the *BamHI A* fragment.[205] However, advances in this area have been hampered by lack of simple *in vitro* systems for analysis of EBV effects on normal human epithelial cells in culture. Interestingly, the latency type II NPC pattern rather than the latency type III lymphoblastoid B-cell gene expression pattern is typical of the malignant Reed–Sternberg (RS) cells of HD, cells that are likely B lymphoid in origin.[206]

DIAGNOSIS

Infectious mononucleosis due to EBV may be difficult to differentiate from other infectious diseases without serologic testing for heterophile antibody and in heterophile-negative cases (in young children) for specific EBV antibody (anti-VCA). In most cases, the clinical presentation of a rapidly growing jaw or abdominal mass in a child in an endemic area is virtually diagnostic of Burkitt's lymphoma. Because of the rapid and specific clinical presentation of endemic Burkitt's lymphoma, EBV serology has not proved useful in the diagnosis of Burkitt's lymphoma. On the other hand, the predominance of nonspecific manifestations (nasal stuffiness and nosebleeds) in the early stages of NPC may delay the clinical diagnosis. Fortunately, large-scale screening in susceptible populations for elevated anti-VCA or anti-early antigen (EA) IgA antibody titers has proved very useful in early detection of the disease and the recurrence of NPC. Recent efforts have focused on the use of BZLF1 IgG, EA IgG, and antibody-dependent cellular cytotoxicity tests in prognosis.[207] The clinical diagnosis of post-transplant lymphoproliferative disease (PTLD) should be suspected if fever, lymphadenopathy, tonsillar enlargement, allograft failure, or abdominal mass is detected. Given the high rate of EBV seropositivity and viral reactivation in the transplant populations, serologic studies generally are not useful. An increase in EBV load, as assessed by quantitative EBV PCR of peripheral blood, has been shown to herald the emergence of PTLD.[208–210] EBV may be detected rapidly in tumor cells from tissue biopsies by immunostaining for the EBV LMP1 protein, by *in situ* hybridization for highly abundant EBV EBER1 or EBER2 RNA, or by detection of EBV DNA by PCR. Cell culture isolation of EBV is technically difficult and is therefore not routinely performed in the clinical laboratory.

TREATMENT AND PROGNOSIS

Treatment of Burkitt's lymphoma and NPC with antiviral drugs is not effective; instead these malignant tumors require standard antineoplastic therapy. For NPC, radiotherapy alone often leads to 5-year survival rates of 50–60%.[211,212] Although the addition of chemotherapy leads to higher initial remission rates, no improvement in survival has been shown.[213] In the post-transplant setting, prophylaxis in seronegative patients with hyperimmune globulin may be useful. The nucleoside analog acyclovir has been used in some cases to inhibit EBV replication and blunt disease, but is incapable of eradicating latent virus. In patients with severe acute complications of EBV infection, such as airway obstruction from tonsillar enlargement, corticosteroids may be useful. Appropriate treatment of PTLD should be individualized to the specific case. Options include reduction of immunosuppressive medication, interferon-α, intravenous immunoglobulin, acyclovir, localized radiotherapy, and conventional chemotherapy. Reduction of immunosuppressive therapy in the early stages of PTLD often leads to clinical remission and cure but should be carefully titrated to prevent organ transplant rejection.[214] Immunosuppressive withdrawal may be accompanied by acyclovir therapy, which, although ineffective in inhibiting tumor cell growth, should prevent further active viral infection. Interferon-α-2b with intravenous immunoglobulin may induce remissions in both polyclonal and monoclonal PTLD and may be considered in those in whom immunosuppressive withdrawal has failed.[215,216] Radiotherapy should probably be limited to treatment of unresectable, highly localized processes. Cytotoxic chemotherapy should probably be limited, as a last resort, to refractory cases owing to the severe life-threatening complications.[217] More experimental approaches with some promise include donor leukocyte transfusion and transfusion of *in vitro* expanded autologous EBV-specific cytotoxic T cells in bone marrow transplant recipients.[218,219] Oral hairy leukoplakia is effectively treated with high-dose oral acyclovir or desciclovir, although recurrence following cessation of therapy is common.[220,221] Recent *in vitro* results suggest that vidarabine and foscarnet may be useful in treatment of EBV-positive NK large granular lymphocyte (LGL) disorders.[222]

PREVENTION AND CONTROL

As with the other herpesviruses, hygienic measures are not very effective in preventing EBV infection. The large number of healthy seropositive viral excreters in the population provides a constant source of infectious virus, and measures to minimize contact with infectious saliva are impractical. Since congenital EBV infection is not a clinical problem, isolation of seronegative mothers from seropositive excreters is not warranted. Although unproven, measures to curb holoendemic malaria may be useful in prevention of Burkitt's lymphoma in central Africa, and avoidance of salted fish in southern China may be useful in prevention of NPC. Ultimately, the development of an EBV vaccine may lead to decreased rates of Burkitt's lymphoma and NPC if administered to seronegative children in the endemic areas. Vaccine development has focused on the 350 kDa major envelope glycoprotein (gp350), which is the major target of neutralizing antibodies *in vivo*.[223] Gp350 subunit vaccines, as well as vaccinia and adenovirus recombinant gp350 vaccines, are undergoing evaluation.[224]

HUMAN HERPESVIRUS 6

THE AGENT

HHV-6 was first identified as a herpesvirus growing from primary lymphocyte cultures of patients with AIDS-associated lymphoproliferative disease.[225] The virus has subsequently been isolated from adults with AIDS[226,227] and children with a febrile illness called exanthem subitum (or roseola infantum, pseudorubella, or sixth disease).[228] The electron microscopic appearance of the virus is typical of herpesviruses with a prominent tegument.[229] Within 3–5 days of culture, infected lymphocytes display characteristic cytopathic effects with ballooning enlargement somewhat similar to that seen with CMV.[230] Although the *in vitro* host cell range differs among different isolates, most can be propagated in normal T cells and T-cell lines, while some isolates infect the fibroblast cell line MRC-5 and EBV-infected B cells.[231–234] *In vivo*, the major target cell in peripheral blood appears to be the $CD4^+$ $CD8^-$ T lymphocyte.[235] The animal host range of the virus has not been clearly established. Serologic studies in nonhuman primates have yielded mixed results, with one study detecting serologic positivity in 8 of 10 species, whereas others detected no positivity in any species tested.[225,236,237]

The HHV-6 genome is 160–170 kb in length with a long unique region flanked on both ends by terminal repeats.[238–240] Sequence analysis demonstrates that HHV-6 is a betaherpesvirus with closest homology to HHV-7 and CMV and likely encodes 80–100 proteins.[241] Genetic, serologic, and biologic evidence suggests two distinct subtypes termed HHV-6A (represented by prototype strains GS and U1102) and HHV-6B (represented by prototype strain Z29).[242,243] The U1102 strain genome contains an interesting gene encoding a protein with close homology to the transregulatory rep 68/78 protein of the human parvovirus AAV-2 strain.[244] Transfection of NIH3T3 cells with HHV-6 DNA induces phenotypic changes associated with cell transformation, including the ability of these transfected cells to grow as tumors in nude mice.[245] Although a transmissible virus-like agent was demonstrated in children with exanthem subitum as early as 1950,[246] it was not until 1988 that HHV-6 was shown to be the cause of the disease.[228] It was subsequently shown that exanthem subitum is associated in almost all cases with the HHV-6B subtype.[190,242,247,248]

EPIDEMIOLOGY

Like the other herpesviruses, HHV-6 is ubiquitous, with greater than 80% seropositivity in US adults detected with a sensitive enzyme-linked immunosorbent assay (ELISA).[249] Primary infection most often occurs in early childhood with seroprevalence rates exceeding 80% by 2 years of age in Japan, Italy, and Thailand.[250–252] HHV-6, like HHV-7, appears to persistently infect the salivary glands where it is shed into the saliva.[253,254] Although high rates of HHV-6 presence in saliva of healthy adults have been reported by some researchers, others have reported much lower rates.[255–260] It has been suggested that the high rates of salivary HHV-6 reported in some studies may be complicated by the cross-reactivity of some reagents and assays with HHV-7.[261] Intrauterine infection appears to be fairly common, with nearly 30% of healthy newborns positive for HHV-6 DNA in blood. Sexual and perinatal transmission is also likely to be common given that up to 30% of women have uterine cervical secretions containing HHV-6 DNA.[262] Primary infection in children younger than 2 years old is often characterized by a syndrome of high fever and evanescent rash (exanthem subitum; ***Fig. 56.2E***). Indeed, exanthem subitum is the most common exanthem in children under 2 years of age. Nearly half of all first febrile episodes after birth and up to 40% of all pediatric emergency room admissions for febrile illness may be due to HHV-6 infection. In one recent study, 10% of all febrile episodes in infants were due to either HHV-6A or HHV-6B infection.[263] In a tropical Brazilian study, primary HHV-6 and HHV-7 infections in children were often misdiagnosed as measles.[264]

THE DISEASE

A high fever for 4–5 days is followed in up to 70% of cases by a diffuse evanescent (fewer than 2 days) maculopapular rash on the chest and abdomen with relative sparing of the face and extremities. Febrile convulsions, splenomegaly, and cervical lymphadenopathy are common. Manifestations may include hepatitis, thrombocytopenia, hemophagocytic syndrome, meningitis, and encephalitis. An association with a specific form of massive cervical lymphadenopathy of childhood, sinus histiocytosis with massive lymphadenopathy, has been reported.[265] Symptomatic primary infection in adults is neither common nor well described but may present as heterophile-negative mononucleosis or hepatitis.[266,267] Although HHV-6 has been suggested as a possible factor in chronic fatigue syndrome, a prospective study did not establish any correlation between HHV-6 seropositivity and chronic fatigue syndrome.[268] HHV-6 has been implicated in some cases of idiopathic acute liver failure.[269] In the post-transplant setting, serologic evidence of reactivation is commonly observed and may be associated with a variety of symptoms, including fever, rash, hepatitis, pneumonitis, neurologic dysfunction, and marrow suppression.[235] Although HHV-6 DNA has been detected in some cases of lymphoproliferative disease,[270–272] the lack of consistent positivity in any specific type of lymphoproliferative disease would argue against a causal link. HHV-6 has also recently been directly implicated in the pathogenesis of multiple sclerosis.[273,274]

DIAGNOSIS

Clinical diagnosis of classic roseola infantum in childhood is not usually difficult and does not require serologic confirmation. Due to the high seroprevalence, single-point IgG titers are not useful. Diagnosis of active infection serologically requires either detection of increased IgM or a greater than fourfold rise in IgG titers from paired acute and convalescent serum specimens using indirect immunofluorescence (IFA), anticomplement immunofluorescence, or ELISA. Virus culture systems have been described. However, caution in interpretation of positive results is warranted owing to the high rate of viral isolation from the normal population. Given the availability of HHV-6 DNA sequence information, the most rapid and sensitive assays for direct detection of HHV-6 are PCR-based assays, which can distinguish between HHV-6A and HHV-6B strains.[247,275]

TREATMENT AND PROGNOSIS

The susceptibility of HHV-6 to antiviral drugs is likely similar to that of the related herpesvirus CMV. The nucleoside analog ganciclovir and viral DNA polymerase inhibitors, cidofovir and foscarnet, may be useful in severe infection, as in the post-transplant setting, but have not been tested in a controlled manner. Although uncomplicated primary infection in childhood is self-limited, infection in immunocompromised patients such as after organ transplantation may lead to life-threatening complications.

PREVENTION AND CONTROL

Given the high infection rate in infancy and childhood and the high rate of asymptomatic oral shedding, preventive measures are unlikely to be effective.

HUMAN HERPESVIRUS 7

THE AGENT

HHV-7 (strain RK) was first isolated from peripheral blood CD4 T lymphocytes of a healthy 26-year-old subject during attempts to isolate and propagate HHV-6.[276] Several additional isolates were obtained from normal healthy persons.[277] Another strain (JI) was isolated from a patient with chronic fatigue syndrome.[278] The ultrastructural appearance of the virus is characteristic of a typical human herpesvirus with a very prominent tegument similar to that of HHV-6. The HHV-7 genome contains 145 kbp with sequence homology to other betaherpesviruses HHV-6 and CMV.[279,280] Antigenically, HHV-7 is similar to HHV-6 since both serologic[281,282] and T cell–mediated[283] cross-reactivity has been described. HHV-7 appears to preferentially infect CD4 T cells, although infection of CD8 lymphocytes has also been demonstrated.[278] Virus is present not only in peripheral blood but also in saliva, salivary glands, and uterine cervical secretions. Transmission likely occurs most commonly through the oral route, but may also occur via the genital tract.

EPIDEMIOLOGY

HHV-7 infection is very common, with adult seroprevalence ranging from over 80% in western Europe and the United States to 60% in Japan.[251,278,281,284] The virus actively replicates in the oral region with salivary isolation rates of 55–96% of normal healthy adults.[250,256,260,261,285] Primary infection is common in early childhood – 42% of children are seropositive by 2 years of age and 82% by 4 years of age – but appears to occur later than primary HHV-6 infection.[252,286]

THE DISEASE

Primary HHV-7 infection in children is a febrile illness that may be complicated by seizures.[287] HHV-7 has been isolated from some patients with exanthem subitum, chronic fatigue syndrome, chronic mononucleosis, hepatitis, and CMV-like disease in the post-transplant setting.[288–292] It has been suggested both from *in vitro* and clinical observations that under some conditions, such as post-transplant or AIDS settings, HHV-7 may act to exacerbate other betaherpesvirus infections (CMV and HHV-6) by reactivation from latency.[292,293]

DIAGNOSIS

Serologic, culture, immunohistologic, PCR, and *in situ* hybridization techniques for the detection of HHV-7 infection have been described but are not widely available for clinical use. However, given the high prevalence of virus infection in the normal population and the absence of clearly defined clinical disease associations, the clinical utility of viral detection or antibody measurement is unclear. Assays should certainly be carefully designed and tested to avoid cross-reactivity with the related betaherpesviruses HHV-6 and CMV.

TREATMENT AND PROGNOSIS

Although controlled studies are unavailable, it is likely that HHV-7 infection, like the betaherpesvirus CMV, will respond to treatment with the nucleoside analog ganciclovir as well as the viral DNA polymerase inhibitors foscarnet and cidofovir.

PREVENTION AND CONTROL

It is likely that, like HHV-6, the high infection rate in childhood and high rate of asymptomatic oral shedding in adults would preclude effective preventive measures, even if prevention of this mild infection was deemed justifiable.

HUMAN HERPESVIRUS 8

THE AGENT

Infectious virus recovered from both the EBV-positive primary effusion lymphoma (PEL) cell line BC-1 and from a Kaposi's sarcoma (KS) biopsy specimen have been cloned and sequenced.[294,295] Although the viral genome was originally reported as 250–270 kb, a more recent estimate is 150–160 kb.[296,297] DNA sequence analysis has revealed close sequence homology to the gammaherpesviruses, herpesvirus saimiri and EBV.[294,298] A striking feature of the viral genome is the presence of genes with homology to cell cycle regulatory and signaling proteins including complement binding proteins, bcl-2, IL-6, IL-8 receptor, nerve cell adhesion molecule (N-CAM) family protein, macrophage inflammatory proteins (MIP-1, MIP-2), cyclin D, and interferon regulatory factor 1, some of which may be important in cell transformation.[294–299] No genes with homology to the known transforming genes of EBV (EBNA, LMP) or herpesvirus saimiri (ORF1) are present. However, it is interesting to note that EBV infection of B cells induces increased expression of some of the same cellular genes (cyclin D, complement receptor 2, bcl-2, IL-8 receptor-like protein, and IL-6) for which HHV-8 encodes a homolog.[295] This suggests that both gammaherpesviruses use the same strategy for successful infection, but in the case of EBV the elements of the program remain within the human host cell while with HHV-8 the program has been acquired by the virus from the host cell.

EPIDEMIOLOGY

PEL cell lines have been utilized as targets for the development of IFA and ELISA assays for detection of anti-HHV-8 antibodies in human serum. Assay variations have included IFA on unstimulated cells or phorbol ester or *n*-butyric acid-stimulated cells for more sensitive detection of antibody to lytic antigens,[300–303] isolated cell nuclei for detection of antibody to nuclear antigens,[300,304,305] and ELISA using recombinant antigens.[305] As expected, nearly all patients with KS are seropositive using any of the preceding methods. Also, not surprisingly, a variable proportion of AIDS patients without KS are seropositive. Both seroconversion and detection of HHV-8 DNA by PCR precede development of KS in HIV-infected patients.[304,306,307]

Immunosuppressed renal transplant recipients exhibit both serologic and molecular evidence of HHV-8 activation,[308] a phenomenon that may be at least partially due to steroid effects on viral replication.[309] Transmission of HHV-8 in transplant recipients may occur by blood transfusion or by allograft.[310,311] Tremendous geographic variation in HHV-8 seroprevalence has been noted. In central Africa, the seroprevalence is approximately 50%, while in southern Europe it ranges up to 20% and is about 5% in northern Europe and in the United States.[312] Seroprevalence rates reported from different laboratories on normal healthy persons from nonendemic regions have varied tremendously (0–24%).[301–305]

Although some variations in results may be due to real geographic or demographic differences, some variability is also likely due to differences in the sensitivity of assay signal detection and the selection of antigen substrate.[313] Seroprevalence studies designed to detect the age of infection have revealed that as contrasted with an early age of infection in Africa,[314] in the United States infection appears to be delayed until adolescence.[315]

THE DISEASE

The clinical characteristics of primary HHV-8 infection have not yet been described. In addition to KS, HHV-8 has also been detected by PCR in high-grade large B-cell lymphomas arising in body cavities, that is, primary effusion lymphoma,[316–318] multicentric Castleman's disease,[319] angioimmunoblastic lymphadenopathy (AILD),[320] non-KS skin tumors in allograft transplant recipients,[321] angiosarcoma,[322] and multiple myeloma.[323]

KS was first described by Kaposi as an indolent tumor of the lower extremity in elderly males of Mediterranean or eastern European descent.[324] KS is a dermal spindle cell neoplasm, likely of endothelial cell origin, which in the skin is manifest as irregular discolored patches, plaques, nodules, or umbilicated tumors (***Fig. 56.2F***). Although most investigators regard KS as a malignant disease, the indolent behavior of classic KS with spontaneous regression in some cases has led some to suggest a reactive process.[325,326] Analysis of DNA of KS lesions has yielded inconsistent results, with some studies suggestive of a nonclonal process and other studies suggestive of a clonal process.[327,328] Pathologically, the early lesion (the patch stage) consists of irregular branching ectatic vascular channels in the upper dermis lined by plump relatively normal-appearing endothelium (***Fig. 56.5***). At this stage, the pathologic changes may be subtle, and distinction from hemangioma or granulation tissue difficult. The late lesion (the plaque stage) consists of an irregular nodular spindle cell proliferation with mitotic figures in both the upper and lower dermis, vascular slits, extravasated erythrocytes, hemosiderin deposition,

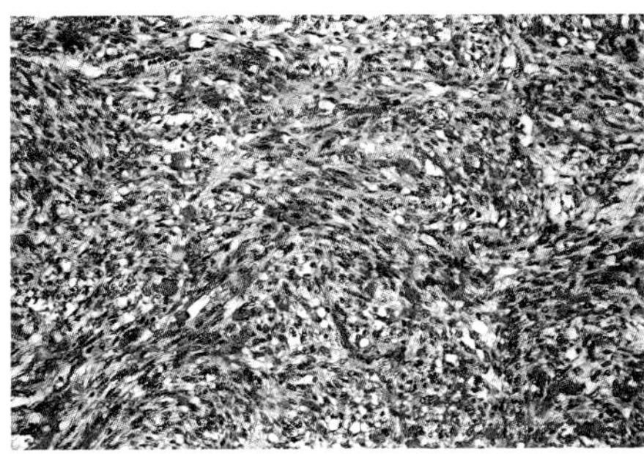

Figure 56.5 Histopathology of Kaposi's sarcoma. (Courtesy of Joanna Borkowski, MD, Department of Pathology, UTMB, Galveston, TX.)

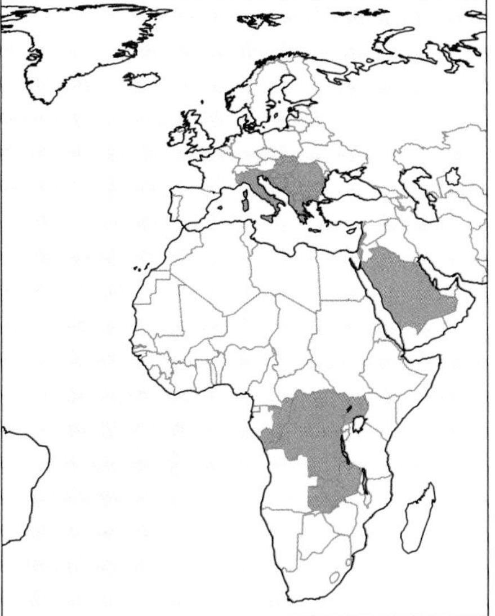

Figure 56.6 Map of geographic distribution of endemic HHV-8 associated Kaposi's sarcoma.

so-called hyaline bodies, and admixed inflammatory cells. At this stage, the pathologic changes are quite characteristic, although in some cases distinction from angiosarcoma may be difficult. KS has been described in four different clinical settings – classic Mediterranean, endemic African, epidemic AIDS-associated, and iatrogenic.[329] Classic KS presents as a chronic, generally indolent, cutaneous disease of the lower extremity, most often in elderly white males (male-to-female ratio, 3:1; mean age, 68 years) of Mediterranean, eastern European, or Jewish ancestry.[324] Interestingly, up to 35% of these persons may develop second tumors, especially malignant lymphoma. Endemic African KS occurs in the sub-Saharan equatorial regions (***Fig. 56.6***) and presents most often in young adult black males (male-to-female ratio, 14:1; mean age, 35 years) with either a florid form (40%), a benign nodular form (25%), or an aggressive form (15%), as well as in young black male children (mean age, 3 years) with a lymphadenopathic form.[330] Endemic KS is often an aggressive disease with a fatal outcome. Iatrogenic KS occurs in persons following chronic treatment with drugs with immunosuppressive effects administered for solid organ transplantation,[331] autoimmune disease,[332] and malignancy. Iatrogenic KS is a generally indolent disease with complete remission in up to 24% of cases following immune restoration. Epidemic AIDS-associated KS is the most common malignant neoplasm in AIDS patients in the Western world.[333] The risk of development of KS in AIDS appears to be directly related to the degree of immunodeficiency and is strongly inversely correlated with the absolute CD4 count. Sexual transmission of HHV-8 is suggested by the much higher incidence of KS in HIV-infected homosexual or bisexual males than in other risk groups such as HIV-infected females and IV drug users. AIDS-associated KS is an aggressive disease closely resembling endemic African KS, with widespread dissemination to lymph nodes and viscera.

Although HHV-8 is nearly always detected in KS lesions within the KS spindle cells, the role HHV-8 plays in the pathogenesis of KS is unclear. Prior to the discovery of HHV-8, work was presented implicating CMV as the causative agent of KS.[334–336] Also, inflammatory cytokines (basic fibroblast growth factor, oncostatin M, and IL-6) from activated T cells and the HIV-1 tat protein have been shown to induce KS-like spindle cell transformation of normal endothelium both *in vitro* and *in vivo*.[337–343] Results of DNA analysis of KS spindle cells are not consistent, with some reporting diploidy and others aneuploidy.[343–346] Although no consistent KS-specific chromosomal abnormality has been described, chromosome X inactivation analysis reveals that AIDS KS is a monoclonal tumor.[347] Analysis of HHV-8 terminal repeats by Southern blotting in a KS biopsy are consistent with monoclonal virus, a finding most consistent with tumor cell monoclonality, as would be expected if KS were a malignant neoplasm.[294] Despite these findings, the absence of HHV-8 in spindle cell cultures derived from KS biopsies is puzzling.[348,349] Perhaps HHV-8 is lost from cells after serial passage *in vitro*.

Castleman's disease is a peculiar lymphoproliferative disorder which presents either as a solitary or multicentric form.[350,351] The more common solitary form usually presents asymptomatically as an anterior mediastinal or neck mass with hyaline vascular histology. The less common multicentric form usually presents with fever, anemia, and generalized lymphadenopathy with plasma cell histology. Patients with the solitary form have an excellent prognosis and in fact are often cured of disease by surgical excision of the mass. On the other hand, patients with the multicentric form have a poor prognosis. Lymph node biopsies of multicentric Castleman's disease may contain HHV-8 DNA by PCR.[319] However, the significance of these findings is unclear since only a minority of cases contain viral DNA.[352] Regarding non-KS vascular lesions, in one PCR study of 155 vascular lesions (including 17 cases of KS and 15 cases of angiosarcoma), HHV-8 DNA was present only in the KS cases, while in another study HHV-8 was found in angiosarcoma (7 of 24) and hemangioma (1 of 20).[322,353] The significance of these findings is unclear since only a minority of cases contain viral DNA.

PEL is a high-grade malignant lymphoma most often seen in homosexual males with AIDS.[317,318,354,355] The tumor presents as a malignant effusion of pleural, pericardial, or peritoneal cavities and tends not to disseminate but to remain confined to the body cavity. Despite the lack of dissemination, these patients do not tolerate chemotherapy well and succumb within a few months of diagnosis. The malignancy is composed of large anaplastic cells with a null cell immunophenotype (negative B- and T-cell markers, CD30-positive) and a B-cell genotype (Jh rearranged) and are usually coinfected with both EBV and HHV-8.[315] Interestingly, up to one-third of PEL cases may be associated with KS.[356] Although usually seen in males with AIDS, rare HHV-8-positive PELs have been described in HIV-negative males and females.[315,356,357]

Multiple myeloma, a malignant plasma cell neoplasm which arises in the bone marrow, is the second most common malignancy of the blood in the United States.[358] Monoclonal gammopathy of undetermined significance (MGUS) is an even more common related condition characterized by a monoclonal proliferation of plasma cells but accompanied by much less severe clinical findings. However, up to 25% of patients with MGUS progress to multiple myeloma.[359] Although HHV-8 DNA had previously been shown to be absent from myeloma cells, HHV-8 DNA was recently reported within the dendritic cell compartment of the bone marrow of 15 of 15 patients with myeloma and two of eight patients with MGUS, while absent from 10 normal bone marrow samples and 16 samples from patients with other malignancies.[323,360] The investigators suggest that the role of the infected dendritic cells may be in stimulating growth of the abnormal plasma cells by elaboration of HHV-8 vIL-6, a factor shown to support the growth of a murine plasmacytoma cell line.[296]

PATHOGENESIS AND IMMUNITY

HHV-8 was first detected as a unique DNA sequence from an AIDS KS skin biopsy using PCR-based representational difference analysis.[361]

Subsequently, this DNA sequence was detected by PCR in nearly all lesional skin biopsies from patients with all forms of KS – classic, endemic African, iatrogenic, and epidemic AIDS associated.[361–365] Virus has been localized within the KS tumor cells by *in situ* hybridization.[366,367] However, viral DNA has also been detected in other tissues as well, including nonlesional skin,[299] non-KS skin tumors,[321] peripheral blood,[368] lymphoid tissue,[369] saliva,[370–372] sensory ganglia,[373] semen,[374,375] and prostate tissue. However, some of these findings have been disputed by others.[365,376,377] HHV-8 DNA has been found not only in KS patients but also in human immunodeficiency virus (HIV)-infected persons without KS as well as HIV-negative healthy controls. Within the blood, the virus has been localized largely to the CD19 B-cell compartment, although it may also be found in some T cells.[378] HHV-8 DNA has also been detected in some cases of AIDS-associated primary effusion B-cell lymphoma, where it may be accompanied by EBV.[316,352,379] Infectious virus obtained from the PEL cell line BC-1 has been shown *in vitro* to infect normal peripheral blood B cells.[380] HHV-8 DNA has been detected in biopsy material from non-KS skin lesions (squamous cell carcinoma, basal cell carcinoma, actinic keratosis, Bowen's disease) and also from normal skin of HIV-negative persons.[381] HHV-8 has also been found in some cases of AIDS-associated multicentric Castleman's disease.[319] In another study, HHV-8 DNA was detected by PCR only occasionally in biopsy material from patients with HIV-negative reactive lymphadenopathy (4 of 23 patients), HIV-negative angioimmunoblastic lymphadenopathy (3 of 15), lymphoma (1 of 43), multicentric Castleman's disease (0 of 5), and HD (0 of 45).[320] The HHV-8-positive reactive lymphadenopathy changes were characterized by florid follicular hyperplasia with increased vascularity resembling HIV-related lymphadenopathy and multicentric Castleman's disease. Normal healthy controls have also been shown to harbor HHV-8 DNA albeit at a lower rate.[320,375] In one study, HHV-8 DNA was found in 6% of normal skin tissues, in 7% of peripheral blood samples, in 44% of prostate tissues, and in 91% of semen samples from healthy immunocompetent Italian males.[382] It has been reported that not only HHV-8 but also EBV and CMV may be detected in African KS biopsies, and CMV, HHV-6, HHV-7, and human papillomavirus in AIDS KS biopsies.[383–385] However, the lack of consistent positive results in these studies argues against these other viruses playing an etiologic role. The increasing number of reports of HHV-8 PCR positivity in normal and abnormal tissues from patients without KS strongly suggests that viral infection may not be strictly limited to persons with KS. It is possible that HHV-8, like the related gammaherpesvirus EBV, will prove to be present not only in patients with virus-associated neoplasms but also in normal persons and serve as an important cofactor in human tumorigenesis, especially in a setting of immunodeficiency.

Coculture of KS spindle cells with a variety of endothelial and epithelial cell lines led to lytic infection of approximately 1% of the cells of the embryonal kidney epithelial cell line 293 from which virus could be serially passaged.[386] Interestingly, virus obtained from an HHV-8-positive, body cavity-based lymphoma cell line did not induce any evidence of infection. Infection of primary microvascular endothelial cells by HHV-8 has been reported and in two cases was associated with cellular transformation.[387–389] Like all herpesviruses, the virus appears to reside within infected cells either in the latent state as a circular episomal form or in the lytic state as a linear form. In one report, it was shown that linear lytic virus is found in the peripheral blood, whereas only episomal latent virus is present within the KS skin lesion itself.[368]

DIAGNOSIS

Because of the very strong correlation of HHV-8 positivity with KS, diagnosis of KS is presumptive evidence of HHV-8 infection. Rapid and specific confirmation of HHV-8 infection, however, may be accomplished by both qualitative and quantitative PCR methods performed on DNA isolated from body fluids or tissue.[361,390] Serologic assays (IFA nuclear antigen assay, IFA lytic antigen assay, ELISA recombinant antigen assay) are currently under development and will likely prove very useful in seroprevalence studies, in characterization of the immune response, and in detection of primary infection (IgM-specific assays). Although an *in vitro* culture method has recently been described, the technical complexity of the method in its current form makes it unlikely to be useful in the clinical laboratory setting.[386]

TREATMENT AND PROGNOSIS

Although HHV-8 infection may not respond to treatment with the nucleoside analogs acyclovir and ganciclovir as well as the other herpesviruses, long-term remission of KS has been reported following treatment with foscarnet,[391] and HIV-infected patients treated with foscarnet or ganciclovir have a decreased risk of KS development.[392] Also, clearance of HHV-8 DNA from the peripheral blood of an HIV-positive patient following treatment with the HIV protease inhibitor indinavir has been reported.[393] The use of HAART in AIDS-related KS is associated with a dramatic clinical response. Local therapy of KS has included cryotherapy, surgical excision, intralesional vinblastine, vincristine, or interferon-α, and radiotherapy. Systemic therapy has included both single- and multiple-agent chemotherapy and interferon-α.[394] Antineoplastic agents such as liposomal anthracyclines and paclitaxel, as well as antiangiogenic agents such as retinoic acids, AGM 1470 (TNP 470), thalidomide, and glufanide disodium (IM 862), have shown some promise in patients with KS.[395]

PREVENTION AND CONTROL

At this time there is no specific information regarding methods of prevention or control of HHV-8 infection. However, the best preventive advice is to reinforce the more general safe sex practices that have been promoted to prevent HIV and other sexually transmitted diseases.

Access the complete reference list online at
http://www.expertconsult.com

Access the complete reference list online at http://www.expertconsult.com

CHAPTER 57

Smallpox and Related Orthopoxviral Infections

Peter B. Jahrling

INTRODUCTION

Viruses classified as *Poxviridae* include the significant human pathogens, variola, the agent of smallpox, and monkeypox virus. During the twentieth century, smallpox is estimated to have caused over 500 million human deaths.[1] Yet the disease and the naturally circulating virus itself were eradicated by the World Health Organization's (WHO) global eradication campaign, which was declared a success in 1980.[2] This program, which involved vaccinating all humans in a ring surrounding every suspected case of variola infection, was successful in part because smallpox is solely a human disease; there are no animal reservoirs to reintroduce the virus into the human population. Despite the eradication of naturally occurring smallpox, variola virus remains a concern because of the possibility that clandestine stocks of the virus may be in the hands of bioterrorists.[3] The impact of reintroduction of smallpox virus into the human population now would be even more catastrophic than during the last century; vaccination programs were abandoned worldwide around 1976, the prevalence of immunosuppressed populations has grown, and mobility, to include intercontinental air travel, has accelerated the pace of viral spread worldwide. As an example, monkeypox virus, which persists in endemic foci in western and central Africa, was recently imported inadvertently into the United States via a shipment of rodents originating in Ghana.[4–6] More than 50 human infections were documented as a consequence of close contact with infected animals traced back to this shipment.

THE AGENTS

Classification

Poxviruses infect most vertebrates and invertebrates, causing a variety of diseases of veterinary and medical importance. The poxvirus family is divided into two main subfamilies: (1) the *Chordopoxvirinae*, which infect vertebrates; and (2) the *Entomopoxvirinae*, which infect insects. *Chordopoxvirinae* are divided into eight genera, one of which is *Orthopoxvirus*, which includes the human pathogens variola, monkeypox virus, and other species that infect humans such as cowpox and vaccinia viruses. Members of the *Orthopoxvirus* genus are mostly zoonotic pathogens.

Morphology

Orthopoxviruses are oval, brick-shaped particles with a geometrically corrugated outer surface. Their size ranges from 220 to 450 nm long and 140 to 260 nm wide.[7] The outer envelope consists of a lipoprotein layer embedding surface tubules and enclosing a core described as biconcave because of an electron microscopy fixation artifact. The core contains the viral DNA and core fibrils and is surrounded by the core envelope and a tightly arranged layer of rod-shaped structures known as the palisade layer. Between the palisade layer and the outer envelope are two oval masses known as the lateral bodies. Two infectious forms of orthopoxviruses result from the replication cycle, as described below.

Phylogenetic Relationships

A more precise definition of the evolutionary relationships among the orthopoxviruses has been facilitated by the recent availability of complete DNA sequences for over 30 species augmented by those for some 50 isolates of variola.[8] Phylogenetic analysis reveals that variola is most closely related to two tightly host-restricted orthopoxviruses, the camel-specific camelpox virus and taterapox, specific for gerbils. Vaccinia is most closely related to cowpox virus strain GRI-90[9,10] and more distantly to cowpox virus strain Brighton, suggesting that at least two separate species are included under the name cowpox virus. Monkeypox virus does not group closely with any other orthopoxvirus, including variola, indicating that it diverged from the rest of the genus long ago. Yet vaccination prevents monkeypox. Virulence or attenuation may hinge on a few genetic determinants. For example, variola major (associated with a 30% case-fatality rate) and variola minor (<1% case-fatality rate) are greater than 98% identical over the length of the 185 000 kilobase (kb) genome.[8,11] Concern has been raised in the arena of biodefense that minor modifications in the camelpox genome might result in a virus with the attributes of variola.

As anticipated from the genomic homologies, members of the *Orthopoxvirus* genus are antigenically related. Serum absorption and monoclonal antibody studies have identified cross-reacting and species-specific neutralizing antigens.[12] Nine neutralizing epitopes have been identified among the intracellular mature virion (IMV) particles of different species of orthopoxviruses;[13] additional epitopes, believed to be critical in protection against infection *in vivo*, exist on extracellular enveloped viral particles.[14,15] Viral antigens in the virus envelope are important for eliciting protective antibody responses. Historically, inactivated smallpox vaccines proved to be ineffective, and their failure was attributed to the absence of envelope antigens in the virion suspensions used.[16,17]

Replication

Orthopoxvirus genomes are linear, double-stranded DNA approximately 200 kb long. The genomes encode about 176–266 proteins, including enzymes and factors that are necessary for self-replication and maturation. The central region of the genome contains highly conserved genes that are essential for viral replication, and the terminal regions contain less conserved genes that are important for virus–host interactions. The virus contains a number of virus-encoded enzymes, in particular a DNA-dependent RNA polymerase that transcribes the viral genome.[7] Replication occurs in cytoplasmic factories referred to as B-type inclusions, in which virions at various stages of assembly are present. Whether host cell nuclear factors are involved in viral replication or maturation is unclear.

Viral replication begins with attachment of viral particles to the host cell surface, most likely through cell receptors which remain to be identified, and involves expression of early, intermediate, and late genes.[7] Initial uncoating occurs during entry, followed by synthesis of early mRNAs, which are translated to facilitate further uncoating and transcription of intermediate mRNAs. Intermediate mRNAs, in turn, are translated to allow transcription of the late mRNAs. The late mRNAs are translated into structural and enzymatic components of the virions. These components, along with DNA concatamers that are formed during the early phase of replication, are assembled into genomic DNA and packaged into immature virions, which then evolve into brick-shaped infectious IMVs. IMVs are infectious only when they are released by cell lysis. IMV particles, which can acquire a second membrane from an early endosomal component to form the intracellular enveloped virion (IEV), migrate to the cell surface via microtubules and fuse with the cell membrane to form cell-associated virions (CEVs). CEVs induce polymerization of actin to form filaments that effect the direct transfer of CEVs to adjacent cells. If CEVs become dissociated from the cell membranes, they are called extracellular enveloped virions (EEV). Although IMVs are produced in greatest abundance in cell culture and are the most stable to environmental degradation, CEVs and EEVs probably play a more critical role in cell-to-cell spread in the intact animal.[18]

Many of the *Orthopoxvirus* gene products interact with and modulate essential functions of the host cells and immune processes.[7,19,20] The limited host range of variola may relate to the unique association of viral gene products with various host signaling pathways.[21] Therefore, strategies that block such key pathways in the replication and maturation of poxviruses provide potential targets for therapeutic intervention.[22]

THE DISEASES: CLINICAL MANIFESTATIONS OF ORTHOPOXVIRUS INFECTIONS

Smallpox

Variola virus is stable and retains its infectivity for long periods outside the host.[23] Variola virus is infectious by aerosol,[3] but natural airborne spread other than among close contacts is unusual.[24,25] Approximately 30% of susceptible contacts became infected during the era of endemic smallpox,[26] and the WHO eradication campaign was predicated upon the requirement of close person-to-person proximity for reliable transmission to occur. Nevertheless, two hospital outbreaks demonstrated that the variola virus can be spread through airborne dissemination in conditions of low relative humidity.[27] The patients in these outbreaks were infectious from the onset of their eruptive exanthem, most commonly from days 3 through 6 after fever onset. If the patient had a cough, then chances of transmission were greatly increased. Indirect transmission via contaminated bedding or other fomites was infrequent. Some people in close contact with patients harbored virus in their throats without developing disease and may have been responsible for secondary transmission.[28]

After exposure to aerosolized virus, variola travels from the upper or the lower respiratory tract to regional lymph nodes, where it replicates and gives rise to viremia, which is followed by a rash.[29] The incubation period of smallpox averages 12 days (range 9–14 days). During global eradication, those who came in contact with infected patients were quarantined for a minimum of 16–17 days following exposure. Similar recommendations pertain to the Centers for Disease Control and Prevention (CDC) response plan for the reemergence of smallpox (www.bt.cdc.gov/agent/smallpox/response-plan). Following infection via the respiratory route and replication in local lymph nodes, variola virus disseminates systemically to other lymphoid tissues, spleen, liver, bone marrow, and lung. During this asymptomatic, prodromal period, variola virus can be recovered from the blood, but the yield is lower than later in the illness. Clinical manifestations begin acutely with malaise, fever, rigors, vomiting, headache, and backache; 15% of patients develop delirium. Approximately 10% of light-skinned patients exhibit an erythematous

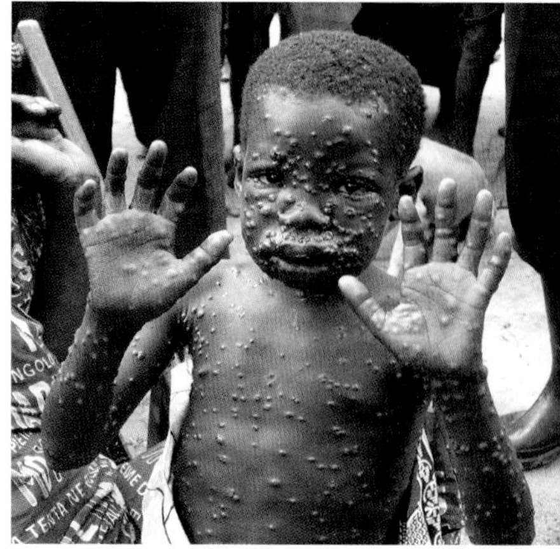

Figure 57.1 Typical presentation of smallpox and monkeypox with synchronized eruption of lesions on the face and extremities and lower densities of lesions on the trunk (centrifugal distribution). This patient was a 7-year-old boy in a recent monkeypox virus outbreak in the Democratic Republic of the Congo.

rash during this phase. After 2–3 more days, an enanthem appears concomitantly with a discrete rash on the face, hands, and forearms. Because of the lack of a keratin layer on mucous membranes, lesions shed infected epithelial cells and give rise to infectious oropharyngeal secretions in the first few days of the eruptive illness, and occasionally 24 hours before eruption.[30] These respiratory secretions are the most important but not the sole means of virus transmission. Following subsequent eruptions on the lower extremities, the rash spreads centrally during the next week to the trunk. Lesions quickly progress from macules to papules and eventually to pustular vesicles (***Fig. 57.1***). Lesions are more abundant on the extremities and face, and this centrifugal distribution is an important diagnostic feature. In contrast to the lesions seen in varicella, smallpox lesions on various segments of the body remain generally synchronous in their stage of development. From 8 to 14 days after onset, the pustules form scabs, which leave depressed depigmented scars on healing. Although variola titers in the throat, conjunctiva, and urine diminish with time,[2] virus can readily be recovered from scabs throughout convalescence.[31] Therefore, patients should be isolated and considered infectious until all scabs separate.

Two distinct forms of smallpox were recognized in the last century of smallpox occurrence. Variola major, the highly virulent, prototypical, and historically significant form of the disease, remained prevalent in Asia and parts of Africa during the twentieth century. Variola minor was distinguished by milder systemic toxicity and more diminutive pox lesions.[29] However, Dixon reported many cases that were indistinguishable from variola major in his extensive comparison of lesion types.[32] Korte first described variola minor, originally in Africa, in 1904. Chapin found a similar mild form known as alastrim that occurred in North America as early as 1896 and subsequently was reported in South America, Europe, and Australia. Two distinct viral strains of reduced virulence caused variola minor and alastrim, and both typically caused 1% mortality in unvaccinated individuals.[11,29]

The Rao classification specified five clinical presentations of variola.[33] Three-quarters of variola major cases were designated classic or ordinary type. After prodromal fever and constitutional symptoms appeared, patients developed the typical variola rash, centrifugal in distribution, with synchronous progression from macules to papules, to vesicles to pustules, and then to scabs. The fatality rate was 3% in vaccinated patients and 30% in unvaccinated patients. Other clinical presentations of smallpox occurred less frequently, probably because of the difference in host immune response. Flat-type smallpox, noted in 2–5% of smallpox patients, was characterized by both severe systemic toxicity and the slow evolution of flat, soft, focal skin lesions that did not resemble the classical variola exanthem. This syndrome caused 66% mortality in vaccinated patients and 95% mortality in unvaccinated patients. Fewer than 3% of smallpox patients developed hemorrhagic-type smallpox, which was accompanied by extensive petechiae, mucosal hemorrhage, and intense toxemia; death usually occurred before typical pox lesions developed.[34] However, on occasion, hemorrhagic smallpox also occurred in the classic type later in the disease. Both hemorrhagic-type and flat-type smallpox may have indicated underlying immunodeficiency; hemorrhagic forms occurred more commonly in pregnant women and young children.[35] The modified type, which occurred typically but not exclusively in previously vaccinated individuals, was characterized by moderation of constitutional symptoms, typically reduced numbers of lesions, and rapid evolution of lesions, with scabs formed by the ninth day of the illness. *Variola sine eruptione* was characterized by prodromal fever and constitutional symptoms. These patients, most of whom had been vaccinated, never developed a rash.[33] In actuality, the manifestations of variola infection fall along a spectrum, and classification is primarily for the purpose of prognosis.

Bacterial superinfection of pox lesions was relatively common in the pre-antibiotic era, especially in the absence of proper hygiene and medical care and in tropical environments.[2] Arthritis and osteomyelitis developed late in the disease in about 1–2% of patients, occurred more frequently in children, and often manifested as bilateral joint involvement, particularly of the elbows.[36] Viral inclusion bodies could be demonstrated in the joint effusion and bone marrow of the involved extremity. Cough and bronchitis were occasionally reported as prominent manifestations of smallpox, with implications for spread of contagion; however, pneumonia was unusual.[2] Pulmonary edema occurred frequently in hemorrhagic-type and flat-type smallpox. Orchitis was noted in approximately 0.1% of patients. Encephalitis developed in 1 in 500 cases of variola major. Keratitis and corneal ulcers were important complications of smallpox, progressing to blindness in slightly less than 1% of cases. Disease during pregnancy precipitated high perinatal mortality, and congenital infection was also recognized.

Partial immunity caused by vaccination resulted in modified-type smallpox, in which sparse skin lesions evolved variably, often without pustules, and quickly, with crusting occurring as early as the seventh day of illness. When exposed to smallpox, some fully immune individuals developed fever, sore throat, and conjunctivitis (called contact fever), which lasted several days but did not give rise to the toxicity or minor skin lesions that signify *variola sine eruptione*. Persons who recovered from smallpox possessed long-lasting immunity, although a second attack may have occurred in 1 in 1000 persons after an intervening period of 15–20 years.[36] Both humoral and cellular responses are thought to be important components of recovery from infection. Neutralizing antibodies peak 2–3 weeks following onset and last longer than 5 years,[37] up to several decades in some individuals.[15]

Monkeypox

The clinical features of human monkeypox are classically described as being similar to those of smallpox.[38] Disease begins with a 2- to 4-day phase with high fever and prostration. The rash develops and progresses synchronously over 2–4 weeks, evolving from macules to papules, to vesicles and pustules, to scabs. Lesions are usually umbilicated, have a centrifugal distribution, and involve the palms and soles. Sore throat and frank tonsillitis frequently occur during the eruptive phase of human monkeypox.[38,39] Lymphadenopathy is a common finding that differentiates monkeypox from smallpox. Lymphadenopathy, which has been documented in up to 83% of unvaccinated persons with monkeypox, arises most frequently early in the course of infection, involving the submandibular and cervical lymph nodes and less frequently the axillary and inguinal nodes.

Clinical manifestations of human monkeypox are likely more diverse and not as stereotypical as those of smallpox. Mild infections were frequent in the first recognized African cases, with 14% of patients having fewer than 25 lesions and no incapacity.[38] In a series of 282 patients, the exanthem first appeared somewhere other than the face in 18% of the vaccinated patients; 31% of vaccinated patients had pleomorphic or "cropping" appearance of rash lesions, and 9.4% had centripetal distribution.[40] All of these features are inconsistent with a mimic of smallpox. Patients in the recent US outbreak tended to have fewer mild lesions than most African patients. Patients were hospitalized in only 19 of 78 suspected cases in the United States, and only two had significant illness requiring some form of medical intervention.[41] None of the initial cases was suspected as a smallpox-like disease. A *sine eruptione* form of monkeypox has not been described, but the number of serologically diagnosed infections without consistent rash illness suggests that it is a possibility.[42] A hemorrhagic form of human monkeypox has not been documented.[43,44] The low incidence of serious disease in the US outbreak is related to the West African origin of the virus; West African monkeypox strains are believed to be less virulent than those from the central African clade.[45] Complications of monkeypox are more common in unvaccinated persons and children.[46]

During intensive surveillance in the Democratic Republic of the Congo between 1980 and 1986, secondary bacterial superinfection of the skin was the most common complication (19.2% of unvaccinated patients), followed by pulmonary disease/pneumonia (11.6% of unvaccinated patients), vomiting/diarrhea/dehydration (6.8% of unvaccinated patients), and keratitis (4.4% of unvaccinated patients). With the exception of keratitis, the incidence of these complications in vaccinated persons was at least threefold less. Alopecia has been noted in some cases.[47] Encephalitis was detected in at least one monkeypox case in the Democratic Republic of the Congo and in one of the cases in the US outbreak of 2003.[40,41] As in smallpox, permanent pitted scars are often left after scabs separate. Monkeypox is now established in endemic sites in the Democratic Republic of the Congo, and on occasion chains of transmission over six generations have been documented.[48,49]

Severity of disease and death are related to age and vaccination status, with younger unvaccinated children faring worse.[38,47,50] The case-fatality rate in Africa varied in different outbreaks and periods of increased surveillance. The fatality rate was 17% from 1970 through 1979, 10% from 1981 through 1986, and 1.5% from 1996 through 1997.[51] No fatalities occurred among 72 suspected cases in the recent US outbreak. The presence of comorbid illnesses, such as measles, malaria, or diarrheal disease, may have a significant impact on mortality in children.[46] Cause of death in monkeypox is not universally clear, although 19 of 33 fatalities in one series of patients involved pulmonary distress or bronchopneumonia, suggesting superimposed bacterial pneumonia.

Other Orthopoxviruses Infecting Humans

Cowpox virus (CPXV) is found primarily in Europe and is maintained in a rodent reservoir that includes voles, mice, and possibly rats. Although CPXV is enzootic in rodents, it has a particularly broad host range, with humans, cats, cows, and exotic zoo animals all serving as incidental hosts for infection.[52,53] CPXV infections in humans are rare and most commonly associated with exposure to infected domestic cats and rodents.[54–57] Cowpox is primarily a localized, cutaneous disease. Baxby, Bennett, and Getty reviewed 54 cases of cowpox infection with a detailed discussion of clinical manifestations.[58] Disease usually consists of a single pock-like lesion on the hands or face, although multiple lesions are seen in roughly one-quarter of cases. Typical lesions progress from macule to papule to vesicle to pustule to dark eschar, with a hemorrhagic base being common in the late vesicular stage. Progression from macule to eschar is slow, often evolving over 2–3 weeks. Local edema, induration, and inflammation are common and can be pronounced. Lesions are painful and are accompanied by regional lymphadenopathy. Complete healing and scab separation usually occur within 6–8 weeks after onset, but may take 12 weeks or longer. A majority of patients experience some constitutional symptoms before the eschar stage.

The majority of human cowpox infections are self-limited and without complication. Ocular involvement, including the cornea, can occur, but usually resolves without permanent damage. A few severe generalized cowpox infections have been reported, including one fatality.[58] Three of these four described cases included a history of atopic dermatitis, indicating a risk of increased severity of disease analogous to vaccinia.

Buffalopox infection in humans has not been extensively described. Limited data suggest that human infection usually occurs on the hands and consists of inflamed and painful pustular lesions progressing through a Jennerian evolution.[59,60] Regional lymphadenopathy and fever can accompany local disease.[60,61]

PATHOGENESIS AND IMMUNITY

Persons who recovered from smallpox possessed long-lasting immunity, although a second attack could occur in 1 in 1000 persons after an intervening period of 15–20 years.[36] Both humoral and cellular responses are important components of recovery from infection. Neutralizing antibodies peak 2–3 weeks following onset, and last longer than 5 years,[37] and perhaps several decades in some individuals.[15]

Most knowledge about smallpox pathogenesis is inferred from animal studies of mousepox,[62,63] rabbitpox,[63] and monkeypox[64,65] in their respective hosts, and from vaccinia in humans. Studies using primates infected with variola[66] corroborate these findings and lend further insight into human smallpox and monkeypox infections. In both natural and experimental infections, the virus is introduced via the respiratory tract, where it first seeds the mucous membranes, including membranes of the eye, and then passes into local lymph nodes. The first round of replication occurs in the lymph nodes, followed by a transient viremia, which seeds tissues, especially those of the reticuloendothelial system, including regional lymph nodes, spleen, and tonsils. A second, brief viremia transports the virus to the skin and to visceral tissues immediately before the prodromal phase. Characteristic skin lesions develop following viral invasion of the capillary epithelium of the dermal layer. The virus may also be present in urine and conjunctival secretions.[67] At death, most visceral tissues contain massive virus concentrations.

In a review of all pathology reports published in English over the previous 200 years,[68] Martin suggested that generally healthy patients who died of smallpox usually died of renal failure, shock secondary to volume depletion, and difficulty with oxygenation and ventilation as a result of viral pneumonia and airway compromise, respectively. Degeneration of hepatocytes might have caused a degree of compromise, but liver failure was not usually the proximate cause of death.

Much of the pathogenesis of smallpox remains a mystery because of the limited tools available when it was an endemic disease. Detailed analysis of the pathophysiology of the disease course using the monkeypox and variola primate models and in comparison with limited clinical and pathology data from human smallpox victims suggests a role for dysregulation of the immune response involving the production of proinflammatory cytokines, lymphocyte apoptosis, and the development of coagulation abnormalities. High viral burdens, which were identified in numerous target tissues in the animal models, were probably associated with organ dysfunction and multisystem failure. Immunohistochemistry studies showing the distribution of viral antigens as well as electron microscopic evidence of the replicating virus correlated with pathology in the lymphoid tissues, skin, oral mucosa, gastrointestinal tract, reproductive system, and liver (***Figs 57.2 and 57.3***). Apoptosis was a prominent observation in lymphoid tissues, with a striking loss of T cells observed. The cause of this widespread apoptosis remains unknown. However, strong production of proinflammatory cytokines at least in part likely contributed to the upregulation of various proapoptotic genes. The strong upregulation of cytokines may also have contributed to the development of a hemorrhagic diathesis. The detection of D-dimers and other changes in hematologic parameters in monkeys that developed classical or hemorrhagic smallpox suggests that activation of the coagulation cascade is a component of both disease syndromes. In human populations, however, hemorrhagic smallpox occurred in approximately 1–3% of the total cases observed. While the majority of hemorrhagic cases died early before the evolution of classic skin lesions, a few died later after classic disease.

From these recent studies of variola and monkeypox virus infection in primates, the "toxemia" described by clinicians for human smallpox[2] may be fundamentally related to the processes underlying septic shock.[69]

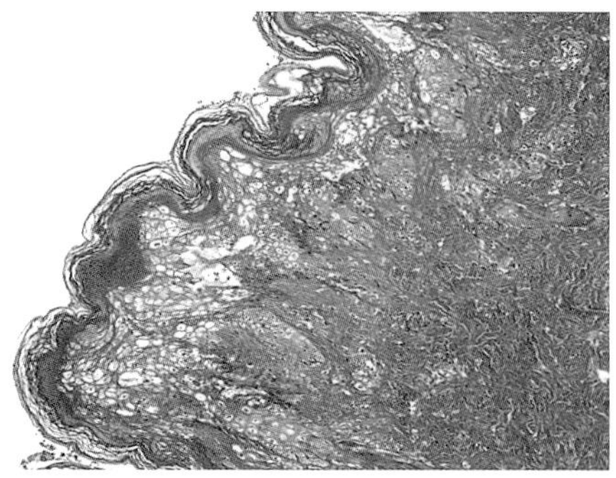

Figure 57.2 Vesicular lesion with epithelial ballooning and degeneration in skin of a human smallpox victim. (Hematoxylin and eosin, ×10.)

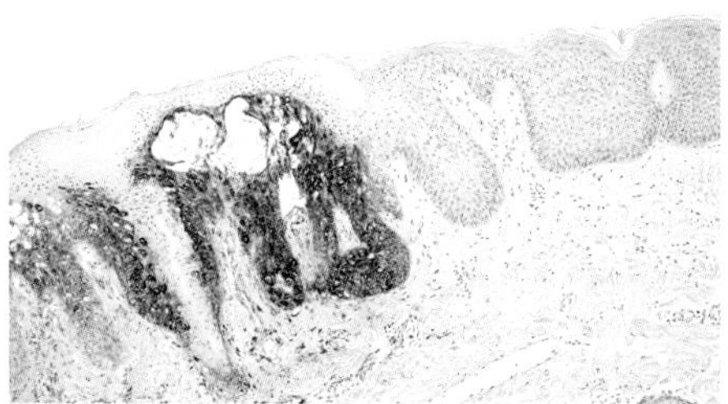

Figure 57.3 Immunohistochemical staining of orthopoxviral antigens in association with epithelial ballooning degeneration and vesiculation in the skin of a smallpox victim. (Immunohistochemistry, ×10.)

Common denominators include lymphocyte apoptosis; proinflammatory cytokines (exuberant production of type I interferon (IFN), interleukin-6 (IL-6), tumor necrosis factor-α (TNF-α), and IFN-γ measurable in plasma); and disseminated intravascular coagulation. Aberrant activation of these pathways, which contributes to toxic shock, is a hallmark of pathological activation of the innate immune system.

To facilitate viral replication, orthopoxviruses generally modulate their host's immune response to the pathogen's advantage. Poxviruses encode proteins that target or interrupt the natural inflammatory response and interfere with apoptosis, synthesis of steroids, and initiation of the complement system. In general, either these proteins block extracellular immune signals (by mimicking or interfering with cytokine/chemokine proteins and/or receptors), or they work intracellularly by interfering with apoptosis, targeting of the virus by the immune system, or intracellular immune cell signaling. A combination of these mechanisms may allow the virus to overcome immunologic surveillance and establish clinical disease in the host.[19,22,70]

DIAGNOSIS

Clinical Diagnosis

The clinical presentation of smallpox is similar to that of many vesicular and pustular rash illnesses, including varicella, herpes simplex, drug reactions, and erythema multiforme. Although the index of suspicion for an eradicated disease may be low, the failure to recognize a case of smallpox could result in the exposure of hospital contacts and the seeding of an outbreak. The Smallpox Diagnosis and Evaluation page on the CDC website (www.bt.cdc.gov/agent/smallpox/diagnosis) is an essential resource to assist a clinician in evaluating a febrile patient presenting with a rash. This site contains an algorithm to quickly determine the likelihood of clinical smallpox and a standardized worksheet to classify the risk of smallpox using the CDC criteria.

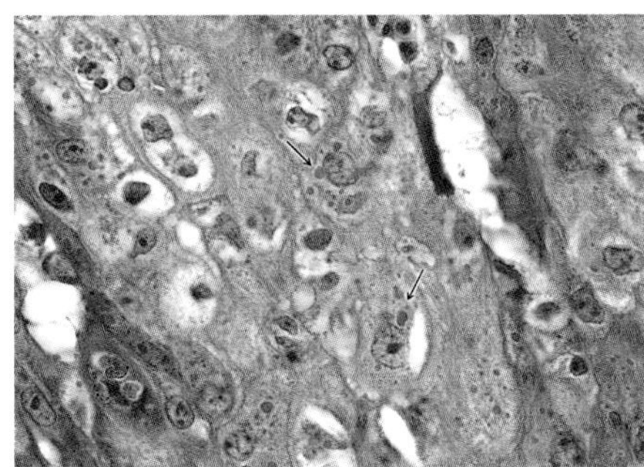

Figure 57.4 Human smallpox skin lesion with intracytoplasmic viral inclusions or Guarnieri bodies (arrows). (Giemsa stain, ×40.)

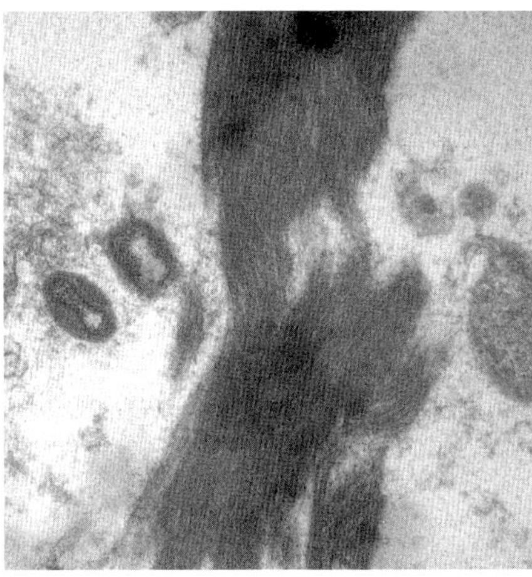

Figure 57.5 Electron microscopic visualization of the characteristic brick-like virion with a dumbbell core typical of orthopoxvirus infections. Virus was visualized in association with fibrin in dendritic cells in this thin section obtained from the spleen of a monkey experimentally infected with variola.

Laboratory Diagnosis

Collection of appropriate specimens is paramount for accurate laboratory diagnosis of *Orthopoxvirus* infection. For virologic diagnosis, specimens from skin lesions are most important because when viremia does occur in *Orthopoxvirus* infections, it is an early phenomenon.[29] Ideally, cutaneous tissue and blood are sent for diagnostic testing, with other samples being sent at the request of public health officials or experts in the field.[43] Detailed instructions for specimen collection can be found in the Department of Defense Smallpox Response Plan (http://www.bt.cdc.gov/agent/smallpox/response-plan/index.asp) or on the CDC website (http://www.cdc.gov/ncidod/monkeypox/diagspecimens.htm). Briefly, vesicles or pustules should be unroofed, the detached vesicle skin sent in a dry tube, and the base of the lesion scraped to make a touch-prep on a glass slide. Biopsy specimens should be split (if possible) and sent in formalin and in a dry tube. If scabs are collected, two scabs should be sent in a dry tube. Dacron or polyester swabs should be used for oropharyngeal specimens and transported in dry tubes. Blood should be collected in a marble-topped or yellow-topped serum separator tube (which is then centrifuged to separate serum) and in a purple-topped anticoagulant tube for whole blood. Clinical specimens potentially containing orthopoxviruses other than variola virus, including monkeypox virus, may be handled in a biosafety level 2 hood using biosafety level 3 practices.[71] Many phenotypic and genotypic methods involving virologic, immunologic, and molecular approaches have been used to identify *Orthopoxvirus*.

Phenotypic Diagnosis

In the past, a presumptive diagnosis of orthopoxviruses required a laboratory with capabilities and expertise in viral diagnostics. Microscopists with experience in poxvirus infections can often recognize the characteristic inclusion bodies (Guarnieri bodies, corresponding to B-type poxvirus inclusions) (***Fig. 57.4***) in tissue samples under light microscopy. These cytoplasmic inclusions are hematoxylinophilic, stain reddish purple with Giemsa stain, and contain Feulgen-positive material. Microscopy alone cannot differentiate members of the *Orthopoxvirus* genus, yet the epidemiologic setting can suggest which species is involved. The orthopoxviruses with pathogenicity for humans (with the exception of molluscum contagiosum) can be grown on the chorioallantoic membranes of 12-day-old embryonated chicken eggs, where they form characteristic pocks. These viruses also grow readily in easily obtained cell cultures, including monkey kidney cell lines, Vero, BSC-1, and A549. Variola can characteristically be differentiated from other viruses by a strict temperature cut-off at 39°C. Methods for isolation and identification of individual virus species have been reviewed.[72] Electron microscopy reveals the unmistakable brick-like morphology of orthopoxviruses in thin sections of infected materials (***Fig. 57.5***). Immunogold stains permit more precise identification to the species level.

Immunodiagnosis

Serologic testing for anti-*Orthopoxvirus* antibodies is an old technique, and various assays were used extensively in the study of smallpox.[29] However, significant serologic cross-reactivity exists among all the *Orthopoxvirus* species; therefore, species differentiation is not possible with conventional serologic assays. Techniques developed in the 1980s to detect monkeypox-specific antibodies are complex and considered unreliable by some experts.[42,73] Although complement-fixation tests detect antibodies that disappear within 12 months of infection, other traditional techniques, such as immunofluorescence assay, radioimmunoassay, enzyme-linked immunosorbent assay (ELISA), hemagglutination-inhibition and neutralization assay, detect immunoglobulin (IgG) antibodies that are persistent. Thus, differentiating antibodies because of acute infection from antibodies resulting from prior vaccination can be difficult with single specimens.

Recently, immunofluorescence assay and ELISAs have been used to detect IgM in acute infection directed against cowpox and monkeypox, respectively.[73] Because IgM seems to disappear within 6 months, ELISAs can be used to detect recent infections but cannot be used after lesions have healed and scabs have separated. In the investigation of the 2003 US monkeypox outbreak, the CDC relied on anti-*Orthopoxvirus* IgG and IgM ELISAs for serologic diagnosis.[41] More recently, a combination of T-cell measurements and a novel IgG ELISA was used to enhance epidemiologic follow-up studies to this outbreak.[74,75]

Nucleic Acid Diagnosis

The molecular diagnostic approaches, including DNA sequencing, polymerase chain reaction (PCR), restriction fragment-length polymorphism (RFLP), real-time PCR, and microarrays, are more sensitive and specific than the conventional virologic and immunologic approaches. Of these techniques, sequencing provides the highest level of specificity for species or strain identification, but current sequencing techniques are not yet as practical as rapid diagnostic tools in most laboratories. RFLP analysis[76,77] and microarray genotyping[78] also provide high levels of specificity, and when combined with PCR, these approaches can offer high levels of sensitivity. Real-time PCR methods provide exquisite levels of sensitivity and specificity.[77]

Successful performance of PCR-based diagnostics requires extraction of DNA from body fluid and tissue samples, careful design of oligonucleotide primers and probes, and optimization of amplification and detection conditions. There are numerous commercial nucleic acid purification methods for various sample types, which involve cell lysis and protein denaturation followed by DNA precipitation or fractionation by reversible binding to an affinity matrix. Selection of appropriate primers, probes, and optimization of assay conditions require knowledge of genome sequences and molecular biology techniques.

One of the basic techniques used in PCR-based diagnostics is gel analysis, in which PCR-amplified regions of the genome are separated on agarose gels by electrophoresis, and the amplicon sizes are used to identify the sample. Several PCR gel-analytic assays have been used to identify cowpox, monkeypox, vaccinia, and variola viruses from clinical specimens.[72,79–81]

Large fragment PCR-RFLP (LPCR-RFLP) analysis requires amplifying large DNA fragments with high-fidelity DNA polymerase enzymes. The amplified LPCR products are purified on agarose gels and digested with a restriction enzyme. The digested DNA fragments are then separated electrophoretically on polyacrylamide gels for a constant period at constant voltage and stained with ethidium bromide. The restriction pattern is then visualized and photographed with a digital camera. The positions for all DNA fragments in each restriction pattern are determined and digitized by appropriate fingerprinting software. From this pattern, a similarity coefficient is calculated for every pair of restriction patterns and used as an index for species differentiation.

Recently developed real-time PCR assays, which can be performed in a few hours, can test clinical specimens for all orthopoxviruses or for specific species such as vaccinia, variola, or monkeypox.[41,77,82,83] Real-time PCR was one of the diagnostic techniques used in the investigation of the 2003 US monkeypox outbreak.[41] Because of its sensitivity, rapidity, and ease, real-time PCR will likely become the primary method of preliminary diagnosis of *Orthopoxvirus* infection, with isolation and growth in a high-level containment laboratory reserved for confirmation.

PREVENTION AND CONTROL

Attempts to use infected material to induce immunity to smallpox date to the first millennium; the Chinese used scabs or pus collected from mild smallpox cases to infect recipients usually via insertion of bamboo splinters into the nasal mucosa. This procedure produced disease in a controlled situation that was typically milder than naturally occurring disease and allowed for isolation or controlled exposure of nonimmune individuals. The practice spread to India and from there to Istanbul, where Europeans encountered it in the early eighteenth century. In Europe the inoculation of the skin with infected pock material was later referred to as variolation to distinguish the procedure from vaccination. The practice of variolation, which was never widely accepted, was outlawed at times because many of those inoculated developed grave clinical illness. Variolation often caused a 1–2% mortality rate, and the individuals who died had the potential to transmit natural smallpox. In 1796 Jenner scientifically demonstrated that inoculation with material obtained from a milkmaid's cowpox lesions would result in immunity and protection from infection with smallpox when introduced by inoculation. He published his findings in 1798 and in 1801 reported that 100 000 persons had been vaccinated in England. By the 1820s vaccination had become widespread throughout Britain and much of Europe. Although derivation of current vaccinia strains is uncertain, it is not a form of cowpox, and because Jenner lost his original material used for vaccination, the specific source of current vaccinia strains remains unknown.[32] The United States began regulating production of the vaccine in 1925. Since then, the New York City Board of Health strain of vaccinia has been used as the primary US vaccine strain. Smallpox vaccination, as part of the global WHO program, eventually led to the disease's eradication, with the last case of natural serially transmitted smallpox reported in 1977. Routine vaccination of children in the United States ceased in 1971, and vaccination of hospital workers ceased in 1976. Because of the perceived risk of bioterrorism, smallpox vaccination in at-risk military personnel and civilian health care workers was resumed in 2003.[84,85]

During the WHO global eradication program, most of the human population received vaccinia virus by scarification. Although there were multiple manufacturers worldwide, and vaccine lots varied with respect to potency and purity, almost all vaccinia administered was derived from one of two lineages, the New York Board of Health and Lister strains.[29] Live vaccinia virus suspension was placed as a drop on the skin or drawn up by capillary action between the tines of a bifurcated needle; the nominal dose of live vaccinia was about 10^5 virions. Usually, primary vaccination is uneventful; following introduction into the skin, the virus replicates in basal layer keratinocytes, spreads cell-to-cell, and leads to discrete vesicle formation. Within a week, the vesicle evolves into a pustule surrounded by inflammatory tissue. This lesion scabs over within 10–14 days; eventually, the scab is shed. Vaccinees in the global campaign often experienced tender axillary lymph nodes, fever, and malaise for brief periods. Occasionally, however, complications arose with varying degrees of severity. Accidental transfer of vaccinia from the inoculation site was common, but of little consequence unless transferred to the eye. Generalized vaccinia, which involved systemic spread of the virus and eruption of multiple pocks at distant sites, was more serious; in individuals with eczema or atopic dermatitis, however, it sometimes led to extensive inflammation and secondary bacterial infection. More serious, life-threatening complications arose in vaccinees with defects in cell-mediated immunity; the vaccination site frequently enlarged to form an ulcer, secondary ulcers appeared, and the infection cleared slowly or not at all. The most serious event was postvaccinial encephalitis. Although rare, this condition was frequently fatal. Death occurred in approximately one in 1 million primary vaccinations.[86,87] Adverse events may be more frequent and severe if mass immunization were to be resumed in an unscreened general population that now includes transplant recipients on immunosuppressive drugs, HIV-infected individuals, and geriatric patients.

Recent Vaccination Campaigns

The requirement that any alternative vaccine must not be inferior to live vaccinia sets a high standard. The successful immunization or "take rate" has been greater than 95%, both historically and in a more recent series of over 450 000 military vaccinees.[84] In this recent series, one case of encephalitis and 37 cases of myopericarditis were documented in a prescreened, healthy, young adult population. Although the incidence of myopericarditis was below the historical average and the cases were mild, this adverse event contributed to the general reluctance of the civilian health care population to accept vaccination.[85] Recently, a potential replacement vaccine was prepared in massive quantities (>300 million doses) by selection of plaque-purified progeny virus from the New York Board of Health strain, which was amplified in Vero cell cultures. This vaccine is more purified and free of adventitious agents in comparison with its predecessor, which was prepared on calf skin. Phase I safety and immunogenicity trials for ACAM 2000 indicate greater than 95% take rates and adverse events comparable to those of live vaccinia.[88] Historically, live (replicating) vaccinia immunization has also been used as postexposure prophylaxis and is believed effective if administered within 4 days of exposure.

The recent immunization of modest numbers of military and civilian individuals has provided an opportunity to study the nature of adverse events using modern tools of immunology. A strong association was established between adverse events and increased systemic cytokines, in particular, IFN-γ, TNF-α, IL-5, and IL-10.[89] Some researchers have speculated that cardiac events, although rare, may be related to dramatic alterations in cytokine profiles.

Protective immunity elicited by live vaccinia is thought to depend on a combination of humoral and cellular immune responses. Using a monkey model in which animals are immunized with vaccinia and challenged with monkeypox, Edghill-Smith has shown that vaccinia-specific B cells are critical for protection.[90] Antibody depletion of B cells, but not $CD4^+$ or $CD8^+$ T cells, abrogated vaccinia-induced protection. Modified Vaccinia Ankara (MVA) is an alternative vaccine that has promise as a nonreplicating immunogen. MVA, which was used in Germany in the later stages of global eradication, was shown to be safe and immunogenic, but its protective efficacy has not been established in humans.[91] MVA was generated by over 500 serial passages in chick embryo fibroblasts, which resulted in multiple deletions and mutations and an inability to replicate efficiently in human and most other mammalian cells.[92] Ultrastructural examination of purified MVA reveals that most of the particles are enveloped; the host restriction occurs at a late stage of maturation. The presence of enveloped particles is believed to be important to the elicitation of protective immunity. Experimentally, MVA was demonstrated to protect monkeys against monkeypox virus challenge, after one or two doses of MVA or MVA followed by Dryvax.[93] Surprisingly, a single dose of MVA also protected when challenge followed immunization by as few as 10 days, although protection was not absolute; a modest number of pocks and low-level viremia occurred in the MVA recipients following challenge.

An alternative vaccine, licensed in Japan, is LC16m8, which was derived from the Lister strain of vaccinia by passaging multiple times, with selection for an attenuated phenotype. In contrast to replication-deficient vaccines such as MVA, LC16m8 retains the majority of the vaccinia genome[94] and is capable of replication at the site of inoculation, hence producing a "take" lesion in vaccinees. This vaccine has been demonstrated to protect cynomolgus monkeys against monkeypox challenge[95] and is associated with fewer common or serious adverse events than Dryvax or ACAM 2000.[96]

Current recommendations for the administration of ACAM 2000 in the event of a recurrence of smallpox in the United States are provided at www.bt.cdc.gov/agent/smallpox/response-plan. In brief, vaccination is performed with a bifurcated needle onto which the reconstituted vaccinia preparation has been drawn, using 15 jabs in the skin, with enough strength to produce a visible trace of bleeding. The resulting vaccination lesion is then kept covered with a nonadherent and nonimpervious dressing. Care must be taken to prevent inadvertent inoculation of the vaccinee or others. In primary vaccinees, a papule forms within 5 days, developing into a vesicle on the fifth or sixth day post vaccination, which signifies a major reaction, or take. The vesicle subsequently becomes pustular, swelling subsides, and a crust forms, which detaches in 14–21 days. At the height of the primary reaction, known as the Jennerian response, regional lymphadenopathy usually occurs, which may be accompanied by systemic manifestations of fever and malaise. Primary vaccination with vaccine at potency of 100 million pock-forming units per mL elicits a 97% response rate both by major reaction and neutralizing antibody responses.

Outcome

During global eradication using a variety of vaccinia-based vaccines, successful smallpox vaccination provided high-level immunity for the majority of recipients for 3–5 years followed by decreasing immunity. In Mack's review of cases in Europe from 1950 through 1972, he provided epidemiologic evidence of some relative protection from death, if not from disease severity, in individuals who had been immunized over 20 years before exposure. However, for the older population, in particular, vaccination within 10 years of exposure did not prevent all cases but did prevent smallpox deaths.[97] Multiple vaccinations are thought to produce more long-lasting immunity. Vaccination has been effective in preventing disease in 95% of vaccinees. Vaccination also was shown to prevent or substantially lessen the severity of infection when given as secondary prophylaxis within a few days of exposure.[2]

Contraindications

Smallpox vaccination is contraindicated in the pre-outbreak setting for individuals with the following conditions or those having close contact with individuals with the following conditions: a history of atopic dermatitis (eczema); active acute, chronic, or exfoliative skin conditions that disrupt the epidermis; pregnancy or the possibility of becoming pregnant; or a compromised immune system as a consequence of HIV infection, acquired immunodeficiency syndrome, autoimmune disorders, cancer, radiation treatment, immunosuppressive therapy, or other immunodeficiencies.

Adverse Events

Vaccinia can be transmitted from a vaccinee's unhealed vaccination site to other persons by close contact, and the same adverse events as with intentional vaccination can result. Adverse reactions to smallpox vaccination are diagnosed by a clinical examination. Most reactions can be managed with observation and supportive measures. Self-limited reactions include fever, headache, fatigue, myalgia, chills, local skin reactions, nonspecific rash, erythema multiforme, lymphadenopathy, and pain at the vaccination site. Adverse reactions that require further evaluation and possible therapeutic intervention include inadvertent inoculation involving the eye, generalized vaccinia, eczema vaccinatum, progressive vaccinia, postvaccinial central nervous system (CNS) disease, and fetal vaccinia.[98]

Inadvertent inoculation generally results in a condition that is self-limited unless it involves the eye or eyelid, which requires an ophthalmologist's evaluation. Topical treatment with trifluridine or vidarabine is often recommended, although treatment of ocular vaccinia is not specifically approved by the Food and Drug Administration (FDA) for either of these drugs. Most published experience is with use of vidarabine, but this drug is no longer manufactured.

Generalized vaccinia is characterized by a disseminated maculopapular or vesicular rash, frequently on an erythematous base and typically occurring 6–9 days after primary vaccination. Treatment with vaccinia immune globulin (VIG) is restricted to those who are systemically ill or have an immunocompromising condition or recurrent disease that can last up to a year. Contact precautions should be used to prevent further transmission and nosocomial infection.[98]

Eczema vaccinatum occurs in individuals with a history of atopic dermatitis, regardless of current disease activity, and can be a papular, vesicular, or pustular rash. This rash may be generalized, or localized with involvement anywhere on the body, with a predilection for areas of previous atopic dermatitis lesions. Mortality ranges from 17% to 30% and is reduced by use of VIG.

Progressive vaccinia is a rare, severe, and often fatal complication of vaccination that occurs in individuals with immunodeficiency conditions and is characterized by painless progressive necrosis at the vaccination site with or without metastases to distant sites. This condition carries a high mortality rate; therefore, progressive vaccinia should be aggressively treated with VIG, intensive monitoring, and tertiary medical center level support. Anecdotal experience has shown that despite treatment with VIG, individuals with cell-mediated immunity defects have a poorer prognosis than those with humoral defects. Infection control measures should include contact and respiratory precautions to prevent transmission and nosocomial infection.[98]

CNS disease, which includes postvaccinial encephalopathy and postvaccinial encephalomyelitis, occurs rarely after smallpox vaccination. Postvaccinial encephalopathy occurs more frequently, typically affects infants and children younger than age 2, and reflects vascular damage to the CNS. Symptoms that typically occur 6–10 days post vaccination include seizures, hemiplegia, aphasia, and transient amnesia. The cause for CNS disease is unknown, and no specific therapy exists. Therefore, intervention is limited to anticonvulsant therapy and intensive supportive care. Fetal vaccinia, which results from vaccinial transmission from mother to fetus, is a rare but serious complication of smallpox vaccination during or immediately before delivery.[98] Recently, antiviral drugs including cidofovir and ST-246 have been used either alone or sequentially to treat serious adverse events associated with vaccinia infection.[99]

In the Department of Defense 2002–2003 vaccination program involving 540 824 vaccinees, 67 symptomatic cases of myopericarditis were reported, for a rate of 1.2 per 10 000. Mean time from vaccination to evaluation for myopericarditis was 10.4 days, with a range of 3–25 days. Reports of myocarditis in vaccinees in 2003 raised concerns of carditis and cardiac deaths in individuals undergoing smallpox vaccination. That year, 21 cases of myopericarditis out of 36 217 vaccinees were reported, with 19 (90%) occurring in revaccinees. The median age of those affected was 48 years, and they were predominantly women. Eleven of the individuals were hospitalized, but there were no fatalities. Of the 540 824 total vaccinees over the 2 years, 449 198 were military personnel (the rest were civilians), and of these there were 37 cases of myopericarditis, for an occurrence rate of 1 per 12 000 vaccinees.[4] Although no clear association has been found, history of ischemic heart disease and significant cardiac risk pose relative contraindications for smallpox vaccination.[100]

Smallpox Biothreat Policy

In a smallpox release from a bioterrorist event, individuals would be vaccinated according to the current national policy, which recommends initial vaccination of higher risk groups (individuals directly exposed to the release and those with close contact to smallpox patients) and medical and emergency transport personnel. Vaccination of the general population would then be extended in concentric rings around the initial cases to impede the spread (www.bt.cdc.gov/agent/smallpox/response-plan). There are no absolute contraindications to vaccination for individuals with high-risk exposure to smallpox. Persons at greatest risk of complications of vaccination are also those for whom smallpox infection poses the greatest risk. If relative contraindications exist for an individual, the risks must be weighed against the risk of a potentially fatal smallpox infection.

Postexposure prophylaxis with vaccine offers protection against smallpox but is untried in other *Orthopoxvirus* diseases.[29] Despite a lack of hard evidence, postexposure vaccination is likely efficacious against other orthopoxviruses, and was recommended during the 2003 US monkeypox outbreak for potentially exposed persons.

TREATMENT AND PROGNOSIS

Passive Immunization

VIG is available from the CDC as an investigational new drug in two formulations, intramuscular and intravenous. VIG may be beneficial in treating some of the adverse effects associated with vaccination. VIG has no proven benefit in smallpox treatment, and its efficacy in treatment of monkeypox infections is unknown. Monoclonal antibodies have been shown to be beneficial in animal models under certain conditions, but further development will be required before potential application in humans.

Antiviral Drugs

Antiviral drugs would be useful for treatment of orthopoxviral diseases including smallpox and monkeypox, as well as adverse effects associated with vaccination. Two antiviral drugs are available for treating orthopoxviruses, cidofovir and ST-246, which have been offered under emergency use protocols maintained by both the Department of Health and Human Services and the Department of Defense.[99]

The first drug used to empirically treat progressive vaccinia and smallpox was Marboran, a compound of the class of *N*-aminomethylisatin-beta-thiosemicarbizones. As with most early treatment strategies, controlled clinical trials were not reported. Marboran administration was also associated with severe nausea and vomiting in the majority of patients. Through combinatorial chemistry, potent and more selective analogs have now been discovered and are in preliminary testing.[101]

Initial studies to identify effective antiviral agents for orthopoxviruses tested drugs that had been developed for other viruses and share molecular targets with poxviruses.[102] The effort to discover effective drugs against DNA viruses initially focused on treatment of herpes infections, leading to the discovery of acyclovir. While inactive against some other DNA viruses such as cytomegalovirus, the dCMP analog,[103] cidofovir was subsequently shown to be active and is licensed for treatment of CMV-associated retinitis under the trade name Vistide. Cidofovir protects monkeys against severe disease in both the monkeypox and authentic smallpox primate models, when administered within 48 hours after intravenous exposure to the virus.[104] Although the drug formulation used in these studies is less than optimal since it requires intravenous administration, patients with advanced disease would already be receiving intravenous fluids as part of their supportive care, and once weekly cidofovir administration would not significantly increase the health care burden. Because cidofovir has been associated with nephrotoxicity, primarily in dehydrated patients, careful attention to fluid management is important, and patient hydration and coadministration of probenecid is required. Cidofovir would not be practical for use in a mass casualty situation or public health emergency.

Oral formulations of cidofovir analogs with better bioavailability and lower toxicity, designed to overcome the lack of an active transport pathway for unmodified cidofovir into cells, are under development.[104] Cidofovir requires bolus dosing to allow drug entry into cells by pinocytosis; however, bolus dosing results in transiently high concentrations in the kidney. The primary design paradigm for oral formulations is the creation of a lipid mimic that allows drug to enter cells via the chylomicron pathway. This formulation dramatically reduces transient drug levels in the kidney and eliminates nephrotoxicity in toxicology studies using mice. However, an oral formulation of cidofovir is not yet available for human use.

A number of essential viral enzymes have been targeted using a homology-based bioinformatics approach, such as that used to develop a structural model of vaccinia virus 17L proteinase. A unique chemical library of 51 000 compounds was computationally queried to identify potential active site inhibitors.[105] Through this effort several potent lead structures for optimization were identified including ST-246. ST-246 is potent (EC_{50} =0.010 mmol), selective (CC_{50} >40 mmol), and active against multiple orthopoxviruses, including monkeypox, camelpox, cowpox, ectromelia (mousepox), vaccinia, and variola viruses *in vitro* and cowpox and ectromelia *in vivo*.[106] ST-246 has been employed on several occasions under compassionate use authorization by the FDA to treat life-threatening vaccinia virus infections, either alone or in conjunction with IVIG and cidofovir.[99,107]

The elaborate replication strategy of poxviruses offers a number of potential targets for therapeutic intervention.[108] Although inhibition of viral replication may be necessary to halt the pathogenic disease course, it may not be sufficient; it may also be necessary to reverse the effects of the mounting damage that increasingly appears to be the result of a cytokine storm, which accounts for the "toxicity" of systemic orthopoxvirus infection.[66] In this regard, cytokine antagonists developed to treat bacterial sepsis and other conditions may play a role in effective management of smallpox- and monkeypox-infected patients.

Alternative therapeutic approaches include peptide mimetics of IFN-γ that play a direct role in the activation of STAT1 alpha transcription factor.[109] These mimetics do not act through recognition of the extracellular domain of the IFN-γ receptor; rather, they bind to the cytoplasmic domain of the receptor chain and thereby initiate the cellular signaling. It is hypothesized that mimetics would bypass the poxvirus virulence factor, B8R protein, that binds the intact IFN-γ and would prevent interaction with its receptor. Experimentally, these mimetics, but not intact IFN-γ, inhibit replication of vaccinia in BSC-40 cells. Thus these mimetics can avoid the B8R virulence factor and have potential activity against poxviruses *in vivo*.

Gleevec, a drug licensed for use in chronic myeloid leukemia, has been shown to block the egress of vaccinia virus from infected cells.[110] Smallpox virus includes an epidermal growth factor-like domain that targets human Erb-1, inducing tyrosine phosphorylation of certain host cell substrates, thereby facilitating viral replication. Poxviruses migrate to the cell membrane via the polymerization of actin tails to produce EEV, which facilitates viral dissemination. The rationale is that low molecular weight inhibitors of Erb-1 kinases might function as antiviral agents. CI-1033, one such inhibitor, blocks variola replication in BSC-40 and Vero cells, primarily at the level of secondary viral spreading. CI-1033 protects mice exposed to a lethal vaccinia challenge via the aerosol route. In conjunction with a monoclonal antibody directed against L1R, CI-1033 clears the mice's lungs of virus within 8 days. Gleevec is also a small molecule that inhibits the Abl-1 family of tyrosine kinases, thereby inhibiting the release of EEV from infected cells. Gleevec inhibits the vaccinia virus spread from the mouse peritoneum to the ovaries and protects the mice from lethal intranasal challenge. The advantage of Gleevec over other tyrosine kinase inhibitors such as CI-1033 is that it is already approved for human use. The potential success of Gleevec suggests that strategies that block key host signaling pathways have merit and augment the approaches that target classical viral replication enzymes. An alternative approach to inhibiting the polymerization of actin, which in turn inhibits the propulsion of viral particles along actin filaments toward the cell membrane, is small interfering RNA directed against the Arp2/3 complex.[111]

Lastly, treatment strategies may be developed to target the toxemia or clinical manifestations of smallpox. In particular, modulation of the systemic immune response to orthopox infection, specifically the prevention of organ damage caused by vascular leakage and fibrin deposition, may provide a useful therapeutic target. Uncontrolled or inappropriate immune responses can contribute to multiple organ failure and death; in this respect the "toxemia" associated with fatal orthopox infections resembles severe sepsis. Several treatment strategies for targeting the manifestations of septic shock,[112] such as activated protein C and inhibitors of the tissue factor pathway,[113] are under consideration for testing in the non-human primate model for smallpox.

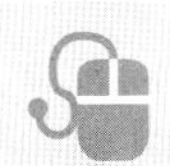

Access the complete reference list online at
http://www.expertconsult.com

CHAPTER 58

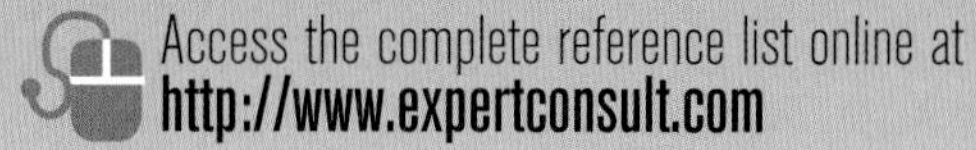
Access the complete reference list online at
http://www.expertconsult.com

Respiratory Viral Infections

José Luiz Proença-Módena • Gustavo Olszanski Acrani • Cynthia B. Snider • Eurico Arruda

INTRODUCTION

Acute respiratory infections (ARIs) are prevalent worldwide[1] and rival diarrhea as the leading cause of death in developing countries (***Fig. 58.1***).[1,2] Unlike pathogens restricted to tropical areas, the respiratory viruses are distributed globally, are efficiently transmitted from person to person, and have impact on all age groups. In impoverished urban populations in South America, ARI symptoms may be present on an almost continuous basis, making it difficult to determine symptom-free days and estimate attack rates.[3,4] The most striking disparity between developing and developed countries with regard to ARI epidemiology is the case-fatality rate of lower respiratory infection (LRI), mainly pneumonia, bronchiolitis, and influenza,[5,6] in children under 5 years of age, which may reach 16% in some areas.[1]

Several community-based studies have established the importance of common respiratory viral infections in tropical countries[7] (***Table 58.1***). In impoverished populations LRI may occur simultaneously with measles, diarrhea, and malnutrition, and can potentially become life-threatening.[1,13]

In most health care facility-based LRI studies conducted in tropical countries, human respiratory syncytial virus (HRSV) has been the virus most frequently detected (11–33%), followed by human metapneumovirus (7–43%), parainfluenza viruses (1–13%), human bocavirus (2–19%), adenoviruses (2–34%), and influenza viruses (1–4%) (***Table 58.2***). Except for a few more recent reports, human rhinovirus (HRV) and human coronaviruses (HCoV) have not been tested in prospective studies conducted in tropical countries. A pathogenic role has been well established for most respiratory viruses, but there is considerable overlap of clinical and pathological features between different viral diseases. Therefore, a direct role of certain viruses in the pathogenesis of a specific respiratory illness is not possible to establish on clinical grounds, which is further complicated when multiple respiratory viruses are detected simultaneously in the same specimen.[22] Detecting viral genomes in respiratory secretions does not necessarily correlate with viral replication and may reflect latency or prolonged shedding unrelated to the current symptoms. Therefore, approaches based on the detection of viable viral progeny or markers of active viral replication should be used in studies of pathogenesis of respiratory viruses.

Saffold virus, a cardiovirus in the family *Picornaviridae*, initially detected in stools from a febrile infant,[23] was recently detected in respiratory samples of children with ARI.[24,25] However, since very little is known regarding the pathogenic role of this agent in respiratory disease, it will not be further discussed here.

Few specific interventions have become available to reduce the impact of viral ARI,[2] and their application may be further hampered by epidemiologic conditions in equatorial regions. Poor housing and crowding, lack of clear seasonal outbreaks in some tropical areas, and insufficient resources to provide influenza immunization or antiviral treatment or HRSV immunoprophylaxis prevail in most developing nations.[26,27] In addition, nutritional and educational interventions, such as reinforcing breastfeeding,[28] vitamin A supplementation for measles,[29] and access to oral rehydration therapy,[30] may have significant effect on the morbidity and mortality due to LRI in its interface with diarrhea.

This chapter addresses the most common viral respiratory infections (***Table 58.3***), highlighting features unique to the developing world.

INFLUENZA VIRUSES

In tropical countries influenza activity may occur year-round, as well as in outbreaks more typical of temperate regions. Twice yearly outbreaks are noted in some areas of Southeast Asia. These infections can have high impact on morbidity and mortality, since impoverished populations have limited access to medical care, including vaccination and antiviral treatments.[31] Influenza virus is considered a prototypic emerging virus, because it undergoes antigenic drift and shift. Antigenic drift occurs by the accumulation of point mutations, where host antibodies from previous circulating strains are ineffective. Antigenic shift, usually caused by reassortment of genes from viruses of animal origin, or sometimes by the crossing of species barriers by animal influenza viruses, generates emerging influenza virus strains that may cause localized outbreaks or pandemics, with enormous potential impact for health on a global scale.[32]

Since the 1997 outbreak of avian influenza A/H5N1 and the 2003 epidemic of SARS coronavirus, global surveillance programs have been implemented to identify emerging infections. In April 2009, such programs identified infections in patients from Southern California, Texas, and subsequently Mexico with a novel influenza A(H1N1). This previously unknown virus was rapidly identified to be a reassortant with gene segments from avian, swine and human viruses[33] and quickly circulated throughout the world, affecting more than 213 countries and being responsible for at least 16 713 deaths as of March 2010[34] (see ***Fig. 14.1***).

THE AGENT

Influenza viruses of the family *Orthomyxoviridae* are pleomorphic, enveloped with segmented negative-strand RNA genomes, distributed in three genera: *Influenzavirus A*, *B*, and *C*, based on the antigenicity of the nucleoprotein (NP) and matrix protein. The type species influenza A virus is further classified in subtypes based on the two surface glycoproteins, hemagglutinin (HA) and neuraminidase (NA).[35] Among the 16 HA and 9 NA recognized subtypes, 6 HA (H1, H2, H3, H5, H7, and H9) and 3 NA (N1, N2, and N7) have been detected in humans.[32] However, only three subtypes of HA (H1, H2, and H3) and two of NA (N1 and N2) have caused pandemics and sustained circulation in human populations.[33] The genomes of influenza viruses consist of eight negative-strand RNA segments in influenza A and B viruses, and seven RNA segments in influenza C.[35]

The viral HA binds to sialic acid-containing cell receptors, and mediates fusion and penetration. Proteolytic cleavage of HA by cellular serine proteases exposes hydrophobic fusion domains that mediate membrane fusion. The NA cleaves terminal sialic acid from glycoconjugates present on respiratory mucins, cells, and progeny virions. This action destroys receptors recognized by HA and allows budding virus to be released from infected cells and to spread within the respiratory tract. Influenza C virus contains a single surface glycoprotein, which binds to receptor, promotes fusion of membranes, and also cleaves sialic acid.[35]

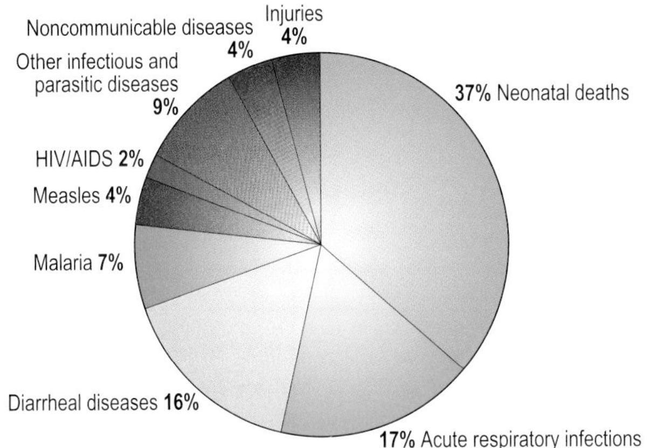

Figure 58.1 Causes of death in children under 5 years of age in the world. (Data from WHO. The global burden of diseases: 2004 update. Geneva: WHO; 2008.)

Virus-receptor binding is followed by internalization into endosomes, acid-dependent fusion of viral and endosomal membranes, and release of genome in the cytoplasm, from where it is transported to the nucleus. In influenza A viruses, the envelope M2 protein serves as an ion channel that facilitates RNA release. Transcription of the negative-strand genomic RNA into positive-strand messenger RNA (mRNA) and complementary RNA (cRNA) is mediated by a viral RNA polymerase complex in the nucleus. cRNA serves as a template for the synthesis of negative-strand RNA genome segments, and mRNA directs viral protein synthesis. Newly assembled nucleocapsids acquire an envelope as they bud through the cell surface and only viruses with a full set of genome segments are infectious.[35]

Influenza A viruses are primarily viruses of aquatic birds, particularly ducks and shore birds, that harbor all of the subtypes recognized to date. Selected subtypes naturally infect a range of terrestrial (swine, horses, humans) and aquatic (seals) mammals; influenza B virus infects humans and uncommonly seals, dogs, cats, and swine; and influenza C virus is primarily a virus of humans. Depending on the virus type and subtype, experimental infection can be induced in mice, ferrets, chickens, swine, and primates, and the viruses can be propagated in primary cultures of

Table 58.1 Detection of Common Respiratory Viruses in Six Representative Community-Based Studies in Tropical Countries

		Respiratory Viruses in Children with Acute Respiratory Infection (%)[a]						
Country	**No. of Samples**	**HRSV**	**HADV**	**HPIV**	**Flu**	**HRV**	**HMPV**	**Reference**
Nepal	919	15.1	–	11	11.2	–	4.2	8
Brazil	1052	–	3.6	5.9	2.1	16.7	–	3
Philippines	311	13.0	3.5	5.1	2.2	–	–	9
Thailand	799	4.4	2.0	4.6	1.7	1.7	–	10
Colombia	506	13.2	1.0	4.7	2.0	–	–	11
The Gambia	221	1.8	8.1	6.3	6.3	–	–	12

[a]Viruses were detected by isolation in cell culture or by antigen detection with immunofluorescence or PCR.

HADV, human adenovirus; Flu, influenza virus; HMPV, human metapneumovirus; HPIV, human parainfluenza virus; HRV, human rhinovirus; HRSV, respiratory syncytial virus.

Table 58.2 Detection of Common Respiratory Viruses in Eight Representative Hospital-Based Studies in Tropical Countries

		Children with Viral Infection (%)[a]							
Country	**No. of Samples**	**HRSV**	**HADV**	**HPIV**	**Flu**	**HRV**	**HMPV**	**HBoV**	**Ref**
Iran	109	12.9	5.9	22.2	10.9	–	–	–	14
Vietnam	659	23	5	–	15	28	4.5	2	15
Malaysia	180	10.5	1.1	2.2	5.5	4.4	–	–	16
Kenya	822	12.0	1.9	2.3	1.0	6.5	–	–	17
Pakistan	1492	32.9	1.9	0.9	1.3	–	–	–	18
Thailand	596	20.3	6.7	13.2	4.2	–	–	–	19
India	809	20.0	4.0	12.0	4.0	–	–	–	20
Philippines	537	11.2	4.0	5.2	2.8	–	–	–	21

[a]Viruses were detected by isolation in cell culture or by antigen detection with immunofluorescence or PCR. Serology for some viruses was used in addition to viral isolation.

HADV, human adenovirus; Flu, influenza virus; HMPV, human metapneumovirus; HBoV, human bocavirus; HPIV, human parainfluenza virus; HRV, human rhinovirus; HRSV, respiratory syncytial virus.

Table 58.3 Common Viral Respiratory Infections

Virus	Types	Principal Syndromes	Virus Detection Method	Specific Therapy	Vaccines
Influenza	A, B, C	Classic "flu," bronchitis, URI, pneumonia, bronchiolitis, croup	Culture, Ag detection, RT-PCR	Oseltamivir, zanamivir (A, B), amantadine/ rimantadine (A)	Inactivated viruses, subunit,[a] cold-adapted, live-attenuated virus, DNA with adjuvant[a]
HRSV	A, B	URI, bronchiolitis, croup, bronchitis, pneumonia	Culture, Ag detection, RT-PCR	Ribavirin, immunoglobulin, palivizumab for prophylaxis, RNAi	(subunit;[a] live attenuated[a])
HPIV	1, 2, 3, 4	URI, croup, bronchiolitis, bronchitis, pneumonia	Culture, Ag detection, RT-PCR	Ribavirin[a]	Live attenuated;[a] recombinant virus[a]
HRV	>100	URI; otitis media; exacerbation of asthma/ COPD	Culture, RT-PCR	Pleconaril;[a] pirodavir[a]	None
HADV	53	URI; PCF; bronchitis; pneumonia	Culture, Ag detection, PCR	Cidofovir[a]	Live oral vaccine (types 4 and 7)
HCoV	OC43, 229E, NL63, HKU1	URI, bronchitis, pneumonia	Culture, RT-PCR	None	None
HMPV	A, B	URI; bronchitis; pneumonia; wheezing	Culture, RT-PCR, ELISA	Ribavirin,[a] immunoglobulin, NMSO3[a]	Live recombinant virus[a]
HBoV	1, 2, 3	URI; bronchitis, pneumonia, wheezing, bronchiolitis, gastroenteritis, tonsillar chronic inflammation	RT-PCR	None	None

[a]Investigational use.

Ag, antigen; COPD, chronic obstructive pulmonary disease; HADV, human adenovirus; HBoV, human bocavirus; HCoV, human coronavirus; HMPV, human metapneumovirus; HPIV, human parainfluenza virus; HRV, human rhinovirus; PCF, pharyngoconjunctival fever; HRSV, respiratory syncytial virus; RT-PCR, reverse transcription-polymerase chain reaction; SARS, severe acute respiratory syndrome; SARS-CoV, coronavirus associated with SARS; URI, upper respiratory infection.

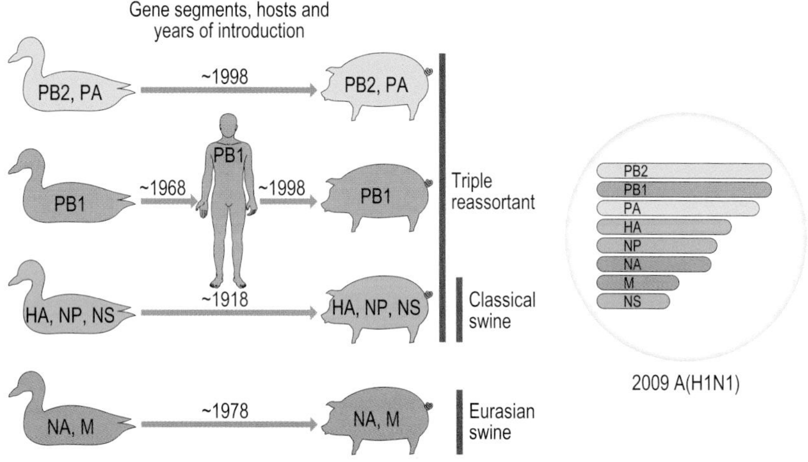

Figure 58.2 Lineage origins for the gene segments of the A/California/04/2009 virus. Phylogenetic analysis shows that six gene segments (PB2, PB1, PA, HA, NP, and NS) were similar to those found in a triple-reassortant swine influenza virus circulating in pigs in North America, with cases previously reported in humans. The NA and M genes entered the Eurasian swine population circa 1979, and that lineage recently combined with the swine triple reassortant. The HA, NP, and NS gene segments are in both the swine triple reassortant and classical swine, which is similar to the human 1918 A(H1N1) lineage. The polymerase PB2 and PA gene segments entered the swine triple reassortant in 1998.[33] The polymerase PB1 gene segment originally entered human population circa 1968 and was seeded into swine from humans in 1998, becoming part of the triple reassortant. (Redrawn from Garten RJ, Davis CT, Russell CA, et al. Antigenic and genetic characteristics of swine-origin 2009 A(H1N1) influenza viruses circulating in humans. Science. 2009;325:197.)

kidney cells, continuous cell lines, and also in embryonated hen's eggs.[36] Influenza viruses are inactivated by temperatures above 50°C, and by lipid solvents, acid, formaldehyde, ionizing radiation, and ultraviolet (UV) light.[36]

The 2009 pandemic influenza A(H1N1) virus contains a unique combination of gene segments not previously reported in swine or human influenza viruses, all with an origin traceable to avian viruses (*Fig. 58.2*). Phylogenetic analysis of the genome of A/California/04/2009 showed that its gene segments come from a triple-reassortant swine influenza virus circulating in pigs in North America, combined with a Eurasian swine virus (*Fig. 58.2*). Antigenically this virus is similar to North American swine A(H1N1) viruses, and distinct from seasonal human influenza A(H1N1).[33]

EPIDEMIOLOGY

Influenza virus infections occur throughout the world, causing highly contagious respiratory infections, with high morbidity and excess mortality, particularly in infants and the elderly. In tropical developing countries, influenza has been associated with an average of 5% of ARIs leading to physician contact.[6,37] These are only the most severe cases, and 30–50% of children under 5 years of age in tropical Africa seroconvert in one outbreak.[37] Previously healthy infants are hospitalized for influenza at rates similar to those for adults at high risk for influenza, and influenza accounts for a great number of outpatient visits and courses of antibiotic therapy in children of all ages.[38] When human influenza virus is introduced into a malnourished population with limited access to health care, high morbidity and mortality rates can occur.[39]

Peaks of influenza activity are associated with excess mortality in tropical and subtropical areas.[40,41] Contrary to the sharp seasonality of influenza A outbreaks in temperate countries, seasonal patterns in tropical countries are variable for reasons that are not clear. In Southern India[20] and Thailand[10] influenza has caused sporadic outbreaks throughout the year, but with consistent outbreaks in June–July and November–January with no apparent association with meteorological factors. In the Philippines, influenza has been more frequent between November and January,[9] while in Senegal, Nigeria, and Taiwan there was a clear association with the rainy season.[27] In southeastern Brazil,[42] Argentina,[43] and South Africa,[44] seasonal outbreaks of influenza A occur from May through August in association with cooler temperatures but not with rainfall. Recent studies show that temperature and humidity play a central role in the timing of influenza circulation in Brazil, where the seasonal wave of influenza activity travels southward from the sparsely populated equatorial region to the densely populated southeast.[45] High temperature and humidity tend to reduce aerosol transmission of influenza virus[46] and thus the reproduction number of influenza outbreaks in tropical regions is reduced as compared to temperate areas.[47]

Influenza B outbreaks occur periodically, yet less frequently than influenza A, both in temperate and tropical regions,[27,36] whereas influenza C is generally nonseasonal.[36]

Ecologists have analyzed migration patterns of influenza viruses throughout the years and have found that there is an East–Southeast Asia seeding of H3N2 spreading to temperate latitudes annually.[48] Interestingly, it has been shown that influenza virus A(H3N2) regularly migrates bi-directionally across hemispheres between seasons.[49] Furthermore, modeling of influenza genealogy suggests there may be North–South transmission where gene flow comes across the Pacific, incorporated into strains in Central America that subsequently migrate to the United States.[50]

Influenza viruses B and C are less prone to antigenic drift. Antigenic shifts occur by the acquisition of genes for novel subtypes of HA or NA, to which humans lack significant immunity.[32] This is typically caused by genetic reassortment in a reservoir host infected simultaneously by human and animal (mostly avian) viruses. Adaptation of such novel influenza A subtypes has led to catastrophic pandemics, including three in the last century. The 1918 H1N1 "Spanish flu" pandemic is estimated to have caused up to 100 million deaths worldwide,[32] while the 1957 H2N2 "Asian flu" and the 1958 "Hong Kong flu" caused an estimated 1–3 million deaths.[32]

Since 1997, clusters of human infections due to highly pathogenic avian influenza viruses H5N1 in Asia have raised concern about new pandemic threats. H5N1 resulted from exposure of humans to infected poultry, but the virus was transmitted inefficiently from person to person.[32,36,51] Other avian viruses, H9N2, H7N7, and H7N3, have also caused mild human disease.[32]

Influenza virus is transmitted from person to person by large droplets and small-particle aerosols, and by fomites with hand contamination and subsequent self-inoculation. Secondary attack rates may be higher than 70% in semi-closed populations, especially among school children and subjects with underlying conditions living in confinement, such as nursing home residents.[36] Children play a major role in influenza outbreaks with respect to propagation of the epidemic virus in families and community.[36]

In March 2009, a previously undescribed influenza virus A(H1N1) quickly spread throughout the community of La Gloria, Veracruz, Mexico with clinical attack rate in children younger than 15 years old twice that in adults, 61% versus 29%.[52] Attack rate of pandemic influenza was estimated at 11%. By July, there were nearly 90 000 laboratory confirmed cases and 382 confirmed deaths globally. The 2009 pandemic A/H1N1 displaced seasonal influenza A(H1N1) and generated fear that its crude mortality rate could surpass that of seasonal influenza in a population lacking neutralizing antibodies. However, total mortality was comparable to that attributed to seasonal influenza, with most deaths associated with predisposing conditions, such as obesity and underlying pulmonary disease, although severe disease was seen with unusually high frequency in younger ages and pregnant women, with a case-fatality rate less than 0.5%.[53]

CLINICAL FEATURES

Classic influenza starts abruptly after an incubation period of 1–4 days, with fever, chills, malaise, headache, myalgia, and prostration, often accompanied by nonproductive cough, sore throat, and mild rhinorrhea. Systemic complaints last 3–5 days, whereas sore throat, hoarseness, and cough, with substernal discomfort, may increase in severity as the systemic symptoms subside. Cough and asthenia often persist for 2 weeks or longer. Respiratory symptoms may be minimal, especially in elderly people or infants. In frail elderly persons, lassitude, lethargy, confusion, low-grade fever, and occasional gastrointestinal complaints may be the primary findings. Influenza B tends to be milder than influenza A, and influenza C typically causes colds or bronchitis.[36] Influenza may also present as unexplained fever, croup, vomiting, diarrhea, and neurologic manifestations in young children.[54] Up to 50% of influenza virus infections in adults are subclinical.[36]

For 2009 H1N1 strain, the incubation period ranged from 1 to 7 days, the most common presenting symptoms were fever, cough, and sore throat, and 25–39% of patients had diarrhea and vomiting, especially children.[55,56] Lymphopenia, and elevated liver transaminases were more common in severely ill patients.[56] Bacterial coinfections were present in 31% of postmortem examinations.[57,58]

Influenza causes a variety of respiratory complications, including otitis media, sinusitis, tracheobronchitis, and pneumonia. Secondary bacterial infections, especially pneumonia, are common complications and should be suspected in relapses of fever, chest pain, and cough.[36] Other complications include meningococcal infections, exacerbations of asthma, chronic bronchitis, and congestive heart failure. In general, pregnant women, HIV-infected patients and other immunocompromised hosts are at higher risk for severe disease and complications.[36] Reye's syndrome occurs in fewer than 1 per 100 000 cases of influenza in patients under 18 years of age, following the use of salicylates. In contrast to seasonal influenza, which leads to increased hospitalization of elderly and children under the age of 5, almost half the hospitalized patients in the A(H1N1) pandemic were persons under the age of 18 and over one-third were between 18 and 49 years old.[56] Risk factors for severe disease associated with 2009 pandemic A(H1N1) were similar to those for seasonal influenza but also included severe obesity.[56]

PATHOGENESIS AND IMMUNITY

The virus infects the respiratory mucosa causing lysis and desquamation of respiratory epithelium, mononuclear cell infiltrates, and altered mucociliary clearance. Tracheobronchitis is a typical feature, often associated with prolonged abnormalities in small airways pulmonary function and airway hyperreactivity. Primary influenza viral pneumonia results in diffuse alveolar damage, alveolar hemorrhage and exudate, hyaline membranes, and reactive fibrosis. Fatal cases of 2009 pandemic influenza A(H1N1) showed pathological changes of multiorgan dysfunction syndrome, such as brain congestion and swelling, myocardial inflammation, fibrinoid changes in arterioles, thrombosis in branches of pulmonary and splenic arteries, leading to wedged splenic infarcts.[36,58]

Viral replication in the upper respiratory tract generally peaks within 1 or 2 days of symptom onset and, depending on age and prior immunity, continues for about 3–8 days. The severity of illness broadly correlates with upper respiratory tract viral loads. Constitutional influenza symptoms are due in part to the release of proinflammatory cytokines and chemokines. Levels of interferon (IFN-α and IFN-γ), tumor necrosis factor (TNF-α), interleukins and chemokines (IL-1β, IL-6, IL-8, IL-10, MCP-10, MIP-1α and MIP-1β) are increased in nasal secretions, and IFN, IL-6 and TNF-α are increased in blood in human influenza.[36] The tissue tropism of a strain of influenza virus depends, among other factors, on a combination of susceptibility of its HA to be cleaved by, and tissue availability of, proteases, thus rendering the virus infectious.[59] Extrapulmonary dissemination of virus has been uncommonly documented in humans, but systemic spread is a regular feature of highly pathogenic avian viruses in chickens and sometimes in rodents or other mammalian hosts. Serum and secretory antibodies directed to HA and NA appear 10 days post infection and correlate with durable protection against reinfection by homologous strain. Vaccine-induced protection may last for up to 2–3 years against homotypic virus. Infection also induces cell-mediated immunity detectable 3–6 days later, which seems to be important for recovery.[36] Cytotoxic T-lymphocyte response against internal proteins may provide some degree of heterosubtypic immunity.

Seasonal influenza A(H1N1) replicates mainly in upper airways, whereas 2009 influenza A(H1N1) replicates in both upper and lower respiratory tracts.[60] Postmortem findings in patients with pandemic A(H1N1) were similar to those with A(H5N1) infection, including diffuse alveolar damage, hemophagocytosis, lymphoid atrophy, and elevated levels of inflammatory markers such as IL-6 and MCP-1 in lung parenchyma. Significant correlation was found between disease severity and levels of proinflammatory cytokines, such as IL-6, IL-10, and IL-15.[60]

DIAGNOSIS

During seasonal outbreaks, the diagnosis of influenza is frequently suspected on clinical grounds. A higher index of suspicion, and laboratory diagnostics are needed in sporadic individual cases or outbreaks of febrile respiratory illness. Viral isolation from respiratory specimens can be done in several cell lines (e.g., PRMK, MDCK, LLC-MK2), with confirmation by hemadsorption or immunofluorescence. Rapid detection of conserved influenza antigens (M or NP) in clinical samples can be done by one of several techniques (e.g., IF, EIA), and multiple point-of-care kits are commercially available with turnaround times of 15–30 minutes. The sensitivities of these assays are higher in children (up to 90%) than in adults (generally 50–70%), and depend on the duration of illness and sample type.[36]

Several formats of reverse transcription–polymerase chain reaction (RT-PCR) assays have been used for the detection of influenza A and B RNAs in clinical samples, with the advantage of detecting genomes of noninfectious virus.[36] Real-time RT-PCR has enabled the development of assays that provide rapid quantitative detection of influenza A and B with high sensitivity.[61–63] These assays have great potential to replace other methods, because they are simultaneously rapid, highly sensitive, quantitative, and amenable to being used in multiplex format, which might include probes for several different respiratory pathogens.[62,63] For the 2009 A/H1N1, real-time and conventional RT-PCR assays were the diagnostic assays of choice.[64] Serologic diagnosis of influenza using paired acute and convalescent serum can be done retrospectively by a variety of techniques, but mainly for serologic survey purposes.[36]

TREATMENT AND PROGNOSIS

There are two classes of antiviral drugs currently licensed for human use: M2 ion channel inhibitors known as adamantanes (amantadine and rimantadine) and neuraminidase (NA) inhibitors (oseltamivir and zanamivir). The adamantanes inhibit influenza A virus replication at the uncoating step.[36] In uncomplicated influenza A in adults without underlying diseases, treatment with either drug can reduce the duration of influenza illness by approximately 1–2 days if started early after the onset of symptoms. Amantadine is excreted in an unchanged state in the urine, while rimantadine is extensively metabolized after absorption and less than 10% of the dose is excreted unchanged in the urine. Elderly persons need only half the dose to achieve similar plasma levels. Amantadine or rimantadine may cause gastrointestinal upset and central nervous system (CNS) side effects. CNS intolerance is more common with amantadine and, when severe, can be manifested as agitation, psychosis, seizures, and coma. Mild complaints include insomnia, dizziness, anxiety, dry mouth, anorexia, and nausea and are reversible upon discontinuation. Amantadine and rimantadine are marketed as 100 mg tablets and 10 mg/mL syrup. The recommended dose is 100 mg twice daily for adults <65 years of age (100 mg per day for patients ≥65 years). For children under 10, a rimantadine dose of 5 mg/kg per day (maximum, 150 mg per day) has been suggested.[37] Dose reductions proportional to the creatinine clearance (ClCr) are suggested for patients with renal insufficiency (amantadine for ClCr less than 60–80 mL/min/1.73 m^2; rimantadine for ClCr less than 10–20 mL/min/1.73 m^2). Resistance of seasonal influenza A viruses to adamantanes, due to single nucleotide mutation in the M2 gene, is widespread,[65–67] leading the CDC to recommend the suspension of their use in the United States in 2006.

The neuraminidase inhibitors (NAIs), zanamivir and oseltamivir, inhibit both influenza A and B viruses by blocking the viral neuraminidase active site and inhibiting cleavage of sialic acid and virus release from infected cells.[68] In adults and children older than 5 years, inhaled zanamivir (10 mg twice daily for 5 days) provides 1- to 2.5-day reduction in illness[69] and reduces antibiotic use for lower respiratory complications by 40%. Zanamivir is generally well tolerated, but may rarely induce bronchospasm, particularly in those with influenza and preexisting airways disease.[37] Oral oseltamivir treatment dosage for adults and children older than 12 months and weigh more than 40 kg is 75 mg twice a day for 5 days, but may need an extended period if the patient is immunocompromised. Oseltamivir dosing is reduced to 60 mg twice a day for children weighing 23–40 kg; for 15–23 kg, dosing is 45 mg twice a day; if <15 kg, then 30 mg twice a day. For infants 3–12 months of age, the recommended oseltamivir dose is 3 mg/kg twice a day. For infants <3 months, data are limited in this age group, but a 3 mg/kg dose twice a day would be recommended in the severely ill. The goal of early implementation of antiviral treatment is to reduce illness severity, shorten time to resumption of daily activities by 1–3 days, and reduce complications leading to antibiotic prescription and hospitalizations by 50% in adults. In children 1–12 years of age, oseltamivir reduces the frequency of otitis media and, consequently, antibiotic prescriptions. Side effects include mild nausea or emesis. Dosage of NAIs does not need to be adjusted for the elderly;[36] however, a dosage reduction is required for patients with creatinine clearance <30.

In the first few years after introduction of NAIs (1999–2001) rates of resistance were low, observed in <0.5% of circulating influenza viruses A/H1N1 and A/H3N2. During the 2007–2008 influenza season, unexpectedly high rates of primary resistance to oseltamivir were detected predominantly in Europe, associated with H274Y mutation in the NA gene. Oseltamivir-resistant viruses remain susceptible to zanamivir and adamantanes.[70–73] For 2008–2009 seasonal influenza A(H1N1), treatment recommendations should include zanamivir or combination treatments for those at high risk for sequelae of influenza.[74] In 2009, the CDC recommended that zanamivir, or a combination of oseltamivir and rimantadine, are more appropriate options than oseltamivir or amantadine alone for the treatment of seasonal influenza A(H1N1).[75] The majority of the 2009 A(H1N1) pandemic viruses were susceptible to NAI; but there are sporadic cases of oseltamivir resistance, 80% of them in viruses from patients with prior exposure to oseltamivir therapy or prophylaxis.[34] Recommendations for the clinical management of 2009 H1N1 infections have been proposed by the WHO.[76] In addition to H274Y mutation, a mutation at amino acid 136 of the influenza virus A(H1N1) NA protein has been linked to reduced susceptibility to zanamivir.[77] Rapidly emerging influenza viruses resistant to NAI highlight the need for development of novel antiviral agents for the treatment and prevention of influenza virus infections. Peramivir, a new NAI for parenteral use, is currently undergoing clinical trials with promising results.[78] Novel therapeutic approaches currently under study are T-705, a selective inhibitor of influenza virus RNA-dependent RNA polymerase,[79] and DAS181, a sialidase fusion protein.[80,81]

Antipyretic-analgesic drugs may be used for influenza-induced fever and aches, but aspirin should be avoided, because of its association with Reye's syndrome.

PREVENTION AND CONTROL

Immunization with formalin-inactivated or live-attenuated multivalent vaccines and chemoprophylaxis are methods available for preventing influenza. Inactivated influenza vaccine is used prior to the influenza season and currently includes one strain of influenza B, and two strains of influenza A viruses, subtypes H3N2 and H1N1, chosen by the WHO among the viruses most likely to circulate in the next influenza season.[82] It has 70–90% efficacy in preventing illness in healthy children and adults, and reduces hospitalizations and mortality in elderly and high-risk patients.[82] The CDC recommendations applied to the United States have been expanded to include not only elderly and high-risk patients but also all children, and now basically recommend universal immunization. During the influenza season when patients often seek medical care, another important group to immunize is health care workers. There is an increasing movement towards mandatory influenza vaccination amongst health care workers, or at least prioritizing those with the most patient contacts in cases of vaccine shortages.[36,82] The inactivated vaccine, administered as a single intramuscular (IM) dose shortly before influenza season (two doses in previously unimmunized children <9 years), is safe during pregnancy but should be avoided in persons with a history of anaphylactic reactions to eggs.[82] Vaccine has a favorable safety profile with 77–91% efficacy in 1- to 15-year-old children. Inactivated vaccine is not currently recommended for children younger than 6 months since the vaccine efficacy is lower in infants; however, vaccination of household contacts and caregivers reduces the risk of these high-risk children contracting influenza. Healthy people aged 2–49 years who are not contacts of immunosuppressed patients can receive either inactivated or intranasal live-attenuated vaccines.[82]

The composition of the inactivated influenza vaccine given in tropical countries is based on viruses that circulate in the southern hemisphere and is given prior to the influenza peak season, which for most countries in the South is between May and July.[83] In South America, annual vaccination of the elderly has reduced hospitalizations and mortality for respiratory diseases.[84]

Live-attenuated, cold-adapted vaccines administered intranasally are well tolerated, genetically stable, rarely transmissible, and have the advantage of inducing local secretory IgA responses.[36] This vaccine was licensed in the United States in 2003, as an option for healthy persons aged 5–49 years, including those in close contact with groups at high risk and those wanting to avoid influenza.[82] This vaccine is not recommended for persons with asthma and other chronic disorders of the pulmonary or cardiovascular systems; persons with underlying medical conditions, including diabetes, renal dysfunction, and hemoglobinopathies; or persons with known or suspected immunodeficiencies or who are on immunosuppressive therapies; children or adolescents receiving aspirin or other salicylates; persons with a history of Guillain–Barré syndrome; pregnant women; and persons with a history of hypersensitivity to eggs.[82] The inactivated vaccine has been more efficient than the live attenuated vaccine in preventing influenza in healthy adults, but appears less effective in young children.[85]

A promising live attenuated influenza vaccine lacking the NS1 protein was shown to be effective in animal models, and induced significant levels of lineage-specific and cross-reactive neutralizing antibodies in healthy volunteers.[86] Other investigational approaches have been explored in influenza vaccine development, including recombinant HA produced in insect cells, virosomes incorporating surface glycoproteins, M2 protein conjugated with hepatitis B virus core, and naked DNA encoding influenza virus nucleoprotein or HA.[36] Cell culture-based vaccines (MDCK, Vero) have been approved in Europe and may offer an alternative to the limitations of the current egg-grown vaccines.

Chemoprophylaxis with antivirals should be considered for nonvaccinated elderly people, immunodeficient patients, patients in chronic care institutions during influenza outbreaks, people with contraindications for vaccination, and those who received a vaccine strain different from the one causing the outbreak. Approved prophylaxis dose is once daily (i.e., one half of treatment dose) for oseltamivir or zanamivir which should be started as early as possible and continued for 7–10 days for post-exposure prophylaxis.[76] However, reports of high rates of influenza resistance to antiviral drugs should prompt more rigorous judgment in the decision to use antiviral prophylaxis. Antiviral agents, especially the neuraminidase inhibitors, could significantly help in the control of a future pandemic of influenza, by reducing lower respiratory complications, hospitalizations, and person-to-person transmission. Availability of antivirals also pose a limitation in resource-constraint settings.[87] Therefore, policies to ensure a stockpile of these drugs, as well as directions to optimize their use, are important issues to be considered.[32]

More emphasis should also be placed upon non-pharmaceutical interventions such as handwashing and use of facemask to curtail the spread of influenza. These measures appear to reduce household transmission of influenza virus as long as they are implemented within 36 hours of the onset of symptoms in the index case.[88]

HUMAN RESPIRATORY SYNCYTIAL VIRUS

Human respiratory syncytial virus (HRSV) is the single most important viral etiology of LRI and a major cause of morbidity and mortality in children worldwide. HRSV is the leading cause of hospitalization in young children[77] and has been the most frequently detected virus in hospital-based ARI studies of children in tropical areas.[7]

THE AGENT

HRSV, the only known human pathogen of the genus *Pneumovirus* in the family *Paramyxoviridae*, is a negative-strand RNA virus with helical nucleocapsid and a lipid-containing envelope. The 15.2 kb HRSV genome encodes 11 distinct viral proteins, and the antigenic differences in the G, F, and SH envelope proteins permit classification of HRSV into groups A and B, each with subgroups.[89] The G glycoprotein interacts with host cell receptors and mediates adsorption to the cell surface,[90] resulting in fusion of virus and host cell membranes mediated by the F glycoprotein.[89] The expression of F protein on the cell surface results in fusions of adjacent cells forming syncytia, the hallmark of paramyxovirus cytopathic effect.[89]

HRSV is sensitive to ether, chloroform, detergents, and pH less than 5, is inactivated at 55°C, survives poorly on porous surfaces, and loses infectivity by slow freezing and storage at temperatures above 4°C.[89]

EPIDEMIOLOGY

HRSV occurs worldwide, causing annual outbreaks in temperate climates in the winter and early spring, with sporadic cases throughout the year.[90] In tropical regions, where temperature fluctuates less, HRSV outbreaks occur in the rainy seasons, as in Malaysia, Hong Kong, India, Papua New Guinea, Colombia, Kenya, and The Gambia.[27] In southeast Brazil, HRSV occurs from February through July, after the rainy season, when temperatures tend to be cooler.[91] In regions with colder winter temperatures, such as Sao Paulo city and the southernmost parts of Brazil, as well as in Argentina and Chile, HRSV peak activity tends to occur in July–August.[92–96] The duration of HRSV season is longer in overcrowded areas with larger families.[97]

HRSV from both groups A and B may co-circulate during a seasonal peak.[98] A recent long-term study in Brazil[99] showed that several amino acid residues in immunodominant epitopes of HRSV G protein undergo back and forth positive selection between seasons, generating a "flip-flop" variation pattern. Changes in herd immunity may select mutants within a limited repertoire of functionally viable HRSV variants. A new variant of HRSV B with a conspicuous 30 amino acid duplication in the G protein has become the dominant genotype in several regions, including Argentina, Brazil, and India.[99–101] HRSV co-circulates with other respiratory viruses and sensitive molecular methods show that coinfections of HRSV with other viruses are common,[102] without evidence of increased severity of the HRSV disease.[103]

Most children develop anti-HRSV antibody by age 2, although reinfections are common throughout life.[104] HRSV transmission occurs by large-particle aerosols or by contamination of hands and subsequent inoculation into the eyes or nose. Transmission to siblings and adults occurs efficiently in household settings. It is estimated that 30% of all infants will have HRSV infection requiring medical attention and up to 2% of them will be hospitalized.[77] An estimated 10% of all children will have bronchiolitis in their first year of life, and 60–90% of those are caused by HRSV.[105]

In southeast Brazil HRSV is responsible for up to 85% of child hospitalizations for LRI during HRSV peak months.[96]

CLINICAL FEATURES

After an incubation period of 3–7 days,[106] HRSV symptoms start, usually with mild upper respiratory infection (URI),[107] but may progress to severe LRI, including pneumonia, bronchiolitis, tracheobronchitis, and croup. Most commonly bronchiolitis follows URI symptoms, with tachypnea, dyspnea, cough, expiratory wheezing, air trapping and, in more severe cases, intercostal muscle retractions and cyanosis. Half of the patients have fever, and chest X-ray may show lung hyperaeration and segmented atelectasis.[107] Blood counts usually show lymphocytosis and increased neutrophils suggest bacterial superinfection, the most common being acute otitis media.[108] HRSV RNA can be detected in up to 75% of middle ear effusions in children with HRSV infection and acute otitis media.[108] While serious bacterial infections are rare in previously healthy infants with HRSV in developed regions,[109] such infections are more likely to occur in tropical areas among children previously debilitated by other diseases and malnutrition.

Those at risk for severe and fatal HRSV infections include: premature infants, infants with congenital heart disease or underlying pulmonary conditions such as cystic fibrosis or bronchopulmonary dysplasia, as well as immunocompromised hosts of any age. HIV-infected children with HRSV infections have a higher rate of pneumonia, prolonged illness and virus shedding, but no increase in severity of the HRSV disease.[107] Differential diagnosis of acute bronchiolitis includes asthma, pneumonia, congenital heart and lung diseases, and cystic fibrosis. The most frequent HRSV illness in children over 3 years of age and adults is characterized by symptoms of URI often with low-grade fever. Exacerbations of chronic pulmonary diseases and wheezing episodes can also be seen in adults.[110] Neurological complications including seizures and encephalopathy occur rarely in severe HRSV infections requiring intensive care.[111] HRSV, as well as influenza and parainfluenza, also contributes to wheezing and asthma exacerbations in infants.[112–115] HRSV has also been increasingly recognized in LRI in the elderly, mainly interstitial pneumonia, with prolonged cough and dyspnea in patients with chronic pulmonary conditions.[116]

PATHOGENESIS AND IMMUNITY

HRSV replicates in respiratory epithelium, reaching titers of 10^6 $TCID_{50}$ (tissue culture infectious dose for 50% of the test units per milliliter) per mL in nasal secretions of infected babies, with virus shedding as prolonged as 3 weeks after symptoms disappear.[89] HRSV spreading from cell to cell may involve the entire respiratory tree, reaching bronchioles 1–3 days after the onset of rhinorrhea. Replication in the bronchiolar epithelium causes necrosis of ciliated cells, syncytia formation, peribronchiolar inflammation with abundant lymphocytes and macrophages, impairment of secretion clearance, small airway obstruction and lung hyperaeration.[89] HRSV nonstructural proteins NS1 and NS2 counteract production of type I interferon (IFN), contributing to pathogenesis.[117] HRSV may also modulate surfactant expression in human pulmonary epithelial cells, which can contribute for disease severity.[118] Pneumonia frequently coexists with bronchiolitis, evidenced by interstitial mononuclear infiltrate, eosinophilic cytoplasmic inclusions in epithelial cells, and multinucleated giant cells. The innate immune response to HRSV is triggered by recognition via Toll-like receptor (TLR)4, TLR3, TLR2 and RIG-I, resulting in expression of proinflammatory cytokines and chemokines.[119] HRSV infects dendritic cells (DCs), causing them to lose their ability to stimulate HRSV-specific T cells.[120] B-lymphocyte-stimulating factors derived from infected DC and epithelial cells are determinants of the mucosal antibody response and disease progression.[121]

Immunity to HRSV is incomplete and short-lived, but reinfections tend to be less severe. Local secretory IgA correlates better with protection than does serum antibody level and age. Cell-mediated immune response is important for recovery from HRSV infection, and patients with suppressed cell-mediated immune response are at risk of severe pulmonary disease and fatal outcome.[89,107]

The type of immune response to the virus is probably a major factor in the development of wheezing. A bias towards a Th2 cytokine profile seems to be associated with more severe disease, whereas a Th1 profile leads to effective viral clearance and milder illness. It has been suggested that HRSV bronchiolitis at early age may predispose to wheezing or asthma later in life.[122]

DIAGNOSIS

HRSV isolation from respiratory samples is usually done in cultures of HEp-2 cells, in which HRSV induces syncytia in 3–5 days. Various assays for HRSV antigen detection directly in respiratory secretion are available, some requiring equipment such as immunofluorescence microscope or EIA readers, and others requiring no equipment, such as the membrane-based immunochromatographic assays ideal for field studies.[123] Such rapid tests may have very low sensitivity for HRSV detection in samples from adult patients.

Detection of HRSV RNA by conventional or real-time RT-PCR is becoming widely available, with the added convenience of being quantitative and amenable for simultaneous detection and subtyping of HRSV directly in clinical specimens.[124] Recently, an ultrasound-based RNA extraction method combined with a multicomponent nucleic acid enzyme amplification procedure was developed to detect HRSV in difficult respiratory samples, as noted in elderly respiratory samples which often bear low viral loads.[125] HRSV serology has limited value for case management, but may be useful in epidemiologic surveys.[107]

TREATMENT AND PROGNOSIS

URI caused by HRSV requires no specific treatment and the use of antibiotics is recommended only in the presence of bacterial otitis media or sinusitis.[107] The supportive treatment of infants with HRSV bronchiolitis consists in preventing hypoxemia and electrolyte imbalance, in addition to aerosolized bronchodilators. Chest X-ray should be recommended only for severely ill or deteriorating infants.[105] To prevent hypoxemia, requirements may vary from simple removal of respiratory secretions and proper positioning of the infant, to mechanical respiratory assistance and even extracorporeal membrane oxygenation (ECMO). Pulse oximetry has been advocated to assess oxygen needs, but in tropical developing areas oximeters may not be available and serial clinical assessment is essential to monitor disease progression. For this purpose, crackles and cyanosis seem to correlate better with hypoxemia than tachypnea and intercostal retraction.[105] Correction of hypoxemia can be accomplished with 40% or lower oxygen concentrations.[107] Oxygen should be humidified with saline and delivered by mask if head boxes or tents are unavailable. The role of corticosteroids remains unclear, with a variety of evidence showing they are not beneficial.[105]

Ribavirin, delivered by small-particle aerosol via a mist tent, mask, oxygen hood, or ventilator, is recommended only for infants and young children with an underlying condition, such as congenital heart disease, cystic fibrosis, or immunosuppression. Premature infants, infants younger than 6 weeks of age, and those severely ill may also be considered for therapy.[126] This treatment requires a specific nebulization device and generates potential exposure of health care workers to a teratogenic agent. Humanized monoclonal antibodies to HRSV, which are beneficial for prophylaxis, have shown no benefit in treatment of HRSV infections.[107] Recently, the use of small interfering RNAs (siRNAs) has become a promising strategy to treat HRSV infections. One such siRNA to the nucleocapsid protein had anti-HRSV activity both *in vitro* and *in vivo*[127] and an inhaled preparation is undergoing clinical testing.[128]

PREVENTION AND CONTROL

Disease enhancement caused by a formalin-inactivated HRSV vaccine in the 1960s and results of more recent unsuccessful trials of live attenuated vaccines have significantly slowed progress toward an HRSV vaccine.[2] However, there is recent evidence that the lack of protection of the formalin-inactivated vaccine of the 1960s was due to reduced antibody affinity resulting from poor stimulation of TLR. This suggests that the efficacy and safety of inactivated HRSV vaccine may be improved by inclusion of TLR agonists in the formulation.[129] An HRSV-A subunit vaccine containing F, G, and M proteins was tested in elderly patients and elicited potentially protective neutralizing antibody.[130]

Passive immunization of high-risk infants with monthly doses of HRSV humanized monoclonal antibodies during the HRSV season reduces incidence and severity of infections in high-risk children.[131] Although the commercially available preparations palivizumab and motavizumab are much too expensive to be routinely used in underprivileged tropical regions, their judicious use for high-risk premature babies, children with congenital heart disease, and children less than 2 years of age with bronchopulmonary dysplasia, may result in net cost savings for some health care systems.[132]

Hospitalized infants with HRSV should be isolated or grouped together to prevent cross-infection. Handwashing, use of eye–nose goggles, gowns, and gloves, and decontamination of surfaces and fomites are additional nosocomial infection control measures.[107]

HUMAN PARAINFLUENZA VIRUSES

Human parainfluenza viruses (HPIVs) are leading causes of croup in infants and children worldwide, and are among the most frequent causes of LRI in infants.[133,134] HPIVs can be detected in up to 13% of children in hospital-based LRI studies in developing countries.[37,135]

THE AGENT

The HPIVs are distributed in two genera of the family *Paramyxoviridae*, sharing structural and biological characteristics of HRSV. HPIVs are classified antigenically into types 1 to 4, with HPIV-4 subdivided into subtypes A and B. HPIV types 1 and 3 are classified in the genus *Respirovirus*, while HPIV types 2 and 4 are in the genus *Rubulavirus*. HPIV-1 and -3 are the types most frequently associated with LRI in children, the immunocompromised, the chronically ill and the elderly, whereas HPIV-4 causes mostly URI both in children and adults.[133]

Binding of HPIV to sialic acid in the cell membrane is mediated by the viral glycoprotein HN, which contains both hemagglutinin and neuraminidase activities. Fusion of viral and cell membranes is mediated by the viral F protein, which is cleaved by cellular proteolytic enzymes.[136] Once inside the cell, the replication cycle is similar to that of HRSV. HPIV budding is finalized when the neuraminidase function of the HN protein cleaves sialic acid, permitting the release of virions from the cell.[137]

EPIDEMIOLOGY

Primary HPIV infection occurs early in childhood, and by age 5 virtually all children are seropositive for one or more HPIVs.[133] Up to one-third of all viral LRIs in children in the United States are caused by HPIV-1 and HPIV-3.[133,138] In tropical areas HPIVs may account for up to 15% of hospital admissions of children due to LRI.[37] In temperate regions HPIV-1 and HPIV-2 cause epidemics in the fall of alternate years, either in co-circulation or alternating with one another. The biennial pattern of HPIV-1 circulation has been found in both hemispheres.[133] HPIV-1 causes most croup outbreaks, whereas HPIV-2 more frequently causes mild illness, although it also causes croup.[133] HPIV-3 occurs endemically throughout the year, with sporadic spring outbreaks mainly among infants, and HPIV-4 occurs sporadically throughout the year in children and adults.[133] In an emergency room study in Fortaleza, northeast Brazil, HPIVs were detected in 4% of children with ARI and HPIV-3 was the most frequently detected and occurred seasonally, with most cases observed from September to November, in inverse relationship to the rainy season.[139] However, community-based ARI studies in children under 5 years of age have shown higher HPIV activity during rainy seasons in tropical countries.[3,10]

HPIVs spread mainly within families and closed communities, such as nurseries, daycare centers and pediatric wards, with high secondary attack rates. In a longitudinal ARI study conducted in children less than 2 years of age in daycare for low-income families in northeast Brazil, HPIVs represented 11% of the viruses detected.[140]

HPIVs are transmitted mainly by large droplets and fomites[107] and virus shedding lasts 3–10 days, but HPIV shedding for months has been reported in very young children and immunosuppressed hosts.[141]

CLINICAL FEATURES

Primary HPIV infection may cause rhinitis, pharyngitis, laryngotracheobronchitis (croup), bronchiolitis, and pneumonia.[133] Approximately two-thirds of HPIV infections in children result in febrile URI, frequently associated with otitis media, and the remaining one-third are cases of croup, bronchiolitis, and pneumonia.[133] HPIVs, principally types 1 and 2, cause up to 74% of all cases of croup,[133] mainly between 6 and 36 months of age.[142] Croup is manifested by inspiratory stridor, barking cough, and hoarseness caused by subglottic edema, preceded by rhinorrhea, mild cough, and low-grade fever.[142] Most children recover in 2–5 days, but some may develop bronchiolitis and pneumonia.[142]

Immunity to HPIV is incomplete and infections occur throughout life, but adults present only nonspecific URI, commonly with hoarseness.[107] HPIVs are detected in 5.8% of cases of influenza-like illness (ILI) in the United States[143] and in 3.2% in Peru.[144]

HPIVs can cause severe disease in immunocompromised hosts, especially children with severe combined immunodeficiency and recipients of bone marrow transplants, reaching mortality rates of 10–20%.[107,145]

PATHOGENESIS AND IMMUNITY

HPIVs cause epithelial cytolysis, spreading from the upper respiratory tract down the respiratory tree. Similar to influenza, the extent of HPIV infection depends on viral F protein cleavage by tissue proteases.[107] Larynx and trachea are mostly involved in the croup syndrome, and extensive involvement of the lower respiratory tree may be present in tracheobronchitis, bronchopneumonia, and bronchiolitis.[133,141,142]

Host immunity is largely directed to the two surface proteins HN and F, and secretory antibody to the HN glycoprotein is the best marker of protection,[141] but such protection is limited and repeated infections occur. T-cell immune response is involved in both the clearance of virus and inflammation, with edema and excess mucus secretion.[133]

In the lungs HPIVs cause mononuclear interstitial infiltrate, epithelial necrosis, alveolar exudate, and hyaline membrane formation.[107]

DIAGNOSIS

HPIV can be recovered from respiratory secretions up to 8 days from the onset of symptoms in several continuous cell lines and virus isolation can be confirmed by immunofluorescence.[133,141] Immunofluorescence done directly on exfoliated respiratory epithelial cells has produced disappointing results due to low sensitivity.[133] Detection of HPIV RNA by real-time RT-PCR is quite sensitive and has become a standard diagnostic method.[146,147]

TREATMENT

At present, only supportive and symptomatic treatment is available for HPIV infections. Management of croup includes supplemental oxygen and racemic epinephrine nebulization in hospitalized patients. Mist therapy, although traditional, has no proven value.[142] Short-term, high-dose systemic corticosteroids may reduce the need for intubation, and nebulized budesonide has a rapid effect and is as safe and efficacious as nebulized epinephrine in moderately severe croup.[142] There is no approved antiviral treatment for HPIV infections, but compounds designed to bind and inhibit the functions of HN protein have been effective *in vitro* and in an experimental animal model.[148,149]

PREVENTION AND CONTROL

No interventions are licensed for the prevention of HPIV infections. Recently, a live attenuated cold-adapted HPIV-3 vaccine was found to be safe and immunogenic in children, with a seroconversion rate of 79%.[150] More recently, a Sendai virus vaccine, with extensive homology with HPIV-1, was found to be naturally attenuated in humans and induced high-titer specific neutralizing antibodies.[151]

HUMAN METAPNEUMOVIRUS

Human metapneumovirus was initially detected in children with ARI in the Netherlands in 2001. The agent is a paramyxovirus of the subfamily *Pneumovirinae*, closely related to avian pneumovirus of the genus *Metapneumovirus*, and is now recognized by serological studies as having circulated for at least five decades.[140,141]

THE AGENT

HMPV is enveloped, pleomorphic, with negative-sense single-stranded RNA contained in a helicoidal nucleocapsid, surrounded by an envelope with glycoproteins that mediate attachment (G), and fusion (F).[152,153] HMPV glycoprotein (F) binds to $\alpha v\beta 1$ integrins on the cell surface to mediate cell entry.[154]

HMPV isolates cluster into two main subgroups, named A and B, and based on the sequence of the F and G genes the two subgroups can be subdivided into two genetic sub-lineages named A1, A2 and B1, B2;[153,155] the A2 sublineage is further divided into two sub-clusters, A2a and A2b.[156]

EPIDEMIOLOGY

HMPV is globally distributed and a frequent cause of ARI in all continents. At the age of 5 virtually all children have become seropositive for the agent.[157–159] HMPV infections are more frequent in the colder months in temperate regions and different strains of both subgroups A and B co-circulate during the same year.[160] However, little is known of HMPV seasonality in tropical countries. In South Africa, HMPV peak activity occurs in the winter season.[161]

Rates of HMPV detection in respiratory samples from ARI patients in tropical countries are quite variable. Hospital-based ARI studies in children have recorded frequencies of HMPV of 7.4% in South Africa,[162] 5.4% in Thailand,[163] 7% in Yemen,[164] and 15.7% in South Korea.[165] In northeast Brazil, HMPV was detected alone or simultaneously with HRSV in 24% of children younger than 3 years of age, in April and May 2002,[157] whereas in the following year it was not detected by the same method.[166] In contrast, in southeast Brazil, HMPV was detected in 5.6% of infants hospitalized for ARI.[167] A 4-year study also done in southeast Brazil found an average frequency of 11.4% in children with ARI, with the two HMPV subgroups co-circulating, with peak frequency in winter or spring.[168]

CLINICAL FEATURES

Clinically, HMPV infections resemble those caused by HRSV, ranging from mild upper ARI to severe bronchiolitis and pneumonia. The median age of children hospitalized for HMPV is higher than that of those with HRSV. The most frequent symptoms are fever, dyspnea, cough, wheezing/stridor, rhinitis, and sore throat.[160,169] All infected children in one study had pneumonia or bronchiolitis, frequently accompanied by otitis media.[160,170,171] HMPV may cause more serious infections in immunocompromised patients, those with previous conditions, the very young and the elderly.[160] HMPV infection in adults may present as influenza-like illness, acute bronchitis, or URI.[160]

HMPV has been increasingly recognized as cause of acute wheezing in children. A study from Finland found HMPV in 8% of wheezing children; in addition, a significantly higher level of IL-8 was found in nasal secretions of those cases.[172] In Brazil, 47% of children with HMPV had wheezing and 31% had chest indrawing.[157] Previous history of asthma has been more frequently associated with HMPV than with HRSV infection; HMPV-infected patients are more often treated with bronchodilators and corticosteroids than are HRVS-infected patients.[169] Remarkably, HMPV was detected in 8.3% of children younger than 5 years with community-acquired alveolar pneumonia in Israel.[173]

PATHOGENESIS AND IMMUNITY

HMPV infection occurs at young age, but reinfections remain common at later ages.[152] Knowledge about HMPV pathogenesis is still limited, but it is clear that it infects both upper and lower respiratory tracts[160] and both subgroups A and B are equally pathogenic.[174] Experimental infections in animal models indicate that peak viral shedding occurs from 2 to 8 days following infection.[153] In humans, HMPV infections are associated with increased levels of IL-8, and reduced levels of inflammatory cytokines IL-12, TNF-α, IL-6 and IL-1β in the upper respiratory tract, as compared with HRSV infections.[175,176]

Interestingly, in experimentally infected animals HMPV replicates in respiratory epithelial cells, and migrates to neuronal processes in the lungs, where it may persist when infection of epithelial cells is no longer detectable. Whether this happens in humans and may contribute to later wheezing is not known.[177]

A common finding in epidemiological studies is the coinfection with HMPV and HRSV and some studies reported that this correlates with increased severity of HRSV disease.[178,179]

DIAGNOSIS

HMPV can be isolated from respiratory samples in LLC-MK2 cells, with late cytopathic effect characterized by syncytia formation or cell rounding and detachment.[160] Sensitive RT-PCR assays for HMPV have rapidly become standard for diagnosis.[180] A real-time RT-PCR assay for HMPV was more sensitive than conventional RT-PCR[180] and other non-molecular methods, such as direct fluorescence assay.[181] A rapid immunochromatography assay for HMPV antigen has been developed which can be completed in approximately 15 minutes and does not require equipment.[182]

TREATMENT, PREVENTION, AND CONTROL

Other than supportive measures, such as oxygen therapy, bronchodilators, corticosteroids, and mechanical ventilation, there is no specific antiviral treatment for this agent.[169] Ribavirin is inhibitory for HMPV *in vitro*[183] and there have been anecdotal reports of its successful use in association with immunoglobulin for HMPV pneumonia in immunocompromised patients.[184] Although an HMPV vaccine is not available, promising preclinical studies have been done with a live recombinant human parainfluenza virus expressing HMPV F protein,[185] and with a chimeric bovine/human parainfluenza virus 3 expressing HMPV F protein.[186] Other approaches successfully tested in animal models were soluble recombinant F protein, DNA vaccine, and live attenuated vaccines.[187] Humanized neutralizing monoclonal antibody to F protein is active in experimentally infected animals.[188,189]

HUMAN RHINOVIRUSES

Human rhinoviruses (HRVs) are the most frequent respiratory pathogens of humans.[190] They were the most frequently isolated viruses in children under 5 years old with ARI in an urban slum in tropical northeast Brazil.[3]

THE AGENT

HRVs are small, nonenveloped, positive-strand RNA viruses in the genus *Enterovirus*, family *Picornaviridae*,[191] with over 100 identified serotypes.[187] HRVs comprise three different species named *Human rhinovirus A* (with 75 serotypes), *B* (25 serotypes), and the recently described group *C*.[192,193]

HRV serotypes are also classified by receptor-specificity into two groups: the major group includes 90% of the serotypes, whose receptor is intercellular adhesion molecule-1 (ICAM-1), and the minor group contains the remaining serotypes, whose receptor is the low-density lipoprotein receptor (LDLR). HRVs are acid-labile, which distinguishes them from other enteroviruses.[190] Genomic analysis of HRVs indicates that a large number of genotypes co-circulate in a short period, causing a high frequency of reinfections. Recombinations between serotypes may be a driving force in rhinovirus evolution.[194]

The HRV genome is a positive single-stranded RNA packed in an icosahedral capsid. Receptor binding destabilizes the capsid, triggering internalization and exposure of the viral genome to the cytoplasm, where the whole replicative cycle takes place, leading to production of mature virions released by cell lysis.[190]

HRVs are stable for days on environmental surfaces, are resistant to ethanol, ether, chloroform, and nonionic detergents, but are sensitive to UV light, pH <5, halogens such as chlorine, bromine, and iodine, and phenolic disinfectants.[190]

EPIDEMIOLOGY

HRV infections occur in people from all continents, including remotely located populations, such as Bushmen from the Kalahari Desert, native Alaskans, and isolated Amazon Indian tribes.[195] HRV causes up to 80% of all colds in adults in temperate climates[196] but very few community-based studies of ARI have included HRV detection methods in the tropics.[3] HRV is frequently associated with ARI in children in tropical Brazil, where it was isolated in 46% of samples from children under 5 with ARI in Fortaleza, and detected by RT-PCR in 52% of toddlers with ARI in a daycare center for the underprivileged in Salvador.[3,140] In southeast Brazil, HRV represented 36% of the respiratory viruses in adults with ARI in Sao Paulo, with seasonality similar to that of influenza virus.[197] Health care facility-based studies of young children with ARI have detected HRV in 30% in Thailand,[198] and 35.4% in Hong Kong,[199] highlighting its importance as a frequent cause of ARI worldwide.

HRV transmission requires close exposure, occurs mainly by hand contact with self-inoculation into the eyes or nostrils, but also by droplet spread, and children play an important role spreading HRV in households.[200] Once HRV reaches the nasal cavity, infection occurs in virtually all exposed susceptible subjects, with 75–80% of the infected developing illness after a 1–4-day incubation.[106]

CLINICAL FEATURES

HRV is responsible for the majority of common colds, which are clinically indistinguishable from colds of other viral causes, consisting of nasal discharge, nasal obstruction, sneezing, sore or scratchy throat, hoarseness, cough, headache, and uncommonly feverishness and malaise. The symptoms last for approximately 7 days, but may persist for up to 2 weeks in 25% of cases. Infants and toddlers may display only nasal discharge, being otherwise asymptomatic.[190] The use of the RT-PCR method has revealed that approximately 20% of HRV infections are asymptomatic.[201]

Most patients with HRV have obstruction and mucosal abnormalities of the sinus cavities, eustachian tubes, and middle ear, which predispose to secondary bacterial sinusitis and otitis media, complications found in approximately 2% of all colds.[202] HRV RNA may be detected in maxillary sinus brushings in 40% of adults presenting with acute sinusitis[203] and in 25% of middle ear fluid samples from children with acute otitis media.[204,205]

HRV infections frequently trigger exacerbations of chronic obstructive pulmonary disease and asthma.[114,206] In adults, HRV is associated with 60–70% of asthma exacerbations.[207] Furthermore, it was recently shown that the HRV species C is more closely related to lower respiratory tract infections, causing febrile wheezing and asthmatic exacerbation in children.[192,193]

PATHOGENESIS AND IMMUNITY

HRV infects only higher primates, causing illness only in humans. It replicates mainly in ciliated cells of the nose and nonciliated cells of the nasopharynx.[208] HRV infection induces little tissue damage, although it appears that viral replication and the associated host pro-inflammatory and neurogenic responses drive the illness.[209] The localized viral replication triggers release of cytokines, chemokines, and inflammatory mediators which, together with stimulation of the local parasympathetic nerve endings, results in cold symptoms. Kinins, prostaglandins, and proinflammatory cytokines and chemokines contribute to vasodilation, increased vascular permeability, influx of leukocytes, exocrine gland secretion, and nerve ending stimulation, resulting in nasal obstruction, rhinorrhea, sneezing, cough, and sore throat.[190]

In addition to the upper airways, HRV can cause LRI, inducing local inflammatory response.[210] Lower respiratory symptoms may also result from the inflammatory response to rhinovirus infections of the upper airways.[211] In this regard, individuals with asthma develop T-cell infiltration of the airway epithelium and submucosa upon experimental HRV infection,[212] suggesting a role for these cells in the pathogenesis of asthma exacerbations caused by HRV.

Serotype-specific mucosal IgA can be detected by day 3 post infection, followed by IgM, and finally by IgG, 7–8 days later.[213] Protection from infection is correlated with both mucosal and serum antibody. Although detectable, the importance of cell-mediated immunity for recovery from infection is unclear, except perhaps for cases of severe lung disease in transplant patients.

DIAGNOSIS

HRV shedding in nasal secretions peaks around 48 hours post infection, declining rapidly thereafter, but remaining at low levels for up to 3 weeks.[190] HRV can be isolated from respiratory secretions in cells kept at 33–35°C, with cytopathic effect developing in 10–14 days. RT-PCR, either by conventional or real-time techniques, is more sensitive and less tedious than HRV isolation,[214,215] and revealed that coinfections of HRV with other respiratory viruses can be documented in 50% of all HRV-positive samples.[22,216]

Novel multitarget molecular methods for HRV detection include multiplex PCR with tagged primers associated with tag-specific colored microspheres and flow cytometry, which allows for the rapid detection of 17 different respiratory viruses in clinical specimens.[217] MassTag is another technique that can identify viral PCR products with the advantage of detecting novel HRV sequences.[218]

TREATMENT

There are no licensed antiviral treatments for HRV infections. Several capsid-binding antiviral compounds inhibit *in vitro* replication of most rhinoviruses and enteroviruses,[219] and one such compound, pleconaril, when used orally reduced the duration and severity of natural colds in adults.[220]

Symptomatic relief from cold symptoms can be obtained with a broad variety of nonprescription medications. Systemic sympathomimetic decongestants, such as pseudoephedrine, may reduce nasal obstruction, first-generation antihistamines may reduce sneezing and rhinorrhea, and nonsteroidal anti-inflammatory drugs, such as naproxen or ibuprofen, may reduce headache, cough, and systemic symptoms.[190] However, these treatments have side effects, such as sedation with the antihistamines and CNS toxicities with the sympathomimetics, which are contraindicated in infants and young children.

PREVENTION AND CONTROL

The large number of HRV serotypes with minimal cross-antigenicity hampers the development of an HRV vaccine. It is possible to reduce HRV exposure by handwashing or virucidal hand treatment after contact with a cold sufferer or objects contaminated with respiratory secretions.[221] Short-term postexposure prophylaxis with intranasal IFN-α significantly reduced the incidence of HRV colds in household contacts of an index case,[222] but is investigational and causes mucosal irritation with sustained use.

HUMAN CORONAVIRUSES

Four species of human coronaviruses (HCoV) cause ARI: 229E, OC43, and the more recently discovered NL63 and HKU1.[223] The known HCoVs are distributed in two of the three known genera of coronaviruses: HCoV-229E and NL63 belong to the *Alphacoronavirus* genus, while HCoV-OC43 and HKU1 are members of the *Betacoronavirus* genus. The other known human coronavirus, discovered in 2003 as the agent of severe acute respiratory syndrome (SARS) is discussed in Chapter 59.

THE AGENT

HCoVs are enveloped viruses with long and widely spaced peplomers on the surface, resembling a crown (*corona*) and a 27–32 kb positive-strand RNA genome, which is the largest known viral RNA genome.[224] The envelope S glycoprotein contains neutralizing antibody and T-cell epitopes and attaches to the cell surface receptor, which for HCoV-229E is the aminopeptidase N and for HCoV-NL63 is the angiotensin-converting enzyme 2 (ACE2).[225] The hemagglutinin (HE) of group 2 HCoVs binds to the receptor 9-*O*-acetylated sialic acid.[226] Coronavirus replication occurs in the cytoplasm and new virions assemble by budding through intracellular membranes, being released through vesicles of the secretory pathway.[224]

EPIDEMIOLOGY

HCoVs are second only to rhinoviruses as causative agents of common colds and may cause up to 35% of mild URI in temperate climate regions,[227] but rates may vary significantly from year to year. In temperate areas HCoV infections occur mainly in the winter and spring months, but summer activity has also been documented.[227,228] However, their impact in tropical countries has not been well studied. HCoV-NL63 has been found in 2–4% of patients with ARI and pneumonia in Hong Kong and Australia[229,230] and HKU1 in 0.3–4.4% of patients with ARI in Hong Kong.[231,232]

In Brazil, the role of HCoV-229E in causing nonhospitalized respiratory infections in children in the community was first documented by serology in the early 1970s, with seropositivity of 26% in adults.[233] A recent study found that 5.7% of adult patients with ARI tested positive for 229E or OC43 in nasal secretions by RT-PCR.[197] A hospital-based study in Thailand detected HCoV-229E and -OC43 in respectively 3.5% and 1% of young children with LRI.[234] Hospital-based studies of children with ARI have detected HCoV-NL63 in 1.3% in Taiwan[235] and 2.4% in South Africa.[236]

CLINICAL FEATURES

Children seroconvert to HCoV-OC43 and -229E in the first 5 years of life, but symptomatic reinfections occur.[224] Clinical manifestations of HCoV infections are typical of common colds, with average incubation period 1 day longer than for HRV, and duration of 6–7 days. Low-grade fever may be present in up to 20% of patients, and cough and sore throat occur frequently. More serious infections of the lower respiratory tract have been documented.[227] In addition, HCoVs have been detected in 8% of influenza-like illnesses in frail elderly people in the United States.[237]

HCoV has been associated with exacerbations of asthma, chronic bronchitis, and recurrent wheezing in children in several parts of the world, including tropical countries such as Brazil, West Indies, and Trinidad.[112,227,238] HCoV infections frequently complicate with otitis media and maxillary sinusitis in children and adults. HCoV were detected by RT-PCR in the middle ear and/or nasopharyngeal aspirate from 16 out of 92 (17%) children presenting with acute otitis media in Finland,[205] and in nasal swabs from 3 out of 20 adults presenting with acute maxillary sinusitis.[203]

HCoV infections cause mostly symptoms of URI, but HCoV-NL63 has been implicated in LRI, including bronchitis and pneumonia,[239] and was detected in 15% of cases of croup in children in Taiwan.[235] HCoV-HKU1 has also been associated with LRI in elderly patients and children with underlying disease.[232]

PATHOGENESIS AND IMMUNITY

There are no convenient animal models to study HCoV pathogenesis, and humans naturally or experimentally infected have been the only source of information. HCoVs are transmitted by the respiratory route and virus shedding begins 48 hours post infection, coincident with onset of symptoms, and in adults lasts approximately 5 days.[227] Both entry and release of HCoV-229E happen on the apical surface of epithelial cells[240] and the virus causes cell damage and loss of cilia on day 3 post infection.[241]

DIAGNOSIS

Except for HCoV-NL63, which can be cultured in LLC-MK2 and Vero cells, isolation of HCoVs in cell culture is tedious.[226] RT-PCR-based assays for HCoVs have become the best alternative for clinical studies.[223] Serology by EIA is sensitive and specific, and is useful in epidemiologic surveys.[224]

TREATMENT AND PREVENTION

Studies with RNAi[242] and broad-spectrum protease inhibitors[243] have been reported, but no specific antiviral therapy is available for HCoV. No vaccines are currently available for HCoV.

RESPIRATORY ADENOVIRUSES

Human adenoviruses (HAdV), the first respiratory viruses isolated, were obtained from cultured adenoid tissue, in which they may remain quiescent for a long time. Respiratory illnesses are among the most frequent consequences of adenoviral infections, particularly in children younger than 5 years.[243] Adenovirus-caused disease may present a wide spectrum of clinical manifestations, including respiratory symptoms, gastroenteritis, and conjunctivitis. HAdV have been frequently detected in ARI studies in tropical countries.[135]

THE AGENT

HAdV are nonenveloped, icosahedral DNA viruses of the genus *Mastadenovirus*, family *Adenoviridae*,[244] grouped into seven species (A–G), based on biological properties and phylogenetic relationships.[245] HAdV are distinguished antigenically into 53 types, which can be further classified into genomic subtypes.[244] HAdV types 7, 3, 4, and 21 are most frequently associated with severe disease.[246]

Adenovirus capsids are formed by three morphologically, antigenically, and functionally distinct types of capsomers: hexons, penton bases, and fibers that project from the penton bases. The hexon and penton bases contain complement-fixing, group-specific antigens common to all human adenoviruses, and the fibers, which are the virus-receptor binding domain, contain the neutralizing and hemagglutinating, type-specific antigens.[244] The adenovirus genome consists of linear double-stranded DNA of almost 36 kb, encoding approximately 40 genes.[244] A small single-stranded DNA parvovirus named adeno-associated virus is commonly detected concurrently with adenovirus, but does not seem to cause disease.[247] The virus fiber binds to a cell surface protein named CAR (Coxsackie and adenovirus receptor), but class I MHC and heparan sulfate serve as receptors for HAdV 5 and 1, respectively.[244,248] Receptor binding facilitates interaction of penton bases with cell surface integrins, triggering entry.[249] Upon endocytosis, double-stranded genomic DNA is transported to the nucleus, where "early" and "late" sets of viral genes are transcribed into mRNAs coding for structural and nonstructural proteins. Early genes encode mostly nonstructural proteins that orchestrate gene expression to maximize progeny production, while late genes encode structural proteins.[250]

Virus assembly takes place in the nucleus, releasing up to 1 million virions by cell lysis.[244] HAdV replicates well in continuous epithelial cell lines, such as HEp-2, HeLa, and A549, and can be adapted to grow in human embryonic lung fibroblasts.[244] HAdV are stable over a wide pH range (5–9), resistant to alcohol, ether and chloroform, stable for weeks at room temperature, and can be lyophilized. They are inactivated by sodium hypochlorite and by 2 minutes of heating at 60°C.[251]

EPIDEMIOLOGY

Respiratory transmission of HAdV occurs at all ages worldwide. Outbreaks happen in military recruits and sometimes in other semi-closed populations such as boarding schools and chronic care facilities. HAdV ocular transmission is associated with swimming pools or clinics where instrument sterilization or handwashing have been inadequate. Asymptomatic HAdV infection and prolonged shedding are common.[244]

HAdV species C, serotypes 1, 2, 3, and 5 are more frequent in children younger than 5 years, accounting for 5–20% of URI cases and approximately 5% of LRI cases in children.[244] In adults, HAdV occurs sporadically and causes mostly URI. Infections by HAdV types 4 and 7 are usually epidemic, with attack rates of 6–16% per week in newly assembled confined groups, such as military recruits, whose HAdV carriage rate may be as high as 18%.[244] In this group adenoviral syndromes vary from mild colds to severe LRI, with attack rates of up to 80%, with 20–40% of individuals requiring hospitalization.[244]

In temperate climates adenoviral infections are more frequent in late winter, spring and early summer, while in tropical northeast Brazil they seem to occur year-round,[135] being detected in 11% of ARI in children younger than 2 years in daycare.[140] In tropical areas the incidence of HAdV infections in military recruits is lower, and different serotypes may be involved.[244]

Adenovirus type 14 had not been associated with severe disease until 2006, when a cluster of severe disease was reported in military recruits, likely due to lack of preexisting immunity.[252] This agent is now known to occur in the general population.

Pharyngoconjunctival fever, commonly caused by HAdV types 3 and 7, may be epidemic or endemic among children in the summer in temperate climates, commonly associated with inadequate chlorination or filtration of swimming pools.[253] The incubation period of HAdV infections averages 10 days.[244]

CLINICAL FEATURES

HAdV respiratory diseases may involve all parts of the respiratory tract, but up to 50% of nonepidemic HAdV infections are asymptomatic. In fact, adenoviruses were discovered because of their propensity for latency in adenoids.[244]

Most HAdV illnesses are febrile colds, but children may have prolonged high fever. Pharyngitis is common and may be associated with fever, pharyngeal exudate, granular appearance of the mucosa, and anterior cervical adenopathy, similar to streptococcal pharyngitis.[244] HAdV can be detected in up to 20% of small children with pharyngitis. In addition to pharyngitis, pharyngoconjunctival fever caused by HAdV types 3 and 7 includes conjunctivitis, which may last 1–2 weeks, with preauricular adenopathy, cough, rhinitis, malaise, and fever.[253] The most frequent complication of HAdV ARI is acute otitis media, which occurs in up to 30% of cases.[254]

Adenovirus LRIs are mainly bronchitis and pneumonia, and may account for more than 10% of childhood LRIs in temperate areas.[255] HAdV may cause permanent lung parenchymal damage, especially when concurrent with measles.[255] Epidemic HAdV infections in military recruits have a spectrum of clinical manifestation including severe pneumonia. Typically, however, the manifestations are fever, pharyngeal symptoms, cough, chest pain, headache, and malaise.[244] More severe clinical manifestations have more recently been associated with infections of adults by an emerging mutant of HAdV type 14.[246]

Overwhelming pneumonitis may be part of disseminated HAdV infections in newborn infants and patients with immunodeficiencies including AIDS. However, frequent coinfections with other respiratory pathogens in patients with AIDS make an association of disease severity with HAdV uncertain.[256]

HAdV is also an important cause of epidemic keratoconjunctivitis.[244] HAdV 7 and 19 were the predominant serotypes associated with conjunctivitis in Brazil.[257]

PATHOGENESIS AND IMMUNITY

Respiratory disease caused by HAdV results from necrosis of cells of the airway epithelia, with viremia that may lead to disseminated infection in immunocompromised persons. Bronchiolitis, interstitial pneumonia, and mononuclear cell infiltrates are part of the inflammatory process in the lungs. The severity of HAdV diseases in children correlates with detection of higher levels of IL-6, IL-8 and TNF-α in the serum.[258] It remains unclear why certain HAdV strains are more virulent than others. For example, the genomic variant B7h was associated with fatal lower respiratory disease in a study in South America.[259] Adenoviruses may cause persistent infection in epithelial and lymphoid cells and this helps to keep viral circulation in the population.[244] HAdV glycoprotein E3 interferes with expression of class I MHC molecules, reducing display of viral epitopes on cell surface and contributing to persistence.[260] In addition, HAdV protein E1A inhibits interferon response and reduces HAdV-induced apoptosis of infected cells.[261]

Protection from HAdV infection and disease is mainly due to type-specific neutralizing antibodies, but reinfections, mostly asymptomatic, may occur. T-cell-mediated immunity is important for recovery from HAdV infection and immunocompromised patients are at higher risk for severe disease.[261]

DIAGNOSIS

HAdV can be detected in several kinds of clinical samples, but clinical correlation is required, since asymptomatic shedding is common. HAdV is amenable to isolation in human cell lines, but the direct detection of viral antigens by IF, or viral DNA by PCR, are attractive alternatives.[244] Rapid antigen detection is around 95% sensitive and easy to use in point-of-care diagnosis. However, conventional or real-time PCR are more sensitive than other methods.[262] HAdV serology has limited clinical utility.[245]

TREATMENT

At present, there is no licensed antiviral treatment for adenovirus infections.[263] Cidofovir has shown some efficacy in the rabbit model of ocular HAdV infection, while iododeoxyuridine and adenine arabinoside have been unsuccessful in treatment of keratoconjunctivitis.[244]

PREVENTION AND CONTROL

A live vaccine consisting of wild-type adenovirus packaged in capsules for enteric release induces immunity without infection of the respiratory tree. This approach has been successful in military recruits immunized with HAdV types 4 and 7.[244] Proper sterilization, handwashing, and chlorination can avoid adenovirus spread through tonometers, hands, and swimming pools.

HUMAN BOCAVIRUS

Human bocavirus (HBoV) was first detected in 2005 by an elegant viral metagenomic survey in nasopharyngeal aspirates from Swedish children with ARI.[264] Since then HBoV has been detected by PCR in children and adults with ARI essentially worldwide.[214,265]

THE AGENT

HBoV is a small, nonenveloped, icosahedral single-strand DNA virus of the family *Parvoviridae*, genus *Bocavirus*,[264] with a 5.3 kb genome encoding four proteins: non-structural proteins NS1 and NP-1, and capsid proteins VP1 and VP2.[264] HBoV capsid proteins bind to unknown cell receptors and the replication of HBoV occurs in the nucleus, where viral DNA replication is mediated by the host cell DNA polymerase.[265] After assembly the viral progeny may be released by exocytosis or by cell lysis.[265] Since DNA synthesis occurs in the S phase of the cell cycle, parvoviruses replicate more efficiently in actively dividing tissues, such as the bone marrow and respiratory and digestive epithelia.[266] Like other parvoviruses, HBoV is resistant to porous environmental surfaces, slow freezing, storage at temperatures above 4°C, or treatment with alcohol.[267]

EPIDEMIOLOGY

Three species of HBoV are recognized: HBoV1, the main species, was detected in most studies prior to 2009; HBoV2 and 3, which differ from HBoV1 by 23% at the nucleotide level, were initially detected in 2009 in stools from children with acute gastroenteritis in Pakistan and Australia, and later also in China and South Korea.[268,269]

HBoV has been detected mostly in children with respiratory and/or gastrointestinal symptoms, with frequencies ranging from 2% to 30%, and often found as a co-pathogen.[270] Its transmission may happen by respiratory and oral routes[270] and the virus can be detected in river water, suggesting potential waterborne transmission.[271]

In temperate climates HBoV is more frequent in winter and spring,[270] but in tropical areas it occurs year round.[217] Serological surveys suggest that most people are infected by HBoV early in life and in Japan 94% of people have been infected by age 6.[272]

CLINICAL FEATURES

HBoV is often detected in samples from patients with ARI[273] most often associated with wheezing, cough, rhinorrhea, and fever.[270] The most frequent clinical diagnosis of patients with HBoV infections are bronchiolitis, pneumonia, common cold, bronchitis, exacerbation of asthma, and croup.[274,275] Symptoms usually last 1–2 weeks, but occasionally may be prolonged.[276] Importantly, HBoV has been detected in association with symptoms of ILI and pneumonia. In a study conducted in Thailand, HBoV was detected in 4% of 512 patients with ILI and in 4.5% of 1168 patients with community-acquired pneumonia.[275] In approximately 90% of the patients, HBoV was present in coinfection wtih other respiratory viruses. When only children younger than 5 years were considered, HBoV was detected in 12% of those with pneumonia, highlighting its importance as a cause of LRI in that age group.[275]

HBoV has also been detected in feces of children with diarrhea.[277] Although not yet firmly established, a causative role of HBoV in diarrhea has been suggested by its detection as a single agent in studies of diarrhea, including one in Brazil.[278] Diarrhea with HBoV is more common in young children, with watery stools, nausea and vomiting.[279]

PATHOGENESIS AND IMMUNITY

Case-control studies consistently find HBoV more frequently in ARI patients than in asymptomatic controls.[274,275] In addition, HBoV viral loads are significantly higher in symptomatic patients than in asymptomatic ones.[280] Little is known about HBoV pathogenesis, including routes of infection, portal of entry, replication sites, mechanisms of tissue injury, duration of shedding, and protective efficacy of immune response. Pathogenesis studies have been hampered by the lack of growth of the virus in routine cell cultures and of experimental animal models of infection, hence Koch's postulates have not been fulfilled. Furthermore, detection of HBoV in asymptomatic individuals or in association with other respiratory viruses with established pathogenic potential complicates the diagnosis.[217,281] However, similar to other parvoviruses, HBoV may cause persistent infection with prolonged shedding.[282] HBoV causes viremia, which is uncommon in other respiratory viral infections.[274] HBoV DNA has been found in 32% of tonsils and adenoids removed from children.[283] HBoV DNA has been detected as single agent in feces from 0.8–7.8% of children with gastroenteritis without ARI symptoms.[277,278,284,285] The role of immune response in pathogenesis and protection against infection remains unclear; but both Th1 and Th2 cytokines are increased in children with bronchiolitis and HBoV.[286]

DIAGNOSIS

HBoV replicates in primary cultures of respiratory cells,[287] but cannot be propagated in common cell lines, and rapid antigen detection methods have not become available. Real-time PCR assays have become the standard for HBoV diagnosis, but with limited availability in most developing countries.[288]

TREATMENT, PREVENTION, AND CONTROL

The actual clinical impact of HBoV respiratory and digestive infections is still uncertain, and no specific therapeutic or prophylactic approaches are available for this agent.

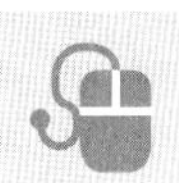

Access the complete reference list online at
http://www.expertconsult.com

CHAPTER 59

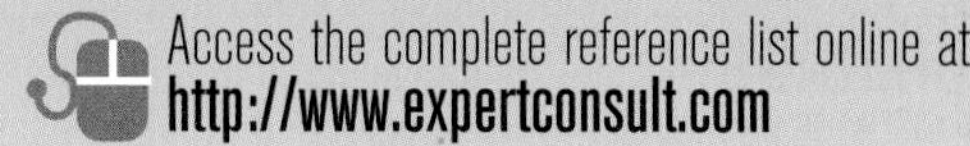
Access the complete reference list online at
http://www.expertconsult.com

Severe Acute Respiratory Syndrome (SARS)

Mei-Shang Ho

INTRODUCTION

> *Initially "that disease" had no name, then we called it atypical pneumonia in China. Later the rest of the world would name it severe acute respiratory syndrome, or SARS ...*[1]

Severe acute respiratory syndrome (SARS) is a newly emerged infectious disease manifested mainly as a severe form of bronchopneumonia that is caused by a novel coronavirus – SARS-CoV.[2,3] The virus was later shown to have jumped host species from horseshoe bat to infect humans via masked palm civets or possibly other mammals sold in live animal markets.[4–9] First having occurred in November 2002 in Guangdong Province of southern China,[10,11] the SARS epidemic that spread to 29 countries in five continents over a few weeks showed its potential to have a pandemic health impact in the absence of precautionary control measures (***Fig. 59.1***).[12] Recognition of the SARS epidemic quickly prompted a global response orchestrated by the World Health Organization (WHO) that effectively facilitated the identification of the etiologic agent, the development of diagnostic tests, and the development and evaluation of treatment protocols aiming to reduce morbidity and mortality. With the successful estimation of key epidemiological parameters affecting epidemic dynamics of transmission, appropriate public health interventions were promptly formulated and implemented on a global basis that ultimately brought the epidemic under control; by July 5, 2003, WHO declared the recovery of the last patient and the successful interruption of the chain of SARS transmission in humans.

In the following winter in Guangzhou between December 16, 2003 and January 8, 2004, four more community-acquired SARS patients were identified, manifesting only a mild flu-like syndrome with no secondary transmission.[13] Information indicated that three of the patients were epidemiologically linked to a restaurant where palm civets were served. The remaining palm civets in the restaurant and in a live animal market that supplied civets to the restaurant were later shown to harbor SARS-CoV that shared near identical nucleotide sequences of the S genes as that detected in specimens collected from some of the patients.[7–9] Following the reemergence of human SARS cases in the winter of 2003–2004, Chinese authorities once again banned trading of live civets in markets, as well as culling all the infected civets in farms, as an attempt to prevent further interspecies transmission to humans. These cases resulted in no grave epidemic impact and provided an opportunity for detailed investigation into an interspecies jump of animal viruses into the human population. It served as a reminder that naturally existing SARS-CoV-like virus may reemerge to cause outbreaks in human populations when given the opportune setting of transmission via interspecies jumping, mutation, and adaptation of the virus to the new host.

The most recent small cluster of two SARS cases that occurred in China in April 2004 originated from a research laboratory. Such an event illustrates another possible source of SARS resurgence in the future.

THE AGENT

SARS-CoV is a newly identified human pathogen that appears to be phylogenically distinct from the two human pathogenic coronaviruses, 229E and OC43, previously known to cause mostly mild upper respiratory tract infections and more severe influenza-like illness in children and the elderly.[14,15] SARS-CoV has since been classified as antigenic group II coronaviruses that, along with group I, are mainly harbored in bats and mammals, in contrast to group III, that are from birds (for detailed phylogeny, see recent review)[16] (***Fig. 59.2***). Coronaviruses are enveloped, single- and positive-stranded RNA viruses which, by nature, carry a high mutation rate that in essence serves the purposes of genetic diversity, plasticity, and adaptability of the virus to a wide host range.[16] The RNA genome, the largest among all RNA viruses, encodes a nonstructural replicase polyprotein and several structural proteins, including spike (S), envelope (E), membrane (M), and nucleocapsid (N) proteins.[17] The S1 subunit of SARS-CoV S protein plays pivotal roles in viral infection and pathogenesis, i.e., it recognizes and binds to host receptors, and the binding brings about subsequent conformational changes in the S2 subunit of the S protein to facilitate fusion between the viral envelope and the host cell membrane.[18] Among all structural proteins of SARS-CoV, S protein is the main antigenic component responsible for inducing host immune responses, neutralizing antibodies, and possibly providing protective immunity against viral infection. The S protein has therefore been suggested as an important target for vaccine and antiviral development.

Animal Reservoir

Initiatives to track SARS-CoV back to the animal origin were inspired by the epidemiological information indicating that several food handlers, especially those who handle, kill, or butcher "exotic" animals for food, were among the first index cases of SARS in late 2002 in Guangdong.[10,19] Further serological studies of animal traders from several live animal markets during the time of the SARS outbreak in Guangzhou (Guangdong, China) in 2003 also showed a higher prevalence of immunoglobulin G antibodies against SARS-CoV than vegetable traders,[10,11] and viruses related to human SARS-CoV were subsequently isolated from a number of animals sold in the markets, including Himalaya palm civets.[4] However, the palm civets were deemed not to be the natural animal reservoir of SARS-CoV based on the observations that all SARS-CoVs identified from palm civets at that time shared >99.6% nucleic acid sequence identity with one another, implying a recent entry of the virus into the palm civet population in the live animal market. Furthermore, a general absence of antibodies against SARS-CoV among palm civets raised in the farms supplying animals to the markets further corroborates the theory of a wet market-perpetuated transmission of SARS-CoV.[4,20,21] Subsequently, several SARS-CoV-like viruses, sharing 88–92% nucleotide homology with that of the human SARS-CoV, were detected in species of Chinese horseshoe bats existing in the wild in Hong Kong and southern China.[5,6]

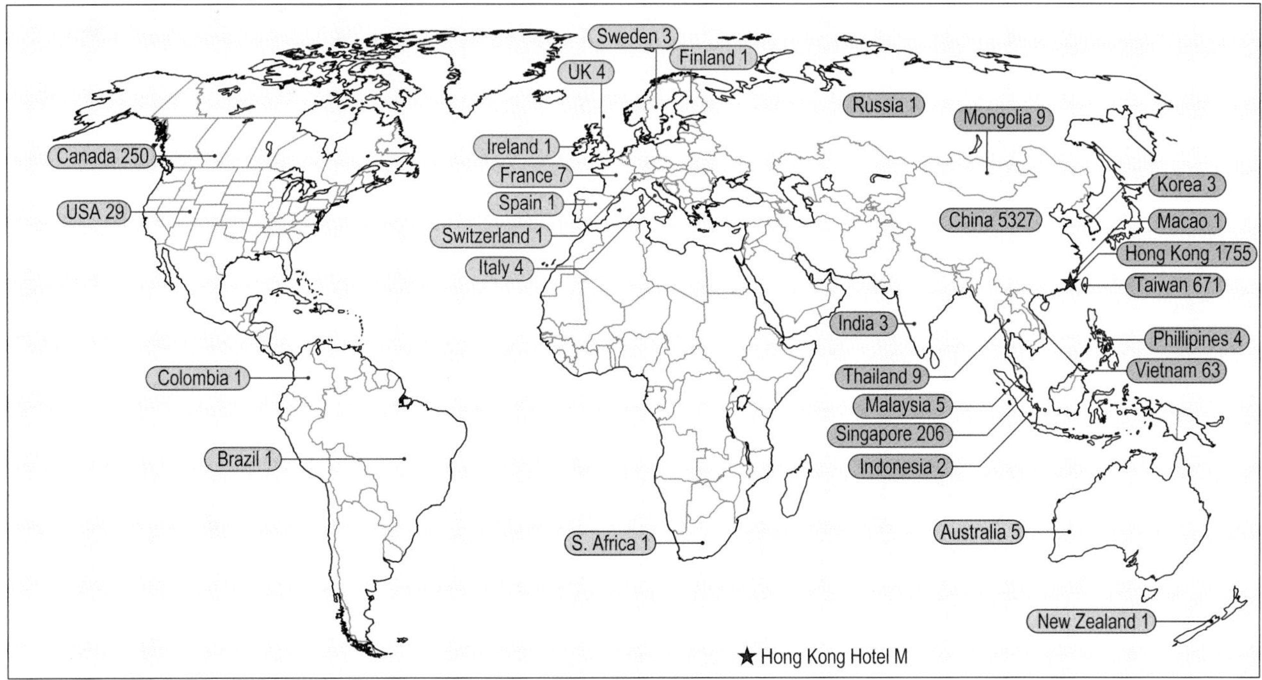

Figure 59.1 Cumulative number of severe acute respiratory syndrome (SARS) patients by country in 2003. The star designates a Hong Kong hotel in which a SARS patient from southern China infected 10 guests, whose subsequent international movements spread the virus outside China, causing multicountry outbreaks of SARS in 2003.[12]

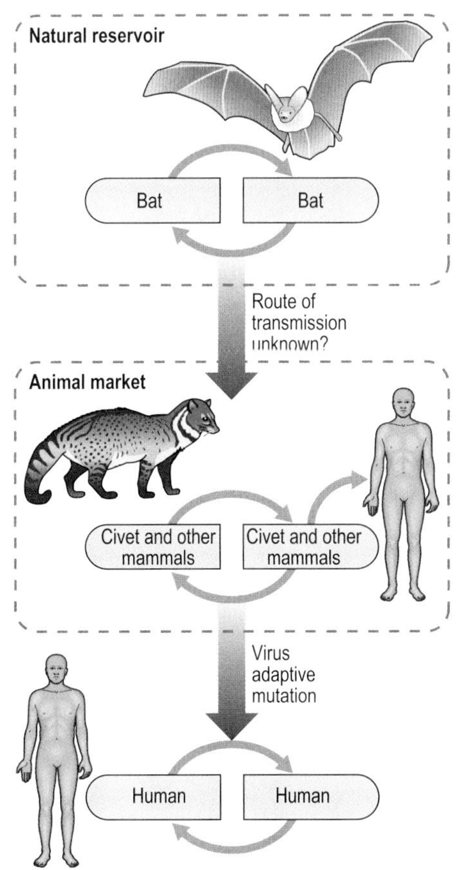

Figure 59.2 Life cycle of severe acute respiratory syndrome (SARS)-coronavirus (CoV). Cross-species transmission of the 2003 SARS-CoV from the natural reservoir of horseshoe bats to a large-scale human outbreak occurred via several mammalian species sold as exotic food in live animal markets; in the animal market, the virus-infected animal handlers were asymptomatic or exhibited a mild clinical picture. The virus acquired the capacity for efficient human-to-human transmission, and also possibly severe pathogenicity, only after adaptive mutations of the viral genome took place.[4–6,10,11,19–22]

These findings culminated in adding SARS-CoV to the long list of viruses that are naturally harbored in a variety of bat species, i.e., rabies, Hendra, Nipha, Ebola, and St Louis encephalitis viruses. Apart from Himalaya palm civets and bats, many other mammalian animal species have also tested positive for SARS-CoV, suggesting a promiscuous nature of SARS-CoV in hosts and the ability for host adaptation (*Fig. 59.2*) (see reference 22 for detailed review).

EPIDEMIOLOGY

Genetic Evolution

The continuing genetic evolution of SARS-CoV serves as a means for temporal and geographic tracking of viral transmission. Molecular analyses of all available (>100 GenBank deposits) SARS-CoV sequences indicate that most of the genetic diversity of SARS-CoV occurred among the earliest human isolates from Guangdong province, China, and that these human isolates were phylogenically clustered along with the isolates from civets in the live animal markets.[4,19,23] The rest of the "panglobal isolates" were clustered with viruses epidemiologically linked to the so-called "superspreading event" associated with the Hong Kong hotel transmission by the SARS patient from Guangzhou. The human "panglobal" isolates as a whole all contain a 29-nucleotide deletion (residues 27869 to 27897) that is 246 nucleotides upstream of the start codon of the N gene; this deletion set apart the human isolates from the civet isolates.[4,23] Whether the generation of these "panglobal isolates," which has clearly demonstrated viral fitness in efficient transmission among human population, is due to the occurrence of critical adaptive mutation(s) of the viral genome to become a human pathogen or as a result of the "superspreading event" occurring by random chance remains to be studied.

EPIDEMIOLOGICAL PARAMETERS

Retrospective investigation identified possibly 11 index SARS cases in Guangdong Province, China, with the earliest case occurring in mid-November 2002. SARS remained a local disease until February 21, 2003, when a physician infected with SARS-CoV traveled to Hong Kong while still in the early course of illness. Through contact in a Hong Kong hotel, 10 guests were infected. The subsequent movements of these international travelers effectively spread the virus outside China where the patients sought medical care and large-scale nosocomial outbreaks ensued (*Fig. 59.1*).

The incubation period estimated in cases with well-characterized events of exposure and the onset of illness is between 2 and 10 days, with a mean around 4–5 days.[24–26] The rate of spread of an epidemic largely depends on the basic reproduction number (R_0), defined as the average number of secondary cases infected by one primary case in a susceptible population. Mathematical modeling of the early phase, based on the epidemiological data collected before the implementation of any control measures when transmission was occurring mainly in the hospital setting, estimated the R_0 to be 2.2–3.7.[27,28] The spread of SARS illustrates two important stages of disease transmission in the modern era: the first stage of the long-distance spread via international travelers and the second stage of establishing the chain of local transmission at each local epicenter. The R_0 must be >1 in order for the disease to establish sustainable local transmission. However, a highly heterogeneous potential of transmission from individual index cases is usually observed, i.e., a "superspreading event," which entails an index case capable of infecting multiple household members and health care workers in both social/family and hospital settings, and these "superspreading events" most often serve to ignite subsequent explosive SARS outbreaks at the local site. The attack rate for SARS-CoV ranges from 10.3% to 60% or 2.4 to 31.3 cases/1000 exposure-hours, depending on the setting and the unit of measurement.[25] The overall case-fatality rate was ~15%, but can be as high as 60% in elderly patients with a high virus load.[29]

Route of Transmission

The virus can be readily detected in the blood and excreta of infective individuals. Transmission occurs mainly via respiratory droplets generated by coughing or sneezing or through contaminated environmental surfaces[30] and fomites.[24,25] Under rare and special circumstances, aerosolized human excreta, exemplified by the fecal–oral or fecal–aerosol transmission in the large outbreak in an apartment complex due to a faulty sewage system, may also contribute to transmission.[31] The infectivity of SARS patients begins a few days after the onset of disease symptoms, most notably fever (*Fig. 59.3*); the infectivity increases, correlating with increasing virus shedding, during the first 10 days of disease.[32,33] The key epidemiological parameter that renders the control of SARS epidemic conducive to isolation and quarantine strategies is that the infectivity of SARS is preceded by the onset of recognizable clinical symptoms in infected patients (*Fig. 59.3*).

THE DISEASE

On Presentation

While SARS is mainly a respiratory disease, the clinical features (*Table 59.1*) on initial presentation are generally indistinguishable from that of influenza infection or atypical pneumonia of other causes (i.e., *Mycoplasma*, *Chlamydia*, or *Legionella*). The most common features at onset of illness include fever, chills, myalgia, malaise, nonproductive cough, headache, and dyspnea.[34,35] Less common symptoms include sputum production, sore throat, rhinorrhea, nausea/vomiting, and diarrhea. During the epidemic period, elderly persons with chronic illness may seek medical care of the underlying disease and have atypical clinical presentation of SARS, i.e., seeming without fever or respiratory symptoms.[36] Watery nonbloody diarrhea, along with recurrent fever, was the predominant extrapulmonary symptom during the first week of illness among patients infected in an apartment complex where fecal–aerosol or fecal–oral transmission was thought to have occurred.[32]

Progression and Clinical Spectrum

A majority of patients have a mild to intermediate clinical course that resolves with bed rest and nasal oxygen supplement (*Fig. 59.3*). About 20–36% require intensive care, and 13–26% progress into acute respiratory distress syndrome (ARDS), necessitating invasive ventilatory support.[24,32,37–39] The clinical course follows a typical biphasic pattern that presumably is linked to events of an initial phase of viral replication and a second phase of immunopathological response (*Fig. 59.3*).[29,32] During

Table 59.1 Frequency of Clinical Features in Severe Acute Respiratory Syndrome on Presentation[24,28,29]

Symptom	Patients with Symptom (%)
Fever >38°C	100
Chills/rigors	55–73
Nonproductive cough	29–57
Myalgia	38–61
Headache	11–56
Dizziness	43
Malaise	35
Coryza	32
Sputum production	15–29
Sore throat	7–23
Diarrhea[a]	1–20
Nausea and vomiting	20
Dyspnea[a]	0–10

[a]By day 8, diarrhea occurred in 73% of patients, and respiratory symptoms worsened in 45% of patients.[27]

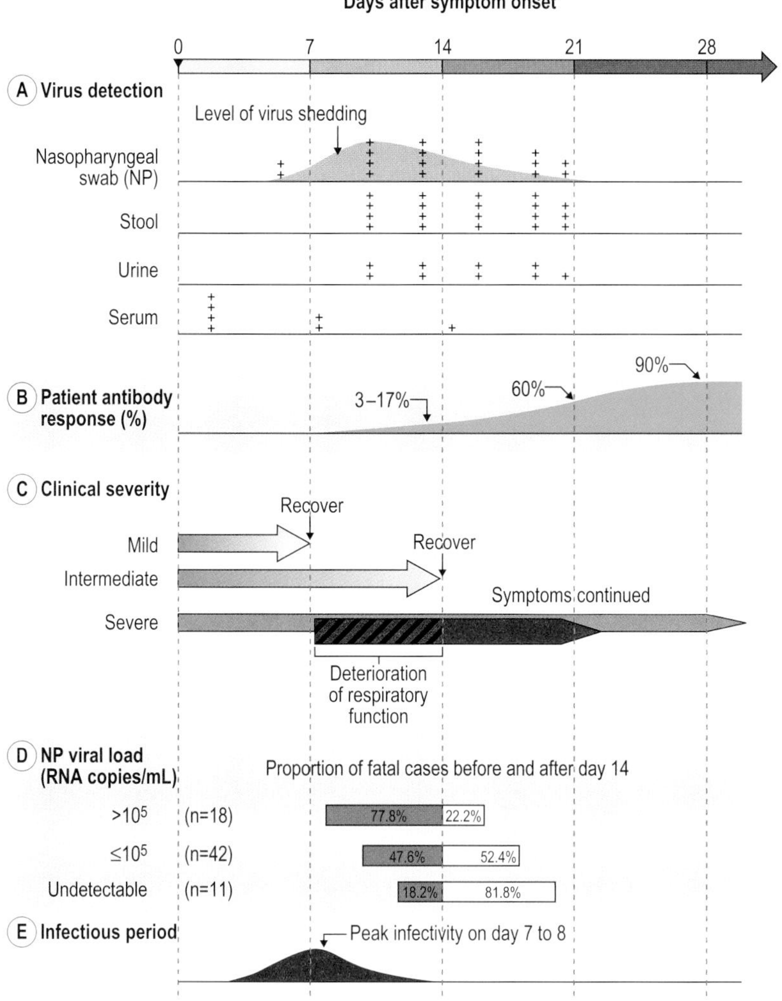

Figure 59.3 Summary of events corresponding to the clinical course of SARS infection (days after symptom onset). (**A**) Relative rate of virus detection and (**B**) antibody response, (**C**) time of clinical deterioration and recovery in patients of various severity, (**D**) time of death in relation to virus load, and (**E**) the approximate infection period.[29,31,36,39,65,66]

the initial clinical phase of up to 10 days, the increasing viral load is associated with clinical features of mainly systemic symptoms, including, most notably, fever and myalgia, which generally improve within days among patients having a short mild to intermediate clinical course. In some patients, despite the falling viral load during the second through the third week, immunopathological damage may ensue with persistent or recurrent fever, oxygen desaturation, and radiologic progression of pneumonia.[12,24,32,37,38] For those in whom ARDS (up to 20%) later ensues, pulmonary function begins to show progressive worsening in the second week of illness.

Retrospective analyses of serial chest radiographs in all 1373 SARS patients in Hong Kong[40] and of high-resolution computed tomographic scan of 14 patients[41] corroborate the progression of radiographic opacities or bilateral fibrotic lung changes during week 2 to be useful prognostic predictors of the ultimate clinical severity. Furthermore, disease severity was intensified by slower and prolonged recovery with complications of pulmonary fibrosis occurring in the third week in some patients.[42]

Chest Radiological Findings

Up to 25% of SARS patients have normal chest radiographs on presentation.[24,35,43,44] While radiographic appearances of SARS, sharing common features with atypical pneumonia of other causes, in general, are characterized by ground-glass opacities and focal consolidations, the abnormalities tend to be localized in the periphery and subpleural regions of the lower zones and are mostly devoid of cavitation, hilar lymphadenopathy, or pleural effusion.[24,42,44] Progression from unilateral to bilateral involvement is not uncommon in SARS patients[42,44] and sometimes with shifting of radiographic shadows, i.e., resolving opacity in one area while a new opacity occurs in another area of lung, and spontaneous pneumomediastinum (12% in one series).[32,45] High resolution computed tomography of the thorax is useful in detecting lung opacities early in cases with unremarkable chest radiographs.[46]

Extrapulmonary Involvement

SARS is a systemic disease, especially in severe cases, in which a wide spectrum of tissue and cell types is directly infected by virus or is affected indirectly. Diarrhea is the most common extrapulmonary manifestation during the early phase, presumably due to viral replication in the gastrointestinal tract.[32] Elevated liver transaminases suggest that hepatic dysfunction is common, though virus is not found in liver; dizziness may be related to central nervous virus invasion; the left ventricular ejection fraction may be decreased though the pathogenic mechanism is unclear[47]; petechiae, myositis, neuromuscular abnormalities, and seizures have also occurred.[47,48] Circulating lymphocytes are widely infected,[49] and lymphopenia is very common.[50] Orchitis was observed in a series of autopsies of fatal SARS patients, suggesting that reproductive function in male patients who recover from SARS should be monitored.[49]

Laboratory Findings

Peripheral absolute lymphopenia (reduction in both CD4 and CD8 lymphocytes) is a prominent feature, occurring in 98% of patients. Features of low-grade disseminated intravascular coagulation (thrombocytopenia, prolonged activated partial thromboplastin time, raised D-dimers), and elevated lactate dehydrogenase, alanine transaminases, and creatine kinase are frequent laboratory features of SARS.[24,35,37,43]

PATHOGENESIS AND IMMUNITY

Tissue tropism of SARS-CoV is stipulated by a specific receptor-facilitated process; angiotensin converting enzyme 2 (ACE2) has been identified as the cellular receptor that binds directly to the viral S protein.[51] ACE2 is expressed in alveolar epithelial cells and in surface enterocytes of the small intestine, both of which are the primary target cells of SARS-CoV infection.[32] ACE2, which acts as a negative regulator of the local renin–angiotensin system and is down-regulated by viral infection, can protect the lung against external damage in experimental animal models. In addition, the S protein of SARS-CoV can also bind to C-type lectins, i.e., CD209 (also known as dendritic cell-specific intercellular adhesion molecule-grabbing nonintegrin, or DC-SIGN) and CD209L, and gain access to cell entry.[52] Although SARS-CoV particles and genomic sequence are detected in a large number of circulating lymphocytes, monocytes, and lymphoid tissues during the early phase of infection,[49] no virus has been found in dendritic cells. Viremia, with or without cell association, occurs early in the clinical course, thus contributing to the spread of virus to organs other than the site of entry.

The intestinal tract is an important extrapulmonary site of viral replication; specimens taken by colonoscopy or at necropsy reveal evidence of active viral replication within both the small and large intestinal mucosa but with minimal pathological changes,[32] and SARS-CoV RNA may be detected by reverse transcriptase polymerase chain reaction (RT-PCR) from gastrointestinal specimens for up to 10 weeks after onset.[53] In an autopsy series of 18 patients who died between days 14 and 62, epithelial cells of the digestive tracts of all patients were virally infected but displayed only mild inflammatory changes.[49] The most obvious lesion in the digestive tract is depletion of the submucosal lymphoid tissues. The minimal pathology in the gastrointestinal tract contrasts sharply with the diffuse alveolar damage in the lung, while both organs serve as primary sites of viral replication. Thus, the pathogenesis must involve tissue-specific host responses, which are most likely intensified during week 2 of illness when pulmonary function worsens with concomitant decreasing viral load in the airways (Fig. 59.3).[32,54] Clinical studies of cytokines during the acute phase[55,56] suggest that activation of Th1 cell-mediated immunity and an excessive innate inflammatory response, rather than direct damage from uncontrolled virus growth, are responsible for the pathogenic process in severe cases who survive through week 2.[32]

A protracted clinical course was intensified by slower and prolonged convalescence due to complications of pulmonary fibrosis occurring in week 3 in some patients.[42] Results of high-resolution computed tomographic scans in follow-up of SARS patients corroborate this observation, with a strong correlation between bilateral fibrotic lung changes and clinical severity.[41]

Based on analysis of 18 autopsies on patients who died between days 14 and 62, SARS-CoV infects multiple cell types in several organs other than the epithelial cells of the respiratory tract and the mucosa of the intestine, i.e., the epithelium of the renal distal tubules, showing focal hemorrhage, neurons of the hypothalamus and cortex in all patients, and infiltrating macrophages in other organs.[49] Clinical manifestations correlate directly with the sites where viral infection occurs, such as higher viral shedding in the stool associated with diarrhea, and a higher urine viral load associated with abnormal urinalysis, probably due to renal involvement.[48,57,58] Status epilepticus in two SARS patients whose cerebrospinal fluid and serum samples contained SARS-CoV was most likely due to central nervous system infection.[59,60] Involvement of other organs includes hepatocellular injury in the centrilobular zone in five out of eight patients with no detectable virus, and the testes of seven male patients displayed focal atrophy with no virus detected. Organs with no pathologic change include heart, pancreas, adrenal gland, thyroid gland, and skeletal muscle, though SARS-CoV-laden lymphocytes and monocytes were present in some of these organs. Immune cells and pulmonary epithelium are the main sites of injury.

Viral Load and Mortality

Viral shedding in the nasopharynx, measured by quantitative RT-PCR, peaks on day 10 (***Fig. 59.3***).[32] However, analysis of 265 laboratory-confirmed SARS patients in Taiwan demonstrates that, on any given day of the clinical course, SARS-CoV shedding in the nasopharynx varies widely from individual to individual, ranging from below the detection limit to as high as 10^8 RNA copies/mL; male patients and elderly patients are more likely to have detectable virus shedding,[29] suggesting that individual host differences in viral shedding surpass the variation during the clinical course for each individual.

Higher nasopharyngeal and serum viral loads are associated with oxygen desaturation, mechanical ventilation, and mortality;[29,48,57] furthermore, a higher nasopharyngeal virus titer is associated with early death occurring within the first 2 weeks of illness (***Fig. 59.3***).[29]

Genetic Predisposition

Individual differences are genetically attributed to single base differences (single nucleotide polymorphisms, SNPs) of genes. Several studies have been carried out to search for genetic predisposition to severe clinical outcomes of SARS in the hope of understanding the pathogenesis through the function of the polymorphism gene with predisposing risk. Human leukocyte antigen (HLA)-B*4601 was associated with both predisposition to infection and severity of illness among both Taiwanese and Hong Kong patients.[61,62] HLA-B*0703, which is an allele of very low frequency in ~3% of the general population, is a predisposition allele.[62] One SNP of FGL2, of nonsynonymous (G53E) nature, was associated with SARS-CoV shedding in the nasopharynx, as well as with a prolonged clinical course of Taiwanese SARS patients;[29,63] FGL2, an interferon-γ-inducible protein expressed by lymphocytes, macrophages, and endothelium, is a prothrombinase that is reported to contribute to fibrin deposition during viral hepatitis, and its expression is associated with a number of pathological conditions. The SNP in the promoter region of CXCL10/IP-10 and heme oxygenase 1, both of which play roles in modulating inflammation, is associated with the SARS clinical outcome.[63] Other SNPs of interleukin (IL)-1α, IL-18 and RelB, all gene products related to innate immunity and interferon pathway, are also associated with nasopharyngeal virus shedding.[29] More studies are needed to determine the biological significance of these genetic determinants in relation to susceptibility to infection and to the host–pathogen interaction contributing to the clinical outcome of the infection.

DIAGNOSIS

Virus Detection

Nasopharyngeal and oral pharyngeal mucosa is the site of viral entry, as well as the major site of viral replication for SARS-CoV; after infection, virus may be detected in nasopharyngeal aspirate, stool, serum/plasma, and urine with variable sensitivity during the clinical course (***Fig. 59.3***). Virus isolation is not routinely carried out for SARS-CoV in the clinical setting as it requires a high containment laboratory for biosafety and biosecurity considerations. Instead, detecting viral nucleic acids based on primers of various segments of the viral genome by conventional RT-PCR or by quantitative RT-PCR is routinely used as the standard diagnostic method. With optimized RNA extraction methods and applying quantitative real-time RT-PCR techniques, the sensitivity for diagnosis of SARS in the first 3 days of disease is as high as 80% when nasopharyngeal aspirate specimens were tested,[64] which is a tremendous improvement when compared with the generally low detection rate by conventional RT-PCR during the first week of illness. In a longitudinal follow-up study of 20 SARS patients with detectable nasopharyngeal SARS-CoV virus by

RT-PCR, the virus load increased from day 5 to day 10 and decreased by day 15 of illness.[32] On day 14 of illness, the sensitivity of detection in urine, nasophargyngeal aspirate, and stool specimens is 42%, 68%, and 97%, respectively.[32]

Viremia occurs early in the clinical course. Testing of serum by quantitative RT-PCR showed a detection rate of 80% on the first day of hospital admission, dropping to 75% and 42% on days 7 and 14, respectively.[65,66]

Serological Diagnosis

Antibody against SARS-CoV may be detected, by either neutralization testing or enzyme-linked immunosorbent assay, by the second week of illness in some 17.4%,[39] but usually requires 4 weeks to reach a detection rate above 90%; the antibody level peaks between weeks 5 and 8, then declines thereafter.[32,39] A short survival, i.e., mortality within 2 weeks of onset, was noted among those who developed neutralizing antibody early in the clinical course.[39] Thus, the level of neutralizing antibody response correlates with the severity of illness.

TREATMENT AND PROGNOSIS

Supportive Care

Since oxygen desaturation and respiratory failure, associated with ARDS and alveolar destruction, represent the majority of decompensating and terminal events in SARS patients, supportive management of pulmonary function to maintain oxygen saturation is imperative. Nasal oxygen supplementation with strict bed rest to reduce oxygen demand is a general practice, and noninvasive positive-pressure ventilation has been used with success in severely ill cases of SARS patients.[67] However, due to the potential risk of viral transmission via positive-pressure mask leakage and flow compensation, causing dispersion of contaminated aerosol, health care workers should adhere to appropriate precautionary practices in wearing personal protective equipment, including mask, gown, and gloves, before noninvasive positive-pressure ventilation is initiated, preferably in a negative-pressure hospital isolation ward or in an isolation room with adequate air exchange.

Antiviral Agents

Treatment of SARS during the outbreak in 2003 was mostly empirical and at times anecdotal owing to the novel nature of the newly emerged SARS and a lack of understanding of the pathogenesis and clinical course. A number of anti-human immunodeficiency virus (HIV) agents were tried. The combination formulation of lopinavir/ritonavir when used in the initial phase was shown in a retrospective multicenter analysis to be associated with a reduction in the overall death rate to 2.3% and intubation rate to 0%, as well as a lower rate of treatment with methylprednisolone when compared with historic controls or with a matched cohort without antiviral treatment.[68,69] The use of ribavirin, on the other hand, appears to be associated with hemolysis and a decrease in hemoglobin, as well as a rise in transaminases.[43]

Immunomodulators

Intravenous high dose (0.5 g daily) of methylprednisolone was given with the intention of preventing immunopathological lung injury based on the rationale that progression of the pulmonary disease may be mediated by the host inflammatory response during week 2, when progressive worsening of radiological findings and hypoxemia occurs.[24,32,68] The use of high-dose pulse methylprednisolone during clinical progression was reported to be associated with more favorable clinical improvement.[68] Intravenous immunoglobulin 1 g/kg/day for 2 days was routinely used as standard therapy in many patients in Taiwan based on the rationale of possibly suppressing an overly elevated cytokine response, though no control group was available for comparison of its effects.[70]

In an uncontrolled trial in Toronto, interferon alfacon-1 plus corticosteroids was reported to reduce disease-associated impaired oxygen saturation, to achieve a more rapid resolution of radiographic lung opacities, and to lower levels of creatine kinase.[71] It should be noted, however, that in the future event of SARS resurgence, any treatment regimen should undergo clinical trials of randomized placebo-controlled design. New antiviral agents and immunomodulating agents such as hyperimmune globulin and monoclonal antibody have been developed and are awaiting the opportunity for clinical evaluation.

Clinical Prognostic Indicators

Advanced age and presence of comorbidities, notably diabetes mellitus and chronic hepatitis B carriage, are poor prognostic indicators associated with higher SARS mortality;[24,32,43] pregnancy also carries significant risk for mortality.[72] Infections in children appear to be milder than those in adults.[73]

Low counts of CD4 and CD8 T lymphocytes at presentation are associated with adverse clinical outcome.[50] Among the abnormal laboratory findings, elevated lactate dehydrogenase level, hypouricemia, acute renal failure, more extensive pulmonary radiological involvement, and a high neutrophil count on presentation are all poor prognostic indicators.[16,24,38]

Patients having higher nasopharyngeal and serum viral loads are more likely to experience oxygen desaturation, require mechanical ventilation, and die.[29,48,57] Furthermore, higher nasopharyngeal viral shedding was associated with early death occurring within the first 2 weeks of illness (***Fig. 59.3***).[29] The correlation between high viral loads in specific specimens and the clinical manifestations suggests that viral replication during the initial phase contributes to the clinical manifestations.[58]

Long-term Prognosis

Abnormalities in the nature of restrictive pulmonary function due to residual lung fibrosis are common.[74] Pulmonary function testing of SARS survivors 1 year after recovery showed a reduction in diffusion capacity and a lower exercise endurance capacity than the healthy population.[75]

PREVENTION AND CONTROL

The global responses have successfully broken the chain of human transmission of the 2003 SARS epidemic that occurred in 29 countries in five continents.[12] Now that several winter seasons have elapsed since the 2003 SARS outbreak without the occurrence of any further SARS case, we can exert a much higher level of confidence that the human population is truly free of SARS-CoV transmission even in a covert manner, though potential resurgence remains in the future either via reintroduction of the virus from a natural animal reservoir (***Fig. 59.2***) or spillage from a research laboratory. SARS is zoonotic in origin, and establishing the capability for early detection in initial human cases is the key to preventing large-scale human transmission. In light of the disease carrying a considerable need for surge capacity of health care services, continued vigilance in determining diagnoses of all cases of atypical or severe respiratory infection in a timely manner, as well as stringent practices to minimize nosocomial infection in general, is imperative.

Access the complete reference list online at
http://www.expertconsult.com

CHAPTER 60

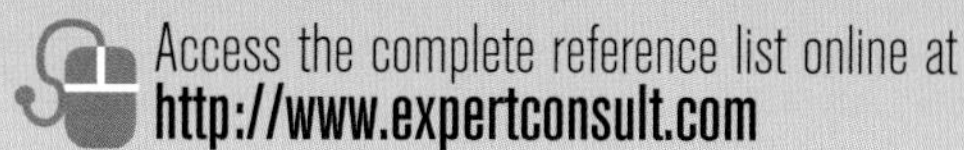
Access the complete reference list online at
http://www.expertconsult.com

Enterovirus Infections, Including Poliomyelitis

Mark A. Pallansch

INTRODUCTION

Enteroviruses are among the most common of human viruses, possibly infecting a billion or more persons annually worldwide. Most infections are largely inapparent, but enteroviruses cause a wide spectrum of acute disease, including mild upper respiratory illness (common cold), febrile exanthem (hand, foot and mouth disease and herpangina), conjunctivitis, aseptic meningitis, pleurodynia, myocarditis, encephalitis, acute flaccid paralysis (paralytic poliomyelitis), and neonatal sepsis-like disease.[1,2] Enterovirus infections result in hundreds of thousands of hospitalizations per year in the developed world, with aseptic meningitis accounting for the vast majority of these cases. The disease burden in the developing world of the tropics is poorly estimated, with the exception of poliomyelitis. Enteroviral infections are more common in most developing countries, so it is reasonable to assume that significant morbidity can be attributed to these viruses globally.

Poliomyelitis is the best described enteroviral disease in the tropics and is probably a disease of antiquity. It was only by the mid-nineteenth century, however, when the Industrial Revolution brought increased urbanization to Europe and North America, that larger and more frequent outbreaks of poliomyelitis began in these regions. From the late 1800s, outbreaks occurred in several European countries and in the United States, and they remained a dominant public health problem in the developed world for the first half of the twentieth century. It was later that the disease burden due to polio in the tropics was fully appreciated. At the time that polio vaccines became available in the 1960s, possibly more than 500 000 children were paralyzed by poliovirus infection every year, mostly in the developing countries of the tropics.

Knowledge about the nature of enteroviruses and the spectrum of clinical disease largely has followed progress made with studies of polioviruses. Despite this progress, much remains to be learned about the differences in epidemiology and disease burden in the tropics.

THE AGENT

Viruses of the genus *Enterovirus*, in the family *Picornaviridae*, are among the simplest in genetic complexity and size. All are small, round, 30 nm particles with icosahedral symmetry and no lipid envelope.[3] The infectious particles are relatively heat-resistant, acid-resistant (distinguishing them from rhinoviruses), and also resistant to many common detergents and disinfectants, including most soaps, nonionic detergents, ethanol, ether, chloroform, and other lipid solvents. The virus is stable for weeks or more at 4°C and for days at room temperature; however, the virus is readily inactivated by desiccation, ultraviolet light, heat, formaldehyde, and free chlorine.[4,5] The genomic RNA is infectious and serves as messenger RNA for viral protein synthesis. The RNA is translated in a single open reading frame into one large polyprotein, which is then processed through proteolytic cleavage by two distinct virus-encoded proteases into the functional viral proteins.[6]

Historically, classification of enteroviruses into polioviruses, coxsackieviruses A and B, and echoviruses was based on their association with clinical syndromes, tissue tropism, nature of disease in suckling mice, growth in certain cell cultures, and antigenic similarities.[7] Using these criteria, 64 different serotypes were recognized and classified, despite the fact that several antigenically related viruses had different pathogenic properties in mice. This last discrepancy eventually led to the last four viruses being designated only as enteroviruses 68–71.[8] A more satisfactory and completely new classification followed from comprehensive genetic studies. The complete RNA genetic sequences for all the recognized enteroviruses[9] have allowed a more detailed comparison among these viruses.[10] The human enteroviruses have been reclassified into four species, A–D, with polioviruses now classified as members of species C (**Table 60.1**).[11,12]

Continued characterization of enteroviral clinical isolates has identified many members of the genus, continuing from enterovirus 73 sequentially.[13–17] These have been assigned to one of the four species (**Table 60.1**). Very little is known about any distinctive clinical or epidemiologic features of these new viruses, but there are likely to be many more described with application of sequencing to viruses from the developing world. Also as a part of these studies, it was demonstrated that echoviruses 22 and 23 are genetically distinct from the enteroviruses,[18] and they have been reclassified as members of the new picornavirus genus, *Parechovirus*, and renamed human parechoviruses 1 and 2, respectively. In addition to the genera *Enterovirus* and *Parechovirus*, at least three more genera in this family have members that infect humans: *Kobuvirus*, *Cosavirus*, and *Hepatovirus* (hepatitis A virus).

The genetic diversity and groupings evident from genomic sequence analysis also correlate with the antigenic properties. Antigenic groupings form the basis of serotype definition and are the primary means of distinguishing different enterovirus isolates and are also important for immunity. Antisera to each of the viruses raised in animals are usually type specific and provide reference reagents for serotype determination of isolates.[19] Antigenic differences among isolates of the same serotype can be very complex, but variation at one or several epitopes does not change the serotype as determined by polyclonal antibodies or host response. The great diversity of serotypes presents considerable problems for laboratory diagnosis and epidemiologic investigations, but the serotype usually has minimal importance to the diagnosis and clinical management of an individual patient.

EPIDEMIOLOGY

The patterns of virus shedding and routes of transmission for enteroviruses are consistent with few exceptions.[20] Virus is isolated in the highest titer and for the longest time, often several weeks, in stool specimens but can also be isolated from respiratory secretions. Therefore, both fecal-oral transmission and spread by contact with respiratory secretions (person-to-person, fomites, and large-particle aerosol) are considered the

Table 60.1 Proposed Species Taxonomy for Enteroviruses

Species	Serotypes
Enterovirus A (EV-A)	CAV2–8, 10, 12, 14, 16
	EV71, 76, 89–92
Enterovirus B (EV-B)	CAV9, CBV1–6
	E1–7, 9, 11–21, 24–27, 29–33
	EV69, 73–75, 77–88, 93–95, 97, 98, 100, 101
Enterovirus C (EV-C)	CAV1, 11, 13, 17, 19–22, 24
	EV96, 99, 102
	PV1–3[a]
Enterovirus D (EV-D)	EV68, 70

[a]Proposed.
CAV, coxsackievirus A; CBV, coxsackievirus B; E, echovirus; EV, enterovirus; PV, poliovirus.

most important modes of transmission for these viruses. The relative importance of the different modes probably varies with the virus and the environmental setting. In addition, enteroviruses that cause a vesicular exanthem can, presumably, be spread by direct or indirect contact with vesicular fluid that contains infectious virus. Exceptions are the agents of acute hemorrhagic conjunctivitis: enterovirus 70 (EV70) and coxsackievirus A24 variant (CAV24v), which are less commonly isolated from respiratory tract or stool specimens and are probably spread primarily by direct or indirect contact with eye secretions, including fomites.[21]

Enteroviruses are efficiently amplified and transmitted among humans without arthropod vectors or other animal reservoirs. Although several species of nonhuman primates may become experimentally or naturally infected with some human enteroviruses,[22] including poliovirus, they do not play any significant role in virus circulation or constitute an animal reservoir.

In tropical regions, especially where sanitation is poor, the efficiency of transmission is high. Consequently, the overall prevalence of enterovirus infections is higher, and the average age of infection is younger. During infancy and preschool age, children are frequently infected with enteroviruses.[23–25] It is not uncommon in these areas to detect two or three simultaneous infections of different enterovirus serotypes, often causing no serious disease. Since children likely become infected with nearly all enteroviruses in the tropics, most adults are immune and nearly all babies are born with maternal antibodies to most enteroviruses.[26,27] Normally, neonates not protected by maternal antibodies are at risk for serious illness when infected by enteroviruses. Because of protective maternal antibodies, neonatal enterovirus disease is extremely rare in the tropics, despite the high prevalence of enterovirus infections in older children. In contrast, in temperate regions where the overall prevalence of enterovirus infections and maternal antibodies is much lower, neonatal enteroviral diseases are relatively more common.[28]

Viral shedding may be intermittent and is affected by the immune status of the individual. Past natural infection with the same enterovirus serotype and immunization for poliovirus significantly reduce the extent and duration of virus shedding.[29,30] Immunity will protect against disease but does not absolutely prevent future infection. Therefore, immune individuals can also contribute to virus transmission, while not being at risk for significant disease. This makes it difficult to track the extent of virus transmission by only observing disease incidence.

Enteroviruses are prevalent worldwide, but in communities with clean food and water, good hygiene, and safe disposal of excreta, transmission is less; therefore, the incidence is lower, and infections occur over a broader age range, including adults.[2] In temperate regions a seasonal pattern is prominent, with increased prevalence in summer and autumn and low prevalence in winter and spring. In the tropics the prevalence is also higher during the warm and wet seasons than in the cooler months; however, seasonal differences can be less prominent and infections are prevalent throughout the year.[23,24,31,32]

An important concept in the epidemiology of enteroviruses is serotypic, temporal, geographic and clinical variation. This concept is illustrated in surveillance studies of nonpolio enterovirus infections.[20] There are two primary patterns of enterovirus prevalence: endemic and epidemic. The epidemic pattern is characterized by sharp peaks in isolations followed by periods with few isolations. Peaks of activity may be a single year or a few years. By contrast, viruses with an endemic pattern are isolated in similar numbers every year, with only rare peaks. Where surveillance data exist, similar endemic and epidemic patterns are seen for most enteroviruses, but are only seldom reflected in changes of disease incidence.

Studies of the prevalence of antibodies to enteroviruses in specific populations[33,34] reveal that many persons have neutralizing antibody to any given enterovirus, indicating a high incidence of past infection. Infections with one serotype can boost antibody titers to other serotypes measured by immunoglobulin M (IgM) or neutralization. The pattern of the heterotypic response varies by serotype and among individuals. The antibody prevalence by serotype varies by geographic location, time, and age. Thus, prevalence data from different years and locations are not directly comparable.

The epidemiology of poliovirus infection has been radically altered by the widespread use of inactivated polio vaccine (IPV) and oral polio vaccine (OPV). Recent activities of the Polio Eradication Initiative have eliminated endemic poliovirus from most of the world.[35] Since 1988, poliomyelitis from wild poliovirus has declined dramatically, and since 2006 remains endemic in only four countries in Africa and southern Asia (***Fig. 60.1***). Three regions of the world – the Americas, Western Pacific, and Europe – have been certified free of endemic poliovirus transmission.[36] It is also highly likely that one of the three serotypes of wild poliovirus (type 2) has been eliminated from the world.[37] The only remaining wild type 2 viruses are in laboratories and vaccine manufacturing facilities.

Even in areas that are no longer endemic or suffering outbreaks, poliomyelitis can still be observed associated with exposure to OPV, either among vaccine recipients (usually with the first dose) or their contacts.[38–40] The incidence of disease associated with OPV is estimated to be 1 case for every 750 000 doses among first-dose recipients and 1 case for every 6.4 million doses (all doses) among contacts.[41] Many developed countries have switched to IPV to eliminate this vaccine-associated paralytic poliomyelitis.[42]

In the past decade, ten outbreaks of poliomyelitis have been documented that were caused by Sabin OPV strains that had acquired the capacity to cause paralysis and be transmitted among human populations (see section on polio eradication, below). Polio-free countries that have populations with low OPV immunization rates are at risk of importation and spread of wild poliovirus as well as emergence of vaccine-derived polioviruses.

Any area with outbreaks or endemic wild polioviruses can serve as a reservoir for reintroduction of poliovirus to areas that have no endemic poliovirus circulation.[43] Since 2003, in addition to several long-range importations over the past 25 years, wild poliovirus has spread from endemic reservoirs in Nigeria and India to cause cases in 25 additional countries and likely re-established virus circulation in four of these.[44] International travel probably results in frequent introduction of wild poliovirus into all regions of the world. High rates of polio vaccine coverage are necessary to prevent poliomyelitis epidemics.

A powerful tool for tracking the circulation of wild poliovirus strains is genomic sequence characterization of isolates. By comparing genetic changes among poliovirus isolates, their geographic and temporal origins can be determined. For example, sequence analysis traced the circulation of particular poliovirus strains throughout endemic countries, elucidated pathways of transmission during outbreaks, and documented importations from endemic regions into polio-free countries.[45–48] The WHO Poliovirus Laboratory Network of 145 formally accredited laboratories provides critical information about wild poliovirus circulation, allowing immunization efforts to be targeted to virus reservoir areas.[49] In addition, improved sequencing technology has facilitated analysis of complete

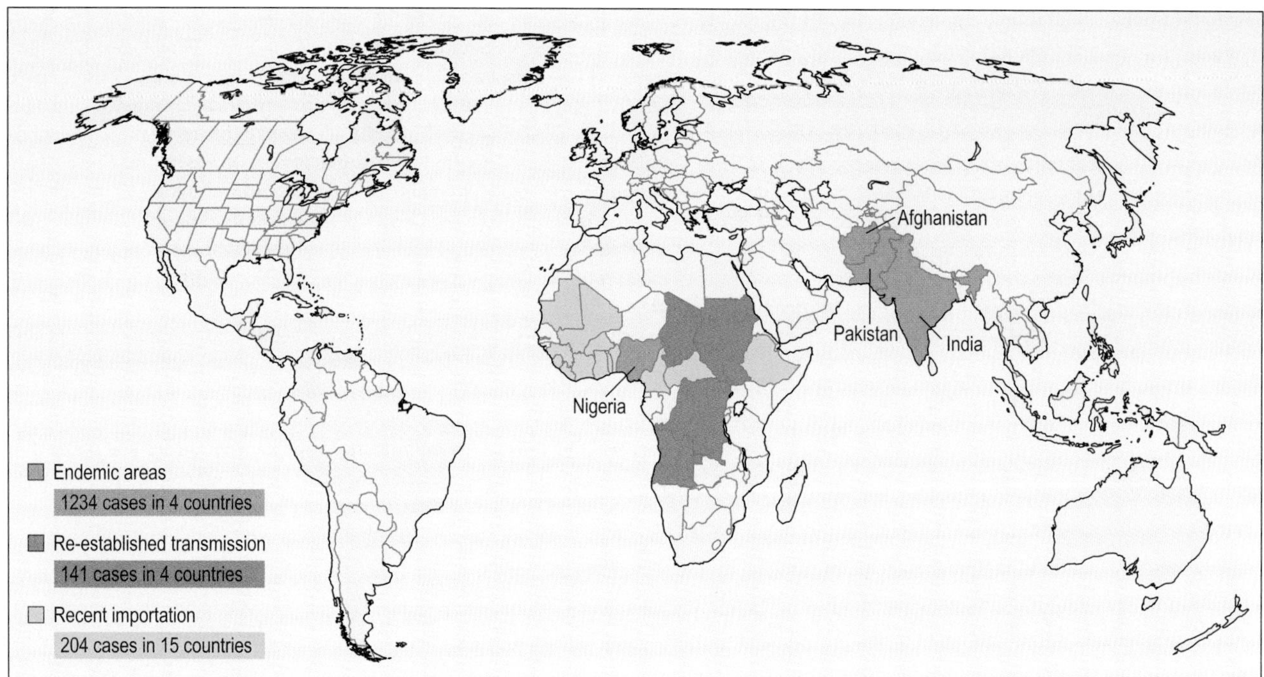

Figure 60.1 Global distribution of wild polioviruses. The map indicates which countries were endemic for wild poliovirus circulation in 2009. Several countries that were previously polio-free suffered importations of wild poliovirus and circulation was likely re-established for a period of at least 12 months.

genomes of circulating polioviruses. This approach has expanded understanding of the mutations that occur, including frequent exchange of genetic material between poliovirus and other enteroviruses.[46,50,51] Similar studies, although with less comprehensive surveillance activities, are also applied to nonpolio enterovirus outbreaks.[52,53] The result of this molecular epidemiology is a more refined understanding of the complexities of enterovirus transmission and epidemiology.

THE DISEASES

Enterovirus infections can result in a wide variety of disease syndromes. The most common result of enterovirus infection is either no symptoms or mild upper respiratory tract symptoms.[2,20] Other mild enteroviral illnesses consist of fever, headache, malaise, and occasionally mild gastrointestinal symptoms. Gastrointestinal symptoms may be the effect of enteric infection without viremia. Much less frequently, serious illness brings the patient to the attention of a physician.

The link between enterovirus infection and a disease syndrome should be made with caution. Inapparent infections and prolonged excretion of virus, especially in stools, are common. A definitive link cannot be made between infection and disease based solely on isolating virus from the stool of an individual. A link can be inferred if virus is isolated from a site that corresponds to the clinical symptoms and if that site is normally sterile. Most associations between enterovirus infection and disease have been made from studies of outbreaks in which a large number of persons with the same clinical signs and symptoms have evidence of infection with the same serotype. Such studies have clearly demonstrated that enterovirus infection can cause aseptic meningitis, pericarditis, pleurodynia, myocarditis, acute hemorrhagic conjunctivitis (AHC), and encephalitis. When an individual has a syndrome clearly associated with enterovirus infection and there is no evidence of involvement by another agent, infection implies probable causation.

The most commonly recognized serious manifestation of enterovirus infection is central nervous system (CNS) disease, usually aseptic meningitis, but sometimes encephalitis or paralysis.[2,19] Although the association between myocarditis and pericarditis and enterovirus infection is clearly established, it is not yet clear how often enterovirus infections are responsible for these syndromes. Several studies suggest, but do not clearly show, that enterovirus infection may be associated with a large fraction of cases of acute myocarditis.[54,55] By contrast, different studies have failed to show conclusive evidence for significant involvement of enterovirus infection in idiopathic dilated cardiomyopathies.[56]

A limited number of viruses cause a few clinically distinct diseases (e.g., poliomyelitis, AHC, and herpangina). They are relatively easily recognized, and etiologic confirmation by laboratory tests, if required, can be directed at a few specific enteroviruses. Certain syndromes have varied causes, including some enteroviruses. In such cases etiologic diagnosis is important for giving appropriate treatment or avoiding inappropriate treatment (e.g., meningitis, encephalitis, and myocarditis). In general, with notable exceptions, most enteroviruses are capable of causing a variety of clinical manifestations, and for any specific disease it is difficult to predict the serotype from signs and symptoms.

Poliomyelitis

The term *poliomyelitis* refers to inflammatory damage (due to infection) of anterior horn cells of the spinal cord, recognized clinically as acute-onset lower motor neuron paralysis (or paresis) of one or more muscles. When its viral cause was recognized, the agent was called poliovirus, thereby redefining poliomyelitis as spinal cord disease caused specifically by a poliovirus serotype. Polioviruses may cause other diseases, such as aseptic meningitis, but muscle paralysis due to myelitis is the most serious. Until poliovirus infections were controlled by immunization, they were the most common cause of acute flaccid paralysis (AFP). This is no longer the case in most countries.

Poliomyelitis may vary widely in severity, from paresis of one or a few muscles, or paralysis of one or more limbs, to quadriplegia and paralysis of muscles of respiration (diaphragm, intercostal muscles). In infants and young children, severe paraspinal muscle weakness (head lag) and localized abdominal muscle paralysis causing a bulge (pseudohernia) when the child cries are diagnostic features, irrespective of the severity. Tendon reflexes of the affected limbs are lost; in others they may be sluggish. The illness usually starts with fever and myalgia, which may last up to a week, followed by sudden onset of paralysis that progresses to its maximum within 4 days, and is typically asymmetric. Cerebral functions are not altered usually, unless hypoxia occurs. In such cases, drowsiness and occasionally mild muscle rigidity or an extensor plantar response in the unparalyzed limbs may be mistaken for upper motor neuron involvement. These signs disappear with oxygen or assisted ventilation. During the acute phase of illness, cerebrospinal fluid (CSF) shows predominantly lymphocytic pleocytosis with moderate elevation of protein concentration. Nerve conduction studies show lower motor neuron involvement without sensory neuropathy.

Most children recover from the acute illness, but 70% continue to have residual motor weakness, which varies from mild impairment to complete flaccid paralysis. The permanent loss of motor neurons results in denervation atrophy of affected muscles. With growth, relative shortening of the limb and deformities such as talipes equinus or equinovarus develop. If the paraspinal muscles are paralyzed, severe scoliosis may develop.

During acute illness, cranial nerve nuclei of the medulla or higher levels may be involved, with paralysis of muscles of deglutition or central paralysis of respiration. This condition is *bulbar poliomyelitis.* When spinal muscle paralysis and bulbar disease occur together, the term *bulbospinal poliomyelitis* is applied. Occasionally facial (seventh cranial nerve) paralysis occurs, either isolated or in combination with spinal or bulbar poliomyelitis. While the vast majority of poliovirus infections are asymptomatic or nonspecific febrile illnesses, the case-fatality rate of poliomyelitis is 2–5% and in some outbreaks as high as 10%. Death is most often due to respiratory paralysis or arrest in children with bulbar poliomyelitis.

Poliomyelitis should be considered in the differential diagnosis for all cases of pure motor paralysis and is usually associated with a normal or slightly elevated CSF protein, normal glucose, and moderate mononuclear pleocytosis. Early in the illness polymorphonuclear cells may predominate in the CSF, followed by a shift to mononuclear cells. Defects in the ventral horns of the spinal cord can be observed by magnetic resonance imaging (MRI). The MRI lesion corresponds to the innervation pattern of the affected extremity. Electromyography and nerve conduction velocities (NCVs) generally fail to show a conduction block.

The differential diagnosis includes spinal cord compression, stroke, neuropathy, and Guillain–Barré syndrome (GBS). Spinal cord compression is unlikely in the absence of central involvement in neural imaging. Lack of sensory involvement would exclude neuropathies. For stroke in the setting of meningoencephalitis, flaccid paralysis sometimes occurs, but the classic spasticity of upper motor lesions should follow. In GBS, protein concentration is markedly elevated in the CSF, and pleocytosis is mild or absent. Fever is usually absent, and paralysis is usually symmetric and ascending with evidence of conduction block by NCV.

Delayed progression of neuromuscular symptoms (postpolio syndrome) may occur 20 years or longer after the initial paralysis due to poliovirus.[57] Postpolio syndrome is characterized by new muscle weakness associated with dysfunction of surviving motor neurons. The illness is usually associated with deterioration of those nerves involved in reinnervation during recovery from the original poliovirus infection. Inflammation is sometimes present in association with degenerating neurons.[58] It is believed that the life span of these nerves has been shortened by the process of reinnervation. This syndrome is not a form of amyotrophic lateral sclerosis. It does not appear that reactivation or replication of poliovirus is involved, but data are inconclusive.[59,60]

Paralytic Myelitis Caused by Other Enteroviruses

AFP may be caused infrequently by certain enteroviruses other than polioviruses. In children, EV71 may cause AFP sporadically or in small outbreaks.[61–63] Several other enteroviruses are associated with AFP on rare occasions. The clinical picture is usually a mild disease, occasionally with paralysis of a single muscle such as the deltoid, often with complete recovery. In a few cases, particularly adults, EV70 has been associated with meningomyelitis and AFP affecting one or more limbs.[64] Although most patients recover completely, some have residual paralysis, as in poliomyelitis.

Viral Meningitis

Fever, headache, and nuchal rigidity, often with Brudzinski's sign, are characteristic of meningitis. CSF is usually clear and under normal or mildly to moderately increased pressure with mild-to-moderate pleocytosis (usual range, 100 to 1000 cells/μL). Although on the first or second day of illness CSF cells may be predominantly neutrophils, they are predominantly lymphocytes 1 or 2 days later. Enteroviral meningitis usually occurs sporadically while other children are infected with the same virus without neurologic disease or even asymptomatically. Occasionally it occurs as small outbreaks. Enteroviruses are by far the most frequent cause of viral meningitis in most locations.

In the tropics, enteroviral meningitis occurs almost exclusively in children under 10 years of age, similarly to poliomyelitis. In temperate regions, it occurs in children or adults, reflecting the delayed age pattern of enterovirus infections in general. Onset is usually sudden, with fever. Sometimes fever is biphasic – a short (1 or 2 days) febrile period accompanied by few or no other signs and symptoms and then, after a day or two, the typical features of meningitis. In older children and adults, headache is common, along with photophobia in some. In infants and young children, febrile convulsions may occur at the onset, in which case careful examination is necessary to exclude encephalitis or other CNS disease. Vomiting, anorexia, rash, cough, pharyngitis, diarrhea, and myalgia are frequently present. Before its closure, the anterior fontanelle may bulge as a sign of raised intracranial pressure.

Many other viruses may cause viral meningitis, such as mumps, herpes simplex, Epstein–Barr virus, arenavirus, and arboviruses. The clinical picture and the CSF laboratory findings lead to diagnosis of aseptic meningitis. Viral isolation from CSF in cell culture or suckling mice is successful only early in the course of illness, and therefore negative culture does not rule out a viral etiology. Virus isolation and detection by molecular methods are the only definitive agent-specific diagnostic results.

Treatment is essentially supportive, and the course of illness is nearly always benign, usually lasting less than a week. Complete recovery is the rule. Although some data suggest that neurologic, cognitive, or development or language abnormalities may follow enteroviral meningitis in infancy, other studies indicate that prognosis is benign.

Encephalitis

Infection of the brain parenchyma is a relatively rare manifestation of enteroviral infection. The encephalitis may be global or focal. It is probably more common in children than adults in both tropical and temperate regions. Illness starts with fever and constitutional symptoms. After a few days, confusion, irritability, lethargy, or drowsiness develops and usually progresses rapidly to generalized convulsions and coma. In some children, focal encephalitis is characterized by focal seizures, as in herpes simplex virus encephalitis. Other clinical manifestations are related to elevated intracranial pressure and cranial nerve or cerebellar involvement. Occasionally myelitis occurs, with lower motor neuron paralysis.

During the previous decade, fatal brainstem encephalitis has been described in countries of Southeast Asia associated with EV71 infection.[61,62] Although sporadic cases and two larger outbreaks have been described since the virus was first recognized in 1971, deaths usually have occurred during widespread hand, foot and mouth disease (HFMD) outbreaks. The fatal outcome has few predictive symptoms but is specifically associated with young children, mostly less than 2 years of age. The onset of neurologic symptoms is particularly rapid, and death occurs often within 24 hours as a result of cardiopulmonary failure, presumably neurogenic.[65,66]

The CSF is usually clear with predominantly lymphocytic pleocytosis in the range of 5–200 cells/μL. CSF protein concentration is normal or slightly elevated, and the glucose concentration is normal or slightly decreased. As a rule, CSF culture does not yield an enterovirus. Brain biopsy is seldom obtained for virus isolation.

Efforts to understand the pathogenesis of rapid progression to a fatal outcome identified possible differences in cytokine expression.[67] Clinical management of severe cases has improved survival; however, neurologic sequelae are common. Because of limited effectiveness of clinical interventions and widespread public concern during HFMD outbreaks, efforts to develop vaccines have been initiated.[68]

Acute Myocarditis and Pericarditis and Chronic Sequelae

Acute myocarditis with or without pericarditis caused by several enteroviruses occurs in infants, children, adolescents, and young adults. The most common implicated serotypes are coxsackie B viruses.[69] Myocarditis usually starts with fever and mild symptoms followed after a short interval by palpitations, chest pain, shortness of breath, and congestive cardiac failure. Occasionally, arrhythmia may be the only manifestation. Pericarditis may accompany myocarditis; often a pericardial rub is heard, but occasionally there is frank pericardial effusion. Investigation usually confirms cardiomegaly and electrocardiographic evidence of myocarditis. The case-fatality rate warrants caution in predicting prognosis.

Treatment is supportive. Most patients recover; however, sequelae have included chronic myocarditis, dilated cardiomyopathy, and chronic relapsing or constrictive pericarditis.[70,71]

Acute Hemorrhagic Conjunctivitis

Mild conjunctival hyperemia is noted with many enterovirus diseases. However, severe conjunctivitis, usually occurring in rapidly spreading epidemics and characterized by subconjunctival hemorrhage in nearly half the subjects, is caused primarily by two enterovirus serotypes. This disease differs from other enteroviral illnesses, having occurred in global pandemics since 1969, when both EV70 and CAV emerged as causes of acute hemorrhagic conjunctivitis (AHC).[72,73] AHC epidemics have recurred in many regions at periodic intervals, with several years in between. To date they have occurred largely in the tropical and subtropical countries of Asia, Africa, and Latin America. Only sporadic cases or small outbreaks have occurred in temperate climates.

The illness has a sudden onset. The incubation period is shorter than for other enteroviruses (24–72 hours), systemic illness much less common, and conjunctival replication of virus is the rule. Spread is mainly through direct contact, via fingers or fomites. Eye pain, photophobia, excessive lacrimation, and conjunctival congestion are almost always present. In most cases, ocular discharge is nonpurulent but may be mucoid in severe cases. The characteristic subconjunctival hemorrhage in a proportion of cases in the epidemic is an important diagnostic feature. The disease is usually bilateral. Adults and school-age children are more affected than infants and preschool children, although household spread is efficient regardless of age. After a few days, symptoms abate, but hemorrhage resolves slowly. Soothing eye drops, such as sterile saline or mild decongestants, ameliorate the symptoms. Recovery is complete in 5–10 days.

During EV70 epidemics, a small proportion of subjects develop acute paralysis of muscle groups of one or more limbs, usually within a few days after onset of eye disease, resembling poliomyelitis, but in reality radiculomeningomyelitis.[63] The only other common complication is secondary bacterial infection.

Pleurodynia (Bornholm Disease)

A distinct illness with mild or high fever of short duration and chest pain located on either side of the sternum or retrosternally occurs sporadically or in outbreaks. Pain is usually intermittent or spasmodic, sometimes excruciating, often exacerbated by deep breathing. Intercostal muscle tenderness and pleural rub, when present, are important signs distinguishing the illness from myocardial infarction, which is often suspected in adults. The chest radiograph and electrocardiogram are normal. Symptoms usually last for a few days to more than 2 weeks, with occasional relapses. In children severe abdominal pain, apparently arising from the diaphragm, may occur.

This syndrome has primarily been associated with coxsackie B viruses,[74] particularly CVB3 and CVB5, although sporadic cases may be caused by other enteroviruses. Rarely, pleurodynia may be accompanied by another clinical manifestation of enterovirus infection, such as aseptic meningitis, or even myocarditis.

Hand, Foot and Mouth Disease

The distinguishing feature of this illness is the vesicular eruption of the hands, feet, and mouth. The oral lesions, mostly on the buccal mucosa, become shallow ulcers. Coxsackievirus A16 is the most frequent etiologic agent, occasionally causing outbreaks. Other enteroviruses, especially coxsackievirus A10 and EV71, may also cause HFMD outbreaks. The etiologic agent can be isolated from the vesicles and from the throat and feces. Occasionally, HFMD may occur with other enterovirus involvement such as meningitis.

Herpangina

This illness is characterized by a typical crop of vesicles on the soft palate, uvula, other parts of the oropharynx, or tongue. Each vesicle is about 1–2 mm in diameter, with a red areola. Herpangina occurs usually in children younger than 10 years old. Fever and sore throat are common symptoms. Careful examination of the oropharynx reveals 1–12 discrete lesions, which usually subside without ulcerating.

Short Fever with Maculopapular Rash

Many enteroviruses may cause a short febrile illness with maculopapular rash resembling rubella or mild measles, particularly in infants and very young children. The distribution of the rash on the face, neck, and chest, and occasionally on the arms and thighs may mimic other well-recognized exanthems. Sometimes there are mild upper respiratory symptoms, adding to difficulty of accurate clinical diagnosis. Outbreaks of enterovirus exanthem have also been called Boston exanthem.

Diarrhea

Mild diarrhea is a common symptom in many enteroviral diseases. However, occasionally enteroviruses cause a short diarrheal illness. Although occasional outbreaks of diarrhea without other typical enterovirus symptoms have been attributed to enteroviral infections, these are uncommon.

Neonatal Enterovirus Diseases

Neonates are more vulnerable to invasive enterovirus diseases than are older children and adults. In the tropics, where most adults are immune to enteroviruses, neonates are protected by maternal antibodies. Therefore, paradoxically, neonatal enteroviral diseases are more common where the general transmission potential is less intense than in the tropics. Infection may occur *in utero* or, more commonly, perinatally.

Many of the clinical features of self-limited illness, as well as the more sinister lesions in the CNS or the heart, may cluster together in the sick neonate.[75,76] Such illnesses resemble other severe systemic infectious diseases such as bacterial septicemia. Thus, the infant may present with lethargy, feeding difficulty, vomiting, tachycardia, dyspnea, cyanosis, jaundice, and diarrhea, with or without fever. Clinical evidence for aseptic meningitis, encephalitis, myocarditis, hepatitis, or pneumonia may be present in any combination. The case-fatality rate is high. Sometimes death occurs rapidly.

PATHOGENESIS AND IMMUNITY

Enteroviruses are cytopathic, and much of the associated disease presumably results from tissue-specific cell destruction. Some disease manifestations, enteroviral exanthems and myocarditis, for example, are thought to result from the host immune response.[2] The mechanisms of virus-induced disease, however, are not well characterized. Typically, the primary site of infection is epithelial cells of the respiratory or gastrointestinal tract and lymphoid follicles of the small intestine, followed by viremia that may lead to secondary sites of infection. Infection of the CNS results in aseptic meningitis or, rarely, encephalitis or paralysis. Other tissue-specific infection can result in pleurodynia or myocarditis. Disseminated infection can lead to exanthems, nonspecific myalgias, or severe multiorgan disease in neonates.

Virus infection is dependent on specific receptors. Five receptors for different nonpolio enteroviruses have been identified in human cells, two integrins, decay-accelerating factor (DAF), the "coxsackievirus-adenovirus receptor" (CAR), and intracellular adhesion molecule 1 (ICAM-1). The receptor for poliovirus (PVR; CD155) is a member of the immunoglobulin superfamily. Some enteroviruses use more than one receptor, and other unidentified receptors may also exist. These receptors may contribute to host specificity. Studies of virus–receptor interactions should improve understanding of the pathogenesis of enteroviral disease and, possibly, advance prevention or treatment strategies.[77]

Once attached to the host cell, virions are thought to be transferred into the cell by pinocytosis. Poliovirus and possibly other enteroviruses are endocytosed by M cells in the gut. After virus entry into the host cell, the virus genome is released into the cytoplasm and functions as messenger RNA. Translation leads to synthesis of viral structural proteins, two proteases and the viral replicase. Sites of viral replication are cytoplasmic membranes that are increased during infection.[78] Along with newly formed capsid proteins, replicated genomic RNA is assembled into progeny virus particles, which are released by cell lysis or apoptosis.[79] A single virion is thus replicated to generate tens of thousands of progeny virions within a few hours.

The sequence of events following viral infection is generalized from experimental infection of polioviruses in chimpanzees and monkeys, partially corroborated by fragmentary data in children. After multiplication at and near the site of entry, virus reaches adjacent lymphoid follicles and draining lymph nodes. Viral multiplication continues at these sites, and virus is shed into the pharyngeal and intestinal lumina for many days to several weeks. Transient viremia occurs in some cases. When primary viremia disseminates infection to distant sites, susceptible organs may become infected. A second amplification resulting from infection and release of virus from these sites may result in more intense secondary viremia and further dissemination. Disease may manifest following primary or secondary viremia. Primary viremia starts 1–3 days after virus inoculation and lasts 1–5 days. Secondary viremia starts soon thereafter and may also last for a few days. The appearance of virus-neutralizing antibody in blood coincides with, and may be responsible for, cessation of viremia, although other factors may also limit viremia in the absence of antibody.

The exact pathway of enteroviruses to reach the CNS is not clearly understood. Viremic spread across the blood–brain barrier or entry via peripheral nerves are possibilities.[80,81] The relatively broad range of the incubation period (5–30 days) suggests that one pathway may operate in some cases and the other pathway in others. The route of viral spread may, in part, determine the site of lesions and the consequent disease. It is also possible that the second pathway is only used by poliovirus. For unclear reasons, there is predilection to poliovirus infection and neuronal damage in the lumbar enlargement of the spinal cord, leading to lower limb paralysis in a majority of cases.

Polioviruses exhibit the greatest neurovirulence among enteroviruses; others have varied but lower neurovirulence. Neurotropism and neurovirulence are, in part, genetically determined properties of the virus. The specific neurotropism in poliomyelitis correlates with the specific poliovirus receptor.[82,83] The RNA sequences of neurovirulent and attenuated vaccine strains of polioviruses show only a very limited number of base changes and indirectly suggest viral determinants affecting neurovirulence. Sequence similarities within the 5′ noncoding region among polioviruses and other enteroviruses that result from recombination suggest that potential neurovirulence of some other enteroviruses may be greater than previously recognized,[12] or that vaccine attenuation is a distinct process not the converse of neurovirulence. Regardless, the reason CNS disease is not more common among infected children is unclear.

In myelitis caused by polioviruses, anterior horn neurons are infected. While many cells are killed and removed by neuronophagia, others regain their function. Paralysis is due to damage to many motor neurons. Neuronal recovery is reflected in recovery of muscle function. It is not generally appreciated that a large number of scattered neurons may be destroyed without paralysis. Perivascular lymphocytic cuffing and interstitial microglial infiltration are usually also observed.

There is a marked increase in the risk of developing paralysis when intramuscular injections are given during the incubation period.[84] This "provocation poliomyelitis" may be explained by possible enhancement of viral entry into the peripheral nerves via the nerve endings in the injected muscle.[85] In such cases the limb in which the injection was given is significantly more frequently affected by paralysis. In experimental animals, poliovirus injection into the ulnar nerve has consistently caused AFP, clinically closely resembling the human disease.

Infection with enteroviruses elicits a strong humoral immune response. Infection with one serotype provides long-term protection from disease by that serotype but usually little protection from disease by other serotypes. Often this response is heterotypic; that is, infection with one serotype induces an immune response to several other serotypes.[86,87] Young children develop a more homotypic antibody response, whereas older children and adults develop a more heterotypic response. This age difference in specificity of the antibody response to enteroviral infection probably reflects exposure to more serotypes with advancing age. The basis of this heterotypic response is not known, but may reflect shared epitopes in multiple serotypes.

Although both humoral and cell-mediated responses occur, the former is probably more important and certainly better understood. The role of cell-mediated immunity in recovery or protection, other than supporting the humoral response, is not clear. Antibodies are usually detected and quantitated by virus neutralization, by which virus is rendered noninfectious following antibody binding. Virus-binding antibody can be detected and quantitated by enzyme-linked immunoassay (EIA). This method is easily adapted to class-specific (IgM, IgG, and IgA) antibodies. Although antibody must bind virus for neutralization, only antibodies directed at certain surface epitopes render the virus noninfectious. Antibodies directed at many non-neutralizing sites are also detected by EIA. While neutralizing antibodies are highly serotype-specific, antibodies detected by EIA are usually more broadly reactive and less specific.

Within 7–10 days after primary infection, IgM antibodies subsequently rise in titer, and persist for up to 3–6 months. IgG antibodies appear shortly thereafter, rise in titer over 2–3 weeks, and remain at relatively high levels for a few years. They persist at detectable levels for one or more decades. IgA antibody appears after 2–4 weeks, both systemically and at mucosal surfaces. Local immunity, which inhibits reinfection, is due partly to mucosal IgA and partly to serum IgG transudate. Humoral immunity is believed the major factor in recovery and clearance of enterovirus infection, as well as protection from disease or infection itself upon reexposure. Vaccine-induced humoral immunity to reexposure polioviruses protects against invasive disease and to a lesser extent against reinfection and replication. Children with agammaglobulinemia do not develop antibodies; hence, they are highly susceptible to disease and chronic infection with prolonged virus shedding. Despite widespread transmission of wild poliovirus and extensive use of OPV in areas with high incidence of HIV infection, surveillance does not suggest that persons with HIV infection or AIDS are at higher risk of poliomyelitis or prolonged excretion of polioviruses. One study found that HIV-infected children were more likely to shed enteroviruses; however, two other studies in Africa did not detect prolonged excretion of poliovirus among children or adults with HIV infection or AIDS.[88-90]

Like other gastrointestinal infections, local immunity is neither absolute nor long-lasting. Reinfections do occur, but the duration of viral shedding is shortened. There is no risk of disease in reinfection, since systemic immunity prevents viral dissemination, even long after primary infection. In other words, risk of invasive infection and disease occurs only during primary infection. However, reinfections contribute to continued circulation of polioviruses in spite of high immunization coverage in regions with high force of transmission.

DIAGNOSIS

The key to laboratory confirmation of enterovirus infection is collection of appropriate clinical specimens for direct detection by molecular methods, virus isolation, or serologic studies.[91] Enterovirus infection cannot be inferred from the clinical syndrome alone, since many infectious agents can cause similar illness. Isolation of poliovirus also makes possible determination of whether the virus is wild or vaccine-related.[92] In areas considered to be free of wild poliovirus, this information may be important to public health officials, who must decide whether intervention is needed to prevent further cases of poliomyelitis.

Enterovirus isolation is accomplished by inoculation of appropriate specimens onto susceptible cultured cells. The best specimens for isolation of virus, in order of sensitivity, are stool or rectal swabs, throat swabs or washings, and CSF. Fecal specimens should always be obtained, since virus is excreted longest and in the highest titer in the intestinal tract. Throat swabs or washings and CSF are most likely to yield virus isolates if they are obtained early in the acute phase of illness. For acute hemorrhagic conjunctivitis, the best specimens, in order of sensitivity, are conjunctival swabs and tears. Virus is detected in cell culture by cytopathic effect and classically identified as a specific enterovirus by neutralization with type-specific antisera,[93] but serotyping remains a time-consuming and expensive procedure.[91]

For poliomyelitis, WHO has established a standard procedure for investigation that is applied to all cases of AFP, not only suspected poliomyelitis. Most countries have adopted this approach, referred to as AFP surveillance.[94] The laboratory procedures are extensively documented and implemented in all 145 laboratories that make up the Global Poliovirus Laboratory Network. Stool specimens from any child can be sent to one of these laboratories to be tested for the presence of poliovirus. In addition, this information is then shared immediately with public health officials for an appropriate response (see later discussion).

Polymerase chain reaction (PCR) to detect enterovirus genomes in cell culture, clinical specimens, and tissues continues to significantly improve the detection of enteroviruses.[95,96] This technique is more rapid than isolation and has the potential for providing timely diagnostic answers for patient management. Molecular serotyping systems offer many advantages and may eventually supplant antigenic typing as global stocks of serotype-specific antisera are depleted.[97] PCR methods for rapid detection and characterization of polioviruses, including determination of the virus serotype, have been developed.[98] Nucleic acid probes, PCR, EIA, and monoclonal antibodies can be employed to determine whether the isolate is vaccine-derived or wild.[99] The methods have different sensitivities and specificities for the various strains of viruses.[92]

Serologic studies can be used in certain circumstances for detecting infection. Classically, infection has been demonstrated by rise in titer of neutralizing antibody between acute and convalescent sera. Poliovirus infection may occasionally be confirmed by rise in titer of neutralizing antibody to one poliovirus serotype, but because of widespread use of vaccine this is often compromised. Enzyme immunoassays have been developed, such as those to detect CVB-specific IgM antibodies.[100] In most cases, IgM antibody tests are not serotype specific. Depending on the configuration and sensitivity of the test, from 10% to nearly 70% of serum samples show a heterotypic response due to other enterovirus infections. A positive result with this method indicates recent enteroviral infection, although with IgM assays the infecting serotype may not be the same one determined by the assay. In general, serology is more valuable as an epidemiologic tool than for clinical diagnosis.

A general diagnostic caveat, however, is shared among enteroviruses. Since enterovirus infections are quite common, especially in childhood, and since most infections are noninvasive and prolonged, the detected enterovirus infection need not be the cause of the illness under investigation. It is an issue of probabilities. If the clinical syndrome is already known to be associated with the detected agent, then infection is taken as reasonable evidence of causation. If the presence of the agent is found in diseased tissue or a relevant body fluid (such as CSF), that constitutes concrete evidence of invasion, hence causation.

TREATMENT AND PROGNOSIS

Since no antiviral therapy is available for enterovirus infections, treatment is directed toward alleviating symptoms. Drugs have been identified that exhibit antiviral activity against several enteroviruses including poliovirus in cell culture and experimental animals.[101,102] These drugs, however, have not completed clinical trials. Interferon has been proposed for treatment of acute hemorrhagic conjunctivitis, but awaits further evaluation.

Treatment of acute poliomyelitis consists principally of supportive therapy and reduced physical activity. Mechanical ventilation is sometimes required in severe cases. In patients with agammaglobulinemia, chronic enterovirus infections have been treated with γ-globulin, and in some cases this has controlled the infection. Use of γ-globulin in other clinical illnesses has not been systematically evaluated.

PREVENTION AND CONTROL

No vaccines are available for nonpolio enteroviruses. General preventive measures include enteric precautions and good personal hygiene. Enteroviruses cause nosocomial infection. Life-threatening infection is most common in newborns, although persons with compromised immune systems are also at higher risk. Hospital staff can inadvertently carry the virus between patients or become infected themselves and spread the virus. Patients with suspected enterovirus infection should be managed with enteric precautions. Patients and staff can be cohorted during outbreaks. During several newborn outbreaks in hospitals, neonatal nurseries were closed to new admissions.

Prevention of Disease by Immunization

By the 1950s, two approaches to the prevention of poliomyelitis by vaccination were developed. The first successful polio vaccine, inactivated polio vaccine (IPV), was produced by Salk and Youngner in 1954 by formaldehyde inactivation of cell culture-propagated virus.[103] This vaccine was completely noninfectious, yet following injection elicited an immune response that was protective against paralytic disease. During the same period, many laboratories sought to produce live, attenuated polio vaccines. The OPV strains of Sabin were licensed in 1961, and widespread mass immunization campaigns in the United States began in 1962.[104] Both IPV and OPV contain three components, one for each immunologically distinct poliovirus serotype. The majority of countries use OPV exclusively, and some, mostly developed countries, use only IPV. A limited number use both in sequence. Recommended vaccination schedules vary among countries, and debate continues about the relative merits. The immunogenic and protective efficacies of OPV show geographic variation, and multiple doses are often required in some of the least developed countries of the tropics. Whereas in North America and Europe, almost all infants seroconvert to all three types of polioviruses with three doses of OPV, in tropical developing countries, 72% and 65% of infants develop antibodies to types 1 and 3 polioviruses, respectively, in response to three doses of OPV, and additional doses are necessary to get equivalent seroconversion rates.[105,106] Nevertheless, polio has been eliminated from the Americas and the Western Pacific region, as well as tropical

South Asia, including Bangladesh and Indonesia, using OPV exclusively. The reason for low seroconversion rates is not fully known, although recent studies strongly implicate diarrheal disease at the time of OPV administration as an important factor.

While OPV is extremely safe, it induces paralytic myelitis in a few instances. In primary vaccinees, vaccine virus-associated paralysis occurs at a rate of less than 1 in 500000. The probability of vaccine-induced paralysis is higher in hypogammaglobulinemic children given OPV and in nonimmune adults in close contact with a recently immunized infant. In tropical regions, when the risk of poliomyelitis due to wild polioviruses was 1 in 200–1000, the paralytic risk of OPV was not an important concern.

Contemporary IPV is highly immunogenic, and primary immunization consists of a minimum of two doses 8 weeks apart or an optimum of three doses, preferably at 8-week intervals. When given as two doses, the first dose should be at or after 8 weeks of age; the three-dose regimen may start at 6 weeks of age or thereafter. The effect of age and dose interval on seroconversion is under active investigation. Booster doses are recommended during the second year of life and around 5 years of age to achieve a total of four doses, and this should suffice for long-term protection. Several IPV-containing combined vaccines are currently available to avoid separate injections.

Polio Eradication

Poliomyelitis is targeted for global eradication and has achieved remarkable progress in all regions of the world. The aim is to terminate transmission of polioviruses and thereby protect all infants and children, rather than protect each child by immunization. The eradication goal is attainable because humans are the only known reservoir. The current global eradication program launched by WHO relies exclusively on OPV for mass vaccination. WHO recommends for developing countries that three routine doses of OPV be given at 6, 10, and 14 weeks of age and an additional dose at birth in endemic regions where exposure of very young infants to wild virus can be expected. To achieve high vaccine coverage in all regions, the Poliovirus Eradication Initiative also relies on supplemental immunization campaigns and aggressive investigation of all suspected cases of AFP to identify wild poliovirus circulation. To ensure that no case of poliomyelitis is missed, every case of AFP in every location in every country must be detected through clinical surveillance and investigated virologically. Two stool samples should be collected on consecutive days, within 2 weeks after the onset of paralysis, and processed for virus isolation in an accredited laboratory.

At least ten poliomyelitis outbreaks have been associated with circulating vaccine-derived polioviruses (cVDPV): on the island of Hispaniola in the Americas in 2000–2001, in the Philippines in 2001, Madagascar in 2002, China in 2004, Cambodia in 2005–6, Indonesia in 2005, Myanmar in 2006–7, Nigeria from 2006 to 2009, Ethiopia in 2008–9, Democratic Republic of the Congo in 2009, India 2009–10, and Egypt from at least 1988 to 1993.[107] The outbreak strains were unusual because their capsid sequences (encoding antigenic properties) were derived from OPV. These viruses had recovered the capacity to cause paralytic poliomyelitis in humans and to be transmitted efficiently among human populations.[108] Intense investigations suggest that circulation of vaccine-derived virus is an uncommon event, occurring only in populations with absence of wild poliovirus of the same type, low immunization rates, and high population densities. The recent discovery of cVDPVs has created urgency in planning a comprehensive post-eradication immunization strategy and emphasizes that risk of polio will not be eliminated until OPV vaccination stops. As a consequence, the eradication effort needs to address issues of future vaccination policy, containment of laboratory and vaccine production strains, and coordinated strategy to achieve cessation of OPV immunization as vital parts of the eradication effort following successful elimination of wild virus circulation.[109]

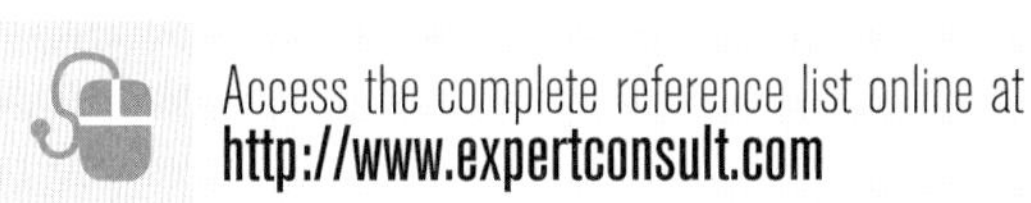

Access the complete reference list online at
http://www.expertconsult.com

CHAPTER 61

Access the complete reference list online at http://www.expertconsult.com

Rotavirus Infections

Juana Angel • Manuel A. Franco • Harry B. Greenberg

INTRODUCTION

Rotaviruses are the most important cause of severe dehydrating diarrhea in young children in both developed and less developed countries (***Box 61.1***). In tropical countries (mostly developing countries), rotavirus infection has several unique characteristics: (1) It is a major public health problem, being responsible for the deaths of approximately 1600 children each day.[1] This presumably occurs because of inadequate access to timely rehydration therapy against a backdrop of poor nutrition and limited access to health care in general. (2) In countries within 10 degrees of the equator infection occurs throughout the year, as opposed to countries with more temperate climates where it presents as a seasonal disease.[2] (3) In tropical countries simultaneous infections with multiple rotaviruses are relatively common (especially during rainy seasons or severe flooding conditions), children become infected at a somewhat earlier age, and the serotype diversity of the viral strains circulating in tropical settings seems to differ to some degree from what is seen in developed countries.[3] (4) Two new safe and effective live virus vaccines available against rotaviruses appear to show lower efficacy in some developing tropical countries; however, they are highly beneficial in terms of cost-effectiveness and are expected to significantly reduce mortality, if issues of delivery are overcome.

THE AGENT

Rotaviruses belong to the family *Reoviridae*. Viruses in this family are icosahedral, nonenveloped, with a segmented double-stranded RNA genome and a multiple-layered protein coat.[4]

Rotaviruses are classified into groups (A through G) depending on the presence of cross-reactive antigenic epitopes and on the overall genetic similarity of their genomes. This chapter concentrates on rotaviruses of group A, which are the principal pathogen of humans and many other species. Group B and C rotaviruses also infect humans and animals, while groups D through G have only been documented in animals (primarily avian species). The group B rotaviruses have been associated with periodic epidemics of diarrhea in adults in China (see ***Fig. 61.1***),[5] but their prevalence seems to be increasing in children.[6] Seroepidemiologic studies for group C rotaviruses show that up to 50% of children over 3 years old and adults[7] have been infected by this virus. However, these viruses appear to be a much less common cause of severe diarrheal illness in humans than the group A viruses.[8]

Detailed structural analysis of the viral particle has been performed by cryoelectron microscopy and several viral proteins have now been crystallized and their structures determined at the atomic level.[4,9] The complete 1000 angstrom viral particles consist of three protein layers with spike structures extending beyond the outer layer. Each particle has 11 RNA segments surrounded by the innermost protein layer. Each RNA segment is monocistronic with the possible exception of genes 9 and 11.[4] The gene-coding assignments and many of the properties of the 11 genome segments of rotavirus have been extensively studied. The virus has eight structural proteins designated by the prefix VP, and six nonstructural proteins designated by the prefix NSP. The outer viral layer is composed of a major structural calcium-binding glycoprotein VP7, and a spike protein VP4. This latter protein is cleaved *in vivo* by trypsin into VP5 and VP8, a process that greatly enhances infectivity. The middle viral layer is composed of VP6 and the inner layer is composed of VP2. On the inner side of VP2, VP1, the viral polymerase, and VP3, the guanyl transferase, are associated with the viral dsRNA genome. Antibodies against VP7 and VP4 were found to neutralize rotavirus growth *in vitro*, and the generation of these neutralizing antibodies has been used to evaluate the effectiveness of vaccination strategies. This finding led to the further serotypic classification of rotaviruses into G (glycoprotein, VP7) and P (protease-sensitive, VP4) serotypes.

Viral replication appears to take place primarily in the enterocytes on the tips of intestinal villi, except in immunodeficient children in whom infection of the liver and kidney has also been documented.[10] Recent studies, however, have shown that viremia is very common and that low level extraintestinal replication frequently takes place, at least in some animal models.[11] Viral attachment to the host cell is mediated primarily by VP4 but likely also involves VP7.[4] The process of entry of the virus into the cell is not completely elucidated and is preceded by interaction with several putative binding and post-binding receptors.[12] Replication occurs in the cell cytoplasm, following partial uncoating of parental viral particles due to the disassembly of VP7 in the low calcium environment of the cytoplasm. Assembly of new viral particles is a multistep process in which unique transient enveloped particles are present inside the endoplasmic reticulum of the infected cell. Mature virions, without an envelope, can be liberated from infected live cells by exocytosis or after cell lysis.[4]

Transfected purified genomic or + sense rotavirus RNA has not been shown to be infectious in the absence of helper virus, which has hampered molecular manipulation of the rotavirus genome.[4] However, a helper virus-driven reverse genetics system has been recently described,[13] and although it has limitations, it opens the possibility of developing better reverse genetics systems. Since the rotavirus genome is segmented, it is capable of undergoing gene reassortment at high frequency during mixed infections. Genetic reassortants have been used to develop "modified jennerian" vaccine candidates, in which attenuated animal viruses carry one or two human rotavirus genes encoding the rotavirus surface proteins.

EPIDEMIOLOGY

Before the introduction of the rotavirus vaccines, this virus was estimated to be responsible for 611 000 annual deaths (range 454 000 to 705 000).[1] Although the mortality caused by rotavirus is very low in developed countries, the incidence of rotaviral disease is similar in children in both

Box 61.1 Key Features of Rotaviruses

The Virus

Icosahedral, nonenveloped, with triple-layered protein coat

Genome consists of 11 RNA segments

Purified rotavirus RNA is not infectious

Gene reassortment during mixed viral infections

Epidemiology and Seasonality

Principal cause of severe dehydrating diarrhea in infants worldwide

Causes the death of 1600 infants daily, mainly in developing countries

Year-round infection in countries within 10 degrees of the equator

Winter peaks in all other regions of the world

Important host range restriction

The Disease

Viral infection mostly limited to the enterocyte

Diarrhea affects principally children aged 2–24 months

Asymptomatic infection and reinfection are common

Diagnosis and Treatment

Rapid diagnosis by viral antigen detection in stool with enzyme-linked immunosorbent assay (ELISA)

Treatment is supportive aimed at preventing dehydration

Two new rotavirus vaccines have been recommended for use by the WHO

(Data with modifications from the previous edition and from Estes MK, Kapikian AZ. Rotaviruses. In: Knipe DM, Howley PM, Griffin DE, et al, eds. Fields Virology. 5th ed. Philadelphia: Lippincott Williams & Wilkins; 2007:1917–1974.)

developed and developing countries, suggesting that common public health measures, such as access to clean water, will not replace the need for an effective vaccine.[14] Moreover, in developed countries rotavirus is still a very important public health problem and has an enormous health cost-impact.[15] Before the introduction of vaccines in the United States, between 1 in 67 and 1 in 85 children were hospitalized with rotavirus-mediated gastroenteritis by 5 years of age.[16]

In the temperate zones of the world rotaviral infection occurs primarily during epidemic peaks in the cooler months of the year.[2] This pattern is not seen in countries within 10 degrees of the equator, where infection occurs in an endemic fashion year-round,[2] and local factors seem to play an important role in determining the occurrence of rotavirus. A recent meta-analysis concluded that in these countries rotavirus disease also occurs related to low temperatures,[17] while a study in Bangladesh concluded that it was related to relatively high temperatures.[18] In the United States, a yearly wave of rotaviral illness spreads across the country, originating in the southwest in the fall, and ending in the northeast in the spring.[19] A similar pattern of distribution was also reported in Europe.[20] An explanation for this interesting phenomenon has recently been proposed.[21]

Rotaviruses are usually transmitted by the fecal–oral route, but some indirect evidence suggests that they could also be transmitted by the respiratory route.[19] The number of babies experiencing their first infection is a primary driver of rotavirus epidemics. Also, feces from asymptomatic older children or adults may provide a vehicle for the transmission.[22] Waterborne outbreaks of rotavirus are probably rare due to their relative instability at high relative humidity,[4] although this is somewhat controversial and may depend on rotavirus strain and other

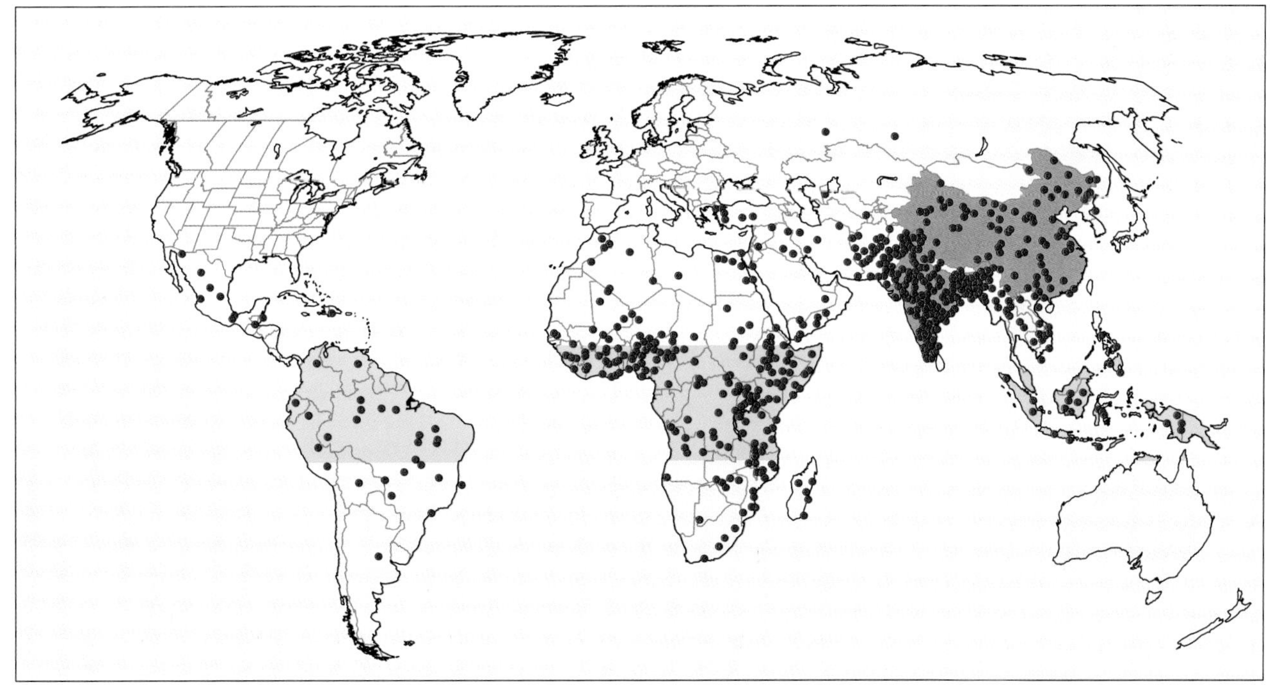

☐ Occurrence year round within 10 degrees of the equator
■ Epidemics of group B rotavirus infection
☐ Temperate climates where rotavirus infection occurs seasonally
• Estimated global distribution of annual deaths in children caused by rotavirus diarrhea. One dot = 1000 deaths

Figure 61.1 Estimated global distribution of annual deaths in children caused by rotavirus diarrhea. (Based on data from the previous edition and from Parashar UD, Gibson CJ, Bresse JS, and Glass RI. Rotavirus and severe childhood diarrhea. Emerg Infect Dis. 2006;12:304–306.)

factors.[23] Foodborne outbreaks are also rare, although oyster and mussel samples can be heavily contaminated by rotavirus.[24] Although animal and human group A rotaviruses can reassort *in vitro*, substantial host range restriction barriers inhibit widespread intraspecies transmission and persistence *in vivo*.[4] However, several studies show that some strains isolated from humans, especially in less developed countries, are reassortants between human and animal strains[3] and recent phylogenetic analyses support the notion of occasional interspecies rotavirus transmission.[25]

Worldwide, most human infections are caused by rotavirus group A of five serotypes: P[8]G1 is by far the most common (approximately 53% of strains), followed by P[8]G3, P[4]G2, P[8]G9, and P[8]G4.[3] In some areas of India, Brazil, and Africa, P[6]G9, G5, and G8 rotaviruses, respectively, are more frequent than elsewhere.[3] Other unusual strains currently circulate and can arise sporadically in both developed and developing countries, but especially in the latter.[26] The number of mixed infections reported has recently increased, mostly in developing countries.[25] Emerging strains and mixed infections could represent an important challenge for rotavirus vaccines, although currently available data do not support this concern.

THE DISEASE, PATHOGENESIS AND IMMUNITY

The pathophysiology of human rotavirus-induced diarrhea has not been fully elucidated.[27,28] Using a semi-quantitative polymerase chain reaction (PCR) assay, a direct correlation was found between the levels of viral RNA in stool and the severity of diarrhea,[29] but this observation needs confirmation. The pathologic changes in the intestines of children with severe rotavirus infection include shortening and atrophy of the villi, mononuclear infiltration in the lamina propria, and distension of the cisternae of the endoplasmic reticulum.[30] A direct relationship between the extent of intestinal histopathology and disease has not been demonstrated[4] and various animal species appear to vary substantially in the degree of histopathologic abnormalities, despite the fact that they all respond to rotavirus infection with diarrhea. This discrepancy could be explained by the fact that rotavirus can cause diarrhea by multiple mechanisms at different times after infection.[27] During the initial phases of the disease, secretory,[31] altered intestinal motility and altered paracellular permeability components could all be playing roles in the pathophysiology of diarrhea. Late in the disease a malabsorption component due to destruction of enteroctyes or defective turnover of microvillar membrane disaccharidases could be causing an osmotic diarrhea.[27] Rotaviral NSP4 was the first viral enterotoxin described[32] and has been proposed to be mediating (at least partially) all of the early mechanisms previously mentioned. It has been postulated that viral infection (NSP4 being implicated or not) induces secretory diarrhea and probably increases intestinal motility by stimulating the enteric nervous system.[31] Whether the toxic effect of NSP4 is clinically relevant in children or other animal species remains to be determined.

The factors that determine virulence seem to be multiple and depend on both viral and host elements: studies using reassortants have identified NSP1, VP4, VP3, VP7, NSP4, VP6, NSP2, and NSP3 as proteins affecting viral virulence.[4] In a study in Mexico the severity of rotavirus-associated diarrhea was related to different P serotypes rather than to G serotypes.[33] Studies of virulence in humans are confounded by a variety of factors including, but not limited to, heterogeneity in the immune status (both passive and active) of affected children.

The severity of the disease is age dependent and the peak incidence of rotaviral illness in children is between 2 months and 2 years of age, and occurs at a lower age in developing countries.[34] Rotavirus infection is frequently asymptomatic in neonates, suggesting either infection with specific attenuated strains during the neonatal period and/or protective maternal immune effects.[35,36] In adults, infection is generally asymptomatic, presumably due to acquired immunity, but disease is seen occasionally in the elderly and in adults who take care of sick children.[37,38]

The clinical features of rotavirus illness are not distinguishable on an individual basis from other enteric infections and do not permit a diagnosis based only on physical examination and history.[4] In general, however, rotavirus diarrhea and dehydration tend to be more severe than illness caused by the other enteric pathogens. Typically, rotavirus-induced diarrhea is watery, lasts for approximately 5 days, is preceded by the sudden onset of vomiting and is frequently accompanied by significant fever and dehydration.[39] The incubation period of rotavirus is estimated to be less than 48 hours. Viral excretion in feces lasts 10 days in the majority of children and up to 57 days in small subgroups, especially when assessed by PCR-based assays.[40]

Although in all species examined to date rotavirus infection appears to be highly restricted to the mature villus tip cells of the small intestine, there is increasing evidence of extraintestinal spread and replication of the virus, and viremia, in humans and other different species.[10,41,42] The role played by extraintestinal rotavirus spread as a cause of the frequently elevated fever or in fatal cases is unclear.[43] Seizures have been reported in association with rotavirus infection and the virus has been detected in cerebrospinal fluid samples by PCR.[44] Electrolyte abnormalities and fever associated with infection could also explain some of the seizures, and a firm conclusion concerning the mechanism of seizures cannot be drawn at present.

Many innate mechanisms participate in the host's defense against rotavirus: age-dependent gastric inactivation of heterologous rotavirus has been shown in mice.[45] Intestinal mucins, as well as certain cytokines and chemokines have also been proposed as innate intestinal factors that may play a role in modulating rotavirus infection.[28] Of note, rotavirus NSP1 has been shown to degrade interferon regulatory factor (IRF) 3, 5, and 7,[46,47] and interferon signaling deficient mice are susceptible to a fatal systemic disease after oral administration of some rotavirus strains.[48] Hence it seems likely that interferon plays a role in modulating acute rotavirus infection.

The acquired immune system has been shown to be crucial for eliminating rotavirus infection, since immunodeficient mice and children do not resolve primary infection and become chronically infected.[10] Studies in mice have shown that both antibody and cytotoxic T cells can mediate viral clearance and protection from rotavirus reinfection. Cytotoxic T lymphocytes are probably the initial effector mechanism that mediates viral clearance, whereas antibodies are the principal mechanism of protection from reinfection.[49]

The observation that children infected with rotavirus as neonates were later protected against severe rotavirus disease,[35] and the fact that in animal models primary infection protects against reinfection indicated that vaccination against rotavirus was feasible. Natural rotavirus infection can protect against reinfection: recurrent episodes of rotavirus disease are less severe than the first episode, one episode of rotavirus infection had a protective efficacy of 77% against rotavirus-induced diarrhea, and two infections, either symptomatic or asymptomatic, completely protected against moderate to severe disease of any serotype.[50]

One explanation for recurrent rotavirus infections is that protection from reinfection is mediated by intestinal rotavirus-specific IgA, which is not long-lasting.[51] Secondary infections will generally boost the fecal IgA response and in many but not all children, induce protective fecal anti-rotavirus IgA levels.[51] Another explanation is that protective antibodies are primarily directed at serotype-specific regions on the rotaviral outer proteins VP4 and VP7.[4] This latter possibility has been supported by some animal and clinical studies but not by others.[52] Moreover, protective efficacy following human and murine vaccination has not been strictly dependent on the serotype of the vaccine strain, nor has it correlated well with the titer of serotype-specific serum antibody,[53] and at present there is not a precise and reliable marker of protection induced by vaccination.[52] These observations have suggested that local antibody levels might be the critical determinant of protection or that antibody levels to nonserotype-specific regions of VP4, VP7 or other proteins, or T cells may play an important role in immunity. Notably, in mice, non-neutralizing antibodies to VP6 can also induce protection,[54] probably by inhibiting intracellular viral replication.[55] Additionally, suckling pups nursed by dams vaccinated with an NSP4-derived peptide can be partially protected from heterologous rotavirus diarrhea.[32] Of note, the monovalent P[8]G1 vaccine induces significant protection from multiple G and P serotypes not included in the vaccine, supporting the conclusion that immunity to rotavirus infection is, in part, heterotypic.[56,57]

DIAGNOSIS

Diagnosis of rotavirus infection in the clinical setting is not strictly essential when diarrhea is of mild or moderate intensity. During the rotavirus "season" in developed countries, well over 50% of the moderate to severe diarrheal episodes in young children will be due to rotavirus. In tropical countries, because of the presence of other enteric pathogens and the absence of seasonal occurrence of rotaviral disease, it is more difficult, without a diagnostic assay, to determine which diarrheal episode is caused by rotavirus. Numerous solid phase immunoassays (ELISA) for rotavirus are now commercially available and these are generally sensitive, specific, and easy to use under most conditions. An inexpensive method of detecting and characterizing rotaviruses is silver staining of electrophoretically separated viral RNA extracted from stool samples.[4] Tissue culture of human rotaviruses is a relatively efficient way to identify rotaviruses as well, since rotaviruses grow well in tissue culture when trypsin is added to the culture medium.[4] However, this technique, like electron microscopy, is time-consuming and requires specialized equipment and/or reagents. Finally, the use of PCR has increased the sensitivity of assays for detecting rotavirus, and has permitted typing of viruses by gene sequence.[58] However, since this is a more sensitive rotavirus detection method and up to 29% of healthy children below 1 year of age may be positive by RT-PCR,[59] it becomes difficult to associate the detection of the virus with the gastroenteritis; for this reason the authors propose to continue using the ELISA for diagnosis of rotavirus-induced disease.[60]

TREATMENT AND PROGNOSIS, PREVENTION AND CONTROL

A review of the treatment of gastroenteritis in children has been performed by a US Centers for Disease Control and Prevention team[61] and is available on the web at http://www.cdc.gov/mmwr/preview/mmwrhtml/rr5216a1.htm. Because rotavirus disease resolves within 1 or 2 weeks without treatment, the basic therapeutic goal is to prevent dehydration. The oral hydration solution (ORS) until recently recommended by the World Health Organization (WHO) was derived from the formula initially created to treat secretory cholera diarrhea, and thus had a high sodium concentration and an osmolarity of 331 mmol/L. After detailed analysis that indicated that the high sodium concentration formula was associated with an increased incidence of transient, asymptomatic hypernatremia, and that rehydration formulas with reduced osmolarity (245 mmol/L) were equally as effective as those with high osmolarity for the treatment of children with cholera diarrhea, the WHO has changed its recommendation to a lower osmolarity ORS (http://www.who.int/child_adolescent_health/documents/fch_cah_06_1/en/index.html).

After rehydration, rapid age-appropriate refeeding is recommended.[61] Rotavirus disease has been shown to induce self-limited intestinal lactase deficiency.[62] Nonetheless, many studies show that withholding lactose-containing products, particularly maternal milk, is not warranted.[61]

Several studies have indicated that passive oral immunotherapy can shorten the duration of rotavirus infection,[63] but will probably only be economically feasible for special cases: immunodeficient patients[64] or low birth-weight infants.[65] Recent studies[66] suggest that *Lactobacillus* (a bacteria present in yogurt) is safe and effective as a treatment for acute rotavirus gastroenteritis. Nonetheless, the potential exists for great variability among different preparations of lactobacilli and a general recommendation on their use has not been issued.[61] Although several studies in developing countries have shown that zinc supplementation is useful for the treatment and prevention of diarrhea,[67] further studies are needed to know if this will be the case in nourished children from developed countries. At present no pharmacologic treatment of rotavirus diarrhea is recommended. Racecadotril, an enkephalinase inhibitor that acts on the enteric nervous system, has been shown in one study to be useful as an adjunct to treat rotavirus diarrhea.[68] Ondansetron, a serotonin antagonist, was effective in reducing the emesis from gastroenteritis during the phase of oral rehydration.[69] More studies are needed before these preparations can be generally recommended for treatment of rotavirus diarrhea.

Acute or chronic complications of rotavirus disease other than dehydration are very rare. Malnutrition, low birth weight and prematurity are all predisposing factors for the severe, life-threatening dehydration associated with rotavirus disease.[70,71] In developing countries, diarrhea is directly related to linear growth retardation during childhood, a determinant of short stature and impaired capacities in adults.[72] Associations of rotavirus infection with necrotizing enterocolitis, hemorrhagic gastroenteritis of neonates, and pneumatosis intestinalis in infancy have been reported, but a causal relationship has not been established.[4] HIV-infected children do not seem to be more susceptible to rotavirus and it will probably be safe to give them the live rotavirus vaccines being developed.[56] Although several reports have suggested that group A and C rotaviruses could be implicated in extrahepatic biliary atresia of children, recent evidence suggests that this is not the case.[73]

Very few years after the discovery of rotaviruses the feasibility of a rotavirus vaccine was established.[74] Studies of the cost-effectiveness of a rotavirus vaccine have clearly established the potential usefulness of this approach.[75] Since rotavirus reinfection occurs even after natural infection, the primary aim of anti-rotavirus vaccination strategies is to prevent severe rotavirus disease rather than prevent rotavirus infection or mild illness. Based on the observation that animal rotaviruses appear to be substantially restricted for growth, pathogenicity, and transmission in humans (host range restriction), the most-studied strategy for vaccination has been the jennerian or modified jennerian approaches using bovine or simian viruses or reassortants as vaccines. In some cases of strict jennerian vaccine failure, the vaccine and the wild-type human strain did not share G serotype specificities.[76] Because of this observation, the jennerian strategy was modified to include animal virus reassortants that contained genes encoding the four most common human VP7 (G) serotypes. A vaccine of this type, the quadrivalent rhesus vaccine (RotaShield, Wyeth/Lederle), was the first effective vaccine licensed for use in the United States, but was subsequently withdrawn from the market because of its association with intussusception.[77] However, the impact of this vaccine on the total attributable risk of intussusception, especially if initially administered at 2 months, remains controversial.[77]

Two second-generation vaccines were subsequently shown in very large field studies to be both safe and effective and are now marketed worldwide: RotaTeq (Merck), a modified jennerian pentavalent vaccine made of bovine virus reassortants containing human G1, G2, G3, G4 (VP7) and P[8] (VP4), and Rotarix (GlaxoSmithKline),[75,78] a monovalent vaccine containing a human tissue culture attenuated strain 89-12 (P[8] G1). Protection rates provided by both vaccines have been very similar and varied from 70% to 80% against any rotavirus disease and 90% to 100% against severe gastroenteritis.[75] Large pre- and post-licensure studies have shown that these vaccines are not associated with intussusceptions.[75,79] Since efficacy and/or immunogenicity trials in all continents have been recently completed, a WHO global recommendation for the use of these vaccines was issued in June 2009.[56] There are some indications that, as for other rotavirus vaccines,[27] these new vaccines are somehow less efficacious (49.5–76.9%) against severe diseases in the poorest developing countries.[56,57,80] However, they are still very cost-effective in terms of number of severe rotavirus-induced diarrheas prevented: overall in African trials, Rotarix prevented 3 out of 5 episodes of severe rotavirus-induced disease per 100 vaccinated children.[56]

An attenuated lamb rotavirus vaccine has been licensed in China and a recent case-control efficacy study was published.[81] A bovine reassortant vaccine developed by the US National Institutes of Health provided high levels of protection in Finland in a phase II trial, and it was licensed to several companies in developing countries, where it is currently under evaluation.[52] Two vaccines derived from neonatal rotavirus strains (the Indian 116E and the Australian RV3 P[6]G3) are also under evaluation.[52,82]

Rotaviruses have been shown to be highly resistant to many commonly used disinfectants.[83] A spray composed of 0.1% *o*-phenylphenol and 79% ethanol has been shown to be highly effective at decontaminating surfaces thought to be contaminated with rotavirus.[84]

ACKNOWLEDGMENTS

This work was supported by funds from the Pontificia Universidad Javeriana, Bogota, Colombia, and grants from the US National Institutes of Health and the US Veterans Administration.

Access the complete reference list online at
http://www.expertconsult.com

Access the complete reference list online at
http://www.expertconsult.com

CHAPTER 62

Calicivirus Infections

Gagandeep Kang • Mary K. Estes • Robert L. Atmar

INTRODUCTION

Until the early 1970s, the cause of most gastroenteritis was unknown. Cases were attributed to the known infectious agents, mainly bacteria, and many other causes, including teething, weaning, diet, old age, drugs, and malnutrition. In 1972, immune electron microscopy of fecal specimens derived from an outbreak at a school in Norwalk, Ohio, USA, resulted in the identification of Norwalk virus, the first time a viral agent was shown to cause gastroenteritis.[1] Subsequently, electron microscopy of stools of young children in the United Kingdom and Japan identified viruses morphologically similar to animal caliciviruses.[2,3] Intensive investigation over the next three decades led to the identification of several viral agents of gastroenteritis and the development of new assays to identify the viral etiology of sporadic episodes and epidemics of gastroenteritis. In 1990, the Norwalk virus genome was cloned and, with the development of reverse transcription–polymerase chain reaction (RT-PCR), many genetically related but antigenically diverse viruses were identified and placed into groups called the "Norwalk-like viruses" and "Sapporo-like viruses."[4,5] In 2001, these groups were given the genus names of *Norovirus* and *Sapovirus*, respectively.

With the identification of new viral agents of gastroenteritis, it has become clear that viruses cause a significant proportion of the enteric illnesses that did not earlier have a defined etiology. Improvements in sanitation and hygiene and better standards of living resulted in a decrease in the proportion of diarrheal disease attributed to bacteria, and an increase in the proportion of cases associated with viral infections. Human caliciviruses are now acknowledged as one of the most frequent causes of gastroenteritis in developed countries and are being increasingly recognized in developing countries and/or tropical regions.[6]

THE AGENT

The name calicivirus is derived from the Latin *calyx*, meaning cup or goblet, and refers to the cup-shaped depressions visible by electron microscopy. These cup-like depressions are more prominent in sapoviruses, earlier called classic human caliciviruses. Viruses now classified as noroviruses often lack the distinct surface depressions and were previously called small, round-structured viruses (***Fig. 62.1***).[7,8] Caliciviruses (family *Caliciviridae*) are nonenveloped, icosahedral 27–40-nm viruses with one major capsid protein enclosing a single-stranded, positive-sense RNA genome. Currently, caliciviruses are classified into four recognized genera, *Norovirus*, *Sapovirus*, *Vesivirus,* and *Lagovirus,* and two other genera that contain bovine viruses (*Nebovirus*) and a rhesus macaque virus (provisionally *Recovirus*) (***Fig. 62.2***). The calicivirus genome is 7.5–7.7 kilobases and has two or three open reading frames (ORFs). In Norwalk virus, the first ORF encodes a nonstructural polyprotein that is processed in infected cells to generate several proteins, including the viral helicase, VPg, protease, and RNA-dependent RNA polymerase. The second ORF encodes VP1, the major capsid protein, and the third encodes VP2, a small, basic protein of unknown function.[9] In sapoviruses, the nonstructural polyprotein and major capsid protein are both encoded in ORF1 and the small basic protein encoded in ORF2.[10] Noroviruses can be genetically classified into five different genogroups (GI, GII, GIII, GIV, and GV), and further divided into different genetic groups or genotypes defined by a minimum amino acid sequence identity over the complete capsid sequence of 85% (***Fig. 62.2***).[11] Genogroup II, the most prevalent human genogroup, presently contains 19 genotypes. Genogroups I, II and IV infect humans, whilst genogroup III is associated with bovine infections and genogroup V infects mice.

A numeric classification system has been proposed based upon numbering genogroups with Roman numerals and genotypes with Arabic numbers.[11,12] For example, the genogroup II norovirus, Lordsdale virus, is a member of genotype 4, and therefore is classified as a GII.4 norovirus. GII.4 viruses currently account for the majority of outbreaks of adult gastroenteritis and the availability of sequencing and modeling techniques has resulted in a better understanding of the evolution and spread of this strain across the globe during the last decade.[13] Sapoviruses are also divided into five genogroups, four of which contain viruses detected in humans in 13 different genotypes.[14] Noroviruses have been found in dogs, lions, and pigs.[15,16] These strains have not been found in human infections, although human strains can infect cows and pigs.[17,18] Serologic data suggest that zoonotic transmission may occur in individuals who have close or prolonged contact with animals.[19]

An understanding of the mechanisms of replication has been limited by the inability to grow these strains in culture. Following the cloning of Norwalk virus in 1990, it became possible to produce virus-like particles (VLPs) by expression of the capsid protein in insect cells. The expressed capsid proteins self-assemble into VLPs with morphologic and antigenic properties similar to native viruses. This resulted in an increased understanding of structure, antigenicity, and, more recently, host susceptibility factors to infection, with the VLPs being used as antigens for detection of antibodies, to generate specific antisera, and for binding assays to identify receptors.[20–24]

EPIDEMIOLOGY AND THE DISEASE

Clinical disease due to the noroviruses has an average incubation period of 24–48 hours and is characterized by acute onset of nausea, vomiting, abdominal cramps, myalgias, and nonbloody diarrhea. Illness usually resolves in 2–3 days, but can be longer – up to 4–6 days in hospital outbreaks and in young children. Vomiting is relatively less prevalent in infants than in older children and is a characteristic feature of gastroenteritis outbreaks in adults.[25,26] Fever is reported in 30–40% of patients and resolves within 24 hours.[25,27,28] Deaths have been reported in the elderly during outbreaks in nursing homes and noroviruses have recently been reported in necrotizing enterocolitis in neonates.[29,30]

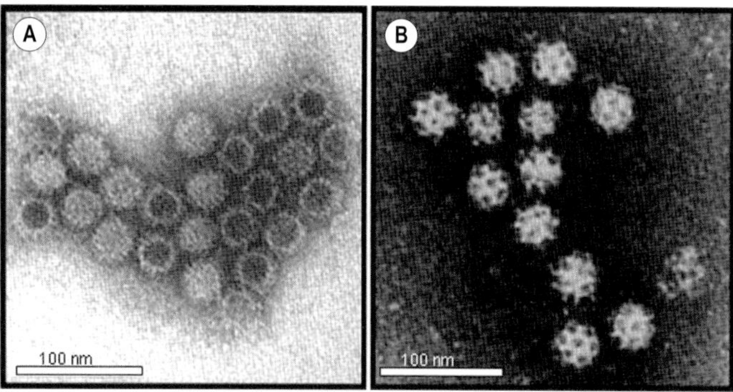

Figure 62.1 Electron micrographs of human caliciviruses. **(A)** Norwalk virus particles from the stool of an ill volunteer. (Reproduced from Guix S, Asanaka M, Katayama K, et al. Norwalk virus RNA is infectious in mammalian cells. J Virol 2007;81:12238–12248.) **(B)** A sapovirus from the stool of a child with gastroenteritis. (Reproduced from Nakata S, Estes MK, Chiba S. Detection of human calicivirus antigen and antibody by enzyme-linked immunosorbent assays. J Clin Microbiol 1988;26:2001–2005.)

Noroviruses are highly infectious and are transmitted primarily through the fecal-oral route, either by consumption of contaminated food or water, or by direct person-to-person spread. Aerosolization of vomitus has also been shown to be a mode of transmission.[31] The ability of the virus to survive in the environment suggests that environmental contamination and fomites are an important source of infection.[32,33] The four distinct patterns of viral gastroenteritis – endemic childhood diarrhea, outbreaks in closed communities, other food- or water-borne outbreaks among wider communities, and viral gastroenteritis in immunocompromised patients – are all seen in caliciviral infections.

In developed countries, diarrhea is mainly seen in children less than 5 years of age, but the peak incidence of diarrhea in developing countries occurs in children less than 2 years of age. In most studies from developed countries, noroviruses are the second most common cause of gastroenteritis in children, following rotaviruses, and, increasingly, studies from tropical countries are reporting patterns similar to those seen in developed countries.[6] There are few community-based studies, but they indicate that in developed countries almost a quarter of all episodes in young children may be due to noroviruses.[34] A summary of 21 studies published in the last 10 years from tropical countries, which identified noroviruses mainly in children hospitalized with dehydrating gastroenteritis, shows a mean prevalence of 11.7% (***Table 62.1***).[35–55]

Studies over the last 30 years, mainly in developed countries, have shown that noroviruses cause large outbreaks of acute gastroenteritis in many settings. Attack rates in outbreaks can be over 50%, and there is often substantial secondary spread. Outbreaks are common in winter, but can occur year-round in closed and semiclosed settings such as nursing homes, hospitals, hotels, and cruise ships.[56] Cruise ship outbreaks can recur even after thorough cleaning and changes of passengers, indicating the ability of the virus to survive in the environment. Nosocomial outbreaks are a particular concern in Europe, where they have led to the closure of wards and significant economic impact, but there are limited data on noroviruses in health care settings in developing countries.[57] Transmission of viruses in such settings can occur from person to person or through fomites, emphasizing the need for hygiene and good infection control practices to limit spread of infections.

Most other outbreaks are believed to be linked to contaminated food and water. A report from the Centers for Disease Control and Prevention (CDC) showed that 39% of 264 confirmed norovirus outbreaks were associated with restaurants or catered events.[58] Foods implicated in outbreaks of norovirus gastroenteritis are usually those contaminated either directly with fecal matter at the source, such as shellfish harvested from sewage-contaminated waters or fresh produce irrigated with sewage or fecally contaminated water, or by infectious food handlers. Shellfish concentrate viruses through filtration and, although depuration reduces fecal coliform contamination, it does not remove noroviruses. In outbreaks identified to be associated with fresh produce, noroviruses were responsible for about 25% of the outbreaks. Most foodborne outbreaks where food handlers are a source of transmission result from foods that require handling, but not cooking, such as salads and sandwiches. Asymptomatic infections and prolonged shedding for several weeks after infection are risk factors for virus transmission if individuals do not maintain high levels of hygiene.[59,60]

Waterborne outbreaks of norovirus gastroenteritis in developed countries have been associated with different forms of recreational water[61] and contamination of drinking water.[62] Although few studies have reported outbreaks in developing countries, it is likely that, given lower standards of hygiene and poor quality of drinking water, such transmission does occur. Although a rapid and accurate diagnostic assay is not widely available for diagnosing norovirus disease, Kaplan et al proposed the presence of four epidemiologic features for confirmation of norovirus as a cause of outbreaks: (1) vomiting in 50% or more of affected persons; (2) incubation period of 24–48 hours; (3) symptoms for 12–60 hours; and (4) absence of bacterial pathogens on culture, which have recently been validated as being sensitive and specific.[26,63]

The few studies that have looked at norovirus infections among immunocompromised individuals have reported both symptomatic and asymptomatic infections in transplant receipients and some increase in viral shedding in persons infected with human immunodeficiency virus.[64–66] Infection in highly immunocompromised transplant recipients can lead to symptomatic diarrhea lasting months to years.[67,68]

Strain characterization studies have suggested that there are differences in the strains detected in outbreaks and in sporadic cases, and some differences in geographic distribution. Analyses of norovirus detected in outbreaks and sporadic cases suggest that infections with GII strains are severalfold more common than those of GI strains. GII.4 norovirus strains have become the predominant cause of epidemic disease in the past decade.[69] Norovirus evolution may be driven by immune selection pressure, with the exposed viral capsid protein that binds carbohydrates in the human gut evolving because of the antigenic drift in the receptor-binding regions of the P2 subdomain.[70]

Seroprevalence studies using recombinant antigens or VLPs of genogroups I and II have been used to assess exposure to infection and have shown that exposure is common, even in isolated populations.[71] However, given the lack of longitudinal data on the persistence of antibodies and the variability in host susceptibility to different viruses, it is difficult to draw meaningful conclusions based on serosurveys in populations that are not well characterized.

PATHOGENESIS AND IMMUNITY

Other than a murine norovirus, noroviruses have not been grown in culture, making studies of pathogenetic mechanisms difficult. In studies carried out on volunteers, infection by Norwalk virus requires a low infectious dose and produces blunting and broadening of the intestinal villi, vacuolation of the villus epithelial cells, and mononuclear cell infiltration into the lamina propria of the proximal small intestine.[72,73] The small intestinal mucosa remains intact and lesions have not been found in biopsies of the colonic and gastric mucosa, suggesting that viral replication may be limited to the upper small intestine.[74] The cause of diarrhea is unknown, although several mechanisms have been proposed, including reduced absorptive capacity of the disrupted epithelium, proliferation of the secretory crypt cells, and reduced expression of certain digestive enzymes, resulting in an osmotic diarrhea. The nausea and vomiting have been attributed to delayed gastric emptying and altered gut motility, although there is no direct evidence to support these proposed mechanisms.

Early volunteer studies showed that infected volunteers developed a short-lived (6–14 weeks) immunity after a Norwalk virus challenge.[75] Symptomatic volunteers could be reinfected with the same virus when challenged 2–3 years later.[75] A second group of volunteers could not be

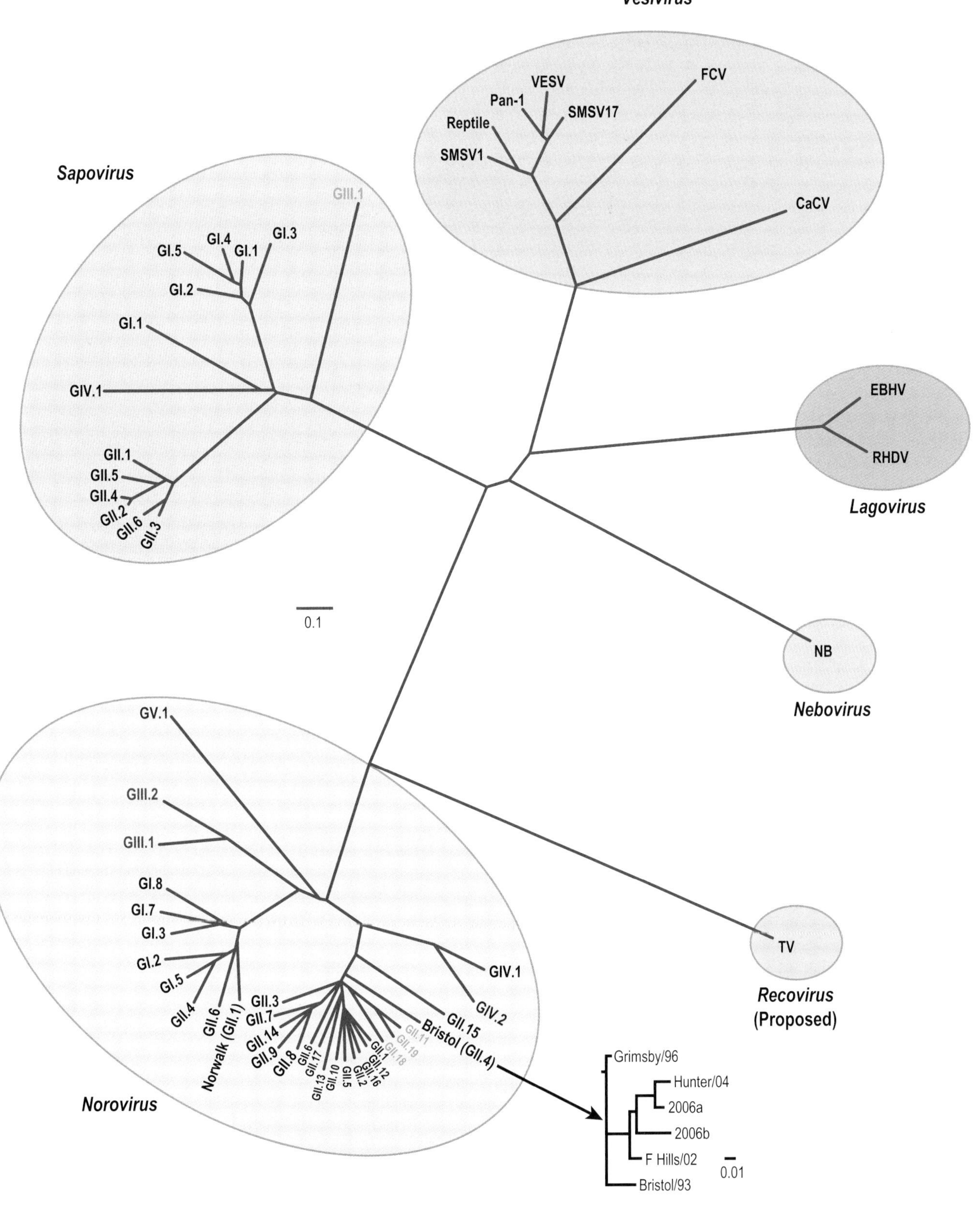

Figure 62.2 Phylogenetic analysis of caliciviruses. A multiple alignment of 57 calicivirus VP1 amino acid capsid sequences was performed using Clustalw (http://www.ebi.ac.uk/Tools/clustalw2/index/html) and the phylogenetic analyses were performed with programs in the PHYLIP v3.6 package. The scale bar represents the unit for expected number of substitutions per site. Within the *Norovirus* and *Sapovirus* genera, human prototype viruses are listed in black, porcine viruses are shown in green, bovine viruses are shown in blue, a murine virus is shown in purple, and a lion virus is shown in red.

Table 62.1 Noroviral Gastroenteritis in Tropical Countries. Studies Published between 2000 and 2009, which Tested >100 Patients Admitted with Dehydrating Gastroenteritis Were Included

Site	*n*	Age in Years	Positive *Norovirus*	Predominant Genogroups	Reference
Dhaka, Bangladesh	917	Children	4.5%	GII.4	35
Delhi, India	226	<5	15.9%	GII	36
Pune, Nagpur, Aurangabad, India	830	<7	6.3–12.6%	GII.4, recombinants	37
Pune, India	236	<5	11.9%	GII.4, GIIb	38
Vellore, India	350	<5	15.1%	GII.1	39
Karachi, Pakistan	517	Children	9.9%	GI, GII	40
Indonesia	218	Children	21%	GII	41
China	1110	<5	10.3%	GII.4	42
Hong Kong, China	995	All ages	16.7%	GII	43
Chiang Mai, Thailand	296	<5	8.1%	GII.4	44
Chiang Mai, Thailand	248	<5	14.1%	GII.4	45
Ho Chi Minh City, Vietnam	502	Children	6.4%	GII	46
Cairo, Egypt	230	<1.5	26%	GII.4	47
Tamale, Ghana	367	<11	7.3%	GII	48
Blantyre, Malawi	398	Children	6.5%	GII.3	49
Leon, Nicaragua	542	<5	12%	GII.4	50
Recife, Brazil	233	Children	15%	ND	51
Rio de Janeiro, Brazil	289	Children	14.5%	GII, GI	52
Rio de Janeiro, Brazil	318	<5	20%	GII.4, GII	53
Goinia, Brasilia, Brazil	1006	Children	8.6%	ND	54
São Paulo, Brazil	234	Children	33.3%	GII.4	55

infected initially or on repeated challenge years later. Recent research has shown that host factors are an important determinant of susceptibility norovirus infections in that Norwalk virus infection depends on the presence of specific human histo-blood group antigen (HBGA) receptors in the gut.[76] Further investigations of the binding of different noroviruses have found that H type 1 and Lewis[b] carbohydrate antigens bind strongly to Norwalk virus VLPs.[77] Persons who express a functional $\alpha(1,2)$-fucosyltransferase-2 (FUT2), which is necessary to make H type 1 and Lewis[b] antigens, are called secretors, and secretors can be infected with Norwalk virus. Individuals who are homozygous recessives for the FUT2 gene and do not express H type-1 oligosaccharide (nonsecretors) are resistant to infection with Norwalk virus.[77,78] Norovirus strains belonging to different genotypes may have specific binding properties to different blood group antigens.[79–81] The combination of the strain-specific binding, the variable expression of the HBGA receptors, and acquired immunity may explain the differences in host susceptibility observed in outbreaks and in volunteer studies.[82]

DIAGNOSIS

Electron microscopy was initially used for identification and continues to be used by some laboratories to screen stools for potential viral pathogens, despite the lack of sensitivity.[5] Early antigen detection assays used reagents derived from human volunteers, but had low sensitivity.[83] Recently, commercial stool enzyme immunoassay detection methods mainly based on monoclonal antibodies have been developed and are available in Europe, and they appear to be useful in outbreaks when the outbreak strain is within the range included in the assay.[84] Serologic assays also have been developed using recombinant-expressed norovirus capsid proteins to detect immune responses to infecting norovirus strains, but are used more in epidemiological studies than for diagnosis in individual patients.[85,86]

Currently, RT-PCR assays are the most common approach for establishing a diagnosis of norovirus infection. Virus-specific primers are used to amplify conserved regions of the genome, usually in the polymerase or capsid genes.[5] No single primer pair can detect all norovirus or sapovirus strains because of the high sequence diversity, but, in most geographic regions, more than 90% of currently circulating strains can be detected using separate primer pairs for genogroup I and II noroviruses and sapoviruses. Highly sensitive assays based on real-time RT-PCR have been developed and evaluated for both noroviruses and sapoviruses, and these assays may be useful both for diagnosis and to study patterns of viral shedding.[87–89]

TREATMENT AND PROGNOSIS

Most viral gastroenteritis is self-limiting and no specific therapy is available or required. However, in children, diarrhea, especially with vomiting, can result rapidly in dehydration, which should be corrected immediately. Oral rehydration solutions providing essential electrolyte replacement are given as first-line therapy. Patients with significant dehydration and those unable to tolerate oral fluids require intravenous rehydration. There is no limitation on food intake. In experimentally infected adults, oral administration of bismuth subsalicylate reduced abdominal cramps and gastrointestinal symptoms;[90] but bismuth compounds and antimotility agents, such as diphenoxylate or loperamide, should be avoided in children.[91]

PREVENTION AND CONTROL

Outbreaks

The prevention of outbreaks of viral gastroenteritis relies on the control of contamination of food and water, maintenance of strict hygiene by food handlers, and reduction of secondary transmission through person-to-person spread. Measures to avoid contamination of waters in oyster-harvesting areas are necessary to prevent shellfish-associated outbreaks. Monitoring of food and water for noroviruses is not yet available routinely, although methods have been developed to detect noroviruses directly from food and water.[87,92]

Strict personal hygiene and the proper disinfection of environmental surfaces are critical to prevent food handler-associated transmission. Food handlers should be excluded from work for 2–3 days after recovery from norovirus illness and perhaps be reassigned to jobs not directly involving contact with food.[93] Similarly, in the care of the sick individuals at home or in hospitals, maintenance of strict hygiene, avoidance of contact with, and appropriate disinfection of, environmental surfaces contaminated with vomitus and feces are required.[83] In situations in which the epidemic is extended by periodic renewal of the susceptible population, such as hospitals, camps, and cruise ships, the facility or institution may have to be closed to interrupt transmission.[94]

Sporadic Disease

Standard hygienic precautions, including frequent hand-washing, careful disposal of waste and thorough cleaning, should help prevent calicivirus infection in all settings. In the absence of a cell culture system for human caliciviruses, it has not been possible to study disinfectants directly, but use of chlorine solutions at a concentration of 1000 parts per million on hard surfaces is recommended in the United Kingdom.[95]

Vaccine Development

With increasing recognition of the widespread incidence and clinical importance of noroviruses, the need for specific prevention strategies, such as vaccines, is becoming apparent. Recombinant VLPs expressed either in baculovirus or in transgenic plants have been shown to be safe and immunogenic when given orally to volunteers.[96,97] These vaccines could be used in settings where it is important to have at least short-term immunity to noroviral gastroenteritis, such as the military, travelers, and the elderly in hospitals or nursing homes. However, the relative roles of mucosal, systemic, and cell-mediated immunity are not understood. Recent reports indicate that noroviruses may not be limited to the intestine, in which case it may be necessary to have both systemic and mucosal responses in order to induce protection.[98,99] An incomplete understanding of the immune correlates of protection, lack of persistent long-term and cross-protective immunity, and the existence of multiple genetic and antigenic types of virus all present challenges to the development of vaccines directed at inducing protection against disease caused by these important agents of viral gastroenteritis.

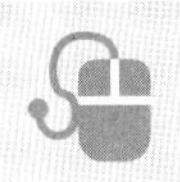

Access the complete reference list online at
http://www.expertconsult.com

CHAPTER 63

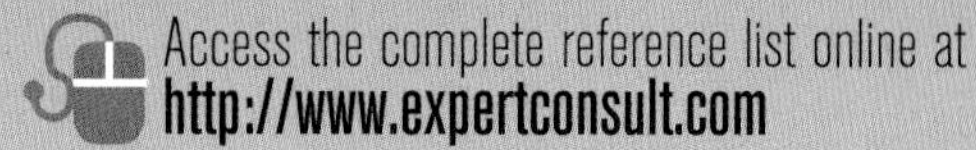
Access the complete reference list online at
http://www.expertconsult.com

Astroviruses, Enteric Adenoviruses, and Other Gastroenteritis Viral Infections

Roger I. Glass • Joseph S. Bresee

INTRODUCTION

Diarrheal disease remains one of the most common causes of morbidity and mortality in developing countries. The problem is particularly acute among young children, who will have an estimated 10–15 episodes of diarrhea in the first 5 years of life[1] and among whom 1.5–2.5 million deaths will occur each year.[2,3] For up to half of all episodes, an etiologic agent cannot be found. The importance of viral agents as causes of diarrheal disease has been increasingly appreciated, beginning with the discovery of rotavirus[4] and caliciviruses[5] in the 1970s. More recently, advances in detection methods for some other viruses, such as astroviruses and enteric adenoviruses, have led us to appreciate their role as causes of diarrheal disease. In addition, a variety of other viruses, such as picobirnaviruses, coronaviruses, toroviruses, parechoviruses, bocaviruses, and even influenza (H1N1) have been associated with gastroenteritis, but their clinical and public health importance remains unclear (***Table 63.1***). Many of these viruses may be responsible for the fraction of illness for which a pathogen cannot be found. A better understanding of their epidemiology will have implications for programs to decrease morbidity and mortality in developing countries.

ASTROVIRUSES

THE AGENT

Astroviruses were first identified in 1975[5,6] and named based on a characteristic five- or six-pointed appearance noted by electron microscopy. Since 1990, improvements in diagnostic methods, including the adaptation of astrovirus to grow in continuous cell lines,[7] sequencing and elucidation of the structure of the genome,[8–10] and development of improved methods of detection such as enzyme immunoassays and reverse-transcription polymerase chain reaction,[11–14] have led to new insights into the role of astrovirus in human disease. It is now clear that astroviruses are a common cause of sporadic gastroenteritis among children and may be associated with large-scale outbreaks of diarrhea as well.

Astroviruses are 28–30 nm, spherical, nonenveloped viruses with a positive sense ssRNA genome and have been classified in their own family, *Astroviridae*.[15] Eight serotypes of human astroviruses have been identified.[16,17] Of these, type 1 is predominant in most studies, accounting for more than half of strains isolated;[16,18,19] types 2, 3, and 4 each account for 10–16% of astrovirus detections; and types 5, 6, 7, and 8 are less uncommonly detected.[16,17] The relative distribution of types seems to vary by geographic location and by year,[20] and more variability may be found in developing countries.[21,22]

EPIDEMIOLOGY

Gastroenteritis associated with astroviruses has been reported worldwide, both as sporadic disease and as outbreaks. Cases of astrovirus-associated gastroenteritis are most common among children less than 2 years of age,[19,21–32] and are less frequent among older children and adults.[33,34] In volunteer studies, most adults neither became infected nor developed diarrhea.[33,35] However, in large outbreaks among schoolchildren,[36,37] teachers became ill as well, perhaps as a result of a large dose of virus in this type of setting or a different mechanism of spread. In addition, outbreaks have been reported among elderly people, probably due to waning immunity with increasing age.[38–40]

Gastroenteritis associated with astrovirus, like rotavirus, occurs in both developed[19,23,24,27–30,41–43] and developing countries,[32,44–48] suggesting that improvements in water and sanitation are unlikely to decrease disease incidence. In temperate climates, astrovirus diarrhea cases peak in winter,[17,19,24,29,31] whereas the seasonality is less clear in tropical settings.[32,44,46] With improvements in detection methods, astrovirus represents an important cause of community-acquired and nosocomial illness and may be the most common viral cause of gastroenteritis in children after rotavirus and possibly Norwalk-like viruses.[19] In developing countries, astroviruses have generally been detected in less than 10% of young children treated for gastroenteritis in outpatient clinics or in hospitals, and the lower proportions reported from some studies (<1%–3%) may reflect insensitive detection methods rather than true prevalence.[19,21,42,45,47–50] Even so, one study in rural Mexico has found astrovirus to be the most common cause of diarrhea in the first 3 years of life, causing 26% of diarrheal episodes in a prospectively followed cohort.[32] Outbreaks of astrovirus gastroenteritis have been reported in schools,[36,37] day-care centers,[25,51,52] hospitals,[26,29,39,53,54] nursing homes,[38,40] and households.[32,55] Nosocomial spread of astroviruses may be common.[56] While the modes of transmission are still unknown, the primary mode of spread of virus is likely to be through fecal-oral contamination via person-to-person contact,[33,35,36,53] although the stability of the virus in water may indicate that waterborne spread is possible.[57]

THE DISEASE

Astroviruses cause gastroenteritis characterized by 2–5 days of watery diarrhea, often accompanied by vomiting and less often by high fever, abdominal pain, and other constitutional symptoms.[23,29,44,46] It is generally milder than rotavirus, less commonly resulting in dehydration,[19,23,26,39,44] and rarely associated with death.[45] Lactose intolerance[43,58] and poor weight gain[46] have been reported following astrovirus infection, and children with poor nutritional status may develop more severe disease[46] or

Table 63.1 Summary of Virologic and Epidemiologic Features of Certain Viruses Associated with Gastroenteritis

Virus	Family	Taxonomy	Detection	Epidemiology	Comment
Astrovirus	*Astroviridae*	28–30 nm, ssRNA, N-env; 10% have 5–6-point star appearance; 8 serotypes	EM, IEM, EIA, RT-PCR	Endemic, most disease in children <2 years; epidemic, children and adults, including elderly; daycare, schools, hospitals	No clear seasonality in tropical countries; fairly common cause of viral diarrhea in children; less severe than rotavirus
Enteric adenovirus	*Adenoviridae*	70–80 nm, dsRNA, icosahedral, N-env; 2 main serotypes	EIA, EM, IEM, RT-PCR, culture, DNA probes, hybridization	Endemic disease in children <2 years	No clear seasonality; disease as severe as rotavirus, but less common
Picobirnavirus	*Birnaviridae*	35 nm, dsRNA, bisegmented genome	EM, PAGE, RT-PCR	Associated with diarrhea in HIV-infected adults; no clear association with diarrhea in healthy persons	Possible association with *Cryptosporidium* infection
Coronavirus	*Coronaviridae*	60–200 nm, ssRNA, pleomorphic, env, with club-shaped projections give a halo appearance	EM	Not known	May cause diarrhea in children and adults; possible association with tropical sprue and necrotizing enterocolitis
Torovirus	*Coronaviridae*	100–150 nm, ssRNA pleomorphic, env, with club-shaped projections	EM	Not known	Possible cause of diarrhea in humans

EIA, enzyme immunoassay; EM, electron microscopy; env, enveloped; IEM, immune electron microscopy; N-env, nonenveloped; PAGE, polyacrylamide gel electrophoresis; RT-PCR, reverse transcription–polymerase chain reaction.

chronic diarrhea.[50] Illness among adults is generally mild and of short duration.[33,35,39] However, in studies of immunocompromised persons, astrovirus is often the most common virus detected in persons with diarrhea and associated with prolonged shedding of virus.[59–61] HIV infection was associated with more severe astrovirus disease in children with HIV in Malawi.[21] Indirect evidence suggests that immunity to astrovirus develops early in life.[25,33,35]

Astrovirus infects intestinal epithelial cells. The incubation period is 3–4 days,[33,35] but may be shorter in outbreak settings.[37] Children may shed virus 1–2 days prior to illness and for 4–5 days following illness,[25,29,51] but shedding for 3 weeks has been reported when more sensitive detection methods have been used. Since most illness with astroviruses is found in young children and elderly persons, it is assumed that protection from illness is conferred by infection, and that the protection is relatively durable. Like many other enteric viruses, the immunologic correlates of protection are poorly understood for astroviruses.

DIAGNOSIS

Astroviruses were first detected by electron microscopy but this method has proven relatively insensitive compared to newer assays.[9,24,26,31,36,37,40,47,53,58,62,63] Enzyme immunoassays are commercially available[11,42] which are more sensitive, easier, and less expensive to use.[23,25,30,36,42,44,46,64] Molecular diagnostic methods – reverse transcription–polymerase chain reaction (RT-PCR) and probes – are the most sensitive and can also be used to type virus. Finally, the virus can be grown in cell culture.[65]

TREATMENT, PROGNOSIS, AND PREVENTION

Therapy for astrovirus diarrhea includes rehydration with oral or intravenous fluids. Illness is generally mild and self-limited, but malabsorption and lactose intolerance have been reported following infection. Death associated with astroviruses is rare.[43,45,58]

In outbreaks, identification of the source of infection, such as food or contact with ill persons, may be helpful in preventing further illness. Sporadic cases are common in children and no methods of prevention have been identified. Since the infection may be spread through close personal contact, enteric precautions including appropriate hand-washing practices and isolation of ill persons may be advisable.

ENTERIC ADENOVIRUS

THE AGENT

When adenoviruses were first identified in fecal specimens of children with diarrhea, their etiologic role was questioned because adenoviruses are common causes of other illnesses (e.g., upper respiratory tract infections) in children and are excreted in the stool. But unlike the common respiratory adenoviruses, enteric adenoviruses were difficult to grow and were therefore distinguished as the fastidious enteric adenoviruses (FEAs). Eventually, these FEAs were placed in their own group and found to belong to two predominant serotypes, 40 and 41. Besides these serotypes, serotype 31 has occasionally been causally associated with gastroenteritis and newer serotypes 42–49 have been identified in HIV patients with chronic diarrhea. Like astroviruses, the development of rapid, sensitive diagnostic assays for the detection of EAs has increased our appreciation of their role as causes of diarrhea in children.

Adenoviruses are members of the family *Adenoviridae* and of the genus *Mastadenovirus*. The 49 defined serotypes are divided into six subgroups (A–F); serotypes 40–49 are members of subgroup F (called EAs because they have been associated with gastroenteritis in humans).[66,67] EAs are nonenveloped, icosahedral, double-stranded DNA viruses, and are 70–80 nm in size.

EPIDEMIOLOGY

Like rotavirus and astrovirus diarrhea, diarrhea associated with EAs occurs primarily among children less than 2 years of age. Infection is probably universal, and the age-specific incidence does not appear to differ between temperate and tropical countries, suggesting that improvements in water and sanitation will not decrease the incidence of disease.

Compared to other viral agents in developing countries, EAs appear to account for a smaller proportion of diarrheal disease than in developed countries. EAs generally have been detected in 1–4% of children with diarrhea in many studies,[19,49] although they have been detected commonly in some studies. EAs were more common than rotavirus in a rural outpatient setting in Guatemala (14% of children with diarrhea had EA detected in stool compared to 5% with rotavirus), and were associated with 31% of hospital admissions for diarrhea.[68] In two South African studies, 6.5–13.2% of hospital admissions for diarrhea were associated with EAs;[69,70] in one study,[70] EAs were detected as often as rotaviruses. In the few studies that have examined the role of EAs in an adult population, they appear to be less important causes of gastroenteritis than in children. No seasonality of EA infections was apparent in studies in temperate[31,71–73] or tropical countries,[68,74] but few studies have reviewed multiple seasons.

THE DISEASE

Infections with EA can range from being mild or asymptomatic to producing profuse, nonbloody, watery diarrhea and vomiting.[71,72,75–79] Children often have 6–10 stools per day, and the mean duration of illness is 5–9 days.[68,71,72,75–78] Abdominal pain[71,76] and 2–3 days of low-grade fever (<38.5°C) are also frequently present, whereas temperatures greater than or equal to 39°C occur in less than 10–25% of children.[71,75] Mild isotonic dehydration may occur in 15–50% of children,[71,72,76] and only severe cases require hospitalization. Respiratory symptoms, including pneumonia, have been associated with EA infections but are present less commonly than with other adenoviruses.[72,75,77] Asymptomatic infections have been documented in 8% and 17% of children in day-care center studies.[23,68,71,72] Serum electrolytes are usually normal, and a slight leukocytosis may be present in a minority of children.[71]

Gastroenteritis associated with EAs has a similar presentation among patients in developed and developing countries. However, enteric adenoviruses may be associated with chronic diarrhea and less common serotypes in HIV-infected subjects.[59,80–84] Deaths from EA gastroenteritis are uncommon, but have been reported, particularly among immunocompromised children.[75,85,86] Long-term complications appear to be rare, but lactose intolerance[71] and malabsorption[87] have been reported and may exacerbate disease among children in developing countries where malnutrition is prevalent.

Differentiation of EA-associated gastroenteritis from other causes of viral gastroenteritis is difficult. EA-associated diarrhea may be more severe and prolonged than viral gastroenteritis caused by other agents[71,72,88] and is commonly associated with a high fever and dehydration similar to rotavirus.[71,88]

Like other viral agents of gastroenteritis, the exact mode of transmission is unknown. EAs are probably transmitted by fecal-oral spread, by person-to-person contact, or by respiratory droplets. No food- or water-borne outbreaks have been described.[89]

The incubation period of the disease is 3–10 days,[77,78,90] and viral shedding may persist for 10–14 days.[90] Mechanisms of diarrhea and immunity associated with EA are poorly understood. Type 40- and 41-specific antibodies develop following infection[71,91,92] and can be detected in the absence of recent diarrheal illness.[69,92] Children can become ill when reinfected with EA.[93] However, illness among adults is uncommon, even in outbreak settings where they have a high likelihood of exposure.

DIAGNOSIS

Electron microscopy (EM) was first used to detect EAs in fecal specimens when they are shed in large amounts (as many as 10^{11} particles/gram of feces). Since EM cannot distinguish EAs from non-enteric serotypes,[94] immune electron microscopy (IEM) can enhance sensitivity and specificity of EA detection.[95–98] Enzyme immunoassays using monoclonal antibodies to types 40 and 41 and to the adenovirus hexon common to all serotypes have been developed.[98–102] These are the easiest, most rapid methods for detection[103] and have proven to be highly sensitive and specific compared to IEM.[98] There are currently no commercial kits using DNA detection methods. EAs grow in Graham 293 cells, a cell line transformed by adenovirus type 5.[104] Viruses can then be identified using one of the preceding methods or by use of restriction enzyme analysis.

TREATMENT, PROGNOSIS, AND PREVENTION

No specific therapy is available for EA gastroenteritis, so therapy is directed towards treatment of dehydration. Oral rehydration solutions are effective in treating diarrhea with mild and moderate dehydration, and severe dehydration may require use of intravenous fluids.

Prevention of illness is currently not possible due to lack of understanding of risk factors for transmission. Attention to good handwashing when caring for ill persons seems reasonable.

NOVEL VIRUSES ASSOCIATED WITH GASTROENTERITIS

PICOBIRNAVIRUS

First identified in 1985,[105] picobirnaviruses (PBVs) have since been detected in a variety of animals,[106–111] as well as in human fecal specimens from patients with and without diarrhea.[59,112–115] It has been associated statistically with disease only in a study of HIV-infected adults in the United States[59] and Argentina.[116]

PBVs are small (pico), bisegmented (bi-RNA) viruses that are members of the family *Birnaviridae*. Atypical PBVs have been detected with three segments of RNA.[112] On electron microscopy, the virus is a 35 nm, discrete virus with no distinctive surface structure.

Little is known about the distribution or incidence of PBVs. In two studies, PBVs have been detected from diarrheic stools of adults with coexistent *Cryptosporidium* infection, and in one study, HIV-infected patients with chronic diarrhea excreted the virus for 7 months.[59,113] PBVs appear to have a global distribution and are relatively rare, with detection rates usually below 2% of children with diarrhea and less in immunocompromised adults.

No serologic immune response, measured by IEM, was detected in a group of adults with HIV,[59] although serum antibody has been detected by solid-phase IEM in infected rabbits.[110]

Although PBVs may be seen by EM, the virus has most often been identified by the distinct presence of two segments of RNA by polyacrylamide electrophoresis from a stool specimen.[59] The virus has been fully sequenced so RT-PCR has become a reliable method to detect and characterize the virus.

CORONAVIRUSES

Coronaviruses were first reported in association with diarrhea in adults[117] and tropical sprue among children and adults in India in 1975.[118] While subsequent reports documented detection of coronavirus-like particles (CVLPs) in stools of persons with diarrhea, they could not associate CVLPs with diarrhea.[119,120]

Coronaviruses are pleomorphic, 60–200 nm, ssRNA viruses that belong to the family *Coronaviridae*. Because of their pleomorphic appearance, misdiagnosis is problematic and no confirmatory test is available. Consequently, the prevalence of human enteric coronaviruses (HECVs) is unknown, and while they have been detected in studies in several countries,[16,24,45,62,121–129] they are not clearly associated with disease. In studies that have compared rates of HECV detection in stools from patients with diarrhea versus controls, the results are mixed. Because of the long duration of shedding and the possibility for asymptomatic infection, the pathogenicity of HECVs may be difficult to prove by comparing rates of detection between well and ill persons. Many studies have reported the majority of viral detections among young children and infants,[24,121,126–128,130] but detections among adults are common.[24,84,119,127,131] With some exceptions,[45,126,130] most studies have reported no differences in detection by time of year.[127] Mode of spread of HECVs is unknown.

Illness descriptions from outbreaks thought to be associated with coronaviruses have included the occurrence of vomiting and diarrhea of short duration, often accompanied by fever.[117,130] Besides gastroenteritis, HECVs have been reported in association with other gastrointestinal diseases including necrotizing enterocolitis,[132,133] and neonatal diarrhea[122] in infants, and tropical sprue.[118,134] In several reports of clinical signs and symptoms associated with the new severe acute respiratory syndrome (SARS)-associated coronavirus, diarrhea has been a common symptom, reported in around a quarter of patients[135,136] It is not clear whether patients with the SARS coronavirus can have diarrhea without respiratory symptoms.

HECVs may be identified with EM by their distinctive 20 nm, clublike projections.[137] Enteric coronaviruses are distinct from respiratory coronaviruses and do not cross-react by enzyme-linked immunosorbent assay (ELISA) or immunoblots, although there is cross-reactivity on IEM.[129]

TOROVIRUSES

Toroviruses are members of the family *Coronaviridae* and the genus *Torovirus*. They are pleomorphic, 100–150 nm, ssRNA viruses with 20 nm, clublike projections extending from the capsid.[138–140]

The epidemiology of these infections remains unclear. Toroviruses have been detected in stools of children and adults with diarrhea in developed countries.[49,140–142] However, in these studies there was no epidemiologic association with illness, and the detections could not be confirmed using additional tests. In an EM survey of diarrhea among children in Toronto, torovirus-like particles were detected in 224 (8%) of 3800 stool specimens. The particles in some of these stools were later confirmed as torovirus by an ELISA incorporating bovine and human antibodies.[143]

A serum response to infection can be measured in infected cows, which develop IgM and IgG following gastrointestinal infection,[144] but no serum immune response has been reported in humans. Electron microscopists can identify torovirus-like particles in human specimens but cannot confirm the detection.[145] Several additional methods including ELISA,[144,146] cDNA probes for hybridization,[142] and RT-PCR[143] have been used successfully in animals and hold promise for detection of human disease.

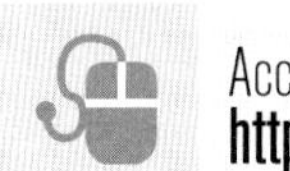

Access the complete reference list online at **http://www.expertconsult.com**

OTHER VIRUSES

A variety of other viruses have been implicated in gastroenteritis to some degree, including parvoviruses, enteroviruses, reoviruses, and pestiviruses, and have been reviewed in detail elsewhere. Parvoviruses, reoviruses, and pestiviruses may cause diarrhea in nonhumans, and there are reports of human cases of gastrointestinal illnesses.[147–153] However, the data are inconclusive, and they are not currently thought to be causes of gastroenteritis in humans.

In 2004, echovirus types 22 and 23 were reclassified as human parechoviruses (HPeV) which are small, nonenveloped, positive-sense single-stranded RNA viruses in the family *Picornaviridae*.[154–158] In an investigation in Thai children with gastroenteritis in whom no other pathogen could be found, HPeV were found in 15% of fecal specimens examined. The full sequence of these viruses is known, which has facilitated detection and characterization by RT-PCR.

Early identification of parvoviruses as a putative cause of diarrhea in animals and humans led to the discovery in 2005 of two members of the parvovirus family, human bocavirus HBoV2 and HBoV3, to be newly recognized agents of diarrhea.[159–166] These DNA viruses have been detected from stool and respiratory samples from patients with acute diarrhea, and in one study were present in 37% of patients tested and were significantly associated with diarrhea. However, no controls were used and prolonged shedding might account for this high rate of detection. The virus has been found in a global distribution and has often been detected in the presence of other pathogens.

Finally, the recent epidemics of influenza (H1N1) have led to the recognition that up to one-third of these patients have diarrhea as part of their clinical presentation.[167,168] While we do not normally consider influenza virus to be a cause of diarrhea, the high prevalence of gastrointestinal symptoms should encourage clinicians to consider this possibility during the flu season when no other enteric pathogens can be found in a patient with a respiratory illness.

CHAPTER 64

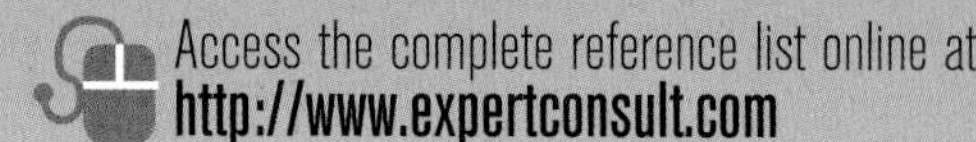
Access the complete reference list online at
http://www.expertconsult.com

Enteric Viral Hepatitis A and E

Shahid Jameel • Rakesh Aggarwal

INTRODUCTION

Viral hepatitis, or inflammation of the liver due to a viral infection, is an important cause of morbidity and mortality worldwide. It is caused by infection with one of the hepatotropic viruses, which predominantly affect the liver (see also Chapter 133). In addition, the liver can also be prominently involved in systemic infection with viruses such as cytomegalovirus, Epstein–Barr virus, and dengue virus that affect several organs. Despite significant overlap in the clinical manifestations caused by them, the five currently known hepatotropic viruses, named as hepatitis A, B, C, delta, and E viruses, differ widely in their morphology, genomic organization, taxonomic classification, and modes of replication. These viruses enter the host by one of the two major routes, enteral or parenteral. This chapter focuses on two enterally transmitted hepatitis viruses, i.e., hepatitis A virus (HAV) and hepatitis E virus (HEV). These infections are more common in tropical areas where opportunities for enteral transmission of pathogens are more frequent. They generally persist in the host for a shorter duration than the parenteral viruses and predominantly cause acute disease with few long-term sequelae. The associated clinical illnesses, named as hepatitis A and hepatitis E, respectively, can each occur either as epidemics, or as sporadic cases in the absence of a recognized outbreak.

HEPATITIS A

Epidemiological and volunteer studies during World War II led to identification of "infectious hepatitis" and "serum hepatitis" as two distinct disease entities, which were then named "hepatitis A" and "hepatitis B", respectively. Further studies showed that hepatitis A was caused by a filterable agent, presumably a virus, had a short incubation period and was spread predominantly by the fecal-oral route. In the 1970s, the agent was successfully transmitted to primates, resulting in development of serological tests for this disease. Success in growing the virus in cell culture paved the way for development of effective vaccines.

THE AGENT

Hepatitis A virus (HAV) is a member of the family *Picornaviridae* (pico = small; RNA virus), which includes other important human pathogens such as polioviruses and human rhinoviruses.[1] It is a nonenveloped virus of 27–32 nm that is stable at low pH and at 60°C for up to one hour, but is destroyed by autoclaving, boiling for about 5 minutes, or exposure to ultraviolet radiation, formalin, β-propiolactone, iodine, chlorine or chlorine-containing compounds.[1]

The virion consists of a capsid of three or four proteins and a single-stranded, positive sense RNA genome of about 7.5 kb (***Fig. 64.1***). Like the genomes of all picornaviruses, the HAV genome is linear and includes: (1) a 5′ noncoding region (NCR) of about 750 nucleotides linked at its 5′ end to the viral protein VPg; (2) a single open reading frame that encodes all the viral proteins; and (3) a short 3′ NCR terminating in a poly(A) tract.[1] The open reading frame is divided into three regions, P1, P2, and P3, of which P1 encodes the four viral structural proteins VP1 to VP4, and P2 and P3 encode the nonstructural proteins with biochemical activities that support viral genome replication and protein processing (***Fig. 64.1***).

Though all HAV strains correspond to a single serotype, genetic analysis has shown the existence of at least seven genotypes, of which genotypes I, II, III, and VII have been isolated from human patients, with genotype I being the most common worldwide.[2] Besides mutations commonly found in RNA viruses, genetic recombination resulting in novel HAV strains has also been observed.

HAV enters target cells by binding to HAVcr-1, a cell surface glycoprotein with immunoglobulin (Ig)- and mucin-like domains.[3] Following entry and uncoating, the genomic RNA is translated into a polyprotein, which is subsequently processed into 11 different proteins through the actions of the viral 3C protease and unidentified cellular proteases (***Fig. 64.1***).[4] Translation is aided by the internal ribosome entry site (IRES), a highly structured RNA element within the 5′ NCR.[4] The viral 2C (helicase) and 3D (RNA polymerase) proteins replicate the genomic plus-stranded RNA through an amplification cycle that involves an antigenomic minus-stranded RNA intermediate.[4] Late in the replication cycle, the capsid proteins package the genomic RNA, and the newly formed virions are secreted across the apical surface of hepatocytes into a biliary canaliculus, passing into the bile and small intestine, and are excreted in the stool of an infected person.[1]

Various primary and continuous cell lines of primate origin support the culture of HAV. These include primary African green monkey kidney (AGMK) cells, primary human fibroblasts and MRC5 human diploid lung cells. Many HAV strains have been characterized, of which HM175 has been adapted to different cell types to yield a range of attenuated, persistent, cytopathic and neutralization-resistant viral variants.[5] The HAV genomic RNA was molecularly cloned as a cDNA copy, and RNA transcripts produced *in vitro* from this copy are infectious when transfected into cultured cells.[6]

EPIDEMIOLOGY

Humans are the only host, and hence the only source, of HAV. The virus is excreted in large amounts in feces of infected persons, and is transmitted by the fecal-oral route. The most important mode of transmission is close contact with an infected person, usually in a household or a school. Rates of transmission to contacts of hepatitis A cases are high even in developed countries with good personal hygiene, indicating that this route is highly efficient.[7] Many cases do not have an identifiable contact; these may be related to contact with an asymptomatic case.

Contaminated food and water are important modes of transmission. Contaminated food products implicated in hepatitis A outbreaks have

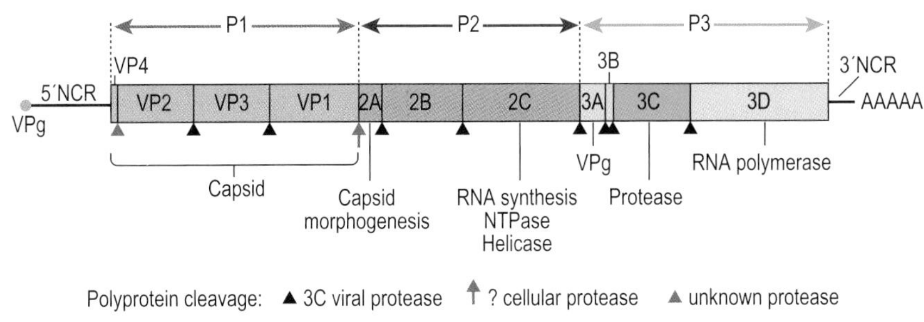

Figure 64.1 HAV genome. The boxed region represents the polyprotein coding segment. The polyprotein is processed into P1, P2, P3 regions and individual proteins by viral (3C), cellular and unknown protease activities as indicated. The functions of individual proteins are indicated. NTPase, nucleoside-5′-triphosphatase; NCR, noncoding region.

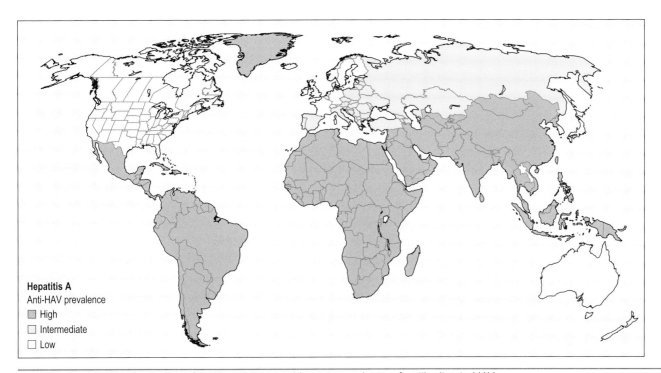

Figure 64.2 Geographic distribution of HAV as determined by seroprevalence of antibodies to HAV.

included seafood,[8,9] farm products,[10] milk, hamburgers, ice-slush beverages, and salads.[11] Some outbreaks have been very large, as in China in 1988, which affected nearly 300 000 persons and was believed to be related to ingestion of raw clams.[9]

Although blood or blood products can also transmit HAV, such events are uncommon. Outbreaks of HAV infection have been reported among injection drug users,[12] but the transmission is believed to have been multifactorial. Sexual transmission of HAV has been reported, especially among men having sex with men.

HAV infection is distributed worldwide (***Fig. 64.2***). However, its epidemiological characteristics vary, determined primarily by socioeconomic development. In developing countries with poor sanitary and living conditions, such as those in Africa, Asia, and parts of South America, transmission rates are high and most infections occur in early childhood. Since HAV infection confers strong protection against reinfection, infection and disease among adults is uncommon in these regions. In contrast, in developed countries, HAV transmission during childhood is much less frequent.

The likelihood of disease following HAV infection increases with age. Thus, infection among children below the age of 6 years is most often either asymptomatic or associated with mild and nonspecific symptoms. In contrast, most older children and adults with HAV infection have liver-specific symptoms such as jaundice.[13] The risk of complications and case-fatality rate also increase with age.[14]

Because of the above factors, three major epidemiological patterns of HAV infection have been described.[15] In highly endemic countries, high transmission rates lead to near universal exposure to HAV during childhood, and only infrequent clinical cases. In areas of intermediate endemicity, the virus circulates at a fairly high rate in the population, which has susceptible older children and young adults. Since HAV infection is frequently symptomatic in these age groups, these areas show a high incidence of clinical disease. This results in large outbreaks, related either to person-to-person transmission, or to common-source contamination of food or water. In areas with low endemicity, disease rates are low even though most of the older children, adolescents, and young adults are susceptible to HAV infection, because of fewer opportunities for exposure. The cases in these regions arise from travel to endemic areas, person-to-person spread or common-source contamination of food. Even within a country or population, rates of antibody prevalence may vary widely, depending on the socioeconomic status, family size, and hygienic practices.

THE DISEASE

Infection with HAV may be asymptomatic or may result in acute hepatitis of variable severity, including fulminant hepatitis.

The symptoms and signs of acute hepatitis A are similar to those for the other types of viral hepatitis. The incubation period is 2–6 weeks.

The illness usually begins with a variable combination of non-specific, systemic symptoms, such as fatigue, malaise, low-grade fever, headache, myalgias, arthralgias, loss of appetite, nausea, vomiting, altered taste sensation, and aversion to fatty foods and smoking. This phase lasts for 1–7 days. Hepatitis is first suspected when specific symptoms, such as dark urine, right upper quadrant pain, jaundice, or light-colored stools appear. Some patients also have pruritus. Appearance of the icteric phase is often accompanied by abatement of systemic symptoms. Physical examination usually reveals icterus, mild tender hepatomegaly, and sometimes splenomegaly.

The illness generally lasts a few weeks. In some patients, the course is protracted, lasting 12–18 weeks; these patients often have prominent cholestatic features (clay stools, marked pruritus, and deep jaundice), which may cause much concern, but almost always recover uneventfully.[16]

In occasional cases, clinical relapses, characterized by reappearance or exacerbations of liver test abnormalities, and less frequently of symptoms and fecal viral shedding, can occur weeks to months after the onset of the initial illness; however, complete resolution is the rule even in these cases. No chronic carrier state, chronic viral excretion, chronic hepatitis, or long-term sequelae such as cirrhosis or hepatocellular carcinoma are associated with HAV infection.

Extrahepatic manifestations, believed to be caused by formation of antigen–antibody complexes, can occur, but are quite rare in hepatitis A. These include joint pains, cutaneous vasculitis, cryoglobulinemia, and neurologic syndromes such as Guillain–Barré, myelopathy, mononeuritis, or meningoencephalitis.

Fulminant hepatitis A occurs in approximately 1 : 1000 cases of acute hepatitis A, and may be fatal. Irritability, alterations in sleep rhythm and confusion may herald the onset of fulminant hepatic failure. The risk of fulminant disease increases with age, being particularly high in those older than 30 years. Persons with preexisting chronic liver disease are at an increased risk for fulminant disease.

PATHOGENESIS AND IMMUNITY

Following entry into the host, HAV presumably replicates in the small intestinal epithelium, from where it reaches the liver through the portal circulation. The major site of HAV replication is the hepatocytes, but this tissue tropism is not fully understood. Replication is followed by virus secretion from hepatocytes through a poorly understood pathway, but one that likely involves cellular vesicles. The virus is shed into the liver sinusoids and bile canaliculi[17] from where it enters the small intestine and is excreted in feces. Unlike other picornaviruses, which are cytopathic, there is little evidence to support a cytopathic nature for HAV. Most HAV isolates are not cytopathic in cell culture, and liver injury is possibly due to the host's immune response.[18] Although there is some correlation between disease severity and HAV shedding in stools,[19] the latter usually peaks before liver injury and ALT elevation (***Fig. 64.3***).

During acute infection, viremia and fecal shedding of the virus appear within days of infection; while viremia typically persists till the appearance of symptoms, stools remain infectious for another 1–2 weeks (***Fig. 64.3***). In nonhuman primates experimentally infected with HAV, viral antigen and/or RNA have been detected in the spleen, kidneys, tonsils and saliva, and occasionally in the intestinal mucosa.[1] This pattern of replication and shedding is supported by the observation that stools of HAV patients are about 100 000 times more infectious than serum, which in turn are about 10 000 times more infectious than saliva.[1]

The host immune response to HAV infection is marked by the appearance initially of anti-HAV IgM, followed by anti-HAV IgG (***Fig. 64.3***). Both function as neutralizing antibodies *in vitro*.[18] Whereas anti-HAV IgM titers wane in 4–6 months, anti-HAV IgG persists throughout life and confers protection against reinfection. Anti-HAV IgA has also been observed in feces and sera, but its role in protection is not fully understood.[18] Virus-specific, HLA-restricted $CD8^+$ cytotoxic T cells have been described in the liver during acute hepatitis A.[20] These cells secrete

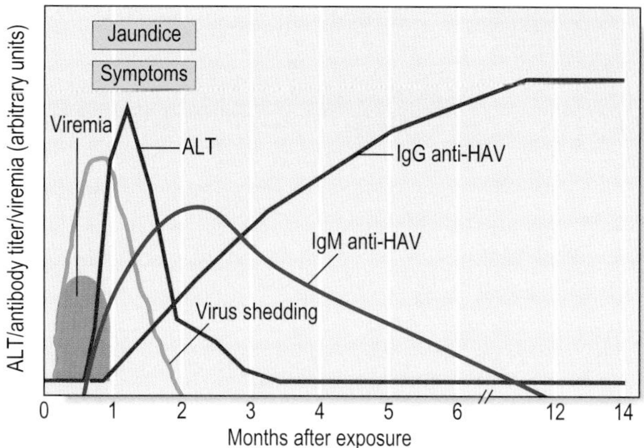

Figure 64.3 Clinical course of hepatitis A. ALT, alanine aminotransferase; HAV, hepatitis A virus; anti-HAV, antibody to HAV; IgG, immunoglobulin G; IgM, immunoglobulin M.

interferon-γ, which is likely to recruit nonspecific inflammatory cells to the sites of viral replication to aid in viral clearance, but may also cause liver injury.[4]

During the incubation period, HAV replicates to high titers in the liver, with viremia and fecal shedding (***Fig. 64.3***), suggesting that HAV may regulate host pathways for virus recognition and clearance. Innate immunity to limit the spread of viral infection is based primarily on interferon production by infected cells, which relies upon double-stranded RNA (dsRNA) recognition by toll-like receptor 3 (TLR3) or an RNA helicase, retinoic acid-inducible gene I (RIG-I).[21] *In vitro*, HAV was shown to inhibit dsRNA-mediated antiviral defense by suppressing the RIG-I-mediated signaling pathway.[4] The hepatitis C virus (HCV) also displays similar effects on innate immunity; however, unlike HCV, infection with HAV induces a robust adaptive immune response, which is sufficient to clear the virus.

DIAGNOSIS

Elevation of alanine and aspartate aminotransferase (ALT, AST) levels is a sensitive, but nonspecific, indicator of liver damage. There is no correlation between the degree of aminotransferase elevation and disease severity. Other factors such as prolonged prothrombin time, especially when accompanied by changes in mental status, may indicate severe disease. In cholestatic hepatitis, alkaline phosphatase levels are elevated. Specific diagnosis of hepatitis A is based on serology. Testing for anti-HAV IgM is the most appropriate since its levels rise early in the acute phase of disease and disappear in 4–6 months, unlike anti-HAV IgG, which persists for life (***Fig. 64.3***). The HAV RNA has also been detected by reverse transcription-polymerase chain reaction (RT-PCR) in the blood and stools of patients in the acute phase of infection, and sequencing of the amplification products has been used for genotyping viral isolates. From a clinical viewpoint, the presence of anti-HAV IgM antibodies is sufficient to confirm hepatitis A.

TREATMENT AND PROGNOSIS

Patients with HAV, including those with cholestatic or relapsing variants, do not need any specific treatment, since the disease is self-limited. Management is thus primarily supportive. Restriction of diet or of physical activity has no proven benefit. Avoidance of alcohol appears prudent. Paracetamol, nonsteroidal anti-inflammatory drugs or antiemetic drugs may be used for symptom control. Cholestyramine may be tried if pruritus is severe. Hospitalization is needed only for patients with another serious medical problem, inadequate oral intake, or incipient liver failure. Patients with fulminant disease need treatment in an intensive care unit or a specialized liver unit. Failure to improve should lead to consideration of liver transplantation.

PREVENTION AND CONTROL

Improvement in hygiene is central to hepatitis A prevention. In endemic areas, provision of a clean, safe water supply, adequate disposal of human waste and improvements in living conditions can reduce the opportunities for HAV infection. Hand washing and avoidance of uncooked or inadequately cooked foods or foods with potential for contamination with water (e.g., salads, iced drinks) help reduce the risk of infection.

Passive transfer of antibodies before or shortly after exposure to HAV provides protection against clinical disease. This can be done by intramuscular administration of human immunoglobulins (Ig). Prepared by cold ethanol fractionation of large plasma pools, Ig preparations contain sufficient amounts of anti-HAV antibodies and are free of risk of transmission of HBV, HCV, HIV, or other viruses. When administered prior to exposure, intramuscular (IM) doses of 0.02 mL/kg and 0.06 mL/kg provide protection for about 3 and 5 months, respectively. The only accepted indication for passive pre-exposure prophylaxis of hepatitis A is travel to endemic areas, the usual recommended dose being 0.02 mL/kg IM within the preceding 2 weeks. When more time is available before travel, the use of hepatitis A vaccine may be preferred (see Chapter 124). The efficacy of Ig in post-exposure prophylaxis depends on the time interval between exposure and its administration, reaching 85–95% following a single dose of 0.02 mL/kg IM given within 2 weeks following exposure to HAV. Later administration reduces efficacy, but may still attenuate disease severity. Post-exposure prophylaxis is recommended for close personal contacts such as household and sexual partners, regardless of age. It is not recommended for casual contacts of hepatitis A patients (i.e., at school or work).

Two different vaccines are currently available against hepatitis A[22,23] – Havrix (GlaxoSmithKline) and VAQTA (Merck). Both contain formalin-inactivated attenuated strains of HAV and are highly immunogenic and safe. For each vaccine, two IM doses separated by at least 4 weeks are recommended. These vaccines offer protection against HAV infection when given before, and even a few days after exposure. Protective antibody levels persist for 10–20 years (see Chapter 124).

Indications for the use of vaccines are similar to those for Ig. However, these have advantages of providing active, long-term protection, without interference with other childhood immunizations or the risk of transmission of bloodborne infections. Thus, in recent years, these vaccines have gradually replaced Ig for prevention of hepatitis A. In addition, their use is recommended in persons with preexisting chronic liver disease, particularly hepatitis C, in whom HAV infection may be associated with a particularly severe disease.[24]

A combined vaccine against both hepatitis A and B is also available – Twinrix (GlaxoSmithKline), for use in persons 18 years or older. It contains protective components of both the single-antigen vaccines, and offers protection against each of these diseases equivalent to individual vaccines. Though its use reduces the number of injections required for protection against these two diseases, it does not fit well into the childhood immunization schedule since the optimum ages for administration of vaccines against hepatitis A and B are quite different.

The current high cost of these vaccines remains a major limiting factor, especially in endemic areas, which are also resource-limited.

HEPATITIS E

The first well-documented report of this disease was a large epidemic of waterborne hepatitis in New Delhi, India during 1955–56. Though initially believed to be due to HAV, testing of stored sera from this epidemic and another outbreak during 1978–79 in Kashmir, India revealed the absence of serological markers for hepatitis A and hepatitis B, suggesting the existence of another viral agent, which was then provisionally named as enterically-transmitted non-A, non-B hepatitis virus.[25] This suspicion was confirmed in 1983 when virus-like particles were identified using immune electron microscopy in the feces of a volunteer who had ingested fecal matter from patients with non-A, non-B hepatitis.[26] The virus was subsequently named hepatitis E virus (HEV), based on its enteric route of transmission and propensity to cause epidemics.

THE AGENT

HEV is a single species in the genus *Hepevirus* of family *Hepeviridae* (http://www.ictvonline.org/virusTaxonomy.asp?version=2009). With availability of the first HEV genome sequence in 1990[27] and subsequently the sequences of several geographically distinct isolates, HEV appears not to be closely related to any other known virus. Besides human HEV, closely related viruses that infect pigs (swine HEV) and a more distantly related virus that causes splenomegaly in chickens (avian HEV) have also been characterized.

Compared to HAV, HEV is less heat-stable. In a cell culture infectivity assay, at least two of three human HEV strains were stable up to 56°C, but lost infectivity when kept at 60°C for one hour.[28] There are no reports on the effects of pH on HEV stability, but being an enteric virus, it is likely to be stable at low pH.

The 27–34 nm nonenveloped HEV particle includes a capsid composed of a single protein and a single-stranded, positive sense RNA genome of about 7.2 kb (***Fig. 64.4***). The HEV genome is linear and includes: (1) a short 5′ NCR of about 25–30 nucleotides, with a 7-methylguanine cap at its 5′ end; (2) a protein-coding region with three open reading frames *orf1*, *orf2*, and *orf3*; and (3) a short 3′ NCR terminating in a poly(A) tract (Fig. 64.4). The ORF1 nonstructural polyprotein is predicted to contain regions with methyltransferase, papain-like protease, RNA helicase, and RNA-dependent RNA polymerase activities to aid in viral genome replication.[29] The ORF2 protein is proposed to encapsidate the viral RNA genome and was shown to bind it.[30] The protein is glycosylated,[31] and this modification is important for virus infectivity.[32] In some expression studies, a truncated capsid protein self-assembles into virus-like particles (VLPs), which have also been explored as a recombinant subunit vaccine against hepatitis E.[33] The ORF3 protein is required for virus infection *in vivo*, but not for replication in cultured cells.[34] It is proposed to optimize the host cell environment for viral replication through its interaction with various cellular proteins and intracellular pathways.[29]

Though all HEV strains correspond to a single serotype, there are at least four genotypes, which include human and swine HEV isolates that are dominant in a particular geographic area, but not limited to it.

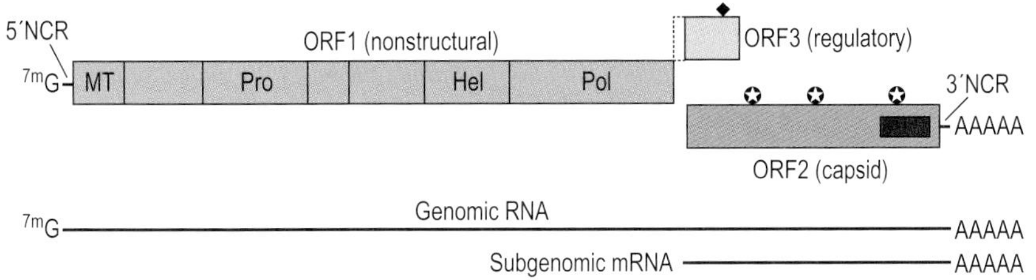

Figure 64.4 HEV genome. The positive sense HEV genomic RNA and a subgenomic RNA produced during replication are shown. The genomic RNA has three open reading frames, which encode ORF1, ORF2 and ORF3 proteins. MT, methyltransferase; Pro, protease; Hel, RNA helicase; Pol, RNA-dependent RNA polymerase; NCR, noncoding region; black diamond, phosphorylation; white stars, glycosylation.

Genotype 1 includes Asian and African strains, genotype 2 includes the single Mexican strain and few isolates from Africa, genotype 3 includes human and swine HEV strains from industrialized countries, and genotype 4 includes human and swine HEV strains from Asia. Viruses of genotypes 1 and 2 are associated with outbreaks due to efficient human-to-human fecal-oral transmission, while genotype 3 and 4 viruses are maintained in animal species and show inefficient cross-species transmission.[35] Some reports suggest that compared to genotype 3, the genotype 4 viruses are more virulent with higher viral loads in infected patients.[36]

The entry of HEV into target cells has not been characterized, and a replication model is based on analogy to similar viruses.[29] Following entry and uncoating, the *orf1* on genomic RNA is translated into a polyprotein, which also includes the viral replicase. From the genomic RNA template, this replicase produces a negative-stranded RNA intermediate, which in turn produces genomic RNA as well as a subgenomic RNA (***Fig. 64.4***); the latter is translated into the ORF2 (and possibly also the ORF3) proteins. *In vitro* transcripts of full-length HEV cDNA clones are infectious for cell lines,[37] nonhuman primates,[38] and pigs,[39] suggesting that the subgenomic RNAs are not required to initiate an infection, and must be synthesized as part of the replication process. The assembly and egress of virions has not been characterized.

Only limited success has been achieved in propagating HEV *in vitro* in 2BS, A549, FRhK, and PLC/PRF/5 cells, and in primary cynomolgus hepatocytes. Recently, HEV genotype 3 was successfully passaged for multiple generations in PLC/PRF/5 cells, and was used to assess the infectivity of HEV shed in patient stools.[40]

EPIDEMIOLOGY

HEV is transmitted predominantly from contaminated drinking water by the fecal-oral route.[41] Foodborne transmission is also possible. Neonates born to mothers with hepatitis E have detectable HEV RNA or anti-HEV IgM antibodies, indicating that maternofetal (vertical) transmission is possible.[42] In regions where hepatitis E is endemic, the presence of HEV viremia among healthy blood donors and transmission of this infection through blood transfusion have been documented. However, the contribution of such transmission to the overall disease burden remains unclear and may be small.

Hepatitis E is endemic in several parts of the world, including south, southeastern and central Asia, northern and western Africa, and the Mediterranean region.[41] In these regions, outbreaks of hepatitis E occur. The unimodal or multimodal outbreaks can be fairly large, affecting several hundred to several thousand people. These are often related to contamination of drinking water supplies with human fecal matter. Smaller outbreaks in urban areas may be related to contamination of water flowing through leaky pipes that pass through soil contaminated with sewage.

In HEV-endemic regions, the disease most commonly affects young adults.[41] Children are likely spared because of a higher proportion of asymptomatic infections. Men are more often affected than women. Characteristically, the infection seems to have worse consequences in pregnant women, and is associated with a high attack rate as well as an increased severity of illness. The disease mortality rates in this group of patients can reach as high as 15–25%. Hepatitis E during pregnancy also adversely affects obstetric and fetal outcomes. The reason for this predilection remains unknown.

In endemic areas, HEV infection also accounts for a large proportion of acute sporadic hepatitis in all age groups. Cases with sporadic hepatitis E closely resemble those with epidemic disease in age distribution, severity and duration of illness, and propensity for worse prognosis during pregnancy. As opposed to hepatitis A, person-to-person transmission of HEV is uncommon.[43] The role of zoonotic transmission of HEV in endemic regions remains unclear, and may be limited. Genotype 1 virus, which is the most prevalent outbreak type, has not been isolated from animals and has not yet been transmitted to non-primate animal species in laboratory studies. The reservoir of HEV in these regions is not known, but may lie in a pool of persons with subclinical infection.

In non-endemic regions, no outbreaks have been reported, and the disease accounts for only a minority of acute viral hepatitis cases. Until a few years ago, most such cases were among travelers to disease-endemic areas. However, in recent years, indigenous transmission of hepatitis E has been reported either as single case reports or small case-series from the United States, Europe, Australia, and Japan.[44] In several cases, the mode of transmission cannot be identified; in others, zoonotic transmission is believed to be responsible. This is based on close genetic relationships between sequences of HEV isolates from autochthonous human cases and swine HEV isolates, with both usually belonging to genotypes 3 and 4. Further, in experimental studies, cross-species transmission of human HEV isolates from these regions to pigs, and swine HEV isolates to primates has been possible.[45] Most convincing evidence has come from a cluster of Japanese cases that developed hepatitis E a few weeks after consumption of inadequately cooked deer meat; genomic sequences of HEV isolated from these cases and the left-over frozen meat were identical.[46] Demonstration of HEV genotype 3 in pig liver meat sold for human consumption in several developed countries suggests that consumption of pig meat or contact with pigs may be responsible for cases in non-endemic regions.[47]

Anti-HEV IgG antibodies, generally taken as evidence of prior exposure to HEV, have been found in healthy persons from all geographical areas. The prevalence rates are generally higher in HEV-endemic regions. In several endemic countries, the age-specific seroprevalence rates of anti-HEV antibodies are much lower than those for antibodies against other enterically transmitted infections, such as HAV and *Helicobacter pylori*.[41] This is in contrast to the situation in Egypt, with anti-HEV detection rates among adults of above 70%, despite absence of disease outbreaks though sporadic disease is known to occur. In developed countries, anti-HEV prevalence rates range from 1% to >20%. These appear to be higher than those expected from the low rate of clinically evident hepatitis E disease in these areas, and could be related to occurrence of subclinical HEV infection, serological cross-reactivity with other agents, false positive serological tests, zoonotic transmission, or a combination of these.[41] Veterinarians and swine farm workers with frequent contact with pigs appear to have higher anti-HEV seroprevalence rates.

THE DISEASE

The incubation period of hepatitis E varies from 2 to 10 weeks, with a mean of around 40 days (***Fig. 64.5***). As with hepatitis A, the clinical consequences of HEV infection vary widely from asymptomatic infection, through typical acute viral hepatitis, to fulminant hepatic failure. Acute viral hepatitis and fulminant hepatic failure caused by HEV are indistinguishable from those caused by other hepatitis viruses, except for the epidemiological setting or serological tests. The disease is usually self-limiting.

As indicated earlier, pregnant women, especially those in the third trimester, are particularly likely to have severe disease. In animal studies, viral inoculum dose determines the severity of liver injury, with lower doses leading to subclinical infection;[48] whether this happens in humans has not been studied.

In endemic areas, HEV infection in patients with preexisting chronic liver disease of any etiology may present with acute-on-chronic liver disease.[49]

Cases reported from non-endemic areas either have icteric illness resembling that seen with other hepatitis viruses or are anicteric with nonspecific symptoms or asymptomatic transaminase elevation.[44] Most of these cases are middle-aged or elderly men, often with another coexistent disease accounting, at least partially, for the somewhat poorer outcome in these patients than those in disease-endemic areas.

Although HEV infection is thought to be self-limiting, recently HEV genotype 3 infection was reported in 14 French solid-organ transplant recipients receiving immunosuppressive drugs who had a recent onset of transaminase elevation.[50] Some of these cases had persistent HEV viremia, prolonged liver enzyme elevation, and liver biopsy showing portal hepatitis, dense lymphocytic infiltrate and variable degrees of piecemeal

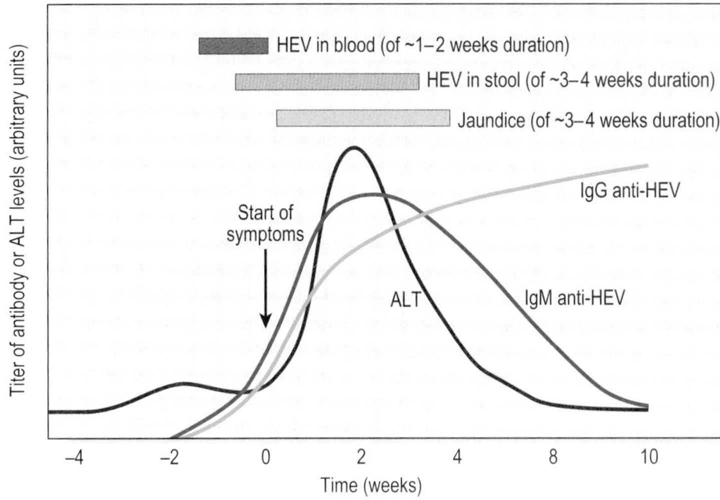

Figure 64.5 Clinical course of hepatitis E. ALT, alanine aminotransferase; HEV, hepatitis E virus; anti-HEV, antibody to HEV; IgG, immunoglobulin G; IgM, immunoglobulin M. (From Jameel S. Molecular biology and pathogenesis of hepatitis E virus. Expert Rev Mol Med 1999;1:1. With permission of Cambridge University Press.)

necrosis and fibrosis. This and some additional case reports of prolonged transaminase elevation, persistent viremia with genotype 3 HEV, and chronic hepatitis and cirrhosis on liver biopsy suggest that chronic HEV infection may lead to cirrhosis. However, it remains unclear whether genotype 1 HEV, the predominant disease-causing strain worldwide, can cause persistent infection in otherwise healthy persons.

PATHOGENESIS AND IMMUNITY

Following fecal-oral entry into the host, the initial site of replication is presumably the intestinal epithelium, from where it reaches the liver through the portal circulation. The major site of HEV replication is the liver, where it replicates in hepatocytes. The tissue tropism of HEV is not fully understood.

Several observations suggest that HEV is not directly cytopathic, but like other hepatitis viruses, liver injury may be mediated by the host immune response. Analogous to HAV, viremia precedes the elevation of serum aminotransferases (*Fig. 64.5*) and histopathologic changes in the livers of experimentally infected animals.[51] In infected animals, liver injury coincides with decreasing HEV antigens in hepatocytes and increasing anti-HEV titers.[48] Further, cytotoxic lymphocytes infiltrate the liver tissue of infected animals.[48]

Viremia in blood and fecal shedding of the virus occur up to 2 weeks prior to and up to 2–4 weeks following the onset of symptoms (*Fig. 64.5*). Prolonged fecal shedding is uncommon, suggesting that this may not be responsible for environmental reservoirs of HEV. The host immune response to HEV infection is marked by the appearance initially of anti-HEV IgM, which is followed by anti-HEV IgG (*Fig. 64.5*). While the IgM titers wane in 4–6 months following exposure, IgG persists for longer periods[52] but its protective efficacy for longer periods is in question. Unlike HAV, the highest prevalence of hepatitis E in endemic areas is in young adults (15–40 years), suggesting that following subclinical infection in childhood, protection wanes with time. Passive immunization studies in experimentally infected animals[53] as well as clinical studies with a candidate vaccine[54] show a definitive role for antibodies in protection against clinical disease.

The cellular immune responses to HEV infection are poorly characterized. One recent study suggests that natural killer (NK) cells might be involved in HEV pathogenesis, and there may be an inherent defect in T-cell activation in HEV-infected persons.[55] These observations with peripheral blood cells may also be due to the migration of immune cells to the liver following infection. Elispots were recently used to estimate B and T cell memory in individuals living in an HEV-endemic area. Even in anti-HEV IgG-negative individuals, B and T cell memory could be detected, suggesting that subclinical HEV infection is more widespread than predicted from antibody studies (S. Naik, personal communication).

The pathogenesis of hepatitis E during pregnancy is not understood. A role for endotoxin-mediated injury to hepatocytes has been proposed, and an increased T-helper type 2 response was observed in pregnant women with hepatitis E compared to nonpregnant women.[56]

DIAGNOSIS

Since an anti-HEV IgM response, viremia, and fecal shedding of HEV are associated with acute hepatitis E (*Fig. 64.5*), these markers are used for its diagnosis. Serological tests for anti-HEV antibodies utilize parts of the ORF2 and ORF3 proteins, which are either recombinant or synthetic. Two commercial tests for measuring anti-HEV IgG are available from Genelabs Diagnostics (Singapore) and Abbott Labs (Germany), and an anti-HEV IgM test is available from Genelabs Diagnostics. Whereas in an endemic area, the IgM test is of more value in ascertaining the cause of acute hepatitis, in non-endemic areas the IgG test is also used.

TREATMENT AND PROGNOSIS

No effective treatment for HEV infection is currently available. Since the disease is self-limiting, no treatment may really be necessary in most cases. It is limited to general supportive measures, as with acute hepatitis A. Patients with fulminant hepatitis need measures to control cerebral edema and consideration of liver transplantation. No data are available on the beneficial effect, if any, on liver function of termination of pregnancy in pregnant women with hepatitis E and fulminant hepatic failure. Because of coagulopathy, these patients are at particular risk of postpartum hemorrhage; hence, prophylactic steps including injection of uterine muscle-constricting drugs must be instituted immediately after delivery. Fresh frozen plasma infusions are helpful if bleeding supervenes. Isolation of infected persons is not indicated, because person-to-person transmission is uncommon.

PREVENTION AND CONTROL

Proper treatment and safe disposal of human excreta, provision of a safe drinking water supply, and improvement in personal hygiene are the mainstays of hepatitis E prevention. Sanitary food handling practices, and avoiding consumption of undercooked or uncooked meat and vegetables should be recommended. In epidemic settings, boiling and chlorination of water supplies may be useful. In non-endemic areas where zoonotic transmission is believed to be the main route, proper cooking of pig and deer meat may be useful.

Administration of immunoglobulins has not been shown to protect humans against hepatitis E, despite its neutralization ability in laboratory studies.

A 56-kDa truncated HEV ORF2 protein, when produced in insect cells infected with a recombinant baculovirus, forms highly immunogenic virus-like particles.[57] An alum-adjuvanted vaccine containing this protein has undergone safety and efficacy studies in humans, and induces protective antibodies in a dose-dependent manner. A phase II–III efficacy trial was conducted in over 2000 volunteers from the Nepalese Army who lacked detectable anti-HEV antibodies. The study subjects received either 20 µg of alum-adjuvanted recombinant HEV protein or a matched placebo, each given as three doses at 0, 1, and 6 months, and were followed up for more than 2 years.[54] The vaccine showed no adverse effects and protective efficacy of 88% or 95% after one or three doses, respectively. More data are needed on its efficacy among pregnant women and children, and in special groups such as persons with chronic liver disease, and the duration of protection. The vaccine is not yet commercially available.

Initial results of another hepatitis E vaccine, the HEV 239 vaccine, have been reported and appear encouraging.[58] A phase III trial with this vaccine is currently in progress.

The exact role of HEV vaccines remains unclear. These should be useful for travelers to HEV-endemic areas, as well as to residents of endemic areas who are at particularly high risk of severe disease following HEV infection, such as pregnant women and persons with preexisting chronic liver disease. A more widespread use in endemic regions will depend on cost considerations, the duration of protection afforded by the vaccines, and their ability to interrupt the transmission of infection.

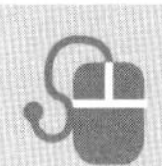

Access the complete reference list online at
http://www.expertconsult.com

Access the complete reference list online at http://www.expertconsult.com

CHAPTER 65

Viral Hepatitis C

Miriam J. Alter

INTRODUCTION

Hepatitis C virus (HCV) is a bloodborne virus whose target organ is the liver. It causes both acute and chronic hepatitis, and contributes substantially to chronic liver disease and liver cancer morbidity and mortality worldwide. Geographic differences in HCV epidemiology, current and future HCV-related disease burden, and the potential for antiviral therapy to reduce that burden reflect the relative time period during which most of the population was infected.

THE AGENT

HCV has been classified within a separate genus, *Hepacivirus*, in the family *Flaviviridae*. This classification is well supported by phylogenetic comparisons of viral sequences.[1] HCV has much in common with the flaviviruses and pestiviruses, two other major genera within the *Flaviviridae,* in terms of their replication mechanisms and life cycle. However, HCV has a number of unusual biological features that distinguish it from other flaviviruses. These include most notably the ability to establish persistent infections in most infected persons.

Like all positive-strand RNA viruses, HCV possesses an error-prone RNA replicase. However, HCV strains show extraordinary genetic diversity, even for an RNA virus. This is true both in terms of the extent of quasispecies variation within infected individuals, as well as in the genetic distances between viruses infecting different persons.[2] The extent of genetic diversity among different strains of HCV considerably exceeds that evident among different strains of human immunodeficiency virus (HIV). Among the six major recognized HCV genotypes, pair-wise differences in the nucleotide sequences are on the order of 31–33%.[3] This approximates the genetic distance between members of the classical flavivirus serogroups, such as the four dengue viruses and members of the Japanese encephalitis serogroup that represent serologically and genetically distinct viruses.[4]

The extent to which these genetic differences reflect important antigenic and serologic differences among HCV genotypes is unknown. While the genetic distance between some genotypes is large enough to suggest that there are biologically significant serotypic differences, only low-level homologous protection is evident when chimpanzees are challenged twice with the same strain of HCV.[5] There are important differences between HCV genotypes in their response to interferon-based therapies; differences among various genotypes in their capacity to establish long-term persistence or to cause liver disease are less certain.[6,7]

The distribution of HCV genotypes varies geographically.[3] Genotype 1 has a worldwide distribution, accounting for 75% of infections in the United States and the majority of infections in Europe, Japan, and many other parts of the world. In Europe there is a higher proportion of non-1 genotypes, particularly subtype 3a, than in the United States. Certain genotypes have a relatively restricted geographic distribution, such as genotypes 4 (Egypt), 5 (southern Africa), and 6 (Southeast Asia).

HCV possesses a single-stranded, positive-sense RNA genome approximately 9.6 kb in length. The RNA contains a single large open reading frame encoding a polyprotein of approximately 3000 residues, flanked by relatively short 5′ and 3′ nontranslated RNA (NTR) segments (***Fig. 65.1A***).[8] The polyprotein can be functionally divided into three segments: (1) the NH_2-terminal region, which comprises the structural proteins (core, E1, and E2); (2) a central region including two proteins (p7 and NS2) that are not required for RNA replication nor likely part of the viral particle, but probably play essential roles in viral morphogenesis and release; and (3) the COOH-terminal region that comprises the nonstructural proteins (NS3, NS4A, NS4B, NS5A, and NS5B) required for RNA replication (***Fig. 65.1A***).

As with other positive-strand RNA viruses, the genome of HCV serves as messenger RNA following its release into the cytoplasm. This is followed by cap-independent translation of the open reading frame under control of an internal ribosome entry site (IRES) located within the 5′NTR. The lengthy polyprotein is co- and post-translationally processed by both cellular and viral proteases (***Fig. 65.1B***).[8] The nonstructural proteins extending from NS3 to NS5B assemble as a macromolecular replicase complex on cytoplasmic membranes, forming a membranous web-like structure and directing the synthesis of a negative-strand RNA intermediate from which subsequent positive-stand progeny genomes are produced. Virus assembly is likely to occur in close association with these membranes, but these processes are still ill defined, as is the process of virus release from the cell.

The 5′NTR is one of the most highly conserved segments of the genome. Overlapping RNA elements within the 5′NTR are essential for both translation of the downstream polyprotein and RNA replication.[9] Because of its high degree of sequence conservation and critical role in replication/translation, the IRES has been a favored target for development of candidate antisense oligonucleotides and other small-molecule therapeutics. The nucleocapsid and envelope proteins of the N-terminal segment are major structural components of the virion. Both E1 and E2 have C-terminal transmembrane domains with endoplasmic reticulum retention activity and heavily glycosylated ectodomains.[10] A hypervariable domain near the N-terminus of E2 (HVR-1) is the most variable part of the viral polyprotein and is likely a target for neutralizing antibodies.[11] While virus in which this domain was deleted is infectious in chimpanzees, it appears to have reduced replication capacity.[12]

At least six nonstructural proteins are derived from the remainder of the polyprotein; these proteins are involved in polyprotein processing and viral RNA replication. They include two viral proteases (activities associated with NS2/NS3 and NS3/4A) and an RNA-dependent RNA polymerase (NS5B) adjacent to the 3′ end. NS3 has both helicase and protease activity. Efforts to develop effective antiviral inhibitors of HCV replication have driven extensive studies of these proteins.[8]

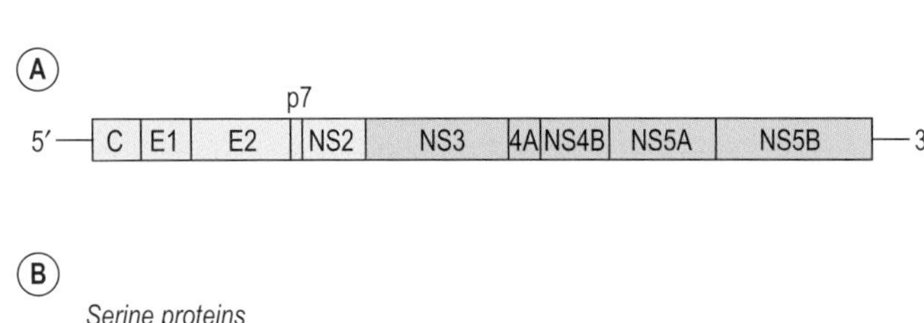

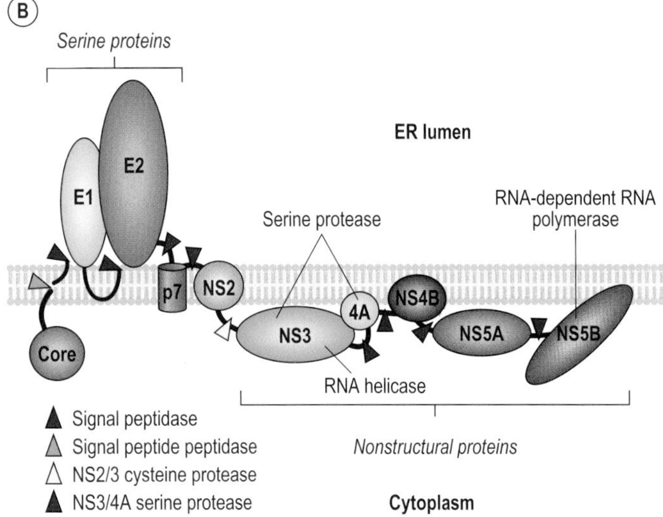

Figure 65.1 Organization of the hepatitis C virus (HCV) genome and polyprotein. (**A**) Organization of the HCV genome with nontranslated RNA segments shown as lines and the open reading frame as a box; the region encoding the nonstructural proteins required for replication is shaded. (**B**) Functional organization and processing of the viral polyprotein, showing approximate membrane topologies of the mature HCV proteins. Sites of cleavage by host cell and viral proteases are indicated by triangles. (Redrawn from Lemon SM, Walker C, Alter MJ, et al. Hepatitis C virus. In: Knipe DM, Howley PM, eds. Fields' Virology, 5th ed. Philadelphia: Lippincott Williams & Wilkins; 2007:1253.)

The development of HCV replicons, first reported in 1999, significantly enabled the study of viral RNA replication in cultured cells.[13] These autonomously replicating HCV RNAs typically contain an in-frame fusion of sequence encoding a selectable antibiotic marker (e.g., neomycin phosphotransferase) within the amino-terminal core sequence, followed downstream by a heterologous IRES from encephalomyocarditis virus, a picornavirus, to drive internal translation of the downstream HCV open reading frame. The 5′ and 3′ NTRs are derived from HCV. Inclusion of sequence encoding the nonstructural proteins from NS3 to NS5B is required for replication, but replication-competent dicistronic RNAs have also been described that encode the entire HCV polyprotein and express all of the viral proteins.[13–16] Replicons have proven invaluable for studies of HCV RNA replication as they appear faithfully to recapitulate events occurring during replication of the viral RNA *in vivo*. However, they do not generate infectious virus particles, even when they encode and express the entire viral polyprotein at high abundance.[14,15]

EPIDEMIOLOGY

HCV infection is distributed worldwide. The estimated prevalence is 2.2%, corresponding to about 130 million HCV-positive persons worldwide (***Fig. 65.2***).[17] HCV prevalences range from <0.05% in northern Europe to >2.9% in selected countries in northern Africa. HCV prevalences are not uniformly high in tropical countries.

The most efficient transmission of HCV is through large or repeated direct percutaneous exposures to blood (e.g., transfusion or transplantation from infectious donors, injecting drug use).[18] HCV is less efficiently transmitted by single small-dose percutaneous exposures (e.g., accidental needlesticks)[19] or by mucosal exposures to blood or serum-derived fluids (e.g., birth to an infected mother, sex with an infected partner).[20,21]

There is evidence that an environmentally mediated mode of transmission exists for HCV. HCV transmission by inapparent percutaneous exposures has been caused by cross-contamination from reused needles and syringes, multiple-use medication vials, infusion bags, and environmental surfaces, including injecting-drug use paraphernalia.[22,23] In addition, an experimental study demonstrated the infectivity of HCV after exposure to drying and storage in typical environmental conditions.[24]

In contrast to infection patterns of hepatitis A virus and hepatitis B virus, the prevalence of HCV is not particularly high in tropical countries,

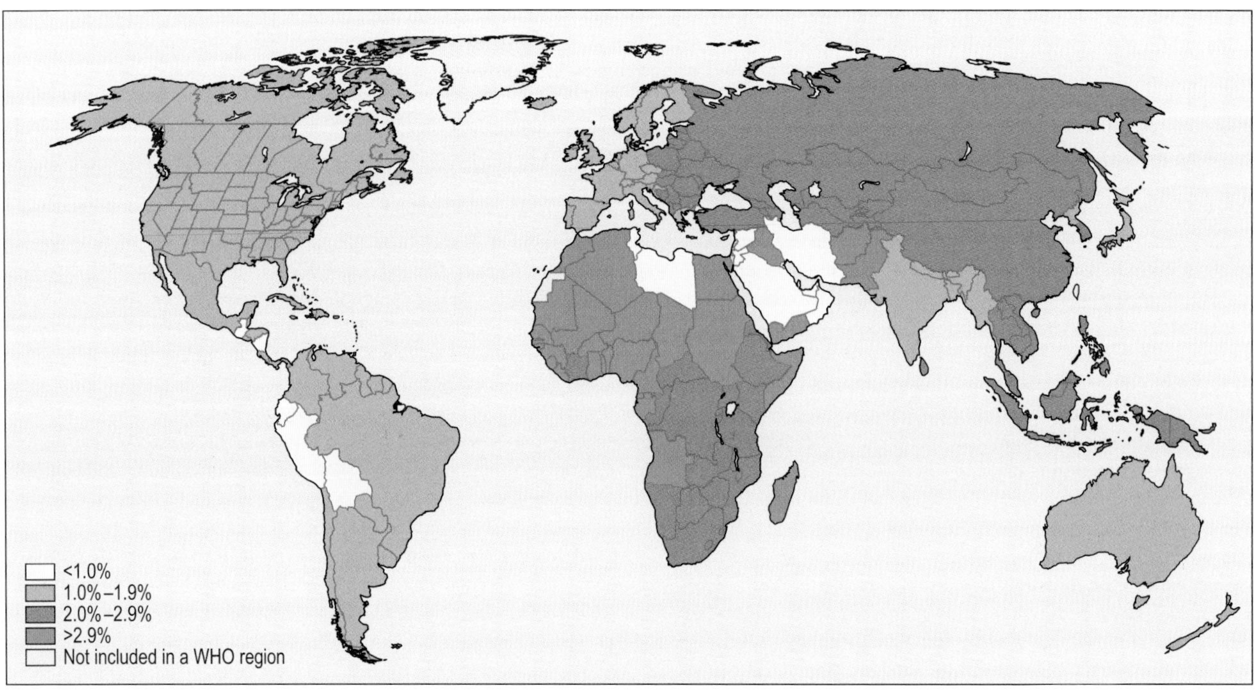

Figure 65.2 Estimated prevalence of hepatitis C virus infection by geographic region.

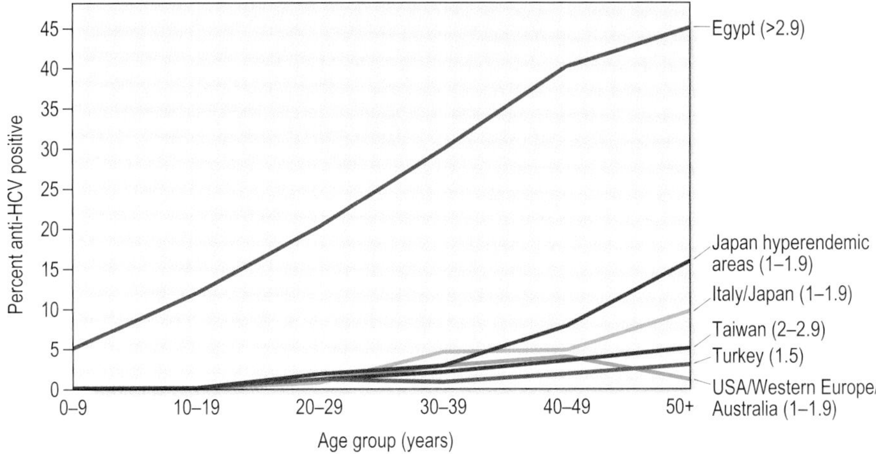

Figure 65.3 Age-specific prevalence of antibody to hepatitis C virus (HCV) infection in selected countries. Numbers in parentheses refer to region-specific prevalences (see ***Fig. 65.2***).

and similarities in average HCV prevalence by country or region do not consistently reflect similar epidemiologic patterns of infection. Instead, there appear to be three distinct patterns of age-specific HCV infection prevalence that indicate geographic differences in the time periods during which there was an increased risk for acquiring HCV infection and in the relative contribution of different modes of exposure (***Fig. 65.3***).[25] For example, vastly different countries, including the United States, Australia, Turkey, Spain, Italy, and Japan, belong to regions of the world that have a similar average overall prevalence of HCV infection (1.0–1.9%), but have different patterns of age-specific prevalence. In the United States, prevalence is highest among persons 30–49 years old, who account for two-thirds of all infections, and lower than average among persons less than 20 and greater than 50 years old.[26] This pattern indicates that most HCV transmission occurred in the last 30–50 years, and primarily among young adults, a pattern similar to that observed in Australia.[27] In the United States, Australia, and countries in western and northern Europe with similar HCV epidemiology, the greatest variations in prevalence occur among persons with different risk factors for infection; those with histories of injection drug use or repeated exposure to untreated plasma products produced from unscreened donors have the highest prevalence.

In Turkey, Spain, Italy, Japan, and China, the age-specific prevalences of HCV infection increase steadily with age (***Fig. 65.3***).[25] In these countries, persons >50 years old account for most infections, which suggests a cohort effect in which the risk for HCV infection was higher in the distant past, i.e., 40–60 years previously. In many countries with this pattern, the greatest variations in HCV prevalence occur geographically. In Italy, Japan, and China, for example, there are hyperendemic areas of the country in which older persons have an HCV prevalence 20-fold greater than the average overall and 1.5–2-fold greater than the prevalence among older persons in other areas of the country.[28–30] HCV transmission in these areas mostly occurs through iatrogenic exposures.

The highest HCV prevalence in the world occurs in Egypt, where prevalence increases steadily with age, and high rates of infection are observed among persons in all age groups (***Fig. 65.3***).[31,32] This pattern indicates an increased risk in the distant past followed by an ongoing high risk for acquiring HCV infection, although there are regional differences in average overall prevalence.

Determining the incidence of HCV infection (i.e., the rate of newly acquired infections) is difficult because most acute infections are asymptomatic, available assays do not distinguish acute from chronic or resolved infection, and most countries do not systematically collect data on cases of acute disease. Even in countries with well-established surveillance systems, acute disease-reporting systems underestimate the incidence of HCV infection. For several countries, mathematical models have been used to infer trends in incidence, which rely on the assumption that current age-specific prevalence reflects the cumulative risk of acquiring infection.

In the United States, modeling showed a large increase in the incidence of newly acquired HCV infections from the late 1960s to the early 1980s. The estimated annual incidence was low (18 per 100 000) before 1965, increased steadily through 1980, and remained high (130 per 100 000) through 1989, corresponding to an average of 240 000 infections per year in the 1980s.[33] Since 1989, the incidence of HCV infection has declined by more than 80% based on reported cases of disease, consistent with the finding that the national seroprevalence of infection remained unchanged between 1988 and 2002.[26] The rate of new HCV infections also declined in Italy and France, and, like in the United States, most newly acquired infections are in young adults (30–35 years old).[34–36] In Australia, however, there has been a steady increase in new HCV infections.[27]

During the past decade, several countries have measured HCV infection incidence by determining the rate of seroconversions in HCV-negative cohorts followed over time. Cohort studies conducted in hyperendemic areas in Taiwan and Japan found incidence rates of HCV infection of 110/10 000 and 28–36/10 000 persons, respectively.[29,37,38] The mean age of persons with newly acquired HCV infection was 50 years in the Taiwan cohort and 40 and 60 years, respectively, in the two Japan cohorts, suggesting that older persons remain at higher risk for HCV even in recent times. Cohort studies in Egypt found incidence rates of 0.8/1000 person-years in an area of upper Egypt, where the background prevalence was 9%, and 6.8/1000 in the Nile delta, where the background prevalence was 24%.[39] Sixty-seven percent of the incident infections were in persons <20 years old, and having an anti-HCV-positive family member was the strongest predictor of infection. In previous prevalence studies of HCV in Egypt, the strongest predictor for past infection was a history of receiving injectable therapy (with reused glass syringes) for schistosomiasis.[32]

Reuse of glass syringes during the early campaign to treat schistosomiasis in Egypt appeared to be responsible for the largest outbreak of iatrogenic transmission of a bloodborne pathogen ever recorded.[32] In fact, the ongoing risk for HCV infection in most resource-poor countries has been attributed to iatrogenic exposures from traditional and conventional medical procedures. An estimated 2 million HCV infections are acquired annually from contaminated health care injections.[40] Unsafe injections performed by both professionals and nonprofessionals may account for up to 40% of all HCV infections worldwide. In many developing countries, supplies of sterile syringes may be inadequate or nonexistent, nonprofessionals often administer injections outside the medical setting, and injections are often given to deliver medications that could otherwise be delivered by the oral route.[41]

Occupational transmission of HCV infection is largely confined to health care workers who have sustained contaminated needlestick injuries; average incidence of anti-HCV seroconversion from an HCV-positive source is 1.8%; transmission has been associated with hollow-bore needles and deep injuries.[42] Transmission rarely occurs from mucous membrane or nonintact skin exposures to blood,[43] and no transmission to health care workers has been documented from intact skin exposures to blood. Furthermore, the prevalence of HCV infection among health care workers, including orthopedic, general, and oral surgeons, is no greater than adults in the general population, averaging 1–2%, and is 10 times lower than that for HBV infection. Even more rarely, HCV-infected health care workers have transmitted the infection to patients, and the risk was extremely low – averaging about 0.5%, even for those episodes involving surgeons.[44]

The rate of perinatal transmission of HCV is 4–7% per pregnancy and occurs only when HCV RNA is detectable in maternal serum at delivery.[20] Transmission may be related to higher levels (above 10^6 copies/mL), although data on the effect of virus concentration have been inconsistent. Prolonged labor after membrane rupture and internal fetal monitoring have been associated with perinatal infection.[20,45] There has been no association with vaginal delivery, cesarean section or breast-feeding. Coinfection with HIV increases the rate of transmission four- to fivefold.[46]

The extent to which HCV is transmitted by sexual activity and under what circumstances is one of the most controversial aspects of the epidemiology of hepatitis C.[21] The strongest evidence for heterosexual activity as a risk factor for HCV infection came from case-control studies of persons with acute non-A, non-B hepatitis (now known as hepatitis C) in the United States during the 1970s and 1980s, which identified sex with an infected partner or with multiple partners as independently associated with acquiring disease. Since then, 15–20% of cases of acute hepatitis C in the United States have reported no other risk factor except one of these sexual exposures.[18] In contrast, no association was found with male homosexual activity, and HCV prevalence is low among men who have sex with men (MSM) and heterosexual persons in long-term monogamous relationships with a partner with chronic HCV.[18,21] One possible explanation for these apparent inconsistencies is that HCV is more likely to be transmitted by sexual intercourse when the infected partner is in the early phase of acute infection; virus concentration is high and there is no antibody to complex with antigen. Recent reports of clusters of acute HCV infections among HIV-positive MSM may support this hypothesis.[47,48]

Because of the wide variety of human activities that involve the potential for percutaneous exposure to blood or blood-derived body fluids, there are numerous other biologically plausible modes of transmission besides those with clearly demonstrated epidemiologic associations with infection. These include cosmetic procedures (tattooing, body-piercing), intranasal drug use, and religious or cultural practices such as ritual scarification, circumcision, acupuncture, and cupping. In most regions of the world, there are insufficient data to determine whether these risk factors make any measurable contribution to overall HCV transmission. In those countries where adequate studies have been done, none of these activities have been consistently associated with HCV transmission (***Fig. 65.4***).[49]

Thus, most of the HCV-related disease burden in developed countries has resulted from injection drug use, receipt of transfusions before donor screening, and high-risk sexual activity. In contrast, most of the disease burden in developing countries is related to receipt of unsafe therapeutic injections and transfused blood.

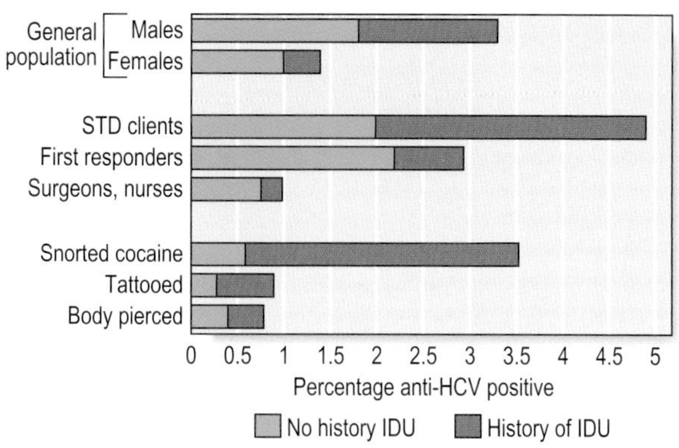

Figure 65.4 Prevalence of antibody to hepatitis C virus infection (anti-HCV) in selected groups of adults by history of injection drug use (IDU), United States. STD, sexually transmitted disease.

THE DISEASE

Persons with acute HCV infection typically are either asymptomatic or have a mild clinical illness: 60–70% have no discernible symptoms; 20–30% have jaundice; and 10–20% have nonspecific symptoms (e.g., anorexia, malaise, or abdominal pain).[18,50] Clinical illness in patients with acute hepatitis C who seek medical care is similar to that of other types of viral hepatitis, and serologic testing is necessary to determine the etiology of hepatitis in an individual patient. Average time period from exposure to symptom onset is 6–7 weeks.

The course of acute hepatitis C is variable, although elevations in serum alanine transaminase (ALT) levels, often in a fluctuating pattern, are its most characteristic feature. Normalization of ALT levels might occur and suggests full recovery, but this is frequently followed by ALT elevations that indicate progression to chronic disease. Fulminant hepatic failure following acute hepatitis C is rare.

After acute infection, 15–25% of persons appear to resolve their infection without sequelae as defined by sustained absence of HCV RNA in serum and normalization of ALT levels.[50] Chronic HCV infection develops in most persons (55–85%), with persistent or fluctuating ALT elevations indicating active liver disease in 60–70% of chronically infected persons. No clinical or epidemiologic features among patients with acute infection have been found to be predictive of either persistent infection or chronic liver disease. Moreover, various ALT patterns have been observed in these patients during follow-up, and patients might have prolonged periods (≥12 months) of normal ALT activity even though they have histologically confirmed chronic hepatitis. Thus, a single ALT determination cannot be used to exclude ongoing hepatic injury, and long-term follow-up of patients with HCV infection is required to determine their clinical outcome or prognosis.[51]

The course of chronic liver disease is usually insidious, progressing at a slow rate without symptoms or physical signs in the majority of patients during two or more decades after infection. Frequently, chronic hepatitis C is not recognized until asymptomatic persons are identified as HCV-positive during blood donor screening, or elevated ALT levels are detected during routine examinations. Natural history studies indicate that 55–85% of individuals who develop acute hepatitis C will remain HCV-infected and 5–20% will develop cirrhosis.[50] Lower rates of chronic infection and progression to cirrhosis have been reported from prospective studies of persons infected at age 30 years or younger than among persons infected when they are older. Retrospective studies of patients referred to tertiary care facilities document higher rates of cirrhosis, 20–25%, but this figure may be inflated by referral bias.

Progression to cirrhosis may be accelerated in persons who are of older age, obese, immunosuppressed (e.g., HIV coinfected), and consume more than 50 g of alcohol per day, although the precise quantity of alcohol associated with fibrosis progression is unknown.[50,52] Persons with HCV-related cirrhosis are at risk for the development of hepatic decompensation (30% over 10 years) as well as hepatocellular carcinoma (1–3% per year). Infection with HCV can also cause extrahepatic diseases, including mixed cryoglobulinemia, types II and III.

Because chronic liver disease often develops many years after infection, the past incidence is a major determinant of the future burden of HCV-associated complications.[53] In the United States and other countries where the emergence of HCV infection is a more recent event, the full magnitude of the burden of HCV-related chronic liver disease has yet to be realized as the duration of infection among most infected persons has not reached the point at which complications from chronic liver disease typically occur.[33,36] In countries where the emergence of HCV infection occurred in the distant past (such as Japan and Italy), the burden of HCV-related chronic disease already might have reached its highest magnitude,[54] but changes in disease transmission patterns that result in younger persons acquiring infection could result in future increases in chronic disease as this cohort ages. In Egypt, where there has been an ongoing high risk for decades, the high magnitude of the current burden of HCV-related chronic disease is likely to be sustained.

PATHOGENESIS AND IMMUNITY

Recent depletion experiments in chimpanzees have defined important roles for both $CD4^+$ and $CD8^+$ T lymphocytes in protection against HCV infection but have not resolved long-standing questions concerning the mechanisms exploited by the virus in establishing persistent infections. HCV-specific $CD4^+$ T cells are detected in both the liver and peripheral blood of HCV-infected patients.[55] The $CD4^+$ T-cell response to HCV is sustained and vigorous in patients with acute, self-limited HCV infection, and is weak and delayed in patients who become chronically infected.[56] The potential protective role of HCV-specific CD4 T cells is suggested by studies showing accelerated liver disease progression in patients coinfected with HIV, who have generalized impairment in $CD4^+$T cells. $CD4^+$ T-cell help is required for the development of an effective $CD8^+$ response, and it has been suggested that interferon-α (IFN-α) secreting $CD8^+$ T cells play an important role in clearance of the virus from liver.[57] However, the $CD8^+$T-cell response in HCV infection demonstrates several puzzling features. HCV-specific $CD8^+$T cells are present and activated within the liver in patients with chronic hepatitis C, but they are incapable of eliminating the infection. Some patients appear to have a "stunned" phenotype, and do not secrete IFN-α in response to antigen stimulation. The HCV-specific $CD8^+$ T-cell response is remarkably variable, and more work is needed to characterize these responses in chronic HCV infection.

It appears that the antibody response, at least as measured by currently available assays, is of limited importance in clearing HCV.[58] The quasi-species nature of the virus confers a survival advantage, allowing rapid selection of mutants that are capable of escaping antibody-mediated neutralization. Finally, recent evidence suggests that HCV is capable of disrupting important innate immune responses that not only have direct intracellular antiviral effects but also play a role in shaping subsequent adaptive T-cell immunity.[59] The NS3/4A protease acts to disrupt the signaling pathways that lead to induction of endogenous interferon synthesis in response to virus infection by blocking the virus-induced activation of IFN-regulatory factor 3. Moreover, the NS5A protein appears to block one of the IFN-mediated effector mechanisms by binding to protein kinase R (PKR) near its catalytic site, and preventing the dsRNA-activated PKR-mediated shutdown of viral and cellular protein translation. The disruption of innate immune responses to the infection may thus be very important in determining persistence of the infection, while also perhaps contributing to resistance to interferon therapy.

DIAGNOSIS

The diagnosis of acute or chronic HCV infection generally requires testing of serum for both antibody to HCV (anti-HCV) using standard immunoassays and for HCV RNA by qualitative or quantitative nucleic acid tests.[60,61] The differentiation of acute from chronic HCV infection depends on the clinical presentation: namely the presence of symptoms or jaundice, and whether or not there was a prior history of ALT elevation and its duration.[51] After acute exposure, HCV RNA is usually detected in serum before antibody; HCV RNA can be identified as early as 2 weeks following exposure whereas anti-HCV is generally not detectable before 8–12 weeks. These two markers of HCV infection may be present in varying permutations, requiring careful analysis for interpretation (*Table 65.1*).

Table 65.1 Interpretation of Test Results for Diagnosis of Hepatitis C Virus (HCV) Infection

Anti-HCV	HCV RNA	Interpretations
Negative	Not done or negative	Absence of HCV infection
Positive	Positive	Acute or chronic HCV depending on the clinical context
Positive	Negative	Resolution of HCV; acute or chronic HCV infection during period of low-level viremia
Negative	Positive	Early acute HCV infection; chronic HCV in setting of immunosuppressed state; false-positive HCV RNA test

Two patterns are particularly common. One is the identification of both anti-HCV and HCV RNA in a person with recent elevation of the ALT value. This scenario is consistent with (1) acute HCV infection when there is a recent known risk exposure; (2) exacerbation of chronic HCV infection; or (3) an acute hepatitis of another etiology in a patient with chronic HCV infection. The other pattern is the detection of anti-HCV and a negative test result for HCV RNA. This may represent acute or chronic HCV infection during a period of transient clearance of HCV RNA, a false-negative HCV RNA result, or recovery from HCV infection; in asymptomatic persons at low risk of infection, this pattern is most likely a false positive anti-HCV result. Re-testing for anti-HCV and HCV RNA 4–6 months later is recommended to confirm the diagnosis.

TREATMENT AND PROGNOSIS

Identifying individuals at risk for developing progressive disease is difficult and presently requires a liver biopsy to assess the degree of fibrosis, using a validated staging system such as the Ishak, IASL, Metavir or Batts-Ludwig staging systems.[51] Persons with no or minimal fibrosis (Ishak stage 0–2; Metavir, IASL, and Batts-Ludwig stage 0–1) have a low risk for liver-related complications and liver-related death (over the next 10–20 years); in contrast, the presence of bridging fibrosis (e.g., Metavir stage 3) is an important predictor of future progression to cirrhosis.

Liver biopsy was previously regarded as routine for defining the fibrosis stage in persons being considered for antiviral therapy, especially those with genotype 1 infection. Because of the high cost of therapy and relatively low sustained virological response (SVR) rates, treatment might be delayed in those with minimal to moderate disease. However, liver biopsy is not mandatory for deciding on treatment, and efforts are underway to seek alternative means of establishing information on the extent of fibrosis by focusing on noninvasive blood marker panels. These markers are useful for establishing the two ends of the fibrosis spectrum (minimal fibrosis and cirrhosis) but are less helpful in assessing the mid-ranges of fibrosis or for tracking fibrosis progression.[62] A liver biopsy may be unnecessary in persons with genotypes 2 and 3 HCV infection, since more than 80% of them achieve a SVR to standard-of-care treatment. Because of limited data on SVR, there is uncertainty as to whether there is need for a liver biopsy in persons infected with genotypes 4 through 6.

The currently recommended therapy of chronic hepatitis C is the combination of a pegylated IFN-α and ribavirin.[51] There are multiple manufacturers of pegylated IFNs among which the dosing recommendations differ. For some, the dose is determined based on patient weight; for others, there is a fixed dose for all patients. For ribavirin, the dose is based on patient weight, although the specific dosages depend on which pegylated IFN is being given concomitantly. Therefore, the package labeling for each drug should be carefully reviewed before therapy is initiated. Patients with genotypes 1 or 4 infection should be treated for 48 weeks, whereas patients with genotypes 2 and 3 can be treated for 24 weeks.[63] There are insufficient data to make specific recommendations regarding dosage or duration for patients with genotypes 5 and 6.

To date, the two major predictors of a SVR among all populations studied are the viral genotype and pretreatment viral titer.[64–66] SVR rates were higher in patients infected with genotype non-1 infection (mostly genotypes 2 and 3) and in those with a viral titer of fewer than 600 000 IU/mL. On average, SVR rates have been about 50% in genotype 1 patients treated with the currently recommended regimen and 85–90% in genotype 2 and 3 patients.

There is consistent evidence that treatment of persons with acute hepatitis C reduces their risk for developing chronic infection. Data from multiple studies that evaluated IFN treatment of patients with acute hepatitis C demonstrated an average SVR of >80%.[67] When combined with the percentage who resolved spontaneously, <10% of these patients developed chronic infection. Although the optimal regimen has not been established, experts believe it is reasonable to consider treating patients with acute HCV infection with IFN-based monotherapy, and treatment can be delayed for 8–12 weeks after acute onset of hepatitis to allow for spontaneous resolution. Because of rapidly emerging data in this field, physicians considering treating patients with acute or chronic hepatitis C should consult the most recent standards of practice in their countries.

PREVENTION AND CONTROL

There is a large global reservoir of HCV-infected individuals who can serve as a source of transmission to others and are at risk for HCV-related chronic diseases. There is no vaccine to prevent hepatitis C, and vaccine development is impeded by the extensive heterogeneity of the virus and its rapid rate of mutation. To prevent new infections, public health programs should focus on ensuring a safe blood supply, implementing appropriate infection control practices, and preventing initiation of high-risk drug and sexual behaviors.

In resource-poor countries where donor screening and testing policies for HCV have not been implemented, transfusions continue to be a major source for HCV infection, and improving the safety of the blood supply should be the highest priority. Programs should also be initiated to reduce the extent to which HCV is transmitted by unsafe injection practices and reuse of contaminated equipment. Such programs should include efforts to modify injection practices of professionals and nonprofessionals, including educating practitioners of conventional and folk medicine, rituals, and cosmetic procedures about the risk for transmission of bloodborne pathogens from nonsterile instruments or objects used in these procedures. Assistance for implementing such programs is available from the World Health Organization Safe Injection Global Network (SIGN), a coalition of governments, international health agencies, corporations, and individuals that advocate for safer injection practices worldwide.[68]

Those countries with more developed economic, medical, and public health infrastructures also should develop programs to identify, counsel, and provide medical management for persons already infected. Such secondary prevention programs are aimed at reducing HCV-related morbidity and mortality through provision of antiviral therapy. However, the price of current regimens is high – US$30 000 for a typical 48-week course of therapy for HCV genotype 1 infection. Given the exponential rise in HCV-related liver disease predicted during the next 10–20 years, there is obvious concern as to whether treatment regimens can be made affordable to most HCV-infected people and prevent the steep rise in HCV-related morbidity and corresponding health care expenditures.[68]

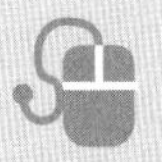

Access the complete reference list online at
http://www.expertconsult.com

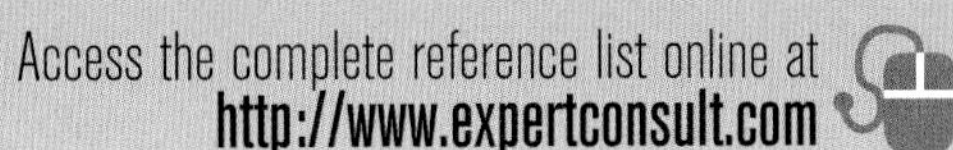
Access the complete reference list online at
http://www.expertconsult.com

CHAPTER 66

Hepatitis B and Deltavirus Infections

Ding-Shinn Chen • Pei-Jer Chen

HEPATITIS B

INTRODUCTION

Hepatitis B virus (HBV) infection is one of the most common and important human viral infections. The infection can cause acute and chronic liver disease, ranging from fulminant hepatitis to cirrhosis and eventually hepatocellular carcinoma (HCC).[1,2] Worldwide, as many as 360 million people are chronically infected with HBV, and around 1 million deaths annually are attributed to this infection. Hence, control of HBV infection is extremely important. Strategies to combat HBV infection comprise interrupting transmission, treating chronically infected patients, as well as providing susceptible individuals with immunoprophylaxis.[3]

THE AGENT

HBV is a double-stranded DNA virus of 3200 base pairs and is the prototype virus of the *Hepadnaviridae* family. The intact virions are 42 nm in diameter (Dane particle). In the serum, intact virions are found in association with more abundant 20-nm, DNA-free, spherical and tubular particles containing the hepatitis B surface antigen (HBsAg) and host-derived lipids.[4]

The viral genome encodes four overlapping open reading frames (ORFs): S, C, P, and X.[4] The S ORF encodes the viral surface envelope proteins, HBsAg, which can be divided into the pre-S1, pre-S2, and S regions. The C (core) gene has the precore and core regions. The C ORF encodes either the viral nucleocapsid hepatitis B core antigen (HBcAg) or hepatitis B e antigen (HBeAg), depending on whether translation is initiated from the core or precore region, respectively. The core protein can self-assemble into a capsid-like structure. The precore ORF codes for a signal peptide that directs the translation product to the endoplasmic reticulum, where the protein is further processed to the secreted HBeAg. The function of HBeAg remains largely undefined, although it has been implicated as an immune tolerogen facilitating persistent HBV infection. The polymerase is encoded by the P ORF and is functionally divided into three domains: (1) the terminal protein domain, which is involved in encapsidation and initiation of minus-strand synthesis; (2) the reverse transcriptase (RT) domain, which catalyzes genome synthesis; and (3) the ribonuclease H domain, which degrades pregenomic RNA and facilitates replication. The HBV X ORF encodes a 16.5-kDa protein (HBxAg), which is required for HBV transcription, but also has multiple cellular functions, including signal transduction, transcriptional activation, and inhibition of protein degradation. HBxAg may contribute to the oncogenic potential of HBV.

EPIDEMIOLOGY AND MOLECULAR EPIDEMIOLOGY

HBV is transmitted via parenteral or percutaneous exposure to infected blood or other body fluids. Risk factors for infection include sexual promiscuity, sharing of syringes among injection drug users, tattooing, working or residing in a health care setting, and long-term household or intimate nonsexual contact with an HBsAg-positive individual.[1,2,5] However, in endemic areas, the perinatal exposure of newborns or toddlers to mother or family members with high HBV DNA becomes the key transmission route.

The prevalence of chronic HBV infection is about 5% worldwide, but differs geographically (***Fig. 66.1***).[5,6] The prevalence is low (0.1–2.0%) in the United States, western Europe and Japan, intermediate (2.0–8.0%) in Mediterranean countries, and high (8.0–20.0%) in Southeast Asia and sub-Saharan regions.

HBV genome evolves and the estimated rate of nucleotide substitution is around $1.4–3.2 \times 10^{-5}$/sites per year. Following human migrations, eight genotypes of HBV have been generated, by sequence divergence >8% in the entire HBV genome, and designated by capital letters from A to H in the order of documentation. Worldwide, HBV genotypes have a distinct geographic distribution.[7] Current evidence suggests that HBV genotype correlates with the hepatitis B disease severity in different areas, and may be associated with the response to antiviral therapy (***Table 66.1***).[7,8]

In a significant proportion of patients with chronic hepatitis B (CHB), the wild-type HBV evolves into new variants under host selection. There are two major HBV variants: the precore stop codon and basal core promoter variant. To follow their evolution in patients, the proportion of precore and basal core promoter variants in HBV carriers was investigated in different age cohorts. In young children, almost 95% of CHB patients harbor wild-type HBV. In adolescents to young adults, the proportion with wild-type HBV decreases to 30–60%, while the remaining 40–70% of CHB patients contain either or both variants. In the 60-year-old cohorts, only about 15% of CHB patients maintain wild-type HBV, but the majority of CHB patients harbor variants. It is clear that genetic drift of HBV occurs in a given CHB population (***Fig. 66.2***).

Precore and basal core promoter mutation may decrease or abolish the production of HBeAg. The percentage of patients with HBeAg-negative CHB is 80–90% in Mediterranean areas, 30–50% in Southeast Asia, and less than 10% in the United States and northwestern Europe. HBV precore variant occurs most frequently in genotype D, followed by genotypes C and B, and is seen least frequently in genotype A. Overall, the precore variant was detected in a median of 60% (range 0–100%) of HBeAg-negative patients, 92% in the Mediterranean, 50% in Asia Pacific, and 24% in the United States and northern Europe.[9] There are few data on the prevalence of basal core promoter variants outside Asia, where its median prevalence among HBeAg-negative patients is 77%.

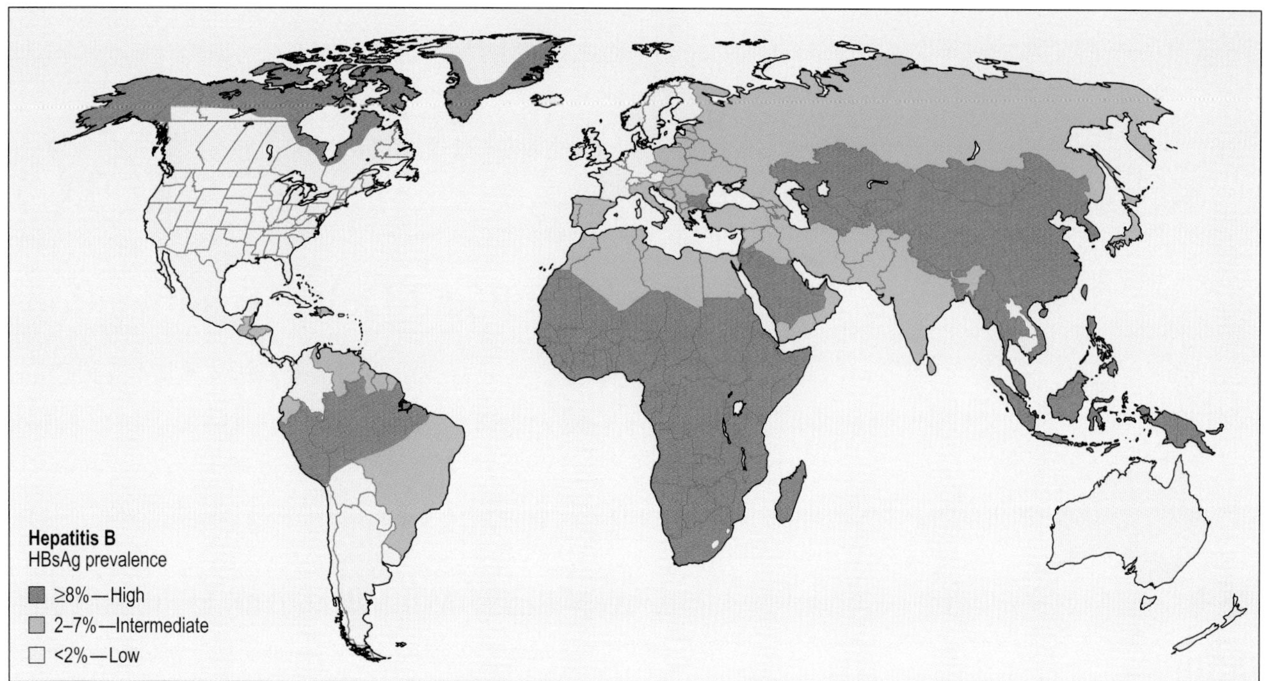

Figure 66.1 Hepatitis B surface antigen (HBsAg) prevalence.

Table 66.1 Changing Epidemiology of Hepatitis B Surface Antigen (HBsAg) Carriage after Hepatitis B Immunization

	HBsAg Carriage Rate (%)		
Country	Before Immunization	After Immunization	Protection Efficacy (%)
China (rural)	14.6	1.4	90.4
China (Shanghai)	11	0.63	94.3
Egypt (Alexandria)	2.2	0.8	63.6
Gambia	12	0.9	92.5
Indonesia (Lombok)	6.2	1.4	61.1
Italy (Afragola)	13.4	0.9	93.3
Japan (Iwate)	0.9	0.03	96.7
Japan (Shizuoka)	0.3	0.03	90.0
Korea	7.5	0.38	94.9
Malaysia	2.5	0.4	84.0
Micronesia	12	2.9	75.8
Polynesia	6.5	0.7	89.2
Saipan	9	0.5	94.4
Samoa	7	0.5	92.9
Saudi Arabia	6.7	0.3	95.5
Senegal	19	2	89.5
Singapore	4.1	0	100
South Africa	12.8	3.0	76.6
Taiwan (Taipei)	10	0.7	93.0
Taiwan (Taichung)	14	1.2	91.4
Taiwan (Hualin)	9.3	1.9	79.6
Thailand	4.3	0.7	83.7
Turkey	1.9	0	100
United States (Alaska)	16	0	100

THE DISEASE

Acute HBV Infection

The spectrum of acute HBV infection ranges from asymptomatic infection to self-limited hepatitis and fulminant hepatitis. Symptomatic hepatitis is rare in neonates (less than 1% of infections) and occurs in about 10% of infected children 1–5 years old. A third of acute infections in adults are symptomatic, and fulminant hepatitis occurs in less than 1% of cases, with a mortality rate of about 70%.[5]

Resolution of HBV infection with HBsAg seroclearance occurs in more than 95% of adult patients. However, small amounts of HBV DNA can still be detected by polymerase chain reaction (PCR) in serum, peripheral mononuclear cells, or liver biopsy tissue years after serological recovery, indicating a state of occult infection. The clinical significance of occult HBV infection is not clarified yet.[10]

Chronic Hepatitis B

The risk of chronicity correlates closely with the patient's age. Infection persists in about 90% of infants infected immediately at birth, 20–30% of children infected between the ages of 1 and 5 years, 6% of infection in children aged 5–15 years, and only 1–5% of patients infected as adults.[5]

The clinical outcomes of chronic HBV infection are determined by the interplay between virus replication and host immune response. The natural course of the majority of chronic HBV infections acquired perinatally or during infancy consists of three distinct phases: (1) immune tolerance phase; (2) immune clearance phase; and (3) inactive hepatitis B phase.[1] HBV reactivation can occur in some patients with inactive disease and again trigger immune-mediated liver injury. Such patients, therefore, enter a variant phase of immune clearance. Adult-acquired chronic infection has a similar clinical course, except that there is no obvious immune tolerance phase.

Patients in the immune tolerance phase are usually young, asymptomatic, HBeAg seropositive, and have high viral loads, but with normal

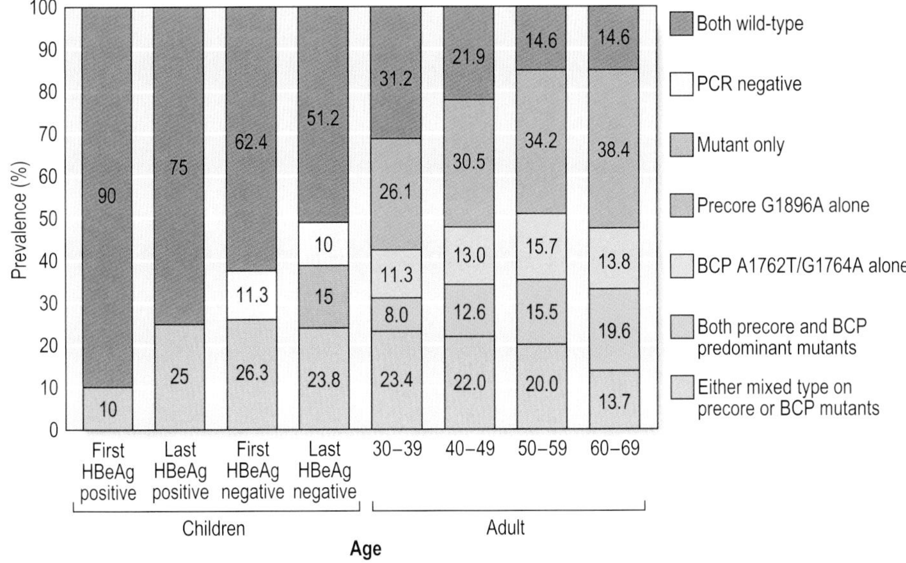

Figure 66.2 Prevalence of hepatitis B virus precore G1896A and basal core promoter A1762T/G1764A mutants by age. PCR, polymerase chain reaction; HBsAg, hepatitis B surface antigen; BCP, basal core promoter.

serum alanine aminotransferase (ALT) levels and nearly normal liver histology. There is usually no or only minimal disease progression. The immune tolerance phase usually lasts between 10 and 30 years, with a low rate of spontaneous HBeAg seroclearance.[11]

During the immune clearance phase, hepatitis activity and intermittent flares (serum ALT level increases to over five times the upper limit of normal) are common.[5] The hepatitis flares are the result of the resurgence of host immunity against HBV; hence the flares can be followed by reduced HBV replication and an HBeAg seroconversion to anti-HBe. However, sometimes severe hepatitis flares can be complicated by hepatic decompensation and facilitate the development of cirrhosis. The estimated yearly rate of spontaneous HBeAg seroconversion is 2–15%.[12] HBeAg seroconversion is usually followed by clinical remission (inactive state) with an excellent outcome. In some cases, even HBsAg can be cleared. A longitudinal study in 1965 Taiwanese patients showed that HBsAg seroclearance occurred at a rate of 1.2% per year, and the rate rose to 1.8% per year in individuals over age 50.[13]

Some CHB patients suffer from repeated hepatitis flares without HBe seroconversion. Even after HBeAg seroconversion, 10% of patients have HBeAg-negative hepatitis. These patients may progress into end-stage liver disease, namely cirrhosis or HCC.

A large population-based study of mostly (85%) HBeAg-negative, HBsAg-positive people older than 30 years demonstrated that the risk of cirrhosis, HCC, and mortality increases proportionally with increasing HBV DNA concentrations, starting with at least 10 000 copies/mL. These findings suggest that HBV replication with subsequent immune-mediated liver injury is the main driver of disease progression.[14–16]

At least a third of patients with cirrhosis have HBV DNA in their blood at presentation, and disease progression can continue even after the development of cirrhosis.[5] The 5-year probability of hepatic decompensation in patients with established cirrhosis is 15–20%, and is fourfold higher in patients with active viral replication than in patients without. The estimated 5-year survival rate of patients with compensated cirrhosis is 80–85% and 30–50% in patients with decompensated cirrhosis. The yearly rate of HCC occurrence is 3–6%. Viral and environmental factors, gender, and family history contribute to hepatocarcinogenesis.[14–19]

PATHOGENESIS AND IMMUNITY

The mechanisms of viral clearance and persistence are incompletely understood. During acute, self-limited HBV infection, innate immunity is activated and may represent the early, noncytolytic, cytokine-mediated viral reduction phase.[20] This is followed by vigorous adaptive immune responses, especially the CD4 T-cell response directed against multiple epitopes within HBcAg, HBeAg, and HBsAg.[21] After HBV infection of the hepatocyte, HBcAg and other viral peptides are presented on the cell surface in association with human leukocyte antigen (HLA) class I protein. This HLA class I–HBcAg complex is recognized by specific cytotoxic CD8 T lymphocytes, which trigger hepatocyte death. Under most circumstances, HBV and its proteins are not directly cytopathic to the hepatocytes. Liver injury in acute hepatitis B is thought to be mediated by cytotoxic T lymphocytes, which attack HBV-infected hepatocytes.

Immunopathogenesis of chronic persistence of HBV remains unclear. The development of HBV tolerance in young children is postulated to be secondary to transplacental exposure of secreted HBV proteins (e.g., HBeAg). The causes of the inability of the infected host to clear HBV include weak and oligoclonal HBV-specific CD4 and CD8 T cells, which are thought to result from T-cell exhaustion, high antigenic load, and viral escape.[21] Recent studies revealed that factors such as regulatory T cells, immunosuppressive cytokines, and inhibitory receptors also contribute to the impairment of virus-specific T-cell responses in chronic infection. Futile but repeated cycles of immunity against infected hepatocytes eventually lead to end-stage liver damage without clearing the HBV.

DIAGNOSIS

The clinical course of acute or chronic HBV infection is indistinguishable from other forms of viral hepatitis, and the diagnosis usually relies on serologic or virological markers. Chronologically, HBsAg is detectable in serum prior to the increase in aminotransferases or the development of symptoms. It remains detectable for 4–6 months following its appearance. Persistence of HBsAg beyond 6 months defines CHB. As HBsAg levels decline, anti-HBs appears in serum. The presence of anti-HBs indicates recovery and immunity after acute infection. It is also the marker of a successful vaccination against HBV.[22]

HBcAg is a particulate antigen that is detectable in liver tissue in patients with acute or chronic hepatitis B but is not found in serum. When detected in liver tissue, HBcAg is an indicator of active viral replication in CHB. HBeAg is soluble and becomes detectable in serum when HBsAg appears, and its presence also correlates with active viral replication as well as a high degree of infectivity. HBeAg disappears from serum several weeks before HBsAg does in acute, self-limited infection, and it is not detectable in serum without HBsAg. In contrast, HBeAg may remain detectable in chronically infected individuals from months to years.[22]

Anti-HBc appears at the onset of symptoms or aminotransferase elevations in acute hepatitis B and persists for life. Immunoglobulin M (IgM) anti-HBc is detected at the beginning of acute hepatitis B and persists for 3–12 months. The presence of IgM anti-HBc in patients with acute hepatitis suggests acute hepatitis B. Detection of IgG anti-HBc only suggests previous exposure to HBV. HBV vaccine recipients do not develop anti-HBc, so the presence of this antibody helps in the differentiation between successful vaccination and HBV infection. In cases of severe CHB flares, low-titer IgM anti-HBc levels may appear, but only to the extent barely detectable by conventional immunoassay.[22]

Antibody to HBeAg (anti-HBe) is detectable as HBeAg disappears from the serum. Its presence during early acute infection is a reliable predictor of spontaneous resolution of acute infection. In CHB, the loss of HBeAg and acquisition of anti-HBe are associated with biochemical and histologic improvement.

HBV DNA is detectable in serum during acute and chronic HBV infections. Clearance of HBV DNA from the serum indicates resolution of active viral replication.

Liver biopsy plays a central role in treatment algorithms in patients with CHB and remains the gold standard for evaluating hepatic pathology.[1] Liver biopsies can also identify additional pathology that may contribute to liver disease, such as steatohepatitis, iron overload, autoimmune hepatitis, and drug-induced injury.

The hepatic lesions in acute viral hepatitis are characterized by hepatocyte necrosis in conjunction with acute and chronic inflammatory cellular infiltrates. The histologic spectrum of CHB is wide. Piecemeal necrosis is defined as the appearance of destroyed hepatocytes and lymphocytic infiltration at the interface between the limiting plate of periportal hepatocyte, parenchymal cells and portal tracts (interface hepatitis). Immunostaining for HBsAg and HBcAg is widely used and can help determine the phase of infection.

In addition to traditional serologic, virologic, and histologic examinations, there are several noninvasive techniques such as serum panels and fibroscan under active investigation for evaluating the grade of inflammation and the stage of fibrosis in the liver compartment. The sensitivity and specificity of these new techniques for these purposes are around 60–90%.[23]

TREATMENT AND PROGNOSIS

Acute hepatitis B in adults is self-limiting in more than 95% of cases; therefore, whether antiviral therapy is indicated only for patients with protracted severe acute hepatitis or fulminant hepatitis B needs further studies. Management of patients with CHB infection includes thorough assessment and counseling, dietary and lifestyle advice, control of alcohol use, avoidance of risky behaviors that lead to superinfection by other viruses, and preventive measures against transmission of hepatitis B to intimate contacts.

CHB patients have to be followed regularly and advised as to the potential benefits of antiviral therapies. Viremic patients with an ALT level of twice the upper limit of normal or greater, or substantial liver disease, are candidates for anti-HBV therapy.

Approved and widely used agents are conventional interferon alfa (IFN) and pegylated interferon-α_{2a} (PEG-IFN); the nucleoside analogs, lamivudine, entecavir, and telbivudine; and the nucleotide analogs, adefovir dipivoxil and tenofovir.[24–27] Drug therapy should be selected according to the patient's condition, the drug's mechanism and resistance, rapidity of action, potency, convenience of administration, adverse reactions, and cost, as indicated by clinical guidelines.

Clinical and Surrogate Endpoints

HBV replication is the key driver to liver injury and disease progression; therefore, the main goals of treatment are to suppress virus replication, to achieve HBeAg seroconversion or both; and to stop or reduce hepatic necroinflammation.[5] Long-term goals are to prevent the development of HCC, and ultimately to extend survival (clinical endpoints).

From another aspect, for chronic HBV infection, it usually takes decades to reach clinical endpoints. Thus, in studies of hepatitis B therapy, loss of HBsAg, HBV DNA level, HBeAg or antibody status, ALT level normalization, and improvement in liver histology have been adopted as short-term endpoints.[28]

Review of the natural history of HBV infection suggests that the elimination of HBsAg may be the best surrogate of clinical outcome because it indicates immunity to HBV, decreased risk for development of cirrhosis and HCC, and improved survival. Thus, although such seroconversion does not occur frequently in response to current treatments, any new anti-HBV strategy, including combination therapy, should aim at clearance of HBsAg. Several studies have identified an elevated HBV DNA level as a predictor of development of cirrhosis and HCC. Suppression of HBV DNA, another commonly used surrogate endpoint, has been associated with improvement in ALT level and improved histology.

IFN/PEG-IFN Therapy

IFN/PEG-IFN is the only worldwide licensed drug for CHB with immunomodulatory as well as antiviral properties. The advantages of IFN/PEG-IFN therapy include a lack of drug resistance, a finite and defined treatment course, durable response posttreatment, and a higher likelihood for HBsAg clearance compared with nucleos(t)ide analogs.[29] Long-term follow-up of virological responders to either IFN or PEG-IFN has demonstrated a progressive increase in the rate of HBsAg clearance. Besides, results from follow-up studies suggest that IFN therapy has long-term benefits by promoting cumulative HBeAg seroconversion, increasing HBsAg loss, reducing development of cirrhosis and HCC, and extending survival, especially in the responders.[30] Based on these findings, IFN/PEG-IFN is recommended as a first-line curative therapy in eligible patients with a high likelihood of response according to serum HBV DNA, ALT, and HBV genotype.

However, IFN-based therapy is associated with several adverse events, including influenza-like symptoms, fatigue, anorexia, weight loss, hair loss, thyroid dysfunction, emotional instability, and bone marrow suppression. Patients may need symptomatic treatment or dose modification.

Nucleos(t)ide Analogs

Nucleos(t)ide analogs act through inhibition of HBV polymerase and reverse transcriptase activity. Five oral agents have been approved for the treatment of chronic hepatitis B, ranging in virological potency, clinical efficacy, barrier to resistance, and adverse effect profile.[24–27] Data from a 1-year registration trial for oral antiviral agents (not head-to-head comparison) suggest that entecavir is the most potent, followed by tenofovir, telbivudine, lamivudine, and adefovir dipivoxil. However, the antiviral potency of these drugs does not guarantee an increased rate of HBeAg seroconversion (up to 20% after 1 year of treatment), and HBsAg loss occurs rarely. *Post hoc* analysis suggests that patients with pretherapy high serum ALT values respond better to lamivudine or telbivudine therapy compared to those with low serum ALT values. More importantly, nucleos(t)ide analogs proved their highest benefit in patients with decompensated cirrhosis by improving liver function, prolonging survival, and decreasing the need for transplantation. In patients with advanced fibrosis or cirrhosis, results of a large randomized controlled trial showed the benefits of long-term therapy after 3 years of lamivudine therapy with reduced disease progression and HCC development.[5] A recent 6-year treatment study using entecavir found a regression of advanced fibrosis in the majority of CHB patients.[31]

Relapse after nucleos(t)ide analog therapy is a critical issue awaiting further studies.[24–27] About 20–50% of patients who have HBeAg seroconversion will relapse with HBeAg reversion within 6–12 months off therapy. The risk of relapse is even higher if the duration of consolidation therapy after HBeAg seroconversion is fewer than 6 months. In HBeAg-negative patients, there is no reliable surrogate endpoint like HBeAg seroconversion. Stopping drug therapy after 1 year is associated with an 80–90% relapse rate.

The emergence of drug-resistant genotypic mutations of HBV in patients receiving long-term therapy is another major problem.[24–27] Clinically, emergence of drug resistance is indicated by viral breakthrough (an increase of serum HBV DNA to more than 10-fold higher than the nadir of the initial response). Subsequent biochemical breakthrough (elevated ALT values) occurs in more than 90% of such patients. Hepatitis flares develop frequently and may be associated with hepatic decompensation despite continued antiviral therapy. Afterwards, the initial clinical and histological benefits of the antiviral therapy diminish.

The incidence of drug resistance rises with increasing therapy duration. Drug resistance occurs most frequently after treatment with lamivudine, followed by telbivudine and adefovir dipivoxil, and rarely with tenofovir and entecavir. Studies have shown that suppression of the HBV to an undetectable level at 24 weeks of telbivudine and lamivudine therapy is associated with a low incidence of drug resistance at week 96. Rescue therapy for drug resistance is now available; therefore, monitoring HBV DNA levels during treatment to detect drug resistance early enough to start rescue therapy before the serum HBV DNA surge is critical. In patients with drug resistance, add-on therapy without cross-resistance should be instituted. Switching to IFN-based therapy is another option.

Drug Treatment Strategies

The currently available evidence does not permit concrete recommendations regarding selection of a particular therapeutic course. Health care providers should discuss the risks and benefits of treatment options with patients to reach the best possible decisions.[24–27] Oral antiviral agents with fast and potent HBV-suppressive effects are preferred for patients with threatening or overt hepatic decompensation. IFN-based therapy is preferred in patients with compensated liver disease – particularly in young patients, women of child-bearing age, and those with low ALT values – because of the finite duration of treatment, sustained response, and long-term benefits, including prevention of HCC. For oral antiviral agents, the benefit of long-term therapy should be weighed against the risk of drug resistance, the durability of treatment response, and the cost. If long-term therapy is anticipated, the drug with the lowest rate of resistance is preferable, although cost may affect choice.

Drug therapy is usually not recommended for children and women of child-bearing age, because of uncertainties associated with long-term therapy. When treatment is absolutely indicated, IFN-based therapy is preferred for nonpregnant women, and pregnancy is discouraged during treatment. Women who become pregnant while receiving oral antiviral agents can continue treatment with telbivudine or tenofovir, which are pregnancy category B agents.

In patients with concurrent hepatitis C or D virus infection, the dominant virus should be determined and treated accordingly. A recent randomized controlled trial study from Taiwan demonstrated that combination therapy of PEG-IFN and ribavirin appears to be just as effective and safe for the treatment of HBsAg-positive patients chronically infected with active chronic hepatitis C as it is in patients with HCV monoinfection.[32]

In patients with HIV coinfection, decisions regarding when to initiate anti-HBV therapy require consideration of the HIV treatment status because several of the nucleoside analogs are active against both HIV and HBV.[33]

HBV reactivation is a serious complication in patients undergoing transplantation, immunosuppression, or cancer chemotherapy. Patients should be screened for HBsAg and, if positive, prophylactic therapy with an antiviral agent should be started before the beginning of, and continue until at least 12 weeks after the end of, the immunosuppressive treatment or cancer chemotherapy.

PREVENTION AND CONTROL

Although current antiviral treatments using PEG-IFN or nucleos(t)ide analogs are effective for suppressing HBV replication, they only achieve a very modest level of HBV eradication. Even among those who have responded well to the available treatments, the majority still carry HBsAg. On the other hand, from the very beginning, the hepatitis B vaccine has prevented HBV infection effectively.[3] Vaccination of infants against hepatitis B, especially those born to HBV carrier mothers, is the most effective way of controlling the spread of HBV. And thus, universal infant vaccination will be the key to the elimination and subsequent eradication of hepatitis B.

HBV vaccine has been available since the early 1980s.[3] Worldwide, there are different strategies of universal hepatitis B vaccination in newborns. Each country chooses its own strategy depending on its needs after considering epidemiology, disease burden, readiness of the public health system, and economic constraints. Any approach in implementing hepatitis B vaccination will help to control hepatitis B in the country. Considering that more than 1 billion doses of vaccine have been used since 1982, the safety record is remarkable. There are currently no data that support the necessity of booster doses of hepatitis B vaccine among immunocompetent individuals who have responded to a complete (3 doses) primary vaccination. Additional information is still needed to establish if booster injections are needed beyond 20 years after hepatitis B vaccination of children and adults. Booster doses may be necessary for immunocompromised individuals.

Since the introduction of hepatitis B vaccination, the worldwide rates of infection in this cohort have fallen (***Table 66.1***). For example, the HBsAg carrier rate in Taiwanese children decreased from 10% in 1984 to less than 1% in 2004,[34] with a resultant 68% reduction of fulminant hepatitis in infants (0–1 year), and a 75% decline in HCC in children (aged 6–14 years).[35,36]

Despite these remarkable results, there are still 0.1–1% of children becoming HBV carriers after completing the regular vaccination protocol.[37] Many logistical problems of vaccination in developing or developed countries have to be overcome. Elimination and eradication of hepatitis B will require long-term commitment all over the world.

HEPATITIS D

INTRODUCTION

Hepatitis D virus (HDV) is a satellite and defective RNA virus, requiring HBV to complete its life cycle. It was discovered in 1977 when a new delta antigen (HDAg) was recognized by immunofluorescence staining in hepatocytes of patients with HBV infection.[38] Subsequent studies disclosed the transmissibility of HDAg to HBV-infected chimpanzees and confirmed that HDAg belongs to a novel and distinct infectious agent – HDV.[39]

THE AGENT

HDV, in the genus *Deltavirus*, is the smallest animal virus, with a spherical shape approximately 36 nm in diameter. The HDV virion uses HBsAg as an envelope to package HDAg and its genome, which is a single negative-sense circular RNA of 1700 nucleotides with a high G + C content, resulting in intramolecular base pairing with a partially double-stranded rod-shaped structure. In addition, both the genomic (negative) and antigenomic (positive) strands of HDV RNA contain a ribozyme motif, serving to self-cleave and self-ligate the circular HDV genome.[40]

HDV genome contains a single ORF, encoding a 195 amino acid protein, the small HDAg (S-HDAg). The ORF is edited by a cellular adenine deaminase at the termination codon to extend translation of 19 more amino acids, producing another 214 amino acid protein, the large HDAg (L-HDAg).[41] Both HDAgs are further modified by cellular enzymes catalyzing phosphorylation, acetylation, methylation, or prenylation and refining their specific functions. For example, the phosphorylation of S-HDAg promotes HDV antigenomic RNA replication,[42] while the prenylation of L-HDAg helps viral assembly.[43]

The replication cycle of HDV begins with the viral attachment to unidentified receptor(s) on the hepatocyte membrane through the help of HBsAg, and its genome is directed into the nucleus by nuclear localization signals. After uncoating, the HDV RNA replicates by a double-rolling-circle mechanism, probably by using the host's RNA polymerase II for two types of RNA: a 0.8-kb mRNA and a 1.7-kb circular antigenomic RNA template. First, the transcription passes through the polyadenylation and self-cleavage sites to release mRNA that travels to the cytoplasm for HDAg translation. Second, the transcription continues beyond the self-cleavage site to release a linear full-length antigenomic RNA, and, subsequently, it self-ligates into another circular configuration, as a template for further replication.[44] The small genomic size, folded RNA loops, and presence of ribozyme make HDV a mimic of the RNA viroids or satellite RNAs of higher plants rather than in an animal virus.

EPIDEMIOLOGY

HDV infection occurs exclusively in subjects with HBV infection; however, the prevalence between HDV and HBV infection is not parallel. Overall, the prevalence of HDV infection is around 1–2 % among all HBV carriers worldwide and accounts for approximately 10–15 million HDV carriers. Highly endemic areas include South America, Middle East, West Africa, Pacific Islands, and Eastern Europe (***Fig. 66.3***).[45]

HDV is transmitted primarily through contact with infected blood or body fluids parenterally. Intravenous drug use (IVDU) is the most common route of transmission in nonendemic areas, such as North America and northern Europe. Transmission through blood transfusion is decreasing after HBsAg screening; however, the risk is still higher in patients receiving multiple transfusions, such as hemophiliacs. Sexual contact is another important route, especially among prostitutes and whoremasters. Cohabitation is a risk of transmission in southern Italy. Unlike HBV, perinatal transmission of HDV is rare.[45]

HDV has eight genotypes, with up to 40% heterogeneity of genomic sequences in various geographic areas. These genotypes may be determined by restriction fragment length polymorphism analysis, direct sequencing or immunohistochemical staining by genotype-specific anti-HDV antibodies on hepatocytes. Different genotypes may account for variation in pathogenicity and interactions with different HBsAg types. For example, HDV genotype 1 is the most common worldwide, and a recent study revealed that genotype 1 HDV and genotype C HBV infection account for more adverse outcomes, including cirrhosis, HCC, and hepatic failure.[46] Genotype 2 infection, predominant in Taiwan and Japan, is associated with a less severe outcome. Genotype 3 infection, found exclusively in northern South America, is associated with fulminant hepatitis with coexisting genotype F HBV infection.

HDV prevalence has declined in several endemic countries, such as Italy, Spain, Turkey, and Taiwan,[41] possibly owing to the successful control of HBV by universal vaccination, using disposable needles and improved precautions in sexual behaviors. However, the decline was offset in Europe because of new immigrants harboring higher rates of HDV infection,[41] and this poses a new threat to the secondary spread of HDV.

Natural History

The clinical spectrum of HDV infection ranges from asymptomatic carrier to end-stage liver disease, similar to other chronic viral hepatitides. HDV infection should be suspected in patients with severe hepatitis B and low HBV replication. HDV carriers appear to have a fourfold higher risk of liver damage than inactive HBsAg carriers.[47]

There are two scenarios of acute HDV infection: concurrent HDV and HBV infection (coinfection) or a subsequent HDV infection in an established HBsAg carrier (superinfection) (***Table 66.2***). The natural histories are different, with more chronic and severe disease in the latter. In patients with HDV–HBV coinfection, a biphasic increase of serum aminotransferase is commonly observed, which may help to differentiate it from acute HBV infection. Usually, patients with HDV–HBV coinfection will recover completely without sequelae and the percentage of chronicity is less than 5% because the helper HBV rarely becomes chronic in acute infection of adult patients.

On the other hand, HDV superinfection can be divided into three phases[48] (***Fig. 66.4***). In the acute phase, the patient may develop severe or even fulminant hepatitis, and an accelerated course to cirrhosis was observed in Italy.[49] Around 70–90% of patients surviving the acute phase progress to chronicity.[48] A study in southern Italy observed that 10% of

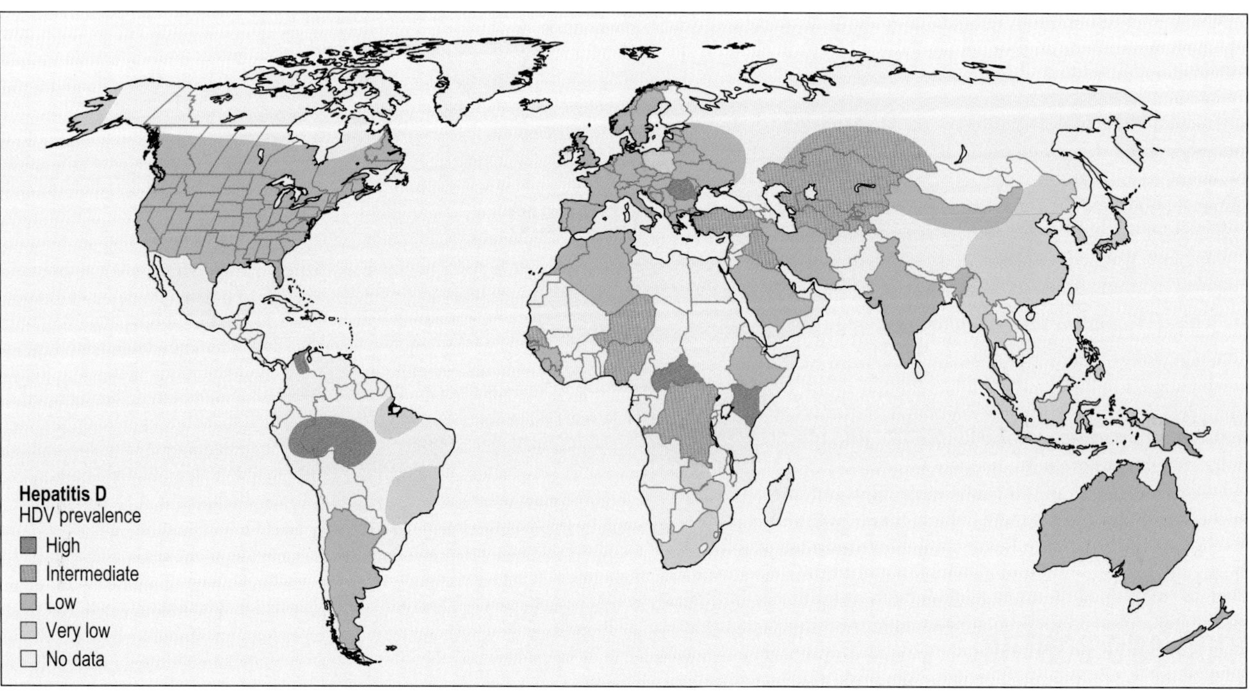

Figure 66.3 Hepatitis D virus (HDV) prevalence.

Table 66.2 Clinical Features of Hepatitis D Virus Coinfection and Superinfection in Hepatitis B Virus Carriers

	Coinfection	Superinfection
HBV infection	Acute	Chronic
HDV infection	Acute	Acute
Serum markers		
HBsAg	Positive and transient	Positive and persistent
IgM anti-HBc	Positive	Negative
Anti-HBs	Positive in recovery phase	Negative
Anti-HDV	Late acute phase, low titer	Rapidly increasing, high titer
IgM anti-HDV	Positive, transient	Rapidly increasing, high titer
HDV RNA	Positive, early and transient	Positive, early and persistent
ALT level	Biphasic elevation	Monophasic elevation
Chronicity	<5%	70–90%
Outcomes	Recovery with seroclearance	Usually persistent infection

HBV, hepatitis B virus, HDV, hepatitis D virus, HBsAg, hepatitis B surface antigen, IgM anti-HBc, IgM antibody to hepatitis B core antigen; Anti-HBs, antibody to HBsAg; Anti-HDV, antibody to HDV; ALT, alanine aminotransferase.

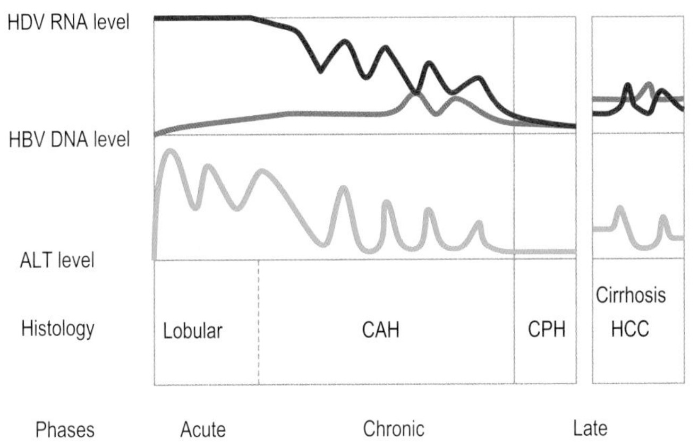

Figure 66.4 Natural course of hepatitis D virus (HDV) superinfection. (1) Acute-phase, active HDV replication and suppression of hepatitis B virus (HBV). The serum alanine aminotransferase (ALT) levels are very high. (2) Chronic phase, reactivating low levels of HBV with decreasing HDV. Serum ALT levels are moderately elevated. (3) Late phase, development of cirrhosis and HCC. CAH, chronic active hepatitis; CPH, chronic persistent hepatitis; HCC, hepatocellular carcinoma.

patients in the chronic stage had a mild, nonprogressive course, while the rest entered a progressive course to compensated cirrhosis in 9 years, and then disease progression slowed for more than a decade.[50] During the late phase, the development of cirrhosis and HCC is caused by replication of either virus. The reduction or clearance of both viruses results in remission.[48] A rare form of HBV-independent latent HDV infection occurs in liver transplantation. The hepatic HDAg of the allograft is occasionally found shortly after the transplantation; meanwhile, serum HBV is cleared by HBV immunoglobulins. During this phase, there is only limited liver disease without HDV viremia. After reinfection with HBV, the HDV regains its infectivity.[51]

The clinical course of subsequent HCC varies between dual HDV–HBV and single HBV infection. In Italy, where most HDV infection occurs at a younger age due to family contact or IVDU, HCC develops earlier than in those with HBV infection alone, indicating more severe necroinflammatory liver damage with subsequent malignant transformation of dual infection.[52] However, in Taiwan, the age of HCC development is similar in these two scenarios because of the older age of HDV patients infected by sexual transmission.[48]

PATHOGENESIS AND IMMUNITY

The pathogenesis of HDV infection, though still unclear, depends on two main mechanisms: direct cytotoxicity in the acute phase and immune-mediated hepatitis in the chronic phase. The HDV infection is usually not directly cytopathic. Only in the extreme situation is the large amount of S-HDAg or HDV RNA production directly cytotoxic to the hepatocyte membrane with subsequent cellular destruction.[53] In the chronic phase, inflammatory cells surround hepatocytes and various autoantibodies (e.g., liver-kidney-microsomal type 3 antibodies) have been detected, suggesting the role of immunopathogenesis.[54] Additionally, the interplay between HDV and HBV influences the natural course: a persistent HDV infection can suppress HBV replication with subsequent HBeAg and HBsAg seroclearance.[55] On the other hand, the persistence of serum HBV DNA poses a higher risk of end-stage liver disease.[50]

DIAGNOSIS

HDV antibody (anti-HDV) is the serological hallmark of HDV infection and can be measured by radioimmunoassay or enzyme-linked immunosorbent assay. The most important diagnostic marker for active HDV infection is IgM anti-HDV, which corresponds to concurrent hepatic necroinflammation and predicts disease progression[56] or resolution of chronic HDV infection.[57] IgM anti-HDV is not diagnostic of acute HDV infection as in hepatitis A or B, because the titer is often high in patients with active chronic HDV infection. By using IgM anti-HBc, one can differentiate between patients with coinfection and superinfection: in HBsAg-positive patients, the presence of both IgM anti-HBc and IgM anti-HDV suggests HDV–HBV coinfection; in those having IgM anti-HDV alone, a superinfection with HDV is likely. The low levels of HDV antigenemia can be detected by sensitive Western blot analysis with radiolabeled antibody. In addition, real-time reverse transcription PCR assay can directly detect HDV viremia as low as 100 copies/mL.[58] The serum HDV RNA level is associated with liver damage and elevated ALT levels in the chronic phase.[48] Liver biopsy remains the most definitive method to assess the disease severity, and the presence of HDAg in the nuclei of hepatocytes is the gold standard for the diagnosis of chronic HDV infection.

TREATMENT AND PROGNOSIS

Currently, IFN-based therapy with 3 million units (mU) 3 mU thrice weekly for 1 year is the only effective regimen; though the virus eradication rate is only about 20–36% at the end of treatment (EOT), and relapse rate is nearly 100% at the end of follow-up.[41,45] Generally, a higher dosage (9 mU) and longer duration of IFN are more effective. The rate of ALT normalization and HDV RNA negativity at EOT was 71% in the high-dose group compared with 29–36% in the low-dose group,[59] though a delayed relapse is common. Although rare, sustained clearance of HDV has been documented and is accompanied by clearance of HBsAg and appearance of anti-HBs.[59] A higher dose of IFN significantly improves the long-term outcome, liver histology, and survival.[60]

The PEG-IFN offers a better outcome and convenience to patients. In one study of patients who failed standard IFN therapy, using weekly PEG-IFN-α_{2b} 1.5 µg/kg for 1 year achieved a sustained virological response (SVR) rate of 43% (n = 6).[61] However, in two other similar studies, the SVR rate was only 17–21%;[62] therefore, the long-term effect of PEG-IFN remains unsettled because of small case numbers and the lack of control groups. Adding ribavirin to IFN or PEG-IFN regimens did not improve HDV clearance.[62]

Since HDV requires HBV to complete its life cycle, using regimens against HBV for chronic HDV infection is reasonable. Nevertheless, antivirals against HBV such as famciclovir, lamivudine, and adefovir dipivoxil are ineffective against HDV, both as monotherapy and in combination with IFN.[41] These HBV polymerase inhibitors indeed rapidly reduce HBV viral load but have limited effects against HBsAg production, therefore not affecting the virion assembly of HDV.

Several studies have demonstrated the deletion, mutations, or conformational change of HBsAg blocking HDV virion assembly or entry into hepatocytes. A recent study reported that lamivudine-resistant HBV failed to support HDV secretion in cell cultures.[63] This finding suggests potential targets for HDV therapy.

Other potential therapies, including the prenylation inhibitors and RNA silencing tools targeting HDV ribozymes, are under investigation. The prenylation of the last four amino acids (Cys-Arg-Pro-Gln, CXXX box) of the L-HDAg is essential in the assembly of ribonucleoprotein into the HBsAg envelope. The prenylation inhibitors (e.g., FTI-277 and FTI-2153) decrease HDV virion production both *in vitro* and *in vivo*.[64] RNA interference has been utilized against viral infection, and the mRNA of HDAg can be successfully targeted by small interfering RNA in cell culture.[65] Liver transplantation provides another treatment option for HDV-related end-stage liver disease. The reinfection rate with HDV after liver transplant is lower than HBV or HCV, and the hepatitis is milder.[51]

No effective vaccine for HDV is available at present. A previous study failed to show any protection by HDV vaccination using a preparation of HDAg in a woodchuck hepatitis model.[66]

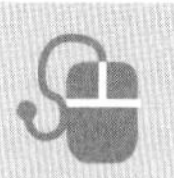

Access the complete reference list online at **http://www.expertconsult.com**

Access the complete reference list online at
http://www.expertconsult.com

CHAPTER 67

Overview of Viral Hemorrhagic Fevers

C.J. Peters • Sherif R. Zaki

INTRODUCTION

Several viruses regularly cause a syndrome that is referred to as hemorrhagic fever (HF). They belong to four different families of RNA viruses, but all are lipid-enveloped and zoonotic in their maintenance strategies. The taxonomy is helpful in understanding their natural history and pathogenesis but does not accurately predict the clinical syndromes following infection with a given family member. For example, virtually all the arenaviruses are maintained by chronic infection of a single rodent host and spread to humans by aerosols of rodent excreta and related mechanisms, with the details of the human epidemiology mainly predictable by rodent dynamics and human behavior. However, several other arenaviruses are not associated with any disease. The best known American arenavirus is lymphocytic choriomeningitis virus, which came to the Americas when the common house mouse, *Mus musculus*, was introduced in post-Columbian times. Lymphocytic choriomeningitis virus infection of humans mainly causes subclinical infection, acute undifferentiated febrile disease, and febrile central nervous system illnesses such as aseptic meningitis, but two cases have resembled the HF syndrome.

THE AGENT

The HF viruses occur worldwide (***Table 67.1***), and the geographic site of infection is an important determinant of the risk to an individual patient. The geography and knowledge of the incubation period are important in suspecting an exported viral HF (VHF). The syndrome characteristically begins with fever, myalgia, and malaise, which then progress to prostration, gastrointestinal and other system involvement, and signs of vascular damage. Involvement of the vascular system is usually manifest by vascular dysregulation (mild hypotension, postural hypotension, flushing, and injected conjunctivae), vascular damage (nondependent edema and organ dysfunction), and hemorrhage. Hemorrhage is usually diffuse in microvascular beds throughout the body and occurs particularly in patients with thrombocytopenia or marked platelet dysfunction. Many patients have little or no bleeding, but some present with extensive cutaneous and mucosal hemorrhage. Severe cases will have shock, central nervous system involvement, or extensive hemorrhagic phenomena. The clinical findings in the different HFs vary in a characteristic way for each virus, but any individual patient is difficult to classify without virologic diagnosis (***Tables 67.2 and 67.3***). The detailed manifestations of each VHF are often based on fragmentary clinical observations and lack proper appreciation of the entire spectrum, which in some cases includes such manifestations as pancreatitis.

PATHOGENESIS AND IMMUNITY

Although there are common themes, the different viruses also differ in their pathology and pathogenesis (***Table 67.4***). Usually, hemorrhages are present in many organs, and effusions are commonly found in serous cavities, but they may be minimal or absent in some patients. There is widespread necrosis, which may be present in any organ system and varies from modest and focal to massive in extent. Liver and lymphoid systems are usually extensively involved, and the lung regularly has varying degrees of interstitial pneumonitis, diffuse alveolar damage, and hemorrhage. Acute tubular necrosis and microvascular thrombosis may also be seen. The inflammatory response is usually minimal. These changes, which may be a direct effect of viral infection or a consequence of cytokine secretion, vary considerably among the different viruses (see ***Table 67.4***).

DIAGNOSIS

Correct diagnosis in most of the diseases depends on demonstration of the infecting virus or one of its products in acute serum samples (***Table 67.5***). Reverse transcription polymerase chain reaction (RT-PCR) is usually the most sensitive test but also is more subject to artifact and contamination. RT-PCR has a unique role in providing an amplicon that can be sequenced for genetic analysis, although this very genetic variation may be a source of difficulty in ensuring that appropriate primers are applied to unknown samples. Viral antigens are readily demonstrable, and often an antigen detection enzyme-linked immunosorbent assay (ELISA) is the best test for identifying patients because of its rapidity and robustness; it is particularly likely to be positive in the more severely ill patient, who is in greatest need of therapy and who may provide the greatest risk of dissemination. In general, viremia and antigenemia are readily detected during the acute phase and disappear as the patient improves. RT-PCR is usually positive during the same period and perhaps 1 or 2 days longer. IgM antibodies may be detectable during illness and usually appear early in convalescence, providing a sensitive, specific method of diagnosis, particularly if they are measured by an IgM capture ELISA technique. Diagnosis of initial patients in any outbreak, particularly if there are unusual features, benefits from study of virus isolates and classic serologic responses, particularly the neutralization test, animal pathogenicity, and genomic analysis. Most of the viruses are hazardous and should only be isolated or studied under biosafety level 4 containment. Hantaviruses are an exception to the generalizations: patients typically present with an ongoing immune response and are best diagnosed with the IgM capture ELISA; virus isolation is difficult, but RT-PCR on acute blood clot may give valuable genetic information about the infecting virus.

Ideally, blood samples from HF patients should be collected early in the course of the illness, and both serum and blood clot should be frozen as soon as possible. A second sample should be obtained before discharge or death for comparative serology, and this can be supplemented by a later follow-up blood sample. In fatal cases, a full autopsy should be performed with a complete set of organs collected in formalin for diagnostic studies; spleen, liver, and lymph nodes should be collected frozen for virus isolation.

Table 67.1 Geography and Epidemiology of Hemorrhagic Fever Viruses

Virus	Disease	Geography	Vector/Reservoir	Human Infection
Arenaviridae				
Junin	Argentine HF	Argentine pampas	Chronic infection of small field rodent, *Calomys musculinus*	Infects agricultural workers disproportionately. Major transmission in fall: aerosol transmission to humans
Machupo	Bolivian HF	Bolivia, Beni province	Chronic infection of small field rodent, *C. callosus*	Rural residents and farmers main target; rodent can invade towns to cause epidemics. Aerosol transmission to humans. Interhuman transmission not usual, but occurs
Guanarito	Venezuelan HF	Venezuela, Portuguesa state	Chronic infection of field rodent, *Zygodontomys brevicauda*	Rural residents in recently developed area with small farms
Sabia	Brazilian HF	Rural area near São Paulo, Brazil	Presumably chronic infection of unidentified rodents	Single infection observed in nature: little information on potential
Chapare	Chapare	Bolivia, Beni province	Presumed chronic infection of rodents	Unknown
Lassa	Lassa fever	West Africa	Chronic infection of rodents of the genus *Mastomys*	The reservoir rodent is very common in Africa, and the disease is a major cause of severe febrile illness in West Africa. Spread to humans occurs by aerosols and by capturing the rodent for consumption, as well as occasional person-to-person transmission Lassa fever is the most commonly exported HF
Lujo	Lujo	Zambia	Presumed chronic infection of rodents	Single infection in nature; interpersonal transmission
Bunyaviridae				
Rift Valley fever	Rift Valley fever	Sub-Saharan Africa	Vertical infection of flood water *Aedes* mosquitoes. Epidemics occur from horizontal transmission by many different mosquito species between domestic animals, particularly sheep and cattle	Humans acquire virus by mosquito bite; contact with blood of infected sheep, cattle, or goats; and aerosols generated from infected domestic animal blood. No interhuman transmission observed
Crimean-Congo HF	Crimean-Congo HF	Africa, Middle East, Balkans, southern Russia, western China	Tick–mammal–tick infection. Vertical infection occurs in ticks. *Hyalomma* ticks are thought to be the natural reservoir, but other genera may become infected and transmit	Tick bite; squashing ticks; and exposure to aerosols or fomites from slaughtered cattle and sheep. (Domestic animals do not show illness but may become infected when transported to market or when held in pens for slaughter.) Nosocomial epidemics observed on numerous occasions
Hantaan, Seoul, Puumala, and others	Hemorrhagic fever with renal syndrome (HFRS)	Worldwide depending on rodent reservoirs	Horizontal infection in a single rodent genus or species typical of the virus. Viruses associated with HFRS have been obtained from *Muridae* (subfamilies *Murinae* or *Arvicolinae*) rodents (rats, mice, and voles)	Aerosols from freshly shed urine of infected rodents. Some infections may be acquired from secondary aerosols or droplets from previously shed rodent excreta and secreta or from rodent bites. Interhuman transmission never documented
Sin Nombre, Black Creek Canal, Bayou, Andes and others	Hantavirus pulmonary syndrome (HPS)	Americas	As for hantaviruses causing HFRS. All viruses associated with HPS have come from *Muridae* (subfamily *Sigmodontinae*) rodents, where the reservoir is known	As for hantaviruses causing HFRS. Entering abandoned, closed buildings may be a particular risk in some settings. Interhuman transmission rarely observed with Andes virus

Table 67.1 Geography and Epidemiology of Hemorrhagic Fever Viruses–cont'd

Virus	Disease	Geography	Vector/Reservoir	Human Infection
Filoviridae				
Marburg, Ebola	Marburg HF Ebola HF	Africa, Philippines	Unknown. Likely to be bats	Infection of index case occurs from unknown source. Infected nonhuman primates sometimes provide link to humans. Later spread among humans or nonhuman primates by close contact with another case
Flaviviridae				
Yellow fever	Yellow fever	Africa, South America	Mosquito–monkey–mosquito maintenance with occasional human infection when unvaccinated humans enter forest. Large epidemics among humans with *Aedes aegypti* as mosquito vector	Mosquito infection of humans entering forest and encountering infected sylvatic vector. Emergence of epidemics into African savannas via specific *Aedes* mosquito vectors. In cities or villages, interhuman transmission by *Ae. aegypti*. Fully developed cases are no longer viremic, and direct interhuman transmission is not believed to be a problem although the virus is highly infectious (including aerosols) in the laboratory
Dengue (types 1–4)	Dengue HF (DHF), dengue shock syndrome (DSS)	Tropics and subtropics worldwide	Maintained by *Ae. aegypti*–human–*Ae. aegypti* transmission with frequent geographic transport of viruses by travelers	DHF/DSS is a major problem in areas where multiple dengue viruses are being transmitted. With the increased worldwide distribution of *Ae. aegypti* and movement of dengue viruses in travelers, this zone is enlarging. The disease was first noted in Southeast Asia but is now common in the Americas and the Caribbean, as well as the Pacific rim countries
Kyasanur Forest disease (KFD)	KFD	Karnataka state, India	Tick–vertebrate–tick	Most infections occur from tick bite acquired in rural areas of the endemic zone. Monkey die-offs may accompany increased virus activity
Omsk HF (OHF)	OHF	Western Siberia	Poorly understood cycle involving ticks, voles, muskrats, and possibly waterborne and mosquito transmission	Few cases in recent years
Alkhurma		Middle East	Unknown. Surmised to involve tick–domestic livestock–tick cycle by analogy to genetically related tick-borne flaviviruses	Transmitted to humans working in livestock-related occupations by unknown route. Six of 9 initial patients were butchers. Little definitive information available

HF, hemorrhagic fever.

Table 67.2 Clinical Features of the Viral Hemorrhagic Fevers

Disease	Incubation Period (Days)	Case Infection Ratio	Case Fatality	Characteristic Features
Arenaviridae				
South American HF	7–14	Most (>1/2) result in disease	15–30%	Typical cases have hypotension, shock, obvious bleeding, and neurologic symptoms such as dysarthria and intention tremor. Some cases have virtually pure neurologic syndrome
Lassa fever	5–16	Mild infections probably common	~15%	Prostration and shock; fewer hemorrhagic or neurologic manifestations than South American HF except in severe cases. Thrombocytopenia less common and less severe. Deafness develops in convalescence in 20%
Bunyaviridae				
Rift Valley fever	2–5[a]	~1%	~50%	Severe disease associated with bleeding, shock, anuria, and icterus. Encephalitis and retinal vasculitis also occur, but not necessarily overlapping with HF syndrome
Crimean-Congo HF	3–12	20–100%	15–30%	Most severe bleeding and ecchymoses of all the HFs
HF with renal syndrome	9–35	>3/4 Hantaan virus 1/20 Puumala virus	5–15% Hantaan <1% Puumala	Febrile stage followed by shock and renal failure. Bleeding during febrile stage, shock, and renal failure. Puumala infections have similar course but much milder
Hantavirus pulmonary syndrome	7–28[b]	Very high for most recognized viruses	40–50%	Febrile stage followed by acute pulmonary edema and shock. Manifestations largely limited to thoracic cavity
Filoviridae				
Marburg or Ebola HF	3–16	High (particularly Zaire subtype of Ebola)	25–90%	Most severe of the HFs. Marked weight loss and prostration. Maculopapular rash common. Patients have had late sequelae (hepatitis, uveitis, orchitis) often with virus isolation from biopsy or aspiration
Flaviviridae				
Yellow fever	3–6	80–95%	20%	Acute febrile period with defervescence accompanied in severe cases by jaundice and renal failure
Dengue HF (DHF), dengue shock syndrome (DSS)	3–15[a]	0.007% of nonimmune and 1.0% of heterologous immune	Probably <1%	High fever for 3–5 days with the development of shock lasting 1–2 days. DHF is not equated to DSS. DSS is the most dangerous manifestation and is due to an acute vascular leak. Attack rates, mortality quite variable with epidemic virus strain and surveillance
Kyasanur Forest disease (KFD), Omsk HF (OHF), Alkhurma	3–8	Variable	0.5–9.0%	Typical biphasic disease with a febrile or hemorrhagic period often followed by central nervous system involvement. Similar to tick-borne encephalitis except hemorrhagic manifestations are not characteristic of first phase of tick-borne encephalitis

HF, hemorrhagic fever.

[a]Uncomplicated disease; incubation for HF may differ.

[b]Not known with certainty; estimated from available data.

Table 67.3 Specific Clinical Findings in Different Hemorrhagic Fevers

Disease	Hemorrhage	Thrombocytopenia	Leukocyte Count	Rash	Icterus	Renal Disease	Pulmonary Disease	Tremor, Dysarthria	Encephalopathy	Deafness	Retinal Lesions
Arenaviridae											
South American HF	+++	+++	⇑⇑⇑	0	0	0	+	+++	++	0	0
Lassa fever	+/S	+	0	++	0	0	+	+	+/S	++	0
Bunyaviridae											
Rift Valley fever	+++	+++		0	++	+		0	E	0	Retina
Crimean-Congo HF	+++	+++	⇑⇑ / ⇑	0	++	0	+	0	+	0	0
HF with renal syndrome	+++	+++	⇑⇑⇑	0	0	+++	+	0	+	0	0
Hantavirus pulmonary syndrome	+	++	⇑⇑	0	0	+	+++	0	+	0	0
Filoviridae											
Marburg and Ebola HF	++	+++		+++	++	0	+	0	++	+	Uveitis Retina?
Flaviviridae											
Yellow fever	+++	++	0/⇑⇑	0	+++	++	+	0	++	0	0
Dengue HF (DHF), Dengue shock syndrome (DSS)	++	+++	⇑⇑	+++	+	0	+	0	+	0	0
Kyasanur Forest disease (KFD), Omsk HF (OHF)	++	++	⇑⇑	0	0	0	++	0	E	0	Retina

HF, hemorrhagic fever.

+ occasional or mild; ++ commonly seen, may be severe; +++ characteristic and usually marked. S, characteristic, seen in severe cases. ⇑ occasionally or mildly increased; ⇑⇑ commonly increased, may be marked; ⇑⇑⇑ characteristically increased and usually marked. O, within normal range or not present; E, develop true encephalitis but either after HF (KFD, Omsk) or in other patients (RVF).

Table 67.4 Viral Tropism and Pathologic Features of Viral Hemorrhagic Fevers

Disease	Pathologic Features[a]
Arenaviridae	
Argentine HF Bolivian HF Venezuelan HF Lassa fever	Multifocal hepatocellular necrosis with minimal inflammatory response, interstitial pneumonitis, myocarditis, and lymphoid depletion; extensive parenchymal cell and reticuloendothelial infection, more than morphologic lesions would suggest
Bunyaviridae	
Rift Valley fever	Widespread hepatocellular necrosis and hemorrhage, sometimes with midzonal distribution, minimal inflammatory response, disseminated intravascular coagulation, lymphoid depletion; Rift Valley fever antigens in few individual hepatocytes; encephalitis and retinal vasculitis also occur
Crimean Congo HF	Widespread hepatocellular necrosis and hemorrhage with minimal or no inflammatory cell response and lymphoid depletion; hepatic and endothelial cell infection and damage
Hemorrhagic fever with renal syndrome (HFRS)	Retroperitoneal edema in severe HFRS, mild to severe renal pathologic changes; congestion and hemorrhagic necrosis of renal medulla, right atrium of the heart, and anterior pituitary; extensive endothelial infection mainly in renal and cardiac microvasculature
Hantavirus pulmonary syndrome (HPS)	Large bilateral pleural effusions and severely edematous lungs, mild to moderate interstitial pneumonitis, immunoblasts, and atypical lymphocytes in lymphoid tissues and peripheral blood; extensive infection of endothelial cells in pulmonary microvasculature
Filoviridae	
Ebola HF	Extensive and disseminated infection and necrosis in major organs such as liver, spleen, lung, kidney, skin, and gonads; extensive hepatocellular necrosis associated with formation of characteristic intracytoplasmic viral inclusions; lymphoid depletion, microvascular infection, and injury
Marburg HF	Similar to Ebola HF
Flaviviridae	
Yellow fever	Midzonal hepatocellular necrosis; minimal inflammatory response; Councilman bodies and microvesicular fatty change; hepatocellular and Kupffer cell infection; lymphoid necrosis (nodes, spleen); focal myocarditis; acute renal tubular necrosis
Dengue HF, dengue shock syndrome	Centrilobular and midzonal hepatocellular necrosis with minimal inflammatory response; Councilman bodies and microvesicular fatty change; hyperplasia of mononuclear phagocytic cells in lymphoid tissues and atypical lymphocytes in peripheral blood; widespread infection of mononuclear phagocytic and endothelial cells
Kyasanur Forest disease (KFD)	Focal hepatocellular degeneration, fatty change, and necrosis; pulmonary hemorrhage, depletion of malpighian follicles, sinus histiocytosis, erythrophagocytosis, mild myocarditis, and encephalitis
Omsk HF	Little known; scattered focal hemorrhage, interstitial pneumonia, and normal lymphoid tissues

HF, hemorrhagic fever.

[a]These features represent the characteristic pathologic findings in the different viral HFs. More general findings seen to variable degrees in all HFs are not listed.

Table 67.5 Diagnosis of Viral Hemorrhagic Fever in the Laboratory

Disease	Acute Serum Antigen ELISA	Acute Serum RT-PCR	Acute Serum Virus Isolation
Arenaviridae			
South American HF	Usually positive	Usually positive; has been successfully applied	Usually positive
Lassa fever	Usually positive; if negative, IgM usually positive	Has been sucessfully applied; geographic variation in primers	Usually positive if patient still ill
Bunyaviridae			
Rift Valley fever	Positive in severe cases	Usually positive	Readily isolated in a few days
Crimean-Congo HF	Positive in severe cases	Useful; several primer sets needed	Usually positive if patient ill
HF with renal syndrome	Negative. IgM is test of choice	May be positive; primers must be carefully selected	Difficult to isolate
Hantavirus pulmonary syndrome	Negative. IgM is test of choice	Usually positive on clot first few days; primers must be carefully selected	Difficult to isolate, even if RT-PCR positive
Filoviridae			
Marburg HF	Usually positive	Positive	Readily isolated
Ebola HF	Usually positive. IgM may be present later	Positive	Most strains readily isolated
Flaviviridae			
Yellow fever	Variable. IgM is test of choice	Experimental	Readily isolated first 4 days
Dengue HF (DHF), Dengue shock syndrome (DSS)	Variable. IgM is test of choice	Positive	Virus readily isolated if early specimens inoculated into mosquitoes
Kyasanur Forest disease (KFD), Omsk HF (OHF), Alkhurma	Little experience	Little experience	Usually isolated during the acute hemorrhagic phase

HF, hemorrhagic fever; ELISA, enzyme-linked immunosorbent assay; RT-PCR, reverse transcription polymerase chain reaction; IgM, immunoglobulin M antibodies.

Classic histopathology is often useful in suspecting yellow fever, Rift Valley fever, or a filovirus infection and in diagnosing some of the confounding diseases. Immunohistochemistry on fixed tissues can usually establish a definitive diagnosis. Precautions appropriate to each virus should be taken to prevent infection while processing samples or performing a necropsy. Frozen samples should be appropriately packed and, whenever possible, shipped on dry ice, although diagnoses can sometimes be made on mishandled specimens. The receiving laboratory should be advised of the shipment, its estimated time of arrival, and the waybill number to allow for tracing the materials if, as often happens, there is a delay en route. Diagnostic expertise and consultation are available from several laboratories.

TREATMENT AND PREVENTION

Approaches to the prevention and treatment of the viral HFs vary with the infecting virus (***Table*** *67.6*). Barrier nursing and avoidance of parenteral exposure of hospital staff are important in the management of all these diseases, but they are particularly important in Crimean-Congo HF and the filovirus diseases because of the regularity with which nosocomial transmission has occurred. The general principles of therapy are similar for all the HFs and require rapid hospitalization, careful maintenance of fluid balance to avoid overhydration in the face of fragile systemic and pulmonary capillary beds, as well as probable myocardial compromise, management of the bleeding diathesis according to the usual principles, and the specific therapy appropriate to each disease (see ***Table*** *67.6*). It is extremely important to exclude or empirically treat the conditions that may be most important in the differential diagnosis, particularly malaria, rickettsial infections, leptospirosis, relapsing fever, typhoid, and shigellosis.

Table 67.6 Prevention and Treatment of Viral Hemorrhagic Fevers

Disease	Prevention	Treatment
Arenaviridae		
Argentine HF	Safe, effective vaccine used for high-risk residents of endemic area	Infusion of convalescent plasma during first 8 days of illness reduces mortality from 15–30% to <1%
Bolivian HF	Elimination of specific reservoir rodents from towns practical and effective; sporadic cases due to exposure outside towns, person-to-person transmission in families and institutions cannot be prevented; Argentine HF vaccine protects experimental animals against Bolivian virus	Ribavirin likely to be effective and should be used in this and other arenavirus diseases unless proven effective; alternative therapy available
Lassa fever	None; intensive village-based rodent control may reduce risk	Ribavirin effective in reducing mortality; use in higher-risk patients, e.g., if aspartate transaminase >150 U/L
Bunyaviridae		
Rift Valley fever	Vaccination of domestic livestock prevents epizootics/epidemics but not sporadic, endemic infections of humans; human vaccine safe and effective but limited supply; veterinarians and virology workers in sub-Saharan Africa are candidates for vaccine	Ribavirin and antibody therapy should be tried in HF patients based on studies in experimental animals
Crimean-Congo HF	Tick avoidance; no slaughter of acutely infected animals (apparently healthy but viremic and therefore an undetected threat); barrier nursing of suspected patients particularly important	Ribavirin should be used based on *in vitro* sensitivity and on uncontrolled South African experience
HF with renal syndrome (HFRS)	Rodent control and avoidance impractical in most cases; investigational vaccines deserve further evaluation	Early diagnosis and supportive care lifesaving; ribavirin has positive effect during initial 4 days of illness and should be used in severe HFRS if available
Hantavirus pulmonary syndrome (HPS)	Rodent avoidance useful; care should be taken before entering or cleaning closed buildings with potential rodent infestations	Early diagnosis and supportive care potentially lifesaving; avoidance of hypoxia and excessive hydration coupled with careful management of shock
Filoviridae		
Ebola/Marburg HF	Barrier nursing and needle sterilization in African hospitals particularly important; avoid close contact with suspected patients; do careful evaluation of sick nonhuman primates	None other than supportive, which may be of limited utility; antiviral therapies urgently needed
Flaviviridae		
Yellow fever	Vaccine is probably the safest and most effective in the world; control of *Aedes aegypti* would eliminate urban transmission but sylvatic transmission remains	None other than supportive
Dengue HF	Reduction of dengue transmission by *Ae. aegypti* control; investigational vaccines will probably be available soon; possibly useful in travelers but may be limited in solving hyperendemic dengue transmission that leads to dengue HF	Supportive care effective and greatly reduces mortality
Tick-borne virus-specific IgG	Avoidance of ticks; vaccination; postexposure prophylaxis with flaviviruses	Supportive care

HF, hemorrhagic fever.

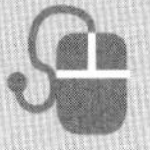

Access the complete reference list online at
http://www.expertconsult.com

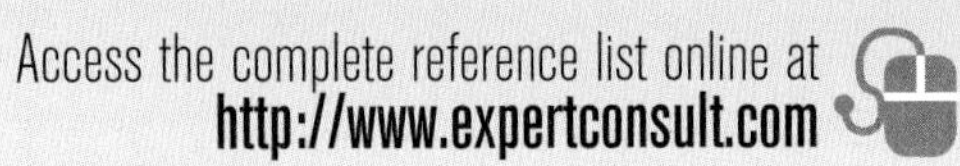
Access the complete reference list online at
http://www.expertconsult.com

CHAPTER 68

Arenavirus Infections

Delia A. Enría • James N. Mills • Dan Bausch • Wun-Ju Shieh • C.J. Peters

INTRODUCTION

Arenaviruses are rodent-borne pathogens that are important causes of hemorrhagic fever (HF) in Africa and South America. Lymphocytic choriomeningitis (LCM) virus occurs in Europe, the Americas, and elsewhere, causing febrile disease, sometimes with central nervous system (CNS) involvement, and congenital infections. Several South American viruses result in HF, but the geographic distribution of each disease is limited.[1–7] In Africa, the major HF is Lassa fever, found only in West Africa,[8] but recently a cluster of HF cases originating in Zambia was identified and attributed to a new African arenavirus, Lujo virus.[9] There are many arenaviruses in Africa and the Americas that are not associated with human disease. Arenaviruses cause chronic, inapparent infections of their rodent hosts, sometimes with prolonged or lifelong viremia and vertical transmission. Human epidemiology is determined by the distribution of infected rodents and their contact with humans, although in some cases interhuman infection has occurred. Thus these diseases occur in rural environments where humans and rodents come into particularly close contact. Their aerosol infectivity and stability have put them in the first rank of bioterrorist threats.[10] Overt damage to infected cells by arenaviruses is minimal or modest, but they alter cell function and induce mediators of shock, directly or by immunopathologic mechanisms. They are sensitive to the antiviral drug ribavirin, and there is a safe, effective vaccine against Argentine HF.

THE AGENTS

There are currently more than 20 recognized members of the *Arenaviridae*. The major agents are shown in ***Figure 68.1*** along with their known distribution and putative hosts. Their associated diseases are described in *Table 68.1*.

Virion Morphology and Structure

Arenaviruses derive their name from the Latin *arenosus* (sandy) from the granular or sandy appearance of virions when viewed by thin-section electron microscopy.[11] Virions are spherical to pleomorphic, have a mean diameter of 110–130 nm (range 50–300 nm), and are enveloped in a lipid bilayer derived from cell membranes (***Fig. 68.2***). Embedded in the lipid bilayer are club-shaped projections, 8–10 nm in length, which are composed of the viral glycoproteins, GP1 (molecular mass, 40–64 kDa) and GP2 (35–44 kDa). A GP1 tetramer forms the head of the spike, whereas a GP2 tetramer forms the stalk. GP1 and GP2 are derived by post-translational cleavage of a precursor molecule, GPC. The most abundant viral protein is the nucleoprotein, NP (63–78 kDa), which associates with genomic RNA in circular nucleocapsid structures.[12,13] The viral L protein (200–250 kDa) has transcriptase and replicase activity and is a minor component of nucleocapsids.[14] The Z protein (10–14 kDa) is a small structural protein with a zinc-binding domain (RING finger motif). In its myristolated form it serves as a matrix protein analog and is a driver of budding at the plasma membrane.[15–17] By interacting with the viral polymerase, it inhibits transcription and replication.[18,19] It also binds to cellular promyelocytic leukemia protein, but this is of unknown significance *in vivo*.[20] Finally, it can serve as an interferon antagonist.[21] The electron-dense granules that give arenaviruses their sandy appearance have been identified as host cell ribosomes.[22] The function of these ribosomes, if any, has yet to be determined.

The lipid envelope of arenavirions makes them susceptible to organic solvents and detergents. Virus infectivity can also be inactivated by exposure to temperatures above 55°C, acidic or basic pH, ultraviolet light, and gamma irradiation. Disinfectants containing phenolic compounds, hypochlorite, or quaternary amines effectively inactivate arenaviruses.[23]

Genomic Organization

The arenavirus genome consists of two single-stranded RNA molecules designated S (small) and L (large), the lengths of which are approximately 3.4 kb and 7.2 kb, respectively. Two genes are encoded on each RNA in an ambisense orientation. The NP gene is encoded at the 3′ end of the S RNA in the complementary sense, whereas the glycoprotein precursor (GPC) gene is encoded at the 5′ end of the S RNA in message sense. In a similar manner, the L protein is encoded at the 3′ end of the L RNA, and the Z protein gene is found at the 5′ end of the L RNA. The 19 nucleotides at the 3′ end of each genomic segment are similar in all arenaviruses and are partially inverted complements to the 19 nucleotides at the 5′ end of each RNA. This sequence complementarity allows genomic RNAs to form a circular conformation with short base paired "panhandle" structures necessary for efficient RNA synthesis. The conserved sequences at the ends of each genomic RNA are speculated to function as a binding site for the L protein. The genes on each viral RNA segment are separated by noncoding intergenic regions in both S and L segments. These intergenic regions have the potential to form several distinct stem-loop structures that are thought to play a role in transcriptional termination.[24]

Replication

Arenaviruses gain entry into cells by attachment of the GP1 glycoprotein to one or more cellular receptors. One of these serves for Old World and clade C arenaviruses and is a 120–140 kDa protein (α-dystroglycan) found on primate and rodent cells.[25,26] Another, human transferrin receptor 1, serves as the receptor for the human pathogenic clade B arenaviruses, Junin, Machupo, Sabia, and Guanarito; the specificity of these and related clade B arenaviruses for their rodent host molecule also appears to be related, at least in part, to their rodent species specificity.[27–30] Virus is then taken into large, smooth-walled vesicles where, in an acid environment, the GP2 glycoprotein mediates fusion between the virion

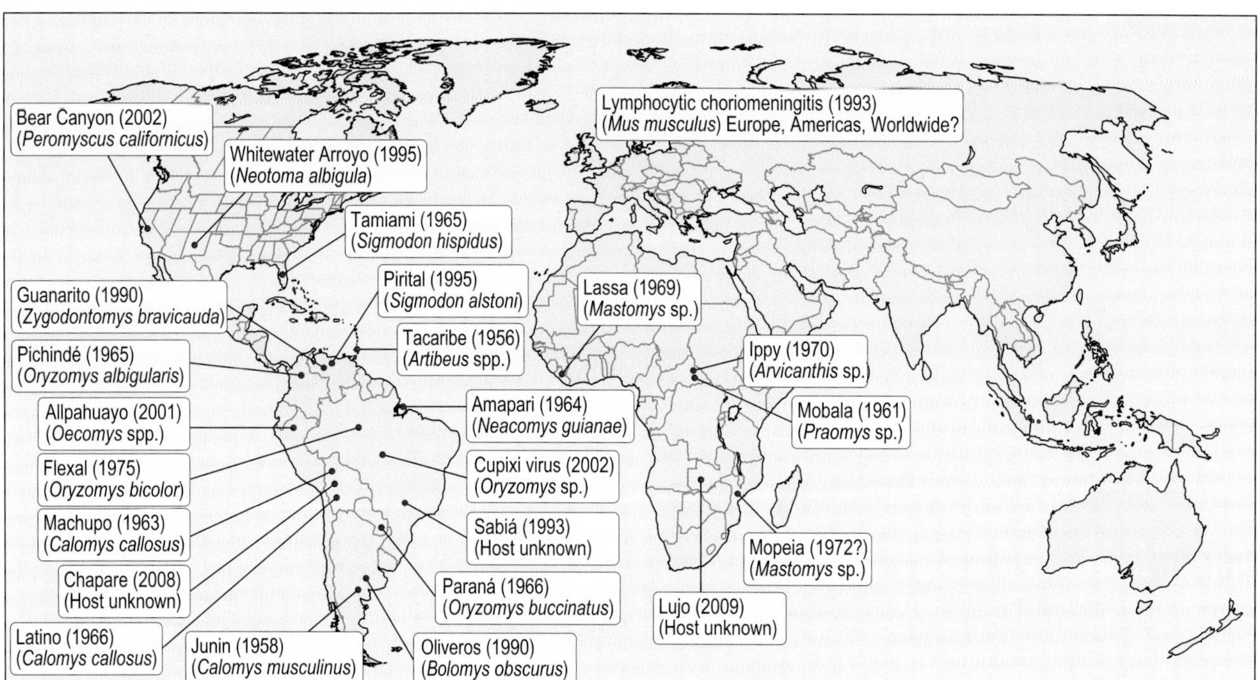

Figure 68.1 Recognized arenaviruses and their geographic distribution. Reservoirs are shown below the viruses in *italics*.

Table 68.1 Arenaviruses and Their Diseases

Virus	Disease	Clinical Manifestations
New World Viruses or Tacaribe Complex		
Junin	Argentine HF	Severe systemic disease with hemorrhage, prominent neurologic manifestations
Machupo	Bolivian HF	Resembles Argentine HF
Guanarito	Venezuelan HF	Resembles Argentine HF
Sabia	–	Limited experience suggests resemblance to Argentine HF but one case with prominent liver necrosis as well
Chapare	–	Severe VHF; few clinical data
Flexal	–	Two symptomatic laboratory infections observed; disease spectrum not defined
Pichinde	–	Asymptomatic
Amapari, Pirital, and others	–	Human infections not yet identified, pathogenicity unknown
Old World Viruses		
LCM	LCM	Acute febrile illness with thrombocytopenia and leukopenia; sometimes associated with orchitis; aseptic meningitis often follows the initial febrile period. Encephalitis rarely occurs; maternal infection may result in fetal hydrocephalus and chorioretinitis
Lassa	Lassa fever	Severe systemic illness; hemorrhagic manifestations or neurologic involvement sometimes seen
Lujo	–	Severe VHF; limited clinical data
Mopeia, Mobala	–	Human infection never observed, but laboratory animal studies suggest less pathogenic than Lassa virus
Unnamed new isolates	–	Human infection never observed

HF, hemorrhagic fever; LCM, lymphocytic choriomeningitis; VHF, viral hemorrhagic fever.

membrane and the endosomal membrane. This process releases nucleocapsids into the cytoplasm where replication takes place.[24]

The ambisense arrangement of arenavirus genes appears to provide a unique mechanism for regulating gene transcription, with genes lying at the 3′ end of each genomic vRNA (i.e., NP, L) being expressed first. Genes residing at the 5′ end of each genomic segment (i.e., GPC, Z) cannot be expressed in the absence of protein synthesis. To initiate gene expression, the viral L protein, which has RNA-dependent RNA polymerase activity and possibly endonuclease activity, is thought to cleave the cap and one to seven bases from cellular messenger RNAs (mRNAs) and use these primers to initiate transcription of subgenomic mRNAs ("cap snatching"). These mRNAs, which are not polyadenylated, are then translated by host cell ribosomes to produce NP and L proteins.[31,32]

Genes at the 5′ ends of genomic RNAs (i.e., GPC, Z) are not translated directly though they are in the proper coding sense. Viral genomic RNAs must go through the first stages of replication to obtain expression of these genes. In this process, the L protein is thought to initiate RNA replication using a dinucleotide template (pppGpC) rather than a capped primer, and a full-length, genome-complementary RNA species termed an antigenome is transcribed.[33] Newly synthesized RNAs are assumed to associate with NP and L proteins in the cytoplasm to produce nucleocapsids.

The zinc finger protein is required for viral and messenger RNA synthesis[34] and participates in viral particle formation. The protein serves as a matrix protein and interacts with the N protein, as well as driving particle formation.[24,35–37]

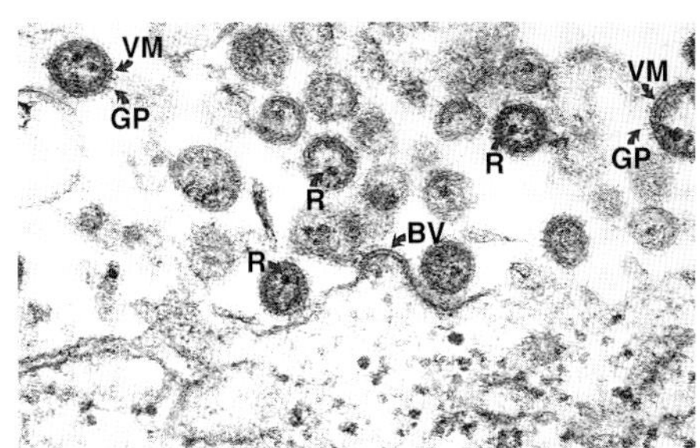

Figure 68.2 Electron micrograph of Machupo virions. Glycoprotein spikes (GP) are embedded in the virion membrane (VM). Electron-dense ribosomes (R) are present in the interior of the virions. A virion budding from a cell membrane (BV) is visible. (Courtesy of C. Goldsmith, Atlanta, GA; S. Zaki, Atlanta, GA; and F. Murphy, Galveston, TX.)

The GPC undergoes considerable processing that is only partially understood. After translation, GPC is truncated by cleavage of a signal peptide from the N-terminus, glycosylated, transported from the endoplasmic reticulum to the Golgi network, cleaved into GP1 and GP2, and transported to the plasma membrane where budding occurs[24] (***Fig. 68.2***). The cytoplasmic tail of GP2 interacts with NP, which, with the Z protein, may play a critical role in assembly and budding.[38]

Virology

Arenaviruses can replicate in a variety of cultured vertebrate cell lines including Vero, Vero E6, BHK-21, mouse L, pig kidney, rabbit kidney, human diploid, and HeLa cells.[4,39] In culture, arenavirus-infected cells usually appear normal. In some cell–virus combinations, cytopathic effect (CPE), characterized by cell rounding and detachment of cells from the culture vessel surface, can be observed. Different isolates of the same virus can differ in their ability to cause CPE in culture. Arenaviruses are somewhat slow growing in cell culture and will form plaques in 4–9 days when grown under a semisolid medium containing a vital stain such as neutral red.

Laboratory animal systems for isolating and propagating arenaviruses include mice, hamsters, and guinea pigs. Pathogenicity varies among viruses and can also differ among strains of the same virus. For example, low-passage isolates of Junin virus differ in their pathogenicity for guinea pigs and nonhuman primates.[40,41] In addition, the age of the animal host, host genotype, and the route of inoculation affect the outcome of infection.[42] New World arenaviruses are generally nonpathogenic for adult mice but may cause immunopathologic encephalitis after intracranial inoculation of weanling or newborn mice.[43–45] Most New World arenaviruses are pathogenic for suckling hamsters.[46]

Of the animal models using Old World arenaviruses, the infection process of LCM virus in mice has been the most intensively studied. Adult mice inoculated intracerebrally with LCM virus develop fatal, T-cell-mediated choriomeningitis whereas intraperitoneal inoculation results in an immunizing infection with viral clearance.[24] Suckling mice or immunosuppressed adults, on the other hand, develop a lifelong, persistent infection after inoculation, as do immunocompetent adults infected with the immunosuppressive Cl-13 strain of LCM virus.[47,48] With most LCM virus–mouse strain combinations, there is no acute disease in the newborn mouse, even after intracerebral inoculation, but chronic immune complex renal disease may develop if host–virus genetics result in antibody formation.[49] In mice and guinea pigs, the pathogenicity of other Old World arenaviruses is more variable, with the outcome of infection depending highly upon host genotype and virus strain.[42]

Persistence and Defective Interfering Virus

In natural rodent hosts, as well as in cell culture, arenavirus infections can shift from an acute phase, in which there is active viral replication and virus production, to a persistent phase characterized by a reduction in the amount of infectious virus produced. In persistent infection, most cells remain infected for life, and there are alterations in transcription, replication, and expression of viral proteins. In cell cultures, a small population of cells may be transiently infected, providing a constant pool of cells for reinfection.[50] A reduction in expression of the viral glycoproteins has been observed in cultured cells and mice persistently infected with LCM virus.[51–53] In persistently infected cells, there is an increase in the number of S genomic RNAs relative to the number of L genomic RNAs.[54,55] In addition, increased levels of NP mRNA can be detected, as well as populations of subgenomic length fragments of genomes and antigenomes.[56,57]

Even in the absence of CPE, arenavirus infections can impair normal cellular functions. Infection of murine endocrine cells with LCM virus decreases levels of growth hormone and thyroid hormone production.[58–60] This viral perturbation of cellular physiology appears to be selective for "luxury" functions, but "housekeeping" functions appear to be minimally affected. Chronic brain infection with LCM virus affects murine behavior, which has some correlates with transcriptional profiling results.[61–63]

Defective interfering (DI) virus, which is able to interfere with the infectivity of standard virus, is produced during acute and persistent arenavirus infections. When LCM virus stocks are passed at high multiplicity of infection in cell culture, the titer of infectious virus rises and falls with passage.[22] Peak titers can exceed trough titers by more than 1000-fold. This interference effect is presumably due to increased production of DI virus after high-titer inoculation, which competes with standard virus for viral packaging proteins in the subsequent passage. Infection of cultured cells with DI virus prior to challenge with standard LCM virus inhibits the replication of the standard virus.[64] Concurrent intracranial injection of DI virus with standard LCM virus inhibits cerebellar disease in a suckling rat model.[64] The potential participation of DI virus in establishing or maintaining chronic infections or in recovery from acute infections *in vivo* has yet to be established.

Antigenic and Genetic Relationships of Arenaviruses

Serologic assays, primarily the complement fixation (CF) test, indirect immunofluorescent antibody (IFA) test, neutralization assay, and enzyme-linked immunosorbent assay (ELISA), have been used to define the antigenic relationships of viruses within the *Arenaviridae*.[65–69] The CF and IFA tests, which primarily recognize epitopes on the NP, were first used to divide the arenaviruses into two groups, the Old World group and the New World group or Tacaribe complex, and disclosed that there is low-level antigenic relatedness between the two groups.

More refined IFA, ELISA, and neutralization tests further defined relationships among arenaviruses. Studies using monoclonal antibodies showed that epitopes on NP and GP2 are shared by Old World and New World arenaviruses[70] and demonstrated close antigenic relationships among Amapari, Junin, Machupo, and Tacaribe viruses and among Pichinde, Parana, and Tamiami viruses.[71] Within the Old World arenaviruses, Ippy, Lassa, Mobala, and Mopeia share certain antigenic determinants that distinguish the African arenaviruses from LCM virus.[72–74]

Analysis of genetic sequence data has provided the most complete picture of arenavirus relationships. New World arenaviruses comprise three evolutionary lineages that are designated lineages A, B, and C[75] (***Fig. 68.3***). Within the New World arenaviruses, lineage A contains Flexal, Parana, Pichinde, Pirital, Tamiami, and Whitewater Arroyo viruses. Lineage B contains the five agents of arenaviral HFs in the New World – Guanarito, Junin, Machupo, Sabia, and Chapare – as well as Amapari and Tacaribe viruses. Latino and Oliveros viruses compose lineage C. The newly discovered human pathogen, Lujo virus, is the most distant of the Old World viruses and lies closest to the New World viruses.[9] Among the other Old World arenaviruses, LCM virus is the next most closely related to the New World arenaviruses. Ippy virus occupies an intermediate position, whereas Mobala, Mopeia, and Lassa viruses make up the most distantly related group. Considerable sequence

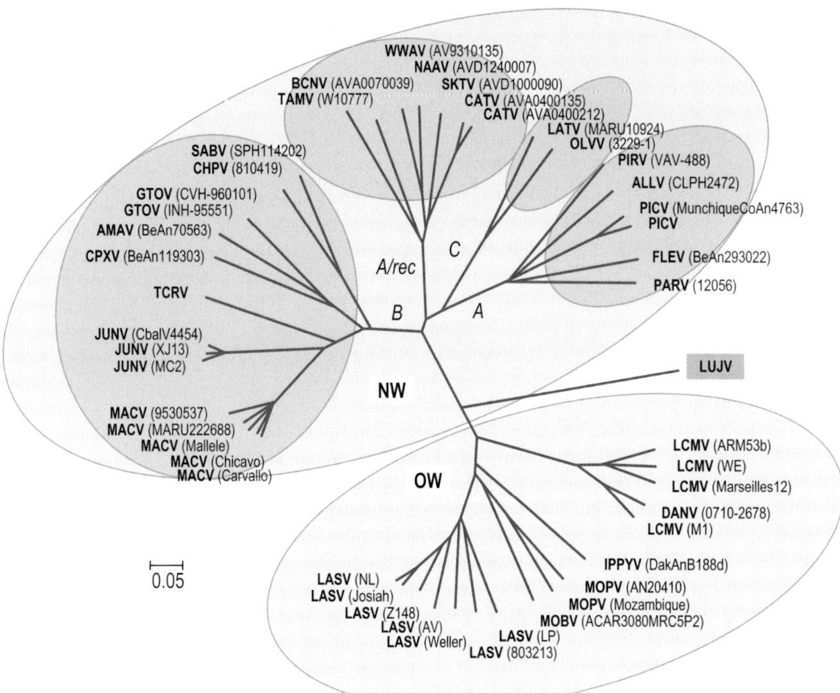

Figure 68.3 Phylogenetic relationships were inferred based on full S segment nucleotide sequences. Phylogenies were reconstructed by neighbor-joining analysis applying a Jukes–Cantor model; the scale bar indicates substitutions per site; not shown are similar phylogenies constructed from nucleotide sequences of L and amino acid sequences of other proteins with similar topology. Note the A, B, and C clades of the New World (NW) arenaviruses and the Old World (OW) arenaviruses are delineated. Note also that LUJV is an outlier between New World and Old World arenaviruses but appears to be closest to the Old World viruses, thus corresponding to its site of isolation in Zambia. (See Briese T, Paweska JT, McMullan LK, et al. Genetic detection and characterization of Lujo virus, a new hemorrhagic fever-associated arenavirus from southern Africa. PLoS Pathogens. 2009;5(5):e1000455.)

diversity, up to 25% nucleotide divergence, is observed among Lassa virus strains and some divergence is evident among Mopeia virus strains and strains of LCM virus. Within the pathogenic American arenaviruses, Guanarito has considerable (up to 17%) divergence.[5] Thus the relationships established by antigenic characterization are confirmed and further refined by analysis of genetic sequence data.

EPIDEMIOLOGY

Transmission Cycle

A hallmark of the *Arenaviridae* is the specificity of the host–virus relationship and the chronic, inapparent infection of the rodent host (***Fig. 68.4***). The Old World arenaviruses are associated with rodents of the family *Muridae*, subfamily *Murinae* (Old World rats and mice) and the New World viruses with the subfamily *Sigmodontinae* (New World rats and mice). This specific host–virus association appears to be a highly evolved form of parasitism, which may be the result of thousands of years of coevolution between each virus and its established rodent host species.[76,77] Receptor considerations may account for some of the specificity (see above and Abraham et al).[28] Maintenance of infection within reservoir populations may be via horizontal or vertical routes.[78] The chronically infected host is usually healthy and shows normal growth, behavior, and intraspecific interactions. As it moves through its environment and contacts other animals, the infected host may shed large quantities of virus in urine, feces, and saliva. Shed virus may be infectious to other animals via aerosol.[79,80] Venereal transmission between rodents may be highly efficient in some cases.[81] Transmission by bite, especially between adult males, may also be an important mechanism maintaining virus within reservoir populations.[82] However, the most important mechanism of virus perpetuation in some virus–host combinations is vertical transmission.[78,83–86]

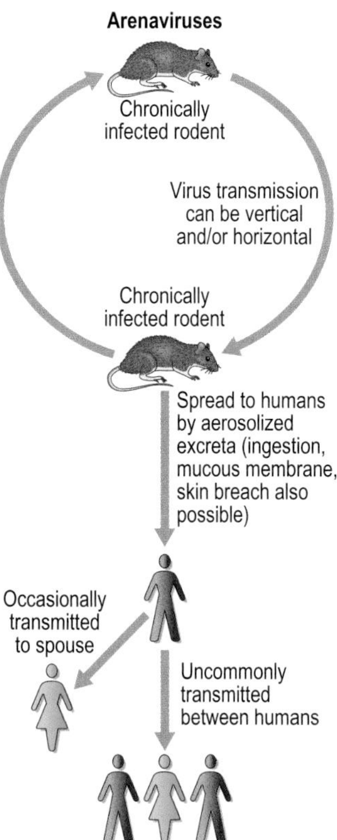

Figure 68.4 Transmission cycle of arenaviruses. These viruses chronically infect rodents. In some rodent–virus combinations there is lifelong viremia, and vertical transmission is very important in maintenance; in others, chronic virus shedding without persistent viremia occurs, or more complicated patterns are seen (see Childs and Peters).[78] In any case, humans are a dead-end host except in rare situations.

The actual mechanism of human infection from rodents is unknown. There is quite strong evidence that these viruses are aerosol infectious and that they readily spread from rodents to humans by this route. Aerosols of LCM, Lassa, and Junin viruses are all stable and infectious to nonhuman primates.[10,39,87,88] In addition, several studies clearly implicate aerosols as one route of human infection.[89–91] It is very likely that rodents shedding urine generate primary aerosols that are inhaled by humans to provide the major source of arenavirus disease. The survival of arenaviruses in rodent urine will be markedly affected by the pH (diet) and other components, particularly protein (some rodent species normally have proteins present in urine).

Other routes of human contamination are less likely but cannot be excluded. Although virus is readily detected in rodent throat swabs and feces, the quantity of virus output is much less, and the mechanisms that would generate aerosols are less apparent. Secondary aerosol generation is notoriously inefficient so disturbing shed urine is also a less likely source of infection. Conjunctival or other mucous membranes, ingestion, and occult cuts are possible routes of entry but similarly are less likely given the relative susceptibility to inactivation of arenaviruses in the environment, although virus survival in the dried state is not well defined. Oral infection, perhaps with a gastric portal, has clearly been demonstrated in the mice and macaques,[92,93] and it is well known that arenaviruses are highly infectious on scarified skin.[94] In some circumstances, humans may come into direct contact with reservoir rodents (see later Lassa fever discussion) and be intensively exposed by several routes.

Geography

The distribution of each arenavirus is limited to that of its rodent host, but it is often less than the range of the host, particularly in the Americas (see ***Fig. 68.1***). Within endemic areas, infection in host populations is often highly focal, and antibody prevalences in host populations vary considerably in both time and space. Factors in emergence are poorly understood, but one common theme with Bolivian[95] and Venezuelan HF[5,96–99] has been conversion of forest to cultivated fields, which has often resulted in "new" arenavirus diseases from viruses of the colonizing savanna rodents infecting humans. The human risk is particularly high if the rodent species enters towns and houses. Cleared forest areas in Africa are also at risk of Lassa fever from savanna-adapted reservoirs of the genus *Mastomys*.[100,101]

Argentine HF occurs in the humid pampas, the most fertile area of a country, which depends on agriculture for its prosperity. The Argentine HF endemic area includes only a part of the geographic range of the primary host species, the drylands vesper mouse (*Calomys musculinus*), which is common and widely distributed in central and northwestern Argentina.[102] A striking epidemiologic characteristic of Argentine HF is the steady and progressive geographic extension that occurred rapidly in the years after its discovery and has continued until the present. In 1958, cases were limited to an area of approximately 16 000 km^2, with the population at risk estimated to be 270 000 persons. At present, the endemoepidemic region covers an area of approximately 150 000 km^2 where an estimated 3 million people live. The incidence of Argentine HF is not the same in different areas of the pampas or in different years. In general, it is higher during a period of 5–10 years in the newly involved areas, and it later declines. Geographic extensions in the past decade have been smaller than those seen earlier.

Nevertheless, there is some continuing northward extension, as well as reemergence in historical areas that have not reported clinical disease in recent years.[2,103,104] The disease is both dramatic and characteristic so it is likely that the patterns based on clinical disease (confirmed by laboratory means after 1965; ***Fig. 68.5***) do indeed represent a valid measure of virus activity, particularly when the virologic data on rodents are considered.[82,105] The elucidation of the factors behind the spread of Argentine HF is the most important issue confronting our understanding of the epidemiology of arenavirus disease.

Bolivian HF is restricted to the Beni Department of Bolivia, although the range of *C. callosus* is much wider, including northern Argentina and

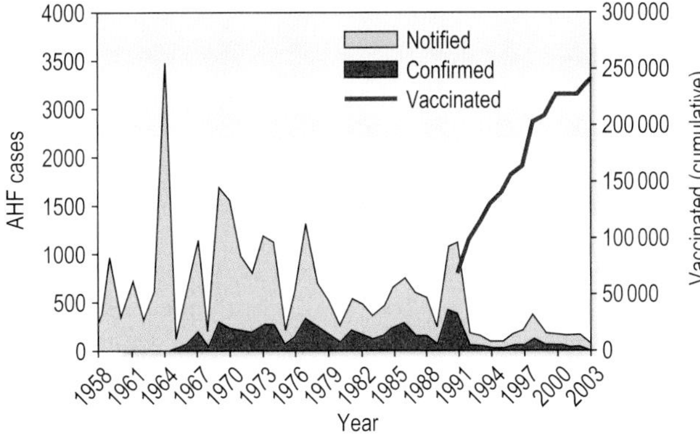

Figure 68.5 Annual cases of Argentine hemorrhagic fever (AHF) showing the decline in cases with vaccination of the critical at-risk adult population. After 1965, laboratory confirmation of cases began and, after 1977, the Instituto Nacional de Enfermedades Virales Humanos was responsible for laboratory confirmation of all cases with samples submitted.

Paraguay, through eastern Bolivia to east-central Brazil. Recent evidence suggests that this discrepancy may be explained, at least in part, by improvements in our understanding of the taxonomy of *Calomys*. The reservoir for Machupo virus appears to be a distinct species of *Calomys*, *C. hildebrandii*, not *C. callosus*, with a more restricted distribution.[106]

Venezuelan HF has been restricted to the municipality of Guanarito, in the southern tip of Portuguesa state, on the Venezuelan llanos.[96,99,107] The reservoir of Guanarito virus, *Zygodontomys brevicauda*, is a savanna species found from southeastern Costa Rica through Brazil north of the Amazon. Recent surveys have demonstrated the presence of Guanarito virus genotypes (some closely matching genotypes from case patients in the disease-endemic area) in host populations over a wide area of the Venezuelan llanos, including areas in five states up to several hundred kilometers from the disease-endemic area.

Lassa fever is a West African disease. The countries most often associated with it are Sierra Leone, Guinea, Liberia, and Nigeria. The extent of Lassa fever transmission in the intervening countries is not known with certainty, but there is evidence to suggest its presence in Côte d'Ivoire, Burkina Faso, Senegal, and related areas.[8,108–110] This broad geographic distribution in an area that enjoys considerable tourism from the United Kingdom and other developed countries makes Lassa fever the most exported of the viral HFs.[111–113] At least eight *Mastomys* species occur in Africa south of the Sahara, and their systematics and distribution are complex. Recently, molecular diagnostics for the species has clarified that Lassa virus is carried by *Mastomys natalensis*.[100,101,114–116] Infection in *Mastomys* populations varies by season and ecosystem, is focal within villages and between villages, and often correlates with human infection and disease.[86,115,117–119]

Several other Old World arenaviruses are known from African rodents (see ***Table 68.1 and Fig. 68.3***), but only one recently isolated virus, Lujo virus from Zambia, is pathogenic for humans.[9] It seems likely that with further research the patterns seen with the several African viruses will come to resemble those of their American relatives with a sprinkling of highly pathogenic agents among a number of apparently nonpathogenic viruses from other rodent species.[120]

LCM virus has a broad distribution wherever the common house mouse (*Mus musculus*) is found, including Europe, the Americas, Australia, and Japan.[83,121–129] *Both Mus m. domesticus* and *M. m. musculus* have yielded virus. The phylogenetic relationships of the viruses and the possible infection of other subspecies of *Mus* are unknown.

Transmission to Humans

Argentine Hemorrhagic Fever

Epidemics occur predominantly during the major harvesting season in Argentina, with a peak incidence in the month of May. The disease is four times as prevalent in males as in females, and is more prevalent among rural workers than in urban populations. Children under 14 years of age constitute about 10% of cases annually, but disease is uncommon in those less than 4 years old and exceptional in those less than 2 years of age. The seasonal distribution of the illness and the prevalence in male rural workers reflect occupational exposure of humans and the habits of the rodent host of Junin virus. Annual incidence within the endemic area may be as low as 1 in 100 000, but in the areas of highest activity it reaches 140 per 100 000 population and 355 per 100 000 adult males.

The Argentine HF endemic area is largely a patchwork of crop fields, which is crisscrossed by linear islands of relatively stable border habitats (roadsides, fence lines, and railroad rights of way). The primary host for Junin virus, the drylands vesper mouse (*C. musculinus*), is a habitat generalist. Although it is most frequently captured in stable border habitats, it ventures into mature and postharvest crop fields where it supplements its diet with grain from corn and soybeans. The drylands vesper mouse is rarely captured in or around human dwellings, although it may enter parklands and undeveloped areas adjacent to the surrounding pampas.[82,130,131] In the early years of Argentine HF, the men affected worked in close contact with the land and harvested crops by hand. Later, mechanized agricultural practices became common, but the workers in the field, especially tractor drivers, have continued to become infected. Cases may be associated with inhalation of infectious aerosols generated during the mechanized harvesting process, or with exposure to primary aerosols of rodent urine or contact with contaminated nesting materials in border habitats. The annual incidence of Argentine HF is positively correlated with local population densities of the reservoir. This epidemiologic pattern is being further modified through vaccination of high-risk populations (see ***Fig. 68.5***).

Argentine HF is not usually contagious, although person-to-person transmission can occur. A special situation is represented by a small number of women who are thought to have acquired the disease from their convalescent spouses through intimate contact.[108]

Bolivian Hemorrhagic Fever

The reservoir for Machupo virus is a species of the genus *Calomys* closely related but not identical to *C. callosus*. The host species resides in habitats where grassland intergrades into forest and, unlike *C. musculinus*, thrives in villages and near human habitations, which are found on high ground in seasonally inundated areas of the Beni Department. Bolivian HF tends to be a seasonal disease, with more cases occurring in the dry season, at the peak of agricultural activity. Most sporadic cases have involved adult men in rural areas, probably via contact with the rodent host in agricultural settings or in isolated small cottages.

However, family and community clusters of Bolivian HF cases affecting both sexes and all age groups have been centered around towns or hospitals. Epidemics in towns may occur during epizootic conditions when rodent densities reach unusually high levels and rodents invade towns or villages. In 1963–1964, a Bolivian HF epidemic occurred in the village of San Joaquin that resulted in 637 cases and 113 deaths among the town's 3000 residents. The outbreak ended abruptly after 2 weeks of continuous trapping in homes, during which 3000 *C. callosus* rodents were captured.[95,132,133] Transmission to humans under these conditions is likely from inhalation of infectious aerosols concentrated within confined spaces of houses and outbuildings, but direct contact of broken skin or mucous membranes with rodent excreta or contaminated fomites such as food is also a consideration. Disease fell to low levels after trapping in towns was instituted and consisted mostly of cases associated with agriculture. Recently, however, there has been a marked upsurge in cases.[134]

Person-to-person transmission, likely via direct contact with infectious body fluids, may occur in familial or nosocomial settings. For example, five health care workers who were exposed to the index case or a secondary case contracted Bolivian HF in a hospital in Cochabamba in 1971,[135] and in 1994 a farm worker transmitted fatal Bolivian HF to six of eight family members.[4] Transmission by intimate contact during convalescence is also possible.[136]

Venezuelan Hemorrhagic Fever

In 1989, a severe HF was recognized by clinicians in the municipality of Guanarito, Portuguesa State, Venezuela. At first, efforts toward laboratory diagnosis centered on dengue viruses, but the causative agent was soon isolated, shown to be an arenavirus, and named Guanarito virus. Guanarito virus is specifically associated with *Z. brevicauda*, while a second arenavirus, Pirital virus, is associated with co-occurring *Sigmodon alstoni*. Within the Venezuelan HF endemic area, both rodent species are commonly captured in crop fields, borders, and roadside habitats, and they are only rarely captured in the peridomestic environment.

While cases have been observed throughout the year, epidemics appear to have a seasonal peak in November to January, coinciding with maximum agricultural activity in the endemic region. Although children and adults of both sexes suffer disease, the highest risk is among adult male agricultural workers. Thus transmission to humans likely occurs most frequently outside the home and may be related to agricultural activities.[5,6,97–99,137,138] Person-to-person transmission or nosocomial infection has not been observed in spite of the fact that Venezuelan HF patients, like other South American HF patients, are usually admitted to open wards with minimal isolation precautions.

Chapare Virus Disease

This virus was isolated from a case of classic viral HF occurring in 2004 as part of a cluster of cases in a village near the Chapare River near Cochabamba, Bolivia on the eastern slopes of the Andes. There is little additional information available.[139]

Lymphocytic Choriomeningitis

The natural rodent reservoir of the virus is the cosmopolitan house mouse, *M. musculus*, although outbreaks of human disease have also been traced to pet hamsters (*Mesocricetus auratus*) in the United States,[140] Germany,[141] and France.[142,143] As its name implies, the house mouse frequently lives in close association with humans within homes and other man-made structures in both rural and urban situations. Infection with LCM virus in house mouse populations can be highly focal. In inner-city Baltimore, antibody-positive mice were clustered within residential blocks; infection varied from 0% (0/753) to 27% (214/594) of mice on four farms in California.[144,145]

The incidence of human disease peaks in the fall and winter, presumably reflecting the seasonal invasion of homes by mice. As expected, human disease is associated with the prevalence of mouse infection and can vary by region or even by house.[121,146,147] Risk of infection is higher among rural dwellers and, in the United States, in low-income groups.[148] Human seroprevalence to LCM virus has often been found to range from 5% to 10% in the United States and elsewhere.[83,121,148,149] An antibody survey using hospital patients in Birmingham, Alabama, showed a prevalence of IgG antibody to LCM virus that was much lower in younger patients than in patients over 30 years of age, although it was not known whether this represented a secular decrease in risk of infection in recent decades or a lower risk in children. The number of acute LCM cases annually is not known because diagnostic testing is not commonly performed; during the period 1941–1958, LCM was the confirmed diagnosis in about 10% of patients with febrile CNS disease admitted to a tertiary care hospital in Washington, DC.[150,151]

Lassa Fever

Lassa fever is an extremely common infection among adults in endemic areas of West Africa. In a heavily affected region such as Sierra Leone's Eastern Province, the disease may be responsible for more than one-fourth of medical admissions and of medical deaths.[119] In the same area it is also common among pediatric admissions.[152] Because of the similar incidence of disease among men and women and the frequent involvement of children, peridomestic exposure is likely to be important.[117] Indeed, rodent density may be higher in houses than in the surrounding agricultural or bush areas. In this setting, transmission to humans may occur via inhalation of primary aerosols from rodent urine, by contact with contaminated fomites, or by ingestion of contaminated food. Human infection is also enhanced by the practice of hunting and consuming rodents as a food source, as well as the high levels of rodent infestation, open food storage, and closed shutters during the day – a practice that favors prolonged rodent activity.[119] These factors are exacerbated in the diamond-mining areas of Sierra Leone and during civil disruption. In Guinea, cases are clustered during the dry season and early part of the rainy season, coinciding with the period of maximum infection in *Mastomys* populations.[87,116–118] The breakdown of living patterns associated with wartime activities in West Africa has also resulted in an increase in Lassa fever incidence.[153,154]

Interhuman transmission of Lassa fever occurs, but it is difficult to quantitate because of the frequent presence of infected *Mastomys* in houses. At least one outbreak provided evidence of person-to-person transmission of Lassa virus without confounding infected rodents or reported needle use.[155–157] Although rare, devastating hospital outbreaks have occurred and have been attributed to aerosols[158,159] or to lack of sterilization of parenteral injection equipment.

Lujo Virus Disease

This virus was isolated from an index case presumably infected near Lusaka, Zambia and four contact cases. Little is known about the distribution or natural host of the virus. This cluster of cases included an air evacuation attendant, a nurse, and a cleaner in Johannesburg. Later a second nurse who cared for the other Johannesburg nurse became ill and was the only survivor. The epidemiology raises the question of aerosol transmission, but barrier nursing was not uniformly practiced. It should be remembered that the initial isolation of Lassa virus occurred in a similar episode, but subsequent studies showed much lower interpersonal transmissibility.[160–162]

Maintenance of the Virus in Rodent Host Populations

Argentine Hemorrhagic Fever

Junin virus is likely maintained in *C. musculinus* reservoir populations primarily via horizontal transmission. When transmitted vertically, the virus may have important deleterious effects on fitness. Newborn *C. musculinus* infected with Junin virus in the laboratory have high mortality (70%), and survivors show stunting and greatly reduced fecundity.[163,164] Animals infected in the laboratory as adults showed a split response. Half of the animals developed antibody and cleared virus; the remainder had chronic viremia and persistent shedding of virus in urine and saliva; there was no obvious deleterious effect on these chronically infected adults. Field studies of natural populations demonstrated that infection with Junin virus among wild *C. musculinus* was more frequent among males than females and was positively correlated with age and the presence of wounds or scars. These data suggest that aggressive encounters between adult males may be an important mechanism of transmission within reservoir populations.

Bolivian Hemorrhagic Fever

As with Junin virus, vertical transmission of Machupo virus would have a severe effect on host reproductive fitness of its reservoir rodent. In the laboratory, females inoculated at birth were chronically infected and sterile. Also, as was later shown to be the case with Junin virus and *C. musculinus*, colonized *Calomys* rodents infected with Machupo virus as adults showed a split response: half developed antibody and cleared viral infection, while half showed chronic viremia and viruria. Longitudinal field studies are needed to assess the mechanisms of transmission of Machupo virus in natural populations.

Venezuelan Hemorrhagic Fever

Laboratory experiments indicate that the maintenance pattern for Guanarito virus in *Z. brevicauda* may be different from either the Junin or Machupo models.[137] Newborn *Z. brevicauda* inoculated subcutaneously with Guanarito virus developed a chronic infection with persistent shedding of virus in urine and saliva. There was no detectable effect of infection on growth of these animals (after 3 weeks). Subcutaneous inoculation of adult animals resulted in a split response. Four of 12 animals showed only transient viremia, followed by the development of high-titer neutralizing and immunofluorescent antibody. The remainder showed chronic viremia and persistent shedding of virus in urine and saliva. Eleven females that had been inoculated with Guanarito virus as adults had only two apparently normal litters after being paired with males, while 11 sham-inoculated females had 10 litters. Thus, horizontal transmission of virus has an apparent negative effect on reproductive fitness. The presence of virus in the blood of one of three pups born to an infected female indicates that vertical transmission is possible, but the fecundity of females infected as newborns has not been studied.[135]

Chapare Virus

This virus is only known from a human isolate, and the rodent reservoir is not identified. The habitat is different from that of *Calomys hildebrandii* so, in keeping with the usual rule for arenaviruses, it probably does not share a rodent host with Machupo virus.[139]

Lassa Fever and Lymphocytic Choriomeningitis

In contrast to the pattern with the New World arenaviruses, LCM and Lassa viruses are thought to be maintained by vertical transmission within reservoir populations. All pups born to chronically infected females are themselves chronically infected (perhaps transovarially).[165] Conversely, inoculation of adult hosts with LCM or Lassa virus results in an immunizing infection; young born to immunized animals are also protected by maternal antibody. This pattern was observed in field studies of Lassa virus in Guinea; most animals trapped were naïve, or chronically infected, with only occasional antibody-positive rodents.[84,166] Thus, strict horizontal transmission of virus within host populations would likely result in its rapid extinction.

THE DISEASES

Clinical Manifestations

The South American HFs resemble one another, and Argentine HF is the best described. Lassa fever has a similar pathogenesis, but neurologic involvement, thrombocytopenia, leukopenia, and bleeding manifestations are less prominent.

Argentine Hemorrhagic Fever

The incubation period is usually 6–14 days with outer limits of 4–21 days. The onset of illness is insidious, with chills, malaise, anorexia, headache, myalgias, and moderate hyperthermia (38–39°C). After several days, this gives way to further constitutional, gastrointestinal, neurologic, and cardiovascular signs and symptoms. Low backache, retro-orbital pain, nausea or vomiting, epigastric pain, photophobia, dizziness, and constipation or mild diarrhea are common symptoms. An almost constant absence of productive cough, sore throat, or nasal congestion is helpful in distinguishing the initial symptoms of Argentine HF from those of influenza or other acute respiratory infections.

During the first week of illness, physical examination reveals flushing of the face, neck, and upper chest. Conjunctival congestion and periorbital edema may also occur. The oropharyngeal membranes are congested, and there is congestion of the vessels bordering the gums, which may bleed spontaneously or under slight pressure. An enanthem characterized by petechiae and small vesicles is almost invariably found over the soft palate if carefully sought.[167] Most patients have cutaneous petechiae in the axillary regions, upper chest, and arms. Lymph nodes become enlarged, particularly in the lateral cervical regions. There are no signs of pulmonary abnormalities. Relative bradycardia and orthostatic hypotension are common. Generally, there is no hepatomegaly or splenomegaly, and jaundice is very rare.

At the end of the first week of evolution, oliguria and different degrees of dehydration occur. Neurologic signs are very common. The patient may be irritable and lethargic, with a fine tremor of the hand and tongue. Moderate ataxia, cutaneous hyperesthesia, and a decrease in deep tendon reflexes and muscular tonicity are present. In females, mild to moderate metrorrhagia is constantly present and, in some cases, is the first sign of the disease.

During the second week of illness, 70–80% of the patients begin to improve. In the remaining 20–30%, severe hemorrhagic or neurologic manifestations, shock, and superimposed bacterial infections appear between 8 and 12 days after the onset of symptoms. Profuse bleeding may occur in the form of hematemesis, melena, hemoptysis, epistaxis, hematomas, metrorrhagia, or hematuria. The severe neurologic manifestations generally begin with confusion, marked ataxia, increased irritability, and intention tremors; these are followed by delirium, generalized convulsions, and coma. Acute renal failure is uncommon, but may occur in terminal cases or after prolonged periods of shock, and is secondary to acute tubular necrosis. Superimposed bacterial infections such as pneumonia and septicemia or thrush can also complicate the clinical course.

Patients begin to improve by the third week of illness and experience a prolonged convalescence. Temporary hair loss is common. Many patients have asthenia, irritability, and memory changes, but these disappear gradually over a period of 1–3 months. During convalescence, 10% of Argentine HF patients treated with immune plasma develop a late neurologic syndrome. This late neurologic syndrome appears after a period of 7–80 days (mean, 20 days) free of symptoms, differs from the neurologic manifestations of the acute period of Argentine HF, and is characterized by fever and cerebellar signs as well as cranial nerve palsies.[168–170]

Clinical laboratory studies are quite helpful in establishing an early clinical diagnosis in South American HF. During the acute phase, there is progressive leukopenia and thrombocytopenia, with counts falling to 1000–2000 white blood cells (WBCs) and 50 000–100 000 platelets per μL. The sedimentation rate is normal or decreased. Almost invariably, there is proteinuria and urinary sediment containing hyaline-granular casts and red blood cells. Round cells with cytoplasmic inclusions are also found, but are not diagnostic. Serum creatinine and urea are normal or increased in proportion to dehydration and shock in the severely ill patient. In Argentine HF, aspartate transaminase (AST), creatine phosphokinase (CPK), and lactate dehydrogenase (LDH) elevations are common but mild, and hyperbilirubinemia or hyperamylasemia is rare. During the acute illness, cerebrospinal fluid (CSF) is normal, even in patients with severe neurologic disease. However, during the late neurologic syndrome following immune plasma therapy, the CSF may have tens to hundreds of cells with normal sugar and normal or slightly increased protein concentration.

Argentine HF during pregnancy is uncommon, but in the last trimester more than half of patients die, at least in part due to tardy recognition of the disease and failure to administer specific treatment. Congenital malformations, fetal death, and death of neonates have also been seen.[171] Children tend to have a milder clinical course, but severe and even fatal disease has occurred.

Other South American Hemorrhagic Fevers

Bolivian HF[95] and Venezuelan HF[172,173] have clinical characteristics similar to those of Argentine HF. Bolivian HF cases from a nosocomial outbreak occurring at high altitude had jaundice and a high mortality, but the reason was not determined. Patients with Venezuelan HF frequently complain of sore throat among their initial symptoms, and hearing loss in convalescence has been reported.

Only a single naturally acquired infection with Sabia virus has been identified, and it resembled other South American HFs except for extensive liver necrosis and jaundice. One laboratory infection appeared to be a mild case of HF, and a second was treated, apparently successfully, with ribavirin and developed only mild disease.[174]

Lassa Fever

Lassa fever occurs in both sexes and all age groups. Typically, after an incubation period of about 10 days (range, 3–21 days), the patient notes the insidious onset of fever, headache, generalized weakness, and malaise.[118,162,175–180] Within a few days, these may be followed by sore throat with or without visible pharyngitis, cough, retrosternal chest pain, conjunctivitis, abdominal pain, and a variety of other generalized symptoms. The minority of patients with florid Lassa fever may then manifest facial and neck swelling, subconjunctival hemorrhage, and bleeding. The bleeding is typically mild oozing from the nose, mouth, or genitourinary or gastrointestinal tract and, with the exception of vaginal bleeding in pregnant women, is unlikely to be hemodynamically significant. Maculopapular or petechial rashes have been observed in white-skinned, but not black-skinned patients. Whether this difference reflects ease of observation or different manifestations of Lassa fever based on host genetic makeup is uncertain.

Elevated respiratory rates, with or without mild rales on lung auscultation, are frequently noted. Hypotension and tachycardia may be present, especially in more severe cases. Pleural effusions are common, and pericardial effusions are occasionally seen late in the course of the disease, particularly in males. A variety of encephalopathic and other neurologic manifestations have been noted in severely ill patients, but it is not clear to what extent these represent direct effects of Lassa virus on the CNS, secondary immune-mediated effects, or nonspecific metabolic ones common to any critically ill patient.[181]

Surviving patients generally begin to defervesce within approximately 10 days of onset. With the exception of sensorineural deafness (see following discussion), recovery is usually complete. Conversely, patients with severe illness may deteriorate rapidly, progressing to shock, delirium, respiratory distress, coma, seizures, and death. The contributions of poor fluid balance, nutritional status, and degree of patient monitoring in this setting of limited resources are unknown. Other underlying health problems such as malnutrition, tuberculosis, and acquired immunodeficiency syndrome (AIDS), as well as nosocomial infections, may affect the clinical course of Lassa fever as well.

Lassa fever in pregnant women carries a significantly elevated risk for both the mother and the fetus. Maternal mortality is particularly elevated during the third trimester, when fetal death approaches 100%.[182,183]

Pediatric Lassa fever is less well described but produces a spectrum of disease ranging from undifferentiated febrile illness to severe Lassa fever.[152,176,184] A "swollen baby syndrome" consisting of anasarca, abdominal distension, and bleeding with high mortality has been described in several Liberian infants. Whether this syndrome is a general feature of Lassa virus infection of infants or related to other concomitant health risks or therapies specific to the area of study is not clear.

Abnormalities in clinical laboratory measurements are usually mild to moderate. Thrombocytopenia, usually not less than 100 000/μL, may be seen. Although often normal, a mild diminution in the WBC count with lymphopenia may occur.[178,180,185] Severely ill patients are more likely to be thrombocytopenic, are usually lymphopenic, and may have an elevated WBC count with neutrophilia. Moderate hemoconcentration and proteinuria are usually present with an elevated blood urea nitrogen (BUN).[162,175,177,178] These are likely a result of capillary leak, fever, and decreased fluid intake resulting in loss of intravascular volume. The AST is often elevated, and higher values are predictive of a poor prognosis, as is the level of viremia.[186] The disproportionate elevation in AST compared to the alanine transaminase (ALT) suggests that its source is not solely the liver but rather may result from diffuse ischemic end-organ damage. Disseminated intravascular coagulation (DIC) is not part of the pathogenesis of Lassa fever. A variety of nonspecific electrocardiographic changes have been reported.[187] Based on limited observations, radiographic studies are usually nonspecific and correlate with the physical examination.

Sensorineural deafness is the major chronic sequela of Lassa fever and may occur in up to one-fourth of those infected. Typically, the deafness presents during convalescence. There is no correlation with the severity of the acute febrile illness, level of viremia, or AST. It may be uni- or bilateral and is permanent in approximately two-thirds of cases.[188,189] Depression and cerebellar ataxia have been reported during recovery, but are relatively uncommon. Lassa virus can often be isolated from CSF; however, a systematic correlation with any of the neurologic manifestations of the disease is not available.[181]

Although a broad range of case-fatality rates from Lassa fever has been reported, about 15% is a good estimate in the patient seeking medical treatment. Nigerian outbreaks have often been associated with a higher mortality than those in countries further west in Africa. Community investigations conducted in Sierra Leone found milder infections to be common, but the role of preexisting immunity is unresolved. The presence of bleeding, high viremia or antigenemia, and elevated AST independently confer a poor prognosis.[119,180]

Lujo Virus Infection

Little is known except for the cluster of nosocomial cases. The disease seems to resemble Lassa fever. There was severe disease in the Lujo infections with four fatalities among five cases. There was relatively little hemorrhage.[190]

Lymphocytic Choriomeningitis

Typical LCM is characterized by two phases, a period of fever and viremia followed by a CNS phase in which virus no longer circulates, antibodies are found in serum, but virus is still present in the CNS[89,90,142,143,149–151,191–193] (reviewed in Lehmann-Grube[83] and Peters).[194,195] Neurologic disease is presumed to be immunopathologic and mediated by $CD8^+$ T cells, as is the process seen in the intracranially infected adult mouse.[24,196–198] Immunosuppressed patients inoculated with LCM virus did not develop CNS signs, although virus grew in the brain. A substantial proportion of infections are subclinical, some of the remainder consist of fever alone, and others show both the initial febrile phase and the CNS disease, often with a short afebrile remission between the two.

The disease may begin with abrupt onset of fever, malaise, and myalgia with additional weakness, gastrointestinal symptoms, and occasionally sore throat or cough. Arthralgia, testicular pain, parotid pain, or even frank inflammation may occur. During this phase, which may last from a few days to 2–3 weeks, leukopenia, lymphopenia, thrombocytopenia, and elevation of LDH and AST are seen.

The neurologic phase begins with aseptic meningitis, usually after a short period of defervescence, but possibly continuous with the initial febrile stage or even without preceding fever. The findings are those of aseptic meningitis, but headache may be severe and disturbances of consciousness may be seen. Signs of nervous system involvement may last 1–4 weeks and virtually always resolve without sequelae. Rarely, LCM may present as encephalitis with a very occasional fatal outcome; in the latter case, cerebral neuronal invasion can be demonstrated.[199] The CSF may have normal or low glucose, and cell counts often reach hundreds to thousands of lymphocytes per μL.

Convalescence may be delayed for several weeks with asthenia, febrile sensations, difficulties in memory, poor cognitive function, headaches, or arthralgia.

Occasionally, LCM virus infection has been associated with ascending paralysis, Parkinson's syndrome, transverse myelitis, or myocarditis, but a causal link remains to be established. Deafness has rarely been reported with LCM[200] and may be a feature, based on the similarity to Lassa fever. Rarely, LCM virus has caused a syndrome resembling viral HF.[201]

As in other arenavirus diseases, LCM virus can cross the placenta, with fetal infection or death.[202–204] The most common manifestation identified has been hydrocephalus with chorioretinitis. This was first reported from Lithuania[203,205,206] but has been confirmed in Germany,[121,202] France,[207] and more recently by several cases in the United States.[208–214] This is probably a much more common problem than appreciated.[215]

An emerging problem is the occurrence of LCM viral infection in transplant donors. It has been known for some time that the virus can infect tumors and be carried over into recipients, even after prolonged storage of the tumor in liquid nitrogen, and this has been a notable problem in nude, athymic mice because their immunodeficiency prevents their recognizing and possibly rejecting the tumor.[91,216,217] It is also known that immunosuppressed tumor patients inoculated with LCM virus in hopes of inducing a remission develop a severe viremic illness resembling Lassa fever.[196] Thirteen recipients from three different organ donors developed serious disease with fever, thrombocytopenia, coagulopathy, and multiorgan failure.[218,219] The single survivor was treated with ribavirin as his immunosuppression was carefully decreased. Only one of the donors had a suspicious contact with a rodent; a hamster was shown to be infected with the same strain of LCM virus, and the supplier's colony was also infected.[220]

PATHOLOGY

Animal Models

Natural and experimental infection of different animals, including guinea pigs, rats, hamsters, and nonhuman primates, has provided useful information on the comparative pathology of arenavirus infections. Lassa virus infection of rhesus monkeys, squirrel monkeys, and guinea pigs demonstrated a wide spectrum of organ tropism involving liver, spleen, lymph nodes, heart, lungs, pancreas, kidneys, and adrenal glands at early stages of infection. The common pathologic findings include hepatocellular necrosis and regeneration, lymphoid necrosis in spleen and lymph nodes, myocarditis, focal arteritis, renal tubular necrosis, and late mononuclear choriomeningoencephalitis.[84,166,221–223]

LCM virus infection of marmosets and tamarins can induce a highly fatal disease (callitrichid hepatitis). The histopathologic lesions are similar to those in human Lassa fever and consistently show focal necrosis in the liver, spleen, lymph nodes, adrenal glands, intestine, and pancreas.[224] In addition, LCM virus causes a viral HF syndrome in rhesus monkeys,[42,225–227] so it is not surprising that rarely human infection by LCM virus may also produce manifestations resembling HF.[201]

Machupo virus infection of rhesus and African green monkeys causes hemorrhage and necrosis in multiple organs. The hemorrhages are present in the skin, heart, brain, and nasal mucosa; necrosis is observed in the liver, adrenal cortex, myocardium, gastrointestinal mucosa, lymphoid tissue, and epithelial cells of the tongue, mouth, esophagus, and skin. Animals that die late in the course of Machupo virus infection frequently have meningoencephalitis and bronchopneumonia.[228,229]

Junin virus infection of rhesus monkeys, marmosets, and guinea pigs produces lesions similar to reported human cases of Argentine HF. The common findings include hemorrhage, bone marrow necrosis, mild hepatocellular necrosis, polioencephalomyelitis, and autonomic ganglioneuritis.[230,231]

Guanarito virus infection of guinea pigs results in focal epithelial cell necrosis of the gastrointestinal tract, interstitial pneumonia, and lymphoid and hematopoietic cell necrosis. Viral antigen is present in lymphoid tissues, macrophages, endothelial cells of multiple organs, pulmonary epithelium, epithelium of the gastrointestinal tract, and other tissues. Intact virions and typical arenavirus inclusions are visualized by immune electron microscopy in these same tissues.[232]

Human Pathology

Pathologic descriptions of arenavirus infections in humans are limited to a few necropsy series.[84,222,233–235] Gross and microscopic pathologic findings in these human cases are generally similar among different arenavirus infections.[84,236] Common gross findings at postmortem examinations include ecchymoses and petechiae involving skin, conjunctivae, mucous membranes, and internal organs. The degree of hemorrhage varies, and sometimes can be minimal or absent. Conjunctival suffusion, pleural effusion, pericardial effusion, and ascites are frequently present.

Microscopically, congestion and variable degrees of necrosis are usually observed in multiple organ systems. Necrosis is most prominent in the liver (***Fig. 68.6***) and spleen, but is also frequently found in adrenal gland, kidney, and gastrointestinal mucosa. The most consistent histopathologic feature is seen in the liver and comprises multifocal hepatocellular necrosis with cytoplasmic eosinophilia, Councilman body formation, nuclear pyknosis, cytolysis, and fatty metamorphosis. Inflammatory cell infiltrates in necrotic areas are usually minimal and, when present, consist of a mixture of mononuclear cells and neutrophils. The spleen usually shows depletion of follicles and focal necrosis. Other pathologic features that may be present in arenavirus infections include mild interstitial pneumonitis, diffuse alveolar damage, myocardial necrosis, and acute renal tubular necrosis.

Because none of these pathologic features are specific, a confirmatory assay such as immunohistochemistry or *in situ* hybridization is essential to establish a definitive tissue diagnosis, and such assays can also delineate the spectrum of tissue tropism as well as elucidate possible pathogenic mechanisms.

In Lassa fever, the localization of viral antigens can be summarized as: (1) hepatocytes, especially those in the areas of necrosis (***Fig. 68.7***); (2) cells of the mononuclear phagocytic system such as Kupffer cells in hepatic sinusoids, alveolar macrophages, and endothelial cells; (3) mesothelial cells lining the pericardium, pleura, peritoneum, and serosal surfaces of other organs; and (4) specialized cells involved in hormone secretion, including those in the adrenal gland, ovary, uterus, placenta, and breast.

In Argentine HF, ultrastructural and immunohistochemical studies reveal characteristic intracellular viral inclusions that are more prominent in lymphoid tissues, coincident with the presence of Junin virus antigens. Macrophages are usually the cell type involved, although there is often necrosis in adjacent lymphocytes.[237–239] In the kidney, a large number of virus-like intracytoplasmic particles are found in distal and collecting tubules coincident with severe tissue necrosis and large quantities of Junin virus antigen as demonstrated by immunofluorescence. Morphologic studies of the bone marrow indicate that an acute and transient arrest of hemopoiesis occurs, with bone marrow hypocellularity, but without permanent hematologic sequelae in survivors.

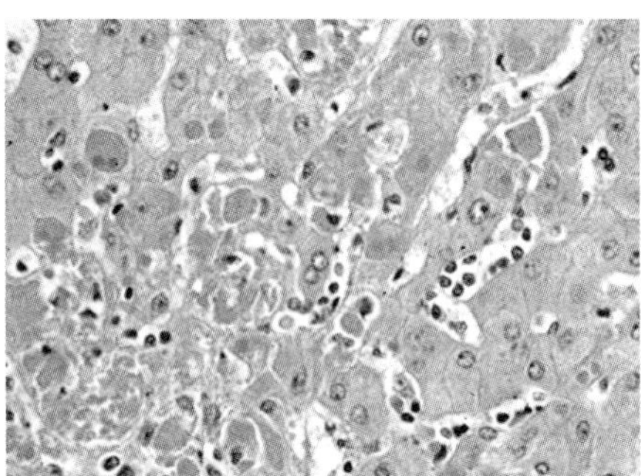

Figure 68.6 Lassa virus infection in the liver, showing multifocal hepatocellular necrosis with cytoplasmic eosinophilia, nuclear pyknosis, cytolysis, and fatty metamorphosis. (Hematoxylin and eosin stain.)

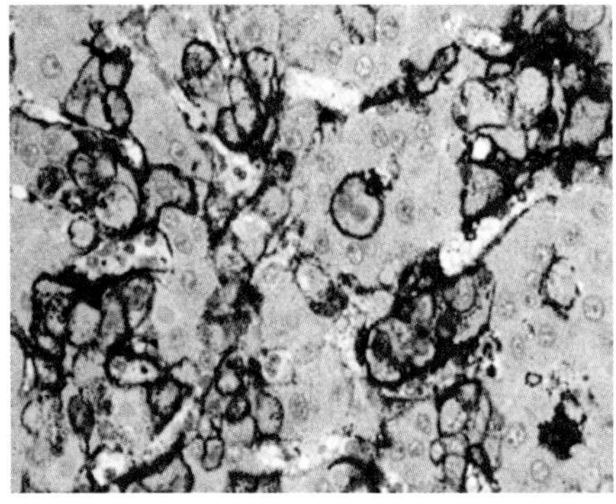

Figure 68.7 Antigens of Lassa virus are present in hepatocytes and sinusoidal lining cells, including Kupffer cells and endothelial cells. (Immunoalkaline phosphatase staining, naphthol fast red substrate with light hematoxylin counterstain.)

Although further study is needed, some possible pathogenetic mechanisms in arenavirus infections can be suggested from these findings.

1. The presence of abundant Lassa virus antigens in or adjacent to the necrotic hepatocytes and Junin virus particles near necrotic foci in the kidney suggests that cellular necrosis can be a consequence of direct viral infection. Although hepatocellular necrosis is the most consistent histopathologic feature in arenavirus infections, it alone is insufficient to explain the fatal outcome in most instances.
2. Lymphoid tissues are the main sites of viral replication, as evidenced by the large amount of viral antigen present, high virus titers, lymphocytopenia and lymphocyte depletion in spleen and lymph nodes.
3. The widespread hemorrhages in arenavirus infections do not appear to be a result of DIC or clotting factor abnormalities; instead, the interactions of viral antigens with platelets, inflammatory cells, macrophages, and endothelial cells may play a more critical role in pathogenesis. The infection of macrophages and endothelial cells may induce secretion of physiologically active substances, including cytokines and other inflammatory mediators, and subsequently cause microvascular instability leading to capillary leak syndrome.
4. The involvement of mesothelial cells can explain serous effusions commonly seen in patients with arenavirus infections.
5. The presence of viral antigens in hormone-secreting cells suggests that an interaction between arenaviruses and hormone receptors may exist. This interaction may further enhance the pathogenicity of the virus and cause more severe pathophysiologic effects. These effects might contribute to the higher mortality of pregnant women with Lassa fever and Argentine HF.

PATHOGENESIS AND IMMUNITY

The paucity of histologic lesions to explain disordered organ function and death is a common characteristic of all arenavirus infections, particularly arenaviral HFs. Studies of LCM virus have shown that the infected cell may have altered function without morphologic changes, but this has not been examined in the HFs. In South American HF, the altered pathophysiology seems to be the result of direct viral action in contrast to the better-known and better-studied mouse models of LCM virus infection in which immunopathologic T-cell action causes acute encephalitis, and B-cell products result in chronic immune complex disease. Several studies failed to demonstrate immune complexes, complement activation, or DIC as relevant pathogenic mechanisms in Argentine HF.[170,240–242] Immunosuppression of the Junin virus-infected guinea pig or the hamster undergoing systemic LCM virus infection failed to ameliorate disease.[42,243–245] Mediators released or activated as a result of the virus–cell interactions, such as cytokines, vasoactive mediators, and proteolytic enzymes, may also explain some of the alterations.

In Argentine HF, bleeding itself seems to be a joint outcome of thrombocytopenia, abnormal platelet function induced by a plasma component, and alterations in blood coagulation with activation of fibrinolysis. Hemostatic abnormalities include prolongation of activated partial thromboplastin time (APTT); low levels of factors VIII and IX; increased values of factor V, von Willebrand factor, and fibrinogen; and mild decreases in antithrombin III as well as plasminogen. Endothelial cell involvement is also suspected considering that Junin virus replicates well in cultured endothelial cells, a feature supported in human disease by increased levels of von Willebrand factor.[240,241,246–250]

Argentine HF is also characterized by an acute transitory immunodeficiency. There is a lag in the humoral immune response, with antibodies appearing during the second week of illness, coincident with recovery. During the acute phase, cell-mediated immunity is also depressed as measured by delayed-type hypersensitivity to nonviral recall antigens and lymphocyte proliferation stimulated by mitogens, as well as marked changes in the T-cell subpopulations; all return to normal values in early convalescence.[2,170,251] Both cellular immunity and antibody are important in recovery by Junin virus-infected guinea pigs and in protection of vaccinees.[252,253]

Very high titers of endogenous interferon (IFN) have been demonstrated in serum samples of Argentine HF patients during the acute period of the disease and are significantly higher in fatal cases.[254–256] The levels of IFN-α decrease after the transfusion of immune plasma. Tumor necrosis factor-α (TNF-α) levels are also markedly elevated, particularly in fatal cases.[257] Lassa fever probably has a similar pathogenesis as South American HF. Major differences are less severe thrombocytopenia, minor neurologic involvement, and the mechanism of recovery from acute disease. Although platelet counts do not fall to the low levels found in South American HF, there are soluble serum factors that mediate a profound but reversible inhibition of platelet aggregation, and extensive inhibition is associated with clinical bleeding. Signs of neurologic disease are less frequent in Lassa fever, but may have been underestimated; indeed, Lassa virus has been isolated from CSF on several occasions, in contrast to Argentine HF in which virus has never been isolated from CSF or CNS tissues in spite of the frequent appearance of brain dysfunction. Cytokine activation is also present in Lassa fever.[258,259] In humans and in animal models, recovery from Lassa fever is not mediated by antibody, as judged by the low, late, and variable levels of *in vitro* neutralization by convalescent serum and the lack of protection in passive transfer experiments.[260] Spleen cell transfers in strain 13 guinea pigs suggest that cellular immunity is responsible for clearing viremia and survival.

The role of cellular immunity in recovery may also be relevant to the severity of Lassa fever in pregnant women. The placenta does not express maternal major histocompatibility complex (MHC) antigens, but in Lassa fever it is highly infected (W.-J. Shieh, unpublished data); by analogy with the situation that holds for LCM virus-infected neurons, which do not express class I MHC and cannot be lysed by host $CD8^+$ T lymphocytes,[261] it seems likely that maternal T cells cannot control placental infection.

The Pichinde virus guinea pig infection has been explored in detail as a model of severe arenavirus infection, and results suggest that many of the same mediators activated in septic shock are involved in the pathogenesis of Lassa fever.[262] Sulfidopeptide leukotrienes, catecholamines, platelet-activating factor, endorphins, and TNF-α are all activated.[263–266] Excessive sodium loss occurs in the face of extensive infection of the mineralocorticoid-secreting zones of the adrenal cortex, although serum corticosteroid levels are somewhat elevated. One potentially important finding is the decrease in cardiac index and increase in peripheral vascular resistance present from the outset, and the poor response to fluid infusion. This resembles the situation in hantavirus diseases but contrasts with the usual situation in septic shock. These results, combined with the pulmonary infection and interstitial infiltrates observed in humans and animal models, recommend that fluids be used with caution in supporting the circulation.

Although little is known about the pathogenesis of sensorineural deafness, its occurrence during convalescence, as well as lack of association with severity of the acute febrile illness, peak AST level, or antiviral therapy, suggests possible immune-mediated injury. Auditory patterns resemble idiopathic nerve deafness.[267]

DIAGNOSIS

Differential Diagnosis

During the first week of illness, the clinical manifestations of South American HF are nonspecific and can be confused with several acute febrile conditions. Among the infectious diseases, the differential diagnosis includes typhoid fever, hepatitis, infectious mononucleosis, leptospirosis, hantavirus pulmonary syndrome, dengue, dengue HF, and rickettsioses. Malaria should also be considered in endemic areas. Diseases presenting with hematologic or neurologic alterations such as intoxications, rheumatic diseases, and blood dyscrasias may also be mistaken. In the respective endemic areas or in patients with a history of travel to the specific geographic regions, a febrile syndrome with proteinuria, leukopenia and thrombocytopenia is suspicious of one of the South American HFs.

As with the South American diseases, the initial presentation of Lassa fever is often very nonspecific, and the differential diagnosis includes most febrile illnesses found in West Africa. Malaria, typhoid, and bacillary dysentery are important conditions to rule out or treat empirically. Combinations of clinical variables have been examined to facilitate determination of both clinical diagnosis and outcome of patients with Lassa virus infection.[180] Although statistically significant positive predictive values can be obtained, they apply only to areas of high prevalence (41% of all adult febrile hospital admissions in this example), a condition unlikely to be met except in selected epidemic settings or in relatively uncommon areas of intense endemic transmission. The pharyngitis often seen in Lassa fever can be a confusing feature.

LCM virus infection should be suspected in any acute febrile disease associated with myalgia, thrombocytopenia, and leukopenia. Orchitis may occur, and CNS manifestations sometimes develop later. The classic presentation of LCM virus infection is aseptic meningitis occurring in the fall, particularly if an initial prodromal period of fever, perhaps with a remission, occurs before the CNS phase. High lymphocyte counts and low glucose values may be found in the CSF, leading to confusion with granulomatous meningitis. History of mouse or hamster contact may also be elicited but is often not present. If toxoplasma, rubella, cytomegalovirus, and herpesvirus testing is negative or doubtful in cases of neonatal hydrocephalus or chorioretinitis, LCM virus testing should be done.

Laboratory Diagnosis

In the arenaviral HFs, viremia occurs throughout the acute febrile period, and the viruses can readily be isolated from blood and from lymphoid tissues of fatal cases.[39] Isolation is usually performed in Vero cells. The presence of virus can also be detected by ELISA for viral antigen or reverse transcription–polymerase chain reaction (RT-PCR). Fatal cases can also be diagnosed by immunohistochemistry on fixed tissues. Antibodies are usually measured by IFA[67] or increasingly by ELISA.[268] Neutralization tests are extremely valuable for confirming specificity of reactions provided the arenavirus species is sensitively neutralized by convalescent serum.

In Argentine HF, cocultivation of peripheral blood mononuclear cells improves the sensitivity of virus recovery.[269] Viral isolation can also be performed in guinea pigs or suckling mice. ELISA is the method of choice for serologic diagnosis. RT-PCR has been successfully applied and can play a role in establishing an etiologic diagnosis in patients dying before the appearance of the specific antibodies.

Recent Bolivian HF cases[4] have been diagnosed by antigen detection ELISA and immunoglobulin M (IgM) ELISA, although the classic approach employs suckling hamster inoculation for virus isolation and IFA with confirmatory neutralization tests for serology.

In Africa, acute Lassa fever is best diagnosed by the combined ELISA for Lassa IgM antibody and antigen, which yields a sensitivity over 90% within 48 hours of admission.[268,270,271] Sensitive RT-PCR assays exist, but even in developed countries strain variation and problems of cross-contamination pose practical problems.[272–274] Lassa antigen is usually present in blood within a few days of infection and becomes undetectable after the appearance of IgM ELISA antibody, which typically appears a few days after the onset of illness and peaks by about 10–12 days. IgG ELISA antibodies typically take longer to develop, but are present in almost all patients by approximately 3 weeks and last for a period of years. It is unclear whether reinfection takes place, although its occurrence is suggested by the finding of significant sharp IgG IFA titer elevations in individuals previously shown positive, sometimes in association with mild febrile disease. Lassa virus can be isolated from serum early in the disease course in about two-thirds of surviving and virtually all fatal cases. In survivors, this viremia is typically cleared by about 2 weeks. Conversely, in fatal cases, viremia persists unabated until death. Virus has also been isolated from serous effusions and a wide array of tissues.

Other serologic tests may be applied to Lassa fever, including IFA, which, like the IgM ELISA, may detect antibodies while patients are still acutely ill. In contrast, neutralizing antibodies appear late in Lassa fever, often several weeks after disease resolves.[260] Furthermore, the final response is low in titer, best seen with a constant serum-varying virus test, and intensely complement-dependent. In monkeys and guinea pigs this neutralizing titer correlates with the ability to transfer protection.[42]

LCM virus circulates in the blood before the onset of CNS symptoms and later can be isolated from CSF by inoculation of adult mice intracranially or by use of Vero cells.[23,275] After the onset of CNS disease, ELISA IgM capture antibody tests in serum and CSF should be positive.[276] The antibody response to LCM virus resembles that to Lassa virus in that the neutralizing antibody response is greatly delayed, complement-dependent, and of poor quality.[277] An RT-PCR procedure with sufficient sensitivity to detect LCM virus in clinical samples has been described, potentially simplifying future viral diagnosis.[278]

TREATMENT AND PROGNOSIS

General Supportive Treatment

Supportive treatment consists of adequate hydration, symptom relief measures, and proper management of the neurologic alterations, blood loss, shock, and superimposed infections. There is no indication for the use of steroids or INF-α. Medication should be given by the oral or intravenous route. Intramuscular and subcutaneous injections are contraindicated because of the risk of hematomas.

In the Argentine HF endemic area, several observations have been made. Pneumonia is the most common secondary bacterial infection and is often accompanied by radiographic changes and an increase in fever but not by leukocytosis; it usually responds to antibiotics. Platelet transfusions have been used, but the complex nature of the coagulopathy and clinical experience suggest they are not useful. Strategies such as desmopressin or activated factor VII have not been evaluated. Transfusions are needed occasionally, but most of the severe forms are neurologic. It is useful to sedate agitated patients with diphenhydramine or diazepam; diazepam also gives some protection against seizures. Cerebral edema may require both steroids and mannitol.

Virus-Specific Therapy

For Argentine HF, a specific treatment is available: the transfusion of immune plasma within the first 8 days of onset of symptoms.[2] This treatment reduces the case-fatality rate, from 15%–30% to less than 1%, and is now standardized based on the amount of neutralizing antibodies to Junin virus infused. Immune plasma is of no benefit to patients when it is initiated after 8 days of illness.

For the other South American HFs, the specific treatment suggested is intravenous ribavirin, which should be considered for off-label use unless a proven alternative effective therapy is available.[2,279] This may be increasingly important as human immunodeficiency virus (HIV) and hepatitis C infections increase in the pampas, making donor selection more difficult, and because plasma-treated patients develop lower titers in convalescence, requiring more plasma for effective therapy of subsequent patients.

Lassa fever can be treated effectively with the nucleoside analog ribavirin. The drug is highly effective *in vitro* and in a monkey model, leading to trials in West Africa that established its utility in human Lassa fever.[280,281] Patients with poor prognostic indicators (e.g., AST >150 units/mL) should be treated with intravenous ribavirin given in a dose of 30 mg/kg initially, 15 mg/kg every 6 hours for 4 days, and 7.5 mg/kg every 8 hours for 6 more days (this is not a licensed drug). The drug should be diluted in 150 mL of 0.9% saline and slowly infused over a 30-minute period.[282] Modest anemia should be expected, both from hemolysis and from a fully reversible normoblastic maturation arrest.

Uterine evacuation appears to improve survival significantly in pregnant women with Lassa fever.[182] Although contraindicated in pregnancy, the elevated maternal mortality rate, along with the almost universal fetal loss, suggests that ribavirin could be used as well, especially in the third trimester when maternal mortality is particularly high.

Neutralizing antibodies have been effective in laboratory models of Lassa fever, but this therapy should not be used unless the infused material is standardized by laboratory assays. Only supportive management is available for LCM.

PREVENTION AND CONTROL

Containment of Patients

Acutely ill patients with South American HF or with Lassa fever are viremic during the acute phase of their illness, and the viruses are infectious by parenteral inoculation. Needle precautions should be emphasized, and transmission of Lassa fever within hospitals by inadequate parenteral precautions has caused serious epidemics in African hospitals. Person-to-person transmission of Lassa fever is uncommon in the medical care setting, but has occurred in the hospital as well as in the community so that barrier nursing precautions should be strictly enforced. Airborne transmission of Lassa fever has not been suspected to be a nosocomial problem except in a single hospital epidemic in Nigeria.[159]

The South American HFs have not been regarded as highly contagious in the endemic areas where they occur, and person-to-person transmission is uncommon. Nevertheless, there are unusual patients who have disseminated both Junin (J.I. Maiztegui, unpublished observations) and Machupo[135] viruses to hospital staff and to families, in some instances suggesting aerosol transmission. Although the major focus should be on proper patient care using basic precautions that will prevent parenteral and droplet exposure to blood and body fluids, the authors believe that, when possible, it is prudent to implement small-particle aerosol precautions once patients with arenavirus HFs are identified.[174,283]

Clinically well patients leaving the hospital are not generally contagious. HF patients have transmitted virus to spouses in convalescence so that intimate contact should be cautious and condoms should be used during sex for 2–3 months. Lassa virus has been isolated from urine for several weeks, and the use of disinfectant in the toilet bowl before voiding is advised. Breastfeeding is thought to be a risk factor for transmission from mother to infant and should be temporarily avoided unless there is no other way to support the baby.

It is not known if arenaviruses could adapt to rodents outside the endemic area. The striking rodent species specificity of arenaviruses seen to date would argue that this is unlikely, but the ability of LCM virus to maintain itself within hamster colonies and of Lassa virus to chronically infect newborn laboratory mice[195] suggests that precautions should be taken to minimize the discharge of exotic arenaviruses to the environment. For these reasons, we also recommend the sterilization of all materials leaving a patient's room in nonendemic areas, including adding disinfectant to toilets before use.

Barrier nursing in African hospitals should be emphasized, both because of the possibility of transmission and the potential presence of other viral HFs. Locally applicable methods for such activities have been developed.

Rodent Control

Rodent control has been successful in the control of Bolivian HF epidemics occurring in towns of the Beni Department,[284] but sporadic cases still occur after rural exposure or contact with a case. For Argentine HF, rodent control or the control of human contact with infected rodent populations is impractical.

The fecundity and ubiquity of the *Mastomys* species complex across West Africa make widespread elimination of rodents unfeasible as a control measure for Lassa fever. Intense trapping in towns may be indicated during epidemics, although care should be taken to ensure that disposal of the trapped rodent does not inadvertently lead to exposure to potentially Lassa virus-infected blood, urine, or feces. Educational campaigns to appropriately store foodstuffs and avoid rodents as a food source, a practice common in some areas of West Africa, may have some impact.

LCM prevention depends on the exclusion of wild mice from dwellings, workplaces, and areas where colonized rodents are housed. The last is particularly important because of the risk of dissemination of infected animals to the pet trade or to laboratories. The occult infection of mouse colonies has been a recurring theme ever since LCM virus was first recognized.[23,285–287] In addition, the virus can be maintained in colonies of hamsters and possibly other rodents, and pet rodents could be infected if wild mice gain access. Pregnant women, in particular, must be protected from infection because of the risk of fetal damage.

Vaccination

A live attenuated Junin virus vaccine (Candid #1) with proven safety, immunogenicity, and efficacy in preventing Argentine HF is now available for use in high-risk populations.[103,253] Administration of 175 000 doses targeted to the maximum risk groups has resulted in a major reduction in morbidity and mortality from Argentine HF (see *Fig. 68.5*). With sufficient supplies of vaccine to protect the whole population at risk, Argentine HF would be definitively controlled. Candid #1 may also be effective in the prevention of Bolivian HF, as suggested by preclinical studies, but the vaccine does not cross-protect against infection with Guanarito or Sabia viruses in experimental studies (P.B. Jahrling, personal communication, 1995).

Definitive control of Lassa fever in Africa urgently requires an effective vaccine. Immunization with the vaccinia-vectored GP gene of Lassa virus has consistently spared guinea pigs and nonhuman primates from death and given partial protection from disease and viremia, suggesting the feasibility of a Lassa vaccine.[288,289] Another promising immunogen employs the Lassa GP expressed on the backbone of the 17D yellow fever vaccine.[290–292] Other approaches have also protected laboratory animals, but the use of killed vaccines has not generally been successful in preventing arenavirus disease.[293]

Bibliographic note: Many original references have been omitted in favor of reviews, particularly in the area of basic virology. The interested reader should consult standard texts[24,39] or recent reviews.[294,295]

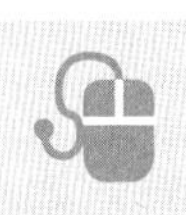

Access the complete reference list online at
http://www.expertconsult.com

CHAPTER 69

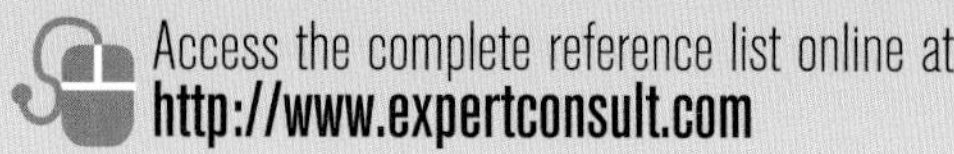
Access the complete reference list online at
http://www.expertconsult.com

Rift Valley Fever

C.J. Peters • Shinji Makino • J.C. Morrill

INTRODUCTION

Rift Valley fever (RVF), caused by a *Phlebovirus* (*Bunyaviridae*), is naturally transmitted by mosquitoes. RVF virus (RVFV) is maintained in nature by vertical transmission in floodwater *Aedes* mosquitoes, and in epidemics by horizontal transmission utilizing various mosquito genera. Additionally, it is highly aerosol infectious, likely to be a major route of spread to humans. Horizontally spread epidemics are usually associated with high rainfall and extensive disease in sheep and cattle accompanied by abortion storms. Human infection usually results in febrile illness but may also cause viral hemorrhagic syndrome (VHF), encephalitis, and ocular disease. The wide variety of mosquitoes that transmit the virus, ubiquity of the vertebrate amplifier, and extension of the virus geographic range suggest the possibility for spread to distant sites either through accident or malign intent.

THE AGENT

Phleboviruses cause acute, immunizing infections in vertebrates and are genetically and antigenically related but distinct.[1–4] RVFV is unusual among its relatives in causing lethal disease in adult laboratory vertebrate hosts, including mice, hamsters, certain rat genotypes, and some *Sigmodon* species. All establish chronic infections in ticks (Uukuniemi group, *Nairovirus* group), sandflies, or mosquitoes; and vertical transmission in the arthropod reservoir is common.

The RVFV genome is composed of three RNA segments: L. M, and S. L, which encodes the 240 kDa L protein that contains typical RNA virus polymerase motifs, is required for replication, and forms an oligomer to function.[5,6] M potentially encodes five nested transcription origins which produce at least three polypeptides, NSm, a 78 kDa protein, and a glycoprotein precursor that is cleaved into G2 (or Gn) and G1 (or Gc). The processed glycoproteins self associate into heterodimers. The Golgi retention signal on G1 is important for transport to membrane maturation sites.[7] The NSm protein is not necessary for replication in mammalian or mosquito cells[8–10] and functions to suppress apoptosis.[11,12] S encodes a nucleocapsid protein and a nonstructural protein NSs.[13] All genes are coded in negative sense except for NSs, which is positive sense. Some RVF virions contain antiviral sense RNA segments, including antiviral S RNA to transcribe mRNA encoding NSs immediately after infection, presumably serving to suppress early cellular defenses.[14]

The virus is very sensitive to interferon pretreatment of cells *in vitro* or *in vivo*.[15–17] NSs directly suppresses interferon gene expression through binding to Sin3A-associated protein 30, which is important for maintaining the repressor complex containing histone deacetylate 3 on the interferon (IFN)-β promoter, and suppresses the IFN-β promoter activation early in infection.[18–20] NSs also interacts with the p44 subunit of TFIIH, an essential transcription factor for cellular RNA polymerase II to suppress general cellular transcription.[18] Furthermore, NSs promotes the degradation of protein kinase R to promote viral translation. NSs' function is reflected in poor replication of NSs deleted viruses in interferon competent cells.[21,22]

RVFV matures within vesicles in the cytoplasm and is exocytosed via fusion of the vesicles with the cell membrane or released with cell lysis; 5 nm diameter by 10–18 nm long peplomers are inserted in the viral unit membrane.[4,23] High resolution cryo-electron microscopy and tomography of the MP-12 vaccine strain show uniform morphology with a median diameter of 103 nm and with peplomers in an icosahedral T = 12 symmetry.[24] Further high resolution exploration of single particles reveals heteromers in the surface membrane (***Fig. 69.1***).[25,26]

Most infections in mammalian cells are highly cytopathic within 1–3 days.[27,28] Carrier cultures have been established under special circumstances.[29] Mosquito cells in culture are readily infected without cytopathic effect,[27] and neither NSs nor NSm is required for vigorous growth.[10,22]

EPIDEMIOLOGY

Transmission Cycle

The first isolates of RVFV were made in 1931 during a Kenyan outbreak involving sheep and humans; mosquitoes were indirectly implicated as vectors.[30] The virus recurred in Kenyan epidemics and appeared in epidemics in southern African countries in the 1950s.[28,31–33] Subsequently virus activity has been detected in most countries in Africa.[28,33–35] The epidemics occur in times of high rainfall.[36]

RVFV transmission dropped to low levels after the 1950s in South Africa, further reinforcing the association with rainfall by inter-epidemic virus isolations in mosquitoes trapped in and around the humid forested areas of Natal.[28] The geography of RVFV transmission in Kenya also revealed a forest edge pattern.[37] Veterinary diagnostics demonstrated that during the rains there was a more or less synchronous eruption of disease.[38] Furthermore, the disease showed congruence with depressions in the ground that are referred to locally as vlies and in East Africa as damboes. These depressions only flood when extensive rains occur. The hypothesis of floodwater mosquitoes and survival during dry season as desiccated eggs was found to be correct in Kenyan damboes (***Fig. 69.2***).[39,40] Virus was isolated from female and male *Aedes mcintoshii* mosquitoes reared from larvae dipped from naturally and artificially flooded damboes, suggesting transovarial transmission. The *A. mcintoshii* emerged first from the dambo followed by other species, particularly *Culex*, suggesting that the vertically infected floodwater species *A. mcintoshii* could initiate transmission and other more numerous vectors could then perpetuate horizontal spread of the virus.[41] High viremias in sheep and cattle and the relative susceptibility of many mosquito species are essential for large epidemics in the African context.[42] This hypothesis explains the large number of different species from which RVFV has been isolated.[43] The vertical cycle has not been definitively initiated in the laboratory, even with field-caught material, presumably because of the inability to colonize the mosquitoes.[44]

Careful surveillance shows tick-over of virus transmission in domestic animals, wildlife, and humans during inter-epidemic periods in sub-Saharan Africa.[36,38,45–47] When there is exceedingly high rainfall then epidemics of various sizes occur (***Table 69.1***).[28,36,48,49] Remote sensing from satellites can detect rainfall and other features that can predict the possibility of RVFV outbreaks,[49–53] particularly in East Africa.

In West Africa prior to 1989, the only sign of RVFV was the presence of a low prevalence of neutralizing antibodies in asymptomatic residents of Senegal. Then there was a period of increased rainfall and collapse of the right bank of the Senegal River when the dam at the river mouth was closed with subsequent flooding of the Mauritanian side. There was a massive swarm of mosquitoes and extensive RVF transmission in humans and livestock. There was also an increase in transmission in the areas not flooded directly, including upriver and south and as far as The Gambia.[54–59] Continuing transmission, usually at a relatively low level, has been mapped in part by remote sensing.[60–63] Other mosquitoes than East African species are involved, but the same pattern seems to hold: floodwater *Aedes* vertically maintain the virus, depressions are an important part of their ecology, and *Culex* species are important horizontal transmitters.

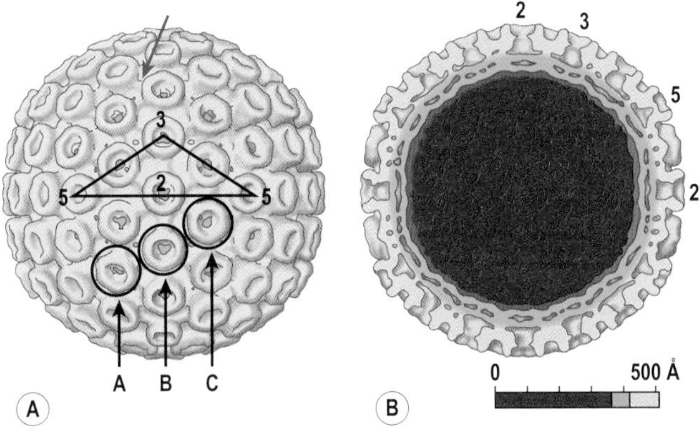

Figure 69.1 Cryo-electron microscopic three-dimensional of Rift Valley fever virus (RVFV) MP-12. **(A)** Surface-shaded representation of the map rendered at 1 standard deviation (1 σ) showing glycoprotein protrusions organized with T = 12 icosahedral symmetry, so far unique to the *Bunyaviridae* family. The black triangle demarcates an asymmetric unit with 5-, 3- and 2-fold axes indicated. There are 12 pentons in the map and 110 quasi-equivalent hexons of three types: A, B, and C, occupying locations at 2-, 3- and quasi-3-fold axes, respectively. The blue arrow points to a ridge connecting two capsomers. **(B)** Surface-shaded representation as in panel **A** with front half of the map removed to reveal interior features. The map is colored by radius, and the structure consists of an outer glycoprotein layer (gold), a lipid envelope (green), and a ribonucleoprotein core (red). Icosahedral two- (2), three- (3), and five-fold (5) axes are labeled. The core is separated from the envelope by a 20 Å gap, and details in the core are not resolved because of its asymmetry. Images are colored radially, according to the scale bar. (From Sherman MB, Freiberg AN, Holbrook MR, et al. Single-particle cryo-electron microscopy of Rift Valley fever virus. Virology. 2009;387:11-15.)

Geography

Epizootic/epidemic RVF can occur virtually anywhere in sub-Saharan Africa where the rainfall is sufficient and the virus is present. If the virus is not present, it can be introduced. This first occurred in Egypt in 1977 when the virus was introduced from Sudan and a massive epidemic occurred on virgin soil.[64–68] Subsequently RVF activity has been found repeatedly in Egypt,[69–71] and RVF epidemics have occurred on the Arabian peninsula and in the Comoros Islands.[72–79]

Distant spread seems a distinct risk. Competent vertebrate amplifiers (sheep and cattle) are widely distributed. Competent arthropod vectors are widely distributed in the United States and other areas such as Australia.[42,80–83] Human viremias are sufficiently high[67] to infect mosquitoes, reaching $10^{4.2}$–$10,^{8.6}$ and therefore sick or incubating humans could be a conduit even to North America. Chronically infected mosquitoes could easily be transported in airplanes or luggage as regularly occurs in "airport malaria."

Transmission to Humans

RVFV can be transmitted to humans by mosquito bite. However, humans in the endemic area are also exposed to contact with blood, aerosols, and tissues from infected animals (necropsy by veterinarians, assisting

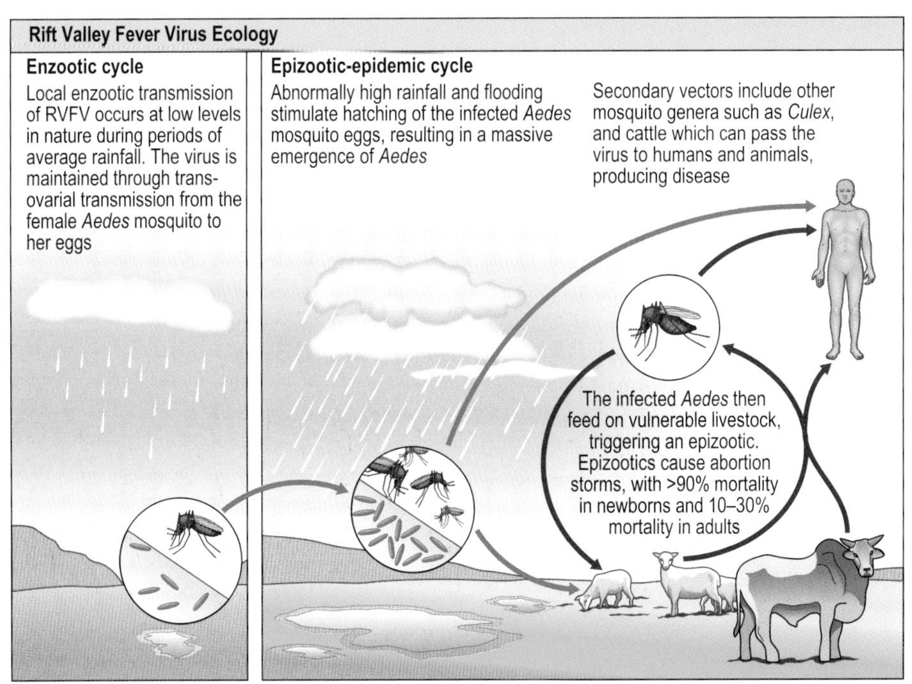

Rift Valley Fever Virus Ecology
Enzootic cycle
Local enzootic transmission of RVFV occurs at low levels in nature during periods of average rainfall. The virus is maintained through trans-ovarial transmission from the female Aedes mosquito to her eggs
Epizootic-epidemic cycle
Abnormally high rainfall and flooding stimulate hatching of the infected Aedes mosquito eggs, resulting in a massive emergence of Aedes
Secondary vectors include other mosquito genera such as Culex, and cattle which can pass the virus to humans and animals, producing disease
The infected Aedes then feed on vulnerable livestock, triggering an epizootic. Epizootics cause abortion storms, with >90% mortality in newborns and 10–30% mortality in adults

Figure 69.2 Illustrated cycle of Rift Valley fever virus (RVFV). (From Special Pathogens Branch, Centers for Disease Control and Prevention, Atlanta, GA.)

Table 69.1 Notable Rift Valley Fever Outbreaks

Year	Location	Significance
1918	Lake Naivasha region, Kenya	Earliest epidemic of ovine hepatitis later regarded as probably RVF
1930–1931	Kenya	Major RVF epidemic, isolation of agent, shown to be filterable, same agent causing sheep and human disease
1950	South Africa	First major epidemic in southern Africa; first description of ocular lesions
1974	South Africa	Return of epidemic RVF, recognition of VHF and encephalitis caused by RVFV
1977	Egypt	Massive epidemic in Egypt, first epidemic recognized outside sub-Saharan Africa
1987	Mauritania, Senegal	First major West African epidemic. Coincided with damming Senegal River and higher rainfall
1990	Madagascar	Large epidemic; possibly related more with ecological change than rainfall
1993	Recurrent epidemic RVF in Egypt	After absence of detectable virus circulation since 1980, disease recurs. Likely that subsequently continued at low level until at least first decade of 2000
1997	East Africa	El Niño led to rainfall and biggest RVFV epidemic recorded[15,16]
2000	Arabian Peninsula	Strain previously active in East Africa spreads to Saudi Arabia and Yemen with possible persistence and also threat to the Hajj
2006–2008	Comoros Islands	RVFV epidemic in 2006 and some activity with human cases 2007–2008
2006+	Kenya	Continuing activity
2008–2010	South Africa	Low level but important activity resumes

RVF, Rift Valley fever; RVFV, Rift Valley fever virus; VHF, viral hemorrhagic fever.

abortions by owners). In the field it is difficult to distinguish between mosquito, contact with animal tissues, or aerosol exposure.

RVFV fulfills the major requirements of an aerosol-infectious virus. It is stable in aerosols and highly infectious in small controlled doses for laboratory animals.[84–87] The aerosol lethal dose for mice or hamsters is as low as one infectious unit and for immature cats and dogs or monkeys is only slightly higher. Inter-cage infections among laboratory animals also implicates aerosol infections.[88] Field data from humans are very suggestive of aerosol infectiousness[65] and numerous laboratory infections without other defined exposures also indicate aerosol transmission.[89–92]

When extensive transmission is occurring among sheep or cattle, humans and domestic animals are exposed to biological transmission by infected mosquitoes, mechanical transmission by partially fed arthropods,[93] aerosols from aborting or dying animals, contact with abortuses or dead animal tissues, or perhaps even the minuscule levels of virus in animal secreta.

THE DISEASE

Clinical Manifestations

The incubation is short, perhaps only 2 days to less than a week. The rapid onset of disease is usually ushered in by a shaking chill. The patient is typically severely myalgic, anorexic or even vomiting, complaining of severe headache, photophobia, retro-ocular pain, and arthralgia without arthritis. Patients have few physical findings but may have epigastric tenderness, flushing, epistaxis, or scattered petechiae. In uncomplicated disease, defervescence and general improvement occurs within 4 days to a week. The fever and symptoms may follow a biphasic curve. The illness may be followed by prolonged convalescence. The disease is not "flu-like" in that coryza and cough are not characteristic. It appears that three-quarters of infections are symptomatic.[94,95]

A small proportion of patients with apparently uncomplicated illness within a few days progress to a state of severe disease with bleeding and hepatic damage. The clinical description and understanding of pathogenesis is poorly understood.[96] The incidence of this syndrome is probably around 0.5–1% of infections. There does not seem to be a single virus or host determinant that can be identified for this VHF syndrome, which was first described in South Africa[97,98] and subsequently in Zimbabwe,[99] Egypt,[100] and other RVF epidemics.

RVFV encephalitis usually begins as the acute uncomplicated disease resolves or several days later. Over a period of 1–2 weeks this condition gradually resolves with variable sequelae and mortality.[66,101–103] The usual clinical picture in full-blown cases includes confusion progressing to hallucinations, delirium, stupor, and coma; focal signs include monoparesis, hemiparesis, hypersalivation, and bruxism. Meningismus is common, and neurological involvement may be manifest only as aseptic meningitis. Cerebrospinal fluid shows modest increase in protein and lymphocytes with normal glucose.

Ocular disease occurs in about 5% of cases, both typical and complicated RVFV. Abrupt onset usually occurs at or shortly after the end of the initial febrile period.[28,104–107] It can be bilateral or unilateral, and the signal lesion is hemorrhage and exudate in or near the macula. The exudate is resorbed or turns into scar tissue, leaving a visual field defect ranging from undetectable to virtual blindness in that eye. Optic atrophy and anterior uveitis may also result.

The incidence of the different complications is inconsistent among different clinical studies.[96] There are no prospective studies on the true incidence, the epidemics occur in areas with poor infrastructure, and the skill and time available from clinicians is highly variable. For example, renal disease had not been mentioned in conjunction with RVF before the Saudi outbreak; at that outbreak severely ill patients sent to tertiary hospitals with more equipment for clinical chemistry and hematology revealed isolated renal failure in some cases and hepatic and neurological syndromes associated with renal failure.[108–110]

A skilled infectious disease physician, during 2 weeks in Kenya at a small hospital, observed an identifiable clinical syndrome suggestive of severe RVF, characterized by fever, large joint arthralgia, and gastrointestinal complaints, followed by jaundice, right upper quadrant pain, and delirium, often with hemorrhagic manifestations.[96] None of the usually reported clinical syndromes were seen, and this syndrome had not been previously described.

PATHOGENESIS AND IMMUNITY

Very few human autopsies have been performed on cases of RVF. Nonhuman primates resemble the human disease in their clinical and pathogenetic manifestations[16,111–118] and other animal models shed light on the processes involved.[27,28,112,119–121]

The determinants of the outcome of RVFV infection in the mammalian host are largely related to innate immunity modulating virus replication and the onset of the humoral immune response. For example, in macaques early onset (not the height) of the interferon response seems to determine the severity of disease.[16,122] Serum viremia levels are not indicative of severity of disease. Thus, the likely action of interferon is at the cellular level. The more severe the illness, the more severe the abnormalities including disseminated intravascular coagulation (DIC).[115]

Further evidence for DIC includes angiopathic hemolytic anemia, thrombocytopenia, fibrin deposition in the kidneys of infected monkeys, and high concentrations of fibrin split products in the plasma.

Hepatocyte infection and death, glomerular capillary infection, and other evidence of widespread infection occur in experimentally infected macaques. Rarely a macaque develops encephalitis after clearing viremia, and a very limited number of human and macaque autopsies reveal neuronal infection, mild polymorphonuclear and lymphocyte infiltration, and perivascular lymphocytic cuffing.[119,120,123]

DIAGNOSIS

Differential Diagnosis

The first signs of an RVF epidemic may be animal or human disease; and veterinary and medical public health authorities rarely communicate effectively even in the developed world. On the animal side there will be high rainfall with a high density of mosquitoes, spreading disease with deaths in sheep and cattle, extensive death of lambs and calves, and abortion storms. There may be delay in diagnosis. On the human side, there will be cases of VHF initially, encephalitis later, retinitis, and nonspecific febrile illness, but suspicion of RVF and diagnostic resources may be lacking. The VHF cases may be diverted to acute care hospitals, encephalitis to neurological wards, and ocular cases to ophthalmological hospitals. These brusque epidemics may run their course in only 6–10 weeks.

Sporadic cases or early in the epidemic, human cases will be confused with other VHF or viral encephalitides, and the retinal lesions may not be attributed to RVF.[124] There is no characteristic that would single RVF out from other VHF; DIC and/or extensive hepatic necrosis would be suspicious for RVF or Congo-Crimean hemorrhagic fever.

Laboratory Diagnosis

The laboratory diagnosis of RVF in humans is easy if suspected and appropriate reagents are available. ELISA antigen detection in sera is effective, and even agar gel diffusion can be effective with serum or liver. The virus is readily isolated from serum or organs using cell culture, suckling mice, or hamsters with subsequent identification via several methods.[28,125] Antigenemia/viremia/RNA is followed by the appearance of antibodies that can be detected readily by hemagglutination inhibition, immunofluorescence, neutralization, and ELISA. The most effective strategy is use of RT-PCR plus IgM capture and IgG ELISAs; if antigen capture ELISA is available, it also aids in early diagnosis.[108,126]

TREATMENT AND PROGNOSIS

General Supportive Treatment

There is no established protocol for dealing with any of the syndromes associated with RVF. VHF should be monitored in an intensive care unit. Nosocomial infection has not been seen in spite of the fact that blood contains RVFV; however, bloodborne precautions should be observed with all patients, and manipulations that generate aerosols should only be performed with personal protective gear. Treatment of DIC should follow established guidelines.

Virus Specific Therapy

No antiviral therapy is available for human use. There are several approaches which are effective for prophylaxis or even therapy in mice and nonhuman primates. These include an immunostimulator (poly ICLC), interferon, ribavirin, and neutralizing antibodies.[16,113,127–133]

PREVENTION AND CONTROL

Ecological Control

It seems unlikely that local modification of the environment can completely control the disease. Some experiments have shown promise in the field to limit hatches of the vertical floodwater *Aedes* reservoir.[134,135] If the local horizontal reservoir can be identified and its habits and insecticide sensitivity are known, perhaps local mosquito control could be useful.

Vaccination of Livestock

Epidemics have been rural, and sheep and cattle have been the most important amplifiers. If they were vaccinated to limit spread to other mosquito vectors, the epidemic could presumably be controlled. The available vaccines cannot achieve this goal. In particular, the inactivated bovine vaccine has been very limited in its field utility,[136] and the Smithburn neurotropic vaccine is excessively teratogenic in sheep.[33,137–139] A live attenuated candidate vaccine that has been developed for humans (MP-12)[13,140–142] and has shown considerable promise in sheep and cattle is under commercial development.

Vaccination of Humans

Human vaccine would be extremely useful for deployment in residents of endemic/epidemic areas, diagnostic laboratorians, veterinarians, and researchers. The first formalin-inactivated vaccine was extremely effective in protecting laboratory workers from disease,[143–145] but stocks were not maintained, three injections were required in the primary series, and boosters as soon as 6 months later were recommended.

The live-attenuated candidate vaccine developed for human use[5] has passed preclinical tests, including monkey neurovirulence testing.[111] More than 60 volunteers were vaccinated with excellent neutralizing antibody response in >95% of recipients and no significant adverse events.

A number of other approaches to vaccination against RVF for humans and animals have been reviewed.[146]

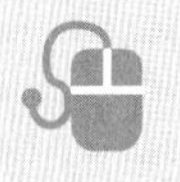

Access the complete reference list online at **http://www.expertconsult.com**

CHAPTER 70

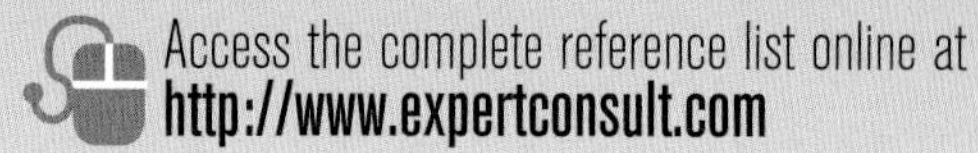
Access the complete reference list online at
http://www.expertconsult.com

Crimean-Congo Hemorrhagic Fever

Onder Ergonul • Michael R. Holbrook

INTRODUCTION

A hemorrhagic disease outbreak occurred in Crimea in the mid-1940s. Although a virus was neither isolated nor specifically identified, the agent associated with the hemorrhagic disease was maintained by the Soviets by passaging the agent through human "volunteers."[1] In 1956, a hemorrhagic disease was identified in the Belgian Congo (now the Democratic Republic of the Congo). Filtration analysis determined that the causative agent of the disease was a virus, and subsequent analysis in 1959 determined the virus to be novel, and it was named Congo hemorrhagic fever virus. In the late 1960s the agent that caused hemorrhagic disease in Crimea was identified as Congo hemorrhagic fever virus. After some negotiation, the virus was renamed Crimean-Congo hemorrhagic fever virus (CCHFV) to represent the two localities where the virus was first identified. Conveniently, unlike many viruses named on the basis of the specific location of initial isolation, the name CCHFV suggests endemicity in a broad spectrum of ecological environments and widespread viral distribution. The wide geographic distribution has turned out to be correct as, to date, CCHFV has caused outbreaks in southeastern Europe, southwestern Asia, the Middle East and large regions of Africa (***Fig. 70.1***). The most recent significant outbreak was in Turkey where more than 5000 cases were reported from 2002 through 2009.[2]

CCHFV is a tick-borne bunyavirus (family *Bunyaviridae*, genus *Nairovirus*) that is typically transmitted by *Hyalomma* spp. ticks although the virus has been isolated from a number of tick species. Viruses within the *Nairovirus* genus also associated with human disease include Dugbe virus and Nairobi sheep disease virus. Following its initial identification, CCHFV has been found across a vast area ranging from southwestern Asia, into southeastern Europe, the Middle East and across Africa. Although the total cases identified to date do not represent a staggering number, the increased frequency of large outbreaks among agricultural workers is concerning, especially in areas where CCHF had not been previously identified.

THE AGENT

CCHFV is an enveloped virion approximately 90–100 nm in diameter with pleomorphic, nearly spherical, morphology. The virus encapsidates a tripartite negative-sense ~19 kb RNA genome consisting of small (S), medium (M), and large (L) segments that each consist of a single open reading frame. The CCHF genome is markedly larger than viruses within other genera of the *Bunyaviridae*. The viral genome encodes four proteins: the viral RNA-dependent RNA polymerase (RdRP) and an ovarian tumor-like protease are encoded by the L segment (12 108 nt)[3]; the viral surface glycoproteins G_n and G_c are encoded by the M segment (5360 nt); the viral nucleocapsid protein is encoded by the S segment (1672 nt). Unlike the phleboviruses, tospoviruses or orthobunyaviruses, there is no evidence of overlapping or ambisense coding strategies that would indicate the presence of small nonstructural proteins such as the NSs or NSm proteins in other bunyaviruses. Each segment of the viral genome also has very short 5′- and 3′-terminal non-coding regions (NCRs). The NCRs are thought to contain promoter elements for transcription and replication as well as encapsidation signal elements for association with the viral nucleocapsid protein and subsequent viral genome packaging.[4–7]

The viral particle consists of a lipid envelope with the viral G_n and G_c proteins integrated into the membrane to generate spike-like structures on the surface of the virus. The nucleocapsid protein is closely associated with the viral RNA within the viral particle, as is the viral RdRP. Upon viral attachment and entry, most likely through clathrin-dependent receptor-mediated endocytosis,[8,9] the viral envelope presumably fuses with the host endosomal membranes to release the viral RNA, nucleocapsid, and RdRP into the host cell cytoplasm. Bunyaviruses are processed through the endoplasmic reticulum and through the Golgi apparatus where they are assembled to generate mature particles. The G_n and G_c are both glycosylated in the Golgi region, although the specific nature of the sugar moieties has not been defined for CCHFV. Glycosylation of one of the two predicted N-linked glycosylation sites (577N) of G_n appears critical to targeting of viral M segment proteins to the endoplasmic reticulum.[10] Glycosylation of G_c of CCHFV does not appear to be critical to virus processing and assembly, but may have a role in virus attachment.

EPIDEMIOLOGY

CCHFV is the most widespread tick-borne virus that causes disease in humans. The virus is distributed across a large part of southern Asia, the Arabian peninsula into the Middle East and Africa. Genetic sequencing and phylogenetic analysis of the viral S segment initially identified seven separate viral lineages while analysis of the L segment has identified five lineages.[11] Recent analysis of complete virus genomes has identified six distinct lineages of S and L segments and seven M segment lineages[12,13] (***Fig. 70.2***). As with all multipartite viruses, reassortment among viruses during concurrent infections does occur with CCHFV. Data from several studies suggest that the S and L segments are closely associated during reassortment events, with the M segment having a higher rate of reassortment.[12,14] There are some discrepancies when comparing S and L phylogenetic data, suggesting that reassortment of these genome segments can occur, albeit at a much lower rate than M segment reassortment.[12] Reassortment of L and S segments appears to be largely restricted within phylogenetic groups while M recombination can occur between groups, potentially resulting in a new virus subtype.[14]

Genetic recombination events can also occur within CCHFV genome segments; these events appear to be largely associated with the S segment rather than the L or M segments.[15]

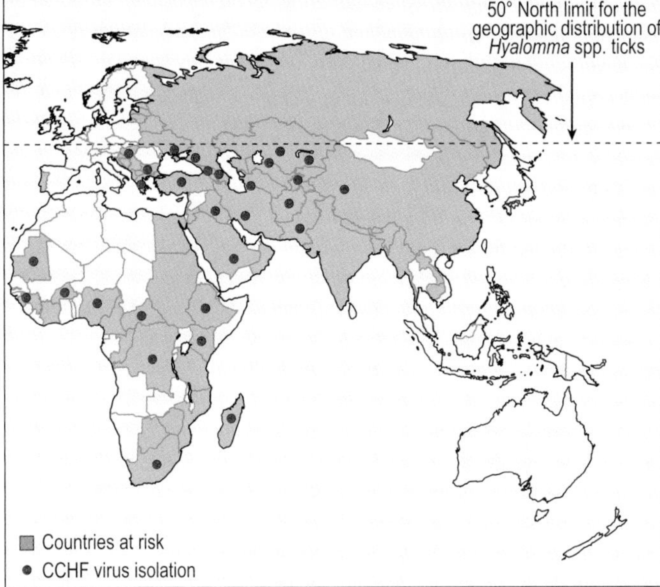

Figure 70.1 Worldwide distribution of CCHF cases indicating countries at risk for CCHF and those where virus isolations have been made. (Adapted from Ergonul O. Crimean-Congo haemorrhagic fever. Lancet Infect Dis 2006;6(4):203.)

THE DISEASE

The initial diagnosis of CCHF in the "pre-hemorrhagic" phase is complicated by the presence of other pathogens in endemic areas that are also associated with the development of febrile disease. These include malaria, brucellosis, sandfly fevers, rickettsial diseases and other viral hemorrhagic fevers. Like these diseases, initial onset of CCHF is typically characterized as a febrile disease with patients displaying malaise, myalgia, nausea, vomiting, headache, and diarrhea. Fever, while generally present, is not typically severe (>40°C). The onset of symptoms follows a 3–7-day incubation period following a tick bite and indicates the onset of the "pre-hemorrhagic" phase of disease during which peak viremia occurs. The "pre-hemorrhagic" phase lasts 1–7 days and is followed by the 2–3-day hemorrhagic phase of the disease. Onset of more severe symptoms is rapid and is characterized by bleeding from the mucosa, petechiae, and large hematomas in the skin. The nose, gastrointestinal tract, urinary tract, and respiratory tract are the most common sites of bleeding. Cases of internal bleeding have also been described,[16] but are atypical. The convalescence period is typically non-eventful, with most survivors recovering fully. There have been reports of cardiovascular and neurological complications,[16] but these sequelae are atypical and may have divergent etiologies. CCHF has a case-fatality rate of 3–30%.[17] Interestingly, the disease in children is milder and of shorter duration than that seen in adults.[16] Documented cases of CCHF in pregnant women resulted in fetal deaths or severe bleeding complications in the newborns.[18]

Clinical characterization of the disease course of CCHF has been studied fairly extensively; in fact, clinical hematological analysis is critical for early diagnosis of disease. Thrombocytopenia is characteristic of CCHF while most patients also have leukopenia and elevated levels of aspartate aminotransferase (AST), alanine aminotransferase (ALT), lactate dehydrogenase, and creatine phosphokinase. In CCHF patients the serum AST levels are typically higher than ALT concentrations, with significantly elevated levels of these enzymes being an indicator of a poor outcome.[19,20] Decreased platelet count and fibrinogen levels along with increased activated partial thromboplastin time are also indicators of a poor outcome.[19,20]

PATHOGENESIS AND IMMUNITY

As with all arboviral infections, the principal route of CCHFV infection is via deposition of the virus into the skin of the host by an infected arthropod. Once the virus is deposited, it is most likely phagocytosed by dermal dendritic cells, Langerhans cells, or macrophages where initial virus replication and antigen presentation are thought to occur.[21] The virus would then spread to draining lymph nodes, where further replication is believed to occur, and subsequently into the venous circulation and disseminated to target organs.

Specific mechanisms of pathogenesis during CCHFV infections are unclear, but similarities to other viral hemorrhagic fevers (VHF) allow for some direct comparisons. Like infection with Ebola, Marburg, and dengue viral infections, disseminated intravascular coagulation (DIC) is a hallmark of disease progression. This immediately differentiates CCHF from yellow fever virus infection where DIC is not characteristic. An extensive amount of work with dengue hemorrhagic fever (DHF) cases and additional limited studies with Ebola virus infection in both humans and nonhuman primates have allowed for a better understanding of virus-induced DIC. This condition is largely associated with an overactive proinflammatory response that induces a loss of vascular integrity and plasma leakage. Major effectors in DIC include circulating macrophages, interleukin (IL)-6, IL-8, tumor necrosis factor (TNF)-α, monocyte chemoattractant protein (MCP)-1 and nitric oxide (NO). Interaction of these components induces vascular damage, increase of tissue factor (TF) expression, and release and increased production of soluble TF. Proinflammatory cytokines including TNF-α, IL-1, and IL-6 are significantly higher among the fatal CCHF cases than in survivors.[22] The production of cell surface TF leads to induction of the extrinsic coagulation cascade and local deposition of fibrin, fibrinolysis, consumption of coagulation factors, and further perpetuation of DIC. The presence of D-dimers, a byproduct of fibrinolysis, is considered a hallmark of DIC and Ebola virus infection, and is a useful indicator of disease status. Once a patient has developed DIC, the disease course is extremely difficult to manage, and death typically occurs.

DIAGNOSIS

CCHFV is classified as a biosafety level 3 or 4 pathogen (country-dependent), which makes clinical diagnosis of CCHFV infections potentially hazardous, particularly if the patient is still in the viremic phase of disease. Most common clinical diagnostics include IgM- and IgG-specific ELISAs or PCR-based assays. Antibodies can be detected 4–5 days after onset of clinical disease,[23] making the ELISA a useful diagnostic tool for hospital use. In cases of known or likely CCHFV infections, more rapid diagnosis may be possible with PCR-based assays where the viral genome would be detectable in the serum of viremic patients. The most conclusive diagnostic tools include immunofluorescence assays utilizing infected cells, plaque reduction neutralization tests (PRNTs) and virus isolation and characterization. However, these assays require work with live virus and maximum containment laboratories, which are not available in most settings.

TREATMENT AND PROGNOSIS, PREVENTION AND CONTROL

There are currently no licensed vaccines or treatment protocols for the effective prevention and treatment of CCHF. Formalin inactivated vaccines were developed and tested in Eastern Europe and the former Soviet Union, and both vaccines stimulated the development of virus-specific antibodies[24]; however, further development of the vaccines was apparently not pursued.

Current approaches for prevention of CCHF are largely focused on control of the tick vector and reducing potential exposure to infected ticks. Control of accidental infections within the health care system relies

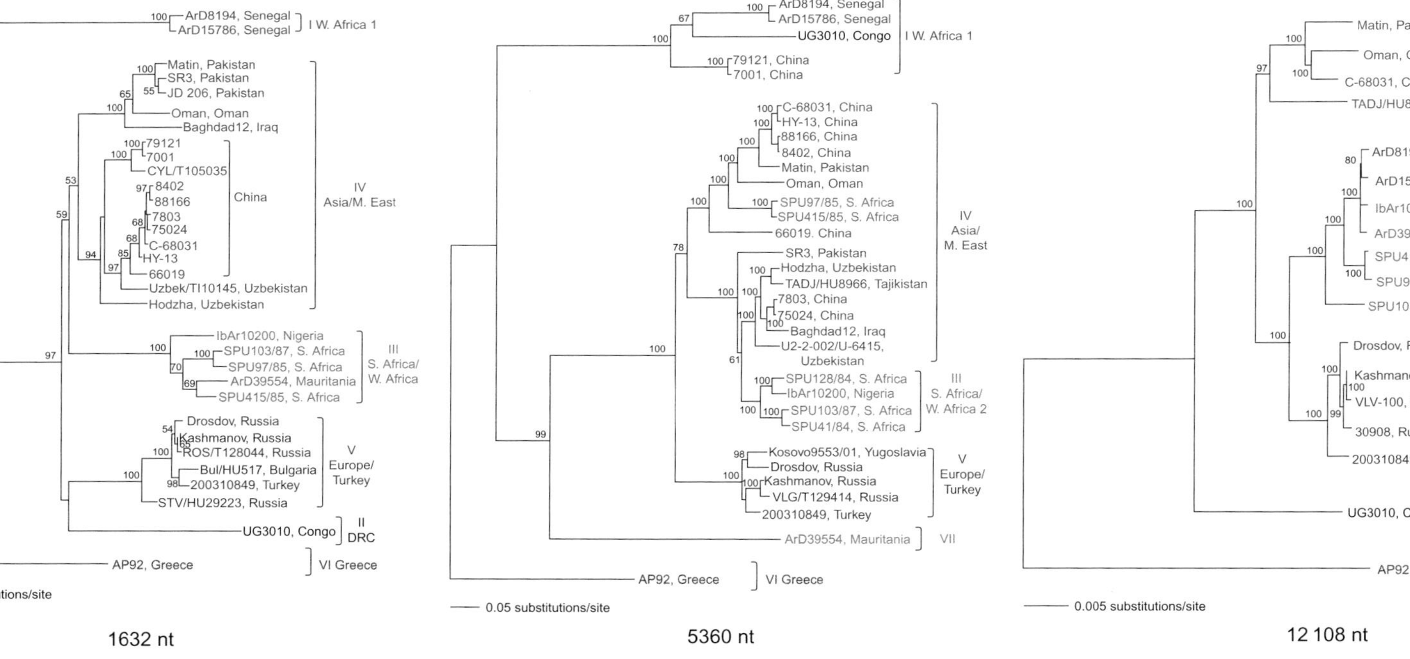

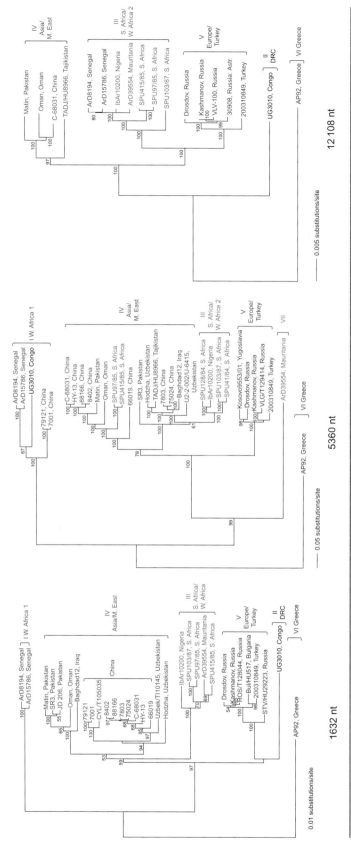

Figure 70.2 Phylogenetic analysis of CCHFV S, M, and L segments showing the different lineages of virus. Groups are: I, West Africa 1 (red); II, Democratic Republic of the Congo (DRC) (black); III, South Africa/West Africa 2 (green); IV, Asia/Middle East (blue); V, Europe/Turkey (purple); VI, Greece (yellow). The M segment analysis also identified lineage VII, Mauritania (also shown in green). (Adapted from Deyde VM, Khristova ML, Rollin PE, et al. Crimean-Congo hemorrhagic fever virus genomics and global diversity. J Virol 2006;80(17):8834.)

on the implementation and effective use of barrier nursing practices and safe handling of sharps.

Ribavirin is the only drug currently available to treat CCHF, although its effectiveness in limiting disease is unclear. Ribavirin is effective *in vitro* and was considered beneficial in clinical studies.[25] Its early use was reported to be promising.[26] As with most VHF, supportive care is the principal treatment approach. Recent work with Marburg virus in nonhuman primates suggests that regulation of TF through the use of rNAPc-2 may help limit the effects of DIC,[27] and in dengue patients the control of blood volume has met with some success, although whether these treatment protocols would be effective for the treatment of CCHF is unclear.

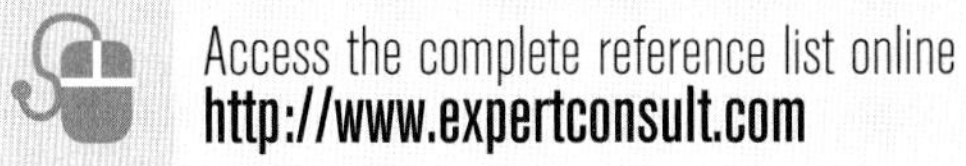
Access the complete reference list online at
http://www.expertconsult.com

CHAPTER 71

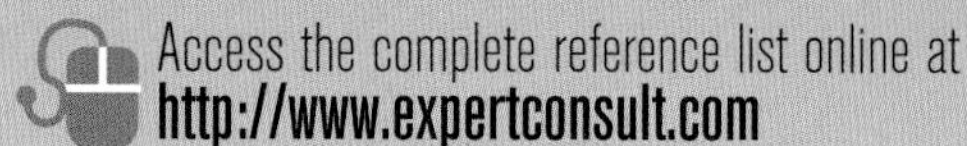
Access the complete reference list online at
http://www.expertconsult.com

Hantavirus Infections

Charles F. Fulhorst • Frederick T. Koster • Delia A. Enría • C.J. Peters

INTRODUCTION

Hemorrhagic fever with renal syndrome (HFRS) and hantavirus pulmonary syndrome (HPS) are rodent-borne zoonoses, caused by members of the virus family *Bunyaviridae*, genus *Hantavirus*,[1] and endemic in the Old World and New World, respectively. Both syndromes are characterized by a long incubation period, febrile prodrome, systemic infection in association with microvascular endothelial cells, thrombocytopenia, leakage of fluid from capillaries, and shock. The endothelial cell dysfunction that leads to extravasation of plasma and, in some cases, hemorrhage has been associated with the cellular immune response in infected tissues. Carefully managed supportive care is critical to recovery from severe disease. Prevention of HFRS and HPS currently rests on avoidance of infected rodents.

THE AGENT

The virus family *Bunyaviridae*, genus *Hantavirus* comprises 23 species.[1,2] Eleven species and 12 other named entities in the genus *Hantavirus* have been associated with human disease (***Table 71.1 and Fig. 71.1***).

Hantavirions are pleomorphic, average 100 nm in diameter (range: 70–120 nm), and possess a lipid-bilayer envelope that surrounds an electron-dense core (***Fig. 71.2***).[1,3] The core contains ribonucleocapsids – segments of single-stranded genomic RNA complexed with L protein (an RNA-dependent RNA polymerase) and nucleocapsid (N) protein. Spikes, approximately 6 nm in length, protrude from the lipid envelope. These spikes are formed from the virus glycoproteins, Gn and Gc.

The genomes of hantaviruses comprise three single-stranded, negative-sense RNA segments, designated large (L, 6.5–6.6 kb), medium (M, 3.6–3.8 kb), and small (S, 1.6–2.1 kb).[1,4] Analyses of L, M, and S segment sequences have revealed high levels of genetic diversity between strains of different hantaviral species. Undoubtedly, the major source of this diversity has been the accumulation of point mutations (i.e., base substitutions, insertions, and deletions). There is natural and experimental evidence for homologous recombination between phylogenetically closely related hantaviruses.[5–7] Laboratory studies suggest that genetic reassortment likely is restricted to phylogenetically closely related hantaviruses.[8,9]

The L, M, and S genomic segments encode the L protein (240 kDa), glycoprotein precursor (GPC), and N protein (48 kDa), respectively.[1] The S segments of Puumala virus, Tula virus, and perhaps some of the other hantaviruses encode a nonstructural (NSs) protein.[10,11] The NSs proteins of Puumala virus and Tula virus inhibit the expression of interferon (IFN)-β mRNA in cultured cells.[10]

The GPC is cleaved cotranslationally to yield Gn (72 kDa) and Gc (54 kDa). Both glycoproteins (Gn and Gc) are class 1 proteins, with the N-terminus exposed on the surface and the C-terminus anchored in the lipid envelope of the virion.[4] The mature glycoprotein spike is a Gn-Gc heterodimer and contains the binding site(s) for cellular receptor(s) and epitopes for antibody-mediated neutralization of infectivity.

Hantaviruses primarily infect endothelial cells. Other cell types infected by hantaviruses include alveolar macrophages, follicular dendritic cells, and renal tubular epithelial cells. Infection is initiated by attachment of the virion to the cell surface. Entry of Sin Nombre, New York, Seoul, and Puumala viruses is mediated by β3 integrins,[12,13] entry of Hantaan virus is mediated by β3 and possibly β1 integrins,[13,14] and entry of Prospect Hill virus (a hantavirus that is not pathogenic in humans) is mediated by β1 integrins.[12] Viral replication is initiated after the ribonucleoprotein complexes are released into the cytoplasm of the host cell. Each RNA segment is transcribed by the virion-associated L protein (RNA-dependent RNA polymerase). The L mRNA and N protein mRNA are translated on free ribosomes, and the GPC mRNA is translated on membrane-bound polysomes. The mechanism(s) involved in the switch from transcription of viral mRNA to replication of genomic RNA are not known. Virion assembly begins when sufficient amounts of the structural proteins and genomic RNA have been synthesized. Highly conserved nucleotide sequences in the termini of the genomic RNA segments may be critical to initiation of encapsidation. Hantaviruses mature through the Golgi apparatus. Sin Nombre virus and some of the other hantaviruses may also mature by budding directly from the plasma membrane (***Fig. 71.2***).[3]

Natural Host Relationships and Ecology

Specific members of the order Rodentia are the principal hosts of the hantaviruses for which natural host relationships have been well characterized. For example, the striped field mouse (*Apodemus agrarius*) is the principal host of Hantaan virus, and the North American deer mouse (*Peromyscus maniculatus*) is the principal host of Sin Nombre virus (***Table 71.1***). Other natural hosts of hantaviruses include shrews and moles (order Soricomorpha).[15–17] None of the hantaviruses associated with shrews or moles are known to cause human disease.

Hantaviruses have no known intermediate host(s) and do not persist in the inanimate environment for extended periods. As such, the principal host and reservoir of a hantavirus are synonymous.

The rodent-borne hantaviruses are associated with members of the family Muridae, subfamily Murinae (Old World rats and mice), family Cricetidae, subfamily Arvicolinae (voles and lemmings), and family Cricetidae, subfamilies Neotominae and Sigmodontinae (New World rats and mice). Murine rodents and voles are the principal hosts of the hantaviruses known to cause HFRS. Neotomine and sigmodontine rodents are the principal hosts of the hantaviruses known to cause HPS. Many of the rodent-borne hantaviruses, particularly those associated with voles, have not been linked to human disease.

Phylogenetically closely related hantaviruses are generally associated with rodents that are themselves phylogenetically closely related. For example, Hantaan virus and Dobrava-Belgrade virus (usually called

Table 71.1 The Hantaviruses Known to Cause Disease in Humans

Virus	Natural Host[a]	Disease[b]	Disease Distribution
Amur	*Apodemus peninsulae*	HFRS	Far eastern Russia
Dobrava-Belgrade	*Apodemus flavicollis*	HFRS	Balkans, European Russia
Hantaan	*Apodemus agrarius*	HFRS	China, Korea, Russia
Puumala	*Myodes glareolus*	HFRS	Europe, European Russia
Saaremaa	*Apodemus agrarius*	HFRS	Northern Europe
Seoul	*Rattus norvegicus*	HFRS	Asia, USA
Bayou	*Oryzomys palustris*	HPS	Southeastern USA
Black Creek Canal	*Sigmodon hispidus*	HPS	Southeastern USA (Florida)
New York	*Peromyscus leucopus*	HPS	Northeastern USA
Sin Nombre	*Peromyscus maniculatus*	HPS	Canada, USA
Choclo	*Oligoryzomys fulvescens*	HPS	Panama
Andes	*Oligoryzomys longicaudatus*	HPS	Southwestern Argentina, Chile
Anajatuba	*Oligoryzomys fornesi*	HPS	Northern Brazil
Araucária	(not known)	HPS	Southern Brazil
Araraquara	*Bolomys lasiurus*	HPS	Southern Brazil
Bermejo	*Oligoryzomys flavescens*	HPS	Northern Argentina, southern Bolivia
Castelo dos Sonhos	(not known)	HPS	Central Brazil
Central Plata	*Oligoryzomys flavescens*	HPS	Uruguay
Hu39694	(not known)	HPS	Argentina
Juquitiba	*Oligoryzomys nigripes*	HPS	Southeastern Brazil
Laguna Negra	*Calomys laucha*	HPS	Paraguay
Lechiguanas	*Oligoryzomys flavescens*	HPS	Central Argentina
Orán	*Oligoryzomys chacoensis*	HPS	Northwestern Argentina

[a]*Apodemus agrarius* (striped field mouse), *A. flavicollis* (yellow-necked field mouse), *A. peninsulae* (Korean field mouse), and *Rattus norvegicus* (brown rat) are murine species (family Muridae, subfamily Murinae); *Myodes glareolus* (bank vole) is an arvicoline species (Cricetidae, Arvicolinae); *Peromyscus leucopus* (white-footed deermouse) and *P. maniculatus* (North American deermouse) are neotomine species (Cricetidae, Neotominae); *Bolomys lasiurus* (hoary-tailed akodont), *Calomys laucha* (little laucha), *Oligoryzomys chacoensis* (Chacoan colilargo), *O. flavescens* (flavescent colilargo), *O. fornesi* (Fornes' colilargo), *O. fulvescens* (fulvous colilargo), *O. longicaudatus* (long-tailed colilargo), *O. nigripes* (black-footed colilargo), *Oryzomys palustris* (marsh oryzomys), and *Sigmodon hispidus* (hispid cotton rat) are sigmodontine species (Cricetidae, Sigmodontinae).

[b]HFRS, hemorrhagic fever with renal syndrome; HPS, hantavirus pulmonary syndrome.

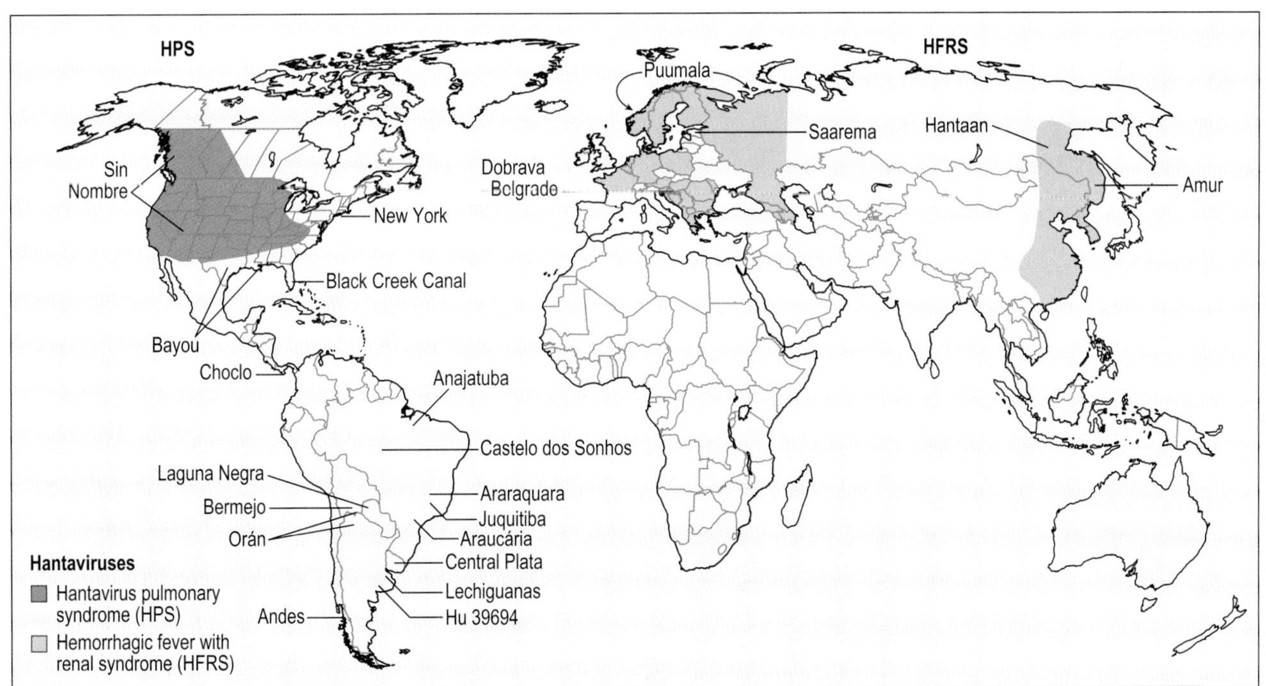

Figure 71.1 Map showing the geographic distribution of hantavirus pulmonary syndrome (HPS) caused by Sin Nombre virus, and hemorrhagic fever with renal syndrome (HFRS) caused by Puumala or Hantaan virus.

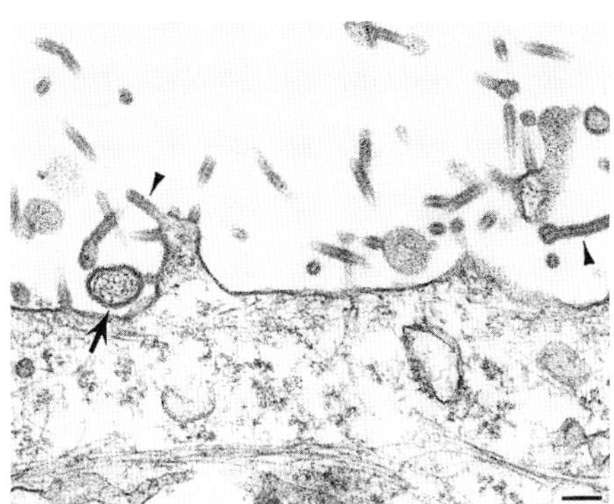

Figure 71.2 Electron micrograph of Sin Nombre virus (SNV) propagated in a monolayer of Vero E6 cells, showing virus particle budding from the cell surface (arrow). Tubular projections that contain specific SNV antigens (arrowheads) extend from the plasma membrane of infected cells. Bar = 100 nm. (Courtesy of C.S. Goldsmith and L.H. Elliott.)

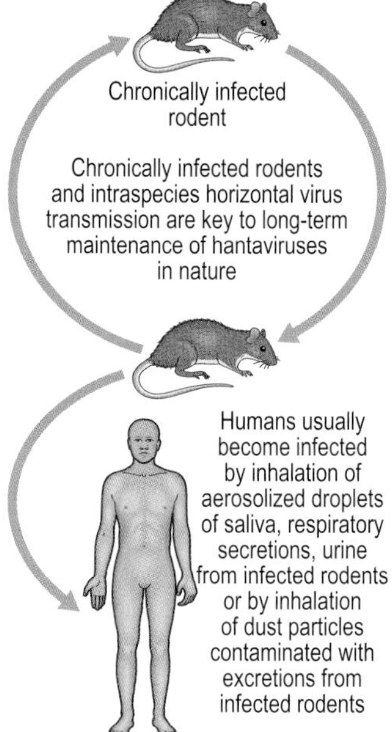

Figure 71.3 Transmission cycle and rodent-to-human virus transmission of a hantavirus. Infected rodents shed virus in saliva, respiratory tract secretions, and – perhaps most importantly – urine. There is limited evidence that infected rodents shed virus in feces. Intraspecific horizontal virus transmission and chronically infected rodents are key to long-term maintenance of hantaviruses in nature. Horizontal virus transmission may occur during aggressive encounters, allogrooming, mating, and other activities that entail close physical contact between rodents. Humans usually become infected by inhalation of aerosolized droplets of saliva, respiratory secretions, or urine from infected rodents or by inhalation of dust particles contaminated with secretions or excretions from infected rodents. The results of experimental studies suggest that the highest titers of virus in secretions and excretions occur during the first month of infection; thus, newly infected rodents may pose a greater risk of infection to humans than chronically infected rodents. Humans usually are a dead end in virus transmission; however, there is evidence for person-to-person transmission of Andes virus in South America. Person-to-person transmission of hantaviruses other than Andes virus has never been documented.

"Dobrava virus") are phylogenetically more closely related to each other and to other hantaviruses associated with murine rodents than to the hantaviruses associated with arvicoline, neotomine, or sigmodontine rodents. Knowledge of these relationships has proven useful in the design of assays for detection of hantaviral RNA in clinical specimens and rodents.

Hantaviruses have been identified on every continent except Antarctica. In accordance with the high specificity of the natural host relationships of the rodent-borne hantaviruses, each hantavirus is restricted to the geographic range of its principal host. Undoubtedly, Seoul virus (an agent of HFRS) is the most widely distributed rodent-borne hantavirus. This virus appears to have been introduced into the New World along with its principal host, the brown rat (*Rattus norvegicus*).[18]

Sympatry of multiple hantaviruses is not uncommon. For example, Dobrava virus and Saaremaa virus coexist in the Balkans, Hantaan virus and Amur virus are sympatric in Far East Russia, and Sin Nombre, El Moro Canyon, Limestone Canyon, and other hantaviruses are sympatric in the southwestern United States. Sympatry of multiple hantaviruses can confound interpretation of serological data because hantaviruses can be highly cross-reactive in enzyme-linked immunosorbent assays (ELISA), indirect fluorescent antibody tests (IFAT), other antibody-antigen binding assays, and even neutralization assays.

The results of field and laboratory studies on the biology of hantaviruses in their respective principal hosts indicate that the vast majority of infected animals seroconvert and shed virus in saliva, respiratory tract secretions, or urine. Some infected animals shed virus for months and maybe even longer periods. Chronic infections in individual rodents are key to long-term maintenance of hantaviruses in nature.

Horizontal virus transmission appears to be the dominant mode of intraspecific virus transmission in nature (***Fig. 71.3***). Aggression, allogrooming, mating, and other activities that entail close physical contact between conspecifics may facilitate virus transmission within reservoir species. Interspecific virus transmission is a dead end in the ecology of a hantavirus because infections in rodents other than the principal host usually are transient and presumably not accompanied by shedding of significant amounts of virus.

The geographic distribution of infected rodent populations may be highly focal. As an example, the prevalence of antibody to Sin Nombre virus ranged from 0% to 50% in deer mouse (*P. maniculatus*) populations sampled nearly simultaneously in the southwestern United States.[19] The number of infected rodents in an enzootic region typically varies from season to season and year to year. In some instances, the number of infected rodents in an enzootic region cycles over multi-year periods.

Hantavirus transmission dynamics in rodent populations are associated with rodent population dynamics. The results of long-term studies in the southwestern United States indicate that hantavirus transmission dynamics in reservoir populations and subsequent risk of human infection are associated with a "trophic" cascade.[20] Favorable climatic conditions result in improved environmental conditions and, in turn, improved reproductive success. Stress and increased interactions associated with crowded conditions lead to increased virus transmission and higher prevalence of infection in host populations.

Human disturbance of native ecosystems may create conditions that favor certain opportunistic species, some of which are reservoirs of hantaviruses that are pathogenic for humans.[21,22] Situations that increase the abundance of infected rodents or intensity of contact between infected rodents and humans may increase the risk of human infection.

It is widely assumed that hantaviruses in their respective principal hosts are nonpathogenic; however, New York virus and Sin Nombre virus have been associated with pulmonary edema and hepatitis in naturally infected white-footed mice (*Peromyscus leucopus*) and deer mice (*P. maniculatus*), respectively,[23,24] Black Creek Canal virus can cause a transient, moderately severe pneumonitis in experimentally infected juvenile hispid cotton rats (*Sigmodon hispidus*),[25] Puumala virus has been associated with reduced winter survival of bank voles (*Myodes glareolus*) in Finland,[26] and Sin Nombre virus has been associated with reduced survival of deer mice (*P. maniculatus*) in the western United States.[27] Whether hantaviruses significantly affect population dynamics in reservoir species and, ultimately, the absolute number of infected rodents in reservoir populations has not been rigorously investigated.

Carnivores that feed on infected rodents may become infected themselves.[28] Infections in predators of infected rodents presumably do not result in disease and likely are not epidemiologically significant.

EPIDEMIOLOGY

Humans usually become infected with hantaviruses by inhalation of aerosolized droplets of urine, saliva, or respiratory secretions from infected rodents or inhalation of virus-laden particles of dust. Aerosol transmission of hantaviruses from rodents to humans has been well documented.[29,30] Other means of transmission include bite wounds from rodents, contamination of cutaneous injuries or mucous membranes with infectious virus, ingestion of food contaminated with infectious rodent secretions or excretions,[29,31–35] and – only in the case of Andes virus in Argentina – contact with an HPS case during the acute phase of illness.[36–40] Rodent bite wounds are potentially very dangerous because hantaviruses are significantly more infectious by parenteral injection than aerosol exposure.[41] Human-to-human transmission of Andes virus was first documented when physicians who treated an HPS case in 1996 became ill themselves.[39] Andes virus has been isolated from urine from an HPS patient, and Andes virus antigen has been found in urine from other HPS patients.[42]

The results of several laboratory studies suggest that recently infected rodents pose a greater risk of infection to humans than do chronically infected rodents.[25,43–45] For example, the concentration of Hantaan virus in urine from striped field mice on days 12 and 15 post-inoculation is 100-fold higher than the concentration of Hantaan virus in urine from striped field mice on day 160 post-inoculation.[44] Also, the ability of Puumala virus-infected bank voles to transmit their infections to naïve bank voles is greatest 14–28 days post-inoculation.[45]

The risk of infection in humans in nature depends upon occupational or recreational activities, ecological factors which affect the abundance of infectious rodents, and other variables that affect the frequency and intensity of human contact with infected rodents and their excreta. The cleaning of closed quarters occupied by infected rodents (e.g., outbuildings on farms or ranches, vacation homes, livestock feed containers, and storage sheds) has been associated with an increased risk of infection.[46–49] As examples, the peak incidence of HFRS cases in Scandinavia usually occurs in summer, when people enter vacation homes and disturb bank voles that have entered these homes during winter,[50] and the risk of infection in military personnel in Korea was associated with living in primitive field conditions, sighting rodents around their quarters, and occupying dusty environments.[51]

The geographic distribution and seasonal occurrence of HFRS and HPS can be understood most easily in terms of the habitat associations of infected rodents, ecological factors that affect the population dynamics in infected rodent populations, and circumstances that bring infected rodents into contact with humans or vice versa. HFRS caused by viruses other than Seoul virus and HPS are diseases of rural areas. Disease caused by Seoul virus occurs mostly in urban areas and in winter, reflecting the habits of the brown rat (*R. norvegicus*).

Hantaan virus is the most important cause of severe HFRS in the Russian Far East, Korea, and China. Amur virus is another cause of HFRS in eastern Russia.[52] Seoul virus is a cause of a moderately severe form of HFRS. The most convincing reports of HFRS caused by Seoul virus in nature come from Korea and China.[33,53–55] Human disease caused by Seoul virus has been associated with infected laboratory rat colonies in Belgium, the United Kingdom, Japan, and other countries, and immunocytomas derived from infected laboratory rats.[56,57] There is a single, well-documented case of hemorrhagic fever caused by Seoul virus in the United States.[58] The infrequent diagnosis of disease caused by Seoul virus in many areas of the world where the brown rat (*R. norvegicus*) occurs has not been explained. Dobrava virus is the cause of a severe form of HFRS in Albania, Croatia, Greece, Slovenia, and other countries of the Balkan Peninsula.[59–61] Puumala virus is the cause of nephropathia epidemica (a mild form of HFRS) and the most common cause of HFRS in Scandinavia, Europe, and European Russia.[62–65] Saaremaa virus is a cause of a mild form of HFRS in northern Europe.[66] Approximately 150 000 HFRS cases occur each year worldwide.[67] Most of these illnesses are caused by Hantaan or Seoul virus and occur in China. Between 50 000 and 100 000 HFRS cases are hospitalized in China each year.[54,68] The case-fatality rate of HFRS ranges from 0.2% (Puumala virus) to 15% (Hantaan virus).

There are reports that suggest that hantaviruses native to India cause HFRS.[69,70] The results of a recent study suggests that Sangassou virus, a hantavirus associated with the African wood mouse (*Hylomyscus simus*),[71] is a cause of HFRS in West Africa.[72]

The geographic range of HPS includes western Canada, 31 states in the contiguous United States, Panama, Argentina, Bolivia, Brazil, Chile, Paraguay, and Uruguay. Undoubtedly, Sin Nombre virus is the major cause of HPS in North America, and Andes virus is the major cause of HPS in South America. Hantaviruses have been discovered in Mexico,[73] Honduras,[74] Costa Rica,[75] Venezuela,[76,77] and Peru[78] in association with neotomine or sigmodontine rodents, but the human health significance of these viruses has not been rigorously investigated. The apparent absence of HPS in these and other countries in the Americas may be related to case-finding. The number of HPS cases that occurred in North and South America in the period from 1993 through 2009 is not known with certainty but likely is on the order of 3000.[79] Although there are far fewer HPS cases than HFRS cases each year, outbreaks of HPS caused by Sin Nombre virus or Andes virus are usually highly lethal, with case-fatality rates as high as 60%.

Almost all Sin Nombre virus infections are clinically evident based on studies of contacts of index cases during the 1993 epidemic in the southwestern United States,[80] intensive searches for milder disease forms in clinics,[81,82] and the very low prevalence of antibody to Sin Nombre virus in normal populations in the United States[83,84] and in mammalogists who had worked extensively with sigmodontine rodents in North America.[85] The majority of Andes virus infections likely result in severe respiratory disease, too. The prevalence of IgG antibody against Andes virus in regions in Chile in which HPS is endemic is less than 2.0%.[86]

Choclo virus is the only virus that has been associated with HPS in Panama.[87,88] The prevalence of neutralizing antibody to Choclo virus in rural communities in western Panama typically exceeds 30%.[89] Yet hospitalizations due to respiratory illnesses resembling HPS are rare in this region of Panama.[88,89] Collectively, these observations suggest that the majority of persons infected with Choclo virus do not develop HPS. Studies done in rural communities in Salta Province of Argentina suggest that the majority of persons infected with hantaviruses enzootic in this region also do not develop severe HPS.[90]

The occurrence of HFRS and HPS is usually sporadic, but small clusters of cases are not uncommon, and there have been large epidemics of HFRS in small geographical regions. A significant number of HFRS epidemics occurred during periods of political strife or armed conflict.

THE DISEASES

The severity of disease and case-fatality rates in HFRS and HPS are dependent upon virus genetics and may be affected by inoculum dose, route of exposure, and host genetics.[91,92] Differences between cases caused by the same virus may be as great as differences between cases caused by strains of different viruses.

Hemorrhagic Fever with Renal Syndrome

HFRS has been known by many names, including hemorrhagic nephrosonephritis and Churilov disease in the Russian Far East, Korean hemorrhagic fever on the Korean peninsula, epidemic hemorrhagic fever in China, and nephropathia epidemica in Europe. The name "hemorrhagic fever with renal syndrome" was recommended in 1983 to consolidate these and other febrile illnesses that are caused by hantaviruses and characterized by hemostatic and renal disturbances.[93]

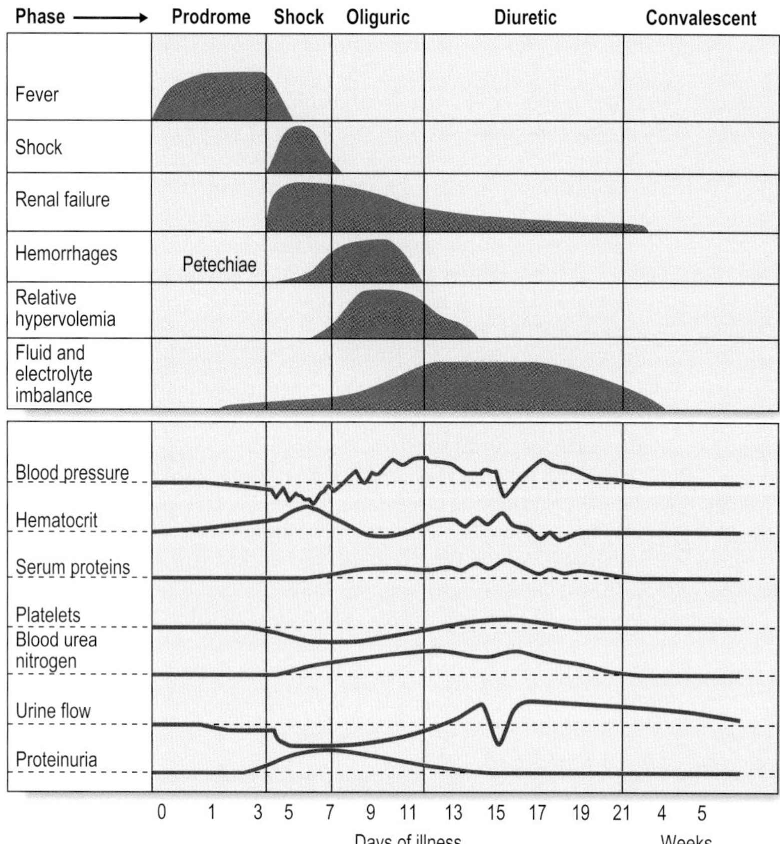

Figure 71.4 Schema of clinical course of severe hemorrhagic fever with renal syndrome (HFRS). (Modified from Sheedy JA, Froeb HF, Batson HA, et al: The clinical course of epidemic hemorrhagic fever. Am J Med 16:619–628, 1954.)

The incubation period of HFRS is usually 2–4 weeks but has ranged from 1 to 8 weeks.[94–96] The clinical course of severe HFRS can be divided into five phases: prodrome, hypotensive (shock), oliguric, diuretic, and convalescent (*Fig. 71.4*). Death, when it occurs, usually is due to renal failure in the oliguric phase or shock in the hypotensive, oliguric, or diuretic phase.

HFRS Caused by Hantaan Virus

Description of the five phases in severe disease caused by Hantaan virus provides a framework for understanding the pathogenesis of HFRS caused by other hantaviruses; however, the spectrum of disease caused by Hantaan virus includes very mild disease that is not readily identified as HFRS, disease that "skips" one or more phases, and fulminant disease with early death.[97]

The prodrome in severe HFRS usually lasts 3–7 days, begins with abrupt onset of high fever and chills, and then includes headache, blurred vision, myalgia, and thirst. Anorexia, abdominal pain, nausea, vomiting, mild cough, hiccough, and dizziness are frequent. Capillary dilatation is evidenced by flushing of the face and neck, and conjunctival and pharyngeal injection. Increased capillary permeability is generalized and typically results in retroperitoneal edema accompanied by severe backache. Low-grade disseminated intravascular coagulation (DIC), thrombocytopenia, and hemorrhage (e.g., petechiae and epistaxis) may occur late in the prodrome.[98] Sudden onset of extreme albuminuria late in the prodrome is usually the first sign of renal involvement.

The hypotensive phase begins with defervescence to a low-grade fever or normal body temperature, lasts hours to several days, and is marked by thrombocytopenia, nausea, and vomiting. Proteinuria and back pain increase, the urine (which contains red blood cells, white blood cells, and casts) decreases in volume, the specific gravity of the urine moves to 1.010, hemoconcentration may result in a hematocrit of 55% or higher, and platelets may fall below 70 000/μL. White blood cells in peripheral blood are increased, often above 30 000/μL, and occasionally reach leukemoid levels. Severe shock occurs in about 15% of patients.[98] Careful management with Trendelenburg's position, pressors, and inotropic agents usually results in survival; but some patients die in severe shock during this phase. The administration of large quantities of fluids in the hypotensive phase can be dangerous because of the hyperpermeability of the microvasculature, especially in lung. Cardiovascular measurements in HFRS cases in Korea showed that patients had a low cardiac output and a high peripheral resistance.[99] Patients in frank shock with peripheral vasoconstriction were often given one to two units of albumin with apparent improvement.

In the oliguric phase, severe hemorrhage (hemoptysis, gastrointestinal bleeding, and hematuria) may become troublesome, urinary output falls dramatically, concentrations of serum creatinine and blood urea nitrogen increase, and fluid is resorbed. The circulation may become overexpanded, leading to a high-output state, hypertension, and sometimes fatal pulmonary edema. Dialysis for treatment of overhydration may be urgently required because of the risk of intracranial hemorrhage and pulmonary edema. Approximately half of the fatalities in HFRS occur during the oliguric phase, with fatalities primarily due to renal failure.

Spontaneous diuresis, with polyuria greater than 3 liters per day, heralds the onset of recovery. Dehydration and electrolyte imbalance may threaten the well-being of the patient during this phase. Urine specific gravity is fixed around 1.010 from 3 weeks to 3 months. The convalescent phase may last weeks to months. Recovery is usually complete, but residual inability to concentrate urine has been documented in a small proportion of patients.

The results of other clinical laboratory tests may be informative. Aspartate transaminase (AST) levels usually are increased. Electrocardiograms are often abnormal with sinus bradycardia, low voltage, or nonspecific ST-T wave findings.[100,101] Atrial arrhythmias are not uncommon; however, there usually are no specific changes in the electrocardiogram in spite of the hemorrhagic lesion usually seen in the heart at autopsy. The kidneys usually are not discernible in survey radiographs because of retroperitoneal edema. The renogram often shows patterns consistent with obstruction or tubular damage.[100] Magnetic resonance imaging may suggest renal hemorrhage because of the low T2-weighted signal intensity along the outer medulla.[102] Pulmonary infiltrates are not common except in the face of overhydration; however, pulmonary edema and pleural effusions may be present even early in disease.[100]

A number of complications of HFRS have been observed. Renal rupture may occur in the oliguric or diuretic phase.[103] Transient hypopituitarism and frank intrapituitary hemorrhage have been associated with pituitary apoplexy, abnormal anterior pituitary hormonal responses, delayed diuresis, and late appearance of Sheehan's syndrome.[104]

HFRS Caused by Seoul Virus

The overall mortality in HFRS caused by Seoul virus acquired from wild rats (*R. norvegicus*) in Asia is approximately 1%.[105,106] Macroscopic hemorrhagic manifestations are rare. Liver involvement in HFRS caused by Seoul virus is more prominent than in HFRS caused by Hantaan virus.[29,53] Recovery is usually complete; however, a minority of patients may not regain their ability to concentrate urine. Also, an extensive study done in the United States linked hypertensive chronic renal failure to the presence of IgG antibody to Seoul virus.[107]

HFRS Caused by Puumala Virus

Illness is usually mild, typically begins with sudden onset of fever, chills, myalgia, and headache, frequently followed by gastrointestinal symptoms, abdominal tenderness, and back pain.[62,108] Myopia, blurred vision, and even glaucoma have been reported in a significant proportion of patients and are very suggestive of the diagnosis.[109–111] Thrombocytopenia often develops late in the prodrome.[62] Mild mucosal bleeding in the gastrointestinal tract can be gastroscopically detected in almost all cases, but petechiae and other manifestations of bleeding (e.g., visible hematuria and melena) are observed in less than one-third of patients.[108] Urinalysis late in the prodrome reveals proteinuria and hematuria in almost 100% of cases. Hypotension is reported in up to 40% of patients but is generally mild.[62] Escalating abdominal pain, perhaps associated with nausea and vomiting, may lead to suspicion of a surgical emergency, but the onset of oliguria, rising concentrations of serum creatinine and blood urea nitrogen, and proteinuria and hematuria usually avert operative intervention.[62,63,108] Less than half of patients become oliguric, and severe hypertension, blood volume overload, or life-threatening electrolyte imbalance occur in only a minority of patients. Fatal cases have been associated with marked leukocytosis and shock.[112,113] Diuresis and hyposthenuria may be notable and persist into convalescence. Sequelae are uncommon and include hypertension in convalescence.[114,115]

Some persons infected with Puumala virus have had notable disease with no apparent renal involvement.[63,108,116] Occasionally, patients have shown a dominant neurological picture suggestive of viral encephalitis or other neurological disorders, including Guillain–Barré syndrome.[109] The ratio of clinical to subclinical (or mild or atypical and undiagnosed) Puumala virus infections ranges from 1 : 5 to 1 : 10.[117,118]

HFRS Caused by Other Hantaviruses

Case-fatality rates in HFRS caused by Dobrava virus have ranged from 7% to 12%.[119,120] The clinical course of disease caused by Dobrava virus may include severe thrombocytopenia, DIC, hemorrhagic manifestations, oliguric renal failure requiring dialysis, pleural or abdominal effusions, and electrocardiographic abnormalities. Hypopituitarism may be a complication of Dobrava virus infection.[121,122] Saaremaa virus is the cause of a mild form of HFRS in northern Europe.

Hantavirus Pulmonary Syndrome

HPS was first recognized in 1993 in the southwestern United States.[123] The original description of HPS was modified to include mild infections

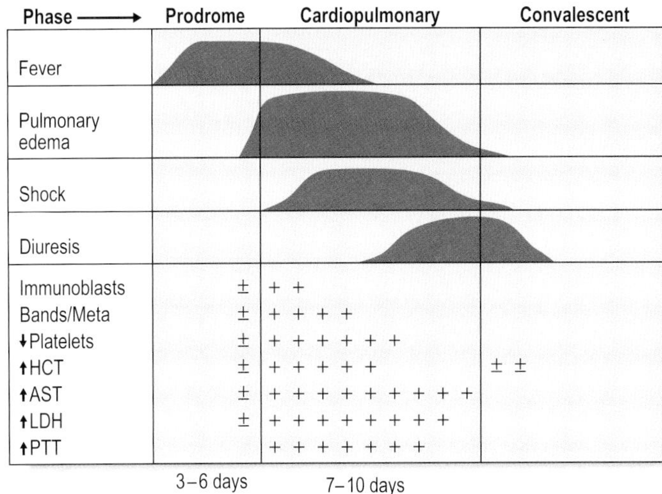

Figure 71.5 Schema of clinical course of severe hantavirus pulmonary syndrome. Meta, metamyelocytes; HCT, hematocrit; AST, aspartate transaminase; LDH, lactate dehydrogenase; PTT, partial thromboplastin time. (Prepared by Li Lien Yang.)

that do not result in radiographic evidence of pulmonary disease.[124] It is now recognized that HPS sometimes includes renal impairment, myocardial depression, and – particularly in South America – bleeding manifestations.[125,126] The incubation period in HPS is usually 2–4 weeks but has ranged from a few days to 6 weeks.[127] The clinical course can be divided into three phases: prodrome, cardiopulmonary, and convalescent (*Fig. 71.5*).

HPS Caused by Sin Nombre Virus

The prodrome typically lasts 3–5 days (range, 1–10 days) and begins with abrupt onset of fever, myalgia, and malaise, often accompanied by chills, anorexia, and headache.[128–130] Other symptoms may include dizziness, abdominal pain, nausea, vomiting, and diarrhea.[131,132] Pharyngitis, coryza, rhinorrhea, conjunctival injection, and rash usually are absent. The patient may seek medical attention during the prodrome because of extreme physical discomfort. In the absence of objective findings and despite the absence of cough, the diagnosis at this time most likely will be "influenza-like illness." Nonproductive cough usually marks the beginning of the cardiopulmonary phase.

The patient usually seeks medical attention at the end of the prodrome because of shortness of breath. Objective findings include tachypnea, mild hypotension, and arterial oxygen desaturation (measured by oximetry or blood gas analysis). The chest radiograph early in the cardiopulmonary phase may be normal or reveal mild interstitial (peribronchiolar) edema, patchy alveolar edema in the basilar portions of the lungs, or Kerley B lines.[129]

Severe HPS is characterized by rapidly progressive (time span, 4–24 h) noncardiogenic pulmonary edema, large volumes of respiratory tract secretions with protein levels even exceeding 80% of those in serum and an electrophoretic pattern resembling that of serum,[128,133] large volumes of pleural fluid, and cardiogenic shock. The chest radiograph in fully developed HPS reveals a marked diffuse alveolar pattern and pleural effusions.[129] The progressive leakage of highly proteinaceous fluid into the pulmonary interstitium and alveoli results in hypovolemia. Hypotension and oliguria, sometimes with delirium, are due to shock. Myocardial depression may occur (see below) and contribute to shock.[91]

Hematological abnormalities that are almost always present at the onset of dyspnea include thrombocytopenia, left shift of the white blood cell count with myelocytosis, and the presence of large, reactive (immunoblastic) lymphocytes.[134,135] Thrombocytopenia is always present at the end of the prodrome in HPS caused by Sin Nombre virus. The white blood cell count in peripheral blood can be normal or elevated on admission and frequently increases to very high values. Other laboratory abnormalities may include hemoconcentration, mildly elevated levels of serum AST, and lactate dehydrogenase, prolonged partial thromboplastin time, hypoalbuminemia, and metabolic acidosis. Severe metabolic acidosis and increased lactate levels above 4 mmol/L are poor prognostic signs.[133] The development of DIC or a clinically significant bleeding diathesis occurs only in a minority of HPS cases caused by Sin Nombre virus.[132,136]

Although the pulmonary findings dominate the initial presentation of the patient, myocardial depression and, ultimately, death due to uncorrectable shock may occur even if hypoxia is properly managed; for this reason, the name "hantavirus cardiopulmonary syndrome" is often used instead of HPS.[133,137] Lactic acidosis reflects the poor tissue perfusion in hypotensive patients with low cardiac output and low stroke work. Unlike septic shock, systemic vascular resistance in HPS is normal or elevated, with only modest elevation of pulmonary artery pressure and pulmonary vascular resistance. The initially low pulmonary wedge pressure increases to high levels as myocardial function worsens and becomes unresponsive to pressor therapy, requiring extracorporeal membrane oxygenation (ECMO) where available. Echocardiography in some patients has shown markedly reduced left ventricular ejection fraction.[138] The etiology of the myocardial depression in HPS is as yet unclear.

Spontaneous diuresis usually marks the beginning of recovery, which is characterized by rapid clearance of pulmonary edema and resolution of fever and shock. Diuresis may exceed 8 liters per day; as such, the patient may require close monitoring for dehydration and electrolyte imbalance. Most patients will have significantly improved cardiopulmonary function within 3–7 days of hospitalization, and respiratory and circulatory support can be discontinued at that time. In the absence of complications, most patients are discharged from the hospital within 10–14 days of admission. Exertional dyspnea is common and may persist up to 3 months after discharge from the hospital. Impaired pulmonary diffusion capacity and reduced small airway expiratory flow rates persist in some patients for up to 2 years, but permanent pulmonary disability has not been identified. Proteinuria and decreased creatinine clearance may develop during convalescence and persist for years after Sin Nombre virus infection in some patients.[139]

HPS Caused by Andes Virus

HPS caused by Andes virus is almost identical to HPS caused by Sin Nombre virus;[140–142] however, hemorrhage and renal involvement are not uncommon in HPS caused by Andes virus.[125,143] Hemorrhage may be severe and from more than one source.[125] Renal failure occurred in 2 (12.5%) of 16 HPS cases caused by Andes virus in Chile.[125]

HPS Caused by Other Hantaviruses

HPS caused by Juquitiba virus in Brazil,[144] Laguna Negra virus in Paraguay,[145] and Lechiguanas virus in Argentina[140] is virtually identical to HPS caused by Sin Nombre virus. In other situations there has been a similar clinical picture with variations. A single nonfatal case caused by Black Creek Canal virus developed modest renal failure (serum creatinine, 4.6 mg/dL) and a markedly elevated serum creatine phosphokinase.[145] Renal failure was documented in three HPS cases caused by Bayou virus in the southeastern United States[147,148] and renal failure occurred in several HPS cases (presumed to have been caused by Orán virus) in northern Argentina near Bolivia.[140,142]

PATHOGENESIS AND IMMUNITY

The pathology in HFRS and HPS appears to be a consequence of microvascular instability: capillary dilatation, leakage, and maybe even hemorrhage. Typical HPS differs from HFRS in that the lesions are primarily confined to the thoracic cavity and – with the exception of HPS caused by Andes virus – not usually associated with hemorrhage.[135,136,149]

In HFRS, large amounts of protein-rich gelatinous edema collect in the retroperitoneal space during the hypotensive (shock) stage. A characteristic triad is congestion and hemorrhagic necrosis of the subcortical renal medulla, anterior pituitary gland, and right atrium.[149–155] Microscopically, the most characteristic changes are observed in kidney, with variable degrees of tubular dilation, necrosis, interstitial hemorrhage, and mononuclear inflammatory cell infiltrates. These changes are severe in HFRS caused by Hantaan virus and relatively mild in HFRS caused by Puumala virus. Interstitial pneumonitis, similar to that seen in HPS, occurs in some fatal cases.

The most striking pathological features of fatal HPS caused by Sin Nombre virus are large amounts of frothy fluid in airways of the lower respiratory tract, congested, edematous lungs, and large volumes of pleural fluid.[136,156] Microscopic abnormalities in lung include vascular congestion, diffuse interstitial pneumonitis, and interstitial and alveolar edema. The inflammatory infiltrate in affected lung comprises $CD4^+$ and $CD8^+$ lymphocytes and activated macrophages, producing an array of inflammatory cytokines.[157] Hyaline membranes in alveoli usually are scant.[136] Other features of diffuse alveolar damage, including alveolar neutrophils and disruption of the cytokeratin-positive basement membrane, typically are absent.[136,156] Lymphoid tissues show an active immune response with variable numbers of immunoblasts present within the red pulp and periarteriolar sheaths of the spleen and sinuses of lymph nodes. Hantaviral antigens can usually be detected in follicular dendritic cells present within germinal centers.[136]

The pathogenesis of HPS is similar to that of HFRS in many ways (***Table 71.2***) even though the viruses that cause HPS are phylogenetically and antigenically distinct from those that cause HFRS. The similarities include long incubation period, widespread infection in endothelial cells of the microvasculature, appearance of anti-hantavirus IgM and activated T cells in peripheral blood early in disease, capillary dilatation, and hyperpermeability of the endothelium of the microvasculature. Together, the immune response early in disease and the presence of activated lymphocytes and activated macrophages in affected tissues suggest that various

Table 71.2 Disease Course Pathogenesis of Typical HFRS from Hantaan Virus Infection and HPS from Sin Nombre Virus Infection

HFRS	HPS
Incubation Period	
Typically 2–4 weeks (1–8 weeks)	Typically 2–3 weeks (1–6 weeks)
Early Signs, Symptoms, and Antibody Response	
3–7 days of fever, myalgia, malaise then gastrointestinal symptoms, flushing of skin, conjunctival injection	3–5 days of fever, myalgia, malaise often accompanied by gastrointestinal symptoms
IgM and immunoblasts already present	IgM and immunoblasts already present
Disease Course	
DIC, kinin, complement activation, bleeding diathesis	Abnormal PTT, platelets
Back pain, retroperitoneal leak	Dyspnea, hypoxemia, pulmonary edema
Hypotension and shock	Hypotension and shock
Defervescence	Fever may continue
Shock lasting 12–48 h	Shock and pulmonary edema worsening up to 48 h
Recovery	
Oliguric renal failure, problems in circulatory status, bleeding, fluid balance	Pulmonary failure and shock management
Diuresis 5–10 days later	Resolution of lung lesion and shock in 3–6 days

DIC, disseminated intravascular coagulation; HFRS, hemorrhagic fever with renal syndrome; HPS, hantavirus pulmonary syndrome; PTT, partial thromboplastin time.

elements of the immune system play an important role in the pathogenesis of HFRS and HPS.

The early events in hantavirus infections in humans are not known with certainty. Viremia is thought to occur subsequent to infection of alveolar macrophages or other cells associated with the lower respiratory tract, leading to infection in endothelial cells in the microvasculature of all major organs. Inflammation in HFRS may occur in multiple organs whereas inflammation in HPS is usually restricted to lung and serosal surfaces in the thoracic cavity. In fatal HPS, the amount of hantaviral antigen in endothelial cells of the pulmonary microvasculature is significantly greater than that in the microvasculature of other organs.[136] The selective distribution of viral antigen in HPS may explain the localization of inflammation to the thoracic cavity.

Morphological changes in the endothelium in HFRS and HPS cases are uncommon and, when present, consist of prominent and swollen endothelial cells, suggesting that the microvascular leak in HFRS and in HPS stems from endothelial cell dysfunction. This dysfunction could be a consequence of a direct, non-lytic effect of infection on endothelial cells, including modulation of cellular function and expression of cell surface proteins that are critical to maintaining the integrity of the endothelial barrier.[158]

Hantaviruses readily infect endothelial cells *in vitro* with no apparent cytopathic effect. Sin Nombre virus infection alone has no measurable effect on the permeability of monolayers of human lung microvascular endothelial cells.[159] Thus, the occurrence of pulmonary edema in HPS likely is dependent upon factors extrinsic to endothelial cells in infected lung tissue. These factors may include antigen-specific $CD8^+$ T lymphocytes,[160] activated macrophages, vascular endothelial growth factor (VEGF),[161] tumor necrosis factor (TNF)-α,[157,162] various other cytokines,[156] and reactive oxygen/nitrogen species.[163]

The fever, capillary dilatation and leak, and shock in HFRS can be attributed to the release of mediators of inflammation during the immune response to infection.[164] Kinin activation occurs during the hypotensive phase and is proportional to the severity of shock.[165] Levels of TNF-α, interleukin (IL)-6, IL-10, interferon (IFN)-γ, IFN-α, and other cytokines usually are elevated;[166,167] but the levels of these cytokines do not consistently correlate with severity of disease. Production of nitric oxide (NO) is increased,[168] endothelial cell adhesion molecules in kidney are increased in association with mononuclear cells expressing TNF-α,[167] and circulating immune complexes and tissue-associated immune complexes have been found in some HFRS cases in Europe.[169–171] The association of specific MHC alleles with the severity of HFRS caused by Puumala virus supports the notion that HFRS is an immunopathological disease.[172]

Renal failure in HFRS is not simply due to shock and acute tubular necrosis since the clinical picture often does not correlate well with histopathological findings.[173] It is possible that metabolically vulnerable sections of the medullary nephrons near the cortical border suffer damage when the renal circulation is compromised by intrarenal factors and circulatory instability.[164] Other factors may be involved, such as intrarenal production of mediators of inflammation and infection of renal endothelial and tubular epithelial cells.[174,175] The extraordinary hyposthenuria during and after the oliguric phase is presumably related to the location of the lesion in the renal tubule. Anterior pituitary necrosis may have a similar pathogenesis involving its portal circulation. The origin of the right atrial necrosis and hemorrhage in HFRS is not known. Bleeding during the early phases of the disease is probably related to vascular infection, with Hantaan virus triggering a procoagulant state in endothelium that leads to DIC. Uremic coagulopathy in the hypotensive or oliguric phase may exacerbate bleeding.

Pulmonary edema in HPS is thought to result primarily from the influx of activated T lymphocytes into lung tissue, activation of macrophages, secretion of various cytokines, adhesion of platelets to endothelial cells, and/or increased sensitization of endothelial cells to the permeabilizing effect of VEGF.[136,176] Direct measurement of T-cell mediators in the circulation has supported this idea.[177] Other evidence in support of the importance of cell-mediated immunity in the pathogenesis of HPS includes the observation that mononuclear cells producing Th1-type cytokines dominate the pulmonary interstitial infiltrate in fatal HPS cases,[157] the description of hantavirus epitope-specific $CD4^+$ and $CD8^+$ T lymphocytes,[178] the observation that circulating hantavirus-specific, tetramer-positive $CD8^+$ T lymphocytes are more abundant in severe cases than in mild cases of HPS,[179] and the results of an *in vitro* study in which hantavirus-specific $CD8^+$ T lymphocytes increased the permeability of monolayer cultures of EA.hy926 endothelial cells infected with Sin Nombre virus.[160]

The severity of HPS correlates positively with level of virus in blood,[180,181] is negatively associated with titer of circulating anti-hantavirus neutralizing antibody,[182] and is associated with specific MHC class I alleles.[177] The association between disease severity and titer of neutralizing antibody on admission to hospital could be interpreted as evidence that HPS patients with delayed or otherwise low-titered neutralization responses may attempt to "compensate" with a more robust T-cell response which, in turn, may lead to greater injury to the microvasculature, especially in lung. The association between disease severity and specific MHC class I alleles could be interpreted as evidence that class I-restricted $CD8^+$ T cells play a critical role in the pathogenesis of HPS.

Myocardial dysfunction contributes to shock in some HPS cases. The heart in fatal HPS cases caused by Sin Nombre virus is grossly and microscopically unremarkable at autopsy.[136] Hantaviral antigen has been found in the endothelium of the microvasculature in the heart of some fatal cases caused by Sin Nombre virus and the heart of fatal cases caused by Andes virus and Brazilian hantavirus(es).[136,183] Further, TNF-α is present in myocardiocytes and macrophages in the hearts of fatal cases caused by Brazilian hantavirus(es).[183] Hypothetically, the myocardial depression in severe HPS may be a downstream effect of the cytokine storm in infected lung or a consequence of infection in heart tissue.

There is pulmonary pathology in HFRS as well as HPS. Careful conventional and CT imaging has demonstrated pulmonary infiltrates or effusions in half of Puumala virus-infected patients.[184] Most patients, even mild cases, have decreased diffusion capacity.[185] Pulmonary edema in HFRS is usually a consequence of overhydration; however, pulmonary edema early in disease may be a consequence of an intense cellular immune response in infected lung tissue.[186–188]

Animal Models of Hantavirus Pulmonary Syndrome

Andes virus in cynomolgus macaques (*Macaca fascicularis*) is infectious but not pathogenic.[189] Laboratory mice (*Mus musculus*) infected with Andes virus, Sin Nombre virus, or other New World hantaviruses do not develop disease that mimics HPS. In contrast, Andes virus in adult Syrian golden hamsters (*Mesocricetus auratus*) is almost invariably lethal,[190] Maporal virus (a hantavirus that is enzootic in Venezuela)[77] in adult Syrian golden hamsters is frequently lethal, and the disease in Andes virus-infected hamsters and Maporal virus-infected hamsters is pathologically highly similar to fatal HPS.[190,191] Other similarities between the disease in hamsters and HPS include long incubation period (9 days to 2 weeks), viremia, infection in endothelial cells in the microvasculature of all major organs, thrombocytopenia and an anti-hantavirus antibody response early in disease, rapid progression of disease following the onset of symptoms, severe dyspnea, and preterminal hypotension and tachycardia.[191–193] The Andes virus-hamster model of HPS has been used to demonstrate that passive antibody transfer before the appearance of disease symptoms may prevent HPS[194,195] and to investigate molecular strategies for prevention of HPS.[196]

Sin Nombre virus and Choclo virus in Syrian golden hamsters are nonpathogenic.[190,196] The failure of Sin Nombre virus to cause HPS-like disease in Syrian golden hamsters is attributed to the inability of the virus to efficiently disseminate from the intramuscular injection site and subsequently infect large numbers of endothelial cells in lung and other solid tissues.[193] In hamsters infected with Choclo virus, large amounts of hantaviral antigen are present in endothelial cells in the microcirculation of lung, and hantaviral antigen is found in endothelial cells in the microvasculature of other major organs.[197] Thus, the reason that Choclo virus is nonpathogenic in Syrian golden hamsters appears to be unrelated to magnitude or distribution of infection in lung.

Subacute interstitial pneumonitis is a prominent feature of HPS-like disease in Syrian golden hamsters and HPS. Choclo virus in Syrian golden hamsters does not evoke an inflammatory response in lung, heart, or other infected tissues.[197] The absence of inflammation and edema in the lungs of Choclo virus-infected hamsters suggests that the cellular inflammatory response in lung tissue plays a key role in the development of the pulmonary edema in the HPS-like disease in Andes virus- and Maporal virus-infected hamsters. Studies to assess the role of hantavirus-specific cytotoxic T cells, macrophages, and vasoactive cytokines in HPS-like disease in hamsters may provide insight into the pathogenesis of the life-threatening pulmonary edema in HPS.

Hantaan virus prototype strain 76–118, Seoul virus strain SR-11, Dobrava virus, and Puumala virus strain K27 are infectious but apparently nonpathogenic in adult Syrian golden hamsters.[198] Whether strains of other Old World hantaviruses (e.g., Amur and Saaremaa viruses) can cause HFRS-like disease in hamsters has not been investigated.

DIAGNOSIS

Differential Diagnosis of Hemorrhagic Fever with Renal Syndrome

Any patient with fever, thrombocytopenia, and laboratory evidence of acute renal dysfunction should be suspected of having HFRS. Diseases that should be included in the differential diagnosis are other viral hemorrhagic fevers, bacterial sepsis, bacterial endocarditis, leptospirosis, murine or louse-borne typhus, and malaria. Poststreptococcal glomerulonephritis, blood dyscrasias, glaucoma, and acute abdominal emergencies also may be important in the differential diagnosis. Severe HFRS cases may resemble fulminant sepsis; milder cases may be mistaken for influenza, hepatitis A, or streptococcal pharyngitis. The leukemoid reaction that occurs in some HFRS cases may suggest leukemia to the inexperienced clinician, particularly with the appearance of myelocytes or atypical lymphocytes in peripheral blood. Hemoconcentration associated with the vascular leak in the febrile, vomiting HFRS patient may be mistaken for dehydration and the ensuing renal failure may be attributed to hypotension or the effects of antibiotics given for the presumed bacterial gastroenteritis. The clinical picture in Puumala virus infection, with its milder presentation and fewer abnormalities of blood and renal function, can be difficult to recognize if the diagnosis is not sought. The most important consideration, also valid for Hantaan virus infection, is disease mimicking an acute abdominal emergency, which should be distinguished by routine urinalysis and blood examination.

Differential Diagnosis of Hantavirus Pulmonary Syndrome

Recognition of HPS during the prodrome is difficult; but, once dyspnea is reported, the finding of thrombocytopenia, left shift (often with leukocytosis and myelocytosis), and/or immunoblasts in peripheral blood is common and helpful.[134] Hypoxemia may be present early, even with a virtually normal chest radiograph.[129] Suspicion of the diagnosis during this phase is critical because oxygenation may fall precipitously over the next few hours. The most common diagnosis in the differential is bacterial sepsis. Plague, tularemia, and endocarditis are not uncommon diseases with similar presentations and may be accompanied by thrombocytopenia. The fever and myalgia in HPS may initially lead to consideration of influenza, but the early symptoms of influenza include cough and coryza whereas HPS patients rarely have respiratory symptoms until the onset of the cardiopulmonary phase. Pneumococcal and other pneumonias can be ruled out because of the symmetric interstitial infiltrates progressing to alveolar pulmonary edema in HPS, although a few cases have had asymmetric findings in the early hours of disease. Abdominal pain and gastrointestinal symptoms may cause confusion of HPS with an acute abdominal emergency. Misdiagnosis of pneumonia has led to excessive fluid loads associated with antibiotic administration. Misinterpretation of the elevated hematocrit as due to dehydration has led to rapid infusion of intravenous fluids.

It should be kept in mind that the flushing of the face and neck, conjunctival injection, and hemorrhagic signs, which are usual in severe or moderate HFRS, have not been seen in North American HPS cases or the majority of South American HPS cases. Further, hemorrhagic signs in HPS are restricted to late stages of the disease, and these cases have signs or laboratory findings of DIC. Renal failure may occur in HPS caused by Bayou virus, Black Creek Canal virus, and some South American hantaviruses, but most infections with New World hantaviruses have only proteinuria and perhaps mildly elevated serum levels of creatinine.

Laboratory Diagnosis

Early diagnosis is critical to the successful management of HFRS and HPS and, in HPS caused by Andes virus, implementation of appropriate isolation procedures to prevent virus transmission to health care providers and others. Fever and severe myalgia, especially in patients who develop thrombocytopenia, should prompt physicians in endemic regions to suspect hantaviral disease.

Serology

Virtually all HFRS and HPS patients have measurable levels of hantavirus-specific immunoglobulin M (IgM) in serum or plasma by the end of the prodrome.[199–202] Many have measurable levels of anti-hantavirus IgG, and some have measurable levels of neutralizing antibody by the end of the prodrome, too.

The diagnosis of hantavirus infection early in the course of disease is best made by IgM-capture ELISA, using an infected cell lysate for the test antigen and an uninfected cell lysate for the comparison (control) antigen. This assay is sensitive and specific for anti-hantavirus IgM but may detect IgM to hantaviruses other than the virus that was used to prepare the test antigen. Other methods for the detection of anti-hantavirus IgM include western blot assay and IFAT. Any "sandwich" method for the detection of IgM suffers from the specificity of the IgM conjugate (a serious problem with IFAT) and inaccuracies related to rheumatoid factor and competition between IgG and IgM. Tests must include a negative control antigen for each serum sample to rule out falsely positive results arising from serum binding to nonviral components of the test antigen (i.e., "sticky" serum).[203]

Measurable levels of anti-hantavirus IgM may persist as long as 6 months after the end of the acute phase of illness in nephropathia epidemica[204] and longer than 2 months after the end of the acute phase of illness in HPS.[205] Thus, anti-hantavirus IgM in an acute phase sample is presumptive evidence that a hantavirus is the cause of a patient's illness. The weight of this evidence will depend, in part, on other laboratory findings (e.g., thrombocytopenia, left shift of the white blood cell count with myelocytosis, and the presence of large, reactive immunoblasts in peripheral blood). The diagnosis can be confirmed by measurement of levels of anti-hantavirus IgG or neutralizing antibody in paired acute-and-convalescent sera, detection of hantaviral RNA in acute-phase blood, respiratory secretions, or other biological specimens, and/or detection of hantaviral antigen in biopsy or autopsy specimens.

The IgM and IgG responses in HFRS and HPS are directed against the N protein and glycoproteins, and the neutralizing antibody response in both syndromes is directed against the glycoproteins.[201,206–209] Neutralization of infectivity has been measured by plaque or focus reduction in monolayer cultures of Vero E6 cells (American Type Culture Collection, CRL-1586).[192,210] The focus-reduction neutralization test is used more widely than the plaque-reduction neutralization test because some hantaviral strains do not consistently produce readily discernible plaques in monolayer cultures of Vero E6 cells stained with neutral red.[211] A drawback of the neutralization assay is that it may entail work with infectious virus at biosafety level 3.

Antibodies (IgM and IgG) from patients infected with one hantavirus may cross-react with the N proteins or glycoproteins of other hantaviruses.[206,212–214] Further, acute- and early convalescent-phase sera may efficiently neutralize strains of several different hantaviruses.[215] Generally, the results of neutralization assays done *in vitro* are more specific than the results of ELISA and other assays for anti-hantavirus antibody.

Levels of hantavirus-specific IgG increase through the end of the acute phase of illness, remain high for months or years, and then decline gradually.[209] Hantavirus-specific IgG may persist as long as 10 years in HFRS cases[209] and longer than 3 years in HPS cases.[216]

Virus Assay

The isolation of infectious hantavirus from clinical specimens, if possible, may require a considerable amount of time and effort. Thus, virus isolation usually is not attempted for the diagnosis of infections in humans even though hantaviruses have been isolated from blood, solid tissue, and/or urine samples from HFRS patients, and Andes virus has been isolated from HPS cases.[42,217] Typically, monolayer cultures of Vero E6 cells are inoculated with the specimen and then maintained under a fluid overlay for 10–14 days. Successful virus isolation may require serial blind passage of inoculated cell culture material. Hantaviruses usually are not cytopathic; consequently, detection of infection in cultured cells requires an indirect method (e.g., IFAT for viral antigen or reverse transcription-polymerase chain reaction (RT-PCR) assay for hantaviral RNA).

Nucleic Acid Detection

Since the 1993 outbreak of HPS in the southwestern United States, RT-PCR assays have been employed extensively to detect hantaviral RNA in clinical or autopsy specimens from HFRS patients and HPS patients. Hantaviral RNA can be detected in acute-phase serum or (even better) clotted blood from HPS patients[218] and from many HFRS patients.[59] Analysis of sequence data enables rapid, accurate determination of the identity of the virus. Sets of primers (oligonucleotides) have been designed that anneal to regions of the S and M genomic segments that are highly conserved among the Old World hantaviruses and highly conserved among the New World hantaviruses. Reverse transcription of hantaviral RNA and subsequent PCR amplification of the resulting cDNA usually can be accomplished by using a "one-step, single-tube" format. Semi-quantitative real-time RT-PCR assays have been developed for some hantaviruses and used for diagnostic purposes.[181,219–221] Real-time assays can match or exceed the sensitivity of nested RT-PCR assays and can provide precise estimates of viral load in clinical samples. RT-PCR assays have been used to detect hantaviral RNA in fixed, paraffin-embedded tissues.[222]

Antigen Detection

Immunohistochemistry has been used to detect hantaviral antigens in formalin-fixed, paraffin-embedded tissues from patients with fatal HPS.[136,155,183,223] Polyclonal antibodies (e.g., immune sera from humans, experimentally infected rabbits or rodents, or naturally infected rodents) and murine monoclonal antibodies have been used as the primary antibodies in immunohistochemical assays for hantaviral antigens.

TREATMENT AND PROGNOSIS

Hemorrhagic Fever with Renal Syndrome

Intensive monitoring in a hospital setting and careful supportive care are extremely important to survival. The experience in the Korean War strongly suggested that early helicopter evacuation improved the outcome relative to prolonged transport over rough roads. Conversely, long medical evacuation flights of seriously ill patients have been associated with adverse outcomes.[187] Management of shock, judicious use of sedation and analgesia, careful monitoring for secondary infections, and appropriately timed dialysis for uremia, hypertension, or electrolyte abnormalities should keep the mortality rate well below 5%.

Ribavirin given intravenously within 4 days of onset was shown in a carefully controlled study in China to reduce mortality, bleeding, and the duration of renal failure in a setting in which hemodialysis was not available.[224] Similar results were obtained in a study done in Korea.[225]

Immunosuppression, immunostimulation, and IFN play no role in therapy. The administration of steroids was reported to have a sparing effect in the Korean War experience.[226] In a randomized study of 48 carefully selected, clinically diagnosed HFRS patients with fewer than 72 hours of symptoms, those treated with 1.1 g of oral cortisone over 5 days had a milder course than those treated with a placebo. The duration of proteinuria and azotemia and the severity of azotemia in the steroid group were statistically significantly less than in the placebo group. It is not clear that the findings in this small study are relevant to the therapy of hantaviral diseases today, given improvements in the ability to support patients, the potency of corticosteroids, and the possible side effects of steroids.

Hantavirus Pulmonary Syndrome

The majority of HPS patients require intensive cardiopulmonary support, and many of these patients decompensate rapidly. Thus, early recognition of HPS and close monitoring in a hospital setting for hypoxemia and shock are crucial to survival. It is imperative that supportive therapy is initiated before irreversible decompensation makes resuscitation difficult.[138,227] Hypoxemia in approximately one-third of North American HPS cases is successfully managed by administration of high concentrations of inspired oxygen through a nonrebreathing or bi-level positive airway pressure mask, monitored by continuous pulse oximetry. Some patents require intubation within a few hours of the beginning of the cardiopulmonary phase.[130,138] Severely ill patients may require the suctioning of more than 1 L of secretions from the endotracheal tube hourly. Mechanical ventilation should be initiated before hypoxemia becomes severe since the loss of adrenergic drive associated with intubation may cause cardiovascular collapse. Vomiting may lead to dehydration in some patients. Initially, fluid support should be restricted to less than 2 L of crystalloid fluids in the first 24 hours of hospitalization, as overhydration will exacerbate the pulmonary edema without improving cardiac function. Early administration of dobutamine is frequently used for inotropic and pressor support. A Swan–Ganz catheter to monitor pulmonary wedge pressure and an arterial line to monitor blood pressure are strongly recommended. Pulmonary wedge pressure will increase as myocardial suppression worsens. The cardiac index may fall below 2.5 $L/min/m^2$ even when blood pressure appears to be maintained. Optimal pressor support has been found to be a combination of dobutamine (5–15 μg/kg/min) and norepinephrine (1–4 μg/min). ECMO should be considered when cardiac index or blood pressure decreases in spite of support.[227,228] The criteria for ECMO are cardiac index <2.5 $L/min/m^2$, PaO_2/FIO_2 <50, or cardiopulmonary deterioration in spite of carefully managed supportive care. Inhaled NO has been proposed based on an anecdotal report,[229] but the lack of high pulmonary artery pressure and the lack of recommendation for use in acute lung injury suggest that further study is needed before administration of NO by inhalation can be recommended.[230] Pending a definitive diagnosis, patients should be administered antibiotics appropriate for plague, tularemia, rickettsial diseases, and other treatable illnesses which could be confused with HPS. Most deaths in HPS occur within 48 hours of hospitalization. Patients who arrive at the intensive care unit in shock have a higher mortality rate than other HPS patients. Late deaths with diffuse alveolar damage may occur.[136] The alveolar damage in some of these cases may be related to prolonged mechanical ventilation and/or secondary bacterial infections.

There is no known specific therapy for HPS. A study done in the southwestern United States suggests that ribavirin initiated in the cardiopulmonary stage is ineffective.[231] The benefit of ribavirin when therapy is initiated immediately after exposure or before the end of the prodrome has not been investigated.

PREVENTION AND CONTROL

Avoidance of Rodents

Reduction of the frequency and intensity of interactions between humans and rodents currently is the key to prevention of hantaviral infections in humans. Guidelines generally emphasize rodent-proofing of houses and outbuildings, removal of cover for rodents near dwellings, and protection of food sources within homes (http://www.cdc.gov/rodents/prevent_rodents/index.htm).[232] In some occupations and in rural areas in Asia and South America, rodent avoidance is not practical and vaccination will be the cornerstone of prevention in the future.

Vaccines

Almost all efforts to develop vaccines have been directed at HFRS. None of the Old World hantaviruses are known to cause frank illness in nonhuman primates or HFRS-like disease in laboratory rodents.[198,233,234] Consequently, protection usually has been measured by the ability to prevent infection. Protective immunity in laboratory rodents usually is highly correlated with antibody-mediated neutralization of infectivity *in vitro*.[79]

Inactivated vaccines have been developed in Asia and used locally in Korea and China for protection against HFRS.[79] These vaccines were prepared from the brains of suckling rats or mice or from cultured cells infected with Hantaan virus or Seoul virus.[235–239] The inactivated vaccines that have been tested in humans yielded only low levels of neutralizing antibodies at 1 year after the last vaccine dose, raising concern about the duration of protection afforded by these vaccines.[240–242] Optimization of vaccination schedules and advances in adjuvant technology may increase the duration of immunity elicited by inactivated vaccines. Other approaches that have been used in the development of HFRS vaccines include recombinant vaccinia viruses that express the S and M genomic segments of Hantaan virus,[243] naked DNA (modified M segment of Hantaan virus and Puumala virus) delivered by gene gun,[79] virus-like particles, and alphavirus replicons.[120,244,245]

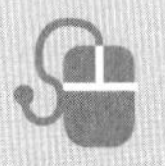

Access the complete reference list online at
http://www.expertconsult.com

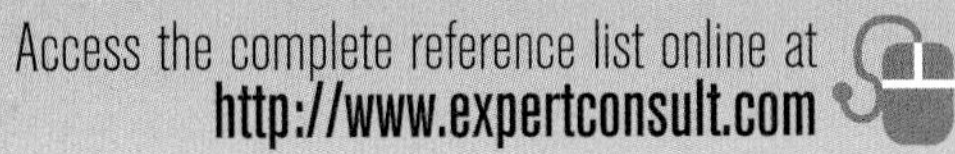
Access the complete reference list online at
http://www.expertconsult.com

CHAPTER 72

Sandfly Fever, Oropouche Fever, and Other Bunyavirus Infections

Robert B. Tesh • Pedro F.C. Vasconcelos

INTRODUCTION

The family *Bunyaviridae* includes more than 300 antigenically distinct members, most of which are transmitted by arthropods.[1] At least 41 of these viruses have been associated with human illness in the tropics. Apart from those members that produce serious and sometimes fatal disease (i.e., the hantaviruses, Rift Valley fever virus, and Crimean-Congo hemorrhagic fever virus), most of the remaining human pathogenic bunyaviruses produce nonspecific febrile illnesses. Because of their nonspecific nature and the limited virus diagnostic capabilities in many tropical countries, these infections are often unrecognized or are misdiagnosed as other common febrile illnesses such as malaria or dengue. This chapter describes some of the more common bunyavirus fevers.

PHLEBOTOMUS (SANDFLY) FEVER

Historically, phlebotomus fever (PF) has been mainly a disease of military importance, since epidemics have typically occurred when large numbers of nonimmune adults enter an area of endemic virus activity. The disease occurred in troops during the Napoleonic Wars, the Austrian occupation of the Adriatic, the British colonization of India and Pakistan, and the North African and Mediterranean campaigns in World War II.[2,3] The largest reported outbreak of PF occurred in Serbia in 1948, when over 1 million persons were affected. PF outbreaks still occur among tourists vacationing in the Mediterranean region.[4–7]

Many of the PF group of viruses appear to be maintained in their insect vectors by vertical (transovarial) virus transmission.[3] Consequently, virus activity is largely correlated with adult sandfly activity rather than by the immune status of the local human or animal populations. During periods of vector abundance (i.e., summer in subtropical or Mediterranean climates and the rainy season in drier tropical climates), phlebovirus activity is continuous. In this situation one sees little illness in the native population, most of whom are already immune, but when a group of nonimmune adults (i.e., tourists, soldiers) enters in the area, an epidemic quickly ensues.[2]

Although more than 40 PF virus serotypes have been described,[2] three virus serotypes (Naples, Sicilian, and Toscana) account for most of the recognized PF cases. This is probably because their sandfly vectors (*Phlebotomus papatasi*, *P. perniciosus*, and *P. perfiliewi*) are highly anthropophilic, readily enter houses, and have a wide geographic distribution in the Mediterranean region and central Asia.[3] In contrast, most of the New World phleboviruses and their vectors have a more focal and sylvan distribution; consequently, PF cases in this region are infrequent and occur mainly in persons who enter forested areas for work or recreation.

After an incubation period of 3–5 days, PF begins suddenly with fever, severe frontal headache, retro-orbital pain, photophobia, malaise, anorexia, nausea, vomiting, and low back pain.[8] The face is often flushed and the conjunctivae are injected, but a true rash is absent. The disease is self-limited, and the symptoms usually disappear within 2–3 days; however, a general feeling of weakness and depression frequently lasts for a week or more after the illness. Marked leukopenia (<4000/μL), consisting of initial lymphopenia, followed by protracted neutropenia, also occurs in PF.[8]

Aseptic meningitis is a relatively common manifestation of Toscana virus infection. Originally described in central Italy, this infection occurs throughout much of the Mediterranean region of Europe and is a frequent cause of summertime meningitis in both adults and children.[9] These cases begin as classic PF, with a nonspecific febrile illness for 2–4 days before the appearance of more serious symptoms, such as nuchal rigidity, positive Kernig's sign, nystagmus, and reduced levels of consciousness.[7] In these cases the hematologic picture is similar to that of classic PF, but the cerebrospinal fluid (CSF) may show increased pressure, but without pleocytosis and with normal glucose and protein levels. The neurologic abnormalities usually resolve in a few days, and most patients recover spontaneously in 1–2 weeks, although headache may persist. The recovery of phleboviruses from patients with PF is uncommon, since the viremia associated with this disease is quite transient (24–36 hours), and most patients do not seek medical care so early. The one exception is patients with neurologic disease due to Toscana virus infection; virus can be recovered from the CSF after it has disappeared from the blood.[6] Culture in Vero cells is the isolation system of choice for most phleboviruses.[2] RT-PCR can also be done on CSF of patients with neurologic symptoms of Toscana virus infection.

A number of serologic techniques can be used for the diagnosis of PF, but each has its limitations. The IgM-capture enzyme-linked immunosorbent assay (ELISA)[10] and plaque reduction neutralization test (PRNT)[2,8,11] are quite specific and sensitive, but one must screen against a variety of phlebovirus serotypes because of their focal and sometimes overlapping distribution. Seroconversion can be demonstrated in paired samples by IgG ELISA and by fluorescent antibody (FA) or hemagglutination-inhibition (HI) tests, but these techniques are not serotype-specific.

Treatment of PF is symptomatic. Except for patients with neurologic symptoms, as in Toscana virus infection, hospitalization is usually unnecessary. The headache associated with PF can be severe, and narcotics are sometimes needed for relief. PF is a self-limited, nonfatal disease, and recovery is complete. One attack of PF confers lifelong immunity against the infecting virus type but not against heterologous serotypes.[8,11] Thus, second cases of the disease can occur among persons living in regions where more than one phlebovirus is active. There are no vaccines for PF. Control measures are directed against the vector and include household spraying with residual insecticides, bednets, and the use of insect repellents.[3]

OROPOUCHE FEVER

Oropouche fever is a midge-borne viral disease that has emerged during the past 50 years as an important public health problem in tropical South America.[12,13] The causative agent, Oropouche virus (genus *Orthobunyavirus*), was first isolated from the blood of a febrile forest worker in Trinidad in 1955. Since 1961, more than 30 outbreaks of Oropouche virus have been reported from the Amazon regions of Brazil and Peru and from Panama. The number of persons affected has varied with each outbreak, but the two largest recorded epidemics (Belem and Manaus, Brazil, in 1980 and 1981) each involved about 100 000 people.[12]

It is postulated that Oropouche virus is maintained in two distinct cycles: (1) an epidemic urban cycle involving the biting midge *Culicoides paraensis*; and (2) a silent maintenance cycle in which forest animals (sloths and possibly monkeys) are the principal vertebrate hosts, and a yet unidentified arthropod serves as the vector.[12] However, the epidemiology of this disease is still not fully elucidated, as it is easily confused with dengue and other acute febrile illnesses, and the true incidence is unknown.

Oropouche fever is characterized by the abrupt onset of fever (up to 40°C), chills, severe headache, mayalgia, arthralgia, anorexia, weakness, dizziness, and photophobia.[12,13] Nausea, vomiting, diarrhea, and epigastric pain may also occur. Some Oropouche fever patients can present with a clinical picture of aseptic meningitis or meningoencephalitis. Rash is rarely present, but leukopenia is a common feature of this disease. The acute clinical illness usually lasts 2–5 days, although a period of asthenia and occasionally dizziness may persist for up to a month. A significant percentage of patients (as high as 60% in some outbreaks) have a recrudescence of their original symptoms within 2–10 days after they become afebrile.[12] The recurrent illness associated with Oropouche fever seems to occur more commonly in persons who quickly resume strenuous activities. No virus can be isolated from the patient's serum during the recurrent illness, and detectable humoral antibodies are usually present.

Oropouche virus can often be recovered from the patient's serum during the first 2–4 days of the disease. The virus can be isolated in newborn mice, adult hamsters, and a variety of mammalian cell cultures. Demonstration of virus-specific antibody can be demonstrated in paired acute and convalescent phase sera by ELISA, IFA, HI, complement fixation (CF), or PRNT. Treatment is symptomatic. No fatalities have been reported with Oropouche fever; and lifelong immunity follows recovery.

There is no vaccine against Oropouche fever. Given our limited knowledge of the maintenance cycle of Oropouche virus, vector control appears to be the best prevention and control strategy. *C. paraensis* is a daytime feeder and, because of its tiny size, readily passes through window screens. Spraying or fogging in and around houses with residual insecticides is of limited value in the control of adult peridomestic populations of this midge vector. Cleaning up rotting vegetation (e.g., banana stalks, decomposing fruit) around houses can help to eliminate *C. paraensis* larval breeding sites. Insect repellent applied to exposed skin also reduces the number of bites.

GROUP C AND GUAMA VIRUS INFECTIONS

Group C and Guama viruses are found throughout the New World tropics and subtropics, including Florida, Mexico, Central America, and the warmer regions of northern South America.[14] At least 25 different virus serotypes have been identified. Most of the serotypes have focal distribution which coincides with forest or forest-fringe habitats, usually in low-lying swampy areas. These viruses are maintained in continuous sylvan cycles involving mosquitoes, mainly *Culex* of the subgenus *Melanoconion*, and small mammals such as rodents and marsupials. Humans are usually infected when they enter the swampy forest habitats where these viruses are endemic and are bitten by infected mosquitoes. Cases are usually sporadic; and because of their nonspecific nature, they are usually not reported, or are misdiagnosed, so their true incidence is unknown.

Persons infected by group C and Guama group viruses develop sudden fever (38–40°C), severe headache, vertigo, myalgia, retro-orbital pain, malaise, and nausea. The fever lasts 2–5 days and is sometimes biphasic. Rash is absent. Patients recover with weakness and anorexia lasting 1 or 2 weeks, but without sequelae.

These viruses can be recovered from patients' sera during the acute febrile phase of the illness. They grow well in a variety of cell cultures and kill newborn mice and hamsters. Antibodies can also be detected in paired acute and convalescent sera by HI, CF, ELISA, IFA, and PRNT. Treatment is nonspecific and supportive. The major risk factor is occupation; avoidance of swampy forest habitats and personal protection against mosquito bites are the only prevention.

BWAMBA, ILESHA, AND TATAGUINE VIRUS INFECTIONS

These three bunyaviruses have been isolated repeatedly from sick persons and mosquitoes in East, Central, and West Africa.[15,16] The diseases associated with them are similar: the acute onset of fever, headache, vertigo, severe mayalgia, and rash, lasting 4–5 days and followed by a week or more of asthenia. No deaths or serious complications have been reported. Most of the mosquito isolations of Bwamba, Ilesha, and Tataguine viruses have been made from *Anopheles* and *Aedes* species.[15] The viruses are thought to be maintained in a mosquito–wild vertebrate cycle, but little other information is available. Given their demonstrated disease potential, wide geographic distribution, and the relatively high antibody rates found in serosurveys among humans in some African countries,[15,16] it seems likely that these agents are of greater health importance to the local populations and to visitors than is currently recognized. But because of the paucity of functioning virus laboratories in Africa and the nonspecific nature of illness associated with them, most of these infections are probably never recognized or reported. Diagnosis can be made by virus isolation from blood during the febrile period or by antibody detection in paired acute and convalescent sera.

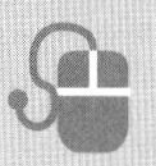

Access the complete reference list online at
http://www.expertconsult.com

Access the complete reference list online at http://www.expertconsult.com

CHAPTER 73

Filovirus Infections

Victoria Wahl-Jensen • C. J. Peters • Peter B. Jahrling • Heinz Feldmann • Jens H. Kuhn

INTRODUCTION

Filoviruses, marburgviruses (MARV) and ebolaviruses (EBOV), are etiologic agents of severe hemorrhagic fevers with unusually high lethality. They are emerging/reemerging zoonotic agents whose natural hosts remain to be identified. The viruses are highly virulent in primates, and the frequency of outbreaks in Africa and Asia as well as their impact on ape populations has been increasing in recent years. Introduction of filoviruses into human populations leads to serious, but limited, epidemics when inadequate sterilization of needles and lack of barrier nursing practices result in nosocomial spread. Interhuman transmission also occurs by direct person-to-person contact and possibly fomites and droplets. The viruses infect, among others, macrophages, dendritic cells, hepatocytes, and endothelial cells. In the infected primate, these infections lead to severe cytokine imbalances that (1) impair the innate and adaptive immune responses; (2) lead to disseminated intravascular coagulation with concomitant hemorrhages, thrombi, and organ necroses; (3) result in multiorgan failure and shock. Currently, there is no FDA-approved treatment or prophylaxis for filovirus infections.[1,2]

THE AGENTS

Taxonomy

The family *Filoviridae*, a member of the order *Mononegavirales*, is divided into two genera. The genus *Marburgvirus* contains one species, *Lake Victoria marburgvirus*, whereas the genus *Ebolavirus* contains one tentative (*Bundibugyo ebolavirus* (BEBOV)) and four accepted species: *Côte d'Ivoire ebolavirus* (CIEBOV), *Reston ebolavirus* (REBOV), *Sudan ebolavirus* (SEBOV), and *Zaire ebolavirus* (ZEBOV).[3]

Virion Structure

Filoviruses are pleomorphic in structure, often forming long filamentous particles. The filaments, which sometimes branch out, can reach 14 μm in length in cell culture. Shorter forms are typical in infected tissues. These particles often appear as U, 6, or circular shapes.[4–6] Filovirions have a uniform diameter of 80 nm but MARV virions recovered from culture fluids are consistently shorter in mean unit length (795–828 nm) than SEBOV (974–1063 nm), ZEBOV (990–1086 nm), or REBOV (1026–1083 nm) particles.[5] The helical nucleocapsid is surrounded by a host cell plasma membrane-derived lipid envelope studded with surface $GP_{1,2}$ spikes.[5,7]

Genome Organization and Replication

The filovirus genome consists of a nonsegmented, single-stranded linear RNA molecule of negative polarity. It contributes 1.1% of the total virion mass with a molecular mass of approximately 4.0×10^6 Da. The average length of a filovirus genome is 19 kb.

Filovirus genomes contain seven genes, *NP*, *VP35*, *VP40*, *GP*, *VP30*, *VP24*, and *L*, which encode the nucleoprotein (NP), polymerase cofactor (VP35), matrix protein (VP40), glycoprotein ($GP_{1,2}$, and in the case of EBOV, also sGP and Δ-peptide), transcriptional activator (VP30), secondary matrix protein (VP24), and RNA-dependent RNA polymerase (L), respectively. Intergenic regions of variable length may exist between adjacent genes; however, gene overlaps are prominent features in filovirus genomes.[8–12] Extragenic sequences at the extreme 3′ (leader) and 5′ (trailer) ends of the genomes of filoviruses are conserved and show a high degree of complementarity. As with other members of the order *Mononegavirales*, these ends play important roles as promoters for the replication and encapsidation of genomic and antigenomic virus RNA.[10,13–15] The seven genes between these promoters are delineated by highly conserved motifs for transcriptional initiation and termination signals.[1,16] Termination of transcription occurs at a consecutive series of five or six uridine residues, where stuttering (repeated copying) by L is thought to result in polyadenylylation of the nascent mRNAs.

The most obvious divergence of MARV and EBOV is manifested in the *GP* gene, which encodes one protein ($GP_{1,2}$) in the case of MARV, but at least three proteins (sGP, Δ-peptide, and $GP_{1,2}$) in the case of EBOV.[17–22] MARV synthesize their spike protein through authentic transcription of the virus RNA. The mechanism used by EBOV involves transcriptional editing by L. Editing occurs approximately in the middle of the *GP* gene at a stretch of seven consecutive uridine residues. The polymerase is thought to stutter over the stretch, and an additional, non-template, adenosine is inserted into the nascent mRNA, causing a shift in the open reading frame and thereby avoiding a translational stop codon downstream of the editing site.[17] Unedited transcripts encode a glycoprotein precursor, pre-sGP, which is proteolytically processed into two secreted proteins, sGP and Δ-peptide.[23,24]

Virus Proteins

Filoviruses produce seven structural proteins. Four of these proteins are associated with the genomic RNA to form the ribonucleoprotein complex (RNP): NP, VP30, VP35, and L. Whereas NP, L, and VP35 are functionally conserved in all members of the *Mononegavirales*, VP30 is thought to represent a unique RNP protein that functions as a transcriptional activator.[25] The genomic position of VP35, when compared to paramyxovirus and rhabdovirus genomes, has led to the hypothesis that it is the functional analog of the phosphoproteins and that it is involved in transcription and replication as a polymerase cofactor.[13,26,27] Additionally, VP35 is a potent suppressor of a host cell's countermeasures against virus infection. ZEBOV VP35 prevents the phosphorylation and dimerization of interferon regulatory factor (IRF)-3 and increases SUMOylation of IRF-7 and thereby inhibits the induction of the host cell interferon (IFN)-β response.

ZEBOV VP35 also inhibits protein kinase R (PKR) activation and, thereby, the antiviral response induced by IFN-α, and serves as a suppressor of the cell's antiviral RNAi machinery.[28,29]

The remaining three structural proteins are all associated with the lipid envelope. VP40 is a membrane-associated protein and the most abundant virus antigen associated with virions.[8,9] The function of VP40 is that of a matrix protein: exclusive expression of VP40 induces the formation of filamentous particles nearly identical in shape to wild-type virions. Co-expression of VP40 and $GP_{1,2}$ results in spiked virus-like particles (VLPs).[30,31] Like VP40, VP24 is localized to the virus membrane. Further studies have shown a specific biochemical interaction among VP24, NP, and VP35.[32] VP24 is believed to be a minor matrix protein that links the membrane-bound proteins (VP40 and/or $GP_{1,2}$) with the RNP, perhaps through interaction with VP35 and NP. VP24 may play a role in virus assembly and budding partially based on evidence that it strongly associates with lipid membranes.[33] In addition to a role in virus budding, VP24 is speculated to play a role in host adaptation.[34] Specifically, VP24 appears to be a "hot spot" for mutations leading to amino acid changes when ZEBOV are serially passed and adapted to cause lethal infection in mice or guinea pigs.[34] Finally, recent experiments suggest that VP24 is another filoviral protein that suppresses the host cell antiviral response by inhibiting IFN-α/β and IFN-γ signaling.[35–37] Interestingly, MARV uses a distinct mechanism to block IFN signaling pathways. Specifically, MARV blocks the phosphorylation of Janus kinases and their target STAT proteins in response to type I and type II interferon and interleukin-6. Unlike EBOV, inhibition is not mediated by the MARV VP24 protein, but by the matrix protein VP40.[38]

Synthesis of $GP_{1,2}$ involves processing of the proprotein by the proprotein convertase furin, a subtilisin/kexin-like convertase localized in the *trans*-Golgi apparatus, at a polybasic cleavage site. Interestingly, furin cleavage is not important for either infectivity or pathogenicity.[15,39] The mature protein is a trimer of a heterodimer, the latter of which consists of the N-terminal fragment GP_1 and the C-terminal fragment GP_2 that are linked by a disulfide bond ($GP_{1,2}$).[19,40,41] During infection, tumor necrosis factor α-converting enzyme (TACE) was shown to be responsible for ectodomain shedding of GP both *in vitro* and *in vivo*.[42] The released protein, $GP_{1,2\Delta}$, may play a role in pathogenicity by binding neutralizing antibodies. $GP_{1,2}$ is heavily glycosylated.[43,44] GP_1, the spike protein ectodomain, contains the receptor-binding domain,[45,46] whereas GP_2 is the functional equivalent of typical class I fusion proteins, such as influenza A virus HA2 or retrovirus TM.[47–49] The primary function of the spike protein is to engage the still unknown filovirus receptor, which seems to be shared among MARV and EBOV, and mediate fusion of the virion membrane with that of the host cell.[45,50] Filovirus cell entry is, mainly due to the unknown identity of the cell-surface receptor, still rather uncharacterized. The endosomal cathepsins B and L, which in turn are modulated by endosomal $\alpha_5\beta_1$ integrins, are key players in filovirus entry.[51–53] $GP_{1,2}$ also counters the cellular antiviral response by inhibiting the IFN-induced action of tetherin/BST-2, which otherwise would tether budding filovirions to the cell membrane.[54]

The sGP proprotein is glycosylated and cleaved at a multibasic amino acid motif similar to GP.[24,55] The larger cleavage product, sGP, is efficiently released as a parallel homodimer.[55–57] In addition to being observed *in vitro*, sGP was detected in the blood of ZEBOV-infected patients.[17,58] It is important to note that while sGP and $GP_{1,2}$ share 295 N-terminal residues, they are structurally distinct. The sGP precursor (ZEBOV) differs from $GP_{1,2}$ in its 69 C-terminal residues. The N-terminal 29 of these amino acids remain within sGP after proteolytic processing.[17,23] The remaining 40 amino acids form a secreted cleavage product termed Δ-peptide, whose function is unknown.[24]

EPIDEMIOLOGY, ECOLOGY, AND TRANSMISSION

Epidemiology

The geographic distribution of filoviruses is best based on actual virus isolation from patients or animals, since most serological surveys have used either unreliable tests or yielded controversial results.[1] BEBOV, CIEBOV, SEBOV, and ZEBOV are endemic in the Central African tropical forest or nearby savanna (Côte d'Ivoire, Democratic Republic of the Congo, Gabon, Republic of the Congo, Uganda, Sudan) and occasionally emerge during the rainy season (***Table 73.1 and Fig. 73.1***). REBOV has repeatedly emerged from a single export facility in the Philippines (1989–1990, 1992, and 1996),[59] before it was recently discovered in numerous domestic swine in the same country (***Table 73.2***).[60] MARV circulates in forested areas of Kenya, Uganda, Democratic Republic of the Congo, Zimbabwe, and Angola, but the epidemiologic information does not permit clear definition of the exact sites. However, contrary to EBOV disease outbreaks, MARV disease outbreaks are almost always associated with caves and mines (***Table 73.3 and Fig. 73.1***).[61,62]

Ecology

The natural host(s) and maintenance strategies of filoviruses remain unknown.[1] This lack of understanding is a major deficit in trying to predict and prevent filovirus transmission to human populations.[60,63,64] Laboratory infections of arthropods, reptiles, and plants, as well as cells derived from arthropods and reptiles, have usually failed.[65] The virologic properties of filoviruses may favor chronic infection of a mammalian reservoir, and indeed it has been possible to experimentally infect certain bats with modest virus persistence.[66] Antibodies against filoviruses and filovirus genomic RNA fragments were detected in several fruit bats in Africa in recent years.[67–69] In 2009, the isolation of infectious MARV was reported from live Egyptian fruit bats (*Rousettus aegyptiacus*).[70]

Transmission

Infection of the index case has always occurred in rural areas of Africa, probably after undefined contact with infected nonhuman primates, other wildlife species, or the unknown reservoir. No common event has been identified among human index cases although proximity to bats, local travel, and a painful "bite" (a single marburgvirus disease case)[61] are often mentioned (***Fig. 73.2***). The Marburg hemorrhagic fever (MHF) outbreaks in Durba/Watsa (Democratic Republic of the Congo) occurred in and/or around a subterranean gold mine where the reservoir(s) seemed to be localized since the outbreaks came to an end after natural flooding of the mine.[71,72] Subsequent spread proceeds readily, particularly to those who care for the patient and are in close contact with body secretions and blood or to those who prepare the body for burial.[73–75] There have been secondary cases among mourners who touched the body or physicians who placed hands on sick patients, but these are the minority. There has been no evidence for aerosol transmission between humans although it is difficult to absolutely exclude any airborne spread.[76] The real engine that drives large Ebola hemorrhagic fever (EHF) outbreaks is the underfunded African hospital that reuses disposable needles and syringes without sterilization and cares for patients without proper barrier nursing precautions. Nosocomial spread combined with intrafamilial infection has led to epidemics of several hundred cases in Sudan and Zaire (see ***Table 73.1***).

The opportunity to formally study cases during a 1995 ZEBOV epidemic in Zaire (now Democratic Republic of the Congo) provided important data.[75,77] General patterns of infection resembled former outbreaks, with medical personnel comprising almost one-third of the cases. Family members were usually infected by direct physical contact with the patient and particularly the patient's body fluids. The overall risk for family members caring for patients was increased fivefold compared with others sharing the same cooking fire. Generally, contact during the early phases of illness carried a low risk with most secondary cases attributable to contact during the later stages of disease and predominantly in the hospital. This correlates with virologic findings in experimental infections of nonhuman primates.[78] Interestingly, touching the cadaver was an important independent risk factor,[75] which may be correlated with the finding of ZEBOV antigen and virions in skin biopsies

Table 73.1 Outbreaks of Ebolavirus Hemorrhagic Fever

Virus	Year(s)	Location	Cases (% Case Fatality)	Epidemiology Remarks
Zaire ebolavirus (ZEBOV)	1976	Yambuku, Zaire	318 (88)	Unknown origin; spread by close contact; nosocomial transmission through contaminated needles; emergence of ebolavirus in Zaire (today Democratic Republic of the Congo) coincidental with emergence of related, but distinct, ebolavirus in Sudan
	1977	Bonduni, Zaire	1 (100)	Unknown origin; single case in missionary hospital
	1994/95	Woleu-Ntem and Ogooué-Invindo Provinces, Gabon	52 (62)	Five independent outbreaks occurred in remote gold-mining camps; originally thought to be yellow fever
	1995	Kikwit, Zaire	317 (77)	Unknown origin; index case thought to have been infected in adjoining forest; epidemic spread through families and hospitals
	1996	Mayibout II, Makokou, Gabon	31 (68)	Outbreak started through handling of dead chimpanzee found in the forest; spread to family members
	1996/97	Ogooué-Invindo and Ogooué-Lolo Provinces, Gabon/Johannesburg, South Africa	62 (74)	Index case was hunter; disease spread through close contact; transport of patients to Libreville; included a medical professional travelling to Johannesburg after being exposed to virus (survived); nurse who took care of the patient in Johannesburg died of EHF
	2001/02	Ogooué-Invindo Province, Gabon/Cuvette-Ouest Region, RC	124 (78)	Eight independent outbreaks occurred across the border of Gabon and RC
	2002	Ogooué-Invindo Province, Gabon/Cuvette-Ouest Region, RC	11 (91)	Outbreak occurred across the border of RC
	2002/03	Cuvette-Ouest region, RC/ Ogooué-Invindo Province, Gabon	143 (90)	Three independent outbreaks occurred across the border of Gabon and RC
	2003/04	Cuvette-Ouest region, RC	35 (83)	Reemergence in the same area of northern RC
	2005	Cuvette-Ouest region, RC	11 (92)	Reemergence in the same area of northern RC
	2007	Kasai Occidental Province, DRC	264 (71)	Index case potentially exposed to fruit bats
	2008	Kasai Occidental Province, DRC	32 (16)	
Sudan ebolavirus (SEBOV)	1976	Nzara, Maridi, Tembura & Juba, Sudan	284 (53)	Unknown origin; spread by close contact; nosocomial transmission; infection of medical care personnel; emergence of ebolavirus in Sudan coincidental with emergence of related, but distinct, ebolavirus in Zaire
	1979	Nzara, Sudan	34 (65)	Unknown origin; recurrent outbreak at same site as 1976
	2000/01	Gulu, Mbarara, and Masindi Districts, Uganda	425 (53)	Most important risk factors associated with infection were attending funerals of EHF victims, contact with patients in family, and medical care provision to case patients
	2004	Yambio County, Sudan	17 (41)	Concurrent outbreak of measles including hemorrhagic cases, which complicated EHF outbreak investigation
Côte d'Ivoire ebolavirus (CIEBOV)	1994	Taï Forest, Côte d'Ivoire/ Basel, Switzerland	1 (0)	Exposure through necropsy on a dead chimpanzee; patient was treated in Switzerland; discovery of a new ebolavirus
Bundibugyo ebolavirus (BEBOV)	2007/08	Uganda	192 (34)	Discovery of a new ebolavirus as the cause of an outbreak in Bundibugyo District of western Uganda

Note: the list does not include ebolavirus laboratory infections or laboratory exposures. DRC, Democratic Republic of the Congo; RC, Republic of the Congo; EHF, ebolavirus hemorrhagic fever.

and surrounding skin appendages.[79] A few patients from the 1995 outbreak had no identifiable risk factor, such as close contact with a patient or an injection.[76]

The exact route of infection and infectious dose are unknown. Nonhuman primates are readily infected by small quantities of injected virus, by low doses of infectious aerosols,[80] and by placing virus suspensions on the conjunctivae.[81] During the Zaire outbreak in 1976, 85 patients had an injection history, and all of these patients died, compared with 89% of the 149 thought to have been infected by contact with other patients.

All EBOV epidemics have ceased, perhaps because of the relatively low transmissibility of the virus once nosocomial spread is prevented. The process is aided by the quarantine practiced by local people once the transmissibility and lethality of the disease are recognized.[73,74] In 1995, the only transmission outside of Kikwit occurred in a nearby town within a hospital; villages without medical facilities often strictly confined patients to their houses, and a single case in Kinshasa in 1976 was managed with barrier nursing without incident.[77,82] The institution of barrier nursing in the hospital in Kikwit clearly stopped transmission to staff while patients continued to be cared for in the medical facility.[77]

The adaptation of virus to interhuman spread has been suggested as leading to the possibility of more efficient transmission[83] or to the virus becoming attenuated.[84] In fact, the secondary transmission rates in

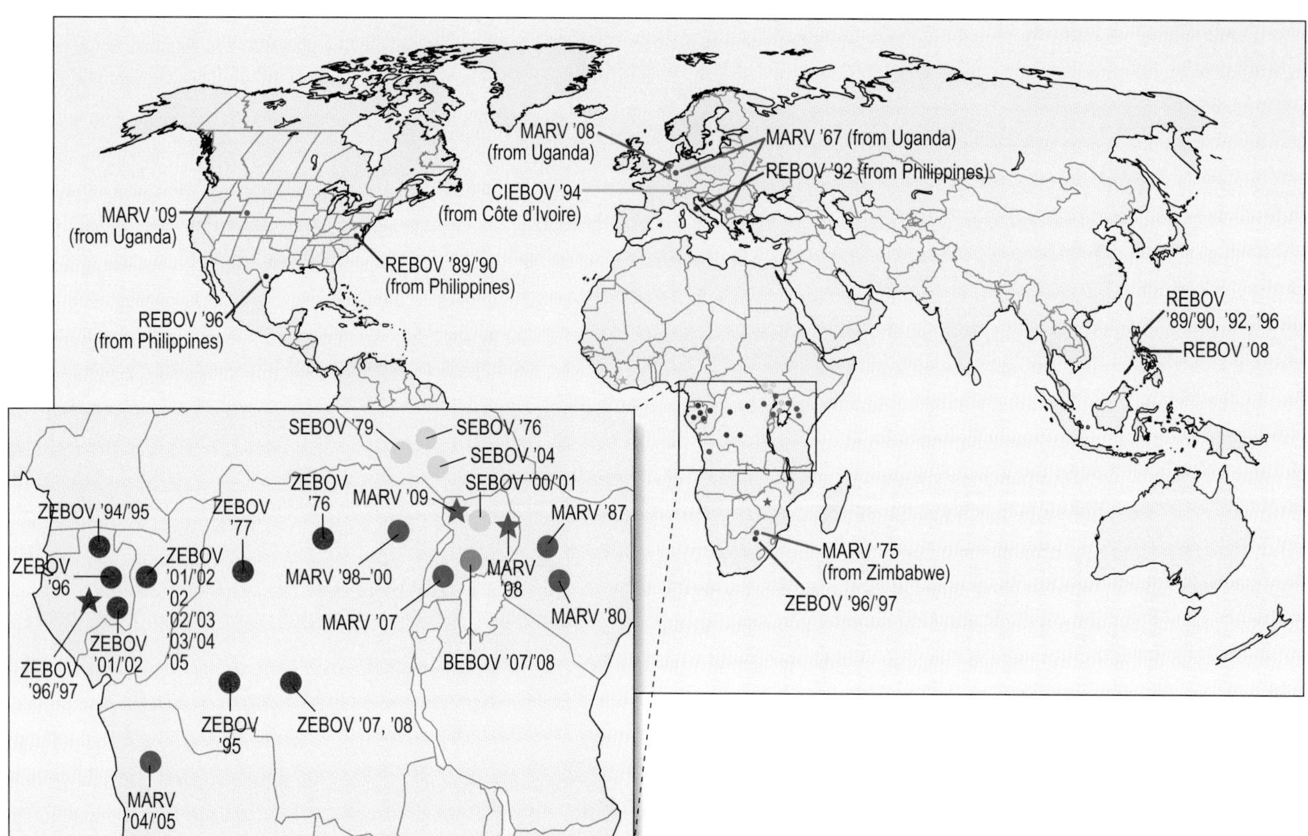

Figure 73.1 Confirmed outbreaks of ebola- and marburgviruses. Outbreaks are depicted as red (ZEBOV), orange (SEBOV), green (CIEBOV), purple (REBOV), turquoise (Bundibugyo ebolavirus, BEBOV), and blue (marburgvirus, MARV). Note that the original site of virus in the case of importations is depicted by a star. ZEBOV, SEBOV, and CIEBOV have occurred exclusively in the tropical forest and adjacent savanna regions of Africa (see insert for location and year of naturally occurring disease). REBOV has been obtained from a single monkey export facility in the Philippines but has been exported to Italy and the United States. An outbreak in the Philippines demonstrated that pigs can serve as a host for REBOV. Exportations of monkeys from Uganda brought MARV to Marburg, Germany and then to Frankfurt, Germany and Belgrade, Yugoslavia, in 1967. In 1975, a traveler infected in Rhodesia (now Zimbabwe) became sick in Johannesburg, South Africa. In 1994, a person infected with CIEBOV was medically evacuated from Côte d'Ivoire to Switzerland. In 1996, a Gabonese physician infected with ZEBOV traveled to Johannesburg, South Africa, for medical care. In 2008, a Dutch woman with a travel history to Uganda was treated for MARV at a hospital in the Netherlands and in 2009 an American woman returned to the United States with febrile illness and was retrospectively diagnosed with marburgvirus hemorrhagic fever. See ***Tables 73.1, 73.2, and 73.3*** for further details on outbreaks.

Table 73.2 Outbreaks of Reston Ebolavirus Disease

Year(s)	Location	Cases (% Case Fatality)	Circumstances of Human Infection
1989–1990	Philippines, USA	7 (0%)	Introduction of virus into quarantine facilities in Virginia and Texas from a single nonhuman primate export facility in the Philippines; four human infections documented in the United States without clinical symptoms. High mortality observed in cynomolgus macaques in export facility responsible for exporting animals to the United States. Workers tested positive for antibodies but had no clinical symptoms
1992	Philippines, Italy	0 (0%)	Introduction of virus into quarantine facilities in Siena from same export facility
1996	Philippines, USA	0 (0%)	Introduction of virus into quarantine facility in Texas from same export facility
2008	Philippines	6 (0%)	First report of Reston ebolavirus in swine. Sequence is closely related to previous Reston ebolavirus isolates. Six workers from the pig farm and slaughterhouse tested positive for antibodies but had no clinical symptoms

families have generally been 3–16% with no change or a small decrease in case-fatality rates over time, and with little to no acquisition of genomic mutations.[73,75,85,86]

Filovirus epidemiology among captive cynomolgus macaques has been studied during the REBOV disease outbreaks. Extensive spread was associated with reuse of needles and syringes and multidose vials for medications and tuberculin testing. Macaques housed in groups with an infected macaque were also at high risk. Spread within quarantine facilities in the United States has not been easily controlled. Even with individual cages, use of sterile injection equipment and precautions by caretakers, one infected monkey in a room has usually led to the eventual infection of others, with more than 80% dying. In US quarantine facilities, which were affected by REBOV spread after they had imported REBOV-infected macaques from the Philippines in 1989–1990, there was spread between rooms sharing common ventilation. It is believed that this movement of virus, the explosive nature of the outbreak in most rooms, the

Table 73.3 Outbreaks of Marburgvirus Hemorrhagic Fever

Year(s)	Location	Cases (% Case Fatality)	Circumstances of Human Infection
1967	West Germany and Yugoslavia	31 (23%)	Imported African green monkeys from Uganda infected humans through contact with the monkeys or primary kidney cell cultures; six secondary cases and no tertiary cases
1975	Rhodesia and South Africa	3 (33%)	A traveler infected in Rhodesia (today Zimbabwe) died in Johannesburg, South Africa; secondary cases occurred in a companion and a nurse infected while providing patient care
1980	Kenya	2 (50%)	Index case was infected in western Kenya and died in Nairobi; a physician was secondarily infected and survived
1987	Kenya	1 (100%)	Expatriate traveling in western Kenya
1998–2000	DRC	154 (83%)	Repeated introductions of multiple viruses and subsequent interhuman spread. Most cases occurred in male workers at a gold mine in Durba
2004–2005	Angola	252 (90%)	A single apparent introduction resulted in nosocomial and close-contact infections. Outbreak began in Uíge Province. Cases were detected in other provinces but could be linked to the outbreak in Uíge
2007	Uganda	3 (33%)	Small outbreak involving workers in a mine
2008	Netherlands ex Uganda	1 (100%)	A Dutch woman with travel history to Uganda was treated at a hospital in the Netherlands. She reported that first symptoms appeared 3 days prior to admission. She succumbed to infection on the 10th day of illness
2009	United States ex Uganda	1 (0%)	An American woman returned to the United States with a febrile illness and was retrospectively diagnosed with MHF

Note, the list does not include marburgvirus laboratory infections or laboratory exposures. DRC, Democratic Republic of the Congo; MHF, marburgvirus hemorrhagic fever.

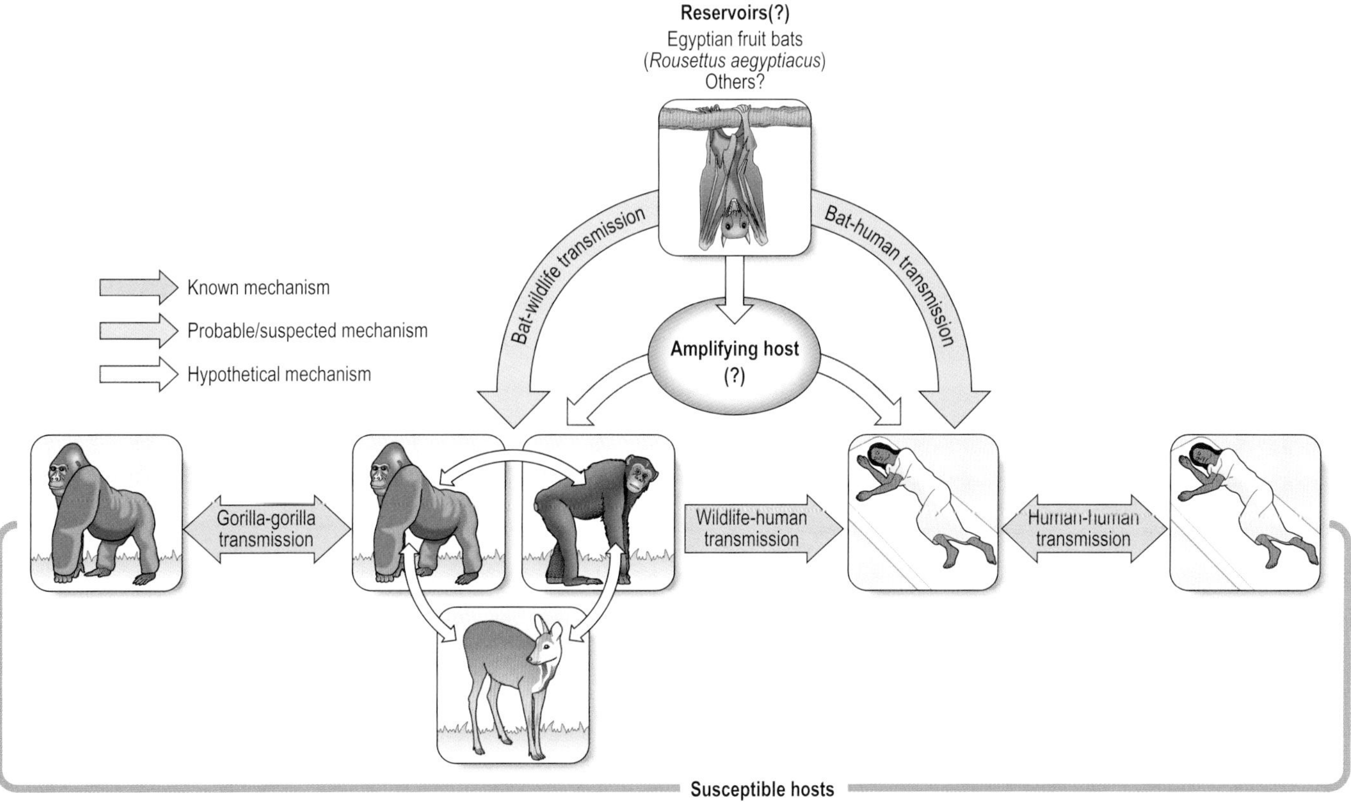

Figure 73.2 Transmission cycle of filoviruses. The viruses are maintained in nature by an unknown mechanism. It is most likely that there is a vertebrate reservoir, and it is possible that there might be an amplifying host. Antibodies against filoviruses and filovirus genomic RNA fragments were detected in several fruit bats in Africa. Additionally, the isolation of infectious marburgvirus was reported from live Egyptian fruit bats (*Rousettus aegyptiacus*), implicating this bat as a potential reservoir. Once the virus is introduced into humans, it is spread by close contact, particularly in the hospital setting. Epidemics have all died out with the institution of quarantine and barrier nursing.

respiratory signs in infected macaques, and the high titer of virus in secretions argued for some component of airborne spread, but evidence is still lacking.[87]

Control of filovirus infections in nonhuman primates in the United States and Europe is achieved by quarantine of imported animals.[88,89] Animals that die during quarantine are tested for the presence of filoviruses, usually by antigen detection enzyme-linked immunosorbent assay (ELISA).[90] Use of antibody tests to detect infection has not been needed because of the high lethality among infected nonhuman primates. During the 1989 and 1990 Reston episodes, numerous confusing titer changes and false positive immunofluorescent antibody (IFA) test results were obtained in primates, including humans,[91] so if antibody testing is deemed necessary to rule out transmission after a member of the cohort is shown to be infected, ELISA should be utilized.[92]

Western chimpanzees are susceptible to EBOV and provide additional epidemiologic data. One animal necropsied in the Taï Forest in Côte d'Ivoire during an epizootic proved to be infected with a filovirus by immunohistochemistry, and was the source of infection of the ethologist who performed the necropsy (only isolation of Côte d'Ivoire EBOV).[93] Western chimpanzee deaths during the epizootic were particularly noted by those hunting red colobus monkeys for meat consumption, and those that were in contact with sick apes.[94]

Since 1994, multiple ZEBOV disease outbreaks have occurred in Central Africa (Gabon, Republic of the Congo), resulting in several hundred human cases and, likely, devastating epizootics among apes (central chimpanzees and western lowland gorillas).[95,96] Epidemiologic observations, confirmed by molecular data, show evidence of multiple outbreaks occurring simultaneously in human and ape populations involving emergence of diverging types of ZEBOV.[97] The patterns of virus transmission between animals or within family groups have not been studied, but surveys of known populations revealed dramatic declines in western lowland gorilla and central chimpanzee populations.[98]

The largest outbreak on record of EHF occurred in Uganda between 2000 and 2001. The outbreak was centered in the Gulu District of northern Uganda (425 presumptive cases), with secondary transmission to other districts, Mbarara (5 presumptive cases) and Masindi (27 presumptive cases).[99] Laboratory confirmation was established for 218 of the presumptive cases with 29 infected health care workers. Sequence and epidemiologic data were consistent with the outbreak having originated from a single introduction into the human population.[100]

Between 1998 and 2000, a large MHF epidemic occurred in Durba and Watsa (Democratic Republic of the Congo) with a total of 73 cases (8 laboratory-confirmed and 65 suspected cases retrospectively identified) (***Table 73.3***). Follow-up surveillance has subsequently identified a total of 154 probable or confirmed cases through December 2000.[101] During this outbreak, all the patients were either working in a gold mine or were taking care of a sick patient who worked in the same gold mine. Data from previous MHF outbreaks have suggested single introductions of virus into the human population with subsequent human-to-human transmission during each outbreak. The largest MHF outbreak to date occurred during 2004–2005 and began in Uíge Province of northern Angola before spreading to an additional seven Angolan provinces. This was the first observation of a MARV outbreak in an urban setting. The geographic location of the Angola outbreak was uncharacteristic for MHF which, until that point, only erupted in the drier and more open areas of Central and East Africa.[102,103] Despite the geographic separation between this outbreak and one in 1967 in Uganda (from where animals were exported to Germany and Yugoslavia), the virus isolates are very closely related.[104] In addition to being the largest outbreak, the case-fatality rate was unprecedented with 227/252 infected individuals succumbing to disease.[105]

THE DISEASE

Clinical Manifestations

Filovirus infection can result in fulminant hemorrhagic disease in human and nonhuman primates.[106] Indeed, among all viral hemorrhagic fevers (VHFs) those caused by filoviruses are regarded as the most severe and are typically associated with hemorrhagic manifestations, coagulation disorders, generalized shock, and hepatic involvement.[107,108] Close observations during human cases of filovirus hemorrhagic fever (HF) have generally been incomplete because of logistics and risk to the health care worker.[4] The incubation period is approximately 4–10 days (range, 3–19) and is followed by abrupt onset of nonspecific influenza-like symptoms including fever, chills, malaise, and myalgia. As disease progresses, more severe and multisystem symptoms are noted such as gastrointestinal (anorexia, nausea, vomiting, abdominal pain, diarrhea), respiratory (chest pain, shortness of breath, cough), vascular (conjunctival injection, postural hypotension, edema), and neurologic (headache, confusion, coma) manifestations.[4] Hemorrhages were observed frequently during the 1976 ZEBOV disease epidemics, but were reported in fewer than half of patients during the 1995 ZEBOV outbreak in Kikwit and even less during the 2000–2001 SEBOV outbreak in Gulu. A maculopapular rash typically appears around day 5. Death is usually associated with fulminant shock that is characterized by fluid redistribution (increased permeability), hypotension, coagulation disorders, and widespread focal tissue destruction.[109] A humoral antibody response in survivors is typically observed between days 7 and 11 and marks a turning point to improvement in health.[110,111] A small percentage of individuals that do not succumb to disease can expect a prolonged period of convalescence with varying degrees of sequelae including arthralgia, uveitis, psychosocial disturbances, and orchitis.[111–114]

The different filoviruses may well cause somewhat different clinical syndromes, but there have been few opportunities for close observation of the diseases under good conditions. Perhaps the best illustration of a varying clinical picture was noted during an outbreak in 2007–2008 in Uganda.[115] The prominent symptoms during the outbreak in Bundibugyo included severe abdominal pain, vomiting, and diarrhea. The presentation led to delays in diagnosis with physicians initially suspecting cholera, malaria, or typhoid fever.[115] The responsible virus was sequenced and recognized as a novel, fifth, ebolavirus (BEBOV) based on its divergence from those already known.[12] The lethality of ZEBOV and MARV infection is high (60–90%), that of SEBOV infection is somewhat lower (50–60%), whereas BEBOV infection ranks on the lower end of the spectrum (34%). The single patient with CIEBOV infection was sick but survived.[4,12,73,74,84,87,116–118] REBOV may be considered nonpathogenic for humans (***Table 73.2***). During the REBOV epizootics in the United States, only four exposures may have caused infections. However, these animal caretakers did not develop symptoms, and infectious virus could only be recovered from one patient with barely detectable titers (P.E. Rollin et al, unpublished observations). More convincingly, REBOV caused extended epizootics among domestic swine between 2007 and 2009 in the Philippines, but human disease was not detected despite numerous exposures of humans to infected live animals or meat products.[60] At least five individuals tested positive for IgG antibodies to REBOV.[119,120] In a serosurvey, 6/141 individuals who either worked on a pig farm or with swine products tested positive for IgG to REBOV, despite a lack of illness.[60]

Because of the vagaries of the fluorescent antibody test, it is difficult to be sure of the case-infection ratios in outbreaks, but in both the 1976[74] and 1995[77] ZEBOV epidemics there was no evidence of mild or subclinical disease in patients or family contacts.

PATHOGENESIS AND IMMUNITY

Pathology

The pathology of EBOV infections has been examined from tissues obtained during human outbreaks in addition to studies using susceptible animal models (mice, guinea pigs, and nonhuman primates). One aspect concerning animal models that should be kept in mind is that they do not always adequately reproduce EHF. Specifically, there are differences in hemorrhagic manifestations, coagulopathy, and bystander apoptosis.

In fatal MHF and EHF cases, hemorrhagic manifestations are usually striking with widespread petechiae and ecchymoses involving skin, mucous membranes, and internal organs; extensive visceral effusions are also present. The histopathologic changes are similar in MARV and ZEBOV infections, and somewhat resemble those seen in other HFs. However, careful study of histopathologic lesions and finding of characteristic virus inclusions in the liver may suggest a specific diagnosis.[4,121]

Focal necrosis is present in many organs and is greatest in liver, spleen, kidney, and gonads. Electron microscopic, immunohistochemical, and *in situ* hybridization studies show strong association of parenchymal necrosis

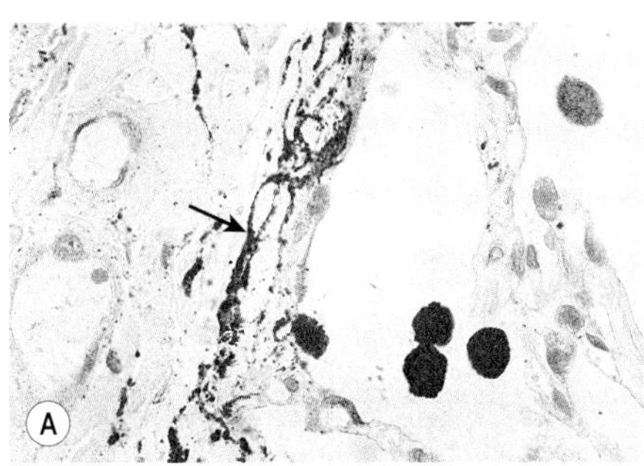

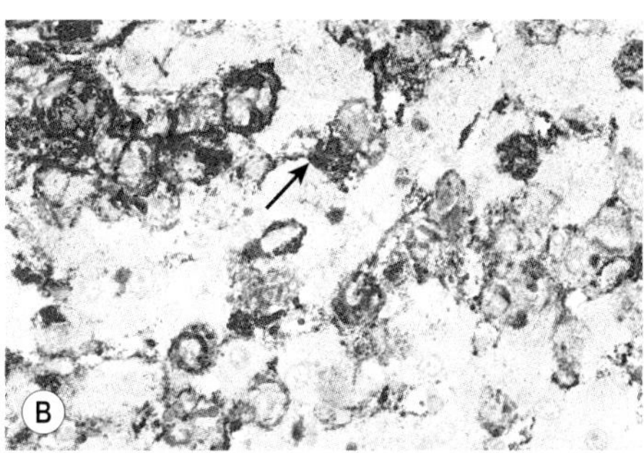

Figure 73.3 Ebolavirus antigen-positive cells in lung and liver of an Ebola patient as determined by immunohistochemistry. **(A)** Lung showing fibroblast and endothelial cell infection (arrow) as well as involvement of several alveolar macrophages. **(B)** Heavy viral burden and necrosis in liver immunostained for ebolavirus antigens. Viral antigens are in hepatocytes and Kupffer cells, many of which are necrotic (arrow). (Immunoalkaline phosphatase staining, naphthol-fast red substrate with light hematoxylin counterstain; **A**, ×158; **B**, ×250.)

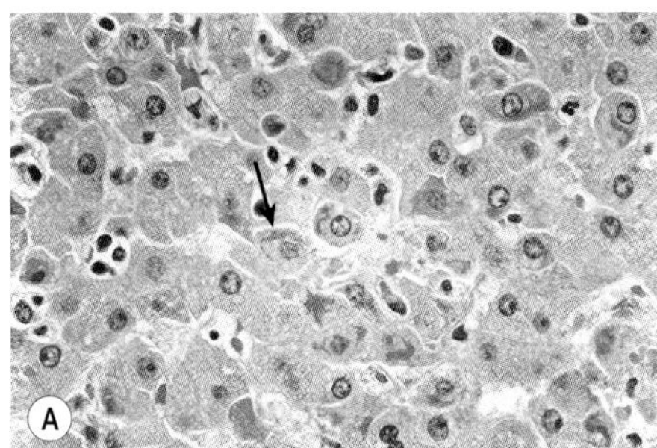

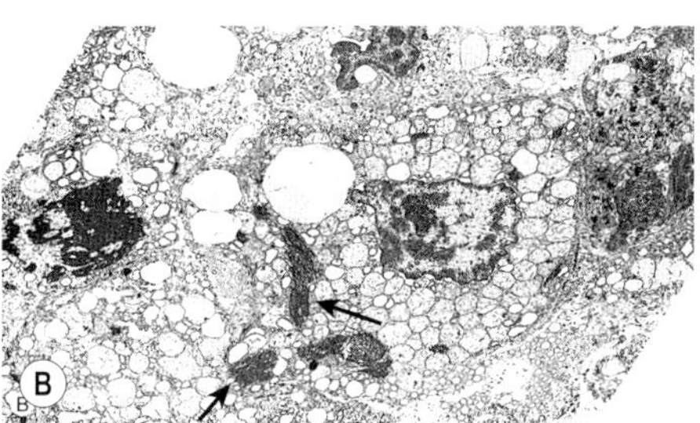

Figure 73.4 Liver in ebolavirus infection. **(A)** Photomicrograph of liver showing hepatocellular necrosis and numerous, eosinophilic, crescent-shaped, intracytoplasmic viral inclusions typical of ebolavirus infection (arrow). (Hematoxylin and eosin, ×158.) **(B)** Thin-section electron micrograph of same liver demonstrating that inclusions (arrows) are composed of aggregates of viral nucleocapsid. (×7000.)

in organs and the presence of abundant virus particles, antigens, and nucleic acids[122,123] (***Figs 73.3 and 73.4***). Filovirus antigens and particles are present in abundance within and in association with (occasionally necrotic) endothelial cells throughout the body. Little or no inflammatory response is associated with necrotic areas. Thus, necrosis appears to be related to both the cytopathic effect of the virus and ischemia. Characteristic histopathologic features in the liver include widespread hepatocellular necrosis, Councilman bodies, microvesicular fatty change, and Kupffer cell hyperplasia. Filovirus inclusions are observed within the cytoplasm of hepatocytes (***Fig. 73.4A***). They are usually numerous in EBOV infections and are eosinophilic, oval, or filamentous, and ultrastructurally consist of aggregates of virus nucleocapsids (***Fig. 73.4B***). Spleen and lymph nodes show extensive follicular necrosis and necrotic debris. The lungs show interstitial edema and are usually hemorrhagic with features of diffuse alveolar damage. Myocardial edema and focal necrosis are not associated with inflammatory infiltrates.

Projected Sequence of Infection

The primary mechanism for human filovirus infection is close contact with skin and secretory products from infected individuals. Filoviruses likely enter via small skin lesions and mucous membranes from which they can acquire direct access to the vascular system or indirect access through the lymphatic system.[106] Monocytes/macrophages and dendritic cells are primary sites of virus replication.[6,121,124–126] Cells of the mononuclear phagocytic system (MPS) located in multiple organs including the liver (Kupffer cells), spleen, lymph nodes, lung (alveolar macrophages), serous cavities (pleural and peritoneal macrophages), and nervous system (microglia) are infected; however, the lymph nodes, liver, and spleen are the three organs consistently affected most severely by filovirus replication.[107] Organ tropism may be enhanced by direct access of particles to sessile cells of the MPS without penetration of cellular or tissue barriers.[127] Subsequent to infection and replication in macrophages, virus particles gain secondary access to lymph nodes and then ultimately the vascular system, which marks a state of viremia.[106] In addition to tissues from fatal human cases and *in vitro* studies, a serial sampling experiment of EHF in cynomolgus macaques has provided a tremendous amount of data regarding the progression of disease in the animal model that most closely resembles human infection.[124,128] Virus was shown to spread from initial infection sites via macrophages and dendritic cells to regional lymph nodes, most probably via lymphatics, and to liver and spleen via blood. Virus infects tissue macrophages, dendritic cells, and fibroblastic reticular cells.[124] Monocytes/macrophages are early and sustained targets of EBOV in both guinea pigs and moribund nonhuman primates.[81,125,129,130] A recent study in cynomolgus macaques confirmed these observations with virus RNA detected in lymphoid monocytes/macrophages as early as 2 days post infection.[124] The interaction between filoviruses and dendritic cells may be critical for the outcomes of EBOV infections. The lymphoid hypoplasia and lack of a detectable immune response in fatal infections could be explained by the early infection of dendritic cells, their increased expression of the TNF-related apoptosis-inducing ligand (TRAIL) and bystander apoptosis of lymphocytes, and the partial suppression of MHC class II in infected immature dendritic cells.[131,132] In tandem with T-lymphocyte depletion, infected monocytes/macrophages release soluble mediators including proinflammatory cytokines.[133] These cytokines usually recruit additional macrophages to infected areas and in EHF could increase the number of target cells available for virus infection and further amplify an already dysregulated host response.[124] Cultured primary human monocytes/macrophages are also activated upon infection, resulting in an increase of TNF-α, interleukin (IL)-1β, IL-6, and IL-8.[134,135] Infection by MARV leads to a significant increase in release of TNF-α by 12–24 hours post infection. Ultraviolet inactivation of virus does not impair the activation and production of cytokines at either the transcriptional or protein level, and noninfectious virus-like particles also activate cells independent of replication.[134,136] EBOV-infected patients also exhibit increased serum levels of various cytokines, and increased levels of IL-10, neopterin, and IL-1 receptor antagonist (IL-1RA) correlate with a fatal outcome, whereas presence of IL-1β and elevated concentrations of IL-6 in the plasma during the symptomatic phase are markers of nonfatal infections.[137–140]

Virus Spreading and Role of the Endothelium

During filovirus infection, the endothelium appears to be affected in two ways: directly by infection with filoviruses, leading to activation and later cell death, and indirectly by a mediator-induced inflammatory response.[108] *In vitro* data suggest that virus-induced cytokine release leads to activation of the endothelium that can be defined as increased expression and/or release of adhesion molecules (intravascular adhesion molecule-1, vascular cell adhesion molecule-1, and E- and P-selectin), as well as a breakdown of the endothelial barrier function.[106,109,141,142] In spite of the *in vitro* upregulation of these molecules, which mediate the binding of leukocytes to the surface of the endothelium and initiate extravasation,[143–145] there is a lack of leukocyte infiltrates in areas of focal necrosis, thereby suggesting a deficient immunoreaction of unknown mechanism.[6] Although the molecular mechanisms for the breakdown of the endothelial barrier function are not completely understood, there is evidence for changes in the protein organization of the adherens junctions, specifically the VE-cadherin/catenin complex.[106,146] Additionally, supernatants from MARV-infected macrophages increase the permeability of human umbilical vein endothelial cell (HUVEC) monolayers, and permeability can be partially inhibited by antibodies that neutralize TNF-α, indicating a critical role for this protein in virus-induced shock.[135] Serial sampling of EHF in nonhuman primates reveals ultrastructural evidence of endothelial cell activation and disruption, but attributes it to indirect mechanisms since the changes were not associated with the presence of intracytoplasmic EBOV antigens. Overall, the data suggest that EBOV affect the function of endothelial cells in the early stages of infection and that EBOV-induced coagulopathy results primarily from vasculopathy induced by factors secreted by infected monocytes/macrophages and dendritic cells (including cytokines and tissue factor); whereas direct virus-induced cytolysis of endothelial cells plays a later, secondary role in hemorrhagic diathesis.[128] The facts that antigen-positive endothelial cells are a hallmark of human infection and that filoviruses readily replicate in HUVEC *in vitro* cannot be dismissed. Whether their infection plays a major role in EHF pathogenesis as compared to indirect effects of mediators remains to be determined. The role of EBOV soluble glycoproteins (sGP and Δ-peptide) in endothelial activation and dysfunction continues to be an active area of research. The ability of sGP to function in endothelial activation is suggested in a model as a third mechanism by which the endothelium is altered during filovirus infection, but interestingly *in vitro* studies reveal that sGP plays an anti-inflammatory role by protecting the endothelial cell barrier function following stimulation with TNF-α.[57,109,142]

DIAGNOSIS

Acute febrile illness with headache, myalgia, and diarrhea can be caused by a variety of different agents, including other hemorrhagic fever viruses. Both occupational and travel history are imperative in narrowing the diagnosis. Rural travel, rainforest or cave exposure, contact with sick humans, contact with sick or dead nonhuman primates, or contact with bats or bat excrement should all raise concern.[4] More common causes of febrile illness that should be ruled out for travelers include rickettsioses, falciparum malaria, typhoid fever, leptospirosis, borreliosis, septicemic plague, and dysentery.[147]

An etiologic diagnosis should be sought at the earliest stages of illness. Virus, virus antigen, and virus RNA in serum or blood should be sought during the acute phase of illness.[147] The most applicable detection methods in the outbreak setting rely on antigen-capture ELISA and reverse transcription-polymerase chain reaction (RT-PCR). Nested RT-PCR was previously utilized (e.g., in Gulu); however, it had limited throughput and was subject to false positive results. Optimized RT-PCR assays were developed and utilized in subsequent outbreaks (e.g., in Angola).[148] Diagnostic assays are performed in mobile field laboratories, local hospitals, and/or reference laboratories.

The most commonly used cell line for both isolation and propagation of filoviruses is the Vero (*Chlorocebus aethiops*, African green monkey kidney epithelial) cell line, particularly the E6 clone.[16] In addition to Vero cells, both MA-104, a monkey kidney cell line, and SW13, a human adrenal carcinoma cell line, have proven useful in primary virus isolation.[149] Filoviruses also infect primary cell cultures, particularly monocytes, macrophages, and endothelial cells.[134–136] Virus can also be demonstrated directly by electron microscopic analysis of tissue culture supernatants, blood or serum, in addition to scanning of cell cultures for cytopathic effects and immunofluorescence assays (IFA) on infected cells. IgM-capture ELISA may only be positive during the early stages of convalescence, and patients can be followed for rising IgG levels to further increase confidence in the diagnosis.

TREATMENT AND PROGNOSIS

There is currently no specific antiviral therapy for EHF/MHF, and patient care is supportive in nature.[4,150] Supportive treatment should include attention to fluid and electrolyte balance, particularly with respect to potassium substitution. In several outbreaks antibiotics were administered (tetracycline, chloramphenicol, penicillin, cephalothin, and streptomycin) but did not alter the fever or course of disease. Neutralizing antibodies specific for the filovirus spike protein ($GP_{1,2}$) were shown to be both protective and therapeutic in rodent models.[151–153] Hamadryas baboons are protected from ZEBOV challenge when large volumes of an EBOV hyperimmune equine serum are administered within 4 hours of infection with a low virus dose.[154] The use of equine serum in humans has been questioned, however, because horses produce a subclass of immunoglobulin (IgG_T) that is highly immunogenic in humans,[108] and the serum was not effective in macaques infected with higher doses of ZEBOV.[155] The use of convalescent sera during an outbreak in Kikwit was reported as protective; however, this report was challenged because the treatment was started relatively late in disease at a stage when most patients are already destined to survive.[86,108,156,157]

The past decade has been a time of rigorous development and testing of candidate therapeutics for EHF/MHF. Therapeutic strategies can be broadly characterized as those that target the virus and/or the host response to virus. Since the coagulation cascade is dysregulated during filovirus HF (leading to disseminated intravascular coagulation), treatments to alleviate microthrombus formation have been attempted. Heparin was used to treat two surviving MARV-infected patients.[147] It has been shown that infection with ZEBOV induces overexpression of the procoagulant tissue factor in nonhuman primate monocytes/macrophages, suggesting that inhibition of the tissue-factor pathway could ameliorate the effects of EHF.[158] In further studies, macaques were administered recombinant nematode anticoagulant protein c2 (rNAPc2), a potent inhibitor of tissue factor-initiated blood coagulation, and post-exposure protection was conferred and provided a new foundation for therapeutic regimens that target the disease process rather than virus replication.[159] Treated animals had increased survival times with 33% survival rates and attenuation of the coagulation and proinflammatory responses. Similarly, partial protection of infected nonhuman primates was reported following treatment with recombinant human activated protein C, a physiological anticoagulant.[160]

A number of other therapeutic candidates have been evaluated *in vitro* and in animal models. Of those, anti-sense technologies such as phosphorodiamidate morpholino oligomers (PMOs) and small interfering RNAs (siRNAs) have shown promise. Both PMOs and siRNAs effectively inhibit filoviruses in cell culture[161,162] and in animal models.[163–165] Interestingly, a small molecule therapeutic, FGI-106, has potent and broad-spectrum antiviral activity *in vitro* and in a mouse model of EHF.[166]

Post-exposure vaccination is also being evaluated for known or high-risk exposures. Administration of recombinant VSV expressing ZEBOV glycoprotein (rVSVΔG-ZEBOVGP) as late as 24 hours post exposure is 100% and 50% protective in mice and guinea pigs, respectively.[167]

Furthermore, rhesus macaques are partially protected (50% survival) when rVSVΔG-ZEBOVGP is given 20–30 minutes after virus exposure. Recombinant rVSV expressing SEBOV glycoprotein fully protects nonhuman primates from a lethal SEBOV challenge,[168] and the rVSV expressing MARV GP, administered 20–30 minutes post exposure, completely protects rhesus macaques in a post-exposure regimen.[169]

PREVENTION AND CONTROL

Initial attempts to develop a vaccine for ZEBOV began soon after the first recognized outbreak in 1976 and used formalin-fixed or heat-inactivated virus in an attempt to confer protection to guinea pigs and nonhuman primates.[108,170] The protection achieved in both studies was inconsistent, and inactivated virus did not induce sufficient immunity to reliably protect hamadryas baboons.[171]

Since the 1990s there has been greater effort on vaccine development. The majority of these attempts have focused on subunit vaccines that are based on one or more of the virus structural proteins. A variety of approaches including naked DNA, replication-defective adenovirus, recombinant vaccinia viruses and VSV, Venezuelan equine encephalitis virus replicons and VLPs have been used to deliver $GP_{1,2}$, NP, VP24, VP30, VP35, and/or VP40.[172–179] The efficacy and specific details of these vaccine strategies have been reviewed recently in great detail.[108,179] The most promising platforms at the moment are those based on adenoviruses,[180] VSV,[181–184] and VLPs,[185,186] all of which have conferred protection in nonhuman primates. These studies, as well as therapeutic studies, have led to an important conclusion about animal models: interventions in the mouse are most successful; success is somewhat more difficult to achieve in the guinea pig; and the primate model is most demanding. The difficulty of obtaining an EBOV vaccine candidate has important implications for vaccine development against viruses that have effective escape hatches against the immune response. There are still formidable problems to overcome in a successful human filovirus vaccine because of the difficulties in defining a target population for efficacy testing. Nevertheless, with today's worldwide travel, the threat of bioterrorism, social unrest in the endemic areas, and the increase in naturally occurring epidemics, a vaccine may well be needed. Possible targets would include apes in endemic areas, medical personnel in Africa, and research workers worldwide.[108]

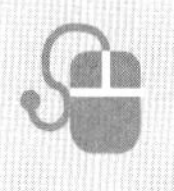

Access the complete reference list online at http://www.expertconsult.com

CHAPTER 74

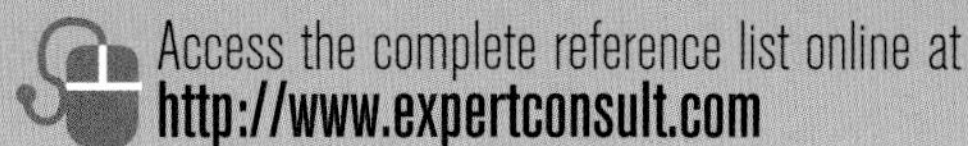
Access the complete reference list online at
http://www.expertconsult.com

Yellow Fever

J. Erin Staples • Thomas P. Monath

INTRODUCTION

Yellow fever is the first-described hemorrhagic fever; in its most fulminant form, it is characterized by severe hepatic and renal injury, hemorrhage, and high mortality. Yellow fever virus transmission occurs in South America and sub-Saharan Africa. Despite this restricted range, it is important for physicians worldwide to consider yellow fever because of its potential to cause large urban outbreaks in areas outside of South America and Africa, because of the risk to travelers in endemic areas, and because of serious adverse events following immunization (AEFI) with live, attenuated yellow fever 17D vaccine.

THE AGENT

Viral Structure

Yellow fever virus is the prototype member of the genus *Flavivirus* (family *Flaviviridae*) that includes ~70 small (40–60 nm), single-stranded, positive-sense RNA viruses, most of which are arthropod-borne. Sequence analysis suggests that yellow fever virus diverged from other mosquito-borne flaviviruses approximately 3000 years ago.[1]

The 10.9-kilobase (kb) genome of yellow fever is organized into a single 10.2 kb open reading frame (ORF) flanked by a short 5′ noncoding region (NCR) and a longer 3′ NCR.[2-4] There are differences in these NCRs between yellow fever virus strains. The 5′ NCR is similar for all strains, but the 3′ NCR includes imperfect repeat sequences of 42 nucleotides. South American strains have one copy of this sequence, East African strains have two, and West African strains have three.[5] There are no known differences in the virulence or replication efficiency associated with the different number of sequences. The ORF consists of three structural protein genes (i.e., capsid (C), premembrane (prM), and envelope (E)) followed by seven nonstructural (NS) protein genes (NS1, NS2A, NS2B, NS3, NS4A, NS4B, and NS5) (***Table 74.1***). These 10 genes are translated into a single polyprotein and then cleaved into individual proteins. The C, prM, and E proteins are present in the mature virion. NS proteins are not present in the mature virion but are produced immediately after infection when they are responsible for replication and polypeptide processing.

The virus envelope is a lipid bilayer derived from the host cell with 90 copies of the E glycoprotein dimers on the surface. The E protein is responsible for attachment to cell receptors and intracellular internalization of the virus; it is the principal target of the host's immune response, and is considered the primary virulence factor. A highly conserved stretch of 14 amino acids in the E protein is responsible for fusion of the virus with the lysosomal membrane of the infected cell. A rearrangement of the E proteins to expose the fusion region is required for the virus to enter the cell cytoplasm. E gene mutations, especially in the fusion domain, greatly alter these biologic functions.[6,7] The E protein contains neutralizing epitopes, and anti-E antibody provides protection by interfering with attachment and, especially, fusion.[8]

NS1 is critical to intracellular virus RNA replication, is released extracellularly, and is expressed on the surface of infected cells (***Table 74.1***). The secreted form has both virus-specific and cross-reactive epitopes. Antibodies to NS1 do not neutralize virus infectivity but provide protection by complement-mediated lysis of infected cells that express the NS1 epitope on their surface.[9] The E, NS1, NS2A, and NS3 proteins contain cytotoxic T-cell epitopes.[10] NS2B and NS3 form a critical enzyme complex that includes a serine protease responsible for post-translational cleavage of the virus polyprotein, an RNA helicase, and an RNA triphosphatase. Mutational studies in the RNA helicase region of NS3 suggest that the protein also may play a role in assembly or release of infectious virus particles.[11] The NS3 gene is highly conserved at the sequence level. The protein is on the host cell surface and, because NS3 contains cytotoxic T-cell epitopes, infected cells are eliminated by cell-mediated immunity.[10,12] NS4A and NS4B are hydrophobic, membrane-associated proteins that regulate RNA replication. NS5 protein is also highly conserved and functions as the RNA-dependent RNA polymerase in virus replication.

Replication

After release of the nucleocapsid into the cytoplasm, the uncoated, positive-sense RNA (i.e., messenger sense) is immediately translated to synthesize RNA-dependent RNA polymerase, RNA helicase, and RNA triphosphatase, which replicate full-length negative RNA strands. These negative strands serve as templates for positive RNA strands that are assembled into virions in the endoplasmic reticulum (ER) and undergo exocytosis.

Genetic Variation

Based on plaque-reduction neutralization assays, the *Flavivirus* genus was divided into eight antigenic complexes and several other antigenically unique viruses, such as yellow fever virus.[13] Gene sequencing confirmed these relationships, grouped yellow fever virus with nine other flaviviruses (Banzi, Bouboui, Edge Hill, Jugra, Saboya, Potiskum, Sepik, Uganda S, and Wesselsbron viruses), and showed that yellow fever virus is most closely related to Sepik virus from New Guinea.[14,15] In addition, these analyses suggest that yellow fever virus is the most distantly related mosquito-borne flavivirus.

Seven genotypes have been distinguished by nucleotide sequencing, but they represent a single serotype. Genomic analyses support the concept that yellow fever virus arose in Africa and that East and West African genotypes diverged prior to the introduction of the virus to the Americas approximately 300–400 years ago.[16-18] Genomic analyses identified two genotypes in West Africa (I and II), a single Central/South

Table 74.1 Functional Description of 10 Genes/Proteins that are Found in Yellow Fever Virus and Other Members of the Genus *Flavivirus*

Gene/Protein	Primary Function	Comments
Capsid (C)	With genomic RNA forms nucleocapsid	
Premembrane (prM)	Stabilizes E protein during exocytosis	Cleaved before release to form pr and M proteins; pr released to extracellular medium, M retained in viral envelope; failure to cleave can affect antigenicity and conformation of E protein and may reduce infectivity of virus
Envelope (E)	Receptor-mediated cell attachment and cell fusion	Forms E protein dimers within lipid bilayer of viral envelope and can be inactivated with organic solvents and detergents
NS1	RNA replication	Monomers released extracellularly and form dimers on surface of infected cells; antibodies to NS1 do not neutralize infectivity but do provide protective immunity through complement-mediated lysis of infected cells
NS2A	RNA replication	Interacts with NS3, NS5, and 3′ NCR to replicate; critical for virion assembly and release
NS2B	See NS3	Forms complex with NS3 to perform functions
NS3	Multifunction: serine protease, RNA helicase, RNA triphosphatase	Serine protease performs post-translational cleavage of the viral polyprotein; RNA helicase and RNA triphosphatase critical to RNA replication; NS3 highly conserved base sequence; target of attack for cytotoxic T cells
NS4A	Regulates RNA replication	Hydrophobic, membrane-associated protein
NS4B	Regulates RNA replication	Hydrophobic, membrane-associated protein
NS5	RNA-dependent RNA polymerase	In addition to polymerase function, functions as a methyltransferase for 5′ cap methylation; like NS3, highly conserved base sequence

African genotype (Angola) and two East African genotypes (East and East/Central).[18,19] Within each African genotype, there is little genetic variation. This is likely due to the yellow fever virus's high-fidelity RNA-dependent RNA polymerase.[20] Unlike the error-prone replication of other RNA viruses that results in one mutation out of every 10^4 bases replicated, yellow fever virus averages two mutations every 10^7 bases. Yellow fever virus has achieved only a modest degree of genetic variation following introduction to the Americas. In the Americas, two genotypes have arisen despite significant geographic overlap.[21] Limited genetic analyses of M, E, NS5, and the 3′ NCR comparing the South American genotypes show that these genotypes represent divergent lineages resulting from geographic and temporal separation and infrequent recombination. There is no difference in the human disease associated with these seven yellow fever variants, but it is unknown whether the highly variable mortality in different epidemics is due to genomic variation.

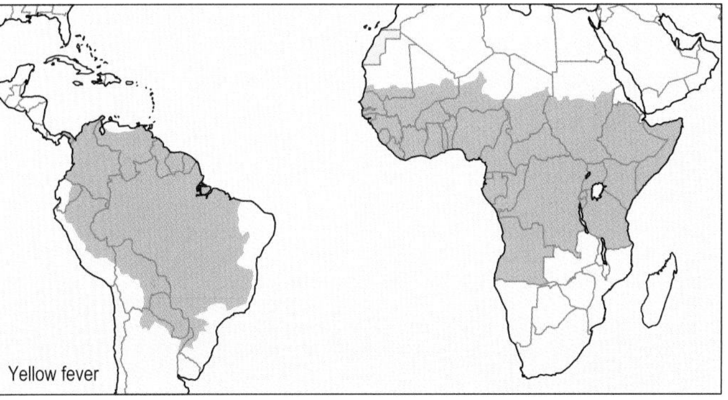

Figure 74.1 Map of yellow fever virus endemic areas (shaded) of South America and Africa. (From International Travel and Health. Geneva: WHO; 2009:96, with permission.)

EPIDEMIOLOGY

Geography

A detailed understanding of the geography of yellow fever virus is critical to the proper utilization of yellow fever vaccine, for indigenous populations, as well as protection of persons at risk of exposure during international travel. A working group of the World Health Organization (WHO) is currently revising the map's delineating endemic areas based on multiple lines of evidence. ***Figure 74.1*** is a preliminary version of this updated map of yellow fever activity.

Transmission Patterns and Ecology

In Africa, three transmission cycles can be distinguished: sylvatic, urban, and savanna cycles (***Fig. 74.2***). In South America, only sylvatic and urban cycles have been identified (***Fig. 74.3***). In all three cycles, yellow fever virus is transmitted between primates by mosquitoes. Neither the virus nor the clinical disease differs in these three cycles, but identifying the type of transmission cycle is important for disease control. The sylvatic (or "jungle") cycle is the predominant transmission cycle in equatorial rainforests in Africa and South America. The cycle is maintained among monkeys by tree hole-breeding mosquitoes. Humans are incidentally infected when they enter the forest or when viremic monkeys exit the forests and infect mosquitoes at the forest fringe. The primary sylvatic vectors are mosquito species that occur in tree canopies – *Aedes africanus* in Africa and *Haemagogus* species in South America. Other African mosquito species implicated in transmission include *Ae. furcifer*, *Ae. vittatus*, *Ae. luteocephalus*, and *Ae. bromeliae* (member of *Ae. simpsoni* complex); in South America, in addition to *Haemagogus* species, *Sabethes chloropterus* may be involved. In a 2008 outbreak extending from Brazil into northern Argentina, a new species *S. albiprivus* was implicated in transmission (D. Enria, personal communication, 2009). Many nonhuman primate species are susceptible to yellow fever. Most African species do not become ill but develop viremia sufficient to infect mosquitoes; however, in South America several species develop lethal infections. Depletion of vertebrate hosts through natural immunization or death during epizootics is a factor in the cyclic disappearance of yellow fever. In many areas, deforestation and hunting have reduced monkey populations, and human beings have become the primary hosts in the transmission cycle. The sylvatic yellow fever cycle may be active but unrecognized in forested areas of countries within the yellow fever endemic zone. Evidence suggests that yellow fever virus will be maintained in one place until the amplifying primates are immune and then reemerge in areas where susceptible primates live. Disease may not be detected for years but then will reappear. Yellow fever virus is maintained through periods during which mosquitoes are absent (e.g., the dry season) by means of transovarial transmission. (i.e., vertical transmission through infected eggs). Sylvatic transmission can most effectively be prevented by vaccination of human populations at risk of exposure.

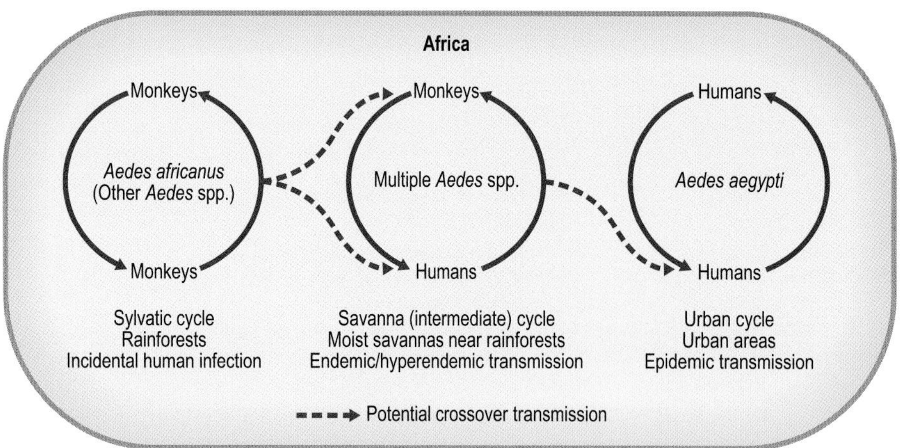

Figure 74.2 African transmission cycles include a sylvatic cycle, a savanna (or intermediate) cycle, and an urban cycle. In each cycle, the mosquito vectors are tree hole-breeding *Aedes* species. The urban cycle, characterized by human-to-human transmission mediated by *Aedes aegypti*, may begin when a viremic human either incidentally infected in the rainforest or infected during endemic transmission in the savanna travels to urban areas.

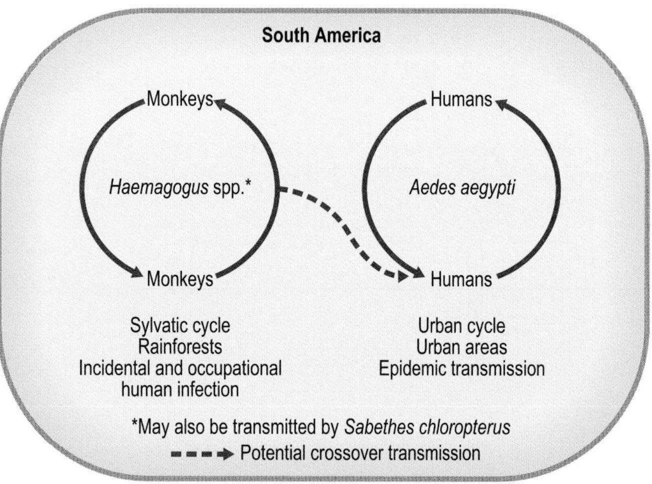

Figure 74.3 South American transmission cycles include a sylvatic cycle and an urban cycle. In the sylvatic cycle, the mosquito vectors are treetop feeding *Haemagogus* or *Sabethes* species. The urban cycle, characterized by human-to-human transmission mediated by *Aedes aegypti*, may begin when a viremic human either incidentally or occupationally infected in the rainforests travels to urban areas. Adapted by Jodi Udd. From the Centers for Disease Control and Prevention: Health Information for International Travellers, 2005–2006 (Yellow Book). A frequently updated version of the CDC's Yellow Book can be found at http://www.cdc.gov/travel/yb/index.htm and should be used to determine a persons' actual need for yellow fever immunization.

Urban yellow fever refers to settings in which human-to-human transmission is mediated by *Ae. aegypti*, a domestic mosquito associated with human habitation and unpolluted collections of water. In areas where *Ae. aegypti* was eliminated, urban yellow fever disappeared. In the mid-1900s, Panama, Brazil, Ecuador, Peru, Bolivia, Paraguay, Uruguay, and Argentina successfully eradicated this vector; no urban epidemics occurred. In other South American countries (e.g., Venezuela, Colombia, Guyana, and Surinam), *Ae. aegypti* eradication never occurred. During the past 30 years, many countries that had previously eradicated *Ae. aegypti* have been reinfested and are at risk for urban outbreaks of the disease.[22–24] The vector is now nearly ubiquitous and present in high density, with the result that dengue (another virus transmitted by the vector) has become endemic and epidemic. The threat of urban yellow fever has thus increased. Two small urban outbreaks have been reported in South America since the 1940s when *Ae. aegypti* control eliminated this threat: one in Santa Cruz, Bolivia in 1998[23] and the second in Asuncion, Paraguay in 2008.[25] In Africa, *Ae. aegypti* eradication was never attempted, and yellow fever epidemics continued to occur in cities, towns, refugee camps, and rural villages where the vector is prevalent.[24,26] Because of an association between population density and the presence of *Ae. aegypti*, massive epidemics have occurred in Africa. In Nigeria in 1987, an epidemic of an estimated 39 000 cases and 8400 deaths occurred in urban areas. Other major *Ae. aegypti*-borne epidemics occurred in 1965 and 1979 in Senegal and in 1971 in Angola.

Because of the mobility of potentially viremic humans, urban yellow fever outbreaks may occur in cities that are remote from sylvatic areas. To eradicate *Ae. aegypti* again will be difficult because of insecticide resistance, urbanization, human population growth, poor sanitation, and other factors increasing vector breeding sites and the high cost of mosquito control. Thus, the scene is set for large urban outbreaks in the Americas. Without reduction of *Ae. aegypti*, urban yellow fever can only be prevented by vaccinating at-risk human populations.

In Africa, a savanna cycle occurs in moist grasslands bordering African rainforests where *Aedes* spp. mosquitoes attain high densities during the rainy season and feed on both humans and monkeys. Interhuman virus transmission can be prominent. In West Africa, the principal vectors are *Ae. furcifer, Ae. vittatus*, *Ae. luteocephalus*, and *Ae. africanus,* which breed principally in the myriad of small collections of rainwater in tree holes. In East Africa, *Ae. africanus* and *Ae. bromeliae* are the principal vectors. During the wet and early dry seasons, high vector density occurs, and mosquitoes readily enter houses. During these periods, virus transmission rates far exceed that found in sylvatic zones.

Mosquito Vectors

Tree hole-breeding mosquitoes are the primary vectors involved in the replication of virus and transmission between vertebrate hosts. Uninfected female mosquitoes become infected when they feed on hosts with a viremia of at least 10^4 PFU/mL. After a 7- to 14-day incubation period in the mosquito, high virus titers are present in the salivary glands. During subsequent blood meals, virus is transmitted to a new vertebrate host. In addition, yellow fever virus can be transmitted transovarially, allowing viral survival in the absence of adult mosquitoes. Field studies during large African epidemics have shown that local strains of *Ae. aegypti* may be inefficient vectors yet sustain intensive interhuman transmission during epidemics.[27] Despite the inefficiency, the anthropophilic nature of the vector and the high densities of the mosquito in urban areas make it an excellent vector for human-to-human transmission. It has been suggested that such inefficiency of mosquito vector strains selects greater virus virulence. For example, the low transmission efficiency of *Ae. aegypti* may select viruses that achieve higher viremia, thus increasing the pathogenicity of the virus strain.

Vertebrate Hosts

Primates are the only vertebrate hosts implicated in the yellow fever transmission cycle. In general, viremia is short (i.e., 2–5 days), although it can be 9 days in colobus monkeys. Infected primates either die or develop lifelong protective immunity. Except for certain bush-baby species (*Galago crassicaudatus*), African primates generally become viremic but do not develop illness. Viscerotropic disease (infection of liver, heart, and kidneys) occurs in neotropical primates, the European hedgehog, laboratory (golden) hamsters, and AG129 mice deficient in α/β interferon receptors. Yellow fever virus causes encephalitis in mice, hamsters, and guinea pigs after intracerebral inoculation. A number of vertebrates (e.g., sloths) have been found to have antibodies against yellow fever virus, but because of their low viremia they are unlikely to be important in maintaining virus transmission.

Geographic Distribution and Incidence

From 1988 to 2007, 26 356 yellow fever cases were reported to the WHO; of these, 23 056 (87%) were reported from sub-Saharan Africa, affecting 33 countries, with the remainder from 14 countries in tropical South America. In Africa, the number of reported cases varied from 0 to 5000 per year and suggests significant inconsistencies in surveillance and reporting. In South America, up to 524 cases per year have been reported to the WHO. Case fatality is highly variable but usually approximately 20%; higher rates have been reported. Because most yellow fever cases are not reported, the WHO estimated that the true incidence may be 200 000 cases and 30 000 deaths annually.[28,29] In addition to underreporting of "classic" yellow fever cases, the number of yellow fever viral infections is not known but believed to be much higher. The ratio of classic yellow fever cases to the number of infections is estimated to be approximately 1 : 10, but this may vary greatly.

In Africa, of the 23 056 cases reported from 1988 to 2007, 4642 (20%) were fatal. The majority of outbreaks have been reported from West Africa; fewer outbreaks have been reported from Central and East Africa. Within Africa, Nigeria has the largest number of reported cases due to a series of epidemics from 1986 to 1994. Since 1995, outbreaks have occurred in many West African countries, including Gabon (1995), Liberia (1995, 1998, 2000–2001, 2004), Senegal (1995–1996, 2002–2003), Ghana (1996), Benin (1996–1997), Guinea (2000–2001, 2005), Côte d'Ivoire (2001–2003), Burkina Faso (2004), Mali (2004), and Togo (2006). During West African outbreaks, up to 3% of the population may develop yellow fever and 20% are infected. Because the population is regularly exposed in and around villages, children without naturally acquired immunity are at highest risk of infection and illness.

In East Africa, outbreaks are less frequent but have been reported from Sudan in 1940, 1959, 2003, and 2005; Ethiopia in 1960–1962 and 1966; and Kenya in 1936 and 1992–1993. Although no human disease was reported in the intervening years, low-level virus transmission occurs sporadically as shown by serological surveys. Since 2008, there have been reports of an increased number of yellow fever cases coming from Central African countries such as Central African Republic, Democratic Republic of the Congo, and Chad. Many of these countries have infrequently reported yellow fever cases in the past, and it is unclear whether the reports of cases in these countries are due to improved surveillance or increased disease activity either locally or by extension from neighboring endemic areas.

In South America, most yellow fever cases are reported from the Orinoco, Amazon, and Araguaia river basins and contiguous grasslands. Between 1988 and 2007, 3300 cases were reported; of these, 1784 (54%) were fatal. The high fatality rate may be due to lower rates of acquired immunity to cross-reactive flaviviruses or to higher genetic susceptibility compared to populations in Africa. This has led to speculation that the true incidence of yellow fever in South America may be 10-fold greater than reported numbers of cases. Peru and Bolivia have had the highest cumulative incidence of yellow fever over the past twenty years. In South America, yellow fever virus is transmitted in the sylvatic cycle, with the highest incidence among males aged 15–45 years who are agricultural and forest workers. In Brazil, most cases are reported from the Amazon and western Brazil; however, starting in 2007 cases have been identified in more southern and eastern states including Sao Paulo, Bahia, Tocantins, Goias, Parana, and Rio Grande do Sul. Areas contiguous with southern Brazil, namely northern Argentina and Paraguay, have also had confirmed cases of yellow fever starting in 2007, the first invasion of these regions since the 1970s. In 1998, the first cases of yellow fever were reported in French Guiana since 1902.[30] In addition to the increased number of cases in recent years, *Ae. aegypti* has reinfested many urban centers in South America, increasing the risk for urban outbreaks of yellow fever in the Americas as occurred in Asuncion, Paraguay in 2007.

Fortunately, yellow fever has never appeared in Asia. Because urban areas in Asia have *Ae. aegypti* that is capable of transmitting yellow fever virus and a large susceptible human population, Asia is vulnerable to the introduction of the virus. Possible explanations for the absence of yellow fever virus in Asia include immunologic cross-protection provided by dengue immunity, low vector competence of local *Ae. aegypti* populations, or the occurrence of yellow fever in remote African and South American areas populated by people who do not travel by air and are unlikely to spread infection.

Seasonality

The ecology of yellow fever virus is complex, and many factors contribute to viral transmission. In general, virus activity increases when temperature, humidity, and rainfall increase through effects on mosquito abundance. In South America, yellow fever incidence is highest during months of high rainfall, humidity, and temperature (January to May). This corresponds to periods of increased activity and reproduction of *Haemagogus* mosquitoes, a mosquito dependent on accumulated water in tree hole-breeding sites. During this time, human exposure to potentially infected mosquitoes is also increased during agricultural activities.

In the savanna zone of West Africa, yellow fever cases begin to appear during the mid-rainy season (August). Peak occurs during the early dry season (October), a period that corresponds to the period of maximum longevity of mosquito vectors. Because *Ae. aegypti* breeds in receptacles used for water storage, its activity and reproduction patterns are less dependent on rainfall. As a result, when *Ae. aegypti* is involved in virus transmission, yellow fever may also occur in the dry season.

Disease Susceptibility and Risk Factors for Human Infection

Age, sex, and occupation affect the distribution of yellow fever cases and differ in Africa and South America. In South America, *Haemagogus* mosquitoes that previously fed on viremic monkeys in the rainforest canopy transmit virus to humans. Human infection is linked to occupational activities such as forest clearing, lumbering, and road construction; up to 90% of yellow fever cases are young men.[31] The age and sex distribution of sylvatic yellow fever cases differs from that observed during the *Ae. aegypti*-borne epidemics in South America. During these epidemics, because *Ae. aegypti* breeds around houses, a higher prevalence of infection occurred among children and women.

In Africa, sylvatic *Aedes* species reach high densities in the moist savanna and enter villages. During outbreaks, children are at highest risk for infection and disease. A high attack rate in children (>70%) typifies areas where older people are protected by preexisting immunity from naturally acquired infections or yellow fever vaccination campaigns.

THE DISEASE

Clinical manifestations of yellow fever viral infection are broad and include asymptomatic infection; abortive infection with nonspecific symptoms (i.e., low-grade fever, myalgia, and headache); and classic

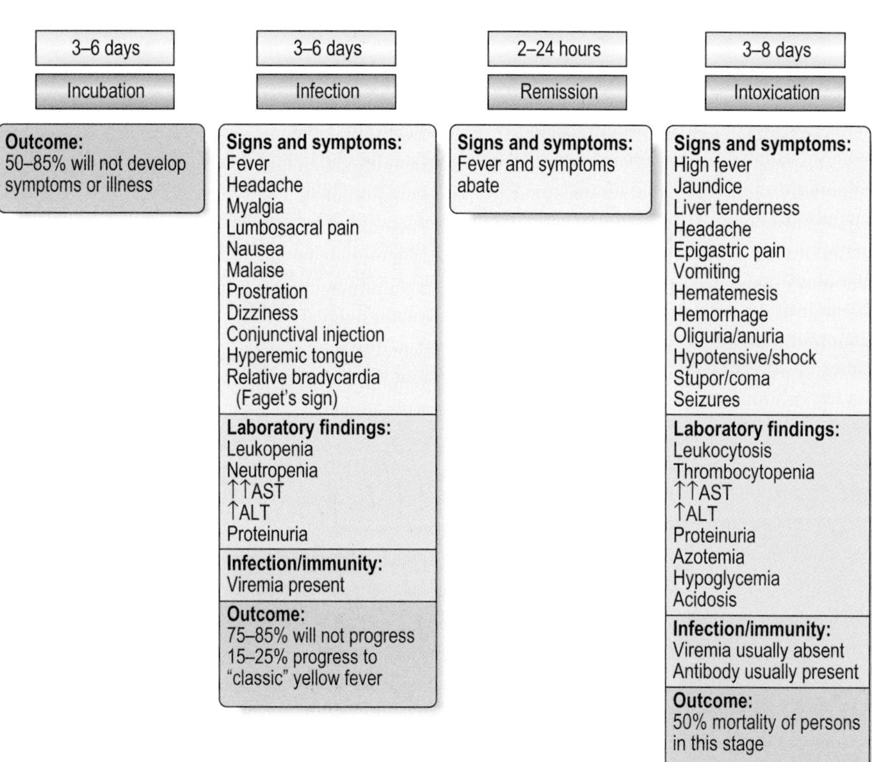

3–6 days
Incubation
Outcome:
50–85% will not develop symptoms or illness
3–6 days
Infection
Signs and symptoms:
Fever
Headache
Myalgia
Lumbosacral pain
Nausea
Malaise
Prostration
Dizziness
Conjunctival injection
Hyperemic tongue
Relative bradycardia (Faget's sign)
Laboratory findings:
Leukopenia
Neutropenia
↑↑AST
↑ALT
Proteinuria
Infection/immunity:
Viremia present
Outcome:
75–85% will not progress
15–25% progress to "classic" yellow fever
2–24 hours
Remission
Signs and symptoms:
Fever and symptoms abate
3–8 days
Intoxication
Signs and symptoms:
High fever
Jaundice
Liver tenderness
Headache
Epigastric pain
Vomiting
Hematemesis
Hemorrhage
Oliguria/anuria
Hypotensive/shock
Stupor/coma
Seizures
Laboratory findings:
Leukocytosis
Thrombocytopenia
↑↑AST
↑ALT
Proteinuria
Azotemia
Hypoglycemia
Acidosis
Infection/immunity:
Viremia usually absent
Antibody usually present
Outcome:
50% mortality of persons in this stage

Figure 74.4 Stages of yellow fever infection showing the duration, major clinical and laboratory findings, and outcome of each stage. AST, aspartate aminotransferase; ALT, alanine aminotransferase. (Modified from Monath TP. Yellow fever: an update. Lancet Infect Dis. 2001;1:11–20.)

yellow fever syndrome of multiple organ system failure (MOSF) with hemorrhage, liver failure, and renal failure (*Fig. 74.4*). These variable manifestations make the diagnosis of less severe and sporadic infections difficult, resulting in an underestimate of morbidity and an overestimate of case-fatality rates.

Triphasic Disease

After a 3- to 6-day incubation, it is estimated that 15–50% of infected people develop illness, with the abrupt onset of fever, chills, and headache. Of those who develop any illness, approximately 75–85% will abort their infection and recover without developing classic yellow fever. The remaining 15–25% who become ill develop the syndrome known as yellow fever.[31] Following incubation, classic yellow fever is characterized by three clinical stages: infection, remission, and intoxication (see *Fig. 74.4*).

The first clinical period, the period of infection, lasts 3 or 4 days and is characterized by viremia and the pathophysiologic response to viremia. Illness onset is abrupt, with fever of 39°C or higher, chills, malaise, headache, low back and knee pain, generalized myalgia, nausea, and dizziness. On examination, the patient has a heart rate lower than would be expected for the degree of fever (Faget's sign) and erythema of the conjunctivae, tongue, and face. Temperatures up to 40.5°C are associated with severe illness and poor outcome. Children 5 years old or younger may experience febrile convulsions. Laboratory abnormalities include leukopenia ($1.5–2.5 \times 10^3$/mL) with relative neutropenia. Jaundice or hepatocellular enzyme elevation is rarely present during this period but may begin 2 or 3 days after illness onset.[32] In addition, proteinuria may be severe and is one of the few specific clinical findings during this early phase. Peak viremia occurs on the second or third day of illness, and infected people may serve as a source of infection for mosquitoes that poses a public health risk.[33]

The period of infection may be followed by a distinct period of remission when fever and other constitutional symptoms abate for up to 48 hours. Viremia may still be present during this period but is usually waning. Most patients will recover from the acute illness. Because they remain anicteric and the specificity of these early clinical signs is poor, it is difficult to diagnose these milder yellow fever viral infections clinically. In patients who do not abort their infection, fever will reappear, and the patients will progress to the more fulminant period of intoxication.

Approximately 15–25% of people who develop any clinical symptoms (or 10% of all infected people) progress to the period of intoxication. This generally occurs 3–6 days after illness onset and lasts for approximately 3–8 days. During this period, viremia disappears, antibodies appear, and the signs of classic yellow fever (jaundice, renal failure, and hemorrhage) appear. It is heralded by the return of fever, relative bradycardia, nausea, and vomiting. In addition, patients develop epigastric pain, jaundice, oliguria, and hemorrhagic signs and rapidly progress to MOSF dominated by hepatic, renal, hematologic, and cardiovascular involvement. Serum concentrations of hepatocellular enzymes, aspartate aminotransferase (AST) and alanine aminotransferase (ALT), peak early in this phase. AST levels are generally greater than ALT levels, in contrast to viral hepatitis, in which the reverse is true. In fatal yellow fever cases, the AST and ALT levels are usually greater than 2700 and 600 U/L, respectively. Direct bilirubin levels are typically between 5 and 10 mg/dL and higher in fatal cases compared to nonfatal cases.[34,35]

Renal dysfunction is characterized by albuminuria, microscopic hematuria, reduced urine output, and rising blood urea nitrogen and creatinine. As a result of increased glomerular permeability, albumin concentrations in the urine are typically in the nephrotic range (3–5 g/L) and may reach 20 g/L. Serum creatinine levels are three to eight times normal. Despite the severity of the renal disease and albuminuria, the extravascular fluid accumulations that accompany many hemorrhagic fever viruses (i.e., edema, ascites, and pleural effusion) are not seen in yellow fever. Also, despite the apparent severity of renal failure, dialysis is not usually needed.[36]

In addition to the pathologic changes in the liver and kidneys, there are widespread petechiae and hemorrhages on mucosal surfaces, in the skin, and within other organs. The hemorrhagic signs include hematemesis, melena, hematuria, metrorrhagia, petechiae, ecchymoses, epistaxis, and oozing of blood from the gums and needle puncture sites. Laboratory findings reflect marked dysfunction of the hematologic system and coagulation cascade that contributes to the hemorrhagic signs. These include thrombocytopenia, prolonged clotting and prothrombin times, and reductions in clotting factors synthesized by the liver (factors II, V, VII, IX, and X). Some patients develop disseminated intravascular coagulation (DIC).

Myocarditis presumably due to virus replication and direct viral injury occurs in many patients and may contribute to cardiovascular dysfunction and shock. The electrocardiogram may show sinus bradycardia and ST-T abnormalities.

Although central nervous system (CNS) signs, such as delirium, seizures, and coma, may be present, there is little to suggest direct viral invasion of the CNS. In the most severe cases, no pleocytosis is present, although there may be modest elevations of protein in the cerebrospinal fluid (CSF). Pathologic examination reveals no inflammatory changes in the brain. Because true encephalitis is rare, it is likely that the CNS signs are the result of poor cerebral perfusion, cerebral edema, cytokine dysregulation, or metabolic abnormality.

Risk Factors for Illness

Older people and males are at risk for a more severe clinical course. Studies of the clinical course among immunosuppressed people are not available. Protein-calorie malnutrition has been associated with failure to respond immunologically to yellow fever vaccine, but there are no reports that malnourished people have more severe disease caused by wild-type yellow fever virus. While one study did find a lower antibody response in pregnant women versus non-pregnant women vaccinated against yellow fever, pregnancy has not been reported as a risk factor for more severe disease. Human immunodeficiency virus (HIV) infection may be an important risk factor for increased yellow fever viremia following infection, disease severity, and risk for AEFI after yellow fever vaccination. A poor immune response has been noted following yellow fever 17D vaccination of HIV-infected travelers and children,[37,38] but there has been only a single published report of a severe AEFI in an HIV-infected person.[39]

Mortality

Nearly 50% of patients who develop hepatic and renal failure and anuria die. Disease severity and mortality are highest in older adults.[40] Death is preceded by profound hypotension and shock that are difficult to manage with fluids and vasopressors. This condition appears to be due to an outpouring of proinflammatory cytokines. In addition to hypotension, worsening jaundice, and acute renal failure, signs of cerebral edema (e.g., hypothermia, coma, and Cheyne–Stokes respirations) are associated with impending death. Other signs include hypoglycemia, uncorrectable acidosis, leukocytosis, hyperkalemia, agitated delirium, intractable hiccups, and seizures.

Complications of yellow fever among survivors include superimposed bacterial pneumonia, parotitis, and sepsis. Late deaths during convalescence have been attributed to myocarditis, arrhythmia, or heart failure. Convalescence may be associated with weakness and fatigability lasting weeks, but healing of the liver and kidney is typically complete without postnecrotic fibrosis. In some cases, jaundice and elevated hepatocellular enzymes may persist for months.

PATHOGENESIS AND IMMUNITY

Pathogenesis and Pathophysiology

Although yellow fever has features in common with other hemorrhagic fevers, the severity of hepatic and renal injury is pathologically distinct.[41,42] Kidney, liver, and myocardial damage is due to the direct injury of viral replication. In addition to the virus-induced pathologic changes in the liver and kidneys, there are profound ischemic changes in other organs resulting from widespread hemorrhages and the resulting shock. In addition, there may be mitochondrial damage that results in increased membrane permeability and apoptotic cell death. Studies of yellow fever virus infection in hamsters also suggest a role for various cytokines in the pathologic changes with significant variations in the level of proinflammatory cytokines based on the organ and time following the initial infection.[43] Interestingly, most of this injury occurs during the period of intoxication, when yellow fever viremia is usually absent and virus-specific antibodies are developing.

Pathogenesis of Hepatic Failure

The liver destruction of yellow fever results from apoptosis[44–46] and is associated with minimal inflammatory cell infiltration, and characterized by Kupffer cells, natural killer (NK) cells, dendritic cells, $CD4^+$, $CD8^+$, and activated $CD45RO^+$ T cells in the midzone and periportal areas.[45,46] Expression of cytokines, including tumor necrosis factor (TNF)-α, interferon-γ (IFN-γ), and transforming growth factor (TGF)-β, is also localized in these areas of the liver lobule. The five central features of yellow fever liver pathology are eosinophilic degeneration of hepatocytes and Kupffer cells, midzonal (zone 2) hepatocellular injury, the absence of inflammation, microvesicular fatty change, and retention of the reticulin structure with return to normal histology in survivors. A unique feature of hepatic injury in yellow fever is the midzonal distribution, with sparing of cells around the central vein and portal tracts. Yellow fever virus antigen and RNA have been observed disproportionately in the hepatocytes in the midzone, suggesting that these cells are more susceptible to virus replication.[42,47] Although, on average, up to 80% of hepatocytes may be destroyed, the livers of survivors heal without postnecrotic fibrosis.

Pathogenesis of Renal Failure

The pathogenesis of renal injury in humans is poorly understood but appears multifactorial. In studies of nonhuman primates, although viral antigen can be detected in the kidney parenchyma, the initial oliguria does not appear to be due to direct renal injury by the virus.[47] Instead, the initial injury appears to be due to renal ischemia that is out of proportion to the degree of hypovolemia and is more likely attributable to TNF and other proinflammatory cytokines. At death, immunohistochemistry (IHC) can detect antigen in glomeruli and renal tubular cells, suggesting a role for direct viral injury. In addition, renal failure may be due to the severe hepatic injury (i.e., hepatorenal syndrome) that alters salt and water regulation and can be present in the absence of renal pathology. Prior to death, oliguria worsens and is often accompanied by proteinuria, azotemia, acidosis, shock, hyperkalemia, and severe tubular necrosis.

Pathogenesis of Myocardial Injury

Myocardial injury in yellow fever appears to be due to viral replication within the myocardial cells, where viral antigen can be demonstrated by IHC. Myocardial cells undergo similar apoptotic changes as seen in liver and kidney, as well as microsteatosis. There is no significant inflammatory response, the reticulin structure is preserved, and no fibrosis occurs after recovery. Lesions have been noted in the conduction system. When bradycardia is present, it may contribute to the physiologic decompensation associated with hypotension, reduced perfusion, and metabolic acidosis in severe cases. The pathologic changes in these major conduction pathways suggest a basis for late deaths attributed to cardiac arrhythmias.

Coagulation Defects and Other Hematologic Abnormalities

In studies of yellow fever virus-infected monkeys, severely ill animals have depressed levels of all clotting factors, particularly fibrinogen and factors V, VII, VIII, and X, as well as platelet dysfunction. This situation suggests that yellow fever virus does not specifically activate the intrinsic pathway, and that the major cause of bleeding is decreased synthesis of clotting factors.

Leukopenia, particularly neutropenia, is an early finding in yellow fever infection. IFN may contribute to leukopenia and thrombocytopenia by bone marrow suppression and induction of a wide array of cytokines. The spleen and lymph nodes undergo profound changes in yellow fever infection, characterized by the appearance of large mononuclear or histiocytic cells and the disappearance of small lymphocytes.

Hypotension and Shock

The terminal events occur precipitously and are characterized by cardiovascular shock and multiorgan failure. The features of this phase strongly suggest that they are mediated by an inflammatory cascade (***Fig. 74.4***), although few patients have been directly studied. In one series of fatal and nonfatal naturally acquired disease, pro- and anti-inflammatory cytokines (IL-6, IL-8, TNF-α, monocyte chemoattractant protein-1, IL-1-receptor antagonist, IL-10), resembling bacterial sepsis were significantly elevated in fatal cases,[48] and similar findings were reported in a fatal case of yellow fever vaccine associated viscerotropic disease (YEL-AVD).[49] An overlooked feature of yellow fever is the marked granulocytic leukocytosis observed in the terminal stage of disease. Given the elevated serum levels of IL-8 and TNF-α, it is likely that these granulocytes are activated, with consequent release of platelet-activating factor (PAF), elastase and other proteases, and leukotrienes, which may modify endothelial integrity, particularly in the presence of proinflammatory cytokines, causing capillary leak. The syndrome in yellow fever thus resembles many elements seen in overwhelming sepsis.

Yellow fever vaccine and wild-type viruses infect endothelial cells and wild-type virus activates proinflammatory cytokine genes, including IL-6 and RANTES;[50] it is possible that these *in vitro* effects contribute to the pathogenesis of yellow fever shock or coagulation defects.

Encephalopathy

In the terminal stage of infection, humans and nonhuman primates develop stupor and coma, which is probably metabolic in origin. Contributing factors include hypoglycemia (due to the liver's impaired gluconeogenesis), decreased perfusion, and acidosis. Changes in tissue concentrations of water and electrolytes in various compartments of the CNS have been described, including intracellular dehydration of medulla, cerebellum, and spinal cord. In addition, the encephalopathy appears to be partially due to the hepatorenal syndrome that frequently accompanies fatal cases of yellow fever. CNS invasion by yellow fever virus is rare. Even in fatal cases, in which seizures and coma are present, inflammatory changes are not present in the brain.

Innate Immunity

Although there are few yellow fever-specific studies, it is assumed that the first line of host defense is a nonspecific, innate immune response. This includes the NK cell response and other resistance factors that interfere with virus replication before the appearance of virus-specific cytotoxic T cells and antibodies. Many studies of dengue show the importance of type 1 IFNs in this nonspecific, innate immune response to flavivirus infection. IFN activates several host defense mechanisms, including increasing NK cells, CD14-bearing monocyte/macrophages, major histocompatibility complex class I (MHC-I) proteins on the host cell surface, Th1-dependent immunoglobulin synthesis, and cytotoxic T-lymphocyte activity.[51–53] Monkeys treated with IFN-γ had lower yellow fever viremia and liver injury,[54] and IFN-α/β deficient mice showed poor yellow fever viral clearance and a poor cellular inflammatory response after intracerebral inoculation compared to parental mice.[55] It is uncertain whether these effects were due to a direct antiviral effect, immunomodulation by IFN, or induction of other cytokines. In addition to IFN, a variety of other proinflammatory cytokines and markers of T-cell activation have been found during the viremic period after yellow fever vaccination in humans, including TNF-α, IL-1, neopterin, β_2-microglobulin, and circulating CD8 T cells.[56,57] Studies of human and mouse dendritic cells *in vitro* showed that yellow fever 17D vaccine activates multiple toll-like receptors (TLR2, 7, 8, and 9) and elicits proinflammatory cytokine responses which strongly drive adaptive immune responses.[58] It is likely that similar responses occur in people infected with wild-type yellow fever virus. Profound innate immune activation likely plays a role in the strong, lifelong adaptive immunity observed after yellow fever vaccination or natural infection.

The genetic constitution of the host is one of the most important factors influencing the outcome of viral infection. This has been investigated using inbred strains of mice that differ in their resistance to flaviviruses including yellow fever virus.[59] In some cases, resistant mice appear to be more susceptible to the antiviral action of IFN, although at least one resistance gene (*flv*) confers flavivirus-specific resistance by an IFN-independent mechanism.[60] In general, susceptibility to disease correlates with increased levels of viral replication in tissues. Protein kinase R (PKR) and 2′-5′-oligoadenylate synthase (OAS) proteins appear to influence susceptibilty of mice to infections with West Nile virus.[61] PKR activation by flavivirus leads to the attenuation of protein synthesis, while OAS activates RNase L that in turn cleaves viral and host RNA. It is uncertain whether these proteins or mechanisms contribute to severe yellow fever disease.

Since approximately 10% of infected people develop classic yellow fever, it is clear that the innate immune system or other mechanisms may fail to protect the host. This may be due to viral mechanisms that reduce immune clearance by NK cells. Unlike many viruses that decrease the density of MHC-I proteins on the infected cell surface, flaviviruses increase their density through the increased supply of related peptides to the ER through the action of IFN.[62] Since MHC-I proteins protect cells against attack by NK cells, flavivirus-infected cells avoid clearance by the innate activity of NK cells.

Adaptive Immune Response

Up to 10^4 yellow fever virions are inoculated into extravascular tissues during probing by an infected female mosquito. In an immune host, virus first encounters yellow fever virus-specific neutralizing antibodies in the extracellular transudate and lymph.

In a nonimmune host, the nonspecific, innate immune response is followed by a specific immune response characterized by the development of neutralizing antibodies and cytotoxic T cells. In addition, cytolytic antibodies against viral proteins on the surface of infected cells and antibody-dependent, cell-mediated cytotoxicity contribute to viral clearance. The humoral response to yellow fever virus is characterized by the appearance of IgM antibodies in the first 7 or 8 days following infection (i.e., 4 or 5 days after illness onset). IgM levels peak 7–14 days after illness onset and decline rapidly over 30–60 days but may persist for years at low levels. Neutralizing antibodies persist for many years, if not lifelong, after natural yellow fever infection and provide complete protection against disease on reexposure to the virus. No documented case of a second clinical yellow fever infection has been reported. Antibodies against NS1 expressed on the infected cell surface lead to complement-mediated cytolysis and may contribute to clearance of infected cells early in recovery. It is not known whether this anti-NS1 antibody protects against reinfection or only plays a role in virus clearance during recovery from infection.

People with preexisting antibody to other flaviviruses (i.e., heterologous antibody) develop broadly cross-reactive antibody responses following yellow fever virus infection. In contrast to dengue, in which such heterologous antibody may enhance disease, this antibody protects against yellow fever. Nonhuman primates actively immunized with Zika, Wesselsbron, or dengue viruses are protected against a subsequent yellow fever virus challenge.[63,64] Other studies show that humans with broadly reactive antibody to unspecified African flaviviruses have a lower incidence of yellow fever disease than people with primary yellow fever infections.[65]

Yellow fever vaccine elicits strong and rapid effector $CD8^+$ T-cell responses, and strong T-cell memory.[66] Cytotoxic T lymphocytes kill flavivirus-infected cells and contribute to viral clearance and recovery from primary infection. In studies of yellow fever viral encephalitis in T- and B-cell knockout mice, $CD4^+$ cells are important for protection.[55] There are no data on human cellular responses to wild-type yellow fever virus.

DIAGNOSIS

The differential diagnosis of classic yellow fever includes severe malaria with rapid hemolysis, severe hepatitis E in pregnancy, hepatitis D superinfection, other viral hemorrhagic fevers that may rarely have jaundice (e.g., dengue hemorrhagic fever and Crimean-Congo hemorrhagic fever), leptospirosis, and relapsing fever due to *Borrelia recurrentis*.[67] Most hemorrhagic fever viruses, such as Marburg, Ebola, and Lassa fever viruses, are not usually associated with jaundice but may still cause diagnostic confusion. Milder clinical cases or the early, anicteric phase of yellow fever resemble many other febrile illnesses.

Specific laboratory diagnosis relies on serology or, during the early, anicteric phase, on detection of virus, viral antigens, or viral RNA in blood. None of these methods are commercially available. In clinical samples, yellow fever virus-specific real-time quantitative reverse transcription polymerase chain reaction (RT-PCR) assays can detect titers as low as 0.1 PFU/mL and much lower than standard RT-PCR (lower limit, 1 PFU/mL) or virus isolation in cell culture (lower limit, 10 PFU/mL).[68] In addition to increased sensitivity, both PCR methods give a definitive result in a much shorter time than virus isolation in any system. Because clinical suspicion of yellow fever is low during the early, anicteric phase of infection when viremia is present, isolation, genomic amplification, and antigen detection have played a minor role in yellow fever diagnosis to date.

Serology is the most important diagnostic test, and yellow fever virus-specific IgM enzyme-linked immunosorbent assay (ELISA) is the most widely used serological method. The presence of IgM antibodies in a single serum sample taken on or after day 7 of clinical illness or during the early recovery phase provides a presumptive diagnosis, and demonstration of a fourfold increase in antibody titer in paired sera (using ELISA, neutralization, or hemagglutination inhibition assays) is confirmatory. The specificity of IgM ELISA is high in primary infections and in most secondary flavivirus infections. Despite this high specificity, cross-reactions between yellow fever virus and other flaviviruses frequently complicate serological diagnosis.

In fatal cases, the characteristic histopathologic liver changes (e.g., midzonal necrosis and Councilman's bodies) are diagnostic. IHC with polyclonal or monoclonal antibodies to yellow fever virus to detect antigen in tissue is diagnostic and more specific than standard histopathology. Despite the high potential for a specific diagnosis, liver biopsies in living patients should not be performed because fatal hemorrhage may occur.

TREATMENT AND PROGNOSIS

The management of patients with yellow fever has not been optimized because disease occurs in areas with rudimentary medical services and the hemodynamic instability of these patients often precludes transport. Because there is no yellow fever virus-specific therapy, intensive supportive care to maximize tissue perfusion, reduce hemorrhagic complications, maintain adequate glucose levels, and provide nutritional maintenance is necessary to reduce the mortality of yellow fever. In addition, the following have been recommended: nasogastric suction to prevent gastric distension and aspiration, intravenous agents to reduce gastric acidity and prevent gastric bleeding, fluid replacement with normal saline or Ringer's lactate, vasopressors if needed, administration of oxygen, correction of metabolic acidosis, treatment of bleeding with fresh-frozen plasma, and treatment of secondary infections with antibiotics. Unfortunately, patients with yellow fever do not respond dramatically to fluid replacement or vasopressors; this is likely due to irreversible pathophysiologic processes and the unchecked effect of TNF or other cytokines. Heparin should only be used to treat DIC when there has been documented consumption of clotting factors and activation of fibrinolytic mechanisms and when there is adequate laboratory support to monitor heparin's effects. If available and needed, dialysis should be used in cases of renal failure or anuria. Other medical considerations may include orthotopic liver transplantation or the use of extracorporeal support systems.[69] In the future, other possible nonspecific treatments may include anticytokine therapies or cytokine receptor blockers to prevent cell apoptosis.

There is no specific antiviral treatment. Although ribavirin has activity against yellow fever virus at high (potentially cytotoxic) concentrations *in vitro*, ribavirin monotherapy has generally not been successful in animal studies.[70] Passive antibody, IFN, and IFN inducers are only effective if given before infection or during incubation.[70] There is no current indication for their use, and passive antibody protection should only be considered in the setting of postexposure prophylaxis (i.e., after known infection and before illness onset), such as after a laboratory exposure. Corticosteroids have not been evaluated for the treatment of yellow fever, but a retrospective study of patients with yellow fever vaccine-associated viscerotropic disease found that stress doses of steroids appear to improve survival.[71] Studies of newer antiviral agents, pyrazine nucleoside analogs and related compounds (T-1106 and T-705), have shown promise with improvements in survival and disease parameters in the hamster model of yellow fever virus infection.[72]

PREVENTION AND CONTROL

Travelers to yellow fever-endemic countries should be advised of the risks of disease, the importance of personal protective measures to reduce the risk of mosquito bites, and the use of yellow fever vaccine to reduce the risk of disease.

Personal Protective Measures

All travelers should take precautions to avoid mosquito bites to reduce the risk of yellow fever and other vector-borne infectious diseases. These precautions include using insect repellent, permethrin impregnated clothing, and bednets, and staying in screened or air-conditioned rooms. Additional information on protection against mosquitoes and other arthropods can be found at http://wwwn.cdc.gov/travel/yellowbook/ch2/insects-arthropods.aspx.

Yellow Fever Vaccine

During the 1930s, two wild-type yellow fever virus strains, Asibi and French, were attenuated to derive live vaccines known as 17D and the French neurotropic vaccine, respectively.[73] Currently, 17D is the only strain of yellow fever virus used for vaccination. During vaccine production from 1937 to 1941, two different 17D substrains, 17D-204 and 17DD, were developed in parallel; these are used for current vaccine production. Although they differ with respect to 17D substrain and other production qualities, they are both produced in embryonated eggs and meet the same WHO standards for safety and potency. In addition, their biologic performance is similar with respect to seroconversion rate, quality of the immune response, durability of immunity, safety, and tolerability. 17D vaccines are heterogeneous mixtures of multiple virus subpopulations. Not surprisingly, differences have been found in plaque size, oligonucleotide fingerprints, and nucleotide sequences. There is no evidence that such variations affect safety or efficacy.

Four manufacturers located in Brazil, France, Senegal, and Russia produce WHO-prequalified vaccine that can be used in the Expanded Programme of Immunization (EPI) and mass vaccination campaigns. Sanofi Pasteur exports vaccine for the traveler's market. Since 1937, 500–600 million doses of the vaccine have been administered worldwide.

Immune Response

Between 95% and 99% of vaccinated people develop neutralizing antibodies within 10–14 days of immunization. Race and age do not appear to influence response rates. In one study, males had lower antibody titers than females.[74] In the majority of cases, antibody titers following vaccination are lower, and their appearance is delayed compared to natural yellow fever virus infections. This is likely due to less virus replication and antigen expression by the 17D strain. The minimal protective level of neutralizing antibodies induced by 17D vaccine has been estimated by dose-response studies in rhesus monkeys that are subsequently challenged after immunization with virulent yellow fever virus. In such studies, log neutralization index (LNI; measured by plaque reduction) of 0.7 or greater is associated with protection. Human clinical trials of 17D vaccine have shown geometric mean LNI values of 2.1 or greater measured within 1 month after vaccination.[74] The International Health Regulations stipulate that the vaccination certificate for yellow fever is valid 10 days after administration of 17D vaccine for primary vaccine recipients, which corresponds to the time at which the majority of vaccinees are demonstrably immune. Immunity following 17D vaccination is remarkably durable and may be lifelong. Although the yellow fever immunization certificate for international travel is valid for 10 years, this interval was based on published studies showing that neutralizing antibodies were present in more than 90% of people 16–19 years after vaccination. Later studies of US military veterans from World War II tested 30–35 years after a single dose of 17D vaccine showed that slightly more than 80% had neutralizing antibody, and in some subgroups more than 95% had it.[73]

T-cell responses to yellow fever vaccination occur rapidly after primary immunization and are critical to clearance of the live virus.[66] From the perspective of vaccine immunity, long-lived functional memory T cells are important and are a hallmark of yellow fever vaccination.

Adventitious Viruses

In 1966, yellow fever 17D vaccines were found to be contaminated with avian leukosis virus (ALV), a potentially oncogenic retrovirus with a high prevalence in chicken embryos. New ALV-free seeds were prepared in the 1970s, and all international manufacturers now use ALV-free seeds as stipulated by WHO. A retrospective study of cancer deaths in World War II veterans revealed that the incidence of all cancers, lymphoma, and leukemia was not significantly different in people vaccinated 5–22 years previously with ALV-contaminated 17D vaccine than in those not vaccinated.

During the original formulation and early use of 17D vaccines, pooled human serum was used as a vaccine stabilizer. This resulted in vaccine contamination with hepatitis B virus and a massive outbreak of jaundice and hepatitis in yellow fever vaccine recipients. Human serum was eliminated from yellow fever vaccines by 1942, and current vaccines are not contaminated with human hepatitis viruses.

Vaccine Dose, Route of Administration, and Preparations

A 17D vaccine dose contains approximately 5×10^4 PFU in 0.5 mL and is given subcutaneously, usually in the upper arm. All yellow fever vaccines are prepared as lyophilized powder but vary with respect to stabilizer additives and salt content. Some contain sodium chloride and buffer salts and are reconstituted with sterile water, whereas others are reconstituted with saline. Because there is no preservative in the vaccine and because the vaccine rapidly loses potency after reconstitution, it must be refrigerated at the point of use, held on ice, and used soon after reconstitution. In the United States, reconstituted vaccine must be discarded within 1 hour; in EPI systems, it must be discarded within 4 hours. Vaccine is supplied in single- and multiple-dose containers. Although combination vaccines have been tested clinically (e.g., yellow fever–measles and yellow fever–typhoid), no such products are available.

Viremia Following 17D Vaccination

Some adult vaccinees have low virus titers in blood (fewer than 100 PFU/mL, which is far below the 4 or 5 logs of virus needed to infect mosquitoes). The low viremia following 17D vaccine may explain the apparent low risk of transplacental transmission in women immunized during pregnancy. Viremia begins 2 to 4 days after vaccination and lasts 1–3 days.[73] The level of viremia following vaccination is high enough to be transmitted through blood products. Transfusion-related transmission of yellow fever vaccine virus has been documented in three persons who received blood products that were collected from persons vaccinated before their blood donation.[75] There are no data on viremia levels in infants or children given 17D vaccine or in people who are immunosuppressed.

Genetic Stability during Replication in the Vaccinated Host

The 17D vaccine is not clonal. It is a heterogeneous mixture of virus variants with varying antigenic, genetic, and biologic properties. Despite this, it is thought to have very little potential for reversion to wild-type, emergence of pathogenic strains, or recombinational events. Isolation of a strain that was more virulent than the parental 17D vaccine strain has been documented only once following routine vaccination. In one fatal human encephalitis case, the viral isolate from the brain had higher neurovirulence in mice than the 17D-204 strain. This isolate caused encephalitis in nonhuman primates, reacted with a wild-type virus-specific monoclonal antibody, and had two amino acid changes in the E protein and one in NS4B. Other studies indicate a high degree of genetic stability of 17D virus during *in vivo* replication. Vaccine virus strains isolated from the sera of people vaccinated with the 17D-204 vaccine contained no mutations in the structural genes and few mutations in the nonstructural protein genes, especially the NS5 protein gene.[76] Other studies have supported the finding that mutations in yellow fever virus tend to accumulate at a significantly lower rate than expected for an RNA virus.[20]

Revaccination

Revaccination or vaccination of people with naturally acquired immunity is followed by a booster antibody response in most vaccinees, although the rise in titer is less than that seen in primary vaccination. This suggests that there is decreased virus replication due to the preexisting immunity. A stronger antibody response following revaccination is more likely in individuals with a low neutralizing antibody titer prior to vaccination.[77] With revaccination, the vaccination certificate for yellow fever is valid the same day as revaccination per International Health Regulations.

Immunization in People with Prior Flavivirus Immunity

Because of cross-reactive antigenic determinants, the primary immune response to 17D vaccine may be qualitatively different in people with preexisting heterologous immunity. Several studies have shown that naturally acquired dengue immunity reduces seroconversion and blunts the immune response to 17D vaccine, whereas preexisting immunity to flaviviruses in the Japanese encephalitis complex does not. There is no clear evidence that prior flavivirus immunity enhances replication of yellow fever 17D virus or the immune response to 17D virus.

Similarly, people with preexisting immunity to the yellow fever 17D vaccine have a qualitatively different immune response to immunization with vaccines against heterologous flaviviruses. In yellow fever-immune individuals vaccinated with an experimental, attenuated dengue vaccine, the antibody response was greater in magnitude and duration than in nonimmune individuals, suggesting that cross-reactive antibodies may be associated with enhanced dengue virus replication *in vivo*. A different mechanism, anamnestic responses to cross-reactive determinants, explains the higher response in recipients of inactivated vaccines (e.g., tick-borne encephalitis vaccine).

People with heterologous flavivirus immunity broadly respond to 17D vaccination with both homologous and heterologous neutralizing antibodies. The phenomenon of "original antigenic sin" has been noted in people previously vaccinated with 17D virus and subsequently infected with another flavivirus. In such cases, an anamnestic response leads to a rapid rise in yellow fever antibodies, but the antibody response to the more recent heterologous infection is delayed and diminished. This phenomenon may lead to diagnostic confusion in patients with clinical syndromes resembling naturally acquired yellow fever.

Yellow Fever Vaccine Efficacy in Humans

The efficacy of yellow fever vaccine has never been tested in controlled human clinical trials. Numerous studies in nonhuman primates have demonstrated that vaccination protects vaccine recipients and that protection is strongly correlated with the development and titer of neutralizing antibody. The importance of neutralizing antibody has been shown by the protection of animals by passive immunization (infusion of serum containing yellow fever virus-specific neutralizing antibody) before or soon after challenge with virulent yellow fever virus.[70]

Several primary observations support yellow fever vaccination as being protective in humans, including the reduction of laboratory-associated infections in vaccinated workers; the fact that in Brazil and other South American countries, yellow fever only occurs in unvaccinated people; and the rapid disappearance of cases during campaign-style vaccination programs initiated during epidemics. One of the greater testaments to the effectiveness of yellow fever vaccination is the disappearance of yellow fever from French-speaking West Africa after institution of mandatory yellow fever immunization with the French neurotropic vaccine in the 1940s. Unpublished reports comparing the yellow fever incidence among the vaccinated and unvaccinated populations during a 1986 epidemic in Nigeria estimate the effectiveness to be approximately 85%.[73] Because there is an effective vaccine available that is now considered the standard of care, it is highly unlikely that a placebo-controlled trial of the 17D or any newer yellow fever vaccines will be performed. Given these constraints, licensure of any new yellow fever vaccine would likely have to be granted based on a combination of animal data and studies using immunologic surrogates and demonstrating noninferiority to the existing vaccine.

Vaccine Failure

Rarely, healthy people fail to develop neutralizing antibodies following 17D vaccination. In controlled clinical trials, the primary failure rate is generally about 1%.[74] This is not an absolute refractoriness; people who fail to develop antibody after their first vaccination may develop antibody upon revaccination. More rarely, a person who was previously vaccinated may develop clinical yellow fever. Although it is uncertain whether all of these people were properly vaccinated with appropriately handled 17D vaccine, there have been five reports of vaccine recipients who developed yellow fever since development of the yellow fever vaccine.[73]

Three host factors (malnutrition, HIV infection, and pregnancy) have been associated with failure to respond immunologically to 17D vaccine. In one study, only approximately 40% of pregnant women seroconverted after vaccination compared to 82–94% among nonpregnant females of childbearing age, male students, and the general population.[78] This difference was attributed to immunosuppression associated with pregnancy and suggests the need to reimmunize at-risk women who were vaccinated during pregnancy. However, a more recent study found 98.2% of 441 women inadvertently vaccinated with yellow fever vaccine during pregnancy developed yellow fever IgG antibodies.[79] Therefore, revaccination may not be necessary in pregnant women, but antibody titers should be checked to ensure an appropriate immune response in women still at risk for the disease.

HIV infection has been associated with a reduced immunologic response to a number of inactivated and live, attenuated vaccines. Some case reports have suggested that vaccinating HIV-infected people without immunosuppression results in seroconversion. However, when 17D vaccine was administered to a small number of adult, HIV-infected travelers with $CD4^+$ counts of 200 or more cells/mL, only 70% seroconverted within 1 month of vaccination.[73] In a more recent retrospective cohort study, 83% of HIV-infected persons developed a reactive neutralization test against yellow fever virus in the first year after vaccination; however, this was significantly lower than vaccinated HIV-uninfected persons.[37] Among HIV-infected infants in developing nations, only 17% developed neutralizing antibodies within 10 months of 17D vaccination compared to 74% of HIV-uninfected controls matched for age and nutritional status.[38] The mechanisms for the diminished immune response in HIV-infected persons are uncertain but appear to be related to HIV RNA levels and $CD4^+$ cell counts. Although an encephalitis case has been reported in an HIV-infected Thai man following yellow fever vaccination, the number of HIV-infected people vaccinated with 17D vaccine is too small to assess safety.[39]

Yellow Fever Vaccine Safety

17D vaccine, the currently approved yellow fever vaccine, has been available since 1937 and widely used during outbreaks in Africa and South America and by the military and travelers operating in or visiting endemic countries.[67,80] In many affected countries, the need for yellow fever vaccination remains and, in fact, may be increasing.[24,81] Because of the vaccine's effectiveness in preventing yellow fever, the lack of virus-specific treatment, and the high mortality of yellow fever, vaccination is an integral strategy for preventing yellow fever-associated mortality and morbidity. In addition, travelers to areas where yellow fever is zoonotic, endemic, or epidemic should be vaccinated if they are at increased risk for infection based on their daily activities or living conditions.[82,83]

General Adverse Events

Reactions to 17D yellow fever vaccine are typically mild. After vaccination, vaccinees often report mild headaches, myalgia, low-grade fevers, or other minor symptoms for 5–10 days. Reactogenicity of 17D vaccine has been monitored in 21 clinical trials conducted from 1953 to 2004. In trials in which vaccinees were actively followed, 18–57% complained of local or systemic adverse events. In one large study, the most common systemic side effects (which did not differ across treatment groups) were headache (~33% of subjects), myalgia (~25%), malaise (~19%), fever (~15%), and chills (~11%).[74] These were generally mild, and few vaccinees curtailed their regular activities. There has been only one placebo control trial done to date, which indicated that the vaccine was responsible for up to 2.5% of local adverse events and up to 7.4% of systemic adverse events when compared to placebo.[84] Immediate hypersensitivity reactions, characterized by rash, urticaria, or asthma, occur principally among people with histories of allergies to egg or other substances and are estimated to occur in 1 out of 55 555 to 131 000 vaccinations.[85,86] Gelatin, used as a stabilizer in yellow fever vaccine, has been implicated as a cause of allergic reactions to other vaccines and may play a role in reactions to yellow fever vaccine.

Yellow Fever Vaccine-associated Viscerotropic Disease (YEL-AVD)

Increasingly frequent reports of YEL-AVD, a syndrome of MOSF following 17D vaccination that pathologically and clinically resembles naturally acquired yellow fever, have raised concern about the safety of this vaccine.[87,88] Fifty-nine cases of YEL-AVD have been reported worldwide.

From 1996 through 2008, the Centers for Disease Control and Prevention (CDC) received reports of 13 recipients of 17D-204 vaccine who developed YEL-AVD in the United States (CDC unpublished, 2008).[73,89] Twelve of these cases were in civilians vaccinated in anticipation of travel, and one was in the military. All 13 people (median age 64 years; range 22–79 years) became ill within 1–5 days of vaccination and developed MOSF requiring intensive care; eight died (case-fatality rate, 62%).[90,91] In addition to fever, hypotension, and respiratory failure, these people had markedly elevated hepatocellular enzymes and bilirubin, lymphocytopenia, and thrombocytopenia. Vaccine-type yellow fever virus was isolated from the blood of two people on the seventh and eighth days after vaccination. Yellow fever antigen was identified by IHC in the liver in one person, kidney in one person, and in multiple tissues (including lung, lymph node, spleen, heart, liver, and muscle) in two fatal cases.

In addition to the 13 US cases, 46 international cases of YEL-AVD have been reported in the literature, at scientific meetings, or to vaccine manufacturers.[82,85,89–92] The first three international cases from Australia and Brazil were reported simultaneously with the first US cases. They were clinically similar to the US cases except that younger people were affected. In these cases, histopathologic changes characteristic of wild-type yellow fever were noted in the liver. Yellow fever antigen and flavivirus-like particles were found by IHC and electron microscopy to be present in the areas of midzonal necrosis. Vaccine-type virus was isolated from all three people. The isolated viruses retained their vaccine phenotype when placed into experimental animals. No genomic changes previously associated with reversion to virulence were detected. Within months of these reports, other cases of hospitalized people with fever, elevated hepatocellular enzymes, and renal abnormalities were identified, suggesting that, like naturally acquired infections, there may be a spectrum of AEFI. These international cases occurred among recipients of 17D-204 and 17DD vaccines.

All but one of the cases of YEL-AVD have occurred since 1996. Three cases, identified retrospectively, occurred in the US in 1973 and 1978,[93] and in Brazil in 1975;[94] it is likely that such cases have occurred all along during the history of use of yellow fever vaccines but were unrecognized. It is not known whether additional cases occurred between 1975 and 1996 but were unrecognized or whether YEL-AVD has newly emerged. No comparable cases were identified in a retrospective review of Vaccine Adverse Event Reporting System (VAERS) reports from 1990 to 1996 (M. Cetron, personal communication, 2004). Interestingly, a report of a vaccine campaign in Nigeria in the 1950s noted a number of cases of sickness which commenced several days after vaccination with the French neurotropic vaccine and exhibited jaundice, vomiting, and albuminuria.[95] While the wild-type virus could not be ruled out, it was felt by the doctor in charge that "vaccination might well be the cause." To date, only underlying thymic disease or history of thymectomy and age >60 years have been associated with increased incidence of YEL-AVD. Attempts to identify underlying genetic mutations that may be related to an increased risk for YEL-AVD have not found common sequence abnormalities between cases though one case had genetic polymorphisms in chemokine receptor CCR5 and its ligand RANTES, which likely influenced the migration of effector T cells and monocytes to tissues.[96] Further research is needed to better quantify the risk and identify risk factors for YEL-AVD.

The estimated incidence of YEL-AVD is 0.4 cases per 100 000 doses administered.[85] However, the incidence of these events increases with age to 2.3 per 100 000 in persons ≥70 years. There is an excess of cases in males. The case-fatality rate is 50%. Recently concepts of the incidence of these serious adverse events were challenged when five cases of suspected YEL-AVD occurred during a mass vaccination campaign in 2007 in Peru, yielding an incidence of 7.9 per 100 000 doses.[97] This was the first time that more than two YEL-AVD cases had clustered within a short time and delimited space. Four of the five persons died. The reasons for this unusual event were not defined, but the vaccine lot used in the campaign was not different at the genome level, and a mutational event was ruled out.

Yellow Fever Vaccine-associated Neurologic Disease (YEL-AND)

The 17D strain of yellow fever virus has retained some of its neurovirulence as demonstrated by intracerebral inoculation of mice and nonhuman primates. In the first decade of vaccine use, vaccine-associated neurotropic disease (postvaccinal encephalitis), primarily among infants, was the most common serious AEFI. The pathogenesis of YEL-AND in these cases is characterized by neuroinvasion (in young infants associated with an immature blood–brain barrier), replication of virus in brain parenchyma, and direct viral injury. A hallmark in these cases is the presence of a local immune response in the brain and IgM antibodies in cerebrospinal fluid. From 1945 through 1991, 21 well-documented cases were reported worldwide. Of these, 16 (76%) occurred in infants aged 9 months or younger.[73] Estimates of the YEL-AND rate among children aged 12 months or younger were elevated and ranged from 0.5 to 4 per 1000 doses. As a result, it was recommended that vaccinating infants younger than 9 months old should be avoided because of the encephalitis risk.[82] A decision to administer vaccine to infants younger than 9 months of age should be based on the risk of exposure to natural infection, but the vaccine should not be administered to infants aged 6 months or younger. The only YEL-AND case in the United States from 1945 to 1991 involved a 3-year-old child who died in 1965.[98]

From the mid-1990s through the mid-2000s, unlike earlier reports, most reported cases of YEL-AND have occurred in adults and have included autoimmune-mediated neurologic disease in addition to neurotropic disease. In a retrospective review of VAERS data from 1990 to mid-2005, a total of 15 cases of YEL-AND were identified among US citizens.[99] Of the 15 cases, 6 were diagnosed with encephalitis, 6 with Guillain–Barré syndrome (GBS), and 3 with acute disseminated encephalomyelitis. Like all YEL-AVD cases, all 15 of these people became ill after their first yellow fever vaccination. In addition to these US cases, 13 international cases have been reported to vaccine manufacturers from 1991 through 2005.[73] The incidence of YEL-AND approximates 0.8 per 100 000, with a strong male predominance.[85] Since 2007, two cases of YEL-AND have been identified in young infants, both approximately 1 month of age (M. Sabourin, personal communication, and reference 100). Neither infant was vaccinated, but their mothers had received yellow fever vaccine and subsequently breastfed their children. Although one case lacks definitive proof that the vaccine virus was the source of the child's encephalitis (finding of yellow fever-specific IgM antibodies in the child's CSF but no virus), in the second case yellow fever vaccine virus was identified by RT-PCR in the CSF. Given these cases, studies are currently ongoing to determine if yellow fever vaccine virus is shed in breast milk and a better estimation of risk. It is noteworthy that other flavivirus infections, such as tick-borne encephalitis, are transmitted by milk of animals ingested by humans. Moreover, there is a potential for direct access to the brain via olfactory neurons in suckling infants who may regurgitate milk through the nasal passages. The olfactory route of yellow fever[101] and other flavivirus infections has been reported in experimental models.

In children, YEL-AND is characterized by the onset of fever and seizures, obtundation, meningismus, and paresis 7–21 days after immunization. In adults, symptoms include severe headache, confusion, and aphasia. Illness in adults varies in onset from 4 to 28 days post vaccination, is similar to that in children, and is longer than that seen with YEL-AVD.[99] In both groups, CSF contains up to 500 cells/mL (predominantly lymphocytic) and elevated protein.

The clinical course is generally brief, recovery is complete, and mortality is low. Of the 15 reported US civilians who developed YEL-AND from 1992 to 2005, all were hospitalized but none died. Similarly, of 21 people who developed YEL-AND from 1945 through 1991, only 1 (5%) died; none of the 16 infants aged 9 months or younger died.[73] Although the risk of death is believed to be low with this syndrome, certain groups of vaccine recipients may be at greater risk of death. In 2002, a fatal case of YEL-AND involving a 53-year-old man with previously unrecognized HIV infection was reported in Thailand.[39]

Risk Factors for YEL-AVD and YEL-AND

Increasing age is a risk factor for serious AEFI.[85,102] Analyses of 2000 to 2006 VAERS data have demonstrated that people aged 60 years or older are at increased risk for both YEL-AVD and YEL-AND. During this period, the all-ages incidence for YEL-AVD in the United States was estimated to be 0.4 per 100 000 doses administered. For vaccine recipients aged 60–69 years and those aged 70 years or older, the incidence was 1 and 2.3 cases per 100 000 doses administered, respectively. According to these same data, the all-ages incidence for YEL-AND was estimated to be 0.8 cases per 100 000 civilian doses administered. For vaccine recipients aged 60–69 years and those aged 70 years or older, the reported incidence was 1.6 and 2.3 cases per 100 000 doses administered, respectively.

Thymus and Autoimmune Disease as a Risk Factor

Although not as defined as age, it appears that removal of the thymus or conditions associated with thymomas are risk factors for YEL-AVD. Of the initial 29 people with YEL-AVD identified worldwide through 2003, four (14%) had undergone thymectomy 2–20 years prior to receiving yellow fever vaccination.[91] Because the incidence of thymomas is low, this observation suggests that a history of thymectomy or conditions associated with thymomas (e.g., myasthenia gravis and hypogammaglobulinemia) may be risk factors for YEL-AVD. Thymomas have been associated with decreased antibody levels, abnormal T-lymphocyte maturation, and several autoimmune conditions. An emerging question is whether systemic lupus erythematosus (SLE), and possibly other autoimmune diseases, represent a risk factor for YEL-AVD. Three persons with SLE and two with Addison's disease have developed YEL-AVD after yellow fever vaccination.

Risk Assessment

The specific mechanisms underlying serious AEFI after yellow fever vaccination are unknown. As a result, defining groups whose risk from vaccination is greater than their benefit is difficult. Notably, all reported YEL-AVD and YEL-AND cases occurred in people who were believed to receive their first yellow fever vaccination. No such cases of people receiving a booster dose have been reported. People receiving booster doses have preexisting immunity to yellow fever.

Increasing age, thymoma, and primary vaccination account for some of the increased number of cases; systematic changes in vaccine administration should also be considered. For example, before 1996, immune serum globulin (ISG) was often given as part of travel immunizations to reduce the risk of hepatitis A. Laboratory studies have shown that ISG used in the United States contains significant titers of neutralizing antibody to yellow fever due to the number of plasma donors previously vaccinated while in the military. Whether introduction of hepatitis A vaccine in 1996, which eliminated the need for ISG, may have inadvertently reduced the number of vaccinees receiving passive antibody protection is unknown.

Yellow fever vaccine has been considered one of the safest live-virus vaccines. Reports of serious AEFI after 17D vaccination require reassessment of vaccine use among travelers, and possibly among residents of endemic areas. Yellow fever remains a serious and potentially fatal disease without an efficacious treatment. As a result, the need to vaccinate travelers and residents of endemic areas remains. Categorically refusing an older person vaccine on the basis of age without assessing his or her true risk for disease is not acceptable. Still, the association of increased AEFI risk with age emphasizes the importance of carefully screening travel itineraries of older travelers, travelers with a history of thymoma, or first-time vaccine recipients and only vaccinating those traveling in yellow fever-endemic areas. For travelers whose risk of serious AEFI is great and administration of vaccine is not considered an option, alternative means of prevention, such as personal protection, should be considered.

Vaccine-associated Adverse Events in Persons Infected with HIV

Yellow fever is endemic across sub-Saharan Africa, where there is a high prevalence of HIV infection. This region has been the site of numerous vaccination campaigns to control yellow fever epidemics. During emergency vaccination campaigns, AEFI surveillance was established in Kenya in 1993 (passive surveillance) and in Côte d'Ivoire in 2001 (active surveillance) (D. Gubler, personal communication, 2002). Surveillance was population-based and not restricted to case investigations among HIV-infected people. Four encephalitis cases (only one of whom was an HIV-infected person) were identified in Kenya,[73] and none were identified in Côte d'Ivoire; no cases of viscerotropic disease were identified during either vaccine campaign. A retrospective study performed in Guinea following a yellow fever vaccine campaign conducted in 2002 found that persons testing positive for HIV did not have a higher risk of developing minor AEFI following vaccination than HIV-uninfected persons.[103] Further studies (e.g., cohort studies of HIV-infected people and case-control studies of the general population) and AEFI surveillance during campaigns in countries with high HIV prevalence are needed to define the risk of serious AEFI in HIV-infected people.

A recent report of a Δ32 mutation in CCR5 in a patient with YEL-AVD[94] and the association of this mutation in determining susceptibility of animals to flavivirus (West Nile) encephalitis raises the question of whether treatment of HIV with CCR5 inhibitors would represent a contraindication to yellow fever vaccination.

CONCLUSIONS

Yellow fever remains a major public health concern in sub-Saharan Africa and tropical South America despite the availability of an effective vaccine that can have tremendous impact on disease control. Because yellow fever is an epizootic disease, the potential for human outbreaks will always remain when vaccination programs are not maintained. Unfortunately, efforts to control disease have not been maintained, largely replaced by a policy of emergency vaccination campaigns after an outbreak is identified. Large preventive vaccine campaigns to improve coverage in persons at risk and integration of yellow fever vaccine into EPI are needed for sustained disease control.

Despite the restricted range of endemic virus transmission, it is important for all physicians to be aware of the clinical manifestations and epidemiology of yellow fever because of its potential to cause large urban outbreaks in areas outside of South America and Africa, because of the risk to travelers to these endemic areas, and because of serious adverse events associated with yellow fever vaccination. Because air travel enables anicteric, viremic travelers to return to their homes from any area of the world in less than 24 hours and because of the possibility that the traveler's home has a potential mosquito vector, there is potential for large urban outbreaks of human disease in new areas.

Access the complete reference list online at
http://www.expertconsult.com

CHAPTER 75

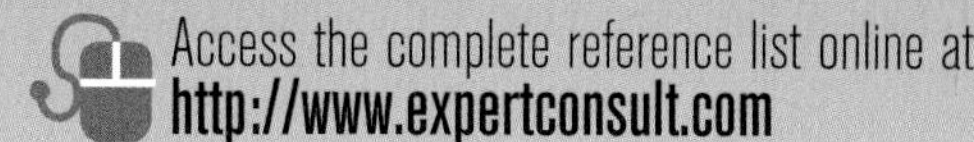
Access the complete reference list online at
http://www.expertconsult.com

Dengue and Dengue Hemorrhagic Fever

Eng Eong Ooi • Duane J. Gubler

INTRODUCTION

The first reports of major epidemics of an illness thought possibly to be dengue occurred on three continents (Asia, Africa, and North America) in 1779 and 1780.[1–4] However, reports of illnesses compatible with dengue fever occurred even earlier. The earliest record found to date was in a Chinese "Encyclopedia of disease symptoms and remedies," first published during the Jin Dynasty (265–420 AD) and formally edited in 610 AD (Sui Dynasty) and again in 992 AD during the Northern Sung Dynasty.[5] The disease was called "water poison" by the Chinese and was thought to be somehow connected with flying insects associated with water. Outbreaks of illness in the French West Indies in 1635 and in Panama in 1699 could also have been dengue.[4,6] Thus, dengue or a very similar illness had a wide geographic distribution before the eighteenth century, when the first known pandemic of dengue-like illness began. It is uncertain that the epidemics in Batavia (Jakarta), Indonesia, and Cairo, Egypt, in 1779 were dengue.[7]

At some point in the past, probably with the clearing of the forests and development of human settlements, dengue viruses moved out of the jungle and into a rural environment, where they were, and still are, transmitted to humans by peridomestic mosquitoes such as *Aedes albopictus*. Migration of people and commerce ultimately moved the viruses into the villages, towns, and cities of tropical Asia, where the viruses were most likely transmitted sporadically by *Ae. albopictus* and other closely related peridomestic *Stegomyia* species.

The slave trade between West Africa and the Americas and the resulting commerce were responsible for the introduction and widespread geographic distribution of an African mosquito, *Ae. aegypti*, in the New World during the seventeenth, eighteenth, and nineteenth centuries. This species became highly adapted to humans and urban environments and was spread throughout the tropics of the world by sailing ships. The species first infested port cities and then moved inland as urbanization expanded. Because *Ae. aegypti* had evolved to become intimately associated with humans, preferring to feed on them and to share their dwellings, this species became a very efficient epidemic vector of dengue and yellow fever viruses. Therefore, when these viruses were introduced into port cities infested with *Ae. aegypti*, epidemics occurred. It was in this setting that major pandemics of dengue fever occurred during the eighteenth, nineteenth, and early twentieth centuries, as the global shipping industry developed and port cities were urbanized in response to increased commerce and ocean traffic. The last major pandemic began during World War II and continues through the present.[8]

The earliest known use of the word "dengue" to describe an illness was in Spain in 1801.[9] However, the most likely origin of the word is from Swahili.[10,11] In both the 1823 and 1870 epidemics of dengue-like illness in Zanzibar and the East African coast, the disease was called *Ki-Dinga pepo*. From this came the name "dinga" or "denga," which was used to describe the illness in both epidemics. Christie[10,11] speculated that the name "denga" was taken via the slave trade to the New World, where it was called "Dandy fever" or "The Dandy" in the St Thomas epidemic of 1827. The illness was first called "dunga" in Cuba during the 1828 epidemic, but later changed to dengue, the name by which it has been known ever since.[12] Most likely, the Spanish recognized the disease in Cuba as the same one that was called dengue in Spain in 1801. If the word dengue did originate in East Africa from "dinga" or "denga", this suggests the disease was occurring before the 1823 epidemics described by Christie. This is not unlikely since epidemics were reported in Africa, the Middle East, and Spain in the late 1700s.

With documentation that yellow fever was transmitted by mosquitoes, many early workers suspected that dengue fever was also mosquito-borne. In the pre-virology era, work was slow and relied on use of human volunteers. Work done by Graham (1903),[13] Bancroft (1906),[14] and Cleland and colleagues (1918)[15] documented dengue transmission by mosquitoes.

Although it had been shown that dengue fever was caused by a filterable agent,[16,17] the first dengue viruses were not isolated until the 1940s, during World War II.[18–21] Dengue fever was a major cause of morbidity among Allied and Japanese soldiers in the Pacific and Asian theaters. Sabin and his group showed that some virus strains from three geographic locations (Hawaii, New Guinea, and India) were antigenically similar.[20,21] This virus was called dengue 1 (DENV-1), and the Hawaii virus was designated as the prototype strain (Haw-DENV-1). Another antigenically distinct virus strain isolated from New Guinea was called dengue 2 (DENV-2), and the New Guinea C strain (NGC-DENV-2) was designated the prototype. The Japanese virus isolated by Kimura and Hotta[18,19] was subsequently shown to be DENV-1 as well. Two more serotypes, dengue 3 (DENV-3) and dengue 4 (DENV-4), were later isolated from patients with a hemorrhagic disease during an epidemic in Manila in 1956.[22] Since these original isolates were made, thousands of dengue viruses have been isolated from all parts of the tropics; all have fitted into the four-serotype classification.

The occurrence of severe and fatal hemorrhagic disease associated with dengue infections is not unique to the twentieth century. Patients with disease clinically compatible with dengue hemorrhagic fever (DHF) have been reported sporadically since 1780, when such cases were observed in the Philadelphia epidemic.[1] Significant numbers of cases of hemorrhagic disease were associated with several subsequent epidemics, including Charters Towers, Australia, in 1897, Beirut in 1910, Taiwan in 1916, Greece in 1928, and Taiwan in 1931.[23–29] However, epidemic occurrences such as these were relatively rare, and the long intervals between them made each a unique event that was not considered important in terms of a long-term, continuous public health problem. Understanding the emergence of dengue and DHF as a global public health problem in the twenty-first century requires a review of the ecological and demographic changes that occurred in the Asian and American tropics during this period. The detailed history of dengue has been reviewed elsewhere.[30]

THE AGENT

There are four dengue virus serotypes: DENV-1, DENV-2, DENV-3, and DENV-4. They belong to the genus *Flavivirus*, family *Flaviviridae* (of which yellow fever virus is the type species), which contains approximately 53 viruses.[31] The flaviviruses are relatively small (40–65 nm) and spherical with a lipid envelope. The flavivirus genome is approximately 11 000 bases and is made up of three structural and seven nonstructural proteins. There are three major subgroups within this family: tick-borne, mosquito-borne, and viruses with no known arthropod vector. The dengue viruses form a complex within the mosquito-borne subgroup. All flaviviruses have common group epitopes on the envelope protein that result in extensive cross-reactions in serologic tests. These make unequivocal serologic diagnosis of flavivirus infections difficult. This is especially true of the four dengue viruses. Infection with one dengue virus serotype provides lifelong immunity to that virus, but there is no cross-protective immunity to the other serotypes. Thus, persons living in an endemic area can be infected with three, and probably four, dengue serotypes during their lifetime.

EPIDEMIOLOGY

Natural History

Humans are infected with dengue viruses by the bite of an infective *Ae. aegypti* mosquito.[32] *Ae. aegypti* is a small, black and white, highly domesticated urban mosquito that prefers to lay its eggs in artificial containers commonly found in and around homes in the tropics, such as flower vases, old automobile tires, buckets that collect rainwater, and trash in general. Containers used for water storage, especially 55-gallon drums and cement cisterns, are especially important in producing large numbers of adult mosquitoes in close proximity to dwellings where people live and work. The adult mosquitoes prefer to rest indoors, are unobtrusive, and prefer to feed on humans during daylight hours. The female mosquitoes are very nervous feeders, disrupting the feeding process at the slightest movement, only to return to the same or a different person to continue feeding moments later. Because of this behavior, *Ae. aegypti* females will often feed on several persons during a single blood meal and, if infective, may transmit dengue virus to multiple persons in a short period of time, even if they only probe without taking blood.[33] It is not uncommon to see several members of the same household become ill with dengue fever within a 24–36-hour time frame, suggesting transmission by a single infective mosquito (D.J. Gubler, unpublished data). It is this behavior that makes *Ae. aegypti* such an efficient epidemic vector. Inhabitants of dwellings in the tropics are rarely aware of the presence of this mosquito, making its control difficult.

After a person is bitten by an infective mosquito, the virus undergoes an incubation period of 3–14 days (average, 4–7 days), after which the person experiences acute onset of fever accompanied by a variety of nonspecific signs and symptoms.[17] During this acute febrile period, which may be as short as 2 days and as long as 10 days, dengue viruses may circulate in the peripheral blood. If other *Ae. aegypti* mosquitoes bite the ill person during this febrile viremic stage, those mosquitoes may become infected and subsequently transmit the virus to other uninfected persons, after an extrinsic incubation period of 8–12 days.[32]

Changing Disease Patterns

The disease pattern associated with dengue, which was characterized by relatively infrequent epidemics until the 1940s, changed with the ecological disruptions in Southeast Asia during and after World War II. Ideal conditions for increased transmission of mosquito-borne diseases were created, and in this setting a global pandemic of dengue began. With increased epidemic transmission, hyperendemicity (the cocirculation of multiple dengue virus serotypes) developed in Southeast Asian cities, and epidemic DHF, a newly described disease, emerged.[30,34–36] The first known epidemic of DHF occurred in Manila, in 1953–54, but within 20 years the disease had spread throughout Southeast Asia. By the mid-1970s, DHF had become a leading cause of hospitalization and death among children in the region.[37] In the 1980s and 1990s, dengue transmission in Asia further intensified; epidemic DHF increased in incidence and expanded geographically west into India, Pakistan, Sri Lanka, and the Maldives, and east into China (***Fig. 75.1***).[30,35] At the same time, the geographic distribution of epidemic DHF was expanding into new regions – the Pacific islands in the 1970s and 1980s and the American tropics in the 1980s and 1990s.[8,30,34,35,38–43]

Epidemiologic changes in the Americas have been the most dramatic. In the 1960s and most of the 1970s, epidemic dengue was rare in the

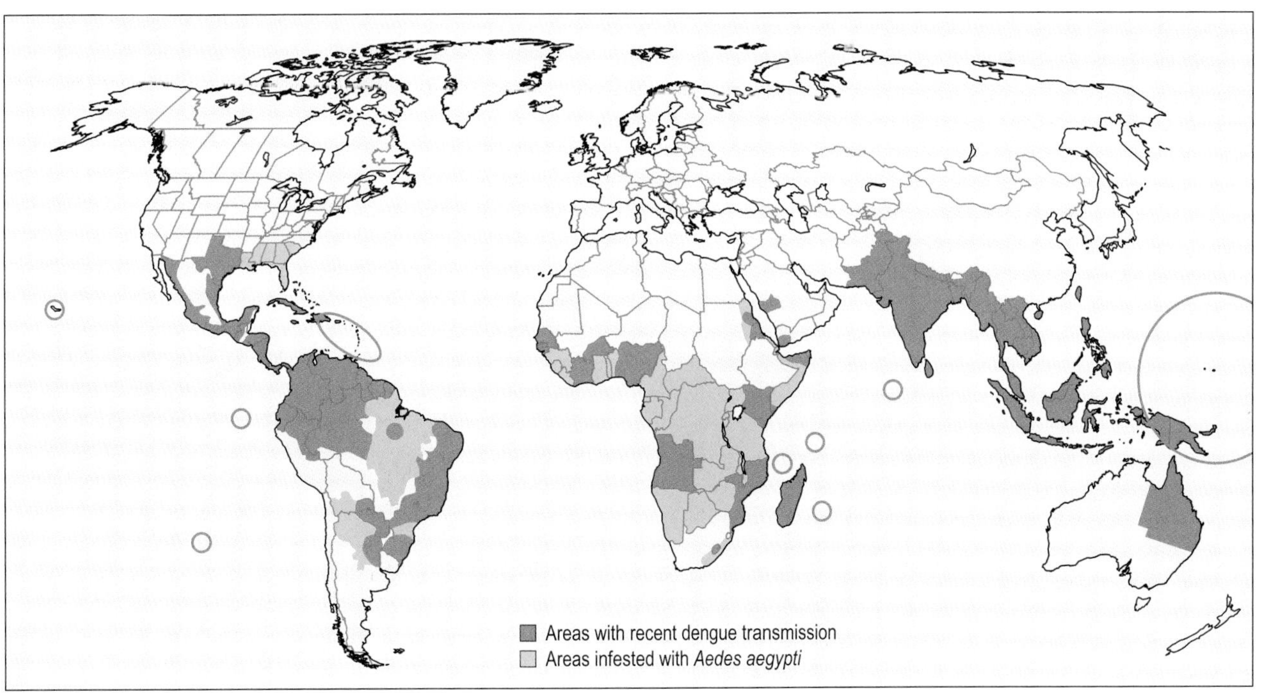

Figure 75.1 The global distribution of dengue/dengue hemorrhagic fever and the principal mosquito vector, *Aedes aegypyti,* 2010. (Adapted from Gubler DJ. Clin Microbiol Rev. 1998;11:480.)

American region because the principal mosquito vector, *Ae. aegypti*, had been eradicated from most of Central and South America.[42,43] The eradication program was discontinued in the early 1970s, and this species then began to reinvade those countries from which it had been eradicated. By the 1990s, *Ae. aegypti* had regained the geographic distribution it had before eradication was initiated (***Fig. 75.2***). Epidemic dengue invariably followed after reinfestation of a country by *Ae. aegypti*. By the 1980s, the American region was experiencing major epidemics of dengue in countries that had been free of the disease for 35–130 years.[34,42,43] With increased epidemic activity came the development of hyperendemicity and the emergence of epidemic DHF, much as had occurred in Southeast Asia 25 years earlier.[42,43] From 1981 to 2009, 28 American countries reported laboratory-confirmed DHF[34,35,43–48] (***Fig. 75.3***).

While Africa has not yet had a major epidemic of DHF, sporadic cases of severe disease have occurred as epidemic dengue fever has increased markedly in the past 30 years. Before the 1980s, little was known of the distribution of dengue viruses in Africa. Since then, however, major epidemics caused by all four serotypes have occurred in both East and West Africa.[35] In the 1990s, transmission was documented in the Horn of Africa and the Arabian peninsula with epidemics in Djibouti in 1991 and Jeddah, Saudi Arabia, in 1994, both of which were the first outbreaks in those countries in over 50 years.[35,49] Since then, there have been multiple outbreaks in East Africa and the Arabian peninsula, including Ethiopia, Yemen, and Saudi Arabia.[50,51]

In 2010, dengue viruses and *Ae. aegypti* mosquitoes have a worldwide distribution in the tropics, with nearly 3 billion people living in

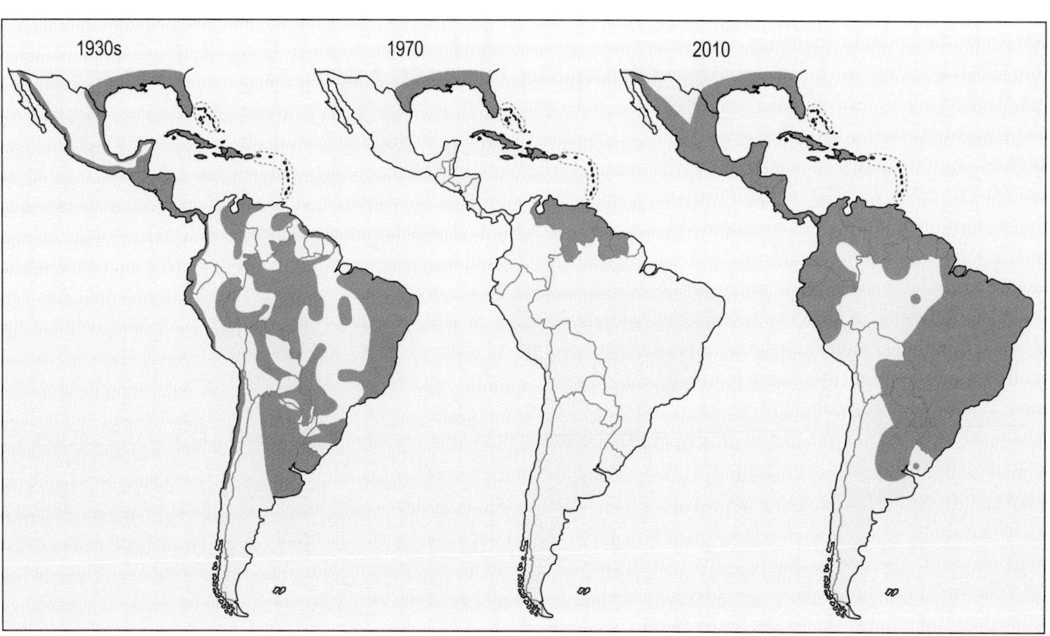

Figure 75.2 *Aedes aegypti:* distribution in the Americas, 1930s, 1970, and 2010. (Adapted from Gubler DJ. Clin Microbiol Rev. 1998;11:480.)

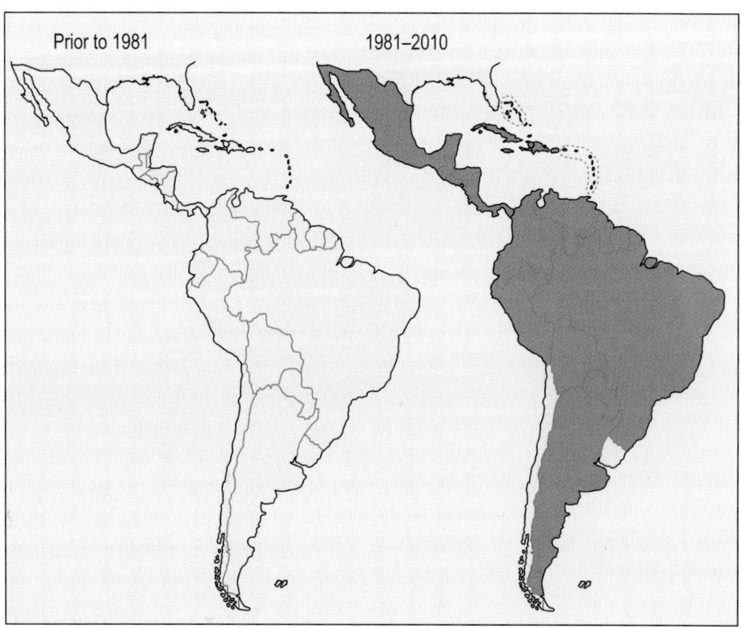

Figure 75.3 Dengue hemorrhagic fever in the Americas prior to 1981 and from 1981 to the present. (Adapted from Gubler DJ. Clin Microbiol Rev. 1998;11:480.)

dengue-endemic areas (see *Fig. 75.1*).[8,34,35,45] Currently, dengue fever causes more illness and death than any other arboviral disease of humans. Each year, an estimated 50–100 million dengue infections and several hundred thousand cases of DHF occur, depending on epidemic activity.[35,45,52,53] DHF is a leading cause of hospitalization and death among children in many Southeast Asian countries.[37]

Factors Responsible for Increased Incidence

The emergence of epidemic dengue and DHF as a global public health problem in the past 30 years is closely associated with demographic and societal changes that have occurred over the past 50 years.[30,34–36] A major factor has been unprecedented population growth and, with that, unplanned and uncontrolled urbanization, especially in tropical developing countries. The crowded human population combined with substandard housing and the deterioration in water, sewer, and waste management systems associated with unplanned urbanization have created ideal conditions for increased transmission of mosquito-borne diseases in tropical urban centers.

A second major factor has been the lack of effective mosquito control in dengue-endemic areas.[34–36] Emphasis during the past 40 years has been on space-spraying with insecticides to kill adult mosquitoes; this has not been effective[54,55] and, in fact, has been detrimental to prevention and control efforts by giving citizens of the community and government officials a false sense of security.[54] Additionally, the geographic distribution and population densities of *Ae. aegypti* have increased, especially in urban areas of the tropics, because of increased numbers of mosquito larval habitats in the domestic environment. The latter include nonbiodegradable plastics and used automobile tires, both of which have increased dramatically during this same period of time.

Another major factor in the global emergence of dengue and DHF is increased air travel by humans, which provides the ideal mechanism for the transport of dengue and other urban pathogens between population centers of the world.[34,35] For instance, in 2006, nearly 4 billion passenger-kilometers were logged by the scheduled airlines globally.[56] Many travelers become infected while visiting tropical areas, but become ill after returning home, resulting in a constant movement of dengue viruses in infected humans to all areas of the world and ensuring repeated introductions of new dengue virus strains and serotypes into areas where the mosquito vectors occur.[57,58] The result is increased epidemic activity, the development of hyperendemicity, and the emergence of epidemic DHF.

A major problem in monitoring the expanding geographic distribution and increased transmission of dengue viruses is the lack of sensitivity and specificity of our surveillance programs.[59–61] Most countries continue to monitor dengue cases by using a passive surveillance approach.[62] Passive surveillance relies on disease notification by health care professionals who have a duty to report all suspected cases to public health authorities. However, passive surveillance systems are uniformly insensitive because of the low index of suspicion for dengue during interepidemic periods.[54,59]

In nonendemic countries, reported dengue cases likewise represent the tip of the iceberg as dengue is often not considered in the differential diagnosis of travelers who return from the tropics with a febrile illness. As a result, many imported dengue cases are never reported. It is important to increase awareness of dengue and DHF among physicians in temperate areas, however, because the disease can be life-threatening. For example, two cases of the severe form of DHF, dengue shock syndrome (DSS), were described in Swedish tourists returning from holiday in Asia.[63] Likewise, in the United States, severe disease does occur among imported cases of dengue.[64] It is important, therefore, that physicians in the United States and Europe consider dengue in the differential diagnosis of viral syndrome in all patients with a travel history to any tropical area.

What is thus needed in both dengue-endemic and nonendemic countries is more effective surveillance for dengue infection. In nonendemic countries, surveillance can be passive, but physicians should be educated about dengue disease. In endemic countries, however, surveillance should be active, systematically sampling the spectrum of illness associated with dengue infection, along with all severe viral illnesses and deaths in the population, with viral isolation, serotyping, and genomic sequencing.[62] These data could be useful for early warning and hence initiating early emergency responses, which are often carried out too little, too late.[61,62]

Finally, the experience in Singapore underscores the need to carry out disease surveillance and prevention at the regional level.[65] Singapore implemented an *Ae. aegypti* control program in 1970 that effectively controlled dengue transmission through the 1970s and most of the 1980s.[65] This resulted in decreasing herd immunity,[66] adaptation of the vectors to the control measures,[67] and a shift from childhood to adulthood infection, where the latter is more likely to result in symptomatic instead of asymptomatic infection.[68] These factors, combined with the increased movement of viruses in viremic hosts, have all contributed to increasing the incidence of disease despite the continued vector control measures in Singapore,[65] underscoring the need for a coordinated regional effort in dengue control.

THE DISEASE

Dengue virus infection in humans causes a spectrum of illness, ranging from inapparent or mild febrile illness to severe and fatal hemorrhagic disease. Infection with all four serotypes causes a similar clinical presentation that may vary in frequency and severity. In dengue-endemic areas, dengue infections are often clinically nonspecific, especially in children, with symptoms of a viral syndrome that has a variety of local names. Important risk factors influencing the proportion of patients who have severe disease during epidemic transmission include the strain and serotype of the infecting virus, the immune status of the individual, the age of the patient, and the genetic background of the human host.[32,37–41,69–71]

Dengue With or Without Warning Signs

A World Health Organization-sponsored study involving clinicians in Asian and American dengue-endemic countries has recently proposed a revised classification of dengue illness that more accurately reflects the global clinical presentation observed in both children and adults.[72,73] The proposed classification includes two major categories, dengue with or without warning signs and severe dengue; the former includes dengue fever, and the latter includes DHF/DSS and other severe forms of infections previously referred to as atypical dengue. The new classification is shown in ***Figure 75.4***.

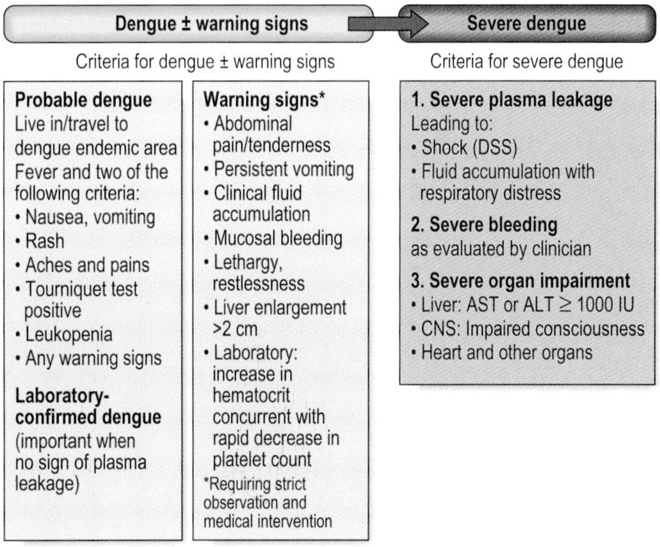

Dengue ± warning signs →		Severe dengue
Criteria for dengue ± warning signs		Criteria for severe dengue
Probable dengue Live in/travel to dengue endemic area Fever and two of the following criteria: • Nausea, vomiting • Rash • Aches and pains • Tourniquet test positive • Leukopenia • Any warning signs **Laboratory-confirmed dengue** (important when no sign of plasma leakage)	**Warning signs*** • Abdominal pain/tenderness • Persistent vomiting • Clinical fluid accumulation • Mucosal bleeding • Lethargy, restlessness • Liver enlargement >2 cm • Laboratory: increase in hematocrit concurrent with rapid decrease in platelet count *Requiring strict observation and medical intervention	**1. Severe plasma leakage** Leading to: • Shock (DSS) • Fluid accumulation with respiratory distress **2. Severe bleeding** as evaluated by clinician **3. Severe organ impairment** • Liver: AST or ALT ≥ 1000 IU • CNS: Impaired consciousness • Heart and other organs

Figure 75.4 The new dengue case classification scheme. DSS, dengue shock syndrome; AST, aspartate aminotransferase; ALT, alanine aminotransferase; CNS, central nervous system.

Dengue Fever

Classic dengue fever is primarily a disease of older children and adults. It is characterized by sudden onset of fever and a variety of nonspecific signs and symptoms, including frontal headache, retro-orbital pain, body aches, nausea vomiting, joint pains, weakness, and rash.[17,21,72,73] Patients may be anorectic, have altered taste sensation and mild sore throat. Constipation is occasionally reported; diarrhea and respiratory symptoms are infrequently reported and may be due to concurrent infections.

The initial temperature may rise to 102–105°F (38.9–40.6°C) and last for 2–7 days. The fever may drop after a few days, only to rebound 12–24 hours later (saddleback).[17] Relative bradycardia may be noted despite the fever. The conjunctivae may be injected and the pharynx inflamed. Lymphadenopathy is common. Rash is variable, occurring in up to 50% of patients as either early or late eruptions. Facial flushing or erythematous mottling may occur coincident with or slightly before onset of fever and disappear 1–2 days after onset of symptoms. A second rash, varying in form from scarlatiniform to maculopapular, may appear between days 2 and 6 of illness.[74] The rash usually begins on the trunk and spreads to the face and extremities. In some cases, an intense erythematous pattern with islands of normal skin may be observed. The average duration of the second rash is 2–3 days. Toward the end of the febrile phase of illness or after the temperature reverts to normal, petechiae may appear; these may be scattered or confluent. Intense pruritus may occur followed by desquamation on the palms of the hands and soles of the feet.

Hemorrhagic manifestations in dengue fever patients are not uncommon and may range from mild to severe. Skin hemorrhages are the most common, including petechiae and purpura, as well as gum bleeding, epistaxis, menorrhagia, and gastrointestinal hemorrhage. Hematuria occurs infrequently, and jaundice is rare.

Clinical laboratory findings associated with dengue fever include neutropenia followed by lymphocytosis, often marked by atypical lymphocytes. Liver enzymes in the serum may be elevated; this is usually a mild elevation but, in some patients, alanine transaminase and aspartate transaminase levels may reach 500–1000 units/dL. In one epidemic of DEN-4, 54% of confirmed patients with data had elevated liver enzymes.[75] Thrombocytopenia is also common in dengue fever; in the preceding epidemic, 34% of confirmed dengue fever patients who were tested had platelet counts of less than 100 000/μL.[75]

Dengue fever is generally self-limited and rarely fatal. The acute phase of illness lasts for 3–7 days, but the convalescent phase may be prolonged for weeks and may be associated with weakness and depression. No permanent sequelae are associated with dengue infection.

Table 75.1 Signs and Symptoms Associated with Laboratory-Confirmed Dengue Hemorrhagic Fever Cases, Jakarta, Indonesia, 1975–77

Sign or Symptom	No.	Percent
Hepatomegaly	297/601[a]	49
Abdominal pain	281/619	45
Vomiting	279/619	45
Cough	142/619	23
Constipation	101/619	16
Nausea	90/618[a]	15
Headache	82/619	13
Sore throat	53/619	9
Rhinitis	50/619	8
Diarrhea	50/619	8
Chills	30/619	5
Myalgia	24/619	4
Joint pain	15/619	2
Stiff neck	15/619	2
Backache	12/619	2
Conjunctivitis	6/619	1
Pruritus	4/619	1
Paresthesias	1/619	1

[a]Data not available on all patients.

Severe Dengue: Dengue Hemorrhagic Fever and Dengue Shock Syndrome

DHF is a vascular leak syndrome and is primarily a disease of children under the age of 15 years, although it can and does occur in adults.[37] It is characterized by sudden onset of fever, usually of 2–7 days' duration, and a variety of nonspecific signs and symptoms. During the acute phase of illness, it is difficult to distinguish DHF from dengue fever and other illnesses found in tropical areas (***Table 75.1***). The differential diagnosis during the acute phase of illness should include measles, rubella, influenza, typhoid, leptospirosis, rickettsioses, malaria, viral hemorrhagic fevers, and any other disease that may present in the acute phase as a nonspecific viral syndrome. Children frequently have concurrent infections with other viruses and bacteria causing upper respiratory symptoms. There is no pathognomonic sign or symptom for DHF (see ***Table 75.1***).

The critical stage in DHF occurs most frequently from about 24 hours before to 24 hours after the temperature falls to normal or below.[37] During this time, hemorrhagic manifestations and, more importantly, signs of circulatory failure usually occur. Blood tests will usually show that the patient has thrombocytopenia (platelet count of <100 000/μL) and evidence of a vascular leak syndrome.

Common hemorrhagic manifestations include skin petechiae, purpura, and ecchymoses. Epistaxis, bleeding gums, gastrointestinal hemorrhage, and hematuria occur less frequently. The tourniquet test, which may be diagnostically helpful, is performed by inflating the blood pressure cuff to the midpoint between the systolic and diastolic pressures for 5 minutes and then releasing the pressure.[37] In persons with increased capillary fragility, a "shower" of petechiae will appear below the cuff. The test is positive if 20 or more petechiae per square inch (2.5 cm) are observed. Some uninfected persons may have a positive tourniquet test; however, if so, it does not mean that a person has DHF when the test is positive. Rather, positive results indicate that the patient has increased capillary fragility, and the physician should do further clinical laboratory tests.

Scattered petechiae are the most common hemorrhagic manifestation observed; they appear most often on the extremities, but also on the trunk, other parts of the body, and on the face in severe cases of DSS. Purpuric lesions may appear on various parts of the body but are most common at sites of venipuncture. In some patients, large ecchymotic lesions develop on the trunk and extremities, and other patients bleed actively at the site of venipuncture, some profusely. More severely ill patients have gastrointestinal hemorrhage, which is manifested by hematemesis or melena or both. Classic hematemesis and melena usually occur after prolonged shock, but patients may develop massive, frank upper gastrointestinal hemorrhage as well, often before the onset of shock. Without early diagnosis and proper management, some patients experience shock from blood loss, which may be mild or severe.[76,77] More commonly, shock is caused by plasma leakage; it may be mild and transient or progress to profound shock with undetectable pulse and blood pressure.[37] Children with profound shock are often somnolent, exhibit petechiae on the face, and have perioral cyanosis.

It is convenient for both clinicians and epidemiologists to classify DHF into four grades of illness based on severity.[37] Grade I DHF is mild; the only hemorrhagic manifestations are scattered petechiae or a positive tourniquet test. Grade II DHF is more severe, with one or more of the overt hemorrhagic manifestations mentioned above. Grades III and IV represent more severe forms of disease (DSS). Grade III illness is characterized by mild shock with signs of circulatory failure; the patient may be lethargic or restless and have cold extremities, clammy skin, a rapid but weak pulse, narrowing of pulse pressure to 20 mmHg or less, or hypotension. Grade IV, the most severe form of DHF or DSS, is characterized by profound shock with undetectable pulse and blood pressure.

In severe cases of DHF and DSS, fever and nonspecific constitutional signs and symptoms of a few days' duration are followed by the sudden deterioration of the patient's condition. During or shortly before or after the fall in temperature, the patient's skin may become cool, blotchy, and congested; circumoral cyanosis is frequently observed, and the pulse becomes rapid and weak. Although some patients appear lethargic at first, they become restless and then rapidly pass into a critical stage of shock. They frequently experience acute abdominal pain shortly before the onset of shock.[37]

In mild cases of DHF, all signs and symptoms abate shortly after the fever subsides. Lysis of fever, however, may be accompanied by profuse sweating and mild changes in pulse rate and blood pressure, together with coolness of extremities and skin congestion. These changes reflect mild and transient circulatory disturbances as a result of plasma leakage. Patients usually recover spontaneously or after fluid and electrolyte therapy.[37] Patients in shock are in danger of dying without appropriate management. The duration of shock is usually short; the patient may die within 8–24 hours or recover rapidly following fluid replacement. Convalescence for patients with DHF, with or without shock, is usually short and uneventful. Even in patients with undetectable pulse and blood pressure, once the shock is overcome surviving patients usually recover within 2–3 days.

As with dengue fever, leukopenia is common; thrombocytopenia and hemoconcentration are constant findings in DHF and DSS. A platelet count of less than 100 000/μL is usually found between the third and eighth days of illness. Hemoconcentration, indicating plasma leakage, is almost always present in classic DHF, but is more severe in patients with shock. Hepatomegaly is a common, but not a constant, finding.[76] In some countries, most patients with confirmed DHF or DSS have been found to have an enlarged liver. In other countries, however, hepatomegaly varies from one epidemic to another, suggesting that the strain or serotype of virus may influence liver involvement.[76] Elevated liver enzymes are common.

The primary pathophysiologic abnormality in DHF and DSS is an acute increase in vascular permeability that leads to leakage of plasma into the extravascular compartment, resulting in hemoconcentration and decreased blood pressure.[37] Plasma volume studies have shown a reduction of more than 20% in severe cases. Objective evidence of plasma leakage includes serous effusions found postmortem, pleural effusion on radiograph or ultrasound, hemoconcentration, and hypoproteinemia. There are no apparent destructive vascular lesions, suggesting that the transient functional vascular changes are due to a short-acting chemical mediator.[37]

Hemostatic changes in DHF and DSS involve three factors: (1) vascular changes; (2) thrombocytopenia; and (3) coagulation disorders.[37] Almost all DHF patients have increased vascular fragility and thrombocytopenia, and many have abnormal coagulograms, suggesting disseminated intravascular coagulation, which is also evidenced by concomitant thrombocytopenia, prolonged partial thromboplastin time, decreased fibrinogen level, and increased fibrin(ogen) degradation products. Gastrointestinal hemorrhage is observed at autopsy in the majority of patients who die.

Some cases of severe disease do not fit the preceding classification and may have a different pathogenesis.[32,71,76–80] These patients generally present with similar signs and symptoms during the acute phase of illness, but develop frank upper gastrointestinal bleeding without evidence of plasma leakage (hemoconcentration) or circulatory failure, as occurs in patients with classic DHF or DSS. Generally, the upper gastrointestinal bleeding occurs 3–5 days after onset of illness and is often the reason the patient is brought to the hospital. All such patients have significant thrombocytopenia. In many cases, bleeding may be severe enough to cause shock from blood loss rather than plasma leakage. In one study in Indonesia, 30% of patients with virologically confirmed fatal dengue infections had this type of severe upper gastrointestinal hemorrhage.[77] Blood transfusions are always indicated for these patients, whose disease is generally more difficult to manage than classic DSS.[77]

Another form of severe dengue disease includes patients who present with neurologic disorders such as convulsions, spastic paresis, and change in consciousness, with or without hemorrhagic manifestations.[71,72,77–82] These patients, who may be admitted to the neurologic ward with a diagnosis of viral encephalitis, may subsequently develop hemorrhagic manifestations and shock. Cerebrospinal fluid findings are normal, and most evidence suggests that the virus does not cross the blood–brain barrier, although some studies suggest that this may occur in some patients.[81,82] Further studies are necessary to identify the underlying pathogenesis of these manifestations.

PATHOGENESIS AND IMMUNITY

The pathogenesis of DHF and DSS is still controversial. Two theories, which are not mutually exclusive, are frequently cited to explain the pathogenic changes that occur in severe dengue disease. The theory most commonly accepted is known as the secondary infection, or immune enhancement, hypothesis.[37,38,69] This hypothesis implies that patients experiencing a second infection with a heterologous dengue virus serotype have a significantly higher risk of developing the vascular leak syndrome (DHF/DSS). Preexisting heterologous dengue antibody recognizes the infecting virus and forms an antigen–antibody complex which is then phagocytosed by macrophages. Because the antibody is heterologous, however, the virus is not neutralized and is free to replicate once inside the macrophage. Thus, it is hypothesized that prior infection enhances the infection of cells of the mononuclear cell lineage by a virus that is not inactivated by neutralizing antibody. Infection of these cells initiates an immunologic cascade of events that produces cytokines and other vasoactive mediators, ultimately leading to increased vascular permeability, leakage, hypovolemia, shock/and death, if not corrected.[83]

The other hypothesis assumes that dengue viruses, like all animal viruses, vary and change genetically as they move through human and/or mosquito populations, and that there are some virus strains that have greater virulence and epidemic potential.[70,71,84] Data suggest that genetic changes in the virus genome occur randomly as the viruses circulate in nature. Some of these genetic changes are advantageous and are propagated through natural selection, resulting in viruses that have increased virus replication and higher viral load, greater epidemic potential, and increased virulence.[85–87]

There is epidemiologic and laboratory evidence to support both of these hypotheses, a discussion of which is beyond the scope of this chapter; most likely, both are valid. While immune enhancement may occur and may be an important factor in the pathophysiologic changes that occur in DHF and DSS, recent studies have questioned the importance of immune enhancement.[88,89] It appears that only certain strains of virus may be involved in producing severe disease by immune enhancement. Moreover, other severe forms of dengue disease appear to have a different pathogenesis.

DIAGNOSIS

A definitive diagnosis of dengue infection can only be made in the laboratory and depends on isolating the virus, detecting dengue virus-specific RNA sequences by nucleotide amplification test, or detecting specific antibodies in the patient's serum.[90–92] An acute-phase blood sample should always be collected as soon as possible after onset of illness, and a convalescent-phase sample should be taken 2–3 weeks later. Because it is frequently difficult to obtain convalescent-phase samples, however, a second blood sample should always be taken from hospitalized patients on the day of discharge from hospital.

Virus can often be isolated from acute-phase blood samples taken in the first 5 days of illness.[90–92] Viral RNA can often be detected by polymerase chain reaction in serum or tissues,[89,90,93] or antigen by immunohistochemistry in tissues.[94] Two serologic tests are used to detect antibodies.

The IgM capture enzyme-linked immunosorbent assay (ELISA) detects IgM antibody, which usually appears by day 5 after onset and persists for 2–3 months.[90–92,95–97] The hemagglutination inhibition test and an IgG ELISA detect IgG antibody, which appears simultaneously or shortly after IgM but persists for life. For this reason, diagnosis using IgG requires paired acute- and convalescent-phase blood samples to demonstrate a fourfold or greater rise in specific antibody, which should be confirmed by neutralization test.[90,91]

TREATMENT AND PROGNOSIS

There is no specific chemotherapy for DHF/DSS. However, early and effective fluid replacement of lost plasma with electrolyte solutions, plasma, or plasma expanders usually results in a favorable outcome.[37] With adequate fluid administration, DSS is reversible. Rapid replacement of fluid will usually prevent disseminated intravascular coagulation. Prognosis depends on early recognition of shock, based on careful monitoring.

In dengue-endemic areas, it is often not possible or necessary to hospitalize all patients with suspected DHF or DSS, since shock develops in only about one-third of the patients.[37] A decrease in the platelet count, which usually precedes the rise in hematocrit, is of great diagnostic and prognostic value. In order to be able to recognize the early signs of shock and thus take preventive action, parents or family members should be advised to bring the patient back for repeat platelet and hematocrit determinations every 24 hours. They should also be instructed to keep a careful watch for any signs of clinical deterioration or warning signs of shock, such as restlessness, lethargy, acute abdominal pain, cold extremities, skin congestion, or oliguria, on or after the third day of illness. Patients with mild DHF can usually be rehydrated orally. An antipyretic drug may be all that is needed. Salicylates and nonsteroidal anti-inflammatory drugs should be avoided.

Patients should be hospitalized and treated immediately if they have any signs or symptoms of shock, such as restlessness; lethargy; cold extremities; circumoral cyanosis; rapid, weak pulse; narrowing of pulse pressure to 20 mmHg or less; hypotension; a sudden rise in hematocrit; or continuously elevated hematocrit despite the administration of intravenous fluids.[37] Frequent recording of vital signs, and hematocrit determinations, and monitoring of urine output are important in evaluating the results of treatment. Blood transfusions are contraindicated in patients with severe plasma leakage in the absence of hemorrhage and, if given, may cause pulmonary edema; however, they may be indicated for patients with significant clinical bleeding. It may be difficult to recognize internal bleeding in the presence of hemoconcentration. A drop in hematocrit of 10% with no clinical improvement, despite adequate fluid administration, suggests significant internal hemorrhage.[37] Transfusion of fresh whole blood is preferable; fresh frozen plasma or concentrated platelets may be indicated in some cases when consumptive coagulopathy causes massive bleeding.

Some controversy surrounds the use of steroids, but the consensus is that they have no beneficial effect in the management of severe DHF or DSS. Although some physicians still use steroids in the treatment of shock cases, two double-blind studies, in Thailand and Indonesia, have shown no increase in survival rates of patients with grade IV DSS who were administered steroids.[37]

PREVENTION AND CONTROL

Prevention and control of dengue fever/DHF currently depend on controlling the mosquito vector, *Ae. aegypti*, in and around the home where most transmission occurs in most endemic countries. Space sprays with insecticides to kill adult mosquitoes are usually ineffective, unless they are sprayed indoors where the mosquitoes are resting. The most effective way to control the mosquitoes that transmit dengue is larval control, including eliminating, cleaning, or chemically treating water-holding containers that serve as the larval habitats for *Ae. aegypti* in the domestic environment.[54,55,59,98]

At present, there is no vaccine for dengue viruses, although several candidates are at various stages of development.[99–103] To be effective, a dengue vaccine must protect against all four virus serotypes, i.e., be a tetravalent formulation. For use in dengue-endemic countries, a dengue vaccine must be safe for use in children 9–12 months of age, must be economical, and should provide long-lasting protective immunity (ideally more than 10 years). Several approaches are being used to develop dengue vaccines. A live attenuated vaccine (LAV) is thought to provide the most complete and lasting immunity, although the development of a tetravalent LAV has proven difficult.[99–106] Several groups have constructed chimeric viruses using various infectious clones as backbones.[99,106–109] There is one subunit vaccine under development.[103] All of these chimeric candidate vaccines look very promising in primate studies. The 17-D yellow fever chimeras are currently undergoing phase II trials in humans, and will soon enter phase III trials. The others are in phase I trials.

There is no completely effective method of preventing dengue infection in travelers to tropical areas. The risk of infection can be significantly reduced, however, by understanding the basic behavior and habits of the mosquito vector and by taking a few simple precautions, such as using aerosol bomb insecticides to kill adult mosquitoes indoors, using a repellent containing diethyltoluamide (DEET) on exposed skin, and wearing protective clothing treated with a similar repellent. The risk of exposure may be lower in modern, air-conditioned hotels with well-kept grounds, and in rural areas.

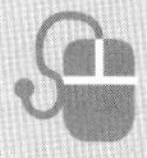

Access the complete reference list online at
http://www.expertconsult.com

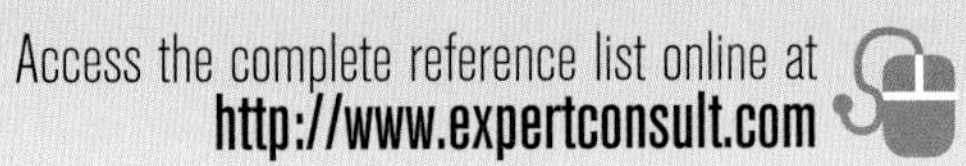
Access the complete reference list online at
http://www.expertconsult.com

CHAPTER 76

Japanese Encephalitis, West Nile, and Other Flavivirus Infections

Robert B. Tesh • Tom Solomon

INTRODUCTION

Four mosquito-transmitted flavivirus diseases are of significant public health importance in tropical and subtropical regions: dengue, yellow fever, Japanese encephalitis, and West Nile virus infection. Other chapters in this book address dengue and yellow fever; this chapter focuses on diseases caused by Japanese encephalitis virus (JEV) and West Nile virus (WNV); Murray Valley encephalitis, Kyasanur Forest disease, Zika and Ilheus virus infections are also described briefly.

EPIDEMIOLOGY

Japanese Encephalitis Virus

JEV is enzootic in rural agricultural areas throughout much of eastern and southern Asia and the Pacific islands.[1–4] The principal enzootic transmission cycle involves *Culex* mosquitoes and vertebrates, with *Culex tritaeniorhynchus* being the most important vector of human infections. These mosquitoes breed mainly in rural areas, especially in flooded rice paddies, and are predominantly exophilic and zoophilic, preferring to feed on swine and birds and to a lesser extent on humans. Domestic swine and ardeid birds, such as herons and other waterfowl, are the most important virus-amplifying hosts. However, the most important source of human infections is linked to the mosquito–swine transmission cycle. JEV infection in avians is usually inapparent, but abortions occur in infected pregnant sows. Humans and equines are believed to be dead-end hosts.

JEV is a leading cause of viral encephalitis in tropical Asia, where it causes an estimated 35 000 to 50 000 clinical cases and 15 000 deaths annually.[3–5] Human infection in temperate zones of Asia and in the northern region of the tropical zone (northern Thailand, northern Vietnam, China, Korea, Japan, Taiwan, Nepal, and northern India) is seasonal, and the incidence varies depending on vaccination practices and climatic conditions. The most common pattern of infection in northern (temperate) regions of Asia is summer epidemics; whereas, in southern (tropical) regions (southern Thailand, southern Vietnam, Malaysia, Singapore, Indonesia, the Philippines, Sri Lanka, and southern India), an endemic pattern occurs with sporadic cases throughout the year and peak case rates appearing after the beginning of the rainy season.[6] In Japan, Taiwan, Korea, and China, the number of Japanese encephalitis (JE) cases has been markedly reduced by the implementation of childhood immunization.[3] However, over the past four decades, the incidence of JE has increased dramatically in central and northern India, Nepal, and the northern region of Southeast Asia.[7] JEV has also expanded its range into other areas of Southeast Asia and eastward to the Australasian zoogeographic region.[8]

The risk of JE is highest among individuals who travel or live in rural areas where rice is grown and swine are raised in close proximity to human dwellings.[3,4,6] In endemic areas, the annual infection rate is about 10% among the susceptible populations, with about 85% of the cases occurring among children under 15 years of age.[4] Most JEV infections are silent; the ratio of symptomatic to asymptomatic infections varies from about one in 25 to one in 1000.[3,4] The lower incidence among adults in Asia has been attributed to high rates of immunity. The case-fatality rate among JE patients admitted to hospital is about 20–30%, and about half of the survivors experience severe neuropsychiatric sequelae.[3,5,9] In contrast to the situation in endemic regions, all age groups are affected during epidemics in nonimmune populations.[3,4] Similarly, when nonimmune individuals (travelers or military personnel) visit endemic areas, they too are at risk.[3,10]

West Nile Virus

WNV is enzootic in Africa, southern and eastern Europe, the Middle East, western Asia, Australia, North America, the Caribbean, and parts of Central and South America. It is now the most widely distributed arbovirus in the world.[11–13] The basic transmission cycle of the virus is similar throughout its range, involving mainly *Culex* mosquitoes as the primary vectors and a variety of passerine birds as the major amplifying hosts. Infection of most avians is benign, although epizootics with high mortality have been documented among certain species of birds (crows, jays, geese). While WNV infection of other vertebrates, including humans and equines, is common, they are generally considered to be dead-end hosts because the level of viremia is thought to be insufficient to infect vector mosquitoes. Experimental and field studies suggest that vertical transmission of WNV in mosquitoes and overwintering of infected adult mosquitoes may be important in the maintenance and transmission cycle of WNV in some temperate and subtropical regions.[14] The primary source of human infections is generally the bite of infected mosquitoes, although WNV can also be transmitted by other routes, including transplanted organs, transfusion of blood products, transplacental spread, possibly breast milk, and accidental laboratory exposure.[13] Since 2003, screening of blood donations in North America has greatly reduced the risk of infection via blood products.

Until the mid-1990s, WNV was usually associated with sporadic cases and infrequent outbreaks of an acute febrile illness with headache, arthralgia, weakness and rash, designated "West Nile fever," and occasionally with more severe central nervous system (CNS) disease.[12,13] Recently, however, the epidemiology has changed to a pattern of more frequent and widespread outbreaks, with an increase in the incidence of neuroinvasive disease, particularly among older adults and immunosuppressed individuals. The most surprising spread of WNV was to the New York City metropolitan area during 1999.[13] Although the mechanism of introduction is unknown, nucleotide sequence data revealed that the New York strain is closely related to a viral strain isolated from a goose in Israel the year before.[15] Since 1999, WNV has spread throughout North America and into parts of the Caribbean, Central and South America. The pattern of spread has been rapid and extensive; 62 human cases were documented in the United States during 1999 and 9862 cases in 2003, with annual cases since then.[11,13]

It is assumed that the virus will continue to spread in Central and South America. However, the risk of severe disease among persons living in these tropical regions may be less than among residents of temperate North America (United States and Canada), because of the higher prevalence of heterologous flavivirus immunity in tropical residents. Experimental studies in animals suggest that prior infection with other flaviviruses (JEV, St Louis encephalitis, dengue, and the yellow fever 17D vaccine viruses) provides protection against severe disease and death upon challenge with WNV.[16–18] A similar phenomenon has been observed with JEV in Southeast Asia; one of the most important factors for developing severe JE appears to be the absence of other flavivirus antibody prior to JEV infection.[4]

Experience in the United States, where relatively few lifetime residents have been infected with other flaviviruses, indicates that only about 20% of persons infected with WNV will develop clinical illness and that overall less than 1% of infections will result in severe neuroinvasive disease (encephalitis, meningitis, or flaccid paralysis).[19,20] Among people who develop neuroinvasive WNV disease, the mortality ranges from about 10% to 12%; but many of the survivors have significant long-term morbidity.[21–23] While the age-specific WNV infection rates are similar, the risk of more severe disease and death increases significantly among persons >55 years of age and in people who are immunosuppressed. Hypertension and diabetes are also risk factors for neuroinvasive disease.[24]

THE DISEASE

Japanese Encephalitis

JEV infection of humans can result in an asymptomatic infection with antibody seroconversion, mild febrile illness, aseptic meningitis, or an acute encephalomyelitis.[4] After an incubation period of 1–2 weeks, patients who develop encephalitis typically present with a history of 1–3 days of fever, headache, stupor, and especially in children, generalized tonic clonic seizures. Physical findings at this time may be limited to a depressed state of consciousness. Some patients have a rapid recovery, but most will develop a variety of neurologic manifestations. The case-fatality rate can be as high as 30%. In some instances, abnormal behavior is the only presenting symptom, without fever, weakness, diarrhea, vomiting, confusion, and rigors. Upper motor neuron weakness is noted in 30–50% of patients,[25] with poliomyelitis-like flaccid paralysis occurring in up to 15% of patients.[26] This poliomyelitis-like syndrome may present with an altered level of consciousness progressing to encephalitis and respiratory paralysis in 20–60%, with poor prognosis for recovery.[5,25] A parkinsonian syndrome occurs in up to 25% of patients, typified by cogwheel rigidity, mask-like facies, and bradykinesia. Other movement disorders consist of myoclonic jerks and haunting orofacial dyskinesias (grimacing, chewing, and lip smacking) noted in up to a third of patients during recovery.[27]

Seizures occur in 85% of children and 10% of adults.[25] Uncontrolled seizures and elevated intracranial pressure demonstrated by opening pressure of greater than 25 cmCSF during lumbar puncture are predictive of poor outcome.[28] The mortality rate in patients with such findings was 62% compared with 14% overall in one study including adults and children.[28] The long-term outcome of JE is grim, with survivors sharing a variety of deficits including 20% with severe cognitive and language impairment, 20% with subsequent seizures, 30% with flexion or extension contractures, and learning/behavioral disorders.[5] Bilateral lesions in the thalamus, basal ganglia, and brainstem on brain MRI and CT scan correlate with the clinical manifestations.[29,30] In the right clinical context, their presence is highly specific for JE, though their absence does not exclude it.

Pathology

JEV is found in lungs, liver, kidneys, and myocardium as well as various regions of gray matter such as the thalamus, basal ganglia, and midbrain. A distinguishing feature of JE is predominant gray matter infection that spares white matter, unlike WNV.[5,29,31] Prolonged viremia may occasionally occur for weeks to months,[32] and has been postulated to lead to rare chronic progressive CNS infection.

West Nile Disease

The range of human clinical disease associated with WNV infection is also broad, ranging from asymptomatic infection to a relatively mild febrile illness to severe and sometimes fatal neurologic disease.[33–35] The usual incubation period for WNV clinical illness is 2–6 days from exposure, although in some cases it can be as long as 14–21 days, especially in individuals with compromised immune systems. The most common clinical manifestation of WNV infection is an acute self-limited febrile illness, "West Nile fever," which is characterized by headache, myalgia, eye pain, malaise, nausea and/or vomiting, and sometimes a generalized maculopapular rash. In this regard, West Nile fever is similar to and can easily be confused with a number of other acute viral illnesses such as influenza and dengue fever. Although West Nile fever was generally considered to be a relatively benign illness, recent studies indicate that some convalescent patients have prolonged symptoms of headaches, muscle weakness, fatigue, dizziness, and depression.[21–23]

Up to 1% of persons with WNV infection will develop neuroinvasive disease; the risk increases among persons >55 years of age. These patients may or may not have manifested symptoms of West Nile fever. Signs of WNV neuroinvasive disease appear 8–14 days after the initial infection and usually take the clinical form of meningitis, encephalitis, and less commonly flaccid paralysis or a Guillain–Barré-like syndrome.[34,35] These patients may suffer headache, altered mental status, stiff neck, convulsions, ataxia, muscle weakness, spasms, tremors, or paralysis. Occasionally ocular symptoms, myocarditis, and fulminant hepatitis have been reported. About 10–12% of WNV neuroinvasive disease patients die either as a result of acute neurologic involvement or from complications resulting from prolonged intubation and ventilatory support.

Pathology

Fatal cases reveal variable amounts of neuronal necrosis in the gray matter, microglial nodules, polymorphonuclear leukocytes, perivascular and leptomeningeal chronic inflammation, and neuronophagia.[31] Viral antigens are present in neurons, neuronal processes, and areas of necrosis in the brain and spinal cord. In immunosuppressed patients who die of WNV neuroinvasive disease, the pathology is more diffuse, and viral antigen can also be detected in organs such as the lung, liver, spleen, and kidney.[36,37]

PATHOGENESIS AND IMMUNITY

The pathogenesis of JEV and WNV infections is similar, with interplay between direct viral damage and the pathologic effects of the host immune response.[38] Infection is believed to begin with the replication of virus in the skin and regional lymph nodes to produce a primary viremia, which leads to infection of the reticuloendothelial system.[33,39] A secondary viremia follows, which may result in systemic infection involving other organs and the CNS. The viremia in both JEV and WNV infections is transient, lasting for only a few days, and then ceases with the onset of symptoms and concurrent development of IgM and IgG antibodies. Immunocompromised individuals may have prolonged viremia and delayed development of symptoms and IgM antibody. The increased incidence and higher mortality rate of WNV neuroinvasive disease in the elderly and immunocompromised individuals suggest that host factors, such as immune competence or changes in the blood–brain barrier, are important determinants of the outcome of infection.[33] The associations between neurocysticercosis in JE[38] and hypertension in WNV neuroinvasive disease[24] suggest a potential role for factors that make the blood–brain barrier vulnerable to invasion. The capability to mount an early immune response plays a critical role in containing viral replication and dissemination.[40]

DIAGNOSIS

The etiologic diagnosis of most flaviviral infections cannot be determined clinically. A high index of suspicion, however, can be gleaned from the geographic area of exposure, history of arthropod abundance, and season of the year. In addition, specific clinical features, such as flaccid paralysis, unusual movement disorders, or subtle motor seizures may provide an additional clue. Leukopenia, when present, may be an indication of a viral illness. Encephalitis cases usually have CSF pleocytosis between 5/µL and greater than 1000/µL. Initially this may be characterized by polymorphonuclear cells, but subsequently lymphocytes predominate; there is usually a normal cerebrospinal fluid to plasma glucose ratio, and an increased concentration of protein in the cerebrospinal fluid.[41]

The laboratory diagnosis of JEV or WNV infection can be made by a variety of tests. Blood samples should be obtained as early as possible from suspected febrile cases. They can be tested for virus in cell culture or for genomic sequences by the polymerase chain reaction (PCR) assay, but in most cases of encephalitis, the period of viremia has ceased by the time the patient seeks medical care, so virus isolation from the blood is usually not possible.[41] Attempts can be made to isolate virus from the cerebrospinal fluid in cases of suspected JE and WN encephalitis, by intracerebral inoculation of newborn mice or culture in Vero (African green monkey kidney) or C6/36 (*Aedes albopictus* mosquito) cells. In general, PCR of blood or cerebrospinal fluid tends to be more sensitive than virus isolation. Isolation of virus from cerebrospinal fluid signifies a poor prognosis. Most patients with JE and WN disease are diagnosed serologically. In persons who have not had previous flavivirus infections, a serologic diagnosis can be made by showing a fourfold rise or fall in IgM and/or IgG antibody titer between an acute serum and a convalescent sample collected 1 or 2 weeks after the onset of illness, by neutralization, hemagglutination inhibition, immunofluorescence, or enzyme-linked immunosorbent assay (ELISA). The IgM capture ELISA is especially useful in primary flavivirus infections because virus-specific IgM is usually present at the time the patient seeks care for encephalitis; antibody can be detected in both the serum and the cerebrospinal fluid.[42,43] IgM capture ELISA detection of antibodies on a single specimen generally indicates a recent infection, usually within the prior 6 weeks. In persons who have experienced prior flavivirus infections, the IgM response to the second or subsequent infection may be minimal or negative. Caution must also be exercised in the interpretation of IgM antibody results for WNV infection because IgM antibody may persist in the serum of some patients for longer than 500 days.[44] Therefore, detection of IgM antibody in a single sample or in the absence of a rise in titer may be unrelated to the current illness. Diagnosis can also be established by virus isolation or by immunostaining of brain collected at biopsy or postmortem examination.

Interpretation of serologic results, especially in the tropics, is complicated by cross-reacting flavivirus antibody.[45] A second flavivirus infection leads to an anamnestic response that is characterized by the rapid development of antibody that is so cross-reactive among flaviviruses that it may not be possible to determine the specific infecting flavivirus.[45,46] In fact, the antibody titer to the first infecting flavivirus may be higher than the titer of antibodies to the more recent agent.[46]

TREATMENT AND PROGNOSIS

At present, no specific therapy has been approved for use in humans with JEV or WNV infections, so current treatment is supportive. Supportive treatment of encephalitis cases includes intravenous fluid, electrolyte management, assisted respiration if needed, anticonvulsants, management of cerebral edema, prevention of secondary bacterial infections, and nursing care.[47] Physical and psychological rehabilitation is important in surviving patients, because sequelae are common and can result in major disability.

The development of specific therapeutic agents and treatment of WNV infection has been challenging, since patients with the most severe form of the disease (neuroinvasive) often are elderly or are immunosuppressed, consequently they often already have underlying immune deficits and other chronic disease problems. Also people with neuroinvasive disease usually do not develop symptoms and not seek medical care until the second week of infection; by this time, the virus is already present in the CNS, and destruction of neurons has already begun. A number of therapeutic agents and therapies have been evaluated for treatment of JEV and WNV neuroinvasive disease, usually in animals or *in vitro*, but none has yet been approved for use in humans.[48] The most promising results with WN disease have been in animal studies using human polyclonal and monoclonal antibodies.[49]

Risk factors predictive of a poor outcome in case of WNV neuroinvasive disease include profound weakness or flaccid paralysis, deep coma, lack of production of IgM antibody, immunosuppression, diabetes, and hypertension. Neurologic sequelae are common in survivors of neuroinvasive disease, and clinical abnormalities can persist for a year or more after the initial illness. Symptoms of fatigue, headache, and mild depression may persist for several months after the acute illness. Recent findings indicate that the frequency and type of seizures and status epilepticus are important predictors of a poor outcome of JE in children.[50] Importantly, in many children, subtle motor seizures, such as twitching of a digit or eyebrow, are the only signs of status epilepticus that can be confirmed by electroencephalography. Awareness, appropriate attention, and management of these manifestations may lead to a better outcome.

PREVENTION AND CONTROL

Japanese Encephalitis

A formalin-inactivated mouse-brain derived JEV vaccine was licensed for human use in the United States and in countries of Asia, but it is now being phased out. It is safe, and was shown, in Thailand, to be efficacious;[50] however, it was too expensive for use in most Asian countries, and at one stage was associated with rare late-onset hypersensitivity reaction adverse events.[51] In the United States, it has been used primarily for military personnel and tourists visiting Asia. This vaccine was produced in Japan, Taiwan, Korea, and Thailand; but in Japan it has been replaced with a Vero-cell derived vaccine. A field trial in Thailand demonstrated greater than 91% efficacy after two inoculations,[51] but three inoculations are recommended in the United States.[52]

A JEV formalin-inactivated vaccine is produced in China in primary hamster kidney cells[53] and has been used for decades to immunize schoolchildren; but it is not available outside of China. The JEV formalin-inactivated vaccine produced in Vero cells is replacing the mouse-brain derived vaccine in Japan. More recently, the SA14-14-2 live attenuated JE vaccine, produced by serial passage in mice, hamsters, and primary hamster kidney cell culture, has been widely used in China. Efficacy is 80% after one dose, but antibody wanes rapidly, and a booster dose at 12 months is recommended to achieve effective protection of 97.5% of recipients.[54] However, when administered just before the start of the JE season, the efficacy of a single dose of vaccine is 99%.[55] Until recently, the use of this vaccine outside of China has been restricted by regulatory concerns over its origins and production. The World Health Organization subsequently described guidelines for the production of live attenuated JE vaccines, and the vaccine has now been used in Korea, Nepal, and India.

An inactivated vaccine, based on SA14-14-2, is also now available internationally under the name of Ixiaro. It was successful in a series of safety and immunogenicity trials, including a multinational observer-blinded, randomized, controlled phase III non-inferiority comparison with the Biken vaccine JE Vax in more than 800 adults.[56,57]

A live attenuated vaccine, ChimeriVax-JE, was prepared by replacing the prM-E genes of yellow fever 17D vaccine with the corresponding JEV genes.[58] A recently completed randomized, double-blind, placebo-controlled phase II clinical trial showed that this vaccine was well tolerated with no adverse side effects.[59] In addition, the vaccine elicited high neutralizing antibody titers in more than 90% of the 87 volunteers within

30 days following a single inoculation of a range of doses. A single dose of Chimeri-Vax-JE induces neutralizing antibodies to JEV at levels comparable to or greater than the standard three-dose vaccination by the inactivated JE Vax.

Other measures to help control JE, including immunization of pigs and vector control, have not proved to be very successful. While personal protective measures against mosquito bites are encouraged, most agree that widespread immunization offers the best hope for future disease control.

West Nile Virus

Since the introduction of WNV into North America, a number of different vaccine approaches have been developed; but to date, none has yet been approved for use in humans. One of the problems in developing a WNV vaccine is that the groups most at risk for severe disease are the elderly and the immunocompromised. Since safety and complete attenuation have been major concerns, the development of a live attenuated WNV vaccine has largely been discarded as a vaccine strategy. Instead, other approaches such as recombinant subunit vaccines, chimeric flavivirus vaccines, non-infectious DNA and novel nucleic acid-based vaccines have been attempted. A recent review of vaccine development for WNV was published by Khromykh et al.[60] These include a recombinant subunit vaccine developed by Lieberman et al,[61] the ChimeriVax-WN vaccine produced by Acambis,[62] dengue 2/WN virus chimeras (DEN2/WNV) developed by Huang et al,[63] and several DNA-based noninfectious replicating vaccines.[60] Each of these candidate vaccines has advantages and disadvantages. The issues that drive the final selection and approval of a WNV vaccine for humans will be safety, efficacy, convenience, and cost.

While a safe and effective vaccine is needed, it is unlikely that vaccination of a large component of the population will be feasible and cost-effective. Therefore, an effective therapeutic agent is also needed for treatment of WNV infection among those at an increased risk of severe disease. In the meantime, until vaccines are available, efforts to prevent WNV disease should be targeted at reducing the risk to humans exposed to infected mosquitoes by using personal protective measures and by instituting appropriate surveillance and vector control measures.[64]

OTHER FLAVIVIRUSES

Murray Valley encephalitis (MVE) virus, which is closely related to the JEV and WNV, is limited to Australia, Papua New Guinea, and part of the eastern Indonesian archipelago.[2] MVE virus causes sporadic outbreaks of severe encephalitis and is transmitted by *Culex* mosquitoes among the resident bird populations. Like JEV and WNV, many MVE cases are asymptomatic, but among patients who develop neurologic disease, case-fatality rates are 22–24%, and >50% of survivors experience neurologic sequelae.[2]

Kyasanur Forest disease (KFD) virus and its close relative Alkahurma virus produce a severe hemorrhagic febrile illness; the pathology of the disease in humans is characterized by liver and kidney damage, hemorrhagic pneumonitis, erythrophagocytosis and meningoencephalitis.[2] Both viruses are transmitted by *Haemaphysalis* ticks. KFD seems to be largely restricted to persons entering forested areas of Karnataka State, India, while Alkahurma cases have occurred in Saudi Arabia among animal handlers and butchers. Clinically, KFD and Alkhurma patients present with a febrile syndrome accompanied by hemorrhages.[2,65] Some patients experience a biphasic course with signs of meningoencephalitis. The case-fatality rate for KFD is 3–5%; survivors do not experience sequelae.[3]

Zika virus produces a dengue-like illness characterized by fever, rash, arthralgia, headache, and myalgia.[66] It has generally been associated with *Aedes* mosquitoes. Serologic surveys suggest that Zika virus is widely distributed in humid areas of tropical Africa, Southeast Asia, the Philippines and Zap Island in the South Pacific. The disease is probably more common than currently recognized, because of its clinical similarity to dengue and the high prevalence of heterologous flavivirus antibodies where it occurs.

Ilheus virus is also mosquito-borne and produces a self-limited febrile illness characterized by headache, myalgia, arthralgia, photophobia, and occasionally CNS symptoms of encephalitis.[67] Ilheus virus has been isolated in Central and South America and in Trinidad; it has generally been associated with rural or forested areas. Like Zika, many Ilheus virus infections are probably unrecognized or misdiagnosed.

A formalin-inactivated vaccine for KFD has been used in India.[68] There are no vaccines for MVE, Ilheus or Zika viruses, and vaccines for these agents are unlikely to find commercial backing because of the small demand.

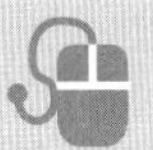

Access the complete reference list online at
http://www.expertconsult.com

Access the complete reference list online at **http://www.expertconsult.com**

CHAPTER 77

Tick-borne Encephalitis and Omsk Hemorrhagic Fever

Christian W. Mandl • Michael R. Holbrook

INTRODUCTION

Tick-borne encephalitis (TBE) and Omsk hemorrhagic fever (OHF) are caused by viruses of the TBE serocomplex (family *Flaviviridae*, genus *Flavivirus*). This complex consists of viruses that cause encephalitis in humans, several viruses that cause hemorrhagic fever, and at least one virus that is largely nonpathogenic in humans. Members of the TBE serocomplex are transmitted primarily by hard ticks in the genera *Ixodes*, *Dermacentor*, or *Hyalomma*, and the distribution of viruses is closely related to the geographic distribution of their tick vectors. The encephalitic viruses are grouped into three principal subtypes based on genetic diversity and geographic distribution. These subgroups include European subtype TBE virus (TBEV-Eu), Siberian subtype TBEV (TBEV-Sib), and Far Eastern subtype TBEV (TBEV-FE)[1] (***Fig. 77.1***). Viruses within the TBE serocomplex associated with development of hemorrhagic fever include: OHFV, Kyasanur Forest disease virus (KFDV), the closely related Alkhurma virus, and a more recently identified KFDV-related virus from China, Nanjianyin virus.[2] Other viruses within the TBE serocomplex include Powassan virus in the northeastern United States and parts of northwestern Russia, and viruses primarily associated with animal illness, including louping ill virus.

THE AGENT

Flaviviruses are small (~50 nm diameter) enveloped viruses with a small, positive-polarity single-stranded RNA genome. The viral genome encodes 10 proteins that are generated by co- and posttranslational cleavage of the viral polyprotein. The virus particle consists of three structural proteins, capsid (C), premembrane/membrane (prM/M), and envelope (E) proteins, which are encoded in the 5′ third of the genome. The 3′ two-thirds of the viral genome encodes seven nonstructural proteins, NS1, NS2A, NS2B, NS3, NS4A, NS4B and NS5. The viral particle is assembled on or in close association with the endoplasmic reticulum and initially consists of C, prM, and E proteins. PrM is cleaved by furin during the exocytic process to generate the mature viral particle. This cleavage event puts the virus into a metastable state that is sensitive to low pH. During infection, the virus binds to a receptor and is internalized via clathrin-mediated endocytosis. During the endocytic process, the endosomal pH decreases and triggers conformational change and rearrangement of the viral E protein. This process facilitates fusion between the viral envelope and the endosomal membrane and subsequent release of viral RNA into the host cell.[3–7]

The viral E protein is the major surface antigen and target of a neutralizing antibody response. NS1 can also generate a protective immune response, albeit much poorer than the E protein. The E protein is also the receptor-binding protein and contains the viral fusion peptide.[8–11]

EPIDEMIOLOGY

TBEV and OHFV are transmitted by hard ticks, although there has been some suggestion that soft ticks may also transmit these viruses.[12] Horizontal transmission of the virus occurs through cofeeding of uninfected ticks in close proximity to infected ticks on the vertebrate host. The viruses are also transmitted transovarially and transstadially allowing for maintenance of viruses in tick populations. The principal vectors for all TBEV subtypes are *Ixodes* spp. ticks. The principal vector for OHFV is *Dermacentor reticulatus*, but this virus has also been found in other genera and species of tick. OHFV has also been found in mosquitoes, but it is unlikely that mosquitoes are competent vectors for tick-borne flavivirus transmission. Members of the TBEV serocomplex typically circulate in nature between ticks and small mammals, particularly rodents. Larger animals, such as deer and cattle, can be infected, although these are likely to be dead-end hosts.

TBEV-FE is found in eastern Asia, including northern Japan throughout the range of its tick vector *Ix. persulcatus* (***Fig. 77.2***). There is also evidence of TBEV-FE in far eastern Europe in the Ural mountains, but these cases are sporadic. Most reports of disease are from eastern Russia, however, TBEV-FE likely occurs in northern and northeastern China.[13]

TBEV-Eu ranges from central Europe to the Ural mountains and is typically transmitted by *Ix. ricinus* ticks. However, the earliest documented outbreaks of TBE in Europe were associated with consumption of contaminated unpasteurized milk from goats or sheep and called biphasic milk fever. Similar recent cases were linked to acute infection of the animal excreting the virus into the milk. Interestingly, the endemic range for *Ix. ricinus* is larger than the range for TBEV-Eu. In the southern and western regions of the *Ix. ricinus* range, TBEV serocomplex viruses such as louping ill, Turkish TBE, and Greek goat encephalitis viruses do not typically infect humans. Possible competition for vectors and small mammalian hosts limits the southern range of TBEV-Eu. TBEV-Eu continues to expand northward[14,15] where there is less competition for vectors and hosts.

TBEV-Sib is typically found in the central and western range of *Ix. persulcatus* with evidence of this virus in Siberia and westward into the Ural mountains. It is also likely that TBEV-Sib exists in north-central China, although this has not been documented.

OHFV is found in a localized region of the Omsk and Novosibirsk Oblasts in central Russia (***Fig. 77.2***). OHFV is transmitted through the bite of *Dermacentor* spp. ticks[16] and is maintained in nature through mechanisms similar to other TBE serocomplex viruses. OHFV is endemic in a region where there is a high population of muskrats, which is a source of human infection when the animals are slaughtered for their fur.

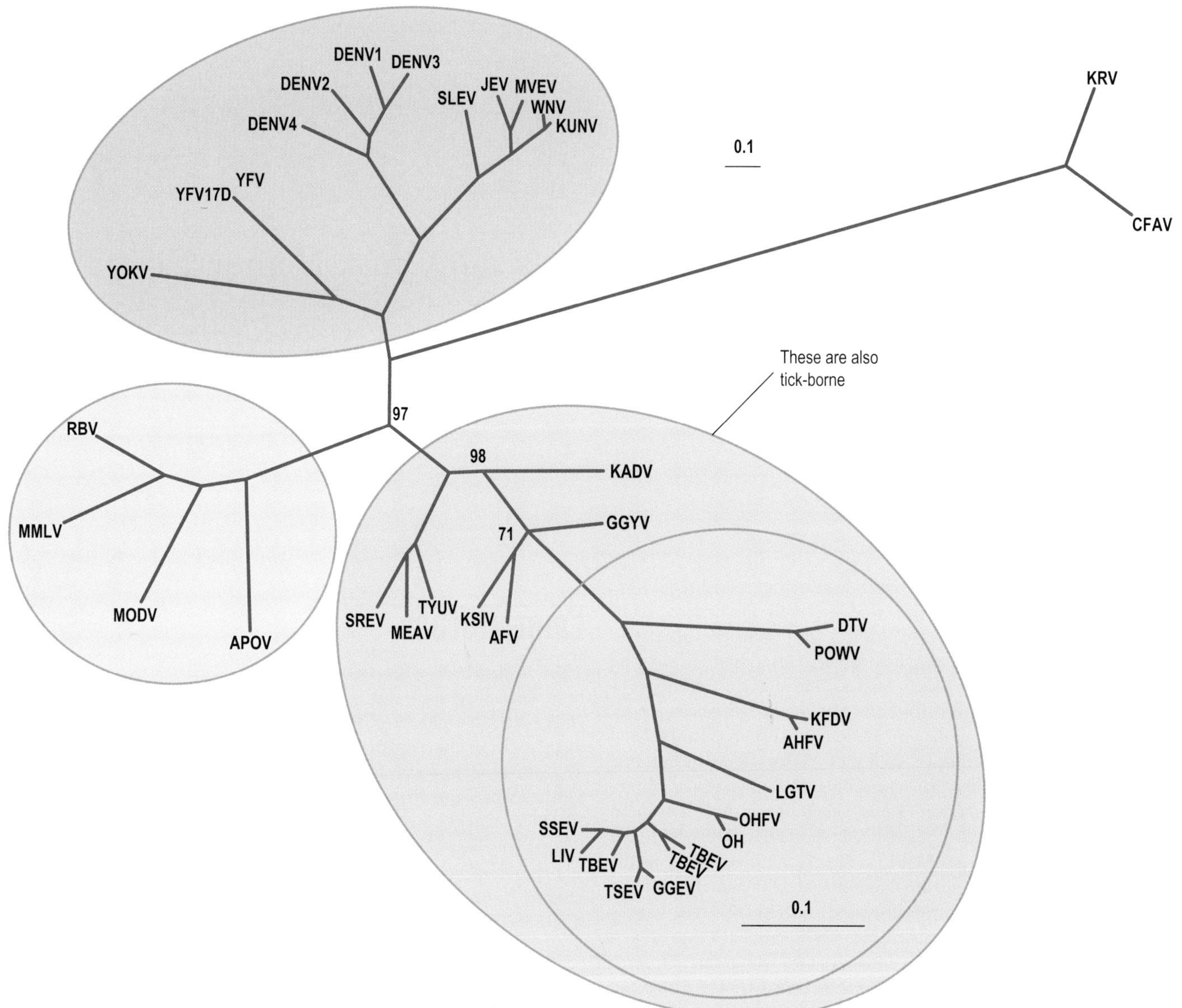

Figure 77.1 Maximum likelihood phylogenetic analysis of the flaviviruses, with the tick-borne encephalitis viruses highlighted in green. Abbreviations: dengue virus 1-4 (DENV1-4), St Louis encephalitis virus (SLEV), Japanese encephalitis virus (JEV), Murray Valley encephalitis virus (MVEV), West Nile virus (WNV), Kunjin virus (KUNV), yellow fever virus (YFV), Yokose virus (YOKV), Rio Bravo virus (RBV), Montana myotis leukoencephalitis virus (MMLV), Modoc virus (MODV), Apoi virus (APOV), Saumarez reef virus (SREV), Meaban virus (MEAV), Tyuleniy virus (TYUV), Karshi virus (KSIV), Kadam virus (KADV), Gadgets Gully virus (GGYV), deer tick virus (DTV), Powassan virus (POWV), Kyasanur forest disease virus (KFDV), Alkhurma hemorrhagic fever virus (AHFV), Langat virus (LGTV), Omsk hemorrhagic fever virus (OHFV), tick-borne encephalitis virus (TBEV), Greek goat encephalitis virus (GGEV), Turkish sheep encephalitis virus (TSEV), louping ill virus (LIV), Spanish sheep encephalitis virus (SSEV). (Adapted from Grard G, Moureau GN, Charrel RN, et al. Genetic characterization of tick-borne flaviviruses: new insights into evolution, pathogenetic determinants and taxonomy. Virology 2007;361:80–92.)

THE DISEASE

TBEV infections can range from asymptomatic infection or mild disease to severe neurological disease and death, which usually occurs within 5–7 days of onset of neurological symptoms[17] (***Table 77.1***). TBEV-Eu and TBEV-FE have been reported to cause clinically distinct diseases, although there is debate regarding the reporting and specific characterizations of each disease. Infections with TBEV-Eu often result in milder disease that may be biphasic, with approximately 65% of patients recovering at the end of the first febrile phase. Of the remaining ~35% of patients, most progress to neurological involvement. The first phase of TBEV-Eu infection begins 2–18 days postinfection as a febrile illness with headache, myalgia, fatigue, nausea, and general malaise. This phase lasts 1–8 days and is followed by an afebrile remission that can last up to 3 weeks. In patients who progress into the second phase of disease, there is rapid onset of high fever and neurologic disease, including meningitis, meningoencephalitis, meningoencephalomyelitis, or meningoencephaloradiculitis.[18] In most instances the disease resolves, although long-term sequelae are not uncommon. The case-fatality rate for TBEV-Eu infections is 1–2%.

Infections with TBEV-FE are typically more severe than TBEV-Eu infections. Following an incubation period similar to TBEV-Eu infections, there is rapid onset of high fever, headache, vomiting, myalgia, and indications of neurologic infection, including photophobia and sensorial and visual changes. Unlike TBEV-Eu, patients with TBEV-FE infections more frequently progress to neurological complications, including paresis, paralysis, seizures, and coma, without an intermittent lucid phase.[19,20] Paralysis typically begins in the upper extremities, and the disease can be complicated by lower motor neuron paralysis, which is indicative of a poor outcome.[19,21] The case-fatality rate for TBEV-FE infections is

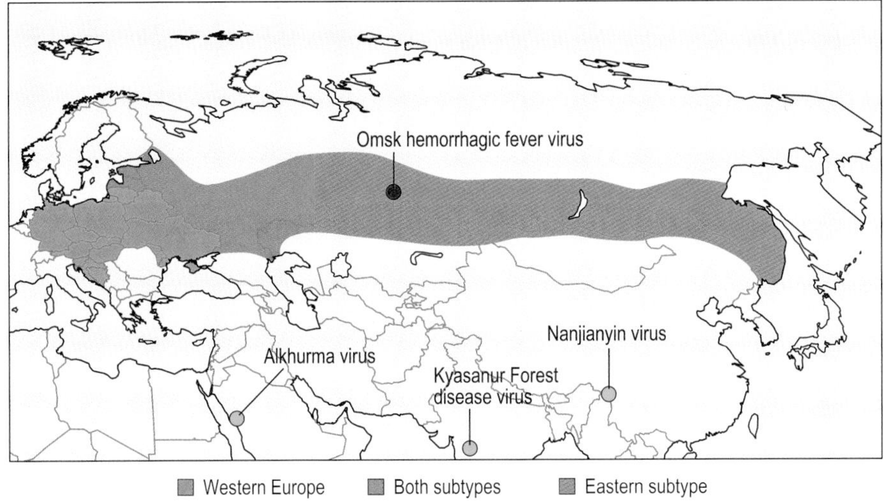

Figure 77.2 Epidemiology of tick-borne encephalitis and Omsk hemorrhagic fever. (Adapted from International Scientific Working Group on TBE/Baxter.)

Table 77.1 Clinical and Pathologic Characteristics for the Three Subtypes of Tick-borne Encephalitis Virus and Omsk Hemorrhagic Fever Virus

	Disease Characteristics in Human			
	TBEV-Eu	**TBEV-Sib**	**TBEV-FE**	**OHFV**
Incubation period	2–18 days	2–18 days	2–18 days	6–14 days
Disease course	Biphasic	Biphasic	Biphasic, although intermittent lucid phase may be very short or nonexistent	Biphasic
Onset	Rapid onset, febrile, myalgia, nausea, malaise, headache	Rapid onset, febrile, myalgia, nausea, malaise, headache	Rapid onset, headache, high fever, vomiting, myalgia, photophobia, sensorial and visual changes	Fever, headache, myalgia, cough, dehydration, hypotension, gastrointestinal symptoms
Neurologic involvement	Photophobia, headache, high fever, encephalitis, meningoencephalitis	Photophobia, headache, high fever, encephalitis, meningoencephalitis	Paresis, paralysis, seizures, and coma; flaccid paralysis of motor neurons; ascending paralysis indicative of a poor outcome	Occasional diffuse encephalitis
Visceral disease	None	None	None	Papulovesicular or petechial cutaneous rash, mucosal hemorrhage, scattered visceral hemorrhages
Convalescence	Generally unremarkable, polio-like flaccid paralysis is seen occasionally, much less frequent then in TBEV-FE cases	Chronic or persistent disease has been noted, occasional neurologic sequelae, otherwise unremarkable	Atrophy and paresis of arm and neck muscles; polio-like neurologic sequelae in the arms and occasionally legs are not uncommon	Unremarkable
Case fatality	1–2%	6–8%	20–60%	<3%

TBEV, tick-borne encephalitis virus; OMFV, Omsk hemorrhgic fever virus; TBEV-Eu, TBEV European subtype; TBEV-Sib, TBEV Siberian subtype; TBEV-FE, TBEV Far Eastern subtype.

20–30%, and survivors frequently develop permanent neurological sequelae, including paresis and atrophy of the neck muscles and paresis in the lower extremities, resulting in polio-like sequelae.[18]

The Siberian subtype of TBEV typically causes a disease that is more severe than TBEV-Eu and less severe than TBEV-FE. However, TBEV-Sib has been associated with chronic infections whereas the other two subtypes have not.[22–25]

OHF is a fairly nonspecific febrile disease with some patients developing hemorrhagic manifestations with petechiae of the soft palate, nose, gums, uterus, lungs, or urinary tract or gastrointestinal bleeding.[26,27] The case-fatality rate is less than 3%, and survivors have an uneventful recovery with no long-term sequelae. There have only been about 1400 cases of OHF identified to date, but there is a relatively high seroprevalence,[16,26] suggesting subclinical or mild disease.

PATHOGENESIS AND IMMUNITY

Under normal circumstances, TBEV and OHFV are transmitted to humans through the bite of an infected tick. The virus is deposited in the skin where it may reproduce locally and/or infect Langerhans cells or resident macrophages and be transported to draining lymph nodes. The virus is believed to replicate in lymphatic tissues and be released into the lymphatic system and subsequently into the venous circulation for dissemination. Disease characteristics and studies in small animals indicate that TBEV and OHFV have differing tissue tropism with TBEV targeting neural tissues and OHFV appearing to target visceral organs.[21,28]

TBEV rapidly penetrates the blood–brain barrier. The mechanism is unclear but depends on significant levels of viremia. Pathologic characteristics of TBEV-FE suggest peripheral penetration near the brachial plexus resulting in death of neurons in this region and resulting paralysis. Magnetic resonance imaging indicates damage to anterior horns of cervical and thoracic vertebrae, lumbar nerve roots, basal ganglia, and the thalamus.[29–31] Studies with TBEV-Eu suggest targeting of neurons in the anterior pons, medulla oblongata, dentate nucleus, and Purkinje cells.[32] Studies in mice with OHFV indicate penetration of the blood–brain barrier with localization in Purkinje cells of the cerebellum.[28,33]

Natural infection with TBEV or OHFV produces lifelong protective immunity in survivors. Both IgM and IgG are produced, with levels of IgM presumably elevated during the prodromal phase and IgG levels becoming elevated 5–7 days postinfection. IgM and IgG levels are also elevated in the cerebrospinal fluid of TBE patients.[34,35] Natural TBEV infections induce a cell-mediated response. Although it is likely that cell-mediated immunity plays a role in the protective response,[36–38] it is becoming apparent that CD8 T cells are also associated in the pathogenesis of TBEV infections[32,39] where recruitment of T cells is driven by chemokines produced by infected cells within the central nervous system[40] and resulting CD8 T cell infiltration and cell death.

DIAGNOSIS

The principal means for diagnosing TBEV or OHFV infection is by enzyme-linked immunosorbent assay (ELISA) or polymerase chain reaction (PCR). Most cases of TBEV infection present at hospital a week or more after the initial infection with the onset of illness. In this case, ELISAs are effective as the patient should have circulating virus-specific IgM and IgG in the serum. PCR is less than ideal as the virus is typically cleared before the onset of severe symptoms. TBEV infection of the central nervous system can be confirmed by collection of cerebrospinal fluid for ELISA and PCR. A more stringent and species-specific serologic test for TBEV or OHFV infection is the plaque reduction neutralization test, but this assay requires use of live virus and specialized facilities that are not typically available in hospital settings.

TREATMENT AND PREVENTION

There are no effective treatment strategies for the tick-borne flaviviruses. However, there are licensed and highly effective vaccines available in Europe and Russia for prevention of infection and disease. The available licensed vaccines all use formalin-inactivated virus adsorbed to alum adjuvant and induce strong protective antibody responses. The typical regimen requires two initial vaccinations with an interval of 2–4 weeks followed by a third booster vaccination after 9–12 months with a protection rate of about 98%. A rapid vaccination schedule involving three doses over a 21-day period is also available with a booster 12–18 months later.[41] Boosters are required every 3–5 years, although age and vaccination compliance may also affect the booster schedule.[42,43] These vaccines are generated using TBEV-Eu strains, but the close antigenic relatedness of the viruses within the TBEV serocomplex suggests that inactivated TBEV vaccines should protect against infection by many members of the TBE serocomplex. Animal studies in mice have shown cross-protection against OHFV (M. Holbrook, unpublished studies). A number of live-attenuated and subunit vaccines are in development, though none has reached clinical trials.[44]

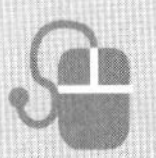

Access the complete reference list online at http://www.expertconsult.com

Access the complete reference list online at
http://www.expertconsult.com

CHAPTER 78

Alphavirus Infections

Scott C. Weaver • David W. Smith

INTRODUCTION

The alphaviruses comprise a genus (*Alphavirus*) in the family *Togaviridae* of enveloped RNA viruses (***Table 78.1***). All are maintained primarily in cycles between insect vectors and rodents, primates, or birds, although a few infect fish and seals. Human disease occurs when people intrude on enzootic foci and are bitten by infected mosquitoes, or when alphaviruses emerge to cause epizootics and epidemics via host range changes or amplification, followed by simple spillover. Five alphaviruses commonly infect people in the tropics: Venezuelan equine encephalitis (VEEV), chikungunya (CHIKV), Ross River (RRV), o'nyong-nyong (ONNV), and Mayaro (MAYV) viruses. Others including eastern and western equine encephalitis and Sindbis viruses cause human disease primarily in temperate regions and are not discussed here.

THE AGENT

Alphavirus virions are about 70 nm in diameter and include an icosahedral nucleocapsid with T=4 symmetry, surrounded by a host cell-derived lipid envelope embedded with glycoprotein spikes.[1] The spikes are consist of 240 heterodimers of the E1 and E2 envelope glycoproteins arranged in 80 trimers that are determined by interactions between the cytoplasmic tails of E2 with underlying capsid proteins.[1] The E1 glycoprotein lies nearly parallel to the envelope while E2 projects outward to form the spikes. The RNA genome is approximately 11 400–12 000 nucleotides in length (***Fig. 78.1***).[1] Like cellular messenger RNA, alphavirus RNA contains a 5′ methylguanylate cap and 3′ polyadenylate tail. The nonstructural proteins coded by the 5′ two-thirds of the genome are translated directly from the open reading frame (ORF) upon entry into the cytoplasm. Structural proteins are encoded by subgenomic RNA that is identical to the 3′ one-third of the genome and is also capped and polyadenylated. Minus-strand RNA synthesis is favored early during replication by the sequential processing of the nonstructural proteins, which are initially synthesized as two polypeptides (nsP123 and nsP1234), or as a single nsP1234 that favors minus-strand synthesis (some alphaviruses contain a terminating codon between nsP3 and nsP4, and others contain arginine or cysteine codons at this position). The nonstructural polyproteins are later cleaved by a protease domain of nsP2 into individual proteins that favor plus-strand synthesis.

The functions of the nonstructural proteins are not completely understood.[1] nsP1 serves as a guanine-7-methyltransferase and a guanyltransferase for capping of RNAs, and is involved in binding of replicative complexes to cytoplasmic membranes. The N-terminus of nsP2 has a helicase function, and the C-terminus is a protease that regulates processing of the nonstructural proteins. nsP3, the least understood, appears to be involved in the functioning of the subgenomic promoter, is transported to the nucleus, and affects cytopathology in some vertebrate cells. nsP4 is the RNA-dependent RNA polymerase for minus- and plus-strand RNA synthesis.

Alphavirus genomes contain several conserved *cis*-acting elements (CSE) required for replication: (1) a 19 nt CSE that immediately precedes the 3′ terminal poly(A) tract and is a promoter element for minus-strand RNA synthesis; (2) a 24 nt CSE promoter for the subgenomic RNA; (3) a 51 nt CSE (approximately nt 155–205) located within the nsP1 coding sequence that is predicted to form two short stem-loop structures, and which functions as a replication enhancer; and (4) the 5′ untranslated region that contains a promoter (on the complementary strand) for initiation of plus-strand RNA synthesis. The 5′ and 3′ ends of alphavirus genomic RNAs probably interact with the help of translation initiation factors to initiate genome replication.

Alphavirus structural proteins are translated from the subgenomic RNA as a polypeptide.[1] The capsid protein possesses a serine protease activity and cleaves itself in the cytoplasm from the polypeptide chain immediately following its translation. The E3 and E2 proteins (precursors called PE2 or P62 before their cleavage) are translocated into the endoplasmic reticulum (ER) where they remain anchored to membranes via hydrophobic amino acids near the C-terminus. The C-terminal part of a small peptide called 6K serves as the signal peptide required for transport of the E1 envelope glycoprotein into the ER, where it is attached to membranes via a hydrophobic anchor on the C-terminus. Proteolytic cleavages between PE2, 6K, and E1 are performed by cell signalases. The E3/E2 cleavage is accomplished last by a furin-type cellular protease and is required for efficient viral infectivity. During transport to the cell surface via the secretory pathway, the envelope proteins are modified via glycosylation, palmitoylation, and heterodimerization.

For virion assembly, the capsid protein recognizes encapsidation signal(s), generally located in the nonstructural protein genes of the genomic RNA.[1] This initiates nucleocapsid formation, involving 240 molecules of the capsid protein, in the cytoplasm. The capsid protein molecules within the nucleocapsid then interact with the cytoplasmic domain of E2 within E1–E2 heterodimers on the plasma membrane, leading to budding whereby the nucleocapsid incorporates its envelope and glycoprotein spikes, resulting in release of virions from the cell surface.

The glycoprotein spikes function both in attachment to cellular receptors and in fusion with endosomal membranes for entry into cells.[1] E2 includes the major antigenic determinants and probably interacts with cellular receptors, while E1 includes the conserved fusion peptide responsible for hemagglutination. E2 is an important determinant of alphavirus virulence in vertebrates and infectivity for mosquitoes. Many of the biologically important epitopes on the envelope glycoproteins are conformational, making the design of subunit or peptide vaccines challenging. The capsid protein elicits broadly cross-reactive antibody and is a major complement-fixing antigen.

Most alphaviruses infect a wide variety of hosts and cell lines of vertebrate and invertebrate origin. Several receptors have been identified and include highly conserved proteins such as the high affinity laminin

Table 78.1 Alphaviruses[a]

Antigenic Complex	Species	Antigenic Subtype	Antigenic Variety	Human Clinical Syndrome	Distribution
Barmah Forest	Barmah Forest (BFV)			Febrile illness, rash, arthritis	Australia
Eastern equine encephalitis (EEE)	Eastern equine encephalitis	I–IV		Febrile illness, encephalitis (rarely recognized in Central, South America)	North, Central, South America
Middelburg	Middelburg (MIDV)			None recognized	Africa
Ndumu	Ndumu virus (NDUV)			None recognized	Africa
Semliki Forest	Semliki Forest (SFV)			Febrile illness	Africa
	Chikungunya (CHIKV)			Febrile illness, rash, arthritis	Africa, Asia
	O'nyong-nyong (ONNV)			Febrile illness, rash, arthritis	Africa
	Getah (GETV)			None recognized	Asia
	Bebaru (BEBV)			None recognized	Malaysia
	Ross River (RRV)	Sagiyama		Febrile illness, rash, arthritis	Australia, Oceania
	Mayaro (MAYV)			Febrile illness, rash, arthritis	South, Central America, Trinidad
	Una (UNAV)			None recognized	South America
Venezuelan equine encephalitis (VEE)	Venezuelan equine encephalitis (VEEV)	I	AB	Febrile illness, encephalitis	North, Central, South America
			C	Febrile illness, encephalitis	South America
			D	Febrile illness, encephalitis	South America, Panama
			E	Febrile illness, encephalitis	Central America, Mexico
	Mosso das Pedras virus (MDPV)		F (strain 78V3531)	None recognized	Brazil
	Everglades (EVEV)	II		Febrile illness, encephalitis	Florida (USA)
	Mucambo (MUCV)	III	A	Febrile illness, myalgia	South America, Trinidad
			C (strain 71D1252)	None recognized	Peru
			D (strain 407660)	Febrile illness	Peru
	Tonate (TONV)	III	B	Febrile illness, encephalitis	Brazil, Colorado (USA)
	Pixuna (PIXV)	IV		Febrile illness, myalgia	Brazil
	Cabassou (CABV)	V		None recognized	French Guiana
	Rio Negro (RNV)	VI		Febrile illness, myalgia	Argentina
Western equine encephalitis (WEE)	Sindbis (SINV)			Febrile illness, rash, arthritis	Africa, Europe, Asia, Australia
		Babanki		Febrile illness, rash, arthritis	Africa
		Ockelbo		Febrile illness, rash, arthritis	Europe
		Kyzylagach		None recognized	Azerbaijan, China
	Whataroa (WHAV)			None recognized	New Zealand
	Aura (AURAV)			None recognized	South America
	WEEV	Several		Febrile illness, encephalitis	Western North, South America
	Highlands J (HJV)			None recognized	Eastern North America
	Fort Morgan (FMV)	Buggy Creek		None recognized	North, South America
Trocara	Trocara (TROV)			None recognized	South America

[a]Alphaviruses isolated from fish and seals are not included.

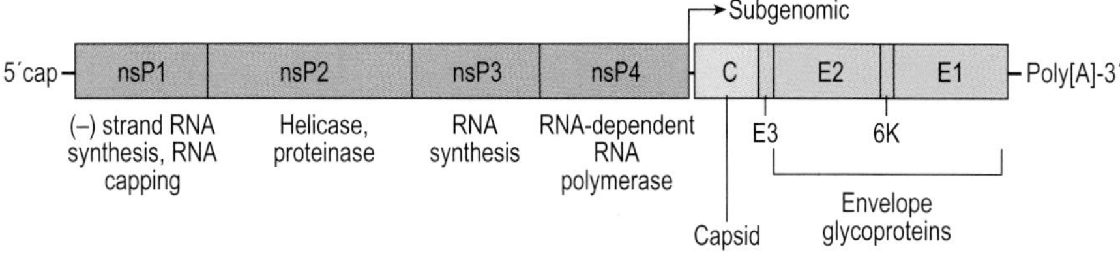

Figure 78.1 The alphavirus gene.

receptor.[1] However, multiple receptors and perhaps coreceptors probably explain the wide host range, especially for vertebrates, as well as the specificity that is sometimes exhibited for mosquito vectors. E2 amino acids 180–220 probably comprise a major receptor-reactive domain. Alphaviruses enter both vertebrate and arthropod cells via receptor-mediated endocytosis, followed by fusion with endosomal membranes after conformational changes in the glycoprotein spikes at acidic pH. Fusion, mediated by a conserved peptide (amino acids 80–96) in E1, leads to the release of the nucleocapsid into the cytoplasm, followed by disassembly in association with ribosomes.

Alphavirus replication in vertebrate cells is accompanied by inhibition of cellular protein, RNA and DNA synthesis. For several Old World alphaviruses, this inhibition of cellular function appears to be regulated by nsP2, while some New World viruses use the capsid protein to inhibit host cell transcription.[2] Transcriptional shutoff may play an important role in the inhibition of interferon (IFN) production by infected cells and more efficient dissemination of the infection. Apoptosis appears to be a major cause of death in alphavirus-infected cells.

PATHOGENESIS AND IMMUNITY

In vertebrates, initial sites of alphavirus replication include skeletal muscle, fibroblasts, osteoblasts, and macrophages in the skin, often leading to infection of the draining lymph node.[3] Viremia is probably the main form of dissemination to other tissues and organs. Some Old World alphaviruses such as CHIKV that cause a rash replicate in the skin and in striated muscle. Infection of macrophages may mediate the pathology in some infections that lead to an arthritic syndrome. Invasion of the central nervous system (CNS) by the encephalitic alphaviruses generally follows initial virus replication in various peripheral sites and a period of viremia exceeding a threshold for CNS entry. CNS entry through the olfactory tract has been demonstrated for VEEV in mice, while pathogenesis in humans is very poorly understood.

Type I and II IFNs are induced soon after alphavirus infections. Type I IFN, which is considered more important, limits early stage alphavirus replication before acquired immunity appears.[3] IFN and other cytokines may also contribute to disease by causing a shock-like disease. Alphaviruses are highly immunogenic for vertebrates but VEEV is also immunosuppressive. Although humoral immunity is believed to be more important for protection, both cellular and humoral mechanisms contribute to recovery following infection and to protection from challenge following vaccination. IgM is usually elicited within 5–10 days of infection and persists for several months. IgG is first detected within a few weeks of infection and remains at least for years and probably for life following many alphavirus infections.

In mosquitoes, alphaviruses generally infect and replicate first in posterior midgut epithelium.[4] Dissemination into the hemocoel then results in infection of secondary target organs including the salivary glands. Transmission via infectious saliva can occur within a few days of mosquito infection when a subsequent blood meal is taken from a susceptible host. The number of midgut epithelial cells infected and the amount of virus transmitted is very small in some cases, suggesting bottlenecks during transmission. Alphaviruses can also cause pathology in their mosquito vectors, though vector pathogenesis has only been investigated in a few cases. Cytopathic effects have been detected in the midgut, muscles, and salivary glands of mosquitoes.[4]

EPIDEMIOLOGY

Venezuelan Equine Encephalitis

VEE was first recognized in Venezuela in 1936, and has caused periodic equine epizootics and epidemics in many regions of tropical America[5] (***Fig. 78.2***). The last major epidemic in northern Venezuela and Colombia in 1995 involved approximately 100 000 persons.[6] VEE complex alphaviruses (***Table 78.1***) occur in two distinct transmission cycles: enzootic and epidemic/epizootic. Enzootic cycles involving small mammalian hosts and *Culex* (*Melanoconion*) spp. mosquitoes that occur in forest and swamp habitats ranging from Florida to Argentina (***Fig. 78.3***). Enzootic viruses (subtypes ID–F, II–VI) are generally avirulent for equids, but are pathogenic for humans and can cause fatal disease.[5] These enzootic strains are increasingly recognized as important human pathogens that are undiagnosed because they typically cause dengue-like illness.[7] In contrast, epidemic/epizootic VEEV (subtypes IAB, IC) are virulent for both equids and humans, but have no known interepizootic maintenance cycles. Their transmission involves mammalophilic mosquitoes, including

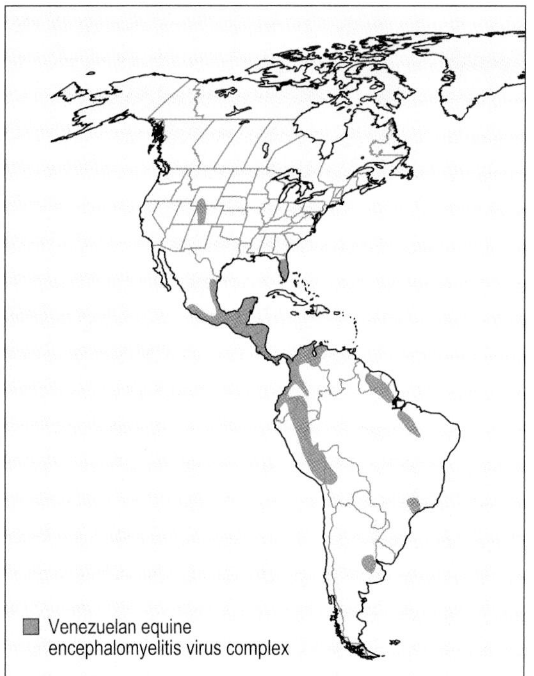

Figure 78.2 Distribution of Venezuelan equine encephalomyelitis complex.

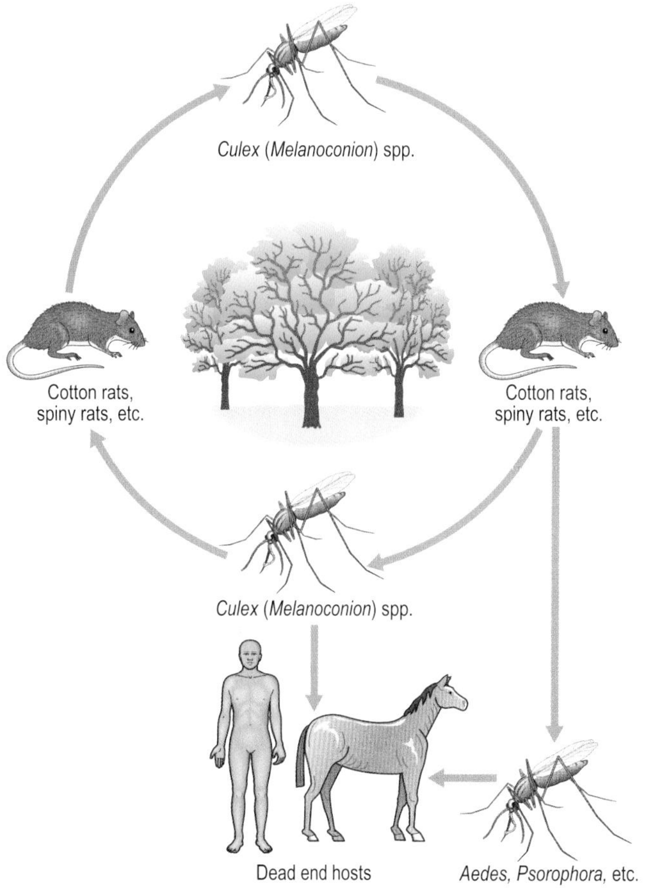

Figure 78.3 The enzootic transmission cycle of Venezuelan equine encephalomyelitis complex viruses.

Aedes (*Ochlerotatus*) and *Psorophora*, which rapidly transmit the virus among equids that develop high levels of viremia (***Fig. 78.4***). A large supply of susceptible equids and large numbers of mosquitoes, usually emerging following heavy rainfall during the wet season, are prerequisites of epizootics. Most have occurred in Venezuela, Colombia, Ecuador, and Peru,

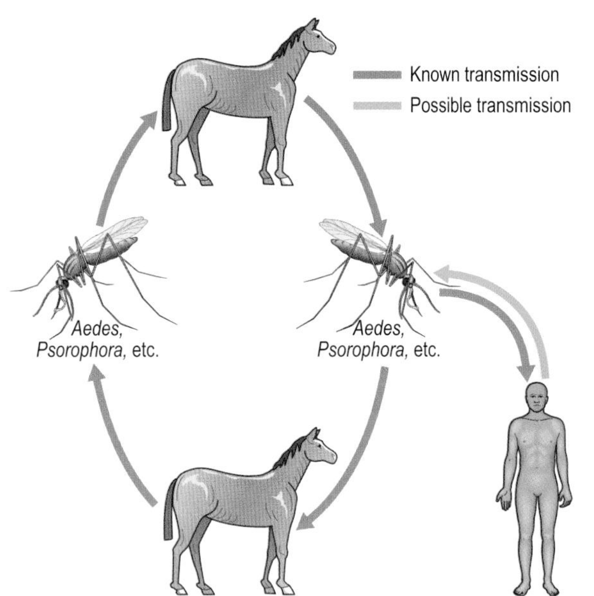

Figure 78.4 The epidemic and epizootic transmission cycle of Venezuelan equine encephalomyelitis viruses.

although one spread from El Salvador through much of Central America, reaching Mexico and Texas in 1971. VEE outbreaks are believed to occur following mutations of enzootic subtype ID viruses that result in the transformation to an equine-virulent IAB or IC phenotype.[5] People become infected by mosquitoes that previously engorged on viremic equids. Human–mosquito–human transmission, although not documented, is possible based on human viremia titers and the competence of anthropophilic mosquitoes such as *Ae. aegypti*.

Mayaro Virus

MAYV, first isolated in 1954 in Trinidad from forest workers, has been detected in lowland tropical forests of Suriname, French Guiana, Colombia, Panama, Brazil, Peru, and Bolivia.[8] Infections usually occur in people living near or working in tropical forests; for this reason, most reported cases have been in adult males. Although the virus has been recovered from a variety of mosquitoes, forest-dwelling *Haemagogus* spp. are thought to be the principal vectors, and nonhuman primates probably serve as the principal reservoirs. As the vectors have a sylvatic distribution, human infections with MAYV usually occur as sporadic cases of febrile illness or small focal outbreaks. Due to its sporadic occurrence, rural distribution, and nonspecific nature, most cases of MAYV disease are probably unrecognized or misdiagnosed. MAYV shares several important characteristics with other arboviruses known to evolve urban transmission cycles, such as CHIKV and yellow fever viruses: (1) it can infect and be transmitted by anthropophilic vectors including *Ae. aegypti* and *Ae. albopictus*, which can efficiently transmit arboviruses in a human–mosquito–human cycle; (2) it probably uses nonhuman primates as its principal reservoir hosts; and (3) it is closely related to CHIKV, which has a history of urbanization in islands of the Indian Ocean and in Asia. These characteristics suggest the possibility that MAYV could emerge to establish an efficient human–mosquito–human cycle, leading to major endemic and epidemic disease in cities of the New World.

Ross River Virus

RRV infection occurs in Australia and the South Pacific. In Australia, most cases occur during summer and autumn in temperate regions, with several thousand reported annually. However, the highest individual risk occurs in the tropical northern areas during the wet season, from December to May. RRV is maintained in Australia primarily in a cycle between mosquitoes (mainly *Culex annulirostris, Ae. camptorhynchus*, and *Ae. vigilax*) and marsupial macropods (kangaroos, wallabies, and euros). Human infection also occurs in Papua New Guinea, the Solomon Islands, New Caledonia, Fiji, American Samoa, and the Cook Islands.[9] In 1979/80 a large epidemic swept across the South Pacific, with 40–60% infection rates on some islands, which was believed to have been initiated by a viremic traveler and maintained in a human–mosquito–human transmission cycle involving *Ae. polynesiensis*.[9]

Chikungunya Virus

Chikungunya comes from Swahili, meaning "that which bends up," and refers to the characteristic posture assumed by patients suffering severe, incapacitating joint pains. CHIKV was first isolated during a 1952 epidemic in Tanzania,[10] but had probably occurred sporadically in India and Southeast Asia for at least 200 years. Prior to the 2005 epidemic in the Indian Ocean, the known geographic distribution of the virus included most of sub-Saharan Africa, India, Southeast Asia, Indonesia, and the Philippines (***Fig. 78.5***).

CHIKV has two distinct transmission cycles: (1) a sylvatic African cycle between wild primates and arboreal *Aedes* mosquitoes, similar to that of yellow fever virus in the same region; and (2) urban, *Ae. aegypti*- and *Ae. albopictus*-borne transmission among humans.[11] Urban outbreaks are sporadic but explosive. During the past 50 years, extensive epidemics have occurred in many large cities of India and Southeast Asia, affecting up to millions people. As it is clinically similar to dengue in signs and symptoms, CHIKV infections are undoubtedly underdiagnosed.

Beginning in 2005, CHIKV was introduced into several immunologically naïve islands in the Indian Ocean and caused major epidemics. On La Réunion Island, approximately 300 000 cases occurred with an attack rate of 35%, including excess mortality associated with CHIKV infections. Then, in 2006, CHIKV was independently introduced from Africa into India and Sri Lanka, where a massive epidemic began that continues at present (***Fig. 78.5***). Many excess deaths were also reported in India, suggesting that CHIKV may cause fatal disease. Subsequently, there has also been a resurgence of CHIKV in Malaysia and Indonesia. The Indian Ocean, Indian, Sri Lankan, and Malaysian epidemics apparently benefited from a mutation in the E1 envelope glycoprotein that enhanced infection of *Ae. albopictus*.[12] This adaptation may have augmented these epidemics because *Ae. albopictus* is more common than the usual vector, *Ae. aegypti*, in many of the outbreak locations. An especially troubling situation has been the exportation of CHIKV-viremic travelers to North and South America, Australia, Europe, and Southeast Asia; in the last two locations, importation resulted in local, mosquito-borne transmission, including in temperate Italy.[13] This dispersal of CHIKV may serve as a harbinger of its future spread throughout the tropics and subtropics, and possibly to temperate regions, with increasing incidence and, possibly, severity of infection.

O'nyong-nyong Virus

The epidemiology of ONNV remains poorly understood 44 years after its discovery. Its name is derived from the description by the Acholi tribe, meaning "joint breaker."[14] ONNV was first isolated during a 1959–1962 epidemic involving about 2 million people in Uganda, Kenya, Tanzania, Mozambique, Malawi, and Senegal. Attack rates were high, and all age groups were infected.[14] Igbo-Ora virus is a closely related genetic variant of ONNV that was isolated from febrile patients in Nigeria in 1966.[15] The transmission cycle of ONNV involves *Anopheles funestus* and *An. gambiae* mosquitoes during epidemics, but the presumed enzootic cycle remains uncharacterized. In June 1996, an outbreak of ONNV infection involving more than 2 million cases began in the Rakai district of southwestern Uganda.[16] The epidemic later spread into the neighboring Mbarara and Masaka districts of Uganda, and the bordering Bukoba district of northern Tanzania, with estimated attack rates of 29–41%.

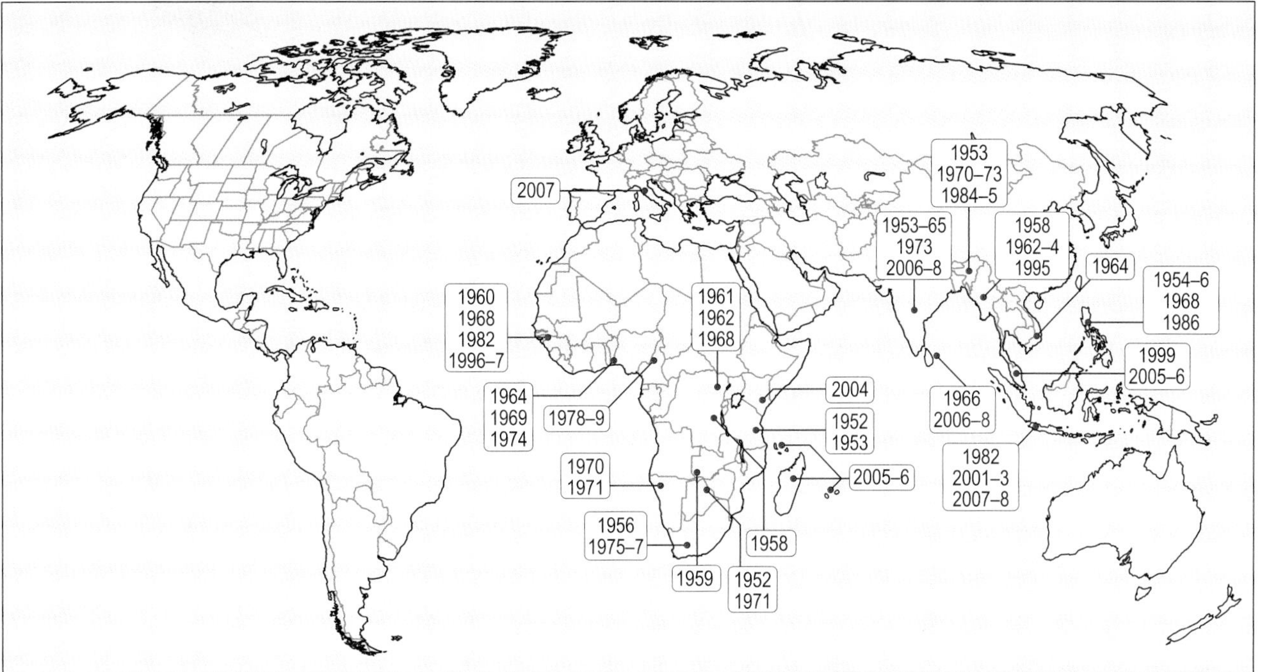

Figure 78.5 Chikungunya virus. Prior to the 2005 epidemic in the Indian Ocean, the known geographic distribution of the virus included most of sub-Saharan Africa, India, Southeast Asia, Indonesia, and the Philippines.

THE DISEASE

Venezuelan Equine Encephalitis

Human VEEV infection causes a disease spectrum ranging from inapparent infection to acute encephalitis, with attack rates of about 30%.[6] Following an incubation period of 1–4 days, signs and symptoms typically include fever, lethargy, headache, chills, dizziness, body aches, nausea, vomiting, and prostration.[3] Inflammation of the throat, cervical lymphadenitis, and abdominal tenderness are also common.[17] Symptoms usually subside after several days, but may recrudesce. VEE occurs in all age groups and both sexes. Severe neurologic signs including convulsions and seizures occur in 4–14% of cases, primarily in children, and often late in the illness. Case-fatality rates in patients who develop encephalitis have been estimated at 10–25%.[3] Laboratory findings include leukopenia during the first few days of illness followed by a lymphocyte rebound and neutrophil decline. White blood cells, predominantly lymphocytes, and elevated glucose have been reported in the cerebrospinal fluid (CSF). CSF protein is occasionally slightly elevated, along with serum aspartate transaminase.[17] Although far more cases are diagnosed during epizootics/epidemics involving subtype IAB and IC VEEV strains, endemic spillover from enzootic transmission cycles is greatly underappreciated as a major cause of febrile disease, sometimes fatal, in the Neotropics.[7]

Mayaro Virus

MAYV disease has an incubation period of up to 12 days and is characterized by a sudden onset of fever, chills, headache, eye pain, generalized myalgia, joint pain and swelling, diarrhea, vomiting, and rash of 3–5 days' duration.[3,8,18] Although MAYV disease is considered self-limiting, the joint disease, which usually involves the wrists, ankles, and toes, and less commonly the elbows and knees, can be incapacitating and persist for months.[3] Approximately two-thirds of patients develop a fine maculopapular rash on the trunk and extremities, appearing around the fifth day of illness and lasting about 3 days. Leukopenia, with moderate lymphocytosis, occurs in most patients during the first week of illness, and may be accompanied by mildly abnormal liver function tests.

Ross River Virus Infection

The reported incubation period of RRVI ranges from 3 to 21 days (mean, 9), and disease begins suddenly with headache, malaise, myalgia, and joint pain.[3,9,19] Multiple joints are involved, most commonly the ankles, fingers, knees, and wrists. Pain and loss of function usually last for several weeks, but some patients have persistent or recurrent fatigue, myalgia, arthralgia, and arthritis for a year or more. About half of patients develop a maculopapular rash, usually lasting 5–10 days, and half have low-grade fever. Disease incidence peaks in the 20–70 years age range, and is uncommon in children. The skin rash and joint swelling appear to be due to a local cell-mediated immune response rather than to immune complexes or a complement-mediated reaction.[3,9] The synovial fluid shows a mononuclear cell predominance, with persistence of viral antigen and RNA for a few weeks.

Chikungunya Virus Infection

CHIKV infection is characterized by the sudden onset of fever, chills, headache, photophobia, backache, arthralgia, and conjunctivitis. Patients are quite sick, although the acute illness only lasts about 3–5 days, with recovery usually in 5–7 days.[3] The incubation period is about 2–4 days, and the most common complaint is the severe arthralgia and joint swelling, usually involving multiple joints, which is seen in 70% of cases. As with RRV and MAYV infections, some patients have persistent or recurrent joint pain and stiffness for a year or more. The rash associated with CHIKV is maculopapular and mainly involves the trunk, but may spread to the limbs. Hemorrhagic manifestations (petechiae, purpura, epistaxis, bleeding gums, hematemesis, and melena) have been reported rarely, associated with thrombocytopenia.[20] Recent CHIKV epidemics have included many deaths and, while many deceased patients had other underlying conditions, there is ongoing concern about CHIKV encephalitis and death. In India alone from August to November 2006, nearly 3000 excess deaths occurred during an epidemic.[21] Disability-adjusted life year (DALY) estimates during the 2006 Indian epidemic were as high as 265.62 per million in some states, which accounted for up to 69% of the total DALYs.[22]

O'nyong-nyong

Disease due to ONNV infection is clinically indistinguishable from CHIKV, including fever, joint pains, rash, and lymphadenopathy.[14]

DIAGNOSIS

Confident clinical diagnosis of alphavirus infections can be difficult unless an outbreak of disease of known etiology is ongoing. For example, the combination of fever, arthralgia, and lymphadenopathy has a specificity of 83% and a sensitivity of 61% in the identification of ONN cases during epidemics.[23] Generally, the arthritogenic viruses cause very similar illnesses, though CHIKV is typically more severe, and can also resemble dengue and a range of other infections. Similarly, VEE clinically resembles the flavivirus encephalitides, such as West Nile and Japanese encephalitis viruses, herpes simplex virus and other infectious agents. Therefore, definitive diagnosis of alphavirus infections generally requires virus detection or serologic confirmation.[3] Alphaviruses may be recovered from blood taken during the first 2–4 days of illness and, for VEEV, from pharyngeal swabs; most alphaviruses readily kill newborn mice after intracerebral inoculation, and produce cytopathic effect in a variety of mammalian and avian cell lines. More recently, detection of viral RNA has been applied to clinical samples and appears to be useful for detection of VEEV in serum and pharyngeal swabs,[6] and for the detection of CHIKV in serum early in illness.[24] VEEV serotypes can be identified using monoclonal antibodies and enzyme-linked immunosorbent assay (ELISA),[25] and phylogenetic studies have been used to delineate the source of outbreaks.[5]

A rapid presumptive diagnosis can be achieved using virus-specific IgM ELISA, though IgM commonly persists for months and does not always indicate recent infection. Cross-reactions with other alphavirus antibodies are uncommon. The exception is CHIKV and ONNV antibodies which are difficult to distinguish due to antigenic cross-reactivity.[14] Seroconversion or rising levels of IgG between acute and convalescent serum samples drawn 1–3 weeks apart is very useful for confirming recent infection. A variety of serologic tests can be used to detect alphavirus antibodies (ELISA, immunofluorescence, hemagglutination inhibition, and neutralization), but the availability of diagnostic tests is often restricted, especially for those that are uncommon or exotic to the area in which the laboratory is located.

TREATMENT AND PROGNOSIS

Treatment for VEEV encephalitis is symptomatic and supportive.[3] Control of convulsions and treatment of secondary bacterial infections, especially pneumonia and gastrointestinal infections, are important. Neurologic sequelae are common following severe VEE and include headache, forgetfulness, nervousness, and motor impairment.[3,6]

For the alphaviruses primarily causing arthritis (MAYV, RRV, CHIKV, ONNV), illness can be debilitating but is usually self-limiting. As there are no established specific therapies, symptomatic treatment with rest, heat, gentle exercise, simple analgesics, and nonsteroidal anti-inflammatory drugs (NSAIDs) is routine. Aspirin is better avoided in acute CHIKV infection due to the risk of exacerbating hemorrhagic disease. Persisting joint symptoms are common with a number of these viruses and are managed in a similar way to the acute pain. Steroid therapy is not recommended.[3]

PREVENTION AND CONTROL

No licensed human vaccines are available for alphaviruses, and control generally relies on interruption of transmission using vector control, vaccination of animal amplifying hosts, avoiding outdoor activities during peak mosquito biting times, use of protective clothing (including permethrin-impregnated clothes, nets, and bedding), and regular application of repellents containing either diethyltoluamide (DEET) or picardin. DEET can cause neurotoxicity, especially in children, and should be used strictly according to instructions.[3] Preventive measures are particularly important when people enter areas of known activity, such as the sylvatic habitats that support VEEV circulation, and are also most effective for vectors that tend to have crepuscular or night-time biting peaks, including *Culex* (*Melanoconion*) spp. that transmit VEEV and the *Anopheles* mosquitoes that transmit ONNV. Unfortunately these control measures may not be suitable for people who live and work in humid tropical areas. Protective clothing is uncomfortable, bednets are not effective for viruses such as MAYV that are transmitted by daytime-biting mosquitoes, and indefinite repeated application of insect repellents is impractical.

Vector control measures can be used where ecologically acceptable. Adulticide fogging to control adult mosquitoes can provide rapid, but temporary, control during epidemics. However, better results are achieved with manual or aerial application of insecticides such as malathion. These are optimally applied soon after floodwater species emerge from the aquatic immature stages, prior to dispersal, infection, and incubation required for transmission, and have been used successfully for control of VEEV and RRV outbreaks.[3] The live-attenuated TC-83 strain of VEEV has been used as a vaccine to protect the equine amplification hosts, and "barriers" of immunized equines may control the spread of outbreaks.

CHIKV is transmitted by urban *Ae. aegypti* and, in some locations *Ae. albopictus*, so control must focus on limiting contact with these species, which often lay their eggs in artificial water containers, prefer to rest indoors in the adult stage, and feed during the daytime. Therefore, treatment of water storage containers or barriers to access by mosquitoes, the use of persistent insecticides on interior walls, and insecticide and/or repellent impregnated window curtains may be more effective than typical vector control measures.

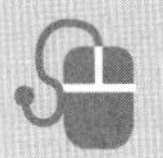

Access the complete reference list online at
http://www.expertconsult.com

Access the complete reference list online at http://www.expertconsult.com

CHAPTER 79

Rabies

Thomas P. Bleck

INTRODUCTION

Rabies is a viral disease producing an almost uniformly fatal encephalitis in humans and other mammals.[1] It has been known throughout recorded history and stands apart as the most nearly uniformly fatal of all viruses. Rabies remains one of the most common viral causes of mortality in tropical countries.[2]

Exposure to potentially rabid animals has profound economic and medical implications; about 4 million people receive postexposure treatment (PET) annually to prevent rabies.[3] Despite technology that permits the production of safe agents for PET, economic considerations frequently lead to the use of older, more dangerous vaccines in the developing world, with catastrophic neurologic complications as a result.

The word rabies comes from the Latin *rabere*, to rage. Rabies is also related to the Sanskrit word for violence, *rabhas*. The Greek term for rabies, *lyssa*, madness, is the source of the taxonomic name of the viral genus, *Lyssavirus*. The Babylon Eshnuna code (twenty-third century BCE) probably contains the first mention of rabies.[4,5] The Greek philosopher Democritus provided the first clear description of animal rabies in about 500 BCE. Wound cauterization was mentioned in the first century CE and remained the only real treatment until Pasteur introduced immunization in 1885. St Hubert, a medieval European healing saint, is depicted with a large key that was heated and used for cautery. In the twelfth century, Maimonides advised thorough wound cleansing, suction, cautery, and rest. Wound cautery remained part of most suggestions for potentially rabid animal bites into the middle of the twentieth century.

The diagnosis of rabies was purely clinical until 1903, when Adelchi Negri described cytoplasmic inclusions (Negri bodies) in this disorder.[6] He initially thought that the inclusion body was part of the life cycle of a parasite.[7] This was the only pathologic marker until the introduction of fluorescent antibody techniques for rabies in 1958.[8]

THE AGENT

The family *Rhabdoviridae* are negatively stranded RNA viruses consisting of two genera that infect animals (*Lyssavirus* and *Vesiculovirus*) and the plant rhabdovirus group.[9] The type species of the subfamily *Lyssaviridae* is rabies (serotype 1),[10] and that of the subfamily *Vesiculoviridae* is vesicular stomatitis virus. Rabies is enzootic, and sometimes epizootic, in many mammals, most commonly wild and domestic canids (e.g., dogs, foxes, coyotes), mustelids (e.g., skunks, badgers, martens), viverids (e.g., mongooses, civets, genets), procyonids (e.g., raccoons and their allies), and insectivorous and hematophagous bats. The five other members of the *Lyssavirus* genus are rare causes of human disease (***Table 79.1***).

The rabies virus is bullet-shaped, with an average length of 180 nm (range, 130–200 nm) and an average diameter of 75 nm (range, 60–110 nm).[11] The complete virus contains a helical nucleocapsid with 30–35 coils with a length unwound between 4.2 and 4.6 μm.[12] The nucleocapsid is enclosed in a 7.5–10-nm-thick lipoprotein envelope; from this envelope, glycoprotein (G protein) spikes project out another 10 nm. The spikes cover the entire surface of the virus except for part of the blunt end.

The rabies viral genome is a single negative strand of RNA weighing 4.6 MDa, and contains a sequence of 11 932 nucleotides.[13] This RNA encodes five genes, named N, NS (or M_1), M (or M_2), G, and L. The N nucleoprotein binds to the RNA and is probably involved in the control of viral RNA replication; it is a potential immunogen.[14] The purpose of the NS phosphoprotein is less clear, but it may control the L protein, which is the polymerase for replication.[15,16] The M (matrix) protein is the major structural protein and is probably located between the nucleocapsid and lipoprotein envelope[17]; its role is uncertain.[11] The G protein is involved in cell surface reception, and it is the only antigen that induces virus-neutralizing antibodies. Variability in this protein accounts for serotypic differences among lyssaviruses,[18] and mutations at arginine 333 cause loss of virulence.[19] This arginine residue is required for G protein-mediated fusion of the viral envelope with neurons.[20] Molecular modifications of the G protein can increase its antigenicity[21] and may aid in the search for better vaccines.

The nicotinic acetylcholine receptor is an important viral binding site, but it is probably not the only one. Once bound to the receptor, receptor-mediated endocytosis allows the virus to enter the neuron. This forms a coated pit, which then fuses with a lysosome, where enzymes release the nucleocapsid into the cytosol.[22] Five messenger RNAs (mRNAs) for production of the viral proteins are transcribed, and a full-length, positively stranded RNA is produced as the template for the viral progeny.[23] The envelope forms from host cisternal membranes into which the G and M proteins are inserted.[24] In natural infections the virus accumulates in cytoplasmic cisterns from which it is released either by membrane fusion or dissolution of the cell.[22]

The virus does not tolerate pH below 3 or above 11, and it is inactivated by ultraviolet light, sunlight, desiccation, or exposure to formalin, phenol, ether, trypsin, β-propiolactone, and detergents.

EPIDEMIOLOGY

Human Rabies

Rabies occurs throughout the world except in Antarctica and a few island nations. In 1999 (the last year for which global data are available), 99 of 151 nations reported the presence of rabies.[25]

The epidemiology of human rabies is that of animal rabies in the community.[26] In developing areas where canine rabies is common, most cases of human rabies result from dog bites. Conversely, rabid wild animals are usually responsible for human rabies in regions where dogs are vaccinated. The spectrum of animals implicated in rabies transmission to humans continues to expand.[27] Transmission via organ donation from a

Table 79.1 Members of the *Lyssavirus* Genus

Rabies Virus	Serotype	Reservoir	Comments	Cross-Protection with Vaccine
Rabies	1	Found worldwide except for a few island nations, Australia, and Antarctica. The vast majority of human cases occur in areas of uncontrolled domestic dog rabies		Not applicable
Lagos bat	2	Probably enzootic in fruit bats. At least 10 cases have been identified, including three in domestic animals, in Nigeria, South Africa, Zimbabwe, Central African Republic, Senegal, and Ethiopia. No reported human cases	First isolated in 1956 from brains of Nigerian fruit bats. Some cases initially diagnosed as rabies, but displayed weak immunofluorescence and later distinguished by monoclonal antibody or nucleotide sequence analysis	Marginal
Mokola	3	Probably an insectivore or rodent species. Cases identified in Nigeria, South Africa, Cameroon, Zimbabwe, Central African Republic, and Ethiopia. At least 19 known cases, including 11 domestic animals and 2 human cases	First isolated from shrews in Nigeria in 1968	None
Duvenhage	4	Probably insectivorous bats. Cases identified in South Africa, Zimbabwe, and Senegal. Four cases known, including one human death. No cases in domestic animals	First identified in 1970 in a man with a rabies-like encephalitis in South Africa (virus named after the patient). Negri bodies were present, but immunofluorescent stains were negative	Marginal
European bat lyssavirus 1 (EBLV1)	5	European insectivorous bats (probably *Eptesicus serotimus*). Over 400 bat cases and one confirmed human death and another suspected. No known domestic animal cases	Suspected as early as 1954 but not identified until 1985. Almost all cases are in the common European house bat	Marginal
European bat lyssavirus 2 (EBLV2)	6	European insectivorous bats (probably *Myotis dasycneme*). Five known cases, including one human death. No known domestic animal cases	First identified in a Swiss bat biologist who died in Finland	Marginal

(Adapted from Rupprecht CE, Smith JS, Fekadu M, et al. The ascension of wildlife rabies: a cause for public health concern or intervention? Emerg Infect Dis. 1995;1:107–114.)

donor not known to have rabies underscores the need for a higher index of suspicion for rabies.[28]

In 1999, 1866 cases of human rabies were reported to the World Health Organization (WHO).[25] These reports represent a substantial underestimate of the worldwide incidence of the disease, which probably causes as many as 100 000 deaths annually. The methods used for the diagnosis of rabies and their corresponding validities vary considerably across the globe. In Africa and Asia, more than 85% of cases are diagnosed on clinical grounds alone, and the source of exposure is not reported for more than half of these. An estimated 4 million persons receive PET annually; the vast majority of these patients are treated with vaccine types carrying a substantial risk of neurologic complications.[29]

Animal Rabies

Animal rabies throughout the world occurs in two types of clusters. In the developing world, rabies predominantly affects domestic or feral animals, with infection of wild animals less important in transmission of disease to humans. In more developed nations, animal control procedures have substantially eliminated rabies from domestic animal populations, and wild animals are the group most affected. For example, bat rabies is the most rapidly increasing source of human infections in the United States.[30] The relative susceptibilities of different animal species to rabies are shown in ***Table 79.2***.

Table 79.2 Approximate Mortality Rates in Nonvaccinated Patients after Exposure to Rabid Dogs

Location	Type	Extent	Mortality (%)
Face	Bite	Multiple, deep	60
Head (other than face)	Bite	Multiple, deep	50
Face	Bite	Single	30
Fingers or hand	Bite	Severe	15
Face	Bite	Multiple, superficial	10
Hand	Bite	Multiple, superficial	5
Trunk or legs	Scratch	Superficial	3
Exposed skin	Bleeding	Superficial wound	2
Skin covered by clothing	Wound	Superficial	0.5
Recent wound	Contamination by saliva		0.1
Wounds >24 hours old	Contamination by saliva		0.0

(Data from Whitley RJ, Middlebrooks M. Rabies. In: Scheld WM, Whitley RJ, Durack DT, eds. Infections of the Central Nervous System. New York: Raven Press; 1991:127–149.)

PATHOLOGY

The appearance of the brain at autopsy is generally unremarkable,[31] except for the vascular congestion expected in patients dying after prolonged mechanical ventilation. The histologic study of rabies typically shows an encephalitis with Negri bodies. However, not all specimens show perivascular lymphocytic cuffing and necrosis (which characterize encephalitis), and some cases have the histology of meningitis.[32]

Negri bodies are concentrated in hippocampal pyramidal cells and somewhat less frequently in cortical neurons and cerebellar Purkinje cells.[31] These eosinophilic cytoplasmic inclusions are round or oval and measure between 1 and 7 μm across. Immunofluorescent and ultrastructural analyses confirm that they contain rabies viral nucleocapsids.[33] The acidophilic lyssa body is ultrastructurally identical to the Negri body.[34]

Paralytic rabies expresses the majority of its pathologic changes in the spinal cord, with severe inflammation and neuronal necrosis;[35] the brainstem is less involved, and a minority of cases have cortical Negri bodies. Segmental demyelination of peripheral nerves is common in these patients, which may explain the resemblance of paralytic rabies to acute inflammatory polyneuropathy (the Guillain–Barré syndrome).

The most important systemic finding in rabies is myocarditis, present in a large number of cases.[36] Its cause is uncertain, but it resembles the myocarditis of other hypercatecholaminergic states (e.g., pheochromocytoma, subarachnoid hemorrhage, and tetanus). However, the hearts of some patients demonstrate Negri bodies, suggesting a more direct pathogenic role for the virus.[37] The discovery of atrial ganglioneuritis suggests that the virus reaches the myocardium via spread from the nervous system.[38] Other postmortem findings reflect the complications commonly seen during a critical illness, such as upper gastrointestinal tract bleeding.

THE DISEASE

Human Rabies

Transmission

Many variables affect the risk of rabies, as well as the incubation period, after exposure to a rabid animal.[39] The viral inoculum must play an important role, expressed in clinical practice as a relationship of rapidity with the extent of exposure to the saliva of a rabid animal (*Table 79.3*). Exposures in which large amounts of saliva contaminate a wound are more likely to produce rabies than a bite through thick clothing, which removes most of the saliva; and multiple bites are more likely to transmit the disease than a single one. The location of the bite is also an important determinant of the likelihood of developing disease (e.g., bites on the face are more likely to produce disease than those on the extremities). Salivary contamination of a preexisting wound, mucous membranes, or the respiratory tract (with aerosolized virus)[40] may also spread virus. Direct human-to-human transmission has been documented only in cases of transplants; one recipient was treated with standard PET plus interferon and did not become ill.[37,41]

Table 79.3 Durations of Different Stages of Rabies

Stage	Type (% of Cases)	Duration (% of Cases)	Associated Findings
Incubation period		<30 days (25%)	None
		30–90 days (50%)	
		90 days–1 year (20%)	
		>1 year (5%)	
Prodrome and early symptoms		2–10 days	Paresthesias or pain at wound site, fever, malaise, anorexia, nausea and vomiting
Acute neurologic disease	Furious rabies (80%)		Hallucinations, bizarre behavior, anxiety, agitation, biting, hydrophobia, autonomic dysfunction, syndrome of inappropriate antidiuretic hormone
	Paralytic rabies (20%)	2–7 days	Ascending flaccid paralysis
Coma		0–14 days	Death[a]

[a]Rare recoveries have been reported.

(Data from Fishbein DB. Rabies in humans. In: Barr GM, ed. The Natural History of Rabies, 2nd ed. Boca Raton: CRC Press; 1991:519–549.)

Incubation

The reported incubation period varies from days to more than 19 years, with 75% of patients becoming ill within 90 days of exposure (*Table 79.4*).

Prodrome

The initial symptoms of rabies resemble those of other systemic viral infections, including fever, headache, malaise, and upper respiratory and gastrointestinal tract disorders.[42] Neurologic problems include changes in personality and cognition, and paresthesias or pain near the exposure site. Because these complaints are so common, rabies is rarely considered early in the differential diagnosis. In one series, rabies was considered in only 3 of 21 patients during the first visit to a physician, despite an exposure history.[42] The prodrome usually lasts about 4 days, but as many as 10 days may elapse before more specific findings develop.[39,43] Myoedema (mounding of a part of the muscle struck with a reflex hammer) develops during the prodrome and persists thereafter.

Established Disease

Human rabies is typically seen in two forms: furious and paralytic (or dumb). Furious rabies (80% of cases) is dominated by encephalitis and presents with hydrophobia, delirium, and agitation. Paralytic rabies shows little clinical evidence of cerebral cortical involvement until late. The pathologic distinction between these forms is primarily quantitative: the spinal cord and brainstem are more involved in the paralytic form. The reasons underlying the two types of rabies are unknown but do not appear to involve virologic or antigenic differences[44] or identified host factors.

Both forms of symptomatic rabies usually last between 2 and 14 days before the onset of coma, and death follows about 18 days after the onset, with a broad range described.[42] Critical care services prolong survival by about 50% but do not appear to change the outcome.[45]

Furious Rabies

Hydrophobia is the symptom most identified with furious rabies; it implies more than simple difficulty swallowing water and produces fear even of the sight of water despite strong thirst (*Fig. 79.1*). Hydrophobia probably represents an exaggerated irritant reflex of the respiratory tract, perhaps due to viral involvement of the nucleus ambiguus.[46] Other manifestations of the furious form include hyperactivity, seizures, and aerophobia. Hyperventilation is frequently present, presumably reflecting brainstem infection. When coma supervenes, pituitary dysfunction, especially disordered water balance (either inappropriate antidiuresis or diabetes insipidus), frequently develops. More serious forms of ventilatory dysfunction replace hyperventilation, including periodic and ataxic respiration,[46] and eventually apnea may end the patient's struggles. Cardiac arrhythmias, mostly supraventricular tachycardias and bradycardias,[47] occur frequently, as a consequence of either brainstem dysfunction or myocarditis.[48] Other autonomic abnormalities include pupillary dilation, anisocoria, piloerection, increased salivation and sweating, and priapism,[49] including spontaneous ejaculation as well as erections.[50]

Table 79.4 Susceptibility of Various Animal Species to Rabies

Very high	High	Moderate	Low
Wolf	Hamster	Dog	Opossum
Fox	Skunk	Primate	
Coyote	Raccoon		
Kangaroo rat	Domestic cat		
Cotton rat	Rabbit		
Jackal	Bat		
Vole	Cattle		

(Data from Sixth Report of the Expert Committee on Rabies. World Health Organ Tech Rep Ser. 1973;523.)

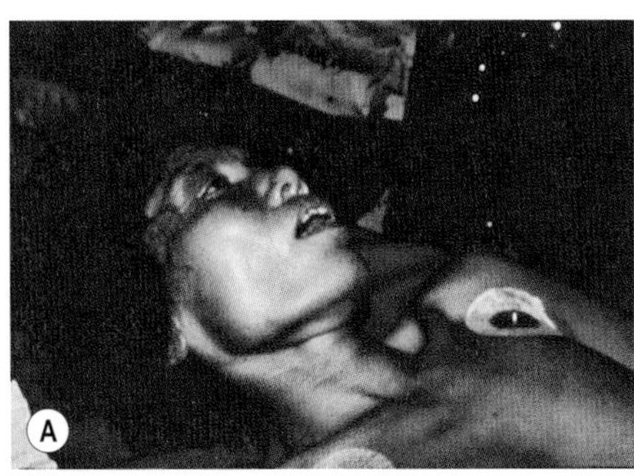

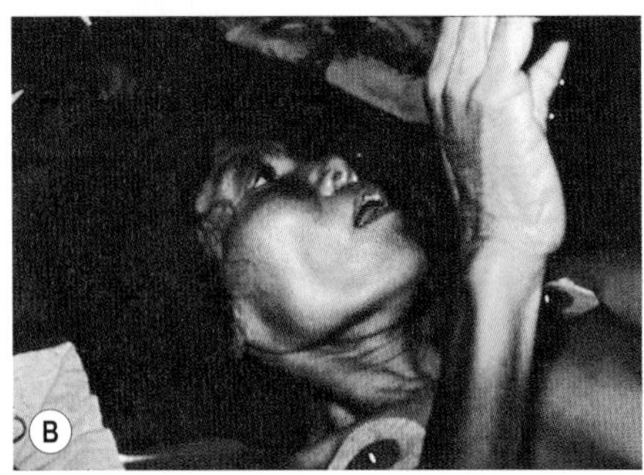

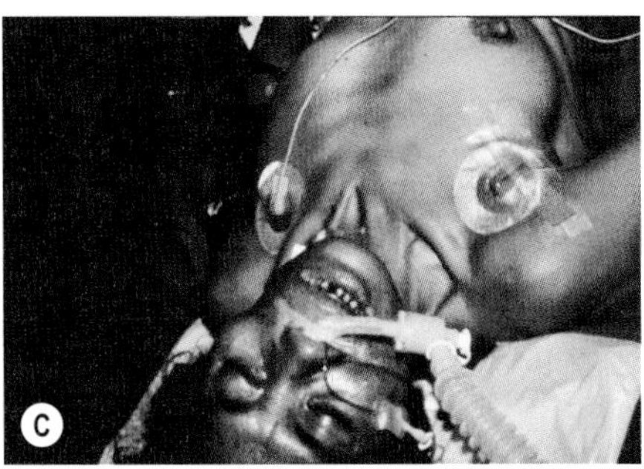

Figure 79.1 Clinical features of furious rabies. **(A)** The grimace and stare which accompany the pharyngeal spasms of hydrophobia. **(B)** Aerophobia provoked by air movement across the patient's face. **(C)** Inspiratory spasm. (Reproduced from Hanley DF, Glass JD, McArthur JC, et al. Viral encephalitis and related conditions. In: Bleck TP, ed. Atlas of Infectious Diseases, Vol. 3: Central Nervous System and Eye Infections. New York: Churchill Livingstone; 1995:3.28.)

Most furious rabies patients entering coma die within 1–2 weeks despite maximal supportive care. Those receiving maximal intensive care support and surviving for a longer-than-expected period pass through the paralytic phase prior to death.[45]

Paralytic (Dumb) Rabies

In contrast to furious rabies, paralytic rabies patients lack signs of cortical irritation (hydrophobia, aerophobia, hyperactivity, seizures). They may present with ascending paralysis or symmetrical tetraparesis. Weakness may be most severe in the exposed extremity. Headache and neck stiffness may be prominent despite a normal sensorium. As the condition progresses, the patient becomes confused and then comatose.

Nonneurologic Findings

In addition to the cardiac arrhythmias mentioned previously, the systemic complications of rabies are similar to those of other critically ill patients. Although the virus disseminates to many organs, its role in nonneurologic organ dysfunction is uncertain. Hypoxemia often develops and is frequently attributed to atelectasis, aspiration pneumonia, or congestive heart failure from myocarditis. Hypotension probably reflects volume depletion but may also follow brainstem involvement. Gastrointestinal complications, in addition to bleeding, include vomiting, diarrhea, and ileus.[51] Those who do not succumb to these complications usually die of rabies myocarditis, manifested as cardiac arrhythmia, or congestive heart failure.[52]

Animal Rabies

WHO has established a ranking of animal rabies susceptibility (see *Table 79.4*).[53] Rabies in dogs and cats is similar to the human disease. Dogs display subtle behavioral changes during the prodromal phase, then enter an excitative (furious) phase; they are agitated, are restless, and may bite without provocation. Paralysis of laryngeal muscles produces a high-pitched bark.[54] Animals in the paralytic (dumb) phase display a "dropped jaw" from masseter weakness. Up to 24% of experimentally infected dogs in one study died without showing any signs of illness but were pathologically demonstrated to be rabid, making symptoms an unreliable guide to diagnosis.[55] The canine incubation period may last 8 months.[56] Other studies suggest that the incubation period depends on the inoculum and strain involved; experiments simulating natural infection suggest a period between 7 and 125 days,[55] and other experimental studies suggest that between 0% and 20% of infected dogs may recover without treatment.[54]

Cats have a 2–3-day prodrome, with subtle behavioral changes, slight fever, pupillary dilation, and impaired corneal reflexes. Most rabid cats then become furious, frequently scratching or biting without provocation. During the next 2–4 days, hypersalivation, tremor, and incoordination are common. Paralysis then ensues, and convulsions may develop; death usually follows in a few days. A description of behavioral changes in wild animals may be found in Baer.[57]

PATHOGENESIS

Virus can enter both motor and sensory nerves. Murphy and colleagues first deciphered the pathogenesis of rabies infection in exquisite studies.[31,58] The process begins with movement of the virus through peripheral nerves to the central nervous system (CNS), CNS viral proliferation, and subsequent spread via peripheral nerves to many other tissues. The virus initially replicates in muscle cells, infecting the muscle spindle, then the nerve innervating the spindle, and subsequently moves centrally through the axons of these neurons. It appears in dorsal root ganglia within 72 hours of inoculation, prior to its appearance in spinal cord neurons. Other studies suggest that the neuromuscular junction may be another site of neuronal invasion.[59] A partial homology between rabies virus glycoprotein and several snake neurotoxins that bind specifically to the nicotinic acetylcholine receptor may explain this phenomenon.[60]

Natural rabies infection seems to require a period of local replication, possibly to increase the inoculum, before nervous system infection occurs. During this period, passive and active immunization can prevent spread of the virus into the nervous system and thus prevent the disease. Once the virus enters peripheral nerves, current therapies do not seem to prevent replication and spread. However, antibody delivery across the blood–brain barrier may allow more effective later treatments.[61]

Once the virus invades peripheral nerve cells, it moves via retrograde axoplasmic flow to their central processes,[62,63] in contrast to herpes simplex virus or tetanus toxin, which use microtubular transport.[64] Once in the spinal cord or brainstem, the virus spreads throughout the CNS, with virtually every neuron infected.[24] After CNS infection, the virus spreads to the rest of the body via the peripheral nerves. Direct viral replication occurs in the salivary glands, but the high concentration of virus in saliva also reflects shedding from sensory nerve endings in the oral mucosa.

The mechanisms by which rabies virus produces CNS dysfunction are obscure; in many cases pathologic evidence of neuronal necrosis is minimal. Interference with neurotransmission may be important,[65,66] and a nearly 30-fold increase in nitric oxide production suggests an excitotoxic mechanism.[67]

Immune Response

The human response to natural rabies infection is insufficient to prevent disease. This may be a consequence of an insufficient antigenic load,[42] but this contention is disputed.[49] Viral replication at an immunologically "privileged" site (the CNS) may also limit the host response. Rabies virus can produce immunosuppression;[68] only a few unvaccinated rabies patients develop measurable antibody.[69] Interleukin-1 production in the CNS during infection may explain the immunosuppressive effect.[70] Those who develop a cellular immune response to the virus tend to have the encephalitic form rather than the paralytic form, and they die sooner than those who do not mount such a response.[71]

Rabies virus may be able to persist in macrophages and may later emerge to produce disease.[72] This may explain the occasional cases with very long incubation periods.

DIAGNOSIS

The diagnosis poses little difficulty in a nonimmune patient with hydrophobia after a bite by a rabid animal, but the presentation of rabies in places where domestic animals are immunized is seldom this straightforward. As the disease becomes less common, physicians are less apt to consider the diagnosis. In some countries, an increasingly large percentage of cases are not associated with a known exposure to a potentially rabid animal (virologic studies frequently indicate that these cases are due to bat rabies viruses).

No diagnostic studies in the patient are useful during the incubation period; exposure to a potentially rabid animal should prompt prophylactic treatment rather than laboratory testing. Once symptoms begin, standard testing does not help distinguish rabies reliably from other encephalitides. The cerebrospinal fluid (CSF) is normal in the majority of patients but may reveal a lymphocytic pleocytosis (5–30 cells/μL), normal glucose, and modest protein elevation (less than 100 mg/dL).[73] Imaging studies are not specific, except to exclude other potential causes such as herpes simplex encephalitis. Magnetic resonance imaging may show lesions involving basal structures of the brain.[74,75,76]

The most important early diagnostic test in symptomatic patients is immunofluorescent staining of a skin biopsy obtained from the nape of the neck, above the hairline because the virus localizes in hair follicles.[77] Approximately 50% of samples reveal rabies virus in the first week of symptoms, and this percentage increases thereafter.[78] This test has been supplanted by reverse-transcription-polymerase chain reaction (RT-PCR) analysis of saliva for viral RNA (see http://www.cdc.gov/rabies/diagnosis.html).[79] The corneal impression test for infected cells is no longer commonly used.

The rapid fluorescent focus inhibition test (RFFIT) is the most commonly employed serologic test for neutralizing antibody.[80] In those receiving neither PET nor immunologic therapies, serum antibody is detectable in a small number of patients by day 6 of illness, in 50% by day 8, and usually in 100% by day 15. Any CSF levels are diagnostically valuable, including those of patients who received PET. CSF may also reveal the presence of specific oligoclonal antibodies not found in the serum as a method of confirming CNS infection.[81]

RT-PCR can be performed on CSF, saliva, or tissues of patients,[82,83] permitting more specific determination of the geographic and host species origin of a particular rabies virus.[83,84] It can be successfully performed on decomposed brain material,[85] a situation in which older techniques failed.[86] Other molecular techniques have been described, and may eventually complement or replace RT-PCR.[87]

Differential Diagnosis

The major differential diagnosis of furious rabies is that of another encephalitis. Lacking a known exposure to a rabid animal, and in those cases in which hydrophobia and hyperactivity are not prominent, it is difficult to distinguish between these possibilities.[88] Since rabies occasionally mimics herpes simplex encephalitis, some patients receive empirical therapy with acyclovir pending a more secure diagnosis. While no data are available concerning this approach, anecdotes regarding the use of vidarabine in rabies do not suggest that it alters the course of the disease.[73]

Tetanus may be confused with rabies, since opisthotonic posturing occurs in both.[64] However, the other findings in rabies (e.g., hydrophobia) are not seen in tetanus, and the CSF is normal in tetanus. The spasms of rabies lack the marked stimulus sensitivity of tetanus, and patients with rabies lack the persistent rigidity of tetanus patients. Strychnine poisoning should be considered.

The paralytic form may variously resemble acute inflammatory polyneuropathy, transverse myelitis, or poliomyelitis. Electromyographic studies may distinguish rabies from polyneuropathy. The complaint of aching pain at the level of the lesion suggests transverse myelitis, as does a high T2 signal lesion in the spinal cord on magnetic resonance imaging. Sensory function is typically normal in rabies patients,[49] whereas a sensory-level abnormality is characteristic of transverse myelitis. A high fever typically precedes the weakness of poliomyelitis, and the resolution of fever with the onset of neurologic findings may be a useful clue favoring this diagnosis over rabies. A history of poliomyelitis or immunization against it should be sought.

CNS reactions to the rabies vaccines available in more developed countries are exceptionally rare, but patients receiving older vaccine forms containing myelin determinants can develop acute disseminated encephalomyelitis (ADEM; also called postvaccinial encephalomyelitis; see Prevention). ADEM has many other known precipitants and may also be cryptogenic. ADEM may seem like a typical encephalitis or may present as a mass lesion resembling a brain abscess. It typically begins 10–14 days after vaccine exposure, an unusually brief incubation for rabies. In the absence of viral isolation, a high RFFIT titer in spinal fluid is evidence of rabies rather than of ADEM, even in patients who have been immunized.[89]

Some persons exposed to a potentially rabid animal may suffer a psychological reaction termed rabies hysteria.[90] They may refuse to attempt to drink, in contrast to those with rabies whose attempts to drink are halted by pharyngeal spasms.

TREATMENT AND PROGNOSIS

There is no established treatment for rabies once symptoms have begun; almost all patients succumb to the disease or its complications within a few weeks of onset. Three survivors have been reported, two of whom apparently made a full recovery.[39,43] Each had undergone some form of PET, which probably modified their courses. Partial recovery occurred in another who received rabies vaccine without immunoglobulin.[81] A working group has published suggestions for the treatment of rabies victims.[91] Using some of these recommendations, a single case of survival without PET has been reported.[92]

Supportive therapy includes intubation, sedation, mechanical ventilation, fluid and electrolyte management, nutrition, and management of intercurrent illnesses and complications.[45] However, none of the patients reported has survived more than 17 days despite aggressive antirabies treatment and symptomatic care.

PREVENTION AND CONTROL

Rabies vaccination for prevention and PET was introduced in the nineteenth century, first by Galtier and later by Pasteur.[93]

While the control of animal rabies is central to the prevention of human disease, only a few nations have succeeded in eliminating rabies, and these maintain quarantine procedures lest the disease reappear. Thus, prophylaxis (for domestic animals and selected humans) and PET remain essential to the prevention of clinical rabies. Cat and dog rabies prophylaxis is mandated by law in many countries; for example, in the United States, 1–3-year vaccines are permitted (although only 3-year vaccines are recommended by the National Association of State Public Health Veterinarians).[94] Vaccination should be supervised by a veterinarian; improper administration can lead to lack of immunity.[95] Some vaccines lack potency; in developing countries, measuring animal seroconversion rates may be considered to ensure protection.[96] Immunizing livestock is recommended in areas of increasing prevalence.

Table 79.5 World Health Organization Guide to Postexposure Prophylaxis

Category	Type of Contact with a Suspect or Confirmed Rabid Domestic or Wild Animal or Animal Category Unavailable for Observation	Recommended Treatment
	Rabid domestic or wild[a] animal, or animal	Unavailable for recommended treatment
I	Touching or feeding of animals; licks on intact skin	None, if reliable case history is available
II	Nibbling of uncovered skin; minor scratches or abrasions without bleeding; licks on broken skin	Administer vaccine immediately;[b] stop treatment if animal remains healthy throughout an observation period[c] of 10 days or if animal is euthanized and found to be negative for rabies by appropriate laboratory techniques
III	Single or multiple transdermal bites or scratches; contamination of mucous membrane with saliva (i.e., licks)	Administer rabies immunoglobulin and vaccine immediately;[b] stop treatment if animal remains healthy throughout an observation period[c] of 10 days or if animal is killed humanely and found to be negative for rabies by appropriate laboratory techniques

[a]Exposure to rodents, rabbits, and hares seldom, if ever, requires specific antirabies treatment.

[b]If an apparently healthy dog or cat in or from a low-risk area is placed under observation, it may be justifiable to delay specific treatment.

[c]This observation period applies only to dogs and cats. Except in the case of threatened or endangered species, other domestic and wild animals suspected as rabid should be euthanized and their tissues examined using appropriate laboratory techniques.

(Reproduced from World Health Organization, Emerging and Other Communicable Disease Branch. WHO Recommendations on Rabies Post-Exposure Treatment and the Correct Technique on Intradermal Immunization Against Rabies. Geneva: World Health Organization. Available online at http://whqlibdoc.who.int/hq/1996/WHO_EMC_200_96.6.pdf. Accessed 11/09/09.)

Wild-animal vaccination can be an effective veterinary public health measure. Vaccines that are effective after ingestion allow vaccination of free-ranging animals.[97] An intensive 4-year campaign in Belgium nearly eliminated rabies from the fox population. Veterinary vaccines prepared in continuous cell lines cost about $0.50 per dose in the United States, in contrast to the Semple-type human vaccines costing about $5 for a course; Vero cell vaccine in France costs about $160 per course, and human diploid cell rabies vaccine (HDCV) in the United States costs more than $500 per course.[98]

Pre-exposure Prophylaxis

Pre-exposure prophylaxis is indicated for those with a relatively high risk of rabies exposure. This includes veterinarians, workers in laboratories using the virus, spelunkers, and those planning to visit countries with a high prevalence of dog rabies for more than 30 days. Recommendations for international travelers are available at http://www.cdc.gov/diseases/rabies.html. A series of three intramuscular (or intradermal, if using a vaccine prepared for this route) injections over a 3-week course are sufficient; antibody response determination is not required in normal hosts. A four-dose intradermal scheme has recently been described.[99] Booster doses are recommended every 2–3 years for persons remaining at risk of exposure. If antibody titers are checked, an adequate response is generally considered to be complete neutralization at the 1:5 level by RFFIT, which is equivalent to the 0.5 IU/mL concentration suggested by WHO.

Postexposure Treatment

After exposure, rabies prevention begins with good wound care, which reduces the risk of rabies by up to 90%.[100] Wash the wound thoroughly with a 20% soap solution; this is as effective as the previously recommended quaternary ammonium compounds.[101] This should be followed by application of 70% ethanol or an iodine-containing solution. Wounds should not be sutured prior to a decision about PET; if a wound must be sutured, rabies immunoglobulin should be instilled into the wound and infiltrated around it (see later discussion). Failure to infiltrate wounds with rabies immunoglobulin, or surgical closure of wounds prior to immunoglobulin infiltration, has been associated with the development of rabies in patients despite otherwise proper PET.[102]

Following wound care, the clinician must decide whether to institute passive or active immunization. Prompt consultation with public health officials is advised, since this decision is based on the current incidence of rabies in the animal species involved in the exposure.[103] WHO recently summarized its recommended approach (***Table 79.5***).[104] The most recent report of the Immunization Practices Advisory Committee is also an important source of information.[105] A decision analysis model may be useful in deciding who should receive prophylaxis.[106]

In general, a healthy dog or cat in countries of low prevalence that has transferred saliva to a human is observed for 10 days. If the animal's behavior remains normal, the patient need not receive PET beyond proper wound care. If its behavior changes, it should undergo immediate pathologic examination for evidence of rabies infection; there is still adequate time to institute PET if rabies is confirmed. Wild mammal exposure, especially if the animal exhibits uncharacteristic behavior, warrants PET in most circumstances. If the animal is available for pathologic examination, and direct fluorescent antibody testing of the brain does not indicate the presence of rabies virus, PET may be discontinued. PET appears safe in pregnant women and should not be withheld for this reason.[107]

Antirabies immunoglobulin is available in both human (HRIG) and equine forms (pooled antirabies serum, and purified antirabies serum of equine origin (equine rabies immunoglobulin, ERIG)). These immunoglobulins are purified from donors that were hyperimmunized with rabies vaccine. The need for immunoglobulin administration with currently available vaccines is uncertain, but the consequence of vaccine failure indicates its routine employment. HRIG is given in a dose of 20 IU/kg, with half injected in the vicinity of the wound (see earlier discussion), and the remainder injected intramuscularly in the gluteal region. The dose of ERIG is 40 IU/kg.

Many different rabies vaccines have been produced since 1882. In some developing countries, vaccine prepared from virus grown in adult animal nerve tissue (Semple vaccine) is still employed, but it carries a risk of central and peripheral neurologic complications in the range of 1 in 200 to 1 in 1600 vaccinees.[43] Its efficacy is uncertain. Production of vaccine in sheep CNS, a common method of Semple-type vaccine production, also carries the theoretical risk of transmitting the scrapie prion.[108] Although these reactions are often assumed to be a consequence of an immune reaction to myelin basic protein in the vaccine, only a minority of patients appear to develop antibody against this constituent of myelin.[109] Suckling mouse brain vaccine is effective and safer, with a neurologic complication rate approximating 1 in 8000.

The currently employed human vaccines in the United States include HDCV and a vaccine grown in rhesus monkey diploid cell cultures (rabies vaccine, adsorbed, RVA). These vaccines are remarkably safe and immunogenic. Local reactions (pain, swelling, or induration) may be common, but systemic complaints (fever, headache, malaise, nausea, abdominal pain, or adenopathy) occur in a minority of patients. Serious reactions have been exceedingly rare, with Guillain–Barré syndrome reported in a few patients[110] and a chimpanzee.[111] Corticosteroids should not be given to patients experiencing a vaccine reaction unless that reaction is life-threatening because they interfere with the development of immunity. Immunocompromised patients may not respond adequately to vaccination and should undergo measurement of antibody titers 2–4 weeks after immunization to ensure adequate immunization.[105]

In other countries, other PET vaccines and regimens are often employed. Consultation with the rabies officer of the state health department may be helpful in the management of patients in whom PET has been initiated with a vaccine not approved for use in the United States.

The usual dose of HDCV or RVA for PET is 1.0 mL intramuscularly on the day of exposure (or as soon as possible thereafter), repeated on days 3, 7, 14, and 28. If possible, the vaccine should be administered in the deltoid muscle. Gluteal injections, which may miss the muscle, have been associated with some vaccine failures. In small children, the vaccine may be given in the lateral thigh. The vaccine must not be given in the same region as the immunoglobulin. The intradermal vaccine was previously indicated only for pre-exposure prophylaxis, but current WHO recommendations include schedules for its use in PET (***Fig. 79.2***). Patients who have been previously vaccinated receive 1.0 mL on days 0 and 3 only, without rabies immunoglobulin.

A single case of a transient false-positive enzyme-linked immunosorbent assay for human immunodeficiency virus after HDCV immunization was reported in 1994.[112] Subsequent screening of samples from 50 patients recently immunized against rabies revealed no similar cases,[113] but in view of a similar phenomenon with other vaccines, physicians administering rabies vaccines should be aware of this possibility.

The limited extent of cross-protection among different lyssaviruses, and the possibility that antigenic differences in lyssaviruses from different locales may impair vaccine efficacy, should prompt future efforts to produce a vaccine effective against all *Lyssavirus* variants. The nucleic acid vaccine approach is promising.[114] Further research in these areas may produce a stable, inexpensive vaccine that could lead to simple, safe, and effective prophylaxis and PET.

Standard WHO intramuscular regimen

Dose: one IM dose (0.1 or 0.5 mL) into deltoid

Day 0 3 7 14 28

5 vials

5 visits

Rabies immunoglobulin

Reduced multisite intramuscular regimen (2-1-1)

Dose: one IM dose (0.1 or 0.5 mL) into deltoid

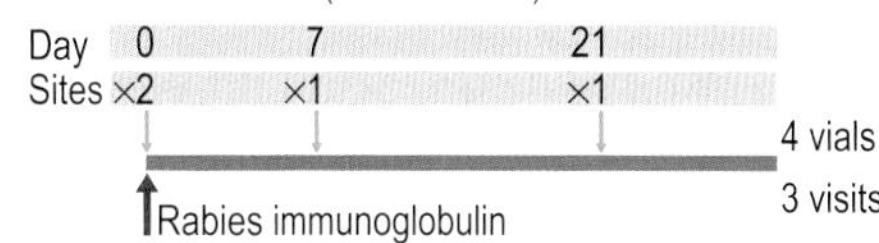

8-site intradermal regimen (8-0-4-0-1-1)

Dose: 0.1 mL ID per site

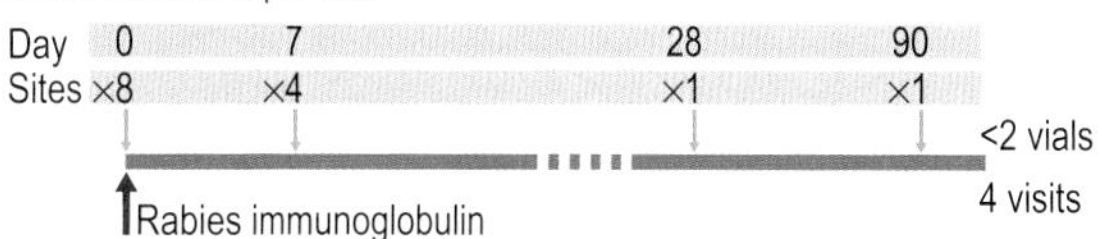

2-site intradermal regimen (2-2-2-0-1-1)

Dose: one ID dose = one fifth of IM dose (0.1 or 0.2 mL), ID per site

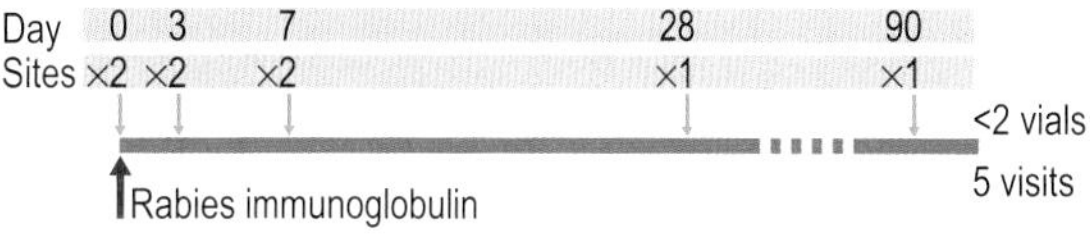

Figure 79.2 World Health Organization (WHO) recommendations for vaccine schedules. IM, intramuscular; ID, intradermal.

Personnel caring for rabies patients should practice standard universal and respiratory precautions. In addition, they should receive a pre-exposure immunization sequence (see earlier discussion) and maintain a serum antirabies antibody titer of 0.5 IU/mL.[115] Exposures to potentially contaminated secretions or tissues should lead to standard PET.

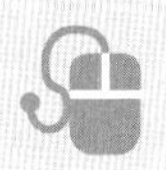

Access the complete reference list online at
http://www.expertconsult.com

CHAPTER 80

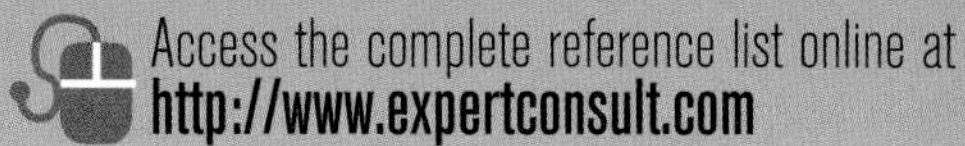
Access the complete reference list online at
http://www.expertconsult.com

Human Papillomavirus Infections

William Bonnez • Gerhard Lindeque

INTRODUCTION

Starting in 1977, it was recognized that there is in fact more than one human papillomavirus (HPV) type, and that each new type isolated is from lesions with a different anatomic distribution (***Table 80.1***). It quickly became apparent that the HPV types associated with cutaneous warts (hand, plantar, and facial flat warts) are different from those retrieved from genital warts. HPV types 6 (in 1980) and 11 (in 1982) were recovered from genital warts. Later, HPV types 16 (in 1983) and 18 (in 1984) were found in cervical cancer. Thus began the pursuit of a causal link between some genital HPV types and cervical cancer, a major cause of morbidity and mortality in women living in the developing world. HPV probably accounts for the largest share of human cancers caused by an infectious agent. Since 2006 effective vaccines have become available that are expected to reduce the rate of HPV-associated cancers.

THE AGENT

Papillomaviruses belong to the family *Papillomaviridae*, genus *Papillomavirus*. All papillomaviruses share an identical structure of a naked, icosahedral capsid 55 nm in diameter, composed of 72 capsomeres. Each capsomere contains five major capsid proteins (L1), which represent 80% of the capsid mass. A minor capsid protein (L2) occupies the center of the pentamer. L2 is dispensable for formation of the capsid *in vitro*. The capsid contains circular, double-stranded, supercoiled DNA of 7900 bp, associated with histone proteins.

All papillomaviruses share the same general genetic organization, with all the regulatory and coding sequences (open-reading frames (ORFs)) located on the same strand. Many of the viral proteins are made from polycistronic spliced messages. The coding regions of the genome are organized according to expression during the viral cycle into early (E) and late (L) ORFs. L1 and L2 ORFs code respectively for major and minor capsid proteins. The other six to seven ORFs encode nonstructural proteins. E1 controls viral plasmid replication in collaboration with E2, which also modulates viral transcription. There are no HPV E3 ORFs. E4 encodes the most abundant viral proteins, which colocalize with cellular intermediate filaments. E5 protein is a cytoplasmic membrane-associated protein that causes acidification of the endosome, stimulates the transforming activity mediated by epidermal growth factor, and contributes to oncogenicity and immune evasion of HPV. E6 and E7 proteins have central roles in HPV oncogenicity through binding cellular factors and major tumor suppressor proteins.

Papillomaviruses are host-specific. The stratified epithelia of the body, namely the skin and mucous membranes, and the transitional glandular epithelium of the cervix are targets of HPV infection. The viral replicative cycle is tightly dependent on differentiation of epithelium, and the virus cannot be grown in monolayer cell culture by standard virologic techniques. Only complex organotypic culture systems and human epithelial xenografts in immunodeficient mice allow experimental propagation of the virus. Taxonomy is based on genotyping. At least 150 HPV types share less than 90% of the nucleotide sequence of the L1 ORF. Subtypes have between 90% and 98% sequence homology. HPVs belong to five of the 18 *Papillomaviridae* genera. There is a general association between HPV genotype and anatomic location of the infection. Therefore, it is convenient, if not strictly correct, to distinguish three groups of HPVs associated with: (1) cutaneous infections such as the warts that develop on the hands, feet, and face; (2) a rare genodermatose, epidermodysplasia verruciformis; and (3) genital infections. The HPV-induced skin lesions in genodermatosis epidermolysis verruciformis have the propensity by the fifth decade to evolve in sunlight-exposed areas into squamous cell carcinomas (SCCs). Genital HPVs belong to the alpha-papillomavirus genus comprising 15 species, some also containing cutaneous HPVs.

EPIDEMIOLOGY

Incidence and Prevalence

HPV infections are ubiquitous throughout the world, from the urban centers of the developed world to the most isolated regions of the Amazon.[1] World Health Organization (WHO) data (http://www.who.int/hpvcentre/en/) indicate that, among women with normal cervical cytology, the HPV prevalence is 14.3% in the less developed regions of the world and 10.3% in the more developed regions. In both areas, the peak prevalence is observed in women younger than 25 years of age, but while prevalence decreases three- to fourfold in older age strata of more developed areas, the decrease is approximately twofold in the less developed regions. In women aged 35–50 years the maximum HPV prevalence varies across the different continents.[2] Prevalence of HPV in male genitalia varies greatly, from 6% to 72%, according to the population screened, sites sampled, and methodology used, but the information is too limited to conclude about geographic variations.[3] Most of the sexually active population is estimated to be infected during a lifetime.[4]

The prevalence of external genital warts in the less developed world is approximately 1%.[4] A history of genital warts is found in 5.6% of 18–59-year-old Americans[5] and about 10% in the female population younger than 45 years of four Nordic countries.[6] HPV types 6 and 11 account for 80–90% of these lesions.[7] Recurrent respiratory papillomatosis (RRP), caused by the same HPV types (6 and 11) as external genital warts, is rare, with an estimated annual incidence in the United States of 4.3 per 100 000 children and 1.8 per 100 000 adults.[8] No data are available for the developing world.

Adequate descriptive epidemiologic information on squamous intraepithelial lesions (SIL) or cervical intraepithelial neoplasias (CIN), precursors to cervical cancer, is not available for the developing world, because it is derived from screening programs based on cervical cytology, colposcopy, and biopsies that are often lacking. Overall, 2–3% of women

Table 80.1 Human Papillomavirus Types and Their Disease Associations

Disease	HPV Types: Frequent Association	HPV Types: Less Frequent Association
Condylomata acuminata	6, 11	16,[a] 18,[a] 31,[a] 33,[a] 35,[a] 40, 42, 43, 44, 45,[a] 51,[a] 52,[a] 53,[a] 54, 55, 56,[a] 58,[a] 59,[a] 66, 68,[a] 70
Intraepithelial neoplasia, unspecified		26,[a] 30,[a] 34, 39,[a] 40, 53,[a] 57, 59,[a] 61, 62, 67,[a] 68,[a] 69, 71, 81, 83
Low-grade	6, 11	16,[a] 18,[a] 31,[a] 33,[a] 35,[a] 42, 43, 44,[b] 45,[a] 51,[a] 52,[a] 54, 61, 70, 72, 74
High-grade	16,[a] 18[a]	6, 11, 31,[a] 34,[b] 33,[a] 35,[a] 39,[a] 42, 44, 45,[a] 51,[a] 52,[a] 56,[a] 58,[a] 66[a], 67[a]
Cervical carcinoma	16,[a] 18[a]	31,[a] 33,[a] 35,[a] 39,[a] 45,[a] 51,[a] 52,[a] 56,[a] 58,[a] 59,[a] 66,[a] 67,[b] 68,[a] 73,[a] 82[a]
Other genital lesions		30,[a] 84,[a] 85, 86,[a] 87, 89, 90, 91, 97, 101, 102, 103, 106
Recurrent respiratory papillomatosis	6, 11	16,[a] 18,[a] 31,[a] 33,[a] 35,[a] 39[a]
Focal epithelial hyperplasia of Heck	13, 32	18,[a] 33,[a] 45[a]
Conjunctival papillomas and carcinomas	6, 11, 16[a]	

Note: The frequency distribution of the different human papillomavirus (HPV) types is not necessarily fully established for the different diseases listed, and some HPV types have been looked for or identified only once. Therefore, this table is only to give a general indication.

[a]Types with high malignant potential or isolated in only one or a few lesions that were malignant.

[b]HPV-64 is a variant of HPV-34, and HPV-55 is HPV-44.

screened will have low-grade SIL (LSIL), and less than 2% will have high-grade SIL (HSIL).[9,10] HPV-16, -58, and -18 are the three top-ranked types, accounting for 32% and 60% of HPV types found in LSIL and HSIL, respectively, in the developing world (http://www.who.int/hpvcentre/en/).

Cancer of the uterine cervix is, after breast cancer, the most commonly diagnosed (age-adjusted incidence rate of 16.2 per 100000) and lethal (age-adjusted mortality rate of 9.0 per 100000) cancer in women worldwide.[11,12] The developing world bears the greatest burden with incidence and mortality approximately five times greater than in the developed world.[11,13] Cancer of the penis with age-adjusted incidence rate of 1 per 100000 in the Western world is more common in Southeast Asia, India, Latin America, and Eastern and Southern Africa. Other cancers associated with HPV affecting the vulva, vagina, and anus do not appear to segregate geographically. Their incidences are under 1.5 cases per 100000.[12]

Coinfection by human immunodeficiency virus (HIV) is associated with increased incidence, prevalence, and persistence of HPV infections, and the level of immunosuppression, measured by CD4 T-lymphocyte counts, is related to HPV-related intraepithelial neoplasias.[14] The risk of cervical, anal, and oropharyngeal cancer increases after the diagnosis of AIDS.[15] The role of immunosuppression is emphasized by the observation that HPV-related cancers of the cervix, vulva, vagina, penis, anus, and oropharynx also occur in excess among immunosuppressed transplant recipients.[16] A large study of patients with diagnosis of AIDS made since 1980 documented a rise in the risk of *in situ* cancers of the cervix and anus, as well as invasive cancers of the oropharynx and anus.[17] The rate of increase and duration of immunosuppression were associated with increased incidence of anal cancer in men. Nevertheless, this evidence is still inconclusive because associations are moderate in strength, not seen for all HPV-related cancers, and not affected by highly active antiretroviral therapy (HAART). Moreover, in developing countries the relationship between HIV/acquired immunodeficiency syndrome (AIDS) and HPV-related cancers is weaker than in developed countries and, if observed, is limited to cervical cancer.[18,19]

TRANSMISSION

HPV infections are transmitted through close personal contact. For infections of the anogenital area, this means sexual contact that is typically part of sexual play, although not necessarily involving penile insertion.[20] The evidence includes age of onset of HPV infection that is the same as other sexually transmitted diseases (STDs), development of genital warts in at least two-thirds of affected sexual contacts, excess association or history of other STDs in patients with anogenital warts, and positive correlation between the number of sexual partners and the presence of genital warts or cervical HPV infections.[21] In sexually active males and females, the acquisition of genital HPV is relatively rapid, with approximately half becoming infected within 2–3 years.[22,23] Although the number of sexual partners is important, the risk of contracting an HPV infection is not trivial, even with the first partner.[24] The transmission from female to male seems to be about three times more efficient than the reverse.[25]

Young children may acquire HPV anogenital infections from HPV types not associated with anogenital infections, and conversely mucosal HPV types, such as HPV-6, occur in cutaneous warts of family contacts of children with anogenital warts, suggesting that in prepubertal children genital warts do not necessarily imply sexual abuse.[26,27]

Young children with RRP apparently acquire infection during delivery through an infected birth canal.[8] There are rare instances of neonates born with mucosa-associated disease. In adult-onset disease, transmission most likely originates from oral sex.[8] The disease is not transmitted horizontally, and no special precautions are recommended for family members and close contacts. Oral sex and open-mouth kissing are linked to oropharyngeal HPV infections.[28]

Although HPV DNA can be recovered from fomites, such as underwear of infected women, it is not a proven source of transmission. However, virus might be acquired through use of shared sex toys.

Association Between HPV and Anogenital Malignancies

The cottontail rabbit (Shope) papillomavirus and several bovine papillomaviruses were established to cause cancer starting in the 1930s. By the 1980s, HPV types such as 16 and 18 were found in many cervical cancers, and the ability of their E6 and E7 genes to induce malignant transformation and immortalization *in vitro* was well established.[29] HPV-16 virions could experimentally induce in human skin macroscopic and microscopic features of intraepithelial neoplasia.[30]

The strength of the association with cervical cancer is extremely high, with odds ratios ranging from 100 to 900 for HPV-16 and SCC, and HPV-18 and adenocarcinoma.[31] HPV DNA is present in 99.7% of cervical cancer worldwide.[32] The fraction attributable to HPV for other cancers is 70% for vagina, 40% for vulva, 84% for anus, 48% for penis, and 26% for head and neck, with at least 37% for oropharynx.[33–35]

Only 15 of the 40 mucosal HPV types are considered to have significant oncogenic potential, not only for the cervix, but also for other sites. Thus, HPV-16 or -18 accounts for 79% of cervical cancers, 73% of vaginal cancers, 56% of vulvar cancers, 79% of anal cancers, and 95% of oropharyngeal cancers.[33,35,36] HPV genotypes vary in oncogenicity, but even within a given genotype variants carry different risk. For example, New World strains of HPV-16 are more oncogenic than Old World strains.

HPV infection always precedes the development of cervical abnormalities and cancer. Overall, about 90% of cervical infections are transient. Those caused by high-risk HPV last longer than those caused by low-risk HPV – 13.5 versus 4.8 months. CIN 2 or 3 has a 20–30% chance of developing in a woman with normal cytology, but infected with high-risk HPV, while it is highly unlikely to develop if she is HPV DNA-negative. The number of sexual partners of the patient and husband are risk factors for both cervical infections and cancer, the latter following the former. Some studies support the concept of higher viral load predicting higher risk of cervical cancer.

If HPV infection is the necessary condition for the development of cancer, it may not be a sufficient one. Among potential cofactors are use of oral contraceptives, higher parity, smoking, presence of other STDs (herpes simplex type 2, *Chlamydia*), and nutrition (vitamins A, C, E, carotenoids, folic acid).[4]

THE DISEASE

External Anogenital Warts and Recurrent Respiratory Papillomatosis

External genital warts, also called venereal warts or condylomata acuminata, are well-demarcated, firm papules ranging from less than 1 mm to several centimeters, but typically 2–6 mm in diameter. They can be sessile, joining normal skin at a slightly acute angle and having a mulberry-like surface, or, especially on mucosal surfaces, a pointed or jagged hyperkeratotic surface. Color ranges from flesh-like to hyperpigmented. Individuals average 5–6 warts, but the number of lesions can vary from 1 to more than 50 and can coalesce into large plaques. They may then entrap hairs, which are otherwise completely absent within a wart.

In the noncircumcised male, the preputial cavity is the site of predilection, while it is the penile shaft in circumcised males. The urethral meatus is involved in a minority of patients. Since lesions only exceptionally extend beyond the fossa navicularis, they are easy to visualize by eversion of the meatus or use of an ear speculum. Lesions are occasionally present in the pubic area, groin, and rarely the scrotum.[21] Men having sex with men are prone to developing perianal and anal warts, with HIV coinfection approximately doubling that risk.[37] However, heterosexual men can also have lesions in that location without anal sexual play.[38]

In women, warts are typically on the vulva, especially around the posterior introitus, fourchette, labia minora, labia majora, and clitoris. The perineum, vagina, anus, and urethra are much less frequently affected.[21]

At least three-quarters of patients are asymptomatic. Symptoms may include discomfort, burning, itching, pain or tenderness, and bleeding. It is important to note that many patients report a significant psychological impact with the diagnosis of genital warts.[39,40]

The natural history of genital warts is not well understood, but controlled clinical trials indicate spontaneous remission in approximately 10% within 4 months.[41] Transformation of genital warts into invasive SCC, a variant being verrucous carcinoma, is rare. Very large warts may in fact show on biopsy local invasion but no metastasis. They have been called Buschke–Löwenstein tumors, an entity that groups verrucous carcinomas and giant condylomas, which are some of the verruciform tumors of genital skin.[42]

In RRP the proliferation of papillomas on the vocal cords causes hoarseness, or an altered cry in infants.[8] The near occlusion of the airway can cause respiratory distress or stridor. A younger age of onset correlates with a more aggressive course and may require very frequent surgical excisions. The disease may extend down the trachea into the lungs. At this stage, the disease can cause obstruction, infection, and respiratory failure. The risk of malignant transformation is high after irradiation of laryngeal papillomas or when lung involvement is present.

Penile, Vulvar, Vaginal, and Cervical Intraepithelial Neoplasias and Cancers

Condylomas occur in the vagina or on the cervix and are best observed after application of 3% acetic acid and using a colposcope. In the vagina they appear as multifocal, small, spiky growths. On the cervix, they are barely raised, typically single papules with well-defined margins, smooth surface contour, white appearance, and normal blood vessels.

Precursor lesions to HPV-associated SCC are the intraepithelial neoplasias. In the cervix, they are called CIN, on the penis, PIN, on the vulva, VIN, and in the vagina, VAIN. Their appearance on the external genitalia is typically multicentric, aggregated papules that are often pigmented. They may grow rapidly, or be recalcitrant to treatment for warts. Such lesions, especially in HIV-infected individuals, should be biopsied. Bowenoid papillomatosis is a combination of lesions with a condylomatous cytoarchitecture, but with the presence of intraepithelial neoplasia. Such a lesion can evolve to a variant of carcinoma *in situ* called Bowen's disease, distinguished by flat, scaly, red to brown plaques. The same condition on the glans penis is called erythroplasia of Queyrat.

Other Diseases Associated with Mucosal HPV

Warts can occur on the mucosal surfaces of the oral cavity and upper aerodigestive tract. The appearance is similar to that in the genital area, but tending to be flatter and difficult to visualize. The patient usually will notice discomfort. The histology of these lesions distinguishes squamous cell papillomas from condylomata acuminata and verruca vulgaris. The first two entities are mostly associated with HPV types 6 and 11, while the last is mostly associated with HPV types 2, 4, and 57, found in cutaneous warts. Focal epithelial hyperplasia (Heck's disease) is a unique, benign condition, found largely in the Indian population of the Americas. It presents as flesh-colored, flat papules that may coalesce, carpeting the buccal and jugal mucosa. It is associated with HPV types 13 and 37. The lesions may persist for years, but typically disappear spontaneously.

Among the mucosal structures of the head and neck, the oropharynx, which includes the palatine and lingual tonsils, is a site of predilection for the development of SCCs. An increasing percentage of these tumors is associated with HPV infections and have a different epidemiologic profile than the HPV-negative cases. While the latter are associated with alcohol and tobacco, oral sex is the main risk factor for the former.[43] HPV-16 or -18 infections account for 95% of these cancers.

The presence of perianal warts, most common in homosexual males, is accompanied by the presence of an intra-anal lesion in up to two-thirds of patients. A history of genital or anal warts increases by at least 10-fold the risk of anal cancer.[44] Therefore, anal symptoms (discomfort, itching, burning, or bleeding), history of anal receptive intercourse, use of anal toys, and presence of perianal warts require a digital anal examination followed by anoscopy.

The conjunctiva can be the site of mucosal HPV-associated condylomas and SCCs. Sun exposure may play an additional role since these uncommon malignancies have been reported mostly in Africa.[45]

PATHOGENESIS AND IMMUNITY

The stratified squamous epithelia contain basal cells resting on a basement membrane that are the only ones dividing in the epithelium. This division causes one of the two daughter cells to move upward and start differentiating. Different layers correspond to stages of differentiation. Immediately above the stratum basale is the stratum acanthosum (the prickle cell layer), the stratum granulosum, and on the surface the stratum corneum that constantly sheds dead cells. For the epithelium to become infected, the virus must reach a basal cell, likely through microabrasions or microtrauma, mostly during sexual intercourse. Furthermore, a thin and immature epithelium, as in the adolescent female cervix, facilitates that breach.

Entry of the virion involves at least one receptor, probably a syndecan. The basal cell is suspected of being the target of HPV because viral DNA replication needs the cellular replicative enzymes, the virus being devoid of DNA polymerase.[46,47] Replication can be at a low level, the infection remaining latent, or it can be associated with abundant protein expression, causing active infection. The early proteins E1, E2, E5, E6, and E7 are

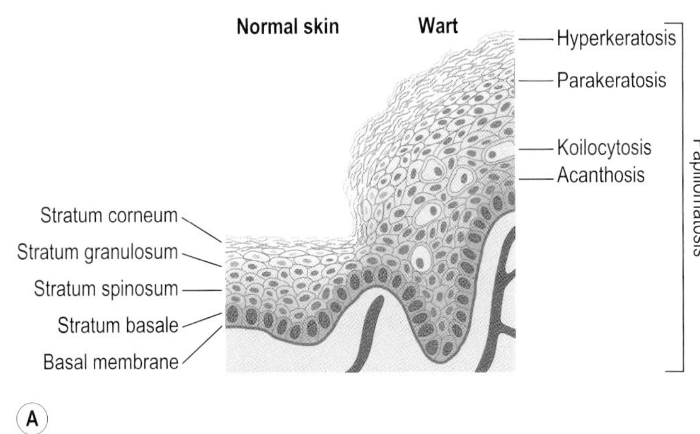

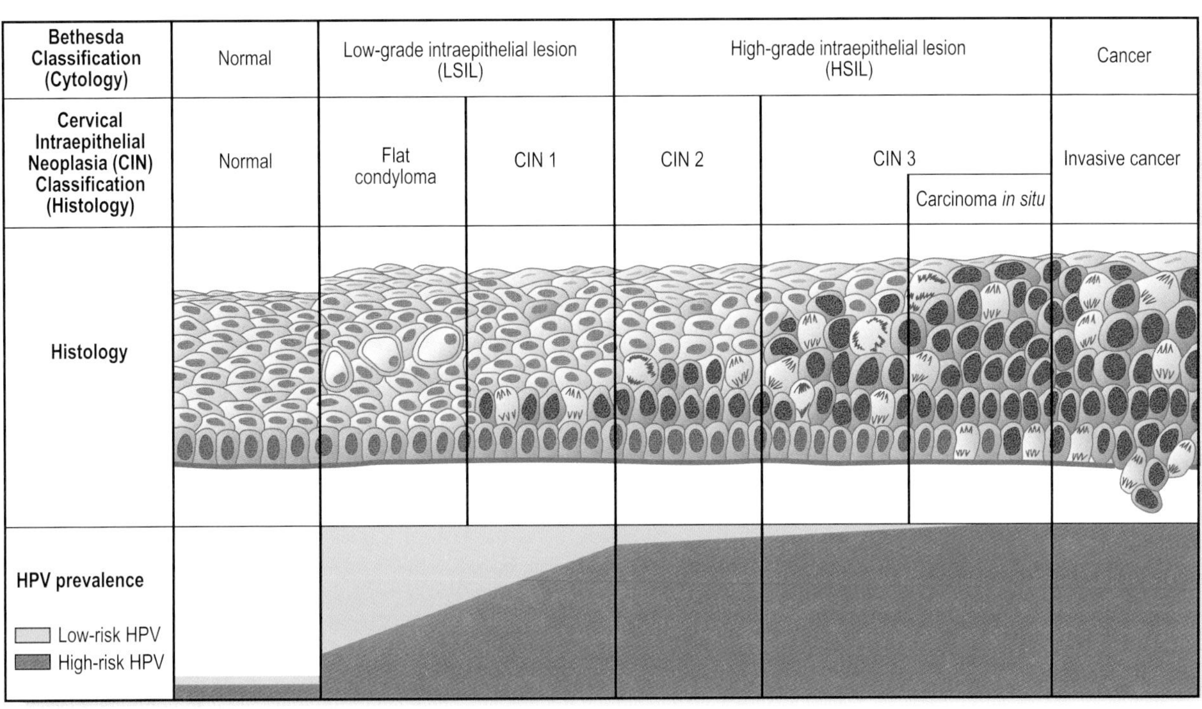

Bethesda Classification (Cytology)
Normal
Low-grade intraepithelial lesion (LSIL)
High-grade intraepithelial lesion (HSIL)
Cancer
Cervical Intraepithelial Neoplasia (CIN) Classification (Histology)
Normal
Flat condyloma
CIN 1
CIN 2
CIN 3
Carcinoma in situ
Invasive cancer
Histology
HPV prevalence
Low-risk HPV
High-risk HPV
B

Figure 80.1 **(A)** Histologic features of a genital/cutaneous wart. **(B)** Histopathogenesis of cervical human papillomavirus (HPV)-associated lesions (see text for details). (Reproduced from Bonnez W. Human papillomavirus vaccines. In: Stanberry LR, Barrett ADT, eds. Vaccines for Biodefense and Emerging and Neglected Diseases. London: Elsevier; 2009:469–493. Copyright Elsevier 2009.)

found in the deeper layers of the epithelium, while E4, L1, and L2 are present in the superficial layers, where viral particles are assembled in the cell nucleus. Virions are released with desquamating cells.

These viral changes of active infection are associated with formation of a wart or papilloma by proliferation of the stratum spinosum (acanthosis), stratum granulosum (parakeratosis), and stratum corneum (hyperkeratosis) (*Fig. 80.1A*).[48,49] This proliferation, called papillomatosis, extends upwards, but also downwards with deepening of the normal scalloping of the basal membrane. One feature is quasi-pathognomonic, the presence in the upper stratum spinosum of large cells with a nucleus surrounded by a halo, koilocytes, which in a cytological sample signal the presence of HPV. A high-risk HPV infection may cause intraepithelial neoplasia (*Fig. 80.1B*).[48,49] In that instance, there is proliferation of the basal layer. The cells start acquiring features associated with malignancy, including high nuclear-to-cytoplasmic ratio and greater number of mitoses. The presence of this basaloid proliferation confined to the lower third of the epithelium is grade 1. Grade 2 extends to the lower two-thirds, and grade 3 goes further. Involvement of the full thickness of the epithelium is carcinoma *in situ*, and breach of the basal membrane by this process defines invasive SCC. Dyskeratosis is also present.

The body sites where squamous epithelium meets glandular epithelium (squamocolumnar junction, SCJ), such as cervix, anus, and pharynx, are particularly susceptible to HPV infections and HPV-induced malignant transformation. In the cervix, under the influence of factors that include hormones and acidification, this SCJ moves from the exocervix to the endocervix from birth to adulthood, thus defining a transformation zone where SCC arises. The glandular epithelium adjoining the CSJ is also susceptible to HPV-induced malignant transformation leading to cervical adenocarcinoma. Because the glandular epithelium is a monolayer, there are no precursor states other than adenocarcinoma *in situ* (AIS).

Among the many molecular events leading to malignant transformation, at least two appear essential because they are directly linked to the virus.[48,50] They are degradation of the p53 protein by E6 and inactivation of the retinoblastoma protein (Rb) by E7. p53 and Rb are key tumor suppressor proteins that regulate the cell cycle and prevent its acceleration. In addition, E6 inhibits cellular apoptosis, preventing abnormal cells from dying. Before the tissue evolves into an invasive cancer, there is an opportunity for the lesion to regress spontaneously. For example, the chances of regression for CIN grades 1, 2, and 3 are 60%, 40%, and 30%, respectively, while for the same lesions the chances of progression to invasive cancer are 1%, 5%, and greater than 12%, respectively.[51] Progression involves additional events such as hypermethylation of viral and cellular DNA, telomerase activation, and development of chromosomal instability and deletions. In addition, the viral genome tends to become integrated as intraepithelial neoplasia progresses. This integration disrupts E2, which changes the viral expression pattern with overexpression of E6 and E7. E5, E6, and E7 appear to contribute in different ways to inhibition of the immune response.[52,53] Regressing warts are notable for the presence of a lymphomononuclear epidermal infiltrate.

The humoral and cellular immune response that develops after HPV infection is neither uniform nor predictive of the severity or behavior of the infection or associated diseases.[54] E6, E7, and L1 are the more potent antigens. The presence of antibodies to L1 is a good marker of past or present infections that can be used for seroepidemiologic surveys. The cellular immune response after vaccination to peptides derived from E6 and E7 of HPV-16 seems capable of inducing regression of HPV-16-associated vulvar intraepithelial neoplasias.[55]

DIAGNOSIS

Visual Examination

External genital warts are usually diagnosed with the naked eye. They are most often confused with molluscum contagiosum. Molluscum contagiosum lesions are skin-colored or lighter papules and have a central dimple. The lesions are more likely to be present over the pubis than the penile shaft, and they can extend to the trunk. Acrochordons or skin tags, another source of confusion, are recognized by their lax elastic texture. In the male, the urethra should be everted to assure that no intraurethral warts are present.

Lesions on the cervix may show condylomatous characteristics or turn white on application of 3% acetic acid. Visual inspection after acetic acid (VIA) is used in some developing countries to detect CIN or to downstage cervical cancer.[56,57] Although not recommended by the WHO for general screening programs, many trials are assessing the place of VIA as a screening tool.[58] The sensitivity and specificity are approximately 50%. Visual inspection of the cervix using Lugol's iodine (VIL) also has the same limitations.[58] VIA and VIL can be used on the penis.

Colposcope-Assisted Examination

Colposcopy is a visual assessment technique allowing magnification with a strong light source. Colposcopy is currently not used as a diagnostic technique but as an aid in assessment of site, spread, appearance, and borders of vaginal and in particular cervical lesions.[59] Treatment for VAIN and CIN lesions is practically always aided by colposcopy. Its main utility is in directing the sites to biopsy on the cervix.

Cytology

Ever since Papanicolaou developed the staining method for detecting cellular abnormalities in cancerous cells, cytology has offered good secondary prevention of cervical cancer and is responsible for detection of large numbers of CIN lesions around the world. The WHO recommends cytology for large-scale screening programs if a country has the resources and infrastructure.[58] Cytology carries a high cost as all slides need individual assessment by a trained technologist and tests are repeated regularly. While annual recall programs have been successfully implemented in developed countries, the cost has forced less frequent screening. In developing countries the recall gap is as long as 10 years, as evidenced by the South African governmental policy on cervical screening. The effectiveness of such a program is less than with more frequent examinations. If long intervals are associated with poor coverage of the population, these programs are doomed to fail.[60]

Cytology is a screening test that requires confirmation of diagnosis by biopsy. Koilocytes indicate the presence of HPV infection. However, koilocytes can be absent in the presence of HPV infection, particularly with high-risk oncogenic types. Therefore, current practice is to be able to test for the presence of HPV by HPV DNA or RNA tests. Cytology is most useful in screening for CIN and cervical cancer but recently has also been used for screening for anal cancer.

Cervical cytopathologic abnormalities are usually reported using the Bethesda 2001 system[61] and revisions (http://nltnlibrary.wordpress.com/2008/05/16/bethesda-system-website-atlas/). The range of abnormalities is described as: abnormal squamous cells of undetermined significance (ASCUS), that can be infectious or precancerous; squamous intraepithelial lesions (SIL), that can be low-grade or high-grade; squamous carcinoma; abnormal glandular cells of undetermined significance (AGUS); AIS; and adenocarcinoma. Women having such abnormalities are recommended to undergo repeat testing (in cases of ASCUS and LSIL) or colposcopy and biopsy (in cases of HSIL or glandular abnormalities).

Histology

While the diagnosis of external genital warts is made clinically and can be confirmed histologically, the diagnosis of all intraepithelial lesions of the genital tract in both males and females must be made by histology. Agreement between surgical pathologists is far from perfect, especially for CIN2.[62]

Nucleic Acid Detection Tests

The cultivation of HPV requires highly complex and fastidious techniques that are too expensive and insensitive for clinical use. There is no commercially available serologic assay for diagnosis of HPV infection. Thus demonstration of HPV in a clinical specimen uses commercially available molecular techniques based on the detection of HPV nucleic acids. The first assay, now updated, available to diagnose HPV in cytologic samples is the Hybrid Capture II, or Digene HPV test (Qiagen Corp., Valencia, CA). It is based on liquid hybridization of the denatured sample DNA to RNA probes, each specific for high-risk HPV (types 16, 18, 31, 33, 35, 39, 45, 51, 52, 56, 58, 59, or 68). This assay is not based on amplification of the target HPV DNA, and is not hampered by cross-contamination, a potential failing of the assays based on the polymerase chain reaction.[63] An advantage of the Hybrid Capture assay is that it has been prospectively validated for screening using clinical outcomes as endpoints. For all other available and more recent assays, only the assay biologic performance has been studied.[63,64]

Program for Appropriate Technology in Health (PATH, Seattle, WA), an international nonprofit organization that sponsors the development of health technologies, has partnered with Qiagen (Gaithersburg, MD) to develop a rapid HPV DNA assay, the *care*HPV test (previously called FastHPV test), which is based on liquid hybridization and capture.[63,65] PATH has also partnered with Arbor Vista Corp. (Sunnyvale, CA) to detect in cervical specimens with a lateral flow strip assay (AVC AVantage HPV E6 Test) the E6 of oncogenic HPV.[63] These assays are designed for regions that do not have effective screening programs.

TREATMENT AND PROGNOSIS

Treatment Methods

The great variety of treatment methods available for the treatment of anogenital HPV diseases reflects the absence of a modality clearly superior in all respects. Therefore, to a great extent selection of a particular treatment option is based on availability, cost, and convenience in an environment with limited resources. The methods available are either chemical or physical. Data on efficacy of those most relevant in the developing world vary greatly as they are often derived from small, noncomparative and nonrandomized studies.

Podophyllin, for at least 50 years used for the treatment of genital warts,[66] is prepared from the rhizome of *Podophyllum peltatum* or the more potent *P. emodi*, usually as a 25% solution in benzoin tincture, liquid paraffin, or industrial methylated spirit. The principal active molecule, podophyllotoxin, a lignan, binds to tubulin, inhibits its polymerization, and prevents formation of the mitotic spindle. Capable of damaging HPV DNA, the main effect is probably nonspecific and related to the high mitotic activity of HPV lesions. The compound is applied directly on the wart with an applicator or swab. Great care has to be exercised not to smear the surrounding healthy skin, which may be shielded with protective ointment in zinc oxide paste. The medication should be washed off by the end of the day, and should never stay on more than 24 hours. The total volume applied in a given patient should not exceed 0.9–1.2 mL for the *P. peltatum* preparation and 0.4–0.5 mL for the *P. emodi* preparation. Mucosal surfaces should be treated cautiously. Application can be repeated at 7–14-day intervals, but response is unlikely if it has not occurred after four sessions. Complete response rates vary greatly, but one typically expects a 30–50% chance of complete resolution. The relapse rate is unfortunately high, 60–85%.[41]

Extensive application or ingestion of podophyllin can cause severe reactions, including death. The toxicity of the compound requires a health practitioner for its application. Because it is a mutagen and abortifacient, it is contraindicated in pregnancy. It should also be avoided in the nursing mother. It is important not to biopsy a lesion that has been treated with podophyllin in the 3 days previously because the histologic changes could be confused with a carcinoma *in situ*.

Although podophyllin is inexpensive, its substantial toxicity makes it much less desirable than podofilox, which is chemically defined, of standardized potency, and less toxic on a weight basis.[66–68] It is appropriate for self-use. It is typically available as a 0.5% solution or gel, the latter being easier to apply without spilling on healthy skin. Applied twice daily for 3 consecutive days for up to 4 weeks, one can expect rates of complete response ranging from 33% to 91%.[41] The toxicity is similar to that of podophyllin, but milder.

Trichloroacetic acid (TCA) (bichloroacetic acid is also sometimes used) as a 50–90% solution does not need to be washed away. It is thus easy to use on mucosal surfaces of the vulva and anal canal, making it favored by many gynecologists. Acids destroy tissue by hydrolysis and may bind covalently to cellular proteins. TCA also destroys HPV DNA. The solution is applied directly on the lesion with a cotton tip applicator. The surrounding tissues should be protected with a thin layer of petrolatum jelly or something equivalent. If there is spillage on to healthy tissue, the acid can be neutralized with talcum powder or sodium bicarbonate. Treatment can be repeated weekly, up to 6–10 times. In comparative trials, TCA has yielded complete response rates similar to those of cryotherapy, 65–90%.[41,69,70] Recurrence rates of 40–55% have been reported. Other than immediate, sharp pain on application, the most common adverse reactions, occurring in about two-thirds of patients, include discomfort, ulcerations, and scabbing. TCA is not contraindicated during pregnancy.

5-Fluorouracil is a pyrimidine antagonist that blocks synthesis of DNA, and to a lesser degree RNA. Regimens for the 5% cream topical formulation vary widely, from twice a day to weekly, and from a few days to 10 weeks. Complete response rates vary from a third to 80% and appear to be better than podophyllotoxin. One favored indication is the treatment of vaginal and meatal warts. However, side-effects are common. Local pain, itching, burning, and hyperpigmentation are noted in about half of the patients. Systemic adverse reactions include contact and allergic dermatitis, leukocytosis, and thrombocytopenia. It is recommended not to use it during pregnancy.

Imiquimod, an imidazoquinolineamine, acts as an agonist of Toll-like receptor 7, and activates the immune system by upregulating the expression of cytokine genes, including interferon-α, interleukins 1, 5, 6, 9, 10, and 12, tumor necrosis factor-α, and macrophage chemotactic factor.[71] It is available as a 5% cream (Aldara) that is applied directly to lesions by the patient, three times a week, every other day, for 8–16 weeks. The complete response rate of genital warts varies from 35% to 60%, with women responding twice as well as males; warts on mucosal surfaces respond better than warts on hairy skin.[41,71,72] Daily delivery increases the response rate, but the side effects are significantly worse. Recurrence rates are approximately 15%. Imiquimod is used in HIV patients for treatment of anogenital and intra-anal warts. For the treatment of genital warts, it does not appear to be superior to placebo.[41,72] The most common side effects are mild to moderate erythema and erosions in two-thirds and one-third of patients, respectively. Edema, scabbing, induration, and vesicles can occur. There is no information on the risk of imiquimod in pregnant women and nursing mothers. Imiquimod is an attractive first-line treatment because it is self-applied. However, cost may be a deterrent.

There are several additional medical approaches to the treatment of HPV disease, but they are less likely to be available in a tropical practice.[41,69,70,73]

Genital warts can be excised with scissors.[74] This is particularly effective if the warts are few, and complete response rates of 90% and upwards are achieved, while the recurrence rate is approximately 20–30%.[41,69] The side effects, mostly pain, are minor and short-lived. Scarring is not a problem, and the technique can be employed in pregnant women. Traditional conization of the cervix for treatment of HPV disease is done with a scalpel blade.

Electrosurgery includes an array of techniques, including electrocautery, electrodiathermy, electrodesiccation, electrofulguration, electrocoagulation, and electrosection, designed to ablate tissue with electric current. Electrocoagulation of genital warts has been reported to be 60% effective. Electrodesiccation has been compared to podophyllin and cryotherapy and cleared half of the patients of their genital warts, an outcome more than three times superior to podophyllin and similar to cryotherapy.[75] Electrocautery also appears to be equal to cryotherapy.[41] Electrosurgery is painful, and local anesthesia is desirable. The prior (30–60 minutes) application of lidocaine and prilocaine cream is effective.[76] The main drawback of electrosurgery is the possibility of scarring, which is higher than with cold-blade surgery or cryotherapy.

Loop electrosurgical excisional procedure (LEEP), or large-loop excision of the transformation zone (LLETZ), is a method of choice for the treatment of HPV disease of the cervix and allows mini-conizations. It is associated with increased rate of preterm labor.[77]

Using cold to treat genital warts and other HPV lesions is a common approach, but the requirement for a cryogenic agent limits use in tropical or rural areas of the developing world. Liquid nitrogen (boiling point –196°C) is the favored cryogenic and is usually delivered as a spray. Other cryogenics such as nitrous oxide (boiling point –89.5°C) or carbon dioxide (boiling point –78.5°C) can be delivered with cryoprobes, cryogenic pencils, or dipped cotton swab applicators. Complete clearance rates ranging between 50% and 100% are reported, and pregnancy is not a contraindication.[41,70] The side effects are a sharp and brief pain easing into a burning and longer discomfort at the site of treatment. This can be prevented by the application of lidocaine and prilocaine cream. An erosion or ulceration follows as the necrotic area repairs itself. Any hypo- or hyperpigmentation usually disappears within 3–12 months, and scars should not be a complication. Cryotherapy can be applied to the cervix.

Heat is another mode of destruction. For example, an infrared coagulator provides an 80% clearance rate for anogenital warts and has been used for the treatment of intra-anal warts and intraepithelial neoplasia in the HIV population.[78]

The CO_2 laser treats HPV disease by vaporizing intratissular water. The cost of the instrument and the need to provide either local or general anesthesia limit this approach to large, urban referral centers. Furthermore, laser therapy has not been submitted to rigorous evaluation of its efficacy, and nothing indicates that it is substantially superior to other approaches.[41,69] The results, especially the complications, which can include severe scarring, are dependent on the skill of the operator. Laser surgery can be applied to external and internal HPV lesions, and used during pregnancy. It is particularly convenient for the management of large, bulky lesions. It is one of the favored approaches, with LEEP, for CIN.

Treatment Approaches

The choice of treatment method of genital warts varies largely according to the resources available, convenience, adverse reactions, and location of the lesions. The lesions may be treated with imiquimod cream if small and isolated. This may be better and safer than podophyllin, which carries a risk in pregnancy. Conglomerate lesions are treated with electrocauterization, cryotherapy, or excision. Follow-up is necessary. Penile HPV lesions are treated in the same way as in females. Persons with immune deficiency may experience recurrent condylomata and require treatment on several occasions.

Treatment of CIN lesions with locally destructive techniques such as cryotherapy or local excisional techniques such as LLETZ/LEEP has a high success rate.[59] Factors associated with recurrence include advanced age, wide lesions (both factors leading to involved margins) and presence of HPV at first follow-up.

Persons with HIV infection are at increased risk for HPV infection, to develop CIN lesions, to have more rapid progress to cancer, and to have recurrent lesions. Thus surveillance of persons with HIV should be even stricter than in the general population. Treatment is the same, but response rates are lower. When surgery is contemplated, the $CD4^+$ lymphocyte count and HIV viral load measurement should be determined as patients with very high viral loads and very low $CD4^+$ counts do not tolerate surgery well.

VIN is commonly treated by surgical resection of lesions. Treatment of VAIN lesions is more difficult and may include resection, topical chemotherapy with 5-fluorouracil, or brachyradiotherapy. These disorders are much more common in HIV patients, contributing heavily to their suffering and having major implications for screening, diagnosis, and treatment.

In pregnant women with genital warts, rapid growth may occur, and the entire vulva and vagina may be obscured by warts. Treatment during pregnancy is not associated with good outcomes in most cases and is often postponed until after delivery. If a woman has severe genital warts, cesarean section is recommended, because of concerns about laryngeal HPV lesions in the newborn, local perineal lacerations and bleeding, and even delayed labor.

Children with genital warts may have been victims of sexual molestation. Such children should be counseled, and social workers and psychologists may be needed to assist. Genital warts in children should always be treated under anesthesia so that the entire genital tract can be assessed.

RRP should be treated by an otorhinolaryngologist. Laser surgery is the mainstay, but various adjuvant therapies are used, such as injection of interferon-α or cidofovir.[8]

PREVENTION AND CONTROL

Environmental Precautions

HPV virions are relatively resistant to degradation by desiccation, ether, acid, and heat. Boiling for 1 minute at 100°C will destroy infectivity. Therefore, methods designed for viruses in general sterilize surgical instruments exposed to HPV-infected tissues. Disposable equipment should be discarded after single use. One should wear gloves during examination or treatment. The plume of smoke generated by laser surgery or electrosurgery ideally should be properly evacuated to reduce the possible risk of operator exposure to HPV infection. The use of mask and face shield or goggles is encouraged. To decontaminate surfaces or shared fomites such as sex toys, one can use household bleach diluted 1 : 10.

Circumcision and Condoms

Male circumcision diminishes the risk by a third to a half for male genitalia being infected with HPV, apparently by increasing clearance of infections.[79–82]

Male condoms reduce transmission of HPV. In a prospective study of virgin females, the risk of contracting HPV infection was inversely proportional to the rate of condom use.[83] Reduction of the risk of developing SIL did not reach statistical significance. Among another group of couples in which the woman had SIL or CIN and randomized to condom use or not,[84] there was a greater rate of clearance of CIN (1.5-fold) and HPV DNA (5.7-fold) in the women with condom use. Furthermore, in males with HPV-associated penile flat lesions, at entry, these lesions cleared faster (1.9-fold) in the condom group. These effects were likely related to the protective effect of condoms because they were observed only in couples with concordant HPV types.[84]

Vaccination

Since June 2006, two vaccines have been available worldwide for the prevention of several genital HPV diseases, especially cervical cancer. These vaccines are based on the ability of major capsid protein (L1) to assemble into an empty capsid without the need for the minor capsid protein (L2). This virus-like particle (VLP) has the same antigenic characteristics as the capsid of the infectious virion. HPV-11 L1 VLPs induce neutralizing antibodies that block the development of HPV infection.[85] Noninfectious HPV VLPs successfully protect animals against their papillomaviruses.[85] The humoral response of neutralizing antibodies confers protection. The cellular immune response is not contributory.

The efficacy of the vaccine was studied in women aged 16–23 years who had had five or fewer lifetime sexual partners,[86] a normal cervical cytology, and no cervical HPV-16 infection. The subjects were randomized to receive an intramuscular injection at months 0, 2, and 6 of either 40 µg HPV-16 L1 VLP with aluminum adjuvant or placebo of adjuvant alone. At a median follow-up of 17.4 months, none of the 768 women who received the vaccine developed persistent HPV-16 cervical infection (primary endpoint) or HPV-16 CIN (secondary endpoint), while 41 of 765 (5.4%) in the placebo group became infected, and 9 (22%) developed HPV-16 CIN. The difference was highly statistically significant. From this original study 290 women have now been followed for a mean of 8.5 years.[87] None in the vaccine group has developed HPV-16 CIN, while 5 in the placebo group have.

Two vaccines are currently available (***Table 80.2***). Gardasil (Merck, West Point, PA), the first available, contains VLPs of HPV-6 and -11 to prevent genital warts, and of HPV-16 and -18 to prevent cervical cancer. This vaccine has been evaluated in randomized, placebo-controlled clinical trials, which involved over 17 000 women, ages 16–26 years.[88] After a mean follow-up of 3 years, the vaccines showed 100% efficacy for preventing CIN of any grade, AIS, VIN 1 and VAIN 1, external genital warts caused by the vaccine HPV types, and VIN 2/3 and VAIN 2/3 caused by HPV types 16 and 18.

The immunization age varies from country to country, ranging from 9 to 15 years. The risk of genital HPV infection or disease is too low in that population to determine efficacy. A surrogate marker of protection, neutralizing antibody levels, was higher than in older women after vaccination.[85]

Neutralizing antibody levels after immunization decrease with the age of the patient.[89] Nevertheless, age does not affect vaccine efficacy substantially. A randomized placebo-controlled trial of nearly 4000 subjects demonstrated vaccine efficacy of 90.5% at a mean follow-up of 2.2 years using as combined endpoint of disease CIN of any grade or external genital warts or persistent HPV infection caused by any of the vaccine types. In a randomized controlled study of 4065 men aged 16–26 years immunized with either Gardasil or the placebo,[90] at a mean follow-up of 29 months, the vaccine had efficacy of 89% to prevent external genital warts.

Adverse events following immunization were similar in the vaccine (59%) and placebo (60%) recipients and included headaches (vaccine, 28.2%; placebo, 28.4%), fever (13% versus 11.2%), and nausea (6.7% versus 6.5%).[91] Pain and swelling at the injection site were common, but only 2.2% were rated as serious in the vaccine group, compared to 0.9% in the placebo group. Postmarketing monitoring[91] revealed that the rates

Table 80.2 Available Human Papillomavirus Vaccines

Name	Gardasil	Cervarix
Manufacturer	Merck and Co.	GlaxoSmithKline Ltd (GSK)
Composition	HPV-6, -11, -16, and -18 L1 VLPs made in *Saccharomyces cerevisiae*	HPV-16 and -18 L1 VLPs made using a baculovirus in insect cells
Content	1 dose is 0.5 mL HPV-6 protein: 20 μg HPV-11 protein: 40 μg HPV-16 protein: 40 μg HPV-18 protein: 20 μg Adjuvant Proprietary amorphous aluminum hydrophosphate sulfate, 225 g	1 dose is 0.5 mL HPV-16 protein: 20 μg HPV-18 protein: 20 μg Adjuvant AS04: 3-*O*-desacyl-4′-monophosphoryl lipid A, 50 μg, adsorbed on hydrated aluminum hydroxide ($Al[OH]_3$), 500 μg
Preservation	Contains no thimerosal Needs to be refrigerated (+4°C) until use, but can be left at ambient temperatures less than 25°C for no more than 72 hours	Contains no thimerosal Needs to be refrigerated (+4°C) until use
Route and schedule of administration	Intramuscular injection (deltoid muscle area) at day 0, month 2, and month 6	Intramuscular injection (deltoid muscle area) at day 0, month 1, and month 6
Populations approved for vaccination	Varies by country but at least some efficacy data available in 9–45-year-old females, and 16–26-year-old males	Varies by country but at least some efficacy data available in 9–45-year-old females
Contraindications	Hypersensitivity to any of the vaccine components and yeast Moderate or severe acute illness	Hypersensitivity to any of the vaccine components Severe acute febrile illness
Special populations	Pregnancy: contraindicated Breastfeeding: not contraindicated, but no data Immunosuppression: not contraindicated, but immune response may be reduced Abnormal Papanicolaou smear or positive cervical HPV DNA test is not contraindicated	Pregnancy: contraindicated Breastfeeding: not contraindicated, but no data Hormonal contraceptives not contraindicated
Booster immunization	Not indicated at this time	Not indicated at this time
Cervical cancer screening	Should be continued if available	Should be continued if available

HPV, human papillomavirus; VLP, virus-like particle.

of adverse events following immunization, including hypersensitivity reactions, autoimmune disorders, and Guillain–Barré syndrome, were not different from the background rates. However, syncopal episodes and thromboembolic events were more common than expected. It is not proven that these events were due to vaccination. The excess of syncopes might have been due to the fact that the vaccine was administered to females only (it is now recommended to observe the patients for 15 minutes after immunization). Also, 90% of patients who developed thromboembolic disease had risk factors.

Cervarix (GlaxoSmithKline, GSK, London, UK), the second available HPV L1 VLP vaccine, is directed at HPV-16 and -18 and contains an AS04 adjuvant. The main efficacy trial (PATRICIA) enrolled about 16 000 women aged 15–16 years.[92] They were randomized to receive at 0, 1, and 6 months either vaccine or placebo, hepatitis A vaccine containing AS04 adjuvant. At a mean follow-up of about 3 years, vaccine efficacy against CIN 2 or greater caused by HPV-16 or -18 was 93%. The vaccine offered some cross-protection (efficacy 54%) against CIN 2+ caused by 12 nonvaccine oncogenic types.

A comparative trial of safety and immunogenicity of Gardasil and Cervarix was conducted with analysis of the immune response 1 month after the last immunization.[93] Cervarix induced significantly higher neutralizing antibody titer than Gardasil. It is unclear if this difference would be sustained or result in a difference in efficacy. The rates of local side effects (pain, redness, and swelling) were 20–70% higher in the Cervarix recipients. The difference was less pronounced for general side effects.

The cost of the vaccine is currently the main obstacle to use in the developing world. Econometric modeling shows that HPV-16 and -18 vaccination could be very cost-effective, even in the poorest countries, if the cost of a dose were $2, with vaccine coverage of 70%.[94] Experience with recombinant hepatitis B vaccine has shown that recombinant vaccine costs do eventually decrease. Both Merck (www.merck.com/corporate-responsibility/access/access-vaccines-immunization/approach.html) and GSK (www.gsk.com/responsibility/preferential-pricing.htm) have pledged to make vaccine available at cost or at a reduced price to developing countries where it is most needed. Novel HPV vaccines in development could also reduce manufacturing costs.[95]

Screening Strategies

In order to use cytology as a tool for a population-wide cervical cancer screening program the following prerequisites must be met: (1) wide coverage of target population; (2) availability of health workers to take smears; (3) recall; (4) infrastructure for analysis of the specimens; and (5) infrastructure for managing referrals.

In developing countries these prerequisites are in most cases not met, and programs of this sort are not likely to succeed.[60] In order to overcome health worker and coverage problems, self-sampling has been introduced where patients place tampons intravaginally and then deposit the tampon at a collecting site. The same principles are applied when performing HPV testing. The correlation between results from self-sampling specimens and taken specimens is very good.[96]

There are possible solutions for the infrastructure problems: firstly VIA was tested, but specificity remains low.[56] This gave rise to the VIA-and-treat plan in which all abnormal cervices detected by VIA (that do not appear cancerous) are treated with cryotherapy on the spot. This is a questionable approach at present, as there is no histology or cytology available and under- or overtreatment may commonly take place. To avoid this, a two-stage approach was suggested in settings with low resources: to perform VIA and then take cytology from those with abnormal cervices.[97] The downside is that this adds to the total number of visits for those with the highest risk and does not remove pressure on health care workers. The most likely solution at present is to use HPV DNA testing as first-line screening.[98] This can be done on self-collected samples, reduces the need for technologists as testing is automated, and specificity is very high. The downside is cost. Thus there is no clear single solution for screening in the developing world, although HPV DNA testing is the most promising possibility.

Once HPV vaccination has been introduced, cervical screening should be continued, but the program may start cytological screening later (in the 20s) and less frequently, and consider using HPV DNA testing rather than cytology.[99]

In developed countries the practice of cytology with recall should be continued as it decreases the incidence of invasive cervical cancer.[100] Greater availability of HPV testing will force changes on to regular screening programs. At present the role of HPV testing in a setting where cytology is used is as follows: (1) HPV as primary test and cytology for those with high-risk HPV positivity; (2) HPV as adjunct test to triage those with ASCUS smears; and (3) HPV as co-test for all with a double negative as the safest possible result.

There is no regular screening program for anal cancer and it is also not likely that such a program will develop as the disease is rare and the detection of abnormalities per test is very low. In high-risk populations (HPV infection of the genital tract: in particular anal warts, persons with a history of same-sex, heterosexual, or sex-toy simulated anal intercourse, and persons with immune suppression), cytology detects cellular abnormalities from endoanal swabs. However, this screening approach is yet to be validated.

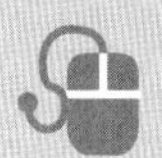

Access the complete reference list online at
http://www.expertconsult.com

Access the complete reference list online at
http://www.expertconsult.com

CHAPTER 81

Human Retroviral Infections in the Tropics

Steven J. Reynolds • Pascal O. Bessong • Thomas C. Quinn

INTRODUCTION

Shortly after the recognition of the acquired immunodeficiency syndrome (AIDS) in homosexual men in North America in the early 1980s, similar cases of immunodeficiency were identified in heterosexual men and women in tropical areas such as the Caribbean and sub-Saharan Africa.[1–6] Subsequent epidemiologic and virologic investigations demonstrated that the human immunodeficiency virus (HIV) was the etiologic agent of AIDS and that HIV was widely prevalent in both the developing and developed world.[7,8] During these early years it became clear that AIDS, which was originally believed to be restricted to a highly selected population of homosexual men in the United States, was in fact a global pandemic, spreading relentlessly to all countries of the world and becoming one of the leading causes of mortality in young adults.[9] In the first decade of the epidemic, 10 million people became infected with HIV, and now more than 33 million people are living with HIV.[10,11]

The pandemic comprises distinct epidemics among different populations and is now disproportionately affecting the developing world. Although the incidence of HIV has apparently leveled off in much of the developed world, it nevertheless continues to increase dramatically in populations of the Caribbean, Latin America, sub-Saharan Africa, Asia, and eastern and central Europe.[11] Despite having only 10% of the world's population, sub-Saharan Africa contains almost two-thirds of all people living with HIV.[11] Because of the overwhelming immunosuppression associated with HIV infections, it is also anticipated that many endemic bacterial and parasitic diseases in these regions will increase dramatically. Diseases such as tuberculosis, toxoplasmosis, cryptosporidiosis, isosporiasis, and fungal infections, including cryptococcosis and *Penicillium marneffei*, will become more prevalent and result in increasing morbidity and mortality (see Chapter 139).[12,13]

This chapter addresses the basic biology of human retroviruses, including HIV infection, the magnitude of HIV infections throughout the world, and the subsequent global response, with particular emphasis on the developing countries of the tropics. Chapter 139 further discusses the clinical presentation of HIV infection in people living in the tropics.

THE AGENT

History

The beginning of the AIDS epidemic is often marked as 1981, when the cases of five young homosexual men with puzzling manifestations of immunodeficiency were reported from the city of Los Angeles. Because the epidemic was first recognized among homosexual men, the acronym GRID ("gay-related immune deficiency") was initially proposed. However, when it became apparent that the disease was also affecting intravenous (IV) drug users and blood transfusion recipients, the term AIDS was adopted. It is remarkable that heterosexual intercourse, now by far the most common mode of transmission worldwide, was not widely recognized as a risk factor for AIDS until several years later.

After an intensive hunt for an etiologic microbe, the lentivirus HIV-1 was shown to be the causative agent of AIDS in 1983–1984. The virus was originally called LAV for lymphadenopathy virus in France and HTLV-III for human T-cell lymphotropic virus type 3 in the United States. Subsequently, the International Committee for the Taxonomy of Viruses recommended the current designation, HIV.[14,15] Serologic tests for antibodies to HIV became widely available in 1985. Only then, after serosurveys were conducted in at-risk populations around the globe, was the staggering impact of the pandemic in tropical regions appreciated.

It is now clear that HIV infections were present among humans in equatorial Africa long before the clinical AIDS epidemic was first recognized. There are sporadic case reports of Europeans, such as physician-missionaries who provided medical care in sub-Saharan African countries, who developed mysterious AIDS-like conditions after their return home. In some cases stored specimens were recently tested to establish a diagnosis of HIV infection. One case was that of a young Norwegian sailor who had traveled extensively, including to "African ports," before he first became ill in 1966.[16] By 1976 he had apparently transmitted HIV and AIDS to his wife and their newborn daughter. Serum specimens from all three family members were HIV-1-positive. Another confirmed case is that of a Portuguese man who lived in Guinea-Bissau between 1956 and 1966 and who developed AIDS in 1974.[17] Serologic tests on multiple stored specimens showed that he was HIV-2-infected. In these cases there was a travel history compatible with having become infected in Africa, clinical disease compatible with AIDS, and good enzyme-linked immunosorbent assay (ELISA) and Western blot serologic evidence of HIV infection. However, such reports of rare early HIV/AIDS cases must be interpreted cautiously, for in other touted early cases of HIV in travelers the diagnosis was proved to be erroneous.

Retrospective serologic studies on stored serum samples have also identified early (pre-1981) cases of autochthonous transmission of HIV in sub-Saharan Africa. One positive specimen was a plasma sample that had originally been obtained as part of immunogenetic studies from a donor in Leopoldville (now Kinshasa, Democratic Republic of Congo) in 1959.[18] When thawed and tested 27 years later, the sample was strongly positive by ELISA, immunofluorescence, Western blot, and immunoprecipitation for HIV-1 antibodies, and tests were negative in appropriate control assays. Even more solid evidence for early prevalence of HIV in Africa was obtained by a retrospective study of serum specimens that had coincidentally been collected in 1976 from apparently healthy persons in northern Zaire (now Congo) as part of a survey for Ebola virus antibodies. When these frozen serum specimens were thawed and tested a decade later, five were found to be antibody-positive for HIV. Three of these patients were then relocated, and all were again confirmed to be HIV-seropositive. HIV-1, genotype A (the Z321 strain), was obtained by blood culture from one of these patients.[19–21]

Collectively these studies show that HIV viruses – strains not dissimilar from contemporary HIV strains – were present, probably at low levels, in equatorial Africa in the 1950s, 1960s, and early 1970s. However, it was not until the late 1970s and early 1980s that the AIDS epidemic became clinically apparent in Africa. Because there were no rare and unique "marker" opportunistic infections in Africa – a role served by *Pneumocystis carinii* infections in Los Angeles – it is more difficult to date the onset of the African AIDS epidemic. Only by reconstructing epidemic curves for certain readily diagnosed but less common infections, such as cryptococcal meningitis (in Kinshasa) or herpes zoster (in Lusaka, Zambia), was it possible to bracket roughly the onset of the African AIDS epidemic. We now know that by the time the AIDS epidemic was first recognized, it had been preceded for several years by a silent HIV epidemic.

By the end of 1984, a global pattern had emerged in which most AIDS cases among Africans and Haitians, whether they lived in their home countries or abroad, were associated with heterosexual intercourse, whereas most cases among North Americans, Europeans, and South Americans (largely Brazilians) were associated with homosexual sex or IV drug use. Early reports of a relatively high AIDS incidence regrettably led to irrational discrimination against Haitians in the United States.

Taxonomy of HIV and Other Lentiviruses

HIV, like all other retroviruses, is an enveloped, positive-stranded RNA virus. Particles are approximately 110 nm in diameter and contain a cone-shaped core of nucleoprotein. The virus is "diploid" in that the genome consists of two essentially identical dimerized full-length strands of approximately 10 000 ribonucleotides. Viral particles also contain reverse transcriptase, the enzyme that copies the RNA into double-stranded DNA (complementary plus and minus strands) that becomes integrated into the host cell genome as a provirus. Genome sequencing has clarified the phylogenetic relationships between the lentiviruses of nonprimate mammals, of nonhuman primates, and of humans.[22]

There are two major lentiviruses of humans – HIV-1 and HIV-2 – in addition to two groups of less well-defined assortments of viruses loosely related to HIV-1, informally referred to as HIV-1-O (outlier) group, HIV-1-N (non-M, non-N), and HIV-1-P.[23–26] HIV-1 and HIV-1-O strains also roughly cluster with the simian immunodeficiency virus (SIV_{CPZ}) branch of primate lentiviruses, while HIV-2 strains cluster tightly with the SIV_{SMM} branch. These phylogenetic relationships of humans with simian lentiviruses have obvious implications regarding the origin of human HIV and AIDS.[27]

Thus far, HIV-1-O and HIV-1-P viruses have been found only in persons from Cameroon, Gabon, or Equatorial Guinea. The designation "HIV-1-M (main) group" has informally been used to distinguish the globally predominant HIV-1 genotypes from viruses in the geographically restricted and incompletely characterized HIV-1-O, HIV-1-N, and HIV-1-P. Nucleotide sequences have been determined for thousands of HIV strains from around the world, and these have been placed into phylogenetic clusters. Different research groups have sequenced and analyzed different regions of the viral genome.[28,29] With a few important exceptions, the phylogenetic relationships based on different regions of the genome, such as *gag* or *env*, are closely congruent. Within each of the HIV types (HIV-1 and HIV-2) there are a number of discrete genotypes or clades. By convention these are given letter designations, in an order that roughly reflects the order of their discovery. At least nine genotypes of HIV-1 group M have been identified, termed HIV-1 A–D, F–H, J, and K. This classification uses phylogenetic and distance analyses of at least three regions of the genome.[30,31] All clades are roughly equidistant from each other in a "star" phylogeny; no virus or clade is an obvious candidate as the progenitor virus for other clades. Maximum *env* gene differences between HIV-1 strains within a clade are no more than 15%, whereas differences between strains of different clades may be as great as 20% or 30%. The oldest known HIV-1 isolate, Z321 virus from the then Zaire in 1976, is an HIV-1 A clade virus. Five genotypes of HIV-2 have been identified, HIV-2A through E. As with HIV-1, no HIV-2 virus or clade is a clear progenitor.[32]

The taxonomy of primate lentiviruses has been complicated by the finding that many strains appear to be naturally occurring recombinants. A variant formerly designated as subtype E based on the *env* gene sequence was later shown to be a recombinant between clades A and E,[33] though a nonrecombinant clade E (pure clade E) has not been found. Interclade A/E possesses *gag* and *pol* genes, which are homologous to clade A viruses, but the *env* gene comes from an as yet undetected clade E. Consequently, clade E is not recognized as a separate cluster of closely related viruses. In a similar vein, previously tagged clade I based on the C3V3 sequence[34] has been shown to be a complex recombinant comprising clades A, G, and regions that do not fall within any presently known defined clade.[35,36] These interclade recombinants have been termed circulating recombinant forms (CRFs), since they contribute significantly to the global epidemic. As a result, previously known subtypes E and I are now referred to as CRF01_AE and CRF04_cpx, respectively. Other CRFs include CRF02_AG, which represents a recombination between clades A and G and circulates in West and Central Africa,[37,38] and CRF03_AB, which represents a clade A/B recombinant form that has mostly been responsible for the epidemic among IV drug users in Kalinigrad.[39] There are now 46 CRFs described in the literature and selected representative lentiviruses and CRFs are shown in ***Figure 81.1***.

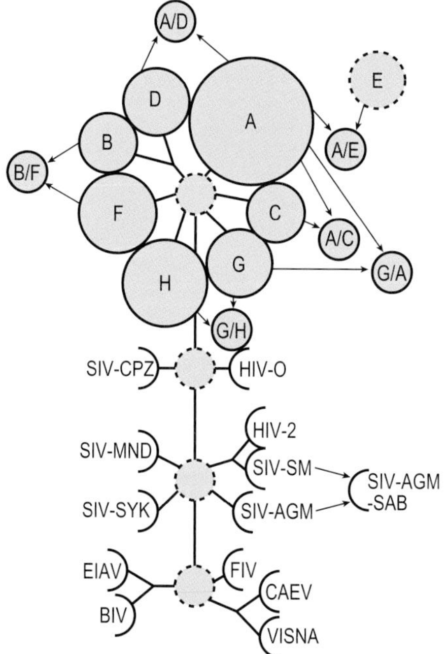

Figure 81.1 Schematic diagram of the lentivirus phylogenetic tree showing the known lentiviruses of nonprimate mammals (BIV, bovine immunodeficiency virus; CAEV, caprine arthritis and encephalitis virus; EIAV, equine infectious anemia virus; FIV, feline immunodeficiency virus), of nonhuman primates (AGM, African green monkey; CPZ, chimpanzee; MND, mandril; SAB, sabaeus monkey; SIV, simian immunodeficiency virus; SM, sooty mangabey; SYK, Sykes' monkey), and the human viruses (HIV, human immunodeficiency virus types 1 and 2 and type 1 "outlier" strains, which are shown at HIV-O). For the human HIV viruses, the clades are shown as circles with the size of the circles roughly proportional to the known genetic diversity of the viruses within each clade. Recombinant strains are shown as the convergence points of arrows from defined clades. The parent E clade virus that contributed genes to the widely prevalent E/A recombinant clade is only hypothetical and therefore shown as a dashed circle.

Scientific Evidence on the Origin of HIV and AIDS

Several lines of evidence suggest that HIV-2 entered the human population directly from sooty mangabeys. Key observations are the following. SIV is a benign, highly prevalent virus in sooty mangabeys; SIV_{SMM} grows well in human cells *in vitro* and can infect humans *in vivo* (laboratory workers); the natural habitat of sooty mangabeys in West Africa corresponds closely to the regions of highest human HIV-2 prevalence; and most important, HIV-2 is essentially genetically indistinguishable from SIV_{SMM} (given a viral isolate with no additional information, it would be impossible to be certain whether it was obtained from a sooty mangabey or a human). Even more suggestive are recent molecular epidemiologic studies showing that HIV-2 strains from a given West African country are more similar to SIV_{SMM} strains from that country than they are to other HIV-2 strains from other countries. These data suggest not only that SIV_{SMM} emerged from sooty mangabeys into humans, but that it may even be "continuously emerging" through repeated cross-species transmissions. The exact mechanism of transmission remains uncertain. Mangabeys that are kept as pets may infect humans through bites or scratches, and hunters or food preparers may become infected through direct contact with blood when mangabeys are killed as a food source.

How HIV-1 may have originated in human populations is not so clear. Reasoning by analogy with HIV-2, one possibility is that HIV-1 simply represents a nonhuman primate virus that became "humanized" after a cross-species transmission. Data indicate that HIV-1 emergence resulted from three independent cross-species transmission events that gave rise to HIV-1 groups M, N, O, and P. All HIV-1 groups are closely related to SIVcpz,[40] and recent sequence and phylogenetic analyses strongly tie the origin of HIV-1-N to SIVcpz.[25] Again, additional sampling in this region might provide crucial information.

One clue to the origins of HIV-1 may be the remarkable genetic diversity of HIV-1, HIV-1-O, HIV-1-N, and HIV-1-P viruses among humans in the equatorial African countries that encompass the Congo river basin rainforest. Eight HIV-1 clades and at least three HIV-1-O clades can be found in this region, whereas in all other parts of the world no more than one or two clades are highly prevalent and autochthonously transmitted. Furthermore, a high proportion (perhaps 25%) of the HIV-1 viruses in this geographic region are interclade recombinants.[41] The high level of diversity and frequent recombination suggest that HIV-1 and related viruses may have been prevalent in equatorial Africa for quite a long time. Instead of a simple recent direct emergence (as occurred for HIV-2), it appears more likely that the current epidemic HIV-1 strains emerged some time ago and have been continuously evolving in human populations. Successively more transmissible forms may have arisen and propagated among humans through natural selection. Careful molecular epidemiologic studies of HIV-1, HIV-1-O, HIV-1-N, HIV-1-P, SIV_{CPZ}, and other primate lentiviruses in the African rainforest could shed considerable light on the emergence and evolution of HIV-1.

Viral Genome Organization

Like all retroviruses, the life cycle of HIV is characterized by alternating stages in which the genetic information is carried by DNA or by RNA: the proviral (intranuclear) stage and the viral (extracellular) stage, respectively. Proviral DNA – viral genetic information that is integrated into the host cell genome in the form of DNA – is transcribed and translated, and full-length plus-strand RNA transcripts are packaged into virions, using conventional cellular machinery. Genetic information is routed back from free viral RNA to the host cell proviral DNA form by unique viral enzymes for reverse transcription and integration.

All retroviruses have in common three major genes: the *gag, pol,* and *env* genes.[42] The *gag* gene was so named because in early serologic studies cross-reactions were most readily detected with these antigens, hence "group-specific antigen," or gag. The *pol* and *env* genes encode polymerase and envelope proteins, respectively. The large precursor proteins expressed from all three of these major genes are subsequently cleaved into smaller functional proteins. In HIV-1 the gag p55 precursor is cleaved into the p17 matrix protein and the p24 capsid, p7 nucleocapsid, and p6 proteins. The latter three proteins collectively form the viral core. The *pol* gene is translated as part of a *gag-pol* frameshift read-through polyprotein, which is cleaved into a p15 protease, a p66/p51 heterodimer with reverse transcriptase and RNAase H activity, and a p32 integrase. The *env* gene encodes a p90 protein that is heavily glycosylated to become gp 160, which is cleaved into surface gp 120 and a transmembrane gp41. Protein sizes and cleavages differ somewhat between human and primate lentiviruses, but overall the coding and expression patterns are similar (*Fig. 81.2*).

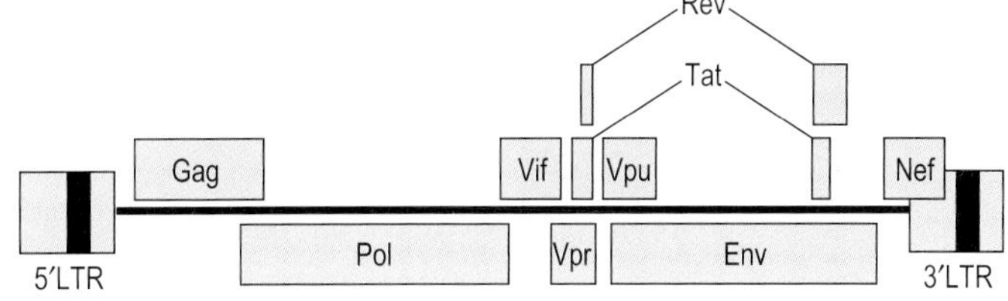

Figure 81.2 Genome organization of human immunodeficiency virus type 1 (HIV-1). Long terminal repeats (LTRs) are shown as broad rectangles at the 3′- and 5′-terminals of the genome. Open reading frames are shown as narrower rectangles with their designated gene names. See text for full names and functions of genes.

The genomes of HIV and related viruses contain genes that encode viral regulatory proteins – *tat* (transactivator of transcription) and *rev* (transport of structural protein messenger RNA (mRNA), especially *env*) – which are important in governing viral transcription and translation. In addition, HIV-1 has four open reading frames from which proteins are expressed *in vitro* and probably *in vivo*, commonly called the "accessory genes": *vif* (viral infectivity factor), *vpr* (viral protein R), *vpu* (viral protein U), and *nef* (negative factor). *Vif* and *vpr* are particle-associated, whereas *vpu* and *nef* are not. These accessory genes are highly conserved in nature but are not essential to replication *in vitro*, and although much is known about the biochemical properties of these gene products, their vital functions remain uncertain.

The suggestion has been made that the lentiviruses, along with the bovine leukemia virus (BLV) and HTLV group of viruses, be classified as "complex retroviruses" because of their unique ability to regulate expression of their own genes through feedback loops.[43] This self-regulating property may be important in the establishment of chronic infections in long-lived hosts.

Viral Life Cycle

The primate lentiviruses all share essentially the same replication cycle (*Fig. 81.3*).

Attachment, Penetration, and Uncoating

When a free virion comes into contact with a cell surface, the first specific attachment is made between a specific region of the HIV gp120 surface envelop glycoprotein and the 58-kDa cell surface CD4 molecule.[44] The CD4 molecule is a member of the immunoglobulin superfamily that is expressed on the surface of T lymphocytes (and at lower levels on other cells) and normally serves as a corecognition factor for major histocompatibility complex (MHC) class II in antigen presentation. The gp120–CD4 interaction initiates conformational changes in gp120, which then permits interaction of gp120 with a second cell surface receptor, the CXCR4 chemokine receptor molecule (on T lymphocytes) or the similar CCR5 molecule on macrophages.[45] Fusion of the viral lipid bilayer membrane with the cell membrane is mediated by a specific hydrophobic region fusion domain of the viral gp41 transmembrane protein. Sequential

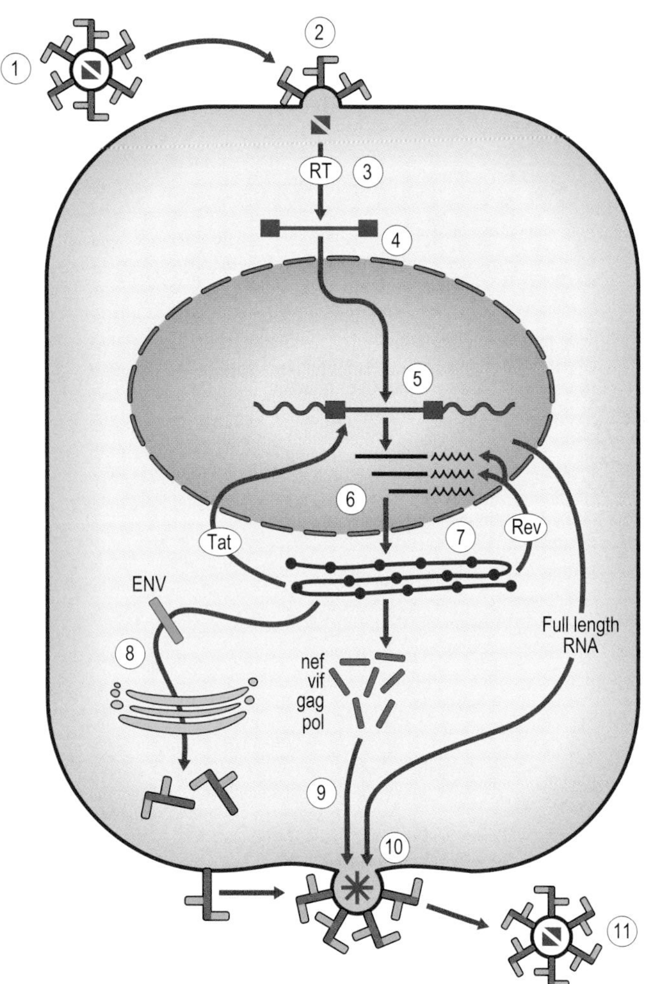

Figure 81.3 Schematic representation of the life cycle of human immunodeficiency virus (HIV) in a cell. The outer boundary is the cell membrane, and the inner boundary is the nuclear membrane. 1, free virus; 2, binding and entry; 3, reverse transcription (RT); 4, nuclear transport; 5, integration; 6, transcription and splicing; 7, translation; 8, glycosylation; 9, membrane transport; 10, assembly and budding; 11, virion release and maturation.

binding of gp120 to CD4 and CXCR4 (or CCR5) is thought to trigger gp41 to "harpoon" the cell membrane lipid bilayer. The process then repeats with many virion gp120 molecules interacting with the cellular receptors until fusion is complete. Fusion can proceed at neutral pH typical of extracellular fluids.

DNA Synthesis, Nuclear Transport, and Integration

Once the virus has inserted itself into the cytoplasm, the reverse transcriptase becomes activated and DNA proviral synthesis begins.[46–48] The initial event in reverse transcription – copying of virion RNA into DNA – is primed by cellular lysine transfer RNA (tRNA) (other retroviruses use other tRNA primers). The HIV reverse transcriptase molecule carries out three distinct enzymatic functions: (1) synthesis of a complete DNA negative strand using the virion RNA template; (2) degradation of the virion RNA template as the DNA strand is synthesized; and (3) synthesis of a DNA positive strand using the newly synthesized complete DNA negative strand. The net product is double-stranded DNA synthesized from an RNA template.

The sequences of the virion RNA and the proviral DNA are identical in their mid-genome (protein-coding regions) but differ in the arrangement of repeat and unique noncoding sequences at their terminals. In viral RNA, the order is repeat, 5′ unique, *gag-pol-env*, 3′ unique, repeat. As a consequence of a somewhat complicated series of head-to-tail jumps of the transcriptase that occur in synthesis of both the negative and positive DNA strands, this order becomes altered such that in the final double-stranded DNA provirus it becomes unique 3′, repeat, unique 5′, *gag-pol-env*, unique 3′, repeat, unique 5′. The U3-R-U5 sequence at both terminals is called the long terminal repeat, or LTR. When viral RNA is forward-transcribed, the outer unique regions of the proviral LTR DNA are not copied. This overall schema is thought to be necessary to provide for efficient priming and complete copying of both terminals. Occasionally aberrant reverse transcription occurs, leading to covalently closed DNA circles containing either one or two LTRs, but these forms are dead-end.

In contrast to other retroviruses, HIV and the lentiviruses do not require that the newly infected cell undergo mitosis for integration to occur. The synthesized double-stranded DNA copy of the viral sequences is transported to the nucleus as a preintegration complex (PIC), probably through microtubules. The nucleophilic behavior of PIC is thought to be influenced by import signals under the control of integrase, viral protein R (vpr), the DNA flap, and the p17 matrix protein.[49–51]

Integration is not site-specific in the host cell chromosome; apparently it can occur anywhere. However, chromosomal sites that are transcriptionally active are more likely, presumably because the chromatin structure is more open and accessible. Proviral integration is catalyzed by the viral integrase and involves 3′ end processing of both viral DNA strands, and strand transfer of both host cell DNA strands to the activated 3′ proviral ends.[52,53] Because the activated 3′ viral DNA strands invade the host cell DNA strands at sites a few nucleotides apart, there is a characteristic short duplication of host cell sequence flanking both ends of the newly integrated provirus.

Gene Expression

The LTRs are organized such that the integrated provirus has a built-in 5′ promoter-enhancer and a 3′ polyadenylation site. The key activator on the HIV-1 5′ LTR promoter is the NF-κB binding site. Since NF-κB serves as an important cell activation factor, HIV transcription is unregulated concurrently with cell activation. The virus-encoded tat protein also increases viral transcription by binding to the tat RNA secondary structure in the 5′ LTR promoter region. An important consequence of this feedback loop is that HIV transcription is autocatalytic.[54–56] HIV transcripts are typically spliced into a large number of RNAs of different lengths. Spliced RNAs are efficiently transported from the nucleus and translated. However, long and unspliced RNAs (those containing the mid-env rev-responsive element, or RRE) are not transported unless the early viral protein rev is present in abundance.[57,58] Transport is mediated by rev binding to the RNA secondary structure formed by the RRE sequence.

Particle Assembly and Budding

Uncleaved gag precursor protein molecules and a much smaller number (5%) of gag-pol read-through proteins are targeted to the interior surface of the cell membrane by their myristoylated N-terminals. Viral core proteins are thereby aligned from outermost to innermost according to their position in the polyprotein: p17 matrix, p24 capsid, and nucleocapsid from the gag precursor, and then protease, reverse transcriptase, and integrase from the pol precursor. Cleavages are self-catalyzed by the viral-encoded protease.[59] HIV protease is an aspartic protease which is active only as a dimer; virion assembly is thought to activate the protease. The nucleocapsid protein, the innermost of the gag proteins, interacts directly with a packaging site on full-length viral RNA via a complex of cystine residues (similar to a zinc finger motif in DNA binding proteins) and thereby guides genome encapsidation.[60] Independently, full-length gp160 envelope protein is oligomerized, glycosylated, and cleaved by cellular protease in the endoplasmic reticulum (ER) and Golgi apparatus into gp120 and gp41.[61,62] Envelope protein on the outer cell surface interacts with the p17 matrix (gag) protein via an internal cytoplasmic region of the gp41 transmembrane protein.

Genetic Organization of Human Lentiviruses from Tropical Regions

The genetic structures of HIV-1, HIV-2, HIV-1-O, HIV-1-N, and HIV-1-P strains thus far studied are quite similar. The most obvious difference is that *p16 vpu* is found only in HIV-1, while *p16 vpx* is found only in HIV-2 (and primate SIV strains). These two genes (of uncertain function) are present in different locations in the mid-genomic accessory gene region. Among the HIV-1 strains the genomic structure is highly conserved despite substantial nucleotide sequence variation. Potentially significant variations between HIV-1 strains have been observed in the number of SP-1 and NF-κB binding sites in the LTR promoter regions, particularly among non-B clade viruses, but these have not been systematically studied. Few attempts have been made to compare the molecular biology of clades, and no clear differences have been found.

Cell Tropism

Human and primate lentiviruses can infect a variety of cell types *in vitro* under relatively artificial laboratory conditions, but there is no convincing evidence that any cells except those of the mononuclear leukocyte lineages are infected *in vivo*. CD4+ T lymphocytes were the first cells found to be infected (hence the originally proposed name HTLV-III), but a variety of macrophage-related cells (blood monocytes, skin Langerhans cells, lymph node dendritic cells) also appear to be infected.[63,64] The presence of the two receptors – CD4 and CXCR4 (or CCR5) – appears to define the population of human cells that are permissive to HIV infection.

HIV-1 strains collected from blood early in infection are genetically homogeneous and uniformly display a characteristic "macrophage-tropic" envelope sequence.[65,66] As infection progresses over months and years, genetic variation in the blood increases so that the viral population becomes a quasispecies of genomes that may differ by 5% or more in their nucleotide sequences. Variation occurs in all genes, including the envelope, where mutations occur that change the affected virions from a macrophage-tropic to a "T-cell tropic syncytium-inducing" phenotype. The reason for this change in phenotype is not very clear, though it could be attributed to changes in the V-3 loop and V-2 region of the envelope protein, since these regions appear to determine coreceptor usage.[67,68] However, these altered viruses could as well be vertically transmitted.[69] The importance of CCR5 as a coreceptor is highlighted in the high degree of resistance to HIV-1 infection by certain individuals who show a 32-base pair deletion in the CCR5 gene. The prevalence of this mutation is estimated to be about 16% in Caucasians, and 1% are homozygous for this trait.[70] Because most new infection initiates with a macrophage-tropic variant, these observations are consistent with a viral life cycle in which macrophage-tropic viruses are the person-to-person transmissible forms and T-cell tropic viruses are the immunologically destructive forms. This suggests a "queen–drone" relationship between the transmission-competent macrophage-tropic genomes and the host-confined T-cell tropic genomes. Based on the type of HIV-1 target cells, the cytopathic effect produced, and the coreceptor preferred, the majority of HIV-1 strains could be classified as three types of viruses: CCR5 viruses (R5) that use CCR5 as coreceptor, infect macrophages, and do not cause syncytia; CXCR4 viruses (R4) that use CXCR4 as coreceptor, infect T cells, and cause syncytia, and CCR5/CXCR4 viruses (R5X4) that are dual tropic.[71,72] M-tropic viruses predominate at the onset of infection and throughout the asymptomatic and symptomatic phases. However, evidence suggests a switch from CCR5 usage to CXCR4 for certain viruses in some individuals in the late symptomatic phase of HIV-1 infection (AIDS). As a result, there is a pool of R5, X4, and R5X4 viruses.[73,74]

Other Human Retroviruses (Including Human T-Cell Lymphotropic Viruses Types I and II)

Transposable Elements and Endogenous Retroviruses

The normal eukaryotic genome is studded with a large number of genetic elements that show similarity to retroviruses.[75] These "normal" mobile genomic regions, called transposons or retrotransposons (depending on whether they encode a reverse transcriptase), can undergo limited replication and reinsertion within the genome but cannot be transmitted from one host cell to another. Other genomic elements show even closer homology to full retroviruses and are thought to represent defective remnants of retroviruses that became stably integrated into the genome in the recent evolutionary past. These endogenous retroviruses can rarely become activated, or they can recombine with other related retroviruses to yield replication-competent chimeric progeny retroviruses. Transposable elements and endogenous retroviruses are thought to be the cause of a number of genetic abnormalities, malignancies, and autoimmune diseases.[76–78]

HTLV-I and HTLV-II

The first isolation of HTLV-I was reported in 1980 in a T-cell line from a patient with a T-cell leukemia/lymphoma. The viruses were found to be similar in morphology and genomic organization to the BLV, a retrovirus that causes B-cell lymphomas in cattle.[79] Shortly thereafter, another related virus, HTLV-II, was identified in a T-cell line from a patient with hairy cell leukemia. These and related viruses are now collectively classified as the HTLV-BLV group. HTLV-I and -II have an overall genomic structure typical of retroviruses, with LTRs and *gag, pol,* and *env* genes. The HTLV-BLV group viruses are similar to the lentiviruses in that they are complex retroviruses with specific viral-encoded mechanisms for transactivation and RNA transport; the *tax* and *rex* genes of HTLV-I and -II are analogs of the HIV *tat* and *rev* genes. HTLV-I and -II share about 65% similarity in their nucleotide sequences. Within HTLV-I, strains from different parts of the world are genetically much less diverse than are HIV-1 strains, showing only about 7% sequence divergence. Clade or subtype systems have been proposed for HTLV-I and for HTLV-II in a manner similar to HIV. It is often possible to reconstruct the epidemiologic spread of HTLV-I epidemics using genetic sequence data.[80]

HTLV-I is proved to be causally associated with adult T-cell leukemia (ATL) and neurologic diseases of spinal cord known in the Caribbean as tropical spastic paraparesis (TSP) and in Japan as HTLV-associated myelopathy (HAM).[81,82] There have been clinical reports of HTLV-I and -II associated with chronic arthropathy and with uveitis, but a causal relationship remains unproved. HTLV-I can present at a variety of stages: asymptomatic, with no symptoms, signs, or laboratory evidence of disease; "smoldering" or chronic T-cell leukemia, with an elevated percentage of abnormal lymphocytes; and full-blown ATL, with an elevated white blood cell count, anemia, and hypercalcemia. The overall natural history of disease in HTLV-I infection is slow, with an average of 20–30 years from the time of infection to the onset of ATL. Although less common, TSP and HAM can develop within a few years after infection. Although HTLV-II has been detected in a number of patients with lymphomas and other malignancies, it is still uncertain whether HTLV-II causes significant disease.

The prevalence of HTLV varies substantially in different parts of the world.[83] Highest prevalence, on the order of 35%, has been reported from Okinawa.[84] HTLV-I is also endemic in East Asia, Papua New Guinea, the Caribbean, and equatorial Africa, where prevalence of 1–10% is common. As with other chronic bloodborne infections, HTLV can be transmitted from males to females or to other males by sexual intercourse, from mother to infant at the time of birth, and by blood transfusion or the use of contaminated needles.[85] High prevalence of

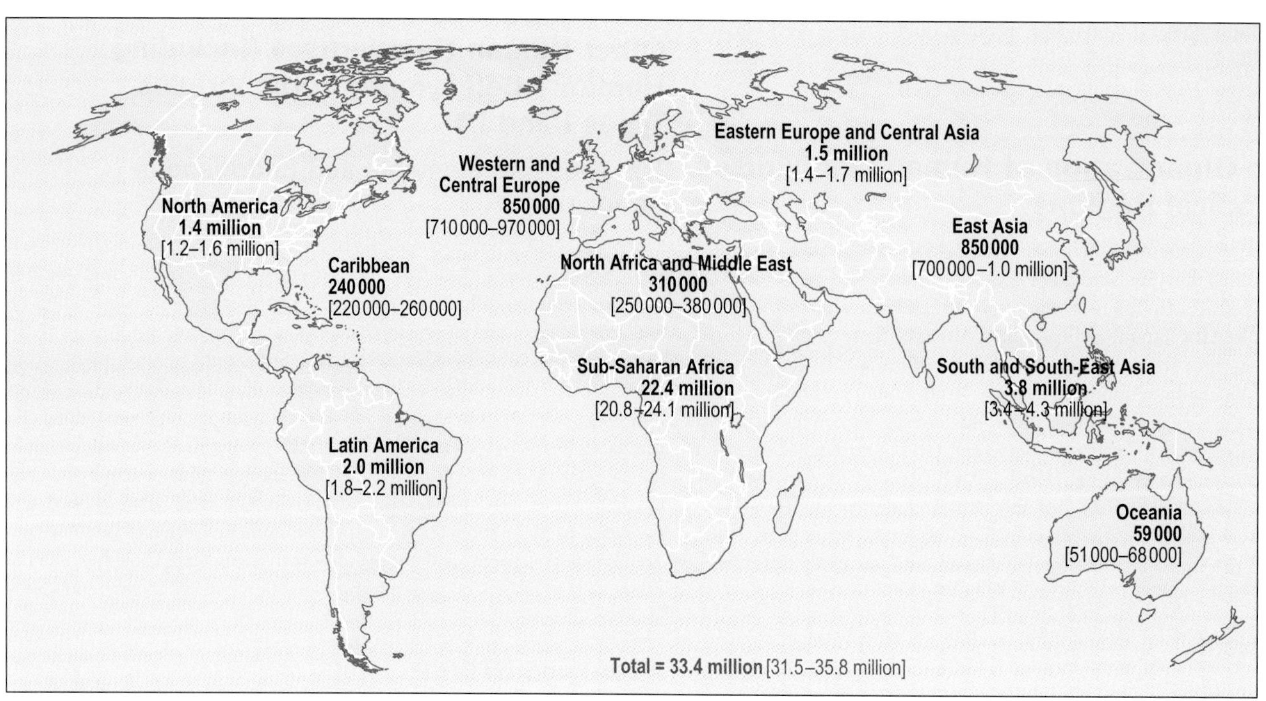

Figure 81.4 Estimated number of adults and children living with human immunodeficiency virus (HIV) as at the end of 2008. (Data from 2009 Report on the Global AIDS Epidemic. Geneva: UNAIDS; 2009.)

HTLV-I and -II has been found in populations of IV drug users in the United States and Europe.[86] A variety of promising antiviral agents have activity against HTLV-I and -II *in vitro*, but none has proved beneficial in ATL, TSP, or HAM. Treatment of ATL is directed at induction of leukemia remission, and for TSP and HAM it is largely supportive.

Magnitude of the HIV Pandemic

In 2008, 2.7 million people became infected with HIV. Globally, 33 million people are currently living with HIV, and women now represent 50% of all infections and over 60% of cases in sub-Saharan Africa due to increasing heterosexual transmission in both the developing and developed world[11,87,88] (***Figs 81.4 and 81.5***). The number of deaths due to AIDS continues to be alarmingly high with an estimated 2.0 million people dying of AIDS in 2008.[11] In many countries, AIDS is erasing decades of progress in improving life expectancy. In sub-Saharan Africa, life expectancy is now 47 years instead of the 62 years expected without AIDS (***Fig. 81.6***). In this setting, the death toll continues to rise with an estimated 68 million people dying earlier than they would have in the absence of AIDS in the 45 most affected countries. AIDS has a particularly strong impact on under-5-year mortality with most children who are infected at birth or through breastfeeding dying of AIDS before age 5. The majority of newly infected adults are under 25 years of age, and 90% of all new infections are occurring in developing countries. With an associated mortality rate greater than 90% and with the current lack of vaccine or curative drug, it is clear from these estimates that the HIV pandemic will continue to escalate worldwide and have an enormous impact on public health over the next several decades.[10]

Currently, the largest number of HIV-infected persons is in sub-Saharan Africa, totaling 22 million, and in Asia and the Pacific, totaling 5 million[11,12] (see ***Fig. 81.4***). The epidemic in South Asia continues to be dominated by India, where 3.8 million infections were noted as of 2008.[89] The magnitude of the epidemic continues to be staggering, with the number of new infections outnumbering the number of individuals on treatment; for every two people started on treatment, five are infected with the virus.[90]

Modes of Transmission

HIV infections are transmitted through unprotected sexual intercourse, including heterosexual and homosexual transmission; parenteral transmission, via blood through use of inadequately sterilized needles, syringes, or other skin-piercing instruments and transfusion of infected blood; and perinatal transmission from an infected mother to her fetus or infant during pregnancy, delivery, or breastfeeding.

Sexual Transmission

Globally, between 75% and 80% of all HIV infections in adults are transmitted through unprotected sexual intercourse.[91] Heterosexual intercourse accounts for more than 70% of global adult HIV infections and homosexual intercourse for a further 5–10%, though in specific regions these proportions differ. For example, the proportion of sexual transmission due to homosexual spread is much greater in North America, Europe, and Australia, whereas heterosexual transmission is by far more common in the developing countries.[10,86,87,92,93] As a result of heterosexual transmission in Africa, the male-to-female ratio of HIV infection is 1 : 1.4. Urban populations with consistently high rates of sexually transmitted diseases (STDs) and prostitution have the highest rates of HIV infection. Rates of infection among female sex workers range from 40% in Kinshasa, Zaire, to 80% in Nairobi, Kenya, and 88% in Butari, Rwanda.[94] In rural areas that are culturally more conservative, and where the incidence of STDs is much lower, there appear to be lower rates of HIV infection also, although rural rates of HIV infection are rising in some areas of Uganda, Tanzania, and other countries.[94–96] Certain risk factors, such as promiscuity, anal intercourse, sex with infected persons, prostitution, and other behavioral factors appear to be responsible for an increased risk of heterosexual transmission.[97]

An epidemiologic synergy has been demonstrated between HIV and STDs that is related to both behavioral and biologic factors.[98] Epidemiologic studies from sub-Saharan Africa, Asia, Europe, and North America suggest that there is approximately a fourfold greater risk of becoming HIV-infected if a genital ulcer caused by syphilis, chancroid, or herpes is present, and a two- to threefold greater risk if other STDs, such as

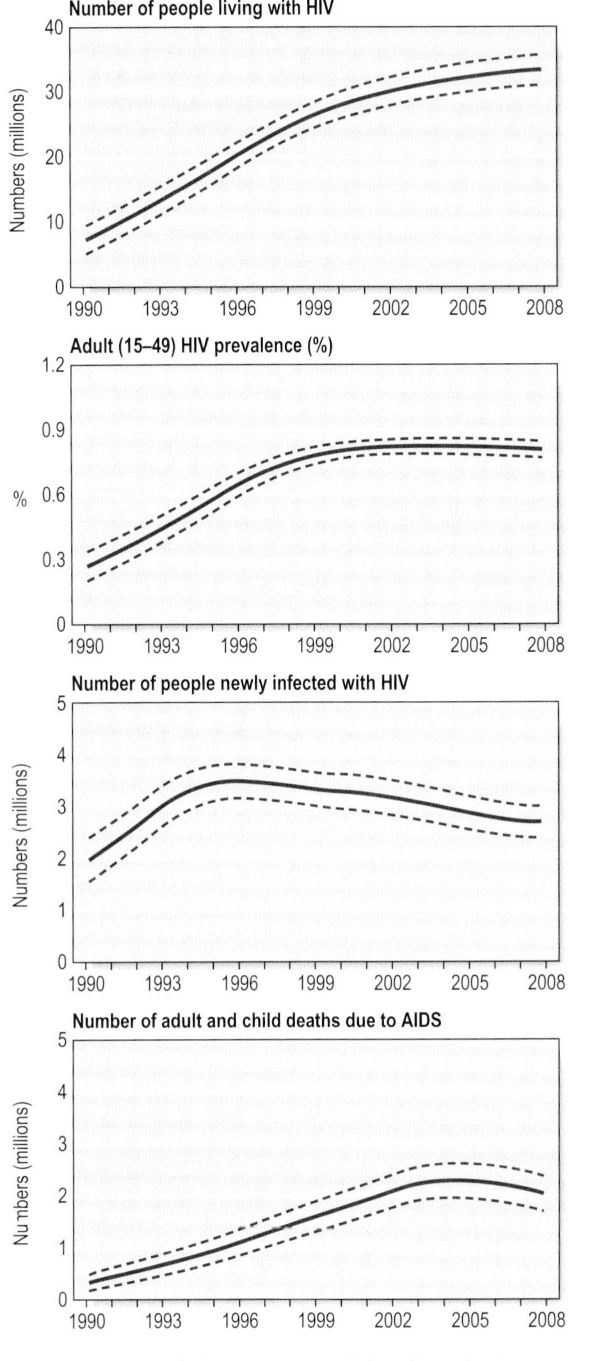

Figure 81.5 Growth of the global acquired immunodeficiency syndrome (AIDS) epidemic between 1990 and 2008 by prevalence and by number of people living with human immunodeficiency virus (HIV)/AIDS. (Data from 2009 Report on the Global AIDS Epidemic. Geneva: UNAIDS; 2009.)

gonorrhea, chlamydia infection, and trichomoniasis, are present.[99–106] Despite the prevention efforts of the past decade, STDs continue to be significant public health problems in developed and developing countries. In 1995 it was estimated that 333 million new cases of curable STDs, including gonorrhea, chlamydia infection, syphilis, and trichomoniasis, occurred.[107] An even greater number of cases may have occurred among the viral STDs, which include human papillomavirus, herpes simplex virus, and hepatitis. Of note, the greatest number of these STDs occur in Southeast Asia and sub-Saharan Africa, the two regions with the highest rate of HIV infection.

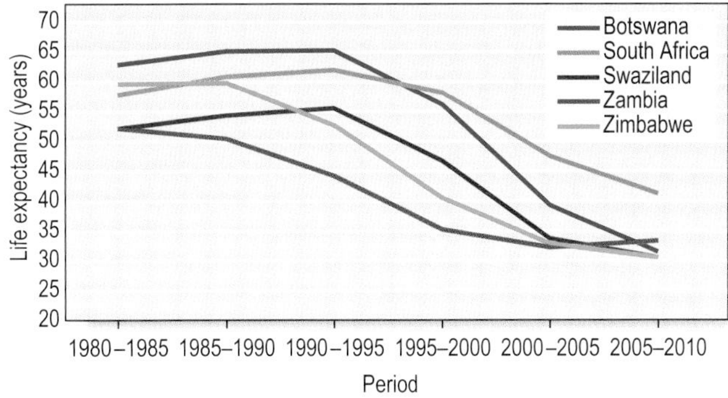

Figure 81.6 Impact of human immunodeficiency virus on life expectancy in selected countries between 1980–1985 and 2005–2010. (Data from 2009 Report on the Global AIDS Epidemic. Geneva: UNAIDS; 2009.)

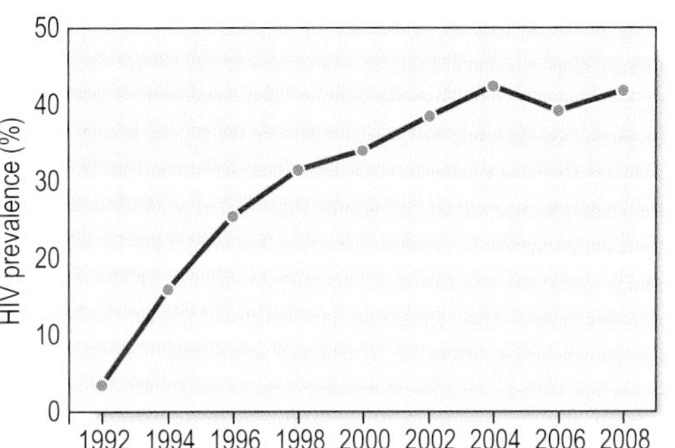

Figure 81.7 Median human immunodeficiency virus prevalence in pregnant women attending antenatal clinics in Swaziland, 1992–2008. Data are from consistent sites. (Data from 2009 Report on the Global AIDS Epidemic. Geneva: UNAIDS; 2009.)

Perinatal Transmission

With the increased incidence of HIV infection among women, perinatal transmission (which can occur *in utero*, during delivery, or postnatally via breastfeeding) is becoming increasingly common.[108] Serologic surveys, particularly in urban centers of sub-Saharan Africa, have found HIV infection rates of 5–30% in pregnant women[109] (***Fig. 81.7***). Transmission rates from mother to infant have been highly variable but range from 13% to 52%, with an average of 30%.[110] Factors associated with increased perinatal transmission include advanced maternal stage of disease, increased viral titers, decreased maternal serum vitamin A levels, chorioamnionitis, placental malaria, maternal anemia, maternal smoking, and low neutralizing antibody titers to the V3 loop of the glycoprotein gp120 of HIV.[108,111–115] The more common use of breastfeeding in developing countries may also contribute to the observed increased perinatal transmission in those countries compared with that observed in developed countries; data suggest that up to 15% of infants breastfed by HIV-infected mothers may become infected through breastfeeding.[116] Although bottle-feeding is recommended for HIV-infected women in developed countries, this has not been recommended in developing countries, where breastfeeding helps prevent diarrhea and provides important nutrients for infants.[98]

Parenteral Transmission

The sharing of HIV-infected injection equipment by illicit drug users results in about 5–10% of all adult infections.[117] In some areas of the world this is the dominant mode of HIV transmission, but in most developing countries, transfusion of HIV-infected blood or blood products still accounts for some adult HIV infections.[118] In many parts of the developing world, HIV screening of the blood supply is still severely limited because of cost. In areas where universal screening of blood donations has not been implemented, progress toward a safer supply of blood and blood products can be achieved through appropriate selection and retention of voluntary, nonremunerated, low-risk donors and through more rational use of blood aimed at decreasing the number of people receiving transfusions, as well as using blood substitutes and plasma expanders wherever possible.[118–122]

Other modes of transmission are more infrequent. For example, the risk of HIV transmission in a health care setting through accidental exposure to HIV-infected blood is estimated to be 0.3%, and the risk after mucocutaneous exposure is much less.[122] Household transmission may also occur when there is contact with blood or other body secretions or excretions from a person already known to be infected with HIV.[123,124] However, surveys done in Africa, Europe, and North America have shown that aside from sexual transmission within the household, nonsexual contact results in very few transmitted cases.[124–126]

Biologic Factors Influencing Transmission

Most humans are fully susceptible to HIV infection. Some persons lack the second (chemokine receptor CCR5) cellular receptor for HIV attachment and appear to be naturally resistant to infection.[65] Such homozygous naturally insusceptible persons are rare in the United States; surveys have not yet been done among populations in tropical regions. Other persons may acquire immunity: some highly exposed, but apparently uninfected, individuals have measurable cellular immunoresponsiveness to HIV, suggesting that they have been immunized through repeated exposure to low levels of antigen or virus, but it is unknown whether they are truly immune to challenge.[127,128]

The co-occurrence of other STDs, such as syphilis, herpes, chancroid, gonorrhea, and chlamydia infection, increases both the risk of acquisition and the risk of transmission of HIV infection. The exact mechanism of this increased risk is uncertain. Several clinical trials evaluating the impact of STD treatment to reduce HIV acquisition and transmission have unfortunately produced disappointing results. Other local genital tract factors, such as male lack of circumcision, intercourse during menses, use of vaginal desiccants, and use of oral contraceptives, have in some studies[129–132] been associated with an increased risk of sexual transmission.

The level of virus in the blood and in genital secretions is probably an important biologic determinant of transmissibility. Some asymptomatic persons with low levels of infection (less than 100 genomes/mL of plasma) may never or only rarely transmit infection, while others with high levels (100 000 or greater) may be relatively efficient transmitters. In maternal–infant transmission studies, maternal viremia is a good, but not perfect, predictor of transmission risk. Genital tract excretion of virus has been reported to be inconsistent and intermittent in HIV-infected persons. However, the relationships between blood viremia levels, genital tract virus levels, and transmissibility are not well established.[133–137]

Viral genotype is another potential determinant of transmissibility. Biologic differences between genetic types have been most convincingly demonstrated in comparative studies of HIV-1 and -2 in West Africa. Blood viral loads, disease progression, and maternal–infant transmission are all much lower for HIV-2 than for HIV-1, but direct comparative studies of virus in genital tract or heterosexual transmission have not yet been done.[138,139] Other studies have focused on the possible differences between HIV-1 genotypes. Because the HIV-1 B clade is regularly associated with World Health Organization (WHO) pattern I transmission (men who have sex with men and IV drug use), whereas the HIV-1 E clade (CRF01_AE) is associated with pattern II (heterosexual sex), one study was done to compare the growth of HIV-1 B clade versus E clade virus strains in skin Langerhans cells cultured *in vitro*. Langerhans cells are thought to be the initial cells infected in the genital tract. E clade viruses were reported to grow preferentially in the Langerhans cells, whereas B clade viruses grew well in T lymphocytes.[140]

GLOBAL MOLECULAR EPIDEMIOLOGY

Molecular epidemiology of HIV genotypes reveals that the global pandemic comprises multiple, genetically distinct virus subepidemics.

The first clue to the nonrandom distribution of HIV strains around the world came from studies of HIV-2. Prevalence is highest in the contiguous West African countries of Guinea-Bissau, Gambia, Senegal, and the Cape Verde Islands (in the Atlantic Ocean 500 km off the western tip of Africa). Other countries with relatively high HIV-2 prevalence are Angola, Mozambique, Southwest India, Brazil, and Portugal.[103,104,141,142] All these countries were the sites of former Portuguese colonies. Portuguese sailors established a settlement just off Dakar, Senegal, in the 1400s, which remained in Portuguese control until it was taken over by the French in the 1600s. The Cape Verde Islands were uninhabited until settled in 1460 by the Portuguese, who then brought West Africans as slaves to the islands. Slave trade to the colonies was an important commercial activity in the Cape Verde Islands throughout the sixteenth and seventeenth centuries. It is uncertain when HIV-2 disseminated through the social networks built on the former Portuguese connections. It is possible that global dissemination of HIV-2 may have occurred as long as 400 years ago at the height of the slave trade, but there are no reliable data to resolve the issue.

More recent studies of genotyping of HIV-1 strains collected from around the world show that the prevalence of different clades in different countries is strikingly nonuniform.[143] Clade B predominates in western Europe and in North America; clades A and D predominate in most of sub-Saharan Africa; clade C predominates in southern Africa, the Horn of Africa, and West India; and clade E/A predominates in Southeast Asia. HIV-1 genotypes A through H have all been detected in the equatorial African region bounded by Congo, Cameroon, Gabon, and the Central African Republic. The "cosmopolitan" clade B predominates in other regions of the world, where prevalence is for the most part lower and transmission is largely associated with men who have sex with men and IV drug users, such as South America, Australia, Japan, and China. HIV-1-O and HIV-1-N strains have been detected only in Cameroon, Gabon, and Equatorial Guinea and from persons with direct ties to these countries.

The Southeast Asian epidemic of the E/A clade was detected and studied relatively quickly. The earliest viral specimens from persons infected in northern Thailand (collected in 1990) all showed remarkable genetic homogeneity, consistent with a clonal epidemiologic origin (i.e., introduction by a single person).[144] This clonal epidemic has rapidly expanded to involve over 2 million persons. Clade E/A recombinants are also prevalent in equatorial Africa, where the genetic diversity of these viruses is substantial. These data suggest that the E/A epidemic in Southeast Asia was introduced from Africa.[145] Other studies of the diversity of the C clade viruses in western India, and F viruses in Brazil and Romania, suggest clonal epidemic origins.

Collectively these data show a pattern of global spread of HIV-1 that is irregular and unpredictable. The global epidemic cannot be characterized as a single emergence in Africa and steady gradual worldwide spread. A number of genetic variants have evolved in equatorial Africa, and at least five of these variants have seeded major clonal epidemics outside this region.

Global Statistics and Projections

A total of 2 million deaths due to AIDS was formally reported to the WHO and the Joint United Nations Programme on HIV/AIDS (UNAIDS) by the end of 2008, compared with 1.7 in 2001.[11] Southern Africa accounted for one-third of all deaths due to AIDS globally. Underdiagnosis and underreporting both contribute to the low total of reported AIDS cases. More effort has gone into monitoring the prevalence and incidence of HIV infection rather than AIDS. From an epidemiologic point of view, this makes more sense, since AIDS cases are HIV infections that occurred 5–15 years earlier. HIV prevalence is determined by collecting data from serosurveys among a variety of high- and low-risk populations and extrapolating to the entire population of the country. Serial surveys in similar populations over many years – such as blood donors, military recruits, and women attending antenatal clinics – can also provide rough information about local incidence rates. Using all available data, including household surveys, to arrive at HIV estimates ensured the best possible quality. On the basis of such data from hundreds of surveys worldwide, WHO–UNAIDS estimated that there were approximately 33 million HIV-infected persons worldwide, with incidence and prevalence rising most rapidly in East and Central Asia and eastern Europe. While HIV-1 prevalence is continuing to increase in many tropical countries, infections have reached a plateau and may be declining in some industrialized countries.

Because the global epidemic is expanding most rapidly in Asia, where HIV-1 clades C and E/A predominate, clades C and E/A are rapidly becoming the most common genotypes worldwide. Clade B viruses, prevalent in North America and Europe (and consequently the virus clade on which most laboratory research has been done), are among the less common variants worldwide.

Over the past two decades, the benchmark reporting systems for AIDS and HIV have changed radically. In the 1970s the epidemic spread silently and nothing was measured; in the 1980s clinically manifest AIDS cases were counted; and in the 1990s HIV prevalence and incidence were widely measured. Public health responsiveness during each of these decades changed correspondingly: in the 1970s ignorance prevailed because no one was aware that an epidemic had begun; in the early 1980s the response was arguably backward-looking, since decisions were driven by the number of AIDS cases; and not until the late 1980s and 1990s was the public health response fully informed in real time by the use of HIV-1 testing. It seems likely that as national and international public health systems continue to evolve, they will become forward-looking so that truly preventive steps will be routinely implemented in high-risk populations even before HIV-1 epidemics erupt.

Regional Epidemics

There are wide variations in HIV prevalence throughout the world. Countries in sub-Saharan Africa and the Caribbean have the highest national rates of adult HIV prevalence.[146] At the end of 2001, adult prevalence ranged from approximately 0.1% in East Asia and the Pacific to more than 20% in seven African countries (Botswana, 38.5%; Zambia, 21.5%; Zimbabwe, 33.7%; Namibia, 22.5%; South Africa, 20.1%; Swaziland, 33.4%; and Lesotho, 31.0%).[147] Part of this disparity can be attributed to the maturity of the epidemics in Africa and the more recent introduction of HIV into central and eastern Asia; often the age of the epidemic in a given country can be gauged by the level of HIV seropositivity in that country. The high prevalence of HIV infections in Latin America, the Caribbean, and sub-Saharan Africa is also reflected in the distribution of AIDS cases in these regions. The United States has the highest reported number of AIDS cases, but underreporting in many developing countries makes the actual reports more unreliable from these regions. Consequently, the estimate of the number of AIDS cases is frequently based on the seroprevalence of HIV infection in these regions. Unfortunately, data regarding incidence or spread of HIV are scarcer but are urgently required to estimate better the future scope of the epidemic. The following section reviews HIV prevalence data for countries in the tropics.

Sub-Saharan Africa

By the end of 2008, 22 million adults in sub-Saharan Africa were living with HIV infection[11] (see ***Fig. 81.4***). Sub-Saharan Africa accounts for only 10% of the world's population but nearly two-thirds of the people living with HIV.[11] Three broadly defined geographic areas, which include countries with severe epidemics and others with epidemics at intermediate stages, account for almost 90% of all current HIV infections in adults and adolescents in Africa.[146] There is tremendous diversity across the continent with respect to HIV prevalence rates with the lowest rates observed in West Africa, with no country having a prevalence rate above 10%. All countries in southern Africa by contrast have prevalence rates above 17%, with Botswana and Swaziland having some of the highest prevalence rates on the continent, both over 35%. Population mobility, patterns of sexual behavior, and societal factors have likely influenced the diversity in HIV rates observed across the African continent.[97,143]

Within each country the HIV epidemic has progressed differently in various population groups. Early in the evolution of the epidemics, urban populations and rural communities located along highways were more rapidly affected. Urban and trading centers continue to have substantially higher prevalence of HIV infection than rural areas, but this pattern is by no means universal; population displacement, armed conflicts, and proximity to highways where intense migration and population mobility occur for economic reasons have strongly influenced the spread of HIV.[97,143] Some rural communities in Kenya, Tanzania, and Uganda have infection rates similar to those observed in neighboring urban populations. Following similar patterns of spread and intensity, HIV epidemics have recently expanded in Botswana, Lesotho, Swaziland, Namibia, Zimbabwe, and South Africa.[11,146] In other countries, perhaps with poorer transport networks, this has not been the case.

HIV seroprevalence surveys have generally been conducted on high-risk populations and pregnant women attending antenatal clinics; the latter provide a better assessment of the general dissemination of HIV in the population (see ***Fig. 81.7***). As of 2004, 17 African countries had prevalence rates above 10% in women attending the antenatal clinics surveyed in urban settings, with rates exceeding 40% in some sites.[147] In other sub-Saharan countries the HIV epidemic is in the intermediate stage, with between 1% and 10% of women attending antenatal clinics being infected with HIV. A few of these countries still have relatively low levels of HIV prevalence, but these have begun to rise in several countries such as Nigeria and Cameroon.[11,146]

The observed high rates of HIV in women of reproductive age have resulted in high numbers of HIV-infected newborns. Of the 3 million infants in the world born with HIV infection since the beginning of the pandemic, over 90% have been born in Africa.[146–152] Typically, most of these children develop AIDS and die within a few years.

In addition to HIV-1 infection, HIV-2 is primarily found in West Africa with the exception of its presence in Angola and Mozambique.[153,154] The highest prevalence of HIV-2 infection is in Guinea-Bissau and in southern Senegal. In contrast to the increasing spread of HIV-1 throughout all of sub-Saharan Africa, the prevalence of HIV-2 has remained rather stable in West Africa and nonexistent in most other countries of Central and East Africa.[155–157] This has been partially explained by the higher infectiousness of HIV-1 compared with HIV-2.[158] The likelihood of transmission of HIV-1 through heterosexual intercourse is estimated to be about three times higher per exposure than for HIV-2. In addition, perinatal transmission rates of HIV-2 are reported to be significantly lower, less than 4%, than for HIV-1 (25–35%).[159]

AIDS has emerged as the leading cause of death worldwide, surpassing tuberculosis for the first time in 1999. In 1998, 19% of all deaths in Africa were due to AIDS.[160–163] Excess deaths attributable to HIV infection are highest in 25–35-year-olds, an age group that usually has a low mortality. Nearly 90% of deaths in this age group were in excess of background rates and were attributable to HIV infection. The fact that many AIDS deaths occur in children and young adults has resulted in a substantial reduction in life expectancy, by more than 20 years in several countries (see ***Fig. 81.6***). It is projected that population growth will decline more rapidly than expected and the size of the African population in the year 2025 will certainly be smaller than it would have been without AIDS.[147,152] However, because many adults bear children (often without AIDS, thus destined to be orphaned) before dying of AIDS, the population growth continues at an alarming 2–3% per year (i.e., doubling every 29 years or so). The increasing number of HIV infections and AIDS cases has already overwhelmed the capacity of urban health systems in some countries. In this regard, it is estimated that 80% of hospital beds in an infectious disease hospital in Abidjan, Côte d'Ivoire, and 50% in a hospital in

Kampala, Uganda, are occupied by people with HIV infection. Demands for care will increasingly fall on poorly equipped and underfunded rural services, households, and individuals.

Demographic surveys in several countries have already noted significant increases in infant and child mortality.[164–166] Owing to high levels of fertility, populations will generally continue to grow, but the critical deficits will be seen in the economically active ages. In countries where 8% of the adult population is HIV-infected, surveys have measured a doubling of mortality due to HIV and a decrease of at least 5 years in life expectancy. In 1995, UNAIDS examined the demographic impact of HIV infection and AIDS in 15 sub-Saharan African countries with a prevalence of HIV infection of more than 1% of the adult population.[91] Below that level of prevalence, the epidemic's impact on the national demographic picture is insignificant. In the 15 countries analyzed, the combined population was estimated to be 2 million people smaller than expected. In the year 2005 it will be 11.6 million smaller (291.8 million versus 303.4 million). As a result of the high fatality rate due to HIV infection and AIDS, life expectancy at birth decreased in these 15 countries from 52.8 to 49.6 years. In the 45 most affected countries, it is projected that, by 2020, 68 million people will die earlier than they would have in the absence of AIDS.[147] Average life expectancy in sub-Saharan Africa has fallen to 47 years compared to an expected 62 years in the absence of AIDS. These HIV epidemics will have severe effects on the population age structure, indenting the population pyramid in the main contributors to social and economic development, namely, young adults.

Since AIDS kills people in their most productive years, it ranks as the leading cause of potential healthy life-years lost in sub-Saharan Africa.[160] In Abidjan, Côte d'Ivoire, it was estimated that 15% of adult male deaths and 17% of male years of potential life lost (YPLL) resulted from AIDS, whereas in women AIDS accounted for 13% of deaths and 12% of female YPLL.[161] In two community-based rural studies in the Masaka and Rakai districts of Uganda, mortality among HIV-infected adults was over 100 per 1000 person-years of observation (PYO), an order of magnitude higher than among adults not infected with HIV.[162,163] In both districts, the adult prevalence of HIV infection was 8% and 13%, respectively, and HIV infection was found to be the leading cause of death. In this regard, more than 80% of deaths in the 20–29-year-old age group occurred among those who were HIV-infected. As a result, AIDS will double or triple the adult mortality rate in sub-Saharan African countries from levels that were already eight times higher than in developed countries. In countries such as Uganda, with an estimated 1.3 million infected persons out of a total population of 17 million, AIDS looms as the predominant health problem of the entire population.

With regard to children, it is estimated that the HIV pandemic resulted in 280 000 childhood deaths in 2008.[11] Additionally, as of the year 2001, more than 14 million children under age 15 years have been orphaned as a result of the premature death of HIV-infected parents.[146] In a survey of child mortality in 10 central and eastern African countries, the death toll from AIDS in children under 5 years of age was found to be likely to rise from 159 to 189 per 1000 by the year 2000. Even for those children who escaped perinatal infection, survival rates will decrease because of the loss of one or both parents to AIDS. For each woman dying of AIDS in Africa, an average of two children are orphaned. Overall, infant and child mortality rates have increased by as much as 30% more than previously projected as a direct consequence of perinatal HIV infection. Consequently, pediatric AIDS is now threatening much of the progress that has been made in child survival in developing countries during the past 20 years.[164]

Care of and support for children orphaned by AIDS will be a growing concern throughout the region, and the social, economic, and demographic impact of AIDS will be enormous. For a country with a current prevalence of HIV infection of 8%, the expected increased demand for health care services ranges from 2.3% to 9.3%, depending on the state of development of its health care sector.[165,166] The strong association of HIV with a burgeoning tuberculosis epidemic combined with the excess mortality associated with HIV infection underscores the critical importance of the HIV epidemic in Africa.[167]

North Africa and the Middle East

This region represents 20 countries, with an estimated 480 000 individuals living with HIV.[11] Information on HIV infection in this region is limited, particularly among high-risk groups such as IV drug users. The highest prevalence of HIV infection in this region has been observed in Sudan, with 2.6% HIV prevalence representing almost 90% of the infections in this region.[147] The majority of infections in this regions appear to be focused on injection drug users (IDUs), although there is concern that HIV may be spreading undetected among men who have sex with men, as homosexuality is highly condemned and illegal in many places. The future size and trends of the epidemic in this region are difficult to predict because of several factors: recent introduction of the virus, the status and disempowerment of women in society with associated decreased access to health care, the highly stigmatizing nature of STDs and the difficulties in their diagnosis and treatment, and the difficulty of conducting effective sexual health programs, often because of religious beliefs.

Asia

Asia, where HIV has more recently been introduced, is in the early phases of an explosive HIV infection and AIDS epidemic. Since more than 60% of the world's population lives in Asia, the HIV epidemic could affect more people in this region than in any other area of the world.[21,22] For example, despite the fact that HIV was introduced into this region in the late 1980s, there were already 4.6 million people living with HIV infection or AIDS in 2008.[11] The overall adult prevalence of HIV infection, however, is less than 1.0% because of the large population of these countries.[147] Thus, on a per-population basis, although more people may actually be infected with HIV in Asia, AIDS may still have a greater impact in sub-Saharan Africa. The epidemic, however, is spreading rapidly in some areas with sharp increases in new infections in Pakistan, Indonesia, and Vietnam and an estimated 360 000 new infections occurring in the region in 2008.[11] Countries such as the Philippines, Singapore, North Korea, and South Korea have had only limited spread to date and the rate of growth appears to be substantially lower.[10]

The pattern of HIV spread in Asia appears to be mainly concentrated among IDUs, men who have sex with men, sex workers, clients of sex workers, and their immediate partners. HIV infection was initially noted among IDUs in Thailand and in Manipur, northeastern India; seroprevalence rose from 55% to 80% in IDUs.[168–172] Data in the Yunnan province of China bordering Burma and Laos and considered part of the "golden triangle" of heroin exportation also demonstrate an alarming prevalence of HIV infection of 43–82% in IDUs.[173] Data from Malaysia and Vietnam show similar increases in IDUs. Concomitant with this rise of HIV infection among IDUs, HIV infection was noted among female sex workers; although highly variable by region, prevalence rates of 30–65% have been reported among female sex workers in various cities of Thailand and India.[172,174] Successive waves of heterosexual transmission from these sex workers to their male clients, and subsequently to other sex partners, including spouses, have resulted in the rapid spread of HIV to the general population.[168,169] Across Asia, effective prevention efforts have been hampered partly because of stigma and discrimination of the affected groups. HIV seroprevalence in India is high in the south and west. For example, in Mumbai (formerly Bombay), prevalence increased from 2% in STD clinic attendees before 1990 to 36% in 1994.[172] The prevalence in sex workers rose from 1% to 51% between 1987 and 1993, and 2% of women attending antenatal clinics were positive in 1994.[146] In Pune, the overall HIV seroprevalence in 2800 STD clinic attendees was 23.4%.[175] Among initially seronegative persons, the subsequent incidence of HIV infection was 26.1 per 100 PYO for female sex workers, 9.4% for men, and 8.4% for women who were predominantly spouses of the men attending these clinics.[176] Unsafe sex between male–male sex partners has emerged as an additional important risk factor in the Indian epidemic.[177] As in Africa, recurrent genital ulcer disease, urethritis, or cervicitis was independently associated with an increased risk of seroconversion.

There is great geographic variation of HIV infection in India. Studies among sex workers in Kolkata (formerly Calcutta) have consistently demonstrated a low prevalence of 1.2%; in Vellore, women attending antenatal clinics have a prevalence of 0.1%. Many factors, including the prevailing sexual practices, a large population of HIV-infected female sex workers, the low social status of women, male patronage of sex workers, high rates of STDs, low rates of condom use, and the high number of IDUs in the north, make it likely that HIV will continue to spread in India and Thailand, as well as in many other populous countries.[10] India has the highest burden of infection in Asia, with an estimated 5.1 million adults and children infected with HIV, making it second only to South Africa in terms of absolute burden of infections.[89] As in Africa, the HIV epidemic is strongly associated with increasing spread of tuberculosis.[178–181] In India an estimated 1–2 million cases of tuberculosis occur every year. In Mumbai 10% of the patients presenting with tuberculosis are now HIV-positive. Tuberculosis is also the presenting symptom of AIDS in more than 60% of AIDS cases. In Thailand public health authorities have noticed a marked increase in tuberculosis cases compared with a steady decline in previous years.[182]

The epidemic in China has raised alarm, since it appears to be spreading into new groups of the population. Despite sketchy surveillance data, it is estimated that 850000 Chinese were living with HIV/AIDS in 2001.[147] Several localized HIV epidemics are being observed among certain population groups across China, highlighting the need for swift action if a more serious epidemic is to be prevented. The majority of early reported HIV infections have been among IDUs in Yunnan province (about 70%).[174] However, China is currently in what has been termed the expansive phase of its epidemic with infections spreading to partners of IDUs and blood donors and a steady rise in rates observed among sex workers.[183] Men who have sex with men, ignored in the official statistics, have also emerged as a high-risk group for HIV transmission. The number of infections in China more than doubled between 1999 and 2002.

THE DISEASE

Pathogenesis and Natural History

After many years of debate on the hypothesis that AIDS is fundamentally an autoimmune disease, it is now clear that autoimmunity is not an essential component of the pathogenesis. Instead, disease progression is a direct reflection of virus replication.[184,185] In the absence of active viral replication, or when viral replication is low (blood viremia levels less than 100 genome copies/mL), HIV infection does not progress to clinical immunodeficiency. Conversely, when viral replication is rapid (viremia greater than 100000 genome copies/mL), disease progression is correspondingly rapid. Treatments with antiviral drugs slow disease progression in proportion to their effect in lowering viremia levels. The course of HIV infection can be quite variable. The initial infection is followed by an eclipse phase in which neither viremia nor an antibody response can be found. A virologic "primary infection" with high levels of viremia then appears and persists for several weeks.[186] Up to 30% of HIV-infected persons are reported to experience a mononucleosis-like syndrome of fever, pharyngitis, rash, and depressed $CD4^+$ cell counts during this primary infection. However, in many careful studies the proportion showing symptoms during primary infection is much lower than this.[187,188] Among HIV-infected patients studied in the United States and Europe, most progress from infection to AIDS in 5–15 years. A fraction of patients, about 5–10%, progress more rapidly (rapid progressors), and another fraction, perhaps 5%, show no evidence of progression over many years (nonprogressors).[189–191] In HIV-1–HIV-2 studies, HIV-2 infection invariably produces a lower viremia than does HIV-1 and HIV-2 also shows a much higher proportion of nonprogressors. Few rigorous natural history studies have been done in tropical countries or in regions where HIV-1 genotypes other than clade B predominate. One study of HIV-1 infections among commercial sex workers in Kenya showed rapid progression to AIDS (within 5 years) in 50%.[192] It is uncertain whether the high proportion of rapid progressors in this study in Africa can be attributed to the prevalent viral genotypes (probably clade A and clade D), to the high prevalence of aggressive opportunistic infection (e.g., tuberculosis), to the lack of optimal medical care, or to poor nutrition or other host factors.

There is no evidence that the virus in rapid progressors is more virulent than average. Instead, natural history studies suggest that rapid progressors mount an inadequate immune response. Most patients show low or absent antibodies or cellular responses. Rarely, rapid progressors have been described who appear to be completely but selectively unresponsive to HIV antigens. Because these patients lack HIV antibodies, they can pose a diagnostic challenge.

Nonprogressors typically have low plasma viral titers. In some nonprogressors, low viral titers are due to infection with grossly replication-defective virus, but in most patients it is uncertain whether low viral titers reflect viral factors (poor replication), host genetic factors, or an unusually strong immune response.[193] Nonprogressors do routinely show strong immune responses to HIV proteins, including antibody and cellular responses, but it is unclear if this is cause or effect.

Mechanism of Immune Dysfunction

Depletion of $CD4^+$ T lymphocytes is the central mechanism of immune dysfunction by HIV. Progressive depletion is a consequence of a furious rate of viral replication in these cells. The turnover rate of $CD4^+$ T lymphocytes – their destruction and replenishment – is correspondingly turbulent. Each day in an infected patient, up to 10^9 new virions are made and about 10^9 $CD4^+$ T lymphocytes are killed and replaced.[194,195] Loss of $CD4^+$ T cells results in a loss of recognition of antigens that are presented on class II MHC molecules. Th1 function is especially damaged with loss of cell-mediated immune functions. Th2 functions are impaired as well with gradual loss of humoral responsiveness to newly presented foreign antigens. Loss of *in vivo* delayed-type hypersensitivity skin test reactivity to recall antigens such as *Candida*, mumps, and tetanus parallels the loss of cell-mediated immunity and the appearance of opportunistic infections.

Three major mechanisms of $CD4^+$ T-lymphocyte killing by HIV have been suggested: direct virus-mediated cytolysis, virus-induced apoptosis, and indirect killing through immune effector mechanisms. Direct virus-mediated cytolysis has been demonstrated *in vitro*. Syncytium formation may accelerate the cytolytic process. Syncytium-inducing isolates appear in blood in the late stages of illness and are a poor prognostic sign when present in earlier stages. However, the presence of syncytium-inducing virus isolates strongly covaries with blood viral titer, so cause-and-effect relationships remain uncertain. Apoptosis may also contribute to cell destruction *in vivo*.[196,197] $CD4^+$ T lymphocytes from infected patients undergo apoptotic death when stimulated *in vitro*. However, uninfected $CD8^+$ as well as $CD4^+$ cells from HIV-infected patients show increased apoptotic death. Apoptosis probably reflects the high rate of ongoing immune activation in HIV-infected persons and probably is not a principal cause of immune depletion. Immune destruction of infected cells also is not likely to be a central mechanism of $CD4^+$ T-lymphocyte depletion: persons with weak immune responses show more rapid depletion and more rapid clinical disease progression. Other pathogenic mechanisms have been proposed, including induction of anergy by circulating soluble gp120 or by superantigen stimulation of lymphocytes, and autoimmunity induced by HIV antigens cross-reactive with normal cell proteins.[198] These *in vitro* mechanisms have not been established to be important *in vivo*.

Anti-HIV Immunity

Unlike in other infectious diseases, there is as yet no direct evidence that humans can become "immune" – in the classic sense – to HIV. Infection becomes chronic in everyone infected; no adults have spontaneously cleared their infection. Also, there is as yet no direct evidence that any candidate HIV vaccine can render a person protected against subsequent challenge. Most HIV-infected adults do mount a vigorous antibody and cellular immune response to HIV. It is thought that this immune response, although insufficient to clear infection, is nonetheless sufficient to impede viral replication.

Serum antibodies to env, gag, pol, and nef appear in the blood of most HIV-infected patients within a few weeks to months after exposure to infection. Antibodies to tat, rev, and the other accessory proteins are also detectable in a variable proportion of patients. Antibody titers to all viral proteins fall as disease develops, and low anti-HIV antibody titer is a poor prognostic sign. *In vitro*, antibodies can block HIV replication through antibody-dependent cellular cytotoxicity, killing of infected cells, or virus neutralization.[199] HIV-neutralizing antibody activity can be measured by mixing dilutions of serum with a small dose of virus, then monitoring viral replication when the mixtures are inoculated into cultures of $CD4^+$ T lymphocytes. HIV antienvelope antibodies effectively neutralize viral growth. Neutralization serotypes of HIV-1 strains have been described, and these correspond to the genotypic clusters. Paradoxically, anti-HIV serum antibodies can increase the replication of HIV-1 in cultures of macrophages and other Fc receptor-bearing cells by facilitating the initial viral binding to the cell surface. It is uncertain whether this "antibody-dependent enhancement" of HIV-1 growth has *in vivo* significance.[200,201]

HIV-reactive lymphocytes are present in the blood of essentially all infected patients. Cultured patient $CD4^+$T lymphocytes proliferate when exposed *in vitro* to HIV envelope or gag proteins. The vigor of proliferation is maximal in the early, asymptomatic stages of infection and decreases as disease progresses. $CD8^+$ anti-HIV class I MHC-restricted cytotoxic T lymphocytes (CTLs) with activity against HIV core, envelope, polymerase, and nef proteins are also present in blood. Class II-restricted CTLs are also found. Appearance of $CD8^+$ blood CTL activity correlates temporally with the initial fall of viremia, so it is thought that CTLs are important in control of replication through killing of infected cells.[202–204] $CD8^+$ cells also release soluble factors that inhibit HIV replication through noncytolytic mechanisms.

Once established, HIV infection never spontaneously disappears completely in adults. However, spontaneous "cures" have been reported in a few infected infants.[205] It is hypothesized that passively acquired maternal immunity was important in partially suppressing the infection in these infants. Self-curing abortive and suppressed infections have also been observed in SIV-vaccinated and -challenged monkeys.[206]

Clinical Manifestations

A substantial proportion of patients with acute primary HIV infection (up to one-half) may experience a mononucleosis-like illness characterized by fever, pharyngitis, and a slight morbilliform rash. Rarely, patients experience neurologic manifestations. In 80–90% of patients, the illness is so mild that medical care is not sought. Primary HIV infection is rarely seen in medical care facilities in tropical countries.

The early stage of chronic HIV infection is usually asymptomatic, with the $CD4^+$ cell count remaining above 500 cells/mL. About half of patients have modest generalized lymphadenopathy. Autopsies on early-stage HIV-infected patients who die of non-HIV-related causes (e.g., automobile accidents) show HIV-1-infected cells in lymphatic tissues throughout the body.[207] At this stage a number of dermatologic conditions of uncertain cause may be present, especially seborrheic dermatitis, psoriasis, and folliculitis.[208]

Intermediate HIV disease, defined by $CD4^+$ counts between 200 and 500 cells/mL, is also usually asymptomatic or at least without serious manifestations. Skin and mucosal opportunistic infections are common, including herpes zoster (shingles), herpes simplex, oral or vaginal candidiasis, oral hairy leukoplakia, and cervical dysplasia.[209,210] Bacterial infections caused by common respiratory tract organisms such as *Streptococcus pneumoniae* are increased, as is pelvic inflammatory disease. Patients may begin to experience fever, diarrhea, and weight loss. The occurrence of these intermediate manifestations, but without an AIDS-defining opportunistic infection or cancer, has historically been referred to as "AIDS-related complex."

Late-stage HIV disease, AIDS, is defined by a CD4 cell count below 200 cells/mL. The list of AIDS-defining conditions issued jointly in 1993 by the Centers for Disease Control and Prevention and WHO is shown in ***Box 81.1***.[211] This revision included three new AIDS-defining conditions that are more common in heterosexual patients: recurrent bacterial pneumonia, cervical carcinoma, and pulmonary tuberculosis. This listing, while an improvement, still omits several HIV-related infections that are more prevalent in tropical countries. These include parasites (*Cryptosporidium*, microsporidia, *Cyclospora*, *Leishmania donovani*, and *Trypanosoma cruzi*); fungi (*Penicillium marneffei*); and bacteria (*Bartonella, Rhodococcus*). The issue is not merely academic, for in many countries the availability of social benefits and access to medical care depend on a diagnosis of an AIDS-defining illness.[212]

Box 81.1 1993 US Centers for Disease Control–World Health Organization Classification of Acquired Immunodeficiency Syndrome (AIDS)-Defining Conditions

CD4 cell count <200/μL	Isosporiasis
Candidiasis, pulmonary or esophageal	Kaposi's sarcoma
Cervical cancer	Lymphoma
Coccidioidomycosis	Mycobacterial disease
Cryptosporidiosis	*Pneumocystis carinii* infection
Cytomegalovirus infection	Pneumonia, bacterial
Herpes esophagitis	Progressive multifocal leukoencephalopathy (polyomavirus)
Human immunodeficiency virus (HIV) encephalopathy	Salmonellosis
Histoplasmosis	

Many common tropical infections, including malaria, schistosomiasis, filariasis, onchocerciasis, cholera, yellow fever, and dengue have not been identified as HIV-related opportunistic infections. Two very prevalent diseases, malaria and African trypanosomiasis, have been studied and shown to have no relationship.[213,214] Nonetheless, the range of HIV-related opportunistic infections does vary in different regions of the world. Certain AIDS-defining infections common in the United States are diagnosed much less frequently in Africa and Asia, particularly *Pneumocystis carinii* pneumonia (PCP), *Mycobacterium avium-intracellulare* (MAI), and cytomegalovirus disease. Other infections are more common in tropical countries, depending on the locally prevalent microbes.

In sub-Saharan Africa, diarrhea from cryptosporidiosis, isosporiasis, or microsporidiosis is common. In Latin America, cerebral toxoplasmosis, cryptosporidiosis and isosporiasis, Chagas' disease, and cutaneous and visceral leishmaniasis are common. Cases of HIV-associated disseminated strongyloidiasis and paracoccidioidomycosis have also been reported. In Southeast Asia, disseminated infections with the dimorphic fungus *Penicillium marneffei* are common.[215]

Mycobacterium tuberculosis (MTB) is the most common serious opportunistic infection worldwide. Clinically apparent tuberculosis can occur at any stage of HIV infection, but the risk increases with immunoincompetence. Each year 5–10% of persons coinfected with HIV and MTB develop active tuberculosis. The prevalence of tuberculosis in persons with AIDS in Latin America has been reported to be 17–30%; in Africa, 25–44%; and in Asia, 23–68%. Almost half of patients with the end-stage HIV wasting syndrome (slim disease) in Africa are shown at autopsy to have disseminated MTB.[216]

DIAGNOSIS AND PROGNOSIS

Disease from HIV becomes clinically apparent only after years of asymptomatic infection, and clinical signs, when they do occur, are usually unspecific. Consequently, laboratory assays are essential to diagnosing HIV infection.

HIV Antibody Assays

HIV antibody assays on blood serum or plasma are used to establish a diagnosis. The most common test is the ELISA. A variety of configurations have been developed and marketed, but plastic microtiter plates or beads are most often used as the solid-phase surface for adsorption of viral antigens. Patient antibodies that bind to viral antigens are detected with antihuman immunoglobulins tagged with enzymes. Readouts are obtained by color changes in a substrate fluid catalyzed by the enzyme.

Several rapid and simple HIV antibody assays have been developed that are intended for use outside laboratory settings. There are a variety of configurations, including agglutination of latex beads or red blood cells, or dot blots on dipsticks. Antibodies are also present in body fluids other than blood serum, but at lower titers, and test kits have been developed and marketed that use urine or saliva. The sensitivity and specificity of these alternative assays can be quite good but are generally below those of serum ELISA testing.

HIV antibody testing is most effective when an algorithm for assay use is thoughtfully designed and scrupulously followed. A variety of algorithms have been proposed, each appropriate for a particular health care setting. Optimal algorithm design will vary according to many local factors: the true prevalence of HIV infection in the population to be tested, the expected ratio of HIV-1 to HIV-2 infections, the availability of laboratory facilities, speed requirements, and cost constraints. Most algorithms include the following steps: (1) a screening assay; (2) repeat testing of specimens with positive screening assay results on the same specimen; and (3) supplemental testing with a second assay of different design. In very low prevalence populations, it is advisable to verify results by obtaining and testing a new serum specimen before a diagnosis is considered established. To avoid confusion, it has been customary to describe individual assay results as "nonreactive" or "reactive" and to reserve the terms "negative" and "positive" for the algorithm bottom-line conclusion.

Diagnosis of HIV infection in infants presents special problems owing to the presence of passively acquired maternal antibodies. One approach is to wait until maternal antibodies have waned (1 year) and then test for antibodies. Another is to test directly for HIV virus, antigens, or genome with viral cultures, p24 antigen assays, or DNA polymerase chain reaction (PCR).

Measurement of HIV Nucleic Acids

The PCR, in which strands of nucleic acid are amplified exponentially one strand to two, then four, then eight, and so on, has revolutionized the diagnostic approach to the HIV-infected patient. PCR can be used to amplify HIV sequences from cellular proviral DNA, from cellular RNA, or from HIV virions.

DNA PCR is useful in establishing a diagnosis of HIV infection in situations in which antibody testing gives ambiguous results.[217] Testing of infants of infected mothers (all of whom passively acquire maternal antibodies) is the most important use. DNA PCR can also be used to confirm HIV infection in persons with indeterminate Western blot results.

HIV RNA measurement with PCR requires an initial conversion of the viral RNA sequences to complementary DNA (cDNA). This is done by addition of exogenous reverse transcription (RT), followed by PCR amplification and then quantification of the specific DNA product.[218,219] Because errors can be magnified exponentially, RT-PCR must be carefully standardized and controlled. Measured quantities of control nucleotide sequences can be added directly into each test specimen tube, as in quantitative competitive RT-PCR, or controls can be run in parallel in separate tubes in each run. Both approaches have been optimized. Commercial RT-PCR test kits are designed to quantitate genomic HIV RNA in plasma, but the technique can be modified in research laboratories to measure various splice classes of HIV RNA in cells or to measure HIV RNA in other fluids such as semen or cervical secretions.

More recently, real-time PCR assays have been introduced on the market which allow for a single, closed system of amplification and detection. Dried blood spot collection methods have also been introduced which have proven useful in settings where centralization of services is advantageous such as many locations in rural Africa.

The plasma HIV RNA level is a direct measure of *in vivo* HIV replication and is therefore a powerful prognostic tool. For any given untreated patient, the plasma viremia level remains relatively constant, or increases slightly, over several years. It appears that the "virologic script" for the disease course is "writ" very early after primary infection.[220,221] Patients with low viremia levels (100–1000 genome copies/mL) after seroconversion do well and are often nonprogressors, whereas patients with high viremia levels (100 000 genome copies/mL or greater) do poorly and are often rapid progressors. Levels are typically quite low in HIV-2-infected patients compared with HIV-1-infected patients.

Immunologic Assessment of HIV-Infected Patients

The $CD4^+$ T-lymphocyte count is the most widely used measure of HIV-induced damage to the immune system. In the United States, absolute counts of less than 200 cells/mL or a $CD4^+$ percentage of less than 14% is strongly associated with an increased risk of opportunistic infections and is now accepted as definitional for AIDS.[222,223]

The $CD4^+$ count can be performed manually and read visually, but usually it is done with an automated fluorescence-activated flow cytometer. $CD4^+$ cell counts are vulnerable to biologic and technical errors. The main biologic error in $CD4^+$ cell counts is attributable to a pronounced diurnal variation that can be up to 150 cells/mL in healthy adults but is usually less in patients with lower T-cell counts. This effect can be minimized by performing counts at a fixed time of day. Another common contributor to inaccurate $CD4^+$ cell counts is simple errors in measuring the percentage of lymphocytes on a standard differential white blood cell count. Normal values for total CD4 cell counts, the percentage of lymphocytes that are $CD4^+$ cells, and $CD4^+/CD8^+$ count ratios may differ among adults in different countries. Ideally, every clinician managing HIV-infected patients should know the local laboratory $CD4^+$ count standard values and variability.

TREATMENT AND PROGNOSIS

Optimal medical management of the HIV-infected patient includes therapy with antiretroviral (ARV) agents, prevention of opportunistic infections and cancers, and treatment of complications as they arise. Complete medical care includes counseling of patients and their families.

Antiretroviral Therapies

The first class of drugs proved to have clinically significant anti-HIV activity was the nucleoside analog reverse transcriptase inhibitors (NRTIs): zidovudine (AZT), didanosine, zalcitabine, stavudine, lamivudine, and abacavir (listed here in order of their approval by the US Food and Drug Administration (FDA)).[224,225] These drugs are phosphorylated by cellular enzymes to their respective triphosphate forms, which block reverse transcriptase by substrate competition with natural nucleosides, and by chain termination of the growing DNA strand. As monotherapy these drugs show only modest clinical and antiviral effects. Major problems include prompt emergence of drug resistance and significant toxicities.[226]

The second major class of anti-HIV drugs is the nonnucleoside reverse transcriptase inhibitors (NNRTIs), such as nevirapine, delavirdine, efavirenz. Added to this list are tenofovir and emtricitabine, nucleotide reverse transcriptase inhibitors. These drugs do not require modification by cellular enzymes but act by direct binding to sites on the reverse transcriptase. As monotherapy the NNRTIs show the same problems as the nucleoside analogs.[227] Recently, a second-generation class of NNRTIs has entered the treatment arena with etravirine receiving early FDA approval in 2008 for the treatment of individuals with resistance to first-generation NNRTIs.[228] Clinical trials are currently under way on a number of newer-generation NRTI and NNRTI compounds targeting individuals who are resistant to the first-generation drugs in these classes. The third class of ARVs, the inhibitors of HIV protease (saquinavir, indinavir, ritonavir, nelfinavir, amprenavir, lopinavir/ritonavir, atazanavir, tipranivir, and darunivir) have demonstrated clinical efficacy.[229–232] These drugs act by binding to and blocking the HIV protease enzyme that is essential to cleaving the gag-pol polyprotein. Combination therapy, usually referred to as highly active ARV therapy (HAART), of two NRTIs and either a protease inhibitor or NNRTI is synergistic, and some combinations have lowered plasma HIV RNA levels to undetectable levels. A recent analysis of 14 cohort studies in resource-rich settings revealed that combination ARV therapies had such an impact on improving survival that life expectancies for a 20-year-old patient could expect to approach two-thirds that in the general population.[233] Three newer drug classes have recently been introduced and have expanded treatment options. Enfuvirtide (Fuzeon), in the class of fusion inhibitors (FIs), is now in use.[234] Maraviroc is also an entry inhibitor but works by blocking the CCR5 coreceptor and was approved for use in previously treated patients with R5 HIV-1 infection.[235] Integrase strand transfer inhibitors are another novel class of ARV agents now being introduced, with raltegravir being the first to receive FDA approval.[236] Most studies of ARV therapy of HIV have been done in industrialized countries, particularly North America and Europe. Limited *in vitro* screening of HIV isolates from other countries, and in particular genotypes other than clade B, has not found any obvious patterns of naturally occurring resistant viruses within the major group of HIV-1. Nevertheless, strains of HIV-1 group O and HIV-2 are naturally resistant to most NNRTIs. However, the price of chronic therapy with ARVs with proven efficacy is high but falling worldwide, making the introduction of lifesaving ARV treatment programs a reality in many resource-limited settings. The search for effective low-cost ARV therapies must continue and be intensified in all countries.

As with other antibiotics, low or intermittent dosing with ARVs as a cost-saving measure is to be discouraged because it has no therapeutic benefit and may lead to community spread of resistant virus. Short-term administration of ARV drugs is warranted only for certain, clearly defined prophylactic indications, such as prevention of maternal–fetal transmission or prevention of needlestick infection in health care workers.

Specific Antiretroviral Recommendations: Who, When, and How

Rapid advances in HIV/AIDS research continue to modify and refine the guidelines for whom to treat, when during the course of infection treatment should be begun, and which therapeutic regimen should be used. Recent recommendations are presented here.[237]

- **Who?** The International AIDS Society USA panel recommends therapy for any patient with established HIV infection who is committed to the complex, long-term therapy.
- **When?** Therapy is usually begun when the $CD4^+$ cell count drops below 350 cells/μL (with consideration at higher $CD4^+$ levels and symptomatic disease).
- **How?** Initial therapy should be with a combination of ARV drugs, usually a minimum of three drugs. Nucleoside or nucleotide reverse transcriptase inhibitors (tenofovir plus emtricitabine are preferred with zidovudine, didanosine, stavudine, lamivudine, abacavir as alternatives) are used in combination with NNRTIs (nevirapine, efavirenz) or ritonivir-boosted protease inhibitors (atazanavir/ritonavir, lopinavir/ritonavir, fosamprenavir/ritonavir, or saquinavir/ritonavir), or raltegravir.

As new results become available, these recommendations will be modified.

Drug Resistance

HIV rapidly develops resistance to ARV drugs *in vivo*. Drug-resistant variants have been found in blood after monotherapy with every ARV thus far evaluated.[238,239] Emergence of resistance does not require patient exposure to an exogenous source of resistant virus; mutation and natural selection can evolve a population of resistant viruses within a single patient in a matter of weeks or months. Resistant HIV can be subsequently transmitted to uninfected persons. Resistance to an antiviral drug is typically generated through mutations affecting amino acids in the HIV target enzyme that are near the drug active site. Many different mutations can lead to resistance to a single drug, and these different mutations are often synergistic in conferring resistance.

Two biochemical mechanisms abrogate the incorporation of triphosphorylated NRTIs, thus leading to drug resistance. The first mechanism is mediated by a mutation that allows reverse transcriptase to discriminate against NRTI during DNA synthesis, as a result preventing their addition to the primer DNA chain. The second mechanism is mediated by mutations in the enzyme that increase the rate of hydrolytic removal of the chain terminating NRTI and enable the continuous synthesis of viral DNA.[240,241] The NNRTIs, which bind to a hydrophobic pocket in reverse transcriptase, close to, but not contiguous with, the active site, inhibit HIV-1 replication allosterically by displacing the catalytic aspartate residues relative to the polymerase binding site. A single mutation in the hydrophobic pocket can result in high-level resistance to one or more NNRTIs. Resistance to NNRTIs appears to emerge by the selection of a preexisting population of mutant viruses in an individual. This is linked to the fact that resistance rapidly develops when NNRTIs are administered as monotherapy or in the presence of incomplete virus suppression. Resistance to protease inhibitors is mediated by structural changes that reduce binding affinity between the inhibitor and the mutant protease molecule. Resistance to protease has also been attributed to mutations at the cleavage sites.[242–244] Mutations occurring outside the active site appear to induce resistance by other mechanisms such as alterations in enzyme catalysis, effects on dimer stability, alterations in inhibitor binding kinetics, or active site reshaping through extensive structural disturbances.[245,246]

In any given patient, the rapidity with which resistance emerges is directly related to the viral replication rate: a high replication rate generates mutants at a high rate. Combination therapies of two or three ARV drugs with different mechanisms of action may lower the replication rate sufficiently to retard the breakthrough of drug-resistant variants. Although this has yet to be proved, early results are encouraging. Recent reports that combinations of ARVs can sterilize blood and perhaps lymphoid tissue of detectable virus have raised hopes that HIV infection may be not just treatable but curable. Studies are under way to determine whether long-term combination chemotherapy of HIV can lead to cure just as long-term combination chemotherapy of MTB can lead to cure of tuberculosis.

Drug resistance can be monitored at three levels: clinical, phenotypic, and genotypic. Clinical unresponsiveness to therapy suggests resistance. For example, a rapid fall in the $CD4^+$ count with a rise in the plasma HIV RNA level strongly suggests emergence of resistance in a treated patient. This can be verified by virus isolation followed by drug sensitivity testing in virus-infected cell cultures, but this process is complicated and expensive. For those drugs where the principal resistance mutations are well characterized, PCR amplification and screening of the viral genome can detect common mutation patterns.

Prevention of Opportunistic Infections and Cancers

Prevention of opportunistic infections in HIV-infected patients can be accomplished in three ways: (1) preventing exposure to pathogens in the environment; (2) preventing an initial episode of disease through chemoprophylaxis or vaccination; and (3) preventing disease recurrence through chemoprophylaxis. Opportunistic cancers can be prevented by screening and treatment of precancerous lesions.

Prevention of exposure to opportunistic pathogens requires knowledge of their environmental sources. For many common opportunistic infections, e.g., PCP, the exact environmental sources are still uncertain. In some, such as *Penicillium marneffei* infection, the sources (thought to be moldy sugar cane or bamboo) are unique to certain geographic regions.[247]

Some universal practical measures include avoidance of contact with known tuberculous patients in health care facilities; avoidance of raw or uncooked eggs, poultry, or dairy products that might harbor *Salmonella*; and avoidance of undercooked meat that may be a source of *Toxoplasma*. Some waterborne opportunistic infections, such as intestinal parasites and possibly MAI, may be difficult to avoid, but where possible only clean water sources should be used.

Chemoprophylaxis with trimethoprim-sulfamethoxazole (TMP-SMX) with one double-strength tablet daily has been proved to reduce the occurrence of PCP and to prolong survival in HIV-infected patients in North America.[248] In South America and Asia, where PCP appears to be a common opportunistic infection, daily TMP-SMX prophylaxis is recommended for patients with advanced infection. Recent studies from Uganda and Zambia in HIV-infected adults and children, respectively, have shown a marked reduction in morbidity and mortality following the introduction of TMP-SMX.[249,250] The incidence of other opportunistic infections is also reduced, including cerebral toxoplasmosis and some bacterial infections.[251] Daily TMP-SMX costs about US$60 per year.

Chemoprophylaxis with isoniazid has been proved to prevent clinical tuberculosis in HIV-infected persons.[252] Ideally, prophylaxis should be used in HIV-infected persons who are shown to be tuberculin skin test-positive but without active tuberculosis. However, the reality in many developing countries is that many HIV-infected patients are already anergic at the time of diagnosis. Furthermore, in many countries skin test reactivity may reflect childhood bacille Calmette-Guérin immunization. Consequently, some have suggested that in regions where MTB prevalence is high, isoniazid prophylaxis should be considered for all HIV-infected patients who do not have active tuberculosis.[253] WHO and the International Union Against Tuberculosis recommend that prophylaxis be given for 6–12 months. This costs about US$60 per year. Several studies of prophylaxis against tuberculosis are currently under way in Africa and Asia.

Bacterial infections, particularly *Streptococcus pneumoniae*, are an important cause of morbidity and mortality among HIV-infected patients in developing countries. The polyvalent pneumococcal vaccine costs US$10 and should be considered.

Human papillomaviruses play an etiologic role in cervical cancers in women and penile and anal cancers in men. Routine screening of HIV-infected patients for perineal and genital dysplasias and precancers with treatment of early lesions is suggested.

Treatment of Opportunistic Infections

Management of the clinically ill, late-stage HIV patient is difficult in any setting, but it is particularly challenging in developing countries where diagnostic and therapeutic options are limited. Experienced physicians often use syndrome-based diagnoses to choose therapies from locally available alternatives. The approach to patients with tropical infectious disease complications of HIV infection is presented in Chapter 139.

Counseling of Patients and Families

A diagnosis of HIV/AIDS can be a devastating psychological blow. In all societies, patients require ongoing emotional support and access to factual, up-to-date information. This can be provided by medical professionals or, alternatively, by trained paraprofessionals or volunteers. Information about prognosis and treatment options is the most obvious need. However, HIV-infected patients usually need assistance with a variety of important life decisions: whom to inform about their illness; how to avoid transmitting infection to others; childbearing options; coping strategies; and custody and death planning, to name a few.

PREVENTION AND CONTROL

HIV prevention efforts can focus either on reducing transmission from already infected patients or on reducing risk in uninfected persons.

HIV Testing as a Public Health Tool

One approach to HIV epidemic control is test-linked interventions: HIV testing coupled with efforts to reduce transmission by those found to be infected.[254–256] This approach reflects the traditional public health philosophy of communicable disease control. During the 1980s a vigorous international debate ensued over the potential benefits of HIV testing, reporting, contact tracing, and quarantine versus the negative impact of such steps on human rights. When aggressive HIV testing systems were implemented in several countries, WHO became concerned about the threat of stigmatization and discrimination and led a laudable international movement to ensure that nondiscrimination was an integral part of global HIV/AIDS control. WHO also condemned mandatory HIV control programs and put a low priority on testing and counseling. The WHO campaign to minimize discrimination appears to have been successful. Public health programs in which HIV testing is linked to treatment and behavioral counseling to reduce transmitting behaviors should also be considered to slow the global spread of HIV.

In at least one specific setting, test-linked interventions to reduce transmission do have near-universal support. This is in maternal-to-infant transmission. Chemoprophylaxis with AZT around the time of delivery was shown to reduce the risk of maternal-to-infant transmission substantially. The field of mother-to-child prevention has advanced tremendously in recent years with frequent breakthroughs prompting guideline changes aimed at preventing transmission at delivery, preventing transmission through breastfeeding, and minimizing the risk of ARV resistance. Pregnant women are advised to be HIV-tested, and there have been calls for mandatory testing in this setting.

Among certain groups of at-risk adults, test-linked interventions may be the only practical way to prevent infection. For example, the common public health recommendation to limit the number of sexual partners is irrelevant advice for a monogamous spouse, although use of condoms may not be. In high-incidence regions where infection of males by commercial sex workers is common, the only way a monogamous married woman may reduce her own risk is to find out if her husband is infected and make difficult – but informed – choices.

Although the ethical issues are complex, test-linked public health programs can be considered if the following conditions apply: (1) testing is accurate; (2) medical treatment is available; (3) legal rights are secure; and (4) cost–benefit calculations are favorable.

Behavioral Prevention in At-Risk Populations

Public health efforts to change human behavior are never simple.[257] In the words of a highly regarded Ugandan HIV training video, "It's not easy." Health education – conveying a knowledge of the facts – is just one step toward behavior change.[258] The full sequence of steps to reach behavior change is often abbreviated as KABP – for knowledge, attitude, belief, and practice. Many individuals become HIV-infected even though they have substantial knowledge about what HIV is, how it is transmitted, and how it can be prevented. A receptive attitude is crucial. Unless the subject believes that this is an issue of personal importance and that the changes can be of personal value and is willing to put into practice risk avoidance skills, then knowledge alone is insufficient.

Behavioral interventions intended to prevent sexually transmitted HIV infections can be designed to reach one at-risk person at a time, small groups of at-risk persons, or larger community or societal groups. Interventions targeted at individuals or small groups permit focusing of resources to those most at risk and minimize political reaction by restricting discussions of sensitive issues and avoiding public forums. However, they are highly personnel-intensive and expensive. Individual counseling has been recommended for persons who seek HIV testing. Community- and societal-level interventions through mass media can be highly effective in reaching many people at once, but the heterogeneity of risks in large groups means that only the most basic messages enjoy widespread public acceptance. Public discussions of "safe sex" have been vigorously opposed in some quarters.

Efforts to control HIV in populations of IDUs have reconfirmed the lesson that knowledge-only programs are not very effective in bringing about long-term behavior change. Changes in attitudes and beliefs typically require a social change process, so newer control efforts have targeted the social settings for drug use.[259] Peer influence is an important factor in social change, and two-way programs that involve current drug users are more effective than one-way, top-down policies. Providing the means for safe injection practices is another proven control method. Data from several countries suggest that over-the-counter sale of needles and syringes reduces the use of contaminated injection "works," and reduces HIV transmission. However, this approach has encountered intense political resistance.

Progress Toward an HIV Vaccine

There is no HIV vaccine with proven protective efficacy. Given the current state of progress and level of effort, a globally available and affordable HIV vaccine is at least a decade away. Despite great advances in our understanding of the immunology of HIV/AIDS made during the last 20 years, we are still not close to a safe, effective HIV vaccine. The recent closure of the large international phase IIb clinical trial of the adenovirus 5-HIV gag, pol, nef vaccine was a stunning blow to the field and has resulted in calls for a return to the laboratory before moving forward with clinical trials.[260] Some of the scientific, political, and economic obstacles to global HIV vaccine development are reviewed here.[261]

Scientific Obstacles

The key unsolved scientific problem in HIV vaccine research is the mechanism of immunity. Although vaccine-induced protection has been demonstrated in SIV analog vaccine models, there is uncertainty whether protection is primarily humoral or cellular and which epitopes are crucial. A parallel problem is how to measure correlates of immunity in vaccine trials. For example, many candidate vaccines induce HIV-neutralizing antibodies but only against selected laboratory-adapted viruses, not against fresh "street virus" isolates.

Political Obstacles

Most incident HIV infections today occur in developing countries, where the prevalent HIV strains differ from those in candidate vaccines. Until recently, there had been no coordinated international effort to produce candidate vaccines that would be suitable for testing in developing countries. Furthermore, vaccine testing capabilities in many regions are still suboptimal despite serious efforts by WHO to strengthen research infrastructures. Recent efforts by the US National Institutes of Health and other international donors have addressed this issue through an effort to create laboratory infrastructure and clinical trial capacity in developing countries. Concern about exploitation (the "guinea-pig issue") is one example of a host of important political issues that must be overcome through community involvement.

Economic Obstacles

Vaccines in general are not a highly profitable venture for industry, especially compared to therapeutics. Liability is an ever-present threat. Other economic disincentives that are unique to private-sector HIV vaccine research and development include the following: vaccine demand is greatest in populations least able to pay; different vaccine types may be necessary for developing countries; and calls for "distributive justice" by activists may force price ceilings.

With global cooperation, none of these obstacles is insurmountable. An effort under the sponsorship of the Rockefeller Foundation called the International AIDS Vaccine Initiative has been building global partnerships that directly involve all parties: scientists, manufacturers, at-risk populations, developing and industrialized countries, and international organizations.

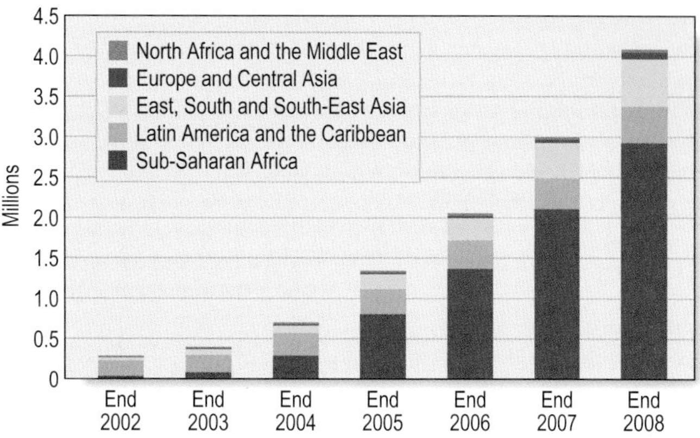

Figure 81.8 Number of people receiving antiretroviral therapy in low- and middle-income countries by region 2002–2008. (Data from 2009 Report on the Global AIDS Epidemic. Geneva: UNAIDS; 2009.)

Turning The Tide on the AIDS Pandemic

The provision of ARV therapy treatment for AIDS in resource-limited settings has become a reality in recent years thanks to increases in donor support, political will, and a gradual reduction in the cost of ARV drugs. More than 3 million people are now receiving ARV therapy in resource-limited settings as a result of the tremendous international efforts to scale up treatment during the last decade, a global health accomplishment thought to be unimaginable only 5 years ago[11] (*Fig. 81.8*). Resource-limited countries affected by the AIDS pandemic still face tremendous challenges to scale up ARV programs that are sustainable and can meet the tremendous demands that will be placed on existing health care institutions.

Global HIV/AIDS Funding

The amount of global AIDS funding has increased 15-fold from US$300 million in 1996 to US$13.8 billion in 2008.[11] Unfortunately, the funding gap has grown as more money is made available, and estimates for 2010 indicate that US$25 billion will be required for HIV prevention and care in low- and middle-income countries. This amount will not be met with current domestic and international development agendas and represents an enormous challenge to donor countries.

Several key milestones have occurred in response to the AIDS pandemic, making the possibility of ARV treatment a reality in resource-limited settings. The Global Fund to Fight AIDS, Tuberculosis and Malaria (GFATM) was created to increase the global resources available to combat these major killers affecting developing countries. GFATM has now gone through eight rounds of funding and more than US$15.6 billion has been allocated for HIV/AIDS projects in 140 countries.[262] The GFATM money will support 2.3 million individuals to receive life-saving ARV treatment through its various programs.[11] In the State of the Union address of January 2003, President George W. Bush announced an unprecedented 5-year, US$15-billion Emergency Plan for AIDS Relief (PEPFAR) to provide HIV care, prevention, and treatment in 15 countries severely affected by the HIV/AIDS pandemic.[263] Currently 15 countries supported through the PEPFAR program are implementing programs focused on ARV treatment, prevention of mother-to-child transmission, HIV prevention, and support for orphans and vulnerable children. The original goal of this program was to treat 2 million people with ARVs, prevent 7 million infections, and care for 10 million HIV-infected individuals by 2007, which has been revised upward to treat 3 million people with ARVs, prevent 12 million new infections, and care for 12 million HIV-infected individuals by 2013. WHO in collaboration with UNAIDS and UNICEF has embarked on an ambitious plan to mobilize support for universal access to care for HIV-infected individuals by 2010 with a focus on urgency, equity, and sustainability. Increasing support from these agencies coupled with growing private-sector involvement has provided a platform for universal access to HIV care in many countries, a goal that was seemingly impossible only 5 years ago. Most countries worst hit by the HIV pandemic have now developed national AIDS plans incorporating ARV treatment and basic HIV care. Several countries in Latin America and the Caribbean now offer universal ARV coverage. Brazil was the first developing country to implement a universal HIV/AIDS treatment policy, and by the end of 2006, 184 252 patients were receiving ARVs free through the public health system. The Brazilian government estimates that, from 1997 to 2003, more than 60 000 new AIDS cases, 90 000 deaths, and 633 200 AIDS-related hospital admissions have been avoided.[264] The overall cost savings from this program is estimated at US$200 million, not taking into account the social benefit of this program. The Brazilian experience has demonstrated that, with government political will and the involvement of other key players in health delivery, it is possible to turn the tide on the AIDS pandemic.

The Challenges Ahead

The complexity of HIV care warrants a dramatic effort to strengthen human capacity to deliver ARVs. Thirty ARV drugs are now approved by the FDA for the treatment of HIV infection and have an array of potentially serious side-effects and drug interactions.[265] Decisions about which drugs to start with, when to start, and when to change therapy have become increasingly complex as the number of available choices increases. The training demands imposed by the complexity of HIV treatment is magnified by the reality of the scarcity of health workers in many resource-limited settings. In many settings, the current health work force must triple or quadruple to achieve the ambitious goal of universal ARV coverage. In countries most affected by AIDS, vacancy rates remain high: Malawi for example has only been able to fill half of its public-sector nursing posts in recent years.[11] As countries expand HIV care programs to meet the current expanded access goals, training and recruitment of health sector workers will be necessary to provide the platform to build sustainable programs.

Current North American and European clinical care guidelines incorporate measurements of plasma HIV viral load and $CD4^+$ T lymphocytes as essential tools in managing patients on HAART.[265] In addition, testing for viral resistance has become a key tool in managing patients with evidence of virologic failure on HAART. Many countries faced with the challenge of delivering ARVs in resource-limited settings lack the laboratory infrastructure and trained technicians to perform the routine chemistry and hematology assays necessary to monitor patients receiving HAART. The more sophisticated virologic tests that have become standard of care in the North American and European settings remain prohibitively expensive for most countries developing HIV treatment programs. The WHO has responded to this challenge by publishing treatment guidelines aimed at resource-limited settings (***Table 81.1 and Box 81.2***). Alternative, low-cost methods for monitoring patients receiving HAART have become a public health priority, but early results have failed to reveal a low-cost alternative that performs as well as the more expensive immunologic and virologic tests.[266]

The threat of ARV resistance looms over the many countries scaling up ARV delivery programs. ARV resistance could be devastating to resource-limited countries, resulting in early treatment failure and potentially abrogating the effectiveness of zidovudine, lamivudine, and nevirapine for the prevention of mother-to-child transmission of HIV. Countries embarking on ARV treatment programs need to ensure sustainable drug supplies in order to avoid the early pitfalls seen in the Côte d'Ivoire, Gabon, and Uganda, where erratic therapy resulted in high levels of drug resistance.[267–269] Effective adherence strategies combined with stable drug supply in resource-limited settings has been shown to result in high levels of viral suppression, which hopefully will avoid widespread development of ARV resistance.[270]

Table 81.1 World Health Organization (WHO) Recommendations for Initiating Antiretroviral Therapy in Adults and Adolescents with Documented Human Immunodeficiency Virus (HIV) Infection and Possible First-Line Antiretroviral Regimens

- Start all patients with WHO stage III or IV disease, irrespective of CD4
- Start all patients with CD4 <350, irrespective of clinical symptoms
- CD4 testing required to identify patients with HIV and WHO stage I or II disease

	Usage in Women (of Childbearing Age or Pregnant)	Major Potential Toxicities
TDF/FTC or 3TC/NVP	Yes	NVP-related hepatotoxicity and severe rash AZT-related GI intolerance, anemia, and neutropenia
AZT/3TC/NVP	Yes	NVP-related hepatotoxicity and severe rash
TDF/FTC or 3TC/EFV	No[a]	EFV-related CNS toxicity and potential for teratogenicity AZT-related GI intolerance, anemia, and neutropenia
AZT/3TC/EFV	No[a]	EFV-related CNS toxicity and potential for teratogenicity

TDF, tenofovir; FTC, emtricitabine; 3TC, lamivudine; NVP, nevirapine; GI, gastrointestinal; AZT, zidovudine; EFV, efavirenz; CNS, central nervous system.

[a]For women in whom effective contraception can be assured, EFV remains a viable option.

(Reproduced from Antiretroviral therapy for HIV infection in adults and adolescents: recommendations for a public health approach (2006 revision). Available at http://www.who.int/hiv/pub/guidelines/adult/en. Accessed 06/01/10; and from Rapid advice: antiretroviral therapy for HIV infection in adults and adolescents. Available at http://www.who.int/hiv/pub/arv/advice/en/index.html. Accessed 06/01/10.)

The current expansion of ARV delivery to some areas hardest hit by the HIV pandemic provides hope and optimism for the future. The experiences of Brazil, Haiti, Thailand, Uganda, Senegal, and South Africa provide a wealth of information to design high-quality HIV treatment programs to improve greatly the health of nations facing the current HIV pandemic.[271–275] We have learned about secondary benefits of these programs from the findings in South Africa that HAART reduced the incidence of tuberculosis associated with HIV by 80%.[276] It is clear from evidence from North America, Europe, and Australia that adherence to therapy is difficult, and suboptimal ARV regimens that are not as effective as HAART may result in the rapid development of drug resistance. As access to HAART expands, it is imperative that programs be supported with the necessary infrastructure to ensure high levels of adherence to build on the success demonstrated in the early treatment programs.

Enthusiasm over the expansion of ARV treatment programs throughout resource-limited settings should not overshadow the importance of basic HIV care and HIV prevention. Basic care and prophylaxis for the prevention of opportunistic infections remain low-cost interventions having the potential to reduce morbidity and mortality greatly among HIV-infected individuals.[250] Efforts to provide access to HAART that do not incorporate other low-cost interventions into a primary care plan could limit the potential effect of these programs on reducing morbidity and mortality among HIV-infected patients in resource-limited settings. Finally, prevention methods must be emphasized as treatment programs expand, to limit the number of new HIV infections and avoid any potential risk disinhibition that could result from the introduction of HAART into communities.

Box 81.2 World Health Organization Classification System for Human Immunodeficiency Virus (HIV) Infection

Clinical Stage 1

- Asymptomatic infection
- Persistent generalized lymphadenopathy
- Acute retroviral infection

Performance Stage 1

- Asymptomatic, normal activity level

Clinical Stage 2

- Unintentional weight loss <10% body weight
- Minor mucocutaneous manifestations (e.g., dermatitis, prurigo, fungal nail infections, angular cheilitis)
- Herpes zoster within previous 5 years
- Recurrent upper respiratory tract infections

Performance Stage 2

- Symptomatic but nearly fully ambulatory

Clinical Stage 3

- Unintentional weight loss >10% body weight
- Chronic diarrhea >1 month
- Prolonged fever >1 month (constant or intermittent)
- Oral candidiasis
- Oral hairy leukoplakia
- Pulmonary tuberculosis within the previous year
- Severe bacterial infections
- Vulvovaginal candidiasis

Performance Stage 3

- In bed more than usual but <50% of daytime during the previous month

Clinical Stage 4

- HIV wasting syndrome
- *Pneumocystis carinii* pneumonia
- Toxoplasmosis of brain
- Cryptosporidiosis with diarrhea >1 month
- Isosporiasis with diarrhea >1 month
- Cryptococcosis, extrapulmonary
- Cytomegalovirus disease of an organ other than liver, spleen, or lymph node
- Herpes simplex virus infection, mucocutaneous
- Progressive multifocal leukoencephalopathy
- Any disseminated endemic mycosis (e.g., histoplasmosis)
- Candidiasis of the esophagus, trachea, bronchus, or lung
- Atypical mycobacteriosis, disseminated
- Nontyphoid *Salmonella* septicemia
- Extrapulmonary tuberculosis
- Lymphoma
- Kaposi's sarcoma
- HIV encephalopathy

Performance Stage 4

- In bed >50% of daytime during previous month

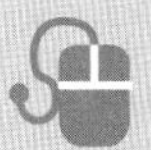

Access the complete reference list online at
http://www.expertconsult.com

Access the complete reference list online at http://www.expertconsult.com

CHAPTER 82

Dermatophytosis

Michael B. Smith • Michael R. McGinnis

INTRODUCTION

Dermatophytosis is a term used to describe mycotic infections caused by a group of fungi that usually remain localized to the superficial layers of the skin, hair, or nails. Despite their propensity to infect the exterior aspects of the host, the dermatophytes prefer a warm, moist environment for growth, and as a consequence, infections are common in tropical regions.[1] Dermatophyte infection of the skin and hair of the scalp (tinea capitis) is exceedingly common in Africa, with a prevalence of 14–86% in children, depending on geographic location and the method of making the diagnosis.[1]

In many tropical regions, dermatophyte infection of the glabrous skin (tinea corporis) is the most common skin disease found.[1] The rate of infection for those not native to a tropical area is usually higher than that of the indigenous population and can reach epidemic proportions. Both US combat forces in Vietnam during the 1960s and British forces several decades earlier in Malaysia and Hong Kong experienced high rates of dermatophyte infections. In Vietnam, up to 73% of US combat infantrymen became infected with dermatophytes.[2] These infections were disabling enough that the soldiers were unable to capably perform in the field, and the deleterious effect on US combat capability was sufficient to warrant the creation of a special medical research team to address the problem.[2]

THE AGENTS

Dermatophytes are a closely related homogeneous clade of keratinophilic filamentous fungi[3–6] and are associated with the stratum corneum of the skin, as well as hair and nails on the living host. They possess similar appearance, physiology, antigenicity, growth requirements, infectivity, and pathology. These fungi are classified in the anamorphic genera *Epidermophyton*, *Microsporum*, and *Trichophyton*. Some dermatophytes may reproduce sexually when the opposite mating types are crossed with each other. The single ascomycete genus *Arthroderma* accommodates the known sexual forms of all of the dermatophytes.[7]

Even though the term dermatophytosis refers to an infection caused by a dermatophyte, not all dermatophytes may cause infection. The fungus colonizes the stratum corneum and then grows in a radial manner without penetrating viable tissue. Invasion of hair, which is nonliving tissue, is an example of colonization. If the fungus enters viable tissue and continues to grow, then infection is present. Colonization or infection may result in disease if there is structural or functional harm. These may be evident as damaged or destroyed hair and nails, hyperhidrosis, pruritus, inflammation, or alopecia. Contamination, the presence of nonreplicating dermatophytes on keratinized tissue, does not occur.

In addition to dermatophytes, other species of fungi that do not colonize or invade the stratum corneum, hair, and nails on the living host are classified in the same anamorphic genera owing to their similar microscopic and colonial characteristics. Some of these species may break down keratin in substrates such as feathers and hooves; however, these keratinophilic species are not dermatophytes. The term dermatomycosis[8] differs in that it encompasses colonization and infection of keratinized tissue by fungi not classified in the genera *Epidermophyton*, *Microsporum*, and *Trichophyton*. In addition, when their sexual forms are known, they are classified in genera other than *Arthroderma*.

EPIDEMIOLOGY

Based on their principal ecologic niches, dermatophytes are categorized as either anthropophilic (people-loving), geophilic (soil-loving), or zoophilic (animal-loving). Several dermatophytes may be associated with more than one ecological niche. The major advantage of this classification scheme resides in determining the source of the dermatophyte causing an infection. Clinically, geophilic and zoophilic dermatophytes typically cause more severe, inflamed, self-limiting lesions. In contrast, as a general rule, anthropophilic species often cause chronic lesions with less inflammation.

Transmission of dermatophytes occurs by contact with hyphal fragments and arthroconidia, usually associated with skin scales or hair fragments deposited on fomites such as combs or towels. Arthroconidia, formed by the fragmentation of hyphae, are infectious propagules that can easily disseminate from one host to another. Animal studies have shown that arthroconidia are more infective than macro- and microconidia and are probably the primary inoculum that causes new infections.[9] Arthroconidia can remain viable for several years on skin scales or hair shed into the environment.[10]

There is variability with respect to the geographical distribution of individual species (***Table 82.1***). Some species are found worldwide, while others are quite localized. The prevalence of an individual species in a given geographic location, and hence the disease it causes, is dependent on a number of factors including population migration patterns, lifestyle practices, primary host range, secondary host susceptibility, standard of living, and climatic preference.[11,12]

THE DISEASES

Dermatophyte infections are clinically characterized by the body site that is involved. The term tinea, which is Latin for "larva" or "worm," is used to refer to dermatophyte infections on the body. The term is thought to be based on the correlation by the ancient Romans of skin lesions on humans with holes in wool blankets caused by the larvae of moths. The major clinical syndromes include tinea capitis, tinea corporis, tinea cruris, tinea pedis, and tinea unguium or onychomycosis.[13–16] The natural history of these clinical syndromes is similar.

Colonization by a dermatophyte begins in the stratum corneum. The outcome depends on the fungal strain and species, host, and anatomical site. For example, if glabrous skin is involved, the fungus grows radially

Table 82.1 Source in Nature and Geographic Distribution of Selected Dermatophyte Species in the Tropics

Species	Anthropophilic	Zoophilic	Geophilic	Tropical Area: Africa	Central/South America	Asia	Australia/Oceania
Microsporum							
M. audouinii	X			±	±	±	+
M. canis		X		+	+	+	+
M. ferrugineum	X			+	–	+	+
M. gypseum			X	–	+	+	–
Trichophyton							
T. concentricum	X			–	+	+	+
T. mentagrophytes	X	X		+	+	+	+
T. rubrum	X			±	+	+	+
T. schoenleinii	X			+	±	+	±
T. tonsurans	X			–	+	+	–
T. verrucosum		X		+	+	+	+
T. violaceum	X	X		+	+	+	+
T. soudanense	X			+	–	–	–
T. megninii	X			+	–	–	–
T. yaoundei	X			+	–	–	–
T. gourvilii	X			+	–	–	–
Epidermophyton							
E. floccosum	X			–	+	+	–

–, absent or rare; ±, uncommon; + common.
(Modified from Shrum JP, Millikan LE, Bataineh O. Superficial fungal infections in the tropics. Dermatol Clin 1994;12:687.)

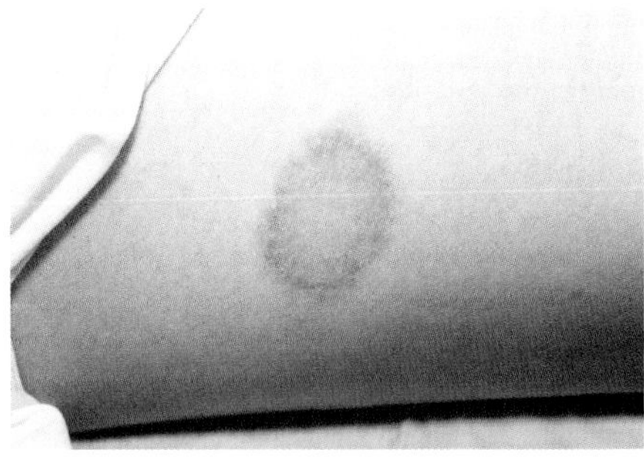

Figure 82.1 Circular lesion of tinea corporis, commonly referred to as ringworm. (Courtesy of Edgar Smith, MD.)

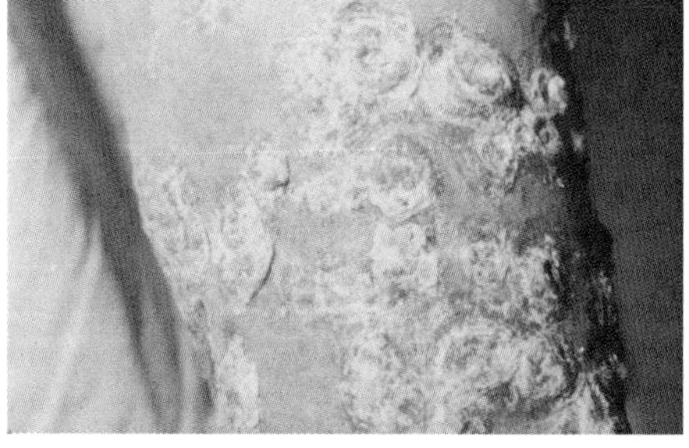

Figure 82.2 Scutula in a case of favus. (Courtesy of Libero Ajello, PhD.)

to form distinctive circular lesions called ringworm (***Fig. 82.1***). Initially, the clinical appearance is patchy scaling or erythematous eruptions. As the fungus and host interact, inflammation of varying degrees occurs. If the etiologic agent is anthropophilic, the clinical symptoms may disappear, and the host typically develops a subclinical infection.

Tinea Capitis

Tinea capitis is a common disease found worldwide, primarily in children, in which dermatophytes cause scaling of the stratum corneum, with or without inflammation (in most patients). Invasion of scalp hair follicles by the fungi results in alopecia. Tinea capitis is caused by species of either *Trichophyton* or *Microsporum*, with the most common etiologic agent varying geographically.[12] Initially, an erythematous scalp papule develops, and during the anagen phase of the hair cycle hairs are invaded, becoming gray, discolored, and lusterless, hence the alternative term gray patch ringworm. Itching may become intense and alopecia follows. Ulceration with kerion formation (a crusted, oozing lesion composed of pus and keratin debris overlying granulation tissue) and scarring may occur.

The fungus grows into the hair bulb and forms hyphae in the cortex of the hair shaft. When the hyphae mature, they either form arthroconidia or decompose. Ectothrix invasion is characterized by the presence of arthroconidia both within and around the hair shaft. This is easily recognized by the destruction of the hair cuticle. Ectothrix tinea capitis may be caused by anthropophilic species such as *Microsporum audouinii*, which once caused large epidemics in Europe and America. Once griseofulvin was used to treat infections caused by *M. audouinii*, the fungus declined markedly in frequency in developed nations.[12] Anthropophilic ectothrix tinea capitis is typically spread by child-to-child contact and resolves after several years when the infected telogen hairs are shed. Ectothrix tinea capitis caused by geophilic and zoophilic species such as *M. canis* and *M. gypseum* results in more severe inflammation. Zoophilic species like *T. mentagrophytes* var. *mentagrophytes* and *T. verrucosum* can result in suppurative folliculitis. Kerion formation and scarring with permanent alopecia are typical with resolution of the infection.

Endothrix invasion is characterized by the production of arthroconidia within the hair shaft with an intact hair cuticle. A special form of endothrix invasion, without the production of arthroconidia, is known as favus. The disease (favus means "honeycomb" in Latin) is characterized by yellow, crusted honeycomb-like masses (scutula) on the scalp, composed of hyphae and keratin debris (***Fig. 82.2***). The hyphae within the hair cortex break down to form long channels. When these hairs are placed in a

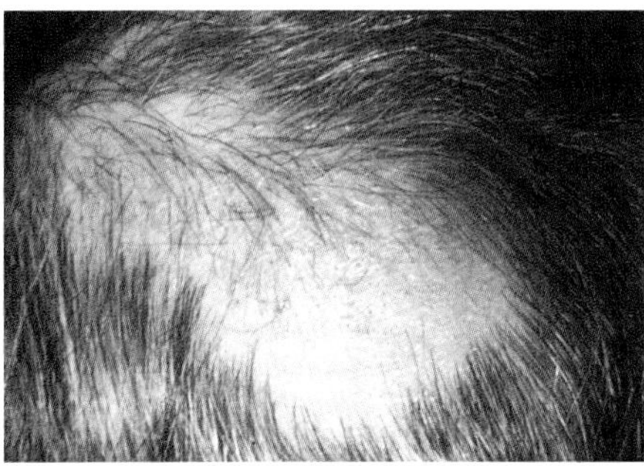

Figure 82.3 Tinea capitis caused by *T. tonsurans.* (Courtesy of Libero Ajello, PhD.)

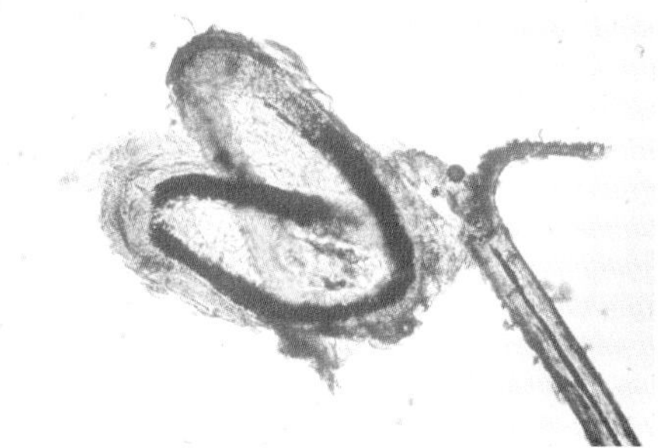

Figure 82.4 Curled "black-dot hair" in endothrix tinea capitis. (Courtesy of Libero Ajello, PhD.)

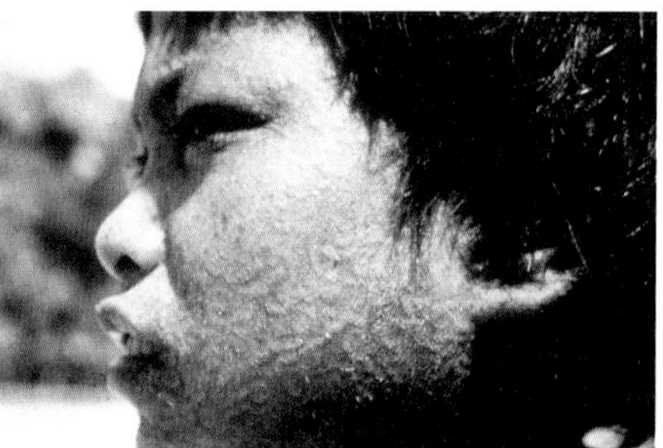

Figure 82.5 Polycyclic rings of papulosquamous scales of tinea imbricata. (Courtesy of Carolyn Halde, PhD.)

mounting fluid such as potassium hydroxide, air bubbles can be seen racing down the channels owing to capillary action. Favus is caused by *T. schoenleinii*, the prevalence of which has been declining in most areas of the world, although it remains an important pathogen in both Africa and Asia.

Trichophyton tonsurans, common in Europe, Russia, the Near East, Mexico, the United States, Puerto Rico, and northern South America, and *T. violaceum*, common in Central Asia, parts of Africa, and the Far East, are the major anthropophilic etiologic agents of endothrix tinea capitis (***Fig. 82.3***). Typically, these fungi tend to cause more severe infections than those caused by anthropophilic ectothrix agents. These two species cause "black-dot ringworm," which is characterized by infected hairs that break off at the follicular orifice resulting in a "black dot" on the scalp (***Fig. 82.4***). The infection is chronic, often continuing into adult life. The host reaction is variable, for while inflammation is minimal in populations living in endemic areas, severe inflammation, kerion formation, scarring, and permanent alopecia can also occur. Unlike ectothrix tinea capitis, not all of the hairs within the area of endothrix tinea capitis are infected, and hairs must be selectively collected for microscopic examination and culture. Because they can be subsurface, a scalpel may be required to epilate the hair stubs for examination.

Tinea Corporis

Tinea corporis results from colonization of the glabrous skin by a dermatophyte. The fungus grows principally in the stratum corneum and usually does not enter viable tissue. While species of *Trichophyton*, *Microsporum*, and *Epidermophyton* all can produce tinea corporis, *T. rubrum* and *T. mentagrophytes* are the most common etiologic agents.

Transfer of epithelial scales containing hyphae, arthroconidia, or a combination of both originating from an infected person or animal, transmits the fungus to the skin of a susceptible person. The fungus enters the layers of cells composing the stratum corneum and spreads radially. After 1–3 weeks, clinical signs appear as the margin of the lesion expands. The fungus is eliminated from the central portion of the lesion, with concurrent formation of concentric zones of inflammation at the lesion's edge. Tinea corporis exhibits two basic types of lesions: annular and vesicular.

Anthropophilic dermatophytes such as *T. rubrum* and *E. floccosum* cause small, dry, scaly, spreading, annular patches with elevated areas of inflammation and red margins. The central areas heal as the fungus spreads radially. The lesions may resolve or remain as a chronic problem.

The second type of lesion, vesicular, is similar to the annular lesion. Vesicles form behind the advancing elevated lesion margin with subsequent crust formation. Hair invasion results in pustules. The lesions typically resolve in a few weeks; chronic lesions are uncommon. Vesicular lesions are characteristic of zoophilic dermatophytes such as *T. mentagrophytes* var. *mentagrophytes* and *T. verrucosum*. Pustular, well-circumscribed, elevated, crusted lesions are known as Majocchi's granuloma. Secondary bacterial infection can result in severe inflammatory lesions that can be disabling.[2]

A special form of tinea corporis known as tinea imbricata is caused by *Trichophyton concentricum* in people living on the Pacific islands of Oceania and in Southeast Asia and Central and South America. The lesions consist of polycyclic rings of papulosquamous scales (***Fig. 82.5***) that can be scattered over as much as 70% of the body. It is believed that the fungus is transmitted by direct, intimate contact. Genetic susceptibility to infection inherited in an autosomal recessive pattern has been demonstrated.[17]

Tinea Cruris

Tinea cruris involves the groin, perineum, and perianal region. It is prevalent in people living in tropical regions, where heat and high humidity contribute to skin maceration. It is more common in males and often occurs in conjunction with tinea pedis. The major pathogens are *T. rubrum* (the most common etiologic agent worldwide), *E. floccosum*, and *T. mentagrophytes*.

The initial lesion is circinate and becomes serpiginous. Lesions associated with *E. floccosum* develop distinct margins and raised borders with randomly dispersed vesicles or vesiculopustules containing serous exudate. The center of the lesion is brownish to red, with branny furfuraceous scales. In males, the infection typically begins on the thigh where it contacts the scrotum. A pruritic, erythematous rash develops with the infection extending downward on the inner thighs, often on the left side. The gluteal and pubic areas are often involved. Acute infections are associated with intense itching.

Tinea Pedis

The interdigital spaces and soles are typically the sites of infection, with lesions varying from mild, chronic scaling to exfoliative and pustular. Tinea pedis occurs in 30–70% of the world's population, making it the most common dermatophytosis. The absence of sebaceous glands and their fungistatic lipids in feet, residence in warm, humid climates, removal of protective surface lipids by sweating, and the wearing of shoes predispose feet to tinea pedis. The infection rarely occurs in populations that do not wear shoes.

Intertriginous-interdigital tinea pedis is the most common clinical form. Peeling, maceration, and fissuring of the skin with dead, white

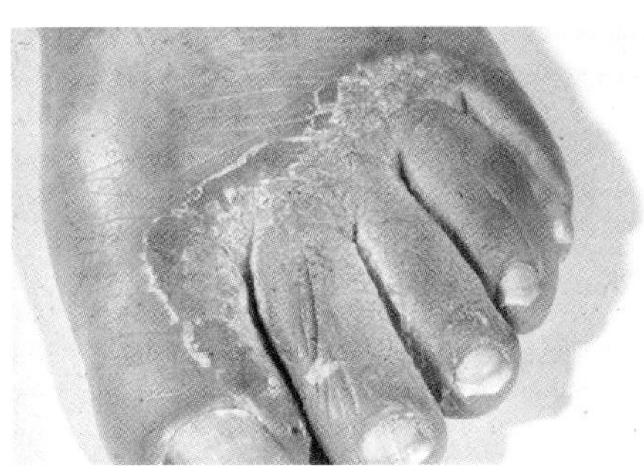

Figure 82.6 Chronic hyperkeratotic form of tinea pedis. (Courtesy of Libero Ajello, PhD.)

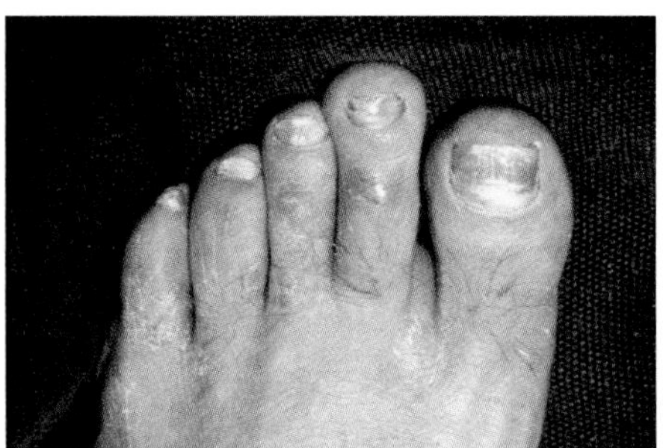

Figure 82.7 Proximal subungual onychomycosis and tinea pedis in an AIDS patient. (Courtesy of Raza Aly, PhD.)

epidermis and debris, and odor characterize this infection. Hyperhidrosis and exacerbation of the infection may result in the fungus spreading to the sole, heel, arch, and dorsal surface of the foot.

A chronic, papulosquamous, hyperkeratotic form tends to be bilateral with areas of pink skin and fine silver-white scales on a thickened red base (*Fig. 82.6*). When the lesions involve the entire foot, the term moccasin foot is used. This variant is frequent in patients who have atopic dermatitis. *Trichophyton rubrum* and *T. mentagrophytes* var. *interdigitale* are the principal agents of moccasin foot.

When zoophilic dermatophytes such as *T. mentagrophytes* var. *mentagrophytes* cause tinea pedis, a vesicular form of the disease develops. Vesicles, vesiculopustules, and occasional bullae occur in the intertriginous areas and spread to the dorsal foot, instep, and sometimes the heel and anterior areas. The fungus can be seen growing in the inner surface of the vesicle roof. Progression can result in a severe ulcerative eczematoid vesiculopustular process complicated by secondary bacterial infection that can lead to cellulitis, lymphangitis, and lymphadenitis.

Dermatophytid (id) reactions, which are allergic manifestations at sites distant from the infected site, are associated with both tinea pedis and tinea capitis. The id reaction site consists of sterile groups of vesicles that itch and are sometimes painful. Id reactions on the fingers and palms are associated with tinea pedis, whereas those on the trunk develop when patients have tinea capitis.

Tinea Unguium (Onychomycosis)

Tinea unguium occurs when a dermatophyte invades the nail unit. Strictly speaking, onychomycosis refers to invasion of the nail unit by nondermatophytic molds and yeasts; however, in common usage, onychomycosis is used to describe all fungal nail unit infections. Only dermatophyte involvement is considered here. Approximately 2–13% of the general population may have nail unit invasion by fungi.[18] Preexisting tinea pedis and trauma that weakens the union of the nail plate and nail bed allow the dermatophyte to penetrate the nail unit. Other factors such as aging (slower nail growth rate, increased trauma to the nail plate, decreased circulation, and foot size changes), heat and moisture, immunosuppression, and genetic predisposition predispose to the occurrence of onychomycosis.

The most common form of onychomycosis is distal lateral subungual onychomycosis, most commonly caused by *T. rubrum*, and occasionally by *T. mentagrophytes*, *T. tonsurans*, or *E. floccosum*.[18] In this form, the nail plate is yellow-brown with onycholysis and subungual hyperkeratosis. Superficial white onychomycosis occurs when a dermatophyte, most frequently *T. mentagrophytes*, invades the nail plate creating a white, crumbly appearance. Involvement of the entire nail surface, nail dystrophy, and invasion of the cornified layer of the nail bed and hyponychium may occur. Proximal subungual onychomycosis (*Fig. 82.7*) was an uncommon entity until the era of human immunodeficiency virus (HIV) infections began. In a study of 62 acquired immunodeficiency syndrome (AIDS) patients, 54 (87%) had proximal subungual onychomycosis.[19] The fungus, usually *T. rubrum*, penetrates the proximal portion of the nail, which results in hyperkeratosis and onycholysis. A white hue extending distally under the proximal nail fold is characteristic. Fingernails are also frequently involved in these patients.

Tinea Infections and AIDS

While early in the AIDS epidemic the prevalence of tinea infections did appear to be increased in this population, with the advent of improved antiretroviral therapy this no longer appears to be the case. Approximately 20% of AIDS patients with CD4 counts less than or equal to 200/μL have either tinea pedis or onychomycosis, a rate not dissimilar to the immunocompetent population.[20] Although the number of tinea infections seen in AIDS patients approximates that seen in non-AIDS patients, the severity of infections and the variability of clinical presentation are increased.

Generalized infection can occur, usually in patients with low CD4 counts, and while many times the disease is responsive to therapy, prolonged treatment, usually with oral therapy, is required, and in some cases the patients are unable to clear the infection.[21,22] Occasionally, infection with unusual species or infection by a species not commonly associated with a particular anatomic site, such as cases of *M. canis* tinea capitis or onychomycosis, is seen.[22,23]

Tissue invasion by dermatophytes in these patients is often sudden in onset, not necessarily associated with a hair follicle, encompasses larger areas, and extends deeper into tissue than with localized invasive lesions seen occasionally in immunocompetent persons (i.e., Majocchi's granuloma). Systemic invasion with a fatal outcome in AIDS patients has been reported, but appears to be infrequent.[24]

It should be noted that the medical literature addressing dermatophyte infections and AIDS originates primarily from the developed world, and that reports and studies addressing this subject in some developing nations, where the prevalence of AIDS is high and where tinea infections are common, are lacking.

PATHOGENESIS AND IMMUNITY

Dermatophyte infection is initiated by adherence of arthroconidia to corneocytes, with rapid germination and production of germ tubes (within 4–6 hours), which grow through layers of keratin in both a horizontal and vertical direction.[10] These pathogens are able to produce and secrete keratinases, lipases, proteases, and phosphatases, all of which aid the spread of the developing hyphae through the keratin layer.

Host resistance is a combination of nonspecific, innate immune mechanisms and an acquired immune response. The intact keratin layer inhibits penetration into deeper layers of the epidermis, at least initially, and allows exposure of the fungus to lethal ultraviolet light in some anatomic locations. The skin surface has a low moisture content and a relatively high temperature, which are not ideal conditions for fungal proliferation. Cytokine production in keratinocytes is stimulated by dermatophytes, and the release of factors such as interleukin-8 by keratinocytes results not only in an influx of neutrophils, but also stimulates increased proliferation of epidermal cells and increased keratinization, which encourages shedding of the fungi.[25] Dermatophytes have been shown to activate complement, with a resultant release of chemotactic factors.[25] Unsaturated fatty acids and lipids present in adult sebum are fungistatic and may serve as a primary resistance mechanism against dermatophytes.[26] This may explain, in part, the resolution of many cases of dermatophytosis at puberty when the composition of lipids in sebum changes.

Dermatophytes are not, however, without their own defense mechanisms. The rapid germination time of these fungi makes elimination by rapid epidermal turnover less effective. Some species of dermatophytes can destroy complement-derived chemotactic factors.[25] Mannan, a cell-wall glycoprotein of fungi, not only inhibits the proliferation of keratinocytes, but, most importantly, has been demonstrated to inhibit the development of cell-mediated immunity against the infecting dermatophyte, a primary factor in clearing an infection.[20]

Infected individuals who are able to produce a decisive delayed-type hypersensitivity reaction are often able to clear their infections. The clinical course of a dermatophyte infection is related, at least in part, to the relative proportions of CD4 (T-helper) lymphocytes and CD8 (T-suppressor) lymphocytes generated in the immune response. Those patients who have decreased CD4 lymphocytes relative to CD8 lymphocytes tend to develop chronic dermatophyte infections.[10] Because 10–20% of the "immunocompetent" world population is thought to have chronic dermatophytosis, a selective as yet undefined cell-mediated immunodeficiency to dermatophytes may be prevalent. Humoral antibodies are not thought to play any role in immunity to dermatophytes.

DIAGNOSIS

The clinical differential diagnosis is extensive.[13] Tinea capitis must be distinguished from seborrheic dermatitis, psoriasis, lupus erythematosus, lupus vulgaris, alopecia areata, pseudopelade, impetigo, trichotillomania, staphylococcal pyoderma, folliculitis decalvans, and secondary syphilis. Tinea corporis may be confused with psoriasis, pityriasis rosea, nummular eczema, granuloma annulare, annular secondary syphilis, lichen planus, seborrheic dermatitis, discoid lupus erythematosus, fixed drug eruption, pityriasis versicolor, candidiasis, and erythema annulare. Tinea cruris must be differentiated from candidiasis, erythrasma, seborrheic dermatitis, psoriasis, lichen planus chronicus, and contact dermatitis; and onychomycosis can be confused with various nail abnormalities such as nonmycotic leukonychia, clubbing, Beau's lines, pachyonychia congenita, contact irritants, and other skin diseases that cause dystrophic nails.

The diagnosis of dermatophytosis is based on the clinical presentation and the demonstration of hyaline, septate, branching hyphae in the stratum corneum, nail, or hair. The demonstration of dermatophyte hyphae in clinical specimens is accomplished by mounting the material in 10–20% potassium hydroxide, allowing the specimen to become clear, and observing the hyphae with a microscope. There is, however, nothing pathognomonic about the appearance of dermatophyte hyphae, and their appearance is similar to other hyaline hyphae formed by such common environmental fungi as *Scopulariopsis*, *Fusarium*, or *Scytalidium* species.

Isolation of the fungus is the only definitive method to identify the etiologic agent. The identification of dermatophytes in culture is based on their colonial characteristics when grown on Sabouraud glucose agar, conidia and their anatomy, temperature ranges for growth, a few limited nutritional tests, and their resistance to cycloheximide.[27] Even though DNA probes and the polymerase chain reaction have been developed, they are not currently a practical method of identifying dermatophyte species in the clinical laboratory.[28]

There are no distinctive histopathologic changes associated with dermatophytes. The epidermis may appear unaffected to mildly hyperkeratotic with patchy parakeratosis. Spongiosis and microabscesses in the stratum corneum may be seen. A perivascular infiltrate of varying severity composed of lymphocytes with scattered histiocytes, plasma cells, eosinophils, and neutrophils can be present in the upper dermis, depending on the infecting species. No or a minimal dermal infiltrate may be seen in infections due to anthropophilic species. Branching, septate hyphae can be demonstrated in the stratum corneum with a suitable stain such as periodic acid–Schiff with diastase predigestion. In ectothrix tinea capitis, arthroconidia can be demonstrated on the surface of the hair, while in endothrix infection, arthroconidia will be demonstrated within the hair shaft.

TREATMENT AND PROGNOSIS

Topical antifungal drugs are the most commonly recommended treatment for most dermatophytoses, excluding tinea capitis and onychomycosis, although oral agents are often necessary in difficult cases. The major compounds utilized include the imidazoles, triazoles, morpholines, and allylamines.

The imidazoles (clotrimazole, ketoconazole, and miconazole) and triazoles (fluconazole, itraconazole), and also the allylamines (terbinafine), inhibit the ergosterol biosynthetic pathway. The pathway is necessary for cell membrane formation by the fungi, and inhibition of the pathway results in the accumulation of toxic metabolites in the fungal cell. Griseofulvin acts by inhibiting fungal mitosis through disruption of the mitotic spindle.

Tinea capitis must be treated with oral antifungals because topical agents are unable to penetrate the hair shaft. Griseofulvin, because of its efficacy, safety, and low cost, is still considered by many to be the drug of choice.[29] The long course of treatment (8–12 weeks) required is a disadvantage, particularly where compliance is a concern. Additionally, increased doses over those required several decades ago are now necessary, and dose and duration of therapy are also dependent on species of the infecting dermatophyte.[30] Pulse therapy, with periods of treatment alternating with periods of no treatment, have been used to address issues related to cost, compliance, and side effects.[30] Terbinafine is considered the second choice, except if the infection is caused by *M. canis*, for which it appears relatively ineffective (although it seems to be more effective for *T. tonsurans* than griseofulvin).[29,30] Itraconazole is efficient but expensive, and ketoconazole does not appear to offer any advantage and has more side effects than other options.[29] Adjuvant topical therapy with either 2% ketoconazole or 1% selenium sulfide shampoo may help to reduce infectivity.[29]

Griseofulvin is relatively poor in eradicating onychomycosis with only a 50% cure rate after 12 months of therapy.[31] Terbinafine, itraconazole, and fluconazole have all shown utility, although long-term follow-up has suggested that terbinafine may be superior in preventing relapse, and that cure with fluconazole may not occur until up to one year after completion of therapy.[31] Chemical, surgical, or laser ablation of the nail may be necessary in addition to antifungal therapy.

For tinea cruris, tinea corporis, and tinea pedis, topical antifungals for 1–6 weeks are usually curative. Patients with the moccasin foot form of tinea pedis, widespread disease, disease that does not respond to topical therapy, or recurrent disease require oral therapy. There have been many clinical trials that have evaluated the comparative effectiveness of allylamines and azoles, with the allylamines overall appearing more effective, and with no detectable difference between individual allylamines or azoles.[32]

Treatment of dermatophytosis in the setting of AIDS is problematic not only because the patient is immunocompromised, but also because many patients have concomitant hepatic disease, predisposing them to hepatotoxicity, a complication of some antifungals. Inhibition of the cytochrome P450 (CYP3A4) enzyme system by the azoles results in dosing problems with some protease inhibitors and precludes the administration of necessary anti-lipemics.[20] Finally, some aspects of AIDS itself can interfere with effective therapy. Oral itraconazole, which requires an acidic environment for maximal absorption, may not achieve therapeutic serum levels at normal dosage due to the hypochlorhydria sometimes found in advanced AIDS.[20] Oral terbinafine appears to be helpful in many cases and is associated with fewer side effects than many other antifungals in this setting.[20]

PREVENTION AND CONTROL

Prevention of dermatophyte infections requires good hygiene to reduce transmission, exposure, and make the skin environment less conducive to dermatophyte growth. Clothing, towels, bedding, and combs should not be shared. Skin, especially the groin and feet, should be kept clean and dry, and exposure to soil or animals requires cleaning as soon as possible. Animal sources of zoophilic fungi need to be located and treated. Effective vaccines against dermatophytes have been developed and used in the cattle industry.[33] LTF-130, a live vaccine against *T. verrucosum*, has been used successfully to reduce infections in cattle herds in Europe.[34] Immunity appears to be dermatophyte species-specific, and live attenuated vaccines appear necessary, as an inactivated vaccine against *M. canis* studied in cats did not prevent disease.[35] No effective vaccines for dermatophytes are currently available for humans. Finally, tight, constrictive clothing or shoes should be avoided, especially in warm, tropical environments.

Access the complete reference list online at
http://www.expertconsult.com

Access the complete reference list online at http://www.expertconsult.com

CHAPTER 83

Mycetoma

Ahmed Hassan Fahal

INTRODUCTION

Mycetoma is a chronic, progressive, granulomatous, inflammatory disease. It commonly involves the subcutaneous tissue, most probably after traumatic inoculation of the causative organism; it then spreads to affect the skin and deep structures resulting in destruction, deformity, and loss of function. Mycetoma is caused by true fungi or by higher bacteria, and hence it is usually classified into eumycetoma and actinomycetoma, respectively.[1]

THE AGENTS

A variety of organisms cause mycetoma. The main agents of eumycetomas are *Madurella mycetomatis*, *M. grisea*, *Neotestudina rosatii*, *Pyrenochaeta mackinnonii*, and *Pyrenochaeta romeroi*. The main agents of actinomycetomas are the aerobic filamentous Actinomycetes, *Streptomyces somaliensis*, *Actinomadura madurae*, *A. pelletieri*, *Nocardia brasiliensis*, *N. otitidiscaviarum*, and *N. transvalensis*. Recently *S. sudanensis* was isolated.[2,3]

EPIDEMIOLOGY

The true incidence and the geographic distribution of mycetoma throughout the world are not precisely known due to the fact that mycetoma is a badly neglected disease. The nature of the disease, which is usually painless and slowly progressive, and late presentation of the majority of patients owing to lack of health education, have contributed to that. Consequently, most of the data on mycetoma is related to advanced hospital patients.[4,5]

Mycetoma has a worldwide distribution that is enormously uneven. It is endemic in many tropical and subtropical areas. It prevails in the mycetoma belt which stretches in a band between the latitudes of 15° south and 30° north and includes Sudan, Somalia, Senegal, India, Yemen, Mexico, Venezuela, Colombia, Argentina, and others. Mycetoma is reported in many temperate regions, possibly owing to the increase in international travel and mobility.[1,5]

The geographic distribution of each individual mycetoma organism shows considerable discrepancy that can be convincingly explained on an environmental basis.

THE DISEASE

Male predominance with a sex ratio of 3 : 1 is a common observation. This was attributed to the greater risk of exposure to organisms in the soil during outdoor activities. This explanation is not convincing as in endemic areas both sexes are involved in outdoor activities.[1,4,5]

No age is exempted. Mycetoma commonly affects adults between 20 and 40 years of age, the earning members of society. However, in endemic regions children and elderly persons may also be affected.

Mycetoma is seen more conventionally in farmers, field laborers, and herdsmen but also occurs in others.[1,4,5]

The clinical presentation of mycetoma is almost identical irrespective of the causative organism. However, the rate of progression is more rapid with actinomycetomas. In eumycetomas, the lesion grows slowly with clearly defined margins and remains encapsulated for a long period; whereas in actinomycetoma the lesion is more inflammatory, more destructive, and invades the bone at an earlier stage.[1,5]

The characteristic triad of a painless subcutaneous mass, sinuses, and discharge is pathognomonic of mycetoma. The swelling has a gradual onset and course. Multiple secondary swellings may evolve as well. They frequently suppurate and drain through multiple sinuses.

The discharge is serous, serosanguineous, or purulent. Secondary bacterial infection is common, and *Staphylococcus aureus* is isolated most frequently. Lesions usually discharge grains, which contain a colony of microorganisms, through the sinuses. The grains can be black, white, red, or yellow and are of variable size and consistency according to the causative organism. Their color may suggest the causative organism but is not conclusive.

As the mycetoma granuloma enlarges, the overlying skin becomes attached, stretched, smooth, and shiny with areas of hypo- or hyperpigmentation. Local hyperhidrosis at the mycetoma site is observed in some patients; however, the mechanism is not clear.

Varicose veins occur occasionally in the affected limb owing to the increased venous return because of the increased vascularity of the mycetoma. For obscure reasons, the tendons and the nerves are curiously spared until very late in the course, possibly explaining the rarity of neurologic and trophic changes in mycetoma.[1,2,4,5]

Mycetoma is usually painless. It was suggested that the organisms produce substances which have an anesthetic action. In a few patients, pain is a presenting symptom because of bone expansion by the lesions or more commonly is due to secondary bacterial infection.[1,4]

The regional lymph nodes are commonly enlarged, potentially due to secondary bacterial infection, genuine lymphatic spread of mycetoma or immune complex deposition as part of a local immune response to mycetoma.[1,4,5]

The infection remains localized, and constitutional disturbances are rare. When they occur, they are generally caused by secondary bacterial infection. Cachexia and anemia may occur in late mycetoma, often due to the infection, malnutrition, and mental depression. Mycetoma, although not commonly a fatal disease, can produce many disabilities, distortions, and deformities. Cranial mycetoma is difficult to treat and can be fatal.[1,2] In general, the clinical picture of mycetoma is influenced by the disease duration, causative organism, infection site, and host immune responses.

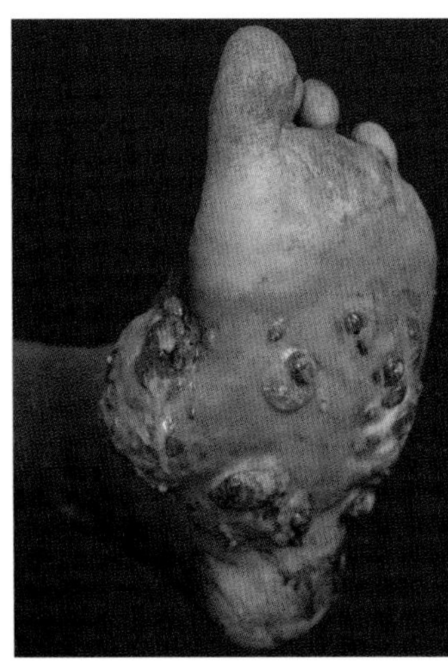

Figure 83.1 Massive eumycetoma of the foot.

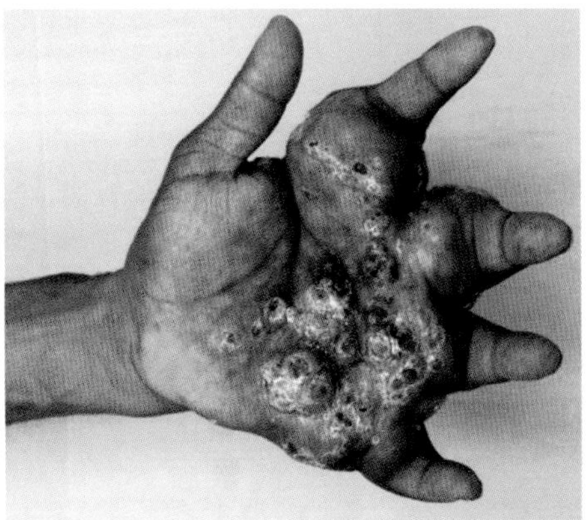

Figure 83.2 Massive actinomycetoma of the hand.

Mycetoma Site

The foot is predominantly affected and is involved in 70% of patients (*Fig. 83.1*). Most of the lesions are present on the dorsal aspect of the forefoot. The hand is the next most common site, seen in 12% of patients (*Fig. 83.2*), and the right hand is more often affected. In endemic areas, other body sites may be involved but less frequently. Intra-abdominal visceral mycetoma has not been reported.[1,2,4,5]

PATHOGENESIS AND IMMUNITY

In the subcutaneous tissue, the organism multiplies and forms grain colonies, which gradually spread along the fascial planes to involve the skin, deep structures, and bones. Actual spread of the mycetoma agents through the lymphatics to the regional lymph nodes is observed in some patients. During the active phase of the disease, these lymph node foci may suppurate and discharge. Lymphatic spread is more common in actinomycetoma than eumycetoma, and its incidence is augmented by repeated inadequate surgical excisions. Nowadays, there is strong evidence that mycetoma can spread by the blood.[1,2,4–6]

Both eumycetomas and actinomycetomas have a similar macroscopic appearance. In eumycetoma, the lesion is well encapsulated by a fibrous wall. Initially the normal anatomy and surrounding structures are not disturbed. As the infection proceeds, the tissue becomes disorganized, and distorted. Mycetoma tends to spread along the fascial planes to form new satellites. There are numerous sinus tracts connecting the various

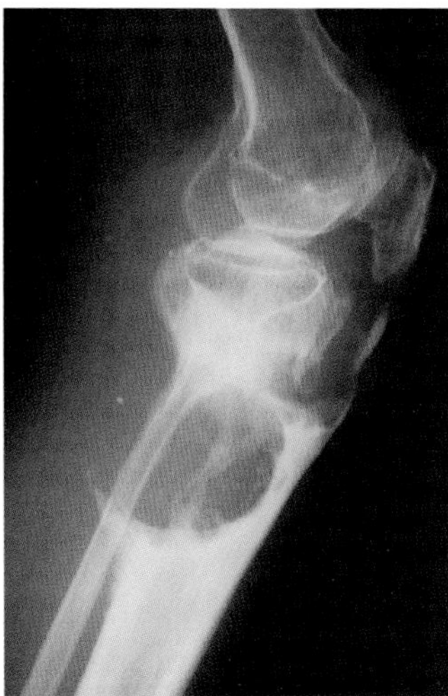

Figure 83.3 X-ray of the knee joint showing soft tissue swelling, periosteal reaction, and multiple bone cavities typical of eumycetoma.

lesions together with the skin and deep structures. Muscles, joints, synovial membranes, and bones are usually involved but at a later stage.

In actinomycetoma the lesion is diffuse, ill defined, unencapsulated and merges with the surrounding tissue. The bone may be absorbed and replaced by fibrous tissue forming a fibrocartilaginous mass. Secondary bacterial infection usually leads to more tissue damage.

Mycetoma usually produces multiple bone cavities. They usually contain solid masses of grains and fibrous tissue, which provides bone support. This may explain the rarity of pathologic fractures in mycetoma.[7]

Microscopically, there are three tissue reaction types in mycetoma.[8] Type I reaction is characterized by the presence of an admixture of neutrophils, lymphocytes, plasma cells, macrophages, and foreign body giant cells. The grains are closely surrounded, and occasionally infiltrated, by neutrophils causing their fragmentation. In type II reaction, the neutrophils have largely disappeared and are replaced by macrophages and multinucleated giant cells. Type III reaction is characterized by formation of a well-organized epithelioid granuloma with Langhans giant cells.

DIAGNOSIS

Differential Diagnosis

In endemic areas any swelling must be considered as mycetoma until a diagnosis is verified. The differential diagnosis of mycetoma includes many soft tissue tumors including Kaposi's sarcoma, fibroma, and malignant melanoma. Foreign body and thorn granulomas must be considered as well. Bone destruction in the absence of sinuses tends to favor the diagnosis of tuberculosis. The radiologic features of advanced mycetoma are similar to those of primary osteogenic sarcoma. Primary osseous mycetoma needs to be differentiated from chronic osteomyelitis, osteoclastoma, or bone cysts.[1,4]

Mycetoma Imaging

Mycetoma has distinct radiologic features (*Fig. 83.3*). A soft tissue shadow is commonly evident in the early stage. Calcification and obliteration of the fascial planes may sometimes be observed. As the disease progresses, the cortex may be compressed from outside by the granuloma, leading to bone scalloping; this is followed by a variable degree of periosteal reaction in a form of sun-ray appearance and Codman triangle, which are indistinguishable from osteogenic sarcoma. Late in the disease, multiple cavities may develop. These cavities are few and large with well-defined margins in eumycetomas, whereas in actinomycetomas they are

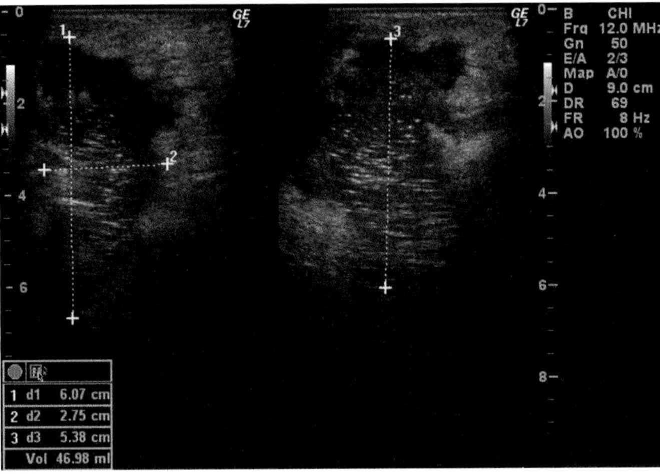

Figure 83.4 Ultrasound showing numerous sharp bright hyperreflective echoes and multiple thick-walled cavities with absent acoustic enhancement typical of eumycetoma ultrasonic appearance.

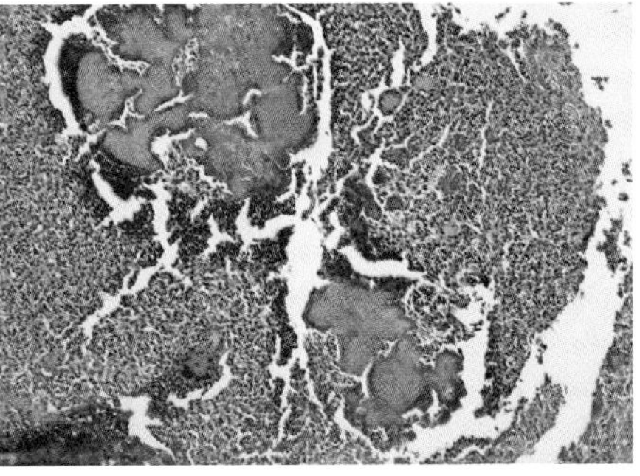

Figure 83.5 Histologic section from a cell block obtained by FNA stained with hematoxylin and eosin. Note the presence of polymorphous inflammatory cells and *Actinomadura madurae* grains closely surrounded by neutrophils.

usually smaller, numerous, and have no definite margins. The bony changes in the skull are unique; they are purely sclerotic with dense bone formation and loss of trabeculation. Osteoporosis of the affected bone is also observed in mycetoma owing to disuse atrophy.[1,5]

The use of MRI and CT scan for diagnosis of mycetoma is increasing; however, the findings are not specific but can accurately determine the extent of the lesion.

Ultrasonic Imaging

The mycetoma grains, capsule, and accompanying inflammatory granuloma have characteristic ultrasonic appearances. In eumycetoma lesions, the grains produce numerous sharp bright hyperreflective echoes, consistent with the black grains. The grain cement substance is most probably the origin of these sharp echoes. There are multiple thick-walled cavities with absent acoustic enhancement. In actinomycetoma lesions, the findings are similar, but the grains are less distinct. This may be due to their smaller size, consistency, individual embedding, or the absence of the cement substances.

The ultrasonic diagnosis of mycetoma is more precise and accurate in lesions with no sinuses. The size and extent of the lesion can be accurately determined ultrasonically, and this is useful in planning surgical procedures (***Fig. 83.4***).[9]

Fine Needle Aspiration Cytology

Mycetoma can be accurately diagnosed by fine needle aspiration cytology (FNA) and cell block technique. Grains have a distinctive appearance in cytology smears similar to that observed in histologic sections, allowing morphologic identification and classification according to its causative agent. The technique is simple, sensitive, inexpensive, rapid, and can be tolerated by patients. It provides appropriate samples for culture and material for investigation.[10]

Culture

The mycetoma-causing organisms can be identified by their colonial morphology and biological activities in pure culture. Grains are the source of the culture. Surgical biopsy is commonly required as grains extracted through the sinuses are usually contaminated and not viable.

Many culture media are in use, and the commonest are Sabouraud, blood, glucose nutrient, malt extract and Lowenstein–Jensen agar. The culture technique is cumbersome and time-consuming, and requires experience, and contamination is common.[1,4,5]

Molecular Diagnosis

Conventional mycological techniques are not sufficient to determine precisely the specific causative species as is clearly noted with a number of species such as *M. grisea*, *M. mycetomatis*, and *P. romeroi*, which do not sporulate readily. The common molecular techniques are sequencing of the rDNA internal transcribed spacer (ITS) and region rDNA restriction fragment length polymorphism and specific ITS polymerase chain reaction.[11,12]

Molecular diagnosis of mycetoma agents is rapid and specific and can be used for both epidemiologic studies and patient management. The technique can assist the discovery of new mycetoma agents.[11]

Serodiagnosis

The common serodiagnostic tests are counter-immunoelectrophoresis and enzyme-linked immunosorbent assays. They have many advantages over culture and histopathology, which require surgical biopsy that may enhance the spread of the organism. However, preparation of the antigen is time-consuming, and cross-reactivity between the different organisms is common. They are useful tools in community seroepidemiologic surveys for disease distribution and prevalence.[1]

Histologic Diagnosis

Histologic and immunohistochemical examinations of mycetoma lesions are attractive as neither aseptic techniques nor rigid time schedule are required. Histopathology usually shows the grain morphology and tissue reaction to the organisms. The surgical biopsy or cell block of FNA containing grains is required for histologic diagnosis (***Fig. 83.5***). The most common stains are hematoxylin and eosin and periodic acid–Schiff.[1,13]

TREATMENT AND PROGNOSIS

The Management of Mycetoma

The treatment of mycetoma depends mainly on its etiologic agent and the extent of the disease. Until recently the only available treatment for mycetoma was amputation of the affected part or mutilating surgical excisions. No case of self-cure has ever been reported in the medical literature. However, spontaneous regression was observed in some patients. Combined medical and surgical treatment is the standard.[14]

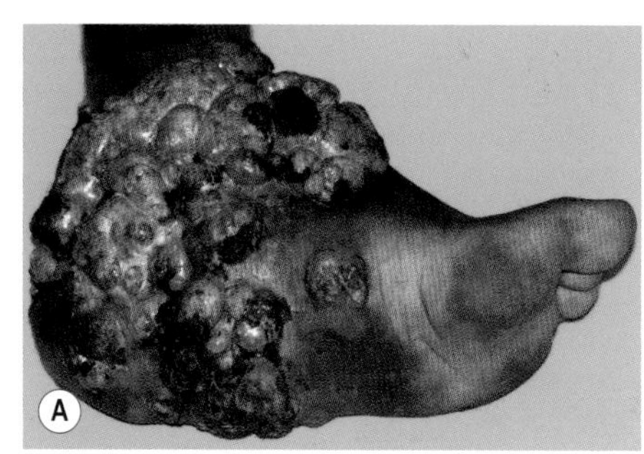

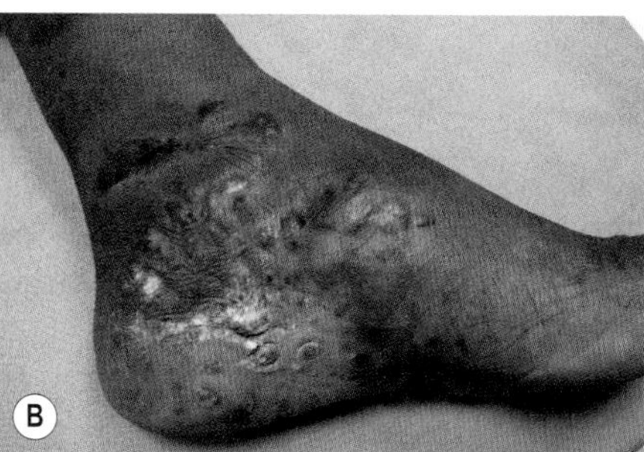

Figure 83.6 The foot of a patient with massive actinomycetoma treated with amikacin sulfate and co-trimoxazole, **(A)** before treatment and **(B)** after treatment.

Treatment of Actinomycetoma

Actinomycetoma is amenable to treatment with a combination of antibiotics. Combined drug therapy is mandatory to avoid drug resistance and to achieve eradication of infection. There are many reports of excellent clinical response to the combination of amikacin sulfate and co-trimoxazole given in cycles. Each cycle consists of amikacin sulfate (15 mg/kg twice daily for 3 weeks) and co-trimoxazole (1.5 mg/kg twice daily for 5 weeks); the cycles are repeated until the patient is cured.[15,16]

In resistant cases, rifampicin, dapsone, and streptomycin are given; however, they are less effective. These drugs have many side effects; hence the patients should be followed closely clinically and biochemically. The cure rate varies between 60% and 90% (*Fig. 83.6*).[14]

Treatment of Eumycetoma

Reports on medical treatment of eumycetoma are few and disappointing. Various antifungal agents have been tried with little success.[17,18] The current drugs in use are ketoconazole (200–400 mg twice a day) and itraconazole (100–200 mg twice a day). However, treatment for a long duration is required to attain cure with an average of one year. There are high recurrence rates and many side effects.[19]

Surgery for Mycetoma

Surgery is indicated for localized mycetomas resistant to medical treatment or for better response to medical treatment in patients with massive disease. The surgical options range from wide local and debulking excisions to amputations. Local anesthesia is contraindicated as the disease extending along tissue planes is unpredictable. A bloodless operative field using a tourniquet is mandatory to identify margins of the lesion.

In advanced mycetoma not responding to medical treatment for a prolonged period, nothing short of amputation is likely to succeed. The amputation rate ranges from 10% to 25%.[1,4]

The postoperative recurrence rate varies from 25% to 50%. This is due to the disease biology, inadequate surgical excision associated with the use of local anesthesia and insufficient surgical experience, and drug noncompliance because of financial reasons and/or lack of health education.

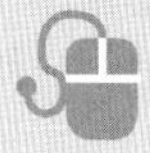

Access the complete reference list online at
http://www.expertconsult.com

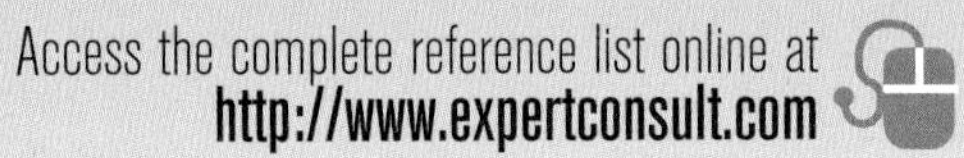
Access the complete reference list online at
http://www.expertconsult.com

CHAPTER 84

Chromoblastomycosis and Phaeohyphomycosis

Tadahiko Matsumoto • Chester R. Cooper • Paul J. Szaniszlo

INTRODUCTION

Human and animal infections caused by fungi having mycelia or cells that are dark-colored (brown to black) in tissue are often separated into categories of superficial, cutaneous, subcutaneous, and systemic diseases. The term "dematiaceous," which had been used to describe dark-colored fungi, was replaced by a new term, "phaeoid" (Greek *phaios*, dusky).[1]

The pigment in the hyphal and conidial walls of the medically important phaeoid fungi is typically a melanin, specifically dihydroxynaphthalene (DHN) melanin.[2–4] Compared with what is known about the role of fungal melanins in phytopathogenic fungi, current knowledge of their role in infections of humans and lower animals is at an early stage of development. However, results obtained with the human pathogen *Wangiella dermatitidis* have unequivocally confirmed that DHN melanin contributes to the virulence of at least one phaeoid fungus.[5–7] Fungal melanins apparently contribute to virulence by functioning as a deterrent against host defense mechanisms and antifungal drugs.[8,9]

The cutaneous and subcutaneous mycoses with etiologic agents that have phaeoid invasive forms are chromoblastomycosis (CBM), eumycotic mycetoma (in part), and phaeohyphomycosis (PHM). "Chromomycosis" is a complete synonym for CBM and should not be used in any other wider meaning(s) of phaeoid fungus infections. Visceral or systemic infections also occur as disseminated cases of PHM of the internal organs. Phaeoid fungal infections have become significant to both physicians and microbiologists because they exhibit a broad spectrum of clinical features.[10–15]

Although most cases of CBM have occurred in tropical and subtropical areas, the disease has been reported from the temperate zones in the world. Africa and Latin America have very high prevalence rates of this disease.[12,15] The highest incidence of CBM has been reported to occur in Costa Rica.[16] However, partly because of the rise in global temperature and increase in emigrants, immigrants, and travelers, cases of CBM apparently are spreading from tropical and subtropical areas to temperate regions. In contrast to CBM, cases of PHM have occurred with equal frequency in tropical, subtropical, and temperate areas, partly because of the opportunistic nature of its etiologic agents.[12–14]

Previously, the distribution of the pathogenic phaeoid fungi was believed to be limited to tropical and subtropical areas. However, isolations of potentially pathogenic phaeoid fungi from nonclinical sources have appeared recently. They have provided new ecologic insights into the global distribution of this group of fungi.[11,17–19]

CHROMOBLASTOMYCOSIS

THE AGENT

CBM is a mycotic infection of cutaneous and subcutaneous tissues characterized by the development in tissue of phaeoid muriform cells. The term "sclerotic cells," as used for the characteristic cells seen in tissue in CBM, has been replaced by the term "muriform cells."[20] A comprehensive review of this mycosis was published recently.[15]

The principal etiologic agents of CBM are *Cladophialophora carrionii*, *Fonsecaea compacta*, *F. monophora*, *F. pedrosoi*, *Phialophora verrucosa*, and *Rhinocladiella cerophilum*. *F. pedrosoi* is the most frequently occurring of these, followed by *C. carrionii* and *P. verrucosa*. *F. pedrosoi* is predominant in warm and humid areas, whereas *C. carrionii* occurs in arid and semi-arid zones. In addition, *F. pedrosoi* and *P. verrucosa* have been reported as etiologic agents of PHM, and the latter also as an etiologic agent of black grain mycetomas. Although *F. compacta* is sometimes considered as a dysgonic variety of *F. pedrosoi*, *F. monophora* was recently segregated from *F. pedrosoi* as a new species, based on ribosomal DNA internal transcribed space (ITS) sequence data.[21] These fungi are present in soil, decaying wood, and decomposing vegetation.[11,12]

In culture, all of these species produce dark colonies with short aerial hyphae, and gray, green, brown, or black velvety surfaces. These agents are differentiated by their conidiogenous morphology, physiology, serology (exoantigen tests), and molecular biology.[3,11,21–24]

THE DISEASE

CBM is a cosmopolitan disease that is most prevalent in tropical and subtropical zones. Generally it affects the exposed areas of the skin, mostly the distal part of the legs of male outdoor laborers who often work barefooted. The primary lesion is a small, pink, scaly papule that occurs at the site of inoculation of the etiologic fungus. The initial traumatic injury could be very minor and may have occurred many years previously, then subsequently forgotten. The papule gradually enlarges to form a superficial erythematous or purplish plaque. The lesion at first may be scaly or verrucous in appearance, but subsequently progresses to a verrucous nodule. Occasionally, the lesion is pruritic, and may become painful when secondarily infected with bacteria. Satellite lesions may develop by way of the superficial lymphatics, or by autoinoculation through scratching. New lesions resemble the primary ones and frequently merge to form a verrucous, sometimes cauliflower-like mass. On the surface, hemopurulent black dots are often observed. Ulceration may occur when a secondary infection or a localized injury to the lesions coexist. Secondary infections also lead to lymphatic stasis, which may result in elephantiasis. Scars may be formed in the center of the lesions when they enlarge centrifugally (***Fig. 84.1***).

Although CBM is generally localized at the site of the primary inoculation, the fungus can break through cutaneous tissue and disseminate to other organs, including the central nervous system, following metastasis into the subcutaneous lymphatics or blood vessels. Early diagnosis of metastasis is of utmost importance in the treatment of patients. The tissue response in CBM is not specific for establishing a histopathologic diagnosis. Fundamentally, it is a purulent and granulomatous inflammatory reaction, which may also occur in other mycoses.

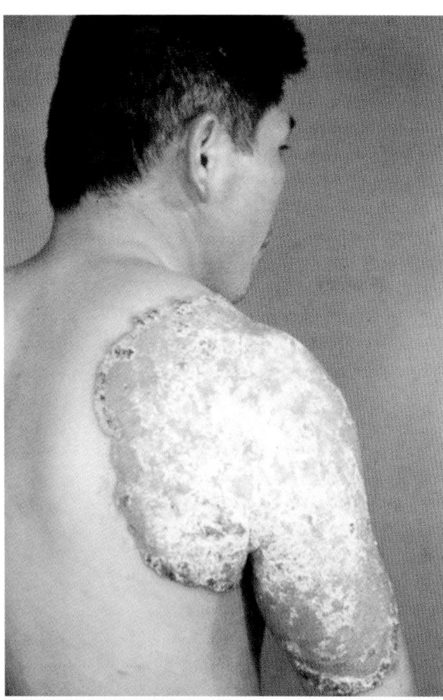

Figure 84.1 Chromoblastomycosis caused by *Fonsecaea pedrosoi*. The patient subsequently died from this infection.

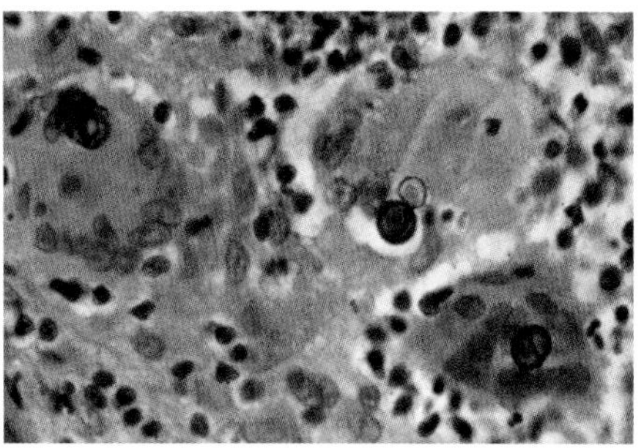

Figure 84.2 Photomicrograph of phaeoid muriform cells in chromoblastomycosis caused by *Fonsecaea pedrosoi* (periodic acid–Schiff stain).

Small granulomatous nodules consisting of epithelioid cells and multinucleated giant cells are often found in the dermis or in subcutaneous tissues. Wood splinters are occasionally encountered *in situ*. The granulomas may have microabscesses containing polymorphonuclear leukocytes and necrotic debris. The surrounding stroma, infiltrated with lymphocytes, plasma cells, macrophages, and polymorphonuclear leukocytes, may show marked fibrosis, especially in older lesions. In the epidermis, either acanthosis or pseudoepitheliomatous hyperplasia or both are recognized. The hyperplastic epidermis may extend into the affected dermis, forming lips around the necrotic tissue. The stratum corneum is frequently distorted and shows hyperkeratosis and parakeratosis. Cellular infiltrates in the epidermis, consisting of polymorphonuclear leukocytes, may occasionally form keratinolytic microabscesses.

In tissue, the phaeoid, round to polygonal, thick-walled, and multicellular muriform cells are the characteristic and diagnostic features of CBM. The muriform cells represent an intermediate vegetative form arrested between yeast and hyphal formation. Based on evidence from *in vitro* experiments, the suggestion has been that calcium limitation may trigger the formation of muriform cells *in vivo*.[25] The muriform cells occur free in tissues or may be contained in giant cells or in microabscesses, as well as in the epidermis, and even in the stratum corneum (***Fig. 84.2***). The wide distribution of muriform cells could be explained, in part, by a phenomenon called "transepidermal (or transepithelial) elimination."

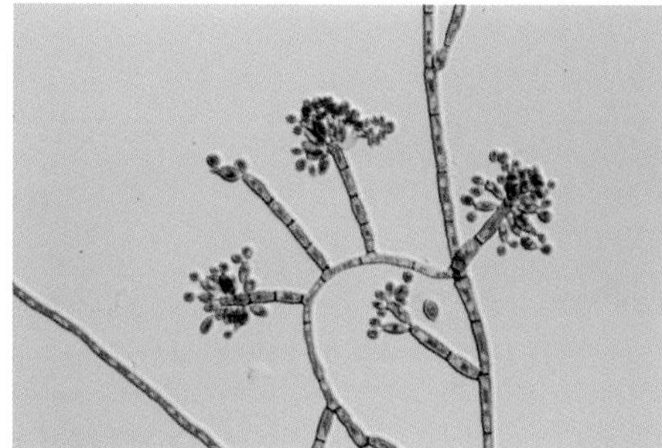

Figure 84.3 *In vitro* micromorphology of *Fonsecaea pedrosoi*.

This phenomenon causes foreign material (e.g., fungal cells) in the dermis to be eliminated via transepidermal passage without causing any major structural alteration or epidermal degeneration.[26]

A morphologic study of the host–parasite interaction in CBM revealed that some of the phagocytosed fungal cells are damaged, but that intracellular killing of the fungus is rare. These findings suggested that the tissue form of the etiologic agents of CBM resist the fungicidal activity of the cutaneous macrophages that possess the ultrastructural features of stimulated phagocytes.[27]

DIAGNOSIS

Diagnosis is based on the characteristic clinical appearance of CBM, by the presence of phaeoid muriform cells in tissue, and by the isolation and identification of the etiologic fungi (***Fig. 84.3***). The exoantigen test is applicable to identification of cultures in some species. However, none of the reagents are commercially available. Several efforts have been made towards the development of identification systems for clinical specimens of phaeoid fungi through the molecular analysis of ribosomal DNA sequences.[23,24,28,29]

TREATMENT AND PROGNOSIS

The treatment of choice is surgical excision of small lesions and antifungal chemotherapy with itraconazole, terbinafine, or a combination of the two. Voriconazole and posaconazole have potential for use in CBM among the second-generation triazole agents. For long-term therapy, itraconazole 200–400 mg/day effectively controls the disease, and a report involving terbinafine (500 mg/day for 6–12 months) treatment of 42 Malagasy patients with CBM described promising results (a global efficiency of about 75%).[30] Agents of CBM are sensitive *in vitro* to the new triazoles, voriconazole and posaconazole, and also to some of the echinocandins.

Local heat therapy, using a pocket warmer or an electric pad, has been tried successfully in some cases of CBM. A study of the mechanisms underlying the effectiveness of topical heat therapy suggests that heat killing of the causative organism is unlikely to have been the sole reason for the effectiveness of this modality.[18,31,32]

Despite success in treating many cases of CBM, the disease is often recalcitrant to therapy, thereby making its management quite frustrating. Clinical type, etiologic species, duration of disease, site of infection, underlying condition of the patient, and experience of the physician are primary factors dictating the type of treatment and the patient's prognosis.

PREVENTION AND CONTROL

The incidence of CBM can be reduced through education, economic development, and early diagnosis and treatment. The low incidence of infections does not justify the development of vaccines, assuming such an approach were feasible.[33]

PHAEOHYPHOMYCOSIS

THE AGENT

PHM is an infection of humans and other animals caused by a number of phaeoid fungi, characterized by the development of dark-colored hyphae and other types of fungal elements, depending on species, in invaded tissues. The term PHM encompasses distinct mycotic infections regardless of the site of the lesion, the pattern of tissue response, granuloma or abscess, or the taxonomic classification of the etiologic agents.[34] Two recent reviews of PMH, one focused on deep-seated infections, have been published recently.[13,14]

With the increasing number of immunocompromised patients, the number of genera and species of fungi causing PHM has been growing. As of 1998, the phaeoid fungi, verified as causing PHM, comprised 109 species classified in 60 genera. Certainly, this number has increased over the past decade. The most common etiologic agents are *E. jeanselmei* and *W. dermatitidis*, followed by such phaeoid fungus species as *Alternaria alternata*, *Bipolaris spicifera*, *Curvularia lunata*, *E. moniliae*, *E. spinifera*, *Exserohilum rostratum*, *Phaeoacremonium parasiticum*, *Phialemonium obovatum*, and *Phialophora repens*.[13,14] Deep-seated cases of PHM have been caused by more than 40 species classified in at least 27 genera. In particular, 44% of cerebral PHM infections are caused by *Cladophialophora bantiana*.

THE DISEASE

PHM is a cosmopolitan disease. Patients are usually adults, and about half of them seem to be immunologically compromised by associated underlying diseases such as diabetes mellitus, tuberculosis, leprosy, acquired immunodeficiency syndrome (AIDS), lymphoma, and leukemia. Some patients appear to be locally compromised because of the application of topical corticosteroids. PHM lesions may occur anywhere in the body, often in exposed parts, especially the upper arms. Frequently, but not exclusively, inoculation of the agent is by wounds made by contaminated materials.

The most common and typical lesions are cutaneous or subcutaneous cysts or abscesses, frequently caused by *E. jeanselmei*. The primary lesion occurs as a single, discrete, asymptomatic small nodule. This is palpable under the smooth and slightly elevated skin. The nodule gradually evolves to become an encapsulated, fluctuant abscess with a liquefied center (***Fig. 84.4***). The overlying epidermis is hardly affected, and formation of a sinus tract or ulceration is rarely observed. Occasionally, a granulomatous, slightly elevated plaque may appear when the main site of the lesion is in the epidermis and dermis. Less frequently, it is manifested as a small verrucous nodule or plaque consisting of coalesced nodules, which resembles the clinical appearance of CBM.

Lymph node involvement and dissemination are rare. However, PHM may occur in the central nervous system or other internal organs, such as the liver, lungs, or pancreas. It may appear as a hematogenous metastasis from cutaneous or subcutaneous infections, or without any visible lesions. Human infections caused by *W. dermatitidis* have been equally distributed between cutaneous and subcutaneous infections and systemic involvement.[35] *W. dermatitidis* should be regarded as a dermotropic and neurotropic pathogen.[20,36] Because of this, its designation as a paradigm for phaeohyphomycosis is appropriate.[37]

Cyst or abscess formation is mainly confined to the dermis and adjacent subcutaneous tissue. Three stages have been described: (1) a tuberculoid phase, (2) a stellate abscess, and (3) a fluctuant abscess. In the primary lesion, a hypercellular tubercle composed mainly of epithelioid cells and foreign body giant cells is formed. Scattered foci of necrosis follow, accompanied by acute and chronic cellular infiltrations, and stellate abscesses develop. The stellate abscesses coalesce to transform themselves into a fluctuant abscess.[38]

A thick wall surrounds the abscess. The inner layer is made up of a combination of epithelioid cells, macrophages, giant cells of foreign body and Langhans types, and neutrophils. The middle layer is composed predominantly of vascularized scar tissue surrounded by an outer layer of hyaline fibrous tissue. The center of the abscess contains necrotic debris mixed with polymorphonuclear leukocytes. Foreign plant material, as in CBM, may be present. The granulomatous lesions in the middle to upper dermis mainly consist of epithelioid cells and giant cells that are covered by the necrotic epidermis. Pseudoepitheliomatous hyperplasia, hyperkeratosis, parakeratosis, and acanthosis overlying the upper dermal granuloma are recognized in PHM. These appear clinically as verrucous plaques resembling CBM.

The pigmented fungal elements show a variety of morphologies in the PHM-infected tissue. They may be dark-walled, short, septate, branched or unbranched hyphal elements, catenulate spherical cells (toruloid or moniliform hyphae), isolated spherical cells that have divided by budding or by septation in a single plane, or combinations of any of these (***Fig. 84.5***). The spherical yeast-like cells occasionally resemble the muriform cells of CBM, but differ by having thinner cell walls, septation in only one plane, and frequently a catenulate morphology. It is important to note that mycoses caused by phaeoid fungi are variable and that a single species may cause more than one type of disease. CBM and PHM represent extremes of a continuum of infections caused by phaeoid fungi.[10,33]

The brown color of the fungal elements, generally easily observable in hematoxylin and eosin-stained tissue slides, is lighter than that of CBM and is often overlooked. Periodic acid–Schiff, Gomori methenamine silver, or other stains for fungi may be required to detect the fungal elements in such a case. If questions should arise concerning the pigmentation of the mycelium in tissue sections, the Fontana–Masson silver stain, specific for melanin, may be used to advantage. Mycelium that appears to be hyaline in sections stained with hematoxylin and eosin may give a positive reaction for melanin.[39]

DIAGNOSIS

Diagnosis of PHM is based on the presence of phaeoid hyphae in tissue and by the isolation and identification of compatible etiologic fungi (***Fig. 84.6***). The exoantigen test is applicable to identification of cultures

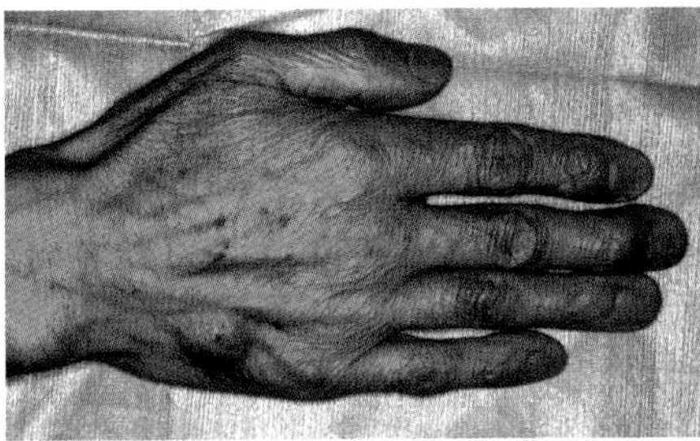

Figure 84.4 Subcutaneous phaeohyphomycosis caused by *Exophiala jeanselmei.*

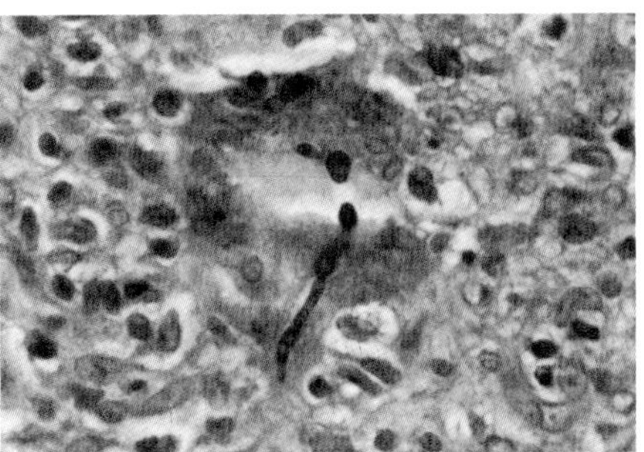

Figure 84.5 Photomicrograph of septate mycelium in cutaneous phaeohyphomycosis caused by *Wangiella dermatitidis* (periodic acid–Schiff stain).

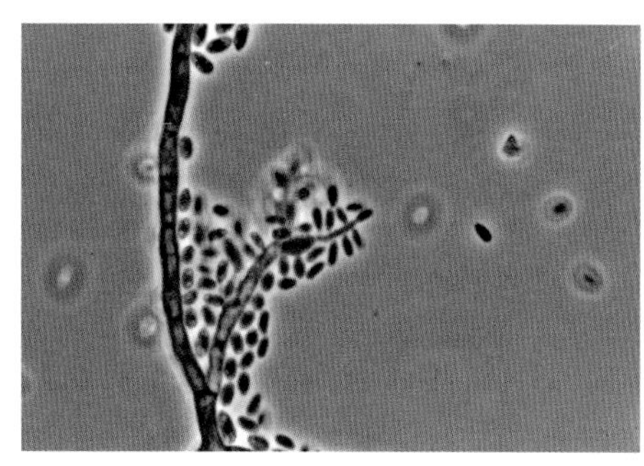

Figure 84.6 *In vitro* micromorphology of *Exophiala moniliae.*

in some phaeoid fungi. However, none of the reagents are commercially available. Molecular-based methodologies have been developed for some agents of PHM, but their application is generally restricted to well-equipped clinical laboratories.[23,24,28,29]

TREATMENT AND PROGNOSIS

Successful treatment of cutaneous and subcutaneous PHM is achieved by simple surgical excision. However, cases of systemic and disseminated PHM are serious and have a high mortality rate. Antifungal chemotherapy is not easy because of the huge variety of etiologic agents. Amphotericin B or flucytosine or combination therapy with these agents, and treatment with fluconazole, itraconazole, ketoconazole, or terbinafine has been reported with mixed results.[13,14] Clinical responses are well correlated with *in vitro* susceptibility test results; however, resistance does not preclude clinical response.

As in cases of CBM, new antifungal agents may prove important in the treatment of PHM. Most fungi causing PHM are sensitive *in vitro* to the triazole voriconazole, as well as itraconazole, an imidazole antifungal agent. Many agents of PHM that cause superficial infections are susceptible to terbinafine in addition to the echinocandins. In contrast, the pathogenic agents of PHM appear less sensitive to fluconazole *in vitro*.

Local heat therapy, using a pocket warmer or an electric pad, may also be applied to cutaneous and subcutaneous PHM, even though some of the etiologic fungi possess considerable thermotolerance.[31,32]

PREVENTION AND CONTROL

Prevention and control are not practical for PHM. Owing to the cosmopolitan, ubiquitous nature of the fungi causing PHM, it is not feasible to attempt their eradication.[33]

ACKNOWLEDGMENT

The authors gratefully dedicate this chapter in memory of the late Dr Libero Ajello, former Director of the Division of Mycotic Diseases at the Centers for Disease Control and Prevention, Atlanta, Georgia.

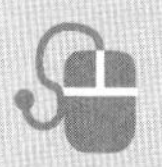

Access the complete reference list online at **http://www.expertconsult.com**

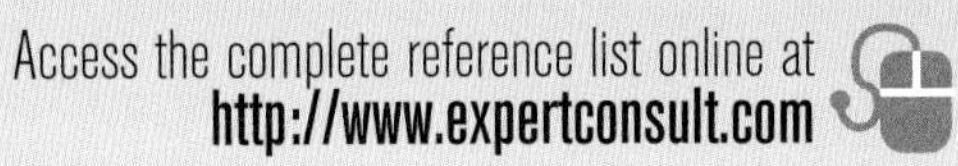
Access the complete reference list online at
http://www.expertconsult.com

CHAPTER 85

Histoplasmosis, Blastomycosis, Coccidioidomycosis, and Cryptococcosis

Gregory M. Anstead • Tihana Bicanic • Eduardo Arathoon • John R. Graybill

HISTOPLASMOSIS

INTRODUCTION

Histoplasmosis is caused by the dimorphic soil fungus *Histoplasma capsulatum*, which has two varieties, *H. c.* var. *capsulatum* and *H. c.* var. *duboisii*. The former is endemic primarily to the United States and Latin America. Histoplasmosis due to var. *capsulatum* presents as acute, subacute, or chronic pulmonary disease, and as disease disseminated to the reticuloendothelial and central nervous systems.[1] Var. *duboisii* endemic to Africa spares the lungs and attacks the sketetal system, skin, and soft tissues.[2]

THE AGENT

H. capsulatum produces a sexual state, *Ajellomyces capsulatus*, when two compatible isolates are paired on soil extract agar. On primary isolation at 25–30°C, small hyphal colonies appear after several days to a week. The mould produces two conidial types: spherical tuberculate macroconidia (8–15 μm) and oval microconidia (2–4 μm). The yeast appears in mammalian tissues or when conidia are inoculated at 37°C for 7–14 days in brain heart infusion (BHI) with blood agar. The yeasts are oval (2–4 μm) with thin walls, multiply by budding, with a narrow isthmus between mother and daughter cells. The budding yeast of var. *duboisii* differs from var. *capsulatum* in larger size (8–15 μm), thicker wall, and prominent bud scar or isthmus.[3]

EPIDEMIOLOGY

The habitat of the mycelia of *H. capsulatum*, soil contaminated with bird and bat guano, is associated with bird roosts, caves, and dilapidated buildings, with outbreaks occurring with exposure to these reservoirs.[1] High-risk activities for histoplasmosis include spelunking (caving), mining, construction, roofing, farming, and gardening.[4,5] In human immunodeficiency virus (HIV)-infected persons, exposure to guano-contaminated soil has a 3.3 times greater risk of histoplasmosis.[6] Immunocompromised patients and children are more prone to develop symptoms after primary infection. Reactivation occurs in immunosuppressed persons, such as cancer patients receiving chemotherapy, persons receiving tumor necrosis factor (TNF)-α antagonists, pregnant women, and persons with acquired immunodeficiency syndrome (AIDS).[3,7] In endemic areas, 2–5% of HIV-infected patients develop disseminated histoplasmosis.[8] In the United States, histoplasmosis is three times more common than tuberculosis in patients receiving TNF-α antagonists.[7]

The most highly endemic areas for *H. capsulatum* var. *capsulatum* include the Ohio, Mississippi, and St Lawrence River valleys and parts of Latin America (***Fig. 85.1***). Histoplasmosis is the most prevalent respiratory mycosis in the United States, affecting 500 000 persons per year.[9]

The epidemiology of histoplasmosis in Latin America is poorly defined, with prevalence estimates based on histoplasmin skin test studies done decades ago. In Guatemala, the rate of histoplasmin sensitivity was 57%, much higher than in other Latin American countries,[10] and histoplasmosis is more common among HIV patients than mycobacterial infection.[11] In Mexico, 1065 cases of histoplasmosis were reported from 1988 through 1994, mostly from the states of Veracruz, Oaxaca, Campeche, Colima, and Tabasco.[12] In Venezuela, prevalence is increasing, including in urban areas.[13] Histoplasmosis also occurs sporadically in Asia, Africa, Australia, and Europe.[4]

In Africa, *H.c.* var. *capsulatum* occurs primarily in South Africa as well as in Zimbabwe and Tanzania. Rates of histoplasmin skin sensitivity in Africa have ranged from 0 to 28% (although skin testing cannot differentiate var. *capsulatum* from var. *duboisii*).[14]

African histoplasmosis, caused by var. *duboisii*, is endemic in central and western Africa, and Madagascar, between the latitudes 15° N and 10° S, with the majority of reported cases from Nigeria.[15] The ecology of the var. *duboisii* is not well determined, but it is present in bat caves.[15]

THE DISEASE

More than 95% of immunocompetent persons remain asymptomatic following infection with *H. capsulatum* var. *capsulatum*. In symptomatic cases, self-limited pulmonary illness usually manifests with fever, malaise, cough, and chest pain. Chest radiographs show focal infiltrates with hilar or mediastinal lymphadenopathy.[16] The degree of exposure and host immunocompetence determine the severity of illness. In cases with heavy exposure or severe immunosuppression, symptomatic disease is common, including severe pneumonia and adult respiratory distress syndrome (ARDS)[17,18] with a miliary radiographic pattern. Rheumatologic manifestations, such as arthritis and erythema nodosum, may occur with primary infection. Uncommonly, granulomatous mediastinitis develops persistently, with enlarged lymph nodes coalescing into an encapsulated mass which may caseate, or impinge on other structures, causing pneumonia, esophageal diverticula, or tracheoesophageal and cutaneous fistulae. Progression to fibrosis may entrap the great vessels or trachea and cause superior vena cava syndrome.[1]

Chronic pulmonary histoplasmosis is a progressive or recurrent pneumonia, with night sweats, fatigue, productive cough, and apical lung infiltrates with fibrosis and cavitation. It often occurs in the setting of chronic obstructive pulmonary disease. Although patients may succumb to pulmonary disease, dissemination is rare.

Disseminated infection presents as prolonged fever, wasting, mucocutaneous lesions, hepatosplenomegaly, lymphadenopathy, pneumonia, meningoencephalitis, adrenal insufficiency, intestinal masses or ulcerative lesions and, occasionally, acute sepsis-like illness.[1,17] Skin lesions, uncommon in US patients with histoplasmosis (~10% of cases), occur more frequently (38–85%) in Latin America (***Fig. 85.2***) possibly owing to

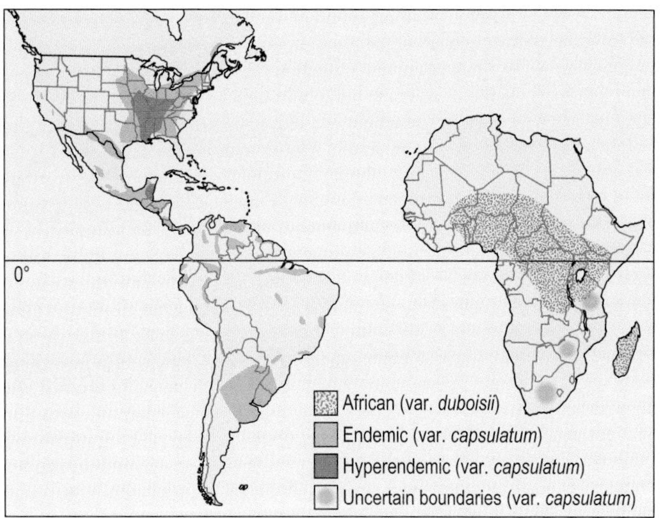

Figure 85.1 Map of the endemic area of histoplasmosis. (Adapted from: Wheat LJ. Histoplasmosis. In: Kauffman CA, ed. Atlas of Fungal Infections. 2nd ed. Philadelphia: Current Medicine 2006:1; Anstead GM, Graybill JR. Histoplasmosis, blastomycosis, coccicioidomycosis, cryptcoccocis. In: Guerrant JR, Walker DH, Weller PF, eds. Tropical Infectious Diseases. 2nd ed. Philadelphia: Elsevier; 2006:903; Laniado-Laborin R. Coccidioidomycosis and endemic mycoses in Mexico. Rev Iberoam Micol. 2007;24:249; Gugnani HC. Histoplasmosis in Africa. Indian J Chest Dis Allied Sci. 2000;42:271.)

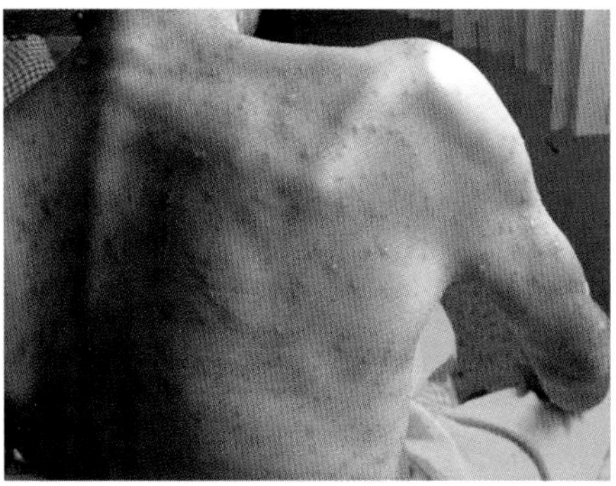

Figure 85.2 Skin lesions in an AIDS patient from Guatemala with disseminated histoplasmosis. Wasting is also apparent.

genetic differences in the fungi.[19] Uncommon presentations include endocarditis, pericarditis, choroiditis, hemophagocytic syndrome, and central nervous system (CNS) mass lesions.[1,20] Laboratory abnormalities include anemia, leukopenia, thrombocytopenia, and elevated liver enzymes and lactate dehydrogenase (LDH). In AIDS patients with pneumonia and high serum LDH levels, histoplasmosis and pneumocystosis are the leading diagnostic considerations.[21]

African histoplasmosis (var. *duboisii*) is characterized by cutaneous ulcers and/or nodules and lytic bone lesions of the axial skeleton and extremities, often with chronic sinus tracts from the bony lesions to the skin.[2] There is no clear correlation between compromised host immune status and infection with var. *duboisii*.[22]

The prognosis is excellent for acute pulmonary disease in the immunocompetent patient. Fibrosing mediastinitis is slowly progressive and often fatal. Acute disseminated disease is usually fatal if untreated. In AIDS patients with histoplasmosis, fungemia, renal insufficiency, older age, dyspnea, thrombocytopenia, and LDH level twice the upper limit of the normal range are associated with death.[23,24] The overall mortality among persons with AIDS and histoplasmosis in the United States is 11–39%, but as high as 50% in HIV patients with fever of unknown origin in Guatemala.[24,25] Delayed recognition and treatment of histoplasmosis accounts for the higher mortality rate in developing countries, especially among patients residing in rural areas with limited access to clinical care. In Guatemala, HIV-infected persons from rural areas often do not seek

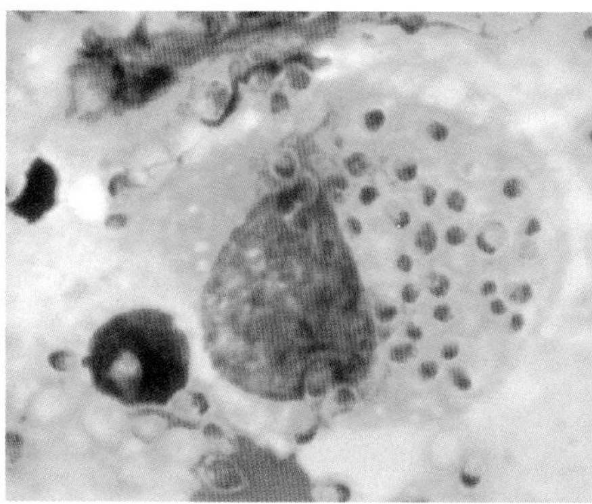

Figure 85.3 Macrophage containing numerous intracellular yeast forms of *Histoplasma capsulatum* var. *capsulatum*. Giemsa stain, ×1000. (From: Pfaller MA, McGinnis MR. The laboratory and clinical mycology. In: Anaissie EJ, McGinnis MR, Pfaller MA, eds. Clinical Mycology. 2nd ed. Elsevier; 2008:55.)

treatment until symptoms render them unable to work.[25] Furthermore, symptoms of disseminated histoplasmosis are nonspecific and similar to those of other opportunistic infections.[26,27]

PATHOGENESIS AND IMMUNITY

Microconidia of *H. capsulatum* are inhaled, reaching the alveolar spaces and transforming into yeasts.[28] Neutrophils and alveolar macrophages engulf the organisms. Yeasts multiply within macrophages, leading to their lysis and infection of new cells.[29] A major determinant of virulence is α-1,3-glucan, which protects the yeast in the macrophage phagolysosome.[30]

CD4 T lymphocytes are crucial to resolving the infection, whereas CD8 lymphocytes are required for optimal fungal eradication.[31–33] In murine models, TNF-α, interferon-γ, granulocyte-macrophage colony-stimulating factor, and interleukin (IL)-1β are necessary to prevent a lethal infection, whereas IL-17 is not.[34]

Following pulmonary infection, organisms spread via lymphatics to regional lymph nodes and hematogenously to other organs. In immunocompetent persons, the pathologic findings resemble tuberculosis, with granulomas occasionally evolving to caseous necrosis. These granulomas heal with fibrosis and may calcify. An immunologic reaction to the fungus is likely responsible for the rheumatologic manifestations associated with the primary infection. Patients with AIDS show minimal inflammatory response, and masses of organisms are commonly found.[17]

DIAGNOSIS

The diagnosis of histoplasmosis based on cultures suffers from low sensitivity and slow growth (2–6 weeks). In disseminated disease, the organism can be recovered from blood, urine, and biopsies of bone marrow, lung, and liver. Isolator blood cultures provide higher yield. Biopsy specimens stained with Gomori methenamine silver (GMS) have high sensitivity and provide a more rapid diagnosis than cultures; however, *Histoplasma* may be difficult to differentiate from *Blastomyces dermatiditis*, *Candida glabrata*, *Cryptococcus neoformans*, *Pneumocystis jirovecii*, *Leishmania*, and artifacts.[35] In overwhelming infection, as occurs in AIDS, demonstration of the organism in the buffy coat by Giemsa stain provides a simple method of diagnosis that is effective in up to 80% of patients (***Fig. 85.3***). Histopathologically in var. *duboisii* infection, the organism has thick, doubly-contoured walls and may show chain formation and "figure-eight" budding.[2]

Serologic techniques, such as immunodiffusion and complement fixation antibody tests (CF), are useful for diagnosis of histoplasmosis in immunocompetent patients and are often still used outside the United States. A CF titer ≥1 : 32 is suggestive of infection. Titers from 1 : 8 to 1 : 16 are less specific, and histopathology or culture may be necessary to establish the diagnosis.[35] Immunodiffusion is less sensitive, detecting antibody later in the infection. These antibodies cross-react with antigens of blastomyces, paracoccidioides, and coccidioides. Also, because antibody titers are usually low in patients with immunosuppression, antibody-based methods have been replaced in the United States by assay for *Histoplasma* antigen.[35] Detection of antigen by enzyme immunoassay in urine is highly sensitive (>85%) and specific in disseminated histoplasmosis in AIDS patients.[35]

Laboratory methods used to detect *H. capsulatum* infections in resource-limited countries are labor-intensive, expensive, and slow, often precluding a timely diagnosis. Reliance on culture and histopathologic methods sometimes delays diagnosis and treatment by weeks. Under these circumstances, persons with AIDS presenting with histoplasmosis may die before the diagnosis is established.

The commercial *Histoplasma* antigen assay is proprietary and thus is generally not available in resource-limited countries. The availability of an inexpensive, rapid method to detect *H. capsulatum* infection in developing countries could dramatically decrease the time to diagnosis and treatment of histoplasmosis. In a study from Guatemala, a simpler antigen-capture enzyme immunoassay demonstrated 81% sensitivity and a 95% specificity for detection of *Histoplasma* antigen in urine.[11]

TREATMENT AND PROGNOSIS

Management guidelines were published in 2007.[36] In severe acute pulmonary histoplasmosis, liposomal amphotericin B (3–5 mg/kg daily for 1–2 weeks), followed by itraconazole (200 mg thrice daily for 3 days, then 200 mg twice daily) is recommended as initial therapy. Amphotericin B (0.7–1 mg/kg daily) is an alternative for patients at low risk for nephrotoxicity or where liposomal amphotericin is not available. Amphotericin B has a response rate of more than 75% in HIV- and non-HIV-infected patients. Methylprednisolone (0.5–1 mg daily) during the first 1–2 weeks of therapy is recommended for patients with significant respiratory distress.[36]

In mild or moderate acute pulmonary histoplasmosis, therapy is usually unnecessary. For symptoms longer than one month, standard doses of itraconazole for 6–12 weeks are recommended. In chronic cavitary pulmonary histoplasmosis, itraconazole (standard doses) for a minimum of one year is the suggested treatment, although 18–24 months of therapy may decrease the risk of relapse.[36]

In rheumatologic syndromes, including pericarditis, nonsteroidal anti-inflammatory drugs may be used. In severe cases, prednisone and itraconazole (standard doses for 6–12 weeks) are used.[36]

In mediastinal lymphadenitis symptomatic for more than one month, itraconazole and prednisone are used. In contrast, in mediastinal fibrosis, antifungal therapy is not recommended. In cases of pulmonary vessel obstruction, intravascular stent placement may be necessary.[36]

In severe progressive disseminated histoplasmosis, liposomal amphotericin B (3 mg/kg daily) is given for 1–2 weeks, followed by oral itraconazole (standard doses) for 12 months.[36] Blood cultures and antigen become negative more rapidly in patients given liposomal amphotericin than itraconazole.[37] Liposomal amphotericin B is also more effective than amphotericin B in treating disseminated disease in AIDS patients (response rate 88% versus 64%; mortality rate 2% versus 13%).[36]

For mild-to-moderate disseminated disease, itraconazole (standard doses) is given for 12 months. Lifelong suppressive therapy is required in patients in which the immunosuppression cannot be reversed or in patients who relapse despite appropriate therapy.[36]

For CNS histoplasmosis, liposomal amphotericin B (5 mg/kg daily; total dose 175 mg/kg) is given over 4–6 weeks, followed by itraconazole (200 mg two to three times daily, with therapeutic drug monitoring) for at least 1 year until resolution of cerebrospinal fluid (CSF) abnormalities.[36] In pregnancy, liposomal amphotericin B is recommended because of azole teratogenicity. Infected infants and children are treated with amphotericin B. Children can also receive itraconazole at 5–10 mg/kg daily; the suspension is preferred.[36]

Serum itraconazole levels should be monitored after steady state is achieved (2 weeks of therapy), with a goal ≥1.0 μg/mL.[36] One problem is that itraconazole levels are decreased by concurrent use of non-nucleoside reverse transcriptase inhibitors.[38] Antigen levels should be measured during and for 12 months after therapy to monitor for relapse.[36] Immune reconstitution inflammatory syndrome, with worsening lung infiltrates and focal lesions, has occurred after initiation of antiretroviral therapy (ART).

For patients unable to take itraconazole, because of intolerance or drug interactions, fluconazole can be used, but it is less effective. Posaconazole and voriconazole have *in vitro* activity against *H. capsulatum*, but clinical data are limited.[36] High-level fluconazole resistance and development of fluconazole resistance and voriconazole cross-resistance while on therapy have been documented.[39,40] Itraconazole can be discontinued after one year of therapy in HIV patients who have achieved immune reconstitution on continuing ART to a CD4 cell count >150/μL with negative blood cultures and urine antigen levels <2 ng/mL.[36] African histoplasmosis is responsive to amphotericin B, ketoconazole, and trimethoprim/sulfamethoxazole.[2]

PREVENTION AND CONTROL

Human-to-human transmission of histoplasmosis does not occur, and there is no vaccine. Prophylaxis with itraconazole (200 mg daily) is recommended in HIV patients with a CD4 cell count <150/μL who reside in endemic areas where the incidence of histoplasmosis is >10 cases per 100 patient-years.[36]

BLASTOMYCOSIS

INTRODUCTION

Blastomycosis is caused by the dimorphic fungus *Blastomyces dermatitidis*, which is found along river basins in the eastern United States, in Canada bordering the Great Lakes and St Lawrence River, and sporadically in Africa, Europe, Asia, and Latin America (***Fig. 85.4***). Blastomycosis presents as acute or chronic pulmonary disease, and may disseminate to skin, bones, prostate, and central nervous system.[41]

THE AGENT

Blastomyces dermatitidis is the asexual stage of *Ajellomyces dermatitidis*. At 25–30°C, fluffy white colonies develop after 1–3 weeks of growth on routine mycological medium. The mould form of *B. dermatitidis* produces 2–10 μm conidia on hyphae and conidiophores. The conidia may be indistinguishable from *H. capsulatum*, having only hyphae, conidiophores, and microconidia. In mammalian tissues, broad-based budding yeasts, 8–30 μm in diameter, with thick refractile walls, are observed. The yeast is also produced *in vitro* at 37°C on blood agar, inhibitory mould agar, or BHI agar.[3]

EPIDEMIOLOGY

Human activities near waterways are risk factors for blastomycosis.[42–44] There are also hyperendemic foci where conditions favor *Blastomyces* growth: sandy, acidic soil, low elevation, and multiple bodies of water.[45] Exposure to soil containing the fungi is associated with large outbreaks.[46] Dogs are susceptible and may act as sentinels in point-source outbreaks.[47]

The prevalence in the North American endemic area is 0.3–1.8 cases per 100 000 persons[41]; however, there are hyperendemic areas, such as the Kenora area of Ontario, with an annual incidence of 117 per 100 000.[48] In the United States, the highest prevalence states are Mississippi, Arkansas, and Kentucky.[49] Diabetes, smoking, and African-American and Amerindian race have been reported as risk factors.[45,50,51]

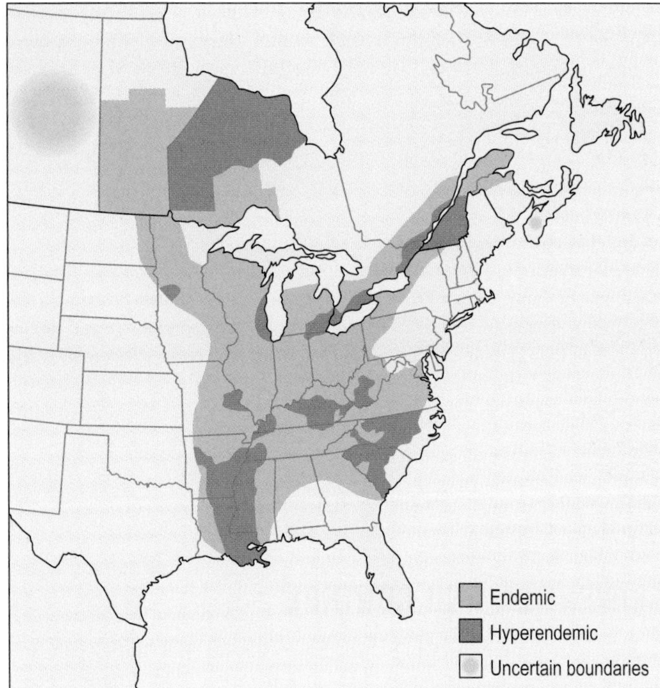

Figure 85.4 Map of the endemic area of blastomycosis in North America. (Adapted from Pappas PG. Blastomycosis. In: Kauffman CA, ed. Atlas of Fungal Infections, 2nd ed, Philadelphia: Current Medicine; 39; Crampton TL, Light RB, Berg GM, et al. Epidemiology and clinical spectrum of blastomycosis diagnosed at Manitoba hospitals. Clin Infect Dis. 2002;34:1310. Reed KD, Meece JK, Archer JR, Peterson AT. Ecological niche modeling of *Blastomyces dermatitidis* in Wisconsin. PloS ONE 2008;3:e2034.)

Southern Africa is the most common area for blastomycosis outside of North America, with most cases reported from Zimbabwe and South Africa; however, blastomycosis is widespread on the continent.[52] The apparent low prevalence in Africa may be a reflection of limited resources to identify the pathogen. The African and North American strains differ in morphology, antigenic structure, and ease of mycelial-yeast conversion.[52]

THE DISEASE

Infection typically occurs by inhalation. Most infections are asymptomatic or mild, and resolve without treatment.[41] Other patients may develop pneumonia over several weeks, associated with lobar or segmental alveolar infiltrates. Resolution may occur over several weeks, or disease may progress to more severe pneumonia, with weight loss, night sweats, sputum production, and chest pain. Patients with miliary disease, diffuse pneumonitis, or ARDS have a mortality of 50–89%.[53]

Chronic pneumonia is the most frequent presentation, with nodular and lobar infiltrates, and often cavitation. Nodular, ulcerative, or verrucous skin lesions are the second most common presentation, occurring in 60% of patients (***Fig. 85.5***).[41] Other sites of dissemination include the bones and genitourinary system, especially the prostate. Typical sites of osseous involvement are the legs and axial skeleton; septic arthritis is less common and usually monoarticular.[51] In spinal blastomycosis, destruction of the disk spaces and anterior vertebral body causes collapse with skipped spinal segments.[51] Less commonly, laryngeal and oropharyngeal nodules, ocular infection, meningitis, and intracerebral abscesses occur.[54] African patients have more frequent bone involvement and chronic skin lesions, but less frequent CNS involvement.[52,55]

In transplant patients or those undergoing chemotherapy, blastomycosis may cause severe pulmonary disease with high mortality.[41] In HIV infection, blastomycosis is uncommon, occurring in patients with a CD4 cell count <200/μL. Diffuse pulmonary disease and CNS involvement are more common in HIV patients. In the pre-ART era, mortality rates

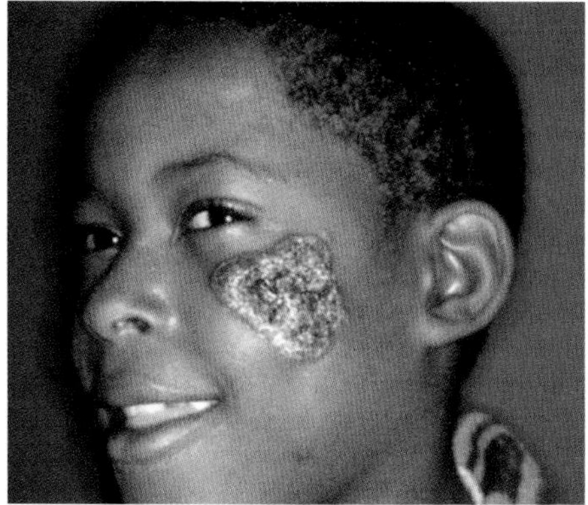

Figure 85.5 Skin lesion in a patient with blastomycosis. (From Raugi GJ. Fungal and yeast infections of the skin, appendages, and subcutaneous tissues. In: Stevens DL, ed. Atlas of Infectious Diseases. Vol. II. Skin, soft tissue, bone and joint infections. Philadelphia: Current Medicine, 1995).

approached 40% in this group, with most deaths occurring within 3 weeks of presentation.[56]

In a Canadian series, the mortality rate of blastomycosis was 6.3%,[57] but in Missouri the rate was 44%.[45] Mortality is strongly influenced by factors that delay diagnosis, such as initial lack of recognition of the disease.[45] Older age and Amerindian race are also risk factors for death.[53]

PATHOGENESIS AND IMMUNITY

The usual route of infection is inhalation of conidia. The organism has also been transmitted sexually and by dog bite.[58,59] In the alveoli, the conidia transform into yeasts and induce an inflammatory response with mixed abscess/granuloma. Alveolar macrophages can inhibit the transition of conidia into yeasts, and neutrophils are also active.[60,61] Yeasts are relatively resistant to phagocytosis and killing.[58]

The BAD1 yeast cell wall protein mediates cellular adhesion and is an indispensable virulence factor and the main target for cellular and humoral immunity. BAD1 suppresses phagocyte release of TNF-α through transforming growth factor-β-dependent and -independent mechanisms.[62] Melanin, another virulence factor, protects the fungus from the leukocyte oxidative burst.[63]

In athymic mice, neutrophils provide an early defense against transition from conidia to yeasts. However, once transition to yeasts has occurred, athymic mice are more susceptible than immunocompetent mice, emphasizing the importance of cell-mediated immunity[64]; the humoral immune response is not significant.[58]

DIAGNOSIS

With its myriad clinical presentations, the diagnosis of blastomycosis is often delayed. In a study from Mississippi, blastomycosis was suspected at the initial evaluation in only 18% of cases.[50] Diagnoses may be made by examination of wet mounts of the sputum digested with potassium hydroxide and by culture. Pulmonary cytology is the most useful diagnostic method; culture is negative in one-third of cases.[49] Histopathology of tissue specimens also provides the diagnosis.[41] On Sabouraud dextrose agar, *B. dermatitidis* grows as mycelia at 25°C after 10–18 days and as yeast at 37°C.

Due to poor sensitivity and specificity (especially cross-reactivity with *Histoplasma*), serologic testing using the complement fixation and immunodiffusion techniques is not useful.[41] Radioimmunoassays and enzyme-linked immunoassays are more sensitive, but are not commercially available.[41] A *B. dermatitidis* antigen assay for urine and serum has a sensitivity of 93%, but cross-reacts with *Histoplasma*. Serial antigen assays permit monitoring the course of infection.[41] In Africa, blastomycosis may be misdiagnosed as tuberculosis or pyogenic infection because of inadequate facilities for identification.[52,55]

TREATMENT AND PROGNOSIS

Management guidelines were published in 2008.[65] For severe pneumonia or disseminated blastomycosis or in immunocompromised patients, amphotericin B (0.7–1 mg/kg daily) or a lipid formulation of amphotericin B (3–5 mg/kg daily) is recommended.[65] After the patient stabilizes, switching to oral itraconazole is appropriate (200 mg three times per day for 3 days, then 200 mg twice a day, for a total of 6–12 months (12 months in disseminated disease)).[65] Lifelong suppressive therapy with itraconazole (200 mg daily) is required when the immunosuppression cannot be reversed or for patients who relapse despite appropriate therapy.

For disease of mild-to-moderate severity, itraconazole can be used as initial therapy, using the doses described for severe disease for 6–12 months. Osteoarticular disease should be treated for 12 months.[65] For CNS blastomycosis, a lipid formulation of amphotericin B (5 mg/kg daily) for 4–6 weeks, followed by oral fluconazole 800 mg daily, itraconazole 200 mg two or three times per day, or voriconazole 200–400 mg twice a day should be given for at least 12 months and until resolution of CSF abnormalities.[65]

During pregnancy, azoles should be avoided, and a lipid formulation of amphotericin B is recommended. For newborns, amphotericin B is the drug of choice (1 mg/kg daily). Children with severe blastomycosis should be treated as above using itraconazole at 10 mg/kg.[65]

For itraconazole treatment, serum levels should be measured after 2 weeks.[65] A serum level ≥500 μg/L is considered appropriate.[66]

Excellent clinical responses (>90%, with few relapses) are achieved with itraconazole at 200 mg/day for 6 months in immunocompetent patients.[67] Amphotericin B affords cure rates of 97% in uncomplicated disease.[41] The efficacy of fluconazole is dose-related; there is a 65% response rate at 200–400 mg/day, and an 87% response rate at 400–800 mg/day.[68]

PREVENTION AND CONTROL

There is no specific avoidable environmental reservoir. Early diagnosis and prompt treatment are key to decrease the morbidity and mortality.

COCCIDIOIDOMYCOSIS

INTRODUCTION

Coccidioidomycosis is caused by dimorphic fungi of the genus *Coccidioides*, *C. immitis* (California isolates) and *C. posadasii* (isolates outside California).[69] There are no differences in disease by these species. *Coccidioides* is endemic to semi-arid to arid zones in the Americas (***Fig. 85.6***).[70] Coccidioidomycosis typically presents as acute or chronic pulmonary disease. The infection may disseminate, with the most common sites of involvement being the skin, bones, and CNS.[71]

THE AGENT

At 25–30°C the fungus grows as a mold and the colonies are usually white. The hyphae are thin, septate, and hyaline. Side branches produce unicellular, barrel-shaped arthroconidia (3–4 × 3–6 μm), alternating with empty disjunctor cells. At 37°C, in tissue or media, the arthroconidia enlarge and develop into spherules (20–60 μm) containing many endospores (2–4 μm) (***Fig. 85.7***).[3]

EPIDEMIOLOGY

Coccidioides occurs naturally only in the Western hemisphere, primarily in the southwestern United States (Arizona; parts of California, New Mexico, Utah, Nevada, and Texas) and northern Mexico (primarily

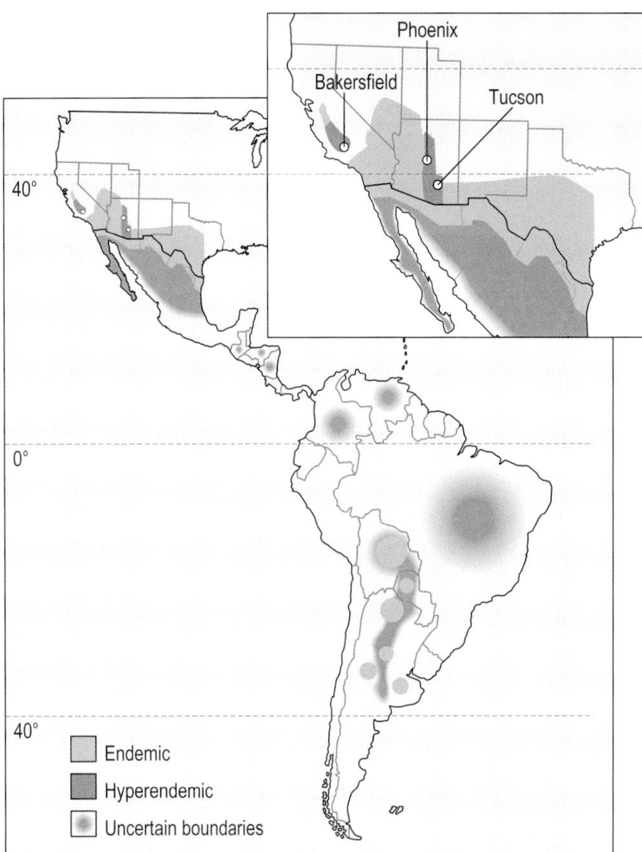

Figure 85.6 Map of endemic range of coccidioidomycosis. (Adapted from: Ampel NM, Einstein HE, Galgiani JN, Pappagianis D. Coccidioidomycosis. In: Kauffman CA, ed. Atlas of Fungal Infections, 2nd edn. Philadelphia: Current Medicine, 2006:23; Laniado-Laborin R. Expanding understanding of epidemiology of coccidioidomycosis in the Western hemisphere. Ann N Y Acad Sci 2007;1111:19.)

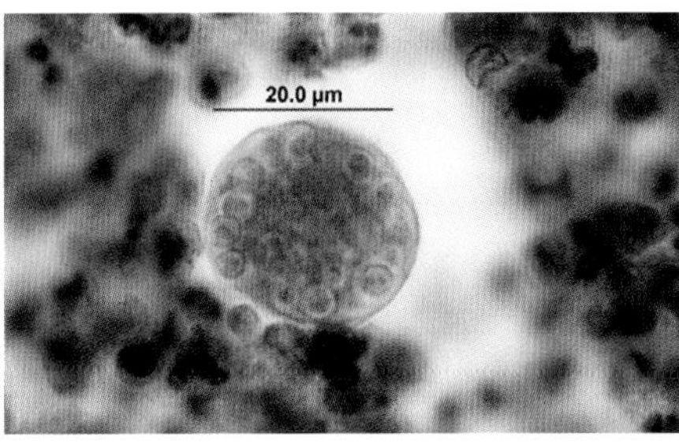

Figure 85.7 Spherule of *Coccidioides* sp., the characteristic tissue form. (From Schnadig VJ, Woods GL. Histopathology of fungal infections. In: Anaissie EJ, McGinnis MR, Pfaller MA, eds. Clinical Mycology, 2nd edn. Elsevier; 2009:79.)

Nuevo León, Coahuila, Sonora, Chihuahua, Baja California; also in Colima, Durango, Guanajuato, Guerrero, Jalisco, Michoacán, Nayarit, San Luis Potosí, Sinaloa, Tamaulipas, and Zacatecas).[72,73] The endemic areas have arid to semi-arid climates, hot summers, low altitude, alkaline soil, and sparse flora. Hyperendemic areas include Kern, Tulare, and Fresno counties in California and Pima, Pinal, and Maricopa counties in Arizona.[70] *Coccidioides* also occurs in Guatemala, Honduras, Nicaragua, Argentina, Bolivia, Paraguay, Venezuela, Brazil, and Colombia.[72,73] In the United States, an estimated 150 000 cases occur annually.[74]

Cycles of rain and drought enhance dispersal of the organism because rains facilitate its growth in soil, and subsequent drought conditions favor aerosolization of arthroconidia.[70] An increase in American cases occurred in the 1980s and 1990s because of the AIDS epidemic.[6,75] California experienced a second rise in incidence from 2000 to 2007, increasing from 2.4 to 7.4/100 000, with 76% of the 16 970 cases occurring in the San Joaquin Valley.[76] Rates in Arizona also increased dramatically, from

7/100 000 in 1990 to 75/100 000 in 2007.[77] Factors responsible for the increase are the influx of older, nonimmune persons with comorbidities, heightened awareness of the disease, climatic changes, and soil disruption due to construction.[76,77]

Knowledge of the epidemiology in Latin America is based primarily on skin test surveys indicating fungal exposure. Surveys performed in northern Mexico have rates of 10–93%.[73] Data on rates of clinical coccidioidomycosis are sparse. From 1978 to 1988, hospitals in Monterrey, Mexico, reported 150 cases; 111 of these were from Nuevo León.[78] In Central America, 21% and 25% of skin-tested subjects in the Motagua River Valley of Guatemala and the Comayagua Valley of Honduras, respectively, were reactive.[73]

In South America, there is a focus in the semi-arid Gran Chaco region of Bolivia, Paraguay, and northern Argentina. In Argentina, skin test positivity rates of 19%, 16%, and 14.8% were observed in the provinces of Santiago del Estero, Catamarca, and San Luis, respectively.[73] Coccidioidomycosis is also endemic in Paraguay (Boqueron and Olimpo departments), Brazil (Bahia, Ceará, Piauí, and Maranhão states), and Venezuela (Falcon, Lara, and Zulia states).[73]

Outbreaks follow events that result in atmospheric soil dispersion, such as dust storms, earthquakes, and droughts.[71,79,80] Persons with soil exposure are at the greatest risk.[81,82] In Brazil, armadillo hunting is a risk factor.[80] Immunocompromised persons are at high risk, including patients with AIDS, transplant recipients (especially those who receive *Coccidioides*-infected organs), persons treated with TNF-α antagonists, cancer patients, and pregnant women.[73] However, maternofetal transmission is rare.[83] Persons of Filipino or African-American descent and those with blood group B are at high risk to suffer disseminated disease.[81,84]

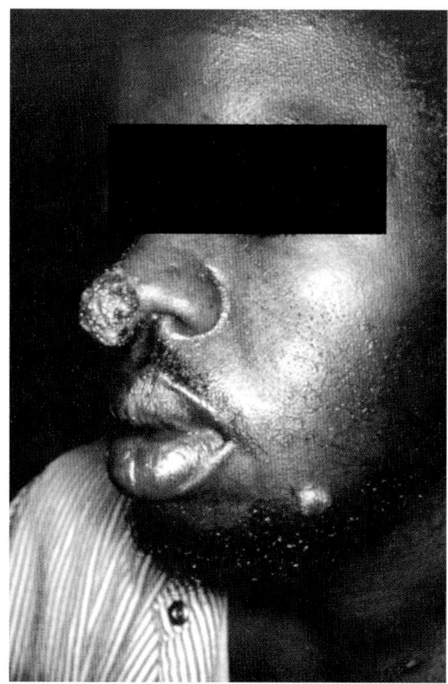

Figure 85.8 Verrucous skin lesions on the face of a patient with coccidioidomycosis.

THE DISEASE

Coccidioidomycosis is asymptomatic in 60% of infected individuals, who are detected only by a positive skin test. In the remaining 40%, a flu-like illness, with dry cough, pleuritic chest pain, myalgias, arthralgia, fever, sweats, anorexia, and fatigue, develops 1–3 weeks after exposure. Primary infection may be accompanied by immune complex-mediated complications, including arthralgias, macular rash, erythema multiforme, or erythema nodosum. Acute infection usually resolves spontaneously, although symptoms may persist for weeks. In 5% of these patients, asymptomatic pulmonary residua persist, including pulmonary nodules and cavitation. Immunocompromised patients are more prone to develop chronic progressive pulmonary infection, with thin-walled cavities that may rupture causing bronchopleural fistula and empyema.[71,85,86]

Symptomatic extrapulmonary disease develops in 1 in 200 patients and can involve the skin, soft tissues, bones, joints, and meninges. The most common cutaneous lesions are verrucous papules or plaques (***Fig. 85.8***). The spine is the most frequent site of osseous dissemination, although lytic lesions also occur in the skull, hands, feet, and tibia. Joint involvement is usually monoarticular, involving the ankle or knee.[71,85,86] *Coccidioides* fungemia, often fatal, occurs in immunocompromised patients.[87] In coccidioidal meningitis, the basilar meninges are usually affected. CSF findings include monocytic pleocytosis (often with eosinophilia), hypoglycorrhachia, and elevated protein levels.[88] The mortality is >90% at one year without therapy, and chronic infection is common.[89] The presence of hydrocephalus, with or without infarction, is associated with a higher mortality rate.[90]

Coccidioidomycosis is a "great imitator," with presentations including immune thrombocytopenia, massive cervical lymphadenopathy, laryngeal or retropharyngeal abscess, endocarditis, pericarditis, peritonitis, hepatitis, and urogenital involvement.[86]

PATHOGENESIS AND IMMUNITY

The usual route of entry of *Coccidioides* arthroconidia is inhalation, although cutaneous inoculation also occurs.[91] In tissue, the arthroconidia germinate to produce spherules, which rupture and release endospores that form new spherules.[92] Neutrophils and macrophages surround these spherules, and form granulomas. Spherule size may inhibit effective phagocytosis.[93] Dendritic cells phagocytose the spherules via mannose receptors, and present antigen.[94] Both B and T lymphocytes are essential host defenses against this pathogen, suggesting that a balanced Th1/Th2 response is necessary for protective immunity.[93]

The resistance of arthroconidia, endospores, and spherules to phagocytosis is mediated by components of the outer cell wall, such as spherule outer wall glycoprotein (SOWgp).[92,93] SOWgp promotes a Th2-biased immune response, thereby compromising cell-mediated immune pathways.[93]

Other virulence factors include melanin, which protects *Coccidioides* from the leukocyte oxidative burst,[63] and extracellular urease, which generates an alkaline microenvironment that impairs granuloma formation.[95] Pulmonary infection with *Coccidioides* alters surfactant production, which may promote disease progression.[96]

DIAGNOSIS

Residence in or travel to endemic areas provides an important clue to the diagnosis, which may be delayed in travelers to endemic areas because physicians lack familiarity with this mycosis.[5]

Diagnosis may be achieved by direct microscopic demonstration of the fungus by staining of tissue or wet mounts of sputa or exudates processed with potassium hydroxide or calcofluor (***Fig. 85.7***). The observation of spherules with endospores is pathognomonic. However, mycelia may also be found in cytologic and histologic specimens.[97]

Unlike *H. capsulatum* and *B. dermatitidis*, *Coccidioides* grows rapidly (usually in 3–5 days). Sporulation may be observed after 5–10 days. Clinicians should notify the laboratory when coccidioidomycosis is suspected to ensure proper biosafety practices (manipulation in a biological safety cabinet).[71] Definitive identification is established by DNA probe or exoantigen testing.[71]

Serological testing is useful in establishing the diagnosis and in monitoring the course of disease. Serological tests demonstrate antibodies in up to 90% of cases of coccidioidomycosis, but the sensitivity is lower in patients with AIDS.[35] Antibodies may be undetectable during the first 3 months after acute infection.[35] IgM antibodies may be present soon after infection or relapse, but subsequently wane, and the titer does not correlate with severity.[35]

IgG antibody appears later and persists for months. IgG antibodies fix complement when combined with coccidioidal antigen and can be detected by immunodiffusion (the IDCF assay). Increasing IgG titers are associated with progressive disease, whereas declining titers are associated with resolution. IDCF titers ≥1 : 16 indicate increased likelihood of disseminated coccidioidomycosis. Detection of antibodies by IDCF in the CSF is diagnostic of meningitis; serology is much more sensitive than culture.[35]

The enzyme-linked immunoassay is no more sensitive than immunodiffusion, and is less specific. The results correlate poorly with complement fixation titers and do not reflect prognosis.[35] A *Coccidioides* urinary antigen assay has a sensitivity of 71% in moderate-to-severe disease, versus 87% for culture.[98] Patients with acute coccidioidomycosis may have a false positive *Histoplasma* urinary antigen test.[99]

TREATMENT AND PROGNOSIS

Guidelines for management were published in 2005.[100] In most patients, primary pulmonary infection resolves without treatment. However, all patients require observation for at least 2 years to document resolution of infection and to promptly identify complications. For patients with risk factors for disseminated disease, treatment is necessary. Other indications for treatment are severe disease (infiltrates involving both lungs, greater than half of one lung, or hilar or mediastinal lymphadenopathy; CF titers >1 : 16; highly symptomatic disease (weight loss >10%; night sweats for more than 3 weeks, symptoms longer than 2 months)). For diffuse or severe pneumonia, therapy with amphotericin B, 0.5–1.5 mg/kg daily, or a lipid formulation of amphotericin B (2–5 mg/kg daily), should be given for several weeks, followed by an oral azole (itraconazole (200 mg twice a day) or fluconazole (400–800 mg per day)). The total duration of therapy should be at least one year; for immunosuppressed patients, oral azoles should be maintained as secondary prophylaxis. In HIV patients whose CD4 counts have risen above 250 cells/μL who had focal pneumonia that responded to azoles, antifungals may be discontinued. Azole therapy may be used initially for less severe disease. During pregnancy, amphotericin B is preferred because of azole teratogenicity.[100]

An asymptomatic patient with a solitary nodule or pulmonary cavitation due to *Coccidioides* does not require antifungal therapy or resection. However, the development of complications due to the cavitation, such as hemoptysis or bacterial or fungal superinfection, necessitates initiation of azole therapy. Cavity resection (particularly if >5 cm in diameter) is an alternative. Rupture of a cavity into the pleural space requires closure by lobectomy with decortication, in addition to antifungals. For chronic pneumonia, the initial treatment should be an oral azole for at least one year. If disease persists, one may switch to another azole, increase the dose if fluconazole was initially selected, or switch to amphotericin B.[100]

The treatment of disseminated infection without CNS involvement employs azoles, such as itraconazole or fluconazole (400 mg per day). If there is little improvement or vertebral involvement, treatment with amphotericin B is recommended (dosage as for diffuse pneumonia). Surgical débridement or stabilization of the spine is a critical component of therapy. In patients who have failed fluconazole, itraconazole, and amphotericin B, treatment with posaconazole (200 mg four times per day or 400 mg twice daily) has been successful.[101]

For coccidioidal meningitis, lifetime treatment with azoles is indicated. Fluconazole, at doses of 800 mg or greater per day, is recommended, affording responses in 79%.[102,103] There are a few reports of successful treatment of meningitis with voriconazole (200 mg orally twice daily after loading dose).[104] Itraconazole is not recommended because of its irregular oral absorption. Obstructive hydrocephalus requires shunting. Intrathecal amphotericin B is typically reserved for meningeal coccidioidomycosis refractory to high-dose azoles.[102]

Itraconazole and fluconazole, both given at 400 mg per day for up to 2 years, produce 57% and 65% response rates, respectively.[105,106] A study comparing oral fluconazole (400 mg/day) to itraconazole (200 mg twice a day) for non-meningeal coccidioidomycosis found equivalency; however, itraconazole showed superior efficacy in skeletal infections.[107] In all patients with disseminated coccidioidomycosis, treatment should be prolonged as much as several years after resolution of lesions. Prolonged post-treatment surveillance is recommended.

In a study from California, the mortality rate of non-HIV-infected patients hospitalized for coccidioidomycosis was 8.2%, whereas for HIV patients the rate was 24%.[108] Thus, coccidioidomycosis can be very difficult to treat because underlying host factors are so important in determining prognosis.

PREVENTION AND CONTROL

Among the endemic mycoses, coccidioidomycosis has generated the most interest in the development of a vaccine, because prior infection engenders immunity and the disease exists in a well-defined zone with a growing population.[109] Many vaccine candidates have been proposed, but no vaccine is commercially available.[109,110]

Azole prophylaxis should be considered for transplant recipients with a history of coccidioidomycosis or a positive serology or those who received organs from a donor with a history of coccidioidomycosis. The risk to transplant recipients visiting or relocating to an endemic area is low, and prophylaxis is not recommended.[111] For workers with soil exposure in endemic areas, there are guidelines to decrease risk.[72]

CRYPTOCOCCOSIS

INTRODUCTION

Cryptococcosis, primarily caused by infection with *Cryptococcus neoformans*, has a worldwide distribution and can infect both immunocompetent and immunocompromised hosts. In recent decades, emergence as an important opportunistic pathogen in immunocompromised hosts worldwide is a result of the HIV pandemic and immunosuppressive treatment of cancer or organ transplantation. Since the introduction of antiretroviral therapy (ART) for HIV, the incidence has declined substantially in North America and Western Europe.[112,113] At the same time, in sub-Saharan Africa, due to high HIV prevalence and inadequate access to ART, *C. neoformans* has become the most common cause of meningitis.[114,115]

THE AGENT

Cryptococci are the only encapsulated fungi, spherical yeast cells that reproduce by budding and are ubiquitous in soil and avian guano. *Cryptococcus neoformans* can transform into a mycelial form (*Filobasidiella neoformans*) and mate sexually. Two species, *Cryptococcus neoformans* (serotypes A, D, and AD) and *Cryptococcus gattii* (serotypes B and C; mycelial form: *F. bacillispora*) are important human pathogens.[116]

EPIDEMIOLOGY

The Centers for Disease Control and Prevention (CDC) estimates that nearly 1 million cases of cryptococcal meningitis occur globally each year, resulting in over 600 000 deaths by 3 months after infection. Approximately 70% of cases and 80% of the deaths occur in sub-Saharan Africa, where cryptococcal meningitis is the fourth most common infectious cause of death.[117] Cryptococcal meningitis is also a major opportunistic infection in HIV patients in Thailand, India, and Brazil.[118–120]

C. gattii was previously thought to be confined to tropical regions, Australia in particular, where it is associated with the tree *Eucalyptus camaldulensis*.[121] Since 1999, *C. gattii* has been responsible for a large epidemic of cryptococcosis among mostly immunocompetent individuals in the Pacific northwest of North America.[122] *C. gattii* (serotype C) was also reported to cause 13–14% of cryptococcal infections in AIDS patients in Botswana and Malawi as well as occurring in California, Thailand, Brazil, Mexico, and Colombia.[123]

THE DISEASE

In immunocompromised patients, the organism causes pneumonia and/or disseminates to the meninges, skin, and bones. Primary cryptococcal pneumonia has been very well described in immunocompetent as well as in immunocompromised persons. In immunocompetent hosts, pulmonary infection is usually mild with productive cough, pleuritic chest pain, and fever. Chest radiographs show single or multiple lung nodules, mediastinal lymphadenopathy, and occasionally pleural effusion. Dissemination is rare.[124] However, in the immunocompromised patient, cryptococcal pneumonia is more severe, with prominent alveolar and interstitial infiltrates; moreover, nodules and cavitation may occur.[125] In these patients, dissemination to the CNS is frequent, especially in those with AIDS.[116]

Meningitis is the most frequent presentation of cryptococcosis in the immunocompromised host and occurs almost exclusively in this population. Typically, cryptococcal meningitis is subacute, with progressive headache, fever, lethargy, personality changes, or memory loss. Signs of meningeal irritation are usually absent.[126] Blindness and deafness are possible presentations or sequelae.[116,127,128] Skin involvement takes the form of papules, acneiform rash, cellulitis, abscesses, ulcers, molluscum contagiosum-like lesions, vesicles, and nodules, and usually indicates disseminated disease (***Figs 85.9 and 85.10***).[126] Bone, eye, and prostate gland are other potential sites of involvement.[116] *C. gattii* infection occurs primarily in immunocompetent persons, and has an increased propensity to form cryptococcomas in the brain and lungs. It produces greater neurologic morbidity and is less responsive to treatment than *C. neoformans*.[129]

PATHOGENESIS AND IMMUNITY

Strain virulence, inoculum size, and host immunocompetence determine the likelihood of developing clinical disease after exposure to *C. neoformans*. In the Bronx, New York, serological testing indicates that 70% of children have been exposed to the fungus, though few suffer symptomatic disease.[130] Defective cell-mediated immunity is the major risk factor for cryptococcosis. Impaired phagocytosis, opsonization, and complement activity are also contributors.[131]

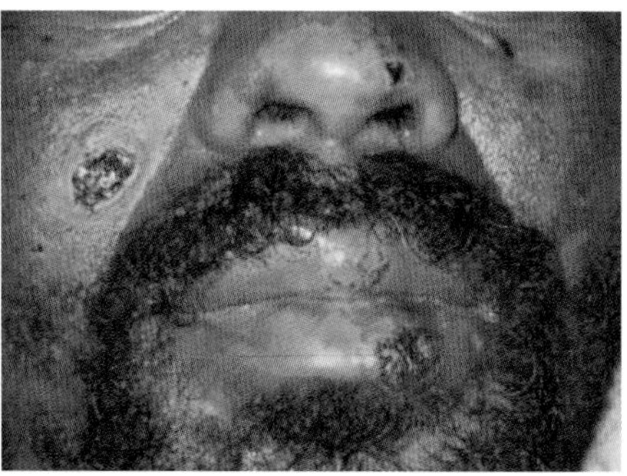

Figure 85.9 Crusted skin lesions in an HIV patient with cryptococcosis.

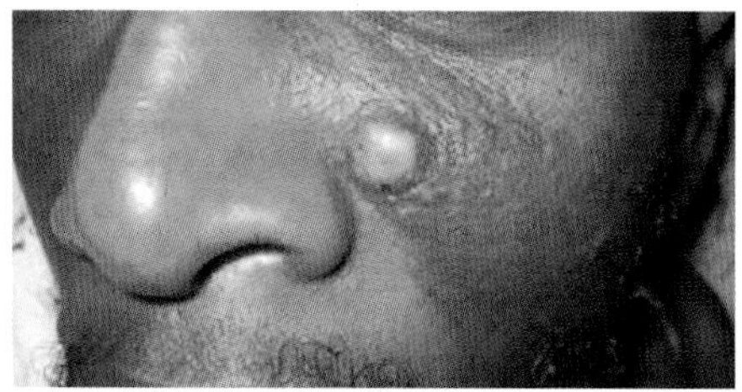

Figure 85.10 Papular skin lesion in an HIV patient with cryptococcosis.

Cryptococci are inhaled and, in most persons, are contained and killed by neutrophils and alveolar macrophages. An effective immune response to *C. neoformans* in murine models includes IL-12 and IL-18 acting synergistically to stimulate early interferon-γ production by natural killer (NK) cells and gamma delta T cells, which stimulates macrophage killing of intracellular cryptococci, decreasing fungal burden in lung and brain[132] associated with Th1-type immune response[133] and granuloma formation.[134] Humoral immunity also contributes to host defense against *Cryptococcus*, by providing opsonins for effective phagocytosis, enhanced NK cell function, and reactivity with capsular polysaccharides.[134] Under conditions of deficient cell-mediated immunity, there is defective granuloma formation, decreased numbers of intracellular yeasts, and the presence of extracellular fungi.[134]

The most important virulence factor of *C. neoformans* is its polysaccharide capsule. The principal capsular component, glucuronoxylomannan, displays immunomodulatory activities, including reduction of neutrophil anticryptococcal activity, induction of monocyte IL-10 production, and disruption of dendritic cell maturation and activation.[135] *C. neoformans* produces melanin from phenolic substrates in the brain, which protects the fungus from phagocytosis, reactive nitrogen and oxygen species, and amphotericin B.[136] Superoxide dismutase and thiol peroxidase protect the fungus from host-derived oxidants.[137,138] *C. neoformans* also displays phenotypic switching, whereby colonial variants differ in morphology and capsular characteristics, facilitating evasion of the immune response.[139]

DIAGNOSIS

Demonstration of cryptococci in tissue or normally sterile body fluids by microscopy and culture is diagnostic. In histopathologic specimens, GMS stain demonstrates the yeast nonspecifically, while the mucicarmine stain is specific for the capsule.

In cryptococcal meningitis, the CSF leukocyte count ranges from normal to markedly elevated, with predominance of lymphocytes. CSF protein is usually mildly elevated (0.5–1 g/L), and CSF glucose may be low. In HIV patients, all these parameters can be normal. The India ink or nigrosin stains are simple to perform and demonstrate the encapsulated yeast in CSF with a sensitivity of 50–80%.[134]

Detection of the capsular polysaccharide antigen in serum and CSF has a sensitivity and specificity >90%, equivalent for both the latex agglutination test and enzyme immunoassay methods.[116] A titer of ≥1 : 8 in serum is indicative of active disease, and if detected in CSF, makes the diagnosis of cryptococcal meningitis highly likely. In asymptomatic HIV-infected patients, serum antigenemia identifies early cryptococcal disease, necessitating CSF examination and treatment.[140] High initial CSF titers (≥1 : 1024) correlate with a high fungal burden, and indicate a poor prognosis.[141] CSF antigen titers fall with successful treatment, but are of little value in management as they remain elevated for months after successful treatment.[142]

C. neoformans grows well on Sabouraud agar and routine media with white- to cream-colored colonies developing in 36–72 hours. Standard automated blood culture systems will detect cryptococcemia. Serotyping is performed using monoclonal antibodies.[116]

TREATMENT AND PROGNOSIS

Treatment guidelines were revised in 2010.[143] For CNS disease, an induction/consolidation/maintenance approach is used. Induction therapy is amphotericin B (0.7–1 mg/kg daily) plus 5-flucytosine (5-FC, 25 mg/kg every 6 hours) for 2 weeks in HIV coinfection and 4–6 weeks in non-HIV patients.[143,144] The addition of 5-FC to amphotericin B results in faster fungal clearance, is an independent predictor of treatment success at 3 months, and leads to a lower incidence of relapse.[145,146] Induction is followed by an 8-week consolidation using fluconazole (400 mg/day; alternative: itraconazole 400 mg/day) and subsequently maintenance therapy with fluconazole 200 mg/day for 6–12 months (non-HIV) or, in HIV, until persistent immune reconstitution on ART (CD4 count >100 cells/μL and suppression of HIV viral load for ≥3 months).[143]

Cryptococcomas are more resistant to therapy and may require prolonged induction (4–6 weeks) and maintenance therapy (up to 18 months). Surgery may be considered for large lesions not responding to antifungal therapy.[143]

For treatment of mild or moderate pulmonary disease, fluconazole 400 mg/day for 6–12 months is sufficient in non-HIV patients, or until immune restoration in HIV patients. Severe disease (diffuse infiltrates, ARDS, evidence of dissemination) has high mortality and should be treated as for meningoencephalitis. Patients with serum antigenemia only and no CSF antigen can be treated with fluconazole 400 mg/day until immune restoration.[143]

Amphotericin B is nephrotoxic and may cause anemia, and 5-FC is myelosuppressive. Pre-treatment with normal saline decreases amphotericin B nephrotoxicity. Liposomal amphotericin B (dose 3–6 mg/kg daily IV) is less nephrotoxic and may be substituted for amphotericin B among patients with or predisposed to renal dysfunction.[147]

5-FC is not available in many countries. Suitable alternatives are amphotericin B monotherapy at 1 mg/kg daily,[148] or in combination with fluconazole (800 mg/day).[149] For remote hospitals in developing countries where amphotericin B cannot be safely administered or monitored, the best oral regimen is high dose fluconazole (800–1200 mg/day), combined with 5-FC.[150]

Voriconazole and posaconazole have good *in vitro* activity against *C. neoformans*. Voriconazole has excellent CSF penetration. Both azoles have only been evaluated in salvage settings[151,152] and are acceptable alternatives in case of fluconazole intolerance, toxicity, or treatment failure, although interactions with antitubercular and antiretroviral drugs warrant caution.

Elevated CSF opening pressure (>25 cmH_2O) occurs in more than 50% of cases of HIV-associated cryptococcal meningitis and is associated with increased neurologic morbidity and short-term mortality.[153] Management consists of daily lumbar puncture for patients with elevated opening pressure, with removal of sufficient CSF (up to 20–30 mL) to reduce opening pressures by 50% or to <20 cmH_2O, continued until opening pressure has normalized.[143,154] For cases of persistently elevated and symptomatic CSF pressure, CSF diversion using a temporary lumbar drain, or permanent shunting, is recommended.[143] Corticosteroids and acetazolamide are discouraged.[153,155]

In HIV-infected patients, rapid rise in CD4 count and fall in HIV viral load within days to months from start of ART may lead to cryptococcal immune reconstitution inflammatory syndrome (IRIS) in up to 30% of patients, manifesting most commonly as CNS symptoms or signs.[156,157] There are two forms: (1) "unmasking" IRIS in patients with subclinical previously undiagnosed cryptococcal disease, with first appearance of symptoms after the start of ART and *Cryptococcus* cultured from CSF; and (2) "paradoxical" IRIS in patients previously diagnosed and treated for cryptococcal infection, with recurrence of symptoms after initiation of ART and usually with negative cultures.[157,158] IRIS is a diagnosis of exclusion for which there is no diagnostic test, and must be distinguished from treatment failure or alternative infections. ART and antifungal therapy should be continued, with corticosteroids for patients with severe or progressive manifestations.

In patients presenting with symptomatic relapse and positive cultures, fluconazole resistance (minimum inhibitory concentration ≥16 μg/mL) may be a factor. Resistance is rare in the United States, but has been reported in some developing countries following fluconazole monotherapy.[159] Weekly amphotericin B at 1 mg/kg daily is an alternative, though inferior, maintenance regimen.[160] Fluconazole-resistant strains may remain sensitive to voriconazole or posaconazole.[161]

The most important indicators of poor prognosis in HIV-associated cryptococcal meningitis are abnormal mental status (confusion, seizures, or depressed level of consciousness) and high fungal burden at the time of diagnosis.[145] Elevated CSF opening pressures and low CSF leukocyte counts are also associated with poor outcome. Although the 10-week mortality rate, even with access to ART, remains 25–50%,[162,163] the long-term prognosis for patients surviving to 6 months on ART is good.[148]

PREVENTION AND CONTROL

There are no vaccines for cryptococcosis. *C. neoformans* is widely distributed in nature, making it difficult to prevent contact with it. Human-to-human transmission does not occur, except from organ transplantation, and rare cases of nosocomial and maternofetal transmission.[116] Transmission from pet psittacine birds has been reported.[164] Thus, it may be prudent to advise immunocompromised patients to avoid birds and their guano.

Fluconazole at 200 mg/day is effective for primary prophylaxis against cryptococcal meningitis in AIDS patients,[165] but was prohibitively expensive. Recent reductions in the cost of fluconazole mandate a reconsideration of targeted fluconazole prophylaxis in areas, such as sub-Saharan Africa, where asymptomatic cryptococcal antigenemia before the start of ART is very common.[166]

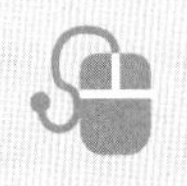

Access the complete reference list online at
http://www.expertconsult.com

CHAPTER 86

Access the complete reference list online at http://www.expertconsult.com

Paracoccidioidomycosis

Ricardo Negroni • Gregory M. Anstead • John R. Graybill

INTRODUCTION

Paracoccidioidomycosis (South American blastomycosis) is a systemic mycosis endemic to the moist tropics of Latin America, caused by the fungus *Paracoccidioides brasiliensis.* Paracoccidioidomycosis takes one of two general forms: acute (juvenile) form or the chronic (adult) form. The juvenile form (occurring in children and immunocompromised patients) is characterized by dissemination to multiple sites, predominantly in the reticuloendothelial system. In the adult form, progressive pulmonary lesions are the hallmark, although lymphadenopathy, hepatosplenomegaly, and cutaneous and mucosal lesions may occur.[1]

THE AGENT

P. brasiliensis is a multinucleated, dimorphic fungus that grows as a yeast in host tissue and culture at 37°C and as a mold in culture at lower temperature.[1–3] Soft, wrinkled, cream-colored colonies of the yeast appear after 1 week of incubation in brain heart infusion (BHI) agar at 37°C. The yeasts are spherical, 20–40 μm in diameter, with thick, double, refractile walls, and several buds resembling a "pilot wheel" (***Fig. 86.1***).[1–3]

At 19–28°C, *P. brasiliensis* grows as a mold; cottony colonies are seen after 3–4 weeks of incubation. Microscopic examination reveals branched, septate, hyaline hyphae 2–3 μm in diameter with intercalated or terminal chlamydoconidiae.[1,4]

P. brasiliensis isolates exhibit significant genetic variability, and there may be a correlation between genotype and geographical isolation, drug resistance, and virulence. Based on recent genetic analyses, the genus *Paracoccidioides* contains two divergent groups: the Pb01-like cluster and the S1/PS2/PS3 clade; for Pb01-like isolates (found in the Brazilian states of Mato Grasso and Goiás) separation into a new species has been proposed, *P. lutzii.*[5]

EPIDEMIOLOGY

Paracoccidioidomycosis occurs from southern Mexico to northern Argentina and Uruguay.[1] The disease is most common in Brazil, followed by Colombia, Venezuela, Argentina, Ecuador, and Paraguay (***Fig. 86.2***).[1] The climate of the endemic area is humid, and the average annual temperature ranges from 17 to 24°C.[4] The environmental niche of *P. brasiliensis* is not well defined; it has been isolated from soil, bat, and penguin feces, and dog food, but these isolations could not be repeated.[6,7]

Most people living in the endemic area acquire the infection at an early age.[2,4] The majority of these infections are asymptomatic and can be detected only by the paracoccidioidin skin test. Because of the long latency period (about 15 years), infection may be acquired in a locality different from where the patient presents.

An estimated 10 million persons in Latin America are infected with *P. brasiliensis*, 2% of whom will develop progressive disease.[8] However, exact rates of progressive paracoccidioidomycosis are not known.[1–4,9] More than 250 new cases are registered each year; 80% are from Brazil.[1,2,4] Agricultural occupation, rural residency, low income, smoking, and alcoholism are all predisposing factors.[1–3]

The chronic form of paracoccidioidomycosis is most commonly observed in 30- to 60-year-old persons.[1,4] The male : female ratio varies between 14 : 1 and 70 : 1.[1] Children represent only 3–5% of the cases, with no difference in incidence between the sexes.[1,4,9] Host genetics, including tumor necrosis factor-α and interleukin (IL)-10 gene polymorphisms and specific HLA alleles, influence susceptibility.[10,11]

THE DISEASE

The acute form (juvenile type) of paracoccidioidomycosis occurs in children or young patients of both sexes. It presents acutely or subacutely, with fever, asthenia, anorexia, weight loss, eosinophilia, and anemia. Adrenomegaly, hepatosplenomegaly, skin nodules, and cold subcutaneous abscesses are frequently detected. Small, ulcerated skin papules and scrofuloderma of the neck and upper chest are also observed (***Fig. 86.3***). Mucosal lesions are rarely present. Although *P. brasiliensis* may be found in the sputum, chest radiographs are often normal.[1]

Intra-abdominal lymphadenopathy and gastrointestinal ulceration occur in severe cases. Diarrhea, abdominal pain, weight loss, and malabsorption with steatorrhea are frequently observed. Jaundice is rare, but may be produced by granulomatous hepatitis or obstruction of the common bile duct by lymphadenopathy. Bony involvement manifests as subacute osteomyelitis.[1,4]

The chronic progressive form (adult type) of paracoccidioidomycosis presents primarily in men >30 years old. In 20–30% of patients, only pulmonary disease is seen.[1,9] Signs and symptoms include anorexia, weight loss, asthenia, productive cough, hemoptysis, dyspnea, thoracic pain, and low-grade fever.[1] Radiologic findings include symmetric bihilar lesions, small nodules, infiltrates, and linear interstitial shadows (***Fig. 86.4***).[1,12] Hilar lymphadenopathy, mass lesions, and pulmonary cavitation may be visualized by computed tomography.[12]

More than 70% of cases of chronic progressive paracoccidioidomycosis develop multifocal lesions beginning with mucocutaneous or pulmonary involvement. Lesions often occur on the oropharyngeal mucosa and consist of ulcers with a granulomatous base, microabscesses, and punctate hemorrhages. Ulcerative gingivitis, partial uvular amputation, tooth loss, and ulcers of the tongue (***Fig. 86.5***), lips, gums, and palate are common findings. Indurated violaceous infiltration of the lips is a very characteristic lesion of this clinical form. Laryngeal involvement may cause dysphonia, dyspnea, and dysphagia.[1]

Nodular or papular lesions often occur near the mouth or nostrils. These ulcerate after some months with a fungating base.[1,4] On the limbs,

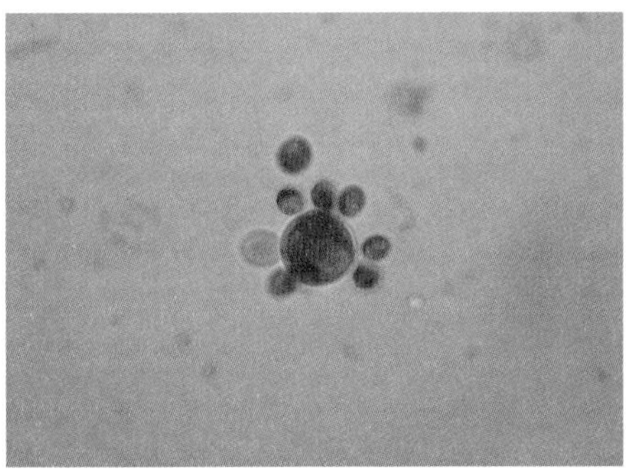

Figure 86.1 Yeast-like form of *Paracoccidioides brasiliensis* showing several peripheral buds (the pilot wheel), culture incubated at 37°C, lactophenol cotton-blue, ×400.

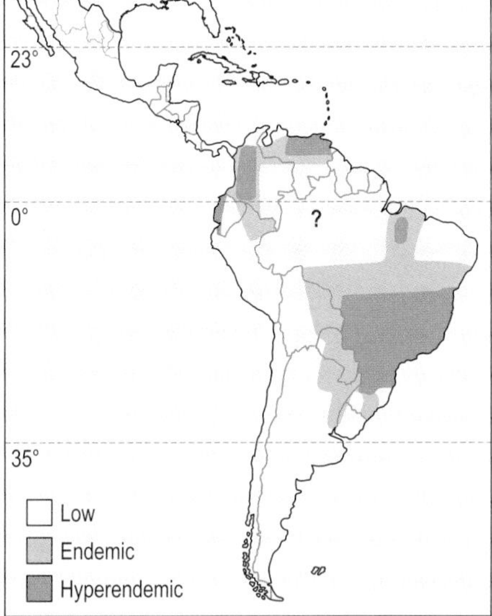

Figure 86.2 Map of endemic area for paracoccidioidomycosis. (Adapted from Graybill JR, Anstead GM, Quieroz-Telles F. Diagnosis of endemic mycoses. In: Maertens J, Marr K, eds. Diagnosis of Fungal Infections. New York: Informa Healthcare, 2007:291–354; and data in Laniado-Laborín R. Coccidioidomycosis and endemic mycoses in Mexico. Rev Iberoam Micol. 2007;24:249.)

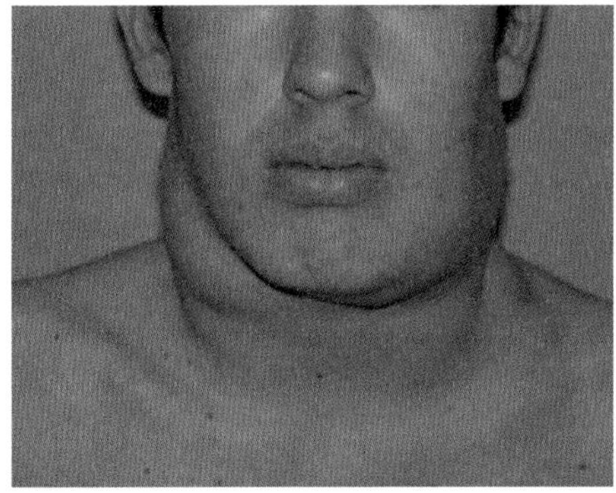

Figure 86.3 Subacute disseminated paracoccidioidomycosis in a 17-year-old male, showing bulky lymphadenopathy of the neck.

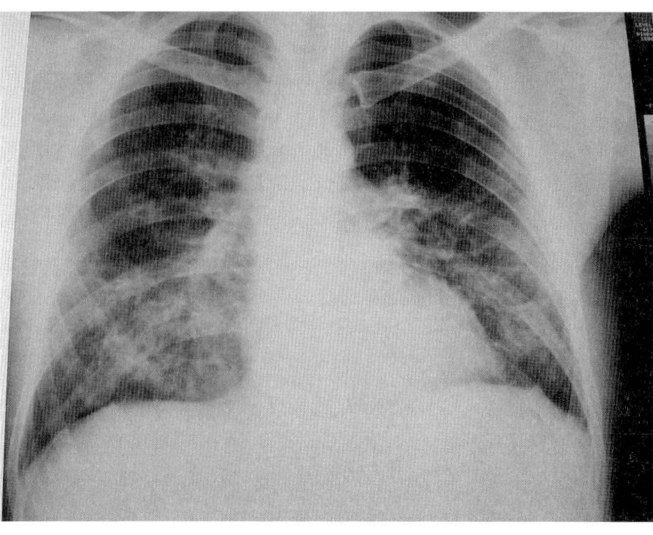

Figure 86.4 Chest radiograph showing bilateral interstitial infiltrates in a patient with paracoccidioidomycosis.

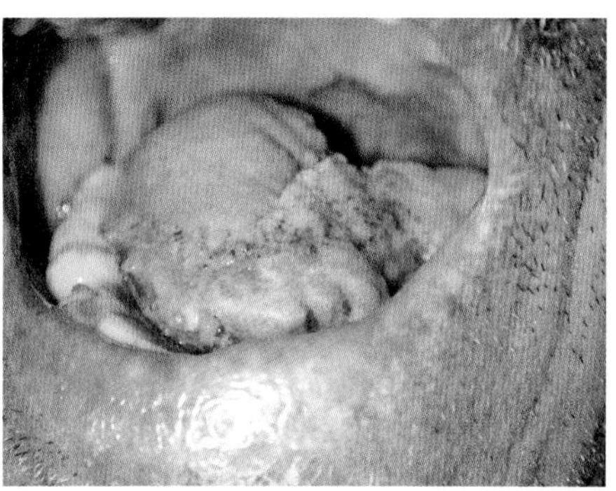

Figure 86.5 Granulomatous ulcerative lesion of the tongue (mulberry stomatitis) in a patient with paracoccidioidomycosis.

cutaneous lesions consist of plaques of various sizes with papular and crusted edges. In the perianal area, the base of the ulcers is often fungating and exudative. Scrofuloderma of the neck and upper chest may be present.[1,9] Adrenal involvement occurs in 40% of severe cases, ranging from minimal impairment to Addison's disease.[6,9] Central nervous system (CNS) infection occurs in <10% of patients, presenting as granulomatous brain abscesses or chronic meningoencephalitis.[1] Other sites of mycotic involvement include the testes, epididymis, prostate, bones, joints, liver, spleen, and arteries.[1,9] Untreated chronic paracoccidioidomycosis is uniformly fatal after several years; most of the patients die of cachexia or respiratory failure.[1]

Medical conditions associated with paracoccidioidomycosis include tuberculosis (10–12% of cases)[1,4,6] and cancer, especially of the lung.[9,13] AIDS-related paracoccidioidomycosis is uncommon, except in Brazil; the majority present with the acute or subacute juvenile type, but there is greater pulmonary involvement.[14] In Brazil overall, paracoccidioidomycosis is the most frequent mycosis causing death, but for AIDS patients, cryptococcosis is a much more common fungal cause of mortality.[15]

Treatment of paracoccidioidomycosis is highly effective, but relapses may occur.[16] Healing may result in intense fibrosis, due to leukocyte secretion of transforming growth factor-β, and may cause tracheal or laryngeal stenosis or pulmonary fibrosis, resulting in cardiorespiratory impairment.[1,2] The overall mortality rate is 3%.[14]

PATHOGENESIS AND IMMUNITY

Paracoccidioides brasiliensis infection follows inhalation of conidia, resulting in a primary pulmonary lymph node complex and acute pneumonitis.[17,18] Traumatic cutaneous inoculation also occurs.[1]

Paracoccidioides gain entry into alveolar macrophages via Toll-like receptors (TLR2, TLR4). Inside macrophages, conidia convert into yeast.[19] The primary inoculation complex with satellite lymphatic lesions is followed by hematogenous dissemination with multiple metastatic foci. These alterations may occur without clinical manifestations other than development of a reactive skin test. Approximately 25% of the people living in the endemic area have a positive paracoccidioidin skin test. *Paracoccidioides brasiliensis* has been found in fibrotic or calcified lung nodules and lymph nodes.[4] Primary infection may also rarely present as a pulmonary focus in a surgical specimen, acute pneumonia, or a mild respiratory syndrome.[9]

Adult females are resistant to the disease, but not from infection, because of β-estradiol, which inhibits the transformation of mold into yeast, a critical step in the pathogenesis.[20] The mold-to-yeast transition is controlled by calcineurin.[21]

Antigens of *P. brasiliensis* are responsible for immune modulation and elicit a specific cellular and humoral immune response. Glycoprotein gp43, the immunodominant antigen secreted by *P. brasiliensis*, is proteolytic and capable of hydrolyzing collagen and elastin, facilitating fungal tissue invasion. Gp43 also mediates binding to laminin, a component of the extracellular matrix,[8] and inhibits macrophage phagocytosis and intracellular killing.[22] Other virulence factors include α-1,3-glucan and melanin.[1,2]

Cell-mediated immunity is the main host defense. Resistance against *P. brasiliensis* infection appears to be controlled by a dominant gene (Pb gene).[23] In susceptible mice, CD4 cells secrete predominantly Th2 cytokines (IL-10, IL-4, IL-5), resulting in a decrease in delayed hypersensitivity, polyclonal B-cell activation with high levels of antibody production, deficient macrophage activation, and defective granuloma formation.[20,22] In patients with HIV infection, paracoccidioidomycosis typically occurs when the CD4 count is <200 cells/μL, again supporting the importance of cell-mediated immunity as defense against the fungus.[14]

When the fungal burden is heavy, there is a high antigen concentration, which downregulates Th1 responses, favors Th2 cytokine expression, and inhibits phagocytosis and the production of nitric oxide and hydrogen peroxide.[2] Antimycotic therapy reduces fungal burden and facilitates restoration of the cell-mediated immune response, with higher Th1 cytokine production, especially interferon-γ.[2]

The interferon-γ-activated macrophage is the final effector of the immune response against *P. brasiliensis*. These cells inhibit fungal growth through the production of reactive oxygen intermediates, nitric oxide, and cytokines, such as IL-1β and granulocyte-macrophage colony-stimulating factor.[2,24] Neutrophils, non-activated macrophages, and antigen-presenting cells participate in the innate immune response.[24] Antibodies are produced, but are not protective.[1,2,6]

Paracoccidioides brasiliensis is pathogenic in several laboratory animals, including guinea pigs, hamsters, mice, rats, and the chicken embryo.[1,4] Natural infections are observed in armadillos (*Dasypus novemcinctus* and *Cabassous centralis*).[5]

DIAGNOSIS

Microscopic observation of the yeast form of *P. brasiliensis* in clinical specimens (using saline or 10% potassium hydroxide) and its isolation in culture are the most important diagnostic techniques. Specimens useful for culture include exudates from ulcers, abscesses, and lymph nodes; sputa; bronchial washings; and tissue from mucocutaneous or pulmonary lesions.[2,4,9] Because of the difficulty of cultivating *P. brasiliensis* from clinical samples, cultures should be performed in multiple media (Sabouraud, Borelli's lactrimel, yeast extract-agar with chloramphenicol-cycloheximide) incubated at 28°C for at least 4 weeks. In enriched media (BHI agar with chloramphenicol or blood-agar), cultures are incubated at 37°C for 10 days.[1,2] Histopathologic examination is also of great diagnostic value. Periodic acid–Schiff and Gomori–Grocott methenamine-silver stains facilitate visualization of the fungus, especially when organisms in the specimen are sparse.

Identification of the mycelial phase of *P. brasiliensis* is often difficult due to the absence of sporulation. Identification methods include exoantigen testing, transformation into the yeast, or inoculation into laboratory animals. A polymerase chain reaction assay is not available.[2] Blood cultures may be positive in severe disease, especially in AIDS patients; lysis-centrifugation is the technique of choice.[25]

Serologic testing is an important tool for diagnosis and monitoring the activity of paracoccidioidomycosis. Immunodiffusion and counter-immunoelectrophoresis using paracoccidioidin or the gp43 glycoprotein are specific for the diagnosis of this mycosis.[1,2,4,17] Complement fixation (CF) is less specific, with cross-reactions with histoplasmin in over 25% of cases.[1] CF titers are high in severe cases and decline after clinical remission. Occasionally, there is persistence of low CF titers. The enzyme-linked immunosorbent assay, using the gp43 antigen, has a high rate of cross-reactions with other fungal antigens.[17] False negative serologic tests can occur in immunocompromised patients and in localized disease.[8]

TREATMENT AND PROGNOSIS

Azoles, amphotericin B, and sulfonamides have been used successfully for treatment of paracoccidioidomycosis.[2,16] Itraconazole is the drug of choice, given at 100–200 mg/day, orally for 6 months. Relapses occur in <5% of cases treated with itraconazole. Patients with relapsed disease respond favorably to itraconazole retreatment. Maintenance therapy is not necessary.[16] Itraconazole failures are rare and are usually due to malabsorption associated with mesenteric adenopathy, which is more common in the juvenile form.[1,9,16] In these patients, intravenous trimethoprim-sulfamethoxazole and amphotericin B are appropriate alternatives. These patients should also receive a low-fat diet.[16]

In meningoencephalitis, intravenous trimethoprim-sulfamethoxazole (240–480 mg/day) is the treatment of choice; alternatives are amphotericin B (0.8 mg/kg daily) or fluconazole (400–800 mg/day). Patients with adrenal insufficiency should also receive hydrocortisone (30 mg/day).[1,16] In paracoccidioidomycosis-tuberculosis coinfection, trimethoprim-sulfamethoxazole or amphotericin B are preferred, due to the interaction of rifampin with azoles.[2,9,16] In patients with paracoccidioidomycosis and AIDS, malabsorption and drug interactions may compromise the use of itraconazole. These cases are treated with amphotericin B alone or in combination with trimethoprim-sulfamethoxazole. Trimethoprim-sulfamethoxazole is also effective in the initial treatment of paracoccidioidomycosis. Sulfonamides are also recommended in adult chronic disease and for less severely ill patients.[4,16] Long-term maintenance therapy is required when sulfonamides are used. Also, in HIV coinfection, sulfa drugs are less effective.[14]

Amphotericin B (0.7 mg/kg daily; total dose: 1.5–2.0 g) is indicated in severe paracoccidioidomycosis; it produces rapid improvement, but does not prevent relapses. After clinical improvement, sulfonamides are prescribed as maintenance treatment. Fluconazole is less active than itraconazole in paracoccidioidomycosis, but may be useful in cases with renal and brain involvement.[2,9,16] It is given at a dose of 400 or 800 mg/day for 6–12 months. In Brazil, fluconazole is often used in the treatment of HIV-paracoccidioidomycosis coinfection because it is available free of charge.[14] In an uncontrolled study, fluconazole treatment resulted in improvement or remission in 93% of HIV-coinfected patients.[14] Ketoconazole is also effective, but requires 1 year of treatment and periodic assessment of hepatic and gonadal function; the daily dose is 200–400 mg.[2,9,16] Due to the teratogenicity of azoles, pregnant women with paracoccidioidomycosis should receive amphotericin B or trimethoprim-sulfamethoxazole (considered safe after the fourth week of pregnancy until 1 week before childbirth).[8]

With the available treatments, most patients with paracoccidioidomycosis survive.[2] However, the acute juvenile form and CNS or adrenal involvement portend a poorer outcome.[1] The use of azoles has made relapses less common than in the past when sulfonamides were the standard therapy.[1,16]

PREVENTION AND CONTROL

Human-to-human transmission of paracoccidioidomycosis does not occur, and the reservoir of infection is the soil. Currently, there is no human vaccine for paracoccidioidomycosis. In the absence of socioeconomic progress, the impoverished agricultural workers of Latin America will continue to contract paracoccidioidomycosis. However, modernization of agriculture, improved nutrition, and decreased alcohol and tobacco abuse may reduce the rates of this destructive and disabling disease.

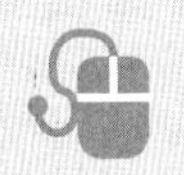

Access the complete reference list online at
http://www.expertconsult.com

CHAPTER 87

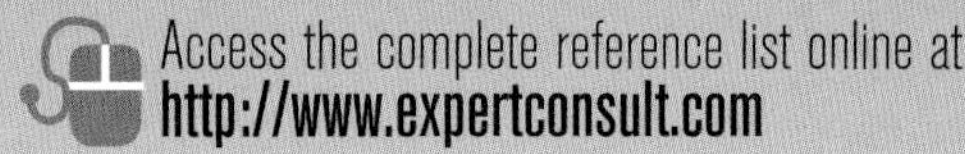
Access the complete reference list online at
http://www.expertconsult.com

Penicilliosis Marneffei

Khuanchai Supparatpinyo • Gregory M. Anstead • John R. Graybill

INTRODUCTION

Approximately 225 species of the fungus *Penicillium* are described.[1] They are widely distributed in the environment, mainly in the soil and decomposing organic matter, and are common laboratory contaminants. *Penicillium marneffei* is the most common *Penicillium* species causing human infection. Penicilliosis marneffei is most frequently found in patients with immunodeficiency, especially HIV infection. In northern Thailand, penicilliosis marneffei is the fourth most common AIDS-related opportunistic infection after tuberculosis, cryptococcosis, and *Pneumocystis* pneumonia.[2] Penicilliosis marneffei has also been reported in HIV patients from other countries following visits to the endemic area.[3]

P. marneffei was first isolated in Vietnam in 1956 from the viscera of a bamboo rat (*Rhizomys sinensis*).[4] The first natural human infection was reported in the spleen of a missionary with Hodgkin's lymphoma who had been living in Asia several years before presentation.[5] The first case of penicilliosis marneffei in an HIV patient was reported in 1989 in Bangkok, coinciding with the beginning of the HIV epidemic in the region.[6] The number of cases has increased markedly since that time.

THE AGENT

P. marneffei is the only species of the genus that is dimorphic. It grows in mycelial form at 25°C and in yeast-like form at 37°C, dividing by binary fission. This dimorphism may be a factor in its greater pathogenicity compared to other members of the genus.[7]

EPIDEMIOLOGY

P. marneffei is endemic to Southeast Asia (Thailand, Vietnam, Taiwan, Malaysia, Cambodia), southern China (Hong Kong, Guangxi and Guangdong provinces), and India (Manipur State) (***Fig. 87.1***).[8,9] Between 1991 and 2004, >6000 cases of penicilliosis marneffei in HIV-infected patients were reported to the Thai Ministry of Public Health. Penicilliosis marneffei was the AIDS-defining illness in 6.8% of HIV patients from northern Thailand but less frequently elsewhere.[2]

P. marneffei infects four species of bamboo rats, *R. sinensis*, *R. pruinosus*, *R. sumatranensis*, and *Cannomys badius*, and the geographic ranges of these rats correspond to areas where human cases of penicilliosis marneffei are found.[10] However, attempts to link bamboo rats and human infection have been unsuccessful.

THE DISEASE

The majority of penicilliosis marneffei cases are observed in AIDS patients with a CD4 cell count of <100 cells/μL.[11] Patients commonly present with signs and symptoms of infection of the reticuloendothelial system, including fever, lymphadenopathy, hepatomegaly, and splenomegaly.[8] Clinical manifestations associated with advanced HIV infection, such as anorexia, asthenia, anemia, weight loss, and cachexia, occur in the majority of the patients. Cough, dyspnea, chest pain, and pulmonary infiltrates may reflect the inhalational route of infection. Skin lesions, arthritis, and osteomyelitis occur secondary to dissemination. Papular skin lesions, usually on the face, chest, and extremities, occur in >70% of patients and, when present, are useful clues to the diagnosis. The center of the papule subsequently becomes necrotic, giving an umbilicated appearance (***Figs 87.2 and 87.3***). Mucosal lesions have also been reported in the oropharynx, stomach, colon, and genitalia.[8,12] Laboratory abnormalities include elevation of liver enzymes and bilirubin, anemia, and leukocytosis or leukopenia. Chest radiographs may show diffuse reticulonodular, localized alveolar, or diffuse alveolar infiltrates. The presentation in children is identical to that of adults.[13]

PATHOGENESIS AND IMMUNITY

Though the disease can be localized, dissemination is likely in both immunocompetent and immunocompromised hosts. The exact mode of transmission of *P. marneffei* is still unknown. It is likely that *P. marneffei* conidia are inhaled from an environmental reservoir. A case report involving an HIV-infected physician who never visited Asia suggests the airborne route of infection; he developed penicilliosis marneffei shortly after entering a mycology classroom in which a specimen of *P. marneffei* was being manipulated. However, air sampling within the building did not yield *P. marneffei*.[14]

In the body, the conidia are engulfed by macrophages, in which they transform into yeast and multiply intracellularly. Melanin is produced by both conidia and yeast and acts as a virulence factor.[15] Dissemination of infection occurs through the lymphatics or hematogenously. The reticuloendothelial system is predominantly involved. The infection can remain dormant and reactivate at a later time. In the immunocompetent host, the cell-mediated immune response is prominent, with the formation of epithelioid granulomas similar to tuberculosis.[16] In a murine model of infection, wild-type mice control the infection with granuloma formation and a Th1 immune response.[17] There is no evidence for a role of humoral immunity in the resolution of infection. In patients with HIV infection, the histopathologic features depend on the degree of immunosuppression.[18] At lower CD4 cell counts, the disease is more invasive. The blunted immune response results in an absence of granulomas and extensive proliferation of extracellular yeast and intracellular forms within foamy macrophages.[19]

DIAGNOSIS

A history of travel to or residence in the endemic region is the most important diagnostic clue. The diagnosis of penicilliosis marneffei is based on the isolation of organisms in cultures of blood or other clinical

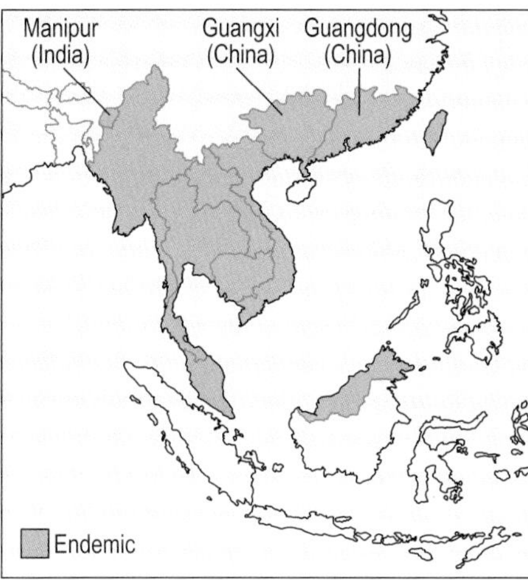

Figure 87.1 Endemic area for *Penicillium marneffei* (Adapted from Supparatpinyo K, Sirisanthana T. *Penicillium marneffei* infections. In: Kauffman CA, ed. Atlas of Fungal Infection, 2nd edn. Philadelphia: Current Medicine; 2006:191–202.)

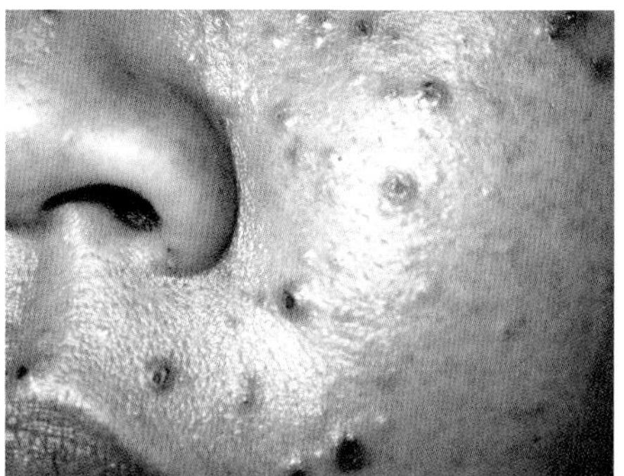

Figure 87.2 Skin lesions on the face of a Thai patient infected with HIV and *Penicillium marneffei.*

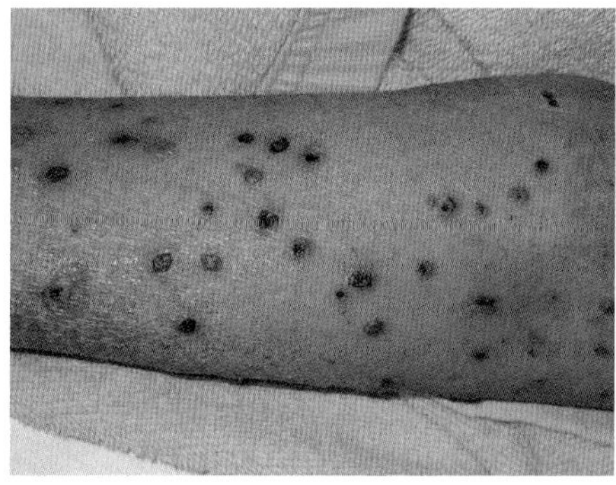

Figure 87.3 Skin lesions on the forearm of a Thai patient infected with HIV and *Penicillium marneffei.*

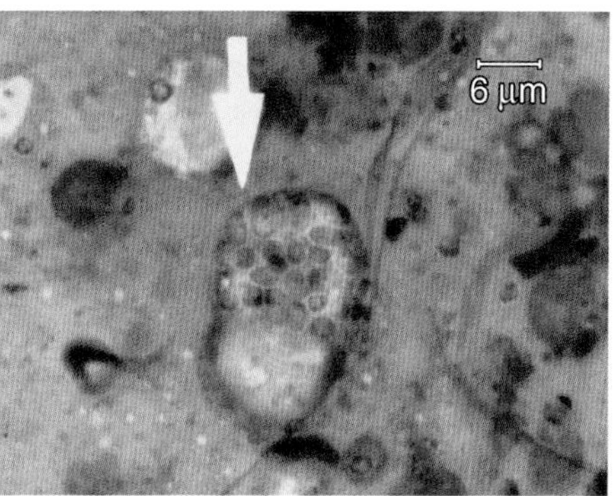

Figure 87.4 A Wright-stained skin smear showing yeast-like organisms with intracellular septa characteristic of *Penicillium marneffei.*

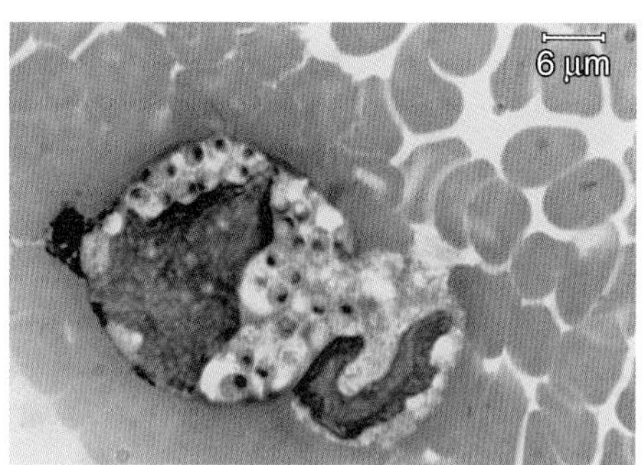

Figure 87.5 A Wright-stained peripheral blood smear from a Thai patient infected with HIV and *Penicillium marneffei.*

specimens or by histopathological demonstration of organisms in biopsy material. In disseminated disease, rates of culture positivity approach 100% from bone marrow and lymph nodes, about 75% from blood,[8] and more variably from skin, liver, bone, joints, lung, and urine specimens. Sabouraud dextrose agar is the culture medium of choice. The fungus grows rapidly within 2–5 days in its mycelial form at 25°C, producing characteristic features that include a flat green surface with surrounding red pigment. Mold-to-yeast conversion can be achieved using brain-heart infusion agar and incubation at 37°C. Demonstration of this thermal dimorphism is generally required before the definitive identification of *P. marneffei* can be made.

Histopathologic diagnosis can be made by demonstration of characteristic organisms in tissue sections stained with Gomori methenamine silver (GMS) or periodic acid–Schiff (PAS) methods.[14,20] However, it is more difficult to document infection in immunocompetent patients in whom granulomatous inflammation may be the only finding, with negative fungal stains.

A rapid presumptive diagnosis can be made by microscopic examination of the Wright-stained samples of skin scrapings, bone marrow aspirate, or lymph node biopsy/fine needle aspirate touch smear, which reveals intracellular and extracellular basophilic, spherical, oval, and elliptical yeast. Some of these cells have a clear central septum, which is characteristic of *P. marneffei* (***Fig. 87.4***).[8,21] In addition, the fungus can be identified by examination of the Wright-stained peripheral blood smear in patients with heavy fungemia (***Fig. 87.5***).[22] *P. marneffei* resembles *Histoplasma capsulatum*, and it can be difficult to distinguish between them. However, *P. marneffei* forms more elongated yeast cells, and it divides by central septate fission rather than budding as for *H.* capsulatum (***Figs 87.4 and 87.5***).

More recently applied diagnostic techniques include: specific fluorescent antibody examination of tissue samples;[23] polymerase chain reaction on skin biopsy specimens;[24] and various serologic assays (immunodiffusion,[25] indirect fluorescent antibody test, enzyme-linked immunosorbent assay of a purified recombinant mannoprotein of *P. marneffei*, and Western immunoblot).[26] Methods to detect *P. marneffei* antigens in serum or urine have also been described.[27] However, none of these molecular diagnostic tests is commercially available.

TREATMENT AND PROGNOSIS

The high mortality rate of HIV patients with penicilliosis marneffei has primarily been due to delayed diagnosis.[8] Outcome has been much better in hospitals where physicians are aware of the clinical features of the mycosis, and the presumptive diagnosis is early. A study of 30 isolates from Thailand revealed that all were highly susceptible to itraconazole, ketoconazole, miconazole, and 5-flucytosine. Amphotericin B had intermediate activity, while fluconazole was the least active.[21] Clinical response to treatment correlated with *in vitro* susceptibility, with high failure rates for fluconazole. An open label noncomparative study confirmed the efficacy and safety of the combination of 0.6 mg/kg daily of amphotericin B intravenously for 2 weeks followed by 400 mg/day of itraconazole orally for 10 weeks.[28] A study by Supparatpinyo et al showed that patients with mild disease can be initially treated with oral itraconazole 400 mg/day for 8 weeks.[29] In a report of 46 patients, treatment with oral itraconazole was effective in 98% of cases.[9] Thus, oral treatment with 400 mg/day of itraconazole for 8–12 weeks is recommended in patients with less severe disease. Antiretroviral therapy should be initiated in all HIV patients with penicilliosis marneffei who are clinically stable after 2–8 weeks of antifungal therapy.

Relapses of penicilliosis marneffei can occur in more than 50% of patients within 6 months after discontinuation of antifungal therapy.[29,30] A double-blind, placebo-controlled trial found that itraconazole 200 mg orally once daily could effectively prevent relapses of penicilliosis marneffei after completion of antifungal treatment.[30] Therefore, suppressive therapy after successful antifungal therapy is required for life or as long as significant immunodeficiency persists.

No randomized controlled studies have demonstrated the safety of discontinuation of secondary prophylaxis for penicilliosis marneffei. However, an open-label, historically controlled trial showed that there was no relapse of penicilliosis marneffei after discontinuation of itraconazole in patients receiving antiretroviral therapy and achieving a CD4 count >100 cells/μL for at least 6 months.[31] Secondary prophylaxis should be reintroduced if the CD4 count decreases to <100 cells/μL[3] or if penicilliosis marneffei recurs.

PREVENTION AND CONTROL

There is no evidence of human-to-human transmission. Primary prevention may be considered in areas where systemic mycoses are common AIDS-associated opportunistic infections. A double-blind, randomized, controlled trial of 129 HIV patients who had a CD4 cell count of <200 cells/μL showed that itraconazole 200 mg/day orally was effective in the prevention of systemic mycoses, including penicilliosis marneffei.[11] The current national guidelines recommend using itraconazole 200 mg orally once daily for primary prophylaxis of systemic fungal infections in all HIV patients with CD4 cell count of <100 cells/μL in northern Thailand.

Several experimental vaccines based on the secreted cell wall antigen Mp1p (DNA by intramuscular administration; DNA vaccine delivered orally via live-attenuated *Salmonella typhimurium*; recombinant protein administered by intraperitoneal injection) were shown to be protective in a murine model of penicilliosis marneffei, but no human studies have been undertaken.[32]

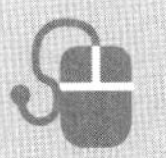

Access the complete reference list online at
http://www.expertconsult.com

Access the complete reference list online at http://www.expertconsult.com

CHAPTER 88

Mucocutaneous and Deeply Invasive Candidiasis

Shmuel Shoham • Marcio Nucci • Thomas J. Walsh

INTRODUCTION

Candidal infections are an important cause of illness worldwide. *Candida* species, particularly *Candida albicans*, are frequent human commensals, but a diverse range of infections can occur when host defenses break down or are breached. Mucocutaneous infections are common in all climates. In hot, humid tropical regions macerated skin often becomes infected, resulting in cutaneous candidiasis. Mucosal candidiasis can involve the lower genital tract, oropharynx, or the esophagus. Vulvovaginal candidiasis is one of the most common genital problems of women in both industrialized and developing countries. Extensive use of antibiotics, diabetes mellitus, local genital immune factors, and human immunodeficiency virus (HIV) all contribute to the widespread prevalence of vulvovaginal candidiasis. Oropharyngeal and esophageal candidiasis are typically encountered in association with local mucosal injury, or as a result of defects in cell-mediated immunity, particularly HIV. With globalization, illnesses previously associated with wealthier societies are assuming an increasingly important role in developing nations. In that regard, in newly industrialized countries, deeply invasive candidiasis occurring in the setting of, or as a consequence of, medical progress have emerged as new challenges. Examples include oropharyngeal and esophageal candidiasis among recipients of cytotoxic therapies, bloodstream infection in persons with indwelling vascular devices, and disseminated candidiasis in highly immunocompromised hosts such as neonates and transplant recipients. Expansion of populations at risk, changes in distribution of colonizing and infecting species, and the impact of widespread use of antifungal agents upon the evolution of resistant organisms are now experienced in an increasing number of regions worldwide. Studies designed to optimize use of existing antifungals and to aid in the development of novel agents continue to be crucial. Perhaps even more important is expansion of our knowledge of regional and global epidemiological patterns, candidal pathogenesis, and host defenses, and the translation of this information into a better understanding of the fungus as it relates to patients in a diversity of environments.

THE AGENTS

The genus *Candida* encompasses over 150 species, but only a small number are human pathogens. In nature, *Candida* species are principally associated with plants and rotting vegetation. Most are unable to grow at temperatures of 37°C and require vitamins produced mainly in plant materials.[1,2] Of the species known to cause human disease, *C. albicans*, *C. glabrata*, *C. parapsilosis*, *C. tropicalis*, *C. krusei*, *C. lusitaniae*, *C. guilliermondii*, and *C. dubliniensis* are the most commonly encountered.[3–8] Because *C. dubliniensis* shares many characteristics with *C. albicans*, it may be misidentified in clinical specimens.[9]

Laboratory identification relies on morphological and biochemical features of the fungus. *Candida* species grow as ovoid budding yeasts (blastoconidia), typically 4–6 μm in diameter. Most species also produce pseudohyphae. Microscopic examination is facilitated by 10% potassium hydroxide (KOH), which digests epithelial cells. Fluorescence microscopy of specimens stained with calcofluor white and Gram staining (*Candida* species stain Gram-positive) are also useful.

Phase transition from yeast to filamentous forms may be an important virulence factor. Germination can be induced by serum, specific carbon sources, hemin, temperatures over 35°C, and pH of 6.5–7.0 or slightly alkaline. Conversely, lower temperatures and an acid environment favor yeast growth.[2,10] During hyphal formation, an outgrowth develops from the yeast cells termed a germ tube. Diagnostic laboratories commonly test for the presence or absence of a germ tube in order to differentiate *C. albicans* and *C. dubliniensis* from other *Candida* species. The germ tube is highly suggestive, but not absolutely diagnostic for these two species. Additionally, *C. albicans* and *C. dubliniensis* can produce large (8–12 μm), thick-walled cells termed chlamydospores. Chlamydospores are occasionally encountered in host tissue and can be induced by various culture media including corn meal agar, rice extract agar, chlamydospore agar, Tween 80-oxgall-caffeic acid and diluted milk.[2,11,12]

Clinically important species of *Candida* grow well in routine blood culture systems and on common media including Sabouraud glucose agar, sheep blood agar, and horse blood agar.[13] At 25–37°C on Sabouraud agar *Candida* species form white-to-beige colonies that are smooth-to-wrinkled. Corn meal agar is a relatively inexpensive medium by which *Candida* spp. can be distinguished based upon microscopic morphology.

Media containing chromogenic compounds such as CHROMagar (CCM) can differentiate *Candida* species based on the formation of various colored colonies with different morphologies, which result from the cleavage of chromogenic substrates, by species-specific enzymes.[14] In a study exploring the usefulness of CCM in a developing country, over 90% of isolates from clinical specimens were identified to species level within 48 hours, and the assay was determined to be cost-effective in a resource-poor environment.[15] Definitive identification of *Candida* species is facilitated by metabolic tests available in commercial kits. Identification of species directly from blood culture bottles using peptide nucleic acid (PNA) fluorescent *in situ* hybridization (FISH) probes is emerging as an important diagnostic modality.[16] *C. albicans* can also be differentiated from *C. dubliniensis* by the latter's inability to grow at 45°C and by DNA fingerprinting probes.[17,18]

PATHOGENESIS AND IMMUNITY

Candida species, particularly *C. albicans*, colonize the human gastrointestinal, respiratory, and reproductive tracts and the skin. Invasion occurs when host defenses break down or are breached. A variety of adhesins facilitate attachment of the fungus to epithelial and endothelial surfaces.[19] The ability of *Candida* species to form biofilms on medical devices has contributed to the emergence of these fungi as major pathogens. Biofilm-associated infections are frequently refractory to antifungal therapy. This resistance could be due in part to changes in candidal sterol composition and upregulation of drug efflux pumps.[20,21] Production of hydrolytic enzymes including secreted aspartic proteinases, phospholipases and lipases have all been linked to virulence of *C. albicans*.[22–24] Morphological transitions among yeast, pseudohyphal, and hyphal forms and the phenomena of phenotype switching contribute to virulence in *C. albicans*.[25,26] Other virulence factors include production of a hemolytic factor that facilitates fungal acquisition of iron and expression of complement receptors that inhibit phagocytosis.[27,28]

Candidiasis can be broadly divided into two categories: mucosal and systemic disease. Innate immunity is the dominant protective mechanism against disseminated disease. Neutrophils, monocytes, endothelial cells, dendritic cells, platelets, opsonins, cytokines, chemokines, and complement all participate in protection against systemic infection.[29,30] The role of cell-mediated immunity and antibodies in disseminated disease is less clear. Cell-mediated immunity is the predominant protective mechanism against non-genital mucosal candidiasis. Clinically, patients with abnormal cell-mediated immune responses due to HIV or corticosteroids are at increased risk for mucosal infections. In the lower genital tract, locally acquired mucosal immunity appears to be more important than systemic cell-mediated immunity against *C. albicans*, and the majority of women with candidal vaginitis do not have a discernible systemic immune defect.[31,32]

Antifungal Agents: Mechanisms, Resistance, and *In Vitro* Susceptibility

Antifungal agents belonging to four major classes (azoles, polyenes, echinocandins, and pyrimidine analogs) are used to treat most infections. Azoles and polyenes target ergosterol, a major component of the fungal cell membrane. The echinocandins impair fungal cell wall synthesis. Flucytosine, a pyrimidine analog, impairs fungal nucleic acid synthesis.

The azoles primarily act on the fungal cytochrome P450 enzyme complex, inhibiting conversion of lanosterol to ergosterol and fungal respiration chain enzyme function.[33] Azole resistance may be intrinsic, as in some isolates of *C. krusei*, or acquired. Resistance mechanisms include reduced affinity of 14-α-demethylase to fluconazole, enhanced 14-α-demethylation, alteration of the ergosterol biosynthetic pathway, and upregulation of multidrug efflux transporters.[34–37] These mechanisms frequently operate simultaneously. Under antifungal pressure clinical isolates can undergo minor genetic alterations that over time lead to azole resistance through the accumulation of multiple mechanisms.[38]

C. albicans is the most common species in mucocutaneous candidiasis. Most isolates are susceptible to all antifungals. The most common species in candidemia are *C. albicans*, *C. glabrata*, *C. parapsilosis*, *C. tropicalis*, and *C. krusei*. Although *C. albicans*, *C. tropicalis*, and *C. parapsilosis*, account for over two-thirds of bloodstream infections, and remain susceptible to fluconazole and itraconazole, resistance among *C. glabrata* and *C. krusei* is a clinically relevant issue.[39] A breakpoint for fluconazole susceptibility has been set when the minimum inhibitory concentrations (MICs) are ≤8 μg/mL. Isolates for which the MIC of fluconazole is 16–32 μg/mL are considered susceptible dependent upon dose (S-DD), and isolates are resistant when the MIC is ≥64 μg/mL.[40] S-DD isolates may be treated successfully with higher dosages of fluconazole.

The vast majority of *C. albicans*, *C. tropicalis*, and *C. parapsilosis* are susceptible to fluconazole.[5] In a recent survey 1.2% of *C. albicans* isolates were resistant to fluconazole compared with 6% of *C. tropicalis*.[39] In a worldwide study 60% of *C. glabrata* isolates were susceptible to fluconazole, 32% S-DD, and 8% resistant.[41] In that study only 5% of *C. krusei* isolates were susceptible to fluconazole, 50% S-DD, and 45% resistant. *C. albicans*, *C. tropicalis*, and *C. parapsilosis* have generally remained sensitive to itraconazole, but over one-third of *C. glabrata* and *C. krusei* isolates have decreased susceptibility to that agent.[42] Nearly all isolates of *C. krusei* are susceptible to voriconazole (MIC <1 μg/mL), irrespective of their level of resistance to fluconazole.[41] However, fluconazole-resistant isolates of *C. albicans* and *C. glabrata* can have substantial *in vitro* cross-resistance to voriconazole.

The frequency of azole resistance varies by locale. Among 1000 *Candida* bloodstream isolates recovered at four tertiary care hospitals in Brazil, the rate of fluconazole resistance was 0.2%, and was restricted to *C. glabrata*. S-DD to fluconazole was observed in 2.3% of *C. glabrata* isolates and 3.3% of *C. guilliermondii* isolates. Despite the low rates of resistance to fluconazole, cross-resistance to voriconazole was observed.[43]

Amphotericin B (AmB) primarily acts by binding to ergosterol with subsequent formation of ion channels and concentration-dependent cell death.[44,45] Resistance has been reported in *C. lusitaniae*, *C. tropicalis*, *C. glabrata*, and *C. albicans*.[36,46,47] Mechanisms of resistance include loss or marked depression of ergosterol in the cell membrane and increased catalase activity with resultant protection against polyene-induced oxidative damage.[47,48] Clinical isolates of *C. albicans* with mutations in the delta-5, 6-sterol desaturase gene, lack of ergosterol in the cytoplasmic membrane, and reduced susceptibility to AmB and fluconazole have been described.[49] In epidemiological studies the majority of *Candida* species remain sensitive to AmB.[41,50]

The echinocandins act by noncompetitive inhibition of the synthesis of 1,3-β-glucan, a polysaccharide in the cell wall of many pathogenic fungi. Together with chitin, the rope-like glucan fibrils are responsible for the cell wall's strength, shape, and osmotic integrity and play a key role in cell division and growth.[51,52] The echinocandins have excellent activity against *Candida* species, but resistant *C. albicans* mutants have been created under laboratory conditions.[53] MIC of ≤2 μg/mL is associated with susceptibility. The MICs of caspofungin for *C. parapsilosis* tend to be higher than for other species, but the clinical significance of this observation is unknown.

Flucytosine (5-fluorocytosine; 5-FC) impairs fungal nucleic acid synthesis.[54] Resistance occurs due to decreased cellular uptake or impaired intracellular metabolism.[37,55] Primary resistance is uncommon except in *C. krusei*.[56] Acquired resistance is far more prevalent. Because resistance can occur during monotherapy, 5-FC is generally used in combination with other antifungal agents. Given its dose-dependent toxicity of myelosuppression and diarrhea, 5-FC is seldom used for invasive candidiasis. Careful attention to dosage, renal function, and serum drug levels can minimize toxicity.

THE DISEASES, THEIR DIAGNOSIS AND TREATMENT

Skin and Nails

Candida species, particularly *C. albicans* and *C. parapsilosis*, are frequent skin colonizers.[57] Colonization is associated with antibiotic therapy, parenteral nutrition, low birth weight infants, endotracheal intubation, duration of hospitalization, intravenous catheters, malignancies, diabetes mellitus, surgery, aging, and obesity.[58,59] Superficial infections regularly involve intertriginous or occluded areas, large skin folds, glabrous skin, and nails.[60] Warm, moist surfaces and macerated skin favor superficial infection. Affected sites include the groin and perianal region, skin under pendulous breasts or large abdominal folds, and the axilla. Environmental conditions such as hot, humid weather, crowding, and poor personal hygiene predispose to candidal intertrigo.[61] Diabetes mellitus is a major risk factor for superficial candidiasis and has emerged as a problem in some tropical regions.[62] Obesity, treatment with antibiotics or steroids, inflammatory skin diseases, and HIV and human T-lymphotropic virus I (HTLV-I) predispose to cutaneous candidiasis.[63–65] These cutaneous lesions consist of pruritic and sometimes painful, moist, erythematous plaques or macules. The involved skin may be eroded, and whitish scaling is often present at the borders of lesions. Erythematous vesiculopapular or pustular satellite lesions are common. The latter may coalesce to extend the infection.

C. albicans of gastrointestinal origin can lead to diaper dermatitis.[66,67] Candidal diaper dermatitis is more common with non-disposable diapers.

The rash, which typically presents as a sharply marginated area of erythema, starts at the perianal region but may extend to involve the anterior thighs, genital creases, abdomen, and genitalia.[68] *Candida* miliaria, which begins with vesiculopustular lesions, affects the backs of bedridden patients, particularly those who are sweating profusely.[69] *Candida* may cause mastitis in lactating women and may be a cause of premature weaning.[70] Angular cheilitis presents with macerated skin, pain, erythema, and fissures at the angles of the mouth. It can be unilateral or bilateral, and is often caused by *C. albicans*.[71] *Candida* may infect hair follicles in the beard area causing erythematous plaques, papules, or pustules. Predisposing factors include use of steroids and antibiotics.[72,73]

Candidal interdigital infections and paronychia are common in the tropics and frequently occur following prolonged immersion in water or wearing of occlusive gloves. Dishwashers, laundry workers, and gardeners are at risk.[74] They appear as painful, erythematous, eroded areas between the fingers or toes. Paronychia presents with redness, swelling and tenderness at the nail fold that may extend beneath the nail and can progress to involve the nail. Candidal onychomycosis may occur without antecedent paronychia. *Candida* species play a relatively minor role in toenail onychomycosis but are frequently found in fingernail infections.[75,76] *C. albicans* and *C. parapsilosis* are the predominant species of *Candida* causing onychomycosis.[77,78] *Candida* onychomycosis may be a manifestation of concomitant HIV infection.

Cutaneous infections generally respond well to topical nystatin or imidazole derivatives.[79,80] Measures that promote dryness are important, and nystatin and miconazole powders are useful options. Topical corticosteroids can provide rapid symptomatic relief.[81,82] Extensive involvement may require systemic therapy. Infections of the nail fold can usually be managed with modification of the predisposing occupational factors, drainage, and topical antifungals. Systemic therapy is required in recalcitrant cases or when the nail itself is involved.[83] Candidal onychomycosis responds well to oral itraconazole.[84]

Congenital cutaneous candidiasis presents at birth or soon thereafter, likely secondary to contamination of skin from the mother. Typically there are generalized erythematous macules, papules, and/or pustules that sometimes evolve to vesicles and bullae. Involvement of the palms and soles is frequent. Very low birth weight infants may develop desquamating and/or erosive dermatitis. There is often evidence of an intrauterine infection with *Candida*.[85] Topical therapy is generally sufficient.[86,87] Some infants may present with respiratory distress or clinical signs of sepsis during the first 2 days of life.[88] Such patients should be treated with systemic antifungals. Hematogenously disseminated candidiasis is far more common in neonates weighing less than 1000 grams. Consequently, low birth weight neonates or infants with prolonged rupture of membranes who demonstrate clinical findings of disseminated neonatal cutaneous candidiasis should be treated with systemic antifungals.[89–91] Invasive fungal dermatitis is characterized by erosive, crusting lesions that develop 1–2 weeks after birth in extremely low birth weight neonates. *C. albicans* is the most common pathogen, and dissemination is common.[92]

Chronic mucocutaneous candidiasis (CMC) refers to a group of disorders that typically present during childhood and are characterized by recurrent and persistent candidal infections. These may involve the skin, nails, and mucosal surfaces. Patients have impaired anti-candidal responses.[93–98] In some patients infections are limited to the nails, whereas in others candidiasis is extensive and disfiguring. Local or diffuse dermatophytosis may coexist with cutaneous candidiasis.[99] Mucosal manifestations include vulvovaginitis and infections of the oropharynx, larynx, and esophagus.[100] CMC can occur alone or in association with endocrine, autoimmune, and infectious disorders.[101]

Deeply invasive candidiasis is rare in CMC. Recurrent and severe non-candidal infections are common and include septicemia, bacterial pneumonia, bronchiectasis, and opportunistic infections, including cryptococcal meningitis and disseminated histoplasmosis.[102–104] An adult form of CMC that typically presents after the third decade of life is associated with thymoma, myasthenia gravis, hypogammaglobulinemia, and abnormalities of the bone marrow and circulating blood elements.[105]

Treatment requires systemic antifungal drugs. Clinical responses may be slow, and infections often require months of treatment to clear. Long-term therapy should be individualized, and most patients require treatment intermittently or chronic suppression in order to remain in remission. Relapses while on treatment and acquisition of resistance to azole antifungals can occur.[106–111] Patients with early manifestations of CMC should be evaluated for HIV infection.

Hematogenously disseminated candidiasis can present with cutaneous manifestations.[112–115] The characteristic lesions are single or multiple 0.5–1.0 cm erythematous or purpuric papulonodules with pale centers. In highly immunocompromised hosts these may be the initial manifestation of candidemia. Disseminated candidiasis with extensive folliculitis has been described in injection heroin abusers.[116,117] Less commonly, disseminated infection presents as ecthyma gangrenosum or purpura fulminans.[118–120] Skin biopsy often establishes the diagnosis prior to growth in blood cultures.[121]

Oropharyngeal Candidiasis (OPC)

Candida species, particularly *C. albicans*, frequently colonize the oral cavity. Multiple factors affect colonization including HIV status and viral load, increasing age, dentures, antibiotic treatment, malnutrition, and poor oral hygiene.[122–130] Development of infection depends upon both systemic and local determinants. Systemic risks include extremes in age, poorly controlled diabetes mellitus, nutritional deficiencies, and immunosuppression. Local factors include inadequately fitting dentures, inhaled steroids, radiotherapy, and cytotoxic chemotherapy.[131–138] HIV is one of the most important predisposing conditions worldwide. Oropharyngeal colonization with *Candida* species is more prevalent among seropositive persons and correlates with serum HIV-1 RNA levels.[128,139]

Oral colonization was assessed in a cross-sectional study involving 331 HIV patients receiving long-term highly active antiretroviral therapy (HAART) at a tertiary care center in Brazil. A total of 161 *Candida* isolates were detected among 147 (44%) patients. *C. albicans* accounted for 85% of the isolates, and were susceptible to all tested antifungal drugs. By contrast, six non-*albicans* isolates were S-DD to fluconazole and nine to itraconazole. *Candida* was more likely to colonize the oropharynx of patients with HIV-treatment failure.[140]

OPC is a leading cause of oral pathology in HIV and is significantly associated with lower CD4 lymphocyte counts, especially below 200/μL.[141–143] Unless HAART is initiated, the presence of oral candidiasis predicts the development of other serious opportunistic infections.[144,145] HAART significantly decreases the prevalence of OPC due to immune reconstitution, decreased viral load, and perhaps antagonism of candidal virulence factors by protease inhibitors.[146–148]

OPC is almost always due to *C. albicans*; however, non-*albicans* species have emerged as both colonizing and infecting species in recipients of radiotherapy, patients with HIV, and those with extensive past antifungal exposure.[149–153] *C. dubliniensis* is increasingly recognized in OPC and may be misidentified as *C. albicans*. Some isolates of *C. dubliniensis* have decreased susceptibility to azoles.[154–156] *C. albicans* with reduced susceptibility to fluconazole can colonize or infect severely immunosuppressed individuals, especially when there has been extensive exposure to azoles. Such isolates may be transmitted person to person.[153,157,158] In mucosal candidiasis refractory to clotrimazole, strains of *C. albicans* with cross-resistance to other azoles have been observed.[159]

The clinical manifestations of OPC are diverse, and multiple forms frequently present concurrently. Pseudomembranous candidiasis or thrush is the most commonly encountered type. It is characterized by curd-like, white patches on the buccal mucosa, gingiva, palate, and tongue. The pseudomembranes may be scraped off leaving raw, erythematous undersurfaces. Microscopically, yeast, hyphae, and pseudohyphae are evident on KOH smear or Gram stain. Erythematous candidiasis (acute atrophic candidiasis) occurs by itself or in association with pseudomembranes.[145,160] In some cases erythematous candidiasis occurs from sloughing of the pseudomembranes. The flat, red, and occasionally painful lesions are typically present on the dorsal surface of the tongue. The erythematous form is more difficult to recognize and likely underdiagnosed. Median rhomboid glossitis, which presents as a smooth, sometimes raised, erythematous lesion at the midline of the dorsal surface of the tongue, was previously thought to be a developmental abnormality, but is now recognized as candidiasis. Chronic atrophic candidiasis presents with mucosal erythema and edema, and affects areas of persistent local trauma due to denture wear. A related condition, *Candida*-associated palatal papillary hyperplasia, has been described in HIV.[161] Angular cheilitis, an inflammation at the angles of the mouth, can be precipitated by candidal infection. The lesions of chronic hyperplastic candidiasis (candidal leukoplakia) typically present as adherent, firm, elevated white patches on buccal mucosa or tongue. This condition can be resistant to treatment and on rare occasions may develop into carcinoma.[162] *C. albicans* is also associated with black hairy tongue, hypertrophy of the filiform papillae on the surface of the tongue following antibiotic use. Patients may complain of a tickling sensation, and treatment consists of débridement and good oral hygiene.[69]

The major therapeutic options for oral candidiasis are topical azoles (clotrimazole troches), oral azoles (fluconazole, ketoconazole, or itraconazole), oral polyenes (nystatin or AmB), intravenous AmB, and intravenous echinocandins (caspofungin).[89] Topical clotrimazole troches 10 mg five times daily or nystatin 500 000 units in suspension or pastille form four times daily are generally effective for mild to moderate disease. Systemic fluconazole may be associated with higher rates of mycological and clinical eradication and fewer relapses.[143,163,164]

Fluconazole is more effective than ketoconazole in HIV-associated OPC.[165,166] Itraconazole cyclodextrin solution achieves higher serum concentrations than the capsule and, if available, is preferred.[167] Itraconazole oral solution at 100 and 200 mg daily is well tolerated and as effective as fluconazole 100 mg tablets.[168,169] In a study of children over 5 years old and adolescents with HIV-associated OPC, itraconazole solution 2.5 mg/kg twice daily was well tolerated and efficacious.[170] In that study all patients with fluconazole-resistant isolates responded to itraconazole. Furthermore, there was no clear correlation between itraconazole MIC and response to therapy.

In the 1990s fluconazole-refractory OPC emerged in HIV-infected patients and was associated with poor overall prognosis (median survival after diagnosis 32.6 weeks).[171–178] Various therapeutic options are available. In cases refractory to fluconazole tablets, the drug may be given topically in swish and swallow formulation.[179] For OPC due to strains with reduced fluconazole susceptibility, increasing the dose to 800 mg daily and treating with longer courses of therapy may work.[180] Itraconazole solution 100–200 mg twice daily in adults and 2.5 mg/kg twice daily in children can also be effective.[170,181] Additional options include oral AmB, intravenous echinocandin, combination therapy with fluconazole and terbinafine (250 mg daily), or sargramostim (GM-CSF: 2.5 μg/kg daily).[182–186] AmB oral suspension, although well tolerated, has limited efficacy for fluconazole-refractory OPC.[178]

Antifungal prophylaxis with clotrimazole or systemic fluconazole may be employed in high-risk patients with cancer, transplantation, or very advanced HIV, but can lead to antifungal resistance.[187–192]

Some regions in developing countries with limited resources may not have access to standard therapy for OPC. In such settings, gentian violet may be as effective as nystatin or ketoconazole.[189] A randomized open label study of the treatment of oropharyngeal and esophageal candidiasis was conducted in Kinshasa among 141 inpatients with AIDS and OPC, of whom 136 also had esophageal candidiasis. The study compared the efficacy of gentian violet mouth washes (1.5 mL of 0.5% aqueous solution twice daily), oral ketoconazole (200 mg daily, after a meal) and nystatin mouth washes (200 000 units oral suspension four times daily). Patients enrolled in this study had very high mortality (probability of death: 41.6% after 14 days). After 14 days, 72 patients could be evaluated. At that time, oropharyngeal lesions had disappeared in similar proportions of patients treated with gentian violet (11/26, 42%) and ketoconazole (10/23, 43%), and in a lower proportion of patients treated with nystatin (2/23, 9%; $P < 0.05$). In esophageal candidiasis, ketoconazole seemed more effective than both other treatments. This study suggests that gentian violet is an effective and relatively inexpensive alternative treatment for OPC. However, some patients express concern that the purple discoloration of their lips may signify to their community that they are being treated for an HIV-related infection.

Esophageal Candidiasis

C. albicans is a frequent esophageal colonizer.[193,194] Risks for esophageal candidiasis include HIV, organ transplantation, alcoholic liver disease, antibiotics, proton pump inhibitors, inhaled steroids, esophageal carcinoma, and defects in cell-mediated immunity.[195–201] Candidiasis is the most common etiology of esophageal symptoms in HIV, and risk factors include low CD4 count, high HIV viral load, antibiotic use, and concurrent or previous OPC.[202,203]

Esophageal candidiasis usually causes odynophagia, dysphagia and retrosternal pain, but it can be asymptomatic and discovered only on endoscopy. Infection is generally limited to the mucosa. Complications include volume depletion, cachexia, esophageal stricture, and rarely, esophageal perforation.[204,205]

Radiological findings include edematous esophageal folds with subsequent development of plaques and diffuse ulceration.[206] Less common are discrete ulcers, or innumerable, tiny round lucencies that appear like a layer of foam.[207,208]

Endoscopy allows direct examination and sampling of the esophagus. The most common findings are white mucosal plaques, which consist of desquamated epithelium and inflammatory cells with infiltration by fungal elements and superinfecting bacteria. With increasing severity, the scattered mucosal plaques coalesce to form circumferential lesions which can result in luminal impingement.[209] The presence of white plaques in HIV-infected patients with dysphagia and odynophagia is highly predictive of esophageal candidiasis.[210]

Fluconazole can be used presumptively in AIDS patients with esophageal symptoms. However, clinical responses should be monitored closely, and endoscopy pursued in patients who do not improve promptly.[211–213]

Fluconazole, 100 mg daily for 2–3 weeks, is the mainstay of therapy, and response rates typically exceed 80%.[214,215] Fluconazole is superior to ketoconazole, flucytosine and itraconazole capsules and comparable to a combination of itraconazole and flucytosine.[216–219] Voriconazole, 200 mg twice daily, is as effective as fluconazole and may have a role in fluconazole-resistant infections, but is associated with more adverse reactions.[220]

Itraconazole, voriconazole, and posaconazole have comparable efficacy to fluconazole, and have been used successfully in fluconazole-resistant cases.[220–224] For azole-refractory cases, intravenous AmB and echinocandins are options.[182,215,225–228] Esophageal candidiasis generally responds well to antifungal therapy. However, in persons with advanced AIDS, recurrences are common.[229] Prophylactic fluconazole, 100 mg daily, is effective in preventing recurrences.[230]

Vulvovaginal Candidiasis

C. albicans commonly colonizes the lower female genital tract.[231,232] Colonization declines with aging.[233] Antibiotics, diabetes mellitus, pregnancy, wearing of poorly ventilated clothing, and possibly oral contraceptives facilitate transformation from colonization to symptomatic vaginitis.[234–236] Most women will have at least one attack of vulvovaginal candidiasis (VVC) in their lifetime. VVC is most common before menopause, but rarely occurs before menarche. HIV is associated with increased vaginal colonization, but the incidence of candidal vaginitis is not significantly elevated in this population.[142]

Clinical findings include irritation, pruritus, erythema, edema, fissures, dysuria, and dyspareunia. Inflammation may extend throughout the vulva and into the perineum. A discharge, which can be thick, is typically present. Often the patient will make a self-diagnosis of "yeast" vaginitis. However, this may be unreliable and can lead to overuse of topical antifungals. The presence of hyphae, pseudohyphae, and blastoconidia on microscopic evaluation of a 10% KOH-treated sample in association with vaginitis symptoms is highly suggestive of candidiasis. Estimation of pH, the amine test, and saline microscopy are not sensitive or specific, but are useful in suggesting an alternative or concomitant etiology for the symptoms. Vaginal cultures do not distinguish colonization from infection, but may be useful for confirming negative diagnoses, detecting microscopy false-negatives, and identifying non-*C. albicans* isolates.[237]

Sporadic mild to moderate disease usually responds to short courses of topical azole or nystatin. Alternatively, one dose of oral fluconazole 150 mg, 3 days of itraconazole 200 mg or 5 days of ketoconazole 200 mg twice daily can be effective.[238–241] In severe cases a week or more of topical therapy or two sequential 150 mg doses of fluconazole given 3 days apart may be necessary.[91,242] Solution of boric acid or gentian violet may also have a role.

Some women develop recurrent VVC. With the exception of poorly controlled diabetics, these patients rarely have recognizable precipitating or causal factors. This condition likely occurs due to local immune dysregulation.[243] The vast majority of recurrent infections are caused by azole-sensitive *C. albicans* even in the setting of long-term exposure to azoles.[244] Rarely, the infection is due to *C. glabrata* or *C. krusei*, and such patients have significantly reduced responses to azoles.[242] Otherwise, the clinical syndromes caused by these organisms are generally indistinguishable from *C. albicans* infections.[245] For patients with chronic *C. glabrata* or *C. krusei* vaginitis unresponsive to conventional therapy, topical boric acid 600 mg daily for 14 days and flucytosine cream may be options.[246–249] Although no definitive cure for recurrent VVC exists, long-term maintenance regimens with oral or topical azoles can effectively control symptoms in some patients.[243]

Candidal Balanitis

Candida species are a common cause of balanitis.[69,250] The lesions start as small papules and papulopustules that may slough, leaving erythematous erosions with associated whitish scales. Infection can spread to involve the scrotum and inguinal areas. There is often pruritus and burning, particularly following sexual intercourse.[251] In diabetics or immunosuppressed patients, there can be extensive cutaneous invasion with severe edema and ulceration.[69,252] Topical therapy with azole antifungals for 7 days or a single 150 mg dose of fluconazole is generally effective, but in patients with advanced immunosuppression or uncontrolled diabetes mellitus the infection can be refractory to treatment.[253,254]

Respiratory Tract Infections

Candida frequently colonizes the respiratory tract.[255–259] Lower respiratory tract infection is uncommon and overdiagnosed. Pneumonia may be secondary to aspiration or hematogenous spread, and occurs in patients with malignancies, lung transplant recipients, and neonates.[258,260,261] With hematogenous spread, involvement is often observed in multiple organs. In lung transplant recipients infection can occur at the bronchial anastomotic site with dehiscence of the anastomosis.[262] Among very low birth weight neonates, infection may be acquired postnatally or antenatally due to chorioamnionitis.[263,264]

Radiographic manifestations include disseminated nodules in cases due to hematogenous spread and nonspecific patchy infiltrates in endobronchial infection.[258,265] Isolation of even a large number of organisms on bronchoscopic specimen does not necessarily reflect infection, and the only accepted criterion for definitive diagnosis is histologic demonstration of the fungus in lung tissue. Mortality of actual candidal pneumonia is high and may exceed 80%.[258]

Candida can cause epiglottitis and laryngitis in immunocompromised patients.[266–268] Laryngitis can be diagnosed by fiberoptic or indirect laryngoscopy, and untreated it can lead to airway obstruction and respiratory compromise. *Candida* frequently colonizes voice prostheses and can lead to their early deterioration.[269,270] Prophylactic miconazole decreases this colonization and increases device lifetime.[271]

Cardiac Infections

Candida is the most common cause of fungal endocarditis. *Candida albicans*, *C. parapsilosis*, *C. glabrata*, and *C. tropicalis* account for the majority of cases.[272,273] Risk factors include injection drug use, indwelling vascular devices, and abnormal or prosthetic valves.[274–276] Prosthetic valve endocarditis (PVE) typically occurs in the first year after valve replacement.[277] *Candida* PVE may only become clinically evident several months after an initial episode of transient candidemia.[278] The large and friable vegetations have a propensity to produce systemic emboli, and patients regularly present with major embolic events.[279–282]

Large dense heterogeneous vegetations are typically seen on echocardiogram. Transthoracic echocardiography may be adequate, but transesophageal echocardiography has superior sensitivity for PVE and allows for optimal assessment of the valvular and paravalvular structures.[279,283] Due to the high risk for devastating embolic events, poor response to medical therapy alone and frequent recurrences, valve replacement is generally necessary.[284] With a combined medical and surgical approach, in-hospital survival is over 80%, but relapses can occur.[279,285,286] Commonly used initial regimens are an echinocandin or AmB followed by long-term fluconazole.[89] The required duration of therapy after surgery is not known, but a minimum of 6 weeks and possibly much longer has been advocated in order to prevent recurrences. The optimal management of patients for whom valve replacement is not possible is unknown, but AmB followed by long-term fluconazole has been successful.[287,288] Lifelong fluconazole may be advisable.

Candidal myocarditis may occur rarely with or without concurrent valvular infection.[283] Pericarditis is rare, but may occur following cardiothoracic surgery, or disseminated candidiasis. Pericardiocentesis, operative drainage, and systemic antifungals are the usual treatment.[289–292] Ventricular assist devices, implantable defibrillators and pacemakers may all become infected with *Candida*.[293–297] Complete device explantation and prolonged antifungal therapy are the recommended treatment.

Urinary Tract Infection

Candida species are frequent colonizers of the lower urinary tract. *C. albicans* represents approximately half of the fungal isolates in urine, but non-*albicans* species of *Candida* may also cause funguria, especially in patients previously treated with antifungal agents.[298–300] Fluconazole use may be associated with selection for resistant species.[301]

Predisposing factors include diabetes mellitus, urinary tract abnormalities, length of hospitalization (particularly in the intensive care unit (ICU)), malignancy, antimicrobial use, older age, and urinary catheters.[298,302,303] In an ICU surveillance study, candiduria developed in 22% of patients admitted for more than 7 days.[304] In a neonatal ICU study *Candida* species were identified in 42% of urinary tract infections, and over half of these patients had associated candidemia.[305]

In adults, candidemia rarely complicates candiduria.[298] In a study of patients with candidemia secondary to a urinary tract source, 88% had urinary tract abnormalities, predominantly obstruction, and 73% had undergone urinary tract procedures before the onset of bloodstream infection.[306] Conversely, with systemic candidiasis, hematogenous dissemination to the kidney may lead to cortical abscesses or obstructive masses termed “fungal balls,” usually at the ureteropelvic junction.[307,308] Ultrasonography may reveal this finding in up to a third of neonates with candidal urinary tract infection (UTI), which may develop weeks after the discovery of candiduria.[305,309] Other complications include papillary necrosis, emphysematous pyelonephritis, and emphysematous cystitis.[310–313]

The diagnosis of *Candida* UTI can be challenging. Candiduria does not necessarily signify true infection and may instead represent colonization or contamination of the urinary sample. The lack of specific signs and symptoms complicates the process of diagnosing fungal UTI, and some infected patients are asymptomatic.[314,315] The presence of pyuria and colony counts of 10 000–15 000 *Candida* species/mL of urine suggest infection; however, the predictive value of these findings when urinary catheters are in place is not known.[316–318] Studies of experimental renal candidiasis have questioned the reliability of colony-forming units for predicting renal candidiasis.[308]

Candiduria may represent colonization or low-grade infection that often resolves without specific therapy or with removal of the urinary catheter. All indwelling urinary instrumentation should be removed if possible. Candiduria should be treated in symptomatic patients, low birth weight infants, patients with neutropenia, and persons expected to undergo urinary tract instrumentation. Antifungal therapy should be given for 7–14 days.[89] Oral fluconazole 200 mg was compared with placebo daily for 14 days in asymptomatic or minimally symptomatic candiduric hospitalized patients. Clearance with fluconazole was significantly greater among those patients receiving fluconazole (50% versus 29%); however, recurrences were common, and long-term candiduria rates were similar in both groups.[319] Intravenous AmB at various doses has been used successfully. In patients with intact renal function, flucytosine 25 mg/kg daily may be an option; however, resistance can develop rapidly when used as monotherapy.[320,321] AmB bladder irrigation is another option, but it is cumbersome and patients may complain of bladder fullness.[89,91,322]

Meningitis and Meningoencephalitis

Candida meningitis and meningoencephalitis are uncommon. Infection can be secondary to hematogenous dissemination or direct inoculation. Neurosurgery, recent antibiotics, and corticosteroids are predisposing factors. Fever, meningismus, elevated CSF pressures, and localizing neurologic signs are commonly noted. Delays in diagnosis, hypoglycorrhachia, intracranial hypertension, and focal neurological deficits are associated with a poor prognosis.[323,324] Clinical manifestations of ventriculoperitoneal shunt-associated candidiasis include hydrocephalus, fever, meningoencephalitis, and abdominal symptoms.[325] The cerebrospinal fluid (CSF) may show a neutrophilic pleocytosis that is indistinguishable from bacterial meningitis or a predominance of lymphocytes. Sometimes the clinical significance of the presence of *Candida* in CSF of patients with shunts is difficult to assess. Ideally the diagnosis of infection is established by repeated cultures from both the indwelling device and lumbar puncture.[326] However, potentially lifesaving therapy should not be withheld while waiting for a confirmatory CSF culture. *Candida* meningitis may be subacute, presenting with fever and headache of several weeks' duration and lymphocytic pleocytosis. Neurological manifestations can range from normal examination to signs of brain infarcts or hydrocephalus.[327–329] Infection may also present as intense granulomatous and necrotizing basal meningitis with cranial neuropathies or basilar artery thrombosis and resultant brainstem and temporo-occipital infarction.[330,331]

Hematogenous *Candida* meningoencephalitis is frequently associated with systemic candidiasis in very low birth weight neonates.[332–335] The initial clinical features are indistinguishable from those of other systemic infections in neonates. CSF commonly shows hypoglycorrhachia, but pleocytosis is inconsistent and Gram stain is generally unrevealing. Therefore, normal CSF parameters do not exclude meningitis.

Successful treatment of candidal meningitis requires systemic therapy and removal of any infected hardware.[325] Therapy with AmB (with or without 5-FC) has been successfully used in children and adults.[334,336,337] In a series of 17 patients with candidal meningitis, the combination of AmB and 5-FC led to cure in 14 patients.[338] Because of its superior safety profile and comparable efficacy in animal models, liposomal AmB is an attractive option.[339] Liposomal AmB was successful in five of six preterm infants with candidal meningitis.[340] *C. lusitania* can be resistant to AmB, and fluconazole has been used successfully in two children with meningitis due to that pathogen.[341]

Joint and Bone Infection

Candidal arthritis and osteomyelitis occur following direct inoculation or hematogenous seeding from a distant source. The knee is most commonly involved.[342] Infection may occur following joint injections and in association with prosthetic joints.[343–346] Injection drug users may also develop infection at vertebrae, sacroiliac joints, and costal cartilage.[347–349] In neonates joint infection typically occurs following disseminated candidiasis.[350,351] The arthritis generally occurs concomitant with, or shortly after, fungemia but in some cases may not manifest until much later.[352,353] Treatment consists of joint aspiration, systemic therapy, and removal of any infected hardware.[354–360] Intra-articular AmB has been utilized in refractory cases and may be a useful adjunct to systemic therapy.[361]

Osteomyelitis may occur following direct inoculation or with hematogenously disseminated disease.[362] Candidal mediastinitis can complicate surgical sternotomy.[363] Common manifestations are chest wall erythema, drainage, fever, and sternal instability. Most patients present within a month of sternotomy. Treatment is prolonged and relapses are common.[364] Surgical débridement and removal of sternotomy wires are often required. Spinal infections can occur following surgery or epidural catheterization or with disseminated candidiasis.[365–368] Most patients present with subacute back pain that may develop months after a transient episode of candidemia.[369,370]

Treatment often requires a combined medical and surgical approach with drainage of abscesses, débridement of devitalized tissue and prolonged courses of systemic antifungal therapy.[371–376]

Endophthalmitis

Endogenous candidal endophthalmitis occurs in association with disseminated candidiasis and may be the initial manifestation of candidemia. In addition to the typical risk factors for disseminated candidiasis, endogenous endophthalmitis has been reported in the postpartum period and in association with induced abortions.[377,378] Patients often complain of eye pain and may have blurred vision or spots in their visual fields. On examination there can be inflammation in the anterior chamber with a hypopyon. Fundoscopic exam may show one or more creamy-white, well-circumscribed lesions of the choroid and retina. These are often accompanied by inflammatory infiltrates in the vitreous.[379] The infection likely begins in the choroid and progresses anteriorly to the retinal layers.[379] In a rabbit model the ocular lesions are focal chorioretinitis with both granulomatous and acute suppurative reactions.[380] In a study of enucleated globes from patients with candidal endophthalmitis, the vitreous was the primary focus of infection.[381]

Studies evaluating candidemic patients have reported widely varying rates for lesions consistent with candidal endophthalmitis. Recent reports have shown a decline in the percentage of cases of candidemia-associated endophthalmitis from nearly 30% in 1989 to less than 2% in 2002.[382–386] The reasons for such disparities are not clear, but may be related to differences in the stringency of case definitions used in the studies. Observation of the pathognomonic three-dimensional retina-based vitreal inflammatory lesions is uncommon, whereas nonspecific findings that may be attributed to candidal endophthalmitis (such as cotton wool spots, retinal hemorrhages, and Roth spots) are frequent.[387] Alternative explanations for the decline are the more aggressive antifungal therapies currently in use and the changing epidemiology of candidemia. Of note, in a rabbit model of endogenous endophthalmitis ocular tissues were found to have increased resistance to hematogenous infections with species other than *C. albicans*.[388] Because candidal endophthalmitis can lead to significant visual loss or blinding, it is reasonable to assess for this complication with fundoscopic examination in patients with disseminated candidiasis.

Infections of the cornea and the intraocular structures following direct inoculation trauma or surgery have been described.[379,389] An outbreak of postsurgical *C. parapsilosis* endophthalmitis was traced to a contaminated lot of irrigating solution.[390]

Treatment depends on the extent of infection. When infection is limited to choroiditis or very minimal endophthalmitis, systemic antifungal treatment may suffice; however, if symptoms of vitritis persist or progress, a vitrectomy may be necessary.[391] Systemic therapy with AmB or fluconazole in conjunction with vitrectomy (with or without intravitreal AmB) has been used successfully in cases of advanced endogenous endophthalmitis.[392,393] In one reported series success was achieved with oral fluconazole 100–200 mg daily for approximately 2 months.[394] In cases of vitritis, early vitrectomy may improve outcomes.[395] Regardless of the therapy, final visual acuity outcomes depend most on the site of initial choroiditis, such that if the macula is spared and preretinal membranes can be effectively removed, visual acuity results can be good.[391]

Intra-Abdominal Infections

Candidal peritonitis most commonly occurs with continuous ambulatory peritoneal dialysis (CAPD) or gastrointestinal injury. Rarely, spontaneous infections occur in patients with chronic liver failure and ascites. CAPD has emerged as an acceptable form of dialysis in some developing countries.[396,397] *Candida* species account for 2.5–6% of CAPD-associated peritonitis.[398–400] Risk factors include recurrent bacterial peritonitis and antibiotic exposure.[400–403] Clusters of infection have been described including an outbreak of *C. tropicalis* peritonitis that was traced to contaminated water baths.[404] Manifestations include abdominal pain, fever, cloudy dialysate, and elevated fluid white blood cell count with a predominance of neutrophils.[405,406] Treatment requires antifungal therapy and removal of the infected catheter.[402,407–410]

Candida species may be isolated from the peritoneal fluid of patients with injury to the gastrointestinal tract.[411,412] Positive peritoneal cultures do not always indicate infection. In a series of patients with *Candida* species isolated from the peritoneum, less than 40% had evidence of infection (intra-abdominal abscess and/or peritonitis).[413] In neonates *Candida* species may be present at the site of intestinal perforation (candidal enteritis of the newborn) or in the peritoneum in necrotizing enterocolitis.[412,414–417] In patients with liver disease and ascites, candidal peritonitis may be spontaneous or secondary to gastrointestinal perforation.[418–420] Pancreatic abscesses due to *Candida* species can occur in association with pancreatitis and pancreatic pseudocysts and as a complication of endoscopic retrograde choledochopancreatography.[421–423]

Chronic Disseminated Candidiasis

The syndrome of chronic disseminated candidiasis (CDC) occurs in neutropenic patients, particularly those receiving therapy for acute leukemia.[424] Multiple organs, including the lungs, kidney, liver, and spleen, can be involved. The diagnosis is typically made after resolution of the neutropenia. Clinical and laboratory features include fever, abdominal pain, hepatomegaly, and elevated serum alkaline phosphatase levels. Abdominal ultrasound or CT scans showing low-density lesions of the liver, spleen and kidneys, hepatomegaly, and hepatosplenomegaly are diagnostic.[425,426] Magnetic resonance imaging can assist in distinguishing acute, subacute treated and chronic healed CDC.[427–429] Laparoscopy typically shows yellowish nodules which can then be biopsied.[430] The histopathology may show large granulomas with yeasts and pseudohyphae.[431] Systemic antifungal treatment has been successful, but needs to be prolonged, sometimes for months, until resolution of the lesions.[424,427,432–434] The presence of CDC does not preclude further chemotherapy and does not constitute a contraindication to marrow transplantation provided that antifungal therapy is continued.[435,436]

Bloodstream Infections

Candida species constitute an important pathogen in bloodstream infections. The vast majority of cases occur in hospitalized patients, and 25–50% are in ICUs.[437,438] ICU and burn/trauma patients have numerous risk factors and increased incidence of candidemia.[439] As a whole *Candida* species are the fourth most common cause of nosocomial bloodstream infections in children and adults.[314,440]

The incidence of candidemia seems to be higher in Latin America than in the northern hemisphere. A multicenter prospective laboratory-based survey conducted in 11 tertiary care centers in Brazil showed a rate of 2.49 cases per 1000 admissions and 0.37 episodes per 1000 patient-days.[441] These rates are 2–15 times higher than those reported in centers in the northern hemisphere, including the United States (0.28–0.96 per 1000 admissions), Canada (0.45 per 1000 admissions), and Europe (0.17–0.81 per 1000 admissions) but similar to those reported at a single center in Taiwan.[441–451] The reasons for these differences are not clear, but may be due to a combination of multiple factors including differences in resources available for medical care and training programs, difficulties in the implementation of infection control programs in hospitals of developing countries, limited number of health care workers to assist patients in critical care units, and less aggressive practices of empirical antifungal therapy and prophylaxis in high-risk patients. Crude and attributable mortalities of approximately 60% and 40%, respectively, have been reported for nosocomial candidemia.[452,453]

C. albicans is the most common cause of nosocomial candidemia, but nearly half of cases are due to other species.[42,454] Clusters of infection and outbreaks may occur in high-risk settings such as neonatal and surgical ICUs.[455–460] These may be facilitated by transmission of yeast between patients, presumably via health care workers' hands.[458] Autoinfection after previous colonization with *Candida* species of gastrointestinal tract origin has also been demonstrated.[461]

Intravenous lines, drains, and intracranial pressure monitors can serve as conduits for introduction of yeast to the bloodstream. Broad-spectrum antibiotics leading to candidal overgrowth are another risk.[462] The anesthetic agent propofol has been implicated in several outbreaks due to extrinsic transmission by anesthesia staff.[463,464] Pressure-monitoring devices (transducers) can provide a portal of entry for systemic infections and have been implicated in several outbreaks.[465–467] The mechanism of infection was attributed to the lack of proper disinfection of reusable transducers. No further outbreaks have been reported since the use of disposable systems.

The incidence of nosocomial *Candida* infections, including outbreaks, in neonatal intensive care units (NICUs) has been increasing.[455–457,460,468–471] Acquisition of *Candida* may be from the mother or exogenous sources such as contaminated fluids, the NICU environment or health care worker's hands.[456,457,459,460,472,473] Risk factors include prematurity, especially very low birth weight neonates, use of broad-spectrum antibiotics, prolonged mechanical ventilation, coagulopathy, parenteral nutrition, catheterization of central vessels, antacids, and prolonged NICU stays.[474] Clinical manifestations include abdominal distension, poor peripheral perfusion, and fever.[475] *C. albicans* remains the most common species in this setting, but rates of non-*albicans* species, especially *C. parapsilosis*, are increasing.[460,475,476] In general, *C. parapsilosis* is less virulent than *C. albicans*. However, in neonates the overall mortality rate is comparable for both pathogens.[477,478]

C. parapsilosis candidemia is frequently associated with vascular devices, and rates vary widely across studies and geographic locales.[454,479–481] *C. tropicalis* is usually associated with cancer and neutropenia. It accounts for 2–10% of candidemias in Europe, 10–12% in the United States and Canada, and 15–40% in Asia, the Middle East and South America.[482–498] The wide use of fluconazole in Europe and North America may have contributed to a recent decrease in incidence of *C. tropicalis* candidemia.[499]

Blood cultures are primary means for establishing the diagnosis of candidal bloodstream infection, and positive cultures should be considered significant unless proven otherwise. Blood cultures are often negative despite disseminated disease. In an autopsy series *Candida* species were isolated from blood in 11 of 19 patients (58%) with disseminated infection.[500] Non-culture-based diagnostic tests are urgently needed, and assays for fungal D-arabinitol, mannans, glucans, anti-candidal antibodies and PCR are currently in various stages of development.

Choice of therapy for candidemia depends upon patient status and antifungal susceptibility pattern of the infecting isolate. The echinocandins appear to be the most effective agents for the treatment of candidemia. They are fungicidal for *Candida*, are active against virtually all *Candida* species, and have a very good safety profile. AmB is another option. AmB lipid complex (ABLC) and liposomal AmB (LAMB, AmBisome) are suitable for treatment of serious infections and have less toxicity than AmB deoxycholate. In stable patients in whom azole resistance is not a concern, fluconazole is a very good option.[501]

Recommendations regarding the choice of antifungal therapy have recently been published by the Infectious Diseases Society of America.[89] In stable patients who have not received previous therapy with an azole, treatment with fluconazole at a loading dose of 12 mg/kg followed by 6 mg/kg daily seems to be appropriate. Alternatively, intravenous treatment with an echinocandin (caspofungin: loading dose of 70 mg, then 50 mg daily; micafungin: 100 mg daily; anidulafungin: loading dose of 200 mg, then 100 mg daily) can be used as primary therapy.[502–504] In clinically unstable or neutropenic patients infected with an unknown species, an echinocandin is the initial drug of choice. AmB at ≥0.6 mg/kg daily, a lipid formulation of AmB (3 mg/kg daily) and voriconazole at 6 mg/kg for two doses, followed by 3 mg/kg daily are also options for such patients, but are associated with more toxicities and potential drug interactions than the echinocandins. For infections due to *C. parapsilosis*, fluconazole is recommended, but this agent should be avoided in cases of *C. krusei*. Treatment of candidemia should be continued for 2 weeks after the last positive blood culture and clinical resolution of infection. Patients may be transitioned to fluconazole during therapy providing that they have become stable and the isolate is susceptible to this drug. In non-neutropenic patients with positive blood cultures, rapid identification of *Candida* to the species level with PNA-FISH facilitates transition to fluconazole. Neonates with disseminated candidiasis are usually treated with AmB.

Whether all central venous catheters (CVCs) should be removed in patients with candidemia is an area of controversy. The catheter may be the primary source of infection, secondarily infected, or not infected at all. If feasible, removal of catheters is generally recommended in non-neutropenic patients with candidemia. In patients with catheter-related candidemia, mortality is higher when the catheters are retained (41% versus 21%, $P < 0.001$).[505] Removal of catheters results in more rapid clearance of the bloodstream.[506] In neonates, removal of the CVC within 3 days of the first positive blood culture reduces the duration of candidemia and mortality.[507] The situation is less clear in patients with implanted CVC and candidemia that is not obviously related to the device. For example, candidemia occurring in the setting of neutropenia is likely due to translocation of yeast across the gut wall. In such patients removal of the catheter, which is frequently tunneled, may be unnecessarily risky, and many authorities recommend retaining it if the patient is clinically stable.[89] For patients in whom the vascular catheter is infected but cannot be removed, salvage of the device may be attempted with medical therapy alone and with instillation of antibiotic lock solutions containing AmB.[91,508–510]

Additionally antifungal prophylaxis may have a role in selected patients at high risk for invasive candidiasis, such as those with leukemia, recipients of bone marrow and liver transplants, and very low birth weight neonates.[511–515] The role of antifungal prophylaxis in critically ill adults is less clear. In patients with recurrent gastrointestinal perforation or anastomotic leakage, fluconazole can reduce intra-abdominal candidal infections.[516] In high-risk, critically ill patients, fluconazole prophylaxis reduces the incidence of candidiasis, but does not appear to impact survival.[517–519] The role of echinocandins for prevention of invasive candidiasis in high-risk, critically ill patients is the subject of an ongoing prospective, multicenter study.

Early initiation of antifungal therapy in critically ill patients with invasive candidiasis may decrease mortality.[520] However, identification of such patients has proved challenging. In a prospective study of critically ill adults with risk factors for invasive candidiasis and fever, empirical fluconazole was no better than placebo.[521] Recent work has focused upon better identifying subsets of patients for targeted prophylaxis or empirical treatment. Risk stratification strategies include clinical prediction rules, measurements of the intensity of fungal colonization, and early fungal detection assays.

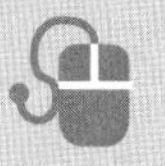

Access the complete reference list online at
http://www.expertconsult.com

Access the complete reference list online at
http://www.expertconsult.com

CHAPTER 89

Mucormycosis

Thomas J. Walsh • Emmanuel Roilides • John H. Rex • Michael R. McGinnis

INTRODUCTION

The class of Zygomycetes includes the medically important orders Mucorales and Entomophthorales. Infections caused by members of the class of Zygomycetes are broadly termed "zygomycosis," while those caused by the members of the order Mucorales may be termed "mucormycosis" and those cause by members of the order Entomophthorales are designated by the term of "entomophthoramycosis" (see Chapter 90).

The Mucorales cause most known cases of human disease.[1–5] Zygomycosis caused by the Mucorales ("mucormycosis") is characterized by a rapidly evolving course, angioinvasion, and tissue necrosis in immunocompromised hosts worldwide. As the term "Zygomycetes" is currently being reassessed and as advances in molecular taxonomy are revealing new mycological relationships, the term "mucormycosis" is used when referring to the infections caused by members of the order Mucorales.

MICROBIOLOGY

Among 465 cases of microbiologically documented cases of zygomycosis, *Rhizopus oryzae* is the most commonly reported single species.[5] Other medically important *Rhizopus* species include *R. rhizopodiformis* and *R. microsporus*. After *Rhizopus*, the genus *Mucor* is the second most commonly reported. *Rhizopus* spp. and *Mucor* spp. are followed by *Cunninghamella bertholletiae*, *Apophysomyces elegans*, and *Absidia* spp. (*Mycocladus* spp. or *Lictheimia* spp.) in frequency of reporting.

Members of the order Mucorales are identified to the genus or species level according to colonial morphology, microscopic morphology, and growth temperature. Microscopic characterization of non-septate hyphae, rhizoids, columellae, sporangia, and sporangiospores help to define genus and species within the order Mucorales. A detailed microbiological description of the Mucorales is reviewed in-depth.[6]

Identification of the Mucorales to the genus or species level carries valuable epidemiological, therapeutic, and prognostic implications. For example, *R. oryzae* is the most common Zygomycete recovered from clinical specimens but tends to be resistant to posaconazole; *M. circenelloides* is less commonly isolated but is more susceptible to posaconazole. *Cunninghamella* tends to have higher minimal inhibitory concentrations (MICs) to amphotericin B (AmB) and a higher overall mortality.

In order to optimize growth, clinical specimens should be inoculated onto appropriate media such as Sabouraud glucose agar and incubated at room temperature. Grinding or homogenization of tissue specimens may destroy the delicate hyphae, rendering cultures negative.[7] Recovery in culture is enhanced if tissue is sliced into small pieces before inoculation onto media. Close collaboration between clinicians and the microbiology laboratory is essential to ensure proper handling of the specimen. Although the Mucorales are angioinvasive, blood cultures are rarely positive unless there is involvement within the lumen of a vascular catheter.

Colonies typically appear within 24–48 hours unless residual antifungal agents, such as AmB are present which can suppress growth. Most mucoraceous species fill a culture dish within 3–5 days and demonstrate a grayish white, aerial mycelium with a woolly texture. The colonies readily separate from the agar surface. There are currently no biochemical, nucleic acid, or serological means to aid in species determination in routine operations of clinical microbiology laboratories.

PATHOGENESIS AND HOST-PATHOGEN INTERACTIONS

The principal mode of acquisition of the fungal elements of the Mucorales is inhalation of sporangiospores from environmental sources. Following inhalation, sporangiospores are deposited in the nasal turbinates, paranasal sinuses, and pulmonary alveoli where they can precipitate allergic sinusitis and interstitial pneumonitis in immunocompetent hosts[8–11] or invasive sinus infection and pneumonia in immunocompromised patients.[12]

In diabetic and other immunocompromised patients the inhaled fungi invade tissues, causing destructive sinus and pulmonary infections. Percutaneous exposure following traumatic implantation of sporangiospores may lead to necrotizing cutaneous infection in immunocompromised hosts.[13] Needle sticks,[14] catheter exit sites,[15,16] and tattoos[17] have all been implicated in local or disseminated disease. Mucormycosis in areas of skin breakdown, most commonly surgical sites and burn wounds, has been associated with use of adhesive products, arm boards, and elastic bandages.[18–21] Ingestion of contaminated milk, vegetables, bread, and herbal remedies has been implicated in gastrointestinal mucormycosis in neonates and other immunocompromised hosts.[22] Further underscoring the introduction of sporangiospores through contaminated fomites, oropharyngeal mucormycosis has been related to contaminated tongue depressors in immunocompromised patients with cancer.[23]

Functional effector cells, including tissue macrophages and neutrophils in sufficient quantity, are needed to mount an effective response to the sporangiospores and hyphal elements of the Mucorales. Pulmonary alveolar and other tissue macrophages ingest and then kill sporangiospores by non-oxidative mechanisms, thereby preventing their germination to hyphae.[24,25] If germination of sporangiospores evades or escapes this first line of defense, functional neutrophils are required to damage hyphae and prevent their invasion of surrounding tissue.[26]

Qualitative and quantitative abnormalities of neutrophils, monocytes, and macrophages increase the risk for development of mucormycosis. Infections typically occur when several layers of innate host defenses are simultaneously impaired due to intrinsic or iatrogenic abnormalities. For example, in patients with diabetes mellitus, monocytes and macrophages fail to suppress germination of sporangiospores. Diabetic ketoacidosis is associated with impairments in neutrophil function including chemotaxis, adherence, and oxidative burst.[27–31]

In addition to defective neutrophil and monocytic cell function, altered iron metabolism is a critical factor in the pathogenesis of patients with diabetes mellitus. There is an increased availability of unbound serum iron, which can then be utilized by the organism, in ketoacidosis, and possibly in other metabolic acidoses.[32–36] As patients with adult-onset type 2 diabetes mellitus without metabolic acidosis are increasingly observed as presenting with mucormycosis, other mechanisms for releasing free iron are hypothesized.[5] The excessive glycosylation of proteins, such as transferrin and ferritin, also results in decreased affinity for iron and its availability as the free ion to *R. oryzae* and other Mucorales. The crucial role of iron in the pathogenesis of mucormycosis is further underscored by an increased susceptibility to infection during chronic deferoxamine therapy and in iron overload states.[37–39] Deferoxamine acts as an iron chelator in humans but as a siderophore for *R. oryzae*, thereby facilitating iron uptake and enhancement of fungal growth.[40]

Angioinvasion with thrombosis and tissue necrosis is a key pathophysiological feature of human Mucorales infections.[41,42] *In vitro,* living and even nonviable germinated *R. oryzae* sporangiospores adhere to and are phagocytosed by endothelial cells, resulting in endothelial damage.[43]

EPIDEMIOLOGY

Mucormycosis is a relatively uncommon infection, occurring approximately 10-fold and 50-fold less frequently, respectively, than invasive candidiasis or aspergillosis. The annual estimated incidence of zygomycosis in the United States is 1.7 cases/million.[44] The male to female ratio of affected patients is approximately 2 : 1.[5] The pathophysiological basis for this predilection of zygomycosis for males is not currently known.

The most common underlying illnesses of mucormycosis are diabetes mellitus, hematological malignancies, and hematopoietic stem cell transplantation (HSCT) and solid organ transplantation.[5] Among these populations, the possible risk factors for mucormycosis include prolonged neutropenia, corticosteroid use, and graft versus host disease (GVHD).

Patients with hematological malignancy, solid organ or hematopoietic stem cell transplantation comprise an increasingly greater proportion of patients with mucormycosis since the 1980s.[5] This trend coincides with improved control of hyperglycemia in diabetics and a concurrent increase in the incidence of mucormycosis at many large cancer centers.[45–47] Among other biologically plausible hypotheses accounting for this evolving pattern are (1) improved post-transplantation survival rates and changes in transplant procedures, (2) use of more aggressive immunosuppressive regimens that include high doses of corticosteroids, (3) voriconazole prophylaxis creating a mycological vacuum in which the Mucorales may emerge, and (4) a direct modulating effect of voriconazole on the fungal pathogen to increase virulence. Laboratory and epidemiological data from several studies support the hypotheses that voriconazole use and high intensity immunosuppression have contributed to this increase.[48–53] As voriconazole is increasingly used prophylactically in HSCT recipients, it likely exerts selective pressure for growth of resistant fungi, such as Mucorales, in high-risk patients. That a large multicenter, blinded clinical trial comparing voriconazole with fluconazole for prophylaxis in HSCT recipients did not demonstrate a difference in breakthrough mucormycosis may be related to the moderate risk for invasive fungal infections in this population and to the protocol-defined use of empirical antifungal therapy with lipid formulation of AmB, which would have activity against *Rhizopus* spp. and other Mucorales.[54]

Mucormycosis also may develop in patients who are not diabetic and who are not pharmacologically immunosuppressed. Among these patients are intravenous drug users and chronic recipients of the iron-chelating agent deferoxamine. Consistent with advances in management of chronic renal disease that have reduced the need for iron and aluminum chelation, there has been a dramatic decline in the frequency of reported cases of deferoxamine-associated mucormycosis.[5] Moreover, the expanded use of deferasirox, which does not increase the risk of mucormycosis, also would also reduce the need for desferrioxamine.

The Mucorales may infect apparently immunocompetent individuals without any known risk factors.[5,54–58] Whether such patients may have undetected haplotypes of allelic polymorphisms in genes encoding innate host defense molecules is not well understood. Mucormycosis also may develop in hospitalized populations including those in high-risk nurseries,[59] general surgical wards,[60,61] cardiac surgery,[62] and burn and trauma units.[63–66] The Mucorales also may cause occupational illnesses in workers in the malt and lumber industries.[67]

The epidemiological trends of zygomycosis may differ by country.[68] Diwakar and colleagues reported that among 461 cases of zygomycosis in India, rhino-orbito-cerebral infections, occurring in 269 (58%), were the most common manifestation. Cutaneous disease in 66 cases (14%) was the second most common form.[68] In contrast to cases from North America and Europe, where transplant recipients and patients with hematological malignancies are increasingly reported with zygomycosis, the most common risk factor in India was uncontrolled diabetes mellitus.

CLINICAL MANIFESTATIONS

The clinical manifestations of mucormycosis may be classified as sinus (localized or extended to the orbit and/or brain), pulmonary, cutaneous, gastrointestinal, miscellaneous, and disseminated infection. Sinus infection is the most common presentation.[5] Patients with diabetes mellitus most commonly present with sinus disease but seldom with pulmonary infection; whereas, neutropenic patients frequently develop pulmonary infection, as well as sinus disease.[5] As the clinical manifestations of invasive mucormycosis may be nonspecific, an otherwise unexplained infection in the appropriate setting should alert physicians to the possibility of this infection.

Sinus Mucormycosis

Mucormycosis frequently presents as invasive sinusitis.[69,70] Approximately two-thirds of cases occur in diabetics, often with ketoacidosis; however, sinus infection may also occur in association with other forms of immunosuppression, including neutropenia, HSCT, and solid organ transplantation. The process can remain within the paranasal sinuses or progress to the orbit (sino-orbital) and/or brain parenchyma (rhinocerebral). Progression of infection with extension to neighboring tissues from the sinuses may be rapid and constitutes a medical and surgical emergency in compromised hosts. The ethmoid sinus is a critical site from which infection may extend through the lamina papyracea into the orbit, extraocular muscles, eye, and optic nerve. The brain may be seeded by invasion of the ethmoidal and orbital veins, which drain into the cavernous sinuses.

The initial clinical features of sinus mucormycosis include nasal congestion, dark blood-tinged rhinorrhea or epistaxis, sinus tenderness, retro-orbital headache, fever, and malaise.[71] More advanced sinus infection may present as facial or periorbital swelling and numbness, blurred vision, lacrimation, chemosis, diplopia, proptosis, and loss of vision in the affected eye.[72,73] A painful black necrotic ulceration may develop on the hard palate, indicating extension from the maxillary sinus into the oral cavity.

Nasal endoscopy may reveal necrotic ulcers along the nasal mucosa or turbinates.[71] Infection can extend to adjacent bone and ultimately to the skull base. Progression to the central nervous system occurs via the optic nerve or from the ethmoid sinuses by way of the cavernous sinus. Abnormal mentation often signifies cerebral involvement. Vision loss, ophthalmoplegia, corneal anesthesia and facial anhidrosis may indicate cavernous sinus thrombosis,[74,75] which may be further complicated by internal carotid artery thrombosis with contralateral hemiplegia.[76,77]

Sinusitis with acute onset of blurred vision or diplopia in a diabetic or otherwise immunocompromised patient should prompt careful clinical and radiological evaluation for mucormycosis, as well as rapid therapeutic intervention. One should note that the clinical manifestations of cavernous sinus thrombosis may precede radiological findings in the central nervous system. Thus, medical interventions and surgical consultation should not be delayed when cavernous sinus thrombosis is clinically evident but not yet apparent in diagnostic imaging studies.

Computed tomography (CT) and magnetic resonance imaging (MRI) of the sinuses are superior to plain films for delineating the extent of infection and can guide surgical débridement. The principal radiographic findings of mucormycosis of the sinuses are opacification of the paranasal sinuses, fluid levels, bone destruction, and osteomyelitis.[78–80]

Pulmonary Mucormycosis

Lower respiratory tract infection develops most frequently in severely immunocompromised patients, particularly those with hematological malignancies and allogeneic HSCT. Key factors associated with development of pulmonary mucormycosis include prolonged and profound neutropenia, corticosteroid use, and GVHD.[81–84] Pulmonary disease also develops in solid organ transplant recipients.[85–87]

Pulmonary mucormycosis may appear radiologically as solitary lung nodules, segmental or lobar consolidation, halo signs, and cavitary or bronchopneumonic lesions. Persistent fevers and pulmonary infiltrates refractory to broad-spectrum antibacterial agents in a compromised patient should suggest fungal pneumonia. As the presentation of pulmonary mucormycosis is similar to that of invasive pulmonary aspergillosis, a diagnostic procedure such as bronchoalveolar lavage (BAL) is important.

The pulmonary lesions of mucormycosis typically are rapidly progressive in compromised hosts. Invasion of pulmonary vessels may lead to thrombosis and pulmonary infarcts. Infection may extend across tissue planes to involve the chest wall, pericardium, myocardium, superior vena cava, and diaphragm.[88,89] Invasion of the great vessels may lead to aneurysm formation with fatal hemoptysis,[90–93] as well as endobronchial disease with airway obstruction.[94,95] High-resolution CT is superior to plain chest radiographs for early diagnosis and for delineating the extent of pulmonary and mediastinal involvement. The air crescent and halo signs, which are typically associated with invasive pulmonary aspergillosis, may also be observed in pulmonary mucormycosis. As lower respiratory tract infection may occur alone, concomitant with sinus disease, or as part of a disseminated process, radiological assessment of extrapulmonary sites should be considered in the initial evaluation.

There are some features in pulmonary mucormycosis that may be helpful in distinguishing this infection from pulmonary aspergillosis. The reversed halo sign, which was seen in approximately 4% of patients with pulmonary mycoses, is most frequently observed in patients with mucormycosis.[96] A review of clinical features and CT findings observed that patients with cancer and pulmonary mucormycosis ($n = 16$) in comparison to contemporaneous patients with cancer and pulmonary aspergillosis ($n = 29$) have a higher frequency of concomitant sinusitis (odds ratio (OR), 25.7; 95% confidence interval (CI), 1.47–448.15; $P = 0.026$), history of voriconazole prophylaxis (OR, 7.76; 95% CI, 1.32–45.53; $P = 0.023$), presence of multiple (≥10) nodules (OR, 19.8; 95% CI, 1.94–202.29; $P = .012$) and pleural effusions (OR, 5.07; 95% CI, 1.06–24.23; $P = 0.042$).[97]

Cutaneous Mucormycosis

Cutaneous mucormycosis may be confined to the skin and subcutaneous tissues, extend into adjacent soft tissue and even bony structures, or serve as a source for disseminated infection.[98–103] Unlike cutaneous fusariosis, cutaneous mucormycosis seldom disseminates to the skin from a distant site with multiple lesions.[104] Cutaneous mucormycosis most commonly occurs after primary inoculation of the skin. With direct inoculation of the organism in a compromised host, infection usually presents with signs of acute inflammation with edema, induration, and necrosis. The lesions are initially erythematous and indurated, but often progress to form necrotic eschars. The eschars are typically dark and firm with a woody consistency in more advanced stages. Necrotic tissue may also ulcerate.[105–108] While primary cutaneous infections disrupt the epidermis and may invade adipose tissue, muscle, fascia, and bone, cutaneous lesions developing from disseminated mucormycosis tend to be nodular with only minimal destruction of the epidermis.

There are important prognostic implications to the staging of lesions of cutaneous mucormycosis. Among 176 patients with cutaneous mucormycosis, patients with localized infection had an overall mortality of 10% and deep extension in 26%, while those with cutaneous lesions as part of a disseminated process had a 94% mortality.[5] Recognizing that most cases of cutaneous mucormycosis are the result of direct inoculation provides a rationale for urgent local surgical control in order to prevent dissemination to other sites in immunocompromised hosts.

Recognition and removal of an environmental source of cutaneous inoculation may help to prevent recurrences in immunocompromised patients. Although *R. oryzae* is the most frequently recovered organism from lesions of cutaneous mucormycosis, *Apophysomyces elegans* is particularly prevalent in the subset of patients with a history of skin and soft tissue trauma in subtropical arid and desert regions.[109]

Gastrointestinal Mucormycosis

Gastrointestinal infection is an uncommon form of mucormycosis. Typically occurring after ingestion of sporangiospores by malnourished patients, premature neonates, or immunocompromised hosts,[56,110–119] gastrointestinal mucormycosis carries a reported mortality of 85%.[5] While the stomach, ileum, and large intestine are the most commonly infected sites, virtually any part of the gastrointestinal tract may be affected. As the organisms may invade the mucosa, submucosa, and vascular structures, bowel wall perforation and peritonitis caused by mixed flora of Mucorales and bacteria may ensue. Early recognition of the clinical manifestations of gastrointestinal mucormycosis, including fever, nausea, vomiting, hematemesis, abdominal pain and distension, and hematochezia, may allow for prompt surgical and medical interventions.[116,119]

Other Forms of Mucormycosis

Endocarditis and isolated cerebral, renal or peritoneal infection are uncommon but potentially lethal manifestations of mucormycosis. Endocardial mucormycosis occurs typically in the setting of prosthetic valves or other cardiac surgery, but may also develop in immunosuppressed patients, hemodialysis recipients, and intravenous drug users.[120–124] Infected emboli may disseminate from large, valvular vegetations and cause distal infarctions. Endocardial infection also may extend transmurally to involve the myocardial wall and pericardium with substernal chest pain and tamponade.

Isolated mucormycosis of the central nervous system (CNS) may develop in immunocompromised patients and in users of illicit intravenous drugs.[125–128] Focal neurological deficits, including hemiparesis, loss of visual fields, seizures and cranial nerve deficits, may be the earliest clinical manifestations of isolated CNS mucormycosis. Cerebral mucormycosis is clinically indistinguishable from CNS aspergillosis.[129] Patients sustaining open head trauma may suffer direct inoculation of fungi into CNS tissue.[130]

Solitary renal mucormycosis occurs in the setting of illicit intravenous drug use or contamination of a central venous catheter.[131–134] The lesions of solitary renal zygomycosis may expand to occupy a large portion of the renal parenchyma before they elicit symptoms. Fever, flank pain, and hematuria may be present. Cytological analysis of the spun sediment of a 24-hour urine collection may establish an early diagnosis, especially in resource-limited settings where transcutaneous needle aspirate technology may not be readily available.

Disseminated Mucormycosis

Disseminated mucormycosis is defined by involvement of at least two non-contiguous sites. Roden et al described the crude mortality of disseminated mucormycosis as 94% to 100%.[5] Disseminated mucormycosis typically occurs in severely immunocompromised patients and in those receiving deferoxamine.[37,45,127,135–137] Although hematogenous dissemination may originate from any site, the lungs are the most common primary source of infection. That pulmonary mucormycosis may be complicated by fatal hematogenous dissemination underscores the importance of early diagnosis and therapeutic intervention.

DIAGNOSIS

The importance of early diagnosis and therapeutic intervention was recently demonstrated by Chamilos and colleagues, who found that a delay in initiation of AmB was associated with a significant increase in overall mortality.[138] As the symptoms, signs, and radiographic manifestations of mucormycosis are nonspecific, a definitive diagnosis requires direct identification of characteristic hyphae and/or recovery of the organism in culture from specimens obtained from the site of infection. Direct examination of sputum, paranasal sinus secretions, or BAL fluid is frequently nondiagnostic, but recovery of Mucorales from these specimens from a susceptible host should be considered as compelling evidence for infection.[139–141] Establishing a diagnosis of pulmonary mucormycosis may also reveal concomitant infections caused by other organisms, including *Aspergillus* spp. and other fungal pathogens.[142]

Samples for direct microscopy by wet mount, cytopathological studies, or histopathologic examination may be collected by radiographically guided percutaneous needle aspirate, transbronchial, or direct biopsies of infected lesions. Histopathology reliably establishes the diagnosis of mucormycosis, but obtaining biopsy material from deep tissue sites is frequently difficult in patients with thrombocytopenia or coagulopathies.

Direct Examination and Histopathology

Direct microscopic examination is performed on all materials sent to the clinical laboratory. Where possible, BAL fluid should be submitted for examination by clinical microbiology and cytopathology laboratories. Hyphae of the Mucorales are typically broad (6–16 µm in diameter), ribbon-like and irregularly shaped, non-septate (coenocytic) or sparsely septate, with branches often arising non-dichotomously at "right angles." Hyphae of the Mucorales may be difficult to observe on an unenhanced potassium hydroxide (KOH) wet mount and may not stain well with conventional Gram stain. The use of chitin-binding stains, such as calcofluor, fungifluor, or blancofluor, may be used with a fluorescence microscope to identify hyphal elements on KOH wet mounts.[143] McDermott and colleagues recently reported the use of calcofluor-stained tissue as a rapid technique for intraoperative diagnosis and assessment of clean resected margins in lieu of frozen sections by pathology.[144] Molecular diagnostic assays for rapid and early detection of mucormycosis are being developed but remain investigational at this time.[145]

The Mucorales are usually distinguishable histologically from other filamentous fungi, such as *Aspergillus* spp, *Fusarium* spp, and *Pseudallescheria boydii,* which typically appear as slender dichotomously branching septate hyphae.[146] Distinction by direct examination may allow AmB and other potentially lifesaving therapeutic interventions to be initiated.

TREATMENT AND PROGNOSIS

Current therapy requires a multidisciplinary approach that relies on prompt institution of appropriate antifungal AmB, reversal of underlying predisposing conditions, and, where possible, surgical débridement of devitalized tissue. Outcomes are highly dependent upon the degree of immunosuppression, site and extent of infection, timeliness of therapy, and type of treatment provided.[5,147–149]

Antifungal Therapy with Amphotericin B

Amphotericin B (AmB) is the drug of choice for primary treatment of mucormycosis. The efficacy of AmB has been reproducibly demonstrated in both laboratory (*in vitro* and *in vivo*) investigations and clinical studies.[150–159] Although interpretive breakpoints for determination of *in vitro* susceptibility to AmB have not been determined, apparent *in vitro* resistance, with elevated MICs, may be observed in clinical isolates, especially among *Cunninghamella* species.[160–163] These *in vitro* properties are consistent with the poor prognosis of mucormycosis caused by *C. bertholettiae*, where among 34 reported cases, overall mortality was 76%.[5]

Underscoring the important therapeutic role of AmB in treatment of mucormycosis, a recent review demonstrated by multivariate analysis that antifungal therapy and surgery were significantly associated with survival, that survival was similar (61% versus 69% respectively; $P > 0.05$) for patients treated with conventional ($n = 532$) or lipid formulation AmB ($n = 116$), and that mortality was nearly uniform (97%) for those who received no treatment at all ($n = 241$).[5] Among the lipid formulations of AmB, including colloidal dispersion (ABCD), lipid complex (ABLC) and liposomal (LAmB), all have been used for treatment of mucormycosis.[5,159,164–181] The lipid formulations of AmB are at least as active as deoxycholate AmB and have less nephrotoxicity. Nonetheless, the efficacy of a lipid formulation of AmB versus deoxycholate AmB has not been evaluated in prospective randomized controlled studies of mucormycosis. As with many antifungal agents and mycoses, the optimal dosage for AmB and its formulations against mucormycosis has not been determined.

Selection of the highest dosage possible of AmB does not necessarily result in a more favorable outcome compared to a lower and less toxic dosage. The dosage of AmB for treatment of mucormycosis has ranged from 0.5 to 1.5 mg/kg per day. A dosage of 0.75–1.0 mg/kg per day is used by many physicians; however, these dosages may incur dose-limiting nephrotoxicity. Selection of a dosage is based upon published reports as well as careful assessment of individual patient tolerability of adverse effects. Where possible, a lipid formulation of AmB is preferable to deoxycholate AmB. However, in resource-challenged environments, deoxycholate AmB may be the only option available.

If a lipid formulation of AmB is available, the initial dosage of this class may be 5.0 mg/kg per day. ABLC at 5 mg/kg per day has been used as salvage treatment with complete or partial responses in 17/24 (71%) patients.[180] Dosages of LAmB as high as 15 mg/kg per day have been tolerated without substantial renal or infusion-related toxicity;[182] however, as plasma concentrations in that study peaked at 10 mg/kg per day, justification of higher daily dosages does not seem tenable. Therapy with LAmB at 10 mg/kg per day has been reported,[183] but such dosing has not been systematically compared with a standard dosage of 5 mg/kg per day. Daily dosages beyond 5 mg/kg (e.g., 7.5 or 10 mg/kg) may be considered on an individual basis, especially if there is CNS involvement. The length of therapy also should be individualized according to a patient's response and underlying condition. In the absence of definitive comparative studies of duration, continuation of antifungal therapy until complete resolution of signs and symptoms, particularly in immunocompromised patients, seems reasonable.

Antifungal Therapy with Posaconazole

Among the antifungal triazoles, fluconazole, voriconazole and itraconazole have little or no activity *in vitro* against the Mucorales.[160,161,163,183,184] Sporadic success has been reported with itraconazole for *Rhizopus* and cutaneous *Cunninghamella* infections.[185–187]

By comparison, posaconazole has more activity *in vitro* against the Mucorales than do the other aforementioned triazoles.[160,161,163,184,188] Laboratory animal studies, however, demonstrate variable activity against the Mucorales, depending upon the species. Experimental infections produced by *Mucor* spp. are most responsive to posaconazole, and those caused by *Rhizopus* spp. are unresponsive in most studies.[188–191] In contrast, individual case reports and several case series report that posaconazole is active in salvage therapy of patients with mucormycosis who are refractory to and/or are intolerant of AmB therapy.[3,192–196] A recent review concluded that based upon the current laboratory and clinical data, orally administered posaconazole may be useful as salvage therapy, but cannot be recommended as primary therapy for mucormycosis.[197] Further studies are needed to understand the pharmacokinetics and pharmacodynamics of this agent, particularly in the parenteral formulation, in order to better understand its potential role in primary treatment of mucormycosis.

Combination Antifungal Therapy with Echinocandins

By targeting different biochemical pathways, combination antifungal therapy may increase efficacy of AmB regimens. Although, the echinocandins *per se* have minimal activity against the Mucorales, when combined with AmB in a murine model of disseminated mucormycosis they augment antifungal activity and improve survival.[157,158] A retrospective clinical study of patients with mucormycosis was consistent with these experimental observations; i.e., patients receiving an echinocandin plus AmB had improved response rates.[159] A prospective clinical trial is warranted in order to ascertain whether the combination of AmB and echinocandin versus AmB alone is more effective as primary therapy in treatment of mucormycosis.

Combination Antifungal Therapy with Deferasirox

Deferoxamine increases the risk for development of disseminated and localized mucormycosis by serving as a false siderophore.[40] By comparison, hydroxypyridinone iron chelators, such as deferasirox, do not act as siderophores for the Zygomycetes and consequently are not associated with increased susceptibility to mucormycosis. Instead, deferasirox protects mice from mucormycosis through deprivation of iron from *R. oryzae*.[198] A recent case report of a patient with rhinocerebral mucormycosis illustrates the potential benefit of this combination therapy with deferasirox.[199] A randomized trial assessing the safety and efficacy of deferasirox with AmB versus AmB alone is necessary in order to further define the role of iron chelation as primary therapy for mucormycosis.

Hyperbaric Oxygen

Hyperbaric oxygen (HBO) is sometimes used as adjunctive therapy in management of mucormycosis. The laboratory foundation for treatment of mucormycosis with HBO includes the early observations that extended exposure to high pressures (10 atmospheres absolute, ATA) of 100% oxygen is fungicidal for some Mucorales and other fungi *in vitro*.[200–202] Shorter exposures and lower oxygen pressures retain a fungistatic effect on *Rhizopus* spp. and are achievable with clinically relevant doses of HBO. The antifungal effects of HBO are likely related to generation of oxygen-based free radicals. HBO also reduces tissue hypoxia and acidosis, and enhances neutrophil function and fibroblastic collagen production. However, results of laboratory animal studies are inconsistent, there are no randomized trials, and the potentially beneficial clinical effects of HBO are confounded by concomitant surgery and antifungal therapy. Favorable outcomes have been reported when HBO is used in conjunction with surgery and amphotericin B for sinus, cutaneous, and soft tissue mucormycosis.[200–205]

Among the potential adverse effects of HBO are pneumothorax, seizures, nausea, tinnitus, and visual abnormalities. As the chamber pressures of HBO were 2–2.5 ATA of 100% oxygen in most reported cases, CNS toxicity is uncommon at these doses. However, because of the uncontrolled nature of the clinical observations, HBO therapy cannot be recommended for routine primary treatment of mucormycosis.

Reversal of the Underlying Host Impairments

Correction of a patient's underlying host impairments is a critical condition for successful management of mucormycosis. For example, hyperglycemia and metabolic acidosis (particularly diabetic ketoacidosis) should be aggressively corrected. Among transplant recipients and patients with hematological malignancies, reduction or temporary discontinuation of corticosteroids or other immunosuppressive agents should be considered until the infection is controlled. When mucormycosis complicates deferoxamine therapy, that drug should be discontinued. As with other infections in neutropenia, response to therapy of mucormycosis hinges upon neutrophil recovery. With the exception of the single patient with severe aplastic anemia treated with granulocyte colony-stimulating factor (G-CSF), in a review of 26 neutropenic (≤500 cells/mm^3) patients with histologically documented disseminated mucormycosis occurring from 1959 through 1994, infections were uniformly fatal.[167] Granulocyte transfusions may also provide a temporizing strategy while supporting neutropenic patients until recovery from neutropenia.[206]

Immune recovery may be accelerated by treatment with G-CSF, granulocyte-macrophage colony-stimulating factor (GM-CSF), and interferon-γ (IFN-γ). G-CSF and GM-CSF stimulate production of neutrophils and/or monocytes and enhance their antifungal activity.[207–209] IFN-γ directly enhances the antifungal activity of host effector cells and induces development of Th1 responses, which further augment innate defenses against fungi.[210] *Ex vivo* incubation of neutrophils derived from transplant recipients with G-CSF enhances the oxidative respiratory burst against *Rhizopus* sporangiospores.[211] Similarly GM-CSF and IFN-γ augment the antifungal activity of neutrophils against *R. oryzae*, *R. microsporus*, and *Absidia* (*Mycocladus* or *Lichtheimia*) *corymbifera*.[209]

Both G-CSF and GM-CSF reduce the depth and duration of chemotherapy-induced neutropenia and diminish the frequency of infections and are included in many antineoplastic protocols for hematological malignancies and HSCT.[212–214] Individual reports of adjuvant therapy for mucormycosis with G-CSF, GM-CSF and IFN-γ have been published.[167,215,216] As a general principle, the use of recombinant cytokines G-CSF or GM-CSF for acceleration of recovery from neutropenia is biologically sound and supported by randomized trials. However, the efficacy of recombinant cytokines in non-neutropenic patients with mucormycosis has not been evaluated through adequately powered randomized controlled trials. Their use in such conditions should be individualized for each patient.

Granulocyte transfusions are an alternative approach for augmentation of innate phagocytic host defenses against invasive fungal infections.[206,217] Early studies of this therapeutic modality were limited by difficulties in collecting adequate doses of leukocytes from healthy steroid-mobilized donors. At this time efficacy data for neutrophil transfusion in mucormycosis are limited, and potential benefits should be weighed against known complications, including respiratory distress, alloimmunization, and anaphylaxis. Nonetheless, granulocyte transfusions with cytokine augmentation may provide critical support to a neutropenic host with a life-threatening infection until recovery from neutropenia ensues.[218] In resource-challenged environments, granulocyte transfusions and recombinant cytokines may not be available as adjunctive modalities.

Surgical Therapy

Surgical débridement is fundamental for successful management of mucormycosis. Infection is associated with angioinvasion and extensive necrosis, and thus antifungal therapy alone may be inadequate for control of infection. Surgery should be considered early in the course of treatment with the goal of removing all necrotic tissue. Repeated débridements are frequently necessary, and the extent of surgery should ideally be guided by evaluation of frozen tissue sections examined histologically or by fresh homogenized specimens stained by calcofluor.[144,219]

Compared with antifungal therapy alone, survival is enhanced with a combined medical/surgical approach.[5,70,149,220–222] The type of surgical procedure is dictated by the extent of the patient's infection. For maxillofacial infection, there is increasing emphasis on using less disfiguring surgical procedures while simultaneously controlling the infection with medical interventions.[144,197,199,223] For infections of the lung, resection of a solitary pulmonary lesion may be preferred if immune reconstitution is not imminent. For infections of the gastrointestinal tract, removal of the infected segment is necessary to prevent or treat life-threatening peritonitis. Infections of skin, soft tissue, muscle, and bone warrant débridement to viable tissue.

PREVENTION AND CONTROL

The most important strategy for prevention of mucormycosis consists of maintaining adequate host defenses. These include but are not limited to maintaining appropriate blood glucose in diabetics, shortening duration of neutropenia, and using corticosteroids and other immunosuppressive agents judiciously. Instructing patients to avoid aerosols of soil, dust, and debris may reduce exposure to large respiratory inocula of sporangiospores. Similarly, maintaining appropriate environmental control measures within health care facilities may also help to prevent acquisition of organisms.

Outbreaks and pseudo-outbreaks of nosocomial *Rhizopus* infections have been associated with construction, contaminated elastic bandages, wooden stick applicators, and tongue depressors.[15,18,19,60,84,224–231] Daily monitoring of skin covered by bandages or boards is an important component of meticulous wound care in immunocompromised patients. Construction activity in hospitals can increase the burden of airborne sporangiospores and the risk of sinopulmonary mucormycosis.[232,233]

Control of environmental transmission during hospital construction and renovation can be established with floor to ceiling impervious barriers.[84] Air conditioning and ventilation systems should be monitored for microbial contamination. While the use of high-efficiency particulate air (HEPA) filters in hospital rooms of profoundly immunosuppressed patients reduces the risk of development of aspergillosis and mucormycosis, financial constraints preclude many centers from routinely using these devices. Whether AmB formulations or posaconazole can prevent mucormycosis is conceptually plausible but has not been definitively demonstrated in clinical studies.

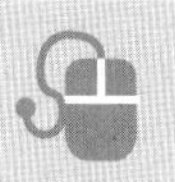

Access the complete reference list online at
http://www.expertconsult.com

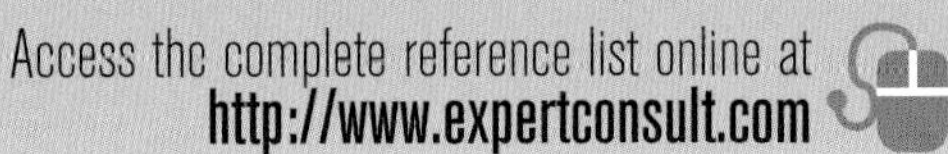
Access the complete reference list online at
http://www.expertconsult.com

CHAPTER 90

Entomophthoramycosis, Lobomycosis, Rhinosporidiosis, and Sporotrichosis

Duane R. Hospenthal

INTRODUCTION

Entomophthoramycosis, lobomycosis, rhinosporidiosis, and sporotrichosis are four diseases that are either restricted to, or occur predominantly in, tropical regions of the world. Each of these most commonly presents as lesions of the skin or mucous membranes. Though all were previously believed to be mycoses, the etiologic agent of rhinosporidiosis is now considered a protistan parasite. Entomophthoramycosis presents as a painless, firm, circumscribed subcutaneous mass, either involving the nose and surrounding face or a single area of the skin elsewhere. The overlying skin is usually normal, but may be reddened and shiny. Lobomycosis presents as a single, sharply circumscribed, painless, verrucous cutaneous papule or plaque. Rhinosporidiosis commonly presents as a single, soft, fleshy polyp of the nasal mucosa or palpebral conjunctiva. Sporotrichosis most often presents as one or more red nodules on the exposed skin that may ulcerate or have intermittent serosanguineous drainage.

ENTOMOPHTHORAMYCOSIS

Diseases caused by species of the genera *Basidiobolus* and *Conidiobolus* are recognized by many names. Together, they are most often denoted by the term entomophthoramycosis, reflecting the order Entomophthorales to which they belong. Unfortunately, this nomenclature appears in jeopardy, as recent molecular study has suggested that *Basidiobolus* should be moved out of the order Entomophthorales.[1] Individually, disease caused by *Basidiobolus ranarum* is termed basidiobolomycosis, and that due to *Conidiobolus coronatus*, conidiobolomycosis.

EPIDEMIOLOGY

Basidiobolomycosis is a subcutaneous infection that predominantly affects children and adolescents and has its highest prevalence in tropical Africa and Southeast Asia. It was first reported by Joe and colleagues in 1956 affecting three Indonesian children.[2] In one of the largest series, Mugerwa reported 80 cases of basidiobolomycosis from Uganda, in which a 5 : 3 male : female predominance was noted.[3] Although disease was observed in persons aged 1–58 years, 76% of those affected were under 10 years of age (and almost half were under 5 years old). Conidiobolomycosis is a submucosal rhinosinusitis occurring most frequently in adults in the tropics (especially in the tropical rainforests of West Africa). It was first described by Emmons and Bridges in 1961 as causing nasal polyps in horses.[4] The first human case was reported in 1965 by Bras and associates.[5] Until 1992, approximately 100 human cases had been reported.[6] *B. ranarum* and *C. coronatus* are found in nature in soil, decaying vegetation, and the intestinal tracts of amphibians, reptiles, and other animals.[7,8] Although these fungi can be recovered throughout the world, they favor warm, humid climates. *C. coronatus* requires 95% humidity to produce conidia, with maximal conidiation occurring at 100% humidity.[9]

THE DISEASE

While the fungi causing these diseases and their respective clinical manifestations differ, the pathologic findings in the two entomophthoramycoses are similar. Both cause indolent infection with granulomatous changes in the skin and subcutaneous tissues without bony or systemic involvement. Basidiobolomycosis presents with a solitary, asymptomatic, circumscribed, hard, subcutaneous mass usually located in the buttock or extremities. Sixty-five percent of patients in one report had disease confined to either the buttock (28 of 75) or thigh (21 of 75).[3] These lesions do not commonly involve muscle and may not involve overlying skin. Conidiobolomycosis most frequently begins in the submucosa of the nose, spreading to involve bilateral skin of the nasal region, the paranasal sinuses, and pharynx. The skin is firmly attached to underlying subcutaneous tissues and may appear normal, or reddened and shiny. Conidiobolomycosis may be asymptomatic or may be diagnosed after symptoms of nasal obstruction, rhinorrhea, or epistaxis. Bacterial sinusitis from obstruction of drainage may also lead to presentation. Entomophthoramycosis is most often slowly progressive, resulting in cosmetic disfigurement. Occasionally, long-standing infection may be complicated by obstruction of the lymphatics in basidiobolomycosis or the facial structures in conidiobolomycosis. More recently, cases of basidiobolomycosis affecting and confined to the gastrointestinal tract have been reported, including from Brazil, the United States, Saudi Arabia, and Kuwait, rarely with fatal outcome.[10–15] A handful of disseminated cases of *Basidiobolus* and *Conidiobolus* species (including one due to *C. coronatus*) have been reported.[15–21] Disease caused by *C. coronatus* similar to that in humans has been observed in sheep, llamas, horses, mules, dolphins, and a chimpanzee. More severe disease with associated dissemination has been reported in sheep, including a *C. incongruus* outbreak in Australia associated with 700 deaths,[22,23] and widespread disease in the Brazilian state of Piauí.[24] *B. ranarum* also causes granulomatous skin lesions in horses.

PATHOGENESIS AND IMMUNITY

Little is known about the pathogenesis of these diseases. Both *Basidiobolus* and *Conidiobolus* possess the ability to grow *in vitro* at 37°C and elicit specific antibodies in humans and animals. Their described *in vitro* production of extracellular proteases and lipases has been postulated to play a role in the limited virulence of these organisms.[25,26]

DIAGNOSIS

Diagnosis of entomophthoramycosis is based on biopsy with microscopic examination of tissue and culture of the etiologic agent. Clinically, basidiobolomycosis can be confused with soft tissue sarcoma. Fibrosing panniculitis and bacterial cellulitis are almost always painful and are thus not difficult to differentiate from this disease. On microscopic examination of biopsy material, both of these organisms are seen as short, aseptate, or sparsely septated wide hyphae with surrounding eosinophilic material in subcutaneous granulomas. The surrounding material stains strongly with periodic acid–Schiff (PAS) stain in what is referred to as the Splendore–Hoeppli phenomenon (see explanation under Sporotrichosis).[27] In addition to observation in tissue sections, these fungal elements may be visualized by direct observation in potassium hydroxide (KOH) wet mounts. Definitive diagnosis is made by culture. Culture of these organisms is usually performed on Sabouraud glucose agar containing antibacterial antibiotics at 25–30°C. Both genera grow well at temperatures of 25–37°C, producing mycelial growth in several days. Conidia that are forcibly discharged are characteristic of the Entomophthorales. In cultures of *B. ranarum* and *C. coronatus*, these conidia may be seen on the covers of Petri plates as the cultures mature. *B. ranarum* produces wide (8–20 μm) hyphae, which become progressively more septate with time. Forcibly discharged conidia, adhesive conidia, and beaked thick-walled zygospores are produced by this species. *C. coronatus* produces phototropic discharged conidia and villose conidia, but no zygospores. No commercially available serologic tests are available to diagnose the entomophthoramycoses. Studies have shown that the genera induce production of a specific antibody response, which may be demonstrated by immunodiffusion. Studies using *B. ranarum* have shown precipitin bands of antigens specific to the species as well as one shared with *C. coronatus* and *Pythium insidiosum*.[28,29]

TREATMENT AND PROGNOSIS

Basidiobolomycosis and conidiobolomycosis differ in their response to therapy. Limited *in vitro* susceptibility data have shown high minimum inhibitory concentrations (MICs) for amphotericin B and flucytosine for both species, obtainable MICs for the azoles against *Basidiobolus*, and mixed results for *Conidiobolus* with the azole antifungals.[30,31] Both have responded to extended therapy (6–12 months) with potassium iodide (**Table 90.1**; see description of potassium iodide use in Sporotrichosis section). In basidiobolomycosis, successful therapy with ketoconazole or trimethoprim-sulfamethoxazole has been reported.[32] Spontaneous resolution occasionally occurs in both diseases, but surgical excision is rarely curative in either. No consistently effective therapy for conidiobolomycosis has yet been found. Mixed results have been reported with therapies including iodide, amphotericin B, trimethoprim-sulfamethoxazole, ketoconazole, and surgery.[6,33] Both successful and unsuccessful results of therapy with ketoconazole have been reported.[34–36] Improvement of disease with fluconazole therapy has been reported in two patients.[37,38] Response to combination therapy with fluconazole and itraconazole has been reported in one person.[39]

Table 90.1 Therapy of Entomophthoramycosis, Lobomycosis, Rhinosporidiosis, and Sporotrichosis

Disease	Primary Therapy	Alternative Therapy
Entomophthoramycosis		
Basidiobolomycosis	SSKI	Ketoconazole, itraconazole
Conidiobolomycosis	SSKI	Ketoconazole, itraconazole
Lobomycosis	Surgery	None
Rhinosporidiosis	Surgery	None
Sporotrichosis		
Cutaneous	Itraconazole (200 mg daily)	Itraconazole (200 mg bid), terbinafine, SSKI, or heat[a]
Osteoarticular	Itraconazole (200 mg bid)	Amphotericin B
Pulmonary	Amphotericin B, then itraconazole	Adjunctive surgery
Disseminated	Amphotericin B, then itraconazole	Itraconazole

[a]For cutaneous plaque lesions.
SSKI, saturated solution of potassium iodide; bid, twice daily.

LOBOMYCOSIS

Lobomycosis (Lobo's disease, keloidal blastomycosis, lacaziosis) is a chronic cutaneous disease found only in Central and South America, caused by the fungal pathogen *Lacazia loboi*. First described by Lobo in 1931, the disease was initially thought to be an atypical presentation of paracoccidioidomycosis.[40] In describing the second reported case in 1938, Fialho thought the histopathology of these first two cases was clearly different from paracoccidioidomycosis, and coined the term Lobo's disease to describe the new entity.[41] The etiologic agent of lobomycosis, previously denoted *Loboa loboi* or *Paracoccidioides loboi*, has been renamed *Lacazia loboi*.[42] Although a mouse foot-pad model has been developed in which to study this disease, our inability to isolate and cultivate the organism from patients and the environment has greatly limited our understanding of its habitat and life cycle.[43,44]

EPIDEMIOLOGY

Epidemiologically, the disease is limited to the tropical and subtropical forests of Central and South America. Occasional cases occur outside the endemic area, typically in association with previous travel to or residency in Latin America. This disease shows no predilection for race, gender, or age, but occurs in persons who work outdoors in rural, hot, humid areas. Cutaneous trauma is thought to be the initiating event in this disease, but cases following insect stings have been reported. Apart from human disease, lobomycosis appears to only occur naturally in dolphins.[45] Isolated reports of probable acquisition in a veterinarian who worked with experimentally infected mice and in an attendant of a dolphin also diagnosed with the disease have been published.[46,47]

THE DISEASE

Lobomycosis is a chronic granulomatous disease of the dermis which produces plaques, nodules, verrucoid lesions, or ulcerated lesions. Beginning as a well-circumscribed papule, the disease is otherwise asymptomatic and spreads by local extension, autoinoculation, and possibly via the lymphatic system. Common sites of initial lesions include the extremities and the ears. The lesions grow slowly for years to decades before most patients seek medical attention. Typical features include indurated lesions with sharp, lobulated margins, which are painless and not attached to underlying structures. The skin is usually shiny, discolored, and atrophic. Complications of disease, including ulceration and bacterial superinfection, are rare. Squamous cell carcinoma has been reported in extremely chronic lesions in three patients.[48]

PATHOGENESIS AND IMMUNITY

The rare prevalence of this disease and the inability to grow *L. loboi* in culture has limited our understanding of the pathogenesis and immunity of lobomycosis. Study has revealed an association of disease with depressed cell-mediated immune (CMI) function and cell populations, in both humans and dolphins.[49] Increased transforming growth factor-β in the lesions of this disease has been postulated to inhibit CMI and induce fibrosis.[50]

DIAGNOSIS

Diagnosis is made by the direct observation of *L. loboi* in lesional biopsy material. Clinically, the lesions of lobomycosis may be similar to those seen in chromoblastomycosis, paracoccidioidomycosis, leishmaniasis, mycosis fungoides, dermatofibrosarcoma protuberans, Kaposi's sarcoma, and squamous cell carcinoma. Microscopically, the dermis is replaced by histiocytic granulomas that contain organisms and remnants of organisms. Disease does not extend deeper than the subcutaneous tissue. Globose to elliptic or lemon-shaped cells approximately 10 μm in diameter, strung together by small tubular connections (resembling a pearl necklace), are typically seen in tissue. The cell walls of the organisms may be quite thick (up to 1 μm). These may be seen with standard hematoxylin and eosin (H&E) stain, but are often better appreciated with PAS or Gomori methenamine silver (GMS) stain. Direct observation of biopsy material mounted in KOH may also yield the diagnosis.

TREATMENT AND PROGNOSIS

The only effective therapy is early wide excision of lesions. Surgical removal of chronic lesions can be effective, but recurrence is common. Medical therapy has been ineffective in the treatment of lobomycosis. The overall prognosis in this disease is very good as the mycosis spreads very slowly and is associated with limited morbidity.

RHINOSPORIDIOSIS

Rhinosporidiosis is a chronic granulomatous submucosal or subcutaneous disease seen most commonly in India and Sri Lanka. This disease was first described in an Argentinean man by Seeber in 1900.[51] In 1923, Ashworth produced a classic monograph on the morphology and clinical manifestations of rhinosporidiosis.[52] As with *L. loboi*, study of this disease has been hampered by our inability to reproducibly culture or maintain it in the laboratory. Recent studies of 18S small-subunit ribosomal DNA sequences of the organism have removed *Rhinosporidium seeberi* from the fungal kingdom and placed it into a novel group of aquatic protistan parasites.[53,54]

EPIDEMIOLOGY

The ecological niche of the organism is not known, although disease has been associated with bathing in stagnant water, river diving, and rice paddy cultivation. Disease has been reported worldwide, with areas of increased incidence in India, Sri Lanka, South America, and Africa. Indigenous cases have been reported from many countries, although the greatest numbers of cases outside India and Sri Lanka are in persons originally from those countries.[55–57] Disease occurs most frequently in children and young adults (aged 15–40 years) with a male predominance. A 4 : 1 male : female ratio was noted in one study of 255 cases.[58] In addition to human disease, infection in the nasal passages of cats, cattle, dogs, goats, horses, mules, ducks, parrots, and swan has been described.

THE DISEASE

Patients most frequently present with friable polypoid nodules in the nose, nasopharynx, or conjunctiva. Approximately 70% of rhinosporidiosis is limited to the nasal mucous membranes, with the conjunctiva being the next most common site of infection. Submucosal and subcutaneous lesions of the face, scalp, ear, lacrimal sac, larynx, trachea, urethra, penis, vagina, scrotum, and rectum have been reported.[59–61] Rarely, isolated bone lesions and disseminated cutaneous lesions have been reported.[62–65] Presenting symptoms are usually those of unilateral nasal obstruction or epistaxis. Cough secondary to postnasal discharge can occur. Occasionally the disease can be complicated by bacterial sinusitis if sinus drainage becomes obstructed. Localized disease is the rule, with disseminated disease of deep organs and tissues noted in only three of several thousand reported cases.[66]

PATHOGENESIS AND IMMUNITY

Rhinosporidiosis has been shown in limited studies to elicit a cell-mediated immune response. Immunohistochemistry has shown that the cell infiltration in human infection includes suppressor lymphocytes and natural killer cells; lymphoproliferation assays have revealed the development of specific immune suppression to *R. seeberi*.[67] Specific delayed-type hypersensitivity has been demonstrated in a mouse foot-pad model.[68]

DIAGNOSIS

Rhinosporidiosis may be suspected in subjects with polypoid lesions that contain white dots on close inspection. Nasal polyps need to be differentiated from those in allergic disease. Vaginal and penile lesions may resemble condylomata, while rectal lesions may mimic prolapsed internal hemorrhoids. Diagnosis is based on the direct observation of the organism in tissue. Culture and serology are not currently available. Microscopic examination can be performed with KOH mounts of macerated tissue or stained histologic sections of lesions. Direct observation of biopsy material may reveal subepithelial white dots, which are the large sporangia of *R. seeberi*. These sporangia, which may contain thousands of endospores, can grow to diameters of 350 μm. Though similar in structure to the spherules of *Coccidioides immitis*, both the sporangia and endospores are larger in rhinosporidiosis. The sporangium wall of *R. seeberi* is also much thicker. Structures of the organism stain well with GMS and PAS stains, but its size allows the diagnosis to be made easily with standard H&E staining. Histopathologically, an inflammatory response with neutrophils, lymphocytes, plasma cells, and multinucleated giant cells is present in the submucosa underlying normal columnar or squamous epithelium. Papillomatous hyperplasia and increased vascularity may also be seen in these lesions.

TREATMENT AND PROGNOSIS

Surgical excision is the only known effective therapy for rhinosporidiosis. Recurrence is common following surgical excision and has led to the practice of wide surgical excision of lesions followed by electrocoagulation of their bases. Medical therapy has not proved effective, although reports of success with dapsone (100 mg/day for one year) have been published.[69]

SPOROTRICHOSIS

Sporotrichosis is a chronic, usually cutaneous, fungal infection caused by *Sporothrix schenckii*. The disease is most commonly limited to cutaneous and subcutaneous tissue, although osteoarticular, pulmonary, and other deep infections can occur. Cutaneous sporotrichosis is caused by inoculation during minor trauma, although the incident is often not remembered. Extracutaneous infection is thought to be initiated via inhalation of the organism with or without dissemination. Sporotrichosis was first described in 1898 by Schenck for whom the organism was later named.[70] Study of sporotrichosis in France by Beurmann and Gougerot in the early twentieth century produced the monograph *Les Sporotrichoses*, and led to the use of potassium iodide as an effective therapy for this mycosis.[71]

THE AGENT

S. schenckii is a temperature-dependent dimorphic fungus, which is found in the environment, usually on living or decaying plants. In this niche and in culture at room temperature, *S. schenckii* is a filamentous fungus (mold). In host tissue and at 37°C in culture, the morphology of the organism is that of a yeast.

EPIDEMIOLOGY

Though worldwide in its distribution, sporotrichosis occurs most commonly in tropical and subtropical climates. This disease usually has a focal distribution, occurring endemically and in small epidemics in temperate and tropical environments. In clustered cases it has been associated with the distribution of sphagnum moss, hay, and with mine timbers. Disease has also been associated with zoonotic transmission from domesticated animals, especially cats. An ongoing epidemic among humans, cats, and dogs has been described in Brazil.[72] The common cutaneous form is usually seen in young adults, without predilection for sex or race. Infection occurs in immunocompetent persons, often those who work outdoors in contact with vegetation or soil. An epidemiologic survey employing skin testing has shown a higher incidence of positive delayed cutaneous hypersensitivity in plant nursery workers than in hospitalized patients or prisoners (32.3% versus 11.2%).[73] Pulmonary disease has a male predominance and an association with alcohol dependence. In a case series of 66 patients, a male : female ratio of 6 : 1 was reported, with 30 of 51 patients having impaired host defenses, and 19 with alcohol dependence.[74] Disseminated disease is more common in patients who are immunosuppressed.[75–77] In the unimpaired host, the incidence of disseminated disease is thought to be quite low. Lurie found only five cases of disseminated disease in over 3000 cases of sporotrichosis in a South African mine outbreak.[78] Sporotrichosis occurs in armadillos, birds, camels, cats, cattle, dogs, dolphins, goats, horses, mules, and rats.[79]

THE DISEASE

Cutaneous disease begins as a relatively painless papule, which enlarges slowly and then drains spontaneously. Infection remains localized or spreads slowly via the lymphatic system to involve proximal sites on an extremity. Although infection may reach the axillary or inguinal lymph nodes, hematogenous dissemination from skin inoculation has not been described. Rarely, lesions may also be solitary and fixed, presenting as plaques which wax and wane for years without resolution. Although minor (often insignificant) trauma is thought to be the common mode by which cutaneous disease is initiated, disease following or associated with insect stings, fish handling, bites or scratches of dogs, cats, parrots, and wild rodents has been reported. Pulmonary sporotrichosis typically presents in the fifth decade of life with productive cough and upper pulmonary radiographic findings.[74] Most commonly, chest radiography reveals a solitary upper lobe thin-walled cavity with surrounding parenchymal infiltrate. Untreated pulmonary sporotrichosis is usually associated with progressive disease and death. Osteoarticular sporotrichosis is an indolent disease usually involving the joints of the knee, elbow, wrist, or ankle.[80,81] Infection presents like osteoarthritis or rheumatoid arthritis with gradual onset of pain, stiffness, and decrease in range of motion. Localized swelling is often present. Laboratory studies usually show an elevated erythrocyte sedimentation rate and synovial fluid with decreased glucose, increased protein, and leukocytes. Hematogenous spread from the lungs or occult sites may lead to chronic meningitis, endophthalmitis, brain abscesses, or disseminated skin lesions.

PATHOGENESIS AND IMMUNITY

The virulence factors and pathogen–host immunity interaction of *S. schenckii* are not currently well understood. *S. schenckii* has limited pathogenicity in laboratory animals, with large inocula being required to establish infection. Virulence of strains of *S. schenckii* can be subdivided by thermotolerance as those strains which grow at 37°C are better able to cause disseminated disease. Antibody to yeast cell wall antigens is produced in some infections. The role of this antibody in controlling infection is not believed to be critical, although agglutinating antibody response in a hamster model is associated with protection against challenge.[82] Cell-mediated immunity (CMI) likely serves a more important role in host defense, especially in humans. Human neutrophils phagocytose and kill *S. schenckii*. This killing requires halide, myeloperoxidase, and peroxide.[83] Opsonization with human serum is thought to enhance this interaction via activation of the alternative complement pathway. Athymic mice are unable to clear an intravenous challenge of *S. schenckii* when compared with euthymic mice, further supporting a role for CMI.[84]

DIAGNOSIS

Diagnosis of cutaneous sporotrichosis is suspected with observation of typical lesions, often with supporting history of likely exposure (e.g., gardening, forestry work, cat scratch). This diagnosis is then confirmed by culture or further supported by microscopic tissue examination. The differential diagnosis of cutaneous sporotrichosis includes disease caused by *Nocardia* species (especially *N. brasiliensis*), *Mycobacterium* species (*M. marinum*, *M. chelonae*, *M. fortuitum*, and *M. kansasii*), leishmaniasis, tularemia, cat-scratch disease, chromoblastomycosis, blastomycosis, and paracoccidioidomycosis. An incorrect diagnosis of squamous cell carcinoma may be made from biopsy specimens that manifest hyperkeratosis and are not cultured appropriately. Pulmonary sporotrichosis should be differentiated from *Mycobacterium avium-intracellulare* complex infection, coccidioidomycosis, tuberculosis, and histoplasmosis. In addition to chronic bacterial osteomyelitis, osteoarticular sporotrichosis should be differentiated from mycobacterial infections. Diagnosis of pulmonary disease is usually made when *S. schenckii* is cultured from sputum, bronchoalveolar lavage, or biopsy. Osteoarticular disease may be diagnosed by culture of joint fluid or fungal stain of synovium. Blood culture is not usually helpful in the diagnosis of sporotrichosis. Although both localized and disseminated disease has been diagnosed by blood culture, these represent only a handful of cases. *S. schenckii* is best recovered on brain-heart infusion agar incubated at 25–30°C for up to 3 weeks.[85,86] Histopathologic examination reveals a pyogranulomatous reaction with neutrophils and necrotic debris surrounded by epithelioid cells. In more chronic lesions, pseudoepitheliomatous hyperplasia is seen. Commonly, skin lesions have a paucity of fungal organisms, making the correct diagnosis difficult to establish without culture. It is often very difficult to find *S. schenckii* in routine H&E-stained histopathologic sections in any tissue. PAS and GMS stains improve visualization of the organism in tissue. Usually seen as oval- to cigar-shaped yeasts in tissue, *S. schenckii* may also form asteroid bodies or appear as spherical yeasts with what appears to be a capsule. The asteroid body is a central rounded yeast structure with radiating eosinophilic substance in tissue.[87] Deposition of eosinophilic material about the infecting organism was first described by Splendore in a 1908 study of sporotrichosis,[88] and then in 1932 by Hoeppli in the study of schistosomiasis in a rabbit model.[89] Classically, the Splendore–Hoeppli phenomenon is believed to be an immune complex (antibody–antigen) deposition. Electron microscopy appears to demonstrate that the asteroid bodies of sporotrichosis may actually be composed of disintegrated immune cells.[90] This phenomenon also occurs in schistosomiasis, actinomycosis, botryomycosis, entomophthoramycosis, mycetoma, and onchocerciasis. In its atypical spherical form with a PAS-positive capsular-appearing structure, *S. schenckii* may be confused with *Cryptococcus neoformans*. Serologic and immune testing is generally of limited value in the diagnosis of sporotrichosis. Although many testing formats have been developed, the availability of these tests and perceived need for them has limited their usefulness.

TREATMENT AND PROGNOSIS

The treatment of sporotrichosis is based on the clinical presentation of the disease.[91] Treatment of all forms of this disease is associated with relapse. The duration of therapy for cutaneous disease is usually 6–12 weeks, 2–4 weeks after lesions resolve. Itraconazole (200 mg daily) is currently the preferred treatment for cutaneous disease based on effectiveness and tolerability. Alternatives include higher dose itraconazole (200 mg twice daily) or terbinafine (500 mg twice daily). Potassium iodide in saturated solution (SSKI) can be used as well and prior to itraconazole had been the mainstay of therapy of cutaneous sporotrichosis since the beginning of the twentieth century. First used by Beurmann for the treatment of cutaneous disease, potassium iodide remains an inexpensive, effective therapy. Iodide therapy can be poorly tolerated and associated with adverse effects. It is a bitter solution, which should be slowly titrated up to treatment doses to minimize adverse effects and increase tolerance.[92] These effects include excessive tearing and salivating, parotid enlargement, acne, and gastrointestinal upset. SSKI (~1 g/mL or 47 mg/drop) can be begun at a dose of 5–10 drops three times daily, usually with juice or water. The dose can be increased slowly (5 drops per dose each week) to 25–40 drops thrice daily in those under 10 years of age and 40–50 drops thrice daily in those 10 years old or older. In those patients with plaque sporotrichosis, topical heat may be beneficial. Hyperthermic therapy using a variety of modalities has been used successfully in these cutaneous infections. Successes with liquid nitrogen and fluconazole have also been reported in cutaneous diease.[93,94] The new broad-spectrum azole voriconazole is less active than itraconazole against *S. schenckii*.[95] Both itraconazole and amphotericin B are effective in osteoarticular disease, although itraconazole is currently favored.[96,97] Intra-articular injection with amphotericin B has been reported to lead to improvement in several patients with disease recurring after parenteral therapy.[81,98] Doses ranging from 0.1 mg to 10 mg of amphotericin B injected every day to every 2 weeks have been used. Pulmonary sporotrichosis has been treated with amphotericin B, iodide, ketoconazole, miconazole, and itraconazole, all with some reported successes. Unfortunately, pulmonary disease does not respond regularly to antifungal therapy and is known to relapse. Currently, amphotericin B (in lipid formulation) followed by itraconazole is suggested for this disease form. Surgical resection of localized disease can also be helpful. Disseminated sporotrichosis is most often treated with parenteral amphotericin B. As with pulmonary disease, this is typically followed by a prolonged course of oral itraconazole. Itraconazole monotherapy has been shown in several reports to lead to a favorable response, but is usually employed in those patients not responding to amphotericin B.[96,99]

PREVENTION AND CONTROL

Prevention of sporotrichosis is based on avoidance of traumatic inoculation of the fungus. Fungicide treatment of timbers was used to bring a halt to the epidemic in South African gold mines in the 1940s. The US outbreak involving conifer saplings packed in sphagnum moss led to suggestions of using chipped wood or shredded paper as packing material for these plants.[100] People who work in forestry or horticulture and others who are engaged in gardening should be encouraged to wear gloves and clothing that covers their extremities, preventing scratches and other minor trauma. Similar recommendations can be made for veterinarians and others handling pets with skin lesions.

Disclaimer The views expressed herein are those of the author and do not reflect the official policy or position of the Department of the Army, Department of Defense, or the US Government. The author is an employee of the US Government. This work was prepared as part of his official duties and, as such, there is no copyright to be transferred.

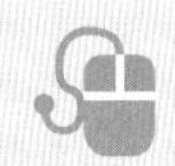

Access the complete reference list online at
http://www.expertconsult.com

CHAPTER 91

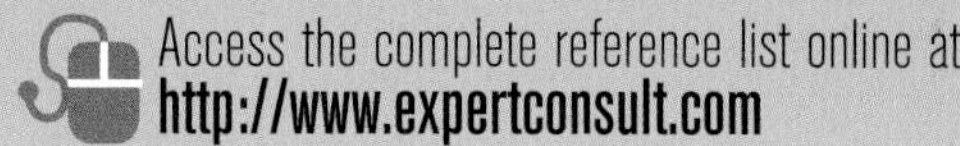
Access the complete reference list online at
http://www.expertconsult.com

Pneumocystosis

Peter D. Walzer • A. George Smulian • Robert F. Miller

INTRODUCTION

Pneumocystis was discovered by Chagas in 1909 during his studies of American trypanosomiasis. The organism was established as a separate genus and species a few years later by the Delanöes, who named it in honor of Dr Carini. Organisms within the *Pneumocystis* genus are of low virulence and reside in the lungs of humans and many animals in nature.

THE AGENT

Although *Pneumocystis* isolates from these hosts are morphologically indistinguishable, molecular, antigenic, and experimental transmission studies have demonstrated a high degree of genetic diversity and host specificity. This information has resulted in new nomenclature that has established the following *Pneumocystis* species: *P. carinii* and *P. wakefieldiae* in rats, *P. murina* in mice, *P. octolagii* in rabbits, and *P. jirovecii* in humans.[1] *Pneumocystis* was first recognized as the pathogen that caused interstitial plasma cell pneumonia in premature, malnourished infants in European orphanages following World War II. However, the disease can occur wherever these conditions exist. More recently, *Pneumocystis* has been found to be a leading cause of pneumonia in immunocompromised patients, such as those infected with the human immunodeficiency virus (HIV).

Knowledge of the basic biology of *Pneumocystis* has been limited by the lack of a continuous *in vitro* culture system.[2] The developmental stages that have been identified include the 5–8 μm cystic form or ascus, which has a thick wall and contains up to eight intracystic bodies or ascospores; the 1–4 μm trophic form, which is the most numerous stage; and the precyst or sporocyte, an intermediate stage. A proposed life cycle is presented in ***Figure 91.1***.[3] The cystic form (ascus) is thought to develop through a sexual cycle that culminates in the release of the intracystic bodies (ascospores), which then become trophic forms; the trophic forms replicate asexually by binary fission. The taxonomic status of *Pneumocystis* has clearly established the organism as a member of the fungi.[1]

EPIDEMIOLOGY

Serologic studies have revealed that *Pneumocystis* has a worldwide distribution, and that exposure to the organism occurs early in life.[4–6] Evidence suggests that *Pneumocystis* remains in the lungs for limited periods of time and that people may be transiently infected at different times in their lives. The HIV pandemic changed pneumocystosis from a sporadic disease to a problem of major medical and public health importance. Although the incidence of *Pneumocystis* pneumonia has fallen with widespread chemoprophylaxis and antiretroviral therapy, the organism remains the leading cause of opportunistic infection in HIV patients in industrialized countries.[7] Despite difficulties in obtaining accurate incidence rates in developing countries because of a lack of access to medical care and the higher frequency of more virulent infections such as tuberculosis, *Pneumocystis* is now recognized with increasing frequency in tropical and developing countries.[8] Recently, a high frequency of pneumocystosis has been reported in pediatric HIV patients in developing countries.[9] Other factors affecting the epidemiology are geography and season of the year.[10,11]

Studies in animal models have demonstrated that *Pneumocystis* is communicable via the airborne route. Young animals acquire *Pneumocystis* infection soon after birth and play an important role in spreading the infection.[12] Molecular studies in humans support the findings from these experimental models.[6] The incubation period is approximately 4–8 weeks.

THE DISEASE

Risk factors for pneumocystosis include prematurity and malnutrition; primary immunodeficiency disorders, particularly severe combined immunodeficiency disease; infection with HIV; and cytotoxic or immunosuppressive drugs for the treatment of cancer, transplantation, and collagen vascular disorders. Studies of HIV/AIDS patients have documented a significant risk of pneumocystosis when CD4 lymphocyte counts fall below 200 cells/μL; other factors associated with a higher risk for *Pneumocystis* pneumonia include $CD4^+$ T-cell percentage <14%, previous episodes of pneumocystosis, oral thrush, recurrent bacterial pneumonia, unintentional weight loss, and high plasma HIV RNA concentration.[13,14] Corticosteroids are by far the most commonly used immunosuppressive drugs that predispose to *Pneumocystis* pneumonia in non-HIV-infected patients.[15] Symptoms often begin after the steroid dose has been tapered.

Pneumocystis pneumonia is characterized by the triad of dyspnea, nonproductive cough, and fever.[16] Although a productive cough and chest tightness may occur, purulent sputum should raise suspicion of bacterial infection. HIV-infected patients frequently have prolonged prodromal periods with subtle clinical manifestations; other immunocompromised hosts are usually ill for 1 or 2 weeks before they seek medical attention.[17] However, the clinical picture varies in individual patients. Physical examination reveals varying degrees of respiratory distress. Lung auscultation is nonrevealing, although basilar rales may occasionally be present. The chest radiograph typically reveals diffuse infiltrates with symmetric reticular or granular opacities emanating from the perihilar regions (***Fig. 91.2***).[18] Unusual manifestations include focal infiltrates, lobar consolidation, nodules, cavities, effusions, pneumatoceles, and lymphadenopathy.[19] An increased frequency of pneumothorax and apical infiltrates has been noted with the administration of aerosolized pentamidine.[20] Patients with early disease may have a normal chest radiograph, but patchy ground-glass opacification may be detected on high-resolution computed tomography (HRCT) (***Fig. 91.2***).[21,22]

The principal laboratory abnormality is arterial hypoxemia with an increased alveolar–arterial (PAO_2–PaO_2) gradient; this is often accompanied by respiratory alkalosis.[18,23] Blood oxygenation may be normal early in the course of pneumocystosis but will desaturate with exercise. Pulmonary function tests are characterized by alterations in lung volumes and spirometry (e.g., reversible airway obstruction and airway hyperreactivity). The diffusing capacity for carbon monoxide (DL_{CO}) sensitively detects alveolar–capillary block. Serum lactate dehydrogenase (LDH) levels, which reflect the degree of lung injury, increase with progression of pneumocystosis and decrease as the disease is treated.[24]

The spread of *Pneumocystis* beyond the lungs is well recognized. Patients at highest risk are those in the late stages of HIV infection who have received aerosolized pentamidine or have not taken prophylaxis.[25,26] The most common sites of extrapulmonary infection are the lymph nodes, spleen, liver, and bone marrow, although most organs in the body have been involved. Clinical features range from incidental findings at autopsy to focal involvement and systemic disease.

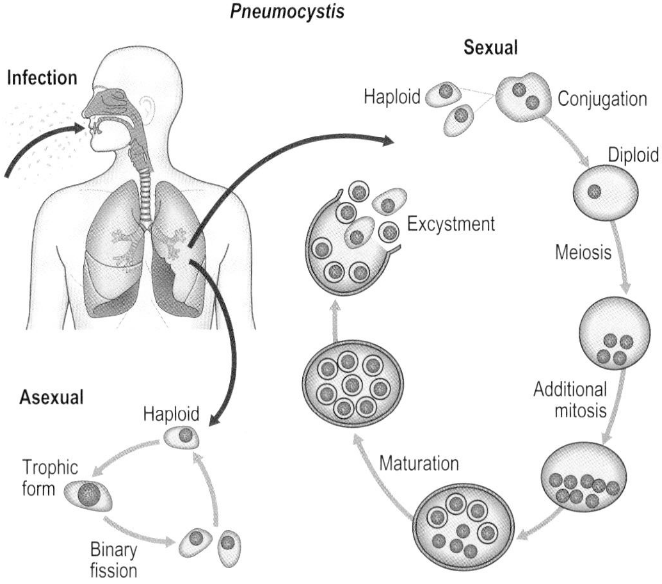

Figure 91.1 Proposed life cycle of *Pneumocystis*. In the asexual phase, the trophic forms replicate by mitosis and cell division. In the sexual phase, the haploid trophic forms (mating types) conjugate to form a diploid zygote (early phase) that undergoes meiosis and subsequent mitosis to form eight haploid nuclei (late phase). The spores are formed by compartmentalization of nuclei and cytoplasmic organelles (e.g., mitochondria). The spores exhibit different shapes, including spherical and elongated forms. It is postulated that the elongation of the spores precedes release from the ascus. Release is thought to occur through a rent in the ascus wall. After evacuation, the empty ascus usually collapses but retains some residual cytoplasm. (From Beck JM, Cushion MT. Pneumocystis workshop: 10th anniversary summary. Eukaryotic Cell. 2009;8:446–460. Copyright 2009 American Society for Microbiology.)

The natural history of untreated *Pneumocystis* pneumonia in HIV-infected and other immunocompromised patients is one of progressive respiratory impairment ending in death.[27] Since recovery from pneumocystosis does not confer immunity, patients are at risk of recurrence as long as the predisposing conditions exist; HIV-infected patients are at highest risk for this complication. Other problems that can complicate recovery include bullous lesions, cavities, and pneumothorax, which appear to result from the tissue destruction and inflammation that accompany the infection. Similarly, chronic airway disease can develop and may be further complicated by bacterial infections.[28]

Histopathologically, *Pneumocystis* pneumonia is characterized by the presence of foamy, vacuolated material filling alveoli in lung sections stained with hematoxylin and eosin (***Fig. 91.3***). The use of stains such as methenamine silver reveals masses of *Pneumocystis* cystic forms (***Fig. 91.4***).[29] With severe disease, there may be interstitial fibrosis, edema, and the development of hyaline membranes. Hypertrophy of type II alveolar cells, which suggests tissue repair, is often present; however, other aspects of the host inflammatory response in HIV-infected and other immunocompromised patients are mild and nonspecific. In contrast, premature or malnourished infants display an interstitial plasma cell infiltrate, which was responsible for the early name of the disease. Extrapulmonary lesions of pneumocystosis display the typical foamy material found in the lungs.

PATHOGENESIS AND IMMUNITY

The mechanisms by which *Pneumocystis* causes disease are poorly understood. Although several different enzymes have been identified, evidence that these enzymes are virulence factors is lacking. Among the antigens that have been identified, two have received the most attention: the major surface glycoprotein (Msg or gpA) and kexin (Kex1).[30,31] Both antigens are highly immunogenic and contain protective B- and T-cell epitopes.[32–35] Other roles for Msg are to facilitate interaction of *Pneumocystis* with the host cells, and because of its ability to undergo antigenic variation, it plays a role in evasion of host defenses.[30,36] Pneumocystosis develops when there are impairments in cellular or humoral immunity.[37] Predisposing T-cell defects can result from the underlying disease (HIV infection) or immunosuppression (corticosteroids). The central role of CD4 cells in host defenses against *Pneumocystis* has been shown by cell depletion and reconstitution experiments.[38,39] Additional factors that participate in host defenses include the CD40–CD40L pathway, which aids the interaction of T cells and B cells; CD8 T cells, which are cytotoxic and secrete cytokines; and T-cell costimulatory molecules.[40–42] The importance of humoral immunity is evidenced by the occurrence of pneumocystosis in patients or animals with B-cell defects, and the beneficial effects of passive immunotherapy and active immunization.[32,35,43] Antibodies do not have a direct lethal effect on *Pneumocystis* but probably function as opsonins.

After being inhaled, *Pneumocystis* eludes the upper airway defenses and lands in alveoli, where it takes up residence. Alveolar macrophages constitute the first line of defense and are the principal host effector cell

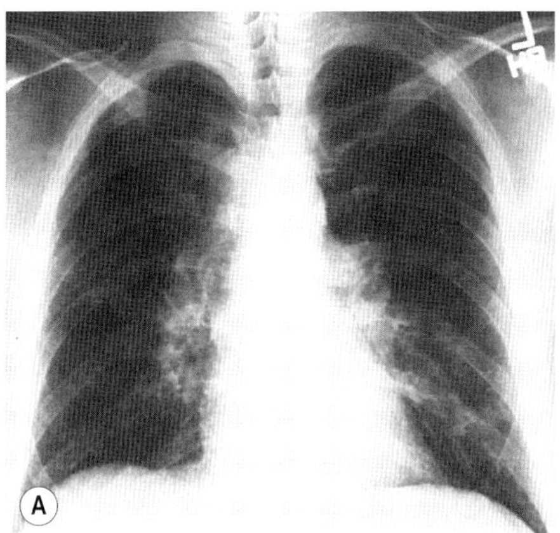

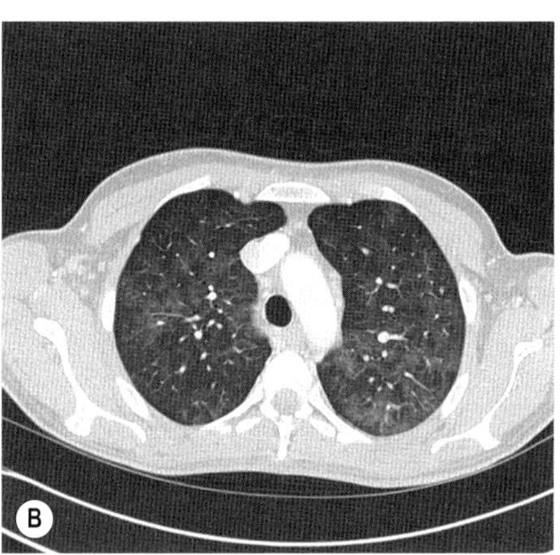

Figure 91.2 **(A)** Chest radiograph from an HIV-infected patient with pneumocystosis. Note the typical bilateral infiltrates. (From Walzer PD, Kim CK, Cushion MT. *Pneumocystis carinii*. In: Walzer PD, Genta RM, eds. Parasitic Infections in the Compromised Host. New York: Marcel Dekker; 1989:83-178.) **(B)** High-resolution computed tomogram (HRCT) of the lung demonstrating diffuse ground-glass opacification compatible with *Pneumocystis* pneumonia. (HRCT from Dr R.F. Miller.)

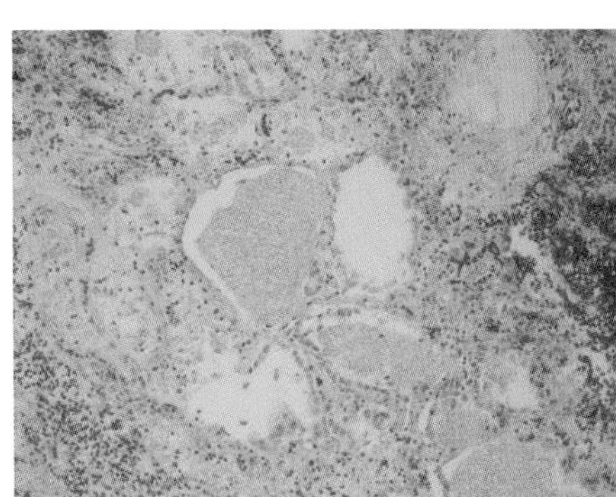

Figure 91.3 Lungs from a patient with pneumocystosis displaying the characteristic foamy, vacuolated alveolar content (H&E; ×300). (Courtesy of Dr Melanie Cushion, Cincinnati, OH.)

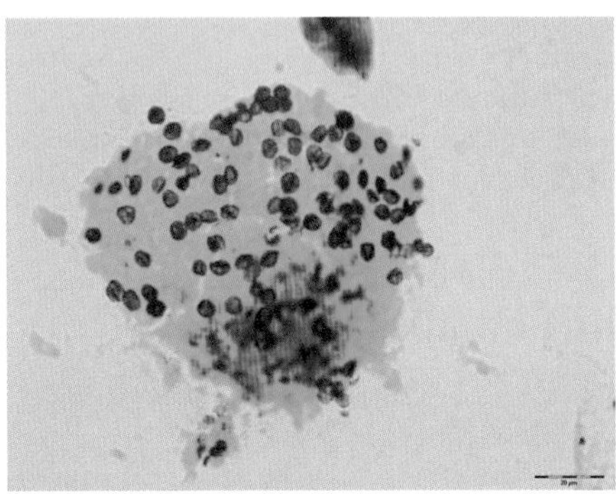

Figure 91.4 A cluster of *Pneumocystis jirovecii* cystic forms in an alveolar "cast" (methenamine silver stain; ×1000). (Courtesy of Dr Melanie Cushion, Cincinnati, OH.)

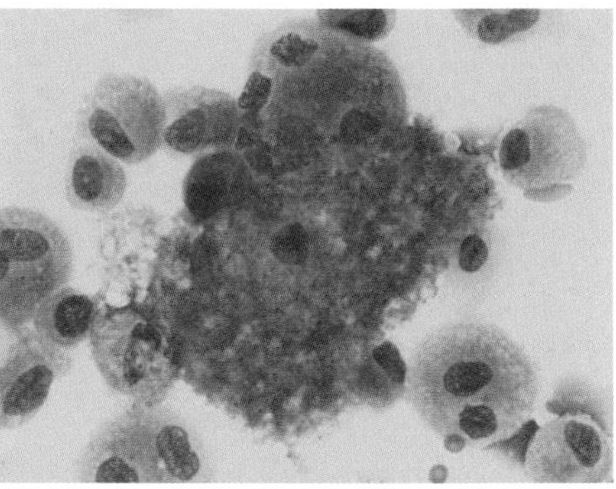

Figure 91.5 Clusters of *Pneumocystis jirovecii* trophic forms and cysts with intracystic bodies (Diff-Quik stain; ×1000). (Courtesy of Dr Melanie Cushion, Cincinnati, OH.)

against *Pneumocystis*.[44] Recognition and adherence of the organism occur by several pathways, including *Pneumocystis* cell surface or cell wall Msg and β-glucan, extracellular matrix proteins (e.g., fibronectin), surfactant proteins A (SP-A) and D (SP-D), Dectin-1, mannose, and Fc receptors.[36,45–48] *Pneumocystis* infection also increases intracellular polyamine levels, which enhance apoptosis.[49] HIV downregulates the mannose receptor, which leads to reduced binding and uptake of *Pneumocystis*.[50] Interaction with macrophages stimulates an oxidative burst and cytokine production. Once the organism is engulfed by the macrophage, it is rapidly killed. Of the cytokines produced in response to *Pneumocystis*, tumor necrosis factor-α, interleukin (IL)-1, IL-12, IL-23, interferon-γ, and granulocyte-macrophage colony-stimulating factor have roles in host defenses against the infection.[36,51–53]

Within the alveolus, *Pneumocystis* adheres tightly to the alveolar type I cell, which plays an important role in the host–parasite relationship in this infection. *Pneumocystis* colonization elicits local and systemic inflammatory responses.[54] These alterations lead to a decline in respiratory function in HIV and chronic obstructive pulmonary disease patients. If the host becomes more immunosuppressed (e.g., by the progression of HIV), *Pneumocystis* organisms slowly propagate and gradually fill the alveoli. Accompanying changes include disruption of the alveolar–capillary membrane, impaired gas exchange, and ventilation–perfusion abnormalities similar to the changes seen in adult respiratory distress syndrome.[55] Alterations in the surfactant system and the host inflammatory response are major contributors to these lung abnormalities.[56,57] There is a decline in surfactant phospholipids SP-B and SP-C, with a concomitant increase in SP-A and SP-D levels.[58,59] In experimental models, there is a hyperinflammatory response mediated by subsets of CD4 and CD8 T cells with a rise in proinflammatory cytokines and chemokines.[60,61] In humans with pneumocystosis, elevated levels of IL-8 and neutrophils in bronchoalveolar lavage (BAL) fluid have been associated with more severe disease and worse prognosis.[62,63] HIV patients experience clinical deterioration soon after beginning treatment for *Pneumocystis* pneumonia. This problem can be ameliorated by the administration of corticosteroids, but the mechanism of action of these drugs is unclear.

DIAGNOSIS

The clinical manifestations of pneumocystosis can be mimicked by a wide variety of infectious and noninfectious agents. Optimal management requires that a specific diagnosis be made by identification of the organism in properly obtained specimens. *Pneumocystis* is rarely present in spontaneously expectorated sputum. However, induced sputum, obtained by breathing in a hypertonic saline mist, has utility as a simple and inexpensive screening technique.[64] Induced sputum is best obtained by specially trained personnel; its sensitivity varies widely among different health care facilities and patient populations.[65]

Fiberoptic bronchoscopy with BAL remains the mainstay of *Pneumocystis* diagnosis, with a yield ⩾90% and a low rate of complications.[66,67] The diagnostic yield of BAL can be increased if multiple lobes are sampled or if the procedure is directed toward the site of greatest radiographic abnormality.[68] Bronchoscopy with BAL also provides information not obtainable from induced sputum about the *Pneumocystis* burden, the presence of other opportunistic infections, the host inflammatory response and presence of tracheobronchial Kaposi's sarcoma (KS).[65,69] Bronchoscopy with transbronchial biopsy can sometimes provide information not obtainable with BAL, but it is more invasive and has a higher rate of complications.[68] Open lung biopsy is reserved for situations in which a diagnosis cannot be made by bronchoscopy or where the patient's clinical course is at variance with findings from induced sputum/BAL.[67,66,70]

Several histologic stains have been used to identify *Pneumocystis*. Those that selectively stain the wall of the cystic form of the organism (e.g., methenamine silver, toluidine blue O, and cresyl violet) are popular because they are versatile and easy to interpret (see ***Fig. 91.4***).[29,71] Stains that demonstrate the nuclei of all *Pneumocystis* developmental stages (e.g., Wright–Giemsa and Diff-Quik) can provide a diagnosis within minutes but require expertise in interpretation (***Fig. 91.5***). Other staining methods, such as Papanicolaou and calcofluor white, a chemiluminescent agent, are used by some laboratories. Immunofluorescent staining with *Pneumocystis*-specific monoclonal antibodies is more sensitive than histologic stains, but it is more expensive and requires specialized laboratory facilities.[71,72] Soluble *Pneumocystis* antigens have been detected in BAL fluid by immunoblotting, but this technique remains investigational.[73] DNA amplification by the polymerase chain reaction (PCR) is the most sensitive method of detecting *Pneumocystis*.[74–78] Although PCR is not licensed for diagnosis, several clinical laboratories use the method applied to noninvasive sampling techniques (e.g., oropharygeal washes) for diagnosis of *Pneumocystis* pneumonia.[76] The clinical significance of a detected PCR product in the absence of respiratory symptoms or other confirmatory tests is unclear.[74] Elevated serum levels of 1,3-β-D-glucan (a component of the fungal cell wall) have been described in patients with *Pneumocystis* pneumonia; diagnostic sensitivity and specificity have not been defined.

Definitive diagnosis of pneumocystosis is best made using a coordinated approach that involves several different clinical services. Several institutions, such as San Francisco General Hospital, have developed algorithms that have been highly successful (***Fig. 91.6***).[64,77] Patients with clinical and radiologic manifestations compatible with pneumocystosis first undergo sputum induction. If this measure reveals the organism, treatment is begun. If induced sputum is nondiagnostic, BAL is performed. If BAL reveals *Pneumocystis*, treatment is begun. A BAL that fails to detect *Pneumocystis* results in a search for alternative causes. Patients with a normal chest radiograph undergo either HRCT or DL_{CO} determination. An HRCT with ground-glass opacities or DL_{CO} less than 75% suggests pneumocystosis; patients then undergo sputum induction. If HRCT or DL_{CO} does not suggest pneumocystosis, patients are observed, and a search for alternative causes is undertaken. Empiric therapy, which is routinely used for treatment of bacterial respiratory infections in HIV-infected and noninfected populations, is also used for diagnosis of *Pneumocystis* pneumonia in areas of the world with few diagnostic facilities; this approach has been controversial in industrialized countries.[79,80] Empirical therapy may be considered if a patient with a CD4 cell count of <200/μL is willing and able to undergo treatment, has mild disease with typical radiologic features, is not receiving anti-*Pneumocystis* prophylaxis, and has a low probability of other diseases (e.g., active or latent tuberculosis).[79,80] Such patients should be followed closely and hospitalized for definitive diagnostic evaluation if they fail to respond to empiric therapy.[80]

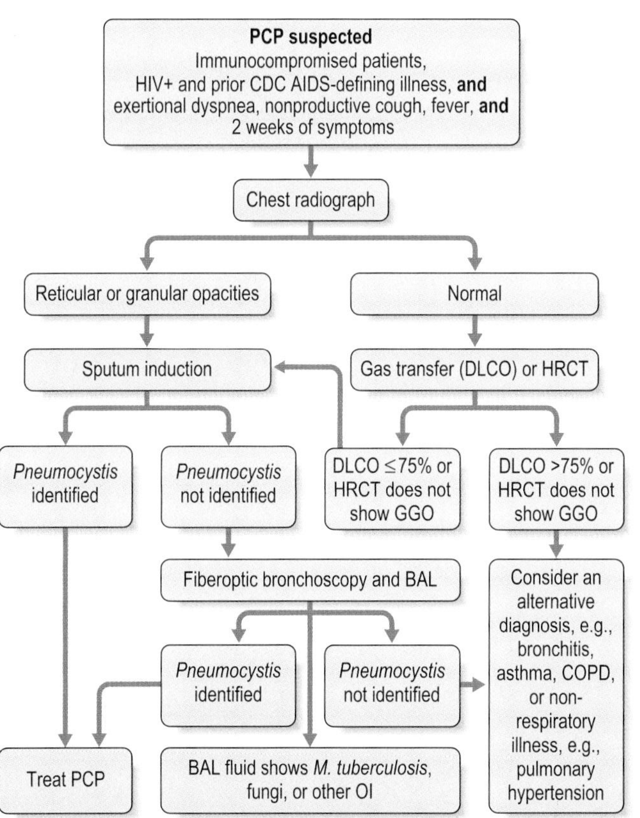

Figure 91.6 A diagnostic algorithm for evaluation of adult HIV-infected persons with suspected *Pneumocystis* pneumonia (PCP), based on a care pathway used at San Francisco General Hospital, USA. CDC, Centers for Disease Control and Prevention; HRCT, high-resolution computed tomography; DLCO, single breath diffusing capacity for carbon monoxide; GGO, ground-glass opacities; COPD, chronic obstructive pulmonary disease; OI, opportunistic infection. (Redrawn from Davis JL, Huang L. *Pneumocystis* pneumonia. In: Volberding PA, Sande MA, Lange J, Greene WC, eds. Global HIV/AIDS Medicine. Saunders/Elsevier; 2008.)

TREATMENT AND PROGNOSIS

Over the past decade the outcome for HIV-infected patients with pneumocystosis has improved due to a combination of earlier detection of the disease, prompt institution of therapy, and better management of complications. In the era of antiretroviral therapy, mortality from *Pneumocystis* pneumonia is 9.7–11.6%.[81,82] The most widely used prognostic indicator has been the degree of hypoxemia (arterial oxygen pressure, PaO_2)[83] (***Fig. 91.7***). This laboratory test has been interpreted in the following way when breathing room air: a PaO_2 greater than 70 mmHg indicates mild disease, and a value of less than 70 mmHg indicates moderate to severe disease. Similarly, the PAO_2–PaO_2 on room air has been categorized as mild (<35 mmHg), moderate (35–45 mmHg), or severe (>45 mmHg). Other prognostic factors present at admission include patient's age, lack of knowledge of HIV status, presentation with a second or subsequent episode of pneumocystosis, medical comorbidity, pregnancy, low hemoglobin, low serum albumin, peripheral blood leukocytosis, elevated serum LDH, and extent of abnormalities on chest radiography. Factors identified after admission and investigation associated with poor outcome include presence of a co-pathogen (e.g., cytomegalovirus or bacteria), neutrophilia (>5%) and high level of IL-8 in BAL fluid, the presence of fibrosis and edema on transbronchial biopsy, pulmonary KS, and serum LDH levels that do not fall in response to treatment.[55,67,81,82] Admission to the intensive care unit (ICU), a high APACHE (Acute Physiology and Chronic Health Evaluation) score, need for mechanical ventilation and/or development of a pneumothorax are also associated with mortality.[81,82,84,85] The prognosis for severe *Pneumocystis* pneumonia requiring ICU admission has improved over the past decade likely because of improvements in management of acute lung injury, rather than improvements in management of pneumocystosis.[84,85] The drug of choice for all forms of pneumocystosis is trimethoprim-sulfamethoxazole (TMP-SMX).[27] This drug combination, which has been used for two decades, works by inhibiting the synthesis of folic acid. The drug is given orally or intravenously at a dose of 15–20 mg/kg per day for TMP and 75–100 mg/kg per day for SMX in a fixed-dose combination, in three or four divided doses, for 21 days. The parenteral preparation is indicated for patients who have difficulty taking oral medications or who are seriously ill. Despite its superior efficacy, the major limitation of TMP-SMX is the high frequency (up to 80% or higher) of adverse drug reactions (ADRs) that necessitate discontinuation of the drug in up to half

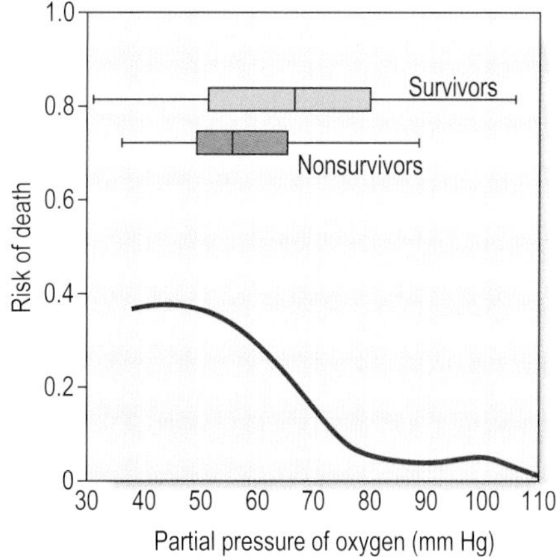

Figure 91.7 Risk of death according to the partial pressure of oxygen in room air at admission of 278 HIV-infected patients with pneumocystosis at the San Francisco General Hospital. Box plots represent the 25th centile, the median, and the 75th centile with survivors and nonsurvivors, with bars extending to the 5th and 95th centiles. (From The National Institutes of Health-University of California Expert Panel for Corticosteroids as Adjunctive Therapy for *Pneumocystis carinii* Pneumonia. Consensus statement on the use of corticosteroids as adjunctive therapy for *Pneumocystis* pneumonia in the acquired immunodeficiency syndrome. N Engl J Med. 1990;323:1500–1504 © 1990 Massachusetts Medical Society. All rights reserved.)

of HIV-infected patients.[27,83] These ADRs, which usually begin during the second week of treatment, consist of rash, fever, neutropenia and other cytopenias, nausea and vomiting, hepatitis, hyperkalemia, pancreatitis, nephritis, and central nervous system manifestations. The mechanisms of TMP-SMX toxicity are incompletely understood but may be related to elevated serum concentrations of the drug, formation of toxic intermediate (hydroxylamine) metabolites, glutathione deficiency, hypersensitivity, CD4 cell count, and its action as a potassium-sparing diuretic.[86]

Several strategies have been devised to minimize these ADRs. One approach is to adjust the dose of the drug to achieve serum concentrations of 5–8 μg/mL for TMP and 100–50 μg/mL for SMX.[86] However, other investigators have not found this to be helpful.[87] The use of folinic acid (leucovorin) does not prevent myelosuppression,[88] and appeared to be associated with treatment failure in one study.[89] In some patients, mild ADRs, such as fever or skin rash, may disappear spontaneously or respond to conservative measures. However, in other cases these ADRs progress to the point where they require discontinuation of the drug. Desensitization protocols have been effective in patients who have suffered non-life-threatening reactions to TMP-SMX, but caution is advised.[90] Corticosteroids may also be helpful.[91]

Several alternative oral regimens are available for the treatment of mild to moderate cases of *Pneumocystis* pneumonia.[92] TMP 15 mg/kg daily in three divided doses combined with dapsone 100 mg daily was shown in one trial to be equally as effective as TMP-SMX, but less toxic.[93] Many patients intolerant of TMP-SMX can safely take TMP plus dapsone. However, caution is advised in using this combination because it is difficult to predict who might experience an ADR. Side effects of TMP and dapsone include hemolysis (especially in patients with glucose-6-phosphate dehydrogenase (G6PD) deficiency), methemoglobinemia, neutropenia, nausea, vomiting, fever, and rash.[86] Another regimen that has shown promising activity against *Pneumocystis* in several trials is clindamycin (oral dose is 300–450 mg four times a day) plus primaquine base (15–30 mg/day).[94,95] The mechanisms of action of these drugs are unknown. Principal side effects include rash, methemoglobinemia, hemolysis (G6PD deficiency), gastrointestinal disturbances, and transient neutropenia. A large, double-blind, randomized trial compared TMP-SMX, TMP plus dapsone, and clindamycin plus primaquine for therapy of mild to moderate pneumocystosis.[96] Similar rates of dose-limiting toxicity, therapeutic failure, and survival were observed among the three regimens, although there were differences in the types of ADR encountered.

Other regimens that have been studied are atovaquone and aerosolized pentamidine isethionate. Atovaquone is a hydroxynaphthoquinone that acts against plasmodia by inhibiting mitochondrial electron transport. Analysis of mutations in *Pneumocystis* isolates in patients who failed atovaquone suggests a similar site of action. In comparative studies, atovaquone was less effective but better tolerated than TMP-SMX or parenteral pentamidine.[97,98] The major side effects of atovaquone are fever, rash, gastrointestinal disturbances, and abnormal liver function tests. Atovaquone is a highly lipophilic compound with poor bioavailability; it is administered as an oral suspension at a dose of 750 mg twice a day with food.[99] Pentamidine is a diamidine that has been used to treat African trypanosomiasis and pneumocystosis for several decades. Its mechanism of action against *Pneumocystis* is unknown. Pentamidine is ordinarily administered intravenously and is highly toxic. The administration of pentamidine via aerosol is attractive because it should produce high concentrations of the drug in the lungs. Although aerosolized pentamidine has been used in the therapy of pneumocystosis, it is not as effective as the oral drugs and thus cannot be recommended.[100]

Pentamidine is the principal drug used to treat patients intolerant of TMP-SMX who have moderate to severe pneumocystosis. Pentamidine is administered as a daily dose of 4 mg/kg intravenously over at least one hour to minimize the risk of hypotension.[27,92] After injection, pentamidine pharmacokinetics follow a three-compartment model with rapid distribution to tissues, secondary distribution, and a long elimination half-life.[86,101] Only a small fraction of pentamidine is excreted in the urine. Autopsy studies have suggested that it takes at least 5 days for pentamidine to reach therapeutic concentrations in the lung.[102] Adverse reactions to pentamidine occur in more than 80% of patients and require discontinuation of the drug in approximately half the cases.[103–105] The principal ADRs are azotemia, cardiac arrhythmias (e.g., torsades de pointes), neutropenia, hypoglycemia, pancreatitis, hypocalcemia, hypomagnesemia, and hepatic abnormalities. Hypoglycemia is due to insulin release with pancreatic islet damage. It typically occurs early and may be followed by diabetes mellitus. The frequency of hypoglycemia and azotemia increases with pentamidine serum levels greater than 100 ng/mL, total drug dose, and duration of therapy.[106,107] Hyperkalemia due to pentamidine toxicity as a potassium-sparing diuretic has also been reported.[108] A dose of 3 mg/kg daily appears to be better tolerated, but controlled studies are lacking.

Alternative therapy for patients with moderate to severe *Pneumocystis* pneumonia who fail or cannot tolerate treatment with TMP-SMX or pentamidine is the combination of clindamycin plus primaquine.[27,92,109,110] Clindamycin 600–900 mg every 6–8 hours intravenously plus primaquine base 15–30 mg/day orally has been used successfully in patients with moderate to severe pneumocystosis.[94,111] Because of limited clinical experience and because primaquine is only available as an oral preparation, this combination should be used with caution in patients who are acutely ill.

During the first few days of treatment, HIV patients with *Pneumocystis* pneumonia frequently experience a worsening of their respiratory status. In patients with marginal blood oxygenation, this deterioration may require intubation. The underlying mechanism is thought to be the host inflammatory response to products released from dying *Pneumocystis* organisms and/or surfactant changes that exacerbate lung injury. Several studies have shown that corticosteroids administered within the first 72 hours of treatment can prevent this deterioration and improve survival; however, administration of corticosteroids after 72 hours was of no benefit. These data led a National Institutes of Health expert panel to recommend corticosteroids for all patients with moderate to severe pneumocystosis (PAO_2 <70 mmHg, PAO_2–PaO_2 >35 mmHg) using an oral regimen: prednisone 40 mg twice daily on days 1–5; 40 mg once daily on days 6–10; and 20 mg once daily on days 11–21.[83] Although a later study questioned whether corticosteroids improved the rate of recovery,[112] a meta-analysis supported the value of these drugs.[113] The ADRs of corticosteroids are primarily metabolic alterations such as hyperglycemia and exacerbation of infections such as thrush and mucocutaneous herpes simplex; nevertheless, concerns about other complications (e.g., pneumothorax) emphasize the need for judicious use of these drugs and careful patient follow-up.[55,114,115] It is not known whether corticosteroids are beneficial in patients with mild pneumocystosis and in pediatric patients.

In contrast to HIV-infected patients, the prognosis of pneumocystosis in other immunocompromised hosts has not changed appreciably during the past two decades. Although there have been few prospective studies, retrospective surveys of non-HIV-infected patients treated at tertiary care facilities have revealed mortality rates of 30–50%.[116–118] All non-HIV-infected patients with suspected *Pneumocystis* pneumonia should be admitted to a hospital for definitive diagnosis because the disease progresses more rapidly in this population than in those with HIV infection. For non-HIV-infected patients TMP-SMX administered for 14 days is the treatment of choice and is well tolerated; the principal ADRs are gastrointestinal disturbances and rash. The choice of alternative drugs is guided by the severity of the pneumocystosis and the clinical status of the patient. Pentamidine, the other major drug used in non-HIV-infected patients, is about as effective as TMP-SMX but is more toxic. Although it is likely that the other regimens described for HIV-infected patients will work in non-HIV-infected patients, clinical experience is limited. Additional studies are needed to determine whether corticosteroids have a place as adjunctive agents in the treatment of pneumocystosis in non-HIV-infected patients.

The clinical response to anti-*Pneumocystis* drugs is slow, particularly in HIV-infected patients. It is usually prudent to wait at least 5 days before deciding that treatment has failed and considering a change in therapy.[110]

Substitution of a drug is preferable to adding a second agent as there is no evidence that two drugs are more effective than a single agent. It is recommended that HIV-infected patients should begin antiretroviral therapy as soon as possible after starting treatment for *Pneumocystis* pneumonia.[119] The optimal start time has not been determined; some clinicians begin antiretroviral therapy once there is evidence of sustained clinical and radiologic recovery. An immune reconstitution inflammatory syndrome, with clinical deterioration, may be precipitated following early institution of antiretroviral therapy; patients require careful follow-up.

Local complications in the management of pneumocystosis, such as bullae and pneumatoceles, require careful attention and follow-up. These lesions lead to a pneumothorax, which presents difficult problems for management.[55,115] A chest tube is helpful but may not fully expand the lung, especially if a bronchopleural fistula develops. Other approaches include pleurodesis with talc or antibiotics and thoracostomy with stapling. Patients with chronic airway disease develop recurrent bacterial pneumonias requiring broad-spectrum antibiotics. Extrapulmonary pneumocystosis is treated with parenteral drugs.

PREVENTION AND CONTROL

Prevention of pneumocystosis can be directed either toward the first episode (primary) or toward recurrent episodes (secondary) of the disease. Chemoprophylaxis became widely accepted as the principal preventive measure in HIV-infected patients and other immunocompromised hosts when prospective, controlled clinical trials demonstrated its safety and efficacy. As a general rule, chemoprophylaxis should be continued as long as the risk factors for *Pneumocystis* pneumonia exist. An expert panel developed by the US Public Health Service, Infectious Diseases Society of America, and the HIV Medicine Association has published guidelines for the prevention of opportunistic infections in HIV-infected patients.[119] Primary prophylaxis is indicated for all adults and adolescents (including those who are pregnant) infected with HIV who have CD4 cell counts less than 200/μL, unexplained fever (>100°F) for more than 2 weeks, or oropharyngeal candidiasis. Individuals with a history of an AIDS-defining illness or a CD4 cell percentage of less than 14% should also be considered for prophylaxis. Secondary prophylaxis is indicated for all adults and adolescents who have recovered from an episode of pneumocystosis.

TMP-SMX is the drug of choice administered as one double-strength tablet (160 mg TMP plus 800 mg SMX) per day. Alternative regimens with one single-strength tablet (80 mg TMP plus 400 mg SMX) per day or one double-strength tablet three times per week are also satisfactory. In addition to its anti-*Pneumocystis* activity, TMP-SMX prevents bacterial infections and toxoplasmosis. The major problem with TMP-SMX is that up to 40% of HIV-infected patients experience ADRs requiring discontinuation of the drug; however, some patients can tolerate reintroduction of TMP by measures such as desensitization.[90]

If TMP-SMX cannot be tolerated, suitable alternatives are dapsone administered at a dose of 100 mg per day or dapsone 50 mg per day plus pyrimethamine 50 mg once a week and leucovorin 25 mg once a week.[119] Other regimens of these drugs have also been effective. Atovaquone suspension given at a dose of 1500 mg per day is approximately as effective as the dapsone regimens in *Pneumocystis* prophylaxis. Another option is aerosolized pentamidine (300 mg administered via Respirgard II nebulizer once a month). Aerosolized pentamidine is more expensive and less effective than the other regimens (particularly in patients with CD4 cell counts less than 100/μL), requires negative pressure rooms with adequate ventilation, may increase the frequency of atypical presentations, pneumothorax or extrapulmonary spread of *Pneumocystis* infection, and should not be used in patients with tuberculosis. Despite these limitations, aerosolized pentamidine is better tolerated than the other regimens. The side effects are cough and bronchospasm, which can be controlled with a β-agonist. Although other anti-*Pneumocystis* drugs (e.g., clindamycin plus primaquine) have also been considered for prophylaxis, insufficient information is available to make recommendations about their use.

Primary prophylaxis is indicated for children born to HIV-infected mothers, beginning at 4–6 weeks of age.[119] Prophylaxis may be discontinued if the child is found not to be infected with HIV, but it should be continued through the first year of life if HIV infection is diagnosed. After this, the need for prophylaxis is based on age-adjusted CD4 cell counts.

Antiretroviral therapy often results in an increase in CD4 cell counts. Primary and secondary *Pneumocystis* prophylaxis may be discontinued in adults if the CD4 cell count remains above 200 cells/μL for more than 3 months.[119] However, HIV patients with a CD4 cell count greater than 200/μL who have had a prior episode of pneumocystosis should continue chemoprophylaxis indefinitely.

Despite the availability and effectiveness of drugs to prevent pneumocystosis, about 20% of HIV patients who are at risk for pneumocystosis do not receive appropriate chemoprophylaxis.[120,121] Non-adherence occurs more commonly in Hispanic people, women, drug users, people with mental health problems, or who are poorly compliant with antiretroviral drugs. Patients with CD4 cell counts <100/μl are especially vulnerable to pneumocystosis.

Guidelines for chemoprophylaxis in non-HIV patients are less well developed because of the heterogeneous nature of these patient populations. However, recent review articles have developed some general guidelines.[122,123] Chemoprophylaxis is indicated for hematological malignancies and solid organ transplantation. Other potential populations include primary immune deficiency diseases, persistent CD4 cell counts <200/μl, severe protein malnutrition, and immunosuppressive or cytotoxic therapy for diseases such as cancer and rheumatologic disorders. If corticosteroids are the sole drug, a reasonable guide to the need for prophylaxis is the equivalent of prednisone 20 mg per day for more than 1 month. Whether prophylaxis is needed for patients given corticosteroids for asthma is controversial. Secondary prophylaxis is recommended for all patients as long as the immunosuppressive conditions persist. TMP-SMX is the drug of choice in all non-HIV patients. Although other agents have not been well studied, it is assumed that they will work as well in these patients as they do in HIV patients.

There are no uniform guidelines about isolating patients with pneumocystosis in health care facilities. However, in light of increasing evidence supporting the communicability of pneumocystosis infection in humans, it seems prudent to prevent *Pneumocystis* patients from having direct contact with other immunocompromised hosts.

ACKNOWLEDGMENTS

This work was supported by the Medical Research Service, Department of Veterans Affairs, and by Public Health Service Contract AI 25467 and grants R01A1-06492 and RO1 HL-090335 from the National Institutes of Health.

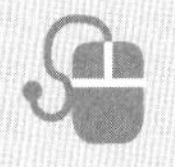

Access the complete reference list online at
http://www.expertconsult.com

CHAPTER 92

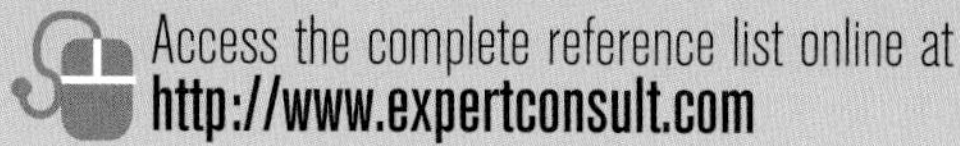
Access the complete reference list online at
http://www.expertconsult.com

Enteric Amebiasis

Kristine M. Peterson • Upinder Singh • William A. Petri, Jr

INTRODUCTION

Entamoeba histolytica is the cause of amebic colitis and liver abscess. *E. dispar* and *E. moshkovskii* are nonpathogenic parasites that are genetically distinct but identical morphologically to *E. histolytica*. Other amebae are less a source of diagnostic confusion as they are morphologically differentiated from the *E. histolytica/moshkovskii/dispar* group and include *E. hartmanni*, *E. coli*, *E. polecki*, *E. gingivalis*, *Iodamoeba butschlii, Endolimax nana*, and *Blastocystis hominis*.

Taxonomy

Entamoeba histolytica is a pseudopod-forming nonflagellate protozoan parasite. The invasive species *E. histolytica* and the noninvasive species *E. moshkovskii* and *E. dispar* can be differentiated by isoenzyme analysis, typing by monoclonal antibodies to surface antigens, and polymerase chain reaction (PCR) (***Box 92.1***).[1–14]

Life Cycle

The *E. histolytica* life cycle consists of an infective cyst and an invasive trophozoite form (***Fig. 92.1***). The cyst is 10–15 μm in diameter and contains four or fewer nuclei (***Fig. 92.2B***). Infection with *E. histolytica* most commonly occurs when cysts are ingested from fecally contaminated food or water. Sexual transmission has also been reported through oral–anal sexual practices.[15] Excystation occurs in the bowel lumen, forming trophozoites. The invasive trophozoite form is 10–60 μm in diameter and has a single nucleus with a central karyosome (***Fig. 92.2A***).

Trophozoites may form new cysts in the intestinal mucin layer. Formation of the cyst appears to involve quorum sensing mediated in part by the parasite cell surface Gal/GalNAc lectin.[16,17] Other processes involved in cyst formation include signaling via beta-adrenergic receptors[18] and autophagy (a method of degrading damaged or unnecessary proteins and organelles).[19] A total of 672 cyst-specific genes and 767 trophozoite-specific genes have been identified.[20,21]

Cell Biology and Biochemistry

E. histolytica is a eukaryotic organism but lacks organelles that morphologically resemble rough endoplasmic reticulum, the Golgi apparatus, or mitochondria[22–25] (***Box 92.2***). The presence of nuclear-encoded mitochondrial genes, such as pyridine nucleotide transhydrogenase and *hsp*60, is consistent with *E. histolytica* having contained mitochondria at one time. Mitosomes, which are mitochondrion-related remnant organelles, have also been identified.[26] Despite the lack of rough endoplasmic reticulum or Golgi apparatus, cell surface and secreted proteins contain signal sequences, and tunicamycin inhibits protein glycosylation.[23] Ribosomes form aggregated crystalline arrays in the cytoplasm of the trophozoite. Remarkably, more than 100 transmembrane kinases are present in the *E. histolytica* genome. These kinases are part of the family of Gal/GalNAc lectin-related proteins that share the extracellular CXXC and CXC motifs of the lectin intermediate (igl) subunit.[27]

E. histolytica is unique among protists in that it possesses both the phosphorylated and nonphosphorylated serine metabolic pathways.[28] The cysteine biosynthetic pathway is also important in *E. histolytica*.[29] Although the synthesis of adenosine triphosphate (ATP) in *E. histolytica* is primarily carried out by the glycolytic pathway, observations from the genome sequence have revealed that amino acids may also play a role in ATP generation.[30,31]

Gene Structure and Organization

E. histolytica genomic organization and promoter elements appear to be distinct from both metazoan and better-characterized protozoan organisms.[23–25]

The size of the *E. histolytica* genome is currently estimated to be ~24 million base pairs and contains a predicted 14 chromosomes and 10 000 genes.[27,32] Ribosomal RNA makes up appoximately 20% of the total cellular DNA, and an unprecedented 10% of the total DNA comprises tRNA genes organized in repetitive linear arrays. Thirty percent of genes are predicted to contain introns,[33] and 6% contain two or more introns.[32] Recently, approximately 7% of the predicted amebic genes were analyzed using an expressed sequence tag library. Evidence to support the splicing of 60% of introns and molecular evidence for U2, 4, and 5 snRNAs was found.[33,34]

Both transient and stable DNA-mediated transfection of *E. histolytica* with heterologous gene expression has been accomplished (***Fig. 92.3***). Deletion and replacement analysis has been conducted on the promoter of the *E. histolytica* gene encoding the heavy subunit of the *N*-acetyl-β-D-galactosamine-specific adhesin (*hgl*5).[35] Four positive upstream regulatory elements and one negative upstream regulatory element were identified in the 200 bases upstream of the start of transcription (***Fig. 92.4***). The transcription factors that control gene expression by these upstream regulatory elements have been identified in two cases. Both transcription factors are novel, with one containing RNA-binding motifs and the other EF-hand motifs.[36,37] Strikingly, the ability of the EF-hand-containing transcription factor to bind to its cognate DNA motif is controlled by calcium.[37,38] Core promoter elements, including a TATA element at 30 base pairs upstream of the transcription start site, the novel conserved sequence GAAC, which is located between the TATA and initiator elements, and the conserved sequence at the transcription start site (putative initiator), have been demonstrated to regulate gene expression and control the site of transcription initiation.[39,40]

Box 92.1 Differentiation of *Entamoeba histolytica* vs *E. moshkovskii* and *E. dispar*

Biochemical Characteristics	Clinical Characteristics
Discrimination by isoenzyme migration	*E. dispar* and *E. moshkovskii* have not been associated with tissue invasion
Immunologic Characteristics	
Monoclonal antibodies	
Genetic Characteristics	
Restriction fragment pattern comparisons	
Repetitive DNA sequences	
Riboprinting	

(Reproduced from Petri WA Jr. Recent advances in amebiasis. Crit Rev Clin Lab Sci. 1996;33:1. Copyright Lewis Publishers, an imprint of CRC Press.)

Box 92.2 Some Unusual Features of the Cell Biology and Biochemistry of *Entamoeba histolytica*

- Lack of mitochondria, rough endoplasmic reticulum, or Golgi apparatus
- Presence of crystalline arrays of aggregated ribosomes
- Ribosomal RNA genes on multicopy circular DNA molecules
- Lack of glutathione and enzymes of glutathione metabolism
- Use of pyrophosphate instead of adenosine triphosphate at several steps in glycolysis
- Inability to synthesize purine nucleotides *de novo*

(Reproduced from Petri WA Jr. Recent advances in amebiasis. Crit Rev Clin Lab Sci. 1996;33:1. Copyright Lewis Publishers, an imprint of CRC Press.)

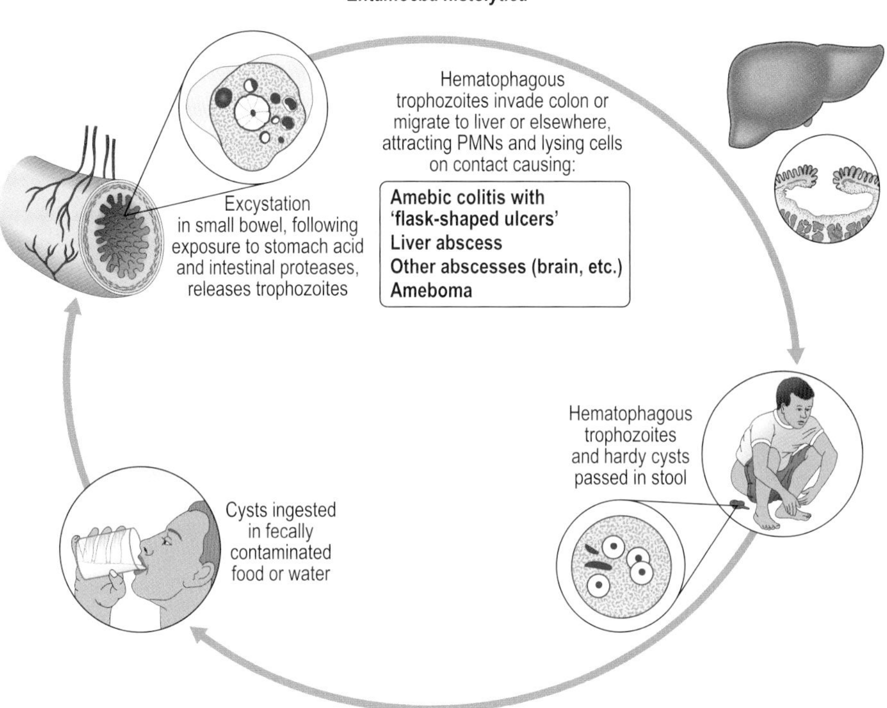
Entamoeba histolytica
Hematophagous trophozoites invade colon or migrate to liver or elsewhere, attracting PMNs and lysing cells on contact causing:
Amebic colitis with 'flask-shaped ulcers'
Liver abscess
Other abscesses (brain, etc.)
Ameboma
Excystation in small bowel, following exposure to stomach acid and intestinal proteases, releases trophozoites
Hematophagous trophozoites and hardy cysts passed in stool
Cysts ingested in fecally contaminated food or water

Figure 92.1 *Entamoeba histolytica* life cycle. PMNs, polymorphonuclear leukocytes.

EPIDEMIOLOGY

The preponderance of *E. histolytica* infection, morbidity, and mortality is experienced in Central and South America, Africa, and the Indian subcontinent. *E. moshkovskii* has been detected from human specimens in Bangladesh,[41] India,[42] Australia,[13] and Tanzania.[43] Serologic surveys reflect the incidence of *E. histolytica* infection, as *E. dispar* and *E. moshkovskii* infection do not result in a positive serologic test.[44]

Studies from the developing world using modern diagnostic tests have highlighted the burden of amebic disease. In Dhaka, Bangladesh, preschool children had a 2.2% annual frequency of amebic dysentery as compared to a 5.3% rate of *Shigella* dysentery during 3 years of prospective community observation.[45] An annual incidence of amebic liver abscess of 21 cases/100 000 inhabitants was observed in Hue City, Vietnam.[46] The 1987–1988 Mexican national survey of 67 668 serums (acquired by a probabilistic sampling technique from a representative cross-section of the country) demonstrated an 8.4% seropositivity for *E. histolytica* as measured with the indirect hemagglutination assay (IHA).[47] Peak seropositivity was 11% in the 5–9-year-old age group. In the year of the serosurvey there was an estimated 1 million cases of amebiasis and 1216 deaths due to *E. histolytica* infection in Mexico.[48]

Residents of developed nations that are at higher risk of developing amebiasis include, most importantly, immigrants from or travelers to countries where amebiasis is endemic.[49–52] One study of 2700 German citizens returning from tropical areas demonstrated a 4% incidence of *E. histolytica*/*E. dispar* infection.[52] Diarrhea and detection of *E. histolytica* only (no other intestinal pathogens present) occurred in 80% of travelers with pathogenic *E. histolytica*.[53] Other groups at higher risk include sexually active male homosexuals (who are predominantly infected with *E. dispar*[54,55]) and institutionalized individuals.[56]

A total of 2970 cases of amebiasis in the United States were reported to the Centers for Disease Control and Prevention (CDC) in 1993 (the last year that it was a reportable disease): 33% of the patients were Hispanic and 17% Asian or Pacific Islanders.[57] Amebic liver abscess is 7–12 times more common in men, although in children the sex distribution is equal.[58,59] The typical patient in the United States with amebic liver abscess is a Hispanic male between the ages of 20 and 40 years. Infection with *E. histolytica* generally presents clinically within a year of immigration to the United States, although it is not rare for presentation to lag immigration by up to 12 years. More severe disease is seen in the very young and old, the malnourished, and pregnant women.[60–63] *E. histolytica* infection in human immunodeficiency virus-infected children was

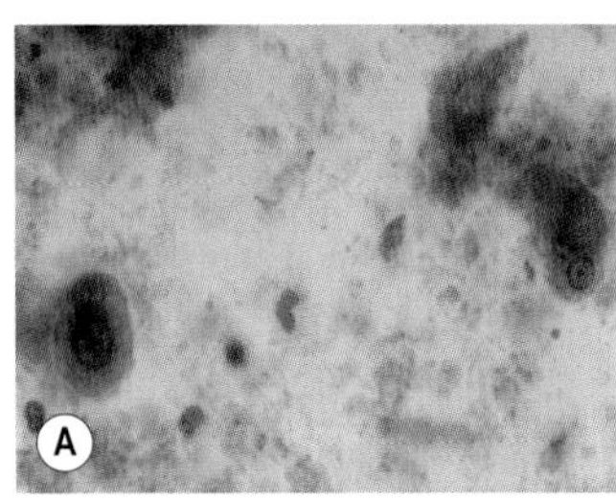

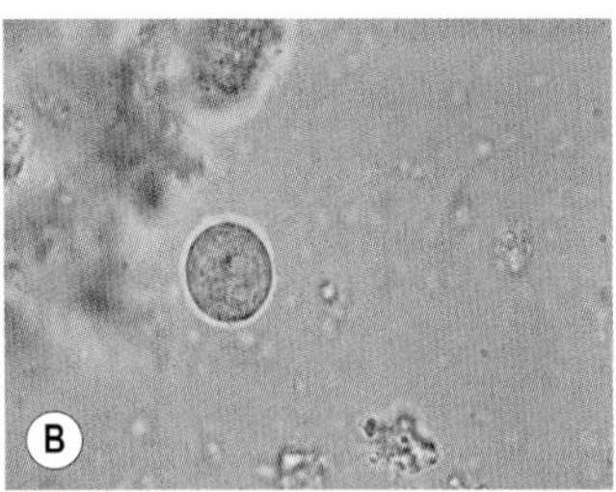

Figure 92.2 *Entamoeba histolytica* trophozoite and cyst. (**A**) The motile and invasive trophozoite form contains a single nucleus and is 10–60 μm in diameter. (**B**) The infectious cyst form is 10–15 μm in diameter and contains four nuclei. Note that it is not possible to distinguish *E. histolytica* from *E. dispar* morphologically. (Courtesy of Centers for Disease Control and Prevention, Atlanta, GA.)

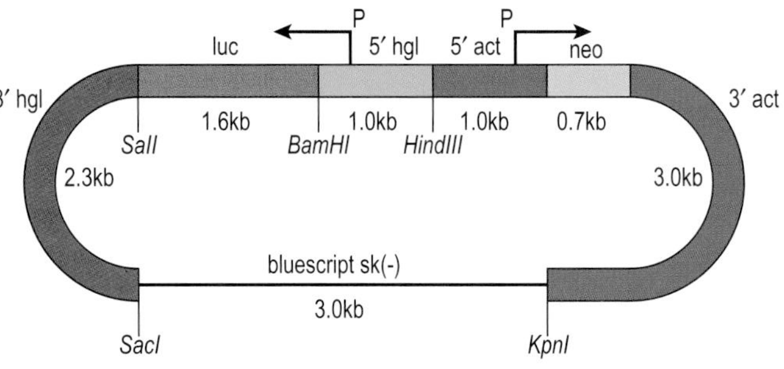

Figure 92.3 The two-promoter transfection vector pTCV3. The actin promoter is used to express neo, enabling selection of stably transfected parasites with the antibiotic G418. The lectin hgl promoter is used to express a gene of interest in the stably transfected amebae, which in this case is firefly luciferase.

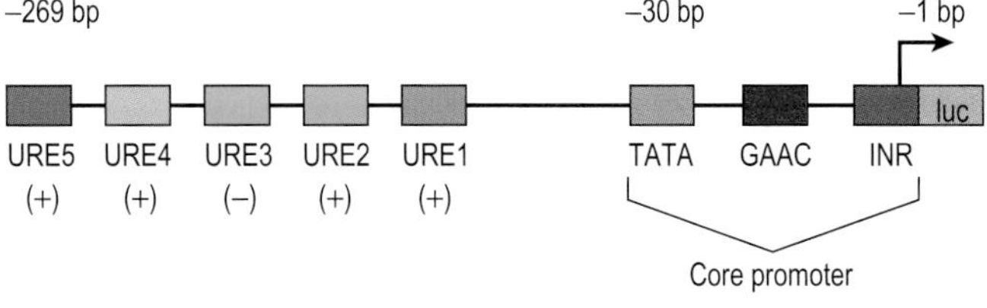

Figure 92.4 Structure of the promoter of the hgl5 gene of *Entamoeba histolytica*. Four positive and one negative upstream regulatory regions have been identified by linker scanner mutagenesis and transient transfection system using the reporter gene luciferase. Three regions have also been identified in the core promoter which appear to control gene expression.

clustered in the most severely malnourished children with chronic diarrhea in a study from Tanzania.[64]

THE DISEASE

Asymptomatic Colonization

Noninvasive intestinal infection is presumed to be the only presentation of *E. dispar* and *E. moshkovskii* infection and is also a common presentation of *E. histolytica* infection (***Box 92.3***). Colonization with *E. dispar* and *E. moshkovskii* does not require intervention on the part of the physician, as these amebae have not been shown to be a cause of colitis or abscess. In contrast, patients colonized with *E. histolytica* are at risk of future (months to even years later) development of invasive disease and should be treated if coincidentally diagnosed.[65] Antigen detection tests to distinguish *E. histolytica* from *E. dispar* and *E. moshkovskii* infection are commercially available for clinical use (see Diagnosis, below).

Box 92.3 Clinical Manifestations of *Entamoeba* Infection

Asymptomatic Colonization	Extraintestinal Amebiasis (*E. histolytica* Only)
E. histolytica	Amebic liver abscess
E. dispar	Splenic abscess
E. moshkovskii	Brain abscess
Intestinal Amebiasis and Its Complications (*E. histolytica* Only)	Empyema
Amebic colitis	Pericarditis
Ameboma	
Toxic megacolon	
Peritonitis	
Cutaneous amebiasis	

(Reproduced from Petri WA Jr. Recent advances in amebiasis. Crit Rev Clin Lab Sci. 1996;33:1. Copyright Lewis Publishers, an imprint of CRC Press.)

Amebic Diarrhea

Diarrhea is the most common disease manifestation of *E. histolytica* infection. Amebic diarrhea is defined as diarrhea in an *E. histolytica*-infected individual. The presence of mucus or visible or microscopic blood in the stool is not required for the diagnosis of amebic diarrhea. In a community-based study of a cohort of preschool children in Bangladesh, the annual incidence of amebic infection, diarrhea, and dysentery was 45%, 9%, and 3% respectively.[66]

Dysentery and Colitis

The major concern of the physician confronted with a patient with dysentery (diarrhea that contains visible or microscopic blood) is to differentiate between infectious causes (including amebiasis, *Shigella, Salmonella, Campylobacter*, and enteroinvasive and enterohemorrhagic *Escherichia coli*) and noninfectious causes (including inflammatory bowel disease, ischemic colitis, and gastrointestinal bleeding secondary to arteriovenous malformations or diverticulitis).[67] It is at times difficult to make the diagnosis of amebic colitis, as the presentation of the illness may be insidious or chronic, bleeding may occur without diarrhea, and fever is an unusual finding. A single stool examination for parasites is insensitive, histopathologic confirmation of infection on biopsy specimens may be difficult, and serologic tests for anti-amebic antibodies are not always positive in the acute setting (***Table 92.1***).

In a developed country such as the United States, most patients with amebiasis will be immigrants or travelers from areas with endemic amebiasis. Patients with amebic colitis typically present with a history over several weeks of gradual onset of abdominal pain and tenderness, diarrhea, and bloody stools. In one series, patients with amebic colitis had an average duration of prehospital illness of 21 days, compared with 4 days for patients with shigellosis.[68] Because of the gradual onset, weight loss is a common finding. Surprisingly, fever is present in only the minority (8–38%) of patients with amebic colitis.[68,69] Examination of stools reveals that they are uniformly positive for occult blood.[69] Colonic lesions can vary from only mucosal thickening, to flask-shaped ulcerations, to necrosis of the intestinal wall (***Fig. 92.5***).

Unusual manifestations of amebic colitis include acute necrotizing colitis, ameboma (granulation tissue in colonic lumen mimicking colonic cancer in appearance), cutaneous amebiasis, and rectovaginal fistulas. Acute fulminant or necrotizing colitis is the most feared complication,

Table 92.1 Symptoms and Signs of Amebic Colitis

Symptoms and Signs	Percentage
Gradual onset	Most
History of symptoms >1 week	Most
Diarrhea	94–100
Dysentery	94–100
Abdominal pain	12–80
Weight loss	44
Fever >38°C	10
Heme (+) stools	100
Male-to-female ratio	1:1
Immigrant from or traveler to endemic area	Most

(Reproduced from Petri WA Jr. Recent advances in amebiasis. Crit Rev Clin Lab Sci. 1996;33:1. Copyright Lewis Publishers, an imprint of CRC Press.)

Table 92.2 Symptoms and Signs of Amebic Liver Abscess

Symptoms and Signs	Range
History of symptoms >4 weeks	21–51%
Fever	85–90%
Abdominal tenderness	84–90%
Hepatomegaly	30–50%
Jaundice	6–10%
Diarrhea	20–33%
Weight loss	33–50%
Cough	10–30%
Male-to-female ratio	9:1
Immigrant from or traveler to endemic area	Most

(Reproduced from Petri WA Jr. Recent advances in amebiasis. Crit Rev Clin Lab Sci. 1996;33:1. Copyright Lewis Publishers, an imprint of CRC Press.)

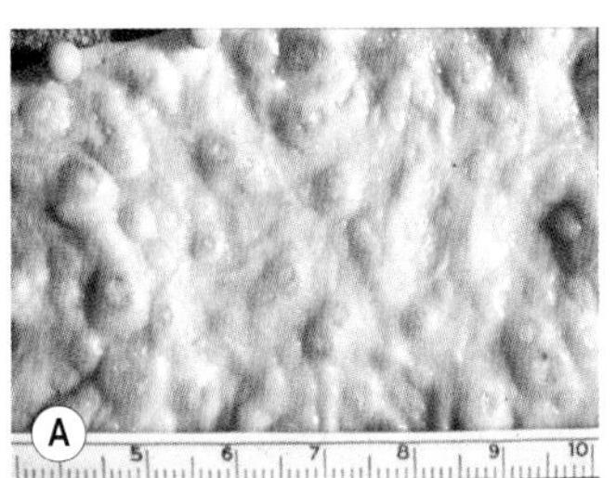

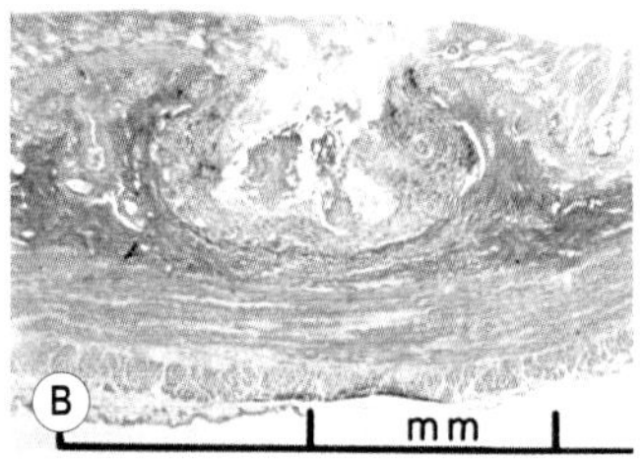

Figure 92.5 Amebic colitis.
(A) Multiple mucosal ulcers are visible in the resected section of the colon (the smallest division of the scale is 1 mm). (**B**) Mucosal ulceration of amebic colitis, with extension of the ulcer into the submucosa. (Hematoxylin and eosin stain.) (From the collection of the late Harrison Juniper.)

occurs in about 0.5% of cases, may require surgical intervention, and has a mortality greater than 40%.[70,71] Abdominal pain, distension, and rebound tenderness are present in most patients with fulminant colitis, although frank guarding is uncommon.

Liver Abscess

A typical patient with an amebic liver abscess is an adult male, age 20–40, from a country with endemic amebiasis. A 1–2-week history of fever and abdominal pain is common. Signs of amebic liver abscess include right upper-quadrant pain, fever of 38.5–39.5°C, leukocytosis, abnormal serum transaminases and alkaline phosphatase, an elevated right hemidiaphragm, and a defect on hepatic imaging study[58,59,72,73] (*Table 92.2 and Fig. 92.6*). A more chronic presentation of 2–12 weeks of weight loss, fever, and abdominal pain has been reported in a subset of patients with single abscesses.[59] Roughly 90% of patients with liver abscess are males, although in children (especially infants)[74,75] the sex distribution is equal. The abscess is single and in the right lobe of the liver 80% of the time. However, the most common location for a pyogenic abscess is also in the right lobe, so the location is not helpful in distinguishing the cause of an abscess.[76,77] Patients with pyogenic, as opposed to amebic, liver abscesses are more likely to be older than 50 years, present with jaundice, pruritus, sepsis, or shock, and have a palpable mass.[78]

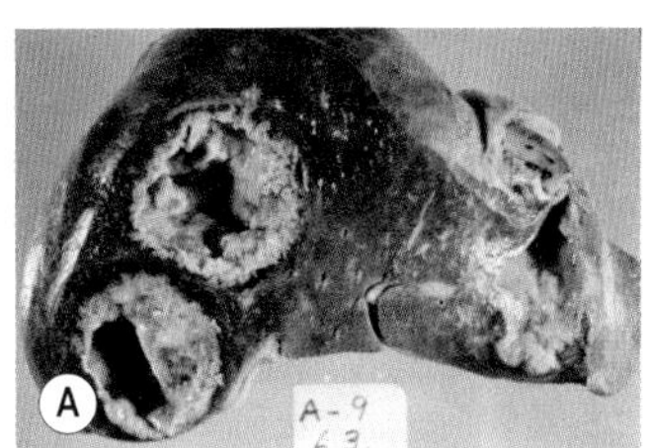

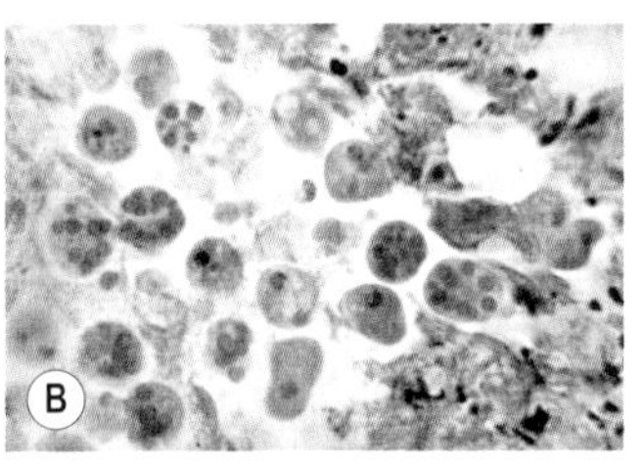

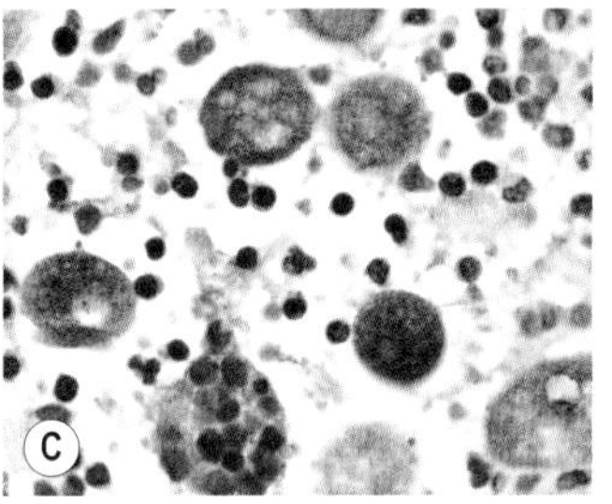

Figure 92.6 Amebic liver abscess. Gross (**A**) and microscopic (**B** and **C**) pathology of amebic liver abscess. (**B**) *Entamoeba histolytica* trophozoites (arrowheads) are surrounded by amorphous eosinophilic debris. (Hematoxylin and eosin stain.) Host inflammatory cells are present only at the periphery of the lesion, most likely a reflection of the parasite's ability to lyse macrophages. (**C**) Periodic acid–Schiff stains amebic trophozoites darkly, with a characteristic surrounding halo which is an artifact of fixation. (Immunoperoxidase stain of amebic trophozoites.) (A, B from the collection of the late Harrison Juniper.)

Most patients with liver abscess do not have concurrent colitis, although a history of dysentery within the last year can sometimes be obtained. Amebae are infrequently identified microscopically in the stool (18% of cases) at the time of diagnosis of liver abscess, although they can be identified in the stool by culture in the majority of patients. Liver abscess can present acutely with fever, right upper abdominal tenderness and pain, or subacutely with prominent weight loss, fever, and abdominal pain. The peripheral white blood cell count and alkaline phosphatase level are often elevated. Chest radiograph demonstrates elevation of the right hemidiaphragm in most patients.[79,80] Early evaluation of the hepatobiliary system with ultrasound, computed tomography (CT), or magnetic resonance imaging (MRI) is essential to demonstrate the abscess in the liver. Direct extension of the liver abscess to the pleura or pericardium may rarely occur.

The differential diagnosis of the lesion in the liver would include pyogenic abscess (less likely if the gallbladder and intrahepatic ducts appear normal), hepatoma, and echinococcal cyst (unlikely to present acutely with fever and abdominal pain). Aspiration of the abscess is occasionally required to diagnose amebiasis. The lack of bacterial infection in the abscess fluid is most helpful in ruling out a pyogenic abscess; amebae are rarely visualized in the pus in only the minority of cases but PCR for *E. histolytica* appears to be very sensitive. Antibodies to *E. histolytica* are present in the serum of 92–97% of patients on acute presentation with amebic liver abscess, and therefore are very useful diagnostically. Because a significant proportion of the population in developing countries is seropositive, antibody tests are less specific in residents or immigrants from the developing world (see Diagnosis, below).

Metastatic Amebiasis

The lung is the second most common extraintestinal site of *E. histolytica* disease after the liver, and most commonly occurs from extension of a hepatic abscess. Pulmonary consolidation, abscesses, or bronchohepatic fistulas may be seen, and an empyema may develop from rupture of a liver abscess into the pleural space. The right lower lobe of the lung is most commonly involved, although any lobe can be affected.[81] Pulmonary amebiasis as a result of haematogenous spread without liver abscess has been described in a patient presenting with superior vena cava syndrome.[82] Pericardial amebiasis is a rare form of thoracic amebiasis. This usually occurs by direct extension from an amebic abscess in the left lobe of the liver, but can occur from infection of the right lobe of the liver, lungs, or pleura. Symptoms may include chest pain and dyspnea. Pericarditis, pericardial effusion, and cardiac tamponade can result from amebic involvement of the pericardium.[81]

An amebic brain abscess due to *E. histolytica* can present without evidence for *E. histolytica* disease elsewhere,[82] although it most commonly presents in individuals with an amebic liver abscess.[83]

Recently the first case of *E. histolytica* encephalitis was diagnosed by PCR of cerebrospinal fluid. The patient was successfully treated with metronidazole.[84] Cutaneous amebiasis presents with painful ulcers, laden with amebae. It most commonly occurs in association with amebic colitis, and involvement of the perianal area and genitalia is most frequent.[85] Rare cases of amebic involvement of other organs, including the kidneys[86,87] and spleen,[88] have been reported.

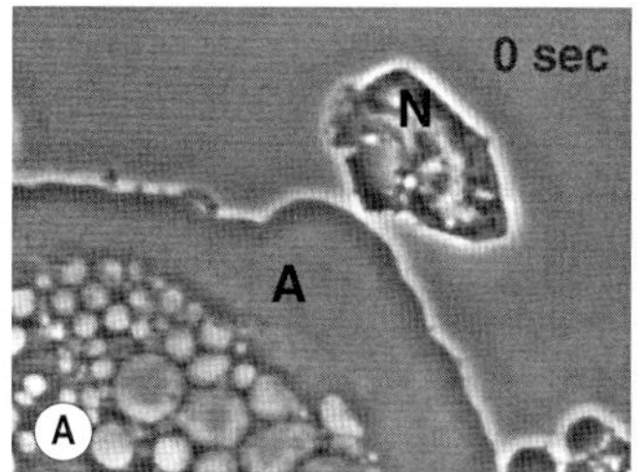

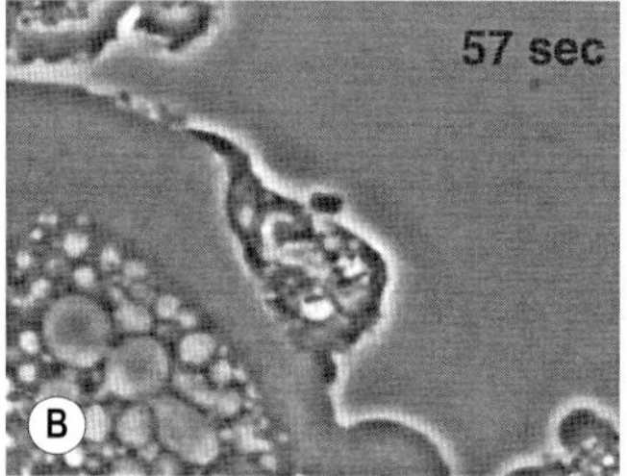

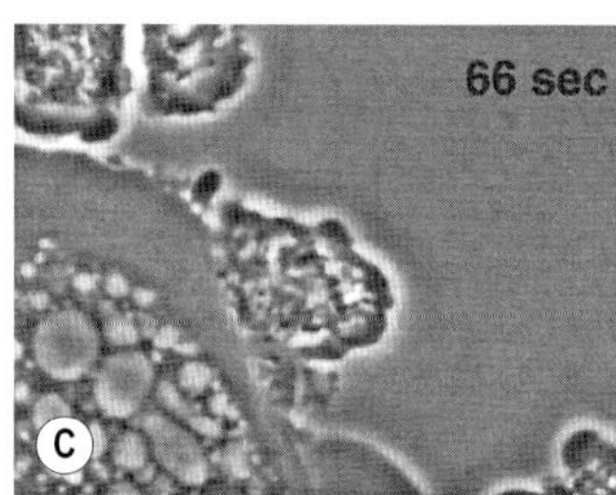

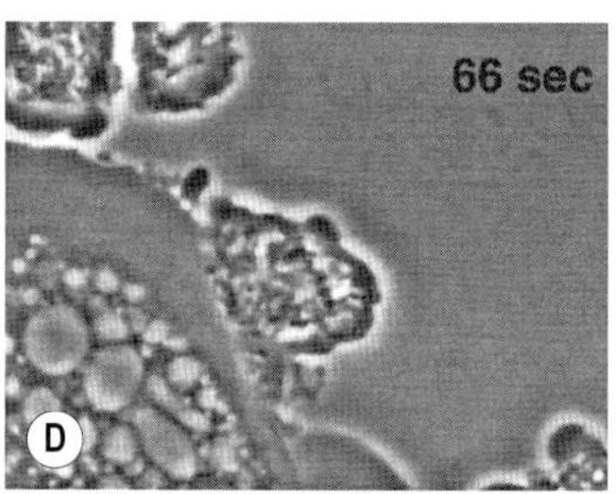

Figure 92.7 Killing of a human polymorphonuclear neutrophil (N) by an ameba (A). On establishing contact with the ameba, the neutrophil undergoes membrane blebbing and loss of granules and cytoplasmic integrity. (Magnification ×2000.) (Reproduced from Ravdin JI, Guerrant RL. Current problems in diagnosis and treatment of amebic infections. Curr Clin Top Infect Dis. 1996;7:82–111.)

PATHOGENESIS

Carbohydrate–protein interactions play a key role in human infection by *E. histolytica*.[89] Killing of host cells by *E. histolytica* trophozoites *in vitro* occurs only on direct contact (***Fig. 92.7***), which is mediated by an amebic adhesin which recognizes N- and O-linked oligosaccharides.[90–96] This amebic Gal/GalNAc lectin is a heterodimer of heavy and light subunits noncovalently associated with an intermediate subunit, all of which are encoded by multigene families, designated *hgl*, *lgl*, and *igl*, respectively.[90–96]

The first receptor encountered by the lectin may be the human colonic mucin layer of the large intestine.[97] Interaction of trophozoites with colonic mucins appears to be a dynamic process, with trophozoites both inducing the secretion of, and degrading, colonic mucins.[97] The mucin layer may protect the host from contact-dependent cytotoxicity of the parasite by binding to and neutralizing the lectin. However, cysteine proteases secreted by *E. histolytica* have the ability to dissolve mucus gels by targeting the C-terminal cysteine-rich domains of MUC2, decreasing the protective ability of the mucus layer.[98] The colonic mucins also serve as a site of attachment for the parasite to colonize the large bowel.

The Gal/GalNAc lectin functions in multiple processes. The lectin is localized to lipid rafts, which are cholesterol-rich domains in the plasma membrane. In *E. histolytica*, rafts play a role in endocytosis as well as adhesion of *E. histolytica* to both host cells[99] and extracellular matrix components.[100] Disruption of the Gal/GalNAc lectin function by expression of a dominant negative mutant in a hamster model resulted in lower penetration of trophozoites into hepatic tissue, decreased hepatic abscess formation, and weak attraction of neutrophils and macrophages to infiltrated areas.[101] Interference with Gal/GalNAc lectin signaling also blocks chemotaxis towards the proinflammatory cytokine tumor necrosis factor-α.[102] In addition, the Gal/GalNAc lectin plays a role in evasion of the host immune defenses by inhibiting the formation of the complement membrane attack complex via a remarkable mimicry of human CD59.[103,104]

Rhomboid protein is another potential example of how *E. histolytica* may evade immune defenses. *E. histolytica* encodes one rhomboid protein (EhROM1) with necessary residues for protease activity. In *E. histolytica* trophozoites, EhROM1 was shown to co-localize with a lectin in vesicles during phagocytosis and the base of the cap during surface receptor capping. Surface receptor capping is used for immune evasion, during which surface receptors that have been recognized by host immune components are rapidly polarized to the posterior of the cell and released. Therefore, EhROM1 appears to be capable of cleaving lectins and releasing them from the cell surface, explaining observations of both membrane-bound and soluble forms of the Gal/GalNAc lectin.[105]

Intracellular calcium in target cells rises approximately 20-fold within seconds of direct contact by an amebic trophozoite and is associated with membrane blebbing.[106] Cell death occurs 5–15 minutes after the lethal hit is delivered. Extracellular ethylenediaminetetraacetate and treatment of the target cells with the slow sodium-calcium channel blockers verapamil and bepridil[107] significantly reduce amebic killing of target cells in suspension. Isolation of an amebic pore-forming protein, similar in function to pore-forming proteins of the immune system, has been reported.[108] A purified 5-kDa amebapore and a synthetic peptide based on the sequence of its third amphipathic α-helix have cytolytic activity for nucleated cells at high concentrations (10–100 μM).[109]

Amebic killing of host cells is a consequence of parasite-activated apoptosis. Cells killed by *E. histolytica* undergo nuclear chromatin condensation, membrane blebbing, and internucleosomal DNA fragmentation. However, the apoptotic process in *E. histolytica* is unusual. Overexpression of the Bcl-2 protein that inhibits apoptosis resulting from cell stresses did not prevent murine cell DNA fragmentation following exposure to *E. histolytica*.[109] *E. histolytica* also caused hepatocyte apoptosis in mice deficient in the Fas/Fas ligand and TNR-R1 signaling pathways.[110] *E. histolytica* apoptosis is also unique in that it can easily kill both caspase-8-deficient cells and caspase-8-deficient cells treated with caspase-9 inhibitor.[111] These findings suggested that the classical upstream caspases were not involved in *E. histolytica*-mediated apoptosis. *E. histolytica* is now known to initiate host cell apoptosis by directly activating the host cell's distal apoptotic components. Caspase 3 is activated within minutes of *E. histolytica* adherence, and its inhibitor blocked *E. histolytica* killing, as measured by both DNA fragmentation and Cr^{51} release. This indicates that caspase 3 is required for *E. histolytica* killing via both apoptosis and necrosis.[112]

Amebae have been shown to ingest erythrocytes and nucleated host cells only after the cells are killed,[113] suggesting that changes on the host cell surface resulting from apoptosis are necessary for phagocytosis. Phosphatidylserine is exposed on the surface of erythrocytes killed by *E. histolytica*, and its inhibitors prevented *E. histolytica* ingestion of erythrocytes.[114] Inhibition of endocytosis by galactose and phosphatidylserine is additive, suggesting the Gal/GalNAc lectin and a currently unidentified phosphatidylserine receptor may act as co-receptors for ingestion. Recently, collectin family members (mannose-binding lectin), the structurally related C1q protein, and serine-rich *E. histolytica* protein have been shown to have roles in phagocytosis as well.[115,116] Importantly, amebae that are defective in phagocytosis are also defective in virulence.

IMMUNITY

During the acute phase of amebic invasion, neutrophils are commonly the earliest infiltrating cells observed.[117,118] Depletion of neutrophils with anti-Gr-1 neutralizing antibodies resulted in severe intestinal pathology in mice, suggesting a protective role for neutrophils in early resistance to amebiasis.[119] *E. histolytica* trophozoites can induce NADPH oxidase-derived reactive oxygen species which activate ERK1/2 (a MAPK subtype) and trigger neutrophil apoptosis.[120] However, neutrophil destruction can subsequently lead to the release of cytotoxic oxidase and lytic peptidases, resulting in host tissue damage.

Macrophages acquire amebicidal activity *in vitro* after stimulation with interferon-γ (IFN-γ), tumor necrosis factor-α, or colony-stimulating factor-1.[117] Macrophages exposed to the surface Gal/GalNAc lectin of *E. histolytica* upregulate TLR-2 expression, which leads to NF-κB activation and proinflammatory cytokine production.[121] Macrophages are also able to recognize *E. histolytica* lipopeptidophosphoglycan (LPPG), which is a highly immunogenic molecular pattern exposed on the trophozoites' surface. LPPG induces NF-κB activation and cytokines of the innate immune response, and macrophages lacking TLR-2 and TLR-4 showed impaired response to *E. histolytica* LPPG.[122]

Nitric oxide is secreted by phagocytes (monocytes, macrophages, and neutrophils) and can inhibit virulence factors of *E. histolytica*, including cysteine proteinases.[123] Mice lacking inducible nitric oxide synthase were also shown to be more susceptible to amebic liver abscess and *E. histolytica*-induced apoptosis of hepatic cells.[124] However, *E. histolytica* has developed multiple responses to counter the effects of nitric oxide, including suppressing the respiratory burst within macrophages[125] and inhibiting nitric oxide production.[126]

Activation of natural killer (NK) and natural killer T (NKT) cells leads to the production of IFN-γ and cytolytic peptides. The cytotoxic activity of NK cells was found to be elevated in mice infected with pathogenic ameba compared to those infected with nonpathogenic strains.[127] Hepatic amebic abscesses are much more common in males than females, and NKT cells may be partially responsible for these gender differences. During the early phase of amebic liver abscess development, spleen cells from female mice were found to elicit higher IFN-γ levels than spleen cells from male mice. The use of IFN-γ-neutralizing antibody or NKT knockout mice dramatically increased the size of amebic liver abscesses in female mice, suggesting the source of the early IFN-γ is NKT cells.[128] Recently, a purified phosphoinositol moiety of *E. histolytica* membrane LPPG was found to induce IFN-γ production in NKT cells. This suggests that EhLPPG may play an important role in limiting the development of amebic liver abscess.[129]

Cysteine proteases of *E. histolytica* trophozoites activate the alternative complement pathway via cleavage of C3 and C5. The resulting C3a and C5a act as chemoattractants to the site of infection. The Gal/GalNAc lectin of *E. histolytica* inhibits the assembly of C8 and C9 into the C5b-9 membrane attack complex, preventing complement-mediated lysis of the parasite.

Immunity to infection is associated with a mucosal immunoglobulin A (IgA) response against the carbohydrate recognition domain of the Gal/GalNAc lectin: children with this response had 86% fewer new infections over 1 year of prospective observation[130,131] (***Fig. 92.8***). In contrast, serum IgG is not associated with protection. An increased frequency of new *E. histolytica* infections was seen in children with serum IgG antibodies to the lectin.[132]

Several lines of evidence suggest an important role for cell-mediated immunity (CMI) in the killing of amebae.[133–137] A CD4 T-cell-mediated immune response may not always be protective, and may depend on the pattern of the $CD4^+$ T-cell response. In the murine model of amebic colitis, depeletion of CD4 T cells has been shown to ameliorate inflammation and colonic ulceration. However, an increase in mast cell activation and infiltration was associated with elevated Th2 cytokines in the colitis model at 10 weeks postchallenge, implying mast cells and a Th2 response have a role in the progression of amebic colitis during the chronic phase.[138]

The association of antiparasite IgA antibody with *in vivo* resistance to infection, as well as the ability of proinflammatory cytokines to activate protective immunity *in vitro*, suggested that major histocompatibility complex class II alleles could affect both the acquisition of amebiasis and

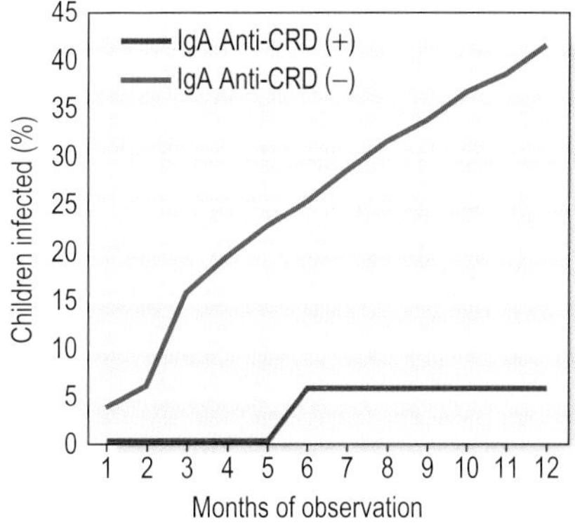

Figure 92.8 Acquired immunity to amebiasis in children. Children who developed stool immunoglobulin A (IgA) anti-CRD (lectin carbohydrate recognition domain) antibodies in the first year of the study (*n* = 81) had a lower incidence of new *Entamoeba histolytica* infections in the second year compared to children who remained IgA anti-CRD-negative (*n* = 149). The two groups are statistically significantly different ($P \leq 0.04$) at every time point. (Reproduced from Haque R, Duggal P, Ali IM, et al. Innate and acquired resistance to amebiasis in Bangladeshi children. J Infect Dis. 2002;186:547–552.)

Table 92.3 Sensitivity of Tests for Diagnosis of Amebiasis

Test	Colitis	Liver
Microscopy (stool)	25–60%	10–40%
Stool antigen detection	>90%	~40%
Serum antigen detection	65% early	~100% prior to treatment
Microscopy (abscess fluid)	N/A	≤20%
Abscess antigen detection	N/A	~40%
Serology (indirect hemagglutination)		
Acute	70%	70–80%
Convalescent	>90%	>90%

(Reproduced from Haque R, Huston CD, Hughes M, et al. Current concepts: amebiasis. N Engl J Med. 2003;348:1565–1573.)

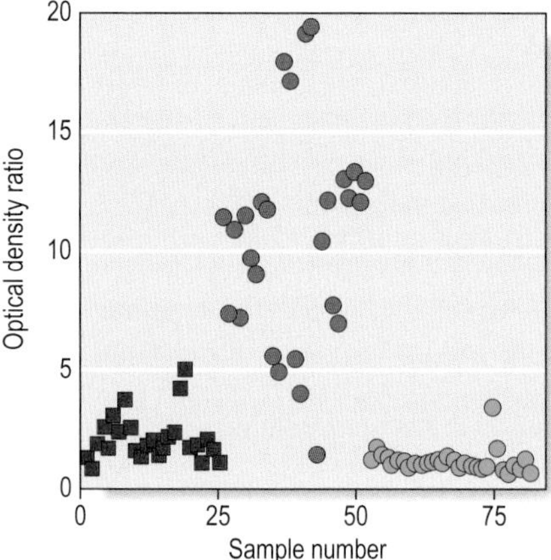

Figure 92.9 Antigen detection test for *Entamoeba histolytica* in stool. Stool specimens with culture-confirmed *E. dispar* (red squares) or *E. histolytica* (blue circles) infection, or stools with no detectable *Entamoeba* detected by microscopy (green circles), were assayed using an enzyme-linked immunosorbent assay containing monoclonal antibody specific for *E. histolytica*.

its disease burden. To test this hypothesis, class II genotype frequencies were determined among a cohort of unrelated Bangladeshi children who had been followed every other day for 3 years for *E. histolytica* infection. Individuals heterozygous for the DQB1*0601/DRB1*1501 haplotype were 10.1 times (95% confidence interval 2.02, 50.6) more likely not to have been infected with *E. histolytica*. Other DQB1 and DRB1 alleles (DQB1*0202, DQB1*0301, DRB1*0701) showed no evidence of association with any of the clinical outcomes related to amebiasis. This potential protective association may offer insight into why amebiasis does not occur in some children exposed to the parasite, and implicates class II restricted immune responses in protection from *E. histolytica* infection.[139]

DIAGNOSIS

See ***Table 92.3*** for a summary of test sensitivities for amebiasis diagnosis.

Microscopy

Microscopic identification of the parasite in stool, liver abscess pus, or colonic biopsies is neither sensitive nor specific and should be replaced with *E. histolytica*-specific diagnostic tests (see following discussion).[140] Erythrophagocytic amebae are more likely to be *E. histolytica* than *E. dispar*, but *E. dispar* trophozoites have also been found to contain ingested red blood cells. Repeated stool examinations in patients with amebic liver abscess were able to detect the parasite in only 8–44% of cases.[76] Identification of the parasite in aspirated pus from liver abscesses, even in the most experienced hands, is only 20% sensitive.[67]

Antigen Detection

The TechLab *E. histolytica* II enzyme-linked immunosorbent assay is the only fecal antigen test able to distinguish *E. histolytica* from *E. dispar* and *E. moshkovskii* (***Fig. 92.9***).[69] This test, based on detection of the Gal/GalNAc lectin in stool, has proven sensitive and specific in several studies in areas both endemic and nonendemic for *E. histolytica*,[69,141–144] although one study has reported a discrepancy between PCR and antigen detection.[145]

Antigen detection is also useful in the diagnosis of amebic liver abscess. In one study, the TechLab *E. histolytica* II assay detected Gal/GalNAc lectin in the sera of 96% (22/23) of patients with amebic liver abscess prior to receiving antiamebic therapy. The sensitivity was 41–74% for detection of the parasite from liver abscess pus.[69]

Polymerase Chain Reaction

Real-time PCR (qPCR) is comparable in sensitivity to stool antigen detection. qPCR is more sensitive than conventional PCR, and is a sensitive test for the detection of *E. histolytica* DNA in both stool and liver abscess pus.[146–148] PCR can also be used to distinguish among isolates of *E. histolytica*, which should prove useful for epidemiologic purposes as well as in determining the virulence characteristics of different isolates.[131,149,150]

Serology

The IHA test for anti-amebic antibody is 70% sensitive early in the illness, to greater than 95% sensitive on convalescence, for the diagnosis of amebic liver abscess and amebic colitis.[67] A major problem with current serologic tests is that they remain positive for years after an episode of amebiasis. As a result, a substantial number (between 10% and 35%) of residents of developing countries have anti-amebic antibodies detected by current serologic tests.[151–153] Since the vast majority of patients with invasive amebiasis in developed countries are immigrants from developing nations, serologic tests may not be as specific as one would hope. For example, in five recent series of patients in the United States with amebic liver abscess, between 80% and 96% of patients were immigrants. Therefore current serologic tests may be inadequate for the differentiation of acute from past amebiasis, even in developed nations, and one should not make the diagnosis of amebiasis in a native of a country where amebiasis is endemic on the basis of a serologic test alone.

Colonoscopy

Colonoscopy is preferable to sigmoidoscopy because disease may be localized to the cecum or ascending colon. Cathartics or enemas should not be used to prepare the patient because they will interfere with the identification of the parasite. Wet preparations of material aspirated or scraped from the base of ulcers should be examined for motile trophozoites and tested for *E. histolytica* antigen. The appearance of amebic colitis may resemble that of inflammatory bowel disease, with granular, friable, and diffusely ulcerated mucosa. Large geographic ulcers and pseudomembranes may also be present.[154–156] The detection rate of trophozoites upon histopathologic examination of colonic biopsy specimens from patients with amebic colitis varies in different reports from all to only some of the patients.[155–157] Biopsy specimens should be taken from the edge of the ulcers. Periodic acid–Schiff stains the parasites a magenta color (see ***Fig. 92.6***), increasing the ease of detection in biopsies. *E. histolytica* has been shown to invade carcinomas, causing diagnostic confusion.[157]

Imaging Procedures

Ultrasound, CT, and MRI studies of the liver are equally sensitive at detecting amebic abscesses (***Fig. 92.10***). All three techniques are

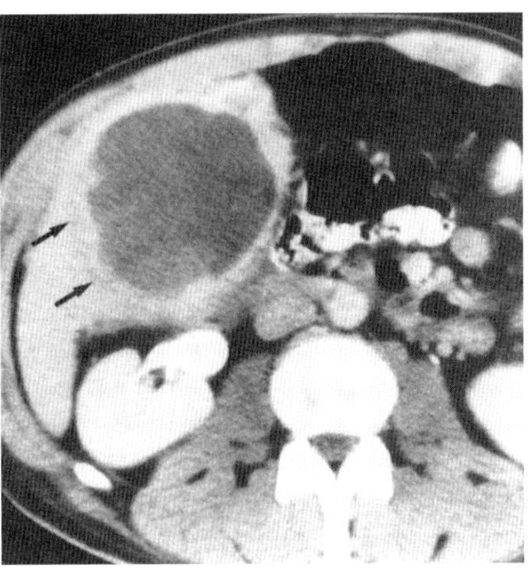

Figure 92.10 Computed tomography of hepatic amebic abscess.

incapable of differentiating an amebic from a pyogenic abscess.[158–161] At 6-month follow-up, only one-third to two-thirds of amebic liver abscesses had disappeared upon repeat ultrasonography.[158–161]

TREATMENT AND PROGNOSIS

Colonization with *E. histolytica* should be treated with a luminal agent alone; *E. dispar* and *E. moshkovskii* infection does not require treatment. Drugs effective against luminal infection include iodoquinol, paromomcyin, and diloxanide furoate. The recommended duration of treatment with iodoquinol is 20 days, paromomycin 7 days, and diloxanide furoate 10 days.[162–164]

Invasive amebiasis (colitis, liver abscess, etc.) should be treated with a nitroimidazole (metronidazole and tinidazole are available in the United States) followed by a luminal agent. The luminal agent is required since intestinal colonization persists in approximately 50% of individuals who receive nitroimidazoles, and relapse of infection can occur months later.[66] The recommended duration of treatment with metronidazole is 7–10 days, and for tinidazole is 3–5 days for mild/moderate to severe disease respectively.[164] A review of 37 trials with 4487 participants compared different drug treatments against amebic colitis. Tinidazole reduced clinical failure compared with metronidazole and was associated with fewer adverse events.[165]

The majority of patients with amebic liver abscess defervesce after 3–4 days' treatment with metronidazole. In most cases, percutaneous drainage is not required and does not speed recovery.[166,167] However, percutaneous drainage of the liver abscess is occasionally necessary as an adjunct to antiparasitic therapy. Drainage of the abscess should be considered in patients who have no clinical response to drug therapy within 5–7 days or those with a high risk of abscess rupture, as defined by cavity with a diameter of more than 5 cm or by the presence of lesions in the left lobe.[168] A prospective randomized study of 39 patients in Vietnam compared treatment of amebic liver abscess with metronidazole alone or in combination with ultrasound-guided needle aspiration. Inclusion criteria were an abscess size of 6–10 cm and abscess in the right lobe of the liver. Only improvement in liver tenderness was significantly faster in the aspiration group during the first 3 days, while other clinical and laboratory parameters did not differ between groups.[169]

Other potential treatment options in need of further study include *Saccharomyces boulardii* in combination with a nitroimidazole, and the drug nitazoxanide.[170,171]

Vaccine Development

Prevention of amebiasis at present requires interruption of the fecal–oral spread of the infectious cyst stage of the parasite by improved hygiene, sanitation, and water treatment. Both the Gal/GalNAc adherence lectin and the serine-rich antigen have proved effective in the prevention of liver abscess in the gerbil model of the disease.[172–175] However, as opposed to the highly variable serine-rich antigen, the Gal/GalNAc lectin is highly conserved between isolates of *E. histolytica*.[91] Only the Gal/GalNAc lectin has been demonstrated to prevent intestinal infection with *E. histolytica*.[173] Recently, it was demonstrated using adoptive transfer experiments in a mouse model of intestinal amebiasis that this lectin vaccine protection is mediated by T cells but not serum. The CMI reponse was characterized by significant IFN-γ, interleukin-12 (IL-12), IL-2, IL-10, and IL-17 production. Subcutaneous delivery of LecA with the Infectious Disease Research Institute's adjuvant system EM014 elicited a potent CMI profile and provided significant protection (79% efficacy). When IFN-γ was neutralized in LecA-immunized mice, the protection conferred by vaccination was lost, demonstrating an important role for IFN-γ in protection from amebiasis.[176]

Other Intestinal Protozoa

See ***Figure 92.11*** for a summary of intestinal protozoa. *E. gingivalis* was the first parasitic ameba of humans to be described and has subsequently been isolated from a variety of human body sites, including teeth (pyorrhea alveolaris), tonsillar crypts, mucus, and vaginal and cervical smears in women with intrauterine devices.[177] It has been designated to be nonpathogenic and its presence in any of the aforementioned sites does not require treatment. Morphologically, it is identical to *E. histolytica*, with trophozoites that range from 5 to 25 μm (average 10–15 μm). It has a single nucleus with peripheral chromatin, and a small, well-defined karyosome that is usually centrally located. Ingested leukocytes and epithelial cells are often seen in *E. gingivalis*, which is a unique finding in that it is the only species of ameba to ingest leukocytes. No cyst form of the parasite has been identified.[178]

Entamoeba coli is a nonpathogenic protozoan with a wide human distribution. The presence of this organism in a patient's stool is a useful indication of fecal–oral exposure. The life cycle of *E. coli* is identical to that of *E. histolytica*, and the two organisms can be found concurrently in up to 10–30% of patients in endemic areas. However, *E. coli* is nonpathogenic and requires no specific treatment. The cysts and trophozoites of *E. coli* can be distinguished from those of the pathogenic *E. histolytica* on the basis of nuclear morphology and cyst size. Whereas *E. histolytica* cysts usually have fewer than five nuclei and are 10–15 μm in diameter, the cysts of *E. coli* are greater than 15 μm and often have five to eight nuclei.[179–181]

E. polecki is an intestinal protozoan that can be found in monkeys and pigs. Although in rare instances it has been reported to cause human infections, the pathogenic potential of this protozoan is at present unclear. Studies have reported that up to 19% of children in Papua New Guinea are colonized.[182] Although routine treatment is not currently recommended, good clinical response has been reported with metronidazole and diloxanide furoate. Most infected persons are asymptomatic, but heavy burdens with this parasite can produce nonspecific gastrointestinal symptoms such as diarrhea, cramps, anorexia, and malaise. The trophozoite form of *E. polecki* resembles that of *E. histolytica* and *E. coli* and differentiation from these and other protozoa relies on identification of the cyst stage of the organism, which is characteristically uninucleate with a large karyosome.[177–181]

Endolimax nana is a nonpathogenic commensal parasite with a worldwide distribution that commonly infects humans. It has the same life cycle as *E. histolytica* and is transmitted through oral–fecal spread and poor sanitary conditions. In the tropics it may be identified in the stool of as many as 10–33% of persons but requires no specific treatment. It can be distinguished from *E. histolytica* on the basis of its small size (cyst 6–10 μm; trophozoite 8–12 μm), vesicular nucleus, and large irregular karyosome. The cysts are often quadrinucleate.[179,180]

Iodamoeba butschlii is a nonpathogenic commensal organism. In the past it had been confused with the virulent *Naegleria* spp. It is less commonly encountered in the human gastrointestinal tract, occurring in 5–8% of the population in the tropics. It has a medium-sized trophozoite (9–20 μm) which is highly vacuolated with a large characteristic karyosome.

	Human pathogen	Estimated frequency	Trophozoite (usual size μm [range])	Cyst (usual size in μm)	Characteristic features
Entamoeba histolytica	+	1%–10%	10–20 (10–60)	5–20	Central punctate karyosome, erythrophagocytosis
E. coli	–	3%–20%	15–25 (10–50)	10–30	Larger, to 8 nuclei splinterlike chromatid bodies
E. hartmanni	–	?	<10	4–10	"Small race"
E. gingivalis	–	10%–90% (mouth)	15 (3–35)	None	Oral trophozoite only
E. polecki	±	Rare	16–18	12–14	Uninucleate cyst with large karyosome
Endolimax nana	–	10%–33%	8–12	6–14	Vesiculate nucleus
Iodamoeba butschlii	–	5%–8%	9–20	6–15	"I" cyst
Dientamoeba fragilis	–	4%–10%	4–12	None	Binucleate trophs with connecting thread

Figure 92.11 Amebae that infect the human gastrointestinal tract. (Reproduced from Ravdin JI, Guerrant RL. Current problems in diagnosis and treatment of amebic infections. Curr Clin Top Infect Dis. 1986;7:82-111.)

The cysts of *I. butschlii* are uninucleate and contain a large, dense glycogen mass which stains with iodine; the cysts are identified as I cysts.[178,179]

Blastocystis hominis is an anaerobic protozoan that commonly inhabits the gastrointestinal tract of humans, where it resides in the cecum and large bowel.[182–194] Although it has a worldwide distribution (including infection in animals such as pigs, monkeys, rodents, and poultry), this protozoan is more commonly found in the tropics. The mode of transmission is unclear but, because of the association with unsanitary conditions, is believed to be oral–fecal spread. Prevalence rates are variable, but up to 52% of samples from homosexual males have evidence of infection with this organism in selected regions. The pathogenicity of this organism is poorly understood, but in the last two decades there have been more frequent reports of infection with *B. hominis*. Infected persons may have gastrointestinal symptoms of diarrhea, abdominal pain, nausea, and vomiting, and systemic symptoms of anorexia and malaise. The organism has been shown to have *in vitro* sensitivity to a variety of agents, including emetine, metronidazole, furazolidone, co-trimoxazole, quinacrine, and pentamadine, and there are some *in vivo* data to support sensitivity of *B. hominis* to iodoquinol and co-trimoxazole. At present, the pathogenic potential of this protozoan parasite is unclear, its pathogenicity is poorly understood, and its role in causing human disease remains to be more clearly defined. *Dientamoeba fragilis*, once classified as an ameba, is now considered in the flagellate group and is discussed in Chapter 93.

Access the complete reference list online at http://www.expertconsult.com

Access the complete reference list online at http://www.expertconsult.com

CHAPTER 93

Intestinal Flagellate and Ciliate Infections

David R. Hill • Theodore E. Nash

INTRODUCTION

The most important of the many flagellates that inhabit the large and small bowel of humans is *Giardia lamblia*; *Giardia* is one of the most common pathogenic parasitic infections in humans. In high-income countries, it is a frequent cause of endemic and epidemic diarrhea, and in many low-income regions of the world, where effective sanitation measures are lacking, infection is nearly universal by 2–3 years of age.

Of the other flagellates, only *Dientamoeba fragilis* causes enteric symptoms. *Chilomastix mesnili*, while not uncommonly seen in stool specimens, is a nonpathogen, as is *Pentatrichomonas hominis* (formerly known as *Trichomonas hominis*), and the rarely seen *Enteromonas hominis* and *Retortamonas intestinalis*. The only ciliate of humans and the largest protozoan is *Balantidium coli*, a rare cause of diarrhea and dysentery, primarily in the tropics.

GIARDIA LAMBLIA

THE AGENT

G. lamblia (also known as *G. duodenalis* or *G. intestinalis*) is a flagellate protozoan that inhabits the small intestine of humans and other mammals. The genus *Giardia* belongs to the category of intestinal flagellates in the division Protozoa.[1] It is likely that Antony van Leeuwenhoek described the organism in his own stool in the 17th century, but Vilem Lambl is credited with describing the trophozoite in humans in 1859 and Grassi discovered the cyst form in 1879.[2]

Giardia is one of the most successful parasites. It is highly adapted with simplified metabolic pathways and molecular mechanisms,[3] in part because it depends upon its host to provide some of its essential nutrients. And yet it undergoes highly complex developmental changes such as encystation, and possesses a unique, rigid cytostructure.[4–6] It has two nuclei that are functionally and morphologically identical,[7,8] simplified transcription, and promotors that are unusually short and compact.[9–11] It has no morphologically identifiable Golgi, and no peroxisomes or classic mitochondria.[12] The identification in *Giardia* of a mitochondrial remnant, the mitosome, and mitochondrial genes[13–15] has called into question whether *Giardia* is a simplified ancestor of higher eukaryotes, or if it was once a more complicated organism that has lost many characteristics of higher eukaryotes.[16–18]

Giardia has two morphologic forms, the trophozoite and the cyst (***Fig. 93.1***). The trophozoite resides in the small intestine and is responsible for disease manifestations; the cyst is the infectious, environmentally resistant form responsible for transmission (***Fig. 93.2***). *Giardia* that infects humans is morphologically indistinguishable from that found in a large variety of mammals. The trophozoite is 9–21 μm long, 5–15 μm wide, and 2–4 μm thick. When viewed from above, its shape resembles a pear or teardrop (***Fig. 93.3***). *Giardia* is bilaterally symmetrical, and has two equal-sized nuclei that contain complete copies of the genome with a ploidy of four.[7,19] The genome for the WB strain has been published (http://Giardiadb.org), and is 11.7 megabases on five chromosomes.[3] *Giardia* has four pairs of flagella, one of which is recurrent, and possesses a ventral sucking disk which is used for adherence. Two claw-shaped median bodies consisting of microtubules cross the middle of the parasite. These are typical of *G. lamblia* and contrast with the round median bodies in *G. muris*, a rodent species. The dorsal surface contains peripheral vesicles that have endocytic and lysosomal activities.[20,21] Multiplication of trophozoites in the small intestine is by longitudinal binary fission with mirror image symmetry.[22,23]

Despite the morphologic similarities among *Giardia* organisms that infect humans, analyses using a variety of methodologies including variant-specific surface proteins (VSPs), differences in isoenzymes, and molecular markers at the glutamate dehydrogenase, β-giardin, small subunit ribosomal RNA, and the triosephosphate isomerase genes, indicate that *Giardia* isolates from humans vary.[12,24–28] Human isolates fall into two major groupings, called genotypes or assemblages (A and B), that differ genetically and biologically (***Table 93.1***). Genetic differences between assemblages A and B are so large that it has been proposed that they be considered separate species.[26] Biological differences include variation in growth rates, host specificity,[29] VSP repertoires,[30] and character of infection in animal models.[31]

Further molecular characterization of *G. lamblia* has divided it into seven assemblages (***Table 93.1***), with assemblages A and B infecting

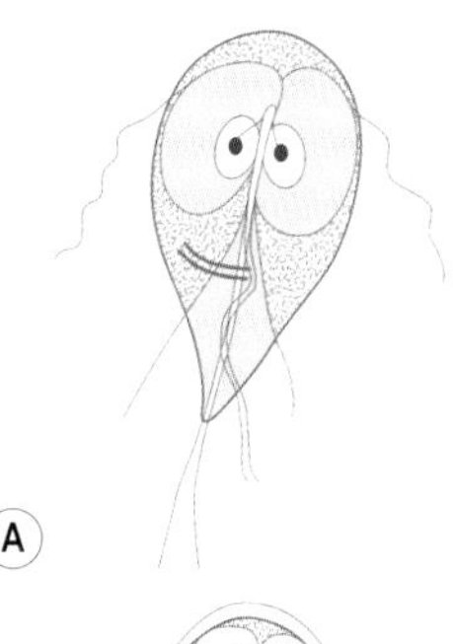

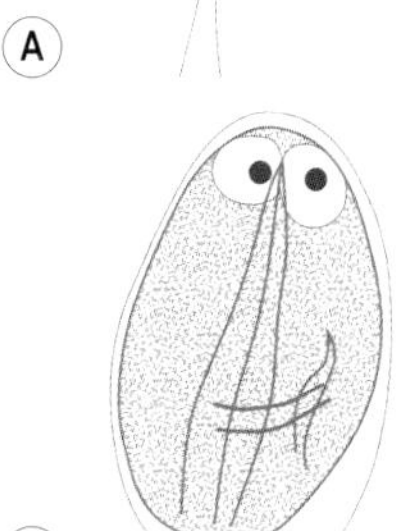

Figure 93.1 Schematic drawing of *Giardia lamblia* trophozoite **(A)** and cyst **(B),** and their key identification points.

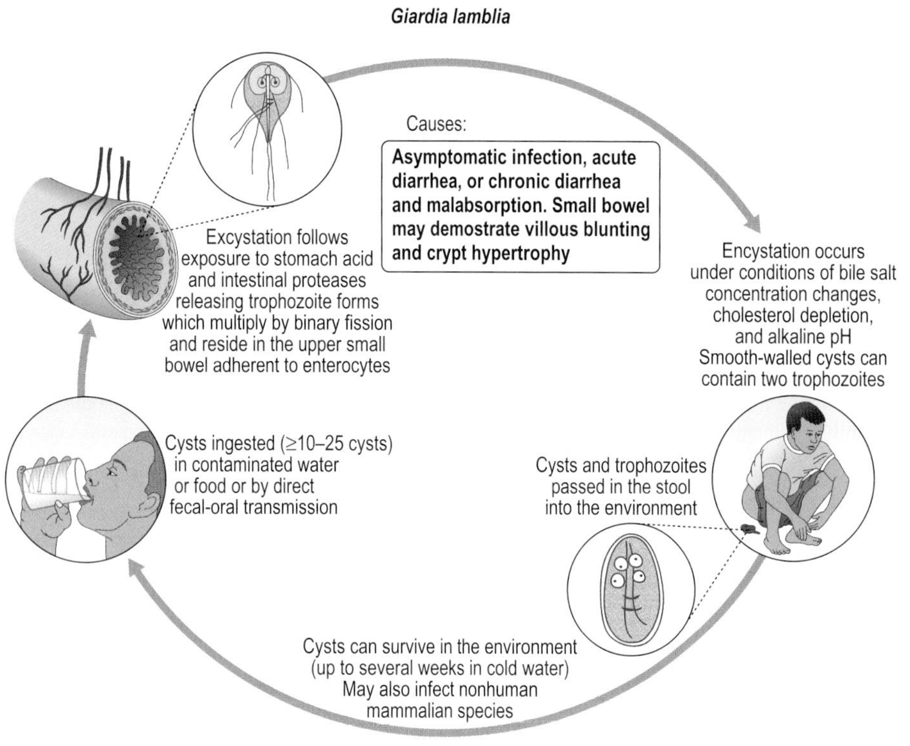

Giardia lamblia

Causes:

Asymptomatic infection, acute diarrhea, or chronic diarrhea and malabsorption. Small bowel may demostrate villous blunting and crypt hypertrophy

Excystation follows exposure to stomach acid and intestinal proteases releasing trophozoite forms which multiply by binary fission and reside in the upper small bowel adherent to enterocytes

Encystation occurs under conditions of bile salt concentration changes, cholesterol depletion, and alkaline pH Smooth-walled cysts can contain two trophozoites

Cysts ingested (≥10–25 cysts) in contaminated water or food or by direct fecal-oral transmission

Cysts and trophozoites passed in the stool into the environment

Cysts can survive in the environment (up to several weeks in cold water) May also infect nonhuman mammalian species

Figure 93.2 *Giardia lamblia* life cycle.

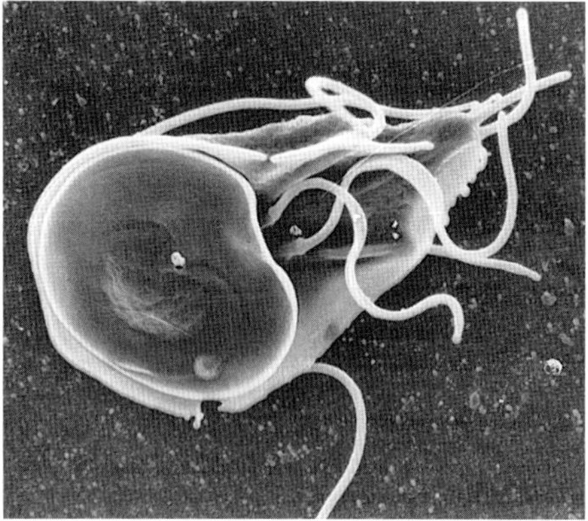

Figure 93.3 Scanning electron micrograph of the ventral surface of a *Giardia lamblia* trophozoite. The ventral adhesion disk and four pairs of flagella are seen. (Courtesy of D. Darwood, Rocky Mountain Laboratory, National Institute of Allergy and Infectious Diseases, National Institutes of Health, Bethesda, MD.)

Table 93.1 Categorization of *Giardia* spp.

Name	Assemblage	Host Range
G. lamblia (duodenalis, intestinalis)	A	Humans, primates, dogs, cats, cattle, sheep, deer, rodents
	B	Humans, primates, dogs, cattle, horses, beavers
	C	Dogs
	D	Dogs
	E	Cattle, sheep, goats, pigs
	F	Cats
	G	Rodents
G. agilis		Amphibians
G. ardae		Birds
G. psittaci		Birds
G. microti		Muskrats, voles
G. muris		Rodents

(Information from: Xiao L, Fayer R. Molecular characterisation of species and genotypes of *Cryptosporidium* and *Giardia* and assessment of zoonotic transmission. Int J Parasitol. 2008;38:1239–1255; Wielinga CM, Thompson RC. Comparative evaluation of *Giardia duodenalis* sequence data. Parasitol. 2007;134:1795–1821; Steuart RF. Proteomic analysis of *Giardia*: studies from the pre- and post-genomic era. Exp Parasitology. 2010;124:26–30.)

humans and other mammalian species such as nonhuman primates, dogs, cats, cattle, and beavers.[25,26,32] Although this suggests the possibility of cross-transmission between mammalian hosts and humans, with the exception of beavers,[33] no epidemics have implicated animals as a source of human infection. *Giardia* from dogs, cats, some hoofed animals such as sheep and cattle, and rodents are placed in assemblages with restricted enzootic potential.[25,26,32,34,35] Different species of *Giardia* are assigned on the basis of morphology, host restriction, and molecular analysis, e.g., *G. muris* in rodents, *G. psittaci* and *G. ardeae* in birds, *G. microti* in muskrats and voles, and *G. agilis* in amphibians (***Table 93.1***).

As trophozoites are swept down the intestine, they begin to form environmentally resistant, oval cysts (***Fig. 93.4***). These measure about 6–10 μm long, have four nuclei, and the anlage of two trophozoites. Encystation can be initiated by a number of ways *in vitro*: the most common method uses a large excess of bile salts.[36,37] A decline in the transfer of cholesterol to the parasite's membrane can also trigger encystation, mimicking decreased cholesterol concentration as the parasite passes through the small intestine.[38] Encystation is a highly coordinated process involving almost all the major cellular processes, including upregulation of encystation-specific genes, and the production and transport to the cell membrane of cyst wall proteins via highly unusual encystation secretory vesicles.[6,39–42]

G. lamblia is the only species that has been cultured *in vitro*.[43] Complex nondefined media are used and the organism grows axenically under anaerobic or microaerophilic conditions. *Giardia* has flavodiiron proteins that may help it scavenge oxygen, enhancing its ability to survive under microaerophilic conditions found in the small intestine.[44] It utilizes

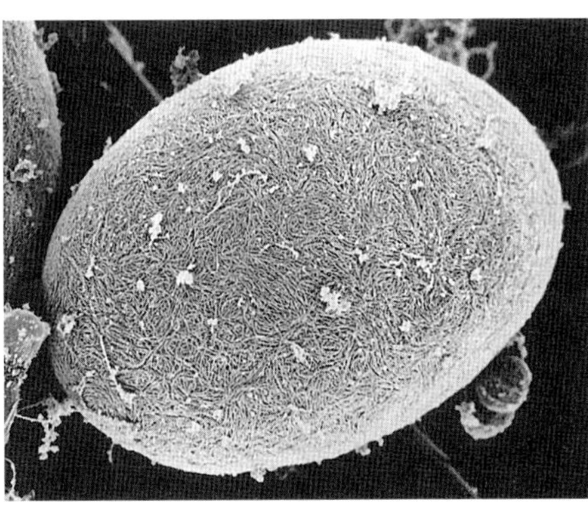

Figure 93.4 Scanning electron micrograph of a *Giardia lamblia* cyst (width 6.8 μm). (Courtesy of S. L. Erlandsen, Department of Cell Biology and Neuroanatomy, University of Minnesota School of Medicine, Minneapolis, MN.)

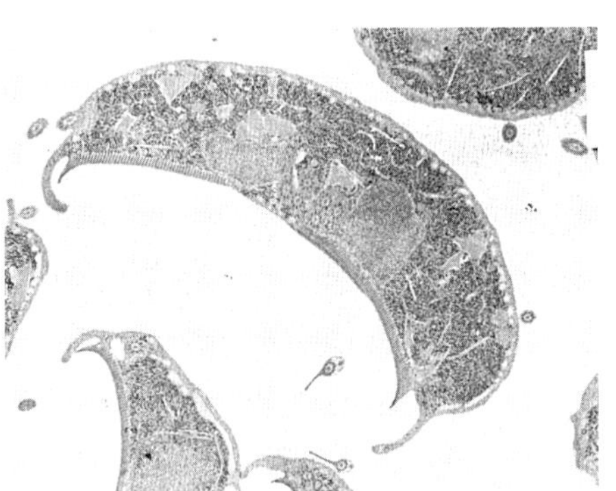

Figure 93.5 Transmission electron micrograph of an encysting trophozoite of *Giardia lamblia*. Two nuclei are readily seen, as well as the axonemes (intracytoplasmic projections of the flagella). Encystment-secretory vesicles are seen lining the dorsal surface. These contain cyst wall antigens. (Courtesy of B. Bowers, Laboratory of Cell Biology, National Heart and Lung Institute, National Institutes of Health, Bethesda, MD.)

glucose as a major source of carbohydrate energy, producing ethanol, alanine, acetate, and carbon dioxide, and generating adenosine triphosphate (ATP) in the process.[12] Another potential mechanism for ATP generation is the catabolism of arginine via the arginine dihydrolase pathway. Exogenous cysteine is essential for survival. *G. lamblia* is unable to synthesize purines or pyrimidines and must salvage these from the intestine. Similar to many protozoans, it is unable to produce cholesterol but can synthesize farnesyl and geranylgeranyl to isoprenylate proteins.[45]

Giardia is used as a model organism to study developmental and cellular processes, including vesicular transport, secretion, cyst wall development, transcription regulation, cytoskeleton organization, and other basic mechanisms present in less complex eukaryotes.[46] The trophozoite is rigid with novel structural components of annexin-like proteins called giardins, some of which are immunodominant.[28,47] Vesicular transport occurs and is G protein-dependent.[48] *Giardia* lacks a Golgi apparatus; it is likely that the the Golgi's function resides in the encystation secretory vesicles.[49] *Giardia* possesses two equally functioning nuclei which are unexpectedly homologous[7,8] because they undergo karyogamy,[50] but it is not known how and if they cooperate and the manner of their communication (***Fig. 93.5***).

Giardia undergoes surface antigenic variation. One of an estimated 250 VSPs is expressed,[30] covers the entire surface of the parasite including the flagella, and changes spontaneously during *in vitro* growth. Antigenic variation with VSP expression is controlled transcriptionally;[51,52] all VSPs are initially transcribed but all but one VSP transcript is inhibited by an RNAi-based mechanism allowing expression of a single VSP. The molecular weight of VSPs varies and some of them have repetitive units.[53] These proteins are cysteine-rich (11–12% cysteine), occurring usually as CXXC motifs.[30,54] A majority have zinc finger motifs,[54] that bind zinc *in vitro*,[55] and possibly *in vivo*.[55,56] The surface location of zinc fingers is highly unusual. VSPs are also able to resist intestinal proteases.[57]

Antigenic variation of VSPs occurs *in vivo* in humans[58] as well as in animal model infections.[29,59] During experimental human infection, a *Giardia* clone (GS/H7) expressing one VSP became replaced by a mixture of other VSPs between 2 and 3 weeks after inoculation.[58] This corresponds to the time when antibody responses to the original VSP are detected. Whether or not antigenic variation allows immunologic escape, causing chronic infections, is unknown. Some regions of VSP differ and impart unique biological characteristics that are favored by or selected against by a specific host, perhaps allowing *Giardia* to expand its host range.

EPIDEMIOLOGY

G. lamblia is one of the most widely distributed protozoan parasites, found in all climates and countries.[60,61] Because transmission of *Giardia* requires oral ingestion of the cyst form of the parasite, the level of sanitation correlates inversely with the distribution of infection. Poor levels of sanitation lead to fecal contamination of water and foods, accounting for high levels of childhood infection in low-income countries, and posing a risk to international travelers. In high-income regions, relative resistance of the *Giardia* cyst to routine water treatment can allow the parasite to escape inactivation and contribute to waterborne outbreaks. The wide distribution of *Giardia* is a major reason why it remains the most frequently found parasite in the United States, found in 4–7% of stools submitted to laboratories[62] and leading to a case rate in 2005 that ranged from 1.4 cases per 100 000 in Louisiana to 30.0 cases in Vermont.[60]

There are three modes of transmission – waterborne, direct fecal–oral, and foodborne. Waterborne transmission of giardiasis was first described in the 1960s from the United States,[63] and has been repeatedly documented.[60,64–68] In the last two decades, as water treatment has improved, *Giardia* has declined as a cause of outbreaks from water intended for drinking.[64,69–72] Outbreaks associated with drinking water often involve *Giardia*-contaminated surface water that has not been subjected to flocculation, sedimentation, and filtration, as well as chlorination. Surface water assessed for the presence of *Giardia* or *Cryptosporidium* has been frequently contaminated with both parasites. Other waterborne outbreaks have occurred because of direct fecal contamination of the water supply when underground pipes carrying sewage and purified water become mixed.[63,66] The association of giardiasis with recreational water often follows a fecal accident or when children wearing contaminated diapers are in the water.[60,66,69,73,74] *Giardia* is relatively resistant to chlorination, a large number of cysts are excreted by infected persons, and there is a low inoculum necessary to establish infection. However, *Cryptosporidium* is now a more common cause of outbreaks associated with treated recreational water, most likely because of the smaller size of the oocyst and higher resistance to chlorination.[69] Historically, mountainous areas of the United States and Canada have been prone to waterborne outbreaks. Survival of cysts in cold lake or river water has been shown for up to 56 days.[75]

Direct fecal–oral transmission occurs in daycare centers, amongst children in low-income countries, in custodial institutions, and with anal–oral sexual practices. Historically, daycare centers have had high infection rates, ranging from 20% to 50%; however, current surveys are lacking.[76,77] While many infected children are asymptomatic, they can transmit *Giardia* to family members and thus contribute to high endemic rates of infection.[78,79] In the United States, Canada, and Scotland most reports are in 1–9-year-old children and in 35–39-year-old adults, supporting this pattern of infection.[60,80,81]

Giardia is near ubiquitous in low-income regions. It is one of the earliest of the enteric parasites to infect infants and has prevalence rates of 10–30% in children less than 10 years old,[61,82–90] and nearly all children will become infected in childhood. In men who have sex with men, older surveys have demonstrated prevalence rates as high as 20%.[91,92]

The third mode of transmission, food, is increasingly recognized. Given the ability of the cyst to survive outside the human host, it is surprising that foodborne outbreaks are not more frequently described. Outbreaks have occurred in restaurants, corporate offices, nursing homes, and churches. They have usually followed ingestion of foods that have not been cooked, such as salads, or cold meats and fish.[93,94] Transmission can occur with as few as 10–25 cysts, so only low levels of contamination are necessary.[95]

Giardiasis occurs year-round, but there is a peak incidence in the late summer and early fall.[60,80] This pattern may be due to increased recreational exposure to water or more frequent international travel during the summer months.[81,96,97] Acquisition of *Giardia* during international travel is increased with travel of longer than a month in duration and with travel to the Indian subcontinent.[81,98,99]

Despite the finding of human assemblages A and B in a variety of mammalian species, with the exception of beavers, there are no epidemics documented from animal sources. An outbreak of beaver-to-human transmission that was waterborne occurred in British Columbia.[100] *Giardia* was detected from the water supplies and from a beaver nesting in the implicated water; the human, water, and beaver isolates were of the same genotype. Other assemblages associated with animal infection (assemblages C–G) have not been found in humans.[25,32,101] Specifically, there is no definitive transmission from dogs or cats to humans, and screening of domestic animals is not warranted.

PATHOGENESIS AND IMMUNITY

A hallmark of giardiasis is clinical variability. Infections can be abortive, transient, or chronic, while accompanying disease manifestations can range from minor or none to fulminant diarrhea, severe malabsorption, and life-threatening malnutrition. Although incompletely defined, both parasite and host factors are important in determining the control and susceptibility to infection and disease.

Infection follows the ingestion of as few as 10–25 cysts.[95] Excystation is initiated with exposure of cysts to stomach acid, intestinal proteases, and the stimulation of a parasite-derived protease.[102] Trophozoites colonize the upper small bowel where they may adhere via the ventral disk or possibly via specific receptor ligands.[103,104] It seems important that parasites are able to adhere to gut mucosa.[105] Gerbils given a high-fiber diet had reduced rates of infection, possibly because of trapping and clearance of trophozoites in the mucous blanket,[106] and humans with asymptomatic giardiasis had decreased parasite excretion following ingestion of wheatgerm agglutinin which could decrease adherence.[107]

The large number of trophozoites present in the bowel suggests a direct effect of the trophozoite on intestinal function. Damage to the brush border and its enzymatic system could be a mechanism for some of the documented changes, particularly disaccharidase deficiencies. In a caspase-3-dependent manner, *Giardia* isolates have caused disruption of tight junctions, increased permeability, and induced apoptosis on intestinal epithelial monolayers.[108–110] These findings have been confirmed on duodenal biopsy specimens from patients with giardiasis.[111] High levels of glucose can protect intestinal epithelial cells against *Giardia*-induced apoptosis by activation of the glucose cotransporter that modulates enterocytic cell death.[112] Nitric oxide is produced by epithelial cells and plays a potential role in the innate protection against *Giardia*.[113] However, *Giardia* can suppress nitric oxide production by consuming arginine, and by releasing proteins that could disable nitric oxide.[114,115]

Small-bowel overgrowth may contribute to diarrhea in giardiasis in some patients; however, it may be associative rather than causative.[116] Mucosal invasion is rare, and there is no evidence of a classic enterotoxin.

Biopsies of the intestine show varying degrees of mucosal inflammation with crypt hypertrophy, villous blunting, and mucosal infiltration with mononuclear inflammatory cells.[117–121] This can rarely be as severe as an entirely flattened, sprue-like gut. The inflammatory response may lead to diarrhea by increasing the number of secretory crypt cells, or initiating a cytokine reaction resulting in diarrhea, similar to proposed mechanisms for other adherent or minimally invasive coccidian enteric protozoa.[122]

Biologic differences have been noted in both animal model infections[31,123] and experimental human infections,[116] suggesting a difference in parasite virulence. For instance, infections with *G. lamblia* isolates differed in their duration, level of cyst excretion, and ability to induce homologous or heterologous immunity. In human experimental infections, only one of two isolates was able to infect volunteers, although both originated from symptomatic donors.[58]

Confirming a clinical difference in *G. lamblia* assemblages A and B has met with conflicting results. Some studies indicate increased intestinal symptoms with assemblage A,[124–127] others have implicated assemblage B,[116,128,129] and still others have shown clinical diversity with genetic similarity.[130] Part of the differences between studies may relate to the predominance of one assemblage over another in different geographic regions of the world.[131–135] A thorough analysis of isolates from all over the world with a careful clinical correlation needs to be undertaken.

In part, the response of the host to *Giardia* determines the course of infection and whether there will be disease.[136] Most understanding of the immune response comes from animal models of *G. lamblia* in gerbils and of *G. muris* or *G. lamblia* in mice. Relatively few data are derived from humans. In animals, an immune response occurs that results in self-cure and resistance to rechallenge.[137,138] However, this response is host- and parasite-dependent, and some animals are less capable of mounting an effective immune response.

In humans, the data are variable. Eighty-four percent of experimentally infected persons self-cured on average 18 days following inoculation while the remainder became chronically infected.[95] Epidemiologic studies suggest partial acquired immunity by demonstrating decreased prevalence of infection in endemically exposed persons compared with those newly exposed.[63,139,140] In low-income regions, there is increased prevalence in the young compared with adults.[82,141,142] However, in highly endemic populations, reinfections are common if not universal in the young,[90] and relatively high prevalence rates continue even in older populations.

The development of an immune response to *Giardia* involves both humoral and cellular mechanisms.[136] Humans and animals produce systemic immunoglobulin G (IgG), IgM, and IgA,[82,116,120,141,143–147] including cytotoxic antibodies.[148,149] There is an important intestinal IgA response to acute infection.[58,150,151] Indirect evidence suggests a role of IgA in control of experimental infections; mouse pups are resistant to infection with *G. muris* when nursed on immune dams,[152] and infection is prolonged in anti-IgM-treated mice.[153] The inability to transport IgA across the murine intestinal epithelium correlated with failure to clear *G. muris*.[154] IgA-deficient mice fail to clear infection with *G. lamblia*; however, they controlled infection better than B-cell knockout mice, suggesting B-cell-dependent, IgA-independent anti-*Giardia* defenses.[155] Responses are dependent on the species of *Giardia* employed, model used, and stage of infection evaluated.[156] Intestinal antibodies could act by interfering with adherence and colonization.

Cellular immune responses are essential. Athymic, nude mice infected with *G. muris* are unable to self-cure,[157,158] but partially control the infection after the administration of immune spleen cells. This control may come at a cost, since following reconstitution the gut developed inflammatory changes[157] that may be mediated through $CD8^+$ cells.[159] Furthermore, elimination of $CD4^+$ T cells in Peyer's patches with anti-CD4 antibodies prevents self-cure in *G. muris*-infected mice.[160] Both nude and anti-CD4-treated mice are unable to mount an intestinal IgA response,[160] suggesting that T cells are essential to the production of specific intestinal IgA.

Interleukin (IL)-6-deficient mice have difficulties controlling early *G. lamblia* infection,[161,162] as do mast cell-deficient mice.[163] Mast cells can produce IL-6 and also contribute to increased intestinal motility that is associated with improved parasite clearance.[164,165] IL-6 may stimulate

T-helper cell-induced clonal expression of IgA-producing B cells and plasma cells.

Specific proliferative responses are found in the Peyer's patches and mesenteric lymph nodes of infected animals,[166,167] as well as in peripheral mononuclear cells from humans.[168] Macrophages and neutrophils can phagocytose *Giardia*.[169–171]

Human host differences are known to contribute to the variability of clinical symptoms; patients who have common variable hypogammaglobulinemia are susceptible to severe and prolonged giardiasis.[172–174] This may be secondary to their failure to produce antibody, but is also likely related to a cellular-based abnormality.[175] Patients with X-linked agammaglobulinemia are also at increased risk.[176] Acquired immunodeficiency syndrome (AIDS) patients with severe cellular immunodeficiency can have giardiasis that is refractory to treatment.[177]

THE DISEASE

Clinical giardiasis is varied and ranges from asymptomatic passage of cysts to chronic diarrhea, malabsorption, and weight loss. Most symptomatic patients experience a characteristic syndrome of diarrhea with foul-smelling stools and gas, bloating, and abdominal cramps (***Table 93.2***). Following cyst ingestion the incubation period is 1–2 weeks before the onset of symptoms. The incubation period can be shorter than the prepatent period (the time from ingestion of cysts to excretion of cysts in the stool), therefore initial stool specimens may be negative.[178] About 50% of patients who have not been exposed previously to *Giardia* will develop symptoms, 15% or more will pass cysts asymptomatically, and the remainder will show no trace of infection.

Malaise and anorexia are common, and weight loss, which occurs in over 50% of patients, averages 4.5 kg (10 lb). It is not clear if weight loss is secondary to the absorptive defects seen in some patients or to the more frequent nausea and anorexia. Vomiting occurs in about one-fourth of patients and low-grade fever is uncommon. Signs of inflammatory diarrhea such as tenesmus and gross blood in the stool do not occur. There are case reports of giardiasis with urticaria,[179,180] Whipple's disease,[181] and a reactive arthritis.[182] Although *Giardia* is generally confined to the small intestine, it has been found in the stomach, almost always in association with atrophic gastritis and occasionally with *Helicobacter pylori*.[183]

The course of giardiasis is frequently prolonged, often 10 days or more.[63] Although many patients resolve infection without treatment, others develop chronic diarrhea,[184] which may alternate with constipation or normal bowel patterns.

While most patients with giardiasis have a benign course, severe illness occurs,[185,186] with US hospitalization rates (2 per 100 000 persons) similar to those for shigellosis. Persons most frequently hospitalized were children under the age of 5 years and women of childbearing age. Volume depletion was the most common reason for admission, and 19% of children less than 5 years old had failure to thrive.

Table 93.2 Symptoms of Giardiasis

Symptom	Percentage (Range)
Diarrhea	90 (64–100)
Malaise	86 (72–97)
Flatulence	75 (35–97)
Foul-smelling, greasy stools	75 (57–87)
Abdominal cramps	71 (44–85)
Bloating	71 (42–97)
Nausea	69 (59–79)
Anorexia	66 (41–82)
Weight loss	66 (56–76)
Vomiting	23 (11–36)
Fever	15 (0–24)
Constipation	13 (0–26)
Urticaria	10 (5–14)

(Data reviewed in Hill DR. Giardiasis: issues in management and treatment. Infect Dis Clin North Am. 1993;7:503–525.)

Malabsorption of fat, vitamins A and B_{12}, protein, D-xylose, and lactose have been documented in chronic infection.[187–189] In some cases, there is a correlation between symptoms, severity of malabsorption, and small-bowel histopathologic changes, with villous flattening and crypt hypertrophy.[118,120] However, severe diarrhea can occur without corresponding pathologic changes, emphasizing the multiple potential mechanisms for the production of diarrhea in giardiasis. Lactase is the most common of the disaccharidase deficiencies, and patients in whom infection is resolved may be lactose-intolerant for several weeks. Development of chronic fatigue and irritable bowel syndrome after giardiasis has also been documented.[189]

Asymptomatic infection is common in children with cyst passage persisting for 6 months or more;[190,191] however, they can introduce *Giardia* to family members and staff in daycare.[78]

In low-income countries, there is ample evidence for the deleterious effect of *Giardia* upon childhood nutrition and development. Reanalysis of Mata's study in Guatemala, as well as other studies, indicates a role for *Giardia* in chronic diarrhea (lasting 2–6 weeks) and malnutrition.[83,142,187,192] Infection with *Giardia* has been associated with stunted growth in children from Ecuador[193] and Turkey,[194,195] increased intestinal permeability and persistent diarrhea in children in Nepal,[196,197] low weight for age and height for age[86] in children in Brazil,[89,198] wasting in Malaysian children,[88] and malnutrition and decreased cognitive function in children from Peru.[85]

In contrast to these findings is documentation of high levels of asymptomatic infection in childen in low-income regions without adverse nutritional consequences, and rapid reinfection following treatment, leading some investigators to recommend not treating young children in these settings.[199,200] A longitudinal study of Peruvian children in a periurban community of Lima found high rates of asymptomatic infection and no adverse effects on growth or nutritional status.[90] Similarly, children followed in Bangladesh who had giardiasis did not demonstrate a deleterious effect on growth.[201]

Therefore, *Giardia* is capable of causing a chronic diarrheal syndrome in children that can be associated with malabsorption and contribute to retarded growth and nutritional deficiency. However, many children are asymptomatically infected or coinfected with other pathogens. These contrasting findings necessitate further study of children in low-income areas with genotyping of organisms.

DIAGNOSIS

Giardiasis should be considered in the differential diagnosis of diarrhea, particularly when illness is prolonged and associated with weight loss. Patients should be asked about risk factors of drinking water source, overseas travel, wilderness camping, daycare, and sexual practices. With a prolonged incubation period the exposure may be remote.[202] Other diarrheal syndromes caused by viruses, noninvasive bacteria, parasites (*Cryptosporidium hominis*, *Cyclospora cayetanensis*, and *Isospora belli*),[203] and tropical sprue should also be considered. Since the epidemiology of *Cryptosporidium* and *Cyclospora* is similar to that of *Giardia* and the clinical presentation and risk factors can overlap, they will need to be distinguished by stool examination.

Stool examination for ova and parasites (O&P) has been the diagnostic standard. However, rapid detection of *Giardia* antigen using immunofluorescence, enzyme-linked immunosorbent assay (ELISA), and nonenzymatic assays are now employed by commercial laboratories because of ease of use and high sensitivity and specificity.[204,205] For the O&P exam, stool aliquots are examined fresh, placed in polyvinyl alcohol, and a third in 10% buffered formalin. The fresh stool can be examined under a saline wet mount or with the addition of iodine that stains the cysts. A loose or watery stool can reveal motile trophozoites. Preserved specimens can be permanently stained, usually with trichrome or iron hematoxylin. Finally, the stool can be concentrated by formalin ether or zinc flotation techniques. Using an O&P exam, *Giardia* should be detected 50–70% of the time following one stool and as often as 90% following three stools.[206]

Antigen detection using polyclonal or monoclonal antibodies directed against cyst or trophozoite antigens is rapid to perform, less observer-dependent than stool O&Ps,[207] and highly sensitive and specific, with specificities in the range of 90–100% and sensitivites of 85–98%.[204,205] Commercial assays include ProSpecT *Giardia* EZ (Remel, Lenexa, KS), which uses ELISA to detect cyst wall protein;[208,209] MERIFLUOR *Cryptosporidium/Giardia* (Meridian Bioscience, Cincinnati, OH), a combination test using monoconal antibodies to detect *Giardia* and *Cryptosporidium*[210]; and ImmunoCard STAT! *Crypto/Giardia* (Meridian Bioscience, Cincinnati, OH), which is a nonenzymatic, immunochromatographic assay.[211] Low parasite levels (≤100 cysts/10 μL) may not be picked up with the immunochromatographic assays.[210,212,213]

These assays should not be done to the exclusion of an O&P in cases when other parasites are in the differential diagnosis. They can be used in screening a population for *Giardia*, such as in an outbreak setting and children in daycare, or for a test of cure. Antigen assays can remain positive for several days following successful treatment due to detection of soluble antigen. Polymerase chain reaction is used to detect and type *Giardia* cysts experimentally, and to detect *Giardia* cysts in water, but is in the development stage as a commercial diagnostic test.[214–216]

With a careful history and a stool properly examined, most cases of giardiasis should be diagnosed without duodenal sampling.[217,218] Early studies indicated that duodenal aspiration, biopsy, or the string test had higher yields than the standard O&P.[219,220] However, new diagnostic tests are likely as sensitive and less invasive. Duodenal aspirates or biopsies can be used in patients for whom the diagnosis of giardiasis cannot be made by stool examinations, when there is a broad differential diagnosis, or when it is important to examine the histology of the small bowel. Small-bowel biopsy can be helpful in patients with human immunodeficiency virus (HIV) infection or AIDS, common variable immunodeficiency, or suspected sprue.

Serology has been used in seroepidemiologic studies and research settings.[82,143,144,221,222] Serology is not used for individual patient diagnosis because of the ease and sensitivity of stool assays and because the serologic response to a noninvasive pathogen can be unreliable for individual diagnosis. Culture of human isolates is possible but is difficult, commonly unsuccessful and limited to research laboratories.[43,223,224]

Radiography is nonspecific and of little use in the diagnosis, but can reveal other lesions when there is a broader differential diagnosis. Findings on upper gastrointestinal studies have included an increased transit time and irregular thickening of the small-bowel folds. Nodular lymphoid hyperplasia has been seen in patients with common variable immunodeficiency. Peripheral white blood cell counts are normal; eosinophilia is not seen. Stools should not contain inflammatory cells.

TREATMENT AND PROGNOSIS

Symptomatic patients with giardiasis should be treated (***Table 93.3***). Because routine culture and sensitivity testing of *Giardia* isolates is not available and *in vitro* results do not always correlate with the clinical picture, treatment protocols have been based on clinical experience.[225,226] Therapeutic classes that have demonstrated efficacy are the nitroimidazoles, nitrofurans, benzimidazoles, and the agent, nitazoxanide.[225,227] A nitroimidazole is the treatment standard.

In 2003 and 2004, two agents were released in the United States for treatment of giardiasis: tinidazole (Tindamax, Mission Pharmaceutical Company, San Antonio, TX) and nitazoxanide (Alinia, Romark Pharmaceuticals, Tampa, FL).[227,228] These agents have expanded treatment options and should permit most patients with giardiasis to be successfully treated. Tinidazole has become the drug of choice: it has a longer half-life

Table 93.3 Treatment of *Giardia lamblia*, *Balantidium coli*, and *Dientamoeba fragilis*

	Dosage	
Drug	**Adult**	**Child**
Giardiasis		
Tinidazole[a]	2 g × 1 dose	50 mg/kg × 1 dose (max. 2 g)
Metronidazole[a,b]	250 mg tid × 5–7 days	5 mg/kg tid × 5–7 days
Nitazoxanide	500 mg bid × 3 days (≥12 years)	100 mg (5 mL oral suspension) q12h × 3 days (age 12–47 months)
		200 mg (10 mL oral suspension) q12h × 3 days (age 4–11 years)
Alternatives		
Albendazole[b]	400 mg qd × 5 days	15 mg/kg/day × 5–7 days (max. 400 mg)
Paromomycin[b]	500 mg tid × 5–10 days	30 mg/kg/day in 3 doses × 5–10 days
Quinacrine[c]	100 mg tid × 5–7 days	2 mg/kg tid × 7 days
Furazolidone[c]	100 mg qid × 7–10 days	2 mg/kg qid × 10 days
Balantidiasis		
Tetracycline[b,c]	500 mg qid × 10 days	10 mg/kg qid × 10 days (max. 2 g/day)
Metronidazole[b]	750 mg tid × 5 days	35–50 mg/kg/day in 3 doses × 5 days
Iodoquinol[b]	650 mg tid × 20 days	30–40 mg/kg/day in 3 doses × 20 days (max. 2 g/day)
Dientamoeba fragilis		
Iodoquinol[b]	650 mg tid × 20 days	30–40 mg/kg/day in 3 doses × 20 days (max. 2 g/day)
Tetracycline[b,d]	500 mg qid × 10 days	10 mg/kg qid × 10 days (max. 2 g/day)
Paromomycin[b]	500 mg tid × 7–10 days	25–30 mg/kg/day in 3 doses × 7–10 days
Metronidazole[a,b]	500–750 mg tid × 10 days	35–50 mg/kg/day in 3 doses × 10 days

[a]Other nitroimidazoles that are not available in the United States, e.g., ornidazole and secnidazole, are effective; see text.
[b]Not a US Food and Drug Administration-approved indication.
[c]No longer produced in the United States. May be obtained from some compounding pharmacies.
[d]Not recommended for use in children younger than 8 years of age.

Table 93.4 Treatment of Giardiasis – Efficacy and Adverse Events

Drug	Efficacy	Adverse Events
Tinidazole	85–98%	As for metronidazole, but may be better tolerated
Metronidazole	80–95%	Gastrointestinal, metallic taste, headache, disulfiram-like effect, rash
		Rare: reversible leukopenia, neuropathy, seizures
		Mutagenic/carcinogenic: *in vitro* and animal studies, not documented in humans
Nitazoxanide	65–85%	Abdominal pain, diarrhea, nausea, headache
Albendazole	85–95%	Anorexia, constipation
		Rare: reversible neutropenia and elevated liver enzymes
Paromomycin	55–90%	Gastrointestinal
Quinacrine	90–95%	Gastrointestinal, headache, yellow discoloration
		Rare: toxic psychosis
		Should not be given to patients with psoriasis
Furazolidone	80–95%	Gastrointestinal, allergic reaction, headache, disulfiram-like effect
		Do not take with tyramine- or tryptophan-containing food or drink, or with tricyclic antidepressants
		Rare: mild hemolysis in G6PD deficiency
		? Carcinogenic

G6PD, glucose-6-phosphate dehydrogenase.

than metronidazole and can be given as a single dose (2 g in adults).[225,229,230] It has more than three decades of experience in the treatment of giardiasis (as well as amebiasis and trichomoniasis) outside the United States.

Metronidazole, never approved by the US Food and Drug Administration (FDA) for use in giardiasis, is also safe and effective,[225] in divided doses over 5–7 days. Shorter courses (1 or 2 days), even at higher doses, are less effective and may be poorly tolerated. Side-effects from tinidazole and metronidazole are similar (***Table 93.4***), but tinidazole may be better tolerated.[231] They should not be taken with alcohol because they can produce a disulfiram-like effect. There has been concern about potential carcinogenicity of metronidazole in children. Although metronidazole can be mutagenic in bacteria and carcinogenic in high doses when given to animals, these findings have never been documented in humans, and the drug has accepted use in children for treatment of anaerobic infections and amebiasis.[232,233] Similar concerns would apply to tinidazole. Ornidazole and secnidazole, nitroimidazoles not available in the United States, have excellent efficacy when given over several days or as a single dose.[225,234,235]

Nitazoxanide is FDA-approved for the treatment of giardiasis and cryptosporidiosis.[227] The drug is active against a wide variety of parasites and bacteria, including some helminths.[236] There is limited experience in patients with giardiasis: trials show 65–85% efficacy when given over 3 days.[236–238]

Of the benzimidazoles, albendazole (Albenza, GlaxoSmithKline) is more effective than mebendazole and, when given in a single daily dose of 400 mg for 5 days, successfully treated 95% of infections in Bangladeshi children.[225,239,240] Other studies have confirmed albendazole's effectiveness, although not always at this high level.[241–243] It needs to be given for 5 days; shorter courses are less effective.[240,244] Because of albendazole's ability to kill other intestinal helminths, it is attractive when considering treatment of intestinal parasitism in low-income regions of the world, as is nitazoxanide.[245]

Quinacrine and furazolidone are no longer available in the United States.[225,246,247] Although quinacrine is highly effective, it may be poorly tolerated, particularly in children. Bacitracin zinc 120 000 units (USP) twice daily was effective in a trial in Tanzania, but this agent is not readily available for use and requires a 10-day course of therapy.[248]

In pregnancy, if a woman has mild disease and is able to maintain adequate hydration and nutrition, treatment can be delayed until after delivery or until the mother has progressed beyond the first trimester. If treatment is necessary, the options usually considered are metronidazole or paromomycin. The safety of metronidazole has been extensively studied; it is probably safe in the last two trimesters,[225,249,250] but should be avoided in the first trimester. Tinidazole is contraindicated in the first trimester.[251] An alternative to nitroimidazoles is paromomycin, an aminoglycoside. There is limited information in giardiasis: efficacy varies from 55% to 90%.[225,252,253] It has the theoretical advantage of not being appreciably absorbed and therefore avoiding potential fetal toxicity.

Drug resistance occurs with *Giardia*, and has been most completely studied with metronidazole. Activation of metronidazole occurs following reduction of the nitro group by acceptance of electrons from parasite protein ferredoxins; binding of activated drug to parasite DNA results in trophozoite death.[254–257] Resistance correlates with decreased parasite pyruvate:ferredoxin oxidoreductase.[254,256]

Patients can fail treatment because of drug resistance, host factors, or simply failure of a single course of treatment. Repeat therapy with the same agent, using a drug of a different class, or combination therapy is usually effective. Combinations found to work are metronidazole with quinacrine and metronidazole (or other nitroimidazole) with albendazole.[177,258–260] Nitazoxanide has also been effective in persons with resistant parasites.[261] Patients who clinically relapse should be documented to have true parasitologically confirmed ongoing giardiasis since many persons have prolonged lactose intolerance that can mimic infection. Irritable bowel disease has been another association with *Giardia* infection.[217,262,263] Repeated failures should be investigated for a potential immune defect such as common variable immunodeficiency.[174,259]

Treatment of asymptomatic *Giardia* infection is controversial, particularly when reinfection is likely to occur, as in children in low-income regions or in daycare settings.[90,199,200,264,265] A case can be made for intermittent antiparasitic treatment of children in low-income regions because of the potentially deleterious effects of acute and chronic giardiasis (as well as other enteric parasites).[142,192] Catch-up growth has been documented following treatment for *Giardia*.[266] Micronutrient supplementation, specifically combination vitamin A and zinc, but not vitamin A alone, reduced the duration of infection with *Giardia* in Mexican children,[267,268] as did lactoferrin in Peruvian children.[269] When considering individual or community treatment one needs to balance the clinical setting, the effect of *Giardia* on the host, the cost and tolerance of treatment, and the ability to obtain a sustained elimination of the parasite. Because of the possibility of transmission in food, all food handlers should be treated.

PREVENTION AND CONTROL

The prevention of giardiasis requires the provision of potable water and adequate sewage treatment for communities and personal hygiene for individuals. Because of widespread contamination of surface water with *Giardia* cysts, treatment of water supplies needs to remove or inactivate these relatively hardy cysts. Water should be treated by multiple purification methods including flocculation, sedimentation, filtration, and then chlorination. Most municipal water supplies use chlorine at levels of approximately 0.4 mg/L. This level of chlorination, when used alone, may not be sufficient to inactivate cysts, so it is important that the other measures are also in place.[270] Solar disinfection methods are being explored for water purification.[271]

In order to purify water for personal use when camping or traveling overseas, it can be brought to a boil (or boiled for a minute if at high altitude), filtered using small-volume water filters (pore size of less than 1 µm), or halogenated with chlorine or iodine preparations.[272] Filters combined with iodine resin should not be used, because uncontrolled release of iodine can lead to high levels of iodine in the water. As single treatments, chlorine preparations can be subject to temperature, pH, and turbidity compared with iodines.[272,273] In the European Union iodine preparations are no longer available for personal use. When using halogens, it is important to increase contact time for cold water and increase the dose of the halogen for turbid water. All halogens may be inadequate for *Cryptosporidium* as well as *Cyclospora*, and therefore filtration or boiling is more reliable,[274] especially when traveling overseas where there is a higher likelihood of acquiring *Cryptosporidium* than from wilderness water in the United States and Canada.[66,275,276] When enteric viruses are a concern and a filter is being used, the water should also be halogenated since viruses will escape the filtration process. Some filters decrease viral contamination through a combination of filtration and electrostatic attraction, but are not able to remove viral contamination completely without additional halogenation or heating.[272]

Prevention of transmission in endemic foci such as daycare centers is challenging.[190,191,277,278] In daycare, symptomatic children, teachers, and family members should be treated. If strict hand washing, separation of diaper-changing areas from play and food areas, and treatment of symptomatic children do not control giardiasis, then consideration can be given to treating all infected children.[279]

Prospects for the control of giardiasis in low-income regions are limited until there are both the financial resources and political and community will to provide for the proper disposal of sewage and the provision of potable water. Sanitary interventions that improve hygiene should be combined with screening and treatment of diarrheal disease. Breastfeeding has been associated with lower rates of infection in developing regions, particularly when maternal milk has contained antibody to *Giardia*.[280–282] Currently, there is no prospect for a vaccine against infection in humans.

BALANTIDIUM COLI

Balantidium coli is the largest intestinal protozoan of humans and the only ciliate (***Fig. 93.6***).[283,284] It is a rare cause of diarrhea and inflammatory colitis. The trophozoite ranges in size from 60 to 70 µm (up to 200 µm), is usually ovoid in shape, and has a large, kidney-shaped macronucleus with a small micronucleus often lying in its concavity (***Fig. 93.7***). Anteriorly at the tapered end it has a tunnel-shaped cytosome or oral apparatus, and posteriorly a small opening in the cell membrane called the cytopyge. Within the cytoplasm, there are numerous vacuoles and occasional intracellular erythrocytes. It is covered by longitudinal rows of cilia, which help propel the organism in a rotary motion. The cyst is also large, 40–60 µm, round to oval, and smooth-walled. The characteristic nucleus may be visible.

Humans are an incidental host to this pathogen, which inhabits the large bowel of several mammalian species. Pigs are one of the main sources of human infection, as they are commonly infected asymptomatically.[284–289] A large outbreak of balantidiasis occurred in the Truk Islands in Micronesia, where it was postulated that the water supplies became contaminated with pig feces after a typhoon.[290] In Iran, where there has been no obvious exposure to pigs, camels or wild boars have been proposed as potential sources.[291–293] Cases in captive lowland gorillas and other primates have been described.[294–296]

While symptomatic infection with *B. coli* has been reported from the Americas, Africa, and Latin America, it remains unusual. In the United States, as in other temperate climates, it was found in less than 0.1% of stools and from only three states.[62,297,298] Manifestations range from asymptomatic, accounting for over 50% of cases, to chronic, intermittent diarrhea and weight loss, to acute dysentery in about 5% of cases.[284,299] Colitis is characterized by several loose stools per day, abdominal pain, and cramps, and may be associated with blood and mucus. Appendicitis, intestinal perforation with peritonitis and death, and disseminated infection to liver and lung have all been reported but are rare.[299–302] Cases of severe extrapulmonary infection have occurred in immunocompromised hosts, including reports in AIDS patients.[303–306]

B. coli appears to cause disease by invasion of mucosa from the terminal ileum to rectum.[297,299,307] The penetration of the mucosa may be aided by a hyaluronidase.[308] Ulcers are usually multiple and superficial, but they can progress to deep ulceration with perforation, and can resemble those formed by *Entamoeba histolytica*.

The diagnosis is made by demonstrating trophozoites in fresh stools or ulcer scrapings from the colon. While cysts may be found in the stool on O&P exam, it is more common to find trophozoites.[284,291,297,299] *B. coli* can be grown on artificial media,[43] but this method is not readily available.

Treatment is effective with tetracycline, metronidazole, and iodoquinol (see ***Table 93.3***).[226,288,297,309] Nitazoxanide also may be effective.[310]

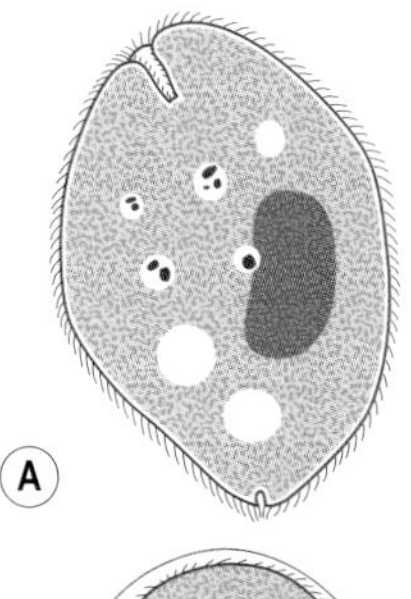

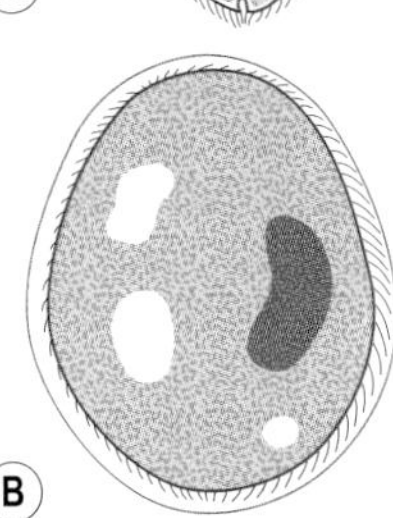

Figure 93.6 Schematic drawing of *Balantidium coli* trophozoite **(A)** and cyst **(B)**, and their key identification points.

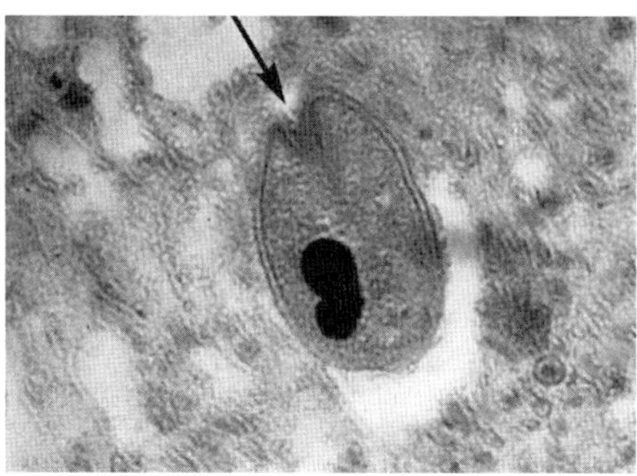

Figure 93.7 Trophozoite of *Balantidium coli*. The large, eccentric, kidney-shaped nucleus is readily seen. The surface is covered with short cilia. The arrow indicates the cytosome. (Reproduced from Baskerville L, Ahmed Y, Ramchand S. *Balantidium* colitis. Report of a case. Dig Dis. 1970;15:727, with permission of S. Karger, Basel.)

DIENTAMOEBA FRAGILIS

Dientamoeba fragilis is an intestinal protozoan of humans. Its pathogenicity has been controversial; however, increasing evidence supports its role as a cause of diarrhea.[311,312] Though originally classified as an ameba,[313] immunologic and ultrastructural studies have placed it in the flagellate group, related to the *Histomonas* and *Trichomonas* genera.[314–316] However, it has no flagella and does not exhibit directed motility in wet microscopy. While a single study of human isolates in England demonstrated two genotypes,[317] other investigators have not found separate genotypes.[318–320] Molecular markers have been idenitifed that could be used in epidemiologic studies.[321] Morphologically, *D. fragilis* exists only in the trophozoite form (***Fig. 93.8***). It is 9–12 μm in size, and usually has two nuclei with a granular appearance, and frequent intracytoplasmic vacuoles.

D. fragilis is found throughout the world. It was identified in 0.5% of US stools: over 50% were from California.[62] In Canada, it was found in 4% of stools from over 40000 people,[322] in 15–17% of stools from patients in the United Kingdom,[323] in 13% in Egypt,[324] and in 5% of stools in Oman.[325] Standard surveys can underestimate its true prevalence as detection of trophozoites in stools can be difficult.[326] In selected populations in the United States the prevalence has been as high as 19–50%.[327,328] In low-income regions it is often seen in conjunction with other intestinal parasites, and has been documented as a cause of diarrhea in returned travelers.[329–331]

Transmission of *D. fragilis* is presumed to be via the fecal–oral route. How it might survive stomach acid is not clear. Because of its association with *Enterobius vermicularis* (pinworm),[322,332,333] some have proposed, but not proven, that the parasite is transmitted in pinworm eggs.[334,335]

The ability of *D. fragilis* to cause gastrointestinal symptoms has been debated because the parasite is seen both in conjunction with other intestinal protozoa and in asymptomatic individuals. Several studies that have surveyed patients with only *D. fragilis* have described symptoms of diarrhea, abdominal pain (frequently epigastric or lower quadrant), increased flatus, anorexia, fatigue, and malaise.[319,320,322,324,325,332,336–339] Abdominal symptoms can be present for weeks.[336,338–340] It has been seen in persons evaluated for irritable bowel disease,[341,342] and a case report describes *D. fragilis* mimicking appendicitis.[343] While it appears to be confined to the large intestine, it has been detected in bile.[344] Reports of severe infection are rare.[345]

The diagnosis of *Dientamoeba* infection requires that stools (preferably three to detect 70–90%) be placed in a fixative, often polyvinyl alcohol, and then permanently stained and examined.[206,311,326] A simple wet mount or iodine stain will miss many infections, and the parasite quickly disintegrates if mixed with water. Although the organism can be cultured in xenic media with rice starch, growth is not sustained.[43,346,347] Detection by immunofluorescence and polymerase chain reaction is investigative.[318,320,348,349] There is an unexplained association with eosinophilia.[350] Many of the cases of eosinophilia have been in patients in whom pinworm was also seen or in immigrant populations in whom other helminth infections were not adequately ruled out.[336,337]

Trophozoite
• 7–12 μm
• rounded
• one or two (80%) nuclei with four to eight symmetrical chromatin granules
• intracellular vacuoles and bacteria
• best identified in permanent stains
• active pseudopods, but sluggish motility
Cyst
No cyst stage

Figure 93.8 Schematic drawing of *Dientamoeba fragilis* trophozoite and its key identification points. *D. fragilis* has no cyst stage.

Successful treatment has been with metronidazole, secnidazole, and ornidazole, iodoquinol, tetracycline, and paromomycin.[226,332,337,350–353] (see ***Table 93.3***). Treatment failures and recurrences occur.

OTHER FLAGELLATES

The other flagellates of humans are considered to be nonpathogens or commensals.[354,355] When they are found in the stool, they are often seen in association with other organisms and are a marker of fecal–oral contamination.[328,356] Rare clinical cases, including extraintestinal infections, have occurred when other pathogens have been ruled out.[357–361] In stool surveys from the United States, *Chilomastix mesnili* (***Fig. 93.9***) and *Pentatrichomonas hominis* (formerly known as *Trichomonas hominis*, and named because a fifth "independent" flagellum is often seen; ***Fig. 93.10***) were found in fewer than 0.5% of specimens.[62] However, in missionaries returning from low-income regions of the world, *C. mesnili* and *P. hominis* were seen in 3% and 2%, respectively,[329] and in a Native American population *C. mesnili* was identified in 20% of stools.[327] In stool O&P, the cyst

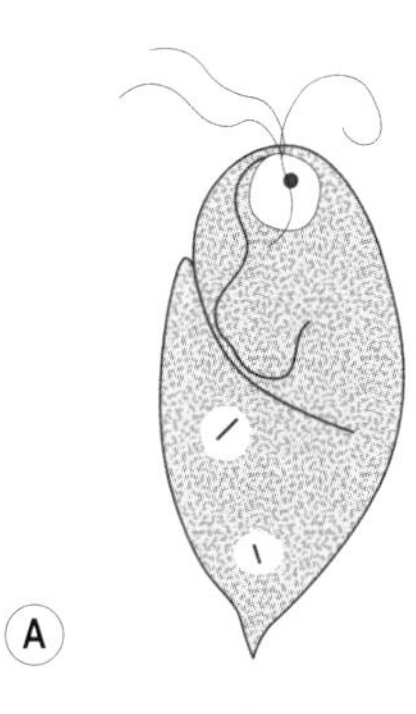

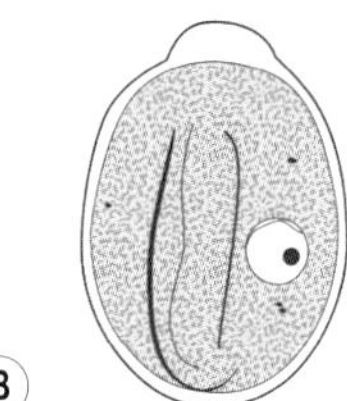

B
Cyst
• 6–10 μm
• unique lemon shape with anterior polar knob
• thick-walled
• single nucleus
• curved cytosomal fibril

Figure 93.9 Schematic drawing of *Chilomastix mesnili* trophozoite (*top*) and cyst (*bottom*), and their key identification points.

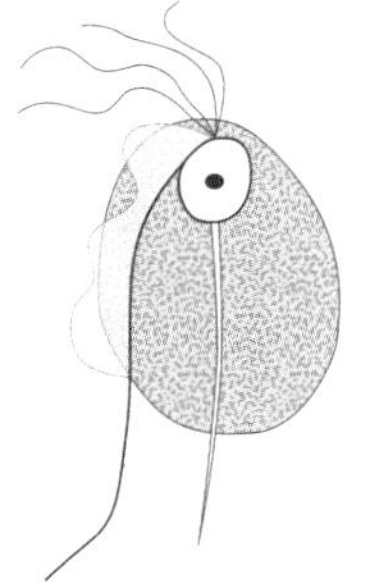

Trophozoite
• 5–8 μm × 10–15 μm
• oval or pear shape
• single anterior nucleus
• four anterior flagella
• undulating membrane with posterior projecting flagellum
• unique costa, or thin rod at attachment of body to membrane
• central axostyle with sharply pointed posterior protrusion
• rapid, jerking movement with wavelike motion of undulating membrane
Cyst
No cyst stage

Figure 93.10 Schematic drawing of *Pentatrichomonas hominis* trophozoite and its key identification points. *P. hominis* has no cyst stage.

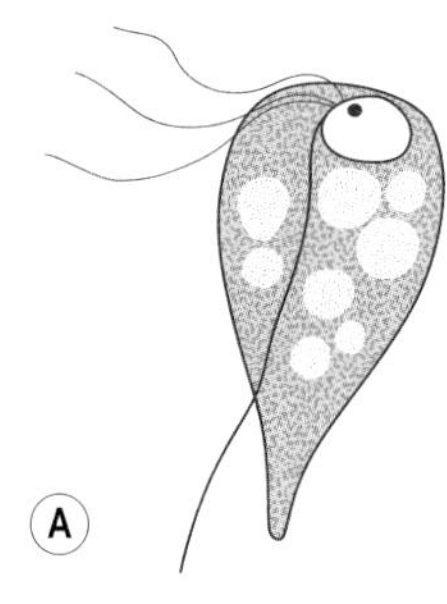

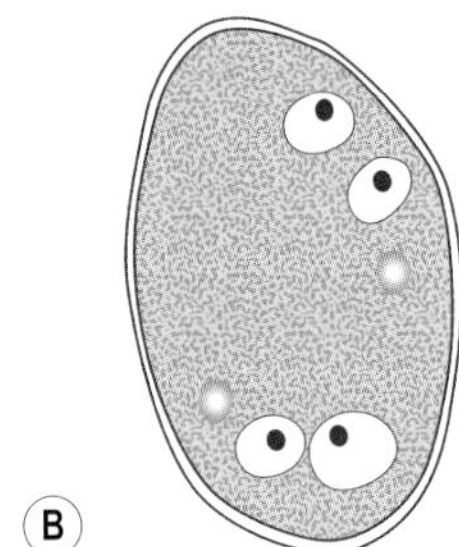

Figure 93.11 Schematic drawing of *Enteromonas hominis* trophozoite (**A**) and cyst (**B**), and their key identification points.

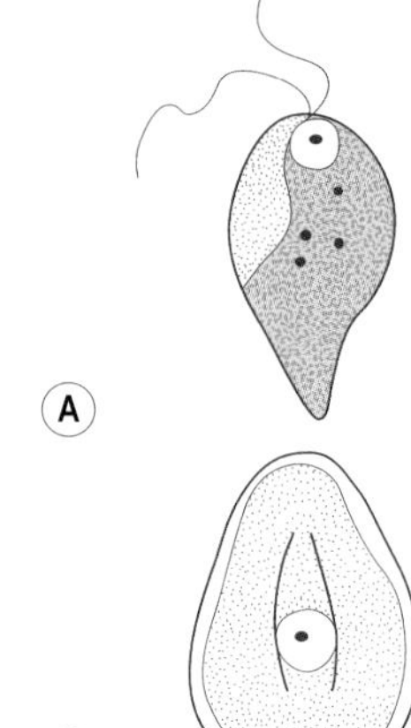

Figure 93.12 Schematic drawing of *Retortamonas intestinalis* trophozoite (**A**) and cyst (**B**), and their key identification points.

of *C. mesnili* has a characteristic lemon-shaped cyst with an apical knob. *P. hominis* has only a trophozoite stage.[362] *Enteromonas hominis* (***Fig. 93.11***) and *Retortamonas intestinalis* (***Fig. 93.12***) are rare infections. *Trichomonas tenax* may be seen in the oral cavity; its role in causing periodontal disease is unclear.[362]

ACKNOWLEDGMENT

Parasite drawings in this chapter are by Linda Tenukas.

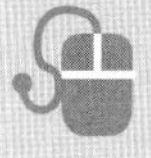

Access the complete reference list online at
http://www.expertconsult.com

Access the complete reference list online at http://www.expertconsult.com

CHAPTER 94

Cryptosporidiosis

Aldo A.M. Lima • Amidou Samie • Richard L. Guerrant

INTRODUCTION

Cryptosporidium, like *Isospora*, *Cyclospora*, and *Sarcocystis*, are intestinal coccidia related to the apicomplexan protozoa infecting humans, including *Plasmodium* species causing malaria. Intestinal coccidia are characterized by the fecal excretion of oocysts, which are the product of a sexual cycle of reproduction in the epithelium of the small intestine.

The coccidian protozoa have long been identified as veterinary pathogens, but their recognition as causes of human diarrheal disease is relatively recent. Although a few sporadic human cases had been reported previously, it was the worldwide spread of human immunodeficiency virus (HIV) in the 1980s that brought these organisms to prominent medical attention, since they tend to produce severe, protracted diarrhea in patients with advanced acquired immunodeficiency syndrome (AIDS). With subsequent increased surveillance and impressive waterborne and occasional foodborne outbreaks, however, *Cryptosporidium* has been identified as a major cause of diarrhea in children, often with long-term developmental impairment, as well as in immunocompetent persons in many settings, especially in tropical, developing areas around the world. Its unique characteristics of chlorine resistance and dependence on cell-mediated immunity for resolution of infection may place it among the most problematic enteric pathogens of the new century.

THE AGENT

History

Cryptosporidium was first described in 1907, primarily as a cause of diarrhea in animal species. The first human cases of cryptosporidiosis were published in two reports in 1976, one in a 3-year-old child with enterocolitis[1] and the other in a 39-year-old patient on cyclophosphamide and prednisolone for severe bullous pemphigoid,[2] and only seven more cases were reported until the early 1980s, when it was recognized as a common and debilitating pathogen in patients with AIDS. Though the first recorded epidemic occurred in 1984,[3] the most memorable one occurred in Milwaukee, when an outbreak affected more than 400 000 people, contributed to the deaths of more than 50 AIDS and chemotherapy patients, and resulted in the loss of more than US$96 million in lost wages and productivity.[4–6] Since then, *Cryptosporidium* has been recognized to occur even more often in immunocompetent persons, and it is a leading cause of endemic childhood diarrhea in developing areas and waterborne diarrheal outbreaks in developed countries.

Taxonomy

The taxonomy of the genus *Cryptosporidium* is incomplete and evolving. The family Cryptosporidiidae belongs to the phylum Apicomplexa characterized by an anterior (or apical) polar complex (with apical rings, micronemes, and subpellicular microtubules), which allows penetration into host cells. The coccidia are further classified based on their life cycles into the class Sporozoasida (locomotion by flexion, gliding, or undulation) and subclass Coccidiasina (sporozoite formation). The vertebrate diarrheal coccidia belong to the order Eucoccidiorida (Eucoccidiida) and suborder Eimeriorina (Eimeriina) based on merogony within vertebrate hosts and independent development of male and female gametocytes. This separates them from other pathogenic apicomplexan protozoa (*Plasmodium* and *Babesia*). The species and genotypes of *Cryptosporidium* are shown in ***Figure 94.1*** and are discussed in the Epidemiology section.

Life Cycle

As shown in ***Figure 94.2***, *Cryptosporidium* is monoxenous (i.e., the complete life cycle occurs in a single host) in contrast to *Plasmodium* spp. and *Sarcocystis* spp., which require two hosts. *Cryptosporidium* oocysts are thick-walled and 3–6 μm, which when ingested by the host, excyst within the lumen of the small intestine to release four infective sporozoites. Sporozoite attachment results in the formation of a unique intracellular but extracytoplasmic parasitophorous vacuole within which they develop into trophozoites and subsequently type 1 meronts (schizonts). These reproduce asexually with three nuclear divisions to release six to eight type 1 merozoites, which invade nearby cells and develop into type 2 meronts or into trophozoites to complete the asexual reproductive cycle. The merozoites are similar in morphology and function to the sporozoites, and are capable of reinfecting other host cells, thereby reinitiating the asexual part of the cycle in the same host. The perpetuation of the asexual stage of the life cycle, a property also shared by *Isospora*, is probably responsible for persistent and severe infections in hosts who do not have repeated exposure to these parasites. Type 2 meronts undergo two nuclear divisions and release four type 2 merozoites, which reinfect the epithelium and develop into male (microgamont) or female (macrogamete) forms. The microgamont releases microgametes, which penetrate the macrogamete to form a zygote, which can then develop into a thin-walled autoinfectious oocyst (approximately 20% of the time) or a thick-walled oocyst (approximately 80%), which is shed in stool. The average incubation period (time from ingestion to disease manifestation) is approximately 1–2 weeks. Remarkably, the entire asexual and sexual phases of development take place just beneath the luminal cell membrane of epithelial cells (in an intracellular but extracytoplasmic parasitophorous vacuole) without deeper cellular or tissue invasion, even in severely immunocompromised patients.[7] Intracytoplasmic invasion has been rarely seen in the Peyer's patches.

EPIDEMIOLOGY

Over 20 species were originally named in the family Cryptosporidiidae based on the host they infected, but these different species were subsequently shown not to be host-specific and are no longer distinguished. On the basis of size and biologic, ribosomal RNA, and genetic studies,

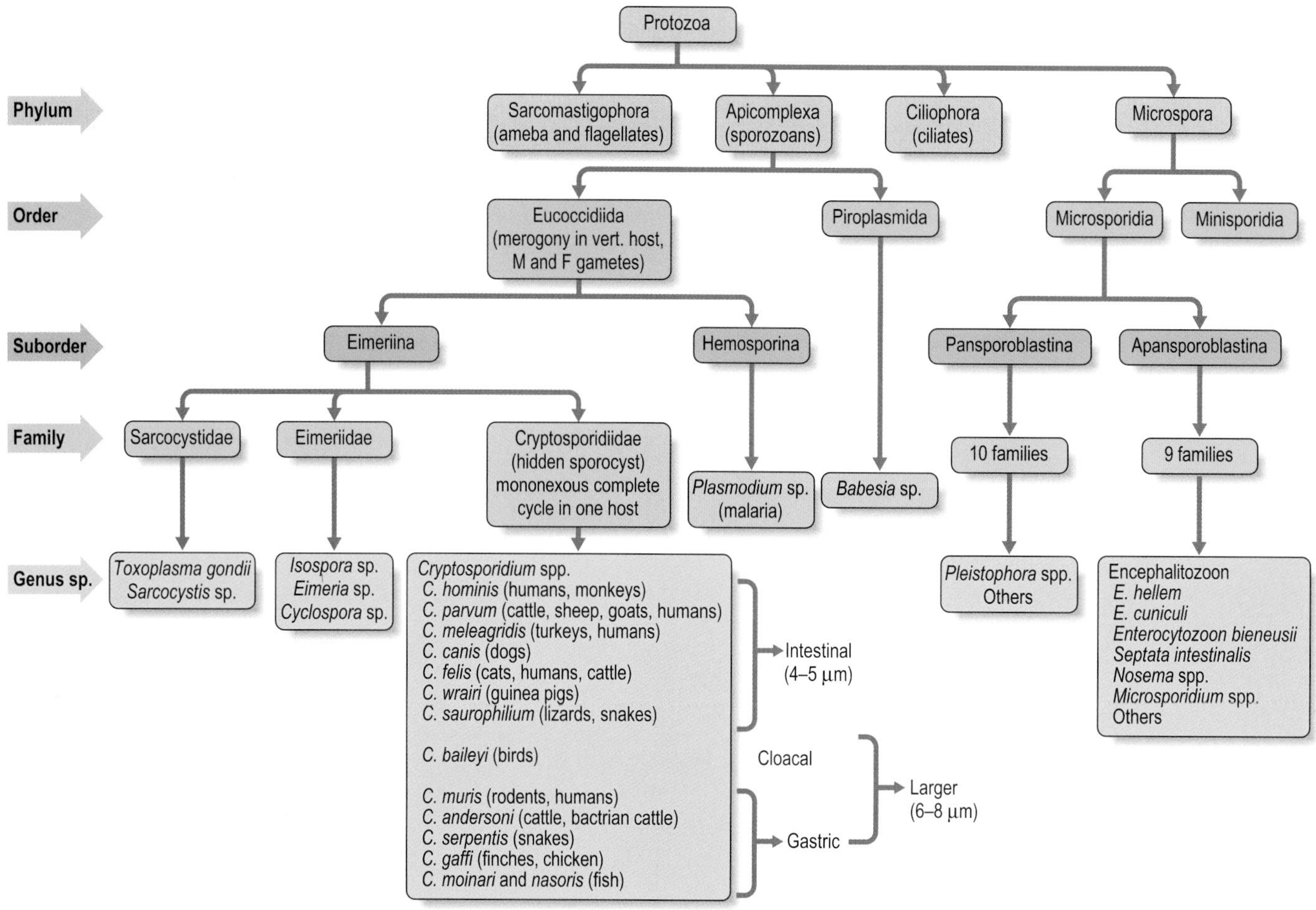

Figure 94.1 Taxonomy of *Cryptosporidium* and related protozoa. *C. hominis* has been responsible for most human outbreaks in Milwaukee, Las Vegas, Atlanta, Washington, DC, Florida, and British Columbia, Canada. Some outbreaks in Minnesota, Pennsylvania, and British Columbia and the United Kingdom have also been with the bovine strain *C. parvum*. (Adapted from Xiao L, Fayer R, Ryan U, et al. *Cryptosporidium* taxonomy: recent advances and implications for public health. Clin Microbiol Rev. 2004;17(1):72–97.)

three larger "gastric" (or cloacal) species (*C. muris*, *C. baileyi*, and *C. serpentis*, predominantly from mice, birds/chickens, and snakes, respectively) can be distinguished from the smaller, intestinal species more closely related to *C. parvum*, including *C. hominis*, *C. parvum*, *C. wrairi* (in guinea pigs), *C. meleagridis* (in birds, especially turkeys), *C. felis* (in cats), and possibly *C. saurophilum* (in snakes), *C. andersoni* (in ruminants), *C. nasorum* (in fish), and others. Species that are known to infect humans are: *C. hominis* (formerly called type 1 or primarily "human" *C. parvum*);[8–10] *C. parvum* (formerly called type 2 or "bovine"), which infects humans and cattle; *C. meleagridis* from turkeys[11,12] and *C. felis* from cats; *C. canis* from dogs as well as rabbit, pig, and monkey genotypes[13–15] (see ***Fig. 94.1*** adapted from Xiao and colleagues).[16,17–19] The significance of the molecular analyses of *C. parvum/hominis* isolates remains to be fully defined; one report suggests no differences in age, antecedent stunting, or association with diarrhea or its duration, but longer shedding with *C. hominis* (type 1) than with *C. parvum* (type 2) in children in Peru.[14] Other reports from Peru, the United Kingdom, Brazil, and Kenya note that *C. hominis* (especially subtype 1b) is associated with more diarrhea, nausea, vomiting, general malaise, and increased oocyst shedding intensity.[20–22] In northeast Brazil *C. hominis* infections were more common, heavier and associated with greater lasting growth shortfalls, even without overt diarrhea, than *C. parvum*.[23]

Cryptosporidium oocysts have been found in 87% of the raw water samples tested from the United States and Canada.[24] A linear regression model found that the presence of oocysts correlated with the level of watershed protection, the amount of coliform bacteria, and the turbidity, pH, and temperature of the water. Domesticated animals are probably the primary reservoir for *C. parvum*, although patients with AIDS and children with cryptosporidiosis may excrete millions of oocysts a day, which can survive for months in sewage.

Cryptosporidium oocysts possess a unique set of five characteristics that make the organism such a common and problematic threat.[25] First, they are highly infectious. The median infectious dose in healthy adult volunteers is 132 oocysts,[26] although a mathematical model based on the Milwaukee outbreak estimated that some people could have been infected after ingestion of as few as 1–10 oocysts. This infectivity probably accounts for the high rate of person-to-person transmission, ranging from 5.4% of household contacts of adults infected in the Milwaukee outbreak developing symptomatic disease to 19% of family members of infected children in Fortaleza, Brazil, developing disease or seroconversion.[5,27] *Cryptosporidium* also may spread among children in daycare centers[28] and among the elderly in hospitals.[29,30]

Second, the size and composition of cryptosporidial oocysts makes them highly resistant to water treatment. The oocysts measure 3–6 μm in diameter, which enables them to pass through most conventional filters. Only water filters capable of removing particles smaller than 1 μm are reasonably effective at removing *Cryptosporidium*, but even these may fail.[31] Effective filters include reverse osmosis filters and those rated as "absolute" at 1 μm but not "nominal" 1 μm filters.[32] Third, *Cryptosporidium* oocysts are highly resistant to chlorination, remaining infectious even after exposure for 30 minutes to 80 ppm chlorine (100 times the acceptable dose for elimination of coliform bacteria).[33] The cysts are inactivated, however, by ozone, freezing, or heating (to 72°C for 1 minute or 45°C for 10–20 minutes).[33,34]

Fourth, the full development of *Cryptosporidium* oocysts by the time they are excreted to a promptly infectious stage means that they can be

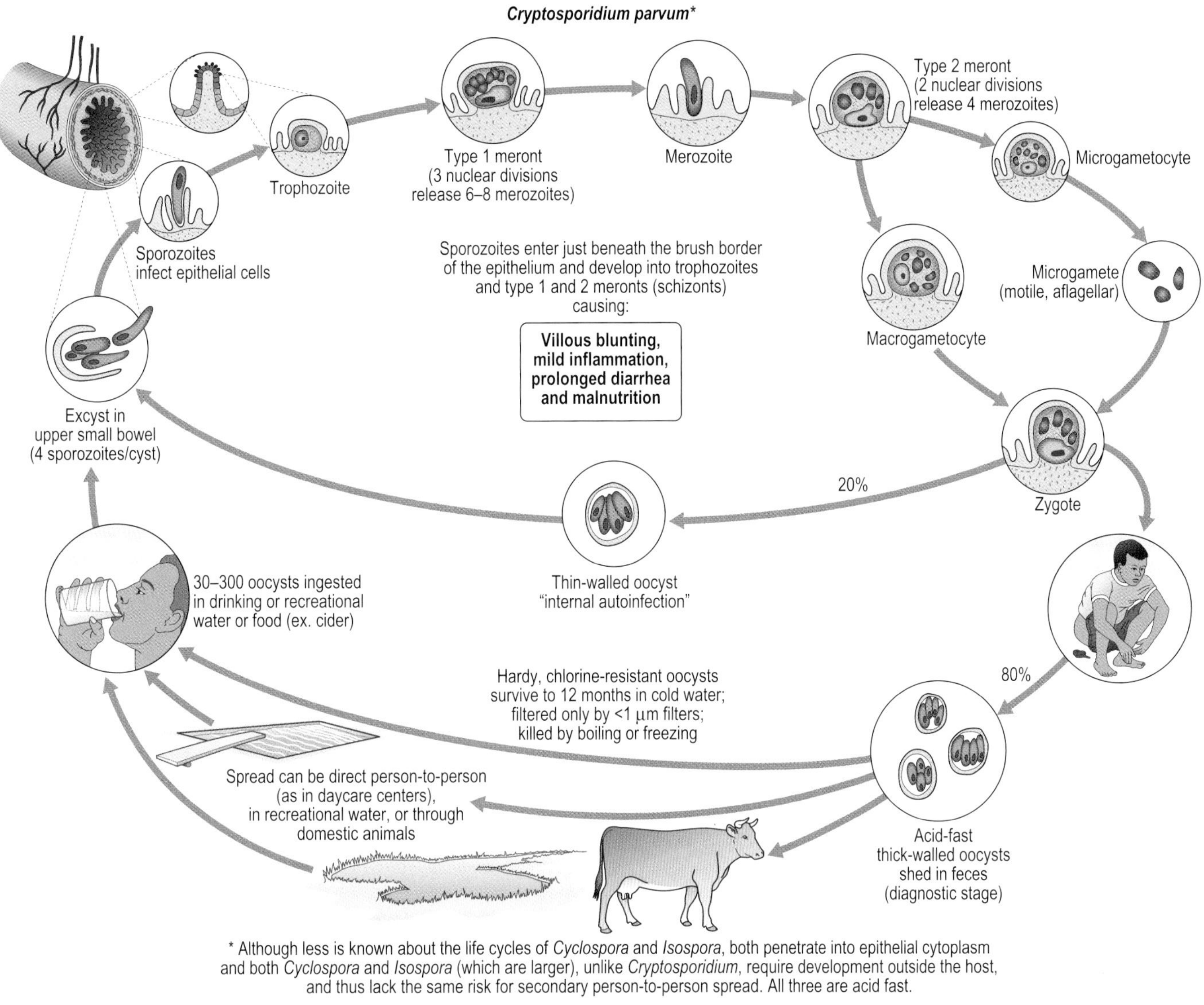
Cryptosporidium parvum*
Type 2 meront
(2 nuclear divisions
release 4 merozoites)
Microgametocyte
Trophozoite
Type 1 meront
(3 nuclear divisions
release 6–8 merozoites)
Merozoite
Sporozoites
infect epithelial cells
Sporozoites enter just beneath the brush border
of the epithelium and develop into trophozoites
and type 1 and 2 meronts (schizonts)
causing:
Villous blunting,
mild inflammation,
prolonged diarrhea
and malnutrition
Microgamete
(motile, aflagellar)
Macrogametocyte
Excyst in
upper small bowel
(4 sporozoites/cyst)
20%
Zygote
30–300 oocysts ingested
in drinking or recreational
water or food (ex. cider)
Thin-walled oocyst
"internal autoinfection"
Hardy, chlorine-resistant oocysts
survive to 12 months in cold water;
filtered only by <1 μm filters;
killed by boiling or freezing
80%
Spread can be direct person-to-person
(as in daycare centers),
in recreational water, or through
domestic animals
Acid-fast
thick-walled oocysts
shed in feces
(diagnostic stage)
* Although less is known about the life cycles of Cyclospora and Isospora, both penetrate into epithelial cytoplasm
and both Cyclospora and Isospora (which are larger), unlike Cryptosporidium, require development outside the host,
and thus lack the same risk for secondary person-to-person spread. All three are acid fast.

Figure 94.2 *Cryptosporidium parvum* life cycle.

readily spread by direct person-to-person contact, a key determinant of the epidemiology of cryptosporidial infections.[25,27] Fifth, there are geographic, seasonal and socioeconomic differences in the distribution of *Cryptosporidium* spp. in humans based on the recent molecular tools developed to detect and differentiate this microorganism at the species/genotype and subtype levels. Recent work suggests that *C. parvum* infection in humans is mostly anthroponotic in developing countries, with zoonotic transmission in developed countries,[35] with *C. hominis* predominating in high density human populations.[20,23,36]

Unlike most outbreak isolates of cryptosporidiosis in the United States and Canada, which are *C. hominis*,[37–39] most sporadic cases and outbreaks in the United Kingdom and Switzerland are with the *C. parvum* genotype, some of which have been associated with ingestion of raw milk or cream.[38–41] Studies in Africa show a higher prevalence of *C. hominis* among children and adults,[22,42,43] although in farm settings *C. parvum* is more common.[44]

Cryptosporidial diarrhea is seen primarily in four settings: endemic childhood diarrhea in developing areas, travelers' diarrhea in visitors to developing areas, protracted diarrhea in immunocompromised patients, and waterborne disease outbreaks in developed countries (***Fig. 94.3***). Seroprevalence studies reflect these settings, with seropositivity ranging from 58% in adolescents in Oklahoma[45] to 50% by 8–10 years of age in China and 95% by age 2 years in a poor community in northeastern Brazil.[46] In all settings, *Cryptosporidium* is strongly associated with diarrhea, although asymptomatic infections do occur. Compiling data from 78 studies published before 1993, Adal and colleagues[19] found an overall prevalence of *Cryptosporidium* in 6.1% of diarrhea patients and 1.5% of controls in developing countries, and 2.15% of patients and 0.15% of controls in developed countries. Recent data from 19 studies published with controls from 1994 to 2003 indicate the overall prevalence of *Cryptosporidium* infection is even higher: 12.7% in immunocompetent patients in developing countries who present with diarrhea and an asymptomatic carriage of 4.5%,[47–62] whereas in developed countries the prevalence is 2.3% in diarrhea cases and 1.2% asymptomatic carriage in controls (***Table 94.1***).[63–65]

The higher rates of cryptosporidiosis in developing areas are likely related to poor sanitation and crowded living conditions. Specific risk factors for acquisition in children include male sex, keeping animals in the house, and weaning.[66] In most studies breastfeeding is protective and children with cryptosporidial diarrhea are less likely to be breastfed.[67] While this may be due in part to passive transfer of immunity, it may also be due to increased exposure to potentially contaminated food and water at weaning.[68]

Those most severely affected by *Cryptosporidium* are immunocompromised patients, especially those with AIDS, in whom the disease can be fulminant and fatal. Adal and colleagues, compiling results from 22 studies published before 1993, found that 13.8% and 24% of patients with AIDS and diarrhea in developed and developing areas, respectively, had *Cryptosporidium* compared with only 0–5% of AIDS patients without diarrhea.[19] In five studies published with controls for 1994 through 2003

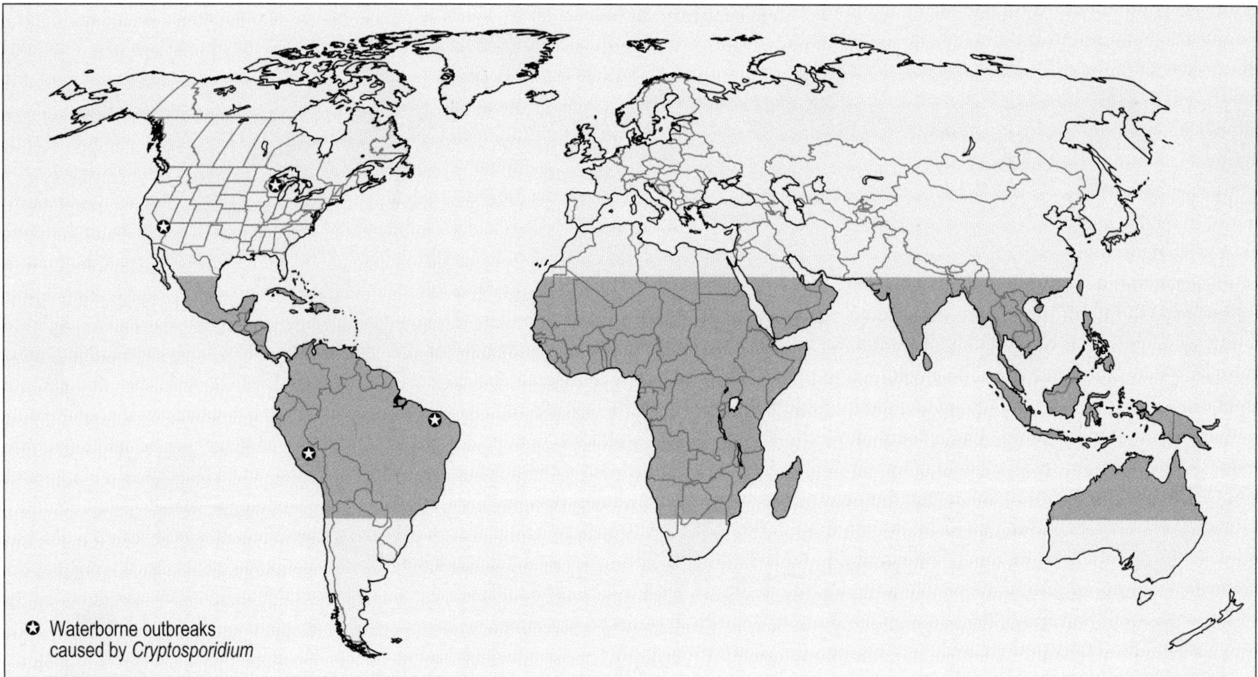

Figure 94.3 Endemic tropical areas and waterborne outbreaks caused by *Cryptosporidium*.

Table 94.1 Frequency of Cryptosporidiosis among Immunocompetent Symptomatic and Asymptomatic Individuals in Developing and Developed Countries 1994–2003

Area	Patients with Diarrhea	Controls without Diarrhea
Asia/Africa/Latin America (16 studies)[47–62]	849/6669 (12.7%)	346/7539 (4.5%)
North America/Europe/Australia (3 studies)[63–65]	25/1049 (2.3%)	67/5624 (1.2%)

Table 94.2 Frequency of Cryptosporidiosis among Immunocompromised Symptomatic and Asymptomatic Individuals in Developing Countries, 1994–2003

Area	Patients with Diarrhea	Controls without Diarrhea
Asia/Africa/Latin America (5 studies)[69–73]	73/453 (16.1%)	7/324 (2.2%)

from developing countries of Africa, Asia, and Latin America, immunodeficient patients (including HIV and malignancies) have a prevalence of 16.1% in cases with diarrhea and 2.2% asymptomatic carriage of *Cryptosporidium* (***Table 94.2***).[69–73]

Patients with AIDS are prone to developing debilitating disease with cryptosporidiosis. In the Nevada outbreak, 61 of the 2270 known HIV-infected patients in the area developed diarrhea, and 32 of these died within 6 months; this is similar to the high mortality in the Milwaukee outbreak, in which 48 of 82 infected patients with AIDS died within a year, with excess mortality largely attributable to the cryptosporidial illnesses.[64,65]

In developed countries, cryptosporidiosis is also sporadic. The prevalence is increased in dairy farmers and other persons who have contact with cattle.[76] Small outbreaks have been reported in daycare centers and veterinary and health care settings. The largest outbreaks, however, have been waterborne. *Cryptosporidium* is the most common cause of recreational water outbreaks due to contaminated lakes and swimming pools. In 1999–2000, *C. parvum* accounted for the largest percentage (44%) of waterborne outbreaks involving gastroenteritis, 61% occurring in treated systems (i.e., pools).[77] Splash water game parks as well as child care centers are also emerging as centers of *Cryptosporidium* transmission in several settings in the United States.[78–80]

Spring is the time of peak incidence, presumably due to the propensity for heavy rains during that season to cause flooding and subsequent contamination of source water.[81,82] Numerous large community-based waterborne outbreaks of *Cryptosporidium* have been reported since 1984, affecting hundreds of thousands of people.[83] By far the largest of these was the 1993 outbreak in Milwaukee, Wisconsin, in which an estimated 403 000 people developed diarrhea due to a combination of source water contamination and transient impairment of prefiltration processing. Of note, the water quality during that outbreak met all US federal drinking water standards at that time.[4] The federal standards for turbidity were strengthened as a result, but a 1994 outbreak affecting over 100 people in Las Vegas, Nevada, occurred even when the water met these tougher standards (i.e., not exceeding 0.17 nephelometric turbidity units).[74]

THE DISEASE

Clinical Manifestations

The clinical manifestations of cryptosporidiosis are indistinguishable from those of giardiasis, isosporiasis, and cyclosporiasis. Clinical illness is characterized by watery diarrhea without red blood cells or leukocytes and may be associated with one or more nonspecific symptoms and signs, such as cramping abdominal pain, anorexia, malaise, flatulence, nausea, vomiting, and low-grade fever. When right upper quadrant pain is present in patients with AIDS, suggesting biliary tract involvement, it should point toward cryptosporidiosis, although similar manifestations are seen with isosporiasis or cyclosporiasis.

The clinical manifestations of cryptosporidial infection vary according to the immune status of the host. In the immunocompetent host, the onset is usually acute, occurs after an incubation period of 2–14 days, and is generally self-limited. The clinical spectrum ranges from asymptomatic passage of oocysts to severe cholera-like gastroenteritis with biliary tract disease. The hallmark of cryptosporidial infection is diarrhea, which is usually described as watery, voluminous, and occasionally explosive and foul smelling. Additional symptoms seen in more than 80% of patients in the Milwaukee outbreak were abdominal cramps, fatigue, and anorexia.[4,5] In addition, more than half of patients may experience weight loss, nausea, low-grade fever (up to 38°C), chills, sweats, myalgias, and headache. The illness may be quite prolonged, lasting 10–14 days, with an average of 12 stools per day during the peak of the illness and often significant weight loss (median 4.5 kg in the Milwaukee outbreak). Although their HIV status is not specified, at Mulago Hospital in Kampala, Uganda, 31% of children hospitalized with persistent diarrhea and 22% with acute diarrhea (versus 8.5% without diarrhea) had *Cryptosporidium* infections, often with wasting and stunting.[84]

Asymptomatic infection can occur in immunocompetent and immunodeficient patients. In one series, as many as 63% of childhood cryptosporidial infections in Peru were asymptomatic, although these "subclinical" infections may have lasting consequences on growth and development.[85–87] In New York, asymptomatic cryptosporidiosis was documented in 6.4% of immunocompetent and 22% of immunodeficient children.[88] Excretion of oocysts after resolution of clinical symptoms can continue for prolonged periods.[86] Relapses of cryptosporidial infection have been considered rare, although 39% of the patients infected in the Milwaukee outbreak had a brief recurrence of diarrhea after a period of normal stools.

In immunocompromised patients, cryptosporidiosis is usually much more prolonged or severe. In particular, patients with AIDS often have chronic intermittent diarrhea, with recurring 3- to 30-day episodes lasting up to 14 months. Those with low CD4 lymphocyte counts are prone to develop protracted, fulminant, and rapidly fatal diarrhea. Cryptosporidiosis in HIV-positive patients can be asymptomatic in 4%, transient in 29%, chronic in 60%, or fulminant (greater than 2 L of stool per day) in 8%. Mean survival in these HIV patients with *Cryptosporidium* coinfection was 25 weeks in the study by Blanshard and associates.[89] Patients who develop fulminant disease usually have fewer than 50 CD4 cells/µL and sharply limited survival of only 5 weeks. Spontaneous clinical remission is associated with higher lymphocyte[90] or CD4 count.[91] In the Nevada outbreak in 1994, two-thirds of the HIV-infected patients with cryptosporidiosis developed chronic disease, with a median weight loss of 13.6 kg, and nausea, vomiting, and abdominal cramping occurred in at least 80%. Over half of these patients died within 6 months of the onset of the outbreak, of whom 60% had cryptosporidiosis listed as a cause of death on their death certificates.[74] Cryptosporidiosis has also been reported as an opportunistic pathogen in patients immunosuppressed due to cytotoxic chemotherapy or congenital immunodeficiencies.

Extraintestinal disease due to *Cryptosporidium* has been seen in immunocompromised patients, especially those in the late stages of AIDS (CD4 counts less than 50/µL). By far the most common site is the biliary tree, manifestations of which include sclerosing cholangitis and acalculous cholecystitis. Direct luminal spread of organisms from the duodenum is believed to be responsible. The hallmark symptom is right upper quadrant pain, which can resemble that of chronic or acute calculous cholecystitis. There have also been reports of respiratory cryptosporidiosis; in one study, 7 of 43 patients with AIDS and cryptosporidial diarrhea had oocysts isolated in sputum, although it was probably nonpathogenic in 6.[92] *Cryptosporidium* was the sole pathogen in a 10-year-old child with nephrotic syndrome on corticosteroids with low-grade fever, breathlessness, and chronic productive cough.[93] One patient with AIDS had cryptosporidial sinusitis that improved during therapy with spiramycin.[94]

Pathology

Cryptosporidium is primarily a pathogen of the small bowel producing villous blunting, submucosal edema, and mononuclear inflammatory infiltrates in the lamina propria. Following excystation, sporozoites with gliding cell motility attach and are internalized in host-derived membrane.[95] *Cryptosporidium* spp. induce actin remodeling which leads to intestinal barrier disruption and malabsorption.[96–99] As shown in ***Figure 94.2***, life cycle forms can be seen in vacuoles with specialized basal membrane folds called "feeder organelles just beneath the apical enterocyte membranes."[99]

Complications

Cryptosporidial enteritis is usually a self-limited, nonfatal illness in normal hosts. As such, the only immediate complication of concern is volume depletion from heavy diarrhea and inadequate fluid intake, especially in young children and elderly people. This is usually treatable with oral rehydration therapy.

Cryptosporidium infections in children have a lasting adverse effect on linear (height) growth and are correlated with impaired cognitive function.[86,87] Infected children who become stunted may not catch up in either weight or height, and exhibit the deficit even 1 year after infection.[86] However, there are more subtle, long-term detrimental effects of childhood cryptosporidiosis, including both an increased overall diarrheal burden over several months following an attack and impaired growth, even with so-called asymptomatic infections.[85,86,100] As such, the public health importance of these infections in developing countries is likely to be far greater than generally recognized.

The life-threatening complications of coccidian enteritis occur most often in chronic disease, which is largely confined to immunocompromised patients. In a recent study in Haiti, chronic diarrhea including *Cryptosporidium* infections among HIV patients at initiation of antiretroviral therapy (ART) was associated with increased mortality (10% among patients with chronic diarrhea compared to 5% in the control group).[101] In these cases severe infection can lead to chronic malabsorption, which may be treated by total parenteral nutrition or novel approaches to enteral, glutamine-based nutrition.[102,103] Supportive therapy is especially important in cryptosporidiosis, which has no uniformly effective antimicrobial treatment at this time. Moreover, extraintestinal disease, especially of the biliary tract, can lead to substantial morbidity from chronic pain and mortality from biliary obstruction.

PATHOGENESIS AND IMMUNITY

A great mystery in the study of cryptosporidiosis is how it disrupts normal absorptive function and causes mild to moderate inflammation without tissue invasion. A simple explanation would be the elaboration of an enterotoxin or cytotoxin, although thorough investigation has failed to discover such a toxin.[104] Guarino and associates[105,106] reported an enterotoxic effect of stool from infected humans or calves on intestinal strips or cells mounted in Ussing chambers, although they were unable to show that this secretagogue was parasite-derived rather than host-derived.

Most research has focused on the direct epithelial effects of infection with *Cryptosporidium*. Several observations on experimental porcine infection suggest that part of the symptomatology of cryptosporidiosis may be due to malabsorption by blunted or inflamed villi coupled with intact fluid secretion from the crypts. Prostaglandins also appear to play a role in this imbalance, but the details of this interaction remain unclear.[102,107] Two studies of intestinal epithelial cells in tissue culture have found destructive effects of *Cryptosporidium* infection, including loss of barrier integrity and moderate cell injury,[99,108] effects that are confirmed *in vivo* by increased lactulose–mannitol excretion ratios in patients with cryptosporidiosis.[81,82] Some of this damage may be due to release of proinflammatory cytokines (such as TNF-α and IL-8) induced by *Cryptosporidium* infection.[67,109] Substance P, a neuropeptide, may also play a role in mediating diarrhea in human cryptosporidiosis.[110] Parasite–host interactions can also upregulate host genes which might influence *Cryptosporidium* organisms to cause infection. A study showed that osteoprotegerin (OPG) gene is upregulated by *C. hominis* and *C. parvum* during early infection and that epithelial cells apoptosis was decreased, allowing *Cryptosporidium* spp. to complete efficiently their life cycle.[111]

Immunity involves both innate and adaptive immune responses. Recent evidence from human studies showed that two chemokines, CXCL-10 and CXCL-8, are involved with the attraction of immune system cells to the site of infection.[112,113] IL-15 is also critical in the early activation of the immune response.[114] Interferon (IFN)-γ is critical for the $CD4^+$ T cell in the human immune memory response.[115] However, the role of $CD8^+$ T cell response in cryptosporidiosis requires further study.

The severe nature of intestinal coccidioses in patients with AIDS suggests that cell-mediated immunity is essential to clearance of these organisms. This is supported by several observations. First, humoral immune responses to *Cryptosporidium* are quite strong in patients with AIDS, perhaps even greater than those in immunocompetent individuals.[116] Second, humoral responses are not associated with clearance of infection. This has been shown in mice,[117] as well as in HIV-infected patients who develop serum and intestinal antibodies but fail to clear infections.[116,118] Third, peripheral blood mononuclear cells (PBMCs) from patients with AIDS do not have normal proliferative responses to cryptosporidial antigens even though they may respond to mitogens.[119] Finally, experimental mice become susceptible to cryptosporidial infection after depletion of functional T-helper lymphocytes or treatment with dexamethasone.[120,121] On the other hand, a role for humoral immunity in the resistance to *Cryptosporidium* is suggested by the severe disease seen in patients with congenital hypo- or agammaglobulinemias but normal T-cell function.[122,123]

One hypothesis is that the cytokine IFN-γ may be required for an effective immune response to *Cryptosporidium*. IFN-γ is produced primarily by the Th1 subset of CD4 lymphocytes, which also release interleukin (IL)-2 but not IL-4, IL-5, or IL-10. Furthermore patients with advanced HIV infections are often deficient in Th1 lymphocytes.[124] Experimental mice can be rendered susceptible to cryptosporidiosis if treated with antibodies to IFN-γ, and mice immunosuppressed with dexamethasone can be protected from the organism by treatment with high doses of IFN-γ.[120,125] Gomez Morales and coworkers[119] found high amounts of IFN-γ released in response to cryptosporidial antigens by PBMCs from immunocompetent patients only if they had a history of transient cryptosporidiosis. In experimentally infected volunteers with *Cryptosporidium*, IFN-γ expression occurs in immunocompetent subjects with self-limited infection and correlates with prior exposure to *Cryptosporidium* and resistance to reinfection.[126] Finally, selective lack of IFN-γ production by lymphocytes in response to cryptosporidial antigens in an HIV-negative child was associated with chronic and ultimately fatal cryptosporidiosis; a thorough immunologic evaluation revealed no other abnormalities.[127]

Naïve volunteers appear to have increased IL-15 expression in their intestinal mucosa when experimentally infected with *Cryptosporidium* and this is correlated with no or low numbers of oocyst shedding.[128] In contrast, TNF-α, IL-1β,[129] and IL-4[128] do not appear to be associated with symptoms or *Cryptosporidium* oocyst shedding in humans. Significant elevations of fecal IL-8, IL-13, and TNF-α receptor 1 have been described in *Cryptosporidium*-infected children in Haiti,[67] and mildly increased fecal IL-8, TNF-α, and lactoferrin in some *Cryptosporidium*-infected children in Brazil.[130]

DIAGNOSIS

Cryptosporidiosis should be suspected in any patient presenting with watery diarrhea, abdominal cramps, and nausea, particularly if symptoms last more than a few days. Although persistent diarrhea (>1–2 weeks) in travelers, those with recreational water exposure, or immunocompromised individuals should raise concern for cryptosporidiosis, no obvious environmental exposure history is necessary, since the organism may be transmitted by so many different means. There are no characteristic findings on physical examination or laboratory or radiologic analysis, although volume depletion, metabolic alkalosis, and hypokalemia may be seen in more severe cases. Children in developing areas as well as patients with HIV respond to *C. parvum* with mild intestinal inflammation with detectable fecal lactoferrin (a sensitive marker for the presence of fecal leukocytes)[67,97,130] and mildly elevated IL-8 and TNF-αR1.[67] In contrast, fecal lactoferrin was not observed in healthy US adults experimentally infected with *C. parvum*.[130]

In immunocompromised patients, the findings are characteristically more severe and prolonged. In addition, if the biliary tree is involved, there may be elevations in alkaline phosphatase and transaminases and irregular ductal strictures and dilations on ultrasound or endoscopic retrograde cholangiopancreatography (ERCP).[131] Pulmonary involvement can produce various infiltrates on chest radiograph.[92]

Oocyst shedding in cryptosporidiosis can be intermittent and up to three stool specimens may be needed for diagnosis.[132,133] The diagnosis can be confirmed by observation of the oocysts in stool or luminal fluids. Using a modified Kinyoun acid-fast stain, oocysts appear as red spheres 3–6 μm in diameter; no other organisms should be confused with *Cryptosporidium* based on size and appearance (***Fig. 94.4***). Unfortunately, acid-fast staining is relatively insensitive, requiring 10 000 oocysts/g of watery stool and 500 000/g of formed stool to make the diagnosis. There are several immunologic techniques, including immunofluorescence and enzyme-linked immunoassays, which are commercially available through several laboratories. These techniques have sensitivity and specificity approaching 100% for *Cryptosporidium*; and require less technician time and experience.[134–136] Serologic testing for antibodies to cryptosporidial antigens is available for epidemiologic surveys, but is of little help in the diagnostic evaluation of patients.

While the immunoassays are adequate for clinical diagnosis of cryptosporidiosis, they are not sensitive enough to detect oocysts in environmental samples or in epidemiologic surveys of asymptomatic contacts, since the oocyst numbers are too low. Various concentration techniques including formalin–ethyl acetate sedimentation and disposable parasite concentrators have been used to increase the efficiency of oocyst recovery for immunoassays; as few as 5000 oocysts/g of stool can be detected by these methods.[137,138] Polymerase chain reaction (PCR) testing is more sensitive, with detection of 50–500 oocysts/mL of liquid stool or less than 1 pg of DNA and less than 10 oocysts from environmental samples.[139–141] Loop-mediated isothermal amplification (LAMP) was recently described and appears to be far more sensitive than PCR methodologies.[142] In a recent study by Bakheit et al,[143] PCR negative samples were detected by LAMP in animal stools and confirmed by sequencing of the LAMP amplified product. Furthermore, this technique does not need sophisticated machines as a simple water bath can be used for the reaction.

TREATMENT AND PROGNOSIS

Cryptosporidiosis in immunocompetent patients is self-limited, and symptomatic therapy should be directed at rehydration and nutrition. Oral rehydration solution should be used as needed to prevent volume depletion. Antimotility agents (loperamide, diphenoxylate, or other opiates) may be used once more invasive conditions (e.g., bacterial enteritis, amebiasis, or pseudomembranous colitis) have been excluded. Glutamine appears to be more effective in driving electrolyte and water absorption in *Cryptosporidium*-infected porcine intestine and has the advantage of enhancing injury repair.[102,103]

The disease is much more problematic in immunocompromised patients, since it is often not self-limited and there is no acceptable antimicrobial treatment currently available for this group of patients.[144] Dramatic improvements in HIV-related cryptosporidiosis after initiation of highly active antiretroviral therapy, including complete eradication of the parasite in patients, have been documented.[145,146] In a survey conducted in France from January 1995 to December 1996, there was approximately a 60% decline in the prevalence of cryptosporidiosis that coincided with the widespread use of protease inhibitors.[147] Recent data suggest that protease inhibitors, particularly indinavir, may directly interfere with the life cycle of *Cryptosporidium*.[148] A study in the northeast of Brazil has indicated a complete elimination of *Cryptosporidium* after the initiation of highly active antiretroviral therapy (HAART), probably due to the reconstitution of cellular immunity as well as the direct action of HAART on the parasites.[149]

Over 100 antibacterial and antiparasitic agents have been tried to no avail. In a small double-blind, placebo-controlled trial, the nonabsorbable aminoglycoside paromomycin has been shown to reduce the frequency and intensity of diarrhea in patients with AIDS and chronic cryptosporidiosis.[150] In addition, inhaled paromomycin was associated with improvement in one reported case of respiratory cryptosporidiosis.[151] The optimal dose has not yet been established. White and coworkers[150]

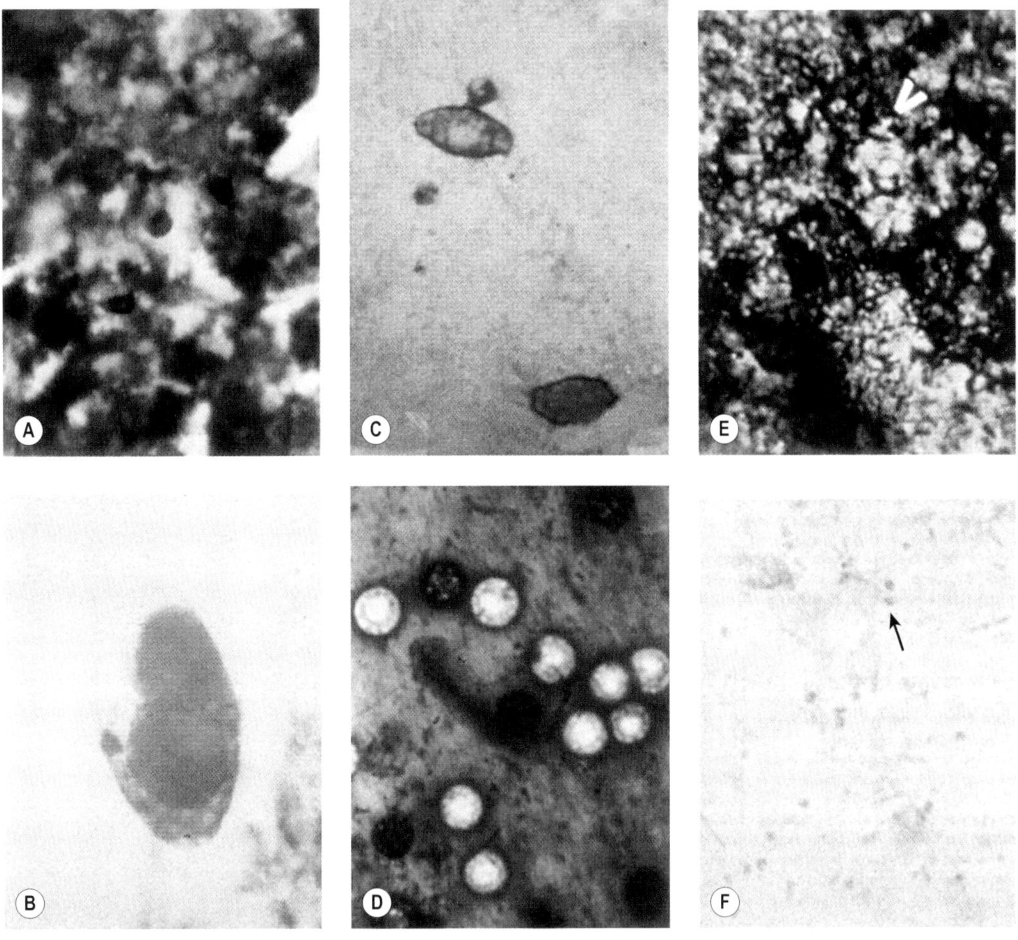

Figure 94.4 Acid-fast protozoan and other causes of diarrhea in patients with AIDS. (*Cryptosporidium* and *Cyclospora* are important causes of diarrhea in immunologically normal hosts as well.) **(A)** Acid-fast *Cryptosporidium* in fecal specimen. **(B)** Acid-fast *Isopora belli* in stool of a Haitian patient with diarrhea. **(C)** *I. belli* and *Cryptosporidium* in a Haitian patient with AIDS and diarrhea. **(D)** Acid-fast *Cyclospora cayetanensis* in the stool of a patient with diarrhea. **(E)** Acid-fast *Mycobacterium avium-intracellulare* in the stool of a patient with AIDS and diarrhea. **(F)** Microsporidia (arrow) in the stool of a patient with AIDS and diarrhea as seen in modified trichrome stain. (**A**, From Guerrant RL, Bobak DA. Bacterial and protozoal gastroenteritis. N Engl J Med. 1991;325:327. © 1991 Massachusetts Medical Society. All rights reserved. **B** and **C**, Courtesy of Drs Rosemary Soave and Medelein Boncy. **D**, Courtesy of Dr Earl Long. **E**, Courtesy of Dr Cynthia Sears. **F**, From Weber R, Bryan RT, Owen RL, et al, for the Enteric Opportunistic Infections Working Group. Improved light-microscopical detection of microsporidia spores in stool and duodenal aspirates. N Engl J Med. 1992;326:161. © 1992 Massachusetts Medical Society. All rights reserved.)

used 25–35 mg/kg per day for 14 days; larger doses (up to 50 mg/kg per day) were shown to be more effective in animal models, but vestibular toxicity has been reported at these doses in humans.[152] Maintenance therapy may be indicated in patients with AIDS and low CD4 counts to prevent relapse. A randomized, controlled trial showed that paromomycin was no more effective than placebo in patients with advanced AIDS.[152]

The most promising new drug for the treatment of cryptosporidiosis is nitazoxanide, a broad-spectrum antiparasitic agent.[153] A search on seven clinical trials involving 169 participants showed that nitazoxanide and paromomycin reduced the duration and frequency of diarrhea, respectively. Nitazoxanide showed a significant evidence of oocyst clearance compared to placebo. In a double-blind, controlled study in pediatric patients with diarrhea, nitazoxanide was associated with the resolution of diarrhea in 88% of children compared to 38% on placebo.[154] In another study of malnourished children with cryptosporidial diarrhea, a significant 56% had a resolution of diarrhea and 52% had parasitological response with 3 days of treatment compared with 23% and 14%, respectively, in controls. In an outbreak of cryptosporidiosis linked to a community swimming pool in Atlanta, the clinical response rate to nitazoxanide was 67%.[155] However, no significant effect was seen in HIV-seropositive pediatric patients.[156] Nitazoxanide elixir is approved for treatment of cryptosporidiosis in children aged 1–11 years in the United States. In children 12–47 months old, a dose of 100 mg every 12 hours is used, and in older children (4–11 years), 200 mg every 12 hours orally is recommended.

Several other agents that have been studied include azithromycin, which at 900–1200 mg/day reduced the severity of diarrhea and oocyst shedding, but only in patients in whom appropriate drug levels were obtained.[157] Azithromycin at 500 mg daily was found to be ineffective compared to letrazuril and paromomycin,[158] while reduced oocyst excretion and modest clinical improvement were noted with open label combination azithromycin (600 mg daily for 4 weeks) and paromomycin (1 g twice daily for 8 weeks).[159] Two phase I trials of letrazuril (50–100 mg/day) have shown modest, short-lived response in 66%; however, clinical relapse and worsening diarrhea occurred in 65% of the responders.[160,161] There are reports of responses to spiramycin, including one patient with extraintestinal disease.[94] In a double-blind, placebo-controlled study of immunocompetent infants in Costa Rica, infants treated with spiramycin had significantly decreased duration of diarrhea and excretion of oocysts.[162] Bovine hyperimmune colostrum (marketed as lactobin) was reported to eradicate the organism in a child with AIDS and chronic cryptosporidiosis.[163] In another case report, a 38-year-old HIV patient with 6–12 L of stool per day for 3 months had resolution within 48 hours of being treated with hyperimmune bovine colostrum and remained asymptomatic for 3 months.[164] Conclusive support for the use of hyperimmune colostrum, however, has not been forthcoming.

Results of non-double-blinded therapeutic studies of cryptosporidiosis should be interpreted with caution. Immunosuppressed patients tend to have intermittent diarrhea that can improve or worsen according to the patient's CD4 count, and clinical responses do not necessarily accompany eradication of oocysts from the stools. Endpoints for successful therapy should include both the cessation of diarrhea and other clinical manifestations, as well as the absence of oocysts in the stools; relapses are frequent.

Symptomatic therapy in patients with AIDS has also been disappointing, since the profound diarrhea may be refractory to antimotility agents. Clinical improvement has been reported with the somatostatin analog octreotide (100–300 μg subcutaneously three times daily), although a placebo-controlled trial found no benefit;[165–168] moreover, this agent is prohibitively expensive for widespread use. The related oral drug vapreotide was found to improve AIDS-related chronic diarrhea, but only in patients without cryptosporidiosis.[169] In biliary cryptosporidiosis, cholecystectomy or papillotomy has provided pain relief for many patients, although the operative morbidity of the former may be high.[75,131]

PREVENTION AND CONTROL

Current Approaches

The only known way to acquire any of the coccidia is to ingest infectious oocysts; the diseases can be completely prevented by elimination of oocysts from food and water and by avoidance of fecal material from infected people. In the case of *Cryptosporidium*, this simple-sounding goal has proved insurmountably difficult to attain. Since effective treatment for cryptosporidiosis is limited, prevention is critical to its control. Two factors make this disease highly infectious by person-to-person transmission: (1) low infectious dose; and (2) large numbers of oocysts excreted by infected host. Guidelines for the prevention of person-to-person spread are thus key.[170] Handwashing and scrupulous personal hygiene and sanitation are necessary to prevent and control person-to-person spread. Persons with cryptosporidiosis should be isolated from other persons or public places such as school, workplace and other type of institutions for at least 48 hours after the last diarrheal episode, which is sometimes difficult to know due to irregular duration and recrudescence of episodes of diarrhea.

The high infectivity and ubiquitous nature of this organism make complete removal of oocysts during water treatment essential to prevent the disease, and to this day even the most technologically advanced systems cannot reliably achieve this. Since oocysts are extremely resistant to chlorination, water treatment plants must rely on mechanical means to remove them: flocculation, sedimentation, and filtration. In theory, these methods should be adequate to prevent waterborne outbreaks, and in general they are quite effective. However, the Nevada outbreak of 1994 proved that these techniques can fail even without obvious malfunction. Conversely, a massive failure of water treatment, as occurred in Washington, DC, in 1993, may not be associated with any increase in human cases of cryptosporidiosis.[171]

The problem of inadequate elimination of *Cryptosporidium* from the water supply in developed countries is minuscule in comparison with the problems in developing areas. As noted earlier, 95% of children in some areas have serologic evidence of infection by age 2 years. Without a source of clean, filtered, or boiled water, improved sanitation, or an effective vaccine, there is no realistic way to prevent cryptosporidial infections in these areas.

Travelers to endemic areas can avoid cryptosporidiosis if they follow the maxim "boil it, cook it, peel it, or forget it." As mentioned earlier, oocysts are easily killed by heat, so hot beverages and boiled water can be considered safe. Because person-to-person transmission occurs through fecal-oral spread, travelers should probably be advised to wash their hands thoroughly before eating and after contact with young children. These precautions are especially crucial in patients with AIDS, especially those who choose to travel to developing areas during the later stages of their illness when CD4 counts are low.

As animal transmission of cryptosporidiosis from livestock, wild animals as well as pets seems to be increasing, care should also be taken to reduce transmission in settings where human–animal contact is common through public education in areas such as parks and zoos.[172]

Because of the ever-present risk of acquisition even in developed countries, patients with AIDS, especially those with CD4 counts less than 100/μL, should be advised of the potentially devastating impact of cryptosporidiosis. Filters that provide the greatest assurance of oocyst removal include those that operate by reverse osmosis, those labeled as absolute 1 μm filters, and those labeled as meeting National Sanitation Foundation (NSF) standard no. 53 for cyst removal. The nominal 1 μm filter rating is not standardized, and many filters in this category might not be capable of removing 99% of oocysts. Some patients may decide that the inconvenience of boiling or filtering (through "absolute" 1 μm filters) all of their drinking water is worth the benefit of protecting themselves from this disease. These patients should also be advised to avoid young farm animals, especially those with diarrhea.

Because of the threat of nosocomial spread of oocysts, strict enteric precautions should be followed when caring for any patient with possible cryptosporidiosis. This includes use of gowns and gloves when fecal soiling is possible and thorough handwashing after all contact. Potentially contaminated medical equipment should be autoclaved. The optimal cleaning compound for contaminated surfaces (e.g., mattresses, toilets) is not known, but hydrogen peroxide is used in laboratories.

Future Approaches

Several new approaches to water treatment have been explored, including ozone, ultrasonic waves, and electrochemical treatment, but these are far from ready for widespread use.[33,173] The Centers for Disease Control and Prevention (CDC) note the need to: (1) assess the public health importance of low-level oocyst contamination of drinking water; (2) develop guidelines and techniques for notification of the public when oocysts are detected (i.e., to know when boil-water advisories are needed); (3) identify options for preventing cryptosporidiosis in immunocompromised patients who use the public water supply; and (4) optimize water sampling techniques to identify *Cryptosporidium* oocysts.[32]

There is considerable interest in vaccine development against *Cryptosporidium*. However, animal models suggest that cell-mediated immunity and intact production of IFN-γ are necessary to prevent infection, so the benefit of immunization in patients with AIDS may be limited. A recent trial of a vaccine made from lyophilized oocysts was moderately protective in a bovine model; vaccinated calves had a shorter duration of diarrhea and excreted fewer oocysts.[174] There have been no vaccines tested in humans yet. A recent study in which previously infected volunteers were rechallenged with *Cryptosporidium* oocysts demonstrated only partial protection against reinfection; although fewer subjects shed oocysts after their second challenge, the rates of diarrhea were the same.[175]

Finally, glutamine, a "conditionally essential" amino acid, is effective in driving electrolyte and water absorption in *Cryptosporidium*-infected porcine intestine and has the advantage of enhancing injury repair.[102,103] Finally, glutamine and its stable derivative alanyl-glutamine have been shown to improve diarrhea and malabsorption in patients with AIDS. These improvements may enhance antiretroviral drug therapy and reduce the emergence of drug resistance[176] as well as ameliorate symptoms associated with severe cryptosporidiosis.[177]

Access the complete reference list online at
http://www.expertconsult.com

Access the complete reference list online at http://www.expertconsult.com

CHAPTER 95

Cyclospora, *Isospora*, and *Sarcocystis* Infections

Ynés R. Ortega • Jean W. Pape

INTRODUCTION

Cyclospora cayetanensis, *Isospora belli*, and *Sarcocystis* spp. are intestinal coccidia associated with gastrointestinal illness in humans. The coccidia belong to the phylum Apicomplexa, subkingdom Protozoa, and order Eucoccidiorida (Eucoccidiida). Coccidia are characterized by an apical polar complex consisting of apical rings, micronemes, and subpellicular microtubules, and this facilitates penetration into host cells.[1,2]

Although some coccidia have been known for decades to be veterinary pathogens, the existence of and pathogenicity for humans were not recognized until recently.[3] The epidemic of human immunodeficiency virus (HIV) infection in the 1980s heightened medical awareness of *Cryptosporidium* spp., *C. cayetanensis,* and *I. belli*, in part because these parasites can cause severe, protracted diarrheal illnesses in patients with the acquired immunodeficiency syndrome (AIDS).[4] Subsequently, large foodborne outbreaks of cyclosporiasis in North America in the 1990s demonstrated that *C. cayetanensis* can also cause diarrhea in immunocompetent persons.[3]

CYCLOSPORA (*Fig. 95.1*)

THE AGENT AND EPIDEMIOLOGY

Cyclospora species were described first in moles and myriapods and subsequently in other animals.[5,6] In 1979, the organism was isolated from the stools of 3 patients in Papua New Guinea. Because of its morphological characteristics it was presumed to be *Isospora*.[7] Other reports described the acid-fast, autofluorescent organism as a fungal spore, a coccidian body, an alga-like organism, and a cyanobacterium-like body (CLB) and it was reported in association with diarrhea in the Caribbean, Nepal, and Chicago.[8–12] In 1994, Ortega and collaborators named the organism *C. cayetanensis.*[5] Later molecular phylogenetic analysis showed that the organism is closely related to *Eimeria* spp.[1,2]

The complete life cycle of *C. cayetanensis* occurs in enterocytes located at the tips of intestinal villi in the small intestine of infected humans.[13] Unsporulated *Cyclospora* oocysts are excreted in stools.[3]

Cyclospora in nonhuman primates was first reported in 1996,[14] and later named *C. papionis* (baboons), *C. colobi* (colobus monkeys), and *C. cercopitheci* (green monkeys). These were morphologically similar but molecularly different from *C. cayetanensis.*[15,16] *Cyclospora* oocysts were also reported in the feces of chickens, ducks, and dogs.[17–20] No histopathological evidence of infection is available but coprophagia by animals may explain the presence of oocysts in their feces. Multiple attempts to infect animal models have been unsuccessful.[21]

C. cayetanensis has been associated with small waterborne outbreaks, notably in expatriates in a military detachment in Nepal,[22] and in a medical dormitory in Chicago.[23] The latter was initially suspected to have been foodborne.[3] *Cyclospora* foodborne outbreaks in the United States have been related to consumption of imported fresh berries and produce.[3,24,25] For example, in 1996 and 1997, more than 2000 cases of cyclosporiasis in multiple US states and Canadian provinces were caused by consumption of fresh raspberries imported from Guatemala.[3,13,14] Foodborne outbreaks associated with mesclun lettuce, basil, and snow peas have also occurred in the United States.[3,24,26–29]

Person-to-person transmission of *C. cayetanensis* is unlikely because the oocysts require at least 7 days to sporulate and become infectious.[6,7] Household clusters have been associated with common-source (e.g., water) exposure.[19]

Cyclospora infections are common and important in tropical and subtropical areas (***Fig. 95.1***).[30] Cases have been reported in travelers returning from or expatriates living in countries or regions such as Mexico, Haiti,[31] Nepal,[8,32] Southeast Asia,[10,11] Puerto Rico,[33] Indonesia,[34] Morocco, Pakistan, and India.[35]

A marked seasonality of *Cyclospora* infection has been observed in endemic regions. In Nepal[36] and Guatemala,[25,30] most cases occur during or near the rainy, hot spring or summer months. In Indonesia, the peak season for cyclosporiasis occurs in the cooler, wetter months of October–May[10] and in Haiti in the cooler, drier months of January–March.[37] In a dry coastal area of Peru, infection occurs predominantly in the warmer months of December–June.[38,39]

Cyclosporiasis may be quite common in areas where it is endemic. During the 1992 rainy season in Nepal,[8] in a clinic-based study, 7% (18/254) of the US embassy expatriate community were infected with CLBs (now *C. cayetanensis*). *Cyclospora* spp. were identified in 11% of 964 patients (travelers to Nepal and foreign residents) with diarrhea and in only 1% of 96 asymptomatic controls.[8] A cohort study in Nepal following 77 expatriates revealed that the annual risk for diarrhea by *Cyclospora* was 32% in the first 2 years of residence in Nepal, second only to 42% for enterotoxigenic *Escherichia coli*.[40]

In the developing world, studies of cyclosporiasis are primarily in children. In a 1994 study,[41] *Cyclospora* was found in 5% of 124 Nepalese children with diarrhea aged 6–60 months. *Cyclospora* was found in only 2% of 103 children with diarrhea but not in 74 children without diarrhea of less than 18 months of age. In two prospective studies (1988–1991) of children living in slums in Peru,[6] 18% of 147 children aged 1–2½ years had *Cyclospora* infection and 6% of 230 children aged 1 month to 1½ years. Diarrhea was present in only 28% and 11% of each group respectively. In 2002, Bern and collaborators[42] determined that in a cohort study of diarrhea, children had an average of 0.2 episodes of cyclosporiasis per year. The incidence was fairly constant in children between 1 and 9 years old and with each episode of cyclosporiasis diarrhea decreased. Cyclosporiasis was frequently associated with ownership of domestic animals, particularly birds, guinea pigs, and rabbits.[42] In Guatemala, at a health care facility, 2.3% of 5552 surveillance specimens were positive for *Cyclospora*. Prevalence increased in May and peaked in June, corresponding to the first 2 months of the rainy season, and infection was

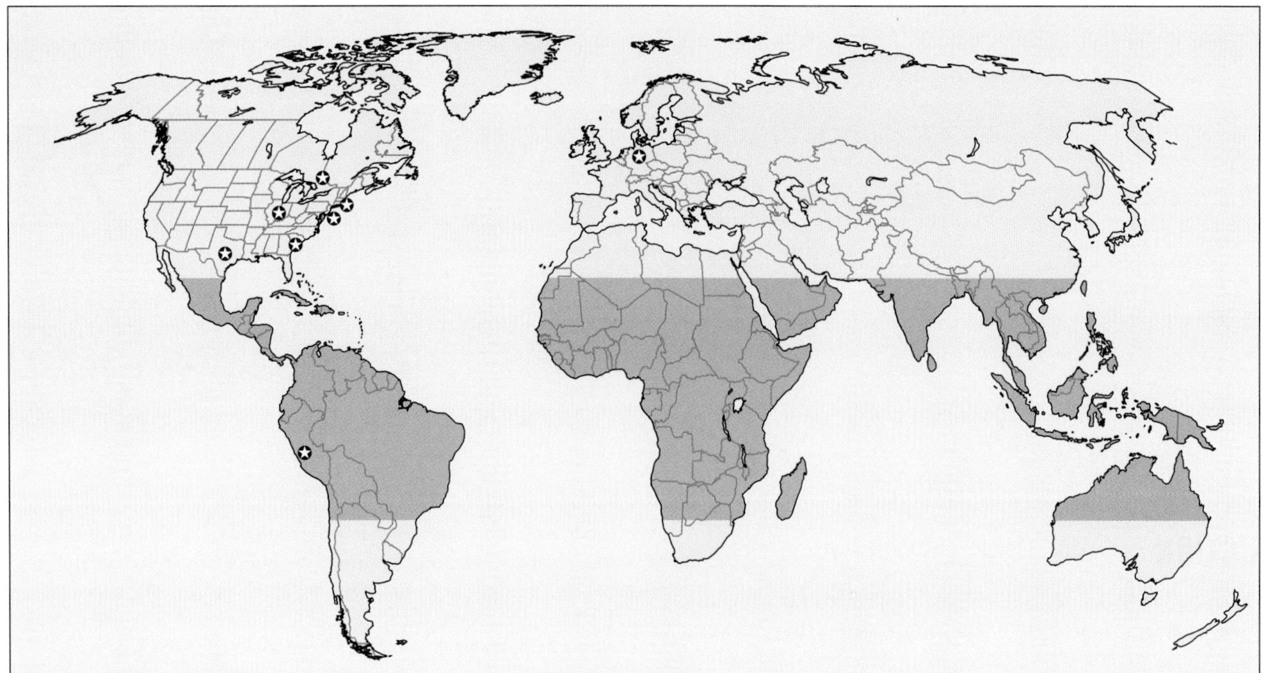

Figure 95.1 Endemic tropical regions for cyclospora infections with ✪ showing outbreaks. ✪ Outbreaks caused by *Cyclospora cayetanensis* (many US states, several Canadian provinces, Germany; other countries have experienced local outbreaks or been affected by widespread "outbreaks").

observed in children aged 5–9 years. Risk factors associated with *Cyclospora* included type of sewage drainage, ownership of chickens and birds, and contact with soil in children under 2 years old.[30] In a community-based survey in Haiti in 1997–1998,[37] similar findings of high prevalence of asymptomatic infection in children were reported. Seasonality was also observed with prevalence of 5–16%. Of the 49 positive samples, 84% were from children less than 10 years of age and only 6–12% had diarrhea. In a community-based study in Venezuela,[43] the highest prevalence of *Cyclospora* infection was 11.5% (7/61) in persons 6–15 years old. All were asymptomatic. In Cuba, *C. cayetanensis* was found in only 5/113 stool samples from hospitalized patients with diarrhea.[44]

AIDS patients with cyclosporiasis can present with prolonged diarrhea. In a 1990–1993 study in Haiti[45] *Cyclospora* was found in 11% of stool samples from 51 of 450 HIV-positive patients with diarrhea, making it the third most commonly identified parasitic pathogen after *Cryptosporidium* spp. and *I. belli*.

THE DISEASE

If symptomatic, *Cyclospora* infection typically is associated with watery diarrhea, abdominal cramps or bloating, nausea, anorexia, and substantial weight loss. Some persons note vomiting and low-grade fever.[3,13,24] Many experience a prodromal flu-like illness and profound, persistent fatigue long after the gastrointestinal symptoms have resolved.[3,46] Infection can persist for weeks to months and can remit and relapse if not treated.[3]

In patients with AIDS, cyclosporiasis can be associated with protracted, fulminant diarrheal illness and weight loss. Acalculous cholecystitis associated with *C. cayetanensis* infection has been reported in AIDS patients.[47–49] Possible associations with Reiter's syndrome and Guillain–Barré syndrome have been reported.[50,51]

C. cayetanensis infection is characterized by villous blunting, crypt hyperplasia, edema, hyperemia, and an inflammatory infiltrate with epithelial disarray, especially prominent at the villus tips.[52] *Cyclospora* is found in an intracytoplasmic parasitophorous vacuole in the apical supranuclear region of the enterocyte.[3,6] Cyclosporiasis is often associated with evidence of malabsorption, such as an abnormal D-xylose test and abnormal lactulose : mannitol permeability ratio.[52]

DIAGNOSIS

Cyclosporiasis should be included in the differential diagnosis for persistent diarrheal illness. Testing for *Cyclospora* spp. should be specifically requested when testing for ova and parasites. Concentration of samples and multiple stool sample testing are recommended.[3]

C. cayetanensis measures 8–10 μm and stains variably with the modified acid-fast method. *Cyclospora* oocysts autofluoresce when observed under epifluorescence microscopy (excitation filter of 360/40 nm, dichroic mirror of 400 nm, and a 420 nm emission filter),[39] allowing for rapid screening of stool specimens.[5,11] By bright-field microscopy, the unsporulated oocysts have an undifferentiated cytoplasm with multiple refractile globules.[3]

Cyclosporiasis can also be diagnosed by histopathology or electron microscopy of jejunal biopsy specimens or aspirates. The histopathological deterioration of the intestinal epithelial cells is not proportional to the number of parasitic vacuoles present in these tissues,[13] as observed in immunocompetent individuals. No serologic tests are commercially available. Molecular methods, including polymerase chain reaction (PCR) for detection of *Cyclospora* in waste water,[2,53] produce[54] and stool specimens,[55] and real-time PCR, PCR-restriction fragment length polymorphism, and an oligonulucleotide ligation assay[56–58] for use with environmental samples, water, and food, have been developed.

TREATMENT AND PROGNOSIS

The treatment of choice for adults with cyclosporiasis is trimethoprim-sulfamethoxazole (TMP-SMX) (160 mg/800 mg) twice daily for a week.[46] In patients with AIDS, TMP-SMX is effective, but maintenance therapy with a single dose of one double-strength tablet of TMP-SMX three times a week is indicated to prevent relapse in HIV-infected patients.[45]

Pediatric cyclosporiasis resolved with TMP-SMX at 5/25 mg/kg/day for 3 days. The mean oocyst excretion was 4.8 days after initiation of treatment, compared to 12 days in untreated children.[38]

To assess an alternative treatment for sulfa-allergic patients, a clinical trial in HIV-infected patients with cyclosporiasis compared patients treated for 7 days with either TMP-SMX (160 mg/800 mg four times a day) or ciprofloxacin (500 mg twice a day). On day 8, all patients (9/9) treated with TMP-SMX had become asymptomatic and *C. cayetanensis* oocysts were not detectable in their stool samples. When treated with ciprofloxacin, 90% (10/11) become asymptomatic and 64% (7/11) had negative stool specimens.[59] Anecdotal experience among immunocompetent patients suggests that ciprofloxacin is not as effective as TMP-SMX for cyclosporiasis.[3]

PREVENTION AND CONTROL

Extensive epidemiologic investigations have identified food items associated with outbreaks in the United States. For example, in 2002, *Cyclospora* was identified in a frozen raspberry-filled wedding cake in an outbreak of diarrhea that implicated Guatemalan raspberries.[27] In 1999 *Cyclospora* was isolated from a basil-containing food item of an outbreak in Missouri.[60] Implementation of measures to prevent contamination of the food in the source country, identification, and decontamination of contaminated food items could prevent *Cyclospora* outbreaks. Chlorinating agricultural or irrigation water is unlikely to help prevent *Cyclospora* transmission, and thorough washing of fresh produce does not eliminate the risk of cyclosporiasis.[3] Studies in Norway failed to identify *Cyclospora* oocysts on imported produce (despite finding *Giardia* cysts and *Cryptosporidium* oocysts),[61] but *Cyclospora* was identified in vegetables and herbs in endemic countries.[62,63] Pesticides commonly used in agriculture failed to prevent sporulation of *Cyclospora* oocysts, thus use of contaminated water could be a source of crop contamination.[64] Highly sensitive PCR-based assays for use in food and water are in development.[58] Gamma irradiation of produce is a possible decontamination strategy but not all produce can withstand irradiation.[55]

Preventing cyclosporiasis in tropical and subtropical areas should also be a priority. The many unanswered questions about the *C. cayetanensis* life cycle and the mechanisms of pathogenesis pose challenges to developing rational environmental or immunologic prevention strategies. To date, infected humans are the only source of oocysts for study.[21,25]

ISOSPORA

THE AGENT AND EPIDEMIOLOGY

I. belli was first identified in US troops abroad during World War I,[65] but it was not studied further until intracellular stages were identified in tissue sections from patients with malabsorptive enteritis.[66] *Isospora* has been reported in residents of and travelers to developing areas, especially those with AIDS.

The oblong oocyst of *I. belli* contains two sporocysts with four sporozoites in each. The asexual phase of the life cycle (from ingested oocyst through sporozoite release and meront formation) is similar to that of *C. cayetanensis*. However, *I. belli* does not form identifiable type 2 meronts; rather, the merozoites develop into either trophozoites or gametocytes. The oocysts of *I. belli* require 24–48 hours after excretion to sporulate, so person-to-person transmission is unlikely. The duration of oocyst passage may last from 21 to 120 days.[67,68]

Humans are the only known hosts for *I. belli* and it is distributed worldwide, with highest prevalence in tropical and subtropical climates. Isosporiasis is acquired by ingestion of food or water contaminated with mature oocysts from human feces. In developing countries *Isospora* rarely causes diarrhea in immunocompetent children. In a 2-year period, the stools of 824 infants in Haiti were examined for the presence of coccidian parasites: 17% had *Cryptosporidium* spp. but none had *I. belli*.[69] In a community-based cohort study of children aged from 3 weeks to 2 years in Guinea (1996–1998), an association between diarrhea and *I. belli* (odds ratio for diarrhea 3.55; 95% confidence interval 1.15–11.0) was suggested, although the incidence was low (11 cases/168.7 child-years at risk).[70] Outside the tropics and subtropics, isosporiasis is usually found only in patients with a history of travel to these areas.[71] In the tropics, immunosuppressed patients are particularly at risk for isosporiasis. In a 1986 study of HIV-infected patients with diarrhea in Haiti, *I. belli* was found in 15% (20/131) of stool specimens.[72] *I. belli* oocysts were not detected in 170 healthy household or heterosexual contacts of HIV-infected patients.[72] In Cuba, of 67 AIDS patients studied, 1 (1.5%) had isosporiasis and 8 (11.9%) had cryptosporidiosis.[73] In Delhi, India, isosporiasis with diarrhea was reported in 2.7% of 75 HIV-1-infected individuals.[74] In Los Angeles County, California, 1% of 16 351 persons with AIDS had isosporiasis. Most of these patients were foreign-born and Hispanics, suggesting more travel exposure and/or recent immigration. It was also more frequent in individuals not receiving *Pneumocystis* pneumonia prophylaxis.[75]

Prophylaxis with TMP-SMX has an impact on the prevalence of isosporiasis and cyclosporiasis in HIV patients. In 2000, prophylaxis with TMP-SMX was implemented in Haiti for HIV-infected symptomatic patients. Since 2001, about 40–65% of HIV-infected patients with diarrhea presenting to the GHESKIO AIDS center had a prior history of TMP-SMX prophylaxis. As a result, the overall prevalence of both cyclosporiasis and isosporiasis has decreased remarkably in patients with diarrhea at the GHESKIO centers, from 12% and 10% respectively in 1999 to 4.5% and 3.5% in 2001. In 2008, out of 1012 HIV-infected patients with diarrhea, 13%, 3.0%, and 1.0% respectively had *Cryptosporidium* spp., *C. cayetanensis,* and *I. belli* identified in stool samples.

THE DISEASE

Isosporiasis generally produces a self-limited diarrheal illness in otherwise healthy persons. The symptoms include watery diarrhea and abdominal pain, usually lasting less than 1 month. Chronic isosporiasis, with malabsorption and weight loss, has been reported in immunocompetent patients. The disease can resemble celiac sprue.[66] Deaths due to chronic isosporiasis in otherwise healthy children under age 2 years have been reported.[67] Diffuse biliary isosporiasis was reported in a West African man with acute illness.[76] In immunocompromised patients, isosporiasis may be prolonged and more severe. The median duration of diarrhea by isosporiasis was 5.8 months and associated with diffuse abdominal cramps and nausea in AIDS patients in Haiti.[72] Dissemination of infection to mesenteric and tracheobronchial lymph nodes as well as dissemination to lymph nodes, liver, and spleen have been reported.[77] Acalculous cholecystitis in patients with AIDS and *I. belli* infection have also been reported.[78,79] *I. belli* can invade beyond the epithelium into the lamina propria.[66] Histopathologic changes are similar to those described in cyclosporiasis but infiltration of large numbers of eosinophils into the lamina propria and dilation of the lymphatics are more common with *I. belli* infection.[67] In immunocompetent individuals with malabsorption, a study reported 1% having isosporiasis.[80]

DIAGNOSIS

Isosporiasis should be considered in residents of or travelers to tropical areas who experience persistent diarrhea, abdominal cramps, steatorrhea, weight loss, and sometimes low-grade fever. Peripheral eosinophilia may explain the presence of Charcot–Leyden crystals in the stool specimens of some patients with isosporiasis.[67,81] Fecal leukocytes are infrequently seen.[72]

Isospora infection is diagnosed by seeing the organism in stool. The oocysts stain with modified acid-fast techniques and may also be autofluorescent. *Isospora* oocysts are elliptical and much larger (10–20 × 20–30 μm) than those of *Cyclospora* and *Cryptosporidium*. Other techniques, including lactophenol cotton blue staining, the auramine-rhodamine technique, Giemsa staining, and the heated safranin-methylene blue technique, have also been used to identify *I. belli* oocysts in stool samples.[67,82] Shedding of oocysts may be intermittent. In a case series of 34 AIDS patients with isosporiasis, diagnosis of *I. belli* in 7 patients required examination of three stool specimens per patient.[83] *Isospora* can also be identified in small-bowel biopsy specimens, duodenal aspirate, or mucus specimen collection by the duodenal string test.[66,67] No serologic tests for *Isospora* are commercially available. A PCR assay[84] was developed to identify *Isospora* in small-bowel tissue but was not validated for stool specimens.

TREATMENT AND PROGNOSIS

Isosporiasis can be treated successfully in patients with or without AIDS with one double-strength tablet of TMP-SMX administered orally two to four times daily for 10 days. The higher dose and longer treatment may be needed for immunosuppressed patients.[85] In a Haitian study, all patients with AIDS and isosporiasis receiving this treatment had complete symptomatic relief and negative stool results. Relapses were common in those receiving placebo therapies for secondary prophylaxis after the initial treatment (50% within 1.6 months of completing the initial treatment). Either maintenance therapy – one double-strength TMP-SMX tablet three times a week or one Fansidar tablet (pyrimethamine 25 mg plus sulfadoxine 500 mg) once a week – prevented all symptomatic relapses. One asymptomatic patient who was receiving TMP-SMX prophylaxis had *I. belli* identified in a routine follow-up stool sample.[83]

Sulfa-allergic patients can receive an alternative regimen of oral pyrimethamine 50–75 mg/day in individual doses (leucovorin 10–25 mg/day).[86,87] Other drugs reported to be effective are roxithromycin 2.5 mg/kg every 12 hours for 15 days and diclazuril.[85,88] The therapeutic efficacy of these drugs needs to be confirmed. Pyrimethamine alone at 25 mg/day can prevent relapses in immunocompromised patients who are sulfa-allergic.[83]

In an extreme case, a 2-year-old child receiving prolonged steroid therapy for systemic vasculitis developed severe debilitating diarrhea due to isosporiasis. Treatment with co-trimoxazole was initially successful but the disease recurred within a few weeks. Four episodes of recurrent isosporiasis followed. The child developed a sulfa allergy. Medical treatment was discontinued and after several diarrheal episodes the child died of severe malnutrition and hepatic falure.[89]

In Haiti 3 hospitalized AIDS patient with isosporiasis with low CD4 counts (below 50 T cells/mm^3) on highly active antiretroviral therapy and 2 with associated tuberculosis therapy did not respond to a 4-week course of high-dose oral TMP-SMX. One was placed on different drugs, including pyrimethamine, roxithromycin, and diclazuril, with no effect. Diarrhea persisted with documentation of *I. belli.* He eventually died of severe malnutrition and probable tuberculosis. The other two were placed on intravenous TMP-SMX with cessation of diarrhea within 7 days.

SARCOCYSTIS

THE AGENT

Sarcocystis spp. belong to the family Sarcocystidae. *Sarcocystis* requires two separate hosts for completion of the life cycle: a definitive host (in which the sexual stage develops, usually a carnivorous predator) and an intermediate host (often herbivorous prey) (***Fig. 95.2***). The cycle in the intermediate host begins with ingestion of infectious sporocysts or oocysts. These excyst in the small intestine to release sporozoites that penetrate the mucosa and develop into schizonts in the vascular endothelium. The schizonts release merozoites that enter the circulation and lodge in skeletal or cardiac muscle to form sarcocysts. When muscle containing sarcocysts is ingested by the definitive host, the cysts rupture to release zoites that invade the intestinal epithelium and differentiate into male or female gametocytes. After fertilization, zygotes undergo encystation and sporulation, and oocysts (with two sporocysts, each with four sporozoites) are excreted in the stool, and the cycle continues.

Humans can be intermediate or definitive hosts for *Sarcocystis* species. However, humans are the definitive hosts for *S. suihominis* and *S. bovihominis* (or *S. hominis*). The intermediate hosts are pigs and cows, respectively. Persons who ingest sporocysts or tissue sarcocysts of these species may develop intramuscular cysts or gastrointestinal symptoms respectively.

EPIDEMIOLOGY

Various *Sarcocystis* species associated with muscle sarcocystosis in humans have been reported in Southeast Asia, India, Africa, Europe, and North and South America (including the United States) (***Fig. 95.3***). Infection may be quite common in some areas. Prevalence rates of 10% and 20–23% were observed in adults in rural areas of Laos and Tibet, respectively. Most of these infections were asymptomatic.[90,91] Infection is thought to be due to consumption of raw beef[92] and undercooked beef or pork.[93]

THE DISEASE

Disseminated sarcocystosis results from the presence of cysts within muscle. However, sarcocysts have been found in biopsy specimens from asymptomatic persons as well as in specimens from patients with myalgias. Other patients with cysts in biopsy specimens had eosinophilia, polyarteritis nodosa, or, in one reported case, cardiomyopathy.[78] It has been difficult to establish whether the sarcocysts *per se* caused such manifestations. Intestinal sarcocystosis can also result in several clinical presentations. Although most infections are asymptomatic, there are reports from Thailand of segmental eosinophilic or necrotizing enteritis requiring resection.[94] One volunteer who ingested experimentally infected beef with *S. hominis* developed anemia, abdominal pain, diarrhea, fatigue, and dizziness 3 days later and shed oocysts for 42 days beginning on day 8.[94] Abdominal distension 5 hours postinoculation with *S. suishominis* in another human volunteer was observed as well as watery diarrhea 8–36 hours postinoculation, vomiting, chilling, and fever (38.5°C), dizziness, headache, joint and muscle ache, epigastralgia, and anorexia. Sporocyst excretion started on day 12. Treatment with acetylspiramycin for 15 days (0.2 g/time, 4 times/day) resolved the infection 30 days later.[95]

DIAGNOSIS AND TREATMENT

Intestinal sarcocystosis is diagnosed by observation of sporulated sporocysts or oocysts in stool. The cysts resemble *Isospora* oocysts; they are acid-fast and contain two sporocysts. *Sarcocystis* sporocysts also autofluoresce when observed by epifluorescence microscopy.[96] However, the thin-walled oocysts usually rupture in the bowel, releasing the sporocysts, which are not seen. Oocysts measure 15.5 × 20 μm and sporocysts 12 × 6 μm. Infection can also be diagnosed by observation of trophozoites or bradyzoites in biopsy tissue, although the organism can be mistaken for *Toxoplasma gondii* (in muscle) or *I. belli* (in the intestine).[92,97,98] Sulfadiazine, tinidazole, and acetylspiramycin have been reported to be active against intestinal *Sarcocystis* infection.[91] In cases of severe enteritis, segmental resection may be necessary. No clinical trials have been conducted to guide treatment of tissue sarcocystosis.

PREVENTION AND CONTROL

Thorough cooking of meat, especially of beef and pork, can prevent intestinal sarcocystosis. The internal temperatures required to guarantee the safety of meat are unknown, as is the effectiveness of alternative preparation techniques (e.g., curing, smoking).

Treating farm animals for sarcocystosis is another possible prevention strategy. However, this has proved difficult. In a survey of beef cattle in New Zealand, all the cattle tested were infected with a *Sarcocystis* species. In 80% of the cattle, the organism resembled *S. hominis*.[99] The prevalence of *S. hominis* infection is difficult to determine[100] because it cannot be distinguished from *S. hirsuta* by microscopic observation.

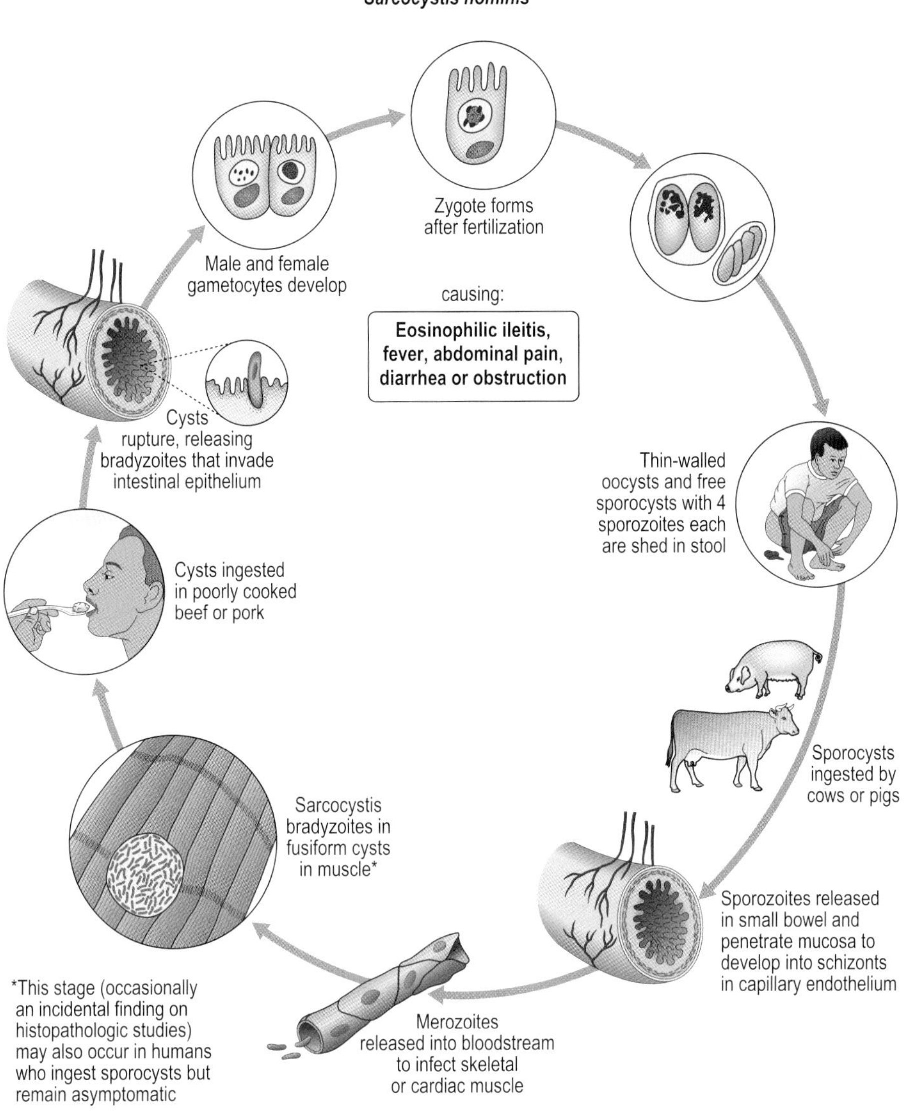
Sarcocystis hominis
Zygote forms after fertilization
Male and female gametocytes develop
causing:
Eosinophilic ileitis, fever, abdominal pain, diarrhea or obstruction
Cysts rupture, releasing bradyzoites that invade intestinal epithelium
Thin-walled oocysts and free sporocysts with 4 sporozoites each are shed in stool
Cysts ingested in poorly cooked beef or pork
Sporocysts ingested by cows or pigs
Sarcocystis bradyzoites in fusiform cysts in muscle*
Sporozoites released in small bowel and penetrate mucosa to develop into schizonts in capillary endothelium
*This stage (occasionally an incidental finding on histopathologic studies) may also occur in humans who ingest sporocysts but remain asymptomatic
Merozoites released into bloodstream to infect skeletal or cardiac muscle

Figure 95.2 *Sarcocystis hominis* life cycle.

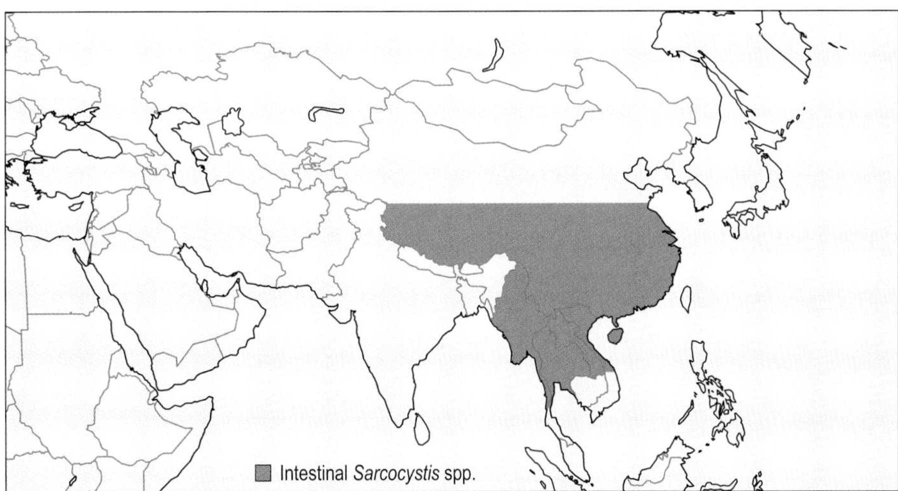
Intestinal Sarcocystis spp.

Figure 95.3 Intestinal *Sarcocystis* spp.

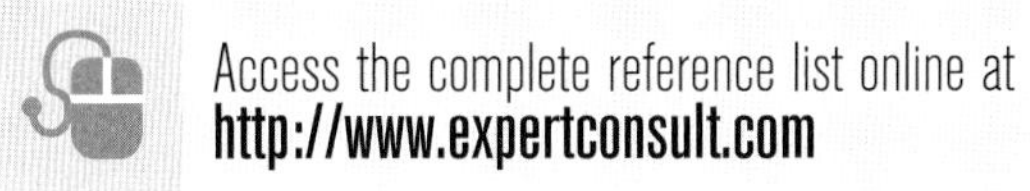

Access the complete reference list online at
http://www.expertconsult.com

CHAPTER 96

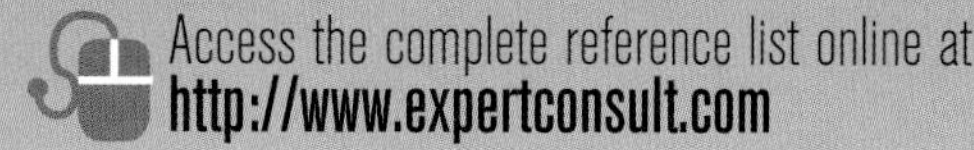
Access the complete reference list online at
http://www.expertconsult.com

Malaria

Stephen L. Hoffman • Carlos C. (Kent) Campbell • Nicholas J. White

INTRODUCTION

Malaria is an acute systemic illness caused by infection with *Plasmodium falciparum*, *P. vivax*, *P. malariae*, *P. ovale*, or *P. knowlesi*, all of which are transmitted to humans by female *Anopheles* species mosquitoes. There are an estimated 500–800 million clinical cases of malaria and 1 million deaths due to malaria annually in the tropics and subtropics (***Fig. 96.1***).[1] The majority of infections and deaths are caused by *P. falciparum* infection of children in sub-Saharan Africa. In fact, *P. falciparum* is responsible for more deaths in children <5 years of age than any other single infectious agent. In Africa, malaria is estimated to result in a minimum economic loss of US$12 billion annually.[2]

All symptoms, signs, and pathologic features of malaria are caused by the asexual erythrocytic stages of the parasite. This stage involves invasion of normal erythrocytes by parasites, intraerythrocytic replication of the parasites over 2–3 days (***Table 96.1***), rupture of erythrocytes, and parasite reinvasion of normal erythrocytes. This exponential parasite replication in the bloodstream can increase parasite densities by 5–30-fold every 1–3 days depending on the *Plasmodium* species.

Malaria caused by any of the five *Plasmodium* species is characterized by fever, chills, diaphoresis, malaise, headache, and other systemic symptoms and signs indistinguishable from illnesses caused by many viral and bacterial pathogens. *P. falciparum* is responsible for almost all malaria deaths. This is in large part due to two unique features of the parasite (***Table 96.1***). Only *P. falciparum* invades erythrocytes of all ages, meaning that the percentage of erythrocytes infected can reach levels as high as 80% (>2×10^6 parasites/μL blood depending on the degree of anemia), thereby increasing the chance that the infection will cause serious disease. Only *P. falciparum* secretes proteins that form knobs on the surface of the infected erythrocyte which then bind to endothelial cells in the microcirculation of the brain, kidneys, intestines, and other organs during the second half of the parasite's 43–52-hour development cycle in erythrocytes. These adherent infected erythrocytes are responsible for microcirculatory obstruction, leading to decreased blood flow and oxygen delivery, and local inflammatory responses critical to the pathogenesis of the severe manifestations of disease that make *P. falciparum* potentially so lethal.

Malaria has had an enormous impact on human health for millennia. Hippocrates described the clinical presentation and complications of malaria in the fifth century BCE. Nearly half a millennium later, Celsus described the distinctions between the clinical manifestations of disease caused by *P. falciparum*, *P. vivax*, and *P. malariae*.[3] In the 1630s it was discovered that the bark of the cinchona tree from Peru could treat the disease. "Peruvian" or "Jesuit's" bark was imported to Europe and became widely used in treatment,[4,5] and Morton and Sydenham in England and Torti in Italy distinguished between fevers that responded to the bark and those that did not.[3] In England, the responsive fevers were called "agues." In the eighteenth century they received the Italian name, malaria (*mal aria*, bad air), because it was believed that the disease was transmitted through the foul air of swampy areas. In 1820 Pelletier and Caventou determined the structure of quinine, the active component of the bark, and the era of modern chemotherapy was initiated despite ignorance regarding the cause of the disease.

In 1880 Laveran, a French military physician working in Algeria, made the first description of malaria parasites in the blood of patients.[6] Transmission of malaria by *Anopheles* mosquitoes was discovered in 1897 by Ross, a British military physician, working in India.[7] Ross found a malaria parasite in a mosquito that had previously fed on a patient with parasitemia. The life cycle in humans was elucidated in 1898–99 by Italian scientists Bignami, Bastianelli, and Grassi.[3] Laveran (1907) and Ross (1902) were awarded Nobel Prizes for their discoveries.

The discovery of the life cycle led to initiation of control efforts aimed at diminishing mosquito populations to reduce transmission of the disease. In some places, such as Panama during the building of the canal, these efforts were highly successful. However, malaria continued to be a problem throughout the world. During World War II, US forces lost 12 million man-days to malaria,[8] and major efforts were initiated to develop better methods of prevention and treatment. By the end of the War, dichlorodiphenyltrichloroethane (DDT), which had been demonstrated to be an insecticide by Mueller in Switzerland in 1939, and chloroquine, a 4-aminoquinolone discovered in Germany in the 1930s, had been shown to be highly effective against the mosquitoes and parasites responsible for malaria. These new tools provided the foundation for dramatic reductions of transmission of malaria in many countries in South and Central America, North Africa, and Asia, but with little impact in most countries of sub-Saharan Africa.[9]

Currently the impact of malaria in many parts of the world is similar to or greater than it was 50 years ago as the campaign of the 1950s and 1960s to eradicate malaria came to a close. *P. falciparum* has become resistant to multiple drugs, and the vector mosquitoes have become resistant to many insecticides. The majority of malaria-related morbidity and mortality is concentrated in the Africa region.

Under the leadership of the Roll Back Malaria Partnership, national scale-up of malaria programs in Africa has accelerated under the framework of Scale-up for Impact. This effort has incorporated high population coverage of insecticide-impregnated bednets (ITNs), selective application of residual insecticide spraying, and expansion of availability of early diagnosis and treatment of malaria, and intermittent preventive therapy for pregnant women.

THE AGENT

Malaria is caused by protozoa of the genus *Plasmodium*, family Plasmodiidae, suborder Haemosporidiidea, order Coccidiida. There are more than 120 *Plasmodium* species that infect mammals, birds, and reptiles. Only four species are known to infect humans consistently: (1) *P. falciparum*; (2) *P. vivax*; (3) *P. malariae*; and (4) *P. ovale*. *P. knowlesi*, a simian malaria parasite, has intermittently been reported to cause human disease.[10]

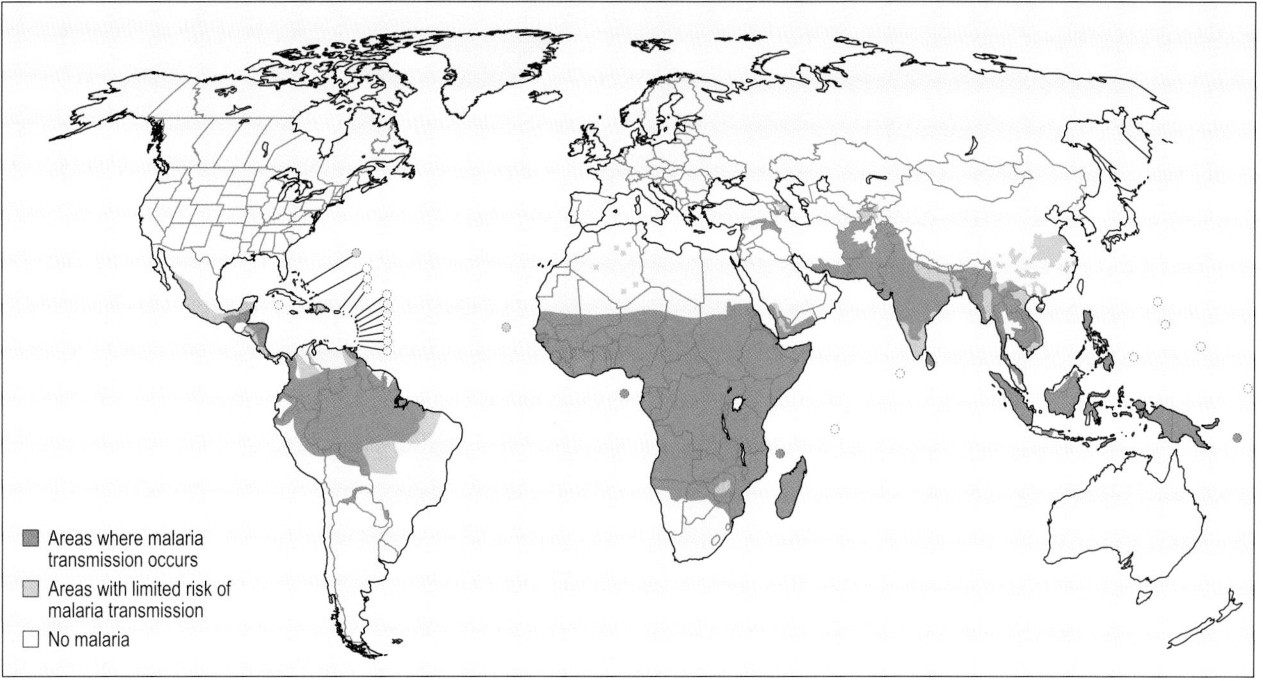

Figure 96.1 Areas of the world where malaria is transmitted, with differentiation between high- and minimal-risk areas. (Reproduced from World Health Organization. Available online at: http://gamapserver.who.int/mapLibrary/default.aspx.)

Understanding malaria (***Box 96.1***) is dependent on understanding the complex life cycle of the parasite in its definitive host in which sexual development occurs – the mosquito – and its intermediate host – the human (***Fig. 96.2***).

Life Cycle of *P. falciparum*

When an infected female *Anopheles* spp. mosquito feeds on a human (***Fig. 96.3A***), she is thought to inoculate an average of 100–500 and as many as 1000–2000 uninucleated sporozoites (approximately 1 × 10 μm) (***Fig. 96.3B***) into the tissues or directly into the bloodstream.[11–13] Sporozoites rapidly pass through the bloodstream to the liver (probably within 2 minutes, but less than 60 minutes).[14] In hepatic sinusoids they penetrate and pass through Kupffer cells[15] and invade hepatocytes through specific receptor–ligand interactions. The primary receptor is thought to be sulfated heparan glycans on the hepatocyte surface; the parasite ligands include the thrombospondin domains of at least two sporozoite proteins – the circumsporozoite protein[16] and a protein known both as the thrombospondin-related anonymous protein (TRAP)[17] and as sporozoite surface protein 2.[18] Sporozoites may invade several hepatocytes before finding the correct hepatocyte in which to develop.[19] Within the hepatocyte, a host cell-derived "parasitophorous" vacuole separates the parasite from the cytoplasm of the hepatocytes. During a minimum of 5.5 days, the uninucleated *P. falciparum* sporozoite develops to a mature liver-stage schizont with an average of 30 000 and range of 10 000–40 000 uninucleated merozoites (***Fig. 96.3C and Table 96.1***).

The hepatocyte containing mature liver-stage schizonts dies or ruptures releasing "sacks" containing merozoites called merosomes containing thousands of merozoites that are about 1.5 μm in diameter, each of which can invade a normal erythrocyte (***Fig. 96.3D***). There are a number of steps in this process (***Fig. 96.3E***),[20] but there is unquestionably a specific interaction between receptors on the erythrocyte membrane and ligands on the merozoite surface. One of these receptor–ligand interactions is between sialic acids and peptides on erythrocyte glycophorin A and the 175-kDa erythrocyte-binding antigen (PfEBA175) on the merozoite.[21] In the erythrocyte, the invading merozoite develops within a parasitophorous vacuole composed of host cell material. During the next 43–48 hours, the uninucleated parasite consumes red cell hemoglobin (Hb) and develops to maturity within the parasitophorous vacuole. First,

Box 96.1 Terminology of Malariologists

Prepatent-period: the time from mosquito inoculation of sporozoites until asexual erythrocytic stage parasites are demonstrated in the bloodstream

Incubation period: the time from mosquito inoculation of sporozoites until the individual first manifests symptoms or signs of malaria

Recurrence: repeat infection causing malaria that is the result of a relapse, recrudescence, or reinfection

- *Relapse:* a recurrent infection caused by development of hypnozoites from the liver. Relapses are thought to occur only with *P. vivax* or *P. ovale* infections
- *Recrudescence:* a recurrent infection caused by a blood-stage infection in which parasitemia declines below the level of detection and then rises above the level of detection. Recrudescence occurs most commonly after inadequate treatment as a result of drug resistance, unusual pharmacokinetics, or incomplete dosage. It can also occur in immunocompromised individuals whose immune systems have been controlling a low level asexual erythrocytic stage infection for years, especially when the parasite is *P. malariae*
- *Reinfection:* a recurrent infection caused by a new exposure to infected *Anopheles* mosquitoes

Classification of endemicity: this classification scheme has been used since the 1950s, but many malariologists do not currently find it useful because of the poor correlation between the number of 2–9-year-olds with palpable spleens and positive blood films and the intensity of malaria transmission in settings where people are fed on by more than 20 infected mosquitoes per year

Type of endemicity:

Palpable spleen (spleen rates) with positive blood film

Holoendemic

- >75% in 2–9-year olds, and low in adults
- >75% in 2–9-year olds

Hyperendemic

- >50% in 2–9-year olds, and >25% in adults
- >50% in 2–9-year olds

Mesoendemic

- 11–50% in 2–9-year olds
- 11–50% in 2–9-year olds

Hypoendemic

- <11% in 2–9-year olds
- <11% in 2–9-year olds

Table 96.1 Differences among *Plasmodium falciparum*, *P. vivax*, *P. ovale*, *P. malariae*, and *P. knowlesi*

Characteristic	*P. falciparum*	*P. vivax*	*P. ovale*	*P. malariae*	*P. knowlesi*[e]
Life Cycle					
Maximum time sporozoites circulate in bloodstream (minutes)	30	60	?	?	?
Primary liver stage (day)	5.5–7	6–8	9	14–16	9–12
Delayed primary liver stage (months)	9[a]	10.5	?	?	?
Relapse from secondary liver stage (hypnozoites)	–	+	+	–	–
Length of secondary liver stage (months)	–	1–36	?	–	–
Liver stage (no. of merozoites/schizont)	30 000	10 000	15 000	2000	
Liver stage (diameter, μm)	55	50	45	40	46
Erythrocyte preference	Young, but all invaded	Reticulocytes or RBCs up to 14 days old	Reticulocytes	Old	
Asexual erythrocytic stage (hours)	43–52	48	48	72	24
Prepatent period (average no. of days)	11	12.2	12.0	32.7[b]	7.2
Incubation period (average no. of days)	13.1	13.4	14.1	34.7	12
Asexual erythrocytic stage (cytoadherence)	+	–[d]	–	–	–[f]
Asexual erythrocytic stage (persistence if inadequately or not treated, years)	1–2	1.5–5	? same as *P. vivax*	3–50	?
Mosquito cycle = sporogonic cycle (gametes to salivary gland sporozoites)	9–13	8–10	12–14	14–16	12–15
Morphologic Findings In Blood Films[c]					
Rings					
Shape	Fine, oval, circular	Irregular, large, thick	Regular, dense	Dense, thick	Fine and dense, circular
Appliqué (squeezed to edge of cell)	Occurs	–	–	–	Occurs
Chromatin dots	1–2	1	1	1	1–2
Parasite density >2%	Frequent	Rare	Rare	Rare	Frequent
Trophozoites					
Band forms	–	–	–	+	+
Schizonts					
Found in peripheral blood	Rare	+	+	+	+
Pigment	Dark brown-black	Orange-brown	Brown	Black	Dark brown-black
No. of merozoites	8–32	12–18	8–14	8–10	10–16
Gametocytes					
Shape	Banana-shaped	Round or oval	Large, round	Large, oval	Round-oval
Male	Light blue	Pale blue (round)	Dense, blue	Pale blue	Blue (round)
Female	Darker blue	Dark blue (oval)	Dense, blue	Dense, blue	Medium pink
Pigment granules	Few blue-black	Few orange	Brown	Large, black	Dark brown
Erythrocyte changes					
Enlarged	–	+	+	–	–
Pale cytoplasm	+	–	–	–	–
Oval with tufted edges	–	–	Frequent	–	–
Crenated	Occurs	–	–	–	–
Red dots in cytoplasm	Mauer's clefts	Schuffner's dots	James' dots	–	Sinton and Mulligan's stippling[g]

[a]In *P. falciparum*, delayed appearance of blood-stage infection has been documented in travelers, but it is unclear whether this results from delayed emergence from the liver or from delayed development in erythrocytes.

[b]Data for *P. malariae* are derived from experimental challenges reported in Boyd MF, ed. Malariology: A Comprehensive Survey of All Aspects of This Group of Diseases from a Global Standpoint. Philadelphia: WB Saunders; 1949.

[c]Preparation of blood films. Thin and thick blood films are routinely prepared on the same slide. Two drops of blood are placed at one end of a clean glass slide. The thin film is made by placing the edge of a second slide into the edge of the more medial drop at an approximately 45° angle and spreading the blood across the entire slide. The thick film is made by placing the corner of a second slide into the drop and circularly spreading the blood to approximately the size of a US penny. The thin-film portion is fixed with methanol, preserving the erythrocytes. The thick-film portion is not fixed, and the erythrocytes are lysed when the slide is stained.

[d]*P. vivax* can cytoadhere to placental cells via attachment to chondroitin sulfate A.

[e]Data for *P. knowlesi* was gathered from Coatney, Contacos, Collins & Warren (1972) The Primate Malarias, Chapter 26 *Plasmodium knowlesi* Sinton and Mulligan, 1932 or CDC Diagnostic Findings Malaria. Accessed 02 September 2010. http://www.dpd.cdc.gov/dpdx/HTML/Malaria.htm.

[f]Partial sequestration was observed for *P. knowlesi* in a single postmortem case. Cox-Singh et al. *Malaria J.* 2010;9:10.

[g]Dots only observed with special stains and with Giemsa stain, only some infected RBCs have dots.

RBCs, red blood cells.

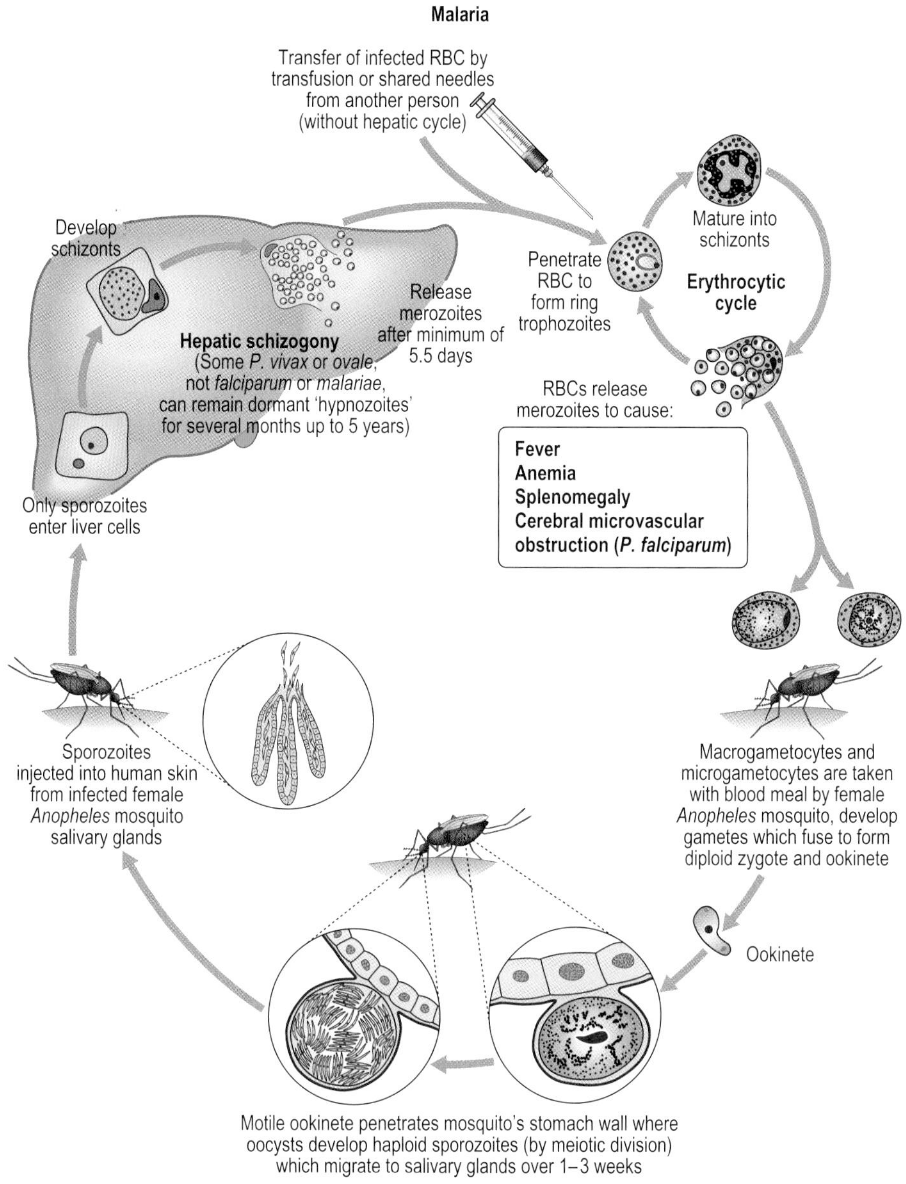
Malaria
Transfer of infected RBC by transfusion or shared needles from another person (without hepatic cycle)
Develop schizonts
Release merozoites after minimum of 5.5 days
Hepatic schizogony (Some P. vivax or ovale, not falciparum or malariae, can remain dormant 'hypnozoites' for several months up to 5 years)
Only sporozoites enter liver cells
Penetrate RBC to form ring trophozoites
Mature into schizonts
Erythrocytic cycle
RBCs release merozoites to cause:
Fever
Anemia
Splenomegaly
Cerebral microvascular obstruction (P. falciparum)
Sporozoites injected into human skin from infected female Anopheles mosquito salivary glands
Macrogametocytes and microgametocytes are taken with blood meal by female Anopheles mosquito, develop gametes which fuse to form diploid zygote and ookinete
Ookinete
Motile ookinete penetrates mosquito's stomach wall where oocysts develop haploid sporozoites (by meiotic division) which migrate to salivary glands over 1–3 weeks

Figure 96.2 Life cycle of *Plasmodium* parasites in humans. RBC, red blood cell.

the parasite becomes a trophozoite and begins to secrete proteins that pass through the parasite membrane and the parasitophorous vacuole membrane and form knobs in the erythrocyte membrane (***Fig. 96.3F***). The proteins in the knobs, especially *P. falciparum* erythrocyte membrane protein 1 (PfEMP1),[22–24] bind to receptors on endothelial cells in capillaries and postcapillary venules, sequestering the infected erythrocyte in the microcirculation for the last 24–34 hours of the parasite's development cycle, when it changes from an immature schizont to a mature asexual erythrocytic-stage schizont with an average of 16 uninucleated merozoites. It is thought that the parasite has developed this mechanism to prevent the increasingly rigid infected erythrocyte from being removed from the circulation when it passes through the spleen. When fully mature, the infected erythrocyte ruptures, releasing the merozoites (***Fig. 96.3F***), which then invade normal erythrocytes, initiating the cycle of intraerythrocytic-stage development, rupture, and reinvasion that leads to a 10–20-fold increase in the numbers of *P. falciparum* parasites in the bloodstream every 43–48 hours and to all the clinical manifestations and pathology of malaria.

Alternatively, erythrocytic-stage parasites can develop to sexual-stage parasites, called gametocytes (***Fig. 96.3G***). In the gut of the mosquito, gametocytes escape from erythrocytes and form gametes. The male gamete fuses with the female, forming a zygote. At ~5 hours after blood-feeding, the zygote undergoes two-step meiosis. By 18–24 hours, the zygote has transformed into an ookinete. The ookinete traverses the midgut wall by passing through epithelial cells and comes to rest adjacent to the basal lamina. Here it begins to transform into an oocyst. From the 6th day onward, the oocyst undergoes cell division that eventually results in the formation of about 8000 daughter cells called sporozoites. By day 12, they are released into the hemocele of the mosquito and migrate to the salivary glands. In the salivary glands, they become infectious for humans and are released into the human host when the mosquito feeds.

Differences Between *P. falciparum* and its Life Cycle and the Other Parasites That Cause Human Malaria

Amongst these differences (***Table 96.1***), one of the most important differences is that *P. vivax* and *P. ovale* can have prolonged (up to 3 years) liver stages. Some populations of *P. vivax* and *P. ovale* sporozoites invade hepatocytes, arrest further development, becoming hypnozoites,[25,26] and then can activate and initiate replication and full development a month to several years after the primary infection. When a patient who was appropriately treated for erythrocytic-stage *P. vivax* or *P. ovale* infection with elimination of both clinical manifestations and all bloodstream parasites

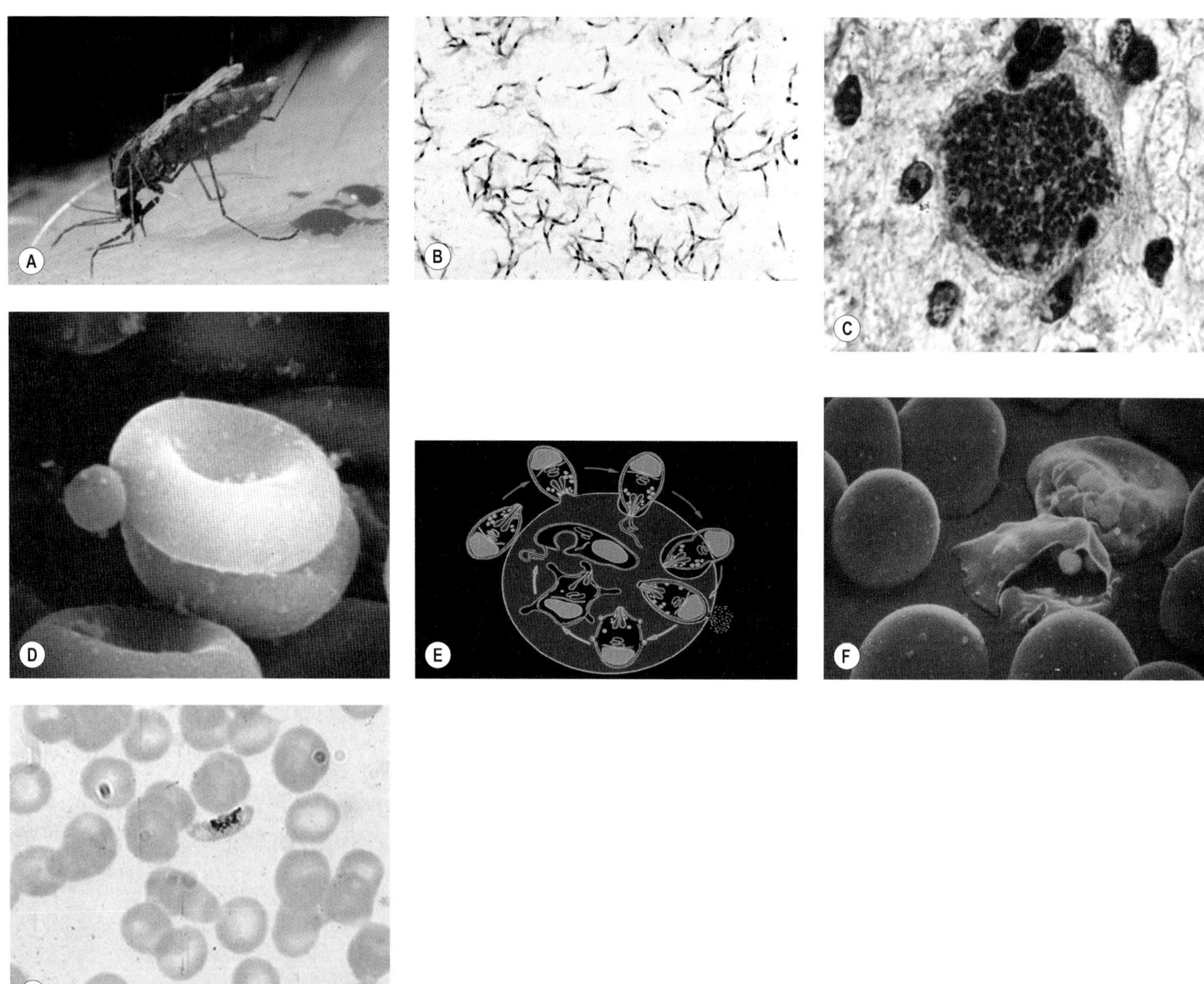

Figure 96.3 Vector and parasites at different stages of the life cycle. **(A)** *Anopheles stephensi* mosquito feeding in characteristic posture. **(B)** *Plasmodium falciparum* sporozoites in a crush preparation of a salivary gland (Giemsa stain). **(C)** Mature liver-stage schizont of *P. falciparum* with thousands of merozoites (hematoxylin and eosin stain). **(D)** *P. falciparum* merozoite attaching to uninfected erythrocyte prior to invasion (scanning electron micrograph). **(E)** Schematic of the process of a *P. falciparum* merozoite invading an erythrocyte. **(F)** *P. falciparum* merozoites rupturing from an infected erythrocyte. Note "knobs" on the surface of the infected, unruptured erythrocyte above the rupturing erythrocyte (scanning electron micrograph). **(G)** *P. falciparum* gametocyte in thin blood smear (Giemsa stain). ((**B**) Courtesy of © Liverpool School of Tropical Medicine, photo by A. Stich, Wellcome Trust International Health Image Collection; (**C**) courtesy of Dr. P. Druilhe, Institut Pasteur, Paris, France; (**D**) courtesy of © L.H. Bannister, Wellcome Trust International Health Image Collection.)

(clinical cure) has a recurrent case of malaria caused by development of hypnozoites, the patient is considered to have a relapse (see ***Box 96.1***). In addition to secondary attacks caused by hypnozoites, some isolates of *P. vivax*, especially those acquired in temperate regions of the world (e.g., Korea, China), cause delayed primary infections owing to persistence in the liver that may occur up to 1 year after inoculation of sporozoites by mosquitoes. These parasites are called *P. vivax* var. hibernans. This phenomenon of delayed primary attacks has been reported with *P. falciparum*[27] but is much less common than with *P. vivax*.

P. vivax differs from the other malarial species in that *P. vivax* merozoites cannot invade erythrocytes that lack the Duffy blood group antigen;[28] this is an erythrocyte membrane receptor for a protein ligand on the merozoite surface called the Duffy-binding protein or ligand.[29]

P. falciparum, *P. vivax*, and *P. ovale* take approximately 48 hours to complete the asexual erythrocytic stage of their life cycle (invasion, development, rupture, and reinvasion), and are called tertian (recurring every 3rd day) malarias. *P. malariae* has an approximately 72-hour cycle and is called quartan (recurring every 4th day) malaria. *P. knowlesi* has a 24 hour cycle.

Genomics of Malaria Parasites

Sequences of chromosome 2 of *P. falciparum*[30] and the entire genomic sequence of *P. falciparum* clone 3D7[31] have been delineated. Because malaria parasites have complex life cycles and are notoriously difficult to study, analyses of the *P. falciparum* genome have provided many insights into parasite biochemistry, cell biology, and pathogenicity. The *P. vivax* genome has also been sequenced,[32] as have those of multiple rodent and simian *Plasmodium* species used as models for human parasites, as well as patient isolates obtained from diverse geographical locations.

The *P. falciparum* genome is ~23 Mb in size and encodes about 5300 genes on 14 chromosomes. Over half of the genes contain introns. On average, the coding regions of *P. falciparum* genes are longer than in other sequenced eukaryotes such as *Schizosaccharomyces pombe* (2.3 kb versus 1.4 kb). The reason for this increased gene length is unknown. Fully 60% of the encoded proteins have little or no similarity to proteins in other organisms and are of unknown function. The proportion of genes encoding these so-called hypothetical proteins is higher in *P. falciparum* than in other sequenced organisms, which is probably a reflection of the greater evolutionary distance between *Plasmodium* and other well-studied eukaryotes.

Analysis of the predicted proteome provides an overview of metabolism and transport in malaria parasites.[33,34] A number of features of parasite metabolism remain unclear because of the absence of some enzymes or enzyme subunits and because the predicted subcellular localization of some enzymes differs from the known localization of the enzymes in other organisms, making it difficult to reconstruct the metabolism of the parasite with certainty. A remarkable feature of this parasite is its relative lack of transcription factors, implying that the parasite relies to a large extent on post-transcriptional control of gene function.

P. falciparum appears to have greatly reduced capacities for metabolism and transport of organic nutrients and ions compared with other free-living organisms. Only 14% of the proteins encode enzymes, a much lower proportion than in other eukaryotes. Similarly, the *P. falciparum* genome encodes a smaller repertoire of membrane transporters in comparison with other free-living eukaryotic microbes such as *Saccharomyces cerevisiae*. The *P. falciparum* genome encodes enzymes for the complete glycolytic pathway from glucose-6-phosphate to pyruvate, and for the conversion of pyruvate to lactate. All enzymes of the tricarboxylic acid (TCA) cycle have been identified, but the function of the TCA cycle is unclear.

Other unusual features of *P. falciparum* metabolism, inferred from the genome sequence, are the absence of gluconeogenesis and the lack of any enzymes for the biosynthesis of amino acids, apart from enzymes required for amino acid interconversions. The lack of amino acid biosynthetic pathways and the apparent absence of clear homologs of known amino acid transporters emphasize the parasite's dependence on the host for amino acids, at least in the erythrocytic stages in which amino acids are obtained by the digestion of Hb in the food vacuole. Overall, the metabolic and transport capabilities of *Plasmodium* are less than those of other free-living organisms, presumably a reflection of its intracellular parasitic life cycle.

Differences between the genome of *P. falciparum* and other malaria parasites versus nonpathogenic eukaryotes are the abundance of genes in malaria parasites that are involved in immune evasion and other host–parasite interactions (3.9% and 1.3%, respectively). The *P. falciparum* 3D7 genome, for example, contains 59 *var* genes that encode highly polymorphic proteins, PfEMP1.[22–24] These proteins are expressed on the surface of infected erythrocytes, mediate cytoadherence of infected cells to host capillary endothelium, and cause sequestration of the infected cells in many organs, including the brain. The PfEMP1 proteins are thought to be the targets of protective antibody responses, but transcriptional switching between different *var* genes provides for antigenic variation and the evasion of the host immune response. The *rif* genes, of which there are 149 in the 3D7 genome, encode proteins called rifins. A third group of proteins called STEVORs (28 in the 3D7 genome) are similar in sequence to the rifins and so far, like the rifins, have no known function. Members of the PfEMP1, rifin, and STEVOR families exhibit extensive sequence diversity, and genes encoding these proteins occur in clusters, most of which are located in subtelomeric regions in association with several kinds of repetitive sequences. The repetitive sequences are thought to facilitate recombination between different alleles of these highly polymorphic proteins and contribute to the generation of antigen diversity. The genomes of other *Plasmodium* species contain their own distinctive polymorphic gene families that are thought to contribute to pathogenesis and immune evasion.[31,35,36]

The availability of *Plasmodium* genome sequences has paved the way for detailed analyses of parasite biology. Technologies such as DNA microarrays,[37,38] proteomics,[33,34] NextGen genome sequencing,[39] metabolomics,[40] and transfection have provided the means to assess how the parasite responds to its environment and how it functions as an organism requiring two such different hosts as humans and mosquitoes. These data have already had a profound effect on our understanding of the biology and biochemistry of the parasite, and are being used to provide clues to developing new interventions against the parasite and the disease it causes.

EPIDEMIOLOGY

Malaria transmission occurs in most of Africa south of the Sahara desert; in many areas of the Indian subcontinent, Southeast Asia, and Oceania; in Central America, Haiti, and the Dominican Republic; and in the Amazon basin of Brazil and contiguous countries in South America (***Figs 96.4 and 96.5***). The global distribution and prevalence of malaria infection have not changed appreciably for the past few decades. While malaria

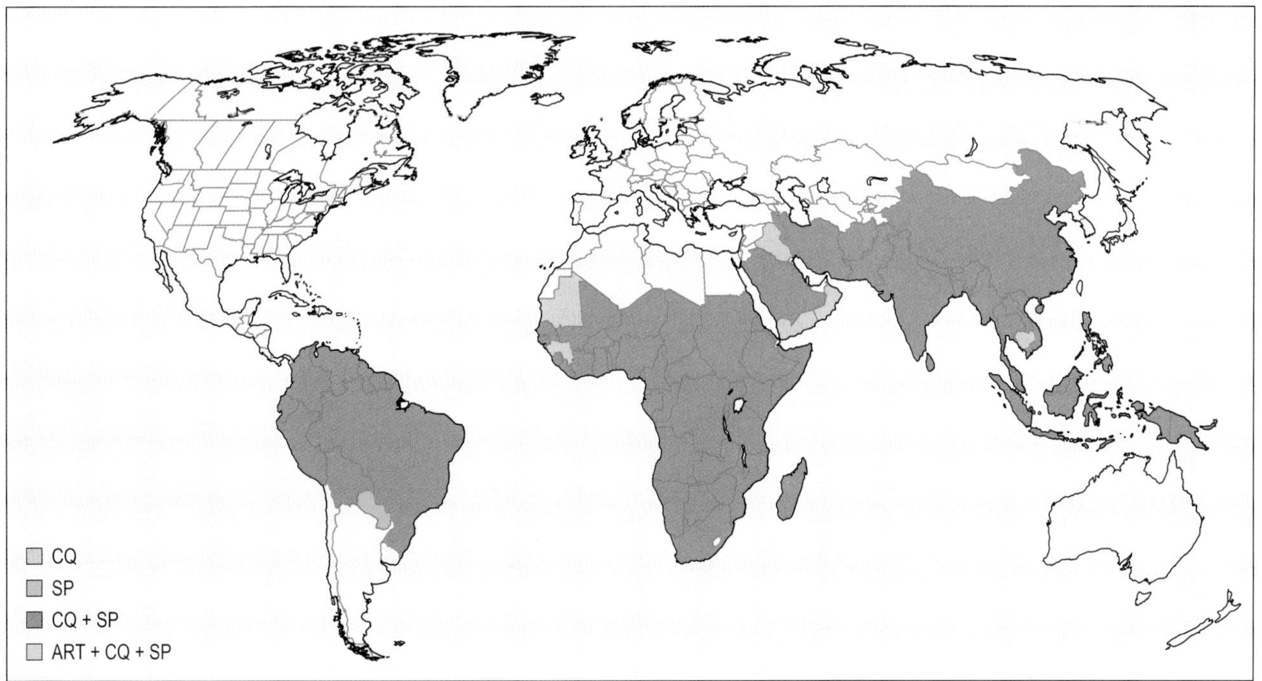

Figure 96.4 Map depicting the global distribution of drug-resistant *Plasmodium falciparum* malaria in 2009, based on literature searches and other publicly available data compiled by the WorldWide Antimalarial Resistance Network (WWARN, www.wwarn.org). CQ, chloroquine-resistant *P. falciparum*; SP, sulfadoxine-pyrimethamine-resistant *P. falciparum*; ART, artemisinin-resistant *P. falciparum*.

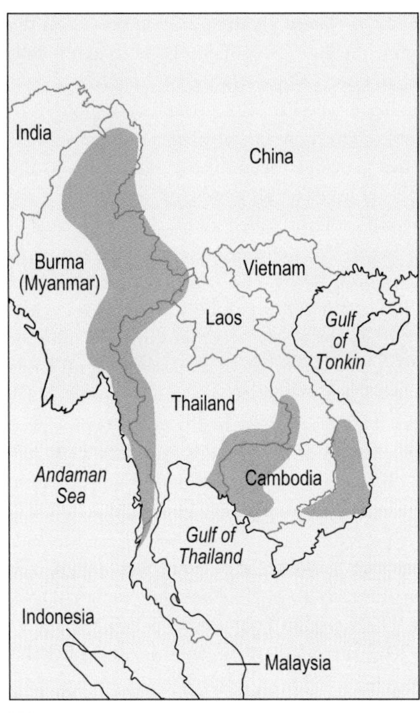

Figure 96.5 Mefloquine-resistant *Plasmodium falciparum* in Southeast Asia. (Courtesy of Centers for Disease Control and Prevention. CDC Health Information for International Travel 2010. Atlanta: US Department of Health and Human Services, Public Health Service; 2009.)

infection is widely distributed, the intensity of transmission of *Plasmodium* is greatest in Africa, where in excess of 80% of new infections globally are estimated to occur annually.

Malaria infection with the four *Plasmodium* spp. that naturally infect humans is characterized by persistence of the blood stage of parasites for intervals of from months to lifelong without therapy. Consequently, in areas, notably Africa, it is difficult to characterize the incidence of new malaria infections since the prevalence of infection is persistently high. It has been estimated that in the range of 500–800 million new malaria infections occur globally each year;[1,41] however, this figure is imprecise, particularly in areas of high levels of transmission in Africa.[42,43]

The major determinants of the epidemiology of malaria infection and disease relate to the *Plasmodium* spp., the transmission intensity, innate and acquired resistance of the human host, and access to and efficacy of control measures. In addition, the immunocompromised states associated with pregnancy and infection with human immunodeficiency virus (HIV) affect the epidemiology of malaria.[44]

Recently it has been documented that the macaque *Plasmodium* parasite, *P. knowlesi*, infects humans in a limited range of Southeast Asia, in particular in areas where humans have close proximity to the macaque natural host. The clinical manifestation of *P. knowlesi* infection in humans is predominately a mild febrile illness. However *P. knowlesi* can multiply rapidly as it has a 1-day erythrocytic cycle and some patients develop severe and potentially lethal malaria. *P. knowlesi* is sensitive to chloroquine.

Plasmodium Species

The species that causes the greatest illness and death in humans, *P. falciparum*, is the predominant infection in Africa south of the Sahara, in the Amazon basin and Haiti, and limited areas of Asia and Oceania. *P. vivax* is widely distributed in the Americas and Asia, and only in very circumscribed areas of Africa. The two less prevalent species, *P. malariae* and *P. ovale*, are transmitted in Africa and the Amazon basin and sporadically in other parts of the world such as Oceania and Southeast Asia. As a consequence of this distribution, most illness and death attributable to malaria occurs in Africa, Asia, and the Amazon region of Brazil.

Transmission Intensity

Plasmodium parasites are transmitted to humans by female mosquitoes of the *Anopheles* genus. Worldwide ~40 anopheline species have been documented to transmit parasites to humans. These species vary remarkably in their capacity to transmit *Plasmodium* to humans. This variability relates to basic habits, including the tendency to seek out humans for a blood meal, types of water sources preferred for laying eggs, and predilection for entering human dwellings, as well as basic biologic capacity to support the development of human *Plasmodium* to development of mature infection that can be transmitted during the taking of a blood meal. Anopheline species with the greatest competence to transmit *Plasmodium* are found in the Amazon (*An. darlingi*) and Africa (the species complex of *An. gambiae*). *An. dirus* is a highly efficient vector in Southeast Asia.

Several identifiable factors characterize the capacity of *Anopheles* mosquitoes to transmit *Plasmodium*. The adult female mosquito can survive under ideal conditions up to 50–60 days. Under field conditions, however, female anophelines survive on the average of 20–25 days, and consequently must be infected by malaria parasites in their early blood meals, taken every 2–3 days. Maturation of the parasites ingested with the blood meal requires 8–12 days, depending on ambient temperatures, before the mosquito has infective sporozoites in her salivary glands. Mathematical modeling of malaria transmission by MacDonald[45] and others incorporates a measure of mosquito density in a defined setting and the probability that an *Anopheles* will feed on a human during a day.

The epidemiologic measure of transmission intensity is the entomologic inoculation rate (EIR), which depends on the proportion of female anophelines with salivary glands infected with *Plasmodium* and the number of potentially infected *Anopheles* mosquitoes feeding on a person in a unit of time (day or year). There is a wide range of documented EIRs by both time and area of the world, and even within regions of a country. In the areas of Africa with the most intense annual transmission, EIRs can reach 3 infected bites per day at the peak of transmission. By contrast, in most malaria-endemic regions of the Americas and Asia, annual EIRs range from <1 to 10 infected bites annually.

Mathematical models of malaria transmission have constructed several composite statistics to quantitate the risk of malaria transmission in defined epidemiologic settings. Vectorial capacity incorporates estimates of mosquito density and human biting rate along with daily survival (longevity) of anopheline mosquitoes to estimate the overall receptivity or intensity of malaria parasite transmission in a defined setting. The estimation of vectorial capacity can be used to compare transmission risk in time and space, and in principle also to monitor the effect of measures used to control malaria transmission.

Black[46] developed the concept of the reproductive rate for malaria transmission: this estimates the number of secondary cases of malaria that are predicted from an infected human in a population susceptible to malaria infection. A reproductive rate greater than 1.0 predicts sustaining malaria transmission in a population. Interruption of transmission requires that the reproductive rate is maintained less than 1.0. These mathematical models were developed and refined during the last century in conjunction with malaria eradication attempts; they have recently been refined further to address malaria transmission dynamics in highly immune populations as encountered in Africa.[47]

In Africa, transmission intensity has a major effect on the clinical manifestations of severe disease and the age at which they are encountered. For example, in areas with extremely high EIRs (100–300 potentially infective bites per year) and long transmission seasons, most severe disease and malaria-associated deaths occur in infants and young children, and the primary cause of malaria-associated death is severe anemia. In these epidemiologic settings, the risk of acutely progressive malaria illness is associated with higher-density parasitemias (>10% of erythrocytes infected). In older children who have survived early infections, higher-density parasitemias are less frequent. In areas with less intense transmission (10–40 infective bites per year) and more limited transmission periods, most cases of severe malaria and deaths occur in older children (e.g., 3–7 years of age), and cerebral malaria is responsible for a high percentage of the deaths.

Innate and Acquired Resistance

Protection from malaria can be expressed as decreased risk of being infected (developing blood-stage parasitemia) or decreased risk of developing higher-density parasitemia and clinical illness due to the parasitemia (clinical immunity). This protection is mediated by innate mechanisms and by acquired adaptive immune responses. In settings of natural transmission, it has been demonstrated that humans do not acquire persisting protection from being infected by mosquito transmission but do develop immune-mediated protection against parasites and disease. It is presumed that under natural conditions the variability of the *Plasmodium* parasite (antigenic variation) is the major factor responsible for persisting susceptibility to infection even after lifelong exposure and infection.

Innate Resistance

Population evolutionary genetics suggests that *Plasmodium* infection has had more impact on the human genome than any other infectious agent. In settings where humans are exposed to high levels of malaria transmission, it has been documented that genetically determined traits have been selected for over generations that mediate protection against either infection or the risk of clinical or severe malaria illness.

A well-characterized protective mutation is in the Duffy erythrocyte surface antigen that, in the homozygous recessive state, is associated with complete protection against *P. vivax* infection.[28] The Duffy antigen is sterically associated with the protein required for attachment and penetration of *P. vivax* merozoites into erythrocytes. The homozygous Duffy mutation is uniform in African blacks, and variable among blacks of African origin in Europe and the United States, and *P. vivax* infection does not occur in homozygous recessive individuals.

The sickle cell mutation in human Hb is a balanced polymorphism that has been selected for in areas of intense *P. falciparum*, mainly in Africa. In the heterozygous state, the sickle trait affords protection against the development of higher-density, life-threatening parasitemia, probably because the variant Hb is a poor substrate for digestion by the parasite and because infected cells are more easily subject to mechanical damage in the circulation.[48,49] The incidence rate of cerebral malaria is reduced by 90% in children with sickle cell trait compared with their peers.[50] There is evidence that a number of other polymorphisms including hemoglobinopathies and erythrocyte membrane variants have evolved and afford survival advantages to affected individuals. For example, recent studies in West Africa have demonstrated that HbC affords protection against a range of malaria illness manifestations.[51] Other erythrocyte disorders associated with an advantage to the host include HbE, HbF, α- and β-thalassemia, glucose-6-phosphate dehydrogenase (G6PD) deficiency, and red cell cytoskeletal abnormalities such as ovalocytosis. These and other red cell abnormalities affecting infection with *Plasmodium* spp. parasites have been summarized.[48]

Reduction of Morbidity and Mortality of Malaria by Adaptive Human Immune Responses

Acquired or adaptive human immune responses occurring on the basis of an individual being exposed to infection with *Plasmodium* spp. parasites can diminish the pathogenic effects of malaria parasites on the human host and also are implicated in the pathogenesis of disease. In areas with the most intense *P. falciparum* transmission in sub-Saharan Africa, the role of host immune responses in ameliorating disease can be viewed as having three different stages during an individual's life.

Neonatal Period and Early Infancy

New infections, especially higher-density parasitemias, and clinical manifestations of malaria are much less common in infants <6 months of age than in older infants and children.[41,51] Newborns have significant protection against high-density parasitemia for periods ranging to 6 months of age. This protective immunity is acquired passively across the placenta *in utero*, and presumably is primarily mediated by maternal antibodies. High erythrocyte concentrations of fetal Hb may also protect against malaria infection.

Late Infancy Through Early Childhood

For several years infants and children are at greater risk of developing repeated infections and life-threatening malaria. However, as they grow older the risk of severe malaria wanes with successive malaria infections. Parasite densities are decreased, as is the incidence rate of severe disease and *P. falciparum*-related death. Immunity to *P. vivax* develops more rapidly than to *P. falciparum* infections. The rate at which clinical immunity is acquired varies in general with the intensity of transmission of *P. falciparum*. In areas with the highest EIRs, if a child survives to the age of 3, he or she may never again develop severe malaria or die directly of severe malaria. In areas with less intense transmission, this clinical immunity against severe disease may not occur until the age of 5, and in areas with even less intense transmission or seasonal transmission it may not occur until the age of 7–10.

Immunity is thought to be primarily mediated by antibodies against asexual erythrocytic-stage parasites and their products. Antibodies against variant surface antigens (such as PfEMP1)[22–24] are thought to prevent sequestration of the infected erythrocytes in the microcirculation and thereby prevent microcirculatory obstruction and severe disease and allow for removal of infected erythrocytes in the spleen, reducing parasite burden. Antibodies against merozoite surface proteins are thought either to prevent invasion of erythrocytes or activate mononuclear cells to release cytokines, free oxygen radicals, and other biologically active substances that inhibit parasite development within erythrocytes, thereby reducing parasite burden. Antibodies against *P. falciparum*-derived "toxins" such as glycosylphosphatidylinositol are thought to inhibit the function of these toxins and limit the clinical manifestations of infection without necessarily affecting the parasites.[53]

Late Childhood Onward

Individuals become infected, probably at the same rate as young children, and may become ill from the infections. However, they have significantly lower densities of parasite-infected erythrocytes in the bloodstream, lower incidence rates of clinical disease, and essentially no severe disease or *P. falciparum*-induced death. The same immune mechanisms thought to contribute to the steady reduction of incidence of severe disease with increasing age in childhood are thought to mediate this antiparasite and antidisease immunity in older children, adolescents, and adults. It has been shown that administration of purified immunoglobulin from adults from areas highly endemic for *P. falciparum* in West Africa reduces *P. falciparum* parasitemia by >95% in children in Africa and Thailand.[54,55] These studies prove that naturally acquired antibodies against asexual erythrocytic stages can have a dramatic effect on *P. falciparum* in infected people. It has been proposed that T-cell responses against liver stages of the parasite life cycle may also play a substantial role in naturally acquired protective immunity,[50] but the fact that adults and children[56–59] become reinfected at the same rate suggests that pre-erythrocytic-stage immunity plays a minor role at best in acquired clinical immunity.

Human Beh avior and Environment

The interactions among humans, parasites, and mosquitoes in malaria transmission are complex. Human behavior not only influences individual risk of being infected, but human behavior and environmental impact can foster conditions that promote malaria transmission and risk. Human activity in clearing and settling land can create conditions that promote breeding of *Anopheles* mosquitoes. Excavation of earth, impounding of water, and the clearing of shade are factors promoting increased mosquito breeding in Africa and areas of the Americas. Housing construction (e.g., the presence of screening and windows) affects the ability of mosquitoes to enter dwellings at night when humans are indoors. Agriculture practices and certain occupations can increase the risk of infection; for example, in Southeast Asia when humans work in forest areas where

Table 96.2 Distribution of Drug-Resistant *Plasmodium falciparum* Malaria

Region	Resistance Reported[a]				Comments
	CQ	SP	AQ	MQ	
	Plasmodium falciparum Infections				
Central America (Mexico, Belize, Guatemalala, Honduras, El Salvador, Nicaragua, Costa Rica, NW Panama)	N	N	N	N	Northwest of Panama canal only
Caribbean (Haiti and Dominican Republic only)	N	N	N	N	
South America (SE Panama, Columbia, Venezuela, Ecuador, Peru, Brazil, Bolivia)	Y	Y	Y	Y	Resistance to MQ and QN, although reported (Venezuela, Ecuador, Peru, Brazil, Bolivia), is considered to occur infrequently
West Africa	Y	Y	N	N	SP resistance can be focally high
East Africa	Y	Y	Y	N	SP resistance is now high-grade in many areas and amodiaquine resistance is increasing
Southern Africa	Y	Y	N	N	Resistance to SP high-grade in KwaZulu Natal, South Africa, and variable elsewhere
Indian subcontinent	Y	Y	Y	N	Amodiaquine resistance in all areas, but SP still effective in some areas
Southeast Asia and Oceania	Y	Y	Y	Y	Border areas of Thailand, Cambodia, and Myanmar highest risk for multiple drug-resistant infections; mefloquine resistance documented in eastern Myanmar, Thailand, Cambodia, and southern Vietnam only
East Asia (China)	Y	Y	Y	N	Resistance greatest problem in southern China where bulk of falciparum transmitted

CQ, chloroquine; SP, sulfadoxine/pyrimethamine; AQ, amodiaquine; MQ, mefloquine; QN, quinine.
[a]Reduced sensitivity to quinine occurs in parts of Southeast Asia and South America, but high-level resistance is extremely unusual.
(Adapted from Bloland PB. Drug resistance in malaria. WHO/CDS/CSR/DRS/2001.4. Geneva: World Health Organization; 2001.)

malaria transmission occurs because those areas are the habitat of the predominant mosquito vector species.

Use and Efficacy of Control Measures

The predominant measures either to prevent or treat malaria infection are the use of antimosquito interventions (ITNs, indoor residual insecticide spraying (IRS)) and the use of antimalarial drugs either to prevent or treat infection. The level of use of these interventions (coverage) as well as their efficacy has a major impact on the epidemiology of malaria as well as programmatic impact.

The efficacy of these interventions substantially alters individual risk of either infection or severe disease. For example, from large-scale trials of ITNs it can be estimated that there is up to a 74% reduction in malaria-associated malaria fevers requiring therapy when ITN coverage exceeds 70–80% at the community level.[60] Conversely, when efficacy is compromised, for example, when drug or insecticide resistance emerges, significant increases in malaria infection risk and disease may occur.[61]

Prompt treatment of malaria illness can substantially reduce the risk of progression to severe disease, and drug therapy can largely prevent the development of severe anemia that is a prominent consequence of malaria infection in children and pregnant women in Africa. The emergence and geographic expansion of drug resistance (***Table 96.2***), mainly in *P. falciparum*, have compromised the effectiveness of prompt therapy to control malaria illness and risk of severe and chronic disease. In some areas of Southeast Asia and the Amazon basin, and increasingly in Africa, resistance to multiple drugs has resulted in ineffectiveness of most available and affordable drugs. The spread of chloroquine resistance across much of Africa south of the Sahara in the 1980s–90s was a major factor in the increase in incidence of severe pediatric anemia in many countries.

Immunocompromised States Including Pregnancy and HIV Infection

In settings where transmission of *P. falciparum* occurs, individuals who are immunocompromised may be at increased risk of malaria. Two such conditions are pregnancy and HIV infection. In these settings adults generally will have experienced repeated malaria infections and acquired some immune protection prior to becoming pregnant or acquiring HIV infection. In neither condition is there complete reversal of the protection that has been acquired, although the immune mechanisms involved have not been defined.

P. falciparum infection during pregnancy produces a range of disease consequences. In settings of low-intensity transmission, notably Southeast Asia and the Americas, pregnant women are at greater risk of high-density parasitemia and severe disease compared with nonpregnant women having comparable prior malaria infection experience.[62]

In settings of more intense transmission, notably Africa, the accumulation of parasitized erythrocytes in the placenta has consequences for the pregnant woman and her fetus. Low birth weight (LBW) is the main fetal complication in all endemic areas, with maternal and fetal anemia also prominent consequences of maternal malaria infection in Africa. The risk of higher-density parasitemia, anemia, and LBW is most pronounced in first and second "malaria-exposed" pregnancies.

Malaria infection has not proved to be an opportunistic infection on the scale of tuberculosis in HIV-infected individuals in Africa. However, several clinically relevant interactions have been documented. Recently in southern Africa there have been reports that in adults living in areas with only sporadic malaria transmission, increased risk of severe malaria disease has been documented when HIV infection has progressed to AIDS. Further, in pregnant women, HIV infection does increase the risk of higher-density parasitemia, and this would appear to be independent of parity.[62] Therapy for severe pediatric anemia, largely a result of malaria infection, has been associated with HIV transmission via blood transfusion in Africa, if blood is not screened for infectious agents.

THE DISEASE

Malaria is a common cause of fever in tropical countries. The first symptoms of malaria are nonspecific: a lack of a sense of well-being, headache, fatigue, abdominal discomfort, and muscle aches are followed by fever. These symptoms are similar to those of a minor viral illness. In some instances, headache, chest pain, abdominal pain, arthralgia, myalgia, or diarrhea may suggest another diagnosis. Nausea, vomiting, and orthostatic hypotension are common. Although headache may be severe in malaria, there is no neck stiffness or photophobia as in meningitis. Myalgia may be prominent, but it is not usually as severe as in dengue fever, and the muscles are not tender as in leptospirosis or typhus. The classic malarial paroxysms, in which fever spikes, chills, and rigors occur at regular intervals, are unusual and suggest infection with *P. vivax* or *P. ovale*. The fever is usually irregular at first (in falciparum malaria it may never become regular). Although febrile convulsions in childhood may occur with any of the malarias, generalized seizures are specifically associated with falciparum malaria and may herald the development of coma (cerebral malaria). Most patients with uncomplicated infections have few abnormal physical findings other than fever, malaise, mild anemia, and in some cases palpable splenomegaly. Anemia is common among young children living in areas with stable transmission, particularly where there is resistance to available antimalarials. Splenic enlargement is common among otherwise healthy individuals in malaria-endemic areas and reflects repeated infections (spleen rates (***Box 96.1***) in healthy subjects are used to assess the intensity of malaria transmission); however, in nonimmune individuals with malaria, the spleen takes several days to become palpable. Slight enlargement of the liver is also common, particularly in young children. Mild jaundice frequently occurs in adults; it may develop in patients with otherwise uncomplicated falciparum malaria and usually resolves over 1–3 weeks. Petechial hemorrhages in the skin or mucous membranes – features of viral hemorrhagic fevers and leptospirosis – develop only rarely in severe falciparum malaria. There is no rash.

Severe Falciparum Malaria

When promptly treated with an efficacious drug, uncomplicated falciparum malaria in nonimmune individuals carries a mortality rate of ~0.1%. However, once vital organ dysfunction occurs or the proportion of erythrocytes infected increases above 3%, mortality rises steeply.[64] The relationship between parasitemia and disease severity depends on the malaria transmission intensity. For example, in one large prospective study in a low transmission area of Thailand, patients with parasitemias greater than 4% but no signs of vital organ dysfunction had a mortality rate of 3%[65] (i.e., 30 times higher than that of other patients with uncomplicated malaria but 5–6 times lower than that of those with vital organ dysfunction). Clinical, clinical laboratory, and parasitologic findings associated with poor outcome are outlined in ***Box 96.2***.[64] Coma is a characteristic and ominous feature of falciparum malaria (called cerebral malaria; ***Figs 96.6 and 96.7***) and, despite treatment, is associated with death rates around 20% among adults and 15% among children.[64] Lesser degrees of decreased level of consciousness, including delirium, obtundation, and stupor, should also be taken seriously. The onset may be gradual or sudden following a convulsion. Cerebral malaria is a diffuse symmetric encephalopathy; focal neurologic signs are unusual. There are no signs of meningeal irritation (***Fig. 96.6A***). The eyes may be divergent, and a pout reflex is common, but other primitive reflexes are usually absent. The corneal reflexes are preserved except in deep coma. Muscle tone may be either increased or decreased. The tendon reflexes are variable, and the plantar reflexes may be flexor or extensor; the abdominal and cremasteric reflexes are absent. Flexor or extensor posturing may occur. Approximately 15% of patients have retinal hemorrhages on direct ophthalmoscopy (***Fig. 96.6B***); with pupillary dilatation and indirect ophthalmoscopy, this figure increases to 30–40%. Other funduscopic abnormalities include discrete spots of retinal opacification (30–60%), papilledema (8% of children, rare in adults), cottonwool spots (>5%), and decoloration of a retinal vessel

Box 96.2 Clinical and Laboratory Findings that Predict a Poor Prognosis and Indicate that the Patient should be Hospitalized in an Intensive Care Unit

Clinical

Abnormal level of consciousness
- Cerebral malaria; Glasgow coma scale <11, Blantyre coma scale ≤3
- Deep coma has the worst prognosis, but delirium, obtundation, and stupor are associated with poor outcome

Retinal hemorrhages

Repeated seizures (≥3 in 24 hours)

Respiratory distress (rapid, deep, labored, stertorous breathing)

Heavy bleeding (unusual)

Shock

Jaundice with other vital organ dysfunction

Parasitologic

>500 000 parasites/μL blood (~10%)

>10 000 mature trophozoites and schizonts/μL blood (parasites with pigment)

>20% parasites with visible pigment

>5% neutrophils with malaria pigment

Laboratory

Elevated serum creatinine (>250 μmol/L)

Acidosis (plasma bicarbonate <15 mmol/L)

Hyperlactatemia (venous lactate >4 mmol/L)

Hypoglycemia (blood glucose <2.2 mmol/L)

Elevated liver enzymes (>3 × normal)

Elevated total bilirubin (>50 μmol/L)

Severe anemia (hematocrit <15%)

Disseminated intravascular coagulation (with bleeding)

(Reproduced from World Health Organization. Division of Control of Tropical Diseases. Severe and complicated malaria. Trans R Soc Trop Med Hyg. 1990;84 (suppl. 2):1–65.)

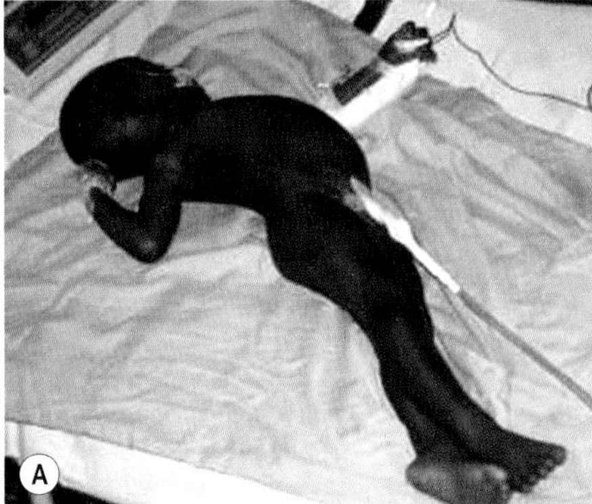

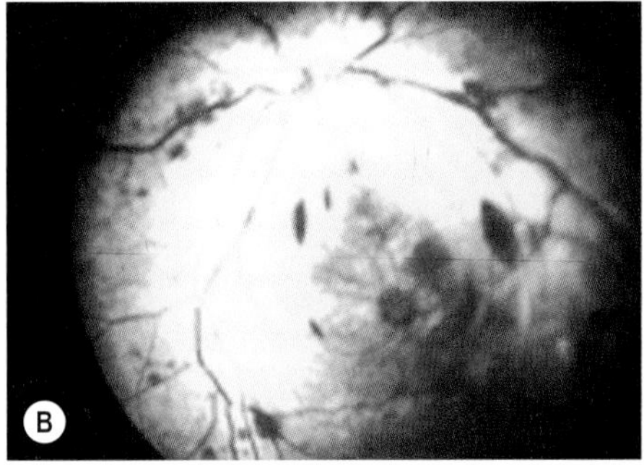

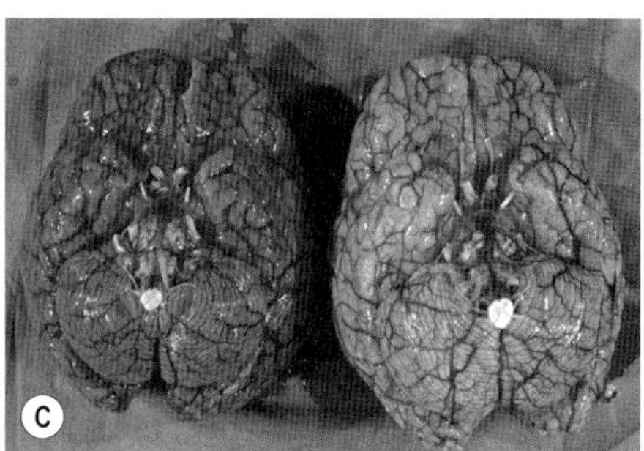

Figure 96.6 Clinical and gross pathologic findings in cerebral malaria. **(A)** Child comatose with cerebral malaria with opisthotonus. **(B)** Retinal hemorrhages (photomicrograph). **(C)** Basal view of the brains of two children. On the left is a brain from a child with cerebral malaria. It is very congested and has a brown-gray color due to heavy hemozoin (malaria) pigment deposition in the blood vessels. On the right is a normal brain, which is relatively pale. It has terminal meningeal congestion only. (**(A)** Courtesy of © J. Crawley, Wellcome Trust International Health Image Collection; **(B)** courtesy of N. White; **(C)** courtesy of © S. B. Lucas, Wellcome Trust International Health Image Collection.)

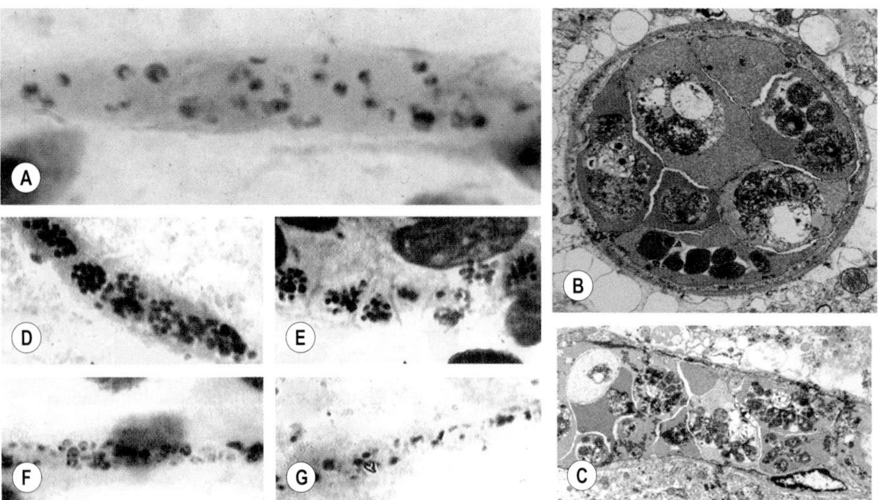

Figure 96.7 Microscopic pathologic findings in cerebral malaria. **(A)** Brain smear (Giemsa) showing sequestration of parasitized erythrocytes. **(B)** and **(C)** Electron micrographs showing venules packed with parasitized erythrocytes; cross-section **(B)** longitudinal section **(C)**. **(D–G)** Different parasite stages sequestered in different venules (reflecting asynchronous upregulation of endothelial adhesion receptors, mainly intercellular adhesion molecule). (Reproduced from Silamut K, Phu NH, Whitty C, et al. A quantitative analysis of the microvascular sequestration of malaria parasites in the human brain. Am J Pathol. 1999;155:395–410. Courtesy of E. Pongpongratn and D. Ferguson.)

or segment of vessel (occasional cases). Convulsions, which are usually generalized and often repeated, occur in up to 50% of children with cerebral malaria. Covert seizure activity is common, particularly in children, and may manifest as repetitive tonic-clonic eye movements. Whereas adults rarely (<3%) suffer neurologic sequelae, approximately 15% of children surviving cerebral malaria – especially those with hypoglycemia, severe anemia, repeated seizures, and deep coma – have some residual neurologic deficit when they regain consciousness; hemiplegia, cerebral palsy, cortical blindness, deafness, and impaired cognition and learning – all of varying duration – have been reported.

Hypoglycemia is a common complication of severe malaria associated with a poor prognosis and is particularly problematic in children and pregnant women. Hypoglycemia in malaria results from a failure of hepatic gluconeogenesis and an increase in the consumption of glucose by both host and parasite. Quinine and quinidine – drugs used commonly for the treatment of severe chloroquine-resistant malaria – are also powerful stimulants of pancreatic insulin secretion. Hyperinsulinemic hypoglycemia is a particular problem in pregnant women receiving quinine treatment. In severe disease, the clinical diagnosis of hypoglycemia is difficult: the usual physical signs (sweating, gooseflesh, tachycardia) are absent, and neurologic impairment caused by hypoglycemia cannot be distinguished from that caused by malaria.

Acidosis is a major feature of severe malaria and an important cause of death. Lactic acidosis is an important component and commonly coexists with hypoglycemia. In adults, coexisting renal impairment often compounds the acidosis, and in children ketoacidosis may also contribute. Acidotic breathing, sometimes called respiratory distress, is a poor prognostic sign. It is often followed by circulatory failure refractory to volume expansion or inotropic drugs, or by respiratory arrest. The plasma concentrations of bicarbonate or lactate are the best biochemical prognosticators in severe malaria. The prognosis of severe acidosis is poor.

Adults with severe *P. falciparum* malaria, and sometimes with *P. vivax* or *P. knowlesi* malaria, may develop noncardiogenic pulmonary edema even after several days of antimalarial therapy. The pathogenesis of this variant of the adult respiratory distress syndrome is unclear. The mortality rate in falciparum malaria is high. This condition can be aggravated by overly vigorous administration of intravenous (IV) fluid.

Mild hemolytic jaundice is common in malaria. Severe jaundice is associated with *P. falciparum* infection, is more common among adults than among children, and results from hemolysis, hepatocyte injury, and cholestasis. When accompanied by other vital organ dysfunction (often renal impairment), liver dysfunction carries a poor prognosis. Hepatic dysfunction contributes to hypoglycemia, lactic acidosis, and impaired drug metabolism. Occasional patients with falciparum malaria may develop deep jaundice (with hemolytic and cholestatic components) without evidence of other vital organ dysfunction.

Renal impairment is common among adults with severe falciparum malaria, and may occur in *P. knowlesi* infections, but is very rare among young children. The pathogenesis of renal failure is unclear but may be related to erythrocyte sequestration interfering with renal microcirculatory flow and metabolism. In patients with severe intravascular hemolysis, hemoglobinuria (blackwater fever) may also cause renal injury. This results in "acute tubular necrosis" although renal cortical necrosis never develops. Acute renal failure (ARF) may occur simultaneously with other vital organ dysfunction, in which case the risk of death is high, or may progress as other disease manifestations resolve. In survivors, urine flow resumes in a median of 4 days, and serum creatinine levels return to normal in a mean of 17 days. Early dialysis or hemofiltration considerably enhances the likelihood of a patient's survival, particularly in acute hypercatabolic renal failure.

Anemia is a prominent feature of malaria. Anemia can develop rapidly, and transfusion is often required. In many areas of Africa, children may develop severe anemia resulting from shortened survival of noninfected erythrocytes, masked dyserythropoiesis, as a consequence of repeated malarial infections, and hemolysis of infected erythrocytes. Anemia is a common consequence of antimalarial drug resistance, which results in repeated or continued infection.

Slight coagulation abnormalities are common in falciparum malaria, and mild thrombocytopenia is usual. Fewer than 5% of patients with severe malaria have significant bleeding with evidence of disseminated intravascular coagulation (DIC). Hematemesis, presumably from stress ulceration or acute gastric erosions, may also occur.

Aspiration pneumonia following convulsions is an important cause of death in cerebral malaria. Chest infections and catheter-induced urinary tract infections are common among patients who are unconscious for more than 3 days. Septicemia may complicate severe malaria; in endemic areas, *Salmonella* bacteremia has been associated specifically with *P. falciparum* infections.

Malaria in Pregnancy

In hyperendemic and holoendemic areas, falciparum malaria especially in primigravid and secundigravid women is associated with LBW (average reduction, ~170 g) and consequently increased neonatal mortality. In general, infected mothers in areas of stable transmission remain asymptomatic despite intense accumulation of parasitized erythrocytes in the placental microcirculation. Maternal HIV infection predisposes pregnant women to malaria and predisposes their newborns to congenital malaria infection and LBW.

In areas with unstable transmission of malaria, pregnant women are particularly vulnerable to developing severe malaria with high-density parasitemias, anemia, hypoglycemia, and acute pulmonary edema. Fetal distress, premature labor, and stillbirth or LBW are common. Congenital malaria occurs in <5% of newborns whose mothers are infected and is related directly to the parasite density in maternal blood and in the placenta. *P. vivax* malaria in pregnancy is also associated with a reduction in birth weight (average, 100 g), but, in contrast with the situation in falciparum malaria, this effect is greater in multigravid than in primigravid women.

Malaria in Children

Most of the estimated 0.8–1 million persons who die as a consequence of falciparum infection each year are young African children. In endemic areas there is considerable diagnostic overlap between septicemia and severe malaria. Convulsions, coma, hypoglycemia, metabolic acidosis, and severe anemia are more common among children with severe malaria than in adults, whereas deep jaundice, ARF, and acute pulmonary edema are unusual in childhood. Severely anemic children may have labored deep breathing, which in the past has been attributed incorrectly to "anemic congestive cardiac failure" but is caused by metabolic acidosis, often compounded by hypovolemia. In general, children tolerate antimalarial drugs well and respond rapidly to treatment.

Transfusion Malaria

Malaria can be transmitted by blood transfusion, needlestick injury, sharing of needles by infected drug addicts, or organ transplantation. The incubation period in these settings is often short because there is no pre-erythrocytic stage of development. The clinical features and management of these cases are the same as for naturally acquired infections. Radical chemotherapy with primaquine is unnecessary for blood-transmitted *P. vivax* and *P. ovale* infections.

Hyperreactive Malarial Splenomegaly

Chronic or repeated malarial infections produce hypergammaglobulinemia; normochromic, normocytic anemia; and, in certain situations, splenomegaly. Some residents of malaria-endemic areas of tropical Africa and Asia exhibit an abnormal immunologic response to repeated infection that is characterized by massive splenomegaly, hepatomegaly, marked elevations in serum titers of IgM and malarial antibody, hepatic sinusoidal lymphocytosis, and (in Africa) peripheral B-cell lymphocytosis. This syndrome, which is called hyperreactive malaria splenomegaly (HMS) (formerly called tropical splenomegaly syndrome), has been associated with the production of cytotoxic IgM antibodies to suppressor ($CD8^+$) lymphocytes, antibodies to $CD4^+$ T cells, and an increase in the ratio of $CD4^+$ T cells to $CD8^+$ T cells.[66] These events may lead to uninhibited B-cell production of IgM and the formation of cryoglobulins (IgM aggregates and immune complexes). This immunologic process stimulates reticuloendothelial hyperplasia and clearance activity and eventually produces splenomegaly. Patients with HMS feel an abdominal mass or a dragging sensation in the abdomen and occasional sharp abdominal pains suggesting perisplenitis. Anemia and some degree of pancytopenia are usually evident, but in many cases malarial parasites cannot be found in peripheral blood smears. Vulnerability to respiratory and skin infections is increased; many patients die of overwhelming sepsis. Persons with HMS who are living in endemic areas should receive antimalarial chemoprophylaxis; the results are usually good. Splenectomy has been used for refractory cases with apparent success.[67] In nonendemic areas, antimalarial treatment is advised. In some cases refractory to therapy, clonal lymphoproliferation may develop and then evolve to a malignant lymphoproliferative disorder.

Quartan Malarial Nephropathy

Chronic or repeated infections with *P. malariae*, and possibly other malarial species, may cause soluble immunocomplex injury to the renal glomeruli, resulting in the nephrotic syndrome. Other unidentified factors must contribute to this process, since only a small proportion of infected patients develop renal disease. The histologic appearance is that of focal or segmental glomerulonephritis with splitting of the capillary basement membrane. Subendothelial dense deposits are seen on electron microscopy, and immunofluorescence reveals deposits of complement and immunoglobulins; in samples of renal tissue, *P. malariae* antigens are often visible. A coarse granular pattern of basement membrane immunofluorescent deposits (predominantly IgG_3) with selective proteinuria carries a better prognosis than a fine granular, predominantly IgG_2 pattern with nonselective proteinuria. Quartan nephropathy usually responds poorly to treatment with either antimalarial agents or glucocorticoids and cytotoxic drugs.

Burkitt's Lymphoma and Epstein–Barr Virus Infection

It is possible that malaria-related immunosuppression promotes infection with lymphoma viruses. Burkitt's lymphoma is strongly associated with Epstein–Barr virus. The prevalence of this childhood tumor is high in malarious areas of Africa.

Laboratory Findings

Normochromic, normocytic anemia is usual in acute malaria. The leukocyte count is generally normal, although it may be raised in very severe infections, and lowered in early mild infections. The erythrocyte sedimentation rate, plasma viscosity, and levels of C-reactive protein and other acute-phase proteins are high. The platelet count is usually reduced to approximately $10^5/\mu L$. Severe infections may be accompanied by prolonged prothrombin and partial thromboplastin times and by more severe thrombocytopenia. In uncomplicated malaria, plasma concentrations of electrolytes, blood urea nitrogen, and creatinine are usually normal, or minimally altered. Findings in severe malaria may include metabolic acidosis, with low plasma concentrations of glucose, sodium, bicarbonate, calcium, phosphate, and albumin together with elevations in lactate, blood urea nitrogen, creatinine, urate, muscle and liver enzymes, and conjugated and unconjugated bilirubin. Hypergammaglobulinemia is usual in immune and semi-immune subjects, and urinalysis generally gives normal results. In adults and children with cerebral malaria, the mean opening pressure at lumbar puncture (LP) is approximately 160 mm of cerebrospinal fluid (CSF); the CSF is usually normal or has a slightly elevated total protein level (<1.0 g/L (100 mg/dL)) and cell count (<20/μL).

PATHOGENESIS

The pathophysiology of malaria results from destruction of erythrocytes (both infected and uninfected), the consequent liberation of parasite and erythrocyte material into the circulation, and the host reaction to these events. *P. falciparum* malaria-infected erythrocytes specifically sequester in the microcirculation of vital organs, interfering with microcirculatory flow and host tissue metabolism.

Toxicity and the Role of Cytokines

No potent malaria toxin has been identified, but malaria parasites do induce release of cytokines in much the same way as bacterial endotoxin does.[68] A glycolipid material, derived from the GPI anchor that covalently links malaria parasite surface antigens to erthrocyte membranes, with some similarities to bacterial endotoxin is released on schizont rupture. Malaria antigen-related IgE complexes also activate cytokine release. These malaria parasite products induce activation of the cytokine cascade, but they are considerably less potent than bacteria. For example, an *Escherichia coli* bacteremia of 1 bacterium/mL carries an approximate mortality of 20%, whereas in falciparum malaria only parasitemias of well over 10^9/mL have such a lethal effect. Cells of the macrophage–monocyte series, γ/δ T cells, α/β T cells, $CD14^+$ cells, and possibly endothelium, are stimulated to release cytokines in a mutually amplifying chain reaction. Initially, tumor necrosis factor-α (TNF), which plays a pivotal role, interleukin (IL)-1, and γ-interferon are produced and in turn induce release of a cascade of other "proinflammatory" cytokines, including IL-8, IL-12, and IL-18. These are balanced by production of the "anti-inflammatory" cytokines IL-6 and IL-10. Cytokines are responsible for many symptoms and signs of the infection, particularly fever and malaise. Plasma inflammatory cytokine concentrations are elevated in both acute *P. vivax* and *P. falciparum* malaria.[69] In established vivax malaria, which tends to synchronize earlier than *P. falciparum*, a pulse release of TNF occurs at the time of schizont rupture and is followed by the characteristic symptoms and signs of the "paroxysm," i.e., shivering, cool extremities, headache, chills, a spike of fever, and sometimes rigors followed by sweating, vasodilatation, and defervescence. For a given number of parasites, *P. vivax* is a more potent inducer of TNF release than *P. falciparum*, which may explain why it has a lower pyrogenic density.

There is a positive correlation between cytokine levels and prognosis in severe falciparum malaria and a disturbed balance between pro- and anti-inflammatory cytokines.[69] Acute malaria is associated with high levels of most cytokines, but the balance differs in relation to severity. IL-12 and transforming growth factor-β1, which may regulate the balance between pro- and anti-inflammatory cytokines, are higher in uncomplicated than in severe malaria. IL-10, a potent anti-inflammatory cytokine, increases markedly in severe malaria but, in fatal cases, does not increase sufficiently to restrain the production of TNF.[69] A reduced IL-10/TNF ratio has also been associated with childhood malarial anemia in areas of high transmission.

Does TNF play a causal role in cerebral dysfunction or death from severe malaria? Genetic studies from Africa indicate that children with the 308A TNF2 allele, a polymorphism in the TNF promoter region, have a relative risk of 7 for death or neurologic sequelae from cerebral malaria.[70] A separate polymorphism in this region that affects gene expression was associated with a fourfold increased risk of cerebral malaria. On the other hand, the clinical studies in cerebral malaria with anti-TNF antibodies and other strategies to reduce TNF production to date have shown no convincing effects other than reduction in fever. Furthermore the 308 polymorphism is not associated with fatal cerebral malaria in Asian adults.[71] There is no direct evidence that systemic release of TNF or other cytokines causes coma in humans (although mechanisms involving release of nitric oxide within the central nervous system (CNS) and consequent inhibition of neurotransmission can be hypothesized). In adults with severe malaria, elevated plasma TNF concentrations have been associated specifically with renal dysfunction,[68,69] and TNF levels were actually lower in patients with pure cerebral malaria compared with those with other manifestations of severe disease. Severe malarial anemia has been associated with a different TNF promoter polymorphism (238A; odds ratio 2.5).

Cytokines are probably involved in placental dysfunction, suppression of erythropoiesis, and inhibition of gluconeogenesis, and do cause fever in malaria. Tolerance to malaria, or premunition, reflects both immune regulation of the infection and also reduced production of cytokines in response to malaria ("antitoxic immunity"). Cytokines may also be important mediators of parasite killing by activating leukocytes, and possibly other cells, to release toxic oxygen species and nitric oxide, and by generating parasiticidal lipid peroxides and causing fever. So, whereas high concentrations of cytokines may be harmful, lower levels probably promote parasite clearance and thereby benefit the host.

Sequestration and Cytoadherence

Erythrocytes containing mature forms of *P. falciparum* adhere to microvascular endothelium ("cytoadherence") and thus disappear from the circulation. This is called sequestration, and it starts at ~12 hours of asexual development. The process is accelerated by fever. Sequestration does not occur to a significant extent with the other human malaria parasites. Sequestration is thought to be central to the pathophysiology of falciparum malaria, since it interferes with microcirculatory flow (***Fig. 96.7***).[72] Once infected, erthrocytes adhere and do not enter the circulation again, remaining stuck until they rupture at merogony (schizogony). As a consequence, whereas in the other malarias of humans, mature parasites are commonly seen on blood smears, these forms are rare in falciparum malaria and often indicate serious infection. It was thought that ring-stage infected erythrocytes do not cytoadhere at all, but recent pathologic and laboratory studies show that they do, although much less so than more mature stages. Sequestration occurs predominantly in the venules of vital organs. It is greatest in the brain, particularly in the white matter; prominent in the heart, eyes, liver, kidneys, intestines, and adipose tissue; and least frequent in the skin. Even within the brain, the distribution of sequestered erythrocytes varies markedly from vessel to vessel,[72] presumably reflecting differences in the local expression of endothelial receptors. Cytoadherence and the related phenomenon of rosetting lead to microcirculatory obstruction in falciparum malaria. The consequences of microcirculatory obstruction are activation of the vascular endothelium and reduced oxygen and substrate supply, which leads to anaerobic glycolysis, lactic acidosis, and cellular dysfunction.

Cytoadherence is mediated by several different processes. The most important parasite ligands are a family of strain-specific, high-molecular-weight, parasite-derived proteins, PfEMP1. These proteins are encoded by *var* genes, a family of over 50 genes distributed throughout the parasite's genome.[22–24] PfEMP1 are transcribed, synthesized, and stored within the parasite and, beginning at around 12 hours of development, are then exported to the surface of the infected erythrocyte. These accretions cause knobs on the surface of the red cell, and these are the points of attachment to vascular endothelium. PfEMP1 expression is greatest at the middle of the asexual cycle. PfEMP1 also appears to be a major antigenic determinant for the blood-stage parasite. As in other protozoal parasites, the immunodominant surface antigen undergoes antigenic variation to "change its coat" and avoid immune-mediated attack. *P. falciparum* "switches" to a new variant of PfEMP1 at a rate of at least 2% per cycle.[73] In the chronic phase of untreated infection, this results in small waves of parasitemia approximately every 3 weeks. The central role of parasite-derived proteins in cytoadherence is not accepted by all. It has been suggested that cytoadherence is mediated by altered red cell membrane components such as a modified form of the red cell cytoskeletal protein band 3 (the major erythrocyte anion transporter). In culture, most parasites lose the ability to cytoadhere after several cycles of replication. *In vivo*, cytoadherence may be modulated by the spleen. In splenectomized patients who develop falciparum malaria, all stages of the parasite can be seen in peripheral blood smears.

Vascular Endothelial Ligands

Several different sticky proteins present on the surface of vascular endothelium have been shown to bind parasitized red cells. The interaction between these proteins and the variant surface adhesin of the parasitized red cell is complex. Probably the most important protein is CD36;[74] nearly all freshly obtained parasites bind to CD36. Binding is increased at low pH (<7.0) and in the presence of high calcium concentrations. CD36 is constitutionally expressed on vascular endothelium and monocytes/macrophages, although usually it is not present on the surface of cerebral vessels. CD36 is expressed on platelets, and platelets may form a bridge between infected erythrocytes and vascular endothelium. The intercellular adhesion molecule (ICAM1) appears to be the major cytoadherence receptor in the brain.[75] Expression of ICAM1, but not CD36, is upregulated by cytokines (notably TNF). At physiologic shear rates (i.e., those likely to be encountered in the human microcirculation) the binding forces ($\approx 10^{-10}$ N) are similar for CD36 and ICAM1. Binding to the two ligands is synergistic.[76] Once stuck, parasitized erythrocytes remain attached until schizont rupture, and then the residual erythrocyte ghost's membranes (sometimes with attached malaria pigment) often remain tethered within the vessel. Thrombospondin (a natural ligand to CD36) also binds to some parasitized red cells (probably to modified band 3), and other endothelial adhesion proteins, VCAM, PECAM, E-selectin, and α/β integrin, have also been shown to bind in some circumstances.[76] P-selectin has been shown to mediate rolling. The relative importance of these molecules and their interactions are still not clear. Chondroitin sulfate A (CSA) appears to be a major receptor for cytoadherence in the placenta.[77] Hyaluronic acid also has been proposed as a candidate for placental adhesion. Antibodies that inhibit parasitized red cell cytoadherence to CSA are generally present in multigravidae in endemic areas but not in primigravidae.[78] This may explain why the adverse effects of pregnancy on birth weight are greater in primigravidae. Thus, ICAM1 appears to be the major vascular ligand in the brain involved in cerebral sequestration, CSA is the major ligand in the placenta, and CD36 is probably the major ligand in the other organs and also in platelet-mediated cytoadherence. Other as yet unidentified vascular receptors are also present, since sequestration also occurs in vessels expressing none of the potential ligands identified so far. Severity is related to the number of parasites in the body and distribution of cytoadherence within the vital organs. The relative importance of parasite phenotype and the various potential vascular ligands in the pathophysiology of severe falciparum malaria and the precise role of the spleen remain to be determined.

Rosetting and Aggregation

Erythrocytes containing mature parasites also adhere to uninfected erythrocytes.[79] This process leads to the formation of "rosettes" seen when suspensions of parasitized erythrocytes are viewed under the microscope. Rosetting shares some characteristics of cytoadherence. It starts at around 16 hours of the asexual life cycle development (slightly after cytoadherence begins) and is trypsin-sensitive. However, parasite species that do not sequester do form rosettes, and, unlike cytoadherence, rosetting is inhibited by certain heparin subfractions and calcium chelators. Furthermore, whereas all fresh isolates of *P. falciparum* cytoadhere, not all rosette. Rosetting is mediated by attachment of specific domains of PfEMP1 to the complement receptor CR1, heparan sulfate, blood group A antigen, and probably other red cell surface molecules. Attachment is facilitated by serum components. Rosetting has been associated with severe malaria in some studies but not in others.[80] It has been suggested that rosetting might encourage cytoadherence by reducing flow (shear rate), which would enhance anaerobic glycolysis, reduce pH, and facilitate adherence of infected erythrocytes to venular endothelium. Rosetting tends to start in venules, and this certainly could reduce flow. The adhesive forces involved in rosetting could also impede forward flow of uninfected erythrocytes as they squeeze past sticky cytoadherent parasitized red cells in capillaries and venules. The mechanical obstruction, or "static hindrance," would be compounded by the lack of deformability of the adherent and circulating parasitized red cells. Another adherence property of parasitized red cells has been characterized and associated with disease severity in African children and Thai adults.[81] This is the platelet-mediated aggregation of parasitized erythrocytes and is mediated via platelet CD36. These cells clump together in *ex vivo* cultures. Aggregation could also contribute to vascular occlusion.

Erythrocyte Deformability

As the parasite matures inside the erythrocyte, its normally flexible biconcave disc becomes progressively more spherical and rigid. The reduction in deformability results from reduced membrane fluidity, increasing sphericity, and the enlarging and relatively rigid intraerythrocytic parasite. Loss of normal, uninfected erythrocyte deformability has been recognized recently as a major contributor to disease severity and outcome. Increased erythrocyte rigidity measured at the low shear stresses encountered in capillaries and venules is correlated closely with outcome in severe malaria.[81] When assessed at the shear rates encountered on the arterial side, and importantly in the spleen, reduced red cell deformability correlates with anemia. This is a malaria-specific phenomenon, since it is not found in severe sepsis.

IMMUNOLOGIC PROCESSES

It is unlikely that severe malaria, in particular cerebral malaria, results from specific immune-mediated damage. In relation to the degree of parasitized erythrocyte sequestration, relatively few leukocytes are found in or around the cerebral vessels in fatal cases (although there are more in African children than in adults studied in Southeast Asia). Thus, there is little pathologic evidence in humans for widepread cerebral vasculitis or inflammatory infiltrates. Indeed, fatal falciparum malaria is remarkable for the lack of extravascular pathology. Despite the enormous intravascular antigenic load in malaria, with the formation and deposition of immune complexes and variable complement depletion, there is little evidence of a specific immunopathologic process in severe malaria.

Acute malaria infections are associated with malaria antigen-specific unresponsiveness. This selective paresis is one of the factors contributing to the slow development of an effective and specific immune response in malaria. Acute malaria is characterized by nonspecific polyclonal B-cell activation. There is a reduction in circulating T cells with an increase in the γ/δ T-cell subset, but other T-cell proportions usually are normal. Although residents of hyperendemic or holoendemic malarious areas have hypergammaglobulinemia, most of this antibody is not directed against malaria antigens. In nonimmune individuals, the acute antibody response to infection often comprises mostly IgM or IgG_2 isotypes, which are unable to arm cytotoxic cells and thus kill asexual malaria parasites. These observations have led to the suggestion that malaria induces an immunologic "smoke screen" with broad-spectrum and nonspecific activation that interferes with the orderly development of a specific cellular immune response. In severe malaria there is evidence of a broader immune suppression, with defects in monocyte and neutrophil chemotaxis, reduced monocytic phagocytic function, and a tendency to bacterial superinfection.

In the nephrotic syndrome associated with chronic *P. malariae* infections, malaria antigen and immune complexes can be eluted from the kidney, indicating a role for quartan malaria in this condition. Why some children are affected while the majority are not is unresolved.

Cerebral Malaria

In the past it was suggested that cerebral malaria resulted from an increase in cerebral capillary permeability, which led to brain swelling, coma, and death. There is evidence of a mild generalized increase in systemic vascular permeability in severe malaria, but it is now clear from imaging studies that the majority of adults and children with cerebral malaria show no evidence of cerebral edema. However, the role of raised intracranial pressure in cerebral malaria remains unclear. Whereas 80% of adults have opening pressures at LP that are in the normal range (<200 mm CSF), 80% of children have elevated opening pressures (>100 mm CSF; the normal range is lower in children), and intracranial pressure may rise transiently to very high levels. Some patients with cerebral malaria die of acute respiratory arrest with neurologic signs that are compatible with brainstem compression. However, these signs are also common and may persist for many hours in survivors.[83] The elevation in opening pressure usually is not great (in general it is much lower than in bacterial or fungal meningitis), and there is no difference between these LP opening pressures in surviving children and fatal cases. Studies of computed tomography or magnetic resonance imaging generally show slight brain swelling in cerebral malaria (compatible with an increased intracerebral blood volume).[84] Immunohistochemical studies on autopsy brain tissues indicate focal disruption of endothelial junctions and endothelial activation in areas of intense sequestration, but clinical investigations have failed to detect major alterations in blood–brain barrier permeability. Thus, raised intracranial pressure probably arises from an increase in cerebral blood volume, independent of permeability.[85] This results from the circulating blood required to maintain cerebral perfusion and a considerable sequestered static biomass of intracerebral parasites. Children may be particularly vulnerable, since after the skull sutures have fused, there is less space for cranial expansion than in adults. The possibility that a sudden rise in intracranial pressure accounts for some deaths cannot be excluded.[85]

The cause of coma in cerebral malaria is not known. Undoubtedly there is an increase in cerebral anaerobic glycolysis with cerebral blood flows that are inappropriately low for the arterial oxygen content, increased cerebral metabolic rates for lactate, and increased CSF concentrations of lactate; but these changes do not provide sufficient explanation for coma. Presumably the metabolic milieu created adjacent to the sequestered and highly metabolically active parasites and their attachment to the activated cerebral vascular endothelium interfere with endothelial and blood–brain barrier function. But how this interferes with neurotransmission is not known. Recent studies point to a disruption of axonal transport as the most likely explanation for rapidly reversible neurologic deficit. Cytokines increase production of nitric oxide, a potent inhibitor of neurotransmission, by leukocytes, smooth-muscle cells, microglia, and vascular endothelium through induction of the enzyme nitric oxide synthase. Inducible nitric oxide synthase expression is increased in the brain in fatal cerebral malaria.

Renal Failure

There is renal cortical vasoconstriction and consequent hypoperfusion in severe falciparum malaria. In patients with ARF, renal vascular resistance is increased. The renal injury in severe malaria results in acute tubular necrosis. The oxygen consumption of the kidneys is reduced in ARF, and it is not improved by dopamine-induced arteriolar vasodilatation and consequent increase in renal blood flow, suggesting a fixed injury.[85] Acute tubular necrosis presumably results from renal microvascular obstruction and cellular injury consequent upon sequestration in the kidney and the filtration of free Hb, myoglobin, and other cellular material. Significant glomerulonephritis is rare. Massive hemolysis compounds the insult in blackwater fever complicating malaria, and hemoglobinuria may itself lead to renal impairment. Mild renal impairment occurs in young children with severe malaria, but established ARF is almost confined to older children and adults.

Pulmonary Edema

Despite intense sequestration in the myocardial vessels, the heart's pump function is remarkably well preserved in severe malaria. Pulmonary edema in malaria results from a sudden increase in pulmonary capillary permeability that is not reflected in other vascular beds.[87] The pulmonary capillary wedge pressure is usually normal, and the threshold for the development of pulmonary edema is relatively low. Whereas ARF, severe metabolic acidosis, and coma are seen only in falciparum malaria, acute pulmonary edema may also occur in vivax and knowlesi malaria. The cause of this increase in pulmonary capillary permeability is not known.

Fluid Space and Electrolyte Changes

Following rehydration, the plasma volume is increased in moderate and severe malaria. Total body water and extracellular volume are usually normal or slightly reduced, even in children who are acidotic. Plasma renin activity, aldosterone, and antidiuretic hormone concentrations are elevated, reflecting an appropriate activation of homeostatic mechanisms to maintain adequate circulating volume in the presence of general vasodilatation and a falling hematocrit. Mild hyponatremia and hypochloremia are common in severe malaria, but serum potassium concentrations usually are normal. Occasionally hyponatremia is severe. Studies in Kenyan children indicate inappropriate antidiuretic hormone secretion in two-thirds of cases,[88] although this has not been confirmed in Bangladeshi adults.[89]

Anemia

The pathogenesis of anemia is multifactorial. There is obligatory destruction of red cells containing parasites at merogony, accelerated destruction of nonparasitized red cells that parallels disease severity, and bone marrow dyserythropoiesis. In severe malaria, anemia develops rapidly; the rapid hemolysis of unparasitized red cells is the major contributor to the decline in hematocrit.[90] Bone marrow dyserythropoiesis persists for days or weeks following acute malaria, and reticulocyte counts are usually low in the acute phase of the disease. The cause of the dyserythropoiesis is thought to be related to intramedullary cytokine production. Serum erythropoietin levels are usually elevated, although in some series it has been suggested that the degree of elevation was insufficient for the degree of anemia.

In falciparum malaria, the entire red cell population (i.e., both infected and uninfected red cells) becomes more rigid. This loss of deformability correlates with disease severity and outcome and, when measured at the high shear rates encountered in the spleen, with the degree of resulting anemia. The mechanism responsible has not been identified, although there is evidence in acute malaria for increased oxidative damage, which might compromise red cell membrane function and deformability.

The role of antibody (i.e., Coombs'-positive hemolysis) in anemia is unresolved. The majority of studies do not show increased red cell immunoglobulin binding in malaria, but, in the presence of a lowered recognition threshold for splenic clearance, this might be difficult to detect. The splenic threshold for the clearance of abnormal erythrocytes, whether because of antibody coating or reduced deformability, is lowered. Thus, the spleen removes large numbers of relatively rigid cells, resulting in shortened erythrocyte survival, particularly in severe malaria. This is unaffected by corticosteroids.

In the context of acute uncomplicated malaria, the anemia is worse in younger children and those with protracted infections. Loss of unparasitized erythrocytes accounts for approximately 90% of the acute anemia resulting from a single infection. Iron deficiency and malaria often coincide in the same patient, and in some areas routine iron supplementation following malaria promotes recovery from anemia.

Coagulopathy and Thrombocytopenia

There is accelerated coagulation cascade activity with accelerated fibrinogen turnover, consumption of antithrombin III, reduced factor XIII, and increased concentrations of fibrin degradation products in acute malaria. In severe infections, the prothrombin and partial thromboplastin times may be prolonged, and in occasional patients (<5%) bleeding may be significant. The coagulation cascade is activated via the intrinsic pathway. Despite this, intravascular thrombus formation is observed rarely at autopsy in fatal cases, and fibrin deposition is sparse and platelets are strikingly unusual.

Thrombocytopenia is common to all human malarias and is caused by increased splenic clearance. Platelet turnover is increased.[91] The role of platelet-bound antibody in malarial thrombocytopenia is controversial. There is evidence of platelet activation in some studies but not others. Erythrocytes containing mature parasites may activate the coagulation cascade directly, and cytokine release is also procoagulant. It was suggested in the past that DIC is important in the pathogenesis of severe malaria, but detailed prospective clinical and pathogenesis studies have refuted this. Coagulation cascade activity is directly proportional to disease severity, but hypofibrinogenemia resulting from DIC is significant in less than 5% of patients with severe malaria, and lethal hemorrhage (usually gastrointestinal) is quite unusual.

Blackwater Fever

This is a poorly understood condition in which there is massive intravascular hemolysis and the passage of Coca-Cola-colored urine. Blackwater (urine) occurs in three circumstances: (1) when patients with G6PD deficiency take oxidant drugs (e.g., primaquine or sulfonamides) irrespective of whether they have malaria; (2) occasionally when patients with G6PD deficiency have malaria and receive quinine treatment; and (3) in some patients with severe, quinine-treated falciparum malaria who have normal erythrocyte G6PD levels. How quinine causes blackwater in these last two situations is not known, since it is not an oxidant drug. G6PD-deficient red cells are particularly susceptible to oxidant stress because they are unable to synthesize adequate quantities of NADPH through the pentose shunt. This leads to low intraerythrocytic levels of reduced glutathione and both alterations in the erythrocyte membrane and increased susceptibility to organic peroxides. Blackwater fever may be associated with ARF, although in most cases renal function remains normal.

The Spleen

There is considerable splenic enlargement in malaria and an increased capacity to clear red cells from the circulation both by Fc receptor-mediated (immune) mechanisms and by recognition of reduced deformability (filtration). The increased filtration of the spleen and the reduced deformability of the entire red cell population result in the rapid development of anemia in severe malaria. The spleen may also modulate cytoadherence. It plays a central role in limiting the acute expansion of malarial infections by removing parasitized erythrocytes, and this has led to the suggestion that a failure to augment splenic clearance sufficiently rapidly may be a factor in the development of severe malaria. The spleen is capable of removing damaged intraerythrocytic parasites and returning the once-infected red cells to the circulation (a process known as "pitting"),[92] where they have shortened survival. This is an important contributor to parasite clearance following antimalarial drug treatment (particularly treatment with artemisinin derivatives).

Gastrointestinal Dysfunction

Abdominal pain may be prominent in acute malaria. Minor stress ulceration of the stomach and duodenum is common in severe malaria. The pattern of malabsorption of sugars, fats, and amino acids suggests reduced splanchnic perfusion. This results from both sequestration of parasites in the microcirculation of the gut leading to decreased oxygen delivery and visceral vasoconstriction. Gut permeability is increased, and this may be associated with reduced local defenses against bacterial toxins or even whole bacteria in severe disease. Antimalarial drug absorption is remarkably unaffected in uncomplicated malaria, except for those drugs which have fat (i.e., food)-dependent absorption (halofantrine, atovaquone, lumefantrine).

Liver Dysfunction

Jaundice is common in adults with severe malaria, and there is other evidence of hepatic dysfunction, with often moderate increases in transaminases, reduced clotting factor synthesis, reduced metabolic clearance of the antimalarial drugs, and a failure of gluconeogenesis, which contributes to lactic acidosis and hypoglycemia. Nevertheless, true liver failure (as in fulminant viral hepatitis) is unusual. There is sequestration in the hepatic microvasculature, and although many patients with acute falciparum malaria have elevated liver blood flow values,[93,94] in very severe infections liver blood flow is reduced. Liver blood flow values less than 15 mL/kg/min are associated with elevated venous lactate concentrations, suggesting a flow limitation to lactate clearance and thus a contribution of liver dysfunction to lactic acidosis. Direct measurements of hepatic venous lactate concentrations in severe malaria confirm that the hepatosplanchnic extraction ratio is inversely correlated with mixed venous plasma lactate (i.e., hyperlactatemia is associated with reduced liver clearance of lactate). There is no relationship between liver blood flow and impairment of antimalarial drug clearance. Jaundice in malaria appears to have hemolytic and cholestatic components. Cholestatic jaundice may persist well into the recovery period.

Acidosis

Lactic acidosis results from several discrete processes: the tissue anaerobic glycolysis consequent upon microvascular obstruction; a failure of hepatic and renal lactate clearance; and the production of lactate by the parasite. Lactate turnover in both adults and children with severe malaria is increased approximately threefold compared with values obtained in healthy adults.[95] Studies in children using stable isotope techniques indicate that increased lactate production (resulting from anaerobic glycolysis) rather than reduced clearance is the main cause of lactate accumulation, although in adults reduced clearance is certainly a contributor. Hyperlactatemia is associated with hypoglycemia and is accompanied by hyperalaninemia and elevated glycerol concentrations, reflecting the impairment of gluconeogenesis. Lactate, glutamine, and alanine are the major gluconeogenic precursors. Triglyceride and free fatty acid levels are also elevated in acute malaria, and plasma concentrations of ketone bodies are raised in patients who have been unable to eat. Ketoacidosis may be prominent in children. Sequestration has recently been visualized and quantified *in vivo* in severe malaria[96] and the degree of microvascular obstruction correlated with hyperlactatemia.

Acidosis is a major cause of death in severe falciparum malaria. Recent studies indicate that the main acid (i.e., the main contributor to the anion gap) is unidentified. There is commonly a lactic acidosis, although ketoacidosis (and sometimes salicylate intoxication) may predominate in children, and the acidosis of renal failure is common in adults.[97,98] In severe malaria, the arterial, capillary, venous, and CSF concentrations of lactate rise in direct proportion to disease severity. In bacterial sepsis there is hyperlactatemia, but unless there is profound shock, the lactate-to-pyruvate ratio is usually less than 15. This indicates that hypermetabolism is the source of lactate accumulation in sepsis. In severe malaria the pathogenesis is different; lactate-to-pyruvate ratios often exceed 30, reflecting tissue hypoxia and anaerobic glycolysis.

In severe malaria there is dysfunction of all organ systems, particularly those with obligatory high metabolic rates. The endocrine glands are no exception. Pituitary–thyroid axis abnormalities result in the "sick euthyroid" syndrome and also parathyroid dysfunction. Mild hypocalcemia is common, and hypophosphatemia may be profound in the very seriously ill. The pituitary–adrenal axis, however, appears normal in acute malaria.

Hypoglycemia

Hypoglycemia, associated with hyperlactatemia, shares the same pathophysiological etiologies: an increased peripheral requirement for glucose consequent upon anaerobic glycolysis, the increased metabolic demands of the febrile illness,[95] the obligatory demands of the parasites that use glucose as their major fuel (all of which increase demand), and a failure of hepatic gluconeogenesis and glycogenolysis (reduced supply).[99] Hepatic glycogen is exhausted rapidly: stores in fasting adults last approximately 2 days, but children have enough for only 12 hours. Healthy children have approximately three times higher rates of glucose turnover compared with adults, but in severe malaria turnover is increased by >50% (to values 5 times higher than those in adults with severe malaria). The net result of impaired gluconeogenesis, limited glycogen stores, and greatly increased demand results in a hypoglycemia in 20–30% of children with severe malaria.[100,101] In patients treated with quinine, this is compounded by quinine-stimulated pancreatic β-cell insulin secretion.[99] Hyperinsulinemia is balanced by reduced tissue sensitivity to insulin, which returns to normal as the patient improves. This probably explains why quinine-induced (hyperinsulinemic) hypoglycemia tends to occur after the first 24 hours of treatment, whereas malaria-related hypoglycemia (with appropriate suppression of insulin secretion) is often present when the patient with severe malaria is first admitted. Hypoglycemia contributes to CNS dysfunction, and in cerebral malaria is associated with residual neurologic deficit in survivors.

Placental Dysfunction

Pregnancy is associated with an increased frequency of a spectrum of *P. falciparum* pathologies. This is probably caused by a suppression of systemic and placental cell-mediated immune responses. There is intense sequestration of *P. falciparum*-infected erythrocytes in the placenta, local activation of proinflammatory cytokine production, and maternal anemia. This leads to placental insufficiency and fetal growth retardation. Illness close to term results in prematurity. In areas of intense transmission, a malaria-attributable reduction in birth weight (≈170 g) is confined to primigravidae.[102] There is no convincing evidence that malaria causes abortion or stillbirth in this context. With lower levels of transmission (i.e., less immunity) the risk extends to other pregnancies, and there is a propensity to develop severe malaria with a high incidence of fetal death. The documentation that *P. vivax*, a parasite originally not thought to cytoadhere, also reduces birth weight (by about two-thirds the amount caused by *P. falciparum*) has questioned the primary role of sequestration in the pathogenesis of placental insufficiency.[103] However, recent evidence suggests *P. vivax* infected red cells do adhere to chondroitin sulfate A in a similar manner to *P. falciparum*.

Bacterial Infection

Patients with severe malaria are vulnerable to bacterial infections, particularly of the lungs and urinary tract (following catheterization). Postpartum sepsis is common. Spontaneous bacterial septicemia may also occur. It is relatively unusual in adults (probably <1% of cases) but is much more common in young children. In malaria-endemic areas, where parasitemia is common in children, it may be difficult to distinguish bacterial infections with coincident parasitemia from infections complicating malaria. *Salmonella* septicemias are an important complication of otherwise uncomplicated falciparum malaria in African children.

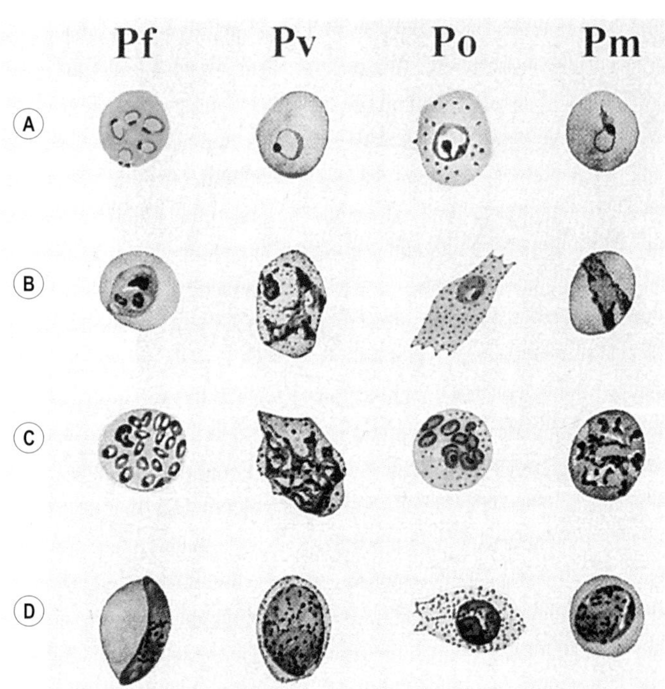

Figure 96.8 Diagnostic forms of malaria in Giemsa-stained thin blood films. Thick smears (not shown) would show parasite forms after lysis of red blood cells. Columns: Pf, *Plasmodium falciparum*; Pv, *P. vivax*; Po, *P. ovale*; Pm; *P. malariae*. Rows: **(A and B)** young and old trophozoites; **(C)** schizonts; **(D)** gametocytes. (Adapted from drawings by Inez Demoney in Brown HW, Neva FA. Basic Clinical Parasitology, 5th ed. Norwalk, CT: Appleton-Century-Crofts; 1983; and World Health Organization. Bench Aids for the Diagnosis of Malaria. Geneva: World Health Organization; 1983).

DIAGNOSIS

Prompt and accurate diagnosis of malaria is the key to effective disease management. Since malaria cannot be diagnosed clinically, blood must be examined either by microscopy, after staining thick and thin films (Giemsa at pH 7.2 is preferred; Wright's, Field's, or Leishman's can also be used), or by rapid antigen detection tests (RDTs). Staining of parasites with the fluorescent dye acridine orange is an alternative that allows more rapid diagnosis of malaria (but not speciation of the infection) in patients with low parasitemias.[104] Polymerase chain reaction (PCR) is more sensitive than other methods of diagnosis but is still a research tool.[104]

In many endemic areas, a high percentage of individuals (often 95% of children and 50% of adults) have low densities of *P. falciparum* in their blood during transmission seasons. Thus, the presence of parasites in a blood smear does not ensure that clinical symptoms and signs such as elevated temperature are due to malaria. Furthermore, in high-transmission areas, parasitemias of up to 10 000 parasites/μL may be tolerated without symptoms or signs in partially immune individuals. In these cases, an absolute density of parasites in the blood (often 5000–20 000 parasites/μL blood) is used to make the clinical diagnosis of malaria, and patients with lower levels of parasitemia must be investigated for other causes of their symptoms and signs. Nonetheless, clinicians should not withhold antimalarial treatment from a patient with clinical symptoms and signs and any level of parasitemia.

Blood Films

The gold standard for diagnosis of malaria is the blood film. Thick films are optimal for diagnosis, particularly at low parasitemias, because 20–40 times more blood is examined. Determination of the species of parasite can often be done by an expert on a thick film but is best done on a thin film (***Fig. 96.8***). In a patient suspected of having malaria with a negative blood film, the blood film (***Table 96.1 and Fig. 96.9***) should be examined every 12 hours for 36–48 hours before considering it to be negative.

Estimation of Parasite Density

Since one criterion for diagnosing severe malaria is the density of parasitemia (***Box 96.2***), it is important, particularly in *P. falciparum* infections, to determine the parasite density. This is expressed as the percentage of erythrocytes parasitized, or as the numbers of parasitized erythrocytes/μL blood. Percent parasitemia is estimated by determining the number of parasitized erythrocytes/1000 red cells in a thin blood film. At low densities of parasitemia percent parasitemia is extremely difficult to determine, and the number of parasites/μL blood is estimated. The number of parasites/μL blood is derived from the number of parasitized erythrocytes/200 white blood cells (WBCs), generally in a thick blood film. If the WBC count is known, then one can calculate the parasite density per microliter. For example, if there are 100 parasites/200 WBCs and the WBC count is 6000/μL, the parasite density is (100 parasites/200 WBCs) × 6000 WBCs/μL = 3000 parasites/μL blood. If the WBC count is not known, it is generally assumed to be 8000 WBCs/μL. The number of parasites/μL blood can also be estimated by knowing the percent parasitemia and the number of erythrocytes/μL blood. If there are 5×10^6 erythroctyes/μL blood, then a 1% parasitemia corresponds to 50 000 parasitized erythrocytes/μL blood. An expert microscopist who examines 200 fields of a thick blood film at 1000× magnification can detect approximately 5 parasitized erythroctyes/μL blood, which for an individual with 5×10^6 erythroctyes/μL blood is a percent parasitemia of 0.0001%. In routine practice densities less than 50/μL are usually reported as negative.

In the nonfalciparum malarias (where sequestration is considered not to occur), the number of parasites in the body may be estimated simply by multiplying the parasite density by the estimated blood volume. In *P. falciparum* malaria the microscopist can see only part of the first half of the asexual life cycle. In the second half of the asexual cycle the parasitized cells are sequestered. As a consequence there may be large discrepancies between the number of parasites in the peripheral (circulating) blood and the number of parasites in the body (the parasite burden). This is the

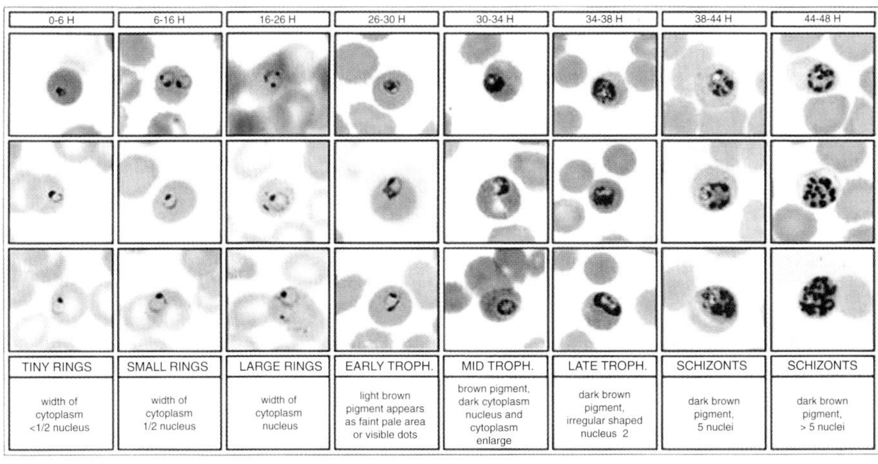

Tiny rings (0-6 H) | Small rings (6-12 H) | Large rings (12-18 H) | Early trophozoites (18-28 H) | Late trophozoites (28-36 H) | Early schizonts (36-42 H) | Mature schizonts (42-48 H)

Ring form. RBC normal or slightly enlarged. | Amoeboid form occupies < 1/3 of RBC RBC enlarged. | Irregular, polymorphic cytoplasm, uneven staining, size > 1/3 of RBC. RBC enlarged, appears paler. | Light brown pigment first visible. Dark polymorphic cytoplasm, size 1/2 of enlarged RBC. | Brown pigment. Cytoplasm coalescing to large, irregular shape, dark staining. | Brown pigment 2-5 nuclei. Large, spherical dense cytoplasm. Large pale RBC. | Brown pigment > 5 nuclei. Large, very pale RBC.

Plasmodium vivax (in vitro culture) Wellcome Unit, Bangkok 2000

B

Figure 96.9 Characteristic features in Giemsa-stained blood smears. **(A)** *Plasmodium falciparum.* **(B)** *P. vivax.* (**(A)** Reproduced from Silamut K, Phu NH, Whitty C, et al. A quantitative analysis of the microvascular sequestration of malaria parasites in the human brain. Am J Pathol. 1999;155:395–410. **(B)** Reproduced from Chotivanich K, Silamut K, Udomsangpetch R, et al. Ex-vivo short-term culture and developmental assessment of *Plasmodium vivax.* Trans R Soc Trop Med Hyg. 2001;95:677–680.)

reason why, in a febrile patient suspected of having malaria, negative blood smears are repeated every 12 hours for 36–48 hours. If all of the parasites are synchronous (at the same stage of development) and sequestered, a patient with a negative blood smear read by an inexperienced microscopist, or a low parasitemia read by an experienced microscopist, could have a high parasitemia 12–24 hours later.

Rapid Diagnostic Tests

Rapid, simple, sensitive, and specific antibody-based diagnostic stick or card tests (RDTs) detect *P. falciparum*-specific, histidine-rich protein (HRP) 2[106,107] or lactate dehydrogenase[108] antigens. Some of these tests incorporate a second antibody, which allows falciparum malaria to be distinguished from the less dangerous malarias. *P. falciparum* HRP2-based tests may remain positive for several weeks after acute infection. This is a disadvantage in high-transmission areas where infections are highly prevalent but is of value in the diagnosis of severe malaria in patients who have taken antimalarial drugs and cleared peripheral parasitemia. The World Health Organization (WHO) has assessed the performance of available RDTs.[109] There is wide variation in the performance of current commercially available tests. Although an expert microscopist can detect as few as 5 parasites/μL blood, in general, microscopy and RDTs have similar levels of detection at ~50 parasites/μL. A parasitemia of 50/μL corresponds to a total body parasite burden in an adult of >100 million parasites and a percent parasitemia of 0.001%.

Blood Film Findings Useful in Identifying Patients with Poor Prognoses

Parasite Density

The relationship between parasitemia and prognosis in falciparum malaria is complex. Patients with >3% parasitemia (approximately 1×10^5 parasites/μL in a patient with anemia) are at increased risk of dying,[65,110] but individuals with a history of repeated infections (semi-immunes) may tolerate parasitemia levels many times higher with only minor symptoms, and some patients, especially nonimmunes, may die with much lower counts. The clue to the discrepancy lies both in the immune status of the host and in the stage of development of parasites on the peripheral blood smear.

Mature Parasites

A predominance of more mature parasites indicates that a greater proportion are sequestered and carries a worse prognosis for any parasitemia than does a predominance of younger forms.[111] In severe malaria, a poor prognosis is indicated by a predominance of more mature *P. falciparum* parasites (i.e., >20% of parasites with visible pigment) in the peripheral blood film (***Box 96.2***).

Malaria Pigment in Polymorphonuclear Leukocytes

Another simple estimation is the number of polymorphonuclear leukocytes (PMNs) that contain malaria pigment.[111] This reflects the amount of recent schizont rupture. Patients with >5% PMNs containing malaria pigment have an increased risk of dying (***Box 96.2***).[111] Phagocytosed malarial pigment seen inside peripheral blood monocytes also provides a clue to recent infection if malarial parasites are not detectable. After the clearance of the parasites, malarial pigment often is evident for several days in peripheral blood phagocytes, bone marrow aspirates, or smears of fluid expressed after intradermal puncture.

Presence of Gametocyes (Sexual Erythrocytic-stage Parasites) in Blood Films

In *P. falciparum* infection, gametocytemia peaks 1 week after the peak in asexual parasites. In the other malarias gametocytes emerge synchronously with the asexual stages. Gametocytes are not involved in the pathogenesis of malaria. The mature gametocytes are not affected by most antimalarial drugs, so their persistence does not constitute evidence of drug resistance.

Antiparasite Antibodies

In endemic areas the presence of antiparasite blood-stage antibodies is used as an epidemiologic tool but in general cannot be used to determine whether an individual is infected, because virtually all individuals have such antibodies. In the past, the presence of antiasexual erythrocytic-stage parasite antibodies was used to determine whether an individual with persistent clinical manifestations consistent with malaria, but negative blood films, might in fact have malaria. In general, the same laboratories that can assess anti-blood-stage antibodies can perform PCR, and PCR has replaced antibodies in the diagnosis of cryptic infections because it detects parasite material, not the host's immune response to the parasites.

TREATMENT

Antimalarial Drugs

The objective of treating severe malaria is to save lives, and that of treating uncomplicated malaria is to prevent the development of severe complications and cure the infection. In general, antimalarial drugs are more toxic than antibacterials, i.e., the therapeutic ratio is narrower, but serious adverse effects are rare. Available antimalarials fall into four broad groups: (1) quinoline-related or quinoline-like compounds; (2) antifolates; (3) artemisinin compounds; and (4) atovaquone.

Quinoline-related or Quinoline-like Compounds

The quinoline-related or quinoline-like compounds (quinine, quinidine, chloroquine, amodiaquine, mefloquine, halofantrine, lumefantrine, piperaquine, pyronaridine) chemically interfere with intraparasitic heme detoxification, preventing the dimerization process that results in the formation of hemozoin (malaria pigment). Primaquine and tafenoquine are structurally related 8-aminoquinolines that kill liver and sexual stages of *P. falciparum* and all stages of *P. vivax*, *P. malariae*, and *P. ovale*. These are also the only drugs that kill the persistent liver stages of *P. vivax* and *P. ovale*, but their mechanism of action is unknown.

Antifolates

The antifolates (pyrimethamine, cycloguanil, chlorcycloguanil, trimethoprim) competitively inhibit plasmodial dihydrofolate reductase. They are synergistic with sulfonamides and sulfones. Cycloguanil and chlorcycloguanil are the active metabolites of proguanil and chlorproguanil, respectively.

Artemisinin Compounds

The artemisinin compounds (artemisinin, dihydroartemisinin, artemether, artesunate, artemotil) are endoperoxides naturally extracted from the naturally occurring *Artemisia* plant. They have the broadest time window of action on the asexual malarial parasites, from young rings to early schizonts, and produce the most rapid therapeutic responses. Their mechanism of action is not known.

Atovaquone

Atovaquone is a potent inhibitor of cytochrome-mediated electron transport. It is synergistic with proguanil (in this case, the parent compound, not its antifolate metabolite cycloguanil).

Several antibacterial drugs also have antiplasmodial activity, although in general their action is slow and they are used only in combination with the antimalarial drugs. Those used are the sulfonamides and sulfones, tetracyclines, lincosamides, macrolides, and chloramphenicol. Significant resistance has been reported to the sulfonamides but not to the other classes of antibiotics. Drugs that are active against sensitive *P. falciparum* are also active against the other malaria species. The most effective antimalarial drugs are combinations of an artemisinin derivative with a slowly eliminated antimalarial drug (artemisinin combination (ACT) treatments).[113,114]

Pharmacokinetics

The antimalarial drugs vary considerably in their pharmacokinetic and pharmacodynamic properties (***Table 96.3***). Oral absorption ranges from good (quinine, chloroquine, amodiaquine, sulfadoxine–pyrimethamine (SP), artemisinin derivatives, primaquine) to variable (mefloquine, lumefantrine, halofantrine, atovaquone). These latter drugs are lipophilic hydrophobic compounds; oral absorption is increased by coadministration with fatty food or drinks. Acute malaria may cause reduced oral antimalarial absorption. Elimination rates also vary considerably from the artemisinin derivatives, which have terminal elimination half-lives ($T_{1/2}$) of less than an hour; quinine, proguanil, and chlorproguanil ($T_{1/2}$ <1 day); pyrimethamine, lumefantrine, and atovaquone ($T_{1/2}$ <1 week), through to mefloquine, chloroquine, and piperaquine, which have $T_{1/2}$ values of several weeks. Although acute malaria may impair metabolic clearance, with the exception of quinine and quinidine in severe malaria, this does not significantly affect dosing or treatment responses. Plasma concentrations of many antimalarials are reduced in late pregnancy.

Some antimalarial drugs have active metabolites that contribute most of the antimalarial activity. *In vivo* artesunate is almost completely hydrolyzed to dihydroartemisinin (DHA), which is the most potent artemisinin derivative. After oral administration, artemether and artemotil are also largely converted to DHA. Amodiaquine is almost completely converted to desethylamodiaquine, and most of the antimalarial activity of proguanil and chlorproguanil derives from their antifolate triazine metabolites cycloguanil and chlorcycloguanil, respectively.

Drugs that are eliminated rapidly (artemisinins, quinine) must be given for at least 7 days to ensure high cure rates, unless they are accompanied by a more slowly eliminated partner. This why, in most ACTs, the artemisinin derivatives are partnered with slowly eliminated compounds, and the treatment course can be shortened to a total of 3 days (***Fig. 96.10***).[113] Shorter ACT treatment courses (i.e., 1 or 2 days) are less effective, may be more prone to resistance, and are not recommended.

Drug interactions among the antimalarials are generally inconsequential. The exception is the potentially dangerous exacerbation of halofantrine's effect in prolonging ventricular repolarization (QT prolongation)

Table 96.3 Summary of Pharmacokinetic Properties of Antimalarial Drugs

Drug	Absorption: Time to Peak (Hours) PO	IM	Oral Dose (mg/kg)	Peak Drug Level (mg/L)	Plasma Binding (%)	V_d/f^a (L/kg)	Cl/f (mL/kg/min)	$T_{1/2}^b$ (Hours or Days)
In Malaria								
Quinine	6	1	10	8	90	0.8	1.5	16
Quinidine	1		10	5	85	1.3	1.7	10
Chloroquine	5	0.5	10	0.12	55	100–1000	2.0	30–60 days
Piperaquine	6		19.2	0.6		600–900	25	28 days
Pyronaridine	3		12.4	0.3				6.6[f]
Artesunate	1.5	0.5	4	0.5		0.15	50	0.8[b]
Artemether	2	3–18	4	1.5	95	2.7	54	1
Dihydroartemisinin	3		2.4	0.7		1.5	20	0.8
Mefloquine	17		25		>98	20	0.35	14 days
Halofantrine	15		8	0.9[c]	>98[d]		7.5	113
Lumefantrine	6		9	3.5[c]	>98[d]	2.7	3.0	86
Pyrimethamine	6	41	1.25	0.5	94		0.33	87
Atovaquone	6		15	5[b]	99.5	6	2.5	30
Healthy Subjects[e]								
Primaquine	3		0.6	0.15		3	6	6
Proguanil (chlorguanide)	3		3.5	0.17	75	24	19	16
Pyrimethamine	4		0.3	0.35		2.9	0.4	85

[a] V_d/f and Cl/f are the total apparent volume of distribution and the clearance respectively, both divided by f, the fraction of drug absorbed.
[b] $T_{1/2}$ of the active metabolite dihydroartemisinin.
[c] Absorption increased significantly by fats.
[d] Binds to lipoproteins.
[e] Pregnancy is usually associated with lower drug concentrations and higher treatment failure rates.
[f] This reported value for the pyronaridine half-life is highly likely to be a considerable underestimate.
PO, oral; IM, intramuscular.

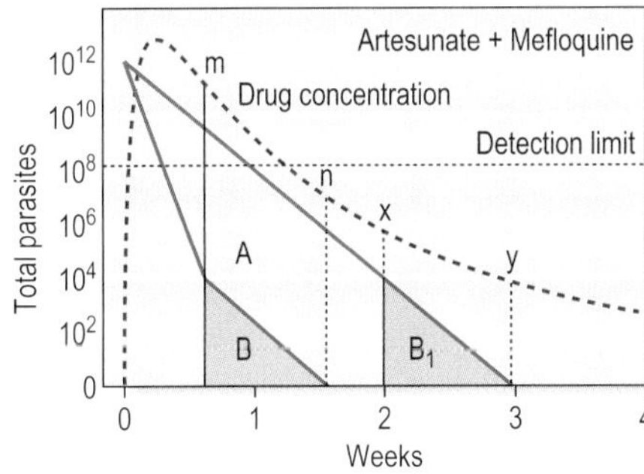

Figure 96.10 Pharmacodynamic rationale underlying artemisinin combination treatment (artesunate + mefloquine). Vertical axis (logarithmic scale) shows total number of parasites in the body of an adult with approximately 2% parasitemia. Artesunate given for 3 days covers two asexual cycles and reduces the parasite numbers by a factor of 10^8. Residual parasites (10^4) are killed by high concentrations of mefloquine (*m* – *n*) (B). If mefloquine alone is used, parasite numbers reduce more slowly and are not eliminated completely for approximately 3 weeks. Thus, in combination treatment, no parasite is exposed to artesunate alone, and only 0.0000001% of the original infecting biomass is exposed to mefloquine alone. (Redrawn from White NJ. Assessment of the pharmacodynamic properties of the antimalarial drugs in vivo. Antimicrob Agents Chemother. 1997;41:1413–1422.)

when given following mefloquine treatment. This may increase the risk of sudden death from ventricular tachyarrhythmias.[114] There is insufficient information on interactions of antimalarials with other drugs (e.g., antiretrovirals).

In some areas of the world there are increased numbers of deaths due to malaria, and the increased death toll has been attributed to drug resistance.[116] *P. falciparum* has developed resistance to all classes of antimalarial drugs, including the more recently introduced artemisinin derivatives.[117] The other human malarias are generally more drug-sensitive, although they have developed antifolate resistance rapidly in some areas. Chloroquine resistance in *P. vivax* in Oceania or Island of New Guinea, and parts of Indonesia is a substantial problem.[118,119] Elsewhere *P. vivax* remains generally chloroquine-sensitive.[120] There has been one report of chloroquine-resistant *P. malariae*.[121]

Classification of Patients for Treatment

It is critical that the care provider determine whether a patient with malaria has uncomplicated or complicated malaria based on clinical, laboratory, or parasitologic findings (***Box 96.2***).

TREATMENT OF UNCOMPLICATED *P. FALCIPARUM* MALARIA

The goal of treatment of uncomplicated malaria is to cure the infection rapidly and reliably. This means achieving a prompt clinical response and preventing recurrence from either recrudescence or relapse. Effective treatment dramatically lowers the risk of progression to severe disease and the additional morbidity associated with treatment failure. Reduction of transmission and prevention of resistance are both important additional considerations for patients treated where malaria is transmitted. In falciparum malaria there is a continuum from mild to severe malaria. Young children with malaria may deteriorate rapidly. Many patients are intolerant of oral medication and require parenteral or rectal administration for 1 or 2 days until they can swallow and retain oral treatment reliably, even though they never show signs of severity. They should receive the same dose regimens as in severe malaria.

Patients without physical signs of severity, but who on examination of the blood film are found to have a high parasitemia, can be treated with oral antimalarials if their condition can be monitored closely. These patients are at increased risk of developing severe malaria and thus have an increased mortality rate. These patients should be treated with rapidly acting antimalarials such as the artemisinin derivatives and should be immediately switched to parenteral therapy if signs of severity develop.

After it has been established whether the patient has uncomplicated or complicated malaria, treatment is dependent on the care provider's estimation of how good follow-up will be, whether the patient is returning to a malaria-endemic area, and the availability of specific antimalarials. Several drugs that are recommended in tropical countries (e.g., piperaquine) are not available in some temperate countries (e.g., the United States). Drug regimens, including single drugs, with expected cure rates of 100% are used for treating patients in whom there will be good follow-up, such as returning travelers, in nonendemic areas. In malaria-endemic areas, it is now recommended that antimalarials should be used in combinations, to augment cure rates (which should be at least 90%) and to prevent the emergence of resistance.

Combining two or more antimalarial drugs with different modes of action (and thus drug targets) provides two main advantages: (1) cure rates are usually increased; and (2) in the rare event that a mutant parasite that is resistant to one of the drugs arises *de novo* during the course of the infection, it will be killed by the other drug. Mutual protection prevents the emergence of resistance.[113] This is the same principle underlying the multidrug combination treatments of tuberculosis and HIV infections. Prevention of resistance is necessary to ensure that antimalarial treatment remains highly effective. Both partner drugs in a combination must be independently effective. ACTs, the most rapidly and reliably effective antimalarial drugs, have the advantage of inhibiting gametocyte development and thus reducing transmissibility. Artemisinin and its derivatives (artesunate, artemether, artemotil, dihydroartemisinin) produce rapid clearance of parasitemia and rapid resolution of symptoms. They reduce parasite numbers by a factor of ~10 000 each asexual cycle,[114] which is more than other antimalarial drugs (which reduce parasite numbers by between 100- and 1000-fold/cycle). Artemisinin is 5–10 times less potent than its derivatives and has generally given way to the derivatives. When given alone or in combination with rapidly eliminated compounds (tetracyclines, clindamycin), a 7-day course of treatment with an artemisinin compound is required, but when given in combination with slowly eliminated antimalarial drugs, shorter courses of treatment (3 days) are highly effective.

The artemisinin compounds are active against all five species of malaria parasites infecting humans. Although reduced susceptibility to artesunate has been reported recently in western Cambodia, elsewhere the artemisinin derivatives are rapidly and reliably effective. The artemisinin derivatives are remarkably well tolerated. The only significant adverse effect to emerge from extensive clinical trials has been rare (≈1 : 3000) type 1 hypersensitivity reactions (manifested initially by urticaria). They also have the advantage from a public health perspective of reducing gametocyte carriage and thus the transmissibility of malaria. This contributes to malaria control.

Specific Drugs and Drug Regimens (Table 96.4)

ACTs are now the first-line recommended treatments for falciparum malaria in all malaria-endemic areas.

Atovaquone–Proguanil

This combination of a naphthaquinone and biguanide is effective against all malarias, including multidrug-resistant falciparum malaria. Atovaquone–proguanil is given in a 3-day, once-daily regimen. Atovaquone–proguanil is well tolerated with no serious adverse effects. The main problem is the high cost of atovaquone. While it continues to be useful for the treatment of travelers and in prophylaxis, it is too expensive for large-scale deployment in endemic areas. It may be combined with artesunate to provide an ACT.

Mefloquine

Mefloquine alone is highly effective against *P. falciparum* from most parts of the world except specific areas of Southeast Asia (***Table 96.4***). A dose of 25 mg base/kg is given in two or three divided doses 8–24 hours apart. The principal problems with mefloquine are nausea and vomiting in young children, and CNS adverse effects (dizziness, dysphoria, nightmares, and less commonly seizures, encephalopathy, or psychosis). Mefloquine is better tolerated when combined with an artemisinin derivative. A fixed-dose 3-day mefloquine ACT is now available in some countries.

Sulfadoxine–Pyrimethamine

Although resistance to SP has spread rapidly in recent years (***Table 96.4***), compromising the efficacy of the combination, there are still some areas, notably in West Africa and Pakistan, Afghanistan, and northwest India, where this combination is very effective. A major advantage of SP is that it is delivered as a single dose and is generally well tolerated. SP should not be used alone for treatment; it should be combined with a 3-day course of artesunate to provide an ACT regimen.

Chloroquine

Chloroquine is still the treatment of choice for *P. vivax*, *P. ovale*, *P. malariae*, and the occasional *P. knowlesi* malaria that is transmitted to humans, but for *P. falciparum* there are now very few places where chloroquine can be relied upon. If one is confident of the response in a locale with presumed chloroquine-sensitive *P. falciparum* (***Table 96.4***), then chloroquine can be used. If uncertain, one should choose another antimalarial.

Quinine

Quinine continues to have an important role in malaria treatment. Although there is reduced susceptibility to quinine in parts of Southeast Asia and South America, these reductions are not large and quinine is still effective in these areas. It is still the drug of choice for uncomplicated falciparum malaria in the first trimester of pregnancy regardless of location. Quinine may also be part of second-line treatment regimens, but it is not standard first-line treatment in endemic areas, because it must be given 3 times daily and is poorly tolerated (bitter taste, nausea, tinnitus, dysphoria, giddiness – a symptom complex termed cinchonism – and hypoglycemia). Poor tolerance reduces adherence to the 7-day regimens needed to achieve high cure rates where there is resistance. In most cases quinine should be combined with either a tetracycline (e.g., doxycycline or tetracycline) or, in children, clindamycin. These antibiotics are given for 7 days. Oral quinine is also often given to complete a full 7 days of treatment following parenteral treatment for severe malaria. Quinine has been associated with immune thrombocytopenia, and very rarely the hemolytic-uremic syndrome, but serious adverse effects from oral quinine are unusual in uncomplicated malaria, although severe and refractory hypoglycemia may occur in late pregnancy.

Treatment with Artemisinin Derivatives and Another Antimalarial

Artesunate–Mefloquine

This 3-day combination treatment is effective against all malaria everywhere. The side effects are similar to mefloquine alone, although early vomiting is reduced by the combination. The fixed-dose regimen comprises 4 mg/kg artesunate and 8.8 mg/kg mefloquine administered daily for 3 days.

Artemether–Lumefantrine

This is a 3-day, six-dose regimen. Provided that there is adequate absorption of lumefantrine, this combination would also be expected to be effective against all malaria everywhere. The principal problem with artemether–lumefantrine is variable oral absorption of lumefantrine,

Table 96.4 Dosage Regimens of Antimalarials for Treatment of Uncomplicated Malaria[a]

Type	Malaria-Endemic Area	Outside Malaria-Endemic Area
Plasmodium vivax, P. malariae, P. ovale, known chloroquine-sensitive *P. falciparum*[a]	Chloroquine phosphate (1 tablet contains 250 mg salt, equivalent to 155.3 mg base). 10 mg/kg base at 0, 24 hours followed by 5 mg/kg base at 48 hours May be combined with artesunate 4 mg/kg/day for 3 days	Chloroquine phosphate (1 tablet contains 250 mg salt, equivalent to 155.3 mg base). 10 mg/kg base at 0, 24 hours followed by 5 mg/kg base at 48 hours
P. falciparum[a] known to be sensitive to sulfadoxine–pyrimethamine (SP)	Oral artesunate 4 mg/kg daily for 3 days + pyrimethamine 1.25 mg/kg + sulfadoxine 25 mg/kg (single dose), 3 tablets in an adult	Pyrimethamine 1.25 mg/kg + sulfadoxine 25 mg/kg (single dose) 3 tablets in an adult
P. falciparum[a] known to be sensitive to amodiaquine	Oral artesunate 4 mg/kg daily for 3 days + amodiaquine 10 mg base/kg/day for 3 days	Amodiaquine 10 mg base/kg/day for 3 days
P. falciparum known to be sensitive to mefloquine (see ***Table 96.2 and Fig. 96.5*** for known mefloquine-resistant areas)	Combination only (see below)	Mefloquine 25 mg base/kg (single dose or divided into 2 or 3 doses given 8–24 hours apart)
	Treatments Effective Everywhere in the World	**Treatments Effective in Infections Acquired Anywhere in the World**
Chloroquine-resistant *P. vivax*[b] and multidrug resistant-*P. falciparum*[a]	1. Oral artesunate 4 mg/kg daily for 3 days + mefloquine 25 mg base/kg (15 mg/kg on day 2, 10 mg/kg on day 3)	1. Atovaquone 20 mg/kg/day, proguanil 8 mg/kg/day for 3 days; this should be combined with artesunate in endemic areas
	2. Artemether–lumefantrine 1.5/9 mg/kg twice daily for 3 days with food	2. Quinine 10 mg salt/kg 3 times daily + doxycycline 3 mg/kg once daily or clindamycin 10 mg/kg twice daily for 7 days
	3. Dihydroartemisinin–piperaquine 2.5/20 mg/kg daily for 3 days	

[a]In endemic areas, only combination treatments should be used for falciparum malaria, whereas outside the endemic area highly effective monotherapies may be used.

[b]This refers to truly resistant infections, which are a significant problem only in Oceania and Indonesia, and should not be confused with relapses.

General Points

1. Pregnancy: artemisinin and derivatives should not be given in the first trimester of pregnancy. Halofantrine, primaquine, and tetracycline should not be used at any time in pregnancy, and sulfadoxine should not be used very near to term. Mefloquine has been associated with an increased risk of stillbirth in one study but not in another. Atovaquone–proguanil and artemether–lumefantrine have not been evaluated adequately in pregnancy.
2. Vomiting may be less likely if the patient's temperature is lowered before oral drug administration.
3. Contraindications to mefloquine treatment include use of the drug in the previous 63 days, epilepsy or neuropsychiatric disorder, history of allergy, or following cerebral malaria.
4. Short courses of artesunate or quinine (<7 days) alone are not recommended.
5. In renal failure the dose of quinine should be reduced by one-third to one-half after 48 hours, and doxycycline but not tetracycline should be prescribed.
6. The doses of all drugs are unchanged in children and pregnant women.
7. Oral treatment of uncomplicated hyperparasitemic infections should include an artemisinin derivative and be prolonged to minimize the chance of recrudescence, e.g., artesunate loading dose of 4 mg/kg initially followed by 2 mg/kg/day on the following 6 days, in combination with mefloquine, clindamycin, or doxycycline as in the table.
8. Patients with *P. vivax* and *P. ovale* infections should also be given primaquine 0.5 mg base/kg (up to 30 mg base) daily for 14 days to prevent relapse (see ***Table 96.5***). In mild glucose 6 phosphate dehydrogenase deficiency, 0.75 mg base/kg should be given once weekly for 6 weeks.
9. Use of tetracyclines in pregnant women or children under 8 years of age is contraindicated.
10. Quinine has been associated with immune thrombocytopenia, and very rarely hemolytic-uremic syndrome bouts.

which may give rise to treatment failure as a result of inadequate blood concentrations. Absorption of lumefantrine is increased by coadministration with fats (food, milk) and improves as the patient recovers from illness. The combination is remarkably well tolerated and rapidly effective.

Artesunate–Amodiaquine

Amodiaquine is more effective than chloroquine against *P. falciparum* in Africa, parts of South America, and Oceania, but not in Asia. Artesunate–amodiaquine is effective in some areas of Africa and South America, but resistance to amodiaquine is increasing. There is insufficient information on the pharmacokinetics of amodiaquine, and there are still uncertainties over the true incidence of clinically significant leukopenia, agranulocytosis, and hepatitis when it is used for treatment. All three adverse effects were observed when amodiaquine was used in antimalarial prophylaxis, and leukopenia may be a particular problem in HIV-infected patients. Oral amodiaquine is considered more palatable than chloroquine by young children. The 3-day fixed dose ACT is generally well tolerated.

Artesunate–Sulfadoxine–Pyrimethamine

A 3-day artesunate–SP combination is well tolerated and effective where sensitivity to SP is retained.

Chlorproguanil–Dapsone

This antifolate–biguanide combination is given in a 3-day, once-daily regimen. It is more effective than SP against antifolate-resistant *P. falciparum*, but it is not effective against parasites with the I164L mutation in *Pfdhfr*. Chlorproguanil–dapsone has been withdrawn recently because it is associated with an increased risk of anemia, probably resulting from dapsone-induced hemolysis.

Dihydroartemisinin–Piperaquine

This is a fixed-dose combination of dihydroartemisinin and piperaquine, a bisquinoline compound with structural similarities to chloroquine. The treatment course is once daily for 3 days. Piperaquine is considerably more active than chloroquine against resistant *P. falciparum*. It is eliminated slowly (terminal half-life, ≈1 month). The combination is highly effective and well tolerated in large treatment trials and has been recommended as a first-line treatment for acute falciparum malaria by the WHO.

Antibacterials with Antimalarial Activity

Many antibiotics that target protein or nucleic acid synthesis are effective against *Plasmodium*. In general these drugs are relatively weak antimalarials that clear parasitemia slowly if used alone, so they are always combined with a specific antimalarial drug. The main exception is trimethoprim–sulfamethoxazole, which has good antimalarial activity (since trimethoprim has the same mode of action as pyrimethamine) but has to be given for 5–7 days. Unfortunately, resistance to SP means resistance to trimethoprim–sulfamethoxazole, and continued use of the antibacterial may also select for SP resistance. Thus, trimethoprim–sulfamethoxazole is not recommended for antimalarial use. The tetracyclines, clindamycin, and sulfonamides are all used in antimalarial treatment. Rifampicin, chloramphenicol, and azithromycin all have significant antimalarial activity. Fosmidomycin is being investigated as an antimalarial. Pending further information, these latter drugs are not recommended for general use.

In the assessment of antimalarial drug efficacy, a follow-up period of at least 28 days is required for rapidly eliminated drugs, but for drugs that are more slowly eliminated (terminal half-life >24 hours; ***Table 96.3***), the follow-up period should be ≥42 days.

TREATMENT OF MALARIA CAUSED BY *P. VIVAX*, *P. OVALE*, OR *P. MALARIAE*

P. vivax is still generally sensitive to chloroquine, although chloroquine resistance is increasing in some areas, notably Oceania, East Asia, and parts of South and Central America. Resistance to pyrimethamine is prevalent in many areas, and SP is consequently ineffective. Proguanil or chlorproguanil is also ineffective in these areas. In general *P. vivax* is sensitive to all the other antimalarial drugs, is more sensitive than *P. falciparum* to the artemisinin derivatives, and is less sensitive to mefloquine (although mefloquine is still effective). In contrast to *P. falciparum*, asexual stages of *P. vivax* are susceptible to primaquine. Thus, chloroquine plus primaquine can be considered a combination treatment. The only drugs with substantial activity against the hypnozoites are the 8-aminoquinolines (primaquine, tafenoquine).[120,122] Simple methods for short-term culture of *P. vivax* have been developed, allowing *ex vivo* assessment of asexual-stage drug sensitivity. *In vivo* assessment suggests that *P. vivax* in East Asia and Oceania is less susceptible to primaquine than elsewhere. There are few data on the *in vivo* susceptibility of *P. ovale* and *P. malariae*. Both are regarded as sensitive to chloroquine, although there is a single report of chloroquine resistance in *P. malariae*.[121] Experience indicates that *P. vivax*, *P. ovale* and *P. malariae* are susceptible to currently available ACTs except in some areas to artesunate SP. For chloroquine-sensitive vivax malaria (i.e., in most places where *P. vivax* is prevalent) the traditional 25 mg base/kg dose of chloroquine is well tolerated and effective. Some have suggested lower total doses, but this is not recommended, since it may encourage the emergence of resistance. Chloroquine is given in an initial dose of 10 mg base/kg followed by either 5 mg/kg at 6, 24, and 48 hours or more commonly as 10 mg/kg on the second day and 5 mg/kg on the third day. The treatment duration can be shortened to 36 hours. It is also clear that if ACT treatment is given, then *P. vivax* will respond as well as or better than *P. falciparum*. The exception is a regimen containing SP. *P. vivax* has developed resistance to SP more rapidly than has *P. falciparum*.

There are relatively few data on treatment responses in chloroquine-resistant vivax malaria. Studies from Indonesia indicate that dihydroartemisinin–piperaquine, artemether–lumefantrine, atovaquone–proguanil,[122] halofantrine,[119] mefloquine, and amodiaquine are all efficacious. Atovaquone–proguanil (3 doses over 3 days), or an ACT combined with primaquine should be given for chloroquine-resistant vivax malaria.

To achieve radical cure of vivax or ovale malaria, relapse must be prevented by giving primaquine.[121] However, the frequency and pattern of relapses vary geographically. It has become clear in recent years that whereas 50–60% of *P. vivax* infections in Southeast Asia relapse, the frequency is lower in Indonesia (30%) and much of the Indian subcontinent (15–20%). Thus, the preventive efficacy of primaquine must be set against the prevalent relapse frequency. The total dose of 8-aminoquinoline given is the main determinant of liver-stage curative efficacy. There is no evidence that short courses of primaquine widely recommended (such as 5 days of treatment) have any efficacy. Primaquine should be given for 14 days. The usually recommended adult dose has been 15 mg base (0.25 mg/kg/day), but in Southeast Asia, particularly Indonesia, and in Oceania, higher doses (0.6 mg base/kg/day) are required, and both the WHO and the Centers for Disease Control and Prevention now recommend the 0.6 mg/kg dose up to an adult dose of 30 mg base/day (***Table 96.5***). Primaquine causes abdominal discomfort when taken on an empty stomach; it should always be taken with food.

The inherited sex-linked deficiency of G6PD is associated with some protection against falciparum and vivax malaria but increased susceptibility to oxidant hemolysis. The prevalence of G6PD deficiency varies but can be a high as 20%. There are a large number of different genotypes, each with different levels of deficiency. Primaquine is an oxidant and causes variable hemolysis in G6PD-deficient individuals. Fortunately, primaquine is eliminated rapidly, so hemolysis is self-limiting provided no further drug is taken. Screening for G6PD deficiency is not generally available outside hospitals, although rapid stick tests are under development. Many people are unaware of their G6PD status. If a patient is known or suspected (individuals of Mediterranean and Asian descent) to be severely G6PD-deficient (≈5–10% of normal G6PD activity), then primaquine should not be given. For the majority of patients with mild variants (≈20% of normal G6PD activity), often found in black Africans, primaquine can be given in a dose of 0.75 mg base/kg once weekly for 6 weeks. If significant hemolysis occurs on treatment, primaquine should be stopped. Primaquine is not given during pregnancy because G6PD status of the fetus is unknown. Tafenoquine, an 8-aminoquinoline in development, is more active and more slowly eliminated. It also causes oxidant hemolysis.

TREATMENT OF SEVERE MALARIA

Death from severe malaria often occurs within hours of admission to hospital or clinic, so it is essential that therapeutic concentrations of antimalarial drug be achieved as soon as safely possible. This is why a loading dose of certain drugs is essential, particularly quinine, quinidine, and artemether. Nearly all cases of severe malaria result from *P. falciparum* infection. Many patients with malaria, including those with species other than *P. falciparum*, cannot take oral medications initially because of repeated vomiting. They do not fulfill the criteria of severe malaria but do require parenteral (or rectal) administration of antimalarials. In practice if there is uncertainty the patient should be treated as having severe malaria until able to swallow medications reliably. Delays in reaching a hospital or health center may be fatal for patients who cannot swallow oral medications reliably. The pre-referral administration of a rectal formulation of artesunate has been shown in a large trial to reduce the mortality from malaria in children under 5 years by 25%.[124]

Management of severe malaria comprises four main areas: assessment of the patient, specific antimalarial treatment, adjunctive therapy, and supportive care.[64]

Severe malaria is a medical emergency. The airway should be secured in unconscious patients and breathing and circulation assessed. The patient should be weighed or weight estimated so that drugs, including antimalarials and fluids, can be given on a body weight basis. An IV cannula should be inserted, and immediate measurements of blood glucose, hematocrit, parasitemia (parasite count, stage of malaria parasite development, and proportion of neutrophils containing malaria pigment), and, in adults, renal function (blood urea or creatinine) should be assessed. The degree of acidosis is an important determinant of outcome; the plasma bicarbonate or venous lactate should be measured if possible. If facilities are available, arterial or capillary blood pH and gases should be

Table 96.5 Drugs used in the Prophylaxis of Malaria as Recommended by the US Centers for Disease Control and Prevention				
Drug	**Usage**	**Adult Dose**	**Pediatric Dose**	**Comments**
Atovaquone/ proguanil (Malarone)	Prophylaxis in all areas	Adult tablets contain 250 mg atovaquone and 100 mg proguanil hydrochloride. 1 adult tablet orally, daily	Pediatric tablets contain 62.5 mg atovaquone and 25 mg proguanil hydrochloride. 5–8 kg: ½ pediatric tablet daily; >8–10 kg: ¾ pediatric tablet daily; >10–20 kg: 1 pediatric tablet daily; >20–30 kg: 2 pediatric tablets daily; >30–40 kg: 3 pediatric tablets daily; >40 kg: 1 adult tablet daily	Begin 1–2 days before travel to malarious areas. Take daily at the same time each day while in the malarious area and for 7 days after leaving such areas. Contraindicated in persons with severe renal impairment (creatinine clearance <30 mL/min). Atovaquone/proguanil should be taken with food or a milky drink. Not recommended for prophylaxis for children <5 kg, pregnant women, and women breastfeeding infants weighing <5 kg. Partial tablet dosages may need to be prepared by a pharmacist and dispensed in individual capsules, as described in the text
Chloroquine phosphate (Aralen and generic)	Prophylaxis only in areas with chloroquine-sensitive malaria	300 mg base (500 mg salt) orally, once/ week	5 mg/kg base (8.3 mg/kg salt) orally, once/week, up to maximum adult dose of 300 mg base	Begin 1–2 weeks before travel to malarious areas. Take weekly on the same day of the week while in the malarious area and for 4 weeks after leaving such areas. May exacerbate psoriasis
Doxycycline (many brand names and generic)	Prophylaxis in all areas	100 mg orally, daily	≥8 years of age: 2 mg/kg up to adult dose of 100 mg/day	Begin 1–2 days before travel to malarious areas. Take daily at the same time each day while in the malarious area and for 4 weeks after leaving such areas. Contraindicated in children <8 years of age and pregnant women
Hydroxychloroquine sulfate (Plaquenil)	An alternative to chloroquine for prophylaxis only in areas with chloroquine-sensitive malaria	310 mg base (400 mg salt) orally, once/ week	5 mg/kg base (6.5 mg/ kg salt) orally, once/week, up to maximum adult dose of 310 mg base	Begin 1–2 weeks before travel to malarious areas. Take weekly on the same day of the week while in the malarious area and for 4 weeks after leaving such areas
Mefloquine (Lariam and generic)	Prophylaxis in areas with mefloquine-sensitive malaria	228 mg base (250 mg salt) orally, once/ week[b]	≤9 kg: 4.6 mg/kg base (5 mg/ kg salt) orally, once/week; >9–19 kg: ¼ tablet once/week; >19–30 kg: ½ tablet once/ week; >31–45 kg: ¾ tablet once/ week; ≥45 kg: 1 tablet once/week	Begin 1–2 weeks before travel to malarious areas. Take weekly on the same day of the week while in the malarious area and for 4 weeks after leaving such areas. Contraindicated in persons allergic to mefloquine or related compounds (e.g., quinine, quinidine) and in persons with active depression, a recent history of depression, generalized anxiety disorder, psychosis, schizophrenia, other major psychiatric disorders, or seizures. Use with caution in persons with psychiatric disturbances or a previous history of depression. Not recommended for persons with cardiac conduction abnormalities
Primaquine	Prophylaxis for short-duration travel to areas with principally *P. vivax*	30 mg base (52.6 mg salt) orally, daily	0.5 mg/kg base (0.8 mg/kg salt) up to adult dose orally, daily	Begin 1–2 days before travel to malarious areas. Take daily at the same time each day while in the malarious area and for 7 days after leaving such areas. Contraindicated in persons with G6PD[a] deficiency. Also contraindicated during pregnancy and lactation unless the infant being breastfed has a documented normal G6PD level
Primaquine	Used for presumptive antirelapse therapy (terminal prophylaxis) to decrease the risk for relapses of *P. vivax* and *P. ovale*	30 mg base (52.6 mg salt) orally, once/day for 14 days after departure from the malarious area	0.5 mg/kg base (0.8 mg/kg salt) up to adult dose orally, once/day for 14 days after departure from the malarious area	Indicated for persons who have had prolonged exposure to *P. vivax* and *P. ovale* or both. Contraindicated in persons with G6PD[a] deficiency. Also contraindicated during pregnancy and lactation unless the infant being breastfed has a documented normal G6PD level

[a]G6PD, glucose-6-phosphate dehydrogenase. All persons who take primaquine should have a documented normal G6PD level before starting the medication.
[b]Tablets outside the United States usually contain 250 mg base.

measured in patients who are unconscious, hyperventilating, or in shock. Blood should be taken for cross-match, and (if possible) full blood count, platelet count, clotting studies, bacterial culture, and full biochemistry. IV fluids may then be started. The assessment of fluid balance is critical in severe malaria. Acidotic breathing or respiratory distress, particularly in severely anemic children, often indicates hypovolemia and requires prompt but careful rehydration and, if available, rapid blood transfusion. In adults there is a thin dividing line between overhydration, which may produce pulmonary edema, and underhydration contributing to shock and worsening acidosis and renal impairment. Nevertheless most patients tolerate prompt rehydration well. Careful and frequent evaluations of the jugular venous pressure, peripheral perfusion, venous filling, skin turgor, and urine output should be made. When there is uncertainty over the jugular venous pressure, and if nursing facilities permit, a central venous catheter should be inserted and the central venous pressure (CVP) measured directly, although the relationship between intravascular volume, cardiac index, and filling pressures in malaria is very variable.

When these immediate measures have been completed, a more detailed clinical examination should be conducted, with particular note of the level of consciousness and record of the coma score. Several coma scales have been advocated. The Glasgow coma scale is suitable for adults, and the simple Blantyre modification or children's Glasgow coma scale can be used for children.[125] Unconscious patients must have a diagnostic LP to exclude bacterial meningitis. The opening pressure should be recorded and the rise and fall with respiration noted. CSF should be sent for microscopic analysis, culture, and measurement of glucose, lactate, and protein. After rapid clinical assessment and confirmation of the diagnosis of severe malaria, full doses of antimalarial treatment should be started without delay.

Specific Antimalarial Treatment of Severe Malaria

Currently four commonly used parenteral drug treatments are recommended for severe malaria: artesunate, artemether, quinine, and quinidine (*Box 96.3*). Artemotil is also used in some areas. It is now increasingly accepted that parenteral artesunate is the treatment of choice for severe malaria. Artesunate, artemether, artemisinin, and quinine have also been formulated for rectal administration. Although chloroquine is available in parenteral formulations, it is no longer recommended because resistance is too widespread to rely on it. Even in a patient considered to need parenteral treatment for *P. vivax, P. ovale*, or *P. malariae* infection, it is best to treat for falciparum malaria because there may be a mixed infection. The IM preparation of SP should not be used to treat severe malaria, since resistance is widespread and responses are slow.

Large multicenter trials conducted in Southeast Asia have shown that parenteral artesunate reduces the mortality of severe malaria by 35% compared with quinine and is also safer and easier to use.[126]

Artemether proved superior to quinine in Southeast Asian adults but not African children, and artesunate is under evaluation. Thus there remains uncertainty over which antimalarial is preferable in this important group of patients. For all other patient groups, including pregnant women, parenteral artesunate is now the treatment of choice. Quinidine is more toxic than quinine and should be used only when no other effective parenteral drugs are available.[64]

Pharmacologic Considerations

In severe malaria it is essential that parasiticidal concentrations of antimalarial drug are attained as soon as safely possible.

Artesunate

Parasiticidal levels are attained immediately following IV injection and within minutes of IM injection. No dose adjustments are needed in liver or renal dysfunction. Artesunate is rapidly hydrolyzed to DHA *in vivo*. The therapeutic range of DHA is unknown but by extrapolation from *in vitro* data is exceeded considerably by current dose regimens.

Box 96.3 Treatment of Severe Malaria

Artesunate is the treatment of choice
Artesunate IV: 2.4 mg/kg stat, at 12 and 24 hours, then daily

If unavailable:
Artemether IM: initial dose of 3.2 mg/kg followed by 1.6 mg/kg every 24 hours until oral medication is tolerated[a]

or
Quinine IV: loading dose 20 mg salt/kg given over 4 hours, then 10 mg salt/kg given 8 hours after the loading dose was started, followed by 10 mg salt/kg every 8 hours[b]

or
Quinine IM: loading dose of 20 mg salt/kg is given as two simultaneous injections in the anterior thigh (10 mg salt/kg in each) after dilution of the quinine in sterile water to a concentration of 60–100 mg/mL; maintenance dose of 10 mg salt/kg is given as one IM injection every 8 hours using the same dilution

or
Quinidine IV: 10 mg base/kg infused over 1–2 hours followed by 1.2 mg base/kg per hour by constant infusion
Electrocardiographic monitoring necessary[c]

Total treatment duration for all regimens = 7 days

- Once the patient has recovered sufficiently to tolerate oral medication reliably, the parenteral treatment can be discontinued and a second drug should be added, such as doxycyline 3 mg/kg for 7 days, clindamycin 10 mg/kg bid for 7 days, or artemether–lumefantrine 1.5/9 mg/kg twice daily or atovaquone 20 mg/kg/day + proguanil 8 mg/kg/day for 3 days[d]
- Sulfadoxine–pyrimethamine (SP) single dose can be used if parasites are known to be sensitive

[a] *Absorption of IM artemether may be inadequate in a subgroup of patients with shock.*
[b] *If QTc (on electrocardiogram) is greater than 25% of baseline or exceeds 600 ms or hypotension occurs temporarily, reduce or stop infusion.*
[c] *Some authorities recommend a lower dose of 6.2 mg base/kg initially over 1 hour followed by 0.012 mg base/kg/hour.*
[d] *Mefloquine should not be used because of the increased risk of postmalaria neurologic syndrome (Mai NTH, Day NPJ, Chuong LV, et al. Post-malaria neurological syndrome. Lancet. 1996;348:917–921).*

Artemether and Artemotil

These oil-based formulations are slowly and erratically absorbed following IM injection (there is no IV formulation), and some patients may not achieve parasiticidal concentrations within the first few hours after starting treatment. Absorption is particularly poor in children and adults with poor peripheral perfusion. Artemether is also converted to DHA *in vivo*, but concentrations of the parent compound exceed those of DHA, so artemether contributes the majority of antimalarial effect *in vivo*. No dose adjustments are needed in liver or renal dysfunction.

Quinine

A full loading dose (20 mg quinine dihydrochloride salt/kg) should always be given irrespective of the degree of vital organ dysfunction unless there is clear evidence that the patient has already received adequate quinine treatment (>40 mg salt/kg in the past 48 hours). For quinine there is considerable variability in apparent volume of distribution, so the full loading dose is necessary to ensure that the majority of patients do have adequate blood concentrations. In the past there was too much concern over the dangers of potential quinine toxicity and insufficient concern over the dangers of undertreatment in severe malaria. The risk-to-benefit ratio changes as treatment progresses. The majority of deaths from malaria occur within the first 48 hours following admission to hospital; undertreatment may have fatal consequences. In practice, quinine toxicity in the first 24 hours of treatment is rare. The maintenance dose is 10 mg/kg every 8 hours. After 48 hours of treatment, if there is no clinical improvement in severe malaria, or if the patient is in ARF, the dose should be reduced by one-third to avoid continued accumulation to potentially toxic concentrations. The therapeutic range has not been well defined, but total plasma concentrations of between 8 and 15 mg/L are thought to be safe and effective. Toxicity is increasingly likely with plasma concentrations >20 mg/L (free quinine >2 mg/L).

Quinidine is more toxic than quinine. Both hypotension and prolongation of ventricular repolarization (QTc interval) are common when parenteral quinidine is used in the treatment of severe malaria. There have been only two small studies of quinidine in severe malaria so dose recommendations rest on limited information. Ideally patients receiving quinidine should have careful cardiovascular monitoring and frequent measurement of plasma concentrations to guide dosing. As with quinine, the dose should be reduced if there is no clinical improvement within 48 hours. Currently an 8-hour interval is recommended. Dose reduction by one-third to one-half is recommended.

Where Parenteral Treatment Cannot be Given

In most areas of the rural tropics, severe malaria occurs far from medical attention. Since delay in starting treatment can have fatal consequences, rectal formulations of artemisinin have been developed and shown to reduce mortality. These should be given by village health workers pending transfer to a facility where parenteral treatment and supportive care can be given.[127–129]

Adjuvant Treatments

Many adjuvant treatments have been evaluated in severe malaria, but none has proved beneficial and several were harmful. Exchange blood transfusion in severe malaria has been recommended by some on the basis of uncontrolled studies which showed benefit. There is insufficient evidence to provide a clear recommendation.

Supportive Care

Patients with severe malaria require intensive nursing in an intensive care unit if possible. Following initial assessment and commencement of antimalarial treatment, clinical observations should be made as frequently as possible, including recording of vital signs, with an accurate assessment of respiratory rate and pattern, assessment of the coma score, and urine output. The blood glucose should be checked, with rapid stick tests every 4 hours if possible, particularly in unconscious patients. Convulsions should be treated promptly with anticonvulsants such as IV or rectal benzodiazepines or IM paraldehyde.

Each patient's fluid requirements should be assessed individually. Although many patients with severe malaria are dehydrated on admission and need immediate rehydration, adults with severe malaria are vulnerable to fluid overload and the physician may tread a narrow path between underhydration, and thus worsening renal impairment, and overhydration, with the risk of precipitating pulmonary edema. If the patient becomes oliguric (<0.4 mL of urine/kg/hour) despite adequate rehydration and the blood urea or creatinine are rising or already high, fluids should be restricted to replace insensible losses only and hemofiltration started as soon as possible. Children, on the other hand, are more likely to be dehydrated and usually respond well to a rate-controlled bolus of fluid. The fluid regimen must also be tailored around infusion of the antimalarial drugs. The CVP should be maintained between 2 and 5 cm. If the CVP is significantly elevated (usually because of overenthusiastic fluid administration), the patient should be nursed with the head at 45° and IV furosemide given if necessary.

If blood glucose is <4 mmol/L, then a 10% glucose infusion should be started following saline replacement; if it is <2.2 mmol/L, then hypoglycemia should be treated immediately (0.3–0.5 g/kg 50% glucose or 5 mL/kg 10% dextrose as an IV bolus). Hypoglycemia should be suspected in any patient who deteriorates suddenly. Stick tests may overestimate the frequency of hypoglycemia, so laboratory confirmation may be necessary.

Patients with acute pulmonary edema should be nursed upright and given oxygen, and the right-sided filling pressures should be reduced with whatever treatments are available (loop diuretics, opiates, venodilators, hemofiltration, dialysis). The right-sided pressure should be reduced to the lowest level compatible with an adequate cardiac output. Positive-pressure ventilation should be started early (if available) if the patient becomes hypoxic.

Less than 2% of patients with severe malaria develop clinically significant DIC. These patients should be given fresh blood transfusions and vitamin K. In endemic areas it is often difficult or impossible to distinguish bacterial sepsis with coincident parasitemia from severe malaria. If there is any possibility that the patient has a severe bacterial infection, then empirical broad-spectrum antibiotics should be given in addition to antimalarial treatment. Patients with secondary pneumonia should be given empirical treatment with a third-generation cephalosporin unless admitted with clear evidence of aspiration, in which case penicillin or clindamycin is adequate. Children with persistent fever despite parasite clearance may have a systemic *Salmonella* infection, although in most cases of persistent fever after parasite clearance no other pathogen is identified. Urinary tract infections are common in catheterized patients. Antibiotic treatments should depend on likely local antibiotic sensitivity patterns.

Severe Malaria in Pregnancy

Pregnant women in the second and third trimesters are more likely to develop severe malaria than are other adults, often complicated by pulmonary edema and hypoglycemia.[64] Maternal mortality from severe malaria approximates 50%, which is over twice that in nonpregnant adults. Fetal death and premature labor are common. The role of early cesarean section for the viable live fetus is unproven but is recommended by many authorities. Obstetric advice should be sought at an early stage, the pediatricians alerted, and the blood glucose checked frequently. Hypoglycemia should be expected and is often recurrent if the patient is receiving quinine. The antimalarial drugs should be given in full doses (***Boxes 96.3 and 96.4***). Severe malaria may also present immediately following delivery. Postpartum bacterial infection is a common complication

Box 96.4 Treatment of Uncomplicated Malaria in Pregnancy

Quinine 10 mg salt/kg tid for 7 days. This should be combined with clindamycin (10 mg/kg bid) for 7 days in the second and third trimesters of pregnancy[a]	Artemisinin derivatives should not be used in the first trimester of pregnancy. In the second and third trimesters of pregnancy, artesunate (2 mg/kg/day for 7 days) may be given with clindamycin 10 mg/kg twice daily for 7 days, or artemether–lumefantrine 1.5/9 mg/kg given twice daily with food for 3 days
or if the infection is known to be from an area with sulfadoxine–pyrimethamine sensitivity, pyrimethamine 1.25 mg/kg + sulfadoxine 25 mg/kg (single dose) 3 tablets in an adult	The role of mefloquine in the treatment of malaria in pregnancy remains uncertain; in one large study, there were no adverse effects,[b] but in another, there was an increased risk of stillbirth[c]
or if the infection is known to be from an area with chloroquine sensitivity to *P. falciparum* or for infections with *P. vivax*, *P. ovale*, or *P. malariae*, chloroquine phosphate (1 tablet contains 250 mg salt, equivalent to 155.3 mg base)[a] 10 mg/kg base at 0, 24 hours followed by 5 mg/kg base at 48 hours	

[a]*Quinine has been shown to be safe in all trimesters. There is no evidence for an increased risk of abortion, stillbirth, or congenital abnormality, but in the third trimester there is an increased risk of iatrogenic hypoglycemia with quinine treatment.*

[b]*Steketee RW, Wirima JJ, Slutsker L, et al. Treatment and prevention in pregnancy: indications for use and adverse events associated with use of chloroquine or mefloquine. Am J Trop Med Hyg. 1996;55(1 suppl):50–56.*

[c]*Nosten F, Vincenti M, Simpson JA, et al. The effects of mefloquine treatment in pregnancy. Clin Infect Dis. 1999;28:808–815.*

in these cases. Falciparum malaria has also been associated with severe midtrimester hemolytic anemia in Nigeria. This often requires transfusion in addition to antimalarial treatment and folate supplementation.

Follow-up Treatment of Severe Malaria

When the patient with severe malaria has recovered sufficiently, oral medication should be substituted. Infections resulting in severe malaria are more likely to recrudesce than milder infections. They are a potentially important source of resistance, and it is correspondingly important that a full course of curative treatment be completed. There has been only one comparative evaluation of consolidation treatments and no studies in which recrudescence rates were documented. A randomized comparison of oral quinine plus SP versus mefloquine (following parenteral artemether or quinine) was conducted in Vietnam. Mefloquine recipients had a significantly increased risk of neuropsychiatric reactions (absolute risk of 5% compared with 0.1–1% in uncomplicated malaria). In a nonrandomized study of doxycycline pharmacokinetics following severe malaria, it was suggested that the current dose regimen (3–3.5 mg/kg/day) may be insufficient.

Current practice for oral treatment following severe malaria is either to complete a full 3-day course of ACT (except for artesunate–mefloquine) or to continue the same drug orally as given parenterally to complete 7 days of treatment. In nonpregnant adults, doxycycline is added to quinine, artesunate, or artemether also to complete 7 days of treatment. Doxycycline is preferred to other tetracyclines because it can be given once daily and does not accumulate in renal failure. Since doxycycline only starts when the patient has recovered sufficiently, the doxycycline course finishes after the quinine, artemether, or artesunate course. Where available and affordable, clindamycin may be substituted in children and pregnant women because doxycycline cannot be given to these groups.

PREVENTION AND CONTROL

Malaria Prevention in Visitors to Malaria-Endemic Areas

Malaria poses a health risk to visitors to malaria-endemic regions. Annually millions of travelers from nonendemic countries travel to areas where there is a malaria risk. As well, many residents of nonendemic regions of countries that have areas of malaria transmission are at risk of infection during short-term visits. Prevention and suppression of infection are far more effective than reliance on treatment of malaria illness in these visitors, owing to the unpredictability of the availability and quality of medical care in many settings. The prevention of infection and disease relies largely on the prophylactic use of malaria drugs (***Table 96.5***).

Several general principles should guide the protection of visitors to regions with risk of malaria transmission. First and foremost, individuals should be protected optimally if there is any risk, since a single infected mosquito bite may result in a fatal malaria infection. If the area to be visited has any *P. falciparum*, the choice of drug for prevention should be based on an assumption of drug resistance unless the travel is to Haiti or Central America. Finally, while the use of efficacious drugs (chemoprophylaxis) can afford a high degree of protection, it is important for visitors to use mosquito protection, including bednets and repellents, and to be aware of how to secure safe and effective medical attention in the event of a potential malaria illness.

Malaria drugs for use in prevention among visitors have several distinct modes of action. Most drugs used for chemoprophylaxis are blood schizonticides (killing only blood-stage parasites). These include chloroquine, other 4-aminoquinolines, and mefloquine. These drugs do not prevent primary infection of the liver but kill parasites once they erupt from the liver and invade erythrocytes, thereby preventing disease progression.

A limited number of drugs have activity against parasites developing in hepatocytes and are termed tissue schizonticides and causal prophylactic drugs. The 8-aminoquinolones, primaquine,[130] and the longer-acting tafenoquine[131] (in development) kill liver-stage parasites. Primaquine has only modest activity against the asexual erythrocytic stages of *Plasmodium vivax*, and tafenoquine probably has more activity against blood stages. The main activity of atovaquone/proguanil,[132] tetracycline, and doxycycline is against the asexual erythrocytic stages (blood schizonticidal activity); but these drugs also have activity against pre-erythrocytic liver stages. Atovaquone/proguanil[132] and doxycycline are considered first-line drugs. Primaquine is now being recommended more often for chemoprophylaxis because it can be taken a few days before arrival in a malarious area and for only 5–7 days afterwards[130,133] and is much less expensive than atovaquone–proguanil, which can also be discontinued 1 week after leaving the malarious area.

Drug Safety and Contraindications

The risk of being infected during visits to malaria-endemic areas is highly variable but is low in the vast majority of settings. Furthermore, most travelers are healthy, and avoidance of travel and risk also is an option. Consequently, drugs used for chemoprophylaxis need to be well tolerated and should not pose a substantive health risk. The current standard chemoprophylactic drugs are within acceptable levels of safety, yet each has a spectrum of potential and nonlife-threatening adverse side effects that must be appreciated by travelers and their medical advisors. The Centers for Disease Control and Prevention[134] and WHO have excellent information on these risks and advice for special populations.

Pregnant women and young children pose special challenges in the chemoprophylactic use of drugs. For several drugs there are specific contraindications for these populations (e.g., tetracycline). Licensure of most drugs by the US Food and Drug Administration does not generally address the safety of drugs during pregnancy and in infancy (e.g., mefloquine); consequently, their use for short-term travel needs to be considered carefully. Ancillary prevention methods (bednets) and the delaying of travel should always be considered. The safety of long-term (i.e., >1 year) prophylaxis with currently recommended prophylactic drugs has not been clearly established.

Malaria Drug Prophylaxis for Residents of Malaria-Endemic Areas

The routine use of malaria drugs for suppressing malaria disease lost favor during the 1970s–80s due principally to the presumption that the use of drugs on a mass basis at subtherapeutic doses would encourage drug resistance to valuable therapeutic drugs, notably chloroquine. In recent years selective use of malaria drugs in a preventive mode but at therapeutic doses (intermittent preventive treatment, or IPT) has been documented to be effective in reducing the adverse effects of malaria in pregnant women, infants, and children.

Malaria Control in Malaria-Endemic Areas

During the past 5 years there has been a renewal in the global commitment to control the enormous health and economic burden that malaria extracts. Under the banner of the Roll Back Malaria (RBM) partnership, national governments and financing and technical agencies such as WHO and UNICEF have mobilized, with a focus on the enormous malaria burden in the Africa region. The malaria control landscape in mid-2010 reflects the remarkable mobilization of resources, players, commitment, and national programming action that has occurred around malaria over the past 3–5 years.

Underlying this accelerated effort is a highly cost-effective set of malaria control interventions that, despite technical limitations such as drug resistance, have been demonstrated to control both malaria transmission and disease. While the treatment of malaria illness remains a constant component of malaria control, prevention has become the predominant cost-effective approach. The major challenge to the control of malaria has been the development of effective program delivery systems to attain and sustain high population coverage with these robust interventions.

Based on malaria epidemiology and the capacity of local health system infrastructures to deliver malaria control interventions, there are currently several distinct settings for malaria prevention and control efforts. In areas where malaria transmission is either highly seasonal or of low intensity, principally in the Indian subcontinent and Southeast Asia and most of the Americas, malaria control focuses around the prompt and effective treatment of malaria illness and selective use of antimosquito measures. In many of these areas there is a continuation of control methods developed during the malaria eradication programs of 1950–75, with the use of the indoor spraying of residual insecticides (currently limited use of DDT and more typically use of less environmentally threatening chemicals) to interrupt malaria transmission.

Malaria control programming and funding have in recent years focused on developing national-level programs to stem the health and economic burden in Africa. Based on WHO and RBM guidance, the following are the key malaria control and prevention interventions advocated for the Africa region.

Insecticide-Treated Nets

Based on evidence from five randomized controlled trials and population-based program effectiveness studies in different malaria transmission settings, ITNs can reduce the number of under-5 deaths from all causes by about 20% and clinical episodes of malaria by about half[135] (***Fig. 96.11***). Since malaria causes approximately 20% of under-5 mortality in Africa, the protective efficacy of nets on malaria-specific mortality in children less than 5 years of age is estimated at 80%, in the range of the protective efficacy of most childhood vaccines.[136,137] Recent evidence shows that ITNs protect not only those who sleep under them but also those in the same dwelling and those living nearby. Current ITNs, termed long-lasting or wash-durable, are effective in community usage for 3–5 years. ITNs are less effective in parts of Asia, where the main malaria vectors bite outdoors early in the evening.

Indoor Residual Spraying

IRS has been a highly effective intervention in many parts of the world, and in particular in the Americas, in Asia, and in Southern Africa. IRS, through its house-to-house, publicly funded and managed approach, can achieve very high coverage and thus have a major impact on malaria disease burden. IRS programs are most feasible in urban areas in countries with stable malaria endemicity, especially those where there has been no tradition of managing programs of such logistic complexity.[138]

Intermittent Preventive Treatment

IPT is the preferred approach to reduce the adverse consequences of malaria during pregnancy in high-transmission areas where *P. falciparum* is SP-sensitive; it involves the administration of full curative treatment doses of SP at predefined intervals during pregnancy, beginning in the second trimester after quickening. Where effective, IPT with SP reduces the incidence of severe anemia in the mother and lowers the proportion of LBW babies.[139,140] There is uncertainty how to deploy IPT in the increasing areas of SP resistance and whether IPT should be deployed in low-transmission settings.

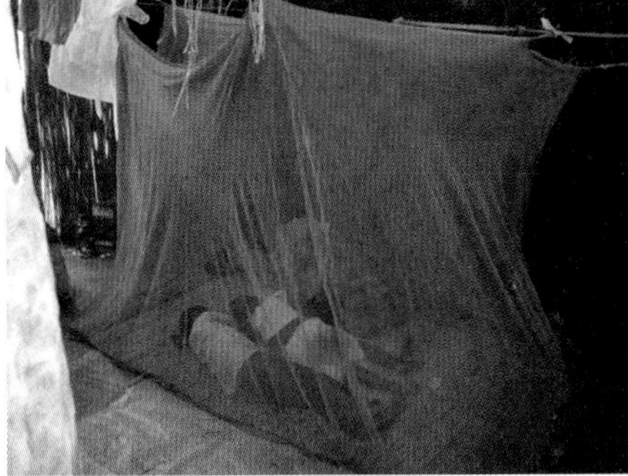

Figure 96.11 Children sleeping under an insecticide-impregnated bednet. (Courtesy of C. Campbell.)

Prompt and Effective Case Management of Malaria Illness

The prompt recognition that a febrile illness could be *Plasmodium* infection is the key to limiting the risk of progression to severe or fatal disease. In most of the malaria-endemic world, malaria is self-diagnosed and treated; many episodes of fever not caused by malaria are therefore self-treated with antimalarials. Standard microscopy – and increasingly, rapid diagnostic tests (see section on diagnosis) in certain settings – allow for an accurate diagnosis of malaria and increase the potential that antimalarial drugs are used for the correct purpose and not simply in response to an unspecified fever episode.

While drug efficacy should be the principal determinant of which drugs are used to treat malaria infections, in many settings there are many substandard and counterfeit drugs in the market place and the majority of malaria drugs come from commercial outlets without the advice of a health care provider.

A major effort has been to extend the availability of rapid diagnostics and certified drugs to the community and household level, through community health workers. While this strategy should increase the promptness and effectiveness of malaria and fever management, it also raises concerns about quality control and the widescale deployment of malaria drugs and the risks of drug resistance.

Program Goals for Malaria Control

In the Africa region currently at least a dozen African nations are at some stage of scaling up at national level malaria control programming. There is an increasing evidence base on these national efforts. A consistent profile emerging is that in the hands of national program partnership the delivery of program to cover 60% with ITNs can happen in 2–3 years, and the national programs are achieving or exceeding the impact on under-5 mortality (20–26% reduction) documented in earlier trials of ITNs.[141]

The Global Fund against AIDS, Tuberculosis, and Malaria (GFATM) has in a decade become the predominant financing agency for malaria control programming. Through GFATM alone, over US$1 billion have been allocated for malaria programming since 2000.

Development of New and More Effective Malaria Control and Prevention Tools

The 2007 call for malaria eradication by the Bill and Melinda Gates Foundation has energized ambitions, constructively. The global community has rallied around the call for a long-term goal of eradicating malaria. In 2008 the RBM partnership launched the Global Malaria Action Plan (GMAP), which mapped a programming sequence from scale-up to elimination.[142] The GMAP will serve as a consensus platform for partners in coordinating investments, and assuring investments in research and development logically linked to programming priorities.

Although there are highly efficacious interventions for malaria control and intervention, continued emphasis on the development of new and more efficacious methods is required since the evolution of drug and insecticide resistance is assumed. In the context of the GMAP, a consensus strategic plan for investments in research, termed MalERA, is being developed.[143]

Response to Drug Resistance and the Development of New Malaria Drugs

Since the early 1960s, there has been increasing resistance of malaria parasites to antimalarial drugs (***Table 96.2***). Resistance has had a profound impact on malaria control and prevention efforts globally. The development of novel malaria drugs has received renewed attention in recent years, notably under the guidance of several multinational initiatives such as the Medicines for Malaria Venture (www.mmv.org), and the Drugs for Neglected Diseases Initiative, public–private partnerships devoted to malaria drug development. There are promising leads, but cost and the long lead time required to move efficacious compounds to licensure remain serious impediments to the control and prevention of malaria globally.

Development of Malaria Vaccines

Malaria vaccines could benefit those living wherever there is malaria and travelers to those areas. The primary goal, however, must be to prevent the enormous numbers of deaths and cases of severe malaria in infants and young children in Africa caused by *P. falciparum*. Thus, most malaria vaccine development efforts are focused on *P. falciparum*.

There are no commercially available vaccines for human parasites. Parasites present a greater challenge than do the viruses and bacteria for which we have vaccines because they are more complex. They have much larger genomes coding for more proteins. They have multistage life cycles in which they express many different proteins at different times (***Fig. 96.12***). As a result, protective immune responses against the extracellular sporozoites that enter during the bite of a mosquito may have no direct effect on the parasites that later emerge from the liver and infect red blood cells (the asexual erythrocytic-stage merozoites). The *P. falciparum* parasite in particular has enormous variability in its proteins. These characteristics are critical to the parasite's survival because they enable it to evade host immune defenses. They also mean that a vaccine containing just a single sequence of a single protein, or a few proteins, may fail to have a large, sustainable impact on the disease. A truly effective malaria vaccine may need to induce both antibody and T-cell responses.

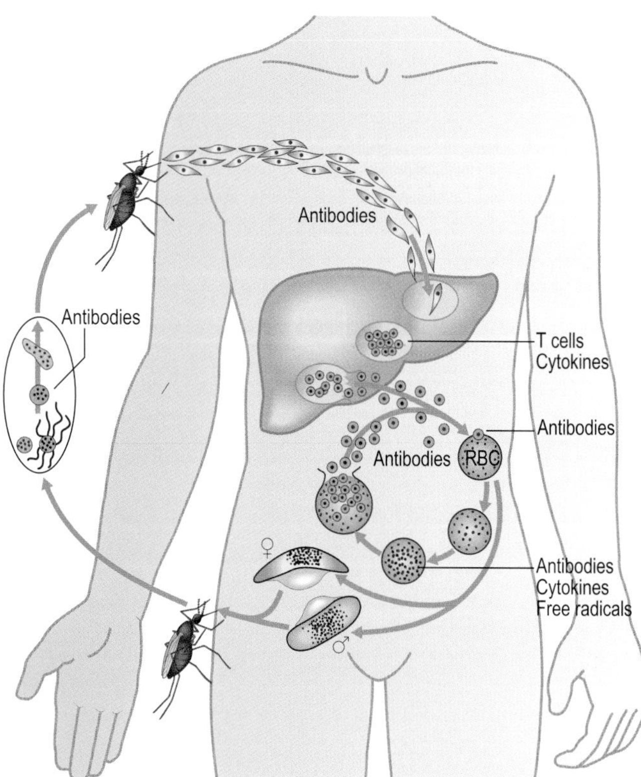

Figure 96.12 Schematic of the life cycle of *Plasmodium falciparum* with indication of which immune responses can affect which stage of the life cycle. RBC, red blood cells. (Reproduced from Hoffman SL (ed.) Malaria Vaccine Development: a Multi-Immune Response Approach. Washington, DC, ASM Press, 1996. Courtesy of the American Society of Microbiology.)

Antibodies have the potential to block sporozoites as they enter the body (***Fig. 96.12***) but have to act within minutes to block entry into the liver. They can also prevent infection of red blood cells, help destroy those that are already infected, and prevent infection of mosquitoes. T cells have the potential to kill infected liver cells, thereby controlling and even eliminating infection and potentially, through release of soluble mediators, have an impact on infected erythrocytes. Both types of response may have to be directed against multiple different proteins, at different stages of the complex parasite life cycle, and at the same time.[144–147] If so, malaria vaccine developers face a technical problem that has never been solved.

Scientists attempting to develop a malaria vaccine have generally kept two observations in mind. The first is that most malaria-associated deaths and severe disease in sub-Saharan Africa occur in infants, young children, and pregnant women. Nonpregnant adolescents and adults who have had multiple previous infections rarely develop severe disease or die when infected with *P. falciparum*. They have presumably developed natural immunity that limits parasite replication and severe forms of malaria but does not prevent infection, resulting in milder symptoms.[42] Pregnant women, especially with their first child, apparently lose this immunity. This observation has led to the idea that a vaccine would be worthwhile even if it only limited the severity of disease for those most at risk without preventing infection or moderate disease. Such a vaccine would probably not be useful for travelers, and as malaria control efforts become increasingly effective in reducing severe disease and death, may be less useful for other populations in endemic areas. The second observation is that when volunteers are exposed to more than 1000 bites from *P. falciparum*-infected *Anopheles* mosquitoes that have been irradiated to weaken the sporozoites they carry, they develop protective immunity against multiple strains of *P. falciparum*. If these volunteers are exposed to normal sporozoites, more than 90% are completely protected against developing erythrocytic-stage infection.[148] This is the strongest evidence that development of a highly effective malaria vaccine is possible, and accordingly there are efforts to develop vaccines that prevent all infections with *P. falciparum* in a majority (>85%) of recipients.[149]

During the last few years control efforts have had a profound effect on malaria in a number of areas of sub-Saharan Africa and the rest of the world. This has led to the call for elimination of malaria from defined geographic areas and eventual eradication of malaria. However, until elimination/eradication is accomplished, as the transmission intensity of *P. falciparum* decreases, it is likely that immunity in the population will decrease, and the susceptibility of a population to *P. falciparum* will increase. Thus, to prevent severe disease and death, paradoxically, more of the population may need to be immunized than has always been anticipated. While transmission will undoubtedly be interrupted in a number of malaria-endemic areas in the next decade, new tools will be needed to eliminate malaria caused by *P. falciparum* in the areas of the world where transmission is most intense. A pre-erythrocytic-stage vaccine that prevents transmission by preventing asexual erythrocytic-stage infection will be the ideal vaccine.[150]

There are three main strategies by which it may be possible to achieve the preceding goals. The first is to create vaccines that counter sporozoites as they enter the body and invade and reproduce in the liver (pre-erythrocytic-stage vaccines). These have the potential to limit or prevent infection altogether, and thereby prevent transmission entirely. The second is to limit parasite invasion of erythrocytes and subsequent multiplication and pathologic effects (asexual erythrocytic-stage and antitoxin vaccines). Such vaccines would limit only severe disease – they would not prevent infection or mild disease, and be unlikely to have a major impact on transmission. The third strategy is to prevent the spread of viable parasites to other people with sexual and mosquito-stage vaccines. These stimulate the production of antibodies that are ingested with the parasite and destroy the parasite within the vector's gut (***Fig. 96.12***), thereby reducing or preventing transmission without having any effect on disease manifestations in the immunized individual. It may be necessary to combine all three strategies to have maximum success. Current vaccine candidates in clinical trials, however, contain just one or a few proteins.

In contrast, the protective immune responses elicited by natural exposure to malaria or by immunization with radiation-attenuated sporozoites could be directed at many – perhaps hundreds or even thousands – of the proteins encoded by the 5300 genes in the *P. falciparum* genome.

According to WHO (http://www.who.int/vaccine_research/links/MaVa/en/index.html), in 2008 more than 50 subunit malaria vaccine candidates were in different stages of development. Despite these efforts only one *P. falciparum* protein, the *P. falciparum* circumsporozoite protein (PfCSP),[151] has been repeatedly evaluated in clinical trials and shown to provide complete protection in a portion of volunteers. The protein was discovered in 1979 by the Nussezweig group, shown to be protective in mice in 1980, and first shown to protect humans as a vaccine in 1987. The lead candidate[152] based on this protein has been RTS,S/AS02A, and it protects approximately 30–45% of nonimmune volunteers against experimental challenge with *P. falciparum* for 2–3 weeks.[151,153] In 1–4-year-old children[154] in Mozambique during 6 months, it reduced the incidence of new clinical attacks of malaria by 22.6%, new *P. falciparum* infection by 10.4%, and the incidence of severe disease by 58%.[155] Subsequently, the adjuvant has been changed from AS02A to AS01E and it appears that this improves the protective efficacy of the vaccine.[154,156] Phase III studies of this vaccine, which does not prevent malaria but reduces the rate at which malaria is acquired by 30–50%, have been initiated in multiple countries in sub-Saharan Africa. Initial trial results should be available in the next 1–2 years.

In addition to the modern subunit vaccine approaches, there is a major effort to develop a nonreplicating, metabolically active whole sporozoite *P. falciparum* vaccine.[149,157] This pre-erythrocytic-stage vaccine is intended to achieve the high level of protection demonstrated when volunteers were immunized by the bite of irradiated, *P. falciparum* sporozoite-infected mosquitoes. The first such vaccine, the PfSPZ Vaccine, has been manufactured, and is now being assessed in clinical trials.

It currently costs US$0.5–1 billion to bring a vaccine to market. There are large numbers of vaccine candidates in preclinical and clinical development, and many more candidates are likely to enter efficacy field trials in the next 5 years. Furthermore, emerging genomic and proteomic studies of *P. falciparum* will lead to the development of even more candidate vaccines.[158] It will unquestionably take creative and committed public–private partnerships to bring a malaria vaccine to the populations who need it most. We look forward to the time when a malaria vaccine is widely used to successfully prevent the morbidity and mortality of *P. falciparum* in the 20–25 million infants born annually in sub-Saharan Africa, and to eliminate and eventually eradicate malaria.

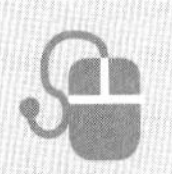

Access the complete reference list online at
http://www.expertconsult.com

CHAPTER 97

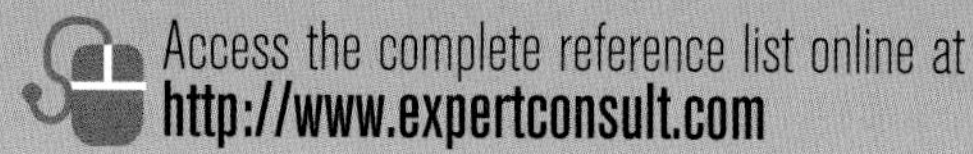
Access the complete reference list online at
http://www.expertconsult.com

Babesiosis

Sam R. Telford III • Peter F. Weller • James H. Maguire

INTRODUCTION

Babesiosis, a tick-borne malaria-like zoonosis, appears to have plagued humans since antiquity in its veterinary form. Human babesiosis has been reported mainly from Europe and the eastern or western United States, but cases are increasingly being reported from Asia. The prevalence of babesiosis afflicting domestic animals in tropical regions suggests that human infection is not rare in the tropics and perhaps is mistaken for falciparum malaria.[1]

THE AGENT

The genus *Babesia* was named after the Romanian bacteriologist Victor Babes, who in 1888 attributed "hemoglobinuric fever" of cattle to inclusions he detected within erythrocytes. *Babesia* are obligately intraerythrocytic in vertebrates but, unlike plasmodia, replicate by budding rather than schizogony, and do not produce hemozoin. Currently *Babesia* are classified as apicomplexans of the order Piroplasmidora and family Babesiidae.[2,3] Over 100 species of *Babesia* have been described from domestic and wild mammals on the basis of morphology and life cycle.[3] Recent molecular taxonomic analyses suggest that there is even greater diversity than what has previously been recognized.[4–7] The powerful new methods of molecular phylogenetics will eventually stimulate the development of a new classification for the piroplasms.

Life Cycle

In 1893, Theobald Smith[8] described the life cycle of *Babesia bigemina,* the agent of bovine red-water fever, and demonstrated for the first time transmission of an infectious agent by arthropods. All piroplasms for which life cycles have been described require a tick as the definitive host (***Fig. 97.1***). Upon ingestion of infectious blood from a vertebrate host, babesiae undergo syngamy and replicate in the intestinal epithelium of the tick vector and develop further in the salivary glands, ovaries, and other tissues. Sporozoites in salivary glands are deposited in the skin of vertebrate hosts during the tick's blood meal. Because of transstadial transmission, ticks infected as larvae generally remain infected as nymphs and adults. Transovarial transmission in the tick has been documented for some species such as *B. bigemina* but not for others such as *B. microti*; such a major life history difference has long been considered to represent a significant phylogenetic divergence.

The common belief that sporozoites enter erythrocytes directly (no pre-erythrocytic phase) has not been critically examined. Exoerythrocytic forms, demonstrated in lymphocytes with *B. equi* and the closely related *Theileria* species,[9,10] may occur in infections with *B. microti.*[10] The process by which extracellular merozoites invade erythrocytes (induced endocytosis) is similar to that of the plasmodia. In the rat babesia, *B. rodhaini,* complement facilitates invasion by modification of either the erythrocyte surface or that of the merozoite; with *B. divergens*, sialic acid appears to be an important ligand for erythrocyte invasion.[11]

Following entry into erythrocytes, pear-shaped trophozoites (piroplasms) replicate by asynchronous budding rather than by schizogony as occurs in malarial parasites. During replication, double-membraned segments develop and pinch off from the parental piroplasm, resulting in both asexually reproducing merozoites and nonreplicating sexual parasites (gametocytes).[12] Asexual forms appear as simple rings, pairs, or tetrads and are difficult to distinguish from sexual stages by light microscopy.

EPIDEMIOLOGY AND DISTRIBUTION

Two major epidemiologic patterns of human babesiosis are apparent. The first involves splenectomized or otherwise compromised persons and diverse babesiae, some of which have been distinguished only by molecular phylogenetic methods. A bovine-infecting species then identified as *B. bovis* (perhaps conspecific with *B. divergens*)[13] was the cause of the first well-documented case of human babesiosis in 1957. A 33-year-old splenectomized farmer living in Yugoslavia and who had been exposed to cattle died as a result of hemolytic anemia, hemoglobinuria, and renal failure.[14] Since then, more than two dozen sporadic cases have been reported from Ireland, Yugoslavia, France, the British Isles, Spain, the Canary Islands, Portugal, Germany, Sweden, and Russia.[15] All cases were severe and often fatal despite treatment. The vector, *Ixodes ricinus*, also transmits Lyme disease, granulocytic ehrlichiosis, and tickborne encephalitis. Reservoirs of *B. divergens*, other than ticks, include cattle and perhaps deer.

In 1992, a splenectomized man living in rural Missouri with an unspecified exposure history died of infection with a parasite closely related to *B. divergens,* designated MO-1.[16] A splenectomized Kentucky resident, potentially exposed while hunting rabbits, recovered from a similar infection[17] with a species whose sequenced 18S rDNA demonstrated 99.8% identity with sequences of bovine-derived *B. divergens* and 100% identity with an agent maintained among cottontail rabbits.[18] A third case was reported in a splenectomized resident of Washington.[19] Although the degree of DNA sequence similarity between the American divergens-like parasites and the European cattle and deer parasites is within that which might be expected due to geographic variation of a single species, the former fails to propagate by subinoculation into gerbils or cattle whereas the latter readily does so.[20] Although European "divergens babesiosis" has heretofore been solely attributed to infection by *B. divergens*, molecular analysis suggests that another closely related babesia, designated EU-1[21] and perhaps representing *B. capreoli* (an agent maintained by *I. ricinus* among red or roe deer),[22] also parasitizes humans and could be mistaken by inexperienced microscopists for *B. divergens* infection. Thus, it appears that "divergens babesiosis" may be due to diverse parasites that are geographically widespread.

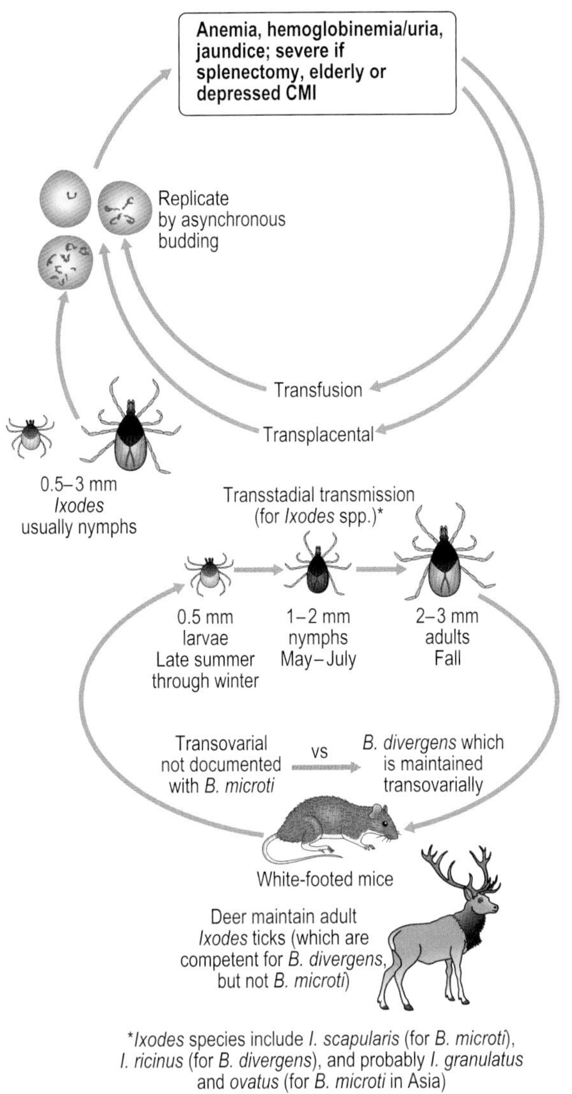

Figure 97.1 All piroplasms for which life cycles have been described require a tick as the definitive host. CMI, cell-mediated immunity.

A variation on this epidemiologic pattern has emerged along the Pacific Coast of the United States. *B. duncani* (previously known as WA-1) is closely related by DNA sequencing to the canine pathogen *B. gibsoni*.[23,24] CA-type (DNA sequences designated CA-1, CA-2, etc.) agents[25] are most closely related to parasites of mule deer and bighorn sheep.[6] Both agents cause a similar disease and appear morphologically indistinguishable on blood smears, with abundant Maltese-cross forms within parasitized erythrocytes. Of 9 reported cases of *B. duncani* or CA-type babesiosis, 4 occurred among splenectomized persons, and 1 involved an apparently healthy 41-year-old man. The others were transfusion-induced cases involving a spleen-intact elderly man with multiple medical problems[26] and a premature infant.[27] It appears that most infections are subclinical because surveys have shown seroprevalences of 3.5–20% among persons with exposure in rural and semirural areas of California.[28] As with *B. divergens*, splenectomized or otherwise compromised individuals appear at risk for more severe infections and cases are sporadic.

The second major epidemiologic pattern is that of endemic infection due to the widely distributed rodent *B. microti*.[29] The risk of human infection with this organism is not increased in the absence of a spleen, although infected persons without spleens are at high risk of becoming severely ill. The global distribution of *B. microti* parallels that of *Borrelia burgdorferi* and other agents transmitted by ticks in the *Ixodes persulcatus* species complex.[30] Human babesiosis due to *B. microti* has been reported from Taiwan, Japan, and Germany.[31–33] Additional sporadic cases of babesiosis due to *B. microti* likely will be detected from Eurasia, given the wide enzootic distribution of this babesial species complex,[7] greater physician awareness, and increasing availability of molecular diagnostic tools.[34]

In the United States, *B. microti* babesiosis largely remains limited to the terminal moraine islands of New York, Massachusetts, and Rhode Island, and focal areas in Massachusetts, Connecticut, New Jersey, Wisconsin, and Minnesota.[35] Because most cases are asymptomatic or mildly symptomatic, the incidence is difficult to estimate and differs from year to year due to fluctuations in the densities of the rodent reservoir and tick vectors. While there have been only several hundred reported cases of symptomatic infection with *B. microti* since the first reported case in 1969, serologic surveys indicate that in highly endemic areas as many as 9–21% of persons have been infected.[36] The incidence of babesiosis has been rising in parts of southern New England since the 1990s, and on Block Island, Rhode Island, there may be as many as 900 cases per 100 000 residents per year.[37] There have been at least 70 cases of babesiosis acquired from blood products from asymptomatically infected donors,[38] most commonly packed erythrocytes, but also platelets and frozen-deglycerolized erythrocytes and 1 case of vertically transmitted infection.[39]

Few cases of babesiosis have been reported outside the United States and Europe, but this may be changing due to the wider diagnostic use of polymerase chain reaction (PCR). There have been case reports demonstrating active infection (a photomicrograph of a blood smear) in China,[40] India,[41] and South Africa,[42] and serosurveys suggesting human babesial infection in Latin America and West Africa. An unusual case of babesiosis due to a *Babesia* sp. most closely related to those that infect sheep was reported from a 75-year-old, splenectomized female Korean resident who was treated and survived.[43] Because of the ubiquity of ticks and the diversity of *Babesia* species and animal hosts, it is likely that transmission to human beings occurs wherever humans are greatly exposed to ticks.

Seasonality and Ecology

Human *B. divergens* cases occur mainly in cattle-raising regions during summer months when the presumed vector, *I. ricinus,* is most active and the incidence of red-water fever in cattle is greatest.[15] The only known reservoir hosts for *B. divergens* are cattle and reindeer, although deer are also suspected as potential hosts. The American *B. divergens*-like agent (MO-1) is most likely transmitted by *I. dentatus*.[18] Although long thought to be specific for rabbits and birds, this tick appears to feed on humans more frequently than appreciated. *B. capreoli* (EU-1) is maintained by *I. ricinus*, probably with roe and red deer as amplifying hosts.[22]

The few reported cases of *B. duncani* and CA-type babesiosis had their onset between June and August. Vectors and reservoirs remain to be described although canids, ungulates, and their associated ticks are suspected given the genetic relatedness of these agents to *B. gibsoni* and the mule deer or bighorn sheep babesias, respectively.[6] Vectors for KO-1 or other agents reported from India or South Africa remain undescribed.

In contrast, the ecology of *B. microti* has been well studied.[44] Its enzootic cycle in the northern United States depends on the interaction of subadult deer ticks, *I. dammini* (thought by some to be an aggressively human-biting variant of *I. scapularis*) and their main source of blood meals, the white-footed mouse. Deer are the hosts on which adult ticks primarily feed, but are incompetent reservoirs. Adult ticks feed during the fall, and lay eggs during the spring. Eggs hatch in late July, and emergent larvae feed mainly during August and September, at which time they may acquire babesial infection from an infected mouse. Fed larvae overwinter and molt to the nymphal stage during the spring. The life cycle of the tick is complete when nymphs that have fed on a mouse or other host during the summer molt to the adult stage in the fall.

Humans become infected primarily by the nymphal ticks (***Fig. 97.2***) rather than adults, because survival of *B. microti* during the nymphal to adult tick molt is poor.[45] In addition, people are likely to discover the larger adult deer tick (albeit smaller than the dog tick) and remove it before the tick has fed long enough (>60 hours for *B. microti*) to deliver

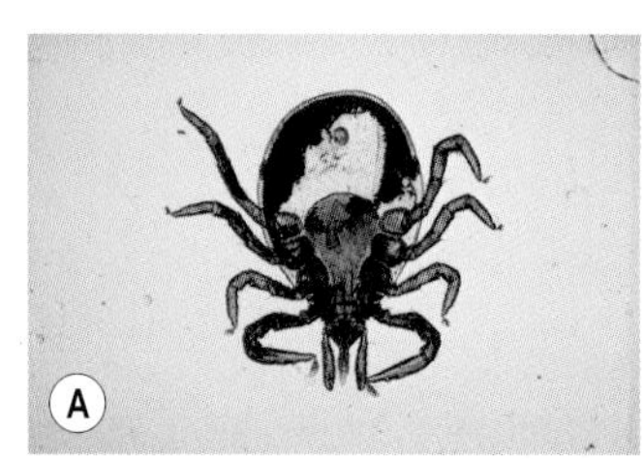

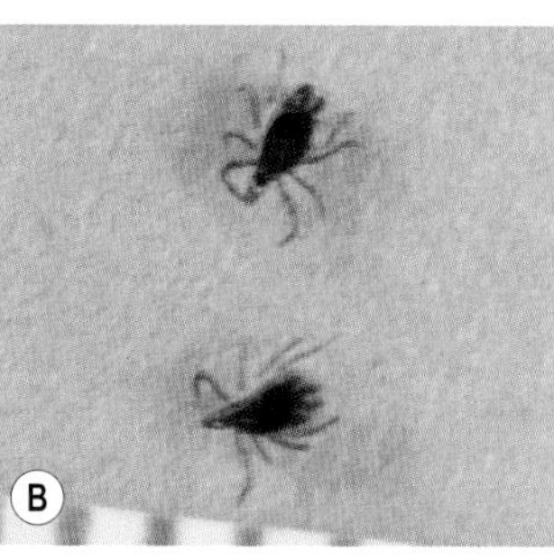

Figure 97.2 *Ixodes dammini* (deer tick) vector of *Babesia microti*. *Ixodes ricinus*, the European vector of *B. divergens*, is morphologically very similar. **(A)** Berlese fluid-cleared nymphal tick demonstrating heavily sclerotized legs and articulations as well as capitulum ("head"). The backward-facing spikes (denticles) of the mouth parts (hypostome) can be seen; this structure helps to anchor the tick and is the basis for the difficulty with which ticks can be removed from the skin. **(B)** Two nymphal deer ticks with a millimeter scale. Most babesiosis cases do not remember the infecting tick bite. Note that in living specimens of unfed or partially fed nymphs, prominent dark gut diverticula are seen through the body wall, giving the impression of an external color pattern.

an infectious inoculum of sporozoites. Accordingly, in >80% of reported cases, onset of illness occurred between May and August, when nymphs are most abundant.[46]

In Taiwan and Japan, zoonotic vectors of *B. microti* remain to be described, although *I. granulatus* and *I. ovatus* are probably enzootic vectors. Various small rodents (*Apodemus* spp., *Rattus* spp.) are frequently parasitized.[47,48] In the German case of *B. microti* babesiosis, acquired from a transfusion, the likely vector is *I. ricinus*. *B. microti* appears to be part of a characteristic microbial assemblage with the agents of Lyme disease, granulocytic ehrlichiosis, and tick-borne encephalitis virus throughout the Holarctic.[30,49]

PATHOGENESIS AND IMMUNITY

Lysis of parasitized erythrocytes leads to anemia, hemoglobinemia, hyperbilirubinemia, and, in severe cases, intense jaundice, massive hemoglobinuria, and renal shutdown. Electron microscopy shows parasite-mediated damage to erythrocyte membranes with perforations, protrusions, and inclusions.[50,51] There is reduced deformability of infected erythrocytes that enhances their removal by the spleen. In experimental *B. bovis* infections, increased peroxidation of membrane lipids appears to be responsible for a further decrease in erythrocyte survival and adherence of infected erythrocytes to the microvascular endothelium. However, endothelial adherence was not observed in tissues of a *B. microti* fatality.[52]

In several European cases, autopsies showed parasites in erythrocytes in congested capillaries of various organs, especially in hepatic sinusoids.[53,54] Other findings in these cases and in fatal cases due to *B. microti* suggest a cytokine-mediated shock syndrome. Indeed, laboratory studies of rodents infected by *B. microti* or *B. duncani* demonstrate overproduction of the proinflammatory mediators tumor necrosis factor-α (TNF-α) and interferon-γ.[55] Mice with a genetic disruption in the TNF-α pathway were less likely to die of fulminating *B. duncani* infection, as were CD4 and CD8 gene knockout mice, whereas in γδ T-cell knockout mice and control mice *B. duncani* infection terminated fatally. Thus, $CD8^+$ T cells may contribute to *B. duncani*-induced pathology.[55] In addition, depletion of macrophages and natural killer cells seems to increase susceptibility.[56] In humans, acute tubular necrosis, ischemic necrosis of liver, spleen, pancreas, and heart, noncardiac pulmonary edema, and swelling and congestion of the brain and other organs have been demonstrated, even in cases in which parasites had been cleared by treatment.[57] Other findings at autopsy have included hemophagocytosis, hypercellularity of the bone marrow, extramedullary hematopoiesis, and hemosiderin deposits in the Kupffer cells and the kidneys, which correspond to findings in histopathologic studies of rodent infections.[58,59]

Asplenia, advanced age, and depressed cellular immunity are associated with severe clinical illness.[60,61] The spleen phagocytizes parasitized erythrocytes, thus limiting parasitemia, particularly early in infection. Nevertheless, persons with intact spleens have died of overwhelming infections, and persons without spleens have recovered from babesiosis, even without specific therapy.[61] Severity of illness is greater in persons older than 50 years than in younger adults, and overt illness in children seems unusual.[36] As a rule, younger persons who become ill are asplenic or immunocompromised or have other underlying medical conditions.[62]

B. microti infections may be severe in persons who are infected with human immunodeficiency virus-1 (HIV) or are receiving corticosteroids or other immunosuppressive therapy, particularly rituximab (anti-CD20 B-cell monoclonal antibody).[63] Similarly, hamsters that receive antilymphocyte serum and athymic mice experience high parasitemias and mortality when exposed to *B. microti*.[64,65] CD4 gene knockout mice sustained *B. microti* parasitemias for longer periods of time than did congeneic controls.[55] Humoral immunity appears to be less important than cellular immunity in controlling infection. Passive transfer of immune serum to immunodeficient severe combined immunodeficient (SCID) and nude mice fails to protect them from *B. microti* infection.[66] B-cell-deficient mice remain less susceptible to *B. microti* infection, whereas T-cell receptor-deficient mice are readily infected.[67] Whether sterilizing immunity develops is questionable. Human infection may last over a year, even in the absence of underlying illness.[68] Reinfection has not been reported and would be difficult to distinguish from recrudescence of an earlier infection.

THE DISEASE

Depending on the species of *Babesia* and host factors, infection can be subclinical, cause a self-limited febrile illness, produce a moderate to severe illness resembling malaria, or progress rapidly to death. Infection with *B. divergens* occurs almost always in splenectomized persons and runs a fulminant, usually fatal, course without treatment.[15] After an incubation period of 1–4 weeks, *B. divergens*-infected patients become acutely ill with high fevers, prostration, rigors, diaphoresis, headache, myalgia, jaundice, and hemoglobinuria. Nausea, vomiting, and diarrhea are prominent, and the liver may be enlarged and painful. Most patients develop acute respiratory distress. Renal failure induced by intravascular hemolysis and hypotension ensues and is followed by coma and death, usually within a week of onset of symptoms. The 3 patients with the American *B. divergens*-like infection, 1 of whom died, presented with fever, headache, and rigors; thrombocytopenia, hemoglobinuria, and proteinuria developed.

Most infections with *B. microti* and likely also with *B. duncani* or CA-1 are subclinical. Subclinical infections have been detected during serosurveys and investigation of blood donors following transfusion-induced cases.[26,27,69] Animal inoculation has confirmed viable parasites in smear-negative asymptomatic persons with positive serologic tests for antibodies to *Babesia*.[27,36] Subpatent parasitemia in the absence of symptoms may last over a year.[70]

Because of the small number of reported cases, the spectrum of illness among persons with *B. duncani* or CA-type infections remains to be defined. Four of 7 persons with symptomatic infections had been splenectomized, including 2 patients who had severe disease with high parasitemias and multisystem organ failure, 1 of whom died.[25] The index case, a healthy, spleen-intact man, had a moderately severe illness with a 3% parasitemia, high fevers, and a slow recovery.[23] A similar illness occurred in an elderly man with multiple medical problems who acquired infection from a blood transfusion.[26]

Persons with symptomatic *B. microti* infections typically experience an influenza-like illness 1–4 weeks after a tick bite or 4–9 weeks following transfusion. There is a gradual onset of malaise, anorexia, and fatigue followed within a week by sustained or intermittent fever as high as 40°C, drenching sweats, and myalgia.[69] Nausea, vomiting, headache, shaking chills, dark urine, emotional lability and depression are not uncommon.[71] Physical examination may show mild splenomegaly and, less often, hepatomegaly. Most patients have mild to moderate anemia, thrombocytopenia, a normal or depressed white blood cell count, mildly elevated hepatic enzymes, and evidence of hemolysis, including hyperbilirubinemia, elevated serum lactate dehydrogenase, and decreased haptoglobin levels. Parasitemias may range from 1% to 20% in spleen-intact persons.

After several days to weeks, fever and more intense symptoms may resolve spontaneously, but weakness, malaise, and fatigue persist for months.[71] In other persons, largely the elderly, those without spleens, and those who are immunosuppressed or have other underlying medical problems, illness can be severe with intense hemolysis leading to jaundice, severe anemia, and renal failure. Parasitemias can reach 85% in asplenic patients.[50] Severe pancytopenia in some cases is due to hemophagocytosis.[72] Disseminated intravascular coagulation, hypotension, and adult respiratory distress syndrome have been seen in fatal cases. Noncardiac pulmonary edema, at times requiring mechanical ventilation, may occur in persons with less severe illness several days after beginning therapy. No relationships are apparent with parasitemia, splenectomy antibody or immune status; onset may be either early or late in the infection; and pulmonary edema resolves with supportive care.[73]

In an early series of 136 patients with babesiosis due to *B. microti*, mortality was 5% despite treatment.[60] Babesiosis in persons with acquired immunodeficiency syndrome (AIDS) is characterized by a prolonged duration and frequent relapses. There have been five reports of *B. microti* infection in persons with advanced HIV infection.[63,74–77] Two splenectomized persons had parasitemias in excess of 40% and more severe illness than the 3 who were spleen-intact, who had up to 20% parasitemia. Recrudescences occurred in 4 patients and lasted as long as 400 days after the initial episode; further recurrences were prevented by continual administration of antimicrobial agents.

Borrelia burgdorferi (see Chapter 44) or the agent of human granulocytic ehrlichiosis (*Anaplasma phagocytophilum*) (see Chapter 52) may coinfect ticks with *Babesia microti* and may be concurrently transmitted.[78,79] Persons with *B. microti* infection who are coinfected with *Borrelia burgdorferi* experience more symptoms and longer duration of illness than persons infected with either organism alone.[80] In a fatal case of a man with coexistent babesiosis and Lyme disease, the cause of death appeared to be related to pancarditis caused by the Lyme disease spirochete.[81] Another man with coinfection developed a more severe case of transverse myelitis than that which is seen with Lyme disease alone.[82] Coinfection with *B. microti* and *Ehrlichia chaffeensis* led to multiorgan failure and death in an 85-year-old man.[83] The differential diagnosis for babesiosis includes other tick-borne diseases, including Lyme disease, ehrlichiosis, typhoidal tularemia, and Rocky Mountain spotted fever, all of which may be endemic in the same region, as occurs in New England. Other illnesses that may be confused with babesiosis include viral hepatitis, bacterial sepsis, infectious mononucleosis, leptospirosis, malaria, and relapsing fever.

DIAGNOSIS

The nonspecific symptoms and absence of a history of a tick bite in most cases preclude the ability to make a diagnosis of babesiosis on clinical grounds alone. The definitive diagnosis usually follows demonstration of organisms parasitizing erythrocytes on conventional Giemsa-stained thin films. The small nucleus of *Babesia* can be difficult to identify on thick films, particularly when parasitemia is sparse. As with malaria, sequential blood smears may be required to detect organisms when the level of parasitemia is low.

Babesia is distinguished on blood smear from *Plasmodium falciparum* by a combination of criteria, including the demonstration of basket-shaped and frequently extracellular merozoites (***Fig. 97.3***) with white or light-colored cytoplasm, erythrocytes containing two or more parasites, and the presence of tetrad forms (Maltese crosses). Tetrad forms, however, are rarely encountered with *B. microti* infection, in contrast to acute *B. divergens* (***Fig. 97.4***), *B. duncani*, and MO-1 (***Fig. 97.5***) infections, in which they are frequent. The absence of hemozoin (malarial pigment) is considered diagnostic for the piroplasms, but early ring stages of the plasmodia also lack pigment. The presence of schizonts, gametocytes, or erythrocyte stippling may be characteristic of malaria but not of *Babesia*. *B. divergens* and related infections may be identified by the presence of accole forms and paired divergent pyriforms occupying no more than 20–25% of the erythrocyte area, along with small single oval or round merozoites; high parasitemias are often apparent. Although it is difficult to identify *Babesia* spp. specifically by morphology inasmuch as host cell factors influence this, there are discriminating features for mature infections. Note that for all species, simple ring forms may be all that is observed on a thin blood smear.

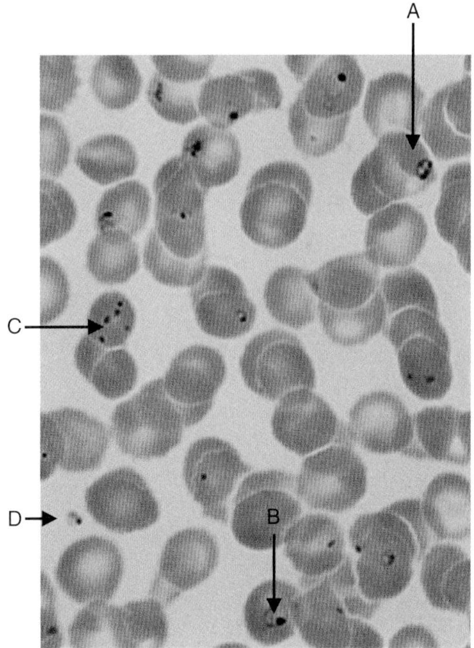

Figure 97.3 *Babesia microti*, human infection, Nantucket Island. Pleomorphic parasites with high parasitemia, multiple parasite infection of single cells, and range of developmental forms from newly invaded merozoites to mature trophozoites. A, mature trophozoite with prominent dark chromatin that extends nearly around the circumference of the cell; whitish cytoplasm; and threadlike band of chromatin across the middle of the parasite cytoplasm. B, mature trophozoite with prominent chromatin dot; white cytoplasm, and threadlike chromatin band across the cytoplasm. C, five small merozoites, perhaps comprising four daughter cells from one tetrad, with an additional newly invaded merozoite. D, extracellular merozoite. In heavy infections clumps of extracellular parasites may be observed; the presence of a discrete nucleus for each such parasite distinguishes them from platelets.

Serologic testing is useful, particularly in diagnosing chronic *B. microti* infections in which the parasitemia is subpatent. The indirect fluorescent antibody test using antigen derived from infected hamster erythrocytes[84] is sensitive and specific, and is currently the serologic method of choice. In cases in which parasitemia is difficult to detect, detection of specific IgM confirms a clinical diagnosis of babesiosis.[85] Absence or low titers of specific antibodies against *B. microti* when blood smears contain parasites suggests an infection by another *Babesia* sp. or an immunocompromised patient (splenectomy, HIV, recent infusion of anti-B-cell antibody). The sensitivity and specificity of serology for *B. duncani* are not known. Because specific antibodies do not become detectable until at least 1 week after onset of illness, serology is not reliable for diagnosis of the rapidly fulminating *B. divergens* babesiosis.[15] Serology for divergens-like babesiosis (EU-1, MO-1) may be accomplished by the use of *B. divergens* antigen because these parasites are cross-reactive.

Inoculation of a sample of patient blood into hamsters or SCID mice facilitates diagnosis of *B. microti* or *B. duncani* infection when smears are

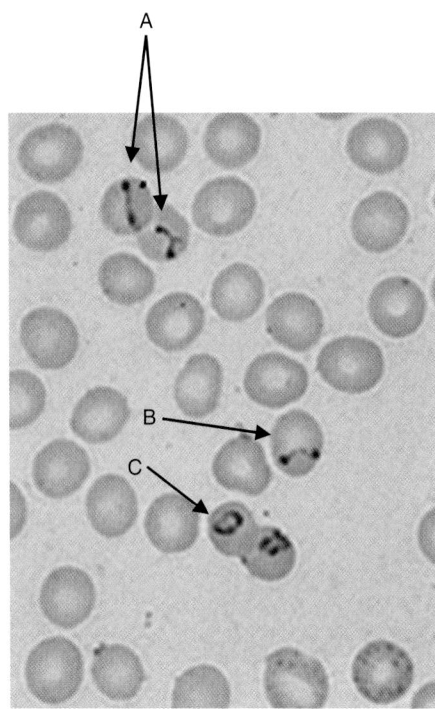

Figure 97.4 *Babesia divergens*, gerbil. The chromatin of this parasite usually appears thick and well stained. A, B, classic paired pyriforms. C, mature trophozoite with prominently staining chromatin that extends around the circumference of the parasite. Compared with *B. microti* and *B. duncani*, *B. divergens*-like parasites tend to produce two pairs of daughter cells as opposed to a tetrad.

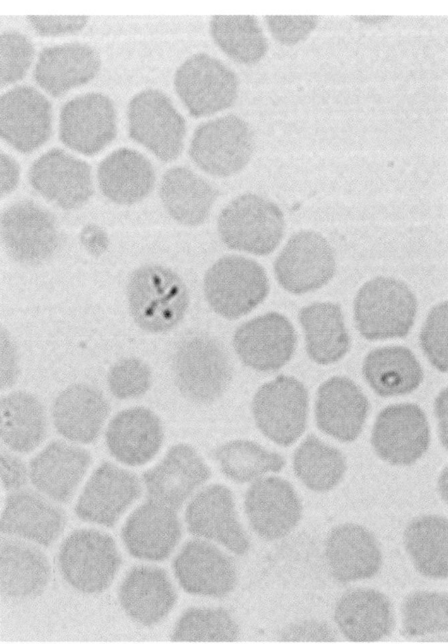

Figure 97.5 *Babesia duncani*, hamster. The classic Maltese-cross form is more frequently seen in *B. duncani*, with daughter cells typically a third of the diameter of the erythrocyte. In contrast, *B. microti* tetrads have "short leaves" with daughter cells shorter and more compact. *B. divergens*-like infections in the United States demonstrate a mixture of paired pyriforms with classic Maltese crosses.

negative. Approximately 300 parasites are sufficient to induce persistent parasitemia, which becomes detectable 1–6 weeks following inoculation. *B. divergens* can be isolated by inoculation of gerbils, but this procedure is only retrospectively useful for confirming the diagnosis of this rapidly progressive infection. PCR-based assays, which can detect *Babesia* DNA corresponding to three parasites in a 100-μL sample of blood, have the advantage of yielding a diagnosis in less than a day.[86] In addition, sequencing of the amplification products may provide more rapid specific identification than immunological analysis or animal inoculation studies when the identity of the infecting parasite is questioned.

TREATMENT AND PROGNOSIS

The combination of quinine (650 mg orally tid and clindamycin, either 1.2 g intravenously bid or 600 mg orally tid) can be used to treat babesiosis due to all species.[87,88] Pediatric doses are quinine 30 mg/kg/day and clindamycin 20–40 mg/kg/day, both in three divided doses.[87] Treatment should be continued for at least 7 days or until parasitemia remits. Evidence of excellent *in vitro* efficacy and the successful resolution of the index case for KO-1 babesiosis suggests that clindamycin alone warrants further study as an effective treatment for babesiosis.[43,89,90]

Because *B. divergens* parasitemias increase very rapidly, any case of babesiosis acquired in Europe should be regarded as an emergency requiring prompt treatment and frequent monitoring of blood smears.[91]

Exchange transfusion should be considered in severely ill patients with parasitemias in excess of 10% and evidence of severe hemolysis or organ failure.[92] In particularly severe cases of *B. divergens* and *B. microti* babesiosis, complete blood exchange transfusion (2–3 blood volumes) should be undertaken, followed by treatment with clindamycin and quinine.[91] Given that patients may be disproportionately ill even with virtually undetectable parasitemia, a one-log reduction of preprocedure parasitemia, rather than a targeted universal recommendation for posttransfusion parasitemia, has been suggested.[93]

Babesiosis due to *B. duncani* appears to respond to the combination of quinine and clindamycin, but the small number of cases that have been treated to date does not permit strong conclusions about the efficacy of this regimen. Because illness due to *B. microti* is often mild and short-lived, not all cases require treatment, with the caveat that such patients be deferred from donating blood. For persons with *B. microti* infections that are not life-threatening, the combination of atovaquone (750 mg PO bid × 7–10 days) and azithromycin (600 mg PO daily × 7–10 days) may be used.[87] A prospective randomized trial demonstrated that patients treated with atovaquone and azithromycin cleared parasitemia as effectively as did those receiving clindamycin and quinine, and with fewer side effects.[94] Combination therapy including all four of these drugs has been used as an alternative for treating human babesiosis when other regimens have failed or patients have developed side effects while receiving standard therapy.[63] Quinine and clindamycin should be given if the symptoms are sufficiently severe or if the patient is elderly, splenectomized, or immunocompromised. Treatment may occasionally fail, especially in such high-risk patients, or in those who must discontinue quinine due to side effects such as severe tinnitus. In most patients who complete the full regimen, parasite DNA seems to become undetectable by PCR within a month.[68] In a minority of cases, particularly in immunocompromised patients, symptoms may resolve, but parasitemia persists.[63] Following treatment, patients with AIDS should remain on suppressive therapy to prevent relapses.[63,95] The ideal regimen and duration of suppression have not been determined, but combinations of quinine, clindamycin, and other drugs have been used for periods of 6 months or maintained for life.

A variety of other agents, including chloroquine, co-trimoxazole, and pentamidine, have been tried without success for treating infected humans. Doxycycline in combination with other agents appears to have efficacy in refractory cases in persons with AIDS,[63] but patients who are treated with a tetracycline for Lyme disease appear to require specific antibabesial treatment if they are coinfected (T. J. Lepore, personal communication).

PREVENTION AND CONTROL

Repellents or arthropod toxicants are useful for personal protection. Permethrin-based formulations applied to shoes, socks, and pants are particularly active against ticks although ticks may attach and feed briefly before succumbing to permethrin intoxication. Common diethyltoluamide (DEET)-based repellents will also repel most ticks, but may require frequent reapplication. Preventing ticks from crawling underneath clothing by simply tucking pants cuffs into socks reduces the risk. Because delivery of an infectious inoculum usually requires more than a day of tick attachment (>60 hours for *B. microti*), the body surface of persons who have visited a site where transmission is intense should be examined daily and all ticks should be removed promptly with forceps.

Various public health strategies may be followed to protect human populations against zoonotic babesial infection. Acaricidal spraying of vegetation, host-targeted acaricides, and reduction of the reproductive hosts for the vector ticks (mainly deer) are all effective community-level interventions.[96–98]

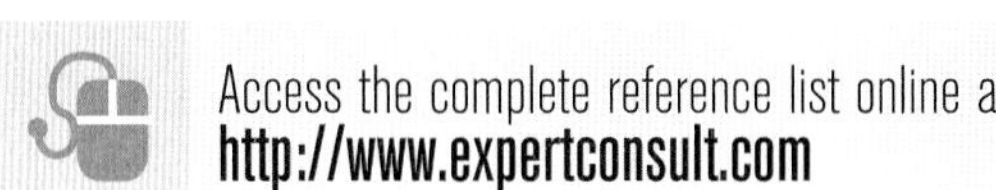
Access the complete reference list online at
http://www.expertconsult.com

CHAPTER 98

Access the complete reference list online at http://www.expertconsult.com

African Trypanosomiasis (Sleeping Sickness)

Jacques Pépin • John E. Donelson

INTRODUCTION

Human African trypanosomiasis (HAT), or sleeping sickness, is a purely African disease caused by two morphologically identical subspecies of trypanosomes – *Trypanosoma brucei gambiense* and *Trypanosoma brucei rhodesiense* – transmitted to humans by tsetse flies. Clinically, *T. b. gambiense* HAT is characterized by an early stage during which trypanosomes are found in the blood or lymph node aspirates of mostly asymptomatic persons and by a late stage during which there is involvement of the central nervous system (CNS) with somnolence, other neurologic symptoms, and trypanosomes in the cerebrospinal fluid (CSF). *T. b. rhodesiense* HAT, which is sometimes seen in short-term visitors to eastern and southern Africa, is a much more acute febrile illness occurring within days of the infective bite and which, if untreated, can be fatal in a matter of weeks.

THE AGENT

T. b. gambiense and *T. b. rhodesiense* are morphologically identical to a third salivarian trypanosome, *Trypanosoma brucei brucei*, which infects domestic and wild animals but does not survive in humans because it is lysed by specific components in the high-density lipoprotein fraction of human serum.[1,2] This group of three subspecies is often referred to as the *T. brucei* complex. Several other African trypanosome species are important pathogens of domestic livestock and wildlife in Africa but do not infect humans and are not discussed here.

The genus *Trypanosoma* occurs within the order Kinetoplastida. The single large mitochondrion of these organisms contains an appendage called the kinetoplast that lies in close proximity to the basal body at the base of the flagellum (***Fig. 98.1***). In the *T. brucei* complex, the kinetoplast contains as much as 10% of the total DNA of the organism. This DNA is organized into homogeneous maxicircle DNA molecules (about 20 000 base pairs each), which are equivalent to mitochondrial DNAs of other organisms, and heterogeneous minicircle DNA molecules (about 1000 base pairs each). A unique feature of organisms in the order Kinetoplastida is that some of their kinetoplast DNA genes are transcribed into RNAs that must be extensively edited by insertions or deletions of uridine nucleotides at many locations along the messenger RNA (mRNA) molecule before the correct mitochondrial proteins can be synthesized.[3] In the *T. brucei* complex, as many as 50% of nucleotides in some kinetoplast mRNAs are added or deleted after the initial synthesis of the RNA molecule. The reasons for the existence of this kinetoplast RNA editing and, indeed, the need for the kinetoplast itself are unknown, but this distinctive property of trypanosomes and related organisms offers an attractive target for future drug development. The sequence of the 35 million base-pair DNA genome in the nucleus of *T. b. brucei* has been determined[4] and also provides the foundation for identification of unique trypanosome enzymes and metabolic pathways that are potential new drug targets.

During their life cycle members of the *T. brucei* complex cycle between the mammalian bloodstream and several species of tsetse flies of the genus *Glossina*. When a tsetse fly bites an infected person, or an animal in the case of *T. b. rhodesiense*, trypanosomes in the bloodstream can be ingested with the blood meal (***Fig. 98.2***). In the fly, the infected blood moves to the lumen of the midgut, where the bloodstream trypanosomes transform during a 2- to 3-day period into the procyclic stage. This transformation is accompanied by many developmental changes including an increase in body length, a switch from anaerobic to aerobic metabolism, and a change in the main nutritional carbon source from glucose to proline, which is also used as the predominant energy source by the tsetse fly itself during flight.[5,6] In addition, the major protein on the surface of bloodstream trypanosomes, the variant surface glycoprotein (VSG), is replaced by an invariant surface protein called procyclin. After 2–3 weeks of multiplication in the midgut, the procyclic trypanosomes migrate to the salivary gland, where they undergo several additional developmental changes, culminating in the formation of the mature metacyclic stage. Metacyclic trypanosomes reacquire a VSG coat and stop multiplying. An infected tsetse fly can harbor as many as 10 000 to 20 000 metacyclic trypanosomes, of which one is potentially sufficient to initiate the mammalian infection if transmitted during the fly bite. Each trypanosome of the mature metacyclic population is completely covered with about 10^7 copies of a single VSG, but the population as a whole expresses 10–15 different metacyclic VSGs.[7] Moreover, one study showed that these metacyclic VSGs gradually diverged over a 20-year period,[8] indicating that a vaccine directed against the metacyclic VSGs would not be successful.

The tsetse fly injects the metacyclic trypanosomes into the connective tissue of the skin, where a temporary local inflammation, called a chancre, often develops. From this initial portal of entry, parasites enter the draining lymphatics, pass into the bloodstream through the thoracic duct, begin to multiply by binary fission and transform back into the bloodstream form, returning to anaerobic glycolysis as the main source of adenosine triphosphate (ATP). They continue, however, to express the metacyclic VSGs on their surface for about 5 days after the initiation of infection. They then switch from the expression of metacyclic VSGs to the bloodstream VSGs, one of which is sometimes the same VSG as on the surface of trypanosomes ingested by the fly.[9] The slender bloodstream form of the parasite actively divides every 5–10 hours, whereas the shorter, stumpy form does not divide but has a more developed mitochondrion and is thought to be more infective to the insect. These bloodstream forms can traverse the walls of the blood and lymph capillaries to the connective tissues and eventually enter the CSF and the brain. The parasite's life cycle is completed when a tsetse fly takes up the bloodstream forms while feeding on an infected mammal (***Fig. 98.2***).

Extracellular trypanosomes, in constant contact with their host's immune system, have evolved sophisticated mechanisms to evade immune attack. The VSG is a crucial component of one of these evasion

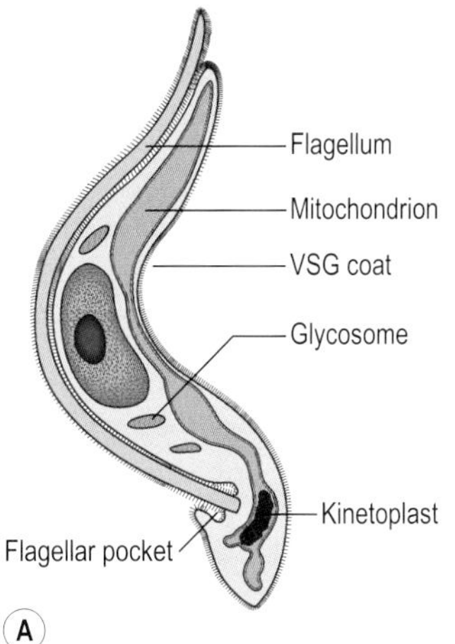

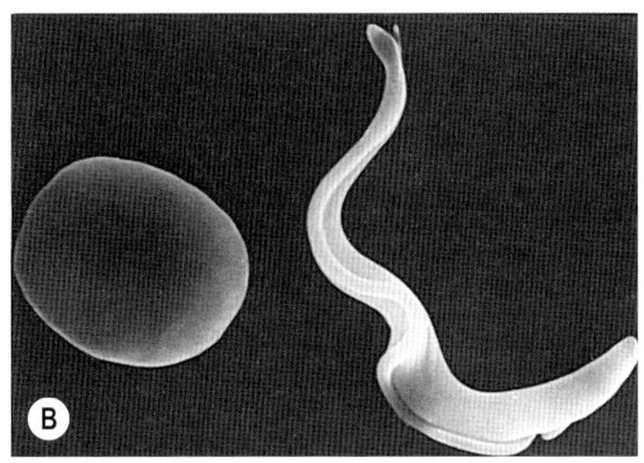

Figure 98.1 **(A)** Schematic diagram of a bloodstream trypanosome showing some of its subcellular organelles and the location of the variant surface glycoprotein (VSG). **(B)** Scanning electron micrograph of a bloodstream *Trypanosoma brucei rhodesiense* adjacent to a rat red blood cell (×5500).

mechanisms, a phenomenon called antigenic variation. As early as 1910, HAT was reported to be characterized by successive waves of parasites in the blood.[10] It is now well known that these peaks of parasitemia are due to trypanosomes expressing antigenically different VSGs.[11] The nuclear DNA of the *T. brucei* complex contains as many as 1000 different VSG genes.[4] Usually each trypanosome expresses one, and only one, of these VSGs at a given instant. The 10^7 copies of a VSG on a trypanosome represent about 5% of the total protein of the organism. The major function of all this protein on the surface of the living trypanosome is to serve as a barrier to protect other invariant constituents of the organism's outer membrane from attack by the immune system.

The three-dimensional structures of two different VSGs have been shown by X-ray crystallography to be cylindrical, allowing them to pack very closely together on the parasite's surface. During infection, antibodies are continually raised against the VSG, but trypanosome populations manage to escape total destruction because individual parasites occasionally undergo antigenic variation by switching spontaneously from the expression of one VSG to another. New antibodies must be directed against the VSG of the switched parasite and its descendants, enabling the population as a whole to stay one step ahead of this humoral (B-cell) immune response. The switch rate of the bloodstream trypanosome's antigenic variation ranges between 10^{-2} and 10^{-6} per parasite per doubling time.[12] The switch itself is often associated with spontaneous VSG gene rearrangements that maneuver duplicated copies of silent VSG genes into special gene expression sites located near the ends of some chromosomes, where they are transcribed into mRNA. Sometimes these rearrangements result in the formation of new VSG genes that are mosaic or mutated versions of preexisting genes.[13,14] This ability to create new VSG gene versions during the DNA rearrangements likely means that bloodstream trypanosomes have the potential to express sequentially a much larger repertoire of VSG proteins than they have VSG genes. Hence, the development of a HAT vaccine directed against bloodstream VSGs is also unlikely.

The tsetse fly vector belongs to the *Glossina* genus, found only in Africa, which contains 22 species, only a few of them being involved in the transmission of HAT: the riverine palpalis group (*G. palpalis*, *G. tachinoides*, and *G. fuscipes*) for *T. b. gambiense*, and the morsitans group (*G. morsitans*, *G. pallidipes*, and *G. swynnertoni*) for *T. b. rhodesiense*. Tsetse flies live in hot, humid, and dark ecologic niches, and their distinct requirements relate to epidemiologic differences between Gambian and Rhodesian HAT. The palpalis group is found mostly in forests on the banks of a river and humans are a variable source (10–40%) of their blood meals, while the more zoophilic morsitans group is seen in the woodland and thickets of East African savannas. Once infected with trypanosomes, tsetse flies remain infected for the rest of their lives (a few months). Less than 5% are infected in epidemic areas.

EPIDEMIOLOGY

HAT is endemic only in sub-Saharan Africa between latitudes 15° N and 15° S, corresponding to the distribution of its vector.[15,16] Its incidence increased considerably at the beginning of the twentieth century as a consequence of population migrations brought on by colonization. In some areas HAT caused half of the overall mortality. Trypanosomiasis control was organized around mobile case-finding teams that regularly examined the population of endemic foci through cervical lymph node palpation and aspiration to detect and then treat infected but asymptomatic persons. The goal was to reduce transmission by shortening the duration of infectiousness. In the late 1940s and 1950s, millions of people were given pentamidine "chemoprophylaxis" twice a year, but it probably corresponded more to early treatment than to prevention. Such initiatives were highly successful, and the incidence of HAT decreased dramatically. After the end of colonial rule, HAT remained at a low level or disappeared in countries able to maintain some case-finding activities, but increased considerably when such programs were interrupted for just a few years at the end of the twentieth century. As a result, the distribution of sleeping sickness ten years ago paralleled that of wars or civil conflicts that devastated parts of Africa, the highest incidences occurring in the Democratic Republic of Congo (DRC), Angola, and Sudan. Once more, substantial investment into its control proved successful: in 2006, a total of 11 382 cases of *T. b. gambiense* trypanosomiasis were reported to the World Health Organization (WHO), down from 37 385 cases in 1999.[17] *T. b. rhodesiense* trypanosomiasis is much less common, with about 500 cases reported annually.[17] Even though there is some degree of underdiagnosis and underreporting,[18] the burden of HAT is now currently less than what was estimated in 2003 (48 000 deaths per year and 1.5 million disability-adjusted life-years lost).[19]

Gambian HAT is endemic in western and central Africa and Rhodesian HAT in eastern and southern Africa (***Fig. 98.3***). Uganda is the only country in which both subspecies are present. In West Africa, the disease has disappeared from Senegal, The Gambia, Guinea-Bissau, Sierra Leone, and Ghana for ecologic reasons that are poorly understood, since significant tsetse fly populations remain. A few dozen cases are diagnosed each year in Ivory Coast, Guinea, and Nigeria. The country with by far the highest incidence is the DRC, where 8023 cases were reported in 2006, followed by Angola (1105 cases), Sudan (809 cases) and the Central African Republic (460 cases). Within the DRC, the epidemic reached Kinshasa, where almost 1000 cases were diagnosed in 1999, mostly acquired in its peri-urban areas.[20]

In southeast Uganda, an epidemic of Rhodesian HAT has been successfully controlled by tsetse fly trapping and case-finding, but Gambian HAT persists in northwest Uganda. In 2006, 245 cases of Rhodesian HAT were reported in Uganda, 125 in Tanzania, 58 in Malawi, 57 in Zambia, and only a handful in Kenya and other countries of the region.[17] Each year, ~30 cases of Rhodesian HAT are diagnosed in tourists, especially visitors to the Serengeti,[21] where this risk has now been reduced through

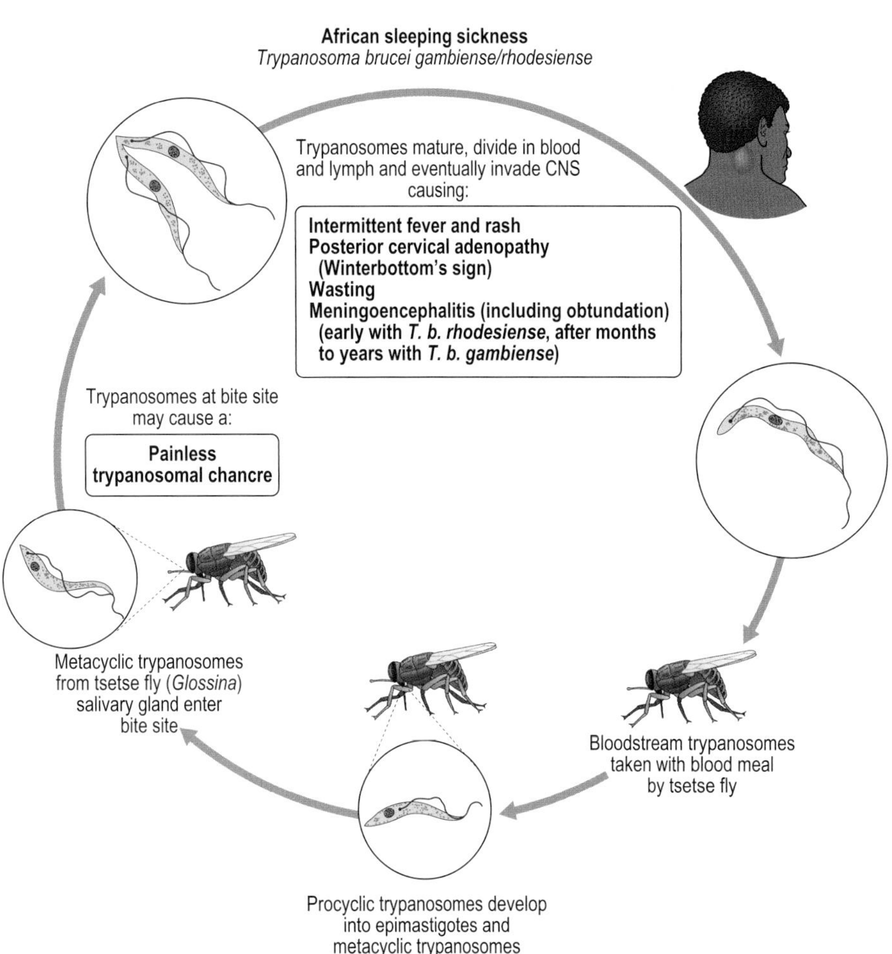
African sleeping sickness
Trypanosoma brucei gambiense/rhodesiense
Trypanosomes mature, divide in blood and lymph and eventually invade CNS causing:
Intermittent fever and rash
Posterior cervical adenopathy (Winterbottom's sign)
Wasting
Meningoencephalitis (including obtundation) (early with T. b. rhodesiense, after months to years with T. b. gambiense)
Trypanosomes at bite site may cause a:
Painless trypanosomal chancre
Metacyclic trypanosomes from tsetse fly (Glossina) salivary gland enter bite site
Bloodstream trypanosomes taken with blood meal by tsetse fly
Procyclic trypanosomes develop into epimastigotes and metacyclic trypanosomes in tsetse salivary gland

Figure 98.2 Life cycle of *Trypanosoma brucei gambiense/rhodesiense* infections (African Sleeping Sickness).

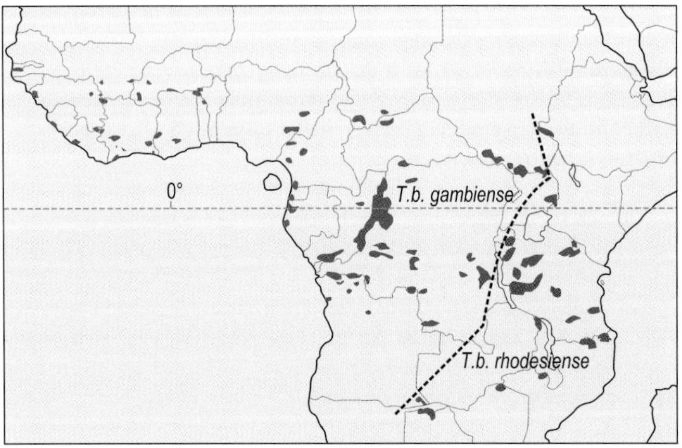
0°
T.b. gambiense
T.b. rhodesiense

Figure 98.3 Distribution of African trypanosomiasis. (Redrawn from World Health Organization. Control and surveillance of African trypanosomiasis. Report of a WHO expert committee. World Health Organization Technical Report Series No. 881, 1998.)

vector control. About 20 cases of Gambian HAT are diagnosed annually in Africans who have migrated outside the endemic areas.[22]

The major determinants of the epidemiology of Gambian HAT are (1) the long duration (up to several years) of infection in human hosts, with cycles of intermittent parasitemia; (2) human–fly contact and infection rates among tsetse flies; and (3) the efficacy of passive and active case-finding.[15] Human–fly contact can be enhanced by changes in tsetse fly density, distribution, and feeding habits or in human behavior that results in people spending more time in areas of high fly density. Breakdowns in active case-finding and, to a lesser extent, in passive detection by multi-purpose health facilities allow the human reservoir to expand and increase the percentage of infectious tsetse flies. Significant immunity appears after an adequately treated first episode of Gambian HAT,[23] which might explain the resurgence of HAT in the same foci as 50 years earlier. After years of high incidence and successful treatment of most cases, a large proportion of the population becomes immune and decades are necessary before the pool of immunologically naïve persons is large enough to sustain an epidemic. Familial clustering is also observed, the risk of HAT in a child being higher if the mother (but not the father) had had HAT before, presumably reflecting shared exposure or congenital infections rather than a genetically determined susceptibility.[24] There seems to be little or no interaction between HAT and human immunodeficiency virus (HIV) infection.[25] Because of the long incubation period, there is no seasonal variation in Gambian HAT incidence.

Domestic animals (pigs, goats, dogs, sheep, cattle, and even chickens) can be infected with *T. b. gambiense*. The importance of these animal reservoirs is probably marginal in high-incidence countries of central Africa, but they might play a role in the persistence of the disease in low-incidence countries, where the size of the human reservoir is much smaller.[15] In contrast, Rhodesian HAT is a zoonosis and to some extent an occupational disease, with many species of game animals and cattle harboring the parasite and sustaining sporadic transmission to humans.[15] Person-to-person spread occurs only during epidemics, but this subspecies offers less potential for large-scale epidemics because of its acute nature. Changes in agricultural practices and movements of cattle have been incriminated as favoring the spread of the parasite.[26]

THE DISEASE

In Gambian HAT, the asymptomatic phase can last many months, if not years. Intermittent fever then appears with nonspecific symptoms such as headache, myalgia, and malaise. These symptoms last a few days before subsiding and reappearing weeks later, and correspond to successive waves of antibodies produced in response to antigenic variation of the VSGs. Eventually weight loss and asthenia become significant, and pruritus can be troublesome. Transient edema, mostly of the face, is seen in fewer than 10% of patients. After months of nonspecific symptoms, evidence of CNS involvement makes the diagnosis obvious. Somnolence is seen in 80% of late-stage patients, and only the occasional patient experiences both diurnal somnolence and nocturnal insomnia. Most patients then complain of constant and severe headaches unresponsive to analgesics. Behavior change or psychosis is seen in 5–10% of cases. If untreated, the somnolence progresses to stupor and coma, and the ultimate cause of death is often a bacterial superinfection such as aspiration pneumonia. Convulsions are rare in adults but more common in children (up to 30%), among whom retardation in psychomotor development, language, or walking, and irritability can be the presenting symptoms. In children, lymphadenopathy is less prominent and the disease progresses more rapidly to overt CNS involvement than in adults. Various endocrine disorders have been reported: hypogonadism, amenorrhea, infertility, and low triiodothyronine (T_3) or low thyroxine (T_4) syndromes but rarely frank hypothyroidism. There are exceptional cases of healthy carriers who remained parasitemic and asymptomatic for years without treatment, but untreated HAT is ultimately fatal to almost all infected persons.

An inoculation chancre is rarely recognized in persons repeatedly bitten all year long by various insects but is more frequent in the rare white individuals who acquire Gambian HAT.[22,27] Fewer than half of asymptomatic patients actively detected during surveys, but up to 85% of those passively detected in a hospital, have the classic Winterbottom cervical lymphadenopathies: soft, painless, 1–2 cm in diameter, numerous, and rather mobile. Lymphadenopathy can be less typical, and in persons from high-incidence areas, any lymph node large enough to be aspirated should be aspirated. As the disease progresses, lymphadenopathy regresses. Cutaneous lesions, the trypanids, are seen only in white people. Modest splenomegaly occurs in 10–20%; hepatomegaly is rare (1%). On neurologic examination, patients do not have neck stiffness apart from the occasional patient with a very high CSF white blood cell (WBC) count. Focal signs (hemiparesis, hemiplegia) are unusual, but in a patient from a high-incidence community, any neurologic sign should be considered as potentially caused by HAT until proved otherwise. The hand–chin reflex can be elicited in half the patients. Tremors are not unusual; choreoathetosis is seen mostly in patients with multiple relapses. Despite *in vitro* evidence of immunosuppression, superinfections seen in HAT patients relate to the altered level of consciousness rather than to opportunistic pathogens.

In Rhodesian HAT, the clinical presentation is similar but much more acute. Most patients have been sick for less than a month when the diagnosis is made.[28] Inoculation chancres are more common than in Gambian HAT, and trypanosomes can sometimes be seen microscopically in fluid expressed from them. Lymphadenopathy is less frequent than in Gambian HAT and is often submandibular, axillary, or inguinal rather than cervical.[28] Myocarditis is an uncommon complication. In tourists from nonendemic countries, the inoculation chancre is often present when the patient develops an acute disease that, if untreated, can rapidly progress to multiorgan involvement and disseminated intravascular coagulation.[29]

PATHOGENESIS AND IMMUNITY

The immune response and pathogenesis that develop during HAT are complex and poorly understood. From an immunologic perspective, a trypanosome may be regarded as a package of thousands of nonvariable antigens surrounded by 10 million copies of a variable antigen, the VSG.[5] Since bloodstream trypanosomes are destroyed during an infection, the immune system is continually exposed to massive amounts of invariant antigens and VSGs, but the immune responses to these foreign antigens are not protective because the invariant antigens inside the living trypanosome are inaccessible and the readily accessible VSGs periodically switch via antigenic variation. Hence, many of the immune events observed in HAT are likely the result of the perpetual presence of ever-changing VSGs combined with many other invariant antigens, a scenario that mimics successive infections by related but nonidentical organisms.

In experimental laboratory animals, the immune responses to a trypanosome infection are dominated by three overwhelming phenomena: nonspecific polyclonal B-cell activation, macrophage activation and generalized suppression of some humoral (B-cell) and cellular (T-cell) immune functions.[30,31] The massive polyclonal B-cell activation results in a large production of immunoglobulin M (IgM), the first class of antibody to be generated by the appearance of new foreign antigens. This activation is not triggered entirely by the continually changing epitopes of the different VSGs, however, since the newly synthesized antibodies do not react solely with VSGs and other trypanosome antigens. They frequently are heterospecific in their reactivity and can be autoantibodies directed against the proteins and nucleic acids of the host. It has been proposed that VSGs or unknown non-VSG molecules of trypanosomes cause this massive nonspecific expansion of B cells and the subsequent increase in immunoglobulin concentration.[30] The greatly elevated levels of antibody and resultant antigen–antibody complexes in turn cause hyperplasia of the reticuloendothelial system, especially the spleen and lymph nodes, and are likely responsible for many of the pathogenic characteristics of the disease.

The other striking immune features of HAT are activation of macrophages and subsequent suppression of immune responses other than the initial B-cell activation, which affects a large variety of both B-cell and T-cell functions and seems to inhibit many secondary immune events.[30,31] The concentrations of the cytokines interferon-gamma (INF-γ) and tumor necrosis factor are greatly increased in experimental animals infected with *T. brucei*. Macrophage activation may be triggered by increases in INF-γ, and the elimination of trypanosomes by antibodies is thought to be mediated by opsonization and destruction by liver macrophages, rather than by complement-mediated lysis. Levels of some other cytokines (e.g., interleukin-2) decrease during trypanosome infections, which may contribute to the lack of T-cell proliferation. Although the coexistence of polyclonal B-cell expansion, macrophage activation, and significant immunosuppression appears at first glance to be counterproductive, these phenomena obviously generate an environment conducive to perpetuation of the infection. Much remains to be learned about the myriad of complex immune events occurring during HAT.

HAT is often accompanied by anemia, which may be caused by hemolysis induced by the immune complexes, although other mechanisms are involved.[32] Platelet destruction and increased vascular permeability occur, and the parasites readily infiltrate the interstitial spaces and lymphatic system, where they continue to multiply. There is widespread lymphadenopathy due to increased lymphocyte proliferation, which can be followed by fibrosis. The spleen is sometimes enlarged, with generalized cellular proliferation, congestion, and focal necrosis. The spleen and lymph nodes can both develop endarteritis with perivascular infiltration by trypanosomes and lymphocytes. The heart can also be affected, particularly in Rhodesian HAT, in which a pancarditis can develop that involves all cardiac structures, including valves and the conduction system, resulting in cardiac failure and electrocardiographic changes.[33]

The late-stage of HAT is defined by the detection of trypanosomes in the CSF via lumbar puncture (LP) or CSF pleocytosis (which appears earlier in CSF obtained by cisternal puncture than by LP). The pressure and total protein content of the CSF are increased, and there is infiltration by immune complexes, white blood cells, and sometimes small numbers of eosinophils and morular (Mott) cells, which are thought to be IgM-containing plasma cells that fail to secrete their antibodies. In the brain, the parasites are found mainly in the frontal lobes, the pons, and the medulla, where they are associated with diffuse meningoencephalitis, parenchymal edema, and dura–arachnoid adhesions. Lymphoid cells often infiltrate the brain through the space surrounding the blood vessels, and hemorrhages can occur. Widespread multifocal white matter degeneration develops, especially during the final stages of the disease, but there are no structural nerve cell alterations.[34] The actual cause of the cerebral damage in late-stage HAT remains uncertain but the lesions may be mediated by immunologic reactions that occur around the blood vessels and affect the brain parenchyma.

DIAGNOSIS

Anemia, thrombocytopenia, an increased erythrocyte sedimentation rate, hypergammaglobulinemia, and hypoalbuminemia are frequent but nonspecific. Eosinophilia is not seen, but an elevated serum IgM (up to 16 times the normal concentration) is suggestive of HAT. The diagnosis requires, however, the detection of trypanosomes. Examination of lymph node aspirates is the classic detection method in Gambian HAT. A 25-gauge needle is inserted in the node, which is massaged for 1 minute while the needle is rotated, the needle is withdrawn and with a syringe the lymph node "juice" is pushed out onto a slide, which must be examined immediately at ×400. Trypanosomes can be seen moving for 15–20 minutes afterwards and are more numerous on the edges of the coverslip. In the absence of lymphadenopathy or if the aspirate is negative, the diagnosis can be made on a wet smear (a drop of unstained blood between slide and coverslip) or a Giemsa-stained thick smear. The latter is more sensitive, but a microscopist who must examine 50 smears per day usually prefers the wet smear in which trypanosomes can be readily detected by their high mobility. Because of the low level of parasitemia and its fluctuation over time, repeated examinations on consecutive days may be necessary before a trypanosome is seen. Patients in whom HAT is suspected but for whom those assays are negative should be tested with other techniques. The most sensitive is the mAECT (miniature anion-exchange centrifugation technique). Blood is filtered through a resin that retains blood cells but not trypanosomes. The eluate is centrifuged, followed by a direct microscopic examination of the pipette in a viewing chamber. The hematocrit centrifugation technique for an examination of the buffy coat is an alternative. The lower limits to the number of parasites detectable by the different methods are 10^4/mL for the wet smear, 5×10^3/mL for the thick smear, 5×10^2/mL for the hematocrit centrifugation, and 10^2/mL for the mAECT. The quantitative buffy coat technique using acridine orange stain is also sensitive.[35] The polymerase chain reaction remains a research tool unavailable in endemic countries.[36]

As the disease progresses, it becomes more difficult to find parasites in the blood and lymph nodes, and more likely that only CSF will reveal trypanosomes. An LP should be performed on all patients for whom parasites have been documented in any of the preceding tests, and on patients with symptoms of sleeping sickness but negative assays. The most sensitive techniques for detecting CSF trypanosomes are the double centrifugation (6–8 mL of CSF is obtained and, after a first centrifugation, the sediment drawn into a capillary tube, centrifuged again, and examined immediately) or simple centrifugation in a sealed Pasteur pipette.[35,37] The CSF WBC is measured; patients with a WBC higher than 5/mm^3 are arbitrarily considered to be in late-stage. Many patients without neurologic symptoms have a slightly elevated CSF WBC; those with overt somnolence usually have a WBC between 100 and 500/mm^3. The CSF is clear, and its white blood cells are mononuclear. Measuring CSF proteins adds little information because they are elevated along with the WBC. Large eosinophilic plasma cells (Mott cells) "typical" of HAT are rarely seen. In endemic areas, clinicians sometimes treat patients with a presumptive diagnosis: no trypanosomes have been found but the typical symptoms, residence in a known focus, positive serologic reactions, and elevated CSF WBC make the diagnosis virtually certain.

Many serologic techniques have been developed for Gambian HAT to improve the efficacy of case-finding surveys by identifying serologically positive persons on whom parasitologic assays are selectively performed. Because of drug toxicity, treatment is generally given only to patients in whom trypanosomes are subsequently documented. The CATT (card agglutination test for trypanosomes, Institute of Tropical Medicine, Antwerp, Belgium), can be performed without electricity, and results are available within 10 minutes. It has good (90–98%) sensitivity and a specificity of ~95% (owing to cross-reactivity with animal trypanosomes).[35] Depending on the prevalence of HAT in the population to be tested, its positive predictive value is 66–89% in passive case-finding in a hospital but only 20–30% in active case-finding surveys. Using the CATT on diluted (1 : 10) serum rather than whole blood increases specificity but decreases sensitivity.[38] The CATT can be reliably performed using a micromethod on filter paper or diluted blood, reducing the cost of screening.[39]

In Rhodesian HAT, parasitemia is higher and trypanosomes easier to find in the blood using the above methods. Lymph node aspirates are rarely feasible or necessary. Since the disease progresses rapidly, an abnormal CSF WBC or CSF trypanosomes are frequent. There are no antibody-detection assays.

Rare patients diagnosed with late-stage African trypanosomiasis in industrialized countries and investigated with modern tools have been found by magnetic resonance imaging to have hyperintense signal changes in the basal ganglia and deep within gray and white matter as well as meningeal thickening.[40,41] Mediastinal, hilar, and para-aortic lymphadenopathy can be seen on CT scan.[40]

Differential Diagnosis

The differential diagnosis of early-stage HAT is that of prolonged fever, associated with a long list of other diseases in the tropics: malaria, HIV infection, typhoid, tuberculosis, etc. The cervical lymphadenopathy of HAT is softer and smaller than in tuberculous lymphadenitis and cancer but similar to HIV-associated lymphadenopathy. In late-stage HAT, other causes of chronic lymphocytic meningitis must be considered, especially tuberculous meningitis and HIV-associated cryptococcosis. In tourists with *T. b. rhodesiense* trypanosomiasis, the disease needs to be distinguished from severe malaria and African tick bite fever.

TREATMENT AND PROGNOSIS

There are few diseases for which most recommended drugs have been used for so long: suramin since 1925, melarsoprol and pentamidine since the 1940s.[42] Eflornithine, the only new drug, is now widely available through the generosity of Sanofi-Aventis. To select the best treatment for a patient in whom trypanosomes have been found, two questions must be answered: (1) Is it *T. b. gambiense* or *T. b. rhodesiense*? (2) Is the patient in early-stage or late-stage? The first is easily addressed by geographic considerations. For the rare traveler potentially exposed to both subspecies, detection of the serum resistance-associated gene can confirm that the infection is caused by *T. b. rhodesiense*.[43,44] To answer the second, an LP must always be performed. Patients with a CSF WBC >5/mm^3 or with CSF trypanosomes are in late-stage, all others are in early-stage. Intrathecal IgM synthesis and interleukin-10 have been proposed to diagnose late-stage disease[45] but are generally unavailable.

Pentamidine is the standard treatment for early-stage Gambian HAT; suramin is less effective and melarsoprol, though very effective, is avoided because of toxicity. Pentamidine isethionate, given intramuscularly or intravenously (IV), cures 93% of early-stage patients. Its efficacy has remained remarkably uniform over space and time. Pentamidine injections are exquisitely painful and may cause sterile abscesses. During pentamidine treatment, 1% of patients die. In rural African hospitals, the causes of such deaths are difficult to determine, but potentially severe adverse effects include hypotension, hypoglycemia (during treatment), diabetes (after treatment), hypocalcemia, hyperkalemia, renal failure, neutropenia, and ventricular arrhythmias. As soon as the CSF WBC count increases, the efficacy of pentamidine decreases: it should not be used in patients with >5 WBC/mm^3.[46]

For late-stage Gambian HAT, eflornithine, a selective and irreversible inhibitor of ornithine decarboxylase, remains the drug of choice for clinicians working in developed countries. It is as effective as melarsoprol but less toxic. The 14-day regimen cures ~95% of new cases and 98% of post-melarsoprol relapses, presumably because of higher CSF eflornithine levels in the latter.[47,48] For new cases, a 7-day course is clearly inferior to the 14-day regimen.[47] Eflornithine is less effective in HIV-seropositive patients, who should be treated with melarsoprol,[42] and in children, who should be given higher doses (125–150 mg/kg every 6 hours for 14 days). Eflornithine is less effective in patients from Uganda, for unclear reasons.[47] For relapsing cases, a 7-day course (same dosage) seems adequate and could be considered in conditions of drug shortage.[47] Anemia, leukopenia, and thrombocytopenia are common adverse effects but not clinically significant. Convulsions (6–8%) are related to high CSF drug levels, usually subside when eflornithine is withheld, and do not recur when resumed after 24–48 hours. Fatalities (~2%) during eflornithine treatment are related to advanced HAT rather than toxicity. Oral eflornithine is less effective than IV eflornithine owing to its 55% bioavailability and the osmotic diarrhea it induces.

Nifurtimox cures at most two-thirds of patients[49] and cannot be recommended as monotherapy. However, there has been much interest in using it as a component of combination therapy. In small case series, encouraging results were documented when nifurtimox was combined with low-dose melarsoprol or a 7-day course of eflornithine.[49–51] A recent multicenter randomized trial documented that the combination of oral nifurtimox (5 mg/kg every 8 hours for 10 days) and intravenous eflornithine (200 mg/kg every 12 hours for 7 days) was as effective as the standard eflornithine 14-day regimen described above.[52] The combination shortens the duration of treatment and decreases the number of intravenous injections to be administered, which makes it an attractive option for hospitals in endemic areas, where it should be considered now as the treatment of choice. Nifurtimox carries substantial toxicity (mostly anorexia and nausea, sometimes tremors) and it is recommenced that each dose should be administered under direct supervision.

The trivalent arsenical derivative melarsoprol should be used in cases of late-stage Gambian HAT if eflornithine is not available. It is remarkably effective (94–97% cure rate) but very toxic (4–6% death rate). It should be given as 10 daily IV injections on successive days, rather than the traditional scheme of three series of three daily injections separated by drug-free intervals. A randomized trial has shown that these two regimens had comparable efficacy and toxicity.[53] A graded regimen of melarsoprol was less effective and more toxic.[54] Reactive encephalopathy (4–8%, 15% if CSF WBC is >100/mm^3) with grand mal seizures, coma, or behavior changes can be a severe, unpredictable complication of melarsoprol treatment, with a case-fatality ratio >50%. Prednisolone, which reduces by two-thirds the risk of encephalopathy without increasing the risk of treatment failure,[55] should be given to all melarsoprol-treated patients, as well as ivermectin or albendazole to avoid disseminated strongyloidiasis. Pretreatment with pentamidine or suramin has been given for decades in the hope of reducing the risk of encephalopathy, but this remains unproved. Encephalopathy should be treated with anticonvulsants and dexamethasone to reduce cerebral edema. Dimercaprol, a heavy metal chelator, is useless in the treatment of encephalopathy whose pathogenesis is an immunologic reaction. Polyneuropathy (up to 10%) is a toxic effect of arsenic, which if neglected can progress to paraplegia or quadriplegia. When a patient complains of paresthesias, melarsoprol should be withheld for a while and thiamine (100 mg three times a day) administered. Tremors respond well to β-blockers. Fever can be caused by lysis of trypanosomes, but superinfections should be sought, especially pneumonia. Cutaneous reactions (1%) can be troublesome. Phlebitis and cellulitis at the injection sites are caused by the propylene glycol solvent.

After treatment, all patients should be followed with an LP every 6 months for 2 years, or sooner if symptoms recur. A relapse is certain if trypanosomes are found in the CSF (rarely in blood or lymph nodes), but most relapses are characterized only by an elevated CSF WBC. Patients should be considered as having post-eflornithine or post-melarsoprol relapse if their CSF WBC is >50/mm^3 and higher than the previous determination, or 20–49/mm^3 and higher than the previous measurement with recurrence of symptoms. When in doubt, the LP should be repeated after 1–2 months. The trend in the CSF WBC is more important than the absolute value, since many genuinely cured patients have a slightly elevated CSF WBC 6 months after treatment. Patients who relapse after eflornithine should be given melarsoprol (and vice versa). Patients with a CSF WBC greater than 10/mm^3 after pentamidine treatment of early-stage Gambian HAT are considered to be relapsing and should be treated with eflornithine or melarsoprol. Those with borderline results (6/mm^3 to 9/mm^3) should be retested earlier than the routine interval. Most late-stage adults cured by melarsoprol or eflornithine, even if comatose before treatment, develop no obvious sequelae, but children do so more frequently (poor school performance).

In early-stage Rhodesian HAT, suramin is the treatment of choice and is superior to pentamidine (melarsoprol would be effective but is avoided because of the risk of encephalopathy). A test dose is traditionally given although anaphylaxis is rare. Several regimens are recommended,[16] but this probably does not matter given the drug's half-life of ~50 days. Suramin is 99.7% protein-bound and has no CSF penetration. The failure rate with suramin varies from 0% to 31%.[42] Adverse effects include fever, proteinuria, and urticaria. *T. b. rhodesiense* is intrinsically resistant to eflornithine. Melarsoprol is the only effective treatment for late-stage Rhodesian HAT patients, having a 95% cure rate. Several regimens are used; ***Table 98.1*** lists one of those recommended by WHO[16] which favors starting with a small dose of melarsoprol and increasing it progressively. However, a similar regimen was more toxic in patients with Gambian HAT[54] and a clinical trial is under way evaluating a regimen of 10 consecutive daily injections. Pretreatment with suramin is generally advocated on the theoretical grounds that it might prevent seeding of the CSF when the LP is conducted. Melarsoprol-induced encephalopathy is more common in Rhodesian (5–18%) than Gambian HAT, and mortality during treatment is higher (3–12%). It seems reasonable to administer prednisolone at the same dosage as in Gambian HAT. Encephalopathy should be treated along the same lines. Follow-up LPs should be carried out every 3 months during the first year, and every 6 months during the second year. Most patients who relapse after melarsoprol treatment of Rhodesian HAT are cured by a second course of melarsoprol. For those who relapse a second time, a combination of melarsoprol and nifurtimox might be considered.

Given the lack of financial incentives, it appears unlikely that novel drugs will be developed in the near future. Orally administered pafuramidine (DB289) unfortunately failed in clinical trials.

PREVENTION AND CONTROL

For Gambian HAT, case-finding remains the cornerstone of disease control. Infected individuals can remain asymptomatic and contagious for months or years before developing overt sleeping sickness, becoming less contagious when CNS involvement progresses since trypanosomes are then found more in the CSF than in the bloodstream. The only way to break the chain of transmission is to identify and treat asymptomatic persons. Populations of endemic foci should be examined twice a year by mobile teams. Previous case-finding surveys based only on detection and aspiration of cervical lymphadenopathy gave excellent results when 95% of the inhabitants were present. If only 50% of the population participates, as is often the case nowadays,[56] and if only this traditional method is used, not enough carriers will be identified to modify the epidemic dynamics. However, using the CATT to identify suspects on whom parasitologic assays are concentrated doubles the number of parasitemic persons detected (half of whom have no lymphadenopathy) and compensates for the lower participation. The best approach is to perform the CATT on all inhabitants. CATT-positive subjects should have blood examinations, and lymph node aspiration if feasible. Most control programs treat only persons in whom trypanosomes have been seen. Whether the systematic treatment of individuals with a positive CATT and negative parasitologic assays would lead to more rapid disease control is unknown, but many such individuals have merely transiently positive CATT assays as a result of infection with animal trypanosomes.[57] Pentamidine

Table 98.1 Treatment Regimens for Gambian and Rhodesian Trypanosomiasis

	Trypanosoma brucei gambiense	*Trypanosoma brucei rhodesiense*
Early stage	Pentamidine IM 4 mg/kg up to 300 mg/day for 7 days	Suramin IV 5 mg/kg on day 1, then 20 mg/kg (up to 1.0 g) on days 3, 5, 12, 19, 26
Late stage	First choice in endemic countries: eflornithine IV 200 mg/kg q12h for 7 days plus nifurtimox 5 mg/kg q8h for 10 days First choice in non-endemic countries: eflornithine IV 100 mg/kg q6h for 14 days Alternative: melarsoprol IV 2.2 mg/kg daily for 10 days	Melarsoprol IV (dose in mg/kg): 1.80 mg/kg (day 5), 2.16 (day 6), 2.52 (days 7, 14), 2.88 (day 15), 3.24 (day 16), 3.6 mg/kg up to 180 mg (days 23, 24, 25)
Pretreatment before melarsoprol	None	Suramin IV 5 mg/kg on day 1, 20 mg/kg on day 3
Other drugs	Ivermectin or albendazole	Ivermectin or albendazole
Melarsoprol-induced encephalopathy		
Prevention	Prednisolone 1 mg/kg up to 40 mg/day, started 1–2 days before first dose of melarsoprol, continued until last dose, tapered over 3 days (30 mg, 20 mg, 10 mg)	As in *T. b. gambiense*
Treatment	Anticonvulsants, IV dexamethasone	As in *T. b. gambiense*
Relapses	Post-pentamidine: eflornithine or melarsoprol as above Post-eflornithine: melarsoprol as above Post-melarsoprol: eflornithine as above	Post-suramin: melarsoprol as above Post-melarsoprol: second course of melarsoprol IV, 3 × 4 daily injections, all doses at 3.6 mg/kg (up to 180 mg)

IM, intramuscular; IV, intravenous; q12h, every 12 hours; q8h, every 8 hours; q6h, every 6 hours.

"chemoprophylaxis" of the whole population of endemic areas would not be acceptable today because of its adverse effects and the risk of transmission of bloodborne pathogens. Certainly no traveler is at sufficiently high risk of HAT to warrant consideration of individual chemoprophylaxis.

To what extent HAT case-finding can be integrated within the activities of multipurpose health centers has been long debated.[58] Most cases passively detected by health centers already have an abnormal CSF, and their treatment must have only a modest impact on transmission. Vector control by tsetse fly trapping is a useful but costly adjuvant, to be considered only for high-incidence villages. Given the lack of commercial potential and the capacity of the parasite to undergo continuous antigenic variation, it is unlikely that a vaccine will ever be developed. For Rhodesian HAT, the experience of Uganda showed that an epidemic can be controlled through surveillance and case detection by sleeping sickness orderlies, combined with intensive tsetse fly trapping.

The international public health community will need to address whether *T. b. gambiense* trypanosomiasis can be eliminated. Such a strategy would imply that for many years donors must be willing to pay a very high cost for each case detected and treated, with the understanding that these expenditures would be reimbursed over time should elimination be accomplished. The contribution of the animal reservoir of *T. b. gambiense* will need to be understood before elimination can be contemplated, and modern molecular biology diagnostics will need to be deployed in endemic countries so as to identify and treat the residual human reservoir. *T. b. rhodesiense* infection is a zoonosis and its elimination may not be feasible, unless at least the cattle reservoir can be controlled.

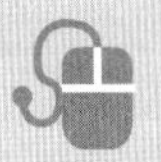

Access the complete reference list online at
http://www.expertconsult.com

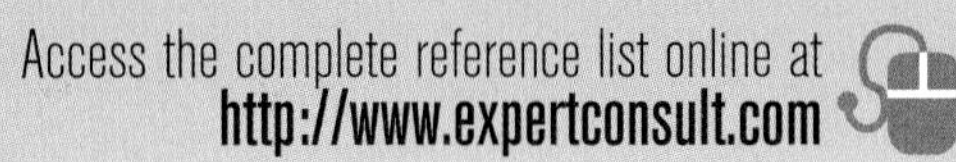
Access the complete reference list online at
http://www.expertconsult.com

CHAPTER 99

American Trypanosomiasis (Chagas Disease)*

Louis V. Kirchhoff

INTRODUCTION

American trypanosomiasis (Chagas disease) is a zoonosis caused by *Trypanosoma cruzi*, a protozoan parasite found only in the Americas. The geographic range of *T. cruzi* infection in humans and other mammalian hosts is primarily determined by the distribution of the various species of blood-sucking triatomine insects that act as its vectors. This range extends from the southern United States to Central Argentina (***Fig. 99.1***).

THE AGENT

The genus *Trypanosoma* contains several dozen species, but only *T. cruzi* and the two African trypanosome subspecies (see Chapter 98), *Trypanosoma brucei gambiense* and *T. b. rhodesiense*, cause disease in humans.[1] *T. rangeli*, found only in the Americas, can be transmitted to humans, but does not cause a persistent infection and is not pathogenic.[2] *T. cruzi* was first described in 1909 by the Brazilian physician Carlos Chagas, who saw the motile parasites while doing microscopic examinations of dissected intestines of triatomine insects.[3] The complex life cycle of *T. cruzi* involves insect vectors as well as mammalian hosts (***Figs 99.2 and 99.3***). Vectors become infected when they ingest blood from mammals that have circulating trypomastigotes, which are nondividing but infective forms of the parasite (***Fig. 99.4***). Once inside the midgut of an insect host, the parasites undergo transformation to epimastigotes, which are flagellates having a distinct morphology, and these organisms then multiply extracellularly. After migration to the hindgut, epimastigotes transform into nondividing metacyclic trypomastigotes, which are then discharged with the feces around the time of a subsequent blood meal. Transmission to a second mammalian host occurs when breaks in the skin, mucous membranes, or conjunctivae are contaminated with insect feces containing the infective metacyclic forms. Inside the new host, these parasites enter a variety of host cell types and, after transformation into amastigotes, multiply intracellularly. When proliferating amastigotes fill the host cell, they differentiate into trypomastigotes and the cell ruptures. The parasites released invade adjacent tissues and spread hematogenously to distant sites where they initiate further asynchronous cycles of intracellular multiplication, thus maintaining a parasitemia infective for vectors. *T. cruzi* can also be transmitted by transfusion of blood donated by infected persons,[4–6] from mother to fetus,[7–10] and in laboratory accidents.[11,12]

*All the material in this chapter is in the public domain, with the exception of the borrowed figures.

EPIDEMIOLOGY

Distribution of *Trypanosoma cruzi*

Epizootiology

Infection with *T. cruzi* is a zoonosis, and involvement of humans in the cycle of transmission is not necessary for perpetuation of the parasite in nature. *T. cruzi* is found only in the western hemisphere, where it primarily infects wild and domestic mammals and insects.[13] Triatomine vectors that transmit *T. cruzi* are found in spotty distributions, from central Argentina to the southern half of the United States. Hollow trees, burrows, palm trees, and other animal shelters are places where transmission of *T. cruzi* occurs among infected vectors and nonhuman mammalian hosts. Piles of wood, old vegetation, and stacks of roof tiles near houses have also been found to harbor large numbers of insects.[14,15]

T. cruzi has been found in more than 100 species of domestic and wild mammals,[16] from the southern United States to Central Argentina.[17–22] Opossums, wood rats, armadillos, raccoons, dogs, and cats are typical hosts, but *T. cruzi* is not a problem in livestock. Nontypical hosts can become infected when held in zoos in areas in which *T. cruzi* is enzootic.[23,24] This lack of species-specificity, combined with the fact that infected mammals have lifelong parasitemias, results in an enormous domestic and sylvatic reservoir in enzootic areas.

Epidemiology of Chagas Disease in Latin America

Historically, humans have become part of the cycle of *T. cruzi* transmission as farmers and ranchers open up land in enzootic regions. When this development takes place, vectors such as *Triatoma infestans*, *Rhodnius prolixus*, and *Panstrongylus megistus* invade the nooks and crannies of the primitive wood, mud-walled, and stone houses that are typical of rural Latin America. In this manner the vectors become domiciliary, establishing a cycle of transmission which involves humans and peridomestic mammals and is largely independent of the sylvatic cycle.[25–27] For the most part, Chagas disease has been a problem of poor people living in rural areas. In recent decades, however, large numbers of infected people have migrated to cities, thus urbanizing the disease and resulting in frequent transmission by blood transfusion prior to the implementation of effective serologic screening.[4,28]

Early reports indicated that most cases of acute Chagas disease that came to medical attention occurred in children.[29] Prevalence data support this view, but few age-specific and geographic incidence data have been available because most cases of the acute illness go undetected due to its mild nature and the lack of access to medical care among those at highest risk. The endemic range of human Chagas disease includes Mexico,[5,30,31] as well as all the countries in Central and South America. There is no Chagas disease in the Caribbean islands. The Pan American Health Organization (PAHO) has estimated that 8 million people are infected

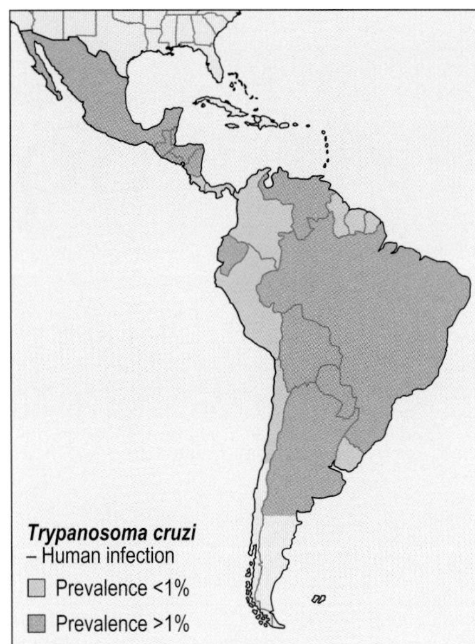

Figure 99.1 Geographic distribution of human infection with *Trypanosoma cruzi* (Chagas disease). Endemic countries in which the overall prevalence rate is ≥1% are shown in pink and those in which the prevalence rate is less than 1% are shown in yellow.

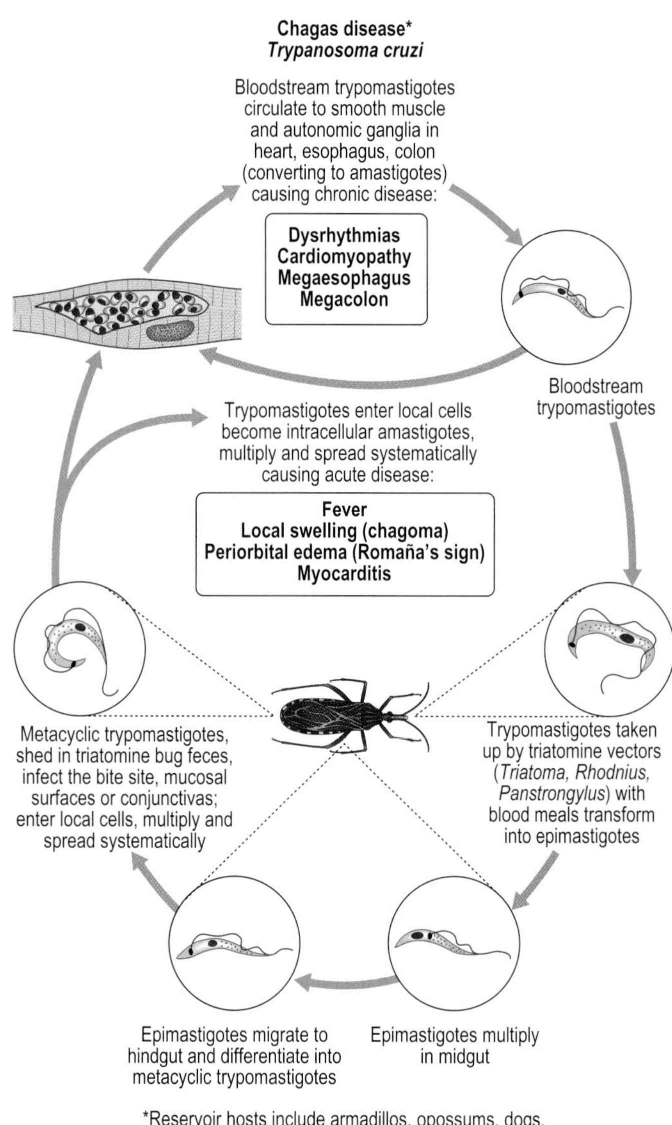

Figure 99.2 Life cycle of *Trypanosoma cruzi*.

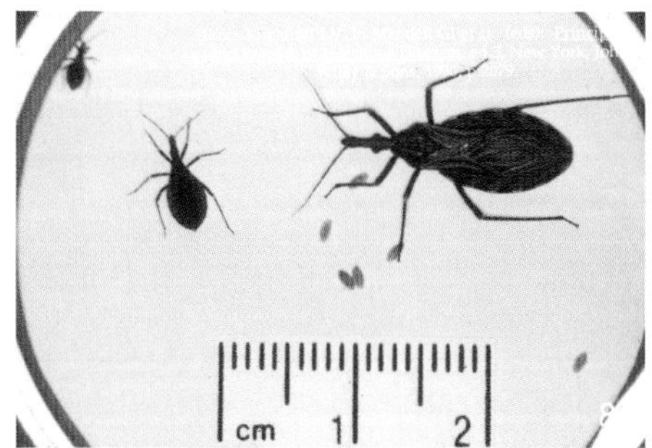

Figure 99.3 Eggs, first and second instar nymphs, and adult of *Rhodnius prolixus*, a triatomine vector of *Trypanosoma cruzi*.

with *T. cruzi* and that roughly 20 000 deaths each year are attributable to Chagas disease.[32] In 2000 the aggregate cost of the morbidity and death associated with Chagas disease was estimated to be more than US$8 billion.[33] Despite this enormous public health burden, however, in recent years the epidemiology of *T. cruzi* infection has improved markedly in much of the endemic range, as vector and blood bank control programs have achieved striking successes. As a consequence, prevalence rates in younger age groups have been decreasing in many areas.[34–37] A major international eradication program in the "southern cone" countries of South America (Brazil, Paraguay, Uruguay, Argentina, Chile, and Bolivia) has provided the framework for much of this progress. Uruguay, Chile, and Brazil were certified as transmission-free in 1997, 1999, and 2006 respectively, and marked reduction of transmission has been achieved in Argentina.[38] Similar control programs have been established in the Andean countries[39] and in Central America.[40] In Mexico, expansion of vector control and blood donor screening for Chagas disease are being implemented.[30,41,42] In the context of these successes, nonetheless, 41 200 instances of vector-borne transmission were estimated to have occurred in 2005 in the endemic range.[32] Moreover, several outbreaks of oral transmission of *T. cruzi* through contaminated food or drink have been reported, and increased transmission in the Amazon basin has been documented.[43–49] The obstacles hindering the elimination of *T. cruzi* transmission to humans throughout the endemic range are economic and political, and no major technological advances are necessary for its completion. The only caveat to this broad statement is that there is no clearly effective approach for blocking congenital transmission, which occurs in 2–10% of pregnancies in women with chronic *T. cruzi* infection.[50,51] An estimated 14 385 instances of congenital transmission occurred in the endemic countries in 2005.[8,32]

The epidemiology of symptomatic chronic Chagas disease is noteworthy. Roughly 70–90% of persons who harbor *T. cruzi* chronically never develop associated cardiac or gastrointestinal (GI) symptoms. In the past, however, the relatively high frequency of sudden death among young adults in some areas was attributed to arrhythmias due to chronic Chagas disease, and several decades ago in one highly endemic area of Brazil chagasic cardiac disease was found to be the most frequent cause of death in adults.[52] Taking a broader perspective, however, the annual disease-specific death rate among all *T. cruzi*-infected persons may be about 1 in 400, or 0.25%.

Interestingly, there is considerable geographic variation in the relative prevalence of cardiac and GI megadisease in patients with chronic Chagas disease. In most South American countries, megadisease is nearly as common as chagasic cardiac disease, but in Colombia, Venezuela, Central America, and Mexico megadisease is virtually unknown. Parasite strain differences (e.g., genotypes TcI and TcII) may play a major role in this variability of clinical penetrance, and host factors likely are important as well.[53,54]

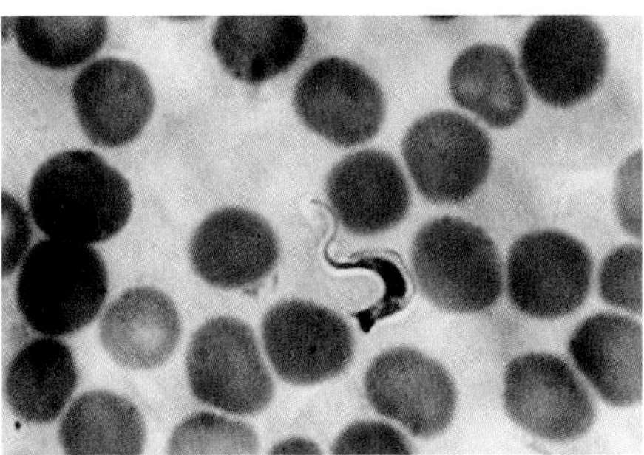

Figure 99.4 *Trypanosoma cruzi* trypomastigote in human blood (Giemsa stain, ×625). (Courtesy of Dr. Maria Aparecida Shikanai Yasuda, São Paulo, Brazil.)

Epidemiology of Chagas Disease in the United States

Despite the presence of the sylvatic cycle of *T. cruzi* in many parts of the southern and western United States, only six instances of autochthonous transmission have been reported there: three in Texas and one each in Louisiana, Tennessee, and California.[55–57] Moreover, the blood donor screening program that started in January 2007, in which more than 35 million donations have been tested, has uncovered only a small number of *T. cruzi*-infected donors who appear to have acquired the infection here. Our relatively high housing standards and low overall vector density probably underlie the rarity of transmission of *T. cruzi* to humans in the United States. In the past three decades only about 15 imported and laboratory-acquired cases of acute Chagas disease have been reported to the Centers for Disease Control and Prevention (CDC), but none in the latter group occurred in returning tourists. Three instances of tourists returning to Europe from Latin America with acute *T. cruzi* infection have been described.[58,59]

In contrast, the number of persons in the United States with chronic *T. cruzi* infections has grown enormously in recent years. It is currently estimated that 23 million persons born in countries in which Chagas disease is endemic currently live in the United States. Approximately 17 million of these individuals are from Mexico,[60] where the overall prevalence of *T. cruzi* infection may be 0.5–1.0%.[5] Moreover, a large proportion of these immigrants have come from Central America, a region in which *T. cruzi* prevalence is relatively high (e.g., 3.4%, 3.1%, and 2.0% in El Salvador, Honduras, and Guatemala).[32] *T. cruzi* infection rates of 1 in 5995 and 1 in 3285 were found in blood donors in Tucson and Los Angeles,[61] and a *T. cruzi* prevalence of 1.0% was found in 782 Hispanic immigrants attending health fairs in Los Angeles (personal communication, Dr Sheba Meymandi).

Recently it was estimated that 300 000 *T. cruzi*-infected persons currently live in the United States.[62] Before blood donor screening began in 2007, the presence here of infected immigrants posed a risk of transfusion-associated transmission of *T. cruzi*,[63] and seven such instances in the United States and Canada had been reported.[64,65] All these cases occurred in immunosuppressed patients in whom the diagnosis of *T. cruzi* infection was made because of the fulminant course of the illness. Since most transfusions are given to immunocompetent persons in whom acute *T. cruzi* infection would be a mild illness, it is reasonable to infer that other cases have occurred here but have not been noticed. The question as to how best to avoid transmission of the parasite via transfusion in the United States has been debated since the first known instance occurred in 1988, although prior to December 2006 this was done in the context of a lack of a Food and Drug Administration (FDA)-approved screening test. Common sense suggested that if screening is warranted in the endemic countries from which the 23 million immigrants living here have come, then they should be tested when they present for donation here. At the end of the day governmental and blood industry authorities adopted this perspective; and shortly after the Ortho *T. cruzi* ELISA Test System (Ortho-Clinical Diagnostics, Raritan, NJ) was approved for donor screening by the FDA, near-universal screening began. To date more than 1200 *T. cruzi*-infected donors have been identified and deferred permanently from donation, and the confirmed rate of *T. cruzi* infection among donors has been about 1 in 29 000.[6] No cases of transfusion transmission of *T. cruzi* have been detected since screening started. In an effort to reduce the enormous cost of universal screening ($100–200 million per year) a selective screening protocol based on negative test results on a prior donation is being implemented in some areas. Sizable numbers of persons have also emigrated from the countries in which Chagas disease is endemic to Europe, and *T. cruzi* infection in these people has been studied.[66,67]

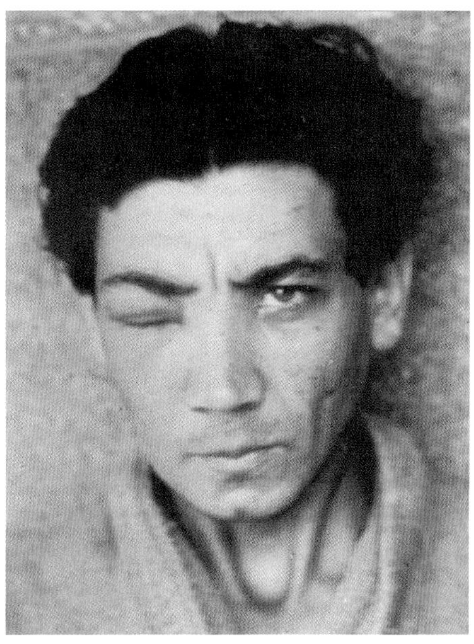

Figure 99.5 Romaña's sign (unilateral painless periorbital edema) in a Brazilian patient with acute Chagas disease. (Courtesy of Dr Mário Shiroma, São Paulo, Brazil.)

Finally, the transplantation here of organs from three persons with chronic *T. cruzi* infections resulted in acute infection in five recipients, one of whom died of the acute illness.[68,69]

THE DISEASE

The clinical manifestations of acute and chronic Chagas disease are different and are described separately. Acute Chagas disease results from a host's first encounter with the parasite whereas chronic symptomatic Chagas disease involves late sequelae resulting from persistent infection.

Acute Chagas Disease

Acute Chagas disease usually occurs in children but can occur at any age. The first sign can be a chagoma, which is an erythematous and indurated lesion at the site of parasite entry that appears a week or two after transmission has occurred.[70] When the conjunctiva is the portal of entry, the patient may develop Romaña's sign, which is unilateral and painless periorbital edema (*Fig. 99.5*). Romaña's sign is found in only a small proportion of patients with acute *T. cruzi* infection and similar findings can be the result of several other processes.

Systemic spread of the parasites from the site of initial multiplication may be accompanied by malaise, fever, and edema of the face and lower extremities, as well as hepatosplenomegaly and generalized lymphadenopathy. A peripheral lymphocytosis may accompany the high parasitemias of acute Chagas disease, and mild elevation of transaminases may also be present. Muscles, including the heart, can be heavily parasitized, and

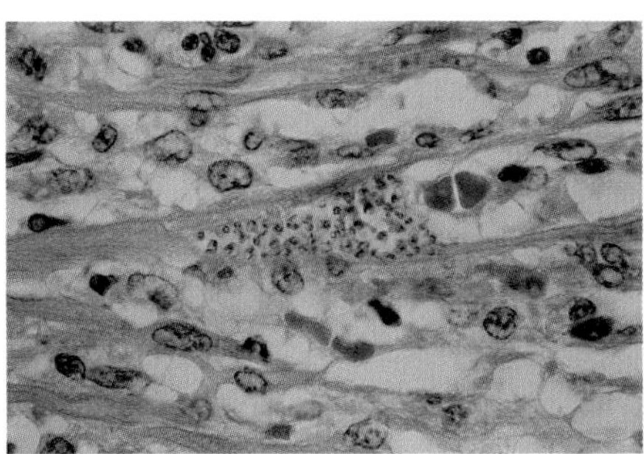

Figure 99.6 *Trypanosoma cruzi* in the heart muscle of a child who died of acute Chagas disease. The infected cardiomyocyte shown contains several dozen amastigotes.

severe myocarditis with functional impairment occasionally causing death develops in a small proportion of patients[29,55,71] (***Fig. 99.6***). Nonspecific electrocardiographic (ECG) changes can occur, but the life-threatening conduction defects common in chronic cardiac Chagas disease are usually not seen. *T. cruzi* also can invade the central nervous system (CNS),[72] but neurologic findings are not common. Rarely, meningoencephalitis develops, and it is associated with a poor prognosis.[73] In the vast majority of patients, the acute illness resolves spontaneously in 4–8 weeks and they then enter the indeterminate phase of the infection, which is characterized by a lack of symptoms, subpatent parasitemias, and generally detectable antibodies to a variety of *T. cruzi* antigens.

Chronic Chagas Disease

Chronic Chagas Cardiopathy

Although most persons chronically infected with *T. cruzi* remain in the indeterminate phase for life, approximately 10–30% develop symptomatic chronic Chagas disease, usually years or even decades after the infection was initially acquired. Cardiac problems are the most frequent complications of chronic Chagas disease.[74–79] Hearts obtained at autopsy from patients who died of chagasic heart disease usually have a global appearance due to chamber enlargement, and mural thrombi are frequently present, often in the right atrium and the apex of the left ventricle. Left ventricular apical aneurysm is typical in patients with advanced cardiac Chagas disease. At a cellular level, the process that underlies these gross pathologic lesions is a chronic inflammation with mononuclear cell infiltration and diffuse fibrosis that affects the conduction system as well as the cardiac muscle.[80–82] Parasites are rarely seen on histological examination, but they can often be detected by polymerase chain reaction (PCR) assays.[83–85] The process results in a variety of dysrhythmias, including atrial bradyarrhythmias and fibrillation; premature ventricular contractions; bundle branch blocks, often of the right bundle (RBBB); and complete atrioventricular block. Most instances of sudden death in persons with chronic *T. cruzi* infection probably result from complete atrioventricular block, ventricular tachycardia, or ventricular fibrillation.

The symptoms associated with chronic cardiac Chagas disease reflect the congestive failure, rhythm disturbances, and thromboembolism that result from the fibrosing cardiopathy.[86–88] The arrhythmias can cause dizziness and syncope, and sudden death is a common occurrence. The cardiomyopathy frequently affects the right side of the heart more than the left, and thus symptoms of right-sided failure are often present.

Chronic Gastrointestinal Chagas Disease (Megadisease)

Dysfunction of the GI tract is the second most common consequence of chronic *T. cruzi* infection.[89,90] As in the case of chagasic cardiopathy, GI Chagas disease usually occurs years or even decades after infection with *T. cruzi* is acquired. Dysfunction related to megaesophagus (***Fig. 99.7***) is the most typical clinical manifestation, but symptoms due to megacolon

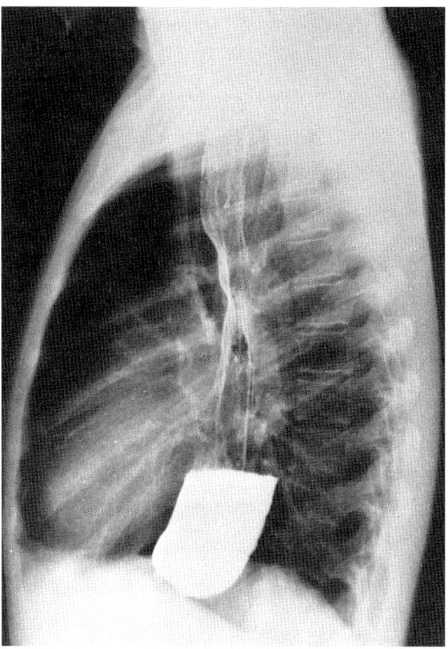

Figure 99.7 Barium esophagogram in a Brazilian patient with dolichomegaesophagus caused by chronic Chagas disease. Contrast material is pooled in the distal esophagus, which is markedly enlarged. (Reproduced from Neva FA, Brown HW. Basic Clinical Parasitology, 6th ed. Norwalk, CN: Appleton & Lange; 1994.)

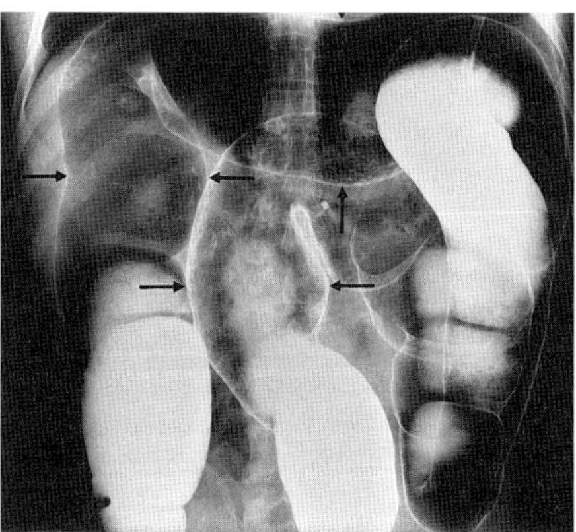

Figure 99.8 Barium enema examination of a patient with megacolon caused by Chagas disease. Markedly increased diameters of the ascending, transverse, and sigmoid segments of the large bowel are marked with opposing arrows.

(***Fig. 99.8***) are also frequent. The process underlying megadisease is a loss of neurons in the gut.[91] Quantitative assessments of this degenerative process have shown that in severely affected patients as many as 85% of the neurons in the esophagus and 50% of those in the colon may be lost. The factors that determine the rate and pattern of the neuronal destruction are not known.

Pathologic examination of esophageal specimens obtained surgically or at autopsy from patients with megaesophagus have shown dilatation and varying degrees of thickening of the muscular wall. As in the case of cardiac tissue, microscopic examination shows mononuclear cell infiltration and fibrosis, but finding parasites is unusual. The most common symptom associated with chagasic megaesophagus is dysphagia. Many patients experiencing this sense the accumulation of swallowed food in the esophagus and take in water or more food, or even eat in a standing position, to facilitate its passage into the stomach. Pain, typically starting in the lower substernal area and spreading upward, is also a frequent symptom in patients with megaesophagus. In patients with severe degrees of megaesophagus, regurgitation can become a problem, and if the underlying problem is not treated, it can lead to intermittent aspiration with associated chronic cough, bronchitis, and pneumonia.

As in the case of chagasic megaesophagus, colonic disease is manifested by dilatation and typically the sigmoid colon is the most affected segment. As the disease progresses, the colon can become markedly enlarged in both length and diameter, and the thickening of the wall can become less pronounced. The pathologic changes evident on microscopic examination of affected colonic tissue are similar to those found in the esophagus. The cardinal symptom associated with Chagas disease of the colon is constipation. Pain is also a common symptom, resulting from accumulation of feces and flatus, as well as ineffective and recurrent colonic contractions.

Other GI and urinary viscera can be affected in persons with chronic Chagas disease, but this is much less common.[92] The most frequent occurrence is hypertrophy of the parotid glands, which is present in as many as 25% of patients with chagasic megaesophagus. The stomach may also be affected, and hypoperistalsis, hypotonia, decreased acid secretion, and delayed emptying of the stomach have been documented in patients with megaesophagus, but dilatation of the stomach is not found frequently.[93]

The pathogenesis of the cardiac and GI lesions of chronic Chagas disease has been debated for decades. Recently, convincing evidence has accumulated supporting the concept that the low-level presence of parasites in chronically affected cardiac tissue, detectable by molecular methods, stimulates a chronic inflammatory response that over time leads to the pathologic changes observed microscopically.[82 85,94,95]

Trypanosoma cruzi Infection in Immunosuppressed Patients

Immunosuppression of persons who chronically harbor *T. cruzi* can lead to a recrudescence of the infection, frequently with an intensity that is atypical of acute Chagas disease in immunocompetent patients.[96–99] The incidence of reactivation of *T. cruzi* in patients who become immunosuppressed is not known. Persons immunosuppressed by the human immunodeficiency virus (HIV) and infected with *T. cruzi* are also at risk for reactivation of the latter. To date, dozens of such cases have been described,[100–103] and it is noteworthy that many of these patients developed *T. cruzi* brain abscesses, which do not occur in immunocompetent persons with acute or chronic Chagas disease, and may be difficult to distinguish radiographically from those of cerebral toxoplasmosis.[104]

DIAGNOSIS

The approaches used to diagnose acute and chronic Chagas disease are quite different and will be considered separately.

Acute Chagas Disease

The first step in diagnosing acute Chagas disease is determining that the patient has a history consistent with exposure to *T. cruzi*. Risk factors include residence or a blood transfusion in an endemic country, birth to a mother known or suspected of being infected with *T. cruzi*, or a laboratory accident involving the parasite. Patients with acute Chagas disease may develop a variety of local and systemic signs, but these are usually mild. Occasionally, severe myocarditis develops, leading to nonspecific ECG changes, radiographic signs of cardiomegaly, or pericardial effusion. Invasion of the CNS by the parasites can lead to abnormal cerebrospinal fluid (CSF) values.[72] The differential diagnoses of all of these clinical findings are quite broad, however, and in the absence of a parasitologic diagnosis they can only be viewed as suggestive of acute Chagas disease.

A definitive diagnosis of acute Chagas disease is made by detecting parasites. Serologic assays for *T. cruzi*-specific IgM are not accurate enough to warrant their use.[105] Circulating trypomastigotes are highly motile and frequently can be seen in wet preparations of anticoagulated blood or buffy coat. The parasites often can be seen in Giemsa-stained smears as well. In immunocompetent patients with acute Chagas disease, examination of blood preparations is the cornerstone of detecting *T. cruzi*. In immunocompromised patients suspected of having acute Chagas disease, however, other specimens such as bone marrow, lymph node aspirates, endomyocardial tissue, skin lesion biopsies, CSF, and pericardial fluid should be examined microscopically.

When these direct methods fail to detect organisms in any patient with clinical and epidemiologic histories suggesting a diagnosis of acute Chagas disease, as well as in infants born to serologically positive mothers, samples should be tested in a PCR assay (see below). Considerable data have accumulated supporting the concept that PCR assays are more sensitive for detecting the presence of *T. cruzi* than are the direct methods described above. Another option is to culture blood or other samples in specialized liquid medium,[106–108] but the usefulness of this approach is limited by low sensitivity (50–70% for hemoculture in the best of hands) and by the fact that a minimum of 2–3 weeks is required for cultures to turn positive. In infants who are negative by direct examinations and a PCR assay right after birth, serology for *T. cruzi*-specific IgG should be done 6–9 months later, by which time maternal antibodies will have cleared.[109]

Chronic Chagas Disease

As mentioned previously, patients with chronic cardiac Chagas disease can develop a variety of dysrhythmias, including RBBB, which is the most representative conduction abnormality of Chagas cardiopathy. Nonetheless, it is a nonspecific finding since many persons with RBBB do not have Chagas disease. Echocardiographic and radiographic signs of chronic cardiac Chagas disease are similar to those found in patients with cardiomyopathies caused by other processes. Megacolon and megaesophagus are best diagnosed by barium contrast radiographic tests. It is important to keep in mind, however, that all of these diagnostic studies are useful primarily for defining the degree of associated abnormalities in patients known to be infected with the parasite.

Chronic Chagas disease is usually diagnosed by detecting IgG antibodies that bind specifically to parasite antigens, and in the vast majority of instances isolating the organism is not important. At the present time, more than 30 assays for the serologic diagnosis of *T. cruzi* infection are available commercially. Most of these assays are based on ELISA, indirect immunofluorescence, and indirect hemagglutination formats,[110,111] and they are used widely in the endemic countries for screening donated blood and clinical specimens. Many of the assays have sensitivities and specificities that are less than ideal, and false-positive reactions typically occur with samples from patients having illnesses such as leishmaniasis, paracoccidioidomycosis, syphilis, malaria, and other parasitic and nonparasitic diseases.[112–115] Because of these shortcomings, the PAHO recommends that samples be tested in two assays based on different formats before decisions regarding infection status are made. A number of assays in which recombinant proteins serve as target antigens are available commercially or in development and hold the promise of improved diagnostic accuracy.[116–119] Two FDA-approved assays are available in the United States for clinical testing, but not for screening donated blood (Chagas kit, Hemagen Diagnostics, Inc., Columbia, MD; Chagatest ELISA Recombinante v3.0, Wiener Laboratories, Rosario, Argentina).[120] The Ortho *T. cruzi* ELISA Test System and the Abbott PRISM Chagas (Abbott Laboratories, Abbott Park, IL), which is based on recombinant antigens, have been approved by the FDA for blood donor screening.[117,121] These assays currently are used to screen most of the 15.2 million units of blood donated in the United States each year. A Clinical Laboratory Improvement Amendments-approved radioimmune precipitation assay (Chagas RIPA)[115,122] is used for confirmatory testing of donated units that are repeat positive in the Ortho and Abbott tests and also is available for testing clinical and research samples in my laboratory.

The possibility of using PCR assays for detecting *T. cruzi* infection has been the focus of considerable study. Although the number of parasites in the blood of chronically infected persons is extremely low, PCR assays have the potential for detecting their presence because they have large numbers of highly conserved nuclear and kinetoplast DNA (kDNA) sequences. Two decades ago Moser and coworkers[123] described a PCR assay in which a 188-basepair nuclear repetitive DNA sequence is amplified using primers called TCZ1 and TCZ2. Each parasite contains approximately 100 000 copies of this sequence, and in contrived experiments as little as 0.5% of the genome of a single organism gave a positive result. A study in mice with acute and chronic *T. cruzi* infections indicated clearly that TCZ1–TCZ2 assay is much more sensitive than microscopic examination of blood.[124]

In another PCR assay, described by Sturm et al.,[125] a 330-basepair segment of the *T. cruzi* kinetoplast minicircle is amplified using primers designated S35–S36. It is estimated that each parasite has 120 000 copies of this sequence, and in mixing experiments the authors detected 0.1% of one parasite genome. To date three studies have been published in which the sensitivities of these two assays were compared head to head, and in all three the TCZ1–TCZ2 assay appeared to have an edge in terms of sensitivity.[120,124,126] PCR assays for *T. cruzi* detection based on several other primer pairs have been described, but none appears to have any advantage over tests based on TCZ1–TCZ2 and S35–S36, probably because the parasite has fewer copies of the DNA sequences they amplify.

Since these two original reports were published in 1989, more than 100 articles have appeared that deal with the detection of *T. cruzi* by PCR tests. In nine key human studies published in the 1990s, the sensitivities of the PCR assays ranged from 44.7% to 100%, with most results falling slightly over 90%.[107,108,127] These disappointing results likely are the result of a sampling phenomenon in that the large numbers of amplifiable sequences are not dispersed, but rather are contained in the rare parasites that may or may not be swept up with blood drawn for testing. Clearly the level of sensitivity achieved with PCR assays for *T. cruzi* infection is not high enough to allow their use for confirmatory testing of donated blood.[128] Nonetheless, PCR assays are potentially useful for detecting *T. cruzi* in persons with possible *T. cruzi* infection who have borderline serologic results, in persons suspected of having acute or congenital Chagas disease in whom parasites are not detected microscopically, and in infected patients who have received specific treatment. In all such individuals, only positive PCR results can be taken as truly indicative of infection status. Recently a group of Latin American experts met to standardize a PCR protocol for *T. cruzi* testing with the purpose of increasing accuracy and facilitating comparability of results.

Parasitologic diagnosis of chronic *T. cruzi* infection also can be attempted by hemoculture or xenodiagnosis. Due to technical issues the latter largely has become a thing of the past. As noted, hemoculture may have a sensitivity as high as 50–70% in persons with chronic *T. cruzi* infection.[106] Its use should be limited to the groups of patients listed above in whom PCR assays also may have a role.

TREATMENT AND PROGNOSIS

Antiparasitic Drugs

Treatment for *T. cruzi* infection is unsatisfactory and the need for a parasitologically curative drug regimen is the most important current challenge in Chagas disease research. Many dozens of drugs have been tested for activity against *T. cruzi*, including those active against other parasitic protozoans, and only two have been found to be clinically useful.[129,130]

The first of these is nifurtimox (Lampit, Bayer 2502, Leverkusen, Germany), a nitrofuran derivative with which extensive clinical experience has accumulated during the three decades it has been available.[131] In patients with acute Chagas disease, nifurtimox reduces the severity and duration of the illness and lessens mortality. Parasitologic cures are achieved with nifurtimox only in approximately 70% of these patients. Importantly, the cure rate is greater than 90% in babies with congenital Chagas disease who are treated during the first year of life.[7,132] Those not cured enter the indeterminate phase of *T. cruzi* infection and over time are at risk of symptomatic chronic Chagas disease. In general, cure rates may be <10% in adults with chronic *T. cruzi* infection, but cure rates are much higher in children. Nifurtimox must be taken for long periods and can cause severe side effects, including GI complaints such as nausea, vomiting, abdominal pain, anorexia, and weight loss.[131] Some patients taking the drug also develop neurologic symptoms, such as restlessness, insomnia, twitching, paresthesias, polyneuritis, and seizures. Treatment with nifurtimox should be initiated as early as possible in patients with acute or congenital Chagas disease. Nifurtimox is available in 30- and 120-mg tablets. For adults, the recommended oral dosage is 8–10 mg/kg body weight per day. For adolescents, the dose is 12.5–15 mg/kg/day, and for children 1–10 years of age, it is 15–20 mg/kg/day. The drug should be given each day in four divided doses, and treatment should be continued for 90–120 days. Nifurtimox can be obtained from the CDC Drug Service (770-488-7775).

The second drug available for treating *T. cruzi* infection is the nitroimidazole derivative benznidazole (Rochagan, Radinil, Roche 7-1051; LAFEPE, Pernambuco, Brazil). Cure rates are similar to those of nifurtimox. Side effects can include granulocytopenia, rash, and peripheral neuropathy.[133] Benznidazole is used widely throughout the endemic countries, where experts view it as the drug of choice. For patients of all ages the recommended oral dosage of benznidazole is 5 mg/kg body weight per day for 60 days.

Regarding which groups of *T. cruzi*-infected patients should be given specific treatment, there is a broad consensus that treatment is indicated in all patients with acute infection as well as chronically infected children 17 years or younger. This recommendation is supported by studies indicating that a majority of patients in these groups can be cured parasitologically with a full course of either drug.[7,134–137] By extension, it is reasonable to treat anyone 18 or older who has acquired the infection within the last 17 years, but there are no data that shed light on the usefulness of this approach. An additional important question is whether specific treatment given before pregnancy will reduce the probability of subsequent congenital transmission. Only one limited study has addressed this issue, and the results suggest a protective effect.[50]

There also is a general consensus that persons with chronic symptomatic *T. cruzi* infection should not be treated with nifurtimox or benznidazole. The question of whether adults with long-standing indeterminate-phase infections should be treated is controversial. This is a thorny issue in part because, as noted, the drugs can cause bothersome side effects, the courses of treatment are long, and the rates of parasitological cure in persons with long-standing infections may be as low as 10–20%.[130,137–141] Thus in the majority of such patients the question is whether mere suppression of the parasites for several months, as opposed to cure, affects long-term outcomes significantly. Importantly, there is no convincing evidence from properly structured trials that treatment with either drug reduces the appearance or progression of symptoms or reduces mortality in persons in the indeterminate phase of the infection.[142,143] Unfortunately, addressing this issue is complicated methodologically by the lack of sensitivity of the parasitological assays (i.e., PCR and hemoculture) that must be used to look for failure to cure since anti-*T. cruzi* antibody levels can remain positive for years, even in patients who have been cured. A panel of experts convened by the CDC in 2006 recommended that adults less than 50 years of age with presumably long-standing indeterminate *T. cruzi* infections be offered treatment.[144] A large trial (the BENEFIT Multicentric Trial) designed to assess the parasitologic and clinical efficacy of benznidazole in indeterminate-phase Chagas disease patients is being carried out in Colombia, Brazil, and Argentina, but initial results will not be available until 2011 at the earliest.[145,146]

The activities of allopurinol and the antifungal azoles against *T. cruzi* have been studied extensively in laboratory animals and to a lesser extent in infected persons. Recent studies have focused on posaconazole, ravuconazole, and TAK-187. To date none of these agents has shown a level of anti-*T. cruzi* activity that justifies its use in humans. Other promising drugs are being evaluated.[147–149]

Finally, concern relating to nifurtimox and benznidazole is raised by experiments showing that 33% of rabbits treated with nifurtimox and 42% of those given benznidazole developed lymphomas, whereas none of the control animals developed tumors.[150,151] Although these findings should be a cause for concern, it merits mention that these two drugs have been used for decades in the endemic countries and no reports of an increased incidence of lymphomas have appeared.

Treatment of Clinical Chagas Disease

Beyond the possible use of antiparasitic drugs, the treatment of both acute and chronic Chagas disease is symptomatic. Patients with severe acute chagasic myocarditis should be supported as would any patient with acute congestive cardiomyopathy. In patients with symptomatic chronic Chagas heart disease, therapy is directed at ameliorating symptoms through the use of the cardiotropic drugs and anticoagulants generally used in patients with cardiomyopathies due to other causes.[78,152–155] Pacemakers have been shown to be useful in patients with ominous bradyarrhythmias or heart block.[156] The usefulness of autologous bone marrow cells to ameliorate symptoms associated with Chagas cardiomyopathy is being studied.[157]

Cardiac transplantation is an option in patients with endstage Chagas heart disease, and more than 150 *T. cruzi*-infected patients have undergone the procedure in Brazil and the United States.[158–160] Reactivated acute Chagas disease occurred often in the patients transplanted initially in Brazil due to the postoperative immunosuppression, but this has been less of a problem in the last decade or so as smaller doses of cyclosporine have been used.[159,161,162] Of concern, the usual parasitologic methods for detecting acute *T. cruzi* infection were not sensitive detectors of the reactivations. Moreover, the occurrence of posttransplant malignant neoplasms is an additional problem.[163] Patients who have had a heart transplant for Chagas disease occasionally develop cutaneous lesions containing large numbers of parasites,[164] and this has been observed in *T. cruzi*-infected patients with renal transplants and HIV/acquired immunodeficiency syndrome (AIDS) as well.[97,102] The efficacy and toxicity of long-term prophylaxis with either nifurtimox or benznidazole in *T. cruzi*-infected patients after cardiac transplantation have not been assessed. In spite of these problems, the long-term survival of Chagas patients with heart transplants is greater than that of individuals receiving heart transplants for other reasons, most likely because the lesions of chronic *T. cruzi* infection are generally limited to the heart.[165] The frequency with which *T. cruzi*-infected immigrants in the United States are considered for cardiac transplantation will increase over time as this group increases in size and ages.

Megaesophagus associated with Chagas disease should be treated as is idiopathic achalasia.[166,167] The best initial relief of symptoms is achieved by balloon dilatation of the lower esophageal sphincter. Patients with megaesophagus who fail to respond to repeated balloon dilatation may require surgical treatment. The procedure most often used is wide esophagocardiomyectomy of the anterior gastroesophageal junction, combined with valvuloplasty to reduce reflux. Patients with extreme megaesophagus can be treated with esophageal resection with reconstruction using an esophagogastroplasty.[168,169] In developed countries, laparoscopic myotomy is being used with increasing frequency to treat idiopathic achalasia, and this relatively simple procedure may become the method of choice for both idiopathic achalasia and Chagas disease. A possible role for the injection of botulinum toxin is being evaluated.[170]

Patients in the early stages of colonic dysfunction associated with chronic *T. cruzi* infection can be managed with a high-fiber diet and occasional laxatives and enemas. Fecal impaction necessitating manual disimpaction may occur, as can toxic megacolon, which requires surgical intervention.[171] Volvulus is a complication of chagasic megacolon that requires immediate attention. Endoscopic emptying can be done initially in patients without clinical, endoscopic, or radiographic signs of ischemia in the affected segment. Cases that are complicated should be treated with surgical decompression. In either case, however, surgical treatment of the megacolon is ultimately necessary because of the common recurrence of volvulus. Several surgical procedures have been used to treat advanced chagasic megacolon, and all of them include resection of the sigmoid as well as removal of part of the rectum.[172,173]

PREVENTION AND CONTROL

Since no vaccine or chemoprophylaxis is available for preventing transmission of *T. cruzi*, diminishing the number of new cases in Latin America must depend on reducing contact with insect vectors and on serologic identification of infected blood donors. Elimination of domiciliary vectors is best accomplished by improving housing conditions, spraying of insecticides, and educating at-risk populations. As noted previously, major successes with these approaches have been achieved in several endemic countries.[174,175] Elimination of the sylvatic vectors and reservoirs is not a reasonable goal. In view of the successes of low-technology measures in reducing the transmission of *T. cruzi*, it appears unlikely that the recent major advances in understanding the molecular biology of the parasite and the pathogenesis of Chagas disease will play a substantive role in the eventual elimination of this public health problem.

Since chronic *T. cruzi* infection carries with it the risk of serious cardiac and GI disease, in industrialized countries immigrants from endemic regions and children born to mothers with geographic risk should be screened serologically. Identification of infected persons is important because pharmacologic agents and pacemakers can benefit patients who develop rhythm disturbances. Infected individuals should have ECGs done every 6–12 months with the goal of early detection of rhythm disturbances. The possibility of congenital transmission and the need to search for *T. cruzi* infection in infants born to seropositive mothers is another reason for screening.

Tourists who travel in areas where *T. cruzi* transmission occurs should avoid sleeping in dilapidated dwellings in rural areas and should use insect repellent and mosquito nets to reduce exposure to vectors. Nonetheless, it is important to keep in mind that, as noted above, the risk of acquiring *T. cruzi* infection during short-term residence in an endemic country is extremely low. To my knowledge, no incidents of this type have been reported among tourists returning to the United States. Special precautions for people engaging in outdoor activities in the United States are not warranted. *T. cruzi* is classified as a risk group 2 agent in the United States and as risk group 3 in some European countries, and laboratorians should work with the parasite or infected vectors at containment levels consistent with the risk group designation in their areas.[176,177]

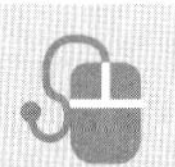

Access the complete reference list online at
http://www.expertconsult.com

CHAPTER 100

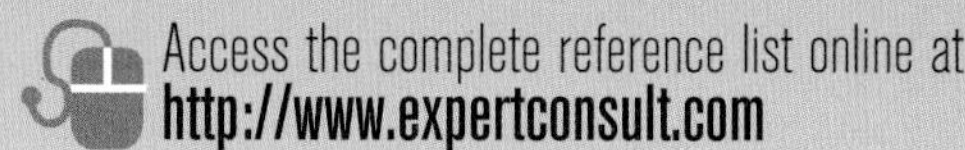
Access the complete reference list online at
http://www.expertconsult.com

Leishmaniasis

Selma M.B. Jeronimo • Anastacio de Queiroz Sousa • Richard D. Pearson

INTRODUCTION

Leishmania species, members of the family Trypanosomatidae, order Kinetoplastida, reside as intracellular amastigotes within macrophages in humans and other mammals and as extracellular promastigotes in the gut of their insect vectors, phlebotomine sandflies. The clinical manifestations of infection vary as a consequence of the virulence of the infecting *Leishmania* species, and the cell-mediated immune responses of their mammalian hosts. Leishmaniasis encompasses a spectrum of findings. It is divided into three major clinical syndromes: (1) cutaneous; (2) mucosal (mucocutaneous); and (3) visceral (***Fig. 100.1***).[1] Although each *Leishmania* species tends to cause a given pattern of disease, the findings can be quite variable. Subclinical, self-resolving infections are common. The persistence of parasites in tissues accounts for a prolonged incubation period in some persons, particularly if they become immunocompromised later in life.[2,3]

Leishmania species are endemic in scattered areas of every continent except Antarctica (***Table 100.1***). The geographic distributions of cutaneous and mucosal leishmaniasis are shown in ***Figures 100.2 and 100.3***. Many *Leishmania* species cause zoonoses involving dogs, other canines, or rodents. They pose a significant problem for residents living in endemic areas as well as refugees, military personnel, visitors, and workers who enter them. Cutaneous leishmaniasis has been acquired by North American travelers to Central and South America and military personnel serving in Iraq and Afghanistan.[4] Mucosal leishmaniasis is encountered primarily among residents of Latin America.[5–7]

Visceral leishmaniasis, also known as kala-azar, poses a major health problem in eastern India and Bangladesh.[8,9] Outbreaks have also been reported among refugees in the Sudan,[10,11] and residents of periurban areas in northeastern Brazil.[12] Visceral leishmaniasis emerged as an important opportunistic disease in people with the acquired immunodeficiency syndrome (AIDS) in Europe in the early 1980s[13–15] and has subsequently been reported in persons with AIDS in Brazil and elsewhere.[16,17] The distribution of visceral leishmaniasis can be seen in ***Figure 100.4***.

THE AGENT

Lainson and Shaw classified *Leishmania* species into two subgenera, *Leishmania* and *Viannia*, based on their development in the gut of the sandfly.[18] The subgenus *Viannia* includes *L. braziliensis* and related species that develop in the hindgut before migrating to the midgut and foregut (peripylaria). The subgenus *Leishmania* includes species that occupy the midgut and foregut only (suprapylaria). Within each subgenus, speciation was historically based on multiple factors including geographic distribution, animal reservoir, and sandfly species.[18]

The sequencing of the *Leishmania major*,[19] *L. braziliensis* and *L. infantum* genomes[20] was a major advance. The three genomes were shown to present strong codon bias and conservation of synteny. Although *L. viannia* spp. and *L. leishmania* spp. have been separated for 20–100 million years,[21] there are only approximately 200 genes with a differential distribution among the three species. Refinements in classification are likely as more information becomes available about the genetic diversity of the *Leishmania* species. The identification of genes involved in pathogenesis should aid in the design of new therapeutic and prophylactic strategies.[22,23]

The life cycle of *Leishmania* is relatively straightforward (***Fig. 100.1***).[24] In mammals, amastigotes reside in mononuclear phagocytes at acid pH within parasitophorous vacuoles. They are oval or round in shape and approximately 2 × 3 μm in diameter. Amastigotes have a relatively large, eccentrically located nucleus; a specialized mitochondrial structure, the kinetoplast, which contains a substantial amount of extranuclear DNA in the form of catenated mini- and maxi-circles; and a flagellar pocket and flagellum, which lie within the confines of the cell. They multiply by simple binary division. A row of subpellicular microtubules is arrayed under the plasma membrane much like the ribs of an umbrella. In the gut of the sandfly, *Leishmania* live and multiply as extracellular, flagellated promastigotes that vary morphologically from short, stumpy forms to elongated ones ranging from 10 to 15 μm in length and 2 to 3 μm in diameter.[25] A single flagellum extends from the anterior pole. Recent evidence indicates that *Leishmania* can undergo genetic exchange in the sandfly gut.[26] After 1 or 2 weeks of development, which varies among species, infectious metacyclic promastigotes migrate to the proboscis.[27,28]

Leishmania species are transmitted by female sandflies of the genus *Lutzomyia* in the Americas and *Phlebotomus* elsewhere. Depending on the species, sandflies live in forested areas, rodent burrows, or debris in peridomestic habitats. They are weak fliers, but they can be carried considerable distances if caught in the wind and have been dispersed more than 200 m from the original focus.[29] The sandfly probes with her proboscis to form a venous pool, from which blood is obtained by capillary action. Metacyclic promastigotes obstruct the proboscis, preventing easy aspiration of blood and stimulating the fly to probe even more. Although not well quantified, a relatively small number of promastigotes, a few to several hundred, are thought to be inoculated.[30]

EPIDEMIOLOGY

The World Health Organization (WHO) estimates that 350 million people are at risk of infection by *Leishmania* species worldwide.[31] The incidence of cutaneous disease is estimated to be 1.0–1.5 million cases per year, and the incidence of visceral leishmaniasis 500 000 cases per year. *Leishmania* species are endemic in 82 countries; 21 in the Americas and 61 elsewhere (see ***Table 100.1 and Figs 100.2–100.4***). Although rare, congenital visceral leishmaniasis has been reported.[32] Transmission has also been reported as a result of blood transfusion,[33] direct person-to-person contact,[34] and laboratory accident.[35]

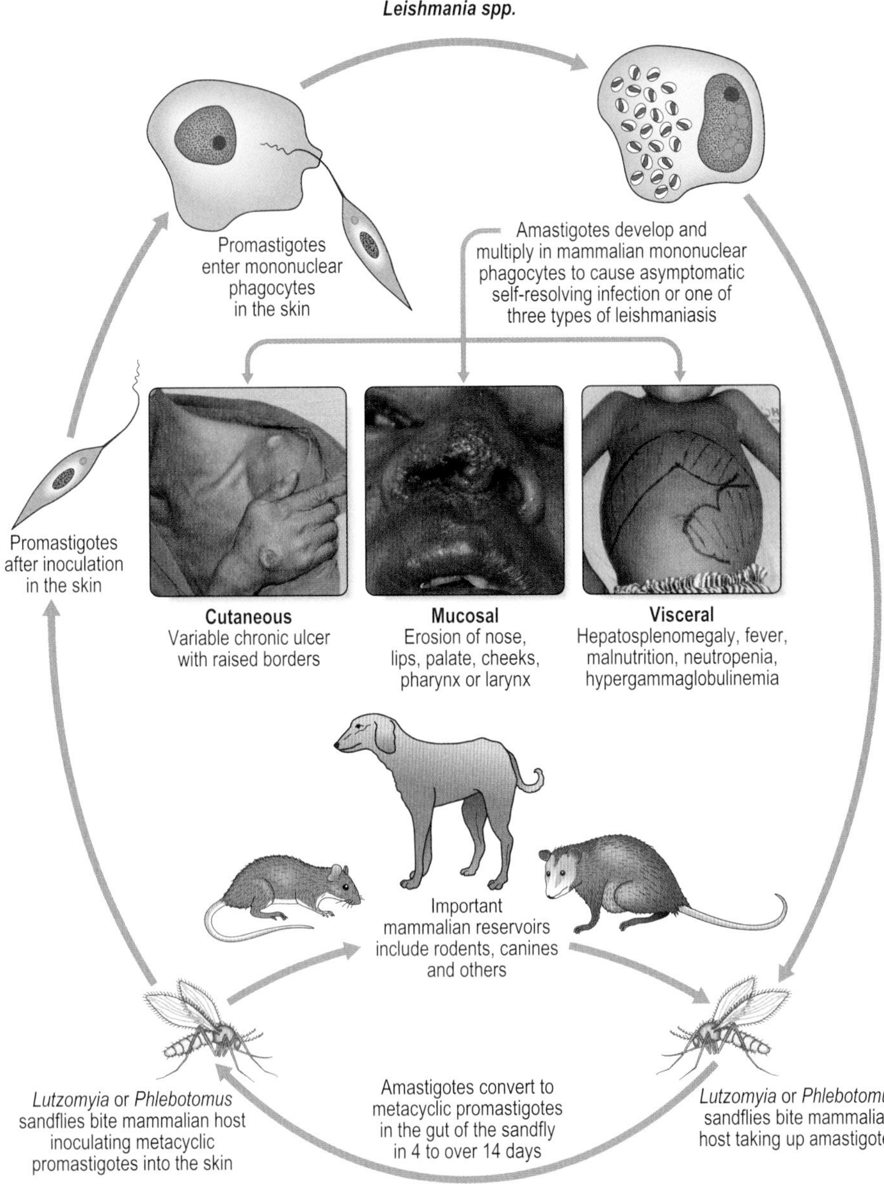
Leishmania spp.
Promastigotes enter mononuclear phagocytes in the skin
Amastigotes develop and multiply in mammalian mononuclear phagocytes to cause asymptomatic self-resolving infection or one of three types of leishmaniasis
Promastigotes after inoculation in the skin
Cutaneous
Variable chronic ulcer with raised borders
Mucosal
Erosion of nose, lips, palate, cheeks, pharynx or larynx
Visceral
Hepatosplenomegaly, fever, malnutrition, neutropenia, hypergammaglobulinemia
Important mammalian reservoirs include rodents, canines and others
Lutzomyia or Phlebotomus sandflies bite mammalian host inoculating metacyclic promastigotes into the skin
Amastigotes convert to metacyclic promastigotes in the gut of the sandfly in 4 to over 14 days
Lutzomyia or Phlebotomus sandflies bite mammalian host taking up amastigotes

Figure 100.1 The life cycle of *Leishmania* spp. with the different clinical forms in humans.

New World Cutaneous and Mucosal Leishmaniasis

Cutaneous leishmaniasis in the Americas is caused by *L. mexicana, L. amazonensis, L. braziliensis, L. panamensis, L. guyanensis, L. peruviana,* and several other species, including *L. infantum chagasi*.[36] For most of the *Leishmania* species in the New World, the reservoirs are forest-dwelling rodents and other mammals. Some have survived agricultural development by adapting to peridomestic habitats.[37] Dogs and other canines are reservoirs for *L. peruviana* and *L. i. chagasi*. The vectors are arboreal or ground-dwelling *Lutzomyia* species.[18] Large outbreaks have occurred among military personnel, road builders, and agricultural workers who enter or clear forested areas.[38] *L. mexicana* is found from Oklahoma and Texas in the north, where a number of autochthonous cases have been reported, to Argentina in the south.[39] *L. braziliensis* is the primary cause of mucosal leishmaniasis in Latin America.[40]

Old World Cutaneous Leishmaniasis

L. major and *L. tropica* are responsible for most of the cases of cutaneous leishmaniasis in the Mediterranean littoral, the Middle East, the Indian subcontinent, and central Asia. *L. aethiopica* is endemic in Ethiopia and adjacent areas of Africa.[41] Cutaneous leishmaniasis has been an important problem for US military personnel serving in Iraq, Afghanistan, and Kuwait.[4] Occasionally, *L. donovani* or *L. infantum* is isolated from cutaneous lesions.[42] *L. donovani* also produces post-kala-azar dermal leishmaniasis (PKDL) in India and Africa, as discussed later.

Visceral Leishmaniasis

The Indian subcontinent accounts for the majority of the world's cases of visceral leishmaniasis. Humans seem to be the only reservoir for *L. donovani* there. Major epidemics have also occurred among refugees in the Sudan as they have moved into endemic zoonotic areas during the civil war.[10,11] *L. infantum* is found in scattered areas extending from France, across the Mediterranean littoral, to the Middle East. Canine species are the major reservoirs. Historically, most cases occurred among children, but in recent decades, visceral leishmaniasis has emerged as an important opportunistic infection among those with AIDS[13,43] and other immunocompromising conditions. Shared intravenous needles have been incriminated in transmission. *L. infantum chagasi* is the principal cause of visceral leishmaniasis in Latin America.[44,45] Genetic data indicate that *L. infantum*

Table 100.1 Clinical Syndromes Caused by *Leishmania* Species and Their Geographic Distribution

Clinical Syndromes	*Leishmania* Species	Location
Visceral Leishmaniasis		
Kala-azar: generalized involvement of the reticuloendothelial system (spleen, bone marrow, liver)	*L. (L.) donovani*	Indian subcontinent, northern and eastern China, Pakistan, Nepal, eastern Africa, Sudan, Kenya
	L. (L.) infantum	Middle East, Mediterranean littoral, Balkans, central and southwestern Asia, northern and northwestern China, northern and sub-Saharan Africa, Latin America
	L. (L.) donovani (archibaldi)	Sudan, Kenya, Ethiopia
	L. (L.) spp.	Kenya, Ethiopia, Somalia
	L. infantum chagasi	Latin America
	L. (L.) amazonensis	Brazil (Bahia state)
	L. (L.) tropica	Israel, India, and viscerotropic disease in Saudi Arabia (US troops)
Post-kala-azar dermal leishmaniasis	*L. (L.) donovani*	Indian subcontinent, East Africa and Sudan
	L. (L.) spp.	Kenya, Ethiopia, Somalia
Old World Cutaneous Leishmaniasis		
Single or limited number of skin lesions	*L. (L.) major*	Middle East, northwestern China, northwestern India, Pakistan, Africa
	L. (L.) tropica	Mediterranean littoral, Middle East, western Asiatic area, Indian subcontinent
	L. (L.) aethiopica	Ethiopian highlands, Kenya, Yemen
	L. (L.) infantum	Mediterranean basin
	L. (L.) donovani (archibaldi)	Sudan and East Africa
	L. (L.) spp.	Kenya, Ethiopia, Somalia
Diffuse cutaneous leishmaniasis	*L. (L.) aethiopica*	Ethiopian highlands, Kenya, Yemen
New World Cutaneous Leishmaniasis		
Single or limited number of skin lesions	*L. (L.) mexicana* (chiclero ulcer)	Central America, Mexico, Texas
	L. (L.) amazonensis	Amazon basin and neighboring areas, Bahia and other states in Brazil
	L. (V.) braziliensis	Multiple areas of Central and South America
	L. (V.) guyanensis (forest yaws)	Guyana, Suriname, northern Amazon basin
	L. (V.) peruviana (uta)	Peru (western Andes) and Argentinean highlands
	L. (V.) panamensis	Panama, Costa Rica, Colombia
	L. (V.) pifanoi	Venezuela
	L. (V.) garnhami	Venezuela
	L. (V.) venezuelensis	Venezuela
	L. (V.) colombiensis	Colombia and Panama
	L. (L.) infantum chagasi	Central and South America
Diffuse cutaneous leishmaniasis	*L. (L.) amazonensis*	Amazon basin and neighboring areas, Bahia and other states in Brazil
	L. (V.) pifanoi	Venezuela
	L. (L.) mexicana	Mexico and Central America
	L. (L.) spp.	Dominican Republic
American mucocutaneous leishmaniasis	*L. (V.) braziliensis (espundia)*	Multiple areas in Latin America
	L. (V.) panamensis	Panama, Costa Rica, Colombia
	L. (V.) guyanensis	Guyana, Suriname, northern Amazon basin

(*L.*), subgenus *Leishmania*; (*V.*), subgenus *Viannia*.

(Modified from Pearson RD, Sousa AQ: Clinical spectrum of leishmaniasis. Clin Infect Dis. 1996;22:1–13; data from Lainson R, Shaw JJ. Evolution, classification and geographic distribution. In: Peters W, Killick-Kendrick R, eds. The Leishmaniases in Biology and Medicine. London: Academic Press; 1987:1–120.)

and *L. chagasi* are the same species.[46] Sporadic cases occur in rural endemic regions, and during the past 30 years epidemics have developed in the urban fringe of cities in Brazil.[12] Visceral leishmaniasis can develop years after exposure in people who are immunosuppressed.[43,47,48]

Occasionally, *Leishmania* species that are primarily associated with cutaneous leishmaniasis, such as *L. amazonensis* in Latin America[49,50] or *L. tropica*[51] in the Middle East and India, are isolated from patients with visceral leishmaniasis. A small number of troops infected with *L. tropica* during Operation Desert Storm developed a viscerotropic syndrome.[52,53] Of note, a canine epidemic of *L. infantum* has occurred among foxhounds in the United States. It is thought to have originated in dogs infected in southern Europe. Transmission has not involved sandflies, and no human cases have been reported.[54,55]

THE DISEASE

A spectrum of findings is observed within each of the three major clinical syndromes: cutaneous, mucosal, and visceral leishmaniasis. Each of these syndromes is associated with more than one *Leishmania* species, and any given species is capable of producing more than one syndrome. Variations on clinical presentation are common, particularly among people with AIDS or other immunosuppressive condition.

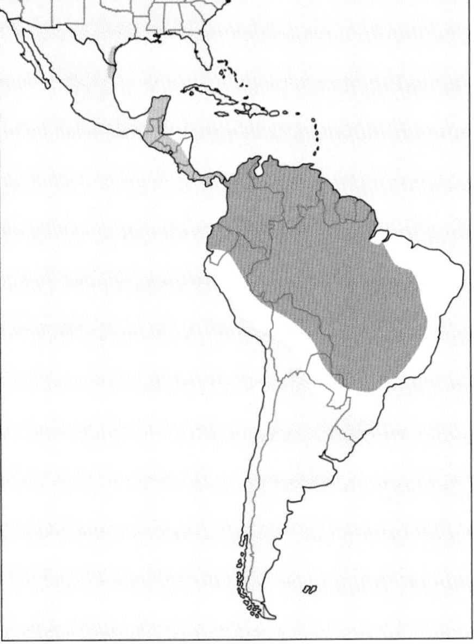

Figure 100.2 The geographical distribution of cutaneous and mucosal leishmaniasis in the New World due to different *Leishmania* spp.

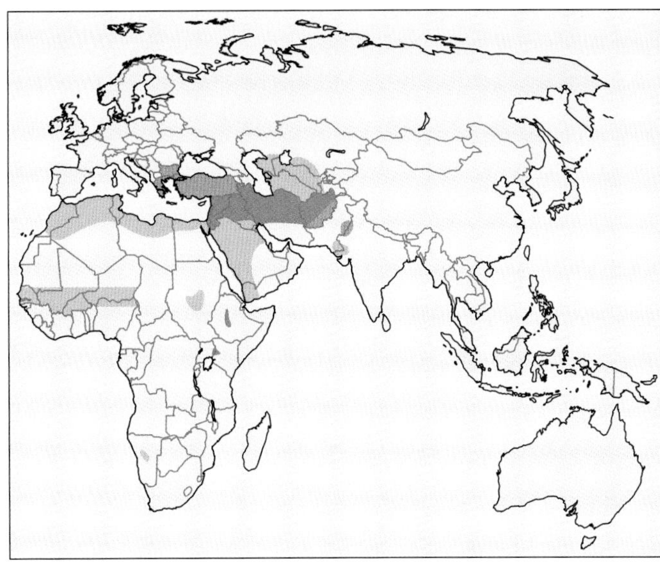

Figure 100.3 The geographical distribution of cutaneous leishmaniasis in the Old World due to different *Leishmania* spp.

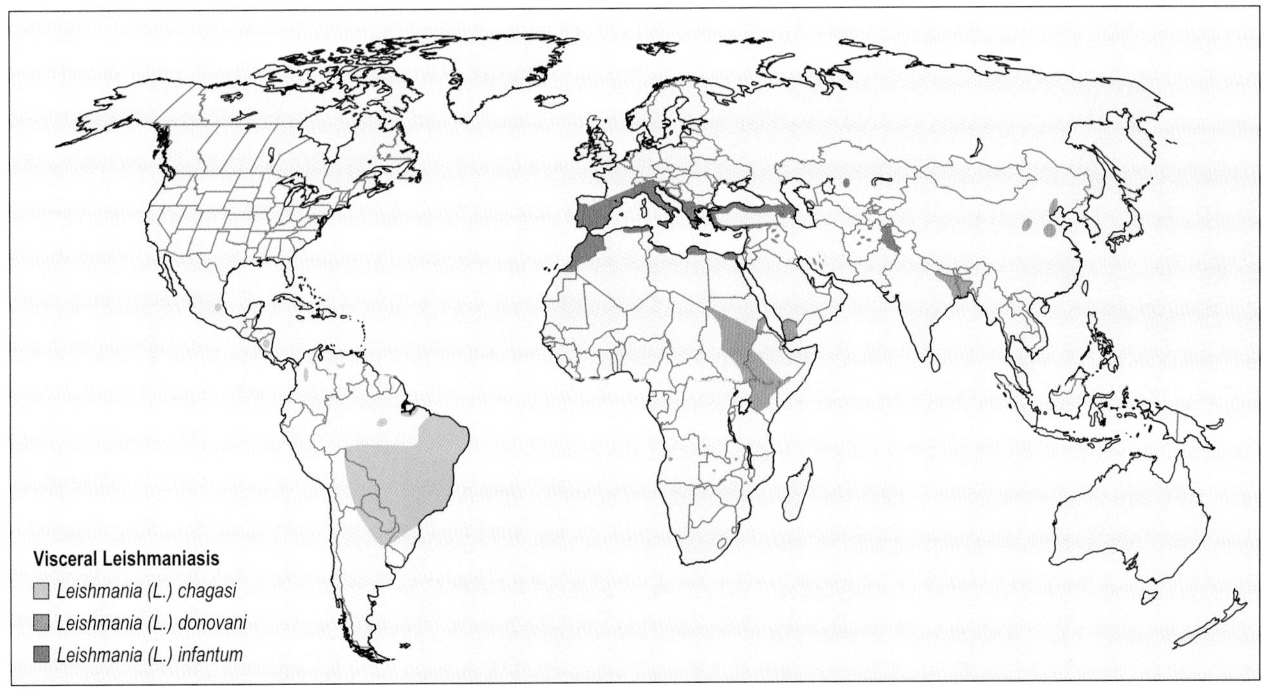

Figure 100.4 The geographical distribution of visceral leishmaniasis due to *Leishmania donovani*, *L. infantum*, and *L. infantum chagasi*.

Cutaneous Leishmaniasis

Depending on the location, Old World cutaneous leishmaniasis is known locally as oriental sore, *bouton d'Orient, bouton de Crète, bouton d'Alep, bouton de Briska*, Aleppo evil, Baghdad boil, and Delhi boil. In Latin America, it is variously known as pian bois (bush yaws), uta, and Chiclero's ulcer.[56] The spectrum includes simple cutaneous leishmaniasis with and without lymphatic involvement, sporotrichoid leishmaniasis, disseminated cutaneous leishmaniasis, diffuse cutaneous leishmaniasis, and post kala-azar dermal leishmaniasis following treatment of visceral leishmaniasis.

Cutaneous leishmaniasis begins at the site where promastigotes are inoculated by an infected sandfly. Single or multiple lesions may be present in the same patient (***Fig. 100.1***). The morphology can be quite variable, even in the same patient with multiple lesions, and it is not possible to make a species-specific diagnosis based on their characteristics.[56] Some lesions are "wet" or "pizza-like," with a raised outer border, granulating base, and overlying white, purulent exudates. This type of lesion is often observed with *L. major* or *L. braziliensis* (Fig. 100.1). Other lesions are "dry" and tend to be smaller and covered with a crust. This is typical of *L. tropica* in the Middle East or India. In some instances leishmanial lesions are papular, acneiform, nodular, or volcano-like with minimal or no ulceration. Cutaneous lesions may be associated with itching, burning, or discomfort, but they are typically not as painful as might be expected given the degree of tissue damage. They may persist for months, and in some cases years, before they heal, leaving flat, atrophic scars as evidence of disease. Once a lesion has resolved, the person is usually left with immunity against the infecting *Leishmania* species.[56] In the case of leishmaniasis recidiva, which is associated with *L. tropica*, skin lesions on the face or extremities enlarge slowly while healing in the center. They can persist or recur over decades. Contiguous mucosal involvement is observed in some patients.

A subset of people infected with *L. braziliensis* develops regional adenopathy, fever, and constitutional symptoms before the skin lesion appears, as seen in ***Figure 100.5***. The constitutional symptoms and adenopathy then resolve as the skin lesion enlarges. In other patients there is involvement of local lymphatic in a sporotrichoid pattern.[57,58] Old World cutaneous leishmaniasis is much less commonly associated with sporotrichoid presentations, but cases have been reported from the Middle East.[59] Necrotizing lymphadenitis has also been reported with *L. major* infection.[60]

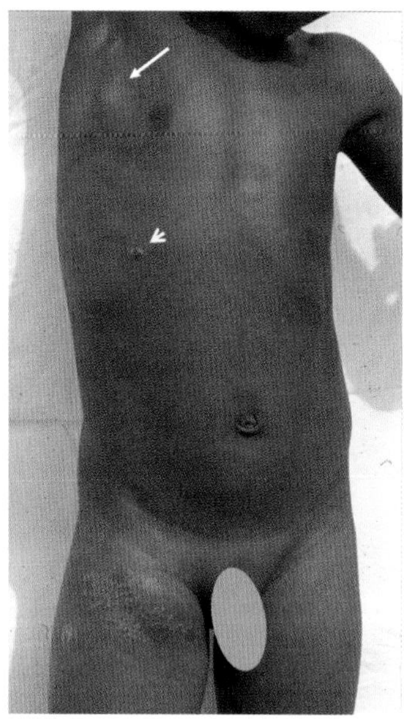

Figure 100.5 Cutaneous leishmaniasis evolving with lymphadenopathy.

Rarely, *L. amazonensis* or *L. braziliensis* disseminates widely in the skin, producing large numbers of cutaneous lesions, often in association with mucosal disease. This syndrome has been termed disseminated cutaneous leishmaniasis. The lesions tend to be small and papular or acneiform. This can occur in persons with no demonstrable immune defect or in those with AIDS.[6,61] Cutaneous dissemination of *L. major* has also been associated with AIDS.[62]

Diffuse cutaneous leishmaniasis is an uncommon, anergic variant of cutaneous leishmaniasis that is associated with *L. aethiopica* infections in Africa,[63] *L. mexicana* or *L. amazonensis* infections in Central and South America,[64,65] and a separate *Leishmania* species in the Dominican Republic. It begins with a localized lesion that does not ulcerate. Amastigotes progressively disseminate to macrophages in other areas of skin, forming cutaneous nodules or plaques.

Cutaneous leishmaniasis should be considered in the differential diagnosis of subacute or chronic skin lesions in people who have lived, worked, or traveled in endemic areas. The differential diagnosis includes cutaneous fungal infections, such as paracoccidioidomycosis, histoplasmosis, sporotrichosis, chromomycosis, lobomycosis; lupus vulgaris,[66] *Mycobacterium tuberculosis*, *M. ulcerans*, and other atypical mycobacterial infections; yaws, syphilis, and leprosy; cutaneous neoplasms; and cutaneous sarcoidosis.[67,68]

Mucosal Leishmaniasis (Espundia)

A small percentage of people infected with *L. braziliensis* and occasionally with related *Leishmania* species develop mucosal lesions in the nose, mouth, pharynx, or larynx months to years after resolution of the primary skin lesion (***Fig. 100.1***). The condition is known in Latin America as espundia.[5,40,69] Patients with active cutaneous leishmaniasis may present with mucosal involvement, but more often mucosal symptoms begin months to years after cutaneous lesions resolve. There seems to be some geographic variation in the clinical presentation associated with *L. braziliensis* strains.[70] Mucosal leishmaniasis often begins with nasal stuffiness and inflammation. Ulceration of the nasal mucosa and septum follows. Of importance is the need to assess closely the extent of damage even if the subject does not show signs of external nasal destruction, as can be appreciated in comparing the physical findings in ***Figure 100.6A*** with those from computed tomography of the head in ***Figure 100.6B***. The lips, cheeks, soft palate, pharynx, and larynx may eventually be involved, resulting in substantial disfigurement and, rarely, aspiration pneumonia

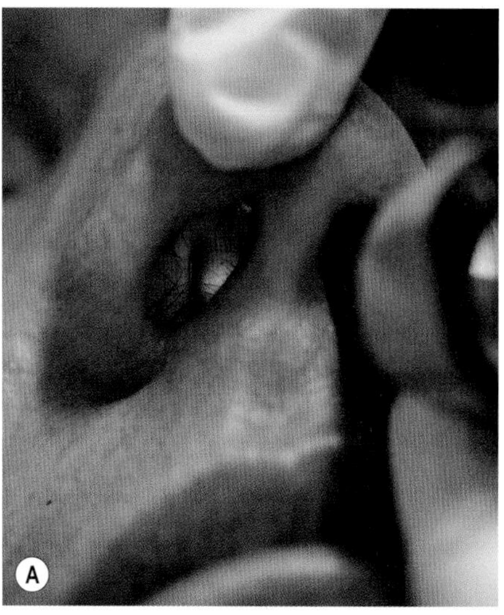

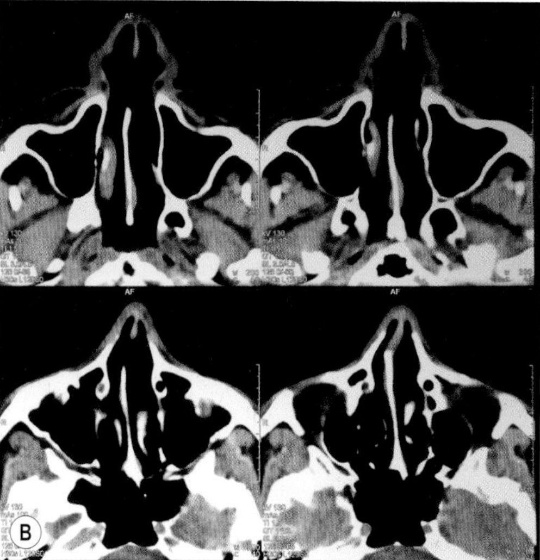

Figure 100.6 Characteristics of mucosal leishmaniasis. **(A)** Perforation of the nasal septum without apparent skin involvement. **(B)** Computed tomography scan indicating the extent of nasal involvement.

and death. Eustachian tube blockage with secondary middle-ear infection has been reported.[71] Involvement of the genitalia occurs on rare occasions.[72,73] Mucosal involvement can be observed with other *Leishmania (Viannia)* species. Therapeutic failures and relapses are common in those treated for mucosal leishmaniasis.

Destructive involvement of the nose and mouth has been reported with *L. tropica* in Saudi Arabia, although the pathophysiology may be different.[74] Mucosal involvement of the upper respiratory tract, larynx, or oral pharynx has been observed in patients with visceral leishmaniasis in the Sudan[75] before and, in some cases, following treatment. In southern Europe, mucosal involvement has been reported rarely in apparently immunocompetent people,[76] but more frequently in those who are immunosuppressed with neoplasms[77] or AIDS.[78] The differential diagnosis of mucosal leishmaniasis includes paracoccidioidomycosis, histoplasmosis, syphilis, tertiary yaws, rhinosporidiosis, leprosy, sarcoidosis, intranasal cocaine abuse, basal cell carcinoma, extranodal NK/T-cell lymphoma, nasal type (midline granuloma), and other neoplasms.

Visceral Leishmaniasis

The outcome of *L. donovani, L. infantum* and *L. i. chagasi* infections is dependent on host factors that affect susceptibility, including genetically determined cell-mediated immune responses, age,[79] and nutritional status.[80] Parasitic virulence factors and heterogeneity are also important.[81] The majority of individuals present with inapparent, self-resolving infection, as documented by the presence of antileishmanial antibodies or delayed-type hypersensitivity responses to leishmanial antigens.[82] A subset smolder with mild symptoms.[45,83] Only a minority progress to full-blown visceral leishmaniasis, or kala-azar.

The incubation period is typically weeks to several months, but it may be as short as 10 days.[45,84] In some cases, symptoms have first become manifest in people who have become immunocompromised years after moving from endemic areas.[85] The clinical findings are similar with *L. donovani, L. infantum,* and *L. i. chagasi*. The onset is usually insidious, but it can be abrupt, with high fever suggesting malaria or another acute infection. The fever pattern may be intermittent, remittent with twice-daily temperature spikes or, less commonly, continuous. Full-blown, progressive visceral leishmaniasis is associated with fever, hepatosplenomegaly, abdominal enlargement, weakness, loss of appetite, and weight loss (***Fig. 100.1***).[79] Symptoms may be present for some time before patients come to medical attention, particularly in impoverished endemic areas. The spleen is firm, nontender, and over time becomes massively enlarged. There is also hepatomegaly; the liver typically has a sharp edge and smooth consistency. Peripheral adenopathy is observed in patients in the Sudan[10] and Egypt.[86] Some patients in India develop hyperpigmentation, which is the basis for the name kala-azar which means "black fever" in Hindi.

The late stages of disease are characterized by malnutrition, severe wasting, and progressive debilitation, which are probably due to secretion of catabolic cytokines such as tumor necrosis factor-α and interleukin-1 (IL-1).[87] Stunting, decreased height for age in comparison to age- and sex-matched neighborhood controls, is observed in children.[45] Peripheral edema may occur late in the disease. Petechiae, ecchymoses, and gingival bleeding may also be observed. Hepatic function can be affected and frank hepatitis has been reported.[88] Death in persons with visceral leishmaniasis is often associated with a secondary bacterial infection, including pneumonia, septicemia, dysentery, tuberculosis, measles, and others.[89]

Laboratory findings include anemia, neutropenia, thrombocytopenia, eosinopenia, and pronounced hypergammaglobulinemia. The anemia is usually normocytic and normochromic, unless there is concomitant iron deficiency. It appears to be due to a combination of factors, including hemolysis, bone marrow suppression, hemorrhage, hypersplenism, and hemodilution.[90] Leukopenia can be profound with white blood cell counts below 1000/mL.[91] Eosinopenia is the rule.[79] The globulin level can reach 9 or 10 g/dL and is due to polyclonal B-cell activation. Circulating immune complexes and rheumatoid factors are frequently present along with the acute-phase C-reactive protein and acid glycoprotein.[92–94] Elevated liver enzymes and bilirubin are noted in some patients.[50,95] The hemophagocytic syndrome has also been associated with visceral leishmaniasis.[96]

The differential diagnosis of visceral leishmaniasis is broad and includes infectious and noninfectious causes. When patients present with a subacute or chronic course and massive splenomegaly, hepatosplenic schistosomiasis, myeloproliferative diseases, and tropical splenomegaly due to chronic malaria must be considered. Other possibilities include miliary tuberculosis, histoplasmosis, brucellosis, subacute bacterial endocarditis, infectious mononucleosis, or prolonged *Salmonella* bacteremia. Patients with more acute presentations must be differentiated from those with malaria, amebic liver abscess, acute Chagas disease, acute schistosomiasis (Katayama fever), typhoid fever, and other acute bacterial or viral infections. Noninfectious diseases, including lymphoma and leukemia, can present with the same clinical features and should also be considered in the differential diagnosis.

Visceral leishmaniasis in people with concurrent AIDS presents in the typical manner in two-thirds of cases, but atypical presentations are common. Splenomegaly may be absent.[13] Amastigotes can be found in macrophages in virtually any organ, including the lung, pleura,[15,97] or larynx;[98] the mucosa of the mouth, esophagus, stomach, or small intestine;[99] kidney[100] or in skin lesions.[101] Aplastic anemia has been the presenting problem in some cases.[102] Asymptomatic leishmanial infections in patients with human immunodeficiency virus infection have also been documented.[103] In addition, *Leishmania* species that commonly cause cutaneous disease, such as *L. braziliensis*, can disseminate to the viscera in the setting of AIDS.[104]

Viscerotropic leishmaniasis was reported in a small group of US military troops infected with *L. tropica* during Operation Desert Storm.[105] They presented with low-grade fever, malaise, fatigue, and in some instances, diarrhea. Although some had enlarged spleens, none demonstrated massive hepatosplenomegaly, wasting, or the progressive deterioration observed in patients with classic kala-azar. Similar visceralizing infections with *L. tropica* have been reported in civilians living in endemic regions and with *L. amazonensis* in Brazil.

Post-Kala-Azar Dermal Leishmaniasis

A subset of persons with visceral leishmaniasis develops PKDL following treatment, most commonly with pentavalent antimonial drugs. The syndrome is seen in India[106] in 5–10% of patients and in the Sudan[107] in 50%. *L. donovani* is the pathogen in these areas. The lesions range from hyperpigmented macules to frank nodules. They typically appear in India 1 or 2 years after treatment and may persist for as long as 20 years. In the Sudan, they usually are seen at the end of therapy or within 6 months and persist for a few months to 1 year. The differential diagnosis includes leprosy.[108] Persistence of lesions beyond 1 year is associated with high antileishmanial antibody titers and a negative leishmanial skin test response.[109] The skin lesions contain amastigotes and are thought to be the reservoir of infection during interepidemic periods in India.[106] In a few instances, visceral leishmaniasis has recurred in patients with PKDL. While the immunopathology is uncertain, the skin lesions may be a consequence of an immune reconstitution inflammatory response to viable amastigotes in the skin. Antileishmanial treatment is indicated for PKDL.

IMMUNOLOGY

The outcome of leishmanial infections is dependent on a series of complex and still only partially understood interactions involving the virulence factors of the parasites, salivary proteins from the sandfly,[110] and genetically determined cell-mediated immune responses of the mammalian hosts.[111] Mosmann and colleagues introduced the paradigm of Th1/Th2 cell-mediated immune responses, which was quickly applied to murine models of leishmaniasis.[112] Th1 cells and the production of interferon-γ (IFN-γ) were found to be associated with protective immunity. Th2 cells and IL-4 appeared to be counterregulatory in infected mice. However, subsequent studies and the characterization of $CD4^+$ T-regulatory cells and effector CD4+ helper cells (Th17) have made it clear that Th2 cells and their cytokines are not necessarily responsible for counterregulation of Th1 responses in leishmaniasis.[113] It is now known that CD4+ cells are characterized by distinctive expression of cell surface receptors and characteristic transcription factors, signaling molecules, that in conjunction determine their phenotype. Abnormal activation of these cells may explain some of the features observed in leishmanial infections.[114–116]

Early insights into the immunology of human leishmaniasis came from studies of the epidemiology and natural history of *L. donovani, L. infantum*, and *L. i. chagasi*.[44,45,117] Observations in Africa, Italy, and Brazil, respectively, indicated that the majority of infections were asymptomatic or mildly symptomatic and self-resolving. Only a minority progressed to classical visceral leishmaniasis. Differences in the ratio of infection to disease varied with age and sex. The incidence of symptomatic diseasae in Brazil is comparable in males and females below age 10 years, but higher in males thereafter.[82,118] After spontaneous resolution of infection or successful treatment, protective immunity develops and is long-lasting. Immunity correlates with the development of *Leishmania*-specific CD4 T-cell responses and the production of IFN-γ in response to parasite antigens. Antibodies are produced in response to *Leishmania*, but they are nonprotective.[119]

The importance of host genetics in the outcome of *Leishmania* infection came with the observation that genetic variability at *Slc11A1* (formerly *Nramp/Lsh/Ity/BCG*) determined resistance to infection with *L. donovani* in mice.[120] A role for *Slc11A1* in human leishmaniasis was subsequently demonstrated in a population from the Sudan,[121,122] and more recently in a Brazilian population with cutaneous leishmaniasis caused by *L. braziliensis*.[123] New strategies such as genome-wide screens and association studies with appropriately powered samples should shed further light on this and other genetic determinants of human leishmaniasis.[124]

The status of the host's immune system is also very important. Visceral leishmaniasis has emerged as an important opportunistic pathogen in persons with AIDS and other immunocompromising conditions with impaired T-cell responses. Relapses after treatment are common in persons with AIDS. Other factors that adversely affect the immune system may also be important. Malnutrition is known to suppress cell-mediated immune responses and has been associated with progression to symptomatic visceral leishmaniasis in some,[80,91] but not all, studies.[45] The potential role of micronutrient deficiencies has yet to be fully assessed.

The role of sandfly salivary antigens in modulating host immune responses to *Leishmania* has also been investigated. Initial studies indicated that sandfly saliva enhanced the infectivity of promastigotes by decreasing the ability of macrophages to present leishmanial antigens to parasite-specific T cells.[125] However, more recent observations indicate a potential role for sandfly salivary gland proteins in protection against *Leishmania* by inducing increased expression of IFN-γ and IL-12.[110,126]

Leishmania–Macrophage Interactions

The initial site of *Leishmania* infection is in the skin where a few to several hundred metacyclic promastigotes are inoculated by an infected sandfly.[127] The primary focus of infection is the macrophage, although the parasite can survive within other cells in mammals, including neutrophils.[128,129] Promastigotes are covered by a glycocalyx layer. The components include lipophosphoglycan (LPG) and the glycoinositol phospholipids to which they anchor.[130] Metacyclic promastigotes can evade complement killing and bind to several macrophage receptors.[131,132] After internalization, promastigotes differentiate into amastigotes in the phagosome. *Leishmania* seem to retard phagosome–endosome fusion via inhibitory molecules like LPG,[133,134] and then they have the ability to inhibit hydrolytic enzymes present in the phagolysosome.[135]

Initial recognition of *Leishmania* and other intracellular pathogens seems to be dependent on cell-surface Toll-like receptors (TLRs). TLRs are one of the early lines of defense against microbial invaders. They are present on macrophages, dendritic cells, and natural killer (NK) cells as well as T and B lymphocytes. TLRs play a crucial role in defending against pathogenic microbial infections through the induction of inflammatory cytokines and type I interferons.[136] For instance, TLR-4 is thought to be important in defense against *Leishmania* through upregulation of nitric oxide production by macrophages.[137] Mice that lack TLR-4 cannot control *L. major* infection. Evolving evidence suggests that activation of TLR-4 is also associated with expansion of IFN-γ producing NK cells and the production of IL-12 by dendritic cells.[138,139] The downstream mechanism of TLR activation is dependent on MyD88 binding, which is involved in transcription of cytokines like IL-1α[140] that contribute to resistance against infection.[141] However, a mixed role for TLR has also been suggested, with signaling through MyD88 hypothesized to result in parasite killing, with signaling independent of MyD88 resulting in a milder inflammatory response and decreased macrophage activation.[142] Of note, MyD88-independent TLR signaling also results in chemokine secretion that may further affect the evolving immune response.

Cytokines produced by macrophages also appear to be important early in infection. IL-12 plays a key role in promoting the development of protective Th1 responses.[143] IL-12 stimulates NK cells,[144] and they in turn produce IFN-γ. In the murine model, CD8+ cytotoxic cells may also contribute to protection by secreting IFN-γ. On the other side of the balance are IL-10 and transforming growth factor-β (TGF-β),[145] which are also produced by macrophages. They can inhibit the development of Th1 cells and stimulate the proliferation of *Leishmania*-specific Th2 cells. Ultimately, cross-talk between innate and adaptive pathways contributes to a successful immune outcome,[146] with IFN-γ activating macrophages to kill intracellular amastigotes through production of nitric oxide[147,148] and reactive oxygen intermediates.[149]

Finally, intracellular *Leishmania* may alter macrophage and immune function in other ways that favor their survival. These include repression of macrophage signaling pathways through activation of tyrosine phosphatases,[150] inhibition of IFN-γ-induced microbicidal pathways, inactivation of transcription factors such as STAT1α, and modulation of NF-κB pathways. *Leishmania* can induce production of suppressive cytokines such as TGF-β and IL-10 by macrophages.[151] *Leishmania* also decrease expression of major histocompatibility complex (MHC) class I and class II molecules on macrophages[152] and increase macrophage secretion of potentially immunosuppressive prostaglandins and leukotrienes.[153]

Cellular and Cytokine Responses in Leishmaniasis

Studies of humans infected with *L. donovani* or *L. i. chagasi* indicate that resolution of infection and protection against reinfection are associated with expansion of *Leishmania*-specific Th1 cells that secrete IFN-γ in response to leishmanial antigens.[154] In humans with progressive visceral leishmaniasis, IL-10 and TGF-β seem to be the dominant cytokines. Messenger RNA (mRNA) for IL-10 has been documented in the bone marrow of people with progressive visceral leishmaniasis, and elevated levels of IL-10 have been found in their serum and in response to cell stimulation.[155]

A discussion of the immunology of leishmaniasis is not complete without a review of the clinical and histopathologic findings observed in cutaneous and mucosal leishmaniasis. Both Th1 and Th2 cells are found in these lesions, but the systemic response is predominantly Th1. Peripheral blood mononuclear cells from patients with cutaneous or mucosal lesions proliferate and produce IFN-γ in response to leishmanial antigens *in vitro*. Those infected exhibit delayed-type cutaneous hypersensitivity responses, as evidenced by positive leishmanin skin tests *in vivo*. Complex chemokine and cytokine responses govern the tissue localization of effector cells and the resulting immune responses.[156]

In some respects, the spectrum of cutaneous leishmaniasis is similar to that of leprosy. In diffuse cutaneous leishmaniasis, disease-enhancing factors seem to dominate, and lesions persist. They are characterized by macrophage predominance and large numbers of amastigotes, analogous to lepromatous leprosy. Patients have negative leishmanin skin tests and their peripheral blood mononuclear cells do not proliferate or produce IFN-γ in response to leishmanial antigens.[157] An increased number of Treg cells has been shown to be associated with the hyporesponsiveness observed in human diffuse cutaneous leishmaniasis.[114] On the other end of the spectrum, persons with destructive mucosal leishmaniasis due to *L. braziliensis* exhibit vigorous delayed-type hypersensitivity responses *in vitro* and *in vivo* and are somewhat analogous to those with tuberculoid leprosy.[158]

In simple cutaneous leishmaniasis, lesions slowly progress from macrophage predominance with relatively large numbers of intracellular amastigotes early in infection to lymphocyte predominance with sparse parasites and granuloma formation later.[105,106] Treg cells isolated from subjects with *L. guyanensis* infection were found to accumulate preferentially in lesions during the early phase of infection. Those Treg cells had suppressive function *in vitro* inhibiting IFN-γ produced by $CD4^+$ CD25−T cells.[159] In addition, active lesions due to *L. braziliensis* have been shown to be associated with a polarized Th2, or a mixed Th1/Th2, response and elevated IL-10 production. Blood monocytes and $CD4^+$ $CD25^+$ T lymphocytes, mostly $Foxp3^+$, were the principal sources of IL-10.[160] In a different study, high levels of IL-17 were found in subjects with cutaneous or mucosal leishmaniasis due to *L. braziliensis*.[161]

Finally, IL-10 has been hypothesized to be involved in the pathogenesis of PKDL caused by *L. donovani*. It was found to be expressed in keratinocytes and sweat glands of patients at the time of the initial diagnosis of visceral leishmaniasis and who went on to develop PKDL.[162] A defect in Treg cells has been suggested based on the finding that there is anergy of circulating lymphocytes and elevation of lesional expression of Foxp3, suggesting their recruitment into the site.[163,164]

The observations from human studies and data from animal models illustrate the complexity of the immune responses elicited by *Leishmania* species and the difficulty of generalizing from one species to another and from animal models to humans. Nonetheless, much has been learned, and new tools resulting from the sequencing of the human and *Leishmania* genomes will certainly help in resolving these complex immunological interactions.

DIAGNOSIS

The diagnosis of leishmaniasis is suggested by the clinical syndrome. Where laboratory facilities allow, parasites can be identified in tissue or isolated in culture. The low titers of antibodies in people with cutaneous leishmaniasis and the presence of cross-reacting "natural" antibodies in the sera of those who have never been exposed to *Leishmania* species make current serological tests useless for cutaneous leishmaniasis. Serological assays are helpful in diagnosing visceral leishmaniasis. The only field-applicable tests now available are based on the identification of antibodies to rk39, a recombinant leishmanial antigen.[165] PCR/DNA based assays are rapidly assuming an important role in the diagnosis of leishmaniasis. However, commercial FDA-approved kits are still not available.

Parasite Identification

The diagnosis of leishmaniasis is often made by identifying amastigotes in a Wright–Giemsa-stained impression smear (touch preparation),[166] dermal scraping, skin slit smears, or tissue section, or by isolating the parasite in culture. The latter is usually performed in reference laboratories. Amastigotes are typically seen in macrophages in tissue sections, but they may appear to be extracellular in touch preparations. They must be differentiated from the fungus, *Histoplasma capsulatum*, which is of similar size but lacks a kinetoplast, and *Toxoplasma gondii*, which typically is smaller.

Leishmania can be grown as promastigotes in a number of culture systems, including Novy, MacNeal, Nicolle (NNN) medium, Schneider's insect medium,[167] and several other tissue culture media to which heat-inactivated fetal calf serum has been added. The cultures are incubated at 24–26°C to approximate sandfly temperatures. In the United States culture media can be obtained from the Centers for Disease Control and Prevention. Promastigotes can be seen in cultures within a few days if the parasite burden is heavy, or they may take several weeks to reach detectable levels if it is light. The growth rate varies among different *Leishmania* species.[168] Speciation is available at WHO reference laboratories using isoenzyme analysis,[169] species-specific monoclonal antibodies,[39] and polymerase chain reaction assays.[170]

In the case of suspected cutaneous leishmaniasis, a biopsy should be obtained from the raised border of the skin lesion after the area is meticulously cleaned with 70% alcohol.[171] The specimen is then divided into pieces for culture, impression smear, and histopathology. Sterile saline without a bacteriostatic agent can be injected into the margin of the lesion, aspirated, and cultured as well. Appropriate cultures and tissue studies should be performed to assess for the possibility of bacteria, mycobacteria, or fungi that are in the differential diagnosis. The sensitivity of blood cultures for cutaneous or mucosal leishmaniasis has not been fully studied. Although it is probably low, cultures have been positive in some cases.[58,172]

In patients with visceral leishmaniasis, fine-needle aspiration of the spleen for culture and touch preparation yields a diagnosis in 96–98% of cases.[173] Although generally safe in the hands of an experienced operator, hemorrhage can occur, particularly in patients who have low platelet counts or prolonged prothrombin time due to liver involvement. Bone marrow aspiration is not as sensitive, but it is diagnostic in more than half of cases and preferred by some physicians. In India, cultures of peripheral blood buffy coat have been positive for *L. donovani* in some persons.

Serology

Antileishmanial antibody titers are typically present in high titer in people with visceral leishmaniasis and at low titer or undetectable in those with cutaneous leishmaniasis. They can be measured by a number of assays. Enzyme-linked immunosorbent assay (ELISA), indirect immunofluorescence tests, and agglutination assays have all been used.[45,165]

The sensitivity and specificity of these tests for visceral leishmaniasis depend on the infecting *Leishmania* species and the leishmanial antigen used in the assay. In general, the highest titers are obtained when the homologous *Leishmania* species is used as the antigen source. The specificity with crude antigen preparations is limited. Cross-reacting antibodies can develop in patients with Chagas disease, African trypanosomiasis, malaria, leprosy, tuberculosis, schistosomiasis, and other diseases.

Recombinant leishmanial antigens have provided comparable sensitivity with greater specificity. Assays using rK39, a recombinant kinesin-like antigen from *L. i. chagasi*, have proven to be both sensitive and specific for the diagnosis of visceral leishmaniasis throughout the world.[165] Antibodies to rK39 are typically not detectable in people with cutaneous leishmaniasis, other infections, or those with self-resolving *L. donovani* or *L. i. chagasi* infections. Both ELISA and immunochromatographic strip tests using rK39 have been reported to have sensitivities greater than 90% and specificities of 98% or higher for the diagnosis of visceral leishmaniasis due to *L. donovani* and *L. i. chagasi*.[174] Antibodies are present at lower titer and not always detectable in people with concurrent visceral leishmaniasis and AIDS, limiting their sensitivity in that setting.

Skin Test

The intradermal leishmanin (Montenegro) skin test becomes positive in the majority of people who have asymptomatic, self-resolving *L. donovani, L infantum* and *L. i. chagasi* infections and in people with cutaneous or mucosal leishmaniasis.[175,176] The skin test is negative in those with progressive visceral leishmaniasis or diffuse cutaneous leishmaniasis. It becomes positive in the majority of people who are successfully treated for visceral leishmaniasis, usually within a few months to a year.[177] The presence of a positive skin test seems to be under genetic control and is a marker for resistance to the development of symptomatic visceral leishmaniasis. The test should not be repeated in less than 6 months because the antigens are immunogenic and capable of inducing a positive response.[178,179] Leishmanin skin test reagents are not approved for use in the United States.

TREATMENT AND PROGNOSIS

Visceral Leishmaniasis

Liposomal amphotericin B is the only drug approved by the US Food and Drug Administration (FDA) for the treatment of visceral leishmaniasis in the United States, and it is generally considered the drug of choice where available.[180,181] Other lipid-associated amphotericin B preparations also appear to be effective, but they have been less extensively studied and are not FDA-approved for this indication.[182] Pentavalent antimony compounds were once the mainstay of therapy, but the development of resistance has limited their use in India and elsewhere.[183] They are still effectively used in Latin America and other areas of the world where *Leishmania* are susceptible. The development of miltefosine, the first orally administered drug for leishmaniasis, has been promising.[184] However, resistance to miltefosine has been documented,[185] and there is concern that it may become widespread in India and other areas where the drug might be available over the counter and may be taken at subtherapeutic doses or inadequate durations.[186,187] Studies are ongoing to assess the efficacy of miltefosine for the treatment of visceral leishmaniasis due to *L. i. chagasi* in Latin America. Relapses are common following treatment with any of these drugs in persons with concurrent AIDS. Recently, combination therapy has been considered, with the goals of decreasing the likelihood of resistance to the few available antileishmanial drugs and possibly decreasing the duration of treatment.[186,188] There is an urgent need for new drug development.[189]

The recommended dosage for liposomal amphotericin B in immunocompetent people with visceral leishmaniasis is 3.0 mg/kg body weight daily on days 1 through 5, 14, and 21. Data from India suggest that a total dose of 15 mg/kg body weight of amphotericin B divided over five injections is 97% effective. The cure rate decreases with shorter courses and lower doses. For immunocompromised people, the recommendation is 4.0 mg/kg body weight on days 1 through 5, 10, 17, 24, 31, and 38. Amphotericin B deoxycholate, 0.5–1.0 mg/kg body weight given either daily or every other day for up to 8 weeks, is effective and less expensive than liposomal amphotericin B, but it is associated with more untoward effects, including more frequent and severe fever, malaise, weight loss, and nephrotoxicity.

Two Sb^v preparations are available: sodium stibogluconate (Pentostam) and meglumine antimonate (Glucantime).[183] Meglumine antimonate is available in Latin America and French-speaking countries, and sodium stibogluconate is available in the United States and elsewhere. Although the bioavailability may vary among lots, these two compounds appear to be comparable when administered on the basis of their Sb^v content. Meglumine antimonate contains approximately 8.5% (85 mg/mL) Sb^v, whereas sodium stibogluconate contains approximately 10% Sb^v (100 mg/mL). The recommended dose is 20 mg Sb^v/kg body weight per day given intravenously or intramuscularly. This dose should not be exceeded. The recommended duration of treatment is 20–28 days.[183] Longer periods of treatment have been used for patients who respond slowly and for the treatment of PKDL.[190]

Although most patients are able to complete a full course of pentavalent antimony therapy, side effects are common and increase with age. They include nausea, vomiting, abdominal pain, anorexia, myalgia, arthralgia, headache, and malaise. Elevated amylase and lipase levels are not infrequent, and clinically apparent pancreatitis can develop.[191] Sb^v causes dose-dependent electrocardiographic changes that include prolonged Q-T intervals and nonspecific ST-T-wave effects that resolve within 2 months after the conclusion of therapy.[192] Sudden death has been observed with doses of Sb^v in excess of 20 mg/kg/day, presumably due to arrhythmias. Renal failure is a rare complication.

Miltefosine was initially developed as an antineoplastic drug. It is a phosphocholine analog and well absorbed after oral administration.[187] It interacts with membrane constituents and affects cell signaling pathways by inhibiting protein kinase C and phospholipase C.[193] Miltefosine, 100 mg daily in adults for 4 weeks, has been reported to cure 97% of people with visceral leishmaniasis in India. A dose of 2.5 mg/kg daily for 4 weeks was 95% effective in children aged 2–11 years. Miltefosine is associated with mild to moderate nausea, vomiting, diarrhea and "motion sickness." Symptoms are more frequent at higher doses. Elevated transaminases, blood urea nitrogen, and creatinine may be observed early in therapy, but typically decrease with continuation of the drug. Miltefosine has potential reproductive toxicity, and it cannot be used during pregnancy. Women taking it must use appropriate contraceptive measures.

A number of other drugs have been used or are under investigation for visceral leishmaniasis. Parenterally administered paromomycin (aminosidine), an aminoglycoside, has been used alone and in combination with other antileishmanial drugs.[194] It appears promising based on studies in India. Pentamidine isethionate 4 mg/kg body weight daily or every other day for 15 doses is a potentially effective, but toxic, alternative.[195] It can cause vascular collapse if infused too rapidly, and it can cause life-threatening hypoglycemia followed by diabetes mellitus due to pancreatic beta-cell injury. The imidazole antifungals also have leishmaniacidal activity. Ketoconazole and itraconazole have been reported to be effective in some cases of visceral leishmaniasis, but failures are also well documented. Recombinant IFN-γ (rIFN-γ) has been used effectively in combination with a pentavalent antimony, but is not curative as monotherapy.[196]

Even with effective antileishmanial chemotherapy, people with visceral leishmaniasis can die of secondary bacterial or viral infections, including sepsis, pneumonia, measles, and others. They should be evaluated and promptly treated for them. Visceral leishmaniasis is often associated with severe malnutrition, which must be addressed. Finally, visceral leishmaniasis may be associated with signs of hypersplenism, but splenectomy is not indicated except in the rare case in which the findings persist following treatment.

There are no rigid criteria of cure in patients treated for visceral leishmaniasis. Improvement in temperature, sense of well-being, and hematological abnormalities, and resolution of hepatosplenomegaly are typically used to assess the response to therapy. The development of a positive leishmanin skin test, which is usually observed within 1 year after successful therapy, correlates with immunity and protection against disease. Treatment does not result in sterile cure, as indicated by clinical relapses, which typically occur within 6 months of the completion of therapy in immunocompetent patients, but can develop years later in persons who subsequently become immunosuppressed.

The treatment of visceral leishmaniasis in persons with AIDS poses special challenges. The initial parasitological cure rates are lower than seen in immunocompetent people, and relapses are common. Secondary prophylaxis with liposomal amphotericin B, pentavalent antimony, or alternative drug(s) seems prudent, but data are lacking to document their efficacy or the optimum regimen. Highly active antiretroviral therapy should be initiated as soon as possible.

Cutaneous Leishmaniasis

The goals of treatment for cutaneous leishmaniasis are to limit tissue damage, and in the case of infection with *L. braziliensis* or related *Leishmania (Viannia)* species, to prevent the later development of mucosal disease. People with cosmetically inconsequential skin lesions can be followed expectantly, provided that the infection is not due to *L. braziliensis* or other *Leishmania (Viannia)* species. Those with involvement of the face, large lesions, diffuse cutaneous leishmaniasis, disseminated cutaneous leishmaniasis, or infected with a *Leishmania (Viannia)* species that can cause mucosal leishmaniasis should be treated.

Pentavalent antimony drugs are often used to treat cutaneous leishmaniasis, but *Leishmania* species vary in their sensitivity. Typically, Sb^v 20 mg/kg/day is given for 20–28 days.[183] Shorter courses and lower doses have been used, but they may predispose to the development of antimony resistance. Even with successful chemotherapy, lesions typically heal slowly over a period of weeks. Cure rates with *L. braziliensis* in residents of Brazil and Colombia have been in the range of 60–70%, but they were greater than 95% in US troops infected with *L. panamensis* in Panama.

In the case of *L. major*, 60% of placebo recipients healed within 20 weeks after seeking medical attention in one study, and 74% of those receiving pentavalent antimony healed within 30 days.

A number of other drugs and approaches have been used for cutaneous leishmaniasis. The imidazole antifungals, ketoconazole, itraconazole, and fluconazole, have been used effectively in some, but not all studies. *Leishmania* species vary in their susceptibility. For example, ketoconazole 400–600 mg/day for 4–8 weeks was reported to be effective in approximately 70% of people with *L. major* and *L. mexicana* infections, but it was less effective against *L. tropica*, *L. aethiopica*, and *L. braziliensis*.[197] Fluconazole (200 mg daily for 6 weeks) was superior to placebo in people with cutaneous leishmaniasis due to *L. major* in Saudi Arabia.[198] At the end of the treatment period, 60% of placebo recipients had healed versus 90% of the fluconazole-treated group. However, the cure rate was similar in placebo control and fluconazole-treated *L. major*-infected travelers in a subsequent series.[199]

Miltefosine holds promise for the treatment of cutaneous leishmaniasis. In a study in Colombia miltefosine,[200] 50–100 mg/day for 21 days, resulted in cure in 66% of recipients; higher doses of 133–150 mg/day cured 94%, but 40% of recipients experienced motion sickness. Vomiting and diarrhea occurred on 2% of treatment days. Further trials of miltefosine are being conducted in Latin America. Allopurinol was reported to be effective in one early study, but its use was subsequently questioned.[201] Other drugs have been reported to have antileishmanial activity based on relatively small studies that were not done in a controlled, blinded manner. Given that spontaneous healing occurs with cutaneous leishmaniasis, it is impossible to formulate recommendations based on them.

Topical and local therapy has been another approach. The application of 15% paromomycin and 12% methylbenzethonium has been used successfully in persons with cutaneous leishmaniasis in Israel and the Middle East and in Latin America.[202] Intralesional injections of antimony have also been used to treat Old World cutaneous leishmaniasis. Typically, 0.5–2.0 mL (100 mg/mL) is injected around all sides of a lesion until it blanches. When 10 such injections were administered on alternate days to Egyptian patients, 85% were cured at 3-month follow-up.

Other approaches, including immunotherapy, local heat, and cryotherapy, have been studied and have their proponents. Cryotherapy has been used for small lesions. Immunotherapy with a combination of *Leishmania* promastigote antigens and live bacille Calmette–Guérin (BCG) has been used effectively in Venezuela and Brazil, but the time to clinical response is relatively long.[203] The combination of pentavalent antimony and granulocyte–macrophage colony-stimulating factor was shown to be effective in treating cases of cutaneous leishmaniasis that were refractory to pentavalent antimony alone.[204] Patients in Guatemala with cutaneous leishmaniasis and those in the Dominican Republic with diffuse cutaneous leishmaniasis have been successfully treated with locally applied heat,[197] although the treatment required close monitoring. In diffuse cutaneous leishmaniasis, an anergic variant that responds poorly to Sb^v, combined therapy with Sb^v and rIFN-γ was reported to be successful.[205]

Mucosal Leishmaniasis

Mucosal leishmaniasis due to *L. braziliensis* is often treated with Sb^v 20 mg/kg for 28 days, but only 60% of patients have clinical responses, and relapses are observed in up to 30% of responders in Brazil.[5,71,206] Amphotericin B has been used as an alternative as well as pentamidine, 2–4 mg/kg once or twice a week until the lesions clear.[180] Both have substantial toxicities. Based on the observation that upregulation of Th-1-type responses is in part responsible for the mucosal damage,[207] treatment of mucosal leishmaniasis has been successfully attained with the combination of pentavalent antimony and pentoxifylline, an inhibitor of tumor necrosis factor-α.[208,209] The combination of Sb^v plus recombinant IFN-γ has been reported to be effective in a limited number of cases. Miltefosine, which is orally administered, seems promising. Administration for 6 weeks increased the cure rate in a study conducted in Bolivia.[210]

Plastic surgery may be necessary for cosmetic purposes in people with mucosal leishmaniasis, but it should be delayed for at least 1 year after clinically successful chemotherapy because skin grafts are likely to be lost if the disease relapses. There is near-universal agreement that well-controlled, long-term studies are needed to assess treatment regimens for cutaneous and mucosal leishmaniasis worldwide in order to improve the quality and standardization of care for these neglected diseases.[211]

PREVENTION AND CONTROL

Leishmaniasis can be prevented by interrupting sandfly transmission. Short-term visitors to endemic areas should use personal protective measures. Sandflies tend to bite from dusk to dawn. The risk of transmission can be decreased by the application of diethylmetatoluamide (DEET)-containing insect repellents to exposed skin and under pants and shirt cuffs, the use of fine-mesh screens or insect nets, and the application of insecticide (usually permethrin or other pyrethroids) to clothing and bednets.[212,213] Improved methods of bonding permethrin to clothing have resulted in long-term protection even after many washings. Unfortunately, while these measures can be used successfully in tourists or military personnel, they are often not practical or affordable for local residents.

Residual insecticide spraying is effective where transmission occurs in the domestic or peridomestic setting, but the use of residual insecticides has been limited by concern for the environment, cost, and potential evolution of resistance among sandflies and other arthropod vectors. It is of historical note that widespread application of residual DDT for malaria control following World War II was credited with a dramatic reduction in the transmission of *L. donovani* in India, Bangladesh, and southern Iran.[214] Epidemics of visceral leishmaniasis subsequently followed the discontinuation of spraying. Residual insecticides have also been used successfully in other locations where transmission is peridomestic. A novel adaptation of this approach has been the use of deltamethrin-impregnated collars for domestic dogs that serve as a reservoir for *L. i. chagasi* in Latin America;[215–217] periodic replacement of the collars is needed and this measure has proven unaffordable for the residents in endemic areas. Obviously, residual insecticides are not useful in rural areas where wild animals serve as reservoirs and arboreal sandflies are responsible for transmission.

Reservoir control programs have also been attempted.[218] In Brazil, where *L. i. chagasi* is endemic and domestic dogs are thought to be a major reservoir, large numbers of seropositive dogs have been killed, but the efficacy of dog eradication has been debated.[45] A major problem has been the delay in identifying infected animals and controlling for their removal. Poisoning rodents and deep plowing have been used in Asia to reduce the reservoir density, with uncertain results. In India and other areas where humans are the reservoir of *L. donovani*, early case identification and treatment of patients with visceral leishmaniasis or PKDL are potentially important elements in control. Finally, humans can be the source of infection, as demonstrated by the transmission of *Leishmania* in donated blood,[219] and the sharing of needles and syringes by intravenous drug users.

While there are still no vaccines to prevent leishmaniasis, clinical experience in humans and studies in animals suggest that vaccines are likely. People who have recovered from leishmaniasis develop high-level immunity against reinfection with the infecting species. In *L. tropica*-endemic areas of the Middle East, mothers have for generations exposed the bottoms of their infants to sandflies to facilitate the development of a lesion at an acceptable site and the development of immunity to protect against disfiguring lesions of the face and extremities. In Russia and Israel, troops were "immunized" with live *L. major* promastigotes injected into the buttocks. This practice was discontinued in Israel because some of the resulting lesions were large and others healed slowly. There was also concern that parasites could persist in the skin even after clinical cure. A vaccine made of killed promastigotes from multiple strains of *Leishmania* was shown to stimulate cellular immune responses in a subset of recipients in Brazil, although its efficacy in preventing cutaneous leishmaniasis was not documented.[220]

One approach in the future would be a defined vaccine composed of recombinant leishmanial antigens and an appropriate adjuvant. Another would be a genetically altered, live vaccine that elicits protective immunity, but carries mutations or gene knockouts that ultimately result in the parasites' death. This concept has been demonstrated in an experimental model of *L. mexicana* infection.[221] The challenge is to find the proper delivery system and antigens that will sustain long-lasting T-cell central memory.[222]

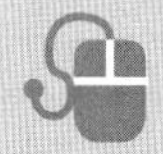

Access the complete reference list online at http://www.expertconsult.com

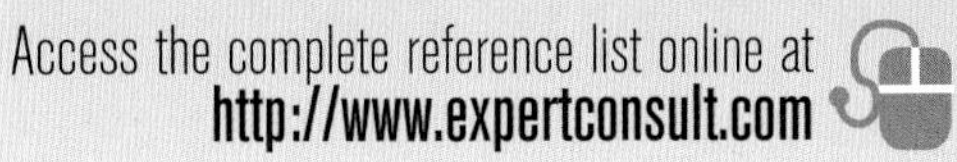
Access the complete reference list online at
http://www.expertconsult.com

CHAPTER 101

Pathogenic and Opportunistic Free-Living Amebae: *Acanthamoeba* spp., *Balamuthia mandrillaris, Naegleria fowleri,* and *Sappinia pedata*

Govinda S. Visvesvara • Sharon L. Roy • James H. Maguire

INTRODUCTION

Infections caused by the pathogenic and opportunistic free-living amebae such as *Acanthamoeba* spp., *Balamuthia mandrillaris*, and *Naegleria fowleri* have been recorded from all parts of the world, including the tropics.[1–39] However, many cases go undetected because of limited resources for diagnosis and low rates of autopsy, the method by which most infections are detected.

THE AGENT

Pathogenic and opportunistic free-living amebae of the genera *Acanthamoeba*, *Balamuthia*, and *Naegleria* are mitochondria-bearing, aerobic, eukaryotic protists. Although they exist as free-living entities in nature, they cause life- and sight-threatening disease in humans and other animals.[1–39] *Acanthamoeba* and *Balamuthia* infecting the central nervous system (CNS) can cause an insidious chronic granulomatous disease known as granulomatous amebic encephalitis (GAE) in both immunocompetent and immunosuppressed persons and animals.[1–21] *N. fowleri* produces a necrotizing, hemorrhagic meningoencephalitis, called primary amebic meningoencephalitis (PAM), principally in healthy immunocompetent hosts who have a history of recent contact with fresh warm water.[1,28,32–39] In 2001 another mitochondria-bearing free-living ameba, *Sappinia*, was identified as causing encephalitis in an otherwise healthy young man.[40,41] Since all these amebae have the ability both to exist as free-living organisms in nature and occasionally invade and parasitize host tissue, they have been called amphizoic or free-living amebae. In contrast to the free-living amebae, *Entamoeba histolytica* is an anaerobic ameba that lacks mitochondria, commonly causes gastrointestinal pathology, and is strictly parasitic.

Acanthamoeba Species

Although the genus *Acanthamoeba* was named by Volkonsky in 1931, Puschkarew in 1913 first isolated the ameba from dust and named it *Amoeba polyphagus*. Page in 1967 redescribed the ameba and renamed it *Acanthamoeba polyphaga*.[42] Sir Aldo Castellani in 1930[32] also isolated an ameba that occurred as a contaminant in a yeast culture plate that was later named *Acanthamoeba castellanii*. In 1958, Culbertson and colleagues demonstrated the pathogenic potential of *Acanthamoeba* when they isolated an ameba, now known as *Acanthamoeba culbertsoni*, contaminating monkey kidney cell culture during production of the poliomyelitis vaccine.[32] It is now well established that several species of *Acanthamoeba* (*A. castellanii*, *A. culbertsoni*, *A. healyi*, *A. polyphaga*, *A. rhysodes*, and *A. lenticulata*) cause GAE, an insidious disease with a protracted course and usually fatal outcome.[1] GAE usually occurs in persons with human immunodeficiency virus (HIV)/acquired immunodeficiency syndrome (AIDS) or who are otherwise immunocompromised, debilitated, or malnourished. In addition to GAE, *Acanthamoeba* can cause a disseminated disease involving skin, sinuses, lungs, and other organs and also a painful, sight-threatening infection of the eye, *Acanthamoeba* keratitis (AK).[1,22–25]

Life Cycle

Acanthamoeba has two stages in its life cycle: a feeding and reproducing trophozoite stage and a resistant cyst stage (***Fig. 101.1***). The trophozoites feed on bacteria present in the environment and multiply by binary fission. A unique and characteristic feature of *Acanthamoeba* is the presence of fine, tapering, thorn-like pseudopodia, called acanthopodia, that emanate from its surface. The trophozoites range in size from 15 to 45 μm and have a single nucleus with a centrally placed, large, densely staining nucleolus. The cytoplasm is finely granular and contains numerous mitochondria, ribosomes, food vacuoles, and a contractile vacuole (***Fig. 101.1A***). Cysts are double-walled and range in size from 10 to 25 μm. The outer cyst wall, the ectocyst, is wrinkled with folds and ripples and contains protein and lipid. The inner cyst wall, the endocyst, contains cellulose and hence is periodic acid–Schiff-positive. It is stellate, polygonal, oval, or spherical. Pores, or ostioles, at the junction of the ectocyst and the endocyst are covered by convex–concave opercula that open at the time of excystation. Cysts also are uninucleated and possess a centrally placed dense nucleolus (***Fig. 101.1B***).[42,43] Cysts can resist desiccation for more than 20 years.[44]

Cultivation

Acanthamoeba spp. can be cultivated easily in the laboratory on nonnutrient agar plates coated with bacteria such as *Escherichia coli* or *Enterobacter aerogenes*. The amebae feed on the bacteria, multiply, and differentiate into cysts when almost all the bacteria have been consumed. *Acanthamoeba* spp. can also be cultured on mammalian cell cultures and in cell-free liquid medium.[45]

Balamuthia mandrillaris

B. mandrillaris, the only known species belonging to the genus *Balamuthia*, causes GAE in both humans and other animals. It was first isolated in 1986 from the brain tissue of a pregnant baboon from the San Diego Wild Animal Park that died of GAE. Initially described as a leptomyxid ameba,[14] it was renamed *Balamuthia mandrillaris* in 1993.[15] GAE due to *B. mandrillaris* has occurred in both immunocompromised and healthy children and adults. *B. mandrillaris* is also known to cause disseminated infections in skin, adrenal gland, kidney, uterus, and possibly respiratory tract similar to that caused by *Acanthamoeba*.[8–21]

Life Cycle

B. mandrillaris, like *Acanthamoeba*, has only two stages in its life cycle (***Fig. 101.2***). The trophozoite is pleomorphic and measures 12–60 μm with a

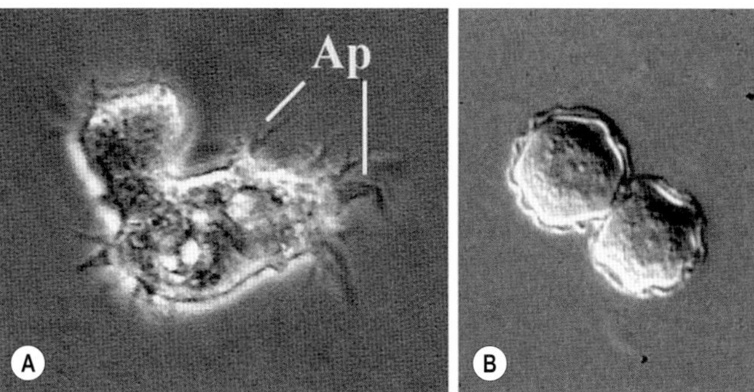

Figure 101.1 *Acanthamoeba castellanii.* **(A)** Trophozoite. **(B)** Cyst. Note acanthopodia (Ap). (Magnification: ×1000.)

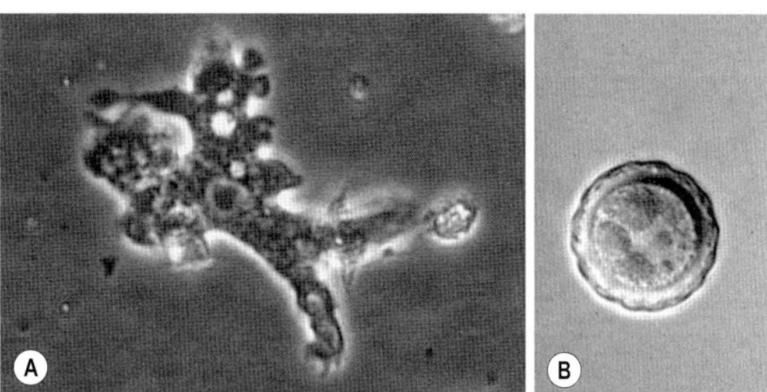

Figure 101.2 *Balamuthia mandrillaris.* **(A)** Trophozoite. **(B)** Cyst. Differential interference contrast. (Magnification: ×1000.)

mean of about 30 μm. The trophozoites usually are uninucleated, but binucleate forms occasionally are seen. The nucleus contains a large, centrally placed, dense nucleolus, and occasionally trophozoites with two or three nucleolar bodies are seen, especially in infected tissues (*Fig. 101.2A*). Cysts are also uninucleated, more or less spherical, and range in size from 12 to 30 μm, with a mean of 15 μm. Under the light microscope, cysts appear to be double-walled, with a wavy outer wall and a round inner wall. Ultrastructurally, however, the cysts possess three walls: an outer thin irregular ectocyst, an inner thick endocyst, and a middle amorphous fibrillar mesocyst (*Fig. 101.2B*).[14,15]

Cultivation

Unlike *Acanthamoeba*, *Balamuthia* cannot be cultured on agar plates coated with bacteria. Although *B. mandrillaris* has recently been isolated from the environment, its food source is not clearly known. It is believed that it feeds on other small amebae that are present in the environment. It can be grown easily in mammalian cell cultures such as monkey kidney (E6) or human lung fibroblasts. It has also been grown axenically in cell-free medium.[45]

Naegleria fowleri

N. fowleri causes PAM, an acute, fulminating, hemorrhagic meningoencephalitis. The infection occurs principally in healthy children and young adults with a history of recent exposure to fresh warm water and is almost always fatal within a week.[1,32–37] Although retrospective examination of brain tissue indicates that PAM due to *N. fowleri* occurred as far back as 1901, it was first described in 1965 in Australia by Fowler and Carter, who attributed the infection to *Acanthamoeba*.[1,32] Butt described the first case of *N. fowleri* infection from the United States in 1966 and coined the term PAM.[32]

Life Cycle

N. fowleri is also called an ameboflagellate, since it has a transitory flagellate stage in addition to an ameboid trophozoite stage and a resistant cyst stage

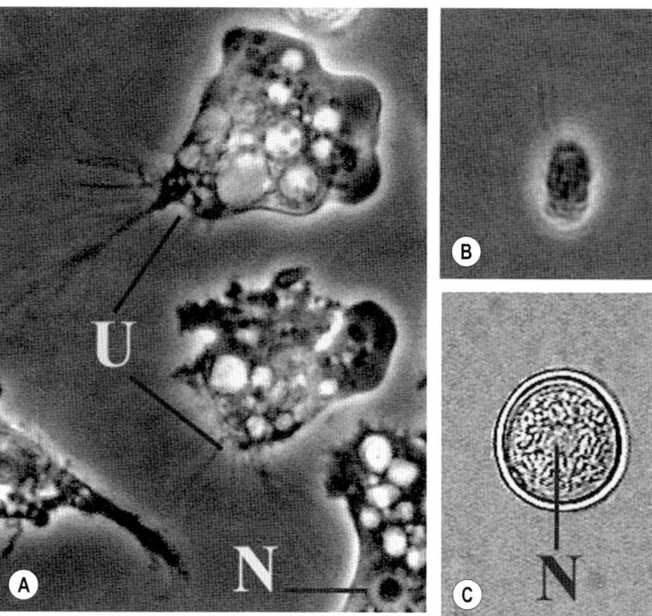

Figure 101.3 *Naegleria fowleri.* **(A)** Trophozoites. **(B)** Flagellate. **(C)** Cyst. N, nucleus; U, uroid with trailing filaments. (Magnification: ×1000.)

in its life cycle (*Fig. 101.3*). The trophozoite moves rapidly by producing hemispherical bulges, called lobopodia, at the anterior end and exhibits active sinusoid locomotion. It measures 10–25 μm, feeds on Gram-negative bacteria, and reproduces by binary fission. It has a single nucleus with a prominent, centrally placed nucleolus that stains densely with chromatic dyes. The cytoplasm is abundant and contains numerous mitochondria, ribosomes, food vacuoles, and a contractile vacuole (*Fig. 101.3A*). The trophozoite transforms into a flagellate stage usually with two flagella when the ionic concentration of the milieu changes. The temporary flagellate stage ranges in length from 10 to 16 μm and reverts back to the trophic stage (*Fig. 101.3B*). The trophozoite transforms into the resistant cyst when the food supply diminishes and environmental conditions become adverse. The cyst, measuring 8–16 μm, is usually spherical and double-walled with a thick endocyst and a closely apposed thinner ectocyst. The cyst wall has pores but might not be noticeable (*Fig. 101.3C*). Both the flagellate and cyst stages possess a single nucleus with a prominent nucleolus.[43]

Cultivation

N. fowleri, like *Acanthamoeba*, grows well on nonnutrient agar plates coated with bacteria, or on monolayers of E6 and human lung fibroblast cells, destroying the monolayers within 2–3 days. Like *Acanthamoeba* and *Balamuthia*, *N. fowleri* can be grown in cell-free axenic medium.[45]

Sappinia pedata

Gelman and colleagues[40] reported the first and only case of amebic encephalitis caused by *Sappinia* in an immunocompetent, previously healthy 38-year-old male. Magnetic resonance imaging (MRI) showed a solitary 2-cm mass in the posterior left temporal lobe. The excised mass on sectioning showed necrotizing hemorrhagic inflammation containing amebic organisms. The patient recovered completely following prolonged antimicrobial and antifungal therapy.[40] Recent molecular sequencing studies carried out on a piece of brain tissue scraped from a slide indicate that the ameba involved belongs to the species *S. pedata* rather than the morphologically similar *S. diploidea,* as initially reported.[40,41] The life cycle of these amebae includes trophic and cyst stages (*Fig. 101.4*). Both trophozoites and cysts are binucleate, with two tightly apposed nuclei. Both *S. diploidea* and *S. pedata* can be cultivated on nonnutrient agar plate coated with bacteria.[40,43,46]

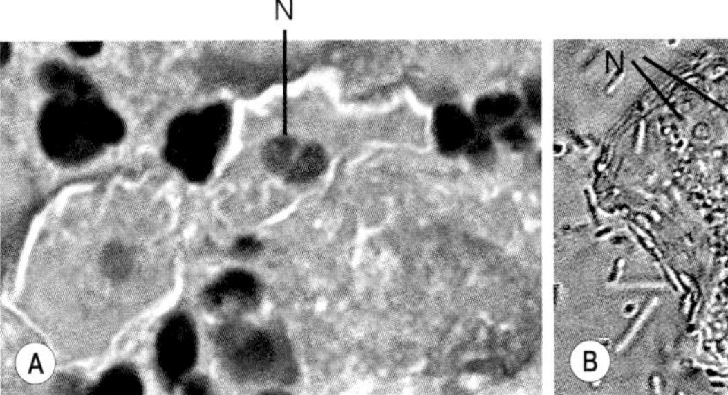

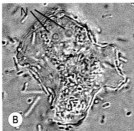

Figure 101.4 **(A)** Central nervous system section of a patient with *Sappinia pedata* infection. Note the two nuclei (N) apposed to one another. (Giemsa stain, ×700.) **(B)** Differential interference contrast image of a trophozoite growing in culture with bacteria. (Magnification: ×1250.)

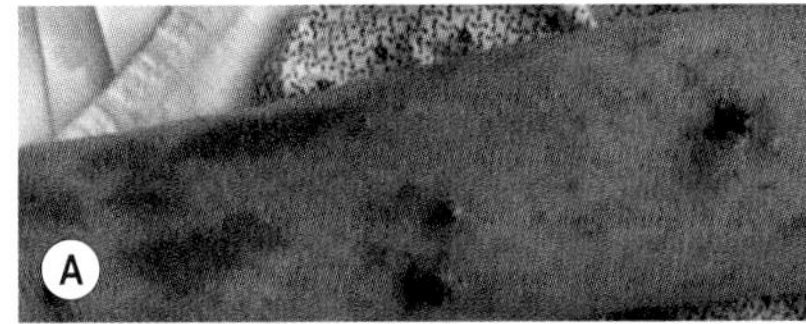

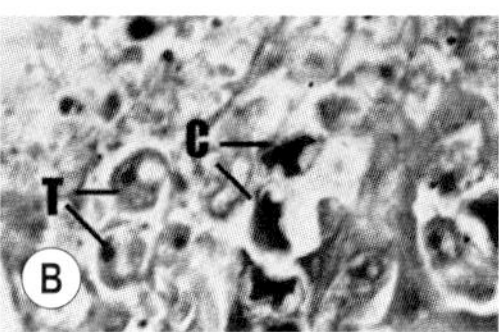

Figure 101.5 **(A)** Patient with human immunodeficiency virus/acquired immunodeficiency syndrome with skin ulcers caused by *Acanthamoeba*. **(B)** A section through the ulcer showing *Acanthamoeba* trophozoites (T) and cysts (C). (Hematoxylin and eosin stain, ×1000.)

Taxonomy and Classification of the Free-Living Pathogenic Amebae

The classical taxonomic classification was based largely on morphologic, ecologic, and physiologic criteria. Thus, *Acanthamoeba* and *Balamuthia*, along with heterogeneous free-living (e.g., *Hartmannella*, *Vahlkampfia*, *Vannella*) and parasitic (e.g., *Entamoeba histolytica*) amebae were classified under phylum Protozoa, subphylum Sarcodina, super class Rhizopodea, class Lobosea, order Amoebida. *Naegleria* was classified under class Heterolobosea, order Schizopyrenida. family Vahlkampfiidae. *Sappinia* was classified under class Lobosea, order Euamoebida, family Thecamoebidae.[43]

EPIDEMIOLOGY

Ecology of Free-Living Amebae

Acanthamoeba is ubiquitous and has a worldwide distribution. It has been isolated from soil; fresh and brackish water; bottled mineral water; cooling towers of electric and nuclear power plants; heating, ventilating and air conditioning units; whirlpool baths; physiotherapy pools; dialysis machines; dust in the air; bacterial, fungal, and mammalian cell cultures; contact lens paraphernalia; and the nose and throat of healthy persons and persons with respiratory complaints.[1,28–30,32,42–45] It has also been isolated from brain, lung, skin, and corneal specimens from infected individuals. Cases of *Acanthamoeba* GAE occur at any time of the year without relation to seasonality.[1] *Acanthamoeba* spp. can harbor pathogenic microorganisms such as *Legionella* spp., *Mycobacteria*, *Francisella tularensis*, *Escherichia coli* 0571, *Burkholderia*, *Parachlamydia*, and mimiviruses and thus might be of greater public health importance than previously believed.[47]

The environmental niche of *B. mandrillaris* was not known until recently, because it had been isolated only from biopsy and autopsy specimens of humans and other animals. *B. mandrillaris* was first isolated in 2003 from the soil of a flowerpot in the household of a person in California who died of GAE;[48] and then from soil[49] and dust in Iran.[50] Cases of *Balamuthia* GAE occur throughout the year.[1]

N. fowleri is widely distributed throughout the world and has been isolated from fresh water; thermal discharges of power plants; heated swimming pools; hot springs; hydrotherapy and remedial pools; aquaria; sewage; and even the nasal passages and throats of healthy individuals.[32,33,43,51,52] Typically, cases of PAM occur in the hot summer months when large numbers of people engage in aquatic activities in lakes, ponds, swimming pools, and other warm, fresh water bodies that might harbor these amebae.[1]

Sappinia spp. have been isolated from soil, fresh water, forest litter, herbivore dung, decaying plant matter, and the rectum of lizards.[40,43,46]

THE DISEASE

Granulomatous Amebic Encephalitis

The clinical manifestations of patients infected with either *Acanthamoeba* spp. or *B. mandrillaris* are similar and will be considered together. The incubation period is unknown, although, in disseminated infections, several weeks or months may elapse between the appearance of cutaneous lesions and the recognition of CNS disease.[11,22,28–32] Peruvian cases of *Balamuthia* GAE show that neurological signs develop 1 month to 2 years (average 5–8 months) after cutaneous manifestations.[11] Neurologic symptoms develop insidiously, and most patients have focal deficits or altered mental status, sometimes with headache, meningismus, nausea, vomiting, lethargy, or low-grade fever. Localizing signs include seizures, hemiparesis, visual disturbances, facial nerve palsy, ataxia, and other cerebellar signs. Over the course of a week to several months, the disease progresses to coma and eventually death from increased intracranial pressure and brain herniation or from secondary infection and multiorgan failure. Initially, MRI shows one or a few lesions, even when computed tomography (CT) scans of the brain are unremarkable. Lesions typically are of low density with peripheral ring enhancement and mass effect.[20,21] Over time, lesions increase in size and number to involve the cerebral hemispheres, cerebellum, brainstem, and thalamus. CT and MRI may indicate hemorrhage within lesions, and angiography may demonstrate occluded blood vessels corresponding to areas of infarction. Examination of cerebrospinal fluid (CSF) shows a predominantly lymphocytic pleocytosis typically with less than 500 cells/mm^3, increased protein, and decreased or normal glucose.[1–3,5–21]

In GAE, there frequently is evidence of infection in the skin, and in cases due to *Acanthamoeba* spp. the lungs or sinuses can be affected as well; any of these sites may be the primary focus of infection that leads to hematogenous dissemination. In the skin, initially minor lesions develop into firm nodules, nonhealing ulcers, and subcutaneous abscesses, mostly on the chest and limbs (***Fig. 101.5***). In the case of infections with *Acanthamoeba*, cutaneous involvement can occur with or without involvement of the CNS.[1,3,6,7] In *Balamuthia* infections, however, cutaneous involvement, especially in Peru, occurs early in the disease. An erythematous plaque of rubbery-to-hard consistency occurs on the face, especially the nose and cheeks, trunk, or the limbs.[11]

Radiographs of the lungs may show focal areas of pneumonitis and consolidation. Chronic sinusitis has been reported in *Acanthamoeba* infections primarily in persons with AIDS, and there have been reports of osteomyelitis, otitis, endophthalmitis, and adrenalitis in immunosuppressed patients with and without AIDS. There are reports of identification of *Acanthamoeba* spp. or *B. mandrillaris* in other organs, such as kidneys, lymph nodes, liver, adrenal, thyroid, prostate, testes, and uterus.

The initial site of infection in GAE, due to either *Acanthamoeba* or *Balamuthia*, probably is the lower respiratory tract, skin, or sinuses, and invasion of the brain and other organs results from hematogenous spread from these sites. Gross pathology shows an edematous brain often with evidence of uncal and tonsillar herniation. Multiple areas of meningeal softening and inflammation overlie necrotic and hemorrhagic lesions in the cortex (***Figs 101.6 and 101.7***), that extend into the white matter in

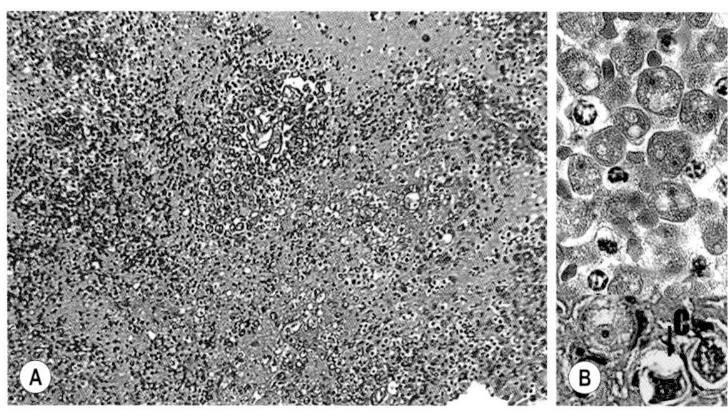

Figure 101.6 Brain section of a patient infected with *Acanthamoeba* (hematoxylin and eosin stain). **(A)** Low-power view (×100) of a central nervous system section showing chronic inflammatory changes. **(B)** Higher magnification (×1000) showing the characteristic nuclear morphology of the trophozoite cysts (C) with double walls.

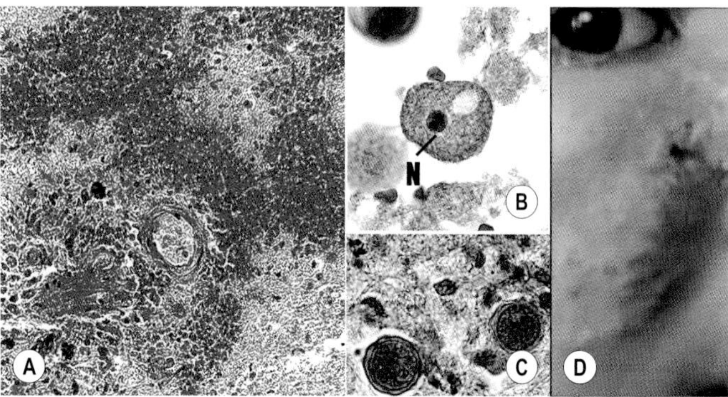

Figure 101.7 Central nervous system section of a patient who died of *Balamuthia mandrillaris* granulomatous amebic encephalitis (hematoxylin and eosin stain). **(A)** Low-power view (×100) depicting intense inflammatory reaction. **(B)** Higher magnification (×1000) of the same section showing a trophozoite with multiple nucleoli (N) and cysts **(C)**. **(D)** Lesion on the skin of a Peruvian case of balamuthiasis. (Courtesy of Drs Bravo and Gottuzo.)

the brainstem, cerebral hemispheres, and cerebellum and have the appearance of hemorrhagic infarctions. Areas of necrosis, hemorrhage, and inflammatory infiltrates consist of neutrophils, mononuclear cells, and multinucleated giant cells. Trophozoites and cysts of *Acanthamoeba* are seen extracellularly or within macrophages, which also contain lipid (***Fig. 101.6B***). In *Balamuthia* infections, the nucleus of the trophozoites may contain two or three nucleoli (***Fig. 101.7B***) which help differentiate *Balamuthia* from *Acanthamoeba*. Blood vessel walls are surrounded and infiltrated with amebae, provoking vasculitis and thrombosis.[1,4,8,12,16,19,32] In some patients, especially those with advanced HIV disease, the inflammatory reaction is sparse and granulomas are not present.

PATHOGENESIS AND IMMUNITY

GAE caused by *Acanthamoeba* spp. typically affects hosts whose metabolic, physiologic, or immunologic integrity is lost, whereas disease due to *Balamuthia* affects both healthy and immunocompromised persons. Predisposing conditions include AIDS, hematologic malignancies, cancer, liver disease, diabetes mellitus, pregnancy, and therapy with corticosteroids and other immunosuppressive drugs following organ transplantation.[1]

GAE etiologic agents enter the skin or reach the respiratory tract through aerosols or dust containing the trophic or cystic stage. Though trophozoites and/or cysts might be temporarily contained at the site of entry by the body's immune system, if the immune system is impaired, the amebae enter the circulation and are carried to the brain and other organs where they proliferate and damage host tissues.[1,28–30,53,54]

Balamuthia, like *Acanthamoeba*, probably invades human tissue by ingesting small pieces of host tissue and producing metalloprotease enzymes. *Balamuthia* induces human brain microvascular endothelial cells to release interleukin-6 and degrades the extracellular matrix to produce CNS pathology.[30,31,54]

Balamuthia GAE has also been reported in a variety of animals including gorillas, baboons, gibbons, monkeys, horses, sheep, and dogs.[1,26,28,31] Severe combined immunodeficient (SCID) mice have been used to study *Balamuthia* GAE.[55] In immunodeficient mice, *B. mandrillaris* adheres to the nasal epithelium, migrates along the olfactory nerves, traverses the cribriform plate of the ethmoid bone, and invades the brain similar to the invasion pathway described for *N. fowleri*.[56] Further, *Balamuthia* amebae migrate to the CNS after oral infection of both immunocompetent and immunodeficient mice; *Balamuthia* antigen but not organisms have been found in mouse fecal pellets.[57]

Acanthamoeba and other small amebae are ubiquitous in nature. Antibodies to *Acanthamoeba* have been found in the sera of healthy soldiers as well as hospitalized patients in Czechoslovakia, adults and children from New Zealand, and patients hospitalized for respiratory disorders.[1,29,30,32,58] Antibodies to *Acanthamoeba* have also been demonstrated in patients who developed GAE.[1,6,7,22,28–30] Schuster et al.[58] demonstrated titers of 1 : 2–1 : 64 in encephalitis patients in California, although no cases of *Acanthamoeba* encephalitis were detected. In another study a survey of antibodies to *Acanthamoeba* revealed that virtually all of the sera tested had antibodies to *Acanthamoeba* and that Hispanics are 14.5% less likely to develop antibodies to *A. polyphaga* than Caucasians.[58] Whether antibody is protective is unclear.

IgG and IgM antibodies to *B. mandrillaris* (with titers from 1 : 64 to 1 : 256) have been demonstrated in sera from healthy individuals as well as in hospitalized patients with encephalitis in South Australia and the United States using immunofluorescence and flow cytometry.[1,9,16,31,58–61] In a group of 290 patients with encephalitis and immunocompetent persons in California, 2% had titers of 1 : 128 for anti-*B. mandrillaris* antibody by immunofluorescence testing and 7 cases were confirmed to be infected with *Balamuthia*, by specific immunostaining of biopsy sections using rabbit anti-*B. mandrillaris* serum.[9,58] Two survivors had acute anti-*B. mandrillaris* titers of 1 : 128 that decreased to 1 : 64 during convalescence.[9,31,60]

In the United States, GAE may be more common among Hispanic Americans. One study, mostly involving California patients, in which serum samples were tested for ameba antibodies, detected 7 patients with antibodies to *B. mandrillaris*; all patients were of Hispanic American ethnicity, even though Hispanics made up only 29% of the study population. This percentage was similar to the percentage of Hispanics in the California population around that time, which was 32%. No patients in this study tested positive for antibodies to *Acanthamoeba* or *Naegleria*.[13,31,58,60] Among 64 confirmed cases of *Balamuthia* infection in the United States reported to the Centers for Disease Control and Prevention (CDC) from 1978 to 2009, ethnicity was known for only 23 patients (36%); 19 (83%) of these patients were Hispanic. Similarly, only 4 of 73 (5%) confirmed cases of *Acanthamoeba* infection in the United States from 1983 through 2007 had known ethnicities; all were Hispanic (CDC unpublished data). Whether these findings are due to surveillance bias, to the innate genetic disposition of Hispanics, or to other factors associated with greater exposure to the pathogens is not evident.[9,13,28,31]

Acanthamoeba Keratitis

AK is a painful, sight-threatening infection of the cornea that may lead to chronic ulceration of the cornea, loss of visual acuity, and eventually blindness and enucleation (***Fig. 101.8***). AK generally affects healthy persons and has been associated with corneal trauma or minor erosion from hard or soft contact lenses and the subsequent use of either contaminated saline solutions or ineffective contact lens disinfection

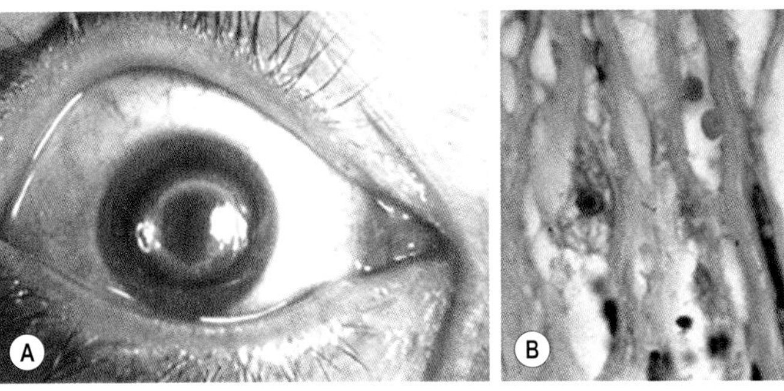

Figure 101.8 *Acanthamoeba* keratitis. Note the concentric ring infiltrate **(A)** and a section of the cornea showing *Acanthamoeba* trophozoite in the corneal stroma **(B)**. (Magnification: ×1000.)

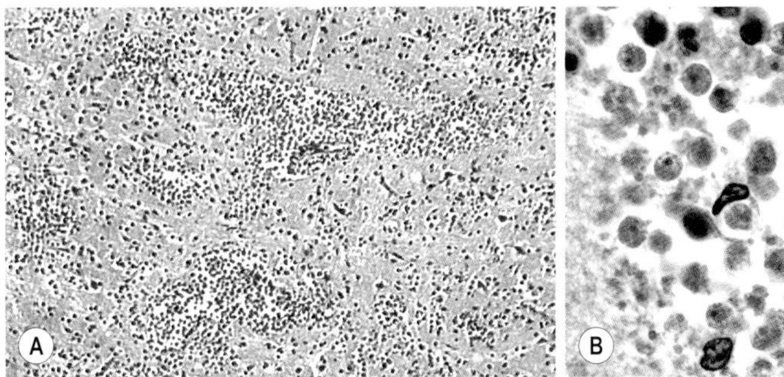

Figure 101.9 **(A)** Central nervous system section of a patient who died of primary amebic meningoencephalitis due to *Naegleria fowleri*. (Hematoxylin and eosin stain, ×100.) **(B)** Higher magnification (×1000) showing numerous amebic trophozoites but no cysts.

solutions. It is characterized by corneal inflammation, severe ocular pain, photophobia, tearing, blurred vision, and refractoriness to the commonly used antibiotic, antifungal, and antiviral agents. Amebae adhere to corneal epithelial cells and secrete proteinases that facilitate invasion of the cornea and the underlying stroma.[1,22–25,28,53] Amebic trophozoites and cysts are seen between the lamellae of the cornea, and inflammatory infiltrates in the superficial and middle layers of the corneal stroma are common (***Fig. 101.8B***). Infiltration of nerves causes radial keratoneuritis, and later a characteristic 360° or paracentral stromal ring infiltrate develops. Anterior uveitis is common. In late stages, AK is characterized by necrosis, ulceration, descemetocele formation, and perforation of the cornea. A nonsuppurative keratitis with recurrent ulceration and a waxing and waning clinical course is a typical history. AK is often misdiagnosed as dendritic keratitis due to herpes simplex virus.[1,24,25]

The first case of AK in the United States was in 1973 in a south Texas rancher following trauma to his right eye.[1,28] Subsequently, the number of cases increased gradually between 1973 and 1984. A case-control study was initiated because of an increase of cases in 1985 and revealed that major risk factors for this increase were the use of contact lenses and homemade saline solution.[22] Because of another increase in AK cases during 2004–2007, a multistate case-control study was conducted in 2007 and revealed that the nationwide increase in the number of cases was associated with the use of Advanced Medical Optics Complete® MoisturePlus™ multipurpose contact lens solution; this finding led to an international recall of this solution by the manufacturer.[24]

Primary Amebic Meningoencephalitis

PAM is an acute, fulminating, rapidly fatal disease that usually affects children and young adults with a history of recent contact with warm fresh water. The time from fresh water contact (e.g., swimming and diving, water skiing, or simply immersing the head in water) to onset of illness is typically 5–7 days. The cause of death usually is increased intracranial pressure with brain herniation leading to cardiopulmonary arrest and pulmonary edema. Early in the illness, patients may experience changes in smell or taste, but usually the first symptoms are sudden onset of bifrontal or bitemporal headaches, high fever, neck stiffness, nausea, and vomiting. Irritability, restlessness, and mental status changes are present at initial presentation, and nuchal rigidity and positive Kernig's and Brudzinski's signs can be demonstrated. Photophobia occurs late in the clinical course followed by neurologic abnormalities including lethargy, seizures, confusion, coma, diplopia, or bizarre behavior. Cranial nerve palsies (third, fourth, and sixth cranial nerves) might indicate brain herniation from brain edema and increased intracranial pressure, often in excess of 600 mmH_2O. Death generally occurs within a week of onset of symptoms. Cardiac rhythm abnormalities and myocardial necrosis are sometimes found.[1,28,32–36]

A CT scan of the head without contrast is often normal or shows cerebral edema with obliteration of the cisterns surrounding the midbrain and the subarachnoid space over the cerebral hemispheres. Marked diffuse enhancement in these regions may be seen after administration of intravenous contrast medium. CSF appears grayish to yellowish-white, tinged red with as few as 250/mm^3 red cells in the early stages. As the disease progresses the red blood cells may increase in number to as high as 24 600/mm^3. CSF white blood cells, predominantly polymorphonuclear leukocytes, vary from 300 to 26 000 mm^3. CSF protein might reach 580 mg/mL or higher, and glucose levels of 10 mg/100 mL or lower are commonly seen.[1,32,37]

On pathology, cerebral hemispheres are usually soft, markedly swollen, edematous, and severely congested, with uncal and tonsillar herniations. The leptomeninges are severely congested, diffusely hyperemic, and opaque, with limited purulent exudate within sulci, at the base of the brain, and around the brainstem and cerebellum. The olfactory bulbs are markedly hemorrhagic and necrotic and are usually surrounded by purulent exudate. The cortex shows numerous superficial hemorrhagic areas, most commonly in the base of the orbitofrontal and temporal lobes, base of the brain, hypothalamus, midbrain, pons, medulla oblongata, and upper portion of the spinal cord.[1,32–37]

Microscopically, the cerebral hemispheres, brainstem, cerebellum, and upper portion of the spinal cord are suffused with fibrinopurulent leptomeningeal exudate containing numerous neutrophils, some lymphocytes, and few eosinophils and macrophages. Pockets of trophozoites without neutrophils are seen within edematous and necrotic neural tissue (***Fig. 101.9***), and are abundant deep in Virchow–Robin spaces, usually around blood vessels, but with no inflammatory response. Trophozoites are characterized by their large nucleus with a centrally located, deeply staining large nucleolus. Amebic cysts are conspicuously absent.[1,32–37]

PATHOGENESIS AND IMMUNITY

The portal of entry into the CNS is the olfactory neuroepithelium. Sustentacular cells lining the olfactory neuroepithelium are believed to phagocytose the amebae that enter the nasal passages of the victims while indulging in aquatic activities. The amebic trophozoites penetrate the cribriform plate of the ethmoid bone, enter the subarachnoid space, and eventually reach the brain parenchyma. *N. fowleri* trophozoites likely possess virulence factors that contribute to the dissolution and necrosis of brain tissue, such as production and secretion of a phospholipase, release of neuraminidase, creation of pores in target cell membranes, and aggressive phagocytic activity. Additionally, amebae possess amebostomes, or food cups, that are capable of pinching off bits and pieces of brain cell cytoplasm.[1,32,33] The incubation period of PAM, which varies from 2 to 15 days, depends on the size of the inoculum and the virulence of the amebae.

Little is known about antibody responses to *N. fowleri* infection, probably because most patients die before serum antibodies become detectable. However, in one patient who survived PAM, an antibody titer of 1:4096 to *N. fowleri* was demonstrated by immunofluorescence in serum samples obtained at 7, 10, and 42 days of hospitalization; antibodies to *N. fowleri* were still present after 4 years.[35] There are reports of antibodies to *N. fowleri* and other *Naegleria* species in serum samples of hospitalized patients in Tennessee as well as in apparently healthy persons.[1,32,33,62] IgG but not IgM antibodies were detected in sera from newborn infants, indicating transplacental transfer.[1,32,33,62] Sera from Pennsylvania residents failed to agglutinate *N. fowleri* and other *Naegleria* spp. when compared with sera obtained from residents of North Carolina, suggesting a higher degree of exposure to *N. fowleri* in persons from the warmer southern region;[62] however, host immunity to *N. fowleri* remains poorly understood.[62]

DIAGNOSIS

Granulomatous Amebic Encephalitis

Neuroimaging

CT and MRI scans of the head demonstrate the presence of single or multiple lesions but are not specific for GAE. The typical enhancing, space-occupying lesions of *Acanthamoeba* or *Balamuthia* infection can mimic a brain abscess, tumor, cerebrovascular accident, and other diseases.[1,2,5,8–10,12,16]

Lumbar puncture is often contraindicated in patients with GAE and large or multiple lesions because of the risk of herniation. When CSF is obtained, analysis usually shows lymphocytic pleocytosis with mild elevation of proteins and normal glucose, but no amebae. Unlike *N. fowleri*, *Acanthamoeba* spp. and *B. mandrillaris* are not readily found in the CSF.

Although in many cases of GAE the diagnosis was made only at autopsy, brain and skin biopsies have yielded *Acanthamoeba* spp. and *B. mandrillaris* in specimens from several patients antemortem.[1,3,5–9,12,16,17] Biopsies in a few patients were lifesaving because they permitted timely administration of specific therapy.[1,3,5–9,12,16,17] In general, *Acanthamoeba* spp. and *B. mandrillaris* are difficult to differentiate in tissue sections by light microscopy because of their similar morphology, although occasionally it may be possible to identify *Balamuthia* based on the presence of multiple nucleoli within the nucleus (***Fig. 101.7B***).[1,8,9,12,14,15] However, they can be differentiated by immunohistochemical analysis of tissue sections using rabbit anti-*Acanthamoeba* or anti-*B. mandrillaris* sera or electron microscopy.[1–4,8,12,14–17] Unlike *Acanthamoeba* spp., *Balamuthia* cannot be easily cultured on nonnutrient agar plates seeded with bacteria. Hence biopsy specimens should be inoculated on layers of mammalian cell cultures.[1,9,14,15] Specimens for culture should be processed as soon as possible.[1,14,15]

Polymerase chain reaction (PCR) has enabled improved taxonomy and understanding of the phylogeny of members of the genus *Acanthamoeba* and in identification of amebae in culture and their genotypes.[1,29,30,63] A PCR probe consisting of a primer pair specific for *Balamuthia* has been developed from sequence data of mitochondrial 16S rRNA genes.[1,31,64–66] Using this specific probe a clinical isolate obtained from the brain of a child was found to be identical to an ameba isolated from flowerpot soil in the home of the child.[65] A real-time multiplex PCR has been developed at CDC for the diagnosis of *Acanthamoeba*, *Balamuthia,* and *Naegleria fowleri* infections.[67]

Acanthamoeba Keratitis

Ocular infections with *Acanthamoeba* can resemble bacterial, fungal, or viral infections, especially those caused by herpes simplex virus. A history of corneal trauma or contact lens use, the characteristic ring infiltrates, and failure of conventional antimicrobial agents should suggest the correct diagnosis.

When microscopic examination or culture of specimens is negative, culturing amebae from contact lenses, lens case, or cleaning solution lends support to a clinical diagnosis of AK. Molecular techniques are employed increasingly in the identification of the amebae in samples of corneal epithelium and tear fluid and in the identification of the genotype of *Acanthamoeba*.[63] Scanning confocal microscopy allows *in vivo* visualization of cysts and trophozoites in the cornea.[68]

Primary Amebic Meningoencephalitis

No distinctive clinical features differentiate PAM from acute bacterial meningitis or meningoencephalitis, although failure of broad-spectrum antibiotics should alert the clinician to the possibility of a nonbacterial cause of the rapidly progressive illness. It is crucial to obtain a history of potential exposure to warm fresh water or hot springs during the past week.

CSF pressure is usually elevated (300 to >600 mmH_2O), and CSF may show a neutrophil-predominant pleocytosis, normal or decreased glucose concentration, and elevated protein content (100–1000 mg/100 mL). A wet mount of the CSF examined immediately may reveal actively moving trophozoites. Smears of CSF should be stained with Giemsa or Wright stain to identify the trophozoite by delineating the nucleus with a centrally placed, large nucleolus. Gram stain is not useful.

CT scans of the head without contrast are unremarkable or show only cerebral edema with PAM. Contrast may show meningeal enhancement of the basilar cisterns and sulci, but these are not specific for amebic infection.[1,20]

Serologic tests usually are of no value in the diagnosis of *N. fowleri* infections, since most patients die too soon in the disease process (within 5–7 days) to mount a detectable immune response.

Molecular techniques such as PCR, nested PCR, and real-time PCR assays have been developed for the specific identification of *N. fowleri* in cultured amebae from patients and the environment as well as *N. fowleri* DNA in the environment.[1,69,70] Sequencing of the 5.8S rRNA gene and the internal transcribed spacers 1 and 2 (ITS1 and ITS2) of *N. fowleri* has shown that the genomic region can be used to identify specific genotypes. Epidemiologic typing of *N. fowleri* has also been done by analyzing the 5.8S rRNA gene and the ITS of clinical isolates.[69,70] For example, *N. fowleri* amebae isolated from two cases who had visited the same hot spring in California at different times belonged to the same genotype (II), and these in turn differed from genotypes of other *N. fowleri* strains examined.[70] A real-time PCR assay provides results in about 5 hours and is currently being used at CDC to identify *N. fowleri, Acanthamoeba* spp., *B. mandrillaris,* and *Sappinia* spp. in CSF or brain tissue.

TREATMENT AND PROGNOSIS

Granulomatous Amebic Encephalitis

Because most cases of GAE have been diagnosed postmortem, or just before, experience with specific treatment is limited, and current recommendations are based on *in vitro* studies of the susceptibility of isolates to different antimicrobial agents and a few cases of successful treatment. Treatment is more likely to succeed with early diagnosis and treatment before the infection disseminates, particularly to the CNS. Several patients with *Acanthamoeba* GAE and *Acanthamoeba* cutaneous infection without CNS involvement have been successfully treated with multidrug regimens consisting of various combinations of pentamidine isethionate, sulfadiazine, 5-flucytosine, fluconazole or itraconazole, trimethoprim–sulfamethoxazole, and topical application of chlorhexidine gluconate for skin ulcers.[1,3,5–7] *In vitro* experiments suggest that azithromycin and miltefosine, a phosphocholine analog, may also be of value in the treatment of *Acanthamoeba* GAE.[71,72] An immunocompromised HIV-negative patient with *Acanthamoeba* GAE and disseminated disease was successfully treated with miltefosine.[7] Cure in a few cases with involvement of the nasal mucosa and paranasal sinuses has included surgical debridement of diseased tissue. Three patients with GAE caused by *B. mandrillaris* also have recovered from the disease following treatment with pentamidine isethionate, sulfadiazine, azithromycin or clarithromycin, fluconazole, and, in two cases, flucytosine as well.[16,17]

Acanthamoeba Keratitis

Unlike GAE, AK often can be cured by prompt aggressive application of topical antimicrobial agents that achieve high tissue levels, and surgery when necessary. In early infections, debridement may remove infectious organisms or improve the penetration of antimicrobial drugs. Medical cure has been achieved with the application of polyhexamethylene biguanide or chlorhexidine gluconate, either alone or in combination, with or without propamidine isethionate (Brolene) or hexamidine. When medical treatment has failed, a combination of debridement and penetrating keratoplasty has been used with good results in some cases.[1,23–25]

Primary Amebic Meningoencephalitis

PAM is almost always fatal. Only a few patients have survived this disease. A well-studied patient, a California girl, who survived the infection was aggressively treated with intravenous and intrathecal amphotericin B, intravenous and intrathecal miconazole, and oral rifampin. At 4 years' follow-up, she was found to be completely healthy and free of neurologic deficits.[35] Miconazole is no longer available in the United States. Another well-documented patient from Mexico also survived PAM.[33]

PREVENTION AND CONTROL

Granulomatous Amebic Encephalitis

Diseases produced by *A. castellanii* spp. and by *B. mandrillaris* have occurred most often in hosts with weakened immune systems, and presently no clearly defined methods are available for the prevention of infection with these amebae.

Acanthamoeba Keratitis

Contact lenses, which are being used not only for vision correction but also for cosmetic purposes, are the major risk factor for AK. During 2004–2007, an outbreak of AK occurred in the United States associated with a particular brand of multipurpose contact lens solution found to have deficient disinfection activity against *Acanthamoeba*.[24] A previous AK outbreak during 1985–86 involving contact lens users implicated contaminated homemade saline solutions.[22,74] Most of the contact lens solutions marketed currently in the United States do not have sufficient disinfection capacity to kill *Acanthamoeba* cysts.[75]

Education of patients regarding the proper care of contact lenses is important in the prevention of AK. Contact lenses should not be used during swimming or while performing water sport activities.

Primary Amebic Meningoencephalitis

As a thermophilic ameba *N. fowleri* proliferates when the ambient temperature exceeds 30°C. Hence global warming might expand the range of *N. fowleri* in the environment.[37] Since *N. fowleri* is susceptible to chlorine at 1 part per million, it can be controlled readily by adequate chlorination of swimming pools. However, unchlorinated lakes and ponds remain a risk. Therefore, people should assume that there is always a slight risk when entering warm fresh water for recreation, such as swimming and waterskiing. Fortunately the risk of infection is very low, with only 33 reported infections in the United States from 1998 to 2007.[75] Only avoidance of water-related activities can prevent *Naegleria* infection. However, one might reduce the risk by limiting exposure to contaminated water through known routes of entry, such as getting water up the nose. These measures include:

- avoiding water-related activities in warm fresh water, hot springs, and thermally polluted water (e.g., water around power plants)
- avoiding water-related activities in fresh water during periods of high water temperature and low water levels
- holding the nose shut or using nose clips during water-related activities in warm fresh water
- avoiding stirring up the sediment during water-related activities in warm, shallow, fresh water.

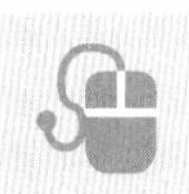

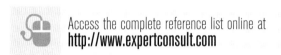

Access the complete reference list online at
http://www.expertconsult.com

CHAPTER 102

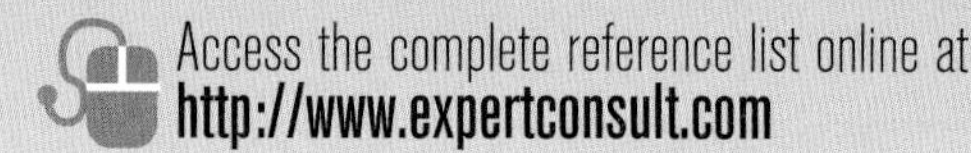
Access the complete reference list online at
http://www.expertconsult.com

Microsporidiosis

Louis M. Weiss • David A. Schwartz

INTRODUCTION

Microsporidia were identified in 1857 as the cause of pebrine, a disease of the economically important silkworm.[1] Microsporidia are worldwide in distribution, with infections reported from all continents except Antarctica (***Fig. 102.1***).[2–10] They are obligate intracellular eukaryotic parasites. Serologic studies of travelers and residents of the tropics suggest that the frequency of infection is higher in tropical countries.[11,12] These organisms are most likely zoonotic and/or waterborne infections. Microsporidia infect nearly every animal phyla including other protists. They are important veterinary and agricultural parasites in insects, fish, birds, laboratory rodents, rabbits, dogs, primates, and many other mammals.[13,14] Some microsporidia have been used as biologic pesticides for the control of destructive insects.[15] Microsporidia were first recognized in mammalian tissue more than 75 years ago[16] and suspected as causing human disease in 1959.[17]

THE AGENTS

The class or order Microsporidia was elevated to the phylum Microspora in 1977,[18] and the phylum was suggested to be renamed Microsporidia in 1998.[19] Although traditionally considered "primitive" protozoa, recent molecular phylogenetic analysis suggests that the Microsporidia are related to the fungi.[20–23] Microsporidia are currently classified on the basis of ultrastructural features, including size and morphology of the spores, number of coils of the polar tube, developmental life cycle, and host–parasite relationship. Excellent overviews describe the history, ultrastructural and structural characteristics, and life cycle differences among taxa of Microsporidia.[18,24–28] Sequence data of rRNA from the Microsporidia have been used to develop diagnostic molecular tests and in the study of phylogenetic relationships.[29]

The genome size of the microsporidia varies from 2.3 to 19.5 Mb,[30] making many Microsporidia among the smallest eukaryotic nuclear genomes so far identified.[31,32] Chromosomal analysis suggest they are diploid.[33] There are almost no introns in the compact 2.9 Mb genome of *Encephalitozoon cuniculi*, the gene density is high, and proteins are shorter than the corresponding genes in *Saccharomyces cervisiae*. There appears to be a high degree of gene conservation among the Microsporidia.[34] A genome sequence survey has been completed for *Enterocytozoon bieneusi*.[35] Genome data on many of the Microsporidia are available at the BioHealthBase Bioinformatics Resource Center (http://www.biohealthbase.org) and on EuPathDB (http://eupathdb.org/eupathdb; and http://microsporidiadb.org).

The phylum Microsporidia contains more than 1100 species distributed in over 150 genera, of which the following have been demonstrated in human disease (***Table 102.1***)[13,28]: *Nosema* (*N. corneum* renamed *Vittaforma corneae*[36] and *N. algerae* initially renamed *Brachiola algerae*[37] and then renamed *Anncaliia algerae*[38]), *Pleistophora*, *Encephalitozoon*, *Enterocytozoon*,[39] *Septata*[40] (reclassified as *Encephalitozoon*[41]), *Trachipleistophora*,[42,43] *Brachiola*[37] (reclassified as *Anncaliia*[38]) and *Microsporidium*.[13] In the immunosuppressed host (e.g., those treated with immunosuppressive drugs or those infected with human immunodeficiency virus (HIV)), microsporidian infection can produce a wide range of clinical diseases. Reports of diarrheal syndromes in patients with acquired immunodeficiency syndrome (AIDS) due to microsporidiosis were first published in 1985.[39] Microsporidia can infect virtually any organ system, and cases of encephalitis, ocular infection, sinusitis, myositis, and disseminated infection are well described.[13,44] These organisms have also been reported in immune-competent individuals. Other intestinal pathogens may occur simultaneously or sequentially with microsporidiosis.[45]

The Microsporidia are eukaryotes containing a nucleus with a nuclear envelope, an intracytoplasmic membrane system, and chromosome separation on mitotic spindles, as well as vesicular Golgi[46] and a mitochondrial "remnant."[47] Microsporidia form characteristic unicellular spores (***Figs 102.2 and 102.3***) that, for the human pathogenic microsporidia, range from 1.0 to 3.0 μm by 1.5 to 4.0 μm in size.[13,48] The spore coat consists of an electron-dense, proteinaceous exospore, an electron-lucent endospore composed of chitin and protein, and an inner membrane or plasmalemma.[49] A defining characteristic of all Microsporidia is an extrusion apparatus consisting of a polar tube that is attached to the inside of the anterior end of the spore by an anchoring disc and coils around the sporoplasm in the spore (***Fig. 102.4***). During germination, the polar tube rapidly everts, forming a hollow tube that brings the sporoplasm into intimate contact with the host cell. The polar tube provides a bridge to deliver the sporoplasm to the host cell. The mechanism by which the polar tube interacts with the host cell membrane is not known, but this may require the participation of the host cell.[50] If a spore is phagocytosed by a host cell, germination will occur and the polar tube can pierce the phagocytic vacuole, delivering the sporoplasm into the host cell cytoplasm. The overall process of germination and formation of the polar tube inoculates the sporoplasm directly into a host cell, functioning essentially like a hypodermic needle.[51,52]

The general features of the microsporidian life cycle are as follows (***Fig. 102.5***):

1. Spores are ingested or inhaled and then germinate, resulting in the extrusion of the polar tube, which injects the sporoplasm into the host cell.
2. Germination is followed by merogony, during which the injected sporoplasm develops into meronts (the proliferative stage) that multiply, depending on the species, by either binary fission or multiple fission with the formation of multinucleate plasmodial forms.
3. Sporogony follows, during which meront cell membranes thicken to form sporonts that, after subsequent division, give rise to sporoblasts that go on to form mature spores without additional

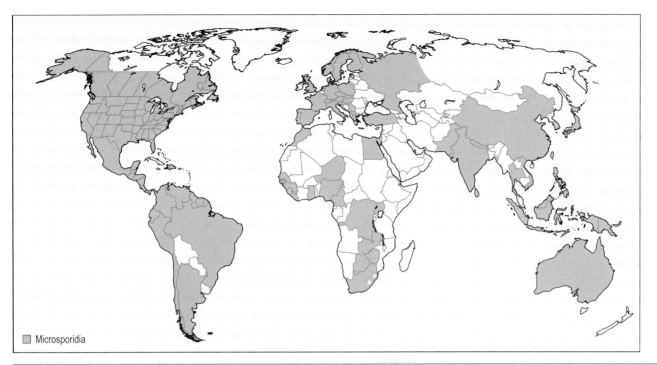

Figure 102.1 The Microsporidia are worldwide in distribution, with infections reported from all continents except Antarctica.

Table 102.1 Microsporidia Identified as Pathogenic to Humans

Genus (Species)	Reported Infections
Encephalitozoon	
Enc. cuniculi	Hepatitis, peritonitis, nephritis, encephalitis,[b] urethritis, cellulitis, prostatitis, sinusitis, keratoconjunctivitis, cystitis, diarrhea,[b] disseminated infection
Enc. hellem[a]	Keratoconjunctivitis, sinusitis, prostatitis, pneumonitis, nephritis, urethritis, cystitis, diarrhea, disseminated infection
Enc. intestinalis[a]	Diarrhea,[b] intestinal perforation, keratoconjunctivitis, cholangitis, nephritis
Enterocytozoon bieneusi	Diarrhea,[b] wasting syndrome, cholangitis, rhinitis, bronchitis
Trachipleistophora	
T. hominis[a]	Myositis, keratoconjunctivitis, sinusitis
T. anthropopthera[a]	Encephalitis, keratoconjunctivitis, disseminated infection
Pleistophora sp.	
P. ronneafiei	Myositis
Pleistophora sp.	Myositis[b]
Anncaliia (Brachiola)	
A. vesicularam	Myositis
A. algerae[a]	Keratoconjunctivitis, myositis, skin infection
A. connori	Disseminated infection
Nosema	
N. ocularum	Keratoconjunctivitis[b]
Vittaforma	
Vittaforma corneae[a]	Keratoconjunctivitis,[b] urinary, tract infection
Microsporidium	
M. africanus	Corneal ulcer[b]
M. ceylonesis	Corneal ulcer[b]

[a]Organism can be grown in tissue culture.
[b]Cases reported in immunocompetent hosts.

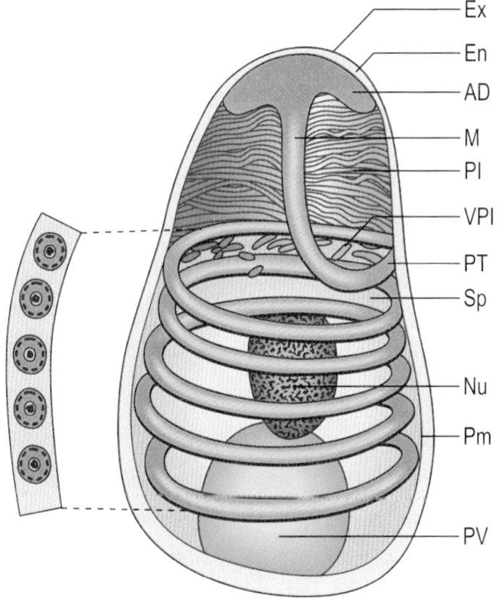

Figure 102.2 Structure of a microsporidian spore. Depending on the species, the size of the spore can vary from 1 to 10 μm, and the number of polar tubule coils can vary from a few to 30 or more. The extrusion apparatus consists of the polar tube (PT), vesiculotubular polaroplast (VPl), lamellar polaroplast (Pl), the anchoring disk (AD), and manubrium (M). This organelle is characteristic of the microsporidia. A cross-section of the coiled polar tube is illustrated. The nucleus (Nu) may be single (such as in Encephalitozoonae and Enterocytozoonae) or a pair of abutted nuclei termed a *diplokaryon* (such as in *Nosema*). The endospore (En) is an inner, thicker, electron-lucent region, and the exospore (Ex) is an outer electron-dense region. The plasma membrane (Pm) separates the spore coat from the sporoplasm (Sp), which contains ribosomes in a coiled helical array. The posterior vacuole (PV) is a membrane-bound structure. (From Chapter 6 "The Structure, Function and Composition of the Microsporidian Polar Tube". Page 199, Figure 4, in Wittner M, Weiss LM, ed. The Microsporidia and Microsporidiosis. Washington, DC: ASM Press; 1999.)

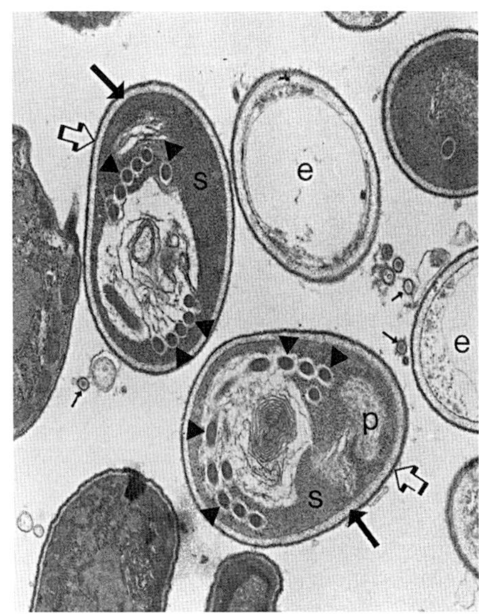

Figure 102.3 Transmission electron microscopy of mature spores of *Encephalitozoon hellem* in a parasitophorous vacuole. The spore wall consists of an electron-dense exospore (open arrows) and an electron-lucent endospore (large solid arrows). The characteristic coiled polar tube, also known as the polar filament, is seen in cross-section (arrowheads). One can also see the polaroplasts (p) within the sporoplasm (s) as well as ribosomes and rough endoplasmic reticulum. Some extruded polar tubules are seen in cross-section (small arrows), and empty spores (e) are also seen that have discharged their contents. (Original magnification ×7000.)

multiplication. Once a host cell becomes distended with mature spores, the cell ruptures, releasing mature spores into the environment and completing its life cycle. The combination of multiplication during both merogony and sporogony results in a large number of spores being produced from a single infection and illustrates the enormous reproductive potential of these organisms.

EPIDEMIOLOGY

Microsporidia appear to be common self-limited or asymptomatic enteric pathogens in immunocompetent hosts.[10,53] Multiple reports describe *Enterocytozoon bieneusi* in travelers and residents of tropical countries,[4,53–62] as well as *Encephalitozoon intestinalis*.[63] Serosurveys in humans demonstrate

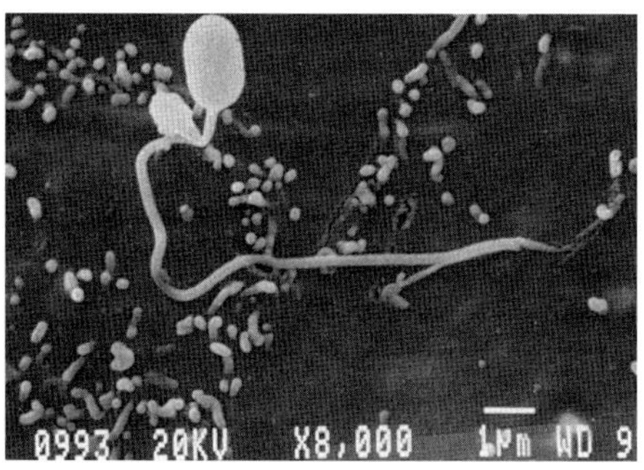

Figure 102.4 Scanning electron microscopy of a single mature spore of *Encephalitozoon hellem* from tissue culture demonstrating an extruded polar tube. (Original magnification ×8000.) (From Schwartz DA, Sokottka I, Leitich GJ, et al: Pathology of microsporidiosis. Emerging parasitic infections in patients with the acquired immunodeficiency syndrome. Arch Pathol Lab Med 120:173–188, 1996.)

Microsporidiosis

Intracellular multiplication via merogony and sporogony

Enc. intestinalis in epithelial cells, endothelial cells, or macrophages

Polar tubule pierces host epithelial cell, injects sporoplasm

Ent. bieneusi in epithelial cell

While *Ent. bieneusi* is primarily in the GI tract other species may invade the lung or eye or disseminate to cause:

Chronic diarrhea
Cholangitis
Sinusitis
Bronchitis
Nephritis
Cystitis/prostatitis
Keratoconjunctivitis

Presumed ingestion or respiratory acquisition of spores

Spore-laden host epithelial cells sloughed into lumina of GI, respiratory or GU tracts

Person-to-person, zoonotic, waterborne or foodborne transmission?

Diagnostic spores present in stool, urine, respiratory fluids, CSF or various tissue specimens

Sloughed cells degenerate; spores shed in bodily fluids

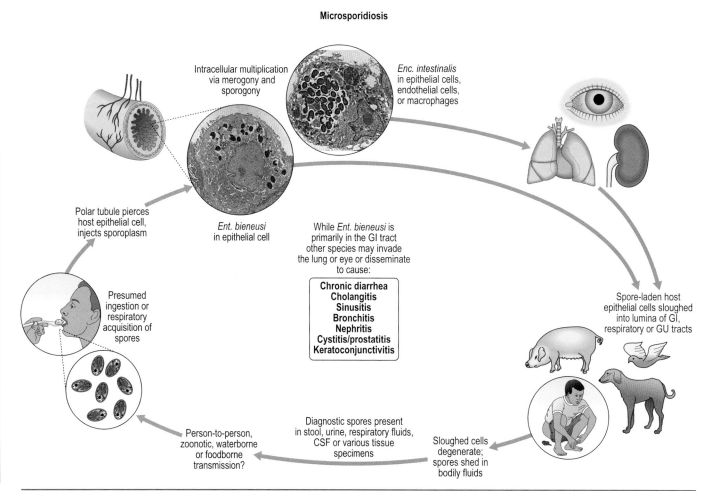

Figure 102.5 The general features of the microsporidian life cycle. CSF, cerebrospinal fluid; GI, gastrointestinal; GU, genitourinary.

a high prevalence of antibodies to *Enc. cuniculi* and *Enc. hellem*, suggesting asymptomatic infection is common.[5,64] In HIV-positive Czech patients, 5.3% were seropositive to *Enc. cuniculi* and 1.3% to *Enc. hellem.*[65] In Slovakia, 5.1% of slaughterhouse workers were seropositive to *Encephalitozoon* spp.[66] Singh and colleagues found positive antibody titers in 8.6% of healthy adults in England, 43% of Nigerians with tuberculosis, 19% of Malaysians with filariasis, and 36% of Ghanaians with malaria.[11] In another study, 12% of travelers returning from the tropics were seropositive and no control nontravelers were positive.[12] Antibodies to *Enc. intestinalis* were found among 5% of pregnant French women and 8% of Dutch blood donors.[67]

Enterocytozoon bieneusi causes the majority of infections in patients with AIDS and presents as diarrhea with wasting syndrome. Infections with *Ent. bieneusi* have been reported in liver and in heart–lung transplantation recipients, and *Encephalitozoon* spp. infections have been reported in patients with kidney, pancreas, liver, or bone marrow transplantation.[68–76] Reported prevalence rates in the 25 studies conducted on patients with HIV infection before the widespread use of highly active antiretroviral therapy (1989–1998) varied between 2% and 70%.[2,8–10,44,77–82] When combined, these studies identify 375 cases of *Ent. bieneusi* among 2400 patients with chronic diarrhea for a prevalence rate of 15% in this population. With immune reconstitution due to highly active antiretroviral therapy, the incidence of microsporidiosis has decreased.

Microsporidian spores are commonly found in surface water, and human pathogenic species have been found in municipal water supplies, tertiary sewage effluent, recreational bathing water, and groundwater.[56,83–87] Water contact has been found to be an independent risk factor for microsporidiosis in some studies[88,89] but not in others.[90,91] *Enc. cuniculi* spores are viable for at least 6 days in water.[92] Most microsporidian infections are transmitted by oral ingestion of spores, with the site of initial infection being the gastrointestinal tract. Microsporidia of the genus *Encephalitozoon* are widely distributed parasites of mammals and birds,[88] and the onset of microsporidiosis has been associated with exposure to livestock, fowl, and pets,[10,14,93–97] suggesting that microsporidiosis may be a zoonosis. *Ent. bieneusi* has been reported in pigs,[98,99] dogs,[100] dairy cattle,[101] chickens,[102] pigeons,[103] simian immunodeficiency virus-infected rhesus monkeys,[104,105] and recently, falcons.[106] A classification system has been published for the description of isolates of *Ent. bieneusi* from different reservoir hosts.[107] Viable infective spores of Microsporidia are present in multiple human body fluids (e.g., stool, urine, and respiratory secretions) during infection.[108] Person-to-person transmission is supported by concurrent infections in cohabiting homosexual men; however, there are no confirmed person-to-person outbreaks of microsporidiosis.[9] It has been possible to transmit *Encephalitozoon* spp. via rectal infection in rabbits, suggesting the possibility of sexual transmission.[109] *Enc. hellem* has been demonstrated in the respiratory mucosa, prostate, and urogenital tract of patients, raising the possibility of respiratory and sexual transmission in humans.[110,111] Although congenital transmission of *Enc. cuniculi* has been demonstrated in rabbits, mice, dogs, horses, foxes, and squirrel monkeys, it has not been demonstrated in humans.[112]

THE DISEASES

Microsporidian Infection in Immunosuppressed Hosts

Although the majority of reported cases of Microsporidia involve diarrhea, the spectrum of diseases caused by these organisms has expanded to include keratoconjunctivitis, disseminated disease, hepatitis, myositis, sinusitis, kidney and urogenital infection, ascites, cholangitis, and asymptomatic carriage.[13,44,113] *Ent. bieneusi* infection usually involves chronic diarrhea of 3–10 bowel movements per day,[44,48,114–116] anorexia, weight loss, and bloating without associated fever. It occurs more commonly in patients with AIDS having $CD4^+$ counts less than 50 cells/mm^3. Diarrhea is often associated with malabsorption, weight loss, and wasting syndrome.[114] The mortality of patients with advanced HIV disease and chronic diarrhea with wasting has been reported to be in excess of 50%.[116,117] In patients undergoing liver and bone marrow transplantation,[68–76,118–121] clinical manifestations have included watery, nonbloody diarrhea, nausea, and diffuse abdominal pain. *Ent. bieneusi* can also invade cholangioepithelium,[117] leading to sclerosing cholangitis, AIDS cholangiopathy, and cholecystitis,[122] with associated abdominal pain, nausea, vomiting, and fever. Imaging studies (abdominal ultrasound, computed tomography, endoscopic ultrasonography, and endoscopic retrograde cholangiopancreatography) usually demonstrate dilated biliary ducts, irregularities of the bile duct wall, and gallbladder abnormalities such as thickening, distension, or the presence of sludge. Systemic dissemination is rare. There is a case report describing this organism in nasal mucosa[123] and reports of respiratory tract involvement with *Ent. bieneusi* associated with chronic diarrhea, persistent cough, dyspnea, wheezing, and chest radiographs with interstitial infiltrates.[114,124]

Enc. cuniculi, *Enc. hellem*, and *Enc. intestinalis* have been associated with gastroenteritis, keratitis, sinusitis, bronchiolitis, nephritis, cystitis-ureteritis, urethritis, prostatitis, hepatitis, fulminant hepatic failure, peritonitis, and cerebritis, as well as disseminated infection.[13,48,113,125–131] An *Encephalitozoon* sp. has also been reported in a case of nodular skin lesions.[132,133] *Enc. intestinalis* most commonly causes diarrhea[134] but can also cause cholangitis,[40,135] keratoconjuctivitis, ostemyelitis of the mandible,[136] upper respiratory infections, renal failure, keratoconjunctivitis, and disseminated infection in patients with AIDS.[135–139] Elimination of this parasite from patients with diarrhea following treatment with albendazole correlates with the resolution of symptoms.[137,140] *Enc. cuniculi* has been associated with hepatitis,[141] peritonitis,[128] hepatic failure,[129] disseminated disease with fever,[130] renal insufficiency, and intractable cough.[142] Cases of encephalitis and seizures due to *Enc. cuniculi* have been reported in AIDS patients.[130,131] These infections have been reported to respond to albendazole.[125,130,131,142] *Enc. hellem* has been reported to cause disseminated disease associated with renal failure, nephritis, pneumonia, bronchitis, sinusitis, and keratoconjunctivitis.[11,143–145]

Most reports of ocular infection due to Encephalitozoonidae, have implicated *Enc. hellem*, including three cases originally classified as *Enc. cuniculi*.[146,147] Patients present with bilateral coarse punctate epithelial keratopathy and conjunctival inflammation resulting in redness, foreign body sensation, photophobia, excessive tearing, blurred vision, and changes in visual acuity. Ocular microsporidial infection in HIV-1-infected patients has been restricted to the superficial epithelium of the cornea and conjunctiva (i.e., superficial keratoconjunctivitis) and rarely progresses to corneal ulceration. Physical examination reveals conjunctival hyperemia with superficial punctate keratopathy, and slit-lamp examination usually demonstrates punctate epithelial opacities, granular epithelial cells with irregular fluorescein uptake, conjunctival injection, superficial corneal infiltrates, and a noninflamed anterior chamber (***Fig. 102.6***). Ocular infection is often associated with disseminated

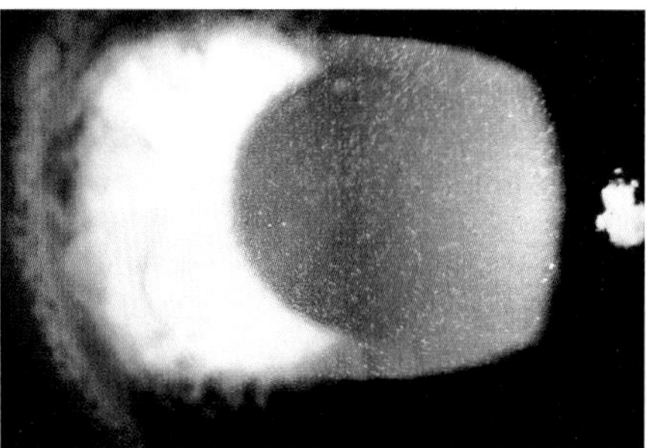

Figure 102.6 Slit-lamp photomicrograph demonstrates punctate epithelial keratopathy in a patient with AIDS and microsporidian keratoconjunctivitis due to *Encephalitozoon hellem*. (From Schwartz DA, Visvesvara GS, Diesenhouse MC, et al. Pathologic features and immunofluorescent antibody demonstration of ocular microsporidiosis (*Encephalitozoon hellem*) in seven patients with acquired immunodeficiency syndrome. Am J Ophthalmol. 1993;115:285–292.)

disease,[143,148–151] and thus urine examination often demonstrates microsporidian spores.[143,148–151]

Trachipleistophora hominis has been described in several patients with AIDS as a cause of disseminated disease,[42] with associated myositis, sinusitis, and keratoconjunctivitis. *T. anthropophthera* was described in several patients with AIDS having encephalitis associated with myositis and keratoconjunctivitis.[43,152] *Anncaliia (Brachiola) vesicularum* was reported as a cause of myositis,[37] as was *Pleistophora* sp. (*P. ronneafiei*).[153–156] The presentation of microsporidian myositis includes myalgias, weakness, elevated serum creatinine phosphokinase and aldolase levels, and abnormal electromyography consistent with inflammatory myopathy.[37,42,154,155] A fatal infection in a 4-month-old athymic male infant with severe diarrhea and malabsorption was due to *Anncaliia (Brachiola/Nosema) connori* at autopsy, where microsporidia were seen in the lungs, stomach, small and large bowel, kidneys, adrenal glands, myocardium, liver, and diaphragm.[157] A case of urinary tract infection and prostatitis due to *Vittaforma corneae* has also been reported in a patient with AIDS.[158] In a child with leukemia, skin infection was due to *Anncaliia (Brachiola) algerae* and spores were seen infecting the cellular elements of the dermis.[159] *A. (Brachiola) algerae* infection also occurred in a patient with rheumatoid arthritis treated with steroids and monoclonal antibody to tumor necrosis factor (TNF)-α.[160]

Microsporidian Infection in Immunocompetent Hosts

In patients with or without HIV infection, the most common symptom of microsporidian infection is diarrhea.[3,4,9,54,58,63,68,69,88,161] *Ent. bieneusi* has been identified as a cause of self-limited diarrhea in immunocompetent patients and travelers[9,53,54,60–63,162,163] and has been found in up to 10% of African children with diarrhea.[2,164,165] *Enc. intestinalis* was found in 8% of the stools of patients in a survey for the etiology of diarrhea in Mexico[88] and has been seen in travelers with chronic diarrhea.[63] Cerebral infections due to *Enc. cuniculi* are described in several mammals but have been reported only rarely in immunocompetent humans. In a 3-year-old boy with seizures and hepatomegaly, *Encephalitozoon* infection was suggested by positive immunoglobulin G (IgG) and IgM indirect immunofluorescence assays (using *Enc. cuniculi* as the antigen).[64] Similarly, *Encephalitozoon* spp. infection was reported in a 9-year-old Japanese boy with headache, vomiting, spastic convulsions, and recurrent fever.[17] An unidentified microsporidium responsive to albendazole was also described as causing multiple cerebral lesions in a 33-year-old man in Japan.[166] *Pleistophora* spp. have been identified in the skeletal muscle of an HIV-negative patient with myositis.[153–155,167]

Ocular infections with ulcer or deep cornea stroma infection associated with eye pain have been reported in immunocompetent patients. In 1981, corneal microsporidiosis due to *Microsporidium africanus*[168] was described, and in 1973 infection due to *M. ceylonesis* was described.[169] Other cases of microsporidian keratitis have since been identified in immunocompetent hosts.[13] One of these organisms was classified as *N. ocularum*[170] and the other, which was successfully propagated *in vitro*, was named *N. corneum*[173] (now *V. corneae*[36]). *A. (Brachiola) algerae* infection of the cornea has also been reported.[159] In these immunocompetent patients with corneal infections, one patient required enucleation,[168] one underwent unsuccessful penetrating keratoplasty,[169] one was successfully treated with a corneal transplant,[170] and the last was maintained on a variety of topical agents without effect until keratoplasty.[172] *Encephalitozoon* spp. and *T. anthropophthera* corneal infections have been described in contact lens wearers.[173,174] In a report from India on 40 immunocompetent patients, epidemic keratoconjunctivitis has been associated with microsporidia.[175]

PATHOGENESIS AND IMMUNITY

Infection of the epithelium of the gastrointestinal tract (small intestine and biliary epithelium) is the most frequent presentation of microsporidiosis. *Ent. bieneusi* infection does not produce active enteritis or ulceration, but infection results in variable degrees of villus blunting and crypt hyperplasia. The organism is located on the apical surface of the enterocytes of the small intestine and epithelial cells of the biliary tract and pancreas. Spores are rarely found on the basal surface or in the lamina propria.[127,176] Infection may be associated with increased intraepithelial lymphocytes and epithelial disarray. *Enc. intestinalis* and other *Encephalitozoon* spp. are invasive; spores are found in the apical and basal sides of infected intestinal enterocytes and in the lamina propria.[177] Histopathology can demonstrate areas of necrosis and mucosal erosion.

Encephalitozoon spp. infect the genitourinary system in most mammals, including humans,[53,127,137,178] in which infection discovered in any organ (eye, gastrointestinal tract, liver, central nervous system, etc.) is often associated with the shedding of spores in the urine. Granulomatous interstitial nephritis composed of plasma cells and lymphocytes is the most frequent pathologic finding. This is associated with tubular necrosis, with the lumen of the tubules containing amorphous granular material. Spores are located in the necrotic tubes and sloughing tubular epithelial cells.[70,74,119,121,148] As spores and infected tubular cells are shed into the bladder, they can infect other epithelial cells of the urogenital tract, causing ureteritis, prostatitis, and cystitis[127] and infection in macrophages, muscle, and supporting fibroblasts of the associated mucosa.

Lower respiratory tract infection due to Encephalitozoonidae has demonstrated erosive tracheitis, bronchitis, and bronchiolitis.[126,148] In most cases, organisms are found in intact or sloughed epithelial cells. Sinus biopsies in AIDS patients with chronic sinusitis and microsporidiosis have demonstrated spores in epithelium as well as in supporting structures.[145,179–185]

Infection with *Enc. cuniculi, Enc. hellem,* or *Enc. intestinalis* can result in punctate keratopathy and conjunctivitis characterized by multiple punctate corneal ulcers (e.g., a superficial epithelial keratitis). Microsporidian spores are present in corneal and conjunctival epithelium that can be obtained by scraping or biopsy of the lesions. The organisms do not invade the corneal stroma but remain limited to the epithelium. Inflammatory cells are rarely present.[93,108,141,186,187] Infections in immunocompetent hosts with other species of Microsporidia have usually involved deeper levels of the corneal stroma with associated necrosis and acute inflammatory cells, with some giant cells in several cases. Clinically, these patients have a corneal stromal keratitis and occasionally a uveitis.

There are scant data on the immune response to microsporidia in humans. It is clear that a strong humoral response occurs during infection and that it includes antibodies that react with the spore wall and polar tube. The immunosuppressive states associated with microsporidiosis (e.g., AIDS and transplantation) are those that inhibit cell-mediated immunity. Microsporidiosis is usually seen in HIV-infected patients when there is a profound defect in cell-mediated immunity (e.g., a $CD4^+$ cell count less than 100/mm^3); spontaneous cure of microsporidiosis can be induced by immune reconstitution with antiretroviral treatment.[188–190] Overall, these data are consistent with observations on the immunology of the mouse model of microsporidiosis in which interferon (IFN)-γ, IL-12, and $CD8^+$ cells have been implicated as critical in the immune response to infection.[191,192] It is possible that, in humans, administration of IFN-γ or IL-12 could be useful adjuncts for treating microsporidiosis.

DIAGNOSIS

Coprodiagnosis

Examination by light microscopy of stool specimens using special stains is the practical method for the diagnosis of gastrointestinal microsporidiosis. Experience is greatest with Weber's chromotrope-based stain.[193] Some laboratories prefer the Ryan modification,[194] which uses aniline blue in place of fast green. Using these chromotrope 2R stains, spores appear as 1–3 μm ovoid light pink structures with a beltlike stripe girding them diagonally and equatorially. *Enterocytozoon* spores are smaller (1.5 μm) than *Encephalitozoon* spores (2.5–3.0 µm). The Gram-chromotrope stain combines chromotrope 2R staining with a Gram-staining step and results in violet-staining spores.[195] Spores can also be visualized by ultraviolet (UV) microscopy using chemofluorescent optical brightening agents such as Calcofluor White M2R (fluorescent brightener 28, Fungi-Fluor)[196] or Uvitex 2B (Fungiqual A),[197] which stain chitin in the spore wall. Chemofluorescent stains also stain fungi, but microsporidian spores can be distinguished from yeast because they have a uniform oval shape and are nonbudding. The limit of detecting microsporidia by these light microscopy techniques appears to be 50 000 organisms/mL.[198] Overall, the sensitivity of the chemofluorescent brightener-based stains is slightly higher than that of chromotrope-based stains (especially when low numbers of spores are present in a sample); however, the specificity of the chemofluorescent stains is lower (90% versus 100% in one study).[198] Microsporidian spores in food can give a false-positive result, but this does not appear to be a common problem in fecal diagnoses.

Because renal involvement with shedding of spores in the urine is common in all of the species of Microsporidia that disseminate, urine specimens should be obtained whenever the diagnosis of microsporidiosis is considered. This has therapeutic implications because the Microsporidia that disseminate (e.g., *Encephalitozoon* spp.) are usually sensitive to albendazole, but those that do not disseminate (e.g., *Ent. bieneusi*) are resistant. Definitive identification of the Microsporidia requires either ultrastructural examination (e.g., electron microscopy) or molecular techniques (e.g., species-specific polymerase chain reaction (PCR)). If stool examination is negative in the setting of chronic diarrhea (more than 2 months' duration), then endoscopy should be performed.

Cytologic Techniques

In body fluids other than stool (e.g., urine, cerebrospinal fluid, bile, duodenal aspirates, bronchoalveolar lavage fluid, and sputum), Microsporidia have been easily visualized using a variety of stains (e.g., chromotrope 2R, chemofluorescent optical brightening agents, Giemsa, Brown–Hopps Gram stain, acid fast staining, and/or Warthin–Starry silver staining).[48,199,200] Since Microsporidia often infect mucosa or epithelium, cytologic preparations are useful for diagnosis.[48,201] Microsporidia have been easily demonstrated in intestinal and biliary epithelium, epithelium of the cornea and conjunctivae, epithelium of the sinonasal and tracheobronchial regions, renal tubular epithelium, and urothelium. Microsporidian keratitis cell samples obtained by gentle rubbing over the conjunctiva and cornea with a tissue swab usually reveal multiple, Gram-positive, oval organisms within epithelial cells (***Fig. 102.7***).

Histologic Techniques

Using routine procedures, microsporidian spores are discernible with a modified tissue chromotrope 2R or tissue Gram stain (Brown–Hopp or Brown–Brenn) in biopsy and autopsy tissue specimens (***Figs 102.8 and 102.9***). In transbronchial biopsies, spores are best identified in bronchial or bronchiolar epithelium, but they can also be found within alveolar spaces. Microsporidia are usually Gram positive and some are also acid-fast positive. Due to their thick wall, unstained spores are refractile and as such can be birefringent in unstained tissue sections. With experience, microsporidia can also be seen on hematoxylin and eosin stain. Other stains that may be useful include periodic acid–Schiff, Giemsa, and Steiner silver stains. Biopsy or autopsy material should, if possible, also be placed in electron microscopic fixative when microsporidiosis is suspected because definitive diagnosis of species requires ultrastructural information. Although molecular methods such as PCR can be performed using formalin-fixed tissue, better results are obtained with unfixed tissue or tissue fixed in ethanol. Similar to its role in the understanding of other emerging infections, the autopsy has proven to be a valuable method for understanding the pathogenesis, mechanism(s) of acquisition, and potential transmission, and organ-based pathology of the emerging microsporidial pathogens.[148,202,203]

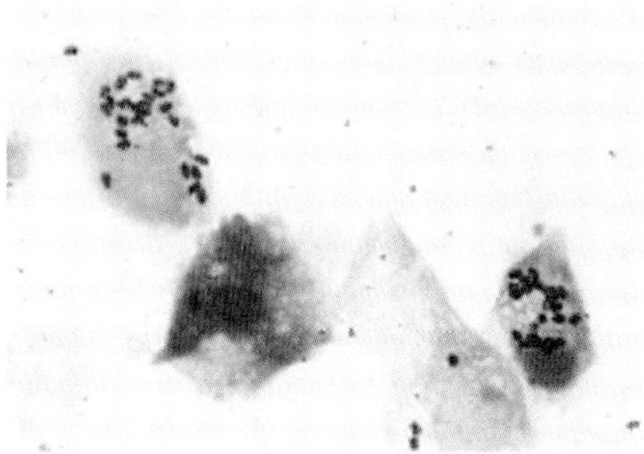

Figure 102.7 Conjunctival smear from a patient with AIDS and *Encephalitozoon hellem* keratoconjunctivitis stained with Gram stain. Numerous Gram-positive microsporidian spores can be seen within the cytoplasm of the epithelial cells as well as outside of these cells.

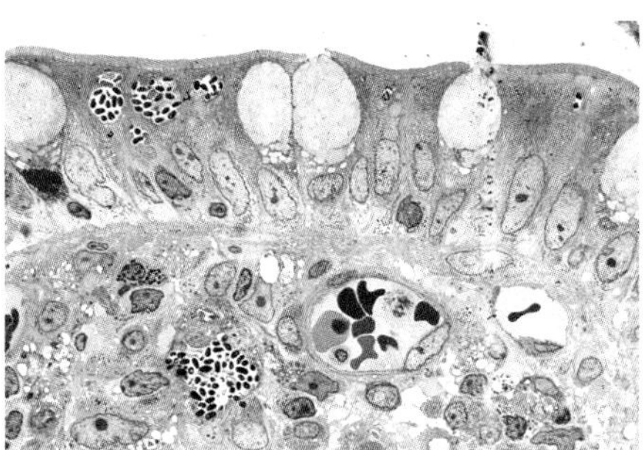

Figure 102.8 *Encephalitozoon intestinalis* in a duodenal biopsy plastic-embedded section stained with toluidine blue. Unlike *Enterocytozoon*, the spores of *Encephalitozoon intestinalis* develop in a vacuole, termed the parasitophorous vacuole, as shown in both superficial enterocytes and in a lamina propria macrophage. (Magnification ×1000).

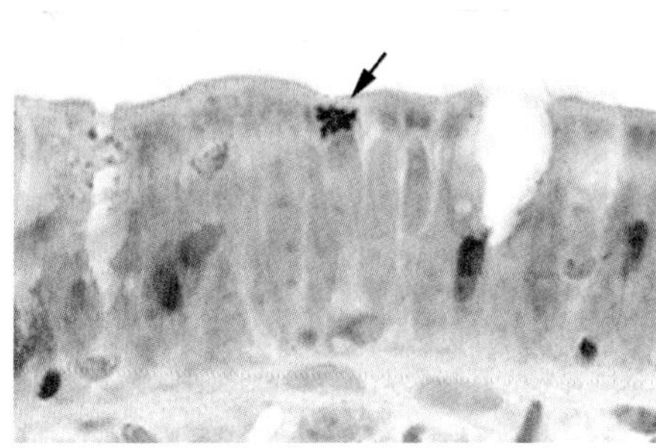

Figure 102.9 *Enterocytozoon bieneusi* in a small intestinal biopsy from a patient with AIDS and chronic diarrhea. Microsporidian spores (arrow) are visible in the apical cytoplasm of an enterocyte in this tissue section stained with Gram stain (Brown and Hopps). (Magnification ×1000.)

Electron Microscopy, Immunofluorescence, Molecular Diagnostic Methods, Serology, and Tissue Culture

Transmission electron microscopy (TEM) is a useful technique for confirmation of microsporidian infection in patient tissues and fluids, as well as for detailed ultrastructural studies of microsporidian life cycles and host–parasite relationships that are required for the description of new species of Microsporidia (see ***Figs 102.2 and 102.3***). TEM should be performed on any new or atypical infections that are diagnosed as being due to Microsporidia. Scanning electron microscopy (SEM), while not as widely available as is TEM, is highly useful in understanding the three-dimensional structure of microsporidia, and their relationship with their host cell.[126,127]

Fluorescent antibody reagents can be used for the species-level identification of various Microsporidia in both cytologic and tissue specimens.[204–208] Monoclonal antibodies to *Enc. hellem*, *Enc. intestinalis*, and *Ent. bieneusi*[209,210] have been described and several of these antibodies have been demonstrated to be useful for the examination of stool specimens and have demonstrated good sensitivity and specificity. Detection kits for microsporidia in stool and environmental samples using antibodies to Encephalitozoonidae and *Ent. bieneusi* are now commercially available (Waterborne, Inc., New Orleans, LA). Serologic tests for the diagnosis of microsporidiosis have been developed and utilized for epidemiologic studies, but they have not been useful for the diagnosis of microsporidiosis in AIDS patients.[211]

Molecular diagnostic techniques such as PCR can dentify Microsporidia at the species level in intestinal biopsies, stool specimens, and other tissues (for a review see Weiss and Vossbrinck[30]).[212–215] Currently, these tests are available in reference laboratories such as the Centers for Disease Control and Prevention. The *in vitro* cultivation of several human-infecting Microsporidia has enhanced our understanding of these pathogens (for a review see Visvesvara[216]). *Vittaforma corneae*,[171] *Enc. cuniculi*, *Enc. hellem*,[186] *T. hominis*,[42] and *Enc. intestinalis*[217] have been cultivated *in vitro*, whereas *Ent. bieneusi* has not. The isolation of Microsporidia from clinical specimens is not a routine procedure and is available only in a few specialized research laboratories.

The Microsporidia are generally considered after the more common pathogens of the gastrointestinal, hepatobiliary, respiratory, genitourinary, ocular, musculoskeletal, and central nervous systems have been considered and ruled out. The index of suspicion for microsporidiosis should be highest in patients with severe immunosuppression, especially, but not exclusively, those infected with HIV or having undergone organ transplantation. Intestinal microsporidiosis should be considered in any patient with chronic diarrhea or hepatobiliary disease of uncertain cause. The differential diagnosis includes other infectious agents characterized by chronic diarrhea. Intestinal microsporidiosis should be considered in cases of presumptive traveler's diarrhea in which other routine pathogens have been excluded. A diagnosis of microsporidiosis should also be considered in cases of unexplained keratoconjunctivitis or corneal ulcers, persistent sinusitis or diffuse lower respiratory disease, unexplained renal insufficiency or abnormalities in urinary sediment, and myositis. Since dissemination can occur, microsporidiosis may affect virtually any organ system, including bone and the central nervous system. Therefore, the identification of Microsporidia in any specimen should prompt a thorough search in all other readily available sources, including stool, urine, sputum, nasal and conjunctival swabs, and possibly cerebrospinal fluid, with consideration of more invasive approaches for those patients requiring a tissue-based diagnosis (e.g., myositis).

TREATMENT AND PROGNOSIS

For a review of drugs used in microsporidiosis in humans and animals, see Costa and Weiss[218] (***Table 102.2***). Although albendazole has significant activity against many Microsporidia, such as the Encephalitozoonidae, it has limited efficacy for *Ent. bieneusi* infection,[219–221] with relapse of symptoms rapidly occurring with the discontinuation of therapy in patients who reported improvement of symptoms with treatment. Other studies have found that albendazole has no efficacy in *Ent. bieneusi* infection.[222] Analysis of the tubulin sequences of *Ent. bieneusi* and *V. corneae* demonstrates that both of these microsporidia have amino acid substitutions associated with resistance to albendazole.[223,224]

Fumagillin is used to treat honeybees infected with the microsporidian *Nosema apis* and has been used to treat microsporidiosis in aquaculture.[225,226] Fumagillin and its semisynthetic analog, TNP-470, were found to have activity *in vitro* and *in vivo* against *Enc. cuniculi, Enc. hellem, Enc. intestinalis,* and *V. corneae*.[227–232] Fumagillin has also been demonstrated in both a dose-escalation trial and a randomized clinical trial to be effective for the treatment of human infection with *Ent. bieneusi* at a dose of 60 mg/day (20 mg three times daily).[227,228] Treatment was associated with resolution of diarrhea, clearance of spores, improvement of Karnofsky scores, and improvement in D-xylose absorption tests. It has also been demonstrated in case reports to be effective in the treatment of *Ent. bieneusi* in

Table 102.2 Treatment Options for Microsporidiosis

Organism	Drug	Dosage and Duration
All microsporidian infections	Restoration of immune function can be critical in control of infection. Patients with AIDS should have highly active antiretroviral therapy optimized	
Ent. bieneusi	No effective commercial treatment	
	Oral fumagillin 20 mg tid (e.g., 60 mg/day has been effective in a clinical trial	
	Albendazole[a] resulted in clinical improvement in up to 50% of patients in some studies; however, it was not effective in other studies	
Encephalitozoonidae infection (systemic, sinusitis, encephalitis, hepatitis, etc.)		
Enc. cuniculi	Albendazole	400 mg bid[b]
Enc. hellem	Albendazole	400 mg bid
Enc. intestinalis	Albendazole	400 mg bid
Encephalitozoonidae (keratoconjunctivitis)	Fumagillin solution[c] (Fumidil B 3 mg/mL, fumagillin 70 µg/mL)	2 drops every 2 hours for 4 days, then 2 drops 4 times a day[d]
	Patients may also need albendazole[a] if systemic infection is present	
Trachipleistophora hominis	Albendazole	400 mg bid
Anncaliia (Brachiola) vesicularum	Albendazole	400 mg bid
	± Itraconazole	400 mg qd

[a]Albendazole 400 mg bid.

[b]The duration of treatment for microsporidiosis has not been established. Relapse of infection has occurred upon stopping treatment. Patients should be maintained on treatment for at least 4 weeks and may require prolonged treatment.

[c]Fumagillin bicylohexylammonium.

[d]Eyedrops should be continued indefinitely; relapse is common on stopping treatment.

bid, twice daily; tid, three times daily; qd, every day.

(Adapted from Costa SF, Weiss LM. Drug treatment of microsporidiosis. Drug Resist Update. 2000;3:384–399.)

the setting of organ transplantation.[76] The main limiting toxicity of treatment was thrombocytopenia, which was reversible on stopping fumagillin treatment. Despite a few case reports that indicated that metronidazole was effective for *Ent. bieneusi* infection, the majority of studies have demonstrated that this drug is not effective.[178,229,233] Other medications used without success in the treatment of gastrointestinal microsporidiosis are azithromycin, paromomycin, and quinacrine.

Clinical studies have demonstrated that improved immune function can result in the clinical response of patients with gastrointestinal microsporidiosis, with elimination of the organism and normalization of the intestinal architecture.[234–238] Relapse has been reported in patients who developed failure of their antiretroviral therapy associated with a decline in immune function and falling CD4+ counts. Overall, these observations suggest that part of the primary treatment of microsporidiosis in the setting of AIDS is the institution of effective antiretroviral therapy. There have been no reports of immune reconstitution syndromes in patients with microsporidiosis treated with antiretroviral therapy.

There are numerous case reports that demonstrate the efficacy of 2 to 4 weeks of 400 mg of albendazole twice daily for the treatment of microsporidian infections due to *Encephalitozoon* spp. A double-blind, placebo-controlled trial of eight patients with AIDS and diarrhea due to *Enc. intestinalis* demonstrated that albendazole (400 mg twice daily for 3 weeks) treatment led to a resolution of the diarrhea and elimination of the organism, similar to observations in case reports.[76,137,138,140,178,182,239,240] In case reports of chronic sinusitis, respiratory infection, and disseminated infection due to *Enc. hellem*, treatment with 400 mg of albendazole twice daily resulted in resolution of symptoms and clearance of the organism.[241,242] In a patient with disseminated *Enc. cuniculi* infection involving the central nervous system, conjunctiva, sinuses, kidney, and lungs, clinical improvement was demonstrated with albendazole treatment.[131] The successful use of albendazole has also been reported in gastrointestinal infection in the setting of organ transplantation[76] as well as in cases of urethritis,[243] renal failure,[244] and disseminated infection[142] due to *Encephalitozoon* spp. In addition, albendazole has been reported to have activity in the treatment of disseminated microsporidian infection with *T. hominis* and in myositis due to a *Anncaliia (Brachiola) vesicularum*.[37,42]

Ocular microsporidiosis can be treated with a solution of 3 mg/mL of Fumidil B, fumagillin bicylohexylammonium, in saline (fumagillin 70 μg/mL);[230,245–248] however, recurrence is known to occur when topical therapy is discontinued. Although clearance of microsporidia from the eye can be demonstrated, the organism is still present systemically and can often be demonstrated in urine or nasal smears. The use of albendazole as a systemic agent is thus also reasonable for the treatment of ocular infection and should probably be used in addition to topical treatment. Polymyxin B, propamidine isethionate 0.1% (Brolene), gramicidin, neomycin sulfate, and tetracycline have limited efficacy and should not be used except as treatment for secondary bacterial infections. Keratoplasty provides temporary improvement in some cases, and debulking by corneal scraping may be useful in cases not responding to medical treatment. Steroids may be useful in decreasing the associated inflammatory response.

PREVENTION AND CONTROL

The presence of infective spores in various bodily fluids suggests that body substance precautions in health care settings and general attention to hand washing and other personal hygiene measures should be useful in preventing primary infections. Hand washing may be particularly important in the prevention of ocular infections, which may occur as a result of inoculation of conjunctival surfaces by fingers contaminated with respiratory fluids or urine. Whether respiratory precautions are necessary for people with spores in sputum or other respiratory secretions is unknown. It is reasonable to screen close contacts of index cases of microsporidiosis. Spores survive and remain infective in the environment for prolonged periods of time.[92] In a typical hospital environment, *Enc. cuniculi* spores can survive and remain infectious for at least 1 month but can be rendered noninfectious by a 30-minute exposure to most common disinfectants and by the methods employed for sterilization. Therefore, the procedures used to clean most hospital rooms should be sufficient to limit infection.

It is likely that these organisms are food- or waterborne pathogens and the usual sanitary measures that prevent contamination of food and water with the urine and feces of animals should decrease the chance for infection. Existing guidelines for the prevention of opportunistic infections that address food, water, and animal contact may be useful in preventing microsporidiosis. Severely immunocompromised patients may wish to consider using bottled or filtered water in some settings. No prophylactic antiparasitic agents have been identified for these organisms. Microsporidiosis has developed in patients on trimethoprim-sulfamethoxazole prophylaxis[249] and those receiving dapsone, pyrimethamine, itraconazole, azithromycin, and/or atovaquone.[250] No studies have evaluated albendazole for prophylaxis, but given its relative lack of efficacy for *Ent. bieneusi* infections, it is unlikely to be effective for prevention. The most effective prophylaxis is a restoration of immune function in immunocompromised hosts. In AIDS patients, several studies have demonstrated that highly active antiretroviral therapy can produce remission of intestinal microsporidiosis.[234–237]

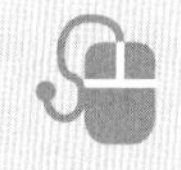

Access the complete reference list online at
http://www.expertconsult.com

CHAPTER 103

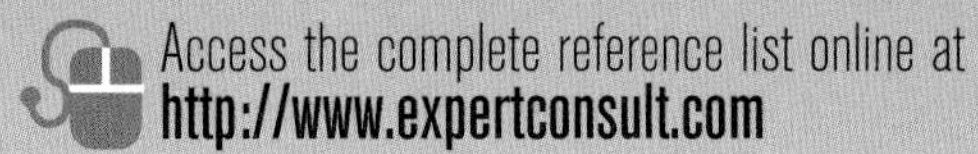
Access the complete reference list online at
http://www.expertconsult.com

Toxoplasmosis

Joseph D. Schwartzman • James H. Maguire

INTRODUCTION

Toxoplasma gondii is a versatile intracellular parasite that has adapted to infect many animal species and is capable of causing a wide spectrum of disease, the preponderance of which is asymptomatic. Invasion of host cells leads to their eventual death; a complex interplay of host cell-mediated immune responses arrests acute infection and maintains continued suppression of the persistent encysted zoites, usually for the life of the host. The wide host range of *T. gondii* is an exception in contrast to other members of the phylum Apicomplexa. *Toxoplasma* also has a wide geographic range: its single species is found worldwide. The ability to infect many species by at least two routes and its broad distribution are responsible for the high prevalence of infections in humans; perhaps a third of the world's people are chronically infected by *T. gondii*. Serious illness is unusual except among persons with deficient cell-mediated immunity and infants infected *in utero*. Toxoplasmosis is an important cause of abortion in sheep, swine, and goats.[1,2]

THE AGENT

History and Taxonomy

In 1908, Nicolle and Manceaux[3] identified *T. gondii* in a laboratory rodent, the North African gondi; and Splendore[4] noted identical forms in a laboratory rabbit. Recognition of the importance of this parasite for humans came in 1937 when it was identified as a cause of "granulomatous encephalomyelitis."[5] The role of chronic infection was appreciated in the 1950s by demonstrating *Toxoplasma* in eyes previously thought to have been involved with tuberculosis or syphilis.[6] The high prevalence of toxoplasmosis was only realized after the serologic dye test was developed by Sabin and Feldman in 1948.[7] Congenital toxoplasmosis in infants was recognized before either generalized disease in adults or the lymphadenitis of primary *Toxoplasma* infections in adults was appreciated.[5] Roles of reactivated latent infections in producing disease in immunosuppressed adults were recognized at the outset of solid organ transplantation.[8] The onset of acquired immunodeficiency syndrome (AIDS) brought recognition of central nervous system (CNS) reactivation causing multifocal encephalitis.[9]

T. gondii is a genetically homogeneous single species.[10] Three genetic types make up 95% of isolates from North America and Europe.[11,12] South American strains appear to harbor more genetic diversity. Type II strains are most commonly recovered from humans with congenital and acquired toxoplasmosis.[11] Type I strains are more virulent in outbred mice, more frequent in congenital infections in some geographic areas,[13] found more frequently in immunosupresssed humans,[14] and, along with "atypical" strains (recombinant genotypes of type I and type II strains), are over-represented in serious ocular infections.[15] Evidence suggests that the genetic lineages were separated between northern continents and South America about 1 million years ago and were introduced into South America approximately 10 000 years ago associated with highly clonal spread, perhaps because of concurrent acquisition of efficient oral infectivity.[16–19]

Life Cycle

Asexual stages of *T. gondii* are pathogenic for humans and animals.[20] Two forms are produced: rapidly dividing tachyzoites invasive in all tissues, and slowly dividing bradyzoites in cysts predominantly found in brain and muscle[21] (***Figs 103.1 and 103.2***). Tachyzoite replication causes acute disease, while bradyzoite cysts are long-lived, with slow turnover, and are responsible for latency and reactivation. Reservoirs of human infection are birds and rodents ingested by cats, as well as human food animals, especially pigs, goats, and sheep, that can carry infectious cysts in meat.[1,2,22] The sexual stage, found in the small intestinal epithelium of both wild and domestic Felidae, yields oocysts that are resistant to environmental conditions, tend to float in watered soils, and thereby may be ingested by contamination of vegetables or hands.[23,24] Oocysts sporulate within 12–24 hours to several days after passage from the cat and are thereafter infectious (***Fig. 103.3***).

ECOLOGY, EPIDEMIOLOGY, AND DISTRIBUTION

Humans may be infected both by eating cysts in meat and by ingestion of oocysts from contaminated soil. The relative risk of infection in industrialized countries is higher from the ingestion of undercooked meat, especially lamb and beef, but in societies with little meat in the diet, oocysts are more important.[25] Birds and rodents are important in picking up oocysts from soil and scavenging bradyzoite cysts from infected animals.[26] Grazing food animals (e.g., sheep) are probably infected by soil oocysts, but swine are omnivores and may also ingest infected rodents.[1,2] The prevalence of *Toxoplasma* in swine is quite variable. Bovine and fowl *Toxoplasma* levels are low.[27,28] Although sexual recombination can take place in cats, it appears to be rare in nature.[15,23,24,29] The distribution of *T. gondii* is worldwide; all genotypes are found on all continents except in Antarctica and on some islands in the Pacific and along the coast of Central America.[25,30,31] Hot, dry climates have a lower incidence of toxoplasmosis than temperate, moist climates, and rates are low at high altitudes.[25,32,33] Geographic foci of transmission by oocysts (cat cycle) have been described in societies that do not consume meat.[34] The role of the cat in the transmission of toxoplasmosis is established, but the epidemiology of transmission includes the possible role of dogs. Dogs may be vectors of oocysts based on associations in epidemiologic surveys and their habit of rolling in or eating cat feces.[26] River water contaminated with oocysts was believed to be the source of an outbreak in a Panamanian jungle.[35] Public water supplies were implicated in an outbreak in British Columbia, and drinking unfiltered municipal and surface water was

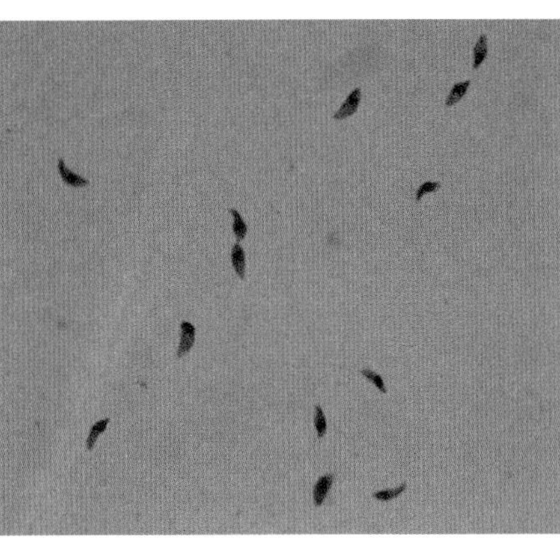

Figure 103.1 *T gondii* tachyzoites from culture, with no other cells (×1000). (Courtesy of Joseph D. Schwartzman.)

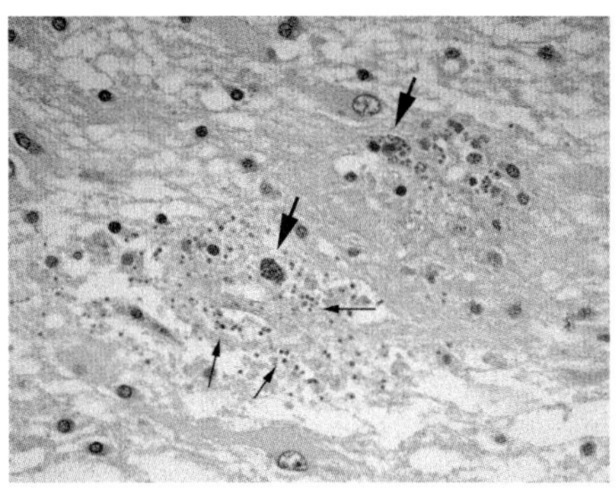

Figure 103.2 Congenital toxoplasmosis. Tissue cysts (large arrows) in uvea of human eye with numerous intracellular bradyzoites (small arrows). (Hematoxylin and eosin, ×1000.) (Courtesy of the Department of Tropical Public Health, Harvard School of Public Health, Boston, MA.)

Toxoplasma gondii

Transmission via blood transfusion or organ donation

with development of immunity

Tissue cysts (10–200 μm) with many bradyzoites form in muscle, myocardium, CNS, et al

Asexual cycle

may reactivate with loss of immunity causing:

Tachyzoites multiply in all nucleated cell types and disseminate through blood and lymphatics causing:

Acute

Lymphadenopathy Hepatosplenomegaly ± fever

Congenital

CNS defects if early Chorioretinitis if late

Immunocompromised patient

CNS lesions Chorioretinitis Pneumonitis Myocarditis

Bradyzoites (from tissue cysts) or sporozoites (from oocysts) are released in intestine and invade surrounding cells becoming fragile 3 × 7 μm tachyzoites

Infection acquired via ingestion of either oocysts from cat feces or tissue cysts in meat

Sheep, pigs, cats, rodents, cows, deer, et al, like humans, are infected from tissue cysts or fecal oocysts and develop throughout their bodies tissue cysts with many bradyzoites

Buoyant oocysts sporulate over 2–3 days to become infectious (>>1 year)

Enteroepithelial sexual cycle in cats

Hardy 10–12 μm oocysts shed over 1–3 weeks in cat feces 3–34 days after cat becomes infected

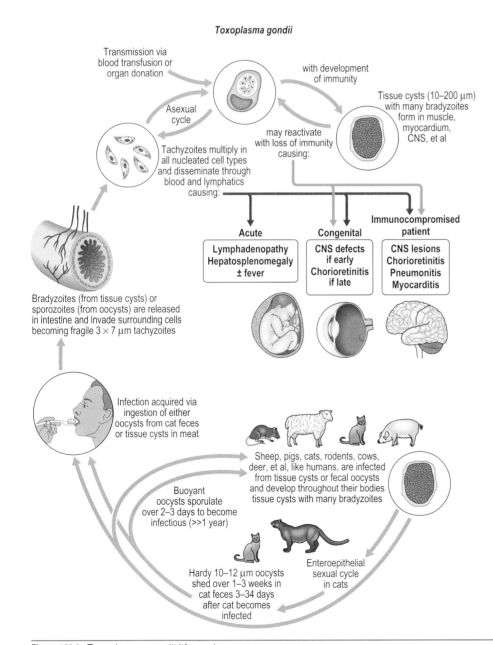

Figure 103.3 *Toxoplasma gondii* life cycle.

associated with a high level of endemicity in Rio de Janeiro State, Brazil.[30] Increased risk of infection has also been associated with ingestion of raw shellfish and raw goat's milk.[36] *Toxoplasma* infection also is acquired by transplacental transmission and, less commonly, through organ transplantation[8] and laboratory accident.[37] Although *Toxoplasma* DNA can be detected by polymerase chain reaction (PCR) in blood from chronically infected persons,[38] transmission of toxoplasmosis by transfusion of banked erythrocytes has not posed a public health problem.[39]

Serologic surveys demonstrate prevalences of infection from <10% to >90% in various geographic locations.[40–50] In parts of France, where rates of infection may exceed 90% by the fourth decade,[40,41] transmission is related to ingestion of rare meat. In contrast, rates in England and Finland are approximately 20%.[42,43] In tropical areas of Latin America and sub-Saharan Africa, where cats are abundant and the climate favors survival of oocysts, prevalences may approach 90%.[25,26,44–48] In comparison, rates in hot, dry regions such as North Africa usually do not exceed 20%.[49] Rates in the United States vary, ranging from 3% in Denver, Colorado, to 17% in Massachusetts, and to 30% in Birmingham, Alabama.[50] The seroprevalence of toxoplasmosis among persons aged 12–49 years in the United States remained stable at around 16% throughout the 1990s.[51]

PATHOGENESIS, PATHOLOGY, AND CLINICAL MANIFESTATIONS

Primary Disease

The primary route of infection is oral, with progression of infection through the gastrointestinal tract to local lymphatics and spread to other organs documented in the mouse, but this has not been documented in humans.[21,50,52] In mice fed bradyzoites, the first step is local invasion of the small intestinal epithelium. The bradyzoite and tachyzoite are both capable of active invasion of many cell types and replicate within a parasite-modified vacuole.[52–58] Bradyzoites rapidly convert to tachyzoites *in vivo*. *In vitro*, the formation of bradyzoite cysts can be stimulated by various maneuvers that stress the infected cells.[59,60] The key step in spreading infection from the localized initial site is likely infection of circulating monocytes in the lamina propria; this cell subset is permissive for *T. gondii* replication in both mice and humans and may therefore be responsible for transport of the parasite widely throughout tissues.[21,52,61]

Tachyzoites are found in all organs in acute infection, most prominently in muscle, including heart, and in the liver, spleen, lymph nodes, and the CNS.[50,52] The initial pathologic lesion is necrosis caused by death of parasitized cells, with a vigorous acute inflammatory reaction. As the disease progresses, more lymphocytic infiltration develops, but true granulomas are not formed. If the host controls the replication of tachyzoites effectively, tissues are restored to anatomical integrity without scarring, and cysts containing the long-lived bradyzoites remain without sign of host reaction.[62] The humoral immune response is rapid and may be capable of killing extracellular tachyzoites (and is of use diagnostically), but it is not protective in the mouse model.[61] Control of disease appears to depend on the elaboration of cytokines including interleukin (IL)-2, IL-12, and interferon-γ (INF-γ)[63–65] followed by a specific cell-mediated immunity, with $CD8^+$ helper T cells apparently the most important subgroup.[66] Virulence of the parasite includes its ability to modulate the host response, a proinflammatory response that may result in increased tissue damage and a higher mortality in experimental infections. Parasite factors responsible for enhanced inflammation have been identified.[67,68]

Subclinical or unrecognized infections are the usual outcome of primary infection in immunocompetent persons.[35,69–74] When symptoms occur, the most common manifestation is painless lymphadenopathy, with or without fever.[50,73] Usually a single cervical node is enlarged, but there may be multiple enlarged nodes at one site or generalized lymphadenopathy. Toxoplasmic lymphadenopathy may persist for 4–6 weeks, raising the suspicion of lymphoma.[73,75] Occasionally, a syndrome of fever, headache, malaise, myalgia, lymphadenopathy, hepatosplenomegaly and atypical lymphocytosis develops after an incubation period of 5–20 days.[35,70–72] The course of illness may last weeks or months, suggesting a diagnosis of infectious mononucleosis. Pneumonitis, myocarditis, meningoencephalitis, polymyositis, and death are rare complications in otherwise healthy persons.[76,77] In Brazil and British Columbia, a high incidence of acute acquired retinochoroiditis has been described.[78,79] Retinochoroiditis in primary acute infection is more common than previously recognized and may be associated with particular genotypes.[80]

Congenital Disease

Primary infection of the mother with consequent infection of the placenta is the mechanism by which almost all congenital disease is transmitted.[33,81–83] The placenta allows transmission to the fetus in 30–50% of infections acquired during pregnancy.[81] Congenital infection is exceptionally rare when the mother acquires infection before gestation,[84,85] and most of the few reported cases have occurred when maternal infection occurred within 3 months of conception or in the setting of maternal immunosuppression due to human immunodeficiency virus (HIV) infection or immunosuppressive therapy.[86,87] Reinfection may rarely be caused by exposure to a new genetic type of *Toxoplasma*.[88] Acute infection is apparent in fewer than 20% of mothers, but both symptomatic and asymptomatic infections place the fetus at risk. The rate of transplacental transmission and the severity of disease vary with time of gestation.[86] If maternal infection occurs during the first trimester, the risk of fetal infection is only around 10%, but disease is usually severe. Rates of congenital infection rise to about 65% for maternal infection during the third trimester and approach 100% at term, but neonatal infection in these instances usually is asymptomatic.[33]

Overall, fewer than 15% of infants with congenital toxoplasmosis have severe impairment of the brain or eyes, and about 80% are asymptomatic at birth or have mild disease that is not detected by routine physical examination.[81,89–93] However, more than 85% of those with asymptomatic infection will develop adverse sequelae of the CNS or eyes in subsequent years.[91,92]

Early fetal infections lead to spontaneous abortion, stillbirth, or severe neonatal disease.[52,83] In the brain, there are foci of necrosis, microglial nodules, and perivascular mononuclear inflammation in association with free and intracellular tachyzoites.[52] Vascular thrombosis may lead to large areas of coagulation necrosis, and necrotic brain may become calcified. Necrosis around ventricles or the aqueduct of Sylvius may lead to hydrocephalus. Neurologic sequelae include seizures, psychomotor retardation, deafness, hydrocephalus, microcephalus, and intracerebral calcifications visible on computed tomography (CT) scan (***Fig. 103.4***). A common feature of severe congenital toxoplasmosis is bilateral retinochoroiditis manifested by necrosis of the retina and granulomatous inflammation of the choroid.[94] Lesions are near to or in the macula, and vitritis and uveitis are frequently present. There may be micro-ophthalmia, strabismus, cataracts, glaucoma, and optic atrophy. Systemic manifestations such as fever, hypothermia, jaundice, vomiting, diarrhea, lymphadenopathy, hepatosplenomegaly, pneumonitis, myocarditis, and rash may be present.[90] Laboratory studies show anemia, thrombocytopenia, high cerebrospinal fluid (CSF) protein, and CSF pleocytosis.

While the majority of infants who acquire infection late in pregnancy appear normal at birth, meticulous examination often shows abnormalities such as retinal scars (***Fig. 103.5***) or abnormal CSF.[89,90] Healthy-appearing infants occasionally develop severe CNS or ocular disease during the first months of life. More commonly, persons with asymptomatic infections at birth experience recurrent episodes of retinochoroiditis or impaired psychomotor development during the first 10–20 years of life.[91,92]

Ocular Disease

Toxoplasmosis may account for one-third of cases of retinochoroiditis.[94–96] Most cases occur in teenagers and young adults and previously were ascribed to reactivation of congenitally acquired infection. Population-based studies in southern Brazil and recent experience with clusters of

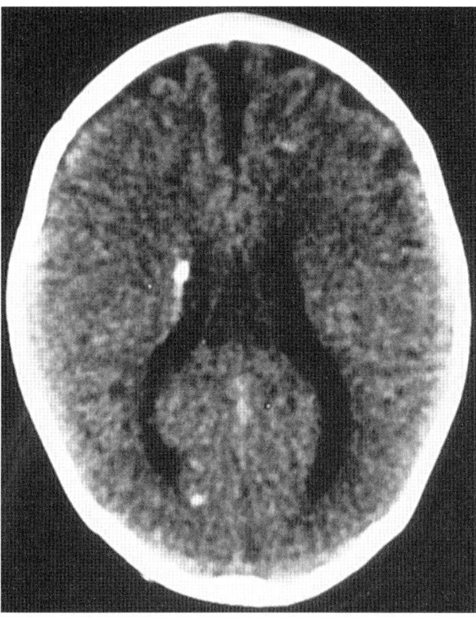

Figure 103.4 Intracerebral calcifications and mild hydrocephalus in an infant with congenital toxoplasmosis. CT scan of the head without contrast.

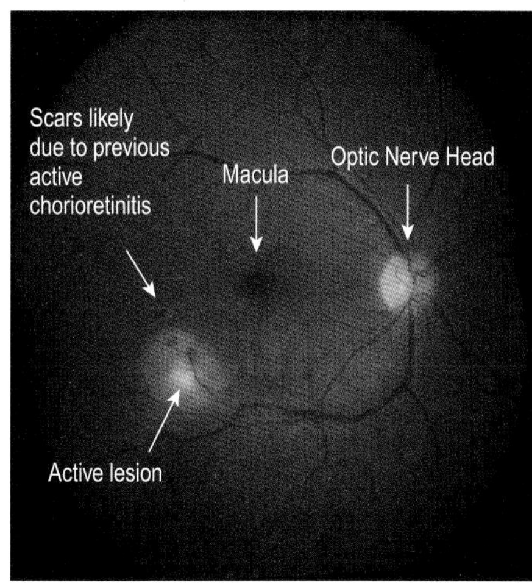

Figure 103.5 Active and healed retinochoroiditis in the periphery of the fundus of the eye of an adult who had documented congenital toxoplasmosis. (Photography by Thomas Monego, Dartmouth Hitchcock Medical Center.)

acute disease in adults have shown that acquired infection may account for more cases of retinochoroiditis than congenital infection.[78–80,97,98] Active disease causes pain, photophobia, and blurred vision in the absence of constitutional symptoms. On funduscopic examination, the vitreous is hazy, and elevated, pale-yellow, or white cotton-like patches are seen in the retina. Healed scars are pale with distinct margins and prominent black spots of choroidal pigment. Recurrent retinochoroiditis usually occurs at the borders of scars and may lead to blindness.

Disease in Persons with AIDS and Other Causes of Immunodeficiency

Toxoplasmosis is life-threatening for persons with impaired cellular immunity, in particular those with HIV infections and $CD4^+$ T-cell counts <100/μL of blood and persons receiving immunosuppressive medications.[8,9,99] Disease in these persons is more commonly due to reactivation of chronic infection than to newly acquired infection.[100,101] Historically, in many AIDS patients with antibodies to *Toxoplasma*

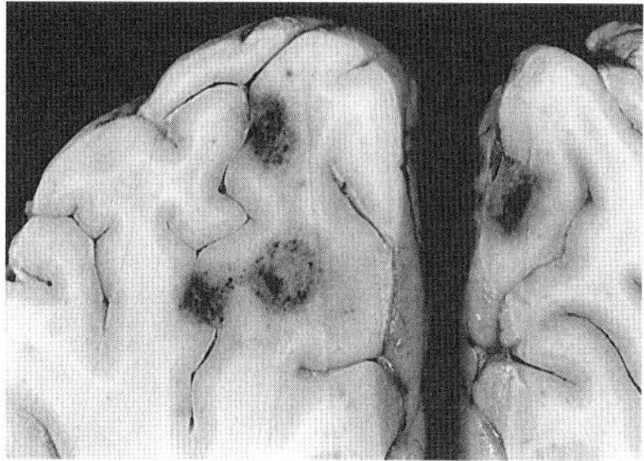

Figure 103.6 Section of brain showing lesions of toxoplasmosis at autopsy of a patient with acquired immunodeficiency syndrome (AIDS).

reactivated latent infections, but with use of antimicrobial drugs to prevent *Pneumocystis jirovecii* pneumonia and highly active antiretroviral therapy, the incidences of reactivation and toxoplasmosis-associated deaths have decreased.[102,103] Because of the high prevalence of chronic *Toxoplasma* infection in tropical climates, reactivated toxoplasmosis is a more frequently observed opportunistic infection among HIV-infected immigrants from developing regions than among HIV-infected natives of industrialized countries.[104] In many tropical regions, reactivation of toxoplasmosis is less common than might be expected because of the short life expectancy of HIV-infected persons due to other causes.[105] Persons who receive chemotherapy for organ transplantation or treatment of lymphomas and leukemia are susceptible to toxoplasmosis, although rates of reactivation in these persons are not as great as those among persons with AIDS.[8,106,107] Transplantation of *Toxoplasma*-infected organs (especially hearts) places antibody-negative recipients at risk of severe generalized toxoplasmosis.[108–110] Immunodeficient persons who receive leukocyte transfusions are also at risk of acquiring toxoplasmosis.[111]

The predominant manifestation of toxoplasmosis in immunocompromised persons is multifocal necrotizing encephalitis[9,99,100] (***Fig. 103.6***). Patients present with altered level of consciousness, headache, focal neurologic deficits, seizures, and often fever. CT and magnetic resonance (MR) scans of the head typically demonstrate multiple low-density lesions at the corticomedullary junction or in the basal ganglia that enhance following the administration of intravenous contrast (***Fig. 103.7***). There is often a mononuclear CSF pleocytosis and mild elevation of protein, but meningeal signs are uncommon. After the brain, the lungs and heart are the next most frequently involved organs in immunocompromised persons. Toxoplasmic myocarditis is frequently subclinical,[112] while a syndrome of rapidly progressive pulmonary infiltrates and shock may evolve when there is pulmonary infection.[113,114] Generalized toxoplasmosis is also seen in immunocompromised patients, and involvement of liver, spleen, lymph nodes, pancreas, intestines, thyroid, peritoneum, testes, retina, and spinal cord has been documented.[99,100,115–117] Without treatment, CNS toxoplasmosis and other severe forms of the disease in compromised hosts are fatal.

DIAGNOSIS

Differential Diagnosis

Because the differential diagnosis of the various forms of toxoplasmosis is broad, diagnostic confirmation in the laboratory is essential in most cases. Acute toxoplasmosis in healthy persons must be differentiated from mononucleosis due to Epstein–Barr virus or cytomegalovirus, acute HIV infection, other viral infections, cat-scratch disease, tuberculosis, fungal diseases, secondary syphilis, tularemia, African and American trypanosomiasis, visceral leishmaniasis, Hodgkin's disease, lymphoma, and sarcoidosis. The differential diagnosis of congenital toxoplasmosis includes congenital infections due to cytomegalovirus, herpes simplex, rubella,

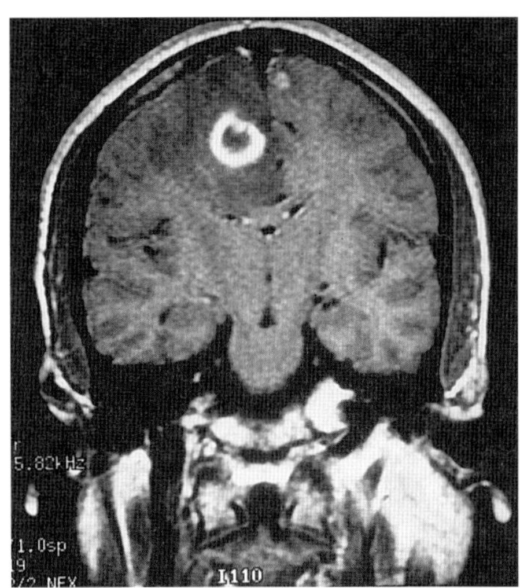

Figure 103.7 MR image of the brain showing a ring-enhancing hypodense lesion and surrounding edema in a patient with CNS toxoplasmosis and AIDS.

Listeria, syphilis, *Trypanosoma cruzi*, and erythroblastosis fetalis. The clinical presentation of acute toxoplasmic retinochoroiditis can be indistinguishable from uveitis associated with syphilis, tuberculosis, leprosy, or sarcoidosis. CNS toxoplasmosis in immunocompromised persons may mimic other causes of enhancing mass lesions such as lymphoma, metastatic carcinoma, tuberculoma and brain abscesses.

Direct Detection and Isolation of Parasites

Toxoplasma may be demonstrated on stained specimens of tissue, blood, sputum, amniotic fluid, and CSF.[118,119] The diagnosis of acute infection requires identification of tachyzoites, since finding tissue cysts does not distinguish acute from chronic infection.[52] Care is needed to distinguish *Toxoplasma* from other intracellular organisms such as *Histoplasma*, *Trypanosoma cruzi*, *Sarcocystis*, and *Leishmania*. Tachyzoites may be difficult to find in tissue sections stained with hematoxylin and eosin, and special techniques such as direct immunofluorescence or the peroxidase-antiperoxidase method may be necessary for their detection.[118,120] Parasites usually are not detected by microscopic examination of lymph nodes in cases of lymphadenitis, but the histopathologic changes may be sufficiently distinctive to permit a diagnosis of toxoplasmosis.[52,73,121]

Parasites may be recovered from both tissue cysts or tachyzoites in tissues and body fluids by inoculation into mice or tissue culture.[52,118–122] Assays based on the PCR[122] are extremely sensitive for the diagnosis of congenital toxoplasmosis when amniotic fluid is examined.[123,124] Such assays are commercially available and can also detect parasite DNA in blood,[38,125] CSF,[126] aqueous humor,[127] and fluid from bronchoalveolar lavage[128] with variable sensitivity.

Serologic Tests

Serologic testing remains an important means of confirming infection with *Toxoplasma*. Various methods are sensitive and specific for the detection of IgG antibody to *T. gondii* antigens.[7,74,118,129–135] Thus, the serologic diagnosis of toxoplasmosis acquired in the distant past is quite reliable. The Sabin–Feldman dye test detects both IgG and IgM antibodies by its ability to lyse live *T. gondii* in the presence of human complement and was for many years the gold standard.[7] Indirect fluorescent and antibody enzyme-linked immunosorbent assay (ELISA) are sensitive tests for the detection of IgG antibody and correlate well with the dye test in adults.[129] Isotype-specific ELISA for IgG, IgM, IgA, and IgE, IgM capture ELISA, immunosorbent agglutination (ISAGA), and others are available from some reference laboratories.[120–134] Results of these tests must be interpreted with age-matched populations. The IgM capture ELISA and IgM-ISAGA are sensitive for detection of specific IgM antibodies, but titers in infants less than 6 months old are lower than in adults.[132,134] While a negative IgM test nearly always rules out a recently acquired infection,[136] a positive test is less useful because commercially available tests have been reported to generate false positive results,[130,133] and specific IgM antibodies may remain detectable for greater than 1 year.[132] Determination of the functional avidity of anti-toxoplasma IgG antibody, by its ability to withstand dissociation from antigen in chaotropic salt solution, is useful in distinguishing recently acquired antibody (low avidity) from that seen in infection more than 4 months old (high avidity).[135,137,138] Avidity measurements are assay dependent and can vary between laboratories, but may be useful in differential diagnosis of lymphadenopathy as well as dating infection in pregnant women,[139] A commercial test based on IgG avidity is available in Europe, but not in the United States. Because low-avidity results may persist for up to a year, a battery of tests including ELISA for IgM, IgA, IgE, the dye test, and differential agglutination test should be employed for interpretation of low or equivocal avidity test results.[140,93]

Diagnosis of Specific Syndromes

The diagnosis of suspected acute acquired toxoplasmosis usually is confirmed by demonstrating rising titers of specific IgG antibodies or by detecting specific IgM antibodies. A single positive IgG test does not distinguish acute from chronic infection because antibodies to *Toxoplasma* persist indefinitely after acute infection, occasionally in high titers. Detection of specific IgM antibody in newborns by IgM-ELISA or the more sensitive IgM-ISAGA indicates congenital infection, but a negative result does not exclude the diagnosis because commonly available assays lack sensitivity to detect the low-avidity IgM antibodies synthesized by young infants.[89,132,134,131,142] Infants with severe toxoplasmosis at birth in particular may have negative IgM tests; in these cases, organisms usually are detected by PCR or by smears or culture of tissue, CSF, or blood.[89]

Specific IgG antibodies are nearly always present in the serum of infants with congenital toxoplasmosis. Uninfected infants born to infected mothers have specific IgG antibodies because of passive transfer of maternal IgG across the placenta, but these antibodies do not persist longer than 6–12 months in the absence of active infection.[142] Examination of the pattern of bands in Western blots between mothers and infants can be used to determine specific fetal antibody production.[136] In active retinochoroiditis, low titers of specific IgG antibodies are usually present, but IgM antibody in the serum is not detected.[94–96] Reference laboratories that can perform PCR and blood/aqueous humor serology ratios may improve diagnostic sensitivity for ocular toxoplasmosis.[143]

Immunocompromised patients with reactivation toxoplasmosis have positive specific IgG tests and negative IgM tests.[9,99] While the absence of specific IgG antibodies weighs heavily against the diagnosis of active toxoplasmosis in these patients, a positive titer does not distinguish active from latent infection. For this reason, the diagnosis of CNS toxoplasmosis in AIDS patients and other severely immunocompromised patients is usually made clinically.[9,99,142] Persons with a suggestive clinical history, positive specific IgG test, and typical radiographic findings are given a trial of anti-*Toxoplasma* chemotherapy. In cases of toxoplasmosis, clinical and radiographic improvement is seen within 7–10 days. A diagnostic brain biopsy is indicated if there is failure to improve within this time.[142] PCR amplification of *Toxoplasma* DNA in CSF has high predictive value, but relatively low sensitivity.[140] Brain biopsy without an antecedent therapeutic trial is indicated for immunocompromised persons with negative specific IgG tests or nonenhancing or single lesions and those who have been receiving prophylactic trimethoprim-sulfamethoxazole, because their CNS lesions are unlikely to be due to toxoplasmosis. Positron emission tomography may help distinguish CNS lymphoma from toxoplasmosis in persons with contrast-enhancing brain lesions.[144,145]

TREATMENT AND PROGNOSIS

Indications and Treatment Regimens

Most immunocompetent persons with primary toxoplasmosis do not require therapy unless there is visceral disease or persistent severe symptoms.[146] The exception is the pregnant mother, in whom early treatment may reduce the risk of fetal infection or may reduce the severity of disease if transplacental transmission has already occurred.[33,124,147,148] Retinochoroiditis is treated for 1–2 weeks after resolution of symptoms with both anti-*Toxoplasma* drugs and corticosteroids to reduce inflammation.[95,136] The frequency of recurrent episodes of retinochoroiditis may be reduced by intermittent therapy with trimethoprim-sulfamethoxazole.[149] Immunosuppressed patients require therapy to control progressive disease, and therapy must be extended for the period of cell-mediated immunosuppression to prevent relapse.[8,9,102,150]

Most drugs for treating toxoplasmosis are active only against the tachyzoite form of the parasite, although atovaquone has activity *in vitro* against tissue cysts as well.[151,152] Treatment even with atovaquone as a rule does not eradicate infection. Standard therapy for most indications is the combination of the oral agent pyrimethamine and a sulfonamide, which are synergistic when given together.[37,146,153] A loading dose of pyrimethamine 200 mg over 1 day in divided doses for adults or 2 mg/kg daily for 2–3 days for young children is followed by a daily dose of 1 mg/kg for adults or every 1–3 days for young children.[83,89,90,141,154] In immunocompromised adults with CNS toxoplasmosis or other severe disease, pyrimethamine 75–100 mg/day is given for 4–6 weeks followed by 25–50 mg/day for the duration of immunosuppression.[9,154,155] Sulfadiazine or triple sulfonamides are preferred over other sulfonamides, which have less activity against *T. gondii*. A loading dose of 50–75 mg/kg for adults or 75–100 mg/kg for infants is followed by daily doses of 75–100 mg/kg in four divided doses for adults or 100–150 mg/kg in four divided doses for infants. Leukovorin (folinic acid) 5–10 mg/day should be administered simultaneously to overcome the bone marrow-suppressive effects of pyrimethamine. Persons who receive pyrimethamine should have a peripheral blood cell and platelet count at least weekly. Clindamycin 600 mg orally or intravenously four times a day in combination with pyrimethamine has been successful in the treatment of adult AIDS patients with CNS toxoplasmosis who could not tolerate sulfonamides.[155–157]

Pyrimethamine is teratogenic and should not be used during the first trimester.[33] The macrolide antibiotic spiramycin (3–4 g/day in divided doses) (not an FDA approved drug in the United States) has been used safely during pregnancy.[33,81,147,148,158,159] It is not as effective as pyrimethamine and sulfonamides, but appears to reduce the rate of transplacental transmission. There is no uniformly accepted treatment regimen for congenital toxoplasmosis. Some authorities recommend standard doses of pyrimethamine and sulfonamides for 1 year, while others employ lower doses of pyrimethamine or give intermittent doses of spiramycin.[89,90,154,155] Other drugs that have activity against *T. gondii* include dapsone, azithromycin, clarithromycin, roxithromycin, atovaquone, minocycline, and rifabutin.[146]

Maintenance and Prophylactic Therapy in Immunocompromised Persons

Following treatment of active toxoplasmosis in immunocompromised patients, suppressive therapy should be continued for the duration of immunosuppression, which often is for life.[9,102,158,160–162] The most effective regimen is the combination of pyrimethamine 25–50 mg/day plus sulfadiazine 2–4 g/day with leukovorin 5 mg/day. This regimen also affords protection against *P. jirovecii* pneumonia. Clindamycin 300–450 mg orally three times a day has been used for persons who cannot tolerate sulfonamides.[9,155] Prophylaxis to prevent reactivation of toxoplasmosis should be given to all HIV-infected persons who have a positive serologic test for antibodies to *T. gondii* and CD4$^+$ T-lymphocyte counts of <200/μL.[163,164] The combination of trimethoprim and sulfamethoxazole is effective in the same doses used to prevent *P. jirovecii* pneumonia. The combination of dapsone 50 mg/day plus pyrimethamine 50 mg/week with leukovorin 10 mg/week[162] or atovaquone 750 mg of suspension twice a day[158] is an alternative for persons who cannot tolerate sulfonamides. The efficacy of azithromycin in preventing reactivation of toxoplasmosis is under study.[146] Suppressive therapy or prophylaxis for toxoplasmosis in HIV-infected patients can be safely withdrawn when the CD4$^+$ T-lymphocyte count has returned to greater than 200/μL and the HIV viral load has remained low for 6 months.[165]

Management of Acute Toxoplasmosis during Pregnancy

A strategy for the management of toxoplasmosis acquired by the pregnant woman has been outlined by French investigators.[124,135,148] When the diagnosis of acute toxoplasmosis is suspected, the mother receives spiramycin 1 g orally three or four times a day while awaiting results of confirmatory serologic tests. The purpose of spiramycin is to prevent fetal infection if this has not yet occurred. If the confirmatory studies indicate that infection may have been acquired after conception, an amniocentesis is performed as soon as possible at 17 weeks or later. Amniotic fluid is examined by a sensitive and specific PCR-based assay for *Toxoplasma*.[124] A positive assay confirms fetal infection, in which case one option is to terminate the pregnancy depending on the stage of gestation and the parents' wishes. If infection appears to have occurred late in pregnancy or if the parents wish to continue the pregnancy, pyrimethamine, sulfadiazine, and leukovorin are given until term. If the PCR assay is negative, the fetus is considered to be uninfected, and spiramycin is continued until delivery. The pregnancy is monitored closely with periodic fetal ultrasonography, and the amniocentesis is repeated if there is suspicion that fetal infection has occurred. The newborn is tested for infection at the time of delivery and treated aggressively if congenital toxoplasmosis is detected. This strategy has been shown to be effective in lowering the rate of severe congenital toxoplasmosis by identifying infections that occur early in pregnancy and that would have devastating consequences if the pregnancy were continued.[124,147,148] It is controversial whether it has otherwise achieved a significant reduction in the overall numbers of cases of congenital toxoplasmosis by reducing the rate of transplacental transmission when compared with historical data.[166,167] By identifying pregnancies in which transmission from the mother to the fetus has not occurred, it also has eliminated the need for considering termination of pregnancy on every occasion of acute maternal infection. In effect, it has spared as many as seven or eight uninfected fetuses from the possibility of therapeutic abortion for every fetus that is infected.

Variations of this strategy are practiced in countries of Europe where rates of maternal infection are high and the infrastructure exists for antenatal serologic screening of pregnant mothers to detect new infections as well as the laboratory expertise to perform accurate examination of amniotic fluid specimens. In countries such as the United States, where rates of acute maternal infection are low, this strategy is not uniformly practiced, and there is ongoing debate about its cost-effectiveness.[168–171] In several states, newborn screening for IgM antibodies to *T. gondii* is practiced to identify subclinical as well as symptomatic congenital infections soon after birth so that treatment can be given in a timely fashion to lower the risk of adverse sequelae.[50,89,134] It is not known, however, whether postnatal treatment is effective, because controlled trials have not been carried out.[172,173] In developing countries, where rates of maternal infections are high, the costs of antenatal screening and diagnosis or newborn screening and treatment are prohibitive.

PREVENTION AND CONTROL

Several studies have shown the efficacy of educational efforts to teach techniques for avoidance of acquisition of toxoplasmosis.[174,175] Seronegative pregnant women or immunocompromised persons should not be exposed to cat feces either in the setting of litter boxes or by digging in soils where cats have defecated.[176,177] Hands should be washed after contact with potentially contaminated soil or meat that may contain tissue cysts. Meat should be thoroughly cooked. In light of recent suggestions that dogs that roll in cat feces may carry infectious oocysts, pet grooming may be a risk factor for transmission.

One strategy for preventing human toxoplasmosis is to reduce the bradyzoite load in food animals. A commercial live vaccine is available in New Zealand and the European Union which reduces the incidence of *Toxoplasma*-induced abortion in sheep, and may reduce the load of parasites in herds under certain management schemes.[178] There is some evidence that careful husbandry practices in swine lower *Toxoplasma* burdens, including cooking feeds and excluding cats from farms.[2,176] A vaccine for cats that prevents oocyst shedding has been developed and tested, but is not commercially available.[179] Should it be marketed, it is not expected to have a major impact on the epidemiology of disease, but could be recommended in situations where cat owners are willing to pay to lower the risk of cat transmission. No human vaccine is available or near development.

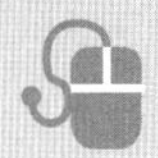

Access the complete reference list online at
http://www.expertconsult.com

Access the complete reference list online at http://www.expertconsult.com

CHAPTER 104

Lymphatic Filariasis

Thomas B. Nutman • James W. Kazura

INTRODUCTION

Lymphatic filariasis is caused by infection with any of three closely related parasitic nematodes – *Wuchereria bancrofti*, *Brugia malayi*, or *Brugia timori*. Unlike most other helminthiases endemic in tropical areas of the world, the burden of infection and disease in lymphatic filariasis occurs primarily during adulthood and not childhood or infancy. The greater impact of lymphatic filariasis on older age groups is due to the fact that infection burdens are determined by the chronicity and intensity of exposure to infective stages of the organisms, which cannot multiply in the mammalian host.

Because disease due to lymphatic filariasis is characterized by disfigurement of the limbs (elephantiasis) and genitalia (hydroceles and other anatomical changes in the male genitalia), it is often perceived as having adverse economic and psychosexual effects as well as medical consequences. This is particularly evident in many tropical countries where physical labor is still the major means of earning money. Indeed, lymphatic filariasis is among the leading health-related impediments to economic and social development in economically disadvantaged areas of the tropics.[1,2]

Lymphatic filariasis can be transmitted in any region of the world where the appropriate mosquito vector breeds. It currently is a significant health problem in tropical Africa, Asia, and the Indian subcontinent, many islands of the western and southern Pacific, and focal areas of Latin America. In the tropics, the geographic distribution of *W. bancrofti* and *B. malayi* infections is expanding due to increased numbers of breeding sites that appear when large numbers of people migrate from rural to urban areas. These pessimistic epidemiologic trends contrast with the recent gains and successes by the Global Program to Eliminate Lymphatic Filariasis using yearly single dose administration of antifilarial chemotherapy.[3]

THE AGENT

The existence of lymphatic filariasis has been recorded in ancient Chinese, Indian, Persian, and Arabic writings, but causative agents and their life cycles were not described until the late nineteenth century.[4,5] Microfilariae of *W. bancrofti*, first discovered by Demarquay in hydrocele fluid from a patient in Cuba in 1863,[6] were later identified in the urine by Wucherer in 1868[7] and in the blood by Lewis in 1872.[8] Manson described the periodicity of microfilariae in the peripheral blood[9] and demonstrated that mosquitoes transmit the parasite.[10] Bancroft first described the adult female worm[11] and Bourne later described the adult male worm.[12] Bancroft in 1899[13] and Low in 1900[14] established the mode of transmission of the parasite. Lichtenstein, Brug and Buckley were primarily responsible for identification of brugian parasites.[15]

W. bancrofti, *B. malayi*, and *B. timori* are threadlike nematodes having five morphologically and biochemically distinct stages in their life cycle (*Fig. 104.1*). Infective or third-stage larvae, transmitted to humans during blood feeding by mosquitoes, are deposited from the mouthparts of the mosquito in the vicinity of the skin puncture wound, and within several minutes make their way through the dermis to enter the local lymphatics. Several hours later, infective larvae shed their cuticle and develop a new surface (a process referred to as molting) that presents novel antigens and other molecules to the mammalian host. These fourth-stage larvae migrate centrally in lymphatic vessels and over a period of approximately 6–9 months develop into sexually mature adult male or female worms. Adult worms are considerably larger than larval stages (male worms are 20–40 mm in length, and female worms 40–100 mm) and have highly differentiated and complex reproductive and digestive systems. This stage of the parasite dwells primarily in the afferent lymphatics. Although all the anatomical areas in which adult lymphatic filariae live in humans are not known with certainty, large numbers are present in the lymphatics of the lower extremities (inguinal and obturator groups), upper extremities (axillary lymph nodes), and, for *W. bancrofti*, male genitalia (epididymis, spermatic cord, testicle). Based on observations of inflammatory reactions elicited by administration of drugs that kill adult worms, it is likely that adult filariae are distributed in subcutaneous tissues more than several centimeters distant from major lymph node groups. The mean life span of adult worms is approximately 5 years.

Following copulation with male worms, fecund female parasites release large numbers (often more than 10 000 per day) of first-stage larvae, microfilariae. Microfilariae are distinguished by their small size (260 mm in length and approximately 10 mm in width). Microfilariae of the lymphatic filariae have an acellular sheath, which is a chitin-containing remnant of the embryonic eggshell or vitelline membrane. Microfilariae of *W. bancrofti* and *B. malayi* differ morphologically from each other in the pattern of nuclei in the cephalic and caudal regions. *W. bancrofti* and *Brugia* microfilariae frequently have a nocturnal periodicity whereby the number present in the peripheral circulation peak at midnight (with large numbers between 10 p.m. and 4 a.m. with few or none present during the day). When absent from the peripheral circulation, microfilariae are sequestered in deep vascular beds of the lung and other organs. This peculiar behavior appears to be an example of adaptation to local ecological conditions in that the time at which peak parasitemia occurs coincides with the time when the local mosquito vectors take their blood meal.[16] The mechanisms that regulate microfilarial periodicity in humans are poorly understood.

After ingestion in a blood meal taken by a female mosquito, microfilariae exsheath within 24 hours, penetrate the chitinous gut wall of the mosquito, and migrate into the thoracic musculature. Over a period of 10–14 days, microfilariae mature to become third-stage larvae capable of infecting another human. The nature of the relationship between filarial larvae and the local mosquito populations has a profound impact on local transmission efficiency. For example, if mosquitoes ingest unusually large numbers of microfilariae, the overall efficiency of transmission may be

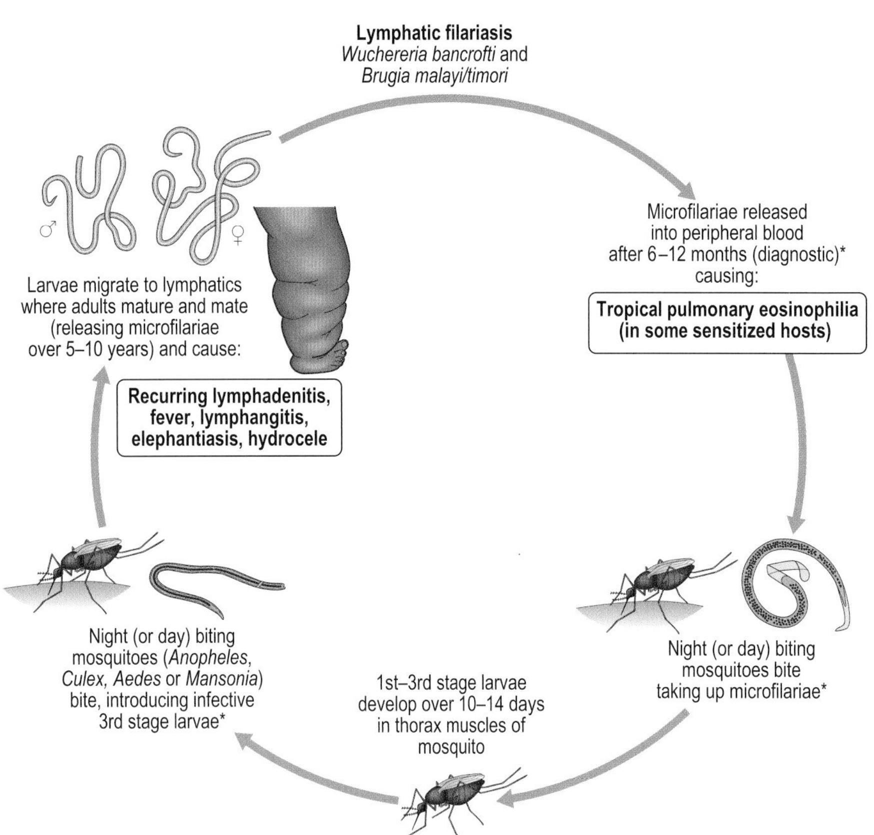

Figure 104.1 Life cycle of lymphatic filariasis. *For many filarial strains (e.g., *W. bancrofti* in Africa), microfilariae become abundant in blood only at night (nocturnal periodicity), when they may be detected by night-biting mosquitoes. For other strains, microfilariae are present by day and are spread by day-biting mosquitoes.

reduced by virtue of the fact that heavily infected mosquitoes have a shortened life span, precluding development of infective larvae. Conversely, in some mosquito–filarial interactions, there may be more efficient transmission at lower microfilarial densities, a phenomenon referred to as facilitation.

An important biologic feature of *W. bancrofti* and *Brugia* species relates to the fact that these nematodes carry an obligate bacterial endosymbiont *Wolbachia*. Ultrastructural studies performed in the 1970s recognized the presence of intracellular bacteria in adult worms and microfilariae;[17,18] but it was not until the late 1990s when molecular probes and genome sequence data became available that *Wolbachia* were definitively identified in human filarial parasites.[19,20] These endosymbiotic bacteria appear to affect filariae in several ways that are pertinent to human filariasis. Incubation of *Brugia* worms with tetracycline and other antibiotics known to kill *Wolbachia* diminishes the release of microfilariae and suppresses larval molting, suggesting that the bacteria are involved in embryogenesis and regulation of the parasite life cycle.[21,22] In the context of human lymphatic filariasis, administration of doxycycline to persons with *W. bancrofti* or *B. malayi* infection augments the suppression of microfilaremia induced by both ivermectin[23] or combination diethylcarbamazine/albendazole.[24] Moreover, 6 weeks of doxycycline has been shown to have macrofilaricidal (killing adult parasites) activity for both *Wuchereria* and *Brugia* infections.[24–26] There is a need, however, to identify anti-*Wolbachia* agents that can be given for short periods of time (and with broader applicability) than the tetracycline antibiotics, which cannot be given to pregnant women or young children.

EPIDEMIOLOGY

It is estimated that 120 million people (in 81 countries) are infected with one of the three genera of lymphatic filariae (***Fig. 104.2***).[27] More than 90% of infections are due to *W. bancrofti*, and, of these, the greatest number are in sub-Saharan Africa, Southeast Asia, and the western Pacific. The infection is prevalent in India, Indonesia, the Philippines, Papua New Guinea, and several Pacific countries such as parts of Fiji and Tahiti. Bancroftian filariasis is also a significant public health problem in many countries of tropical Africa (see ***Fig. 104.2***). Within Africa, *W. bancrofti* infection is not limited to these tropical zones since endemic foci are found as far north as the Nile delta in Egypt and Sudan. In the Americas, endemic foci persist in several islands in the Caribbean (Haiti and the Dominican Republic) and coastal areas of South America (Brazil and Guyana). There are no animal reservoirs of *W. bancrofti*.

Infection with *B. malayi* is limited to Asia (China, India, and Malaysia) and several Pacific island groups (e.g., Indonesia and the Philippines). There are fewer than 10 to 20 million persons in these areas infected with *B. malayi*, which may coexist with *W. bancrofti*. *B. malayi* infection is a zoonosis in that there are feline and primate reservoirs. *B. timori* infection is limited in its distribution to the islands of southeastern Indonesia.

Within a given geographic area, the distribution of lymphatic filariasis is highly focal such that the frequency of infection in some communities is high compared with physically approximate localities. This heterogeneity of infection patterns, both locally and globally, is due in large part to the peculiarities of the ecological relationships between the mosquito vector and the human host, and the impact of filarial parasites on both of these. Unlike other common vector-borne infectious diseases of the tropics (e.g., malaria), several genera of mosquitoes are capable of transmitting lymphatic filariae. *W. bancrofti* is transmitted in many rural areas of Africa and the Pacific by *Anopheles* species.[28] The proximity of human dwellings to breeding sites increases the risk of repeated contact with mosquitoes bearing infective larvae. In many urban areas of the world, including India, *Culex* species is the major vector of *W. bancrofti* and *B. malayi*.[29] Unlike anopheline mosquitoes, larvae of these mosquitoes breed

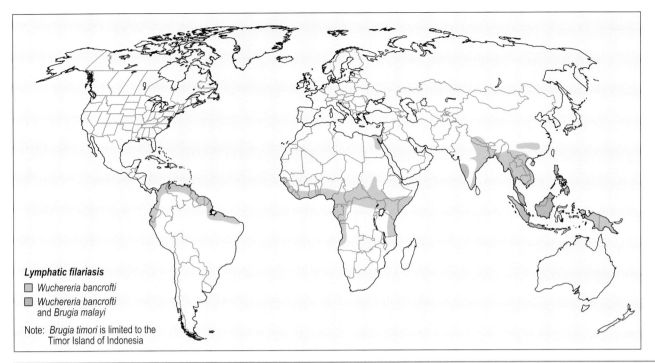

Figure 104.2 World map of lymphatic filariasis infection.

readily in small pools of water that form in discarded tires and cans. Other vectors include *Aedes aegypti* in some Pacific islands (e.g., Tahiti) and *Mansonia*, which transmits only *B. malayi*. These various genera of mosquitoes also differ in their efficiency of transmission. In general, anopheline mosquitoes are more efficient vectors of *W. bancrofti* than are culicine mosquitoes.

The age-related pattern of infection, as judged by the proportion of persons harboring microfilariae in the blood (the "microfilarial carrier rate," see below), increases gradually with age up until the third or fourth decade of life, after which it remains constant or slightly decreases. This epidemiologic pattern is related to the gradual slow accumulation of adult-stage worms over time. The proportion of the entire population or a specific age group with patent infection is remarkably variable in different endemic areas. In addition to these differences in infection patterns, there is remarkable variation in the frequency of various disease manifestations based on age and geographic area. Lymphatic disease, manifest by persistent lymphedema of the lower extremity or genital disease in males (see below), is rare in persons less than 10 years of age, and tends to increase gradually throughout life. Of the total 120 million persons estimated to be infected in all endemic areas, about one-third have clinically overt disease. The likelihood of developing such manifestations appears to be particularly high in some areas of the world, such as India, Pacific islands such as Papua New Guinea, and in equatorial Africa, whereas it is considerably lower in the Caribbean and South America. Local transmission conditions may account for the striking heterogeneity of disease manifestations that may be observed within a given geographic area. Indeed the cumulative exposure to infective larvae may be an important risk factor for lymphatic pathology at the population level.[30]

THE DISEASE

Infection with *W. bancrofti*, *B. malayi* or *B. timori* can cause a wide variety of clinical manifestations, ranging from those without apparent clinical disease to those with lymphedema and/or severe disfigurement of the limbs and genitalia. From the clinical perspective, it should be stressed that there is a great deal of overlap in these symptom complexes, several of which may occur contemporaneously.

Subclinical Patent Infection

The overwhelming majority of filarial-infected inhabitants in endemic areas have few overt clinical manifestations of their filarial infection despite large numbers of circulating microfilariae in the peripheral blood.[31] Although they may be clinically asymptomatic, virtually all persons with patent *W. bancrofti* or *B. malayi* infection (microfilaria- and/or circulating filarial antigen-positive) have some degree of subclinical disease that includes microscopic hematuria and/or proteinuria,[32] dilated (and tortuous) lymphatics (visualized by lymphoscintigraphy[33–35]), and, in men with *W. bancrofti* infection, scrotal lymphangiectasia (detectable by ultrasound).[36–38]

Acute Adenolymphangitis

Acute adenolymphangitis (ADL) is often the first manifestation of lymphatic filariasis. It is characterized by the sudden onset of high fever, painful, lymph node and lymphatic inflammation (lymphangitis and lymphadenitis), and transient local edema. The lymphangitis is retrograde, extending peripherally from the lymph node draining the area where the adult parasites reside – the retrograde nature of the lymphadenitis distinguishes filarial-induced disease from bacterial-induced lymphangitis. Regional lymph nodes (e.g., inguinal, obdurator, axillary, epitrochlear) are often enlarged, and the entire lymphatic channel can become indurated and inflamed. Concomitant local thrombophlebitis can occur as well. In brugian filariasis, a single local abscess may form along the involved lymphatic tract and subsequently rupture to the surface. The lymphadenitis and lymphangitis can involve both the upper and lower extremities in both bancroftian and brugian filariasis, but involvement of the genital lymphatics occurs almost exclusively with *W. bancrofti* infection.[39] This genital involvement can be manifested by funiculitis, epididymitis, scrotal pain, tenderness as well as a condition termed lymph scrotum.[40]

In endemic areas, another type of acute disease – dermatolymphangioadenitis (DLA)[41,42] – is recognized as a syndrome that includes high fever, chills, myalgias, and headache. Edematous inflammatory plaques clearly demarcated from normal skin are seen. Vesicles, ulcers, and hyperpigmentation may also be noted. There is often a history of trauma, burns,

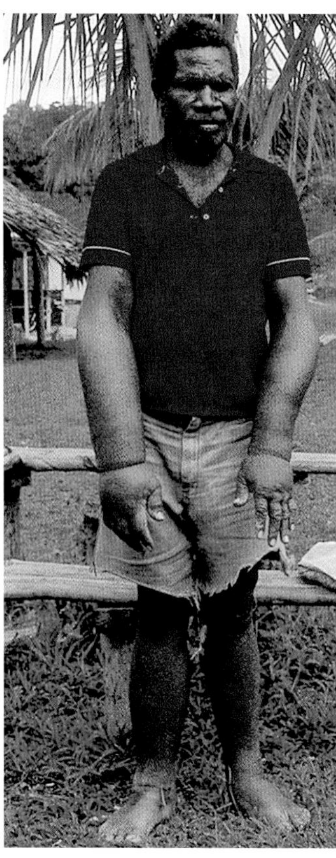

Figure 104.3 Lymphedema of the upper and lower extremities in a 50-year-old man. Swelling had been present for approximately 10 years, and the level of microfilaremia was 1000 parasites per milliliter of blood.

radiation, insect bites, punctiform lesions, or chemical injury. Entry lesions, especially in interdigital areas, are common. DLA is often diagnosed as cellulitis.

Lymphedema of the Arms, Legs, and Breasts

Swelling of the upper or lower extremities is the most common chronic manifestation of lymphatic filarial infection. Disease of the lower extremities is more prevalent.

Leg involvement in bancroftian filariasis may include the entire limb, whereas only the area below the knee is usually involved in brugian filariasis. The World Health Organization has adopted a grading system to quantify the severity of involvement.[43] Grade I indicates pitting edema that is reversible upon elevation of the leg; grade II, non-pitting edema that does not resolve with elevation of the extremity; grade III, non-pitting edema of the limb that is not reversible with elevation and with thickened skin or skin folds; and grade IV, non-pitting edema with fibrotic and verrucous skin changes (elephantiasis), and the presence of skin folds (*Fig. 104.3*). Although both lower extremities may be involved, asymmetrical involvement is the rule.

In some persons with filarial-associated edema, the overlying skin may exude serous fluid suggestive of lymph. Although it is possible that this sign occurs as a result of increased hydrostatic pressure in the lymphatics draining the skin, skin turgor alone cannot reliably be used to distinguish between edema due to lymphatic disease and that from other causes, such as cardiac failure and liver disease.

Unilateral or bilateral involvement of the female breast occurs in adult residents of filarial endemic areas. This should be distinguished from chronic mastitis and other causes of chronic breast inflammation.

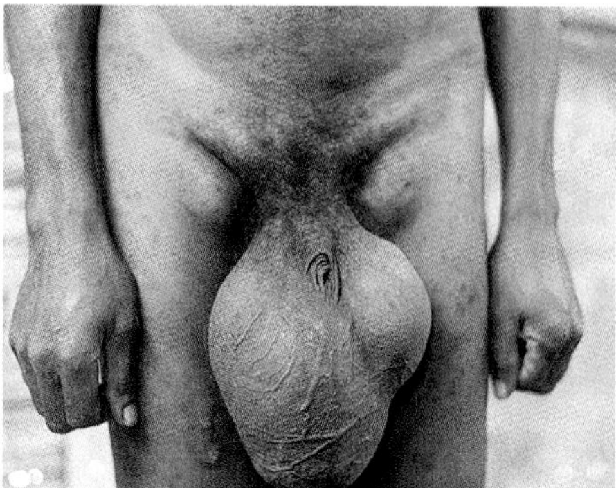

Figure 104.4 Hydrocele and inguinal lymph node enlargement in bancroftian filariasis. The patient is a 40-year-old man who first experienced epididymitis at the age of 20. The hydrocele has been present for 2 years.

Disease Involving the Genitourinary System

Along with lymphatic disease of the lower extremities, disease of the male genitalia is the most common manifestation of bancroftian filariasis. Indeed, in many endemic areas, its prevalence is greater than that of lymphedema. Genital involvement is uncommon in *Brugia* infection. The prevalence of disease of the female genitalia is not known since systematic surveys have not included examination of this anatomical area. Anecdotal evidence suggests that the frequency of vulvar disfigurement is low. Genital disease is usually not experienced until the teenage years. Acute painful episodes of epididymitis or funiculitis last several days and are accompanied by fever and malaise. Involvement is most commonly unilateral.

Hydroceles

Chronic disease of the male genitals mostly produces hydroceles, which vary in diameter from less than 5 cm to over 30 cm (*Fig. 104.4*). As is the case with other causes of hydrocele, the scrotal contents appear translucent when transilluminated. Hydroceles are usually not painful unless they are complicated by acute epididymitis or funiculitis. Thickening of the spermatic cord commonly accompanies hydroceles. The skin of the scrotum may also be thickened and have a "brawny" character on palpation. If hydrocele fluid is drained, it is clear and straw-colored. Parasites are usually not found in this fluid. Inguinal lymph nodes and other nearby lymph nodes may also be enlarged (see *Fig. 104.4*).

Lymphedema of the genitalia

Swelling of the scrotum when accompanied by thickened scrotal or penile skin may have a characteristic "peau d'orange" appearance.[39] In long-standing cases verrucous lesions and lymphorrhea are common,[40] the latter being a condition in which lymph oozes out to the exterior directly from dilated ruptured lymphatic vessels in the scrotal wall. The genitals may be grossly deformed and terms such as "ram horn penis" have been used to describe the gross distortion of the penis seen in this condition.

Chyluria

Chyluria, resulting from obstruction or physiologic impairment of the renal lymphatics with passage of lymph from the lacteals draining the genitourinary tract, is a rare but serious manifestation of lymphatic filariasis. Chyluria may have serious nutritional consequences in that large amounts of fat and protein are lost in the urine. Its precise frequency in filarial endemic areas has not been established, but is exceedingly low compared to lymphedema of the extremities and hydroceles.[44]

Tropical Pulmonary Eosinophilia

Tropical pulmonary eosinophilia (TPE) is a distinct syndrome that develops in some individuals infected with either *W. bancrofti* or *B. malayi*.[45,46] The majority of cases have been reported from India, Pakistan, Sri Lanka, Brazil, Guyana, and Southeast Asia. The main clinical features include paroxysmal cough and wheezing that are usually nocturnal (and probably related to the nocturnal periodicity of microfilariae), weight loss, low-grade fever, adenopathy, and pronounced blood eosinophilia (>3000 eosinophils/μL). Chest radiographs may be normal but generally show increased bronchovascular markings; diffuse miliary lesions or mottled opacities in the middle and lower lung fields. Tests of pulmonary function show restrictive abnormalities in most cases and obstructive defects in half. Total serum IgE levels (10 000–100 000 ng/mL) and antifilarial antibody titers are characteristically elevated. Typically those with TPE do not have microfilaremia. Administration of the antifilarial drug diethylcarbamazine (see below) leads to significant symptomatic improvement with commensurate decreases in eosinophilia and serum IgE. If patients with TPE are not treated appropriately, the disease may progress to chronic restrictive lung disease with interstitial fibrosis.[47]

Lymphatic Filariasis in Expatriates and Travelers

American servicemen returning from prolonged exposure to infectious mosquitoes in the South Pacific during World War II and French soldiers exposed in Indochina (now Vietnam) suffered from acute episodes of acute adenolymphangitis of the legs accompanied by eosinophilia. These acute disease manifestations were apparently caused by immune-mediated inflammatory responses to developing larvae, and resolved on departure from the endemic area.[48] Progression to chronic lymphedema or elephantiasis was rare. Studies of Indonesian transmigrants from nonendemic to endemic regions[49] as well as studies in which volunteers were experimentally infected with infective larvae of *B. malayi*[50] provide corroboration of these early clinical manifestations.

The risk of developing acute or chronic manifestations of lymphatic filariasis for the traveler to endemic areas is extraordinarily small, given the inefficiency of transmission by infected mosquitoes, although it has been seen rarely.[51]

PATHOGENESIS AND IMMUNITY

The precise and likely multiple mechanisms leading to the diverse clinical manifestations of lymphatic filariasis have not been established. However, several factors have been suggested to underlie the development of lymphedema, including parasite-derived factors[52,53] that may be responsible for the lymphatic dilatation seen early in infection, host genetic susceptibility,[54–59] secondary bacterial infections,[60–63] specific host adaptive immune responses to parasite antigens,[64,65] and inflammatory responses to dying or dead parasite material.[39,60,66–69]

Establishing the relative importance of these diverse factors and a central unifying hypothesis to explain the pathogenesis of human lymphatic filariasis has been difficult because the onset of disease occurs over a period of years or decades and because of the marked heterogeneity in transmission and disease in geographically distinct filarial-endemic areas. The immunologic basis for the relative lack of pathology seen in the majority of individuals with patent infection, however, has been reasonably well studied in both cross-sectional and longitudinal population-based studies. Studies in animal models and *in vitro* human systems have suggested that the initial immune response to infective stage larvae (L3) and to the next developmental stages (L4 and early adult stages) are dominated by proinflammatory and a mixed Th1-like and Th2-like T-cell responses.[70,71] With the onset of patency (when microfilariae appear in the blood), there is a marked diminution of the parasite antigen-specific T-cell responses (both proliferation and Th1 cytokine responses)[72–78] that is primarily mediated by interleukin (IL)-10[79–82] and other regulatory cell populations (e.g., adaptive and natural Treg cells, alternatively activated macrophages/monocytes[83–85]).

Examination of protective immunity in lymphatic filariasis in human populations has been extraordinarily difficult. However, population-based studies[86–88] have identified groups of individuals who appear to be infection-free despite long-term exposure to the filarial parasites. When looked at immunologically, on balance cells from these individuals are more likely to respond to parasite antigen than were those with patent infection. The best evidence, however, for the induction of protective immunity has come from studies in animals (jirds, cats, ferrets) permissive for *Brugia* spp. given radiation attenuated L3; in these studies irradiated L3s induced protection to varying degrees (60–95% protection from challenge).[89–92] Attempts with subunit vaccines using recombinant antigens or DNA vaccination have been less successful but levels of protection that range between 30% and 69% have been achieved.[93–97]

DIAGNOSIS

Lymphatic filariasis is diagnosed by a combination of the appropriate epidemiologic history, physical findings, and laboratory tests. In residents of endemic areas, the appearance of lymphedema of the extremities or disease of the male genitalia is most likely due to filarial infection if there is no other obvious other secondary cause, such as trauma to the lymphatics or congestive heart failure.

A definitive diagnosis can be made only by detection of the parasites, parasite antigen, or parasite DNA. Adult worms localized in lymphatic vessels or nodes are largely inaccessible. Examination, however, of the scrotum or the female breast using high-frequency ultrasound in conjunction with Doppler techniques may result in the identification of motile adult worms within dilated lymphatics.[98–101] Worms may be visualized in the lymphatics of the spermatic cord in up to 80% of infected men.[98] Live adult worms have a distinctive pattern of movement within the lymphatic vessels (termed the *filaria dance sign*).[36,98]

Microfilariae can be found in blood, in hydrocele fluid, or (occasionally) in other body fluids. Such fluids can be examined microscopically, either directly using a Giemsa-stained thin blood smear or – for greater sensitivity – after concentration of the parasites by the passage of blood through a polycarbonate cylindrical 3–5 μm pore filter (Nuclepore) or by the centrifugation of fluid fixed in 2% formalin (Knott's concentration technique).[102] The timing of blood collection is critical and should be based on the periodicity of the microfilariae in the endemic region involved.

Many infected individuals do not have microfilaremia, and definitive diagnosis in such cases can be difficult. Assays for circulating antigens of *W. bancrofti* permit the diagnosis of both microfilaremic and amicrofilaremic infection. Two tests are commercially available: one is an enzyme-linked immunosorbent assay (ELISA)[103] and the other a rapid-format immunochromatographic card test.[104] Both assays have sensitivities that range from 96% to 100% and specificities that approach 100%. There are currently no tests for circulating antigens in brugian filariasis.

Polymerase chain reaction (PCR)-based assays for DNA of *W. bancrofti* and *B. malayi* in blood have been developed.[105–110] A number of studies indicate that this diagnostic method is of equivalent or greater sensitivity compared with parasitologic methods, detecting patent infection in almost all infected subjects.

Antibody-based assays for diagnosing filarial infection have typically used crude parasite extract and have suffered from poor specificity. Improvements have been made by the use of detection of antifilarial IgG_4 antibodies[111] in that they have relatively less cross-reactivity to non-filarial helminth antigens. Specificity has also been improved by the use of species-specific recombinant antigens for both brugian and bancroftian infection;[112] indeed a diagnostic dipstick test has been developed for use in areas endemic for brugian filariasis.[113]

In cases of suspected lymphatic filariasis, radionuclide lymphoscintigraphic imaging of the limbs reliably demonstrates widespread lymphatic abnormalities in both subclinical microfilaremic persons and those with clinical manifestations of lymphatic pathology. While of potential utility in the delineation of anatomic changes associated with infection, lymphoscintigraphy is unlikely to assume primacy in the diagnostic evaluation of individuals with suspected infection.

It is important to note, however, that it is not possible to exclude a diagnosis of filarial-induced disease in the absence of circulating antigens or parasites since disease may persist in persons with so-called burned-out infections. This situation may occur in persons who have received multiple courses of treatment or who have left endemic areas.

TREATMENT AND PROGNOSIS

Chemotherapeutic Agents

Diethylcarbamazine (DEC, 6 mg/kg daily for 12 days), which has both macro- and microfilaricidal properties, remains the treatment of choice for the individual with active lymphatic filariasis (microfilaremia, antigen positivity, or adult worms on ultrasound), although albendazole (400 mg twice daily for 21 days) has also demonstrated macrofilaricidal efficacy. The use of a 4- to 6-week course of doxycycline (targeting the intracellular *Wolbachia*) has also been demonstrated to have significant macrofilaricidal activity,[24,26] as has daily DEC/albendazole used for 7 days.[114] Adding diethylcarbamazine to a 3-week course of doxycycline has also recently been shown to be efficacious.[25]

Regimens that utilize combinations of single doses of albendazole (400 mg) and either DEC (6 mg/kg) or ivermectin (200 μg/kg) have all been demonstrated to have a sustained microfilaricidal effect,[115–118] and are the mainstay of control programs in Africa (albendazole/ivermectin) or elsewhere (albendazole/DEC) for the eradication of lymphatic filariasis (see below).

Side effects of DEC treatment include fever, chills, arthralgias, headaches, nausea, and vomiting. In heavily infected patients, painful nodules in the skin, lymph node enlargement, and epididymitis may appear. Both the development and the severity of these reactions are directly related to the number of microfilariae circulating in the bloodstream and likely represent an acute inflammatory reaction to either the antigens being released by dead and dying parasites or *Wolbachia* endosymbionts freed from their intracellular niche. Ivermectin has a side effect profile similar to that of DEC when used in lymphatic filariasis. Albendazole (when used in single dose regimens) has relatively few side effects associated with its use in lymphatic filariasis, but when used in multiday regimens has been associated with painful scrotal nodules.

Pathology Based Therapy

As has already been mentioned, a growing body of evidence indicates that, although they may be clinically asymptomatic, most patients with *W. bancrofti* or *B. malayi* microfilaremia have some degree of subclinical disease (hematuria, proteinuria, abnormalities on lymphoscintigraphy). Thus, early treatment of asymptomatic individuals is recommended to prevent further lymphatic damage.

For ADL, supportive treatment (including the administration of antipyretics and analgesics) is recommended, as is antibiotic therapy if secondary bacterial infection is likely. Similarly, because lymphatic disease is associated with the presence of adult worms, treatment is recommended for microfilaria-negative adult worm carriers.

In persons with chronic manifestations of lymphatic filariasis, treatment regimens that emphasize hygiene, prevention of secondary bacterial infections, and physiotherapy have gained wide acceptance for morbidity control. These regimens are similar to those recommended for lymphedema of most non-filarial causes, and are known by a variety of names, including *complex decongestive physiotherapy* and *complex lymphedema therapy*. Drainage of hydroceles provides immediate relief, though they recur in the absence of drug therapy or surgical removal of the tunica albuginea.

With chronic manifestations of lymphatic filariasis, drug treatment should be reserved for individuals with evidence of active infection; therapy has been associated with clinical improvement and, in some cases, reversal of lymphedema.

In severe cases of deforming elephantiasis, surgical approaches involving lymphatic-venous and nodal-venous anastomoses have been somewhat successful in diminishing the degree of leg swelling,[119] as has reconstructive surgery for genital involvement. The long-term effects of these expert surgical techniques have not been determined.

PREVENTION AND CONTROL

Individual protection against filarial infection may be achieved by avoiding contact with infected mosquitoes. This can be done by use of personal protective measures including bednets, particularly those impregnated with insecticides such as permethrin.

Created in 1997, the Global Programme to Eliminate Lymphatic Filariasis (GPELF) was based on mass drug administration with single annual doses of diethylcarbamazine plus albendazole (non-African regions) or albendazole plus ivermectin in Africa.[116,120–124] Information at the end of 2008 indicates that >695 million persons in 51 countries have thus far participated.[125] Not only has there been success in eliminating lymphatic filariasis in some defined areas, but also collateral benefit in averting disability (estimated 32 million disability-adjusted life-years averted)[122] and treating intestinal helminths and other conditions (e.g., scabies, lice). The strategy of the global program is being refined and guided by ongoing research aimed at understanding the ecology and transmission efficiency of the various mosquito vector species and integration with other mass treatment strategies (e.g., deworming programs, malaria control, trachoma control).[126–132]

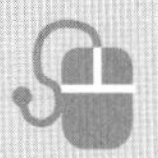

Access the complete reference list online at
http://www.expertconsult.com

Access the complete reference list online at http://www.expertconsult.com

CHAPTER 105

Loiasis and *Mansonella* Infections

Amy D. Klion • Thomas B. Nutman

LOIASIS

INTRODUCTION

Loiasis, infection with the filarial nematode *Loa loa*, is limited to and highly endemic in western and central Africa. Although generally associated with low morbidity, loiasis is the third most common reason for a medical visit in some hyperendemic regions[1] and the most common filarial infection acquired by travelers,[2] affecting as many as 30% of long-term visitors to endemic areas.[3] Characteristic clinical features include Calabar swellings (transient localized angioedema) and subconjunctival migration of the adult parasite (eye worm). Severe complications of infection, including cardiomyopathy, nephropathy, and fatal encephalitis, are rare, but do occur.

THE AGENT

Although extraction of an adult worm from the eye of an African slave was reported in 1770,[4] clinical manifestations of loiasis were not described until 1781.[5] The association between eye worm (synonyms: *Filaria loa*, *F. oculi humani*, *F. lacrimalis*, and *F. subconjunctivalis*), Calabar swellings, and *Microfilaria diurna* (Manson 1891) – a novel species of microfilaria in day blood samples of persons from the Congo – remained debatable until the parasite's life cycle was elucidated in the early 1900s.[6,7]

Infective larvae are transmitted to humans by bites of infected female *Chrysops* species flies.[8] Over 6–12 months, these larvae develop into white, threadlike adult worms that migrate through subcutaneous tissues, including the subconjunctiva (hence eye worm), at a rate of up to 1 cm/minute. Adult worms may live for 17 years.[9] In bisexual infections, offspring microfilariae (***Fig. 105.1***) are released into the bloodstream. Ingestion of microfilariae in a blood meal by the *Chrysops* vector completes the cycle (***Fig. 105.2***). Blood microfilarial levels range from undetectable to >100 000 parasites/mL and are remarkably constant in infected individuals over time.[10]

The diurnal periodicity of bloodborne microfilariae coincides with the temporal feeding patterns of the principal vectors, *Chrysops silacea* and *C. dimidiata*.[11] These day-biting flies living primarily in the canopy of the rainforest,[12] are attracted by movement,[13] dark skin and clothing, and wood smoke,[14,15] and bite most frequently in shaded areas or indoors. With simian strains of *Loa loa*, morphologically similar to human *Loa loa*,[16,17] microfilariae demonstrate nocturnal periodicity and infections are transmitted by night-biting *Chrysops* species that do not bite humans.[18]

Unlike most filarial parasites that infect humans, *Loa loa* does not harbor the bacterial endosymbiont *Wolbachia*.[19–21]

EPIDEMIOLOGY

Loa loa causes an estimated 3–13 million chronic infections in residents of endemic areas in western and central Africa,[22] including the coastal plains of northern Angola, southeastern Benin, Cameroon, Central African Republic, Chad, Republic of the Congo, Equatorial Guinea, Gabon, Nigeria, Sudan, and the Democratic Republic of Congo.[23,24] Rare cases have been reported in the region from Ghana to Guinea[25,26] and in Uganda,[27,28] Mali,[29] Zambia,[23,30] and Ethiopia.[31] The occurrence of *Loa loa*-related encephalopathy following mass treatment of onchocerciasis has led to renewed interest in mapping the distribution of loiasis in Africa, and subsequently to the validated implementation of new epidemiologic techniques, including remote sensing for suitable *Chrysops* spp. habitats[32] and RAPLOA, a rapid assessment method to determine the proportion of community members with a history of eye worm.[33,34]

Most infected people have histories of prolonged exposure (>4 months' residence in an endemic area),[2,35] although infections can occur after repeated short stays,[36] and anecdotally after 1–2 weeks of intense exposure. In hyperendemic areas, exposure, defined by the presence of filaria-specific antibodies, may approach 100%,[37] and up to 40% of residents may be clinically infected (i.e., have clinical symptoms or microfilaremia).[1] Although nonhuman primates can be experimentally infected with *Loa loa*, natural infection is restricted to humans.[38]

Alterations in the ecology of rainforests, primarily due to rubber plantations, which have a lower canopy and scant undergrowth, have led to an increased prevalence of loiasis in some regions.[39] Conversely, village development with replacement of forests with farmland may decrease transmission by reducing vector populations.[40] The need for both

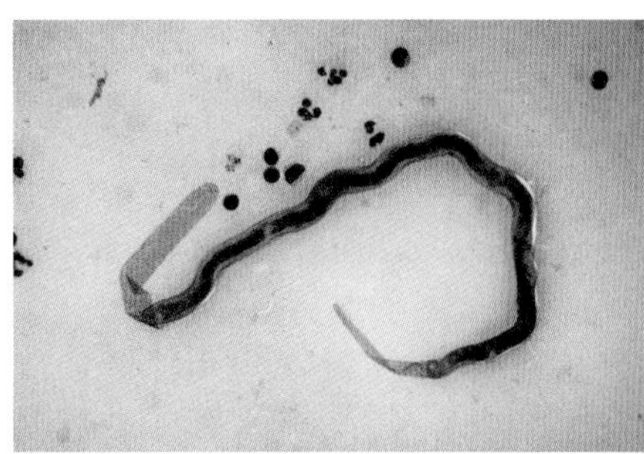

Figure 105.1 Microfilaria of *Loa loa* in a hematoxylin-stained thick smear of peripheral blood (magnification, ×180). (From Armed Forces Institute of Pathology.)

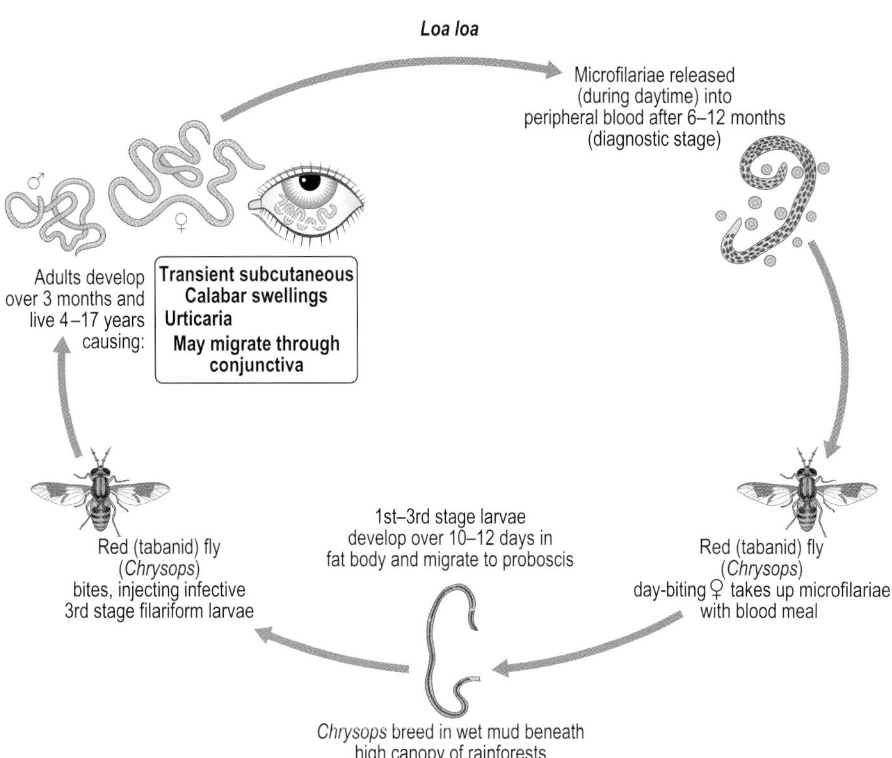

Figure 105.2 Life cycle of *Loa loa*.

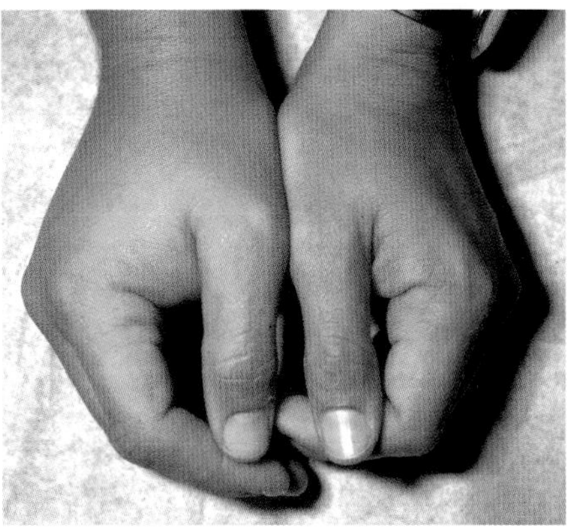

Figure 105.3 Calabar swelling of the right hand.

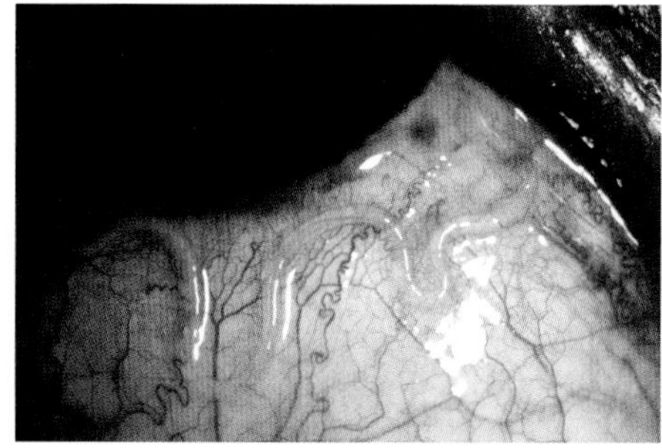

Figure 105.4 Subconjunctival migration of an adult *Loa loa*. (From Armed Forces Institute of Pathology.)

reservoirs of infected persons and conditions that support the insect vector is illustrated by the lack of establishment of endemic foci of loiasis in Cameroon following immigration of numbers of microfilaremic people to a nonendemic region,[41] or in Louisiana (US), where *Chrysops* vectors capable of transmission of loiasis to humans exist,[42] but microfilaremic individuals are exceedingly rare.

THE DISEASE

Whereas the majority of infected persons from endemic areas are asymptomatic despite high levels of microfilaremia, visitors to endemic areas are often symptomatic, with "allergic symptoms," including pruritus, urticaria, and transient, migratory angioedema (Calabar swellings).[35,43] Clinical complications, with the exception of renal abnormalities, are also more common in nonendemic patients, in whom bloodborne microfilariae are rarely detectable. Characteristic laboratory abnormalities in loiasis include eosinophilia (often >3000/μL) and elevated serum IgE, both of which are more pronounced in symptomatic amicrofilaremic patients.

Calabar Swellings

Calabar swellings (*Fig. 105.3*) may occur anywhere on the body, but are most common on the face and extremities, and may be brought on following local trauma. These are evanescent, migratory angioedematous swellings in which edema is often preceded by local pain or itching lasting 1–2 hours after which a 10–20 cm non-erythematous, non-pitting swelling develops. The swelling generally resolves in 2–4 days, but may last as long as several weeks. Recurrences are common in the same site, but may develop anywhere on the body. The precise cause of Calabar swellings remains unproven, although they are thought to represent hypersensitivity responses to antigens or microfilariae released by a migrating adult parasite.

Eye Worm

Migration of the adult worm across the conjunctiva occurs with equal frequency in natives of and visitors to endemic areas[43] (*Fig. 105.4*). Conjunctival migration, often associated with transient intense edematous conjunctivitis, resolves without ocular sequelae.

Complications

Renal involvement, manifest by hematuria or proteinuria, occurs in up to 30% of infected persons and may be transiently exacerbated by treatment.[35,43,44] Proposed mechanisms include immune complex glomerulonephritis or mechanical trauma due to filtration of large numbers of bloodborne microfilariae,[44–47] although microfilariae are rarely seen in the urine.[46,48] Azotemia or progression to renal failure is uncommon.

Encephalitis that may develop after antifilarial chemotherapy is the most serious complication of *Loa loa* infection.[49] It is most common in persons with high levels of microfilaremia (>5000 microfilariae/mL blood) and is associated with the presence of microfilariae in the cerebrospinal fluid (CSF).[50,51] Symptoms range from headache, irritability, and insomnia, to coma and death. In fatal cases, autopsies demonstrated generalized acute cerebral edema or encephalitis with necrotizing granulomas around degenerating microfilariae.[49] More recently, mass distribution of ivermectin in areas where *Loa loa* and *Onchocerca volvulus* are co-endemic has revealed similar posttreatment central nervous system effects.[47,52] Although mechanisms underlying these neurologic sequelae of ivermectin treatment remain unclear,[53] hemorrhages in the palpebral conjunctiva and retina may be an early marker and are more frequent with high levels of *Loa loa* microfilaremia.[54] Perivascular inflammation and vascular wall thickening in the brain parenchyma have been described in a fatal case of post-ivermectin *Loa loa*-related encephalopathy, although no microfilariae were seen, likely due to the delay (54 days) between administration of ivermectin and the fatal outcome.[55]

Other less common complications of loiasis include entrapment neuropathy,[56,57] psychiatric disturbances,[58] arthritis,[59,60] lymphadenitis,[61] hydrocele,[62] pleural effusion,[63,64] retinal artery occlusion,[65] posterior uveitis,[66,67] macular retinopathy,[68] blindness,[69] and endomyocardial fibrosis (EMF).[35,70,71] Circumstantial evidence linking EMF to loiasis includes their similar geographic distribution and the detection of antifilarial antibodies in some persons with EMF.[72] Clinical resolution of biopsy-proven EMF in a nonendemic patient with loiasis following antifilarial treatment provides additional support for this association,[35] most likely secondary to massive reactive eosinophilia and eosinophil infiltration of the endomyocardium.

Other

Microfilariae and adult worms have been detected in pathologic and cytology specimens from various unusual anatomical locations,[73,74] and calcified adult worms may be detected by routine radiography in some infected persons.[75,76]

PATHOGENESIS AND IMMUNITY

Many clinical manifestations of loiasis, including Calabar swellings, are likely immunologically mediated and are more severe in visitors to endemic areas than in the endemic population.[35,43] This clinical hyperresponsiveness is accompanied by hypergammaglobulinemia, marked eosinophilia, increased serum IgE levels, and vigorous humoral and cellular immune responses to filarial antigens.[77] In contrast, asymptomatic persons tend to have high levels of microfilaremia and relatively suppressed immune responses to filarial antigens.[43] Mechanisms underlying these differences, while ill-understood, may involve genetic factors,[78] prenatal sensitization to filarial antigens, or differences in duration or degree of exposure to parasite antigens.[79–81]

As with most helminth infections, *Loa loa* infection elicits eosinophilia (see Chapter 131) and elevations of serum IgE, which are most pronounced in persons with symptomatic infections.[43] Eosinophils in these patients express surface markers associated with cellular activation, suggesting that activated eosinophils may contribute to anti-parasite immunity[82] and/or may mediate pathologic changes. The presence of blood eosinophilia has been associated with secretion of interleukin (IL)-5 by mitogen-stimulated peripheral blood mononuclear cells (PBMCs) from patients with loiasis and other filarial infections.[83] Further, filarial antigens can induce IL-4 and IL-5 secretion from PBMCs or $CD4^+$ T cells *in vitro*.[84,85] Similarly, IgE can also be induced by parasite antigens *in vitro*, and persons with loiasis have markedly elevated numbers of B cells and T cells capable of responding to parasite antigen *in vitro*.[85–88] Complement activation with deposition of C1q on the surface of microfilariae has been described, although a recent study demonstrating that complement regulators, including complement factor H and C4 binding protein, bind to the surface of *Loa loa* microfilariae *in vivo* suggests that inactivation of C3b and C4b may help the parasite down-modulate inflammatory responses.[89]

The presence of long-term residents of hyperendemic areas who have neither detectable microfilaremia nor clinical symptoms of loiasis suggests that protective immunity to loiasis may develop in some people.[90] Definitive proof of naturally occurring immunity will require diagnostic tests sensitive and specific enough to exclude occult infections.

DIAGNOSIS

Loiasis should be suspected in any person returning from an endemic area who presents with urticaria, localized swellings, visualization of an adult worm beneath the conjunctiva and/or eosinophilia.

Definitive diagnosis can be made by extracting an adult worm from subcutaneous or subconjunctival spaces or identifying *Loa loa* microfilariae (or their DNA) in peripheral blood. Adult male worms are approximately 3.5 cm × 0.5 mm and female worms are 5–7 cm × 0.3 mm.[91] The cuticle is thick, unstriated, and covered with irregularly spaced bosses, which are useful in identifying fragments of the worm. *Loa loa* microfilariae, approximately 290 × 7.5 μm in size, are distinguished from microfilariae of other species (most notably *Wuchereria bancrofti*, *Brugia malayi*, and *Mansonella perstans*) by their diurnal periodicity, sheath, and the presence of three or more terminal nuclei.[23] The periodicity of *Loa loa* microfilariae is affected by differing time zones and variations in body temperature,[92] supporting the hypothesis that blood microfilarial levels are linked to the host's circadian rhythm. In those evaluated soon after leaving endemic regions, the optimal time of blood sampling for diurnal periodicity may still reflect timing in the endemic countries.

Serology may be useful for confirming the diagnosis in visitors to endemic areas who have suggestive clinical symptoms or unexplained eosinophilia; however, currently available methods using crude antigen extracts from *Brugia* or *Dirofilaria* species do not differentiate between *Loa loa* and other filarial pathogens.[93,94] The utility of serologic testing in endemic areas is limited by the often high prevalence of species nonspecific antifilarial antibodies.[37] In a small study of patients with parasitologically proven loiasis and/or *M. perstans* infection living in an endemic area, a detectable IgG_4 response to *Loa loa* adult antigen was 92% sensitive and 94% specific for *Loa loa* infection.[95] Cross-reactivities in subjects with onchocerciasis and lymphatic filariasis were not assessed, and difficulties in obtaining adult *Loa loa* worms will limit the use of serologic tests based on extracts of *Loa* antigens. More recently, serologic assays using recombinant *Loa loa* antigens have been developed, including a sensitive and specific rapid assay that uses a luciferase immunoprecipitation system to detect antibodies to the recombinant *Loa loa* antigen LLSXP-1.[96] Diagnostic testing for *Loa loa* antigen has yet to be developed.

The identification of *Loa loa*-specific DNA sequences[97,98] enabled the development of polymerase chain reaction (PCR)-based strategies both for speciation of *Loa loa* from pathologic specimens difficult to identify on morphologic grounds and for sensitive diagnostic strategies. Using different *Loa*-specific targeted sequences, a PCR-based multiplex technique has been developed that is 10 times more sensitive than traditional blood filtration. Further, a colorimetric detection system that can be performed at ambient temperature has simplified the PCR readout, facilitating its use in endemic areas.[99]

Differential diagnosis of Calabar swellings includes angioedema associated with C1 inhibitor deficiency, infection with other filariae (particularly *M. perstans* and *Onchocerca volvulus*), specific nematode and trematode infections (e.g., trichinellosis, gnathostomiasis), and hypereosinophilic syndromes. Although "eye worm" in the setting of a compatible exposure history is extremely suggestive of loiasis, subconjunctival migrations of a few nematodes, including *Dirofilaria repens*, a dog and cat filarial parasite (see Chapter 107), and *Thelazia californiensis*, deer eye worm (see Chapter 112), have been reported.[100,101] Finally, the symptoms of *Loa loa* infection may sometimes be difficult to distinguish from those of often co-endemic onchocerciasis or bancroftian filariasis.

TREATMENT AND PROGNOSIS

Diethylcarbamazine (DEC) is effective against both microfilariae and adult worms and, at a dose of 8–10 mg/kg daily for 21 days, remains the drug of choice for the treatment of *Loa loa* infection in amicrofilaremic patients, including most long-term visitors to endemic areas.[102] Although curative after a single course in 45–50% of such patients, multiple courses of DEC are often necessary and recrudescence may occur up to 8 years post treatment.[103] Mild side effects of treatment are common and include Calabar swellings, pruritus, arthralgias, fever, nausea, diarrhea, right upper quadrant discomfort, and a sensation of creeping under the skin.[35,104] Antihistamines or steroids may reduce the occurrence and severity of these symptoms. Occasionally, adult worms become motile under the skin following DEC treatment and may be removed with forceps through a small skin incision[104] or by excisional biopsy.[105]

More serious treatment-related complications, including renal failure, shock, coma, and fatal encephalitis, are related to microfilarial burden and may be triggered by the massive microfilarial clearance that occurs with DEC treatment.[106,107] Historically, gradual increases in doses of DEC and pretreatment with antihistamines and steroids were advocated to prevent these complications; however, numerous reports demonstrated that these strategies do not prevent encephalitis.[50] The level of microfilaremia that presents a significant risk for serious encephalitic complications is unknown, but 2500/mL blood has been suggested. Alternatives for persons with high levels of microfilaremia include no treatment, removal of circulating microfilariae by cytapheresis prior to DEC treatment,[108,109] and newer drugs, including ivermectin[110–114] and albendazole.[115]

Ivermectin reduces microfilarial levels in patients with *Loa loa* infection, but is ineffective against adult worms.[110,113] Furthermore, side effects secondary to microfilarial clearance occur in 30–70% of patients with high levels of microfilaremia, and, in rare cases, may be life-threatening.[110,111] This has become a major problem for mass drug administration programs using ivermectin as unexpected deaths have occurred in subjects with concomitant loiaisis.[116]

Although reduction in microfilarial levels has been described after prolonged administration of high dose mebendazole in some patients with loiasis,[117,118] clearance of microfilaremia is rare and at least one study has failed to demonstrate any effect of mebendazole on *Loa loa* microfilarial levels.[119] Recently, albendazole, a benzimidazole with better oral bioavailability, has been shown to significantly decrease Loa microfilarial levels in a double-blind, placebo-controlled study when used at a dose of 200 mg twice daily for 3 weeks.[115] Adverse effects were not observed, even in persons with greater than 50 000 microfilariae/mL blood. Unfortunately, shorter higher dose regimens do not appear effective.[120,121] The gradual decrease in blood microfilarial levels over the course of several months suggests that albendazole may have preferential effects on adult parasites, explaining the lack of adverse effects associated with acute microfilarial clearance. Sequential therapy with albendazole and a microfilaricidal agent (DEC or ivermectin) may provide an alternative to pretreatment cytapheresis in patients with high level microfilaremias.

PREVENTION AND CONTROL

Weekly chemoprophylaxis with DEC (300 mg) is effective for prevention of loiasis in long-term travelers to endemic areas.[3] Vector control programs have achieved only limited success, primarily because of the dense vegetation in endemic areas and difficulties accessing *Chrysops* breeding sites.[40]

MANSONELLA STREPTOCERCA

INTRODUCTION

Streptocerciasis, infection with the filarial nematode *Mansonella streptocerca*, is limited to the tropical rainforests of central Africa, although a small focus has been found in western Uganda.[122] Whereas infection can be completely asymptomatic, characteristic clinical features include a chronic, pruritic dermatitis and lymphadenopathy, often indistinguishable from onchocerciasis. Because adult male and female worms have been found in the skin of chimpanzees and because microfilariae have been found in gorillas, streptocerciasis may be a zoonosis.

THE AGENT

Microfilariae of *M. streptocerca* (synonyms: *Dipetalonema streptocerca*, *Tetrapetalonema streptocerca*) were first identified in the skin in 1922.[123] Adult female[124] and male worms were recognized in 1972.[125]

Infective larvae are transmitted to human hosts by bites of infected *Culicoides grahamii* midges.[126,127] Over months to years, these larvae develop into white, threadlike adult worms (males 17–18 mm × 40–50 μm; females 27 mm × 65–85 μm) that live in the dermal layer of the skin. In bisexual infections, microfilariae (sheathless, 2.5–5.0 μm × 180–240 μm) are produced and reside in the upper dermal and collagen layers of the skin.[128]

M. streptocerca has also been found in nonhuman primates,[129] which appear to be additional definitive hosts for this parasite.

EPIDEMIOLOGY

M. streptocerca is present in tropical rainforests of northern Angola, Cameroon, Central African Republic, Republic of the Congo, Equatorial Guinea, Nigeria, Uganda, and the Democratic Republic of Congo. In endemic areas, 40% of people may be infected (i.e., have clinical symptoms or detectable skin-dwelling microfilariae).

THE DISEASE

The major clinical manifestations of streptocerciasis are dermatologic[125,128] and include pruritus, papular rashes, and pigmentation changes. A chronic, pruritic dermatitis, characterized by nonanesthetic, hypopigmented macules, is most common.[125] These macules may be discrete or confluent, and are located predominantly over the shoulder girdle and thorax. Dermal thickening is often present. Papular eruptions occur relatively less frequently. Inguinal adenopathy is extremely common in streptocerciasis; in several studies, often as frequent as 100%.[125] Although massive lymphedema (elephantiasis) has been reported as a result of *M. streptocerca* infection, this causality remains unproven. Infection is associated with blood eosinophilia without leukocytosis.[125,128]

PATHOGENESIS AND IMMUNITY

Most pathologic changes seen in streptocerciasis are dermal and consist of sclerosis of the papillae, edema, fibrosis, and perivascular infiltration with lymphocytes and eosinophils.[125,128] Dermal lymphatics are dilated. Similar to other filariae, *M. streptocerca* is well adapted to human hosts and provokes little inflammatory reaction in the absence of treatment. With filaricidal treatment, however, inflammatory reactions appear around adult worms and microfilariae, potentially due to antigens or constituents released from treated parasites.[125,128]

DIAGNOSIS

Streptocerciasis should be suspected in persons returning from endemic areas who present with pruritus, a rash, or bilateral inguinal adenopathy. Definitive diagnosis is made by identifying *M. streptocerca* microfilariae in skin snips (see Chapter 106). Microfilariae are distinguished from microfilariae of other species (most notably skin-dwelling *O. volvulus*) by a characteristic tapered hook-shaped tail (shepherd's crook) and nuclei extending to the very end of the tail.[125,130,131] Adult worms may be found in skin biopsies, but this is rare. *M. streptocerca* DNA can be identified in skin biopsies using a nested PCR-based assay,[132] which is specific and more sensitive than skin snips for diagnosis of streptocerciasis. Serology is not of diagnostic value.

Streptocerciasis may be confused with onchocerciasis and other chronic dermatitides. Hypopigmented macules can resemble those of lepromatous leprosy. Although the nonanesthetic nature of nodules and their location on the upper body may suggest streptocerciasis, histopathologic evaluation is often necessary to distinguish leprosy from *M. streptocerca* infection.

TREATMENT AND PROGNOSIS

DEC (6 mg/kg daily in divided doses for 14–21 days) is effective in killing both microfilariae and adult worms.[125,128,133,134] As in onchocerciasis, increased pruritus, urticaria, and papular eruptions and systemic findings (arthralgias, myalgias, headaches, fever, nausea, and vomiting) may accompany treatment. Generally these symptoms occur within 24–48 hours of treatment and can be treated symptomatically with antihistamines and anti-inflammatory agents. Nevertheless, because DEC is contraindicated in most of Africa because of concerns with post-treatment reactions in onchocerciasis, its use in this infection is limited. Ivermectin 150 μg/kg is an effective microfilaricide both early (6–12 days)[135] and later (1 year) following treatment.[136]

PREVENTION AND CONTROL

There have been no studies of chemoprophylaxis for prevention of streptocerciasis. Although specific control programs have not been attempted, mass drug administration campaigns for *W. bancrofti* and *O. volvulus* control in Africa may help to dampen transmission of *M. streptocerca*.[136]

MANSONELLA PERSTANS

INTRODUCTION

Perstans filariasis, an infection caused by *Mansonella perstans*, is distributed across the center of Africa, parts of North Africa, the Caribbean basin, and in northeastern South America.[23] Although generally associated with little morbidity, clinical manifestations may include transient angioedema and pruritus of the arms, face, or other parts of the body (analogous to the Calabar swellings of loiasis), fever, headache, arthralgias, and right upper quadrant pain. Occasionally pericarditis and hepatitis occur.

THE AGENT

Microfilariae of *M. perstans* (synonyms: *Dipetalonema perstans*, *Tetrapetalonema perstans*, *Acanthocheilonema perstans*) were first identified in 1890,[137] and the adult form of *M. perstans* was first collected from the mesentery in 1898.[138]

Infective larvae are transmitted to humans by bites of several species of infected midges (*Culicoides* spp.).[139–144] Over 9–12 months, these larvae develop into creamy-white, threadlike adult worms (males, 35–45 mm × 50–70 μm; females, 60–80 mm × 100–150 μm) that live in serous cavities – pericardial, pleural, and peritoneal – as well as in the mesentery and in the perirenal and retroperitoneal tissues. In bisexual infections, microfilariae (sheathless, 3.5–4.5 μm × 100–200 μm) are produced and are found in the blood without any significant periodicity.[145]

Like most filarial parasites that infect humans, *M. perstans* appears to harbor the bacterial endosymbiont *Wolbachia*,[146] although this may not be true for *M. perstans* from all geographic areas.[20,21]

EPIDEMIOLOGY

At least 30 million residents of endemic areas are infected with *M. perstans*.[22] Distributed mainly in sub-Saharan Africa, from Senegal east to Uganda and south to Zimbabwe, and in South America along the northern coast of the entire continent, minor foci have been identified in Tunisia and Algeria. In highly endemic areas, close to 100% of people may have microfilaremia. Although humans are principal reservoirs of infection, nonhuman primates (gorilla[147] and chimpanzee[129]) can also be hosts for the parasite.

The principal vectors of *M. perstans* are *Culicoides milnei* and *C. grahamii*, but *C. austeni*, *C. fulvithorax*, *C. kingi*, and *C. furens* can also transmit infection.[139–144]

THE DISEASE

The clinical and pathologic features of *M. perstans* infection are poorly defined. Although most patients are asymptomatic,[148–151] a wide range of clinical manifestations have been described,[148] including transient angioedema and pruritus of the arms, face, or other parts of the body (analogous to the Calabar swellings of loiasis) and recurrent urticaria.[148,150,152] Less commonly, fever, headache, arthralgias, and right upper quadrant pain can occur.[148,150,152–155] Pericarditis,[72,156] hepatitis[157–159] meningoencephalitis, neuropsychiatric disturbances[148,151,159] and rarely, conjunctival granulomas[160,161] and intraocular (retinal) lesions[162] have been reported.

PATHOGENESIS AND IMMUNITY

Little is known about immune responses or the pathogenesis of symptomatic infections. Whereas blood eosinophilia and IgE elevations are common,[157,160,163–165] inflammatory reactions in this infection have been difficult to document.[163] There is some evidence that, when inflammation occurs, it is granulomatous.[160,161] Live adults induce little host response,[128] and pathologic findings are rare.[166] Although uncommon, secondary complications of hypereosinophilia due to *M. perstans* (e.g., valvular heart disease) have been reported.[165]

DIAGNOSIS

The diagnosis is made by finding microfilariae in blood or serosal effusions. Concentration techniques may be necessary in light infections.[130,167–169] More recently, PCR has been developed for specific identification of *M. perstans*.[146] Rarely, adult worms may be recovered. Occasionally, CSF and urine contain microfilariae. *M. perstans* filariasis is often associated with blood eosinophilia and antifilarial antibody elevations.[153,164,170,171]

TREATMENT AND PROGNOSIS

Treatment protocols have been attempted, including (1) DEC 8–10 mg/kg daily for 21 days,[150,151,154,172,173] (2) mebendazole 100 mg twice daily for 30 days,[114,115,165,169,170,174,175] (3) mebendazole combined with levamisole,[171,176] (4) ivermectin,[114,177–180] (5) albendazole (up to 400 mg twice daily for 10 days),[181] and (6) combination ivermectin/albendazole.[180–182] None has been effective in *M. perstans* filariasis, although some regimens reduce microfilaremia to a small degree. Consistent with the presence of *Wolbachia* endosymbiouts within *M. perstans*, a randomized trial in Mali demonstrated the utility of doxycycline (200 mg daily for 6 weeks) treatment for this infection.[183]

PREVENTION AND CONTROL

There are no studies of chemoprophylaxis for prevention of *M. perstans* infection, and control programs have not been attempted, although repeated doses of ivermectin (used for onchocerciasis control) have reduced the prevalence of *M. perstans* microfilaremia.[184,185]

MANSONELLA OZZARDI

INTRODUCTION

Infection with the filarial nematode *Mansonella ozzardi* is restricted to Central and South America and certain Caribbean islands. Although infected persons are usually asymptomatic, varied nonspecific symptoms have been ascribed to this infection.

THE AGENT

M. ozzardi microfilariae were first described in blood films in 1897,[186] and the adult worm was described in 1898.[192] Infective larvae are transmitted to humans by bites of infected midges (*Culicoides furens*[188–190] and other species[191,192]) or black flies (*Simulium amazonicum*[192–194]). There appears to be no difference between the parasites that are transmitted by the different vectors.[195,196] Over months to years, these larvae develop into slender, threadlike adult worms (females, 32–51 mm × 130–160 μm; males, 24–28 mm × 150 μm), which probably inhabit the thoracic and peritoneal cavities.[187,197] Adult worms have also been found in the lymphatics.[198] In bisexual infections, microfilariae (sheathless, 3–5 μm × 170–240 μm) are produced and are found in the skin and blood, generally without periodicity.[199–203]

EPIDEMIOLOGY

The number of people infected with *M. ozzardi* is unknown.[23] The distribution of *M. ozzardi* is restricted to Central America, South America (Colombia, Venezuela, Guyana, Suriname, Brazil, Argentina, Bolivia) and certain Caribbean islands (Puerto Rico, Antigua, Guadeloupe, Nevis, Dominican Republic, Haiti, Martinique, St Kitts, St Lucia, St Vincent, and Trinidad). In highly endemic areas, 65–70% of people may have microfilaremia.[204] Although nonhuman primates, other mammals, and certain birds and amphibians can be infected with *M. ozzardi*, humans are the only significant reservoir of infection. Like many other pathogenic filariae, *M. ozzardi* contains an endosymbiont of the *Wolbachia* genus.[205]

THE DISEASE

Although *M. ozzardi* is generally thought to cause little or no disease in humans, several reports have clearly associated this infection with urticaria, lymphadenopathy, articular pains, pruritic skin eruptions, edema, headache, and pulmonary symptoms.[171,204,206–213] Blood eosinophilia is commonly found.[171,204,206,211,214–216]

PATHOGENESIS AND IMMUNITY

The pathogenesis of *M. ozzardi* infection is poorly characterized. Evidence from small numbers of expatriates suggests that immediate hypersensitivity may be responsible for some of the pathologic changes, eosinophilia, and IgE elevations seen in this infection.

DIAGNOSIS

Definitive diagnosis of *M. ozzardi* infection is made by identifying microfilariae in blood or skin biopsies or by PCR in skin biopsies.[217]

TREATMENT AND PROGNOSIS

Treatment of *M. ozzardi* infection has been problematic, since DEC[207,218–222] and the benzimidazoles are ineffective against this parasite. In a single case report, ivermectin was effective in reducing symptoms and microfilaremia.[215] In another study, four annual single doses of ivermectin (6 mg) reduced *M. ozzardi* microfilaremia levels by 82%.[223] The presence of *Wolbachia* in *M. ozzardi* suggests that doxycycline may be an effective treatment.

PREVENTION AND CONTROL

There have been no studies of chemoprophylaxis for prevention of *M. ozzardi* infections, and control programs have not been attempted.

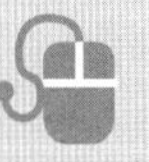

Access the complete reference list online at
http://www.expertconsult.com

Access the complete reference list online at http://www.expertconsult.com

CHAPTER 106

Onchocerciasis

Achim M. Hoerauf

INTRODUCTION

Onchocerciasis, caused by the filarial nematode *Onchocerca volvulus*, is transmitted by black flies within tropical Africa, limited geographic areas of Latin America, and in Yemen. Pathology and disease symptoms such as keratitis, chorioretinitis, and forms of dermatitis are caused by offspring larvae, microfilariae, which migrate through the skin and the eye after release from adult worms that reside in subcutaneous nodules. Apart from this typical pattern of dermal and ocular disease in conjunction with rather high infection loads seen in people from endemic areas with a lifetime of exposure to the worms, a different syndrome develops in short-term visitors, with often stronger immunologic responses and usually light infection.[1,2] In endemic areas, onchocercal disease is an important factor in higher mortality and economic loss.

THE AGENT

O. volvulus is one of eight filarial species infecting humans. Several veterinary *Onchocerca* species not infecting humans but transmitted by the same black fly vector coexist in some endemic areas. When dissected from captured black flies, larvae of *O. ochengi*, *O. gibsoni*, *O. lienalis*, and *O. cervicalis* are morphologically indistinguishable from those of *O. volvulus*, but can be differentiated by polymerase chain reaction (PCR).[3] *O. volvulus* uniformly harbors *Wolbachia* endosymbiotic intracellular bacteria,[4] which are essential for fertility and reproduction[5–8] as well as survival of the parasites.[9] Substances released from dying *Wolbachia* play roles in treatment-induced reactions[7] and in ongoing pathogenesis of human onchocerciasis.

History

O'Neill in 1875 associated microfilariae present in skin with a papular dermatitis in Ghana.[10] Leuckart in 1893 described adult worms in subcutaneous nodules from persons in West Africa. In 1917, Robles, a Guatemalan physician, demonstrated the association between nodules, skin lesions, anterior ocular lesions, and the presence of microfilariae.[11] Several descriptions of ocular pathology including histologic proof of microfilarial presence in ocular tissues were made by Hisette in what was then the Belgian Congo.[12]

Life Cycle (Fig. 106.1)

Humans are the only definitive host for *O. volvulus*, although chimpanzees have served as definitive hosts in experimental onchocerciasis. Black flies of the genus *Simulium* (***Fig. 106.2A***) are obligatory intermediate hosts. *O. volvulus*, like all nematodes, has a five-stage life cycle involving four molts. Infection begins with the bite of an infected *Simulium* vector.[13] Infective larvae (L3 stage) are deposited into the skin of a new host, where 6–12 months is required for two molts and development of mature adult females (L5 stage) capable of producing new L1-stage larvae, called microfilariae. The white, hairlike adult worms live coiled in subcutaneous or deeper intramuscular tissues surrounded by a fibrous capsule (***Fig. 106.2B***) containing blood and lymph vessels. Adult males, which are 3–8 cm long, appear to migrate from nodule to nodule to inseminate the much larger females, which range from 30 to 80 cm in length. Microfilariae (220–360 μm long) are released from nodules to migrate through subcutaneous, conjunctival, and intraocular tissues. Adult females can live for up to 14 (average 9–10) years, each producing on average more than 700 microfilariae per day. Considerable numbers of adult females may lie in deep impalpable nodules.[14] Microfilariae, which live for 6–30 months, are ingested by black flies. The two molts in the vector and maturation of the infective larvae (L3 stage) take 1–3 weeks. Any increase in adult worm burden necessarily implies reexposure to infective L3 from a vector, because *O. volvulus* adult worms do not reproduce within humans.

Vectors

Six species of the *Simulium damnosum* sensu lato complex, identified based on fly morphology and on chromosome banding patterns, are vectors of *O. volvulus* in West Africa. Based on habitats and mitochondrial gene sequences,[15,16] further grouping into a savanna clade (*S. damnosum* sensu stricto, *S. sirbanum*), a rain forest clade (*S. yahense*, *S. squamosum*), and a transition zone clade (*S. leonense*, *S. sanctipauli*) is possible. *S. neavei* is the principal vector in eastern and central Africa;[17,18] *S. ochraceum* is the vector in Central America;[19] and several other species transmit onchocerciasis in South America.

Most *Simulium* species lay their eggs attached to rocks and vegetation submerged in highly oxygenated stretches of rivers and streams, where larval and pupal stages develop. In savanna areas in Africa, the vector breeds in large rivers such as the Volta, while in forest areas of Africa and the Americas the vector breeds in streams and rivulets that are less accessible to larviciding by aircraft. Larvae of *S. neavei* attach to crabs living in small creeks for further development. Flight range of *Simulium* is 12 km, and therefore transmission areas are limited to these distances away from breeding sites.

EPIDEMIOLOGY

Onchocerciasis is endemic in 34 countries: 27 in Africa, 6 in Latin America, and 1 (Yemen) in the Arabian peninsula (***Fig. 106.3***). From data derived from a new mapping technology based on palpation of nodules in randomly selected communities,[20] approximately 90 million people are at risk, with 37 million people infected. About 270 000 individuals developed blindness from onchocerciasis and another 500 000 have severe visual disability.[7,21] Global disease burden in 2002 was 0.95

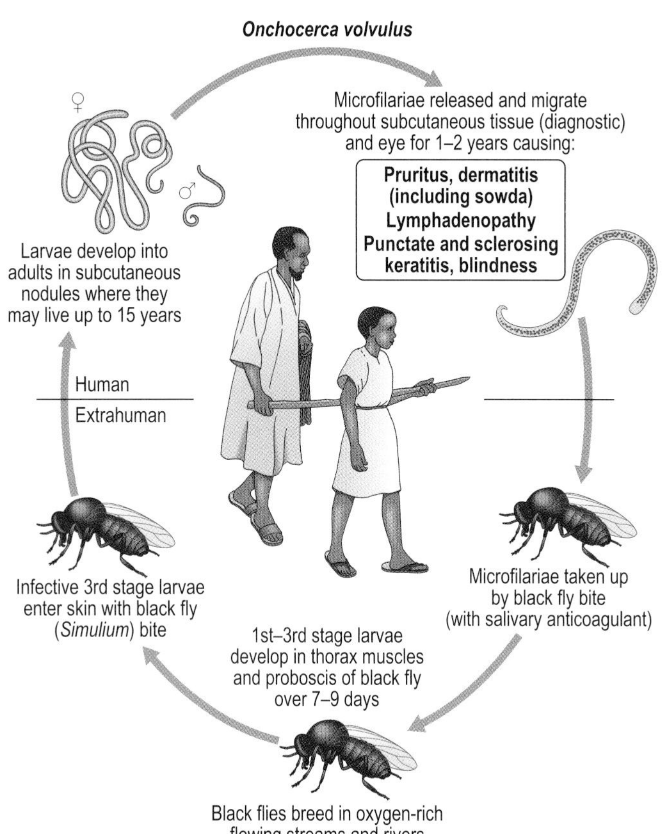

Figure 106.1 Life cycle of *Onchocerca volvulus.*

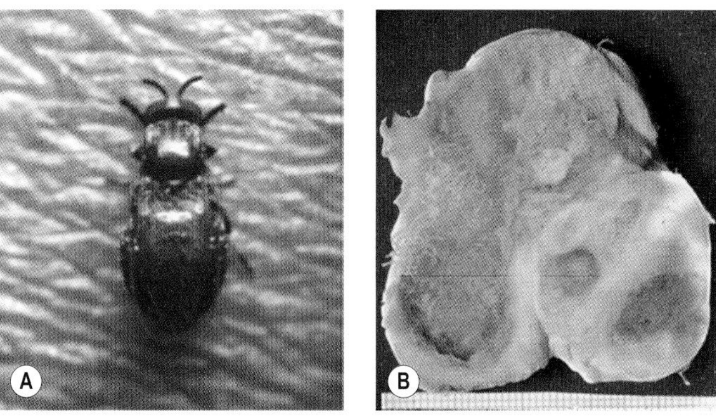

Figure 106.2 *Onchocerca* vector and nodule. **(A)** *Simulium damnosum*, the vector. **(B)** Sliced onchocercal nodule with three adult worm nests.

million disability-adjusted life years (DALYs).[20,22] Over 99% of cases occur in sub-Saharan Africa. In hyperendemic villages of Africa, infection rates commonly approach 100%. In Latin America, distribution is focal and vector transmission is at least 10-fold less intense.[20] Thus, infected individuals in Latin America have low worm burdens and consequently few people develop blindness. Forest-strain *O. volvulus*, found in rainforest coastal regions of sub-Saharan Africa and genetically different from the savanna strain,[23–29] only causes mild ocular diseases but rarely blindness, even in heavily infected persons.[30] In contrast, in endemic savanna regions of Africa, a linear relationship between a derived parameter, the community microfilarial load, and the incidence of blindness in that community exists.[22,30,31] On an individual basis, the likelihood of blindness is positively associated with increasing microfilarial burden.[32]

Other factors influencing the epidemiology of onchocerciasis are less well defined. Host immunity seems to play a role in limiting total worm loads with increasing age. Also, children of *O. volvulus*-infected mothers have a higher risk of infection and become infected at a younger age and with increased microfilaria intensity, suggesting intrauterine *O. volvulus*-specific immunosuppression.[33]

In regions outside the savanna, skin manifestations are the main complications of disease. The profound psychosocial implications of unremitting pruritus and disfiguring skin lesions make onchocercal skin disease a major public health problem and more than 50% of DALYs lost due to onchocerciasis are due not to blindness but to skin disease.[34,35] On a community basis, there is a strong correlation between prevalence of pruritus and *O. volvulus* endemicity in the community. In communities hyperendemic for *O. volvulus* (defined as >60% of people with microfilardermia and >30% with palpable nodules (onchocercomas)), 30–40% have symptomatic skin disease and 50% of children aged 5–9 are already infected. Adult persons may harbor up to 50 adult worms and >100 microfilariae/mg skin. In mesoendemic areas, 30–60% of people and in hypoendemic areas <30% have microfilardermia.

A link between onchocerciasis and epilepsy (thought secondary to erosion of nodules through the skull) has often been suggested[36–39] but lacks statistical significance on meta-analysis,[40,41] although one form of seizure, head-nodding syndrome, is significantly associated.[42] A proposed link to hyposexual dwarfism remains uncertain.[38–41]

The socioeconomic consequences of onchocerciasis are profound. *O. volvulus*-induced blindness is associated with a life expectancy 10 years shorter than that of nonblinded persons in the same area.[43] Microfilarial burden is the single most significant parameter associated with mortality.[44] Consequences of onchocerciasis extend beyond the individual and affect family, community, and country. The common image of young boys holding sticks to guide blind, unproductive men in their twenties and thirties attests to why entire villages, within otherwise fully arable river zones, become economically nonviable and have been deserted when blindness rates reach about 10%.

THE DISEASE

In symptomatic persons, inflammatory responses to microfilariae cause the dermatitis, keratitis and chorioretinitis that are the cardinal manifestations of infection. The subcutaneous nodules containing adult worms evoke no inflammatory response and hence few, if any, clinical symptoms. Of importance to clinicians in non-onchocerciasis endemic areas is that nonspecific dermatitis is usually the sole clinical disease manifestation in short-term visitors to endemic areas.[2] Transmission of onchocerciasis, as with other filarial infections, is highly inefficient when compared with vector-borne protozoan diseases such as malaria. Infection is unlikely after a short stay of a year or less in an endemic area, although it does happen, according to a recent GeoSentinel study, even after short visits of <1 month.[45] In another study of infected expatriates, the median duration of exposure was 2 years (range, 20 months to 6 years), and in these lightly infected persons, a median period of 18 months (range, 3 months to 3 years) from the end of exposure passed before the onset of symptoms.[2]

Subcutaneous Nodules (Fig. 106.4)

Asymptomatic 0.5–3.0 cm subcutaneous onchocercomas usually occurring over bony prominences are freely movable encapsulated nodules that contain coiled masses of adult worms (***Fig. 106.2B***). In Latin America, where the vector *S. ochraceum* bites high, nodules are often located on the head and upper body. In Africa where *S. damnosum* bites lower, nodules are most often over the hips, over the os sacrum and lower limbs, but also on the thorax and near the knee; in children they are often found on the head. Palpable subcutaneous nodules are uncommonly found in lightly infected expatriates.

Dermatitis

The especially intractable pruritus of onchocerciasis is secondary to reactions to microfilariae. In heavily affected persons, scratching and

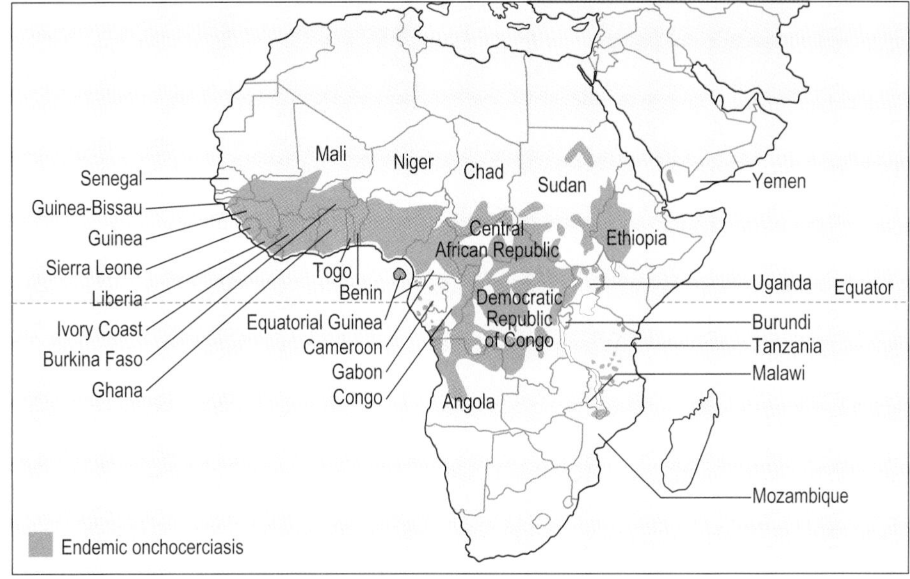

Figure 106.3 Distribution of onchocerciasis in Africa and in Yemen.

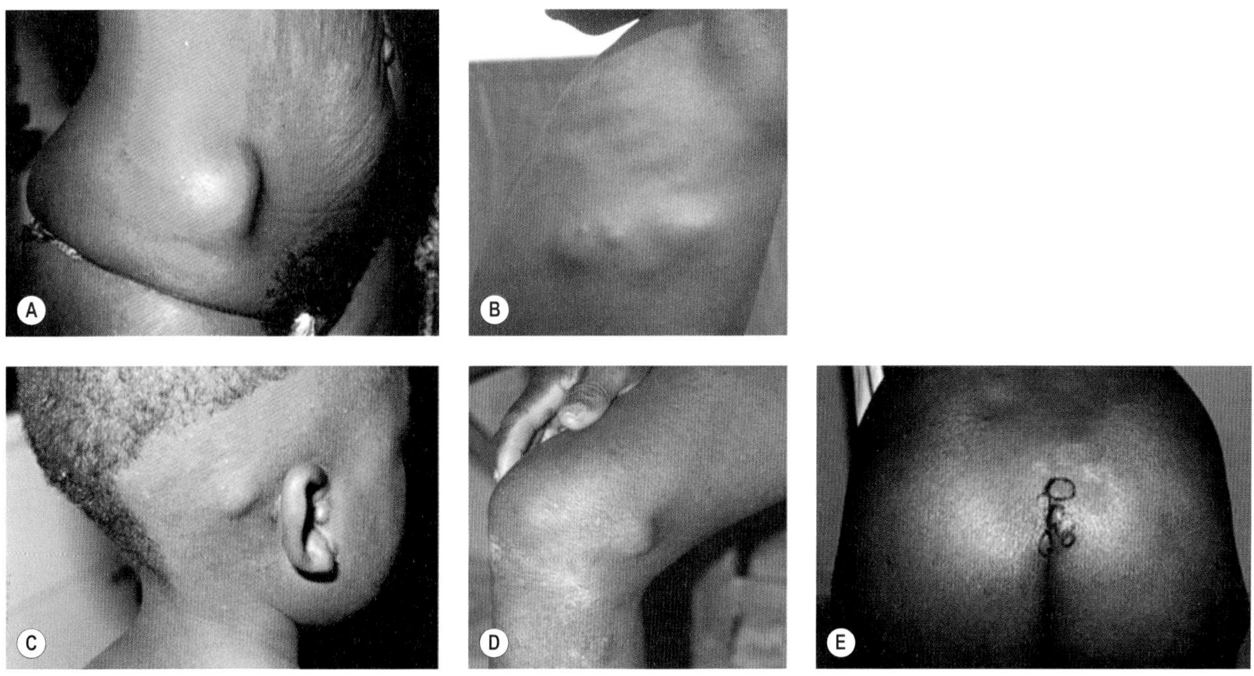

Figure 106.4 Typical locations of onchocercomas at **(A)** the hip, **(B)** thorax, **(C)** head, **(D)** knee and **(E)**, the sacrum.

excoriation to the point of bleeding occurs. Episodes of localized rash, erythema, and angioedema may be superimposed on ongoing dermatologic manifestations at essentially any stage of the disease.[21] A common scheme, categorizing skin disease into five groups, provides a category-specific grading for severity, activity, and distribution.[35,46] Categories are not mutually exclusive in a given patient and clinical findings are not specific for onchodermatitis.

1. **Acute papular onchodermatitis** (*Fig. 106.5A*). Small pruritic papules may be scattered on limbs, shoulders, and trunk. Lesions may progress to become vesicular or pustular and may be spontaneous or occur as a reaction to microfilaricidal treatment. Histologically, papules are intraepidermal microabscesses; microfilariae are inconsistently present. A variable perivascular infiltrate of lymphoid origin is seen in this and most types of onchocercal skin disease. Microfilariae, when found, are in the superficial dermis and are frequently associated with lymphatics.
2. **Chronic papular onchodermatitis** (*Fig. 106.5B, C*). Papules, often flat-topped, are larger but more variable in size than in the acute papular eruption. Dermatitis is usually symmetrical over buttocks, waist, and shoulder areas and less pruritic than in the acute eruption. Clinical hyperpigmentation and hyperkeratosis correlate histologically with epidermal acanthosis and incontinence of pigment. This is the most common skin manifestation in hyperendemic areas.
3. **Lichenified onchodermatitis** (*Fig. 106.5K*). Due to pruritus and scratching, the epidermis becomes hypertrophied, resulting in thickening of the skin and exaggeration of normal skin markings.
4. **Atrophy** (*Fig. 106.5H*). Premature atrophy, due to degeneration of the structural elements of the skin with chronic infection, is

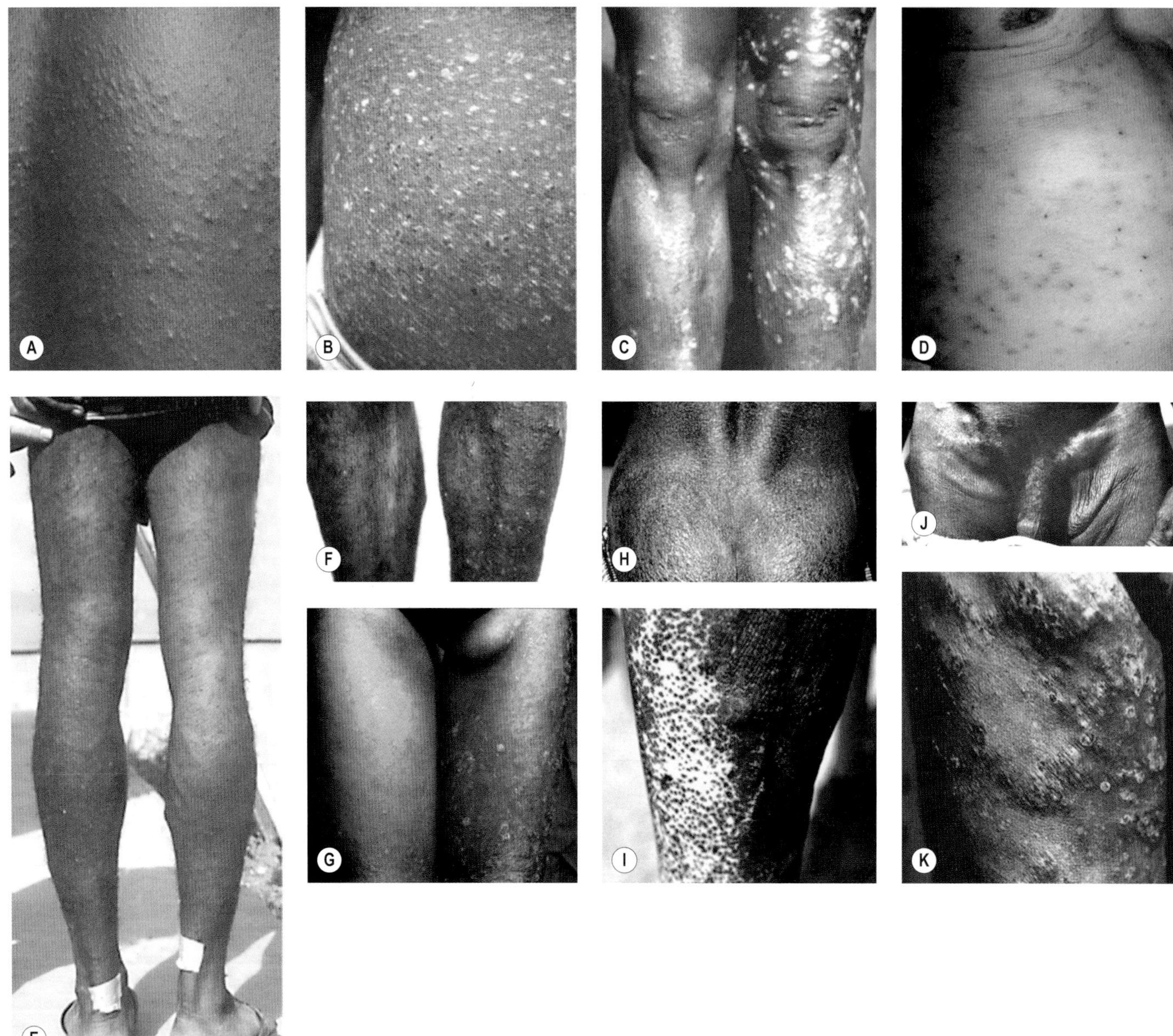

Figure 106.5 Cutaneous lesions in onchocerciasis. **(A)** Acute pustular onchodermatitis. **(B, C)** Chronic onchodermatitis. **(D)** Dermatitis in Guatemala, erisipela de la costa. **(E, F, G)** Sowda with unilateral preference and dark skin as well as swollen femoral lymph node. **(H)** Skin atrophy in a 15-year-old boy. **(I)** Leopard skin. **(J)** Hanging groin. **(K)** Lichenified onchodermatitis.

most common over the buttocks but can occur over limbs. Clinically, fine wrinkles will appear after pushing along the skin surface with one finger. Loss of elasticity can be demonstrated by slow return to position of skin pinched between two fingers. Histologic stains reveal loss of elastic fibers. The diagnosis of onchocercal atrophy should only be made in those under 50 years.

5. **Depigmentation** (*Fig. 106.5I*). Areas of depigmentation over the anterior shin with islands of normally pigmented skin around hair follicles, commonly called "leopard skin," are seen in advanced onchodermatitis.

In Mexico and Guatemala, chronic skin lesions distinct to this region are described. These include erisipela de la costa (*Fig. 106.5D*), a macular rash and edema of the face, and mal morado, a lesion associated with a reddish discoloration, particularly on the trunk and upper limbs.

Moderate to severe pruritus is the major presenting complaint in expatriates; and an evanescent nonspecific maculopapular rash, which may have an urticarial component, is the main physical finding. The rash is often localized to one area of the body, usually the trunk, presumably in proximity to the few adult worms present that have released microfilariae. The long incubation period of onchocercal dermatitis and the unfamiliarity of physicians in the industrialized world with its manifestations make misdiagnosis frequent.

Severe Dermatitis, "Sowda"

An intensely pruritic eruption limited to one limb, usually the leg, sowda consists of hyperpigmented papules and plaques with accompanying edema of the entire limb (*Fig. 106.5E–G*). Regional lymph nodes are enlarged and show prominent follicular hyperplasia, suggesting that sowda is due to an aberrant humoral hyperresponsiveness in affected persons. Bacterial superinfection is common due to excoriation of the intensely pruritic lesion. Histologically, few microfilariae are found and hyperkeratosis, acanthosis, and dermal fibrosis are found. Sowda is most common in Yemen and Sudan but is seen elsewhere in Africa. Immune reactions in sowda patients are clearly distinct from those with generalized onchocerciasis.

Lymphadenopathy

Dead microfilariae, eliminated via the lymphatics, can cause lymphadenitis leading to atrophy of the lymphatic tissue with fibrosis. The so-called hanging groin (***Fig. 106.5J***) results when large fibrotic inguinofemoral lymph node conglomerates build up in a sling of stretched-out atrophic skin.

Eye

Involvement of all tissues of the eye has been described. Host reactions to microfilariae of *O. volvulus* as they migrate through the eye initially present as punctate keratitis or as snowflake corneal opacities. Individual opacities clear spontaneously to be followed by others. Free microfilariae may be visible by slit-lamp examination in the anterior chamber or aqueous humor. Long-standing infection in particular with savanna-strain *O. volvulus* leads to sclerosing keratitis and eventually to blindness. Sclerosing keratitis is characterized by a fibrovascular pannus and an inflammatory infiltrate at the level of Bowman's membrane. The opacity develops around the edge of the cornea and as it becomes vascularized advances toward the center. Iridocyclitis with flare and cells in the anterior chamber leads to development of synechiae, raised intraocular pressure, and secondary glaucoma. Adult *O. volvulus* do not migrate through the subconjunctiva, in contrast to the occasional subconjunctival migration of the adult worm of *Loa loa*, confusingly called the eye worm, that is visible to the naked eye of both patient and observer (Chapter 105).

Inflammatory disturbances of the retinal pigment epithelium leading to chorioretinitis, chorioretinal atrophy, and posterior ocular disease occur in up to 10% of the population of savanna regions. The acute phase can last for a year or more. A postneuritic optic atrophy associated with scarring and retinal pigment disturbance or with vascular sheathing of retinal vessels then ensues. Visual field loss may progress to keyhole vision or even total loss of light perception.

Human Immunodeficiency Virus and Onchocerciasis

Impaired immunoglobulin G (IgG) and IgM responses to *O. volvulus* antigens occur in HIV-positive persons with onchocerciasis. However, no epidemiologic association between HIV infection and onchocerciasis has been demonstrated.[47] Both initial microfilarial densities and efficacy of ivermectin treatment are equivalent in HIV-positive and HIV-negative persons.[48]

PATHOGENESIS AND IMMUNITY

Systemic Immune Responses

Like other helminthic parasites that persist long term in their hosts, *O. volvulus* modulates deleterious parasite-specific immune responses in order to live in relative immunologic harmony with its host. The majority of infected people with so-called generalized onchocerciasis (relatively high parasite loads with more than 10 microfilariae/mg skin but little dermatitis) develop a mixed Th1–Th2 response (dominated by Th2), which is counter-regulated by antigen-specific regulatory T cells, which produce high amounts of interleukin (IL)-10 and/or transforming growth factor (TGF)-β, two cytokines that down-regulate proinflammatory immune responses.[49] Evidence for this can be found by *in vitro* cultures of peripheral blood mononuclear cells from those patients, in which reduced proliferative responses[50,51] can be restored by addition of neutralizing antibodies to these cytokines.[52,53] Down-regulation becomes biologically significant with the start of microfilarial production and is probably mediated by secretory–excretory products of adult microfilariae-producing female worms. Those products, studied in more detail from the related filaria *Brugia malayi*, may down-regulate the ability for proper antigen-presentation by dendritic cells,[54] or monocytes/macrophages. One well-studied molecule secreted from *O. volvulus*[55] with these properties is nematode cystatin, which is able to suppress macrophage immune responses also to other immune stumuli such as allergens.[56] Lower cellular reactivity to BCG as well as to tetanus vaccination was also shown in onchocerciasis patients.[57,58] After microfilaricidal chemotherapy of onchocerciasis, there is a reversal of the immunosuppression[59] and increase of Th2 responses.[60] Suppression by regulatory T cells seems also to affect humoral immune responses: regulatory T cells induce IgG_4. Individuals with generalized onchocerciasis show higher production of antigen-specific subclass 4 IgG (IgG_4).[49,61]

In contrast to generalized onchocerciasis, hyperreactive onchocerciasis, and sowda in particular, are characterized by brisk production of Th2 cytokines (IL-4, IL-5, IL-13) and highly elevated IgE responses even without chemotherapy (reviewed in reference 49). Data from filarial murine infection models indicate that these cytokine responses limit filarial burdens.[62]

Local Immune Responses

Since in onchocerciasis filariae are not present in the peripheral blood, it is important that findings about regulatory responses be corroborated *ex vivo* from sites of infection. Accordingly, FoxP3-positive regulatory T cells have been demonstrated by immunohistology in onchocercomas from generalized onchocerciasis patients[63] and in *in vitro* cultures suppress proliferation of other T cells.[64] Immunohistology also shows that TGF-β is produced by several cell types (macrophages, T cells, plasma cells) in the onchocercomas adjacent to adult worms in higher amounts than in onchocercomas from sowda patients.[65,66]

In summary, proinflammatory responses that dominate in hyperreactive onchocerciasis are thought to lead to the activation of neutrophilic and eosinophilic granulocytes and macrophages, which then can be demonstrated to actively kill skin microfilariae, but at the expense of strong dermatitis, in contrast to generalized onchocerciasis, in which these cells only become activated after microfilaricidal treatment. Why some people develop sowda upon infection while the majority does not is not well understood. Genetics may be important, with clustering of disease in families. A gene variant of human IL-13, leading to higher IL-13 responses, is significantly associated with sowda development;[67] but more genes may orchestrate genetic predispositions.

Protective Immune Responses

People with exposure to *O. volvulus* infective larvae but without active infection (so-called endemic normals or putatively immunes) show a different immunological profile with a strong mixed Th1 and Th2 response,[53,68] which is thought to prevent establishment of active infection. Apart from the few individuals in a hyperendemic community, sterile protection does not regularly develop upon natural exposure to L3, as almost all exposed individuals will become infected. The immune system does seem to limit acquisition of new worms, since they reach a plateau of several dozen adults in the human body, regardless of annual transmission rates that may vary from hundreds to tens of thousands of transmitted L3.[69,70] From these calculations it can be estimated that >99% of transmitted L3 may be destroyed by the immune system.

Role of *Wolbachia* Endosymbionts

O. volvulus harbors endosymbiotic intracellular *Wolbachia* bacteria,[4] essential for fertility, embryogenesis, larval development, and survival of adult worms[5–9] (***Fig. 106.6A***). Depletion of *Wolbachia* (***Fig. 106.6B***) with doxycycline therapy sterilizes adult females and leads to adult worm death.[9] *Wolbachia* released from dying microfilariae after microfilaricidal treatment of infected individuals induces release of tumor necrosis factor and related mediators,[71] which contribute to the sometimes severe post-treatment reactions (the Mazzotti reaction)[66,72] that until recently were attributed solely to systemic release of onchocercal parasite

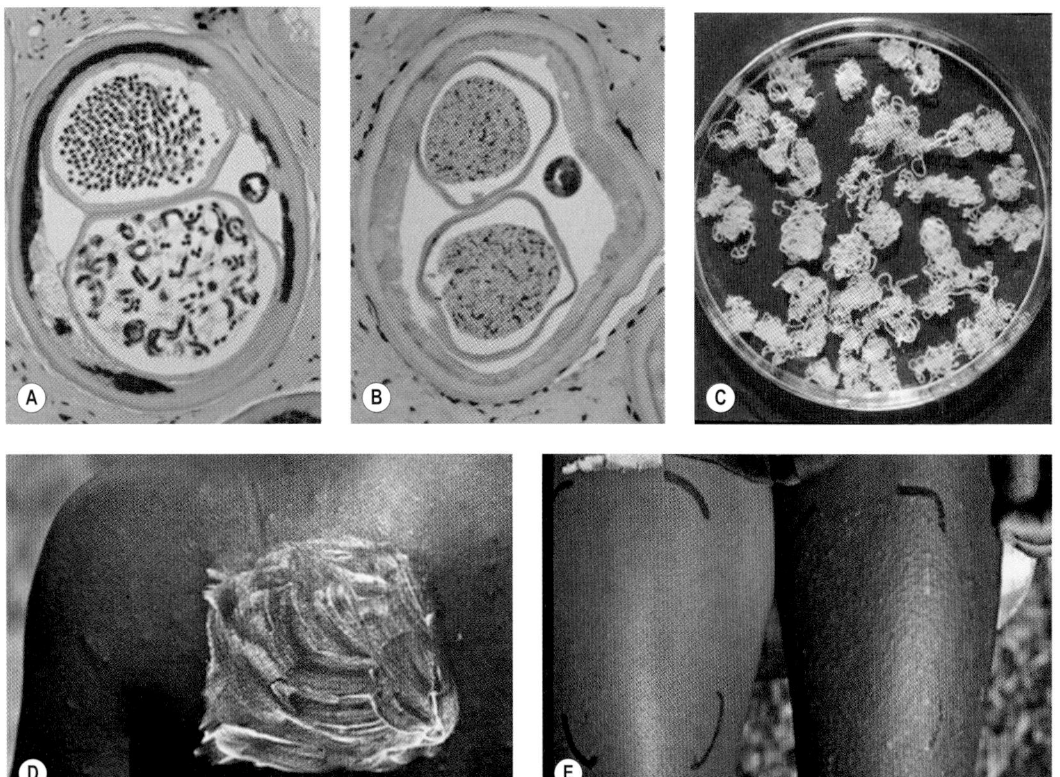

Figure 106.6. **(A)** Transverse section through female *O. volvulus* with red-dotted *Wolbachia* (immunostained using antibodies against *Wolbachia* surface protein), upper uterus tube with embryos, lower tube with coiled microfilariae. **(B)** Depletion of *Wolbachia* (no red dots) and uterus with dead embryos following doxycycline. **(C)** Female worms after collagenase digestion of onchocercoma. **(D)** Topical Mazzotti test with diethylcarbamazine (DEC) cream. **(E)** Acute dermatitis on left leg only, due to Mazzotti reaction.

antigens. *Wolbachia* do not produce endotoxin, but their major surface proteins as well as a peptidoglycan-associated lipoprotein activate the innate immune system through Toll-like receptor 2.[73–75] In a murine model of onchocercal keratitis, *Wolbachia* are capable of inducing the early neutrophilic response and causing corneal opacities.[76]

DIAGNOSIS

Clinical Examination

O. volvulus has a well-defined distribution, but because of its geographic overlap with other filarial parasites, a well-taken travel or residence history by an epidemiologically cognizant physician will reduce unnecessary diagnostic investigations in those with no possible exposure. *O. volvulus*, *Loa loa*, *Mansonella perstans*, *M. ozzardi*, and *M. streptocerca* all may cause overlapping clinical syndromes. In suspected onchocerciasis, the history should focus on duration and intensity of exposure.

A physical examination with the patient completely disrobed is necessary to detect (1) localized dermatitis, preferentially occurring where the onchocercomas and thus the emigrating microfilariae are present (e.g., in the buttock region in adults from Africa), associated with either *O. volvulus* or *M. streptocerca*; (2) subcutaneous nodules; or (3) Calabar swellings of loiasis. A thorough palpation of all lymph node groups, including those in the inguinal region, will aid in the diagnosis of *Wuchereria bancrofti*, *O. volvulus*, or *M. streptocerca*. Slit-lamp examination of the eye is required to work up possible ocular onchocerciasis, although the yield is so low in lightly infected expatriates that it is likely unnecessary. The patient should first sit for 10 minutes with the head forward and bowed to allow microfilariae located posteriorly and inferiorly to become visible. Fluorescein angiography is the most sensitive detector of early chorioretinal lesions.

Laboratory Diagnosis

Definitive diagnosis is often dependent on the parasitologic demonstration of microfilariae from skin snips. In well-equipped clinical settings, biopsy or ultrasound demonstration of adult parasites in nodules may be diagnostic.

Skin Snips

Microfilariae are detected utilizing skin snips taken down to the level of the dermal papillae. This type of limited skin biopsy employs either a razor blade to slice a thin piece of skin which has been tented up with a needle, or a corneoscleral biopsy instrument to obtain 1–2 mg of skin bloodlessly.[77] A microscopic count of highly motile microfilariae migrating out of two to six biopsies, one from over each scapula, iliac crest, and lateral aspect of each calf, is performed after incubation of the skin snips with saline in microplate wells at 37°C. In heavier infections, motile microfilariae will be visible emerging from the skin snip under low-power microscopy in 10–60 minutes, but initially negative snips should be covered to prevent evaporation and checked periodically for at least 24 hours. Sensitivity can be increased if skin snips are put in a 1% collagenase solution.

A heavily infected person may have more than 100 microfilariae/mg of skin. In Africa, the highest yield will be from the iliac crest and in Latin America from over the scapula. In expatriates, the majority of infected persons do not have microfilariae in their skin and those that do have very low counts.

Deep punch biopsy of the skin is not necessary, and multiple skin snips will have a higher yield than one traumatic deep biopsy. Blood contaminating a skin snip may result in other species of the bloodborne microfilariae escaping into the specimen. If the patient has been in an area endemic for *M. streptocerca*, it is necessary to fix the skin and to stain the microfilariae for identification. In contrast to *M. streptocerca*, *O. volvulus* microfilariae are longer and thicker (5–9 μm in contrast to 3–5 μm width and a maximum length of 260 μm for *M. streptocerca*), have anterior nuclei that are side by side, a caudal space free of nuclei, and a tail tapered to a fine point. *M. streptocerca* is most often found in snips taken from the upper trunk.

Blood Examination

Because of geographic overlaps in distributions of filarial parasites that may cause overlapping clinical syndromes, examination for circulating microfilaremia is often necessary (see Chapters 104 and 105).

Urine and Other Fluids

Microfilariae of *O. volvulus* have been found in the urine of some infected persons during mass epidemiologic studies in hyperendemic regions, with microfilarial counts being correlated with skin counts.[78] Examination of the urine, however, has no utility as a general diagnostic technique and is no substitute for skin snips in the diagnostic workup of a single patient. Cerebrospinal fluid microfilariae can be seen in severe *O. volvulus* infection.

Demonstration of the Adult Parasite

A coil of hairlike white worms discovered in an excised nodule in the appropriate epidemiologic setting is diagnostic of onchocerciasis on visual inspection. Most nodules have only three to five adults in them (less in hypoendemic areas), though nodules containing as many as 50 have been found, which can be liberated from tissue by collagenase digestion (***Fig. 106.6C***).

Serology

Serologic testing for *O. volvulus* IgG is not generally available and when done usually utilizes a crude antigenic preparation of a non-onchocercal filarial parasite. A positive result cannot differentiate between the eight filarial species and may cross-react, albeit at lower titers, with other nematode infections such as strongyloidiasis. Despite the lack of specificity, the sensitivity of this type of serology is almost 100%. Most people resident in endemic areas will have antibodies whether or not they are currently infected. Thus, serologic evaluation in filarial disease is helpful only in two situations: (1) in persons exposed to or infected with filarial parasites who are originally from nonendemic areas and were presumably seronegative initially; and (2) to detect a quantitative decrease in antibody levels that may occur as a response to definitive therapy.

Eosinophil Count

The total eosinophil count is not helpful diagnostically as it is often but inconstantly elevated in onchocerciasis.

IgE Levels

Serum IgE levels are usually elevated in onchocerciasis, with highest levels in sowda patients.

Ultrasound Examination

Adult worms in suspected onchocercomas will produce a central, relatively homogeneous echogenic area containing echo-dense particles with a lateral acoustic shadow. Within the onchocercomas, calcifications or fluid may be identified.[79] Occasionally, worm movements are observed, regularly so in cystic nodules. Particularly in these nodules, sequential ultrasonographic monitoring of nodules after macrofilaricidal therapy can provide information on drug effects.

Mazzotti Test

A 50 mg dose of diethylcarbamazine (DEC), the Mazzotti test,[72] can be given to patients suspected of harboring *O. volvulus* but in whom no microfilariae can be detected.[80,81] Since severe reactions in the skin and eye are not totally avoidable, the systemic test has now been replaced by a patch test performed by applying topical DEC (10% in body solutions such as Nivea) to a small area of skin (10 × 10 cm) in order to provoke a localized Mazzotti reaction[82,83] (***Fig. 106.6D***). This is a highly sensitive and specific diagnostic test (pruritus and pustular onchodermatitis develop after 24–48 h) (***Fig. 106.6E***) and is considered for detecting recrudescence of *O. volvulus* infection in a sentinel population of children and young adults within the onchocerciasis-free zone created by the control programs.[83]

DNA Diagnosis of Individual Patients

Detection of parasite DNA in routine skin snips by PCR amplification of O-150, an *O. volvulus*-specific 150 bp repeated genomic DNA family, is more sensitive for detecting low-level infection in individual patients than classical skin snipping, and similar in sensitivity to the DEC patch test.[84,85] PCR assays, available in research settings, are of importance in diagnosing expatriates. Several methods (standard qualitative protocols followed by gel electrophoresis, PCR-ELISA,[86] quantitative PCR with probes) are applied to DNA extracted from skin snips or less painful skin scratches that are fresh, frozen, or preserved in ethanol. PCR is the method of choice in the detection of *O. volvulus* in the *Simulium* vector in large pooled samples.[3]

Diagnostic Difficulties

Scabies, insect bites, hypersensitivity reactions, miliaria rubra, and contact dermatitis enter the differential diagnosis of acute pruritic disease. In expatriates, Calabar swellings (see Chapter 105), clinically similar episodes of localized rash, and mild angioedema can mimic onchodermatitis. Tuberculoid leprosy and eczema should be considered if there are chronic skin changes. Dermatomycoses, previous trauma, and yaws can also cause hypopigmented skin lesions. The differential diagnosis of onchocercomas comprises lipomas, fibromas, lymph nodes, cysticerci, dermoid cysts, foreign body granulomas, exostosis, and ganglia.

Onchocercal chorioretinitis must be differentiated from choroiditis due to syphilis, tuberculosis, or toxoplasmosis. Optic neuropathy in endemic areas may be due to nutritional optic atrophy, syphilis, or primary glaucoma. In expatriates with a suggestive history (i.e., being a travel partner of a skin snip-positive patient) but with negative skin snips and no nodules, presumptive diagnosis can be made by Mazzotti test and/or serology.

TREATMENT AND PROGNOSIS

Because the pathologic sequelae of *O. volvulus* infection are due to microfilariae in skin and ocular tissues, a treatment leading to sustained absence of microfilariae is necessary for morbidity reduction. This can be achieved either by repeated treatment with drugs active against microfilariae for the lifetime of adult worms (up to 14 years),[87] or by killing or removing the adult worms. In principle there are two modes of treatment available for onchocerciasis: nodulectomy, and microfilaricidal or macrofilaricidal drugs.

Ivermectin

Ivermectin[88] elicits receptor-mediated hyperpolarization of cells after an influx of negatively charged ions occurs utilizing a novel glutamate-sensitive chloride channel present in nematodes.[89] Ivermectin is well absorbed orally, excretion is almost entirely in the feces, and its serum half-life is 12 hours.

Large field trials in Africa in the 1980s established ivermectin as the treatment of choice in a single oral microfilaricidal dose of 150 μg/kg administered every 6–12 months.[90,91] Skin microfilariae are decreased within days though maximum reduction may not occur for up to 2 weeks. Because drug effects are so much longer than its half-life, and because histologically, immune effector cells attack the damaged microfilariae after treatment, the immune system is important for the long-term drug effects. Ocular microfilarial counts do not begin to be reduced for at least 2 weeks. Microfilariae are not killed inside the eye, which accounts for the limited ocular inflammatory adverse reactions, thus making the drug safe to use, in contrast to DEC. Further microfilarial production is suppressed for 6 months before once again reaching levels that lead to renewed transmission at about 12 months. Annual treatment effectively reduces progression and rates of ocular disease including blinding and skin disease as manifest by pruritus.[92–95] Advanced eye disease and existing blindness are not reversed. Higher doses of ivermectin given yearly do not have enhanced effect on viability or fecundity of female adult worms but cause significant ocular and dermal side effects.[96–98] Increasing the frequency of ivermectin administration to every 3 months decreases microfilaria production up to threefold and may impair adult fecundity, but not life span long term.[97] There is no evidence for an additive effect of albendazole.[99] Elimination of microfilariae after ivermectin leads to partial reversion of immunosuppressed cellular immune responses.[59,61]

Pruritus in lightly infected expatriates may be refractory to annual or 6-month therapy and repeated treatments with standard doses may be needed for the first 2 years or so.[100–102] Ivermectin administration should be titrated (regarding frequency, not higher doses) to symptoms and may be given as often as every 3 months. Appropriate long-term duration of this intermittent therapy in those without further exposure to transmission is not known. Annual treatment in these cases might theoretically be offered for the possible 14-year life span of the adult worm; however, clinical experience is that most patients stop returning after several years, so likely cease to develop recurrent symptoms after several years of therapy. Combination with a one-time course of 4–6 weeks of doxycycline is an alternative that will reduce the total follow-up time[103] (***Fig. 106.7***).

Ivermectin by itself has no intrinsic pharmacologic effects in humans. Adverse effects correlate with microfilarial loads. At levels above 20–50 microfilariae/mg skin, adverse effects may be considerable (usually not severe) and lead to acute dermatitis, fever, pruritus, urticaria, myalgia, edematous swelling of the limbs and face, tender lymphadenopathy, and postural hypotension; reactions occur mostly within 1–2 days of treatment.[104–106] Symptomatic treatment with analgesics and antihistamines or corticosteroids is generally sufficient. Postural hypotension can be eliminated if patients are instructed to rest in bed if dizziness occurs. Reactions are diminished on subsequent treatments of individuals or

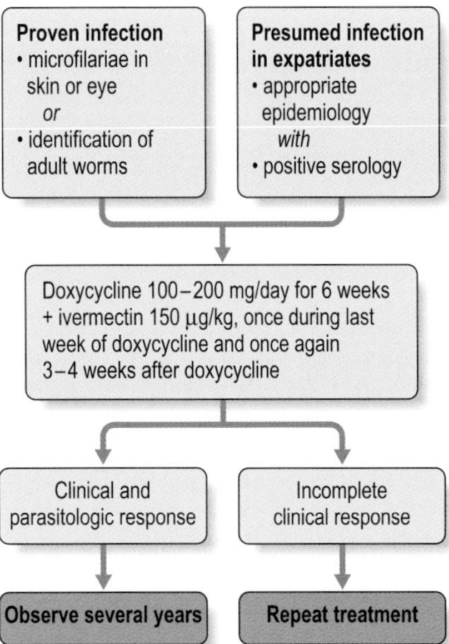

Figure 106.7 Treatment algorithm for individual patients.

populations. Ivermectin appears to be safe in pregnancy but treatment is best postponed until after delivery[107] and should not be given to children smaller than 90 cm.

In coinfected patients with high levels of *Loa loa* microfilaremia, caution must be exercised using ivermectin to avoid causing a rare encephalopathy (see Chapter 105 and below).[108–110]

In 2004, a phenomenon called "suboptimal response to ivermectin" was observed in an area in northern Ghana, which had seen more than 15 consecutive rounds of yearly ivermectin mass treatment.[111–113] Poor compliance was ruled out in subsequent supervised ivermectin administrations.[111,112] Of concern, this may indicate the beginning of a genetically mediated resistance as observed for ivermectin in veterinary use. Notably, genes associated with resistance against veterinary nematodes are selected during ivermectin mass treatment.[114,115]

Moxidectin

This drug, currently in phase II efficacy studies,[116] is structurally similar to ivermectin and has shown more sustained diminution of microfilariae in animal models. The hope is therefore that moxidectin may reduce microfilarial loads and thus transmission better than does ivermectin. Since the drug has the same mode of action and binds to the same sites, it is uncertain whether it could act as a replacement for ivermectin were ivermectin resistance to spread.

Doxycycline

Doxycycline 100 mg/day for 6 weeks leads to depletion of the endosymbiotic *Wolbachia* in *O. volvulus* (***Fig. 106.6A***), followed by long-term or even permanent cessation of early embryogenesis and thus production of transmissible microfilariae.[5–8,103] This contrasts with ivermectin, which kills larvae only at the later stage of intrauterine microfilariae production[6] with the result that early embryos survive to develop again into microfilariae. In placebo-controlled trials, doxycycline at 200 mg/day for 6 weeks killed 60–70% of adult female worms and sterilized the remaining ones.[9] The same dose for 4 weeks has equivalent sterilizing and about 50% macrofilaricidal activity.[9] If followed up for a longer period of over 2 years, the 100 mg daily dose also has 50% macrofilaricidal effects and shows complete sterilization in the remaining female worms.[117] This makes doxycycline the only safe macrofilaricidal drug against *O. volvulus*. Due to the length of treatment and restrictions of its use in pregnant and breastfeeding women and children below age 9, doxycycline is currently not suitable for mass chemotherapy but has its advantages in the treatment of individual patients, for example expatriates and others who leave an endemic region for longer, or patients with severe hyperreactive onchodermatitis whose symptoms would not be controlled with repeated ivermectin therapy. A recommended current regimen comprises 200 mg/day doxycycline for 6 weeks plus 1–2 additional standard doses of ivermectin (150 μg/kg) toward the end of the doxycycline cycle and for 3–4 months thereafter[103] (***Fig. 106.7***), in order to allow a quick removal of peripheral microfilariae that are not killed by doxycycline, since this drug acts only on the early embryogenesis and the adult worms. This regimen will lead to absence of skin and ocular microfilariae for at least 2–3 years (probably however permanent), and thus it effectively clears the patient from the pathology-inducing microfilariae, with excellent improvement of skin diseases. As recent studies demonstrate, doxycycline is also of use in areas with ivermectin resistance.

Diethylcarbamazine

DEC has microfilaricidal but not adulticidal activity and was used before the introduction of ivermectin. Due to frequent unacceptable DEC-elicited reactions to dying microfilariae, ranging from urticaria and angioedema to hypotension and death, and ocular damage,[90] DEC is no longer used for microfilaricidal treatment of onchocerciasis.

Suramin

Before doxycycline, suramin was the only agent adulticidal to *O. volvulus*. Suramin is extremely toxic, necessitating hospitalization for several days with each dose; and its original regimen of weekly 1 g doses given for 6 weeks is clearly unsafe. Toxicity includes a fatal progressive wasting syndrome, exfoliative dermatitis, progression of chorioretinitis, and development of optic atrophy. Better-tolerated weekly escalating dose regimens, which deliver 4 or 5 g total, are still not without risk and have the disadvantage that at least 34% of adult worms are viable 1 year later.[106,118–120] Because of this, and the alternatives available, suramin treatment is rarely if ever used nowadays.

Nodulectomy

Periodic removal of palpable nodules to reduce microfilarial loads and the ensuing pathologies has been successfully pursued in Latin America. In Africa, where many nodules are deeper, and less accessible, and where reinfection is more frequent, this strategy is less effective. Removal of a single nodule in an expatriate with no further exposure anticipated may be considered.

PREVENTION AND CONTROL

Prophylaxis

At present, there are no effective vaccines or approved chemoprophylactic drugs. Since doxycycline was shown, in several animal models, to block the development from infective larvae (L3) to adult worms,[121–125] doxycycline likely also has an equivalent blocking effect on L3 to adult maturation in onchocerciasis and thus might be prophylactic. As onchocerciasis transmission areas often overlap with those of malaria endemicity, travelers may consider using doxycycline as malaria chemoprophylaxis for the added benefit of protection against onchocerciasis. For expatriates or others with sufficient resources, personal mosquito protection using repellents is likely of benefit. As *Simulium* spp. are daytime biters, bednet programs for malaria control have no effect of onchocerciasis transmission.

Protective immunity is induced after inoculation with live radiation-attenuated L3 in animal models[62,126–128] that are not naturally permissive hosts for *O. volvulus*, as well as under natural exposure conditions in bovine onchocerciasis with *O. ochengi*, the species most closely related to *O. volvulus*.[129] Similar degrees of protection, however, could not be achieved following immunization with single recombinant antigens.[128,130] It is hoped that in the post-genomics and proteomics era better vaccine candidates may be identified.

Vector Control

The Onchocerciasis Control Program (OCP) by the WHO extended from 1974 to 2002 over 11 countries of West Africa most affected by blinding savanna-strain *O. volvulus*.[94,131,132] A strategy of aggressive vector control using aerial larviciding of 50 000 km of rivers combined with annual ivermectin treatments (added in 1988) essentially interrupted transmission in the area under control. It is estimated that 35 million people were protected from infection, and about 200 000 people have been prevented from going blind. Because rapid development of new black flies necessitated weekly treatment of the rivers, the program cost over US$550 million and was unsustainable. Since infected black flies will invade from around the perimeter of the controlled region and infected individuals will continue to migrate into controlled areas, maintenance of OCP success will depend on establishment of ongoing ivermectin treatment programs.

Mass Ivermectin Distribution

The Mectizan Donation Program is a unique and generous initiative established in 1988 by Merck, the manufacturer of ivermectin, to provide free drug to any governmental or nongovernmental program that can demonstrate need and capability to distribute it.[133]

The mandate of the African Programme for Onchocerciasis Control, launched in 1995, is to establish by 2015 a sustainable mechanism for eliminating onchocerciasis as a public health problem in African countries where it is endemic.[134] The program assists 19 affected African countries outside the OCP area in establishing sustainable national programs for ivermectin distribution with the hope that national governments will take over after program closure. More than 90 million treatment doses are planned to be distributed annually.[134] The strategy is based on annual mass treatment with ivermectin to communities (primarily those that are hyper- and mesoendemic, but extending to the rest as the program continues) in order to break transmission by eliminating microfilariae. Unfortunately modeling calculations that take into account expected coverage rates and known levels of microfilariae recurring in the skin 1 year after treatment predict that transmission cannot be interrupted with the current strategy,[135,136] so the treatment programs might have to be continued in perpetuity, although more recent data suggest that elimination of onchocerciasis with ivermectin treatment might be feasible in some endemic foci in Africa.[137] Three-monthly ivermectin treatment does affect microfilaria production long term but is likely not a sustainable strategy in the African context.[97] Mass treatment with ivermectin for onchocerciasis is difficult in loiasis endemic areas because of the risk of encephalopathy, in particular in patients with *Loa loa* microfilariae densities of >8000/mL blood (see Chapter 105). Rapid epidemiologic assessment tools have been developed to allow identification of a community as high risk for such occurrence and providing a tool for decision making in co-endemic areas.[138,139] An alternative may be the administration of doxycycline in such communities, which does not affect *Loa* (since *Loa* does not contain *Wolbachia*) and reduces *O. volvulus* microfilariae only slowly; a pilot study is under way in Cameroon.[140]

OEPA (Onchocerciasis Elimination Programme in the Americas) was launched in 1991 and aims, by 2012, to eliminate transmission, which is defined as <1% reversible (= new) morbidity of ocular disease (anterior chamber) and <0.1% of *O. volvulus* antibodies in "exposed" school children (<1 in 1000). The program is using a strategy of biannual ivermectin treatment and 85% coverage of affected communities. Six countries are covered (Brazil, Colombia, Ecuador, Guatemala, Mexico, and Venezuela), and transmission was interrupted in Colombia and half of the foci in Mexico and Guatemala by 2007.[141–143] Lower vector efficiency, a much lower population at risk (less than half a million), biannual treatment and rigid adherence to coverage rates including annual head counts seem to be key to success.

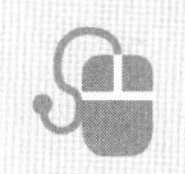

Access the complete reference list online at
http://www.expertconsult.com

CHAPTER 107

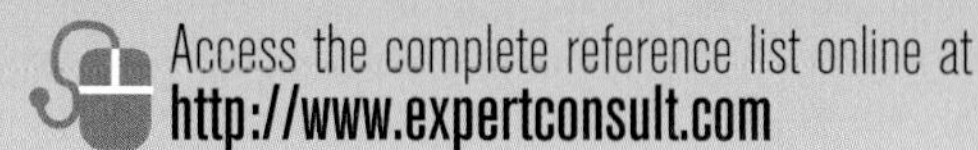
Access the complete reference list online at
http://www.expertconsult.com

Zoonotic Filariasis

Mark L. Eberhard

INTRODUCTION

Zoonotic filariasis is human infection with a filarial parasite that normally parasitizes some other animal host. As is typical of filariae, obligate development occurs in an appropriate arthropod intermediate host and transmission is through the bite of an infected vector. In this regard, transmission of filariasis, including zoonotic infections, has a greater likelihood of occurring in tropical or subtropical climates. This may be due, in part, to a wider diversity of species and greater number of biting insects throughout the year, hence a transmission season that may be year-round. However, as a general rule, a far greater number and range of types of zoonotic infections have been reported in temperate than in tropical regions. Any unique aspects of zoonotic filarial infections limited to the tropics is a reflection only of the geographic distribution of a particular species of parasite involved. Zoonotic filarial infections, therefore, are neither restricted nor unique to the tropics.

THE AGENT

The first well-recognized report of human infection with a zoonotic filaria is attributed to Addario[1] in 1885, who described a case from Italy and called the parasite *Filaria conjunctivae*. It was Desportes,[2] working in Paris in 1939 and 1940, who correctly recognized that *F. conjunctivae* infection was actually caused by species of *Dirofilaria*, and he applied the name *Dirofilaria conjunctivae* to these zoonotic infections. It was not until 1965, however, that Orihel and Beaver[3] concluded that *D. conjunctivae* infection in the United States is most often caused by *Dirofilaria tenuis*, a parasite of raccoons (*Procyon lotor*), whereas in other areas of the world these infections are commonly caused by *Dirofilaria repens*, a natural parasite of dogs in those areas. Since then, several additional species of *Dirofilaria* have been recognized as causes of subcutaneous infection in humans.[4] Subcutaneous infections caused by members of the genus *Dirofilaria* probably constitute the most commonly recognized zoonotic filarial infections in humans.[5–7]

The second most commonly encountered form of zoonotic filarial infection, that caused by the dog heartworm, *Dirofilaria immitis*, was first reported by Faust and coworkers[8] in 1941 from the vena cava of a woman in New Orleans. Infections with *D. immitis* most frequently result in a well-circumscribed lesion in a lobe of the lung, are commonly referred to as coin lesions, and are widely reported from around the world.[4]

More recently, several other genera of filariae have been recognized with some frequency as causes of zoonotic infections. These include *Dipetalonema*-like worms,[9–15] *Onchocerca*,[16–26] and *Brugia*.[27–41] These infections have involved recovery of adult worms in tissue biopsy or surgically excised specimens, although occasionally worms have been recovered free from the surrounding tissues.

On occasion, microfilariae that did not correspond to known human species have been found in skin or blood. These include *Brugia* species,[34] *Mansonella rhodhaini*,[42] *Meningonema peruzzii*,[43,44] *Microfilaria semiclarum*,[45] *Microfilaria bolivarensis*,[46] *Dirofilaria*-like,[47] and *Dipetalonema*-like species.[48] The presence of microfilariae in skin, blood, or cerebrospinal fluid (CSF) indicates the presence of adult male and female worms somewhere in the host tissues.

For ease of review, zoonotic filariae are discussed according to the tissue or organ that they infect in the human host. This information is summarized in ***Table 107.1***.

EPIDEMIOLOGY

The actual, and potential, distribution of zoonotic filariasis is worldwide, depending on the species of filaria. The potential for any given individual to acquire a zoonotic filarial infection is quite low. It would seem that spending an appreciable amount of time outdoors exposed to insect bites is the greatest risk factor. However, there must be other factors besides exposure to infective bites that contribute to infection, since it is likely that nearly everyone who spends time outdoors occasionally will be bitten by an infected insect and exposed to infective filarial larvae. However, in the majority of people, these infective larvae apparently do not survive to undergo development.

Regardless of the type, all zoonotic filariae are transmitted to humans through the bite of infected arthropods similar to the other human filariae (***Fig. 107.1***). As far as is known, transmission of most zoonotic filarial infections has been through mosquito bites, although *Culicoides* and *Simulium* are undoubtedly responsible for transmitting zoonotic *Onchocerca* and *Mansonella* infections.

The geographic distribution of the filariae that are recognized as causes of zoonotic infections is, for the most part, poorly defined, and the distribution of human infections is even more patchy. The continued reports of human zoonotic infections from new geographic areas[49] where there is an absence of information about the occurrence of the parasite in the natural host highlights how little we know about both the natural infections as well as zoonotic infections. More zoonotic infections are detected and identified in North America and Europe than in Latin America, Africa, or Southeast Asia. This is illustrated by the number of zoonotic *Brugia* infections reported from the United States[28,30–32,34,35,38–40] and the large series of zoonotic *D. repens* cases documented by Pampiglione and coworkers[50–53] from Italy. However, this in no way implies that the true incidence of zoonotic infections is higher in temperate than in tropical regions. This disparate distribution of known cases undoubtedly reflects better access to health care and a much different level of health-related concerns on the part of both patient and clinician.

Equally poorly defined are other factors that may contribute to filarial infections. There may well be seasonality to the transmission potential, and this would be more marked in temperate than in tropical areas. Proximity to the natural definitive host also may play an important role in acquisition of infection. In the case of zoonotic infection with *D. immitis*

Table 107.1 Summary of Major Zoonotic Filarial Infections Reported to Cause Infection in Humans

Site	Parasite	Natural Host	Geographic Distribution in Natural Host	Geographic Distribution Site of Reported Human Cases
Lung	*Dirofilaria immitis*	Dog	Cosmopolitan	North and South America, Australia, Japan, Europe
Skin, subcutaneous tissue	*D. tenuis*	Raccoon	North America	North America
	D. repens	Dog	Europe, Russia, Middle East, Africa, Southeast Asia	Europe, Russia, Middle East, Africa, Southeast Asia
	D. ursi	Bear	North America, Japan	North America, Japan
	D. immitis	Dog	Cosmopolitan	North America, Japan
	D. striata	Bobcat, wildcats	North and South America	United States
	Onchocerca spp.	Ungulates	Cosmopolitan	North America, Europe, Russia, Japan
	Mansonella rhodhaini	Chimpanzee	Africa (Gabon)	Africa (Gabon)
Eye	*D. tenuis*	Raccoon	North America	North America
	D. repens	Dog	Europe, Russia, Africa, Southeast Asia	Europe, Russia, Africa, Southeast Asia
	D. immitis	Dog	Cosmopolitan	Australia, Southeast Asia
	Loaina spp.	Rabbit, kangaroo	North America, Australia	South America, Australia
	Dipetalonema-like	?	?	North America
	Onchocerca spp.	Ungulates	Cosmopolitan	United States, Hungary
	Brugia ceylonensis	Dog	Sri Lanka	Sri Lanka
Lymphatics	*Brugia* spp.	Rodents, carnivores	North America, Africa, Southeast Asia	North and South America, Africa
Blood	*Microfilaria bolivarensis*	?	South America (Venezuela)	South America (Venezuela)
	Dipetalonema semiclarum	?	Africa (Congo)	Africa (Congo)

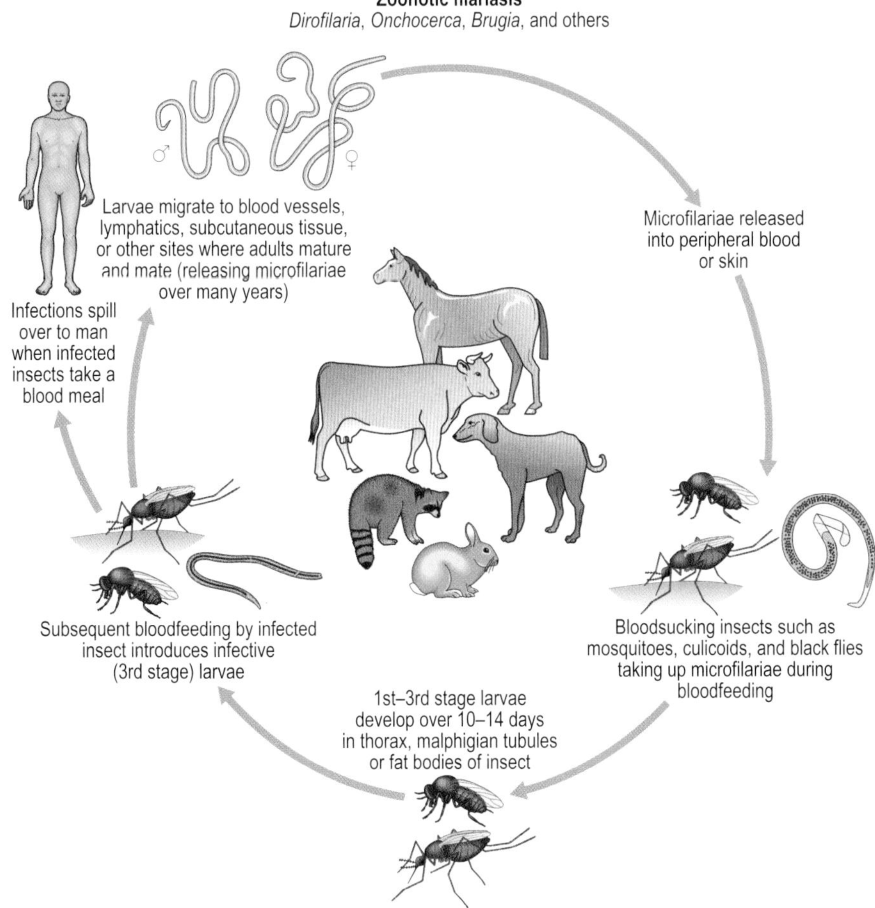

Zoonotic filariasis
Dirofilaria, Onchocerca, Brugia, and others
♂
♀
Larvae migrate to blood vessels, lymphatics, subcutaneous tissue, or other sites where adults mature and mate (releasing microfilariae over many years)
Microfilariae released into peripheral blood or skin
Infections spill over to man when infected insects take a blood meal
Subsequent bloodfeeding by infected insect introduces infective (3rd stage) larvae
Bloodsucking insects such as mosquitoes, culicoids, and black flies taking up microfilariae during bloodfeeding
1st–3rd stage larvae develop over 10–14 days in thorax, malphigian tubules or fat bodies of insect

Figure 107.1 Zoonotic filariasis life cycle.

or *D. repens*, both natural infections of dogs, having an infected dog in the household or in the neighborhood probably increases the risk of exposure to infected mosquito bites. Numerous wild animals, such as raccoons and rabbits, which harbor *D. tenuis* and *Brugia leporis*, respectively, commonly live in residential areas and persons may be exposed in their own backyard or community.

Unfortunately, there is no way to estimate the number of zoonotic filarial infections acquired each year, nor is it possible to gauge the percentage of infections that are detected and diagnosed each year. Many of these zoonotic infections, especially those caused by species of *Dirofilaria*, are now becoming more widely recognized by clinicians and pathologists, and unless there is something unusual about the case, they are not routinely reported in the literature. The more unusual infections, such as those caused by *Brugia* or *Onchocerca*, when recognized, still hold enough interest to merit publication. Overall, however, it is probably safe to say that hundreds of zoonotic infections are attributable to various *Dirofilaria* species each year. On the other hand, no more than about 30 cases of zoonotic *Brugia* infections have been reported, all but one or two occurring in the Western hemisphere. Some zoonotic filarial infections have been recognized on only several occasions. These include 15 reported cases of *Onchocerca*,[16–26] several cases of *Dipetalonema*-like worms,[9–15] three observations of a *Loaina*-like worm,[54,55] and one instance of *Macacanema*.[56]

Although most often caused by a single, infertile worm, zoonotic filarial infections occasionally are recognized to be caused by more than one worm. This has been most evident in cases in which gravid female worms were observed or in which microfilariae were detected. Both instances require not only the presence of a male worm but also that both worms survive long enough to reach sexual maturity and mate. This situation has been reported at least four times in the case of *Dirofilaria* infections,[57–60] three times in *Brugia* infections,[34,35,37] and once in a *Dipetalonema*-like infection.[48] Orihel and colleagues[61] have described a different situation in which two *D. repens* worms, both female and both unmated, were recovered from the same person about 10 months apart. The authors concluded that the worms were from the same inoculum but appeared in the conjunctiva at different times. Multiple worms were reported also in a case of zoonotic onchocerciasis.[26] For some reason, female worms are recorded about three times more often than male worms, although there is no biologic basis for this difference.

THE DISEASE

The disease, its clinical manifestations, and pathologic findings are reflected in the anatomic site of infection and can, for ease of discussion, be broken into four major categories of lesions: subcutaneous, lung, eye, and lymphatic.

Subcutaneous Infections

Several different filarial parasites cause subcutaneous or connective tissue infections, including species of *Dirofilaria*, *Onchocerca*, and *Dipetalonema*-like. In Europe, Africa, and Southeast Asia, *D. repens* is most often incriminated as the etiologic agent and would be at the top of the list of suspected species. In the United States and Canada, *D. tenuis* is most frequently involved. Subcutaneous infection due to one of these *Dirofilaria* species most commonly results in the appearance of a small (0.5–1.5 cm), discrete nodule that is noticed by the patient anywhere from several days to several weeks prior to surgical removal.[4] On sectioning, one or more sections of encased filarial worm are evident (***Fig. 107.2***). These nodules can be either painless or painful and with or without signs of local inflammation. Occasionally, there has been some sensation that a moving worm was present, and in these cases, there tends to be more generalized edema and swelling and a less discrete nodule. There is little systemic sign of infection, although some patients may have an elevated eosinophilia; generally, the presentation is otherwise unremarkable. Zoonotic *Dirofilaria* infections can be expected to occur in almost any anatomic location, but some of the more unusual locations include the bladder,[62] spermatic cord[63–67] or epididymis,[68] liver,[69] and mouth.[70]

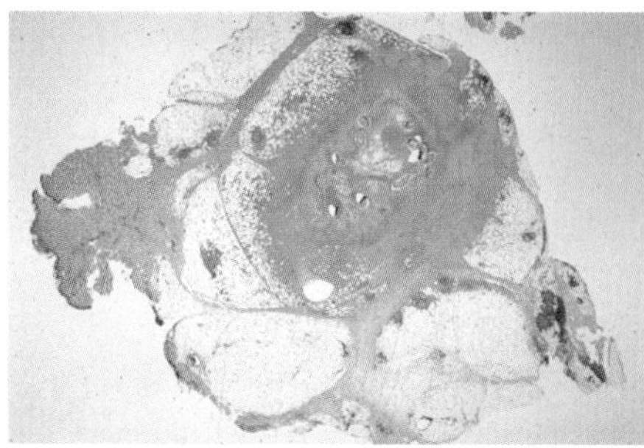

Figure 107.2 A subcutaneous nodule caused by a zoonotic filarial infection due to *Dirofilaria tenuis* from a case in South Carolina. Note the proximity of the nodule to the skin surface and the numerous sections of a single parasite encased in the nodule, which measured approximately 8 mm in diameter. (Hematoxylin and eosin (H&E) stain.)

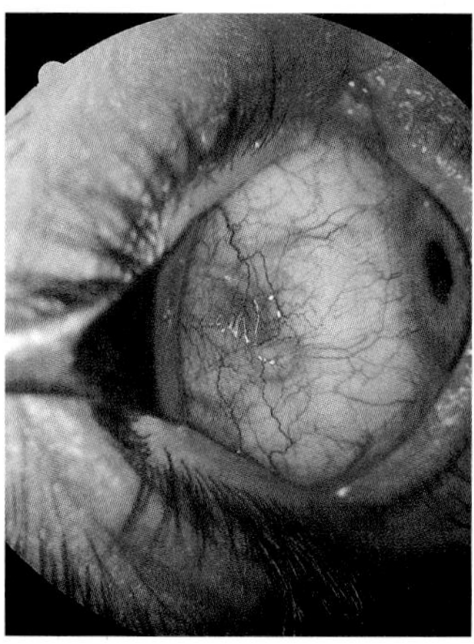

Figure 107.3 Clinical photograph of coiled *Dirofilaria repens* on the conjunctiva. (From Pampiglione S, Canestri Trotti G, Rivasi F. Human dirofilariasis due to *Dirofilaria* (*Nochtiella*) *repens*. A review of world literature. Parassitologia. 1995;37:149–193.)

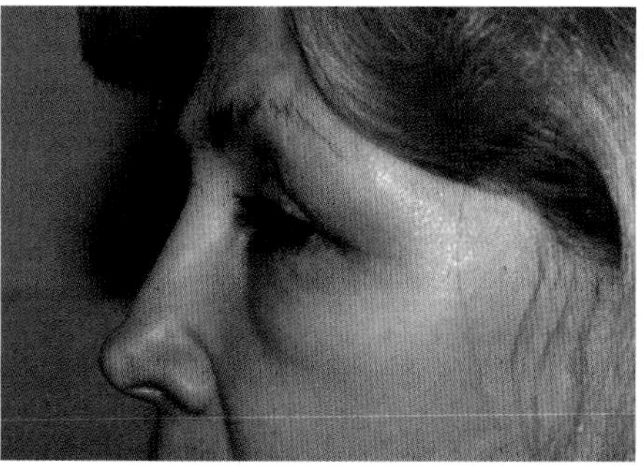

Figure 107.4 Clinical photograph of facial edema in a patient with periorbital soft tissue swelling due to *Dirofilaria tenuis* infection. (From Kersten RC, Locastro AJ, Eberhard ML, et al. Periorbital dirofilariasis. Ophthalmic Plast Reconstr Surg. 1994;10:293–296.)

Eye Infections

A report of a worm in, on, or near the eye of a patient (***Fig. 107.3***) is always a dramatic occurrence for both patient and clinician. Patients frequently report the sensation of "movement of an object" in or near the eye, and the physician can occasionally see the worm in the conjunctiva, on the eye itself, or in the anterior and posterior chambers.[4] The presence of a worm in or around the eye is frequently accompanied by swelling or edema of the eyelid and face (***Figs 107.4 and 107.5***) and a sharp stinging or burning sensation. Worms located in the retina and anterior or posterior chamber of the eye are frequently recognized by the patient because of blurred vision and pain in or behind the eye. In some cases, there is

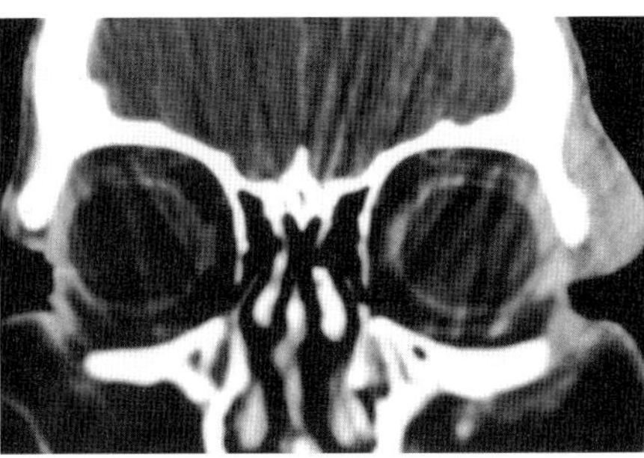

Figure 107.5 Coronal CT scan of the same patient as in Figure 107.4, demonstrating a discrete soft tissue mass without bony or intraorbital involvement. (From Kersten RC, Locastro AJ, Eberhard ML, et al. Periorbital dirofilariasis. Ophthal Plast Reconstr Surg. 1994;10:293–296.)

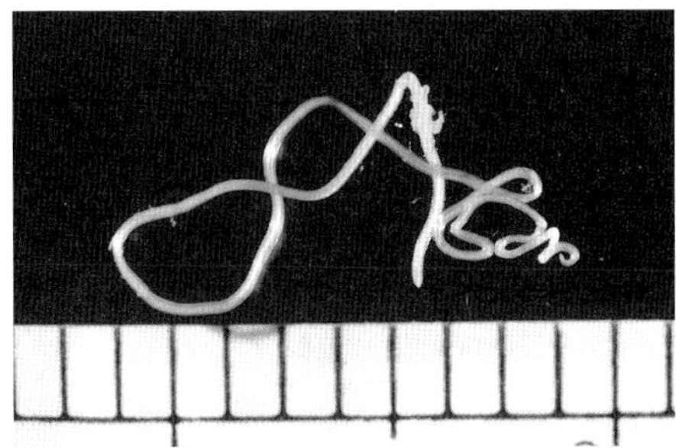

Figure 107.6 Male *Dirofilaria tenuis* worm removed intact from the conjunctiva of a patient in the United States. Scale is in millimeters.

no inflammation, blurred vision, or swollen lids. Reports of a worm in the chamber of the eye often have been attributed to natural human filariae such as *Wuchereria bancrofti*, *Loa loa*, or *Brugia malayi*. However, zoonotic infections due to *Dirofilaria* (*D. repens*, *D. immitis*), *Loaina*, *Dipetalonema*-like worms, *Brugia ceylonensis*, and *Onchocerca* have been described.[23,41,55,71] Many times, worms around or in the eye are recovered free from the tissues (***Fig. 107.6***), while occasionally those in the eye can either be extracted by irrigation-aspiration or destroyed *in situ* using photocoagulation.

Lung Infections

The second most common finding associated with zoonotic filarial infections is discrete lesions in the lung parenchyma resulting in very well-circumscribed, circular nodules (***Figs 107.7 and 107.8***) that on radiographs appear as coin lesions.[4] These lesions are due most often to *D. immitis* but can be caused by *Brugia*-like worms,[14] and recently Pampiglione noted many cases in Europe to be caused by *D. repens*.[72] There is a tendency for these nodules to be solitary and somewhat larger than those due to subcutaneous dirofilariasis. There are cases of multiple nodules[73] as well as reports of transient nodules, suggesting that human infections are much more common than thought.[74] Again, as in the case of subcutaneous dirofilariasis, patients with a lung nodule due to *D. immitis* are often not in bad health, and it is not unusual for the lesions to be detected on chest film as part of a routine medical examination. Over 50% of these patients are asymptomatic, although there are reports of chest pain, low-grade fever, cough, and malaise. Eosinophilia may or may not be a remarkable clinical feature. In direct contrast to subcutaneous dirofilariasis, pulmonary dirofilariasis is almost always confused initially with a malignancy. A large number of reports have addressed the problem of zoonotic filarial infections mimicking pseudotumor or carcinomas, and issues related to differential diagnosis.[75–81] Once the lesion is removed, histologic examination reveals its true nature (***Fig. 107.9***), and the concern of both clinician and patient can be allayed.

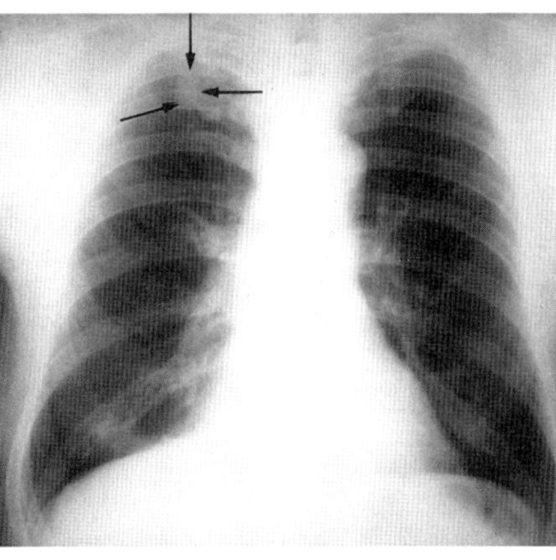

Figure 107.7 Radiograph showing a solitary, subpleural nodule (coin lesion) of the upper lobe of the right lung due to *Dirofilaria* infections. (From Pampiglione S, Canestri Trotti G, Rivasi F. Human dirofilariasis due to *Dirofilaria* (*Nochtiella*) *repens*. A review of world literature. Parassitologia. 1995;37:149–193.)

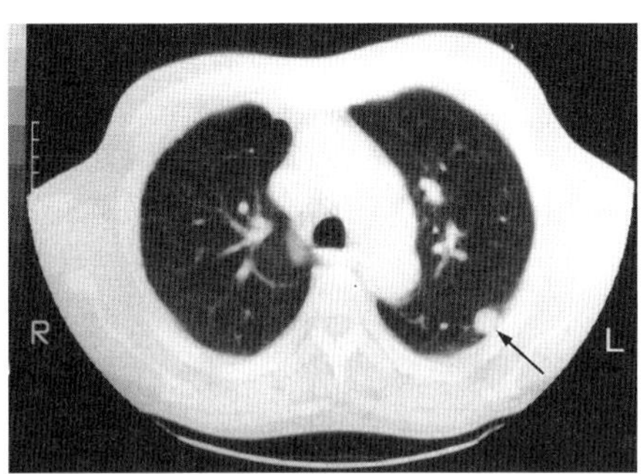

Figure 107.8 CT scan of a solitary nodule in the left lung (arrow) due to *Dirofilaria* infection. (From Pampiglione S, Canestri Trotti G, Rivasi F. Human dirofilariasis due to *Dirofilaria* (*Nochtiella*) *repens*. A review of world literature. Parassitologia. 1995;37:149–193.)

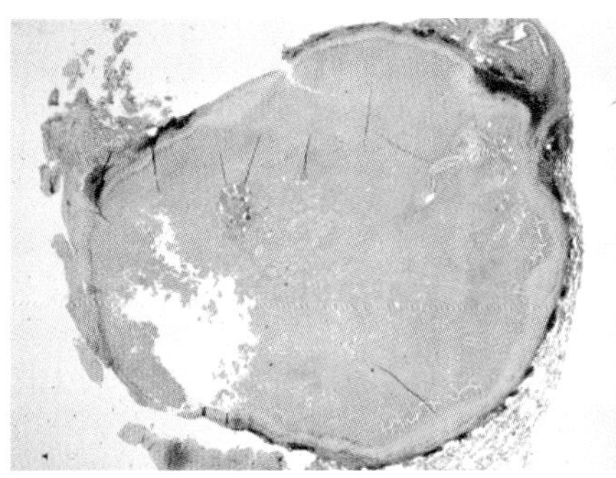

Figure 107.9 Panoramic view of a histologic section of a classic coin lesion in the lung caused by *Dirofilaria immitis* infection. Some normal lung tissue is evident at the lower right-hand corner of the section, and several sections of a worm are evident. Note the well-circumscribed nature of this lesion, which measures approximately 12 mm in diameter. (H&E stain.)

Lymphatic Infections

The location of zoonotic filariae in the lymphatics leads to the classic presentation of a tender, swollen lymph node (***Fig. 107.10***). Although zoonotic *Brugia* infections have been reported from a variety of anatomic locations, the three most common sites are the neck region, groin, and axillary region. The main presenting symptom is an enlarged, painful regional node of one to several weeks' duration. This finding frequently leads to an initial diagnosis of lymphoma or other malignancy. Eosinophilia may or may not be a presenting feature, and occasionally the enlarged node may not be tender. Histologically, the overall presentation is one

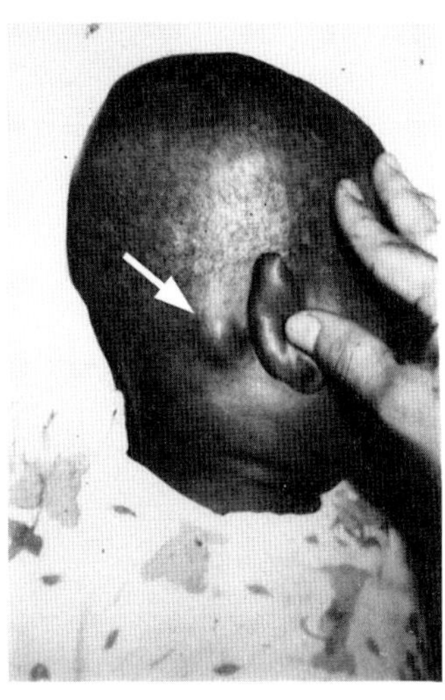

Figure 107.10 Clinical photograph of an enlarged retroauricular lymph node (arrow) in a patient with a zoonotic *Brugia* infection. (From Kozek WJ, Reyes MA, Ehrman J, et al. Enzootic *Brugia* infection in a two-year-old Colombian girl. Am J Trop Med Hyg. 1984;33:65–69.)

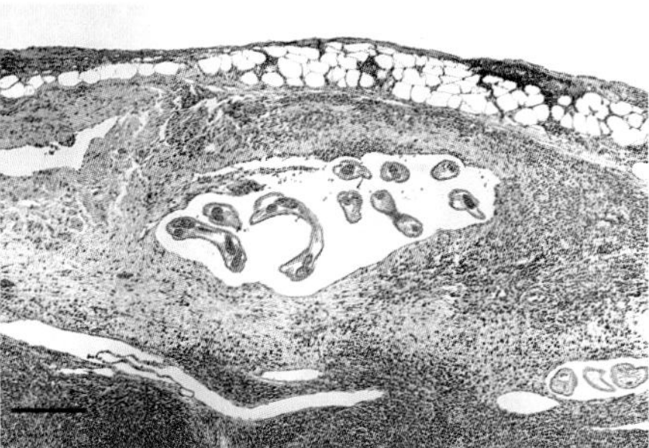

Figure 107.11 Histologic section of a lymph node from a case of zoonotic *Brugia* infection illustrating multiple sections of a worm in lymph channels. Scale bar = 200 μm. (H&E stain.) (From Eberhard ML, DeMeester LJ, Martin BW, et al. Zoonotic *Brugia* infection in western Michigan. Am J Surg Pathol. 1993;17:1058–1061.)

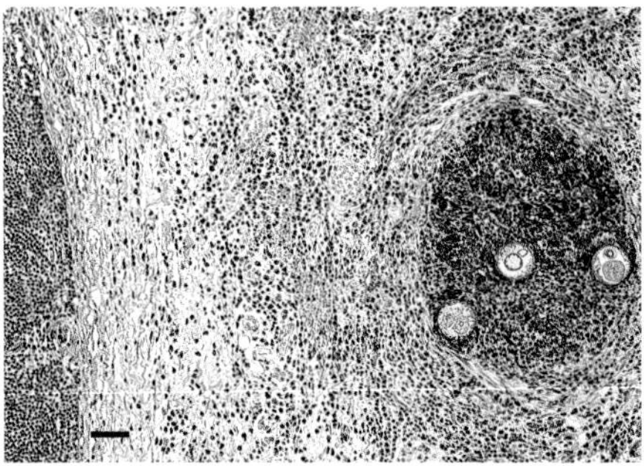

Figure 107.12 Histologic section of a lymph node from a zoonotic *Brugia* infection in which the lymph channel has been obliterated around the worm. Scale bar = 200 μm. (H&E stain.)

of a hyperplastic node with a focal granulomatous reaction. The location of worms in a patent lymph channel is occasionally evident (***Fig. 107.11***), but in more advanced cases, the normal structural architecture of the lymph canal is lost in the inflammatory reaction (***Fig. 107.12***). These differences undoubtedly reflect both the condition of the worm (i.e., alive or dead) and the duration of the host response.

Microfilarial Infections

The detection of microfilariae ascribed to zoonotic filarial infections has not been correlated with clinical symptoms or signs in most cases, although there was clear central nervous system (CNS) involvement in human cases of *Meningonema peruzzii*,[43] and classic signs of lymphatic filariasis, including lymphedema, were noted in a case of zoonotic *Brugia* infection.[34]

PATHOGENESIS AND IMMUNITY

The pathogenesis of zoonotic filariasis is one of localized foreign body reaction around a dead or dying parasite. On the basis of the size of worms seen in these cases and our understanding of the life history of some of these filariae in their natural or experimental hosts, these represent infections of a month to many months' duration. More often than not, these infections are asymptomatic until just prior to the detection of the inflammatory nodule surrounding the worm. Some zoonotic infections, especially those caused by *Dirofilaria* and *Onchocerca*, may represent 6 months or more of asymptomatic growth and wandering by the developing worm. It is believed that only upon the impending death of the worm does a marked tissue reaction occur. Whether the host's response precedes and is responsible for killing the worm, or whether the worm dies because of physiologic incompatibility followed by host reaction to a moribund parasite, is unclear. The fact that many of these zoonotic infections persist asymptomatically for appreciable periods of time suggests that the latter is the case.

Limited studies indicate that the human host produces antibodies directed at the parasite, and that these antifilarial antibodies can be detected in serum samples. In several cases of zoonotic *Brugia* infections, isotype-specific, antifilarial antibodies, as determined by an enzyme-linked immunosorbent assay (ELISA) using adult *Brugia* antigens, have demonstrated elevated responses that markedly diminish by 3 months post surgery.[39,40] Various serologic assays have also been developed to detect *Dirofilaria* infections.[82–88] These assays, although frequently not able to distinguish between different types of infections, could clearly be helpful in suspected cases when no worm was observed in the biopsy but a suggestive granulomatous reaction was present, and in conducting seroepidemiologic surveys. It has been suggested that zoonotic filarial infections result in immunopathologic reactions, such as arthritis.[89]

DIAGNOSIS

The diagnosis of zoonotic filarial infections, for the foreseeable future, will continue to be the recognition and accurate identification of these parasites in excisioned or biopsy histologic sections.[90] This is not to say that good serologic assays would not play a vital role in diagnosis and management. However, because zoonotic filarial infections are constituted of any number of different species, serologic assays that are genus-specific rather than species-specific would be much more valuable as screening tools.

Diagnosis of the genus (and species) of filaria causing the infection is best accomplished by study of the morphologic features seen in tissue sections. Occasionally, intact worms are removed, particularly from in or around the eye, and these can usually be tentatively identified based on comparison with recognized species found in the area where the patient is believed to have acquired the infection.

Location of the lesion containing the worm can frequently provide some guidance in identifying the worm. For instance, a worm associated with the lymphatic system has a high probability of being a zoonotic *Brugia* infection, while the location of a worm in a coin lesion in the lung is likely to be *D. immitis*. The morphology of the worm provides a much greater degree of accuracy (sensitivity) than does the location of the lesion and ensures that a worm in an unusual location is not misdiagnosed. The polymerase chain reaction was recently utilized on tissues to assist with the diagnosis of zoonotic dirofilariasis.[91]

The diagnosis of zoonotic filarial infections is almost always made from stained tissue sections, and there are morphologic features that allow placement of worms into several broad groups.[90,92] These are discussed briefly in the following sections.

Dirofilaria

By far the most common zoonotic infections encountered are caused by species of *Dirofilaria*. Three species are believed to account for the vast majority of recognized cases. *D. immitis*, the dog heartworm, has a nearly cosmopolitan distribution that is continuing to expand; *D. repens* infects dogs and cats in Europe, Africa, Southeast Asia, and possibly elsewhere; and *D. tenuis* is a natural parasite of raccoons in North America. Other species reported from humans include *D. striata* of wildcats in North and South America, and *D. ursi*, which parasitizes bears in North America and Japan. A vast number of other dirofilariae exist, and all probably hold zoonotic potential.

Dirofilaria worms have several consistent features that are recognizable in sections. Generally, they are relatively large worms, up to 400 or 500 μm in diameter; they have a thick cuticle, which, with the exception of *D. immitis* and *D. striata*, has prominent longitudinal ridges; and the musculature is prominent, with numerous muscle cells that extend far into the body cavity (***Figs 107.13–107.18***). It should be noted here that size can be a very useful feature in the determination of possible species. However, one must also use caution, as many of the worms removed in these cases represent immature worms, which makes size comparisons difficult.

Brugia

The recognition of small filariae in close association with lymph nodes or lymph vessels, or on rare occasions the eye, would be suggestive of infection with a zoonotic *Brugia* species (see ***Figs 107.10–107.12***). The species involved in the reported human cases have not been established. A number of species have been described from various animals. In the United States we recognize two species, *B. beaveri* of the raccoon and *B. leporis* of rabbits; from South America, *B. guyanensis* of the coatimundi; *B. tupaie* of tree shrews and *B. pahangi* in dogs, cats, slow loris, leaf monkeys, and wildcats from Malaysia; *B. patei* of dogs, cats, wildcats, and bush babies from Africa; and *B. ceylonensis* from dogs and *B. buckleyi* from hares in Sri Lanka.

In section, zoonotic *Brugia* are small worms, almost always less than 150 μm and occasionally less than 50 μm in diameter. The cuticle is relatively thin but frequently thickens over the lateral chords, and the muscle

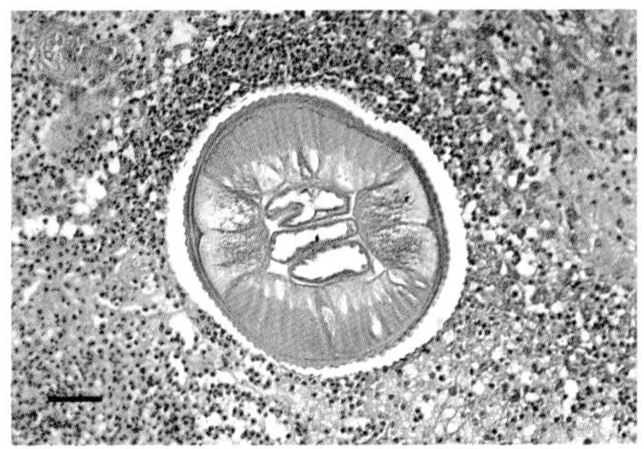

Figure 107.13 High-power photomicrograph of a section of a female *Dirofilaria tenuis* from the same case as illustrated in ***Figure 107.2***. This section clearly illustrates the nature of the thick cuticle with numerous external ridges and two internal lateral ridges in the region of the lateral chords. Tall, heavy musculature, prominent lateral chords, two uterine tubes, and a section of intestine are also evident. Scale bar = 50 μm. (H&E stain.)

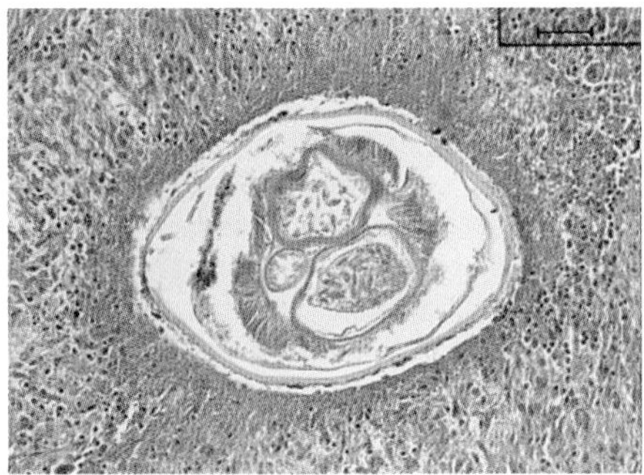

Figure 107.14 High-power photomicrograph of a section of a female *Dirofilaria tenuis* from the case illustrated in ***Figure 107.4***. Although this worm is moribund and has undergone considerable degeneration, the thick cuticle with external ridging, heavy musculature, two uterine reproductive tubes, and a single digestive tube are still evident. Scale bar = 50 μm. (H&E stain.)

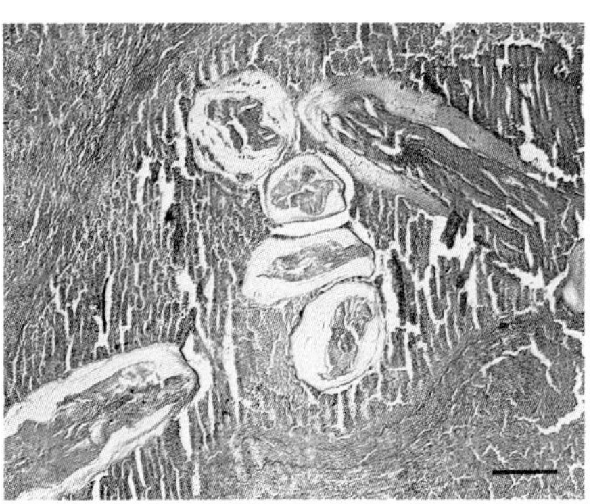

Figure 107.15 Photomicrograph of the coiled *Dirofilaria immitis* worm seen in ***Figure 107.9***. At this magnification, several features of the worm are evident, including the thick cuticle and heavy musculature. Scale bar = 200 μm. (H&E stain.)

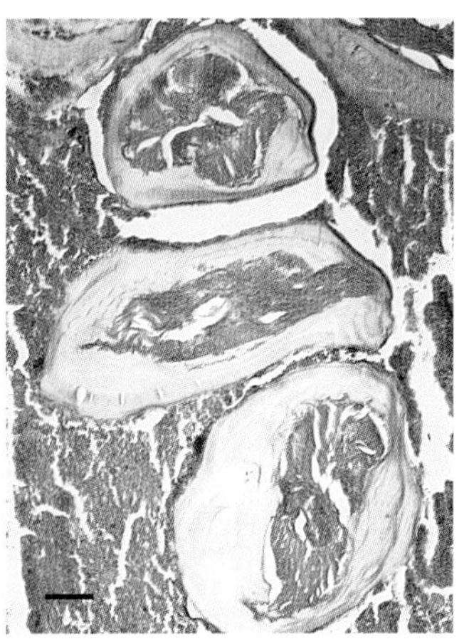

Figure 107.16 High-power photomicrograph of the worm seen in ***Figure 107.15***. At this higher magnification, it is evident that the worm is moribund and has undergone considerable degeneration. The cuticle is considerably swollen and thickened and has a smooth outer surface, and remnants of the heavy musculature are evident. Scale bar = 50 μm. (H&E stain.)

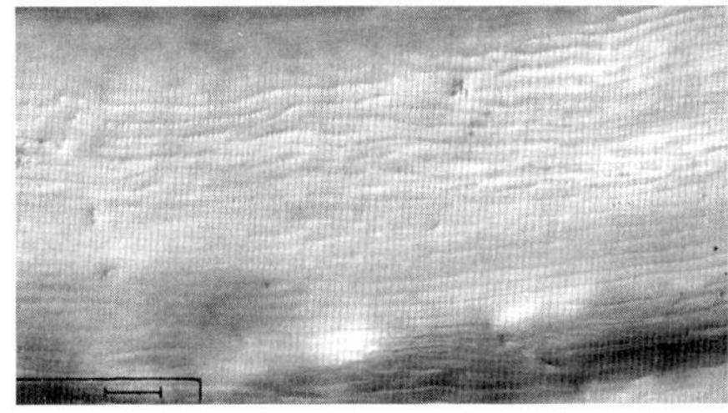

Figure 107.17 Low-power view of the cuticular surface of a *Dirofilaria repens* removed intact from the tissues, illustrating the beaded ridges that run longitudinally along the worm. Scale bar = 50 μm.

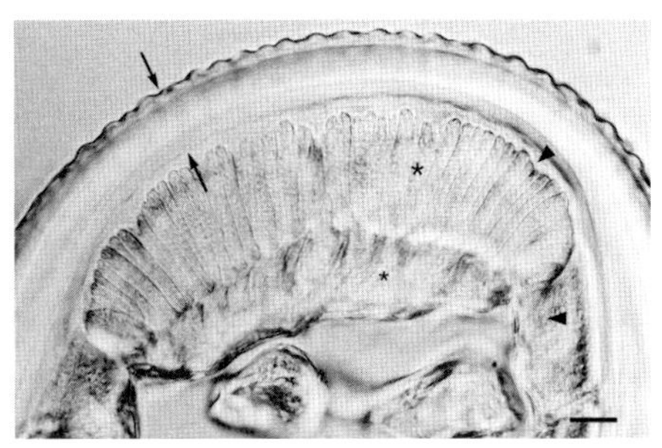

Figure 107.18 Cross-section of an unstained *Dirofilaria repens* (in glycerin), illustrating the typical *Dirofilaria* anatomy. Evident is the thick, multilayered cuticle with external ridging (arrows), the thin inconspicuous hypodermal tissue that greatly expands in the area of the lateral chords (arrowheads), and the tall, heavy muscle cells that are composed of a narrow, basal, fibrillar, contractile portion (large asterisk) and a shorter cytoplasmic portion (small asterisk). Scale bar = 50 μm.

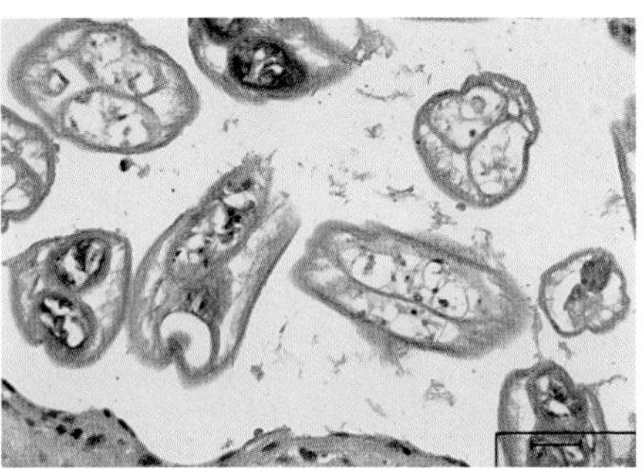

Figure 107.19 High-power view of a coiled female *Brugia* worm in a lymph channel, illustrating the small size of the worm, the thin cuticle, and the small number of low muscle cells per quadrant. Scale bar = 25 μm. (H&E stain.)

cells are few in number, flat, and broad, and do not extend far into the body cavity (***Fig. 107.19***).

Onchocerca

The number of described *Onchocerca* species that might result in zoonotic infections in humans is too great to list here, but the genus is cosmopolitan, and normal animal hosts include a wide range of ungulates, including cattle, horses, camels, various antelope, deer, and sheep. *Onchocerca* species have a predilection for residing in or near connective tissues in their natural hosts, and this has been the case in the majority of zoonotic infections as well. Two cases involving the eye have been reported.[22,25]

In sections (***Figs 107.20–107.24***), *Onchocerca* have several prominent features including, in longitudinal section, a cuticle that bears external ridges and internal striae, and in transverse section, a thick cuticle that is often unevenly thickened; prominent hypodermal tissue not restricted to the lateral chords; and few muscle cells per quadrant, which are distinctive in appearance, being atrophied and wispy.

Dipetalonema-like

Zoonotic filarial infections that do not readily fall into the preceding categories are frequently referred to as *Dipetalonema*-like. Generally, these worms are small and have been reported from several anatomic locations, including the eye and subcutaneous tissue. A number of these cases have resulted in recovery of nearly intact worms from the eye.[55] The morphologic features of *Dipetalonema*-like worms in tissue are nondescript and include small size, the presence of a relatively thin, smooth cuticle, and weak musculature. Assigning a definitive identification to these specimens has been difficult owing in part to their immature state of development and further complicated by the large number of described species and the recognition that there may be a great number of as yet unrecognized species.

Interestingly, one report described recovery of microfilariae similar to *Mansonella interstitium* of squirrels from the blood of a 12-year-old child from Alabama.[48]

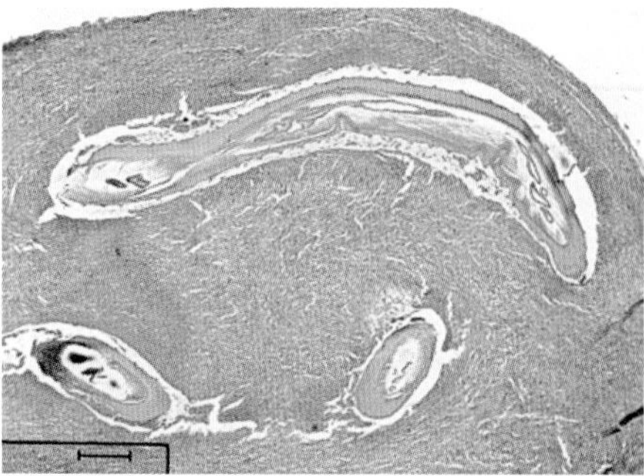

Figure 107.20 Low-power view of connective tissue containing three sections of a female *Onchocerca* species from a case of zoonotic human infection. The coiled nature of the worm, the thick cuticle, and ridging on the surface of the cuticle are evident. Scale bar = 200 μm. (H&E stain.) (From Ali-Khan Z. Tissue pathology and comparative microanatomy of *Onchocerca* from a resident of Ontario and other enzootic *Onchocerca* species from Canada and the United States. Ann Trop Med Parasitol. 1977;71:470–482.)

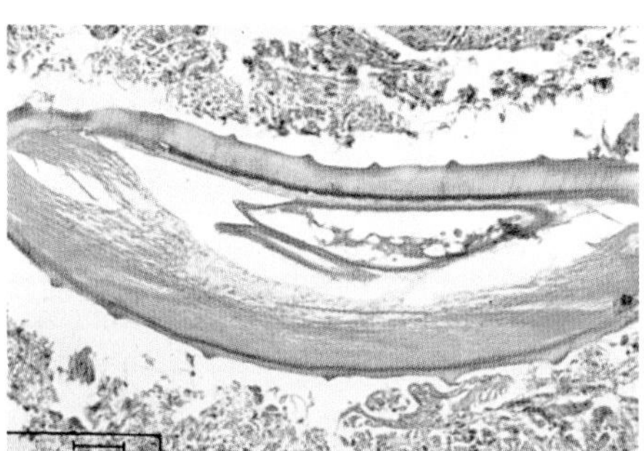

Figure 107.21 Higher magnification of the worm seen in ***Figure 107.20***, illustrating the nature of the cuticle, including external ridges, internal striae, and uneven thickness. Scale bar = 50 μm. (H&E stain.) (From Ali-Khan Z. Tissue pathology and comparative microanatomy of *Onchocerca* from a resident of Ontario and other enzootic *Onchocerca* species from Canada and the United States. Ann Trop Med Parasitol. 1977;71:470–482.)

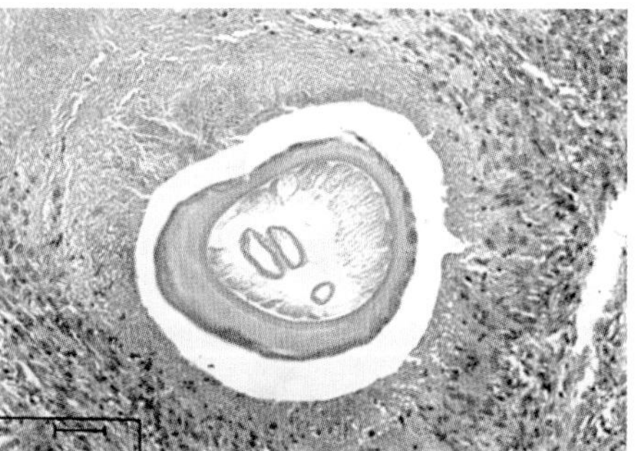

Figure 107.22 Higher magnification of a cross-section of the female *Onchocerca* species seen in ***Figure 107.20***, illustrating the typical features seen in zoonotic infections. The cuticle is thick throughout, but much thicker over the upper part of the worm as a result of an outer ridge. The muscle cells are few per quadrant and weak in nature; they are appreciably taller in the ventral hemisphere, seen here in the lower half of the worm. The hypodermal tissue is most evident in the region of the lateral chords. Two paired uteri are evident, as is the small intestine, which lies to the left. Scale bar = 50 μm. (H&E stain.) (From Ali-Khan Z. Tissue pathology and comparative microanatomy of *Onchocerca* from a resident of Ontario and other enzootic *Onchocerca* species from Canada and the United States. Ann Trop Med Parasitol. 1977;71:470–482.)

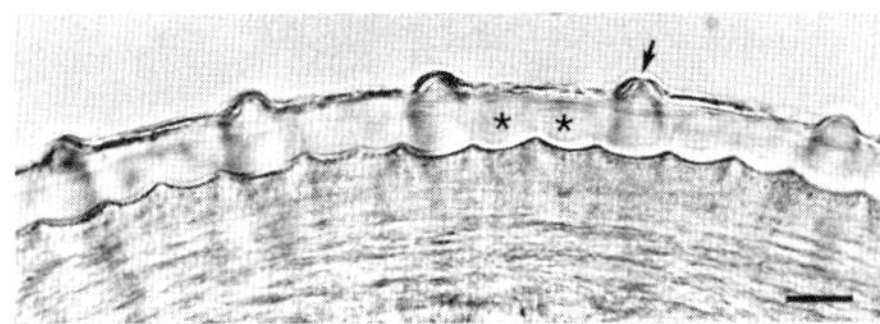

Figure 107.23 Unstained, cleared section of body wall of *Onchocerca stilesi*, a natural parasite of the ligaments of the legs of cattle in the United States, illustrating the external ridging (arrow) and interval striae (asterisks) in the cuticle. Compare the stained section illustrated in ***Figure 107.24***. Scale bar = 15 μm.

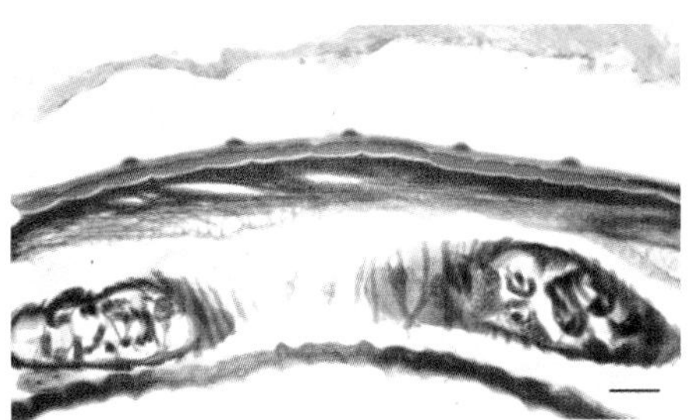

Figure 107.24 High-power photomicrograph of a longitudinal section of a female *Onchocerca stilesi*. This trichrome-stained section illustrates the characteristic features of the cuticle useful in identifying zoonotic onchocercal infections. The outer ridges and inner striae illustrated in ***Figure 107.23*** are evident. Sections of uterus with developing microfilariae also are evident. Scale bar = 15 μm.

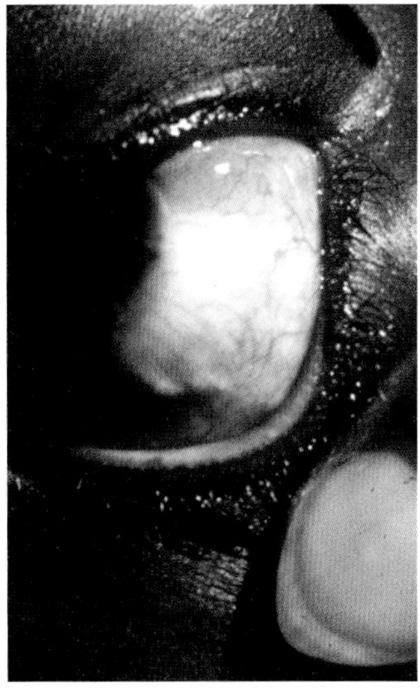

Figure 107.25 Photograph showing two small nodules (lower left hand quadrant) in the conjunctiva of a Ugandan, typical of those seen in cases of bung-eye. (From Baird JK, Neafie RC, Connor DH, et al. Nodules in the conjunctiva, bung-eye, and bulge-eye in Africa caused by *Mansonella perstans*. *Am J Trop Med Hyg*. 1988;38:553-557.)

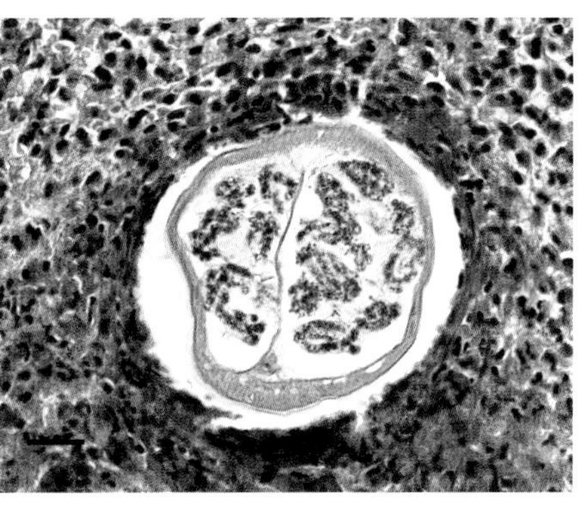

Figure 107.26 High-power photomicrograph of a worm seen in sections of a nodule removed from a case of bung-eye in Uganda. The morphologic features of the parasite include a thin cuticle, numerous muscle cells, which are low and do not extend far into the body cavity, paired uteri containing microfilariae and a very inconspicuous intestine. Scale bar = 20 μm. (H&E stain.) (From Baird JK, Neafie RC, Connor DH, et al. Nodules in the conjunctiva, bung-eye, and bulge-eye in Africa caused by *Mansonella perstans*. *Am J Trop Med Hyg*. 1988;38:553-557.)

Zoonotic Filariae of Uncertain Origin (or Incompletely Described Zoonotic Infections)

There are numerous other reports of zoonotic filarial infections in humans, some of which represent single case reports, while in others only microfilariae have been recovered with no description of the accompanying adult worm. These are briefly discussed as follows:

In 1932, Owen and Hennessey[93] noted 33 cases of an unusual presentation of small (2 mm diameter) yellow nodules containing dead filarial worms located on the conjunctiva of persons living in Uganda. The authors referred to these cases as "bung-eye" or "bulge-eye." Baird and colleagues[94] reviewed eight cases of bung-eye (***Fig. 107.25***) collected from several countries in Africa, and concluded that the majority of cases were caused by aberrant localization of *Mansonella perstans* (***Fig. 107.26***). This determination suggests that these infections were not zoonotic but rather common human infections in an uncommon location. However, a final decision on the identity of these worms awaits a better understanding of the microanatomy of the genus *Mansonella*, which contains a number of species that infect humans as well as animals. It is now clear that bung-eye is not restricted geographically to Uganda.

In 1968, Dukes and colleagues[43] described two cases of microfilariae in the CSF from residents of then Rhodesia (now Zambia and Zimbabwe). The authors attributed the infections to *M. perstans* and provided detailed clinical descriptions. In 1973, Orihel and Esslinger[95] described a new filarial parasite, *Meningonema peruzzii*, from the CNS of African monkeys. The microfilariae of *M. peruzzii*, although sheathed, resemble *M. perstans* microfilariae to a great extent. In that same year, Orihel[44] reviewed original material from the previous human cases reported by Dukes and associates and demonstrated a sheath on the microfilariae, concluding that these were infections due to *M. peruzzii*. Another report of this filaria in humans has been documented.[96] Clinicians and laboratorians must be alert to the presence of microfilariae in CSF or blood and to the morphologic features of the parasite, including the presence of a sheath. An unusual microfilaria with a marked clear region in the posterior body was described by Fain[45] in 1974 from 52 inhabitants of several villages in Zaire; the microfilaria was named *Dipetalonema semiclarum*. *D. semiclarum* resembles *M. perstans* but differs by having, in addition to the clear space in the posterior half of the body, a much longer cephalic space. The adult stage has not been recovered and described, but the microfilaria does not correspond to any recognized species reported from animals of that region of Africa.

In 1980, an unrecognized microfilaria was reported from the blood of American Indians living in the Orinoco River basin in Venezuela.[46] It was given the name *Microfilaria bolivarensis*. The microfilaria superficially resembles that of *Onchocerca volvulus* but is smaller and stouter and has a shorter cephalic space and less compact nuclear column.

Richard-Lenoble and colleagues[42] reported in 1982 the occurrence of microfilariae indistinguishable from *Mansonella rhodhaini* in 14 inhabitants of Gabon. This is a natural parasite of chimpanzees, and the microfilariae measure more than 300 μm in length by only 2–3 μm in diameter, making them clearly distinct from either *Onchocerca volvulus* or *Mansonella streptocerca*.

TREATMENT AND PROGNOSIS

Treatment of zoonotic filarial infections almost always involves surgical removal of the worm or lesion containing the parasite. Frequently, the correct diagnosis is not made until after examination of the specimen or histologic section reveals the identification. However, since most cases involve only a single worm, surgical removal is curative.

The prognosis in most cases is good. Many worms probably die and are absorbed without any clinical signs or symptoms. In those cases in which a marked tissue reaction draws attention to the presence of a foreign body, the lesion, as noted, is frequently removed surgically. If the host tissue reaction were left to run its course without surgical intervention, the parasite would eventually die and be resolved and the inflammatory lesion would subside over time. This scenario would be true for worms in almost all locations, except worms inside the eye (anterior or posterior chamber, retina). In this location, the physical damage caused by the worm itself, as well as a pronounced inflammatory reaction, could result in serious, permanent damage and loss of visual acuity.

PREVENTION AND CONTROL

Prevention and control of zoonotic filarial infections are difficult tasks, further complicated by the insect intermediate host. The surest way to prevent zoonotic filarial infections is to protect oneself from the bite of potentially infected insect vectors. This is easier stated than accomplished, especially given the wide range of potential vectors. Because the majority of filariae that are known to cause zoonotic infections are transmitted by various mosquito species, the greatest risk is through mosquito bites. Protective clothing, use of insect repellents, household screening, and behavior modification geared toward avoidance of insect bites would provide some degree of protection.

Control of zoonotic filarial infections is even more challenging. Clearly, efforts directed at reducing mosquito or other biting insect populations would significantly reduce the risk of exposure. Because of flight ranges, however, these efforts would need to be coordinated and sustained at the community level or higher. Local government efforts directed at mosquito abatement probably indirectly reduce the overall risk of zoonotic filarial infection. Of the species of filariae that are recognized to cause zoonotic infections, only *D. immitis* and *D. repens* occur commonly in a domestic pet population. Putting a household pet dog on heartworm preventive treatment may well reduce the likelihood of acquiring infection from one's own pet, but unless every dog (and wild canid) in the area is treated, a potential risk still exists. However, until there is better understanding of why some individuals exposed to zoonotic filariae develop infection while most others do not, it will be difficult to develop comprehensive prevention and control strategies.

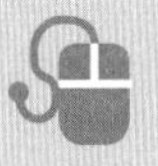

Access the complete reference list online at
http://www.expertconsult.com

Access the complete reference list online at http://www.expertconsult.com

CHAPTER 108

Dracunculiasis

Ernesto Ruiz-Tiben • Donald R. Hopkins

INTRODUCTION

Guinea worm disease (dracunculiasis), caused by the nematode parasite *Dracunculus medinensis*, is a disabling disease of rural people in parts of six countries in Africa.[1,2] Other synonyms for the infection include dracontiasis and dracunculosis. Salient characteristics of this infection are that it manifests by 2–3 foot (~1 meter) long worms emerging directly through a lesion on the skin, and it has an enormous adverse impact on school attendance and agricultural production. Dracunculiasis is also close to being completely eradicated.

THE AGENT

Dracunculus medinensis has been known since at least ancient Egypt. Because differentiation between species of *Dracunculus* requires morphological examination of adult male worms (which are seldom available), efforts are under way to map the genome of the guinea worm's DNA in order to ascertain this parasite's species more precisely and reliably. Although there are several known zoonotic species of *Dracunculus*, only *medinensis* is specific to humans. The life cycle of the parasite was first fully described by Alexei Fedchenko in 1870.[3]

EPIDEMIOLOGY

During the nineteenth and twentieth centuries, dracunculiasis was common in much of southern Asia, and in North, West, and East Africa. When the Dracunculiasis Eradication Program was getting under way in 1986, an estimated 3.5 million cases still occurred in India and Pakistan and 16 African countries.[4] Yemen was discovered to still be endemic in 1994. The World Health Organization (WHO) declared Central African Republic to have indigenous transmission in 1996, making it the 20th endemic country.[5] By 2008, only 4619 cases were reported in the six remaining endemic countries of East and West Africa (***Fig. 108.1***); Asia became free of the disease in 1997.

People become infected when they drink water containing tiny freshwater copepods called "cyclops" or "water fleas," which act as intermediate hosts and harbor infective larvae.[6] When the ingested copepods are killed by the digestive juices in the stomach, larvae are released and move to the small intestine where they penetrate the intestinal wall and migrate to the connective tissues of the thorax.[6] Male and female larvae mature and mate 60–90 days after infection. Over the next 10–14 months, gravid female worms mature, reaching lengths of 70–100 cm (2–3 feet), and slowly migrate to the surface of the body (***Fig. 108.2***). On contact with fresh water, powerful contractions cause a loop of the worm's uterus to break and discharge a swarm of motile larvae. Contraction of the worm and discharge of larvae may be repeated if the lesion is again submerged in water, until the entire brood of larvae is discharged. Motile free-swimming larvae are ingested by copepods and mature in their body cavity in about 2 weeks. Stagnant sources of drinking water, such as ponds, cisterns, pools in dried-up river beds, and shallow unprotected hand-dug wells, commonly harbor populations of copepods, and are the usual sites where infection is transmitted.

The disease's seasonality varies according to location. In endemic areas just below the Sahara Desert (e.g., Mauritania, Mali, Niger, northern Nigeria, Burkina Faso, southern Sudan, and Ethiopia) transmission usually peaks during the rainy season at mid-year (May–September). This is because stagnant surface sources of water are far more common during the 5–6 month-long rainy season in such areas. In areas near the Gulf of Guinea (e.g., Côte d'Ivoire, Ghana, Togo, Benin, and southern Nigeria), the disease peaks during the dry season, from October to March, when mostly stagnant sources of drinking water remain, in contrast to abundant surface water sources during the rest of the year. The seasonal emergence of the worm often coincides with harvest or planting seasons, and thus significantly affects agricultural productivity and also school attendance.

THE DISEASE

Infected persons remain asymptomatic for approximately a year after infection, until the mature female worm approaches the skin and forms a painful papule in the dermis. This papule can become a blister within 24 hours or may enlarge for several days before becoming a blister (***Fig. 108.3***). Eventually the blister ruptures, exposing the worm (***Fig. 108.4***). Shortly before the skin lesion forms, focal and systemic symptoms may occur, including local erythema and an urticarial rash with intense pruritus, nausea, diarrhea, and dizziness. Worms usually emerge from the lower extremities, but they can also emerge from any part of the body, including the head, upper extremities, buttocks and genitalia. As the worm emerges through the skin lesion, the affected person pulls it out slowly and carefully (because of inflammation and pain), usually by winding a few centimeters of the worm each day on a small stick. This very painful process may last many weeks. Pain and other symptoms may lessen with the rupture of the blister, but at this time pyogenic bacterial organisms invariably invade the superficial lesion and worm tract and aggravate the condition. If the worm breaks during extraction and the remaining part retracts into the tissue, an intense inflammatory reaction occurs, with pain, swelling, and cellulitis along the worm tract, and usually the formation of an abscess. The reported period of incapacitation ranges from 2 to 16 weeks (average 8.5 weeks)[6–18] and more than half of a village's population may be affected at the same time. In addition to the blisters and skin lesions, the secondary bacterial infections usually exacerbate local inflammation and often lead to sepsis, abscesses, septic arthritis, contracture of muscles near joints, or even tetanus.

DIAGNOSIS, PATHOGENESIS AND IMMUNITY

The symptoms produced by *Dracunculus* vary in the acute or chronic phases of the infection. The acute manifestations begin about 1 year after

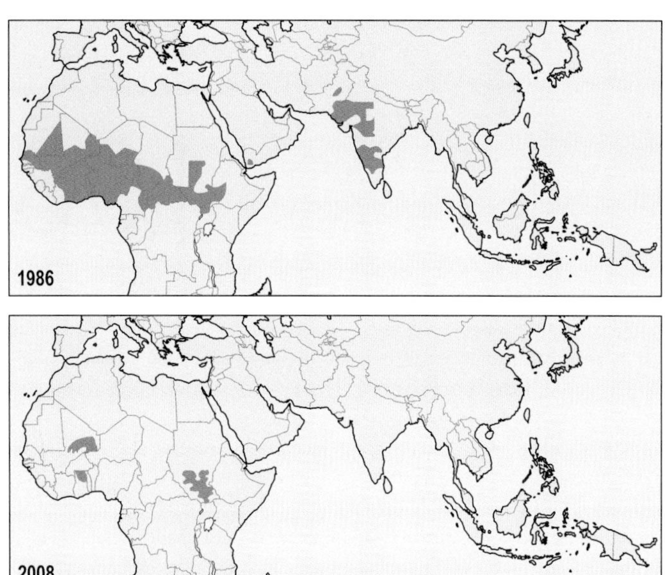

Figure 108.1 Extent of areas affected with endemic dracunculiasis in Asia and Africa during 1986, and during 2008.

infection and are related to the release of the larvae into the water. The initial blister in the skin is accompanied by redness and induration, and is usually preceded by slight fever and allergic symptoms. The lesion is found in 85–90% of cases on the lower extremities, including the ankle, or foot. The blistering lesion produces intense irritation and burning, inducing the patient to seek relief by immersing the affected limb in water, where the blister breaks, allowing the adult worm to discharge larvae into the water. The chronic manifestations are due to inflammation of the joints with clinical symptoms and signs of arthritis,[19] synovitis,[20] and muscle and tendon contractures with resultant ankylosis of the limb.[21] Migration of the worms to the retroperitoneum and from the retroperitoneum to the subcutaneous tissue in the leg sometimes results in aberrant (ectopic) locations of the worm such as in the pancreas,[22] lung,[23] periorbital tissues,[24,25] testis,[26] pericardium,[27,28] and the spinal cord, producing compression[29,30] as well as focal abscess formation.[31]

TREATMENT AND PROGNOSIS

There is no curative drug or vaccine against dracunculiasis. Infected persons do not develop immunity. Applying wet compresses to the lesion may relieve pain during the worm's emergence. Placing an occlusive bandage on the wound keeps it clean and may help prevent the patient from contaminating sources of drinking water. Oral medications to alleviate the associated pain and inflammation, and topical antiseptics or antibiotic ointment to minimize the risk of secondary bacterial infections also help reduce inflammation, and may permit removal of the worm by gentle traction over a number of days.

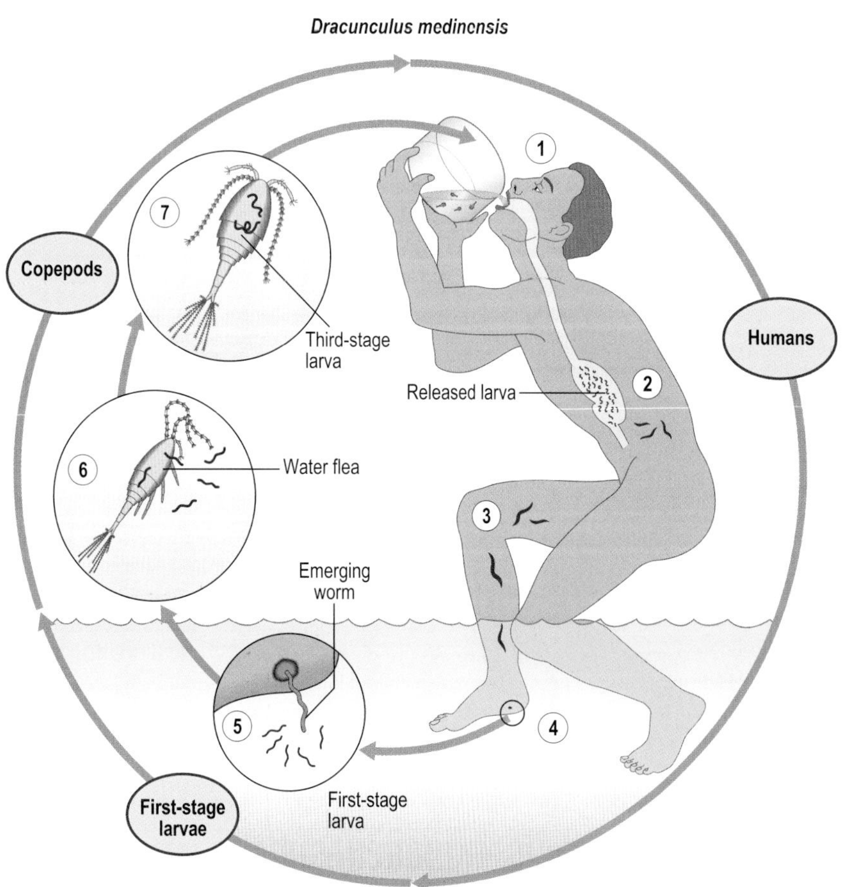

Figure 108.2 Life cycle of *Dracunculus medinensis.* (Redrawn from Encyclopedia Britannica, Inc., © 1996.)

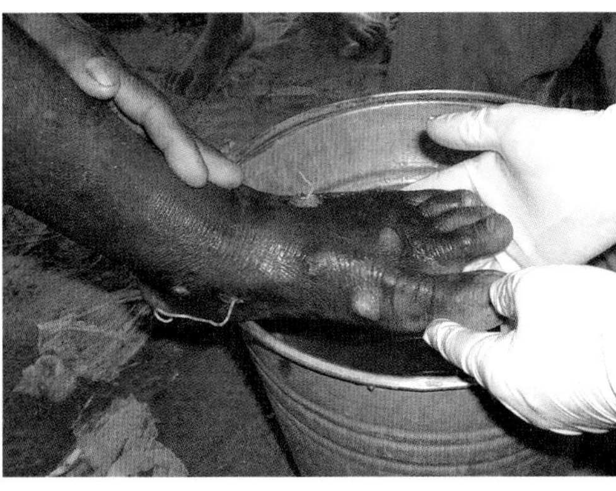

Figure 108.3 Blisters caused by *Dracunculus medinensis* and rupture of blisters resulting in lesions with protruding guinea worms. (Courtesy of Elizabeth Long.)

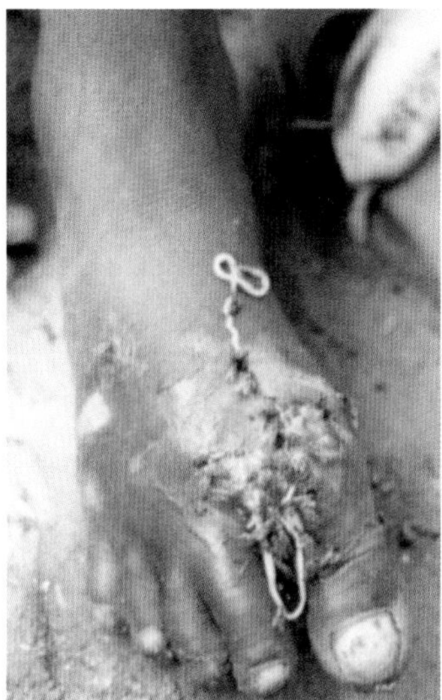

Figure 108.4 Pyogenic organisms invade the superficial lesion and worm tract, aggravating the condition. (Courtesy of WHO Collaborating Center for Research, Training, and Eradication of Dracunculiasis at the Centers for Disease Control and Prevention.)

PREVENTION AND CONTROL

Transmission of dracunculiasis is prevented by educating people about the origin of the disease, teaching them to filter drinking water through cloth to remove the copepods, and never to enter a source of drinking water (or allowing anyone else to do it) when a guinea worm is emerging. The ideal means of prevention is the provision of safe sources of drinking water. Applications of ABATE® larvicide (temephos) in selected unsafe sources of drinking water to control copepod populations is another means of controlling transmission of the disease.

The global Dracunculiasis Eradication Program (DEP) began in 1980, when the Centers for Disease Control and Prevention (CDC)[32] proposed that eradication of dracunculiasis was the ideal indicator with which to measure the success of the International Drinking Water Supply and Sanitation Decade (1981–1990), since this disease is only transmitted via drinking water. In 1981, the steering committee of the Decade adopted dracunculiasis eradication as a subgoal of their efforts. The African ministers of health passed a resolution in 1988 calling for the eradication of dracunculiasis by 1995, and the World Health Assembly endorsed that mandate in 1991.[33] Since 1988 a growing number of agencies, organizations, companies, and other institutions have assisted national programs with their efforts to eradicate dracunculiasis. India began its own independent national dracunculiasis eradication program in 1983.

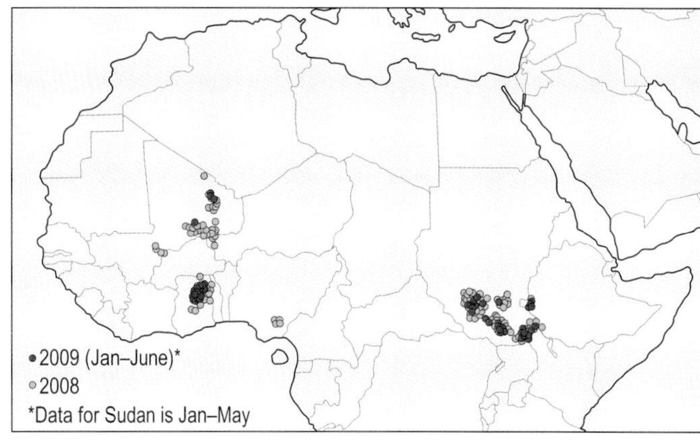

Figure 108.5 Distribution of villages in Africa reporting indigenous cases of dracunculiasis (Guinea worm disease) during 2008 and January–June 2009 (2009 data is provisional).

The strategy for dracunculiasis eradication includes three phases.[34] During phase I national programs conducted nation-wide or area-wide case searches to determine the locations of villages with endemic transmission and the numbers of cases, organized a national secretariat and a program structure at district and village levels, and developed a national plan of action. In phase II, program staff and village-based health workers (village volunteers) were trained to conduct active village-based surveillance using case registers, and to implement interventions against transmission of the disease, by providing health education to mobilize communities to action, providing cloth filters, and educating villagers on their care and proper use. During phase III, when the incidence of disease has been reduced to fewer cases per year and halting transmission is imminent, surveillance is intensified to rapidly detect all persons with emerging worms (preferably before or within 24 hours of worm emergence) and to contain transmission from each case by providing care for the wounds, applying occlusive bandages, and counseling the patient not to enter sources of drinking water. In 2001 most national programs began offering persons with dracunculiasis the option of medical care at "case containment centers."[35] When patients voluntarily attend such case containment centers they are provided a small monetary or in-kind incentive (for agreeing to stay at the center until each guinea worm is successfully pulled out), medical care, food, sanitation, and shelter. Care of the last cases of dracunculiasis at case containment centers or at established public health clinics permits patients to recover from their incapacitation much faster and the program to contain transmission from each emerging worm much more effectively. All other broad-based interventions continue to be employed until transmission is halted.

Attainment of eradication is not certified until the national program requests the WHO to validate the claim that no cases have occurred during at least 3 years since the last indigenous case, and an international certification team confirms that the surveillance system is sensitive and has not detected indigenous cases during the required 3-year period. An International Commission for the Certification of Dracunculiasis Eradication reviews the findings of the certification team and recommends to the WHO whether or not to certify the country free of dracunculiasis.[36]

The 4619 cases of dracunculiasis reported in 2008 from six countries (Sudan, Ghana, Mali, Ethiopia, Nigeria, and Niger) is a reduction of 99.9% from the 3.5 million cases estimated in 1986. ***Figure 108.5*** depicts the location of villages reporting cases of dracunculiasis in 2008 and during January–June 2009 in the six endemic countries. Fourteen of the 20 endemic countries have interrupted transmission of dracunculiasis, and three (Ethiopia, Nigeria, and Niger) of the remaining six countries with endemic disease reported fewer than 100 cases each in 2008.[37] Indigenous cases of dracunculiasis were reported from only 1025 villages in 2008, compared to 23 735 villages in 1993. As of 2008, the WHO had certified 180 countries free of dracunculiasis, including six formerly endemic ones, India, Pakistan, Yemen, Senegal, Cameroon, and Central African Republic.

The Sudan Guinea Worm Eradication Program began in 1992–1993 with a village-by-village search for cases in areas accessible to the government of Sudan. Many endemic areas of southern Sudan were inaccessible to the program because of the then 10-year-old civil war. The program accelerated its progress in 1995, including in armed-conflict areas, under a 6-month "Guinea Worm Cease-Fire" that was negotiated between the two sides in the war by former US President Jimmy Carter.[38] Transmission of the disease in the northern states of Sudan was interrupted in 2003.[39] A political settlement of the war was reached in January 2005 when a Comprehensive Peace Agreement (CPA) between northern and southern Sudan was signed. The CPA allowed the program to implement surveillance and interventions throughout southern Sudan, beginning in 2006 when 20 582 cases of the disease were reported from 3137 villages. During 2008 southern Sudan reported 3618 (78%) of the 4619 cases of dracunculiasis reported globally, from only 947 villages.

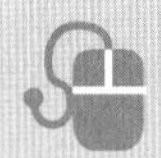

Access the complete reference list online at
http://www.expertconsult.com

Access the complete reference list online at http://www.expertconsult.com

CHAPTER 109

Toxocariasis and Larva Migrans Syndromes

James S. McCarthy • Thomas A. Moore

INTRODUCTION

Toxocariasis is the clinical term used to describe human infection with either the dog ascarid *Toxocara canis* or the feline ascarid *Toxocara cati*. As with almost all other helminthic zoonoses, the infective larvae of these *Toxocara* species cannot mature into adults in the human host. Instead, the worms wander through tissues and organs in a vain attempt to find that which they need to mature into adults. The migration of these immature nematode larvae causes local and systemic inflammation, resulting in the "larva migrans" syndromes. Although human toxocariasis has been studied more intensively in Western countries, the disease has a global distribution, occurring in areas wherever dogs coexist with humans.

The clinical manifestations of toxocariasis (***Table 109.1***) are divided into *visceral larva migrans* (VLM) and *ocular larva migrans* (OLM). Subclinical infection is often referred to as covert toxocariasis. *Cutaneous larva migrans*, on the other hand, is most often caused by hookworms of domestic animals and is a widespread and well-recognized dermatologic problem in the tropics.

This chapter covers toxocariasis (including visceral and ocular larva migrans) and cutaneous larva migrans (CLM). Other helminthic zoonoses that cause similar larva migrans syndromes (e.g., gnathostomiasis, angiostrongyliasis, and anisakiasis) are discussed elsewhere (see Chapter 111).

THE AGENT

Toxocara species are nematodes, taxonomically included within the order and family Ascaridida. The morphology of the adult worms resembles that of *Ascaris lumbricoides*, only they are much smaller: the males measure 4–6 cm long, females 6.5–10.0 cm long. The brown-colored eggs are almost spherical, with superficial pits, and are larger than *A. lumbricoides*, measuring 85 μm × 75 μm.

In the dog, the life cycle of *T. canis* (***Fig. 109.1***) is similar to that of *A. lumbricoides* in humans, but with two important differences: the parasite can undergo developmental arrest within the definitive host (hypobiosis), and vertical transmission occurs from infected pregnant bitches to their pups.[1]

Gravid adult female worms, which are generally found only in young puppies and lactating bitches, excrete up to 200 000 eggs/day in the feces of an infected dog. Freshly passed eggs are unembryonated and develop into infective, embryonated eggs over several weeks at optimum temperature (10–35°C). Lower temperatures delay embryonation. Like other ascarid eggs, *Toxocara* eggs are hardy and relatively resistant to freezing, moisture, and extremes of pH,[2] and retain their infectivity for months.[3] Unembryonated eggs shed in the winter can lie dormant until temperatures rise in the spring.

On the ground, the infective first-stage larvae within these unembryonated eggs molt twice to become third-stage juveniles. However, they do not shed their second-stage cuticle until after ingestion. Infection begins when these now-embryonated eggs are ingested. The eggs hatch in the duodenum; the larvae penetrate the intestinal wall and eventually reach the liver where they increase in size but do not molt. From the liver, the larvae travel to the heart and then to the lungs, where they molt into the fourth stage. In young dogs (under 6 months), the larvae travel from the lungs into the trachea where they are swallowed. The larvae undergo an additional molt in the stomach before maturing into adults in the intestine. Mating then results in release of unembryonated eggs, making the infection patent 60–90 days after egg ingestion. In older dogs (6 or more months), infective juveniles do not exit the lungs via the trachea but are carried through the systemic circulation to somatic tissues where they remain in a state of arrested development for as long as 6 months. This migration to somatic tissue creates the conditions for transplacental and transmammary transmission to pups; latent somatic larvae are reactivated during each pregnancy and migrate either across the placenta to the fetal liver after the 45th day of gestation or to the mammary gland to infect pups in breast milk.[4] Larvae acquired *in utero* by the puppies remain as third-stage juveniles until birth, when they mature in the intestine of the pups. Puppies born with a patent infection shed large numbers of eggs from birth. In contrast, adult dogs excrete few eggs. Dogs born without infection can acquire the infection later by ingesting eggs from the soil or by ingesting embryonated eggs carried by transport hosts such as earthworms, ants, and other soil-dwelling invertebrates.

A wide variety of animals, including humans, can become infected with *T. canis* by ingesting embryonated eggs from contaminated soil, hands, or fomites. In these so-called paratenic, or transport, hosts, the larvae follow a similar developmental path as in older, nonpregnant dogs. The larvae do not develop to maturity, but arrest at the L2 larval stage and migrate for months through host tissues before lodging in a state of arrested development. The larvae do not encyst but remain exposed to the host environment, absorbing nutrients across their cuticle. The larvae can survive in tissues for several years despite vigorous host immunologic responses to parasite antigens.[5]

Humans generally acquire infection with *T. canis* by ingesting embryonated eggs. Exposure to infective eggs generally occurs in areas where dogs defecate, such as public parks.[6] Infection acquired by ingestion of raw snails and raw lamb has also been reported.

The cat roundworm, *T. cati*, has a life cycle similar to that of *T. canis* except that vertical transmission is due to lactation more than transplacental transmission. While in most cases humans are paratenic hosts as in *T. canis*, one report documents four cases of adult *T. cati* intestinal infection in children.[7] *T. cati* causes fewer cases of human infection than *T. canis*, probably because of the defecation patterns of cats, which make environmental contamination less frequent. Although other zoonotic ascarid nematodes may be responsible for some cases of VLM, *T. leonina*, another ascarid parasite of dogs and cats, has not been associated with human disease.

Table 109.1 Clinical Syndromes of Human Toxocariasis

Syndrome	Clinical Findings	Average Age	Infectious Dose	Incubation Period	Laboratory Findings	*Toxocara* Antibody Titer (ELISA)
Visceral larva migrans	Fever, hepatomegaly, asthma	5 years	Moderate to high	Weeks to months	Eosinophilia, leukocytosis, elevated IgE	High
Ocular larva migrans	Visual disturbances, endophthalmitis, retinal granuloma	12 years	Low	Months to years	Usually none	Low
Covert toxocariasis	Abdominal pain, gastrointestinal symptoms, weakness, pruritus	School age to adult	Low to moderate	Weeks to years	Eosinophilia and/or elevated IgE may be present	Low to moderate

(Adapted from Glickman LT, Schantz PM. Epidemiology and pathogenesis of zoonotic toxocariasis. Epidemiol Rev. 1981;3:230–250.)

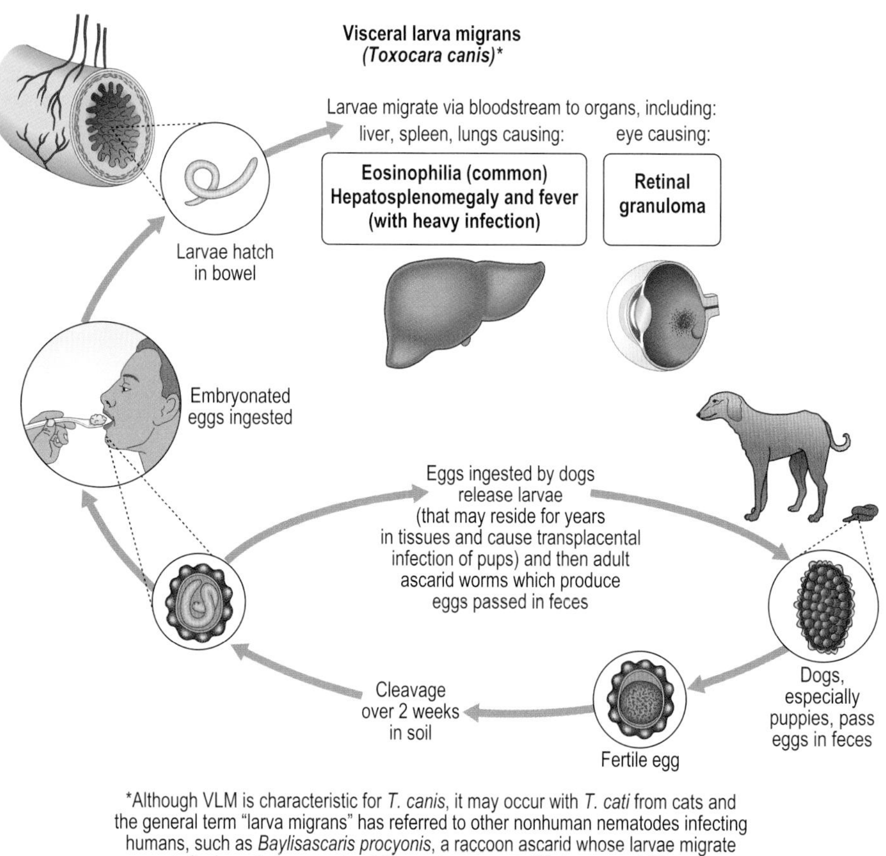
Visceral larva migrans
(Toxocara canis)*
Larvae migrate via bloodstream to organs, including:
liver, spleen, lungs causing:
eye causing:
Eosinophilia (common)
Hepatosplenomegaly and fever
(with heavy infection)
Retinal granuloma
Larvae hatch in bowel
Embryonated eggs ingested
Eggs ingested by dogs release larvae (that may reside for years in tissues and cause transplacental infection of pups) and then adult ascarid worms which produce eggs passed in feces
Cleavage over 2 weeks in soil
Fertile egg
Dogs, especially puppies, pass eggs in feces
*Although VLM is characteristic for T. canis, it may occur with T. cati from cats and the general term "larva migrans" has referred to other nonhuman nematodes infecting humans, such as Baylisascaris procyonis, a raccoon ascarid whose larvae migrate to brain and cause eosinophilic meningoencephalitis in young children

Figure 109.1 Life cycle of visceral larva migrans (*Toxocara canis*).

EPIDEMIOLOGY

The ascarids *T. canis* and *T. cati* are ubiquitous parasites of dogs and cats, respectively, and occur in both temperate and warm climates. These parasites appear to have caused disease for millennia.[8] *T. canis* infection of dogs has been reported worldwide, and canine infection rates vary widely. Not surprisingly, environmental contamination of public grounds with *T. canis* eggs is also widespread.[9–17] Infected rodents have been proposed to constitute a significant reservoir of *Toxocara* larvae.[18]

Toxocariasis in humans is presumed to be contracted through the ingestion of eggs from contaminated soil; children with geophagia (pica) and contact with a litter of puppies appear to be particularly vulnerable.[19] Recent data suggest that dogs infected with *T. canis* may infect people by direct contact.[20] Additional risk factors include intellectual disability requiring institutionalization[21] and ingestion of uncooked infected meat[22] or raw liver from lamb[23] or chicken.[24]

Because patent infection does not occur in human toxocariasis (presence of eggs in stool), estimates of prevalence in humans depend on seroepidemiologic surveys. Such studies show wide differences depending on the population tested. The seroprevalence of toxocariasis in children aged 1–11 years in the United States, as measured by enzyme-linked immunosorbent assay, varies from approximately 4% to 8%,[25] with higher rates in Puerto Rico and the southeastern United States.[26] Even higher infection rates of 16–30% have been reported among socioeconomically disadvantaged African-American[25] and Hispanic[27] children. Similar rates have been reported in Europe.[28,29] In a recently published study of the seroprevalence of *Toxocara* spp. antibodies in the US population, sera from individuals aged ≥6 years who participated in the Third National Health and Nutrition Examination Survey (1988–1994) was reported.[30] Among the 20 395 subjects tested, the age-adjusted *Toxocara* seroprevalence was 13.9% (95% confidence intervals (CI): 12.5, 15.3). Seroprevalence was significantly higher in non-Hispanic blacks (21.2%) than non-Hispanic whites (12%) or Mexican Americans (10.7%; $P < 0.001$). The investigators reported that seropositivity was associated with head of household level of education (low versus high) (odds ratio (OR): 2.2; CI: 1.8, 2.8), poverty (OR: 1.5; CI: 1.3, 1.8), elevated blood lead concentrations (OR: 1.4; CI: 1.1, 1.9), and dog ownership (OR: 1.2; CI: 1.1, 1.4). The prevalence of human toxocariasis in the tropics has been less well studied, but is assumed to be significant since canine infection with *T. canis* is commonly found in these areas,[31,32] veterinary care is less widespread, and routine deworming of domestic animals is less commonly practiced. Significant rates of toxocariasis have been found among populations in the Caribbean,[33] South America,[34–38] Turkey,[39] Iran,[40] India,[41] Sri Lanka,[42] and Southeast Asia,[43] while the prevalence in New Zealand was reported to be less than 1%.[44]

THE DISEASE

Visceral Larva Migrans

In 1952, Beaver and colleagues reported a series of children who presented with high peripheral eosinophilia accompanied by severe, long-term, multisystem disease.[45] Examination of biopsy tissue revealed the causative agents as larvae of either *T. canis* or *T. cati*.

The syndrome of VLM is typically described as being characterized by eosinophilia, fever, and hepatomegaly.[46] It is most commonly seen in toddlers with a history of pica and an association with puppies. However, the spectrum of VLM may also encompass cough, wheeze, bronchopneumonia, and anemia. Although almost any organ can be affected, the liver is the most frequently involved, with hepatomegaly being a common finding. Occasionally, the lesions may be mistaken for neoplastic metastases.[47] A minority of patients can develop splenomegaly or lymphadenopathy. The dermatologic manifestations of VLM have been recently reviewed,[48] and include urticaria, chronic pruritus and miscellaneous eczema. Wheezing is a common presentation of VLM,[49] and severe asthma and hypereosinophilia can develop in intense infections.[50] Pulmonary infiltrates occur on chest radiographs, and toxocariasis can produce acute or chronic eosinophilic pneumonia,[51,52] occasionally progressing to respiratory failure.[53] Monoarthritis, panniculitis, and other rheumatologic manifestations can develop.[54]

Although rarely reported, direct invasion of the central nervous system by *T. canis* larvae can occur, resulting in a variety of neurologic manifestations including eosinophilic meningitis,[55] meningoencephalitis,[56,57] seizures,[58] encephalopathy,[59] arachnoiditis,[60] solitary brain lesions,[61] and myelitis.[62,63] Cardiac involvement with *T. canis* rarely occurs, but can be serious.[64,65]

Ocular Larva Migrans

Nematode endophthalmitis was first recognized in 1950 in a series of eyes enucleated for presumed neuroblastoma.[66] Ocular involvement with *T. canis* larvae results in the clinically distinct syndrome OLM. Patients with OLM tend to be older children without evidence of other organ involvement, suggesting an alternative pathogenic mechanism.[5] *T. canis* larvae that migrate to the orbit become trapped, and an eosinophilic inflammatory mass results. The syndrome takes several weeks to become clinically apparent, but the typical presentation is that of an older child presenting with a unilateral visual deficit, ocular pain, leukocoria, or strabismus.[67] The retinal lesion most commonly presents as a solid tumor often at or near the macula. In the early stages, it is raised above the level of the retina and closely mimics a retinoblastoma (***Fig. 109.2***). After the acute phase has subsided, the lesion remains a well-defined circumscribed area of retinal degeneration. Strabismus due to macular damage is often the presenting symptom. Low-grade iridocyclitis with posterior synechiae may develop and progress to endophthalmitis and retinal detachment.[68] Posterior and peripheral retinochoroiditis as well as optic papillitis have also been reported.[69] The inflammatory response created by ocular involvement may result in epiretinal membrane formation and traction retinal detachment. In contrast to VLM, hypereosinophilia, hepatomegaly, and pulmonary symptoms are typically absent in OLM.

Covert Toxocariasis

Patients with serologic evidence of toxocariasis who have mild or no symptoms of infection have been assigned into a diagnostic category of

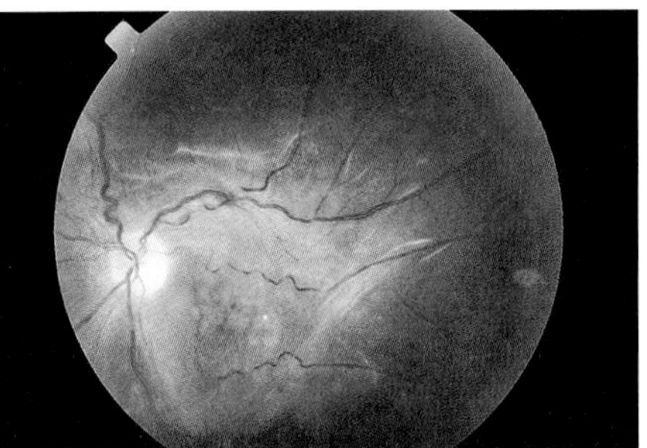

Figure 109.2 Retinal lesion of ocular larva migrans.

"covert" or "occult" toxocariasis.[70,71] The development and commercial availability of serologic tests for toxocariasis have facilitated the identification of such individuals.[27] This diagnostic category has been proposed to describe patients with a range of largely nonspecific clinical manifestations including cough, sleep disturbance, abdominal pain, headache, and behavioral disturbances in association with elevated toxocaral antibody titers.[70,71] Eosinophilia may be present, but at a lower level than that typically observed in VLM. Recurrent abdominal pain is often the sole presenting complaint.[72] Less common findings include anorexia, fever, and cervical adenitis. Covert toxocariasis has been described in adults in the French Pyrenees, where patients demonstrated nonspecific manifestations including weakness, pruritus, rash, difficulty breathing, and abdominal pain.[71] While the association between VLM and respiratory symptoms including an asthma-like illness with cough and wheeze is well recognized,[73] the link between subclinical *Toxocara* infection and allergic asthma is less clear, with some studies suggesting an association[74,75] while this association has not been observed in other settings.[76] The impact of *Toxocara* infection on behavior and learning is not well established, but a link has been suggested in murine models[77] and evidence points to a correlation.[19]

The prevalence of *Toxocara* seropositivity suggests that most human infections are asymptomatic. Indeed, most children with mild eosinophilia and antibodies to *T. canis* do not appear to develop clinically apparent sequelae when evaluated for up to 7 years.[78]

PATHOGENESIS AND IMMUNITY

The mucinous surface coat of *T. canis* larvae is a dynamic structure that turns over quite rapidly and generates large quantities of glycosylated excretory–secretory proteins.[79,80] Many of these proteins constitute a family of highly antigenic mucins[81] that, like most other tissue helminth antigens, induce a Th2-type $CD4^+$ cellular immune response characterized by the production of interleukin (IL)-4 that promotes eosinophilia and the production of immunoglobulin E (IgE).[82] However, the recruited eosinophils adhere to a membranous layer that is frequently detached from the larval epicuticle, allowing the larvae to largely evade the immune response elicited by these antigens.[83] In murine models of infection, the dominant cytokine produced is IL-5,[84] which plays a major role in the induction of eosinophilia; however, overproduction of IL-5 in transgenic mice does not significantly inhibit the life cycle of *T. canis* larvae, suggesting an alternative method by which the parasites are cleared.[85] Investigation into other molecular aspects of the parasite promises further insight into the pathophysiology of toxocariasis.[86]

T. canis larvae elicit both a humoral and cellular response in humans. Tissue damage is due to the host inflammatory reaction more than the infection itself. In both experimental and natural infections, *Toxocara* larval antigens induce granulomatous inflammation with eosinophils, histiocytes, and fibrous tissue (***Fig. 109.3***). Although the granulomas commonly develop where the larvae have come to rest, they do not always contain the larvae themselves. The granulomas are found most often in the liver, but they may be found in any tissue, including the lungs, brain, and eyes. These eosinophil-mediated granulomatous responses are almost exclusively responsible for the clinical manifestations of toxocariasis;

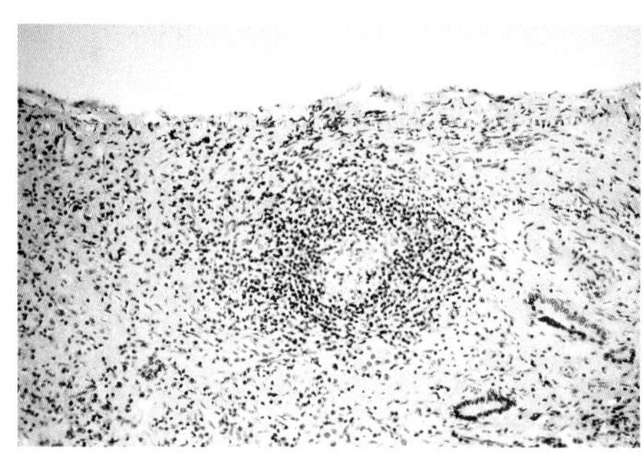

Figure 109.3 Granulomatous lesion of the liver due to visceral larva migrans.

however, it is not clear what factors are responsible for the development of OLM, VLM, or covert toxocariasis. It has been proposed[5] that parasite load is the key determinant of disease severity. Specifically, ingestion of lower doses of infective eggs is more likely to result in OLM or asymptomatic infection, whereas VLM is associated with a larger inoculum.

DIAGNOSIS

Like many parasitic diseases, the diagnosis of toxocariasis is made on clinical grounds, supported by confirmatory serologic testing. The diagnosis should be entertained when a child is found to have eosinophilia (absolute eosinophil count greater than 450 eosinophils/mm^3), especially when accompanied by hepatomegaly, fever, or wheezing. Exposure to dogs, particularly puppies, is an additional clue to the diagnosis. In the absence of hepatomegaly, the symptoms and signs of VLM can mimic tropical pulmonary eosinophilia, as well as other helminth infections characterized by a tissue migration phase such as ascariasis, hookworm infection, and strongyloidiasis (see Chapters 115–117).

Other laboratory findings can include hypergammaglobulinemia and elevated isohemagglutinin titers to A and B blood group antigens. The latter develop as a result of cross-reaction to parasite antigens. Radiographic imaging of involved organs using ultrasound, computed tomography (CT), or magnetic resonance imaging (MRI) can identify focal lesions. If biopsied, these lesions will show granulomatous inflammation; however, larvae are not always found within the granulomas. Biopsy is not recommended to establish the histopathologic diagnosis in an otherwise clinically typical case of toxocariasis.

The diagnosis is most often established by confirmatory serologic testing using an enzyme-linked immunosorbent assay (ELISA). Excretory–secretory (E-S) proteins from second-stage *T. canis* larvae maintained *in vitro* form the substrate for the ELISA.[87] The sensitivity has been estimated to be approximately 78%, with a specificity of approximately 92% at a cutoff dilution value of 1 : 32.[88,89] While limited data indicate no significant cross-reactivity in individuals infected with common helminth infections,[33,90] some have reported increased specificity after adsorbing patient sera with *Ascaris* antigen.[91] An ELISA based on IgE-subclass antibodies appears to be comparably sensitive for detection and post-treatment follow-up of human toxocariasis.[92] A Western blot using toxocaral E-S antigens is more specific,[93] but is more labor-intensive. More recently, the expression cloning of recombinant E-S antigen has enabled the development of immunoblot[94] and ELISA[95] assays with improved diagnostic sensitivity and specificity. The sensitivity of a *Toxocara*-specific IgG_4 ELISA utilizing a combination of three cloned E-S antigens was 100%, with specificity ranging from 92% to 96%.[95] Unfortunately, the ability of these serologic tests to distinguish between past and current infection is not clear. An antigen capture test using a monoclonal antibody to toxocaral E-S antigen offers the ability to distinguish current infection. Preliminary data indicate the test is more than 50% sensitive; however, there is a false positive rate of 25% in patients with filariasis and schistosomiasis.[96]

The diagnosis of OLM is based on typical clinical findings of a retinal or peripheral granuloma or endophthalmitis, plus an elevated antibody titer to *T. canis* larval antigens. Identification of characteristic CT or ultrasonographic findings can facilitate diagnosis.[97,98] Although the finding of elevated *Toxocara* antibodies helps to establish the diagnosis of OLM, patients can sometimes have low or even negative titers.[99,100] Finding elevated *Toxocara* antibodies in the vitreous and aqueous humor can also facilitate the diagnosis.[101,102] Other nematode infections of the eye (e.g., cysticercosis, onchocerciasis, and diffuse unilateral subacute neuroretinitis) should be carefully considered in the differential diagnosis.[103]

Covert toxocariasis should be considered in individuals of any age who present with chronic weakness, abdominal pain, or atopy accompanied by elevated IgE levels and eosinophilia. Finding antitoxocaral antibodies in serum does not necessarily establish the diagnosis but, in the absence of response to skin or pulmonary allergens, would certainly support it.

TREATMENT AND PROGNOSIS

The majority of patients with toxocariasis do not require treatment, since the disease is usually self-limited; nevertheless, the disease can be fatal in severe cases. Treatment is generally reserved for patients with severe disease, although this remains a controversial point.

Acute VLM in children and adults is usually treated either symptomatically or with specific anthelminthic therapy, depending on the severity of clinical disease. Patients with either mild visceral larva migrans or covert toxocariasis and peripheral eosinophilia are often treated conservatively, since these forms of the disease are usually self-limited. Asymptomatic subjects with eosinophilia and those with covert toxocariasis in the absence of eosinophilia do not normally require any specific therapy.

Generalized treatment recommendations are limited by a paucity of controlled clinical data. Thiabendazole, mebendazole, diethylcarbamazine (DEC), albendazole, and ivermectin have been examined as treatments for VLM. Thiabendazole, a benzimidazole anthelminthic, has largely been superseded on account of its poor tolerability profile and the availability of more effective drugs in this class such as albendazole and mebendazole. Thiabendazole appears to be ineffective in asymptomatic children with toxocariasis, as measured by serial eosinophil counts and antitoxocaral antibody titers.[78] While the drug administered in a dose of 15 mg/kg daily appeared to be effective in symptomatic VLM, albendazole therapy resulted in more frequent clinical cure and decrease in eosinophil counts.[104] A dose of 400 mg of albendazole twice a day for 5 days is the currently recommended therapy.[105] While a 21-day course of mebendazole (20–25 mg/kg daily) has also been shown to be effective,[106] the poor systemic bioavailability of this drug would argue that albendazole should be used in preference. For those with severe symptoms treated with anthelminthics, corticosteroids are often administered concomitantly (prednisone 0.5–1.0 mg/kg daily). Several small studies have demonstrated that a 21-day course of DEC (~6 mg/kg daily) results in resolution of clinical symptoms and a decline in antitoxocaral antibody titers, although patients experienced a significantly higher rate of adverse reactions.[94] In the United States, DEC is only available through the Centers for Disease Control and Prevention (CDC) Drug Service. While ivermectin is a highly effective drug for treatment of many human nematode infections, including the related roundworm *A. lumbricoides*, the limited available data accrued in a mouse model of paretenic infection[107] indicates that the drug is less active against the L2 stage of the parasite than the comparator benzimidazole.

Albendazole has been found to be effective in OLM, but higher doses (adults, 800 mg twice daily; children, 400 mg twice daily) have been used in these clinical studies.[108] Albendazole should be administered for 4 weeks, with concomitant glucocorticoids (prednisone 0.5–1.0 mg/kg daily) for 2–4 weeks. Despite the promise of medical therapy, surgery is still sometimes required to treat OLM.[109]

CUTANEOUS LARVA MIGRANS

CLM, also known as creeping eruption, is a zoonosis caused by animal hookworms, most often that of the dog (*Ancylostoma caninum*) or cat (*Ancylostoma braziliense*).

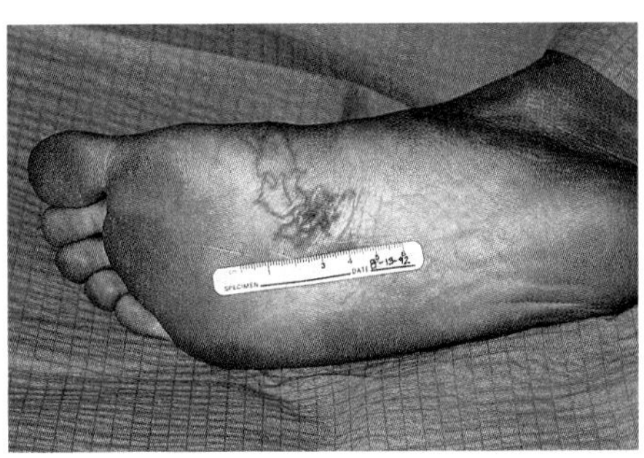

Figure 109.4 Typical lesion of cutaneous larva migrans involving the foot.

Infected animals shed eggs in the stool that subsequently hatch, yielding first-stage larvae that mature into infective third-stage larvae in the soil. As with human hookworms, the infection starts when the worm enters the skin from contaminated soil that is protected from desiccation and temperature extremes, such as on beaches and under houses. As in toxocariasis, the worm cannot complete the infective cycle, so it continues to burrow through the subcutaneous tissues, resulting in the characteristic serpiginous, erythematous, elevated, and pruritic skin lesion (***Fig. 109.4***). The pruritus is sometimes incapacitating. The infection is often seen in travelers who have walked barefoot on beaches frequented by roaming cats and dogs. CLM is the most common dermatologic problem to affect Westerners after travel to tropical countries.[110] Almost one-third of travelers had symptoms for more than 4 weeks before the diagnosis was properly established.[111] In European travelers, the lesions are very few in number and most commonly involve the feet and buttocks. The infection may present as an outbreak as was reported in Florida where 22 individuals contracted infection, likely caused by *A. braziliense* larvae present in a sandbox contaminated by cat feces.[112] In contrast, a study of CLM in an endemic area indicates the clinical presentation is different from that reported in travelers.[113] Lesions were more frequent and spared the feet, most often occurring on the trunk, legs, and arms.

Systemic symptoms and eosinophilia are rare. The diagnosis is made solely on clinical grounds; skin biopsy is of negligible value. Other diagnoses to be considered include larva currens due to *Strongyloides stercoralis*, jellyfish stings, phytophotodermatitis, and myiasis. As with many other tropical diseases presenting in industrialized nations, physicians' lack of familiarity with this entity results in a significant delay in diagnosis and effective treatment. Even without treatment the lesions resolve spontaneously in 2–8 weeks, although longer periods of infection have been occasionally reported,[114] and the patients are often miserable due to pruritus.

Albendazole is well tolerated and quite effective, resolving the infection within 1 week;[115] however, clinical trials have yielded conflicting results with respect to the optimal dosage. It would appear that travelers with CLM should be treated with 400–800 mg/day for 3–5 days.[116] A single dose of ivermectin (200 µg/kg on an empty stomach) is well tolerated and curative in 77% of patients; 97% were cured with one or two supplemental doses, if necessary.[117] The median time required for pruritus and lesions to disappear was 3 and 7 days, respectively.

Topical cryotherapy is not recommended because it does not work and is potentially harmful to the patient.[116] Topical application of a 10–15% thiabendazole solution/ointment to the affected area effects a cure within 10 days in 98% of patients. Thiabendazole is also effective against CLM when given orally, although less so; 89% of patients are cured after four weekly doses. The side effects of oral thiabendazole make topical treatment attractive; however, this treatment has limited value for multiple lesions. Topical thiabendazole preparations are not commercially available in the United States.

PREVENTION AND CONTROL

The association with dogs as a risk factor for the development of toxocariasis is well established.[20,118] Likewise, the association between failure to deworm cats and dogs and the occurrence of CLM is clear. While the prevalence of dog ownership varies throughout the world, most of the world's population shares its environment with *T. canis*-infected dogs. Thus, exposure to canine ascarids is likely to be widespread. In the United States, an estimated 53 million dogs are distributed among 31 million households.[119] This number is not expected to decline for the foreseeable future.[120] While the true incidence of toxocariasis is unknown in the United States, one would assume a significant portion of these animals are infected given the cosmopolitan distribution of the parasite.

While discouraging geophagia in children is a laudable goal for the prevention of toxocariasis, such behavior modification in this age group is unrealistic. Instead, measures to prevent infected dog feces from contaminating the environment are of paramount importance. These include keeping dogs on a leash and excluding pet animals from playgrounds and sandboxes where geophagia occurs. Placing a vinyl covering over sandboxes at night has been shown to reduce the viability of *T. canis* eggs.[121] An education campaign to highlight the risk to humans would be a logical component of any control program.

An effective surveillance and control program would require attention to potentially infected animals. However, pups and kittens are frequently not brought to veterinarians until they are at least 6 weeks old, by which time exposure to environments with extensive contamination with *Toxocara* eggs may have already occurred. Despite this obstacle, the prevalence of canine infection with *T. canis* has declined as a result of animal control measures and the widespread veterinary use of broad-spectrum anthelminthics effective against the adult worms.[122] Using subcutaneous ivermectin,[123] topical selamectin (a macrocyclic lactone similar to ivermectin),[124] or oral fenbendazole[125] at scheduled intervals during pregnancy dramatically reduced the worm burden carried by puppies. Likewise anthelminthic treatment of dogs and cats is the primary means for preventing CLM. Pet owners should be encouraged to treat their pets for intestinal helminths on a biannual or yearly basis.[112] In addition, stray animals should be reported to the responsible authority, and animal feces should be removed promptly from areas of human activity. While potential vaccine candidates have been identified for these zoonotic parasites,[126] none are yet available.

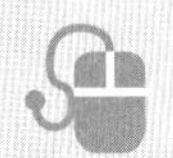

Access the complete reference list online at
http://www.expertconsult.com

CHAPTER 110

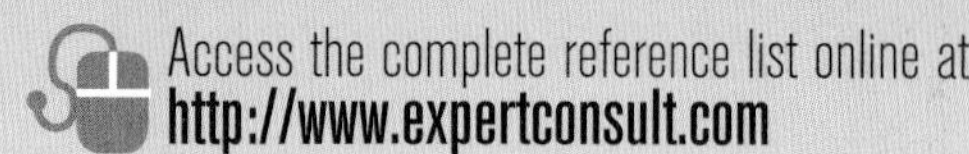
Access the complete reference list online at
http://www.expertconsult.com

Trichinellosis

Fabrizio Bruschi • K. Darwin Murrell

INTRODUCTION

Trichinellosis, the proper term for trichinosis or trichiniasis, results from infection by a parasitic nematode belonging to the genus *Trichinella*. Trichinellosis, though often unrecognized, has been an important disease for thousands of years. Species of *Trichinella* responsible for the infection are widely distributed (see ***Table 110.1***), including the Arctic, temperate lands, and the tropics.[1] Virtually all mammals are susceptible to infection; however, humans appear to be especially prone to developing clinical disease. Infection with various species of *Trichinella* is far more common than is generally recognized. In spite of having a low prevalence worldwide, the parasite remains an important foodborne zoonosis because of its epizootic nature and the economic burden associated with preventing its incursion into the human food chain.[2,3] The prevalence of swine trichinellosis and the incidence of human trichinellosis appear to be greater in countries such as China, Thailand, Mexico, Argentina, and Bolivia, and in some central European countries.[4]

Until recently, the epidemiology and systematics of this parasitic zoonosis were considered relatively simple and straightforward.[1] Human trichinellosis was believed to involve one species, *Trichinella spiralis* (Owen, 1835). During the past two decades, major changes in the understanding of this epidemiology have occurred, yielding a transmission pattern that may involve domestic swine, horses, and especially wild animals (game). Furthermore, new molecular genetic data have led to the creation of a new taxonomy for *Trichinella* that includes eight species rather than one[1] (***Table 110.1***). This revised taxonomy is yielding a greater comprehension of the clinical course of the disease caused by the different *Trichinella* species.[5] Although this parasite was first described more than 160 years ago, both its biology and its complete control remain an unfinished story.

THE AGENT

The parasite's discovery resulted from the microscopic examination of cadaver muscle in London in 1835, and it was named *Trichina spiralis* by Owen. During the mid-nineteenth century, the life cycle and etiology of domestic trichinellosis (human–swine) were elucidated by German scientists, along with its basic epidemiology. Over the succeeding century and a half, the domestic trichinellosis cycle was reported from many countries. In some regions, especially in Europe and the former Soviet Union, the problem of trichinellosis was so severe that mandatory inspection of all pork for muscle larvae (so-called trichinae) was instituted. These measures have been effective and in countries with mandatory meat inspection, trichinellosis has become a low-incidence disease.

The classic and most frequent cause of human trichinellosis, *T. spiralis*, is normally derived from domestic pork, occasionally from wild game; the pig–man epidemiologic pattern is usually referred to as the synanthropic or domestic cycle. All species of *Trichinella* are morphologically difficult to distinguish from one another, but all have a direct life cycle with complete development in a single host; there is a degree of host specificity, but the complete host range for each species is not completely known. The host capsule, when present, surrounds a complex represented by the infective larvae inside a modified striated muscle structure called a nurse cell.[6] The capsule is digested away in the stomach when infected muscle is ingested by the next host.[7] The free larvae (L1 stage) then move into the upper small intestine and invade the columnar epithelial intestinal cells. Within 30 hours, the larvae undergo four molts to reach the mature adult stages, as males and females. After mating, the female begins shedding live newborn larvae (NBL), approximately 5 days post infection; the NBL are early developmental forms of the L1 stage.[4] The persistence of adult worms in the intestine of humans may last for several weeks.[7] The NBL migrate throughout the body via the blood and lymph circulatory system. Although NBL may attempt to invade many different tissues, they are successful only if they can enter striated skeletal muscle cells.[6] The NBL continue to grow and develop during the first 2 weeks of intracellular life until they reach the fully developed L1 infective stage. The longevity of the nurse cell–L1 complex appears to vary by parasite and host species, but it generally persists for one to several years before calcification and death occur.[4] The life cycle (***Fig. 110.1***) is completed when the host's infected muscle is ingested by a suitable host. Three species, *T. pseudospiralis*, *T. papuae*, and *T. zimbabwensis*, form a non-encapsulated clade because a host capsule does not develop around the muscle larvae.[4]

EPIDEMIOLOGY

The most salient feature of this parasite group's epidemiology is its obligatory transmission by ingestion of meat. A second cardinal feature is its existence in two normally separate ecological systems, the sylvatic and the domestic. In certain circumstances, the two biotopes are linked through human activities, resulting in the exposure of humans to *Trichinella* species normally confined to wild animals; only *T. spiralis* is highly infective to pigs. The species most frequently associated with human infection is *T. spiralis*, which is normally found in domestic pigs but frequently detected in rodents and wild mammals.[4] The domestic cycle of *T. spiralis* involves a complex set of potential routes.[4] Transmission on a farm may result from predation on or scavenging other animals (e.g., dead wild animals, synanthropic rodents), hog cannibalism, and the feeding of uncooked meat scraps. Although the frequency of transmission from infected game animals is significant, the importance of wild animal reservoirs is often underappreciated.[4]

The worldwide incidence of human trichinellosis has declined substantially during the past few decades, but outbreaks are still frequent, especially in developing countries[4] (***Table 110.2***). In developed countries, the epidemiology of human trichinellosis is typified by urban common-source outbreaks.[5] In the United States, the largest human outbreaks have

Table 110.1 Biologic and Zoogeographic Features of *Trichinella* Species			
Species	**Distribution**	**Major Hosts**	**Reported from Humans**
T. spiralis	Cosmopolitan	Domestic pigs, wild mammals	Yes
T. britovi	Eurasia/Africa	Wild mammals	Yes
T. murrelli	North America	Wild mammals	Yes
T. nativa	Arctic/subarctic, Palaearctic	Bears, foxes	Yes
T. nelsoni	Equatorial Africa	Hyenas, felids	Yes
T. pseudospiralis[a]	Cosmopolitan	Wild mammals, birds	Yes
T. papuae[a]	Papua New Guinea, Thailand	Pigs, crocodiles	Yes
T. zimbabwensis[a]	East and South Africa	Crocodiles, lizards, lions	No

[a]Non-encapsulating types.

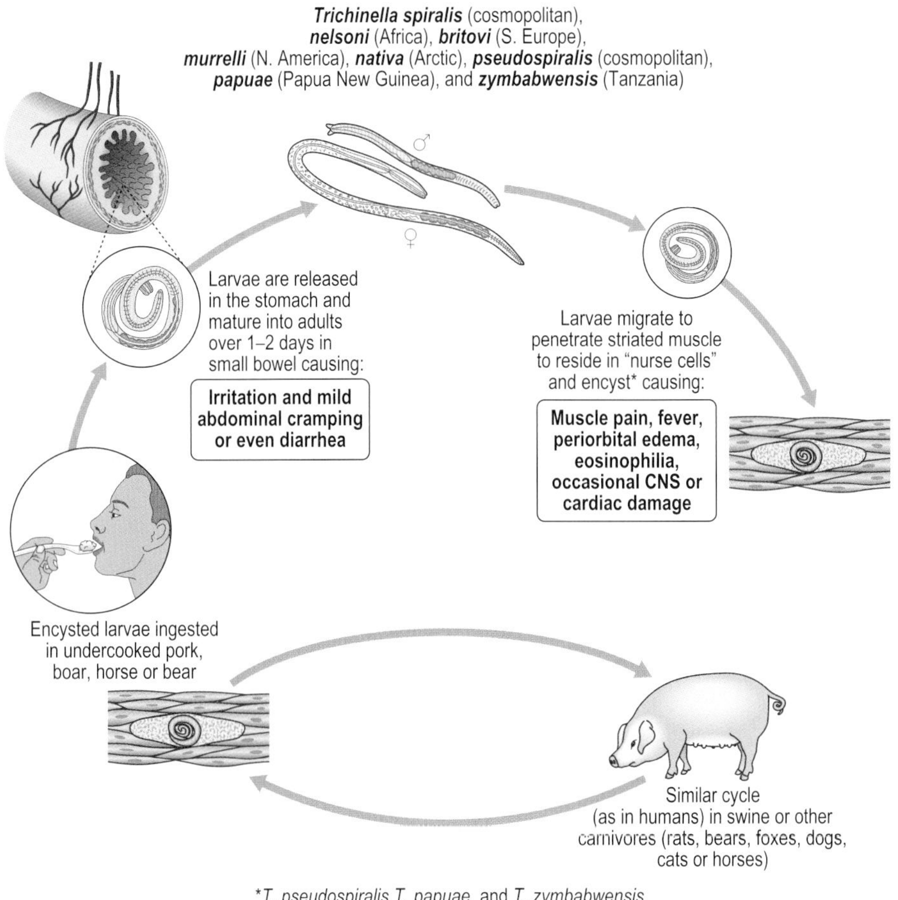

Figure 110.1 *Trichinella* life cycle. *Trichinella spiralis* (cosmopolitan), *nelsoni* (Africa), *britovi* (southern Europe), *murrelli* (North America), *nativa* (Arctic), *pseudospiralis* (cosmopolitan), *papuae* (Papua New Guinea), and *zimbabwensis* (Tanzania).

occurred among ethnic groups with preferences for raw or only partially cooked pork. Infected meat is typically purchased directly from local farmers' butcher shops, or other commercial outlets. However, in recent years, nearly one-third or more of human infections in the United States have been derived from wild game meat.[4,5] In Europe, where the safeguard of pork inspection is mandatory, most recent outbreaks have resulted from infected horse or wild boar meat.[7] The resurgence of trichinellosis in central Europe appears to result from increased transmission from both pork and wild game. In Latin America[8] and Asia, however, domestic pork appears to be the main source of infection.

Surprisingly, during the past 25 years, Europe has experienced six large outbreaks due to infected horse meat, a heretofore unrecognized source of infection.[7,8] Three outbreaks occurred in France in 1976 (125 patients) and two in 1985 (400 and 980 patients), and three occurred in Italy: one in 1976 (96 patients), one in 1984 (13 patients), and one in 1986 (300 patients). Four of the outbreaks were shown to be due to *T. britovi*, one to *T. nativa*, and one to *T. spiralis*.[8] One outbreak in France was due to horse meat infected with *T. murrelli* that was imported from the United States.[2]

Foreign travelers also account for some cases of human trichinellosis: 26 cases occurred from 1975 to 1989 in the United States, most of them after travel to Mexico or Asia.[9] Globally, the prevalence of *T. spiralis* in domestic swine ranges from less than 0.001% (United States) to 25% or more (e.g., some regions of China). The global rise in consumer demand for greater food quality assurance also makes eradication of *T. spiralis* from pork an unavoidable responsibility of both producers and governments.

THE DISEASE

The clinical course of the acute period of infection is characterized by two phases: enteral (the parasite alters intestinal function) and parenteral,

Table 110.2 Worldwide Examples of Recent Human Trichinellosis Cases

Country	Period	Number of Cases	Sources
United States	1996–2005	61	Pork, game
Canada	2005	9	Bear
Mexico	1991–1998	280	Pork
Argentina	1990–2002	6919	Pork, game
Bulgaria	1993–2000	5683	Pork, game
Croatia	1997–2000	1047	Pork
Serbia	1995–2001	3925	Pork
Romania	1990–1999	16712	Pork
Poland	2007	201	Pork
France	1995–1997	27	Game, horse
Italy	1999–2001	164	Pork, horse, game
Spain	1993–1998	290	Pork, game
Germany	1996–2007	99	Pork, game
Russia	1998–2002	864	Game, pork
Israel	2002	30	Pork
Turkey	2004	418	Pork
China	1964–2004	23004	Pork, dog, game, mutton
Thailand	1994–2007	136	Pork
Laos	2005	625	Pork

associated with an inflammatory and allergic response to muscle invasion by the larval parasites.[10] Gastrointestinal signs appear first, a result of mucosal invasion by the first-generation (ingested) larvae. These signs typically last 2–7 days but may persist for weeks. Subsequently, fever, myalgia, periorbital edema, and eosinophilia, which together constitute the so-called trichinellotic syndrome or general trichinellosis syndrome, begin.[11] However, the acute phase, lasting 1–8 weeks, is commonly asymptomatic, especially when the number of ingested larvae is low.

The severity of the clinical course depends on the parasite and host factors,[11] such as immune status; this is particularly evident in patients treated with immunosuppressive drugs for kidney transplantation.[12] In experimental infections, steroids and immunosuppressive treatments delay intestinal worm expulsion,[13] and this probably also occurs in humans.[10] Furthermore, the prolonged diarrhea in the absence of myalgia, reported in elderly Inuit people, may be due to previously acquired immunity against the enteral stage of the parasite.[5] The incubation period ranges from 7 to 30 days, depending on the severity of infection. When the course of infection is severe, the incubation period is brief, although death may also occur with a longer incubation period.[11]

The clinical course may be abortive (symptomatology not complete), mild (complete even if mild), moderate, or severe (often with complications).[7] Malaise, anorexia, nausea, vomiting, abdominal pain, fever, diarrhea, or constipation may occur. Diarrhea is more persistent than vomiting, lasting up to 3 months, and, when excessive, causes dehydration; this, together with enteritis, is an occasional cause of death. Variations in this pattern occur. For example, in outbreaks in the Canadian Arctic caused by the Arctic species *T. nativa*, trichinellosis occurred in two forms: the classic myopathic form and a clinical syndrome featuring prolonged diarrhea without fever and only a brief period of myalgia, affecting primarily elderly patients.[5]

Muscles are mainly affected during the parenteral phase, but other organs, such as the myocardium, central nervous system (CNS), lungs, kidney, and skin, may also be involved. The trichinellotic syndrome is characterized by facial edema, muscle pain and swelling, weakness, and, frequently, fever; anorexia, headache, conjunctivitis, and urticaria occur less frequently. Fever, usually remittent, generally begins at 2 weeks and peaks after 4, with temperatures as high as 40°C or 41°C in severe cases. Despite fever, patients may appear in good condition. Ocular signs at this time may help in diagnosis, in particular edema of the eyelids, chemosis, conjunctivitis, conjunctival hemorrhages, disturbed vision, and ocular pain. Periorbital edema is peculiar to trichinellosis due probably to an allergic phenomenon.[14]

The entire face may also be involved, giving patients a characteristic aspect, often rendering them unrecognizable. At this time, the muscles of the rest of the body usually become painful. Extraocular muscles, masseters, tongue and larynx muscles, diaphragm, neck muscles, and intercostal muscles are most frequently infected. The pain may be so severe as to limit function of the arms and legs, inhibiting walking, speaking, moving the tongue, breathing, and swallowing. Weakness is also a consequence of the muscle involvement. The muscles become stiff, hard, and edematous; the edema may be so intense as to simulate hypertrophy.[7] Edema lasts 1 or 2 weeks and disappears with increased diuresis. In an outbreak in Thailand due to *T. pseudospiralis*, myalgia and asthenia lasted more than 4 months.[15]

Gastrointestinal symptoms, such as vomiting and diarrhea, may also extend into this phase.[11] Dyspnea (even ventilatory failure),[16] coughing, and hoarseness may also be present. Dyspnea is caused primarily by parasite invasion and consequent inflammation of respiratory muscles such as the diaphragm.[7] Bronchopneumonia and infarction may also be responsible. The cough begins in correspondence with the passage of the larvae through the capillary bed of the lungs approximately 1 week after infection.[17]

Neurologic manifestations, more common in severe infections, occur in 10–24% of cases.[18,19] In 55 patients affected by neurotrichinosis (involvement of the CNS), meningoencephalitic signs were observed in almost all cases. Less frequent signs are focal paralysis or paresis, delirium, and psychosis.[20] Headache is very common in trichinellosis, being exacerbated by movements of the head. Myocarditis is the most frequent cardiovascular complication. It is sometimes responsible for heart failure or bronchopneumonia; in some cases, death occurs between the fourth and the eighth week of infection, although sudden death may occur even earlier.[11] Arrhythmias, secondary to myocarditis, may also occur. In one case, it was necessary to use a pacemaker for 1 year to maintain normal cardiac rhythm.[16] Electrocardiographic alterations (premature contractions, prolongation of the P-R interval, small QRS complexes with intraventricular block, and flattening or inversion of the T waves, especially lead II and precordial leads) may be present from the second week and may persist up to the third or fourth week. Blood pressure may be low during the early phase of infection and also during convalescence. Edema due to heart failure has been observed, generally in the later phase of the infection when edema due to myositis has almost disappeared. Vascular signs such as epistaxis, hemoptysis, hemorrhages from the bowel, thrombosis of the femoral or pulmonary artery, and embolism are less common. In one fatal case, the arterioles of different organs were affected by disseminated intravascular coagulation with platelet-fibrin thrombi.[20] Less frequent are petechial hemorrhages, mainly subungual resembling bacterial endocarditis, and roseola and maculopapular exanthems, resembling measles.[17] After the acute period, convalescence follows (lasting from months to years), usually with a complete recovery. During the first few years, muscle larvae are slowly but completely destroyed, followed by calcification.[21] Although this is true for *T. spiralis* infections, the calcification process in infections with other species may occur earlier.[22]

The existence of chronic trichinellosis[23] or "persisting sequelae"[24] (the persistence of myalgia, early fatigability, ocular signs, and headache for decades) is somewhat controversial and requires investigation. Some studies have confirmed the occurrence of these sequelae for periods up to 10 years after clinical recovery.[25,26]

Although death is now rare in trichinellosis, owing to improved therapy, it may result from congestive heart failure due to myocarditis, encephalitis, pneumonitis, hypokalemia, or adrenal gland insufficiency.[11,17] In the United States, during the period 1991 to 1996, in 230 cases of trichinellosis reported to the Centers for Disease Control and Prevention, only 3 were fatal.[9] During an outbreak in Thailand caused by *T. pseudospiralis*, one fatality was reported in 59 patients and it was attributed to the high number of larvae ingested rather than to pathogenicity of the *Trichinella* species involved.[15] In 2006 an outbreak caused by

Trichinella papuae was reported in Thailand, involving 28 patients, 3 of whom were hospitalized, with no fatalities.[27]

PATHOGENESIS AND IMMUNITY

The early phase of infection, associated with the presence of the parasite in the gastrointestinal tract, induces a type 1 hypersensitivity reaction, a result of Th2 cell activation, leading to increased levels of parasite-specific IgE and eosinophils, the protective role of which is still under debate.[28,29] The mechanisms regulating the response to a primary infection, especially in human hosts, are not clear. The prolonged diarrhea observed in the outbreaks in the Canadian Arctic[30,31] suggests adult worms persist in the intestine of people with frequent exposure to infection, a circumstance that arises from possible down-regulation of the intestinal immune response, a premunition state, or a down-regulation of gut physiology.

It has been shown in infected mice deficient in a mast cell-specific protease as well as in interleukin (IL)-9 transgenic mice (mast cells overproduced) that these cells are responsible for the modifications of the intestinal epithelial barrier, including production of a mucosal chymase, occurring during *T. spiralis* infection, which lead to an increased mucosal leakiness.[32] The effect of this protease, increasing gut permeability, could facilitate the passage of antibodies to the lumen.

The parenteral phase is associated with inflammatory and allergic responses to invasion of the muscles by the migrating larvae. This invasion can directly damage the muscle cells or indirectly stimulate the infiltration of inflammatory cells, primarily eosinophils. These cells may damage the muscle tissue.[33] Neurotrichinosis arises mainly from vascular perturbations, such as vasculitis and granulomatous inflammatory reactions that surround invading larvae. The larvae tend to wander, causing damage before reentering the bloodstream, or they remain trapped and are destroyed by the provoked granulomatous reaction.[34] Neural cells may also be damaged by eosinophil degranulation products such as eosinophil-derived neurotoxin and major basic protein (MBP).[35,36] Myocarditis results initially from invasion by the migrating larvae, followed by immunopathologic processes such as eosinophil infiltration (***Fig. 110.2***) and mast cell degranulation, according to results obtained in experimental infections.[37]

The mechanisms responsible for the pronounced eosinophilia, so characteristic of trichinellosis, are not well understood. The involvement of factors specific for eosinophils such as cytokines, including IL-5 produced by the Th2 subset of CD4 T cells, may be involved.[29] The role of IgE in inducing the eosinophilia is controversial.[28] Eosinophils are cytotoxic for newborn larvae in both animal and human antibody-dependent cellular cytotoxicity *in vitro* reactions; they release products such as MBP, peroxidase, or reactive oxygen species.[29] However, their actual role *in vivo* is not understood. Interestingly, suppression of eosinophilia by an IL-5-specific monoclonal antibody *in vivo* does not modify either primary or secondary *Trichinella* infections in mice;[38] but mice genetically lacking the CCR3 (a receptor for eosinophil chemokines), infected with *T. spiralis*, have a significantly higher parasite burden (although evaluated only on histologic sections) compared to wild-type animals.[39]

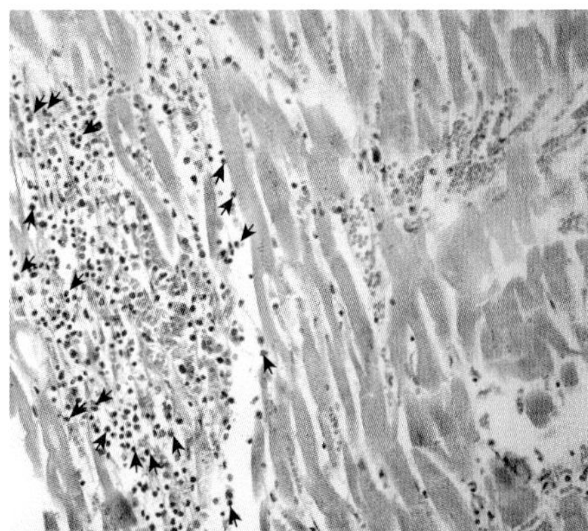

Figure 110.2 Eosinophils infiltrating the myocardial tissue of a trichinellosis patient. Eosinophils are indicated with arrows. This patient died of complications from trichinellosis. Tissue sample provided by Wanda Kociecka. Sample stained with May–Grünwald–Giemsa. Scale bar (bottom left) represents 50 μm. (Reproduced with permission from Bruschi F, Korenaga M, Watanabe N. Eosinophils and *Trichinella* infection: toxic for the parasite and the host? Trends Parasitol. 2008;24:462.)

DIAGNOSIS

The issue of whether trichinellosis is a low-prevalence disease or one that is frequently misdiagnosed cannot be adequately resolved. Diagnosis is difficult in low-level, sporadic infections because the resulting clinical manifestations are common to many other diseases,[17] including chronic fatigue syndrome.[40] Trichinellosis should be considered in the differential diagnosis of myositis in patients with human immunodeficiency virus (HIV) infection.[41] When the infection occurs in epizootic or outbreak form, its diagnosis is easier. Special care must be taken when obtaining clinical histories, giving particular attention to eating habits during the weeks before the onset of symptoms. Ingestion of infected meat (raw or undercooked), the presence of gastroenteritis, myalgia, facial edema, subungual or conjunctival hemorrhages, and an increase in blood eosinophils should suggest trichinellosis.[11] Electromyography (EMG) may help in the diagnosis of moderate and severe infections during the acute period, even if the muscle changes are not pathognomonic.[11] With clinical improvement, EMG changes generally disappear within 2 or 3 months[42] but may persist for many years.[43,44]

A definitive diagnosis may be made when L1 stage larvae are found in a muscle biopsy, generally performed in the more accessible deltoid muscle. Biopsy is recommended only in rare and difficult cases, particularly when serology is not clear. If the result is negative, however, a low-level infection cannot be excluded.[11] Artificial digestion (1% pepsin-HCl) of a muscle sample is more sensitive than direct microscopic observation of the tissue specimen, but, importantly, larvae cannot be isolated from muscle before 17–21 days of infection because of their sensitivity to digestion.[4] A muscle biopsy may help, however, not only in diagnosis but also in evaluating the level of infection, the pathologic changes in the muscle tissue and the infection duration and in the isolation of the parasite and its subsequent genetic typing by molecular techniques;[45] this is important when the source of infection is unknown or no longer available. This technique allowed for the first time the identification of *T. pseudospiralis* in a human trichinellosis case.[46] All such information is useful in deciding on therapeutic strategies.[11]

The histologic examination may reveal modifications of skeletal muscles, including at first a basophilic degeneration of the fibers, fatty metamorphosis, hyaline or hydropical degeneration or both, and interstitial inflammation; sometimes it is possible to observe dead nonencapsulated parasites. Small hemorrhages, the accumulation of inflammatory cells (myositis) such as eosinophils, lymphocytes, and macrophages, among the muscle cells are also visible. Inflammatory cells invade the muscle cells when the sarcolemma is damaged. Vascularity increases near muscle fibers.[47,48] The process of encapsulation of the parasite, with the exception of *T. pseudospiralis*, *T. papuae*, and *T. zimbabwensis*, begins at approximately 2 weeks and is usually completed at 5 weeks of infection, depending on the *Trichinella* species involved.[22] In humans, calcification begins approximately 5 months after infection and is usually completed after at least 18 months.

As previously mentioned, the diagnosis of trichinellosis is difficult in sporadic cases, but it is even more difficult when CNS involvement is present. Neurotrichinosis is sometimes accompanied by multifocal CNS lesions, nodular or ringlike, with a diameter of 3–8 mm, and, in most cases, showing contrast enhancement.[36,49] However, in cases with neurologic manifestations of trichinellosis, computed tomography images of the brain have been reported to be normal.[49,50]

Eosinophilia, leukocytosis, serum muscle enzyme-level increases, and increased immunoglobulin levels, especially total IgE, are the most

Table 110.3 Algorithm for Diagnosing the Probability of Being Infected with Acute *Trichinella* in Humans

Group A	Group B	Group C	Group D
Fever Facial and/or eyelid edema Myalgia	Neurological signs Cardiological signs Conjunctivitis Subungual hemorrhages Cutaneous rash Diarrhea	Eosinophilia (>1000/mm^3) and/or increased total IgE levels Increased levels of muscle enzymes	Positive serology (with a highly specific test) Seroconversion Positive muscle biopsy

The diagnosis is:
Very unlikely: one A or one B or one C
Suspected: one A or two B and one C
Probable: three A and one C
Highly probable: three A and two C
Confirmed: three A, two C, and one D; any of groups A or B and one C and one D
(Reproduced with permission from Dupouy-Camet J, Bruschi F. Management and diagnosis of human trichinellosis. In: Dupouy-Camet J, Murrell KD, ed. FAO/WHO/OIE guidelines for the surveillance, management, prevention and control of trichinellosis. Paris: World Organisation for Animal Health Press; 2007:37.)

characteristic laboratory findings in this disease. Eosinophil levels increase dramatically during trichinellosis (up to 19000/μL).[10] Eosinophilia (based on the absolute number rather than the percentage) occurs in all cases of trichinellosis, even the subclinical; the exception may be very severe infection with eosinopenia, which has a fatal course.[51] Eosinophilia may also be absent when bacterial infections complicate the disease. After steroid therapy, eosinophil levels also decrease.[11] Leukocytosis, up to 24000/μL,[52] occurs in very severe infections, usually early in the infection.

Increased serum creatine phosphokinase (CPK), lactate dehydrogenase (LDH), aldolase, and aminotransferase levels reflect skeletal muscle damage, helping in the diagnosis.[11] Serum CPK levels can increase up to more than 17000 U/L. CPK isoenzyme profiles, however, are not very helpful.[53] LDH should be evaluated together with CPK, even if the former is less specific. When high levels of CPK and LDH are present, a differential diagnosis with myopathies is necessary. Before antibody levels increase, the level of total serum LDH and of the isoenzymatic forms LD_4 and LD_5 may increase in approximately 50% of patients.[54] Hypoalbuminemia is observed mainly in severe cases, in which the amounts of this serum protein can reach 2.5 g/dL.[55]

Immunoglobulin level changes may also occur, the most characteristic being an increase in total IgE, which, however, is not a consistent phenomenon, and it is not possible to exclude trichinellosis by its absence.[11] A poor correlation with specific IgE has been observed for both *T. spiralis* and *T. britovi* infections.[28]

Many serologic tests are available for diagnosis,[11,56] with three objectives: (1) recognizing the acute infection to allow early anthelminthic treatment, (2) making a retrospective diagnosis, and (3) adding information to the epidemiology of the infection.[57] Seroconversion usually occurs between the third and fifth week of infection and serum may remain positive up to 1 year or more after cessation of clinical symptoms. Antibodies have been detected, however, up to 19 years after the end of the acute phase of infection.[11] Antibody levels do not correlate with the severity of the clinical picture[54] or with a particular clinical course.[58]

Indirect hemagglutination, bentonite flocculation, indirect immunofluorescence (IFA), latex agglutination, and enzyme-linked immunosorbent assay (ELISA) are the more commonly used tests, the last of which is the most sensitive.[11] Factors such as sensitivity, specificity, convenience, simplicity, cost, and commercial availability must be considered when choosing a test. However, a diagnostic laboratory should have at least two or more tests available to ensure a correct diagnosis: one to detect the response against a soluble antigen and another for antibodies that react with parasite surface antigens.[57] For the latter, the IFA is performed with whole L1 stage larvae killed with formalin[59] or with unfixed frozen sections of infected muscles[60]; the latter is more sensitive. With this test, all specific immunoglobulins can be evaluated. The ELISA assay,[61] using excretory/secretory (E/S) antigen,[62] is preferable to use of crude extracts of *T. spiralis* muscle larvae for soluble antigen because it is more specific.[56] This is particularly important in tropical regions where cross-reactions with other helminth parasites can give false positive results.[63,64] Cross-reactions with *Trichinella* antigens were observed in patients with autoimmune diseases.[65] It is necessary to standardize as much as possible the antigens used for serological diagnosis.[62] Recombinant[66] or synthetic[67] antigens are now available for diagnostic purposes.

A capture ELISA (cELISA) using TSL-1 antigens (tyvelose-bearing epitopes) immobilized with a specific monoclonal antibody on the plates resulted in a reliable method for serodiagnosis of human trichinellosis compared to other antigens (crude antigen, deglycosylated crude antigen, and affinity purified TSL-1 antigens), giving 100% specificity and 100% sensitivity. The cELISA with TSL-1 antigens was also more sensitive than indirect immunofluorescence or ELISA, allowing earlier detection of infections.[68]

The ELISA can also be used for the evaluation of the different specific immunoglobulin classes (IgA and IgM)[69,70] or IgG subclasses,[71,72] but the sensitivity of these tests is lower than that of the ELISA IgG. The data on specific IgE are contradictory,[63,69,70] and this test cannot yet be recommended. The detection of circulating antigens has also not been completely satisfactory compared to IFA or a competitive inhibition assay.[73] However, it is worthwhile because it may demonstrate early the actual presence of the parasite and may represent an alternative to muscle biopsy.

The study of the cellular immune response in humans[74] is important for research purposes but of little value for diagnosis. Immunoelectrotransfer blot assay[75,76] can be used as a primary or confirmatory test. When E/S antigens are used, it is quite specific and useful for follow-up studies.[46] In accordance with the International Commission on Trichinellosis, the serum reactivity for the TSL-1 antigen family (40–70 kDa in the reduced form) should be considered diagnostic.[56]

An algorithm to identify the probability of acute trichinellosis cases has been recently formulated (see ***Table 110.3***).[7]

TREATMENT AND PROGNOSIS

It is difficult to differentiate the efficacy of drug therapy from natural recovery of infection in mild to moderate cases. Factors such as the *Trichinella* species involved, intensity and length of infection, and host response can aid in deciding on the treatment course.[11] Symptomatic treatment[51] includes analgesic and antipyretic drugs, bed rest, and corticosteroids (prednisolone at 50 mg/day), especially in severe infections to prevent shocklike symptoms. Specific treatment[51] is with mebendazole, which should be administered in adults at a daily dosage of 5 mg/kg in two doses for 10–15 days (the treatment cycle may be repeated after 5 days), or with albendazole. In adults, this latter drug should be administered at a dosage of 15 mg/kg daily in two doses for 10–15 days; in children older than 2 years, the drug is given at 10 mg/kg daily. For severe infection, the treatment may be repeated after 5 days. Blood cell counts and liver function should be regularly monitored, to prevent adverse side effects.[77] Mebendazole and albendazole are contraindicated in pregnant women. Thiabendazole is no longer used because of its side effects.[51] Pyrantel has been proposed for children and pregnant women, but its efficacy is doubtful.[7]

The specific treatment is recommended for intestinal and muscle stages, but light infections do not require treatment. The treatment goal for the very early infection phase is to limit muscle invasion by larvae; when this has already occurred, the goal is to reduce muscle damage, which is responsible for the major clinical manifestations. Therapeutic plasma levels of the drug should be maintained for an extended period rather than high levels for short periods. The success of treatment is evident from clinical improvement of the patient's symptomatology.

Until recently, very few prospective, controlled clinical trials of treatment for trichinellosis have been carried out,[78] and as a consequence, there are several uncertainties in the treatment choices.[7]

As previously mentioned, the prognosis as far as life is concerned is usually good, except in rare, heavily infected cases. The prognosis as far as health is concerned depends on the number of ingested larvae and on the time passed before the diagnosis has been made and treatment begins.

PREVENTION AND CONTROL

Control of swine trichinellosis and prevention of infection in humans have both direct and indirect aspects. Mandatory inspection of pork at slaughter, although common in developed countries, especially Europe,[79] is required in the United States only for the production of certified pork (not commonly performed).[80] In developing countries, testing for trichinellosis as part of routine inspection is rare. Instead, emphasis is placed on educating the consumer on safe handling and cooking of pork and wild game. The US Department of Agriculture has established recommended procedures for devitalizing any muscle larvae present in these meats by cooking or freezing. For example, the consumer should cook pork until all pink color has disappeared, which normally occurs at approximately 137°F (58°C); to allow for a margin of error, however, it is recommended that the internal temperature of meat should uniformly reach 160°F (71°C) throughout, whether by conventional cooking or by microwaving. Care must be taken to avoid cold spots with the latter method.

Fresh pork less than 6 inches (15 cm) thick can be rendered safe if frozen to 5°F (−15°C) for 20 days, −10°F (−23°C) for 10 days, or −20°F (−29°C) for 6 days. Because of the freeze resistance shown by sylvatic species of *Trichinella*, particularly *T. nativa*, freezing of meat from wild game is not uniformly reliable. Because infection from wild animal meat accounts for an important proportion of human trichinellosis, inspection of wild game muscle is either recommended or is mandatory in some European countries. Consumers should also be warned of the danger and advised on proper meat handling and preparation procedures.

The control of trichinellosis in swine relies on good general management practices.[81] For example, US pork producers are encouraged to observe federal garbage feeding regulations in those states where this practice is allowed, to practice stringent rodent control, to avoid exposing pigs to dead animal carcasses of any kind, to ensure that hog carcasses are properly disposed of, and to try to establish effective barriers between domestic swine and wild and domestic animals.

Efforts are under way in both the United States and Europe to develop farm certification systems for the production of *Trichinella*-free pigs.[81] The International Commission on Trichinellosis, the Food and Agriculture Organization (FAO), the World Health Organization (WHO), and the World Organisation for Animal Health (OIE) have published recommended requirements for such certification which could exempt marketed pigs from mandatory inspection.[81]

The management practices required are intended primarily for conventional pig rearing (indoors), and are not easily amenable to outdoor pig rearing. This is of concern because of the expanding production of organic or ecological pig production which increases risk of exposure to wild animal reservoirs of infection.[82]

A modest amount of research has been carried out on the development of a vaccine. Unlike rodents, the typical experimental host, pigs do not develop strong intestinal immunity;[83] hence, muscle larval L1 stage stichocyte antigens are insufficient for a vaccine. The antigens from the NBL have proved highly effective in pigs, and a first generation vaccine has been developed.[84]

Access the complete reference list online at
http://www.expertconsult.com

CHAPTER 111

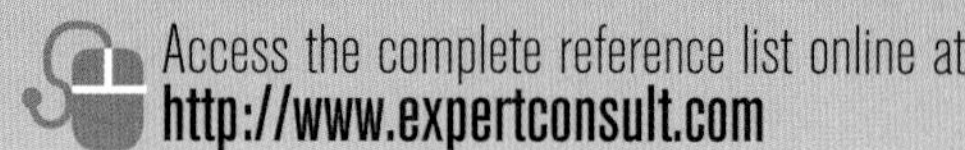
Access the complete reference list online at
http://www.expertconsult.com

Angiostrongyliasis

John H. Cross† • Kao-Pin Hwang

INTRODUCTION

Two species of *Angiostrongylus* (*Parastrongylus*), both natural parasites of certain species of rodents, cause two distinct diseases of importance. The geographic distribution of the nematodes and clinical syndromes are different so they will be discussed separately. *Angiostrongylus cantonensis* causes a meningoencephalitis characterized by a high number of eosinophils in the cerebrospinal fluid (CSF). The disease is called eosinophilic meningitis and is prevalent in Asia and certain tropical Pacific islands and is appearing elsewhere, including the Americas. *Angiostrongylus costaricensis* causes an eosinophilic inflammation of the intestinal tract that can mimic appendicitis and is found mainly in Central and South America.

ANGIOSTRONGYLUS CANTONENSIS

THE AGENT

A. cantonensis, first described from China in 1935,[1] is known as the rat lungworm, living as an adult in the pulmonary arteries of the rat. The life cycle (***Fig. 111.1A***) involves rats and mollusks, with humans being incidental hosts. The first human infection was reported from Taiwan in 1945.[2] In rats, adult worms in the pulmonary arteries produce fertilized eggs that develop into first-stage larvae.[3] These larvae penetrate lung arterioles, move into the respiratory tract, and are then coughed up, swallowed, and passed in the feces. Larvae remain viable in the feces for variable periods, depending on moisture, and can remain infectious for several weeks in fresh water.[4] The life cycle is completed only if these larvae penetrate or are consumed by an appropriate mollusk intermediate host, usually land snails or slugs.[3] First-stage larvae then mature into third-stage larvae that remain infectious for the life of the mollusk. When a rat consumes a mollusk with viable larvae, larvae penetrate its intestinal wall, enter the bloodstream and migrate to the central nervous system (CNS). In the CNS of the rat, larvae mature into the fifth stage (young adults) that then make their way from the subarachnoid space of the CNS into the pulmonary arteries, completing the life cycle in 42–45 days. If a human consumes a mollusk with viable third-stage larvae, larvae likewise migrate to the CNS. However, because humans are abnormal hosts, the parasite is unable to complete its life cycle and dies in the CNS.

EPIDEMIOLOGY

A. cantonensis is now enzootic in many parts of the world.[5,6] The first epidemic outbreaks of eosinophilic meningitis were reported from Ponape, Caroline Islands.[7] Other early reports of eosinophilic meningitis were from French Polynesia, New Caledonia, and Hawaii.[8,9] Subsequently, the parasite has been found almost worldwide from the Pacific Basin, Asia, Africa, India, and more recently from Caribbean islands, Brazil, and North America.[5,6,10,11] Most human infections have been reported from Taiwan, Thailand and more recently from China.[11] The geographic spread of this parasite is related to infected rats being transported to various places aboard ships and/or the introduction of mollusks such as the giant African snail (*Achatina fulica*).[5,6,11] The Amazonian apple snail (*Pomacea caniculata*), introduced into Taiwan and China in the 1980s, is now the major source of infection in these countries.[12]

Purposeful or inadvertent ingestion of uncooked or marinated snails is important to query in the histories of patients. In Thailand, eosinophilic meningitis has been related to the ingestion of sliced, pickled *Pila* snails;[13] and other outbreaks of eosinophilic meningitis have been attributable to consumption of raw *Achatina fulica* snails.[14] However, in many sporadic cases there is no obvious exposure to mollusks. Since cases of eosinophilic meningitis have been reported in vegetarians,[15] it is postulated that larvae can remain viable in the slime of snails or slugs and cause infection when contaminated, unwashed vegetables are eaten. Cases in young children have been attributed to unobserved ingestions of a contaminated snail or slug.[16]

A cold-blooded predator or scavenger (paratenic host) can be an incidental carrier of larvae if it has ingested an infected mollusk.[17] Thus, freshwater shrimp or crabs can carry larvae capable of causing infection if eaten.[17,18] Infectious larvae can remain viable for long periods of time in such hosts, many of which are eaten raw in many tropical cultures. Eating uncooked monitor lizard has been a source of infection in Thailand, India and Sri Lanka; and eating raw frog legs was incriminated as a source of infection in Taiwan.[19] Larvae in paratenic hosts are not capable of completing their life cycle, but can remain viable for long periods of time. Water in wells or cisterns can also be a source of viable larvae, becoming contaminated when released from drowned terrestrial mollusks. Contamination of fingers with larvae during collection and preparation of snails for eating is another potential source of infection.[20]

THE DISEASE

The incubation period is about 2 weeks[14] or as long as 45 days. The most common presentation is that of a nonbacterial meningitis.[20] Patients present with headache, nausea, vomiting, and neck stiffness.[14,21,22] Fever is less common in adults than in children.[11,13,23] The main, and occasionally only, complaint is a headache, which is usually global and severe. In children, in addition to fever, common symptoms include vomiting, headache and somnolence.[11,22] The duration of illness ranges from 2 to 8 weeks.[20,21] Paresthesias are a distinctive complaint; they are asymmetrical and usually noted on the extremities.[20,24] Paresthesias, which can distinguish this form of meningitis from others, can be persistent, lasting months after resolution of the illness.[23,24] Transient cranial nerve palsies, especially of the abducent and facial nerves, can occur, but serious neurologic sequelae are unusual.[20,23,24] Papilledema seems to be more common in children.[23] Most cases resolve spontaneously with complete

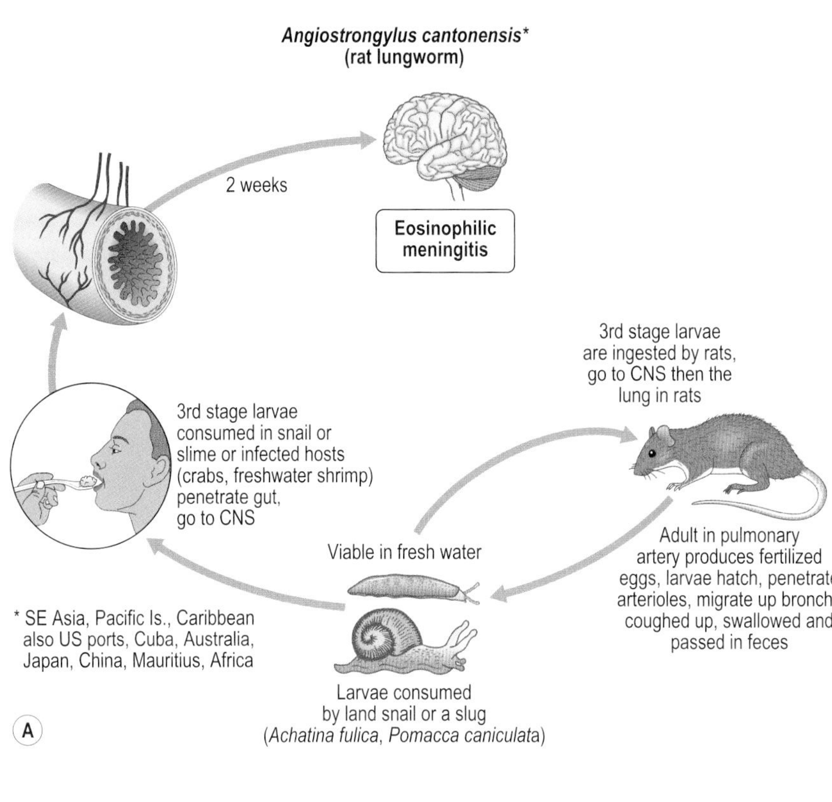
Angiostrongylus cantonensis*
(rat lungworm)
2 weeks
Eosinophilic meningitis
3rd stage larvae are ingested by rats, go to CNS then the lung in rats
3rd stage larvae consumed in snail or slime or infected hosts (crabs, freshwater shrimp) penetrate gut, go to CNS
Viable in fresh water
Adult in pulmonary artery produces fertilized eggs, larvae hatch, penetrate arterioles, migrate up bronchi, coughed up, swallowed and passed in feces
* SE Asia, Pacific Is., Caribbean also US ports, Cuba, Australia, Japan, China, Mauritius, Africa
Larvae consumed by land snail or a slug (Achatina fulica, Pomacca caniculata)
A

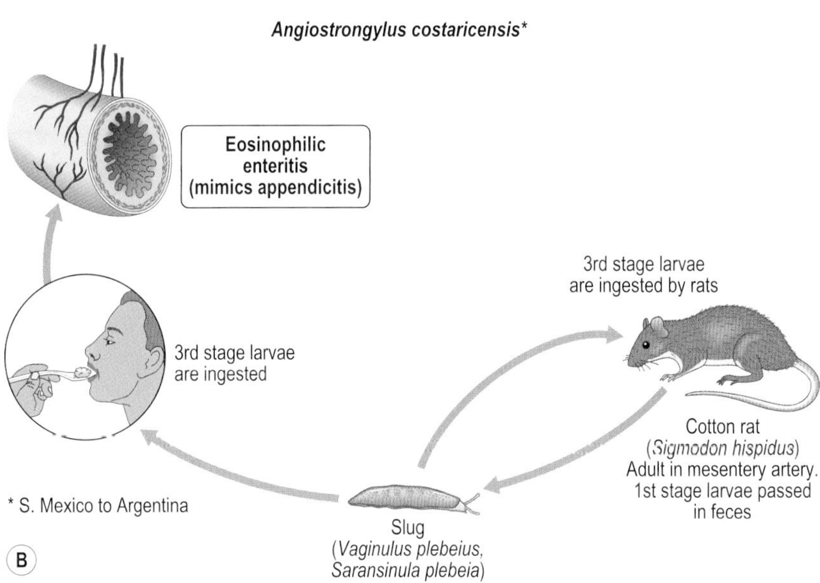
Angiostrongylus costaricensis*
Eosinophilic enteritis (mimics appendicitis)
3rd stage larvae are ingested by rats
3rd stage larvae are ingested
Cotton rat (Sigmodon hispidus) Adult in mesentery artery. 1st stage larvae passed in feces
* S. Mexico to Argentina
Slug (Vaginulus plebeius, Saransinula plebeia)
B

Figure 111.1 Life cycles of *Angiostrongylus cantonensis* **(A)** and *Angiostrongylus costaricensis* **(B)**.

recovery. However, serious complications and death do occur uncommonly, probably resulting from larger numbers of migrating larvae or migration of larvae into critical parts of the brain.[21,25]

PATHOGENESIS AND IMMUNITY

The hallmark of this infection is an eosinophilic CSF pleocytosis that results from larvae migrating through the CNS. Death of parasites in the CNS likely contributes to the eosinophilic response. Since humans are not normal hosts, it is extremely rare for an *Angiostrongylus* adult worm (but never clearly *A. cantonensis*) to be found in the lungs of humans.[26] An episode of infection does confer immunity in rats but not in humans.[8]

DIAGNOSIS

A definitive diagnosis of angiostrongyliasis cantonensis would require finding larva in the CSF or in the anterior chamber of eye,[27,28] although this is not common.[29] Finding high numbers of eosinophils in the CSF and exposure in an endemic area should suggest eosinophilic meningitis (see Chapter 131).[29] Low numbers of CSF eosinophils can be seen in a variety of conditions, but finding greater than 10% eosinophils in the CSF should suggest this disease.[28] Typically, the CSF shows 100–5000 leukocytes/μL, 10–90% of which are eosinophils.[23] The CSF protein is usually elevated, but the glucose is normal or slightly lowered.[23] Although worm recovery from the CSF by lumbar puncture (LP) is rare, larger volumes of CSF collected with pumping after a sitting position may achieve a recovery rate as high as 60%.[22,30] A peripheral eosinophilia is not a consistent finding.

The differential diagnosis of eosinophils in the CSF includes gnathostomiasis, cysticercosis paragonimiasis, schistosomiasis, and strongyloidiasis[29,31] (see Chapter 131). *Gnathostoma spinigerum* is characterized by nerve root pain, paraplegia, spinal cord lesions, and xanthochromic CSF (see Chapter 112). The raccoon parasite *Baylisascaris procyonis* has also been the cause of fatal eosinophilic meningoencephalitis in humans (see Chapter 112). Nonparasitic etiologies, such as coccidioidomycosis and lymphomas of the CNS, may be associated with an eosinophilic pleocytosis (see Chapter 131).[32]

Headaches frequently improve dramatically after an LP.[23] Ventricular dilation, only occasionally seen, is probably due to a transient communicating hydrocephalus caused by inflammation of the arachnoid decreasing the resorption of CSF. *A. cantonensis* larvae have rarely been observed in the eye[27] and CSF.[22,28] A computed tomography (CT) scan of the brain in eosinophilic meningitis is generally nonspecific.[33,34] However, magnetic resonance imaging (MRI) with contrast dye can show meningeal enhancement as well as hyperintense T2 signal lesions in punctate areas of the brain.[11,35] The usual absence of focal lesions on CT scans helps distinguish eosinophilic meningitis from the focal lesions observed with neurocysticercosis and gnathostomiasis.[11] While serologic diagnosis of angiostrongyiasis has been hampered by a lack of specificity and by cross-reactivity with other helminths,[36] purification of antigens and defining IgG subclass antibody responses have improved accuracy;[37–39] but serodiagnosis is not routinely available. Elevated levels of IgE in serum have been reported.[40]

TREATMENT AND PROGNOSIS

There is no specific treatment. Supportive treatments, including repeated LPs and analgesics, can diminish increased intracranial pressures and headaches. Anthelminthics (albendazole, mebendazole) alone and/or corticosteroids have been tried,[41–44] but it is difficult to assess their efficacy when there are no controlled studies and the disease is self-limited.[44] Anthelminthics that cross the blood–brain barrier, such as praziquantel or albendazole, should theoretically work in this disease, but a systemic response to dying worms might make the condition worse. Adjunctive corticosteroids or corticosteroids alone should be considered in more severe cases (i.e., marked encephalitis or cranial nerve damage). In one randomized trial of corticosteroids (60 mg prednisolone daily for 2 weeks) versus placebo control, corticosteroid-treated subjects were substantially improved with shorter durations of headaches, fewer LPs, and less analgesic use.[44,45]

PREVENTION AND CONTROL

Prevention involves educating travelers or persons in endemic areas that snails, slugs, freshwater shrimp, crabs, monitor lizards, and other paratenic hosts must be cooked, not simply marinated or refrigerated, before they are eaten. Vegetables must be washed if eaten uncooked. Commonly infected mollusks such as *A. fulica* and *P. canaliculata*[12] should be handled carefully to avoid contamination of the fingers with larvae. Control of mollusks and planarians and reducing numbers of rats are also potential measures.

ANGIOSTRONGYLUS COSTARICENSIS

THE AGENT

A. costaricensis (*Morerastrongylus costaricensis*), first described from Costa Rica in 1971,[46] has a life cycle similar *to A. cantonensis* in that rodents are the definitive hosts and mollusks are intermediate hosts (***Fig. 111.1B***).[47] *A. costaricensis*, however, develops into its adult form in the mesenteric arteries of rats. Humans are abnormal hosts in whom the parasite is unable to complete its life cycle,[46] and larvae become trapped inside granulomas in the intestinal wall.

EPIDEMIOLOGY

Human infections occur predominantly from southern Mexico to Argentina. Clinical disease was reported in Costa Rica in the 1950s before *A. costaricensis* was described. Following the recognition in 1971 that *A. costaricensis* was the etiologic agent,[46] abdominal angiostrongyliasis in humans has been reported from Honduras, Mexico, Venezuela,[47] Martinique, Dominican Republic, Puerto Rico,[48] Argentina, Brazil,[49] Nicaragua,[50] and rarely in Africa (Democratic Republic of the Congo).[51] In a case reported from the United States (Los Angeles, California), there has been uncertainty whether it was due to anisakiasis or *A. costaricensis*.[52,53] Parasites have been found in rodents in Colombia[54] and Panama[55] without reports of human cases.

At least 12 species of rats and one coati have been shown to be naturally infected.[56] The most important rat is the cotton rat (*Sigmodon hispidus*).[47] Rats pass first-stage larvae in their feces for up to 8 months.[47] *A. costaricensis* in rat definitive hosts live within mesenteric arteries, especially in the ileocecal region. Female worms deposit eggs which are carried by the bloodstream into the intestinal wall where they embryonate. First-stage larvae, hatched from eggs, migrate through the intestinal wall into the intestinal lumen and pass within rat feces to the soil. While many mollusks may serve as intermediate hosts, veronicellid slugs are considered the most important. First-stage larvae enter slugs by oral or cutaneous infections. After penetration larvae are retained in fibromuscular tissue or spread throughout whole slugs via their circulation.[57] These larvae develop by 20 days into third-stage larvae that may remain in the slug for months or may leave the animal in mucous secretions. Upon entering the rat definitive host, larvae go through lymphatic/venous pathways to develop into adult stages. Mature females begin producing eggs at about 15 days.[58] The mode of transmission to humans is not well established. Since people do not eat slugs, it is assumed that infectious larvae from molluskan intermediate hosts, such as *Vaginulus plebeius* and *Saransinula plebeia*, contaminate water or vegetation with infectious larvae, which are inadvertently consumed by humans, as in salads.[47] Although the *V. plebeius* slug is not indigenous to the continental United States, it has been found on imported produce.[52] Most human cases have been described in children between the ages of 6 and 13 years.[59] Higher, rather than lower, socioeconomic status is more common.[59] In general, males outnumber females by 2 : 1.

THE DISEASE

The incubation period for abdominal angiostrongyliasis (called Morera's disease in Latin America) is not known, but is estimated to be 3–4 weeks. Clinical findings mimic those of appendicitis[59] or an inflamed Meckel's diverticulum. Patients have fever, nausea, vomiting, and abdominal pain. Abdominal pain is frequently localized to the right lower quadrant.[56] Occasionally a painful mass in the right lower quadrant can be noted on rectal examination.[59] Symptoms are generally more indolent than those typical of acute appendicitis. Patients tend to have recurrent episodes over several months. There may be hepatic involvement with nodules seen by ultrasound and at laparoscopy yellow spots may be seen on the liver surface.[60] Surgical exploration on the suspicion of appendicitis frequently occurs. Complications can be abscess formation, obstruction, and infarction of the bowel.[59] A few deaths have been reported.[59] Occasionally, the testicular artery can be involved, but this diagnosis is generally not made before surgery, which is usually done for suspected torsion.[61]

PATHOGENESIS AND IMMUNITY

In humans, the parasite usually confines itself to the abdominal cavity. Inadvertent ingestion of slugs, either chopped up in salads or on vegetation contaminated with their mucous secretions, can introduce infectious third-stage larvae into the human gastrointestinal tract. Larvae eventually enter the mesenteric arteries where they mature into adults. Adult parasites in mesenteric arteries can cause arteritis, thrombosis, infarction, and gastrointestinal hemorrhage.[62] Eggs from adults can lodge in capillaries, producing an inflammatory reaction within the intestinal wall. The embryonated eggs do not hatch, but degenerate and cause an eosinophilic granulomatous reaction.[63] The resultant histopathologic changes could be suggestive of an allergic granulomatous angiitis (Churg–Strauss vasculitis).[48] The terminal ileum and appendix are most commonly involved within the intestines, but other parts of the intestine and occasionally regional lymph nodes can be involved.[46,59,63]

DIAGNOSIS

There are no diagnostic tests other than to demonstrate the parasite or its eggs in tissue. Most patients have pain in the right lower quadrant, and a leukocytosis, findings common in appendicitis. In endemic regions suspicion of this parasite should be raised when there is an associated blood eosinophilia, which can range from 11% to 82% with a leukocytosis of 10 000–50 000 white blood cells/μL.[47,59] The worms usually localize to the mesenteric arteries of the ileocecal region, and radiologic examinations of the intestinal tract may show bowel edema and spasticity in that area.[56,59] Stool examinations for parasites are warranted to search for other intestinal nematodes and to exclude heavy infections with *Enterobius vermicularis* that might also cause intestinal inflammation (see Chapter 113). Human anisakiasis or visceral larva migrans due to *Toxocara* spp. can also mimic abdominal angiostrongyliasis.[63] Serologic tests are currently not readily available, although newer ELISA assays are showing promise.[64,65]

TREATMENT AND PROGNOSIS

No specific medical treatment is known. Surgical treatment for acute intestinal inflammation may be necessary. The use of anthelminthics has not been systematically studied. Neither thiabendazole nor diethylcarbamazine was effective.[59] Acute episodes can be uncomplicated and resolve spontaneously. The prognosis is generally good.

PREVENTION AND CONTROL

Avoidance of slugs and the ingestion of raw food and water that might be contaminated by imperceptible slugs or slime from slugs are the cornerstones of prevention and control. Washing fruits and vegetables in vinegar or salt may reduce infection. Control of rats is important in preventing the spread of this parasite.

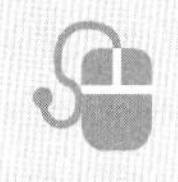

Access the complete reference list online at
http://www.expertconsult.com

CHAPTER 112

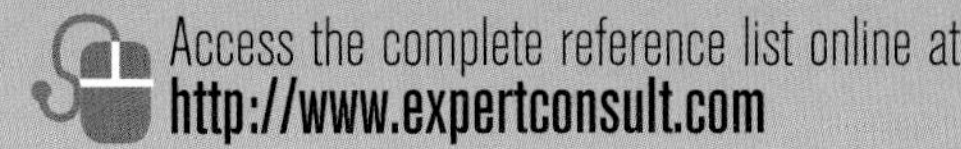
Access the complete reference list online at
http://www.expertconsult.com

Other Tissue Nematode Infections

Yezid Gutierrez

INTRODUCTION

A number of other nematode parasites that can infect humans range from the uncommon to some that are more frequent in specific geographic and epidemiologic settings. These infections are zoonotic. In recent years, there have been many more reports of these infections. That does not signify that they are "newly emerging diseases," but that they are newly recognized. Some of these nematodes have a tropical distribution, others occur in tropical and temperate zones, and as of today, none behaves opportunistically in immunocompromised hosts. Others, for example, the anisakids, are of paramount regional importance in areas like Japan.[1]

RHABDITIDA

The Rhabditida, a group of saprophytic free-living nematodes inhabiting soil, water and decomposing matter, include *Strongyloides* (see Chapter 117), the most important medically. Members of the genera *Halicephalobus* (= *Micronema*), *Rhabditis*, *Pelodera*, *Turbatrix*, and *Diploscapter* have occasionally been described parasitizing humans and animals, and with *Halicephalobus* there have been fatal infections. In general, members of the Rhabditida have direct life cycles in their natural habitats, where males and females produce eggs that hatch, releasing larvae that develop into adult worms. One exception is *Strongyloides*, which in addition to its free-living cycle has a parasitic phase in the small intestine of humans and animals. Development during the parasitic phase is by parthenogenesis.[2]

Halicephalobus (= *Micronema*)

Halicephalobus is an important free-living nematode. There have been at least three fatal human infections, all in North America.[3] In animals, *Halicephalobus* often causes gingivitis,[4] mastitis,[5] or disseminated disease.[6] Fatal human cases have been the result of central nervous system (CNS) involvement (meningoencephalitis) in two cases, and of the CNS plus other viscera in the third.

One child acquired infection during an accident in a manure-spreading machine, resulting in lacerations of the face, buttocks and thigh, fractures of the mandible and femur, and penetrating chest and abdominal wounds. Meningoencephalitis developed after 18 days in the hospital and he died 6 days later. Microscopic examination of the CNS revealed numerous nematodes (***Fig. 112.1***) in various stages and eggs, some with a developing embryo.[7] In another instance, a middle-aged man developed meningoencephalitis and died within 3 weeks of developing the disease. Microscopic examination of his brain demonstrated female nematodes developing parthenogenetically. How the infection was acquired in this patient is unknown.[8] A third man admitted to a Washington, DC hospital, chronically ill, with bilateral decubitus ulcers on the buttocks, died within 10 days of hospitalization. Autopsy revealed similar lesions and nematodes in the CNS, heart, and liver.[3] The parasites in the first two cases were identified as *Micronema deletrix* and in the third only as *Micronema*, suggesting that the species identification (*deletrix*) in previous cases was presumptive.[3] The genus of this parasite has been renamed *Halicephalobus* (= *Micronema*) and the species *gingivalis* (= *deletrix*).[9]

Rhabditis

Species of *Rhabditis* have been encountered sporadically in the stools and urine of humans,[10–12] but there is a consensus that this is usually due to contamination of stools before samples are taken. The worms in fecal samples are developing as they do under natural conditions in decaying matter. A report that appears credible is that of a 5-month-old Brazilian child with gastrointestinal (GI) symptoms, who recovered after treatment with thiabendazole.[13] In the case of an HIV-positive Iranian patient there was GI disease and a large number of eggs and larvae that on culture yielded several generations of *R. axei*.[14] There was suspicion of a relationship between the worms and the patient's symptoms, though this was not demonstrated.

Pelodera

Pelodera strongyloides occurs in dogs, cattle, sheep, and horses, sometimes causing significant dermatitis, but in lemmings and murid rodents the parasite lives in the conjunctival sac producing no ill effects. Four human infections are known, one in an 11-year-old European girl,[15] another in a 6-month-old infant girl in the United States,[16] a third in a 20-year-old man,[17] and a fourth in a mentally disabled 18-year-old Japanese man.[18] However, other cases may be undiagnosed. In the skin, the larvae do not develop further and probably feed on tissue and desquamated cells, producing pruritic papular lesions.[18] The European child had extensive dermatitis (***Fig. 112.2***) and acquired the infection from a pet puppy that succumbed to the disease. The US infant presented with failure to thrive and improved after treatment of her infection with hydrocortisone lotion, but the relationship of the infection and the symptoms remains uncertain. Cure of the 20-year-old man was with oral thiabendazole and of the Japanese man with γ-hexachlorocyclohexane ointment. Cortisone used in the Japanese man initially aggravated the infection. In the veterinary literature, recommendations are to keep the lesions clean and dry, which then resolve spontaneously. The diagnosis is made by study of larvae recovered in skin scrapings or in biopsied tissue sections,[16] or by cultures of the worm.[18]

Turbatrix and *Diploscapter*

Turbatrix aceti, the vinegar eelworm, has been found previously, but not recently, in the vagina of healthy women who used vinegar for douching.[19] Asymptomatic infections of the urinary bladder have been reported.[20]

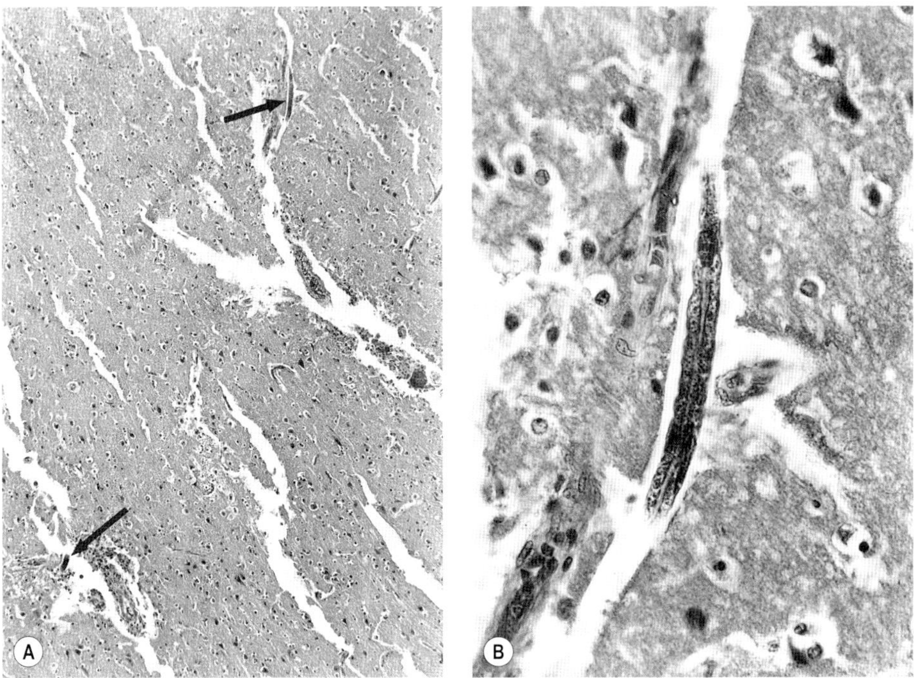

Figure 112.1 *Halicephalobus* in brain. **(A)** View showing some nematodes (arrows), and areas of inflammatory infiltrate. (Hematoxylin and eosin (H&E) originally ×70.) **(B)** Higher magnification of nematode. (H&E stain, originally ×450.)

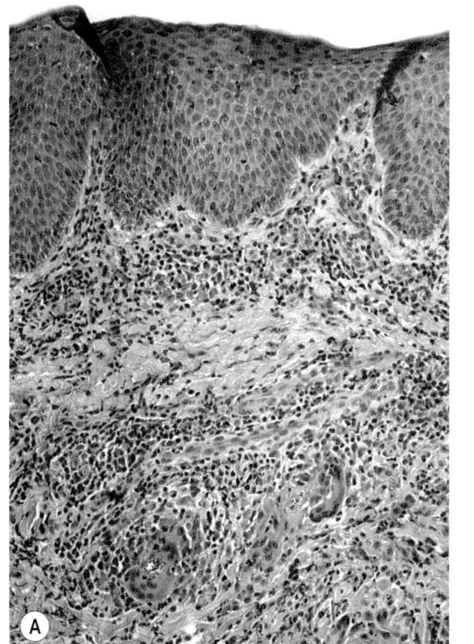

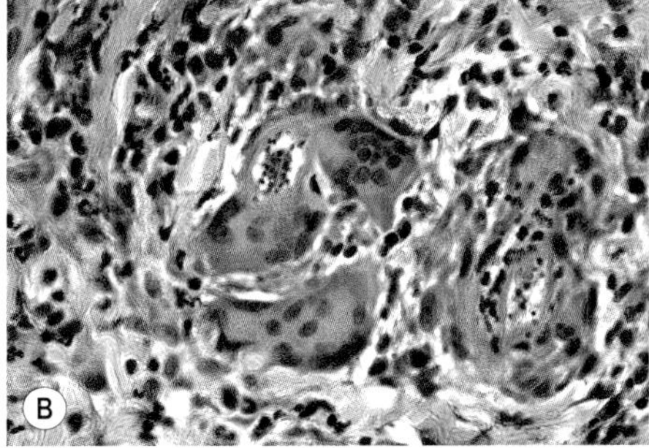

Figure 112.2 *Pelodera strongyloides* in skin. **(A)** View of a section of skin illustrating the granulomatous inflammation. (H&E, originally ×140.) **(B)** Two well-formed granulomas containing larvae. (H&E, originally ×280.) (Courtesy of PC Beaver, PhD, School of Public Health and Tropical Medicine, Tulane University, New Orleans. From: Ginsburgh B, Beaver PC, Wilson ER, et al. Dermatitis due to larvae of a soil nematode, *Pelodera strongyloides*. Pediatr Dermatol. 1984;2:33.)

Diploscapter coronata has been found in the stomach of achlorhydric patients, and in the urine of others.[21,22] Reports also describe a woman from Thailand passing numerous *D. coronata* worms in her stools without ill effects,[23] and in Japan, an 8-year-old girl with Henoch–Schönlein purpura had this infection.[24] Morphological and biological studies of cultured worms suggested that acquisition of infections was likely by ingestion of females, eggs, or both. Adult females do not survive gastric juices, but eggs do and hatch to produce larvae that develop in the intestine.[24]

STRONGYLIDA

The Strongylida, known as the hookworms, are a large group of parasitic nematodes of the intestine, lower and upper respiratory tract, blood vessels, and other sites. The morphologic characteristic of the group is the presence of a bursa in the posterior end of the males.[2] Members of Strongylida producing morbidity and mortality in humans belong to the genera *Ancylostoma* and *Necator* (see Chapter 116), and *Angiostrongylus* (see Chapter 111). Other genera, *Trichostrongylus*, *Mammomonogamus*,

Oesophagostomum, and *Ternidens*, have species responsible for zoonotic infections, which are diagnosed sporadically, are endemic in restricted geographic areas, and have low prevalence rates.

The life cycle of these nematodes can be direct, with fecally passed eggs maturing in soil into infective larvae that enter the skin of the new host and, via the bloodstream, reach the lungs and the intestine where they mature to adults (*Ancylostoma* and *Necator*). Others upon ingestion reach the intestine and grow to adults (*Trichostrongylus*, *Oesophagostomum*). Alternatively, some of these nematodes use an indirect cycle in which an intermediate host, usually a slug or a snail, ingests fecally evacuated larvae. Upon ingestion of the snail/slug by the final host, larvae migrate to their preferred anatomic locations (*Angiostrongylus*).

Trichostrongylus (Trichostrongyliasis)

In terms of prevalence in humans, *Trichostrongylus* is the most important of the four strongylids discussed here, living embedded in the intestinal mucosa of herbivorous animals worldwide. *Trichostrongylus* produce eggs that, after passage in feces reach the soil, mature rapidly and hatch into larvae that become infective. Infection is acquired by the ingestion of larvae with soil or more commonly with infected vegetation (grass).[2]

Trichostrongylus has many species that are difficult to differentiate, of which at least a dozen occur in humans. *T. orientalis*, *T. colubriformis*, *T. vitrinus*, *T. axei*, *T. capricola*, *T. probolurus*, and *T. skrjabini* are responsible for the majority of infections. Their distribution is worldwide, but prevalences are highest in the Middle East, the former southern Soviet republics, India, North Africa, Southeast Asia, Japan, Siberia, Central Africa, and central and southern China. Reported sporadic cases are in Australia,[25] Hawaii,[26] the United States,[27] France,[28] and South America.[29] Prevalence rates are as high as 69% in parts of Iran,[30] 40% in some villages in Japan,[31] 25% in some localities of Iraq,[32] and 2.5% among school children in southern Sudan.[33]

Male and female worms live embedded in the small intestinal mucosa where, if in sufficient numbers, they are capable of producing trauma, desquamation of the mucosa, and hemorrhages. Eosinophilia[25] can be very elevated.[27] Some patients have small amounts of blood in the stools, especially those passing between 100 and 400 eggs/gram of feces.[34] Diagnosis is by identification of the characteristic eggs in stool samples. The infection is underdiagnosed because of the resemblance of *Trichostrongylus* eggs (***Fig. 112.3***) to hookworm eggs. *Trichostrongylus* eggs are larger than those of hookworms, are slightly more elongated, and have a thicker wall.[28,35] The development of a polymerase chain reaction (PCR) for diagnosis based on the internal transcribed spacer (ITS) region ribosomal gene sequence will help clarify the distribution, speciation, and prevalence of *Trichostrongylus* in humans.[35]

Mammomonogamus (Mammomonogamiasis)

Members of the genus *Mammomonogamus* are parasites of the upper respiratory tract of mammals, especially cats and cattle, producing a disease known as "gapeworm" infection or mammomonogamiasis. Earlier references to the disease in humans used the term "syngamiasis," because the worm's erroneous identification was *Syngamus*, a related genus parasitic in birds. The life cycle and mode of transmission are unknown,[2] and <100 infections are known in humans, most from tropical America, including Brazil,[36] Martinique,[37] Puerto Rico,[38] Guadeloupe,[39] Saint Lucia, Trinidad, Jamaica,[40] and other Caribbean islands. There are reports of human infections from Colombia,[41] the Philippines,[2] Thailand,[42] and Korea,[43] as well as in tourists returning to Europe,[44] the United States,[40] Australia,[45] and Canada[46] after travel to the endemic areas.

The clinical manifestations in humans are a dry persistent cough sometimes with hemoptysis and asthma, often at night, produced usually by a single pair of worms firmly attached to the tracheal mucosa. Occasionally, worms were within a cyst[47] and in another in the duodenum.[42] The patient from Korea harbored "many" (but not enumerated) pairs of worms.[43] Some patients complained of weight loss,[45] pleuritic pain[48] or nausea.[49] Worms are sometimes expectorated by the patient after a bout of coughing, revealing a female of ~1 cm in length and a male of ~4 mm permanently attached to the mid-body of the female, somewhat resembling a letter Y, red in color[2] (***Fig. 112.4***). The patient may bring expectorated worms to the physician who, recognizing them as worms, should submit them for proper identification. In other instances, patients presenting with persistent cough undergo bronchoscopy, allowing the physician to see and retrieve the worms. Once worms are removed (only a single pair in most patients), symptoms disappear. Examination of the worms is necessary for their identification and diagnostic confirmation.

Oesophagostomum (Oesophagostomiasis)

Most species of *Oesophagostomum* occur in monkeys and apes with a few in swine and sheep. Human infections are zoonotic.[2] The exception is *O. bifurcum*, which in Togo and northern Ghana[50,51] is maintained in humans, as confirmed by DNA fingerprinting of worms from humans and lower primates, establishing the existence of four genetic clusters, one occurring in humans, the others in nonhuman primates.[52,53] Other foci are mostly in Africa: Uganda,[54] Kenya,[55] Côte d'Ivoire,[56] Ethiopia,[57] Sudan,[58] Guinea,[59] and Nigeria.[60] Isolated cases are known in Brunei,[61] Malaysia,[62] Indonesia,[63] and Brazil.[64]

Estimates of *O. bifurcum* prevalence in Togo and northern Ghana were 250 000 people infected and at least 1 million at risk.[50,65] Some surveys in these areas show that it occurs focally in about 90% of the population,[66] with lower rates in children <5 years of age. Females are more affected than males, but there is no explanation for this gender difference.[67] In other areas, *O. apiostomum*, *O. stephanostomum*, and *O. aculeatum* infect humans.[2]

Adult worms live attached to the mucosa of the colon; eggs passed in feces mature in soil and produce larvae that enter a new host orally and reach the wall of the large intestine to develop in abscess-like cavities (***Fig. 112.5***). Once worms reach adulthood, they leave the abscess and attach to the colonic mucosa.[2]

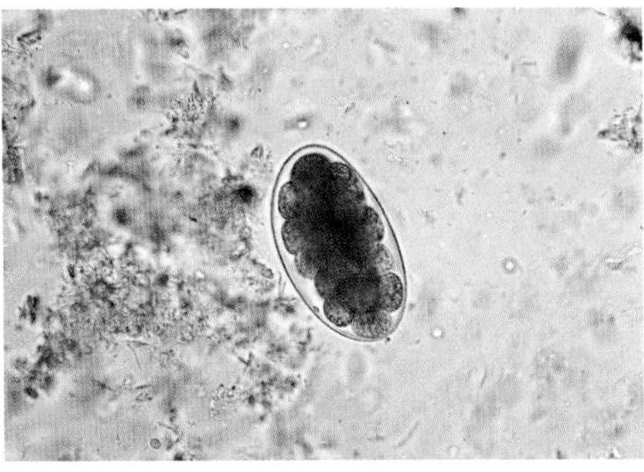

Figure 112.3 *Trichostrongylus* sp. egg in stool sample. (Unstained, originally ×450.)

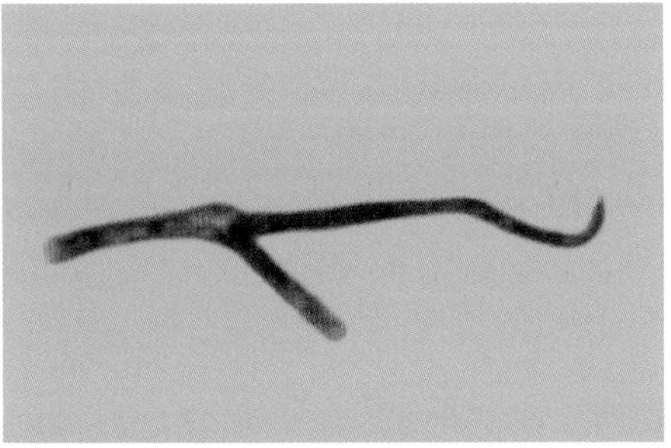

Figure 112.4 *Mammomonogamus laryngeus*; adult worms in copulo. Note the characteristic configuration of a Y. (Courtesy of JS Nosanchuck, MD, Department of Pathology, Tompkins Community Hospital, Ithaca, NY. From Nosanchuck JS, Wade SE, Landolf M. Case report of and description of parasite in *Mammomonogamus laryngeus* (human syngamosis) infection. J Clin Microbiol. 1995;33:998.)

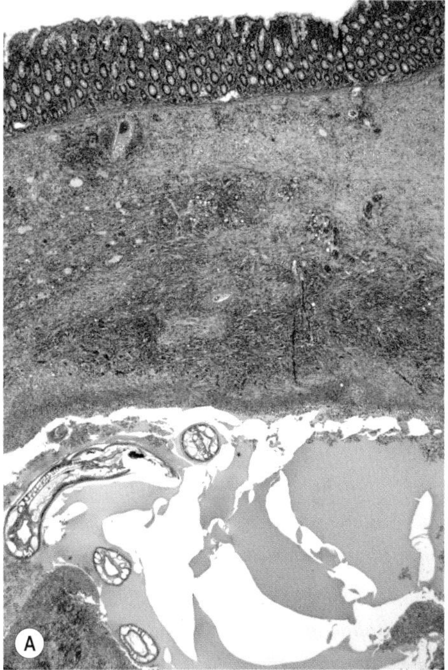

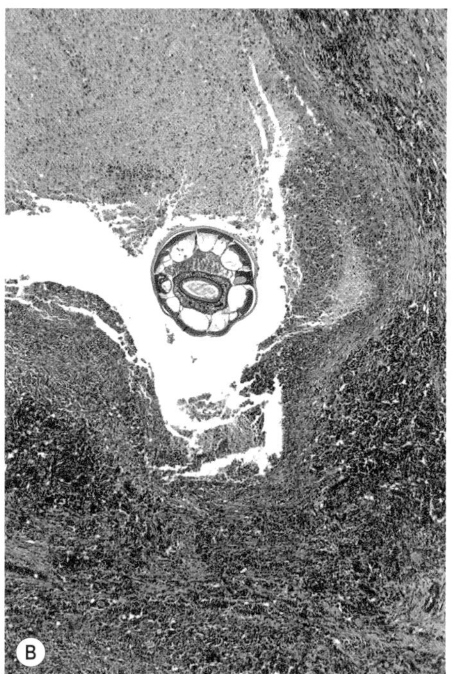

Figure 112.5 *Oesophagostomum* sp. in human colon. **(A)** View of abscess in the wall of the colon, showing sections of the parasite. (H&E, originally ×22.) **(B)** The wall of the abscess and sections of the worm. (H&E, originally ×70.)

The lesions (abscesses) produced by the growing larvae in the colonic wall are visible grossly as nodules, 1–2 cm in diameter. In heavy infections lesions occur on the peritoneal surface, the omentum, kidneys, spleen, and other viscera, producing symptoms and signs of the infection. Sometimes lesions push into the abdominal wall, where they can be seen and felt as well-demarcated painful tumors. Lesions encountered in the periumbilical area are known as "Dapaong tumor."[65]

Clinical manifestations are those of an abdominal mass, sometimes large or painful; others have acute intestinal symptoms, often of obstruction, due mostly to peritoneal adhesions. Asymptomatic persons, mostly children, may present because of a painless or disfiguring abdominal mass.[54] Assessment of patients has improved with the use of ultrasound.[68,69] In acute cases, treatment is often surgical, and diagnosis is confirmed by gross and microscopic examination of the removed specimen. In tissue sections recognition of the worms as strongylid nematodes is easy, although more difficult to the generic level (*Oesophagostomum*). Speciation is possible only by study of male worms *in toto*. In patients with patent colonic infections, the diagnosis is made by morphologic identification of hatched larvae in coprocultures, since the eggs are indistinguishable from those of hookworms.[70] A PCR assay has detected *O. bifurcum* in human feces,[71] and multiplex real-time PCR studies of fecal samples have differentially detected *Ancylostoma*, *Necator*, and *Oesophagostomum* infections.[72] Albendazole, used in the cases from Togo and Ghana, was effective in mixed infections with hookworms against both parasites.[73] Pyrantel pamoate was effective against *Oesophagostomum*, but not against hookworms.[74]

Ternidens

Ternidens deminutus, implicated in human infections,[75] is a parasite that resembles *Oesophagostomum* morphologically and biologically. It inhabits the colon, producing ulcerations and nodular lesions, although a cause–effect relationship between the worms and the lesions remains uncertain.[76] The life cycle of *T. deminutus* is unknown and the mode of infection for humans and animals remains unexplained. Experimental attempts to infect humans percutaneously have failed; thus, it is postulated that there is an arthropod intermediate host.[76] *Ternidens* usually parasitizes monkeys in Africa, India, and Indonesia,[2] and human infections have been recorded in Zambia and Zimbabwe.[77] The prevalence in these countries is variable, but may be up to 87%.[77] A Thai woman has been reported with an omental mass that histologically revealed cross-sections of a worm identified as *Ternidens*.[78]

Ternidens produces nonspecific symptoms in a few patients, but most are asymptomatic. Intestinal blood loss is slight; there is no eosinophilia or diarrhea, though the latter occurs in animals.[77] The explanation for the lack of symptoms is likely due to the low number of worms found in the colon: eight worms in a few cases, but most harbor only three to five. Thiabendazole and pyrantel pamoate have been used to treat patients, curing ~90% of the infections.[79] The diagnosis is made in stool samples by recognition of the eggs, which are easily mistaken for hookworm eggs; careful measurement of the eggs allows proper identification.[2]

ASCARIDINA

The Ascaridina is one of the largest nematode groups. In humans, *Ascaris lumbricoides* is responsible for infections worldwide (see Chapter 115) and *Toxocara* sp, roundworms of dogs and cats, are responsible for visceral larva migrans (see Chapter 109).

Other members of the group are *Anisakis*,[80,81] *Pseudoterranova*, *Baylisascaris*, and *Lagochilascaris*. These ascarids are intestinal parasites of mammals with life cycles requiring intermediate hosts.[2] *Anisakis* and *Pseudoterranova* are parasites of marine mammals with squid and fish as intermediate hosts.[82] *Baylisascaris*, the intestinal roundworms of raccoons, skunks, bears, martens, and other carnivores, uses small rodents, birds and many others as intermediate hosts. *Lagochilascaris* uses wild cats and others as definitive hosts, and rodents as experimental intermediate hosts.[83–85]

Anisakis and *Pseudoterranova* (Anisakiasis and Pseudoterranoviasis)

Anisakiasis ("herring worm disease") and pseudoterranoviasis ("cod worm disease") have similar clinical presentations, and thus the common name "anisakiasis" has been used for both infections. There is confusion in the medical literature because the names of the parasites have changed several

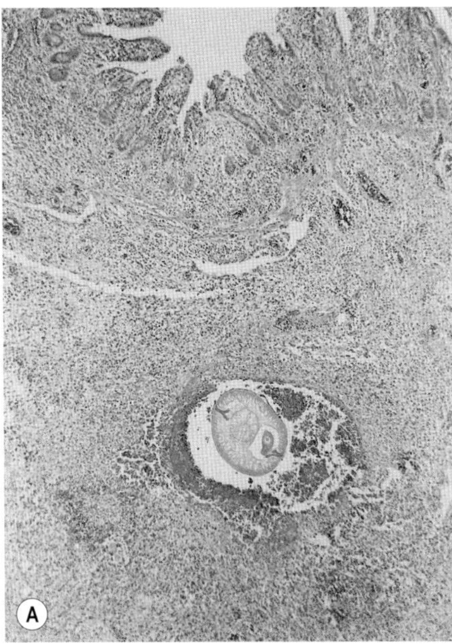

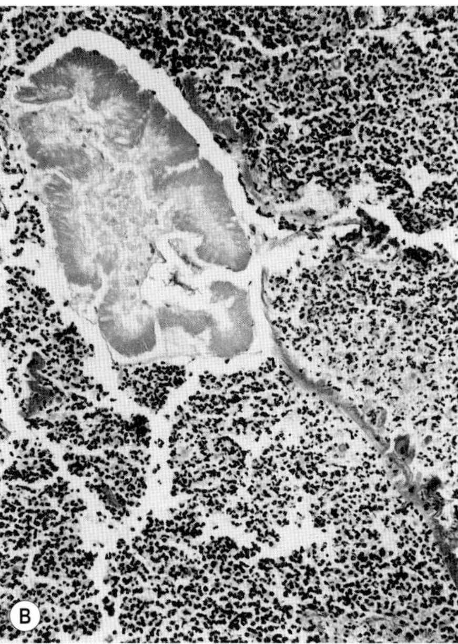

Figure 112.6 *Anisakis* in intestinal wall. **(A)** View of the lesion showing a section of a well-preserved worm. (H&E, originally ×55.) **(B)** Another patient with a similar lesion, but markedly degenerated worm. (H&E, originally ×200.)

times as their relationships and their classification became more defined.[86] *Anisakis*, a parasite of whales, has nine species, *A. simplex* sensu latu – a complex composed of three sibling species *A. simplex* sensu strictu, *A. pegreffii*, and *A. simplex* C – which, together with *A. typica*, *A. zyphydarum*, and *Anisakis* sp. correspond to larva type I. The *A. simplex* complex has similar larval and adult morphologic characteristics, while the other three have adults that are morphologically distinguishable.[87] The other species, *A. physeteris*, *A. brevispiculata*, and *A. pagiae*, correspond to larva type II and are distinguishable morphologically.[87] Advances in speciation of this genus are based on PCR by restriction fragment length polymorphism or sequencing analysis of the ITS region. These species have differences in distribution, preferences for final hosts, and other biologic characteristics.[87,88]

Pseudoterranova (previously known as *Ascaris*, *Porracecum*, *Terranova*, or *Phocanema*) has one species complex, *P. decipiens*, consisting of seven species impossible to speciate morphologically in their larval stages.[89] *Pseudoterranova* parasitizes exclusively pinnipeds.[82,89] Of note, the use of a species name of the worm (i.e., *A simplex*, *P. decipiens* and others) for a clinical disease has justification only when identification of larvae recovered from humans is conclusive (now requisitely based on genetic studies). Pathologists should use the generic "anisakid" to be consistent with the limitations of identifications in tissue sections. Similarly, clinical studies of patients with suspected anisakiasis should not use specific names based on serologic or skin tests with larval antigens. There are too many species and too much uncertainty in serologic tests, because of cross-reactivity among parasite species and the likelihood of previous exposure to the parasite. Genotyping of worms recovered from patients or animals should be the gold standard when using specific names in publications. Work in Japan showed the validity of genotyping larvae recovered from humans, demonstrating that 99% of larvae were *A. simplex* sensu strictu and 1% were *A. pegreffii*.[90]

Anisakids inhabit the stomach of their final hosts with their cephalic ends buried in the GI mucosa. Eggs passed in feces mature and develop into larvae that hatch and become part of the zooplankton. Squid and several other species of macro-invertebrates can ingest the larvae. Fish may also ingest infected intermediate hosts bearing larvae. When the final host ingests infected squid, macro-invertebrates, or fish, it becomes infected. Humans acquire the infection by eating raw marine fish in food such as sushi, sashimi, oka, poisson cru, and ceviche.[91] The disease is important in Japan, where cases number in the thousands, because raw marine fish is a daily staple.[80,81] Infection is found sporadically elsewhere where consumption of raw fish has become fashionable or where fish is a large part of the diet and an occasional larva survives in undercooked dishes. In the United States[92] and in South America[93] there are small numbers of cases. In Europe,[94,95] especially in the Netherlands where the infection was traced in the 1960s to the consumption of raw herring,[96] public health measures have brought it under control. In Spain, a major consumer of fish, the disease was recognized in the early 1990s[97] with reported cases clinically and histologically similar to those in Japan. However, in Spain there are an inordinate number of patients with allergies attributed to *Anisakis* infection on the bases of serologic tests, IgE determinations, skin tests with extracts of *Anisakis simplex* larvae, or histories of consumption of raw fish.[98–101]

Anisakiasis is mostly a GI tract infection, with rare ectopic locations in the peritoneal cavity, other abdominal organs, [80,81] and once in the lungs.[102] In most instances, there is only one larva, uncommonly two and rarely several.[1] The lesion in humans parallels the biologic behavior of the parasite in the final host, burrowing the cephalic end into the GI mucosa.[82] Because humans are abnormal hosts, the parasite dies, producing an abscess characterized by marked inflammation and tissue eosinophilia[2] (***Fig. 112.6***). This abscess occurs anywhere in the GI tract, often of sufficient size to allow clinical palpation or radiographic imaging. Sometimes the larva reaches the peritoneal cavity, producing an abscess in the omentum, occasionally on the surface of other viscera.[80,81] Larvae have been recovered from the peritoneum during exploratory laparotomies and in the effluent of one patient under dialysis.[103] Some persons have symptoms of itching or a scratchy sensation in the mouth or throat during or soon after a meal of raw or insufficiently cooked fish.[104] A sensation of a foreign element in the oral cavity makes the person reach for the bothersome worm or they expectorate it after a coughing paroxysm. Many anisakiasis cases reported in the United States presented in this manner, and were mostly due to *Pseudoterranova*, a worm apparently with lesser tissue invasion capacity.[104] The recovered larva is often submitted to the physician, who should reassure the patient of the benignity of the condition. Other reports in the United States had typical lesions with an anisakid in histologic sections.[92]

Clinically and for diagnostic and therapeutic purposes, the classification of the infection is as gastric, intestinal, or extraintestinal anisakiasis.[82] Often the clinical presentation is acute, but in some it has an indolent course. The main symptoms are abdominal, with epigastric pain accompanied by nausea and vomiting, sometimes with expulsion of the worm. Clinical and radiographic signs and symptoms of intestinal obstruction may be evident,[82,105] accompanied by diarrhea, followed by normal stools or constipation, and blood and mucus in the stools. Palpation may demonstrate a discrete mass, which in contrast radiographs appears as an intestinal wall defect. The mass and symptoms resolve spontaneously in some instances. Mild fever, leukocytosis, and eosinophilia are usually present, as is a certain amount of peritoneal fluid, which is rich in leukocytes and eosinophils. Endoscopic examination of the stomach and duodenum may reveal a red, bleeding, often-ulcerated lesion, sometimes with the worm at the center attached by its cephalic end to the mucosa, the rest of the body extending into the lumen. Extracting the worm cures the condition.[80,81] Worms in the intestine are more difficult to reach by endoscopy and, if the symptoms are acute, surgical resection yields a segment of inflamed bowel. In radiographs, the worm may appear as a negative image in the contrast media, in spite of its relatively small size, 2.0–3.5 cm × 1–2 mm. The pathologist may find the worm on the open bowel segment either grossly or on tissue sections.[1]

Extraintestinal or ectopic anisakiasis is rare and difficult to diagnose clinically, usually requiring exploratory surgery for treatment and diagnosis. The inflammatory mass is usually <4 cm in diameter and located anywhere in the abdominal cavity. Several cases of ectopic anisakiasis diagnosed presumptively or based on Western blot have been reported in Japan.[102] The clinical diagnosis can be difficult especially because *Paragonimus*, *Gnathostoma*, *Fasciola*, *Sparganum*, and others produce similar syndromes. No medical treatment is used, since the disease resolves with removal of the worm.

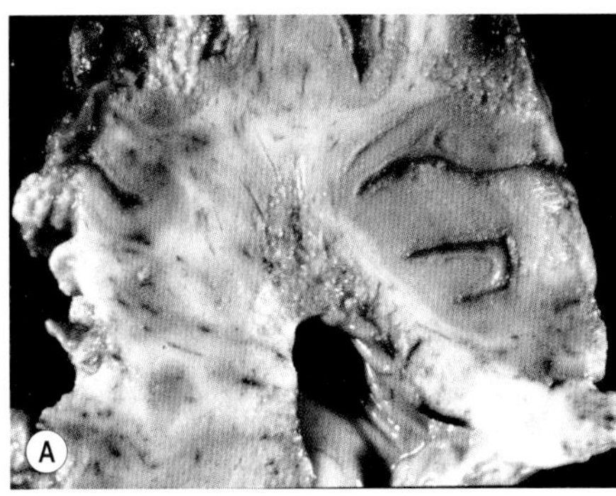

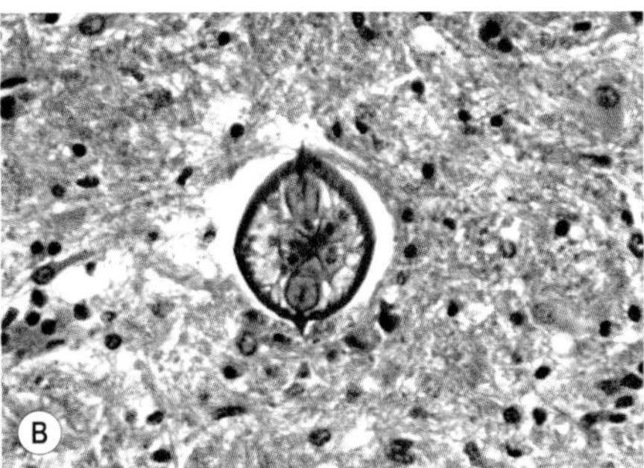

Figure 112.7 *Baylisascaris* sp. in human brain. **(A)** Gross lesion, consisting of areas of necrosis. **(B)** View of a section of the larva. (H&E, originally ×180.) (Courtesy of NS Gould, MD, Department of Pathology, Michael Reese Hospital and Medical Center, Chicago. Case reported in Fox AS, Kazacos KR, Gould NS, et al. Fatal eosinophilic meningoencephalitis and visceral larva migrans caused by the raccoon ascarid *Baylisascaris procyonis*. N Engl J Med. 1985;312:1619.)

Baylisascaris (Baylisascariasis)

Several species of *Baylisascaris* worldwide, which inhabit the intestine of lower vertebrates, are common in raccoons (*B. procyonis*), skunks (*B. columnaris*), martens (*B. devosi*), bears (*B. laevis*), and others with rodents, birds, and other small animals as intermediate hosts.[1] Eggs evacuated in the feces of the final host mature to infective stages in soil, and upon ingestion by the intermediate host, a larva is released and via the bloodstream migrates to the tissues. Larvae eventually encapsulate after producing severe tissue damage and high mortality due to CNS involvement.

Over a dozen cases of baylisascariasis have been reported, some proven by finding larvae in the tissues (autopsy or biopsy specimens) and some diagnosed on serologic tests.[106,107] All cases occurred in the United States, mostly in young children. Two patients illustrate the typical presentations of the disease: a 10-month-old,[108] and an 18-month-old with Down's syndrome.[109] In both, infections started with a mild upper respiratory illness, but each soon developed CNS symptoms due to the migrating larvae in the brain. The 10-month-old infant was lethargic, irritable, obtunded, with lack of spontaneous movements, and semicomatose when brought to the hospital. The other child also presented with CNS involvement, though of a lesser degree. Laboratory data showed moderate leukocytosis, with 37% and 27% eosinophilia, respectively; the cerebrospinal fluid (CSF) contained 5 and 92 cells, respectively. One child died 6 days after hospitalization; the other went home in a decompensated CNS state and died 14 months later.

Other patients presenting with several neurologic complaints were diagnosed with *Baylisascaris* infection based on positive tests to *B. procyonis* larval antigens in serum and CSF.[110,111] These patients were treated with thiabendazole, albendazole, ivermectin, and prednisone in different combinations with some response. Most patients left hospital with severe neurologic sequelae.[110,111] One report of *Baylisascaris* infection based on study of a "presumed" larva, too degenerated for any identification, is doubtful. The presumed larva was eliciting an eosinophilic pseudotumor in the left myocardium, protruding into the left ventricle, resulting in the sudden death of the patient, a 10-year-old boy in Massachusetts.[112]

Examination of tissues recovered at autopsy of fatal cases shows extensive CNS damage (***Fig. 112.7***) varying from acute to chronic. Microscopically, larvae with morphology similar to those of *Baylisascaris* were found encapsulated in every tissue examined.[1] There is no question that *Baylisascaris* was responsible for these infections; and on the basis of circumstantial and epidemiological evidence the species *B. procyonis* is the best candidate. However, speciation of *Baylisascaris* based on larval morphology in tissue sections is impossible today. The best possible interpretation in these cases with larvae seen in tissues would be *Baylisascaris* spp., not *B. procyonis* until genotyping is available.

A diagnosis of ocular baylisascariasis in patients suffering from diffuse unilateral subacute neuroretinitis (DUSN), with or without demonstration of a nematode larva in the retina, has been reported in the literature. Again, although *Baylisascaris* is a good candidate for this lesion, there is still no direct confirmation that this worm is the culprit, and still less that it is *B. procyonis*. Animals experimentally infected with *B. procyonis* may develop retinitis produced by larvae migrating into the eye. In some reported patients, a nematode larva has been found in the retina with the slit lamp, and as well as can be determined, the nematode has a size range consistent with that of *Baylisascaris*. Since species identification of worms based on size alone is not a valid criterion, the role of *Baylisascaris* in the production of DUSN remains possible, but unproven.[113]

Lagochilascaris (Lagochilascariasis)

Fewer than 50 *Lagochilascaris* infections in humans are known, all in Central and South America.[114] The species implicated in these infections is *L. minor*, but the manner in which humans acquire the infection remains obscure, because of the poorly known life cycle. Studies with *L. minor* of human origin have shown a heteroxenous cycle experimentally with cats as final hosts and mice as intermediate hosts.[85,115]

L. minor resides in the upper airways and the oropharynx of its natural host, and the disease in humans parallels both the location and the known development of the parasite in animals. Manifestations of the disease are marked chronic inflammation, edema, and numerous sinus tracts in the neck, face, tonsils (***Fig. 112.8***), throat, mastoid, and paranasal sinuses.[116] The appearance of the lesion is that of a large tumor mass, without fever or pain progressing for months before the patient seeks medical help. Some complain of sinusitis, others of cough and expectoration, which may

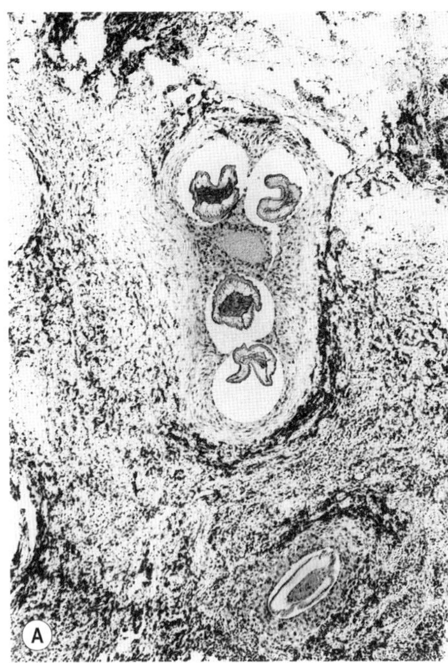
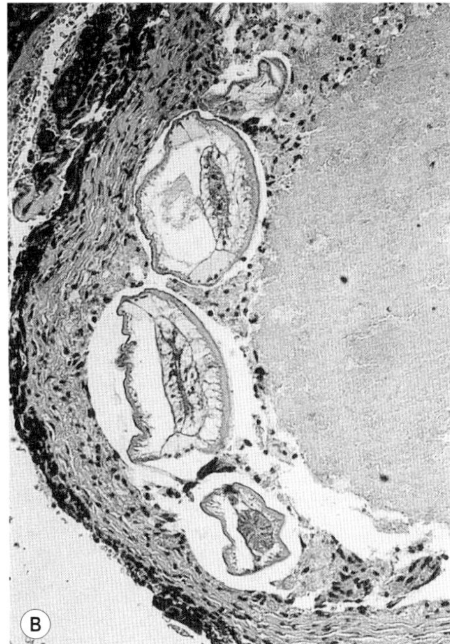

Figure 112.8 (A, B) *Lagochilascaris minor* in human tonsil: views of the abscess, showing cross-sections of the worms (H&E, originally ×70 and ×180, respectively.) (Courtesy of MD Little, PhD, School of Public Health and Tropical Medicine, Tulane University, New Orleans. From: Botero D, Little MD. Two cases of human *Lagochilascaris* infection in Colombia. Am J Trop Med Hyg. 1984;33:381.)

dislodge the worms that then pass with the sputum.[117] Eggs, larvae, and adults are in the discharged pus from the sinuses, and sometimes the eggs are in the stools, where they are often mistaken for *Ascaris* eggs.[118] There are at least two known fatal infections due to migration of the worms, in one case to the brain causing encephalitis,[119] and in the other to the lungs producing abscesses.[120] One report describes involvement of the ocular globes, ears, and meninges.[114] No definitive treatment studies of the infection in humans exist.[36] However, one case with surgical drainage of the abscesses and administration of cambendazole and levamisole did not improve the patient's condition, whereas a course with ivermectin resulted in complete remission.[121] Another patient treated with thiabendazole was cured.[118]

SPIRURIDA

The Spirurida is a large group of nematodes, which use intermediate hosts in their life cycles. Its largest superfamily, the Filarioidea, comprises the filarial worms, some producing important diseases in humans (see Chapters 104–107). Intermediate hosts of species relevant to humans are arthropods for filarial worms, *Thelazia* and *Gongylonema*, and freshwater fish for *Gnathostoma*, which is becoming more frequently diagnosed as awareness of the disease increases. *Gongylonema* remain rare, while reports of *Thelazia* have increased.

Gnathostoma (Gnathostomiasis)

The genus *Gnathostoma* has 11 known species in wild and domestic cats and other carnivores worldwide, each with its own geographic distribution. Most human infections are produced by *G. spinigerum*; rare cases by *G. hispidum*,[122] *G. doloresi*,[123] *G. malaysiae*,[124] and *G. nipponicum* in Southeast Asia and by *G. binucleatum* in Mexico and Ecuador.[125,126] Gnathostomiasis is an infection of individuals with a taste for raw freshwater fish. Imported cases in travelers occur outside of endemic areas.

In their natural hosts, the parasites reside coiled in fibrous tumors formed in the stomach wall; fecally passed eggs reach water to produce larvae that develop further upon ingestion by small crustaceans, *Cyclops*. In small freshwater fishes, frogs, snakes, and other vertebrates that ingest infected crustaceans, larvae become infective and encapsulate in their vertebrate muscles. A non-appropriate host ingesting infective larvae becomes a paratenic host, harboring the larva unchanged in their tissues. Snails infected experimentally act as paratenic hosts.[127] Ingestion of intermediate or paratenic hosts, by the definitive host, produces infection in the stomach. If humans become infected, they behave as paratenic hosts, where the larva migrates through the tissues producing either cutaneous or visceral larva migrans. Any organ can be compromised, sometimes resulting in devastating, often fatal, clinical syndromes.[1]

Human gnathostomiasis occurs mainly in Asia and Southeast Asia: Thailand, India, Japan, China, Malaysia, Philippines, Sri Lanka, Bangladesh, Myanmar, Laos, and Vietnam.[128,129] Foci in the Americas are in Mexico[126] and Ecuador[130]; and there is a single report from Africa (Zambia).[131] In the United States and Europe most cases are in Southeast Asian immigrants or tourists to endemic areas.[128,132]

Symptoms and signs produced by migrating larvae are protean, difficult to diagnose clinically, and may involve any organ system.[1] After ingestion, larvae may reach the liver and from there almost any other organ.[133] Symptoms begin after ingestion of a single larva, rarely two or more, and consist of epigastric pain, nausea, and vomiting lasting sometimes 2–3 weeks, due to migration through the intestinal wall. Eosinophilia is an important laboratory finding that resolves with the extraction of the larva or effective treatment.[134] A larva located in the subcutaneous tissues (***Fig. 112.9***) produces an indurated, pruritic, erythematous lesion. The swelling may resolve, but reappears later in another location; and if it reaches the superficial squamous epithelium it manifests as cutaneous larva migrans[133] (see Chapter 109). The larva is relatively large, visible in the skin, and easily recovered by scarification of the stratum corneum.[2]

The most important clinical manifestations of gnathostomiasis are in the CNS, often with fatal results.[135] The best known syndromes are radiculomyelitis,[136] radiculomyeloencephalitis,[137] and subarachnoid hemorrhage.[138] Marked radicular pain is the result of migration of the larva through the spinal root nerves on its way to the spinal canal and brain. In the spinal canal the larva mimicked an intrinsic tumor or myelitis in one 4-year-old.[139] The pain lasts 1–5 days[135,137] and is accompanied often by paralysis of one or more extremities; paraplegia occurs often, sometimes followed by triplegia and quadriplegia. In the brain, encephalitis manifests

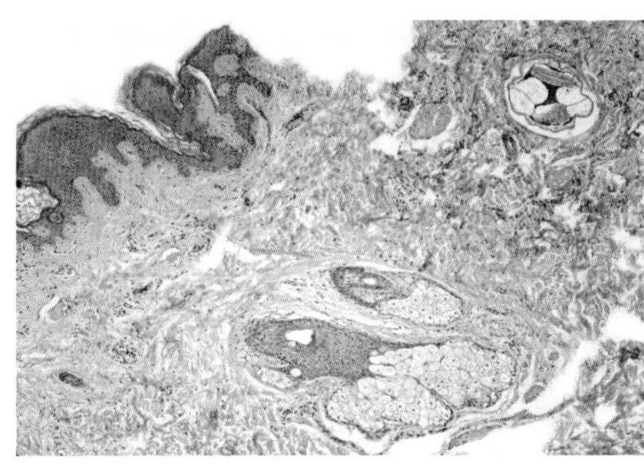

Figure 112.9 *Gnathostoma* sp. in section of human skin, showing the inflammatory reaction and a section of the worm in the subcutaneous tissues. (H&E, originally ×70.)

with cranial nerve symptoms, such as palsies, nystagmus and meningeal irritation, characterized by a changing neurologic picture due to the migration of the larva.[135] Laboratory data are not always helpful, but the CSF is often hemorrhagic or xanthochromic, with an elevated pressure and eosinophilia in all cases.

Other anatomic sites involved by *Gnathostoma* are the eye,[140,141] lungs,[142,143] and GI tract,[144] but any organ can be involved.[1] In endemic areas the clinical condition is suspected by physicians accustomed to dealing with the infection, but diagnosis is difficult in non-endemic ones. The infection has been treated with albendazole 400 mg once or twice a day for 21 days; ivermectin was less effective with a single dose of 200 μg/kg.[145]

Recovery of the larva and study of its morphologic characteristics provide definitive confirmation of the clinical diagnosis. Larvae from humans have measured 2.5–12.5 mm in length by 0.4–1.2 mm in width. Identification of larva to the general group level is possible in histologic sections based on the internal anatomy, but naming the species is difficult, if not impossible. In good sections it is possible to identify some species, based on the larval size and the number of intestinal cells.[146]
Serologic tests can help corroborate a clinical diagnosis. However, these tests do not provide scientific proof for the identity of the parasite species,[147] because all gnathostomids cross-react serologically with each other.[148,149] A 21 kDa antigen prepared from *G. spinigerum* gave 100% positivity with sera from patients with gnathostomiasis, and the IgG_4 was the antibody reacting more readily.[150] DNA sequencing of ribosomal DNA, especially of the ITS1 region, gave good discrimination among five species of *Gnathostoma*;[151] and a multi-dot ELISA readily differentiated eosinophilic meningitis produced by *Gnathostoma*, *Parastrongylus cantonensis*, and *Taenia solium*.[152]

Thelazia (Thelaziasis)

Reports of infections with *Thelazia callipaeda* are expanding as awareness of the disease increases. Known as the "oriental eye worm," the infection is particularly important in Asian countries, producing mild to severe signs of lacrimation, epiphora, conjunctivitis, and sometimes corneal ulcers. *Thelazia* parasitizes dogs, cats, and foxes where it lives in the conjunctiva and the lachrimal sac; human infections are sporadic and zoonotic. Adults produce larvae that are passed within tears, which upon ingestion by flies that feed on lacrimal secretions encapsulate and develop to infective stages in the arthropod.[153] Infective larvae migrate to the mouthparts of the fly to gain access to a new host during feeding on lacrimal secretions.[153]

Human infections occur mostly in rural areas with poor socioeconomic conditions. China has seen an exponential increase in the number of cases in the past two decades and is the country where infections are more common.[154] Study of 179 patients in China showed no gender preference; infections occurred mostly in children <6 years old, were unilateral in 88% of instances, and 4 patients had invasion of the anterior chamber.[154,155] Other cases have been reported from Japan,[156] Korea,[157]

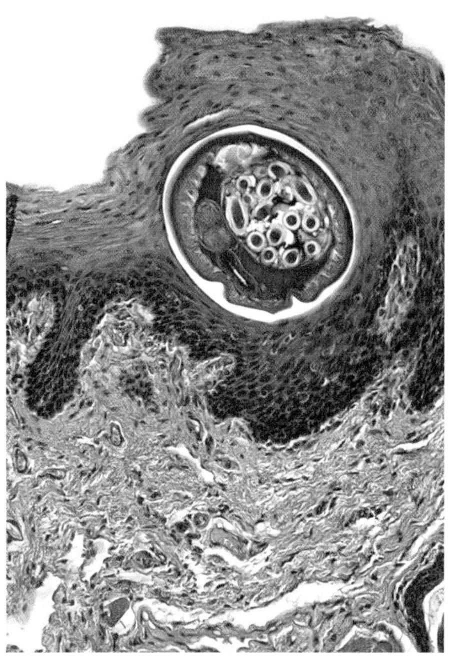

Figure 112.10 *Gongylonema* sp. in section of tongue of infected animal. (H&E, originally ×140.)

India,[158] Russia,[159] Taiwan,[160] and Thailand.[161] Studies in Europe show that transmission is present in Italy and France, as are human infections.[162–164] *T. californiensis* has infected humans in California.[165]

Careful examination of the eye reveals adult worms and/or larvae in the conjunctival sac or medial or lateral canthus; finding worms in the anterior chamber, the vitreous, or the retina signifies a more serious infection. Rinsing of the conjunctiva with sterile saline solution dislodges some worms, and others are mechanically retrieved with forceps; removal of the worms cures the condition rapidly.[154] Specific identification of the worms is important for diagnosis.

Gongylonema (Gongylonemiasis)

Gongylonema pulchrum, a parasite of ruminants, occasionally causes zoonotic infections in humans.[166] Cases have occured in Europe,[167,168] China,[169] Morocco,[170] Russia,[171] New Zealand,[172] Sri Lanka,[173] Iran,[166] Japan,[174] and the United States.[175,176] Worms migrate through superficial tunnels in the epithelium of the esophagus, tongue (***Fig. 112.10***), and other places in the oral cavity. The main symptom is the sensation of something moving in the neck and upper part of the digestive system, often for months, leading the physician to suspect delusions of parasitosis (see Chapter 140).[166,175,176] The majority of worms recovered from humans were in the lips, gums, tonsils, hard and soft palates, and jaw, and were seen as small, migrating threadlike structures under the superficial layers of the squamous epithelium. Human infections are probably by accidental ingestion of an infected cockroach, the intermediate host. In Thailand, an infected Japanese patient passed eggs of *Gongylonema* in the stools[177] and nine similar cases occurred in the same country.[178] In these instances the "infection" is spurious, resulting from ingestion of infected animals, after which the adults are digested and the liberated eggs passed in the stools. Cure of the infection is by removal of the worms; in one instance the use of 400 mg of albendazole made the worms more active, apparent, and easy to retrieve.[166]

ENOPLIDA CAPILLARIDS

The capillarids are common parasites of animals, sometimes causing human infections, usually sporadically, but occasionally in clusters, and rarely in large numbers (*P. philippinensis*). The capillarids belong to a larger group, the Trichinelloidea, with *Trichinella* (see Chapter 110) and *Trichuris trichiura* (see Chapter 114) as representatives in humans. Their distinctive morphologic characteristics are a slender anterior half of the body and the structure of their esophagus, which is made up of gland-like cells.[2]

Calodium hepaticum (=*Capillaria hepatica*) (Hepatic Calodiasis)

This parasite occurs worldwide in small rodents, prairie dogs, monkeys, and other animals, producing marked liver fibrosis known as "parasitic cirrhosis." Adults inhabit the liver, producing eggs that elicit granulomas and fibrosis, which destroys the worms in the process. Eggs remain in the liver, until by predation a carnivore ingests and evacuates them in the feces; the eggs become infective in soil and eventually reach the final hosts, or accidentally humans, to produce a new infection.[2]

Fewer than 40 human infections have been reported worldwide, in the United States,[179] New Zeland,[180] Hawaii,[181] England,[182,183] India,[184] Turkey,[185] Nigeria, South Africa,[186] Mexico,[187] Thailand,[188] Brazil,[189] Italy,[190] Switzerland,[191] Korea,[192] Kosovo,[193] and the former Czechoslovakia.[194] Clinical symptoms vary from acute to subacute, with manifestations of hepatitis that evolve into a picture indistinguishable from visceral larva migrans (see Chapter 109). The only clinical difference with visceral larva migrans is the greater liver enlargement in capillariasis, about 2–3 cm below the costal margin, versus 1 cm in larva migrans. The only positive laboratory test is marked eosinophilia.[195] Liver biopsy or autopsy specimens show different histologic patterns, depending on the stage of evolution of the infection. Early, there are immature worms (***Fig. 112.11A***), granulomas, and extensive eosinophilic infiltrate. Later, a mixture of adult worms and numerous eggs predominate, producing lesions characterized by marked tissue eosinophilia (***Fig. 112.11B***). The final stages of the lesion lack adult worms, and have numerous viable eggs and marked fibrosis.[1] The outcome of the infection apparently depends on the worm load, with some cases progressing rapidly to severe liver disease and death, others following a chronic course, and still others having remission of their illness. In animals fibrotic lesions eventually regress to normal,[196] but there are no data on the evolution of lesions in humans. The basis for the clinical diagnosis is the triad of leukocytosis, eosinophilia, and enlargement of the liver disproportionate for *Toxocara* infections. Confirmation is by needle liver biopsy specimens[197] or open biopsies,[198] which provide rapid and accurate diagnosis. Two cases have been treated with thiabendazole: one recovered completely;[191] the other with a more severe disease, developed IgA nephropathy, and 2 years later his condition was stable, though still with severe liver damage.[197]

One important aspect of hepatic calodiasis in humans is the possibility of spurious (false) infections when humans ingest liver of infected animals; the eggs are freed and evacuated, but may be detected in stool samples,[199] leading to a misdiagnosis. There is an immunofluorescence assay for diagnosis, using frozen sections of infected mice liver.[200]

Paracapillaria philippinensis (Paracapillariasis)

Intestinal capillariasis, produced by *P. philippinensis*, was described in the Philippines in 1964 during an epidemic of GI disease that produced many deaths.[201] Because the original description was incomplete, the parasite was later placed in the genus *Aonchoteca*[202] and more recently in *Paracapillaria*.[203] Infections have been reported in other countries including Thailand,[204,205] Iran,[206] Japan,[207] Egypt,[208] Indonesia,[209] Laos,[210] Korea,[211] India,[212] and Taiwan.[213] In Spain it was diagnosed in a traveler who probably acquired the infection in Colombia.[214] The geographic distribution of intestinal capillariasis is likely greater than currently known because infections are undiagnosed due to the mistaken identification of *P. philippinensis* eggs as *Trichuris* eggs (***Fig. 112.12***, inset). In autopsy material from patients dying in the Philippines epidemic, parasites were in the small intestinal mucosa buried in crypts (***Fig. 112.12***). The life cycle of the parasite involves small freshwater fish as intermediate hosts, which upon ingestion by the final hosts release larvae that grow to adults in the intestine. Mature females produce larvae that grow into adults and enter the mucosa (internal autoinfection, as also uniquely occurs with *Strongyloides stercoralis* – see Chapter 117), explaining the large number of worms in infected persons. This new generation of adult females lays eggs[215] that upon evacuation embryonate in water to infect fish intermediate hosts.[216]

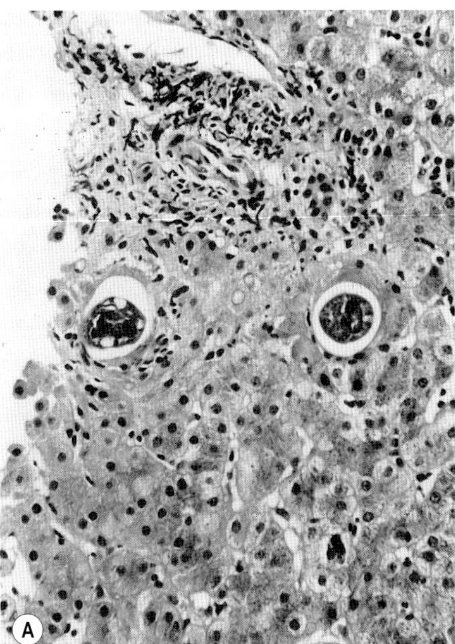

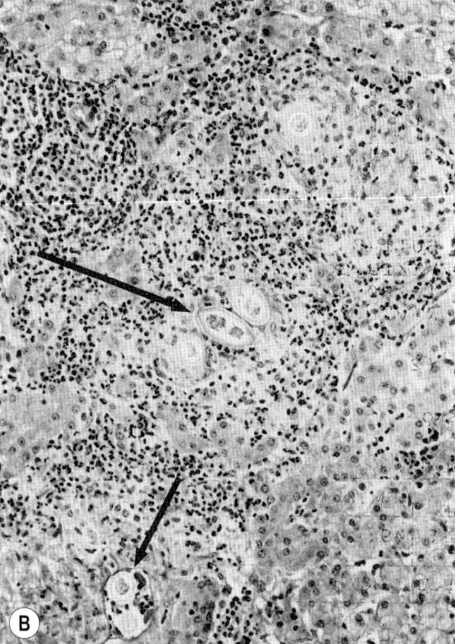

Figure 112.11 *Calodium hepaticum* in human liver. **(A)** View of section of liver biopsy specimen showing sections of immature worms. Note the scant inflammation at this stage. (H&E, originally ×200.) **(B)** Liver section from another case with advanced disease. Note the granulomatous inflammation and the presence of eggs (arrows). (H&E, originally ×180.)

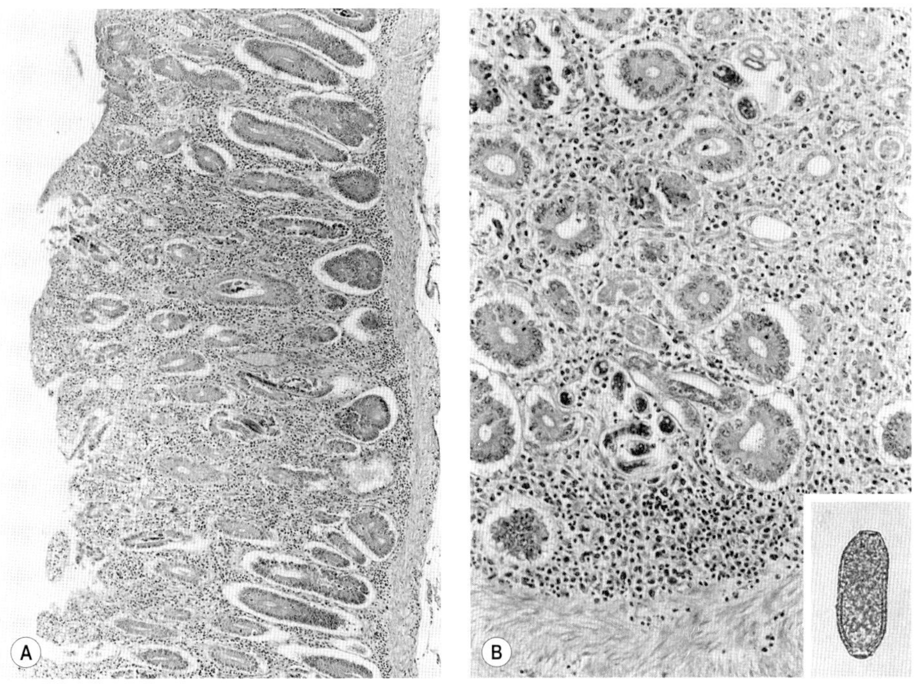

Figure 112.12 *Paracapillaria philippinensis* in human intestines. **(A)** View of section of small intestine showing diffuse inflammatory infiltrate and sections of worms. (H&E, originally ×70.) **(B)** The inflammatory infiltrate and the worms. (H&E, originally ×180.) *Inset*: Egg in unstained stool sample. (H&E, originally ×450.)

The clinical manifestations are watery diarrhea. The patient, usually a 20- to 50-year-old man, acquires infection while working in the fields and supplementing his diet with the small, raw fish. He usually presents days after the beginning of his illness, when the symptoms are more sprue-like, with marked weight loss, dehydration, and malabsorption of fats, vitamins, proteins and carbohydrates. Abdominal pain, slight fever, and anorexia are also found.[217] Laboratory tests demonstrate a slight leukocytosis and increased eosinophilia; stool examinations demonstrate eggs, larvae, and sometimes adult worms.[218] Albendazole 400 mg/day for 21 days, or mebendazole 200 mg twice a day for 20 days are the drugs of choice.[219]

Access the complete reference list online at
http://www.expertconsult.com

CHAPTER 113

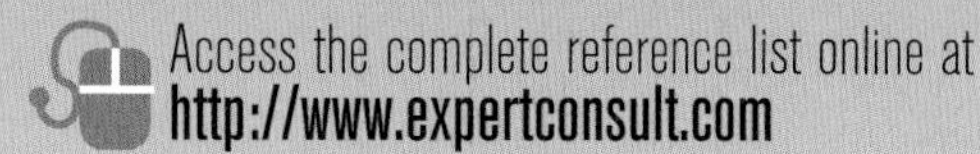
Access the complete reference list online at
http://www.expertconsult.com

Enterobiasis

Thomas A. Moore • James S. McCarthy

INTRODUCTION

Enterobius vermicularis, commonly known as pinworm, is one of the most prevalent intestinal nematodes of humans. However, it differs from other common intestinal nematodes in that it does not disproportionately affect residents of tropical climates or populations with poor hygiene or low socioeconomic status. In addition, the eggs that are deposited on the perianal skin are immediately infective and do not require a period of embryonation in the environment. Thus, transmission is largely from person to person. Infection generally results in irritating but not life-threatening perianal pruritus.

THE AGENT

E. vermicularis is a member of the Oxyuridae class of nematodes. It has been proposed that it should be placed in a subfamily of oxyurid parasites, the Enterobiinae, a group that includes the pinworm parasites of primates and some rodents. The status of a new species proposed to infect humans, *E. gregorii*, remains controversial.[1] Some authors suggest that the distinctive morphologic appearance reported to differentiate this species may instead represent transitional life cycle stages of *E. vermicularis*.[2] Further, no molecular genetic studies have yet established that this separate species indeed exists.

The adult female *E. vermicularis* worm, a small, white roundworm, measuring 9–12 mm in length and 0.5 mm in width (***Fig. 113.1A***), possesses a double-bulbed esophagus and a mouth with a cuticular expansion. It has a long, pointed tail and a slit-like vulva on the ventral surface about one-third of the distance from the anterior end. The adult male is rarely seen in clinical practice, since it has a much shorter life span and is significantly smaller, measuring 2.5 mm in length and 0.2 mm in width. It is curved along its posterior third and has a blunt caudal excretory-copulatory spicule. A detailed morphologic description of the parasite is available.[3] Parasite eggs are the life cycle stage most readily identified for diagnosis. The characteristic eggs are ovoid and measure 50 × 25 μm. The eggs are flattened on one side, giving them the classical bean shape (***Fig. 113.1B***).

Life Cycle

Adult worms inhabit the lumen of the cecum and appendix. The life span of the adult female is 4–10 weeks; the adult male, only about 2 weeks. Following fertilization, the gravid adult female migrates from the large intestine onto the perianal skin (***Fig. 113.2***), where she deposits up to 11 000 eggs by uterine contraction and rupture. The sticky eggs adhere to the anal skin and embryonate rapidly over about 6 hours to reach the infective L3 larval stage, still inside the eggshell. The intense pruritus induced by the adult female and the eggs facilitates fecal–oral transfer of eggs. Alternative modes of transmission of infective-stage eggs include fomites and sexual transmission. The minimum interval between egg ingestion and the next egg deposition is between 3 and 4 weeks. The role of retroinfection (migration of newly hatched larvae from the anal skin back into the large intestine) remains to be established (***Fig. 113.3***).

EPIDEMIOLOGY

Pinworm eggs have been identified in coproliths from the Americas dating back to 7800 BC,[4] from China (206 BC to 220 AD),[5] and from Egyptian mummies (30 BC to 395 AD).[6] Contemporary epidemiologic surveys have documented infection in all populations studied. However, there is a paucity of recent large-scale studies in which the prevalence and intensity of infection have been documented. Furthermore, no recent longitudinal studies have been undertaken to evaluate systematically changes in epidemiology. In a survey of the results of 216 275 stool parasitologic examinations undertaken in state diagnostic laboratories in the United States in 1987, 9597 sellotape test results from 35 states were reported; 11.4% had a documented pinworm.[7] In a number of reports, however, the prevalence of infection in well-recognized at-risk groups such as residents of orphanages and homes for the intellectually disabled appears to be in decline.[7,8] This likely reflects improved sanitation and living standards in such institutions. Likewise, in a report of sellotape test results from a large hospital in New York City from 1971 to 1986, a decline was observed in both the number of tests undertaken annually, from 248 in 1971 to 38 in 1986, and the frequency of positive tests, from 57 (23%) to 0 (0%), respectively.[9] Whether such results reflect a true decrease in prevalence remains to be conclusively established.

Although it is commonly held that enterobiasis, in contrast to other intestinal helminth infections, is more prevalent in temperate than tropical climates, there is a paucity of contemporary data to support this view. Certainly the parasite has been found throughout the developing and developed world when appropriate diagnostic testing has been undertaken. Like other intestinal helminths, a small proportion of the population carries a disproportionate worm burden. For example, in one study undertaken in a fishing village in southern India, the most heavily infected 25% of study subjects harbored more than 90% of the parasites.[10] In this study, a significant aggregation of infection in household units was also observed. In addition, individuals with heavy infection tend to reacquire a disproportionately high parasite burden after curative treatment.[11]

Well-recognized cofactors for increased risk of *Enterobius* infection include overcrowding, poor sanitation, and lack of water for bathing and washing of hands and clothes. While sexual transmission of the parasite also occurs,[12] this route of transmission is likely to be of low significance. Likewise, although eggs have been identified in household dust, the relative role of fomites in transmission remains to be established. While the potential for nosocomial transmission of the parasite exists, such an occurrence is unlikely in hospital environments where good standards of hygiene prevail.[13]

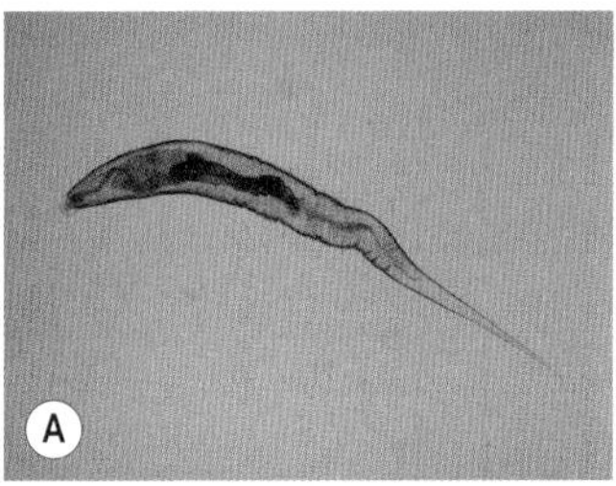

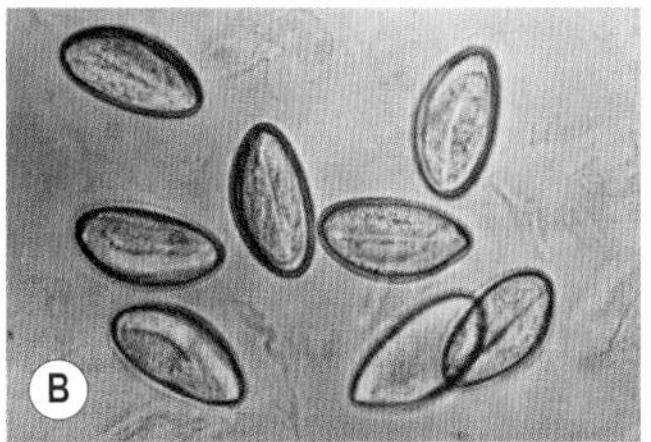

Figure 113.1 **(A)** The adult female *Enterobius vermicularis* worm appears as a small white roundworm, measuring 9–12 mm in length and 0.5 mm in width. **(B)** The characteristic eggs are ovoid in shape and measure 50 × 25 μm. The eggs are flattened on one side, giving them the classical bean shape appearance.

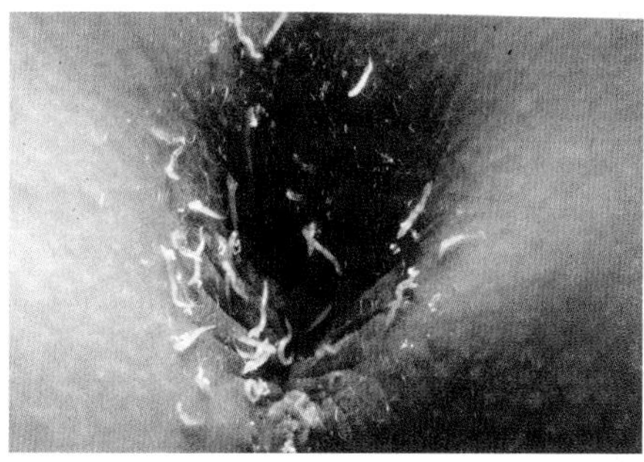

Figure 113.2 Adult *Enterobius vermicularis* worms in the perianal region. (Reproduced from Weber M. Pinworms. N Engl J Med 1993;328:927.)

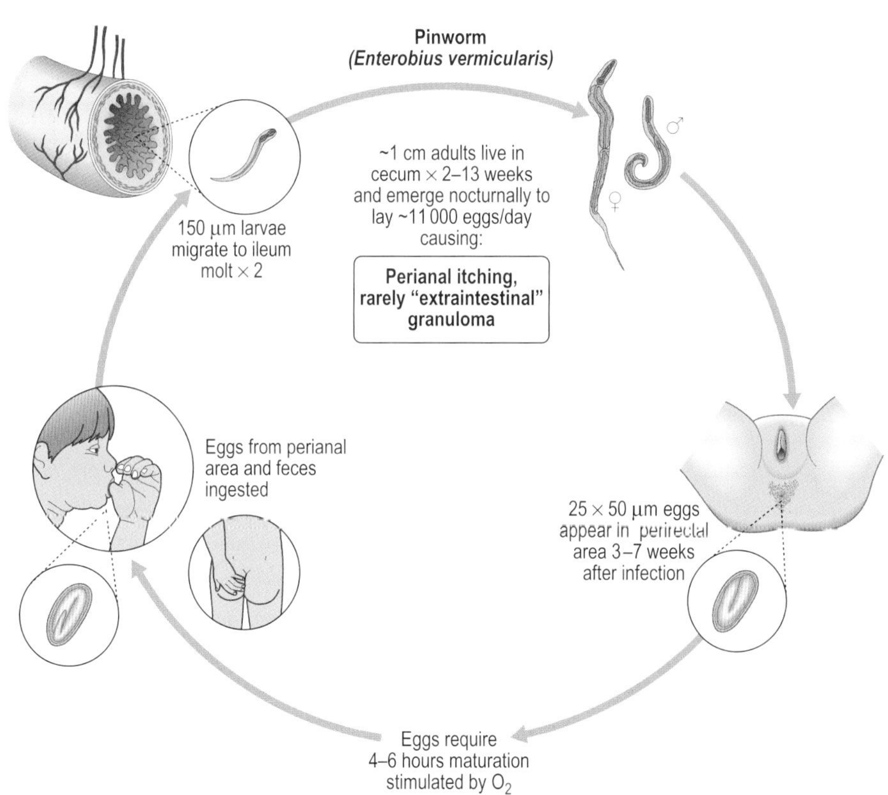

Figure 113.3 Pinworm (*Enterobius vermicularis*) life cycle.

THE DISEASE

The most common clinical manifestation of *E. vermicularis* infection is pruritus ani. This is attributable to the expulsion of eggs by gravid females on to the skin of the anus. When very heavy infection is present, an eczematous reaction with bacterial superinfection may occur. While these symptoms certainly favor spread of infection, the mechanism by which egg deposition causes irritation remains unknown. Other clinical manifestations associated with infection include teeth grinding, enuresis, insomnia, nausea, vomiting, abdominal pain, and appendicitis (*Fig. 113.4*). The association of these manifestations with pinworm infection is unknown, since no well-performed case-control studies have been undertaken. Likewise, the incidence of asymptomatic infection remains unknown. While appendiceal pinworms have been identified in up to 4% of surgical specimens, appendiceal inflammation is not universal in their presence.[14] Furthermore, the role of pinworms in the pathogenesis of appendicitis remains to be defined. Infection of the female genital tract has been well reported, with manifestations including vulvar and cervical granulomas, salpingitis, oophoritis, tuboovarian abscess, and peritonitis. Eosinophilic colitis has also been reported and appears to occur early in

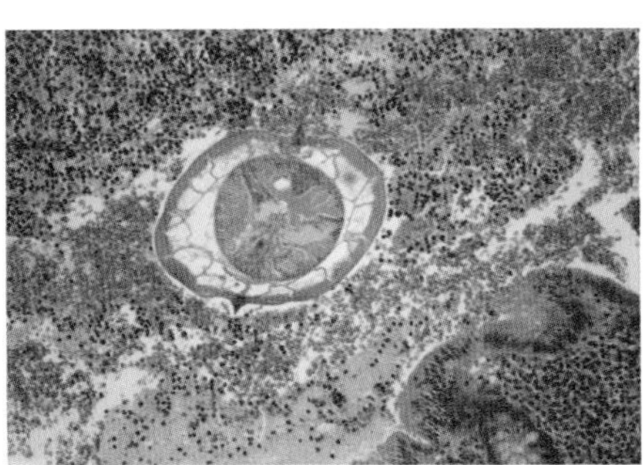

Figure 113.4 Adult *Enterobius vermicularis* seen in cross-section of appendix.

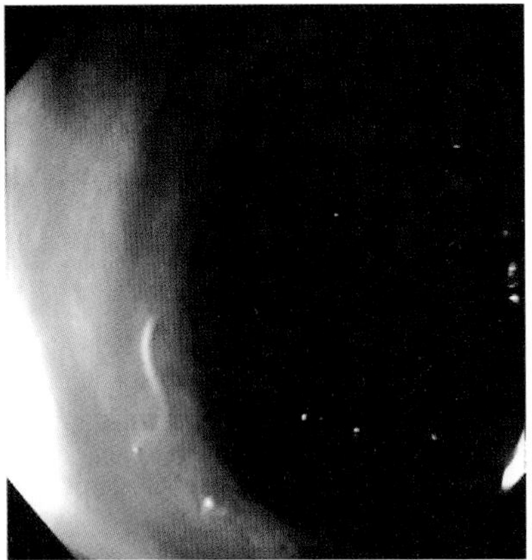

Figure 113.5 Adult *Enterobius vermicularis* worm in colonic mucosa seen on endoscopy.

infection, since only larvae rather than eggs have been identified in such cases.[15] Rare cases of ectopic infection involving other organs, including the breast, liver, and epididymis, and inguinal hernia have been reported. When pinworms are identified in unusual external locations such as the conjunctivae, self-inoculation with infected fecal material is the cause.

DIAGNOSIS

A diagnosis of *E. vermicularis* infection is almost universally established by demonstrating parasite eggs using the sellotape tape (unfrosted Scotch tape) test. Although commercially produced tests are available, the test in essence involves preparing a wooden tongue depressor or swab stick with clear adhesive tape, with the sticky side facing outward. This is then applied to the anal skin; the tape is removed and placed sticky side down on a glass slide. The slide is then examined under a microscope to identify the characteristic eggs (see ***Fig. 113.1B***). As for other parasite infections, the collection of multiple samples has been reported to improve diagnostic sensitivity significantly.[16] Testing at night or first thing in the morning is reported to improve sensitivity. Eggs or adult parasites are rarely seen in fecal samples collected for diagnosis of other intestinal helminth infections such as ascariasis or whipworm or hookworm infections. Adult pinworms can sometimes be seen on the perianal skin (see ***Fig. 113.2***) or in the colon during colonoscopy (***Fig. 113.5***). Likewise, adult worms may occasionally be identified on toilet paper, diapers, or underwear. Infection does not generally result in eosinophilia; no serologic test is available.

TREATMENT AND PROGNOSIS

Although several effective anthelminthics are available, the benzimidazole, mebendazole, is the most widely used efficacious drug. It is generally administered as a single dose of 100 mg, for which a cure rate in excess of 90% is expected.[17] Alternatives include the other widely used benzimidazole drug, albendazole, also as a single dose of 400 mg, and pyrantel pamoate as a single dose of 11 mg/kg (up to a maximum dose of 1000 mg). Ivermectin is less effective with cure rates after a single oral dose of 150–200 µg/kg of only 53%.[18] Older drugs that are now less widely available or used but still are effective include pyrvinium pamoate 5 mg/kg up to a maximal dose of 250 mg and piperazine in a dose of 65 mg/kg for 7 days. A second course of therapy should be readministered 2 weeks after the first dose to cover for auto- or reinfection. Likewise, all individuals sharing a household where the index case is a child should be given empiric treatment.

Infection in pregnancy poses a significant clinical dilemma, with some patients suffering great discomfort. Unfortunately, the safety in pregnancy of most antiparasitic agents has yet to be established, and some drugs have shown teratogenic effects in animal models when administered in high dose. However, in a number of retrospective surveys of women who took mebendazole in the first trimester of pregnancy, the rate of congenital abnormalities, fetal loss, or neonatal death was not significantly higher than in the general population.[19,20] In a large World Health Organization-sponsored study of over 7000 Sri Lankan women who took mebendazole during pregnancy, a beneficial effect was observed overall, with a significantly lower rate of stillbirth and perinatal death observed in those who took the drug in comparison to those who did not, likely reflecting improved iron status due to cure of hookworm infection.[21] However, among those who took the drug contrary to advice during the first trimester there was a trend toward a higher incidence of major congenital defects, with a rate of 2.5% observed in those who took the drug versus 1.5% among those who did not (odds ratio of 1.66; 95% confidence interval, 0.81–3.56).

Studies of single-dose albendazole therapy in pregnant women undertaken in Sierra Leone did not demonstrate any observed increase in frequency of fetal loss or malformation.[22] In a review of 49 cases of albendazole administration to women in the first trimester of pregnancy, no cases of congenital abnormalities were reported.[23] In the two cases studied where neonatal death ensued, the deaths were not likely attributable to the albendazole exposure. Nonetheless, prudence should be observed in the administration of these drugs to pregnant or potentially pregnant women, especially in the first trimester of pregnancy.

PREVENTION AND CONTROL

Reinfection in household and institutional environments is common, and repeated group treatment, usually with single-dose mebendazole, is advised. Other advisable measures include careful attention to hand hygiene, trimming of fingernails, and washing of bedclothes and underwear. Regular vacuuming of house dust has also been advised, despite the lack of evidence supporting a significant role of fomites in transmission. Little is known about host immunity, and vaccine development has not been pursued. Among intestinal helminths, this parasite has not assumed a large place in public health programs in developed or developing countries.

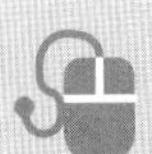

Access the complete reference list online at
http://www.expertconsult.com

CHAPTER 114

Trichuriasis

Nilanthi R. de Silva • Edward S. Cooper

INTRODUCTION

Members of *Trichuris* species are successful nematode parasites of the mammalian bowel, and *Trichuris trichiura* has had much opportunity to coevolve with man. Its human presence is associated with poor hygiene rather than a specifically tropical environment, although warmth and moisture in the soil enhance transmission through promotion of the viability of the infective stages. Until about 35 years ago, four things led to the underestimation of *T. trichiura* as a pathogen:

1. Low-intensity infections, which are by far the most common, are asymptomatic.
2. *Trichuris* is seldom found as the only pathogen, but is commonly just one of multiple health and environmental threats.
3. The onset of significant symptoms is often too slow to alarm the family.
4. It produces a transient, although prolonged, disease of the developing child while seldom causing disability to adults.

However, infections are amenable to treatment with effective anthelminthics that have minimal side effects; this makes case detection and treatment most rewarding and population-based prevention most productive.

THE AGENT

Trichuris trichiura is a member of the nematode superfamily Trichuroidea and is related to *Trichinella spiralis*. The genus was previously often called *Trichocephalus*, logically enough since the hairlike part (tricho-) is in fact the head end (cephalus). However, the original name given by Linnaeus (1771), in the mistaken belief that the hairlike part was the tail (uris), is the official name. Whipworm is a commonly used unofficial name. The adult is shaped like a whip, with the handle representing the wider posterior section containing the reproductive organs and the intestine, while the long, fine anterior part, called the stichosome, contains the long pharynx. The adult is about 4 cm long. The male has a curled posterior end. The eggs are thick-walled and barrel-shaped, about 50 μm long, with a plug at each pole.

Eggs, passed in the feces, contain a zygote and are not infective until embryonation, which takes place in the soil over 2–4 weeks (***Fig. 114.1***). The egg now contains the L1 larva. Following human ingestion, the larva is released in the stomach and passes into the intestine. It penetrates the epithelium in the mucosal crypts of the cecum.[1] The larva develops by molting, and the adult develops from the L4 stage, by now having migrated with the epithelial cells up the sides of the crypts. The anterior part of the adult lies in a tunnel within the epithelium between the mouths of the crypts, while the posterior part is free in the lumen. The stichosome is surrounded by a syncytium and debris of the epithelium. Each female produces 3000–20 000 eggs per day; the life expectancy of a worm within the host has been estimated at 1–3 years,[1] which would imply that some adults live far longer.

EPIDEMIOLOGY

T. trichiura is estimated to infect 600–800 million individuals worldwide.[2,3] However, many helminthic infections have an aggregated ("clumped") distribution among their hosts. This is extreme in trichuriasis, where over 90% of a community may be infected but only 10% or less have intense, symptomatic infections.[4] Familial aggregation occurs.[5] After treatment, there is a tendency for the most heavily infected to become the most heavily reinfected, but there is much crossing over between light and heavy strata too.[6] Evidence to support a possible genetic basis to the predisposition to trichuriasis has been shown. Significant heritabilities for susceptibility to infection have been shown in two independent Asian populations and two quantifiable trait loci associated with susceptibility have been identified in one of these populations.[7,8]

As with *Ascaris lumbricoides*, warm, damp soil provides the best medium for transmission once it is fecally contaminated. *T. trichiura* is found in humid, tropical environments as well as in temperate climates including northern Europe and South Africa. ***Figure 114.2*** shows the estimated prevalence of endemic trichuriasis by country. Although transmission occurs in cool climates, hyperendemicity is correlated with higher temperatures and lower altitudes.[9] *T. trichiura* is observed as a coinfection with *A. lumbricoides* more commonly than might be due to chance, perhaps because of their common mode of transmission.[10]

THE DISEASE

Most infections are asymptomatic. In heavy infections (many adult worms, see next section), stools become loose and frequent and there is tenesmus. Frequency can exceed 12 stools per 24 hours and nocturnal stooling is especially characteristic. Stools consist largely of mucus but may also be watery. There is a characteristic acrid smell. Frank blood is common. Trichuriasis is one of the most frequently identified causes of recurrent rectal prolapse and the worms may be seen on the prolapsed mucosa. Children with this degree of symptomatic infection are almost invariably severely anemic and growth-retarded.[11] They are also geophagic and much of their stool may consist of ingested earth or even small stones. Finger-clubbing is common, correlated in prevalence and severity with the number of adult worms harbored.[12]

PATHOGENESIS AND IMMUNITY

Light infections (20 adult worms or fewer) are not associated with any discernible morbidity. Heavy infections (200 adult worms or more) are

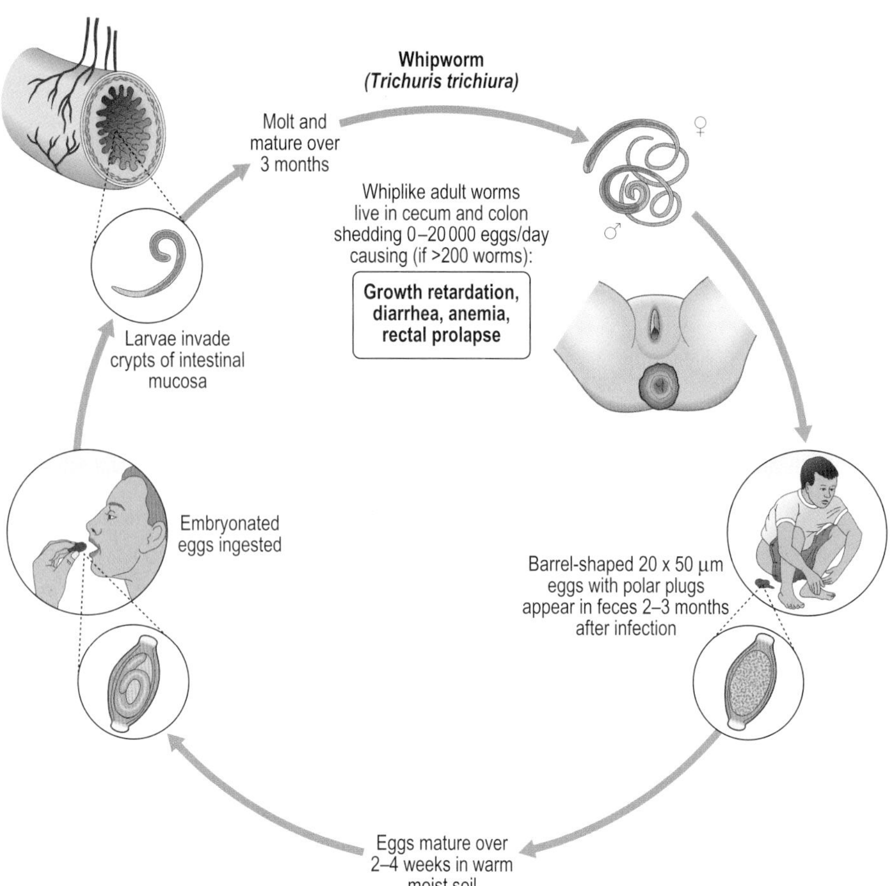
Whipworm
(Trichuris trichiura)
Molt and mature over 3 months
Whiplike adult worms live in cecum and colon shedding 0–20 000 eggs/day causing (if >200 worms):
Growth retardation, diarrhea, anemia, rectal prolapse
Larvae invade crypts of intestinal mucosa
Embryonated eggs ingested
Barrel-shaped 20 x 50 μm eggs with polar plugs appear in feces 2–3 months after infection
Eggs mature over 2–4 weeks in warm moist soil

Figure 114.1 Whipworm (*Trichuris trichiura*) life cycle.

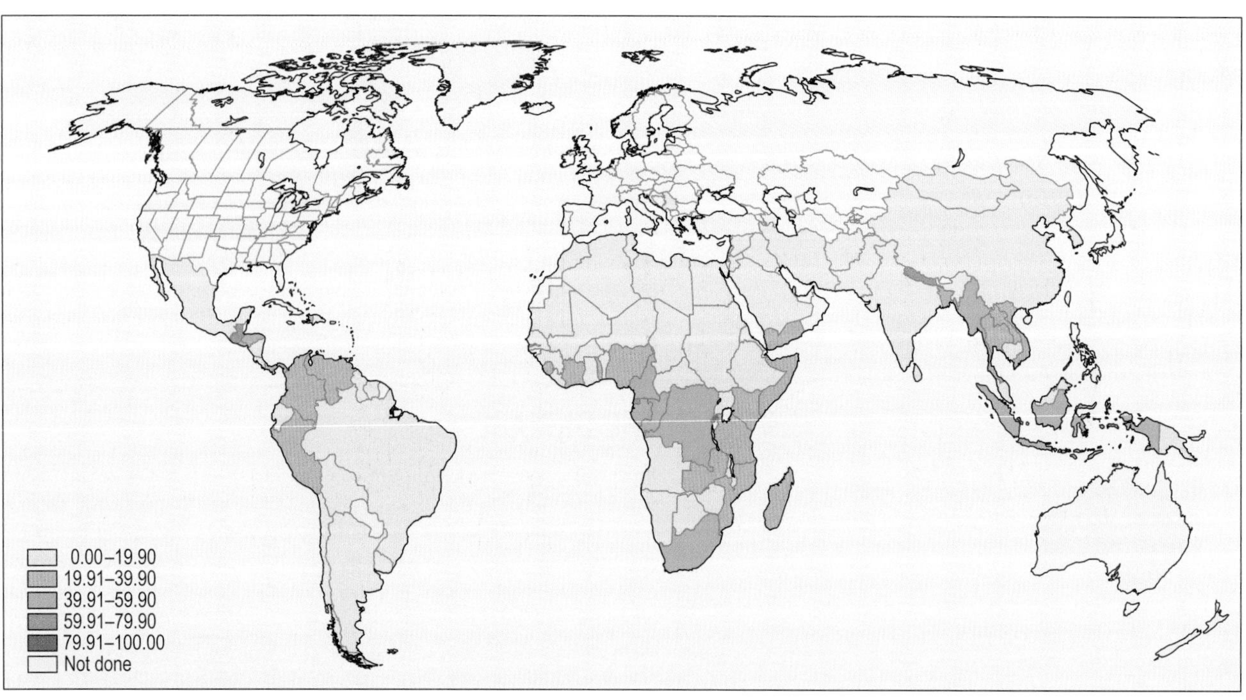
0.00–19.90
19.91–39.90
39.91–59.90
59.91–79.90
79.91–100.00
Not done

Figure 114.2 Estimated prevalence (%) of endemic *Trichuris trichiura* by country.

associated consistently with the clear-cut syndrome described above, which has both colonic and systemic features. The difference is not only one of parasite biomass (in which a 10-fold increase may scarcely be significant clinically), but perhaps more importantly of the site affected: in light infections, the worms are confined to the cecum and the ascending colon, whereas in heavy infections there are adult worms in the distal colon and rectum, and also often in the terminal ileum. The mucosa at these latter sites may have a greater tendency to a local hypersensitivity reaction to *T. trichiura*.

In the inflamed areas, especially the rectum, the mucosa is edematous. At the cellular level, the most significant abnormalities are distended goblet cells, an increased concentration of superficial mast cells, which are degranulating, and an increase in the lamina propria of calprotectin-secreting cells, presumed to be monocytes.[13] Increased tumor necrosis factor (TNF)-α is both produced by lamina propria cells and found circulating in the peripheral blood.[13,14] Bloody mucus commonly exudes from the mucosal surface.

The systemic consequences are anemia and impaired growth.[15] The former is presumed to follow from direct loss from the gut of red blood cells followed by iron deficiency. Recent work has demonstrated fecal occult blood in a significant proportion of children with moderately heavy infections.[16] The mechanism for the impaired growth is not clear but could involve both substrate-limited and substrate-wasting pathways. In support of the former is the finding of protein-losing enteropathy proportional to the worm burden,[15] and of the latter increased circulating TNF-α, which may inhibit appetite as well as having direct effects on cell division and metabolism. Plasma insulin-like growth factor-1 (IGF-1) concentration is found to be correspondingly reduced during the *Trichuris* dysentery syndrome, although it returns to a similar level to that of comparable children from the same community within a month of worm expulsion.[17] The increase in plasma IGF-1 after treatment accompanies a fall in plasma TNF-α, an increase in collagen synthesis as shown by rising plasma procollagen type 1, and an acceleration in physical growth. The elevation of acute phase proteins[18] is further evidence of a systemic component in the response to heavy *Trichuris* infection. Plasma viscosity[18] is also moderately elevated and declines slowly over a period of months, despite the rapid resolution of symptoms after anthelminthic treatment.

Concentrations of immunoglobulin A (IgA), IgM, and IgG antibody to *T. trichiura* are correlated with the host's current worm burden.[19,20] Specific responses of IgG1, IgG4, IgA, and IgE have been shown.[14] As with *Ascaris*, multiple reinfections with *Trichuris* are to be expected,[21] implying that protective immunity must be incomplete. Epidemiologic data combined with serology can be interpreted as consistent with an increase in immunity with age, and as suggesting that both IgA[19] and IgE[14] may be mediators of this.

In mice, it is now widely accepted that protection against *Trichuris muris* is associated with Th2-induced responses and susceptibility with a Th1 phenotype.[22] Th2 cytokines associated with functional resistance in different murine models include interleukin (IL)-4, IL-5, IL-9, and IL-13. In the *T. muris* model, TNF-α is also required for resistance. A recent study suggested that IL-33 plays two independent roles in *T. muris* infections, providing the initial impetus for Th2 polarization upon infection, and also acting as a T cell-independent proinflammatory cytokine at the site of infection, influencing the gut inflammatory response to parasite invasion.[23] However, a recent human study showed that constitutive levels of the regulatory cytokines IL-10 and transforming growth factor β1 were enhanced in direct relation to intestinal worm burden (both *A. lumbricoides* and *T. trichiura*).[24] This elevation in anti-inflammatory cytokine secretion was linked to reduced immune reactivity to worm antigen as well as to unrelated stimuli. These findings suggest a mechanism for the observed lower incidence of autoimmune disease, allergies, and asthma in communities where intestinal nematodes are endemic.

Consistent with the hypothesis that gut nematodes are important mediators of immunoregulation, several studies have confirmed that infection with *Trichuris suis* (a natural parasite of pigs) reduces gut inflammation and induces remission in patients with inflammatory bowel disease.[25] It is thought that the Th2 response induced by the helminth infection prevents or antagonizes the Th1 response that promotes gut pathology in inflammatory bowel disease.[26]

Jamaican children with moderate or high intensities of trichuriasis have been shown to have impaired cognitive function.[27] *T. trichiura* infected Filipino children have also been shown to perform poorly in tests of verbal fluency, regardless of intensity of infection.[28] The strength of association in the latter study was reduced upon adjustment for hemoglobin, suggesting that anemia may play a significant role in the trichuriasis–fluency relationship. The systemic inflammation, especially increased circulating TNF-α, is also a possible mediator between the parasitized intestine and impairment of higher brain function.

DIAGNOSIS

The differential diagnosis is from other causes of infective dysentery or idiopathic colitis. A stool specimen may be examined by any of the techniques for parasites, but the Kato–Katz preparation is recommended for simplicity, reliability, and quantification. Although from a population perspective a count of eggs per gram (epg) of feces is well correlated with adult worm burden, this cannot be applied to the individual. With less than 1000 epg clinically significant trichuriasis is unlikely and with over 10 000 epg it is likely, but severe cases occur with absent eggs on a single stool specimen and some lightly infected children have over 10 000 epg. Proctoscopy showing worms on the rectal mucosa is more reliable evidence of *Trichuris* colitis,[28] and this can be used in the clinic. Colonoscopy sometimes reveals an intense colonic infection, either in a research setting or if the diagnosis has not been made before the procedure. It cannot be justified as a diagnostic procedure: presumptive treatment or a trial of treatment is fully justified in a busy clinic setting.

TREATMENT AND PROGNOSIS

Mebendazole or albendazole by mouth are recommended for treatment of trichuriasis. A recent systematic review of the efficacy of single dose, oral mebendazole, albendazole, levamisole, and pyrantel found that all four showed low cure rates in trichuriasis, whereas higher cure and egg reduction rates were reported when 3-day dosing schedules of mebendazole or albendazole were used.[29] A double blind, placebo-controlled study that examined the efficacy of ivermectin for treatment of trichuriasis found it to be at least as effective as single dose albendazole,[30] but other studies have reported low efficacy.[31] Thus for clinically significant infections, mebendazole 200 mg/day on 3 successive days is recommended, or albendazole 400 mg/day for 3 days. These drugs are contraindicated in the first trimester of pregnancy and not recommended for infants, but clinical judgment must be used in the event of symptomatic infection. Worm expulsion will be followed by clinical cure, but if the environment is unchanged reinfection is likely and retreatment every 3 months,[21] or at least every year,[32] is well justified. Several studies have reported that single dose ivermectin (200–400 μg/kg body weight) in combination with albendazole improves cure and egg reduction rates in trichuriasis.[33]

In veterinary practice, resistance to benzimidazoles is associated with a single amino acid substitution from phenylalanine to tyrosine at position 200 in parasite β-tubulin. A pyrosequence assay has shown this substitution to occur commonly in *T. trichiura* but not *A. lumbricoides*.[34] This could explain why benzimidazoles are much less effective against trichuriasis than ascariasis.

PREVENTION AND CONTROL

Satisfactory fecal disposal using water-seal toilets or good pit-latrines completely interrupts the life cycle of these geohelminths. Hand washing and washing of any vegetables grown in fecally contaminated soil are also useful. In the real-life situation of crowded, poor dwellings, scarce piped water and heavily contaminated soil, mass chemotherapy with cyclical repetition is highly effective.[32] Children of preschool and school age should be targeted.[1]

Access the complete reference list online at **http://www.expertconsult.com**

CHAPTER 115

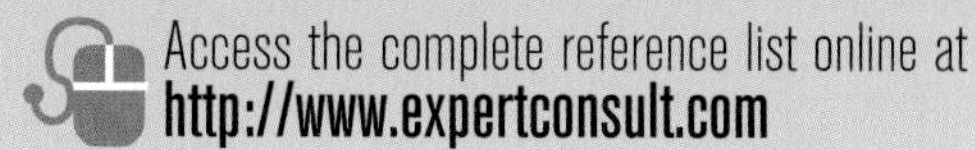
Access the complete reference list online at
http://www.expertconsult.com

Ascariasis

David J. Diemert

INTRODUCTION

Ascaris lumbricoides, or roundworm, is one of three nematodes that are referred to as the soil-transmitted helminths. Infections with *Ascaris* and the other two soil-transmitted helminths, whipworm (*Trichuris trichiura*) (see Chapter 114) and hookworm (see Chapter 116), occur following exposure to parasite eggs or larvae that preferentially develop in the warm, moist soil of the tropics and subtropics. Globally, *A. lumbricoides* is a highly common cause of infection, with over 800 million estimated to be chronically infected worldwide, mostly those living in impoverished rural areas of the developing world.[1]

Although adult *Ascaris* worms survive for over a year within the human gastrointestinal tract, most *A. lumbricoides* infections are clinically asymptomatic. Morbidity and uncommonly mortality can occasionally occur due to intestinal or biliary tract obstruction from adult worms. More insidious are the chronic secondary health effects of infection, especially in school-aged children who experience malnutrition, growth stunting, and delays in cognitive development.[2–4] This morbidity is proportional to the worm burden in an individual host, with the highest rates of complications seen in those – especially children – with moderate- or high-intensity infections. Repeated exposure to eggs in the environment can lead to ever greater numbers of adult *Ascaris* worms in an individual's intestine without induction of a protective immune response. In fact, chronic *Ascaris* infection is associated with a down-regulatory effect on the host's immune system that may have impacts on the prevalence of concomitant allergic diseases and even the progression of infection with the human immunodeficiency virus (HIV).

THE AGENT

Infection with *A. lumbricoides* is acquired by ingesting infective embryonated eggs. In the stomach, gastric acid dissolves the egg's protective outer shell, releasing rhabdoid larvae into the duodenum. After migrating to the cecum, larvae penetrate the intestinal mucosa, enter the portal vasculature and travel first to the liver and then hematogenously to the lungs, where they break through the capillaries into the alveolar space (***Fig. 115.1***). After ascending the bronchial tree, larvae pass over the epiglottis and are swallowed and reenter the GI tract where they develop into adult, egg-laying worms (if fertilized females) approximately 9–11 weeks after egg ingestion.[5]

Adult *Ascaris* worms can reside anywhere within the lumen of the small intestine, where they can live for up to 18 months.[6,7] *A. lumbricoides* is the largest of the intestinal nematodes: adult female worms are 20–49 cm in length (***Fig. 115.2***), male worms are smaller, with a length of 15–30 cm. Fertilized female adult *Ascaris* worms produce prodigious numbers of eggs: a single worm may produce 240 000 eggs per day.[8]

After being passed in the feces, unembryonated eggs require warm, moist, shady soil for embryonation to occur, which takes between 2 and 4 weeks, after which time they become infective. *Ascaris* worms do *not* reproduce within a host. Embryonated eggs are yellowish-brown, ovoid and measure 60–70 μm in diameter; unembryonated eggs are slightly more oblong (***Fig. 115.3***). Eggs are covered by a thick outer shell that protects them from environmental conditions and enables them to remain viable and infectious for up to 10 years. Eggs resist chemical methods of water purification, although boiling will destroy them.

EPIDEMIOLOGY

Humans are the definitive host for *A. lumbricoides*. Human infections with porcine *Ascaris suum* may uncommonly be acquired in developing countries where domestic swine are kept in living quarters.[9] *A. lumbricoides* infections are widely distributed throughout the tropics and subtropics, with an estimated 884–1221 million people infected worldwide.[1] Sub-Saharan Africa, Latin America, and South and Southeast Asia are the most affected regions.

Socioeconomic factors, particularly sanitation and disposal of human waste, are important determinants of the prevalence and intensity of disease in communities. *A. lumbricoides* is highly associated with poverty, illiteracy, and lack of access to adequate sanitation and treatment of sewage.[10] Prevalence is highest in crowded rural areas where subsistence agriculture is the main economic activity, especially where untreated human feces are used as fertilizer. Climate is also an important determinant of disease, as warm temperature and adequate moisture are required for embryonation of eggs in the soil.[11,12] Even within a country, differences in prevalence can be found between regions with varying climactic conditions. For example, in Cameroon schoolchildren living in the north of the country, which has a relatively short rainy season, have low prevalence (<5%) of *A. lumbricoides* infection compared to those living in the south (>60%), where abundant rainfall occurs year round.[13]

In endemic areas, the prevalence of ascariasis increases markedly during the first 2–3 years of life, remains high between the ages of 4 and 15 years, and then declines during adulthood. Reasons for this age dependency are unknown, but may include behavioral factors or variable immune responses that affect resistance to reinfection. Infection with multiple – sometimes hundreds – of worms is common due to continual exposure to infective eggs and the fact that having an active infection does not protect against additional infections. Because clinical disease and morbidity due to *Ascaris*, as well as the rate of transmission, are directly related to the worm burden within a host, intensity of infection is commonly used to describe the epidemiology of this infection.[14] For *A. lumbricoides*, the highest worm burdens are found in children between the ages of 5 and 15 years, with a decline in both intensity and prevalence in adulthood.[15] Furthermore, the infections within an affected community are usually over-dispersed such that the majority of worms are harbored by a minority of individuals.[16] The distribution of infections is also clustered within families and households.[17] Whether this is due to shared

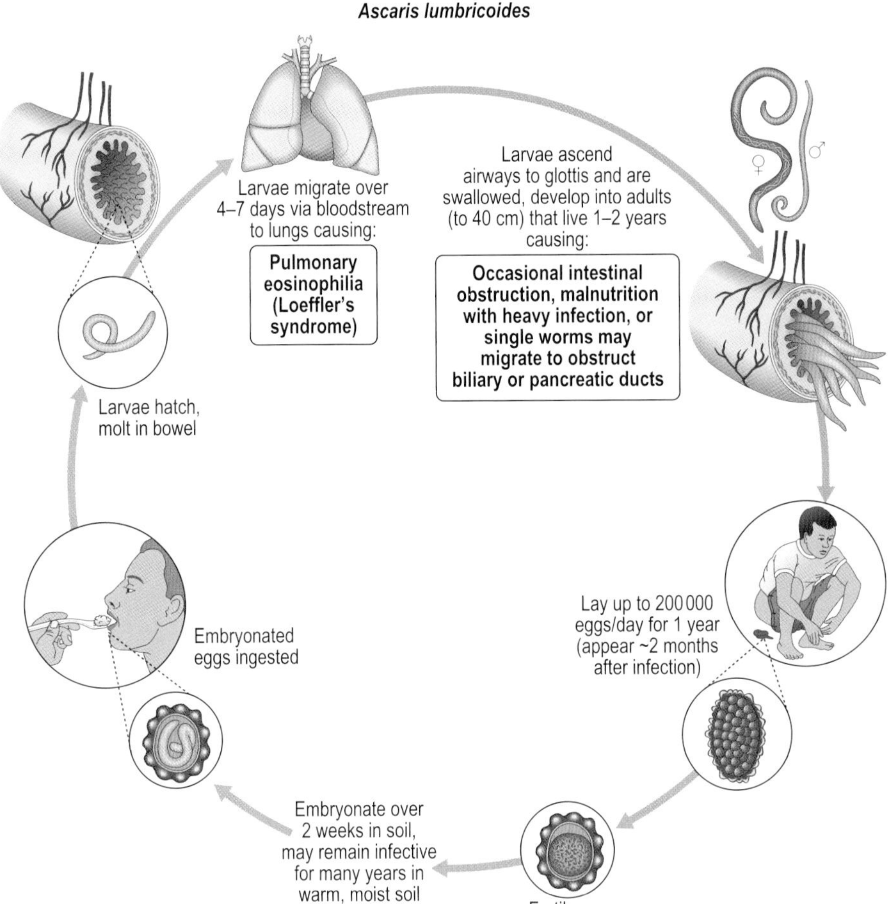

Ascaris lumbricoides
Larvae migrate over 4–7 days via bloodstream to lungs causing:
Pulmonary eosinophilia (Loeffler's syndrome)
Larvae ascend airways to glottis and are swallowed, develop into adults (to 40 cm) that live 1–2 years causing:
Occasional intestinal obstruction, malnutrition with heavy infection, or single worms may migrate to obstruct biliary or pancreatic ducts
♀
♂
Larvae hatch, molt in bowel
Lay up to 200 000 eggs/day for 1 year (appear ~2 months after infection)
Embryonated eggs ingested
Embryonate over 2 weeks in soil, may remain infective for many years in warm, moist soil
Fertile egg

Figure 115.1 Life cycle of *Ascaris lumbricoides*.

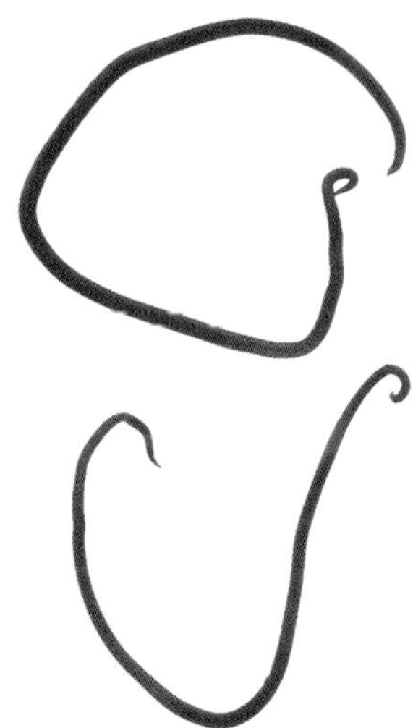

Figure 115.2 Adult female (upper) and male (lower) *Ascaris lumbricoides* worms. (Reproduced with permission from Despommier D, Gwadz RW, Hotez PJ, Knirsch CA. Parasitic Diseases, 5th ed. New York: Apple Tree Productions; 2005.)

susceptibility, for example due to genetic factors, or a common environment and exposure, is not clear.

Ascariasis is uncommonly fatal: estimates range between 3000 and 60 000 deaths directly attributable to *A. lumbricoides* annually.[18,19] Infection results more often in chronic morbidity and disability which is typically assessed by estimating the loss of disability-adjusted life-years (DALYs).[20] The World Health Organization (WHO) has estimated that approximately 1.8 million DALYs are lost annually because of ascariasis.[21]

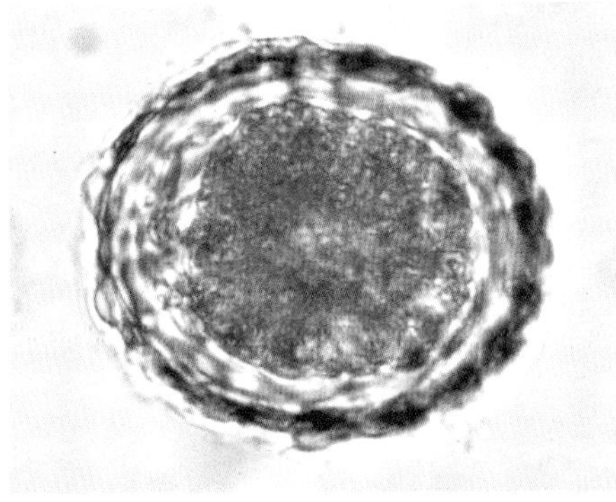

Figure 115.3 Fertilized, unembryonated egg of *Ascaris lumbricoides*. (Reproduced with permission from Despommier D, Gwadz RW, Hotez PJ, Knirsch CA. Parasitic Diseases, 5th ed. New York: Apple Tree Productions; 2005.)

THE DISEASE

The vast majority of infections due to *A. lumbricoides* are asymptomatic. When clinical manifestations occur, they usually affect the small minority of individuals harboring high worm burdens. Clinical disease can be classified into that associated with larval migration through the lungs, and the acute and chronic manifestations resulting from parasitism of the GI tract by adult worms.

More important than the direct effects of infection are the long-term indirect effects on nutrition and the physical and mental development of infected children. *Ascaris* infection contributes to protein energy malnutrition, decreases fat absorption, contributes to deficiency of vitamins A and C, and may lead to lactose intolerance.[22] Either because of these nutritional effects or due to toxic effects of the *Ascaris* worms, moderate and high intensity, *A. lumbricoides* infections have been associated with stunted growth in children and impairment of cognitive development.[3,23,24]

Chronic infection with *A. lumbricoides* may also have detrimental effects on the outcomes associated with other infections. For example, infection with *Ascaris* has recently been associated with more rapid decline in CD4 cell counts in adults who are coinfected with HIV.[25]

Pulmonary Ascariasis

Ascaris larvae migrating through the lungs can induce intense reactions due to the physical disruptions as they transit into alveoli as well as to the dramatic eosinophil-rich inflammatory hypersensitivity responses elicited to larval antigens. Pulmonary ascariasis is more common in children living in endemic areas, especially where transmission is seasonal such as on the Arabian peninsula; in these areas, outbreaks of pneumonitis typically follow the rainy season due to resumption of *Ascaris* transmission.[26] Symptoms begin approximately 1–2 weeks after egg ingestion and last for 2–3 weeks, resolving spontaneously in most cases. Symptoms are more severe with reinfections, likely because the pathogenesis involves a hypersensitivity response to larval antigens due to sensitization from previous infections.

Ascaris pneumonia typically presents with the sudden onset of wheezing, dyspnea, paroxysmal nonproductive cough, and high fever. During heavy infections, blood-tinged sputum may be produced. Respiratory symptoms may coincide with or be preceded by urticarial rash, angioedema, and abdominal pain and vomiting. Affected children occasionally develop status asthmaticus, leading some to hypothesize that *A. lumbricoides* may play an etiologic role in the development of asthma.[27] Chest radiographs usually show diffuse infiltrates that appear to migrate on subsequent films. Peripheral eosinophilia, sometimes high, may be present.

Intestinal Ascariasis

Usually only moderate and high intensity infections in the GI tract produce clinical manifestations, with the highest intensity infections occurring most often in children. The presence of large numbers of adult *Ascaris* worms in the small intestine can cause abdominal distension and vague symptoms such as generalized abdominal pain, loss of appetite, nausea, and episodic diarrhea.

In young children, probably because of the small diameter of their intestinal lumens and their propensity for higher worm burdens, a bolus of worms can accumulate in the ileum and cause partial obstruction.[28,29] If left unattended, potential consequences include intussusception, volvulus, and complete obstruction, leading to bowel infarction and intestinal perforation. The resulting peritonitis is due to both spillage of intestinal bacteria and the granulomatous reaction to adult *Ascaris* worms and eggs. The latter may develop into a chronic granulomatous peritonitis similar to that caused by *Mycobacterium tuberculosis*. Typically, a child with intestinal obstruction due to *Ascaris* presents with colicky abdominal pain, vomiting (sometimes of adult worms) and obstipation. In some cases, a mass may be felt in the right lower quadrant, the usual location of a worm bolus (***Fig. 115.4***).[7]

Adult *Ascaris* worms have the propensity to migrate out of the intestinal lumen, especially in children with high fever, resulting in the dramatic emergence of worms from the mouth, nose, or anus. Occasionally, worms may enter the lumen of the appendix, where they can cause obstruction leading to acute appendicitis.

Hepatobiliary and Pancreatic Ascariasis

Hepatobiliary and pancreatic ascariasis (HPA) results when adult worms in the duodenum enter the ampulla of Vater and either obstruct it or ascend further up the biliary tract to the gallbladder, liver, or pancreas.

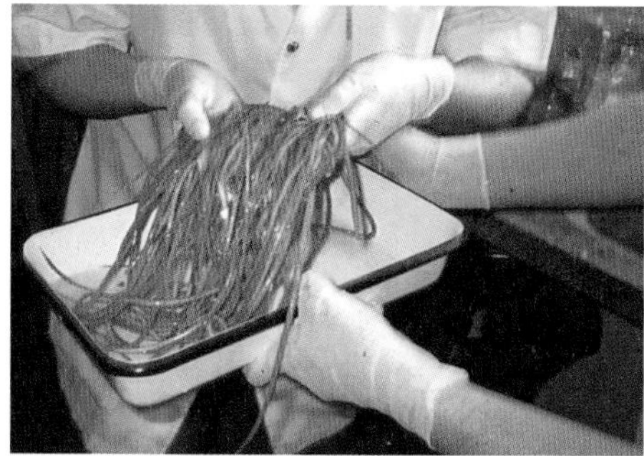

Figure 115.4 Mass of adult *Ascaris lumbricoides* recovered from a child after administration of mebendazole. (Reproduced with permission from Despommier D, Gwadz RW, Hotez PJ, Knirsch CA. Parasitic Diseases, 5th ed. New York: Apple Tree Productions; 2005.)

Resulting complications include biliary colic, cholecystitis, cholangitis, pancreatitis, and hepatic abscess.[30] In endemic areas, ascariasis is the etiology of a significant proportion of biliary and pancreatic disease (see Chapter 133). In contrast to intestinal obstruction, HPA occurs more commonly in adults than in children, presumably because the adult biliary tree is large enough to accommodate a migrating adult worm.[28] Pregnant women are especially at risk, as are those who have had biliary tract surgery or endoscopic sphincterotomy, due to the greater ease of entry of worms into the biliary tree.

PATHOGENESIS AND IMMUNITY

The pathology caused by infection with *A. lumbricoides* is primarily related to the physical presence of adult worms within the lumen of the small intestine or wherever the worms may migrate. In addition to causing mechanical obstruction, worms may interfere with host digestive and absorption processes. In general, the severity of the pathology is proportional to the worm burden in an individual host, although potentially even a single or a few adult worms may result in clinical disease if they migrate into small diameter lumens and result in obstruction, such as in the biliary tract. In addition to the effect of adult worms in the intestinal tract, migration of larvae through tissues, especially the pulmonary parenchyma, can induce granuloma formation with surrounding eosinophils, neutrophils, and macrophages.

A. lumbricoides has a complex life cycle and undergoes a succession of developmental stages with passage through various tissues of the human host, each of which is associated with stage-specific antigens. One of the key features of infection with *A. lumbricoides* is that despite its ability to elicit strong immune responses, it manages to establish chronic infections lasting for months. It is thought that *Ascaris* worms survive within the host not simply by evading the immune system, but also by modulating the immune response away from one that would prove fatal to the parasite.[31]

The immune response to *A. lumbricoides* infection is characterized by high levels of IgE, tissue eosinophilia and mastocytosis, mucus hypersecretion, and T cells that preferentially secrete type 2 (Th2) cytokines, especially interleukin (IL)-4, IL-5 and IL-13.[32,33] The Th2 immune response may have protective effects against *A. lumbricoides* such as eosinophil-mediated destruction of migrating larvae, production of specific and polyclonal IgE against worm antigens, mast cell degranulation, goblet cell hyperplasia, and increased mucus secretion in the intestinal mucosa.[34] Inverse associations between IL-5 and IL-13 secretion and susceptibility to reinfection have been described in individuals who have been treated for *A. lumbricoides* infections.[35–37]

In addition to the Th2 response seen with *A. lumbricoides* infection, abundant production of the regulatory cytokine IL-10 is also observed, which likely plays a role in down-modulating the overall immune response to the adult worm, thus allowing survival of the parasite in the host in addition to protecting the host from excessive tissue damage due to the inflammatory response to the worm.[31,36,38] This down-regulated immune response to *Ascaris* infections may also have effects on bystander antigens, which may explain why chronic infection with *A. lumbricoides* has been associated with reduced prevalence of allergy to common allergens in some endemic areas.[39,40]

DIAGNOSIS

The diagnosis of ascariasis is usually made by microscopic examination of a sample of feces for characteristic *A. lumbricoides* eggs. Given the prodigious number of eggs produced by even a single female adult worm and the fact that eggs are relatively easy to visualize and are morphologically distinct, diagnosis is not difficult. A stool sample may be examined directly for eggs under the microscope by mixing a small amount of feces with a drop of saline solution; stains such as lactophenol cotton blue can be used on wet mounts. Smears can also be fixed and stained with the Wheatley–Gomori trichrome or iron–hematoxylin stains to improve visualization. Additionally, techniques such as the formalin–ethyl acetate sedimentation procedure can concentrate eggs from a fecal sample and thereby increase the sensitivity for detecting even light infections.[5] Although used mostly for epidemiological studies rather than for diagnosis of individual patients, the Kato–Katz and McMaster methods can be used to quantify the intensity of infection by estimating the number of eggs per gram of feces.[41,42]

Because *Ascaris* infections often present without specific signs and symptoms, the clinician typically requires some index of suspicion, such as local epidemiology or country of origin, to request a fecal examination. In some cases, persistent eosinophilia is a common presenting finding.[43] Diagnosis of *Ascaris* pneumonia is made clinically in the context of recent exposure, together with typical symptoms (dyspnea, dry cough, and fever) and peripheral eosinophilia, although the latter finding is not uniform. Chest radiographs may show mottled and transitory infiltrates, and microscopic examination of the sputum may yield *Ascaris* larvae and eosinophils or Charcot–Leyden crystals.[44] Since at this stage of the life cycle adult worms are not present in the intestinal tract (if this is a new infection), examination of the feces will be negative.

Diagnosis of intestinal or biliary obstruction due to *A. lumbricoides* relies increasingly on radiologic evaluation, given a patient with compatible symptoms and a history of exposure in an endemic area. Plain abdominal films reveal air–fluid levels and linear opacities of *Ascaris* worms in dilated bowel loops. Ultrasound has been used to reliably diagnose the presence of adult worms in the intestine, biliary tract, liver, and pancreas.[28,45–47] Endoscopic retrograde cholangiopancreatography (ERCP) is a highly sensitive method for diagnosing hepatobiliary and pancreatic ascariasis and, in addition, allows for removal of worms and relief of acute obstruction.[48,49]

TREATMENT AND PROGNOSIS

The treatment goal for *A. lumbricoides* infections is to eliminate adult worms from the GI tract. Whether as part of mass drug administration campaigns in endemic regions or for the treatment of infected individual patients currently residing in non-endemic areas, management centers on the use of anthelminthic medications. The most commonly used drugs are the benzimidazoles albendazole and mebendazole, which act by binding irreversibly to intracellular tubulin in nematodes, thereby inhibiting its polymerization and assembly into microtubules. The loss of cytoplasmic microtubule formation results in impaired uptake of glucose, leading to depletion of glycogen stores and reduced production of adenosine triphosphate.[50] This disruption of energy production results in starvation of the parasite, causing death of adult worms through a process that can take several days.[51,52]

Both albendazole and mebendazole are broad-spectrum oral anthelminthic agents that are equally effective against *Ascaris* when given as a single dose (400 mg for albendazole and 500 mg for mebendazole), with reported cure rates typically in excess of 90%.[53–55] An alternative recommended dosage for mebendazole is 100 mg twice daily for 3 days, which has demonstrated equivalent efficacy. Systemic toxicity associated with the benzimidazoles (e.g., hepatotoxicity, bone marrow suppression) rarely occurs at the brief, low doses used to treat *A. lumbricoides* infections.[50] However, transient abdominal pain, diarrhea, nausea, dizziness, and headache can commonly occur.

Because the benzimidazoles are embryotoxic and teratogenic in pregnant rats and rabbits, there are concerns regarding their use in children younger than 1 year of age and during pregnancy. Teratogenicity in humans has not been observed, and a study of over 800 women treated with albendazole during the second and third trimesters demonstrated no adverse effects.[56] Use in the first trimester is not recommended. Although the manufacturers do not recommend use of albendazole or mebendazole in children less than 2 years of age due to a lack of formal safety studies in this population, both drugs have been used safely in treating entire communities irrespective of age as part of large-scale mass drug administration programs.[57] Due to the lack of observed pediatric-specific problems, the WHO recommends that albendazole can be used safely as a single, reduced dose of 200 mg and mebendazole at the same 500 mg dose (or 100 mg twice a day for 3 days) in children between 12 and 24 months of age.[58]

Two other medications recommended by the WHO for the treatment of ascariasis are pyrantel pamoate and levamisole, although both are slightly less effective than the benzimidazoles.[2,55] Pyrantel is highly effective against *A. lumbricoides* when administered as a single, weight-adjusted dose.[55] Pyrantel pamoate binds to a nicotinic acetylcholine receptor on the body muscle of nematodes, resulting in depolarization and spastic paralysis of the muscle and passive expulsion of the worm from the GI tract.[59] Levamisole, which has activity against *A. lumbricoides*, is no longer marketed in the United States but is used in several endemic areas.

Treatment of the pulmonary manifestations of *Ascaris* infection is usually not warranted due to their transitory nature, and the unknown activity of anthelminthics against the larval stage of infection. For patients with evidence of obstruction due to intestinal ascariasis, medical management with anthelminthics and fluid resuscitation has been used successfully, provided no signs of perforation or peritonitis are present.[60] Gastrografin solution administered via nasogastric tube has been used to treat subacute bowel obstruction and is hypothesized to act by causing separation of the worms from the intestinal wall due to its hyperosmolarity.[61] Signs of an acute abdomen necessitate surgical intervention, which usually involves laparotomy with manual advancement of the worm mass through the intestine to the colon and rectum; resection of bowel is not required unless signs of infarction or perforation are present.[7]

For patients presenting with complications due to hepatobiliary or pancreatic ascariasis, conservative management with anthelminthics and supportive care may be adequate.[62] In severe cases such as those with cholangitis, ERCP with or without resection of the ampulla of Vater has proven highly successful and obviates the need for surgical intervention.[63,64] Adult worms can be extracted during endoscopy, and anthelminthics should be administered to kill any remaining worms.

PREVENTION AND CONTROL

Use of anthelminthic medications has also become a tool for reducing the burden of disease in endemic countries. Because of the chronic morbidity associated with *A. lumbricoides* and the other soil-transmitted helminths, control programs have been instituted that consist of the periodic mass administration of anthelminthics to children living in endemic areas. In 2001, the World Health Assembly adopted a resolution urging member states to provide regular anthelminthic treatment to high-risk groups with the target of regular treatment of at least 75% of at-risk school-aged children by 2010. Preschool children have also been targeted through national child health days.[65]

Regular treatment of children with benzimidazoles reduces and maintains worm burdens below the threshold associated with disease,[66,67] and leads to improvements in growth and physical fitness, cognitive performance, and school attendance.[4,68] In preschool children, studies have demonstrated improvements in nutritional indicators such as stunting and wasting.[24,69] Large-scale treatment also reduces the number of *Ascaris* eggs that are released into the environment, thereby theoretically leading to reduced transmission.

One limitation of mass drug administration programs is that reinfection occurs rapidly after treatment. Reinfection with *A. lumbricoides* following benzimidazole treatment can reach 55% of pre-treatment levels within 11 months.[70] Another concern with current control programs is the potential development of drug resistance[71,72] similar to that which has already become widespread in nematodes that infect livestock as a result of ubiquitous use of benzimidazoles on farms.[73] Concerns about the sustainability of periodic mass administration of benzimidazoles and the emergence of resistance with widespread use have prompted efforts to develop new control tools. Tribendimidine, a synthetic derivative of amidantel, has been shown to be highly active against *A. lumbricoides*.[74] Originally developed in China, further clinical trials will be necessary before licensure can occur in other countries. Additionally, nitazoxanide is also being explored as a broad-spectrum anthelminthic and has been shown to have excellent activity against *A. lumbricoides* in human studies.[75,76] Finally, combinations of available drugs with different modes of action are being evaluated as a strategy to improve efficacy and delay the emergence of resistance.[77]

Although periodic treatment with anthelminthic medications is effective in reducing the burden of disease due to *A. lumbricoides*, elimination of this parasite as a public health problem will likely not be achieved without significant reductions in poverty and improvements in sanitation and treatment of sewage in endemic areas.

Access the complete reference list online at
http://www.expertconsult.com

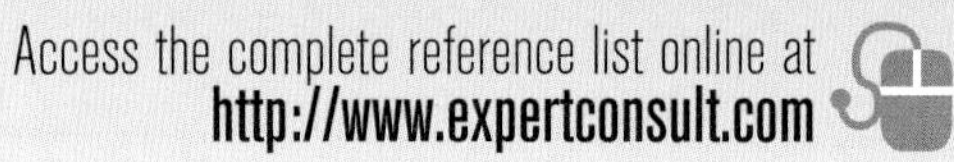
Access the complete reference list online at
http://www.expertconsult.com

CHAPTER 116

Hookworm Infections

Peter J. Hotez

INTRODUCTION

Hookworms are nematode endoparasites that cause intestinal blood loss during a part of their life cycle. An estimated 576–740 million people are infected with *Ancylostoma duodenale*, *Necator americanus*, or both.[1] *N. americanus* is the predominant hookworm worldwide. Moderate and heavy worm burdens can result in hookworm disease, which is characterized by blood loss sufficient to produce iron deficiency and anemia in the human host. Children and women of reproductive age are particularly vulnerable to the effects of hookworm anemia.[2–4] For that reason, there is an increasing awareness of hookworm disease as a problem affecting maternal–child health.[3,4]

Perhaps more than any other nematode parasite, the life cycle of hookworms is intimately connected to rural poverty in warm climates. Hookworm infection is endemic in most developing areas of the subtropics and tropics where sanitation is poor and the environmental conditions, especially adequate moisture and sandy soils, support the survival and hatching of parasite eggs and then the subsequent migrations of larvae. Therefore, unlike *Ascaris* and *Trichuris* infections, hookworm is not usually a public health threat in urban slums. Instead, hookworm occurs primarily in impoverished tropical coastal communities and in areas of intense agricultural activity. In these high-transmission areas, hookworm infection remains endemic even when populations are routinely treated with anthelminthic drugs. In this setting, hookworm reinfection routinely occurs, and the prevalence and intensity of hookworm infection return to pretreatment levels within months.[5] More recently, high rates of drug failure have been reported with one of the two major drugs used to treat hookworm worldwide.[6] Ultimately, the adequate control of hookworm may depend on new advances in biotechnology for the development of a recombinant hookworm vaccine.[7]

THE AGENT

Hookworms are classically identified as adult nematode worms having a buccal capsule armed with teeth or cutting plates. The two major human parasitic species, *A. duodenale* and *N. americanus* (***Fig. 116.1***), and the minor human zoonotic parasites, *A. ceylanicum*, *A. caninum*, and *A. braziliense*, are members of the family Ancylostomatidae, superfamily Strongyloidea (***Table 116.1***). Although most clinicians usually consider the major species as generic "hookworms," there are, in fact, important differences between them[8] (***Table 116.2***). The clinical features of each hookworm infection are also distinct.[4]

N. americanus ("American murderer") was probably discovered by Charles W. Stiles,[9] who identified the parasite as the principal cause of hookworm anemia in the rural southeastern United States. Many historians also credit Bailey K. Ashford of the US Army Medical Corps, who encountered hyperendemic hookworm infection in Puerto Rico at the end of the Spanish–American War.[10] Adult *N. americanus* hookworms are relatively small compared to *A. duodenale*. The males are typically between 7 and 9 mm, and the females between 9 and 11 mm in length. They live attached via cutting plates to the mucosa and submucosa of the small intestine, where they can live for 3–5 years. The blood loss caused by each *N. americanus* has been estimated by ^{51}Cr-labeled red blood cell measurements to be 0.01–0.04 mL per worm per day;[11] in general, it is less than *A. duodenale*-associated blood loss. *N. americanus* is therefore considered better adapted to human parasitism.[7] Each gravid female worm produces 5000–10 000 eggs/day, which exit from the host in feces. The eggs are thin-shelled, hyaline, and ovoid, measuring approximately 60 × 40 μm. Further development of the eggs depends on suitable external environmental conditions. These are usually met by adequate moisture and shade at temperatures of 20–30°C.[12,13] Egg hatching gives rise to a first-stage (L1) rhabditiform larva approximately 250–300 μm in length with a characteristic flask-shaped muscular esophagus. The L1 larva presumably feeds on bacteria and other organic debris prior to undergoing two spontaneous molts over the next week. Transformation to the infective third-stage larva (L3) is accompanied by a number of developmental changes, including elongation to a length of approximately 600 μm and cessation of feeding as a consequence of mouth closure and the buildup of an electron-dense "plug" in the buccal capsule. The infective larva is developmentally arrested and will remain so until it enters a suitable definitive host.[14,15] *N. americanus* infects humans only through the skin. The L3 larvae increase their chances of finding a definitive host by a characteristic questing behavior. The infectious process of all hookworm larvae is intimately linked to the developmental biology of the parasite because host entry is accompanied by the resumption of hookworm larval development.[15] Developing L3 larvae enter into host venules and lymphatics, where they are swept into the pulmonary vasculature. The larvae migrate into the lungs and ascend the respiratory tree and epiglottis before entering the gastrointestinal tract. Entry into the small intestine stimulates the molting of L3 larvae to the L4 stage and then the adult stage. Approximately 49–56 days elapse from the time *N. americanus* L3 larvae enter the host until the adult female hookworm releases eggs.[7,8]

A. duodenale was first identified from the intestine of an Italian woman in 1843 by Dubini. Its life cycle was largely elucidated by a series of impressive investigations in Egypt conducted by Looss.[16] The distinct features of the life cycle and life history stages of *A. duodenale* were a result of human investigations by G.A. Schad and colleagues working in rural West Bengal, India, in the late 1960s and early 1970s.[7,13,17–23] The adult *A. duodenale* is larger and more robust than *N. americanus*. Each adult male is 8–11 mm, whereas each adult female is 10–13 mm in length. Adult *A. duodenale* hookworms live only approximately 1 year in the small intestine. However, during that time they cause greater blood loss (0.05–0.30 mL per worm per day) and produce more eggs (10 000–30 000 eggs/day) than *N. americanus*.[7,11] Egg hatching of *A. duodenale* is faster than that of *N. americanus*.[13] *A. duodenale* L3 larvae are infective via the oral route in addition to percutaneous entry.[7,20] In some endemic areas, oral ingestion of L3 larvae may be the predominant route of infection. Moreover, *A.*

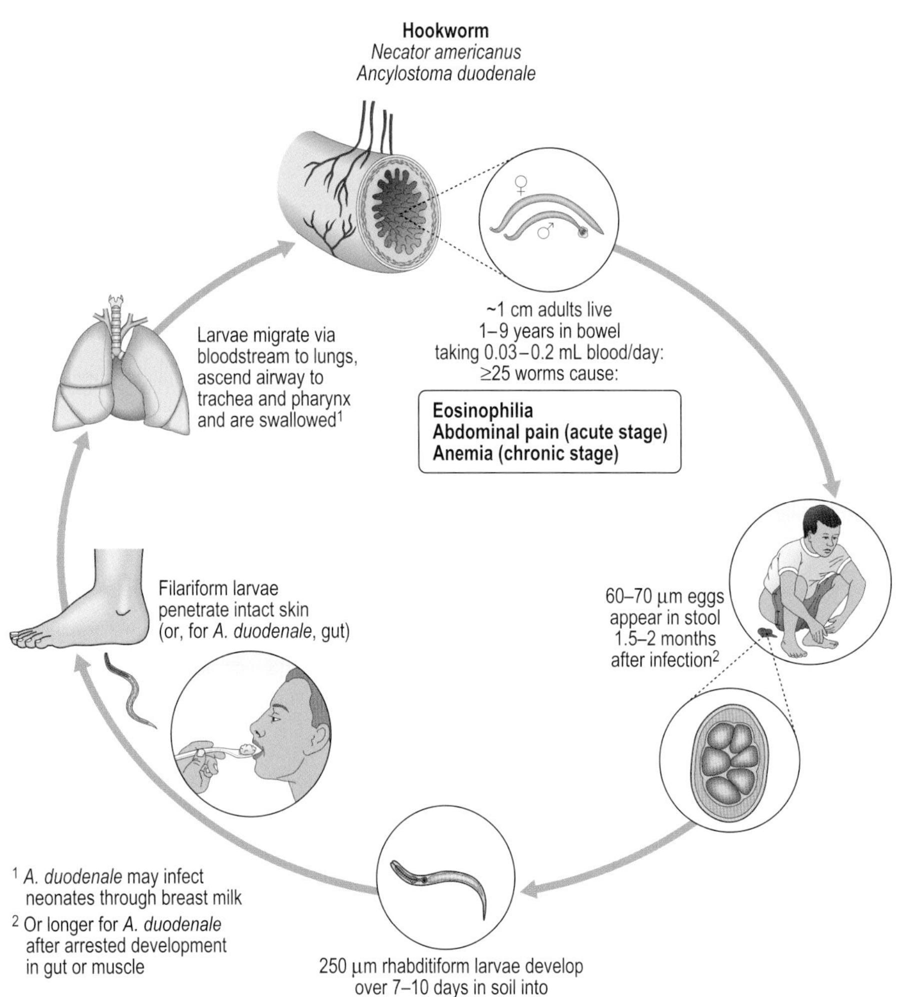
Hookworm
Necator americanus
Ancylostoma duodenale
♀
♂
~1 cm adults live
1–9 years in bowel
taking 0.03–0.2 mL blood/day:
≥25 worms cause:
Eosinophilia
Abdominal pain (acute stage)
Anemia (chronic stage)
Larvae migrate via
bloodstream to lungs,
ascend airway to
trachea and pharynx
and are swallowed1
Filariform larvae
penetrate intact skin
(or, for A. duodenale, gut)
60–70 μm eggs
appear in stool
1.5–2 months
after infection2
1 A. duodenale may infect
neonates through breast milk
2 Or longer for A. duodenale
after arrested development
in gut or muscle
250 μm rhabditiform larvae develop
over 7–10 days in soil into
infective 3rd stage filariform larvae

Figure 116.1 Hookworm life cycle.

Table 116.1 Human Hookworms

Hookworm	Animal Reservoir Host	Disease
Necator americanus	None	Anemia
Ancylostoma duodenale	None	Anemia
A. ceylanicum	Dogs, cats	Enteritis
A. caninum	Dogs	Eosinophilic enteritis
A. braziliense	Dogs, cats	Cutaneous larva migrans
Uncinaria stenocephala	Dogs	Cutaneous larva migrans

duodenale L3 larvae can remain in a developmentally arrested state, even after host entry.[17,23] Larval hypobiosis is considered evolutionarily adaptive because it allows the prolonged survival of the parasite in the host during times when the environment is unfavorable to larval development. For instance, *A. duodenale* L3 larvae probably remain arrested in the host during the hot and dry months of the year in some areas, only to resume development to egg-laying adult hookworms during or soon before the monsoon rains.[17] Arrested development may even explain how *A. duodenale* arrived with prehistoric humans during their early migrations into North America.[24] Arrested *A. duodenale* L3 larvae in maternal somatic tissues may also enter the mammary glands.[23] This phenomenon may account for vertical transmission of human ancylostomiasis to infants.[2,23,25]

Human intestinal infection with *A. ceylanicum* is probably a zoonosis transmitted by L3 larvae from eggs in either dog or cat feces and

Table 116.2 Properties of the Major Species of Hookworm

Property	*Ancylostoma duodenale*	*Necator americanus*
Size of adult (female slightly larger than male)	8–13 mm	7–11 mm
No. of eggs produced daily per worm	10000–30000	5000–10000
Estimated amount of blood removed daily	~0.2 mL (greater draw makes this species more virulent)	~0.02 mL/worm
Mouthparts	Teeth	Cutting plates
Natural adult life span	1 year	3–5 years
Ability to produce infection if ingested	Yes	No
Ability of larvae to lie dormant	Yes	No

(Data from Hoagland KE, Schad GA. *Necator americanus* and *Ancylostoma duodenale*: life history parameters and epidemiological implications of two sympatric hookworms on humans. Exp Parasitol. 1978;44:36–49; Hotez P. Human hookworm infection. In: Farthing MJG, Keusch GT, Wakelin D, eds. Enteric Infection 2: Intestinal Helminths. London: Chapman & Hall; 1995;129–150.)

does not result in host blood loss and therefore is not considered clinically significant. However, zoonotic intestinal infection from the dog hookworm *A. caninum* can occasionally result in a severe eosinophilic enteritis syndrome.[26–31] Nonintestinal cutaneous larva migrans (CLM; "creeping eruption") occurs when L3 larvae of the dog and cat hookworm *A. braziliense* enter the skin but subsequently abort the infection (see Chapter 109).

EPIDEMIOLOGY

As noted in the Introduction, hookworm infections are common throughout the rural areas of the tropics and subtropics. Hookworm is intimately associated with the agrarian practices of societies in developing countries and is one of the most prevalent infections of humans. Coastal communities in the tropics typically have the highest intensity of hookworm infections; presumably this observation reflects the mild humid climate and sandy soils in these regions, which are favorable to transmission.[32] Overall, the highest prevalence and intensity of hookworm infections occur in sub-Saharan Africa and Asia followed by tropical regions of the Americas.[1] Among individual countries, India, Indonesia, Bangladesh, Nigeria, Brazil, and the Democratic Republic of the Congo are believed to currently have the largest number of cases,[33] while the prevalence rates in China have declined considerably over the last two decades in association with rapid economic growth and development.[1] Whether hookworm infection in any given endemic area is due to *A. duodenale* or *N. americanus* is often unknown because differentiation between the two species is not routinely performed in the parasite diagnostic laboratory. Often, endemic hookworm is reported as either "ancylostomiasis" or "uncinariasis" (necatoriasis) when, in reality, no efforts were made to investigate the actual etiologic agent. Worldwide, *Necator* infections are far more common than *Ancylostoma* infections. However, when the worm burdens in a given community are similar, *A. duodenale* infections produce greater blood loss and endemic hookworm anemia than *N. americanus* infections.[34]

Infections with *N. americanus* are found predominantly between the tropics of Cancer and Capricorn (***Fig. 116.2***). *N. americanus* is the predominant hookworm of sub-Saharan Africa, southern China, southern India, and Southeast Asia.[4] *N. americanus* is also the major hookworm in Central and South America, hence the designation "New World hookworm," but in reality this parasite was probably transported from Africa during the Middle Passage of the Atlantic slave trade. *Necator* infections still occur in North America, especially in southern Mexico; rare pockets may even remain in the southeastern United States, although it is no longer a significant public health threat there. Hookworm was reported from rural Georgia in the early 1970s,[35] but there are no published reports of autochthonous hookworm transmission in the United States over the past two decades.[36] Infections with *A. duodenale* frequently overlap *N. americanus* infections in areas of Africa, India, and China. However, they also occur as either the exclusive or predominant hookworm of northern India and China and North Africa (***Fig. 116.3***). Possibly, the ability of *A. duodenale* to undergo arrested development in the host allows the parasite to survive in climatic conditions that are unfavorable for *N. americanus*. Arrested development also accounts for the seasonality of ancylostomiasis. In rural West Bengal, India, and presumably elsewhere, the premonsoon rise in human fecal egg excretion occurs as a consequence of arrested hookworm larvae entering the intestine and developing into adult hookworms.[17,23] Some endemic ancylostomiasis still occurs in Brazil, Paraguay, northern Argentina, and Peru. *A. ceylanicum* is a minor hookworm species of India and Southeast Asia.[8] *A. caninum* has been identified as the cause of an emerging zoonotic eosinophilic enteritis syndrome in Australia.[26–31] Eosinophilic enteritis from *A. caninum* has been reported recently in Louisiana. CLM from *A. braziliense* is found in many areas of the tropics and subtropics, including the Gulf Coast, and southern regions of that Atlantic seaboard. It also occurs commonly in Caribbean tropical beach resorts and is thus a common problem seen in the travel medicine clinic.[37]

Hookworm infection is prevalent in almost all age classes in an endemic area (***Figs 116.2 and 116.3***). The characteristic pattern of age prevalence is one of an initial rise in childhood to a stable asymptote in early adulthood.[2] Rarely, because of infantile disease from vertical transmission, *A. duodenale* infections can also be found in children younger than 1 year of age.[25] Similar to other soil-transmitted helminths (STHs), hookworm exhibits an overdispersed distribution, with the majority (usually between 65% and 85%) of infected individuals in an endemic community exhibiting low-intensity infections, and a minority (usually between 15% and 35%) exhibiting moderate- and heavy-intensity infections. In contrast, there are marked differences in the age-dependent intensity patterns for hookworm compared with other STH infections.[2] Whereas worm burdens with *Ascaris* or *Trichuris* are often heaviest in children older

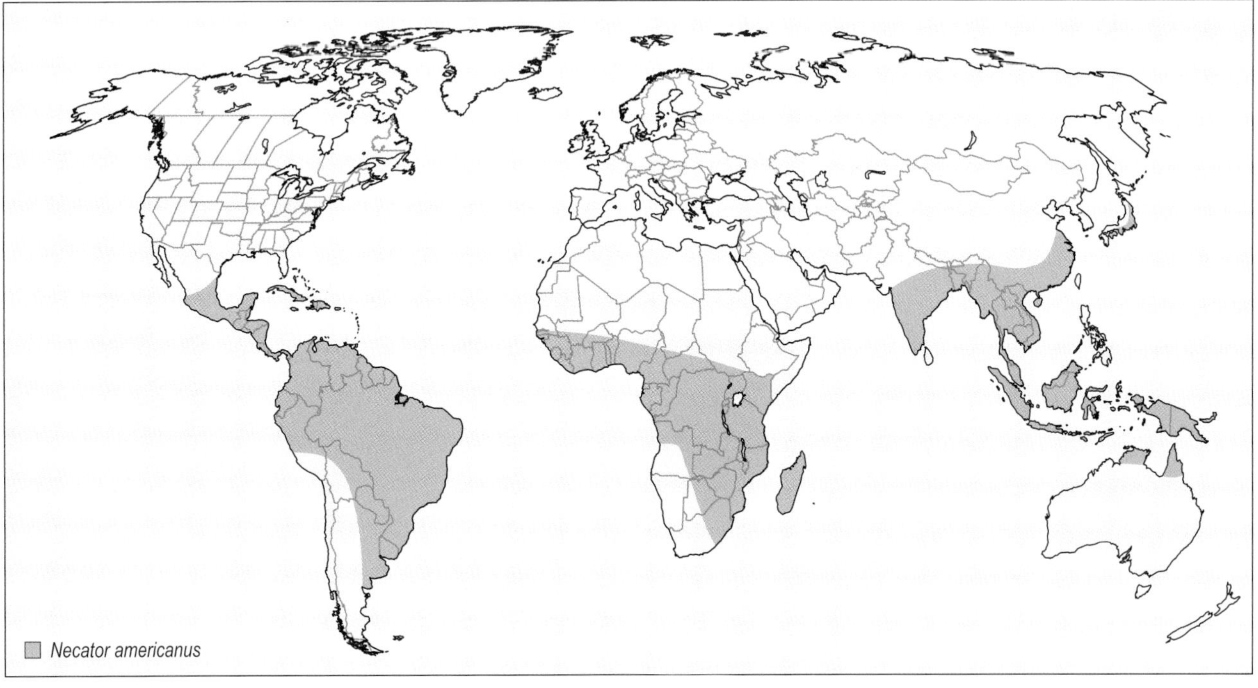

Figure 116.2 Global distribution of *Necator americanus*.

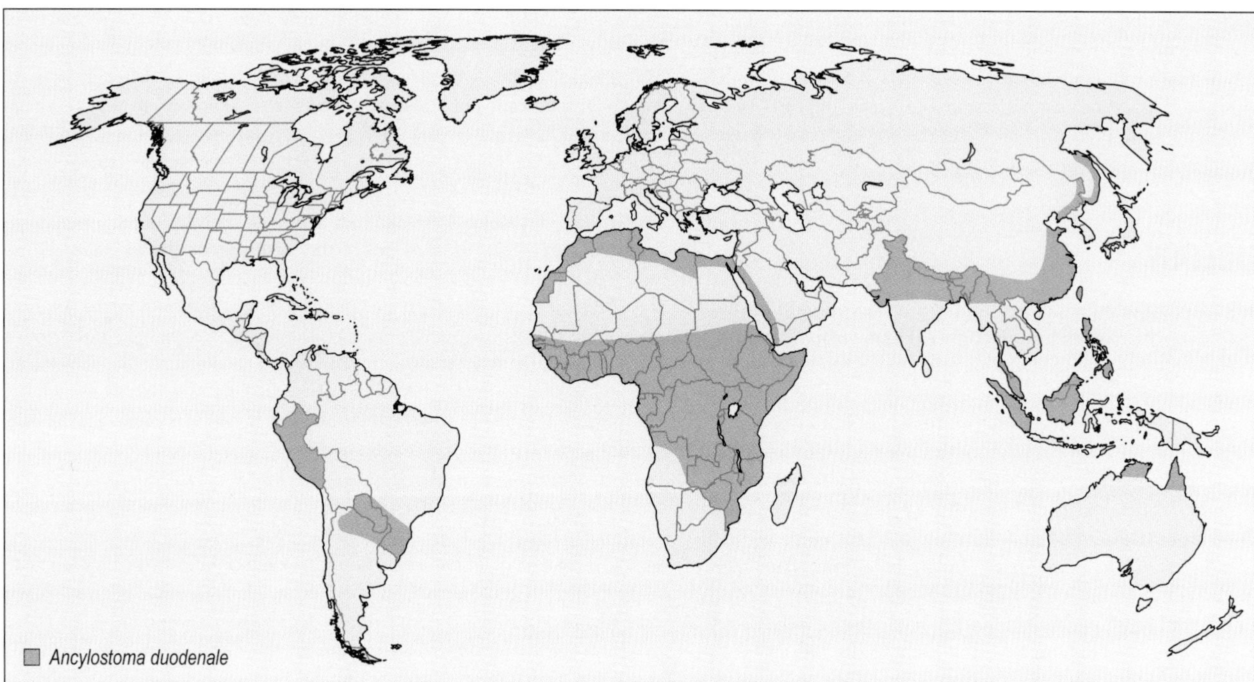

Figure 116.3 Global distribution of *Ancylostoma duodenale*.

than 2 years of age and then decline in adolescence, the worm burdens associated with hookworm infection do not exhibit such a clearcut pattern. It is not uncommon, for instance, for hookworm intensities to decline only slightly in adulthood or even to plateau or increase.[2,38] This observation helps to explain the high rates of hookworm infection and anemia among women of reproductive age, including pregnant women.[3] Studies from several different endemic areas suggest that humans are predisposed to acquire certain hookworm infection intensities so that people who are heavily infected prior to specific anthelminthic drug therapy will often reacquire heavy infections when left in the same environment.[22] Increasing evidence indicates a genetic basis for hookworm predisposition.

THE DISEASE

Repeated percutaneous exposure to infective hookworm larvae of either *A. duodenale* or *N. americanus* results in a papulovesicular dermatitis sometimes referred to as "ground itch." The pruritus and burning associated with ground itch typically are most intense at the site of host entry, usually on the hands and feet, and last less than 1 week. Some species of animal hookworms, including *A. braziliense*, will migrate laterally in the epidermis and give rise to local inflammation that follows the serpiginous migratory pathways of the larvae. This condition, CLM, presents commonly on the lower extremities or buttocks, usually within 2 weeks to several months after exposure to *A. braziliense* L3 larvae. Approximately 20% of patients with CLM will have eosinophilia, and some will develop pulmonary infiltrates (see Chapter 109).[37]

A second, urticarial rash can subsequently occur with the onset of *A. duodenale* or *N. americanus* larval migrations through the lungs. Hookworm pneumonitis occurs as the L3 larvae enter the alveoli and ascend the respiratory tree; it is commonly associated with wheezing, dyspnea, and a nonproductive cough.[4] Hookworm pneumonitis is less severe than other verminous pneumonias caused by *Ascaris* or *Toxocara*. Eosinophilia can begin during the larval migratory phase, but it typically peaks when the L3 enter the small intestine. Oral ingestion of large numbers of *A. duodenale* L3 larvae results one or a few days later in a syndrome (Wakana disease) consisting of nausea, vomiting, cough, dyspnea, and eosinophilia.

Attachment and tissue invasion of adult *A. duodenale* and *N. americanus* hookworms to the intestinal mucosa and submucosa are accompanied by mild abdominal pain, nausea, and anorexia. The gastrointestinal symptoms are more pronounced in patients with eosinophilic enteritis from zoonotic *A. caninum* infection. Intestinal parasitism by hookworms begins approximately 1.5–3 months after host entry by the L3 larvae. The prepatent period can last up to 1 year or possibly even longer if the L3 larvae of *A. duodenale* first undergo a period of arrested development.[18] Hookworm-associated blood loss results from the parasite-mediated destruction of capillaries in the intestinal mucosa. The degree of iron deficiency or anemia is dependent on a number of variables, including (1) worm burden; (2) type of hookworm – *A. duodenale* causes more blood loss than *N. americanus*; (3) iron reserves and diet of the host; and (4) overall host nutritional status.[8] In moderate and heavy infections, hookworm anemia (also known as "hookworm disease") will cause signs and symptoms of iron-deficiency anemia: fatigue, exertional dyspnea, poor concentration, koilonychia (spoon nail deformity), pallor, pale sclerae, and heart murmurs. In addition to presenting with profound iron deficiency, people with heavy hookworm burdens can develop protein malnutrition from chronic plasma protein loss and even the signs and symptoms of kwashiorkor.[4] Some of these patients will also acquire a pasty and sallow appearance, a condition known as chlorosis.[39] In Brazil, China, and elsewhere chronic hookworm infection is sometimes known as the "yellow disease." In childhood, chronic hookworm anemia leads to developmental delays associated with reductions in height and weight, physical fitness, and intellectual and cognitive deficits.[1,4,40] During pregnancy, the anemia resulting from hookworm disease has been linked to increased maternal mortality and several adverse neonatal outcomes, including low birth weight and increased morbidity and mortality.[2,3] Throughout many rural areas of low income countries hookworm disease accounts for a significant percentage (or in some cases a majority) of the iron-deficiency anemia in children and women.[4] In such highly endemic areas hookworm infection can actually thwart economic development.[41]

An extreme form of hookworm anemia, with high mortality, occurs in infants heavily infected with *A. duodenale*, who exhibit melena, diarrhea, pallor, and failure to thrive.[25] Most of the cases of infantile ancylostomiasis, which may result from vertical transmission of L3 via lactogenic transmission, have been reported from Asia.

PATHOGENESIS AND IMMUNITY

Infective larval migrations through tissues usually do not cause severe visceral lesions, although heavy infections can result in hookworm pneumonitis.[8] However, the inflammation associated with skin entry is pronounced and is probably exacerbated by the release of eicosanoids and hydrolytic enzymes from migrating L3 larvae.[42–44] Hookworm larvae also release a family of proteins known as the *Ancylostoma*-secreted proteins (ASPs) of unknown function, which contain amino acid sequences homologous to plant proteins, insect venom polypeptides, and other members of the pathogenesis-related protein superfamily.[6,45,46] CLM occurs when *A. braziliense* L3 larvae fail to penetrate the basement membrane of the epidermal–dermal junction and migrate laterally in the skin.

Hookworm-induced blood loss occurs at the site of adult parasite intestinal attachment. Hookworms use their teeth (*A. duodenale*) or cutting plates (*N. americanus*) to fasten onto the mucosa and submucosa, where they secrete a battery of pharmacologically active polypeptides that prevent blood from clotting and downregulate the host inflammatory response.[4,47–55] Among the peptides identified, cloned and expressed from the adult dog hookworm *A. caninum* (but presumably also released by *A. duodenale*) is a family of serine protease inhibitors that inhibit clotting factor Xa and tissue factor VIIa.[47,48] Adult hookworms also release hydrolytic enzymes.[56–59] The destruction of mucosal capillaries and the resultant extravasation of anticoagulated blood account for hookworm-associated blood loss leading to iron-deficiency anemia. Some red blood cells are lysed and the released hemoglobin is degraded by an orchestrated cascade of hemoglobinases that line the hookworm gut,[59,60] while the released heme is detoxified by one or more parasite glutathione S-transferases.[61] Chronic iron-deficiency is particularly detrimental in childhood and may directly impair cognitive and intellectual abilities by interfering with the development of dopaminergic neurons and the biosynthesis of brain enzymes with iron prosthetic groups.[4,62,63] In addition, in Africa and elsewhere hookworm infection is often co-endemic with malaria[64] and other anemia-associated infections; when these conditions occur simultaneously they can combine to produce profound deficits in hemoglobin.[65–67]

Human immune responses to hookworms are not well characterized. Immunoepidemiologic studies and observations with self-administered *N. americanus* infections suggest that humoral antibodies and cellular responses to hookworm antigens often are not linked to resistance to reinfection.[68–70] It has been hypothesized that hookworms are immunosuppressive and may promote susceptibility to other infections, including malaria and HIV/AIDS.[2,65,71–73] In the laboratory, however, immunity to canine hookworm infections has been produced by administering repeated doses of living larvae or larvae attenuated by ionizing radiation.[74–76] Hookworm immunity generated by living larval vaccines is not sterile but manifests by reduced worm burdens and decreased egg fecundity of the adult hookworms.[75,76] Evidence suggests that the protective effect offered by living larval hookworm vaccines may be reproduced by immunization with genetically engineered recombinant polypeptides.[7,77–83]

DIAGNOSIS

Severe hookworm anemia clinically resembles iron-deficiency anemia, with physical signs and symptoms as outlined previously. A peripheral blood smear from a heavily infected patient will demonstrate the presence of microcytic hypochromic red blood cells. Measurement of hemoglobin concentration will also help to confirm the diagnosis. Eosinophilia is often a prominent feature of the complete blood count. In many endemic areas, other causes of anemia should be excluded, including malaria, HIV/AIDS, and hemoglobinopathies. Hookworm will also exacerbate anemia in patients with underlying nutritional deficiencies. Occasionally, a patient will be diagnosed early in the clinical course of hookworm infection because of a characteristic rash, pruritus, and pulmonary symptoms.

A definitive diagnosis of hookworm infection is established by identifying hookworm eggs from feces under light microscopy. Fecal concentration techniques are not required to diagnose moderate or heavy infections, or even most light infections. Quantitative egg counts are sometimes useful for determining the intensity of infection; this is essential to epidemiologic investigations since prevalence determination provides superficial information. Common quantitative techniques include the Kato–Katz, Beaver direct egg count, Stoll dilutional egg count, and McMaster techniques.[84] Hookworm eggs are easily differentiated from other common human intestinal nematodes, such as *Ascaris* and *Trichuris*. However, the eggs of *A. duodenale* and *N. americanus* are not usually distinguishable by light microscopy. Species assignment of eggs using the polymerase chain reaction is under investigation.[85] Currently, however, species assignment usually requires either recovery of the adult worms from patients treated with an anthelminthic agent or rearing and identifying L3 larvae from eggs by fecal cultures.[84] Human *A. caninum* infections that result in eosinophilic enteritis usually result in negative fecal examinations. Often, a single male or nongravid female adult hookworm living in an ectopic gastrointestinal site can cause eosinophilic enteritis. Therefore, definitive diagnosis may require identification of the parasite by either upper endoscopy or sigmoidoscopy. CLM is most often diagnosed clinically and must be differentiated from scabies.[37] Unlike patients with CLM, the mite *Sarcoptes scabiei* or its eggs can be demonstrated from skin scrapings. Patients with CLM may not have eosinophilia or a rise in IgE titer as they frequently do in systemic helminthic infections (see Chapter 109).[37]

TREATMENT AND PROGNOSIS

The benzimidazole anthelminthic drugs mebendazole and albendazole are the current treatment of choice for removing adult hookworms from the gastrointestinal tract.[6,86] Both agents act on the microtubules of the parasite. Mebendazole is given either in a single 500 mg dose or 100 mg twice daily for 3 days; albendazole is given 400 mg once.[86] However, a recent meta-analysis has revealed high rates of drug failure in patients with hookworm treated with mebendazole, especially when this agent is used in a single dose.[86] The benzimidazoles are teratogenic and embryotoxic in experimental animals and have not been rigorously tested in young children or in pregnancy. However, increasing experience with these agents given during mass chemotherapy programs in developing countries indicates that they are probably safe in children older than 1 year of age and therefore should be given to hookworm-infected preschool children, as well as pregnant women in their second and third trimesters.[6,87,88] In at least one anecdotal report from Papua New Guinea, thousands of children were treated with mebendazole and albendazole with no side effects.[89] Occasional adverse effects of the benzimidazoles include diarrhea, abdominal pain, and the induction of adult *Ascaris* worm migrations to ectopic sites. Rarely, the benzimidazoles will cause leukopenia, alopecia, and an increase in serum transaminases.

The World Health Organization has advocated the use of single-dose albendazole or mebendazole for mass treatment programs of school-age children with STH infections.[87] Both agents will reduce hookworm burdens below the threshold that would otherwise result in disease. Mass treatment of school-age children offers a number of health- and non-health-related benefits to children, including improvement in iron and hemoglobin status, physical growth, cognition, educational achievement, and school absenteeism.[2,6] However, in areas of intense transmission, hookworm-infected children can be expected to reacquire their infections to pretreatment levels approximately 4–12 months after receiving albendazole or mebendazole,[5] and longer in areas with lower transmission rates.[2] In addition to high rates of mebendazole drug failure,[6,86] one study noted diminishing efficacy of mebendazole with repeated use, possibly because of emerging anthelminthic drug resistance.[90,91] There is also no direct evidence that benzimidazole will eradicate populations of arrested, hypobiotic larvae in human tissues. Therefore, patients with latent *A. duodenale* infections could theoretically have positive fecal examinations months after curative treatment, even in nonendemic areas. The prognosis of hookworm infection is dependent on its chronicity, its intensity, and the iron reserves and diet of the host. Many of the sequelae of hookworm anemia are potentially reversible with anthelminthic drugs and iron supplementation.[92,93] However, severe hookworm iron-deficiency anemia in infancy may cause irreversible effects.[4,63] The majority of patients with CLM are cured by oral administration of albendazole (400 mg daily for 3 days) or ivermectin (200 µg/kg daily for 1 or 2 days).

PREVENTION AND CONTROL

Since there are no animal reservoir hosts for *A. duodenale* or *N. americanus*, effective sanitation should interrupt hookworm transmission and prevent reinfection. However, by itself, the effect of sanitation in terms of reducing community hookworm prevalence and intensity is often not realized for decades.[2,94,95] Economic development with improvement in living standards and the introduction of piped water supplies, waterborne sewage systems, mechanized agriculture, and replacement of human feces with chemical fertilizers will control endemic hookworm and are largely responsible for the control of hookworm infection in North America, Europe, Japan, and Korea.[4,41] Presumably, these measures would be effective in many developing countries. Health education to advise on the proper use of sanitation facilities and to avoid using uncomposted human manure is also an essential component of control.[95]

Because of the health and educational benefits of albendazole and mebendazole outlined previously, and because they have become available as low-cost generic drugs, there has been interest in using them to control STH infections worldwide. At the World Health Assembly in 2001, a resolution was put forward (resolution 54.19) urging endemic countries to control STH infections and regularly treat at least 75% of all at-risk school-age children with albendazole or mebendazole (as well as praziquantel in schistosomiasis endemic regions) by 2010.[6,87,91] It has been further proposed that, wherever possible, schools should provide the infrastructure for anthelminthic health care delivery, with trained teachers responsible for administering the drugs.[6,87] Moreover, increasingly preschool children are also being targeted for mass drug administration because of the infrastructure established through child health days for the simultaneous administration of childhood immunizations, antimalarial drugs, bednets, and micronutrients.[6] Neither school-based deworming nor deworming administered as part of child health days will reduce hookworm transmission attributable to heavily infected adults. Moreover, where high-intensity endemic hookworm occurs, reinfection will occur within months necessitating, in some cases, thrice yearly treatments.[4,87,91] There is further concern that such frequent administration of benzimidazoles may promote the emergence of drug resistance.[6,90] For these reasons, there is great interest in developing new tools and strategies to control hookworm infection in developing countries. Through a product development partnership known as the Human Hookworm Vaccine Initiative, several recombinant hookworm proteins formulated with Alhydrogel and other adjuvants are currently entering clinical trials in Brazil.[7,81,82]

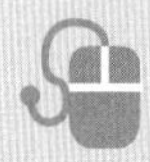

Access the complete reference list online at
http://www.expertconsult.com

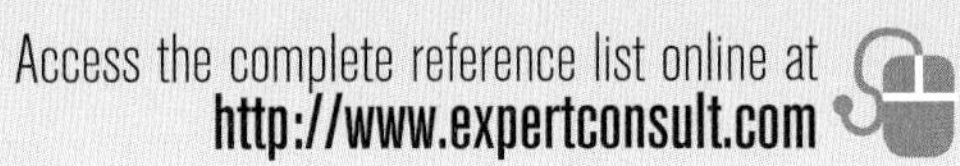
Access the complete reference list online at
http://www.expertconsult.com

CHAPTER 117

Strongyloidiasis

Afzal A. Siddiqui • Robert M. Genta • Ismael Maguilnik • Steven L. Berk

INTRODUCTION

Strongyloidiasis, caused by *Strongyloides stercoralis*, is the fourth most important intestinal nematode infection in the world. Although isolated pockets of low endemicity and indigenous sporadic infections have often been found in many temperate areas of the world, *S. stercoralis* infection is predominantly a problem of humid tropical areas. The specific impacts of chronic infections with *S. stercoralis* on human health are difficult to evaluate in populations with widespread enteric diseases, parasitoses, and malnutrition. Infection of humans with *S. stercoralis* usually produces an often negligibly or minimally symptomatic chronic disease of the gastrointestinal tract that can remain undetected for several decades. However, in immunocompromised patients, especially those receiving corticosteroids, hyperinfection strongyloidiasis can develop with dissemination of larvae to extraintestinal organs, resulting in mortality rates as high as 85%.

THE AGENT

History

In the nineteenth century, French troops deployed in Cochin China (modern Vietnam) often developed persistent severe diarrhea that became known among military personnel as "diarrhée de la Cochinchine." In 1876 Normand discovered small worms in stools of some repatriated soldiers and reported his findings to the Academy of Sciences of Paris.[1] Bavay, a colleague of Normand's, named the worm *Anguillula stercoralis* (from the Latin words for "small eel" and "dung"), and later provided a detailed description of the worm under the new name, *Anguillula intestinalis*. Several parasitologists became interested in the new nematode, and in 1879 Grassi established a new genus which he called *Strongyloides* (Greek *strongylos*, "round") and gave *Strongyloides stercoralis* its current name.[2] In subsequent years the parasite's life cycle was partially described. Although several detailed descriptions of individual patients infected with *S. stercoralis* were published in the early years of the twentieth century,[3] it was not until Napier[4] conducted extensive clinical surveys of British World War II ex-prisoners of war and Galliard[5,6] performed systematic experiments in normal and immunosuppressed dogs that the clinical importance of strongyloidiasis began to be fully appreciated.

Taxonomy

The family Strongyloididae (class Secernentea, order Rhabditida) comprises only the genus *Strongyloides*. The members of this genus, also called threadworms, are heterogenetic, with free-living and parasitic generations, and comprise at least 40 named species.[7] The only species discussed in this chapter is *S. stercoralis*. Another species, *S. fuelleborni*, is a parasite of primates that may also infect humans.[8] Several other species are also important, either because they can cause disease in livestock (*S. ransomi*, *S. westeri*, *S. papillosus*) or because they can be used as models of human strongyloidiasis (*S. ratti* and *S. venezuelensis*).[9]

Life Cycle and Morphology

Infection (***Fig. 117.1***) is acquired when filariform larvae (slender, fast-moving worms measuring ~50 μm in diameter and between 350 and 600 μm in length) penetrate the skin of a susceptible host, enter a venous or lymphatic channel, and are transported to the lungs. Larvae break out of the capillaries into the alveoli (***Fig. 117.2***), migrate to the trachea as they mature, and are eventually swallowed. Parthenogenic females lodge in the lamina propria of the duodenum and the proximal jejunum, where they lay eggs (***Fig. 117.3***). From the hatching eggs emerge rhabditiform larvae. The shorter and slower rhabditiform larvae (~60 μm in diameter and 250–300 μm in length) migrate into the intestinal lumen. The rhabditiform larvae may either directly molt into infective (parasitic) filariform larvae able to repenetrate the colon or pass with the feces. In the external environment rhabditiform larvae can switch to a free-living cycle. In this latter, indirect, or heterogonical, cycle, four molts lead to the development of adult male and female worms (***Fig. 117.4***). These mate and produce a generation of offspring whose filariform stage will have the ability to reenter parasitic life.[9] The crucial characteristic of *S. stercoralis* that sets it apart from all other major human parasitic worms is that rhabditiform larvae can molt within the host's intestine into the filariform stage. These tissue-penetrating infective larvae may penetrate the colonic wall (***Fig. 117.5***) or the perianal skin, complete an internal cycle, and become established as mature adult females in the small intestine. This process, known as autoinfection, represents the mechanism by which *S. stercoralis* can persist virtually indefinitely in infected hosts.[10,11]

EPIDEMIOLOGY

The worldwide prevalence of strongyloidiasis is not known with certainty, with estimates varying between 3 million and 100 million people infected worldwide (***Fig. 117.6***).[12] The unreliability of these estimates is further reflected in the wide range of reported prevalence rates, which vary between less than 1% and 85% in populations living in adjacent regions of the same country.[13,14] With these limitations in mind, *S. stercoralis* is likely present in virtually all tropical and subtropical regions of the world.[15] Areas of known but low endemicity (less than 1% to 3%) still exist in several countries of Europe (e.g., northern Italy, France, Spain, Switzerland, Poland), the United States (e.g., Appalachian region[16] and West Virginia[17]), Japan (Okinawa), and Australia (aboriginal populations).[15] In some areas, for example, in a rural community near Valencia community in Spain, the high prevalence of strongyloidiasis has been attributed to agricultural activities.[18] Strongyloidiasis has also been found intermittently in institutionalized individuals[19] as well as in patients of cancer centers[20] in several North American locations where the parasite is not endemic in the general population. Considering the long

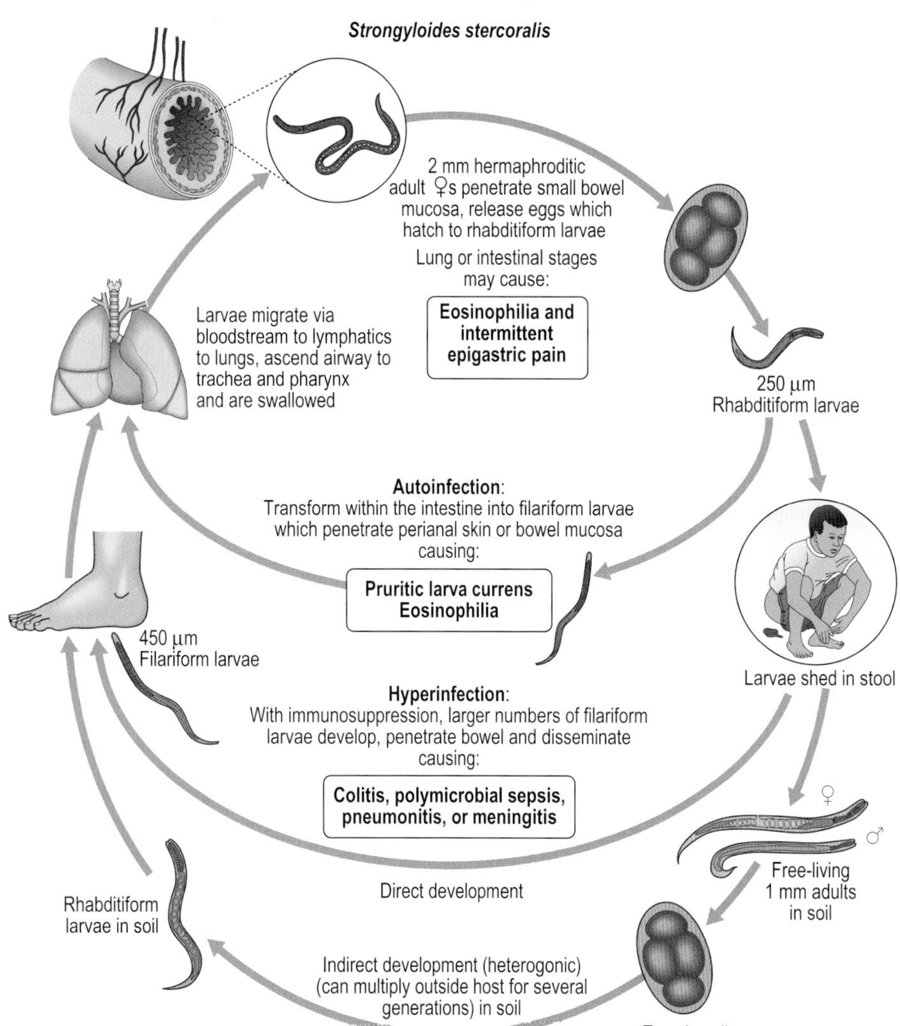
Strongyloides stercoralis
2 mm hermaphroditic adult ♀s penetrate small bowel mucosa, release eggs which hatch to rhabditiform larvae
Lung or intestinal stages may cause:
Eosinophilia and intermittent epigastric pain
Larvae migrate via bloodstream to lymphatics to lungs, ascend airway to trachea and pharynx and are swallowed
250 μm Rhabditiform larvae
Autoinfection: Transform within the intestine into filariform larvae which penetrate perianal skin or bowel mucosa causing:
Pruritic larva currens Eosinophilia
450 μm Filariform larvae
Larvae shed in stool
Hyperinfection: With immunosuppression, larger numbers of filariform larvae develop, penetrate bowel and disseminate causing:
Colitis, polymicrobial sepsis, pneumonitis, or meningitis
♀
♂
Free-living 1 mm adults in soil
Direct development
Rhabditiform larvae in soil
Indirect development (heterogonic) (can multiply outside host for several generations) in soil
Eggs in soil

Figure 117.1 Life cycle of *Strongyloides stercoralis*.

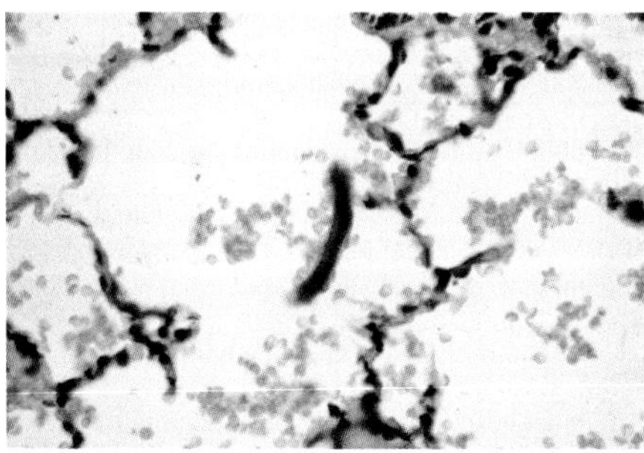

Figure 117.2 Fragment of a *Strongyloides stercoralis* filariform larva in the alveolar spaces of an immunocompetent host. There are scattered blood cells but no significant hemorrhage.

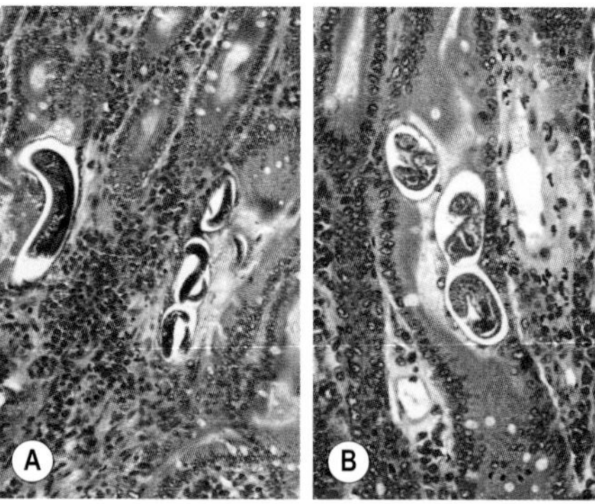
A
B

Figure 117.3 (A, B) Section of an adult *Strongyloides stercoralis* female worm and embryonated eggs in the lamina propria of an immunocompetent subject. There is moderate mononuclear inflammation in the vicinity of the parasites.

persistence of *S. stercoralis* in its host and its relatively high prevalence in some tropical and subtropical populations, physicians practicing in industrialized countries should consider strongyloidiasis in immigrant or refugee patients born in developing regions,[8] as well as in persons from known local areas of endemicity.

PATHOGENESIS AND IMMUNITY

Chronic strongyloidiasis is probably sustained by a relatively low and stable number of adult worms which reside in harmony within their host's intestine and survive by means of well-regulated autoinfection (*Fig. 117.1*).[21] Autoinfection is believed to be regulated by the host immunity.[10,22,23] When immunosuppression impairs the host's regulatory function, increasing numbers of autoinfective larvae complete the cycle, and the population of parasitic adult worms increases (hyperinfection). Eventually, the extraordinary numbers of migrating larvae deviate from the canonical route (intestine → venous circulation → lungs → trachea → intestine) and disseminate to other organs, including meningeal spaces and brain, liver, kidneys, lymph nodes, and cutaneous and subcutaneous

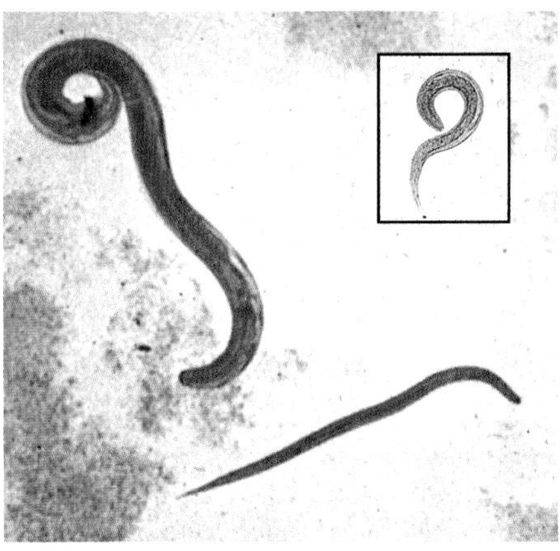

Figure 117.4 Filariform larva (approximately 550 μm in length) and an immature adult worm (1.3 mm) recovered from the feces of an immunocompromised dog experimentally infected with *Strongyloides stercoralis*. It is extremely rare to recover from the stools of immunocompetent patients any *S. stercoralis* stages other than the shorter (approximately 300 μm) and plumper rhabditiform larvae (inset).

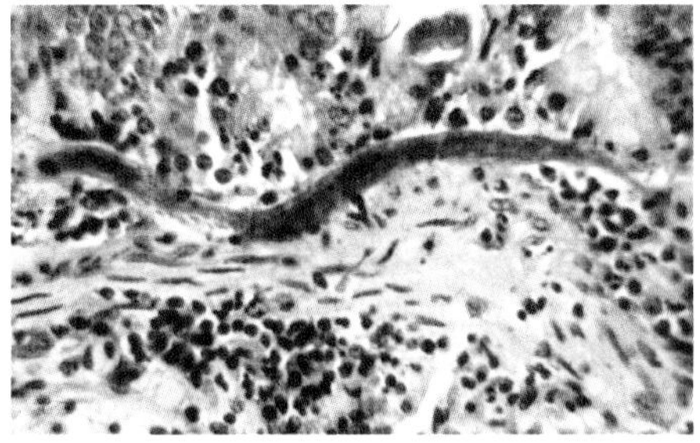

Figure 117.5 Intestinal muscularis mucosae and submucosa with a full-length section of a penetrating filariform larva.

tissues, where they cause hemorrhage and inflammation, and implant Gram-negative bacteria carried from fecal material. The resulting syndrome, known as disseminated strongyloidiasis, is nearly always fatal.[10,23]

The validity of the above model has been questioned by Schad et al[24] and other investigators,[25,26] who used an experimental canine model of disseminated strongyloidiasis to show that only a few larvae could be recovered from the lungs of dogs with massive hyperinfection. Later, in a series of experiments based on the compartmental analysis of radiolabeled larvae and mathematical modeling, they presented convincing evidence that the tracheobronchial route in the dog was not used by the majority of the migrating larvae.[27,28] According to their model, larvae that began their migration in the skin (primary infection) or in the distal ileum (autoinfection) were not more likely to pass through the lungs than through any other organ, suggesting that the migratory pathway involved random dissemination throughout the body. However, this conclusion may not be applicable to the cycle in humans, since large numbers of larvae are frequently identified in bronchoalveolar lavage fluid from hyperinfected patients.[29,30]

We have challenged the accepted paradigm that host mechanisms regulate hyperinfection and dissemination.[15,21] The theory that host immunity alone controls infection fails to consider the role that parasites may play in their own regulation. The adverse impact of increased parasite density on egg production and growth has been demonstrated for several intestinal helminths. Although distinguishing between host resistance and direct parasite-to-parasite effects may be difficult, it seems clear that most parasites reach a particular population size or a critical biomass, after which yet unknown regulatory mechanisms intervene to limit the population.[28]

We have proposed that *S. stercoralis* may have the ability to reach an optimal population size in the human small intestine. If the initial infective dose of larvae is low, a higher rate of intraluminal molting (i.e., autoinfection) occurs until the "optimal" size of the adult population is reached. If *S. stercoralis*, like other nematodes, transmits its molting signal by molting hormones (ecdysteroids),[31] adult females adjust their production of ecdysteroids to levels sufficient to replace the dying adults. During the initial phase of infection, the host mounts an immune response directed

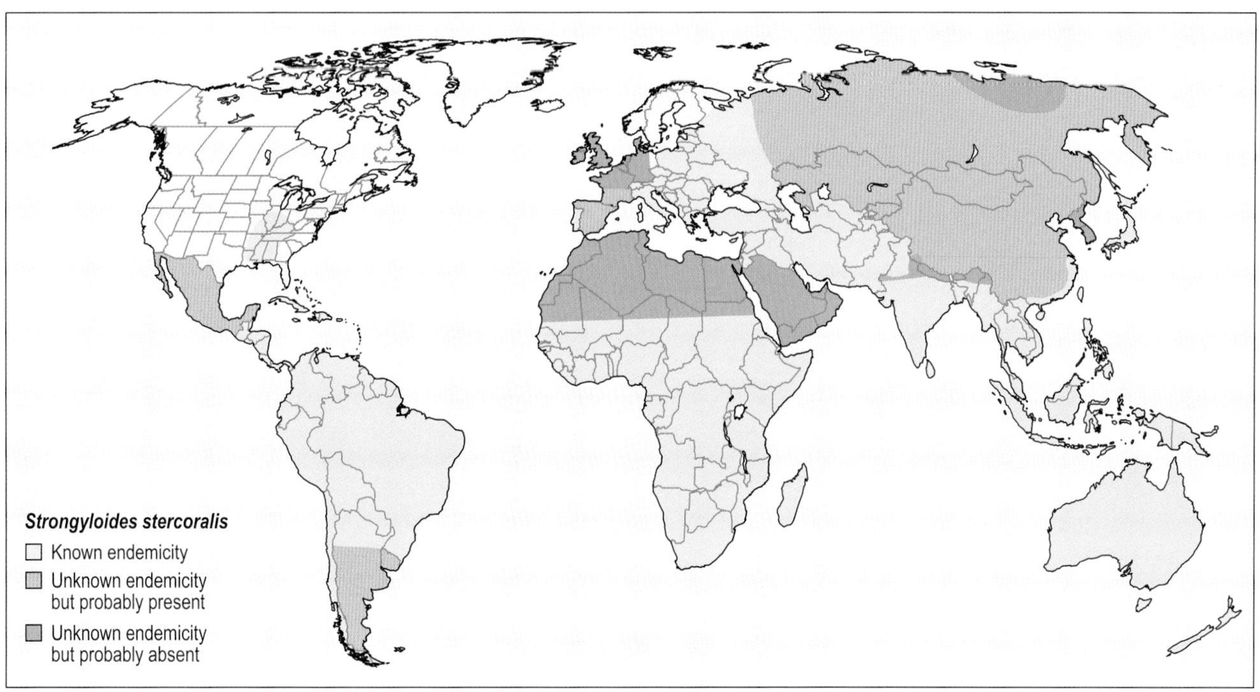

Figure 117.6 Endemicity of *Strongyloides stercoralis*.

at all tissue stages of the parasite.[22,32–35] These responses may not eradicate all parasites, but may limit the size of the parasite population. Impaired immune responses may allow the growth of larger numbers of parasites, as reported in agammaglobulinemic patients,[36] human T-cell lymphotropic virus type 1 (HTLV-1)-infected subjects (see Chapter 81),[37] and severely malnourished children,[38] but total dysregulation of the parasite population does not seem to occur since worms, in part, regulate their own growth.

The level of ecdysteroid-like substances is generally negligible in healthy subjects.[31] The administration of exogenous or endogenous corticosteroids may result in increased amounts of ecdysteroid-like substances in the host's tissues, including the intestinal wall, where adult females reside. These substances may act as molting signals for the eggs or rhabditiform larvae, which transform intraluminally into excessive numbers of filariform larvae. Available data are not sufficient to prove a dose-dependent effect, but it is indeed remarkable that patients who develop fulminating hyperinfection after only a few days of steroid administration are usually those who have received intravenous methylprednisone.[39] Once an intestinal population has become very large (e.g., 100 000 adult worms) it continues to expand rapidly even at low molting rates, and the discontinuation of steroids is not sufficient to arrest the population growth, which leads to the host's death.

Based on our observations, we further postulate that in *S. stercoralis* these developmental processes are regulated via a class of transcription factor(s) that typically regulates genes in response to fat-soluble hormones, such as steroids or fatty acids, as is the case with the free-living nematode *Caenorhabditis elegans*. We have described a gene in *S. stercoralis*[40] which showed significant homology with a number of nuclear hormone receptors including the dauer formation loci (*daf*) gene, *daf-12* of *C. elegans* and ecdysone receptors of insects.[40] The identification of *daf-12* orthologs from *S. stercoralis* and from *Dirofilaria immitis* suggests that this component of the genetic pathway is conserved among nematodes. DAF-12 regulates the dauer diapause and developmental age in *C. elegans*, and it is possible that mechanisms similar to those acting in *C. elegans* also regulate the development in *S. stercoralis*. Furthermore, in an animal model of *S. stercoralis*, it has been observed that when normal male gerbils were infected subcutaneously with 1000 infective filariform larvae, the infected animals harbored moderate numbers (83.6 ± 27.6) of adult worms at 35 days after infection.[41] More interestingly, a low-grade infection persisted for 131 days, mimicking the chronic nature of human infections. Gerbils treated weekly with 2 mg of methylprednisolone acetate developed hyperinfective strongyloidiasis with up to 8000 autoinfective larvae occurring in these animals at post-infection day 21. Autoinfection never occurred in normal untreated gerbils.[41] This animal study coupled with examples from human case reports reinforce our thesis that immune suppression *per se* is not the major cause of hyperinfection but is the direct effect of steroids on the parasite which causes the hyperinfection. Recent experimental evidence has confirmed our hypothesis; specifically, a conserved steroid hormone signaling pathway in parasitic nematodes, including *S. stercoralis*, that is mediated by DAF-12 and controls the progression of the parasite's infectious stage, a process that is homologous to *C. elegans* dauer recovery, has been elucidated.[42] Furthermore in these studies, steroid hormone-like dafachronic acids induced recovery of the dauer-like *S. stercoralis* larvae by activating DAF-12. Administration of dafachronic acid markedly reduced the pathogenic larval populations of *S. stercoralis*, indicating the potential use of DAF-12 ligands to treat disseminated strongyloidiasis.[42]

Pathology

The pathologic lesions associated with chronic, uncomplicated *S. stercoralis* have received little attention, because only rarely have patients with such lesions come to autopsy. However, pathologic descriptions of the lesions in a few patients in whom strongyloidiasis was an incidental finding, our own experience, and animal studies[25,43] indicate that the worms can exist in the intestinal mucosa without causing significant inflammatory responses or tissue damage (see ***Fig. 117.2***). The classic description of the pathologic changes in strongyloidiasis was made by De Paola et al[44] in 1962, and later updated by Genta and Caymmi-Gomes.[45] When present, intestinal lesions range from mild mucosal congestion and abundant mucoid secretions ("catarrhal enteritis") with a mildly increased mononuclear infiltrate in the lamina propria, to a more severe "edematous enteritis," with a grossly thickened intestinal wall. Submucosal edema, flattening of the villi, and parasites scattered throughout the lamina propria may be observed microscopically. The most severe form ("ulcerative enteritis") is almost exclusively seen in association with hyperinfection. The intestinal walls may be rigid due to the edema and fibrosis resulting from long-standing inflammation, and the mucosa may show atrophy, erosions, and ulcerations. An abundant inflammatory infiltrate, most often consisting of neutrophils, as well as all stages of *S. stercoralis*, are present throughout the intestinal mucosa. Jejunal perforation has been reported in patients with the ulcerative enteritis form of strongyloidiasis.[46] Uncommonly, the mucosal damage occurs predominantly in the large intestine, simulating ulcerative colitis and pseudopolyposis.[47,48] A form of eosinophilic colitis associated with strongyloidiasis has been described in older patients.[49] *S. stercoralis* larvae have been found in the appendix, and eosinophilic appendicitis apparently caused by this parasite has been reported.[50,51] In patients with disseminated strongyloidiasis, the intestinal lesions reflect the large number of worms dwelling within the small intestinal mucosa and penetrating the intestinal walls. In addition, the stomach[52,53] (***Fig. 117.7***) and the peritoneal cavity[50,54,55] may be invaded by migrating parasites. However, because most of these patients are receiving immunosuppressive doses of corticosteroids, the inflammatory responses are often minimal in spite of extensive tissue damage.

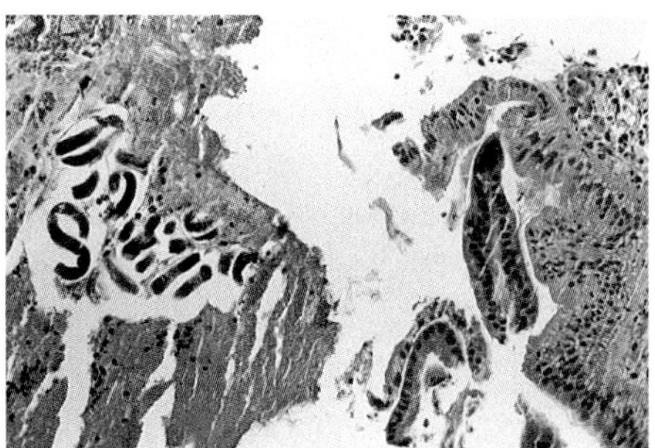

Figure 117.7 Gastric mucosal biopsy with numerous fragments of *Strongyloides stercoralis* larvae in a patient with AIDS and multiple opportunistic infections. The larvae were present in the mucus but were not seen penetrating the gastric mucosa itself.

Migrating parasites may cause mechanical damage as well as inflammation in other organs. As larvae penetrate the large intestine, they create small breaks in the mucosa that facilitate the invasion of the bloodstream by enteric bacteria. The larvae themselves carry bacteria on their cuticles to distant sites. In human patients, the extraintestinal organ most commonly affected by this migratory damage is the lung. In severe disseminated infection, when hundreds of thousands of adult parasites dwell in the intestine and millions of larvae migrate throughout the body, alveolar microhemorrhages may result in massive pulmonary bleeding[56] (***Fig. 117.8***). The widespread dissemination of larvae is almost invariably associated with polymicrobial sepsis, diffuse or patchy bronchopneumonia, pulmonary and cerebral abscesses, and/or meningitis.[23] Filariform larvae, and occasionally rhabditiform larvae and adult worms, also may disseminate to mesenteric lymph nodes and the biliary tract, as well as the liver, pancreas, spleen, heart, endocrine glands, and ovaries.[45] In these locations the parasite may induce a granulomatous response.[57,58]

THE DISEASE

The majority of persons with chronic infection are either asymptomatic or have mild, nonspecific symptoms. In contrast, disseminated strongyloidiasis is a catastrophic event which, if untreated, invariably results in death.

Gastrointestinal Manifestations

Epigastric abdominal pain, postprandial fullness or bloating, and heartburn are among the symptoms most commonly reported, and brief episodes of diarrhea alternating with constipation may also occur.[59,60] Occult blood is occasionally detected in the stools of subjects with chronic infections,[61] and even massive colonic[62] and gastric hemorrhage[63] have been reported. Physical examination of chronically infected patients is normal or reveals only mild abdominal tenderness on palpation. Rarely, chronic strongyloidiasis may resemble inflammatory bowel disease, particularly ulcerative colitis, and the endoscopic appearance may be that of pseudopolyposis.[47] Although malabsorption has been reported frequently in patients with strongyloidiasis,[64] a clear causal relationship between *S. stercoralis* infection and malabsorption in otherwise healthy subjects has not been established.[65]

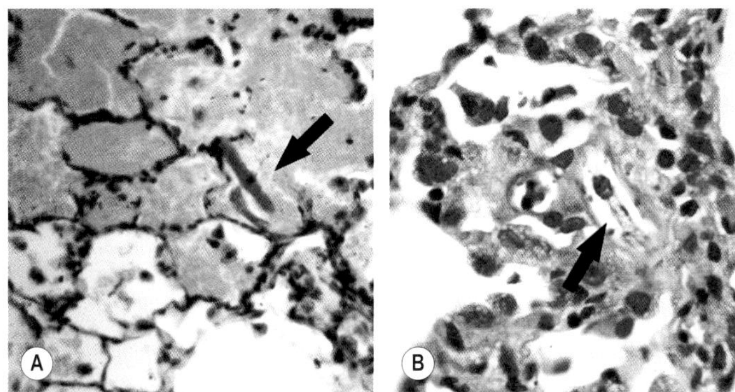

Figure 117.8 **(A)** Severe intra-alveolar hemorrhage and fragment of a larva (arrow) in a patient with disseminated strongyloidiasis. In some patients, larvae may be found within the alveolar walls, where they may form granulomas. **(B)** A possible early granuloma around a fragment of larva (arrow).

In contrast to chronic strongyloidiasis, the gastrointestinal manifestations of disseminated strongyloidiasis are almost invariably serious. Hyperinfection is often heralded by profuse diarrhea, which is a consequence of the erosions, ulcerations, and edema caused by millions of adult worms and filariform larvae in the mucosa of the small and large intestine.[23] Malabsorption, exudation, and altered motility may also result. These mucosal changes predispose the patient to bacterial enterocolitis and, after variable periods of diarrhea, paralytic ileus.[66] Possibly because of the large numbers of larvae migrating from the large intestine into the circulation,[67] polymicrobial (predominantly Gram-negative) sepsis may occur and local infections and abscesses may develop in virtually any organ.[23,67] Larvae have been detected in the liver, stomach, and pancreas of patients with overwhelming infections, but their presence in these locations is not known to be associated with characteristic symptoms.[68]

Pulmonary Manifestations

Although patients with chronic obstructive pulmonary disease may have an increased risk of strongyloidiasis,[15] no respiratory signs or symptoms are associated with chronic strongyloidiasis. In these infections the numbers of larvae passing through the lungs are so small that they do not cause significant tissue damage.[69] However, patients who presented with asthma (most likely unrelated to the infection) and were treated with corticosteroids later developed disseminated strongyloidiasis.[70,71] In these situations, how hyperinfection can develop is illustrated in a conceptual model shown in ***Figure 117.9***. In summary, in patients with disseminated strongyloidiasis, pulmonary manifestations are the rule, particularly diffuse bronchopneumonia. Intra-alveolar hemorrhage, often so severe as to cause the patient's death, is frequent. Filariform larvae and at times rhabditiform larvae and even eggs may be present in respiratory secretions in those with disseminated strongyloidiasis.

Neurologic Manifestations

Uncomplicated strongyloidiasis is not associated with neurologic manifestations. Gram-negative polymicrobial meningitis is the most frequent central nervous system manifestation of disseminated strongyloidiasis, and in some cases, larvae have been identified in the cerebrospinal fluid[72] (***Fig. 117.10***). Less common is the formation of cerebral and cerebellar abscesses containing *S. stercoralis* larvae.[73]

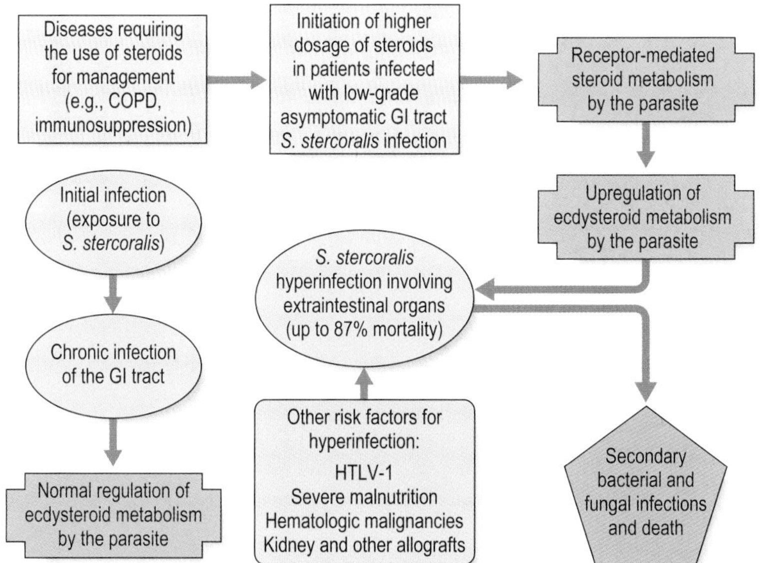

Figure 117.9 Conceptual model of the development of *Strongyloides stercoralis* in patients receiving corticosteroids for treatment of diseases such as chronic obstructive pulmonary disease (COPD).

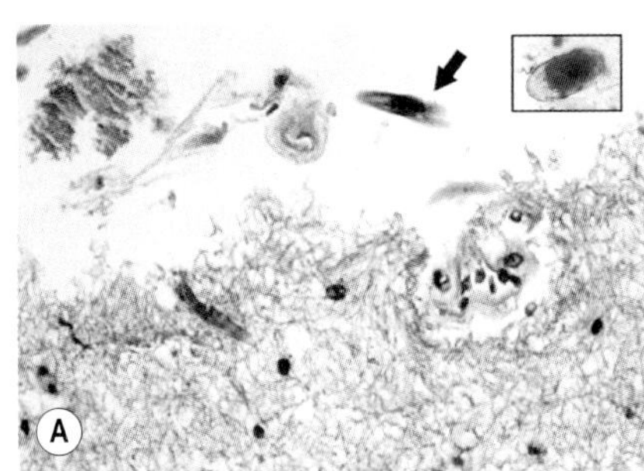
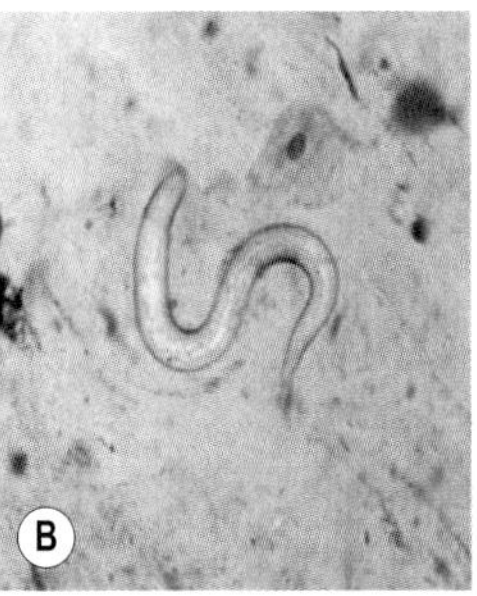

Figure 117.10 (A) Fragment of larva (arrow) in the meninges of a man who died of disseminated strongyloidiasis. The egg in the inset was recovered from the cerebrospinal fluid when the patient was alive; this is a most unusual finding. **(B)** A larva detected during cytologic examination of a bronchoalveolar lavage specimen from the same patient.

Cutaneous Manifestations

Two types of cutaneous manifestations have been described in patients with chronic strongyloidiasis: urticarial rashes, possibly caused by a sensitization to parasite antigens, and a characteristic, migratory serpiginous dermatitis caused by the subcutaneous migration of filariform larvae (larva currens). The latter has been reported more often in white patients infected in the Far East.[74–76] Some patients with disseminated infection, leukopenia, and various degrees of thrombocytopenia may develop generalized or periumbilical cutaneous purpura,[77–80] probably related to the rupture of small vessels caused by filariform larvae migrating in the dermis.[76,79]

Other Systemic Manifestations

Arthritis is an unusual manifestation of strongyloidiasis and is associated with the local deposition of immune complexes containing *S. stercoralis* antigens.[81] Cardiac arrhythmias and arrest are exceedingly rare and have been attributed to direct myocardial damage caused by the migrating larvae[82] or to electrolyte imbalance precipitated by severe diarrhea.[83] The passage of larvae in semen and the presence of genital lesions[84] as well as multivisceral damage has also been attributed to strongyloidiasis.[85]

Strongyloidiasis and Diseases of the Immune System

Since disseminated strongyloidiasis is a disease of the immunocompromised, one would expect persons with either inherited or acquired deficiencies of the immune system to be particularly prone to this severe complication of infection.

Acquired Immunodeficiency Syndrome

Traditionally, impaired immunity was thought to be one of the main factors regulating the development of *S. stercoralis* autoinfection. Therefore frequent and severe infections with *S. stercoralis* were expected to emerge in patients with acquired immunodeficiency syndrome (AIDS). However, this has not happened, even in areas of the world where both *S. stercoralis* and AIDS are endemic, and in general there does not appear to be a higher prevalence of chronic strongyloidiasis with AIDS (see Chapter 139).[86] In Brazil, where both strongyloidiasis and HIV infection have a high prevalence, coinfection is common and cases of hyperinfection in patients with HIV have been reported.[87] Even though cases of strongyloidiasis have been reported in patients with HIV,[87,88] strongyloidiasis was removed from the list of AIDS-defining illnesses by the Centers for Disease Control and Prevention. However, there are some conditions that co-segregate with HIV infection and are known to predispose to hyperinfection syndrome, including inanition and the use of steroids.[89] In fact, the list of immunosuppressive diseases associated with hyperinfection are unified by having corticosteroid as a common denominator of treatment.[89] However, *S. stercoralis* should still be searched for and promptly treated in HIV-infected patients with a suggestive geographic history.

HTLV-1 and Leukemia

Severe strongyloidiasis has often been reported to occur in some patients infected with both *S. stercoralis* and HTLV-1 (see Chapter 81).[90] An epidemiologic association between infection with HTLV-1 and strongyloidiasis was observed on the island of Okinawa[91] and in the West Indies.[92,93] It has been suggested that HTLV-1 infection may predispose to more severe strongyloidiasis and that infection with *S. stercoralis* may promote the progression of HTLV-1 infection to leukemia.[37] Several reports have shown that patients with HTLV-1 infection and no other known predisposition to precipitating factors have developed disseminated strongyloidiasis.[94] The nature of this association remains unexplained, but physicians should be aware of it, particularly when treating patients from areas of the world where there is an epidemiologic overlap between the two infections.

Acquired Immunoglobulinopathies and Immunodeficiencies

No cases of disseminated strongyloidiasis have been reported in children with congenital immunodeficiencies. However, a few adults with acquired agammaglobulinopathy have been reported to have persistent extraintestinal *S. stercoralis* infection refractory to pharmacologic treatment. Although these individuals were producing large numbers of larvae in the stools and the sputum, they neither had symptoms that could be ascribed to strongyloidiasis nor developed the disseminated hyperinfection syndrome.[35,36,95]

DIAGNOSIS

The diagnosis of strongyloidiasis is usually accomplished by the detection of larvae in the stool. However, in a majority of uncomplicated cases of strongyloidiasis, the intestinal worm load is often very low and larval output is minimal.[59,67] Eosinophilia is usually the only indication to the presence of *S. stercoralis* infection but is mild (5–15%) and nonspecific (see Chapter 131).[12,18,59,67,68] In more than two-thirds of cases, there are no more than 25 larvae per gram of stool.[59,67] Single examination of a stool sample has been shown to be negative in up to 70% of cases. Repeated examinations of stool specimens improve the chances of finding parasites;[96] in some studies, diagnostic sensitivity increases to 50% with three stool examinations and can approach 100% if seven serial stool samples are examined.[97] A number of techniques can be utilized to detect larvae in stool samples including direct smear of feces in saline/Lugol's iodine stain, Baermann concentration, formalin–ethyl acetate concentration, Harada–Mori filter paper culture, and nutrient agar plate cultures.[98–101]

The examination of duodenal aspirate is reportedly very sensitive; this invasive method is recommended only in children when it is necessary to achieve a rapid demonstration of parasites.[15,59] Microscopical examination of a single specimen of duodenal fluid was found to be more sensitive than wet mount analysis of stool samples for the detection of larvae, identifying 76% of patients; the parasite was found exclusively in duodenal fluid (and not in feces) in 67% of patients.[102] The "string test," a gelatin capsule containing a string swallowed by the patient and retrieved after a few hours, enjoyed a brief period of popularity three decades ago, but currently it is rarely if ever used.[103] Also, in some cases, histological examination of duodenal or jejunal biopsy specimens may reveal *S. stercoralis* embedded in the mucosa.[15]

Detection of *S. stercoralis* larvae is usually easier in cases of hyperinfection because large numbers of worms are involved in disseminated infections.[15,59,67] The larvae can be identified in wet preparations of sputum, bronchoalveolar lavage fluid, bronchial washings and brushings, lung biopsies, or examination of pleural fluid using either Gram, Papanicolaou or acid-fast (Auromine O and Kinyoun) staining procedures.[15,29,67] Findings on chest films are usually variable; pulmonary infiltrates, when present, may be alveolar or interstitial, diffuse or focal, uni- or bilateral.[104] Lung consolidation, occasional cavitation, and even abscess formation have also been reported.[56] Varying chest X-ray pictures are explained by different types of bacterial super-infection, particularly Gram-negative bacilli.[56,104]

A wide variety of immunodiagnostic assays have been tested over the past three decades with varying degrees of success. The long list includes skin testing with larval extracts, indirect immunofluorescence using fixed larvae, and radioallergosorbent testing for parasite-specific IgE.[15,59,67,68,105–107] The enzyme-linked immunosorbent assay (ELISA) test ("*Strongyloides* antibody") for detecting the serum IgG against a crude extract of the filariform larvae of *S. stercoralis* is currently the principal serologic test.[105,108,109] The sensitivity and specificity of this ELISA test can be improved if the serum samples are preincubated with *Onchocerca* antigens before testing.[110] The "*Strongyloides* antibody" test shows cross-reactivity with other helminths including filariae, *Ascaris lumbricoides* and schistosomes, but for the general population in developed countries these are rarely in the differential diagnosis of symptomatic strongyloidiasis.[15,59,67] However, this does not hold true with respect to armed forces personnel, international travelers, immigrants or residents of geohelminth endemic regions because they may have been exposed to "cross-reactive" antigens of other helminths on their trips to or residence within endemic areas. Furthermore, those helminths which contain "cross-reactive" antigens have the ability for long-term persistence within the host and the tendency to produce circulating antibodies which can be detected for many years after exposure. In comparison with an ELISA assay, a luciferase immunoprecipitation assay using a recombinant *Strongyloides* antigen has been shown to have enhanced diagnostic sensitivity and parasite specificity in serologic testing for *Strongloides* infections.[111] The major value in serology is the provision of a screening test which, if positive, can stimulate further searches for the parasite.[15,67] A positive serology does not distinguish prior from current infection.

In summary, stool examinations are currently the primary technique for the detection of *S. stercoralis*. If special techniques are not available, several specimens collected on different days should be examined if the diagnosis is strongly suspected. Serologic testing can help exclude latent chronic strongyloidiasis, especially in patients likely to receive corticosteroids.

TREATMENT AND PROGNOSIS

Nematodes do not replicate within their definitive hosts (with the very limited exceptions of *S. stercoralis* and *Capillaria philippinensis*; see Chapter 112). Therefore treatment that reduces the worm burden for most nematodes below the level at which clinical disease can develop is usually sufficient.[15,59,68] However, in *S. stercoralis* infection, only the complete eradication of parthenogenic adult females and autoinfective larvae removes the danger of potentially life-threatening hyperinfection.[15,59] Therefore, all patients with strongyloidiasis (even asymptomatic patients) require treatment.[86] The poor sensitivity of diagnostic stool examination makes it even more difficult to determine the effectiveness of the treatment, because a true cure cannot be ascertained based on a negative follow-up stool examination.[59,67] In some instances, serologic tests and changes in eosinophil counts may serve as useful markers of treatment success.[59,67] Generally, three anthelminthics have been used to treat strongyloidiasis with varying degrees of efficacy.[86]

Ivermectin

Ivermectin is derived from β-avermectins (monocyclic lactones) that are produced by *Streptomyces avermitilis*. The mode of action of this orally administered broad-spectrum anthelminthic is through selective binding with glutamate-gated chloride ion channels in nerve and muscle cells that causes hyperpolarization of the nerve and muscle cell membranes, resulting in paralysis and death of the worm.[86] The plasma half-life of this drug is 16 hours, and it is metabolized in the liver.[86] Ivermection is the drug of choice for the treatment of intestinal and disseminated strongyloidiasis.[112–117] Ivermectin has a cure rate of 64–100% after a single dose.[118] The standard dosage is 200 μg/kg per day, given orally for 2 days, for intestinal infections.[117] The same regimen is recommended for adults and children (>15 kg). Although adequate and well-controlled clinical studies have not been conducted to determine the optimal dosing regimen in immunocompromised patients or patients with the disseminated disease, it may be necessary to prolong (e.g., 7–10 days) or repeat the therapy.[117] Ivermectin administered as an enema may be of some benefit in patients with severe strongyloidiasis who are unable to absorb or tolerate oral therapy.[119]

Thiabendazole

Historically thiabendazole has been the drug of choice for the treatment of strongyloidiasis, despite frequent gastrointestinal and neuropsychological side effects and a high relapse rate. Thiabendazole has a cure rate of 50–94% and may not be effective in disease that is disseminated beyond the gastrointestinal tract.[20,117,118] Thiabendazole is a broad-spectrum drug for intestinal nematode and acts by inhibiting helminth-specific mitochondrial fumarate reductase. Thiabendazole is absorbed rapidly and peak plasma concentration is reached within 1–2 hours after the oral administration of a suspension.[86] The standard dosage is 50 mg/kg per day orally in two doses (maximum 3 g/day every 2 days; this dosage is likely to be toxic and may have to be decreased).[117] Pediatric dosages are the same as adult dosages.[117]

Albendazole

This drug is an orally administered broad-spectrum anthelminthic with variable therapeutic efficacy. It is poorly absorbed from the gastrointestinal tract because of its low aqueous solubility, and it has a cure rate of 36–75%.[118,120] Maximal plasma concentrations of albendazole sulfoxide are achieved typically 2–5 hours after dosing.[86] The principal mode of action for albendazole is by its inhibitory effect on tubulin polymerization, which results in the loss of cytoplasmic microtubules.[86] The standard dosage for adults (>60 kg) is 400 mg orally after meals twice a day for 7 days and at least 7–10 days for hyperinfection; for children (<60 kg), 15 mg/kg per day orally after meals in two doses for 3 days, 7–10 days for hyperinfection (maximum total daily dosage 800 mg).[117]

For hyperinfection strongyloidiaisis, the concurrent discontinuation or tapering of corticosteroids is necessary, as is appropriate antibiotic/antifungal treatment of the infections that usually accompany extraintestinal strongyloidiasis. Even with this regimen, more than two-thirds of the patients with dissemination succumb to disease.

PREVENTION AND CONTROL

The strategies for the control of strongyloidiasis in endemic areas are similar to those developed for the control of other geohelminthiases. Appropriate methods of human fecal sanitation and sewage disposal and the use of shoes are of paramount importance. For at-risk individuals, virtually all cases of fatal hyperinfection and dissemination could be prevented by suspecting, detecting, and treating chronic well-regulated infections in patients who are candidates for immunosuppression, particularly from any form of corticosteroid therapy. Unexplained eosinophilia (see Chapter 131), prior, even remote, histories of potential exposures to contaminated soil in *Strongyloides* endemic regions, and/or compatible cutaneous or gastrointestinal symptoms, although often nonspecific, of chronic strongyloidiasis should prompt consideration of underlying strongyloidiasis prior to corticosteroid treatments.

The principal transmission mode of *S. stercoralis* is that of a geohelminthiasis, through the contamination of soil with infected feces. In ordinary hygienic conditions, human-to-human transmission does not appear to occur. Thus, the infection can be prevented by implementing public health measures aimed at ensuring proper disposal and treatment of excrement and by avoiding skin contact with contaminated soil. In institutional facilities caring for those with fecal incontinence or contamination (e.g., people with mental disabilities), filariform *Strongyloides* larvae in feces can cause nosocomial or intrainstitutional spread of infection.

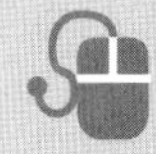

Access the complete reference list online at
http://www.expertconsult.com

Access the complete reference list online at http://www.expertconsult.com

CHAPTER 118

Introduction to Tapeworm Infections

Herbert B. Tanowitz • Murray Wittner • A. Clinton White, Jr

Tapeworm infections are among the oldest recognized afflictions of humanity.[1,2] Phylogenetic studies[2] suggest that the ancestors of modern humans may have acquired taeniid tapeworm infections about 2 million years ago, from the animals they consumed, and eventually passed the infection on to bovine and porcine hosts about 10 000 years ago.

The Cestoda, or tapeworms, are a class in the phylum Platyhelminthes (flatworms) and except for the ciliated embryo of the order Pseudophyllidea are exclusively parasitic for their entire life.[3] Adult stage tapeworms live exclusively in the alimentary canal, including occasionally the bile ducts, gallbladder, and pancreatic duct, and infect all vertebrate classes, although members of the subclass Cestodaria and several neotenic species attain adulthood in invertebrates (oligochaetes). However, cestode larvae often infect both vertebrates and invertebrates.

With few exceptions, the characteristic feature of adult tapeworms is their elongated (i.e., tapelike) dorsoventrally flattened structure. Their outer covering, or tegument, allows the passage of both nutritive and waste material. The absorptive surface of the tegument is amplified by the formation of many cytoplasmic extensions termed microtriches, which function like microvilli of enterocytes to increase the absorptive surface area. Tapeworms actively take up and utilize carbohydrates from the intestinal lumen as their major, if not sole, energy source, with the production largely of lactate, proprionate, and succinate as end products. There is active uptake of α-D,L-amino acids across the tegumental membrane.[4]

Of the various orders of cestodes, there are two that include important parasites of humans and domestic and marine mammals. Their adult stage resides in the lumen of the small intestine and the larval stage in various tissues of the intermediate host. The order Pseudophyllidea is characterized by the presence of a scolex, or attachment organ, containing two sucking grooves. Examples of this group are members of the genus *Diphyllobothrium*, including *D. latum* and *D. pacificum* (fish tapeworms), and worms that infect humans only at the larval stage such as *Spirometra* (i.e., sparganosis). The order Cyclophyllidea, which includes all other tapeworms that parasitize humans, is characterized by a scolex that possesses four suckers. This group includes the genus *Taenia*, examples of which are the beef and pork tapeworms, *Hymenolepis*, *Bertiella*, *Dipylidium*, *Mesocestoides*, *Raillietina*, *Inermicapsifer*, and *Echinococcus*.

The life cycles of the Pseudophyllidea involve a minimum of three hosts. Those of the Cyclophyllidea generally require two, although in some species the definitive host can also serve as the intermediate host. Medically important tapeworms range in size from the minute dog tapeworm, *Echinococcus granulosus*, which generally consists of a scolex and three or four segments, to *Taenia saginata*, which may reach 20–30 feet (6–9 meters) in length.

Adult tapeworms typically possess an anterior scolex or head that may be modified or adorned with structures or organelles that serve as organs for attachment to the small intestinal mucosa. In the Pseudophyllidea, the structures that function for attachment are termed bothria, which are two shallow sucking grooves whose gripping power is feeble.[5] Some species of Cyclophyllidea, in addition to having four sucking disks or acetabula, possess hooklets that encircle the top of the scolex or are mounted on a protrusion known as the rostellum (***Fig. 118.1***). In some species, such as *Hymenolepis*, the rostellum is protrusible. The distal portion of the scolex, termed the "neck," is an area of intense metabolic activity, which in most groups of tapeworms is the zone from which new segments or proglottids proliferate and form a chain of proglottids or strobila. Clinically, the scolex is significant since therapy is aimed at its destruction or elimination, inasmuch as failure to do so will result in regrowth of the entire tapeworm. Usually the most proximal proglottids are immature and contain only the earliest rudiments of the organs that are present in the mature proglottids. More distal are mature proglottids that contain one set, and in some species two complete sets, of both male and female sex organs such that tapeworms are hermaphroditic. The distal most segments are filled with eggs and are termed "gravid proglottids," in which in cyclophyllidean cestodes the sex organs have atrophied, leaving the segment occupied largely by a uterus filled with eggs.[6]

Except for the coracidium, the tapeworm egg is the only stage that interacts with the external environment. For diagnostic purposes, eggs are characteristic. In members of the genus *Diphyllobothrium*, eggs are discharged through a muscular uterine pore and, therefore, they are regularly found in the feces. However, in many cyclophyllidean species, the gravid proglottids split and the eggs are released through rents in the proglottids. The eggs of other tapeworms, such as *Hymenolepis nana* and *H. diminuta*, are found in the stool after disintegration of the gravid prognostics, whereas those of the beef tapeworm, *T. saginata*, are often not found in the stool because they are passed out within intact segments. Consequently, a "Scotch tape" preparation, as used for diagnosing pinworm infection, is more reliable in finding *T. saginata* eggs. Eggs of the diphyllobothriid tapeworms are operculate, resembling those of many trematodes, and hatch in water to release a free-swimming larva, the coracidium. Cyclophyllidean tapeworm eggs all contain a fully developed hexacanth (six-hooked) embryo, the oncosphere. The embryonic envelope that surrounds this oncosphere comprises what is generally referred to as the egg shell, and its morphology is often diagnostic of the species. With the single exception of *H. nana*, tapeworms that infect humans require one or more intermediate hosts to complete their life histories. The life cycle of diphyllobothriid cestodes involves two or more intermediate hosts. First stage larvae (coracidia) are ingested by water fleas or copepods, and develop into procercoid larvae in the body cavity of these hosts which, while retaining their embryonic six hooklets, show evidence of developing bothria. When infected copepods are ingested by appropriate piscine hosts, the procercoid enters the musculature of the fish, where it becomes a plerocercoid or sparganum larva. Interestingly, the latter may have a number of transfer or paratenic hosts. Thus, a plerocercoid that has developed in a minnow may next parasitize a somewhat larger fish, and may even pass through a series of such transitory domiciliary

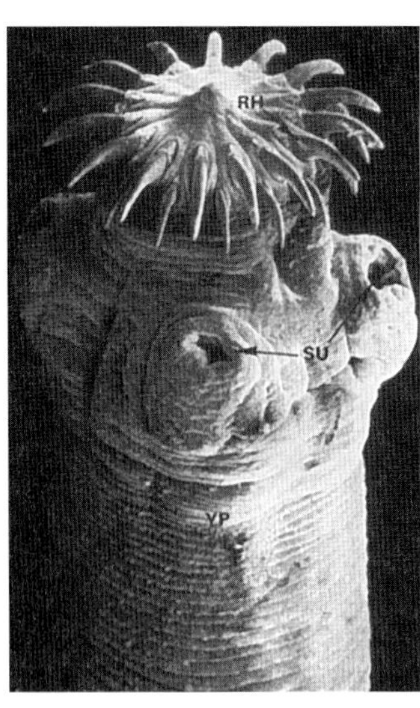

Figure 118.1 *Taenia solium* scolex. RH, rostellum; SU, sucking disks, or acetabula; YP, young proglottids.

relationships until its final piscine host is ingested by a suitable mammal, in which it will become an adult.

Some cestodes infect humans in the larval stage.[7,8] These larval stage infections are primarily zoonoses for which humans are incidental or dead-end hosts. For example, sparganosis is caused by infection with the plerocercoid (sparganum) of *Spirometra mansonoides*, which migrates through various tissues. Other tapeworms can infect humans in both the adult and larval stages.[9] For example, humans are the definitive hosts for the adult intestinal *T. solium* tapeworm; and human ingestion of *T. solium* ova may result in cysticercosis, a larval form. As another example, *H. nana* forms tapeworms in the intestines and cysticercoids in the intestinal walls of individual human hosts. The cysticerci of *T. solium* and *T. saginata* contain only a single invaginated scolex. By contrast, cysticerci of *T. multiceps* and species of *Echinococcus* contain multiple infectious larval forms such that when ingested by a suitable definitive host, large numbers of adult worms may be produced.

Adult tapeworm infections may persist for many years or even for the life of the host. During this period, tapeworm infections, usually well tolerated, may be relatively asymptomatic or cause persistent symptoms and deprive the host of important and/or essential nutriment. Infections with larval stage parasites often cause serious or fatal disease and can be of great economic consequences. Especially in endemic countries, these serious larval infections have often gone undiagnosed.[9]

The diagnosis of tapeworm infections is improving. While examination of stools for parasite life stages (e.g., eggs, proglottids) is important, detection of parasites by immunodiagnostic and molecular approaches promises improved diagnosis of both adult and larval infections.[10] The diagnosis of larval tapeworm infections has been markedly enhanced by imaging techniques including magnetic resonance imaging (MRI) and computed tomography (CT) of the brain for neurocysticercosis and sparganosis.[9,11,12] Similarly, CT, MRI, and ultrasonography have become routine diagnostic procedures for imaging of hydatid disease of the liver and lung.

The management of tapeworm infections is undergoing change (see Chapters 119–121). The medical treatment of both adult tapeworm and larvae with albendazole and praziquantel has become an important adjunct to surgery and in some instances has supplanted invasive procedures.

The development of safe, effective, and inexpensive vaccines to protect against several of the economically important tapeworm infections has been an important area of investigation.[13–15] Recombinant oncosphere-subunit peptide vaccine candidates have been produced or identified for use against several important taeniid cestodes, including *T. saginata* and *T. solium*, and several of these vaccines are undergoing clinical trials.

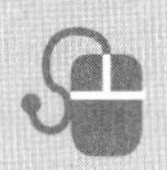

Access the complete reference list online at
http://www.expertconsult.com

Access the complete reference list online at http://www.expertconsult.com

CHAPTER 119

Cysticercosis

Hector H. Garcia • Christina M. Coyle • A. Clinton White, Jr

NEUROCYSTICERCOSIS

INTRODUCTION

Cysticercosis is caused by the larval stage of the tapeworm *Taenia solium*. The ancient Greeks identified larval forms in meat, which they termed cysticerci (meaning "cyst tail").[1] By the early twentieth century, large case series had been published, identifying many clinical manifestations of cysticercosis. Only in the 1980s with the availability of neuroimaging scans did neurocysticercosis (NCC) begin to be recognized as a major cause of neurologic disease. When computed tomography (CT) scans were used, many patients with seizure disorders or hydrocephalus were recognized as having NCC. NCC is a major cause of neurologic disease worldwide.

THE AGENT

Taenia solium has separate adult (intestinal tapeworm) (see Chapter 121) and larval (metacestode or cysticercus) forms. Humans can host both forms of the parasite. The *T. solium* life cycle (***Fig. 119.1***) includes two obligate hosts, each with a different form of the parasite. In the normal life cycle, the larval form (cysticercus) is found primarily in muscles of pigs, the intermediate host. Pigs ingest the ova or proglottids from the tapeworm carrier. Humans are the obligate definitive host for the adult tapeworm form. Humans become infected with the tapeworm (taeniasis) by ingesting undercooked pork infected with *T. solium* cysticerci. After ingestion, the scolex evaginates, converting to the adult tapeworm. The scolex is ~1 mm in diameter and contains four suckers and two rows of hooklets, which facilitate attachment to the small intestines. New proglottids arise at the base of the scolex, and the older proglottids form a chain that can reach a length of up to 15 feet (4.5 m), usually 6–12 feet (1.8–3.6 m).

Human cysticercosis follows ingestion of eggs from a tapeworm carrier (***Fig. 119.1***). Close personal contact with a tapeworm carrier is noted in most cases. Eggs hatch in the upper intestines, releasing oncospheres (invasive larvae) that penetrate the intestinal mucosa using their hooklets and excretory proteases,[2,3] enter the bloodstream, and migrate to the tissues, where they mature into cysticerci. Cysticerci may lodge in skeletal and cardiac muscle, subcutaneous tissue, and even lung tissue, but, in most of these locations, cysticerci cause few symptoms and spontaneously degenerate, which may lead to formation of calcified granulomas. Most disease, NCC, results from the minority of parasites that invade the central nervous system (CNS), including the brain, cerebral ventricles, or eye. While cysticercosis is not acquired directly from eating pork, tapeworm carriers can infect themselves, probably by the fecal–oral route. The fact that pork ingestion is not the direct cause of human cysticercosis is illustrated by cases of cysticercosis that occurred among an orthodox Jewish community in New York City and vegetarians in India.[4–6]

EPIDEMIOLOGY

Definitive diagnosis requires neuroimaging studies not widely available to populations at highest risk. Serodiagnosis has been plagued by poor sensitivity and problems with specificity. Thus, the importance of this infection has been significantly underestimated.[7]

T. solium is endemic in all areas of the world where pigs are raised under conditions in which they have access to human fecal material. Highly endemic areas are in Latin America, Eastern Europe, sub-Saharan Africa, and India.[8,9] NCC is also recognized in Indonesia, Southeast Asia, China, and Korea.[10] Occasional cases are still acquired in eastern and southern Europe. The burden of disease began to be appreciated after the introduction of imaging studies. For example, introduction of CT scanning was followed by a fourfold increase in the number of cases of NCC diagnosed among Latin American immigrants in Los Angeles.[11] Subsequent studies from Latin America documented that up to half of patients with adult-onset seizures had evidence of NCC by neuroimaging studies.[12,13] Population-based surveys in rural villages have documented a high prevalence of infection throughout Latin America, with rates of seizure disorders ranging from 11 to 30/1000 and CT abnormalities consistent with NCC noted in up to 70% of those with seizures.[14–23] Similar studies demonstrated NCC in a high proportion of African patients with seizures, with the disease prevalent throughout sub-Saharan Africa.[24–29] However, CT-based diagnosis of NCC is not widely available in Africa.[7] Consequently, there is a lack of reliable data on the disease burden of cysticercosis. Studies estimating the economic impact due to NCC from sub-Saharan Africa are limited, but suggest that DALYs lost due to the disease are significant and may exceed estimates for some other neglected tropical diseases (NTDs).[24,30] Only recently, the World Health Organization included cysticercosis as part of a neglected zoonosis subgroup for its 2008–15 strategic plan for the control of NTDs.[7,31]

NCC is also prevalent in southern Asia.[32–35] When neuroimaging studies were performed on patients in India with seizures, most patients had focal abnormalities.[36–38] Single enhancing CT lesions were frequently attributed to tuberculosis or to the effects of seizures. However, excisional biopsies demonstrated that nearly all showed histopathologic evidence of NCC.[39] For example, over half of 401 patients presenting with a single enhancing lesion were diagnosed with NCC.[40] NCC is the cause of nearly one-third of all cases of epilepsy in both urban and rural regions of southern India (***Fig. 119.2***).[32–34,41]

THE DISEASE

The clinical presentation, pathogenesis, management, and prognosis of *T. solium* cysticercotic infections vary markedly depending on the location,

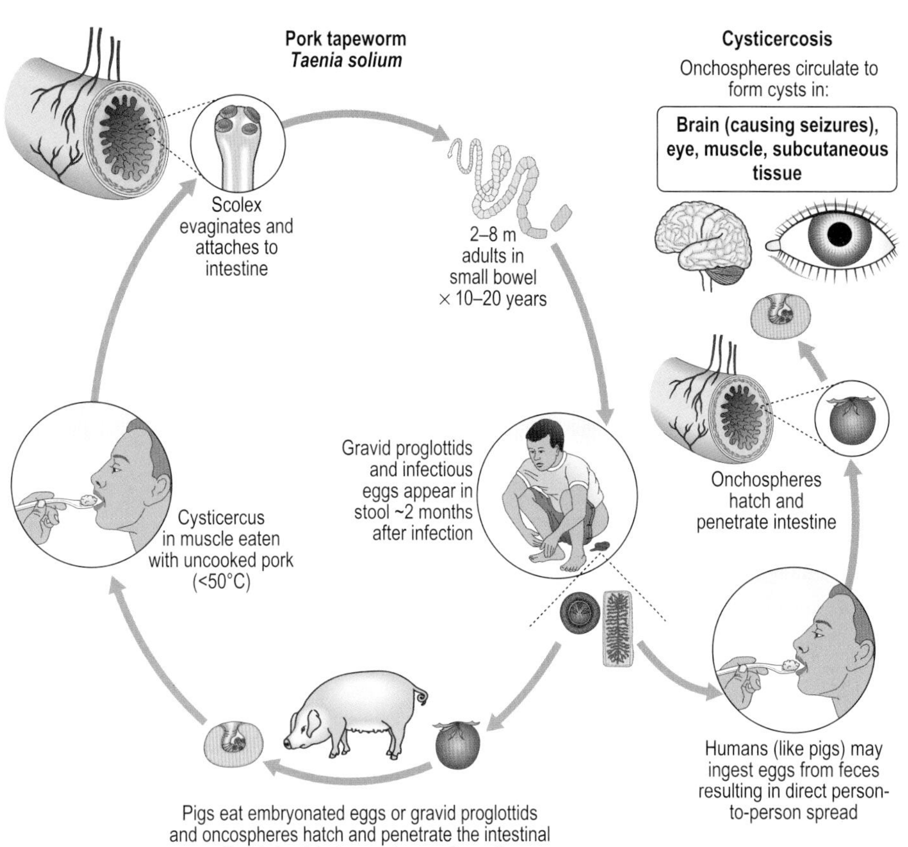

Figure 119.1 Life cycle of *Taenia solium* and cysticercosis.

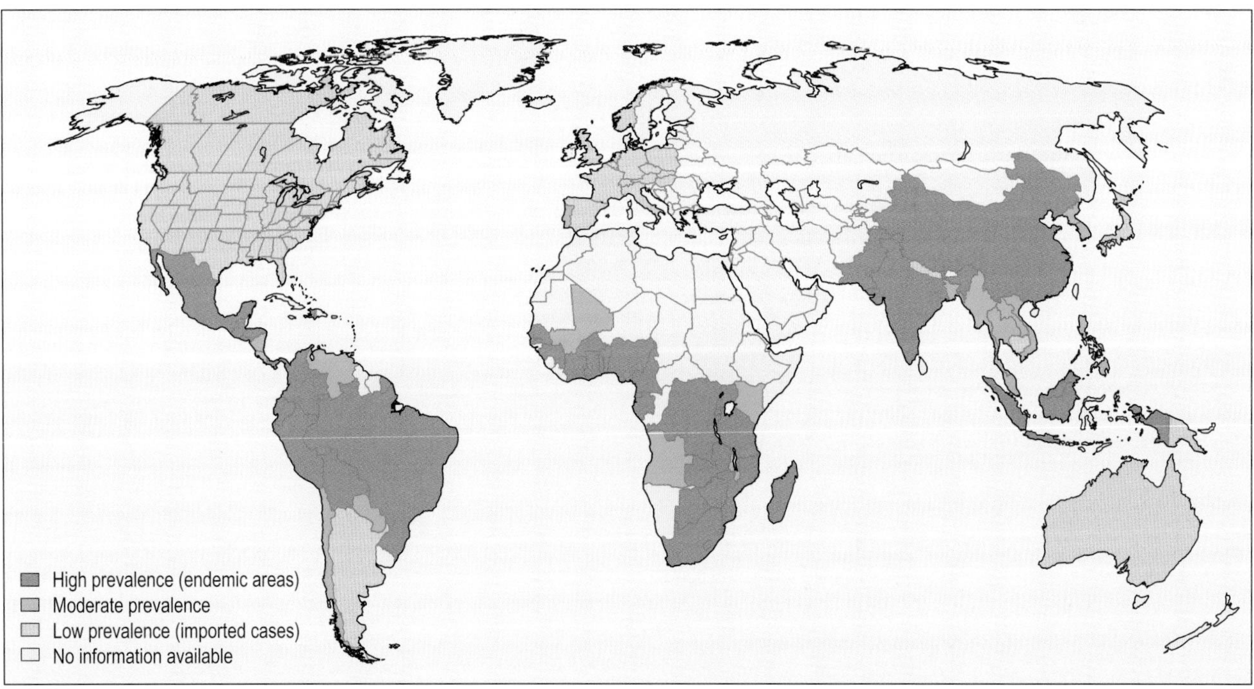

Figure 119.2 Geographic distribution of *Taenia solium*.

number of cysticerci, and the associated host response. NCC should be regarded as a spectrum of illnesses rather than a single disease entity. NCC is typically separated into parenchymal and extraparenchymal disease. Involvement of the subarachnoid space, ventricles, spinal cord, and eye is considered extraparenchymal. Many patients, particularly those with large numbers of parasites, will present with mixed forms.

Clinically, parenchymal NCC usually presents with seizures and carries a favorable prognosis. Seizures can occur early in the disease in the setting of intense inflammation associated with viable or degenerating cysts or in patients with calcified brain lesions observed on CT scans that are typical for NCC. In population-based studies calcified lesions on CT are more common than viable cysts and are more prevalent in patients with epilepsy

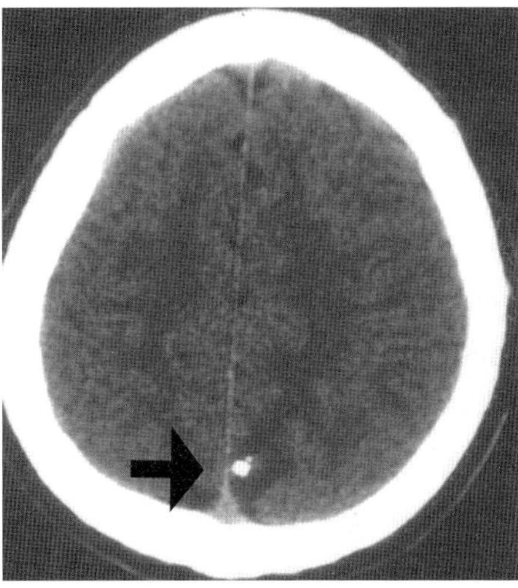

Figure 119.3 Calcified cysticercal lesion with surrounding edema revealed by computed tomography scan (arrow).

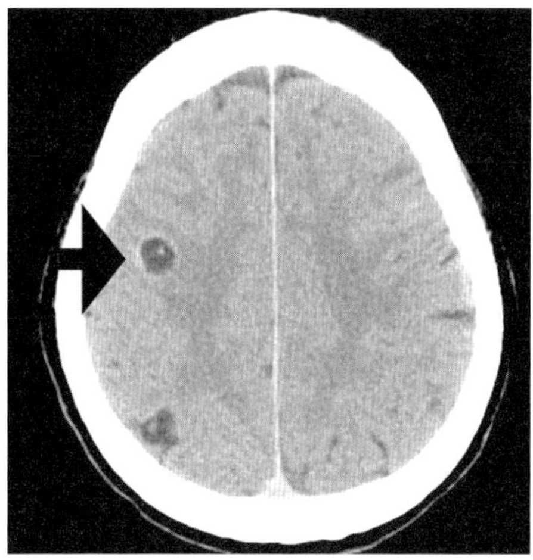

Figure 119.4 Parenchymal cysticercus revealed as a ring-enhancing lesion (arrow).

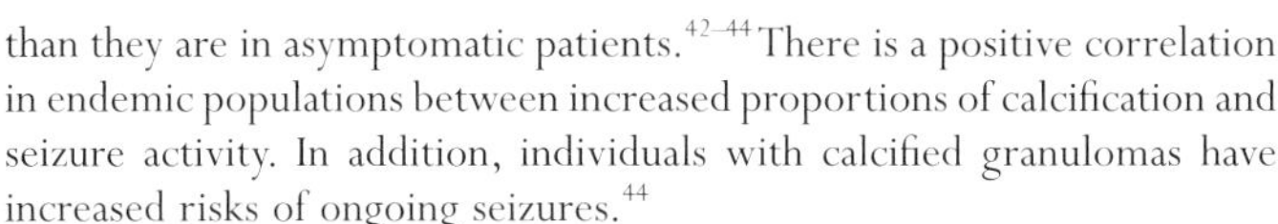

than they are in asymptomatic patients.[42–44] There is a positive correlation in endemic populations between increased proportions of calcification and seizure activity. In addition, individuals with calcified granulomas have increased risks of ongoing seizures.[44]

Most severe or fatal cases of NCC are due to extraparenchymal disease.[45,46] Subarachnoid and ventricular disease are often complicated by increased intracranial pressure. Thus, patients often present with symptoms of increased intracranial pressure.

Parenchymal Neurocysticercosis

Parenchymal Calcifications

Parenchymal brain calcifications are often the only imaging finding in NCC. Calcifications are typically 2–10 mm in diameter, well defined, and solid (*Fig. 119.3*). Such lesions likely represent fibrotic reactions to prior infection that have calcified. Patients frequently present with seizures.[47] Few have focal abnormalities on electroencephalogram (EEG) studies.[48,49] Patients with calcifications are more likely to have recurrences of seizures if antiepileptic drugs are withdrawn, and usually should be treated with antiepileptic therapy indefinitely.[50,51]

Magnetic resonance imaging (MRI) studies have documented that patients with NCC, seizures, and calcified lesions often have associated contrast enhancement and edema.[43,44,52,53] There is increasing evidence that perilesional edema, which occurs episodically, is associated with seizures.[53] The natural history or pathophysiology of perilesional edema is not yet known; but it appears that it recurs and repeated episodes tend to be associated with the same lesions in a patient. In a prospective nested case-control study, 110 patients with seizures or headaches and calcified lesions in an endemic region were followed for recurrent seizures. Of those with recurrent seizures, perilesional edema was noted on MRI in 50% of cases as opposed to 9% of asymptomatic matched controls.[53] This study suggests that perilesional edema is a common, potentially preventable cause of seizures in endemic regions. There is no evidence that these lesions are associated with viable parasites. Instead, enhancement may result from breakdown of the calcified granulomas with antigen release resulting in restimulation of host inflammation.[52]

Parenchymal Cystic and Enhancing Lesions

Parenchymal infection is the most common form of NCC. The vast majority of patients with symptomatic parenchymal NCC and seizures have neuroradiologic evidence of parasite degeneration and/or host inflammation such as edema or contrast enhancement (*Fig. 119.4*).[54] Symptoms likely result from the host inflammatory response, which will eventually subside. By contrast, noninflamed cysts cause few symptoms, even when they are numerous.[55] Thus, symptomatic infection likely occurs when one or more cysticerci can no longer control the host inflammatory and immune responses.

Seizures are the principal clinical manifestation of parenchymal infection.[56] Seizures are often generalized or focal with secondary generalization, but may also be focal.[48,56,57] EEG studies for patients with enhancing lesions may reveal focal abnormalities, particularly in those with single inflamed cysticerci.[48,49] Seizures associated with parenchymal cysts are likely caused by parenchymal inflammation. Seizures can usually be controlled during treatment with antiepileptic drugs and often resolve after normalization of imaging studies as the inflammation subsides.[56–58] Relapse is, however, frequent.

Some patients present with large numbers of inflamed cysticerci, with diffuse cerebral edema, raised intracranial pressure, seizures, and altered mental status. This is termed cysticercal encephalitis.[59,60] This form is more common in children than adults and more common in women than men. Treatment is mainly directed at controlling the cerebral edema.

Extraparenchymal Neurocysticercosis

Ventricular Neurocysticercosis

Between 10% and 20% of patients with NCC have cysticerci in the ventricles.[61] Cysticerci can obstruct cerebrospinal fluid (CSF) flow, causing hydrocephalus, and may be found in any of the ventricles. In most cases, the cysticerci cause symptoms while still viable.[62] Since viable cysticerci have thin walls with cyst fluid isodense with CSF, they may be difficult to detect. CT scanning usually only shows evidence of obstructive hydrocephalus or distortion of the shape of the involved ventricle. Intraventricular cysticerci are frequently visible on MRI (*Fig. 119.5*).[63,64] These patients may also have parenchymal cysticerci.[65]

Patients with ventricular NCC present with symptoms or signs of raised intracranial pressure. Symptoms include nausea or vomiting, altered mental status, visual changes, or dizziness. The onset varies and can be abrupt, intermittent, or gradual. Cysticerci may form a ball valve in the foramina that may come and go with position changes. Cysticerci in the fourth ventricle have been associated with acute obstructive hydrocephalus that can lead to drop attacks.

Subarachnoid Neurocysticercosis

Cysticerci in the fissures (especially the Sylvian fissure) can enlarge to several centimeters in diameter, termed giant cysticerci.[66] Isolated cysticerci in fissures often have a similar prognosis to parenchymal cysts. However, the cysts may be larger, and resolution in response to chemotherapy less reliable. In some cases, however, the cysts may enlarge,

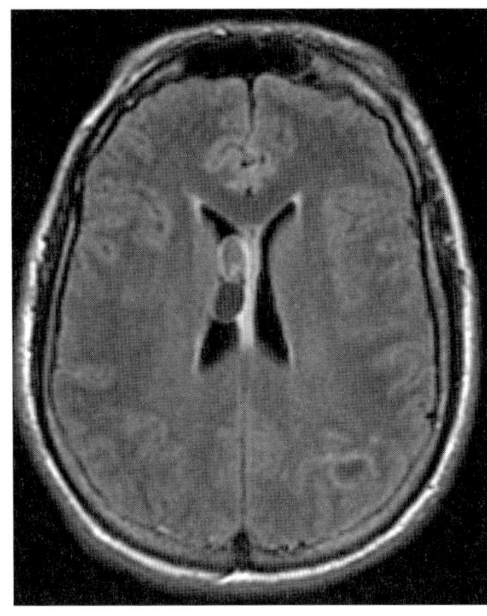

Figure 119.5 Two cysticerci in the lateral ventricle revealed by magnetic resonance imaging.

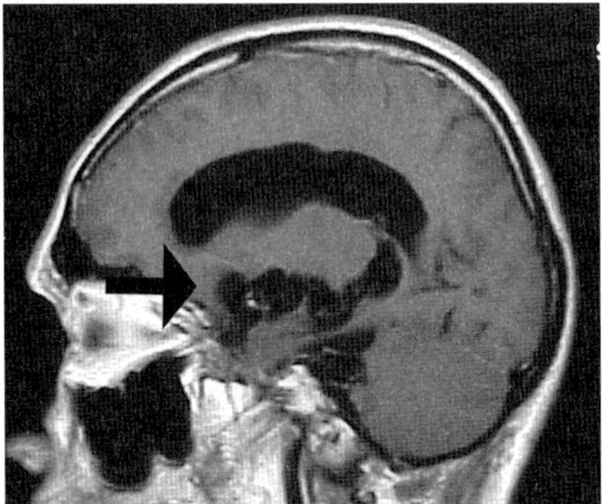

Figure 119.6 Cysticerci in the subarachnoid space (arrow) of the basilar cisterns revealed by magnetic resonance imaging.

causing mass effects such as midline shift. Frequently, giant cysticerci are accompanied by cysticerci in the parenchyma or basilar cisterns. Giant cysticerci are readily visualized by CT or MRI, but the accompanying basilar cysticerci may not be seen as easily.

Cysticercosis of the basilar cisterns carries a grave prognosis. Numerous cysticerci may fill the basilar cisterns (*Fig. 119.6*). Patients so affected can present with communicating hydrocephalus due to CSF outflow obstruction or arachnoiditis. Basilar arachnoiditis appears on imaging studies as focal or diffuse meningeal enhancement or vasculitis and can be complicated by strokes due to vasculitis.[67,68] Cerebrovascular complications of NCC include cerebral infarction, transient ischemic attacks, and brain hemorrhage.[65,67,69] The most common mechanisms by which NCC produces cerebrovascular disease are related to cerebral arteritis, mainly in those individuals with subarachnoid cysticercosis. The frequency of cerebral arteritis in subarachnoid cysticercosis seems to be higher than previously reported, and middle-size vessel involvement is a common finding.[67] The basilar arachnoiditis appears to play an important role in the pathogenesis of this severe form of the disease.

Spinal Neurocysticercosis

Only ~1% of patients with NCC have recognized spinal involvement.[70–72] Most cases of spinal NCC result from cysticerci in the subarachnoid space.[45] Initially, spinal subarachnoid cysticerci are free-floating and may move between levels. When cysticerci degenerate, they eventually become fixed at one level. The accompanying inflammation may cause mass effect with obstruction of flow on myelogram. Clinical manifestations include radicular paresthesias or pain, which may progress to myelopathy with bowel or bladder incontinence and paraparesis. Intramedullary cysterci, although rare, can present with cord compression from mass effect or accompanying inflammations.

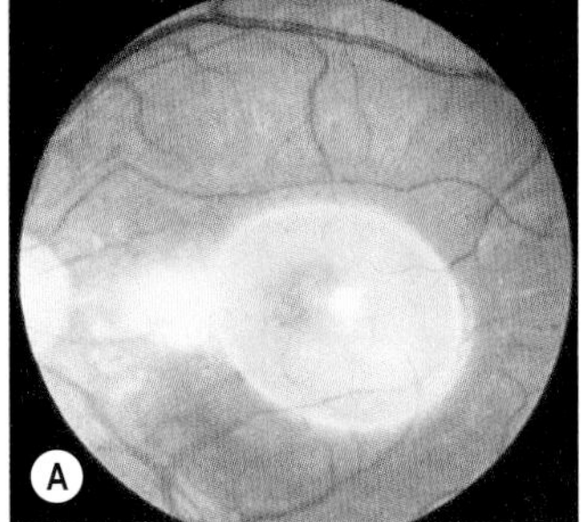

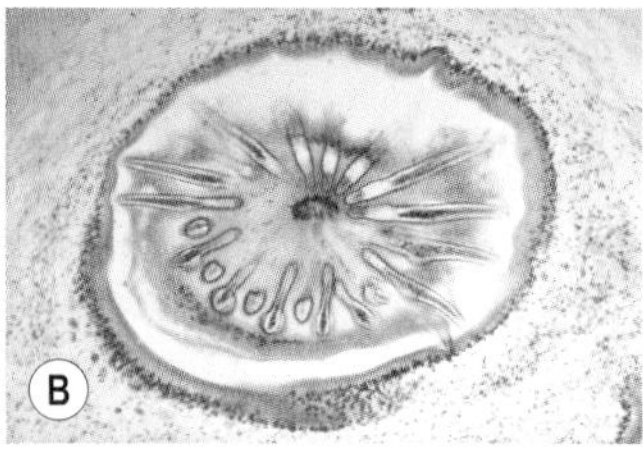

Figure 119.7 **(A)** Subretinal cysticercosis at the macular area with overlying retinal edema. **(B)** Cysticercosis of the eye. ((**A**) Courtesy of Robert Ritch, MD, New York Eye and Ear Infirmary, New York, NY. Reproduced from Teekhasaenee C, Ritch R, Kanchanaranya C. Ocular parasitic infection in Thailand. Rev Infect Dis. 1986;8:350–356.)

Other Forms of Cysticercosis

Cysticercosis can involve the orbit and/or eye. The most common ocular presentation is ptosis related to involvement of the extraocular muscles.[73,74] Ocular involvement is usually subretinal, but can be intravitreal or subconjunctival (*Fig. 119.7*).[74–77] Patients may present with altered vision. Subconjunctival cysts may spontaneously extrude. Intraocular disease usually requires surgical removal.

Cysticerci may involve the muscles but only rarely cause more than minor symptoms. Cysticerci can involve the subcutaneous tissues, where they present as palpable, painless, and mobile cystic lesions that can be confused with sebaceous cysts. As cysticerci degenerate, lesions may become firm nodules that may calcify or later resolve. Subcutaneous disease is rarely noted in the western hemisphere, but is commonly noted in Asia.

Mixed Forms

Clinical cases, especially those involving large numbers of cysticerci, often include more than one of the preceding forms.

Other Syndromes

Headaches are common among patients with NCC and may be seen with parenchymal, ventricular, or cisternal NCC. Headaches may be hemicranial or bilateral.[78,79] The headaches can be confused with uncomplicated migraines or tension headaches. The pathogenesis is also variable. In some cases, headache is the initial symptom of raised intracranial pressure. The association of parenchymal NCC with migraine-like headaches suggests vascular involvement.[78]

Neurocognitive defects have been described with cysticercosis.[80] Infected children are thought to suffer from learning disabilities.[81]

Psychiatric manifestations of NCC, such as depression and psychosis, have been described.[35,82,83] However, it is not clear whether these manifestations were due to NCC or whether these conditions predisposed patients to increased rates of infection. By contrast, acute alterations of mental status usually reflect ongoing seizures or hydrocephalus. In our experience, altered mental status that does not resolve after a reasonable postictal period commonly is usually due to hydrocephalus and is a clue that the patient needs to be evaluated for emergency neurosurgery.

PATHOGENESIS AND IMMUNITY

Cysticerci reach their final size within a few weeks of invasion into the CNS. However, there is a period of several years between infection and onset of symptoms.[35,84] Once a cysticercus has reached the parenchyma of the brain, it undergoes stages of evolution.[85] The vesicular stage is characterized by a cyst with a translucent vesicular wall, clear fluid, and a viable invaginated scolex with little host inflammatory reaction. In autopsy studies of individuals who died of other causes, cysticerci have an appearance similar to viable cysticerci from pigs.[86] In contrast, cysticerci from patients who died with seizures demonstrate a prominent inflammatory infiltrate. After a period estimated to last 2–3 years, the cysticercus loses the ability to control the host inflammatory response. The parasites elaborate a number of molecules that modulate or suppress the host inflammatory and immune response.[87] For example, parasite excretory proteases cleave CD4 from the surface of host lymphocytes, degrading immunoglobulin and cytokines such as interleukin (IL)-2.[88] Parasites also produce prostaglandins that modulate the host response.[89] Parasite secretory protease inhibitors block complement activation and decrease cytokine production and leukocyte chemotaxis.[90–92]

By contrast, an animal model has demonstrated that seizures are induced by the host granulomatous response rather than the parasite *per se*.[93] Clinical studies suggest that cysticerci lose their ability to control the host response and are attacked by host inflammatory cells composed of mononuclear cells, with variable numbers of eosinophils and neutrophils.[94,95] The tissues pass through a series of stages of inflammation.[96,97] These cells elaborate type 1 cytokines such as IL-12, interferon-γ, and IL-2, as well as variable amounts of type 2 cytokines (e.g., IL-4 and IL-5).[94,95,98] Proinflammatory cytokines such as IL-1, tumor necrosis factor (TNF)-α, and IL-6 are also found in the CSF from active cases.[99,100] The wall gradually degenerates, cyst fluid increases in density and agglutinates, and the cyst cavity is invaded by inflammatory cells. Radiographic examination reveals cystic lesions with edema and enhancement at this stage and seizures are common. As the cyst continues to degenerate, it becomes encased by fibrosis with collapse of the cyst cavity. The fibrotic granuloma may calcify. Even calcified lesions can be associated with inflammation. Parts of the degenerating cysticercus (e.g., hooklets) may still be identified in the calcified lesion.[101]

Imaging Findings

Similar steps in progression have been noted on neuroimaging studies.[102,103] A viable cysticercus demonstrates the cyst cavity as an area of decreased density, isodense with CSF. The scolex may be seen as a mural nodule. The cyst wall is thin and isodense with brain parenchyma and lacks surrounding edema or contrast enhancement. When the cysticercus becomes inflamed, the cyst wall density increases. The cyst wall may enhance with contrast, and there may be associated edema and/or enhancement in the surrounding brain parenchyma (see ***Fig. 119.4***). Subsequently, the cyst fluid increases in density. As the cysticercus becomes fibrotic or collapses, neuroimaging studies reveal an area of focal enhancement, suggestive of a granuloma. Finally, the calcified stage is defined by focal areas of calcification. The calcifications are well demarcated, typically several millimeters in diameter. Edema and contrast enhancement often surround calcified lesions associated with symptoms (see ***Fig. 119.3***).[44,53] Breakdown of the calcified granulomas is thought to trigger the host inflammation.

Cysticerci within the cerebral ventricles initially float in the ventricular fluid (see ***Fig. 119.5***). They can become lodged particularly in the foramina and cause mechanical obstruction of CSF flow.[104] This type of obstruction is usually due to viable cysticerci.[62] Inflammation may cause cysticerci to adhere to the ventricular walls or the inflammation may block CSF flow directly (especially in the aqueduct of Sylvius).

Cysticerci in basilar cisterns are associated with subarachnoid cysticercosis (see ***Fig. 119.6***). Some of these cysticerci may enlarge to sizes up to 10 cm in diameter and may form clusters. The older term racemose cysticercosis was used to describe clusters, which lack a scolex, but many of the so-called racemose cysticerci actually contain remnants of a scolex.

Subarachnoid NCC is usually accompanied by a prominent basilar arachnoiditis causing meningeal signs, communicating hydrocephalus, and/or vasculitis.[68] Hydrocephalus is thought to result from CSF outflow obstruction or blocked ventricular outflow.[104] Arachnoiditis often results in vasculitis, which may present as lacunar infarctions or as large-vessel strokes.[67,105]

Cysticerci within the brain parenchyma typically reach a diameter of 1–2 cm. By contrast, cysticerci within the subarachnoid space (and particularly those in the Sylvian fissure) may expand to sizes up to 10 cm in diameter. These enlarged cysticerci may cause mass effects.[66,106] The mass effects are especially prominent when the cysticerci are inflamed either from spontaneous degeneration or after drug treatment.

DIAGNOSIS

Diagnosis of NCC is problematic. The main clinical presentations (e.g., seizures or hydrocephalus) are shared with a wide spectrum of other diseases. Furthermore, the location of the parasites within the CNS limits the usefulness of traditional parasitologic studies. Immunoblot assays, with good specificity, are not widely available, especially in endemic areas. Neuroimaging studies (e.g., CT and MRI) have led to a dramatic increase in case identification. Neuroimaging studies are the mainstay of diagnosis.[107] CT scanning is more sensitive than MRI at detecting calcifications and is usually used initially.[64,108] MRI is better at detecting cysticerci in the ventricles and subarachnoid space.[63,64,108,109] MRI may also reveal the pathognomic scolex, which is usually not visible on CT scans.[109] Either method is adequate for imaging intraparenchymal cysticerci or hydrocephalus.

Parenchymal cystic lesions are the most common neuroradiographic manifestation of NCC.[6,64,107,110] The number of cysticerci varies from one to several thousand. In India and the United States, the majority of cases of parenchymal NCC have only a single degenerating cyst.[6,54,71] By contrast, most studies from Latin America reveal multiple parasites. Whether this is due to biological differences or biases in which patients are scanned is uncertain. On CT or MRI, parenchymal cysticerci appear as round cystic lesions, typically 4–20 mm in diameter. They are usually found in the cerebral cortex or the basal ganglia.[111] Cysts in fissures are often larger, with a diameter of up to 10 cm. They may be either round or lobulated. For viable cysticerci, cyst fluid is isodense with CSF. The cyst wall is thin (<1 mm thick) and is usually not visible. When identified, the scolex is a round or tubular nodule, 1–3 mm long on one side of the cyst wall. The presence of cystic lesions with a mural nodule (scolex) is often considered pathognomonic for cysticercosis.[64,108] The wall of the inflamed cyst wall is denser and may enhance with contrast (ring enhancement). The cyst fluid or surrounding tissues may also enhance. There is often edema surrounding the cysticercus, especially on T2-weighted MRI scans. Later-stage cysticerci appear as focal areas of enhancement or granulomas.

Parenchymal brain calcifications are also a common CT finding in NCC. Calcifications tend to be solid, dense, supratentorial, and 2–10 mm in diameter. In the absence of evidence of other illnesses, calcifications should be considered as highly suggestive of NCC. MRI scans often reveal surrounding edema and/or contrast enhancement in symptomatic cases. The latter may be associated with a residual scolex on gradient refocused echo images.[52,112]

Cysticerci in ventricles are often poorly visualized by CT.[63,109] Most are viable cysts, with cyst fluid isodense with the CSF and thin walls. The presence of ventricular cysticerci can be inferred from distortion of the ventricular shape or the presence of obstructive hydrocephalus.[63,109] In contrast to CT, the increased resolution of MRI frequently allows visualization of the cyst walls and scolex.

Even though imaging studies detect most cases of NCC, the appearance is not always pathognomonic. Del Brutto and colleagues proposed diagnostic criteria based on neuroimaging studies, serologic tests, clinical history, and exposure (***Box 119.1***).[113] Patients with either an absolute criterion or two major criteria alone with two minor or epidemiologic criteria were considered to have a definite diagnosis. One major criterion plus two other criteria or three minor criteria plus exposure were considered to establish a probable diagnosis (***Box 119.1***).

Box 119.1 Diagnostic Criteria for Neurocysticercosis

Absolute Criteria

- Histologic demonstration of the parasite from biopsy of a brain or spinal cord lesion
- Cystic lesions showing the scolex on computed tomography or magnetic resonance imaging
- Direct visualization of subretinal parasites by fundoscopic examination

Major Criteria

- Lesions highly suggestive of neurocysticercosis on neuroimaging studies
- Positive serum immunoblot for the detection of anticysticercal antibodies
- Resolution of intracranial cystic lesions after therapy with albendazole or praziquantal
- Spontaneous resolution of small single enhancing lesions

Minor Criteria

- Lesions compatible with neurocysticercosis on neuroimaging studies
- Clinical manifestations suggestive of neurocysticercosis
- Positive cerebrospinal fluid enzyme-linked immunosorbent assay for detection of anticercal antibodies or cysticercal antigens
- Cysticercosis outside the central nervous system

Epidemiologic Criteria

- Evidence of a household contact with *Taenia solium* infection
- History of frequent travel to disease-endemic areas
- Individuals coming from or living in an area where cysticercosis is endemic
- One major criterion and two other criteria or three minor criteria plus exposure were considered to establish a probable diagnosis

(Reproduced from Del Brutto OH, Rajshekhar V, White AC Jr, et al. Proposed diagnostic criteria for neurocysticercosis. Neurology. 2001;57:177–183.)

Absolute diagnostic criteria for NCC include identification of the parasite by visualization or histology or pathognomonic neuroimaging results.[113] Parasites can occasionally be visualized directly in the eye. Neuroimaging studies revealing a cystic lesion with an associated scolex (demonstrated as a 1–3-mm mural nodule) are thought to be pathognomonic for cysticercosis.[64,108]

Neuroimaging studies highly suggestive of NCC were considered a major diagnostic criterion. These included cystic lesions, single or multiple ringlike or nodular enhancing lesions and typical parenchymal brain calcifications. Ring or nodular enhancing lesions are also highly suggestive of NCC, but tuberculomas, brain abscesses, and tumors can cause similar lesions. Cysticercal lesions are usually <20 mm in diameter and rarely cause midline shift.[40] Clinical and radiologic critieria for NCC among patients who presented with seizures and single enhancing lesions include the combination of a single, round, enhancing lesion, <20 mm in diameter, with no midline shift, in patients without increased intracranial pressure, focal neurologic deficits, or evidence of systemic disease.[40] These criteria were prospectively studied in 401 patients in India with a high sensitivity and specificity.[40] Resolution of the lesion spontaneously or after anticysticercal therapy or precipitation of symptoms by antiparasitic drugs is also supportive of the diagnosis. All of these are major diagnostic criteria.[113]

Serodiagnosis has proven problematic in the diagnosis of cysticercosis due to cross-reactions to other parasites and nonspecific binding. Assays employing unfractionated antigen have poor sensitivity and specificity.[114,115] The enzyme-linked immunotransfer blot (EITB) is an immunoblot assay employing semipurified membrane antigens.[116] Binding to any one of seven bands is considered positive. Studies have confirmed ~100% specificity, but rare false positives have been noted with a single gp50 band.[117] The sensitivity is limited in subjects with either a single lesion or with only calcified lesions.[115,116,118,119] Performance data suggest that the predictive value of the EITB assay for NCC is better with serum than with CSF.[120] Assays to detect parasite antigens may prove to be an important diagnostic tool.[121–123]

Minor criteria (*Box 119.1*) include: (1) lesions on neuroimaging studies that might be NCC, but are less suggestive (e.g., isolated basilar meningitis, hydrocephalus, or filling defects in the spinal subarachnoid space without discrete cysticerci); (2) symptoms suggestive of NCC (e.g., seizures or hydrocephalus); (3) serologic tests for cysticercosis other than the EITB; (4) cysticercosis outside the nervous system (e.g., cigar-shaped muscle calcifications or subcutaneous nodules); and (5) epidemiologic exposure criteria, such as residence or prolonged visits to endemic areas or contact with a tapeworm carrier.[113]

Different antigen detection tests are being developed. Detection of circulating parasite antigen reflects the presence of ongoing viable infection and may permit quantitative verification of successful treatment. Antigen detection assays offer the hope of an improved method for following responses to therapy and might be helpful in drug development.[122,124–128] Garcia and others have used antigen ELISA based on the use of a monoclonal antibody (HP10) that reacts with a repetitive carbohydrate epitope found in excretory/secretory and surface antigens of living cysticerci.[122] This assay had a sensitivity of 86% when tested on CSF samples from 50 Peruvian patients with EITB-positive NCC.[121] The assay specificity was ~96%, and it has been used to follow patients after treatment. Parasite antigen levels fell significantly by 3 months after treatment in patients with "cured" parenchymal disease after albendazole therapy.[122] This study found that the sensitivity is low in intraparenchymal NCC, especially in patients with only a few intraparenchymal cysts.[122] In a study examining patients with hydrocephalus and NCC, the assay was positive in 14 of 29 patients, but negative in patients with calcifications.[123] Drops in antigen levels (serum and CSF) after treatment in subarachnoid disease have been reported in a small number of patients.[129] Management of subarachnoid disease is particularly complicated, and the appropriate endpoint for treatment has not been established. A monoclonal antibody-based ELISA to detect *T. solium* antigens in urine had an overall sensitivity of urine antigen detection for viable parasites of 92%, which decreased to 62.5% in patients with a single cyst. Most individuals with only calcified NCC were urine antigen-negative. This assay could be useful in diagnosis of NCC and evaluating the efficacy of treatment.[130]

TREATMENT AND PROGNOSIS

Antiepileptic therapy, antiparasitic drugs, anti-inflammatory drugs, and surgical therapy are all variously important in the management of NCC patients. Therapy should be individualized based on the pathogenesis of different forms of disease.

Symptomatic Therapy

Symptomatic therapy plays a key role in the management of NCC. Most fatalities are associated with failure to provide effective therapy for complications such as raised intracranial pressure or seizures. Most seizures can be controlled with any of a number of antiepileptic drugs. A single first-line antiepileptic drug such as phenytoin or carbamazepine can successfully control seizures in most patients.[48,56,110,131] Data on newer antiepileptic drugs are limited, but one study suggested that clobazam was superior to phenytoin in patients with single enhancing lesions.[132] Breakthrough seizures often reflect poor adherence, subtherapeutic drugs levels, or coexisting conditions (e.g., alcohol abuse).[57] Among patients in whom neuroimaging studies normalize and seizures are controlled, antiepileptic treatment may eventually be tapered,[48,56–58,133] although seizures may recur in 20–40% of patients. In some studies, the presence of residual calcifications is a marker for high risk of recurrent seizures and is thought to be an indication for continuous antiepileptic use.[50,53]

Hydrocephalus is primarily treated surgically. Definitive therapy for obstructive hydrocephalus is removal of the obstructing cysticercus. However, emergent therapy may include CSF diversion procedures such as placement of a ventriculostomy or ventriculoperitoneal shunting.[61,62] In the past, there was a high rate of shunt failure, in part due to aspiration of the cysticerci into the shunt. Antiparasitic drugs and/or treatment with corticosteroids may decrease the rate of shunt failure.[62,71,134–136]

Corticosteroids

Corticosteroids are used in NCC to control inflammation and are a key component of therapy for severe forms of NCC, including cysticercal encephalitis, subarachnoid NCC, and spinal intramedullary cysticercosis. For patients with NCC in the subarachnoid space, meningitis, vasculitis with stroke, and communicating hydrocephalus can result from the host inflammatory response and accompanying arachnoiditis. Corticosteroid therapy is an essential component in these cases. There are few data available on the optimal dose or duration of therapy. For severe disease, high doses (e.g., 1 mg/kg/day of prednisone or 0.5 mg/kg/day of dexamethasone) are often used initially. Lower doses have been used along with initial antiparasitic drugs to ameliorate inflammatory reactions to dying parasite. One randomized trial suggested that treatment with a short course of prednisolone (1 mg/kg/day for 10 days) led to a marked reduction in seizures and more rapid resolution in patients with single enhancing lesions.[137] Methotrexate has been used with some success as a steroid-sparing agent in patients with prolonged steroid use or intolerable side effects.[138,139]

Antiparasitic Drugs

The role of antiparasitic drugs in the treatment of NCC has been controversial. The first randomized controlled trials were published in the 1990s, and consensus on optimal management is only now emerging.[140–142]

Praziquantel is absorbed well after oral administration, but has extensive first-pass metabolism, which is accelerated by antiepileptic drugs (carbemazepine, phenytoin, and probably phenobarbital) as well as by corticosteroids.[143,144] This induction can be inhibited by cimetidine (e.g., 400 mg PO tid). Coadministration increases levels of praziquantel, but the effect of the increased drug levels on efficacy is unproven.[145–148] Initial dose-ranging studies demonstrated greater effect at doses ≥50 mg/kg/day in 3 daily doses for 14 days. Subsequent studies demonstrated that doses as high as 100 mg/kg/day could be given safely.[149] Studies with praziquantel in parenchymal NCC given in 3 doses of 25 mg/kg separated by only 2 hours along with cimetidine suggest similar efficacy with longer courses of therapy in patients with one or two cysts, but the efficacy may be lower in those with more cysts.[148,150,151] Adverse effects, including worsening neurologic function (e.g., headaches, dizziness, seizures, increased intracranial pressure), are due to the host inflammatory response to the dying parasite. Along with antiparasitic drugs, corticosteroids are recommended to decrease side effects, but routine use of corticosteroids could potentially decrease efficacy of praziquantel by affecting serum levels.

Albendazole, a benzimidazole anthelminthic agent with broad-spectrum activity, is usually used at doses of 15 mg/kg/day in 2 daily doses. Side effects include mild gastrointestinal problems, rarely alopecia and agranulocytosis, and inflammatory responses to the parasites. Imaging studies demonstrated as good or better resolution of parenchymal NCC compared with praziquantel.[152,153] Controlled trials in parenchymal NCC showed no difference in neuroradiologic resolution with treatment for 7 days versus longer courses.[153–155] Albendazole was subsequently studied in cases of extraparenchymal disease and was associated with improvement.[66,134,136,156–158] However, none of these trials was controlled, due to concerns about disease progression.

Eight well-controlled studies of antiparasitic drugs have been performed in different forms of parenchymal NCC.[57,159–165] Overall, the studies demonstrate that patients with parenchymal NCC have a more rapid radiologic response when treated with antiparasitic drugs both in cystic lesions as well as in degenerative (enhancing) lesions.

In vitro, a combination of albendazole and praziquantel induces greater and irreversible damage to a *Taenia* sp. than either drug alone.[166] A prospective, randomized, placebo controlled trial looking at combination therapy with albendazole and praziquantel versus albendazole alone in 110 children with seizures and single enhancing lesions showed more children with resolution and fewer with calcifications in the dual-therapy group, but the differences were not statistically significant.[167] Larger studies are warranted with combination therapy for both parenchymal and extraparenchymal forms of NCC.

Parenchymal Neurocysticercosis with Cystic Lesions

In parenchymal cystic NCC, the clinical response is generally favorable. A randomized trial compared albendazole plus corticosteroids to symptomatic therapy alone and found fewer seizures in the treatment group, although the proportions of patients with at least one seizure relapse were similar.[57] While imaging studies will eventually normalize with or without antiparasitic drugs, Garcia and colleagues clearly demonstrated that spontaneous resolution of the cystic lesions was prolonged (>6 months) unless patients were treated with antiparasitic drugs.[57,159]

Calcified Parenchymal Neurocysticercosis

Antiparasitic drugs are not recommended in calcified disease, since there are no signs of viable parasites. These patients typically present with seizures clustered near the time of diagnosis, but they can recur years later.[48,53,56,58,133] Thus, symptomatic patients with calcifications require chronic antiepileptic therapy. If patients maintain therapeutic levels of the drugs, risks of recurrent seizures are very low.[48] On imaging studies, some patients show contrast enhancement or edema around established calcified lesions.[43,44,52,53] There is no proven effective treatment for perilesional edema associated with calcified lesions aside from symptomatic therapy.

Ventricular Neurocysticercosis

Some patients have hydrocephalus related to scarring from prior infection (e.g., aqueductal stenosis).[106] In this case, hydrocephalus can be corrected by ventriculoperitoneal shunting without the need for antiparasitic drugs. Patients with viable ventricular NCC usually present with obstructive hydrocephalus. Initial management should focus on relieving intracranial hypertension, reversing hydrocephalus, reducing the risk for recurrence, and minimizing treatment-associated morbidity.[61,168–170] In the past, removal of the cysticercus from the ventricle via an open craniotomy was the main approach. Recent studies have demonstrated that cysticerci can usually be removed by endoscopic surgery with less chronic morbidity. When feasible, endoscopic surgery is the preferred approach, but patients should be selected carefully.[61,168,171–176] Lateral and third ventricular cysts can be removed with rigid endoscopes and the fourth ventricle can be approached with flexible endoscopes. Connections between the third ventricle and the basilar cisterns can shunt CSF around obstructions. Patients with significant ependymal enhancement have not been effectively managed surgically due to adherence of the cysticerci to the ependyma and may not be good candidates for endoscopic removal.[168]

An alternative approach, especially in the setting of acute decompensation, is placement of a ventriculoperitoneal shunt. Shunting is associated with a lower perioperative mortality rate than seen with an open craniotomy.[177] Up to 75% of shunts malfunction, requiring shunt revision or replacement if no other treatment is given. Requirements for shunt revision are less frequent among patients who are also treated with antiparasitic drugs.[54,62,136] Similarly, corticosteroids may decrease the risk of shunt obstruction.[135]

Subarachnoid Neurocysticercosis and Giant Cysticerci

Subarachnoid cysticercosis is associated with a poor prognosis. In one series, patients treated with only CSF diversion were noted to have a 50% mortality rate.[178] Complications include mass effect, communicating hydrocephalus, vasculitis with strokes, and basilar meningitis.[66,68,106] There are no controlled trials of management of subarachnoid NCC. Case series in which patients were treated with antiparasitic drugs, corticosteroids, and shunting for hydrocephalus have demonstrated a markedly improved prognosis compared to older studies.[45,61,66,156,157] Thus, most experts consider subarachnoid NCC an indication for antiparasitic therapy.[169] There is no consensus on the dose of antiparasitic agent or length of treatment for this form of NCC. A study of 33 patients with giant cysticerci treated with albendazole (15 mg/day for 4 weeks) found only one single death from aplastic anemia at 59 months, with patients requiring several courses of therapy.[66] Therefore, a single course of 28 days or less in patients with subarachnoid disease is probably inadequate and longer-term therapy over months might be required to treat some patients. The host inflammatory reaction around the cysts may result in occlusion of leptomeningeal vessels, resulting in stroke or hydrocephalus.[67,178] Therefore, high-dose steroids (e.g., prednisone 60 mg/day) must be used in conjunction with antiparasitic therapy and might be required for prolonged periods with a slow taper. The taper should be based on the neuroimaging and the paired antigen response in either the serum or the CSF.[121,129] Methotrexate has been used as a steroid-sparing agent in subarachnoid disease in patients requiring long-term steroids and experiencing intolerable side effects.[138]

Other Forms of Neurocysticercosis

Spinal NCC can be subarachnoid or intramedullar. There is only anecdotal evidence on the effectiveness of any therapies. Intramedullary NCC should usually be approached surgically due to the risk of paralysis from cord swelling.[169] Spinal subarachnoid cysticerci, however, may respond to antiparasitic drugs.[45] Ocular disease may respond to antiparasitic treatment, but the standard therapy is still surgical removal.[169]

PREVENTION

Cysticercosis transmission was eliminated in Europe by improved sanitation, better animal husbandry, and meat inspection.[179,180] Porcine cysticercosis can be prevented by confining pigs and not allowing them access to human fecal material.[181] However, confined pigs must be fed, adding expenses to the cost of raising them. This economic pressure is a major barrier to corralling the pigs as a method of control. Human infection with adult tapeworms can also be prevented by destruction, freezing, or adequate cooking of measly pork. Meat inspection has been unsuccessful in areas where pigs are raised by peasant farmers.[182] Treatment of human tapeworm carriers could potentially eliminate the disease, but current detection methods are suboptimal. Mass chemotherapy of endemic populations results in significant decreases in human taeniasis and porcine cysticercosis, but the effects are of short duration.[179,183,184] In recent years, new tools, including coproantigen detection and effective porcine vaccines,[185] have increased the options and likelihood of control. Cysticercosis is assumed to be one of a few eradicable diseases. A wide elimination program in Peru has recently shown proof of concept of focal elimination of transmission using combined pig and human chemotherapy allied to porcine vaccines and health education.

COENUROSIS

Human infection with the larval form of the canine tapeworm *Taenia multiceps* (*Multiceps multiceps*) is termed coenurosis and is reported from tropical and subtropical areas of the world. Rarely, human disease may be caused by zoonotic infection with *T. serialis*.

THE AGENT

Definitive hosts are dogs, wolves, foxes, and coyotes, where adult *T. multiceps* or *T. serialis* are found in the small intestines.[186] Gravid proglottids passed in the feces of the canid hosts disintegrate and release eggs that are ingested by intermediate hosts, including rabbits and rodents. The larval stage of *T. multiceps* usually develops in herbivores such as sheep, goats, or horses, whereas the larval stage of *T. serialis* is usually found in rabbits and squirrels. Humans may also serve as an accidental intermediate host as a consequence of ingestion of eggs released by proglottids in dog feces. As in hydatid disease, the oncospheres eventually lodge in various tissues of the body, typically the brain and spinal cord of herbivores. The cyst, about the size of a hen's egg, eventually develops. The coeunus is a fluid-filled cyst that measures from a few millimeters to 2 cm or more in diameter; the wall is a thin, delicate membrane to which multiple invaginated scolices (protoscolices) are attached in rows or clusters. External cysts are also formed that remain attached by long stalks to the main cyst.

EPIDEMIOLOGY

The majority of human cases have been reported from Africa, specifically Kenya, Uganda, Nigeria, and South Africa,[187–189] with other cases also reported from the United Kingdom, France, and North America.[190] Subcutaneous, ocular, muscle, and CNS cysts have been commonly described, although it is unclear if all cases were due to *T. multiceps*.

THE DISEASE

Human coenurosis usually involves the CNS, muscles, or subcutaneous tissues.[190] In the CNS coenorosis presents as a cyst and acts as a space-occupying mass causing pressure necrosis as it enlarges. Intracerebral cysts may cause seizures or other localizing signs and symptoms and can be confused with NCC and echinococosis. Intraparenchymal lesions of the spinal cord have been reported as well as meningitis, arteritis, arachnoiditis, ependymitis, and involvement of the eye. Subcutaneous and intramuscular cysts are reported most commonly in Africa and involve the intercostal area and anterior abdominal wall. Allergic symptoms, such as recurrent urticaria, fever, and night sweats, have been reported.

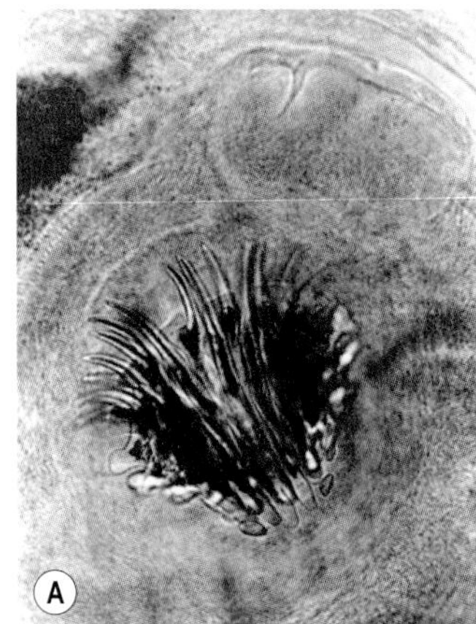

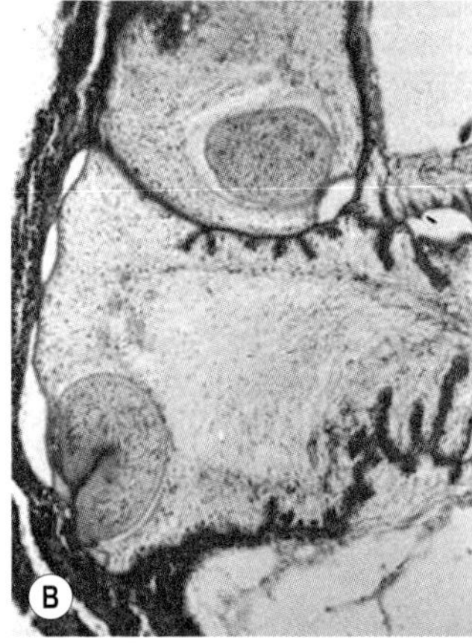

Figure 119.8 (A, B) Pathologic images of coenurosis caused by *Taenia multiceps*.

DIAGNOSIS

Presumptive diagnosis by MRI or CT scan, as well as ultrasound, has been helpful but not definitive.[190,191] The definitive diagnosis is dependent on surgical excision and pathologic identification (*Fig. 119.8*). Fine-needle aspiration of a cyst has been reported to yield a diagnosis.[190] There is no reliable serologic test for this disease.

PREVENTION AND CONTROL

Surgical intervention has been the mainstay of therapy.[192] There are no reliable data on the use of praziquantel or albendazole in this disease. Elimination of adult worms with praziquantel may reduce transmission from dogs to humans.

Access the complete reference list online at
http://www.expertconsult.com

CHAPTER 120

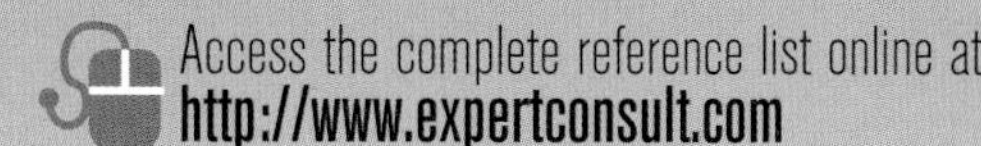
Access the complete reference list online at
http://www.expertconsult.com

Echinococcosis

Peter M. Schantz • Peter Kern • Enrico Brunetti

INTRODUCTION

Echinococcosis is an infection caused by cestodes of the genus *Echinococcus* (Cestoda: Taeniidae), the life cycles of which involve two mammalian hosts. Definitive hosts are carnivores, in which adult worms are present in the intestines. *Echinococcus* eggs, passed in feces of definitive hosts, hatch when ingested by suitable intermediate hosts, including humans, and the liberated embryos migrate to parenteral sites and develop into the metacestode (larval) forms. Under natural conditions, transmission of *Echinococcus* spp. from intermediate to definitive hosts is the result of predator–prey relationships existing between hosts; however, transmission in synanthropic cycles is considerably modified by human behavior. Larval forms are referred to as hydatid cysts, and the diseases caused by them are commonly referred to as cystic, alveolar, or polycystic hydatid disease or echinococcosis.

Aspects of the controversy concerning speciation within the genus *Echinococcus* have been reviewed by Thompson.[1] Until recently, the genus *Echinococcus* had contained four species: *E. granulosus*, *E. multilocularis*, *E. oligarthrus*, and *E. vogeli*, which are morphologically distinct in both adult (***Fig. 120.1***) and larval stages. A fifth species, *E. shiquicus*, has recently been described.[2] The species *E. granulosus* is made up of a number of biologically and genetically distinct entities whose taxonomic positions are in states of flux. These variants are separated ecologically, although not necessarily geographically, by the nature of their respective unique host assemblages. They have been referred to as strains or subspecies; however, recent proposals based on the application of molecular tools have elevated several of them to separate species status, some reflecting much earlier proposals based on morphologic characteristics and host specificities[1] (***Table 120.1***).

Classic cystic echinococcosis (CE) is caused by *E. granulosus*. Alveolar echinococcosis (AE) is caused by *E. multilocularis* and polycystic echinococcosis (PE) is caused by *E. vogeli* and, less commonly, *E. oligarthrus*. The newly described *E. shiquicus*, discovered parasitizing the intestine of the Tibetan fox (*Vulpes ferrilata*) on the eastern Tibetan plateau in China, is morphologically and genotypically distinct from previously described species. Molecular phylogenetic analysis of mitochondrial genes indicates that *E. shiquicus* is the most primitive of the recognized species in the genus, which may imply a Eurasian origin for *Echinococcus* spp.[2] The larval stage has been found parasitizing the black-lipped pika (*Ochotona curzoniae*). Nothing is known of potential infectivity for humans.

Biologic, epidemiologic, and clinical aspects of the echinococcoses were reviewed by international consultants of the World Health Organization's Informal Working Group on Echinococcosis (WHO/IWGE).[3]

CYSTIC ECHINOCOCCOSIS (*ECHINOCOCCUS GRANULOSUS* AND RELATED SPECIES)

THE AGENT

Echinococcus granulosus was the first *Echinococcus* sp. to be described. For many years, considerable morphologic and biologic variabilities have been noted between populations of *E. granulosus* in different geographic regions and in different host assemblages. Described differences have included features such as morphology, biochemistry, physiology, pathogenicity, developmental patterns, and infectivity to humans and domestic animals.[1] Whereas adults consistently infect canids, metacestodes from different "strains" or genotypic variant populations appear to be adapted to distinct species of domestic and wild herbivorous hosts, including sheep, cattle, pigs, horses, and wild cervids. However, the host specificities of a given variant population vary enormously. Molecular characterization has revealed that the genetic differences between what were perceived to be host-adapted strains of *E. granulosus* are conserved and occur consistently in isolates derived from different species of intermediate hosts throughout the world.[1] This has been demonstrated for the sheep, horse, cattle, pig, and camel genotypes in molecular epidemiological studies in Australia, Europe, Iran, Africa, and South America.[1,3]

Current data, based on genome patterns, generally support previous characterizations based on morphologic and biologic criteria. At least 10 genetically distinct populations exist within the complex until recently denoted *E. granulosus*[1] (***Fig. 120.2 and Table 120.1***). Probes characterizing the mitochondrial and genomic DNA of the variant populations provide reliable genetic markers to distinguish them.[1,3] The "sheep" genotype (G1) is maintained in life cycles involving dogs and sheep; it also sometimes infects humans, cattle, goats, buffalo, camels, pigs, macropods (intermediate hosts), and foxes and some other canids (definitive hosts), although development and maturation in some of these hosts are significantly impaired in comparison to those in sheep and dogs. The genetic structure of this strain is highly uniform throughout its nearly cosmopolitan geographic distribution; however, a second sheep genotype (G2), slightly different from the common sheep strain in mitochondrial DNA sequences, has been identified in Tasmania. This isolate is also morphologically distinct and has a significantly shortened prepatent period in dogs than the common sheep strain. The "horse" genotype (G4) is adapted to horses, donkeys, and dogs throughout the United Kingdom, areas of Europe, the Middle East, and possibly South Africa and New Zealand; no human infections with this genotype have been identified. The "cattle" genotype (G5) occurs in cattle and dogs in western Europe and in buffalo

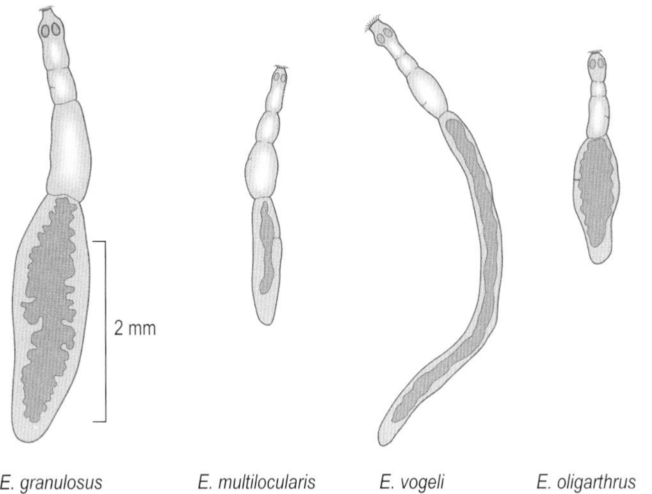

Figure 120.1 Comparative morphology of adult-stage *Echinococcus* species. (From Rausch RL, Bernstein JJ. *Echinococcus vogeli* sp. n. (Cestodea: Taeniidae) from the bush dog *Speothos venaticus* (Lund). Tropenmed Parasitol. 1972;23:25.)

in Sri Lanka and India. Cysts occur mainly in the lungs of cattle and buffalo and, in contrast to those caused by infection of cattle with the sheep genotype (G1), are large and highly fertile. The "camel" genotype (G6) is found in areas of the Middle East and North Africa in cycles involving camels and dogs. The "pig" genotype (G7), adapted to pigs and dogs, has been characterized from isolates in eastern Europe; but it may occur much more widely. Human infections with this genotype are reported from Poland[4] and Mexico.[5] The "cervid" or northern sylvatic genotype (G10) is maintained in cycles involving wolves, dogs and moose, caribou, and other cervids throughout northern North America and does not readily infect domestic ungulates.[6] Human infection with this strain is characterized by predominantly pulmonary localization, slower and more benign growth, and less frequent occurrence of clinical complications than reported for other forms. A distinct genotypic *Echinococcus* sp. (G10) appears to be the variant infecting reindeer and moose in Fennoscandinavia.[7] A limited number of isolates from humans have been typed as the cattle strain and the pig strain.[1] Accumulating data support long-held speculations that the horse strain is noninfective to humans.

It is likely that the *Echinococcus* speciation question will be clarified as additional information is presented. At this time, it is important to recognize that important biologic differences exist between populations currently identified as *E. granulosus*, the causative agent of CE, and that these may account for local differences in patterns of transmission and clinical and public health significance of the disease. The great majority of *E. granulosus* isolates from human patients thus far characterized by genotype have been of the sheep genotype (G1), and this and the worldwide epidemiologic association of high endemicity with sheep raising confirm the paramount public health importance of the sheep genotype.

Comparative details of maturation and growth rates of most of the *E. granulosus* genotypic variants are not available, and the following description applies primarily to genotype G1 in sheep and canid hosts. The adult intestinal forms of *E. granulosus* genotypic variants are small tapeworms approximately 3–7 mm in length when fully mature (***Fig. 120.1***); they attach firmly to the small intestine of the canine host. Following infection by ingestion of protoscolices originating from fertile hydatid cysts, sexual maturity of adult-stage tapeworms is reached within 4–7 weeks. Development from ovum to the oncosphere or hexacanth embryo takes place *in utero* in the adult *Echinococcus*. The oncosphere measures approximately 0.018 mm and is bilaterally symmetrical, possessing three pairs of hooks (hexacanth), muscle fibers, and glands, which aid it in penetration and locomotion within the intermediate host. The oncosphere and its surrounding membranes (0.030–0.036 mm in diameter) are often referred to as the cestode egg. Eggs are fecally shed into the external environment, and when ingested by a suitable intermediate host, the oncospheres hatch and become activated. Lytic secretions may facilitate the passage of motile oncospheres through the intestinal mucosa and into the host's circulatory system (via venous and lymphatic pathways). Oncospheres are distributed to other sites via the host's circulatory system, where post-oncospheral development continues. Within a few days after oncospheres reach their preferred site, cystic development begins. This process involves degeneration of the oncospheral stage and emergence of the vesicular metacestode stage, which grows expansively by concentric enlargement. In general, hydatid cysts increase in diameter from 1 to 5 cm each year, depending on unknown factors. Protoscolex formation occurs as early as 4 months in white mice, but it may require more than 1 year in sheep and other intermediate hosts.

The fully developed metacestode (hydatid or hydatid cyst) of *E. granulosus* is typically fluid-filled and unilocular, but multiple chambers may also occur. Structurally, the cyst consists of an inner germinative layer of cells supported externally by a characteristic acidophilic-staining, acellular, laminated membrane of variable thickness. Cytoplasmic extensions of the germinative layer unite to form a syncytium, which is differentiated into numerous microtriches. The microtriches project peripherally into the laminar layer toward the host tissues surrounding the cyst. Surrounding the parasitic cyst is a host-produced, granulomatous, adventitial reaction of extremely variable intensity. Small secondary cysts, called brood capsules, bud internally from the germinative layer and, by polyembryony, produce multiple protoscolices. A protoscolex is a scolex with the rostellum and suckers deeply withdrawn into the postsucker region. In humans, the slowly growing hydatid cysts may attain a volume of many liters and contain many thousands of protoscolices.

TRANSMISSION, EPIDEMIOLOGY, AND GEOGRAPHIC DISTRIBUTION

Dogs and other definitive hosts become infected upon ingesting organs of other animals that contain hydatid cysts or protoscolices released from recently ruptured cysts. *E. granulosus* has remarkable biologic potential; there may be as many as 40 000 tapeworms in a heavily infected dog, and each tapeworm sheds approximately 1000 eggs every 2 weeks. Dogs infected with *E. granulosus* tapeworms pass eggs in their feces, and humans become infected through fecal-oral contact, particularly in the course of playful and intimate contact between children and dogs. Eggs adhere to hairs around the infected dog's anus and are also found on the muzzle and paws. Indirect means of contact via soil, water, and contaminated vegetables, or through the intermediary of flies and other arthropods, may also result in human infections.

Eggs of *E. granulosus* are capable of surviving snow and freezing conditions, remaining viable for at least 1 year on pasture, but they are susceptible to desiccation and will become incapable of hatching after only a few hours when exposed to direct sunlight. People of both sexes and all ages are susceptible, and opportunities for exposure are mainly related to direct and indirect contact with infected dogs. Socioeconomic and cultural characteristics are defined risk factors for human infection: dogs living closely with people, uncontrolled slaughter of livestock, and insanitary living conditions.[8] Whether it be among Arabs in Tunisia, Quechua Indians in Peru, Turkana tribesmen in Kenya, or Tibetans in China, these common factors are readily discernible. When dogs at risk of infection are maintained close to the family home, all members of the family may be exposed, or, as in certain cultural situations, one sex or the other may take responsibility for feeding and handling the dogs, thus favoring exposure of people of that sex.[9,10] CE imposes serious medical and economic disabilities on affected communities through the economic burden associated with infection in livestock as well as the disability and treatment costs associated with infection in humans.[11,12]

The greatest prevalence of CE in humans and nonhuman animals is found in countries of the temperate zones, including southern South America, the entire Mediterranean littoral, the southern and central areas of the former Soviet Union, Central Asia, China, Australia, and areas of Africa[8] (***Fig. 120.3***). Consistently, highest prevalence is found

Table 120.1 Characteristics of Hosts and Known Geographic Distribution of Recognized and Proposed Species and Strains in the Genus *Echinococcus*

Species Strain/Isolate (Genotype)	Known Intermediate Hosts	Infective to Humans?	Known Definitive Hosts	Probable Geographic Distribution	Proposed Taxonomic Designation
Echinococcus granulosus					
Sheep strain (G1)	Sheep, cattle, pigs, camels, goats, macropods	Yes	Dog, fox, dingo, jackal, hyena	Australian mainland, Europe, United States, New Zealand, Africa, China, Middle East, South America, Russian Federation	*E. granulosus*
Tasmanian sheep strain (G2)	Sheep, cattle?	Yes	Dog, fox	Tasmania, Argentina	*E. granulosus*
Buffalo strain (G3)	Buffalo, cattle?	?	Dog, fox?	Asia	*E. granulosus*
Horse strain (G4)	Horses and other equines	No	Dog	Europe, Middle East, South Africa	*E. equinus*
Cattle strain (G5)	Cattle	Yes	Dog	Europe, South Africa, India, Nepal, Russian Federation, South America?	*E. ortleppi*
Camel strain (G6)	Camels, goats, cattle?	Yes	Dog	Middle East, Africa, Argentina, China	*E. granulosus*?
Pig strain (G7)	Pigs	Yes	Dog	Europe, Russian Federation, South America	*E. intermedius*
Cervid strain (G8)	Moose, caribou, reindeer	Yes	Wolf, coyote, dog	North America, Eurasia	*E. granulosus*
Fennoscandinavian cervid strain (G10)	Reindeer, moose?	?	Wolf, dog	Eurasia	*E. granulosus*?
Lion strain	Zebra, wildebeest, warthog, bushpig, buffalo, various antelope, giraffe? hippopotamus?	?	Lion	Africa	*E. granulosus*?
Echinococcus multilocularis					
European isolate	Rodents, domestic and wild pig, dog, monkey	Yes	Fox, dog, cat, wolf, raccoon-dog	Europe, China?	*E. multilocularis*
Alaskan isolate	Rodents	Yes	Fox, dog, cat	Alaska	*E. multilocularis*
North American isolate	Rodents	Yes	Fox, dog, cat, coyote	North America	*E. multilocularis*
Hokkaido isolate	Rodents, pig, monkey, horse	Yes	Fox, dog, cat, raccoon-dog	Japan	*E. multilocularis*
Echinococcus vogeli					
None reported	Rodents	Yes	Bush dog	Central and South America	*E. vogeli*
Echinococcus oligarthrus					
None reported	Rodents	Yes	Wild felids	Central and South America	*E. oligarthrus*
Echinococcus shiquicus					
None reported	Rodents, lagomorphs?	?	Tibetan fox	Tibetan Plateau (China)	*E. shiquicus*

(Modified from Thompson RCA, McManus DP. Toward a revised nomenclature of *Echinococcus*. Trends Parasitol. 2002;18:452–457; and McManus DP, Thompson RCA. Molecular epidemiology of cystic echinococcosis. Parasitology. 2003;127:S37–S51.)

among populations involved with sheep raising, thus emphasizing the overwhelming public health importance of the sheep genotype *E. granulosus* (G1). In certain regions of the former Soviet Union (e.g., Kazakhstan and Kyrgyzstan), changing agricultural practices and disruptions in regulatory policies have led to increased transmission in both lower animal and human hosts.[13] The cervid genotypes (G7 and G8) also commonly infect humans in northern North America and Eurasia; as with the sheep genotype cestode, it is the synanthropic link through the dog that results in most human exposure.

In many countries of these regions, national diagnostic incidence rates have been reported to range from 5 to 20/100 000 population.[8] "National" rates are misleading, however, because most urban populations are at low risk; in rural endemic areas diagnostic incidence is manyfold higher. Furthermore, surveys of local populations using ultrasound imaging diagnostic techniques often measure CE prevalences of 2–6%.[9,10] In the United States, most infections are diagnosed in immigrants from countries in which hydatid disease is highly endemic; historically, this was mainly Italians and Greeks, but in recent years increasing numbers of cases have been diagnosed in people of Middle Eastern and Asian origin.[9,10] Sporadic autochthonous transmission is currently recognized in Alaska, Arizona, and New Mexico.

THE DISEASE

There are numerous descriptions of the diverse clinical manifestations of CE (hydatid disease) (***Fig. 120.4***).[14,15] Many human infections remain asymptomatic; hydatid cysts are frequently observed as incidental findings at autopsy or detected by abdominal ultrasound screening at rates much higher than the reported local morbidity rates. The severity and nature of the signs and symptoms produced by larval cestodes are extremely variable and never pathognomonic. The particular manifestations are determined by the site of localization of the cysts, their size, and their condition.

The incubation period of human hydatid infections is highly variable and often prolonged for several years. Cysts localized in the liver or

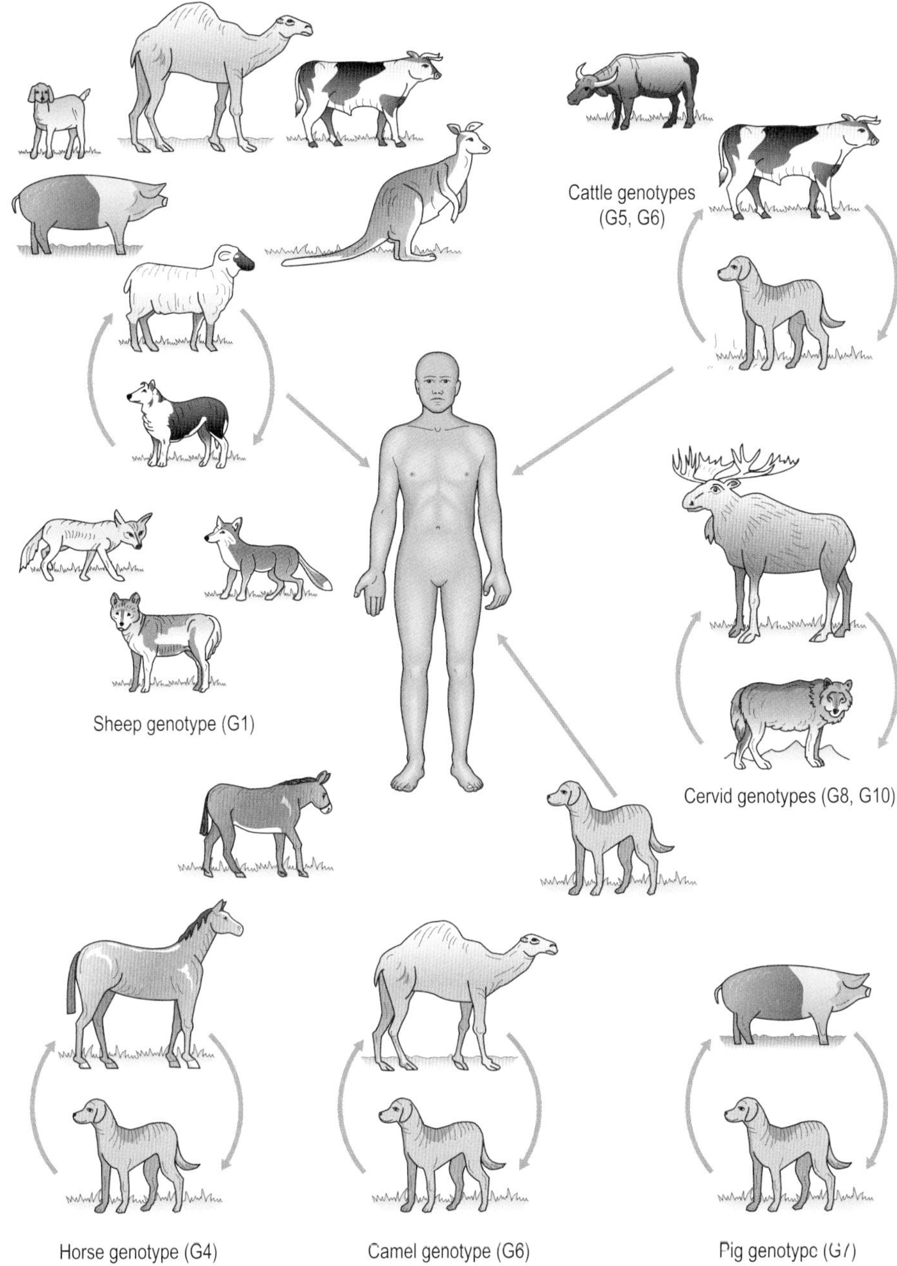

Figure 120.2 Life cycle patterns of principal genotypic variants of the *Echinococcus granulosus* complex and infectivity to humans. Curved arrows designate principal and alternative definitive and intermediate hosts. Straight arrows designate those variants known to infect humans. (See ***Table 120.1*** for complete listing.) (Modified from Schantz PM, Chai J, Craig PS, et al. Epidemiology and control. In: Thompson RCA, Lymbery AJ, eds. Echinococcosis and Hydatid Disease. London: CAB; 1995.)

lung may grow for many years before obtaining enough mass to cause symptoms; in contrast, those located in the brain or eye need reach only very small size before clinical symptoms appear. Age-specific prevalence of liver and pulmonary hydatid cysts increases gradually with age, suggesting that new infections continue to be acquired throughout the human life span. Most primary infections in humans consist of a single cyst; however, 20–40% of patients have multiple cysts or multiple organ involvement. The liver is the most common site of cyst localization (65%), followed by the lungs (25%); hydatid cysts are less frequently seen in the spleen, kidneys, heart, bone, and central nervous system. Cysts of the cervid (G7), or northern sylvatic, form localize predominantly in the lungs; however, the disease caused by this variant has been described as usually more benign and uncomplicated than that caused by the sheep strain.[6] In secondary echinococcosis, new cysts develop from released protoscolices after spontaneous or trauma-induced cyst rupture or during invasive treatment procedures.

The slowly growing hydatid cyst is well tolerated by the human host until it becomes large enough to cause dysfunction. Cyst rupture, often resulting from trauma, may cause a variety of immediate or delayed sequelae. Mild to severe anaphylactic reactions (and occasionally death) may follow the sudden massive release of cyst fluid. In the lungs, ruptured cyst membranes may be evacuated entirely through the bronchi or retained to serve as a nidus for bacterial infection. Dissemination of protoscolices incidental to surgical treatment may result in multiple secondary disease; however, postsurgical chemotherapy reduces this risk.

Hydatid cysts of the liver may become relatively large before producing symptoms because of the large size and the distensible nature of the organ. Signs and symptoms may include hepatic enlargement with or without a palpable mass in the right upper quadrant, right epigastric pain, nausea, and vomiting. Rupture or leakage usually results in acute or intermittent allergic manifestations. Urgent complications existing at the

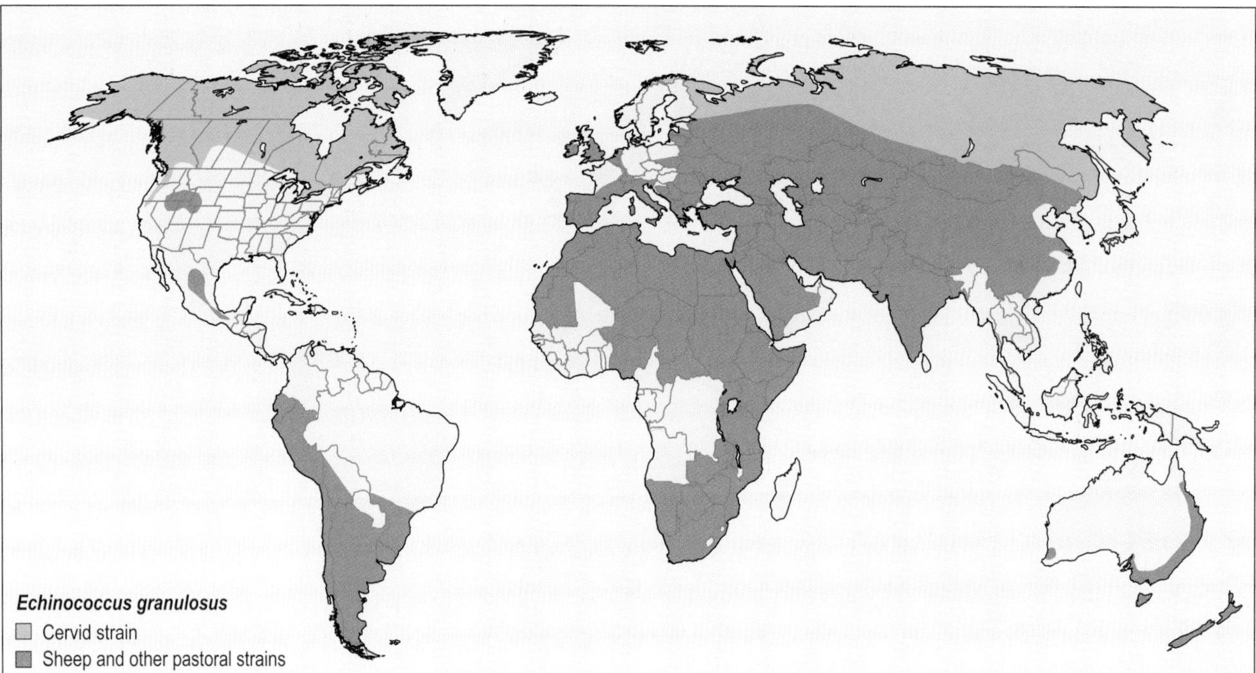

Figure 120.3 Geographic distribution of *Echinococcus granulosus.*

time of initial presentation in patients with hepatic cysts include traumatic or spontaneous rupture, thoracobilia, and biliary fistula.[15]

Intact hydatid cysts in the lungs may cause no symptoms, but leakage or rupture causes chest pain, coughing, dyspnea, and hemoptysis. Hydatid membranes may be coughed up, sometimes resulting in spontaneous cure. Emergency complications existing at the time of initial presentation include cyst rupture and secondary bacterial infection. Around 20–40% of patients with pulmonary hydatidosis can be shown to have liver involvement as well.[14,15]

In most surgical series, 5–10% of cases involve organs other than the lungs or liver.[16,17] The clinical manifestations of cysts in unusual localizations often present special difficulties and delays in diagnosis. The first symptom of cerebral cysts may be raised intracranial pressure or focal epilepsy, whereas renal cysts may be manifested by loin pain or hematuria. Bone cysts are often asymptomatic until pathologic fractures occur, and because of the resemblance, they are often misdiagnosed as tuberculous lesions. Cysts in the heart are especially dangerous because they may rupture and cause systemic dissemination of the protoscolices, anaphylaxis, or cardiac tamponade.

Although mortality rates associated with hydatid disease may appear low in comparison to those for some other infectious diseases, the morbidity associated with each case is considerable. Patients with hydatid disease often require multiple surgical interventions. Extensive secondary hydatid disease often becomes inoperable. Economic losses to affected families include surgical and hospital expenses as well as loss of income.[11] In Uruguay, it was shown that 60% of surgical patients were unable to return to normal activities for 4 months after leaving the hospital, and 40% were incapacitated for 6 months or longer.[17]

PATHOGENESIS AND IMMUNITY

Intermediate hosts mount an early immune response to infection with *Echinococcus* larvae as evidenced by the specific antibody and cellular responses and protective immunity generated by a primary infection.[18] The immune response may be separated into two phases: The first is that directed against the hatched oncospheres attempting to penetrate the gut mucosa and establish themselves in the host tissues. The second phase is aimed at the established metacestode at the site of election. Immune effector mechanisms of the first phase are more successful in destroying the parasites than those of the second because established metacestodes have evolved highly effective mechanisms for evading the host's defenses. Evidence suggests that early oncospheres are highly vulnerable to attack by host defenses, but only briefly, and a race between parasite development and the host response occurs in the critical first few days of infection.[19] The explanation for the ability of larvae to persist indefinitely in the tissues of immunologically competent hosts has been of great interest to parasitologists; but understanding is incomplete.[18,19]

Antibody-mediated, complement-dependent destruction of oncospheres in the gut or at the tissue site of development is the most effective mechanism of host defense. Specifically activated B lymphocytes, eosinophils, neutrophils, and macrophages migrate to and concentrate in the vicinity of the developing larvae; however, the exact roles of cellular mechanisms in the immune response are not known. Once established in the tissues, the metacestode appears well protected from the host immune response. Although direct exposure to complement and immune serum readily causes lysis of protoscolices and other metacestodes in tissues, *in vivo* they somehow evade or counteract these effects. For *E. granulosus* cysts, this protective state appears related to sequestration of the parasite by the laminated and germinative membranes and host capsule, which greatly limit the exchange of high-molecular-weight substances between host and parasite. The host's capacity for developing a parasite-specific cellular response able to eliminate the parasite may be modulated by parasite-derived effector substances. Anticomplementary factors released by the metacestode may contribute to the evasion by causing complement depletion at the host–parasite interface. Larval cestodes may also induce a disturbance of normal immune function. Mice chronically infected with *E. granulosus* exhibit an alteration of the T-cell populations resulting in suppression of normal immune responsiveness; these include a polyclonal B-cell activation, a marked decrease in mean T-cell percentage but increase in suppressor cell activity, direct splenic T-lymphocyte cytotoxicity to the metacestode, and impairment of the host defense potential by the formation of antihuman leukocyte antigen-reactive host antibodies. Other hypotheses proposed to account for prolonged survival of metacestodes include membrane fixation of blocking antibodies, which could interfere sterically with the attachment of protective antibodies or specifically sensitized cells. Several mechanisms may

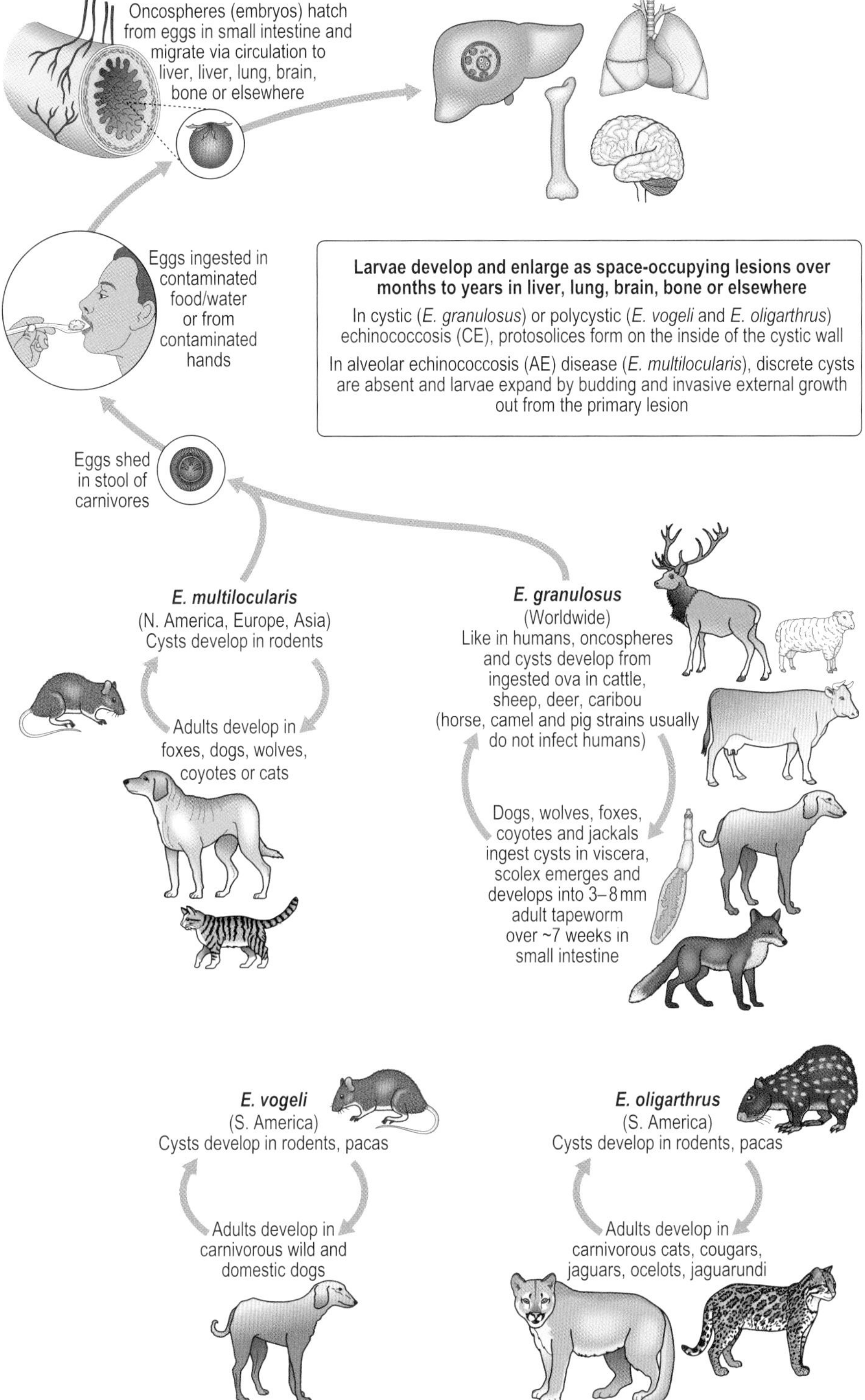

Figure 120.4 Life cycles of *Echinococcus* species.

contribute to the parasite's defense simultaneously or at a different stage of the infection.[19]

Progress in developing effective vaccinations against infection with oncospheres and immunotherapy of the metacestode have been reviewed.[20] The protoscolex appears to contain antigens that may be useful in immunotherapy, whereas the oncosphere contains antigens useful for vaccination against tissue-invading oncospheres. Vaccines based on these antigens may ultimately provide an additional tool for control and prevention of this infection.

DIAGNOSIS

The presence of a cyst-like mass in a person with a history of exposure to sheepdogs in areas in which *E. granulosus* is endemic supports the diagnosis of CE; noninvasive confirmation of diagnosis can usually be obtained by ultrasound or radiologic imaging and immunologic techniques.[14–16] Cystic echinococcosis must be differentiated from nonparasitic cysts, cavitary tuberculosis, mycoses, abscesses, and benign or malignant neoplasms.

Radiography permits the detection of hydatid cysts in the lungs; however, in other organ sites, calcification is necessary for visualization. Computed tomography (CT), magnetic resonance imaging (MRI), and ultrasound imaging are all useful for detecting and defining the extent and condition of avascular fluid-filled cyst(s) in most organs[21,22] (*Fig. 120.5*). These noninvasive imaging techniques have proved valuable for diagnosis and preoperative evaluation by staging the condition of the lesion (intact, unilocular, ruptured, complicated with daughter cysts, or calcified), the extent of the lesion in reference to other organs and vital structures, and identifying the presence of additional, occult lesions. Because of its relatively low cost and portability, ultrasonography has been used widely for screening, clinical diagnosis, and monitoring of treatment of liver and intra-abdominal cysts.[22] WHO/IWGE proposed a standard ultrasound classification of echinococcal cysts based on their ultrasound appearance consistent with the natural history of the disease and response to treatment that is useful for defining the extent and condition of the cyst(s)[23] (*Fig. 120.6*). The standardized classification scheme is intended to promote uniform standards of diagnosis and treatment and may be applied to clinical management of patients as well as to field diagnostic surveys.

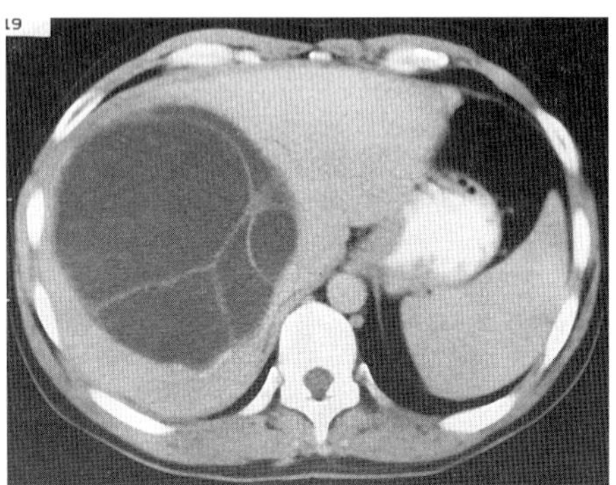

Figure 120.5 Abdominal computed tomography scan showing large primary hydatid cyst (*Echinococcus granulosus*) in the right lobe of the liver. Note multiple internal septations indicating secondary (daughter) cyst formation. (Courtesy of Dr D. Rubin, New York.)

Serologic tests are useful for confirming presumptive imaging diagnoses; however, the limitations of serodiagnosis in CE must be understood to correctly interpret the findings. False-positive reactions, which, with tests using whole hydatid cyst fluid antigens, occur relatively frequently in people with other helminthic infections, cancer, and chronic immune disorders, may be misleading. Detectable specific immune responses have been associated with the location, integrity, and vitality of the larval cyst. Hepatic cysts are more likely to elicit an immune response than pulmonary cysts; nearly 50% of patients with single intact hyaline cysts of the lungs may be seronegative. Cysts in the brain and spleen are associated with lowered serodiagnostic reactivity, whereas those in bone appear to more regularly stimulate detectable antibody. Because fissuring or rupture of cysts is followed by an abrupt rise in titer of antibodies, it appears that the sensitivity of serologic tests is inversely related to the degree of sequestration of the hydatid antigens inside cysts, regardless of the location. Enzyme-linked immunosorbent assay (ELISA) and the indirect hemagglutination test are highly sensitive procedures for the initial screening of serum; diagnostic sensitivity varies from 60% to 90%, depending on the characteristics of the cases. Specific confirmation of reactivity can be obtained by demonstrating echinococcal antigens by immunodiffusion (arc 5) procedures or immunoblot assays (8, 16, and 21 kDa bands).[24–28] These latter serodiagnostic markers are the most *E. granulosus*-specific criteria described, but even they may be detected in serum of patients with other forms of echinococcosis and 5–10% of patients with *Taenia solium* cysticercosis. Circulating antigens are detectable in serum of many patients with CE. The sensitivity of antigen assays is relatively low in comparison with rates of antibody detection. However, since circulating antigens may be detectable in serum of some patients with negative or borderline antibody titers, antigen assays may be useful as a secondary test for clinical diagnosis.[28] Antigen assays are also useful for testing fluid from cysts of unknown origin.

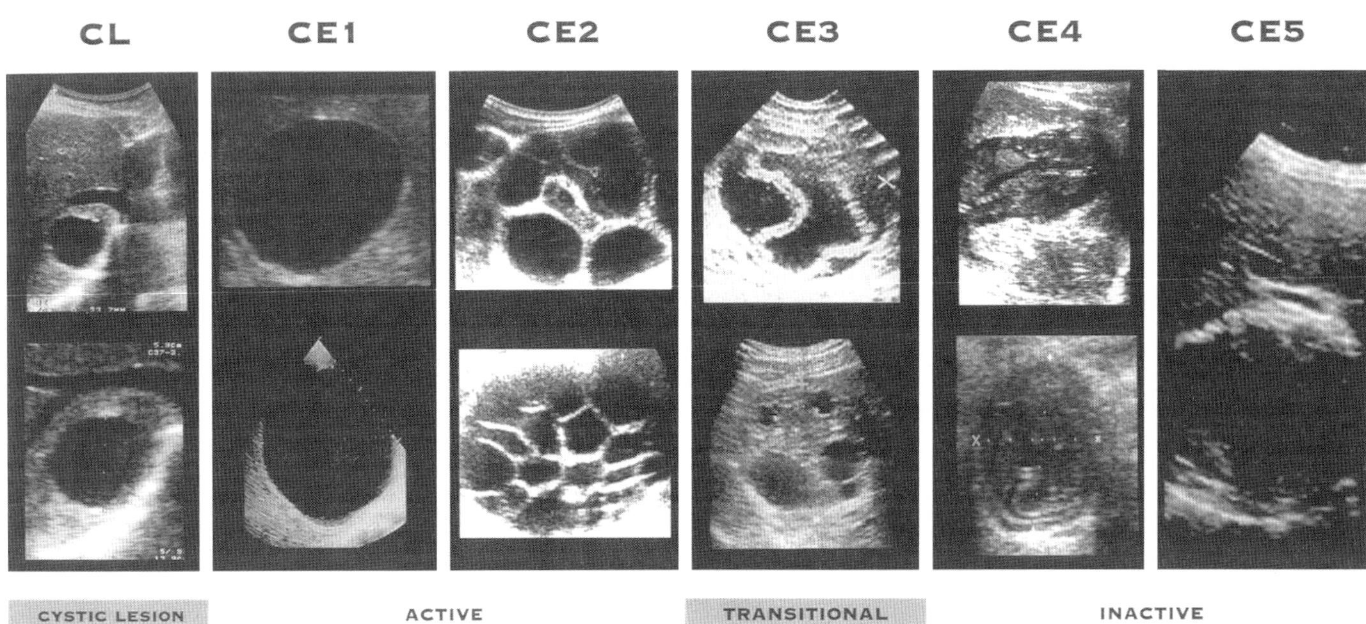

Figure 120.6 World Health Organization/Informal Working Group on Echinococcosis (WHO/IWGE) classification of ultrasound images of cystic echinococcosis. There are six types of cysts: CL are cysts whose parasitic nature cannot be discerned, thus requiring further diagnostic tests to reveal their identity; CE1 and CE2 are active, usually fertile echinococcal cysts; CE3 are transitional in that their membrane integrity has been compromised either by the host reaction or by therapy and may reactivate to CE2 (active) or continue to regress to inactivity; types CE4 and CE5 are solid cysts, with calcified rim in the latter. (From WHO/IWGE. International Classification of Ultrasound Images of Cystic Echinococcosis. Reproduced with the permission of WHO.)

In seronegative patients, a presumptive diagnosis may be confirmed by demonstrating specific antigens,[28] protoscolices, or hydatid membranes in the liquid obtained by percutaneous aspiration of the cyst. Closed aspiration may result in leakage of cyst contents with attendant risks of anaphylaxis or secondary hydatidosis; however, these risks can be minimized if the procedure is guided by ultrasound or CT and followed by benzimidazole treatment. Protoscolices released from cysts can sometimes be demonstrated in aspirates, sputum, or bronchial washings; identification of hooklets is facilitated by acid-fast stains. Eosinophilia is present in <25% of infected people. Although not widely available in clinical centers, polymerase chain reaction (PCR) techniques exist that are capable of differentiating genomic *E. granulosus* DNA from that of other species of *Echinococcus* and other infectious agents.[28]

TREATMENT AND PROGNOSIS

Until recently, surgery was the only option for treatment of echinococcal cysts. However, chemotherapy with benzimidazole compounds and, more recently, cyst puncture, percutaneous aspiration, injection of chemicals, and reaspiration (PAIR) are increasingly used to supplement or even replace surgery as the preferred treatment.[28,29]

Surgery

Surgical removal of intact hydatid cysts, when possible, has the potential to remove cysts and lead immediately to complete cure. The aim of surgery is total removal of the cyst while avoiding the adverse consequences of spilling its contents. Pericystectomy is the usual preferred procedure, but simple drainage, capitonnage, marsupialization, and resection of the involved organ may be used depending on the location and condition of the cyst(s).[14–16,29–32] The more radical the intervention, the higher the operative risk but the lower the likelihood of relapse, and vice versa.[29–33] Surgery may be the preferred treatment when liver cysts are complicated or located in certain organs – i.e., the brain, lung, or kidney. Surgery is contraindicated in patients who refuse, are pregnant, have pre-existing medical conditions that put them at risk, or in those with multiple cysts that are difficult to access. Surgical risks include those associated with any surgical intervention (e.g., anesthesia and infections) and those unique to echinococcosis (e.g., anaphylaxis and secondary recurrence). Operative mortality varies from 0.5% to 4.0% but increases with repeated interventions and in conditions of inadequate facilities.

Conservative surgical management of CE involves injection of protoscolicidal chemical solutions into the cyst(s), followed by evacuation, prior to further manipulations and extirpation of cysts. The use of formalin is no longer acceptable for intracystic injection because of the danger of resultant sclerosing cholangitis.[28,29] Currently used compounds, including 70–90% ethyl alcohol and 15–20% hypertonic saline, have relatively low risk, but all have been reported to cause some complications. Few of these compounds are registered for parenteral or intraoperative use, and it is often difficult to accurately estimate the volume of cysts or determine if an intrabiliary communication exists. Given these considerations, and the current alternatives of peri- or postoperative chemotherapy[30–34] or both, perioperative injection of protoscolicidal chemicals should not be practiced as a routine procedure.

Chemotherapy

Documentation of experience with chemotherapy with benzimidazole compounds is extensive, and the medical approach can be recommended for many patients. Approximately one-third of patients treated with benzimidazole drugs have been cured of their disease (e.g., collapse or solidification of cysts), and higher proportions (30–50%) have responded with significant regression of cyst size and alleviation of symptoms.[35–40] However, between 20% and 40% of cases do not respond favorably. In general, small (<7 cm diameter) isolated cysts, surrounded by minimal adventitial reaction, respond best, whereas complicated cysts with multiple compartments or daughter cysts, or with thick or calcified surrounding adventitial reactions, are relatively refractory to treatment. Both albendazole 10–15 mg/kg body weight per day and mebendazole, 40–50 mg/kg body weight per day for 3–6 months have demonstrated efficacy. Some investigators who have compared both drugs concluded that albendazole has slightly greater efficacy in terms of rates of complete cure and improvement; the more consistent response obtained with albendazole may be related to its superior pharmacokinetic profile that favors intestinal absorption and penetration into the cyst(s).[37] Adverse reactions (neutropenia, liver toxicity, alopecia, and others), reversible on cessation of treatment, have been noted in a minority of patients treated with both drugs. The reported variability in response to medical treatment suggests that the details of treatment, such as dosage, duration, and length of follow-up, must be determined individually for each case; it seems that a minimum duration of treatment is 3 months. The long-term prognosis in individual patients is difficult to predict; therefore, prolonged follow-up with ultrasound or other imaging procedures is needed to determine the eventual outcome.[36–38]

Another important use of chemotherapy is as an adjunct to surgery. Albendazole has been administered to patients prior to surgery for the intended purpose of facilitating the safe surgical manipulation of the cyst(s) by inactivating protoscolices, altering the integrity of cyst membranes, and reducing the turgidity of the cysts. Benzimidazole therapy is recommended for prevention of recurrent disease secondary to the spillage of contents of cysts after spontaneous or accidental rupture.[38,39] Following such accidents, preventive treatment recommendations are 1–3 months continuously of mebendazole or albendazole.[28,29] Praziquantel 40 mg/kg body weight also has high protoscolicidal activity and may be useful for postspillage preventive therapy[34] or as a protoscolicidal agent in the PAIR procedure.[40] Although praziquantel has shown significant destructive activity on cyst germinal membranes *in vitro* and *in vivo*, sometimes greater than that of benzimidazoles, the drug has not been consistently efficacious against established hydatid cysts. Combining praziquantel with albendazole was superior to albendazole alone as preoperative therapy.[38–40]

Contraindications to chemotherapy include patients with chronic hepatic disease and bone marrow depression. Since benzimidazole drugs are teratogenic, they should never be administered to pregnant women. Treatment of pregnant women, unless their disease is life-threatening, probably should be aimed at reducing discomfort until term, after which they can be treated with one of the previously discussed approaches.

PAIR (Percutaneous Aspiration, Injection, Reaspiration)

Another option for the treatment of hydatid cysts in the liver and some other locations is percutaneous puncture using sonographic guidance, aspiration of substantial amounts of the liquid contents, and injection of a protoscolicidal agent (e.g., 90% ethanol or 15–20% hypertonic saline) for at least 15 minutes, followed by reaspiration (PAIR).[41,42] Reported experiences with this approach suggest good results in terms of efficacy and safety.[43–45]

PAIR is indicated for patients with single or multiple cysts in the liver, abdominal cavity, spleen, and kidney. Echinococcal cysts with ultrasound appearances of "liquid cysts" (ultrasound image types CE1 and CE3 with detached endocyst)[23] (***Fig. 120.6***) respond favorably to the procedure.[46–48] PAIR is contraindicated for inaccessible or superficially located liver cysts, in those with multiple daughter cysts ("honeycomb" appearance on imaging), for inactive or calcified cystic lesions, and for cysts with biliary communication. To avoid sclerosing cholangitis, this procedure must not be performed in patients whose cysts have biliary communication; the presence of the latter can be determined by testing the cyst fluid for the presence of bilirubin by endoscopic retrograde cholangiopancreatography (ERCP) or, preferably, by injection of contrast medium following aspiration and prior to injection of the protoscolicidal agent. Complications have included secondary infection of the cavity, acute allergic reactions, and recurrence;[47] however, these have been managed successfully. Applications of PAIR to pulmonary cysts, employed as an alternative in patients who have failed medical therapy, have been associated with frequent complications.[49]

The physician must be prepared to treat an allergic reaction should it occur. The possibility of secondary hydatidosis resulting from accidental spillage during this procedure can be minimized by concurrent treatment with benzimidazoles; indeed, a report suggests that combined treatment (PAIR with albendazole) may improve the results in comparison with either chemotherapy or PAIR alone.[50,51] The recommended treatment course is 4 days prior to and 1 month (albendazole) or 3 months (mebendazole) after the PAIR procedure. For treatment of uncomplicated cysts in the liver, Khuroo and coworkers[51] reported that, in comparison with patients who underwent surgical intervention (cystectomy), patients treated by PAIR followed by 8 weeks of albendazole chemotherapy had comparable rates of cyst disappearance (88% versus 72%) but had reduced hospital stay (4 versus 13 days) and reduced risk of complications (32% versus 84%).

Conventional PAIR, using fine needles, is less effective in treating multivesicular cysts (WHO CE2 and "solid" CE3; ***Fig. 120.6***) than univesicular cysts (CE1 and CE3 with detached endocyst); recurrent cyst growth is common following treatment of these former types of cysts with PAIR.[47] Alternative percutaneous approaches to treatment have been proposed for these types of cysts, including trocar aspiration/drainage of the cyst matrix using large bore catheters or trocar devices[52,53] or inactivation of the germinal layer using a thermal treatment similar to that used for treatment of neoplasms.[54] Data on the long-term outcome of percutaneous treatment of these complex-type hydatid cysts are limited, and long-term follow-up is needed to evaluate effectiveness.[55]

The PAIR procedure should only be performed by experienced physicians with adequate surgical backup support to deal with complications. The procedure is minimally invasive and less expensive than surgery.[55,56] Reported experiences with this approach suggest good results in terms of the absence of acute complications and recurrence. A meta-analysis concluded that in comparison to conventional surgical treatment, PAIR plus chemotherapy was associated with greater clinical and parasitologic efficacy, fewer recurrences, lower morbidity and mortality, as well as shorter hospital stays.[57] The development and use of ultrasound imaging technology for clinical diagnosis and population screening has provided significant improvements for abdominal forms of echinococcosis and has provided new information on the natural history of the disease. It is now clear that many, if not the majority of cases of CE have a benign prognosis. This knowledge has led to new, unanswered questions about the necessity for, criteria for, and selection of appropriate treatments. Further long-term observations and multicenter comparative trials of various interventions and placebo are required to answer these questions.

Monitoring Results of Treatment

It has been observed that in echinococcosis, it is easier to prove treatment failure than treatment success;[15] however, noninvasive methods for monitoring cyst size, consistency, and integrity have substantially improved our ability to assess viability of hydatid cysts. The occult nature of the hydatid cyst confounds post-treatment evaluation. Objective response to treatment, whether surgery or chemotherapy or both, is best assessed by repeated evaluation of cyst(s) size and consistency at 3-month intervals with ultrasound imaging or at longer intervals with CT or MRI. Since the time of appearance of recurrence is extremely variable, monitoring should be continued for 3 or more years. Changes in titers of serologic tests have not by themselves been able to define the outcome of chemotherapy[58] or PAIR, presumably because of continued antigenic stimulation from parasitic tissue. In contrast, following successful radical surgery, antibody titers decline and sometimes disappear; titers rise again if secondary hydatid cysts develop.[16,58]

PREVENTION AND CONTROL

E. granulosus has been viewed as highly vulnerable to the implementation of preventive measures, at least in theory. When only synanthropic hosts under human control are involved, the cestode cycle can be interrupted if dogs are prevented from consuming infected viscera from sheep and other domestic ungulates. Indeed, there are a number of successful examples of echinococcosis control, achieved on a national or regional scale, that confirm that *E. granulosus* is relatively unstable in synanthropic hosts and responds readily to comprehensive and consistently applied measures of intervention.[8]

The earliest successful program was that in Iceland initiated nearly 130 years ago when cystic hydatid disease was recognized as affecting approximately one of every six Icelanders.[8] A uniquely effective health education campaign sensitized the entire population to the disease, and subsequent measures virtually eliminated home slaughter of sheep; the result was gradual elimination of transmission. By the 1950s, echinococcosis was considered eradicated from Iceland. Programs initiated in New Zealand (1959) and Tasmania (1965) were primarily based on education of rural populations and motivating them to change their practices. Strict control and prohibition of farm slaughter were key features in these programs. The initially voluntary nature of the programs was reinforced by legislative acts and strengthened efforts at enforcement as the programs progressed. This policy proved highly successful: the number of infected dogs declined steadily throughout the campaigns. The decline in canine infection preceded decreases in the prevalence of infection in sheep and young cattle and a reduced number of cases in humans diagnosed annually. In New Zealand, the first year when no dogs were found infected was 1985–1986, and hydatid cysts in sheep are now rare. No new human cases of hydatid disease have been reported in children or adults younger than 19 years old since 1977. CE has been declared provisionally eradicated in both Tasmania and New Zealand. A program in Cyprus benefited from very aggressive stray dog elimination and strict control of working dogs and those kept as pets. All used diagnostic purging of dogs with arecholine as a surveillance technique for monitoring the effectiveness of the program and identifying problem farms. Tasmania quarantined infected dogs and infected sheep flocks. Regional programs in Argentina (1970) and Chile (1978) benefited from the advent of the highly effective echinococcicidal drug praziquantel. Monitoring of surveillance data in all these programs documented the reduction of prevalence in dogs, animal intermediate hosts, and humans.[8]

The epidemiologic characteristics associated with the transmission of echinococcosis in the endemic regions where control interventions have been successful were varied, as were the events leading to official commitments to undertake control efforts and the specific technical measures employed. Nevertheless, sustained implementation of control measures resulted in a successful interruption of transmission, and it seems that the fundamental requirements for effective control are now tried and proven in a variety of epidemiologic situations.[59] Control measures with proven usefulness include health education, stray dog control, registration of owned dogs, routine diagnostic testing and treatment of dogs, restrictions or controls on commercial and home slaughter of sheep and other livestock, and enactment and enforcement of legislation supporting the other measures. Since the available technology has improved throughout the years, the degree and the rapidity of demonstrable progress have, in part, reflected the degree of sophistication of the technology. Application of new technology (e.g., a vaccine for sheep[20]) will further improve the technical possibilities for effective control. The immediate prospects for further progress in control of hydatid disease depend on the development of adequate surveillance systems and careful documentation of the disease in all important hosts in order to characterize the quantitative dynamics of transmission and the costs and benefits of different control strategies.[59]

It must be noted that the positive achievements of successful control programs, however significant at the local level, have not markedly changed the global distribution and public health importance of hydatid disease. In most endemic areas, effective control has not been achieved or even attempted. Much remains to be done.

ALVEOLAR ECHINOCOCCOSIS (*ECHINOCOCCUS MULTILOCULARIS*)

THE AGENT

Although there is evidence of variation in morphology, pathogenicity, developmental characteristics, and host specificity between populations of *E. multilocularis* from Europe, Alaska, and central North America, few comparative data are available and the epidemiologic significance of "strain" variation remains unconfirmed.[1,60,61] In comparison to the genetic variability in *E. granulosus*, direct genomic variation in different geographic populations of *E. multilocularis* appears minor.[1,61]

Post-oncospheral development of larval *E. multilocularis* in susceptible rodent hosts is fundamentally the same as that of *E. granulosus*, except that the primary vesicle gives rise to others by continuous exogenous budding, to produce a larval mass composed of hundreds of contiguous vesicles that may occupy more than one-half of the invaded hepatic lobe.

There is no limiting membrane of host or parasite origin. Growth of the larva from the single primary vesicle to the compound multivesicular stage with infective protoscolices may be completed in as short a period as 2 months or as long a time as 7 months, depending on conditions for growth in the host. The rapid rate of development of *E. multilocularis* compared with that of *E. granulosus* is an adaptation to the short-lived rodent intermediate hosts. The number of protoscolices within a larval mass derived from a single embryo is highly variable within and between species of hosts but may number several thousand.

TRANSMISSION, EPIDEMIOLOGY, AND GEOGRAPHIC DISTRIBUTION

The life cycle of *E. multilocularis* involves foxes, coyotes, and arvicolid rodents; *Ochotona* sp., a small lagomorph, is an important intermediate host in Central Asia (***Fig. 120.7***). Domestic dogs and cats also become infected; cats are less efficient definitive hosts, however, and develop fewer, less fecund adult worms in comparison with dogs.[62]

Infection rates in the natural hosts, both intermediate and definitive, are influenced by the numerical densities of these mammals as well as the kind of predator–prey relationship that exists between them. In the northern tundra zone, a strongly defined predator–prey relationship exists between arctic foxes and microtine rodents. The arctic fox feeds almost exclusively on microtine rodents. In studies carried out during different years, infection rates in foxes and voles ranged from 40% to 100% and from 2% to 16%, respectively.[60,63] The variations correlated closely with fluctuations in the host populations; the parasites were least numerous when the populations of hosts were reduced, but infection rates were additionally influenced by habitat and climatic season. The number of worms in infected arctic foxes usually exceeded 100 000–200 000/animal, but they apparently cause no adverse effects. Most worms are eliminated spontaneously 3–4 months after infection, although some may remain for 7 months or longer; however, these are senescent and can no longer produce eggs.[60,63]

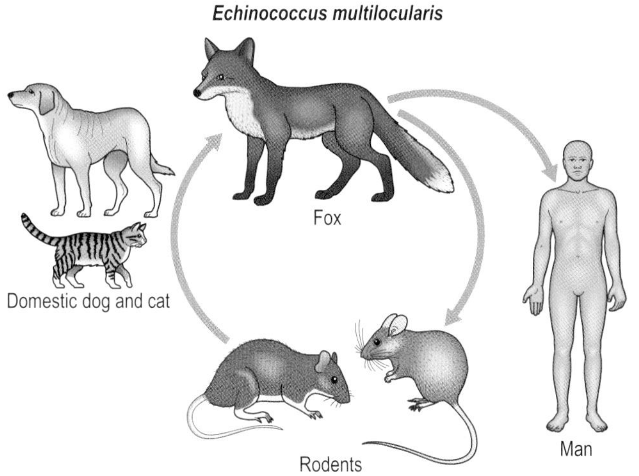

Figure 120.7 Life cycle and principal and alternative hosts for *Echinococcus multilocularis.*

Being largely confined to life cycles involving foxes and arvicolid rodents, in ecosystems generally separate from humans, exposure of humans to *E. multilocularis* is relatively less common than exposure of humans to *E. granulosus*.[8] Fox trappers and other people who work with foxes or their fur would appear to be relatively frequently exposed to eggs of *E. multilocularis*, but these occupations have not been associated with higher rates of infection.[64–67] In most endemic areas, there are few well-defined individual risk factors for infections; however, infection rates are highest in people resident in rural areas where the cestode is endemic. There is ecological overlap to humans because domestic dogs or cats may become infected when they eat infected wild rodents, and infected pets are an important source of infection for humans.[65–67] It remains unclear whether genetic factors in humans play a role. Associations between MHC polymorphism and clinical presentation have been demonstrated.[68,69]

Hyperendemic foci have been described in some Native American villages of the North American tundra[63,67] (now largely disappeared) and in China,[9,10,70] where local dogs regularly feed on infected commensal rodent and lagomorph intermediate hosts. In these circumstances, indirect or direct contamination from feces of infected dogs appears to be the most important source of infection, and human infection prevalence may reach 2–6%.[9,10]

E. multilocularis has an extensive geographic range in the northern hemisphere, widespread and increasing in Europe, most of northern Eurasia, from Bulgaria and Turkey through most of Russia, and the nations of the former Soviet Union, extending eastward to several of the Japanese islands (***Fig. 120.8***).[8] In North America, the cestode is found throughout the northern tundra zone and in a discontinuous zone to the south. In the Middle East, *E. multilocularis* is reported in eastern Turkey and Iran. One human case has been reported in northern India.[71]

Surveys in Central Europe extended the known distribution of *E. multilocularis* from four countries at the end of the 1980s to at least 11 countries in 2000 (***Fig. 120.9***). The incidence of diagnosed disease in humans remains low, 0.02–1.4/100 000 for entire countries or larger regions of endemicity.[72] Between 1982 and 2000, 559 cases of AE in humans were reported voluntarily from nine European countries to the European Echinococcosis Registry.[73] The cestode appears to have spread eastward in Europe in association with increased populations of foxes, and this may herald the emergence of AE in humans in central Eastern Europe. Surveys of foxes in Germany and France carried out in the mid-1990s compared recent data with that collected in the 1970s and 1980s and documented higher fox densities as well as increased prevalences of *E. multilocularis* infection.[74,75] New human cases have been reported in recent years in several European countries previously considered non-endemic: Belgium, the Netherlands, Luxembourg, Czech Republic, Slovakia, Poland, Italy, Slovenia, Hungary, Bulgaria, and Romania.[73] Increasing fox populations, increasing encroachment of foxes into urban areas, and spillover of *E. multilocularis* infection from wild carnivores to domestic dogs and cats might presage increased public health risks of AE.[76,77] The known distribution and prevalence of infection in foxes and coyotes have increased in central North America. Before 1964, there were no reports of *E. multilocularis* in North America south of the Arctic tundra zone, but in that year it was reported in foxes and rodents in North Dakota.[78] Currently, the cestode has been reported in red foxes, coyotes, and deer mice throughout the central United States and Canada, extending south to Indiana and Illinois and east to Ohio.[79–84] To date, only two people are known to have acquired their infections in the endemic region in central North America: a 54-year-old man from Manitoba, Canada, and a 60-year-old woman from Minnesota;[66] however, the potential exists for a more serious public health problem.[8,66]

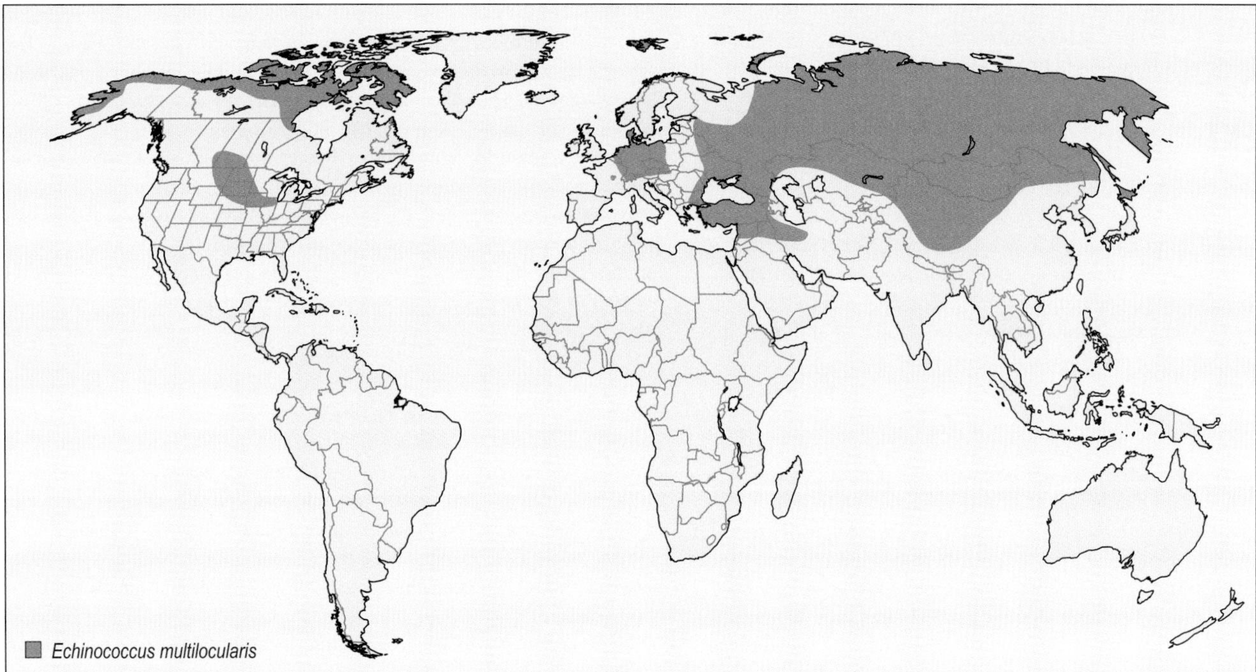

Figure 120.8 Geographic distribution of *Echinococcus multilocularis.*

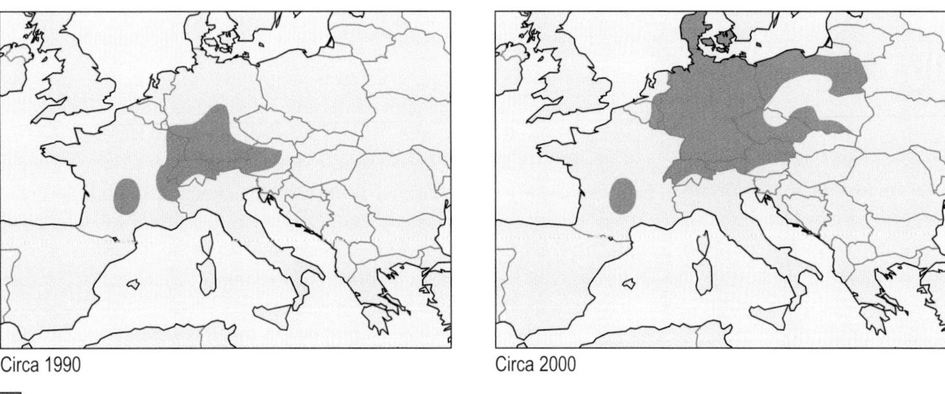

Figure 120.9 Distribution of *Echinococcus multilocularis* in Central Europe.

THE DISEASE

After ingestion, cestode eggs hatch and release embryos (oncospheres) in the small intestine. Penetration through the mucosa leads to bloodborne distribution to the liver and other sites, where larval development begins (*Fig. 120.4*). The primary infection in humans is in the liver, but direct extension to contiguous organs, as well as hematogenous metastases to the lungs and brain, is not uncommon. AE in humans is comparable to that in the natural intermediate hosts (i.e., the primary larval lesion develops in the liver) but differs in that the larval mass is inhibited by the host from completing its development and remains in the proliferative stage indefinitely. The larval mass resembles a malignancy in appearance and behavior; thus, it continues to invade and destroy the hepatic parenchyma and surrounding tissues, and retrogressive stages within the mass result in necrosis of the central portion (*Fig. 120.10*). In AE infections, the lesion consists of a central necrotic cavity filled with a white amorphous material that is covered with a thin peripheral layer of dense fibrous tissue.[85] There are focal areas of calcification and extensive infiltration by proliferating vesicles. Protoscolices are rarely observed in infections of humans. Host tissue is directly invaded by extension of the budding and proliferating cyst wall, causing a pressure necrosis of surrounding host tissue (*Figs 120.11 and 120.12*). A fibrous tissue reaction usually surrounds the larval mass, and a moderate inflammatory reaction is restricted to active lesions. Symptoms are often vague, with presenting complaints of right upper quadrant discomfort or pain, weight loss, and malaise. Occasionally, symptoms related to pulmonary or cerebral metastases may constitute the presenting symptoms.

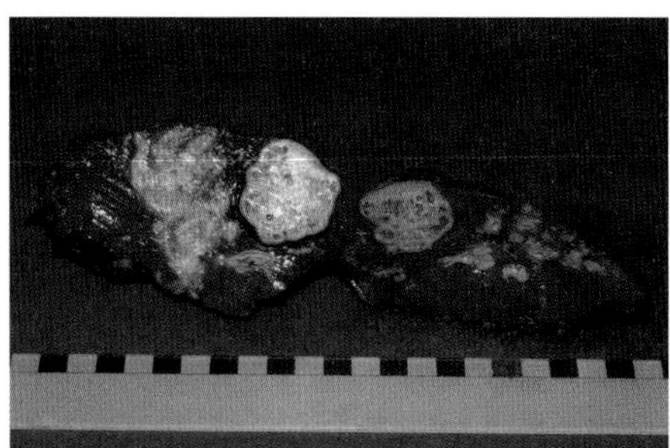

Figure 120.10 Lesions of *Echinococcus multilocularis* metacestode involving liver segments IV to VIII following surgical resection in a 17-year-old woman. Note extensive infiltration of hepatic parenchyma and solid structure with small vesicles.

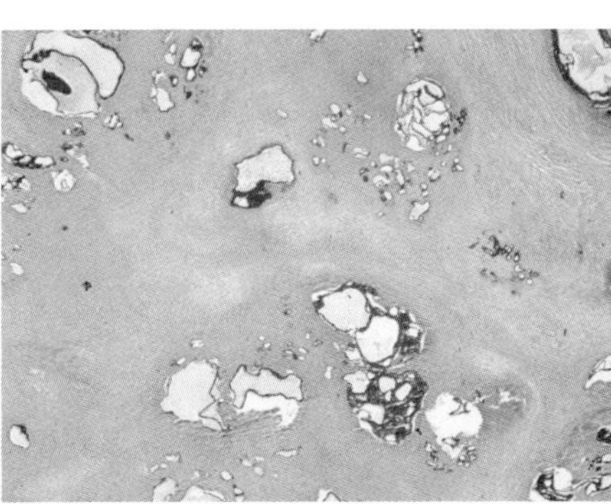

Figure 120.11 Fibrous tissue with numerous small vesicles of *Echinococcus multilocularis* metacestode in the liver of infected patient. Irregular cuticular vesicles are prominently stained by the periodic acid–Schiff reaction.

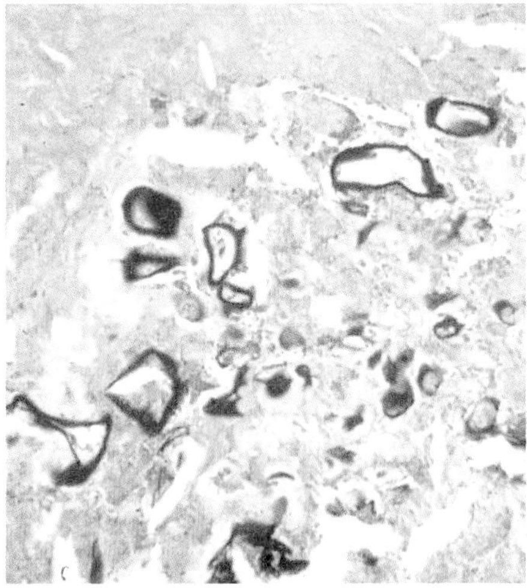

Figure 120.12 *Echinococcus multilocularis* larvae in liver tissue of infected patient. Irregular cuticular vesicles are prominently stained by the periodic acid–Schiff reaction.

Cases of AE are typically characterized by an initial asymptomatic incubation period of more than 10 years and a subsequent chronic course. Because of the natural history of the disease, the nonspecificity of early symptoms, and perhaps because health care providers may not be familiar with the disease, diagnosis is often delayed until an advanced and inoperable stage. AE is a serious disease; although some *E. multilocularis* infections in humans resolve spontaneously in the early stages of the disease,[85–89] the death rate in progressive, clinically manifest cases is high. With or without surgery, reported mortality rates have ranged between 50% and 75%.[16,72] Screening of populations at risk by abdominal imaging (ultrasound or CT scans) followed by specific immunodiagnostic techniques detects cases in the early stages of AE and, consequently, improves the prognosis by reducing complications, morbidity, and mortality.[72] A clinical classification system for human AE has been proposed and designated as the PNM system (P, primary lesion; N, involvement of neighboring organs, including lymph nodes; and M, metastases). The PNM classification follows closely the TNM classification of hepatocellular carcinoma and allows an anatomical description of the lesion at initial presentation as well as a prospective staging of the disease (stage I to stage IV).[88] The PNM system aids a precise description of the disease at diagnosis, providing a baseline for evaluation of treatment strategies.

PATHOGENESIS AND IMMUNITY

Immunologic or constitutional resistance to infection or immunologic resistance to disease following infection may be common features.[90] Although high levels of parasite-specific antibodies are characteristic of infections, antibodies do not appear to restrict the growth of the metacestode. In contrast, T-lymphocyte interactions are of great immunopathologic significance. Periparasitic granulomas – mainly composed of macrophages, myofibroblasts, and T cells – contain a large number of $CD4^+$ lymphocytes in patients with so-called abortive or died-out lesions, whereas in patients with active metacestodes, the number of $CD8^+$ cells is increased.[90] An association between lymphocyte responsiveness and mechanisms of resistance or susceptibility to *E. multilocularis* infections has also been suggested in patients with different courses of disease. Interleukin (IL)-5 and IL-10 were shown to be the predominant cytokines produced by peripheral blood mononuclear cells in patients with AE, indicating the activation of Th2 immune responses in disease.[90–94] Whereas the innate immune system seems to be highly activated, there is no specific memory T-cell response detectable in the chronic state of the disease.[93,94] It seems that viable larvae efficiently suppress specific cellular immune responses which may constitute an immune escape mechanism which reduces inflammatory host responses, prevents tissue destruction and organ demand and may also facilitate parasite persistence.[95]

Clinical observations have allowed discrimination between two groups of people infected with *E. multilocularis*: those who develop disease, thus reflecting susceptibility to unlimited metacestode proliferation, and those in whom metacestode proliferation has ceased, who harbor intrahepatic died-out lesions, and thus reflect resistance to disease. A third group of people demonstrating putative immunologic resistance to infection has become evident in seroepidemiologic surveys. Many apparently exposed people (as evidenced by seroconversion to specific *E. multilocularis* antigen, i.e., Em2) do not permit post-oncospheral parasite development and are assumed to be resistant.[85]

Murine models of AE have shown that a preexisting larval infection can prevent or suppress the development of a secondary infection, but once a primary infection is established in susceptible laboratory rodents, the initial *E. multilocularis* metacestode appears well protected from the host immune response.[93–95] Depletion of T cells enhances metastasis formation in mice. Activated macrophages appear to be key participants in the immune response because they adhere to the metacestode; the cestode grows and metastasizes despite a marked lymphoproliferative activity in the B- and T-cell areas of lymphoid tissue. The parasite may survive by actively impairing cellular mechanisms of recognition and neutrophil chemotaxis in experimentally infected mice. Susceptibility and resistance to infection with *E. multilocularis* metacestodes may depend on genetically based immunologic factors, as evidenced by marked differences in susceptibility to infection in different mouse strains.[96]

DIAGNOSIS

Clinical onset of AE typically occurs in people of advanced age. In the large European Registry, mean age at first diagnosis was 52.5 years, with a range of 5–86 years and a gender ratio of 1 : 1.2.[73] The disease closely mimics hepatic carcinoma and is a challenge to diagnose, even in endemic regions. The most frequent morphological profile of AE is an intrahepatic heterogeneous, infiltrative, and destructive mass, with irregular outlines, and an avascular and necrotic center that appears on abdominal ultrasound as a hypoechoic lesion with a hyperechoic rim. The usual CT image of the same lesion is a hypodense structure with a density of 0-25 Hounsfield units, often showing characteristic hyperdense, plaque-like calcifications.[97] The multivesicular pattern of the lesion is most clearly demarcated on T1-weighted MRI images, whereas the nonhomogeneous character of the lesion is appreciated on T2-weighted images (***Fig. 120.13***). Fluorodesoxyglucose positron emission tomography (FDG-PET) was found to be a reliable method for the determination of metabolic activity in and around *E. multilocularis* liver lesions, thereby allowing the "functional imaging" of infectious lesions.[97,98]

Most patients with AE respond to infection with synthesis of parasite-specific antibodies.[88] Serologic tests are usually positive at high titers. Specific antigens[99–102] have been identified and synthesized which, when

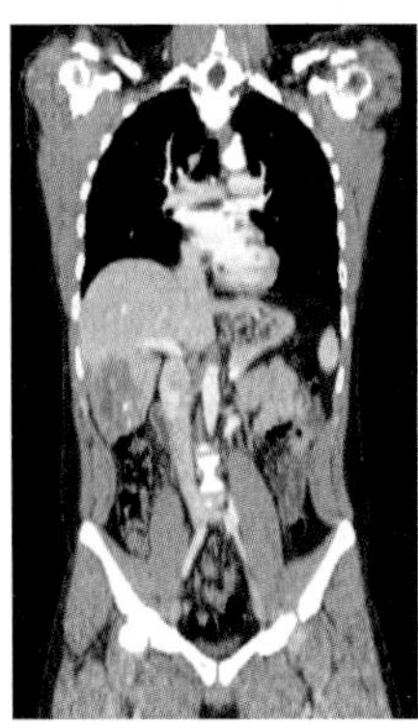
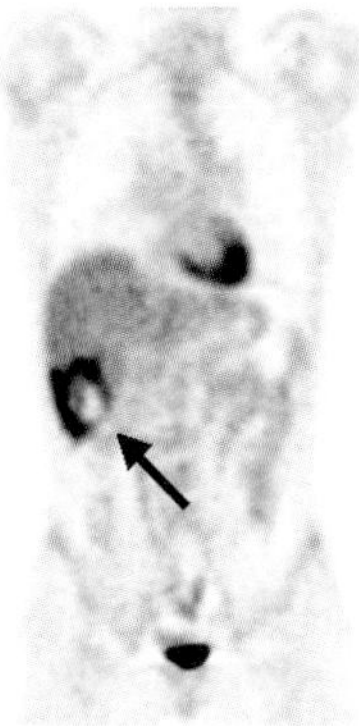
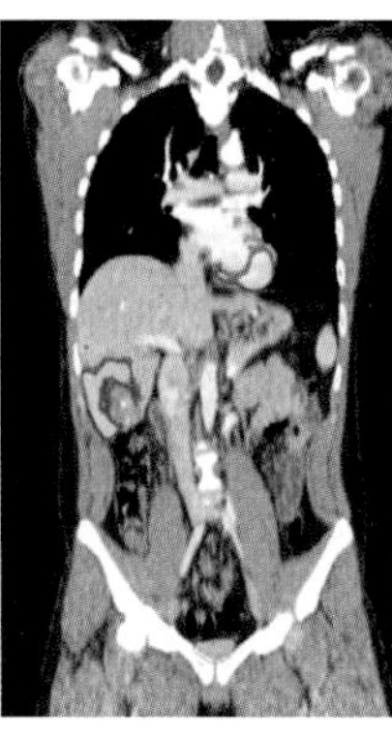

Figure 120.13 Images of alveolar echinococcosis, coronal views. *Left,* Computed tomographic (CT) image of liver of a patient with alveolar echinococcosis. *Middle,* The same lesion visualized by 18-fluordesoxyglucose positron emission tomography (FDG-PET). Note enhancement of the periphery of the image indicating enhanced metabolic activity of host cells in response to the viable *E. multilocularis* larvae (arrow). *Right,* PET-CT; the coloration indicates different intensities of metabolic activity.

used in serologic assays, are highly sensitive and specific for diagnosis of AE and can distinguish this infection from CE (*E. granulosus*) and other forms of echinococcosis. As in CE, serologic tests are more useful for evaluating prognosis following surgery than for determining outcome of pharmacotherapy.[99,103] Antibodies persist indefinitely in the serum of patients managed by anti-infective treatment; however, negative seroconversion occurs within 1 year in patients whose lesion is completely extirpated by surgery. Antibodies of the IgG_1 and IgG_4 isotypes are the most sensitive IgG responses in AE, and monitoring of these isotypes tended to correlate with active versus inactive disease and successful treatment.[103]

In seronegative patients, PCR reactions for detection of echinococcal-specific RNA or DNA in closed or open biopsy specimens have been developed and may confirm the diagnosis.[104–106] Exploratory laparotomy, sometimes performed to confirm the diagnosis and delineate the size and extent of the invasive lesion, should be avoided because of potential spread of larval tissue into the peritoneal cavity.

TREATMENT

Clinicians familiar with this disease emphasize that management of AE, characterized by a malignant-like proliferating cestode, is difficult and usually requires radical surgery, ideally at an early stage, and long-term or lifelong pharmacotherapy with benzimidazoles.[107,108] Choosing from the variety of treatment options requires specific clinical experience; therefore, patients should be referred to recognized national or regional AE treatment centers.[38] Surgical treatment usually requires extensive resection of host tissue (i.e., partial or total resection of the affected hepatic lobe) and should only be performed if a safety margin of 2 cm can be achieved.[108] In cases that are inoperable, in which resection is incomplete or partial, or in cases in which there are metastases to the brain or lungs, treatment with benzimidazoles is required. In clinical trials with patient follow-up of many years, mebendazole administered continuously for up to 10 years at doses of 40–50 mg/kg body weight per day inhibited progression of AE and reduced lesion size in approximately half of treated cases.[109,110] In patients administered albendazole either for repeated periods of 28 days at doses of 10 mg/kg body weight per day with treatment-free intervals of 14 days or given continuously, the results were similar to those described with mebendazole.[110–113] Benzimidazole treatment enhanced length and quality of life; however, in most cases, chemotherapy with either drug was not parasiticidal.[37,110–113] In Europe, postoperative chemotherapy for 2 years is routinely carried out after radical resection, with careful monitoring of the patient for a minimum of 10 years for possible recurrence.[113]

Liver transplantation is not recommended as a treatment option since larval infiltration of the transplant from the surrounding tissue is frequent. However, in patients with terminal liver disease, transplantation may prolong survival.[114]

PREVENTION AND CONTROL

In regions where the infection is enzootic in sylvatic cycles, emphasis should be placed on personal preventive measures, including avoiding contact with foxes and other potentially infected definitive hosts and carefully washing and cooking vegetables and other fresh produce. Control of working and pet dogs and cats must be practiced to prevent them from preying on rodents and, thereby, becoming infected.[8] People living in areas where *E. multilocularis* is enzootic should be educated about the potential dangers, to promote better personal hygiene and sanitation and to motivate them to take effective measures to prevent their pets from eating rodents.

Active intervention for control of *E. multilocularis* presents special difficulties because the primary cycle is almost always sylvatic. In most regions where *E. multilocularis* is enzootic, controlling the cestode by eliminating its sylvatic hosts would be impractical for economic and logistic reasons or unacceptable for ecological reasons.[8] Two approaches to control of infection in sylvatic hosts, one mainly of historical interest and the other experimental, are described next. Where exposure of humans is mainly related to cycles involving synanthropic hosts (i.e., dogs), protection might be achieved by regular taeniacidal treatments of dogs; one such demonstration project is described here.

Control in Sylvatic Life Cycles

Approximately 25 years after its introduction in foxes translocated from the Kuril Islands, *E. multilocularis* was eliminated from Rebun Island in Japan by eliminating the cestode's hosts. Between 1950 and 1955, 2026 foxes and 3224 dogs were captured and killed; without adequate numbers of definitive hosts *E. multilocularis* was soon eliminated. This is the only known instance in which *E. multilocularis* has been eradicated from an area where it was previously enzootic. However, *E. multilocularis* continues to spread on Hokkaido Island and threatens to become established on the mainland of Japan.[115]

Increases in fox populations in areas of Europe have led to introduction of *E. multilocularis* into urban environments. Although this has not been associated with apparent increases in infections in humans, it has raised public health concerns. In Zurich, Switzerland, monthly distribution of praziquantel-containing baits during a 16-month period resulted in significantly decreased prevalence in foxes (from 39–67% to 1.8–5.5%), whereas infection in foxes remained the same in nonbaited control areas.[116]

Control in Synanthropic Cycles

Where it is determined that dogs frequently become infected by preying on commensal rodents, thus contributing significantly to local environmental contamination with eggs and potential human exposure, periodic mass echinococcicidal treatments of dogs is one approach to reducing the risk of human infection. This was evaluated in a 10-year field trial in a village on St Lawrence Island, Alaska, where *E. multilocularis* was hyperendemic.[117] All dogs in this village were given praziquantel 5 mg/kg body weight at monthly intervals. This was effective in reducing egg contamination as evidenced by an average 83% reduction in infection prevalence in voles during the course of the trial; prevalence in locally captured voles declined from an average of 29% at the beginning of the trial to less than 5% at the end. Fluctuations in the annual incidence of infection in voles appeared to be related to the degree that dog owners cooperated in making their pets available for treatment. This control method, which is relatively costly, may be applicable to other regions where synanthropic cycles create a high risk for local human populations; such areas may include recently described endemic foci in Gansu, Qinghai, and Sichuan provinces, China, where surveys showed high rates of infection in domestic dogs.[9,10] The costs and benefits of this approach require further evaluation.

POLYCYSTIC ECHINOCOCCOSIS (*ECHINOCOCCUS VOGELI* AND *ECHINOCOCCUS OLIGARTHRUS*)

THE AGENT

E. vogeli and less commonly *E. oligarthrus* are causes of polycystic echinococcosis (PE) in humans.[118,119] Both species utilize the same intermediate hosts (hystricognath rodents), in which the macroscopic appearance of the larval cysts is similar; however, differentiation of *E. vogeli* and *E. oligarthrus* (as well as other species of *Echinococcus*) can be made on the basis of the length and proportions of the rostellar hooks.[120] The metacestode of *E. vogeli* is fluid-filled, with a tendency to form multichambered conglomerates (polycystic); the predilection site in the intermediate host is the liver.[118,119] Endogenous proliferation and convolution of both germinal and laminated layers leads to the formation of secondary subdivisions of brood capsules and protoscolices.[120,121] The *E. oligarthrus* metacestode is similar; however, there is less subdivision into secondary chambers and the laminated layer is significantly thinner than that of *E. vogeli*. In lower animal hosts and in humans, *E. oligarthrus* metacestodes tend to be localized in the muscles or other extrahepatic sites.

TRANSMISSION, EPIDEMIOLOGY, AND GEOGRAPHIC DISTRIBUTION

The life cycle of *E. vogeli* involves the bush dog and the paca, *Cuniculus paca*, as definitive and intermediate hosts, respectively (***Fig. 120.14***). Domestic dogs are also suitable definitive hosts. *E. vogeli* larvae have also been found in agoutis (*Dasyprocta* spp.) and spiny rats (*Proechimys* spp.).[118,119] Very little is known about the circumstances associated with infection with this species. Bush dogs are rare and avoid human beings, and therefore probably play little role in direct exposure of humans. In endemic areas, human infections are probably acquired from the feces of domestic dogs that become infected when they are fed viscera of infected pacas; this practice has been reported commonly by patients.[118,119]

PE due to *E. vogeli* infection has been reported in most countries within the cestode's known range in neotropical America, including Costa Rica, Panama, Colombia, Argentina, Ecuador, Brazil, Bolivia, and Venezuela.[118,119] Some cases of PE are mistakenly assumed to be *E. granulosus* infection. The natural hosts of *E. vogeli* range throughout neotropical areas of Central and South America, and as local awareness and availability of diagnostic capability increase, it is probable that increasing numbers of cases will be recorded.

The infected bush dog, from which the specimens originally identified as *E. vogeli* were recovered,[122] was housed temporarily in the "children's area" of the Los Angeles Zoo adjacent to an enclosure that housed a variety of infant higher primates, including gorillas, gibbons, orangutans, and chimpanzees. The primates were exposed to eggs in feces of the infected canid and many of them became infected, with at least 15 of them dying of polycystic hydatid disease during the ensuing 10 years.[122] No infections in zoo employees or visitors were ever identified, but this incident illustrates the potential public health hazards associated with housing wild-caught animals that are potential hosts of *Echinococcus* spp.

E. oligarthrus is the only species of *Echinococcus* that characteristically uses wild felids as definitive hosts (***Fig. 120.15***). Naturally acquired infections have been demonstrated in the puma, the jaguarundi, the jaguar, the ocelot, the pampas cat, and Geoffroy's cat.[1] The larval forms of *E. oligarthrus* have been described in agoutis, pacas, spiny rats, and rabbits (*Sylvilagus floridianus*). Presumably, the remote behavior of the definitive hosts limits human exposure. The documented range of *E. oligarthrus* extends from northern Mexico to southern Argentina.[119,123] However, one of the definitive hosts of this species, the puma, ranges from Canada to Tierra del Fuego so that this cestode may be found throughout the Americas. Human infection with *E. oligarthrus* is apparently rare; only three human cases are documented: from Venezuela, Brazil, and Suriname.[119,123–125]

THE DISEASE

Approximately 106 human cases of PE have been recorded, from 12 countries mainly (more than 85%) from Brazil, Colombia, Ecuador, and Argentina.[119,123] Patients' ages at diagnosis have ranged from 6 to 78 years (median, 44), and the most common signs at presentation were hepatomegaly, palpable peritoneal masses, and jaundice (***Fig. 120.4***). PE has characteristics intermediate between the cystic and alveolar forms. Of cases in which the causative agent was speciated, the ratio of *E. vogeli* to *E.*

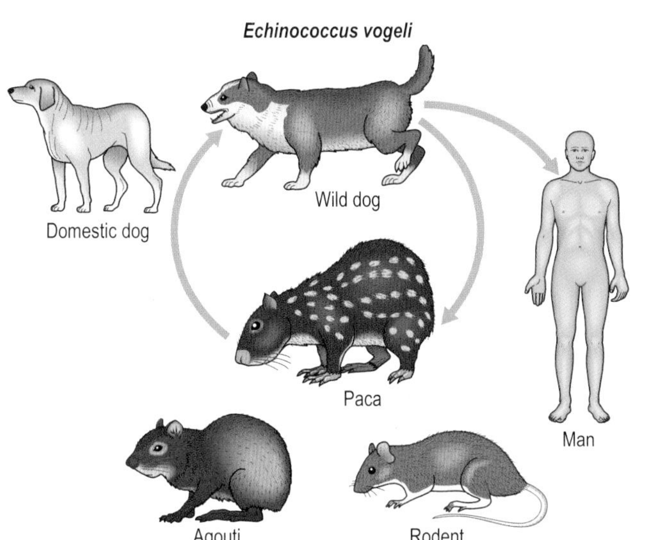

Figure 120.14 Life cycle and principal and alternative hosts for *Echinococcus vogeli.*

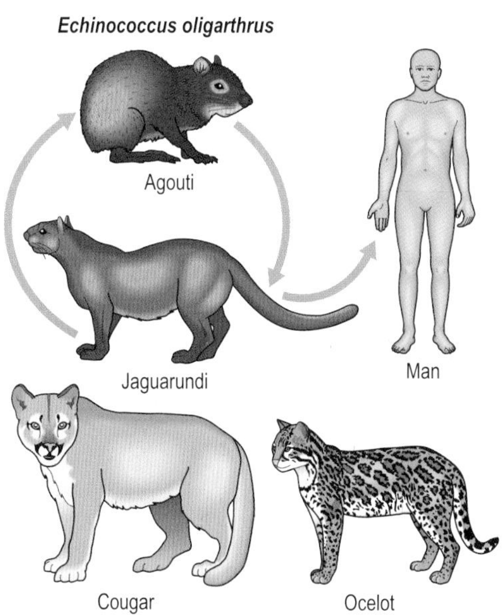

Figure 120.15 Life cycle and principal and alternative hosts for *Echinococcus oligarthrus.*

oligarthrus was approximately 10 : 1. The primary localization of *E. vogeli* infections is the liver, but cysts often invade contiguous sites. In humans and other higher primates, the *E. vogeli* metacestode proliferates by means of a unique process after which extensive spread into the peritoneal cavity and other organs usually occurs.[121]

Hepatomegaly or tumor-like masses in the liver have been typical findings. The lungs are involved in ~15% of cases. Clinical findings may be suggestive of malignancy, and the disease may lead to progressive deterioration of hepatic function, portal hypertension, and biliary cirrhosis. The prognosis for PE caused by *E. vogeli* is poor; approximately 14% of patients die from complications of biliary obstruction and portal hypertension. The three known human cases of *E. oligarthrus* infection have involved the eyes (two cases) and the heart.[119,123]

Macroscopically, the larva of *E. vogeli* appears as a whitish-gray polycystic structure that contains a yellow fluid or gel.[126] The entire cyst may measure only 10 mm in diameter or may form vesicular aggregates that replace most of the liver. The protoscolex with its four circular suckers and rostellum with hooks can be seen in wet mount preparations and tissue sections. The large hooks are 38–46 μm in length, and the small hooks measure 30–37 μm. Microscopically, there are multiple vesicles, varying in size from a few millimeters to centimeters. The vesicles are partitioned by septa formed from the hyaline laminated membrane that is 8–65 μm thick and stains intensely by the periodic acid–Schiff technique. The internal surface of the septa is lined with a germinal membrane that is 3–13 μm thick and contains calcareous corpuscles. The brood capsules bud internally from the germinal epithelium. Externally, the cyst is surrounded by fibrous tissue, with only slight cellular infiltration. Portions of these cysts are frequently necrotic and mineralized, and the only remains of *Echinococcus* may be the hooks and calcareous corpuscles.

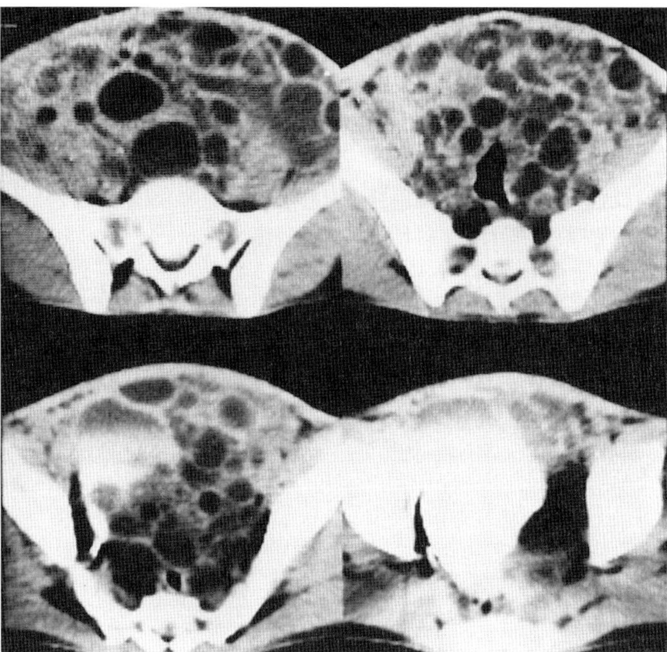

Figure 120.16 Abdominal computed tomography scans showing multiple *Echinococcus vogeli* larvae (polycystic echinococcosis). The lesions are hypodense, round or oval, and scattered in the liver, spleen, and abdominal cavity. (Courtesy of Dr V.G. Meneghelli, São Paulo, Brazil.)

DIAGNOSIS

The diagnosis of PE should be considered in patients who present with abdominal masses and who live or previously lived in rural Central or South American regions where the cestode agents are known to occur.[119,123] Radiologic imaging (ultrasound or CT) is very useful for demonstrating polycystic structures and diffuse mineralization in the liver or other sites (*Fig. 120.16*).

Serologic tests are often, but not invariably, useful for confirming the diagnosis. Specific *E. vogeli* antigens may differentiate hydatid disease due to *E. vogeli* from that caused by *E. granulosus* but not from *E. multilocularis*; however, tests using *E. vogeli*-specific antigens are not widely available.[127] *Echinococcus* species can be distinguished by PCR followed by sequencing or restriction fragment length polymorphism analysis.[126]

TREATMENT

Experience in the treatment of PE is limited. The principles of management of CE and AE also apply to PE. Because the lesions are so extensive, surgical resection may be difficult and usually incomplete. A combination of surgery with albendazole treatment is most likely to be successful.[119,123] Approximately 40% of patients with *E. vogeli* PE improved (reduction or disappearance of cysts for 10–30 months) after receiving albendazole 10 mg/kg daily for different lengths of time from weeks to months.[119,123]

PREVENTION AND CONTROL

In regions where *E. vogeli* and *E. oligarthrus* are enzootic in sylvatic cycles, emphasis should be placed on personal preventive measures, including avoiding contact with wild canids and felids. Raw viscera of animals killed in hunting should not be given to dogs and cats. Control of pet dogs and cats must be practiced to prevent them from preying on rodents and thereby becoming infected. For dogs or cats that cannot be controlled and that habitually prey on local rodents, prophylactic treatment with praziquantel 5 mg/kg body weight can be given. People living in areas where *E. vogeli* and *E. oligarthrus* are enzootic should be educated about the potential dangers, to promote better personal hygiene and sanitation and to motivate them to take effective measures to prevent their pets from becoming infected.

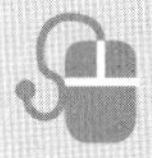

Access the complete reference list online at
http://www.expertconsult.com

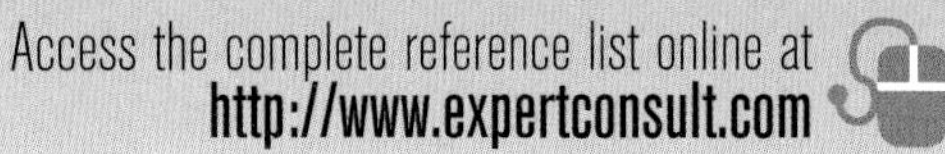
Access the complete reference list online at
http://www.expertconsult.com

CHAPTER 121

Taenia and Other Tapeworm Infections

Murray Wittner • A. Clinton White, Jr • Herbert B. Tanowitz

TAENIASIS

INTRODUCTION

The pork tapeworm, *Taenia solium*, and the beef tapeworm, *T. saginata*, are parasites of humans that have been known since ancient Greece.[1] However, it was not until 1782 that Goeze differentiated the two species. The larval stage was clearly described by Aristotle and Aristophenes from the tongue of hogs, but it remained for Leukart (1856) and Kuchenmeister (1855) to prove that human infection with the adult worm resulted from eating pork containing viable larvae.[1,2] More recently, a third species, *T. asiatica,* has been identified.

THE AGENT (Fig. 121.1)

T. saginata adult worms vary in size from 4 to 12 m and may be composed of 1000–2000 proglottids. When mature proglottids become gravid, the testes, ovaries, and other reproductive organs degenerate and are replaced by the enlarging egg-filled uterus (***Fig. 121.2***). The scolex of *T. saginata* is distinctive, being approximately 1.5–2.0 mm wide and possessing four simple sucking disks, and is "unarmed" (i.e., without hooklets; ***Fig. 121.3***). *T. asiatica* appears similar to *T. saginata*, except that it has a rostellum (also unarmed) and the proglottids have a posterior protuberance. In contrast, *T. solium* is somewhat smaller, varying from 2 to 8 m, with a total of approximately 1000 proglottids. The scolex possesses a well-developed crown or rostellum upon which is a double row of hooklets; that is, it is "armed"[3] (***Fig. 121.4***).

Following the ingestion of viable metacestodes (cysticerci) in insufficiently cooked or raw beef or pork, the scolex evaginates and attaches to the upper jejunum by its well-developed holdfast organs, and strobilation occurs. Infection with adult tapeworms causes few pathologic changes. However, intestinal mucosal biopsies in patients harboring *T. saginata* have shown a minimal inflammatory reaction, suggesting that the worms can have an "irritative" effect, perhaps causing clinical symptoms.

Proglottids, that develop initially from the neck of the scolex, mature further as they are replaced by newer proglottids. Gravid proglottids contain thousands of ova. The ova are 30–40 μm in diameter, radially striated, and, when mature, contain a six-hooked (hexacanth) embryo called the oncosphere. The eggs of the three *Taenia* species are morphologically indistinguishable (***Fig. 121.5***). Cattle or pigs become infected by ingesting mature eggs contaminating pastures or barnyards. Hatching is initiated by the action of gastric juice, intestinal enzymes, bicarbonate, and bile on the eggs. Liberated embryos penetrate the intestinal mucosa, attach to intestinal cells via elongated microvillae,[4] enter the circulation, and are transported throughout the body. Both *T. saginata* and *T. solium* oncospheres produce excretory-secretory peptidases, including serine and cysteine endopeptidases, and aminopeptidase, which may play a role in invasion of the intestinal mucosa.[5,6] Larval encystment usually occurs in a wide range of tissues, but is most commonly identified in striated muscle and the central nervous system; within 8–11 weeks the larvae become infectious. In muscle, cysticerci are ellipsoid, translucent bladder-like cysts in which an inverted scolex has developed. In humans who ingest a cysticercus, the scolex evaginates, attaches to the jejunal wall, and develops proglottids at the base of the scolex. *T. solium* becomes a mature tapeworm in 5–12 weeks, whereas it takes approximately 10–12 weeks for *T. saginata* to mature. The adult tapeworm may live for a few years.[3]

EPIDEMIOLOGY

Taenia infections have worldwide distributions, but there are few reliable data on prevalence due to the insensitivity of available diagnostic tests. *T. saginata* is common in cattle-raising areas of Africa and the Middle East, found throughout Latin America, but rare in the United States and Europe. *T. asiatica* is endemic in much of east and Southeast Asia, including Taiwan, Korea, Indonesia, Vietnam, Thailand, and China. Currently, there are only reliable data on intestinal *T. solium* infections from a relatively small number of nations, especially Mexico, Guatemala, Peru, India, China, and some African countries. Thus, the extent of the endemicity of the infection is largely unknown. More data are available on the prevalences of human and porcine cysticercosis, which are common in Mexico, Central and South America, sub-Saharan Africa, Eastern Europe, China, South Asia, and Southeast Asia[7–10] (see Chapter 119).

THE DISEASE

Most people with taeniasis are either asymptomatic or have minor complaints. The most frequent complaint in *T. saginata* infection is spontaneous egress of proglottids per rectum. Since proglottids of *T. saginata* are motile, the patient may have a sensation of the worms moving. Taeniasis may be associated with abdominal pain, nausea, weakness, loss of appetite, increased appetite, headache, constipation, dizziness, diarrhea, pruritis ani, and hyperexcitability. Children are more frequently symptomatic than adults. Eosinophilia may be present but is usually mild. Serum immunoglobulin E levels may be increased. Only occasionally do these infections result in serious, life-threatening illness from intestinal,[11] biliary, or pancreatic obstruction (***Fig. 121.6***).

DIAGNOSIS

Taeniasis is usually diagnosed by identification of ova or proglottids. Although ova can be identified in stool, stool examination is an insensitive method for diagnosis of intestinal tapeworms. *T. saginata* gravid proglottids often emerge spontaneously per anus, depositing eggs on the perianal and perineal region. Thus, anal swabs, such as the "Scotch tape" method, as usually done for the diagnosis of pinworm (see Chapter 113), may be

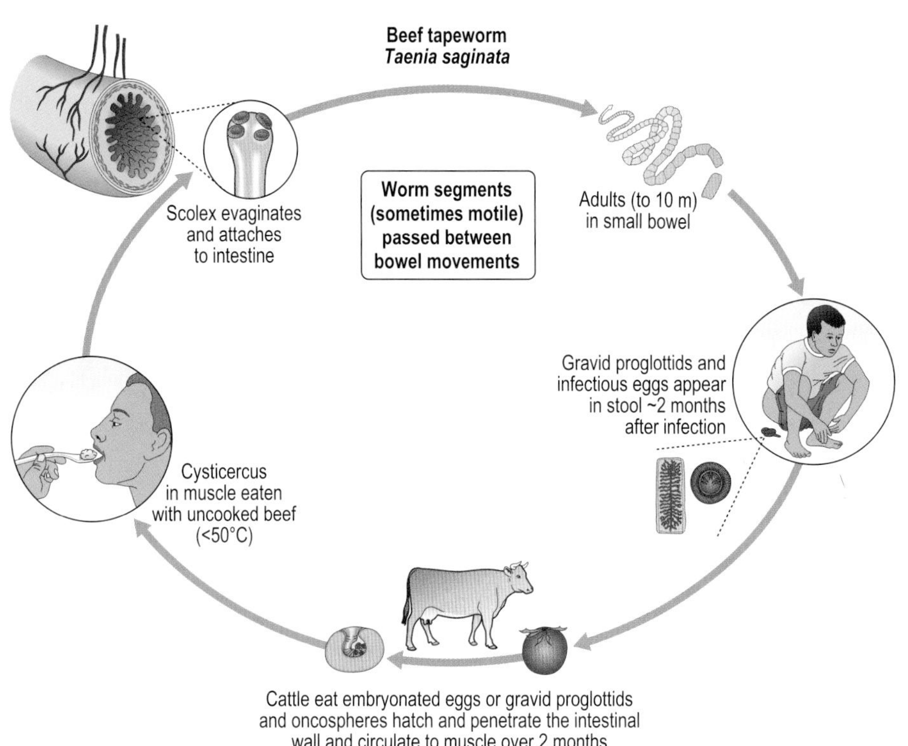

Figure 121.1 Beef tapeworm (*Taenia saginata*) life cycle.

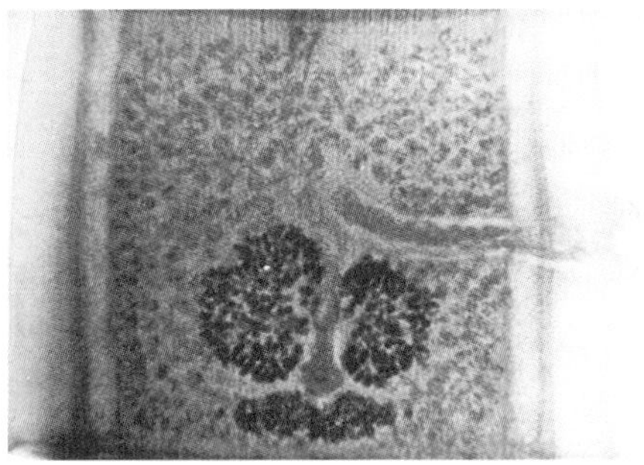

Figure 121.2 *Taenia solium* proglottid. (Courtesy of the American Society of Tropical Medicine and Hygiene/Zaiman: A Presentation of Pictorial Parasites.)

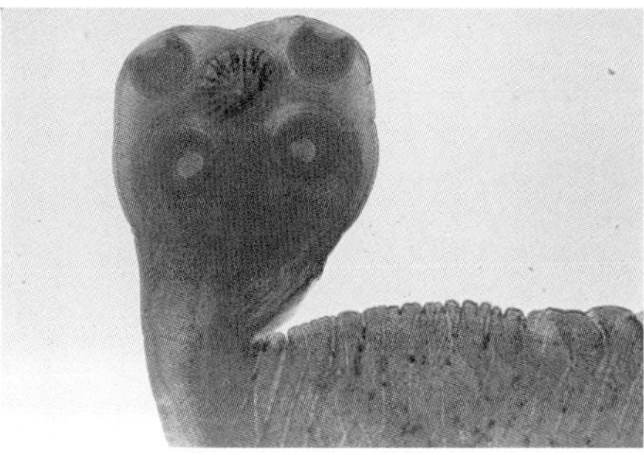

Figure 121.4 *Taenia solium* scolex. Four suckers and hooks are seen. (Courtesy of the American Society of Tropical Medicine and Hygiene/Zaiman: A Presentation of Pictorial Parasites.)

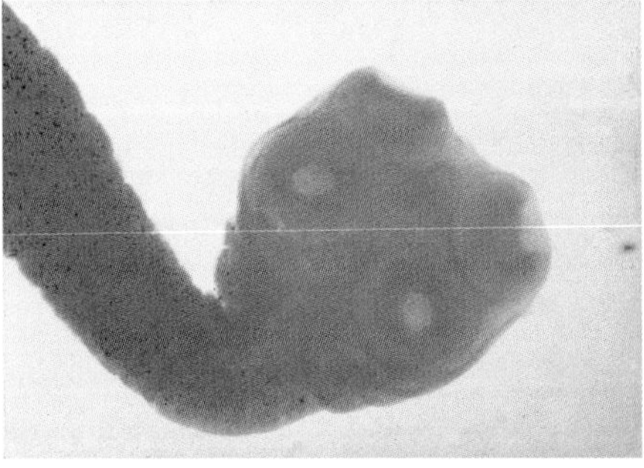

Figure 121.3 *Taenia saginata* scolex. Note the four suckers and no hooks. (Courtesy of the American Society of Tropical Medicine and Hygiene/Zaiman: A Presentation of Pictorial Parasites.)

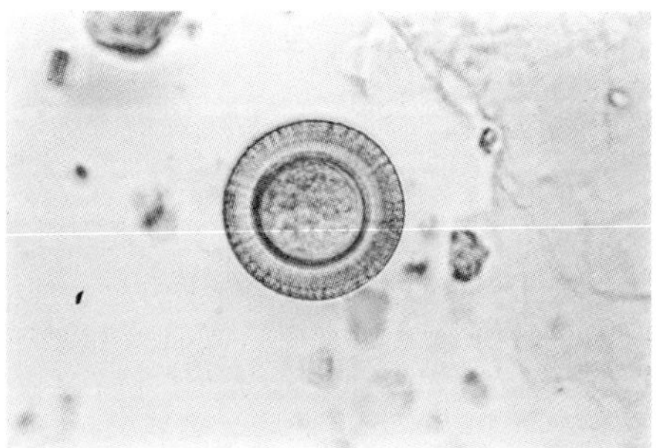

Figure 121.5 *Taenia* ovum. (Courtesy of the American Society of Tropical Medicine and Hygiene/Zaiman: A Presentation of Pictorial Parasites.)

diagnostic. While the morphology of ova of the three species is identical, differentiation of the *Taenia* species can be accomplished based on proglottid morphology by pressing the segment between two glass microscope slides and counting the main lateral branches on one side of the uterus.[12] *T. solium* has fewer primary branches, usually 7–13 on each side; *T. saginata* and *T asiatica* usually have more than 15 lateral primary branches per side[12] (***Fig. 121.7***). An electrolyte-polyethyleneglycol purgative can enhance the recovery of the scolex and proglottids, which could aid in species identification.[13]

Newer immunodiagnostic and molecular approaches have been developed for the diagnosis of taeniasis,[7,14–16] including the detection of coproantigens, copro-DNA, and serum antibodies to adult-stage antigens. Some of these methods were shown to be highly sensitive and specific.[17–20]

TREATMENT AND PROGNOSIS

Treatment of taeniasis, identical for all three species, is with praziquantel (a single dose of 10–20 mg/kg). For treatment of *T. solium*, precautions

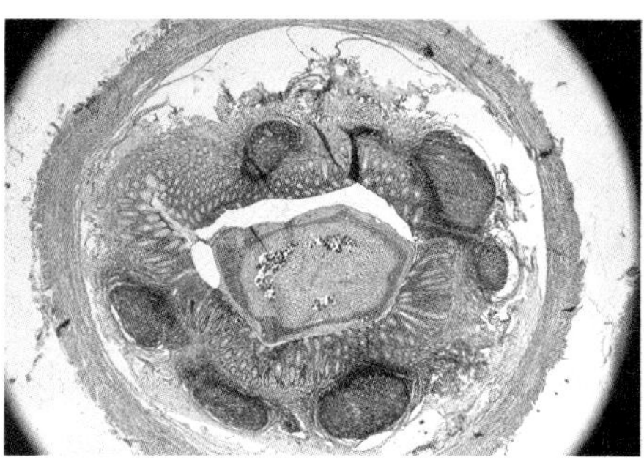

Figure 121.6 *Taenia* proglottid in intestine.

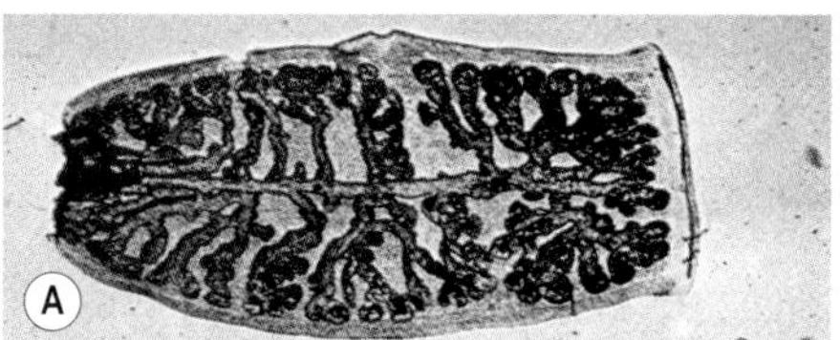

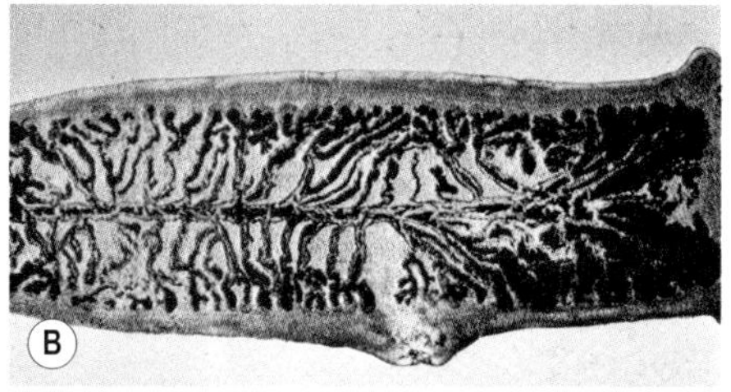

Figure 121.7 (A) *Taenia solium* proglottid and **(B)** *Taenia saginata* proglottid (India ink-stained).

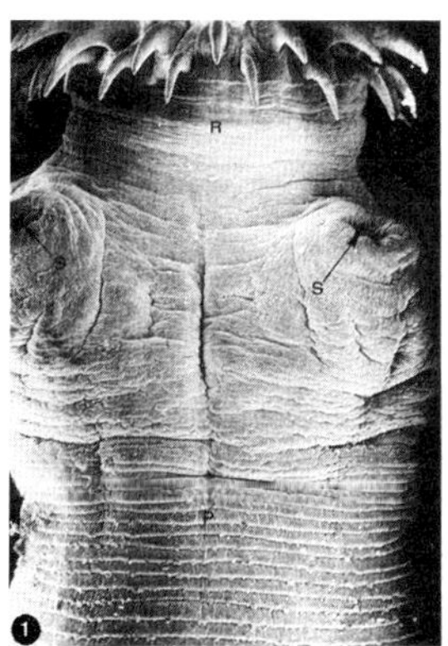

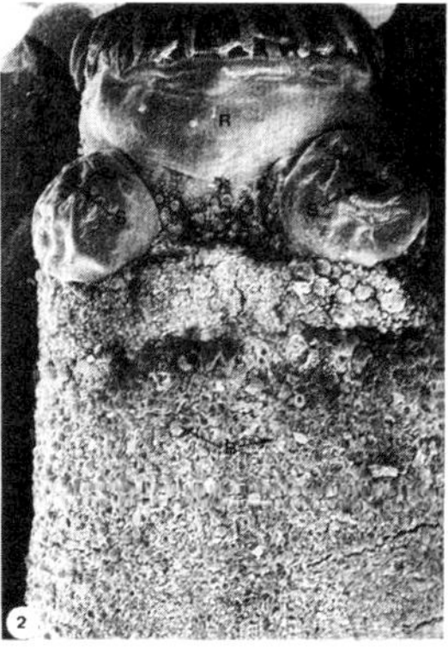

Figure 121.8 Scanning electron microscopy of *Taenia solium* scolex, showing effect of praziquantel. (Reproduced from Thomas H, Andrews P, Mehlhorn H. New results on the effect of praziquantel in experimental cysticercosis. Am J Trop Med Hyg. 1982;31:803–810.)

should be taken to prevent autoinfection or dissemination to others. In addition, since praziquantel kills the worm (***Fig. 121.8***) but does not inactivate the eggs released from the disintegrating gravid segments, cysticercosis is theoretically possible following treatment. Niclosamide, as a 2-g oral dose, is also effective, but less widely available. Nitazoxanide 500 mg twice daily for 3 days has also been used for *T. saginata*. Post-treatment follow-up stool examination should be performed after approximately 5 weeks in the case of *T. solium* and 3 months for *T. saginata* infections. The prognosis of treated taeniasis is excellent.

PREVENTION AND CONTROL

Education is an important aspect of the prevention of taeniasis.[8] Beef and pork tapeworm infection can be prevented by adequate cooking or freezing of beef and pork. *T. solium* cysticerci are killed by moderate temperatures of 65°C (150°F) or if the pork is frozen at approximately −20°C (−38°F) for at least 12 hours, whereas pickling in brine or salting of pork is not always sufficient. *T. saginata* cysticerci are killed by thorough cooking at 56°C (131°F) or freezing at −10°C for 5 days. Pickling of beef in 25% brine for 5–6 days is said to render the beef safe. Treatment of all infected people would eliminate the source of soil and sewage pollution with *Taenia* eggs and therefore reduce porcine and bovine infection. Meat inspection would help reduce transmission to humans who fail to prepare meat properly. Investigations are underway to develop vaccines against cysticercosis in pigs and cattle. Encouraging results have been obtained,[21] but are not yet commercially available.

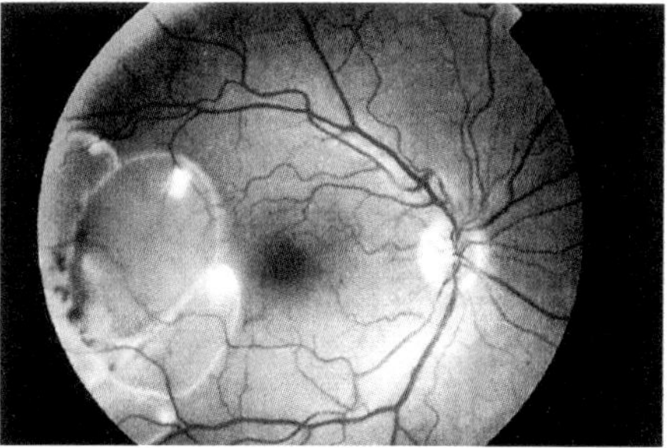

Figure 121.9 Proliferating cysticercus of *Taenia crassiceps* presenting as a large subretinal mass in the right fundus. (Courtesy of Drs GJ Weil, RS Chuck, and RJ Olk, Washington University School of Medicine, St Louis, MO.)

TAENIA CRASSICEPS

T. crassiceps, a tapeworm of canids, is transmitted by the oral–fecal route only rarely to humans. Since humans are not the usual hosts, it presents as a cysticercus in the brain, eye, or subcutaneous tissue.[22–26] Medical therapy has been disappointing. One case of subretinal *T. crassiceps* has been managed by surgery (***Fig. 121.9***).

DIPHYLLOBOTHRIASIS

INTRODUCTION

Diphyllobothriasis occurs in areas where uncooked fresh water fish as well as brackish water and marine fish are consumed.[27–30]

THE AGENT

The distinction between *Diphyllobothrium*, the broad or fish tapeworms, and *Taenia* appears to have been well known to medieval physicians. *Diphyllobothrium* was the earliest tapeworm to be scientifically recognized by Linnaeus in 1758.[1]

The life cycle of *Diphyllobothrium* (***Fig. 121.10***) requires three hosts: (1) the definitive hosts are predominantly humans and fish-eating carnivores; (2) the first intermediate hosts are a large number of copepod species (crustaceans); and (3) the second intermediate hosts are fresh-water, anadromous, and marine fish. *Diphyllobothrium* is a large tapeworm, often consisting of 3000–4000 segments or proglottids measuring from 3 to 12 m, that inhabits the ileum and jejunum. *Diphyllobothrium* tapeworms possess a scolex that is characteristically elongate or spoon-shaped with a ventral and dorsal sucking groove or bothrium (***Fig. 121.11***). Egg production takes place in many proglottids simultaneously over a relatively extended period. The mature proglottid is broader than it is long and contains both testes and uterus. In the center of the mature proglottid is a characteristic dark rosette: the egg-filled uterus that aids in its recognition (***Fig. 121.12***). The uterus leads to a muscular uterine pore through which eggs pass into the feces. Typically, proglottids do not break off and migrate out of the body, but a million eggs are extruded daily into the small intestinal lumen by contractions of the uterine pore.

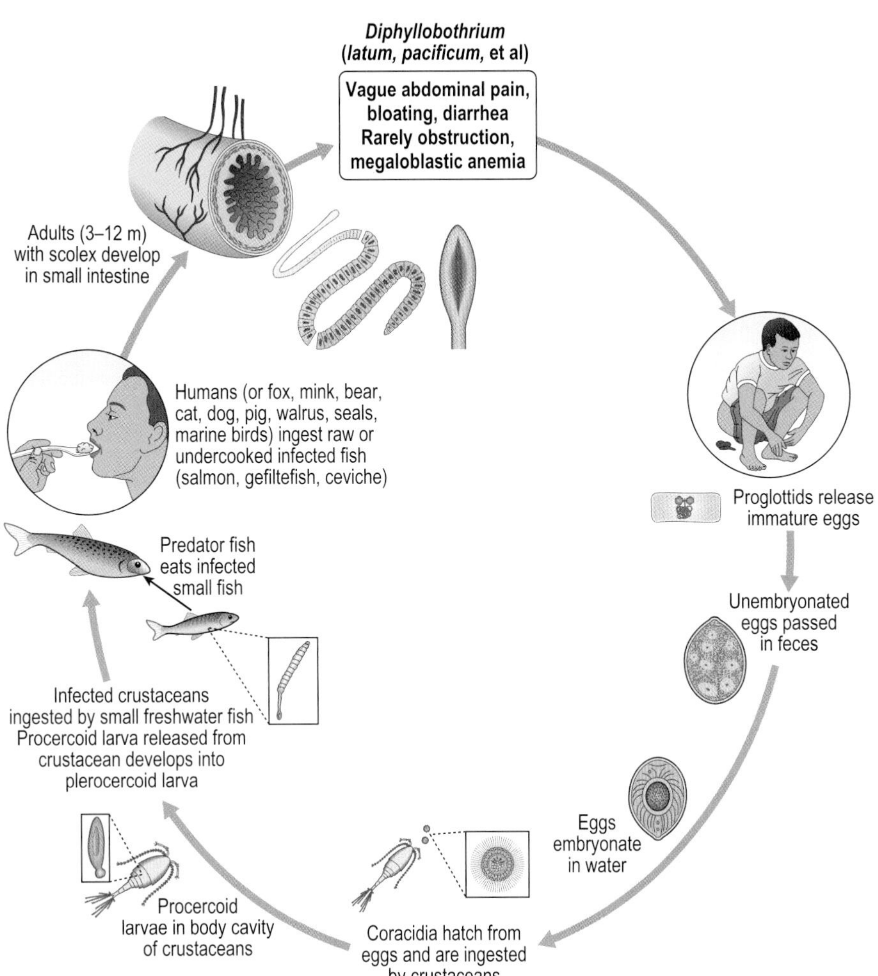

Figure 121.10 *Diphylloborthrium* (*latum*, *pacificum* et al.) life cycle.

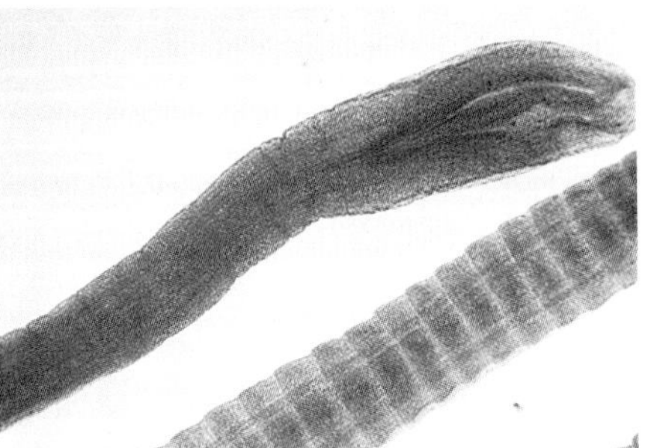

Figure 121.11 *Diphyllobothrium latum*. Immature proglottids and scolex. The scolex bears grooves. (Courtesy of the American Society of Tropical Medicine and Hygiene/Zaiman: A Presentation of Pictorial Parasites.)

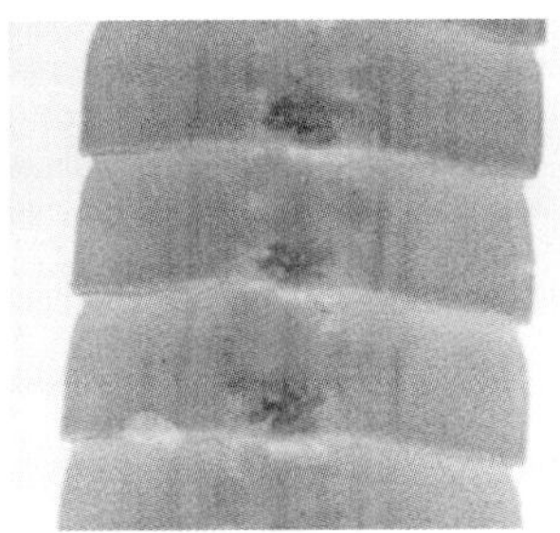

Figure 121.12 *Diphyllobothrium latum*. Proglottid. Note the rosette shape of the uterus. (Courtesy of the American Society of Tropical Medicine and Hygiene/Zaiman: A Presentation of Pictorial Parasites.)

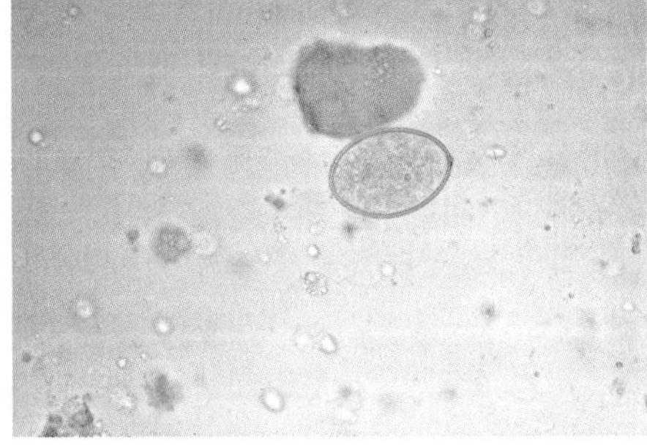

Figure 121.13 *Diphyllobothrium latum*. Ovum. (Courtesy of the American Society of Tropical Medicine and Hygiene/Zaiman: A Presentation of Pictorial Parasites.)

Spent proglottids eventually disintegrate and pass out of the body. Occasionally, a long chain of proglottids is passed with the stool.[12]

The most widely recognized species, *D. latum*, has characteristic light-yellow eggs, which are 42–50 μm wide by 59–75 μm long, with an operculum or lid at one end and a characteristic tiny knob at the aboper-cular end (***Fig. 121.13***).[12] In fresh water, the unembryonated egg requires approximately 10–14 days to mature at 15–25°C. After the operculum opens, a ciliated hexacanth, or six-hooked, embryo (coracidium) emerges; the swimming embryo must be ingested within 6–12 hours by one of many crustacean species of copepods (*Cyclops* sp. and *Diaptomus* sp.) or perish. The larva penetrates the midgut and enters the hemocoel of the copepod and in 10–21 days transforms into an elongated procercoid larva, reaching approximately 0.5 mm in length. It remains in the copepod until ingested by one of many species of small fresh-water plankton-eating fish (second intermediate host). The procercoid larva next makes its way through the tissues of the fish and settles in almost any organ or tissue of the second intermediate host where it transforms into a plerocercoid (sparganum) larva. The latter has the characteristic rudiments of a scolex but is unsegmented. Next, these fish are eaten by larger carnivorous fish, such as perch, wall-eyed pike, or the burbot (paratenic or transport hosts). The plerocercoid larvae later reinvade the tissues of these fish and if consumed raw or inadequately cooked by a suitable host (i.e., humans, carnivorous mammals), the larva attaches to the wall of the small intestine and becomes a mature tapeworm in approximately 5 or 6 weeks.

EPIDEMIOLOGY

D. latum biotypes are mostly shallow fresh-water littorals with vegetation favoring the development of copepods and fish. Infection with this parasite is most prevalent in areas of the north temperate and subarctic zones, where fresh-water fish are commonly consumed.[30–32] The estimated worldwide prevalence is approximately 9–10 million people. In North America, endemic foci have been found among Native Americans in Alaska and Canada. In the United States, fish from the lakes of the north-central region and from Florida and California are found to be infected. In highly endemic regions of Finnish and Russian Karelia, prevalences ranged from 25% to 100%.[28] In North America, human cases have declined, whereas in South America there have been increased reports from fish, especially salmonids. Transmission has been brought under control in western Europe, and only a few cases now occur in Finland, where nearly 20% of the population was infected in the 1950s. However, areas of Sweden, France, Switzerland, northwestern Russia, the Danube and lower Volga basins, and the lake regions of northern Italy and Switzerland contain infected fish. Humans are the primary definitive host and most important reservoir of infection. Secondary intermediate hosts can be species of brackish and fresh-water fish, including anadromous fish that spawn in fresh water (e.g., salmon). Salmon has been the cause of the transmission of this parasite in Japan (*D. nihonkaiense*) and the west coast of the United States where sushi has been prepared with infected salmon.[30]

Eating raw, insufficiently cooked, or lightly pickled fish or fresh roe can transmit infection. In northern Minnesota and Michigan, where large numbers of people of Scandinavian background live, raw and pickled fish are still eaten, although infection with *D. latum* has now become less common. Other diphyllobothriids can cause disease. *D. pacificum* has been reported from Japan and is endemic in coastal areas of Peru. Unlike *D. latum*, infection with this parasite is acquired from eating marine fish that has been prepared in lime juice (e.g., ceviche). *Diplogonoporus grandis*, another member of this group, is found in Japan and thought to be acquired by consumption of raw anchovies and sardines. Other species of *Diphyllobothrium*, such as *D. dendriticum*, *D. klebaanovskii*, *D. cordatum*, *D. dalliae*, *D. ursi*, and *D. nihonkaiense*, are found as occasional human parasites.[31,32]

THE DISEASE

Infection is usually associated with few symptoms or pathologic changes in the intestinal mucosa. Often, infection is first recognized in an asymptomatic patient as a result of a stool examination carried out for other reasons. However, some patients complain of vague abdominal pain and others describe the sensation that "something is moving inside." Others describe bloating, sore tongue, sore gums, allergic symptoms, headache, hunger pains, loss of appetite, or increased appetite. Rarely, mechanical intestinal obstruction may occur as a result of several worms becoming entangled. Diarrhea may also occur. Almost all patients become aware of the infection when spontaneously passing a large section of the spent proglottids; most often this startling event brings the patient to the office or clinic. Unlike the proglottids of *T. saginata*, those of *D. latum* do not spontaneously crawl through the anus.[33]

In a small proportion of patients, *D. latum* causes pernicious anemia, a hyperchromic, macrocytic, megaloblastic anemia with thrombocytopenia and mild leukopenia. The development of pernicious anemia is usually associated with attachment of the tapeworm within 145 cm of the mouth. In this situation, more than 80% of vitamin B_{12} is absorbed by the worm, with a differential absorption pattern of 1000 : 1 in favor of the worm. Anemia associated with diphyllobothriasis is most frequently encountered in Scandinavia, likely due to differences between parasite species. Approximately 40% of people harboring the worm in Scandanavia have reduced serum vitamin B_{12} levels, but fewer than 2% develop anemia. Neurologic lesions due to vitamin B_{12} deficiency include subacute combined degeneration of the dorsal and lateral columns and peripheral nerve degeneration. The anemia and neurologic manifestations respond to vitamin B_{12} and do not recur after the worm has been expelled.

DIAGNOSIS

The infection can be diagnosed readily by finding characteristic ova in the feces (see ***Fig. 121.10***).[12] The eggs can usually be identified without concentration due to the large number of eggs. However, species recognition or differentiation usually requires recovery of the scolex. Molecular methods have been employed for the diagnosis of *Diphyllobothrium* sp.[34] Thus, restriction fragment length polymorphism has been used to speciate *D. latum* from *D. nihonkaiense*. It is not uncommon to find mild eosinophilia in patients with *D. latum* infection.

TREATMENT AND PROGNOSIS

The treatment of choice is praziquantel, which is administered as a single dose of 5–10 mg/kg for both adults and children.[35] Alternatively, niclosamide is given as a 2-g dose once for adults and 50 mg/kg for children. The prognosis for treated individuals is excellent.

PREVENTION AND CONTROL

Careful cooking of fresh-water fish would eliminate all possibility of human infection. The sale of fish originating in heavily infected lakes should be regulated because freezing at −10°C for 24 hours suffices to kill the plerocercoid larva. In the United States, smoked salmon is usually brined before smoking and is not considered a source of infection. Other control measures include the education of cooks regarding the sampling of raw fish during preparation. In addition, sanitary sewage disposal rather than the dumping of raw sewage into fresh-water lakes would prevent viable eggs from contaminating various intermediate hosts.

HYMENOLEPIASIS

INTRODUCTION

Two species of *Hymenolepis* infect humans: *H. nana* and *H. diminuta*. They are cosmopolitan in distribution. *H. nana* is common in warmer climates whereas *H. diminuta* only occasionally infects humans.[36]

THE AGENT (Fig. 121.14)

The adult *H. nana* is approximately 0.5 cm long and is found attached to the mucosa of the ileum by a scolex that has four suckers and a retractable, armed rostellum (***Fig. 121.15***). The entire worm usually consists of a scolex and approximately 200 proglottids. The uterus in a gravid proglottid contains approximately 100–200 mature eggs that are 30–60 μm in diameter (***Fig. 121.16***).[36] The eggs are passed in the feces and ingested by a new human or the same host (autoinfection). The embryo hatches in the small intestine and penetrates a villus, where it becomes a cysticercoid larva (***Fig. 121.17***). Upon maturation, in 3 or 4 days, it emerges from the tissue and attaches to the intestinal mucosa by its scolex. In 2 or 3 weeks, the new worm is producing eggs. Hyperinfection can occur when eggs liberated in the small intestine hatch and

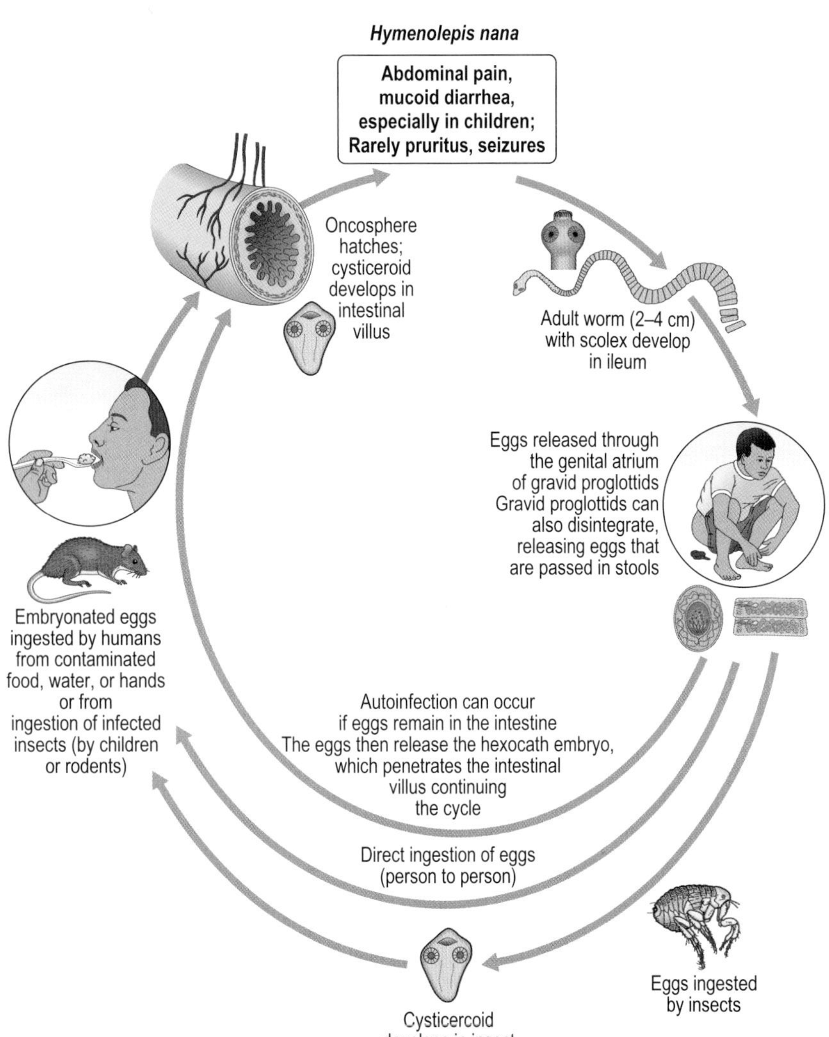
Hymenolepis nana
Abdominal pain, mucoid diarrhea, especially in children; Rarely pruritus, seizures
Oncosphere hatches; cysticeroid develops in intestinal villus
Adult worm (2–4 cm) with scolex develop in ileum
Eggs released through the genital atrium of gravid proglottids Gravid proglottids can also disintegrate, releasing eggs that are passed in stools
Embryonated eggs ingested by humans from contaminated food, water, or hands or from ingestion of infected insects (by children or rodents)
Autoinfection can occur if eggs remain in the intestine The eggs then release the hexocath embryo, which penetrates the intestinal villus continuing the cycle
Direct ingestion of eggs (person to person)
Eggs ingested by insects
Cysticercoid develops in insect

Figure 121.14 *Hymenolepis nana* life cycle.

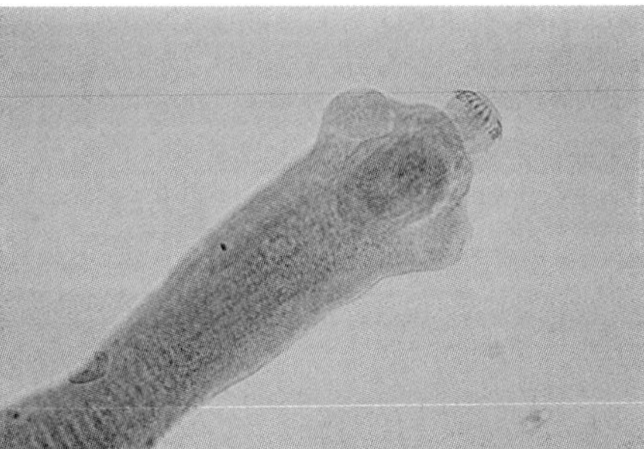

Figure 121.15 *Hymenolepis nana* scolex and proglottids. (Courtesy of the American Society of Tropical Medicine and Hygiene/Zaiman: A Presentation of Pictorial Parasites.)

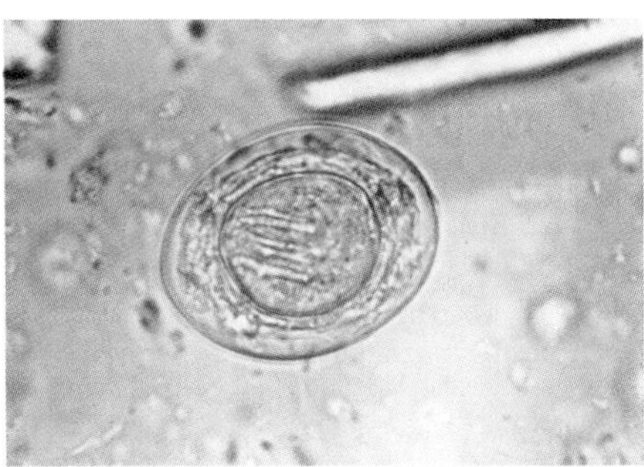

Figure 121.16 *Hymenolepis nana* ovum. (Courtesy of the American Society of Tropical Medicine and Hygiene/Zaiman: A Presentation of Pictorial Parasites.)

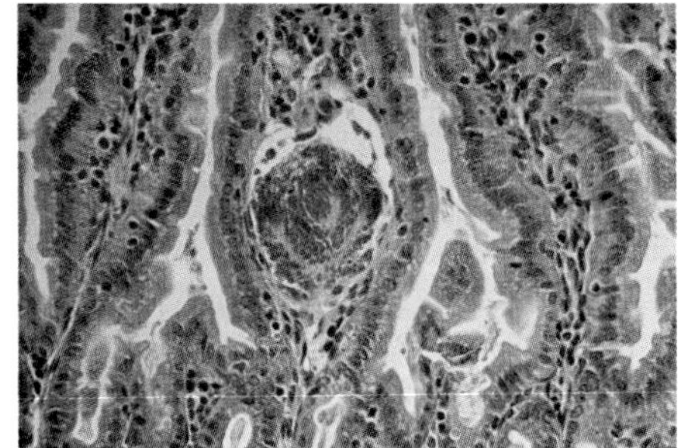

Figure 121.17 *Hymenolepis nana* cysticercoid stage in the small intestine. (Courtesy of the American Society of Tropical Medicine and Hygiene/Zaiman: A Presentation of Pictorial Parasites.)

immediately penetrate a villus to undergo a new cycle. As a result of hyperinfection, children may harbor many hundreds or even thousands of adult worms. The entire life history from ingestion of the egg to adulthood requires approximately 10–14 days. Eggs are first seen in the stools in approximately 25–30 days. *H. nana* is spread from hand to mouth.

The closely related species, *H. diminuta*, which commonly parasitizes the rat and mouse, infrequently infects humans.[36] Most of the more than 200 reported human infections have been in children younger than 3 years of age. The adult worm is 3–5 mm and possesses a club-shaped scolex that has a rudimentary apical unarmed rostellum with four small suckers. The ova are spherical and 60–86 μm in diameter.[12] In contrast to the eggs of *H. nana*, there are no polar filaments. Development of this tapeworm requires an intermediate host. Presumably, infected rat fleas (*Nosopsyllus* and *Xenopsylla*) and mealworms (*Tenebrio*) are accidentally ingested, and the mature adult develops in approximately 3 weeks. Cockroaches may also serve as intermediate hosts and become infected by ingesting eggs passed in rodent feces.

EPIDEMIOLOGY

The dwarf tapeworm, *H. nana*, is found in most warm regions of the world. It is the most common cestode infection worldwide with endemic foci in Latin America, southern Europe, Russia and the former Soviet republics, the Indian subcontinent, and southeastern United States.[36]

THE DISEASE

Most cases are asymptomatic. Young children may develop symptoms when many worms are present.[37,38] These patients may have loose bowel movements or occasionally frank diarrhea with mucus but no blood. Diffuse, persistent abdominal pain is the most common complaint. Pruritus ani and nasi are occasionally encountered. Many children have sleep and behavioral disturbances that resolve after successful therapy. Serious neurologic disturbances such as seizures have been reported. Many patients with hymenolepiasis have a moderate eosinophilia of 5–10% and skin eruptions.[37]

DIAGNOSIS

The diagnosis of hymenolepiasis rests on finding the characteristic ova by stool examination. Stools of the entire family must be checked before therapy is initiated because other members of a household are commonly infected, and they must also be treated for therapy to be successful. Post-treatment stool examinations should be done after 5 weeks and again after 3 months.[1–3]

TREATMENT AND PROGNOSIS

Praziquantel is the drug of choice for the treatment of hymenolepiasis and is highly effective in a single dose of 15 mg/kg. It not only eliminates adult worms but also, unlike other anthelminthics, is efficiently absorbed and kills the larval stages (cysticercoids) in the submucosa.[2] Treated individuals have an excellent prognosis. Niclosamide (2 g in a single dose) and nitazoxanide (500 mg PO twice daily for 3 days) are alternative therapies. Recently nitazoxianide has been evaluated in field trials in Peru.[38]

PREVENTION AND CONTROL

This infection is spread from person to person and therefore extremely difficult to control. Education in hygiene is probably the only practical way to reduce the incidence.

DIPYLIDIASIS

INTRODUCTION

The dog tapeworm, *Dipylidium caninum*, is also a frequent parasite of cats and wild carnivores worldwide. It is an occasional parasite of the small intestine of humans.

THE AGENT (Fig. 121.18)

The adult worm is approximately 15–20 cm long and usually has approximately 60–175 proglottids. The scolex is characteristic, being rhomboid with four oval suckers and an armed retractable conical rostellum containing 30–150 thorn-shaped hooks arranged in transverse rows (***Fig. 121.19***). The proglottids have a double set of reproductive organs with genital pores midway on each lateral margin (***Fig. 121.20***). The gravid proglottids are packed with 15–25 eggs. Each egg is 35–60 μm in diameter and contains an oncosphere with six hooklets. The strobila can migrate several centimeters per hour and pass out of the anus spontaneously or with the feces. Eggs are expelled by contraction or disintegration of the proglottid.[39]

EPIDEMIOLOGY

Most infections occur in children younger than 8 years old as well as infants younger than 6 months of age.[40–44] The ova of *Dipylidium* are ingested by the larval dog or cat flea, in which they become cysticercoid larvae. Infection occurs following accidental ingestion of the infected flea.

THE DISEASE

Infection is often asymptomatic. The most common symptom is noting proglottids in stool, which are similar in size and color to grains of rice. Some children have intestinal disturbances, including abdominal pain and diarrhea (***Fig. 121.21***).[40–42] Allergic manifestations such as urticaria and pruritus ani have been reported; intestinal obstruction has been a rare complication.[1,2]

TREATMENT AND PREVENTION

Treatment is with 5–10 mg/kg of praziquantel once for both adults and children. An alternative therapy is 2 g of niclosamide once for adults and 25 mg/kg once for children. Children should not be allowed to fondle and kiss dogs and cats. Periodic treatment of pets for tapeworm infection and periodic use of insecticides to kill ectoparasites will control the spread of this infection.

SPARGANOSIS

INTRODUCTION

Sparganosis is an uncommon parasitic infection usually caused by the migration of larval tapeworms of the genus *Spirometra*.

THE AGENT

Human sparganosis may occur following ingestion of species of *Cyclops* that are infected with the procercoid larva of various pseudophyllidean tapeworms of the species *Spirometra*.[1,45] The procercoid penetrates the intestinal wall and migrates to various sites, including subcutaneous tissues, the central nervous system, and muscle, where they develop to second-stage larvae or plerocercoids. This condition is called sparganosis. Ingestion, either deliberately or accidentally, of infected uncooked flesh of an amphibian, reptile, bird, or mammal harboring plerocercoid larvae may also be a source of infection. All the spargana are morphologically indistinguishable. Since these worms cannot mature in humans, they migrate into the tissues and remain as plerocercoid larvae. However, in the few instances in which the larvae were allowed to complete their life cycle in dogs or cats, they were identified as members of the genus *Spirometra*. In some cases in the United States, they were identified as *S. mansoni*. Molecular approaches have been applied to this parasite that may aid in the diagnosis of this infection.[46]

EPIDEMIOLOGY

Sparganosis is reported in many areas of the world, including China, Japan, Southeast Asia, and South and Central America, and has occasionally been reported in various areas of the United States and Europe.[47,48]

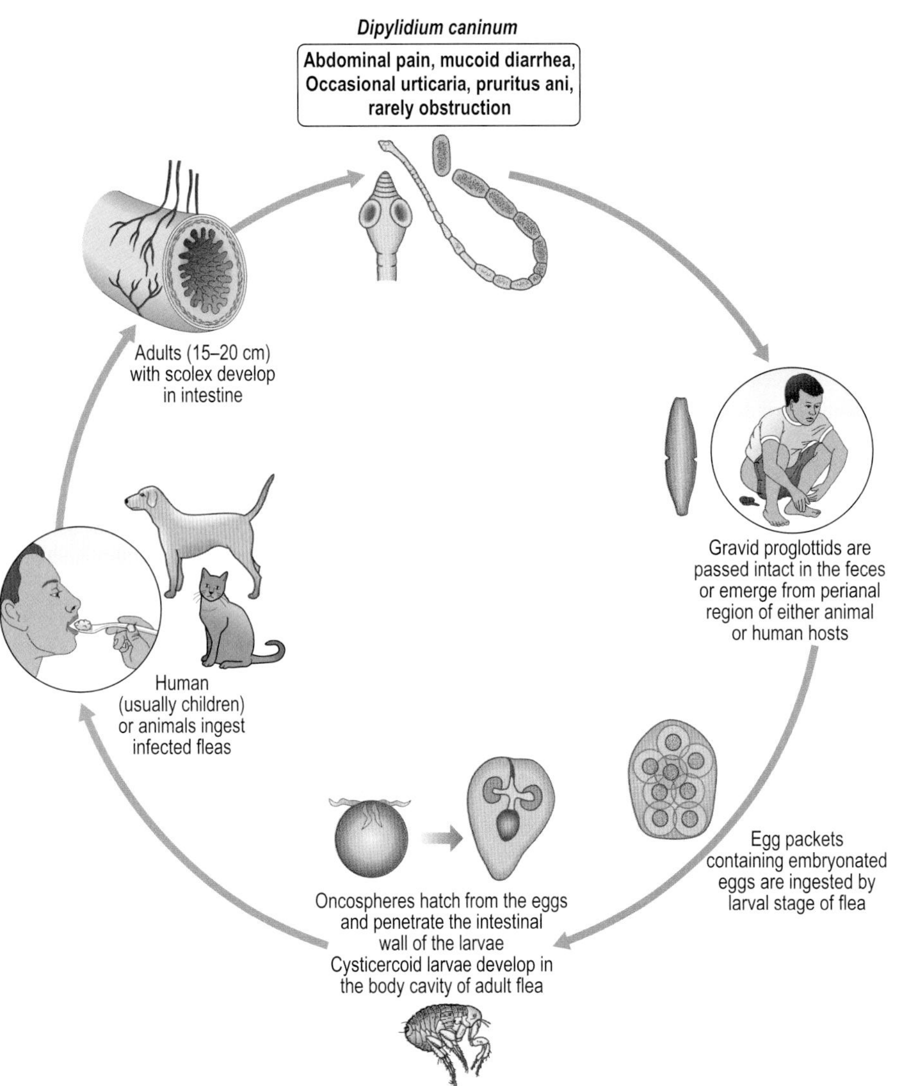

Figure 121.18 *Dipylidium caninum* life cycle.

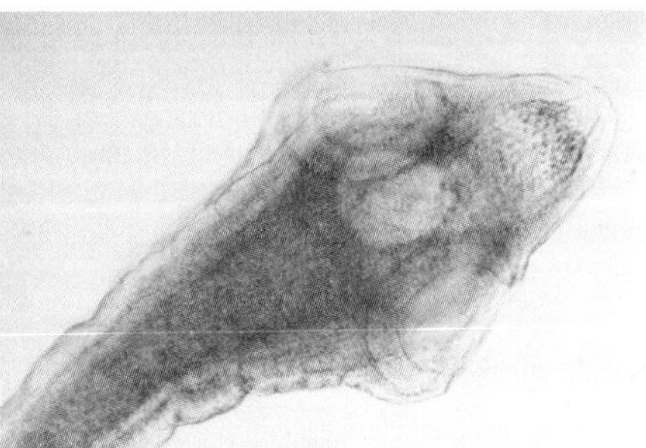

Figure 121.19 *Dipylidium caninum* scolex. Three of the four suckers and the retracted armed rostellum can be seen. (Courtesy of the American Society of Tropical Medicine and Hygiene/Zaiman: A Presentation of Pictorial Parasites.)

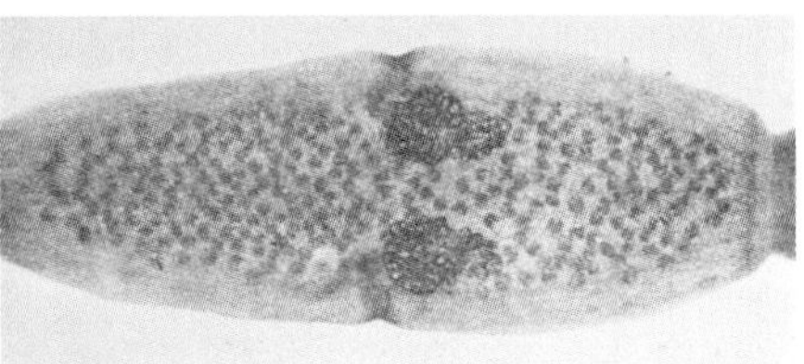

Figure 121.20 *Dipylidium caninum* proglottid. Note the two genital pores and the massing of the ova. (Courtesy of the American Society of Tropical Medicine and Hygiene/Zaiman: A Presentation of Pictorial Parasites.)

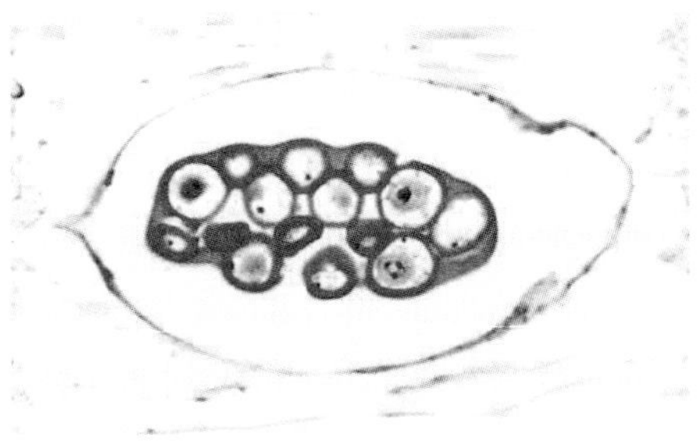

Figure 121.21 Egg pockets of *Dipylidium caninum* in an infant. (Courtesy of Dr Patrick Adegboyega, Department of Pathology, University of Texas Medical Branch, Galveston, TX.)

THE DISEASE

The presence of plerocercoids in subcutaneous tissues is typically associated with a nodular mass consisting of tissue necrosis and a granulomatous inflammation with lymphocytes, plasma cells, and eosinophils (***Fig. 121.22***).[49–51] Swelling and edema are often painful (***Fig. 121.23***). Any part of the body may be involved, including the neck, breast, scrotum, and pleura.[50–55] Raw amphibian poultices harboring plerocercoid larvae applied to the eye have also been a cause of ocular sparganosis and may impair vision.[56,57]

Cerebral sparganosis is a rare complication of this infection. In the brain, the presence of the parasite evokes an intense inflammatory

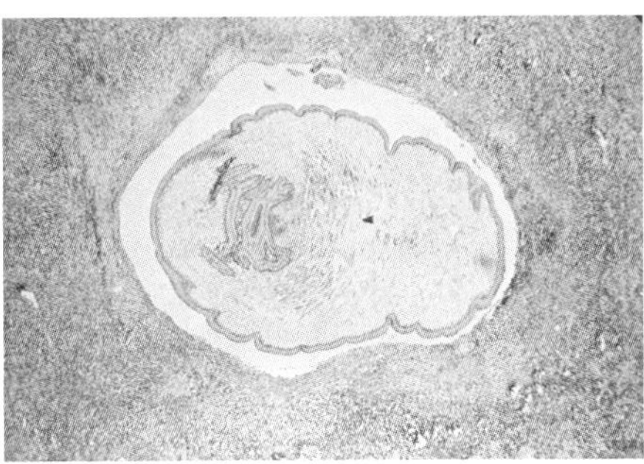

Figure 121.22 Sparganum: abscess in muscle. (Courtesy of the American Society of Tropical Medicine and Hygiene/Zaiman: A Presentation of Pictorial Parasites.)

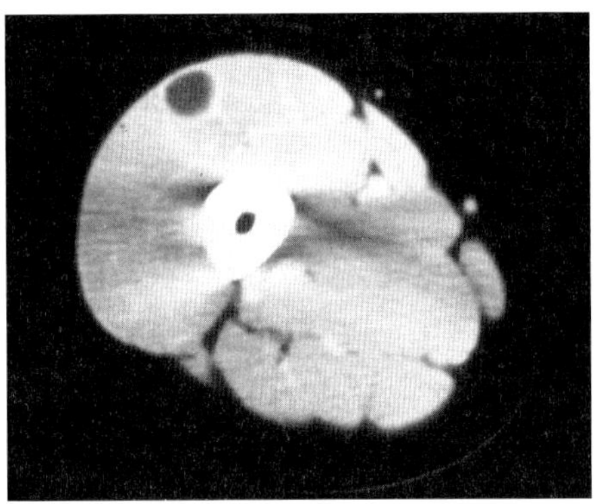

Figure 121.23 Sparganosis: computed tomography scan of the thigh showing a circular hyperlucent lesion with inflammatory response of adjacent tissues. (Courtesy of the American Society of Tropical Medicine and Hygiene/Zaiman: A Presentation of Pictorial Parasites.)

response. Pathological and radiographic (computed tomography and magnetic resonance imaging) studies demonstrate white-matter degeneration, cortical atrophy, ventricular dilatation, punctuate calcifications, irregular or nodular enhancement, vasculitis, and hemorrhage.[58–66]

An unusual manifestation of sparganosis is a condition known as sparganum proliferum, in which larvae of a pseudophyllidean tapeworm of unknown genus and species proliferate in the tissues as independent organisms. In several instances, thousands of spargana have been found in the subcutaneous tissues.[45]

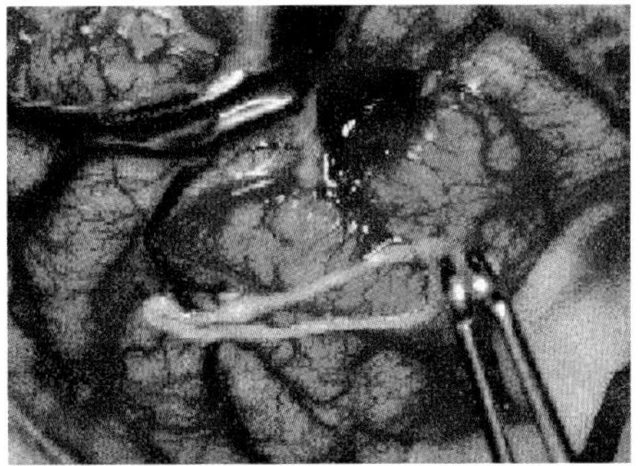

Figure 121.24 Sparganum removed from the right occipital cortex. (Reproduced from Kim DG, Paek SH, Chang KH, et al. Cerebral sparganosis: clinical manifestations, treatment, and outcome. J Neurosurg. 1996;85:1066–1071, with permission of the Journal of Neurosurgery and the authors.)

DIAGNOSIS

In general, the diagnosis is based on pathological examination of biopsy or autopsy specimens and/or direct visualization of the parasite (***Fig. 121.24***). In the case of cerebral sparganosis, magnetic resonance imaging is most helpful in the diagnosis and is usually followed by stereotactic biopsies.[61,62,67] Serodiagnosis using monoclonal antibodies in a competition enzyme-linked immunosorbent assay has been reported.[68,69] False-positive results may occur when *Clonorchis* and *Paragonimus* infections are present.

TREATMENT AND PREVENTION

Treatment of sparganosis has been surgical removal of the larvae. Ocular sparganosis is sometimes treated by killing the larvae and allowing the organisms to resorb, although surgical removal has come into favor. Mebendazole, albendazole, and praziquantel have not been demonstrated to be useful. Spargana are destroyed by flash freezing at 10°C for 24 hours.

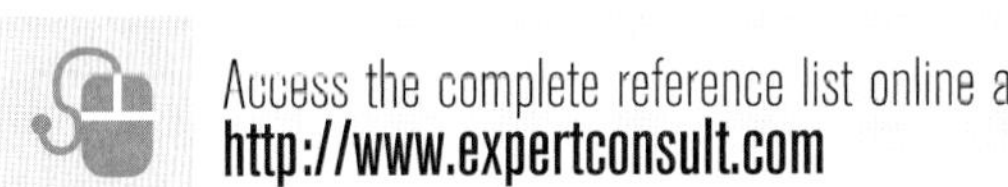

Access the complete reference list online at **http://www.expertconsult.com**

CHAPTER 122

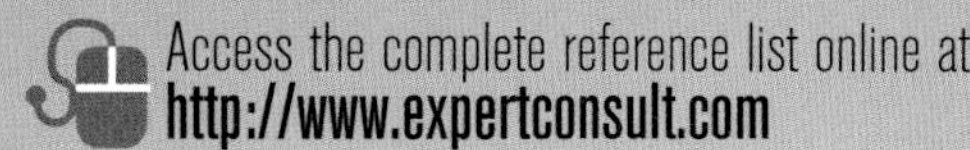
Access the complete reference list online at
http://www.expertconsult.com

Schistosomiasis

Charles H. King

INTRODUCTION

Schistosomiasis remains one of the most prevalent helminthic infections in the world. It is found in tropical and subtropical areas of South America, Africa, the Middle East, East Asia, and the Philippines.[1,2] Recent updates to World Health Organization (WHO) estimates indicate that more than 207 million people are infected worldwide, with over 700 million people at risk of infection.[3] Schistosomiasis is associated with renal and bladder dysfunction (*Schistosoma haematobium*) or liver and intestinal disease (*S. mansoni, S. japonicum, S. mekongi*, and *S. intercalatum*) in endemic areas, and it also is a contributing cause of anemia and growth retardation.

Schistosomiasis is acquired through the skin while wading or bathing in fresh water when the human host comes into contact with the infectious, free-living, cercarial larvae that are released by the parasite's intermediate hosts – aquatic or amphibious snails.[2] Patterns of water supply, sanitation, and human water use are, therefore, critical factors in determining the risk of infection.[3,4] In addition, the geographic distribution of the different *Schistosoma* species is entirely dependent on the distribution of the distinct snail species that serve as intermediate hosts. Climate, water quality, and other ecologic factors that regulate these snail populations also determine the distribution of schistosomiasis on a district as well as a national level.[3,4]

Readily available animal models of schistosome infection have allowed intensive study of the immunology and molecular biology of schistosomiasis. Detailed analysis of host responses to these complex multicellular parasites has provided significant insight into the regulation of cell-mediated and humoral immunity,[5] as well as the resistance pathways available for elimination of macroparasites.[6] Molecular studies of the parasite[7] have provided information on novel modes of genetic expression, as well as leads for the development of vaccines[8] and new pharmaceuticals for control of this widespread chronic infection.

THE AGENT

Schistosomiasis is an ancient human disease. Parasites and their eggs have been identified in early Egyptian mummies and the symptoms described in early papyrus records. In modern times, the parasite cause of schistosomiasis was identified by Theodor Bilharz in 1852 and later by Patrick Manson.

Five species of schistosomes infect humans. The three major species are: (1) *S. haematobium*, found in Africa and the Middle East (***Fig. 122.1***); (2) *S. mansoni*, found in Africa, the Middle East, the Caribbean, and South America (***Fig. 122.2***); and (3) *S. japonicum*, found in China and the Philippines (***Fig. 122.3***). Human infection also occurs with *S. intercalatum*, which is found in central and West Africa, and *S. mekongi*, which is found only in the Mekong river basin of Southeast Asia.

Schistosomal species are distinguished by differences in their morphology, both in their parasite stages and in their eggs (***Fig. 122.4***). The characteristic feature of the *S. mansoni* egg is its lateral spine; of the *S. haematobium* egg, its terminal spine; and of the *S. japonicum* egg, its limited, inconspicuous spine.[2] Further species distinction is made by the species of intermediate host snails found to be supporting transmission of the parasite. These are *Biomphalaria* species snails for *S. mansoni*, *Bulinus* species snails for *S. haematobium*, and *Oncomelania* species snails for *S. japonicum*.[4]

Given the geographic differences reported in local susceptibilities to antiparasitic drugs, there undoubtedly are *Schistosoma* subspecies, as well as intraspecies strain differences that exist between continents and within individual countries.[9,10] Epidemiologic studies in Kenya have focused on significant differences in the pathogenicity of *S. mansoni* infection in different areas of the country.[9] Clinical evidence had suggested that there might be distinct strains of *S. mansoni*, centered in discrete geographic areas, that result in significantly different levels of morbidity when local human populations are infected. Molecular biologic studies are under way confirming the genetic similarities and differences between geographic strains of *S. mansoni* in Brazil and other endemic areas.[11,12] Significant differences have also been reported between the clinical aspects of *S. japonicum* infection in China and *S. japonicum* infection in the Philippines. Recent completion of the *S. mansoni* and *S. japonicum* genome projects will shed further light.[13,14]

EPIDEMIOLOGY

In endemic areas, schistosome infection is first acquired in early childhood. Infection increases in prevalence and intensity with age, peaking in the age group of 15–20 years. In older people, a drastic decline in intensity, but not in prevalence, has been demonstrated.[15–17] The debate is still active over whether the decline represents acquired immunity, a change in water contact, a change in egg production by adult worms, or a combination of these factors.[18] Schistosome infections in human populations of endemic areas follow an overdispersed pattern, in which most infected persons show low egg counts, and a small percentage (1–5%) harbor extremely heavy infection. Susceptibility to high-intensity infection may reflect water exposure patterns or may be related to certain human genetic characteristics.[19,20] The epidemiology of schistosomiasis is further regulated by the duration of the parasite life span (3–7 years) and the multiple immunologic and nonimmunologic responses of the host that participate in regulating infection and disease.

Expression of disease due to schistosome infection is similarly complex. Although adult schistosomes do not replicate in the mammalian host, they produce eggs throughout their life span. These parasite eggs elicit host immunopathologic reactions, which are responsible for most disease manifestations.[21] Pathogenesis may be related, therefore, to intensity of infection and certainly to factors that regulate host response, including genetic influences.[22]

Mathematical modeling that describes schistosome prevalence, intensity, and transmission patterns has been developed.[23,24] Central to these

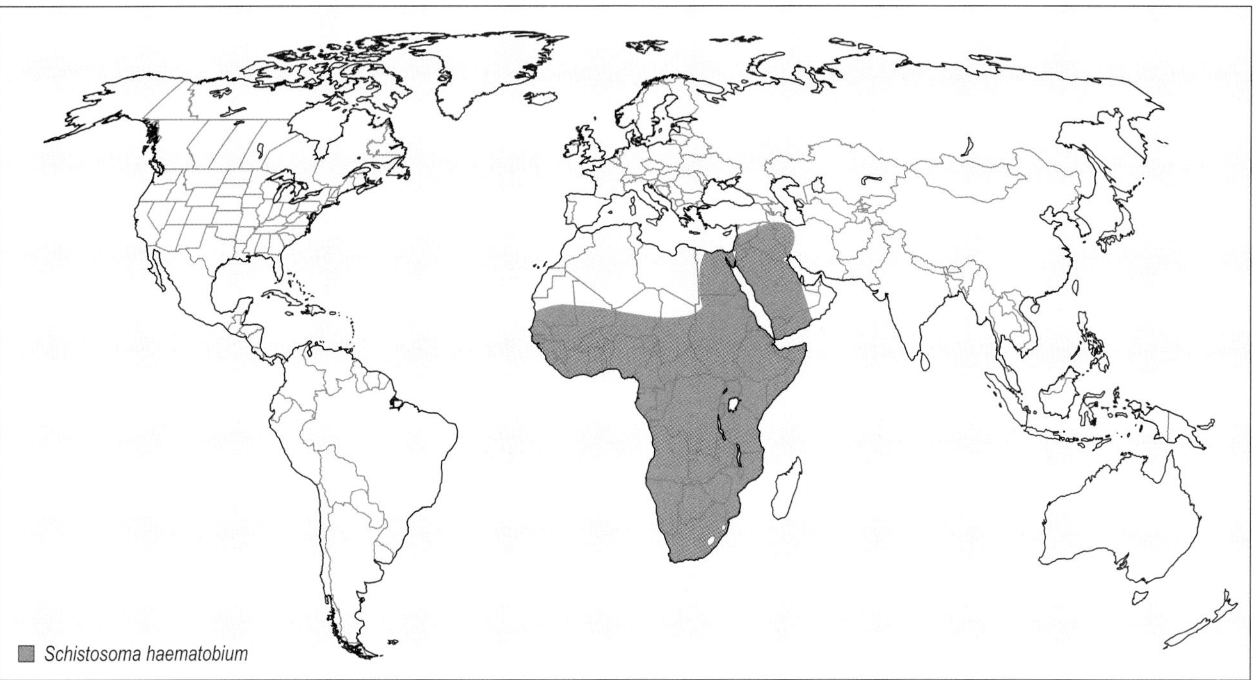

Figure 122.1 *Schistosoma haematobium.*

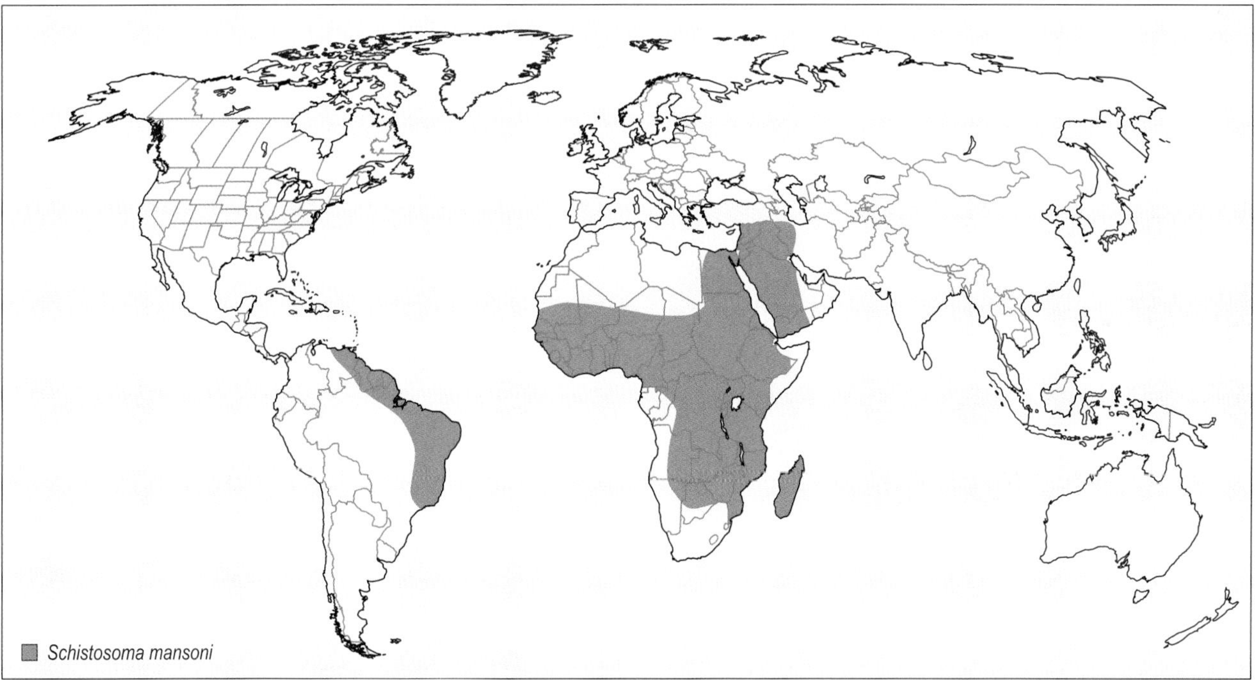

Figure 122.2 *Schistosoma mansoni.*

studies is the concept of quantification of infection, which is possible in helminthic infections because adult worms do not replicate in mammalian hosts. Access to quantitative data on schistosomiasis is mainly based on egg counts in feces or urine. Despite these limitations, however, useful mathematical models have been constructed for schistosome infections, their transmission, and their disease sequelae.[24]

THE DISEASE

Illness due to *Schistosoma* infection differs between the early, or acute, stages of infection and the later disease caused by chronic infection (***Fig. 122.5***).[25] Early manifestations include dermatitis and acute schistosomiasis (Katayama syndrome, or "snail" fever).[26] Initial manifestations are caused by the entry of the parasite's cercarial forms into the skin, which causes a localized dermatitis, then subsequent migration of the developing schistosomulum through the lung and hepatic circulation during its development into a mature schistosome worm. The chronic disease of schistosomiasis, which is much more prevalent in endemic areas, is due to a granulomatous response to parasite eggs, resulting in chronic fibroobstructive sequelae in the intestine or portal veins (*S. mansoni*, *S. japonicum*, *S. mekongi*, and *S. intercalatum*) or the urinary tract (*S. haematobium*).[25]

Cercarial dermatitis is a pruritic, papular rash found on skin exposed to cercaria-containing waters. In northern climates, cercarial dermatitis

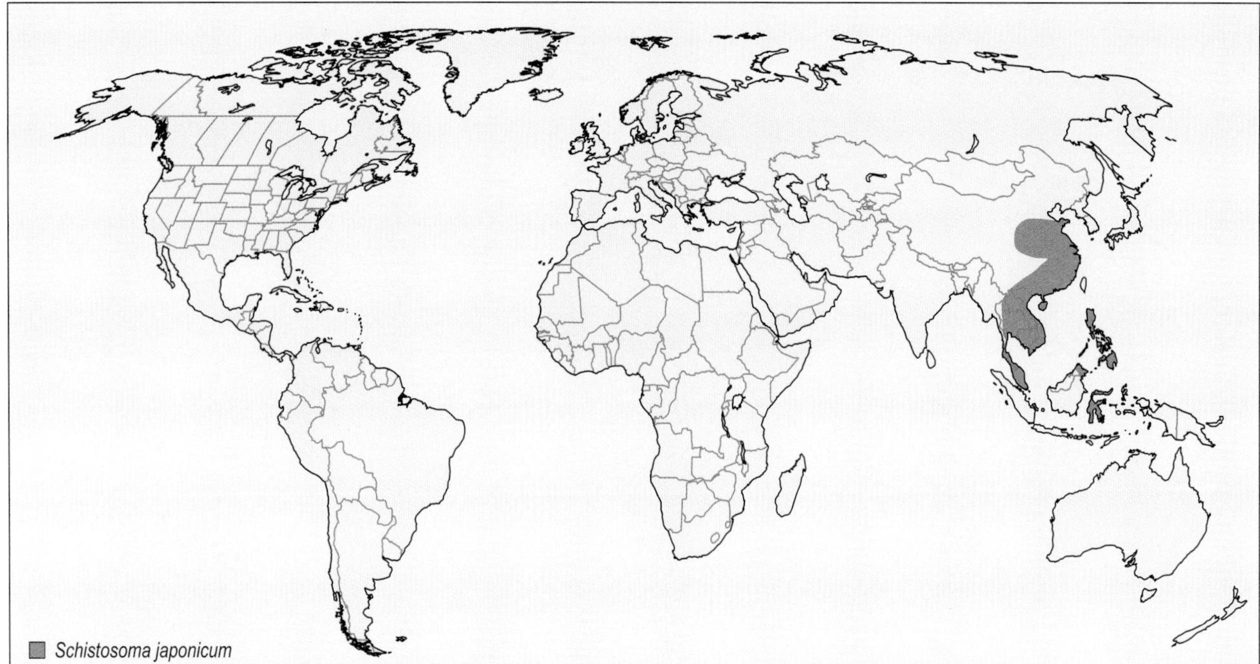

Figure 122.3 *Schistosoma japonicum.*

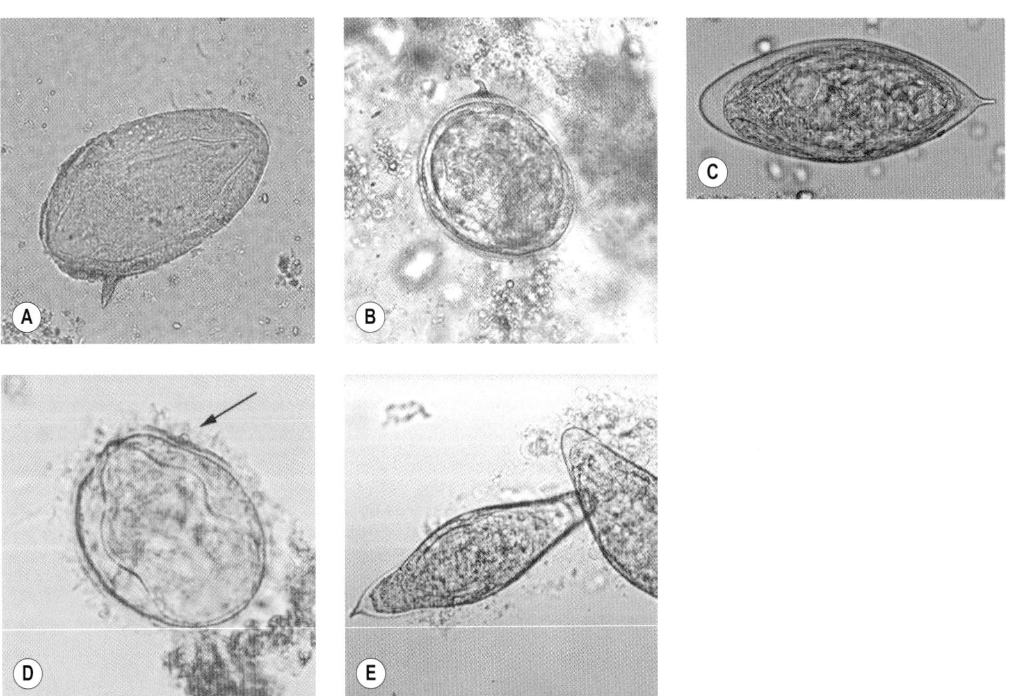

Figure 122.4 Eggs of human schistosomes. Egg of *Schistosoma mansoni* **(A)** has a prominent lateral spine. Egg of *S. japonicum* **(B)** is more rounded and has a less prominent spine. Egg of *S. haematobium* **(C)** is larger with a terminal spine. Egg of *S. mekongi* **(D)** has an inconspicuous spine (arrow). Egg of *S. intercalatum* **(E)**, like *S. haematobium*, has a terminal spine but has a central bulge. (Reproduced from http://www.dpd.cdc.gov/dpdx/HTML/Schistosomiasis.htm. Part A courtesy of the Missouri State Public Health Laboratory.)

is the cause of "swimmer's itch," an eruption that occurs after abortive skin penetration by cercariae of bird schistosomes (*Trichobilharzia* and *Bilharziella*). In areas endemic for human schistosomiasis, cercarial dermatitis is most common in *S. mansoni* and *S. haematobium* transmission areas. It occurs within 24 hours of exposure, appearing as pruritic red papules on the surface of the skin. Because exposure typically occurs by walking or wading in infected ponds or rivers, the rash is usually located on the lower legs. The duration of symptoms depends on the intensity of the local cutaneous inflammatory response.

Acute schistosomiasis develops in some persons with heavy exposure to *S. japonicum* or *S. mansoni* infection. It is rarely seen in *S. haematobium* infection. Originally described in the Katayama valley of southern Japan, acute schistosomiasis is most likely to occur in the previously unexposed traveler or new immigrant to an endemic area.[26,27] While symptoms usually resolve over several weeks, intense infection may result in death. Symptoms develop between 4 and 8 weeks of exposure, coinciding with the maturation of the infecting schistosome and the beginning of oviposition (egg-laying). Symptoms include fever, sweats, chills, cough,

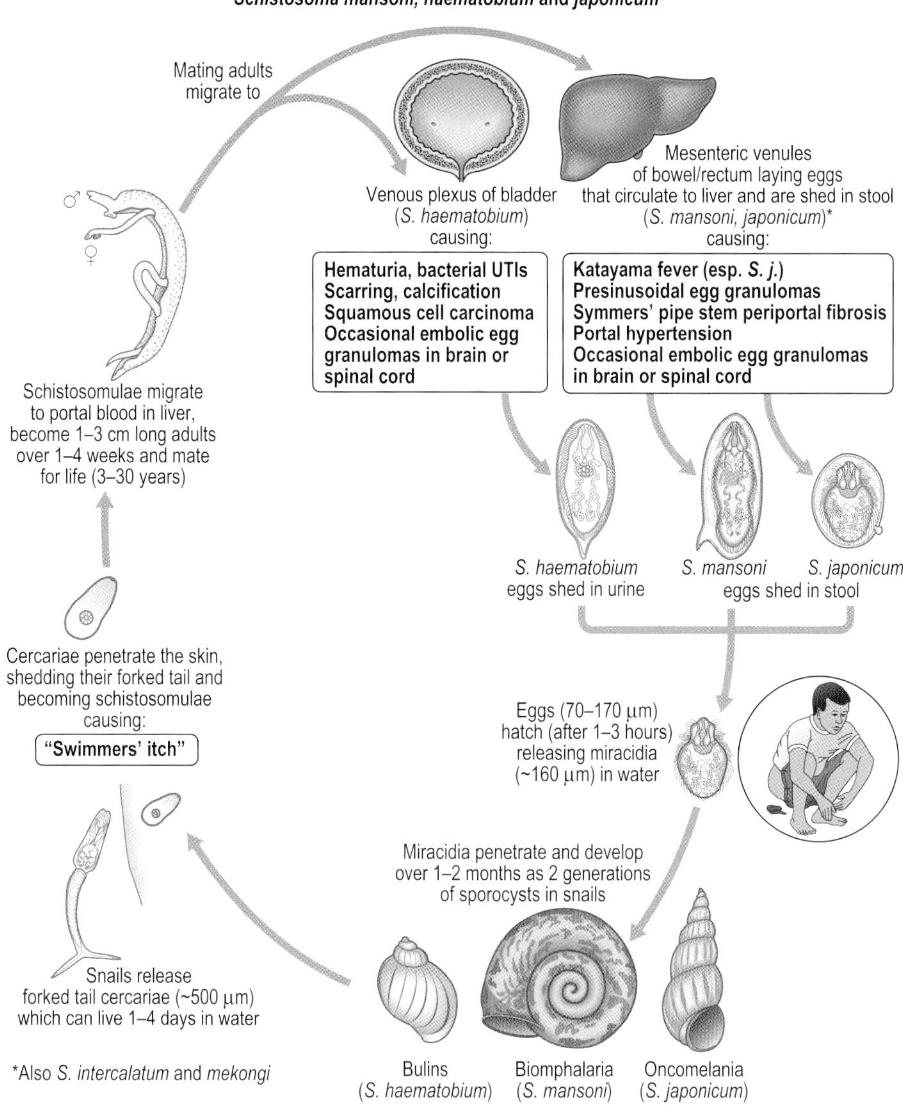

Figure 122.5 Life cycles of *Schistosoma mansoni, S. haematobium,* and *S. japonicum*. UTIs, urinary tract infections.

and headaches. Physical findings include lymphadenopathy and hepatosplenomegaly, and there is associated eosinophilia on laboratory examination. Early in the course of acute schistosomiasis, when egg production is just beginning, routine fecal parasitologic diagnosis is often negative due to the early absence or limited numbers of eggs passed in the stool. Serologic testing or, less commonly, rectal or bladder biopsies may be required to establish the diagnosis. In fatal cases, large numbers of eggs are found in the liver and intestines, and massive infection is the rule.

Chronic schistosomiasis, as seen in endemic areas, is a less dramatic, progressive illness resulting from repeated prolonged tissue injury and fibrosis from deposition of parasite eggs in affected organs: the intestine and liver for *S. mansoni, S. japonicum, S. mekongi*, and *S. intercalatum*, and the bladder, ureters, and kidneys for *S. haematobium*.[2]

The patient with intestinal schistosomiasis may complain of fatigue, abdominal pain, diarrhea, or dysenteric bloody diarrhea caused by granuloma and ulcer formation in the bowel wall.[28] Granulomatous inflammation may result in polyp formation, which can be detected on barium contrast studies or endoscopy. Persistent inflammation of chronic schistosomiasis contributes to anemia of chronic disease in many patients, while, in more advanced disease, ulceration and chronic bleeding may lead to the development of moderate or severe iron-deficiency anemia.[29,30]

In *S. mansoni*, *S. mekongi*, and *S. japonicum* infections, a significant number of parasite eggs are retained in the body and travel to the liver via the portal circulation. These eggs lodge in presinusoidal radicles of the portal vein, where they elicit a granulomatous reaction.[18] Venous flow is affected, first by the presence of the living egg and the surrounding granuloma formation, and later by local scar formation resulting from fibrosis. The net result is portal vein hypertension and the development of portosystemic collateral blood flow. The earliest sign of chronic schistosomiasis is hepatomegaly. As infection progresses, and liver damage becomes more severe, splenomegaly is also seen.[15,31] Portal pressures are markedly elevated, whereas the wedge hepatic pressure remains normal. Liver perfusion is maintained by an increase in arterial flow from the hepatic arteries. Consequently, hepatocellular function remains intact until late in the course of infection, unless alcoholism or coinfection with hepatitis B or C virus also is present.[2]

The major manifestations of *S. haematobium* infection are seen in children and young adults living in endemic areas.[16] Deposition of schistosome eggs around the lower end of ureters and in the wall of the urinary bladder results in hematuria, dysuria, and urinary frequency. The functional consequence of *S. haematobium* infection is bladder neck obstruction with back pressure causing hydroureter and hydronephrosis. Urinary schistosomiasis usually creates a setting for repeated bacterial infection, compromised kidney function, and finally renal failure.[32] In several endemic areas, *S. haematobium* infection is epidemiologically associated with squamous cell bladder carcinoma.[33,34] The relationship is such that the International Agency for Research on Cancer has classified *S. haematobium* as a human carcinogen.[35] While the sequence of events in *S.*

haematobium-related disease seems clear, the natural history and outcome are poorly understood because of the lack of long-term longitudinal population-based studies.

Other clinical manifestations of intestinal and urinary schistosomiasis constitute important aspects of infection and disease. Among the most significant are pulmonary, central nervous system (CNS), renal, and cutaneous manifestations.[36-38] Pulmonary schistosomiasis results from parasite egg deposition, accruing through the collateral vessels that develop in those with substantial hepatic involvement, in the pulmonary vasculature followed by granuloma formation and obstruction of blood flow.[36] The pathophysiologic consequence is pulmonary hypertension and the features of cor pulmonale. This course of events may occur during *S. haematobium* infection (because of the anatomic location of the adult worm) or during chronic intestinal schistosomiasis when eggs may pass to the pulmonary circulation via portosystemic collaterals.

CNS schistosomiasis causes grand mal epilepsy in 1–2% of persons with *S. japonicum* infection. Transverse myelitis is the usual disease entity detected in those with *S. mansoni* or *S. haematobium* infection. Disease usually occurs in chronically infected persons but may happen during the acute phase.[37]

PATHOGENESIS AND IMMUNITY

Schistosome infection presents the host with a complex challenge. Adult worms do not replicate in the host but produce hundreds of thousands of eggs over a life span of 4–7 years. Eggs retained in the host tissue survive for up to 6 weeks. Host reactions are therefore complicated by these overlapping parasite factors, which result in a myriad of immunologic and nonimmunologic responses.[18,28] Central to the cause of disease is the cell-mediated granuloma formation and multiple humoral and cellular regulatory responses.[18] Resistance to infection with any schistosome species is both innate and acquired.[8,39] The role of each in regulating parasite populations is still being examined. Population-based studies suggest strongly that acquired immunity exists in humans.[23] The challenge in examining such a phenomenon is to understand its mechanisms and ultimately succeed in inducing resistance.

DIAGNOSIS

The "gold standard" for identifying an established schistosome infection is to demonstrate parasite eggs in the patient's stool (*S. mansoni, S. japonicum, S. mekongi*, and *S. intercalatum*) or urine (*S. haematobium*).[40] Sensitivity of detection is improved by concentration and clarification techniques. Intensity of infection can be determined by quantitative sampling of defined quantities of stool (Kato template technique) or urine (syringe filtration). It should be noted that parasite eggs are deposited in the wall of the bowel or bladder and may pass into the lumen only some time later. The presence of a patent, active infection is associated with viable eggs (as determined by miracidial hatching when the eggs are placed in fresh water), whereas remote or treated infection is associated with passage of only nonviable eggs. In very heavy infections, the anatomical distribution of eggs may not be typical; that is, *S. haematobium* eggs may be found in the stool, and *S. mansoni* eggs may be found in the urine.

Infection is also defined when parasite eggs are identified in tissues obtained on rectal, intestinal, liver, prostatic, cervical, or bladder biopsy. Unfortunately, standard fixation and staining may not be able to distinguish the viability of these eggs, and may not ascertain whether the infection is current or remote. In ectopic infections (e.g., skin or CNS), or very light infections, the biopsy may be the first clue to the presence of schistosome infection.

Serologic tests have been developed to detect the presence of specific antischistosome antibodies in patients suspected of infection. Species-specific antigens have been identified on Western blotting, allowing some confidence in the determination of the infecting parasite.[41] However, a positive serology does not distinguish between current and past infection. In endemic populations, serology is sensitive but not specific for active infection and is therefore most useful for its negative predictive value; that is, negative serology is useful in excluding infection.[2] However, among travelers from nonendemic areas who have only a recent, brief, defined exposure to the parasite, and most often a low intensity of infection, positive serology strongly suggests an active infection, even in the presence of negative stool and urine parasitologic examinations.

A valuable approach to disease quantification in endemic areas has been ultrasound imaging by means of portable, generator-powered machines.[42] For *S. mansoni* and *S. japonicum* infection, imaging of the liver allows identification of characteristic periportal fibrosis and defines the level of disease associated with parasite infection. In *S. haematobium* infection, ultrasound examination of the kidneys and bladder allows identification of granulomas, hydronephrosis, and other inflammatory changes strongly associated with this parasite.

Recent studies have focused on alternative means of identifying active parasite infection. Workers in the Netherlands have identified two parasite antigens (CCA and CAA) that circulate in the blood during the course of active, patent infection in experimental animal models.[41] In subsequent studies in human populations, the level of circulating antigen was roughly correlated with the intensity of infection, suggesting that antigen detection may be a useful means of identifying and quantifying active infection. To improve the utility of antigen testing, research is progressing on the use of dot enzyme-linked immunosorbent assay techniques, which can be performed using a single drop of blood obtained by the fingerstick method. Studies are also progressing on antigen detection in urine, particularly for patients infected with *S. mansoni*.[43]

Operational research has established the use of observed macro- or microhematuria or even symptom questionnaires as surrogates for the diagnosis of *S. haematobium* infection.[44] Prior experience has identified the labor and material costs of parasitologic screening as significant factors in raising the cost of control programs for this parasite. Further, incomplete adherence with screening limits the participation of a significant proportion of infected persons with the later treatment phase of a control program. Studies in *S. haematobium*-endemic areas have identified that close to 100% of subjects under age 12 years with gross or microscopic hematuria are infected with the parasite. Treatment strategies based on urine dipstick diagnosis of hematuria have been validated in follow-up studies, with expected implementation in other heavily infected endemic areas.

TREATMENT AND PROGNOSIS

Praziquantel is currently the treatment of choice for all forms of schistosomiasis.[45] Praziquantel is a well-tolerated, broad-spectrum oral anthelminthic agent that is given as a single dose of 40 mg/kg for the treatment of *S. haematobium*, *S. mansoni*, and *S. intercalatum* infections, and as two separate 30 mg/kg doses (spaced at least 3 hours apart) for *S. japonicum* and *S. mekongi* infections. Cure rates in field studies have typically been equal to or greater than 85%. Those with infection still remaining typically have their infection intensity reduced by more than 99%, as measured by reduction in parasite egg counts in stool or urine samples. Some side-effects are directly drug-induced (vomiting, dysphoria, abdominal pain), while others are proportionate to the intensity of the parasite load and appear to be related to the host immune response to the dying parasites (abdominal pain, urticaria, diarrhea).[46] Among younger patients, completion of therapy is associated with reductions in egg output, as well as reduced blood loss (gastrointestinal with *S. mansoni* and urinary with *S. haematobium* infection),[47] and regression of granulomatous inflammation in the liver (*S. mansoni* and *S. japonicum* infection) or bladder (*S. haematobium* infection). These latter effects can result in reduction of portal pressure and reversal of hydronephrosis. In older people with more advanced fibrotic tissue injury, *Schistosoma*-associated lesions may not be able to be reversed. Likewise, in patients with the late findings of esophageal varices or cor pulmonale, therapy may or may not improve their hemodynamic values. Symptomatic "ectopic" infection, as in the CNS, may initially worsen with therapy because it provokes a strong local inflammatory response. Coinfection with human immunodeficiency virus-1 does not alter the efficacy of praziquantel therapy for schistosomiasis.

A WHO expert panel has reexamined the issue of praziquantel safety during pregnancy and lactation and determined that minimal risk is associated with treatment.[48] WHO recommendations are that women of child-bearing years should not be routinely excluded from mass treatment campaigns, and further, given the potential risks of infection-associated anemia during pregnancy, that schistosome-infected pregnant women and lactating women should be offered immediate treatment whenever the infection is diagnosed.

Several, sometimes less expensive, second-line drugs have been used in the past for treatment of specific schistosome species. Metrifonate is an older agent for treatment of *S. haematobium* infection. It is given as a single oral dose of 10 mg/kg. Metrifonate efficacy for parasitologic cure varies from 60% to 80%. Repeated use in the same area may be associated with decreased efficacy over time.[49] Oxamniquine is a second-line drug used for treatment of *S. mansoni* infection. Given in doses of 40–60 mg/kg as a single oral dose, it has a reported efficacy of approximately 80% in achieving parasitologic cure in most areas. *S. mansoni* resistance to oxamniquine has been documented in both Brazil and Kenya. There are currently no second-line drugs for *S. japonicum* infection.[2]

PREVENTION AND CONTROL

Given the complex nature of the *Schistosoma* life cycle (see ***Fig. 122.5***), there are, in theory, a number of different ways to prevent transmission of infection or reduce the likelihood of heavy infection.[1,3] These include: (1) reduction or elimination of intermediate host snails; (2) elimination of snail habitats; (3) sanitation measures to prevent human excreta from contaminating local water sources; (4) provision of safe fresh water supplies to reduce contact with snail-infested water sources (this may include provision of communal baths, laundries, and swimming facilities)[50]; (5) use of protective footwear or clothing, or use of protective medicated salves to prevent cercariae from reaching the skin; and (6) use of periodic drugs to limit infection intensity in exposed populations.[24,32] If efficiently applied on a population-wide or targeted subpopulation basis to achieve coverage of the most heavy excreters of eggs, this last approach also results in a significant reduction in parasite transmission as a result of a substantial reduction in parasite eggs reaching transmission sites.

Each of these approaches has been tested under field conditions. Long-term eradication of schistosome transmission has been achieved in Japan and in areas of Venezuela, where water improvements and sanitation measures associated with development have eliminated transmission of *S. japonicum* and *S. mansoni*, respectively. Similarly, water supply projects, including provision of communal swimming pools, were associated with a significant reduction in *S. haematobium* prevalence in southern Iraq before the onset of the first Persian Gulf War. A head-to-head comparison of snail vector control, drug therapy, and water and sanitation measures for control of *S. mansoni* was performed over a 10-year period on the island of Saint Lucia in the Caribbean.[50] Although all modalities were effective in reducing infection, drug therapy was the most effective and least expensive, while provision of piped water was nearly as effective but much more expensive, requiring provision of individual household taps, as well as communal baths and laundries, to achieve comparable levels of control.

At present, the most practical approaches to control appear to be, in the short term, provision of periodic drugs to limit intensity of infection and morbidity,[51] and in the long term, provision of safe water supplies,[4] with continuing integrated health care education[52] to limit high-risk exposure. Repeated drug therapy reduced the prevalence of severe morbidity in longitudinal studies. However, in some cases, particularly with *S. japonicum*, suspension of control measures runs the risk of rapid reemergence of infection prevalence and increased risk of hepatic morbidity and recurrent anemia.[53–55] Sustainability is an essential feature of any planned schistosomiasis control program. This may be difficult to achieve without assistance from vertical health programs owing to the relatively high per capita cost of medication delivery relative to the low priority assigned by some to control of diseases perceived as minimally lethal. Nevertheless, schistosomiasis has a significant impact on chronic morbidity, including malnutrition, anemia, retardation of growth and development, loss of exercise or work capacity, and either urinary tract or intestinal and hepatic disease.[56] Recent social science and health care delivery research is focusing on developing more effective ways to raise awareness of schistosomiasis as a significant health problem and on developing means to incorporate schistosomiasis control into primary health care delivery.

Access the complete reference list online at **http://www.expertconsult.com**

CHAPTER 123

Access the complete reference list online at http://www.expertconsult.com

Liver, Lung, and Intestinal Fluke Infections

Siddhartha Mahanty • J. Dick Maclean† • John H. Cross†

This chapter is dedicated to the memory of J. Dick MacLean, a valued colleague, an outstanding teacher, and an inspiration to a new generation of tropical medicine practitioners.

INTRODUCTION

More than 40 million people are estimated to have trematode (commonly referred to as flukes) infections. These parasites infect liver, lung, and intestine, with 21 million individuals harboring lung flukes, 20 million infected with liver flukes, and unknown millions with intestinal flukes.[1] These trematodes are all foodborne zoonoses, with reservoirs in a wide range of domestic and wild animals, transmitted to humans through freshwater fish, crustaceans, and aquatic vegetation. With a worldwide distribution, the highest prevalences are in East and Southeast Asia, determined as much by local eating habits as by the presence of the obligatory intermediate hosts. All of these flukes can produce serious clinical disease, especially with heavy infections, because of the sites of infection and longevity of the parasite.

These flukes are hermaphroditic, bilaterally symmetrical, and flattened dorsoventrally with an anterior oral and a ventral sucker. Their length can range from 1 mm to 12 cm with shapes described as spatulate, piriform, lanceolate, or leaflike (***Fig. 123.1***). Different fluke species share some common features in their life cycles. In general, adult flukes in the mammalian host produce eggs that, after passage in feces or sputum, are ingested by the appropriate first-intermediate-host snails or hatch and subsequently penetrate the snail host as ciliated miracidia. Within the snail, asexual multiplication through sporocyst, redia, and cercaria stages occurs. Free-swimming cercaria leave the snail and penetrate fish or shellfish or attach to aquatic vegetation to encyst as metacercaria. When eaten by the mammalian final host, the metacercaria excyst, migrate to liver or lungs, or stay in the small intestine and develop into adults.

LIVER FLUKES

Human liver flukes are members of two families, the Opisthorchiidae and the Fasciolidae, distinguished by differences in life cycle and pathogenesis (***Fig. 123.2***). In human Opisthorchiidae there are three major species (*Clonorchis sinensis* in East Asia, *Opisthorchis viverrini* in Southeast Asia, and *O. felineus* in some countries in Europe and the former Soviet Union) and two minor species (*O. guayaquilensis* in North and South America and *Metorchis conjunctus* in North America). In the Fasciolidae the species are *Fasciola hepatica*, which has a worldwide distribution, and *F. gigantica* in South Asia, Southeast Asia, and Africa.

OPISTHORCHIASIS AND CLONORCHIASIS

THE AGENT

The three major Opisthorchiidae species – *C. sinensis*, *O. viverrini*, and *O. felineus* – have similar life cycles and pathogenic processes. Differentiation among species is usually based on adult fluke morphology or geographic distribution, as differences in egg morphologies are small.[2,3] Adults, which live in the intrahepatic bile ducts of their host, are flat, spatulate to lanceolate, aspinous, and reddish to brown in color. *C. sinensis* is the largest (10–25 × 3–5 mm) (***Fig. 123.3A***), in contrast to the smaller *O. viverrini* (5–10 × 1–2 mm) and *O. felineus* (7–12 × 2–3 mm). The adults produce ovoid eggs that are yellowish-brown, have opercula, and are of such overlapping and variable size (*O. viverrini*, 30 × 12 μm; *O. felineus*, 30 × 12 μm; *C. sinensis* 28–35 × 12–19 μm) (***Fig. 123.3B***) that speciation by the egg is very difficult.

The transmission of these trematodes follows the general schema outlined above for flukes, with susceptible freshwater fish species serving as the source of infection in humans. After ingestion in uncooked fish by the final human host, excystation occurs in the duodenum, followed by rapid maturation into adults, and migration through the sphincter of Oddi and up the common bile duct to become wedged in the intrahepatic biliary radicles. The prepatent period is 3–4 weeks, and the life span in the human host can be as long as 30 years.

EPIDEMIOLOGY

C. sinensis is endemic in China, Japan, Korea, Taiwan, Vietnam, and Asian Russia. In China, infection is endemic in 24 provinces, with prevalence rates between 1% and 57%; the greatest number of cases is in the south-eastern province of Guangdong and the southern region of Guangxi Zhuangzu.[4] Hong Kong is not an endemic area for the parasite; infections are acquired by eating fish imported from the mainland of China. In Korea, rates of 8–40% were reported in the past, but prevalence rates in the 1990s dropped to 1.5%.[5] People living along river basins are more commonly infected. This parasitosis is reported from all areas of Taiwan, with the highest infection rates of 52–57% from three widely separated areas in northern, central, and southern counties of the island.[5] Although clonorchiasis was found in up to 3% of the Japanese population prior to 1960, by 1991 the disease had almost disappeared. Endemic areas in Russia are in the Amur river region (***Fig. 123.4***).

Opisthorchis spp. are prevalant in Kazakhstan, Russian Federation, Siberia, Ukraine, Germany, and Italy (for *O. felineus*), and Cambodia, Laos, South Vietnam, and Thailand (for *O. viverrini*). Prevalence rates for *O. viverrini* are reported to be >24% in Thailand, and 40–80% in Laos,[1,6]

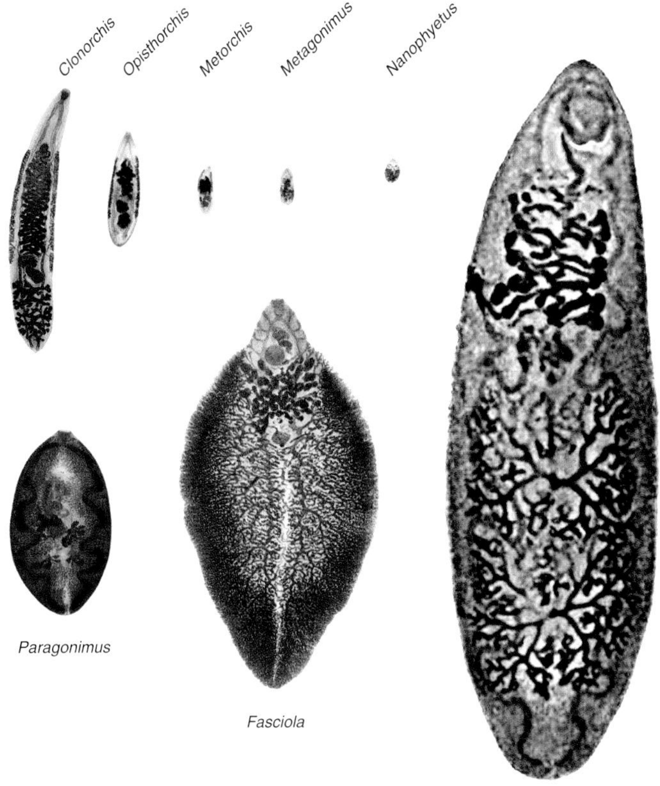

Figure 123.1 Threefold magnification of selected flukes illustrating relative sizes. Actual lengths: *Metagonimus yokogawai* 1.0–2.5 mm, *Nanophyetus salmincola* 0.8–2.5 mm, *Metorchis conjunctus* 1.5–7.0 mm, *Opisthorchis viverrini* 5–10 mm, *Paragonimus westermani* 7–16 mm, *Clonorchis sinensis* 10–25 mm, *Fasciola hepatica* 20–30 mm, *Fasciolopsis buski* 20–75 mm. (*Metagonimus yokogawai* image from Centers for Disease Control and Prevention, Division of Parasitic Diseases, Atlanta, GA; *Nanophyetus salmincola* and *Fasciolopsis buski* images courtesy of Steve J. Upton, Kansas State University; *Opisthorchis viverrini* image from Ash LR, Orihel TC. Atlas of Human Parasitology. Chicago: ASCP Press; 1990: plate 73, 2, p. 213; *Paragonimus westermani, Clonorchis sinensis*, and *Fasciola hepatica* images from Orihel TC, Ash LR. Parasites in Human Tissues. Chicago: ASCP Press; 1995, figures 72, 60, and 58, pp. 272, 268, and 264.)

and ranging from 0.3% to 37% in Vietnam.[7] The epidemiology and clinical presentation of *Opisthorchis* infections are similar to those described for clonorchiasis.[8] *O. felineus* has been reported from Italy[9] and from regions in the former USSR, with endemic foci in western Siberia, the Russian Federation, Kazakhstan, and Ukraine and prevalences in these regions ranging from 40% to 95%.[1]

Other opisthorchiids reported to cause human infections are *O. guayaquilensis* (*Amphimerus pseudofelineus*) and *Metorchis conjunctus*. These have been reported from animals and humans in Latin America and North America. An epidemic of metorchiasis occurred in 19 persons in Canada who had eaten freshly caught white suckers (*Catostomus commersoni*) near Montreal.[10]

A variety of freshwater hydrobid snails, abundant in fish-raising ponds, serve as first intermediate hosts for *C. sinensis*, *O. viverrini*, and *O. felineus*. *Bithynia fuchsiana*, *Parafossarulus manchouricus*, and *Simisulcospica libertina* are important vectors of *C. sinensis* in most endemic areas, while *B. siamensis* is a vector of *O. viverrini* in Thailand; *Melanoides tuberculatus* is an important vector in Vietnam;[7] and *Codiella inflata*, *C. troscheli*, and *C. leachi* are vectors of *O. felineus* in the former USSR.

Over 100 species of fish, many of them synonyms, and most belonging to the carp (Cyprinidae) family, are reported as second-intermediate hosts of *C. sinensis*. *Ctenopharyngodon idellus* in China, *Cyprinus carpio* in Japan, and *Pseudoraspora parva* in Korea are the predominant sources of human infections, often eaten raw. Many of the fish are cultivated in ponds inhabited by snail hosts, and contaminated or intentionally fertilized with human and animal feces. Aquaculture is now playing an important role in transmitting foodborne trematodiasis.[11,12] Twenty-two species of cyprinids are intermediate hosts for *O. felineus* in the former USSR. The fish, such as *Barbus barbus* and *Tinca tinca*, may be eaten raw, dried, salted, and sometimes frozen. In endemic areas of opisthorchiid liver fluke infections, a myriad of mammalian hosts such as dogs, cats, pigs, rats, rabbits, and other wild fish-eating animals serve as reservoir hosts.

THE DISEASE

The biologic and pathologic characteristics of *Opisthorchis* and *Clonorchis* are considered to be essentially the same.[11,13] Variations in clinical presentations seen in different geographic areas are thought to reflect the duration and intensity of infection as well as the genetics and nutrition of the host rather than parasite-specific characteristics. Acute disease has been recognized most frequently in *O. felineus* infections in Russia. The risk of cholangiocarcinoma appears greatest in *O. viverrini* infections in northern Thailand. Intrahepatic pigment stones are reported more frequently in association with *C. sinensis*. Chronic infections are usually asymptomatic, although symptoms may occur in heavier infections. The complications of chronic infection include acute cholangitis, frequently bacterial, and cholangiocarcinoma.

Acute Opisthorchiasis and Clonorchiasis

Acute illness due to new infections with *C. sinensis* has rarely been reported except for a large outbreak of acute clonorchiasis in Shanghai in the 1940s.[14,15] The illness lasted several weeks and was characterized by persistent fever, abdominal pains, fatigue, an enlarged and tender liver, high eosinophil counts, and opisthorchiid eggs in the stool after 3–4 weeks.[15] In Russia acute opisthorchiasis, presenting as fever, abdominal pain, and urticaria, has been seen frequently in migrant populations settling in regions endemic to *O. felineus*.[16,17] In Canada an outbreak of acute illness due to *M. conjunctus* presented with upper abdominal pain, moderate fever, anorexia, high eosinophil counts, and opisthorchiid eggs in the stool late in the second week of illness.[10]

Chronic Opisthorchiasis and Clonorchiasis

Light to moderate infections, lasting for years or decades, are almost always asymptomatic.[18] Case-control and community-based studies have revealed no differences in the signs, symptoms, or laboratory findings between light infections and uninfected controls, but cases with heavy infections (>10 000 eggs/gram) show significantly more abdominal pain, fatigue, dyspepsia, and hepatomegaly.[19–22] There is a correlation between stool egg counts, adult fluke counts, and host disease in *Opisthorchis* infection. But even in heavily infected persons, abdominal symptoms occur in only 10%. These studies are difficult to interpret because raw fish consumption in many communities is frequent and reinfection likely.[21–24] Chronic infection generally reflects the worm burden, and manifests variously as recurrent pyogenic liver cholangitis, cholecystitis, obstructive jaundice, hepatomegaly, cholecystitis, multiple hepatic tumors,[25] and cholelithiasis.[26,27] Many uncontrolled hospital-based studies in endemic regions demonstrate a variety of intermittent symptoms that increase in frequency in those with heavy infections.[28,29] These symptoms include intermittent fatigue, abdominal pain and fullness, anorexia, weight loss, and diarrhea. In these studies, physical signs, such as liver enlargement and tenderness, are more frequent in the heavily infected, and eosinophil counts are higher. Uncontrolled treatment trials with praziquantel have demonstrated a decrease in symptoms of upper abdominal pain, diarrhea, distention, dizziness, fatigue, and insomnia from 72% to 45%.[30]

Ultrasonographic studies have revealed a high frequency of gallbladder enlargement, sludge, dysfunction, and stones in asymptomatic moderately to heavily infected patients. Treatment appears to reverse these parasite-associated gallbladder abnormalities.[31–33]

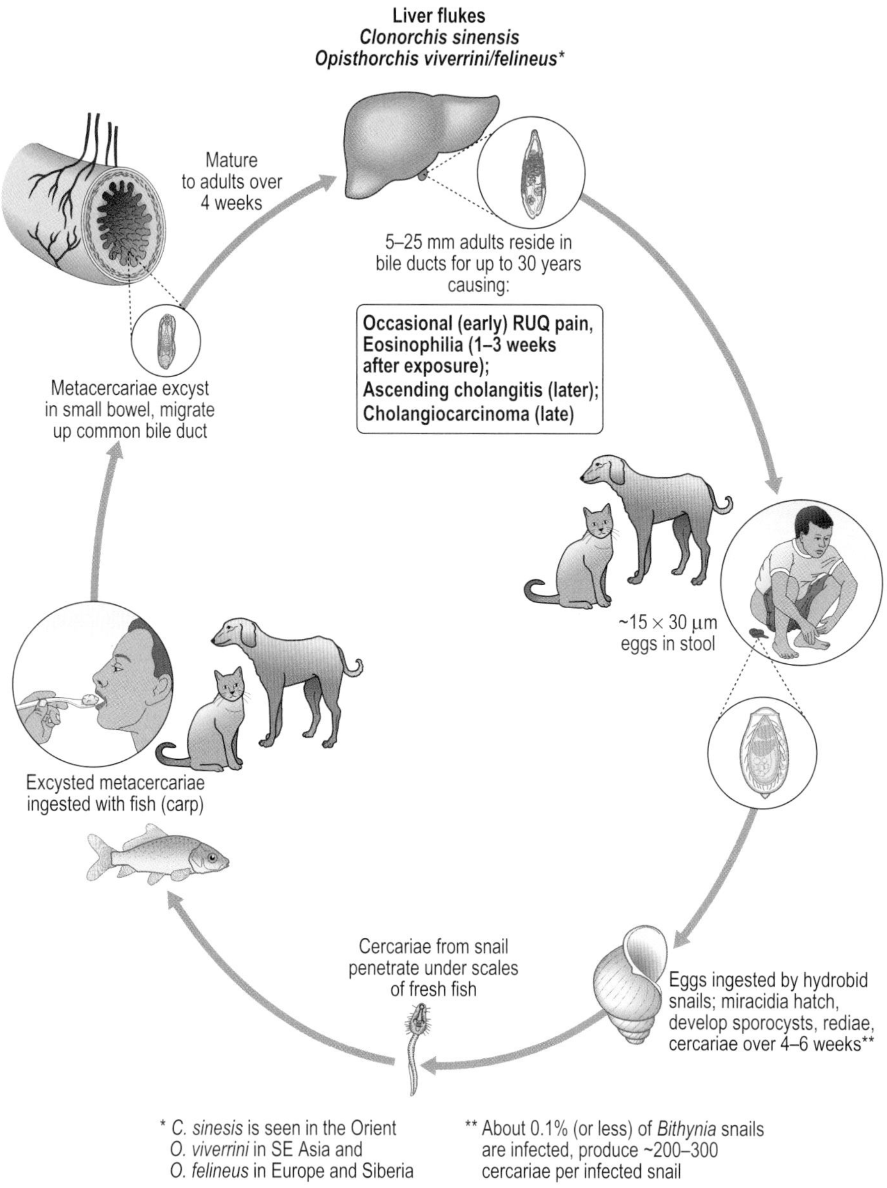

Figure 123.2 Life cycle of *Clonorchis sinensis* and *Opisthorchis viverrini/felineus*. RUQ, right upper quadrant.

Pathologic changes observed on necropsy and biopsy relate to intensity and duration of infection. Early infections reveal bile duct proliferation and pseudostratification of the biliary epithelium. Later, metaplastic squamous cells and glandular proliferation appear, suggesting adenomatous hyperplasia.[34] A small percentage of patients with chronic infection will develop complications, which include recurrent ascending cholangitis, pancreatitis, and cholangiocarcinoma.

Recurrent Ascending Cholangitis and Pancreatitis

Recurrent ascending cholangitis is characterized by repeated episodes of fever, chills, jaundice, right upper-quadrant pain, Gram-negative sepsis, and leukocytosis. Soft, muddy pigment stones are found in the biliary radicles and common bile duct and are associated with dilated intrahepatic bile ducts, ectasia, strictures, and multiple pyogenic abscesses, most notably of the left lobe of the liver.[35] Recurrent exacerbations and remissions can occur over years.[36,37] Pancreatitis at times is found on endoscopic retrograde cholangiopancreatography (ERCP), or at the time of surgery or autopsy, but it is rarely symptomatic or found in isolation without liver involvement.[38,39]

Cholangiocarcinoma

Worldwide, cholangiocarcinoma is much rarer than hepatocellular carcinoma, except for those areas in East Asia where infection with *O. viverrini* or *C. sinensis* is widespread and highly prevalent in humans.[40] An increased frequency of cholangiocarcinoma of the liver is seen in northern Thailand, where case-control studies reveal a fivefold increased risk in those infected.[41] The risk increases to 15-fold in persons with heavier infections. In one endemic province of Thailand, the rate of cholangiocarcinoma in males and females was 10- and six-fold higher, respectively, than in a nonendemic area.[41,42] In animal studies, nitrosamines increase the incidence of cholangiocarcinoma in *Opisthorchis*-infected animals.[43–45] High levels of such substances have been noted in the northern Thai diet.[46] An interesting recent discovery has been of a human granulin homolog in *O. viverrini*, termed Ov-GRN-1, that is secreted by the parasite and is able to promote fibroblast proliferation through a mitogen-activated protein kinase-dependent pathway.[47] In recognizing the role of trematode parasites in the induction of cholangiocarcinoma, the International Association for Research on Cancers has recently listed *O. viverrini* as a group 1 agent, a classification that assigns proven risk to an agent.[48] The mechanism of carcinogenesis is thought to be due to the presence of chronic inflammation at the site of infection, which results in the generation of free radicals and nitrogen species that damage DNA, initiate DNA mutations, and lead to genetic instabilities and malignant transformation.[49]

PATHOGENESIS AND IMMUNITY

The pathologic changes seen in the liver and biliary system in clonorchiasis and opisthorchiasis have been attributed to mechanical injury by the suckers of the flukes and host interactions with their secreted metabolic products,[50–52] such as excess proline production by adult flukes.[53] Eggs probably serve as nidi for biliary stones in the bile ducts and gallbladder.[34,54] Immunohistochemical studies indicate that the excretory-secretory proteins from the digestive and excretory organs (i.e., the intestines and bladder) are the most potent antigens and likely induce the dominant immunologic response.[4] Periductal infiltration with eosinophils and round cells with fibrosis of portal areas – a common finding – implicate immune-mediated tissue damage in the pathogenesis of disease.[4] The local reactions to eggs and migrating parasites are driven by T-lymphocyte effector mechanisms and are regulated by the $CD4^+$ subset of T lymphocytes in infections with related trematodes.[55] The presence of apparently uninfected persons in endemic regions with significantly higher levels of parasite-specific IgM, IgG, and IgA than egg-excreting persons has been used as evidence of protective immunity.[52,56,57]

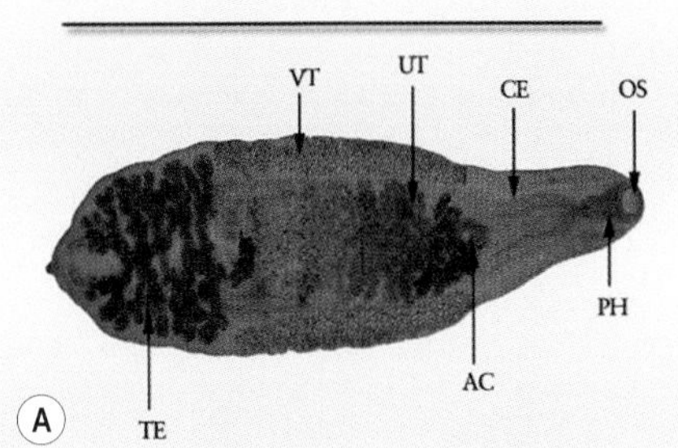

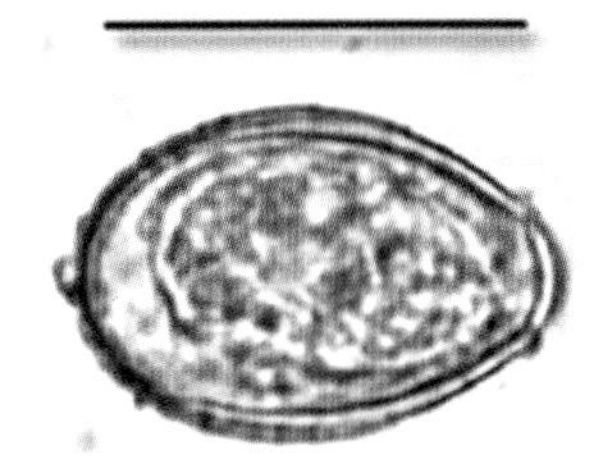

Figure 123.3 *Clonorchis sinensis.* **(A)** Adult of *C. sinensis* stained with carmine. Features of the adult trematode image identified in the photomicrograph include the oral sucker (OS), pharynx (PH), ceca (CE), acetabulum, or ventral sucker (AC), uterus (UT), vitellaria (VT), and testes (TE). The bar represents 1 cm. **(B)** Egg (size 29 × 16 µm). The bar represents 15 µm. (Courtesy of DPDx, Division of Parasitic Diseases, National Center for Infectious Diseases, Centers for Disease Control and Prevention, Atlanta, GA).

DIAGNOSIS

Asymptomatic infections with Opisthorchiidae are diagnosed by the presence of characteristic findings on ultrasound, computed tomography (CT), or magnetic resonance imaging (MRI), or by the detection of eggs in stool. In contrast, acute infection typically presents with a history of raw freshwater fish consumption (salted, fermented, or smoked fish, fish sauces, fish condiments), followed within several weeks by upper abdominal pain, high-grade eosinophilia, liver enzyme elevation, and the appearance of compatible eggs in the stool. The combination of cystic or mulberry-like dilations of intrahepatic bile ducts on ultrasound is pathognomonic of opisthorchiasis. With M-mode ultrasound, numerous spotty echoes and thin linear and moving intraductal echoes may be seen. Examination of multiple stool specimens may be necessary in lighter infections, but in infections of <20 adult flukes, no eggs may be found.[58] While egg counts in stools are relatively stable over time and such egg counts have prognostic significance, paradoxically, low egg counts may be seen in the heaviest infections because of blockage of biliary radicles or because pyogenic ascending cholangitis has killed the adults.[59–61] The eggs of *Clonorchis*, *Opisthorchis*, and *Metorchis* are essentially indistinguishable from one another by routine microscopy and can be confused with other fluke eggs as well. A definitive diagnosis may be made by examining the adult flukes in the stool immediately after a praziquantel treatment and purge or at the time of surgery. Recent advances in molecular

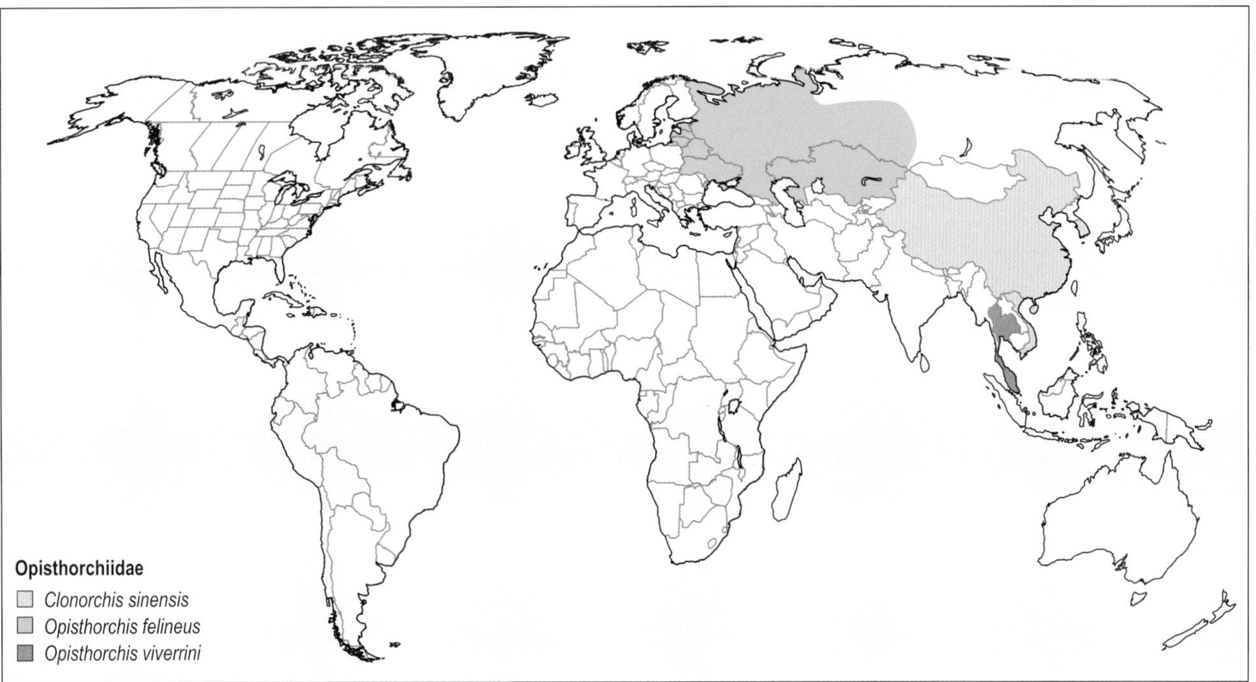

Figure 123.4 Geographic distribution of Opisthorchiidae.

techniques applied to stool samples have allowed considerable improvement in the detection of *Opisthorchis* (and *Clonorchis*) in stool.[62–64] These techniques are at least as sensitive as microscopic examination[63] and have the added advantage of high throughput. While these tests are useful as research tools, they are not yet available for routine use and further work will be required to adapt the techniques to laboratories in endemic regions.

Immunodiagnosis

Immunologic tests generally complement parasitologic testing and until recently have not had a primary role in the diagnosis of opisthorchiasis and clonorchiasis because they do not distinguish between active and old infections.[65] The preferred assay for immunodiagnosis in recent surveys has been enzyme-linked immunosorbent assay (ELISA). When compared with egg-positive stools, sensitivity can be high (79–96%).[4,66] However, use of crude worm extracts in ELISA is associated with significant lack of specificity; antibody positivity is seen in cases of paragonimiasis (33%), schistosomiasis japonica (5–25%), cysticercosis, hepatitis, liver cancer, and tuberculosis. Specificity can be enhanced somewhat by using immune affinity-purified antigens. Monoclonal antibodies have boosted the specificity in an ELISA inhibition test, which has proved to be as sensitive (77%) and more specific (virtually no cross-reactivity with other trematode infections) than the ELISA using crude worm extracts.[4] The use of excretory-secretory antigens as plate antigens has been reported to achieve sensitivities and specificities of >95% in smaller serologic surveys, but their utility in large-scale surveillance is yet to be proven. After treatment, antibody levels return to normal by 6 months in more than half of cases.[67,68] Circulating antigen detection with a monoclonal antibody-based capture ELISA has been reported to detect as little as 30 ng/mL of *C. sinensis* antigen in serum.[69,70] Antigen positivity is seen in 95% of antibody-positive infected patients. This test was reported to be positive in 95% of seropositive infected patients, declining to undetectable levels after 3 months in 81% of those parasitologically cured.[69,70] Stool antigen detection techniques show similar promise.[60]

A metabolic profiling strategy has been utilized successfully for biomarker discovery of the two trematodes, *Schistosoma mansoni* and *S. japonicum*,[71,72] and this has raised hopes for its application in the diagnosis of other trematodes, including *Opisthorchis* and *Clonorchis*. This approach uses a combination of analytical tools, including high-resolution nuclear magnetic resonance spectroscopy and mass spectrometry, with multivariate statistical analysis to measure quantitatively biochemical responses of organisms to physiological or pathological stimuli.[73]

TREATMENT

Praziquantel has been the drug of choice for opisthorchiasis and clonorchiasis since the 1970s because of ease of administration, lack of side effects, and demonstrated effectiveness. Its mechanism of action is thought to be through disruption of calcium homeostasis in parasite cells.[11,12] The recommended dosage of 25 mg/kg three times daily for 2 days has produced cure rates up to 100%, but patients with heavy infections (>5000 eggs/gram of stool) and in some geographic regions where praziquantel cure rates are low (Vietnam) may require retreatment.[1,4,74,75]

Albendazole has produced cure rates of 93–100% at a dosage of 10 mg/kg daily for 7 days.[4,76] Although some studies have suggested that it may not be as effective as praziquantel, it has fewer side effects.

Preliminary studies using rodent models have demonstrated that the artemisinins (e.g., artemether and artesunate) and synthetic peroxides (e.g., synthetic trioxolanes) known for their antimalarial properties,[77] and the Chinese anthelminthic drug tribendimidine[78] show promise for use against foodborne trematodiases.[12] With all treatments, success of therapy is defined as the disappearance of fluke-induced symptoms and fecal egg output, reduction in liver size, and a reversal of biliary tract abnormalities.[31] Recurrent pyogenic cholangitis is primarily a surgical problem, requiring relief of intrahepatic obstructions due to strictures, stones, and sludge, and drainage of the associated abscesses. Antibiotics may be necessary to treat the associated sepsis.

FASCIOLIASIS

Two flukes of the family Fasciolidae infect humans: *Fasciola hepatica*, the most common and widely distributed, and *F. gigantica*, a fluke of much more focal distribution. Both have similar life cycles and produce similar human disease, but *F. gigantica* can be recognized by its larger adult and egg sizes. *F. hepatica* was the first intestinal fluke to be described,[79] causing a significant burden of illness in domestic sheep since antiquity. The life cycle was described in 1883.[79]

THE AGENT

The adult *F. hepatica* is a large fluke (30 × 15 mm), flat and leaflike along the margins, with a cephalic cone (***Fig. 123.5A***). As for other flukes, size, shape, and integumental and internal morphology are species-defining features. The adult fluke lives in the common and hepatic bile ducts of the human or animal host, and eggs reach the exterior via the sphincter of Oddi and the intestine. The eggs are large (130–150 × 60–90 μm), ovoid, and inconspicuously operculate (***Fig. 123.5B***). In water, miracidia hatch from the eggs and penetrate suitable snail hosts where, after multiplying as sporocysts and redia, they leave the snail as free-living cercaria (***Fig. 123.6***). These attach to suitable plants, evolve into metacercarial cysts, and, when ingested by the human final host, excyst in the duodenum. The larvae migrate through the small intestinal wall and through the peritoneal cavity where they penetrate the liver capsule and slowly migrate to the large hepatic ducts. This prepatent period lasts 3–4 months. Anecdotal reports suggest that the life span in the human host can be up to 10 years.

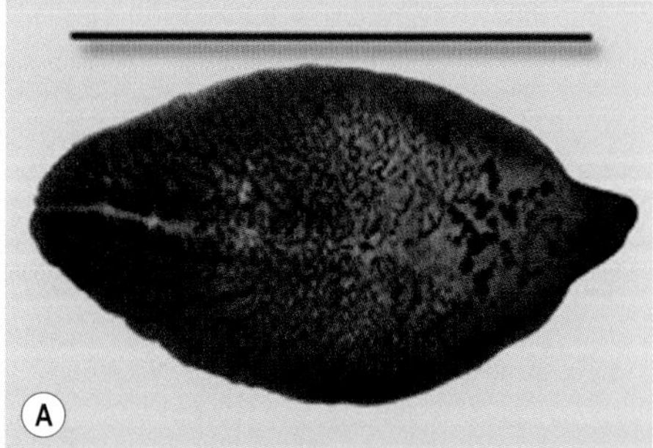

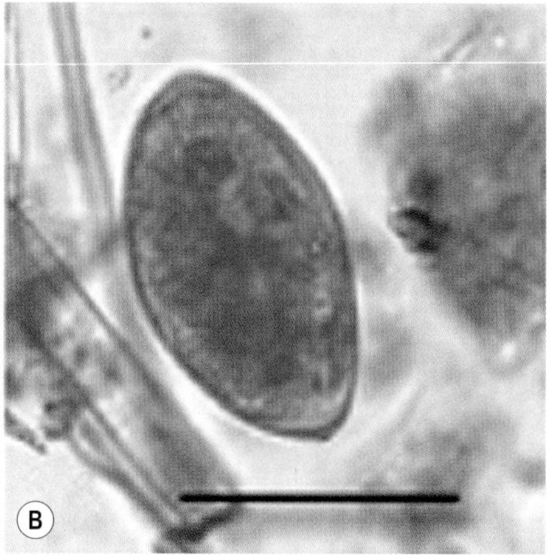

Figure 123.5 *Fasciola hepatica.* **(A)** Adult (size 30 × 15 mm). The bar represents 3 cm. **(B)** Egg (size 130–150 × 60–90 μm). The bar represents 100 μm. (Courtesy of DPDx, Division of Parasitic Diseases, National Center for Infectious Diseases, Centers for Disease Control and Prevention, Atlanta, GA.)

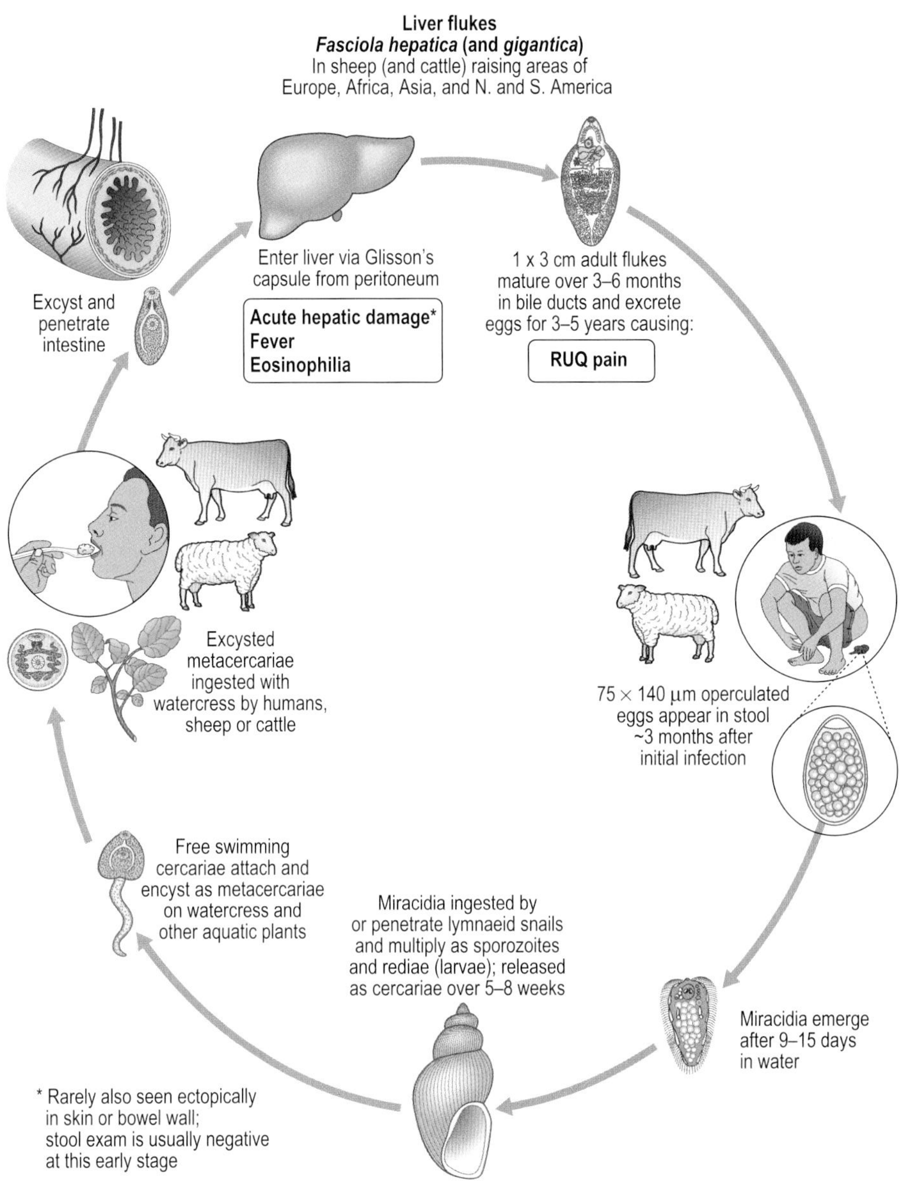
Liver flukes
Fasciola hepatica (and gigantica)
In sheep (and cattle) raising areas of Europe, Africa, Asia, and N. and S. America
Enter liver via Glisson's capsule from peritoneum
Acute hepatic damage*
Fever
Eosinophilia
1 x 3 cm adult flukes mature over 3–6 months in bile ducts and excrete eggs for 3–5 years causing:
RUQ pain
Excyst and penetrate intestine
Excysted metacercariae ingested with watercress by humans, sheep or cattle
75 × 140 μm operculated eggs appear in stool ~3 months after initial infection
Free swimming cercariae attach and encyst as metacercariae on watercress and other aquatic plants
Miracidia ingested by or penetrate lymnaeid snails and multiply as sporozoites and rediae (larvae); released as cercariae over 5–8 weeks
Miracidia emerge after 9–15 days in water
* Rarely also seen ectopically in skin or bowel wall; stool exam is usually negative at this early stage

Figure 123.6 Life cycle of *Fasciola hepatica* (and *F. gigantica*) in sheep (and cattle)-raising areas of Europe, Africa, Asia, and North and South America. It is rarely also seen ectopically in skin or bowel wall; stool exam is usually negative at this early stage. RUQ, right upper quadrant.

EPIDEMIOLOGY

F. hepatica is believed to be of European origin, and remains highly prevalent throughout Europe, but its ability to infect many different species and of the intermediate snail host to adapt to a wide range of ecological niches has allowed the parasite to achieve a cosmopolitan distribution.[80] It is now also found in the southern states of the United States, Mexico, North Africa, New Zealand, and small regions within Australia (***Fig. 123.7***). The parasite primarily infects cattle and sheep, although other domesticated animals such as goats, horses, and pigs can be infected. The major natural reservoirs for *F. hepatica* are cattle, sheep, goats, buffalo, camels, llamas, deer, pigs, horses, rabbits, and other wild animals, with prevalence rates of 25–92% in Bolivia, 20–40% in Ecuador, 10–100% in Peru, and 20–40% in Iran. In humans, stool- or antibody-positive prevalence rates in these countries can be similarly high (65–92% in Bolivia, 24–53% in Ecuador, 2–17% in Egypt, and 10% in Peru).[1,12] Since the introduction of *F. hepatica* to South America by Europeans in the eighteenth century it has become a major problem in Brazil, Argentina, Uruguay and in several Andean countries such as Bolivia, Peru, and Ecuador.[80–82] Fasciolosis is now an important veterinary disease and the cause of significant economic loss to the global agricultural community, estimated at >$2000 million annually, as >600 million animals are infected.[83,84] In terms of human disease burden, more than 2 million people are infected, mostly in Bolivia, Peru, Iran, Egypt, Portugal, and France. A variety of freshwater plants upon which metacercariae encyst, such as watercress, water lettuce, mint, and parsley, are important sources of human infection because they are often eaten raw in salads.[82] Over 25 species of amphibious lymnaeid snails that live in wet mud along the shoreline, and rarely in fast-moving or deep waters, serve as the first intermediate host for *F. hepatica*, the most important being *Lymnaea truncatula*. Climate change and manmade modifications of the landscape may influence the spread of fascioliasis.[85]

THE DISEASE

Acute Hepatic (Invasive) Stage

The clinical presentation of infection with *F. hepatica* reflects its peregrinations in the human host. Hepatic transit, variably called the hepatic, larval, invasive, or acute stage, lasts several months. This is followed by

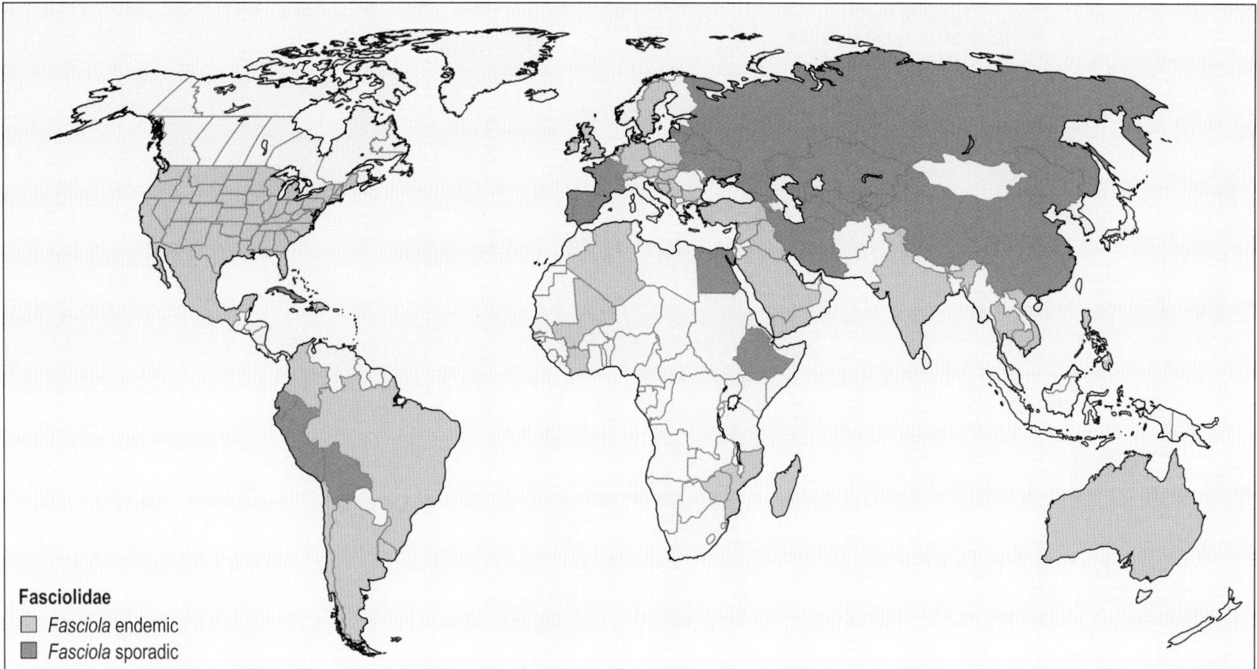

Figure 123.7 Geographic distribution of fascioliasis.

the biliary, adult, or chronic stage, which can persist for years. Where repeated ingestion of metacercaria occurs over an extended period, these two stages can overlap. Within 6–12 weeks of ingestion of metacercariae, symptoms occur that reflect larval migration through the small intestinal wall, the peritoneal cavity, and liver capsule.[86] This acute stage can last for 2–4 months. Typical findings include marked eosinophilia (95%), abdominal pain (65%), intermittent fever (60%), malaise and weight loss (35%), urticaria (20%), and cough, dyspnea, and chest pain (15%). A change in bowel habits, anorexia, and nausea may occur.[87,88] The abdominal pain may be generalized but frequently becomes localized to the right hypochondrium.[12,89] Hepatomegaly is a variable finding, and the liver may be tender on palpation. In some cases, mild elevations of hepatic enzymes are noted. The pulmonary symptoms may be associated with right-sided pleural effusions, which, on aspiration, reveal increased eosinophils.[90] Anemia has been reported.[91,92]

Ultrasound examination of the liver in the acute stage is usually normal, although small amounts of ascites have been found.[90] CT scans frequently reveal single or, more frequently, multiple small hypodense lesions 2–10 mm in diameter.[87] In addition, tunnel-like, branching, hypodense lesions (best delineated with contrast), most frequently situated peripherally within the liver, are relatively specific for fascioliasis, representing the pathologic changes created by the migration of the immature fluke through the liver.[26,93] The hepatic lesions are remarkable in that, on sequential CT scans, the position, attenuation, and shape of the lesions change over time.[94] On laparoscopy, multiple gray-white and yellow nodules 2–20 mm in diameter and short vermiform cords are noted on the liver surface and at times on the adjacent peritoneal surface.[95] Liver biopsies reveal microabscesses and tunnel-like areas of parenchymal necrosis surrounded by inflammatory infiltrates containing abundant eosinophils.[93,96] Necropsies reveal multiple subscapular cavities 5–10 mm in diameter filled with necrotic material from which necrotic tracts radiate. Increasing fibrosis is seen in older lesions.[96,97]

Rarely, immature flukes may migrate to nonhepatobiliary locations such as the skin, lung, intestinal wall, brain, and genitourinary tract, where granulomatous nodules or small abscesses lead to local clinical findings. A variant form of cutaneous larva migrans with migrating erythematous 1.5–6.0 cm cutaneous nodules has been reported.[67,87,97,98]

Chronic Biliary (Obstructive) Stage

F. hepatica has a propensity to migrate to the lumen of the common bile duct, where it reaches maturity. Eggs appear in the stool after a prepatent period of 3–4 months. Clinical findings reflect this new luminal location in that the liver-destructive phase of the infection ends. Fever, anorexia, and abdominal pain resolve, and the patient may become asymptomatic. Eosinophilia is infrequent. An unknown percentage of these cases develop intermittent biliary obstruction presenting with intermittent pain in the epigastrium or right hypochondrium, mimicking biliary colic or acute cholecystitis. At times the presentation is that of ascending cholangitis with fever, jaundice, and upper abdominal pain.[26,27] Ultrasound examination (more sensitive than CT examination) often reveals a soft intraluminal mass obstructing the extrahepatic biliary tree. Lithiasis of the common bile duct and gallbladder is a common sequela.

PATHOGENESIS AND IMMUNITY

Morbidity from *F. hepatica* is dependent on the number of worms and stage of infection.[99] The characteristic hepatic (and extrahepatic) changes of fascioliasis result largely from the anatomic location and large size of the parasite, a foreign body that induces eosinophilic and mononuclear infiltration around the eggs and adult worms.[50] As in other tissue-invasive helminthic infections, fascioliasis is associated with prominent eosinophilia, particularly in the early stages of infection,[87,99] and immune responses to *F. hepatica* appear to be regulated by Th2 subpopulations of T-helper cells, that are characterized by secretion of interleukin (IL)-4, IL-5, and IL-10.[100,101] This subset of T-helper cells also appears to regulate granuloma formation and liver disease in schistosomiasis.[102] IL-10 plays a dominant role in the downregulation of inflammatory responses to *F. hepatica* infection.[103] The role of T cells and other nonantibody-mediated effector systems in killing of the parasite and in the development of pathologic changes in humans is not well understood.[104,105] The role of eosinophils in parasite killing is also unclear, although it has been noted that the invasive phase in the liver is associated with peripheral eosinophilia and eosinophilic infiltrates around the sites of parasites and eggs.[67,96]

Immune evasion mechanisms are likely to play an important role in the survival of this long-lived parasite, and several evasion strategies have been proposed based on observations in animal models.[106,107] The surface glycocalyx may mediate immune evasion in several ways. First, the glycocalyx changes in composition during development of the parasite. Second, the glycocalyx is continuously sloughed off by the maturing juvenile worm, by one estimate every 3 hours, thus presenting a moving target.[108] Third, glycocalyx released from the surface can mop up circulating antibodies, interfering with antibody-mediated immune effector functions, such as antibody-dependent cellular toxicity.[109] Other evasion strategies include migration away from inflammatory cells, inhibition of oxygen radical generation by macrophages, and inhibition of T-cell function.[110] Natural resistance to fatal infection with *F. hepatica* has been observed in sheep and several strains of mice. Relative resistance to infection in mice correlates with type 1 T-cell responses (interferon-γ), whereas type 2 responses are associated with susceptibility.[106] Protection from challenge infection in mice and rats can be transferred by passive transfer of serum, but this protective effect is limited to sera collected 7–8 weeks post donor infection; after 25 weeks, serum from infected rats gave no protection, attributed to a decline in titers that accompanies the entry of the parasite into bile ducts.[108] Recombinant parasite-derived molecules, particularly peptidases of the cathepsin family (type L1 and B), have been demonstrated to induce protective immunity against challenge with infective stages of the parasite in animals.[83,111,112] Several potential vaccine antigens have been identified from animal models of *F. hepatica* infection. These include fatty acid-binding proteins, glutathione-*S*-transferase, cathepsin-L, and fluke hemoglobin.[8,110,113] Two of these molecules, glutathione-*S*-transferase and a 14.7-kDa polypeptide (Fh15) that has significant homology to, and cross-reacts with, *Schistosoma mansoni* fatty acid-binding protein, appear to confer partial resistance to infection in experimental infections.[105,114,115] Vaccination studies, using cocktails of recombinant antigens in animal models of fascioliasis, have shown that significant reductions in worm burdens (31–72%) and egg production (69–98%) can be achieved.[105,116] However, the success of vaccination and advances in our knowledge of immunological responses to *F. hepatica* detailed above have been largely limited to veterinary infections; the immunology of human disease requires further elucidation.

DIAGNOSIS

F. hepatica eggs are not found in stool specimens during the acute phases of infection, so the diagnosis must be based on the clinical findings of persistent pain and tenderness in the right hypochondrium or epigastrium, altered intestinal function, mild to moderate fever, and high levels of eosinophilia, often in the thousands/μL.[94] CT scans (ultrasound is less sensitive) contribute to the diagnosis, since the majority of symptomatic patients have visible hypodense lesions and tracts in the liver that migrate and change contour over time. The differential diagnosis of this clinical and radiologic syndrome includes visceral larva migrans caused by *Toxocara canis*, in which pulmonary symptoms also occur (see Chapter 109). Needle biopsies of the liver have not been helpful in diagnosis, but laparoscopy may reveal elongated nodules in the liver capsule.

In the acute invasive period, lasting 3–4 months, immunodiagnostic techniques are valuable. Tests that have been employed with varying success include complement fixation, immunofluorescence assays, indirect hemagglutination, countercurrent electrophoresis, and ELISA.[4,67,117–122] ELISAs have largely replaced other techniques because they are sensitive, rapid, and quantitative.[120,121,123] The preferred ELISAs employ excretory-secretory products of the adult worm as an antigen.[124,125] Antibodies to excretory-secretory antigens are elevated early in infection (based on studies in animal models) and remain elevated for years after infection, and successful treatment correlates with a decline in ELISA titers.[126,127] More recently, the Falcon assay screening test-ELISA (FAST-ELISA), a simple and rapid assay based on the ELISA and enzyme-linked immunoblot transfer assay, has been used for serodiagnosis, achieving sensitivities of 95–100% compared with parasitologic diagnosis. However, the specificity of this test is not known and may limit its utility.[87]

An ELISA antigen capture technique to detect circulating antigens has demonstrated a sensitivity of 100% and specificity of 98%.[128] Antigen detection techniques can detect parasite antigens in stool specimens 3–4 weeks before the appearance of eggs.[92] Immunodiagnostic tests continue to evolve, and the use of genus-specific antigens is likely to improve diagnostic accuracy.[87,127,129] Other attempts to improve the specificity of immunodiagnosis have used IgG subtype antibody levels instead of total IgG. Subtype analysis of antibody responses to excretory-secretory antigens such as the cathepsin protease (cathepsin L1) demonstrated that the predominant subtypes induced in human infections are IgG_1 and IgG_4, consistent with a predominant type 2 T-cell response.[26,106,127,129–131] The detection of subtype-specific antibodies in ELISAs may improve the specificity of the diagnostic immunoassays and make it possible to distinguish recent from remote infections.[132] A large study using a FAST-ELISA (a cathepsin (L1)-based antibody detection assay) in 634 children from an endemic region in Peru yielded a sensitivity of 92%, specificity of 84%, and a negative predictive value of 97%.[133]

In chronic biliary fascioliasis, the diagnosis is made on finding *F. hepatica* eggs in stool specimens or at the time of surgery for bile duct obstruction when eggs or adult flukes are removed from the biliary tree. Because egg production tends to be low, it is advisable to examine multiple stool specimens using the AMS iii (Tween 80) method or the Weller-Dammin modification method (since the formalin–ethyl acetate concentration technique appears to be less sensitive).[67,134] Eggs of *F. hepatica* can be confused with those of the intestinal flukes *Fasciolopsis buski* and echinostomes. Recovery of adults after anthelminthic treatment often allows species identification. False-positive "spurious" stool results can occur after consumption of liver of infected animals and can be ruled out by repeated stool examinations.

TREATMENT AND VACCINATION

In the past bithionol was considered the drug of choice.[135–137] Although side effects were mild, constituting anorexia, nausea, vomiting, abdominal pain, and pruritus, more than one course was often necessary. Triclabendazole, a benzimidazole, is now the drug of choice as a single 10 mg/kg oral dose or two doses 12 hours apart. Bioavailability is increased when triclabendazole is taken with food.[138,139] Efficacy has been as high as 92% in humans, but significant resistance has been seen both in animal and *in vitro* studies and repeat treatment may be necessary.[140–142] The most frequent side effect was colicky abdominal pain between days 3 and 7 post-treatment, compatible with fluke expulsion through the bile ducts. Unlike other trematodes, *F. hepatica* is frequently resistant to praziquantel, although some studies have shown effectiveness.[26,87,94,99,143–145] Animal studies show a lack of effectiveness of praziquantel against both immature and adult flukes in cattle and sheep.

Acute ascending cholangitis must be treated with antibiotics and surgery. A patient with a severe acute hepatic stage may benefit from the short-term use of systemic steroids. Other drugs used in the past include emitine, dehydroemetine, chloroquine, albendazole, and mebendazole, but all have been dropped because of toxicity or lack of effectiveness. Surgical approaches, such as ERCP, have been successfully used to relieve obstruction of the biliary tract.[146,147]

Fasciola is one of the few trematodes for which vaccines have been developed and used to protect against veterinary disease. The *F. hepatica* cathepsin-L protein, an important virulence determinant that was identified as a dominant antigen in excreted-secreted proteins, is a first-generation vaccine. There have been a number of trials using this molecule in cattle and sheep, with protection against challenge infection ranging from 38% to 79%.[107,112,148,149] In natural and experimental infections, a polarized Th2 response induces the generation of IgG_1 but little or no IgG_2 antibody subtypes, whereas vaccination induces antibody responses to cathepsin-L, the immunogen, that include high titers of both IgG_1 and IgG_2, indicating a mixed Th1/Th2 response.[106,107] These observations have been interpreted to indicate that protection is associated with a Th1 or a mixed Th1/Th2 response.[83,84,106] However, some vaccine trials with the same antigen have demonstrated little or no protection, suggesting that other factors, such as adjuvant and antigen formulation, may be important in generating protective immune responses.[83] No vaccines have yet been developed for human infections.

LUNG FLUKES

INTRODUCTION

Lung flukes are members of the genus *Paragonimus* and, while more than 40 species have been described, only eight are presently considered of human importance. Most of the 40 species are parasites of animals, of which 28 are considered distinct species (the remaining may be synonymous species), with 21 from Asia, two from Africa, and five from the Americas; most are in tropical areas.[150] *P. westermani* is the best-known species and is found in humans and animals throughout the East, from India to Japan and the Philippines. *P. heterotremus* is reported from China and Southeast Asia, *P. skrjabini* and *P. hueitungensis* from China, *P. miyazakii* from Japan, *P. uterobilateralis* and *P. africanis* from central and western Africa, *P. mexicanus* from Central and South America, and *P. kellicotti* from North America.[1,12,151]

THE AGENT

P. westermani was first found in a Bengal tiger that died in an Amsterdam zoo and was named after the zoo director, G.F. Westerman. The first human infection was found in a Portuguese sailor who died in Taiwan in 1879. He had earlier been a patient of Patrick Manson's in Amoy, China, and Manson later concluded that the hemoptysis seen in this man and his Chinese patients was due to this parasite.[152]

Adult *P. westermani* is reddish-brown in color, coffee bean-shaped, 7–16 mm in length, 4–8 mm in width, and 5 mm thick. The integument is spiny, and the anterior and ventral suckers are of equal size (***Fig. 123.8A***).

The eggs are yellow-brown in color, thick-shelled with a large operculum, and measure 80–120 × 50–65 μm (***Fig. 123.8B***). The eggs embryonate in water, and the miracidia hatch in 3 weeks and search for specific snail hosts. Development in snails yields free-swimming cercariae, which penetrate a crab or crayfish as second intermediate host and encyst as metacercariae. When these are eaten raw, partially cooked, pickled, or salted, the metacercariae excyst and penetrate the intestinal wall of the definitive hosts and enter the peritoneal cavity. The larval worms remain here for several days, then cross the diaphragm, and enter the pleural cavity and eventually the lung parenchyma to mature to adults in ~2 months. A fibrotic cyst wall develops around paired (or tripled) adults, but eggs that are produced escape through cyst-bronchial fistulas and are coughed up in sputum or swallowed and passed in the feces.

Other species of *Paragonimus* have life cycles similar to *P. westermani* but develop in different snail and crustacean intermediate hosts. Species differentiation is based on adult fluke rather than egg morphology.

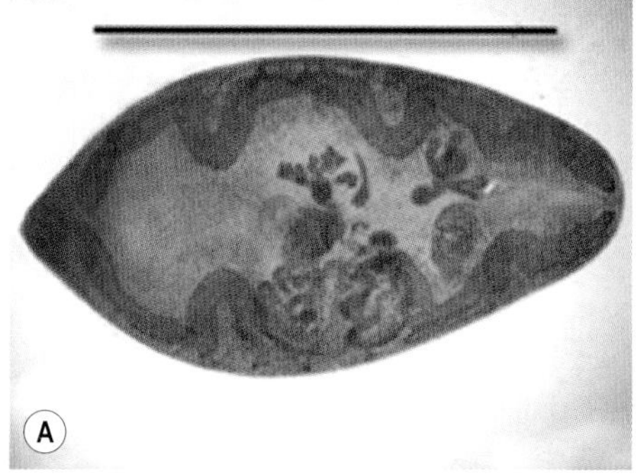

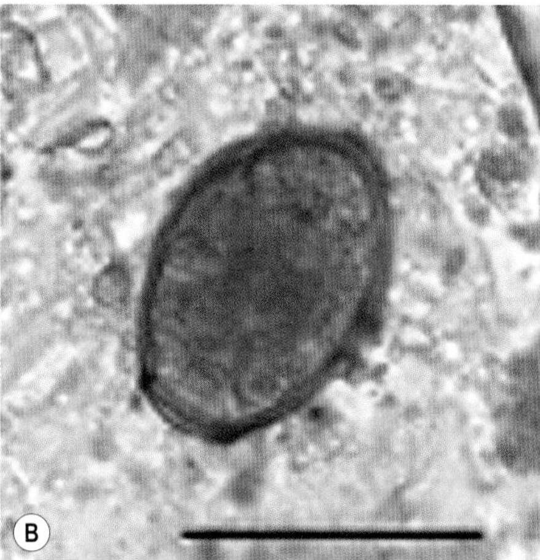

Figure 123.8 *Paragonimus westermani.* **(A)** Adult (size 7–16 × 4–8 mm). The bar represents 1 cm. **(B)** Egg (size 80–120 × 50–60 μm), unstained wet mount. The bar represents 100 μm.
(Courtesy of DPDx, Division of Parasitic Diseases, National Center for Infectious Diseases, Centers for Disease Control and Prevention, Atlanta, GA.)

EPIDEMIOLOGY

Paragonimus transmission occurs worldwide (***Fig. 123.9***), most notably in China (*P. westermani*, *P. skrjabini*, *P. heterotremus*, and *P. hueitungensis*), Korea (*P. westermani*), Japan (*P. westermani*, *P. miyazakii*), Vietnam (*P. heterotremus*), Cameroon (*P. africanus* and *P. uterobilateralis*), Ecuador (*P. mexicanus*), and Peru (*P. mexicanus*).[1,85]

In China, human disease caused by *P. westermani*, *P. skrjabini*, and *P. heterotremus* has been reported from 21 provinces with prevalences of up to 10.4% in some areas. Based upon a national survey the total prevalence was about 1.7% in 2005.[153] In Korea, a national skin test survey revealed an overall prevalence of 13% in 1959; however, recent estimates are that no more than 1000 people are infected.[154] Control measures, disruption of the ecosystem, and pollution have reduced crab and crayfish populations, and only 16 of 16 million stools were egg-positive in 1990.[1] Taiwan had several endemic foci in the past, but today human infections are rare owing to changes in eating habits and the effect of water pollution and industrialization on the intermediate hosts.[155] Fewer than 300 human cases of paragonimiasis have been reported from a few areas of the Philippines, although infected crustaceans are easily found in endemic areas.[153,154] Despite the reductions in Southeast and East Asia, it has been estimated that there are 20.5 million cases worldwide.[1,11,12]

More than 15 species of snails in the families Hydrobiidae, Thiaridae, and Pleurocercidae serve as the first intermediate hosts of *P. westermani*. The important second intermediate hosts are crabs in the genera *Eriocheir*, *Potamon*, and *Sundathelphusa*, and crayfish of the genus *Cambaroides*. Individuals become infected by eating these crustaceans raw or insufficiently cooked. The range of culinary artistry is wonderful. In China there is wine-soaked freshwater crab, crayfish curd, raw crab juice, and crab jam; in Thailand, raw freshwater shrimp salad or crab sauce; in Korea, raw crab in soy sauce; in the Philippines, roasted or raw crabs and crab juice seasoning. Crabs and crab juice have been used for medicinal purposes.[150,156]

Paragonimus species can cause abortive infections in many mammalian species, but when humans consume these paratenic hosts, the larvae survive stomach acid and penetrate the small-intestine wall, completing their life cycle in the human host (***Fig. 123.10***). Paratenic wild boars have served as a source of infection when eaten raw.[156]

THE DISEASE

The spectrum of disease caused by *Paragonimus* is species-dependent (determined by host–fluke compatibility), with *P. westermani* representing one clinical pole, with, most commonly, pleuropulmonary disease and relatively infrequent extrapulmonary disease. *P. heterotremus*, *P. africanus*, and *P. uterobilateralis* appear to be similar in presentation to *P. westermani*.[157–160]

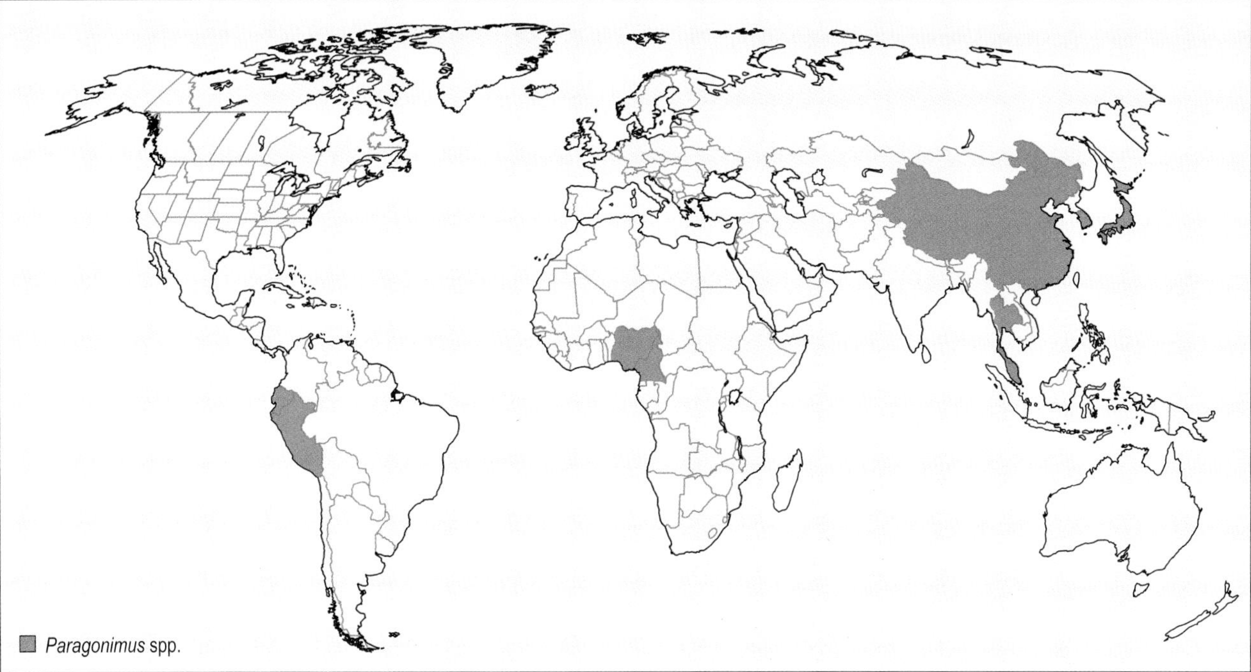

Figure 123.9 Geographic distribution of *Paragonimus* spp.

The other clinical pole, represented by *P. skrjabini*, is mainly extrapulmonary, with cutaneous lesions the most frequent clinical presentation. Pulmonary disease appears to be caused by adult flukes and cutaneous disease by immature flukes.[60,161]

Acute Paragonimiasis

After an incubation period of 2–15 days, the initial symptoms are diarrhea and abdominal pain, followed several days later by fever, chest pain, fatigue, urticaria, eosinophilia, or cough, or any combination of these, lasting several weeks.[12,162]

Pleuropulmonary Paragonimiasis

Although acute paragonimiasis may occur, most infections are either silent or insidious in onset. The initial clinical presentation occurs early in the 5–10-year life span of the adult fluke, but in some cases it may occur many years after acquisition of the infection.[163,164] In *P. westermani* infections, the initial presentation is often an abnormal chest film in an asymptomatic patient. Early clinical symptoms include cough or chest pain. The cough, initially dry, often becomes productive of viscous and rusty-colored or blood-tinged sputum and appears to be worsened by exertion.[165] The sputum may be peppered with rusty-brown flecks consisting of clumps of eggs.[60] Charcot–Leyden crystals are frequent. Occasionally there is profuse hemoptysis following paroxysmal coughing. The chest pain is often pleuritic. Fevers are infrequent and, in spite of a prolonged clinical history, the patient's health usually remains relatively unimpaired. Eosinophilia may be present initially but is usually absent in chronic infections.

Radiographic findings include pulmonary lesions such as focal, segmental, or lobar air space consolidation, small cysts (5–30 mm), calcified spots, linear opacities, or nodules. The earliest infiltrates and nodules may show some limited migration.[161,163,166] About 10–40% of egg-positive patients will have normal chest films.[163] As the fluke matures, cavitary lesions of 1–4-cm diameter are seen; as the fibrotic reaction increases with time they appear as nodules, but their cavitary nature and associated burrow tracts of 0.5–1.0 cm diameter can be visualized by CT scan. Eventually these lesions are replaced by oval to round calcifications.[163] Bronchoscopy, other than as a means of retrieving eggs, does not reveal any diagnostic findings.[163]

Pleural lesions have been found in 5–71% of patients in different clinical series of *P. westermani* infections and include effusions, hydropneumothorax, and pleural thickening, which can be bilateral.[163,167,168] The frequency of pleural disease appears to be greatest in *P. skrjabini* infections.[169] Pleural fluid is sterile, contains a leukocyte count over 1000/μL, many eosinophils, and elevated protein and lactate dehydrogenase, and decreased glucose values. Eggs are rarely found in sputum or pleural fluid.

Excised pulmonary lesions reveal a wide variety of histopathologic changes characterized by the presence of adult worms within fibrous cysts up to 1.5 cm in size, juxtaposed and often communicating with bronchioles or bronchi. Egg-induced granulomas are easily confused with tuberculosis. Adjacent to the cysts are bronchiectases, various pneumonic processes, and vasculitis. Both acute and chronic cellular reactions can coexist within the same lesions.[165,168,170]

Extrapulmonary Paragonimiasis

A small percentage (~1%) of patients with paragonimiasis will develop lesions in locations other than the lung.[154] The frequency is dependent on the species of *Paragonimus*, the intensity of the infection, and possibly the duration. The diagnosis of these ectopic infections depends on the organ involved; cerebral infection produces the most frequent morbidity.

Cerebral Paragonimiasis

Cerebral paragonimiasis is the most frequent form of extrapulmonary disease diagnosed, possibly reflecting the sensitivity of the central nervous system (CNS) to such an insult rather than a predilection of the parasite for that site. Cerebral involvement occurs in <1% of cases in community-based studies and up to 24% in hospital-based studies.[171] Cerebral paragonimiasis most often occurs in younger age groups: 90% of patients are <30 years of age.[172] Clinical findings in cerebral paragonimiasis range from meningitis, arachnoiditis, to cerebral and spinal space-occupying lesions. Meningitis tends to be acute in onset and to be the initial presentation of cerebral paragonimiasis in up to a third of cases. Intracerebral lesions occur usually in occipital or temporal lobes, or both. The clinical presentation, usually insidious in onset, includes a history of seizures (80%), visual disturbances (60%), headache (55%), motor weakness (48%), sensory disturbances (40%), and vomiting

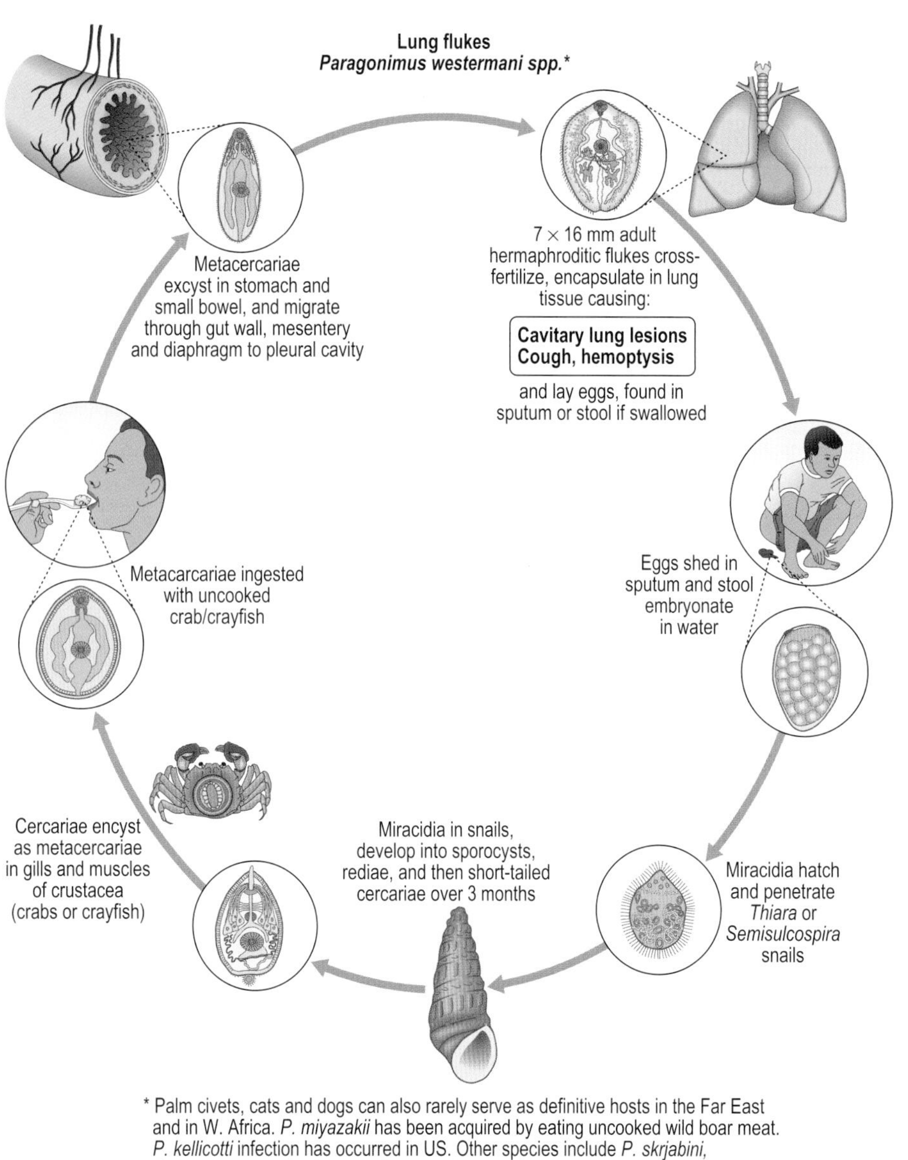
Lung flukes
Paragonimus westermani spp.*
7 × 16 mm adult hermaphroditic flukes cross-fertilize, encapsulate in lung tissue causing:
Cavitary lung lesions
Cough, hemoptysis
and lay eggs, found in sputum or stool if swallowed
Eggs shed in sputum and stool embryonate in water
Miracidia hatch and penetrate Thiara or Semisulcospira snails
Miracidia in snails, develop into sporocysts, rediae, and then short-tailed cercariae over 3 months
Cercariae encyst as metacercariae in gills and muscles of crustacea (crabs or crayfish)
Metacarcariae ingested with uncooked crab/crayfish
Metacercariae excyst in stomach and small bowel, and migrate through gut wall, mesentery and diaphragm to pleural cavity
* Palm civets, cats and dogs can also rarely serve as definitive hosts in the Far East and in W. Africa. P. miyazakii has been acquired by eating uncooked wild boar meat. P. kellicotti infection has occurred in US. Other species include P. skrjabini, P. heterotremus, P. africanus, P. uterobilateralis, P. mexicanus

Figure 123.10 Life cycle of *Paragonimus westermani* spp.

(33%).[172,173] Physical findings include ophthalmologic abnormalities (75%), a decline in mental function (70%), hemiparesis (60%), and hemihypoesthesia (45%). Pulmonary paragonimiasis is seen in the majority of cases of CNS disease and, in fact, precedes CNS involvement in two-thirds of patients.

Plain films show calcifications and characteristically aggregated, round or cyst-like "soap bubbles" in more than 40% of patients. Common CT and MRI findings are conglomerated, multiple ring-shaped enhancing lesions with surrounding edema, described as grape clusters.[174] These rings are usually smooth and round, but may at times be irregular in outline. They are usually 1–3 cm in diameter and have contents with a density equal to or slightly greater than that of cerebrospinal fluid (CSF). At times hemorrhages up to 4 cm in diameter are associated with the ringlike structures, or the lesions may be nodular. Calcifications can be punctate, round, cystic, or amorphous and will increase in frequency with the duration of disease.[171,172,174]

Cutaneous Paragonimiasis

Cutaneous presentation, uncommon in *P. westermani* infections, has been reported to occur in 80% of infections due to other species of *Paragonimus* (e.g., *P. skrjabini*, *P. miyazakii*). The cutaneous presentation, which has been called trematode larva migrans, consists of painless and migratory subcutaneous swellings or subcutaneous nodules on the trunk and proximal extremities,[175,176] often accompanied by high-level eosinophilia.

Miscellaneous Sites

Flukes, usually immature, may come to rest in ectopic intra-abdominal sites such as the liver, spleen, peritoneum, intestinal wall, or mesenteric lymph nodes. The clinical picture reflects the site and can include abdominal pain, diarrhea, and even dysentery.

PATHOGENESIS AND IMMUNITY

As with other tissue-dwelling trematodes, infection with *P. westermani* is also associated with eosinophilia and leukocytosis in the early stages of infection, reflecting activation of the immune system. Eosinophil infiltration around the sites of egg deposition is a consistent pathologic feature, as is eosinophilia and an elevated IgE level, indicative of a Th2 cell-regulated response.[177] IgG_4 antibodies predominate, but the role of Th2 lymphocytes in resistance to the parasite remains to be determined.[177] In rodent models, excreted-secreted products of *Paragonimus* appear to regulate the innate and adaptive immune response in the host, by a number of mechanisms such as attenuating the survival and function of eosinophils, and secreting proinflammatory cytokines and chemokines.[178,179] However, these immune mechanisms have been studied only in rodent and bovine models of paragonimiasis, and their roles in human infections are unconfirmed.

DIAGNOSIS

Pulmonary paragonimiasis must be suspected in persons from known endemic areas when a chronic cough is present; the most important differential diagnoses are tuberculosis, bronchiectasis, and chronic bronchitis. The diagnosis is almost always made by finding the characteristic eggs in sputum, stool, gastric aspirates, or tissue, i.e., by parasitological techniques. Examination of blood-streaked sputum is most likely to yield positive results. Egg detection in sputum may require repeated examinations, and a 24-hour sputum collection can increase the sensitivity.[180] This collection is centrifuged, the sediment dissolved in 3% sodium hydroxide, and then examined for eggs. In children and the elderly, in whom sputum swallowing is more frequent, the examination of stool and gastric aspirate specimens can be more productive.[180] Ziehl–Neelsen stains of specimens for mycobacteria may destroy the fluke eggs, making separate examinations necessary.[166] In patients who have pleural or CNS involvement, it is very uncommon to find eggs in pleural fluid or CSF aspirates.

Immunodiagnosis

The complement fixation test has been a standard test for years. This test is sensitive and becomes negative 6–12 months after cure, making it useful for following therapy.[168,181] Some cross-reactivity with other trematode parasites has been noted, particularly in the chronic phase of paragonimiasis.[182] A skin test using extracts of adult *Paragonimus* is useful for screening in epidemiologic surveys because of its high sensitivity (80–90%), but it remains positive 10–20 years after cure.[183] ELISAs for detection of antibodies to *P. westermani* are both sensitive (92%) and highly specific (>90%), but require longer (4–24 months) to become positive after infection and longer to normalize after cure.[184–187] Crude worm extracts do not provide an acceptably specific ELISA,[188,189] and the most sensitive ELISA to date, using an 8-kDa component of *P. westermani* as the antigen, has been developed by Centers for Disease Control and Prevention (sensitivity, 96%; specificity, 100%).[190] Recently, antigen detection assays have been developed that utilize mixtures of monoclonal antibodies to capture *P. westermani* antigens from serum, with a sensitivity approaching 100% and specificity >95%.[162,191] The utility of these assays in the field remains to be evaluated, but they will likely provide a sensitive measure of active infections in field surveys.

TREATMENT AND PROGNOSIS

Untreated, pulmonary paragonimiasis can resolve in 5–10 years, leaving dysfunction commensurate with the degree of scar tissue produced in the pleura or lungs.[163] Praziquantel is the drug of choice because of minimal side effects and the short course of administration. A regimen of 75 mg/kg/day in three divided doses for 2 days is 90–100% effective.[163,192–194] Symptoms improve within 2–3 days, although radiologic findings may worsen for the first 10 days.[166] Adverse effects are mild and include headache, intestinal symptoms, and transient urticaria. Large pleural effusions may require drainage. Surgical intervention may be required for long-standing effusions (years) or empyemas (months).[163] Triclabendazole, a drug introduced as therapy for fascioliasis, successfully treats pulmonary paragonimiasis at a dosage of 5 mg/kg daily for 3 days or 10 mg/kg bid for 1 day.[195] Bithionol could cure 92% of pulmonary cases at a dosage of 40 mg/kg/day on alternate days for 10–15 doses.[196] Gastrointestinal side effects in 70%, dermatologic side effects in 21%, and the duration of treatment are recognized limitations.

INTESTINAL FLUKES – INTRODUCTION

Little is known about the clinical presentations of 70% of trematode species that inhabit the human intestinal tract, even for those that affect relatively large populations.[12,60,197] The best known are *Fasciolopsis buski*; the Heterophyidae, including *Heterophyes heterophyes* and *Metagonimus yokogawai*; and several *Echinostoma* species. The intestinal flukes are thought to produce no symptoms except when present in very large numbers (a rare occurrence). Few cause serious disease, but community-based and case-control studies have yet to be done. Most of these flukes occur in Asia, but foci of these infections occur in other populations throughout the world. They are usually localized in areas where there are freshwater snail vectors and animal reservoir hosts and occur in people with particular dietary habits.[198]

FASCIOLOPSIS BUSKI

THE AGENT

F. buski, the giant intestinal fluke, was first found, by Busk, in an Indian sailor in London in 1843. The parasite is found in China, Taiwan, Thailand, Laos, Bangladesh, India, Indonesia, Vietnam, Myanmar, and Kampuchea. The worm is elongated, oval, and fleshy, measuring 20–75 × 8–20 × 0.5–3.0 mm. Eggs are large, operculate, and unembryonated when passed, and measure 130–140 × 80–85 μm. The miracidia develop in several weeks, hatch from the eggs, and infect planorbid snail intermediate hosts. Snails of the genera *Segmentina, Hippeutis,* and *Gyraulus* serve as intermediate hosts.[85] After development in the snail, cercariae emerge and encyst as metacercariae on aquatic plants. When the plant is eaten, the attached metacercariae excyst and attach to the small intestinal mucosa. The prepatent period is 3 months, and the worms are known to live for 6 months or more in the human. Pigs and dogs act as reservoirs.

EPIDEMIOLOGY

Several planorbid snails found in muddy ponds and streams, including those found adjacent to slaughterhouses where feces from pigs contaminate the waters, serve as the first intermediate host of *F. buski*. The metacercaria of *F. buski* can attach to most aquatic plants, including water caltrop (*Trapa bicornis*, *T. natans*), water chestnut (*Eliocharis tuberossa*), water bamboo (*Zizania aquatic*), water hyacinth (*Eukhornia crassipes*), water morning glory (*Ipomoea aquatic*), watercress (*Nasturtium officinale*), lotus (*Nymphaea lotus*), and others, that serve as sources of infection, although detached metacercariae can also transmit infection.[1,199] These plants may be cultivated near homes in water contaminated accidentally or fertilized intentionally with human or pig feces. Pigs are a major reservoir host, but there are some areas where humans are infected while pigs are not.[200] Children eating plants during play, especially in rural areas, have the highest prevalence rates.

THE DISEASE

This large fluke attaches to the duodenal and jejunal mucosa and produces focal inflammation, ulceration, and small abscesses at the sites of attachment. However, community-based studies reveal no clinical or biochemical differences between lightly to moderately infected cases and controls.[201] Early symptoms, which begin 30–60 days after exposure, are epigastric pain, mimicking peptic ulcer disease, and diarrhea.[202] Hunger or anorexia, nausea, and vomiting may occur. Rarely, in heavy infections, edema of the face, abdominal wall, and legs, ascites, and severe prostration have been described.[183] The cause of these symptoms is not understood. Large numbers of flukes may cause focal ileus or intermittent obstruction. Eosinophilia is variable but may be marked.[203]

HETEROPHYIDS

There are a large number of small intestinal flukes (less than 2.5 mm long) that have been reported in humans, other mammals, and birds that come from the families Heterophyidae, Plagiorchiidae, Lecithodendridae, Microphallidae, and others. The flukes in the Heterophyidae are the most prevalent and best studied. The importance of these flukes is being increasingly recognized,[204] although their pathogenic potential is as yet unclear.

THE AGENT

Of at least 10 human species of intestinal fluke in the family Heterophyidae, the three most prevalent are *Heterophyes heterophyes*, *H. nocens*, and *Metagonimus yokogawai*. Bilharz described the first, *H. heterophyes*, at the autopsy of a native of Cairo.[50] These are the smallest of the human flukes. They measure 1–2 mm in length, are oval to pear-shaped, and have spiny integuments. The eggs are operculate, ovoid, and yellowish in color, measure 27–30 × 15–17 μm, and are very difficult to speciate. The eggs are embryonated when passed and are ingested by a snail intermediate host. Cercariae from the snail enter freshwater fish, encyst as metacercariae, and, when eaten raw, excyst and complete their development to adult flukes within 1–2 weeks in the small intestine of humans, other mammals, and fish-eating birds. The prepatent period is only 9 days and the parasite may live for a few months to a year in the final host.[12]

EPIDEMIOLOGY

The heterophyids are parasites of fish-eating mammals and birds, and humans acquire the infection by eating raw or incompletely cooked freshwater or brackish water fish. The highest infection rates for *H. heterophyes* have been reported in Egypt, Iran, and Sudan; for *M. yokogawai*, in Korea, China, Taiwan, Indonesia, Russia, and Japan; and for *H. nocens*, in Korea and Japan. *H. heterophyes* infects the gray mullet *Mugil cephalus* in the brackish lagoons of Egypt's Nile delta. Infection rates can reach 65% in children in villages where these fish are traditionally eaten raw. However, reports of these and other heterophyid species in scattered locations around the world (particularly from South and Southeast Asia) are frequent. Distributions of the different Heterophyidae greatly overlap. In Korea, of 19 different intestinal flukes reported in humans, 12 are different heterophyid species.[204,205] Intestinal flukes are common in farmed fish in Vietnam, with dogs, cats, and pigs important reservoir hosts, especially for *Haplorchis* species.[7,200] The overall prevalence of *M. yokogawai* in Japan is low (0.2–0.3%), but in some areas the prevalence is high (51–75%).[206] In Korea, *M. yokogawai* infection rates of 1–2% have been reported for the population as a whole, reaching 29% along some coastal streams.[204] Infection rates of *M. yokogawai* in Taiwan and the Philippines are around 1%.[207]

THE DISEASE

Symptoms begin 9 days following ingestion of the metacercaria, on average, with dyspepsia, and colicky abdominal pain, diarrhea, and eosinophilia.[208,209] A mild focal inflammatory reaction and superficial erosions are produced at the site of attachment.[2] The fluke may penetrate the mucosa, and eggs may embolize from these intramucosal sites via lymphatics to the systemic vascular system. Eggs of three different heterophyid species have been recovered from capillaries of brain, heart, lungs, spleen, and liver, where space-occupying granulomatous lesions induce clinical pathology.[209–212] Myocarditis can follow the occlusion of myocardial vessels by eggs and the resultant granulomatous and fibrotic host reaction. Thickened mitral valves containing ova has been reported.[213]

ECHINOSTOMA SPECIES

THE AGENT

These trematodes are primarily parasites of birds and mammals but are common among certain populations of Asia. Fifteen species have been reported in humans. The parasites are elongate, tapered at both ends, and 5–15 × 1–2 mm in size. The name derives from a collar of spines in two rows surrounding the oral sucker. The anterior integument is also provided with tiny spines. Eggs are operculate, thin-shelled, and vary in size (83–130 × 58–90 μm).[54] The eggs embryonate in freshwater in 14 days, and the miracidia enter the snail host. Cercariae emerge from the snail and encyst in the same snail from which they emerged or in other snails, clams, fish, or tadpoles, which serve as second intermediate hosts. Any of these, if eaten uncooked, infect the human final host.[12,82,213]

EPIDEMIOLOGY

The most common of the 15 reported *Echinostoma* species in humans are *E. ilocanum* in the Philippines and Thailand, and both *E. malayanum* and *E. revolutum* in Thailand.[2,85,214] In northern Luzon in the Philippines, *E. malayanum* infection rates have averaged 10% of surveyed populations, with highs of over 40%.[12,155] In northern Thailand, a variety of echinostomes infect humans, with prevalence rates as high as 50%.[215] These and the other species are found at lower prevalences in Southeast Asia, eastern and South Asia, and also in Egypt and Central and South America.[216] The major source of infection with *E. ilocanum* is the snail *Pila conica*, which is eaten uncooked in parts of the Philippines. Other sources of infections are clams, tadpoles, frogs, and fish, all serving as second intermediate hosts for echinostomes. Rats, dogs, cats, birds, and other fish-eating animals are reservoirs of infection.[12,217]

THE DISEASE

These flukes attach to small intestinal mucosa, producing inflammatory lesions and shallow ulcers at the sites of attachment. A self-infection by ingestion of 113 metacercariae of *Echinochasmus japonicus* resulted, after 10 days, in abdominal pain and diarrhea.[2,12,217] There are no clinical epidemiology studies, but it is generally accepted that symptoms are rare in any but the heaviest infections (approximately 500 flukes), which are uncommon.[54,218] The presentation may include colicky abdominal pain and loose bowel movements and at times diarrhea and eosinophilia.

MISCELLANEOUS INTESTINAL FLUKES

There are many other intestinal flukes within the preceding families – Fasciolidae, Heterophyidae, and Echinostomatidae[12,60] – that have been reported to cause human infections with more limited distributions and are less well studied. Two flukes in two other families, Troglotrematidae and Paramphistomatidae, are worth mentioning.

Nanophyetus salmincola is a small fluke found in eastern Siberia and the northwestern coast of North America. It belongs to the same family, Troglotrematidae, as does *Paragonimus*. Adults are 0.8–2.5 × 0.3–0.5 mm, and eggs are 64–97 × 34–55 μm in size. Fish, such as salmon, are the second intermediate hosts. Intestinal symptoms can occur with heavy infections in a manner similar to that of other intestinal flukes. More unusually, this fluke is a vector for the rickettsial organism *Neorickettsia helminthoeca*, which produces a fatal illness in dogs ("salmon poisoning").[219,220]

Gastrodiscoides hominis is a piriform intestinal fluke that is 8–14 × 5–8 mm in size and produces eggs that measure 150 × 60–70 μm. It is widely distributed from India to the Philippines and north to Kazakhstan. The human colon can be colonized, with resultant mucoid diarrhea. Pigs and rodents appear to be the reservoir.

DIAGNOSIS

Since clinical presentations are nonspecific, infection is often indicated by eosinophilia, a particular dietary history, and the time interval since possible infection; *H. heterophyes* and *M. yokogawai* do not survive in the intestine for more than a year. The diagnosis is made on stool examination or by tissue biopsy or necropsy. Egg identification can be very difficult because many of the intestinal fluke eggs have similar morphology and overlapping sizes. Overlapping "small" fluke eggs include *H. heterophyes* (28–30 × 15–17 μm), *M. yokogawai* (26–28 × 15–17 μm), *Clonorchis sinensis* (28–35 × 12–19 μm), and *O. viverrini* (30 × 12 μm). Overlapping "large" fluke eggs are *Fasciolopsis buski* (130–140 × 80–85 μm), *Echinostoma* spp. (83–130 × 58–90 μm), and *Fasciola hepatica* (130–150 × 60–90 μm). As well, there are many other less common intestinal flukes with focal distribution that produce similarly sized eggs. The eggs of small opisthorchid and heterophyid flukes are difficult to differentiate microscopically and many of the infections are misdiagnosed. Polymerase chain reaction assays targeting ribosomal DNA are being developed to differentiate some species.[221] Examination of stools for expelled adult flukes after treatment with praziquantel (a praziquantel "purge") is often necessary to make a definitive diagnosis. Although praziquantel may damage the integument of the adult fluke, it is still often possible to make a species identification.

TREATMENT AND PROGNOSIS

Although the evidence comes from limited clinical trials, it appears that praziquantel is highly effective against intestinal flukes at 15–25 mg/kg given in a single dose.[12,85,222] The new benzimidazole, triclabendazole, at 5 mg/kg twice daily after a meal at a 6–8-hour interval for 1 day, shows promise in the treatment of intestinal flukes.[223–225] Alternative drugs include for *Fasciolopsis buski*, niclosamide 40 mg/kg/day for 1–2 days (maximum daily dose of 4 g); for *H. heterophyes*, niclosamide 1000 mg in a single dose; and for *Echinostoma* spp., albendazole 400 mg twice daily for 3 days.[54,176,209,226]

Recent studies in rodent models have shown that the artemisinins (e.g., artemether and artesunate) and synthetic peroxides (e.g., synthetic trioxolanes), recognized for their antimalarial properties,[77] and the Chinese anthelminthic drug tribendimidine[78] may be useful against foodborne trematodiases.[176] In one study, a single oral dose of artesunate, artemether, or OZ78 (100–400 mg/kg) resulted in 100% worm burden reductions in a chronic *F. hepatica* infection in the rat model.[227] Artesunate and artemether also showed activities against adult *C. sinensis* flukes in rats, with 99–100% reduction in worm burdens with a single 150 mg/kg oral dose of either drug.[228] In addition, *O. viverrini*-infected hamsters treated with a single oral dose of artesunate and artemether (400 mg/kg) demonstrated 78% and 66% reductions in worm burden, respectively.[228] Trematodes show variable sensitivity to tribendimidine. A single oral dose of tribendimidine (150 mg/kg) administered to rats infected with adult *C. sinensis* flukes resulted in a 99% reduction of worms, and 400 mg/kg caused a 96% reduction in adult *O. viverrini* flukes in hamsters. However, no activity of tribendimidine against *F. hepatica* was observed in the rat model.[229] Scanning electron microscopy indicates that both artemether and tribendimidine disrupt the tegument of adult trematodes.[229] Since treatment options are limited and there is concern about the emergence of resistance, combination chemotherapy may hold promise for the treatment of foodborne trematodiases.[12,225]

PREVENTION AND CONTROL

Public health interventions to prevent these foodborne infections will need to include plans for adequate sanitation, the use of chemical fertilizers, food inspections, and campaigns to disseminate information, education, and communication. The ultimate aim is to change human behavior, specifically to change habits that have been in practice for generations,[230] because the consumption of raw or undercooked freshwater fish and other aquatic products is the key risk factor for acquiring foodborne trematode infections. These habits are variably dependent on attitudes, education, poverty, environmental degradation, food security, and other factors, and control strategies will have to take all these into account. Human vaccines are presently not available for the prevention of foodborne trematodiases, but recent gene discovery efforts may assist in the rational development of vaccines and the next generation of trematocidal drugs.[231] National strategies are necessary to control these parasites. Health education and appropriate regulations, both for water bodies used for pisciculture and aquatic plant crops, can have an impact. Mass treatment programs using praziquantel or triclabendazole may be beneficial but require more experience.[232] Molluscicides for the elimination of the animal host reservoirs do not appear to be realistic over the long term.[1] Irradiation of food may offer an alternative.[233] Preservation by cooking can be difficult in many heavily populated regions where fuel is scarce. On the other hand, some populations prefer to eat raw food, aware of the nutritional value of raw foods.

Access the complete reference list online at
http://www.expertconsult.com

CHAPTER 124

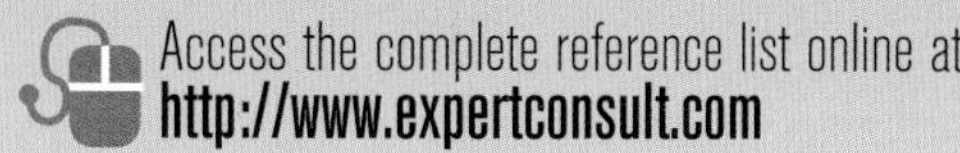
Access the complete reference list online at
http://www.expertconsult.com

Arthropods, Tongue Worms, Leeches, and Arthropod-borne Diseases

Jerome Goddard

INTRODUCTION

Arthropods (phylum Arthropoda), characterized by a chitinous exoskeleton, segmented bodies, and jointed appendages, may negatively affect human health in a number of ways. There may be direct effects, such as bites and stings; indirect effects, such as disease transmission; and perceived effects, such as entomophobia or delusions of parasitosis (see Chapter 140). Only a small percentage of all arthropod species are medically important, most being benign in their association with humans. An even smaller percentage are true human parasites – a few mite and lice species. However, especially in tropical regions, many human illnesses are either caused by or transmitted by arthropods.

Nothing better exemplifies the dynamic nature of the natural world than do the diseases transmitted by insects and other arthropods – the vector-borne diseases. For example, malaria affects hundreds of millions of people annually (see Chapter 96). In fact, the malaria situation has been worsening due to development of insecticide resistance in mosquitoes and drug resistance in parasites. Dengue fever is expanding geographically and inflicts pain and suffering on millions of people annually (see Chapter 75). There are even new or emerging vector-borne diseases. Lyme disease was virtually unknown 40 years ago but now occurs at the rate of about 20 000 reported cases per year in the United States alone (see Chapter 44). Human tick-borne ehrlichiosis (see Chapter 52) in the United States, first reported in 1986, has caused at least 5000 cases since then. Recent evidence indicates that there may be several *Ehrlichia* and tick species involved in this disease.[1]

To understand and control outbreaks of these diseases requires knowledge of ecology and medical entomology not commonly encountered in today's world of molecular biology and medical specialization. This chapter provides classic medical entomology information in a brief accessible overview.

PARASITIC ARTHROPODS

Although most bloodsucking arthropods (e.g., mosquitoes, ticks) could be considered "parasites" since they derive nourishment at the expense of other organisms, in this discussion the term parasitic arthropods is limited to human parasites that live most of their lives on or in the host. Lines of demarcation are not clear, but the parasites chosen to be included here are the human lice, a couple of skin-inhabiting mites, and a few flesh-dwelling fly larvae.

Lice

Two species of sucking lice (insect order Phthiraptera, previously known as Anoplura) are parasites of humans – head and body lice both being varieties of one species, *Pediculus humanus*, and pubic lice, *Phthirus pubis* (***Figs 124.1 and 124.2***). Neither head nor pubic lice are involved in disease transmission, but body lice may carry the agents of epidemic typhus, trench fever, and louse-borne relapsing fever.[2] Body and head lice look almost identical, but head lice remain more or less on the scalp and body lice on the body or in clothing. Head and body lice are tiny (1–4 mm long), elongated, soft-bodied, light-colored, wingless insects with gradual metamorphosis – that is, the young look like the adults, only smaller. They are dorsoventrally flattened (top to bottom, as opposed to fleas, which are flattened side to side), with an angular ovoid head, and a nine-segment abdomen. The head bears a pair of simple lateral eyes and a pair of short five-segment antennae. Head lice live on the skin among the hairs of the patient's head. Eggs (nits) are laid at the base of shafts of hair. Body lice live primarily in the clothing of infested persons, but move to the body occasionally for a blood meal.

Head lice are transmitted among humans by close contact such as hugging or sharing of personal items such as hats, scarves, or combs. Body lice are transmitted also by close contact, but more so by sharing infested clothing. Since neither head nor body lice usually survive more than 24–48 hours off their hosts, pesticidal fogging or spraying of entire homes and schools is not indicated. Pediculicidal lotions or shampoos, combined with washing of garments and bedding, will usually eliminate the infestation.

Pubic lice (crab lice) occur almost exclusively in the pubic or perianal areas, rarely on eyelashes, eyebrows, or other coarse-haired areas. They are not as active as head or body lice, being attached more often to the skin. Thus, pubic lice may often be confused with nymphal (immature) ticks. Pubic lice generally cannot survive more than 24–48 hours off their human hosts and therefore do not inhabit rugs, carpets, pets, or bathrooms. Although it is theoretically possible to obtain the infestation from inanimate objects such as toilet seats, most transmission occurs from sexual contact. In fact, pediculosis pubis is rightly categorized as a sexually transmitted disease (see Chapter 138). One study reported that one-third of patients with pubic lice may have other sexually transmitted diseases.[3] Treatment involves pediculicidal lotions and shampoos for the patient, as well as all family members and sexual contacts of the patient.[4]

Mites

Scabies mites (acarine order Astigmata), *Sarcoptes scabiei*, infest human skin causing intense itching and sometimes a generalized rash. Scabies occurs worldwide, affecting all races and socioeconomic classes. The mites are very tiny (0.2–0.4 mm long), oval, saclike, eyeless specimens with rudimentary legs (***Fig. 124.3***). Scabies mites are transmitted almost entirely by close human-to-human contact with infested persons.[5] The mites burrow under the skin, leaving tiny open sores and linear serpiginous burrows (tracts) that contain the mites and their eggs. Sensitization is the cause of the itching, erythema, and rash.

Scabies should be confirmed by finding the mites in a skin scraping, since other forms of dermatitis may resemble scabies. Finding the mites

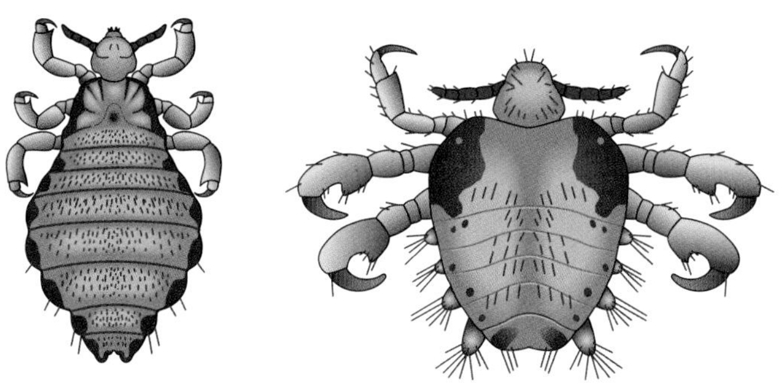

Figure 124.1 Head louse (*left*) and pubic louse (*right*). (From US Department of Health, Education, and Welfare, Public Health Service, Centers for Disease Control and Prevention, pictorial keys.)

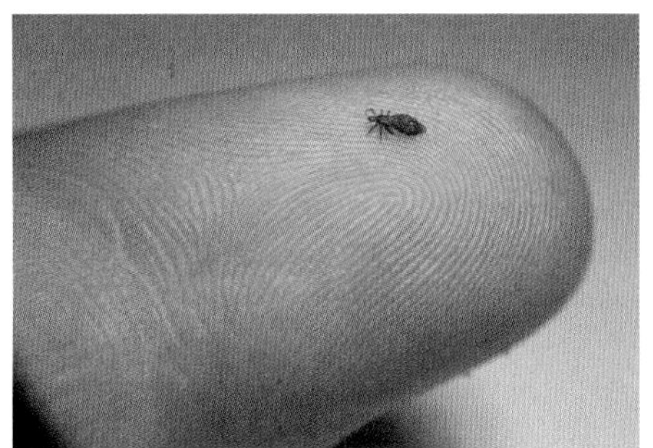

Figure 124.2 Body louse. (Photo copyright 2005 by Jerome Goddard, PhD, Mississippi State University, Starkville, MS.)

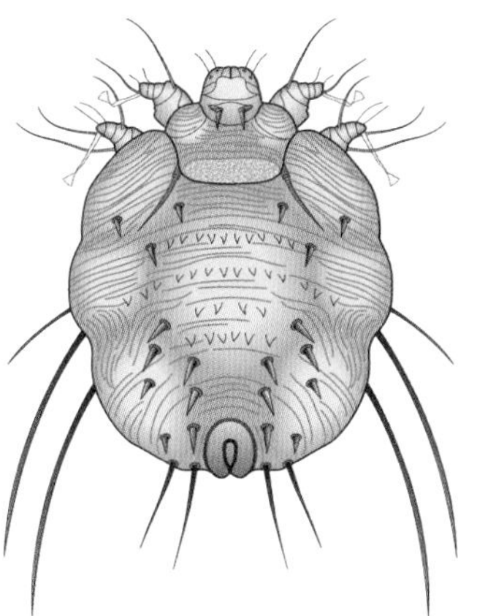

Figure 124.3 Scabies mite.

is often not as easy as it seems and an experienced dermatologist may be needed. Treatment involves scabicidal creams or lotions applied per package instructions. Some commonly used products today are lindane (Kwell), permethrin (Elimite), and crotamiton (Eurax).[2] For crusted or Norwegian scabies developing in immunocompromised patients (see Chapter 139), therapy may involve a single dose of ivermectin given at 200 μg/kg orally and repeated after 2 weeks, if needed.[6] Ivermectin may have specific utility in treating scabies in institutional or community outbreaks.[7] Since the mites cannot live off a human host for more than 24 hours or so, pesticidal treatment of rooms, schools, and so on is unnecessary.

Dog or horse scabies is also caused by races of *S. scabiei*, but these mites cannot complete their life cycle in human skin. Humans can acquire dog scabies, causing itching and papular or vesicular lesions, primarily on the waist, chest, or forearms. However, removal or treatment of the source of infestation (i.e., infested dog or horse) will lead to gradual resolution of the human case.

Follicle mites (acarine order Prostigmata) are minute, wormlike mites that infest humans. Two species may be found. *Demodex folliculorum* lives in the hair follicles and *D. brevis* in the sebaceous glands. Although some researchers have attributed various pathologic conditions to *Demodex* infestation, the mite is basically a harmless saprophyte. They most commonly occur on the forehead, the malar areas of the cheeks, the nose, and the nasolabial fold, but may occur anywhere on the face or around the ears. Most people acquire *Demodex* from maternal contacts in early childhood.

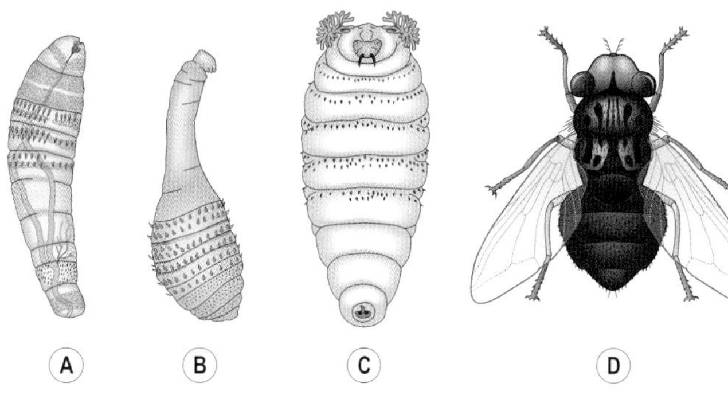

Figure 124.4 Human bot fly. **(A)** First-stage larva. **(B)** Second-stage larva. **(C)** Third-stage larva. **(D)** Adult fly. (From US Department of Agriculture, Miscellaneous Publication No. 631.)

Parasitic Fly Larvae

Myiasis is the infestation of human or animal tissues by fly larvae (insect order Diptera). It may be accidental (e.g., eating eggs or larvae), facultative (e.g., eggs laid on malodorous or festering wounds), or obligate (e.g., necessary for fly development – true parasitism).[8] Accidental myiasis is mostly a benign event, but the larvae could possibly survive temporarily, causing stomach pains, nausea, or vomiting. Facultative myiasis may result in considerable pain and tissue damage as fly larvae leave necrotic tissues and invade healthy tissues. Obligate myiasis can be serious or even fatal, as fly larvae feed in healthy tissues.

Species Involved in Facultative Myiasis

Numerous species of house flies (Muscidae), blow flies (Calliphoridae), and flesh flies (Sarcophagidae) – all in the insect order Diptera – have been implicated in facultative myiasis. Some notorious offenders are the blow fly, *Lucilia sericata*, the rat-tailed maggot, *Eristalis tenax*, the black blow fly, *Phormia regina*, and the house fly, *Musca domestica*.[9] In addition, the latrine fly, *Fannia scalaris*, has often been associated with urinary or rectal myiasis.

Species Involved in Obligate Myiasis

The human bot fly, *Dermatobia hominis*, is a parasite of humans, cattle, swine, cats, dogs, horses, sheep, and other mammals and a few birds in Mexico and Central and South America. The larvae feed under the skin, causing often episodically painful, swollen, draining cutaneous lesions with a typical air-pore. Although this parasite does not occur in the United States, numerous cases are seen by US physicians as a result of people returning from cruises or vacations to endemic areas (see Chapter 132).[10]

The adult bot fly (about 15 mm long) resembles a large bluish blow fly. It has a yellowish or brown head and legs. Adult bot flies catch various bloodsucking flies (often a mosquito) and attach eggs to their sides. The carrier flies subsequently feed on a human, cow, or other host at which time the newly hatched bot fly larvae penetrate the host skin. The larvae vary in appearance depending upon stage of development (***Figs 124.4 and 124.5***), usually do not move laterally within the skin, and may feed for 4–10 weeks. When mature, larvae exit the lesion, drop to the soil, and pupate. Treatment involves direct removal of the maggots (by excision or otherwise) and antibiotics to prevent or control secondary infection.

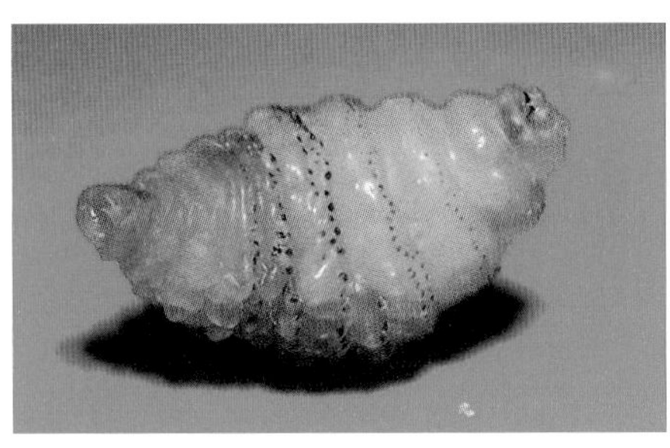

Figure 124.5 Third-stage *Dermatobia hominis* larva. (Photo copyright 2007 by Jerome Goddard, PhD, Mississippi State University, Starkville, MS.)

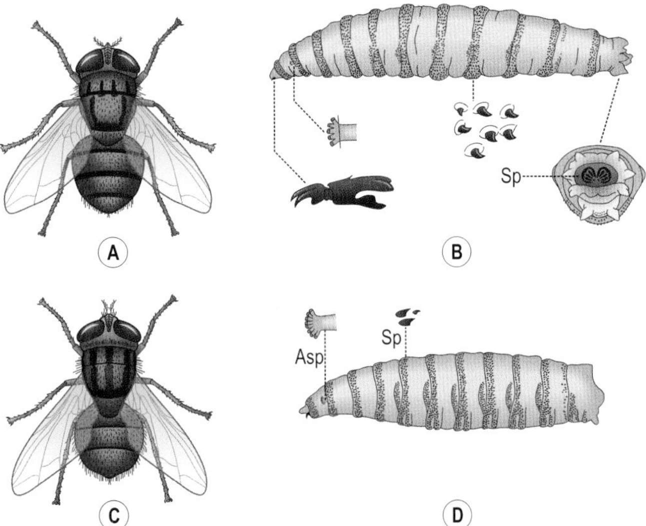

Figure 124.6 Screwworm flies. **(A)** Adult female *Chrysomyia bezziana.* **(B)** Larva of *C. bezziana.* Sp, spiracle. **(C)** Adult female *Cochliomyia hominivorax.* **(D)** Larva of *C. hominivorax.* Asp, anterior spiracle; Sp, spine. (From US Department of Agriculture, Miscellaneous Publication No. 631.)

Screwworm flies are also obligate parasites of living flesh, feeding for the entire larval period inside a host. Natural hosts include domestic and wild mammals, as well as humans. Human infestations have resulted from the flies ovipositing on or near a wound, or sometimes inside the nostril while a person sleeps in the daytime. Upon hatching, the larvae begin feeding, causing extensive tissue destruction. There is an Old World species, *Chrysomyia bezziana*, a species of tropical Africa and Asia, and a New World species, *Cochliomyia hominivorax*, which at one time was distributed from the southern United States to southern Brazil (***Fig. 124.6***).

Fortunately, due to a sterile male release program, the New World species no longer occurs in the United States. Treatment of screwworm myiasis involves removal of the larvae. Surgery may be required if larvae cannot be removed via natural orifices. Since eggs are laid in batches, there could be tens or even hundreds of maggots in a wound.

The tumbu fly, *Cordylobia anthropophaga*, is a major cause of cutaneous myiasis in tropical Africa. The larvae burrow into subcutaneous tissues creating a boil-like lesion with a serous exudate. Children are most commonly affected, with lesions occurring on areas of the body covered with clothing since the flies oviposit on soiled clothing. The adult fly has a yellow-brown body and is about 6–12 mm long. Full-grown larvae are 13–15 mm long. The larvae exit their furuncular lesions after about 8–10 days. Treatment involves direct removal of the maggots, surgically if necessary, and treatment to prevent or control secondary infection. *Wohlfahrtia magnifica*, one of the sarcophagid flies, is an obligate parasite in the wounds and natural orifices of mammals, including humans. It occurs over the warmer parts of Europe, Asia, northern Africa, the Middle East, and the Mediterranean region. *Wohlfahrtia* behavior is similar to that of a screwworm fly, in that it oviposits – actually depositing larvae instead of eggs – on tiny skin lesions such as scratches, tick bites, and such on mucous membranes. The developing larvae feed for 5–7 days, exit the host, fall to the ground, and pupate. *Wohlfahrtia* flies look similar to flesh flies (Sarcophagidae), but instead of a checkerboard pattern on the abdomen they have round spots. *W. magnifica* occurs over the warmer parts of Europe, Asia, northern Africa, the Middle East, and the Mediterranean region.

W. magnifica infestations are difficult to treat because of the (usually) numerous aggressively feeding larvae within the nose or existing wounds. Irrigation or possible surgical exploration to remove the larvae is needed.

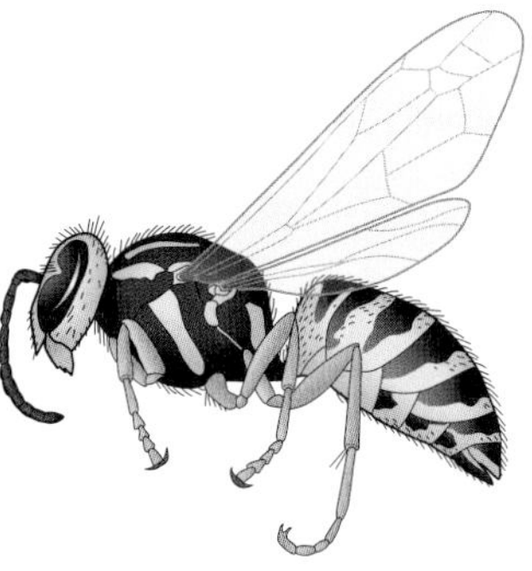

Figure 124.7 Typical stinging insect (yellow jacket). (From US Department of Health, Education, and Welfare, Public Health Service, Centers for Disease Control and Prevention, pictorial keys.)

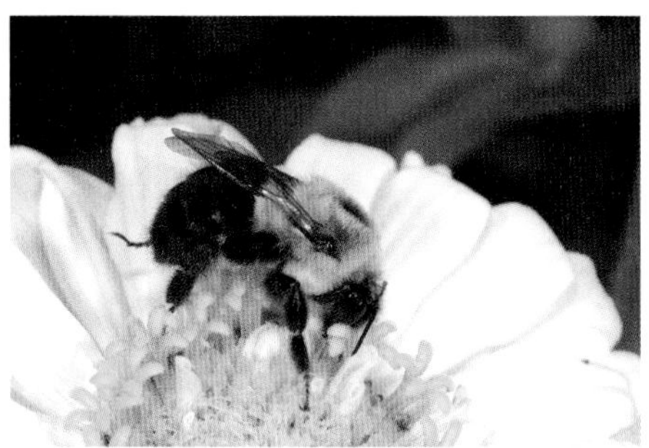

Figure 124.8 Bumble bee. (Photo courtesy of Dr Blake Layton, Mississippi State University, Starkville, MS, used with permission.)

INJURIOUS ARTHROPODS

Stinging Arthropods

The insect order Hymenoptera contains ants, wasps, and bees.[11] Most stinging wasps and some bees are solitary or subsocial insects; they primarily use their stings to subdue prey. Rarely does this offensive use of stinging and venom lead to human envenomization. These venoms do not cause much pain or swelling. Social wasps, bees, and ants, however, sting for defensive purposes, and their venom causes intense pain. Workers of these groups instinctively defend their nests and readily sting intruders coming too close to their nests. Social hymenopterans include yellow jackets, honey bees, bumble bees, paper wasps, and fire ants (***Figs 124.7 and 124.8***). All stings generally cause pain, itching, wheal, flare, and other symptoms, which resolve in a couple of hours unless there are enough stings (several hundred) to produce a direct toxic reaction. Allergic systemic reactions include cutaneous manifestations (e.g., urticaria, angioedema), bronchospasm, edema of the upper airway, and hypotensive shock, and range from mild to life-threatening.[12,13] Even if a person is not allergic to the venom, toxic effects from hundreds of stings can occur, including histamine release (nonallergic), contraction of smooth muscle, increase in capillary permeability, vasodilation with accompanying drop in blood pressure, and hemolysis.[14]

Some caterpillars can sting. Both mechanical irritation and injection of venom by the caterpillar spines or hairs contribute to the urticarial response in humans. Upon exposure, these structures may be broken, allowing venom to either be injected into the skin or to ooze out onto abraded skin. I reported observations from a caterpillar sting case that included erythema, small papules, throbbing pain, and axillary pain resulting from venom travel to local lymph nodes.[15] Allergic reactions from caterpillars may occur just like those from other stinging arthropods.[16]

Urticating caterpillars include the io moth, *Automeris io*; the brown-tail moth, *Euproctis chrysorrhoea*; the buck moth, *Hemileuca maia*; the puss caterpillar, *Megalopyge opercularis*; the saddleback caterpillar, *Sibine stimulea*, and many others (***Fig. 124.9***). Treatment may include ice packs and oral administration of antihistamines to relieve the itching and burning sensation. Acute urticarial lesions may be relieved by application of topical corticosteroids. For severe pain associated with stings, meperidine hydrochloride, morphine, or codeine is sometimes used. Systemic allergic reactions such as hypotension and bronchospasm are treated with epinephrine, antihistamines, and other supportive measures.[17]

Scorpions (arachnid order Scorpiones) are eight-legged, generally flattened arthropods with two apparent body regions – a broad seven-segment mesosoma and a narrow five-segment metasoma terminating in a sting (***Fig. 124.10***). Many scorpions pose no serious health hazard, but several species have venom sufficiently toxic to kill a human (outright, not an allergic reaction). Systemic effects from such stings include drowsiness, spreading partial paralysis, muscle twitching, profuse salivation, perspiration, hypertension, tachycardia, and convulsions. In the United States, the only dangerous species, with the exception of allergic reactions to the venom, is *Centruroides exilicauda* (formerly *C. sculpturatus*) of the southwestern United States, especially Arizona. The fat-tailed scorpion, *Androctonus australis*, is a notoriously dangerous scorpion of northern Africa and the Middle East. Treatment of scorpion stings is somewhat controversial.[18] For the dangerous species, some advocate prompt use of antivenin. Others take a wait-and-see approach since many scorpion sting cases resolve on their own in a few hours. Severe cases usually occur in children and are characterized by agitation and other systemic symptoms. Hospitalization for close monitoring and supportive care is required in such cases.

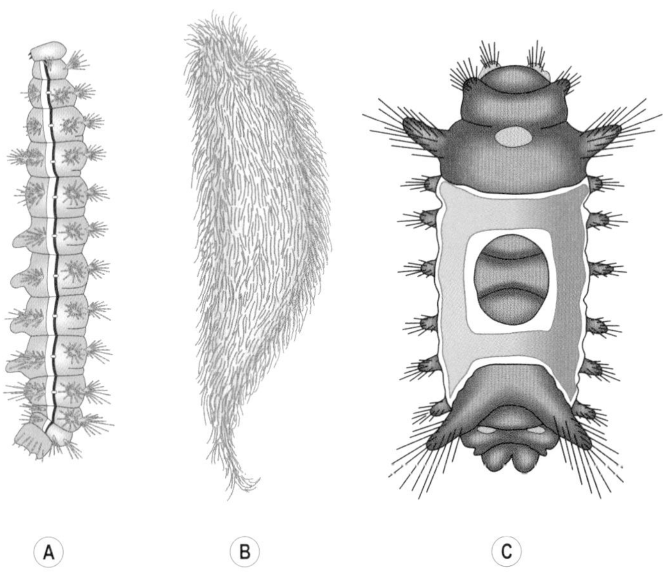

Figure 124.9 Some stinging caterpillars. **(A)** Io moth. **(B)** Puss caterpillar. **(C)** Saddleback caterpillar. (Adapted from US Department of Health, Education, and Welfare, Public Health Service, Centers for Disease Control and Prevention, pictorial keys.)

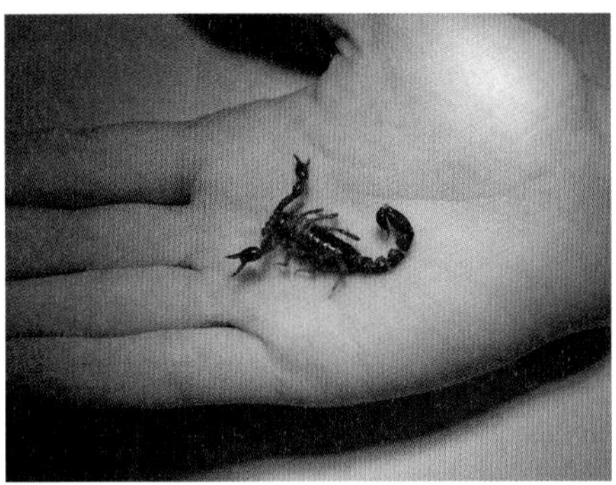

Figure 124.10 Typical scorpion. (Photo copyright 2008 by Jerome Goddard, PhD, Mississippi State University, Starkville, MS.)

Biting Arthropods

The bed bug (insect order Hemiptera), *Cimex lectularius*, is a bloodsucking human pest that may cause itching and inflammation from its bites (***Fig. 124.11***). There has been a tremendous increase in the number of reported bed bug infestations over the past decade.[19] Bed bugs have occasionally been found that are naturally infected with disease organisms such as those causing anthrax, plague, and typhus. However, they are not considered vectors of these disease agents.[20] Adult bugs are oval-shaped (approximately 5 mm long), flattened insects that somewhat resemble immature cockroaches. They are reddish-brown in color; the immature bed bugs are yellowish-white. Bed bugs are found in temperate regions worldwide. A related species, *Cimex hemipterus*, occurs in the tropics. The bugs hide in cracks and crevices during the day, usually on or near the host's bed, and feed at night, taking blood from their host for 5–10 minutes. Bites from bed bugs are generally self-limited and require little specific treatment other than antiseptic or antibiotic creams or lotions to prevent infection.[20]

Horse flies and deer flies (insect order Diptera) are notorious pests of horses, cattle, deer, dogs, and humans. They have scissors-like mouthparts and can inflict painful bites. Although no human illnesses have been associated with horse flies, deer flies can transmit the agents of tularemia and loiasis in Africa (see Chapter 105).[8]

Horse flies look like giant, robust house flies (15–25 mm long) with large prominent eyes (***Fig. 124.12***). Deer flies, also in the family

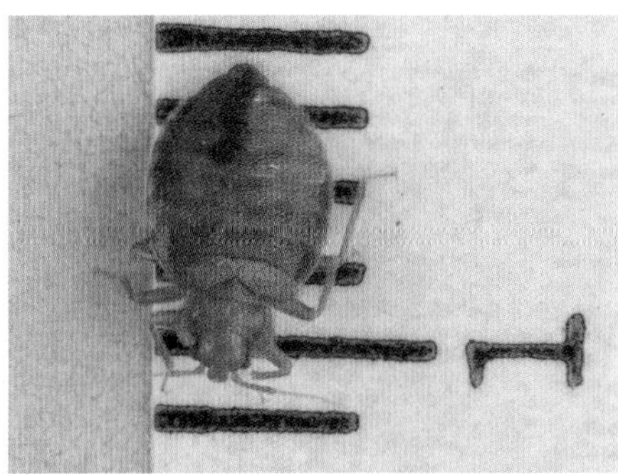

Figure 124.11 Bed bug. (Copyright © 2002 by Jerome Goddard, PhD, Mississippi State University, Starkville, MS.)

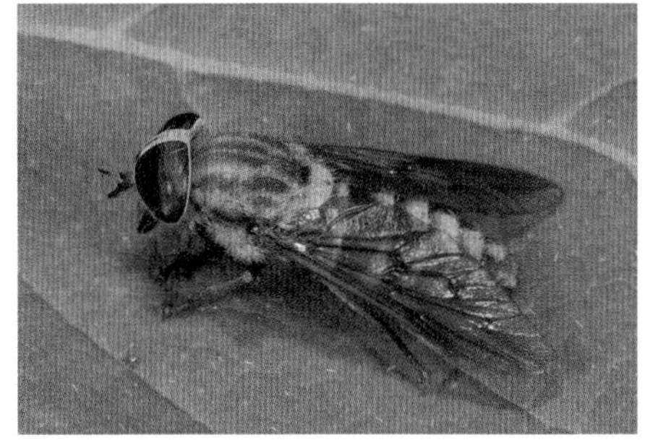

Figure 124.12 Adult horse fly. (Photo courtesy of Dr Blake Layton, Mississippi State University, Starkville, MS, used with permission.)

Tabanidae, are much smaller (8–15 mm long) and have dark patterned wings. Many deer fly species have a gray or yellow-gray body with various arrangements of spots on the abdomen. Numerous species of both groups occur almost worldwide, where they breed in moist or semi-aquatic sites such as margins of ponds, damp earth, or other sites containing mud and water. The wormlike larvae spend their entire developmental time in these muddy habitats. Adult females seek a blood meal, whereas males may feed on flower nectar. Except for secondary infections, requiring appropriate antibiotics, horse fly and deer fly bites are generally few and self-limited.

Biting midges (insect order Diptera) are tiny, delicate flies that bite people, especially near coastal areas. They are also sometimes referred to as "no-see-ums," "punkies," or "biting gnats." Other than the severe biting nuisance, biting midges are generally of no medical significance to humans in the United States. They are usually gray in color, extremely small (0.6–1.5 mm), and may have clear or hairy wings which fold scissors-like over the abdomen at rest. Adults are generally active only in the warmer months of the year. Simple antipruritics are generally the only treatment needed for biting midge bites. Avoidance of midge-infested areas at or near dark (e.g., salt marshes), and repellents containing picaridin or DEET are the best course of action for those affected by biting midges.[21]

Numerous species of spiders (arachnid order Araneae) bite people, but the hobo spiders, violin spiders, and widow spiders may be a medical threat in the United States.[2,22] Violin spiders have a necrotic venom affecting cutaneous tissues. The brown recluse spider, *Loxosceles reclusa*, is perhaps the most important member of the group, although other violin spiders producing necrotic lesions also occur in the United States and elsewhere. Brown recluse spider bites are usually localized, producing necrosis that may result in an unsightly scar (***Fig. 124.13***), although other medical conditions may be misdiagnosed as brown recluse bites.[23] The bite may be painless at first, but becomes very painful within 8 hours. Healing may require several months. Systemic reactions to brown recluse spider bites may occur, including hematuria, anemia, rash, fever, coma, and cyanosis. Death may occur but is rare. The adult spider is tan to dark brown with a 2–4 cm leg span (***Fig. 124.14***). Six eyes, arranged in a semicircle of three pairs, are on top of the head and a characteristic violin-shaped marking (base forward) extends from the eyes to the beginning of the abdomen. The brown recluse spider may be found from Minnesota to Maine, south to Florida, and west to Arizona and Wyoming. It is most common in the south-central United States. Treatment of brown recluse spider bites is symptomatic and quite controversial. Current therapies include ice, antibiotics, and perhaps the leukocyte inhibitor dapsone.[2,24–27] Controlled studies are lacking and dapsone may produce hemolysis, so it should be used under careful supervision.

Widow spiders, in contrast to violin spiders, have a neurotoxic venom that produces systemic pain, weakness, tremor, muscle spasm, and tightness in the chest.[28] Often patients exhibit a rigid, boardlike abdomen. There is rarely a significant lesion at the bite site. Paralysis, stupor, and convulsions may occur in severe cases, with an occasional fatality. Several widow spiders occur in North America – all with similar appearance. *Latrodectus mactans* is the species most generally associated with the name "black widow spider" and the female has a red or orange hourglass-shaped marking on the underside of the abdomen (***Fig. 124.15***). There is considerable variation in these red markings, with some species having red dots or hash marks on the top and bottom of the abdomen. Recently, a related species, the brown widow, has been found expanding its range throughout much of the south-central and southeastern United States.[29] Treatment of *Latrodectus* envenomization includes application of ice, symptomatic treatment of muscle spasms and pain, and (possibly) antivenin in severe cases. Children, the elderly, and persons with other medical conditions of risk may need hospitalization and close monitoring.

Centipedes (arthropod class Chilopoda), sometimes called "hundred-leggers," are long multisegmented arthropods with one pair of legs per body segment (***Fig. 124.16***). They are flattened, fast-moving creatures that can inflict a painful bite. Bites are generally harmless, but often produce two red and swollen puncture wounds. Rarely, systemic symptoms such as anxiety, vomiting, irregular pulse, dizziness, and headache may occur. Most of the smaller centipede species are harmless, but larger species (especially in the genus *Scolopendra*) in the southern United States and tropics can inflict a painful bite. Treatment includes washing the bite site with soap and water, application of ice, and analgesics for pain.

Numerous mite species (arachnid subclass Acarina), while not parasitic on humans, will bite, causing itch or dermatitis (***Fig. 124.17***). Examples are the bird and rat mites, which will bite if in close proximity to people. People may also be bitten as a result of occupational exposure to products containing chicken mites, straw mites, or grain mites (***Fig. 124.18***). One of the most common mites causing human dermatitis in poultry houses, farms, ranches, and markets where chickens are sold is the chicken mite, *Dermanyssus gallinae*. Straw itch mites, *Pyemotes tritici*, will bite people as they come into contact with infested straw, hay, grasses, oats, or peas. The grain and flour mites (several species) may cause grocer's itch, copra itch (coconuts), and other itches. Grain and flour mites occur worldwide.

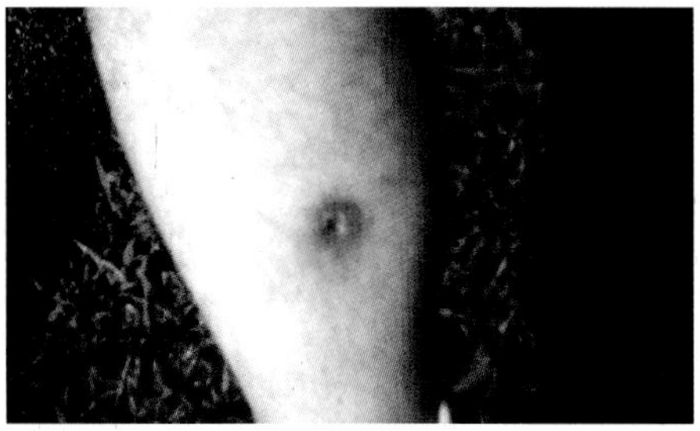

Figure 124.13 Brown recluse spider bite approximately 3 months post bite. (From Jarratt JH, Gaydon DG, and Goddard J, Mississippi Cooperative Extension Service, Publication No. 2154, Mississippi State, MS.)

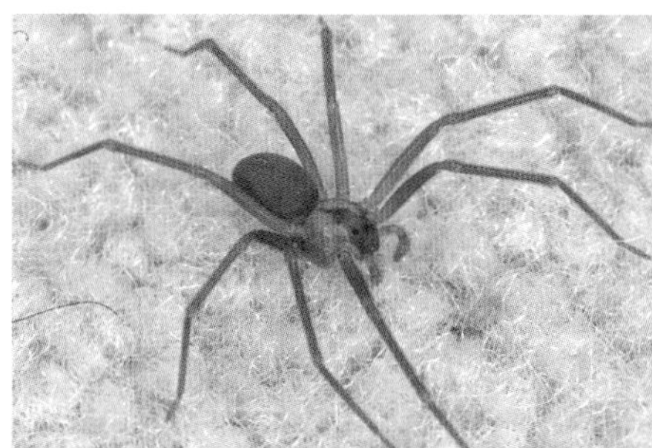

Figure 124.14 Adult brown recluse spider. (Photo courtesy of Dr Blake Layton, Mississippi State University, Starkville, MS, used with permission).

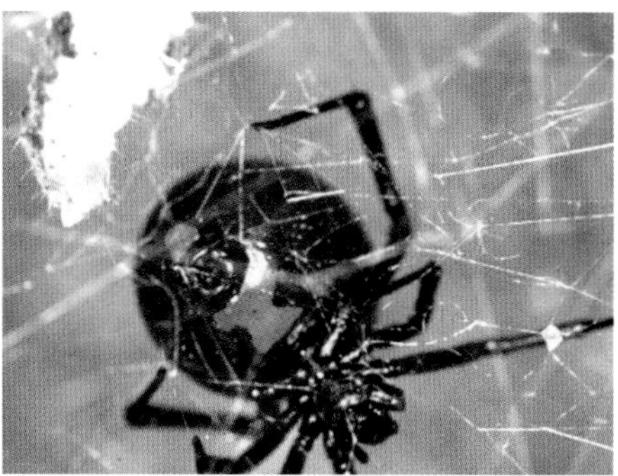

Figure 124.15 Female black widow spider underside showing hourglass-shaped marking. (Courtesy of Dr James Jarratt, Mississippi Cooperative Extension Service, Mississippi State, MS.)

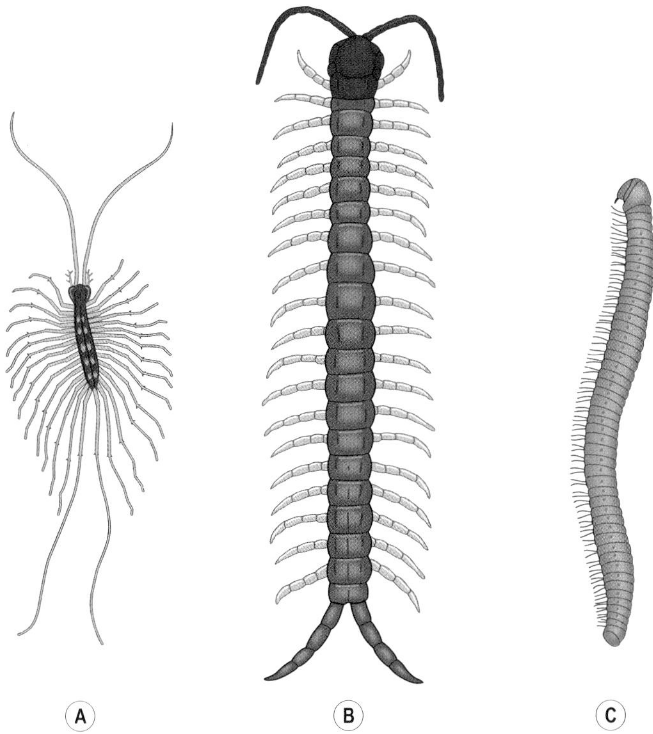

Figure 124.16 Centipedes and millipede. **(A)** House centipede. **(B)** Large southwestern United States centipede. **(C)** Millipede. (From US Department of Health, Education, and Welfare, Public Health Service, Centers for Disease Control and Prevention, pictorial keys.)

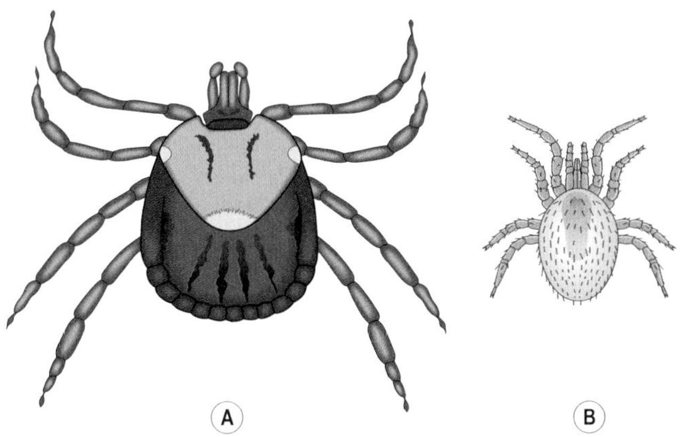

Figure 124.17 **(A)** Tick. **(B)** Mite. (From US Department of Health, Education, and Welfare, Public Health Service, Centers for Disease Control and Prevention, pictorial keys.)

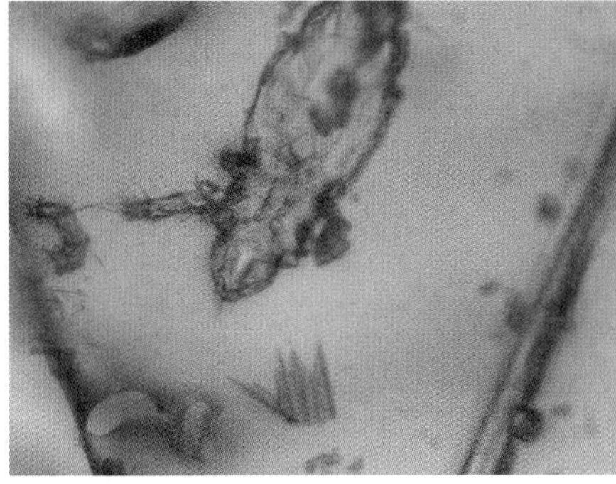

Figure 124.18 Grain mite. (Photo copyright 2005 by Jerome Goddard, PhD, Mississippi State University, Starkville, MS.)

Treatment of mite bites primarily involves alleviation of symptoms, and avoidance or eradication of the mites. Since none of these mite species take up permanent residence on human skin, elimination of the source of mite exposure should be the main objective. Competent pest control operators (exterminators) are often helpful in finding and eliminating bird nests or rat burrows in and around the home.

Chigger mites (acarine order Prostigmata), also sometimes called "harvest mites" or "red bugs," although not truly parasitic on humans, are actually the six-legged larval stage of trombiculid mites. The adults do not bite. Chiggers cause intense itching and irritation, and some species are involved in the transmission of the scrub typhus rickettsia (see Chapter 51) in the Far East.[30] Chigger larvae are very tiny (0.2 mm), round mites with numerous setae. Numerous chigger species occur in various parts of the world, where they utilize a wide range of vertebrate hosts. They reach their hosts by crawling up on blades of grass or leaves. On humans, they generally crawl into and attach to where clothing fits snugly or where flesh is tender. The feeding process is irritating and produces erythematous itchy patches on affected areas of skin. Treatment often includes an antiseptic, hydrocortisone, anesthetic (such as benzocaine) solutions, or ointments to minimize itching and reduce the possibility of secondary infection.

Other Forms of Injury

Blister beetles (insect order Coleoptera) may cause blistering on human skin when touched or handled. The beetles contain the blistering agent cantharidin in their body fluids, which is released when they sense danger. Many species of blister beetles exist in the United States, most in the family Meloidae, although a few beetles in the Staphylinidae family cause blisters. Blisters resulting from blister beetle exposure are usually not serious, with reabsorption occurring in a few days if the blisters are unruptured.[31] The skin may flake if the blisters have ruptured, leaving an area of mild erythema for a week or so. Affected areas should be washed with soap and water and bandaged until the blisters reabsorb. Antibiotic ointments or creams may help prevent secondary infection.

Millipedes (arthropod class Diplopoda), also sometimes called "thousand-leggers," are slow-moving elongate, wormlike arthropods (see ***Fig. 124.16C***). They are somewhat similar to centipedes except they have two pairs of legs on most body segments and are generally rounded instead of flattened. Millipedes are commonly found in soft, decomposing plant materials. Although millipedes neither bite nor sting, some species secrete defensive body fluids that may discolor and burn human skin. Treatment involves washing the exposed area with copious amounts of water as soon as possible. Some medical personnel have recommended using solvents such as ether or alcohol to remove the noxious fluids. Eye exposure from millipedes requires a thorough irrigation with warm water and consultation with an ophthalmologist.

House dust mites (acarine order Astigmata) indirectly affect human health by producing allergic reactions in some people. The mites do not bite or sting, but a considerable amount of allergic rhinitis, asthma, and childhood eczema is attributable to their presence in the human environment.[32] Adult house dust mites are whitish, plump, very tiny (0.5 mm) mites with fine striations on their cuticle. They are most often associated with furniture on which people spend a lot of time – mattresses, sofas, and recliners. House dust mite allergy is often managed by immunotherapy using mite extracts and by minimizing the level of mites in the patient's home. Carpets may need to be replaced with tile or wood floors. Feather pillows should be replaced with synthetic ones. Encasements are available for mattresses.

ARTHROPOD VECTORS OF DISEASE

Arthropods that are capable of transmitting disease organisms to vertebrate hosts are called vectors. For example, mosquitoes in the genus *Anopheles* are vectors of malaria (see Chapter 96). Interestingly, no other mosquitoes are able to acquire and transmit the malaria parasites. In disease outbreaks there are primary vectors (the main species involved in disease transmission) and secondary vectors (the species that may occasionally become involved under certain conditions). An understanding of how disease agents are acquired and transmitted by arthropods is crucial to preventing and managing vector-borne diseases. Mechanical transmission of disease agents occurs when arthropods just physically carry pathogens from one place or host to another host – often via body parts. For example, flies and cockroaches have numerous hairs, spines, and setae on their bodies which collect contaminants as the insects feed on dead animals or excrement (***Fig. 124.19***). When they subsequently walk on food or food preparation surfaces, mechanical transmission occurs. Mechanical transmission may also occur if a bloodfeeding arthropod has its feeding interrupted. For example, if a mosquito feeds briefly on a viremic bird and is interrupted, a subsequent feeding (if immediate) on a second bird may result in virus transmission.

In biologic transmission, there is either multiplication or development of the pathogen in the arthropod, or both (***Fig. 124.20***). Biologic transmission is often classified into three types. In cyclodevelopmental transmission the pathogen must undergo a cycle of development within the arthropod vector, but no multiplication. For example, the filarial worm that causes bancroftian filariasis (see Chapter 104), when first ingested by mosquitoes, is not infective to a vertebrate host; it must undergo a period of development. Propagative transmission means the pathogen must undergo multiplication before transmission can occur. There is no cyclic change or development of the organisms – plague bacteria in fleas, for example (see Chapter 41). Finally, in cyclopropagative transmission the pathogen must undergo both cyclic changes and multiplication. The classic example is malaria plasmodia in *Anopheles* mosquitoes (see Chapter 96). The following discussion relates to some of the arthropod species involved in biologic transmission of disease agents.

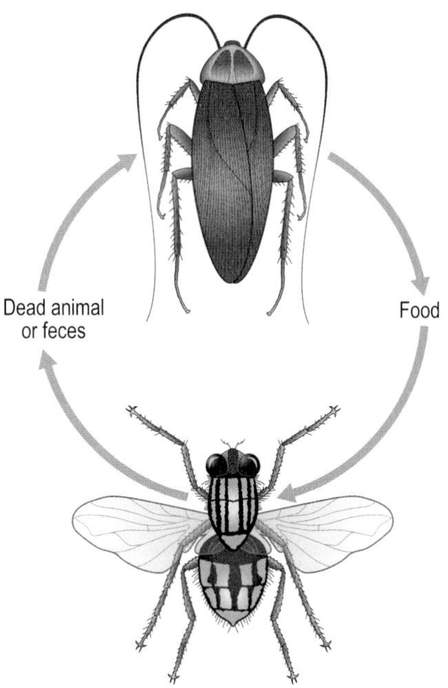

Figure 124.19 One example of mechanical transmission of disease organisms.

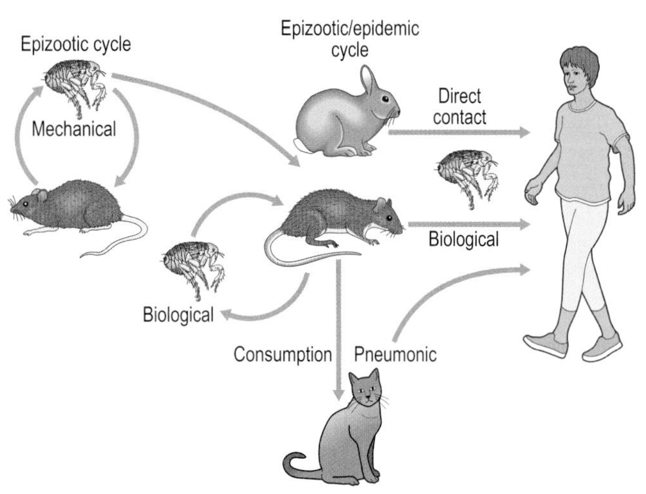

Figure 124.20 Biologic transmission: enzootic and epizootic transmission cycles of plague bacillus. (US Air Force drawing courtesy of Dr Chad P. McHugh.)

Kissing bugs (insect order Hemiptera) have an elongate, cone-shaped head and are often called "cone-nose bugs" (***Fig. 124.21***). They are called kissing bugs because their blood meals are occasionally taken near the lips at night. Other sites of frequent attack are the hands, arms, and feet. Kissing bugs may transmit the causative agent of Chagas' disease, or American trypanosomiasis (*Trypanosoma cruzi*) in Mexico and Central and South America (see Chapter 99). Some cases have occurred in the southern United States.[33] Several species of kissing bugs are capable of transmitting the agent. However, four are considered principal vectors: *Panstrongylus megistus*, *Rhodnius prolixus*, *Triatoma infestans*, and *T. dimidiata*. These bugs occur most commonly in poor, underdeveloped areas with dilapidated or poorly constructed huts or shacks. Infection is not by salivary secretions associated with the bite but by fecal contamination of the bite site. Treatment of kissing bug bites involves washing the bite site with soap and water, and application of topical palliatives. Oral antihistamines may help relieve itching.[34] Occasionally, systemic allergic reactions result from kissing bug bites.[34] Those cases may be treated like any other sting or bite allergic reaction.

Ticks (acarine order Ixodida) are efficient vectors of bacteria, viruses, rickettsiae, and protozoans. At least 14 human diseases are caused or transmitted by ticks (***Table 124.1***). One of the recent additions to this list – American boutonneuse fever – was discovered as a "disease within a disease" because the new clinical entity was apparently hidden within cases diagnosed as Rocky Mountain spotted fever (RMSF).[35–37] Major tick-borne diseases in the United States are Lyme disease (approximately 20 000 cases per year; see Chapter 44), RMSF (approximately 2000 cases per year; see Chapter 49), and ehrlichiosis (approximately 800 cases per year). Two main types of tick-borne ehrlichiosis (see Chapter 52) are now recognized: human monocytic ehrlichiosis (HME), caused by *Ehrlichia chaffeensis*, and human granulocytic anaplasmosis (HGA), caused by *Anaplasma phagocytophilum*.

Two families of ticks occur over much of the world: the hard ticks, Ixodidae, and the soft ticks, Argasidae. Hard ticks resemble huge mites and have anteriorly attached mouthparts visible dorsally (see ***Fig. 124.17A***). They often have white or shiny markings (***Fig. 124.22***); they attach firmly to their hosts for several days. The females are capable of enormous expansion. Soft ticks are leathery without hardened plates, and their mouthparts are not visible dorsally. They do not remain firmly attached to their hosts (as larvae sometimes do), but instead feed only for

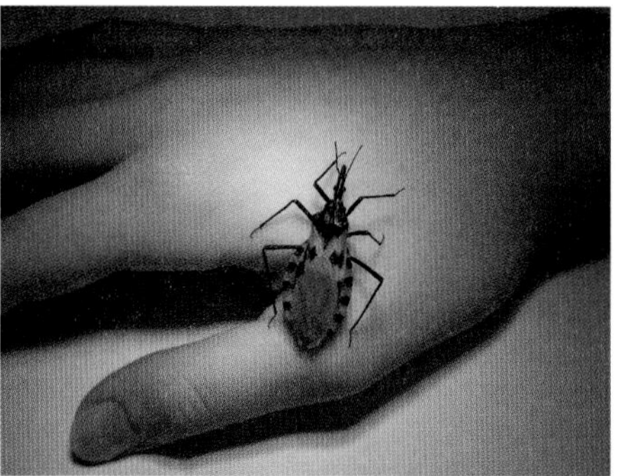

Figure 124.21 Kissing bug on hand. (Photo copyright 2008 by Jerome Goddard, PhD, Mississippi State University, Starkville, MS.)

Disease	Causative Agent	Tick Vectors
Lyme disease	Spirochete	*Ixodes ricinus* complex
Human monocytic ehrlichiosis	Rickettsia	*Amblyomma americanum*
Human granulocytic anaplasmosis	Rickettsia	*Ixodes scapularis*, others
Rocky Mountain spotted fever	Rickettsia	*Dermacentor variabilis, D. andersoni*, others
African tick-bite fever	Rickettsia	*Amblyomma hebraeum*, others
American boutonneuse fever	Rickettsia	*Amblyomma maculatum, A. triste*, others
American babesiosis	Protozoan	*Ixodes scapularis*
Colorado tick fever	Virus	Primarily *D. andersoni*
Tularemia	Bacterium	*A. americanum, D. variabilis, D. nuttalli, Ix. ricinus*
Boutonneuse fever	Rickettsia	*Rhipicephalus sanguineus, R. appendiculatus*, others
Tick paralysis	Salivary toxin	*Dermacentor andersoni, D. variabilis, Ixodes holocyclus*
Tick-borne encephalitis	Virus	*Ixodes ricinus, Ix. persulcatus, Dermacentor marginatus*, others
Relapsing fever	Spirochete	Several soft tick *Ornithodoros* spp.
Crimean-Congo hemorrhagic fever	Virus	*Hyalomma marginatum, H. anatolicum*, others
Siberian tick typhus	Rickettsia	Primarily *Dermacentor marginatus, D. silvarum, D. nuttalli*

Table 124.1 Major Tick-Borne Diseases

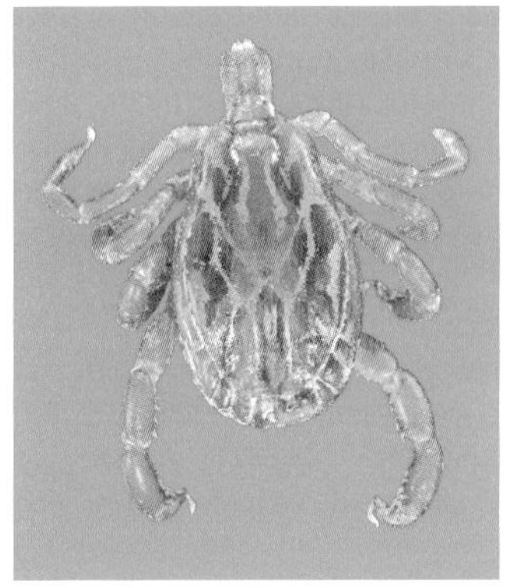

Figure 124.22 Male hard tick showing ornamentation. (Photo courtesy Dr Blake Layton, Mississippi State University, Starkville, MS, used with permission.)

approximately 15–30 minutes. Soft ticks are reclusive and not commonly seen or recognized by people. There are three motile life stages of hard ticks: larva, nymph, and adult. Larvae are extremely small (1 mm) and are often called seed ticks. Seed ticks of some species, especially *Amblyomma americanum* and *A. cajennense*, will feed on a wide variety of animal hosts and often get on people by the thousands, causing itching and irritation. Nymphs (approximately 2 mm in size) also require a blood meal and some species will feed on humans. Adult ticks feed on various vertebrates, depending upon the tick species; some are specific to a certain host, whereas others are indiscriminate.

The Lone Star tick, *A. americanum*, is an important species distributed from central Texas, east to the Atlantic Coast, and north to approximately Iowa and New England. It also occurs in the northern states of Mexico.

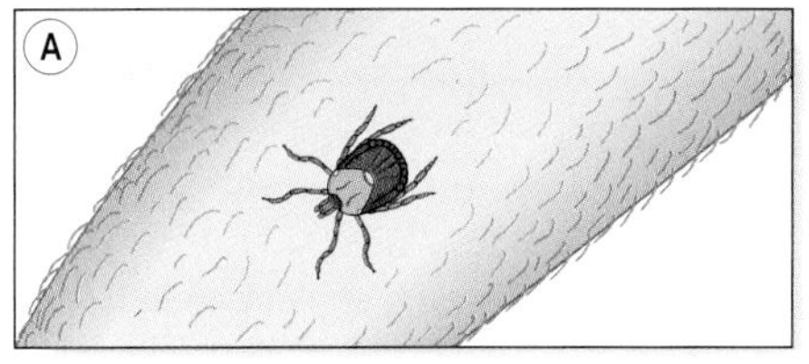

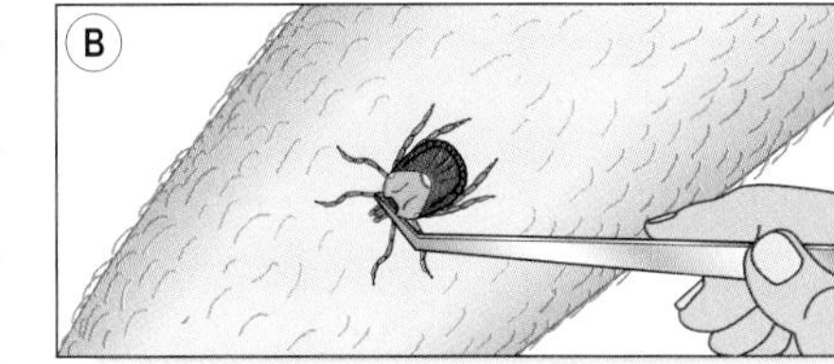

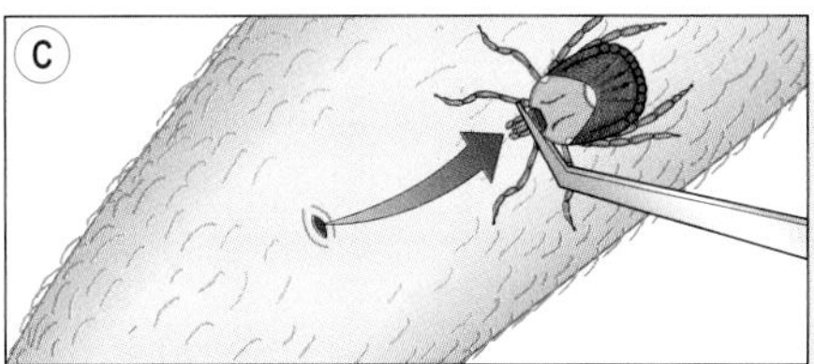

Figure 124.23 Recommended method of tick removal. **(A)** Tick found on skin. Use forceps to grab tick near mouthparts **(B)** and pull straight off **(C)**. (From US Air Force Publication No. USAFSAM-SR-89-2.)

Other than nuisance effects from biting, the Lone Star tick is a known vector of the agents of tularemia and ehrlichiosis (HME).

The deer tick, *Ixodes scapularis*, is the principal vector of *Borrelia burgdorferi*, the causative agent of Lyme disease in the eastern United States. It also transmits HGA and babesiosis. At one time, researchers considered the northern form of this tick, *Ixodes dammini*, as a different species, but evidence was subsequently offered that the two are the same species.[38]

The American dog tick, *Dermacentor variabilis*, is another species of medical importance in the United States. It is the primary vector of the agent of RMSF in the East, a vector of tularemia, and may cause tick paralysis. The American dog tick occurs throughout the United States except in parts of the Rocky Mountains region.

Generally, no treatment is needed for tick bites other than palliatives after tick removal. Tick removal methods vary greatly. A study by J.H. Theis[39] advocated tick removal by the use of tweezers or protected fingers using a steady retracting pressure. Needham[40] evaluated five methods commonly used for tick removal: (1) petroleum jelly, (2) fingernail polish, (3) 70% isopropyl alcohol, (4) a hot kitchen match, and (5) forcible removal with tweezers. He found that the commonly advocated methods are either ineffective, or, worse, actually created greater problems. If petroleum jelly or some other substance causes the tick to back out on its own (and most often it does not), the cement used for attachment surrounding the mouthparts remains in the skin where it continues to cause irritation. Touching the tick with a hot match may cause it to burst, increasing the risk of disease germ exposure. Furthermore, hot objects may induce ticks to salivate or regurgitate infected fluids into the wound. "Unscrewing" a tick is likely to leave broken mouthparts in the host's skin. Needham recommended the following procedure for tick removal: (1) use blunt forceps or tweezers; (2) grasp the tick as close to the skin surface as possible (***Fig. 124.23***) and pull upward with steady, even pressure; (3) take care not to squeeze, crush, or puncture the tick; (4) do not handle the tick with bare hands because infectious agents may enter via mucous membranes or a break in the skin; (5) after removing the tick, thoroughly disinfect the bite site and wash hands thoroughly with soap and water.[40]

Mosquitoes (insect order Diptera) are the most significant, medically important arthropods worldwide, causing annoyance and transmitting disease to humans and a host of other animals (***Fig. 124.24***). Besides the disease threat, the nuisance effect of mosquito bites can be unbearable,

Table 124.2 Some Major Mosquito-Borne Diseases

Disease	Causative Agent	Mosquito Vectors
Malaria	Protozoan	Numerous *Anopheles* spp.
Dengue fever	Virus	*Aedes aegypti, Ae. albopictus*
Filariasis	Nematode	Various *Culex* spp., *Anopheles, Mansonia*
Yellow fever	Virus	Mainly *Aedes aegypti*
Chikungunya	Virus	*Aedes aegypti, Ae. albopictus*
West Nile encephalitis	Virus	Numerous *Culex* spp.
St Louis encephalitis	Virus	*Culex quinquefasciatus, Cx. tarsalis, Cx. nigripalpus*, others
Western equine encephalitis	Virus	Mainly *Culex tarsalis*
Eastern equine encephalitis	Virus	*Aedes (Ochlerotatus) sollicitans, Coquillettidia perturbans*, others
La Crosse encephalitis	Virus	Mainly *Aedes (Ochlerotatus) triseriatus*
Venezuelan equine encephalitis	Virus	*Psorophora columbiae*, others
Japanese encephalitis	Virus	*Culex tritaeniorhynchus*, others

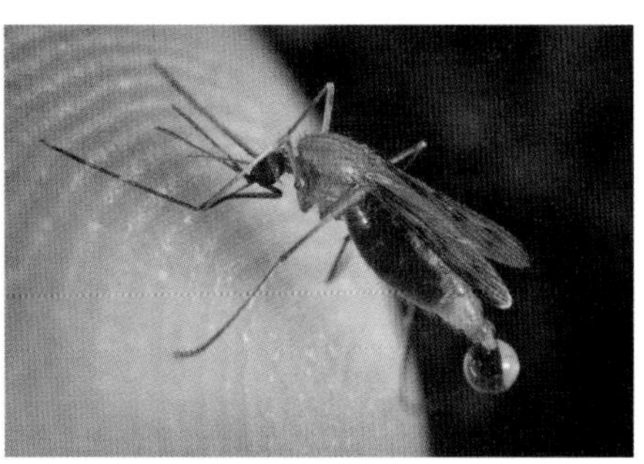

Figure 124.24 Female mosquito taking blood meal. (Centers for Disease Control and Prevention photo, Atlanta, GA.)

leaving many geographic areas undeveloped. Only a relatively few of the 3000 or so mosquito species are significant vectors of human disease, but mosquito-borne diseases are major health problems (***Table 124.2***). Mosquitoes are small flies with long, 15-segment antennae, a long proboscis for bloodsucking, and scales on their wings. Due to the pattern of wing scales, some mosquitoes may appear to have spots on their wings. Female mosquitoes take a blood meal and subsequently lay eggs on or at a water source. The water source varies, depending on the mosquito species, but includes swamps, flooded areas, tree holes, and artificial containers such as cans, discarded tires, and the like. The larvae develop in their aquatic habitat for one or more weeks, after which they pupate and eventually emerge as adult mosquitoes.

Numerous species in the genus *Anopheles* are vectors of the malaria organism. Notorious members of the genus are the *An. gambiae* complex in Africa, *An. albimanus* in Central and South America, and the *An. minimus* complex in Southeast Asia.[2] There are at least three efficient malaria vectors in the United States – *An. quadrimaculatus*, *An. hermsi*, and *An. freeborni*. Other major mosquito-borne diseases are yellow fever, dengue fever, filariasis, chikungunya, and numerous encephalitis viruses. *Aedes albopictus* and *Ae. aegypti* are the primary vectors of yellow fever, dengue, and chikungunya. Various species in the genera *Culex*, *Mansonia*, *Psorophora*, and others transmit the agents of filariasis and mosquito-borne encephalitis, such as West Nile virus.

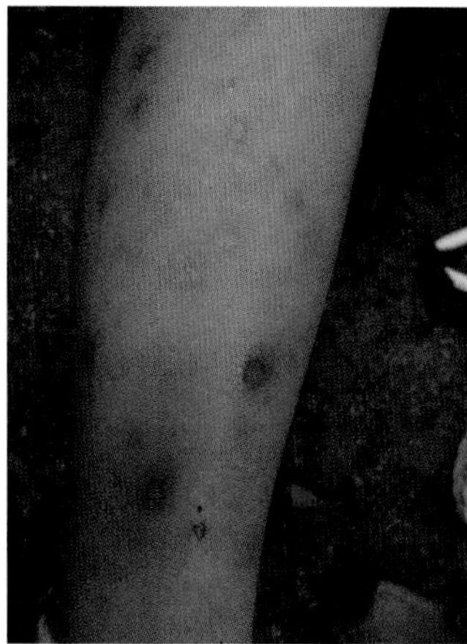

Figure 124.25 Mosquito bites on child's leg. (Photo copyright 2003 by Jerome Goddard, PhD, Mississippi State University, Starkville, MS.)

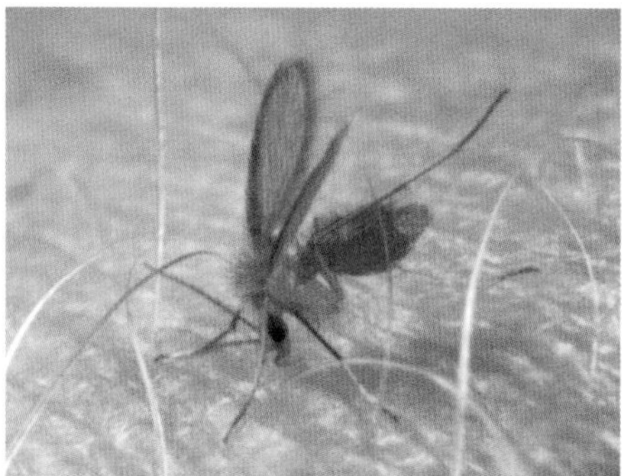

Figure 124.26 Adult sandfly. (From Armed Forces Pest Management Board, Washington, DC.)

Other than the disease transmission threat, treatment of mosquito bites is generally unnecessary. Exceptions may include topical corticosteroids or antibiotic creams to prevent secondary infection from scratching (especially in children), and hypersensitivity reactions to the bites themselves (***Fig. 124.25***). People highly sensitive to mosquito bites may safely reduce the cutaneous reactions to bites by prophylactic treatment with nonsedating antihistamines such as cetirizine[41] and use of picaridin or DEET-containing insect repellents.[21]

Fleas (insect order Siphonaptera) constitute a major human health threat because of their ability to transmit the causative agents of plague (see Chapter 41) and murine typhus (see Chapter 50). They may also serve as intermediate hosts of the dog tapeworm, *Dipylidium caninum* (see Chapter 121). Fleas are small, laterally flattened, wingless insects that take a blood meal from a wide variety of animal hosts. Some species are extremely host-specific, only biting a particular rodent or bat, or other animal. Others are indiscriminate, feeding on almost any mammal (some attack birds also). The cat flea, *Ctenocephalides felis*, is one of the most important fleas in North America, feeding on several domestic and wild animal species, causing severe annoyance. Most fleas found on dogs in the United States are cat fleas. The oriental rat flea, *Xenopsylla cheopis*, is an ectoparasite of Norway rats and roof rats and is the primary vector of plague and murine (endemic) typhus. The chigoe flea, *Tunga penetrans*, burrows into the skin (especially toes) of people in tropical and subtropical regions. Flea bites may be treated with topical corticosteroids and antibiotics if secondary infection is a problem. Tungiasis (tropics) may require excision of the embedded fleas.

Sandflies (insect order Diptera) are small, delicate bloodsucking flies that somewhat resemble tiny mosquitoes (***Fig. 124.26***). Though not commonly recognized by most people, sandflies are significant vectors of the disease agents of leishmaniasis (see Chapter 100), bartonellosis (see Chapter 39), and sandfly fever (see Chapter 72). Sandflies are tiny (3 mm), golden, brown, or gray long-legged flies. They hold their wings

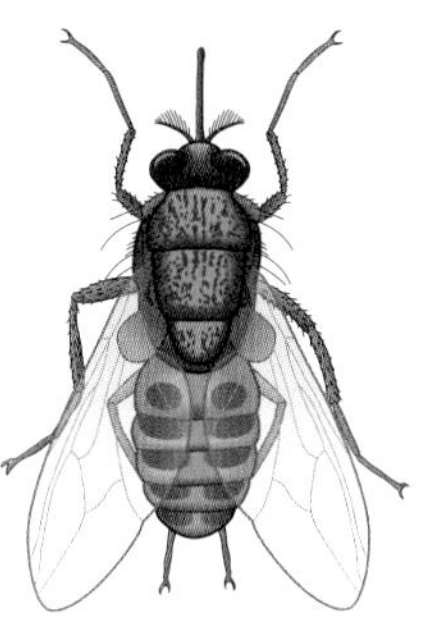

Figure 124.27 Adult tsetse fly. (From Yearbook of Agriculture. Washington, DC, US Department of Agriculture, 1952.)

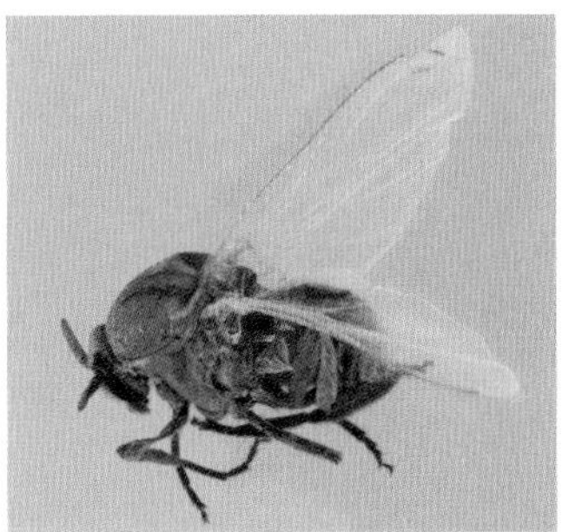

Figure 124.28 Adult black fly. (Photo copyright 2009 by Jerome Goddard, PhD, Mississippi State University, Starkville, MS.)

in a V when at rest. Instead of scales (like mosquitoes) on the wing margins, these flies have hairs. Numerous species occur almost worldwide. Other than disease transmission concerns, treatment of sandfly bites generally only involves palliative antipruritic lotions or creams.

Tsetse flies (insect order Diptera), including several species in the genus *Glossina*, are vectors of trypanosomes of humans and animals in Africa. The Gambian form (*Trypanosoma brucei gambiense*) of African trypanosomiasis, or sleeping sickness (see Chapter 98), is transmitted by *Glossina palpalis*, *G. fuscipes*, and *G. tachinoides*. The East African form (*Trypanosoma brucei rhodesiense*) is primarily transmitted by *G. morsitans*, *G. swynnertoni*, and *G. pallidipes*. Tsetse flies (7–13 mm long) are yellow, brown, or black, and fold their wings scissors-like over their back at rest (***Fig. 124.27***). They superficially resemble honey bees. Contrary to popular belief, people are not the preferred hosts of tsetse flies; these flies feed on a wide variety of mammals and a few reptiles. The effects of their bites are generally self-limited (aside from the disease transmission threat), but hypersensitive persons may react to the saliva, and subsequent bites produce welts and extensive swelling.

Black flies (insect order Diptera), also known as buffalo gnats or turkey gnats, are small flies that are important as disease vectors and nuisance pests (***Fig. 124.28***). The causative agent of onchocerciasis, *Onchocerca volvulus*, is transmitted by black flies in tropical areas of Africa and Central America (see Chapter 106). They are smaller than mosquitoes, are black with a humpbacked appearance, and may attack in swarms, biting viciously. They breed in shallow, fast-flowing streams, mainly in upland regions. Black fly bites may be itchy and slow in healing. Occasionally, people experience systemic reactions to black fly bites such as hives, wheezing, and leukocytosis.

TONGUE WORMS AND LEECHES

Tongue Worms

Pentastomes (phylum Pentastomida), sometimes also classified as members of the Arthropoda because of their chitinous exoskeleton, are wormlike parasites that are found mainly in the respiratory tracts of

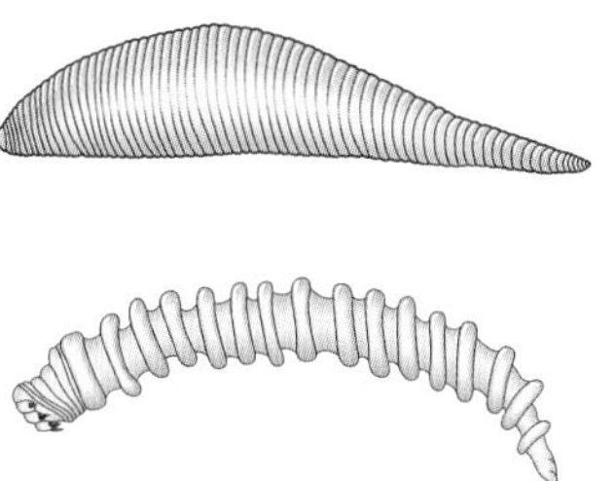

Figure 124.29 Pentastomids: tongue worm, *Linguatula serrata* (*top*), and *Armillifer armillatus*, a common species (*bottom*).

carnivorous mammals, reptiles, and birds.[42] Recent phylogenetic studies place them in a group of modified crustaceans, similar to "fish lice," in the subclass Branchiura.[43] Almost half of the genera parasitize snakes. Human parasitism by pentastomes is called pentastomiasis and may occur in the viscera, where immature forms develop in the liver, spleen, lungs, eyes, and other organs, or in the nasopharyngeal area. Nasopharyngeal pentastomiasis involves infestation of the nasal passages, larynx, or eustachian tubes. Most infestations are asymptomatic and only found by radiography, surgery, or autopsy. However, problems may arise from encysted larvae enlarging, through molting, creating pressure on vital structures.[44]

The worms vary in color and shape, depending upon the species, but are generally colorless to yellow, ringed organisms with no apparent legs or body regions. The body may be cylindrical or flattened. Females may be up to 130 mm long and 10 mm wide; males are smaller, being up to 30 mm long. On either side of the mouth are two pairs of hollow, fang-like hooks, which can be retracted into grooves like the claws of a cat. Two species account for 99% of the infections in humans.[42,45] The tongue worm, *Linguatula serrata*, which occurs worldwide, is often found in the nasal passages and frontal sinuses of several host animals, but especially dogs (***Fig. 124.29***). Human infestations may result in discomfort in the throat, paroxysmal coughing, and sneezing. *Armillifer armillatus* (see ***Fig. 124.29***) ordinarily inhabits the respiratory tract of certain snakes in central Africa. In humans, the free-moving larvae may migrate through many tissues and organs. Encysted larvae are often found in the mesenteries.

The life cycle of *L. serrata* is provided as an example of pentastomid biology.[46] Adults are often found in the nasal passages and frontal sinuses of canines and felines. Eggs are produced and pass out of their host in nasal discharges that are deposited in water or on vegetation. An intermediate host (e.g., rabbit or sheep) swallows contaminated water or vegetation and the eggs hatch into primary larvae, which penetrate the intestinal wall and become lodged in the liver, lungs, or mesenteric nodes. The larvae then pass through two molts resulting in a pupa-like stage. Up to seven more molts may occur before the nymphal stage develops (sometimes called an infective larva). The nymphs then migrate to the abdominal or pleural cavity of the intermediate host where they become encysted. When a definitive host (dog or cat) eats the intermediate host, the nymphs escape rapidly and migrate anteriorly, subsequently clinging to the lining within the host's mouth. From this point they migrate to the nasal cavities where they develop into adults. The adult stage may survive for up to 2 years.

Treatment of pentastomiasis is usually not necessary, but in symptomatic cases surgical removal of the parasites may be needed.[42,45]

Leeches

Most leeches (annelid class Hirudinea) are bloodsucking parasites that attach themselves to vertebrate hosts, bite through the skin, and suck out a quantity of blood. Other than the nuisance effect of their biting, their medical significance is generally minimal. On feeding, leeches secrete an anticoagulant (hirudin) that aids in securing a full blood meal. Leeches vary in shape from elongated cylindrical to broadly ovoid, and may be black, brightly colored, or mottled; they have muscular suckers at both their anterior and posterior ends. Their dorsal side is convex and the ventral side is flattened. Leeches have external annulation (segments) like other annelids, but differ in having neither setae nor appendages. They are hermaphroditic. Length varies from minute (5 mm long) to giant (45 cm long).

Several different groups or types of leeches occur worldwide. The familiar freshwater leeches parasitize people or animals visiting muddy-bottomed rivers or ponds. This external attachment of leeches is often called external hirudiniasis. The famous medicinal leech, *Hirudo medicinalis*, a freshwater worm about 10 cm long, was often used in the eighteenth century as a means of bloodletting. Bloodthirsty land leeches inhabit warm moist areas of South America and Southeast Asia. Land or terrestrial leeches commonly live in tropical rainforests, where they may be found on stones, shrubs, and leaves. Some leeches attach internally when people drink contaminated water, infesting the upper digestive or respiratory tract. "Horse leeches" may attach inside the pharynx or nasal passages of horses or people drinking water from infested pools or streams in the Middle East or North Africa. The internal leech, *Limnatis nilotica*, is found in southern Europe, northern Africa, and western Asia, where it may become attached to the mucous membranes of the pharynx, nasopharynx, and esophagus. Persons with *L. nilotica* infestation often present with epistaxis, hemoptysis, or hematemesis.

Treatment of leech infestation generally involves only mechanical removal of the worms. This is often done by the victim without medical consultation. However, leech infestation of the nasopharynx, respiratory tract, or esophagus is usually remedied by endoscopic removal.

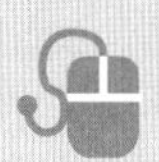

Access the complete reference list online at
http://www.expertconsult.com

Access the complete reference list online at http://www.expertconsult.com

CHAPTER 125

Distinguishing Tropical Infectious Diseases from Bioterrorism

Juan P. Olano • C.J. Peters • David H. Walker

MICROORGANISMS AND TOXINS CAUSING TROPICAL DISEASES WITH POTENTIAL USE AS BIOTERROR AGENTS

Bioterrorism can be defined as the intentional use of infectious agents or microbial toxins with the purpose of causing illness and death, leading to fear in human populations. The dissemination of infectious agents with the purpose of attacking livestock and agricultural resources has similar motives. Many of the agents that could potentially be used in bioterror (BT) attacks are also responsible for naturally occurring infectious diseases in the tropics. Thus naturally occurring outbreaks must be differentiated from BT attacks for public health, forensic, and security reasons. If a BT attack occurs in tropical underdeveloped countries, owing to their weak public health infrastructure, the public health implications would be even more dramatic than in developed nations. An outbreak of smallpox due to a BT attack would probably require vaccination and mandatory quarantine of millions of people in order to control the outbreak and quell global public unrest.

The first step in managing the damage from a covert biological dissemination is recognition of the attack and the organism(s). As in most emerging infections, we predict that in bioterrorist attacks the diagnosis will be made by a clinician or pathologist and the recognition of the event will be through geographic and epidemiologic anomalies. However, we have made important advances in environmental detection capability and point-of-care diagnostics for BT agents. Some diseases such as inhalational anthrax or smallpox may be relatively readily recognized by an alert clinician because of their distinctive presentations. However, the leading edge of a BT epidemic will arrive without prior suspicion. For example, individual cases of pneumonic plague as the earliest harbingers of an attack will presumably present as community-acquired pneumonia and probably die without clinical diagnosis. Given the short window available for successful treatment, the recognition of these earliest cases is paramount. Sartwell[1] has demonstrated empirically that incubation periods follow a log-normal distribution, which results in "front-loading" of cases (***Fig. 125.1***). Delay in recognizing the epidemic through reliance on surveillance or other surrogates will likely result in most cases of diseases such as plague and tularemia being well into their disease course and perhaps unsalvageable.[2]

Bioterrorist events will enlarge our knowledge of tropical diseases. Viral hemorrhagic fevers (VHF) transmitted by aerosol[3] are underrepresented in naturally occurring case series, and a BT attack would provide an opportunity to answer questions about the underlying host factors and pathogenesis.

In October 2001, anthrax spores were distributed covertly in the US Postal Service, leading to 22 cases of human anthrax and billions of dollars spent on controlling a small inhalational anthrax epidemic.[4,5] Ever since the times of Greeks and Romans, humans have tried to inflict damage by the use of contagion on other populations.[6,7] Less than 4% of the groups responsible for terrorist attacks on human populations take responsibility for their actions.[8] The use of biological weapons is ideal to conduct covert attacks. In addition, it has been estimated that to kill the same number of human beings with biological weapons as compared to chemical or nuclear weapons, the cost is far less with biological weapons ($2/human casualty) compared with chemical ($2000/human casualty) and nuclear ($2 000 000/human casualty).[6] Hypothetical BT attacks would range from an overt attack of a large city with a bomb containing several kilograms of an agent (weaponized bacteria, viruses, or toxins) to discrete or covert intentional release of the infectious agent through a delivery system, such as spray devices, postal service, ventilation ducts, water supplies, and food supply.

Based on transmissibility, severity of morbidity and mortality, and likelihood of use (availability, stability, weaponization), potential BT agents are divided into three categories, A–C (***Table 125.1***).

EPIDEMIOLOGY OF A BIOTERROR ATTACK

All potential BT agents are capable of producing illness under natural circumstances. Therefore, the first challenge is to identify the etiologic agent, followed by a thorough epidemiologic and microbiologic analysis of the epidemic. In some circumstances the identification of a BT attack would be obvious. A case of smallpox in any human population is an international emergency that would trigger a massive response of the public health systems around the world. Sophisticated epidemiological investigations would follow in order to characterize the outbreak, identify the source, and possibly label it "intentional." In other cases, the identification of the outbreak as secondary to intentional dissemination of an infectious agent will require use of sophisticated epidemiological and molecular tools, especially for diseases endemic to the area where the outbreak occurs. The need to use genetic sequences as markers has spawned a new discipline, microbial forensics, sister to phylogenetics and "molecular epidemiology."

Differentiation between natural infections and a biological attack rests firstly on disease patterns given by epidemiological clues. They include presence of disease outbreaks of the same illness in noncontiguous areas, disease outbreaks with zoonotic impact, different attack rates in different environments (indoor versus outdoor), presence of large epidemics in small populations, increased number of unexplained deaths, unusually high severity of a disease for a particular pathogen, unusual clinical manifestations owing to route of transmission for a given pathogen, presence of a disease (vector-borne or not) in an area not endemic for that particular disease, multiple epidemics with different diseases in the same population, a case of a disease by an uncommon agent (smallpox, VHF, inhalational anthrax), unusual strains of microorganisms when compared to conventional strains circulating in the same area, and genetically homogeneous organisms isolated from different locations.[9,10] These are a few

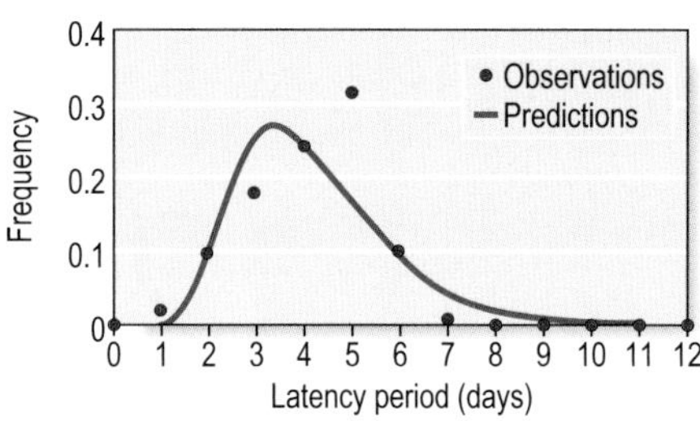

Figure 125.1 Log-normal distribution of incubation periods. (Reproduced from Sartwell P. The distribution and incubation periods of infectious diseases. Am J Hyg. 1950;51:310–318.)

Table 125.1 Potential Bioterror Agents

Category/Agent	Disease
Category A	
Viruses	
Variola major virus	Smallpox
Ebola, Marburg, CCHF, RVF, Lassa, Machupo, and Junin viruses	Viral hemorrhagic fevers
Bacteria	
Francisella tularensis	Tularemia
Yersinia pestis	Plague
Toxins	
Clostridium botulinum toxin	Botulism
Category B	
Viruses	
Alphaviruses (VEE, EEE, WEE)	Various encephalitides
Bacteria	
Rickettsia prowazekii	Epidemic typhus
Brucella spp.	Brucellosis
Coxiella burnetii	Q fever
Burkholderia mallei	Glanders
B. pseudomallei	Melioidosis
Toxins	
Ricin	
SEB	
Food- and waterborne viruses	
Shigella	
Salmonella	
Escherichia coli	
Vibrio cholerae	
Cryptosporidium	
Category C	
Emerging infectious agents such as Nipah virus and hantaviruses; *Mycobacterium tuberculosis*	

CCHF, Crimean-Congo hemorrhagic fever; RVF, Rift Valley fever; VEE, Venezuelan equine encephalitis; EEE, eastern equine encephalitis; WEE, western equine encephalitis; SEB, *Staphylococcus aureus* enterotoxin B.

guidelines that could prove helpful when investigating an outbreak; however, the deduction will not be based on any single finding but rather the pattern seen in its totality. First and foremost, the possibility of an attack must be ever in mind, or differentiation of a covert BT attack and a natural outbreak of an infectious disease may not be made. In fact, the outbreak of salmonellosis in Oregon in 1984 by a covert attack planned by the Rajneeghee leadership was accompanied by distinctive epidemiological clues. It was not labeled as intentional until somebody came forward with the information leading to the responsible group; as in most of medicine, the unsuspected diagnosis is the easiest to miss.[11]

Biosurveillance

Due to the increased awareness of emerging infectious diseases and potential bioterrorist attacks, biosurveillance is now a health care priority. Approximately 70 pathogens have emerged between 1967 and 2009, and the majority of these microorganisms made the "jump" from their zoonotic host into the human species. Infectious disease surveillance has evolved dramatically during the last few years as part of the "molecular revolution" in life sciences. Infectious disease surveillance systems are generally divided into three categories: (1) laboratory-initiated infectious disease notification; (2) syndromic surveillance systems; and (3) genotyping-based surveillance of biothreats.[12] In any of these three complementary systems, the clinical laboratory plays a critical role.

Laboratory-initiated infectious disease notification is mostly based on conventional microbiological techniques for pathogen identification and relies on clinical laboratories for reporting of notifiable diseases to public health authorities. This system is slow, insensitive, but more specific when compared to syndromic sureveillance.[12] The low sensitivity is due to the variable sensitivity of different diagnostic tests used in clinical laboratories to confirm infections and the fact that only a small fraction of human infections are actually confirmed by laboratory means. In essence, the overall sensitivity of the surveillance system depends on the coverage of the laboratory-based surveillance, characteristics of the laboratory tests, screening practices to detect asymptomatic individuals, and the actual reporting system.[12,13]

Syndromic surveillance systems, on the other hand, rely on health utilization patterns and the use of health-related data collected electronically for other purposes. Reporting sources include clinical laboratories, pharmacies, emergency rooms, primary care physicians, intensive care units, and hospital admission and discharge data. Monitoring occurs in real time, and whenever deviations from a "normal pattern" of patients reporting for doctor visits, utilization of laboratory tests or pharmaceuticals occurs, an alarm is triggered suggesting the possibility of an outbreak.[12,14–16] The biggest challenge is the establishment of a baseline above which the system should signal an alarm. Sensitivity and specificity range widely depending on the disease/syndrome and the threshold for triggering the alarm.[16] When syndromic surveillance is used in conjunction with laboratory-initiated surveillance, the low specificity and high sensitivity of syndromic surveillance are potentially compensated by the higher specificity of the laboratory-initiated surveillance system.[12]

Genomic-based surveillance evolved during the past decade with the advent of new molecular techniques and high-throughput diagnostic tests for detection of infectious agents, their markers of virulence, and resistance patterns to antimicrobials.[12] Molecular typing and subtyping have allowed national and international agencies to monitor and initiate early warnings to public health and clinical laboratories. In addition, powerful biosensors using molecular approaches have monitored selected environments to detect potential pathogens before onset of symptoms in exposed persons (BioWatch and Biological Aerosol Sentry and Information System,[12,17] and the Autonomous Pathogen Detection System).[17,18] The current challenge is to integrate all surveillance systems into a system that provides comprehensive information and timely alerts. The vast electronic data collected by syndromic and genomic surveillance require new technologies for data storing, mining, and temporal/spatial analysis of outbreaks. The ultimate goal is the creation of "global laboratories" or global real-time epidemiological surveillance in which all surveillance information is processed along with geographic information systems and a real-time output is rendered regarding infectious threats around the world.[12] Attempts to achieve this goal are represented by the World Health Organization (WHO) Global Outbreak Alert and Response Network and the International System for Total Early Disease Detection (InStedd).

Conventional epidemiological investigations are by no means obsolete. Confirmation of an outbreak is based in many cases on laboratory analysis of patients' samples or autopsy material. A case definition is constructed to increase objectivity of the data analyzed and to enable determination of the attack rate. Other variables are included in the analysis, such as time and place, and an epidemiological curve can be constructed.[10]

Epidemiological curves are important tools to analyze epidemics and suggest the mode of transmission and propagation. A point source epidemic curve is classically log-normal in distribution[1] and suggests a common exposure of a population to an infectious agent.

CATEGORY A

Bacterial Agents

Bacillus anthracis (Anthrax)

B. anthracis (see Chapter 38) is the microorganism that has received the most attention as a BT agent due to its high lethality (inhalational form), ease of propagation, and high environmental stability. Fortunately the disease is not transmitted from person to person. However, the first three characteristics make it an ideal bioweapon.

Anthrax presents in humans as four different clinical syndromes, depending on the portal of entry: (1) cutaneous; (2) gastrointestinal; (3) oral/oropharyngeal; and (4) inhalational. In the event of a BT attack, either overt or covert, the clinical presentation of patients affected by the attack would be that of inhalational anthrax. This form of anthrax is so rare that a single case of inhalational anthrax should raise immediate suspicion, as dramatically demonstrated during the BT attacks in the fall of 2001.[19–21] During those attacks, 50% of cases were cutaneous anthrax, presumably secondary to handling of anthrax-laced mail envelopes or environmental surface contamination in the presence of minor cutaneous lesions, providing a portal of entry for the spores.[5] An outbreak of inhalational anthrax also took place in Sverdlovsk (former Soviet Union) as a result of an accidental release into the air of *B. anthracis* spores from a facility producing anthrax for a bioweapons program.[5,22–28]

Inhalational anthrax should be suspected clinically in any individual presenting with fever and a widened mediastinum on chest radiograph (due to hemorrhagic mediastinitis).[25,26] The incubation period is normally 3–5 days, but in some cases it can be as short as 2 days and as long as 60 days depending on inoculum and the time of germination of the spore.[23] Based on research in rhesus monkeys, the LD_{50} is estimated to be 8000–10 000 spores.[27–29] However, as few as 1–3 spores may be capable of producing a fatal outcome in ~1% of those exposed to these quantities.[30] Mortality is 100% without antibiotic therapy.[26,31–33] Early diagnosis, aggressive treatment with antimicrobial agents to which the bacteria are susceptible, and aggressive supportive therapy decreased the mortality to 40% in 2001 attacks.[5] Pathologic studies performed on the Sverdlovsk victims revealed hemorrhagic tracheobronchial lymphadenitis and mediastinitis. However, many patients also developed hematogenous hemorrhagic pneumonia. Pleural effusions were usually large and frequently led to severe lung atelectasis. In about half of cases, hemorrhagic meningitis led rapidly to central nervous system (CNS) manifestations terminating in coma and death.[22,34,35]

Yersinia pestis (Plague)

Y. pestis (see Chapter 41) is a Gram-negative, aerobic, nonsporulating coccobacillus, member of the Enterobacteriaceae, with a wide host range.[36] The most important reservoirs are urban rats, and its main vector is the rat flea. In rural epizootics, reservoirs include prairie dogs and squirrels in the United States.[37] *Y. pestis* has been responsible for some of the most devastating pandemics in human history during the pre-antibiotic era (sixth, fourteenth, and nineteenth centuries).[38] Public health measures have made this disease a rarity in the United States (around 20 cases/year) and around the world, although approximately 1000 cases are reported to the WHO every year (from Madagascar, Tanzania, and Peru, among others).

Clinical presentation in naturally acquired infections takes five forms: (1) bubonic; (2) septicemic; (3) pneumonic; (4) cutaneous; and (5) meningeal. The pneumonic form is the most likely presentation in a case of plague due to a BT attack. Plague has already been used as a BT agent when Japan dropped thousands of *Y. pestis*-infected fleas over China, leading to small outbreaks of bubonic plague in continental China during World War II.[39,40]

The incubation period for pneumonic plague is short, ranging from 2 to 3 days. It is the rarest form in natural infections (1% or less) but has the highest mortality, reaching 100% in untreated patients. The initial presentation is nonspecific and consists of cough, fever, and dyspnea. Cough may be productive (bloody, purulent, or watery in the initial phases), followed by a rapid clinical course leading to respiratory failure and death if not treated with antibiotics early in the course.[36,37,41]

The factors that led to the severe Manchurian pneumonic plague outbreaks in the early twentieth century are unknown, but weather, hygiene, and crowding were important factors. More recent outbreaks worldwide and in the United States have been much smaller and readily controlled. Pneumonic cases occur in the United States, but secondary transmission has been rare in the last 50 years. Modeling of pneumonic transmission using eight small outbreaks to derive the parameters finds R_0 to be approximately 1 prior to any control measures.[42]

Francisella tularensis (Tularemia)

This was one of the most scientifically neglected microorganisms with BT potential. Tularemia is a zoonotic infection caused by a small strictly aerobic, Gram-negative, nonsporulating coccobacillus. *F. tularensis* subspecies *tularensis* (Jellison type A) is by far more virulent than *F. tularensis* subspecies *holarctica* (Jellison type B) and is present only in North America.[43] Of the bacteria with potential as BT agents, *F. tularensis* has by far the widest host range, including wild and domestic animals, humans, fish, reptiles, and birds. Vectors are also numerous, including ticks, fleas, mosquitoes, and biting flies[43,44] – an impressive range for any human pathogen.

In natural infections the most common sources of infection are tick bite and handling infected animals such as wild rabbits. Six clinical syndromes have been described: (1) ulceroglandular; (2) glandular; (3) oculoglandular; (4) pharyngeal; (5) pneumonic; and (6) typhoidal. Marked overlap exists among all these forms, and for practical purposes two syndromes (ulceroglandular and typhoidal) have been proposed.[45–47] As a BT agent, *F. tularensis* would most likely cause disease with a primary pulmonary component and secondary dissemination (typhoidal/systemic). In natural infections both ulceroglandular and typhoidal forms can have a hematogenous pulmonary component that is more common in typhoidal tularemia. Case-fatality rate approaches 30% if not treated with appropriate antibiotics.[47]

Viral Agents

Smallpox Virus (Variola Major)

Smallpox (see Chapter 57) is the only disease so far eradicated from the face of earth due to human intervention. The WHO declared smallpox eradicated in 1980 after the last case of natural disease was diagnosed in Somalia in 1977,[48] and vaccination ceased around the world, rendering humankind vulnerable to reintroduction of the virus.[49–51] A laboratory accident was responsible for two more cases in 1978 in England. This accident prompted the WHO to restrict the frozen virus to two places: Centers for Disease Control and Prevention (CDC), Atlanta, Georgia and the Institute for Polyomyelitis and Viral Encephalitides in Moscow, later moved to NPO VECTOR, Novosibirisk. However, it is suspected that secret military repositories exist after the fragmentation of the Soviet Union and the subsequent exodus of scientists involved in its bioweapons program (Biopreparat).[52,53] The agent responsible for this disease is an orthopox virus with no known animal reservoir, but high aerosol infectivity, stability, and mortality. Although not a category A agent, monkeypox is responsible for outbreaks in Africa and is the only other member of the *Orthopoxvirus* genus capable of producing systemic disease in humans. Monkeypox is potentially indistinguishable from smallpox, where mortality rates in tropical Central Africa are around 10–15%. In May and June 2003, an outbreak of monkeypox occurred in the United States.[54] Thirty-seven infections were laboratory-documented and involved humans exposed to infected prairie dogs which had become infected because of contact with infected Gambian rats and dormice shipped from Africa earlier that year. Cases included veterinarians, exotic pet dealers, and pet owners. The clinical spectrum in this outbreak ranged from asymptomatic seroconversions to febrile illness with papulovesicular rash, but no deaths. However, phylogenetic analysis of the virus placed it in the less virulent West Africa clade rather than the Central Africa clade, which carries a case-fatality rate of 10–15%.

A single case of smallpox would trigger a massive public health response in order to contain the outbreak. An outbreak in Germany in 1970 resulted in 19 cases with 100 000 people vaccinated to contain the outbreak. In 1972, Yugoslavia underwent an epidemic with a total of 175 cases (35 deaths) and a vaccination program that included 20 million people in order to contain the outbreak and obtain international confidence. Vaccination with vaccinia virus (a related orthopox virus) is the most effective way to prevent the disease and can be administered up to 4 days after contact with ill patients. Strict quarantine with respiratory isolation is also mandatory for 17 days. The newer generation of antivirals developed after the disease was eradicated has never been tested in human populations, but *in vitro* data and experiments in animal models of poxvirus disease suggest some antiviral activity for the acyclic nucleoside phosphonates such as cidofovir.[55] The only vaccine available in the United States is Dryvax, and sufficient doses have been manufactured to cover the entire US population. However, newer vaccines which may have fewer side effects are being developed.

The clinical presentation is characteristic. The incubation period ranges from 10 to 12 days. The initial phase is nonspecific, characterized by abrupt onset of fever, fatigue, malaise, and headaches. During this phase in 10% of patients with fair complexion, a discrete erythematous rash appears on the face, forearms, and hands. The typical smallpox rash has a centrifugal distribution (more abundant on the face and extremities than on the trunk and abdomen). An enanthem also develops with presence of oral ulcerations by the time the exanthem appears. Systemic manifestations begin to subside once the rash appears and can reappear with superinfection of skin lesions or superimposed bacterial bronchopneumonia. Progression of the lesions is synchronous (maculopapules, vesicles, pustules). After pustules rupture, scabs form and detach in 2–3 weeks, leaving depigmented, scarred areas. This form of the disease, variola major, is fatal in up to 30% of unvaccinated patients and 3% of vaccinated individuals. Various hemorrhagic forms exist.[56]

Viral Hemorrhagic Fevers

This syndrome (see Chapter 67) is caused by a heterogeneous group of RNA viruses that belong to three different families: (1) filoviruses (Ebola and Marburg viruses); (2) arenaviruses (Lassa, Junin, Machupo, Guanarito, and Sabia viruses); and (3) bunyaviruses (Crimean-Congo hemorrhagic fever and Rift Valley fever viruses).[57–59]

The common denominator in these infections is the increased vascular permeability in the microcirculation leading to hemorrhagic diathesis and systemic manifestations such as pulmonary and cerebral edema related to leaky capillaries.[60] These viruses usually have a very narrow geographic range determined by their natural reservoirs and vectors. Humans are accidental hosts. These diseases have caught great public attention due to their high mortality. This, combined with their aerosol infectivity, has led to the use of biosafety level (BSL)-4 laboratories for their study.

Clinical presentation is usually nonspecific and consists of fever and malaise, followed by signs of increased vascular permeability and circulatory compromise. VHF usually terminates in shock, generalized mucocutaneous hemorrhages, and multiorgan failure.

Diseases Caused by Toxins

Toxins in the context of BT agents are substances of biological origin that are capable of producing human illness. Toxins are usually proteins synthesized by living bacteria, fungi, or plants. Toxins are generally less dangerous than infectious agents. The most potent biological toxin is that from *Clostridium botulinum,* and it is one-tenth or less lethal than anthrax on a weight basis. Other toxins such as ricin are less than one-thousandth as toxic as botulinum toxin, and sarin is 30-fold less toxic than ricin.

Clostridium botulinum Toxins (Botulism)

There are seven similar toxins produced by seven different serotypes of *C. botulinum* (A–G), all leading to the same clinical manifestations and lethality. The approximately 150-kDa toxins block neurotransmission at the presynaptic level in cholinergic neurons including the neuromuscular junction, leading to progressive palsies of cranial nerves and skeletal muscle. Botulinal toxins are among the most lethal substances known, with LD_{50} of 0.001 μg/g of body weight when administered parenterally.[31,61,62] The aerosol route decreases its lethality 80–100-fold. Both aerosol attacks and contamination of food supplies are potential BT scenarios.

Clinical manifestations consist of progressive bulbar and skeletal paralysis in the absence of fever, including diplopia, dysphagia, blurred vision, ptosis, dysarthria, dysphonia, mydriasis, dry mucosae, and descending paralysis.[31,62]

CATEGORY B AGENTS

All the agents in category A are generally recognized as serious threats for causing extensive casualties. Categories B and C are much more heterogeneous.

Viral Agents

Viral Encephalitides

These are caused by the genus *Alphavirus*, family *Togaviridae* (eastern, western, and Venezuelan equine encephalitis viruses; see Chapter 78). Natural infections are usually transmitted by mosquitoes, but aerosol transmission is the notorious cause of numerous laboratory infections and is the basis of its historic weaponization.[58,63]

Most of these viruses cause systemic illness characterized by fever, myalgias, and prostration.

Clinically apparent involvement of the CNS is present in some cases and varies among the different viruses. Eastern equine encephalitis is by far the most virulent, leading to case-fatality rates of 50–75%, and survivors usually have severe neurologic sequelae.[64,65] Venezuelan equine encephalitis, in contrast, leads to CNS manifestations in no more than 4% of cases, and almost all Venezuelan equine encephalitis infections are symptomatic even in the absence of CNS involvement.[66–68]

Bacterial Agents

Epidemic Typhus (*Rickettsia prowazekii*) and Rocky Mountain Spotted Fever (*R. rickettsii*)

Typhus (see Chapter 50) is another disease that has played a historic role in human populations.[69–72] Millions perished in World Wars I and II due to epidemic, louse-borne typhus. Large outbreaks of the disease still occur in tropical regions around the world in areas stricken by war, famine, and poverty. Rocky Mountain spotted fever, on the other hand, is transmitted by tick bites and occurs endemically in South, Central, and North America. Rickettsiae target the microvascular endothelium leading to leaky capillaries systemically.[73] The main causes of morbidity and mortality are noncardiogenic pulmonary edema and meningoencephalitis. Rickettsiae are remarkably underestimated biothreats as they are highly infectious by low-dose aerosol, possess a stable extracellular form, and are resistant to most empirically administered antibiotics, including β-lactams, aminoglycosides, and erythromycin, and infections are exacerbated by sulfonamides. Case-fatality rates can be as high as 40–50% without antibiotic therapy and 3–5% with adequate antibiotic coverage. Lethal cases are usually due to delayed diagnosis.[70,71,74]

These potent BT agents are often discounted because of their susceptibility to tetracycline and chloramphenicol. However, the severity of the illness, difficulty of clinical diagnosis, exhaustion of antibiotics in the face of a mass attack, and existence of antibiotic-resistant organisms suggest they are still formidable threats.

Coxiella burnetii (Q Fever)

This Gram-negative, obligately intracellular bacterium has a high degree of infectivity (1 organism by inhalation) and low lethality.[75–78] The distribution of Q fever is worldwide and results from exposure to animals such as sheep, cattle, goats, cats, rabbits, and others (see Chapter 53). *C. burnetii* can withstand harsh environmental conditions and be transported by wind. In natural infections, 60% are asymptomatic. In symptomatic cases, the presentation is nonspecific, including malaise, fever, myalgias, cough, chills, headaches, anorexia, weight loss and, in some cases, pleuritic chest pain. Hepatomegaly and splenomegaly are sometimes observed, although not frequently.

Brucella spp. (Brucellosis, Undulant Fever, Mediterranean Fever, Malta Fever)

Four species of these Gram-negative, aerobic, nonspore-forming coccobacilli are pathogenic to humans: *B. abortus, B. melitensis, B. suis,* and *B. canis* (see Chapter 40). Host ranges include goats and sheep (*B. melitensis*), swine and horses (*B. suis*), cattle, bison, elk and horses (*B. abortus*), and dogs (*B. canis*).

Transmission occurs by exposure to infected animal products (meat, milk). Less common routes of infection are inhalational and cutaneous. The clinical presentation is highly variable, even after inhalational exposure. Undulant fever is characterized by relapses of fever, weakness, generalized aching, and headache. Chronic infections may have manifestations related to several organ systems such as the gastrointestinal and genitourinary tracts, CNS, joints, and bones.[75–81]

Food- and Waterborne Pathogens

Developing countries with insufficient water treatment and food security are more vulnerable to enteric BT attack. These agents include *Shigella dysenteriae*, *Salmonella* spp., enterohemorrhagic *Escherichia coli*, *Vibrio cholerae,* and *Cryptosporidium* spp.

Shigella and *Salmonella* have in fact already been used as agents of biorevenge or biopolitics in small-scale attacks: one (*Shigella*) in an office setting by a disgruntled employee and one in Oregon by a religious sect that led to almost 1000 cases of *Salmonella*-related gastroenteritis.[11,82] These agents are indeed ideal for small-scale attacks since large-scale attacks would require contamination of large water supplies, which, because of enormous dilution factors and susceptibility of all these agents (except for *Cryptosporidium* spp.) to standard chlorinating procedures, would decrease the number of bacteria to below that required to infect large numbers of people.[75]

Occasional outbreaks of nontyphoidal *Salmonella* and *Shigella* infections occur in the United States. *Shigella* and *Crystosporidium* are highly infectious organisms that require very low numbers (10^2–10^3 organisms) to provoke clinical disease. Imported cases of *V. cholerae* have been diagnosed in the United States in the past. However, the disease occurs in southern Asia and Latin America as large outbreaks. The clinical illness is characterized by explosive watery diarrhea that leads to rapid dehydration and circulatory collapse.

Cryptosporidium spp. infections are characterized by watery diarrhea and abdominal cramping for 2–3 weeks. The disease is self-limited except in patients with acquired immunodeficiency syndrome (AIDS) or other conditions of compromise; in such cases illness can last for months or years if immune function is not restored. *Cryptosporidium* spp. are resistant to standard chlorine concentrations in water supplies.[83] The main human pathogen is *C. hominis,* followed by *C. parvum*. Other less common pathogens include *C. meleagridis, C. muris, C. felis,* and *C. canis*. The largest outbreak in the United States was in Milwaukee in the early 1990s, and was responsible for thousands of cases and increased mortality among AIDS patients.[75,84,85]

Category B Toxins

Ricin Toxin (Castor Beans from *Ricinis communis* Plants)

The toxin composed of two glycoproteins of approximately 66 kDa[86] inhibits protein synthesis by blocking elongation factor 2 at the ribosomal level. Ricin toxin is not a weapon of mass destruction since its lethal dose in humans is much higher than previously believed. However, the use of the toxin in small BT attacks is possible in the tropics because of its ready availability and relatively easy extraction from the beans. Clinical presentation depends on the route of administration, as does the LD_{50}. When large amounts of toxin are ingested, the manifestations include nausea, vomiting, severe abdominal cramping, rectal hemorrhage, and diarrhea. As the course progresses, anuria, mydriasis, severe headaches, and shock supervene, leading to death in 2–3 days. Clinical manifestations usually appear within 10 hours after ingestion of the toxin. Inhalational exposure leads to prominent pulmonary manifestations 8–28 hours after exposure with fever, dyspnea, cough, cyanosis, and death. Histologically, there is widespread necrosis of pulmonary parenchyma and pulmonary edema. A single case of parenteral intoxication is documented. A defector from Bulgaria was injected with a pellet containing ricin from a weapon disguised in an umbrella, resulting in local necrosis, regional lymphadenopathy, gastrointestinal hemorrhage, liver necrosis, nephritis, and disseminated intravascular coagulation.[87]

Staphylococcus aureus Enterotoxin B

Staphylococcus aureus Enterotoxin B (SEB), a 28-kDa, heat-stable exotoxin produced by certain strains of *S. aureus,* causes food poisoning after ingestion in improperly handled food. In BT scenarios exposure can occur by either inhalation or ingestion, leading to SEB food poisoning or SEB respiratory syndrome. The toxin is highly incapacitating and not very lethal. The doses that cause symptoms in half of exposed persons and LD_{50} differ by a magnitude of 5 log scales for inhalational exposure.[88]

The incubation period after ingestion is short (4–12 hours), followed by explosive vomiting that persists for several hours. Weaponization of the toxin as an aerosol is possible due to its high stability. Manifestations after inhalation of SEB are respiratory and consist of fever, cough, chills, myalgias, chest pain, and pulmonary insufficiency due to alveolar edema. General manifestations consist of multiorgan failure secondary to cytokine storm.[31] These toxins are superantigens that bind to major histocompatibility complex class II molecules on large numbers of lymphocytes and macrophages, leading to hyperactivation of the immune system and massive release of cytokines, including interferon-γ, tumor necrosis factor-α, interleukin-6 and other mediators, such as leukotrienes and histamine.[88]

DIAGNOSIS

The role of the clinical laboratory in the diagnosis of possible cases related to a BT attack is of utmost importance.[89,90] On the one hand, standard clinical microbiology laboratories will be receiving specimens for diagnostic purposes, and communication with clinicians regarding their suspicions is critical. Certain isolates in the laboratory are not pursued further (*Bacillus* spp. is a classic example) unless specifically requested due to the frequent isolation of contaminants with similar characteristics. In addition, handling of certain specimens will require added biosafety level (BSL) requirements due to their infectivity (***Table 125.2***). Certain samples will have to be shipped to highly specialized laboratories for initial or further work-up. Environmental testing is challenging due to the complexity of the samples to be analyzed.[91,92] This type of testing takes place in highly specialized laboratories and is not undertaken by the standard clinical microbiology laboratory.

Table 125.2 Laboratory Response Network for Bioterror Attacks

Level	Functions
A	Community-level laboratories that should recognize the clues of a possible bioterror agent and be able to package samples and ship them for confirmation at the upper-level laboratories
B	State and county public health laboratories with capacity to work with BSL-2 and some with BSL-3 agents. Capable of isolation of some of the agents, presumptive level testing, and antibiotic susceptibility profiles
C	Greater BSL-3 capabilities than level B and molecular testing capabilities for rapid identification
D	Highest level of containment (BSL-4) for isolation and identification of highly pathogenic viruses

BSL, biosafety level.

Table 125.3 Molecular Diagnostic Techniques

Type	Techniques
Nonamplification techniques	Labeled-nucleic acid probes Hybridization protection assay (HPA) *In situ* hybridization
Amplification techniques	
Signal amplification	Branched DNA (bDNA)
	Hybrid capture assays
Target amplification	Polymerase chain reaction (PCR), reverse transcription (RT)-PCR, real-time PCR
	Transcription-based amplification Transcription-mediated amplification (TAM) Nucleic acid sequence-based amplification (NASBA)
	Strand displacement amplification (SDA)
Probe amplification	Cleavase-invader technology
Detection systems	Gel analysis
	Colorimetric microtiter plates
	Hybridization
	Direct sequencing
	Quantitative methods: Diagnostic chips, microarrays Bead-based flow cytometric analysis Gas chromatography/mass spectrometry (GCMS)

Conventional and Molecular Diagnosis of Potential Bioterror Agents

General Principles

The bacterial diseases caused by the BT agents in this chapter, with the exception of *Coxiella burnetii* and *Rickettsia* spp., can be diagnosed by standard isolation techniques in clinical microbiology laboratories. Isolation of rickettsiae and the BT viruses requires specialized laboratories with BSL-3 or BSL-4 biocontainment.[93] Serological assays are available for detection of antibodies against all BT agents. However, for many organisms serological assays require the presence of rising antibody titers, and therefore the serologic diagnosis is usually retrospective in nature. For some viral diseases, a reliable diagnosis can be established based on elevation of IgM titers during the acute stage of the disease.

With the advent of molecular techniques, rapid and sensitive diagnostic tests are becoming available for BT agents during the acute disease.[94–96] This is of utmost importance in a BT event since identification of the first cases would be critical for a rapid and effective public health response. In addition, treatment and prophylactic measures can also be initiated as quickly as possible. Molecular diagnostic techniques can also be applied to potential BT agents as epidemiological and forensic investigations. Postmortem diagnosis is also possible by analysis of frozen or paraffin-embedded tissues by immunohistology or nucleic acid-based amplification techniques. Several molecular techniques have been developed for nucleic acid amplification and detection (***Table 125.3***).

Rapid diagnosis of the initial cases in a BT event requires a high degree of clinical suspicion from the physicians having contact with such patients in the emergency room or outpatient setting. The clinical laboratories would then play a critical role in detecting the suspected agent and/or referring the appropriate specimens to higher-level laboratories for specialized testing (***Table 125.2***).[89,91,97]

Several of the agents cause zoonotic diseases. Therefore, diagnosis of certain zoonotic diseases in animals may be important in identifying some BT attacks. In such situations animals could be seen as either direct victims of the attack or sentinel events in a human outbreak. There are currently efforts to establish a network of laboratories dedicated to diagnosis of veterinary agents.[91]

DIAGNOSIS OF SPECIFIC BIOTERROR AGENTS

Category A Agents

Bacillus anthracis

The diagnosis of inhalational anthrax is based on isolation and identification of *B. anthracis* from a clinical specimen collected from an ill patient. In cases of inhalational anthrax, samples of sputum, blood, or cerebrospinal fluid (CSF) may yield growth of the agent. Demonstration of *B. anthracis* from nasal swabs has more epidemiological and prophylactic implications than clinical importance.

Standard diagnostic techniques are based on visualization and isolation in the clinical microbiology laboratory and serological demonstration of antibodies against *B. anthracis*.[98–102]

Visualization of *B. anthracis* from clinical specimens (blood cultures, CSF, and cutaneous lesions) by Gram stains is not difficult. *B. anthracis* appears as large Gram-positive, spore-forming rods with a bamboo appearance. Isolation is achieved by inoculating standard sheep blood agar plates, and colonies appear as small, gray-white, nonhemolytic colonies. A selective medium (polymyxin-lysozyme-EDTA-thallous acetate agar) is available mostly for environmental samples and inhibits the growth of other *Bacillus* spp., such as *B. cereus*. Growth is rapid (24–48 hours).[99] Confirmatory tests include γ-phage lysis, detection of specific cell wall and capsular antigens, and polymerase chain reaction (PCR) amplification of DNA followed by sequencing.[96]

Serological tests available for clinical diagnosis are based on detection of antibodies directed against protective antigen. Cross-reactive antibodies decrease the specificity of this test. Assays based on toxin detection are available in specialized centers and are based on capture of anthrax toxins by using antibodies. Antibody-coated immunomagnetic beads are then analyzed by electrochemiluminescence technology. The analytical sensitivity of this technique for detection of anthrax toxin is at the picogram to femtogram level (10^{-12} to 10^{-15}).[103,104] Liposome PCR, liposomal technology combined with real-time PCR (for a DNA reporter sequence), has also been developed for cholera and botulinum toxins, with analytical sensitivity in the attomolar to zeptomolar (10^{-18} to 10^{-21}) range.[105] The specificity of this assay is determined by the toxin-capturing antibody.

Nucleic acid amplification techniques (PCR) are also available in both standard and real-time formats. Extraction of DNA from spores is challenging and requires modification of DNA extraction protocols in order to facilitate release of DNA from spores or induction of germination prior to DNA extraction.[96] Real-time PCR tests have been developed by Applied Biosystems (TaqMan 5′ nuclease assay) and Roche Applied Science (LightCycler).[106–108] The analytical sensitivity of both techniques is extremely high, and testing times have been decreased to 1–2 hours.

Portable PCR instruments are being developed for rapid deployment to the field.[109] Examples include the rugged advanced pathogen identification device (RAPID),[106] the Smartcycler (Cepheid, CA),[107] and the miniature analytical thermal cycler instrument (MATCI), developed by the Department of Energy's Lawrence Livermore National Laboratory.[110] This instrument later evolved into the advanced nucleic acid analyzer (ANAA) and handheld advanced nucleic acid analyzer (HANAA).[111] The only commercially available test approved by the Food and Drug Administration (FDA) is the JBAIDS anthrax detection kit (Idaho Technology Inc., Salt Lake City, UT).

Molecular subtyping of *B. anthracis* is also possible by using the 16S rRNA subunit gene, multiple-locus variable number tandem repeat analysis of eight genetic loci, and amplified fragment length polymorphism techniques.[112,113]

Environmental testing also plays a role in the investigation of a BT event. In this setting, detection of *B. anthracis* relies heavily on molecular techniques for confirmation of potentially contaminated samples (e.g., surfaces, air).[114,115]

Postmortem diagnosis is also possible by using Gram stains on paraffin-based tissues or immunohistochemical procedures using polyclonal or monoclonal antibodies against various anthrax antigens.

Yersinia pestis

Diagnosis is based on demonstration of the bacillus in blood or sputa. Standard diagnostic techniques include visualization of Gram-negative coccobacilli, which by Giemsa, Wright, or Wayson stains reveal a "safety pin" appearance. Isolation is performed on blood and McConkey agar plates where colonies appear as nonlactose fermenters. The organisms are identified preliminarily by direct immunofluorescence assay with *Y. pestis*-specific antibodies, with final identification based on biochemical profiles.[116]

Molecular diagnostic techniques based on real-time PCR became available in recent years and involve detection of *Y. pestis* genes such as plasminogen activator (*pla*), genes coding for the Yop proteins and the capsular F1 antigen, and the 23S rRNA gene, which allows distinction from other *Yersinia* spp.[117–119] Assays detect resistance to particular antibiotics. The importance of these diagnostic techniques in a disease such as plague is evident. The log-normal epidemic curve with a narrow dispersion of the incubation periods (***Fig. 125.1***) and the short interval for successful antibiotic therapy mandate recognition of the earliest cases if the bulk of the exposed are to be saved.

Molecular subtyping of *Y. pestis* is also possible by analyzing polymorphic sites in order to identify the origin of strains in the event of a BT attack.

Francisella tularensis

Diagnosis is made by demonstration of the microorganisms in secretions (sputa, exudates) by direct immunofluorescence or immunohistochemically in biopsy specimens. Isolation may be achieved on regular blood agar plates, posing a risk to laboratory personnel not employing BSL-3 facilities and procedures.

The procedure for isolation of *F. tularensis* in the laboratory is very similar to that described for *Y. pestis*. Final identification is based on the biochemical profile.[120]

Molecular diagnostic techniques are based on PCR detection of *F. tularensis* using primers for genes such as outer-membrane protein (*Fop*) or *tul4* and real-time detection systems.[96,121,122] A commercial FDA-approved PCR kit is available (JBAIDS Tularemia Detection Kit, Idaho Technology, Inc., Salt Lake City, UT).

Smallpox Virus

Diagnosis of variola major is suggested by its clinical presentation and visualization of Guarnieri bodies in skin biopsy samples. Preliminary confirmation requires identification of typical brick-shaped orthopox virus by electron microscopy, followed by isolation from clinical specimens and accurate molecular identification to differentiate it from the morphologically (and sometimes clinically) similar monkeypox virus. Confirmation of smallpox is performed only under BSL-4 containment facilities at CDC.[53]

Molecular techniques are based on PCR amplification using real-time or standard technology, followed by sequencing or use of restriction fragment length polymorphism for identification.[123] Techniques developed for smallpox molecular testing include Taqman- and LightCycler-based assays with primers designed for the hemagglutinin gene and A-type inclusion body proteins.[124–127]

Sequencing of the smallpox genome has been completed for some Asian strains of variola major and one of variola minor. Other strains are being sequenced and will provide more information for probe design and treatment targets.[96]

Viral Hemorrhagic Fevers

Diagnosis of these diseases is performed in highly specialized centers in the United States since special isolation procedures and highly contained laboratories are required.

Initial diagnosis of these diseases is suspected on clinical and epidemiological grounds. Laboratory diagnosis involves isolation, electron microscopy, and serological assays. Immunohistochemical detection of hemorrhagic fever viral antigens in paraffin-embedded tissues is also performed in highly specialized centers such as the CDC.[128–132]

Molecular diagnostic techniques have also improved dramatically. Serum or blood is the most common specimen for reverse transcription-PCR amplification of viral nucleic acids.

Design of primers for this heterogeneous group of RNA viruses that are highly variable is one of the limitations.[90] Therefore, multiplex PCR techniques are required to detect as many targets as possible in a single assay.[133,134] Real-time PCR based on detection of the target sequence using fluorescent probes therefore limits the number of targets that can be identified because of the limited wavelength range for fluorescence applications.[134–136] Multiplex has evolved during the past several years, and molecular test combinations are now possible. Both low target number multiplexing (3–6) and highly multiplexed assays (>10 targets) have been developed. The Luminex xTag RVP assay is capable of detecting 16 targets using universal bead array sorting technology. The use of microchips and microarrays containing several thousands of oligonucleotides from all viruses known to be pathogenic to humans is an encouraging development. In fact, the rapid identification and characterization of the novel human coronavirus responsible for the severe acute respiratory syndrome (SARS) outbreak in 2003 are excellent examples of the power of hybridization-based microchips. Chips and microarrays vary in complexity. Some are designed for influenza typing and some others, such as the GreeneChipResp, can identify 15 or more virus families.

Category B Agents

Rickettsia prowazekii (Epidemic Typhus) and *R. rickettsii* (Rocky Mountain Spotted Fever)

Diagnosis of these infections in the clinical microbiology laboratory currently rests on the identification of antibodies in serum during the acute and convalescent periods in order to demonstrate seroconversion or rising titers. The diagnosis is therefore retrospective.[74,137] Detection of rickettsial DNA from blood or skin samples during the acute phase of the disease is possible via PCR assays. However, these assays are not standardized and are not commercially available. Primers have been designed for amplification of several rickettsial genes, including citrate synthase, 17-kDa protein genes, *ompA* and *ompB*.[137–141] The clinical sensitivity and specificity of standard or real-time PCR techniques have not been determined. Real-time PCR is superior due to the higher analytical sensitivity of this technique and low risk of sample contamination with DNA amplicons when compared to standard PCR amplification methods.

Isolation of rickettsiae from clinical specimens is performed in very few specialized laboratories and requires the use of cell monolayers, embryonated eggs, or animals. Detection of rickettsial antigens or whole bacteria in blood specimens is theoretically possible by using ultrasensitive methods, but such assays are currently only in the early phases of development. Immunohistochemical detection of rickettsiae in paraffin-embedded tissue has also been applied pre- or postmortem.[142–144]

Salmonella spp, *Shigella dysenteriae*, *Escherichia coli* O157:H7 and *Cryptosporidium* spp. (Acute Enteric Syndromes)

Diagnosis of *Salmonella*, *Shigella,* and *Vibrio* infections is based on isolation of the offending agent on standard microbiological media followed by specialized confirmatory tests to identify the specific serotype.[145] Diagnosis of *Cryptosporidium* spp. is based on visual identification of the protozoan in fecal specimens using modified trichrome stain.[145] Other methods include antigen detection in fecal specimens using enzyme immunoassay or fluorescence detection methods.

Coxiella burnetii (Q Fever)

The diagnosis rests on serological demonstration of antibodies by immunofluorescence antibody analysis or enzyme-linked immunosorbent assay (ELISA). Antibodies remain elevated for years after the acute infection, and therefore a fourfold rise in titers is the gold standard for diagnosis. PCR detection of *C. burnetii* DNA from blood or tissues also yields a diagnosis of Q fever.[94]

Brucella spp.

Diagnosis of brucellosis requires a high degree of clinical suspicion due to the protean manifestations related to this disease. Laboratory diagnosis is based on isolation of the microorganism from blood, bone marrow, or other tissue samples. Isolation is not easy due to the slow growth of *Brucella* spp. Colonies usually appear after 4–6 weeks, and therefore communication with the clinical laboratory is important so that appropriate media will be used and the cultures will be held long enough for colonies to be detected.[96] Serologic assays for demonstration of rising antibody titers are retrospective. PCR detection is promising, but is not standardized.[146–148]

Alphaviruses (Encephalitic Syndromes: Venezuelan, Eastern, and Western Equine Encephalomyelitis)

Diagnosis is based on isolation of the virus from serum or brain (postmortem specimens) in a BSL-3 environment. PCR detection of viral sequences is also possible. Serologic diagnosis is based on demonstration of antibodies in acute and convalescent sera.[149–151]

Botulinum Toxins

The diagnosis of botulism relies heavily on clinical parameters. An afebrile patient with signs and symptoms of progressive bulbar palsies and descending neuromuscular paralysis is highly suspected of having botulism. Demonstration of the toxin due to ingestion of contaminated food is achieved by examination of gastric samples, feces, blood, and urine. However, detection of minute amounts of toxin would be difficult by current immunoassay systems such as ELISA platforms.[151] Detection techniques based on electrochemiluminescence and immunoliposomes are currently under development.[105,152] PCR assays can be performed in cases of ingestion of bacterially contaminated food in order to detect *C. botulinum*. If weaponized toxin is used in the absence of *C. botulinum* organisms, detection of the genetic material would be difficult and would rely on the presence of residual DNA after toxin purification procedures. If inhalational botulism is suspected, respiratory secretions and nasal swabs should be obtained as early as possible. Postmortem samples of liver and spleen can be used for detection of botulinum toxins.

Ricin Toxin

Diagnosis is based on clinical presentation and requires a high index of suspicion due to the nonspecific signs and symptoms. Laboratory diagnosis rests on detection of the toxin in body fluids by immunoassays (capture ELISA and IgG ELISA).[151] A new generation of tests using more sensitive detection methods is under development (see liposome PCR description, above).

Staphylococcal Enterotoxin B

Diagnosis is suspected on clinical grounds and confirmed by demonstration of the toxin in nasal swabs early in the disease, feces, and, in fatal cases, kidneys and lung tissue. Serum can be analyzed by ELISA, and PCR can be performed for detection of toxin genes of *S. aureus* if present.[151]

Development of Multiplex Detection Systems

The creation of an automated, easily deployable instrument capable of detecting all possible potential BT agents by highly sensitive techniques such as electrochemoluminescence or PCR would be ideal. The nonspecific nature of presenting symptoms is a major problem for several agents. An early diagnosis of the epidemic must be established, particularly for organisms such as *Y. pestis* in which there is only a short window for successful treatment. An example is the automated biological agent testing system (ABATS), that combines the above techniques.[92] The system integrates several commercially available technologies into one single automated, robotized instrument for detection of viruses, bacteria, and parasites considered potential BT agents. The technologies incorporated into this "super system" include automated specimen preparation (both nucleic acid-based and protein-based, such as immunodiagnostics), thermocyclers for PCR detection, electrochemiluminescence detectors for immunobased assays, sequencers, and software programs for sequence analysis. Another powerful system is the Ibis T5000 Universal BW sensor based on broad-range PCR and high-performance mass spectrometry.[153,154] This system is based on technology developed for the Department of Defense and known as TIGER (triangulation identification for the genetic evaluation of risks). Mass spectrometry of amplified products derives the identity of the agent based on the composition of amplicons. This technology has been used successfully to amplify nucleic acids of bacteria, viruses, fungi, and protozoans. Several pairs of broad-range primers are used in a multiplex format, and amplified products are analyzed by mass spectrometry followed by species/strain identification using sophisticated software systems. Liquid-based microassay bead systems (Luminex) are also providing an outstanding platform for development of multiplex detection systems.

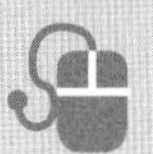

Access the complete reference list online at
http://www.expertconsult.com

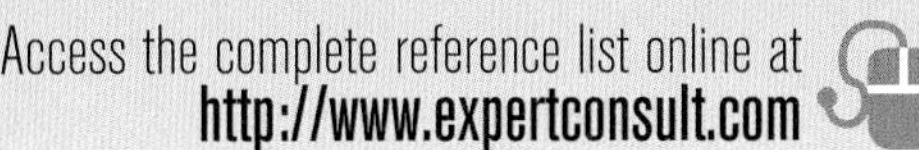
Access the complete reference list online at
http://www.expertconsult.com

CHAPTER 126

Health Advice for International Travel

Jay S. Keystone • Robert Steffen • Phyllis E. Kozarsky

INTRODUCTION

International travel has become increasingly common as travelers search out exotic vacation destinations or conduct business, government, or missionary activities in remote areas of the world. As tracked by the World Tourism Organization (WTO) (www.unwto.org), international tourism has grown from 25 million international arrivals in 1950 to over 600 million in 1998, and to greater than 900 million in 2008. WTO statistics show that travel from industrialized areas to developing countries has also been increasing, with Asia and the Pacific, and Africa and the Middle East now the emerging destinations.[1] In 2007, 51% of all international tourist arrivals was motivated by leisure, recreation and holidays – a total of 458 million. Business travel accounted for 15% (138 million), and 27% represented travel for other purposes, such as visiting friends and relatives (VFR), religious reasons/pilgrimages, and health treatment (240 million). Data from the US Department of Commerce report that the VFR component represents 34% of American travelers abroad. VFRs have some of the highest risks for acquisition abroad of many serious illnesses.

Unfortunately, studies continue to show that between 50% and 75% of short-term travelers to the tropics or subtropics report some health impairment, usually due to an infectious agent.[2–4] Although infectious diseases contribute substantially to morbidity, they account for only 1–4% of deaths among travelers.[5–9] Cardiovascular disease (CVD) and injuries are the most frequent causes of death among travelers, accounting for about 50% and 22% of deaths, respectively. If one excludes mortality due to CVD and preexisting illness, motor vehicle accidents account for >40% of the remaining causes of death. Age-specific rates of mortality due to CVD are similar to those of nontravelers, whereas injury deaths, the majority from motor vehicle accidents and drowning, are several times higher among travelers.[9]

The provision of health recommendations for international travelers is based on individual risk assessments and requirements (e.g., immunizations) according to the traveler's destinations. The estimated monthly prevalence of health problems (***Fig. 126.1***) includes such preventable diseases as traveler's diarrhea (in 30–80%, depending on destination), malaria (in 2.5% of travelers to West Africa without chemoprophylaxis), hepatitis A (0.003%), and typhoid fever (in 0.03% of travelers to India, West Africa, or Peru). The risk of acquiring illness depends on the area of the world visited, the length of stay, activities and location of travel within these areas, and the underlying health of the traveler. In addition, as mentioned above, an increasingly important group at particularly high risk for travel-related problems are VFRs.[10,11] Therefore, it is essential that the health advisor know:

- **Travel-related**
  - The country of origin
  - The itinerary
  - The departure date
  - The length of stay in each country
  - Whether travel will be rural or urban
  - The style of travel (e.g., first-class hotels versus local homes)
  - The reason for travel (including special activities like high-altitude exposures).
- **Host-related**
  - Whether the traveler has any health problems, including any immune deficiency, allergies
  - Does the traveler have any underlying chronic illness?
  - Current use of medication
  - History of seizures, psychiatric/emotional problems
  - History of jaundice
  - History of thymus operation, splenectomy
  - Problems from previous immunizations or adverse event due to antimalarial medications used for prophylaxis
  - In the case of a female traveler, whether or not she is planning pregnancy or is pregnant.

IMMUNIZATIONS

See ***Table 126.1***.

General Considerations

Immunizations for international travel can be categorized as: (1) *routine* childhood and adult immunizations (e.g., diphtheria, tetanus, pertussis, poliomyelitis, varicella, measles, mumps, and rubella, human papillomavirus); (2) *required* – those needed to cross international borders as required by international health regulations (e.g., yellow fever and meningococcal); and (3) *recommended* according to risk of illness (e.g., hepatitis A and B, unless it has become routine, typhoid, and rabies).

Several practical issues are germane regarding vaccine administration:

1. **Interrupted multidose schedules**: regardless of the duration of interruption of a schedule, there is no need to restart a primary series of immunizations. It is sufficient to continue where the series was interrupted.
2. **Simultaneous administration of vaccines**: inactivated and live vaccines can be administered simultaneously at separate sites. Theoretically, live vaccines should be administered simultaneously or 30 days apart because of possible interference of the immune response. Since live virus vaccines can interfere with an individual's response to tuberculin testing, the test should be done on the day of immunization or between 4 and 6 weeks later.
3. **Immunoglobulin administration**: when certain live attenuated vaccines are given with immunoglobulin, the antibody response may be diminished. This caveat does not apply to yellow

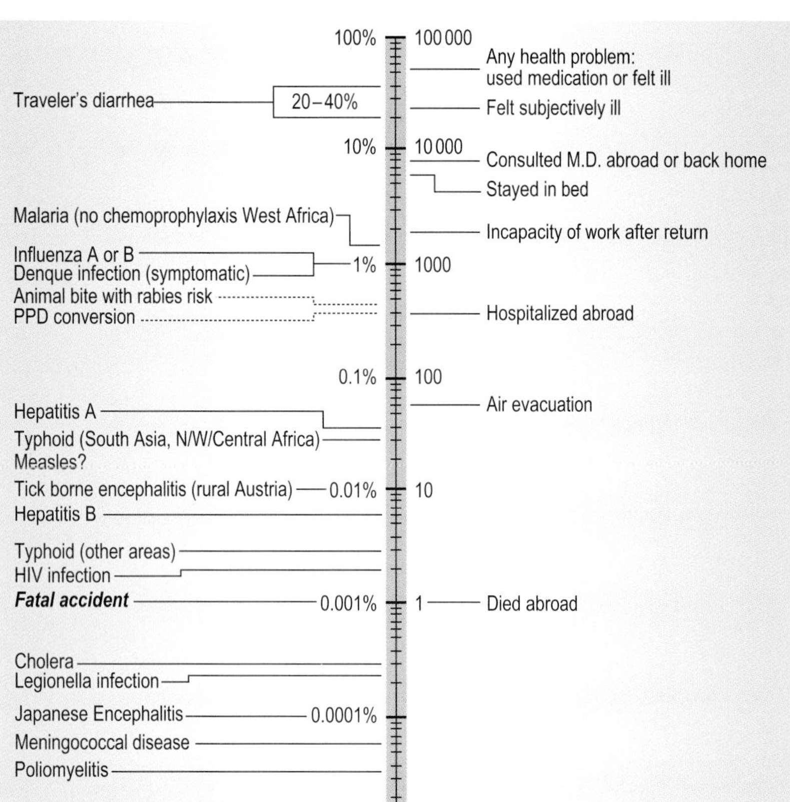

Figure 126.1 Incidence rate per month of infections and fatal accidents among travellers in developing countries (2010). PPD, purified protein derivative. (R. Steffen, unpublished, personal communication.)

Table 126.1 Immunizations for International Travel

Vaccine	Type	Schedule	Indications	Precautions and Contraindications	Side-Effects
Routine					
Diphtheria–tetanus–pertussis, *Haemophilus influenzae b*		See references 12, 13			
Hepatitis A	Inactivated viral (Havrix) GSK	Primary: 1 dose IM; 2nd dose at 6–12 months Booster: not recommended	All non-immunes to developing countries	P – safety data not available; immunize according to risk H – 2-phenoxyethanol	~50% have mild local reactions, ~3–10% have mild systemic reactions (headache, malaise)
	Inactivated (Vaqta) MF	Primary: 1 dose IM; 2nd dose at 6 months Booster: not recommended	All non-immunes to developing countries	P – safety data not available; immunize according to risk H – neomycin	~50% have mild local reactions, ~3% have mild systemic reactions (fever, fatigue, abdominal pain)
Hepatitis B[c]	Recombinant-derived hepatitis B surface antigen (Recombivax HB), MF (Engerix-B), GSK	Primary: 2 doses 1 month apart; 3rd dose 5 months after second Booster: not recommended	Health care workers in contact with blood; persons residing in areas of high endemicity for hepatitis B surface antigen; others at risk for contact with blood, body fluids, or potentially contaminated medical or dental instruments	P – not a contraindication	10–20% have mild local reactions, occasional mild systemic reactions (fever, headache, fatigue)
Influenza	Inactivated and live attenuated influenza A and B viruses	See references 12, 13; one dose annually	All travelers without contraindications	H – eggs, unless cell culture vaccine used	<35% mild local reactions; occasional systemic reactions; rare allergic reactions

Table 126.1 Immunizations for International Travel—cont'd

Vaccine	Type	Schedule	Indications	Precautions and Contraindications	Side-Effects
Measles	Live attenuated virus (available in monovalent form or combined with rubella (MR) or mumps (MMR))	Primary: 2 doses; see text for interval between doses Booster: none	Persons born after 1956 who have not had documented measles infection or have not received 2 doses of live measles vaccine	I – contraindicated (HIV not a contraindication) H – eggs or neomycin	Temperature of ≥39.4°C, 5–21 days after vaccination, in 5–15%; transient rash in 5%; 4–55% have a local reaction
Meningococcal (A, C, Y, W-135)	Polysaccharide conjugate	Primary: 1 dose Booster: 3–5 years Primary: 1 dose Booster: at 3 years if first at <7 years age; at 5 years if first at >7 years age	Required for entry into Saudi Arabia during the Hajj and Umrah Recommended for African meningitis belt during the dry season (December–June) and in regions where meningococcal disease is highly endemic or epidemic	P – safety unknown	Local reactions, fever (2%)
Mumps	Live attenuated virus	Primary: 2 doses (usually given as part of MMR vaccine) Booster: none	Persons born after 1956 who have not had documented mumps	H – eggs or neomycin	Mild allergic reactions uncommon; rarely parotitis
Poliomyelitis	Live attenuated virus, trivalent	Primary: 3 doses PO, the first 2 given at 6–8-week intervals, the 3rd, 8–12 months later Booster: 1 dose PO	Only used in developing countries	Immunocompromised contacts of recipients; not used for primary immunization in persons >18 years	Rarely paralysis
Poliomyelitis	Inactivated virus, trivalent; enhanced	Primary: 2 doses at 4–8-week intervals; 3rd dose 6–12 months after 2nd dose Booster: 1 lifetime dose	Preferred for persons 18 years and older and for immunocompromised hosts[a]	P – safety unknown H – streptomycin or neomycin	Mild local reaction
Rubella	Live attenuated virus	Primary: 1 dose (usually given as part of MR or MMR) Booster: none, unless given as MMR	All persons, particularly women of childbearing age, without documented illness or live vaccine on or after 1st birthday	H – neomycin P – contraindicated I – contraindicated	Up to 40% postpubertal females have joint pains, transient arthritis, beginning 3–25 days after vaccination, persisting 1–11 days; frank arthritis in <2%
Tetanus–diphtheria (Tdap)	Adsorbed toxoids (acellular pertussis)	Primary: 2 doses (0.5 mL) IM, 4–8 weeks apart; 3rd dose 6–12 months later Booster: every 10 years	All adults (Tdap × 1)	P – first trimester contraindicated Hypersensitivity or neurologic reaction to previous doses; severe local reaction	Local reactions, occasional fever, systemic symptoms Arthus-like reactions in persons with multiple previous boosters, rarely systemic allergy
Varicella	Live attenuated virus	Primary: 2 doses 4–8 weeks apart Booster: ?	Persons without a history of varicella	P, I – contraindicated H – neomycin	Fever (10%), rash (8%), local reaction (25–30%)
Required					
Yellow fever	Live attenuated virus	Primary: 1 dose (10 days to 10 years before travel) Booster: every 10 years	As required by individual countries	P – only high-risk travel Prudent to avoid vaccinating infants <9 months I – contraindicated H – eggs	Mild headache, myalgia, fever, 5–10 days after vaccination (2–5%), rarely immediate hypersensitivity
Recommended					
Cholera, oral[b]	*Vibrio cholerae*	Primary: 2 doses 1–6 weeks apart at least 6 days before travel Booster: 6 months	As required by few countries	P – safety unknown Previous severe local or systemic reaction	

Table 126.1 Immunizations for International Travel—cont'd

Vaccine	Type	Schedule	Indications	Precautions and Contraindications	Side-Effects
Encephalitis, tick-borne	Killed vaccine available in Europe and Canada	Depending on vaccine brand used	Exposure in endemic areas	Serious adverse reactions to previous doses	Local reactions, rarely fever
Encephalitis, Japanese	Inactivated	Primary: 2 doses 1 month apart	Rural areas in risk countries of Asia, particularly prolonged exposure	P – avoid in pregnancy unless high-risk travel H – allergic reaction to prior doses (thimerosal)	Local reactions (20%), systemic reactions (10%), allergic reactions (0.1%)
Combined hepatitis A/B	Inactivated viral A and recombinant B surface antigen (Twinrix) GSK	Primary: 2 doses 1 month apart; dose 3, 5 months after second Booster: none Alternate schedule: 0, 7, 21 days + booster at 1 year	As for hepatitis A and B (Havrix and Engerix B)	As for hepatitis A and B (Havrix and Engerix B)	As for hepatitis A and B (Havrix and Engerix B)
Immunoglobulin	Fractionated immunoglobulins	Travel of <3 months duration: 0.02 mL/kg Travel 4–6 months: 0.06 mL/kg	Infants <12 months, allergy to vaccine, immunocompromised		Transient local discomfort; rare systemic reaction
Meningococcal	See Routine				
Pneumococcal	Capsular polysaccharide	Primary: once Booster: 5 years for chronic illness, splenectomy, immunocompromised	Elderly, chronic illness, splenectomy, Hodgkin's disease	P – no studies available Not recommended <2 years of age	Local reactions (71%), rarely fever, arthritis, rash, urticaria, serum sickness
Rabies	Inactivated virus grown in human diploid cells	Preexposure: days 0, 7, and 21 or 28 Booster: 2 doses if possible exposure to rabies	Travel to areas for >1 month where rabies is a constant threat	H – allergy to previous doses P – not contraindicated in high-risk persons; ID route should be completed >30 days before travel; ID route should not be used with concurrent chloroquine or mefloquine administration	~30% have local reactions, ~20% have mild systemic reactions of headache, nausea, aches, and dizziness, rarely neurologic illness, occasional (6%) immune complex reactions with booster doses occurring 2–21 days after vaccination
Typhoid, oral	Live attenuated (Vivotif Berna)	Primary: 1 capsule every other day for 4 doses[d] Booster: same dose every 5 years	Rural or prolonged travel in a risk area, especially VFRs to South Asia	I, P – contraindicated Not recommended <6 years	Infrequent gastrointestinal upset (nausea, vomiting, diarrhea), rash, mild systemic reactions
Typhoid, injectable	Vi capsular polysaccharide (Typhim Vi)	Primary: 1 dose Booster: every 2 years	Rural or prolonged travel in a risk area, especially VFRs to South Asia	Not recommended <2 years Previous severe local or systemic reaction lasting 1–2 days	Local reaction of pain, swelling, and induration, occasional systemic reaction

H, hypersensitivity; I, immunocompromised; ID, intradermal; IM, intramuscularly; P, pregnancy; PO, orally; HIV, human immunodeficiency virus.

[a]Immunocompromised persons include patients with immunodeficiency diseases, leukemia, lymphoma, generalized malignancy or acquired immunodeficiency syndrome, or immunosuppression from therapy with corticosteroids, alkylating agents, antimetabolites, or radiation.

[b]Unofficially required for entry into some countries contrary to World Health Organization recommendations; not available in the United States.

[c]Ideally, all travelers should be immunized.

[d]In Canada: 1 sachet every other day for three doses.

(Adapted from Hill D. Immunizations. Infect Dis Clin North Am. 1992;6:291–312.)

fever vaccine. However, the measles–mumps–rubella (MMR) vaccine and its component vaccines should be delayed after immunoglobulin administration; the duration of delay is dependent on the purpose for which the immunoglobulin was administered – for example, 3, 4, and 5 months for hepatitis A, rabies, and measles or varicella prophylaxis, respectively.

4. **Hypersensitivity to vaccine components**: the most common animal protein allergen is egg protein in vaccines prepared from embryonated chicken eggs (e.g., yellow fever and egg-derived influenza vaccines) or gelatin (e.g., MMR). Screening people by asking whether they can eat eggs without an allergic reaction is a good way to identify those who may be at risk from embryonated chicken egg vaccines. Preservatives such as thimerosal or trace amounts of antibiotics such as neomycin may cause a hypersensitivity reaction to a vaccine; however, thimerosal has been removed from the majority of these products. The package insert should be reviewed carefully if the traveler gives a history of hypersensitivity.
5. **Altered immunocompetence**: inactivated vaccines pose no danger to the immunocompromised host, although the immune response to these vaccines may be suboptimal. Since virus replication after administration of live attenuated vaccines can be

enhanced in the immunocompromised host, live vaccines generally should be avoided in such people. Exceptions apply in the recommendations for yellow fever and measles immunization in some infected with human immunodeficiency virus-1 (HIV) infection.

6. **Pregnancy**: live vaccines are contraindicated during pregnancy, except for yellow fever vaccine in those at very high risk. Detailed travel health recommendations for pregnant women and children are available from the Centers for Disease Control and Prevention (CDC) in *Health Information for International Travel*[12] and from other sources.[13–15] The CDC guide, accessible at www.cdc.gov/travel, also provides a complete discussion of the general principles and specific country-by-country requirements for immunizations.
7. **Infants**: immunization of infants may be started at birth for hepatitis B and injectable polio vaccine; at 4 and 6 weeks for diphtheria–tetanus–acellular pertussis (DTP) and *Haemophilus influenzae* b (Hib) vaccines, respectively; at 6 months for measles; and 1 year for hepatitis A and varicella (followed by full recommended schedules).

Routine Immunizations

Travel is an excellent opportunity to update a person's "childhood" immunizations, such as DTP (or TdaP), MMR, polio, hepatitis B, and varicella. The influenza vaccine should be administered when available to those without contraindications and the pneumococcal vaccine should be considered. Guidance on routine adult immunizations is available in the recommendations of the Advisory Committee on Immunization Practices,[16] in the *Canadian Immunization Guide*,[17] and in other guidelines issued by national expert bodies.

Required Immunizations

Yellow fever vaccination may be a legal requirement for all travelers planning to enter either countries where the disease is present, or countries that are concerned about importation of this viral infection. For the latter, especially some countries in Asia, vaccination may be required for those who have recently transited through countries either known or thought to harbor yellow fever virus. Yellow fever (see Chapter 74) has been reemerging in recent years, and fatalities in tourists have been documented.[18] The risk of yellow fever is highest in sub-Saharan Africa, estimated to be as high at 1 : 250 per 2-week stay during an epidemic and 1 : 2500 between epidemics. The risk in South America is considerably less – approximately 1 : 25 000 for a 2-week exposure.[19]

A World Health Organization (WHO)-sanctioned vaccine must be administered at an approved yellow fever vaccination center.[20] Vaccinees should receive a signed and stamped International Certificate of Vaccination or Prophylaxis, commonly referred to as the "yellow card." The vaccine is recommended for persons 9 months of age or older who are traveling or living in areas at risk for yellow fever transmission in South America and Africa (as specified on WHO and CDC websites: www.who.int/ith and www.cdc.gov/travel). However, a risk:benefit analysis concerning use of the vaccine is important, particularly among senior travelers, because of the risk of severe adverse reactions that may occur in 1 : 200 000–1 : 300 000 vaccinees overall, and in 1 : 50 000 of the elderly.[19–22] Yellow fever vaccine is contraindicated in those with allergy to vaccine components, age <6 months, symptomatic HIV infection or $CD4^{+}$ T lymphocytes <200/mm^3, thymus disorders, primary immunodeficiencies, malignant neoplasms, transplantation, or immunosuppressive and immunomodulatory therapies (including recent radiation treatments) and during breastfeeding.[21] Precautions about yellow fever vaccinations are indicated for those 6–8 months of age, aged ≥60 years, with asymptomatic HIV infection and $CD4^{+}$ T cells counts of 200–499/mm^3, and who are pregnant or breastfeeding.[21]

Although no country officially requires administration of cholera vaccine for entry, documentation of vaccination has been requested at times at few remote borders. The risk of cholera (see Chapter 20) among travelers is extremely low (1 : 500 000 travelers).[23,24] A single available vaccine (oral B-subunit whole-cell cholera vaccine) provides approximately 85% protection for about 6 months, but is not effective against the serotype O139, which has been spreading throughout Asia.[25,26] The vaccine, available in Canada and some European countries, but not the United States, is recommended only for health care workers, backpackers, and other volunteers working in highly endemic areas (e.g., refugee camps) who are likely to be exposed to infection.

Saudi Arabia requires pilgrims to Mecca during the Hajj and Umrah to be immunized with a quadrivalent meningococcal vaccine containing A, C, Y, and W-135 serotypes.[12] Documentation of polio vaccination must be presented for infants and children up to 15 years of age. Proof of influenza immunizations (seasonal and H1N1) may be required.

Recommended Immunization

Hepatitis A (see Chapter 64) is one of the most frequent vaccine-preventable infections of travelers.[27–32] In one study, the incidence of symptomatic infection during a 1-month stay in a developing country ranged from 3 cases per 1000 in resort areas but increased to 20 per 1000 for those who strayed from the usual tourist routes.[27] Recent studies suggest that the risk is lower at 0.003%. Mortality from hepatitis A infection increases with age and reaches 2.1% in those older than age 40 years and almost 3% by the age of 50.[33] Although most infants and young children are asymptomatic when infected, they pose a health risk to others due to the ease of fecal–oral spread of this virus.[33,34] Hepatitis A vaccination is recommended for all international travelers to developing countries. Hepatitis A vaccines are highly efficacious, with seroconversion rates of almost 100% by the second dose.[35,36] Within 2 weeks of the first dose, between 70% and 85% of vaccinees will have protective levels of antibody, but most experts believe that protection against symptomatic infection is achieved even if the first dose is given on the day of departure. However, this may not be the case in older travelers whose immune response may be slower than younger vaccinees.[37]

It is important to note that antibody measurements by routine laboratories following immunization with hepatitis A vaccines have a sensitivity of approximately 50%. Simultaneous administration of serum immunoglobulin may reduce peak antibody levels; however, this has not been shown to interfere with long-term protection.[38] Simultaneous administration of immunoglobulin with hepatitis A vaccine even with imminent travel is not recommended. Following primary immunization hepatitis A vaccines provide lifetime immunity without subsequent booster immunizations.[39]

When assessed prior to routine vaccination, the monthly incidence of hepatitis B infection (see Chapter 66), both symptomatic and asymptomatic, was 80–240 cases per 100 000 for long-stay overseas workers who were at considerable risk for hepatitis B.[40] Canadian, UK, and Australian studies have subsequently shown that about 15–18% of short-term travelers were at risk from blood and body fluid exposure.[41–43] Of pertinence to the risk of acquiring hepatitis B from unsterile equipment, one study reported the likelihood of receiving an injection from unsterile equipment to be as high as 80% in some countries.[44] In one study, 8% of US travelers received medical care abroad, of whom 17% received an injection.[45] Recombinant hepatitis B vaccines are highly effective and likely provide lifelong protection.[46] Some experts believe that hepatitis B immunization, if not recommended as a "universal vaccine," is appropriate for all international travelers regardless of length of stay and style of travel. Moderate- and high-risk areas for hepatitis B include all of Africa, Asia (except Japan), Greenland, Alaska, some islands of the Caribbean, and Latin America.[47,48]

Since 97% of international travelers are repeat travelers, providing both hepatitis A and B immunizations for all travelers regardless of their itinerary is a lifetime investment. Immunizations for both hepatitis A and B can be easily achieved with the combined hepatitis A and B vaccine that provides excellent protection against both viruses and may be administered in an accelerated schedule that can be completed within 21 days for protection lasting at least 1 year. An additional dose 1 year later is recommended for long-lasting protection.[49]

The risk of typhoid fever (see Chapter 16) has been estimated to be 1 per 30 000 per month of stay in the developing world; however, attack rates have been documented to be 10-fold higher in south Asia (India, Pakistan, and Bangladesh).[50,51] Within these areas, rates are particularly high among VFRs and those traveling off the usual tourist routes. Reviews of typhoid fever in the United States and Quebec, Canada reported that 77% and 86% of all cases, respectively, occurred among the VFR population.[51,52]

Typhoid immunization is often recommended for special risk groups, including those with destinations in south Asia, VFRs, travel off usual tourist routes in endemic areas, and long-stay travelers. Recommended typhoid vaccines are the live attenuated multidose oral vaccine developed from the Ty 21a mutant strain of *Salmonella typhi* and the Vi capsular polysaccharide vaccine administered intramuscularly in a single dose. Both vaccines protect 55–75% of recipients, depending in part on the degree of exposure to the organism.[53–55] The oral vaccine appears to provide longer protection when four capsules are taken as marketed in North America (4–5 years versus 2–3 years), but in Europe, where only three packets are sold, protection is more limited. The oral vaccine may be associated with compliance problems because vaccine administration is undertaken by the recipient. A combined hepatitis A/typhoid vaccine has been marketed globally, but is not yet available in the United States.[56]

The risk of meningococcal disease (see Chapter 24) appears to be greatest among travelers who live among indigenous populations in overcrowded conditions in high-risk areas.[57] Meningococcal vaccine is recommended for long-stay travelers to the meningitis belt in sub-Saharan Africa (the savannah region extending from Guinea to Ethiopia) or for short-term travelers to this area during the dry season (December to June). A study in Saudi Arabia showed that although the polysaccharide vaccine protected against disease, a number of travelers transmitted the infection to household contacts on return.[58] Since the conjugate quadrivalent meningococcal vaccine has been shown to reduce nasal carriage of *Neisseria meningitidis*, it would be the vaccine of choice for international travelers.

Japanese encephalitis (JE) (see Chapter 76) is a mosquito-borne, viral encephalitis found throughout much of the rural Indian subcontinent and Southeast Asia.[59] The risk of JE is roughly 1 per 5000 per month of stay in an endemic rural area. Twenty-four cases of JE were reported in travelers from 1978 through 1992 with a similar number reported in the time period from 1992 to 2008.[60] Those more recently reported from the United States were in Asian immigrants who had traveled to rural areas visiting friends and relatives and did not perceive any risk.[61] Among Europeans many were short-term beach vacationers with no obvious risk factors, e.g., in Bali. Although most infections are asymptomatic, among those who develop clinical disease the case-fatality rate may be as high as 30%, with severe neurologic sequelae occurring in 50% of survivors.[63] A new vero cell culture-derived inactivated JE vaccine has been shown to be immunologically noninferior to the prior mouse brain-derived vaccine and to have a better safety profile;[62] it has not been associated with allergic reactions. The only downside is that the schedule requires 2 doses 1 month apart, making it difficult to protect the last-minute traveler. The new vaccine is currently available in the United States except for those under age 17, where the older mouse brain-derived vaccine is still being used.[64] Typically, JE vaccine has been reserved for those with overnight stays in rural endemic areas for greater than 3 weeks;[65] but rather than just the length of travel, circumstances of the traveler and itinerary that affect the risk of illness should dictate the importance of vaccine administration.

Each year a few cases of rabies (see Chapter 79) have been reported in travelers, but there are no data on the risk of infection. The incidence of animal bites per 1000 per month of stay ranges from 1.7 to 3.6. The risk may be as high as 2% per year.[66,67] A study of 815 Israeli travelers showed that the risk of potential rabies exposure from an animal bite was 2.66 per 1000 travelers per month.[68] A 3-year study in Nepal showed that the incidence of possible rabies exposures among tourists was 1.9 per 1000 people per year.[69] From 1980 to 1992, five imported cases of rabies in US citizens were reported; in three of these cases, the source of infection was a bite from a pet dog.[70] Risk is highest among children, who may not report bites and who tend to have a greater affinity for small animals. Approximately 40% of bites are in children, of which the majority are on the head and neck.[71,72] A study utilizing the GeoSentinal database found that almost 50% of potential exposures occurred with the first month of travel; this finding contradicts the usual recommendation that rabies vaccine should be recommended mostly for long-stay travelers.[73]

Travelers to the developing world should be counseled on avoidance of animals, particularly dogs, prompt and thorough cleansing of animal bite wounds, and postexposure rabies prophylaxis. Pre-exposure immunization is recommended for prolonged travel (because of cost considerations), for those with an occupational risk of exposure (e.g., veterinarians and spelunkers), and for participants on bicycle tours (magnets for dogs) in areas where rabies is a significant threat.[71,75] Of note, the Advisory Committee on Immunization Practices with its international consultant group met in June of 2009 and recommended a reduced number of postexposure injections. (For CDC recommendations see http://www.cdc.gov/vaccines/recs/provisional/downloads/rabies-July2009-508.pdf.)

TUBERCULOSIS

People who live for prolonged periods in developing countries and those who have close contact with locals are at increased risk of exposure to tuberculosis (see Chapter 35). For nonmedical travelers the risk of tuberculosis infection is estimated to be approximately 3% per year.[76] The efficacy of bacille Calmette–Guérin (BCG) is still debated, although the vaccine is not currently marketed in the United States. However, WHO and many European countries recommend BCG only for exposed infants younger than 12 months of age, as vaccination is probably ineffective in older children and adults. Side effects, ranging from draining abscesses at the site of immunization (common) to disseminated infection (rare), must be weighed against the risk of exposure to active tuberculosis for the traveler – a risk that varies directly with the intimacy and duration of contact with the indigenous population. If BCG vaccine is not administered, long-stay travelers (>3 months) should have at least one baseline tuberculin skin test placed before travel and repeated at 1- or 2-year intervals (3 months after exposure) if the risk continues.

TRAVELER'S DIARRHEA

Several studies have shown that diarrhea is the most frequent health impairment among travelers to developing countries, affecting one- to two-thirds of all travelers.[77–81] Among those who become ill, 30% will remain in bed and another 40% will have to curtail their activities.[77] In general, countries with higher standards of living present lower risks of traveler's diarrhea.[80–83] Although all age groups are at risk, the incidence is highest among the very young, presumably due to increased fecal–oral contamination;[84] those with decreased gastric acidity;[85] and those in the 15–29-year-old age group, probably because of their adventurous lifestyle and ingestion of larger amounts of potentially contaminated foods.[80,86,87] Bacterial pathogens are the most frequent cause of traveler's diarrhea, particularly enterotoxigenic *Escherichia coli* (ETEC), enteroadherent *E. coli* (EAEC), and *Shigella*, *Salmonella*, and *Campylobacter* species.[88] The prevalence of each organism varies according to season and destination.[83] When counseling travelers about diarrhea, several issues must be considered: food and water precautions, chemoprophylaxis, self-treatment of illness, and immunization.

Food and Water Precautions

Unpeeled fruits, uncooked vegetables, and food that has been cooked or stored at insufficiently hot or cold temperatures, respectively, are believed to be the main sources of enteric pathogens for the traveler. An additional important source is unpurified water and ice cubes made from it. Tap water and ice cubes should be avoided unless there are strong assurances of proper treatment. Organisms in contaminated ice will survive concentrations of alcohol found in drinks mixed with tequila and whisky.[89] Since swallowed water can lead to infection, swimming in water that is potentially contaminated by sewage should also be avoided.[90]

Tea or coffee is safe if consumed hot. Commercially bottled, carbonated beverages are recommended since carbonation results in an acid pH that will effectively kill bacteria over a period of several days.[90] Unpasteurized milk and milk products should be avoided.[91] If safe beverages are not available, travelers may need to disinfect water from potentially contaminated sources. Since almost all enteropathogens are killed at 100°C, bringing water to the boil is sufficient for disinfection.[92] Tap water "too hot to touch" has not been shown to be reliably disinfected; even in situations in which a low inoculum of organisms may be transmitted, such as in toothbrushing, bottled water is preferred.

Although not effective for resistant cysts such as *Cryptosporidium* and *Giardia*, chemical disinfection with the halogens iodine or chlorine is an otherwise effective method of water purification. Two drops (0.1 mL) of 5% chlorine bleach or four drops of 2% tincture of iodine should be added to 1 liter of water and allowed to stand for 30 minutes at room temperature (20°C) before using.[90] Commercial tablets and iodine crystals serve the same purpose; however, it is important to note that colder water temperatures and turbidity will inhibit the purification process, necessitating a longer contact time.[92,93] Chlorine dioxide (Pristine) appears to be more effective and better tolerated than standard halides and, with sufficient contact time, will eradicate *Cryptosporidium* cysts.[94]

Unlike the straightforward approaches to water and beverage precautions, avoidance of contaminated food entails considerably more restrictions. Raw foods are best avoided. Not only should food be well cooked but also it should be served hot, that is at 140°F/60°C. Reheated foods may not be safe because of the presence of preformed heat-stable toxins. Since vegetables are not infrequently grown in "night soil" (human excrement used for fertilizer) or washed with fecally contaminated water before display, they should be well cooked or treated adequately. Only fruit that can be peeled by the traveler should be eaten. Pastries are an excellent source of substrates for bacterial proliferation.

It should be noted that the location where meals are taken is important. Studies from Mexico have shown that the incidence of traveler's diarrhea is higher when food is purchased from street vendors or restaurants or eaten at the homes of locals than when travelers prepare their own meals.[95]

Unfortunately, many studies have shown that education regarding food and water precautions has a decidedly low efficacy in the prevention of traveler's diarrhea. In one study, stricter observance of precautions was associated with a greater likelihood of acquiring diarrhea, explained by a recall bias.[96] In a subsequent prospective study, 98% of international travelers committed dietary indiscretions within 3 days; the incidence of diarrhea was proportional to the number of "mistakes" made.[97] If one considers the standard precautions outlined previously, it is clear that flawless observance may be virtually impossible, particularly among vacationers, who, wanting to relax and indulge in local cuisine, are more likely to be noncompliant with food precautions. As noted by David Shlim, "personal hygiene precautions, when performed under the direct supervision of an expatriate operating his or her own kitchen, can prevent traveler's diarrhea, but poor restaurant hygiene in most developing countries continues to create an insurmountable risk of acquiring traveler's diarrhea."[98] For this reason, the concepts of chemoprophylaxis and self-treatment have gained popularity in recent years. One particularly insightful colleague noted, "Boil it, peel it, cook it, or forget it – easy to remember, impossible to do" (Lawrence Green, personal communication, 1995).

Chemoprophylaxis

A variety of pharmacologic interventions have been evaluated to prevent traveler's diarrhea. Since bacterial pathogens account for the majority of episodes of traveler's diarrhea,[99–101] antibiotics and bismuth subsalicylate (BSS) have been the focus of testing for its prevention. BSS, an insoluble salt of bismuth and salicylic acid, is hydrolyzed in the stomach to bismuth oxychloride and salicylate. The exact mechanism of its action is not completely understood, but it appears to involve both antimicrobial activity linked to the bismuth moiety and antisecretory activity associated with the salicylate portion.[102,103] Studies of BSS have shown a protective effect of up to 65% with the liquid form, 60 mL four times per day (4.2 g/day), or tablet form, two tablets four times daily (2.1 g/day).[104] BSS is generally safe but should be avoided in those with salicylate hypersensitivity or in those already taking salicylates, anticoagulants, or antihyperuricemic drugs. Also, BSS interferes with absorption of doxycycline, which may be used for malaria, rickettsial, and leptospiral chemoprophylaxis and for treatment. Studies of the use of lactobacilli to prevent traveler's diarrhea have shown minimal or no efficacy.[105–109] The protective efficacy of antibiotics for traveler's diarrhea varies with the season and geographic area visited, which in turn determine the likely pathogens and degree of antibiotic resistance.[110] The widespread use and abuse of antimicrobial agents globally have resulted in the emergence of resistant organisms, particularly enteric pathogens.[83] Previously used antibiotics for the prophylaxis of traveler's diarrhea, such as doxycycline and trimethoprim sulfa, are no longer recommended due to significant bacterial resistance in most areas of the world.

In view of their activity against most bacterial enteropathogens, quinolone antibiotics have become the agents of choice for the prevention and treatment of traveler's diarrhea. Protective efficacy has ranged from 88% to 94% in various areas of the world.[111–113] However, reports of quinolone resistance are increasing. In Thailand and Egypt, approximately 90% and 50%, respectively, of *Campylobacter* isolates were resistant to ciprofloxacin but sensitive to azithromycin.[114,115] Quinolone resistance rates among travelers with diarrhea, however, were markedly lower.[88] Although toxicity from quinolones remains low, these agents can cause central nervous system symptoms, which potentially could be aggravated by antimalarials such as chloroquine or mefloquine and may augment xanthine or theophylline toxicity. Also, quinolones may cause tendinitis with subsequent Achilles tendon rupture, especially in those who are immunosuppressed and the elderly. Although quinolones are not recommended for children or pregnant women, a number of travel medicine and pediatric infectious disease experts use very short-term quinolone regimens for self-treatment in children who develop traveler's diarrhea. Rifaximin, a nonabsorbable antibiotic, is another option for the prophylaxis for bacterial diarrhea, though it is only approved by the Food and Drug Administration (FDA) for the treatment of noninvasive strains of *E. coli*.[116,117] Comparative trials have shown that rifaximin is equally effective as quinolone antibiotics for this use and some use it for both prevention and treatment of traveler's diarrhea in general.[118] Although there is no approved indication for prophylaxis, some consider it very helpful, especially since a significant number of travelers may suffer from prolonged postinfectious irritable bowel syndrome, which the drug could prevent.[119–122]

The indications for antibiotic prophylaxis of traveler's diarrhea are controversial since it is well established that self-treatment regimens are highly effective in shortening the course of illness;[123,124] however, they have not been shown to prevent postinfectious irritable bowel syndrome. Routine use of antibiotic prophylaxis in traveler's diarrhea has not been endorsed by the National Institute of Health Consensus Development Conference,[78] and this view was reiterated at a meeting of traveler's diarrhea experts.[125] Even strong advocates of chemoprophylaxis do not recommend its routine use.[126–129] Prophylaxis with BSS, a quinolone antibiotic, or rifaximin may be considered for less than 3 weeks' duration for the following groups of travelers: those who repeatedly develop diarrhea during their travels, those with diminished protective gastric acidity, those who cannot afford incapacity for even 1 day (e.g., athletes, military personnel, and businesspeople), and those with an underlying medical disorder for whom traveler's diarrhea may be poorly tolerated (e.g., those suffering from inflammatory bowel disease, brittle insulin-dependent diabetes mellitus, chronic renal failure, or acquired immunodeficiency syndrome (AIDS), although the last group should take extra care to avoid such potentially devastating infections as cryptosporidiosis, not prevented by antimicrobial agents). Vaccine development against traveler's diarrhea has focused on preventing ETEC since it is responsible for the majority of cases. Because of the similarity between the cholera toxin and heat-labile toxin of ETEC, efficacy studies of the oral cholera B subunit whole-cell vaccine to prevent traveler's diarrhea showed an overall protective efficacy of 23%, which increased to 52% when ETEC was isolated and to 60% when ETEC was associated with another pathogen. This cross-protection was extremely short-lived, lasting less than 3 months.[129] Those receiving this cholera vaccine must still use food and water precautions and carry an antibiotic for self-treatment of diarrhea due to other pathogens.

Self-Treatment

The overriding principle in the management of traveler's diarrhea is the maintenance of an adequate fluid and electrolyte balance. Rehydration can be achieved with tea with sugar, bottled soft drinks, juices, or electrolyte-containing oral rehydration solutions such as those formulated by WHO.[131,132] Because of damage to the intestinal lactase-producing cells by enteric pathogens, dairy products should be avoided during illness.

When dysenteric symptoms are absent, nonantibiotic preparations alone may be useful in the management of traveler's diarrhea. BSS 30 mL every 30 minutes for eight doses reduces diarrhea by 25%.[133] Loperamide up to 16 mg per 24 hours reduces the duration of diarrhea by 42%[134] and is more effective than BSS[135] for diarrhea reduction and abdominal pain but less effective for nausea. However, loperamide should be avoided for monotherapy during bouts of dysentery, pragmatically defined as diarrhea with fever and/or blood admixed to the stools, unless used with an antibiotic. Kaolin- and pectin-containing agents are not very effective.[136] Therapy with lactobacilli or other probiotics has not been shown to be effective in modifying the course of traveler's diarrhea.[137]

Few would disagree that most travelers should carry an antimotility agent and an antibiotic for self-treatment of diarrhea that occurs during travel.[138,139] Many studies have shown that antimicrobial therapy leads to symptomatic improvement and a reduction in the duration of illness, particularly in those infected with ETEC and *Shigella*[123,124] (***Table 126.2***).

Antimicrobial therapy of nontyphoidal salmonellosis remains controversial because of the potential for antibiotics to prolong excretion of the organism, although the duration of illness is decreased with the use of quinolones.[123] A recent multinational study from Asia revealed that reduced susceptibility to ciprofloxacin in nontyphoid *Salmonella* isolates was common in Taiwan (48%) and Thailand (46%) and in *S. enterica* serotypes Choleraesuis (69%) and Virchow (75%) from all seven countries. In contrast, a study among returned Finnish travelers to Thailand and Malaysia showed that reduced fluoroquinolone susceptibility in *S. enterica* isolates had decreased from 65% to 22% from 2003 to 2007. A study of US soldiers in Thailand has led to concern about the continued usefulness of quinolone antibiotics for the management of traveler's diarrhea because of *Campylobacter* resistance.[115] Although azithromycin was an efficacious alternative, the drug was less effective than ciprofloxacin against other pathogens.

Two different studies in Mexico showed that rifaximin and azithromycin were as effective as ciprofloxacin for treatment of traveler's diarrhea.[118,140] More data are needed to confirm these results in different geographic areas.

Thus quinolones and, particularly in Southeast Asia, azithromycin have become the antibiotics of choice for self-treatment; rifaximin may also be considered for noninvasive illness. Studies have shown single-dose therapy and 3–5-day courses to be equally effective, except when *Shigella dysenteriae* is the offending pathogen.[124,141–144] The combination of antibiotics with loperamide for traveler's diarrhea has been shown to be more effective than the antibiotic alone.[145,146]

Table 126.2 Treatment of Traveler's Diarrhea

Drug	Dose	Duration (Days)
Standard Dose		
Rifaximin	200 mg tid	3
Norfloxacin	400 mg bid	3–5
Ciprofloxacin	500 mg qd/bid	1–5
Ofloxacin	300 mg bid	3
Levofloxacin	500 mg qd	3
Azithromycin	500 mg qd	3
Bismuth subsalicylate	30 mL q 30 min for 8 doses	
Single Dose, Standard Therapy		
Azithromycin	1000 mg	
Norfloxacin	800 mg	
Ciprofloxacin	500 mg to 1 g	
Fleroxacin	400 mg	

MALARIA

More than 30 000 cases of malaria (see Chapter 96) were diagnosed in North America and Europe each year.[147] A proportion of these were in immigrants, refugees, and other visitors, but the majority were travelers. Studies have shown that the majority of travelers who acquire malaria are VFRs.[148–150] For a number of reasons VFRs visit travel clinics infrequently for pretravel health advice and usually do not follow recommendations concerning antimalarial chemoprophylaxis. However, they often visit high-risk malarious areas, particularly sub-Saharan Africa. The risk of malaria per month of stay without prophylaxis is highest in sub-Saharan Africa and Oceania (1 : 50 to 1 : 1000) and during the past decade has increased more than fivefold in travelers to Kenya. The risk is intermediate (1 : 1000–1 : 12 000) in travelers to Haiti and the Indian subcontinent, and it is low (<1 : 50 000) in travelers to Southeast Asia and to Central and South America.[151] Declines in the incidence of malaria imported into the UK from West Africa and Latin America have been reported.[152,153] Of the 1200–1500 cases of malaria reported annually in the United States, most of those due to *Plasmodium falciparum* occur in travelers, especially VFRs, returning or immigrating from Africa and Asia.[154] With the worldwide increase in chloroquine- and multidrug-resistant *P. falciparum* malaria, decisions on chemoprophylaxis have become more difficult. In addition, the spread of malaria due to primaquine- and chloroquine-resistant strains of *P. vivax* has added further complexity to the issue of malaria prevention and treatment.[155,156] In addition, *P. knowlesi*, a species of monkey malaria that has the potential to infect and kill humans, is now spreading in Southeast Asia.[157,158]

Compounding these problems are new data showing that *P. vivax* malaria may be responsible for greater mortality than previously recognized, especially in young children.[159–161]

The use of personal protection measures to prevent mosquito bites is the first line of defense; this and antimalarial chemoprophylaxis regimens are keys to prevention.[148] Compliance is paramount. Several studies indicate that only approximately 50% of travelers adhere to basic recommendations for malaria prevention.[162–164] Travelers must be educated about the risk of malaria, personal protection measures against mosquito bites, appropriate chemoprophylaxis, symptoms of the disease, and measures to be taken in case of suspected malaria during travel. This approach is outlined in the checklist for travelers to malarious areas (***Box 126.1***). Travel medicine advisors must conduct a careful review of the itinerary, including whether urban or rural areas will be visited, the length of stay, style of travel, and a medical history, including allergies, previous experience with antimalarials, and the likelihood of pregnancy.

Box 126.1 Checklist for Advising Travelers to Malarious Areas: Key Issues to Be Considered

Risk of Malaria and the Presence of Drug-Resistant *Plasmodium falciparum* in the Area of Destination

Antimosquito measures
Insect repellents
Knockdown insecticides
Bednets
Long-sleeved shirts, trousers
Chemoprophylaxis

Caveats Re Use of Antimalarials

Appropriate drug regimen
Need to start drug before travel, during exposure, and depending on selected chemoprophylaxis for 4 weeks after leaving the malaria-endemic area
If necessary, need for self-treatment
Warning that malaria may develop despite chemoprophylaxis
Warning that fellow travelers or locals may recommend alternative drug regimens that may be less effective
Adverse effects of antimalarials

In Case of Illness, Travelers should be Informed About:

Symptoms of malaria (unexplained fever, with or without headache, muscle aches, chills, weakness, vomiting, or diarrhea)
Need for prompt medical help if malaria is suspected since it may be fatal if treatment is delayed; for diagnosis, a blood sample should be examined on one or more occasions
Self-treatment in special circumstances, the need to take it only if prompt medical care is not available, and the need to seek medical advice as soon as possible after self-treatment
Incubation period is ≥ 6 days

(Adapted from World Health Organization: International Travel and Health. www.who.int.)

Personal Protection Measures

Anopheles mosquitoes, the vectors of malaria, are exclusively nocturnal in their feeding habits; protection from mosquito bites from dusk to dawn is highly effective in reducing the risk of malaria. However, as *Aedes* mosquitoes carrying dengue fever virus bite during the day and *Culex* transmitting JE mainly at dusk, personal protective measures are to be recommended around the clock. When practical, travelers should wear protective clothing, such as long-sleeved shirts and long pants, when outside during evening hours. The most effective method of preventing mosquito bites is to combine a pesticide, such as permethrin, on clothing with an insect repellent containing diethylmetatoluamide (DEET) applied to exposed skin.[165] Although all concentrations of DEET (from 10% to 99.9%) are equally efficacious in preventing mosquito bites, the duration of action is proportional to the concentration (e.g., 30% DEET lasts 4–6 hours, whereas 99% DEET provides 8–10 hours of protection). Newer controlled-release formulations with lower concentrations of DEET provide prolonged protection.[166] DEET is well tolerated, but serious adverse reactions such as toxic encephalopathy have rarely occurred in very young children who were exposed to excessive amounts for extended periods.[167–170] The Environmental Protection Agency and the American Academy of Pediatrics have recommended that 30% DEET may be used in children 2 months of age or older.[171] This recommendation is not uniformly accepted by experts in all countries.[172] Also, DEET has been shown to be safe during the second and third trimesters of pregnancy.[173] Insect repellents should be applied sparingly to intact skin and washed off when there is no longer a risk of mosquito bites. Although the cosmetic product Skin-So-Soft has some repellent activity, it requires frequent (hourly) reapplication.[168,174] Picaridin has been shown to be equally effective as DEET, although there may not be as much data regarding the prevention of bites by malaria-infected mosquitoes.[175–177]

Efficacy rates of up to 80% in the prevention of malaria have been shown by using bednets impregnated with permethrin.[178,179] A pyrethroid-based flying insect spray should be used to clear the bednet and room of mosquitoes. Where bednets are not available, mosquito coils and other preparations of vaporized pyrethrum flowers have been shown to reduce mosquito bites.[180] A number of herbal products that have far less efficacy than DEET are sold in stores or on the internet.

Chemoprophylaxis

Personal protective measures greatly reduce but do not eliminate the risk of malaria. Antimalarials are only suppressives, and they act on the hepatic or erythrocytic stage of the parasite, thereby preventing the clinical symptoms of disease but not infection. No drug guarantees protection against malaria. For this reason, travelers must be informed that any febrile illness that occurs during or soon after travel to a malaria-endemic area should be evaluated immediately by a health care professional for malaria. Since in only one-third of patients in the United States and Canada who died from malaria was the diagnosis considered before death, it is incumbent upon travelers to inform their health care provider of the risk of malaria and the need to have it ruled out regardless of the malaria prophylactic used.[181,182]

The choice of a drug regimen for chemoprophylaxis will be dependent on the individual's itinerary, length of stay, age, pregnancy status, use of other medications, general medical history (including previous experience with antimalarials), cost, and the estimation of the risk of drug side effects compared with the risk of developing malaria.[183–187]

Antimalarials should be started 1 day to 2 weeks prior to entry to a malarious area, during exposure, and for some period of time after departure. Beginning some antimalarials early ensures an adequate blood concentration of the drug and enables travelers to change to alternative drugs should adverse effects occur. The postexposure period of prophylaxis for antimalarials such as chloroquine, mefloquine, and doxycycline is particularly important to enable the antimalarial to eradicate any organisms that are released from the liver into the bloodstream after departure from a malarious area. A postexposure period is similarly recommended for those using atovaquone/proguanil but it is limited to 7 days. *P. vivax* and *P. ovale* infections, however, often have dormant hypnozoites in the liver that may be released many months after the onset of infection. With other medications, such as atovaquone/proguanil and primaquine, this postexposure period may be shortened considerably because these drugs act on the hepatic phase.

The development of resistance to antimalarial drugs has seriously hampered the ability to prevent and treat infections.[188] Chloroquine-resistant *P. falciparum* infections have spread throughout the world except in areas of Central America, Haiti, and the Middle East[189] (***Figs 126.2 and 126.3***). Along the Thailand–Cambodia and Thailand–Myanmar (Burma) borders, and in South-Central Vietnam, *P. falciparum* malaria is resistant to chloroquine and mefloquine (see ***Fig. 96.4***).[190,191] Reports from the Indonesian archipelago and Oceania indicate considerable chloroquine-resistant *P. vivax* and *P. malariae*.[192,193] However, because of chloroquine-resistant *P. falciparum* in these areas, the problem of *P. vivax* resistance does not affect current recommendations for chemoprophylaxis. According to CDC and Health Canada, antimalarials should be continued as long as a traveler is at risk of malaria; however, in some European countries use of certain antimalarial drugs such as atovaquone/proguanil has been restricted to several months.[194]

Antimalarial Drugs

Table 126.3 lists the drugs, doses, and adverse effects of available drugs for malaria chemoprophylaxis and self-treatment.[195–197]

Chloroquine

Chloroquine phosphate is a 4-aminoquinolone that acts by inhibiting heme polymerase.[198] Chloroquine is well tolerated and in appropriate doses may be safely used by young children and pregnant women.[199] Transient nausea or vomiting is seen in a small proportion of individuals and may usually be reduced by taking the drug with food. Occasionally, headaches or blurred vision are reported. Intense pruritus is well documented, almost exclusively in black Africans.[200,201] Although long-term

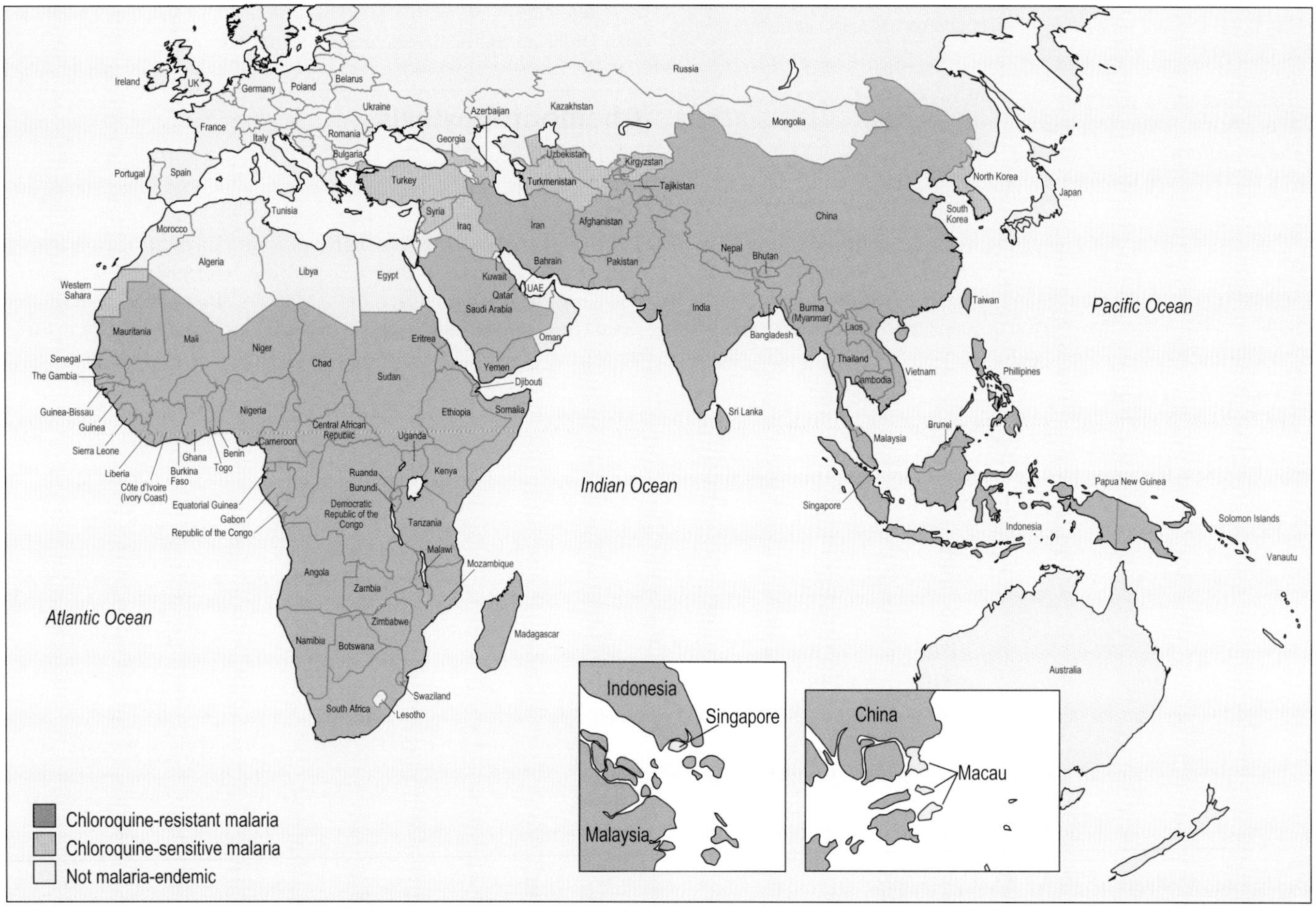

Figure 126.2 Malaria-endemic countries in the eastern hemisphere. (Reproduced from Centers for Disease Control and Prevention. CDC Health Information for International Travel 2010. Atlanta: U.S. Department of Health and Human Services, Public Health Service, 2009.)

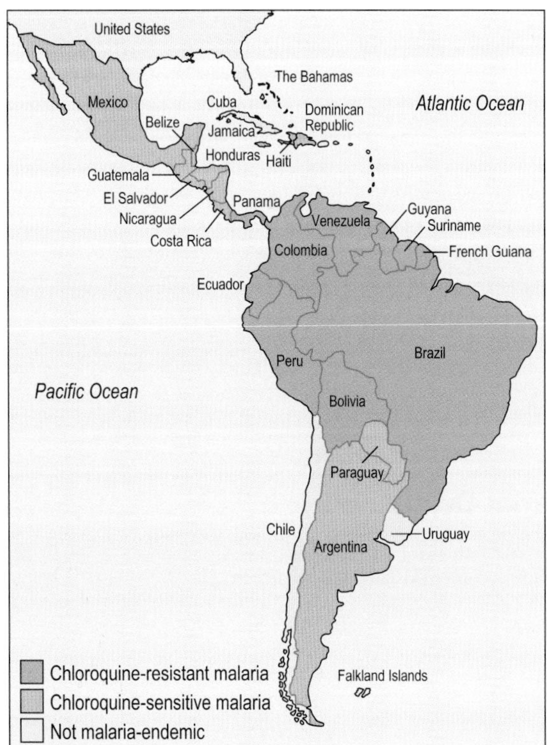

Figure 126.3 Malaria-endemic countries in Central and South America. (Reproduced from Centers for Disease Control and Prevention. CDC Health Information for International Travel 2010. Atlanta: U.S. Department of Health and Human Services, Public Health Service, 2009.)

chloroquine use can produce ocular keratic precipitates, irreversible keratopathy does not occur in the doses used for malaria chemoprophylaxis. Chloroquine should be avoided in people with a history of epilepsy.[202] Chloroquine should be stored in childproof containers because as little as a single tablet can be fatal to an infant; overdosages should be reported to a physician immediately.

Mefloquine

Mefloquine is a 4-quinoline methanol compound that has a prolonged half-life of approximately 30 days;[203] steady-state levels are not reached for approximately 7 weeks, unless a loading dose is used. Comparative studies among travelers have shown that mefloquine is less well tolerated than other antimalarials, although only 5% of users have to stop the drug due to adverse events.[204,205] With mefloquine use, seizures and acute psychosis occur in 1 : 10 000–1 : 13 000 users.[206–208] Mefloquine is safe during the second half of pregnancy, and there is increasing evidence that it is safe during the first trimester as well.[209–213] However, due to increasing concerns about the neuropsychiatric adverse events, the FDA has required that all health providers distribute drug information with all mefloquine prescriptions. Since the majority of adverse effects to mefloquine occur within the first 3 doses, many travel medicine practitioners recommend starting the drug 4 weeks before exposure in order to assess adverse events and to switch the antimalarial if significant side effects occur.

Mefloquine is currently recommended for all age groups, including infants, at a dose of 5 mg/kg weekly (maximum, 250 mg).[214–216] Mefloquine is contraindicated in those with a history of seizures or psychiatric disorder, including depression or anxiety reaction. Neuropsychiatric adverse effects of mefloquine tend to occur more frequently among women[216–218] and appear to be less common in children.[219] The

Table 126.3 Antimalarial Drugs for Chemoprophylaxis and Self-Treatment

Drug	Tablet Size	Adult Dose	Pediatric Dose	Side-Effects
Prevention				
Atovaquone plus proguanil (Malarone)	Adult tablet and pediatric tablets[a]	1 adult tablet daily	5–8 kg: ½ pediatric tablet/day 8–10 kg: ¾ pediatric tablets/day 11–20 kg: 1 pediatric tablet/day 21–30 kg: 2 pediatric tablets/day 31–40 kg: 3 pediatric tablets/day >40 kg: 1 adult tablet/day	Frequent: gastrointestinal upset, headache Occasional: fever, rash, cough, insomnia
Chloroquine phosphate (Aralen)	150 mg base (250 mg salt) or 300 mg base (500 mg salt)	300 mg base (500 mg salt) once weekly	5 mg/kg base PO weekly up to adult dose of 300 mg base	Frequent: pruritus, nausea, headache Occasional: skin eruptions, reversible, corneal opacity, partial alopecia
Hydroxycholoroquine sulfate (Plaquenil)	310 mg base (400 mg salt)	310 mg base once weekly	5 mg/kg base once weekly	See above for chloroquinine
Doxycycline	100 mg	100 mg once daily	<8 years: contraindicated ≥8 years: 2 mg/kg once daily (maximum 100 mg/day)	Frequent: gastrointestinal upset, vaginal candidiasis, photosensitivity Occasional: azotemia in renal disease Rare: allergic reactions, blood dyscrasias
Mefloquine (Lariam)	250 mg	250 mg once weekly	5–10 kg: ⅛ tablet/week 11–20 kg: ¼ tablet/week 21–30 kg: ½ tablet/week 31–45 kg: ¾ tablet/week	Frequent: dizziness, nausea, diarrhea, headache, insomnia, strange dreams Occasional: depression, anxiety, irritability Rare: seizures, psychosis, headache, insomnia, strange dreams
Primaquine				
Prevention of *Plasmodium vivax* relapse	15 mg base	30 mg base/day for 14 days	0.6 mg base/kg/day for 14 days	Occasional: gastrointestinal upset, hemolysis secondary to glucose-6-phosphate dehydrogenase deficiency, methemoglobinemia
Prophylaxis	15 mg base	30 mg base/day	0.6 mg/kg/day	As above
Self-Treatment				
Mefloquine	250 mg base	15 mg/kg in 2 divided doses 12 hours apart (or 1250 mg in 1 dose)	Same as adults	
Atovaquone plus proguanil (Malarone)	Adult and pediatric tablets[a]	2 adult tablets bid × 3 days	5–8 kg: 2 pediatric tablets/day × 3 days 9–10 kg: 3 pediatric tablets/day × 3 days 11–20 kg: 1 adult tablet/day × 3 days 21–30 kg: 2 adult tablets/day × 3 days 31–40 kg: 3 adult tablets/day × 3 days	Frequent: gastrointestinal upset, headache Occasional: fever, skin rash, cough
Quinine sulfate plus doxycycline		650 mg q8h × 3–7 days 100 mg bid × 7 days	30 mg/kg/day in 3 doses × 3–7 days 4 mg/kg/day in 2 doses × 7 days	
Artemether/ lumefantrine		6 doses over 3 days (4 tablets/dose at 0, 8, 24, 36, 48 and 60 hours	6 doses over 3 days at same intervals as adults: <15 kg: 1 tablets/dose 15–25 kg: 2 tablets/dose 25–35 kg: 3 tablets/dose >35 kg: 4 tablets/dose	

[a]Adult tablet: 250 mg atovaquone plus 100 mg proguanil; pediatric tablet: 62.5 mg atovaquone plus 25 mg proguanil.

drug should be used with caution in those who have a known cardiac conduction disturbance. It should not be used in those taking chloroquine or quinine-like drugs, including halofantrine.

Doxycycline

Doxycycline is a tetracycline derivative with a half-life of approximately 16 hours. Its major benefit is that it is effective against multidrug-resistant *P. falciparum* as well as *P. vivax*.

The most common adverse reactions to doxycycline are gastrointestinal (GI) disturbances and phototoxicity (exaggerated sunburn).[220,221] The former can be reduced by taking the drug with extra fluids and meals, and the latter can be reduced by using a sunscreen that absorbs ultraviolet (UV) A as well as UVB radiation. It is estimated that 2–15% of those using doxycycline will develop phototoxicity. Doxycycline should not be ingested while in the supine position because of the risk of esophageal ulceration caused by lodgment of the tablet in the distal esophagus. BSS (Pepto-Bismol) and antacids decrease doxycycline bioavailability. In addition, vaginal candidiasis is a very common and troublesome problem consequent to doxycycline use in female travelers; some advisors suggest carrying fluconazole for self-treatment as necessary. The drug is contraindicated in pregnant women and children younger than the age of 8 years.

Proguanil

Proguanil is a dihydrofolate reductase inhibitor that is not commercially available in the United States. Proguanil is not recommended by the CDC or the Public Health Agency of Canada because of suboptimal protection but is recommended by some European countries and WHO in some areas.

Primaquine

Primaquine is an 8-aminoquinolone that has been shown to be a good alternative for the prevention of all forms of malaria.[222] It has slightly lower protective efficacy against *P. falciparum* compared with other agents (e.g., it has been shown to have 85–95% protective efficacy in studies in East Africa, Colombia, and Irian Jaya, Indonesia).[223–227] Unlike chloroquine, doxycycline, and mefloquine, primaquine acts on the primary exoerythrocytic stage in the liver and eradicates dormant hypnozoites. For this reason, the drug may be discontinued soon after leaving the malarious area.

Primaquine, because it eradicates dormant hypnozoites in the liver, may also be used as presumptive antirelapse treatment (PART), previously called terminal prophylaxis, to prevent relapses of *P. vivax* malaria when taken after departure from a malarious area. PART should be reserved for those who have had prolonged intense exposure outside sub-Saharan Africa where there is little *P. vivax*. Recently primaquine has been recommended by CDC as a prophylactic agent of choice for countries that have >90% *P. vivax* malaria. This would apply to all countries of Central America except for Honduras and some countries of Asia.

Primaquine is a potent oxidizing agent that causes hemolysis in people with glucose-6-phosphate dehydrogenase (G6PD) deficiency. The drug has been shown to produce mild (below toxic levels) methemoglobinemia when used for prolonged periods as prophylaxis in those with normal enzyme levels.[226] G6PD levels should be measured before primaquine is used, especially in those who are likely to be at risk for this enzyme deficiency (blacks, southern Europeans, and Asians). GI side effects may be reduced by taking the drug with food. Primaquine is contraindicated during pregnancy.

Atovaquone/Proguanil (Malarone)

A more recent addition to the armamentarium for the prophylaxis and treatment of malaria is the fixed combination or atovaquone and proguanil (250 mg atovaquone/100 mg proguanil).[228–230] Like primaquine, atovaquone/proguanil targets the liver and blood stages. For this reason, the drug may be discontinued soon after leaving the malarious area. Unlike primaquine, atovaquone/proguanil does not eradicate the dormant hypnozoites, putting travelers at risk of *P. vivax* malaria after the drug has been discontinued. Atovaquone/proguanil is highly efficacious and is equivalent to mefloquine or doxycyline.[231–234] Adverse events include headache, GI upset, insomnia, dizziness, and rash. Side effects are least frequent among current recommended antimalarials; 0.2–1.2% of users discontinued the drug compared with 5% for mefloquine and 2% for chloroquine/proguanil.[204,205,235] The high cost of this excellent antimalarial is prohibitive for some users, especially for VFRs and long-term travelers.

Recommended Regimens

Tables 96.5 and 126.3 list the recommended antimalarial drug regimens for travelers to malaria-endemic areas. For travel to chloroquine-sensitive areas, chloroquine is the drug of choice. Any of the other first-line drugs may be used as alternatives. However, many travelers prefer atovaquone/proguanil because it may be discontinued soon after departure. For travel to chloroquine-resistant *P. falciparum* areas, atovaquone/proguanil, doxycycline, and mefloquine are the first-line drugs of choice. Primaquine is a second-line drug for these travelers because of the need for a G6PD level prior to its use and because it is somewhat less effective. However, as noted above, it is considered a first-line drug for travel to areas where *P. vivax* is the predominant infection. For travel to chloroquine- and mefloquine-resistant areas (the Thailand–Cambodia and Thailand–Myanmar borders), atovaquone/proguanil and doxycycline are the drugs of choice. Regardless of the chemoprophylactic regimen recommended, it is important for travel health advisors to indicate to travelers that globally there is no uniformity concerning recommendations for malaria chemoprophylaxis and therefore they are likely to meet fellow travelers and health care providers overseas who give conflicting advice as to the optimal regimen. Also, in many developing countries, particularly those in Africa, malaria is often overdiagnosed among travelers either as a presumptive diagnosis or due to a high rate of false positivity of blood films.[236] Travelers should be advised to continue their antimalarial regimen even if they are told they have developed malaria while taking a recommended regimen. Travelers are advised not to purchase antimalarials in developing countries due to high rates of the manufacture and sales of counterfeit drugs.[237,238]

Self-Treatment

People who are unable to tolerate effective antimalarials, who are in an area where drug resistance is frequent, or who are unable to obtain medical care in less than 24–48 hours may consider a self-treatment regimen. In many European countries, malaria chemoprophylaxis is not generally prescribed for travelers to most areas of Asia and Latin America where low endemicity prevails; instead, self-treatment regimens are routinely recommended. Unfortunately, however, there is evidence that those who carry self-treatment regimens often use them inappropriately.[239] Also, there is evidence that travelers who use the rapid diagnostic drug kits for malaria do not use them effectively.[240–242]

Few recommend a self-treatment drug in addition to chemoprophylactic medication. Drugs used for self-treatment should be different from the agent used for prophylaxis. Most travel medicine advisors recommend atovaquone/proguanil or artemether/lumefantrine combination as the drugs of choice for self-treatment. If atovaquone/proguanil is being used for prophylaxis and there is a high degree of suspicion for malaria, mefloquine, the combination of quinine and doxycycline, or the artemether/lumefantrine combination may be used for self-treatment. From a global perspective, artemisinin combinations are the most widely used and effective drugs for the treatment of malaria. However, it is worrisome that resistance to these drugs has been recently reported.[243,244]

SEXUALLY TRANSMITTED DISEASES AND BLOODBORNE PATHOGENS

During international travel, people often feel a sense of anonymity, may be less sexually inhibited, and may therefore put themselves at greater risk for the acquisition of sexually transmitted diseases (STDs) (see Chapter 138).[245,246] In a survey of 354 British travelers, 4.8% admitted to having casual sex while abroad compared with 6.4% of 484 Swiss travelers.[247] In another study, 5.6% of short-term travelers to Peru had casual sexual contact; only 70% were protected by condoms.[248] A Canadian study revealed that 5–15% engaged in sex with a new partner during travel lasting approximately 1 month.[41] Long-term overseas workers appear to put themselves at even greater risk of acquiring STDs. Among Belgian men working in central Africa, 51% and 31% reported casual sex with local women or commercial sex workers, respectively.[249]

The most effective ways to avoid STDs during travel are to abstain from sexual activity, have sexual relations with a well-known partner, or use safer sexual practices. These practices will only succeed in preventing infection if applied in each and every sexual encounter, especially when different partners are involved. The highest risk activity is with commercial sex workers: 90% of commercial sex workers in Nairobi and more than 50% of those in Bangkok are HIV-infected.[250] Since precautions may fail because of condom breakage, having "safe sex" with a high-risk partner may still be dangerous. Some of the STDs that are very common in the developing world include gonorrhea, syphilis, chancroid, *Chlamydia* infection, trichomoniasis, and viral infections such as hepatitis B, C, and HIV-1, HIV-2, and human T-cell lymphotropic virus type I.[245,246,251,252]

Since several of the pathogens mentioned previously may also be transmitted by exposure to blood and secretions, safer sexual practices are not the only way to avoid infection. People requiring injections overseas (e.g., travelers requiring updating of their immunizations or those with diabetes mellitus) should consider carrying their own needles and syringes, particularly long-stay travelers who plan to visit remote areas. However, they should carry an official-appearing note from a health care provider to use at international border posts. In case of serious accident or injury, all travelers should know their blood type, particularly if they are traveling with a group, which is considered to be a "safe" source of blood for transfusion. Although no guarantee of safety, blood received from expatriates or staff at embassies, consulates, or international agencies may be less risky with regard to HIV infection. In a study of US travelers to developing countries, it was noted that medical care was sought by 8% of all travelers, of whom 17% received an injection.[45] The significance of this as a risk factor was highlighted by data that showed that in Southeast Asia and in the eastern Mediterranean approximately 80% of injections were given using nonsterile equipment.[44] Where blood products may be necessary, transportation to the home country or nearest developed country should be considered in situations in which blood cannot be accurately screened prior to transfusion. Travelers may wish to purchase medical evacuation insurance before departure to cover the enormous cost of being transported home or to specialized medical centers.

The HIV-Infected Traveler

The HIV-infected traveler is at increased risk of serious infections from a number of pathogens that may be more prevalent at travel destinations than at home. However, the degree of risk depends almost entirely on the state of the immune system at the time of travel. People with AIDS and others with immunodeficiency require special counseling before travel.[253–255]

Several countries continue to deny entry to HIV-positive people, even though there are no data that show that these restrictions decrease rates of transmission of the virus. In general, HIV testing has been required of those people who intend to stay longer than 3 months or who intend to work or study abroad. Some countries accept an HIV serologic test done within 6 months of departure, whereas others require that the test be done at the time of arrival.

Health insurance is highly recommended for HIV-positive travelers. Such policies should include trip cancellation and evacuation insurance in the event of illness.

Immunizations

In general, live attenuated vaccines are contraindicated for people with immune dysfunction. Exceptions to this rule may include some individuals who should obtain protection against measles and yellow fever who must travel to high-risk areas. The HIV-infected person whose CD4 count is less than 200/μL should be discouraged from traveling to areas endemic for yellow fever and should not be given live vaccines.

Gastrointestinal Illness

Traveler's diarrhea is especially problematic in HIV-infected people because of decreased levels of gastric acid and abnormal GI mucosal immunity. Salmonellosis, shigellosis, and campylobacteriosis are likely to be more frequent, more severe, and more difficult to treat.[256–258] Both isosporiasis and cryptosporidiosis are greater risks in developing countries. Because of these potential problems, the HIV-infected traveler must take stringent food and water precautions.

Other Travel-Related Infections

Reports strongly suggest that HIV infection predisposes to more severe malaria infection, which may stimulate HIV replication.[259,260] There are few data on the interactions between antimalarial drugs and antiretroviral drugs, even though protease inhibitors share common hepatic pathways (e.g., cytochrome P-450). One unpublished study of healthy volunteers suggested that plasma levels of ritonavir decreased with concomitant use of mefloquine. Other vector-borne diseases, such as visceral leishmaniasis and Chagas disease, may cause serious illness in HIV-infected travelers.[261–263] Precautions to avoid sandfly bites in the case of leishmaniasis and reduviid bug bites in the case of Chagas disease should be undertaken. Tuberculosis is not usually of concern to the short-term HIV-infected traveler. However, histoplasmosis from caves and coccidioidomycosis in endemic areas are of concern because of their greater morbidity and mortality among HIV-infected people.[264,265]

SPECIAL HEALTH CONSIDERATIONS FOR TRAVELERS

Issues of chronic illness, disability, pregnancy, and travel with young children are beyond the scope of this article. However, excellent reviews of these subjects have been published.[266,267]

Mortality

Despite the emphasis on pretravel advice on prevention of infection, deaths from infection are relatively uncommon.[5–9] In a study of 421 deaths among Australian travelers, only 10 (2.4%) were attributed to infection, and in a Scottish study involving 952 people who died abroad, infection occurred in only 34 (3.6%).[8,9] CVD is the most common cause of death in travelers, accounting for 35–69% of deaths, except in developing countries, where injuries are the number one cause of death.

Motor Vehicle Accidents and Injuries

Trauma is by far the most important preventable cause of death in travelers.[5–9] Injury deaths, particularly from motor vehicle accidents, account for 21–26% of deaths that occur during travel. As expected, when those with CVD are compared with those who had injuries or accidents, there is a marked preponderance of older people in the former group and younger people in the latter. Motor vehicle accidents can be reduced by advising travelers to avoid travel by road in rural areas at night, overcrowded public vehicles, and riding on motorcycles and bicycles – or if they do, at least to wear a helmet.

Bites and Stings

Arthropods and Insects

Although malaria is the most important vector-borne infection in travelers, there are others that require attention. Of these, dengue (see Chapter 75) is an increasing problem. The past decade has seen a dramatic rise globally in dengue, particularly in the Caribbean, Central and South America, and Southeast Asia.[268–270] This has been reflected by a marked increase in travelers.[271] In fact, a study from Sweden reported that 1 : 3500 travelers to the Malay peninsula become infected.[272] The infection is transmitted by the *Aedes* mosquito, which prefers an urban and often indoor habitat. This mosquito bites during the day, particularly in the hours of the early morning and late afternoon. Recently, chikungunya fever (see Chapter 78), another arbovirus infection transmitted by *Aedes* mosquitoes, has spread rapidly across South Asia and Indonesia since a major outbreak occurred in Madagascar in 2005. This dengue-like illness, accompanied by arthritis, has even spread locally in Italy, likely brought there by a traveler from the tropics.[273–275]

In addition to insect precautions, some vector-borne diseases can be prevented by prophylactic medication. For example, loaiasis can be prevented by taking 300 mg (adult dose) of diethylcarbamazine once each week while in a very heavily infected area, such as Central or West Africa.[276] Unfortunately, diethylcarbamazine is no longer available in the United States, except from the CDC drug service, which will provide it to clinicians who are treating documented cases. Tick- and mite-borne typhus, relapsing fever, leptospirosis, bartonellosis, and plague can be prevented by using doxycycline prophylaxis 100 mg/day during exposure.[277] Chagas disease, transmitted by the night-biting reduviid bug, can be prevented by the use of a bednet and by avoiding sleeping in thatched huts and/or those with mud and stick walls.

Travelers who walk through undergrowth or have close contact with animals are at risk of tick infestation. Tick transmitted diseases include Lyme disease, ehrlichiosis, relapsing fever, tularemia, typhus, and Congo-Crimean hemorrhagic fever. The risk of a tick bite can be reduced by wearing long sleeves and pants, tucking the latter into socks, and by using effective insect repellents such as DEET. Permethrin clothing spray will protect against tick bites for 2 weeks or more. Finally, a "tick check" of the entire skin should be performed each night by the traveler.

Venomous scorpions are found in many areas of the developing world. Children are at particular risk of dying from a scorpion bite.[278,279] The risk of a scorpion sting can be reduced by shaking out boots, shoes, blankets, sleeping bags, and clothing before use; consistently and properly using a mosquito net; wearing shoes when walking at night; not putting one's hands blindly into ground holes, wood piles, and so on; wearing gloves when cleaning rocks or debris; and removing debris from around housing and camping areas.

Diseases Transmitted by Soil and Water

Schistosomiasis is a helminthic disease that infects more than 200 million people worldwide in areas of South America, the Caribbean, Africa, the Middle East, and Southeast Asia (see Chapter 122). GeoSentinel data suggest that travelers continue to be infected and it is unclear whether travel health advisors are highlighting preventive measures during pre-travel consultations.[280] To avoid schistosomiasis, travelers should be advised to stay out of fresh water in most developing countries. Swimming in the ocean or fresh water pools without snails is safe. Travelers who cannot control their urge to swim in fresh water should confine themselves to the middle of a lake. After emerging from potentially contaminated water, travelers should dry off quickly in an attempt to prevent skin penetration by the parasite. By allowing infested water to stand for 48 hours, the infectivity of the schistosome larvae in the water will be eliminated. Studies suggest that DEET in a lipid formulation may prevent cercarial penetration and therefore may be a practical approach in the prevention of infection when schistosome-infested water cannot be avoided.[281–283]

Leptospirosis (see Chapter 45) is another risk associated with fresh water flooding and ecotourism. Infection can be prevented in unavoidable high-risk situations by taking doxycycline 200 mg per week.[284]

Walking barefoot exposes the traveler to a variety of hazards, including tungiasis (the sand flea) (see Chapter 124), snakebites, cutaneous larva migrans from larvae of the dog and cat hookworm (see Chapter 109), human hookworm infection (see Chapter 116), and strongyloidiasis (see Chapter 117). Sandals provide only partial protection.

Adaptation to the Environment

Heat Acclimatization

Although the body possesses the mechanics to survive in extremely hot climates, time is required to put the adaptive mechanisms into play.[285] The adaptation process can take from 1 to several weeks depending on the severity of the climate. Children adapt to hot environments very quickly, whereas unfit, obese people, the elderly, and those with cardiovascular problems are at greatest risk of suffering from disorders associated with a hot climate.[286]

In hot climates, the body's main defense against heat is perspiration. In hot weather and in the absence of strenuous exercise, the average person must replace at least 1.5 L of fluid per day. Cold fluids are best, whereas alcohol and caffeinated drinks are poor choices because they tend to increase fluid excretion. Since sweat contains both water and salt, it is important to replace salt by eating salty foods or adding extra salt to food. Finally, appropriate clothing will help to prevent heat illness. Clothing made of natural fibers, such as cotton and linen, allows air to circulate. Light colors reflect light and are preferable to dark fabrics.

Jet Lag

Jet lag, the result of a desynchronization of biologic rhythms, is often experienced by travelers who have not had enough time to adjust to a new time zone during a long journey.[287] It affects nearly all travelers crossing more than three time zones. Symptoms of jet lag include fatigue, insomnia, decreased appetite, disequilibrium, a change in bowel habits, and headache. A variety of practical techniques can be used to reduce jet lag. If possible, one should allow 1 day to adjust to every time zone crossed. It is advisable to readjust one's schedule to local time as soon as possible. Naps during the day may be helpful as long as they are kept to less than 45 minutes to avoid the groggy feeling that occurs on awakening. Travelers on a tight schedule are advised to break up a long journey to reduce the adjustment time required at the final destination. Caffeine and alcohol, especially before and during night flights, should be avoided to reduce the risk of sleep disturbance. It has been suggested that alterations in diet can assist in reducing jet lag, although there are no scientific data to support this.[288]

Studies of zeitgebers (light cues that affect body rhythms) have shown that alteration in the amount of daylight exposure will affect the production of melatonin, which can, in turn, assist in adjusting the body's biorhythms.[289,290] The following regimen has been suggested: west-to-east travelers crossing six or fewer time zones should increase their morning outdoor light for the first few days after arrival, exposing themselves to at least as many hours of light as the number of time zones crossed. Those crossing seven or more time zones should stay indoors early in the morning and get their sunlight later in the day. These schedules should be reversed for those traveling from east to west. This method works only when light comes from an outdoor source, and in general, even if one cannot adhere to the specific recommendations, the greater exposure to the outdoors on arrival appears to be helpful in adjustment. Indoor light can be used to overcome jet lag if the source provides 25 000 lux.[291]

Short-acting mild sedatives have been shown to improve sleep and daytime performance in shift workers.[292] However, prograde amnesia and rebound insomnia may occur.[293] Some consultants recommend zolpidem tartrate (Ambien) instead.[294] A number of studies of airline crews have shown that melatonin has the potential to reduce jet lag.[295–301] It is recommended that, for east-bound travelers, melatonin 3–5 mg should be taken before departure at 2 or 3 a.m. destination time for 3 nights prior to departure and at bedtime for 4 days after arrival. West-bound travelers need not take melatonin prior to departure but only after arrival at bedtime for 4 nights. Since melatonin is not FDA-approved and its manufacture is not standardized, recommendation of this agent is controversial.

High-Altitude Sickness

Rapid exposure to altitudes higher than 10 000 ft (3000 m) above sea level can cause a variety of serious medical problems:[302–308] acute mountain sickness (AMS), high-altitude pulmonary edema, high-altitude cerebral edema, and high-altitude retinopathy. The incidence and severity of high-altitude sickness are related to the altitude achieved, speed of ascent, amount of physical exertion, and degree of acclimatization. The most effective way to prevent AMS is to stay at an intermediate altitude (6000–8000 ft: 1800–2400 m) for 2 days before gradually ascending to higher elevations. Alcohol and sedatives should be avoided. Acetazolamide (Diamox, a sulfa drug) 125–250 mg every 12 hours (or 500 mg of a sustained-release formulation once daily) beginning 1 or 2 days before ascending and continuing at high altitude for 48 hours after reaching the peak can diminish symptoms of AMS in many but not all people.[309–311] The medication can be stopped as soon as descent begins. Dexamethasone (Decadron) 4 mg every 6–12 hours for 48 hours before and after a rapid ascent may also be helpful in preventing the symptoms of AMS.[312,313] Concurrent prophylactic use of both drugs may be more effective than either alone.[314] Nifedipine has been shown to prevent high-altitude pulmonary edema when used prophylactically at a dose of 20 mg of a slow-release preparation taken before ascent in the following way: one dose per day for 2 days, then one dose twice a day for 1 day, followed by three times a day on the day of ascent.[315,316] Ginkgo biloba has not been shown to prevent altitude sickness.[317–319] Zolpidem may be used for insomnia because it does not suppress ventilation at high altitude.

Deep-Vein Thrombosis and Travel

The issue of the risk of development of deep-vein thrombosis (DVT) during travel, particularly air travel, has been highlighted due to several deaths from pulmonary embolism following long-haul flights (usually more than 5–8 hours). Initially, the problem was called "economy-class syndrome," although it appears also to occur in those who fly in the more exclusive cabins.[320] A variety of case-control studies have examined the risk of DVT in airline passengers.[321–324] Two of three studies did show a relation between venous thrombosis and air travel, but the third study, which was the best designed and lacked referral bias, did not.[323] One study revealed that 1 in 10 travelers developed symptomless DVT, and the use of below-the-knee compression hose made a significant difference in flights more than 8 hours.[325]

Venous stasis appears to be the common denominator, although other risk factors have been identified, including previous DVT or pulmonary embolus, congestive heart failure, cancer, obesity, age (the elderly), and estrogen therapy, and some believe that dehydration may play a role as well.[326–328] There is a growing consensus on the basis of a variety of studies,[326–328] including a meta-analysis,[329] that the risk of DVT on prolonged international flights is very low unless additional risk factors are present.[330] It has been recommended that during long flights travelers should occasionally walk the aisles of the aircraft and flex and extend their calves. Certainly, high-risk individuals should do so. In addition, those at high risk should ask their health care provider whether they should take low-molecular-weight heparin for travel, or even warfarin. It is controversial whether antiplatelet drugs, such as aspirin, play a role in prevention. Support hose has been shown to be effective and is recommended for some.[331]

Traveler's Health Kit

Carrying a travel health kit (*Box 126.2*) containing items most commonly required and desired can be very helpful.[332] Furthermore, allowing oneself the time to prepare prior to traveling, as well as time to adjust on arrival, is the key to productive and enjoyable travel.[333–336] In addition, knowing the risks associated with travel and what one can anticipate in the returning traveler who is ill will help the health care advisor develop an appropriate perspective in provision of the pretravel health advice.[337] Finally, the internet may be a very useful source of information for the potential traveler and the individual providing health advice.[338,339]

Box 126.2 First-Aid Kit and Travel Medications

Long-Term and High-Risk Travel

First-Aid Kit

- Absorbent cotton
- Gauze
- Adhesive tape
- Alcohol swabs
- Antiseptic
- Band-Aids, butterfly closures
- Moleskin for foot blisters
- Safety pins, scissors, tweezers (or Swiss army knife)
- Tensor bandage
- Disposable syringes (3–5 mL) and needles (22–25-gauge)
- Thermometer
- Petroleum jelly (Vaseline)

Medications

- Analgesic
- Antihistamines
- Antinausea/-motion sickness
- Antidiarrheal (see Traveler's diarrhea in text)
- Oral rehydration solution
- Antimotility agent
- Antipyretic
- Antibiotic
- Systemic, bowel, bladder: ciprofloxacin, ofloxacin, norfloxacin, rifaximin (the latter two are not systemic)
- Skin, respiratory tract: cephalexin, clarithromycin, azithromycin, levofloxacin
- Topical: mupirocin, fusidic acid
- Antifungal (topical)
- Antimalarial
- Insect repellent
- Laxative
- Sunscreen (sun protection factor ≥15)
- Sunburn cream, spray
- Water purification tablets, cup

Short-Term and Low-Risk Travel

First-Aid Kit

- Band-Aids
- Moleskin (for foot blisters)
- Scissors, tweezers (or Swiss army knife), safety pins

Medications

- Analgesic
- Antidiarrheal
- Oral rehydration solution
- Antiperistaltic (loperamide)
- Antibiotic (ciprofloxacin, ofloxacin, norfloxacin)
- Antibiotic, topical (mupirocin, fusidic acid)
- Antihistamine
- Antimalarial
- Antinausea/-motion sickness
- Laxative
- Insect repellent
- Sunscreen (sun protection factor ≥15)
- Sunburn cream, spray
- Water purification

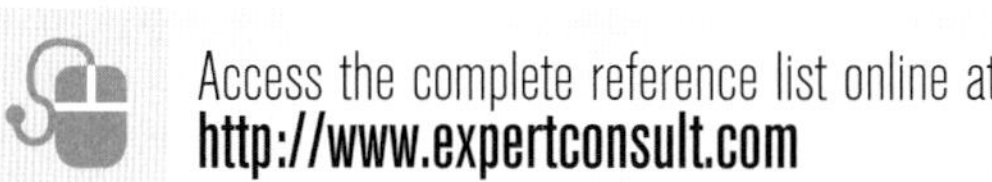
Access the complete reference list online at **http://www.expertconsult.com**

CHAPTER 127

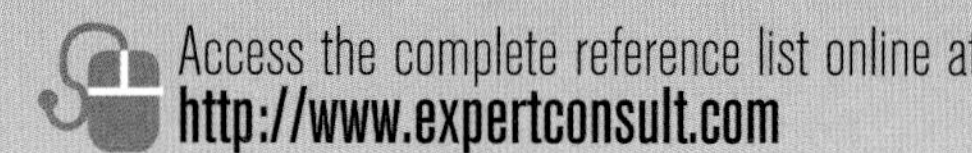
Access the complete reference list online at
http://www.expertconsult.com

Migrant, Immigrant, and Refugee Health

Luis S. Ortega • Rachel B. Eidex • Martin S. Cetron

INTRODUCTION

The global migration landscape has undergone substantial changes in the past quarter century, and the number of population groups contributing to global mobility is steadily rising. The Human Development Report 2009 by the United Nations Development Program estimates 70 million migrants have moved from developing countries to developed ones and more than 200 million migrants have moved between developing countries.[1] Migration is truly a major social phenomenon, with many complex linkages to economic, trade, social, security, and health policies. In the dynamic relationship between migration and health, immigration has long been recognized as having a large impact on disease epidemiology and the use of health services in migrant receiving nations.[2,3] For example, the impact of immigration on disease epidemiology is demonstrated by the global epidemiology of tuberculosis. Tuberculosis (TB) is a major global cause of infectious disease morbidity and mortality; however, rates of TB in most regions of the developing world are many times higher than those in the developed world (the TB prevalence gap) and are decreasing at a much slower rate.[4] Many migrant-receiving countries in the developed world have had stable or increased migration of persons from regions with high TB prevalence, while at the same time having successfully decreased TB incidence in their native-borne population, further exacerbating the prevalence gap. Consequently, the majority of TB cases in migrant-receiving countries such as the United States and Canada are now being diagnosed in foreign-born populations from high-prevalence source countries[5,6] (***Fig. 127.1***). This linkage between migration and TB epidemiology becomes more significant when designing solutions for the control and prevention of multidrug-resistant (MDR) TB and the emerging threat of extensively drug-resistant (XDR) TB.[7–10]

Many migrant-receiving countries have prearrival medical examination requirements and protocols for entering migrants, which vary both by the types of populations screened and by the diseases for which examination is required. The health conditions tested through the medical examination procedures required by countries such as Canada, Australia, New Zealand, and the United States are determined on the basis of the risk or danger that these conditions can represent to public health and safety and the additional costs that may be incurred by national public services expenditures.[11–15] In general, these medical examination procedures include a review of the past medical history, a physical examination, and tests that include a chest radiograph and laboratory analyses. The diseases most frequently tested to determine visa eligibility or admissibility of a migrant are infectious diseases such as tuberculosis, sexually transmitted diseases, and mental or behavioral conditions. Immigration regulations in some countries do allow for the consideration of medical waivers to inadmissible health conditions. Although many migrant-receiving countries in Europe either do not require prearrival health evaluations or have fewer requirements and only limited grounds for refusal of admission based on health grounds, most have provisions for notification and inspection if a communicable or serious health condition is recognized or suspected.[16]

US MIGRATION AND HEALTH SCREENING POLICIES

The number of foreign-born persons living in the United States, almost 38 million in 2007, is greater than ever before in the nation's history representing approximately one-eighth of the total US population.[17] In contrast to the previous twentieth-century US immigration wave, which was dominated by Eastern Europeans who were driven from their countries of origin by such factors as persecution and poverty (so-called "push factors"), the twenty-first century immigration wave, which began in the 1970s, is characterized predominantly by Hispanic followed by Asian migrants who are attracted to the United States for economic opportunities (or "pull factors"). In both waves of migration, migrants have brought with them not only skills and cultural traditions that enriched US economic and social fabric, but also diseases and disease exposures that were different from those existing in US-receiving communities. In addition, twenty-first century migrants are more mobile and remain connected to their countries of birth, typically making several back and forth journeys to visit friends and relatives.[18] New immigrants and refugees, who cross disease prevalence gaps and frequently travel to visit friends and relatives, constitute potentially high-risk populations for translocating communicable diseases of public health significance.

The US Department of Homeland Security has reported more than 175 million nonimmigrant legal admissions, defined as number of entries, not persons, into the United States during 2008.[19] This category includes the approximately 39 million admissions of short-term visitors (tourists, business travelers) and temporary residents (students, specialty workers, diplomats). The majority of these nonimmigrant migrants admitted are not required to undergo health screening prior to US entry. Given the immense numbers of persons crossing US borders and finite resources for evaluation and surveillance, US migrant health screening policy focuses on migrants planning to establish permanent US residence, since this group has the largest potential long-term impact on both disease epidemiology and health care resources utilization. Currently, the US Immigration and Nationality Act (INA) requires that medical screening examinations be performed overseas for all US-bound immigrants and refugees, and in the United States for migrants applying to adjust their visa status to permanent residence (i.e. "green cards").[20,21] In 2008, the over 1 million immigrants (adjustment of status and new arrivals) and refugees admitted underwent medical screening examinations prior to their admission. The remainder of this chapter covers US medical screening issues for immigrants and refugees. Similar issues and regulations apply across developed and developing countries worldwide. Disease transmission among refugees crowded into camps in resource-limited

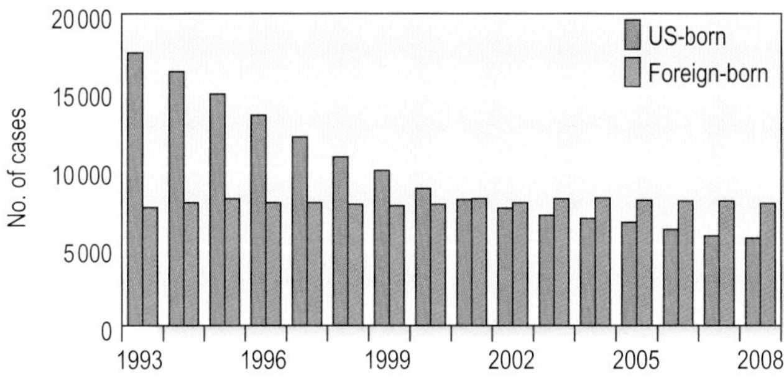

Figure 127.1 Number of tuberculosis cases in US-born versus foreign born persons, United States, 1993–2008. (Data from the Division of Tuberculosis Elimination, Centers for Disease Control and Prevention: www.cdc.gov/tb/statistics.)

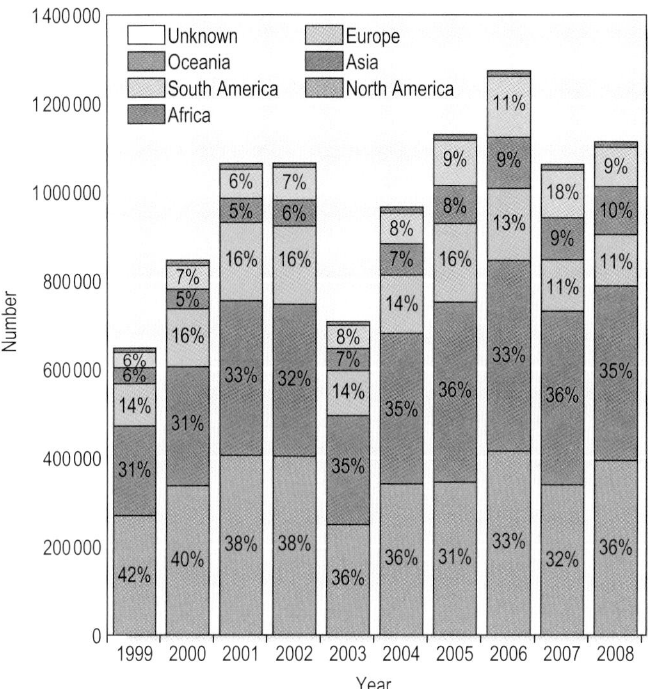

Figure 127.2 US immigrants admitted by region of birth, 1999–2008. (Data from the Division of Global Migration and Quarantine, Centers for Disease Control and Prevention.)

countries further accentuates the huge importance of international refugee public health preparedness.

REQUIRED OVERSEAS MEDICAL SCREENING EXAMINATIONS FOR US-BOUND IMMIGRANTS AND REFUGEES

Over 460000 immigrants and 60000 refugees arrived in the United States during Fiscal Year 2008. Trends in the number and regions of origin for US-arriving immigrants and refugees have important public health implications in determining the medical evaluation and treatment of these two groups, both overseas and stateside.[19,22] From 2006 to 2008, over 1.3 million immigrants arrived in the United States; the number of arrivals and regions of origin remained relatively stable over this 3-year period (*Fig. 127.2*). On average, approximately 450000 immigrants arrived each year, most of these arriving from Asia (majority from China) and the Americas (majority from Mexico), followed by Europe and Africa. From 2006 to 2008, close to 150000 refugees arrived in the United States; in contrast to immigrants, the number of arrivals and regions of origin have changed markedly over this 3-year period (*Fig. 127.3*). In 2006, the majority of arriving refugees (45%) were from Africa, 25% from Europe, and only 20% of arriving refugees were from

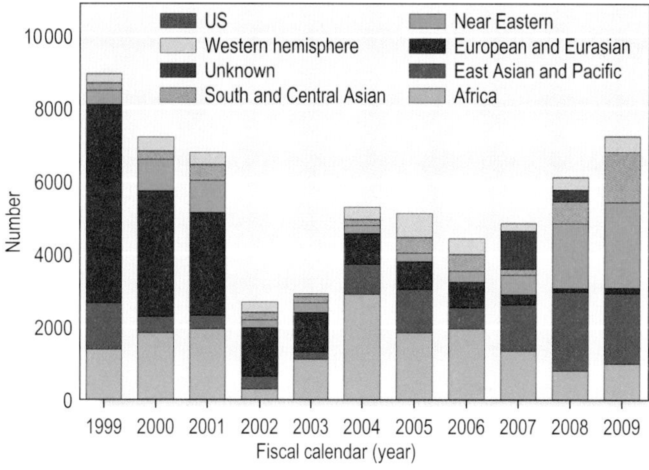

Figure 127.3 US refugee arrivals, 1999–2009. (Data from the Division of Global Migration and Quarantine, Centers for Disease Control and Prevention.)

Asia. In contrast, in 2008, almost 75% (approximately 45000 refugees) arrived from Asia. Trends have important implications for medical evaluation and treatment, both overseas and stateside, as refugees from Africa have relatively high rates of certain diseases, including immunodeficiency virus (HIV) infection, TB, malaria, intestinal helminth infections and other tropical diseases (e.g. schistosomiasis), and likely lack routine vaccinations.[23,24] Similarly, epidemiological information from Southeast Asia, such as reports of artemisinin-resistant *Plasmodium falciparum* are valuable in alerting on the need to invest in preventive and health promotion activities.[25]

All immigrants and refugees migrating to the United States are required to have a medical screening examination overseas, which is performed by local physicians (panel physicians) appointed by the local US embassy. The mandated medical examination as defined by federal regulation focuses primarily on detecting diseases determined to be inadmissible conditions for the purposes of visa eligibility. These diseases include certain serious infectious diseases, mental disorders associated with harmful behavior, and substance abuse.

The definition of communicable diseases of public health significance, amended on October 2009 by the US Centers for Disease Control and Prevention (CDC), with the purpose of adding flexibility to respond in a timely way to unpredictable health threats and outbreaks, divides these into three categories:

1. Active tuberculosis, infectious syphilis, gonorrhea, infectious leprosy, chancroid, lymphogranuloma venereum, and granuloma inguinale.
2. Any quarantinable, communicable disease specified by Executive Orders. The current diseases are pandemic flu, severe acute respiratory syndrome (SARS), viral hemorrhagic fevers, cholera, diphtheria, infectious tuberculosis, plague, smallpox, and yellow fever.
3. A communicable disease that may pose a public health emergency of international concern according to the World Health Organization's 2005 International Health Regulations.[26]

CDC also amended the provisions that describe the scope of the medical examination by incorporating a more flexible, risk-based approach based on medical and epidemiologic factors. This approach will determine which diseases are included in the medical screening and testing of immigrants and refugees in areas of the world that are experiencing outbreaks of specific diseases.[27]

With regard to HIV infection and inadmissibility, in 2008 by federal legislative mandate, the statutory ban on nonimmigrants, immigrants and refugees with HIV from entering the United States was removed. Subsequently on November 2, 2009 the CDC posted a Final Rule removing HIV infection from the list of excludable communicable diseases of public health significance, as it is well established that HIV-infected foreign travelers, immigrants, and refugees entering the United States are not a threat to the public's health.[28]

For the purposes of determining the inadmissibility of an applicant, medical conditions are categorized as class A or B. Class A conditions are defined as those conditions which preclude an immigrant or refugee from entering the United States. Class A conditions require approved waivers for US entry and immediate medical follow-up upon arrival. These conditions include communicable diseases of public health significance, a physical or mental disorder associated with violent or harmful behavior, and drug abuse or addiction. Class B conditions are defined as significant health problems: physical or mental abnormalities, diseases, or disabilities serious in degree or permanent in nature amounting to a substantial departure from normal well-being. Follow-up evaluation soon after US arrival is recommended for migrants with class B conditions. If an immigrant or refugee is found to have an inadmissible condition that may make them ineligible for a visa, a visa may still be issued after the illness has been adequately treated or after a waiver of the visa eligibility has been approved by the US Department of Homeland Security.

In 1996, a new subsection was added to the INA requiring that persons seeking immigrant visas for permanent residency show proof of receipt of at least the first dose of all vaccination series recommended by the American Committee for Immunization Practices (ACIP). Although these regulations apply to all adult immigrants and most immigrant children, internationally adopted children who are younger than 10 years of age have been exempted from the immunization requirements as a consequence of strong objections posed by advocacy groups, who cited safety concerns over immunization practices in several origin countries. In 2009 the CDC proposed that revised criteria be used in determining which vaccines recommended by the ACIP and not specifically listed in immigration law should be required for immigrants seeking admission into the United States or those seeking adjustment of status for permanent residency. Proposed criteria are:

- The vaccine must be age-appropriate, as recommended by ACIP for the general US population.

AND at least one of the following:

- The vaccine must protect against a disease that has the potential to cause an outbreak.
- The vaccine must protect against a disease that has been eliminated from the United States or is in the process of being eliminated in the United States.

These criteria were posted for public viewing in the Federal Register on November 2009 and will allow CDC the flexibility to adapt vaccination requirements for US immigrants based on public health needs.[29] At this time, refugees are not required to meet the INA immunization requirements at the time of initial entry into the United States but must show proof of vaccination at the time they apply for permanent US residence, typically within 3 years of US arrival. This policy is under review.

The US Centers for Disease Control and Prevention (CDC), Division of Global Migration and Quarantine (DGMQ), is responsible for providing technical guidance to the panel physicians performing the overseas medical screening examination.[20] The testing modalities recommended for the medical examination are outlined in ***Table 127.1***, and the algorithm for the required overseas medical screening examination is presented in ***Figure 127.4***. In 2007, CDC DGMQ published the revised requirements for the TB screening section of the overseas medical examination, called 2007 Technical Instruction for Tuberculosis Screening and Treatment[30] (***Fig. 127.5***). This updated version requires:

- sputum smears and mycobacterial cultures for applicants suspected of having TB
- drug susceptibility testing (DST) on isolates positive for *Mycobacterium tuberculosis*
- treatment to be delivered as directly observed therapy (DOT) and completed before traveling to the United States.

Although the 1991 TB Technical Instructions (TB TI) uses a high yield algorithm for identifying tuberculosis, changes were introduced as it was determined that 1991 TB instructions were insensitive and miss smear-negative, culture-positive cases, and inadequate to prevent the importation of MDR TB into the United States.[7,31] The implementation of the 2007 TB TI overseas is being done in phases based on a set of priorities that include: number of immigrants admitted to the United States, number of refugees resettling to the United States, and burden of tuberculosis in the country of origin. The 2007 TB TI have been implemented for US-bound populations from Botswana, China, Dominican Republic, Ethiopia, Haiti, Hong Kong Special Administrative Region (SAR), Japan, Jordan, Kenya, Lesotho, Macau SAR, Malaysia (refugees only), Mexico, Mozambique, Namibia, Nepal (refugees only), Philippines, South Africa, Swaziland, Taiwan, Tanzania, Thailand (refugees only), Turkey, Uganda, and Vietnam.

The CDC DGMQ is also responsible for monitoring the quality of the overseas medical examination process at over 650 panel physician sites (health care staff, radiology facilities, vaccination programs, and laboratories) worldwide, through its Quality Assurance Program (QAP). Owing to limited resources, not all panel physician sites can be visited and assessed annually. Sites are prioritized for monitoring based upon the number of immigrant and refugee visas processed and country-specific prevalence of such diseases as TB and HIV. In addition, DGMQ performs remediation visits when medical screening examination deficiencies have been identified. In an effort to share experiences regarding the optimization of immigration medical processes, technical aspects of the medical screening, the performance evaluation of panel physicians, and review policies, regulations, and practices of the various resettlement nations,

Table 127.1 Testing for Required Overseas Medical Screening Examination

Health Condition	Testing
Tuberculosis	Chest radiograph; sputum smears and cultures if CXR positive. Drug susceptibility testing if culture positive
Syphilis	Serology
Other sexually transmitted diseases	Physical examination
Leprosy (Hansen's disease)	Physical examination
Mental disorders with associated harmful behavior	History
Drug abuse or addiction	History, physical examination
Vaccinations	History/vaccination records serology

(Data from the Division of Global Migration and Quarantine, Centers for Disease Control and Prevention)

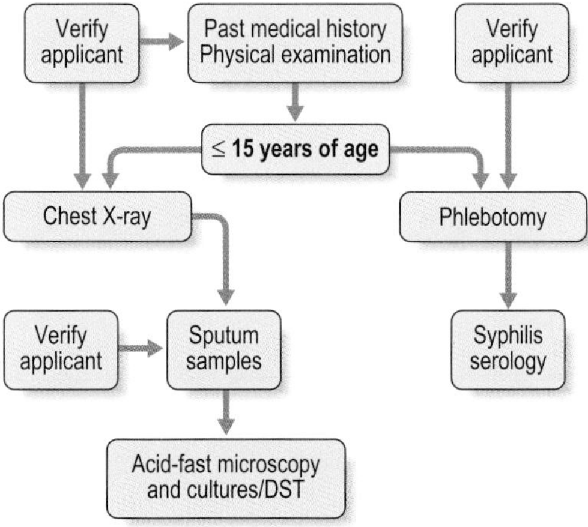

Figure 127.4 Required overseas medical screening examination from the Division of Global Migration and Quarantine, Centers for Disease Control and Prevention. DST, drug susceptibility testing.

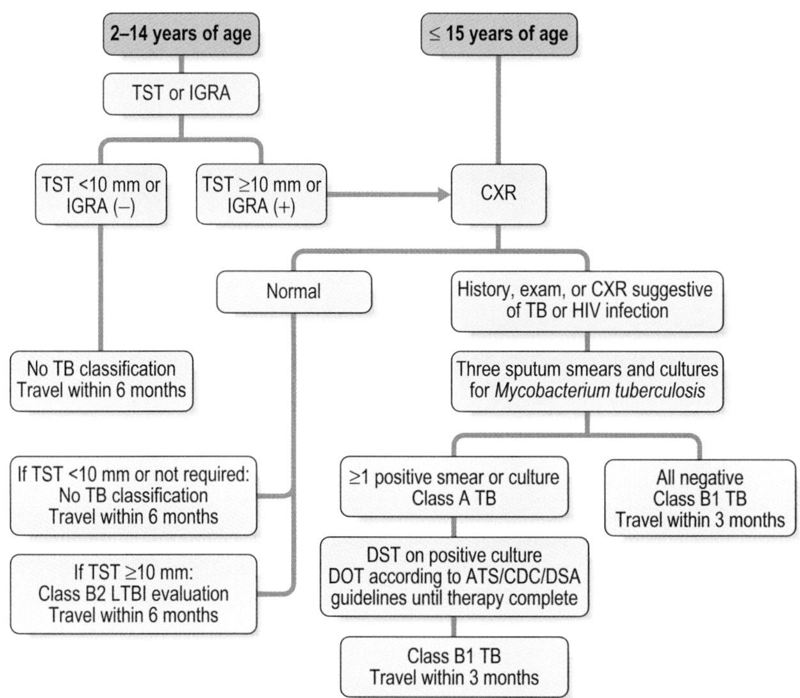

Figure 127.5 Required overseas tuberculosis screening medical examination from the Division of Global Migration and Quarantine, Centers for Disease Control and Prevention (CDC). TST, TB skin test; IGRA, interferon-γ release assay; CXR, chest X-ray; LTBI, latent TB infection; DST, drug susceptibility testing; DOT, directly observed therapy; ATS, American Thoracic Society; IDSA, Infectious Diseases Society of America.

DGMQ meets annually with sister agencies from other countries (Canada, Australia, New Zealand, and the United Kingdom) to discuss possible approaches to common challenges such as health information systems, privacy, confidentiality, and resource utilization and constraints.

HEALTH CONDITIONS IDENTIFIED THROUGH REQUIRED OVERSEAS MEDICAL SCREENING EXAMINATIONS

The number and types of health conditions identified through required overseas medical screening examinations and captured into the CDC Electronic Disease Notification (EDN) database, from 20 000 immigrants and 140 000 refugees who arrived in the United States between 2007 and 2009, are summarized in ***Table 127.2***. For both refugees and immigrants, the most frequent conditions identified were suspected active (B1) and inactive (B2) tuberculosis.

The underlying objective of the overseas TB screening process is to limit the entry of persons seeking long-term or permanent US residence who have infectious (defined as acid-fast bacilli (AFB) smear and/or culture-positive) active TB and who therefore pose an immediate public health risk, and to refer others with suspected active and inactive TB for further evaluation and treatment in the United States. This objective is connected to the facts that, as in previous years, in 2008 approximately over half (58.5%) of the 12 898 new tuberculosis cases in the United States were diagnosed among foreign-born persons and the TB rate in foreign-born persons in the United States was 10 times higher than in the US-born population.[32]

The high rates of TB in newly arrived immigrants and refugees underscore the importance of both revised overseas TB screening requirements and assuring timely and appropriate US follow-up evaluation of immigrants and refugees with suspected active TB. Together with deployment in 2007 of the EDN system, and its nationwide coverage capacity, notification delays have been minimized; and most of the operational potentially negative factors have been reduced.

Table 127.2 Number of Health Conditions Identified through Overseas Medical Screening Examination, among Immigrants and Refugees 2007–2009 (Data from the Division of Global Migration and Quarantine, Centers for Disease Control and Prevention)

Health Conditions	Immigrants	Refugees	Total
Infectious (AFB+) active TB: class A	12	5	17
Not infectious (AFB–) active TB: class B1	8800	4844	13644
Not active TB: class B2	10133	2542	12675
HIV[a]	358	448	806
Syphilis	131	209	340
Leprosy (Hansen's disease)	6	21	27
Mental disorder associated with harmful behavior	67	893	940
Drug abuse or addiction	12	47	59
Total	**19519**	**8989**	**28508**

[a]HIV testing not required after January 4, 2010.
AFB, acid-fast bacilli; TB, tuberculosis; HIV, human immunodeficiency virus.

The number of HIV infections identified during the overseas medical screening examination is relatively small. Early identification of HIV infections among immigrants and refugees is important to assure appropriate notification and linkages to medical services in resettlement communities. Current regulations require that syphilis infections be treated before departure to the United States. During 2007–2009, fewer than 350 immigrants and refuges infected with syphilis were identified overseas and captured into EDN. In reference to other inadmissible conditions listed in ***Table 127.2***, fewer than 30 cases of leprosy (Hansen's disease), fewer than 1000 cases of mental disorder associated with harmful behavior, and 59 cases of drug abuse or addiction were identified among US-bound immigrants and refugees.

The CDC DGMQ notifies state and local health departments of all arriving refugees and those immigrants with health conditions who are resettling in their jurisdiction that need follow-up evaluation and possible treatment in the United States. Under the current system, forms summarizing the results of the overseas medical examination, including classification of health conditions, are manually collected at US ports of entry. This information is then transmitted electronically to state and local health departments. State and local health departments are asked to report to DGMQ the results of these US follow-up evaluations via a web-based system and to report any significant public health conditions occurring among recently arrived immigrants and refugees. This is a way to better understand epidemiologic patterns of disease in recently arrived migrants and to monitor the quality of overseas medical examination.

NEW HEALTH SCREENING PROGRAM INITIATIVES TO IMPROVE IMMIGRANT AND REFUGEE HEALTH

Electronic Disease Notification System

The purpose of the EDN system is to electronically notify state and local health departments of newly arriving immigrants and refugees with a TB condition using the CDC secure data network. The EDN system provides federal and state public health officials with an electronic system to inform other health departments of secondary migration of immigrants and refugees with TB conditions within the United States, data to evaluate the effectiveness of follow-up on TB cases, and the ability to record the results of the domestic TB follow-up examination.[33] In addition, it allows comparison of overseas health assessments with domestic follow-up outcomes as part of a comprehensive quality assessment program for overseas TB screening examinations. The EDN system has a fully functional module that is used by all 50 states and plays a significant role in enhancing TB control and prevention efforts among arriving immigrants and refugees. The EDN system has the capability to interconnect with other data systems, such as the interface created with the International Organization for Migration (IOM) health information system, allowing electronic transmission of refugee medical examination data in a secure and timely manner, eliminating the manual entry of medical information upon their arrival to the United States. Currently, the EDN database contains information for over 150 000 medical records. The next objective for EDN is to be redesigned to include other disease modules, including disease of pandemic or bioterrorism potential, and to develop it into a real-time disease surveillance and response system.

Enhanced Refugee Health Program Initiative

The UN High Commissioner for Refugees (UNHCR) estimated that in 2008, worldwide, there were 15.2 million refugees and a total of 42 million people of concern (including refugees, internally displaced persons, and stateless persons).[34] Every year, the United States provides a safe place and freedom to 50 000–70 000 refugees from around the world who are fleeing political, religious, and ethnic persecution. Between 2007, when an Iraqi resettlement program was started, and 2009 more than 20 000 Iraqi refugees have arrived in the United States.[19]

It has long been recognized that refugees may carry significant disease burdens, which are determined by geographic origin, ethnicity, and living and health conditions in countries of origin or departure.[35,36] Refugees can suffer from a multitude of health conditions, including infectious diseases (such as tuberculosis and many tropical and parasitic diseases), malnutrition, reproductive health needs, physical trauma, and mental health disorders, often caused by tenuous circumstances in their countries of origin or departure.[35–41] Such disease burdens can seriously hamper refugees' ability to successfully integrate and optimally contribute to their resettlement communities and may cause strain on health and social services systems in the United States.[37] Most of these health conditions are not addressed during the required overseas medical examination process.

Refugees do receive stateside evaluation and treatment, usually conducted at state or local health departments, within 3 months of US arrival. However, there is currently no standardized nationwide protocol for postarrival health assessment, and therefore the content of postarrival refugee health evaluations varies from state to state, and funding sources are often noted to be inadequate to provide comprehensive services. CDC DGMQ has made available refugee health guidelines, which include clinical testing and medical treatment options.[42] Further, refugees often have other daily demands to achieve integration into their new living environment that may compete with their need for health evaluations and treatment. Optimizing refugee health prior to resettlement and addressing refugee health needs, such as vaccination and presumptive treatments, early in the migration process can be cost-effective and can prevent larger expenditures later.[43–49]

Realization of this fact has led to the development of the US Enhanced Refugee Health Program (ERHP), an initiative aimed at achieving integration of the health needs of refugee populations with facilities of the host and receiving countries. The US CDC developed the initiative, in collaboration with the US Department of State, Bureau of Population, Refugees, and Migration (PRM), the US Department of Health and Human Services, Office of Refugee Resettlement (ORR), the International Organization for Migration (IOM), and US state and local health departments, to begin to comprehensively address health care needs of US-destined refugees while they are still overseas, and to facilitate and promote appropriate stateside evaluation and treatment. The ERHP currently focuses on refugees for a number of reasons: (1) refugees are vulnerable populations, exposed to a variety of harsh environmental conditions and diverse diseases, with limited access to health care; (2) a unique opportunity exists to address refugee health concerns during required overseas health assessments; (3) the language and charge of the US Refugee Act provide more latitude to address conditions of public health concern among refugees (in addition to inadmissible conditions); and (4) lessons learned from a focus on the smaller number of refugees may be potentially applicable to the larger numbers of immigrants or other migrant groups.

The overseas component of the EHRP addresses five major areas:

- Vaccine-preventable diseases, including the Advisory Committee on Immunization Practices (ACIP)-recommended pediatric vaccinations and selected adult vaccinations.
- Tuberculosis: implement the revised 2007 Technical Instructions for Tuberculosis Screening and Treatment which stipulates improved diagnostic testing with cultures and drug susceptibility testing, directly observed treatment, and expanding tuberculosis screening to all ≥6 months of age.
- HIV infection: with activities that focus on preventing perinatal transmission through the provision of intrapartum antiretroviral therapy for HIV-infected pregnant women, the use of co-trimoxazole for prevention of opportunistic infections and the referral of HIV-infected refugees to Global AIDS Program services, where available.
- Parasitic (malaria, schistosomiasis, strongyloides, roundworms) and waterborne diseases. The proposed parasitic and waterborne diseases component includes presumptive treatment for malaria, and intestinal parasites, such as schistosomiasis, strongyloides, and roundworms, and the use of other measures, such as Safe Water Systems, to prevent waterborne diseases.
- Surveillance for emerging infectious diseases, focusing on the inclusion of US-bound refugees in global surveillance activities for febrile and respiratory illnesses, such as 2009 H1N1 flu and avian influenza.

The ERHP strategy is to utilize the required overseas medical examination process as a unique opportunity to assess and improve the health status of refugees overseas, and to incorporate both required screening components for inadmissible conditions and additional expanded components, which are tailored to specific refugee population needs and targeted to diseases of public health importance. The program ensures quality staffing and infrastructure in the field evaluating, training, and lending resources. For this purpose, in 2007, CDC DGMQ established two international offices located in Kenya and Thailand. Extending health services in the country of origin or transit allows patients to be served by health care providers who are closer geographically and often culturally to the patients' circumstances and health needs. Furthermore, through the development of enhanced and electronic data exchange systems, ERHP promotes more timely transmission of population-based health and medical examination data acquired overseas to US health departments in resettlement communities, facilitating appropriate follow-up and treatment of refugees after arrival in the United States. The domestic component of the ERHP strives to support and standardize follow-up evaluation and treatment of refugees after US arrival by state and local health departments and other community health care providers.

Since 1997, the CDC has undertaken enhanced refugee health programs for at least eight large-scale, emergent movements of refugee populations and one US-based intervention for the Lost Boys and Girls of Sudan. These programs have included components to provide presumptive predeparture treatment for malaria, intestinal parasites, and other tropical diseases, expanded TB diagnosis and treatment, HIV services, appropriate immunizations, dental and mental health assessments, chronic disease evaluations, and postarrival treatment for schistosomiasis and strongyloides infection. These programs have successfully prevented thousands of cases of intestinal parasitosis, malaria, TB, and vaccine-preventable diseases and hundreds of cases of other communicable diseases among US-bound refugees.[50-52] Other integral components of the ERHP initiative have been efforts to provide linkages to US programs in host countries, such as the Global AIDS Program (GAP) and the Global Disease Detection (GDD) Program, which can provide diagnostic, treatment and prevention services to refugees awaiting US resettlement. Such efforts are aimed at assuring refugees access to needed health care services in a prompt manner even while still in asylum countries prior to US resettlement, and to reduce the burden placed on host country resources, since overseas interventions can decrease refugee health utilization once in the United States, reduce treatment cost, and avoid overburdening the domestic health system. Finally, some more recent ERHP programs have included enhanced surveillance and response for emerging infectious diseases, including vector-borne and vaccine-preventable diseases, and most recently, 2009 H1N1 flu and H5N1 avian influenza. As part of the EHRP for Liberian refugees in Côte d'Ivoire, field staff were able to identify O'nyong-nyong fever, an emerging infectious disease in West Africa, and prevent its importation.[53]

Vaccine preventable diseases are a source of significant morbidity and mortality in developing countries, and refugees are known to be under-vaccinated owing to collapsing public health infrastructures in countries of origin or departure and lack of access to health care.[54] In addition, outbreaks of measles, pertussis, and varicella among US-bound Somali refugees in Kenya in 2007, 2008, and 2009, malaria among Burundians in 2007, as well as varicella among Bhutanese refugees in Nepal and measles among Burmese refuges in Thailand in 2008, were identified and controlled during ERHP programs. As a result of these and other disease outbreaks such as cholera (*Fig. 127.6*), the movement of refugees has

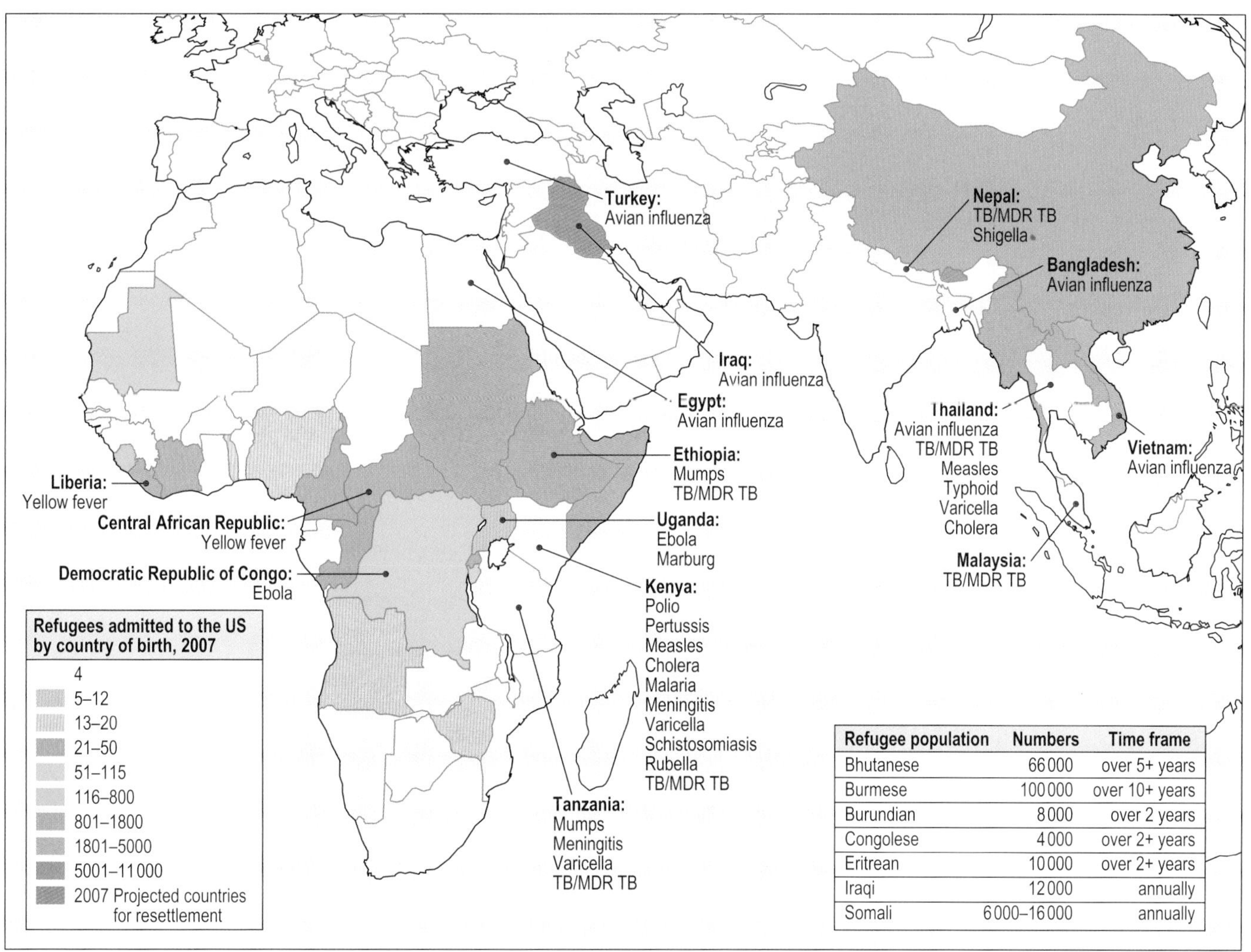

Refugee population	Numbers	Time frame
Bhutanese	66000	over 5+ years
Burmese	100000	over 10+ years
Burundian	8000	over 2 years
Congolese	4000	over 2+ years
Eritrean	10000	over 2+ years
Iraqi	12000	annually
Somali	6000–16000	annually

Figure 127.6 Disease outbreaks and diseases of concern in US-bound refugees, 2006–2008, from the Division of Global Migration and Quarantine, Centers for Disease Control and Prevention.

Table 127.3 Requirements for Routine Vaccination of Immigrants Examined Overseas Who Are Not Fully Vaccinated or Lack Documentation

	Age						
Vaccine	**Birth to 1 Month**	**2-11 Months**	**12 Months to 6 Years**	**7-10 Years**	**11-17 Years**	**18-64 Years**	**≥65 Years**
DTP/DTaP/DT	NO	YES		NO			
Td/Tdap	NO			YES, ≥7 years old (for Td); 10–64 years old (for Tdap)			
Polio (IPV/OPV)	NO	YES				NO	
MMR	NO		YES, if born in 1957 or later				NO
Rotavirus	NO	YES, 2–6 months old	NO				
Hib	NO	Yes, 2–59 months old		NO			
Hepatitis A	NO		YES, 12–23 months old	NO			
Hepatitis B	YES, through 18 years old					NO	
Meningococcal (MCV/MPSV)	NO				Yes, 11–18 years old	NO	
Varicella	NO		YES				
Pneumococcal	NO	YES, 2–59 months old (for PCV)		NO			YES (for PPV)
Influenza	NO		YES, 6 months to 18 years old (annually each flu season)			NO	YES, ≥50 years old (annually each flu season)

DTP, diphtheria and tetanus toxoids and pertussis vaccine; DTaP, diphtheria and tetanus toxoids and acellular pertussis vaccine; DT, pediatric formulation diphtheria and tetanus toxoids; Td, adult formulation tetanus and diphtheria toxoids; Tdap, adolescent and adult formulation tetanus and diphtheria toxoids and acellular pertussis vaccine (Boostrix for persons 10–18 years old; Adacel for persons 11–64 years old); IPV, inactivated poliovirus vaccine (killed); OPV, oral poliovirus vaccine (live); MMR, combined measles, mumps, rubella vaccine; Hib, *Haemophilus influenzae* type b conjugate vaccine; MCV, meningococcal conjugate vaccine; MPSV, meningococcal polysaccharide vaccine; PCV, pneumococcal conjugate vaccine; PPV, pneumococcal polysaccharide vaccine.

(Data from the Division of Global Migration and Quarantine, Centers for Disease Control and Prevention.)

frequently been delayed and necessitated substantial additional per capita investments in the resettlement process (e.g., last-minute cancellation of nonrefundable commercial airline tickets and the need for dedicated refugee charter flights), not to mention the obvious risks to refugee health and threat of importation and spread of disease in receiving communities.

To prevent morbidity, mortality, and the threats of disease importation along with the avoidance of costly delays in refugee resettlement, CDC DGMQ recommends that refugees also receive age-appropriate immunizations listed in the *Technical Instructions to Panel Physicians for Vaccination Requirements* (for immigrants) if the vaccines are available in-country or easily obtained (***Table 127.3***). CDC recognizes that some vaccines may not be available in all host countries, and therefore vaccination with some vaccines may not be feasible. However, common vaccines that can be routinely obtained overseas for use in most host countries include diphtheria and tetanus toxoids and pertussis (DPT), tetanus and diphtheria toxoids (Td), live oral poliovirus (OPV), measles-mumps-rubella (MMR), hepatitis B, and varicella; an initial dose of vaccines in these series should be administered as early as possible before migration to maximize utility and protection.[46] The following vaccinations may not be easily obtained in host countries: *Haemophilus influenzae* (Hib), *Streptococcus pneumoniae*, and influenza. If vaccines are not available in host countries, they should be administered as soon as possible after arrival in the United States.

In Fiscal Year 2008, the total number of adoptions to the United States was over 17 000. The five countries from which Americans adopted the largest number of children were: Guatemala, China, Russia, Ethiopia, and South Korea. Special concerns for internationally adopted children include hepatitis B and C, measles, syphilis, HIV infection, TB, and intestinal parasitic infections, which may warrant screening in addition to a review and update of routine childhood immunizations.[55–57]

FUTURE DIRECTIONS

Migrant, immigrant, and refugee health aims to shift the migration health paradigm away from a focus merely on inadmissible conditions and regulatory exclusion toward integration of migration and health needs, which is advantageous not only for the health of migrant populations but also for those in host countries and the receiving communities. Achieving more integrated and comprehensive migration health programs and policies, includes:

1. Continuing efforts to tailor migration health policies to incorporate the unique needs of migrant populations and to provide flexibility to address emerging global health issues, such as pandemic flu.
2. Expanding the role of migration health assessments in protecting public health of migrants and of receiving and host countries. Priority areas should include the following:
   a. support for delivery of essential preventive and treatment interventions, such as vaccinations and treatment for malaria and other parasitic diseases
   b. creation of effective surveillance systems for emerging infectious diseases
   c. development of emergency response capacity
   d. inclusion of components to address emerging infectious diseases, reproductive and mental health needs, and other diseases of public health importance.
3. Applying new information technology to secure electronic information exchange among numerous international and interagency partners and assuring real-time communication of health data along the migration pathway.
4. Identifying sustainable funding to support migration health programs, in both receiving and host countries.

5. Promoting public–private partnerships to address migrant health issues.
6. Developing international and interagency partnerships to facilitate harmonization of policies and the integration of global migration and health issues.

Ultimately, health and migration are intimately linked and interdependent. Early investment in addressing and integrating the health needs of migrants and of receiving and host communities will facilitate the migration process, improve migrant health, decrease associated morbidity and mortality, and avoid long-term health resource and social costs, and protect global public health.

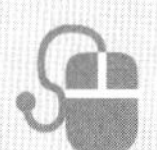

Access the complete reference list online at **http://www.expertconsult.com**

CHAPTER 128

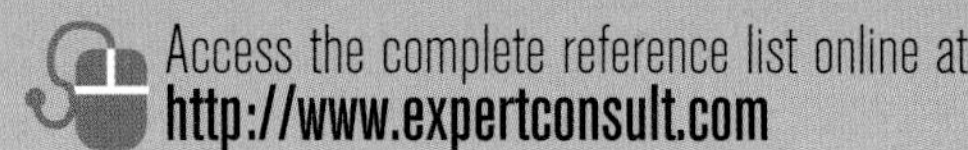
Access the complete reference list online at
http://www.expertconsult.com

Infectious Diseases in Modern Military Forces*

Alan J. Magill • Bonnie L. Smoak • Truman W. Sharp

INTRODUCTION

The modern military forces era can be defined from the end of the Cold War in 1991 to the present. This chapter describes infectious diseases reported in military populations and will help health care providers broaden their differential diagnoses of the ill soldier or veteran. We use the term soldier for brevity's sake to represent all those serving in the armed services, including airmen, sailors, and marines. Military forces from many countries serve outside their homelands in peacekeeping operations and wars. In 2009, over 500 000 US military personnel were operating in at least 150 countries, including two major wars in Afghanistan and Iraq. In 2009, United Nations peacekeeping forces were involved in 17 operations on five continents around the world.[1] This included almost 120 000 military personnel and civilian police from 117 countries. These individuals may be exposed to diseases not endemic in their home countries and may be at even higher risk for acquiring these diseases than other travelers because of their unique living conditions. While training or deployed, military units living in crowded conditions may have increased rates of transmission of pathogens spread by droplets or aerosol, such as *Neisseria meningitidis* or *Streptococcus pneumoniae*, and poor hygienic conditions or uncertain control of food sources, and food preparation in the field may increase the likelihood of diseases transmitted by the fecal–oral route.

Provision of health care to these troops varies by country of origin. Some countries, like the United States, have an extensive military medical system; however, ill reserve soldiers, and even active duty soldiers on leave, may be first evaluated by civilian physicians. Other countries refer all ill soldiers to civilian care.

US military personnel receive immunizations to prevent numerous infectious agents at various time points in their career from entry on active duty through geographic-specific deployments. Current Department of Defense and Service specific immunization policies can be found at the MILVAX website (http://www.vaccines.mil/default.aspx).

DISEASES TRANSMITTED BY DROPLET OR AEROSOL

Deployed troops and military trainees living in crowded conditions are at increased risk of acquiring diseases transmitted by the respiratory route.[2] Of special concern to the US Armed Forces are respiratory illnesses caused by adenoviruses, influenza, *S. pneumoniae*, *S. pyogenes*, and *Mycoplasma pneumoniae*.[3] In the 1950s and 1960s, adenoviruses caused more than 90% of the hospitalized pneumonia cases at training sites during the winter months.[3] Introduction of an oral live vaccine in trainees for adenoviral serotypes 4 and 7, the predominant strains observed in military epidemics, in 1971 largely controlled the problem. Unfortunately, the sole manufacturer of the vaccine ceased production in 1996 and by 1999 respiratory illness rates among trainees increased to levels observed during the prevaccine era. Approximately 10–12% of all recruits became ill with adenovirus infections. In 2000, the first deaths since 1972 associated with adenovirus infection occurred in basic trainees.[4] Frequent adenovirus infections and deaths have continued to occur, prompting the US military to initiate a new adenovirus vaccine program.

A new outbreak of a rare human adenovirus serotype 14 was described in multiple recruit training centers in the spring of 2006.[5] Severe illness requiring hospitalization and one death have been decribed.[6] Although preexisting adenovirus 7 neutralizing antibodies acquired from natural infection were protective against severe disease,[6] it is not known whether the new adenovirus 4 plus 7 vaccine-induced neutralizing antibodies will protect against infection with the adenovirus 14 serotype.

Frequent outbreaks of influenza-like illnesses are reported among US forces even though a mandatory influenza vaccination program occurs each fall. Most outbreaks are the consequences of a lack of vaccination rather than failure of the vaccine and occur when vaccination centers fail to obtain or administer the vaccine in a timely manner,[7] an influenza strain not contained in the vaccine causes infections,[8] or due to other respiratory viruses, such as parainfluenza.[9]

Large outbreaks of pneumococcal pneumonia and group A streptococcal pneumonia occurred among marine recruits in 2000 and 2002, respectively.[10,11] An outbreak of pneumococcal pneumonia occurred among US Army Ranger students undergoing intense training in the winter of 1998–99.[12] Mass chemoprophylactic regimens with two doses of benzathine penicillin (4 weeks apart) as prophylaxis and vaccination have been required to control *S. pneumoniae* and *S. pyogenes* infections in US training forces.

There is always concern that troops may be at increased risk of acquiring tuberculosis (TB), including multidrug and extensively resistant strains, when they are deployed to countries with high prevalence of this disease. This potential risk has been difficult to verify. Sailors and marines appear to be at higher risk of infection because of their close living and working quarters on board ships.[13,14] In 1998, a US marine on an amphibious ship became ill with a dry cough of 1 month's duration.[15] He was treated for atypical pneumonia twice and stayed onboard the ship for 3 months before he was transported to a local naval hospital where active TB was diagnosed. Contact investigation involving 3338 persons identified 712 new latent TB infections and 21 persons who developed active TB. Because of the impact of active disease in closed populations, identification of latent TB infection is a priority in military populations to identify those at risk of active disease so that they may receive presumptive treatment.

Concerns about TB exposure have been raised in recent deployments to Iraq and Afghanistan, which are reported to have among the highest

*The views expressed are those of the authors and should not be construed to represent the positions of the Department of the Army, Department of the Navy, or Department of Defense.

rates of active TB in the world. Therefore universal TB skin testing, including testing both before and twice after deployment, was recommended starting in 2003.[16] The testing of this predominantly low-risk population results in a low positive predictive value of the test. This leads to both a greater proportion and absolute number of false positives among the positive test results. A report of eight pseudoepidemics of tuberculin skin test conversions[17] led to new policies to limit skin testing to only those with clinical or epidemiologic risk factors and also a recommendation preferentially to use Tubersol brand of tuberculin for all military testing in 2008.[18]

Crowded conditions in military populations facilitate the transmission of other respiratory-transmitted diseases, such as meningococcal disease, measles, chickenpox, and rubella. Recruits are at especially high risk for meningococcal disease with its high case-fatality rate and potential sequelae that include limb loss, neurologic disabilities, and hearing loss.[19] Since 1971, vaccines have been effective in preventing disease caused by vaccine-homologous serogroups in US recruits.[19] Similar reductions were seen in French, British, and Israeli recruits after the introduction of vaccination programs in the 1990s.[20–22] Sporadic cases and occasional outbreaks still occur. The public health management of these events is made difficult by the number of close contacts of cases and the mobility of a military population. Large numbers of persons may have had close contact with the case because of crowded living and working conditions. In 1995, 340 persons received prophylactic treatment after the sudden death of a soldier on maneuvers from group B meningococcemia.[23] In 2003, 99 sailors were identified as having close contact with a suspected case of meningococcal meningitis on a US aircraft carrier and received antibiotic prophylaxis.[24]

DISEASES TRANSMITTED BY ARTHROPODS

Malaria continues to cause significant morbidity and mortality in military populations serving around the world (see Chapter 96). A review of malaria cases in the US military between 2002 and 2008 showed 80–150 cases per year, with the majority of the cases acquired in Afghanistan, reflecting the long-term deployment to this region since 2001.[25] In 1993, vivax malaria re-emerged as a threat to military forces and the civilian population in the Republic of Korea. Over 9000 cases were diagnosed in Korean soldiers and veterans from 1993 to 2000.[26] During this same time period, 186 cases were reported in US soldiers who had served in Korea.[27,28] Many of these cases were diagnosed at locations outside Korea because of the long latency of this temperate strain (>6 months) and the short duty assignment (1 year) of the soldiers. The number of cases of vivax malaria acquired in Korea has declined significantly and in 2008 no cases were reported in US military personnel.[25]

Deployments to sub-Saharan Africa are frequently associated with malaria cases. During a 6-month period in 1995–96, Brazilian troops deployed to Angola had an 18% attack rate and three soldiers died of cerebral malaria.[29] French troops had malaria rates of 35.7 cases per 1000 person-months during their first month of deployment to the Ivory Coast in 2002.[30] During 2003, a US military unit operating in Liberia had an attack rate of 35% (80 of 225) after only a 10-day period of exposure (Tim Whitman, personal communication). In each of these incidents, failure to comply with the recommended chemoprophylaxis regimen and the infrequent use of personal protection measures (PPMs) were responsible for high disease rates.[29,30] This is in contrast to the Swedish experience in Liberia from 2004 to 2006 in which no cases of malaria were seen in over 7000 person-months of exposure when PPMs and routine chemoprophylaxis were used.[31]

Relapsing malaria caused by *Plasmodium vivax* is a recurring problem in deployed forces when they return home. Forty-eight cases of malaria occurred among US forces while in Somalia during 1993; most were caused by *P. falciparum*.[32] Several hundred cases of malaria from *P. vivax* infections occurred after they returned home.[33,34] A similar pattern was observed in Italian forces serving in Somalia during this same time period. Among 11 624 soldiers, 18 cases occurred in Somalia, while 147 cases occurred after returning to Italy.[35] The scenario was repeated in 1999, when 11 000 United Nations peacekeepers from 17 countries were sent to East Timor to restore order. During the initial 5 months, the Australian Defence Force deployed 5500 soldiers. Sixty-four cases of malaria occurred in-country, with two-thirds of these infections caused by *P. falciparum*. After returning to Australia, 212 malaria cases, almost all due to *P. vivax*, were treated.[36]

The majority of vivax malaria cases acquired by US personnel in Afghanistan also present after soldiers leave the endemic area.[25] Vivax malaria in particular is problematic for military forces placed on one of the accepted malaria prophylaxis agents such as mefloquine, doxycycline, or atovaquone–proguanil. These agents do not have any effect on the hypnozoite of vivax malaria and thus do not prevent the late relapse, regardless of how compliant soldiers are with the chemoprophylaxis regimen in the field. Primaquine is the only available drug that can prevent late relapse of vivax malaria.

Thus malaria is a common problem for troops deployed to endemic areas, even when preventive measures were recommended and in some cases enforced. Several challenges arise in providing effective protection against malaria to immunologically naïve populations, such as soldiers. First, knowledge about the risk of acquiring malaria is frequently incomplete. The geographic distribution of malaria is uncertain and often increasing secondary to population movements, environmental changes, and decreased control efforts associated with the political events that precede a military intervention or a peacekeeping mission. Determining if re-emergence has occurred before military forces deploy to an area is difficult because generally public health efforts have ceased in these areas. Even in areas of established malaria transmission, evaluating the risk can be difficult because rates of transmission can be very focal within a country and the exact movement of the military unit is not known.

The preceding examples also demonstrate the difficulties in determining when primaquine should be recommended as a terminal prophylactic drug regimen for vivax malaria; predicting the risk of infection is difficult. Endemic population rates may underestimate the risk because troops may operate in more remote areas and local populations may self-treat and not present to medical facilities. Rates observed in troops during the deployment also underestimate the risk when military forces are using an appropriate chemoprophylactic regimen. There were few vivax cases during deployments to Somalia and East Timor, but hundreds of cases after the troops returned to their homelands.

As seen in US troops returning from Somalia, even when primaquine is recommended, the effectiveness of the regimen may be low if the drug is not given under directly observed treatment, thus insuring the drug is taken.[33] Noncompliance with the standard drug regimen – 15 mg (base) daily for 14 days (15 mg × 14 days) – is common and commanders rarely require that it be taken under direct observation. Further, some tropical vivax strains require a higher dose than the 15 mg × 14-day regimen to eradicate the liver stages.[37,38] It is not always known at the time of a policy recommendation if a higher dose regimen should be recommended for a given locale.[34] Given the difficulties in assessing the risk of infection and the generally low effectiveness of the standard 14-day regimen, some military planners decide not to recommend a terminal prophylactic regimen with primaquine. The Dutch did not use primaquine for antirelapse prophylaxis when their troops returned home from Cambodia and estimated that they would have had to treat 100 soldiers presumptively for each vivax case that did occur.[39]

In summary, despite having efficacious chemoprophylactic drugs, personal protective measures, and vector control strategies that would protect the majority of military personnel from disease, malaria continues to cause illness and sometimes death among foreign troops deployed to endemic areas. *P. vivax* is the predominant species causing illness in military forces when appropriate chemoprophylaxis is used during the deployment and occurs most frequently in soldiers after return to their home country. It has been extremely difficult to prevent vivax infection in troops after they return home. Health care providers should always consider malaria in the differential diagnosis of any febrile soldier who has served in a malarious area, especially within the past year.

Dengue infections in troops should be expected when they deploy to dengue-endemic areas (see Chapter 75). During the multinational deployments to Haiti from 1994 to 1997, dengue was a major cause of febrile illness. When US forces first entered Haiti in 1994, dengue was identified in 29% of the hospitalized febrile patients during the first 6 weeks of the deployment.[40] Of 249 hospitalized febrile patients, 32% were infected with dengue.[41] PPMs were not fully utilized. Dengue cases were identified among US forces in Somalia[42] and Italian troops in East Timor.[43] Epidemic transmission occurred in French troops stationed in French Polynesia in 1989, with an attack rate of 47%.[44] The importation of dengue virus back by soldiers returning from duty abroad is a possibility. Nine Australian soldiers returning from duty in East Timor following peacekeeping operations in 2000 were found to be viremic in the home station in north Queensland. Fortunately no civilian cases were reported in the area for the following 4 months.[45]

Other arboviruses have been reported in soldiers: for example, Rift Valley fever in two febrile French soldiers in Chad, 2001;[46] Ross River virus disease ("epidemic polyarthritis") during a joint exercise held in Queensland, Australia, during 1997;[47] and Japanese encephalitis in Okinawa in 1991. Given the short incubation period of most of these diseases (less than 2 weeks), most ill soldiers and veterans presenting to civilian physicians will have recently returned from their deployment. In summary, military personnel are at risk of being infected with endemic circulating arboviruses when they are deployed overseas.

Tick-borne diseases occur in troops deployed or training in rural areas at home or abroad (see Chapters 49–52). There are multiple human pathogens found in ticks to include all *Rickettsia*, *Francisella tularensis*, members of the *Ehrlichia* phagocytophila genogroup, Crimean-Congo hemorrhagic fever, *Borrelia burgdorferi* sensu lato, and the European tick-borne encephalitis virus.

Rocky Mountain spotted fever and human ehrlichiosis have been reported in military forces after field training in endemic areas of the United States. A cluster of tick-borne infections at two US military installations led to a prospective study that resulted in the isolation of *Ehrlichia chaffeensis*, the causative agent of human monocytic ehrlichiosis in 1990.[48] A prospective serological study of 1194 US military personnel following a training exercise in Arkansas indicated a 2.5% seroconversion rate to spotted fever group *Ricksettsia* (SFGR) and a 1.3% seroconversion rate to *Ehrlichia* species, although most infections were not associated with symptoms (73% of SFGR seroconvertors and 67% of the *Ehrlichia* species seroconvertors did not report symptoms).[49]

These rates of infection have importance beyond the health of the individual soldier. In 1997, 10 US National Guard members in Iowa presented with symptoms consistent with tick-borne diseases shortly after a 2-week training exercise in Arkansas.[50] Several of these soldiers, along with others in their unit, had donated blood shortly before becoming ill. Among the 377 blood donors, 12 individuals were found to have confirmed or probable infection with Rocky Mountain spotted fever or ehrlichiosis. Sixty (16%) donors had evidence of asymptomatic seroconversion. A total of 320 units of platelets or packed red blood cells were transfused into 129 recipients in nine states. Seven hundred units were recalled. Ten recipients received units from ill soldiers, although none became ill.

Tick-borne disease can affect the operational readiness of an entire unit. In 1992, a large outbreak of African tick bite fever occurred in a US airborne unit that had deployed to Botswana for 2 weeks.[51] Eighteen percent (31/169 soldiers) were clinically ill and had lab confirmation consistent with *Rickettsia africae* infection. PPMs were not fully utilized.

Scrub typhus is an important disease entity to rural and military populations throughout Southeast Asia, Korea, and Japan. Since 1934, outbreaks have been described among US and Japanese troops training in a camp near Mount Fuji, Japan. Recent outbreaks among US forces were reported in 1995, 2000, and 2001.[52] Attack rates of 1% were observed in each incident. Scrub typhus was once common in north Queensland, Australia, but cases had not been reported for 30 years until 1996.[53] At that time, a soldier was diagnosed with scrub typhus and an investigation followed. Seventeen additional cases were identified. One year later, another outbreak involving 11 cases occurred at the same training site. Based on seroconversion rates, Thai soldiers working near the Thai–Cambodian border during 1992 had an estimated 2.66% annual infection rate.[54]

Infections caused by the protozoan parasite *Leishmania* (see Chapter 100) can cause significant morbidity to military forces worldwide. Numerous outbreaks of cutaneous leishmaniasis (CL) have been associated with military units deployed to jungle training centers. The incubation period of CL varies widely from a few days to many years, but the majority of lesions appear within the first few months after exposure. For short-term training missions, most cases occur after redeployment to their home base. Training-related outbreaks have occurred in Belize,[55] French Guiana, the Brazilian Amazon,[56–58] and at the former US Army-operated Jungle Operations Training Center in Panama.[59] Attack rates can be surprisingly high in nonimmune soldiers, with 80–90% reported from French Guiana.[60] A striking example is a report from 1990 of 17 cases of CL seen in 27 Canadian paratroopers (63% attack rates) on the ground for 6 hours in British Guyana.[61] CL is a serious morale problem for Latin American military organizations. Overall infection rates of 1–2%, with much higher epidemic outbreaks in small units, are not uncommon in units stationed in remote areas to counter antigovernment insurgencies or narco-trafficking.

CL caused by *Leishmania major* was described in soldiers with Middle East peacekeeping duty associated while serving in the Multinational Force and Observers in the Sinai desert.[62,63] Both Israeli and Jordanian soldiers have suffered epidemic outbreaks of CL caused by *L. major* while assigned to duties near the Jordan river valley and the Negev desert.[64,65]

Prior to the deployment of large numbers of troops to Afghanistan for Operation Enduring Freedom in 2001 and to Iraq for Operation Iraqi Freedom in 2002, the US military experience with CL was predominantly related to training missions in Central America, especially Panama.[66–68] The recent deployment to Iraq has resulted in the largest outbreak of CL in US forces since World War II.[69–71] Exact case totals are difficult to know as many cases of CL are not reported, are not sufficiently severe to warrant treatment, or are not parasitologically confirmed. Over 1000 cases of CL caused by *L. major* have been described to date.[72] The majority of cases were acquired in Iraq, with fewer cases of CL caused by *L. tropica* and *L. major* acquired in Afghanistan. The transmission season in Iraq and Afghanistan begins as early as March as temperatures rise and can extend into November depending on local microenvironments. Most clinical presentations occur between August and May, peaking in October through February. In 2003–2004, around 50 cases per month were recorded in US forces with more recent years declining to fewer than 10 cases per month reported.[72] One unit returning from Iraq in 2004 showed an overall 1% case rate (237 confirmed cases of CL and 360 suspected cases from a 20 000-person unit).[73] A wide range of severity was described and multiple interventions were given, to include intravenous sodium stibogluconate (Pentostam), flucaonzole, cryotherapy, and heat treatment with the ThermoMed device. Seventy-two soldiers elected no treatment.

Recent military experience with visceral leishmaniasis (VL) is more limited, most likely due to the fact that military operations have not occurred in areas of the world at highest risk for VL, such as the Ganges river drainage in India, Nepal, and Bangladesh, and southern Sudan. In addition, clinically apparent disease is much less common than inapparent infection in otherwise healthy, nonimmune adults. Sporadic cases of VL have been described in French soldiers, acquired in Chad,[74] and in five US soldiers – two cases acquired in Iraq, one in Oman, and two in Afghanistan.[75,76] Of note, all five cases of VL had a typical presentation of prolonged fever, hepatosplenomegaly or splenomegaly, weight loss, and various cytopenias, but the diagnosis of VL was not considered until the patient reached specialists in infectious disease. In addition, multiple attempts at parasitologic confirmation in bone marrow aspirates and liver biopsies were required. The combination of smears, histopathology, culture, and polymerase chain reaction was needed to confirm the diagnosis.

VL may present differently in healthy nonimmune adults with lower parasite burdens, making parasitological diagnosis more difficult, and more atypical symptoms.[77] For example, 12 cases of systemic illness caused by *L. tropica*, a parasite usually associated with CL, were described in US soldiers following the first Gulf War in 1991.[78,79] None of these patients presented with typical signs and symptoms of VL and instead presented with fatigue, malaise, gastrointestinal symptoms, adenopathy, transient hepatosplenomegaly, and mild laboratory abnormalities. The syndrome was called "viscerotropic" because parasites were isolated from bone marrow, liver tissue, or lymph nodes.

Large groups of American military personnel and their families live in *Leishmania*-endemic areas of the world. The US naval air station in Sigonella, Sicily, is an area long known to be endemic for a zoonotic cycle of *L. infantum*, canine reservoirs, and local sandfly vectors. Occasionally infantile kala-azar is seen in children of assigned military personnel. A study in companion pet dogs showed a 75% subclinical infection rate,[80] suggesting that subclinical human infection occurs more often than recognized.

Prevention of *Leishmania* infection in military populations relies on vector PPMs. The use of permethrin-impregnated uniforms is recommended, but clinical trial data to support such use are limited. Four of 143 (3%) Colombian soldiers wearing impregnated uniforms acquired CL, while 18 of 143 (18%) wearing control uniforms acquired CL.[81] The success in Colombia was not seen in a clinical trial in Iran.[82] Practical insect avoidance measures, combined with treated bednets and DEET-based repellents, can achieve high protection against biting arthropods.[82]

DISEASES TRANSMITTED BY THE FECAL-ORAL ROUTE

Diarrheal diseases continue be an important cause of illness in modern military forces. Rates and etiologies reflect regional and seasonal distributions of enteric pathogens.[83] During conflict or a time of rapid buildup of forces, toilet facilities can be primitive, consisting of open trenches or wooden latrines. Fly control may not be established and adequate levels of personal hygiene and sanitation are difficult to maintain. These factors, together with crowded living conditions, increase the transmission potential of pathogens transmitted by the fecal–oral route.

Campylobacter infections were a leading cause of diarrhea in US troops training in Thailand during the 1990s as quinolone-resistant strains became more prevalent in that area.[84]

In 1990 during the initial months of Operation Desert Shield, outbreaks of watery diarrhea occurred in US troops.[85] This was followed by outbreaks of more severe, bloody diarrhea in the second month. More than 50% of 2022 US combatants surveyed reported at least one episode of diarrhea and 20% of affected combatants reported that it interfered with their work and resulted in a medical visit.[85] In a separate survey, microbiologic studies showed that half of the diarrhea in combatants seeking medical care was of bacterial origins, mostly enterotoxigenic *Escherichia coli* and *Shigella* species.[85] Many of the outbreaks were attributed to ingestion of raw vegetables, especially lettuce, that were procured from countries outside the United States.

Diarrhea control measures among US forces were strongly enforced during Operation Restore Hope in Somalia, 1992–1993. A comprehensive medical surveillance system that included over 85% of all deployed forces was instituted and found that less than 1% of the force each week sought care for diarrhea during the first 2 months.[86] No large diarrhea outbreaks were observed. *Shigella* species (33%) and enterotoxigenic *E. coli* (16%) were the predominant bacterial pathogens isolated.

Self-reported disease prevalence during Operation Iraqi Freedom and Operation Enduring Freedom (Aghanistan) indicated that diarrhea rates may have been high during the initial phase of deployment.[87] Seventy percent of 2389 volunteers reported at least one episode of diarrhea and 56% reported multiple episodes. Seventeen percent of those with diarrhea reported being on bed rest for a median of 2 days.

Diarrhea rates during deployments on humanitarian missions can be high. British (n = 36) and Australian (n = 75) medical teams working among the Kurdish refugees in 1991 had different rates of diarrhea during the first 5 weeks in northern Iraq.[88] Diarrhea rates were higher among the British force (69%), which did not use doxycycline for malaria prophylaxis and did not enforce hand- and plate-washing procedures, than among the Australian group (36%), which did. In 1994 among a 131-person Dutch military unit serving in the refugee camps in Goma, Zaire, 20% reported diarrhea during the first 3 weeks.[89] On the day of departure, 102 servicemen ate at a local hotel and 59% developed diarrhea shortly after returning home.

Norovirus outbreaks are being increasingly recognized among military forces. While outbreaks among civilian ships have received publicity, at least 60–80% of cases occur on land.[90] Outbreaks of vomiting were reported in Operation Desert Shield/Storm among American forces and an attack rate of 4–9% occurred over a 5-month period in one marine unit.[91] Ninety-nine soldiers in an Army trainee unit (12%) were hospitalized during an outbreak at El Paso, Texas, in 1998.[92] In May 2002, 11 British soldiers were air-evacuated from Afghanistan when the initial patients presented with a severe acute illness characterized by headache, neck stiffness, photophobia, obtundation, and gastrointestinal symptoms.[93] Two patients required ventilatory support and one patient's illness progressed to disseminated intravascular coagulation. Norovirus infection was later confirmed by laboratory analyses in England.

Explosive outbreaks have occurred on US Navy vessels, with several hundred sailors becoming ill in a short time period.[94] For the deployed forces, this infection causes a major diagnostic dilemma. Currently, there are no rapid diagnostic field tests to identify norovirus infection from an unknown chemical or biological attack that produces similar clinical symptoms and attack rates.

ZOONOTIC DISEASES

Q fever has emerged as a significant infectious disease among those deployed to Iraq since 2003 in support of Operation Iraqi Freedom.[95–99] Fever, pneumonia, and/or hepatitis are the most common signs of acute infection with Q fever.[100,101] In those in whom chronic disease develops, infective endocarditis is the initial condition in >70% of cases. Asymptomatic infection may occur in >50% of infected patients. Q fever is known to have a multitude of clinical manifestations. Raoult et al. described seven distinct presentations:[102] fever, pneumonia, hepatitis, meningitis, meningoencephalitis, pericarditis, and myocarditis; and Parker et al described >30 clinical syndromes.[100] This broad variation in clinical presentation can result in confusion and much delayed diagnosis. It is recommended that Q fever be considered in the differential diagnosis of any febrile illness acquired in Iraq or Afgahnistan. Empiric treatment with doxycycline should be given while pursuing confirmation of the diagnosis, which is most often accomplished retrospectively by documenting seroconversion with paired acute and convalescent sera. Clinical response to doxycycline should be seen in the first 24–48 hours after the start of treatment if the illness is Q fever. The incidence of Q fever among soldiers is likely significantly underestimated. Most infections present as a nonspecific flu-like illness and are self-limited.

Although uncommon, a possible case of human-to-human sexual transmission of Q fever from a returning soldier to his spouse has been reported.[103] The infective agent of Q fever, *Coxiella burnetii*, is resistant to heat, drying, and most disinfectants. Although the primary method of transmission is via aerosolization, numerous other modes of transmission have been reported, to include ingestion of contaminated food (raw milk), transplacental transmission, blood transfusion, tick bites, handling contaminated clothing (laundry), and sexual transmission.

Hemorrhagic fever with renal syndrome (HFRS), a rodent-borne disease (see Chapter 71), has caused significant casualties during military conflicts. The war in the Balkans during the 1990s was no exception. In Bosnia, more than 300 military and civilian cases were treated in a single hospital during a 1-year period.[104] In 1995, large outbreaks of HFRS occurred at several sites in Croatia. Of the 129 reported cases, 120 were Croatian Army soldiers. Two of the soldiers died.[105] Severe clinical manifestations were reported in many patients. These infections were caused by a newly described hantavirus, Dobrava, rather than the Puumala virus, which also circulates in this area but causes a milder illness.

The association of rodent-borne diseases and war arises from increased numbers of rodents with improperly stored food and garbage in military camps. Military outbreaks have also occurred during field training when the rodent's natural habitat is disturbed. In January 1990, US troops camping in southern Germany during training maneuvers had 16 cases of HFRS for an attack rate in one unit of 8.5%.[106]

In Korea, HFRS affects both civilian and military populations. Of 3000 cases 24% were Korean soldiers, but only 22 cases occurred among American soldiers.[107] Another outbreak occurred in 1986 among 3754 US marines participating in a 5-week joint training exercise with Korean troops.[108] Fourteen cases occurred; two died. Eight of the cases became symptomatic after leaving Korea. Infection can occur without exposure to a field setting. Recently, a case occurred in a soldier; it appeared that the infection was acquired on base in an urban environment.[109]

Leptospirosis (see Chapter 45) is an occupational hazard for soldiers training and operating in aquatic environments. In the early 1980s, some US military units training in Panama had attack rates of 2–8%. In response, military researchers tested and demonstrated the efficacy of weekly (200 mg) doxycycline for chemoprophylaxis.[110] In 1987, two clusters of cases occurred in US military personnel serving in Okinawa, Japan, with attack rates of 47% and 18%.[111] In 1999, 193 Peruvian military recruits trained for 2 weeks in the high jungles near Pichanaqui, Peru.[112] During the subsequent 4 weeks, 78 recruits became ill with an acute undifferentiated febrile illness. Laboratory testing showed 92% of the cases were positive for leptospirosis by the microscopic agglutination test. Like Q fever, this disease is probably underreported because the clinical presentation is quite broad, ranging from asymptomatic infection to severe life-threatening disease, and there is very limited availability and accuracy of laboratory confirmation of acute illness. As in Q fever, empiric treatment of suspected leptospirosis with doxycycline can be life-saving. Retrospective confirmation of leptospirosis is usually accomplished by demonstrating seroconverion between acute and convalescent sera by the microscopic agglutination test.

DISEASES TRANSMITTED THROUGH EXPOSURE TO SOIL AND DUST

Military forces working or training in areas with endemic soil pathogens that can be transmitted through inhalation are at particular risk of acquiring these infections. Military activities that often produce dust – such as the driving of vehicles, construction, helicopter operations, digging ditches, or cleaning of abandoned buildings – increase the risk for exposure.

Coccidioidomycosis has had an impact on the military since the discovery of the causative agent, *Coccidioides immitis,* over a century ago.[113] *Coccidioides* spp. are found in the soil of only certain regions of the western hemisphere (see Chapter 85). Endemic regions in the United States are in the desert southwest. Currently, more than 350 000 military personnel are stationed in endemic areas, with thousands more training in these locales annually. Military bases are situated near or in endemic areas in Arizona, California, Nevada, New Mexico, Utah, and Texas. Cases most often present within endemic areas; however, given troop mobility, hundreds of cases have been diagnosed in nonendemic areas in this country as well as overseas, emphasizing the need for clinicians around the globe to be able to recognize and treat this disease. Given the protean manifestations of chronic or disseminated disease and the nonspecific nature of acute respiratory infections, a high index of suspicion is needed, and travel and exposure histories should be obtained.[114] As noted earlier, the diagnostic challenge is worldwide, not just regional, on account of rapid deployments and mobility of troops.

Sporadic cases, as well as outbreaks of this disease, occur in military populations.[115–119] From 1981 to 1994, 113 US sailors and marines were hospitalized in Navy medical facilities for coccidioidomycosis, with primary pulmonary disease representing the most common form (72%).[118] Failure to obtain an adequate travel history and unfamiliarity with this disease have led to delayed or missed diagnoses.[116,119] In 1992, a 27-man marine reserve unit from Tennessee trained for 3 weeks at Vandenberg Air Force Base, California.[119] A week after returning, one of the reservists developed symptoms of pneumonia and, despite treatment with tetracycline and amoxicillin, his illness persisted. Later during his hospitalization, coccidioidomycosis was diagnosed. Other members of the group (26%) had symptoms consistent with coccidioidomycosis infection. All had sought medical intervention, but only two were diagnosed correctly.

Misdiagnoses are not infrequent. During the fall of 2001, elite Navy Special Forces personnel (n = 23) trained for 6 weeks in Coalinga, California.[116] Six presented to a local medical clinic during the exercise with cough, fever, chills, night sweats, and malaise, but were diagnosed with a "viral illness."[116] Because of persistent symptoms, one Navy Seal was evaluated at a military hospital 6 weeks later and a diagnosis of coccidioidomycosis was made. An investigation of the group found that 45% of the team had serologic evidence of acute coccidioidomycosis and all were symptomatic. In summary, physicians attending to any ill military personnel must be vigilant for this disease. Large numbers of personnel train in desert warfare at Fort Irwin, California, and may present with their illness thousands of miles away from this endemic area. Early detection and treatment can prevent progression to disseminated disease and complications.

Melioidosis (see Chapter 33) is an important infectious disease for military personnel because of its multiple modes of transmission, the severity of illness, latent infections that become clinically apparent years after initial exposure, its intrinsic resistance to many antibiotics, and its high relapse rate.[120,121] It is a bacterial disease which is highly endemic throughout Southeast Asia and caused several hundred hospitalizations in US forces during the Vietnam conflict.[122] US military personnel have presented with disease years after exposure in Vietnam.[123] Between 1987 and 1994, 23 acute cases were diagnosed in the Singapore Armed Forces.[124] Unlike patients from endemic areas who frequently have underlying illnesses or are elderly, soldiers are usually fit. A case of disseminated melioidosis was identified in an otherwise healthy 20-year-old marine following a 2-week training deployment to U-Tapao naval base on the coast of Thailand.[125] A subsequent clinical and epidemiologic evaluation of others in the unit identifed a 38% (13/34) seropositive rate among previously unexposed US marines after their 2 weeks in Thailand. Asymptomatic infection with *Burkholderia pseudomallei* may be common, even from brief exposures. The disease is probably underdiagnosed in soldiers as well as endemic populations because of failure of medical personnel to recognize its many clinical presentations and the lack of access to microbiologic assays.[120]

Parasitic infections that are transmitted by contact with contaminated soil, such as hookworm and strongyloides (see Chapters 116 and 117), have long been associated with deployed soldiers. During World War II, there were 23 300 hospitalizations of US troops attributed to hookworm.[126] In a study of 500 American soldiers returning from Vietnam in 1965, 15% were infected with intestinal parasites (55% had hookworm, 19% had strongyloides, and 14% had both).[127] During 1983 after military intervention in Grenada, over 200 soldiers in different US Army units reported signs and symptoms consistent with soil-transmitted helminthic infections.[128] Hookworm was confirmed in 8.3% of soldiers in one survey. Outbreaks of hookworm and strongyloides infections occurred repeatedly in US troops training at the Jungle Operations Training Center in Panama during the 1980s and 1990s.[129] In 1993, 566 soldiers from an infantry battalion trained for 3 weeks in Panama. Approximately 3 weeks after returning home, soldiers began to seek medical care for abdominal pain, nausea, vomiting, and diarrhea. An investigation identified hookworm infection in 12% of 75 soldiers who submitted a single stool sample and strongyloides in 3%. Eosinophilia (>7%) was detected in 129 of 473 blood samples, suggesting helminthic infection in 27% of the soldiers.

Remarkable attack rates can occur. A total of 153 British soldiers were deployed on a 3-day hostage rescue mission in Sierra Leone in 2006. Fifty percent reported gastrointestinal symptoms and eosinophilia. Hookworm infection was confirmed in 26% and strongyloides in 9%.[130] A similar experience was reported by Singaporean soldiers following a 10-day jungle training exercise in Brunei.[131] Twenty-nine percent (33/113) reported diarrhea, 26% (29/113) reported abdominal pain, 41% (42/103) had eosinophilia, and 17% (18/103) had hookworm eggs in their stool by light microscopy. Most reported exposure to soil or groundwater but the only specific exposure that correlated with acquiring hookworm infection or eosinophilia was not wearing footwear during rest periods. From experimental human challenge, it is important to note that hookworm infections in nonimmune individuals result in mid epigastric abdominal pain about a month after infection, with eosinophilia peaking about a week after onset of symptoms.[132] Diarrhea may be absent or only a minor complaint.

These outbreaks demonstrate the importance of considering helminthic infections in troops exposed to muddy, contaminated soil. Many will present with gastrointestinal symptoms several weeks after exposure, but before eggs are observed in the stool. Soldiers should have a complete blood count with differential to document eosinophilia and uncover asymptomatic infections. Of particular concern to the long-term health of infected soldiers is the ability to detect strongyloides infections, which, if untreated, can lead to lifelong infection and the possibility of life-threatening hyperinfection if the soldier/veteran becomes immunosuppressed.

MULTIDRUG-RESISTANT WAR WOUND INFECTIONS

Arguably one of the most important infectious disease problems arising from the current US military experience in Afghanistan and Iraq since the conflicts began in 2001 is the presence of multidrug-resistant bacteria, especially the *Acinetobacter calcoaceticus–Acinetobacter baumannii* complex (*Acinetobacter*).[133] Because of the nature of injuries in this conflict (wounds caused by improvised explosive devices, mortars, rocket-propelled grenades, and gunshots) and the near-universal use of protective gear, extremity wounds are prevalent. Rapid evacuation to skilled surgical centers, early debridement, heroic attempts at limb salvage, and the early use of broad-spectrum antibiotics have led to late complications with the emergence of multidrug-resistant Gram-negative bacteria as either wound colonizers or true pathogens. Suboptimal debridement of devitalized tissue and environmental contamination may play a role in acquisition of *Acinetobacter* species and infection.

Since 2003, the incidence of multidrug-resistant *Acinetobacter* has increased significantly. Nosocomial transmission of these strains from wounded US service personnel to civilian patients in military treatment facilities[134] and to health care workers[135] has been reported. Intensified infection control measures have been implemented during transit or personnel to the United States. Upon arrival to US military treatment facilities, hospitalized, injured personnel are placed in contact isolation and tested for *Acinetobacter* skin colonization. If axilla and groin skin swab culture results are negative, then the patient is removed from isolation.

CONCLUSION

Although modern war has evolved substantially, and today's battlefield is quite different from previous conflicts, infectious diseases remain a major threat to deployed troops. Presently, large numbers of nonimmune military personnel from many countries are sent to areas with high incidences of infectious diseases. When their working and living conditions are crowded or unhygienic, particularly in times of war and conflict, their risk of infection increases. When appropriate public health and preventive measures are implemented, the incidence of infectious diseases can be greatly reduced. When military and civilian physicians who care for ill soldiers recognize their illnesses and institute appropriate therapies promptly, morbidity from infectious diseases can be lessened. However, even in these optimal circumstances, infectious diseases still occur.

When appropriate preventive measures are not instituted and treatment providers are not adequately prepared, attack rates from malaria, diarrheal diseases, acute respiratory infections, and other contagious infectious diseases can be quite high and deaths do result. Many nations do not have the resources to implement sound public health measures in their troops or to deploy sophisticated medical care. Although developed nations, such as the United States, may have the means to prevent and treat infectious diseases even in the most austere conditions, sometimes they do not implement the most effective preventive and curative services. Furthermore, with the speed of today's travel, deployed troops incubating an infectious illness may return home and present to garrison-based or civilian physicians. All physicians, whether they are with deployed troops or caring for those who returned home, need to be mindful of the exposures to infectious diseases and the illnesses that can occur in military settings. The ill soldier or veteran represents a high-risk traveler who may have been exposed to various pathogens in many different countries.

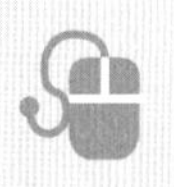

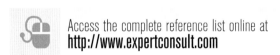

Access the complete reference list online at
http://www.expertconsult.com

CHAPTER 129

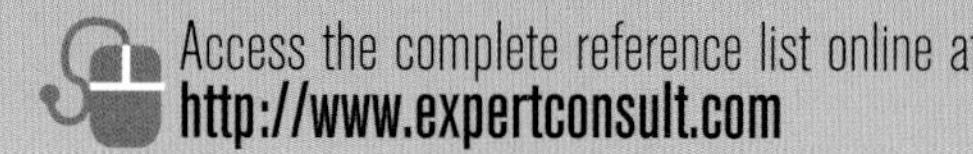
Access the complete reference list online at
http://www.expertconsult.com

Gastrointestinal Symptoms

Luis M. Valdez • Eduardo Gotuzzo • Nathan M. Thielman • Herbert L. DuPont

INTRODUCTION

We live in a changing world where the effects of rural-to-urban migration and international travel to and from tropical areas of the world underscore the importance of recognizing and understanding tropical infections. Because most developing countries are in the tropics, the poor sanitary conditions that exist in these areas favor the acquisition of infections in which the gastrointestinal tract is an important portal of entry for microbes. These infections may manifest in different ways, with signs and symptoms that may or may not be related to the gastrointestinal tract. Although gastrointestinal symptoms are often nonspecific, it is important to recognize them in the context of the patient's environment, exposures, and immune status. The latter has become increasingly important in resource-poor settings which have a disproportionate share of the world's HIV infection burden. Recent data from UNAIDS shows that in some countries in Asia, Latin America and sub-Saharan Africa, the annual number of new HIV infections is falling, and the estimated rate of AIDS deaths is declining as there is expanding access to antiretroviral drugs.[1]

When assessing patients with gastrointestinal symptoms, it is important to remember that although these symptoms are usually related to enteric infections, they may be secondary to systemic infections or to complications from a previously acquired infection. For example, malaria may often present with diarrhea and mislead critical diagnostic evaluation. It is thus essential to obtain a careful history, with emphasis on environmental exposures, dietary habits, contacts, and immunizations (***Box 129.1***). Gastrointestinal symptoms in the tropics are diverse, and although some may be related to "nontropical" conditions, it is also important to remember that some tropical enteric infections may present with predominantly systemic symptoms.

SYMPTOMS AND SYNDROMES

In tropical enteric infections, the presence of symptoms relates to organism virulence, the degree of infection or inflammation caused by the infecting organism, and the host immune response. In the case of some enteric infections, especially in children living in endemic areas, the presence of pathogenic organisms may not correlate with the existence of symptoms.[2] For example, among children with *Giardia* infection in a study in Egypt, there was a failure to show an association between infection and symptomatic illness.[3] The same has been described in longitudinal studies in Peruvian children, where no association was found between a variety of enteropathogens and persistent diarrhea.[4] Evidence suggests that asymptomatic infections with organisms such as enteroaggregative *Escherichia coli*[5] and *Cryptosporidium*[6] may be associated with impaired growth, probably because of inflammatory responses and/or malnutrition caused by these pathogens. Recent studies are showing that in certain populations mass treatment for helminths may be effective in improving certain parameters such as anemia.[7,8]

We have classified gastrointestinal symptoms in the tropics into seven syndromes (***Table 129.1***), and it is important to consider that certain microorganisms may cause more than one syndrome. In many infections, specific therapies are available (***Table 129.2***), but in some diseases, when the symptoms are a result of the host response to the infection, antimicrobial agents are ineffective.

Although systemic symptoms may be even nonspecific, it is important to recognize that some enteric tropical infections may present without a predominance of enteric symptoms. Such is the case, for example, of *Cyclospora cayetanensis* infections,[9] where symptoms of profound fatigue, anorexia, and weight loss often predominate over the diarrheal symptoms, sometimes resulting in a delay in the time of diagnosis.

Enteric Fever

Enteric infections can cause clinical syndromes in which fever is predominant, sometimes associated with abdominal pain, in a protean clinical picture distinctive from other acute enteric processes. Usually the portal of entry in these infections is the gastrointestinal tract, but the differential diagnosis includes other infections and some noninfectious conditions. The classic infections causing enteric fever include typhoid fever, caused by *Salmonella* Typhi (*S. typhi*), and the nontyphoid salmonellosis, brucellosis, yersiniosis, and *Campylobacter* infections. Common characteristics of these infections include gastrointestinal portal of entry, intracellular nature of the infection, and multiplication of organisms in the lymphoid tissue before disseminating.

Typhoid fever caused by *S. typhi* is the classic prototype of enteric fever and still represents an important cause of morbidity and mortality in areas where it is endemic (see Chapter 16).[10] It is estimated that worldwide there are 26 million cases of typhoid fever each year with 200 000 deaths.[11] Although the syndrome classically is characterized as an acute illness with fever, headache, and abdominal pain, the symptoms are relatively nonspecific and the differential diagnosis, especially when there is associated splenomegaly, should include malaria, brucellosis, amebic liver abscess, visceral leishmaniasis, and viral syndromes such as dengue, and sometimes acute HIV, depending on the epidemiologic and geographic history the patient gives. For example, acute HIV infection, presenting with acute febrile illness, headache, leukopenia and elevation of transaminases, and low titers on Widal's test have been misdiagnosed as typhoid. Delays in the diagnosis of typhoid fever should be avoided, since complications occur characteristically during the second week of illness. The complications in typhoid fever may be related directly to direct involvement of the gut resulting in hemorrhage, perforation, and ileus, and to the systemic inflammatory response secondary to the infection (typhoid state), or to dissemination of *S. typhi* (meningitis, endocarditis, bone lesions).[12] Other salmonellae (especially *Salmonella* Paratyphi A and B, *S. choleraesuis*, and other *Salmonella* serotypes) may also cause a typhoidal clinical syndrome.[13]

Acute brucellosis (see Chapter 40) is another cause of enteric fever in which systemic symptoms predominate over those symptoms related to the gastrointestinal tract. In a fever surveillance study in Egypt, 87% of patients with brucellosis were actually diagnosed with and treated for typhoid.[14] Anorexia, abdominal pain, vomiting, and diarrhea or constipation are some of the complaints elicited in patients with brucellosis if the patient is carefully questioned.[15] In areas where brucellosis is endemic, it is important to obtain a detailed history assessing ingestion of unpasteurized milk or cheese, as well as occupational exposures.

Yersinia enterocolitica infections, although found in tropical areas, are rarely a cause of tropical diarrhea,[16] and the septicemic disease is seen mostly in patients with underlying predisposing factors and chronic diseases.

Epidemiologic information may prove critically important in identifying some zoonoses, such as plague and anthrax, that can occasionally present with a clinical picture suggestive of enteric fever. Septicemic plague, for example, may present with prominent gastrointestinal symptoms (nausea, vomiting, diarrhea, and abdominal pain), symptoms that may precede the development of a bubo, or even be part of septicemic plague, in which no bubo is recognized. In a review of 71 human plague cases, gastrointestinal symptoms occurred in 57% of patients, with nausea and vomiting being the most common symptoms and diarrhea and abdominal pain occurring less frequently (28% and 17% of patients, respectively).[17] In disease caused by *Bacillus anthracis* following the ingestion of contaminated food, abdominal anthrax will present after an

Box 129.1 Important Aspects of the History in Patients from Tropical Areas

Environment	Host
Travel history (knowledge of epidemic or endemic diseases in the area)	Recent contact with infected persons
Insect bites	Previous infections
Occupational or recreational exposures	Vaccination status
Contact with animals (domestic and wild)	History of sexually transmitted diseases and risk factors for HIV infection
Dietary history (type and source of food and water)	

Table 129.1 Syndromes (and Their Most Common Causes) in Patients with Gastrointestinal Symptoms in the Tropics

Syndrome	Agent/Condition	Organisms	Differential Diagnosis
Enteric fever	Bacteria	Typhoid fever (*Salmonella* Typhi)	Tuberculosis
		Salmonellosis (non-*Salmonella* Typhi)	Acute schistosomiasis
		Brucellosis	Malaria
		Yersiniosis (rare)	Septicemic plague
		Campylobacter (rare)	Abdominal anthrax
Oral lesions	Bacteria	Noma (children), syphilis (primary or secondary), actinomycosis, oral anthrax	
	Mycobacteria	Tuberculosis, leprosy	
	Fungi	Paracoccidioidomycosis, histoplasmosis, candidiasis	
	Protozoa	Mucocutaneous leishmaniasis	
	Viruses	Herpes simplex	
Dysphagia	Protozoa	Trypanosomiasis	Esophageal cancer
	Fungi	Candidiasis (AIDS)	
	Viruses	Herpes simplex (AIDS), cytomegalovirus (AIDS)	
Bleeding	Upper gastrointestinal bleeding	Esophageal varices: chronic schistosomiasis, cirrhosis (hepatitis B and C)	Stomach cancer
	Peptic ulcer disease	*Helicobacter pylori* infection	
	Lower gastrointestinal bleeding	Typhoid fever, nonspecific colitis, tuberculosis (rare), amebiasis (rare)	Polyps, colon cancer, diverticulosis
Abdominal pain	Peptic ulcer disease	*Helicobacter pylori*	Appendicitis, complicated hernia, intussusception
	Intestinal parasitosis	*Ascaris lumbricoides*, *Strongyloides stercoralis*, *Angiostrongylus costaricensis*, *Anisakis*, hookworm	
	Bacteria	Tuberculosis	
		Typhoid (perforation)	
Abdominal mass	Bacteria	Tuberculosis, actinomycosis	Colon cancer, lymphoma
	Parasites	Ameboma, *Angiostrongylus*	
	Fungi	Histoplasmosis	
Diarrhea	Watery diarrhea and gastroenteritis	ETEC, EAEC, *Vibrio cholerae* O1 and non-O1, *Salmonella*, *Shigella*, *Campylobacter*, *Staphylococcus aureus* and *Bacillus cereus* (toxin-mediated), *Cryptosporidium parvum*, *Cyclospora cayetanensis*, *Isospora belli*, viruses	
	Inflammatory diarrhea	*Shigella*, *Salmonella*, *Campylobacter*, *Entamoeba histolytica*, *Balantidium coli*	
	Persistent diarrhea	EAEC, tuberculosis, *Giardia lamblia*, *Cryptosporidium*, *Cyclospora*, *I. belli*, *S. stercoralis*, *Capillaria philippinensis*	Lymphoma, tropical sprue, Brainerd diarrhea
	Travelers' diarrhea	ETEC, EAEC, *Shigella*, *Campylobacter jejuni*, *Aeromonas*, *Plesiomonas shigelloides*, *Salmonella*, *Giardia*, *Cryptosporidium*, *Cyclospora* and noroviruses	

AIDS, acquired immunodeficiency syndrome; EAEC, enteroadherent *Escherichia coli*; ETEC, enterotoxigenic *E. coli*.

Table 129.2 Recommended Antimicrobial Therapy for Adults Infected by Selected Organisms Causing Gastrointestinal Disease in the Tropics[a]

Organisms	Therapy
Typhoidal syndrome	Ciprofloxacin 500 mg PO bid (or comparable quinolone) for 10–14 days *or*
	Ceftriaxone 2.0 g IV for 10–14 days *or*
	Chloramphenicol 50 mg/kg per day PO divided into approximately 6-hour dosing intervals (max. daily dose 3 g) for 14 days *or*
	Cefixime 200 mg PO q12h for 14 days *or*
	Azithromycin 500 mg q24h for 7 days
Brucellosis	Doxycycline 100 mg PO bid for 3 weeks + gentamicin IM 240 mg qd for 7 days *or*
	Doxycycline + rifampin 900 mg qd *or*
	Doxycycline + streptomycin 1 g IM qd for 2 weeks
Helicobacter pylori	Clarithromycin 500 mg PO bid + omeprazole 40 mg PO qd for 14 days *or*
	Metronidazole (250 mg PO tid) + amoxicillin (500 mg PO qid) + bismuth subsalicylate (2 × 262 mg tablets qid) for 14 days
Vibrio cholerae O1	Tetracycline 500 mg PO qid *or* doxycycline 100 mg PO for 3 days *or*
	Doxycycline 300 mg PO single dose *or* 250 mg PO q12h for 3 days
V. cholerae, non-O1	Tetracycline *or* ciprofloxacin
	Resistant to furazolidone and trimethoprim-sulfamethoxazole
Shigella	Ciprofloxacin 500 mg q12h for 3 days *or*
	Norfloxacin 400 mg q12h for 3 days
Campylobacter	Erythromycin 500 mg PO qid for 5 days *or* other macrolides as above
Salmonella	Therapy not indicated unless severe or in a host susceptible to bacteremic complications; fluoroquinolones for 7–10 days
Giardia lamblia	Metronidazole 250 mg PO tid for 5 days *or*
	Tinidazole 2.0 g single dose *or*
	Quinacrine 100 mg PO tid for 5 days
Entamoeba histolytica	Metronidazole 750 mg PO tid (500 mg IV q6h) for 10 days *or*
	Tinidazole 2.0 g PO qd for 3 days
	Use of above agents should be followed by iodoquinol 650 mg PO tid for 20 days *or* paromomycin 25–35 mg/kg daily in 3 doses for 7 days
Cyclospora cayetanensis	Trimethoprim-sulfamethoxazole 1 double-strength tablet (160 mg/800 mg) bid PO for 3–7 days
Cryptosporidium	No effective therapy demonstrated in adults
	Paromomycin 500 mg PO qid (partial response, used in patients with AIDS)
	Nitazoxanide 500–1000 mg bid for 14 days (response in some patients with AIDS)
Isospora belli	Trimethoprim-sulfamethoxazole 1 double-strength tablet (160 mg/800 mg) PO qid for 10 days then bid for 3 weeks
Balantidium coli	Tetracycline 500 mg PO qid for 10 days *or*
	Metronidazole 750 mg PO tid for 5 days *or*
	Paromomycin 500 mg PO tid for 7–10 days
Ascaris lumbricoides	Mebendazole 100 mg PO bid for 3 days *or*
	Pyrantel pamoate 11 mg/kg PO qd for 3 days *or*
	Albendazole 400 mg PO single dose
Strongyloides stercoralis	Ivermectin 200 μg/kg daily for 2 days *or*
	Albendazole 400 mg PO qd for 3 days *or*
	Thiabendazole 22 mg/kg PO bid for 2 days

[a]Duration of therapy for nonimmunocompromised patients. Duration of therapy will be prolonged in patients with AIDS.
PO, by mouth; IV, intravenously; IM, intramuscularly; bid, twice a day; tid, three times a day; qid, four times a day; qd, every day; q12h, every 12 hours.

incubation period of 2–11 days.[18] Symptoms initially may be nonspecific, with fever, anorexia, nausea, and vomiting. As the disease progresses, abdominal pain, hematemesis, and bloody diarrhea will often develop.

Tuberculosis (see Chapter 35) and schistosomiasis (see Chapter 122) should also be considered in the differential diagnosis of fever and enteric symptoms. In patients with intestinal tuberculosis, although they may have associated pulmonary disease, some series have found evidence of active or remote pulmonary tuberculosis in as few as 25% of cases, the diagnosis being an unexpected finding at exploratory laparotomy.[19] Patients with acute schistosomiasis (Katayama fever) may also present with an enteric fever syndrome. Typically, this occurs in subjects who are not residents of endemic areas, and it is believed to be in relationship to the host response to the parasite.[20] The history of swimming in fresh water during the previous month in areas in which schistosomiasis is endemic favors this diagnosis.

It is important to recognize the endemicity of certain tropical diseases in order to recognize infections such as typhoid fever and those that are unusual in other geographic settings. When approaching patients with enteric fever, it is thus essential to obtain a complete history and to do a complete physical examination looking for clinical clues that may suggest one process or another. Microbiologic diagnosis should be attempted whenever possible, but in some tropical areas this may not be feasible and in the case of typhoid the diagnosis may rely on serologic methods (Widal's test) and a suggestive clinical picture.[21] In an Indian study, Widal's test was acceptable as a diagnostic tool, with a high specificity and positive predictive value when an O-antigen 1:160 dilution defined a positive result in the presence of a suggestive clinical picture.[22] In the same study, the same titer was observed in 10.2% of patients with other febrile illnesses of known cause and in 1.8% of normal children. Studies in nonendemic areas also show that the test can give a significant number of false positives.[23] The diagnosis of typhoid fever by Widal's test alone is prone to error and there are no universally applicable criteria for the serologic diagnosis. In areas where microbiologic diagnosis is not possible, Widal's test should only be considered as a "fever screen" for typhoid, recognizing that it will not identify all cases and that it may give some false positives, particularly in areas with low endemicity for the disease. In areas where malaria is endemic, false positives have been described; in one study, Widal's test was found to be positive in 15% and 10% of malaria patients for *Salmonella* O- and H-antigen titers, respectively.[24] In areas where malaria is also endemic, typhoid fever and malaria always have to be considered in the differential diagnosis of an acute febrile illness, so a thick smear in addition to cultures for *Salmonella* should be obtained. For the microbiologic diagnosis of typhoid fever, blood and stool cultures have been recommended traditionally for the isolation of *S. typhi*, but bone marrow cultures and duodenal string cultures (duodenal string-capsule culture) provide a higher yield. In a Peruvian study in adult patients with documented *S. typhi* infection, duodenal content cultures were as sensitive as bone marrow in providing a diagnosis (86% and 75% sensitivity, respectively) compared with blood (42%) and stool (26%) cultures.[25] Bone marrow and duodenal string cultures also remain positive for a longer period despite antibiotic therapy, and thus may be useful in patients who have received empirical antibiotic therapy and in whom a microbiologic diagnosis is needed.[25,26] In older pediatric patients, the duodenal string method has also been shown to be better than blood cultures,[27] but in smaller children it may not be practical.[27,28]

The treatment of patients with acute enteric fever syndromes should be based on an etiologic diagnosis, but at times empirical therapy may be necessary while awaiting culture results. In the case of typhoid fever, delays in diagnosis and treatment should be avoided because of the impact of therapy on disease mortality and on the incidence of intestinal hemorrhage.[12] When treating patients with typhoid fever one has to consider that strains of *S. typhi* that are resistant to the three first-line antibiotics (chloramphenicol, amoxicillin, and trimethoprim-sulfamethoxazole) have been described in many tropical countries,[29] and the presence of nalidixic acid resistance, which may predict failure for the older quinolones. Thus, it is essential to know the local resistance patterns in each endemic area. Multiresistant organisms are typically susceptible to third-generation cephalosporins and to the newer fluoroquinolones and azithromycin,[30,31] but responses have been slower with the cephalosporins. In an open study comparing ceftriaxone (2 g per day for 5 days) with fleroxacin (400 mg once a day for 7 days), the mean fever clearance times were 160 hours and 81 hours, respectively, and there were two failures in the ceftriaxone group and none in the fleroxacin group.[32] In another study comparing ceftriaxone (3 g per day for 7 days) with ciprofloxacin (500 mg twice a day for 7 days), there were six failures (out of 22 patients) in the ceftriaxone group and none in the ciprofloxacin group.[33] Oral cefixime has been studied in children with multidrug-resistant typhoid in Pakistan, but failures were reported in 3 of 50 patients (6%).[34] Fluoroquinolones are considered the drugs of choice in many areas of the world, but caution has to be advised in areas where there is increased nalidixic acid resistance, as failure has been described with the older fluoroquinolones. Resistance to ciprofloxacin was initially described from India and in travelers returning to the United Kingdom after travel to the Indian subcontinent.[35,36] Fluoroquinolone-resistant strains, which are often multidrug-resistant, are best treated with either azithromycin (which also covers quinolone-resistant *Campylobacter*) or cephalosporins.[37] Gatifloxacin, a useful alternative for nalidixic acid resistant strains, was removed from the market in the United States after some severe episodes of dysglycemia in older adults were described.[38] ***Table 129.2*** summarizes the most accepted regimens for treating typhoid, and the antibiotics should be used based on the knowledge of the local patterns of resistance, cost, compliance, and safety.

Oropharyngeal Lesions

Bacterial, fungal, parasitic, and viral infections can all give rise to oropharyngeal lesions. The first three types present with increased frequency in the tropics.

Among the bacterial infections causing oral lesions seen in tropical areas, one seen with an increased incidence in West Africa is noma (cancrum oris), a severe gangrene of the soft and hard tissues of the mouth, face, and neighboring areas. *Fusobacterium necrophorum*, along with other organisms, has been implicated in its pathogenesis. These opportunistic pathogens invade oral tissues in children whose immune system is weakened by malnutrition, acute necrotizing gingivitis, debilitating conditions, trauma, and other oral mucosal ulcers. Noma occurs in communities characterized by extreme poverty, severe malnutrition, poor sanitation, and limited access to health care. Although African countries are most affected, Latin America and Asia are not exempt.[39]

Considering the increasing prevalence rates for sexually transmitted diseases in developing countries, orogenital contact can result in oral and oropharyngeal lesions of syphilis. Secondary syphilis can also present with painful oral ulcerations or oral condyloma lata lesions.[40,41] In contrast with the oral lesions of primary syphilis, which tend to be solitary, painless, indurated, and punched-out ulcers, oral lesions of secondary syphilis are typically painful and multiple and are accompanied by a generalized rash.

Actinomycosis, anthrax, tuberculosis, and leprosy can also present with oral lesions. Actinomycotic infections of the cervicofacial area are rare, and the most common presentation is an acute painful swelling associated with a soft tissue abscess secondary to dental lesions.[42] Rare cases of oral actinomycosis may mimic neoplasms of the tongue.[43] Oral anthrax is characterized by a mucosal lesion in the oral cavity or oropharynx which can progress to pseudomembranous necrosis, and to cervical adenopathy and edema.[44] Primary tuberculosis of the mouth may present with painless ulcerations of long duration and enlargement of the regional lymph nodes.[45] Lepromatous leprosy can cause oral lesions in 20–60% of patients. Oral lesions are often an extension of disease in the nasal mucous membranes. Oral lesions are characterized as hemorrhagic sessile nodules involving the maxillary incisive papilla, lips, tongue, soft palate, uvula, and glossopharyngeal arches.[46]

Among the fungal infections in the tropics, paracoccidioidomycosis (South American blastomycosis), histoplasmosis, and candidiasis can present with oral lesions. Oral lesions may be the first sign of paracoccidioidomycosis. Patients may present with chronic, proliferative, mulberry-like ulcerated oral lesions. Typically the gingiva or alveolar process is affected, but lesions can be seen on the palate and lip. Most patients with oral lesions have detectable pulmonary involvement.[47] In disseminated histoplasmosis, lesions of the oral mucosa may be found in 30–50% of cases. Oral lesions may involve the lips, tongue, gingiva, and palate.[48] Oral candidiasis can be associated with malnutrition and debilitating diseases, but within the current AIDS epidemic its presence should raise the possibility of HIV infection.

Among the protozoan infections, mucocutaneous leishmaniasis can present with oral lesions (see Chapter 100). Patients with infection by *Leishmania viannia braziliensis* in Latin America may develop mucosal lesions of the nose, mouth, pharynx, or larynx months to years after the primary infection.[49] Other protozoal and helminthic infections may be associated with oropharyngeal lesions on very rare occasions.[50]

Dysphagia

Many of the conditions causing oral lesions in tropical areas can present with dysphagia. In this section, we concentrate on infectious processes that may affect primarily the esophagus.

In areas where *Trypanosoma cruzi* infection (Chagas' disease) is endemic, esophageal symptoms such as dysphagia and regurgitation may be secondary to motor disorders related to this parasitic disease (see Chapter 99).[51] The involvement of the esophagus encompasses a spectrum with mega-esophagus at the most severe end to milder variants without evidence of esophageal dilation in subjects who have documented serologic evidence of infection with *T. cruzi*.

Dysphagia and odynophagia may present secondary to infectious esophagitis, particularly among patients with advanced HIV infection (see Chapter 139).[52] *Candida* esophagitis is the most common cause of esophageal symptoms in patients with HIV infection, accounting for 50–100% of symptomatic patients, and may be a presenting symptom of AIDS among those unaware of their HIV serostatus. The absolute number of HIV-infected patients presenting with this complication has decreased dramatically with greater access to highly active antiretroviral therapy. After *Candida*, the most common causes of esophageal disease in symptomatic patients were cytomegalovirus (CMV), herpes simplex, and idiopathic esophageal ulcers.

Among the noninfectious pathologic conditions, esophageal cancer is unevenly distributed within the tropical regions; its prevalence rate is higher in East and South Africa and in the Far East. In these areas, this must be a consideration when assessing patients with esophageal symptoms.[53]

Gastrointestinal Bleeding

While gastrointestinal bleeding is typically not associated with infection, several infectious conditions in the tropics may present in this way. For example, enterohemorrhagic *Escherichia coli* (EHEC), *Shigella*, *Salmonella*, or *Campylobacter* can cause bloody diarrhea in the tropics (and in sporadic outbreaks in industrialized temperate areas).

Longterm sequelae of infection with *Schistosoma mansoni* and *S. japonicum* include periportal fibrosis, which may lead to portal hypertension and varices with the resultant risk of gastrointestinal bleeding. This represents an important cause of morbidity and mortality in endemic areas due to the large number of infected subjects.[54] In a field study in an area of the Sudan endemic for *S. mansoni*, the prevalence of esophageal varices in subjects undergoing esophagoscopy ranged between 54% and 67%. The varices were usually asymptomatic, with symptomatic varices (with a positive history of hematemesis) occurring in 3–4% of subjects with sonographic evidence of liver periportal fibrosis.[55] Abdominal ultrasound can accurately measure liver and spleen size and configuration and can detect and grade periportal fibrosis and portal hypertension – findings that can help to predict the risk of variceal bleeding in patients with complicated schistosomiasis.[56]

Another infectious condition that may present with gastrointestinal bleeding is typhoid fever, typically resulting from necrotic erosion of a Peyer's patch into an enteric vessel.[37] If untreated, it may result in passage of gross blood in the feces or melena in 10–20% of patients, with severe gastrointestinal bleeding occurring in 2% of patients late in the course of the disease.[12] Early treatment of typhoid fever reduces the frequency of this complication, highlighting the importance of rapid diagnosis and treatment for typhoid in endemic areas.

Gastrointestinal tuberculosis on rare occasions can present with gastrointestinal bleeding. There have been case reports describing upper gastrointestinal bleeding from a tuberculous gastric ulcer and from esophageal tuberculosis.[57,58] Reports of massive rectal bleeding from colonic tuberculosis have also been published.[59,60] Amebiasis, which commonly presents with bloody stools, on rare occasions may present with massive gastrointestinal bleeding requiring surgical therapy.[61]

In patients with lower gastrointestinal bleeding, colonoscopic examination may provide the diagnosis in a majority of patients. In a study of lower gastrointestinal bleeding carried out in a tropical area of India, predominant lesions in 138 adults were nonspecific colitis and ulcers (58%), polyps (19%), cancer (10%), rectal varices (4%), and tuberculosis (3%), with most lesions involving the left colon. Diffuse lesions were seen when nonspecific colitis and ulcers were the source of bleeding.[62] In another study from India, of 166 patients who underwent colonoscopy, a diagnosis could be made in 85%. Major causes of lower gastrointestinal bleeding included idiopathic ulcerative colitis (19.3%), acute colitis (12.0%), colonic polyps (10.2%), radiation colitis (9.0%), solitary rectal ulcer (7.8%), and colonic carcinoma (7.2%). Among the infectious conditions, colonic tuberculosis was found in 4.2% and enteric fever in 3.0%.[63]

Abdominal Pain

Abdominal pain can be acute or chronic, and sometimes may be part of an acute abdominal syndrome that requires a surgical approach. The causes of abdominal pain are diverse; enteric tropical infections should be considered in the differential diagnosis. Epigastric abdominal pain of gastric or duodenal origin can be linked to *Helicobacter pylori* infection (see Chapter 23). There is definite evidence of a link between this organism and peptic ulcer disease and chronic gastritis, and epidemiologic evidence supports its role in gastric cancer and lymphoma.[64] Gastric *H. pylori* infection is very common throughout the tropics, as evidenced by serologic surveys, yet active gastric infection does not always correlate with the incidence of serious upper gastrointestinal changes.[65] In a study of patients examined by gastroscopy for dyspepsia in northern Nigeria, 176 (92%) of 193 with acceptable biopsies had gastritis. *H. pylori* was present in 161 of 192 patients (84%): in 31 of 41 (75%) with chronic gastritis and in 130 of 135 (96%) with active gastritis.[66] Considering the role of *H. pylori* in gastritis, dyspepsia, peptic ulcer disease, and possibly gastric cancer, eradication of this infection should be attempted, although the cost of therapy may be difficult to justify in developing tropical areas.

Abdominal pain can also be a nonspecific symptom of intestinal parasitosis,[67] and in travelers to tropical areas the absence of symptoms should not preclude examination of the stools looking for parasites.[8] Although ascariasis is rarely a cause of abdominal pain, in a study in Nigeria assessing 865 patients with suspected peptic ulcer disease, 175 patients (20%) were found to have *Ascaris* infection, and their symptoms resolved after the use of anthelminthics.[68] Interestingly, the diagnosis of ascariasis was made radiologically as part of the workup for the diagnosis of peptic ulcer disease. In areas with a high prevalence of ascariasis, a stool examination should be part of the assessment in patients with uncomplicated suspected peptic ulcer disease. Hookworm may also be associated with abdominal pain and eosinophilia in the tropics, presenting several weeks before ova are shed to aid in the diagnosis.[69]

Among the causes of chronic abdominal pain in the tropics, when there is an association with ascites, the possibility of tuberculous peritonitis should be considered. The presentation of peritoneal tuberculosis is quite insidious, with most patients having symptoms for weeks or months before seeking medical attention. Marshall,[70] in a review of tuberculosis of the gastrointestinal tract and peritoneum, summarized data from six large series in the literature (two from tropical countries). In his review, abdominal pain was present 58% of the time, and the most common symptom was abdominal distension (about 82% of the cases). Other common symptoms included fever and weight loss. The ascitic fluid is an exudate with a lymphocytic predominance in the white blood cell differential count. The diagnostic yield from smears and cultures from the ascitic fluid is very low, although Singh and colleagues[71] reported 83% positive cultures when culturing 1 L of fluid concentrated by centrifugation. Currently, the best diagnostic test is laparoscopic biopsy of the peritoneum. Simply the gross appearance of the peritoneal cavity during laparoscopy allows a presumptive diagnosis in 85–95% of patients, and caseating granulomas are found from the biopsy specimens in 85–90% of cases.[70,72] The measurement of adenosine deaminase activity has been reported as a sensitive way of making a presumptive diagnosis by some.[73]

When patients present with an acute abdomen in the tropics, apart from the usual pathologies seen in other areas, certain infectious conditions should be considered in the differential diagnosis.

In the case of appendicitis, the most common abdominal surgical emergency in nontropical areas, pathologic studies in tropical areas have shown that in a few cases infection can be detected. In a pathologic study of 2921 appendectomies in a tropical area over a 25-year period, 70 (2.3%) specimens showed typical evidence of tuberculosis. Parasitic infection was detected in 75 (2.5%), including enterobiasis (1.4%), amebiasis (0.5%), ascariasis (0.5%), ascariasis with trichuriasis (0.05%), and taeniasis (0.05%).[74]

Intestinal obstruction in patients living in tropical areas can be caused by external hernia, sigmoid volvulus, intussusception (particularly in children), and ascariasis.[75,76] In a prospective evaluation of acute intestinal obstruction in 3550 consecutive patients in Africa, the majority of patients (75%) had an external hernia.[75] However, *Ascaris* infection in children, volvulus of the sigmoid colon in adults, and intussusception in both children and adults were significant causes of abdominal obstruction in 18% of the patients. In highly parasitized children, a mass of *Ascaris* adult worms can cause acute small bowel obstruction, although in most cases the obstruction is not complete and conservative measures and anthelminthic therapy can obviate the need for surgery (see Chapter 115).[77] *Strongyloides stercoralis* has also been reported, presenting as a subacute intestinal obstruction in two patients from Iraq.[78] Gastrointestinal tuberculosis can sometimes present with a subocclusive or obstructive picture. In a series of 300 cases of abdominal tuberculosis that required surgical therapy, Bhansali[79] found that of 139 patients presenting with abdominal pain, 92 had abdominal obstruction, 23 had perforation, and 19 had peritonitis. In 56 of the patients, the acute episode was the first manifestation of abdominal tuberculosis, while the other 83 had a previous history of chronic abdominal pain for a period of time that ranged from 1 month to more than 10 years. Only 10% of these patients had active pulmonary or pleural tuberculosis; 12% gave a history of previous tuberculosis, or their chest films showed a past, healed focus. Obstruction can be secondary to narrowing of the lumen by hyperplastic cecal tuberculosis, strictures of the small intestine, adhesions, or be related to extrinsic compression of the bowel by mesenteric lymph nodes. In approaching patients with abdominal pain in tropical areas where tuberculosis is prevalent, this diagnostic possibility should always be considered.

One of the most lethal complications of typhoid fever is ileal perforation, which should be considered if an acute abdomen develops in a patient with prolonged fever. The most important sign is pneumoperitoneum on plain abdominal film. This complication requires surgical therapy, usually consisting of simple closure and irrigation of the peritoneal cavity.[80] In a review of the literature published after 1960 on typhoid perforation in different developing countries, information was obtained on a total of 1990 cases of typhoid perforation in 66 157 patients with typhoid fever, published in 52 reports from all over the world.[81] The overall frequency of intestinal perforation in typhoid fever was 3% with an overall mortality rate of 39.6%. In a recent report from Turkey,[82] mortality decreased significantly, from 28% to 10%, with the institution of aggressive fluid resuscitation and appropriate antibiotic therapy in the preoperative period, and total parenteral nutrition to provide adequate metabolic support during the postoperative period. Apart from specific antibiotic therapy against *S. typhi*, broad-spectrum antibiotics should be added to cover enteric flora (mainly anaerobes and Gram-negative organisms).

The tropical spectrum of generalized peritonitis is different from the Western spectrum. In a study in India, of a total 155 cases of generalized peritonitis that were surgically treated, the most common cause of peritonitis was peptic ulcer perforation followed by typhoid perforation. Other causes of peritonitis in the same study were appendicular perforations, tubercular perforations (sometimes with a previous history of subacute intestinal obstruction and evidence of pulmonary tuberculosis), and ruptured amebic liver abscess.[83] Amebic perforation of the colon has also been described in patients presenting with an acute abdomen and a past history of fever, pain, and diarrhea.[84]

It is important in tropical areas to identify nonsurgical infectious causes of abdominal pain that may mimic an acute abdomen. *Angiostrongylus costaricensis* is found in areas of Central and South America and infections in children caused by this organism may present with fever, anorexia, vomiting, and right lower quadrant or flank pain or mass, suggesting a classic case of appendicitis (see Chapter 111). In a study in Costa Rica, more than three-fourths of children found to have *A. costaricensis* underwent surgery.[85] Ileocecal tuberculosis, amebiasis, and salmonellosis may also mimic appendicitis, although a more prolonged story of pain or fever may differentiate them from acute appendicitis. Patients with mesenteric adenitis may also have an illness clinically indistinguishable from acute appendicitis, although this condition has been reported mostly in non-tropical areas. Anisakiasis, although not typical of tropical areas, is a disease caused by the larval nematode *Anisakis marina* ("herring worm") and is associated with eating raw fish. It is a recognized public health problem in Japan, and cases have been reported in Europe. The intestinal burrowing of the larval form causes acute abdominal symptoms clinically resembling acute appendicitis.[86]

Abdominal Mass

Among the infectious conditions that can present with an abdominal mass, tuberculosis should be a leading consideration. Primary intestinal tuberculosis may present with abdominal pain, fever, and a tender, fixed palpable mass in the ileocecal area.[87] Bhansali,[79] in his series of patients with tuberculosis requiring surgery, found 96 patients who had a palpable mass on physical examination, and all of these patients had a chronic presentation. In 75 of these patients, the mass was caused by hyperplastic cecal tuberculosis, in 19 it was due to a mass of enlarged lymph nodes, and in the remaining 2 it was related to rolled-up omentum. Common symptoms in these patients were fever, weight loss, altered bowel habits, and chronic abdominal pain. Although uncommon in nonimmunocompromised persons, tuberculosis can involve the mesenteric lymph nodes and present with abdominal pain, fever, a palpable mass, or symptoms of partial small bowel obstruction.[88] In contrast, in patients with AIDS tuberculosis, mesenteric lymphadenitis is more common and generally more extensive.[89]

Another infectious condition that may present with a mass is abdominal actinomycosis. The cecal area is most frequently the site of abdominal actinomycosis, and it can present as an abscess or as a firm-to-hard mass lesion that is often fixed to the underlying tissue. Sinus tracts may develop, draining through the abdominal wall or perianal region.[90] Amebiasis can present as a chronic localized infection termed *ameboma* (see Chapter 92). An ameboma presents as a painful abdominal mass that occurs more commonly in the cecum or the ascending colon.[91]

Other tropical infectious disease conditions that may present with an abdominal mass are histoplasmosis[92] and *A. costaricensis* infection (described previously). Histoplasmosis involving the gastrointestinal tract usually occurs with disseminated disease. Gastrointestinal histoplasmosis differs from other forms of disseminated histoplasmosis in that pulmonary symptoms are uncommon and gastrointestinal symptoms predominate. Common symptoms, although they may be absent in as many as 50% of cases, include diarrhea, weight loss, abdominal pain, and fever. Clinically, patients may also present with generalized lymphadenopathy and hepatosplenomegaly. Histoplasmosis involving the gastrointestinal tract most frequently is characterized by ulcerations or an intestinal mass, especially when there is involvement of the terminal ileum, cecum, or colon.[92]

Diarrhea

Diarrheal diseases, despite major scientific advances, are a major cause of morbidity, and their frequency in the tropical areas of the world underscores the global impact of tropical diseases.[93] In these areas, diarrhea is a common cause of infant mortality, and diarrheal morbidity and mortality are linked with the poverty and poor sanitation commonly seen in developing areas. For people from nontropical developed areas visiting the tropics, it also represents an important cause of morbidity, affecting 20–50% of travelers.[94]

When approaching patients with diarrhea, it is important to obtain a good history and to define the clinical syndrome: acute watery diarrhea (small bowel disease), profuse vomiting (gastroenteritis), dysenteric disease, febrile dysenteric illness, or persistent diarrhea.

Acute Watery Diarrhea

Acute watery diarrhea is characterized by the presence of large-volume stools and is usually associated with a small bowel secretory process. The causes of acute watery diarrhea are different in temperate climates compared with tropical areas. In temperate climates, the usual causative

Table 129.3 Evaluation of Dehydration in Patients with Diarrhea

	Mild (3–5% Body Weight)	Moderate (6–9% Body Weight)	Severe (≥10% Body Weight)
Blood pressure	Normal	Normal	Normal to reduced
Heart rate	Normal	Increased	Increased[a]
Quality of pulses	Normal	Normal or slightly decreased	Moderately decreased
Skin turgor[b]	Normal	Decreased	Decreased
Mucous membranes	Slightly dry	Dry	Dry
Eyes	Normal	Sunken orbits	Deeply sunken orbits
Tears	Present	Absent	Absent
Extremities	Warm, normal capillary refill	Delayed capillary refill	Cool, mottled
Mental status	Normal	Normal to listless	Normal to lethargic or comatose
Urine output	Slightly decreased	Moderately decreased	Severely decreased to anuric

[a]Bradycardia may develop in severe cases.
[b]May not be reliable in the presence of severe malnutrition.
(Adapted from Bern C, Martines J, deZoysa I, et al. The magnitude of the global problem of diarrheal disease: a ten-year update. Bull WHO. 1992;70:705.)

Table 129.4 The Reduced Osmolarity Formulation

Reduced Osmolarity ORS	Grams/ Liter	Reduced Osmolarity ORS	Mmol/ Liter
Sodium chloride	2.6	Sodium	75
Glucose, anhydrous	13.5	Chloride	65
Potassium chloride	1.5	Glucose, anhydrous	75
Trisodium citrate, dihydrate	2.9	Potassium	20
		Citrate	10
		Total osmolarity	245

(Source: http://rehydrate.org/ors/low-osmolarity-ors.htm.)

organisms are largely undefined, although viruses are suspected in many cases. In the tropics, where most adults live in areas with poor sanitation, several other agents can cause acute noninflammatory diarrhea. Of particular importance are enterotoxigenic *E. coli* (ETEC) (see Chapter 15) and cholera (see Chapter 20). Enteroaggregative *E. coli* (EAEC) is an enteric pathogen of increasingly recognized importance. The watery, nonbloody diarrhea seen with EAEC is mediated by intestinal inflammatory mechanisms and is an important cause of persistent diarrhea in infants in the developing world, travelers' diarrhea, and AIDS-associated diarrhea in many regions.

The seventh cholera pandemic, caused by *Vibrio cholerae* biotype El Tor, has affected most of the continents of the Eastern hemisphere, including Asia, Africa, and the Mediterranean region of Europe. In 1991, the organism appeared in Peru and spread throughout Latin America.[95] Peru alone reported 322 562 cases, half of which occurred during the first 12 weeks of the epidemic. A new strain of the non-O1 serogroup, *V. cholerae* O139 synonym Bengal, was seen in late 1992, beginning in Madras (now Chennai), India, and rapidly spreading to Calcutta (now Kolkata) and Bangladesh in 1993, causing epidemic cholera gravis.[96,97] This may represent the beginning of an eighth pandemic.[98] The hallmark of this disease is a secretory diarrhea induced by an enterotoxin, cholera toxin, which produces water and electrolyte losses in the intestinal lumen resulting in dehydration ranging from mild to severe. In endemic areas, the differential diagnosis in cases of mild to moderate disease should include infections produced by ETEC, food poisoning, and viruses such as rotavirus (especially in children).

Other bacterial pathogens, such as *Shigella*, *Salmonella*, and *Campylobacter jejuni*, which typically cause inflammatory diarrhea, may occasionally present with a clinical picture of acute watery diarrhea. Because it is not possible to differentiate between these infections solely on clinical grounds, the assistance of a microbiology laboratory is advised, although in remote areas in the tropics it is not always possible to access a properly equipped and staffed laboratory facility. To make the diagnosis of cholera bacteriologically, one should culture stool specimens using thiosulfate–citrate–bile salts–sucrose (TCBS) agar.

Initial management of these patients should include assessment of dehydration (***Table 129.3***), adequate fluid replacement, preferably orally with glucose-electrolyte solutions (***Table 129.4***), or if unable to tolerate oral fluids or if severely dehydrated, intravenously with isotonic fluids. Oral rehydration therapy, in conjunction with educational programs on its effective use, allowed Peruvian physicians to achieve a survival rate of more than 99% in the more than 300 000 cholera patients seen during the first year of an outbreak in Peru.[99] Antibiotic therapy with tetracyclines and quinolones is effective in decreasing the duration and severity of the disease and in eradicating the infecting organism.[100,101]

Among the parasitic diseases capable of causing acute noninflammatory diarrhea, two coccidians are becoming increasingly important, especially because of the fact that waterborne outbreaks in the case of *Cryptosporidium parvum*[102] and food- and waterborne outbreaks caused by *Cyclospora cayetanensis*[9] have been recognized with increasing frequency, and because both are capable of causing significant disease in immunocompromised hosts, particularly those suffering from AIDS.[103,104] The fact that chlorination is ineffective in eliminating these organisms adds to their impact.

Cryptosporidiosis can cause acute, noninflammatory, self-limited diarrhea (see Chapter 94). Although not limited to tropical areas, this parasite can be easily transmitted in areas with poor sanitation, with transmission rates similar to other highly infectious enteric pathogens such as *Shigella* species.[105] This coccidian parasite is particularly important in malnourished children and immunocompromised hosts, causing a more severe and prolonged clinical picture than in immunocompetent hosts. In a study in Guinea-Bissau, cryptosporidiosis was associated with excess mortality in children independent of malnutrition, socioeconomic factors, hygienic considerations, or breastfeeding.[106] *Cryptosporidium* has been found in as many as 50% of patients with AIDS and diarrhea in developing countries.[107] The diagnosis is made by the microscopic detection of oocysts in stools using acid-fast stains. Newer methods based on enzyme-linked immunosorbent assay (ELISA) or immunofluorescence are also available, and a study showed that all methods (including acid-fast staining) were equally sensitive and specific in detecting oocysts,[108] but the threshold of detection may not be optimal.[109] Therapy is problematic. Paromomycin has been shown to decrease oocyst excretion and the number of stools in patients with AIDS and cryptosporidiosis,[110] but is rarely curative. Nitazoxanide was found to improve cryptosporidial diarrhea in one study of patients with AIDS in Mexico[111] and in HIV-negative children in Zambia.[112] The most effective intervention in this circumstance, however, remains immunologic recovery mediated by highly active antiretroviral therapy.[113]

Cyclospora cayetanensis has been described in Central and South America, the Caribbean, India, South Africa, Southeast Asia, eastern Europe, and recently from several outbreaks in the United States (see Chapter 95).[9] The disease seems to be endemic in areas of Nepal, Haiti, and Peru, and coincides with the rainy season in those areas. Although diarrhea is a common manifestation of *Cyclospora* infection, it may not be the presenting or predominant symptom in immunocompetent patients with this condition. A flu-like syndrome may precede the onset of diarrhea. *Cyclospora* has been described as a cause of prolonged diarrhea in patients with HIV infection.[104] The diagnosis of *Cyclospora* infection is based on the microscopic detection of oocysts from fecal specimens. Like *Cryptosporidium*, *Cyclospora* oocysts should be stained using acid-fast techniques such as the modified Ziehl–Neelsen stain or the Kinyoun acid-fast stain. *Cyclospora* oocysts are autofluorescent, appearing neon-blue when seen under an ultraviolet fluorescence microscope. Trimethoprim-sulfamethoxazole is the drug of choice for treating *Cyclospora* infection.[114]

In general, the management of acute, noninflammatory diarrhea in adults consists primarily of rehydration. If glucose or sucrose accompanies the isotonic fluid taken orally, the coupled absorption of sodium and water is often sufficient to replace fluid loss. In the absence of a significant febrile or inflammatory process, low doses of antimotility agents may offer some relief with minimum risk if cramping is severe. Symptomatic treatment is more often used in industrialized regions to improve symptoms, allowing persons to return to work or school. In tropical regions drugs play a minor role in the treatment of acute diarrhea. In selected cases, the use of antibiotics may provide a faster resolution of the symptoms.

Gastroenteritis

The syndrome of acute nausea and vomiting, or "viral gastroenteritis" due to rotaviruses or noroviruses, commonly occurs in winter months in temperate climates, whereas this syndrome occurs year-round in tropical and semi-tropical areas. The syndrome may also be caused by ingestion of preformed toxins of *Staphylococcus aureus* and *Bacillus cereus*, yet with a shorter incubation period. In a recent study from Taiwan, 20% and 15% of food poisoning outbreaks were caused by *S. aureus* and *B. cereus*, respectively.[115]

Acute staphylococcal food poisoning typically occurs in foodborne epidemics. Patients will present initially with nausea, vomiting, and acute salivation, followed by abdominal cramps and diarrhea. The short incubation period (2–7 hours) and the existence of similar cases from a common source (meal) will suggest the diagnosis. The diarrhea usually is watery, but rarely can contain mucus and blood. Management consists of rehydration and monitoring and replacement of fluid and electrolyte losses. The symptoms usually resolve after a few hours. The potentially contaminated food should be examined for the presence of *S. aureus* (culture and Gram stain) and enterotoxin. Meat, poultry, or their products (with ham and chicken most frequently implicated) are among the most common vehicles, but other foods, including fish and shellfish and milk and milk products, have also been implicated.[116]

Outbreaks of foodborne disease caused by *B. cereus* have been reported from tropical and nontropical areas. The organism produces an emetic or diarrheal syndrome induced by an emetic toxin and enterotoxin, respectively.[117] The emetic syndrome has a shorter incubation time (1–7 hours) and mimics staphylococcal food poisoning. Typically, the illness is associated with the ingestion of contaminated rice. The diarrheal syndrome has a longer incubation time (10–14 hours) and is usually related to the consumption of meat or vegetables. The diarrhea is profuse, lasting 12–24 hours, and is associated with abdominal pain, tenesmus, and nausea. *B. cereus* foodborne disease is self-limited, and again treatment is symptomatic, with rehydration provided as needed.

Many forms of diarrheal disease present with both watery diarrhea and vomiting. This form of gastroenteritis may be caused by enteropathogens that infect the upper gastrointestinal tract, including enteric viruses, bacterial pathogens such as diarrheagenic *E. coli*, *Shigella* spp., *Salmonella* spp., noncholera vibrios, *Campylobacter jejuni*, *Aeromonas* spp., and the protozoal parasites.

Acute Inflammatory Diarrhea

Acute inflammatory diarrhea is characterized by the passage of many small-volume stools often containing blood and mucus. The causes of acute inflammatory diarrhea include several specific distal small bowel and colonic infections such as shigellosis, salmonellosis, campylobacteriosis, and amebiasis as the most representative organisms. Enteroinvasive *E. coli* has also been described as a foodborne cause of inflammatory diarrhea in tropical areas, but data on its prevalence are scarce.[118,119]

Shigella infection is characterized by the occurrence of an invasive bacterial colitis. It is estimated that *Shigella* spp. are responsible for over 163 million infections annually in developing countries, resulting in 1.1 million deaths (see Chapter 18).[120] The disease can present with acute bloody diarrhea with high fever and systemic manifestations of malaise, headache, and abdominal pain. The incubation period ranges from 8 hours to 9 days but is usually between 14 and 72 hours, and a very low inoculum is required for its transmission, facilitating its spread. This syndrome may be particularly severe in malnourished children, in whom the mortality can be as high as 11%.[121] *Campylobacter* enteritis has been associated with ingestion of contaminated water, raw milk, or poultry, and typically occurs in young children or in travelers visiting tropical areas, and it is recognized as a common pathogen during the rainy seasons (see Chapter 19).[122]

Entamoeba histolytica is an important cause of inflammatory diarrhea (although fecal leukocytes may be pyknotic or absent) (see Chapter 92). It is estimated that infection by *E. histolytica* results in 50 million cases of invasive enteric disease and liver abscess and up to 100 000 deaths per year. High rates of infection occur in the Indian subcontinent, southern and western Africa, in the Far East, and in the tropical areas of Central and South America. Patients with amebic colitis typically present with a 1- to 2-week history of abdominal pain, tenesmus, and frequent loose watery stools containing blood and mucus. Fever can be present, and on occasion the disease can be severe enough to cause extensive colitis with colonic perforation.[123] The diagnosis of intestinal amebiasis is based on examination of the stools or biopsy of mucosal tissue. A direct saline wet mount will reveal motile trophozoites, some containing red blood cells, suggesting invasive disease. In 90% of the cases, three separate stool examinations are required for the diagnosis. Rapid stool antigen detection kits have been developed based on antilectin antibodies, differentiating between *E. histolytica* and the nonpathogenic *Entamoeba dispar* (which morphologically are indistinguishable) in stool specimens.[124] Metronidazole is the drug of choice for the treatment of invasive colitis. A luminal agent is recommended (usually iodoquinol or paromomycin) after nitroimidazole therapy of invasive amebiasis.

Balantidium coli is another protozoan capable of causing inflammatory diarrhea in tropical areas of the world (see Chapter 93).[125] The most common reservoir is swine, and in tropical areas, monkeys. Like *E. histolytica*, this parasite invades the terminal ileum and colon, and may cause appendicitis or a dysenteric syndrome with rectosigmoid ulceration. The diagnosis is made by examination of wet preparations. Tetracycline is the drug of choice, but metronidazole is also active against this ciliated protozoan.[126]

In the management of patients with acute inflammatory diarrhea, it is necessary to perform a stool culture and a parasitologic examination, based on the organisms prevalent in each tropical area. Antimicrobials are essential to those with severe shigellosis and amebiasis, and empirical antimicrobial therapy is indicated in patients with diarrhea who have high fever and systemic toxicity or dysenteric disease.

Persistent and Chronic Diarrhea

Most diarrheal episodes acquired in the tropics subside spontaneously within a few days, but in some patients diarrhea may persist for more than 2 weeks.[127] The problem of persistent diarrhea is particularly important in poorly nourished children living in developing regions. Classic causes of persistent diarrhea include *Giardia lamblia*, EAEC, and *Cryptosporidium* (which can also cause acute disease as described previously). *Cyclospora* can also cause persistent diarrhea.[128] Tuberculosis can also present with chronic diarrhea.[70]

Infection with *G. lamblia* ranges from asymptomatic cyst passage to a chronic syndrome of diarrhea with malabsorption and weight loss (see Chapter 93). Symptomatic giardiasis is characterized by the acute onset of diarrhea, abdominal cramps, bloating, and flatulence. Initially, stools may be profuse and watery, but later are commonly greasy and foul-smelling. Patients may present with periods of diarrhea alternating with periods of constipation or normal bowel habits, and the disease may wax and wane over months until therapy is given or spontaneous resolution occurs. For the diagnosis of giardiasis, repeated stool examinations may be necessary. Immunofluorescent- and ELISA-based methods have also been developed for the diagnosis of giardiasis. The drugs of choice for the treatment of giardiasis are metronidazole and tinidazole. Nitazoxanide, which is available as a liquid and given for 3 days, is another treatment option for children.

Isospora belli infection appears to occur more commonly in tropical and subtropical climates, and although diarrhea due to *I. belli* infection is typically acute and self-limited in the immunologically normal host, prolonged diarrhea can occur in certain patients (see Chapter 95).[129] In immunocompromised hosts, including patients with AIDS, isosporiasis can be protracted, with profuse diarrheal disease. Laboratory diagnosis is done by examination of stained stool specimens by the modified Ziehl–Neelsen method. *I. belli* infection responds promptly to trimethoprim-sulfamethoxazole therapy and recurrent disease can be prevented with either trimethoprim or sulfamethoxazole.

Among the nematodes, *Strongyloides stercoralis*, *Capillaria philippinensis*, *Trichuris trichiura*, and *Schistosoma* have been reported as causing diarrhea.[130] *Strongyloides* can be associated with persistent diarrhea, cramping abdominal pain, and weight loss, particularly when there is hyperinfection or disseminated strongyloidiasis. Eosinophilia is a prominent feature of this infection. Occasionally some patients may complain of nausea, vomiting, and weight loss with evidence of malabsorption or of protein-losing enteropathy. *C. philippinensis* is a nematode that can also cause chronic diarrhea and malabsorption. The infection is seen in the Philippines and Thailand, and has also been reported in India and Egypt. *T. trichiura* can also be a cause of diarrhea (chronic dysentery) in highly parasitized patients. In schistosomiasis, diarrhea may occur due to the resulting granulomatous inflammation of the colon seen during the chronic phase in patients with heavy infections, or during acute schistosomiasis in unexposed patients (Katayama fever). In the latter case, the pathologic findings are completely different from those seen in the chronic form and are likely to be related to a hypersensitivity reaction.

Disseminated histoplasmosis and paracoccidioidomycosis (South American blastomycosis) may unusually present with chronic diarrhea, sometimes as an important symptom, and have to be considered in the differential diagnosis.[92,131]

Postinfective malabsorption (tropical sprue or "tropical enteropathy") was a common cause of chronic small bowel diarrhea, malabsorption, and weight loss in adults, especially in India, East Asia, and Central America. Small bowel bacterial overgrowth seems to play a role in the pathogenesis of tropical sprue. The treatment of tropical sprue with tetracycline and folate for up to 6 months seems to be most effective in symptom resolution and cure of diarrhea, with promotion of weight gain. *Tropical enteropathy* is a term used to describe an increasingly recognized syndrome of reduced absorption (with villous flattening) that is seen in many who live in tropical, developing areas (including Peace Corps volunteers)[132] and in many infections (ranging from *Cryptosporidium*, *Cyclospora*, or microsporidia to viral enteropathies).[133]

A form of persistent diarrhea showing worldwide distribution is Brainerd diarrhea. This is an idiopathic secretory process frequently associated with chronic lymphocytic inflammation in the colonic mucosa. The source is characteristically unpasteurized milk or untreated (well or surface) water. The prognosis is good, with diarrhea generally subsiding after 6 months to 1 year.

Travelers' Diarrhea

Travelers' diarrhea is a syndrome characterized by a twofold or greater increase in the frequency of unformed bowel movements, associated with one or more signs or symptoms of enteric infection occurring during or shortly after a trip away from home (see Chapter 126). The tropical areas of Latin America, Africa, and southern Asia are considered the high-risk areas for travelers' diarrhea.[134] Attack rates are variable, but average approximately 40% for travel from an industrialized region to one of the high-risk areas.

Bacterial enteropathogens cause most cases of travelers' diarrhea regardless of the specific area of risk. ETEC is the single most common bacterial pathogen isolated, followed by EAEC, *Shigella* spp., *Campylobacter jejuni*, *Aeromonas* spp., *Plesiomonas shigelloides*, *Salmonella* spp., and non-cholera vibrios. Parasites such as *G. lamblia* and *Cryptosporidium* occur in approximately 2–3% of cases of travelers' diarrhea. In 20–50% of episodes of travelers' diarrhea, no agents can be identified despite complete microbiologic assessment. Most of this undefinable illness appears to be bacterial in origin in view of the favorable response to antimicrobial therapy.

The management of patients with travelers' diarrhea involves adequate rehydration, followed by dietary management and symptomatic treatment.[94] Evidence-based expert reviews have been published recently with recommendations on the self-therapy and prevention of travelers' diarrhea.[135,136] Treatment is designed to reduce symptoms and shorten the duration of illness and the inconvenience associated with it. For rehydration, increasing fluids and salt-containing foods in the diet is usually enough for hydrating most ill travelers. Restriction of diet during diarrhea appears to have no overt clinical benefit, but it should be useful to consume easily digestible foods. Patients should resume their usual diet once stools retain their shape. Drinks or food containing caffeine or lactose should be avoided while stools are unformed, since they may prolong diarrhea. Commonly used symptomatic drugs include bismuth subsalicylate and the antimotility synthetic opiate drugs such as loperamide. These agents are useful for the symptomatic treatment of mild to moderate cases of travelers' diarrhea.

Antimicrobial therapy shortens the duration of travelers' diarrhea from an average of 59–93 hours to 16–30 hours. For most adults with moderate to severe travelers' diarrhea without fever or dysentery antimicrobial therapy will be effective. Fluoroquinolones, or in South Asia azithromycin, are the preferred agents because of their activity against enteric pathogens in most high-risk parts of the world. When high fever is present or travelers are passing grossly bloody stools, azithromycin is the recommended therapy. Rifaximin, a poorly absorbed oral rifamycin derivative, approved by the Food and Drug Administration for the treatment of travelers' diarrhea caused by noninvasive strains of *E. coli* is appropriate for therapy of watery diarrhea occurring in international travelers. Its use in patients with fever or blood in the stool and for those infected with *Campylobacter jejuni* is discouraged.

With regard to prevention, travelers to high-risk areas should be educated as to the safe foods and beverages to consume. Antimicrobial prophylaxis will prevent 70–80% of the disease that would occur without prophylaxis. If the traveler has an important underlying health impairment, or the trip will be ruined if the traveler has a brief illness that might force a change in itinerary, antimicrobial prophylaxis may be considered. An effective antibacterial drug for prevention of travelers' diarrhea is poorly absorbed rifaximin.[137] Bismuth subsalicylate has also been used as a prophylactic agent, preventing up to 65% of the cases of diarrhea that would occur during travel to high-risk areas if prophylaxis were not employed.[138] High-risk travelers should begin taking the drug to be used for prophylaxis on their first day in the country they are visiting and should continue to take it for 1 or 2 days after leaving the country, but no more than 2 weeks of prophylaxis is advised. Pathogens such as *Cryptosporidium*, which may be devastating in immunocompromised patients, are prevented only by strict food and water precautions.

Immunoprophylaxis may be an alternative in the future, as the whole cell *Vibrio cholerae*/recombinant B subunit cholera toxin–oral cholera vaccine has provided some short-term protection against ETEC diarrhea and cholera diarrhea. Newer experimental vaccines are been tested, including an LT-ETEC patch vaccine, and the results look promising.[136]

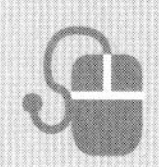

Access the complete reference list online at
http://www.expertconsult.com

Access the complete reference list online at http://www.expertconsult.com

CHAPTER 130

Fever and Systemic Symptoms

Mary E. Wilson • Andrea K. Boggild

INTRODUCTION

Fever in the tropics and after travel is a common response to microbial invasion. Fever can presage rapidly progressive disease or indicate a trivial self-limited infection, the early symptoms of which can be indistinguishable. Several features make evaluation of fever a major and continuing challenge: the causes include diverse infectious and noninfectious diseases; similar signs and symptoms characterize infections caused by unrelated pathogens requiring different interventions; and timing of onset of fever after exposure to a pathogen can range from hours to decades. Interventions may be lifesaving if applied in good time.

This chapter describes the causes of fever in persons with tropical and other diverse geographic exposures. The discussion focuses on recognizing possible causes of fever and on reaching a specific diagnosis and omits details of treatment, which can be found elsewhere in this book. Although the differential diagnosis for the febrile short-term international traveler and the febrile resident of the tropics may be similar, the relative likelihood of specific diseases and their consequences may differ greatly, thus mandating flexibility in the approach to the initial evaluation. Foreign-born residents of industrialized countries and their children who visit relatives and friends (VFRs) in developing countries may receive no pretravel prophylaxis and often have intense local exposures, placing them at greater risk for a wider range of infections than the usual tourist or business traveler.[1] Several key concepts that underlie the evaluation of the febrile patient are listed in ***Box 130.1***.

PATHOGENESIS

The complex interactions of endogenous pyrogens and neural pathways in the pathogenesis of fever are reviewed in several publications.[2–4] Pyrogenic cytokines, such as interleukin (IL)-1β, IL-6, and tumor necrosis factor-α, which result from stimulated mononuclear phagocytes, interact directly with the anterior hypothalamus, which coordinates thermoregulation through a hierarchy of neural structures. Prostaglandin E_2 is a proximal mediator in the preoptic-anterior hypothalamic area. Direct neural pathways from the periphery to the brain also may be involved.[2] Exogenous pyrogens including bacterial cell wall products may act on Toll-like receptors in the hypothalamus and elevate the thermoregulatory setpoint.[5]

EPIDEMIOLOGY

Fever is a common reason for seeking medical care during and after travel. Although risks and types of infection vary greatly depending on the circumstances of travel and the specific time and place, available studies provide general estimates of the likelihood of fever during and after travel. In the classic studies by Steffen and colleagues,[6] 152 of 7886 (almost 2%) of Swiss short-term travelers to developing countries reported "high fevers over several days" on questionnaires completed between 4 and almost 7 months after return from travel. In a study of 784 American travelers who spent 3 months or less in developing countries, 3% reported fever unassociated with other symptoms.[7] Among almost 25 000 ill returned travelers who were seen at 31 different clinical sites as part of the global GeoSentinel surveillance network, 28% cited fever as a chief reason for seeking care.[8]

The likelihood of infection and the specific infections observed are strongly linked to the geographic location of exposure. In a study of GeoSentinel data Freedman et al compared the frequency of multiple diagnoses among ill returned travelers from six developing regions (see ***Fig. 130.1***).[9] They found significant differences by geographic region for 16 of 21 broad syndromic categories. Systemic febrile illness occurred disproportionately among travelers returning from sub-Saharan Africa or Southeast Asia. In most years, risk of dengue was highest in parts of Asia, falciparum malaria in sub-Saharan Africa, and enteric fever in the Indian subcontinent. Estimates of the relative risk of malaria in travelers from 2000 to 2002 based on GeoSentinel data range from 1 (very low risk areas) to >200 in sub-Saharan Africa.[10] Among German travelers who acquired dengue fever in 2002, incidence rate per 100 000 travelers ranged from 27.9 for Thailand to 2.1 for the Greater Antilles islands.[11] Illness in returning travelers reflects only part of the disease burden experienced by travelers. Many infections begin and are treated abroad. In one study of malaria in travelers to Africa, about half of the cases were treated abroad.[12]

Multiple studies have identified malaria as the most common specific infection in travelers with systemic febrile illness after tropical travel. Among 6957 febrile returned travelers seen at a GeoSentinel site between 1997 and 2006, malaria was identified in 21%.[8] In a study of 1743 patients seen at referral centers in Belgium with febrile illnesses within 12 months of a tropical stay, malaria accounted for 28% of the fever episodes.[13] In a Swiss outpatient clinic, among 336 travelers and migrants with a history of fever or malaise, 29% of those who were tested had confirmed malaria.[14] Of 195 consecutive patients hospitalized with fever between November 1992 and April 1993 at the London Hospital for Tropical Diseases, malaria was the most common diagnosis, accounting for 42% of admissions.[15] Other studies of hospitalized febrile returned travelers from Australia,[16] Italy,[17] and France[18] also found malaria as the most common specific diagnosis. Among 153 hospitalized febrile returned pediatric travelers in the UK, diarrheal disease and malaria were the most common diagnoses.[19] Recent papers also highlight the growing importance of dengue fever in tropical areas,[20–24] and as a cause of hospitalization after travel, the specific diagnosis second only to malaria in a study from Israel.[25] Dengue accounted for 6% of patients with febrile systemic illness in the GeoSentinel analysis.[8]

It is worth noting that diseases with a cosmopolitan distribution, such as respiratory infections, hepatitis, diarrheal illness, urinary tract infections, and pharyngitis, are found as the cause of fever in a substantial proportion of febrile returned travelers. In studies by MacLean and

Box 130.1 Key Concepts in the Evaluation of the Febrile Patient

Fever after travel may be unrelated to exposures during travel.	Unfamiliar infections can follow exposures in temperate areas.
A history of fever in a person exposed to malaria should prompt evaluation for malaria, even if the patient is afebrile at the moment seen.	Reexamine the febrile patient if the initial evaluation does not suggest a specific diagnosis.
Always look for malaria. Look again if exposures and clinical findings are consistent with that diagnosis.	Keep in mind the public health implications. Should the infection be reported? Do contacts need treatment or special attention? Are special isolation techniques required?
Exposure to many widely distributed infections is more common during travel than during life at home.	Use electronic networks to supplement and update information from other sources.

associates[26] and Doherty and coworkers,[15] of the top 10 most common causes of fever after tropical travel, more than half are diseases with broad or worldwide distribution. In the study by Bottieau, cosmopolitan infections accounted for 34% of cases of febrile illnesses after stays in the tropics.[13] *Table 130.1* lists the most common causes of fever after tropical travel as described in published series. Many categories define a body site of infection and not a specific pathogen. In large published series, the specific cause remains undefined in about one-fourth of febrile illnesses.[8,13] Although recently published studies have identified malaria, dengue, rickettsioses, and enteric fever as the most common specific diseases, patterns of infectious disease are dynamic and will continue to change.[27,28] A recent example is chikungunya virus, identified as the cause of multiple outbreaks in Africa, many parts of Asia, and even one in Italy.[29–31] More than 1000 travelers visiting outbreak areas have also been infected. Several factors can lead to changes in the types and relative frequencies of diseases diagnosed in persons visiting tropical regions: shifts in the epidemiology of disease; the rising resistance of pathogens to drugs; changes in popular destinations; the availability and use of effective preventive strategies (e.g., vaccines against hepatitis A and B); and new knowledge and techniques that facilitate diagnosis.

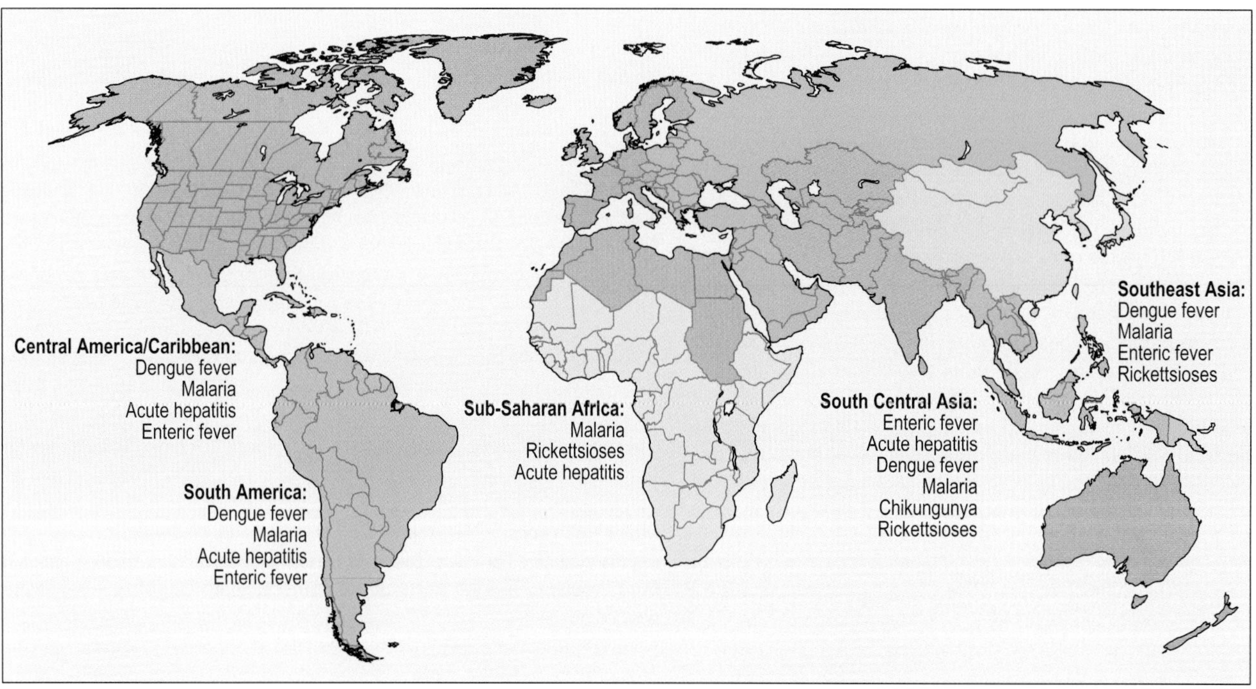

Figure 130.1 Common tropical infectious causes of systemic febrile illness by region of travel. (Information adapted from Freedman DO, Weld LH, Kozarsky PE, et al. Spectrum of disease and relationship to place of exposure in ill returned travelers. N Engl J Med. 2006;354:119-130.).

Table 130.1 Summary Data from Major Studies of Illness and/or Fever in Returned Travelers

Study	Patient Population (Location)	Most Common Specific Infectious Causes of Illness (*or Fever if Reported)	Most Well Represented Regions of Travel (*Among Those Who Reported Illness if Available)
Steffen et al[6]	7886 returned travelers to the tropics >12 years of age, 1168 of whom reported some travel-related illness (Switzerland)	Giardiasis (3.3%) Amebiasis (2.6%) Gonorrhea (2%) Malaria (1%) Hepatitis A (0.7%) Helminthiases (0.6%)	East Africa (29%)* West Africa (26%)* Sri Lanka/Maldives (23%)* South America (11%)* Far East (6%)*
Hill[7]	784 returned travelers, 64% of whom reported some travel-related illness, 93 of whom sought care post travel (United States)	Gastrointestinal illness (31%) RTI (24%) Skin disease (11%) Malaria (2%) Hepatitis (2%) Dengue fever (1%) Mediterranean spotted fever (1%)	Indian subcontinent (21%) Central and East Africa (20%) South America (16%) Southeast Asia (14%) West Africa (10%) Central America (10%)

Table 130.1 Summary Data from Major Studies of Illness and/or Fever in Returned Travelers—cont'd

Study	Patient Population (Location)	Most Common Specific Infectious Causes of Illness (*or Fever if Reported)	Most Well Represented Regions of Travel (*Among Those Who Reported Illness if Available)
Wilson et al[8]	24920 ill returned travelers, 6957 of whom had fever (multicenter, global)	Malaria (21%)* Acute TD (15%)* RTI (14%)* Dengue fever (6%)* Dermatologic illness (4%)* Enteric fever (2%)* Rickettsioses (2%)* Acute UTI (2%)* Acute hepatitis (1%)	Sub-Saharan Africa (37%)* Southeast Asia (18%)* Latin America/Caribbean (15%)* South Central Asia (13%)* North Africa (3%)*
Bottieau et al[13]	1743 outpatients presenting with fever after tropical travel (Belgium)	Malaria (27.7%)* RTI (10.5%)* Bacterial enteritis (6.2%)* Mononucleosis-like syndrome (3.9%)* Skin/soft tissue infection (3.6%)* GU infection/STD (3.4%)* Rickettsioses (3.3%)* Dengue fever (3%)*	Sub-Saharan Africa (68%)* Southeast Asia (12%)* Latin America (7%)* Indian subcontinent (6%)* North Africa (4%)*
Doherty et al[15]	195 inpatients presenting with fever after tropical travel (United Kingdom)	Malaria (42%)* Non-specific viral syndrome (25%)* Dengue fever (6%)* Bacterial dysentery (5%)* RTI (4%)* Hepatitis A (3%)* UTI (2%)* Typhoid (1.5%)*	Sub-Saharan Africa (60%)* Indian subcontinent (13%)* Far East (8%)* South America (3%)* Europe (0.5%)*
O'Brien et al[16]	232 inpatients admitted for management of fever after overseas travel (Australia)	Malaria (27%)* RTI (24%)* Gastroenteritis (14%)* Dengue fever (8%)* Typhoid (3%)* Hepatitis A (3%)* Rickettsioses (2%)* Tropical ulcer (2%)*	Asia (61%)* The Pacific (20%)* Africa (15%)* Latin America (2%)*
Antinori et al[17]	147 inpatients admitted for fever after tropical travel (Italy)	Malaria (48%)* Presumptive viral illness (12%)* Viral hepatitis (9%)* Gastroenteritis (5%)* Schistosomiasis (5%)* Typhoid (4%)* Dengue fever (3%)* RTI (3%)* UTI (1%)*	Africa (61%)* Asia (22%)* Central and South America (13%)* Oceania (2%)* Middle East (2%)*
Parola et al[18]	613 inpatients admitted for fever after tropical travel (France)	Malaria (75%)* RTI (4%)* Food/waterborne infection (4%)* Dengue fever (2%)* Viral hepatitis (1%)*	Indian Ocean islands (55)* West Africa (22%) Central Africa (9%)* Southeast Asia (4%)* Indian subcontinent (3%)* North Africa (2%)* Central America/Caribbean (0.5%)*
West and Riordan[19]	162 pediatric inpatients admitted with fever following travel to tropics and subtropics (United Kingdom)	Viral illness (34%)* Diarrheal illness (27%)* Malaria (14%)* Pneumonia (8.5%)* Hepatitis A (5%)* UTI (4%)* Enteric fever (3%)*	Indian subcontinent (82%)* Middle East (6%)* Africa (4%)* Southeast Asia (2%)*
Klein and Millman (BMJ. 1998;316: 1425)	31 pediatric inpatients admitted with fever after tropical travel (United Kingdom)	Malaria (13%)* Bacillary dysentery (10%)* Dengue fever (6.5%)* Typhoid (6.5%)* Hepatitis A (3%)*	South Asia (61%)* Sub-Saharan Africa (35%)* Caribbean (3%)*

RTI, respiratory tract infection; TD, travelers' diarrhea; UTI, urinary tract infection; GU, genitourinary; STD, sexually transmitted disease.

Studies that describe causes of fever in specific geographic areas help define the pathogens present in that area. The capacity to share data through electronic networks has improved the flow of information.[32] Increasingly, websites with data from surveillance networks provide current information. Exposures differ among short-term travelers, long-term visitors (such as missionaries and Peace Corps workers), local residents, and military troops, but studies from these groups can be useful. Several studies looked at US troops in Vietnam. The most frequent diagnoses in 524 US Marines in South Vietnam with acute fevers lasting at least 4 days included leptospirosis (20.1%), scrub typhus (11.6%), Japanese encephalitis (6.8%), and infectious mononucleosis (5.4%).[33] Another study in Vietnam of febrile American troops (with a negative malaria smear) found dengue to be the cause of fever in 29%, chikungunya in 9%, scrub typhus in 8%, and malaria in 7%.[34] While these studies provide a general idea of the pathogens in that region, most troops have a level of exposure to water, soil, and arthropods unmatched by the usual traveler (see Chapter 128). A recent prospective study of febrile illnesses in Amazonia, Ecuador, an area with known malaria and yellow fever, also identified leptospirosis, rickettsioses, dengue fever, and Q fever, infections previously unknown in this area.[35]

In 876 consecutive febrile adults seen at a general hospital in Nepal in 2001, enteric fever and pneumonia were the most common clinical diagnoses.[36] A putative pathogen was identified in 37%, with the most common specific diagnoses being typhoid and paratyphoid fever, murine typhus, pneumococcal infection, scrub typhus, and leptospirosis. The most common diagnoses in 505 adults in Spain with unexplained fever (with negative chest films and without localizing signs or symptoms) lasting 1–3 weeks were Q fever (21%), brucellosis (19%), spotted fever (murine typhus and boutonneuse fever; 15%), and mononucleosis syndrome (9%).[37]

In northern Thailand, melioidosis, caused by the Gram-negative organism *Burkholderia pseudomallei*, is a major cause of community-acquired sepsis.[38] During a 1-year period, 63 cases of septicemic melioidosis and 206 patients with other community-acquired septicemias were documented. Melioidosis accounted for 20% of all documented cases of sepsis and 40% of all deaths from community-acquired sepsis.[39] Melioidosis is also commonly reported in Malaysia.[40] Reflecting the importance of this pathogen, especially in Southeast Asia, melioidosis (see Chapter 33) is occasionally seen in travelers to and immigrants from these endemic regions.[41,42]

Serologic studies of local residents can provide insights into potential risks to persons who visit that region. A study that measured prevalences of antibodies to *Coxiella burnetii*, *Rickettsia conorii*, and *R. typhi* in seven African countries found wide variations in evidence of past infections. The seroprevalence for *C. burnetii* was generally higher in areas of West Africa, where stock breeding is prominent; prevalences of antibodies to *R. typhi* were higher in coastal regions.[43] In Inner Mongolia, nearly half of the human population tested had antibodies to *R. sibirica*.[44] Rates of positivity varied according to region, with the highest rates being found in desert dwellers. Several reviews discuss the causes and evaluation of persons with fevers after visits to specific geographic regions: the Middle East,[45,46] Africa,[47] Southeast Asia and Oceania,[48] and Latin America and the Caribbean.[49]

APPROACH TO THE PATIENT WITH FEVER

Because unusual infections occur in temperate regions as well as in the tropics, this discussion considers a wide range of possible exposures. Four questions can help focus thoughts on an individual patient with fever:

1. What is possible based on the geographic areas visited?
2. What is biologically plausible given the time of travel and incubation periods?
3. What are more likely diagnoses based on epidemiologic data, activities, host factors, and clinical and laboratory data?
4. What is treatable or transmissible or both?

Initial data will help set the tempo and scope for the workup. Often, therapeutic interventions are called for before a specific diagnosis can be confirmed.

Time

Time can be a powerful tool in refining and limiting the list of diagnostic possibilities. Every pathogen can be characterized by a typical incubation period: the interval between exposure (entry into the host) and the development of clinical signs and symptoms of infection. Incubation periods can range from minutes to decades. Although the time range may be wide, most infections acquired by short-term travelers have incubation periods measured in days or weeks. In contrast, the time lapse between exposure and the first symptoms of filariasis in US military personnel was between 5 and 18 months.[50] How long a pathogen can survive in the human host is relevant when thinking about how far back one must go when inquiring about past travel and exposures.

In the evaluation of a febrile patient who has traveled recently, it is useful to calculate the shortest and longest possible incubation periods, assuming potential exposure at all points during travel.[51] Sometimes this immediately allows the rejection of several diagnoses that had been considered. More complicated are patients who have had multiple, diverse geographic exposures over many months or years, which expands the number of diagnostic possibilities. Time analysis helps one construct a list of diseases in a geographic region that are biologically plausible given what is known about the usual ranges of incubation periods. ***Box 130.2*** lists infections by interval between exposure and onset of symptoms. The clinician should always keep in mind that fever occurring after travel may not be related to exposures during travel. It is also useful to know the most typical time of symptom onset for infections whose incubation periods are characterized by a broad range, such as malaria. Among the cases of malaria reported to the Centers for Disease Control and Prevention (CDC)[52] in 2007, the dates of the person's arrival in the United States and onset of symptoms and the infecting *Plasmodium* spp. were known for 771 cases. For 10.1% of cases, symptoms began before arrival in the United States. As can be seen in ***Table 130.2***, 80% of cases of falciparum malaria became apparent <30 days after arrival in the United States. In contrast, only 35.9% of cases of vivax malaria were identified during the first month after arrival and about 20% were seen more than 6 months after return, including almost 3% seen more than a year after return. Overall 1.6% of all malaria cases had onset greater than 1 year after return. Similar findings come from a study of 482 cases of malaria from Canada in which 87% of cases of falciparum malaria presented within 6 weeks of return from travel, whereas one-third of cases of vivax malaria presented more than 6 months after return.[53] The importance of malaria as a cause of late-onset fevers is underscored by the study by Antinori and associates.[17] Among 147 febrile hospitalized returned travelers, malaria was the diagnosis made in all cases of fever presenting more than 1 month after return from a tropical area (see Chapter 96).

Symptoms of dengue fever typically begin within 10–14 days of exposure. When fevers start 2 weeks or longer after exposure, dengue and most other arboviral infections are no longer biologically plausible. In the study by Bottieau all cases of rickettsioses presented within 1 month of return.[13] In contrast, among patients with acute schistosomiasis acquired during swimming in freshwater pools in the Dogon area of Mali, the median incubation period was 40 days (range, 14–63 days).[54] Other sequelae of schistosomiasis may appear later.[55–58]

History

All stays in a given geographic region are not of similar relevance. Although many infections can be acquired through a single, brief encounter (the bite of an infective vector, ingestion of contaminated food, sexual contact, etc.), the probability of an encounter that leads to disease increases with longer stays. For example, a study of British travelers to West Africa found that if the relative risk of malaria was considered to

Box 130.2 Infections by Interval between Exposure and Onset of Fever or other Symptoms (Lists Are Not Exhaustive)

Incubation <14 days

Undifferentiated fever

Malaria
Dengue fever
Spotted fever rickettsiae
Typhus group rickettsiae
Scrub typhus (*Orientia tsutsugamushi*)
Leptospirosis
Typhoid and paratyphoid fevers
Campylobacteriosis, salmonellosis, shigellosis
Brucellosis
Acute HIV
Tularemia
Relapsing fever
Toxoplasmosis
Ehrlichiosis
African trypanosomiasis (*Trypanosoma brucei rhodesiense*)
American trypanosomiasis
Trichinellosis

Fever and hemorrhage

Meningococcemia, leptospirosis, other acute bacterial infections
Dengue fever
Lassa fever
Yellow fever
Hemorrhagic fever with renal syndrome
Other hemorrhagic fevers
  Africa: Rift Valley fever, Ebola, Marburg viruses
  South America: Junin, Machupo, Sabia, Guanarito viruses

Fever and CNS findings

Meningococcal meningitis
Malaria
Arboviral encephalitis (including Japanese encephalitis, West Nile virus, tick-borne encephalitis, dengue, others)
Rabies
Poliomyelitis
Many other viral and bacterial forms of meningitis and encephalitis
Angiostrongyliasis (eosinophilic meningitis)
African trypanosomiasis (*T. b. rhodesiense*)

Fever and respiratory findings

Influenza
Other common bacterial and viral respiratory pathogens
Legionellosis
SARS
Q fever
Coccidioidomycosis, acute
Histoplasmosis, acute
Hantavirus pulmonary syndrome
Diphtheria
Tularemia
Plague
Anthrax
Melioidosis

Incubation 2–6 weeks

Malaria
Typhoid and paratyphoid fevers
Hepatitis A
Hepatitis E
Acute schistosomiasis (Katayama syndrome)
Leptospirosis
Amebic liver abscess
Q fever
HIV, acute
African trypanosomiasis (*T. b. rhodesiense* and *T. b. gambiense*)
Viral hemorrhagic fever (hantaviruses often have incubation >2 weeks)
Brucellosis
Tuberculosis
Cytomegalovirus infection (acute)
Toxoplasmosis

Incubation >6 weeks

Malaria
Tuberculosis
Hepatitis B
Leishmaniasis, visceral
Schistosomiasis
Amebic liver abscess
Filariasis, lymphatic
Hepatitis E
Rabies
African trypanosomiasis (*T. b. gambiense*)
Fungal infections, including histoplasmosis, coccidioidomycosis, paracoccidioidomycosis, others
Brucellosis
Melioidosis
Bartonellosis
Fascioliasis
Visceral larva migrans due to *Toxocara canis*

Table 130.2 Imported Malaria Cases by Interval between Date of Entry and Onset of Illness and by *Plasmodium* Species, United States, 2007

Interval (days)	*P. falciparum* (%)	*P. vivax* (%)	*P. malariae* (%)	*P. ovale* (%)	Mixed (%)	Total (%)
<0[a]	62 (12.5)	13 (6.3)	1 (3.7)	2 (6.2)	0 (0)	78 (10.1)
0–29	398 (80.1)	74 (35.9)	14 (51.9)	10 (31.2)	8 (88.9)	504 (65.4)
30–89	22 (4.4)	44 (21.3)	8 (29.6)	2 (6.3)	0 (0)	76 (9.8)
90–179	6 (1.2)	33 (16.1)	1 (3.7)	11 (34.4)	1 (11.1)	52 (6.7)
180–364	6 (1.2)	36 (17.5)	2 (7.4)	5 (15.6)	0 (0)	49 (6.4)
>365	3 (0.6)	6 (2.9)	1 (3.7)	2 (6.3)	0 (0)	12 (1.6)
Total	497 (100)	206 (100)	27 (100)	32 (100)	9 (100)	771 (100)

[a]Onset of illness before arriving in the United States.

be 1 for a 1-week stay, it increased to 80.3 for stays that lasted between 6 and 12 months.[59]

The probability of exposure to uncommon infections also increases during a prolonged stay. Residence or extended stays in areas may also be more likely to be associated with greater exposure to local residents, rural or remote areas, and local foods and vectors. The separation between person and microbes that can be maintained during a brief visit seldom can be sustained over a period of months or years.

The type of residence and activities engaged in also affect the risk of infection. The initial history should review the details of living conditions, work, and recreational activities en route and during the stay. Many travelers seek adventures during travels that make it likely they will come into contact with animals, insect vectors, and soil- and water-related pathogens. Of 32 Dutch travelers who were found to have leptospirosis, a history of contact with surface water could be confirmed in all but one case.[60]

Some infections, such as louse-borne relapsing fever[61] and Chagas' disease,[62] pose little risk to most short-term travelers because their living conditions are unlikely to lead to exposure. Although hantaviruses are widely distributed, most travelers have little risk of exposure. In studies of hemorrhagic fever with renal syndrome in two villages in China, risk factors for infection included direct rodent contact, camping in grain fields, living in a house on the periphery of a village, and some kinds of agricultural work – activities in which few visitors to a region would engage.[63] Acquisition of plague during travel has been an exceptional event.[64]

Box 130.3 lists elements of the history that may provide clues to specific exposures. Sources of infection are typically food or beverages, close contact with other persons, or exposure to pathogens in soil and water or pathogens carried by vectors or animal hosts. Although the list is not exhaustive, it indicates the types of exposures that may be relevant. *Table 130.3* lists specific infections that can follow various types of exposures.

Box 130.3 The History

Checklist of Potential Exposures

- When: season/month/year
- Duration of stay
- Area visited: urban or rural; altitude
- Living conditions: e.g., hotel with air conditioning or well-maintained screens, bednets, camping
- Food and drink
  - Raw or undercooked meat or fish
  - Unpasteurized milk, cheese
- Activities
  - Close contact with others
  - Sex or other intimate contacts (dates, nature of sexual contact, with whom)
  - Crowded living and sleeping arrangements
- Medical and other interventions, including regular prescription medications
  - Injections, acupuncture, transfusions
  - Dental work, ear or body piercing
  - Tattoos
  - Shaved with used razor
  - Intravenous drug use/shared cocaine use
- Recreational or occupational
  - Water (swimming, wading, rafting, bathing in streams, etc.)
  - Exploration of caves
  - Digging or soil contact
- Animal exposure
  - Bites or licks to broken skin
  - Direct physical contact with dogs, birds, primates, etc.
  - Proximity to birds, rodents

Host Factors

- Age
- Sex
- Prior residence
- Past infections
- Immunizations
- Chemoprophylactic drugs
- Antibiotics, corticosteroids or other drugs
- Underlying diseases
- Previous surgery (e.g., splenectomy, gastrectomy, insertion of prosthetic material)
- Genetics
- Family history

Casual sex with a new partner is common during travel, occurring in 5–50% of travelers.[65–68] This information may not be offered unless the patient is asked specifically about sexual exposures. A study by Correia and colleagues found that 15% of Canadians traveling internationally reported sex with a new partner or potential exposure to blood and body fluids through other means (e.g., injections, tattoos, dental work, other skin-perforating procedures).[69] Of 782 persons who were seen after travel in 1991 and 1992, 18.6% reported a new sexual partner, almost two-thirds of those did not use condoms consistently, and 5.7% acquired a sexually transmitted disease (STD) during the most recent trip.[70] In a study of known HIV-positive travelers, 23% reportedly engaged in casual sexual activity while traveling, and only 58% reported using condoms "always" during these encounters.[71]

Many infections exhibit striking seasonality in patterns. The risk may be absent during parts of the year for vector-borne infections, especially if there are distinct rainy and dry seasons or the climate is temperate and the winters cold.[72] In German travelers to Thailand the incidence of dengue fever per 100 000 travelers ranged from 2 in January 2002 to more than 70 in April.[11] Infections that are spread from person to person

Table 130.3 Examples of Infections Associated with Specific Exposures

Exposure	Infection
Contacts	
Sex, blood, body fluids	Hepatitis A, B, C, D; CMV, HIV, syphilis, HSV, amebiasis
Fresh water	Leptospirosis, schistosomiasis
Rodents and their excreta	Hantaviruses, Lassa fever and other hemorrhagic fevers, plague, rat-bite fever, murine typhus
Soil	Several dimorphic and filamentous fungi, melioidosis
Animals and their products	Q fever, brucellosis, anthrax, plague, tularemia, toxoplasmosis, rabies, psittacosis, monkeypox, herpes B virus, cat-scratch disease
Ingestions	
Unpasteurized milk and products	Brucellosis, salmonellosis, tuberculosis, Q fever, listeriosis
Raw or undercooked shellfish	Clonorchiasis, paragonimiasis, vibrios, hepatitis A, gnathostomiasis
Raw or undercooked animal flesh	Trichinellosis, salmonellosis, *Escherichia coli* O157, campylobacteriosis, toxoplasmosis, gnathostomiasis
Raw vegetables, water plants	Fascioliasis, fasciolopsiasis, angiostrongyliasis (if in contact with snails or snail slime)
Arthropod Vectors	
Mosquitoes	Malaria, dengue fever, filariasis, yellow fever, Japanese encephalitis, West Nile virus, many other arboviral infections
Fleas	Typhus (and exposure to flea feces), plague
Lice	Relapsing fever, epidemic typhus, trench fever
Sandflies	Leishmaniasis, Oroya fever, sandfly fever
Black flies	Onchocerciasis
Deer flies	Loaiasis
Triatomine bugs (reduviid bugs)	American trypanosomiasis (Chagas' disease)
Tsetse flies	African trypanosomiasis
Ticks or mites	Babesiosis, Crimean-Congo hemorrhagic fever, Colorado tick fever, Omsk hemorrhagic fever, ehrlichiosis, anaplasmosis, Kyasanur Forest disease, Lyme disease, scrub typhus, spotted fevers (rickettsial), tick-borne encephalitis, tularemia

(e.g., influenza) and those associated with soil and water (e.g., melioidosis, cholera) can also show a seasonal pattern. Influenza epidemics typically occur in winter months in temperate regions. They can occur throughout the year in tropical areas, although epidemics often follow changes in weather patterns (e.g., monsoons).[73,74] Melioidosis occurs more often in the rainy season,[75] meningococcal meningitis in Africa in the dry season,[76,77] and leptospirosis during warmer months in temperate areas and during the rainy season in the tropics.[78]

Host Factors

Host factors can affect the probability of exposure, the likelihood of infection if exposure occurs, and the expression or outcome of infection. Hepatitis A is often mild or clinically inapparent in a young child, whereas it causes serious illness and, rarely, death in the older adult. Prior immunizations and chemoprophylactic agents also influence the probability of disease and delay the onset of symptoms or alter clinical expression.[79] A study in the United Kingdom found that persons taking mefloquine had delayed onset of symptoms of falciparum malaria.[80] A history of having received a vaccine or having taken prophylaxis for a specific disease should not lead one to automatically exclude the possibility of that disease. Rather, one must consider the efficacy of the vaccine, compliance with prophylactic regimens, and local drug resistance patterns.[81] Preventive measures vary greatly in efficacy. Failures with yellow fever vaccine have been reported only rarely,[82] whereas protective efficacy with the parenteral Vi capsular polysaccharide typhoid vaccine is estimated to be 60–72% in field trials in endemic regions.[83,84] Typhoid and paratyphoid fever have been reported in visitors to Nepal who received typhoid vaccination.[85,86] A single dose of measles vaccine is about 95% efficacious in preventing measles in preschool-aged children immunized at or after 15 months of age.[87] The protective efficacy of influenza vaccine depends on host factors as well as whether antigens included in the yearly formulated vaccine match the circulating influenza viruses. A complete history should include dates and types of vaccines received. Potentially relevant host factors are listed in ***Box 130.3***.

Malaria chemoprophylaxis can fail because of missed doses, poor drug absorption, and resistant parasites, but even when prophylactic regimens are followed rigorously, breakthrough cases of malaria still occur.[88] Efficacy can vary depending on the drug regimen used, the geographic region, and time. Drugs that were effective in the past may no longer work because of increasing resistance of malaria parasites. Commonly used chemoprophylactic agents act on the blood stage of the parasite, hence do not protect against relapses due to *Plasmodium vivax* and *P. ovale*. In a study of delayed-onset malaria (defined as >2 months after return), approximately two-thirds of patients with vivax or ovale malaria reported taking antimalarials active against the blood stage.[89] If travelers take drugs acquired locally in a developing country, counterfeit or substandard drug is a possible reason for failure of treatment or prophylaxis.[90,91] Doxycycline, one option for chemoprophylaxis for malaria, reduces the risk of certain other infections or may modify the clinical course. Doxycycline has demonstrated efficacy in preventing leptospirosis[92] and scrub typhus.[93] Among other infections that might be prevented or altered are rickettsial infections, relapsing fever, syphilis, and plague. Of note, poor response of scrub typhus (*Orientia tsutsugamushi*) to doxycycline has been reported from Thailand, where rifampin worked better.[94]

A review of the drugs the patient is taking or has recently used should include herbal or traditional remedies and medications obtained without prescription, including injections. Many drugs, including antimicrobials, can be purchased without a prescription in many countries. Recent drug use can influence resistance patterns of infecting organisms and results of diagnostic tests and can also be associated with side effects and adverse reactions. Drug fever[95] and cutaneous reactions can mimic infections or complicate their evaluation if both a drug reaction and infection overlap in time. Antipyretics and anti-inflammatory agents may mask fever and local symptoms.

Underlying diseases or conditions may predispose to infections or influence their severity. Persons who have lost gastric acid because of surgery, H_2 blockers and other drugs, or disease may be more likely to become infected with some pathogens that enter through the gastrointestinal tract. The interaction with human immunodeficiency virus (HIV) and a number of infections is discussed in the following sections.[96,97]

Genetic factors affect susceptibility to and expression of infections (see Chapter 6). Persons whose erythrocytes are Duffy antigen-negative cannot be infected with *P. vivax*. Falciparum malaria is less severe in persons who are heterozygous for sickle cell hemoglobin.[98] Some persons may be genetically resistant to infection with parvovirus.[99] In most instances, genetic determinants are not yet sufficiently well characterized to influence the approach to the patient with fever.

CLINICAL MANIFESTATIONS

Duration and Pattern of Fever

Many textbooks have dedicated long discussions to the diagnostic implications of different patterns of fever. In an era when few patients are hospitalized and monitored regularly with vital signs, little information may exist about their fever patterns. General characteristics of fever that may provide some discriminatory value include onset (abrupt versus gradual), height (high versus low), pattern (e.g., continuous, every 48 hours, biphasic, intermittent), and duration. These characteristics may point to some infections that are more and others that are less likely but should not be interpreted rigidly.[100,101] Few patients with malaria, for example, follow the textbook pattern of fevers. In a study of 482 patients with malaria in Canada, only one-half had fever at the time of presentation.[53] Of nonimmune travelers with fever and malaria, fewer than 50% had the classic synchronous pattern. In a study of 86 patients with malaria, 22 (25%) were afebrile at the initial hospital visit.[102] Absence of fever and systemic toxicity should not deter the clinician from seeking evidence of malaria in the patient with an appropriate exposure history. In some instances patients with fever are unaware of having fever. Self-treatment with antipyretics and antimicrobials can change the natural pattern of fevers.

Undifferentiated Fever

Many infections first manifest with fever and no other signs or symptoms, or only nonspecific associated symptoms such as headache and malaise. With time, focal findings or other clues often emerge, but early interventions may be necessary to prevent serious sequelae or death. When tropical exposures have occurred within the past month, the list of possible diagnoses is long.[103] In general, the most common diagnoses in returned travelers with undifferentiated fever are malaria, dengue fever, rickettsial infections, enteric fever, leptospirosis, and common infections with a global distribution, such as respiratory and urinary tract infections. Chikungunya infection recently has appeared as an important cause of fever in travelers returning from areas with outbreaks.[29,30] The fungal infections histoplasmosis and coccidioidomycosis, which have caused outbreaks in travelers, can begin with a nonspecific acute febrile illness. The presence of polymorphonuclear leukocytosis should lead to studies for bacterial sepsis with common organisms, such as staphylococci, meningococci,[77] streptococci, and other pyogenic organisms. *Campylobacter* infections, legionnaires' disease, and tularemia[104] may begin with undifferentiated fever and an elevated white blood cell (WBC) count. Leptospirosis,[78,105] tick-borne relapsing fever,[106] louse-borne relapsing fever,[107] and amebic liver abscess[108] often cause elevation of the WBC count. The total WBC count is often normal or low in some bacterial infections such as enteric fever (unless complicated by intestinal perforation),[109–112] brucellosis,[113,114] rickettsial infections,[115–122] ehrlichiosis,[123] Q fever,[124–126] many protozoan infections (e.g., malaria, toxoplasmosis, visceral leishmaniasis), and many viral infections (dengue, HIV, chikungunya,[127] Lassa, cytomegalovirus (CMV), Epstein–Barr virus (EBV), and many others). The initial evaluation should include a WBC and differential leukocyte count. The presence of large numbers of atypical lymphocytes or high-grade eosinophilia would shift more attention toward viral and helminthic infections, respectively. A marked left shift can be seen early in many infections (e.g., dengue fever) which later may be characterized by lymphocytosis.

Among the acute undifferentiated (at least initially) fevers that benefit from specific treatment are bacterial (including rickettsial and spirochetal infections), viral (e.g., Lassa fever), and protozoan (e.g., malaria, amebiasis, African trypanosomiasis) and several fungal infections.

Several sexually transmitted infections, including primary HIV infection,[128–130] CMV, syphilis, gonoccocemia, primary herpes simplex infection, and hepatitis B,[131] can present with undifferentiated fever. Among the rare but "cannot miss" diseases are plague, Lassa fever,[132] anthrax, diphtheria,[133] African trypanosomiasis,[134–137] and rabies. In each instance, early recognition can lead to appropriate treatment, isolation, or public health interventions.

ASSOCIATED SYMPTOMS AND CLINICAL FINDINGS

The presence of hypotension, tachypnea, confusion or altered mental status, and evidence of hemorrhage demand urgent evaluation and intervention.

Fever and Hemorrhage

Among the infections that evoke greatest fear are the so-called hemorrhagic fevers. The term describes the shared clinical manifestations, not a specific cause. The globally distributed *Neisseria meningitidis* is a cause of acute hemorrhagic fever (see Chapter 24).[77] Other acute bacterial infections (e.g., leptospirosis, plague, rickettsial infections, vibrio infections), rarely fungi, and other processes can occasionally cause a similar clinical picture. Among travelers, the list of potential causes is vastly expanded and includes some infections for which specific treatment can be lifesaving and others for which only supportive therapy is available but also may save lives. The viruses associated with hemorrhagic fevers include dengue virus,[138] hantaviruses,[139] Lassa fever,[140] Ebola,[141] Marburg, Rift Valley,[142] Venezuelan hemorrhagic fever,[143] yellow fever,[144] Crimean-Congo hemorrhagic fever viruses,[145] and others (see Chapters 67–77).[146,147]

Viruses typically associated with hemorrhagic fever are listed in ***Table 130.4*** along with their known geographic distributions.[146–148] Acquisition most often involves the bite of an infective vector (usually a mosquito or tick) or contact with rodents or their excreta. Because some viral hemorrhagic fevers are treatable (e.g., Lassa fever[149,150] and possibly Crimean-Congo hemorrhagic fever[151,152]) and findings from some bacterial infections (e.g., meningococcemia, leptospirosis) can cause similar hemorrhagic manifestations, it is essential to proceed rapidly with the initial evaluation. Management should always include general support, even when specific treatment is not available. Infection control measures including masks, face shields, gloves, gowns, and appropriate biosafety protocols for handling specimens, should be used in the care of a patient with hemorrhagic fever that may have been acquired in a tropical area, pending more complete information, to protect members of health care and laboratory teams.[150] Nosocomial transmission of dengue virus has been documented after exposure to blood (needlestick and mucocutaneous exposure) from viremic patients[153] in the absence of hemorrhage. If infections that can be spread from person to person (e.g., Lassa fever, Ebola, Crimean-Congo hemorrhagic fever, Marburg, Venezuelan and Argentine hemorrhagic fever viruses) are among those that are plausible based on time and place of exposures, it makes good sense to request input early from public health officials and the CDC or other experts in the field who can advise about the handling of the patient and clinical specimens and can also expedite diagnostic studies. Staff at the Special Pathogens Branch, Division of Viral and Rickettsial Diseases, CDC, can provide assistance. In some instances, prompt recognition of an unusual infection may make it easier to trace contacts and prevent or limit future cases. Endemic hantaviruses vary with geographic region. The clinical manifestations of infection also vary widely and include severe hemorrhagic fever with renal syndrome, hantavirus pulmonary syndrome (with a mortality rate of about 50%), and a milder illness, nephropathia epidemica,[154] found in Scandinavia.[155]

Table 130.4 Hemorrhagic Fever Viruses and their Known Distributions

Virus or Disease	Vector or Reservoir
Americas	
Argentine (Junín) hemorrhagic fever	R, P
Bolivian hemorrhagic fever (Machupo virus)	R, P
Dengue fever	M
Hemorrhagic fever with renal syndrome	R
Hantavirus pulmonary syndrome	R (rare P, South America)
Sabia virus infection	R
Venezuelan hemorrhagic fever (Guanarito virus)	R
Yellow fever	M
Africa	
Crimean-Congo hemorrhagic fever	T, P
Dengue fever	M
Ebola	?, P
Marburg	?, P
Lassa fever	R, P
Rift Valley fever	M
Yellow fever	M
Asia	
Crimean-Congo hemorrhagic fever	T, P
Dengue fever	M
Hemorrhagic fever with renal syndrome	R
Kyasanur Forest disease	T
Europe	
Crimean-Congo hemorrhagic fever	T, P
Hemorrhagic fever with renal syndrome	R
Omsk hemorrhagic fever	T
Oceania and Australia	
Dengue fever	M

M, mosquito transmission; P, person-to-person spread documented or suspected; R, rodent reservoir; T, tick transmission.

Fever and Central Nervous System Findings

The presence of altered mental status, stiff neck, or focal neurologic signs in a patient with fever heralds a range of infections, including many that can result in serious sequelae or death. Neurologic findings can be useful in helping focus the workup but also suggest that the workup should proceed rapidly. High fever alone or metabolic derangements associated with serious systemic infections can lead to an altered mental status in the absence of central nervous system (CNS) invasion. Patients with legionnaires' disease, for example, may be lethargic and confused even though the cerebrospinal fluid (CSF) may be acellular and sterile. Headaches, sometimes severe, may accompany systemic infections such as malaria, rickettsial infections, dengue fever, and enteric fever. It may be necessary to image the CNS and sample spinal fluid to assess CNS signs and symptoms. Common infections with a worldwide distribution, such as meningococcal infections, syphilis, tuberculosis, herpes simplex, and cryptococcus infections, should always be considered and looked for, as appropriate.

Pathogens that may invade the CNS include bacteria, viruses, fungi, helminths, and protozoa, though bacteria and viruses predominate. Many geographically focal arthropod-borne viruses cause meningitis or encephalitis. Among those that threaten travelers is Japanese encephalitis (JE) (see

Chapter 76), the mosquito-borne flavivirus widely distributed in Asia and also found in northern Australia.[156] Imported cases of JE are rare.[157,158] Other flaviviruses that cause encephalitis include West Nile (wide distribution now includes the Americas), St Louis encephalitis (North, Central, and South America), and Murray Valley (Australia and New Guinea). Dengue fever can manifest with neurologic findings, including encephalitis and transverse myelitis, but neurologic presentations are noted in 1% or less of cases.[159] JE virus, as well as West Nile virus and Murray Valley virus, can cause a poliomyelitis-like illness. Patients may present with febrile flaccid paralysis.[160] Neurologic complications have also been reported with chikungunya infections.[30,127,161,162]

Rabies is another cause of encephalitis occasionally acquired in developing areas of the world (see Chapter 79).

Nipah virus, a paramyxovirus, has been identified as a cause of severe, rapidly progressive encephalitis in Malaysia and Singapore in outbreaks first noted in 1998 (see Chapter 55).[163] Since 2001, outbreaks have occurred in Bangladesh related to introductions from the fruit bat, the reservoir host. Secondary transmission to close contacts of Nipah case-patients has also been reported in Bangladesh.[164] Initial outbreaks in Malaysia affected persons having close contact with pigs.

Sandfly fever viruses are occasional causes of fever and headache in travelers to Mediterranean countries and elsewhere.[165–167] Fever and headache are common findings; some serotypes, including the Toscana serotype, have been associated with meningitis or meningoencephalitis and prolonged convalescence.[167] Of eight German tourists diagnosed with acute sandfly virus infection, serotype Toscana, seven acquired infections during visits to Tuscany (Italy) and one to Portugal.

In patients who have visited areas of Africa endemic for African trypanosomiasis (sleeping sickness),[168–171] early diagnosis and treatment of infection can prevent CNS involvement, which complicates therapy and worsens prognosis (see Chapter 98). Patients with African trypanosomiasis must be evaluated for possible CNS infection, since its presence will alter management. Other treatable bacterial infections that can involve the CNS and may be unfamiliar to many clinicians include Q fever,[172] rickettsial infections, relapsing fever, brucellosis, leptospirosis, and bartonellosis. Anthrax and plague, both rare, can cause hemorrhagic meningitis. In patients with cerebral malaria, parasites may be present in small numbers on initial peripheral smears.[173] Other protozoal infections, including primary amebic meningoencephalitis and granulomatous amebic encephalitis, caused by *Naegleria folweri* and *Acanathamoeba/Balamuthia mandrillaris*, respectively, may manifest as fever and signs of meningeal irritation or focal neurologic deficits. CNS manifestations occur in about 20% of patients with ehrlichiosis caused by *Ehrlichia chaffeensis* and include altered mental status, lymphocytic pleocytosis, and elevated CSF protein.[174] Many clinicians are familiar with Lyme disease and ehrlichiosis but may be unaware that they occur in many countries outside the United States.[175]

Few helminthic infections cause fever and neurologic findings. The presence of eosinophilia should suggest one of these infections (see Chapter 131). Angiostrongyliasis due to *Parastrongylus (Angiostrongylus) cantonensis* can cause fever, headache, and eosinophilia in CSF and peripheral blood. In 2000, an outbreak of eosinophilic meningitis occurred in travelers who had visited Jamaica and had shared a meal.[176] Gnathostomiasis and baylisascariasis can also cause febrile eosinophilic meningitis. Disseminated strongyloidiasis in compromised hosts can be associated with bacteremias and meningitis, sometimes years or decades after the host has left the endemic region. Other helminths that reach the CNS (e.g., cysticercosis, paragonimiasis, sparganosis) are generally not associated with an acute febrile illness. When trichinellosis[177] causes fever and CNS findings, it is typically in the setting of other systemic findings, including eosinophilia and myalgia. The neurologic complications of schistosomiasis are typically not observed during the acute febrile illness, Katayama syndrome.[178]

The differential diagnosis of a patient with fever and unexplained meningitis should include the possibility of drug-induced meningitis. Among the drugs that have been implicated are trimethoprim-sulfamethoxazole (TMP-SMX) and several nonsteroidal anti-inflammatory agents, drugs that may be obtained without a prescription in many countries.

Fever and Respiratory Symptoms

The respiratory tract is a common site of infection during and after travel, though the specific cause often remains undefined.[7] Among approximately 22 000 ill returned travelers who presented to a GeoSentinel site for medical evaluation (from September 1997 through August 2001), almost 8% had respiratory tract infections.[179] Among almost 7000 ill returned travelers with fever who sought care at a GeoSentinel clinic (1997 through 2006), 14% had a respiratory illness.[8] In a study of American travelers,[7] 26% reported respiratory tract symptoms during travel and 10% following travel. Patients with pneumonia after travel should be evaluated for common pathogens, such as *Streptococcus pneumoniae*, *Staphylococcus aureus*, *Haemophilus influenzae*, and *Mycoplasma pneumoniae*. Outbreaks and sporadic cases of influenza occur in travelers, including on cruise ships[180] and in pilgrims to the Hajj.[181] One well-studied outbreak documented the spread of influenza on an aircraft.[182] WHO identified >100 cruise-associated outbreaks of influenza between 1970 and 2007.[183] While travelers are at risk for acquiring influenza,[74] they also play an important role in the global dispersal of influenza viruses, clearly demonstrated by the rapid global spread of 2009 H1N1 influenza A, first identified in humans in Mexico and the United States.[184] Highly pathogenic H5N1 continues to circulate in parts of Asia and Africa with occasional outbreaks in avian species in Europe. To date, sustained human-to-human transmission has not occurred. The clinical spectrum may include diarrhea and CNS changes.[185] Outbreaks of SARS in 2002–2003 caused more than 8000 cases and almost 800 deaths and disrupted global travel.[186] Fever is prominent in SARS, often preceding the development of respiratory findings. Transmission also occurred on aircraft.[187] Several clusters have highlighted the acquisition of legionnaires' disease during travel in many regions of the world.[188,189] Between 45% and 65% of cases of legionnaires' disease in England and Wales have been travel-related.

Melioidosis is a common cause of pneumonia, especially in parts of Asia. The fungal infections coccidioidomycosis and histoplasmosis have caused outbreaks in travelers in the Americas.[190–192] Q fever is a common cause of pneumonia in some areas, including Spain.[37]

Risk of infection with *Mycobacterium tuberculosis* is increased by travel to areas highly endemic for tuberculosis, especially with prolonged stays.[193,194] Transmission can also occur on long flights. Infection may manifest months or years after travel.

Other infections that can produce prominent pulmonary findings include hantaviruses, plague, tularemia, and anthrax. In patients with amebic liver abscess, extension of the process to the diaphragmatic surface of the liver may cause pulmonary findings.[108] Severe malaria may be complicated by acute respiratory distress syndrome. Pulmonary infiltrates may be present during the pulmonary migration phase of several helminths, including hookworm, ascaris, and strongyloides (see Chapters 115, 116, 117). Acute schistosomiasis (Katayama syndrome) may cause fever, cough, and pulmonary infiltrates.[195] Pulmonary emboli and infarction can cause fever and pulmonary findings that can mimic respiratory infections including pneumonia.

Fever and Diarrhea

Many infections are acquired via ingestion of contaminated food or drink (see Chapters 15, 17, 19, 22, 129). Enteric infections, such as campylobacteriosis and salmonellosis, may produce an illness with just fever and no, few, or delayed gastrointestinal symptoms. In the GeoSentinel analysis of returned ill travelers with fever, 15% had a febrile diarrheal illness.[8] Workup of the febrile patient with diarrhea should include studies for *Clostridium difficile*. This infection has been reported after many antimicrobials, including doxycycline taken for malaria chemoprophylaxis.[196] Diarrhea and other gastrointestinal symptoms can also be found as part of systemic infections (e.g., malaria, dengue fever, rickettsial infections), hence the workup of the febrile patient with diarrhea should not focus exclusively on enteric pathogens. In a series of 52 patients with amebic liver abscess in Cairo, only 25% gave a history of diarrhea and 6% reported dysentery.[197] Fever and right upper quadrant pain were the most common manifestations. In this series, 42% had an acute illness, characterized by high fever, vomiting, and leukocytosis, and 58% had a more chronic illness, often with low-grade fever, weight loss, and anemia.[197]

Systemic infections can involve the gut and be associated with gastrointestinal symptoms and fever. Some of these include visceral leishmaniasis, histoplasmosis, paracoccidioidomycosis, tuberculosis, nontuberculous mycobacteria, and Whipple's disease.[198]

Fever and Hepatitis

Hepatitis A has been the most common form of hepatitis after travel to developing countries; however, this infection is becoming less common in travelers with the wide use of the hepatitis A vaccine. A relapsing form of hepatitis A has been described, though fever has not been a prominent finding.[199,200] In the GeoSentinel database of ill returned travelers with a final diagnosis of hepatitis A, only 55% had fever as a main reason for seeking medical care; for hepatitis B, only 18% had fever recorded as a reason for seeking care.[8] Hepatitis B assumes a more important role in persons with prolonged stays in developing areas and those who have close contact, including sexual contact, with local residents, receive injections, or have other parenteral exposures.[201] Cases of hepatitis B continue to occur among unvaccinated travelers.[202] In the early 1980s before hepatitis B vaccine was available, serologic studies suggested that 6% of American troops stationed in Korea for 4–12 months became infected with hepatitis B. Among those with acute hepatitis B, 83% gave a history of Korean sexual partners.[131]

Hepatitis D virus (HDV) infection, which requires a helper function from hepatitis B virus (HBV), is a risk for persons already infected with HBV or who become coinfected with HBV and HDV. Hepatitis D can be expressed in the absence of detectable hepatitis B surface antigen (HBsAg).[203] Acute infection can be confused with yellow fever in tropical regions where both can occur. HDV has been a cause of severe and frequently fulminant hepatitis in outbreaks in South America (Amazon Basin).[204] Other geographic areas reported to have a high incidence of infection include parts of Africa, the Middle East, and islands of the South Pacific.[205] Rates of hepatitis D infection in HBsAg carriers range from 30% to 90% in these areas. In Europe, high rates of infection have been reported primarily in the Mediterranean basin, the Balkan peninsula, and in the European part of the former Soviet Union. In North America, Australia, and other parts of Europe, hepatitis D is largely a problem in intravenous drug users.

Travelers occasionally acquire hepatitis E.[206,207] Although hepatitis E viruses (HEV) are widespread,[208] large outbreaks have occurred in areas with poor sanitation, including Mexico, Asia,[206,207] and Africa. The manifestations of acute HEV are similar to those of HAV except in pregnant women, who are at substantial risk of developing severe or fulminant hepatitis. Chronic infection has been documented in immunocompromised patients.[209]

In the evaluation of patients with fever and abnormal liver function, treatable infections such as leptospirosis, Q fever, brucellosis, visceral leishmaniasis, and rickettsial diseases should be considered. Many systemic viral infections, including yellow fever, cause prominent hepatic dysfunction.

Fever and Rash

Skin findings are visible clues that may help suggest or exclude specific diagnoses[210–213] (see also Chapter 132). Although skin lesions are a common reason for seeking medical care after travel (found in 18–23% in some series),[212,213] a smaller percentage of patients with fever have an associated rash or other skin findings.[13] The distribution of a rash, the nature of the lesions, the time of onset relative to other symptoms, and its evolution over time may be helpful pieces of information. The astute clinician will repeat careful examinations of the skin when a patient has persistent fever of uncertain cause. Rashes are not a clinical feature of malaria. A careful history of drugs, including over-the-counter agents, is essential in any patient with a rash. Skin lesions secondary to insect bites, hypersensitivity reactions to topical agents, and dermatitis related to water-associated infestations may occur in patients with an acute systemic infection causing fever. An analysis of 62 patients with fever and exanthema who were seen in a tropical disease unit in Paris in 2006–2007 found that the most common diagnoses were chikungunya fever (35%), dengue fever (26%), and African tick-bite fever (10%).[211] The uncharacteristically high proportion of patients with chikungunya fever reflected the travel patterns (Indian Ocean islands) at a time of major chikungunya outbreaks. Although chikungunya and dengue infections are both associated with fever and rash, prominent polyarthralgia that may be severe, disabling, and persistent is a common feature in chikungunya infections.[30]

Petechial lesions and hemorrhagic findings herald life-threatening diseases and should prompt a search for one of the hemorrhagic fevers (see previous discussion). In the series of patients with African tick-bite fever, 4% of patients with rash had purpuric lesions.[116] A local skin lesion may reflect the portal of entry of the pathogen; for example, tache noire in rickettsial infection, erythema migrans (Lyme disease), cutaneous diphtheria, the eschar of anthrax, chagoma in American trypanosomiasis (Chagas' disease), and the chancre in African trypanosomiasis.[214] Diffuse rashes are seen in many bacterial (including rickettsial) and viral infections. Few are sufficiently distinctive to allow a definitive diagnosis on the basis of the skin findings alone. Characteristic skin lesions, such as those described in rickettsial infections and the rose spots of typhoid fever, may appear late or not at all.[215] Their absence should not lead the clinician to reject the diagnosis if findings are otherwise typical. Rashes that mimic the diffuse erythema of staphylococcal and streptococcal toxic shock syndrome have been reported in other infections, such as dengue fever and ehrlichiosis. Rubella and measles viruses remain endemic in many countries, and these infections can be acquired during travel.[216]

Among the more common infections causing high fevers after tropical exposures, dengue fever produces a rash in 30–50% of cases,[217,218] chikungunya infection in 40–75%,[219,220] typhoid fever is associated with rose spots (though they may be evanescent) in 30–50%, and the rashes of rickettsial infections vary with the infecting rickettsial species. Lymphangitis has also been reported in association with rickettsioses.[221] Ross River fever, also known as epidemic polyarthritis and found in South Pacific islands and Australia, is associated with a maculopapular rash in 40–78% of cases.[222,223] Although dengue fever has become increasingly recognized as a common infection in travelers, all that resembles dengue fever is not dengue. During a 1984 dengue outbreak in Mexico, investigators[224] found that 10% of patients with the clinical diagnosis of dengue fever had serologic evidence of acute rubella infection. Rickettsial infections and leptospirosis can also be misdiagnosed as dengue fever. During a 1993 study in Mexico, 50 patients with clinical findings suggestive of dengue fever but negative serologic tests for dengue infection underwent further study. Twenty (40%) had IgM antibodies reactive with spotted fever group rickettsiosis.[225] During a dengue outbreak in Bangladesh, 18% of dengue-negative patients tested positive for leptospirosis.[226] Dengue and chikungunya coinfections have also been observed.[227] Other treatable infections that can cause skin lesions include leptospirosis, Rocky Mountain spotted fever, relapsing fever, rat-bite fever, syphilis, Q fever, psittacosis, bartonellosis,[228] brucellosis,[229] and tularemia.

Vesicular and vesiculopustular rashes that can resemble varicella are seen in rickettsial infections[230,231] including rickettsialpox.[232] Among 55 patients with African tick-bite fever with rash (46% of the total cases), lesions were maculopapular in 51%, vesicular in 45%, and purpuric in 4%.[116] A number of viral infections, some widespread (e.g., parvovirus, coxsackievirus, enteroviruses) and others focal (e.g., monkeypox, Ockelbo, Sinbis viruses), can cause vesicular rashes. In one study, of 29 travelers who had swum in freshwater pools in the Dogon area of Mali, West Africa, 28 became infected with schistosomiasis. Of those, 10 (36%) had cercarial dermatitis and 15 (54%) later developed Katayama syndrome.[54] In an outbreak of acute schistosomiasis after exposures on safari in Tanzania, 37% developed a rash, usually urticarial (typically beginning 3 weeks or longer after exposure), often with onset prior to development of fever.[233] Among 75 patients with acute schistosomiasis seen in Israel, 71% had fever and 45% had skin lesions, but both were present at the same time in only 26%.[234]

Erythema nodosum and other skin lesions may be present in acute coccidioidomycosis, histoplasmosis,[187] and mycobacterial infections including tuberculosis. Urticarial skin lesions in the person with fever in addition to hypersensitivity reactions related to drugs should bring to mind early hepatitis B and several helminthic infections (e.g., acute schistosomal infection or Katayama syndrome, fascioliasis, trichenellosis, loiasis, gnathostomiasis, and others). Fever is not a prominent finding in many helminthic infections, but of 20 patients with acute fascioliasis diagnosed at a university hospital in Spain, 12 (60%) had fever and 4 (20%) had urticaria. Although patients with fascioliasis can have undifferentiated fever, the presence of abdominal or right upper quadrant pain and eosinophilia are findings that can suggest this infection.[235] Vasculitic skin manifestations are associated with a variety of infections, collagen vascular diseases, and antimicrobial drugs.[236]

Fever and Lymphadenopathy

The presence and location of any enlarged lymph nodes should be noted on initial and follow-up examinations. Localized lymphadenopathy frequently appears adjacent to the entry of a pathogen. Generalized lymphadenopathy more often suggests systemic infection though it does not necessarily indicate infection of lymphoid tissue. Prominent local enlargement of nodes in tularemia, leishmaniasis, plague, cat-scratch disease (*Bartonella*), syphilis, primary herpes simplex, lymphogranuloma venereum (LGV), and some rickettsial or mycobacterial infections may suggest a nearby portal of entry through the skin or genital tract. Generalized lymphadenopathy is found in many viral infections (including infectious mononucleosis and acute HIV infection), rickettsial infections,[237] leptospirosis, brucellosis, and relapsing fever, among others. Of 22 patients with rickettsiosis imported to Germany, lymphadenopathy was found in 14 (64%); an eschar was noted in 55% of patients with *Rickettsia conorii* infection and in one patient with scrub typhus.[238]

Lymphadenopathy can be found in several protozoan infections – trypanosomiasis (both African and American), leishmaniasis, and toxoplasmosis – but not malaria. Acute lymphangitis, lymphadenitis, orchitis, and epididymitis are characteristic features of filariasis.[50] These episodes frequently are recurrent. Local lymphadenopathy can precede the development of skin lesions in *Leishmania braziliensis* infections.

Persistent and Relapsing Fevers

Persisting and recurring fevers present a clinical challenge. Recent reviews of persons with fevers of unknown origin (typically defined as fevers lasting 3 weeks or longer), excluding persons with HIV infection or other immunocompromising conditions, in developed countries have found that noninfectious inflammatory diseases (e.g., connective tissue diseases, vasculitides, and granulomatous disorders) are now more common than infectious diseases as causes of unexplained fevers.[239] In contrast, infectious diseases remain the most common cause of unexplained fevers in developing countries. Neoplasms are identified in 10–30% of cases in most series.[239] Q fever is a prominent cause of prolonged fever in endemic areas, including parts of Spain and France. Q fever has also been reported in short-term travelers.[240] An analysis of causes of fever of undetermined origin in 129 patients hospitalized in Egypt in 1971–1973 found that infections accounted for the majority (60%) of the fevers, and neoplasms for only 14%. The most commonly diagnosed infections were enteric fevers (salmonellosis), tuberculosis, pyelonephritis, sepsis, endocarditis, brucellosis, visceral leishmaniasis, and amebic hepatitis.[241] A 1990 Egyptian study of 133 patients with undiagnosed fever lasting at least 3 weeks again found infectious diseases in the majority (56%).[242]

Among 43 pediatric patients in Egypt with fever lasting at least 3 weeks, 30 (69.7%) had parasitic infections. Schistosomiasis (23.3%), visceral leishmaniasis (16.3%), toxoplasmosis (11.6%), and malaria (4.7) were the most commonly diagnosed parasitic infections. The most commonly identified bacterial infections were typhoid fever (11.6%), tuberculosis (7.0%), and urinary tract infection (4.7%).[243]

Viral infections occupy a less important role in chronic than in acute fevers. CMV infection can cause prolonged fever.[244] Bottieau and colleagues found that 4% of 1842 febrile illnesses in persons with tropical stays within the preceding 12 months had infectious mononucleosis-like syndromes, caused by CMV, EBV, toxoplasmosis, or acute HIV.[245] Patients with these infections were more likely to have prolonged fever (>7 days), lymphocytosis (>40% of white blood cells), lymphadenopathy, and elevated liver enzymes (ALT) as compared with patients with other causes for fever. Among 41 patients with acute illness associated with HIV seroconversion,[130] the most common symptoms were fever, sore throat, fatigue, weight loss, and myalgia. The median duration of symptoms was 14 days though symptoms persisted 4 weeks or longer in 32%.[130] Physical findings in patients with acute HIV infection often include rash (70%) and lymphadenopathy (77%).[246] In the evaluation of a person with prolonged fever, it is important to determine the HIV status, since the range of infections and the probabilities of each will be altered if the person is HIV infected.

Causes of chronic or persistent fevers include protozoa, e.g., malaria, amebic liver abscess, trypanosomiasis (American and African), and visceral leishmaniasis; chronic bacterial infections such as brucellosis,[247] tuberculosis, bartonellosis, Q fever, and melioidosis; fungal infections, such as histoplasmosis, coccidioidomycosis, and paracoccidioidomycosis;[248] and a few helminthic infections, such as visceral larva migrans, fascioliasis, and schistosomiasis.

Visceral leishmaniasis is an important cause of chronic fevers that can be acquired in some temperate as well as tropical areas of the world.[219–251] For example, of 89 patients with visceral leishmaniasis in France in 1986–1987, 70 (79%) had acquired the infection in France. Imported cases came primarily from other Mediterranean countries.[249] In recent years visceral leishmaniasis has emerged as an important opportunistic infection in persons with acquired immunodeficiency syndrome (AIDS) living in southern France, Spain, and Italy.[252]

Melioidosis can reactivate years after the initial exposure. Manifestations are protean. Infection can involve lung, skin, and soft tissues and any part of the body via bacteremic spread. Pulmonary changes, including cavitation, can mimic tuberculosis.[253,254] In a series of 602 patients seen in one Thai hospital, in-hospital mortality was 42%. Among 118 adult patients with long-term follow-up, 23% had culture-proven relapses, occurring 1–290 weeks after discharge (median, 21 weeks).[255] Recrudescent infection has been reported as long as 26 years after initial infection.[256]

Ehrlichiosis is another potentially treatable cause of prolonged fever. In a series of 41 cases of human ehrlichiosis, 6 patients manifested protracted fever (range 15–51 days) as the principal finding.[257]

Chronic or recurrent fevers can be the result of uncommon complications of an infection; for example, Q fever endocarditis, brucella osteomyelitis or endocarditis, and splenic or liver abscesses secondary to melioidosis.[258] In a prospective study of 530 patients with brucellosis in Spain followed for at least 1 year after treatment, 86 patients relapsed (97 relapse episodes). Among recognized relapses, 95% occurred within 6 months of the end of therapy.[259]

Relapsing fevers are commonly seen due to *Borrelia*[260–263] and with malaria. They can also occur with cholangitis (which can be associated with parasites as well as with stones and other biliary disease), chronic meningococcemia,[264] rat-bite fever (*Streptobacillus moniliformis/Spirilum minus*), brucellosis, filariasis, infective endocarditis, visceral leishmaniasis, trypanosomiasis, Whipple's disease,[198] Hodgkin's disease, familial Mediterranean fever, and many other diseases.[265,266] Pyomyositis can cause undifferentiated fever in its early stages. It is usually seen in persons who have lived in tropical areas.

The fever that accompanies acute schistosomiasis (Katayama syndrome) and fascioliasis[235] can persist for weeks. In an outbreak of

Box 130.4 Persistent and Relapsing Fevers[a]

Bacterial

- Bartonellosis
- Brucellosis
- Ehrlichiosis
- Endocarditis (multiple causes)
- Leptospirosis
- Lyme disease
- Melioidosis
- Q fever
- Relapsing fever
- Rickettsial infections (several)
- Syphilis
- Tuberculosis and nontuberculous mycobacteriosis
- Tularemia
- Typhoid fever

Fungal

- Blastomycosis
- Coccidioidomycosis
- Cryptococcosis
- Histoplasmosis
- Paracoccidioidomycosis
- Penicilliosis (*Penicillium marneffei*)

Protozoan

- Amebic liver abscess
- Babesiosis
- Leishmaniasis (visceral)
- Malaria
- Toxoplasmosis
- Trypanosomiasis

Viral

- Cytomegalovirus infection
- Human immunodeficiency virus infection

Helminthic

- Angiostrongyliasis due to *Angiostrongylus costaricensis*
- Clonorchiasis
- Fascioliasis
- Filariasis
- Gnathostomiasis
- Loiasis
- Opisthorchiasis
- Paragonimiasis
- Schistosomiasis
- Toxocariasis
- Trichinellosis

[a]*List includes infections that may cause fevers with duration exceeding 3 weeks. Infections and other illnesses unrelated to tropical exposures (e.g., endocarditis, cholangitis, Hodgkin's disease, others) also can be associated with chronic and relapsing fevers.*

Box 130.5 Sequelae of Infections Acquired more than 10 years earlier: Mechanisms and Examples

Reactivation of Latent Infection or Recrudescence of Inapparent Infection

- Brill–Zinsser disease (*Rickettsia prowazekii*)
- CNS Chagas' disease
- Coccidioidomycosis
- Histoplasmosis
- Leishmaniasis
- Malaria (*Plasmodium malariae*)
- Melioidosis
- Paracoccidioidomycosis
- Strongyloidiasis
- Toxoplasmosis
- Tuberculosis

Persistent Infection and Recurrent Symptoms or Progressive Disease

- Chagas' disease
- Filariasis
- Leprosy
- Loiasis
- Onchocerciasis
- Syphilis

Mechanical Effects; Loss of Normal Function; Scarring, Fibrosis, Tissue Destruction

- Cysticercosis
- Echinococcal cysts
- Liver flukes
- Onchocerciasis (blindness)
- Schistosomiasis
- Tuberculosis (e.g., cavities and bronchiectasis in lungs; scarring and obstruction in urinary tract; adrenal insufficiency)

Malignancy[a]

- *Schistosoma haematobium* (bladder cancer)
- Epstein–Barr virus
- Hepatitis B and hepatitis C viruses (hepatocellular carcinoma)
- Human immunodeficiency virus
- Human T-cell lymphotropic virus type 1
- Liver flukes

Allergic, hypersensitivity reactions

- Rupture of echinococcal cyst

[a]*Papillomaviruses are also associated with cancers, but fever is not a feature of these infections.*

schistosomiasis among travelers, 15 of 29 who were infected developed Katayama syndrome. The median duration of symptoms was 12 days (range 4–46 days).[54] Visceral larva migrans[267] can cause prolonged or intermittent fevers. The associated findings of leukocytosis, eosinophilia, and enlarged liver suggest the diagnosis.

Box 130.4 lists some of the more common causes of persisting and intermittent or relapsing fevers.

Fevers and Remote Residence in Tropical Areas

Some infections can become clinically manifest years or decades after a person has left the place of acquisition. Late manifestations also may result from chronic sequelae of an earlier infection, even if active infection no longer is present. Persons with long residence in tropical areas are more likely to have acquired infections with late sequelae (***Box 130.5***). The mechanisms by which remotely acquired infections can cause disease are several. Latent infection may reactivate, causing fevers and focal or systemic symptoms. Examples include tuberculosis, histoplasmosis, paracoccidioidomycosis, melioidosis, and leishmaniasis. Low-grade, persistent infections may expand (recrudesce), causing symptoms leading to diagnosis (e.g., malaria, Brill–Zinsser disease). The balance between host and microbe may tip in favor of the pathogen in persons whose immunity has been altered by disease, drugs, or age. *Strongyloides* larvae may disseminate widely outside their usual gastrointestinal habitat; for example, in persons with cell-mediated immunosuppression, particularly those taking corticosteroids or coinfected with human T-cell lymphotropic virus type 1.

Salmonella typhi may be carried in the biliary tree and remain inapparent unless mechanical (e.g., biliary obstruction) or other factors alter the local milieu. Worms with long life spans may breach a tissue barrier or cause chronic inflammatory changes leading to acute symptoms. Migration of ascaris can provoke acute pancreatitis or cause biliary obstruction.

Remote infection may cause scarring, obstruction, or alteration in structure that may predispose to superimposed infections or affect function. Scarring associated with renal tuberculosis can increase the risk of urinary tract infection with *Escherichia coli* and other uropathogens, even if tuberculosis is inactive or has been treated and cured. Scarring of the urinary tract secondary to *Schistosoma haematobium* can be associated with bacterial infections and an increased risk of squamous cell carcinoma of the bladder. Late sequelae of schistosomiasis may include portal and pulmonary hypertension, liver cirrhosis, and polyps and fistulas of the bowel. Echinococcal cysts can impinge on the biliary tree, causing acute obstructive symptoms, or erode into the biliary tree and cause symptoms of acute cholangitis. Rupture of an echinococcal cyst can cause acute allergic symptoms, even anaphylaxis. Seizures can occur in patients with cysticercosis, even if parasites are no longer viable. Late complications of Chagas' disease typically do not include fever unless progression of infection occurs (e.g., in persons with AIDS or immunocompromised transplant patients).[268–270]

Clinical findings of hepatocellular malignancy related to remotely acquired, persistent infection with HBV or HCV may include fever secondary to tissue necrosis and the effects of the tumor.

Processes Other Than Infection Causing Fever After Travel

Travel itself may predispose to problems that cause fever. In their series of 24 patients with drug-induced hypersensitivity syndrome requiring hospitalization between 2004 and 2008, Ben m'rad and colleagues demonstrated that 50% of culprit drugs were antibiotics ($n = 8$) or antimalarials ($n = 4$), all of which could be used by the traveling population.[271] One hundred percent of cases had fever and skin involvement, while 58% had peripheral edema, 54% had evidence of hepatic dysfunction, and 42% had hypotension.[271] Pulmonary emboli after prolonged air flights[272,273] may be associated with fever.[274]

Noninfectious diseases also cause fevers and should be considered if studies do not document infection.[239,266,275,276] Biopsy may be necessary to confirm a diagnosis in processes such as inflammatory bowel disease, malignancies, and lymphadenopathy of Kikuchi.[277] Hyperthyroidism may present with fever and diarrhea. In the Belgian study, 2.2% of the fevers after tropical travel were not caused by infections.[13]

Special Patients (HIV-infected, Immunocompromised, Pregnant)

Many infections are more common, more severe, or have altered clinical expression in persons who are immunocompromised. Opportunistic infections, such as tuberculosis, visceral leishmaniasis,[278] American trypanosomiasis, and histoplasmosis and other fungal infections may reactivate and become clinically apparent long after the infection was acquired. An evaluation of 50 HIV-infected patients in Spain with unexplained fever lasting at least 4 weeks found the most frequent diagnoses were tuberculosis (42%), visceral leishmaniasis (14%), and disseminated *Mycobacterium avium* complex (14%).[279] Disseminated infection with the fungus *Penicillium marneffei* is occasionally seen in travelers, typically persons immunocompromised by HIV infection or other disease.[280] In its endemic area in Thailand and Southeast Asia it is an important opportunistic pathogen.[281]

It is important to know during the evaluation whether a female patient is pregnant. The cause of fever may threaten the pregnancy, diagnostic tests and therapies may be harmful to the fetus, some infections can be transmitted transplacentally, and other infections, such as malaria, influenza, and hepatitis E, are more severe in pregnant than in nonpregnant women. Although Q fever is likely to be asymptomatic in pregnant women, infection is significantly associated with fetal morbidity and mortality.[282]

EVALUATION OF THE PATIENT WITH FEVER

Patients with fever and recent tropical exposures always deserve careful evaluation even though similar symptoms might be treated casually in a person without a history of travel. It is helpful to construct a differential diagnosis encompassing potential bacterial, viral, parasitic, and fungal pathogens based on initial history, geographic exposures, and clinical findings. Patients with confusion, hypotension, hypoxemia, or hemorrhagic skin rash need immediate attention and care. A more leisurely pace may be appropriate in patients with subacute or chronic fevers. Any patient with a potential exposure to malaria who is febrile or gives a history of fevers or chills must be evaluated promptly for malaria.[283-286] In general, most infections with the potential for rapid progression and fulminant course (e.g., falciparum malaria, hemorrhagic fevers, meningococcemia, plague, rickettsial infections) become manifest within a month of exposure. In thinking about the causes of fever in a person with diverse geographic exposures, one should always think first about possible diagnoses had the person not traveled, and then expand the differential diagnosis to include infections that may be related to exposures during travel. Omitting the first step can lead to pursuit of obscure or exotic diseases when the patient has a common readily treatable infection, such as acute pyelonephritis or streptococcal pharyngitis.

Initial studies will generally include a complete blood count (CBC) with a differential leukocyte and platelet estimate, thick and thin malaria smears, blood cultures, urinalysis, and liver function tests. Serum should be saved early in the course in the event serologic studies are indicated. Chest radiographs should be obtained in patients with pulmonary symptoms or signs and in persons with persistent, unexplained fever. Serologic studies for HIV infection should be requested in persons with persistent fevers and those with possible exposures during travel. Studies that may yield useful information if initial studies are unrevealing include repeated malaria smears, blood cultures, serial CBCs, differentials, liver function testing, and abdominal ultrasound. Repeated physical examinations may yield new information with the development of new skin findings, lymphadenopathy, or a tender liver or spleen. Although many of these findings may not give the diagnosis, they may help refine the list of considerations, allowing a more focused and efficient path to the diagnosis. Occasionally a patient will have two unrelated infections, both requiring specific interventions.[287] ***Box 130.6*** outlines an approach to patients with fever and a history of tropical exposures.

Box 130.6 Approach to Patient with Fever and History of Tropical Exposure

Initial Evaluation of Acute Fever

Complete blood count with differential

Liver enzymes and function tests

Blood culture: bacterial, viral, fungal (rarely)

Urinalysis (culture if abnormal)

Blood smears for malaria

Other tests

- Serologic tests (save acute serum)
- Urinary antigens (e.g., *Legionella* species, *Histoplasma*)
- Blood smears for *Babesia*, *Borrelia* causing relapsing fever
- Bone marrow aspiration/ biopsy: pathology and culture

Tests to Consider for Focal Symptoms and Findings

Cough: chest film; sputum Gram stain, acid-fast stain, stains for fungi; cultures for bacteria, mycobacterial species, fungi; wet preparation for ova (*Paragonimus* species) or larvae (hyperinfection with *Strongyloides stercoralis*); bronchoscopy

Diarrhea: examination for fecal leukocytes (lactoferrin where available); blood (stool guaiac); toxin and culture for *Clostridium difficile*; ova and parasites, stool cultures; fecal antigens; endoscopy

Sore throat: rapid streptococcal antigen test, culture, infectious mononucleosis absorption test (Monospot) (in appropriate clinical setting)

Skin lesions: aspirate, scrapings, biopsy, Gram stain, acid-fast stain, fungal stain, Wright–Giemsa stain (*Leishmania*); culture for bacteria, fungi, mycobacteria, *Leishmania*

Lymphadenopathy: aspirate or biopsy, acid-fast stain, fungal stain, Wright–Giemsa stain (trypanosomes); culture

Genital lesions or symptoms: pelvic examination, dark-field examination of ulcers, cultures and urine sample for *Neisseria gonorrhoeae* and *Chlamydia trachomatis*, wet preparation for white blood cells, *Trichomonas vaginalis*, *Candida albicans*, and clue cells (bacterial vaginosis), vesicle exudate for electron microscopy

CNS: CT scan, MRI, lumbar puncture with opening pressure and examination of CSF for cells, protein, glucose, bacterial antigens; cultures for bacteria, *Mycobacterium tuberculosis*, fungi, viruses; India ink for *Cryptococcus neoformans* and cryptococcal antigen; VDRL, PCR for specific antigens/ microorganisms; rarely, brain biopsy

Abdominal pain: liver enzymes, amylase, lipase, lactate, stool examination (see above), abdominal radiographic series and/or ultrasound, CT scan, MRI

Arthritis: aspirate – examine fluid for cells, protein, crystals; stains and cultures for bacteria, fungi, *Mycobacterium* species

Cardiac findings: echocardiogram (transesophageal or transthoracic), blood cultures (at least three sets; hold for 21 days; consider lysis centrifugation), serology for Q fever, and brucellosis, PCR for *Tropheryma whipplei*, scan chest and abdomen for other possible foci of infection

CNS, central nervous system; CT, computed tomography; MRI, magnetic resonance imaging; CSF, cerebrospinal fluid; VDRL, Venereal Diseases Research Laboratory; PCR, polymerase chain reaction.

EMERGING DISEASES AND DIFFICULTIES

Diseases are not fixed in distribution, clinical expression, or response to antimicrobials.[28] As the hepatitis A and hepatitis B vaccines are now more widely used, these infections have become uncommon in travelers to developing countries. Conversely, increasing antimicrobial resistance of bacteria and protozoa may increasingly limit choices for prophylaxis, empirical therapy, and treatment. Persons who are older and those with chronic diseases are traveling more regularly and to more remote destinations. Long-term travel is also becoming increasingly popular, and carries its own set of unique risks.[288] Multiple diverse geographic exposures are becoming a common part of the carefully taken medical history. New technologies, such as polymerase chain reaction, may reduce some of the frustrations currently encountered in making rapid specific diagnoses. Even with these advances in diagnosis and communication, evaluation and management of the patient with fever will continue to be a challenge, requiring a thoughtful and systematic approach and broad knowledge or access to it.

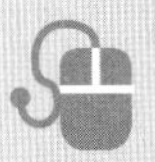

Access the complete reference list online at
http://www.expertconsult.com

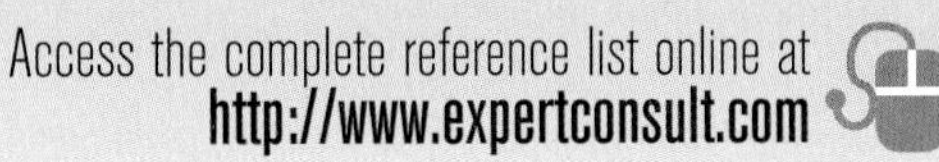
Access the complete reference list online at
http://www.expertconsult.com

CHAPTER 131

Eosinophilia

Mary E. Wilson • Peter F. Weller

INTRODUCTION

Eosinophilia develops as an immunologically mediated response in association with diverse processes, including allergic, neoplastic, and infectious diseases (***Box 131.1***). Eosinophilia is a hematologic marker that warrants attention and serves as a clue to help direct a diagnostic workup. Although many diseases are associated with eosinophilia, the presence of eosinophilia in a person with tropical exposures suggests the possibility of specific parasitic infections. Eosinophilia is notably common in association with helminthic parasites, especially those in tissues.[1] Before embarking on an exhaustive search for parasitic infections in a patient with eosinophilia, however, it is prudent to consider noninfectious causes of eosinophilia, such as allergic diseases and drug-induced hypersensitivity reactions.[2]

Eosinophilia in parasitic infections is the result of dynamic interactions that are influenced by host factors, the stage of parasite development, the location of the parasite within the human host, and the parasite burden, among other factors. Eosinophilia may wax and wane. Parasites often associated with eosinophilia may not provoke an identified eosinophilic response in all patients or at all times. Parasites may elicit a localized eosinophilic tissue response that is not reflected by an increase in peripheral blood eosinophil numbers. This chapter considers the immunobiology of eosinophils, the causes of eosinophilia with special attention to parasitic infections, and the evaluation of patients with eosinophilia.

Overview

Most unicellular pathogens do not provoke an eosinophilic response.[1,2] In contrast, multicellular, helminthic parasites are common, potent stimuli for eosinophilia (***Box 131.2***). Relative to most bacterial and viral pathogens, helminths are large and have a long life span, often measured in years or even decades. Unlike viral and bacterial pathogens that multiply in human hosts, most helminths cannot undergo reproductive cycles in humans; hence the numbers of adult helminths is limited by the number of eggs or larval forms acquired by the human. Prolonged or repeated exposures may be required for a human to acquire sufficient parasites to cause symptomatic infection. Many helminthic infections cause few or no symptoms or only intermittent findings. In addition, because of the lengthy developmental period and longevity of helminthic parasites, symptoms may begin months or years after exposures in endemic regions. Thus, the time period between possibly relevant exposures and the onset of clinical or other evidence of infection may be longer than usually considered in obtaining a medical history for most clinical evaluations.

Most protozoan infections are not associated with eosinophilia. Exceptions are *Isospora belli*[3] and possibly *Dientamoeba fragilis*,[4] which have been reported to be associated with eosinophilia. In some reports of these infections, other causes of eosinophilia had not been excluded. Eosinophilia and eosinophilic myositis have been reported in association with the coccidian parasite *Sarcocystis*.[5] In general, however, the finding of eosinophilia in a patient with a protozoan infection should prompt a search for a concomitant helminthic infection or an alternative noninfectious process to explain the eosinophilia.

Only a few fungal and, rarely, specific viral infections are associated with eosinophilia (***Box 131.3***). Acute bacterial and viral infections characteristically produce eosinopenia.[2] Likewise, acute protozoan infections, including malaria,[6,7] will suppress eosinophilia, including that caused by helminthic infections, during the intercurrent infection. Bacterial superinfections that complicate hyperinfection strongyloidiasis contribute to suppression of eosinophilia that might otherwise be a salient clue to the presence of strongyloidiasis. When eosinophilia is observed in bacterial infections, it may be consequent to hypersensitivity reactions to antibiotics used for treatment. The fungal diseases associated with eosinophilia are: aspergillosis, in the form of allergic bronchopulmonary aspergillosis,[8] coccidioidomycosis,[9] and basidiobolomycosis.[10,11] Blood eosinophilia, peaking during the second or third week of illness, occurs with primary coccidioidomycosis. Eosinophilia also may develop with disseminated coccidioidomycosis.[12,13] Eosinophilia has been reported in children with paracoccidioidomycosis, an infection whose involvement of adrenal glands[14] perhaps is causing eosinophilia due to hypoadrenalism. A few reports note eosinophilia in patients with ectoparasitic infestations caused by myiasis[15] and scabies.[16]

PATHOGENESIS

Eosinophils are bone marrow-derived leukocytes. Eosinophilia develops when three specific cytokines, granulocyte–macrophage colony-stimulating factor (GM-CSF), interleukin (IL)-3, and IL-5 stimulate enhanced eosinophilopoiesis. Of these, IL-5 is principally responsible for increases in eosinophilopoiesis and eosinophilia in helminthic, allergic, and other diseases. In humans, enhanced eosinophilopoiesis within the marrow requires over a week to increase blood eosinophilia. IL-5 also acts more rapidly to increase blood eosinophilia by mobilizing a marginated pool of preformed eosinophils resident within the marrow. IL-5 is produced by Th2-like $CD4^+$ T lymphocytes (as well as other cells, including eosinophils); and eosinophilia is frequent with immune responses characterized by Th2-like T-cell activation, including those elicited by helminthic parasite infections and associated with allergic diseases.[17] In both of these, enhanced immunoglobulin E (IgE) production is usually present.[17] GM-CSF, IL-3, and IL-5 also act on mature eosinophils to prolong their survival by antagonizing apoptosis and to enhance their effector functions. In other diverse diseases associated with eosinophilia (***Box 131.1***), mechanisms leading to eosinophilia are not yet delineated.

Although Th2-like T-cell responses lead to eosinophilia, it remains uncertain how specific parasitic or allergic diseases characteristically stimulate Th2-type responses. Specific features of helminthic antigens, as well as their particulate presentation, may influence the initial antigen presentation process that leads to Th2-like lymphocyte responses and consequent eosinophilia. As noted below, eosinophilia is most prominent

Box 131.1 Eosinophil-associated Diseases and Disorders

"Allergic" Diseases
- Atopic and related diseases
- Medication-related eosinophilias

Infectious Diseases
- Parasitic infections, mostly with helminths
- Specific fungal infections
- Other infections – infrequent

Hematologic and Neoplastic Disorders
- Hypereosinophilic syndromes, including forms of chronic eosinophilic leukemia, lymphocytic variants, and idiopathic forms
- Lymphomas, especially nodular sclerosing Hodgkin's; some T- and B-cell lymphomas
- Tumor-associated: on occasion with large-cell nonkeratinizing cervical tumors, large-cell undifferentiated lung carcinomas, squamous carcinomas (vagina, penis, skin, nasopharynx), adenocarcinomas (stomach, large bowel, uterine body), and transitional bladder cell carcinoma
- Mastocytosis

Diseases with Specific Organ Involvement
- Skin and subcutaneous diseases (e.g., blistering diseases, bullous pemphigoid, pemphigus vulgaris, dermatitis herpetiformis, herpes gestationis, and drug-induced lesions)
- Pulmonary diseases (e.g., acute or chronic eosinophilic pneumonia, allergic bronchopulmonary aspergillosis)
- Gastrointestinal diseases (e.g., eosinophilic gastroenteritis)
- Neurologic diseases (e.g., eosinophilic meningitis)
- Rheumatologic diseases (e.g., Churg–Strauss syndrome vasculitis)
- Cardiac diseases (e.g., endomyocardial fibrosis)
- Renal diseases (e.g., drug-induced interstitial nephritis, eosinophilic cystitis, dialysis)

Immunologic Reactions
- Specific immunodeficiency diseases (hyper-IgE syndrome, Omenn's syndrome)
- Transplant rejection

Endocrine
- Hypoadrenalism

Other
- Atheroembolic disease
- Irritation of serosal surfaces
- Inherited

with helminthic infections when parasites are migrating through or beginning to localize within tissues.

IMMUNOBIOLOGY

Eosinophils are primarily tissue-dwelling leukocytes, normally several hundredfold more abundant in tissues than in blood. Eosinophil numbers are greatest in tissues with a mucosal epithelial interface with the environment, including the gastrointestinal (GI) and lower genitourinary (GU) tracts. The life span of eosinophils is longer than that of neutrophils. Eosinophils probably survive for weeks within tissues.

The immunologic functions of eosinophils remain the subject of intense investigation. In addition to functioning as endstage effector leukocytes, eosinophils likely have additional roles in interacting with lymphocytes and other cells.[18]

As effector cells, eosinophils are capable of releasing specific lipid mediators, such as leukotriene C_4, and are a source of a range of preformed, granule-stored cytokines. In addition, eosinophils uniquely contain specific, highly positively charged ("cationic") proteins within their cytoplasmic granules. These eosinophil granule cationic proteins include major basic protein and eosinophil cationic protein. The release of these granule proteins can damage host tissues and more beneficially can contribute to the killing of helminthic parasites. The extent to which eosinophils are involved in the immune responses to helminthic parasites, and especially their early larval forms, to help kill these parasites *in vivo* is still not certain.[17,19]

Box 131.2 Key Concepts: Eosinophils in Parasitic Infections

- Elevation is caused primarily by helminthic parasites that reside in tissues. Most protozoan parasitic infections are not associated with eosinophilia
- Eosinophils may be prominent during only one stage of parasite development. Migration of parasites within tissues is often associated with high-grade eosinophilia. Chronic parasitic infections in antigenically sequestered sites (e.g., echinococcal cysts) or solely within the gut lumen (e.g., adult *Ascaris* or tapeworms) may not provoke an eosinophilic response. Release of antigenic material when parasites die or when walls protecting parasites are breached may lead to increased eosinophilia
- Eosinophil levels may wax and wane; many factors unrelated to the helminthic infection influence the level of blood eosinophilia. Acute bacterial, viral, and protozoal (e.g., malaria) infections suppress eosinophilia
- High-grade eosinophilia and symptoms may be prominent during the prepatent period and before the diagnosis can be confirmed by finding eggs or diagnostic forms of the parasite in tissues. Serologic tests may help in early diagnosis
- The degree of eosinophilia and other clinical manifestations caused by helminthic infections may differ between long-term residents of endemic regions and short-term visitors, being more prominent in the latter
- Many infections associated with eosinophilia cause no or intermittent symptoms; first symptoms may develop months or years after exposure. Many helminths are long-lived with life spans that can exceed a decade
- Multiple infections may be present, especially in long-term residents of tropical areas. Finding intestinal eggs or certain parasites does not confirm that they are the cause of the eosinophilia. In a patient with *Ascaris* eggs and moderate or high-grade eosinophilia, the search for the cause of eosinophilia should continue
- Absence of eosinophilia does not exclude a parasitic infection typically associated with eosinophilia

Box 131.3 Infections Associated with Eosinophilia

Viral
- Human immunodeficiency virus-1 – on occasion, may be associated with skin eruption

Fungal
- *Aspergillus* – only with allergic bronchopulmonary aspergillosis
- *Coccidioides immitis* – acute and sometimes later disseminated infections
- Basidiobolomycosis
- Paracoccidioidomycosis

Protozoan
- *Isospora belli*
- *Dientamoeba fragilis*

Helminthic
- Many (see Table 131.1)

Infestations
- Scabies
- Myiasis

In patients with marked eosinophilia, eosinophils may cause organ damage, most notably to the heart. The damage to the heart, ranging from early necrosis to subsequent endomyocardial thrombosis and fibrosis, is the same with varied eosinophilic conditions. Thus, endomyocardial thrombosis and fibrosis develop with eosinophilia associated with the hypereosinophilic syndromes,[20] carcinomas and lymphomas, and parasitic infections, including at times trichinellosis, visceral larva migrans, loiasis, or other filarial infections.[21–25] Pathologically, eosinophilic endomyocardial fibrosis[26] is identical to tropical endomyocardial fibrosis.[27,28] While diverse eosinophilic diseases can cause identical forms of cardiac disease, many patients with sustained eosinophilia never develop cardiac disease. Thus, the pathogenesis of eosinophil-mediated cardiac damage involves both the presence of increased eosinophils and other, as yet ill-defined, stimuli for recruitment or activation of these leukocytes.

Box 131.4 Factors that Lower Eosinophil Counts

Acute bacterial and viral infections; acute malaria	Immunosuppressive states (also less elevation of immunoglobulin E; sensitivity of serologic tests may be lower)
Corticosteroids – endogenous and exogenous	Epinephrine (sharp fall after initial transient rise; can be inhibited by β-blockers)
Acute stress	
Pregnancy (counts especially low during stress of delivery)	

Host Factors that Influence Eosinophil Responses

Blood eosinophilia is clearly present when eosinophils are in excess of 450 cells/μL blood. Published studies use cutoffs that range from 350 to 500 cells/μL blood. Increased percentages, but not absolute numbers, of blood eosinophils (pseudoeosinophilia) due to leukopenia in other white blood cell lines can be misleading.

Many host factors and other stimuli influence peripheral blood eosinophil levels (***Box 131.4***). Blood eosinophil numbers vary diurnally, with levels being higher in the early morning and lower at about noon. Levels are higher in the neonatal period and decline with age. Eosinophil levels fall during pregnancy; during the stress of delivery they almost disappear from the peripheral circulation.[29] Epinephrine causes a sharp fall in circulating eosinophils, after a transient increase. Injection of 100 mg hydrocortisone is followed by a decrease in peripheral eosinophils to 35% of control levels within 1 hour, and blood eosinophils are nearly absent 4 hours after the steroid administration.[30] Corticosteroids inhibit tissue accumulation of eosinophils, probably by several mechanisms, including promoting eosinophil apoptosis.[31] Acute bacterial and viral infections and other processes causing acute inflammation are associated with a decline in and transient suppression of blood eosinophilia.[30,32] Eosinophils drop during acute malaria, even if previously elevated.[6,7] Depression of eosinophils in malaria persists beyond the clearance of fever and parasitemia, and is followed by an increase in eosinophils in convalescence.[7] When it is important to know whether a patient has eosinophilia, a blood differential count should be repeated after a patient has recovered from an acute intercurrent infection.

Patterns

Characteristics of the eosinophil response that may be useful in assessing more likely causes of eosinophilia include level, duration, pattern (constant versus intermittent), and associated symptoms. If a person has had tropical exposures, the timing of onset of eosinophilia in relation to those exposures may help in the evaluation. Eosinophilia should be characterized by level, not simply as present or absent. Absolute eosinophil counts of greater than 3000/μL are categorized as marked or high-grade eosinophilia. Several different patterns of eosinophilia may be seen in relation to parasitic infections. Factors that influence these patterns include the type of parasite, the stage of parasite development, the location within the human host, the integrity of barriers between parasite and host, and the viability of the parasite, as well as many attributes of the host. In some helminth infections, eosinophilia is prominent only during one stage of parasite development. An example is the intestinal parasite *Ascaris lumbricoides*, which provokes eosinophilia principally during the initial stage of larval migration through the lungs (see Chapter 115). Adult worms residing in the lumen of the gut typically do not cause an eosinophilic response. Some parasites, such as the tapeworms *Diphyllobothrium latum* and *Taenia saginata*, whose entire life in the human host takes place in the lumen of the gut, cause little or no eosinophilic response even though they can grow to impressive lengths and survive for decades. ***Table 131.1*** delineates the many helminthic infections associated with eosinophilia, the main body site affected by each and candidate diagnostic tests for each; fuller details are found in pathogen-specific chapters.

Several helminthic parasites may induce high-grade eosinophilia (***Table 131.2***) during one stage of development followed by chronic low-to-moderate levels of eosinophilia. Acute schistosomiasis (Katayama syndrome)[33,34] (see Chapter 122) and the larval migration stage of *Ascaris*[35] and hookworms[36] may provoke high-grade eosinophilia, which declines during the chronic stages of infection. In experimental hookworm infections, blood eosinophilia increases progressively after 2–3 weeks of infection and peaks between 5 and 9 weeks before gradually diminishing. In untreated hookworm infections, eosinophilia slowly diminishes but can persist for several years after experimental infection.[37] The blood and pulmonary eosinophilia, often characterized as "transient," associated with the pulmonary migration phases of *Ascaris* and hookworms typically persists for weeks or months.[35,38,39] The eosinophilia with strongyloidiasis (see Chapter 117) often fluctuates over time, being high during pulmonary migration and low to moderate during chronic infection. During hyperinfection syndromes, eosinophilia can be prominent or absent, influenced by host characteristics and suppression due to corticosteroids or concomitant bacterial infection.[40] The dramatic eosinophilia seen with acute trichinellosis usually disappears when a fibrous capsule forms around the larvae in muscles (except with the nonencapsulating species *Trichinella pseudospiralis*, which may cause a prolonged eosinophilic myositis[41]) (see Chapter 110). Parasites encysted in tissues, such as echinococcal cysts and cysticercosis, and physically isolated from the host by cyst walls, typically cause no eosinophilia unless disruption of the barrier allows leakage of antigen-rich material. Intermittent leakage of fluids from echinococcal cysts can transiently stimulate increases in blood eosinophilia and elicit allergic (urticaria, bronchospasm) or anaphylactic reactions.[42,43] Breaching of these barriers or disintegration with death of the parasite can lead to intense tissue reactions, increased eosinophilia, and acute symptoms in the host.

Adult parasites that live and migrate in tissues, such as *Loa loa* and *Gnathostoma spinigerum*, provide an ongoing stimulus to eosinophils.[24,44] Many filarial infections cause persistent eosinophilia (see Chapters 104 through 107).

The magnitude of eosinophilic responses and the presence and intensity of other symptoms may vary greatly depending on age at first exposure, the immunologic state of the host, and the number and timing of subsequent exposures. Temporary residents and long-term residents of endemic regions have different patterns of response to a number of helminths.[23,45,46] Loiasis (see Chapter 105) in temporary residents of endemic regions is characterized by immunologic hyperresponsiveness, high-grade eosinophilia, and more severe symptoms not seen in long-term residents of the same area.[24] Short-term residents are more likely to have Calabar swelling and less likely to have detectable microfilaremia than the native population.[24,46] Among persons diagnosed with filariasis in the GeoSentinel Surveillance Network, those born and raised in filaria-endemic regions were 2.5 times as likely to be clinically asymptomatic compared with those from nonendemic areas.[47] With schistosome infections, previously unexposed and nonimmune persons, and not long-term residents of endemic areas, may experience the Katayama syndrome in acute schistosomal infection.[33,34]

EPIDEMIOLOGY

Published studies provide guidance to the infections more commonly associated with eosinophilia in persons who have visited or resided in tropical regions.[48] Amongst 261 patients with eosinophilia (defined as $>0.5 \times 10^9$/mL) evaluated in London (Hospital for Tropical Diseases), with a standard protocol and all diagnostic studies done at one laboratory, a diagnosis related to tropical exposures was made in 64%, with the most common diagnoses being schistosomiasis (33%), strongyloidiasis (25%), hookworm (5.3%), onchocerciasis (4.2%), loiasis (2.3%), ascariasis (2.3%), and trichuriasis (2.3%).[49] More than one parasitic infection was found in 17%. The predominant diagnoses varied by geographic areas of exposure. Schulte et al. in Germany found blood eosinophilia (defined as ≥8%) in 4.8% of 14 298 patients who were evaluated after return from developing countries.[50] The majority (73.6%) were born in Europe, the

Table 131.1 Helminthic Infections and Eosinophilia

Parasitic Infection	Main Body Site	Diagnosis
Angiostrongyliasis cantonensis	CNS	Serology,[a] rarely larvae in CSF
Angiostrongyliasis costaricensis	GI	Tissue biopsy (ileum, colon)
Anisakiasis	GI	Parasite via endoscopy or biopsy; serology[a]
Ascariasis	GI, lung (larvae)	Eggs in stool; larvae in sputum or BAL for early infection
Capillariasis hepatica	Hepatobiliary	Biopsy of liver
Capillariasis philippinensis	GI	Eggs, larvae, adults: stool, duodenal or jejunal aspirate, biopsy
Clonorchiasis	Hepatobiliary	Stool examination, duodenal aspirate; serology
Coenurosis	Many, including CNS	Parasite in tissue
Cutaneous larva migrans	Skin	Clinical
Cysticercosis	Many, including CNS, soft tissues	Tissue imaging, serology
Dicrocoeliasis	GI	Eggs in stool, duodenal aspirate, bile
Dirofilariasis	Lung, subcutaneous	Morphology in biopsied tissue
Dracunculiasis	Soft tissues, skin	Morphology of worm
Echinococcosis	Liver, lung, CNS, other	Morphology in tissue or aspirate; serology
Echinostomiasis	GI	Eggs in stool
Enterobiasis	GI, perianal	Eggs or worms in perianal area
Fascioliasis	Hepatobiliary	Eggs in stool, duodenal aspirate, serology[a]
Fasciolopsiasis	GI	Eggs in stool
Filariasis		
Lymphatic: *Wuchereria, Brugia*	Blood, lymphatics	Microfilariae in blood; worm in tissue, serology[a]
Loiasis	Subcutaneous, eye	Removed worm; microfilariae in blood, serology[a]
M. ozzardi	Blood, skin, body cavities	Microfilariae: blood, skin biopsy
M. perstans	Blood, body cavities	Microfilariae: blood, fluids; adult in tissue
M. streptocerca	Skin, subcutaneous tissues	Microfilariae: skin biopsy, snips; adult in tissue
Onchocerciasis	Skin, subcutaneous tissues, eye	Microfilariae: skin snips, blood, eyes; adults: tissue, serology[a]
Tropical pulmonary eosinophilia	Lung	Serology
Gnathostomiasis	Subcutaneous, other tissues	Morphology in surgical specimen, serology[a]
Heterophyiasis	GI	Eggs in stool
Hookworm	Skin (transient), GI, lung (larvae)	Eggs in stool
Hymenolepiasis	GI	Eggs in stool
Metagonimiasis	GI	Eggs in stool
Opisthorchiasis	Hepatobiliary	Eggs in stool, duodenal aspirate, bile
Paragonimiasis	Lung, CNS, subcutaneous	Eggs: sputum, BAL, feces, pleural fluid
Schistosomiasis		
Schistosomal dermatitis	Skin	Clinical
S. haematobium	Urinary tract, rarely CNS	Eggs in urine, tissue biopsy; serology
S. intercalatum	Liver, GI (venules of bowel), rarely CNS	Eggs in stool, biopsy
S. japonicum	Liver, GI (venules of bowel), rarely CNS	Eggs in stool, biopsy; serology
S. mansoni	Liver, GI (venules of bowel), rarely CNS	Eggs in stool, biopsy; serology
Sparganosis	Subcutaneous, multiple sites	Parasite in surgical specimen
Strongyloidiasis	GI, lung (larvae), skin (episodic)	Larvae in stool, duodenal aspirate; serology
Trichinellosis	GI (early), muscle, CNS	Muscle biopsy; serology
Trichostrongyliasis	GI	Eggs in stool or duodenal aspirate
Trichuriasis	GI	Eggs in stool, worms on protoscopy
Visceral larva migrans		
T. canis, T. cati	Liver, eye, lung (larvae)	Larvae in tissue; serology
Bayliscaris procyonis	CNS, eye, other	Identification of larva

CNS, central nervous system; CSF, cerebrospinal fluid; GI, gastrointestinal; BAL, bronchoalveolar lavage.
[a]Serologic tests may be available in some specialist laboratories.

median duration of travel was 35 days, and one-third were asymptomatic. A definite diagnosis was made in 36%. In 18.9%, a specific helminth infection was found, with the most common helminth infections being schistosomiasis, hookworm, cutaneous larva migrans, strongyloidiasis, filariasis, and ascariasis. Travelers to Africa were more likely to have eosinophilia than those who visited the Indian subcontinent and Latin America. In returned travelers with higher levels of eosinophils (>16%), a helminth infection was found in 46.6%. In Belgium, of more than 8000 consultations for tropical diseases, 378 patients were found to have eosinophil levels greater than 450/μL. Specific diagnoses were made in 170 patients, and parasites were detected 107 times, most commonly intestinal helminths and filarial and schistosomal species. When serologic tests and the Mazzotti test (see Chapter 106) were added as diagnostic criteria, intestinal helminthic infections were diagnosed in 19%, filarial infections

Table 131.2 Common Parasitic Causes of Marked Eosinophilia

Parasite/Disease	Magnitude	Comment
Angiostrongyliasis	High early	
Ascariasis	Moderate to high (larval migration)	Often absent with adult worms
Clonorchiasis	High early	May wax and wane in chronic infection
Fascioliasis	High early	May wax and wane in chronic infection
Fasciolopsiasis	High early	
Filarial infections		
Loiasis	High	Especially in expatriates
Mansonellosis	Can be high	
Onchocerciasis	Can be high	Normal eosinophil counts in up to 30%
Tropical pulmonary eosinophilia	High	
Gnathostomiasis	May be high	Wax and wane in chronic infection
Hookworm	High during larval migration	Persistent low to moderate
Opisthorchiasis	High early	
Paragonimiasis	High in early infection	Low or absent late
Schistosomiasis	High during early infection	Low or absent in chronic infection
Strongyloidiasis	High during larval migration	Low to moderate in chronic infection
Trichinellosis	High during acute infection	Absent late, except with nonencapsulating species
Visceral larva migrans	High to moderate	May persist months or longer

in 13%, and schistosomal infections in 10% of patients.[51] Among 2224 asymptomatic newly arrived refugees evaluated in Boston, 12% were found to have eosinophilia. Of the 45% who had serologic testing for specific pathogens, 39% were positive for *Strongyloides*, 22% for schistosomiasis, and 51% for filariasis.[52] For African immigrants in Spain with eosinophilia (27% of 788 immigrants) who underwent parasitologic and serologic testing within 6 months of arrival, 75% were asymptomatic.[53] A final diagnosis was made in 77% (55% had one parasitic infection, 14% had 2, and 7% had 3 or more), with the most common identified infections being filariae (30%), schistosomiasis (17%), and hookworms (17%). Predominant parasites varied by country of origin. A limitation of this study was the lack of good materials for the serologic diagnosis of *Strongyloides*. In Indochinese refugees with persistent eosinophilia whose initial comprehensive screening failed to reveal a cause for the eosinophilia, the most commonly implicated infections after further investigation were hookworm (55%) and *Strongyloides* (38%) infections.[54]

As noted above, the prevalence of various helminthic causes of eosinophilia will vary from one population to another depending on their geographic origins, their duration of residence, and their exposure-related activities. Although eosinophilia is a useful marker that suggests the possible presence of certain parasitic infections, many patients with these infections do not have eosinophilia when evaluated.[55] The absence of eosinophilia does not exclude the possibility of schistosomiasis, strongyloidiasis, and other infections commonly associated with eosinophilia. In a study of 1107 travelers with schistosomiasis seen in the United Kingdom, eosinophilia was present in only 44%,[56] and in another study 45% of 92 returned travelers with schistosomiasis had eosinophilia.[50] When persons are known to have had intense exposure to parasites, such as schistosomes,

Box 131.5 Eosinophilia and Remote Tropical or Other Exposures[a]

Clonorchiasis	Onchocerciasis
Coenurosis	Opisthorchiasis (up to 10 years)
Cysticercosis	Paragonimiasis
Echinococcosis	Schistosomiasis
Fascioliasis (rarely >10 years)	Sparganosis (at least 9 years)
Gnathostomiasis	Strongyloidiasis (autoinfection enables persistence for decades)
Hookworm (rarely 6 years or longer)	Tropical pulmonary eosinophilia (filarial)
Hymenolepiasis	Visceral larva migrans
Loiasis	
Mansonelliasis	

[a]*Parasitic infections that can be associated with eosinophilia 10 years or more after exposures in tropical areas. Eosinophilia may wax and wane.*

screening tests for these infections are warranted in the absence of eosinophilia or specific symptoms.[34,55] Many helminthic infections eliciting eosinophilia persist for years or even decades (***Box 131.5***).

In contrast to persons who have not left temperate areas, persons with tropical exposures are more likely to have an infection as the cause of eosinophilia. Although infections associated with eosinophilia, such as visceral larva migrans, trichinellosis, or even strongyloidiasis, can be acquired in temperate regions, these infections account for a small percentage of cases of eosinophilia in nontravelers. Eosinophilia in most temperate regions is more likely to be caused by a process other than infection. As a rule of thumb, one should think first of parasitic infections in persons with eosinophilia and tropical exposures and look first for nonparasitic causes in persons who have always lived in temperate climates.

Many infections associated with eosinophilia are seen primarily in persons with prolonged exposures. In general, cysticercosis, onchocerciasis, loiasis, lymphatic filariasis, paragonimiasis, and clonorchiasis are rare in persons with brief exposures. However, infections have been documented in persons with less than 1 month of exposure.[57] In the GeoSentinel study, among travelers from nonendemic areas who acquired filarial infections, 30% reported trips of 31 days or less.[47] Development of acute schistosomiasis after a single brief exposure to infested water has been described repeatedly. Because of differences in the immunologic response to parasites, a nonimmune visitor to an endemic region may develop severe symptoms and more marked eosinophilia with a small parasite burden relative to that in residents of the region.

COMMON CAUSES

Strongyloides

Among the helminths, the principal parasite that needs to be considered is *Strongyloides* since it frequently elicits eosinophilia of varying magnitudes; is often difficult to detect on stool examination; can persist for decades, even without causing major symptoms; and, importantly, can cause a disseminated, often fatal, disease (hyperinfection syndrome) in patients unsuspectingly given immunosuppressive corticosteroids (see Chapter 117).[40] The capacity of *Strongyloides* larvae to mature within the host into filariform larvae which invade the mucosa of the colon or penetrate the skin (usually in the perianal region) means that ongoing reinfection enables the parasite to persist for the lifetime of the host. In a study from Toronto General Hospital, of 51 consecutive individuals with *S. stercoralis* larvae documented in fecal specimens (and no other parasites found), 83% had eosinophilia (absolute eosinophil count >400 cells/μL) with a mean eosinophil count of 890 cells/μL.[58] Infection was longstanding in many; 22% had immigrated to Canada more than 10 years before diagnosis. Among 76 patients with strongyloidiasis, 25% were asymptomatic, 42% had GI symptoms, and 22% had skin complaints (primarily urticaria or pruritus).[58] In a study from the United Kingdom, eosinophilia was present in 88% of travelers and 76% of immigrants with *Strongyloides* larvae detectable on fecal examination.[59] While low-level or varying eosinophilia may be the only clue to strongyloidiasis,[60] at times the magnitude of hypereosinophilia suggests a hypereosinophilic syndrome.[61]

The importance of specifically considering *Strongyloides* infections, especially in those with eosinophilia, is based on the additional capacity of this infection to develop into disseminated, potentially fatal, disease (hyperinfection syndrome) if patients subsequently receive corticosteroids or become immunocompromised.[40] Thus, clinicians should carefully assess the probability of past exposure to *Strongyloides* in persons who will be given steroids or other immunosuppressive agents or who develop diseases associated with immunosuppression.[40] Cases of hyperinfection and dissemination have been reported more than 50 years after the last known exposure in endemic areas.[62] Patients with hyperinfection and dissemination may present with acute respiratory failure and Gram-negative sepsis.[63] Rarely, disseminated strongyloidiasis has been reported in apparently immunocompetent persons.[64] Persons infected with human T-cell lymphotropic virus type I (HTLV-1) have an impaired immune response to *Strongyloides* that increases the likelihood of hyperinfection and slows clearance of parasites after treatment with ivermectin compared with persons not infected with HTLV-1.[65] Although certain groups of immunocompromised patients (especially those with hematologic malignancies, or on steroids, or with severe malnutrition) appear to be at increased risk for the *Strongyloides* hyperinfection syndrome,[66] this has not been a frequently reported complication in human immunodeficiency virus serotype 1 (HIV-1)-infected persons in geographic areas where both HIV-1 and *Strongyloides* infections are common. Because fecal examinations are insensitive, enzyme-linked immunosorbent assay serology is useful in detecting strongyloidiasis even when fecal examinations are unrevealing, though sensitivity of serologic tests is lower in immunocompromised individuals.[54]

Schistosomes

Eosinophilia frequently accompanies schistosomiasis (see Chapter 122). Travelers who have visited endemic areas may present with acute schistosomiasis, subacute symptoms, or even without symptoms.[67] In one series of returned travelers with acute schistosomiasis, 73% had eosinophilia, 43% had respiratory symptoms, and 45% had skin changes at some point in the clinical course.[34] Many reports document sporadic cases and clusters of nonimmune persons with acute schistosomiasis after brief water exposures in endemic regions. Typical findings are spiking fevers, sweating, diarrhea, skin findings (urticarial rash and angioedema) and dry cough that can persist for a month or longer. Pulmonary symptoms were noted in 8 of 60 nonimmune travelers seen in Israel with acute schistosomiasis, occurring 3–6 weeks after exposure.[68] Chest radiographs showed multiple small nodules and diffuse interstitial infiltrate.[68] Among 31 patients with acute schistosomiasis mansoni in Brazil, all had eosinophilia, 90% had fever, 94% had diffuse abdominal pain, 81% had cough, 52% had dyspnea, and liver enzymes were elevated in 38%.[69] Other symptomatic presentations of schistosomiasis in travelers can include hematuria, hematospermia, or, uncommonly, transverse myelitis.[70–72] Infections can occur after a brief stay;[73] but for many, schistosomiasis develops only after longer-term exposures in endemic regions. A study of expatriates and visitors to Malawi found that serologic evidence of current or past schistosome infection increased directly with the length of stay in Malawi.[74] Seroprevalence was 48% in people resident 4 years or longer, in contrast to 11% for those resident 1 year or less. Recreational fresh-water exposure in Lake Malawi was an important source of infection.[74]

Filariae

Eosinophilia is common in infections caused by filarial parasites (see Chapters 104–106), which differ by geographic regions and vector insects. For lymphatic filariasis, early manifestations may include filarial fevers with lymphangitis.[75,76] Among 271 travelers and immigrants seen in GeoSentinel clinics who were diagnosed with filarial infections, 75% were acquired in sub-Saharan Africa and 10% in South America.[47] The most commonly diagnosed infections were onchocerciasis (37%), loiasis (25%), bancroftian filariasis (25%), and other filarial species in 6%. Two-thirds of those with onchocerciasis sought care for symptoms within 1 month of return.

Human Immunodeficiency Virus Type 1

Occasional reports have noted increased levels of eosinophils in HIV-1-infected persons.[77] In a study of 855 HIV-infected persons in New York examined over 4 years, however, no single, consistent cause of eosinophilia could be identified.[77] Increased eosinophil levels appeared to result from a relative preservation of the eosinophil cell line (while other cell lines declined as the CD4 count decreased) in some patients and in others from the presence of truly increased eosinophils.[77] Increased eosinophil levels in HIV-infected subjects were more commonly associated with rashes, including eosinophilic folliculitis,[78] atopic dermatitis, and prurigo nodularis. One study suggested no extensive evaluation for eosinophilia was warranted.[79] Although some HIV-infected patients with eosinophilia have a definable cause, such as adverse drug reactions or adrenal insufficiency due to cytomegalovirus and other infections, in most instances no obvious cause can be identified, indicating that HIV infection may be associated at times with increased levels of eosinophils.

COMMON SYNDROMES

Pulmonary

Eosinophilic lung diseases are a heterogeneous group of disorders characterized by a common presence of increased eosinophils in inflammatory infiltrates in the airways or parenchyma of the lungs. The clinical presentation of pulmonary eosinophilia usually consists of symptoms referable to the respiratory system accompanied by an abnormal chest radiograph and blood, sputum or bronchoalveolar lavage eosinophilia. While pathogenic mechanisms underlying many of the disorders are undefined, we classify pulmonary eosinophilias based on recognized etiologic agents and distinct clinical and pathologic patterns[2] (*Box 131.6*). Several helminthic infections that can cause eosinophilic lung diseases can be categorized based on the behavior of the parasites.

Transpulmonary Passage of Helminth Larvae

This category, the true Löffler's syndrome, arises from reactions elicited by larvae that pass through the lungs as part of the parasite's initial developmental cycle in the human. For three helminthic intestinal parasites (*Ascaris*, hookworms, and *Strongyloides*), infecting larvae pass through the

Box 131.6 Pulmonary Eosinophilia

1. Drug- and toxin-induced eosinophilic lung diseases
2. Helminthic infection-related eosinophilic lung diseases
   - Transpulmonary passage of larvae (Löffler's syndrome): *Ascaris*, hookworm, *Strongyloides*
   - Pulmonary parenchymal invasion: mostly helminths, paragonimiasis, echinococcosis
   - Heavy hematogenous seeding with helminths: trichinellosis, disseminated strongyloidiasis, cutaneous and visceral larva migrans, schistosomiasis
   - Tropical pulmonary eosinophilia: filaria
3. Fungal-related eosinophilic lung diseases
   - Allergic bronchopulmonary aspergillosis
4. Chronic eosinophilic pneumonia
5. Acute eosinophilic pneumonia
6. Churg–Strauss syndrome – vasculitis
7. Other: neoplasia, hypereosinophilic syndromes, bronchocentric granulomatosis, sarcoidosis

lungs, entering via the bloodstream, penetrating into alveoli, and then ascending the airway to transit down the esophagus into the small bowel. Löffler, who first described this syndrome of migratory pulmonary infiltrates and blood eosinophilia in Swiss patients, subsequently implicated *Ascaris* infection, acquired from the use of contaminated human feces as fertilizer, as the cause of this syndrome.[80] *Ascaris* is especially capable of eliciting eosinophilic inflammatory responses and is prevalent in regions where human feces contaminate soil or are used as fertilizer (see Chapter 115). Although infecting hookworm (see Chapter 116) and *Strongyloides* (see Chapter 117) larvae likewise traverse the lungs, these larvae rarely elicit symptoms of pulmonary eosinophilia in natural or experimental infections.[81]

Since Löffler's syndrome occurs only when developing larvae are transiting the lungs, about 9–12 days after ingestion of *Ascaris* eggs, this cause of pulmonary eosinophilia should be considered only in those with a recent exposure to *Ascaris* eggs (see Chapter 115). In symptomatic patients, common complaints are an irritating, nonproductive cough and burning substernal discomfort, and over half of patients have rales and wheezing. Acute symptoms generally subside within 5–10 days. Chest radiographs show unilateral or bilateral nonsegmental densities with indefinite borders ranging in size from several millimeters to several centimeters. Infiltrates are generally transient and migratory and clear over 1 or more weeks. Blood eosinophilia increases after several days of symptoms and resolves over many weeks. *Ascaris* pneumonia is diagnosed at the time of pneumonic involvement only by detecting *Ascaris* larvae in respiratory secretions or gastric aspirates.[81] At least 40 days must elapse before the larvae responsible for pulmonary infiltrates have matured sufficiently to produce eggs detectable in the stool. Negative stool examinations during or soon after an episode of pneumonitis do not exclude *Ascaris* as the cause, nor do positive stool examinations for *Ascaris* eggs during the stage of pulmonary involvement establish the cause, as these eggs reflect infection acquired 2–24 months earlier.

Pulmonary Parenchymal Invasion with Helminths

In contrast to the parasites that transit through the lungs, a few helminths, such as *Paragonimus* lung flukes (see Chapter 123) and echinococcal species (see Chapter 120), have a predilection to localize within the pulmonary parenchyma, and these may elicit eosinophil-enriched inflammatory reactions.[81] *Paragonimus* larvae undergo maturation in the lungs. Larval flukes can leave hemorrhagic, necrotic tracts; their eggs provoke a granulomatous response. Because the chronic cavitary lesions of paragonimiasis can mimic tuberculosis, and many adults from Southeast Asia have positive tuberculin tests, patients may be misdiagnosed as having tuberculosis.[82] Echinococcal infection can also involve the lungs, though encysted parasites typically do not elicit a peripheral eosinophilia.

Heavy Hematogenous Seeding with Helminths

This disease category includes the eosinophilic pulmonary responses elicited by helminthic larvae or eggs that are carried into the lungs hematogenously in an aberrant fashion. Thus, in contrast to the "normal" transpulmonary migration noted previously, etiologic helminths include abnormal numbers of nonhuman hookworms or ascarids causing cutaneous or visceral larva migrans,[83,84] abnormal numbers of hematogenous larvae in heavy trichinellosis infections,[81] and abnormal spread following chemotherapy of schistosomal parasites via collateral vessels into the lungs.[81,85] Also included in this category is disseminated strongyloidiasis, which develops when the *Strongyloides* autoinfection cycle becomes unbridled, often in association with corticosteroid drug administration (see Chapter 117). Large numbers of larvae traverse the lungs eliciting pulmonary findings. Adult parasites can develop in the bronchial tree, causing bronchospasm mimicking asthma.[86] In disseminated strongyloidiasis, filariform larvae can be found in many sites, including the stool, sputum, and bronchoalveolar lavage. The usual eosinophilia of strongyloidiasis can be suppressed in disseminated disease because of concomitant pyogenic infection or steroid administration.

Tropical Pulmonary Eosinophilia

Tropical pulmonary eosinophilia (TPE) results from a distinct immune response to the normally bloodborne microfilarial stages of lymphatic filariae, *Wuchereria bancrofti*, and, less commonly, *Brugia malayi* (see Chapter 104).[87–89] TPE is prevalent in regions where these filariae are endemic, and residents or immigrants from these regions are those who may experience TPE. Males are affected more often than females in a ratio of about 4 : 1. Dyspnea, cough, wheezing (especially at night), and chest discomfort may be accompanied by weight loss and malaise. Infection is commonly misdiagnosed, with asthma being a common diagnosis.[89,90] In addition to blood eosinophilia, features specific to TPE include high levels of serum IgE and antifilarial antibodies. Total white blood cell count is typically elevated and blood eosinophilia may be extremely high. Bloodstream microfilariae are almost never found. Abnormalities on chest radiographs may be subtle and include diffuse miliary lesions 1–3 mm in size, patchy consolidations, cavitation, reticulonodular infiltrates of the lower lung zones, and an interstitial nodular pattern.[91] Without treatment, TPE can lead to progressive fibrosis and chronic respiratory compromise.[89] TPE is an immunologically mediated disorder with microfilariae trapped in the lungs. Microfilariae are detected in inflammatory foci in biopsies from the lung, liver, and lymph nodes. A related, nonfilarial syndrome of TPE of uncertain cause has been recognized.[92]

Other Pulmonary Eosinophilias

Cases of acute eosinophilic pneumonia occurred in US military personnel deployed in or near Iraq in 2003–2004.[93] The etiology was not determined; an association with recent initiation of cigarette smoking was noted.

Among the drugs reported to cause pulmonary eosinophilia are ones sometimes taken for malaria prophylaxis and hence pertinent in patients who will have had tropical exposures. These include pyrimethamine, and dapsone.[94,95]

Eosinophilic pleural effusions (***Box 131.7***) can have multiple causes.[96] In the setting of someone with potential infectious exposures, several helminthic infections, including toxocariasis,[97] TPE,[98] paragonimiasis,[99] loiasis,[100] and anisakiasis,[101] can cause eosinophilic pleural effusions.

Abdominal Pain or Diarrhea

The gut is the primary or sole residence for many helminthic parasites. Symptoms from these eoosinophilia-associated parasitic infections (***Box 131.8***) may result from several mechanisms, including attachment of the

Box 131.7 Eosinophilic Pleural Effusions

Helminthic Infections	Other Infections
Anisakiasis (rare)	Coccidioidomycosis
Echinococcosis	Tuberculosis
Gnathostomiasis	**Other Causes**
Loiasis	Hemothorax
Paragonimiasis	Hypersensitivity reactions, including drug reactions
Strongyloidiasis (disseminated infection; may also find larvae in fluid)	Malignancy
Toxocariasis	Pneumothorax, including from thoracentesis
Trichinellosis (early weeks of infection)	Pulmonary infarct
Tropical pulmonary eosinophilia	**Rheumatologic Diseases**

Box 131.8 Parasites Causing Eosinophilia and Abdominal Pain or Diarrhea

Helminths	Protozoa
Ancylostoma caninum (eosinophilic enteritis)	*Dientamoeba fragilis*
Anisakis spp. and other genera (anisakiasis)	*Isospora belli*
Angiostrongylus costaricensis	**Other Causes**
Ascaris lumbricoides	Eosinophilic gastroenteritis
Capillaria philippinensis	Dermatitis herpetiformis
Clonorchis sinensis	Churg–Strauss syndrome (vasculitis)
Echinococcus	Regional enteritis
Enterobius vermicularis (eosinophilic colitis)	Ulcerative colitis
Fasciola hepatica	Lymphoma
Fasciolopsis buski	Solid tumors
Gnathostoma	Drug reaction (e.g., eosinophilic colitis from naproxen)
Hookworm (heavy infection)	Hypereosinophilic syndromes
Schistosomes	Allergy (e.g., cow's milk, soy protein in infants)
Strongyloides	
Trichinella	
Toxocara canis, T. cati, other (visceral larva migrans)	

parasite to, or penetration of, the gut mucosa, causing irritation and inflammation; migration through the wall or to other adjacent sites (such as biliary and pancreatic ducts); intraluminal obstruction by a bolus of worms; and entry into the appendix, among others. The canine hookworm (*Ancyclostoma caninum*) has been associated with a syndrome of abdominal pain, sometimes acute and severe, and peripheral eosinophilia.[102] Larvae of the pinworm *Enterobius vermicularis* (see Chapter 113) have also been reported to cause eosinophilic colitis and enteritis.[103] Capillariasis (*Capillaria philippinensis*) (see Chapter 112) can be associated with chronic, severe diarrhea and intestinal tissue infiltration of eosinophils.[104] Helminth-elicited disease must be distinguished from often idiopathic eosinophilic gastroenteritis.[105,106]

Skin

Intermittent and migratory lesions of the skin and subcutaneous tissues can reflect migration of parasites in human tissues (***Table 131.3***) (see Chapter 132). Skin lesions associated with gnathostomiasis (see Chapter 112) may begin as early as 3–4 weeks after ingestion of the parasite or may be delayed until months or even years later. The third-stage larvae cause localized swellings that typically last 1–2 weeks and are associated with edema, pain, itching, and variable erythema. Swellings may recur off and on for 10–12 years. Because a single gnathostome can cause symptoms, cases have occurred after a brief stay in an endemic area or after eating foods, usually raw fish, from those areas. Disease has been most often reported from Southeast Asia. Increases in cases in Mexico, Peru, and Ecuador have been noted.[107,108] In addition to causing cutaneous disease, the worm can also migrate to tissues throughout the body, causing pulmonary, gastrointestinal, genitourinary, central nervous system, ocular, and other localized disease.[44] Loiasis, another disease causing migratory lesions and eosinophilia, follows exposures to *Loa loa* in west-central Africa (see Chapter 105).[57] Symptoms typically do not appear until at least 4 months after exposure and can first appear more than 5 years after exposure. Classic findings are localized areas of angioedema (Calabar swellings), which may be warm, red, itchy, or painful,[24,46] usually disappear within a few days, and may recur multiple times per year.

A pruritic skin rash is a common feature of onchocerciasis (see Chapter 106). Swelling of an extremity should suggest obstruction of lymphatics caused by one of the lymphatic filarial parasites. Patients may experience recurrent lymphangitis (often with retrograde progression) lasting 3–7 days, which may be associated with fever.[76] Orchitis and epididymitis are

Table 131.3 Helminths Associated with Eosinophilia and Skin and Soft-tissue Changes

Parasite/Disease	Manifestation
Ascariasis	Urticaria
Coenurosis	Subcutaneous nodules, usually solitary
Cutaneous larva migrans[a]	Characteristic serpiginous lesions
Cysticercosis	Rubbery, painless cysts; often multiple
Dracunculiasis	Papules, vesicles; rupture and discharge larvae
Echinococcosis	Soft, subcutaneous cysts, varying sizes; urticaria
Fascioliasis	Urticaria; rare painful or itchy subcutaneous nodules
Filariasis	
Brugia zoonotic filariae	Local lymphadenopathy
Zoonotic dirofilariasis	Subcutaneous nodule
Loiasis	Pruritic 5–10-cm Calabar swellings; urticaria; papulovesicular lesions
Onchocerciasis	Subcutaneous nodules; papules and severe itching; urticaria; lizard skin
Wuchereria bancrofti	Recurrent retrograde lymphangitis and lymphadenitis; scrotal mass; hydrocele, elephantiasis
Brugia malayi, B. timori	Recurrent retrograde lymphangitis and lymphadenitis; scrotal mass; hydrocele, elephantiasis
Gnathostomiasis	Urticarial, edematous, recurrent, migratory subcutaneous swellings; creeping eruption; panniculitis
Hookworm	Urticaria; itchy maculopapular rash; may be vesicular
Paragonimiasis	Urticaria (early); subcutaneous nodules
Schistosomiasis	Urticaria, itchy maculopapules (early); papules (ectopic egg deposition)
Sparganosis	Edematous, painful migratory swellings secondary to worm migration
Strongyloidiasis	Itchy papular and migratory serpiginous lesions at points of penetration and dermal migration (larva currens); urticaria; papulovesicular lesions; petechiae and purpuric lesions in hyperinfection syndrome
Trichinellosis	Urticaria; periorbital edema; splinter hemorrhages
Visceral larva migrans	Urticaria; nodules

[a]Eosinophilia usually low-grade or absent.

also characteristic features. Although eosinophilia can occur in patients with cutaneous larva migrans caused by the hookworm *Ancylostoma braziliense* and related nematodes, in one series only 20% had at least 7% blood eosinophilia.[109]

Penetration of schistosomal cercariae is typically followed by the development of an itchy, erythematous, papular rash.[110] Exposures to avian schistosomes elicit a similar skin reaction (swimmer's itch).[110,111]

Hepatobiliary

Helminths that cause eosinophilia and hepatic dysfunction (***Box 131.9***) include several parasites that reside in the biliary tree and cause localized inflammatory changes and can obstruct the bile or pancreatic ducts, leading to a clinical picture that can mimic acute cholangitis or cholecystitis (see Chapter 123). *Ascaris* adult worms can wander from their usual habitat within the gut lumen to enter pancreatic or biliary ducts causing

Box 131.9 Infections Causing Eosinophilia and Hepatic Dysfunction

Angiostrongyliasis cantonensis (infrequent hepatic involvement)	Fascioliasis
Ascariasis (mechanical obstruction of bile ducts by migrating worm)	*Metorchis conjunctus*
Capillariasis due to *Capillaria hepatica*	Opisthorchiasis
Clonorchiasis	Schistosomiasis
Dicrocoeliasis	Strongyloidiasis (with hyperinfection)
Echinococcosis (eosinophilia may be absent with intact cysts; liver function may remain normal despite multiple cysts)	Taeniasis (*Taenia saginata*; rare obstruction of bile ducts)
	Visceral larva migrans (toxocariasis)

Box 131.10 Helminthic Infections Causing Eosinophilia and Prominent Fever[a]

Clonorchiasis	Trichinellosis
Fascioliasis	Visceral larva migrans (toxocariasis)
Gnathostomiasis (early, episodic)	
Onchocerciasis	
Schistosomiasis (Katayama syndrome)	

[a]*Acute, early* Ascaris, *hookworm, or* Strongyloides *may be associated with fever.*

acute symptoms (see Chapter 115). In fascioliasis, young flukes penetrate the capsule of the liver and migrate through liver parenchyma causing local necrosis and inflammation before they enter the bile ducts, where they mature and produce eggs that are released into bile and passed in feces.[112,113] Eosinophilia may wax and wane when infection becomes chronic. Clonorchiasis, endemic in eastern and southeastern Asia, and opisthorchiasis, acquired mainly in Southeast Asia, are other parasites that reside in bile ducts (see Chapter 123). Among 17 immigrants who were found to have ova of *Opisthorchis* spp. or *Clonorchis sinensis* in fecal specimens when evaluated in the US Midwest, 88% had eosinophilia (defined as absolute eosinophil counts >500/μL). Clinical symptoms included vague right upper abdominal discomfort; 24% of those infected had been in the United States at least 5 years.[114]

Fever

Only a few helminthic infections cause eosinophilia and prominent fevers (***Box 131.10***). Fever and eosinophilia can be seen in acute schistosomiasis,[33,115] visceral larva migrans,[116] trichinellosis,[117] fascioliasis,[112] gnathostomiasis,[44] and some other infections. In many instances, focal findings (e.g., localized subcutaneous swellings, muscle tenderness, lymphangitis, cough and pulmonary infiltrates, abdominal pain, and others) provide diagnostic clues. The combination of exposure history (when, where, and what activities) along with clinical findings can help the clinician to focus on more likely diagnoses.

Central Nervous System Findings

Larvae of *Angiostrongylus cantonensis* migrate to the brain, spinal cord, and eye, where the larvae and young adults provoke an intense inflammatory response and cause the clinical picture of eosinophilic meningoencephalitis (see Chapter 111). A number of other parasites or their eggs can be associated with an eosinophilic tissue response and with variable eosinophils in the spinal fluid. Cysticercosis, which commonly involves the central nervous system, typically causes focal neurologic findings, including seizures (see Chapter 119). The cerebrospinal fluid may be acellular and peripheral eosinophilia absent. In addition to helminthic parasites, other infections, drug reactions, and other processes can induce an eosinophilic meningitis[118,119] (***Box 131.11***).

Box 131.11 Causes of Eosinophilia in Cerebrospinal Fluid

Helminths

Nematode (Roundworm) Infections with Migrating Larvae Inherently Neurotropic

- *Angiostrongylus cantonensis*
- *Gnathostoma spinigerum*
- *Baylisascaris procyonis*

Cestode (Tapeworm) Infection with Cysts Developing in the Central Nervous System

- Cysticercosis
- Echinococcosis
- Coenurosis

Trematode (Fluke) Infection with Ectopic Central Nervous System Localization

- *Paragonimus westermani*
- Schistosomiasis
- Fascioliasis

Miscellaneous Infectious Causes

- Coccidioidomycosis
- *Cryptococcus neoformans*
- Toxocariasis (*Toxocara canis*)
- Trichinellosis
- Myiasis (larvae of cattle botflies)

Noninfectious Causes

- Ventriculoperitoneal shunts
- Leukemia or lymphoma with central nervous system involvement (Hodgkin's)
- Drug hypersensitivity reactions: nonsteroidal anti-inflammatory agents, antibiotics (e.g., sulfonamides, ciprofloxacin, vancomycin), phenytoin; myelography contrast agents
- Hypereosinophilic syndromes
- Sarcoidosis

Table 131.4 Examples of Drug-associated Reactions with Eosinophilia

Drug Reactions	Examples
Pulmonary infiltrates	NSAIDs
Pleuropulmonary	Dantrolene
Interstitial nephritis	Semisynthetic penicillins, cephalosporins
Necrotizing myocarditis	Ranitidine
Hepatitis	Semisynthetic penicillins, tetracyclines
Hypersensitivity vasculitis	Allopurinol, phenytoin
Gastroenterocolitis	NSAIDs
Asthma, nasal polyps	Aspirin
DRESS	Antiepileptics
Asymptomatic	Ampicillin, penicillins, cephalosporins

NSAIDs, nonsteroidal anti-inflammatory drugs; DRESS, drug-induced rash, eosinophilia, and systemic symptoms.

NONINFECTIOUS DISEASES

Many processes (***Box 131.1***) associated with eosinophilia may need to be considered if helminthic infections do not explain a patient's eosinophilia. Drug hypersensitivity reactions should always be considered as a potential cause of eosinophilia, even in persons who have visited or lived in tropical regions. The presence of a characteristic rash may suggest a hypersensitivity reaction, but drug-associated eosinophilia can occur in the absence of skin changes. In addition to peripheral eosinophilia, drug reactions may be associated with pathologic changes and dysfunction of other tissues and organs (***Table 131.4***). Any of these findings may predominate, or a combination of several may be seen at the same time or in staggered development. Some medication-related eosinophilic responses (e.g., Stevens–Johnson syndrome, acute anaphylaxis, and drug-induced rash, eosinophilia, and systemic symptoms (DRESS)) can be life-threatening and preclude continued use of or rechallenge with candidate offending medications. Because of the striking blood or tissue eosinophilia, some drug reactions can mimic parasitic infections.

Evaluation of Patients with Eosinophilia

Several key concepts are relevant to the evaluation of a patient with eosinophilia after tropical exposures:

- Multiple parasitic infections may be present.
- Fecal excretion of eggs may be in small numbers or intermittent.
- Examination of stool for eggs is useless during the prepatent period. Symptoms such as fever and eosinophilia may be present for 2 weeks or more before the products of the adult parasite (e.g., eggs or larvae) are passed in the stool.
- Eosinophilia is most prominent with tissue-dwelling helminths, and many of these never enter the intestinal tract. Stool examinations will not detect tissue-dwelling helminths or exclude their presence as a cause of eosinophilia.
- Serologic tests may be negative early in the symptomatic period.

It is necessary to have some idea of the possible infections that might be present in order to focus the evaluation and determine which tests to do and which tissues to examine. Even if the patient is entirely asymptomatic and the physical examination is unremarkable, the presence of eosinophilia should lead to a workup to identify treatable diseases that could cause future problems. Eosinophilia, however, need not be present.[55] Knowledge of the geographic distribution of various parasites and the characteristic time interval between exposure and onset of symptoms and the presence of diagnostic forms of parasites or eggs in tissue or fluids is an essential part of the evaluation (*Box 131.12*).

Even when sensitive and specific serologic tests are available, they may be negative early in the course of infection. In a study of patients with acute schistosomiasis, serologic results were negative in 3 of 8 persons tested during the first week of illness.[33] If suspicion is high, serologic tests should be repeated if initially negative. During the prepatent period, serologic studies may be the only way to confirm the diagnosis.[120]

Timing of obtaining blood to search for microfilariae needs to be done cognizant of the potential periodicity exhibited by the species and strains of filariae (see Chapters 104 and 105).

In general, it is preferable to diagnose infection by identification of eggs, larvae, adults, or other parasitic stages or products in tissues, fluids, or stool. Sometimes diagnostic material is unavailable or its retrieval would entail serious risk to the patient (e.g., brain biopsy, liver biopsy, major surgical intervention). When parasites, eggs, or other products are unavailable, serologic tests are useful in some infections. Problems with serologic tests may include lack of sensitivity, availability, standardization and quality control, and low specificity. Cross-reactivity to related parasites is common for many of the tests.

Acid-fast techniques stain schistosome eggs and hooklets of *Echinococcus granulosus*.

Box 131.12 Eggs or Parasites in Tissues or Fluids

In Urine

- Filariasis (microfilariae, e.g., *Wuchereria bancrofti, Loa loa*)
- Gnathostomiasis (parasite passed in urine; rare)
- Schistosome eggs (*Schistosoma haematobium*)
- Strongyloidiasis (larvae, rare)

In Sputum

- Ascariasis (larvae during early migration)
- Echinococcosis (fragments of larvae and free scolices after rupture of cyst into bronchus: rare)
- Gnathostomiasis (rarely, coughed-up worm)
- Hookworm (larvae, early)
- Paragonimiasis (eggs in sputum)
- Schistosomiasis (eggs)
- Strongyloidiasis (filariform larvae, and, rarely, eggs and adults in sputum in hyperinfection syndrome)

In Pleural Fluid

- Paragonimiasis (eggs)
- Strongyloidiasis (filariform larvae)

On Blood Smears

- Microfilariae of filariasis (e.g., *W. bancrofti, Brugia malayi, L. loa, Mansonella perstans, M. ozzardi*)
- Trichinellosis (rarely observed on blood smears)

In Cerebrospinal Fluid

- Angiostrongyliasis due to *Angiostrongylus cantonensis* (larvae rarely in cerebrospinal fluid)

On Perirectal Skin (Tape Test)

- Pinworm eggs
- Tapeworm proglottids

In Feces[a]

- Strongyloidiasis (20–30% positive with a single examination; 60–70% with three or more; 40–90% positive on duodenal sample or endoscopic aspirate)
- Several intestinal nematodes, trematodes, and cestodes

[a]*Eggs and parasites are not found in feces in patients with many helminthic infections, such as echinococcosis, toxocaral visceral larva migrans, and trichinellosis; stool examinations are often negative at the time of earliest symptoms in patients with many infections, including schistosomiasis, ascariasis, and hookworm infections.*

RESPONSE TO TREATMENT

Several key points should be kept in mind when treating patients with helminthic infections:

- Treatment may not be curative; efficacy may vary depending on the stage of the parasite.
- Symptoms may worsen, usually only transiently, with therapy.
- The level of eosinophilia may be a poor predictor of whether treatment has cured infection.
- Eosinophilia may rise following initiation of treatment which elicited killing of helminths
- Relapses can occur late.

Even when parasitic infections are recognized and treated, anthelminthic drugs may fail to cure infection.

A temporary rise in eosinophilia after treatment has been observed in a number of helminthic infections.[121,122] The magnitude of the posttreatment eosinophilia correlates with the parasite burden prior to therapy.[123] This may be associated with other symptoms, such as pruritus, dermatitis, arthralgia, and myalgia in patients with loiasis.[124] Patients with schistosomiasis may develop respiratory symptoms and new pulmonary infiltrates in association with therapy.[85,122,123] Severe symptoms have been reported when treatment is given during the early Katayama syndrome.[121] These worsening symptoms and the rise in eosinophils may reflect the host immune response to antigens released or exposed from dead or dying larvae or worms. In patients with loiasis treated with diethylcarbamizine, levels of eosinophils usually returned to normal within 6 months.[124] This occurred even in patients who had late relapses of infection.[124] Thus, normalization of levels of eosinophils after treatment does not necessarily indicate that infection has been eradicated. Conversely, however, the persistence of eosinophilia likely indicates that infections persist.

Box 131.13 outlines an approach to the evaluation of the patient with eosinophilia.

Box 131.13 Evaluation of the Patient with Eosinophilia

Eosinophil Determinations

Confirm that the eosinophil count is elevated

Estimate the absolute blood eosinophil count: normal, ≤350 eosinophils/μL; elevated, >450 eosinophils/μL

Categorize eosinophilia as low (<1000/μL), moderate (1000–3000/μL), or high (>3000/μL) (see Table 131.2)

Medical History

Eosinophil History

Inquire from history or medical records if eosinophil counts were previously normal or elevated, and if so for how long

Medication History

Review drug exposure history for recent or current drugs that may be associated with eosinophilia. Discontinue any drugs that are commonly associated with eosinophilia and make a complete list of other medications, vitamins, supplements, or herbal preparations that the patient is taking. If patient is taking drugs that have been associated with eosinophilia, assess for associated serious organ involvement. Note any history of allergies to drugs or other agents

Disease History

Review the medical history for diseases or disorders typically associated with eosinophilia (see Box 131.1). Given their prevalence, allergic and atopic disorders should be noted, although new onset of some allergic manifestations (e.g., urticaria, bronchospasm, wheezing) may be secondary to helminthic infections

Geographic History

Review history of past residence and travel in other countries or regions. Relevant are time periods extending even decades before. Especially relevant are exposures in tropical regions and those with poor sanitation. Note places, dates, and duration of exposures. Some helminths have discrete geographic distributions (e.g., *Clonorchis* in the Far East; *Angiostrongylus cantonensis,* a cause of eosinophilic meningitis, principally, but not exclusively, in the Pacific Basin; *Loa loa* in central-west Africa; *Onchocerca volvulus* in equatorial Africa and elevated regions in Central America). Even nontropical geographic histories are relevant to some helminths and other agents, e.g., the southwestern United States for coccidioidomycosis. Exposures in sheep-rearing areas are pertinent to *Echinococcus granulosus*

Activity History

Review occupational and recreational exposures. Histories of swimming in or contact with fresh water in areas where schistosomiasis occurs are pertinent. Contact with fresh or salt water followed by a rash on water-exposed skin suggests schistosome dermatitis (avian schistosome species). Skin contact with soil potentially contaminated with human or dog feces, walking barefoot, or occupational (military or job-related) exposures are pertinent to the acquisition of cutaneous larva migrans, hookworm, and *Strongyloides* infections

Dietary History

Dietary histories are pertinent to several helminthic infections, including anisakiasis (raw fish), fish tapeworm (fish), *Nanophyetus salmincola* (salmon), *Taenia solium* (pork), *T. saginata* (beef), fascioliasis (watercress), fasciolopsiasis (water chestnut), gnathostomiasis (fresh-water fish, eels, frogs, snakes, and poultry and pigs fed on fish), *Angiostrongylus cantonensis* (land snails or slugs, fresh-water shrimp, crabs, some marine fish), and trichinellosis (pork, boar, bear, horse, walrus, warthog)

Other Epidemiologic History

Helpful in the evaluation is knowledge of whether the patient traveled with others and whether others developed similar illnesses – relevant to common-source water exposures (e.g., schistosomiasis) or foodborne illness (e.g., trichinellosis). In concert with geographic exposures, histories of exposures to insect vectors are pertinent (e.g., filarial infections)

General History

Do a careful review of systems for any current or recent symptoms, including a history of fevers (see Box 131.10), skin lesions (see Table 131.3) that may have cleared, and gastrointestinal illnesses (see Box 131.8)

Physical Examination

Do a careful physical examination, paying close attention to skin and soft tissue for nodules or masses

Initial Laboratory Evaluation

The presence of specific clinical symptoms and physical findings, as well as other information from the history, may begin to direct laboratory testing

As needed, check routine studies to assess organ involvement (e.g., liver function tests, renal function tests, urinalysis, serum troponin for cardaic involvement, chest radiograph (CXR)) or high-resolution chest computed tomography (CT)

Further Diagnostic Evaluations

Symptomatic Patient with Localizing Findings

The evaluation will be guided by the nature of the historical information and results from the physical examination and initial laboratory tests based on the focal findings.

Skin: skin snips, skin biopsy, excision of mass

Central Nervous System

CT and magnetic resonance imaging (MRI); cerebrospinal fluid examination (cell counts, differential, protein, glucose; larvae)

Pulmonary Findings or Abnormal CXR

Sputum examination (routine, acid-fast bacteria, ova and parasites (O&P)), CT or MRI to define lesions better, including those not seen on CXR

Stool O&P; urine O&P; rectal biopsy; other tests (see Box 131.12)

Eosinophilia in a Patient without Other Findings

Stools for O&P (×3 as needed)

Strongyloides serology (if stools negative), toxocara serology

Check serologic studies for schistosomiasis, filariasis, and onchocerciasis if patient may have been exposed

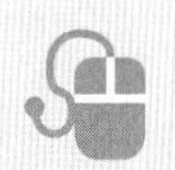

Access the complete reference list online at
http://www.expertconsult.com

CHAPTER 132

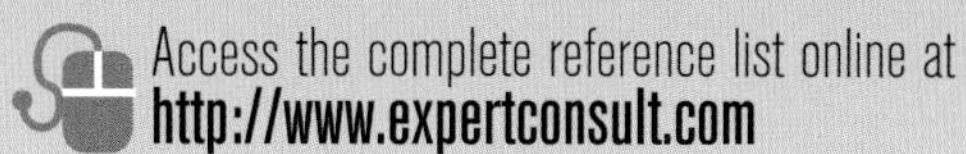
Access the complete reference list online at
http://www.expertconsult.com

Cutaneous Lesions

Steven D. Mawhorter • David L. Longworth

INTRODUCTION

Cutaneous lesions can be cardinal manifestations of diverse infectious diseases wherever they are acquired. Notably, in travelers returning from tropical regions, skin lesions are one of the top five medical concerns.[1–5] The top three dermatologic diagnoses in travelers are cutaneous larva migrans (CLM), bacterial infections (cellulitis, abscess, and pyoderma), and arthropod/insect-related lesions.[5–7] The majority of these lesions develop prior to return home and rarely require hospitalization, although often lead to medical evaluation.[4,5] The skin represents the largest organ of the body and the most accessible to direct examination and observation. As a result, it is often a sentinel for many infectious diseases by being the primary site of involvement; the entry site of parasitic or bacterial pathogens; or by demonstrating lesions that result from toxin-, inflammatory-, or vascular-mediated changes associated with infection.[8]

Specific pathogens and the clinical manifestations of diseases commonly found in people residing in, or traveling to, tropical areas are discussed in detail in pathogen-specific chapters. This chapter considers the pathophysiology of tropical and parasite-associated skin reactions, and focuses on the approach to the patient who presents with cutaneous lesions, to assist in the generation of a differential diagnosis.

THE SKIN AS TARGET ORGAN – PATHOGENETIC MECHANISMS

Although many pathogens can produce cutaneous manifestations, the skin has a limited number of responses to inflammatory or infectious processes. In general, the pathogenesis of skin manifestations of infectious diseases can be considered under six broad categories. The first involves bloodborne dissemination of the actual infectious agent.[9,10] This category can be further subdivided into two areas based on whether the etiologic agent engages in direct interaction with the skin and dermal appendages to produce cutaneous manifestations or mediates the interaction through cellular, humoral, or other immune mechanisms. Examples of organisms that directly involve the skin include *Neisseria meningitidis*, *Rickettsia* spp., endocarditis-related bacterial embolization (e.g., Janeway lesions, Osler's nodes), *Pseudomonas* spp. and other Gram-negative ecthyma lesions, *Bacillus anthracis*, and *Candida* spp. In this setting, Gram stain of the skin lesion may reveal the offending organism.[11,12] Viral pathogens, such as varicella-zoster virus and many enteroviruses, may elicit cutaneous findings following viremic seeding of the skin.[10] Examples of immune reactions involving the skin to bloodborne organisms include *Salmonella* spp. (rose spots), *N. meningitidis* and *N. gonorrhoeae*, measles, and rubella.[10] In these cases, cutaneous manifestations are typically due to local cutaneous immune vasculitis or dermal immune responses, including, but not limited to, immune complex deposition. Since the skin changes are largely immune complex-mediated, direct smears of the lesions are unlikely to reveal a pathogen. Many diseases associated with the bacteremic or viremic pathogenesis of this first category of cutaneous involvement are severe and occasionally life-threatening.[10]

The second category involves local reactions to parasites that gain access to the body elsewhere and migrate to the skin but are not bloodborne. They can elicit a direct or indirect immunologic response to produce the cutaneous changes. This category includes agents such as the filarial parasites *Onchocerca volvulus* (see Chapter 106) and *Loa loa* (see Chapter 105).[13,14] The nodules of onchocerciasis and loiasis often contain adult worms (direct mechanism). However, generalized pruritus and maculopapular eruptions appear to be mediated by immune reactions to dermal-based microfilariae (indirect mechanism).[15] Other helminthic examples include the cutaneous nodules of *Dracunculus medinensis* (see Chapter 108) and *Spirometra* spp. (sparganosis, see Chapter 121).[13,16]

A third category involves cutaneous immune reactions to direct penetration of the organism, which may or may not proceed to the further development of active infection. Examples are primarily parasitic, including human hookworm "ground itch," which occurs at the site of primary penetration.[17] When nonhuman helminths, such as feline or canine hookworms, penetrate the skin, they are unable to complete their life cycle and migrate through the epidermis with characteristic serpiginous tracks, called CLM, created by the worm and the local host immune reaction (see Chapter 109). "Swimmer's itch," caused by avian schistosome cercariae penetrating the skin of sensitized people, is another example of an abortive helminthic infection.[18,19] The immunologic nature of the response (immunoglobulin E (IgE)-mediated histamine response in this case) is shown by the absent or minimal reaction in previously unexposed people.[20,21] Similar pruritic reactions occur in human schistosomiasis at the time of cercarial penetration (see Chapter 122).[19] Myiasis and arthropod infestations, such as scabies and lice, are further examples in this category.[22–25] Arthropod bite and sting reactions are similar in that they usually represent a local immune reaction to deposited salivary contents that many vectors use to facilitate their blood meal. Mosquito saliva-specific IgE antibodies have been detected in humans.[26,27]

The fourth pathogenetic category involves dissemination to the skin of toxins produced by infectious agents.[9] The causative microorganisms are typically localized and distant from the skin. Examples are toxic shock syndrome, streptococcal scarlet fever, and staphylococcal scalded skin syndrome (see Chapter 30).[9,28] Depending on the agent involved and the host response, diffuse erythema or vesiculobullous lesions can be seen, at times with associated hemodynamic instability.

The fifth category relates to mechanical disruption of normal cutaneous homeostatic mechanisms resulting in pathologic changes in the skin and its supporting structures. Lymphatic filariasis, with its inflammatory and physical distortion of the normal lymphatic structures, is a good example of this category.[29,30] The resulting lymphedema and increased susceptibility to bacterial infection contribute to skin changes that can occur over time. Similarly, lesions that form ulcers significantly increase the likelihood of secondary bacterial infection, usually prevented by an intact dermal–epidermal layer. This is often compounded by the limited

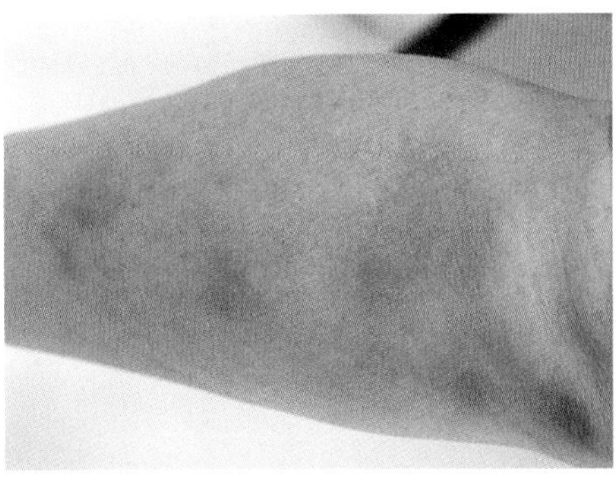

Figure 132.1 Erythema nodosum. (Courtesy of Kenneth J. Tomecki, MD, Cleveland, OH.)

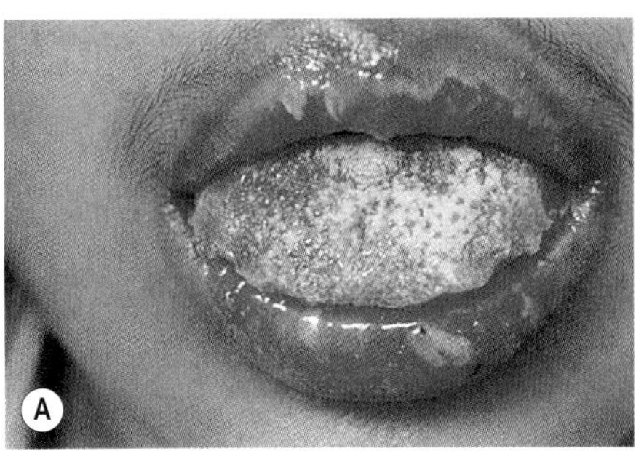

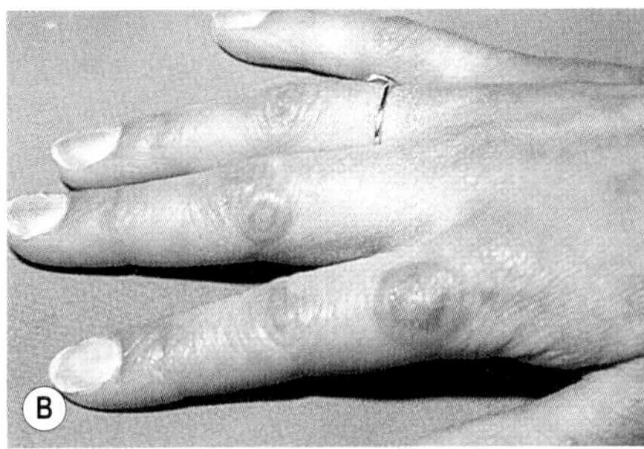

Figure 132.2 Erythema multiforme of the mouth (**A**) and hand (**B**). (Courtesy of Kenneth J. Tomecki, MD, Cleveland, OH.)

hygiene available in many developing countries to both residents and travelers.

A sixth, less well-understood, category involves an apparently systemic immunologic pathogenesis. Examples include erythema nodosum (***Fig. 132.1***), classic erythema multiforme, and Stevens–Johnson syndrome (SJS) (***Fig. 132.2***). In some cases of erythema multiforme, herpes simplex virus or *Mycoplasma pneumoniae* organisms have been found in the skin of such lesions, but most cases lack evidence of demonstrable cutaneous microbial antigen localization or toxin production.[31–38] Infectious, noninfectious, and idiopathic causes are seen in this category. Infectious agents associated with erythema nodosum (***Box 132.1***) and erythema multiforme (***Box 132.2***) include bacteria, mycobacteria, fungi, viruses, and helminths. In addition, many serious cutaneous manifestations due to medications are mediated through this mechanism.[39–41]

Box 132.1 Differential Diagnosis of Erythema Nodosum

Bacteria
- *Bartonella* spp. (cat-scratch disease)
- *Brucella* spp.
- *Chlamydia trachomatis* (lymphogranuloma venereum)
- *Chlamydia psittaci* (psitticosis)
- *Francisella tularensis*
- Streptococcal infections
- *Yersinia* spp., *Campylobacter* spp., *Salmonella* spp. (diarrheal diseases)

Mycobacteria
- *M. tuberculosis*
- *M. leprae*
- *M. marinum*

Viruses
- Cytomegalovirus
- Epstein–Barr virus
- Hepatitis C virus
- Vaccinia (smallpox inoculation agent)

Fungi
- Blastomycosis
- Cryptococcosis
- Coccidioidomycosis
- Histoplasmosis
- *Trichophyton*: deep-seated infection

Protozoa
- *Giardia lamblia*
- Trypanosomiasis, African

Helminths
- *Ascaris lumbricoides*
- Filariases (especially *Wuchereria bancrofti*)

Drugs
- Noninfectious: systemic lupus erythematosus, sarcoid, pregnancy, Crohn's disease, ulcerative colitis, Behçet's syndrome

Idiopathic (up to 40%)

Box 132.2 Causes of Erythema Multiforme[a]

Bacteria
- *Chlamydia* spp.
- *Proteus* spp.
- *Francisella tularensis*
- *Salmonella* spp.
- *Staphylococcus* spp.
- Streptococci, hemolytic
- *Vibrio* spp.
- *Yersinia* spp.
- *Mycoplasma pneumoniae*

Mycobacteria
- *Mycobacterium tuberculosis*

Viruses
- Herpes simplex virus types 1 and 2 (commonly associated)
- Epstein–Barr virus
- Adenovirus
- Coxsackievirus (especially B5)
- Orf virus

Fungi
- Histoplasmosis
- Coccidioidomycosis

Parasites
- Cutaneous larva migrans
- *Trichomonas*

Drugs
- Nonsteroidal anti-inflammatory agents
- Antituberculosis drugs
- Sulfonamides

Case Reports
- Mebendazole, mefloquine, albendazole
- Streptococcal toxic shock syndrome

Idiopathic (up to 50%)

[a]*Important to differentiate from giant urticaria and Stevens–Johnson syndrome (erythema multiforme major).*

GENERAL APPROACH TO THE PATIENT

In approaching patients with rash and tropical exposures, there are three important steps to help define the diagnostic possibilities. First, the patient's general medical and exposure history needs to be obtained.[42] Second, the rash should be accurately defined based on morphology (e.g., macule, papule, vesicle, and nodule), location, and distribution.[43,44] Third, associated clinical information gathered from a complete medical history and physical examination needs to be integrated. Such information includes a medication list, any sensations associated with the rash, pigmentation, migratory nature, duration, and changes in the rash over time. Ancillary clinical information not directly related to the rash must also be considered, including other organ system involvement and the results of laboratory tests.

Patients often present with a specific rash, which provides a starting point for the evaluation and construction of the differential diagnosis.[45,46] The importance of careful characterization of the rash cannot be overemphasized. This chapter is organized to provide important general information regarding the evaluation of patients with rash who have potential infectious diseases exposures and includes tables organized by the character of the specific lesion or primary associated symptom to facilitate the practical usefulness of the information. We focus the text and tables on parasite-associated skin conditions and those nonparasitic conditions that are more prevalent in tropical and subtropical climates.

Most of the tables based on presenting cutaneous manifestations (*Tables 132.6–132.10*) include information about the geographic distribution of the disease entities. They also provide acquisition and incubation information together with parasite survival times to help assess which diagnoses fit the medical history of exposure. Common associated findings are included since cutaneous findings are often not the sole problem but, rather, one aspect of a multisystem disorder. The presence or absence of specific associated findings may also help the provider to focus further evaluation by knowing what other things to look for to rule in or rule out a specific diagnostic consideration.

HISTORY

A detailed history (*Box 132.3*) is the starting point in evaluating a patient with a cutaneous lesion who has traveled abroad. In broad terms, the history has three main components. First is information about the patient, second is information about the patient's exposure to possible pathogens, and third is a detailed history regarding the rash.[47] As a general rule, travel within the past 3 months is more likely to be relevant to the diagnosis of an acute illness than more remote travel.[47,48]

The underlying immune status of the patient also has important implications regarding the differential diagnosis. Immunosuppressed travelers may be at increased risk of acquiring intestinal protozoa, including *Giardia lamblia*, *Isospora belli*, *Entamoeba histolytica*, and *Cryptosporidium*.[49,50] Interestingly, there is little evidence that human immunodeficiency virus (HIV) infection increases the rate of helminthic infection or decreases the efficacy of treatment, with the limited exception of strongyloidiasis.[51] Some infections acquired in the developing world have the potential for reactivation or dissemination years later, especially in the setting of immunosuppression. Examples include coccidioidomycosis, histoplasmosis, hepatitis B, leishmaniasis, strongyloidiasis, and *Trypanosoma cruzi* infection.[52]

Details related to the specific exposures of an individual patient are a crucial aspect of the history. A detailed dietary history is essential. Even if high-risk exposures are not identified, foodborne illnesses such as hepatitis A can be acquired from food preparers who themselves reside in high-risk areas for infections and may contaminate a traveler's food during its preparation.[53]

Because sexually transmitted infections rank high on lists of disease prevalence in travelers (see Chapters 126 and 138), a sexual history is an essential part of the exposure evaluation.[1,54] This should include inquiry regarding the use of condoms. Moreover, many sexually transmitted infections, such as primary HIV, syphilis, and the group of genital ulcerative conditions, have prominent cutaneous findings (*Table 132.1 and Fig. 132.3D*).

Vector exposure related to geography, types of vectors present, and intensity of exposure all need to be considered. Many tropical diseases have very defined distributions (even to regions within countries), making geographic exposure very important. Emerging infections (e.g., dengue, chikungunya, West Nile, Zika virus) and reemerging ones (measles, *Staphylococcus aureus* – including methicillin-resistant *S. aureus*) represent challenging concerns as international travel increases exposure to these pathogens with broader geographic distributions.[55–57] Of note, fever and rash are prominent presentations for most of this group of infections.

Recent exposure is typically most important, especially exposure within the past 3 months.[58] However, as noted in the tables, malaria, many helminths, and other tropically acquired pathogens can persist for months to years in the human host, requiring their consideration in selected clinical settings well beyond the actual time of travel.[42] In such cases, the presentation is typically subacute or chronic, although it may be punctuated by acute episodic illness.

Box 132.3 Important Historical Aspects Regarding Etiologies of Rash

Patient Demographics

- Age, sex, occupation
- Reason for travel (vacation versus business versus other)
- Medications, allergies, immunizations
- Pretravel evaluation (compliance with pretravel recommendations?)
- Medical conditions that may alter immune status
- Time interval from travel dates to onset of symptoms

Exposure Histories

- Geographic location, description of location, duration of exposure
- Vector exposures (precautions taken?)
- Animal exposures (wild versus domestic)
- List of items purchased (e.g., animal hide rugs, nickel-containing jewelry)
- Sexual contact with new partners
- Parenteral exposure (e.g., vaccine or injection abroad, acupuncture, tattoos, poultices on open sores)

If Immigrant

- Country of origin
- Age on arrival in developed country
- Frequency and duration of return visits

Rash-related Information

- Prodromal symptoms
- Character, distribution, progression, including speed and physical pattern
- Relation to fever
- Previous treatment and efficacy

Table 132.1 Dermatologic Manifestations of Sexually Transmitted Diseases

Disease	Ulcer	Nodule	Maculopapular	Pigment Change	Lymphadenopathy	Other
Chancroid	X (p)				X (p, L)	
Donovanosis	X (nt)					
Gonorrhea			If disseminated			
Granuloma inguinale	X (nt)	X			Pseudobubo	Occasional painful necrotic ulcer
HIV			1°		X (nt, G)	
Herpes simplex virus	X (p)					Vesicle ulcerates
Lymphogranuloma venereum	X (nt)	X			X (p, L)	
Syphilis, endemic (bejel)	X (nt)	X		↓ (late)	X (G)	
Syphilis, venereal	X (nt)		2°		2° (L, G)	Occasional oropharyngeal mucous patches
Yaws	X (nt)		X	↓ (late)	X (L)	
Scabies		X	X			

X, lesion develops; G, generalized lymphadenopathy; HIV, human immunodeficiency virus; L, localized lymphadenopathy; nt, nontender; p, painful; 1°, primary disease; 2°, secondary disease; ↓, hypopigmented.

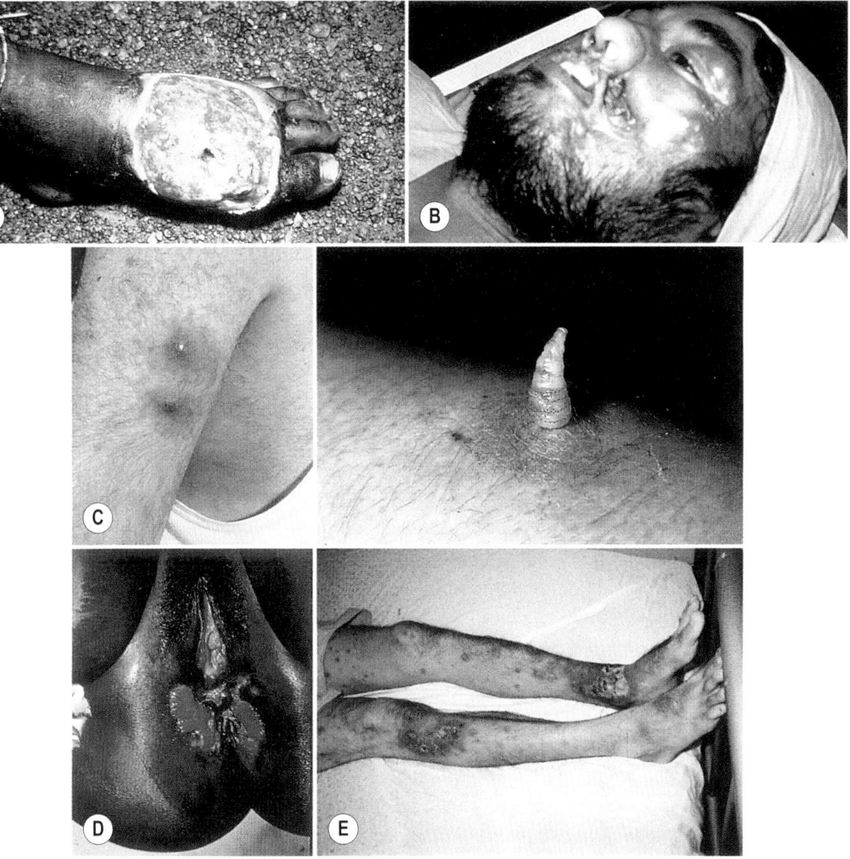

Figure 132.3 **(A)** Tropical phagedenic ulcer. **(B)** Buruli ulcer. **(C)** Myiasis extruding larva. **(D)** Granuloma inguinale. **(E)** South American blastomycosis (paracoccidioidomycosis). ((**A–C**) Courtesy of Jay S. Keystone, MD. (**D** and **E**) Courtesy of R. L. Guerrant, MD, Charlottesville, VA.)

Understanding the life cycles of parasitic pathogens is important when obtaining the history, as the life cycle may predict when a traveler becomes ill. For example, *Loa loa*-associated symptoms often require at least 6 months to appear and can first present as late as 18 months after the last possible exposure (see Chapter 105).[59] Because of an autoinfective cycle, *Strongyloides stercoralis* infections (see Chapter 117) acquired decades earlier can result in risk to people who require immunosuppression many years after their disease exposure and acquisition.[60,61]

Another exposure-related issue is whether the patient is a lifelong resident of a developed country or has emigrated there recently or remotely. Expatriates are more likely to have an allergic-hypersensitivity reaction to *L. loa* infection compared to the local population.[62] The frequency and duration of return visits to tropical areas may be very important information in creating the proper differential diagnosis. Malaria may be more frequent and severe in people who have returned to an endemic area after several years away. People traveling to visit family and relatives in malarious countries are often less rigorous about seeking pretravel advice and using prophylactic medication (see Chapter 126). Rarely, the index patient being evaluated has not had exposures in parasite endemic regions but has become infected via contacts through a friend or worker. For example, cysticercosis in Orthodox Jewish community members in New York who had not traveled outside the United States was attributable to household employees from endemic areas in Central America.[63]

Questioning the patient about unusual situations or risky behaviors may uncover relevant events, such as ingestion of raw seafood or questionable medical interventions. Acupuncture with unsterilized needles carries a risk of hepatitis and HIV transmission. A peculiar route of acquisition of sparganosis is seen when raw frog flesh is used as a poultice (see Chapter 121). Physicians unaware of alternative medical practices of some immigrant populations usually do not consider such a route of exposure when obtaining a history. Asking about souvenirs purchased may reveal exposure to animal products (e.g., animal skin rugs) that carry the risk of disease transmission, such as brucellosis or anthrax, or to new materials (e.g., nickel-containing jewelry) that can result in allergic contact skin reactions.[64]

Occasionally, the history may help to point to an obsessional concern about the presence of parasites without other evidence to support such a diagnosis, and the possibility of delusional parasitosis should be considered (see Chapter 140).[65,66]

Specific questions about the rash and any associated clinical symptoms, such as fever pattern, weight loss, diarrhea, and response to any attempted treatments, are also important. The symptoms related to the rash may, at times, provide important diagnostic clues. For example, patients with myiasis (see Chapter 124), produced by cutaneous invasion by larvae of the bot fly in Latin America (***Fig. 132.3C***) or tumbu fly in Africa often present with papules, nodules, and subcutaneous swellings and will frequently describe a sensation of movement and intermittent pain at the site of the lesion.

PHYSICAL EXAMINATION

A complete physical examination is important since cutaneous manifestations may be only one component of a systemic disorder. The entire skin should be examined with attention to the elements listed in ***Box 132.4***. Repeated examination over time may be necessary. The rapidity of spread of a rash can have implications regarding the aggressiveness of the evaluation. The general level of a patient's toxicity and the nature, tempo, and pattern of the rash dictate the initial evaluation and therapeutic approach. Although only 7% of cases with petechiae and fever will turn out to be meningococcemia,[67] the life-threatening nature of meningococcal disease requires an aggressive evaluation and often empirical therapy when this diagnosis is a consideration (see Chapter 24).[8,9]

The classification of the rash is often the focal entry point into the creation of a differential diagnosis.[4,5,68] As a result, the primary and secondary characteristics of the rash should be carefully determined (*Box 132.4*). Some rashes are fleetingly present, such as *Salmonella* spp. rose spots. Other rashes may evolve in relatively unique patterns over time, such as anthrax, Rocky Mountain spotted fever (RMSF), and dengue.[22,69–73] For example, cutaneously acquired anthrax (see Chapter 38) characteristically evolves from a papule to a vesicle with surrounding brawny, gelatinous edema, and occasional satellite vesicles[69,70] (*Fig. 132.4*). The lesion then progresses to hemorrhage and necrosis, eventually turning into an eschar. RMSF skin changes are often absent in the first few days of clinical illness. Then a macular rash typically starts on the wrists and ankles with centripetal spread (see Chapter 49).[22] During progression, the rash usually becomes petechial or purpuric or both (*Fig. 132.5*). Dengue fever rash often begins as a transient macular exanthem approximately 24 hours after the abrupt onset of fever (see Chapter 75). Three or 4 days later, a generalized maculopapular truncal rash appears, with centripetal spread, sparing the palms and soles (*Fig. 132.6*). This rash may become petechial and may even desquamate.[71–73]

The original and subsequent distribution of the rash, consideration of mucosal (enanthem) or genital involvement, and other associated physical findings may be helpful in establishing a diagnosis. The presence of lymphadenopathy (*Box 132.5*) and splenomegaly or hepatosplenomegaly

Box 132.4 Important Aspects of the Physical Examination in the Patient with Rash

Vital signs	• Size
General appearance	• Scale on surface
• Level of toxicity to establish tempo of evaluation and therapy	• Other
Primary character of the rash	Location of primary lesion, if any
• Petechial or hemorrhagic	Distribution of rash
• Macular	Direction of spread (centripetal or centrifugal)
• Papular	Mucosal or conjunctival involvement
• Migratory	Genital involvement
• Urticarial	Associated physical findings
• Nodular	• Visible parasite at the site of the rash
• Ulcerative	• Lymphadenopathy
Secondary character of the rash	• Splenomegaly or hepatosplenomegaly
• Shape (linear versus circular versus irregular)	

Box 132.5 Differential Diagnosis of Infections with Rash and Lymphadenopathy

Helminths
- Lymphatic filariasis
  - *Brugia malayi*
  - *B. timori*
  - *Wuchereria bancrofti*
- Loiasis
- Mansonelliasis
- Onchocerciasis
- Opisthorchiasis
- Schistosomiasis (Katayama fever)

Protozoa
- Leishmaniasis
  - Cutaneous and mucocutaneous
  - Visceral
- Toxoplasmosis
- Trypanosomiasis
  - African
  - American

Fungi
- Coccidioidomycosis
- Chromomycosis
- Cryptococcosis
- Histoplasmosis
- Lobomycosis
- Paracoccidioidomycosis
- Penicilliosis marneffei
- Sporotrichosis

Bacteria
- Numerous

Viruses
- Numerous, including primary human immunodeficiency virus

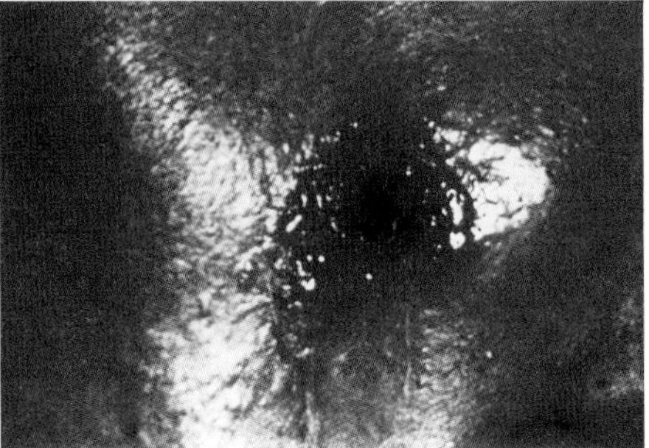

Figure 132.4 Cutaneous anthrax showing characteristic central eschar with surrounding edema and vesicles. (Courtesy of Kenneth J. Tomecki, MD, Cleveland, OH.)

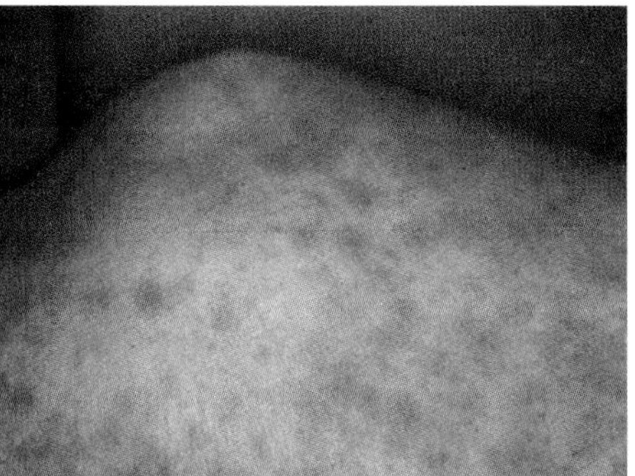

Figure 132.5 Early macular rash of Rocky Mountain spotted fever. Papular and petechial changes are often seen. The rash typically begins around the wrists and ankles.

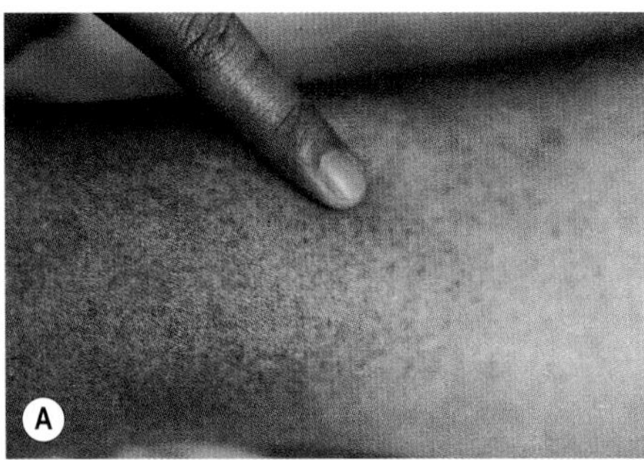

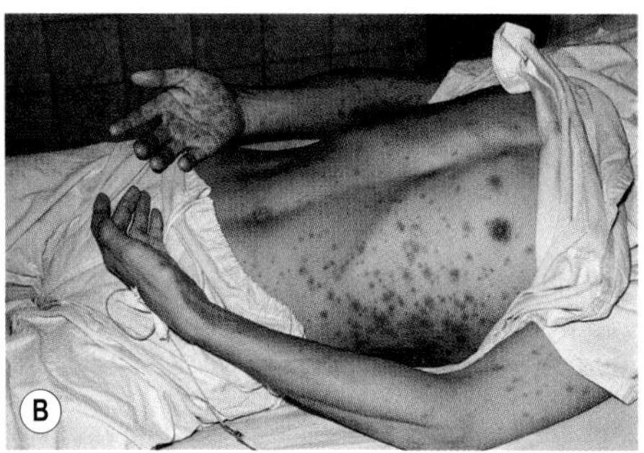

Figure 132.6 Cutaneous manifestations of dengue. **(A)** Early maculopapular nonpruritic rash usually seen at the time of defervescence. **(B)** Late hemorrhagic and purpuric skin changes of a patient with dengue hemorrhagic fever. (Courtesy of James H. Maguire, MD, Centers for Disease Control and Prevention, Atlanta, GA.)

(*Box 132.6*) are examples of findings that may help focus the evaluation. If a primary lesion or an inoculation site can be determined, it should be given careful attention. For example, an eschar would indicate rickettsial disease or anthrax (*Table 132.2*), whereas periorbital swelling in a child soon after a visit to rural Brazil would focus the evaluation on Chagas' disease. Despite these examples in which the appearance of the rash can point to the diagnosis, the appearance of the rash is often not pathognomonic of a single disease entity.

Characterizing the Rash

Careful identification of the primary and secondary characteristics of the rash will facilitate creating a differential diagnosis, especially when integrated with the clinical history and any associated physical findings. After defining the rash, the reader should refer to the table related to that characteristic to help with diagnosing the individual patient. The role of tropical exposures is highlighted here. Significant medical conditions with prominent cutaneous manifestations may be due to common pathogens with worldwide distribution despite exposure to specific tropical pathogens. For example, although petechiae in the recently returned febrile traveler may represent malaria, dengue, or even Lassa fever, it is still crucial to consider meningococcemia, rickettsial disease, and other diagnoses. Life-threatening diagnoses with cutaneous manifestations are seen throughout the temperate and tropical world (*Table 132.3*).[8,9]

Hemorrhage and Petechiae

Hemorrhagic or petechial rashes (*Table 132.4*) must be considered of life-threatening importance and evaluated rapidly.[8,9,22] Although many nonlethal rashes have this presentation, it is difficult, if not impossible, to rule out serious pathogens at the initial evaluation. Worldwide, meningococcemia is the most important cause of life-threatening disease presenting with fever and cutaneous hemorrhage or petechiae (see Chapter 24). Infection-mediated petechial or purpuric lesions may arise directly from infected emboli or via an indirect immunologic mechanism.

Box 132.6 Differential Diagnosis of Rash with Splenomegaly or Hepatosplenomegaly

Organomegaly Commonly Associated	Organomegaly Occasionally Associated
Brucellosis	Cytomegalovirus infection
Ehrlichiosis	Histoplasmosis
Epstein–Barr virus infection	Leptospirosis
Glanders (*Burkholderia mallei*)	Malaria
Leishmaniasis, visceral	Psittacosis
Penicilliosis (*Penicillium marneffei*)	Rocky Mountain spotted fever (*Rickettsia rickettsii*)
Q fever	Typhoid fever
Relapsing fever (*Borrelia recurrentis*)	Scrub typhus (*R. tsutsugamushi*)
Schistosomiasis (*Schistosoma mansoni, S. japonicum*)	**Organomegaly Rarely Associated**
Trypanosomiasis (*Trypanosoma cruzi*)	Babesiosis
	Drug reaction
	Serum sickness

Table 132.2 Diagnostic Considerations in the Patient with an Eschar

Pathogen	Condition (Vector)
Rickettsia africae	African tick bite fever
R. akari	Rickettsialpox (mite)
R. australis	Queensland coastal fever (tick)
R. conorii	Mediterranean spotted fever (tick)
R. sibirica	North Asian tick typhus
R. tsutsugamushi	Scrub typhus (mite)
Bacillus anthracis	Anthrax[a]
Loxosceles reclusa	Brown recluse spider bite

[a]Usually transmitted by contact with infected animals or their products, rarely mechanically via biting flies or insects.

Table 132.3 Life-threatening Conditions with Cutaneous Manifestations

Cutaneous Manifestation	Pathogen	Time to Appearance (after Onset of Illness)	Pathophysiology
Peripheral gangrene	Gram-negative bacteria	12–36 hours	Vascular thrombosis due to shock
Scattered, multiple petechiae and purpura	*Neisseria meningitidis* *Rickettsia rickettsii* Gram-negative bacteria	12–36 hours (later for *Rickettsia*)	Vascular invasion (?) Schwartzman reaction
Ecthyma gangrenosum	*Pseudomonas* spp. Gram-negative bacteria	Days	Vascular invasion, mostly venous
Asymmetrical scattered maculopapular rash	*N. meningitidis* *N. gonorrhoeae*	3–10 days	Immune vasculitis due to immune complex deposition
Polymorphous lesions	*N. meningitidis* *N. gonorrhoeae* *Salmonella* spp.	3–10 days	Immune vasculitis
Rose spots	*Salmonella* spp.	5–10 days	Immune vasculitis
Osler's nodes; small (<1 cm) painful nodular erythema	*Staphylococcus aureus*	Days to weeks	Emboli from endocarditis with microabscesses
Janeway lesions: painless, purpuric or pustular, infarcted lesions	*Streptococcus* spp. *S. aureus*	Days to weeks	Emboli from endocarditis
Diffuse toxic erythema	*S. aureus* *Streptococcus pyogenes*	Minutes	Vascular toxin with peripheral vasodilation
Macronodules	*Candida* spp.	Several days	Vascular invasion of dermis
Progressive petechiae and purpura (distinctive periumbilical purpura)	*Strongyloides stercoralis* (hyperinfection syndrome)	Hours to days from immunosuppression	? Larval skin penetration ? Immune vasculitis
Petechiae, purpura, hemorrhage	Viral hemorrhagic fevers	Within 3 weeks of exposure	Immune vasculitis; disseminated intravascular coagulation, thrombocytopenia, decreased clotting factor synthesis

Table 132.4 Differential Diagnosis of a Petechial or Purpuric Rash after Travel or Tropical Exposure

Organism	Disease	Comment
Bacteria		
Borrelia spp.	Relapsing fever	
Enterococcus, viridans streptococci	Endocarditis	HACEK organisms as well
Haemophilus influenzae, H. aegyptius	Brazilian purpuric fever	Purulent conjunctivitis; mostly children ages 1–4 years
Leptospira interrogans		
Neisseria meningitidis	Meningococcemia	
N. gonorrhoeae	Gonococcemia	
Burkholderia pseudomallei	Melioidosis	
Pseudomonas aeruginosa	Ecthyma gangrenosum	
Streptobacillus moniliformis	Rat bite fever	Different from *Spirillum minus*
Treponema pallidum	Syphilis (especially congenital)	
Yersinia pestis	Plague (septicemic)	"Black death" referred to purpura
Rickettsia prowazekii	Epidemic typhus	
R. typhi	Murine typhus	
R. rickettsii	Rocky Mountain spotted fever	Often on wrists and ankles
Vibrio vulnificus		
Viruses		
Alphaviruses		
Enteroviruses		
Cytomegalovirus		Especially congenital
Colorado tick fever		
Measles	Atypical measles	
Lassa fever		
Dengue		
Junin	Argentine hemorrhagic fever	
Machupo	Bolivian hemorrhagic fever	
Chikungunya		
Crimean-Congo hemorrhagic fever		Tick bite; contact with infected blood
Ebola		
Hantavirus	Hemorrhagic fever with renal syndrome	Aerosol from rodent excreta
Kyasanur Forest		
Marburg		
Omsk hemorrhagic fever		
Rift Valley fever		Mosquito bite; aerosol or contact with fresh carcasses of infected animals
Yellow fever		
Protozoa		
Plasmodium falciparum	Malaria	
Toxoplasma gondii	Toxoplasmosis	Especially congenital
Helminths		
Trichinella spiralis	Trichinellosis	

Thrombocytopenia from a variety of causes, including adverse drug reactions, may also lead to purpuric or petechial lesions.

Macules and Papules

Macules are flat lesions with altered pigmentation less than 1 cm in size. A patch is a macule greater than 1 cm in diameter. A papule is a solid elevated lesion less than 1 cm in diameter, whereas a plaque is used to describe a similar lesion larger than 1 cm or a group of confluent papules.

Macules, papules, and maculopapular eruptions are the most common cutaneous manifestations of infectious diseases and imply an inflammatory response to the inciting pathogen. Viral and bacterial diseases are the most common causes (*Table 132.5*).[74] Some specific tropical bacterial and viral disorders associated with macular, papular, or maculopapular rashes include anthrax, bartonellosis (*Fig. 132.7*), brucellosis, glanders, leptospirosis, Lyme disease, melioidosis, plague, relapsing fever, *Rickettsia*

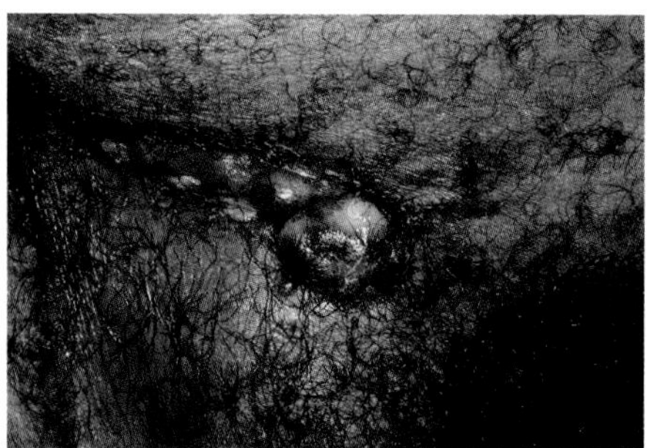

Figure 132.7 Bacillary angiomatosis in a patient with human immunodeficiency virus infection. Typical friable, exophytic papulonodular changes and violaceous hue are noted. (Courtesy of Karim A. Adal, MD, Minneapolis, MN.)

Table 132.5 Differential Diagnosis of Macular and Maculopapular Rashes after Travel or Tropical Exposure

Organism/Agent	Disease
Epstein–Barr virus	Mononucleosis
Dengue virus	Dengue fever[a]
Lassa fever virus	Lassa fever
Marburg virus	
West Nile virus	West Nile fever[b]
Rickettsia typhi	Endemic (murine) typhus
R. prowazekii	Epidemic (louse) typhus
R. quintana	Trench fever
Coxiella burnetii	Q fever
Bacillus anthracis	Anthrax[a]
Spirillum minus	Rat bite fever
Streptobacillus moniliformis	Rat bite fever
Leptospira spp.	Leptospirosis
Yersinia pestis	Plague
Salmonella typhi	Typhoid fever (rose spots)
Borrelia burgdorferi	Lyme disease, erythema chronicum migrans
B. recurrentis	Relapsing fever
Bartonella bacilliformis	Bartonellosis
Brucella spp.	Brucellosis
Treponema pallidum	Syphilis (secondary syphilis)
Coccidioides immitis	Coccidioidomycosis
Toxoplasma gondii	Toxoplasmosis
Strongyloides stercoralis	Strongyloidiasis
Onchocerca volvulus	Onchocerciasis
Leishmania spp.	Leishmaniasis (some with visceral, rare with cutaneous)
Ancylostoma duodenale and *Necator americanus*	Hookworm disease
Human immunodeficiency virus (HIV)	Primary HIV infection
Drug	

[a]Only at onset; later, hemorrhage.
[b]50% rash late in course of 3–6-day fever.

infections (especially typhus and trench fever), tularemia, yaws, meningococcemia, dengue, rat bite fever, secondary syphilis, tuberculosis, and *Vibrio vulnificus* infection. Many other viral pathogens acquired in the tropics are commonly associated with maculopapular eruptions. Most of the viral hemorrhagic fevers progress from macular exanthems to a maculopapular form prior to developing a hemorrhagic appearance.[71,73,75] The acute illness associated with HIV seroconversion may be accompanied by a transient maculopapular dermatitis in approximately 50% of patients.[76,77] Protozoan parasites rarely cause macular or papular rashes. The exceptions are toxoplasmosis, African trypanosomiasis, and some forms of both cutaneous and visceral leishmaniasis[78–83] (***Fig. 132.8***). Fungal infections usually manifest a nodular or ulcerative appearance (***Fig. 132.3E***);[83] however, coccidioidomycosis may have a maculopapular presentation.[84] Helminthic infections rarely have a papular or macular appearance, although some forms of chronic onchocerciasis occasionally present this way.[13,85,86] Arthropod bites (e.g., mosquito bites) and infestations (e.g., scabies), together with water-related exposures to some diatoms, venomous fish, jellyfish, or sea urchins, commonly result in a toxin-mediated papular eruption.[18,22,23] This type of rash is also common in the setting of drug hypersensitivity reactions.[39] Some arthropod bites/exposures may persist for weeks as immunologic reactions (e.g., papular urticaria) beyond the actual exposure, without indicating persistence of the organism. Fever is seen with many, although not all, skin reactions manifesting as macules or papules, possibly reflective of the systemic immune mechanism responsible for many maculopapular rashes.

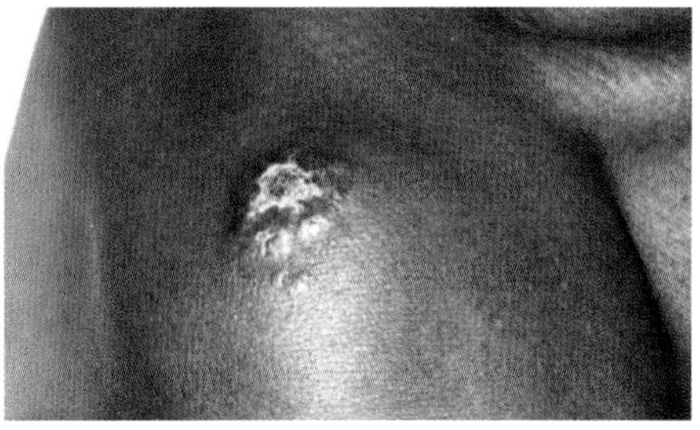

Figure 132.8 Cutaneous leishmaniasis lesion demonstrating characteristic painless papular, nodular, and ulcerative lesions with serum crusting.

Migratory Rash

Migratory lesions are somewhat unique to parasites (***Table 132.6***)[17,87–90] and represent a common cause of cutaneous lesions in travelers to tropical countries.[5] In some cases, such as cutaneous and visceral larva migrans (see Chapter 109),[91] humans are accidental hosts. The parasite is hence unable to complete its normal life cycle, resulting in continued wandering of the infecting larva through the skin.[69] CLM (***Fig. 132.9A and B***) is often due to canine and feline hookworms (*Ancylostoma braziliense* and *A. caninum*) species. Human hookworms (***Fig. 132.9C***) (*A. duodenale* and *Necator americanus*) (see Chapter 116) and *Strongyloides stercoralis* (see Chapter 117) will occasionally manifest skin changes during initial or reinfective cutaneous penetration.[17,92] Other uncommon etiologies of CLM-like rashes include *S. myopotami* (a zoonotic *Strongyloides*), *Gnathostoma spinigerum*, and hookworms of cattle (*Bunostomum phlebotomum*) and European dogs (*Unicinaria stenocephala*). Since parasite-associated eosinophilia is primarily related to the tissue migratory phase of helminths, the above helminth infections causing migratory cutaneous lesions often elicit a marked eosinophilia[93–95] (see Chapter 131). *Dracunculus medinensis* may produce superficial migratory skin lesions at the completion of its life cycle, prior to expulsion of the adult through the skin.[13] Lyme disease (see Chapter 44) may present with an expanding macular rash – erythema chronicum migrans.[96]

Pruritus and Urticaria

A common manifestation of inflammatory skin conditions is pruritus (***Table 132.7***). Often, the inciting pathogen, drug, or irritant causes an immune response characterized by IgE production and subsequent histamine release by mast cells in sensitized people. As a result, pruritus is often accompanied by urticarial lesions. Classic syndromes include the intense itching seen following exposure to avian schistosome cercariae in IgE-sensitized people (swimmer's itch)[18,19] and the pruritic migratory angioedema seen with *L. loa* infections[62] (***Fig. 132.10***). Most helminthic parasites are capable of inducing an urticarial response, although it is uncommon. Helminthic infections where humans are accidental hosts, such as CLM, gnathostomiasis, and sparganosis, are likely to present this way due to the continued presence of the parasite in the skin. Human helminthic infections with cutaneous penetrating or cutaneous resident parasites, such as hookworm, strongyloidiasis, onchocerciasis, and loiasis, also frequently cause pruritus and urticaria. Hence, there is overlap with many of the migratory parasites. Some myiasis infestations are pruritic, especially when the larvae move.[97,98] Pruritus and/or urticaria are rare presentations of *Giardia lamblia*, but its worldwide distribution and relative prevalence reinforce the need for consideration of this parasite in the differential diagnosis. Humans can develop specific IgE antibodies to mosquito saliva and some people may benefit from prophylactic administration of antihistamines, resulting in less intense bite reactions.[25] Travelers to tropical climates may experience a noninfectious condition known as miliaria rubra (prickly heat) with characteristic tiny itchy papules or vesicles on an erythematous base concentrated on the trunk and in flexure areas.[83]

Table 132.6 Differential Diagnosis of Migratory Skin Lesions

Cause of Migratory Lesions	Distribution	Acquisition	Incubation and Time of Symptoms (sx)	Parasite Survival	Common Associated Findings	Additional Information
Cutaneous larva migrans ("creeping eruption") Larval movement of zoonotic nematodes	Worldwide (especially tropics, subtropics)	Skin contact with contaminated soil (especially beaches)	Usually 2–3 days (range, 1–6 days)	Weeks–months	Eosinophilia; serpiginous skin lesions; may migrate up to several cm/day	Dog and cat hookworms, zoonotic *Strongyloides*; larvae cannot mature, wander in skin
Dracunculiasis Adult worm moves below dermis before eruption	Sub-Saharan Africa	Ingestion of copepod in drinking water	~1 year	12–18 months	Eosinophilia; dead calcified worms on radiograph	Adults exit via skin; blisters that rarely ulcerate
Fascioliasis Migratory inflammatory lesions	Worldwide except Oceania; sheep- and cattle-raising areas mostly	Ingestion of metacercariae on watercress or other in-water plants	3–4 months	≥10 years	Eosinophilia, ↑ LFTs, anemia. Early: fever, RUQ pain, jaundice, hepatomegaly	Rare extrabiliary migration; nodules up to 6 cm
Gnathostomiasis Migratory inflammatory lesions	Asia (especially Thailand and Japan); sporadic worldwide	Ingestion of larva in undercooked meat or infected copepod in water; rare skin penetration	GI sx: 1–2 days; soft-tissue swelling in 3–4 weeks Other sx: months to years	≥10 years	Eosinophilia common; can migrate anywhere, including CNS	Larva cannot mature, migrates in tissues at 1 cm/h, or faster when subcutaneous
Hookworm Larval movement during inoculation	Worldwide (especially tropics, subtropics)	Skin contact with contaminated soil	Local skin sx: 1–2 days; lung sx: 1–3 weeks; GI sx: ~4 weeks	*Ancylostoma duodenale*: 1 year *Necator americanus*: 2–6 years	Eosinophilia during tissue migration; anemia	Gross or occult blood in stools; eggs appear in 4–6 weeks
Loiasis Migratory subcutaneous swellings	Central and West Africa	Bite of infected *Chrysops* fly	~1 year (range, 4 months to 8 years)	10 years	Eosinophilia? ↑IgE; expatriates have more hypersensitivity sx	5–6 months until microfilariae seen in blood
Paragonamiasis Subcutaneous migratory swellings or nodules	Sub-Saharan and southern Africa; Americas; East and Southeast Asia	Ingestion of metacercariae in raw or undercooked crustaceans	Lung sx : 6 months CNS sx: 12–16 months	≤10 years	Eosinophilia 80%; CXR very variable	Eggs in sputum, feces, pleural or spinal fluid, first appear in 10 weeks
Sparganosis Larval movement	Worldwide (especially tropics; most cases Southeast Asia)	Ingestion of infected copepod in water or undercooked meat; use of infected flesh as poultice on open wound	Depends on route of acquisition	≥9 years	Eosinophilia and leukocytosis during migration	Larvae cannot mature but can migrate anywhere, including CNS
Strongyloidiasis (*Strongyloides stercoralis*) Migratory, serpiginous lesions of larva	Worldwide (especially tropics, subtropics)	Skin or mucous membrane contact with contaminated soil	Skin and lung sx: days to decades Other sx: days to decades	Indefinite (autoreinfection possible)	Eosinophilia; skin changes (larva currens) even in chronic infection; can migrate up to 5–10 cm/hour	Ex-POWs and others from endemic areas can carry asymptomatically for decades
Myiasis Visible movement of maggot(s) or larva(e)	Worldwide (especially tropics)	Dependent on fly species; contact with infected arthropods, vegetation, food, clothes; direct inoculation	Depends on fly: *Cordylobia anthropophaga* 7–10 days; *Dermatobia hominis* 5–12 weeks	≥2 months	Movement of maggot(s) within the lesion may be visible; larvae of some *Diptera* migrate in soft tissues	Adult leaves host when mature

↑ increased; LFT, liver function test(s); RUQ, right upper quadrant; GI, gastrointestinal; CNS, central nervous system; CXR, chest X-ray film; POWs, prisoners of war.

Table 132.7 Differential Diagnosis of Pruritic and Urticarial Skin Lesions

Cause of Pruritic Lesions	Distribution	Acquisition	Incubation and Time of Symptoms (sx)	Organism Survival	Common Associated Findings	Additional Information
Helminthic						
Cercarial dermatitis; avian schistosome dermatitis	Worldwide (for all species salt and fresh water)	Skin contact with cercariae in water	Hours	Unable to survive in human host		Avian and other schistosomes; sx more severe with repeated exposure
Cutaneous larva migrans	See Table 132.6					
Dracunculiasis	See Table 132.6					
Gnathostomiasis	See Table 132.6					
Hookworm	See Table 132.6					
Loiasis	See Table 132.6					
Onchocerciasis Severe, persistent pruritus	Sub-Saharan Africa, Mexico, Central and tropical South America, Yemen, Saudi Arabia	Bite of infected black fly	1–2 years	Microfilariae: 2–3 years Adult: 10–15 years	Eosinophilia Skin nodules common	Microfilariae reside in skin
Pinworms ("pruritus ani") Perianal adult worm movement	Worldwide	Ingestion of infective eggs	4–6 weeks	≥ Months; autoreinfection common	Nocturnal perianal itching; often not associated rash	Diagnosis by tape test
Schistomiasis (early)	Asia, Africa, Caribbean, tropical South America	Skin contact with cercariae in water	Skin sx: hours; Katayama fever[a] 2–10 weeks	3–10 years	Eosinophilia early	
Strongyloidiasis	See Table 132.6					
Trypanosomiasis, African	Regions in sub-Saharan Africa	Bite of infected tsetse fly	Chancre at bite site starts in 2–3 days, lasts 2–4 weeks; 2–3 weeks to fever	Years	Rash common, mostly on trunk; recurrent fevers; generalized LN; anemia	Diagnosis difficult; elevated IgM in both serum and CSF when CNS involved
Trichinellosis	Worldwide	Ingestion of undercooked meat with larvae	10–20 days (range, 1–76 days)	Cysts viable in muscle 5–10 years	First week: diarrhea, abdominal pain Second week: fever, myalgia, periorbital edema, eosinophilia	Encysted larvae do not cause symptoms; most cases asymptomatic
Protozoan						
Amebiasis	Worldwide	Cyst ingestion from contaminated food or water	1–3 weeks (range, 3 days to months)	Months		Rare presentation
Giardiasis	Worldwide	Cyst ingestion from contaminated food or water	1–3 weeks (range, 1 day to 6 weeks)	Weeks to months	Malabsorption sx predominate; diarrhea; occasional chronic GI sx	Rare presentation; common cause of chronic diarrhea after travel
Bacterial						
Relapsing fevers (*Borrelia* spp. infections)	Louse: Africa, South America, Asia Tick: worldwide except Caribbean and Oceania	Contact with infected louse (hemolymph of crushed louse); tick bite	7–8 days (range, 2–18 days)	Months	Relapsing fevers last 4–10 days; relapses milder Louse: 1–5 relapses Tick: 1–13 relapses	Louse: case fatality in epidemics 40% Louse and tick: mortality with treatment 2–5%

Table 132.7 Differential Diagnosis of Pruritic and Urticarial Skin Lesions—cont'd

Cause of Pruritic Lesions	Distribution	Acquisition	Incubation and Time of Symptoms (sx)	Organism Survival	Common Associated Findings	Additional Information
Pinta	Central and South America	Close contact with an infected person	7–21 days (range, 8–60 days)	≥10 years	Slowly enlarging papules over weeks to months; regional LN; papulosquamous rash 3–12 months later with generalized LN; depigmented macules months to years later with atrophic scars	50% of infections subclinical; VDRL and FTA-ABS used as with syphilis
Typhus fever (*Rickettsia prowazekii*)	Worldwide	Infected louse feces enter mucosal surface or break in skin	10–14 days (range, 5–23 days)	Lifetime of host	Fever, severe HA, myalgias; maculopapular rash starts on trunk on days 4–7, spreads to extremities	Infection of endothelial cells → vasculitis; Brill–Zinsser (recrudescent) disease: milder sx, fever 7–12 days less rash
Secondary syphilis	Worldwide	Contact with infectious lesions; usually sexually transmitted, rarely by blood transfusion	2–4 weeks from onset of primary lesion (range, 10 days to years)	Lifetime of host	Chancre early; skin and mucous membrane lesions weeks to months later	Protean manifestations
Rat bite fever (*Spirillum minus*)	Worldwide	Bite or close contact with infected rat	1–3 weeks (range, 5–40 days)	Months	Bite site heals, then suppurates/ulcerates; rash in 75%, most prominent near bite, reddish brown to purple	Can cause false-positive VDRL: organism, best seen by dark-field examination
Plague	Worldwide except Australia	Bite of infected flea or infected animal; inhalation of fomites from an infected patient	2–3 days pneumonic, 2–7 days bubonic (range, 1–14 days)	No long-term carriage	Abrupt onset of fever, chills, HA, and GI sx; hours later buboes form (no buboes in septicemic form); WBC may reach 50 000; CXR: diffuse interstitial infiltrate; infarcts, hemorrhagic and necrotic nodules common	Fleas infectious for months; can contact disease without travel; hunting and skinning animals a risk
Viral						
Hepatitis B	Worldwide	Sexual contact; blood and blood-contaminated objects; mucous membrane contact with infected material; transplacental	2–3 months	Usually weeks; uncommon chronic carriage	Often no sx; jaundice, anorexia, diarrhea; 5–10% of cases have urticarial rash with arthralgia or arthritis	Chronic infection increases risk of hepatocellular cancer
Arthropod Bite and Infestations						
Myiasis (*Diptera* fly larva)	Worldwide	Deposition of eggs directly, or via arthropod or inanimate vector	Days to weeks	2 months; larvae leave host when adult	Local swelling and redness; occasional 2° bacterial infection	Some forms cause local tissue necrosis
Tungiasis (*Tunga penetrans*)	Tropical Central and South America, Caribbean, Africa, Asia	Skin penetration by larva of female sand flea	8–12 days	Up to 1 month (flea dies after laying eggs)	Local pain and swelling usually on feet; tiny black spot at site of penetration	Inflammatory reaction to dead flea can persist; can result in tetanus and rarely gas gangrene

Table 132.7 Differential Diagnosis of Pruritic and Urticarial Skin Lesions—cont'd

Cause of Pruritic Lesions	Distribution	Acquisition	Incubation and Time of Symptoms (sx)	Organism Survival	Common Associated Findings	Additional Information
Fleas	Worldwide	Flea bite (usually unnoticed)	Hours to days		Urticarial papules; papulovesicles/bullae (can persist for weeks)	Skin lesions often found in clusters
Lice (*Pediculus humanus, Phthirus pubis*)	Worldwide	Close physical contact with infected person	Days to weeks	Months[b] (life cycle: 3–4 weeks)	Papular urticaria; nits (eggs) found on hair shaft; excoriations common; blue-gray macules at bite site	Shaving affected area may facilitate treatment
Mosquitoes	Worldwide	Bite of female mosquito	Immediate and 24 hours		Immediate wheal; delayed (24-hour) papule	Repeated exposure alters cutaneous response
Bedbugs	Worldwide	Bite of *Cimex lectularius*	Hours		Papular urticaria	
Kissing bugs	South America	Bite of *Triatoma sanguisuga*	Hours		Papular urticaria; occasional nodular lesion	Walls of mud homes
Scabies	Worldwide	Skin-to-skin contact with infected person; mite acquisition from infected source, e.g., clothing/bedding	Primary infection: 1 month Repeat infection: hours to days	Months[b] (life cycle: 3–4 weeks)	Severe generalized pruritus; burrows; occasional vesicles or nodules	Hypersensitivity to mite and mite products; nodules often need steroid injections to heal
Tick granuloma	Worldwide	Bite of uninfected tick	Few hours		After tick removal a pruritic, red, papule/plaque seen; lasts 1–2 weeks; occasionally firm nodule "tick granuloma" seen	At times need intralesional steroid or surgery for relief of pruritus

LN, lymphadenopathy; IgM, immunoglobulin M; CSF, cerebrospinal fluid; CNS, central nervous system; GI, gastrointestinal; VDRL, Venereal Disease Research Laboratories; FTA-ABS, fluorescent treponemal antibody absorption (test); HA, headache; WBC, white blood cells; CXR, chest X-ray.

[a]Katayama fever is characterized by fever, chills, cough, malaise, hepatosplenomegaly, diarrhea, eosinophilia, occasional urticaria, and lymphadenopathy. Symptoms last days to 3–4 months.

[b]Symptoms persist from reinfection until treatment given.

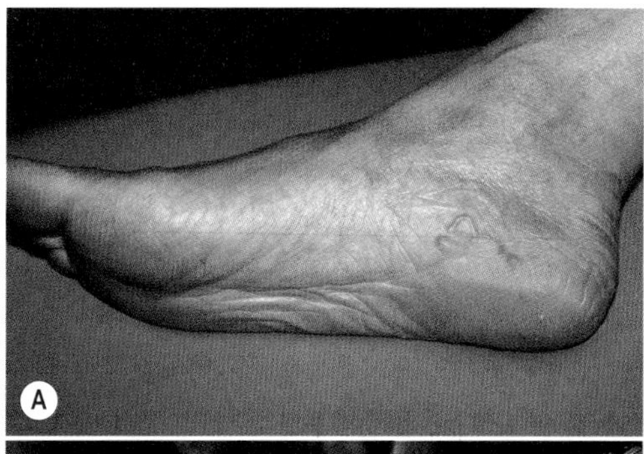

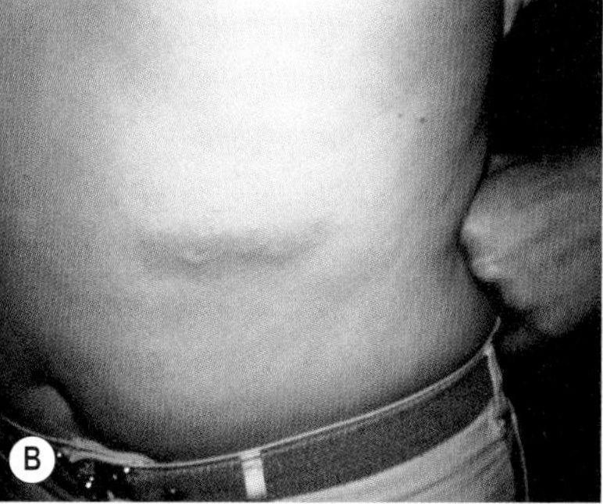

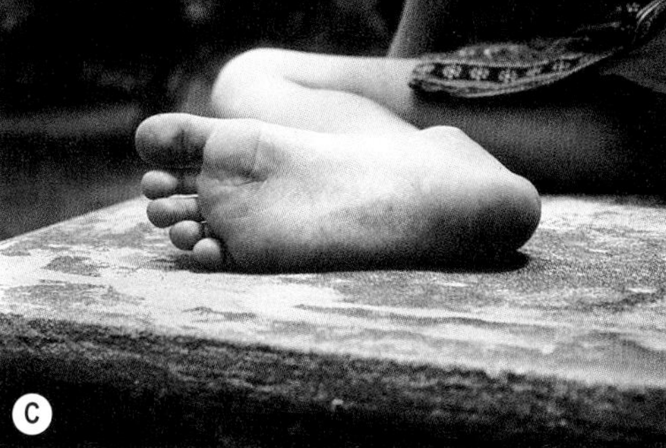

Figure 132.9 Migratory parasitic skin lesions. (**A**) Cutaneous larva migrans due to canine or feline hookworm infection. (**B**) Larva currens due to *Strongyloides stercoralis* infection. Typical distribution near the waistline is shown. (**C**) "Ground itch" from an acute hookworm infection. (Courtesy of Richard Brown, MD, Democratic Republic of the Congo, and Richard L. Guerrant, MD, Charlottesville, VA.)

Nodules and Ulcers

A nodule is a palpable solid lesion greater than 0.5–1.0 cm in diameter. Nodules larger than 2.0 cm are classified as tumors. Most nodules are dermal in location, although occasionally they arise from the epidermis (***Table 132.8***). Adult worms of *O. volvulus* typically reside in nodules (see Chapter 106) (***Fig. 132.11***).[15] Nodules are typically nearer the head in South and Central American disease, but tend to involve the hips in African onchocerciasis. In dracunculiasis (see Chapter 108) adult worms need to leave the human host via the skin to complete their life cycle and form a nodule prior to extrusion.[13] In other examples, such as echinococcosis, CLM, sparganosis, and dirofilariasis, humans represent intermediate hosts where parasites experience developmental arrest at the larval stage, variably in lung, skin, or muscle tissue. An inflammatory nodule eventually forms around the larva.[99,100] In cysticercosis (see Chapter 119), subcutaneous nodules may develop.[101]

Although nodules and ulcers are separate dermatologic entities and can arise individually, there is often an association between the two lesions. In many cases, nodular lesions undergo eventual ulceration if the inflammatory process is intense enough to result in destruction of the overlying epidermis. Ulcers are defined as skin defects with loss of the epidermis and the papillary layer of the dermis (***Table 132.9***; ***Fig. 132.3A and B***). Although ulcers often develop from nodules, the reverse is rarely seen. Fungal skin lesions are typical of infections that show a spectrum of nodular and ulcerative presentations (***Table 132.10***).[82,102] The time sequence of fungal skin lesions is indicated in ***Table 132.10*** by the designation I for initial ulcerating lesions and S for secondary ulceration. Anthrax, cutaneous leishmaniasis, and cutaneous mycobacterial diseases (*Mycobacterium marinum* and *M. ulcerans*) are typical examples of lesions that progress through a nodular phase to develop ulcers in most patients[69,103–105] (***Fig. 132.12***). Chancroid and syphilitic chancres are examples of lesions that directly develop painless ulcers, without a primary nodular phase. Tularemia also presents with an ulcer at the inoculation site, which typically is intensely painful.

Chronic ulcers related to tropical country residence or travel most commonly are due to *Staphylococcus aureus* or group A streptococcal pyoderma (purulent ulcers) or *Leishmania* lesions.[106,107] The pyoderma is in turn usually secondarily infected bites or abrasions acuired during travels. Other infection-related possibilities that may present with chronic ulcers include deep fungal infections, herpes simplex type 2, cutaneous tuberculosis, amebiasis cutis, and brown recluse spider bites.

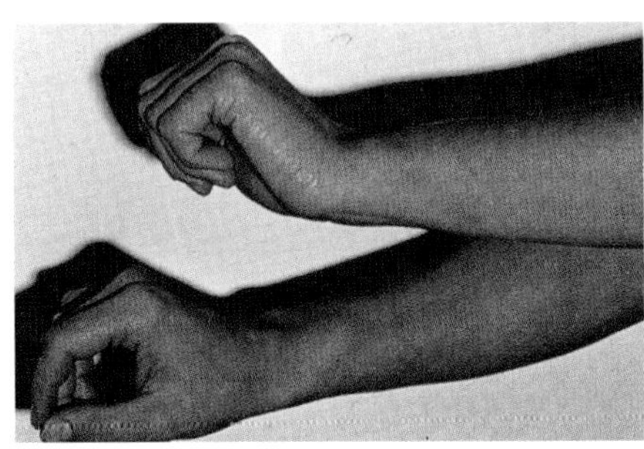

Figure 132.10 Calibar swelling in the left (upper) forearm of an expatriate patient with loiasis. Eosinophilia of 60% was coincident with this rash.

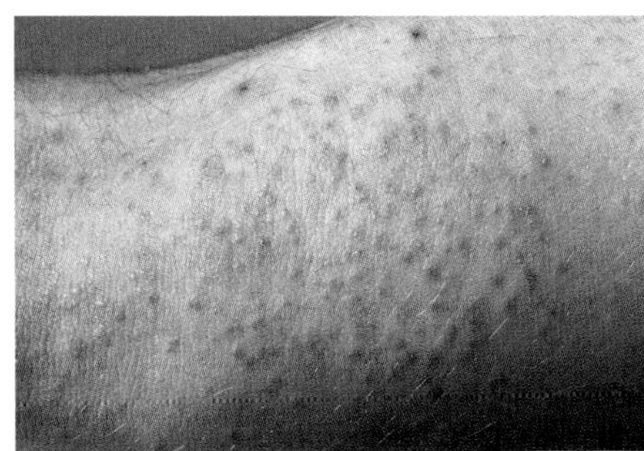

Figure 132.11 Onchocercal dermatitis demonstrating characteristic pruritic papules due to cutaneous microfilaria.

Table 132.8 Differential Diagnosis of Nodular Skin Lesions

Cause of Nodular Lesions	Distribution	Acquisition	Incubation	Organism Survival	Common Associated Findings	Additional Information
Helminthic						
Coenurosis	North America, South America, Europe, Africa, Asia	Ingestion of eggs in food, water, or on fecally contaminated sources	Months	≥15 years	Neurologic sx if CNS involved; painless mass lesion ~2–6 cm cyst	Rare infection, <100 cases; hematogenous spread before encystment
Cysticercosis Cysts, may be multiple	Worldwide	Ingestion of *Taenia solium* eggs in food, water or on fecally contaminated sources	2 years to onset of symptoms (range, months to 30 years)	10–15 years	Usually no eosinophilia; head CT: cysts ± punctate calcifications	Sx can start after parasite dead
Dirofilariasis	Worldwide (rare in Africa)	Bite of infected mosquito	2–3 months	Months to years	No sx; rare hemoptysis; rare subcutaneous nodules; coin lesion on CXR	
Dracunculiasis	see Table 132.6					

Table 132.8 Differential Diagnosis of Nodular Skin Lesions—cont'd

Cause of Nodular Lesions	Distribution	Acquisition	Incubation	Organism Survival	Common Associated Findings	Additional Information
Echinococcosis	Worldwide	Ingestion of eggs with food, fluid, or on fingers	Few years	Up to lifetime of host	Eosinophilia <35%; cyst wall may calcify; liver > lung disease; sx due to mass effect or immune reaction	Hematogenous and lymphatic dissemination
Filariasis (*Wuchereria bancrofti, Brugia malayi*) Mass in scrotum	*W. bancrofti*: Africa, Asia, Pacific islands, Central and South America, Caribbean *B. malayi:* South and East Asia	Bite of infected mosquito	5–18 months	8–10 years	Hydrocele, scrotal mass; lymphedema, lymphadenitis, elephantiasis	Rare tropical pulmonary eosinophilia syndrome
Gnathostomiasis	see Table 132.6					
Loiasis	see Table 132.6					
Onchocerciasis	see Table 132.6					
Paragonimiasis	see Table 132.6					
Schistomiasis (early)	see Table 132.7					
Sparganosis	see Table 132.6					
Visceral larva migrans (*Toxocara canis*, other zoonotic nematodes)	Worldwide	Ingestion of embryonated eggs from contaminated soil	≥1 month (range, weeks to years)	10 years	Eosinophilia, ↑WBC; fever, cough, wheeze, abdominal pain, tender hepatomegaly	Later eye disease uncommon; no eosinophilia, focal eye sx
Protozoan						
Amebiasis, cutaneous	Worldwide	Cyst ingestion in fecally contaminated food or water; uncommon sexual transmission	1–3 weeks (range 2 days to months)	Months to years	Mucous membrane lesions of vagina, anus, or penis similar to carcinomas; skin lesions: painful. Often perineal granulation tissue or ulcers	Cutaneous amebiasis is rare
Leishmaniasis, cutaneous and mucocutaneous	Scattered: Africa, South and Central America, Caribbean, Asia	Infected sandfly bite	Weeks to 2 months; strain-dependent; may take months to years for correct diagnosis	Months to years	Papule → nodule with central crust; crust falls off to reveal painless ulcer with raised border; heals slowly with scar; single lesion → cluster: widespread papules, nodules, plaques; mucocutaneous: more ulcerative and erosive; cutaneous: more nodular	Presentation varies from self-limited to disfiguring; infection can be subacute, chronic, or relapsing; biopsy best diagnostic test
Leishmaniasis, visceral	Africa, Mexico, South and Central America, Mediterranean area, Asia	Infected sandfly bite; rarely blood transfusion	2–6 months (range, 10 days to 1 year)	Years	Bite papule/nodule may persist for months; insidious onset of fever, malaise, weight loss, and sweats; diarrhea and cough may be prominent; nontender HSM and LN; post kala-azar dermal disease starts 1–20 years after apparent cure as nodular skin lesions	Can see profound decrease in CD4 T cells without HIV
Trypanosomiasis, African	see Table 132.7					

Table 132.8 Differential Diagnosis of Nodular Skin Lesions—cont'd

Cause of Nodular Lesions	Distribution	Acquisition	Incubation	Organism Survival	Common Associated Findings	Additional Information
Trypanosomiasis, American	Central and South America	Bite of infected triatomine bug; blood transfusion; ingestion of food contaminated by triatomine feces or uncooked meat of infected animal	Few days → chagoma; 2–3 weeks → systemic symptoms (days to years)	Lifetime of human host	Acute: fever, LN, HSM, and HA. Chagoma at bite site: 1–3 cm red indurated lesion; Romaña's sign (periorbital chemosis). Chronic infection: cardiac and/or GI	Disease, acute, subacute, and/or chronic, ranges asymptomatic to fatal
Bacterial						
Bartonellosis *Bartonella bacilliformis*	South America: along the western slope of the Andes below 3200 m, and Guatemala	Bite of infected sandfly	3 weeks to fever; 1–2 months to eruptive stage	Weeks to years	Multiple nodules, may be verrucous; fever, rigor, myalgia, arthralgias; skin lesions last 3–4 months (range, 1 month to 2 years); jaundice; variable HSM; generalized tender LN and pancytopenia	Fever irregular or remittent; lasts 3–4 weeks; skin lesion may worsen with steroid treatment; can see organism in tissue section of skin lesions
Cat-scratch disease *Bartonella henselae*	Worldwide	Scratch, lick, or bite of infected cat (90%), or dog	5–7 days to 1° skin lesion (range, 3–10 days); 3 weeks to LN (range, 3–50 days)	Months	Local LN; papule or pustule at inoculation site; malaise, HA, weight loss, sore throat	Risk kitten > cat; rare encephalitis; angiomatous nodules with AIDS
Glanders *Burkholderia mallei*	Sporadic in Asia, Africa, South America	Inhalation of aerosolized organism; direct inoculation of mucous membrane; ingestion of contaminated meat or drink	5–14 days (range, 1–3 weeks): aerosol shorter; skin, mucous membrane longer	Weeks to years	CXR can show nodular, lobar, or peribronchial infiltration, especially with inhalation. Percutaneous: nodular lesion; local lymphangitis may → ulcer, gangrene. Mucous membrane: local inflammation. Disseminated: papular/pustular eruption	Can have latent infection; chronic infection → multiple subcutaneous and intramuscular abscesses with sinus tract formation; highly variable clinical presentation, from mild to rapidly fatal
Granuloma inguinale (genital) (*Calymmatobacterium granulomatis*)	Worldwide	Sexual contact	7–30 days (range, 3 days to 6 months)	Years in human host	Insidious onset, papule → nodule → ulcer; lesion painless; tissue response characterized by acanthosis and pseudoepitheliomatous changes	Borders of lesions well defined and irregular; organisms in macrophages seen with Wright's or Giemsa stain (Donovan bodies)
Mycetoma Mixed bacterial and fungal infection; begins as subcutaneous nodule	Worldwide (especially in tropics)	Percutaneous inoculation	Weeks to months	Years (up to 25 years untreated)	Granules may be discharged from wound; sinus tracts common; nodules slowly enlarge and become phlegmonous	Systemic sx usually absent; male:female 4:1; local bone invasion with cortical erosion, lytic lesions; tendons spared; path: granuloma around purulent center

Table 132.8 Differential Diagnosis of Nodular Skin Lesions—cont'd						
Cause of Nodular Lesions	**Distribution**	**Acquisition**	**Incubation**	**Organism Survival**	**Common Associated Findings**	**Additional Information**
Lymphogranuloma venerum (genital) (*Chlamydia trachomatis*)	Worldwide (especially tropics and subtropics)	Direct contact (usually sexual) with infected person	7–10 days to 1° lesion (range, 3–30 days); 10–30 days to inguinal bubo (range, months)	Weeks to years	Painless papule → vesicle → ulcer; heals without scar; prominent, painful, fluctuant inguinal LN (bubo); rectal infection → proctitis with blood, tenesmus, and mucoid discharge; fever, chills, HA, malaise, LN	Male : female: 6 : 1; rare presentation with FUO or erythema nodosum
Rhinoscleroma (*Klebsiella rhinoscleromatis*)	Worldwide sporadic	Uncertain	Uncertain	Months to decades	Nodular nose lesions; usually painless; slow local progression; enlarged cervical LN; can see destruction of bone and cartilage	Path: chronic histiocytic granulomatous changes; characteristic: Mikulicz's cell (large, vacuolated macrophage)
Syphilis, endemic; bejel (*Treponema pallidum* subsp. *endemicum*)	Focal: Africa, Asia (western), Australia	Exposure to contaminated utensils	Weeks (range, 2 weeks to 3 months)	Months to years	1° lesion rarely seen; 2° lesion: papillomas at corner of mouth; mucous patch on oropharynx, tongue, buccal region, later disseminated papillomas; generalized LN; late painful osteoperiostitis of tibia and fibula	Not transmitted by direct or sexual contact; infection usually acquired in childhood; untreated lesions often resolve in 1 year, but may relapse
Mycobacterium ulcerans (begins as nodule)	Focal: Africa, Southeast Asia, Papua New Guinea, Australia, South and Central America	Percutaneous inoculation	6 weeks (range, 3 weeks to 2 months)	Years	Lesions single (98%) and on extremity (90%) or trunk; nodule at onset can be pruritic; nodule → ulcer that enlarges over 1–4 months; extensive undermined edges and necrotic base; usually no redness, LN, or systemic sx	Toxin-mediated process → extensive subcutaneous necrosis. BCG: limited protection. Mostly found in vegetation in swampy lowlands; bony involvement <1%
Leprosy	Worldwide (especially tropics and subtropics)	Person-to-person fomite	3–5 years	Lifetime of host	Mostly subclinical; 75% with single skin lesion that heals spontaneously; disease spectrum tuberculoid (TT) to lepromatous (LL): TT – few anesthetic asymmetrical macules/papules with red rim and hypopigmented center; LL – many bilateral symmetrical lesions (macules, papules, plaques, or nodules). Iritis and keratitis common	50 70% with no known contact of patient with leprosy; erythema nodosum seen occasionally; may worsen with pregnancy; anesthesia → trauma → deformity; ANA, RF, VDRL may be falsely positive
Mycobacterium marinum	Worldwide	After trauma in infected water or from infected fish/crustaceans	2–3 weeks	Not available	Papule → larger nodule with blue/purple hue → suppuration → ulceration; sporotrichoid pattern; usually confined to superficial, cooler body tissue of extremities	Grows best at 25–32°C; pathologic findings range from pus to granulomas

Table 132.8 Differential Diagnosis of Nodular Skin Lesions—cont'd

Cause of Nodular Lesions	Distribution	Acquisition	Incubation	Organism Survival	Common Associated Findings	Additional Information
Leptospirosis	Worldwide (especially tropics)	Ingestion of water or food contaminated by animal urine	7–12 days (range, 2–26 days)	Blood: 3 months Urine: 11 months	Pretibial, red, tender nodules 1–5 cm	Survives weeks to months in soil and water; infection can persist for weeks
Yaws (*Treponema pallidum* subsp. *partenue*)	Focal warm, humid, rural areas; Africa, Asia, Central and South America, Caribbean, Oceania	Direct contact with person with infected lesion	3–5 weeks (range, 10 days to 3 months)	Years to decades	Initial painless papule enlarges to 1–3 cm papillomatous raspberry-like lesion; can ulcerate → fluid teeming with spirochetes; some regional LN; 1° lesion heals without scar in 6 months; 2° lesions months later are disseminated papillomas in moist areas; late lesions cause tissue destruction and scarring	Latent infection:active disease ratio 5:1; variable presentation: self-limited to destructive chronic
Fungal						
All invasive fungal infections can cause nodular skin lesions (see Table 132.11)						
Viral						
Orf (*Parapoxvirus*)	All goat- and sheep-raising countries	Close contact with infected animals with skin break	3–6 days (range, 2–7 days)	Weeks	Papule at entry site → nodule → 1–2 cm plaque/vesicle; weeping ulcer with crust develops; lesions single or multiple; usually painful; local LN, fever seen	Associated with exposure to sheep and goats; heals spontaneously over weeks
Pseudocowpox (*Parapoxvirus*) Milker's nodule	Dairy herds worldwide	Close contact with cow lesion and skin break	5–7 days (range, 5–14 days)	Weeks	Papule → 0.5–2.0 cm nodule; firm, cherry red to red/blue, painless; regional LN; no systemic sx	Associated with milking cows; heals spontaneously over 4–6 weeks without scar
Arthropod						
Myiasis	see Table 132.6					
Scabies	see Table 132.7					
Tick granuloma	see Table 132.7					
Tungiasis (*Tunga penetrans*)	see Table 132.7					

sx, symptoms; CNS, central nervous system; CT, computed tomography; CXR, chest X-ray film; WBC, white blood cell count; HSM, hepatosplenomegaly; LN, lymphadenopathy; HIV, human immunodeficiency virus; HA, headache; GI, gastrointestinal; AIDS, acquired immunodeficiency syndrome; FUO, fever of unknown origin; BCG, bacille Calmette-Guérin; ANA, antinuclear antibody; RF, rheumatoid factor; VDRL, Venereal Disease Research Laboratories.

[a]See Table 132.4.

Cysts

Cysts are similar to nodules but contain fluid. Overall, nodules are much more common than true cysts among tropical-associated infections. In echinococcosis and coenurosis, a true cyst is formed as part of the developmental process of the parasite. However, cutaneous and subcutaneous disease is rare with both of these infections. Some patients with *Gnathostoma spinigerum* form cysts around the parasite as part of the host immune response.[108] Among the filarial parasites, loiasis and onchocerciasis have skin nodules that harbor the adult parasites and occasionally appear cystic due to fluid accumulation around the nodule. Lymphatic filariasis occasionally results in lymphatic obstruction of the scrotal lymphatics in men, resulting in the development of a cystic hydrocele as the presenting manifestation.[109]

Vesicles

Vesicular lesions (***Table 132.11***) can be considered in three clinical categories. The first and most common is single or localized lesions.[10] An example is anthrax, with its evolving cutaneous lesion from painless papule to ulcer with surrounding vesicles. Other examples include herpes simplex and varicella-zoster, contagious ecthyma (orf and parapoxvirus), milker's nodule (pseudocowpox), tanapox, and papulonecrotic tuberculids. In addition, secondarily infected skin lesions with phage group 2

Table 132.9 Differential Diagnosis of Ulcerative Skin Lesions

Entity	Distribution	Acquisition	Incubation	Organism Survival	Common Associated Findings	Additional Information
Bacterial						
Anthrax (*Bacillus anthracis*)	Worldwide, sporadic; Asia, Africa, especially with animal care	Contact with infected animals or their products via skin break, inhalation, or ingestion of contaminated meat; rare biting fly transmission	2–5 seconds (range, 12 hours to 7 days)	Duration of acute illness in human host; spores persist for years in soil	Cutaneous entry (90%) → papule → vesicular with surrounding brawny, gelatinous edema; satellite lesions seen; lesion becomes hemorrhagic → necrotic → eschar; low-grade fever, malaise common	Variable disease: subclinical to rapidly fatal; toxin mediates many sx In septicemic form: hemorrhagic meningitis and severe GI sx
Chancroid (*Haemophilus ducreyi*)	Worldwide (especially tropics)	Sexual contact with infected person	3–10 days (range, 2–21 days)	Weeks to months	Papule/pustule ulcerates in 1–2 (1–2 cm); edges irregular, undermined; painful ulcer; multiple ulcers common; unilateral/bilateral LN painful, prone to rupture	Autoinoculation can occur; 2% urethritis
Diphtheria, cutaneous (*Corynebacterium diphtheriae*)	Worldwide	Close contact with infected person (fomite and direct contact); rarely in contaminated unpasteurized milk	2–5 days (range, 1–10 days)	Usually <2 weeks; rare carriers 6 months	Deep, punched-out ulcers covered by easily removed membrane; can look like impetigo or infected insect bite; nasopharynx infected in 20% with skin infection; cardiac arrhythmias common; cranial and peripheral neuropathies can persist for 2–3 months	Toxin mediates most of disease process; adults immunized as children often lack immunity; can superinfect other skin sores
Glanders (*Burkholderia mallei*)	see Table 132.8					
Granuloma inguinale (*Calymmatobacterium granulomatis*)	see Table 132.8					
Leprosy	See Table 132.8				Neuropathic ulcers, especially in later tuberculoid leprosy	
Melioidosis (*Burkholderia pseudomallei*)	Tropics and subtropics; endemic Southeast Asia	Direct contact with contaminated water or soil via skin break; aspiration of contaminated water	2 days to 3 weeks (range, 1 day to years)	Decades	Percutaneous entry → cellulitis, lymphangitis, bacteremia; pustular rash then due to bacteremic spread → chronic suppuration in skin, bones, CNS, liver, spleen, others; acute disease → many systemic sx	Pulmonary infiltrates on CXR Upper lobes 90% Cavitation 60% Disease can be acute or chronic
Mycetoma	See Table 132.8					
Mycobacterium ulcerans	See Table 132.8					
Plague (*Yersinia pestis*)	Worldwide except Australia	Bite of infected flea; inhalation of airborne bacilli; bite or scratch of infected animal (e.g., cat)	2–7 days bubonic; 2–3 days pneumonic (range, 1–14 days)	No carrier state known	Abrupt onset with severe systemic sx; painful swollen mass/LN (bubo) seen in hours, groin > axilla; red/purple skin lesions; GI sx (>70%)	High mortality if untreated; septicemic form may have no bubo formation
Rickettsia[a]	see Table 132.2					
Syphilis, venereal (*Treponema pallidum*)	Worldwide	Direct contact with infected lesion, usually sexually; transplacental; blood transfusion	2–4 weeks to primary lesion	Lifetime of human host	1° lesion: painless ulcer with indurated edge 2° lesions: protean skin and mucous membrane lesions seen after asymptomatic interval	Serologic tests do not distinguish among treponemes; disease can be acute, subacute, latent, or chronic

Table 132.9 Differential Diagnosis of Ulcerative Skin Lesions—cont'd

Entity	Distribution	Acquisition	Incubation	Organism Survival	Common Associated Findings	Additional Information
Tropical ulcer (mixed bacteria including *Fusobacterium nucleatum*)	Worldwide (especially tropics)	? Minor trauma may play a role	?	Months	Papule/pustule/vesicle → painful ulcer 1–6 cm diameter, circular raised edge and surrounding edema; deeply penetrating and destructive	Male > female; can have 2° tetanus and gas gangrene; multiple and recurrent ulcers seen
Tuberculosis, primary cutaneous	Worldwide	Unusual direct cutaneous inoculation	Months	Lifetime of human host	Inoculation papule can ulcerate	Rare form of tuberculosis
Tularemia	North America, Europe, Asia (scattered)	Bite of infected arthropod or animal; contact with infected animal tissue; inhalation; ingestion of contaminated meat or water	3–5 days (range, 1–25 days)	2–4 weeks in human host; organism can survive prolonged freezing	Clinical sx reflect portal of entry; skin inoculation → local, painful ulcer followed by painful regional LN, fever; rare erythema nodosum	Disease range is asymptomatic to fatal; ulceroglandular form most common; chronic/recurrent fevers and LN seen
Yaws	See Table 132.8					
Fungal	See Table 132.10				All invasive fungal infections can cause ulcerative skin lesions	Deep abscesses and sinus tracts may form
Helminthic						
Dracunculiasis	See Table 132.6				Ulcer at site of worm eruption	
Protozoan						
Amebiasis, cutaneous	Worldwide See also Table 132.8	Cyst ingestion in contaminated food or water; uncommon sexual transmission	1–3 weeks (range, 2 days to months)	Months to years	When cutaneous, painful, rapid-growing ulcers with necrosis	Uncommon sexual transmission: anal > vaginal intercourse
Leishmaniasis, cutaneous and mucocutaneous	See Table 132.8					
Viral						
Orf (*Parapoxvirus*)	See Table 132.8					
Herpes simplex	Worldwide	Type 1: direct contact with infected oral secretions Type 2: contact with genital secretions	2–12 days	Lifetime in human host	Grouped vesicles on erythematous base ulcerate; lesions painful; moderate to severe generalized systemic sx with 1° infection; local LN common	Recurrence due to latent virus in neural cells; autoinoculation possible
Arthropod						
Brown recluse spider bite (*Loxosceles reclusa*)	?	Spider bite	Immediate to hours		Bite → mild sting followed by intense pain in 2–8 hours, bullae and erythema, local ischemic necrosis, deep ulceration Occasional fever, myalgias, and generalized morbilliform rash 24–48 hours after bite	Parenteral steroid use in first 24 hours controversial; heals spontaneously though scars common Can be confused with pyoderma gangrenosum
Myiasis	See Table 132.7					
Tungiasis	See Table 132.7					

sx, symptoms; GI, gastrointestinal; LN, lymphadenopathy; CNS, central nervous system; CXR, chest X-ray film.
[a]Several rickettsial infections are associated with an ulcerative eschar; see Table 132.2.

Table 132.10 Differential Diagnosis of Nodular and Ulcerative Fungal Infections

Entity	Distribution	Acquisition	Incubation	Organism Survival	Common Associated Findings	Additional Information
Primary Skin Infections						
Chromomycosis (several agents)	Worldwide, especially tropics and subtropics	Percutaneous inoculation of nonintact skin	Weeks to months	Years	Nodule I ++++ Ulcer S +++	Lymphatics involved, (e.g., elephantiasis and lymphedema); starts as local papule → painless, irregular, papule → nodule
Entomophthoromycosis (*Basidiobolus baptosporus*)	Tropical Africa, rarely elsewhere	Percutaneous inoculation of nonintact skin	?	Years	Painless subcutaneous nodule → expanding woody swelling Nodule I ++++ Ulcer None	Rare systemic sx or dissemination
Lobomycosis (*Loboa loboi*)	Tropical Central and South America	Percutaneous inoculation of nonintact skin	1–2 years	Years	Starts as painless, small mobile nodules Nodule I ++++ Ulcer S +	Autoinoculation seen; histopathology characteristic
Mycetoma Mixed bacterial and fungal infection; begins as subcutaneous nodule	Worldwide (especially tropics)	Percutaneous inoculation	Weeks to months	Years (up to 25 years untreated)	Granules may be discharged from wound; sinus tracts common; nodules slowly enlarge and become phlegmonous Nodule I +++ Ulcer S ++	Systemic sx usually absent; male:female 4:1; local bone invasion with cortical erosion, lytic lesions; tendons spared; path: granuloma around purulent center
Pityriasis (tinea) versicolor (*Malassezia furfur*)	Worldwide	Direct inoculation of fungal elements	?	?	Circumscribed hypo- or hyper- (brown) pigmented scaly lesions; usually upper chest and back Nodule None Ulcer None	Superficial stratum corneum infection; enzyme of fungus produces pigment changes
Sporotrichosis (*Sporothrix schenckii*)	Worldwide	Direct percutaneous inoculation	3–8 weeks	Months to years	Papule → painless; nodule → may ulcerate; secondary nodules along lymphatic channels Nodule I ++++ Ulcer S ++	25% extracutaneous lung, bone, joints
Tinea imbricata (*Trichophyton concentricum*)	Asia, South Pacific islands; Mexico, Central and South America	Direct contact with infected person	10 days	Lifetime of host	Concentric rings 0.3–1.25 cm apart; no systemic sx except pruritus Nodule None Ulcer None	Hypopigmentation >hyperpigmentation; covers up to 70% of body
Primary Nasal and Oropharyngeal Infections						
Entomophthoromycosis (*Conidiobolus coronatus*)	Tropical Africa; rarely elsewhere	Inhalation of spore usually on to nasal turbinate	?	Years	Painless indurated mass → local insidious spread Nodule I ++++ Ulcer None	Male:female 8:1
Rhinosporidiosis (*Rhinosporidium seeberi*)	Worldwide (sporadic); endemic foci in India and Sri Lanka	Direct inoculation of fungus	Weeks to months	Years to decades	Characteristic, friable, vascular sessile growth or polyps on mucosal surfaces; lesions painless Nodule I ++++ Ulcer None	Treatment surgical, but recurrence common

Table 132.10 Differential Diagnosis of Nodular and Ulcerative Fungal Infections—cont'd

Entity	Distribution	Acquisition	Incubation	Organism Survival	Common Associated Findings	Additional Information
Primary Respiratory Infections						
Blastomycosis (*Blastomyces dermatitidis*)	North America (most); sporadic in Central and South America, Africa, Poland, India, Middle East	Inhalation of infectious conidia; rare percutaneous inoculation; rare STD from men with GU infection	1–2 months inhaled; 2 weeks cutaneous	~15 years in human host	Nodule: I, +++ Ulcer: S, ++	Most hematogenous to skin; 20–80% of patients disseminate to skin, bone, GU tract (male > female), CNS; male : female 3–9 : 1
Coccidioidomycosis (*Coccidioides immitis*)	Southwest United States, Mexico, Central and South America	Inhalation of infectious arthroconidia; rare cutaneous inoculation	2 weeks	Years	1° disease; fever, cough, chest pain, malaise; hypersensitivity reactions (15–20%): erythema nodosum, generalized erythema, maculopapular rash, arthralgias, urticaria, rare erythema multiforme Nodule: + Ulcer: +	Extrapulmonary disease rare (<1%): bone, skin, LN, CNS, joints, GU, GI, eye; eosinophilia common in 1° infection
Cryptococcosis (*Cryptococcus neoformans*)	Worldwide	Inhalation of infectious conidia	?	?	Mostly pulmonary with no sx; skin lesions 10% (hematogenous papule → nodule → ulcer) Nodule: I, ++ Ulcer: S, ++	Can cause CNS, bone, prostate, liver, eye, heart, kidney infections, rarely
Histoplasmosis (*Histoplasma capsulatum*)	Worldwide (but focal and sporadic)	Inhalation of infectious spores	2 weeks	Years	Mostly pulmonary with no sx; skin changes (erythema nodosum) seen with reactions to 1° infection Nodule: I, Often oropharynx, + Ulcer: I, Oropharynx, +	Rare dissemination: metastatic skin lesions Disseminated disease can affect any organ
Histoplasmosis, African (*Histoplasma capsulatum*, var. *duboisii*)	Tropical Africa	Uncertain; suspect inhalation of infected spores	?	Years	Common painless skin lesions from skin and underlying bony disease Nodule: I, +++ Ulcer: I, +++	Lytic bony lesions common
Paracoccidioidomycosis (*Paracoccidioides brasiliensis*)	Central and South America	Inhalation of infectious spores	Months to years	Years to decades	Initial respiratory infection usually no sx; common mucocutaneous oropharyngeal lesions due to hematogenous dissemination (60%) Nodule: I, +++ Ulcer: I, ++	Ratio of disease in males : females 9 : 1; isolated CNS or adrenal involvement seen
Penicilliosis (*Penicillium marneffei*)	East and Southeast Asia	Inhalation/ ingestion of infectious spores; rare percutaneous inoculation	9 days to 1 month	Years	Nodules are subcutaneous abscesses; ulcers from necrosis of nodules/ papules Nodule: I, +++ Ulcer: S, ++	Most patients disseminate; immunodeficiency favors ulcer formation

sx, symptoms; GI, gastrointestinal; LN, lymphadenopathy; CNS, central nervous system; CXR, chest X-ray; I, initial lesion; S, secondary lesion; STD, sexually transmitted disease; GU, genitourinary.

+, scale (1–4) based on frequency when skin lesions present: +, rare; ++, uncommon; +++, occasional; ++++, frequent.

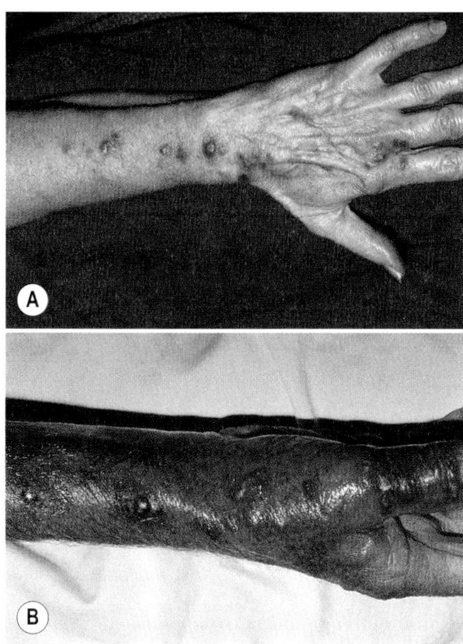

Figure 132.12 **(A)** Sporotrichoid rash of *Mycobacterium marinum* infection showing typical location on the superficial cooler body tissues of the extremities. **(B)** A similar rash in a patient with classical sporotrichosis due to the fungal pathogen *Sporothrix schenckii*.

toxin-producing staphylococci can produce bullous impetigo. Noninfectious plant toxin contact, such as with poison ivy, typically results in a vesicular reaction.[110]

The second category consists of generalized lesions with greatest concentration on the head and scalp. Varicella (chickenpox) is the prototype of this vesicular presentation. The third group includes generalized lesions with greatest concentration on the extremities. Although predominantly peripheral, rickettsialpox lesions are noted to spare the palms and soles.[22] In contrast, coxsackievirus has a very characteristic predilection for those areas, resulting in the name hand, foot, and mouth disease to describe this combination of exanthem and enanthem. Disseminated gonococcal infection is associated with painful peripheral lesions that mature into vesicles, often on a hemorrhagic base (***Fig. 132.13***). Toxic epidermal necrolysis and some drug hypersensitivity reactions can produce vesicles (***Fig. 132.14***). Bullae (large vesicles) are occasionally seen with Gram-negative bacteria (especially *Pseudomonas aeruginosa*)-associated ecthyma lesions.[8,32]

Changes in Pigmentation

Infection-related changes in skin pigmentation are commonly either hypo- or hyperpigmented (***Table 132.12***). In addition, they can be focal, scattered, generalized, or a combination thereof. Finally, the lesion may be noted early or late in the disease process. In general, pigmentation changes early in a disease process are more likely to result in hyperpigmentation, whereas later changes more commonly result in decreased pigmentation. This information is occasionally helpful in differentiating the underlying cause. Pinta is an example in which papulosquamous skin lesions are usually red at onset and then shift to a spectrum of blue, gray, violaceous, yellow, black, and brown, referred to as dyschromic lesions. Over many months to years, the skin lesions become depigmented macules associated with atrophic scars.[111]

Cutaneous jaundice is occasionally seen in patients related to hepatic involvement with various pathogens (***Box 132.7***) (see Chapter 133). The major pathogen causing jaundice in travelers is hepatitis A. The agents associated with jaundice have a wide geographic distribution. The incubation period can be an important clue to the cause. Yellow fever symptoms usually begin within 2 weeks of exposure, whereas the incubation period for the hepatitis viruses is 2–6 weeks. Due to extensive exposure to water among triathletes and eco-challenge participants, they represent a high-risk group for waterborne illness, especially leptospirosis.

The vaccination status of the traveler provides important information in formulating the differential diagnosis of the jaundiced traveler.[112] Rarely, both pigment alteration (e.g., erythroderma) and jaundice (e.g., immune-mediated hepatic involvement of drug hypersensitivity) can be medication-related.[39]

TRAVEL-RELATED MEDICATIONS

The care of patients who travel to or live in the tropics often involves the use of medications not usually prescribed by physicians in the developed world. Although medication reactions are rare, these agents represent a significant new exposure for many travelers to tropical and subtropical climates. Drug reactions can take many forms, with mechanisms both direct and immunologic. Hypersensitivity reaction types 1–4 have been documented with various pharmacologic agents.[58] The actual dermatologic presentation can take any form, from maculopapular to urticarial, vesiculobullous, or vasculitic. Other less frequent manifestations of drug eruptions include toxic epidermal necrolysis, erythema nodosum, and lichenoid reactions.[113,114] In the GeoSentinel review, 0.9% (42) of the nearly 5000 foreign-exposed individuals with a dermatologic condition developed a drug-related rash.[5] With few exceptions, other information related to cutaneous reactions associated with medications in this setting comes from case reports. ***Table 132.13*** is organized by application of the medications (e.g., antimalarials and antidiarrheals). The reactions listed for each medication appear in the approximate order of their reported incidence.

Chloroquine can occasionally induce a pruritic reaction without cutaneous changes, which can be moderately severe in up to 90% of cases. There appears to be an increased risk of a reaction to chloroquine in blacks and in people with a family history of pruritus.[115] If another option exists for malaria prophylaxis, it should be considered in such patients. Chloroquine pruritus is usually not responsive to antihistamines, although a study on chlorpheniramine showed efficacy when given 3 hours after ingestion of chloroquine in 70% of patients compared with 40% when given concomitantly.[116] Prednisolone 5 mg or niacin 50 mg also significantly reduced the pruritus intensity time curve in another study. Chloroquine may also exaggerate existing psoriasis; hence, psoriasis should be considered a relative contraindication to the use of chloroquine. Bleaching of the hair can be seen, although usually after use longer than 1 year.[117]

In patients traveling to tropical and subtropical climates, there is almost always increased exposure to sunlight in both time of exposure and intensity of exposure. Sunscreens are an important part of the cutaneous hygiene in such travelers. In addition, certain medications given to travelers carry potential photosensitization as a side-effect, especially doxycycline, quinine, proguanil, ciprofloxacin, and ofloxacin.[58,118–121] Nonsteroidal anti-inflammatory agents can also photosensitize, and sedentary travelers who are physically active during foreign travel may use them frequently.[122] Travelers who require these medications should be reminded to be especially vigilant about using sunscreens with high sun protection factor ratings. Troubling bullous phototoxic "phytophoto dermatitis" can cause painful erythematous lesions after exposure to funanocoumarins in lime juice and sunlight.[135,136]

Very rarely, travelers will develop serum sickness or serum sickness-like reactions to vaccines or antibiotics administered for travel-related disease prevention.[39] As a type of immune complex disease, a spectrum of reactions can be seen, from mild morbilliform maculopapular eruptions to multisystem organ involvement arising from systemic (including cutaneous) vasculitis.[114] A more common presentation of serum sickness is fever, urticaria, arthralgias, and lymphadenopathy approximately 1–3 weeks after primary antigen exposure or 3 days after reexposure.[123] Rare case reports have described this reaction to bacille Calmette-Guérin, measles, and poliomyelitis vaccines, as well as to tetanus and diphtheria antitoxins.[124] Antibiotics such as penicillin and

Table 132.11 Differential Diagnosis of a Vesicular Rash after Travel or Tropical Exposure

Organism/Agent	Disease
Bacteria	
Bacillus anthracis	Anthrax
Brucella spp.	Brucellosis
Mycobacterium tuberculosis	Papulonecrotic tuberculids
Mycoplasma spp.	
Rickettsia akari	Rickettsialpox
R. tsutsugamushi (?)	
Streptococcus pyogenes (?)	Impetigo
Vibrio vulnificus	
Viruses	
Alphaviruses (chikungunya, O'nyong-nyong, Ross River, Sindbis)	
Enteroviruses (coxsackievirus, echovirus, enterovirus 71)	
Measles	Atypical measles
Mumps (?)	
Monkeypox	
Herpes simplex (type 1 and type 2)	Latent virus with recurrence
Varicella-zoster	Chickenpox: zoster (latent virus with recurrence)
Vaccinia	Progressive vaccinia Eczema vaccinatum Accidental remote inoculation
Variola	Smallpox
Orf	Ecthyma contagiosum
Tanapox	
Parasitic	
Leishmania braziliensis	American cutaneous leishmaniasis
Necator americanus	Hookworm (at site of skin penetration)
Noninfectious	
Toxic epidermal necrolysis	Drug-related
	Vaccine-related: rare case reports with bacille Calmette-Guérin, diphtheria toxoid, measles, poliomyelitis, tetanus toxoid
Plant dermatitis	Poison ivy
Drug hypersensitivity	

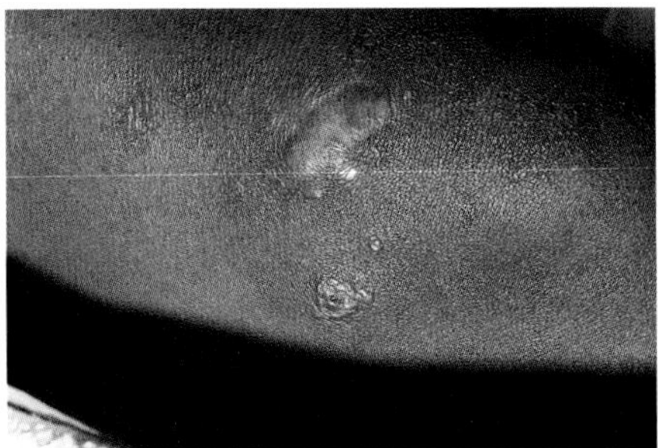

Figure 132.13 Disseminated gonococcal infection. Cutaneous lesions showing characteristic discrete pustules and papules with subcutaneous hemorrhage. (Courtesy of Kenneth J. Tomecki, MD, Cleveland, OH.)

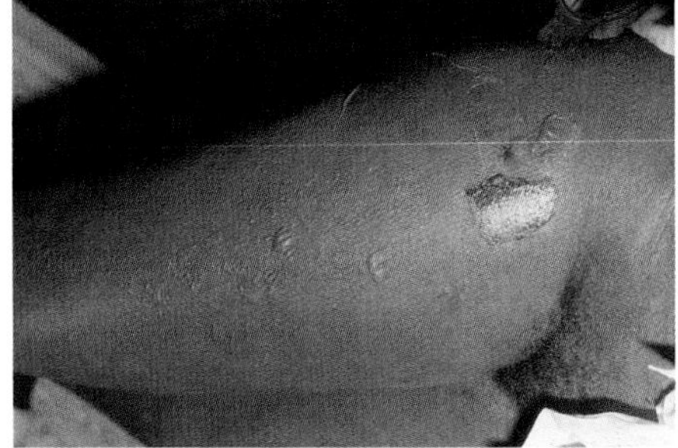

Figure 132.14 Toxic epidermal necrolysis showing large, flaccid bullae and characteristic ruptured bullae with separation of sheets of skin (Nikolsky's sign); can occur with toxin-producing *Staphylococcus aureus*, drug reaction, and viral illnesses. (Courtesy of Kenneth J. Tomecki, MD, Cleveland, OH.)

Table 132.12 Alterations in Pigmentation

	Location			Time	
	Focal	**Scattered**	**Generalized**	**Early**	**Late**
Decreased Pigmentation					
Leishmaniasis, visceral	+ + (face)	+			+ (untreated)
Leprosy	+	+		+	+
Onchocerciasis	+ (pretibial)				+
Pinta	+	+	+		+
Pityriasis (tinea) versicolor (*Malassezia furfur*)		+		+	
Syphilis, venereal, secondary	+ + (neck)				+
Yaws	+ (inoculation site)	+ (hand, wrist, feet)		+	
Increased Pigmentation					
Erythrasma (*Corynebacterium minutissimum*)	+			+	
Pinta	+	+	+	+	+
Loiasis	+			+	
Pityriasis (tinea) versicolor (*Malassezia furfur*)		+		+	
Leishmaniasis, visceral (especially India)			+		+

+, present; ++, common.

Box 132.7 Diagnostic Concerns in the Traveler with Jaundice

Diseases in Which Jaundice is Common

Yellow fever
- Symptom onset less than 2 weeks

Hepatitis A–E
- Incubation to symptoms varies from 2 to 6 weeks

Rift Valley fever
- Zoonotic hepatitis pathogen (arbovirus)
- Sub-Saharan Africa
- Transmission: mosquito, airborne, unpasteurized milk

Diseases in which Jaundice is Uncommon

Leptospirosis
- Animal urine (especially rats) contaminates environment worldwide
- Organism can survive weeks to months in soil and water
- Incubation period 7–12 days
- Symptoms last 2–4 weeks

Dengue fever
- Usually in setting of severe disease

Malaria

Epstein–Barr virus

Q fever

Syphilis

Drug reactions

sulfa-containing drugs can also act as the foreign antigen initiating a cascade immune response very similar to serum sickness.[125] Another rare, but potentially severe, cutaneous reaction was seen with sulfadoxine-pyrimethamine (Fansidar) use in malaria prophylaxis or treatment. Both SJS and toxic epidermal necrolysis have been reported. The antimalarials mefloquine and atovaquone/proguanil (malarone) rarely lead to SJS.[37,126] Development of rash during use is considered an indication to discontinue these medications.

ACKNOWLEDGMENTS

We are indebted to Dr Mary Wilson[42] for gathering an enormous amount of data related to the practical information that bears on the clinical care of patients with health concerns related to international and tropical medicine. We also acknowledge Kenneth Tomecki, MD, for his helpful review and comments. In addition, we thank Vicki Grosh for significant assistance in the preparation of the tables.

Table 132.13 Cutaneous Reactions to Travel Medications

Medication	Reactions	Factors that May Increase Reactions
Antimalarials		
Chloroquine	Hair blanching	Dosing ≥1 year; hair exposed to light
	Pruritus without rash	Black race; family history of reaction
	Photosensitivity	Long-term usage; increased age; female > male
	Worsens psoriasis	
	Rare: hypo- or hyperpigmentation of skin, blue-brown nail bed changes, erythema annulare centrifugum, bullous erythema, toxic epidermal necrolysis (TEN), erythema nodosum	Pyrimethamine use Renal failure
Mefloquine	Rare: itching, varied nonspecific rashes, Stevens–Johnson syndrome	
Proguanil	Rare: mild urticaria, phototoxic reactions, exanthems, periorbital papules	
	Hair loss	Female > male
	Scaling of palms/soles	2 of 6 patients receiving concurrent chloroquine
Primaquine	None reported	
Doxycycline	Photosensitivity	
	Rare: photo-onycholysis, exanthematous pustulosis, urticaria, angioedema, purpura, anaphylaxis, serum sickness	
Quinine	Urticaria, papular rash, scarlatiniform rash, erythema multiforme	
	Rare: fixed drug eruption; urticaria; flushing, sweating, facial edema; photosensitivity	
Halofantrine	Pruritus posttreatment	Incidence 0.3–2.3%; black race; family member with history of pruritus posttreatment
		Family member with history of pruritus posttreatment
Antidiarrheals		
Pepto-Bismol	Salicylate hypersensitivity, erythematous rash, bismuth reaction, transient darkening of tongue	
Trimethoprim–sulfamethoxazole	Diffuse maculopapular rash, allergic/toxic dermatitis	Overall incidence 2.2%; HIV/AIDS higher incidence
	Rare: erythema multiforme	
	Exfoliative eczema exanthems	~1/200 000 doses
	Stevens–Johnson syndrome	~1/200 000 doses
	TEN	
Ciprofloxacin	Generalized skin rash	Incidence of 1.1%
	Rare: pruritus, urticaria, photosensitivity, flushing, angioedema, hyperpigmentation, erythema nodosum, fixed drug eruption, pustulosis, TEN	
Ofloxacin	Generalized skin rash, pruritus, eczema	Incidence up to 14% of patients
	Rare: hypersensitivity vasculitis, phototoxic dermatitis, photo-onycholysis	
Metronidazole	Hypersensitivity reaction, flushing, ± erythematous rash	Alcohol ingestion
	Rare: pityriasis rosea, fixed drug eruption	
Furazolidone	Maculopapular eruptions, vesicular morbilliform, hypersensitivity reaction, pruritic rash, contact dermatitis, erythema multiforme	0.5% incidence rate overall (based on evaluation of 10 433 patients)
Anthelminthics		
Albendazole	Hair loss (reversible)	High-dose chronic therapy
	Rash and pruritus	
	Stevens–Johnson syndrome	
Diethylcarbamazine	Hypersensitivity reaction (Mazzotti reaction)	Onchocerciasis ≫ Loiasis > other filariae
Ivermectin	Rash and pruritus	
Biting arthropod repellent		
Diethyltoluamide	Rare: local irritant reaction, scarring bullous dermatitis	

HIV/AIDS, human immunodeficiency virus/acquired immunodeficiency syndrome. TEN, toxic epidermal necrolysis.
(Data from references 105–117, 119–123, 125–134.)

Access the complete reference list online at
http://www.expertconsult.com

Access the complete reference list online at http://www.expertconsult.com

CHAPTER 133

Hepatobiliary Disease

Mohammad S. Khuroo • Mehnaaz S. Khuroo

INTRODUCTION

A broad group of infections affect hepatobiliary organs in the tropical countries. These include infections prevalent in nontropical zones and those restricted to tropical zones of the world (***Table 133.1***). Amongst the hepatitis viruses, hepatitis E virus (HEV) has the most significant palpable impact.[1] A number of nonviral infectious agents predominantly prevalent in tropical countries affect the liver and biliary tract as primary targets.[2] Commonest amongst these are amebiasis, echinococcosis, schistosomiasis and hepatobiliary and pancreatic ascariasis (HBPA). Tuberculosis and the acquired immunodeficiency syndrome (AIDS) are endemic in tropics and can involve both the liver and/or biliary tree.[3,4] Several viral and nonviral tropical infections such as malaria, typhoid, dengue fever, and leptospirosis may affect the heptobiliary system as a part of multiorgan involvement.[5] Hepatobiliary infections prevalent in tropical countries have a special predilection and distinct pattern for expatriate Western travelers to such countries.[6,7]

DIAGNOSTIC CONSIDERATIONS

Methodology to be followed for proper evaluation of hepatobiliary diseases in tropics is no different than that employed in nontropical countries.[8] This includes a proper history, thorough physical examination, routine blood counts and serum chemistries including bilirubin, alanine aminotransferase (ALT), aspartate aminotransferase (AST), and alkaline phosphatase (ALP). Abnormal liver tests can be classified into definite patterns: (1) hepatocellular (elevated bilirubin; elevated ALT/AST >500 IU; ALT>AST; normal to <3 times normal elevation of ALP); (2) cholestatic (elevated bilirubin, normal to <300 IU ALT/AST; >4 times normal elevation of ALP); (3) haemolytic/Gilbert's syndrome (isolated elevation of unconjugated bilirubin rarely above 5 mg/dL); (4) synthetic liver failure (elevated bilirubin, modestly elevated ALT, AST, and ALP; low albumin, high globulins, and high prothrombin time); and (5) infiltrative (isolated >4 times normal elevation of ALP). Each pattern has different clinical connotations and defines corresponding further workup. Hepatobiliary ultrasound with Doppler is a valued complement to clinical examination for hepatobiliary diseases and is strongly recommended as a part of primary evaluation. Ultrasound with Doppler is useful for detecting gallstones, thickened gallbladder, dilated bile ducts, cysts and masses within the liver, periportal fibrosis, hepatosplenomegaly, and evidence of portal hypertension.[9] Based on findings, further cost-effective, evidence-based laboratory tests, imaging tools such as computed tomography (CT), magnetic resonance imaging (MRI), magnetic resonance cholangiopancreatography (MRCP), endoscopic retrograde cholangiopancreatography (ERCP), or other invasive tests such as liver biopsy or guided fine needle aspiration biopsies may need to be employed.

DISEASES CAUSED BY HEPATITIS VIRUSES

Acute Sporadic Viral Hepatitis

Viral hepatitis (see Chapters 64–66) is highly endemic in tropical countries and is a cause of significant morbidity and mortality. Etiology of acute sporadic hepatitis in these countries is different than in the West. Around half of sporadic viral hepatitis in the tropics is related to HEV. Hepatitis B virus (HBV), hepatitis C virus (HCV), and non-A-E hepatitis constitute around 22%, 9%, and 25% of patients, respectively. Hepatitis A virus (HAV), a dominant cause of acute hepatitis in the West, is an uncommon (<4%) cause of hepatitis in adults in the tropics and is mostly encountered in children below 10 years of age.[10–14]

Acute viral hepatitis affects adults predominantly in the age group of 25–45 years. Male : female ratio is 1.4 : 1. Pregnant women especially in the third trimester are often infected with HEV and constitute around one-fourth of the females infected.[15] The clinical profiles and serum chemistries are typical of acute viral hepatitis as seen in the West. However, around 20% of patients with HEV infection present with prolonged cholestasis. Abdominal ultrasound is usually unremarkable. However, it may show a hypoechoic liver with focal bright spots (starry sky appearance). The gallbladder often shows wall edema and pericholecystic fluid resembling features of acalculous cholecystitis.[16] Recovery takes 4–6 weeks. Acute liver failure develops in around 8–10% of hospitalized patients. However, over 50% of pregnant women with HEV infections develop acute liver failure with high maternal and perinatal mortality.[15]

Patients with sporadic hepatitis need to be evaluated for acute markers of hepatitis viruses (IgM anti-HAV; HBsAg and IgM anti-HBc; anti-HCV; IgM anti-HEV), cytomegalovirus (CMV) and Epstein–Barr virus.[17] Dengue fever, typhoid fever, malaria, and leptospirosis may cause abnormal liver tests of hepatocellular damage; however, these infections cause systemic manifestations and these should be carefully evaluated.[4]

Epidemic Hepatitis

Epidemic hepatitis in tropical countries is exclusively caused by HEV.[18–21] Epidemiological features of HEV infection have several peculiar characteristics, which remain unexplained. HEV presents as repeated large-scale waterborne epidemics of jaundice in highly endemic areas occurring every 10–20 years. HEV is a disease of adult populations, and during epidemics attack rates in adults are higher than in children. HEV has an increased incidence and severity in pregnant women, and the major cause of mortality in epidemics is the high rate of fulminant hepatitis in pregnant women.[22–25]

The clinical and biochemical presentations of HEV are similar to those of infection with other hepatitis viruses and encompass a wide variety of

Table 133.1 Hepatobiliary Diseases Caused by Infectious Agents in Tropical Countries

Disease	Agents	Endemic Areas	Manifestations	Diagnosis	Treatment
Hepatic Disease Caused by Hepatitis Viruses					
Acute sporadic hepatitis	HEV (40%), HBV (22%), HCV (9%), non-A-E (25%), HAV (4%). Children often infected with HAV	Endemic in all developing countries	Adults involved; prolonged cholestasis in 20%; mortality 8–10% (high in pregnant women with HEV)	Acute markers (IgM anti-HEV; HBsAg and anti-HBc IgM; anti-HCV; IgM anti-HEV); Monospot test (CMV). Ultrasound to exclude EHBO	Supportive care
Epidemic hepatitis	HEV	All developing countries with unsafe water supplies and poor sanitation	Repeated large-scale epidemics; adult disease; high incidence in pregnant women; mortality in pregnant women 20%; no chronic liver disease; vertical transmission with severe neonatal HEV	IgM anti-HEV	Safe water and sewage disposal to control epidemics
Acute liver failure	HEV (37%), HBV (18%), HCV (5%), non-A-E (37%), HAV (3%). Antitubercular drugs small percentage	Endemic in all developing countries	Encephalopathy; cerebral edema; coagulopathy; multiorgan failure; GI bleed; death. ALF related to HEV in pregnant women – explosive disease with DIC; may represent a severe manifestation of a Schwartzman-like phenomenon	Acute markers of HV; lab data to assess severity of liver failure and prognostic factors	Intensive care management; early consideration for liver transplant
Subacute hepatic failure	HEV, HBV	Indian subcontinent	Progressive jaundice, ascites, renal failure and SBP, terminal encephalopathy	Acute markers of HV	Supportive treatment
Chronic hepatitis/ cirrhosis	HBV, HCV	All developing countries	Asymptomatic; incidental abnormal liver tests; recurrent jaundice; established cirrhosis presents as signs of liver failure and portal hypertension	Serological markers and NAT for HBV and HCV	Consider antiviral therapy; supportive treatment for established cirrhosis
Acute on chronic liver failure (AOCLF)	HEV superinfection on established HBV/HCV cirrhosis, reactivation HBV and HCV	Indian subcontinent	Rapid decompensation of stable liver disease; presents as jaundice, ascites, renal failure, and GI bleed	Evaluate serologic markers of HV; lab tests to assess severity of liver failure	Supportive treatment; antiviral therapy if indicated
Hepatobiliary Disorders Caused by Nonviral Infections Prevalent in the Tropics					
Pyogenic liver abscess	*Escherichia coli*, *Klebsiella pneumoniae*, enterococci, anaerobes	Worldwide	Insidious onset, fever, RUQ pain and tenderness	Ultrasound or CECT and aspiration	IV antibiotic plus image-guided drainage; surgery in select cases
Amebic liver abscess	*Entamoeba histolytica*	Tropical and subtropical areas	Acute onset, fever, RUQ pain and tenderness	Ultrasound or CECT plus serology	Metronidazole plus diloxanide furoate
Cystic hepatobiliary hydatid disease	*Echinococcus granulosus*	Sheep and cattle raising areas	Incidental, mass lesion, infection, rupture into bile duct causes cholangitis and cholestasis	Ultrasound or CECT plus serology; ERCP to define biliary disease	Surgery or PAIR and albendazole; therapeutic ERCP for biliary disease
Alveolar hepatic hydatid disease	*Echinococcus multilocularis*	Germany, Austria, Switzerland, France, Turkey, Iran, Afghanistan, India (Kashmir), Canada, Japan	Expanding hepatic mass, portal hypertension, liver failure, cholestasis due to bile duct disease	Ultrasound or CECT plus serology; ERCP to define biliary disease	Long-term albendazole, resection, therapeutic ERCP
Polycystic hepatic hydatid disease	*Echinococcus vogeli*, *E. oligarthrus*	Panama, Ecuador, Colombia, Venezuela, French Guiana	Expanding hepatic mass, portal hypertension, liver failure, cholestasis due to bile duct disease	Ultrasound or CECT plus serology; ERCP to define biliary disease	Long-term albendazole, resection, therapeutic ERCP

Table 133.1 Hepatobiliary Diseases Caused by Infectious Agents in Tropical Countries—cont'd

Disease	Agents	Endemic Areas	Manifestations	Diagnosis	Treatment
Hepatobiliary and pancreatic ascariasis	*Ascaris lumbricoides*	Developing countries	Biliary colic, cholangitis, cholecystitis, pancreatitis, liver abscess	Ultrasound and ERCP	Anthelminthic therapy and worm extraction at ERCP
Hepatic schistosomiasis	*Schistosoma mansoni*, *S. japonicum*, *S. intercalatum*, *S. mekongi*	Asia, Africa, South America, Caribbean	Portal hypertension and variceal bleeding	Serology, hepatic imaging, ova in stool/rectal or liver biopsy	Praziquantel therapy and treat portal hypertension
Fascioliasis	*Fasciola hepatica*	Cattle and sheep raising areas	Cholangitis, cholestasis	Eggs in feces/bile ERCP	Triclabendazole/ bithionol, therapeutic ERCP
Clonorchiasis/ opisthorchiasis	*Clonorchis sinensis*, *Opisthorcis viverrini*, *O. felineus*	Southeast Asia	Cholangitis, cholestasis, cholangiocarcinoma	Ova in stool, ERCP	Praziquantel therapy and therapeutic ERCP
Hepatobiliary tuberculosis	*Mycobacterium* spp.	Developing countries	Fever, weight loss, hepatomegaly and elevated liver tests	Tuberculin skin test; serology for TB; liver biopsy	Antitubercular drugs
HIV cholangiopathy (in AIDS with $CD4^+$ <200/ mm^3)	*Cryptosporidium parvum*, Microsporidia, *Cyclospora cayetanensis*, *Isospora belli*; CMV	Worldwide	RUQ pain, fever, jaundice	Elevated ALP; ERCP papillitis and bile duct stricture; duodenal biopsy shows typical organisms	Antibiotics; therapeutic ERCP
Hepatobiliary Involvement Caused by Tropical Diseases as a Manifestation of Multiorgan Disease					
Malarial hepatitis	*Plasmodium* spp.	Asia, Africa, South America	Hepatitis occurs in 11–25% of infections; presents as jaundice, tender hepatomegaly, elevated liver tests, hepatic failure in severe *P. falciparum*	Look for parasites in blood film; lab tests to evaluate severity of liver disease	Antimalarial therapy; supportive treatment
Tropical splenomegaly syndrome	*Plasmodium* spp.	Asia, Africa, South America	Massive splenomegaly	Antimalarial antibodies; high IgM levels; liver biopsy: hepatic sinusoidal lymphocytosis (B cells)	Long-term antimalarial therapy
Typhoid hepatitis	*Salmonella* spp.	Indian subcontinent, South/Central America	Occurs in 1–26%; presents as jaundice, RUQ pain, elevated liver tests, rarely liver failure occurs, typhoid abscess may occur	Blood, urine and stool culture; serology; lab tests to evaluate severity of liver disease	Antibiotic therapy; supportive treatment
Leptospirosis hepatitis	*Leptospira* spp.	Tropical countries (sewage workers)	Hepatic involvement in second week; presents as RUQ pain, severe jaundice, elevated liver tests, rarely liver failure	Isolation of organism from blood or CSF; serologic tests (MAT or ELISA)	Antibiotic (penicillin, ampicillin, or erythromycin) therapy
Hyperinfection syndrome	*Strongyloides stercoralis*	Tropical and subtropical countries (high-risk AIDS and renal transplant)	Jaundice and elevated liver tests	Stool for *S. stercoralis* larvae; liver biopsy shows eosinophilic granulomatous hepatitis with larvae in canaliculi	Ivermectin
Invasive candidiasis	*Candida* spp.	Worldwide (acute leukemia on immunosuppression)	Chronic debilitating illness, RUQ pain, high fever, weight loss, hepatomegaly, elevated ALP	Ultrasound/CECT hypoechoic hepatic masses; guided needle aspiration biopsy of lesions	Amphotericin or fluconazole

ALF, acute liver failure; ALP, alkaline phosphatase; CECT, contrast-enhanced computed tomography; CMV, cytomegalovirus; DIC, disseminated intravascular coagulation; EHBO, extrahepatic biliary obstruction; ERCP, endoscopic retrograde cholangiopancreatography; GI, gastrointestinal; HV, hepatitis virus; MAT, microscopic agglutination test; NAT, nucleic acid amplification testing; PAIR, puncture, aspiration or injection of a scolicidal agent and reaspiration; RUQ, right upper quadrant; SBP, spontaneous bacterial peritonitis.

symptoms. Prolonged intrahepatic cholestasis lasting from 3 to 6 months occurs in about 20% of patients and simulates large bile duct obstruction. A small percentage of patients show a biphasic enzyme elevation; however, no chronic liver disease or chronic hepatitis is known to develop after HEV in immunocompetent hosts.

Acute Liver Failure

Acute liver failure (ALF), a dramatic and challenging syndrome in clinical medicine,[26,27] is characterized by rapid and progressive deterioration of liver function from massive hepatocellular necrosis or infiltration leading to encephalopathy and multiorgan failure. There is little information on the epidemiology of ALF in various regions of the world. Crude estimates suggest that ALF affects approximately 2000 individuals annually in the United States. In contrast, ALF caused by HEV infection is a substantial health problem in developing countries.

Most ALF in the tropics is caused by hepatitis viruses.[25,28,29] Amongst these, HEV is the cause of ALF in over 40% of patients. HBV and non-A-E constitute 17% and 33% of patients, respectively. HAV is an uncommon (<4%) cause of ALF in tropical countries. In comparison, HAV, HBV, and non-A-E cause 14%, 33%, and 53% of viral ALF in the United Kingdom. HEV is an uncommon cause of ALF in developed countries and is either seen in Western travelers to the Indian subcontinent or as a result of recently recognized zoonotic foodborne autochthonous HEV infections. Drugs, especially antitubercular drugs, cause <4% of ALF in developing countries, in contrast to developed countries where drugs, namely acetaminophen and anti-inflammatory drugs, constitute more substantial etiologies of ALF.

A number of transplant centers from the West have defined prognostic criteria in ALF and these criteria can be applied to estimate the probability of spontaneous recovery in a given patient. While one model of prognostic indicators has been developed at King's College Hospital, London,[30] data from India have shown that these prognostic indicators may not be valid for other geographical regions, in view of differences in the etiologic causes, behavior, and clinical profiles of ALF.[25,29] Early predictors of a poor outcome are non-HEV etiology, prothrombin time >30 seconds, grade of coma >2, and age >40 years.

Subacute Hepatic Failure

Subacute hepatic failure is an entity reported from the Indian subcontinent.[31,32] The hepatic failure shows a more protracted illness and is characterized by development of progressive jaundice, ascites, coagulopathy and renal failure during the course of acute hepatitis. Patients often develop spontaneous bacterial peritonitis and gastrointestinal bleeding. Encephalopathy is usually a preterminal event. Liver biopsy reveals extensive bridging, submassive necrosis, and cholestasis. HBV and HEV are the causes in most patients.

Chronic Hepatitis and Cirrhosis

Chronic active hepatitis in the tropics is caused most commonly by HBV and HCV (see Chapters 65 and 66).[33,34] Coinfection with hepatitis delta virus (HDV) may accelerate the course of chronic HBV infection.[35] While failure to resolve infection with these agents may lead to cirrhosis or hepatoma, persons with chronic hepatitis may remain asymptomatic for years, despite persistently elevated hepatic enzymes. Serologic testing and liver biopsy confirm the diagnosis. Macronodular or "postnecrotic" cirrhosis develops in up to 25% of chronic hepatitis B surface antigen carriers and in over 20% of persons infected with HCV for over 20 years. The process may be clinically silent for several years before the appearance of symptoms and signs of hepatocellular dysfunction and portal hypertension such as jaundice, encephalopathy, ascites, and bleeding from esophageal varices. The liver is firm, nodular, and shrunken.

Acute on Chronic Liver Failure

Acute on chronic liver failure (AOCLF) is a recently recognized entity wherein there is rapid hepatic decompensation once acute hepatic insult is superimposed on established stable chronic liver disease.[36–38] Alcoholic cirrhosis constitutes 50–70% of the underlying liver diseases in AOCLF in Western countries, whereas in most of tropical countries HBV constitutes 70% and alcohol only about 15% of the etiologies of AOCLF. Autoimmune liver disease, Wilson's disease, metabolic liver disease, and chronic cholestatic liver disease constitute only a minority of patients. Among the precipitating causes of AOCLF, HEV superinfection has remained a very important acute insult in the Indian subcontinent and is an important cause of mortality in patients with cirrhosis.[38–40] Reactivation of HBV and HCV infections leading to hepatitis "flares" are the other major causes of AOCLF in the Asian region.[41] In contrast to this, sepsis and variceal bleeding play important roles in the sudden decompensation of established chronic liver disease in the West.

DISEASES CAUSED BY TROPICAL NONVIRAL INFECTIOUS AGENTS

Pyogenic Liver Abscess

Pyogenic liver abscess is responsible for 8–20 cases per 100 000 hospital admissions. Pyogenic abscesses most often occur in patients over 40 years of age, with a peak incidence in the sixth decade. No significant gender, ethnic, or geographic differences exist for the development of pyogenic liver abscesses. About one-half of patients have a solitary abscess. Abscesses involve the right lobe in 75%, left lobe in 20%, and caudate lobe in 5% of cases.

Suppurative cholangitis as a result of bile duct stones, benign and malignant biliary strictures, and endoscopic, radiologic, and operative biliary interventions are the major identifiable causes of pyogenic liver abscess in the West.[42–47] In endemic areas, *Ascaris lumbricoides* (see Chapter 115) and *Clonorchis sinensis* (see Chapter 123) can invade the biliary tree, cause cholangitis, and commonly predispose to liver abscesses.[2,45] Liver abscesses can be caused by *Salmonella enterica* serovar Typhi, *Mycobacterium tuberculosis* and *Brucella* spp. (***Fig. 133.1***). Most pyogenic liver abscesses are polymicrobial. The frequently isolated organisms include *Escherichia coli*, *Klebsiella pneumoniae*, *Streptococcus viridans*, *Staphylococcus aureus*, *Enterococcus faecalis*, *Bacteroides* spp., *Fusobacterium* spp., anaerobic streptococci, *Actinomyces* spp., and rarely *Clostridia* spp.

In the past, patients typically presented with acute-onset abdominal pain (89%), high fever with rigors and chills (67%), and right upper

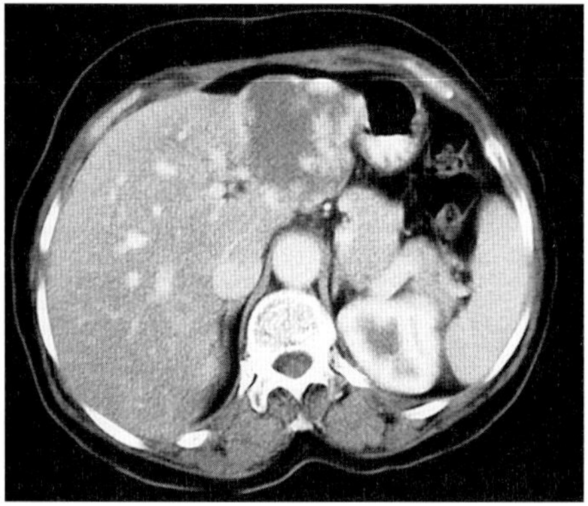

Figure 133.1 Liver abscess caused by brucellosis in a 30-year-old woman who presented with fever, arthralgia, hepatomegaly, and elevated serum alkaline phosphatase. Contrast-enhanced CT scan image of liver shows hypodense mass in the left lobe with thick ring enhancement of the margins. (From Khuroo MS, Khuroo NS. Non-viral infections of the liver. In: Al Knawy B, Schiffman ML, Wiesner RH, eds. Hepatology: A Practical Approach. Amsterdam: Elsevier BV Academic Press; 2004:158, Fig. 1B.)

quadrant (RUQ) tenderness (70%). Since the introduction of antibiotics, the presentation of pyogenic liver abscess has become less acute, often insidious and characterized by malaise, low-grade fever, and dull abdominal pain. Diagnostic imaging studies are essential in making the diagnosis of pyogenic liver abscess. Sonography is highly sensitive (94%) and is the imaging method of choice in patients with suspected biliary disease. Contrast-enhanced computed tomography (CECT) has high sensitivity (100%), and visualizes abscesses better because contrast enhancement highlights the unaffected liver. Treatment of pyogenic liver abscess requires antibiotic therapy and image-guided percutaneous drainage of the abscess. Such treatments are successful in 85–90% of patients. Surgical drainage is reserved in the following situations: (1) percutaneous drainage is unsuccessful, (2) there is coexisting intra-abdominal disease requiring surgery, and (3) abscess is complicated by rupture or extension into adjacent structures.

Amebic Liver Abscess

Amebic liver abscess is the most common extraintestinal manifestation of *Entamoeba histolytica* infection (see Chapter 92) and occurs in approximately 8.5% of such patients. The disease is endemic in many tropical regions namely Mexico, Central America, northern South America, West and South Africa, and India.[48–53]

Amebic liver abscess most often occurs in the age group 20–45 years. Most patients present with an acute illness, and duration of symptoms is usually <2 weeks. Clinical symptoms and signs include low-grade fever and chills, RUQ pain and tenderness, and hepatomegaly. Left lobe abscesses can present with toxemia; epigastric pain, tenderness, and guarding; and a large epigastric mass. Multiple liver abscesses usually present with high fever, toxemia, jaundice, and encephalopathy. Complications of amebic liver abscess include secondary bacterial infection, rupture, and compression of the bile ducts.

Diagnosis is made on hepatic imaging and amebic serology. Ultrasound and CECT are useful in delineating and localizing the abscess as well as to monitor the response to treatment. Amebic serologic tests, (e.g., enzyme immunoassay) can have sensitivities of 99% and specificities >90% in patients with amebic liver abscess. Amebic liver abscess needs to be differentiated from pyogenic liver abscess in endemic areas, especially in view of the different treatment regimens employed in the two entities and different responses to therapy (***Table 133.2***).

Table 133.2 Differentiating Features of Pyogenic and Amebic Liver Abscesses

Feature	Pyogenic Liver Abscess	Amebic Liver Abscess
Distribution of disease	Worldwide	Tropical and subtropical regions
Age of occurrence	Above 40 years	20–45 years
Sex distribution	Equal	3–10 times more in males than females
Number	Often multiple (50%)	Often single (80%)
Location	Either lobe	Often right lobe under dome of diaphragm
Duration of illness	Usually 1 month	Often 2 weeks
Symptoms	Low-grade fever, RUQ pain and tenderness	Low-grade fever, RUQ pain and tenderness
Jaundice	Mild unless associated with biliary disease	Moderate in large and multiple abscesses
Blood culture	Positive (50–90%)	Negative
Hepatic imaging	Mass lesion with fluid component	Mass lesion with fluid component
Amebic serology	Negative	Positive
Treatment	Intravenous antibiotics plus drainage	Metronidazole plus diloxanide furoate
Mortality	16%	2–18%
High-risk groups	Jaundice, low albumin, comorbid disease	Multiple abscesses, left lobe abscess, high bilirubin, encephalopathy, low albumin

RUQ, right upper quadrant.

(Reproduced with permission from Khuroo MS, Khuroo NS. Non-viral infections of the liver. In: Al Knawy B, Schiffman ML, Wiesner RH, eds. Hepatology: A Practical Approach. Amsterdam: Elsevier BV Academic Press; 2004:161.)

Metronidazole, 800 mg three times per day orally for 10 days, is curative in over 90% of patients with amebic liver abscess. Clinical improvement is usually seen within 3–5 days. After clinical cure, the abscess cavity disappears in 6–9 months. Alternative agents include secnidazole 500 mg orally three times per day, and tinidazole 600 mg orally twice per day for 7 days. A luminal amebicide, diloxanide furoate 500 mg three times per day for 10 days, is often used to eradicate intestinal carriage of the organism. Unlike pyogenic liver abscess, needle aspiration or abscess drainage offers no additional therapeutic benefit. Aspiration is indicated in patients with persistent symptoms after 5 days of medical therapy and in those with: (1) very large abscess, (2) abscess involving the left lobe, (3) abscess which shows signs of imminent rupture, and (4) abscess with secondary bacterial infection. Open surgical drainage is indicated when an abscess has ruptured into the peritoneum or adjacent viscera.

Hepatic Hydatid Disease

Hydatid disease, echinococcosis, (see Chapter 120), is a zoonotic infection caused by larval forms (metacestodes) of the tapeworms of the genus *Echinococcus* and is characterized by development of expanding cysts in the liver and other body organs (***Fig. 133.2***).[54–59] Within the genus *Echinococcus*, four principal causes of human disease are recognized. *E. granulosus* causes cystic hydatid disease, *E. multilocularis* causes alveolar hydatid disease, and *E. vogeli* and *E. oligarthrus* cause polycystic hydatid disease. The most clinically relevant form is cystic echinococcosis caused by *E. granulosus*. Uncomplicated liver cysts usually present with dull ache in the RUQ or a feeling of abdominal swelling or distension. A large cyst in the hilar region can compress the common hepatic duct causing cholestasis. Cyst rupture into the biliary tree causes obstruction of the ducts by daughter cysts and laminated membranes and presents as biliary colic, cholangitis, and progressive cholestasis.

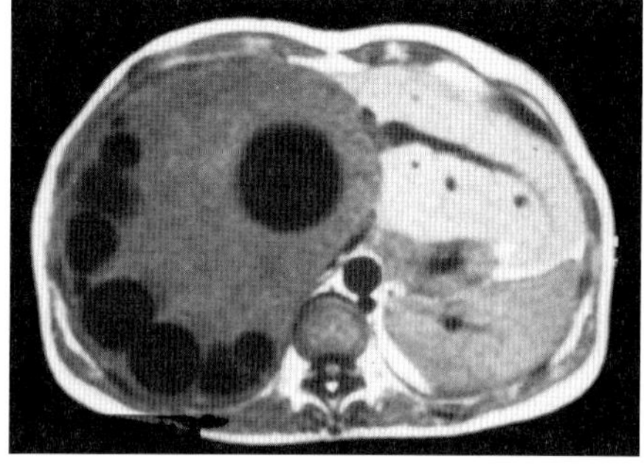

Figure 133.2 Cystic hepatic echinococcosis. A 50-year-old man complained of RUQ discomfort of 6 months' duration. An axial T1-weighted MR image shows a large rounded lesion occupying the whole right lobe of the liver. The lesion reveals multiple rounded low signal lesions (daughter cysts). The remainder of the contents reveal high intensity signal (matrix). (From Khuroo MS, Khuroo NS. Non-viral infections of the liver. In: Al Knawy B, Schiffman ML, Wiesner RH, eds. Hepatology: A Practical Approach. Amsterdam: Elsevier BV Academic Press, 2004:163, Fig. 2.)

Serology and imaging tools can help establish the diagnosis (see Chapter 120). Serology detects specific serum antibodies or circulating antigen by a variety of immunodiagnostic methods. Positive test results need confirmation by the arc-5 immunoelectrophoretic (IEP) test, which detects antibodies against immunodominant and specific antigen (antigen 5) of the cestode. Liver cysts are well visualized by ultrasound. Cysts may appear univesicular, rounded with well-defined margins containing pure fluid or multivesicular (daughter cysts) with pure fluid collection in each vesicle. Cysts may have a hyperechoic solid pattern (pseudotumor appearance) or may have reflective walls suggestive of calcification. Rupture of liver cysts into the bile ducts can be suspected on ultrasound. Ultrasound appearances in such cases include dilated bile ducts, non-shadowing echogenic structures within the ducts, and loss of continuity of the cyst wall adjacent to the bile duct representing the site of communication. However, ERCP is the recommended tool and reveals filling defects of varying shape and size in the dilated bile ducts and leakage of contrast medium into the cyst cavity.

Treatment options for cystic hydatid disease are surgery, drug therapy, and percutaneous drainage (see Chapter 120). Surgery has the potential to remove cysts and lead to complete cure. The surgical procedure of choice is cystectomy with removal of the germinal and laminated layers and preservation of pericyst. Operative mortality varies from 0.5% to 4.0% in centers with adequate medical and surgical facilities. Albendazole and praziquantel can be effective in small cysts (<4 cm diameter), in cysts with thin walls, and in younger patients. Alternatively, percutaneous treatment of hepatic hydatid cysts, known as PAIR (puncture, aspiration, installation of scolicidal agent, and respiration) has been efficacious. The procedure is minimally invasive, cost-effective, involves reduced hospital stay, and has less morbidity and mortality than surgery.

Hepatobiliary and Pancreatic Ascariasis

Ascariasis is caused by the nematode *Ascaris lumbricoides* (see Chapter 115). Hepatobiliary and pancreatic ascariasis (HPA) is one of the most common complications caused by intestinal *Ascaris* infections. Ascarides in the duodenum can enter the ampullary orifice and block it; they can advance further to the bile duct and hepatic ducts (***Fig. 133.3***). While in the common duct, the cystic duct can be blocked by worms entering its orifice. Less often, worms can reach the gallbladder or enter the pancreatic duct.[60–63]

HPA is more common in women than men (female : male ratio of 3 : 1) with a mean age of occurrence being 35 years (range 4–70 years). HPA is more frequent in pregnant women and in patients with previous cholecystectomy, choledocholithotomy, sphincteroplasty, and endoscopic sphincterotomy in whom the widened ampullary orifice facilitates passage of worms into the bile ducts. HPA can cause five distinct clinical presentations, namely intractable biliary colic, acalculous cholecystitis, acute cholangitis, acute pancreatitis, and liver abscesses.

Diagnosis of HPA can be made by ultrasonography and ERCP. Ultrasonography is a highly sensitive and specific method for detection of worms in the biliary tree. This noninvasive investigation can be used in patients with symptoms and repeated frequently to monitor movement of worms in the ducts. ERCP has an advantage as a diagnostic tool in that it permits identification of the worms in the duodenum and those across the papilla and also allows removal of worms from the ducts or the duodenum.

Hepatic Schistosomiasis

Hepatic schistosomiasis is caused by *Schistosoma mansoni*, *S. japonicum*, *S. intercalatum*, and *S. mekongi* (see Chapter 122). Hepatic schistosomiasis is characterized by granuloma formation in the liver with hepatic fibrosis leading to portal hypertension and manifests as splenomegaly, esophageal varices, and portosystemic collateral shunts at other sites (***Fig. 133.4***). Variceal bleeding in hepatic schistosomiasis is better tolerated than variceal bleeding in posthepatitic or alcoholic cirrhosis and encephalopathy is not usually precipitated following bleed. Patients with hepatic schistosomiasis may be coinfected with HBV or HCV that may cause rapid deterioration of liver functions in such patients.[64–66]

Ultrasonography with Doppler is noninvasive, inexpensive, and a sensitive tool to stage the severity of disease and monitor the response to therapy. Liver biopsy is helpful in excluding other causes of liver disease. The presence of schistosome eggs in the biopsy is seen as often as positive findings on stool examination or rectal biopsy.

Hepatic schistosomiasis is managed by antischistosomal chemotherapy and measures to treat portal hypertension and its complications and hepatic failure following standard guidelines. Drug therapy eradicates the infection, prevents progression of disease, and interrupts egg excretion and disease dissemination.

Liver Flukes: Fascioliasis

Fascioliasis is caused by the liver fluke *Fasciola hepatica* (see Chapter 123). Mature flukes reside in the biliary tree and cause chronic obstructive biliary symptoms. Fascioliasis is endemic in parts of Europe and Latin America, North Africa, Asia, the Western Pacific, and some parts of the United States.[67–71]

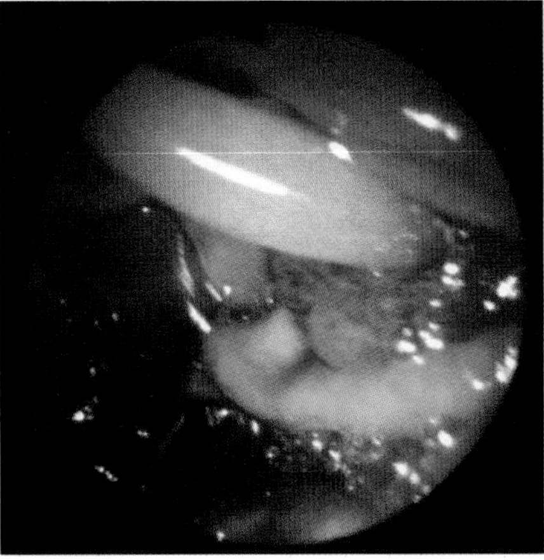

Figure 133.3 Hepatobiliary and pancreatic ascariasis. A 30-year-woman presented to the emergency room with intractable pain RUQ. Duodenoscopy shows a large ascaride entering the ampullary orifice. A cholangiogram (not shown) showed the remaining part of the ascaride in the bile duct. Endoscopic extraction of the worm from the papilla caused immediate relief of biliary pain. (From Khuroo et al. Gastrointest Endosc. 1993;39, 680–685, Fig. 1.)

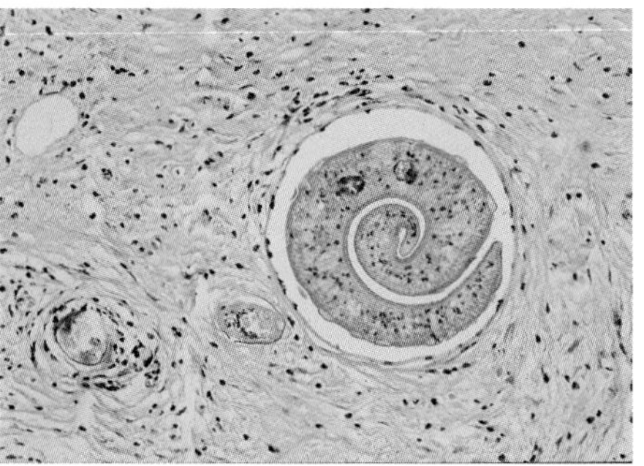

Figure 133.4 Schistosomiasis. Microscopic examination of a mesenteric mass in a 40-year-old male who had a laparotomy for intestinal obstruction. A mesenteric mass with adhesions to the bowel loops was seen at surgery. Histology of the mass shows an adult worm of *Schistosoma mansoni* curled up in the mesenteric vein. Two eggs, oval in shape and with lateral spines (*S. mansoni* eggs), are nearby. (From Khuroo MS, Khuroo NS. Non-viral infections of the liver. In: Al Knawy B, Schiffman ML, Wiesner RH, (eds). Hepatology: A Practical Approach. Amsterdam: Elsevier BV Academic Press; 2004:169, Fig. 4.)

Three clinical syndromes are recognized: acute or invasive, chronic latent, and chronic obstructive. The acute phase corresponds to migration of young flukes through the liver and is marked by fever, RUQ pain, urticaria, hepatomegaly, and eosinophilia. The latent phase corresponds to the settling of the flukes into the bile ducts and can last for months to years. The chronic obstructive phase is a consequence of intrahepatic and extrahepatic bile duct inflammation and hyperplasia evoked by the flukes. Recurrent biliary colic, cholangitis, cholelithiasis, and cholestasis may result. Liver tests reveal features of biliary obstruction. Long-term infection can lead to biliary cirrhosis and secondary sclerosing cholangitis.

Diagnosis of acute infection can be done by serologic detection of antibodies. Chronic infection can be diagnosed by detection of eggs in feces, duodenal aspirate, or bile. Hepatic imaging by ultrasonography or CECT is useful to define biliary dilatation and secondary hepatic changes due to cholestasis. ERCP will demonstrate adult flukes in the biliary tree and can be used to extract the parasites from the ducts.

Liver Flukes: Clonorchiasis and Opisthorchiasis

The liver flukes include *Clonorchis sinensis*, *Opisthorchis viverrini*, and *O. felineus* (see Chapter 123). *C. sinensis* and *O. viverrini* are prevalent in East and Southeast Asia, and *O. felineus* is prevalent in eastern Europe.[72–75]

Clinical manifestations are caused by the presence of adult flukes in the bile duct, which release eggs that cause severe inflammation and fibrosis. Fever, RUQ pain, tender hepatomegaly, and eosinophilia are initial manifestations. Later chronic biliary obstruction can occur. Patients develop cholelithiasis, cholecystitis, and recurrent pyogenic cholangitis. Long-term infection leads to exuberant inflammation, marked biliary epithelial hyperplasia, and dysplasia, and a substantially increased risk of cholangiocarcinoma.

Diagnosis is made by detection of characteristic fluke eggs in the stool except late in the disease. Cholangiography, percutaneously or at ERCP, reveals slender, uniform filling defects within intrahepatic ducts. Bile ducts reveal strictures, dilatation, and sacculation mimicking sclerosing cholangitis.

Hepatobiliary Tuberculosis

Tuberculosis (see Chapter 35) is a disease of developing countries; however, its incidence is increasing in developed countries, mainly in immigrant populations and in patients with AIDS.[3,76]

Hepatobiliary tuberculosis is seen in a number of situations:

1. Incidental. Liver involvement is seen at autopsy in 25–50% of patients dying from active pulmonary tuberculosis.
2. Miliary tuberculosis, due to hematogenous spread of tubercle bacilli, causes multiple granulomas within the liver.
3. Granulomatous hepatitis. Patients present with unexplained fever, jaundice, hepatomegaly, elevated ALP, and abnormalities of other liver function tests. Imaging of the liver may be normal or reveal nonspecific abnormalities. Laparoscopy is useful and shows cheesy white irregular nodules on the liver surface. Biopsy from such lesions reveals caseating granulomas. Granulomatous hepatitis with multiple granulomas in the liver may also be seen following vaccination with bacillus Calmette–Guérin, especially in persons with impaired immune response.
4. Nodular disease. In this entity single or multiple focal masses develop in the liver and are seen as low-density non-enhancing lesions with or without peripheral rim enhancement. Such appearances need to be differentiated from lymphoma, fungal infection, and metastasis. Diagnosis is confirmed by image-guided fine needle aspiration biopsy of the lesion.
5. Tuberculous liver abscess. Tuberculous abscesses in the liver are extremely rare. Clinical picture and imaging resembles pyogenic or amebic liver abscess. Culture of the aspirated material clinches the diagnosis by growth of tubercle bacilli.
6. Tubular disease. These patients present with obstructive jaundice due to involvement of bile ducts. Bile ducts may be involved by an enlarged tuberculous lymph node compressing the bile duct or diffuse involvement of the intrahepatic ducts by tubercle bacilli. ERCP reveals multiple intrahepatic biliary strictures, areas of dilatation, beading and ectasia, resembling sclerosing cholangitis or cholangiocarcinoma. Biliary stricture may occur at the hilar region or distal common bile duct with dilatation of the intrahepatic ducts.

HIV Cholangiopathy

A number of parasites can involve the biliary tree in patients with HIV infection and lead to a spectrum of clinical manifestations including HIV cholangiopathy and acute cholecystitis (see Chapter 139). Among these are included *Cryptosporidium parvum* (see Chapter 94), Microsporidia (see Chapter 102), *Cyclospora cayetanensis* (see Chapter 95), and *Isospora belli* (see Chapter 95). Most patients with cholangiopathy have severe immunosuppression, with $CD4^+$ counts of $<200/mm^3$. HIV cholangiopathy can also be caused by infection with cytomegalovirus (CMV) (see Chapter 56), *Mycobacterium avium-intracellulare* complex infection (see Chapter 35), and *Candida albicans* (see Chapter 88).[4,77]

Typical symptoms are RUQ pain, fever, and elevated serum ALP. Jaundice is uncommon. Diarrhea is common because many of the pathogens infect the small bowel as well. On physical examination RUQ or epigastric tenderness is characteristic. ERCP shows intrahepatic or extrahepatic changes of sclerosing cholangitis. Papillary stenosis is also common.

Diagnosis and treatment of the etiologic infections are considered in the pathogen specific chapters. In addition, endoscopic management of biliary disease may be required. Endoscopic sphincterotomy is adequate in patients with papillary stenosis, while bile duct strictures may need dilation or stenting.

HEPATOBILIARY DISEASE CAUSED BY TROPICAL INFECTIONS AS A PART OF MULTIORGAN INVOLVEMENT

Other systemic tropical diseases that can involve the hepatobiliary tree as a part of multiorgan involvement include malaria, typhoid, leptospirosis, strongyloidiasis, and invasive candidiasis.[5,78,79] ***Table 133.1*** briefly delineates the hepatobiliary disease caused by these agents.

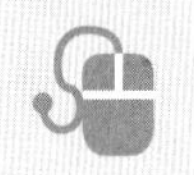

Access the complete reference list online at **http://www.expertconsult.com**

CHAPTER 134

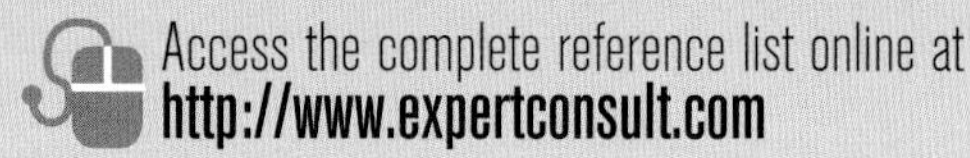
Access the complete reference list online at
http://www.expertconsult.com

Approach to the Patient in the Tropics with Pulmonary Disease

Gregory J. Martin

Pulmonary disease is one of the leading causes of morbidity and mortality throughout the world, and respiratory tract infections are the most frequent infections of humans. Four of the 10 leading causes of global death reported to the World Health Organization (WHO) are attributable to some form of acute or chronic pulmonary disease (***Table 134.1***). Lower respiratory infection (mainly pneumonia) is the leading cause of death in the developing, often tropical, nations.[1]

The viral, bacterial, fungal, and protozoal etiologies of worldwide lung infections are protean. Tropical pulmonary disease includes most temperate climate etiologies as well as a greater incidence and prevalence of tuberculosis (TB), human immunodeficiency virus (HIV)-related disease, and helminthic infections. In addition, a few etiologies are unique to the tropics. Diverse factors such as poverty, crowding, malnutrition, and proximity to animals have additional impacts and are responsible for diseases that are infrequently encountered outside the tropics.

As developing nations make economic transitions, smoking, air pollution, and unregulated occupational and environmental exposures have become significant risk factors for chronic obstructive pulmonary disease (COPD), respiratory tract malignancies, and pneumoconioses. This effect has been most dramatic in large nations with rapid economic changes such as India and China where rates of COPD and respiratory malignancies now exceed those in developed nations.[2,3]

As travel increases, agents responsible for localized outbreaks of disease in remote, undeveloped areas have been more frequently imported to the industrialized world. Vigilance for respiratory illness in the tropics is now recognized as crucial in identifying diseases and trends that will impact health in temperate nations. Most notably in 2003, the ability of a zoonotic coronavirus to infect humans led to the severe acute respiratory syndrome (SARS). SARS rapidly became a public health emergency not only in much of Asia but also in Canada and, to a lesser extent, the United States and Europe, with deaths in 774 of 8098 cases in 29 nations.[4]

Novel influenza viruses have commonly been first discovered in tropical Asian populations where animals, especially chickens, ducks, and pigs, are often kept in close proximity to humans. As outbreaks of avian and swine influenza occur in these areas, sporadic cases of these same strains occur in humans, creating the potential for human–zoonotic recombinations and returning travelers presenting with these "exotic" strains.[5] Novel influenza viruses may be encountered in countries with advanced diagnostics and then later determined to have been circulating in a less well-developed setting for some time, as was demonstrated with the swine–avian–human recombinant H1N1 pandemic strain in 2009.

This chapter aims to facilitate developing a differential diagnosis for patients presenting with pulmonary complaints who are in, or had exposure in, the tropics. Infectious etiologies are more fully considered in pathogen-specific chapters. Emphasis is on those entities found exclusively or more commonly in the tropics or, like respiratory infections in children, those that have a major impact on public health. Common respiratory infections in industrialized, temperate settings are also frequent in the tropics, whereas some pulmonary infections, especially those associated with parasites, are rarely encountered in the temperate setting. Parasitic etiologies associated with respiratory disease from the tropics and their geographic distributions must be considered (***Table 134.2***).[6]

Clinicians evaluate patients' illnesses in geographic areas differently depending on the local disease prevalence and on the resources available. In developing a differential diagnosis for respiratory complaints, it is helpful to consider patients' epidemiologic groups that have considerable differences in their exposures and risk factors:

1. Lifelong residents of the tropics (and those who have recently emigrated from the tropics) who may have established, long-standing infections or infectious sequelae.
2. Travelers from temperate areas who have returned from the tropics after short (less than 3 months) visits; this would include immigrants who return to their tropical home to visit friends and family (generally the highest-risk travelers).
3. Expatriates from temperate areas who are currently living in the tropics or have recently returned from years in the tropics.

The etiologies and diagnostic approaches to each of these groups may be quite different as the intensity of their exposures, potential contact with infected individuals, and access to medical care (and advanced diagnostics) may vary significantly.[7]

ACUTE RESPIRATORY TRACT INFECTIONS, INCLUDING PNEUMONIA

Acute respiratory tract infections (ARIs) include a spectrum of illnesses from colds and influenza to pharyngitis and pneumonia. Upper respiratory illnesses (URIs) are the most common infections in humans in both temperate and tropical climates and are primarily viral in etiology. The frequency of URIs among children is much greater than in adults.[8] Although the frequency of URIs in the tropics appears to be no higher than in temperate climates, children in the tropics often suffer multiple comorbid conditions including chronic malnutrition. Undernourished children experience respiratory infections, coupled with bouts of diarrhea, intestinal helminths, epidemic measles, and more. These comorbidities allow what would be a mild respiratory illness in a healthy child to cause significant morbidity or mortality.[9] The role of viral URIs, particularly influenza and respiratory syncytial virus, in predisposing individuals to subsequent bacterial pneumonia, predominantly with *Streptococcus pneumoniae* and *Haemophilus influenzae,* has emphasized the importance of controlling epidemic influenza in developing nations where vaccines have been historically underutilized.[10]

Acute lower respiratory infections cause most of the respiratory disease-associated deaths worldwide and pneumonia kills significantly more children than any other illness (***Fig. 134.1***).[11] Pneumonia is the primary focus in the WHO's effort to decrease childhood mortality by two-thirds between 1990 and 2015. Although all age groups have some

Rank	Cause of Death	% of Total Deaths
1	Coronary heart disease	12.2
2	Cerebrovascular disease	9.7
3	**Lower respiratory infections[a,b]**	**7.1**
4	**Chronic obstructive pulmonary disease[b]**	**5.1**
5	Diarrheal disease	3.7
6	Human immunodeficiency virus (HIV)/acquired immunodeficiency syndrome (AIDS)	3.5
7	**Tuberculosis[b]**	**2.5**
8	**Cancers of the trachea, bronchus, lung[b]**	**2.3**
9	Road traffic accidents	2.2
10	Prematurity and low birth weight	2.0

Table 134.1 Ten Leading Causes of Death Worldwide, 2004

[a]*Lower respiratory infections are the leading cause of death in lower-income (mainly tropical) nations, causing 11.2% of deaths.*

[b]*Attributable to some form of acute or chronic pulmonary disease.*

(Reproduced from WHO. The top 10 causes of death. WHO Fact Sheet No. 310. Geneva: WHO, 2008.)

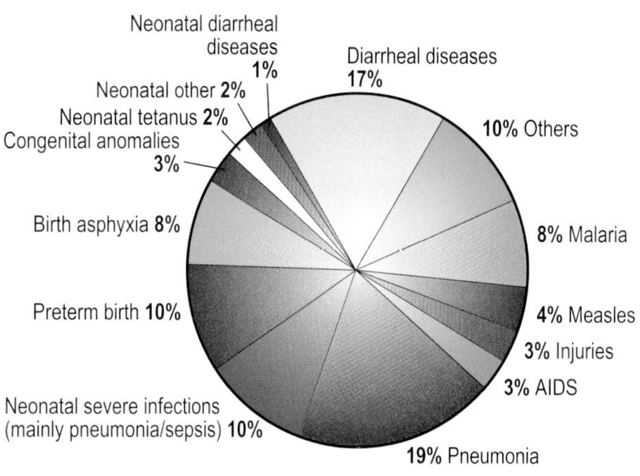

Figure 134.1 Global deaths in children under 5 in 2004. Pneumonia is the leading killer of children worldwide. AIDS, acquired immunodeficiency syndrome.

Box 134.1 Etiologies of Childhood Pneumonia in the Tropics

Bacterial Etiologies

- *Streptococcus pneumoniae* (30–50%)
- *Haemophilus influenzae* b (10–30%)

Other Frequent Bacterial Etiologies

- *Staphylococcus aureus*
- *Salmonella* spp. (nontyphoidal)
- Nontypable *Haemophilus influenzae*
- *Mycobacterium tuberculosis* (causing acute pneumonia)
- *Klebsiella pneumoniae*
- *Bordetella pertussis*
- Group B *Streptococcus*

Viral Etiologies

- Respiratory syncytial virus (15–40%)
- Influenza A and B
- Parainfluenza
- Rubeola (measles)
- Human metapneumovirus
- Adenovirus

Other Agents (Sporadic or Outbreaks)

- *Mycoplasma pneumoniae*
- *Chlamydia* spp.
- *Pseudomonas* spp.
- *Escherichia coli*
- *Pneumocystis jirovecii* (HIV-associated)
- *Histoplasma* spp.
- *Toxoplasma gondii*
- Hantaviruses
- Hemorrhagic fever viruses

(Extracted from: Rudan I, Boschi-Pinto C, Biloglav Z, et al. Epidemiology and etiology of childhood pneumonia. Bull WHO. 2008;86:408.)
HIV, human immunodeficiency virus.

deaths associated with pneumonia, the greatest burden is borne by elderly adults and children (***Fig. 134.2***),[12] especially those younger than 5 years old. One in five deaths worldwide in children under 5 years old is due to pneumonia. These 2 million annual deaths exceed those from acquired immunodeficiency syndrome (AIDS), malaria, and measles combined.[11]

WHO data reveal a marked difference in the proportion of deaths in children less than 5 years old caused by pneumonia and neonatal sepsis (usually pneumonia-associated) in industrialized nations (5%) versus those in tropical sub-Saharan Africa (28%) and South Asia (34%) (***Fig. 134.3***).[13] The role of coinfection with HIV and/or malnutrition in ARI-associated deaths cannot be overemphasized. WHO data from Botswana, currently the nation with the highest prevalence of HIV infection, revealed that approximately 60% of childhood deaths are due to HIV/AIDS, often associated with respiratory coinfections.[14]

S. pneumoniae and *H. influenzae* remain the most important bacterial causes of pneumonia in young children (***Box 134.1***),[15] accounting for 40–80% of the deaths from pneumonia and neonatal sepsis. The use of *H. influenzae* b (Hib) and, more recently, pneumococcal conjugate vaccines, has dramatically decreased the frequency of these infections in developed countries but, due to their cost, they remain underutilized in the developing nations.[10]

The role of pneumonia associated with *Staphylococcus aureus* and nontyphoidal *Salmonella* remains controversial. In one large, prospective, multicentered study in the tropics, *Staphylococcus aureus* was found in 42% of those children with positive cultures and exceeded even *S. pneumoniae*.[14] Another study in Malawi found nontyphoidal *Salmonella* in the blood of children with radiologic evidence of pneumonia.[16] Nontypable *H. influenzae* and *Mycobacterium tuberculosis* have also been found in lung aspirates in children with acute pneumonia in some studies.[17]

Common causes of atypical pneumonia, such as *Mycoplasma pneumoniae, Chlamydia pneumoniae,* and *Legionella* spp., are probably as common in the tropics as they are in temperate areas but have been inadequately studied. There have been numerous reports of outbreaks of legionellosis associated with travel, especially among the elderly. Nearly half of the cases of *Legionella* pneumonia in the United Kingdom are travel-associated.[17]

Fungal etiologies should also be considered if another diagnosis is not readily evident. Although *Histoplasma* sp. infections are not uncommon in many temperate areas, they are also found in much of the tropics and often overlap in distribution with endemic fungal infections such as *Paracoccidioides brasiliensis* in South America and *Penicillium marneffei* in Southeast Asia. Although paracoccidioidomycosis may occur in immunocompetent and HIV-infected individuals, penicilliosis occurs almost exclusively in HIV-infected individuals where, along with cryptococcosis, it is a common opportunistic pathogen. Although each of these mycoses starts with pulmonary disease the progression to a systemic illness with skin, central nervous system (CNS), and other visceral involvement is much more common in the immunocompromised. These infections, common in their endemic zones, should be especially considered in the setting of an "atypical" pneumonia in an immunocompromised host.

Measles, one of the most important viral respiratory diseases, is associated with significant morbidity and mortality in much of the developing world. Since measles vaccination was introduced in 1963, there has been a marked decrease in cases, and the WHO has a goal of worldwide eradication by 2015.[18] Despite a 74% drop in measles deaths globally from 2000 to 2007, there were more than 20 million cases and 197000 deaths in 2007, 95% in children less than 5 years old.[19] Due to recent trends among some groups to avoid childhood immunizations, measles should be considered in the differential diagnosis for fever associated with rash in a returning traveler, especially a child. Death from measles is usually associated with either primary viral pneumonia or secondary bacterial infection with *S. pneumoniae, H. influenzae, S. aureus,* or in some cases secondary viral

Table 134.2 Parasites Associated with Respiratory Illness

Parasite	Distribution
Nematodes	
Roundworms	
Ascaris spp.	Worldwide
Toxocara canis and *T. cati*	Worldwide
Hookworm	
Necator americanus	Southeast Asia, West and Central Africa
Ancyclostoma duodenale	South Europe, North Africa, India, China, Japan
A. caninum	South United States, Mexico, Africa, Asia, South America
Necator brasiliense	South America, Caribbean
Strongyloides stercoralis	Worldwide
Trichinella spiralis	Worldwide
Filaria	
Loa loa	West and Central Africa
Wuchereria bancrofti	Pacific, Asia, Africa, China, Americas
Brugia malayi	Southeast Asia
Dirofilaria immitis	Southeast Asia, America, South Africa, Australia
Other nematodes	
Gnathostoma spinigerum	India, Philippines, Thailand
Strongyloides stercoralis	Worldwide
Trichinella spiralis	Worldwide
Trematodes	
Schistosomes	
Schistosoma mansoni	Africa, South Arabia, South America, Caribbean
S. haematobium	Africa, Middle East
S. japonicum	Far East
S. intercalatum	West and Central Africa
Lung flukes	
Paragonimus westermanii	Far East, China, Japan, Philippines
P. africanus	Africa
P. caliensis	South and Central America
Cestodes	
Hydatid disease	
Echinococcus granulosus	Australia, Africa, South America (endemic)
E. multilocularis	Worldwide
Pentastomes	
Linguatula serrata	Worldwide
Armillifer sp.	Worldwide
Protozoa	
Entamoeba histolytica	Worldwide
Plasmodium falciparum	Africa, South and Central America, Asia
Toxoplasma gondii	Worldwide
Leishmania donovani	Africa, Middle East, South America, Asia
Other	
Pneumocystis jirovecii	Worldwide

(Modified from Savani DM, Sharma OP. Eosinophilic lung disease in the tropics. Clin Chest Med. 2002;23:377.)

infection with herpes simplex or adenovirus. Studies have demonstrated a marked reduction in measles-associated morbidity and mortality after initiation of childhood vitamin A supplementation. This is especially evident in refugee settings where malnutrition with a superimposed measles outbreak may be the leading cause of death.[20]

Particular settings in the tropics may suggest the role of certain bacterial organisms. Examples include staphylococcal pneumonia complicating measles and varicella, pertussis in areas with inadequate childhood immunization, and *Klebsiella* pneumonia in lower socioeconomic rural settings with alcoholism and malnutrition.

Chronic cavitary upper-lobe infiltrates in a patient from Southeast Asia may be misidentified as TB but actually represent melioidosis, an acute or chronic infection with *Burkholderia pseudomallei*, a Gram-negative soil saprophyte endemic to Southeast Asia and part of Australia (see Chapter 33). Melioidosis accounts for 20% of all community-acquired bacteremia in northeast Thailand and is associated with death in 40% of treated patients.[21] It was also the most common cause of fatal, community-acquired pneumonia at a regional referral hospital in the Northern Territory of Australia. In a series of 252 cases of melioidosis in Australia, half presented with pneumonia and one-quarter were bacteremic, 15%

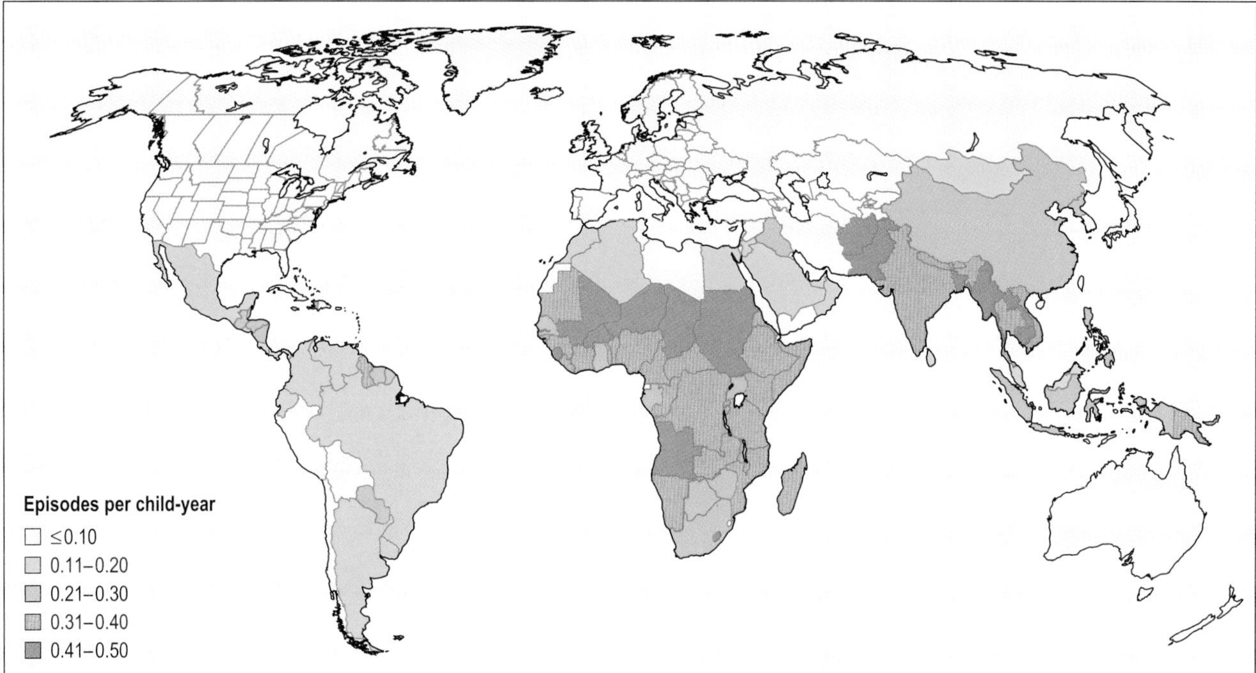

Figure 134.2 Incidence of childhood clinical pneumonia at the country level. (Modified from Rudan I, Boschi-Pinto C, Bilogav Z, et al. Epidemiology and etiology of childhood pneumonia. Bull WHO. 2008;86:408.)

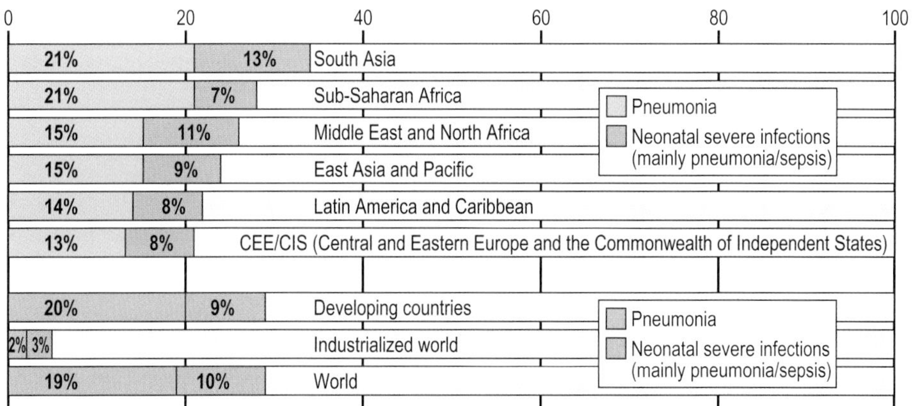

Figure 134.3 Percentage of deaths in children under 5 years old due to pneumonia. (Reproduced from UNICEF/WHO. Pneumonia: The Forgotten Killer of Children. Geneva: WHO, 2006.)

presented with pneumonia and septic shock, and 84% of the septic individuals died.[22] Melioidosis is well documented to occur months to years after exposure and should remain in the differential diagnosis for those with appropriate exposure who present with chronic, subacute, or acute pulmonary disease that may appear to be TB.[23]

Occupational exposures may suggest an etiology for unusual bacterial pneumonias such as anthrax, Q fever, tularemia, and leptospirosis. Outbreaks associated with hantaviruses, pneumonic plague, influenza, and SARS coronavirus are each potential etiologies for pneumonia that may be very regionally specific. Infections with *Paragonimus*, *Echinococcus*, and *Entamoeba histolytica* do not cause typical air space disease but may present like pneumonia and should be considered in the differential diagnosis. Since these rarer etiologies may be encountered sporadically nearly worldwide, it is helpful to query online resources at the time of evaluating a patient. The WHO's Global Outbreak and Alert Response Network (www.who.int/csr/outbreaknetwork/en/) or the US Centers for Disease Control and Prevention's travel notices (www.cdc.gov/travel) have current information on disease outbreaks globally that are helpful when evaluating a returning traveler with pulmonary disease.

There are a number of considerations in treating patients with lower respiratory infections. Bacterial antimicrobial resistance has become an increasing problem worldwide, including in the tropics; however, a lack of antibiotic availability in underserved areas has led to lower prevalence of resistant organisms. Conversely, poorly controlled access to antibiotics and inappropriate use have led to much higher levels of resistance in other areas. One study in Uganda identified 95% of *S. pneumoniae* as penicillin-resistant and 75% of *H. influenzae* as β-lactamase-producing.[24] Despite this resistance, there was a good clinical response to ampicillin, even among HIV-infected individuals.

Availability of antibiotics in developing nations is variable. Many nations have access to less expensive penicillin, ampicillin, chloramphenicol, erythromycin, tetracycline, and aminoglycosides; but more expensive third-generation cephalosporins, fluoroquinolones, and newer macrolides, commonly used in developed nations, are often unavailable. Empiric therapy for adults and children with pneumonia in the tropics has become increasingly difficult with the growing prevalence of HIV infection in many regions. WHO-recommended regimens have, in some studies, been found to be inadequate and recommendations for modifications are imminent.[14]

Availability of oxygen and vaccines may have the greatest impact on respiratory infections in the tropics. Studies have demonstrated a reduction in pneumonia deaths by over one-third with the addition of pulse oximetry and oxygen in hospitals.[24] Additional use of pneumococcal, Hib, measles, pertussis, and influenza vaccines in poorer nations will likely have a significant effect on morbidity and mortality from respiratory infections in the tropics.[25]

CHRONIC COUGH

Cough, a common symptom of URIs, is also frequently associated with pneumonia, COPD, bronchiectasis, sinusitis, and asthma. URIs are among the most common illnesses of travelers but most cough persisting for less than 2 months is associated with relatively benign viral or bacterial etiologies. However, cough may be associated with recent infection with *Ascaris*, hookworm, *Strongyloides*, or schistosomes. Cough persisting for more than 2 months is considered chronic, and a far wider differential diagnosis (***Box 134.2***) should be considered, especially with tropical exposure.[26,27]

In developing a differential diagnosis for chronic cough, indepth inquiry into the patient's travel background and exposure history must be obtained. A knowledge of which infectious agents are endemic to the area is crucial. A short-term traveler to an urban area of the tropics may have only a remote opportunity to have encountered helminths or TB, whereas those with long-term travel to remote areas, and extensive exposure to the local population, have probably had ample opportunity to be exposed to a wide range of endemic infections. Similar exposure considerations should be applied to those who live in the tropics: an urban office worker is much less likely to have had the constant animal, insect, and freshwater contact of a rice farmer in rural areas. Conversely, individuals living in some rural tropical areas may all have some degree of chronic cough due to smoke exposure from indoor fires for cooking and heating.

Box 134.2 Considerations in the Differential Diagnosis of Cough of Greater than 2 Months' Duration, Etiologies Worldwide, and Those More Common in the Tropics

Worldwide

Infection-associated

- Postinfectious inflammation
- Tuberculosis
- Endemic mycoses
- Eosinophilic bronchitis
- HIV-associated opportunistic infections
- Recurrent aspiration

Environment-associated

- Allergic and nonallergic rhinitis
- Reactive airways disease (asthma)
- Pneumoconiosis

Other

- Cigarette smoking
- Chronic obstructive pulmonary disease
- Bronchiectasis
- Congestive heart failure
- Pulmonary neoplasm
- Gastroesophageal reflux
- Sarcoidosis
- Interstitial lung disease
- Angiotensin-converting enzyme inhibitor-associated

Tropics

Infection-associated

- Tuberculosis
- Loeffler's syndrome (helminthic pulmonary transmigration)
- Schistosomiasis (acute or late-stage disease)
- Tropical pulmonary eosinophilia (filarial infection with hypersensitivity)
- Paragonimiasis
- Penicilliosis
- Paracoccidioidomycosis
- Melioidosis
- Chagas disease-associated congestive heart failure

Environment-associated

- Indoor air pollution (heating, cooking)

HIV, human immunodeficiency virus.

TB should nearly always be considered in the differential of chronic cough if there is associated fever, weight loss, and pulmonary infiltrates, particularly in infants and young children. Schistosomiasis and intestinal helminths should be considered in "eco-tourists," campers, and those who report freshwater exposure as well as denizens of the rural tropics. Endemic mycoses, melioidosis, and environmental toxins are potential etiologies that should be entertained in the context of the appropriate geographic region and exposure history. Chest radiographs and serology, as well as sputa and stool microscopy, will usually confirm these diagnoses (if they have been considered).

A complete blood count (CBC) with differential should always be obtained, as cough associated with a helminth infection may have a normal total leukocyte count but a significantly elevated eosinophil count that would guide the diagnostic evaluation (see Chapter 131). Chest radiographs (CXR) are indicated in evaluation of chronic cough as characteristic radiologic findings are seen with many diagnoses. Abnormal CXRs in resource-rich nations are often further evaluated by computed tomography (CT) scan. Although readily available in most developed nations, CT scanners are not available in many tropical countries.[28] Similarly, availability of bronchoscopic evaluation is variable outside developed nations but should be considered if the etiology of cough cannot be determined with less invasive testing. Sputum examination is generally available in most areas and is most important to rule out TB. In contrast to some other diagnostic modalities, microscopists in the developing world are often quite experienced and skilled in reading stains for acid-fast bacteria, protozoa, and helminths. In industrialized nations, routine sputa, and even bronchoscopic samples, are often not examined for fungi, mycobacteria, or parasites. These etiologies, more common in the tropics, should nearly always be considered in the diagnostic evaluation and may require special consideration with technicians and pathologists in the laboratory to ensure specimens are handled appropriately and that the best diagnostic modalities are utilized.

HEMOPTYSIS

Regardless of tropical or temperate exposure, the development of significant hemoptysis nearly always warrants diagnostic evaluation. While trivial hemoptysis with scant streaks of blood is not uncommon with bronchitis, the differential diagnosis should remain broad, especially in those with tropical exposure. While studies of the etiology of hemoptysis vary significantly depending on geographic location (and decade of publication), hemoptysis often indicates an underlying serious disease.

Although bronchiectasis and neoplasia are the most common causes of hemoptysis in developed nations, TB may exceed these noninfectious etiologies in developing nations. Understanding the prevalence of TB in the area of exposure is crucial in developing a differential diagnosis. In a 1997 Israeli study of 208 patients presenting with hemoptysis, only 3 (1.4%) were associated with TB.[29] Similarly, in a 1952 study from Boston, only 2 (1.9%) of 105 cases of hemoptysis were attributed to TB.[30] Conversely, in a 2002 study from Turkey of 108 cases of hemoptysis, 18 (17.4%) were associated with TB[31] and in a 2001 study of 52 patients with hemoptysis from Kuwait, 17 (32.7%) of the cases were attributed to either "old" or active pulmonary TB.[32] A similar study performed in an area with much higher TB rates, such as Afghanistan or sub-Saharan Africa, might find TB in an even greater percentage of patients with hemoptysis.

The role of other infectious etiologies such as *S. pneumoniae*, *Haemophilus*, melioidosis, endemic mycoses, ameba, and helminthic agents (ascaris, hookworm, *Strongyloides*, *Echinococcus*, and *Paragonimus*) should all be considered in the differential diagnosis based on the location of the exposure (***Box 134.3***). Hemoptysis evaluation should start with CXR but may require CT or bronchoscopy with biopsies to make a definitive diagnosis. Advising the microbiology and pathology laboratories of the potential for fungal, mycobacterial, and parasitic disease will ensure that appropriate stains and cultures are performed.

Box 134.3 Considerations in the Differential Diagnosis of Hemoptysis, Etiologies Worldwide, and Those More Common in the Tropics

Worldwide	Tropics
Bronchiectasis	Tuberculosis
Bronchogenic neoplasm	Endemic mycoses
Bronchitis	Paragonimiasis
Congestive heart failure	Pulmonary echinococcal cyst
Tuberculosis	Amebic lung abscess
Endemic mycoses	Leptospirosis
Vasculitides (e.g., Wegener's)	Melioidosis
Blood dyscrasias	

EOSINOPHILIA ASSOCIATED WITH PULMONARY COMPLAINTS

Patients presenting for medical attention in (or after visiting) the tropics not uncommonly (up to 5%) are found to have eosinophilia.[33] Although generally not considered to be clinically significant until reaching an absolute eosinophil count of greater than 1500, a relative increase in eosinophils on a CBC will often lead to pulmonary or infectious diseases consultation. The differential diagnosis and evaluation of eosinophilia are considered in Chapter 131.

Evaluation of patients with eosinophilia can be very difficult, especially in the absence of significant symptoms to help guide the assessment. A thorough account of both domestic and tropical travel must be included in the history as well as a detailed inquiry into use of prescription drugs, over-the-counter drugs, and supplements as the etiology may be a hypersensitivity reaction rather than an infection. There are many nonparasitic and noninfectious etiologies that should be considered in the evaluation (see Chapter 131).[34] Stool, sputa, and serologic assays are frequently negative during the larval stages in the pulmonary vasculature.

The intestinal helminths most commonly associated with transmigration of larvae through the lung leading to eosinophilia, frequently referred to as Loeffler's syndrome, are *Ascaris, Strongyloides,* and the hookworms *Necator* and *Ancyclostoma*.[35] Larvae penetrate into the alveolar spaces, are coughed into the mouth and then swallowed, thereby completing their journey to the intestinal tract where the adult stages live. *Ascaris* is most likely to be associated with development of significant pulmonary symptoms; hookworm and *Strongyloides* usually cause minimal inflammation during pulmonary transmigration. Loeffler's syndrome occurs 10–12 days after ingestion of *Ascaris* eggs (or 5–10 days after penetration of hookworm larva) and, if there are symptoms, is characterized by 5–10 days of nonproductive cough, burning substernal chest pain, and frequently, wheezing and rales. CXR reveals ill-defined, patchy, homogeneous consolidation or, occasionally a fine miliary pattern. Infiltrates may be unilateral or bilateral, have indefinite borders, and range from a few millimeters to 2–3 cm.[33,36]

Migration of *Toxocara canis* or *T. cati* larvae in pulmonary tissues as a manifestation of visceral larva migrans (see Chapter 109) is associated with high levels of eosinophilia, and may be associated with fever, hepatosplenomegaly, and transient reticulonodular infiltrates.[34,37]

Schistosomes may be associated with eosinophilia and chest symptoms (see Chapter 122). Acute schistosomiasis (3–8 weeks after schistosome penetration) may be associated with headache, malaise, dyspnea, wheezing, and nonproductive cough, especially while recumbent in bed. Pulmonary symptoms may coincide with the fever (Katayama syndrome) associated with acute infection, but more commonly present a few weeks after resolution of fever and are associated with marked (30–50%) eosinophilia, mild to moderate leukocytosis, and liver enzyme abnormalities.[38] Pulmonary symptoms are likely an immune manifestation in the lung while the organism has become established elsewhere.[39]

Chronic pulmonary disease is a complication of established schistosomal infections as ectopic migration of schistosome eggs occurs. This becomes more common in late disease as portal hypertension leads to portacaval shunts and deposition of eggs embolized in the pulmonary vasculature. The granulomatous response to eggs in the pulmonary vessels leads to pulmonary hypertension and eventually cor pulmonale. Finally, some helminths (mainly *Paragonimus* and *Echinococcus*) establish their adult stage in the lung and may be associated with years of waxing-and-waning eosinophilia and leading to misdiagnosis as TB or fungal infection[37,40] (see Chapters 120 and 123).

Table 134.3 Considerations in the Differential Diagnosis of Pleural Effusions, Etiologies Worldwide, and Those More Common in the Tropics

Worldwide	Frequency of Diagnosis	Tropics
Heart failure	Common	Tuberculosis
Parapneumonic malignancy	Less frequent	Paragonimiasis
Pulmonary embolus		Cryptococcosis
Cirrhosis		Histoplasmosis
Tuberculosis		Amebiasis
Endemic mycoses		Toxocariasis
Nephrotic syndrome		Echinococcosis
Idiopathic		Sparganosis
Hypothyroidism		Gnathostomiasis
Drug hypersensitivity		
Asbestosis		
Collagen vascular disease		
Pancreatitis		

PLEURAL EFFUSION

The etiologies of pleural effusion are extensive (***Table 134.3***). Common noninfectious etiologies such as malignancies, heart or liver failure, collagen vascular diseases, and others predominate in temperate areas. The differential diagnosis of pleural effusion after tropical exposure is skewed due to the high prevalence of TB and HIV-associated disease and the increased incidence of helminthic and fungal infections. In one study from Zimbabwe of 100 consecutive patients with pleural effusion of unknown etiology, pleural biopsy led to a TB diagnosis in 58.[41] Temperate areas with a high TB incidence may also have TB as a common cause of pleural effusion. A study of 642 pleural effusions in Spain (in an area with TB incidence of 95 per 100 000) found TB responsible for 25%, neoplasia for 23%, and congestive heart failure for 18%.[42,43] In areas with low TB prevalence, pleural effusions are rarely associated with TB and are much more commonly a sign of malignancy.

Evaluation of pleural effusion should involve consideration of the clinical setting. Bilateral pleural effusion in a patient with underlying heart disease returning from the tropics is still likely a pleural transudate related to heart failure. Presence of fever, pleuritic chest pain, and leukocytosis are obvious indicators of potential infectious etiologies and are indications for thoracentesis. In addition to cell count, differential, pH, chemistries, Gram stain, and bacterial culture that are routinely obtained, consideration of mycobacterial or fungal disease should prompt appropriate stains and cultures.[44] If CXR or the clinical scenario is consistent with TB, then a large volume of pleural fluid (at least 10 mL) should be centrifuged and the pellet examined with acid-fast (and fungal) stains and culture to increase the diagnostic yield. Adenosine deaminase levels in the pleural fluid, pleural biopsy, and tuberculin skin testing may also be considered as potentially helpful in determining the diagnosis.

An effusion with eosinophilic pleocytosis at pleurocentesis appropriately prompts consideration of helminthic etiologies (***Table 134.4***).[45–47] Although estimates are that 5–16% of pleural effusions are eosinophilic (greater than 10% of nucleated cells are eosinophils), only a minority of eosinophilic effusions are due to infectious etiologies, and even fewer are due to helminths. In most studies, blood or air in the pleural space is most commonly associated with eosinophilic pleural effusion, but malignancy, infection, pulmonary embolus, drug-induced, and asbestos-associated all

Table 134.4 Etiology and Clinical Features of Eosinophilic Pleural Effusions

Etiology	Clinical Features
Chest trauma or thoracic medical procedure	Presence of air or blood in the pleural cavity Pleural fluid is bloody or straw-colored
Malignancy, either primary pulmonary or pleural or metastatic	Increased eosinophils, even in nonbloody effusions
Parapneumonic effusions	Eosinophils appear a month or more after resolution of infiltrate Gram stain and culture are negative for bacteria
Tuberculosis (TB), either pleural or associated with pulmonary infiltrates or nodule(s)	Although eosinophils are rarely associated with TB, the frequency of pleural effusion due to TB is common in the tropics
Endemic fungi such as coccidioidiomycosis, histoplasmosis, cryptococcisis, penicilliosis	If living in or traveling from an endemic area
Parasitic infections: Paragonimiasis, ascariasis, strongyloidiasis, echinococcosis, filariasis, loiasis, toxocariasis, dracunculiasis, amebiasis, cutaneous myiasis	Travel to or living in endemic areas: Pleural fluid exam may reveal ova, larva, or other parasitic forms Paragonimiasis is the most common parasitic etiology (associated with pleural pH <7.1 and glucose <60 mg/dL)
Medication-associated: Nitrofurantoin, isotretinoin, fluoxetine, warfarin, dantrolene, gliclazide, mesalamine, bromocriptine	Usually weeks to months after drug administration but may be as short as hours or as long as years
Pulmonary embolism	18% of pleural effusions are eosinophilic Pleuritic chest pain and dyspnea greater than would be expected with size of effusion
Asbestosis or other pneumoconioses	History of occupational exposure, Pleural effusion is usually the sole radiographic abnormality Up to 50% of asbestos-associated effusions are eosinophilic
Idiopathic	Most commonly in middle-aged males with small to moderate, unilateral effusion. May be long-standing but associated with a good prognosis Should prompt consideration of undiagnosed parasitic infections

(Modified from Kalomenidis I, Light RW. How to approach a patient with an eosinophilic pleural effusion. J Respir Dis. 2003;24:247.)

occur.[45,46] In a 2009 retrospective study of 2205 patients, 135 with eosinophilic effusions, one-third had malignancy, although the higher the percentage of eosinophils in the effusion, the less likely to be associated with malignancy.[47] Patients in or from the tropics presenting with eosinophilic pleural effusion (who do not have an identified etiology) should also have a sputum examination and culture for fungi and mycobacteria. Sputum and stool should be examined for ova and parasites. Bronchoscopy and/or lung biopsy are considerations if less invasive diagnostic evaluation is unrevealing. If biopsies are performed, it is important to consider evaluating tissue for fungi, mycobacteria, and parasitic etiologies in the microbiology and pathology labs.

Of all the parasitic etiologies, *Paragonimus* infections (see Chapter 123) are the most likely to be associated with a significant eosinophilic pleural effusion. Asian studies have found that approximately 50% of cases of paragonimiasis are associated with pleural effusions.[48,49] Findings of pleural pH less than 7.1 and pleural fluid glucose less than 60 mg/dL are characteristic.[46] Sputa exam with *Paragonimus* ova can confirm the diagnosis.

Despite aggressive evaluation, as many as one-quarter of eosinophilic pleural effusions remain undiagnosed, but the prognosis, even if the effusion has been prolonged, has been shown to be better than for those with a noneosinophilic effusion.[46,47]

TUBERCULOSIS

The importance of including TB (see Chapter 35) in the differential diagnosis of nearly all pulmonary complaints from the tropics cannot be overemphasized. Although prevalence and mortality associated with TB are dropping globally, the increase in global population yields increased total cases. Over 85% of the 9.27 million new TB cases in the world in 2007 were from Africa and Asia and 15% of these individuals were HIV-positive.[50] In children, 90% of TB cases and 95% of TB deaths occur in developing nations. Many of these same nations are also burdened with the highest HIV infection rates. As the two infections act synergistically to cause progression of the other, the effects have been devastating, especially in sub-Saharan Africa (see Chapters 81 and 139).

The incidence of multidrug resistance has been a further complication of TB in the tropics.[51] Inadequate treatment and follow-up have led to gradually increasing levels of drug resistance, thus requiring not only sensitivity testing but also more expensive, and potentially more toxic, therapy.

Numerous studies have documented the frequency of TB in those who have immigrated from the tropics. Concerns about travelers visiting areas of high TB endemicity and potential exposures during air travel are frequently raised.[52] Although the increased emphasis on case-finding has yielded a recent rise in the number of air travel-associated cases, the risk of acquiring TB infection among short-term travelers and on flights is quite low.[53] Despite commonly held misconceptions about aircraft air systems, rapid filtering of air leaving the cabin near the floor and released overhead removes most infectious particles. Transmission of TB on aircraft, although extensively reported by the media, has rarely been documented.[54]

In contrast to short-term travelers, those remaining in areas with a high TB prevalence have infection rates approaching that of local populations. This was seen most dramatically in long-term Dutch travelers to Africa, Asia, and Latin America, where their risk of infection increased from approximately 10 to 2000 infections per 100 000 person-years. Health care workers with direct patient contact had more than threefold greater risk of TB than other travelers.[55] Obviously, in considering TB it is critical to know the TB prevalence in the source nation as well as contacts with TB, the living situation, and the activity of the individual evaluated.

Numerous studies have documented that immigrants to developed nations have a much higher incidence of TB disease than natives of developed nations. In 2007, 58% of incident cases of TB in the United States occurred in the foreign-born, and disease incidence is 10 times greater in foreign- than US-born individuals.[56] Approximately 25% of immigrant TB cases diagnosed in the United States present within the first year of immigration. The incidence of active TB among political asylum seekers in

London was 241 per 100 000, 20 times greater than the overall incidence in England.[57] Clearly individuals from developing nations who present with pulmonary complaints, especially chronic cough associated with hemoptysis, weight loss, and night sweats, should have TB considered as one of the most likely etiologies and have CXR, possibly a tuberculin skin test or interferon-γ releasing assay (for those with a history of prior Bacille Calmette–Guérin immunization), and sputa examination as part of the evaluation.

PLASMODIUM-ASSOCIATED PULMONARY FINDINGS

Plasmodium falciparum and, to a lesser extent, *P. vivax* have been associated with significant pulmonary involvement in a minority of infected patients (see Chapter 96). There is no evidence that malarial infections are associated with a true pneumonitis, but pulmonary edema can develop during the treatment of falciparum malaria, especially more severe cases. Malaria-associated pulmonary edema is noncardiogenic (high cardiac index and low systemic vascular resistance) and is considered by most authorities to be consistent with the acute respiratory distress syndrome (ARDS) and related to the malaria-associated increase in pulmonary permeability.[58] Pulmonary edema occurs in less than 1% of all cases of falciparum malaria.[59] More recently, three of five marines who returned to the United States from Liberia in 2003 with greater than 10% falciparum parasitemia developed ventilatory failure and an ARDS-like presentation 48–72 hours after initiation of antimalarial treatment and clearance of parasitemia (unpublished personal data). Malaria-associated pulmonary disease should be considered in the differential diagnosis of those returning from a malarious region with unexplained pulmonary edema.

HIV-ASSOCIATED PULMONARY DISEASE

Like TB, the prevalence of HIV in many tropical areas, especially sub-Saharan Africa, makes it an important consideration in the differential diagnosis of pulmonary disease (see Chapters 81 and 139). TB coinfection is clearly the greatest threat to HIV-infected individuals in the tropics. In 2007, the WHO reported that HIV-infected individuals in sub-Saharan nations with high HIV rates are 20 times more likely to develop TB than those who are HIV-uninfected, yielding rates of TB/HIV coinfection greater than 250 per 100 000.[50] In a study of African children dying from respiratory illness in Zambia, *Pneumocystis jirovecii* (formerly *P. carinii*) pneumonia was exceeded only by acute pyogenic pneumonia as the cause of death in HIV-infected children who were under a year old. Cytomegalovirus, TB, and interstitial lung disease were all common findings.[60]

Etiologies of HIV-associated infectious pulmonary diseases in the tropics include all those seen in temperate areas and an extensive variety of pathogens (see Chapter 139). A few notable geographic considerations are the prevalence of *Penicillium marneffei* and melioidosis in Southeast Asia and Australia, paracoccidioidomycosis in South America, and blastomycosis in areas of Africa, South America, and Asia. These diseases are often erroneously attributed to TB, even in the areas where they are most common. With the frequency of multiple simultaneous pulmonary infections in HIV infection, even for those diagnosed with TB the possibility of additional diagnoses should be considered.

NONINFECTIOUS ETIOLOGIES OF TROPICAL RESPIRATORY DISEASE

Tobacco Use in Developing Nations

Estimates are that a half billion of the world's current population will be killed by tobacco and, by 2030, 8 million people will die annually from tobacco-related diseases, with 80% of these deaths in the developing world. Tobacco currently is a risk factor for six of the eight leading causes of death and its impact has been increasing annually. Aggressive marketing has led to male smoking prevalence that exceeds 50% in much of Asia and Latin America.[61] This consequence of "development" is the most preventable etiology of pulmonary disease.

Rheumatic Heart Disease Presenting with Pulmonary Symptoms

Currently 12 million people worldwide are affected by rheumatic fever (RF) or rheumatic heart disease (RHD). These sequelae of β-hemolytic streptococcal infection continue to be common problems in the tropics. Two-thirds of those afflicted are between 5 and 15 years of age. RHD incidence rates in most developed nations are <1 per 100 000; in Sudan it is 100 per 100 000 and in China 150 per 100 000. Prevalence rates as high as 77.8 per 1000 (in Samoa) have been described and are many-fold higher than in the developed world. The WHO estimates that up to 1% of all schoolchildren in Africa, Asia, Latin America and the eastern Mediterranean may have signs of RHD.[62] Pulmonary complaints and fever in the tropics may represent acute rheumatic carditis or bacterial endocarditis complicating prior rheumatic heart damage. Fever, cough, hemoptysis, and dyspnea may lead to misdiagnosis of a primary pulmonary infection. Pulmonary hypertension or congestive heart failure with pulmonary edema due to RHD is not uncommon in impoverished countries, where secondary prophylaxis to prevent recurrent RHD episodes is difficult to administer and valve replacements are unavailable. Consideration of RF is almost forgotten in much of the industrialized world but should be considered in adults who grew up in the tropics and in children who have recently arrived or visited areas of the tropics with significant rates of RF/RHD.

Pulmonary Diseases Caused by Occupational and Environmental Exposures

Discussion of pulmonary disease in the tropics cannot ignore the role of environmental exposures in acute and chronic lung disease. Poorly regulated working conditions in agriculture and mining have resulted in substantial burdens of occupationally related and environmental lung disease in many regions. Although good prevalence data are lacking, it is likely there are millions of cases of silicosis worldwide and possibly comparable numbers of other lung disorders due to cotton dust (byssinosis), extrinsic allergic alveolitis caused by microbial contamination of agricultural products such as sugar cane, and airway injury from indiscriminant use and poor control of indoor and outdoor air pollutants.[63,64]

There is a dramatic increase in both TB risk and virulence in populations with silicosis, and in those with exposure to silica without overt silicosis. In areas where large portions of men have been recruited into mining, as in southern Africa, this risk factor is very broadly disseminated and may account in part for very high rates of TB in these regions. In a study of 304 men from Botswana who had been employed in South African mines for a mean of 15 years, 30% had pneumoconiosis and 6.8% had progressive massive fibrosis; additionally 26% had a history of, or current, TB.[65]

While adult males are the primary victims of occupational exposures, children and women face increased risk from indoor, nonoccupational exposures due to the use of dung and other biomass fuels for cooking and heating. When combusted, these materials emit everything from silica and other minerals to hazardous air pollutants such as oxides of sulfur and nitrogen, resulting in various clinical syndromes, including silicosis ("hut lung" in this setting), chronic bronchitis, asthma, and increased risk of respiratory tract infection.[66,67] The most severely affected regions are those with colder climates, such as the South American Andes, mountainous regions of central Asia, and the high plains of Africa.

Ambient air pollution due to rapid urbanization has resulted in levels of ozone, oxides of nitrogen, and other irritants (photo-oxidant pollution) that are much higher than even in the worst cities in Europe and North

America. Data from Latin America, India, and China suggest that very high rates of respiratory infection and asthma may be resulting.[67]

SUMMARY

Developing a differential diagnosis for a patient presenting with pulmonary complaints after exposure in the tropics requires clinicians to consider a broad range of infectious and noninfectious etiologies. Determining a diagnosis compels a careful review of a patient's travel and exposure history, as well as the ascertainment of the geographic ranges of various infectious agents. Recognition that many common etiologies of respiratory illness in temperate areas are also common in developing tropical areas will assist in guiding the diagnostic evaluation.

Access the complete reference list online at
http://www.expertconsult.com

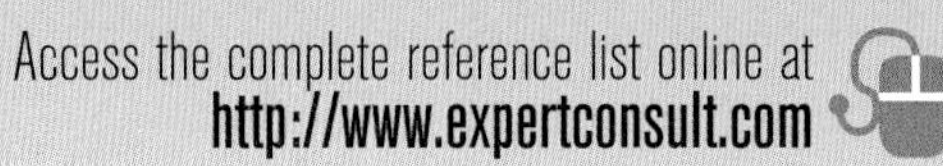
Access the complete reference list online at
http://www.expertconsult.com

CHAPTER 135

Ocular Disease

Edward T. Ryan • Marlene Durand

INTRODUCTION

Many tropical infectious diseases have ocular manifestations that include conjunctivitis, keratitis, uveitis, retinitis, optic neuritis, lesions of the adnexa including ulcerative lesions of the eyelid, Parinaud's oculoglandular syndrome (an ulceronodular conjunctival/corneal lesion with associated preauricular adenopathy), proptosis (a forward bulging of the eye itself), or a conjunctival, intraocular, or orbital "worm." These infections, especially trachoma, onchocerciasis, measles/xerophthalmia, leprosy, are causes of significant visual loss and blindness worldwide.[1,2] Fuller considerations including pathogenesis, non-ocular manifestations, diagnosis, and treatment are found in the cited pathogen-specific chapters.

VIRAL INFECTIONS

Adenovirus – Chapter 58

Worldwide, adenovirus is the most common cause of viral ocular infections. Ocular involvement by adenovirus manifests as one of three clinical syndromes: nonspecific follicular conjunctivitis, pharyngoconjunctival fever, or epidemic keratoconjunctivitis.[3] Nonspecific follicular conjunctivitis, the most common manifestation, occurs with many adenoviral serotypes and is most often mild and self-limited. Adenoviral conjunctivitis may include petechiae or may more rarely present as hemorrhagic conjunctivitis. Pharyngoconjunctival fever, also a self-limited disease, most commonly associated with serotypes 3, 4, and 7, manifests as acute follicular conjunctivitis that is associated with an upper respiratory tract infection, regional lymphadenopathy, and fever. Mild punctate keratitis may appear. The illness, most frequently reported in children, spontaneously resolves over 1–2 weeks.

Epidemic keratoconjunctivitis, which has the most severe ocular manifestations, presents as acute follicular conjunctivitis with a diffuse, superficial, fine "pinpoint" epithelial keratitis. Because of the corneal involvement, ocular pain is a prominent feature. Preauricular lymphadenopathy may be present. By the second week of infection, focal or punctate epithelial keratitis occurs (***Fig. 135.1***), and by the second to third weeks, subepithelial corneal infiltration may develop in 30–80% of affected persons. The infiltrates are thought to represent an immunologic reaction, can persist for months to years, and can result in significant visual disturbances if located within the visual axis. Epidemic keratoconjunctivitis is most frequently associated with adenovirus serotypes 3, 8, 10, 19, 21, and 37. Rarely, a large corneal erosion or conjunctival pseudomembrane can occur. Diagnosis is usually one of clinical recognition. Viral cultures, immunofluorescence studies, serologic examinations, and molecular techniques can be employed. Treatment is usually symptomatic.[4] Topical steroids should be used only to treat severe, symptomatic subepithelial corneal involvement in epidemic keratoconjunctivitis or if extensive pseudomembrane formation has occurred (and only after any herpetic ocular involvement has been excluded). Adenoviral ocular involvement can be explosively epidemic.

Enterovirus – Chapter 60

Ocular manifestations of enteroviral infections (e.g., enterovirus, poliovirus, coxsackievirus, and echovirus[5]) include acute hemorrhagic conjunctivitis, cranial nerve dysfunction in acute enteroviral neuropathy, and possibly retinitis.

Acute Hemorrhagic Conjunctivitis

Acute hemorrhagic conjunctivitis (AHC) may be caused by adenoviruses, but two enteroviruses, enterovirus 70 and coxsackie A24 variant, are the major causes. AHC, first recognized as a clinical entity in Ghana in 1969, was caused by enterovirus 70; a worldwide pandemic ensued. Epidemics of AHC due to coxsackie A24 variant have been reported since 2000 in Spain, Pakistan, Singapore, India, Korea, and China. The 2007 epidemic in Guangdong, China, involved 200 000 people.[6] Viruses are spread by hand-to-hand and fomite-to-hand transfers. Respiratory spread may occur. The incubation period for illness is only 1–2 days. Presentation is one of acute conjunctivitis with eyelid edema and tearing. Affected persons often have conjunctival hemorrhages, usually bulbar. Hemorrhagic involvement may be either petechial or involve the entire conjunctiva (***Fig. 135.2***). Preauricular lymphadenopathy is common. The syndrome is usually short in duration, with resolution beginning within 2–4 days of onset, and with no long-term ocular sequelae.

Diagnosis of AHC is one of clinical recognition (usually during an epidemic), confirmed by viral culture, neutralization assay, or serology assay. Molecular identification techniques are being applied to AHC outbreaks to allow rapid diagnosis, including a reverse transcription-polymerase chain reaction (RT-PCR) assay for detecting enterovirus 70 and coxsackie A24 variant.[6] Non-enteroviral infectious agents (***Box 135.1***), including pneumococci, *Neisseria* species, *Haemophilus* species, *Chlamydia*, herpesvirus, and the poultry-associated Newcastle disease virus, also may cause "hemorrhagic conjunctivitis."

Poliovirus – Chapter 60

Ocular manifestations of poliomyelitis are rare. Some persons with paralytic poliomyelitis experience bulbar involvement. Although involvement of the ninth and tenth cranial nerves (with pharyngeal paralysis) is most frequent, over 10% of patients with bulbar poliomyelitis have cranial nerve involvement that affects the eyes, orbital musculature, or both. Ocular palsies, ptosis, pupillary disturbances, and ophthalmoplegia can occur.

Influenza – Chapter 58

Conjunctivitis may occur as part of influenza viral infection, but other manifestations are rare. Avian influenza A, particularly subtypes H5N1 and H7N7, may cause conjunctivitis in humans; over 90% of patients infected with subtype H7N7 in the Netherlands in 2003 had conjunctivitis.[7] The conjunctivitis is mild and self-limiting.

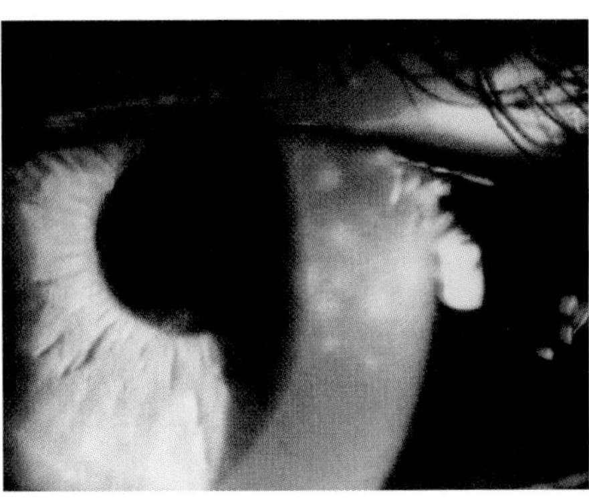

Figure 135.1 Adenoviral keratoconjunctivitis. Note punctate opacities in the cornea. (From Sandford-Smith J. Eye Diseases in Hot Climates, 2nd ed. Oxford: Wright Publishers, Butterworth Heinemann; 1990: plate 4e.)

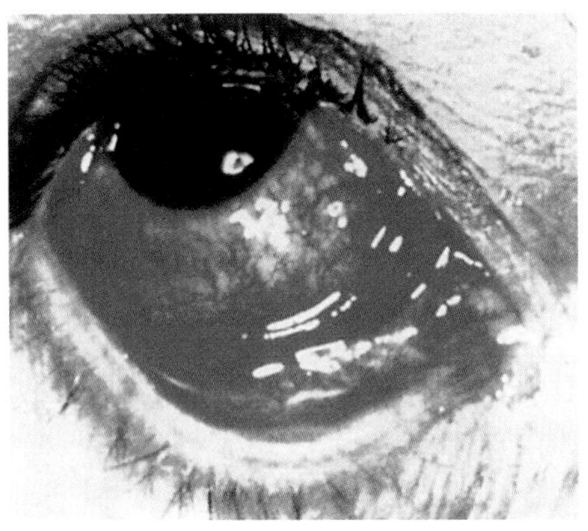

Figure 135.2 Acute hemorrhagic conjunctivitis due to coxsackievirus A24. (From Yin-Murphy M, Goh KT, Phoon MC, et al. A recent epidemic of acute hemorrhagic conjunctivitis. Am J Ophthalmol. 1993;116:213.)

Box 135.1 Causes of Selected Types of Conjunctivitis

Hyperacute Conjunctivitis[a]

- *Neisseria gonorrhoeae*[b]
- *Neisseria meningitidis*[b]
- *Corynebacterium diphtheriae*
- *Streptococcus* species

Membranous/ Pseudomembranous Conjunctivitis

- *Corynebacterium diphtheriae*[b]
- Pneumococci
- *Streptococcus* species
- *Neisseria* species
- *Chlamydia* species
- *Mycoplasma* species (Stevens–Johnson syndrome-associated)
- Adenovirus[b]
- Enterovirus
- *Candida* species

Hemorrhagic Conjunctivitis

- Enterovirus type 70[b]
- Coxsackievirus A24[b]
- Pneumococci
- *Neisseria* species
- *Haemophilus* species
- *Chlamydia* species
- *Borrelia* species
- *Rickettsia* species
- Adenovirus
- Herpesvirus
- Newcastle virus
- Hemorrhagic fever virus (e.g., Ebola virus)
- *Trichinella* species

[a]*Hyperacute conjunctivitis is defined as a rapidly progressive conjunctivitis with copious purulence.*

[b]*Common or classic ocular manifestation of infection.*

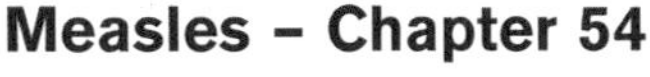

Measles – Chapter 54

Keratitis, which develops in persons with measles, occurs within a few days of the outbreak of the skin rash and may persist for months. Slit-lamp examination discloses punctate epithelial erosions, even in patients with

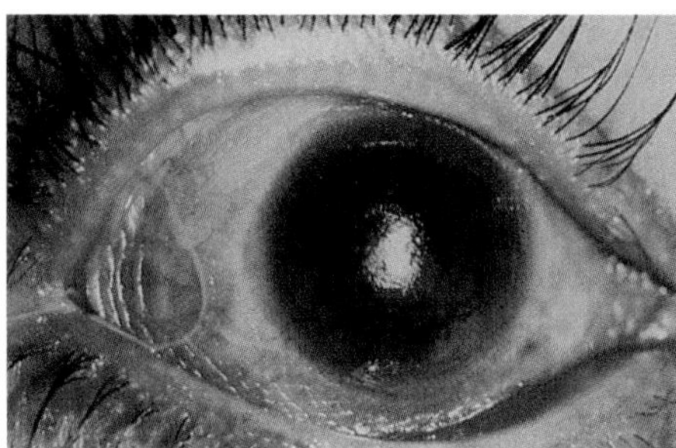

Figure 135.3 Early xerophthalmia. Corneal and conjunctival xerosis secondary to vitamin A deficiency. (From Sandford-Smith J. Eye Diseases in Hot Climates, 2nd ed. Oxford: Wright Publishers, Butterworth Heinemann; 1990: plate 12a.)

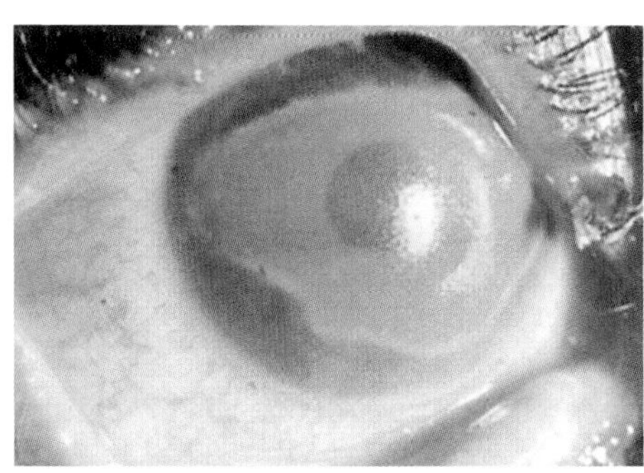

Figure 135.4 Measles-associated corneal ulceration (superficial) stained with fluorescein. The child was deficient in vitamin A. (From Sandford-Smith J. Eye Diseases in Hot Climates, 2nd ed. Oxford: Butterworth Heinemann; 1990: plate 12c.)

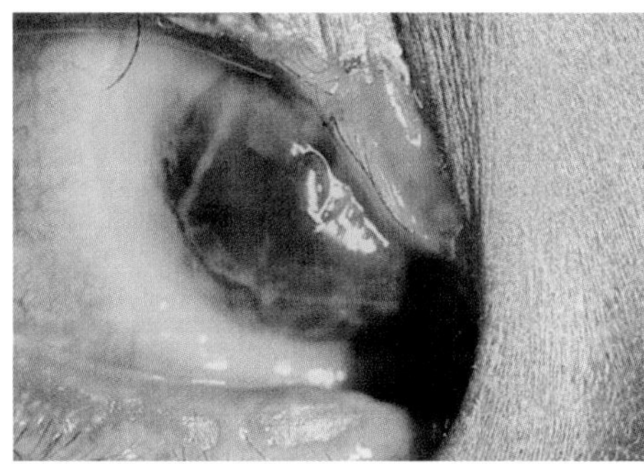

Figure 135.5 Measles-associated keratomalacia in a child with vitamin A deficiency. The cornea has completely melted away and only a thin sheet of fibrin covers the iris. (From Sandford-Smith J. Eye Diseases in Hot Climates, 2nd ed. Oxford: Wright Publishers, Butterworth Heinemann; 1990: plate 12d.)

measles without eye symptoms. Conjunctivitis with tearing and eyelid edema is common and resolves without sequelae.

Vitamin A deficiency results in xerophthalmia (conjunctival/corneal epithelial irregularities and xerosis; *Fig. 135.3*). Acute vitamin A deficiency can be induced by measles in persons with marginal vitamin A stores. Results can be catastrophic. Without adequate vitamin A, the punctate epithelial keratitis of measles can coalesce into larger epithelial ulcers (*Fig. 135.4*) that can become secondarily infected with bacteria or fungi. Corneal scarring may result. Keratomalacia, a marked weakening of the corneal stroma that can result in total melting of the cornea, may occur in persons who are markedly vitamin A deficient (*Fig. 135.5*). Measles-associated corneal ulceration and scarring can result in significant visual loss and blindness (*Fig. 135.6*). Measles and vitamin A deficiency accounted for 20% of childhood blindness in one series from India.[8] Posterior ocular disease associated with measles includes retinopathy, retinal vessel attenuation, retinal edema, and retinal hemorrhages. Visual acuity may be markedly decreased and, even after resolution of acute illness, loss of vision may be severe. Involvement of the central nervous system (CNS) with measles-associated acute encephalitis or subacute

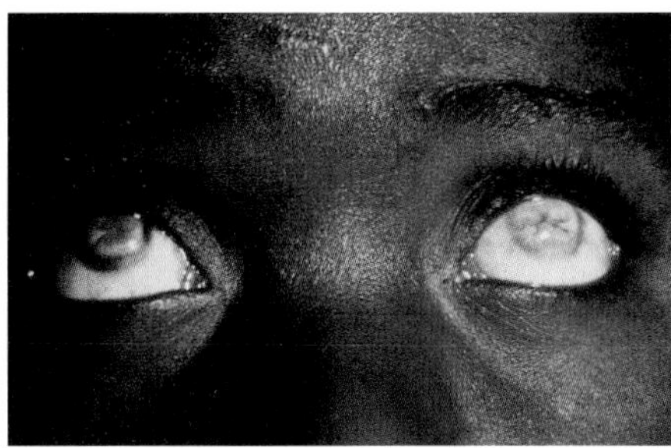

Figure 135.6 Child blinded from corneal scarring secondary to measles and xerophthalmia. (From Sandford-Smith J. Eye Diseases in Hot Climates, 2nd ed. Oxford: Wright Publishers. Butterworth Heinemann; 1990: cover.)

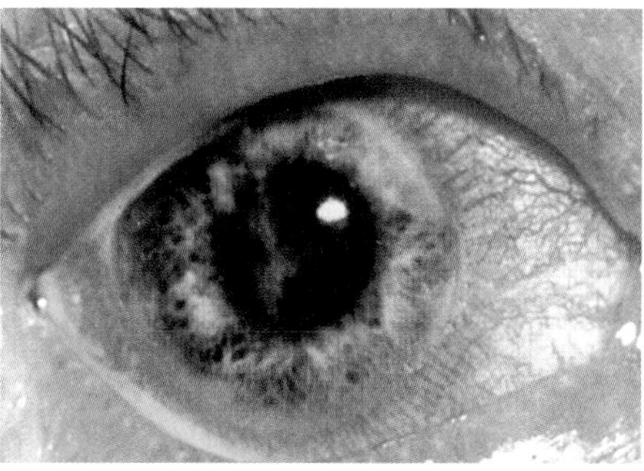

Figure 135.7 Herpes simplex virus-associated dendritic corneal ulcer stained with fluorescein. Prior to the addition of fluorescein, the cornea appeared normal to the naked eye. (From Sandford-Smith J. Eye Diseases in Hot Climates, 2nd ed. Oxford: Butterworth Heinemann; 1990: plate 7e. Courtesy of Mr E. Rosen, Manchester, UK.)

sclerosing panencephalitis can be associated with papilledema, chorioretinitis, optic neuritis, optic atrophy, and extraocular palsies.

Studies in the developing world have demonstrated that routine administration of vitamin A to patients with measles (both among hospitalized individuals and in the community) leads to a 30–80% reduction in measles-associated mortality as well as to a marked reduction in measles-associated morbidity.

Rubella

Infection with rubella virus can be either acquired or congenital. The most common ocular manifestation during acquired rubella infection is conjunctivitis, which occurs in the majority of symptomatic patients. Epithelial keratitis occurs in 5–10% of infected patients.[9] Corneal stromal involvement, iritis, retinitis, and vasculitis have been reported. Rubella infection in a susceptible woman in her first trimester of pregnancy has an 80% chance of affecting the fetus. Ocular manifestations may occur in over half of all such neonates with congenital rubella.[10] Retinopathy, the most common manifestation, is characterized by patchy black retinal pigmentary changes. Visual acuity is often preserved. Cataracts, either unilateral or bilateral, affect 15% of persons with the congenital rubella syndrome. Microphthalmia, glaucoma, buphthalmos, retinal neovascularization, and nystagmus can occur. Acute rubella retinitis may improve with systemic steroids.

Mumps

The most common ocular manifestation of mumps is dacryoadenitis, which occurs in up to 20% of persons with mumps. Dacryoadenitis may present as edema and erythema of the superotemporal lid and conjunctiva. The gland may be visibly enlarged. Involvement is usually bilateral. Optic neuritis, disciform keratitis, iritis, uveitis, scleritis, and acute glaucoma have been reported.

Herpes Simplex Virus - Chapter 56

Worldwide, herpes simplex virus (HSV) ocular infection is a leading cause of visual impairment with an estimated 10 million people having a history of herpetic eye disease. Ocular involvement can result from infection with either HSV-1 or HSV-2. Primary ocular involvement, usually due to HSV-1, in children and adults is uncommon. Such involvement usually presents as follicular conjunctivitis that may be associated with epithelial keratitis. Vesicular formation on the eyelid and ulcerative blepharitis can occur. Primary ocular involvement in neonates is usually due to HSV-2, often resulting from infection during passage through the birth canal. Ocular manifestations occur in 15–20% of infected neonates and usually develop 2–14 days after birth.[11] Almost all HSV-infected neonates with ocular findings have evidence of skin involvement/vesiculation. Neonatal ocular HSV disease usually presents as nonfollicular conjunctivitis. Keratitis, chorioretinitis, acute necrotizing retinitis, optic neuritis, and iritis can occur. Cataracts, chorioretinal scarring, optic atrophy, and microphthalmia may result.

Non-neonatal ocular involvement by HSV can be due to primary infection, but most cases are due to viral reactivation. The most common manifestation is epithelial keratitis, which accounts for 70–80% of all HSV keratitis cases. In most cases, there is a dendritic pattern in the epithelium which may be seen by topical fluorescein (***Fig. 135.7***). Occasionally, HSV epithelial infection presents as a geographic epithelial keratitis (macro-ulcerative). Tearing, photophobia, pain, and blurred vision are common. The epithelial keratitis heals spontaneously within 2 weeks in 50% of patients, but treatment leads to healing in 90% of patients within 1 week. Involvement of the corneal stroma can cause interstitial keratitis, which may lead to scarring. Neovascularization, limbic vasculitis, corneal "ring" immunologic reactions, disciform keratitis, iridocyclitis, corneal anesthesia, and secondary glaucoma can occur.

Posterior ocular HSV disease is more rare than anterior disease. The primary manifestation is acute retinal necrosis, which presents as a rapid decrease in vision. Patients may have eye pain at onset. On funduscopic examination, there is marked destruction of the peripheral retina, occlusive vasculitis, and white blood cells in the vitreous (vitritis). There is often optic nerve swelling. HSV-associated encephalitis or meningoencephalitis can result in papilledema, cranial nerve dysfunction, extraocular palsies, and visual disturbances.

Compared with what is the case in the developed world, ocular HSV disease in the developing world is more likely to present with larger geographic or ameboid corneal epithelial ulcerations than with classic, thin-branching, dendritic, ulcerative patterns, and is more likely to present with bilateral ocular involvement; and is more likely to involve non-neonatal children.[12] These differences may be related to differences in nutritional status and to delay in seeking medical attention. The occurrence of HSV ocular disease has been well associated with both concurrent measles and malaria, possibly because of fever-induced reactivation of HSV disease, concurrent immunologic alterations, or both.

Diagnosis of ocular herpetic involvement is usually one of clinical recognition. The classic corneal dendritic epithelial ulceration pattern may be visualized with fluorescein or rose bengal staining and is most frequently associated with HSV (although it may also occur with herpes zoster). Tzanck preparation of an epithelial scraping can disclose multinucleated giant cells. Seroconversion during primary infection can aid in diagnosis, as can the presence of anti-HSV immunoglobulin M (IgM) antibodies in neonates; however, interpretation of antibody levels in recurrent disease is problematic. Antiviral agents are available for the treatment of ocular HSV disease.[13] The application of topical antiviral agents combined with gentle débridement can be employed in the therapy of simple epithelial HSV involvement. Treatment with oral acyclovir alone is effective in most cases. Patients with HSV stromal keratitis or iridocyclitis may require corticosteroids in addition to oral acyclovir, but corticosteroids may worsen some forms of HSV eye disease and should only be prescribed by an eye physician. Recurrent episodes of HSV stromal keratitis may lead to significant cornea scarring, and long-term oral acyclovir prophylaxis is effective in preventing recurrences.

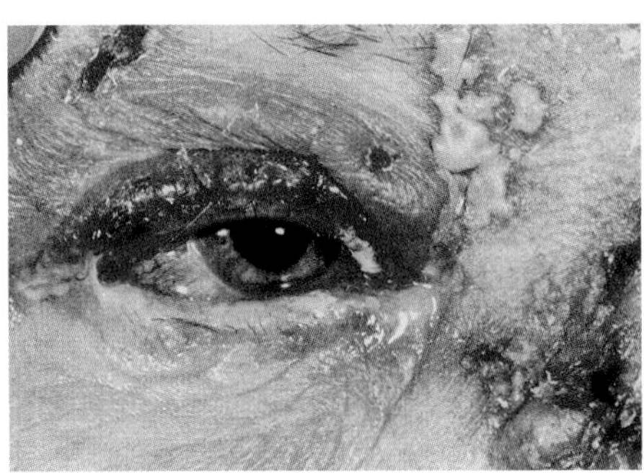

Figure 135.8 Zoster ophthalmicus with involvement of the nasociliary and frontal nerves. Note conjunctival injection and purulent discharge. (From Liesegang TJ. The varicella-zoster virus: systemic and ocular features. J Am Acad Dermatol. 1984;11:170.)

Varicella Zoster Virus - Chapter 56

Infection with varicella zoster virus (VZV) can present in one of two classic patterns: *varicella* (chickenpox) or *zoster* (shingles).

Varicella (Chickenpox)

Ocular involvement during acute varicella, occurring in about 4% of children, is usually one of vesicular lid eruption, conjunctivitis, and keratitis. Varicella vesicles can form on the conjunctiva itself and may be associated with marked edema and injection. Dendritic keratitis, disciform keratitis, stromal keratitis, and uveitis have been reported. Rarely, optic neuritis, retinitis, and cranial nerve palsies occur. Varicella encephalitis can be complicated by papilledema and extraocular palsies. Congenital varicella infection is rare; however, chorioretinitis, cataracts, and microphthalmia can occur.

Diagnosis of acute varicella is usually one of clinical recognition. Tzanck preparation of epithelial scrapings of the base of vesicles can disclose multinucleated giant cells and viral antigenic assays can be employed. Therapy is usually supportive. Systemic antiviral agents should be employed in immunocompromised persons and adults because the incidence of severe complications is increased in these populations. Acute varicella involving the eye may also be an indication for use of systemic antiviral agents. Bacterial superinfection of eyelid vesicles may occur and should be treated; corneal epithelial ulcers should be treated with topical antibiotic drops or ointments in addition to oral acyclovir. Anterior uveitis (iritis, iridocyclitis) may be treated with topical steroids in addition to oral antiviral agents. Acute retinal necrosis (see below) may occur rarely in primary varicella, and should be treated with intravenous acyclovir.

Zoster

When VZV reactivates along a nerve distribution, it is called shingles or zoster. Reactivation, common in thoracic or trigeminal nerve distributions, is most frequent in older or immunocompromised persons. Involvement of the ophthalmic branch of the trigeminal nerve (V_1) is called zoster ophthalmicus. Such involvement is associated with ocular manifestations in 50–70% of affected persons (***Fig. 135.8***). Involvement of the nasociliary branch of V_1 produces vesicles on the lateral aspect of the tip of the nose and is associated with ocular manifestations in 85% of affected patients. As in varicella, most ocular disease in zoster involves the anterior segment of the eye. Eyelid involvement can lead to lid scarring with retraction and complicating ectropion, exposure keratitis, or both. Papillary conjunctivitis, epithelial keratitis, stromal infiltrative keratitis, and disciform keratitis can occur. Corneal anesthesia may be pronounced and persistent and can predispose affected persons to complicating corneal infections and ulcerations. Corneal scarring can occur (***Fig. 135.9***). Iridocyclitis (with secondary iris atrophy and secondary glaucoma), optic neuritis, vitritis, and retinitis have been reported.

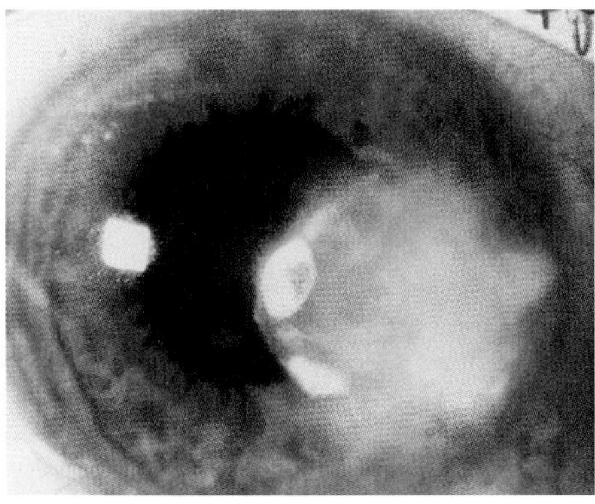

Figure 135.9 Residual corneal scarring, lipid deposition, and corneal thinning after zoster ophthalmicus. (From Liesegang TJ. The varicella-zoster virus: systemic and ocular features. J Am Acad Dermatol. 1984;11:172.)

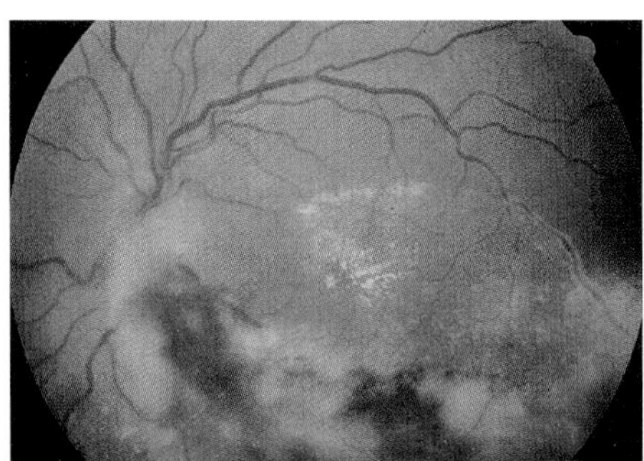

Figure 135.10 Cytomegalovirus-associated retinitis. Note hemorrhagic necrosis of the retina with exudates and periphlebitis. (From Rao NA. Acquired immunodeficiency syndrome and its ocular complications. Indian J Ophthalmol; 1994:42:57.)

VZV can cause acute retinal necrosis (ARN) (described below), often with no associated rash. VZV may also cause branch retinal artery occlusion. Zoster may be the presenting feature of infection with human immunodeficiency virus (HIV), especially in young persons.

Diagnosis of zoster is usually one of clinical recognition and can be supported by a Tzanck preparation of an epithelial scraping, culture, or viral antigenic studies. Systemic acyclovir, valacyclovir, and famciclovir can decrease the time to healing, and may lessen the pain associated with zoster. Intravenous therapy should be considered in immunocompromised patients and employed in patients with acute retinal necrosis or disseminated zoster. Topical steroids may be used for treatment of anterior uveitis, along with oral acyclovir. Cycloplegia can aid in preventing synechial formation in patients with anterior uveitis. Patients with corneal epithelial defects should receive topical antimicrobial agents to prevent bacterial superinfection.

Cytomegalovirus - Chapter 56

Some infants (~40%) born to mothers who sustain primary CMV infection during pregnancy acquire congenital infection. Of such newborns 10–15% have clinical manifestations, and approximately 20–30% of infants with severe cytomegalic inclusion disease have chorioretinitis. Optic atrophy and rarely anophthalmia may occur.

Acute CMV infection acquired after gestation in immunocompetent persons is often asymptomatic. A mononucleosis-like syndrome can occur and can be associated with mild, nonspecific conjunctivitis. Rare cases of retinitis have been reported. Most symptomatic disease occurs in immunocompromised persons, especially in those with AIDS or who have undergone organ transplantation. AIDS-associated CMV ocular disease occurs almost exclusively in persons whose CD4 cell count is ≤50 cells/mL. In such persons, CMV classically involves the eye with hemorrhagic necrotizing chorioretinitis (***Fig. 135.10***). The retinitis, which often follows a perivascular distribution, is progressive and can be bilateral.

Retinal detachments are frequent. Optic neuritis can occur and result in optic atrophy. Punctate keratitis and iridocyclitis can occur. Up to 40% of individuals with untreated AIDS will develop ocular CMV disease.

Diagnosis of ocular CMV disease is usually one of clinical recognition. Systemic CMV disease can be diagnosed by viral antigenic assays, serologic or molecular assays, and culture. CMV retinitis needs to be distinguished from acute retinal necrosis (see below), VZV retinitis, progressive outer retinal necrosis, and toxoplasmosis-associated retinitis, among other entities. CMV retinitis in immunocompromised patients is progressive without therapy. The antiviral agents ganciclovir, valganciclovir, foscarnet, and cidofovir, the mainstays of therapy, are virostatic; and, after an initial course of induction therapy, maintenance therapy must be continued. Even after an initially favorable clinical response is achieved, reactivation of CMV chorioretinitis occurs if the severe immunocompromised state continues. In the case of CMV retinitis associated with advanced HIV disease, immune reconstitution following initiation of antiretroviral therapy has been associated with an immune recovery uveitis.[14] Maintenance anti-CMV treatment has been successfully discontinued in individuals with HIV whose CD4 count increases to at least 100 cells/mL who have been taking highly active antiretroviral treatment for at least 6 months.

Oral valganciclovir may be used for maintenance therapy, as can a sustained-release ganciclovir intraocular implant with oral valganciclovir or intravenous cidofovir. Repeated intravitreal injections of fomivirsen with oral valganciclovir can also be employed in both induction and maintenance therapies of CMV retinitis.

Acute Retinal Necrosis

ARN is a syndrome characterized by occlusive retinal vasculitis, retinal necrosis, and vitritis.[15] The retinitis usually starts in the periphery of the retina (distant from the macula and optic nerve) and involves full-thickness retinal necrosis. There are often several patches of retina involved simultaneously. Optic nerve head swelling is common. Patients with ARN present with decreased vision and ocular pain. One eye is usually involved, but the second eye may become involved days to weeks later if no therapy is given. Most cases of ARN occur in immunocompetent patients, and these are due to HSV, more commonly, and VZV. Rare cases of CMV-associated ARN occur in immunocompromised patients. Visual loss can be severe, and retinal detachments are common. Treatment with intravenous acyclovir should be started promptly, and after the retinitis has stabilized, should be converted to oral valganciclovir for a prolonged period (months), and possibly long-term acyclovir prophylaxis following that. Systemic steroids may be required to control vitritis in acute ARN.[16] Steroids should not be started until after intravenous acyclovir has begun. Intravitreal ganciclovir or foscarnet may be indicated in severe cases. Retinal detachments occur commonly, usually weeks to months later, and these usually require surgical repair. Patients immunocompromised with HIV may have a fulminant form of ARN called progressive outer retinal necrosis (PORN).[17] In PORN, the deepest layers of the retina are involved, and progression to blindness is usually rapid despite prompt intravenous acyclovir therapy. Successful treatment of PORN has been described using combination therapy (intravitreal and systemic antiviral agents) along with highly active antiretroviral therapy (HAART).[18]

Epstein–Barr Virus - Chapter 56

The most common ocular manifestation of Epstein–Barr virus (EBV) infection is transient mild conjunctivitis that is often follicular, can be unilateral, and occurs in 2–40% of persons with infectious mononucleosis. Superficial and stromal keratitis have been reported. EBV infection may be associated with dacryoadenitis and Parinaud's oculoglandular syndrome. EBV-associated Burkitt's lymphoma, a disorder most frequently reported in children in sub-Saharan Africa (but worldwide in distribution), most often manifests as a maxillary/orbital mass and can present with proptosis.

Human Immunodeficiency Viruses - Chapter 81

The majority of patients with untreated AIDS due to HIV-1 and HIV-2 have ocular manifestations. Ocular manifestations of HIV infection can be due to HIV itself or to secondary opportunistic ocular infections.[19] The most common ocular involvement resulting from HIV itself is HIV retinopathy (***Fig. 135.11***) which occurs in over two-thirds of patients with untreated AIDS and is characterized by the formation of retinal cotton wool spots, microaneurysms, and hemorrhages. Cotton wool spots, areas of ischemia in the nerve fiber layer, are usually oriented along vascular arcades. The frequency of HIV retinopathy increases as the level of immunologic suppression increases, but HIV retinopathy usually remains asymptomatic as long as the macula is not affected. Some persons infected with HIV develop large-vessel vasculopathy with consequent retinal vaso-occlusion of central or branch retinal veins and leading to potentially severe visual loss. HIV infection can also be associated with a primary optic neuropathy and an infiltrative lymphocytosis syndrome.

Compared with what occurs with primary HIV eye involvement, HIV-induced ocular opportunistic infections (see Chapter 139) are often symptomatic, may be the presenting feature of infection by HIV, and can result in severe visual loss or blindness. The frequency of specific ocular opportunistic infections varies by geographic location and patient population, but may include CMV, toxoplasmosis, tuberculosis, syphilis, cryptococcosis, histoplasmosis, and HSV infection, among others. Such infections can result in chorioretinitis, uveitis, optic neuritis, and keratitis. AIDS-associated meningitis or encephalitis may be associated with cranial nerve dysfunction and ocular palsies. Involvement of the CNS or orbit by HIV-associated lymphoma may result in papilledema or proptosis, respectively.

A number of distinct ocular entities occur in persons infected with HIV. Infectious multifocal choroiditis describes a choroidal infection, usually caused by a systemic opportunistic infection with *Pneumocystis jirovecii*, *Cryptococcus neoformans*, *Mycobacterium tuberculosis*, *Histoplasma capsulatum*, or *Mycobacterium avium-intracellulare* complex, among others (see Chapter 139). Progressive outer retinal necrosis is a fulminant retinitis that may occur in patients with AIDS (see 'Acute Retinal Necrosis' above). Coinfection with *Molluscum contagiosum* virus can also lead to follicular conjunctivitis. Kaposi's sarcoma of the eyelid, conjunctiva, and orbit may develop in patients with AIDS. Ocular surface squamous neoplasia is associated with HIV infection.[20] Treatment of HIV retinopathy is directed toward systemic anti-HIV therapy, and treatment of opportunistic ocular infections is targeted to the specific pathogenic entity. Initiation of antiretroviral treatment may be associated with ocular immune reconstitution syndromes.[14]

Human T-Cell Lymphotropic Virus Type I - Chapter 81

Persons infected with human T-cell lymphotropic virus type I (HTLV-I) may develop adult T-cell leukemia/lymphoma (ATCLL) or tropical spastic

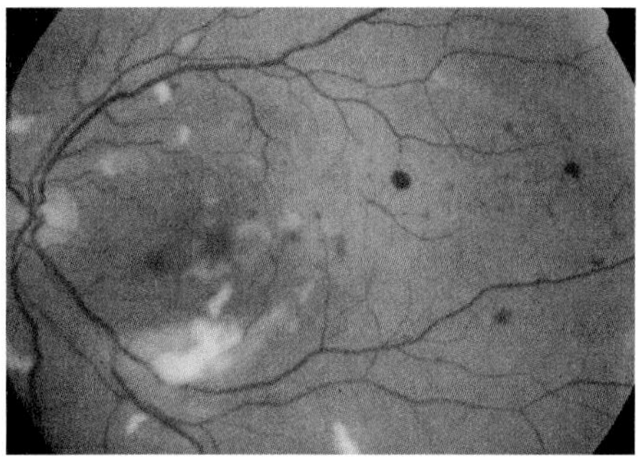

Figure 135.11 Human immunodeficiency virus-associated retinopathy. Note retinal cotton wool spots and hemorrhages. (From Rao NA. Acquired immunodeficiency syndrome and its ocular complications. Indian J Ophthalmol; 1994:42:57.)

paraparesis/HTLV-I-associated myelopathy (TSP/HAM). Similar to those infected with HIV, asymptomatic retinal cotton wool spots and transient retinal exudates and hemorrhages have been observed; and uveitis and interstitial keratitis are the most frequent symptomatic ocular manifestations in patients with HTLV-I infection.[21] Keratoconjunctivitis sicca, vitritis, retinal vasculitis, retinal exudates, and retinal hemorrhages have been reported. Ocular involvement in persons with TSP/HAM can include uveitis and vasculitis as well as neuro-ophthalmologic manifestations. Ocular involvement in persons with ATCLL can include direct lymphomatous or leukemic involvement of the eye. Lymphoma/leukemia of the eyelid, orbit, retina, and vitreous, as well as a lymphoma/leukemia that diffusely infiltrates all ocular structures have been reported.

VIRAL ENCEPHALITIS – CHAPTERS 56, 76, 78

Encephalitis can be caused by a number of viruses, including herpesviruses and arboviruses, the latter including West Nile virus, Venezuelan equine encephalitis virus, western equine encephalitis virus, Japanese encephalitis virus, Murray Valley encephalitis virus, Rocio virus, and Oropouche virus, among others. Ocular manifestations during encephalitis are rarely reported; however, elevated intracranial pressure can result in papilledema. Encephalitis involving brainstem structures can result in disorders of ocular motility, and diffuse encephalitis can result in cortical visual disturbances.

Specific ocular involvement is associated with Rift Valley fever virus.[22] In 1–5% of affected persons hemorrhagic manifestations, encephalitis, or chorioretinitis can occur. Ocular involvement may be immunologically mediated. Clinical features of hemorrhagic fever, encephalitis, and retinitis usually do not overlap in the same individual. Ocular disease includes retinal vasculitis, retinal hemorrhages, and retinitis.[23] Retinal detachment, optic atrophy, vitreal hemorrhages, and blindness can occur. Involvement may be unilateral or bilateral. Conjunctivitis, keratitic precipitates, and uveitis have been reported.

West Nile virus infection has been associated with multifocal chorioretinitis, occlusive retinal vasculitis, optic neuritis, uveitis, and vitritis.[24] Acute flaccid paralysis of facial and ocular muscles can result in diplopia.

Viral Hemorrhagic Fevers – Chapters 67–76

Ocular involvement in hemorrhagic fevers is usually a manifestation of a systemic bleeding diathesis. Endothelial vascular and rheologic abnormalities can lead to hemorrhagic involvement of the conjunctivae and retina. Nonspecific eye pain may be a prominent presenting feature of dengue fever, and hemorrhagic conjunctivitis occurs in patients infected with Ebola virus. A specific ocular association has been recognized with Puumala virus in the Scandinavian hantavirus-associated hemorrhagic fever and renal syndrome, nephropathia epidemica.[25] Transient myopia is the most frequent ocular manifestation and relates to forward movement of the ocular anterior diaphragm and thickening of the lens. Eyelid edema, chemosis, conjunctival injection, conjunctival hemorrhage, iritis, acute glaucoma, and retinal edema and hemorrhages have been reported. Ocular involvement in nephropathia epidemica usually resolves spontaneously.

Chikungunya Virus – Chapter 78

During an outbreak of chikungunya virus in southern India in 2006, a number of cases with ocular manifestations were seen.[26] The most common ocular finding was anterior uveitis, followed by panuveitis and optic neuritis, but retrobulbar neuritis, multifocal choroiditis, and keratitis were also seen.

Hepatitis Viruses – Chapters 64–66

The conjunctiva sensitively reveals the presence of jaundice. Acute viral hepatitides can be associated with immune-complex deposition during the pre-icteric and icteric phases of illness, and posthepatitis polyneuritis has been reported (including Guillain–Barré syndrome). Cranial nerves involved by neuritis can result in extraocular palsies. Immune-complex deposition resulting from chronic active hepatitis B or C infections can result in a variety of clinical vasculitic entities. Uveitis associated with chronic active hepatitis B may occur. Chronic hepatitis C infection is associated with a dry eye syndrome similar to Sjögren's syndrome and/or ischemia retinopathy caused by hepatitis C-induced vasculitis or treatment with interferon.

Rabies – Chapter 79

Rabies secondary to animal bites of the face may be associated with facial paralysis and mydriasis. Retinitis and retinal vasculitis can occur with direct viral destruction of retinal ganglion cells, and inflammation of the ciliary bodies and choroid has been reported. Human-to-human transmission of rabies has occurred through corneal transplantation.

Lymphocytic Choriomeningitis Virus

With lymphocytic choriomeningitis virus (LCM) excreted into the urine and feces of infected rodents, infection in humans may cause an influenza-like illness with concomitant meningitis. Chorioretinitis may be present. Congenital infection with LCM may result in a chorioretinopathy (which mimics that seen in toxoplasmosis) and neurological sequelae.

BACTERIAL INFECTIONS

Chlamydiae – Chapters 46–48

Three chlamydial species infect humans: *Chlamydia trachomatis*, *C. pneumoniae*, and *C. psittaci*. On the basis of antigenic differences, *C. trachomatis* is divided into various immunotypes.

Trachoma – Chapter 46

Trachoma, caused by *C. trachomatis* immunotypes A to C, is a leading infectious cause of blindness worldwide. Active trachoma affects an estimated 84 million people worldwide.[27] Another 7.6 million people have end-stage disease and 1.3 million of these are blind. *C. trachomatis* A to C is transmitted by direct contact, often within families. Unhygienic practices, aridity, crowding, low socioeconomic status, and the presence of flies are important epidemiologic risk factors for developing trachoma. Trachoma occurs predominantly in rural communities of developing nations.

Active trachoma is predominantly a disease of children. Following direct deposition, the organism infects columnar epithelial cells of the conjunctiva. After an incubation period of 5–7 days, chronic follicular conjunctivitis of varying severity can result (***Fig. 135.12B, C***). Inflammation may be intense, with marked conjunctival edema, conjunctival papillae, and lymphoid folliculitis. Rupture and scarring of limbic follicles can lead to a semilunar pattern known as Herbert's pits. Untreated infection may resolve over weeks to months. Long-term ocular sequelae from a single episode of *C. trachomatis* A to C conjunctivitis are often minimal. Ocular pathology and morbidity are due to recurrent episodes of conjunctival infection.[28] The upper tarsal conjunctiva is most severely affected. Recurrent infectious episodes lead to eyelid scar formation and cicatrization (***Fig. 135.12D***) with consequent retraction of the eyelids inward (entropion; ***Fig. 135.13***). Eyelashes then sweep directly over the cornea and conjunctival surfaces (trichiasis; see ***Figs 135.12E and 135.13***). Trichiasis can lead to epithelial breakdown, erosion, ulcerations, inflammatory responses, pannus formation, neovascularization, and scarring (***Fig. 135.12F***). This corneal scarring is the primary cause of trachoma-associated blindness. The World Health Organization's (WHO) categorization system delineates the stages/manifestations of ocular involvement during trachoma (***Box 135.2 and Fig. 135.12***).

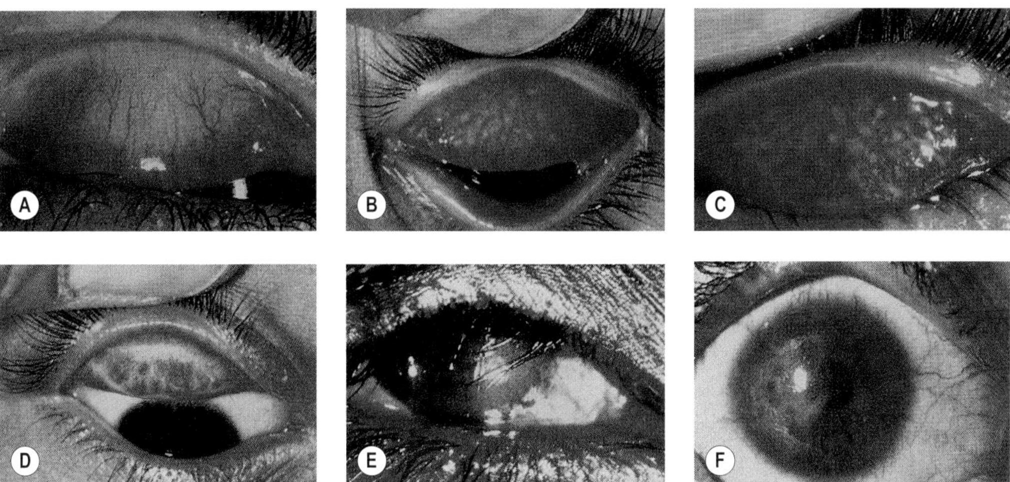

Figure 135.12 Trachoma – World Health Organization classification system. **(A)** Normal tarsal conjunctiva. **(B)** Trachomatous inflammation – follicular (TF). **(C)** Trachomatous inflammation – intense (TI). **(D)** Trachomatous scarring (TS). **(E)** Trachomatous trichiasis (TT). **(F)** Corneal opacity (CO). (From Thylefors B, Dawson CR, Jones BR, et al. A simple system for the assessment of trachoma and its complications. Bull WHO. 1987;65:481.)

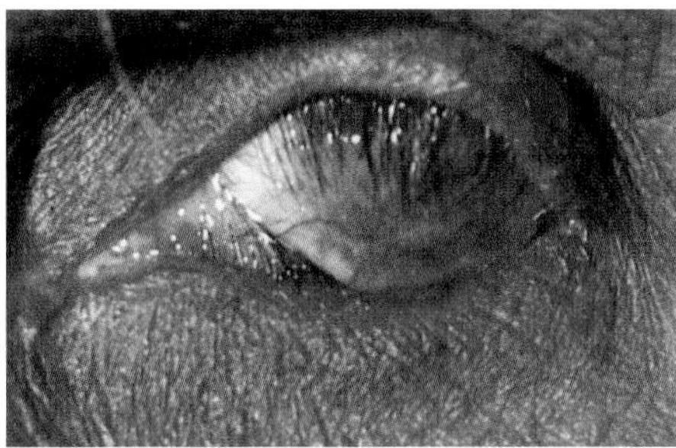

Figure 135.13 Trachoma-associated entropion and trichiasis. Note inturning of the upper and lower eyelids. The eyelashes of the lower eyelid are present, but completely inturned. (From Sandford-Smith J. Eye Diseases in Hot Climates, 2nd ed. Oxford: Wright Publishers, Butterworth Heinemann; 1990: plate 7b.)

Box 135.2 Trachoma: World Health Organization Categorization

Trachomatous inflammation – follicular (TF): Presence of at least five follicles in the upper tarsal conjunctiva (see ***Fig. 135.12B***)	Trachomatous scarring (TS): Scarring of the tarsal conjunctiva (see ***Fig. 135.12D***)
Trachomatous inflammation – intense (TI): Obscuring of at least half of the normal deep tarsal vessels by a pronounced inflammatory thickening of the upper tarsal conjunctiva (see ***Fig. 135.12C***)	Trachomatous trichiasis (TT): At least one eyelid rubbing on an eyeball (or evidence of self-epilation due to trichiasis) (see ***Fig. 135.12E***)
	Corneal opacity (CO): Visible corneal opacity over the pupil (see ***Fig. 135.12F***).

Although most active ocular infections occur during childhood or adolescence, most visual loss and blindness occurs in adults (because of the chronic nature of the ocular damage and the requirement for repetitive acute infections). Bacterial superinfection is not uncommon.

The main global control strategy is called SAFE (surgery for trichiasis, antibiotic treatment for active trachoma, facial cleanliness, and environmental improvement). This was begun in 1998 as a WHO initiative, with the goal of eliminating trachoma by 2020. Treatment of trachoma can be directed toward an individual patient or at a community–mass treatment level.[29]

C. trachomatis Nontrachoma Ocular Disease

Ophthalmia Neonatorum

C. trachomatis immunotypes D to K, common causes of genital disease, including urethritis, cervicitis, and epididymitis, can also cause ocular disease. Neonates can be infected during passage through the birth canal, and *C. trachomatis* is one of the most common causes of ophthalmia neonatorum (along with *Neisseria gonorrhoeae*). Other causes of ophthalmia neonatorum include *Streptococcus*, *Escherichia coli*, and other Gram-negative organisms. Ophthalmia neonatorum occurs in 1–2% of newborns in developed nations, and in 10–20% of infants born in developing nations that do not employ prophylactic measures. Prophylaxis can be achieved with application at the time of birth of topical silver nitrate or tetracycline, and can reduce the incidence of ophthalmia neonatorum by 60–70%. Approximately 20–30% of neonates exposed to *C. trachomatis* during birth develop conjunctivitis, and 10–20% develop pneumonitis. The conjunctival presentation is one of a diffuse papillary reaction with lacrimation that occurs between 5 and 14 days after birth. Eyelids are swollen, and hyperemia is present. Discharge may be purulent, and pseudomembranes can form. The conjunctivitis is nonfollicular because the immature immune system of neonates is unable to generate follicles. After 6–8 weeks, follicles can form, and chronic infection may present at this time as follicular conjunctivitis. Keratitis has been reported. Conjunctival scars and corneal neovascularization can occur.

C. trachomatis is not only present in ocular structures of affected neonates, but may also be found in the nasopharynx, vagina, and rectum. The systemic nature of the infection (and the risk of developing pneumonitis or autoreinoculation) negates topical therapy as a sole therapeutic intervention. Untreated, ocular disease slowly resolves over weeks to months. Diagnosis may be confirmed by conjunctival scrapings with culture and Giemsa staining. Giemsa staining for the detection of chlamydial inclusion bodies may have a sensitivity of over 90% in ophthalmia neonatorum. Immunofluorescence or ELISA antigenic assays can be performed. Molecular techniques may also be employed. Serology is often not helpful.

Adult Inclusion Conjunctivitis

C. trachomatis immunotypes D to K can also cause inclusion conjunctivitis in children, adolescents, and adults. Ocular involvement results from direct inoculation of infectious genital secretions. Genital infection is most frequently asymptomatic. Ocular involvement is often unilateral. Conjunctival involvement is usually follicular, and onset is usually acute.

Preauricular adenopathy may be present. Discharge is minimal, and pseudomembranes that may be present in neonates do not form in adults. Epithelial keratitis, subepithelial opacities, anterior uveitis, and corneal vascularization can occur. Untreated, the conjunctivitis may be chronic and usually resolves over months. Diagnosis can be made by culture or Giemsa staining of conjunctival scrapings; however, a direct immunofluorescent assay is usually employed. Molecular techniques are also available. Examination of the genital tract for chlamydial infection and other concomitant sexually transmitted diseases must be performed. Sexual partners need to be appropriately evaluated and treated.

Lymphogranuloma Venereum

Ocular involvement during lymphogranuloma venereum (LGV), a sexually transmitted disease caused by *C. trachomatis* immunotypes L1, L2, or L3, is rare. Keratoconjunctivitis may include fleshy vascularization of the conjunctiva or marginal cornea. Parinaud's oculoglandular syndrome with preauricular adenopathy, and small corneal ulcerations, episcleritis, iridocyclitis, uveitis, and optic neuritis may occur. Granulomas may involve the orbit or eyelid, and scarring and blockage of lymphatic drainage may result in eyelid elephantiasis. Diagnosis may occasionally be confirmed by culture; however, LGV is usually diagnosed by serologic assay employing complement fixation or microimmunofluorescence.

Chlamydia psittaci – Chapter 48

Uncommon ocular manifestations of psittacosis include follicular conjunctivitis, uveitis, and keratitis that may be epithelial or interstitial.

Chlamydia-Associated Reactive Arthritis Syndrome

The classic triad of this syndrome, formerly termed Reiter's syndrome, includes conjunctivitis or iritis, urethritis, and arthritis.[30] Characteristic skin, mucous membrane, and bone lesions can occur. The syndrome may be accompanied by keratoderma blennorrhagica (red-brown papular/vesicular/pustular skin lesions that usually occur on the feet) or balanitis circinata (moist, well-demarcated erosions with raised borders involving the penis). The syndrome, thought to be immunologically mediated, appears to be initiated by a number of infectious processes. Chlamydial urethritis is a frequent precipitating factor. Synovial tissue samples from patients with reactive spondylarthritis may be positive for *Chlamydia* DNA by PCR assays.[31] Ocular manifestations include the classic conjunctivitis, which is usually nonfollicular, and iritis. Keratitis, iridocyclitis, corneal ulcerations, hypopyon, intraocular hemorrhages, posterior uveitis, and optic neuritis may also occur. Diagnosis is usually one of clinical recognition. Chlamydial involvement of the genitourinary system should be sought and if there is evidence of a sexually transmitted disease, sexual partners should also be evaluated and treated. Treatment involves the use of nonsteroidal anti-inflammatory agents for the arthritis. Topical steroids may be employed in the treatment of anterior uveitis.

Mycobacteria

Leprosy – Chapter 37

Ocular involvement in leprosy is common; and, worldwide, leprosy is a leading infectious cause of visual loss.[32] Ocular involvement in leprosy can be due to direct mycobacterial involvement of the eye or to secondary immunologic or inflammatory manifestations. The eye may be involved during all forms of leprosy, but ocular involvement occurs most frequently during lepromatous leprosy (***Fig. 135.14***). *Mycobacterium leprae* prefers the cool temperatures of the anterior chamber of the eye, and ocular disease is usually anterior in nature. Involvement of the fifth and seventh cranial nerves during type 1 lepra reactions can lead to corneal anesthesia and lagophthalmos (the inability to fully close the eyelids). Such involvement can predispose affected persons to corneal ulcerations, suppurative keratitis, corneal perforation, corneal scarring, and blindness. Staphyloma, a marked bulging of the anterior eye through a weakened corneal wall, may result (***Fig. 135.15***).

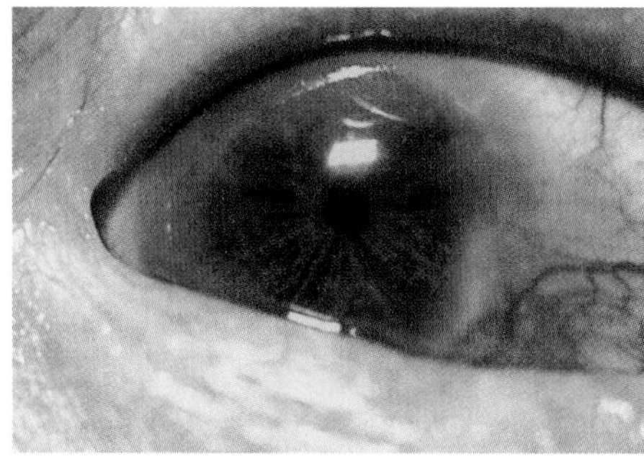

Figure 135.14 Ocular involvement in lepromatous leprosy. Interstitial keratitis is shown by the white appearance of the margin of the cornea. Episcleritis is shown by the dilated episcleral vessels. There is chronic iritis with constriction of the pupil. Note also the loss of eyelashes. (From Sandford-Smith J. Eye Diseases in Hot Climates, 2nd ed. Oxford: Wright Publishers, Butterworth Heinemann; 1990: plate 22f.)

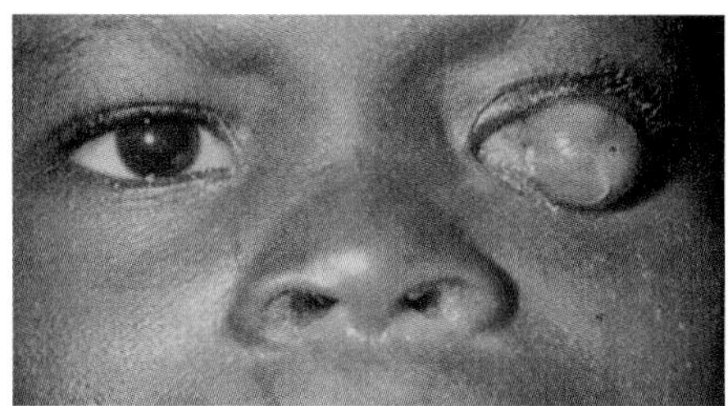

Figure 135.15 Staphyloma secondary to marked weakening of the cornea and sclera. The damage is irreversible. (From Sandford-Smith J. Eye Diseases in Hot Climates, 2nd ed. Oxford: Wright Publishers, Butterworth Heinemann; 1990: plate 9.)

Persons with lepromatous leprosy may also experience erythema nodosum leprosum (type 2 reactions). This form of the disease appears to be immune complex-mediated and may manifest as a serum sickness-type reaction with fever, myalgias, diffuse subcutaneous nodule formation, and arthritis. Iridocyclitis and episcleritis can occur. The iridocyclitis can become chronic, and can lead to iris atrophy, persistent myosis, and posterior synechiae.

Adnexal ocular involvement during leprosy is common. *Madarosis*, a term used to describe leprosy-associated loss of eyelids and eyelashes (the lateral third of the eyelids is most commonly lost), is most common in multibacillary leprosy. Lagophthalmos may be due to either type 1 reactions in paucibacillary disease or to chronic nerve infiltration and inflammation in multibacillary disease. Lagophthalmos may be associated with paralytic ectropion of the lower eyelid. Multibacillary disease may be associated with a marked thickening of the eyelids and can lead to excessive folds of skin (blepharochalasis) and apparent ptosis.

Lepromatous forms of leprosy may be associated with limbic lepromas (focal, nodular mycobacterial lesions). Corneal sensation can be decreased or absent in both tuberculoid and lepromatous forms of leprosy: the former from acute reversal reactions involving the fifth cranial nerve, the latter from direct mycobacterial invasion and chronic low-grade inflammation of corneal nerve fibers. Loss of corneal sensation may precede any other ocular manifestation of leprosy. Beading of corneal nerves, punctate keratitis, interstitial keratitis, and pannus formation may occur. Giant lepromas have been reported. Involvement of the lacrimal gland can lead to dacryoadenitis and keratoconjunctivitis sicca. Nasal collapse in multibacillary disease can lead to obstruction of the nasal lacrimal duct with resulting epiphora (excessive tearing). Acute or chronic iridocyclitis can occur in multibacillary disease. Iris pearls represent iris edge leproma that may be miliary or nodular. Atrophy of the dilatory muscle eventually leads to nonreactive pinpoint pupils and posterior synechiae. Lepromatous choroiditis, retinal pearls, and optic neuritis have all been reported.

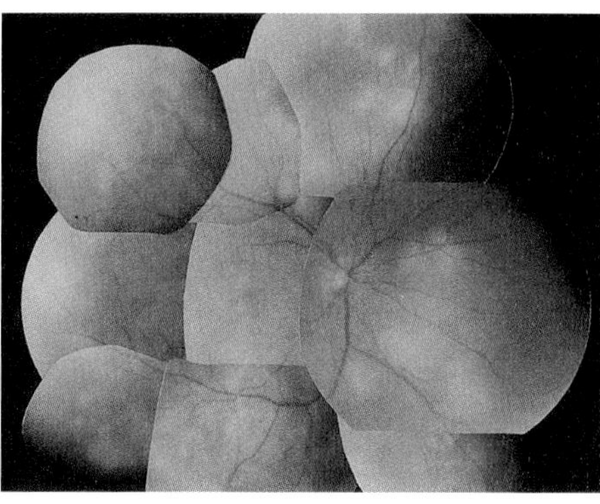

Figure 135.16 Multifocal tuberculous chorioretinitis. Note scattered lesions. (From Barondes MJ, Sponsel WE, Stevens TS, et al. Tuberculous chorioretinitis diagnosed by chorioretinal endobiopsy. Am J Ophthalmol. 1991;112:460.)

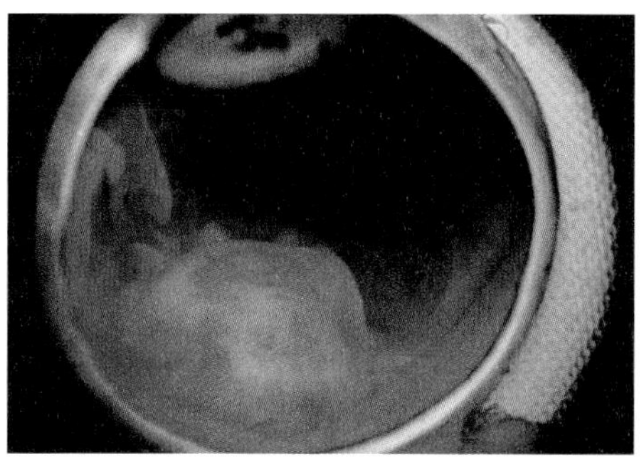

Figure 135.17 Choroidal tuberculoma. Gross section of the left globe. (From Lyon CE, Grimsen BS, Peiffer RL Jr, et al. Clinicopathological correlation of a solitary choroidal tuberculoma. Ophthalmology. 1985;92:847.)

Diagnosis of leprosy rests on clinical recognition and involves demonstration of acid-fast bacilli in skin smears or skin/nerve biopsies. An ocular manifestation can be the presenting feature of leprosy. Treatment of leprosy requires multidrug treatment usually involving dapsone, rifampin, and clofazimine. Specific ocular therapy is tailored to the given clinical manifestation. Type 1 reactions of less than 6 months' duration (including involvement of cranial nerves such as V and VII) indicate the need for immediate institution of systemic steroids. High-dose clofazimine may also be employed. Erythema nodosum leprosum reactions (with associated iridocyclitis) can be treated with systemic steroids, clofazimine, and thalidomide (contraindicated in women of childbearing age). Iridocyclitis, episcleritis, and scleritis can be treated with topical steroids. Cycloplegics should be employed in acute iritis. Mydriatics should be employed in chronic iritis. Chronic ocular manifestations such as lagophthalmos and ectropion may require surgical management, including tarsorrhaphy (suturing of the lateral eyelids together to protect the exposed cornea) and lid suspension.[33] Recognition of ocular involvement, corneal anesthesia, and lagophthalmos should prompt measures to prevent exposure keratitis and progressive ocular disease. Education, eye patches, protective glasses, repeated conscious blinking, antibiotic eye drops, and surgery should all be considered.[34]

Tuberculosis – Chapter 35

Ocular involvement occurs in less than 1% of persons with tuberculosis. The eye can be involved during pulmonary tuberculosis, during systemic extrapulmonary tuberculosis, or as the sole manifestation of systemic tuberculosis.[35] The most common manifestation of ocular tuberculosis is multifocal choroiditis (***Fig. 135.16***). Here, multiple choroidal nodules are seen. Involvement may also manifest as choroidal "tubercles" (***Fig. 135.17***), which are usually one-quarter to several disk diameters in size, are seen in the posterior pole of the eye, and are yellow, white, or gray, with an overlying vitritis in active lesions. Most patients have fewer than five lesions, but the range is 1–60 lesions. Inactive lesions appear as scars.

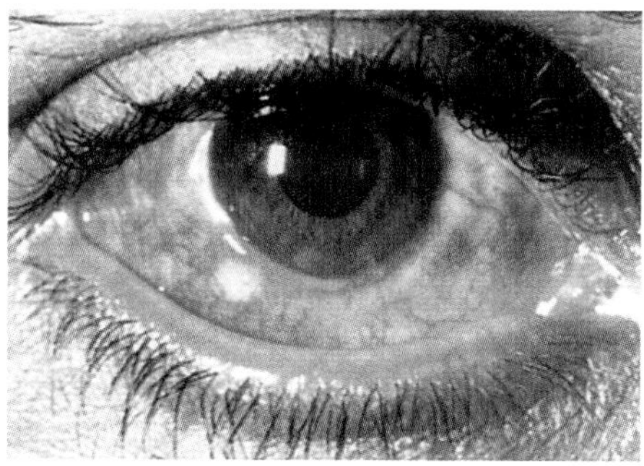

Figure 135.18 Conjunctival phlyctenule in a patient with pulmonary tuberculosis. (From Helm CJ, Holland GN. Ocular tuberculosis. Surv Ophthalmol. 1993;38:229. Courtesy of Dr A.M. Mehta, Los Angeles.)

More rarely, several choroidal tubercles may coalesce and form a large solitary mass (see ***Fig. 135.17***). The second most common manifestation of ocular tuberculosis is a chronic granulomatous anterior uveitis, in which "mutton fat" or "granulomatous" keratoprecipitates coalesce on the endothelial surface of the cornea. These are not true granulomas, but rather clumps of white blood cells. When the eye itself is the site of direct infection of *M. tuberculosis*, disease is most often limited to conjunctival or corneal structures. Preauricular adenopathy is common, and involvement is usually unilateral. Tuberculoid eyelid abscesses can occur from direct deposition or from contiguous spread from sinus structures. Phlyctenular keratoconjunctivitis can occur (***Fig. 135.18***). A phlyctenule first appears as a raised nodule with surrounding hyperemia that becomes necrotic and then sloughs. It is thought to be an immune response to microbial proteins and is associated with a number of infectious processes, including tuberculosis.[36] Involvement is usually at or near the limbus. Infection with *M. tuberculosis* can also result in interstitial keratitis. Involvement of the retina is usually manifested as Eales' disease, an inflammatory retinal periphlebitis (vasculitis involving the retinal veins). There are often peripheral retinal capillary occlusions that lead to retinal hemorrhages and subsequent neovascularization. Eales' disease most often occurs in patients from India, Pakistan, and Afghanistan. Other manifestations of ocular tuberculosis include scleritis, interstitial keratitis, and optic neuritis. Orbital tuberculosis can result from hematogenous dissemination or contiguous spread, and is often unilateral. Panophthalmitis may also occur.

Diagnosis of ocular tuberculosis can be difficult as there may be no signs of systemic disease: the chest radiograph is clear in 50% of patients. A positive purified protein derivative (PPD) test may be helpful, but by itself a positive PPD test has a low positive predictive value for ocular tuberculosis. Ocular tuberculosis responds well to standard systemic multidrug chemotherapeutic regimens. Ethambutol therapy itself, however, may cause optic neuritis, so is often avoided.

Atypical Mycobacteria – Chapter 35

Although atypical mycobacteria are rare causes of ocular infection, *M. fortuitum* and *M. chelonae* (*abscessus*) are the atypical mycobacteria that most frequently affect the eye. Keratitis, corneal ulceration, orbital granulomas, scleral abscesses, iritis, and endophthalmitis have been reported. Such involvement is usually associated with trauma or surgery or occurs in persons who wear contact lenses.[37] *M. gordonae*, *M. marinum*, and *M. flavescens* have more rarely been associated with keratitis. *M. avium-intracellulare*/*M. avium* complex (MAI/MAC) has been associated with corneal ulcerations, preseptal cellulitis, endophthalmitis, and choroiditis (the latter being associated with coinfection with HIV).

Diagnosis of atypical mycobacterial infection of the eye is based on demonstration of organisms by acid-fast staining, culture, and molecular assays. For keratitis, topical therapy with amikacin plus moxifloxacin or gatifloxacin plus clarithromycin may be necessary. Disseminated MAI/MAC disease should be treated with systemic therapy.

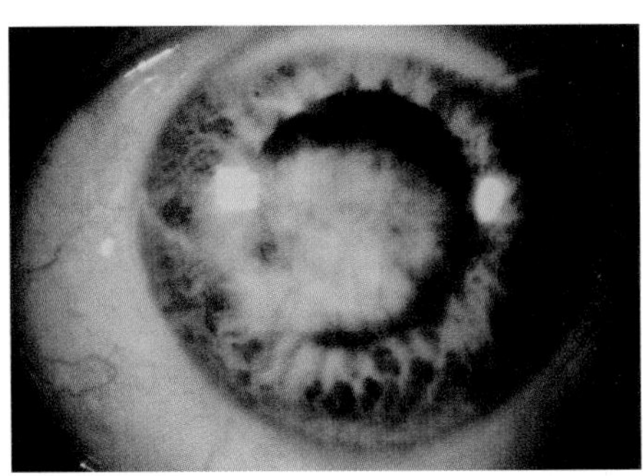

Figure 135.19 Central stromal scarring and ghost vessel formation secondary to late latent syphilitic interstitial keratitis. (From Brooks AMV, Weiner JM, Robertson IF. Interstitial keratitis in untreated latent (late) syphilis. Aust NZ J Ophthalmol. 1986;14:128.)

Spirochetes

Treponemal Infections – Chapter 43

The eye can be involved during all stages of congenital or acquired syphilis, caused by *Treponema pallidum*. During primary acquired syphilis, chancres of the eyelid, conjunctiva, and lacrimal gland have been reported. During the rash of secondary syphilis, conjunctivitis and blepharitis can occur. Approximately 10% of persons with secondary syphilis have ocular involvement. Madarosis (loss of eyelashes and eyebrows) has been reported. Keratitis, iritis, iris hyperemia (roseolae), iris nodules, episcleritis, and scleritis can also occur. Anterior uveitis is the most common ocular finding during secondary syphilis. Keratitis may be unilateral. Chorioretinitis, peripapillary neuroretinitis, pigmentary retinitis, retinal vasculitis, and vitritis may also occur. A "salt-and-pepper" appearance of the retina is often seen. During tertiary syphilis, the eyelid, lacrimal glands, and deep ocular structures can be involved with destructive gummatous lesions. Orbital bones may be involved with periostitis that can be bilateral. Chronic interstitial keratitis is not infrequent (***Fig. 135.19***). The most common ocular manifestations of syphilis are uveitis (iritis, chorioretinitis, retinitis) and optic neuritis, although episcleritis and scleritis can occur. Occlusive retinal vascular disease, neovascularization, aneurysm formation, retinal detachments, and pigmentary retinopathy can also occur.

Neurosyphilis can occur during secondary or tertiary disease. Meningovascular syphilis can be associated with neuro-ophthalmic complications. Nerve palsies can result in ocular dysmotilities. The classic Argyll Robertson pupil, a small, irregular pupil that reacts normally to accommodation, but not to light, may be visible in meningovascular syphilis. Papilledema can also occur. Neuro-ophthalmic findings are possible with parenchymous neurosyphilis, but they are rare. Argyll Robertson pupil and optic atrophy can be seen in tabes dorsalis.

Ocular involvement during congenital syphilis may be mild or even asymptomatic. Clinically evident involvement during the first few months of life can include conjunctivitis, iridocyclitis, uveitis, optic neuritis, salt-and-pepper chorioretinitis, extraocular paresis, and neuro-ophthalmic manifestations. Disease often becomes quiescent, with only pigmentary retinopathy being subsequently evident. The disease can reactivate, however, and an affected patient can present with chronic interstitial keratitis as an adolescent or as an adult. Such involvement, usually bilateral, is often misdiagnosed. Chronic inflammation can lead to scarring, neovascularization, and residual "ghost vessel" formation. Hutchinson's triad includes malformed Hutchinson's teeth, deafness (from eighth nerve involvement during neurosyphilis), and interstitial keratitis. Iritis or kerato-uveitis may occur and can result in secondary glaucoma. Chronic retinitis and pigmentary retinopathy may be evident.

Ocular syphilitic involvement during concurrent infection with HIV is not infrequent. Involvement is possible even in patients previously treated for syphilis. Conjunctivitis, iridocyclitis, uveitis, retinitis, neuroretinitis (***Fig. 135.20***), vitritis, papillitis, optic perineuritis (***Fig. 135.21***), and retrobulbar neuritis have all been reported.

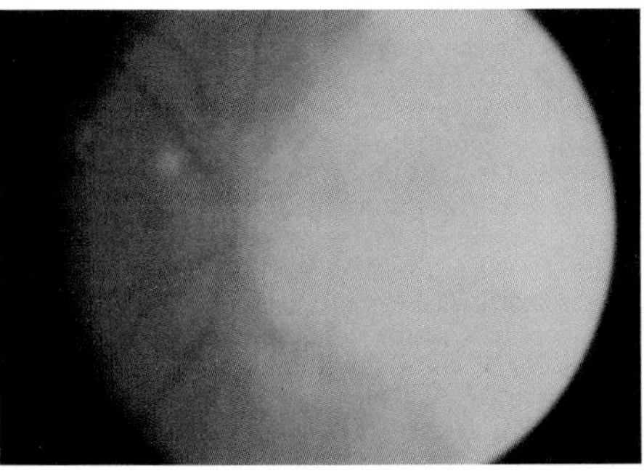

Figure 135.20 A large wedge-shaped area of syphilitic neuroretinitis with small cotton wool spots. (From McLeish WM, Pulido JS, Holland S, et al. The ocular manifestations of syphilis in the human immunodeficiency virus type 1-infected host. Ophthalmology. 1990;97:198.)

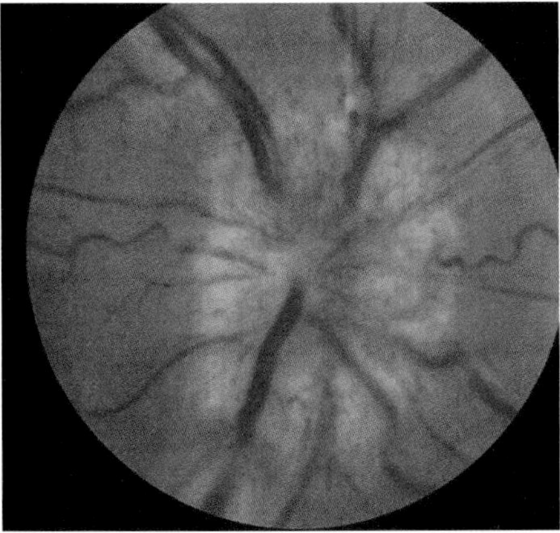

Figure 135.21 Syphilitic optic perineuritis with disk swelling. (From McLeish WM, Pulido JS, Holland S, et al. The ocular manifestations of syphilis in the human immunodeficiency virus type 1-infected host. Ophthalmology. 1990;97:198.)

Diagnosis is usually based on clinical recognition and serologic examination. Both a non-treponemal (such as rapid plasma reagin: RPR) and a treponemal test (such as fluorescent treponemal antibody absorbed: FTA-abs) should be performed to screen for ocular syphilis. A negative RPR does not exclude ocular syphilis, as RPR decreases spontaneously with time and may be negative in up to 50% of patients with tertiary syphilis. A positive FTA-abs should be confirmed with a TPPA (*Treponema pallidum* particle agglutination assay), as false positive FTA-abs results may occur in patients with acute Lyme disease or rheumatologic conditions. A lumbar puncture should be performed to evaluate for concomitant neurosyphilis. However, it should be emphasized that a normal lumbar puncture does not exclude ocular syphilis, as syphilis may involve the eye without involving the CNS. Independent of the evaluation of the CNS, all persons with ophthalmic manifestations of syphilis should be treated with a 10–14-day course of intravenous high-dose penicillin therapy. If the lumbar puncture suggests concomitant neurosyphilis, then a lumbar puncture should be repeated 6 months after completion of intravenous penicillin to ensure adequacy of treatment. Certain immunocompetent persons with an isolated primary chancre of the eyelid or periorbital area could be treated with short, low-level therapy. Follow-up serologic analysis should be performed to monitor post-therapy resolution of disease. Follow-up analysis of cerebrospinal fluid should be performed in patients with neurosyphilitic involvement. Topical steroids, mydriatics, and cycloplegics may also be employed for anterior syphilitic inflammatory ocular disease, including keratitis and uveitis.

Endemic Treponematoses – Chapter 43

Nonvenereal endemic syphilis (bejel) is a nonvenereal treponematosis caused by a variant of *T. pallidum* that is morphologically and serologically indistinguishable from that which causes venereal syphilis. A number of ocular manifestations, including anterior uveitis, choroiditis, and chorioretinitis have been reported to be late manifestations of bejel.[38] Diagnosis is one of clinical recognition in an appropriate demographic setting. Serologic assays cannot distinguish between venereal and nonvenereal syphilis, so it is clinically impossible to firmly ascribe isolated ocular disease to venereal and nonvenereal syphilis. The treatment of ocular disease presumed to be caused by nonvenereal syphilis is the same as that due to venereal syphilis (intravenous penicillin).

Yaws (pian, frambesia), caused by infection with *T. pertenue*, is found in warm tropical areas throughout the world, is spread by bodily contact, and has distinct early, latent, and late-stage manifestations. Yaws has been associated with neuro-ophthalmic abnormalities (including Argyll Robertson-type pupillary responses), sheathing of retinal vessels, perivascular pigmentation, and optic atrophy, but differentiation from infection with venereal syphilis is not possible. Acute skin lesions can involve the eyelid and may result in catarrhal conjunctivitis. Scarred/healed skin lesions of the face may result in ectropion. Massive destruction of the nasal mucosa can result in saddle-nose, and central facial necrosis (yaws gangosa) can result in destruction of the eye and orbit.

Pinta (mal de pinto) is caused by *T. carateum*. No ocular abnormality has definitely been associated with pinta except for scarring skin lesions that have involved the eyelids.[39]

Leptospirosis – Chapter 45

During the acute leptospiremic phase of leptospirosis, a retro-orbital headache can occur. Conjunctival suffusion and photosensitivity are common. During the immune phase, meningitis can occur that may be associated with cranial nerve paresis and optic neuritis. In the severe form of leptospirosis, Weil's disease, scleral jaundice and conjunctival and retinal hemorrhages can occur. Uveitis is the most frequent ocular manifestation after conjunctival suffusion. Uveitis may present from 10 days to many months after the initial infection,[40] which may have been clinically asymptomatic. Uveitis, often acute and bilateral, usually presents as anterior uveitis and iridocyclitis. Anterior chamber involvement, hypopyon, elevated intraocular pressure, and synechiae can occur. Posterior uveitis, vitreal clouding, retinal exudates, and retinal hemorrhages may also occur.

Relapsing Fever – Chapter 44

Epidemic relapsing fever is caused by louse-borne *Borrelia recurrentis*; endemic relapsing fever is caused by tick-borne *B. duttoni*. Ocular manifestations during acute relapsing fever include photophobia, eye pain, and conjunctivitis. During severe episodes of relapsing fever, bleeding diathesis can occur, and conjunctivitis and conjunctival and intraocular hemorrhages can result. Meningoencephalitis and optic neuritis can occur. Involvement of the sixth and seventh cranial nerves can result in disorders of ocular motility and ptosis. Uveitis may be the most frequent ocular manifestation associated with relapsing fever and can occur after several relapses of the disorder. Iridocyclitis is common, and posterior synechial formation can result. Posterior uveitis, vitritis, vitreal exudates, and retinal venous occlusion have all been reported.

Rickettsia – Chapters 49–51

Louse-borne epidemic typhus is caused by *Rickettsia prowazekii*. Flea-borne endemic typhus is caused by *R. moosei* (*typhi*). During acute epidemic typhus, conjunctival suffusion may occur, and can predate the appearance of the body rash. The rash itself may be associated with small, oval, pink-purple, conjunctival lesions. Persons with typhus may appear to have a glassy-eyed "drugged look." Keratoconjunctivitis has been reported, and hemorrhagic manifestations can lead to conjunctival and intraocular hemorrhages. The vascular damage induced by rickettsial infection can lead to vascular thrombosis, retinal vasculitis, retinal hemorrhages, and possibly uveitis.

Tick-borne rickettsial spotted fevers can be caused by many *Rickettsia* species, including *R. rickettsii* (the cause of Rocky Mountain spotted fever), *R. conorii* (the cause of boutonneuse fever), and *R. africae* (the cause of African tick fever). Mite-borne scrub typhus is caused by *R. tsutsugamushi*. An eschar may be evident at the site of the tick or mite bite in boutonneuse fever/African tick fever or scrub typhus, respectively. Eschars can involve the lid and periocular structures. Conjunctival suffusion and photophobia may occur in acute cases of rickettsial spotted fevers or in scrub typhus. Direct ocular inoculation of infectious blood from crushed ticks can result in conjunctivitis, corneal ulceration, and preauricular adenopathy (Parinaud's ocular glandular syndrome). Bilateral anterior uveitis, papilledema, retinal vein engorgement, retinal hemorrhage, retinal vein occlusion, papillitis, and optic neuritis can occur. Meningoencephalitis can result in cranial nerve dysfunction and in ocular palsies.

Mycoplasma

Mycoplasma pneumoniae

Mycoplasma pneumoniae is associated with the development of Stevens–Johnson syndrome/erythema multiforme major (SJS/EMM). With SJS, vesicles and bullae can involve mucocutaneous surfaces, including conjunctivae. Conjunctival involvement is present in 50–80% of patients with SJS/EMM. Catarrhal conjunctivitis, pseudomembranous conjunctivitis, and membranous conjunctivitis can occur. Anterior uveitis has been reported. Residual scarring can lead to keratitis sicca, lid retraction, corneal pannus formation, corneal opacifications, corneal ulcerations, and corneal perforations. Trichiasis and lagophthalmos can occur. Epiphora can result from scarring of lacrimal puncta and canaliculi. Late ocular complications are directly related to the severity of the primary SJS.

Mycoplasma hominis/Ureaplasma urealyticum

Mycoplasma hominis may be present in genital secretions and may be associated with mild neonatal conjunctivitis. *Ureaplasma urealyticum* may be associated with the development of conjunctivitis as part of the presentation of Reiter's syndrome.

Actinomyces

Actinomycosis

Actinomycosis can be caused by a number of species of *Actinomyces*. The organisms are worldwide in distribution and are part of the mouth flora. Ocular manifestations are usually due to *Actinomyces israelii* and are due to direct deposition of organisms or contiguous spread.[41] *Actinomyces* is the most common cause of canaliculitis. The chronic inflammation can lead to obstruction of tear drainage, epiphora (excessive tearing), and chronic conjunctivitis. *Actinomyces* is also a rare cause of chronic dacryocystitis (lacrimal sac infection).

Orocervicofacial actinomycosis is characterized by an expansile cold abscess that begins at the mucosal surface of the oropharynx and does not respect anatomic borders. Sinus tract formation and fistula formation/drainage are common. *Actinomyces* species may also be introduced into ocular structures during ocular surgery or through trauma. Diagnosis of actinomycotic infection is confirmed by culture. Concretions may be expressed from the canaliculi that are typical "sulfur granules," so named for their yellow appearance. These are aggregates of *Actinomyces*. Examination of tissue samples or secreted granules can disclose the characteristic stellate radiations of the organism.

Nocardia

Nocardia species are soil organisms that are worldwide in distribution. Nocardial ocular infections are rare, but they do occur. Ocular involvement in immunocompetent persons is usually related to trauma, introduction of foreign bodies, or surgical manipulation. Involvement in immunocompromised persons is usually secondary to hematogenous dissemination (usually from a pulmonary focus). Dacrocystitis or canaliculitis with concretions (similar to that associated with actinomycosis) can occur. Preseptal cellulitis, catarrhal conjunctivitis, keratitis, or corneal ulcerations may all occur after contaminating inoculation. Nocardial endophthalmitis can occur in immunocompromised persons. Diagnosis is usually based on culture results.

Whipple's Disease

Whipple's disease is caused by *Tropheryma whipplei*, a Gram-positive, non-acid-fast, periodic acid–Schiff-positive bacillus with a characteristic tri-lamellar plasma membrane surrounded by a cell wall. It is related to *Actinomyces*, and is probably fairly ubiquitous in soil. The organism can be identified in the saliva of 10–30% of healthy individuals. In certain individuals (usually white males), the organism is able to cause deep systemic infection. In these individuals, there is a marked absence of any immune or cytotoxic response, and organisms replicate freely within foamy macrophages. The classic manifestations of Whipple's disease include a large joint arthritis, diarrhea, weight loss, and abdominal pain. Rash and neurological and ocular manifestation are common. Ocular manifestations includes uveitis. Ocular movement manifestations pathognomonic for Whipple's disease include oculomasticatory myorhythmia (continuous rhythmic movements of eye convergence with concurrent contractors of masticatory muscles) and oculofacial-skeletal myorhythmia.[42] These abnormalities are usually accompanied by supranuclear vertical gaze palsy. Posterior uveitis may be present. Diagnosis is usually based on identification of organisms on pathology specimens or using molecular techniques.

Brucellosis – Chapter 40

Ocular manifestations of brucellosis during the acute/early stage of infection include endophthalmitis and optic neuritis. There may be marked pain on eye movement. Involvement of the meninges during *Brucella* meningoencephalitis can result in ocular palsies and in papilledema. Ocular manifestations during the chronic phase of infection may include uveitis, which may be granulomatous, as well as episcleritis and nummular keratitis.[43] Isolated iridocyclitis or choroiditis may occur. Uveitis may be the only apparent manifestation of brucellosis and may occur after appropriate antibrucellosis therapy. Less common manifestations may include dacroadenitis, conjunctivitis, corneal ulceration, retinal detachment, papillitis, and retrobulbar optic neuritis.

Diagnosis is usually based on a serologic assay. Direct culture of infected material may be helpful during the early stage of infection.

Tularemia

Tularemia is caused by *Francisella tularensis*. Ocular manifestations usually result from deposition of the organism either through direct inoculation of infectious material on or around ocular structures or through aerolization. The disease may be bilateral. Deposition on the conjunctivae may result in an ulceronodular conjunctivitis that is usually painful. Chemosis, injection, and excessive lacrimation may be present. Painful, local lymphadenopathy may be prominent. Tularemia is a leading cause of Parinaud's oculoglandular syndrome. Nodal suppuration, corneal ulceration, and dacryocystitis can occur. Although the organism may be cultured, the diagnosis is usually confirmed with antibody-based serologic assays or molecular techniques.[44]

Bartonella Infections – Chapter 39

Trench Fever

Bartonella quintana is the cause of trench fever. Ocular manifestations occur only as part of the systemic illness. The headache of trench fever is often localized at the front of the head and behind the eyes. Conjunctival injection and congestion can occur.

Bacillary Angiomatosis

B. quintana and *B. henselae* can cause bacillary angiomatosis. The vascular proliferative lesions of bacillary angiomatosis may involve the conjunctiva, eyelid, and anterior orbit.[45] Lesions may appear superficially similar to those of Kaposi's sarcoma. Diagnosis is usually based on histologic examination of biopsy samples.

Cat-Scratch Disease

B. henselae is also a cause of cat-scratch disease. A common ocular manifestation is Parinaud's oculoglandular syndrome, characterized by unilateral follicular conjunctivitis and adjacent preauricular lymphadenopathy. Cat-scratch disease may also be associated with encephalopathy that may result in cranial nerve dysfunction, and in ocular palsies or dysmotilities. The most common posterior manifestation of cat-scratch disease is neuroretinitis, a syndrome comprising papillitis and a macular star. Neuroretinitis may present as painless, unilateral (rarely bilateral) decrease in vision, with a central scotoma, optic disk swelling, and macular star formation. Inflammation and occlusion of retinal vessels may occur. The retinal star is related to exudative leakage of optic nerve capillaries. Two-thirds of patients with neuroretinitis have positive serology for *B. henselae*. Diagnosis of *B. henselae* infection during cat-scratch disease is usually based on serologic assay.[46] Serologic tests have variable sensitivity and positive predictive value, given the seroprevalence of low titers for IgG in the general population. However, high titers are supportive of the diagnosis in the right clinical setting.

Carrion's Disease

B. bacilliformis is the cause of Carrión's disease, which during its early stage may manifest as Oroya fever and during its late stage may manifest as verruca peruana. Verruca peruana is associated with the formation of vascular proliferative nodular lesions, which are similar to those observed in bacillary angiomatosis. The skin is the most frequently involved site, but mucous membranes (including the conjunctiva) may also be affected.

Q Fever – Chapter 53

Ocular manifestations of Q fever caused by *Coxiella burnetii* are rare; however, cranial nerve palsies and optic neuritis have been reported.[47]

Anthrax – Chapter 38

Anthrax is caused by *Bacillus anthracis*. The eye and periocular structures may be involved by the eschar and edema of cutaneous anthrax. Extensive eyelid scarring can lead to severe ectropion.

Diphtheria – Chapter 34

Ocular diphtheria may occur after or concurrently with nasopharyngeal diphtheria, oropharyngeal diphtheria, or cutaneous diphtheria.[48] Ocular diphtheria can also occur independently of other diphtheric manifestations. Ocular diphtheria usually presents as membranous or pseudomembranous conjunctivitis, nonspecific purulent conjunctivitis, or a corneal process. Affected eyelids and conjunctivae are "hardened," tender, and erythematous. Pain and preauricular adenopathy may be pronounced, and discharge is initially minimal. Conjunctival membranes or pseudomembranes may then appear. Such membranes represent necrotic material/cellular debris and are leather-like and pale gray in appearance. Subepithelial petechiae may be present. Vascular necrosis is common. If the adherent membrane is removed, punctate hemorrhages appear. The membrane eventually sloughs with extensive exudation. Granulation tissue then appears. Healing can lead to extensive scar formation, with such secondary ocular sequelae as entropion, trichiasis, and xerosis. The cornea may also be involved in acute disease. Corneal erosions or ulceration, and a punctate keratitis may occur. Diphtheria toxin that is systemically absorbed from any site (e.g., nasopharyngeal, oropharyngeal) can lead to demyelinating neuritis. Cranial nerve paralysis can then occur and can result in disorders of ocular motility and ciliary function.

Diagnosis is usually one of clinical recognition and culture analysis. If the diagnosis of diphtheria is considered, treatment with systemically administered antitoxin should begin immediately, prior to culture confirmation. The presence of membranous or pseudomembranous conjunctivitis is not pathognomonic for ocular diphtheria (see ***Box 135.1***). Such membranes may be seen with conjunctival infections due to pneumococci, *Streptococcus* species, *Neisseria* species, certain enteroviruses, and adenoviruses. A Gram stain may be helpful; however, large Gram-positive rods may be commensal conjunctival organisms (e.g., *Corynebacterium xerosis*). Long-term sequelae of ocular diphtheria (such as entropion) may require surgical intervention.

Botulism – Chapter 22

Botulism is caused by neurotoxins produced by *Clostridium botulinum*. Blurred vision secondary to mydriasis is often the presenting clinical feature of botulism.[49] Autonomic dysfunction may also manifest as paresis of accommodation and as dry eye. Involvement of cranial nerves may result in ptosis, diplopia, ophthalmoplegia, and nystagmus.[50,51] Pupillary abnormalities may be present and may persist for months. Ocular manifestations may vary, depending on the type of botulism toxin being produced. Diagnosis is usually based on antigenic assays for toxin, culture, and electrophysiologic studies. Therapy involves administration of equine antitoxin with preliminary skin testing. Intestinal purgatives or lavage may be employed if contaminated food is thought to be still present within the intestinal lumen. Persons with wound botulism should undergo débridement. Botulism toxin could be used as an agent of bioterrorism (see Chapter 14), and the simultaneous presentation of many individuals with blurred vision should prompt consideration of intentional or inadvertent intoxication. Systemic penicillin or metronidazole is often coadministered. Administration of antitoxin only limits or prevents additional neuronal damage.

Tetanus – Chapter 42

Ocular manifestations of tetanus can occur during any manifestation of tetanus (generalized, localized, cephalic, and neonatal), but are most frequently observed during cephalic tetanus. Cephalic tetanus usually results from production of toxin from a local head or neck infection. Cephalic tetanus is associated with cranial nerve dysfunction.[52] Ocular involvement during tetanus may include ptosis, ocular palsies, ophthalmoplegia, saccadic eye movements, and supranuclear palsies.[53] Facial palsies may also occur. Ocular structures may themselves also be directly infected by *Clostridium tetani* organisms, usually in the setting of traumatically introduced foreign bodies. Orbital cellulitis, corneal infection, and panophthalmitis have all been reported. Diagnosis is one of clinical recognition. Strychnine poisoning needs to be excluded. Treatment involves the use of passive immunization with human tetanus immunoglobulin. Débridement of wounds is required. Systemic metronidazole or penicillin is usually employed.

Neisseria Species

Neisseria meningitidis – Chapter 24

N. meningitidis can involve the eye in a number of ways. Primary purulent conjunctivitis can occur. The conjunctivitis is hyperacute, with production of extensive purulent discharge.[54] Involvement is usually unilateral and may include subconjunctival hemorrhages. Keratitis can occur, and corneal ulceration and endophthalmitis may result. Ocular structures may also be involved during meningococcemia or meningococcal meningitis. Conjunctival petechiae and hemorrhages, iritis, hypopyon, endophthalmitis, panophthalmitis, and orbital cellulitis may occur. Diagnosis rests on clinical recognition and culture. Gram stain of conjunctival discharge may disclose the presence of Gram-negative diplococci. Treatment should be systemic, even in isolated conjunctival disease.

Neisseria gonorrhoeae – Chapter 25

N. gonorrhoeae is a more common cause of hyperacute purulent conjunctivitis than is *N. meningitidis*. Keratitis commonly leads to corneal perforation. Iritis, panophthalmitis, and lid abscesses can occur. Involvement is usually unilateral. Lymphadenopathy may be present. The disease not only involves sexually active persons, but also affects neonates. Gonococcal ophthalmia neonatorum usually begins between 1 and 13 (usually 2–5) days after birth, is often bilateral, and is often markedly purulent. Corneal ulceration and perforation can occur. Corneal scarring, neovasculization, and blindness may result. Diagnosis is based on microscopic examination of conjunctival smears and culture. Treatment should be systemic. The mother of an affected infant, the mother's sexual partner(s), and adults with *N. gonorrhoeae*-associated conjunctivitis should be examined for the presence of additional sexually transmitted diseases and appropriately treated. Local irrigation and removal of conjunctival purulent material should be performed. Topical therapy may supplement systemic therapy. Prophylactic regimens of topical silver nitrate, tetracycline, and erythromycin should be used at the time of birth to prevent or diminish the chance of ophthalmia neonatorum.

Brazilian Purpuric Fever

Brazilian purpuric fever (BPF), caused by *Haemophilus influenzae* biogroup *aegyptius*, is a hemorrhagic fever that resembles meningococcemia, but affects children almost exclusively.[55] *H. aegyptius* usually causes a self-limited purulent conjunctivitis. In children with BPF, conjunctivitis is followed up to 15 days later by purpura fulminans, characterizd by high fever, abdominal pain, vomiting, vascular collapse, purpura, and necrosis. The mortality rate can be as high as 40–70%, and most patients die within 24 hours. Blood cultures were positive for a particularly virulent clone of *H. influenzae* biogroup *aegyptius*, although the virulence factor or factors still have not been identified. After several outbreaks and sporadic cases in Brazil, no additional cases have been confirmed since 1993.[55,56]

Chancroid – Chapter 26

In chancroid, a sexually transmitted disease caused by *Haemophilus ducreyi*, ocular involvement is rare, but has been reported, presumably secondary to ocular inoculation of contaminating secretions. Involvement of the eyelid, conjunctiva, or both has been reported. The chancroid papule forms a shallow, painful, purulent ulcer. Conjunctivitis can occur. Marked enlargement of preauricular lymph nodes can occur. Diagnosis is usually based on clinical recognition, the presence of characteristic "schools of fish" Gram-negative bacilli on Gram stain of ulcer secretions, and, rarely, culture.

Cholera – Chapter 20

Ocular manifestations during cholera are directly related to the severe volume loss and osmotic/electrolyte disturbances that occur in affected persons. Severe dehydration leads to the characteristic "sunken" eyes of patients with cholera (***Fig. 135.22***). There is a decrease in tear production and in spontaneous blinking. Conjunctivitis and exposure keratitis with subsequent corneal ulceration may result. Fluid and osmotic shifts may result in corneal edema and can precipitate the sudden development of bilateral cataracts.

Typhoid – Chapter 16

In typhoid, rose spots can involve the conjunctiva, and conjunctivitis has been reported. Involvement of the CNS during typhoid can result in cranial nerve dysfunction, pupillary disturbances, and extraocular palsies.

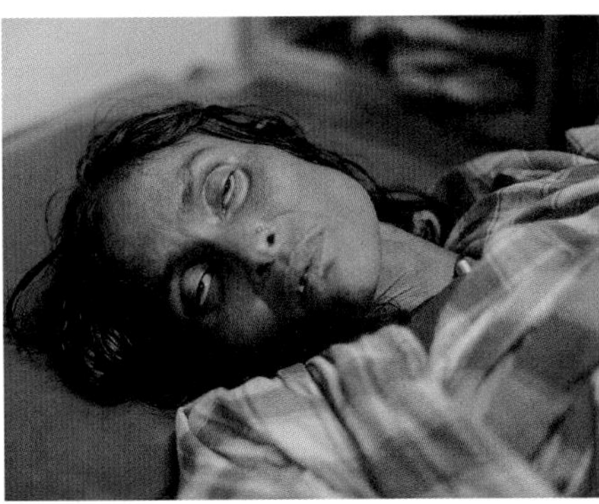

Figure 135.22 Woman with severe dehydration from cholera. Note the sunken and unclosed eyes.

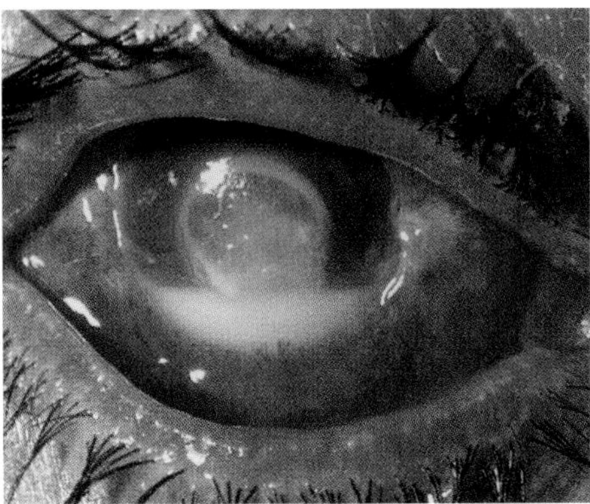

Figure 135.23 Suppurative keratitis with a large hypopyon and corneal ulceration. (From Sandford-Smith J. Eye Diseases in Hot Climates, 2nd ed. Oxford: Wright Publishers, Butterworth Heinemann; 1990: plate 8.)

Bacillary Dysentery - Chapters 15, 17–19

Bacillary dysentery is classically associated with shigellosis, although it may also be caused by a number of other infectious agents. Direct ocular deposition of *Shigella* species can result in conjunctivitis, keratitis, and corneal ulceration. Diffuse orbital inflammation of unclear etiology may occur.

The conjunctivitis associated with the reactive arthritis syndrome may be precipitated by an episode of dysentery-type diarrhea caused by *Shigella* species, *Salmonella* species, *Campylobacter* species, and *Yersinia* species, among others. Such involvement can occur 1–4 weeks after resolution of the dysenteric symptoms. Uveitis and iridocyclitis may be observed. Synechial formation may occur. Non-shigellosis dysenteric pathogens may also more rarely be associated with direct infection of ocular tissues and can result in a conjunctivitis, keratitis, Parinaud's oculoglandular syndrome, and endophthalmitis. Diagnosis is one of clinical recognition, historical questioning, and serologic analysis. Cultures are often unrevealing in cases of postdysenteric ocular disease, although they are helpful in infective ocular cases. Postdysentery immunologically mediated ocular reactions may be managed with topical steroids.

Melioidosis - Chapter 33

Ocular involvement in melioidosis may occur after direct traumatic deposition of the organism or from hematogenous dissemination. Necrotic scleral nodules and orbital abscesses may present with chemosis and exophthalmos. Chronic untreated infections may be associated with the development of a mild iritis. Intracerebral abscesses may form and can lead to papilledema. Diagnosis is usually made by culture.

Bacterial Keratitis and Conjunctivitis

Bacterial infections of the eye may be caused by a number of organisms, including *Streptococcus* species, *Streptococcus pneumoniae*, *Staphylococcus aureus*, *Haemophilus influenzae*, *Moraxella* species, *Neisseria* species, *Pseudomonas* species, and Enterobacteriaceae (including *Escherichia coli* and *Klebsiella* species), among others (***Fig.** 135.23* and ***Boxes** 135.3–135.8*). Keratitis of bacterial origin is a leading cause of visual loss in the developing world. Such conditions as trauma, introduction of foreign bodies, epithelial defects from xerophthalmia/measles, herpetic keratitis, exposure keratitis, and entropion with trichiasis all predispose affected persons to the development of suppurative keratitis. Corneal scarring, neovascularization, and corneal ulceration/perforation may result (***Figs** 135.23 and 135.24*). Diagnosis should include a Gram stain and culture of conjunctival or corneal scrapings.

Treatment of bacterial keratitis needs to be urgent and intense. Topical fluoroquinolones or topical cephalosporins and gentamicin or tobramycin are usually employed. Careful clinical monitoring is required. If the Gram stain or culture result discloses fungal forms, or if the keratitis is progressive despite the use of topical antibacterial agents, a topical antifungal agent should be employed. A mydriatic/cycloplegic is often employed in persons with suppurative keratitis.

Box 135.3 Infectious Causes of Conjunctivitis

Viral
- Adenovirus[a]
- Coxsackievirus[a]
- Measles virus[a]
- Herpes simplex virus
- Herpes zoster virus
- Molluscum contagiosum
- Rubella virus
- Mumps virus
- Cytomegalovirus
- Epstein–Barr virus
- Rift Valley fever virus

Bacterial
- *Streptococcus pyogenes*[a]
- Pneumococci[a]
- *Staphylococcus aureus*[a]
- *Haemophilus influenzae*[a]
- *H. influenzae aegypticus*[a]
- *Moraxella* species[a]
- *Neisseria* species[a]
- *Corynebacterium diphtheriae*
- *Francisella tularensis*[a]
- *Brucella* species
- *Bartonella* species
- *Shigella* species
- *Burkholderia mallei*
- *B. pseudomallei*
- *Actinomyces* species
- *Nocardia* species
- *Treponema pallidum*
- *T. pertenue*
- *Leptospira* species
- *Borrelia* species
- *Mycoplasma* species
- *Chlamydia trachomatis*[a]
- *C. psittaci*
- *Rickettsia* species
- *Coxiella burnetii*
- *Mycobacterium tuberculosis*

Fungal
- *Candida* species
- *Coccidioides immitis*
- *Aspergillus* species
- *Sporothrix* species[a]
- *Rhinosporidium seeberi*[a]

Parasitic
- *Microsporidia* species[a]
- *Loa loa*
- *Dirofilaria* species
- *Mansonella* species
- *Thelazia* species[a]
- *Trichinella* species
- *Gnathostoma spinigerum*[a]
- *Ascaris lumbricoides*
- *Wuchereria bancrofti/B. malayi/B. timori*
- *Dracunculus medinensis*
- *Cysticercus cellulosae*
- *Spirometra* species (sparganosis)[a]
- *Echinococcus* species
- *Schistosoma* species
- Myiasis[a]

[a]*Common or classic ocular manifestation of infection.*

The most common causes of acute bacterial conjunctivitis are *Staphylococcus aureus*, streptococci, and *Haemophilus influenzae*. Bacterial conjunctivitis usually resolves spontaneously over 7–10 days. Topical application of an antibiotic speeds resolution.

Bacterial Endophthalmitis

Exogenous bacterial endophthalmitis may result from introduction of organisms through trauma, surgery, or a perforated corneal ulcer.

Box 135.4 Infectious Causes of Keratitis

Viral

Adenovirus[a]
Herpes simplex virus[a]
Herpes zoster virus[a]
Mumps virus
Measles virus[a]
Rubella virus
Enterovirus
Rift Valley fever virus

Bacterial

Streptococcus species
Staphylococcus species[a]
Haemophilus influenzae[a]
Moraxella species[a]
Klebsiella species[a]
Corynebacterium diphtheriae
Neisseria species[a]
Pseudomonas species[a]
Brucella species
Shigella species
Rickettsia species
Treponema pallidum
Actinomyces species
Nocardia species
Vibrio cholerae (exposure keratitis)
Mycobacterium leprae[a]
M. tuberculosis
Atypical mycobacteria[a]
Chlamydia trachomatis[a] (secondary keratitis)
C. psittaci

Fungal

Aspergillus species[a]
Candida species[a]
Curvularia species[a]
Mucorales species[a]
Sporothrix schenckii
Coccidioides immitis
Fusarium species[a]
Penicillium species[a]
Cephalosporium species[a]
Phaeohyphomycosis
Cryptococcus neoformans[a]

Parasitic

Microsporidia species[a]
Acanthamoeba species[a]
Trypanosoma species
Ancylostoma species
Onchocerca volvulus[a]
Thelazia species
Echinococcus species
Coenuriasis[a] (exposure keratitis)
Myiasis

[a]*Common or classic ocular manifestation of infection.*

Box 135.5 Infectious Causes of Posterior Uveitis, Anterior Uveitis, or Both

Viral

Cytomegalovirus[a]
Herpes simplex virus[a]
Herpes zoster virus[a]
Rubella virus
Mumps virus
Epstein–Barr virus
Enterovirus
Influenza virus
Rift Valley fever virus
Hantavirus
Hepatitis viruses
Human T-cell lymphotropic virus I

Bacterial

Francisella tularensis[a]
Brucella species[a]
Coxiella burnetii
Burkholderia pseudomallei
Neisseria species
Bartonella henselae
Mycobacterium leprae[a]
M. tuberculosis[a]
Treponema pallidum[a]
T. pertenue
Tropheryma whipplei
Leptospira species
Borrelia species
Rickettsia species
Chlamydia trachomatis
C. psittaci

Fungal

Aspergillus species
Candida species
Cryptococcus neoformans[a]
Histoplasma capsulatum[a]
Blastomyces dermatitidis
Paracoccidioides brasiliensis
Sporothrix schenckii
Pneumocystis jirovecii[a]

Parasitic

Toxoplasma gondii[a]
Trypanosoma brucei species
Onchocerca volvulus[a]
Toxocara species
Loa loa
Dirofilaria species
Gnathostoma spinigerum
Coenuriasis
Schistosoma species[a]
Myiasis
Pentastomiasis (*Lingulata serrata*)

[a]*Common or classic ocular manifestation.*

Box 135.6 Infectious Causes of Ulcerative Lesions of the Eyelid

Viral

Herpes simplex virus
Herpes zoster virus
Measles virus

Bacterial

Treponema pallidum
T. pertenue
Mycobacterium tuberculosis
Haemophilus ducreyi
Rickettsia species (eschar)
Bacillus anthracis (eschar and edema)

Fungal

Blastomyces dermatitidis
Paracoccidioides brasiliensis
Sporothrix schenckii

Parasitic

Leishmania species
Entamoeba histolytica

Box 135.7 Infectious Causes of Parinaud's Oculoglandular Syndrome

Viral

Adenovirus
Enterovirus
Epstein–Barr virus
Mumps virus

Fungal

Sporothrix schenckii[a]
Blastomyces dermatitidis[a]
Coccidioides immitis[a]
Paracoccidioides brasiliensis

Parasitic

Trypanosoma cruzi[a]

Bacterial

Bartonella species[a]
Francisella tularensis[a]
Corynebacterium diphtheriae
Pasteurella species
Yersinia species
Burkholderia mallei
Haemophilus ducreyi
Chlamydia trachomatis
Rickettsia conorii
Treponema pallidum
Mycobacterium tuberculosis[a]
Actinomyces species

[a]*Common or classic ocular manifestation of infection.*

Box 135.8 Infectious Causes of Proptosis

Viral

Epstein–Barr virus-associated Burkitt's lymphoma

Bacterial

Orbital cellulitis
Orbital abscess

Fungal

Mucorales species
Aspergillus species
Histoplasma capsulatum var. *duboisii*
Orbital abscess

Parasitic

Angiostrongylus cantonensis
Gnathostoma spinigerum
Echinococcus species
Cysticercus cellulosae
Spirometra species (sparganosis)
Coenuriasis

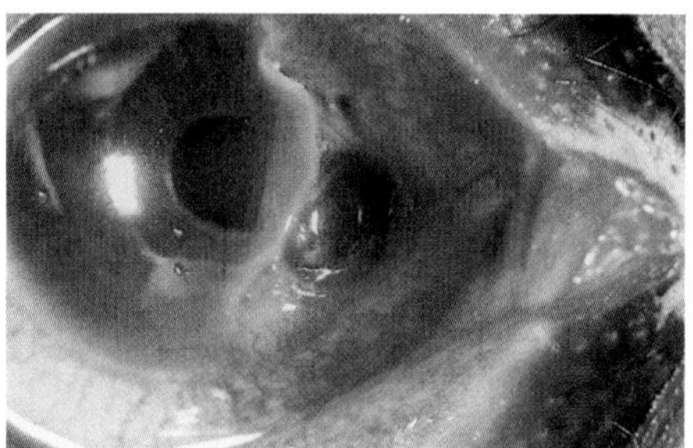

Figure 135.24 Corneal perforation secondary to ulceration. Note prolapse of the iris. (From Sandford-Smith J. Eye Diseases in Hot Climates. 2nd ed. Oxford: Wright Publishers, Butterworth Heinemann; 1990: plate 4e.)

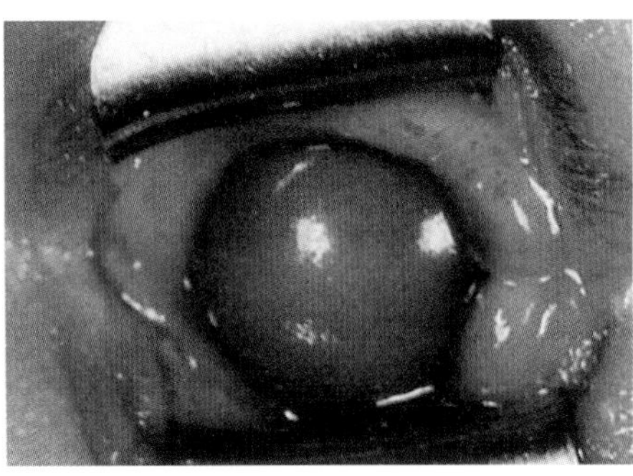

Figure 135.25 Metastatic bacterial endophthalmitis due to group B β-streptococcus. In this patient, inflammation was predominantly anterior. Note the corneal edema and cloudy and inflamed aqueous. Vitreal inflammation was minimal in the case, but can often be quite pronounced. (From Greenwald MJ, Wohl LG, Sell CH. Metastatic bacterial endophthalmitis: a contemporary reappraisal. Surv Ophthalmol. 1986;31:85.)

Endogenous bacterial endophthalmitis is secondary to hematogenous dissemination of a systemic infection (***Fig. 135.25***). Therapy of endophthalmitis must include intravitreal installation of antibiotics (usually vancomycin and either ceftazidime or amikacin). Vitrectomy is beneficial in severe cases. The role of systemic antibiotics in isolated endophthalmitis without systemic infection is controversial.

Bacterial Orbital Cellulitis

Bacterial orbital cellulitis results from infection/inflammation that occurs within the bony orbit. Orbital cellulitis most often results from infection in the adjacent ethmoid or frontal sinus, but may occur after direct inoculation/trauma, or rarely from hematogenous dissemination. The findings of orbital cellulitis include swollen red eyelids, proptosis, limitation of extraocular movements, and sometimes decreased vision. Treatment is with systemic antibiotics. Subperiosteal and orbital abscess may present with identical findings on physical examination, but treatment requires emergency surgical drainage in addition to systemic antibiotics. Concomitant sinusitis may also require surgical drainage.

FUNGAL INFECTIONS

Fungal Keratitis

The cornea is the most common site of fungal infection of the eye. Fungal keratitis (keratomycosis) can lead to corneal ulceration, corneal scarring, visual loss, and blindness.[57] In the tropics, 25–50% of all cases of suppurative keratitis are fungal in origin.[58,59] The most common causes of fungal keratitis are *Aspergillus* species and *Fusarium* species. Others include *Curvularia* species, *Candida* species, *Penicillium* species, and *Cephalosporium* species, among others (see ***Box 135.4***). Keratomycosis may occur after minor corneal trauma, especially trauma involving vegetable matter. The fungal corneal infiltrate typically has a feathery border and satellite lesions. Corneal scrapings by an ophthalmologist should be performed in all cases of suppurative keratitis. Gram stain and potassium hydroxide wet-mount preparations are economic and effective means of preliminarily establishing whether keratitis is bacterial or fungal in origin and in directing initial treatment. Suppurative keratitis of either mycotic or bacterial origin is an ophthalmic emergency, and therapy should be instituted immediately (see ***Fig. 135.23***). Definitive therapy may be guided by culture results of corneal scrapings. Hyphae of molds may only be detected by Giemsa stain or calcofluor white stain: the Gram stain may be falsely negative. If the Gram stain and cultures do not disclose fungal forms but the corneal lesion is progressive despite the administration of appropriate topical antibacterial agents, repeat cultures should be performed. Empiric antifungal agents should be considered in cases with consistent history (subacute presentation) and slit-lamp findings (corneal infiltrates with feathery borders and satellite lesions). Treatment of keratomycosis should be intense and include hourly eye drops with topical amphotericin B (0.15%) and/or topical natamycin. Therapy of keratitis due to *Candida* species may include topical amphotericin or fluconazole, plus oral fluconazole. For keratitis caused by *Aspergillus* species, topical amphotericin or natamycin may be supplemented with topical plus oral voriconazole. Topical voriconazole plus amphotericin or natamycin, plus oral voriconazole is usually effective in *Fusarium* keratitis. Oral posaconazole has been used with success in a few cases of *Fusarium* resistant to other therapies. Topical silver sulfadiazine has also been used in the treatment of keratomycosis, especially that caused by *Fusarium* species. The use of steroids should be avoided. Débridement may improve ocular penetration of drugs. Corneal transplant should be considered in cases with progression of infection despite antifungal therapy.

Aspergillosis

Aspergillosis can be caused by a number of *Aspergillus* species. Ocular involvement by *Aspergillus* species may result in conjunctivitis that may involve the lacrimal duct and can result in tear-flow obstruction. Scleritis with ulceration may occur. *Aspergillus* is a common cause of keratitis worldwide, as noted above. Endophthalmitis may result from posterior progression of keratitis, from traumatic or surgical inoculation, or from hematogenous dissemination (the latter usually occurring in immunocompromised persons or in intravenous drug abusers).[60] Acute invasive fungal sinusitis can be caused by *A. fumigatus* (although more commonly by fungi of the order Mucorales), usually in immunocompromised persons, and may invade the orbit. Orbital involvement with proptosis and chemosis can occur. A more chronic form of invasive fungal sinusitis, often due to *A. fumigatus*, may occur in immunocompetent or immunocompromised persons and is associated with the development of orbital apex syndrome: ptosis, proptosis, ophthalmoplegia, neuralgia of the ophthalmic division of the trigeminal nerve, and visual loss. A more chronic, indolent fungal sinusitis, often caused by *A. flavus* and called granulomatous invasive fungal sinusitis, is most commonly reported in Africa and South Asia.[61] Involvement is usually in immunocompetent persons, who often present with unilateral proptosis. Diagnosis of ocular involvement by *Aspergillus* species is usually based on microscopic examination of tissue preparations and cultures. Blood antigen tests may support the diagnosis of invasive fungal disease. Topical amphotericin (0.15%), intravitreal amphotericin (5–10 μg as an injection), and systemic antifungal agents (or combinations) should be employed, depending on the location of the *Aspergillus* infection. Penetrating keratoplasty may be required for keratomycosis caused by *Aspergillus*; vitrectomy with injection of intravitreal amphotericin is required for endophthalmitis caused by *Aspergillus*. Systemic administration of voriconazole is usually required.

Candidiasis – Chapter 88

Candidiasis can be caused by a number of *Candida* species, of which the most commonly reported is *C. albicans*. Ocular involvement by *Candida* species most commonly manifests as chorioretinitis complicating hematogeneous dissemination (usually in an immunocompromised host). Funduscopic examination reveals multiple fluffy white chorioretinal lesions. These may be asymptomatic, or may progress to involve the vitreous as endophthalmitis. Chorioretinitis or endophthalmitis due to *Candida* may be chronic and may be initially mistaken for a noninfectious uveitis (***Figs 135.26 and 135.27***). Diagnosis of *Candida* chorioretinitis is commonly presumptive, with characteristic eye findings in the setting of blood cultures positive for *Candida* species. *Candida* may colonize the ocular surface, particularly in patients on chronic corticosteroid eyedrops. However, *Candida* keratitis also occurs, and may appear as white infiltrates in the cornea. Diagnosis of *Candida* keratitis may be made by culturing the corneal surface. Candidal keratitis should be treated with topical amphotericin and a systemic azole (e.g., fluconazole if due to a susceptible *Candida* species). Candidal endophthalmitis should be treated with vitrectomy and intravitreal amphotericin B regardless of *Candida* species, plus systemic therapy. Systemic fluconazole may be used for

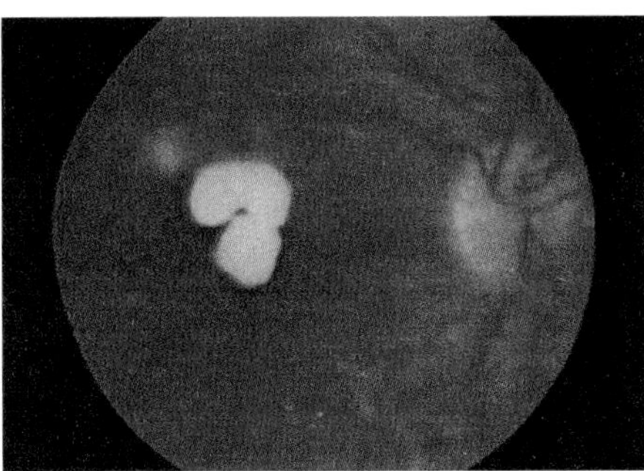

Figure 135.26 Candidal chorioretinal lesion with vitreal extension and overlying vitreal haze. (From Edwards JE Jr, Foos RY, Montgomerie JZ, et al. Ocular manifestations of *Candida* septicemia: review of seventy-six cases of hematogenous *Candida* endophthalmitis. Medicine (Baltimore). 1974;53:48.)

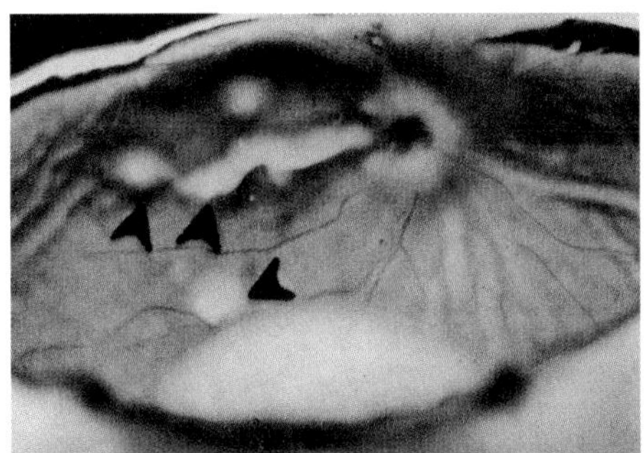

Figure 135.27 Chorioretinal candidal lesions of the posterior fundus (arrowheads). The optic disk is edematous. Gross specimen, right eye. (From Edwards JE Jr, Foos RY, Montgomerie JZ, et al. Ocular manifestations of *Candida* septicemia: review of seventy-six cases of hematogenous *Candida* endophthalmitis. Medicine (Baltimore). 1974;53:48.)

endophthalmitis caused by *Candida* species susceptible to this agent, but should be given in high doses (e.g., 600–800 mg by mouth daily in adults with normal renal function). Voriconazole also achieves excellent intraocular levels when given systemically, and may be helpful for fluconazole-resistant species. The intraocular penetration of systemic echinocandins is unclear. Systemic amphotericin with or without flucytosine may be required in difficult cases.

Cryptococcosis – Chapter 85

Cryptococcosis is caused by *Cryptococcus neoformans* and *C. gattii*, the latter historically reported primarily from tropical and subtropical regions, but with recent extension into the Pacific Northwest of North America.[62] Ocular involvement during cryptococcal infection usually occurs in the setting of disseminated cryptococcosis, usually with cryptococcal meningitis. At least 30% of persons with cryptococcal meningitis have ocular signs or symptoms. The organism can spread directly along the optic nerve sheet, and can result in direct cryptococcal invasion of the optic nerve. Papilledema and visual loss are common. Optic atrophy usually results if the patient survives an acute infection complicated by cryptococcal papilledema. Involvement of the CNS during cryptococcosis may result in cranial nerve dysfunction and extraocular muscle paresis.

Hematogenous spread usually involves the posterior pole of the eye and, when considering *C. neoformans*, usually occurs in immunocompromised persons, such as those with AIDS or those on steroid immunosuppression, while *C. gattii* most frequently affects immunocompetent individuals.[20,63] Involvement may be focal or multifocal, and may be bilateral. Isolated ocular involvement can occur and may precede systemic manifestations. Posterior involvement includes choroiditis, chorioretinitis, neuroretinitis, and endophthalmitis (***Fig. 135.28***). More rarely, anterior uveitis, iridocyclitis, and an iris mass may occur. Direct intraocular inoculation of organisms following trauma or surgery may result in rare cases of keratitis and cryptococcal endophthalmitis.

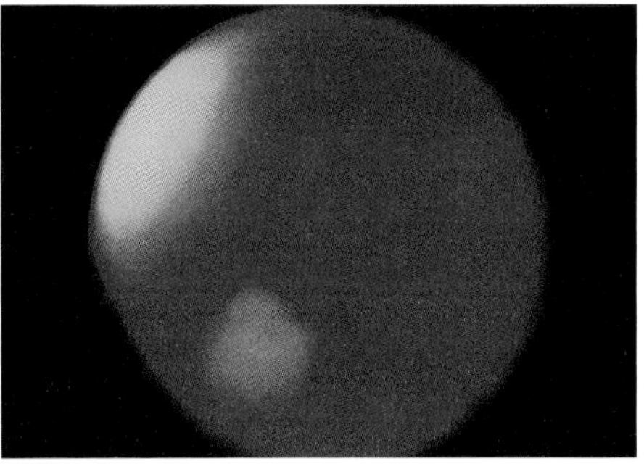

Figure 135.28 Cryptococcal retinovitreal abscess along the inferotemporal arcade, right eye. (From Hiss PW, Shields JA, Augsberger JJ. Solitary retinovitreal abscess as the initial manifestation of cryptococcosis. Ophthalmology. 1988;95:162.)

Diagnosis rests on microscopic and culture analysis of aqueous or vitreal samples. Persons with disseminated cryptococcosis may have positive blood cultures, and cryptococcal antigen assays of blood, cerebrospinal fluid, or urine may be positive. Treatment involves fluconazole and/or intravitreal and systemic amphotericin B. Flucytosine may be added during acute management. Initiation of antiretroviral therapy in individuals with HIV and cryptococcosis can induce an ocular immune reconstitution syndrome.[64] Repetitive (daily) lumbar punctures with removal of cerebrospinal fluid to control intracranial hypertension are often required. Surgical intervention may be required. Once the infection is controlled, oral fluconazole may be employed. Recrudescence is common, especially in immunocompromised persons. Maintenance fluconazole may be required.

Histoplasmosis – Chapter 85

Histoplasma capsulatum

Ocular involvement due to *H. capsulatum* can take one of three forms, depending on the immunologic status of the affected person: chorioretinal granuloma formation, disseminated histoplasmosis, and presumed ocular histoplasmosis syndrome (POHS).[65] Involvement of the eye by *H. capsulatum* occurs predominantly during hematogenous dissemination. Immunocompetent persons may present with a focal chorioretinal granuloma. Such a lesion can present as a tumor-like intraocular mass or as a diffusely infiltrating granulomatous lesion. Conjunctival granulomas have also been reported. Ocular involvement during widely disseminated histoplasmosis is most common among immunocompromised persons, such as those with AIDS. Choroiditis, chorioretinitis, retinitis, optic neuritis, endophthalmitis, iritis, scleritis, and conjunctivitis can occur. Fungal invasion of the central retinal vein has been reported. Inflammatory responses may be minimal in such severely immunocompromised persons.

POHS is characterized by the triad of atrophic choroidal scars in the macula or mid-periphery known as “histo spots,” peripapillary atrophy, and choroidal neovascularization which often leads to severe loss of central vision (***Fig. 135.29***). POHS is most common in areas highly endemic for histoplasmosis, and POHS is thought to occur in persons with strong immunity to *H. capsulatum*.[66,67] The etiology is unknown, and *Histoplasma* organisms have not been found in pathologic specimens. Vision in patients with POHS is often compromised by subfoveal neovascularization; neovascularization may be complicated by retinal hemorrhages. Loss of vision may be pronounced. Diagnosis of POHS is presumptive, based on characteristic funduscopic findings in patients from endemic areas. In POHS, antifungal therapy is not administered. Laser photocoagulation has been demonstrated to lessen loss of vision secondary to choroidal neovascular membrane formation (when such lesions are nonfoveal).[67] Careful ophthalmic monitoring of patients with POHS is required. Intravitreal steroids may be of benefit.[67]

In contrast with POHS, disseminated ocular histoplasmosis occurs in the setting of systemic infection. *H. capsulatum* may be cultured from the blood in severely immunocompromised persons. Blood and urine antigen

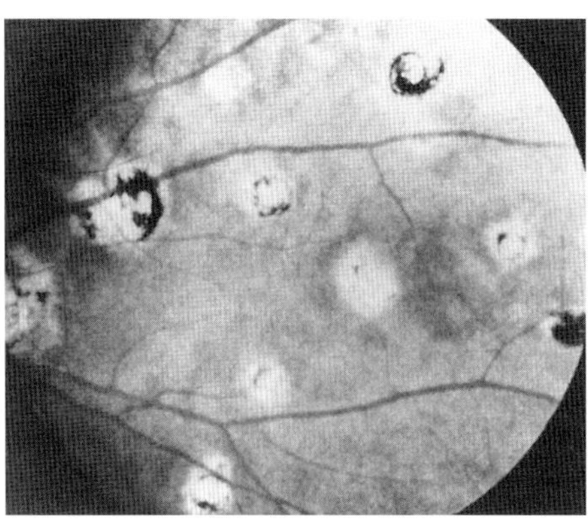

Figure 135.29 Presumed ocular histoplasmosis syndrome-associated atrophic chorioretinal scars. (From McMillan TA, Lashkari K. Ocular histoplasmosis. Int Ophthalmol Clin. 1996;36:181.)

tests are usually positive. Treatment of active ocular histoplasmosis includes the use of a systemic amphotericin preparation. Intravitreal therapy may also be employed. Itraconazole has poor intraocular penetration, and should be used only after control of the active infection has been achieved. Immunocompromised persons may require maintenance suppressive therapy.

H. capsulatum Variety *duboisii*

Infection with *H. capsulatum* var. *duboisii* has been reported from Africa and causes a clinically distinct form of histoplasmosis called African histoplasmosis. Involvement is usually of the skin, soft tissue, and bone. Lesions are chronic and may present as nodules or expansile cold abscesses. Involvement may present as an isolated lesion or, more rarely, as a systemic infection. Involvement of bones is common. Ocular involvement has been reported due to orbital spread from the bones of the face.[68] Diagnosis is based on microscopic and culture analysis of tissue specimens or abscess contents. Treatment of ocular *H. capsulatum* var. *duboisii* has involved surgical intervention supplemented by systemic antifungal agents.

Coccidioidomycosis - Chapter 85

Eye involvement in coccidioidomycosis is often asymptomatic. Funduscopic examination in infected persons may disclose healed inactive chorioretinal scars that are similar to, but distinct from, those associated with previous histoplasmosis. Symptomatic involvement usually occurs during disseminated disease or during chronic coccidioidomycosis. Primary pulmonary coccidioidomycosis may be associated with phlyctenular conjunctivitis, scleritis, episcleritis, or keratoconjunctivitis.[69] Such manifestations may well represent hypersensitivity reactions and may occur in the presence of erythema nodosum. Immunocompromised persons with disseminated disease may present with conjunctivitis and preauricular adenopathy. Granulomas of the eyelid may occur in disseminated disease. Intraocular involvement during progressive systemic coccidioidomycosis may include iridocyclitis, iris nodule formation, choroiditis, chorioretinitis, and endophthalmitis. Involvement is often granulomatous. Choroidal involvement may present as whitish yellow, slightly raised nodular lesions. Such involvement of deeper ocular structures may rarely occur in the absence of apparent systemic coccidioidomycosis. Involvement of the CNS can result in papilledema and cranial nerve dysfunction.

Diagnosis is usually by serology, but when tissue specimens are available, histologic examination and culture are definitive. Ocular involvement usually occurs in disseminated disease, and therapy will be directed against the disseminated disease. Systemic antifungal agents are required. In disseminated disease with intraocular involvement, agents other than itraconazole should be used, as itraconazole does not cross the blood–eye barrier. Chronic suppressive therapy may be required in immunocompromised persons, such as those with AIDS.

Blastomycosis - Chapter 85

Ocular involvement during blastomycosis is rare, usually manifesting as a blastomycotic skin lesion involving the eyelid. The sclera, conjunctiva, and cornea may be involved. Scarring can lead to ectropion. Hematogenous dissemination may result in direct ocular deposition of organisms, usually in the choroid. Choroidal granulomas may present as small subretinal masses or as diffuse granulomatous lesions with vitritis. Iritis, iris nodules, choroiditis, endophthalmitis, or panophthalmitis may occur. Orbital involvement has been reported. Ocular involvement usually occurs in patients with disseminated blastomycosis, although rare persons may present with apparently isolated ocular involvement. The incidence of the disease does not appear to be increased among immunocompromised persons with AIDS.

Paracoccidioidomycosis (South American Blastomycosis) - Chapter 86

Ocular involvement by *Paracoccidioides brasiliensis* usually involves contiguous spread of an ulceronodular skin lesion that rarely involves the eyelid. Parinaud's oculoglandular syndrome has been reported. Disease is often systemic, and choroidal granulomatous lesions have been reported. Chorioretinitis may occur. Involvement of the CNS can lead to granulomatous meningoencephalitis or mass lesions, with resultant cranial nerve dysfunction and ocular palsies. The optic nerves and chiasm may also be involved. The incidence of *P. brasiliensis* infection is apparently not increased in immunocompromised persons, including those with AIDS.

Sporotrichosis - Chapter 90

Involvement of the eye in sporotrichosis usually entails conjunctival, adnexal, or eyelid disease. Orbital infection of deeper ocular structures may occur. Ocular involvement may occur with hematogenous dissemination, after trauma (especially that involving vegetable matter/thorns), or after surgical manipulation. Involvement of sinuses and facial bones can lead to contiguous orbital spread. Scleritis, keratoconjunctivitis, corneal perforation, iridocyclitis, iris nodule formation, necrotizing granulomatous chorioretinitis, granulomatous uveitis, optic neuritis, vitritis, endophthalmitis, and panophthalmitis may occur. Regional lymphadenopathy may be present. Parinaud's ulceroglandular syndrome may occur. The necrotizing chorioretinitis may mimic that occurring in toxoplasmosis; however, the degree of overlying vitreal inflammation may be less pronounced in sporotrichosis. Hematogenously disseminated sporotrichosis may present with isolated ocular disease.

Mucormycosis - Chapter 89

Rhino-orbital-cerebral mucormycosis is a clinical entity that may be caused by a number of Mucorales fungi, including *Mucor* species, *Rhizopus* species, and *Absidia* species, among others. The same organisms can also rarely be a cause of isolated post-traumatic keratitis in immunocompetent persons. Rhino-orbital-cerebral mucormycosis is characterized by necrotizing sinusitis, usually in a person with insulin-dependent diabetes or who is immunocompromised. Ocular involvement results from contiguous spread of the necrotizing and rapidly progressing fungal process. Orbital cellulitis is the most frequent ocular presentation. Chemosis, proptosis, ptosis, ophthalmoplegia, uveitis, optic neuritis, hypoesthesia of the forehead (cranial nerve V_1), central retinal artery inclusion, cavernous sinus thrombosis, and orbital apex syndrome may occur.

Diagnosis is usually one of clinical recognition followed by biopsy of intranasal or orbital tissues. An eschar of the hard palate may be evident. Intranasal examination usually reveals a black eschar due to necrosis of

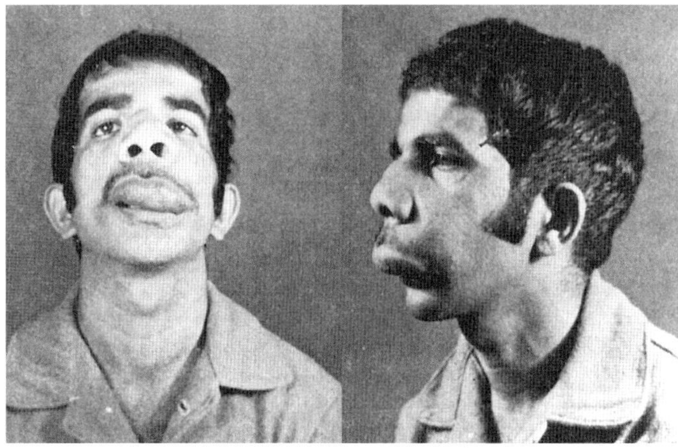

Figure 135.30 Facial rhinoentomophthoromycosis. Facial involvement can extend to the periorbital area and lead to inability to open the eyelids. (From Singh D, Kochlar RR, Seth HN. Rhinoentomophthoromycosis. J Laryngol Otolaryngol. 1976;90:872.)

the mucosa/turbinates. Definitive diagnosis rests on microscopic and cultural analysis of tissue samples or discharge. Treatment is urgent and requires aggressive systemic amphotericin and surgical intervention. If the eye is involved, exenteration of orbital contents may be required. Even in preserved eyes, visual loss is usually pronounced and permanent.

Isolated post-traumatic keratitis due to Mucorales species may be treated as mycotic keratitis. Systemic therapy and corneal transplantation may be required.

Entomophthoramycosis - Chapter 90

Entomophthoramycosis can be caused by *Conidiobolus* species or *Basidiobolus* species. When entomophthoramycosis involves the face, it is characterized by a slowly progressive subacute infiltrative process that usually involves the nose and perinasal sinus areas (***Fig. 135.30***).[70,71] The infiltrative process can become periocular, and can result in inability to open the eyelids. Diagnosis is usually one of clinical recognition and pathologic/culture analysis of subcutaneous tissue samples. Optimal therapy is not known. Surgical resection of infected tissue may be required.

Facial Mycotic Infections and Fungal Sinusitis - Chapters 83, 84, and 90

Rare reports of infiltrative or ulceronodular fungal facial lesions have also been reported with chromoblastomycosis, mycetoma, and lobomycosis. Facial involvement may result in eyelid, conjunctival, or lacrimal canal involvement. Phaeohyphomycosis has rarely been associated with keratitis, and endophthalmitis after trauma or epithelial disruption. Fungal sinusitis may be caused by phaeohyphomycosis and *Aspergillus* species, *Scedosporium* species, *Fusarium* species, and *Penicillium* species. Fungal sinusitis may also occur with mucormycosis, blastomycosis, coccidioidomycosis, histoplasmosis, and paracoccidioidomycosis, among others. Fungal sinusitis may lead to orbital involvement, which can lead to proptosis, diplopia, ptosis, epiphora, or an orbital mass. Diagnosis usually rests on culture analysis of tissue samples. Surgical management supplemented by amphotericin preparations and azole agents is often required.

Rhinosporidiosis - Chapter 90

Rhinosporidiosis, caused by *Rhinosporidium seeberi*, is usually associated with a polypoid (often pedunculated) lesion of the nasal mucosa. The conjunctival mucosa may also be affected (***Fig. 135.31***). Conjunctival involvement is usually unilateral. Scleral melting may result.[72] Lacrimal glands may be involved. Keratitis has been reported. Diagnosis is usually based on histologic examination of resected polyps. Treatment has involved surgical excision and basal cauterization.

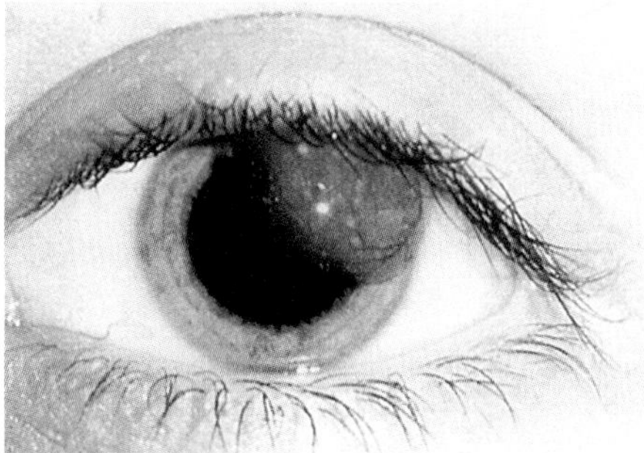

Figure 135.31 *Rhinosporidium seeberi* conjunctival lesion arising from the superior fornix and extending onto the cornea. Note the fleshy pink appearance and the small white spherules of the lesion. (From Reidy JJ, Sudesh S, Klafter AB, et al. Infection of the conjunctiva by *Rhinosporidium seeberi*. Surv Ophthalmol. 1997;41:410.)

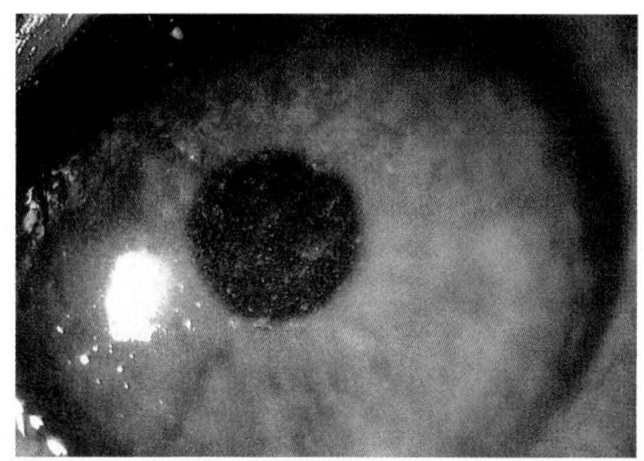

Figure 135.32 Microsporidial epithelial keratopathy: diffuse illumination of the cornea with granular epithelial involvement. (From Yee RW, Tio FO, Martinez JA, et al. Microsporidial epithelial keratopathy in a patient with AIDS. Ophthalmology. 1991;98:198.)

PARASITIC INFECTIONS

Microsporidial Infections: Microsporidiosis - Chapter 102

Microsporidiosis may be caused by *Encephalitozoon* species, *Enterocytozoon* species, *Nosema* species, *Vittaforma* species, and *Pleistophora* species. *Nosema* and *Vittaforma* species can result in stromal keratitis and keratoconjunctivitis after trauma and direct inoculation of organisms in immunocompetent persons.[73] Such involvement usually results in a prominent inflammatory response. Ocular involvement during disseminated microsporidiosis can occur in immunocompromised patients, especially those with AIDS, and is usually due to *Encephalitozoon hellem*.[74] Ocular involvement in disseminated microsporidiosis usually presents as a superficial keratitis with fine to coarse epithelial opacities, mild conjunctivitis, or both (***Fig. 135.32***).[73] Endophthalmitis has been reported. Diagnosis rests on microscopic identification of organisms in corneal/conjunctival scrapings. In disseminated microsporidiosis, the organism may also be present in urine, stool, and nasal mucosal tissue samples.

Protozoal Infections

Toxoplasmosis - Chapter 103

Ocular toxoplasmosis usually presents as recurrence of a previously unrecognized primary infection. Most cases present with a unilateral and painless posterior uveitis, and funduscopic examination reveals a creamy yellow active inflammatory chorioretinal lesion adjacent to an old scar (***Fig. 135.33***). Inflammation in the vitreous (vitritis) is usually intense and may obscure the view of the retina, with only a hint of the active

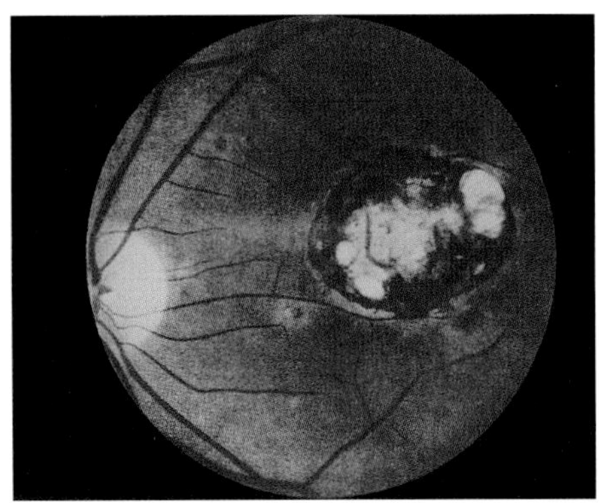

Figure 135.33 A lesion of toxoplasmic chorioretinitis showing a cotton-like patch with hemorrhage. (From Kean BH, Sun TS, Ellsworth DM, eds. Color Atlas of Ophthalmic Parasitology. New York: Igaku-Shoin; 1991:17.)

creamy yellow lesion behind the cloud of vitreous white blood cells ("headlight in the fog" appearance).[75,76] Satellite lesions may surround a central larger lesion. Once the active inflammation subsides, a hypopigmented "punched out" scar with a surrounding area of retinal hyperpigmentation may be present.

Congenital toxoplasmosis is evident in the minority of infected neonates. Ocular involvement in such infections may be bilateral and severe. Chorioretinitis, vitritis, glaucoma, nystagmus, strabismus, ocular muscle palsies, and microphthalmia may occur.[75,77] Infants with congenital toxoplasmosis that is clinically silent at birth often develop clinically evident reactivation chorioretinitis by their second or third decade of life. Reactivation usually occurs along the borders of old lesions or at previously uninvolved sites.

Chorioretinal involvement may be severe, bilateral, and multifocal in immunocompromised persons. In such persons, toxoplasmosis can cause uveitis, scleritis, and optic neuritis; involvement of the CNS can produce space-occupying lesions that may result in ocular palsies, nystagmus, and visual field defects.

The diagnosis of ocular toxoplasmosis is usually clinical, based on the appearance of the eye. Positive *Toxoplasma* IgG titers are supportive; rarely, the case is one of primary ocular toxoplasmosis, in which IgM is positive and there is only the active choroidal lesion, but no adjacent chorioretinal scar. In patients with reactivation ocular toxoplasmosis, the diagnosis may be supported but not confirmed by serology, since many populations have a high baseline seroprevalence rate for toxoplasmosis. The decision to treat ocular toxoplasmosis depends on whether the active lesion is centrally located (i.e., threatens the macula); if so, treatment is indicated. Treatment is also usually given if there is marked vitritis. No treatment may be required if the lesion is peripheral and there is minimal vitritis. Immunocompromised patients with ocular toxoplasmosis should also be treated.

Malaria – Chapter 96

Ocular involvement during malaria occurs predominantly during infection with *Plasmodium falciparum*. The ability of this parasite to cause erythrocyte sludging (***Fig. 135.34***), vascular congestion, local cytokine release, and local tissue hypoxemia is thought to account for its ability to affect the eye.[78] Malarial involvement of retinal vessels can lead to retinal sludging, hemorrhage, edema, and exudates. Involvement may be most prominent in the macular area, and retinal signs and hemorrhage correlate with severity of malaria and risk of death.[78,79] Involvement of ophthalmic and cerebral vessels can result in intraocular ischemia, infarction, hemorrhages, optic neuritis, papilledema, ocular palsies, and cortical blindness. Papilledema during malaria is associated with a marked increase in mortality. An episode of malaria may be complicated by reactivation of herpes simplex keratitis. Diagnosis usually rests on microscopic or antigenic identification of the parasite in blood. Chronic, inappropriate use of the antimalarial agent choloroquine (which is available "over the counter" in

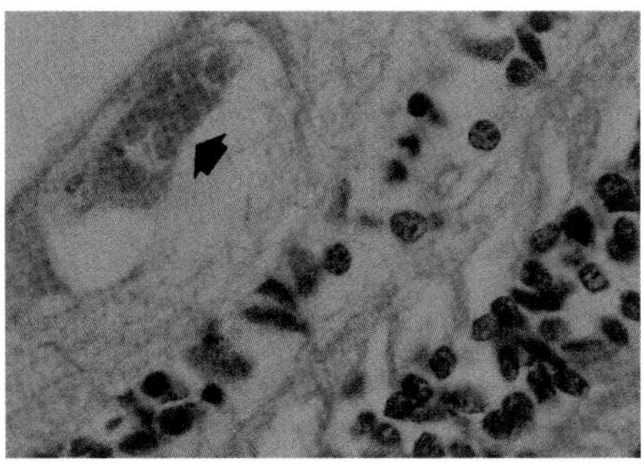

Figure 135.34 *Plasmodium falciparum* malarial involvement of a retinal capillary (arrowhead). Note almost complete occlusion of the vessel lumen by parasitized erythrocytes. (H&E stain; original magnification: ×750.) (From Hidayat AA, Nalbanian RM, Sammens DW, et al. The diagnostic histopathologic features of ocular malaria. Ophthalmology. 1993;100:1184.)

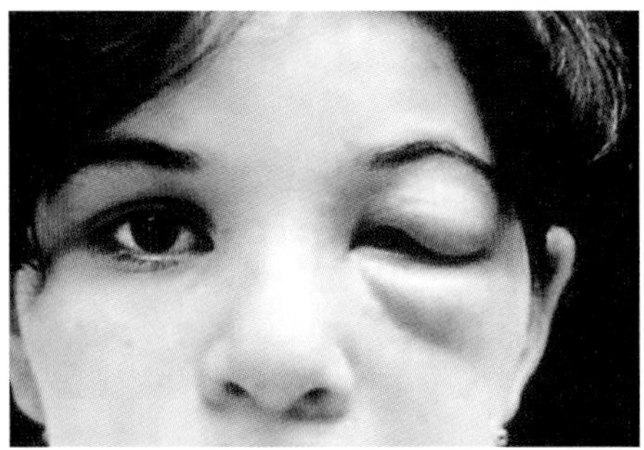

Figure 135.35 Acute Chagas' disease in a young child. The eye sign of Romaña is present. This is frequently seen in acute cases and is presumed to mark the point of entry of the parasite. (WHO/TDR.)

much of the world) can produce a characteristic "bull's-eye" retinal pigmentary maculopathy.

African Trypanosomiasis (Sleeping Sickness) – Chapter 98

Ocular involvement during African trypanosomiasis is secondary to trypanosomal infiltration of ocular tissues and can result in mild eyelid edema, conjunctival injection, interstitial keratitis, and uveitis. Stromal opacification and deep neovascularization may occur. Papilledema, ptosis, ophthalmoplegia, and optic neuritis may complicate neuroencephalitis. Diagnosis rests on identification of trypanosomes in blood, in tissue sections, in aspirated lymph node fluid, or in cerebrospinal fluid.

American Trypanosomiasis (Chagas' Disease) – Chapter 99

The most common and well-recognized ocular feature of American trypanosomiasis is Romaña's sign: a painless, unilateral, pronounced periorbital edema and conjunctivitis that persists for days (***Fig. 135.35***). Romaña's sign results from conjunctival inoculation and penetration of infective trypomastigotes from reduviid bug feces. Lacrimal gland involvement and preauricular and regional lymphadenopathy may occur. Romaña's sign occurs with acute Chagas' disease.

Leishmaniasis – Chapter 100

Ocular involvement can occur during visceral, cutaneous, or mucocutaneous leishmaniasis. Ocular involvement during visceral leishmaniasis is rare. Keratitis, iritis, papillitis, chorioretinitis, and retinal hemorrhages have all been reported during visceral leishmaniasis, and have been noted to improve after the initiation of antileishmanial therapy; however, direct leishmanial involvement of ocular tissues has not been documented. Ocular involvement during cutaneous and mucocutaneous leishmaniasis usually results from direct extension of a leishmanial lesion and usually

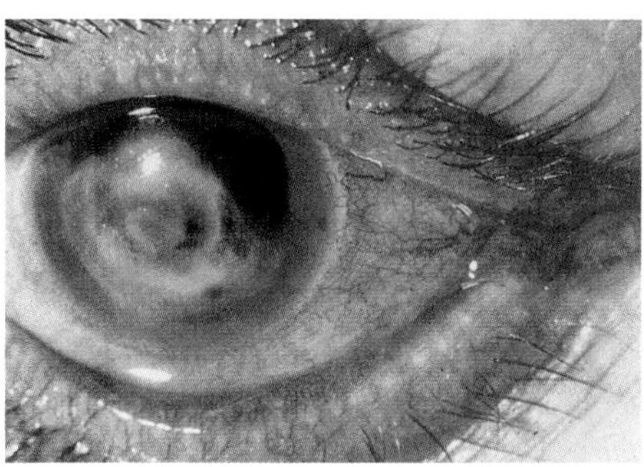

Figure 135.36 *Acanthamoeba* keratitis. Note chemosis, double concentric ring of the corneal infiltrate, and a central corneal epithelial defect. (From Hirst LW, Green WR, Merry W, et al. Management of *Acanthamoeba* keratitis. Ophthalmology. 1984;91:1106.)

involves a nodular or ulcerative lesion of the eyelid that can extend into the lacrimal gland or onto the conjunctiva.[80,81] Total ocular destruction may complicate severe cases of mucocutaneous leishmaniasis. Diagnosis is usually based on clinical recognition and microscopic identification of organisms in tissue scrapings or samples.

Acanthamoeba – Chapter 101

Acanthamoeba is an uncommon but important cause of keratitis in patients who wear contact lenses. *Acanthamoeba* keratitis may also occur after ocular trauma. Acanthamebic keratitis is characterized by pain out of proportion to eye findings. The keratitis is often initially misdiagnosed as herpes simplex keratitis. On slit-lamp examination, a perineural infiltrate may be seen in the cornea in early infection. Later infection usually produces a ring corneal infiltrate (***Fig. 135.36***). There may be a sterile inflammatory reaction in the anterior chamber. Diagnosis is made by special culture of corneal scrapings for *Acanthamoeba*. Examination of the culture plates under the microscope reveals acanthamebic cysts and trophozoites within a few days. Corneal transplantation may be required, but ideally should be delayed until the active infection is controlled.

Amebiasis – Chapter 92

Documented ocular involvement during amebiasis is rare but usually involves an expansile ulcerative lesion of the face. The most frequent site of ocular involvement is the eyelid, but total ocular destruction can occur. Space-occupying amebic lesions of the CNS may result in papilledema, ocular palsies, and visual loss. Diagnosis involves molecular or microscopic identification of organisms in stool, intestinal samples, or aspirates of tissue collections.

Giardiasis – Chapter 93

Direct parasitic involvement of ocular structures during giardiasis has never been documented. Iridocyclitis, choroiditis, retinal and subretinal hemorrhages, and macular changes have been reported in persons with giardiasis and have been noted to improve or resolve after anti-*Giardia* therapy is initiated, but causality has never been established. Such involvement may represent immunologically mediated reactions or may be secondary to nutritional deficiencies due to *Giardia*-induced malabsorption.

Helminthic Infections: Nematodes

(See also *Boxes 135.9–135.11*.)

Onchocerciasis – Chapter 106

Onchocerciasis, or "river blindness," is a leading cause of blindness in central Africa. Onchocerciasis is also present in focal areas in a number of countries in Central and South America, as well as in Yemen in the Arabian peninsula. Microfilariae can migrate freely within the cornea, anterior chamber, vitreous, retina, choroid, and optic nerve. Dead or dying microfilariae provoke a prominent inflammatory response, either relating to microfilarial antigens themselves, or to derivatives from endosymbiotic *Wolbachia*. Live microfilariae provoke a limited inflammatory response. Ocular onchocerciasis may be anterior (keratitis and iritis) or posterior (chorioretinitis, papillitis, and optic atrophy). The type of ocular disease may depend in part on parasitic strain and variability.

Box 135.9 "Worms" that Involve the Conjunctiva[a]

Nematodes
- *Loa loa*[b]
- *Dirofilaria* species[b]
- *Thelazaria* species[b]
- *Ascaris lumbricoides*
- *Mansonella perstans*
- *Dracunculus medinensis*
- *Wuchereria bancrofti/Brugia malayi/B. timori*

Cestodes
- *Spirometra* species (sparganosis)[b]
- *Cysticercus cellulosae* (cystic involvement)
- *Taenia multiceps, T. serialis* (coenuriasis; cystic involvement)
- *Gnathostoma spinigerum*

Trematodes
- *Paragonimus* species

Ectoparasites
- Myiasis[b]

[a]*This list includes ectoparasites and nonmicrofilarial helminths.*
[b]*Common or classic ocular manifestation of infection.*

Box 135.10 "Worms" that Involve Intraocular Structures[a]

Nematodes
- *Toxocara* species[b]
- *Baylisascaris procyonis*[b]
- *Angiostrongylus cantonensis*[b]
- *Gnathostoma spinigerum*[b]
- *Loa loa*
- *Dirofilaria* species
- *Wuchereria bancrofti/Brugia malayi/B. timori*

Cestodes
- *Cysticercus cellulosae* (cystic involvement)[b]
- *Spirometra* species (sparganosis)[b]
- *Echinococcus* species (cystic involvement)
- *Taenia multiceps, T. serialis* (coenuriasis; cystic involvement)

Trematodes
- *Paragonimus* species[b]
- *Schistosoma* species

Ectoparasites/Pentastomids
- *Lingulata serrata*[b]
- Myiasis[b]

[a]*This list includes ectoparasites and nonmicrofilarial helminths.*
[b]*Common or classic ocular manifestation of infection.*

Box 135.11 "Worms" that Involve the Orbital Space/Cavity[a]

Nematodes
- *Loa loa*[b]
- *Angiostrongylus cantonensis*[b]
- *Gnathostoma spinigerum*[b]
- *Dirofilaria* species[b]
- *Thelazaria* species

Cestodes
- *Spirometra* species (sparganosis)
- *Cysticercus cellulosae* (cystic involvement)
- *Taenia multiceps, T. serialis* (coenuriasis; cystic involvement)
- *Echinococcus* species (cystic involvement)

Trematodes
- *Paragonimus* species[b]

Ectoparasites/Pentastomids
- Myiasis[b]
- *Lingulata serrata*[b]

[a]*This list includes ectoparasites and nonmicrofilarial helminths.*
[b]*Common or classic ocular manifestation of infection.*

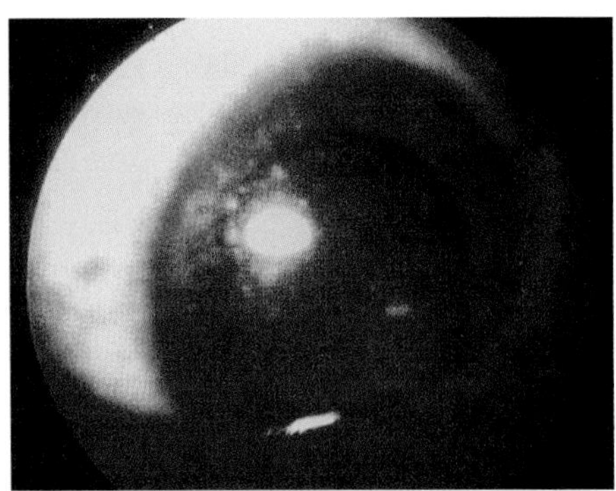

Figure 135.37 Punctate keratitis secondary to onchocerciasis. (Courtesy of Armed Forces Institute of Pathology, Washington, DC, negative No. 75-1622.)

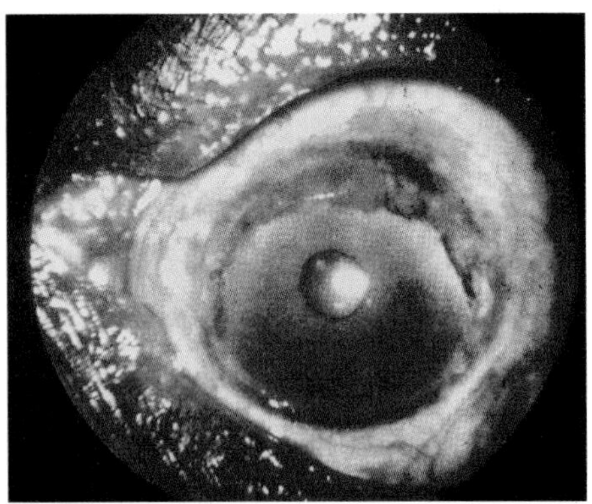

Figure 135.38 Moderately advanced sclerosing keratitis secondary to onchocerciasis. (Courtesy of Armed Forces Institute of Pathology, Washington, DC, negative No. 75-1624.)

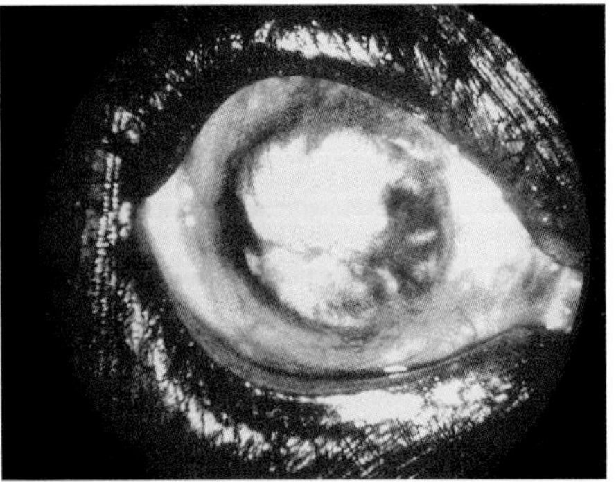

Figure 135.39 Advanced sclerosing keratitis secondary to onchocerciasis. (Courtesy of Armed Forces Institute of Pathology, Washington, DC, negative No. 75-1626.)

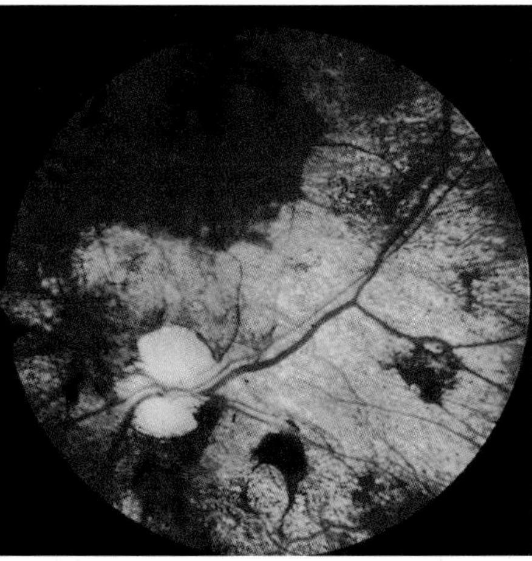

Figure 135.40 Extensive chorioretinal degeneration secondary to onchocerciasis with sparing of the macula and optic atrophy. (Courtesy of Armed Forces Institute of Pathology, Washington, DC, negative No. 75-1632.)

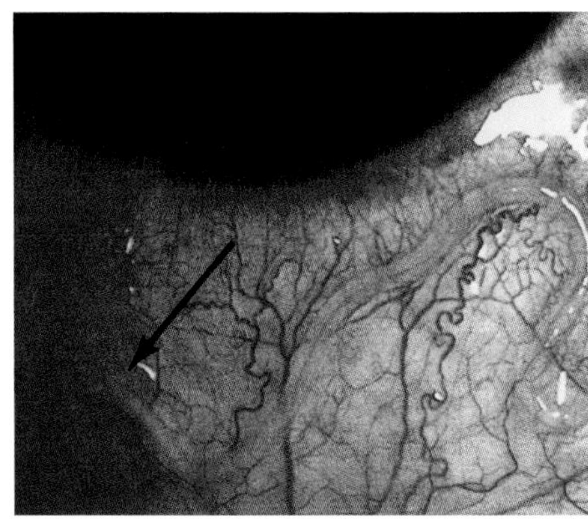

Figure 135.41 Adult worm of *Loa loa* visible under the conjunctiva (arrow). (From Kean BH, Sun TS, Ellsworth DM, eds. Color Atlas of Ophthalmic Parasitology. New York: Igaku-Shoin; 1991:127. Courtesy of Armed Forces Institute of Pathology, Washington, DC, negative No. 73-6654.)

Involvement of the anterior eye can result in punctate keratitis with "fluffy snowflake" corneal opacities that represent local responses to dead or dying microfilariae (***Fig. 135.37***). Such lesions clear without any residua and occur most commonly in young persons. Punctate keratitis can occur spontaneously or after the initiation of anti-onchocercal therapy. Chronic, recurrent, ongoing inflammation may result in a more serious sclerosing keratitis, which usually affects older persons and can result in total loss of vision. Sclerosing keratitis is characterized by a pannus of inflammatory cells and neovascularization that encroaches from the lower, medial, and temporal borders of the cornea (***Figs 135.38 and 135.39***). Anterior inflammation may also include iritis. Secondary glaucoma, cataracts, and synechiae may result. The risk of sclerosis, keratitis, or iritis has been associated with the presence and load of microfilariae in the anterior chamber, cornea, and outer canthus of the eyelid.

The pathophysiology of posterior ocular involvement is less well understood. Chorioretinitis and atrophic changes may occur. Atrophic changes have been associated with filarial load and may be the result of low-level, ongoing host–parasite interactions. Chorioretinitis may be severe, may be unilateral, and may often involve the temporal retina and spare the macula in early disease. Pigmentary hyperplasia and atrophy, fibrosis, and neovascularization may be present (***Fig. 135.40***). Chorioretinitis has not been associated with filarial load. Optic atrophy may be the result of optic neuritis or secondary glaucoma from iridocyclitis.

Diagnosis often involves clinical recognition, skin snip analysis, or serological assays. Surgical nodulectomy and identification of the adult worm may also be employed. Ophthalmic diagnosis rests on slit-lamp and funduscopic examination. Visualized living microfilariae are curved, motile, and transparent, and are visible in the anterior chamber and cornea. Dead microfilariae are straight and opacified.

Loiasis – Chapter 105

Ocular manifestations of loiasis relate to migration of adult worms into and around the eyes. Subconjunctival migration is most common (***Fig. 135.41***). Conjunctival migration results in a foreign-body sensation and conjunctival injection. The worm moves approximately 1 cm/min. Periorbital swelling and pruritus may occur. Migration of the worm can result in Calabar swelling of the eyelid. Adult worms may rarely migrate across or through the anterior chamber, vitreous, or retina.

Diagnosis rests on visualization of subconjunctival worms, a history of Calabar swellings, or demonstration of microfilariae in blood. Eosinophilia may be striking, especially in persons nonendemic to the area of infection. Surgical removal of the adult worm is not necessary, but if performed,

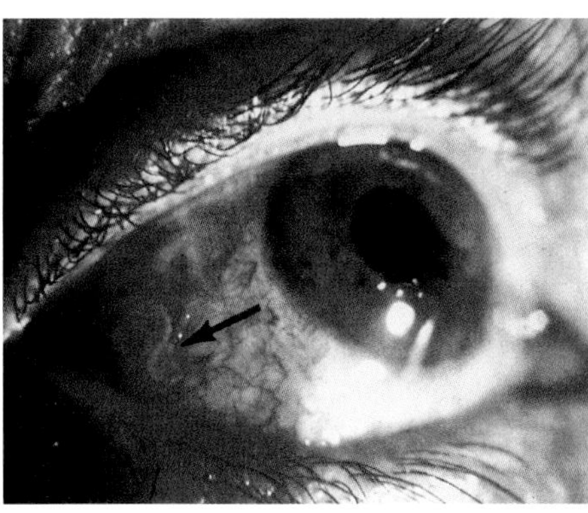

Figure 135.42 A subconjunctival female worm of *Dirofilaria tenuis* (arrow). (From Kean BH, Sun TS, Ellsworth DM, eds. Color Atlas of Ophthalmic Parasitology. New York: Igaku-Shoin; 1991:133. Courtesy of Armed Forces Institute of Pathology, Washington, DC, negative No. 74-6351-2.)

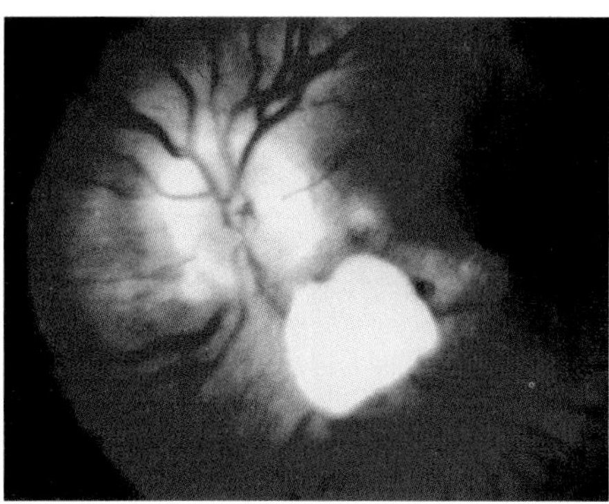

Figure 135.43 A toxocaral granuloma (center) visible on the eye ground. (From Kean BH, Sun TS, Ellsworth DM, eds. Color Atlas of Ophthalmic Parasitology. New York: Igaku-Shoin; 1991:112.)

may involve the application of a topical conjunctival anesthetic, such as lidocaine to numb the conjunctiva and slow or halt the movement of the worm. After a single small conjunctival incision is made, the adult worm may then be grasped gently with forceps and a small suture may be passed beneath the worm and carefully tied. The worm may then be removed by dissection.

Dirofilariasis – Chapter 107

Ocular involvement is most frequently associated with dirofilarial species associated with subcutaneous migration and nodule formation: *Dirofilaria repens*, *D. ursi*, and *D. tenuis* (previously, *D. conjunctivae*). Ocular dirofilariasis usually involves a migrating worm that most frequently invades the eyelid or subconjunctiva or, more rarely, intraocular structures (***Fig. 135.42***). Inflammatory reactions and nodule formation, foreign-body sensation, eyelid swelling, ptosis and pruritus, uveitis, and glaucoma have all been reported. Diagnosis is usually based on pathologic examination. Treatment involves surgical removal of the worm.

Mansonelliasis – Chapter 105

Migrating adult *Mansonella perstans* organisms have been found in subcutaneous tissues and can present with *Loa loa*-like Calabar swellings. Involvement of ocular structures by immature adult *M. perstans* worms can result in conjunctival nodule formation, eyelid swelling, and proptosis.[82] Retinal masses have been reported. Diagnosis involves pathologic identification of adult or immature worms after surgical resection or morphologic identification of microfilariae in blood. Ocular disease has been surgically treated. *M. ozzardi* infections have been associated with keratitis, presumably from migratory microfilariae.[83]

Bancroftian and Brugian Filariasis (Lymphatic Filariasis) – Chapter 104

Ocular involvement during lymphatic filariasis usually results from aberrant adult worm migration to the conjunctiva, resulting in chemosis, pain, and foreign-body sensation. Adult and maturing worms have also been reported in the lacrimal gland, eyelid, anterior chamber, iris, and subretina. Blocked lymphatic drainage may result in chronic elephantiasis of the eyelids. Microfilariae, although usually confined to blood, have also been isolated from the lacrimal gland, anterior chamber, iris, lens, choroid, and retina. Diagnosis involves identification of microfilariae in blood.

Toxocariasis – Chapter 109

Toxocariasis may present as visceral larva migrans or as ocular larva migrans, perhaps depending on the load of infecting organisms. Ocular larva migrans results from infection with only one or a few larvae. It is most common in older children and, more rarely, in adults. Ocular involvement relates to the migration of a wandering larva and the

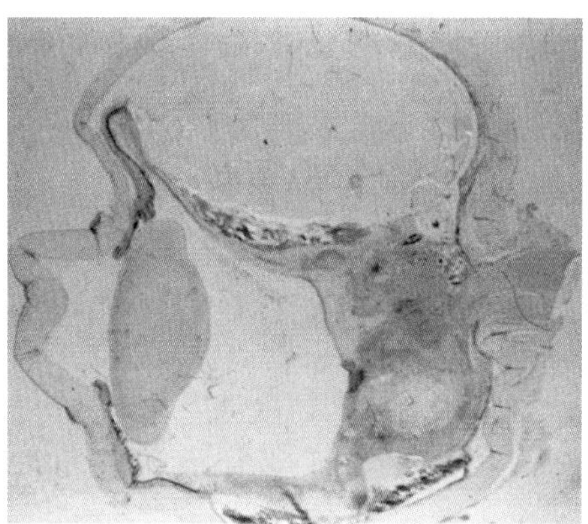

Figure 135.44 A sagittal section of an eye showing a large toxocaral granuloma. (H&E stain; original magnification: ×25.) (From Kean BH, Sun TS, Ellsworth DM, eds. Color Atlas of Ophthalmic Parasitology. New York: Igaku-Shoin; 1991:112.)

granulomatous-inflammatory host response that it provokes (***Figs 135.43 and 135.44***).[84] Peripherally based ocular inflammatory masses may result in visual field defects. Centrally located ocular inflammatory masses can lead to a marked decrease in visual acuity. Retinal inflammation and edema may be severe. Migrating larvae can produce retinal scarring and retinal "track" formation. Retinal traction, retinal hemorrhages, and retinal detachment may occur. Rupture of retinally based inflammatory masses or active migration of larva out of the retina and into the vitreous may result in severe, painless endophthalmitis. Migratory larvae can also result in granulomatous uveitis and secondary glaucoma, keratitis, and optic neuritis. Ocular larva migrans due to toxocariasis often presents as a unilateral, painless, white, retinally based mass in a child and thus must be distinguished from retinoblastoma.

Baylisascariasis – Chapter 112

Baylisascariasis, caused by the raccoon ascarid *Baylisascaris procyonis*, may present with involvement of the CNS with severe neurological sequelae. Isolated ocular involvement may also occur and is one of ocular larval migrans.[85] Larval migration in the eye can cause diffuse unilateral neuroretinitis and multiple choroidal infiltrates, a granulomatous retinal mass, retinal and subretinal track formation, retinal scars, retinal hemorrhages, chorioretinitis, vitritis, and uveitis.[86] Diagnosis of ocular disease is one of clinical recognition. Neurological involvement usually involves serologic evaluation employing *Baylisascaris*-specific antigens.

Ascariasis – Chapter 115

Ocular involvement by *Ascaris lumbricoides* is extremely rare, but young adult *A. lumbricoides* worms have been recovered from the nasolacrimal duct, presumably after migration up the esophagus into the

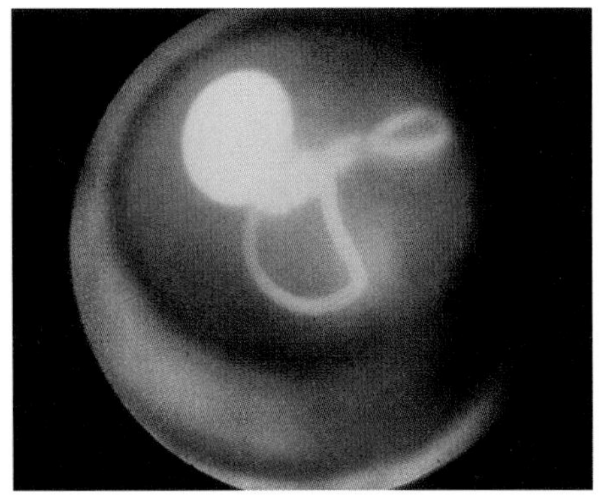

Figure 135.45 *Angiostrongylus cantonensis* in the vitreous cavity. (From Teekhasaenee C, Ritch R, Kanchanaranya C. Ocular parasitic infection in Thailand. Rev Infect Dis. 1986;8:352.)

nasopharynx.[87] Treatment of facial/ocular ascariasis involves mechanical removal of the worm; however, systemic therapy should be employed to treat concomitant intestinal involvement.

Hookworm – Chapter 116

Humans may act as a definite host in hookworm infection caused by *Necator americanus* or *Ancylostoma duodenale* or as a dead-end host for canine hookworms such as *A. braziliense* or *A. caninum*. Infectious filariform larvae of the latter species can migrate throughout the host and can result in a syndrome of cutaneous larva migrans. Migratory hookworm larvae have rarely been reported to involve ocular structures, including the cornea.[88,89]

Thelaziasis – Chapter 112

Thelaziasis is caused by *Thelazia callipaeda* (the oriental eyeworm) or *T. californiensis*. The worms inhabit the conjunctival sac and lacrimal system of various mammals.[90] Humans occasionally become infected.[91] Adult worms residing in the conjunctival sac of mammalian hosts release eggs that are ingested by flies. After maturing in the insect vector, worms are regurgitated during a subsequent ocular secretion meal. Adult worms are approximately 2 cm in length. Ocular involvement in humans results in excessive lacrimation, foreign-body sensation, and local discomfort. Corneal and conjunctival scarification can result.[92] Diagnosis rests on identification of recovered worms. Treatment of the disease in humans involves mechanical removal of the worms.

Dracunculiasis – Chapter 108

The older literature reported orbital involvement during dracunculiasis; however, the only confirmed case of *D. medinensis* involving ocular structures entailed the isolation of an adult female worm from the conjunctiva of a patient with extensive lacrimation and conjunctival irritation.[93] Therapy of ocular disease involves mechanical removal of the worm.

Angiostrongyliasis – Chapter 111

Ocular angiostrongyliasis due to *Angiostrongylus cantonensis* results from ocular migration of worms in various stages of development.[94] Worms can migrate through the anterior chamber and the vitreous and subretinal space, and then can cause eyelid edema, blepharospasm, inflammation of the anterior chamber, iridocyclitis, retinal detachment, and vitritis (***Fig. 135.45***). Vitreal migration can lead to vitreal fibrosis and resultant retinal distortion and detachment (***Fig. 135.46***).[95] Angiostrongyliasis-associated eosinophilic meningoencephalitis may be associated with papilledema (often unilateral) and optic neuritis. Cranial nerve dysfunction can result in ocular palsies and ptosis.[96] Orbital involvement may result in extraocular palsies and exophthalmos. Intraocular angiostrongyliasis may occur without associated meningitis. Diagnosis is usually based on the diagnosis of eosinophilic meningoencephalitis or pathologic examination of migratory worms. Serology tests are available.

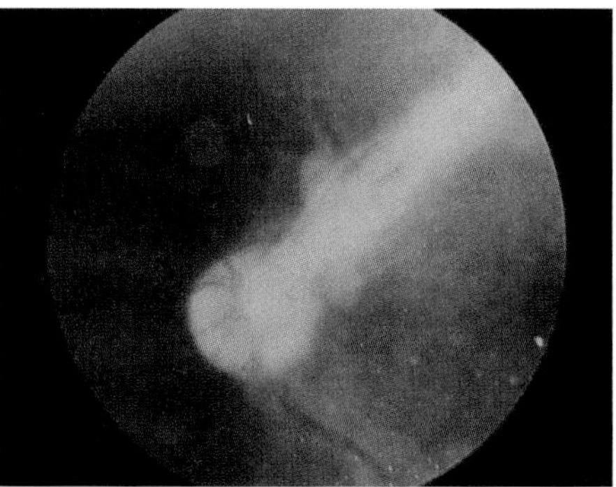

Figure 135.46 *Angiostrongylus cantonensis*: fibrous tract formation from the optic head into the vitreous cavity. (From Teekhasaenee C, Ritch R, Kanchanaranya C. Ocular parasitic infection in Thailand. Rev Infect Dis. 1986;8:352.)

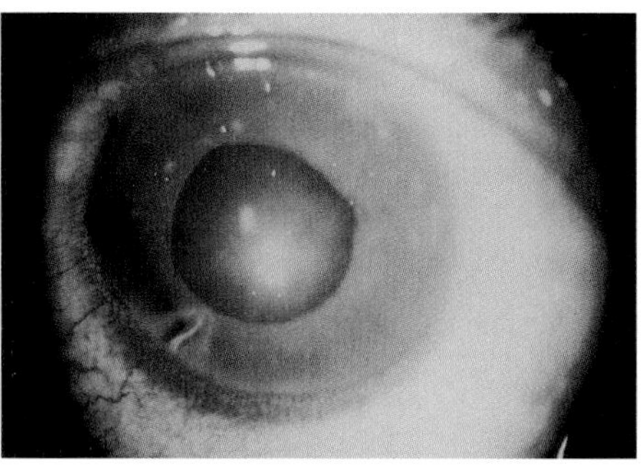

Figure 135.47 Intraocular gnathostomiasis. *Gnathostoma spinigerum* worm in the anterior chamber with the head end attached to the cornea. (From Biswas J, Gopal L, Sharma T, et al. Intraocular *Gnathostoma spinigerum*. Clinicopathologic study of two cases with review of literature. Retina. 1954;14:440.)

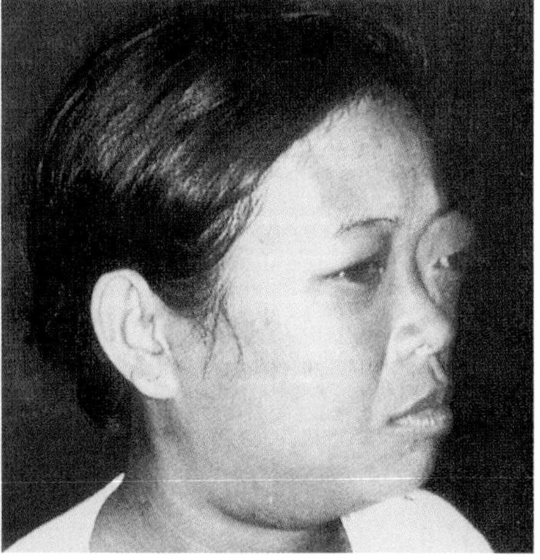

Figure 135.48 Ocular gnathostomiasis in a patient with marked periorbital edema. (From Kean BH, Sun TS, Ellsworth DM, eds. Color Atlas of Ophthalmic Parasitology. New York: Igaku-Shoin; 1991:155.)

Gnathostomiasis – Chapter 112

Ocular gnathostomiasis usually caused by *Gnathostoma spinigerum* results from direct invasion of the eye or surrounding tissues by a migratory larva (***Fig. 135.47***). Direct invasion of ocular tissue may result in corneal ulceration, iris perforation, subretinal hole formation, optic neuritis, and retinal artery occlusion. The inflammatory response may be pronounced, and uveitis, vitreal hemorrhage, vitritis, and secondary glaucoma can occur.[97,98] Edema and hemorrhage of the eyelid and orbital inflammation may also be prominent (***Fig. 135.48***). Fibrous reactions and scarring along worm tracks can result in vitreal fibrosis. Retinal distortion and detachment may result.[99] Worms may invade the CNS, and may provoke

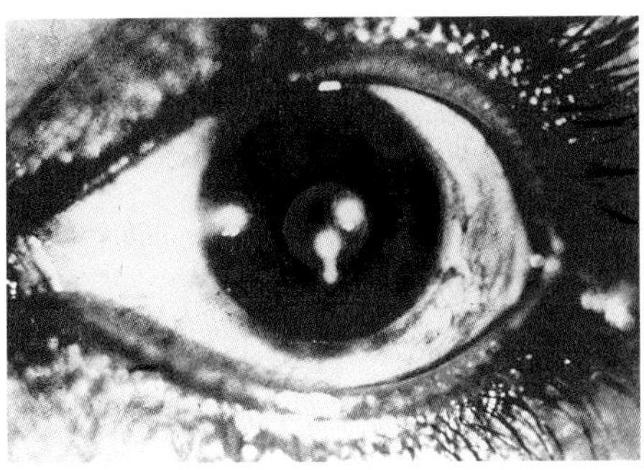

Figure 135.49 Ocular cysticercosis. Three cysticerci, one of them evaginated, are visible in the eye. (From Kean BH, Sun TS, Ellsworth DM, eds. Color Atlas of Ophthalmic Parasitology. New York: Igaku-Shoin; 1991:180.)

eosinophilic meningoencephalitis. Papilledema and cranial nerve palsies may result. Specific diagnosis may be difficult. Inflammation is usually severe. Serologic assays are available. Although optimal therapy is not known, systemic disease has been treated with albendazole, mebendazole, and ivermectin. Ocular disease is usually treated with mechanical removal of the worm. Such a procedure not only treats the ophthalmic disease itself, but also prevents subsequent penetration of the worm into brain parenchyma. In an attempt to decrease inflammation, corticosteroids may be of benefit when used concurrently with surgical intervention.

Trichinellosis – Chapter 110

Ocular involvement in trichinellosis usually occurs during the invasive larval stage and usually manifests as bilateral palpebral edema. Invasion of ocular musculature and structures by larvae may result in conjunctival chemosis and hemorrhage, photophobia, retinal hemorrhages, optic neuritis, and optic edema. Pain on eye movement may be prominent. Trichinellosis should be considered in any person presenting with bilateral palpebral edema, myalgias, and eosinophilia. Diagnosis is usually one of clinical recognition, serologic assay, or muscle biopsy.

Helminthic Infections: Cestodes

Cysticercosis – Chapter 119

Ocular involvement in cysticercosis relates to the intraocular or periocular presence of cysticerci (***Fig. 135.49***).[100,101] The posterior segment of the eye is most frequently involved symptomatically in ocular cysticercosis. Subretinal cysticerci may be quiescent or may provoke prominent inflammatory responses. Retinal edema, hemorrhage, and detachments may occur. Rupture into the vitreal cavity can occur, as can chorioretinitis, vitritis, and vasculitis. Freely floating cysticerci have been noted in the anterior and posterior chambers, and cysticerci may embed on the ciliary body, iris, or optic nerve. Cysticerci may also develop in the conjunctiva, lacrimal glands, and periorbital musculature. Cysticerci within the CNS may result in papilledema, cranial nerve dysfunction, and ocular palsies.

Sparganosis – Chapter 121

In sparganosis, caused by migratory plerocercoid larvae of *Spirometra* species, migratory worms can involve ocular structures. The application of fresh flesh (usually frog or snake flesh) as traditional eye poultices can lead to direct ocular deposition of larvae. Invasion of periocular structures in the anterior chamber may occur; however, ocular worms are usually found in the subconjunctiva. Inflammation may be pronounced and proptosis, lacrimation, periocular edema, pain, and pruritus may be intense. Diagnosis involves pathologic identification of removed worms. Ocular therapy involves surgical removal of the worm. No systemic antiparasitic agent has been shown to be of benefit.

Echinococcosis – Chapter 120

Ocular involvement in cystic hydatid disease due to *Echinococcus granulosus* usually relates to enlargement of a hydatid cyst in the orbital cavity, usually arising from bony structures. Proptosis, exposure keratitis, corneal ulcerations, extensive lacrimation, conjunctival chemosis and injection, impairment of extraocular mobility, optic atrophy, and orbital bone erosion may result.[102] Replacement of the vitreous by intraocular cysts has also been reported. Hydatid disease of the CNS can result in papilledema. Intraocular disease due to invasive alveolar hydatid disease has also been reported. Diagnosis involves clinical recognition, imaging studies, and serologic assays. Ocular hydatid disease should be treated surgically.

Coenuriasis

Coenuriasis is caused by the cystic larval stage of dog *Taenia* species tapeworms. *Taenia multiceps* and *T. serialis* appear to have a tropism for ocular structures and for the CNS. Ocular involvement is usually one of a space-occupying cystic lesion. Ocular cysts may occur in the eyelids, conjunctiva, and extraocular muscles. Intraocular cysts may be located subretinally or intravitreally. Proptosis, exposure keratitis, and corneal ulceration may occur. Older and ruptured cysts can provoke a prominent inflammatory response. Panophthalmitis and blindness may result. Diagnosis involves clinical recognition, imaging studies, and histologic examination. Ocular disease is treated with surgery.

Helminthic Infections: Trematodes

Schistosomiasis – Chapter 122

During acute schistosomiasis (Katayama fever), eyelid edema may be present. Direct ocular involvement in later disease can be due to egg deposition from portosystemic shunting, passive egg transfer via the vesicovertebral-CNS venous plexus, or by an aberrantly migrating worm pair. Ocular eggs elicit a granulomatous response that may be pronounced. Most confirmed cases of ocular involvement in schistosomiasis have involved conjunctival or lacrimal gland egg-related granuloma formation.[103] Choroidal egg-related granulomatous lesions have been reported, and involvement of the optic nerve can lead to optic atrophy.[104] Ocular involvement is most frequently reported with *S. haematobium* infection. Aberrantly migrating worms have been found in the superior ophthalmic vein and in the anterior chamber.[105] Ocular involvement should be treated systemically.

Paragonimiasis – Chapter 123

Ocular involvement in paragonimiasis usually involves aberrantly migrating worms. Mechanical damage can be extensive. Ocular pain due to an actively migrating worm is usually severe and recurrent, but the pain often spontaneously resolves within an hour of onset.[106] Worms can migrate through the eyelid, anterior chamber, and orbit. Retinal hemorrhages and subluxation of the lens can occur. Prominent inflammatory responses can result in hypopyon, uveitis, and secondary glaucoma. Cerebral involvement can result in cranial nerve palsies and papilledema. Ocular disease should be surgically treated.

Ectoparasites

Pentastomiasis – Chapter 124

Ocular involvement in pentastomiasis caused by *Lingulata serrata* involves migratory nymphs that have been recovered from the anterior chamber. Iritis and secondary glaucoma have been reported.[107] Diagnosis involves histologic examination of recovered specimens. Therapy for ocular disease involves surgical removal of the pentastomid.

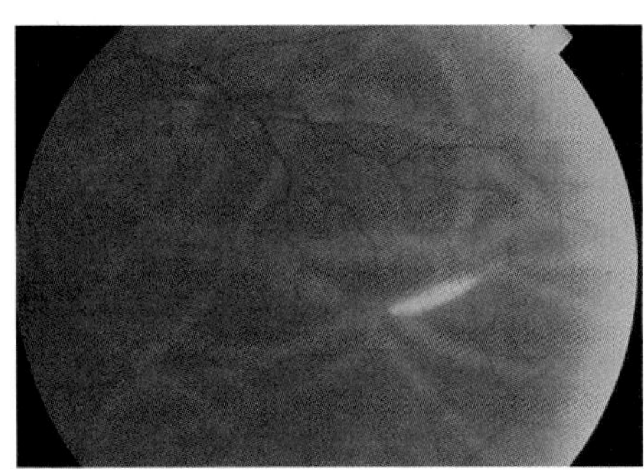

Figure 135.50 Internal ophthalmomyiasis. Funduscopic examination showing a segmented fly larva. Note depigmented, subretinal epithelial tracks. (From Currier RW, Johnson WA, Rowley WA, et al. Internal ophthalmomyiasis and treatment by laser photocoagulation: a case report. Am J Trop Med Hyg. 1995;52:312.)

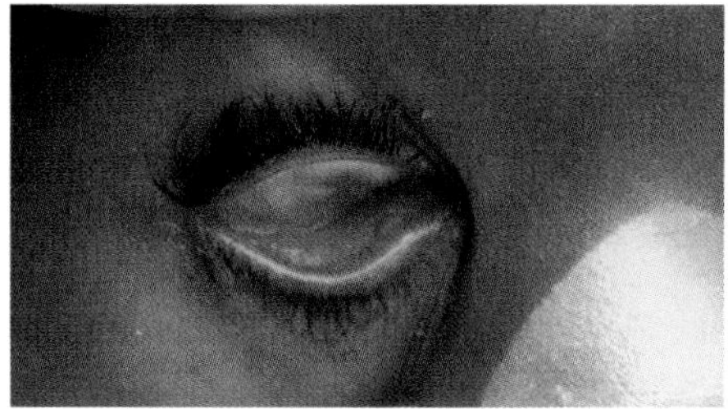

Figure 135.51 Phthisis bulbi. Note shrunken, scarred, blind, end-stage eye. Damage is irreversible. (From Sandford-Smith J. Eye Diseases in Hot Climates, 2nd ed. Oxford: Wright Publishers, Butterworth Heinemann; 1990.)

Myiasis – Chapter 124

Ocular involvement by larvae of flies is called ophthalmomyiasis. Ocular involvement in humans has been reported with a number of fly species, including *Oestrus ovis* ("sheep bot fly"), Gasterophilidae ("horse bot fly" or "horse warble fly"), *Wohlfahrtia magnifica* ("sheep maggot fly"), *Chrysomyia bezziana* ("screwworm fly"), *Cordylobia anthropophaga* ("tumbu fly"), and *Dermatobia hominis*, among others. Ocular disease occurs from deposition of eggs by flies or by secondary vectors, such as mosquitoes. Larvae emerge and penetrate the periocular and ocular tissues. Ocular involvement of the orbit, eyelid, or conjunctiva is called "ophthalmomyiasis externa."[108] "Ophthalmomyiasis interna" implies that larvae have invaded deep ocular structures (***Fig. 135.50***).[109] Such involvement may be either anterior or posterior. Larval migration can result in conjunctivitis, keratitis, scleritis, iritis, vitritis, subluxation of the lens, uveitis, and vitreal hemorrhage. Subretinal involvement may result in retinal detachment and hemorrhages. Retinal scarring and "track" formation may result. Involvement may be bilateral.

Specific diagnosis is confirmed by pathologic examination of recovered larvae or of subsequently matured flies. Treatment of ophthalmomyiasis externa involves mechanical removal of the larva(e) with careful searching for the presence of additional intranasal or intraocular larvae. Ophthalmomyiasis interna may be treated with laser photocoagulation or with surgery. Topical and systemic steroids may be used to minimize local inflammatory reactions.

BLINDNESS AND NONINFECTIOUS TROPICAL OCULAR PATHOLOGY

The WHO estimates that approximately 45 million persons are currently blind worldwide and that over 100 million persons have markedly decreased vision and are at substantial risk of becoming blind. Leading causes of blindness worldwide include cataract, glaucoma, age-related macular degeneration, corneal opacities from infection or trauma, diabetic retinopathy, and trachoma. Trauma is a leading cause of unilateral blindness worldwide. Blindness due to thermal or chemical burns to the eye may be accidental or intentional. The application of traditional eye medicines and poultices in much of the developing world often exacerbates initial ocular pathology. End-stage ocular damage may result in formation of a markedly shrunken, useless eye (phthisis bulbi; ***Fig. 135.51***). End-stage ocular damage may also result in a marked anterior bulging of the cornea due to a severely weakened cornea and sclera (staphyloma; see ***Fig. 135.15***). Although blindness due to infectious diseases is decreasing, blindness due to diabetes and age-related conditions continues to increase.

Sunlight can cause a number of ophthalmologic conditions. Intensive prolonged ultraviolet exposure may be associated with cortical cataract formation. Exposure to ultraviolet sunlight is linked to the development of climatic droplet keratopathy, a degenerative condition in which corneal opacifications form in the superficial corneal stroma. This condition may also be associated with extensive puffiness of the eyelids. Formation of a pterygium (a "fleshy wing" of conjunctival/subconjunctival tissue that encroaches on the cornea laterally and medially) may be related to ultraviolet irradiation. Intense, acute exposure to ultraviolet light may also lead to corneal/conjunctival epithelium damage that can present as photophobia, lacrimation, and ocular pain. Direct observation of the sun or exposure to excessive reflective glare can also result in macular damage that may be permanent.

A number of other conditions that may occur in the tropics may also result in ocular manifestations. Deficiency of vitamin A may result in xerophthalmia. Deficiency of vitamin B complex may result in optic neuropathy. Snake venom from spitting cobras may result in conjunctivitis, keratitis, or both that may be blinding. Argemone–poppy oil intoxication may result in glaucoma and optic nerve atrophy in India and Bangladesh. Local reactions to secretions of blister beetles, millipedes, and centipedes may result in painful conjunctivitis. Improperly prepared cassava can cause cyanide-related peripheral neuritis and optic neuropathy. The vasculopathy of sickle cell disease may result in ocular vascular changes, hemorrhages, scarring, and neovascularization. Reaction to an unknown allergen may result in vernal keratoconjunctivitis, a disorder that is most common in children and results in papillary conjunctivitis involving the tarsal conjunctiva and limbal region.

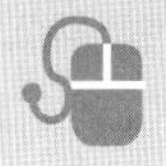

Access the complete reference list online at **http://www.expertconsult.com**

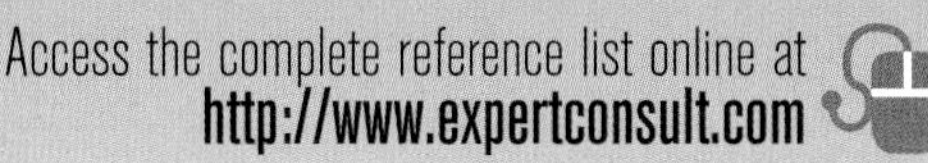
Access the complete reference list online at
http://www.expertconsult.com

CHAPTER 136

Neurologic Disease

Tom Solomon • Mustapha A. Danesi • Frank J. Bia • Thomas P. Bleck

INTRODUCTION

Neurologic presentations are more common in the tropics than in other regions and offer particular diagnostic and management challenges. A variety of factors contribute to this increased incidence, including a climate that favors transmission of insect-borne pathogens (e.g., malaria, arthropod-borne viruses, trypanosomiasis); the increased incidence of vaccine-preventable diseases (e.g., tetanus, diphtheria, polio); the impact of human immunodeficiency virus (HIV) on central nervous system (CNS) infections, particularly tuberculous meningitis; and the poverty, overcrowding, and poor sanitation that are risk factors for so many tropical diseases (e.g., cysticercosis, typhoid). Although this chapter focuses on infectious neurologic diseases, noncommunicable neurologic diseases are also more common in the tropics (e.g., motor vehicle collisions and other forms of trauma). The patterns of cerebrovascular disease in many parts of the tropics are catching up with those in the developed world.

DIAGNOSTIC APPROACHES

Taking a careful history and performing a detailed neurologic and general medical examination are even more important in the tropics than elsewhere because in many tropical settings the availability of diagnostic tools – particularly imaging – is limited. This section concentrates on the approach to the comatose patient, which is often the greatest challenge.

History

Compared with seeing a patient in more developed nations, getting a history from a patient with a neurologic problem in the tropics can be especially difficult. The patient may have traveled a great distance over many days to arrive at the health facility, and the person accompanying the patient may not know the original history. In addition, it may not be clear what drugs were administered along the way; for example, anticonvulsants given at a clinic on the way to hospital. Obtaining an accurate history about possible seizures is particularly difficult because of the range of terms used in different settings and the ways in which abnormal movements are interpreted. Remember that in many settings seizures may be regarded as a sign of mental illness or even of possession by evil spirits.[1] Communication problems are often further compounded by language and translation difficulties. It is worth making a special effort to inquire about possible remedies given by a traditional healer. In many parts of the world, the traditional healer is the first port of call, and referral to conventional health care systems is very much a last resort.

Examination

It is common to be faced with a comatose patient for whom little reliable history is available. There may be important clues to the cause on examination: check the pockets for any drugs or other information about past medical history; examine the skin for rash (meningococcal meningitis), bites (e.g., snakebite), marks of intravenous drug abuse, a healed dog bite (rabies), chancre (for trypanosomiasis); examine the ears and nose carefully for blood or cerebrospinal fluid (CSF) leak consistent with head trauma; feel for lymphadenopathy, particularly in the posterior cervical triangle (Winterbottom's sign in African trypanosomiasis); and smell the breath for alcohol or ketones.

In the neurologic examination, determine the level of consciousness, check for neck stiffness and other signs of meningism (including Kernig's sign – with the patient supine, and the hip and knee flexed, extension of the knee causes pain and neck flexion), and Brudzinski's sign (with the patient supine, flexion of the neck causes spontaneous flexion of the hip and knee); focus on whether there is hemiparesis, brainstem abnormalities (particularly of the pupils, eye movements; spontaneous or elicited), the breathing pattern, or other focal signs.

It should be possible to classify comatose patients into one of four groups (which may overlap):

1. Diffuse encephalopathy (i.e., a reduction in consciousness) with no focal neurologic signs. If the patient is febrile or has a history of fever, think of CNS infection (e.g., cerebral malaria) or a metabolic cause of coma (e.g., diabetic coma, drugs, toxins) with secondary infection such as aspiration pneumonia.
2. Encephalopathy with meningism (neck stiffness, or positive Kernig's sign). If the patient is febrile, a CNS infection (especially bacterial meningitis) is likely, but subarachnoid hemorrhages or posterior fossa vascular disorders should also be considered, especially if the onset was sudden.
3. Encephalopathy with lateralizing neurologic signs (e.g., hemiparesis). This often indicates supratentorial focal damage; think of abscess, tuberculoma, meningitis with a subdural collection, stroke, or if the history is more insidious, tumor.
4. Encephalopathy with brainstem signs. This may indicate pathology within the brainstem itself (caused, for example, by a local infection) or herniation of the brainstem secondary to raised intracranial pressure due to any of the preceding causes.

Investigations

Examination of the CSF is the single most important investigation for diagnosis of a CNS infection. In industrialized nations, if a patient has deep coma or focal neurologic signs, a computed tomographic (CT) scan is usually performed before a lumbar puncture to ensure there is no intracranial abscess or other significant type of brain shift, since if there is incipient herniation of the brainstem, a lumbar puncture can worsen this situation. However, if CT scanning is not readily available, the benefits of a lumbar puncture in terms of obtaining an accurate diagnosis are often felt to outweigh the risks.[2]

A definitive diagnosis may require radiographic confirmation of a neurologic lesion with skull or sinus films, CT scans, magnetic resonance imaging (MRI) or angiographic studies, myelography, electroencephalography (EEG), electromyography (EMG), nerve conduction studies, or histologic study of muscle biopsy specimens. Infections such as bacterial meningitis can be confirmed by Gram stain and culture of the infecting organisms obtained from CSF, though pretreatment with antibiotics before patients come to hospital is common. Distinguishing it from tuberculous meningitis can be difficult, though recent algorithms may prove helpful.[3] In suspected bacterial meningitis, treatment should not be delayed because a lumbar puncture cannot be performed quickly. Blood cultures should be obtained regardless of whether a lumbar puncture is performed, since they may reveal the cause of the meningitis. Parasitic infection may be confirmed by examination of blood films, sputum, stool, or in some cases, CSF obtained for the identification of adult parasites, larvae, or ova. Serologic studies of peripheral blood or CSF can be useful in confirming certain bacterial or viral infections. Simple rapid diagnostic kits are becoming available for a variety of infections. Many viral CNS infections are now diagnosed by using the polymerase chain reaction, particularly encephalitis caused by herpes simplex virus.

SYNDROME-BASED DIAGNOSIS

Syndrome-based differential diagnosis is a convenient way to organize the large number of neurologic infections encountered in tropical medicine (*Box 136.1*). *Table 136.1* presents detailed information on the diagnosis of infections of the CNS.[4–7]

Box 136.1 Tropical Infections and Infectious Disease with Major Neurologic Presentations

Meningitides and Meningoencephalitides

- Acute bacterial meningitis
  - Pneumococcal meningitis
  - *Haemophilius influenzae* type b meningitis
  - Meningococcal meningitis
  - *Listeria monocytogenes* meningitis
- Subacute bacterial meningitis
  - Secondary syphilis with aseptic meningitis
  - Borreliosis
- Tuberculous meningitis
- Fungal meningitis
  - Cryptococcal meningitis
  - *Candida* spp. meningitis
  - Coccidioidal meningitis
- Viral meningitides and meningoencephalitides
  - Arboviruses (e.g., Japanese encephalitis virus)
  - Rabies
  - Herpes simplex and varicella-zoster viruses
  - Enteroviruses
  - Mumps virus
  - Human immunodeficiency virus
  - Epstein–Barr virus
  - Cytomegalovirus
  - Rubeola

Postviral and Postimmunization Meningoencephalitides

- Measles, rubella, varicella-zoster
- Measles vaccine, rabies vaccine, yellow fever vaccine

Parasitic Meningitides and Meningoencephalitides

- Amebic meningoencephalitis (*Naegleria* and *Acanthamoeba* spp.)
- Strongyloidiasis
- Paragonimiasis
- *Angiostrongylus cantonensis*
- *Gnathostoma spinigerum*
- Trichinellosis
- *Toxocara canis* (visceral and ocular larva migrans)
- Trypanosomiasis
  - *Trypanosoma gambiense*
  - *Trypanosoma rhodesiense*
- *Loa loa* (filarial)

Brain Abscesses

- Bacterial (also causing subdural empyema and epidural abscess)
  - Anaerobic bacteria (e.g., mouth flora)
  - Gram-negative enteric and nosocomial organisms
  - *Streptococcus intermedius*
  - Staphylococci
- Fungal
  - Immunologically normal host
  - Coccidioidomycosis
  - Immunologically impaired host
  - Aspergillosis
  - Candidiasis
  - Zygomycosis (e.g., mucormycosis in diabetic ketoacidosis)
- Parasitic mass lesion of the central nervous system (CNS)
  - Toxoplasmosis
  - Cysticercosis
  - Echinococcosis (hydatid cysts)
  - Schistosomiasis (*Schistosoma japonicum*)
  - Amebiasis (*Entamoeba histolytica*)

Infections with Minimal CNS Inflammation

- Malaria
- Leptospirosis
- Borreliosis
- Brucellosis
- Rickettsial infections
- Ehrlichiosis

Infections Producing Brainstem and Spinal Cord Syndromes

- Bacterial
  - Spinal epidural abscess
- Viral
  - Rabies
  - Poliomyelitis
  - Flaviviruses
  - Human T-cell lymphotropic virus type 1-associated tropical spastic paraplegia
- Parasitic
  - *Diphyllobothrium latum* (megaloblastic anemia, vitamin B_{12} deficiency)
  - *Dracunculus medinensis*
  - Schistosomiasis (*Schistosoma mansoni* and *S. haematobium*)
  - Paragonimiasis

Infections Involving the Peripheral Nerves and Muscles

- Leprosy
  - Viruses (e.g., Epstein–Barr virus, varicella, etc.)
  - Bacteria (e.g., *Campylobacter*, causing Guillain-Barré syndrome)
- Toxin-mediated
  - Tetanus
  - Botulism
- Muscle infection
  - Trichinellosis
  - Tropical pyomyositis
  - Diabetes-associated and human immunodeficiency virus-associated pyomyositis
  - Necrotizing fasciitis

Table 136.1 Parasitic Infections of the Central Nervous System

	Distribution	Exposure	Major Manifestations
Protozoan			
Toxoplasma gondii	Worldwide	Rare meat, cat feces	Focal findings, occasionally diffuse encephalopathy, meningoencephalitis in immunocompromised hosts
Plasmodium falciparum malaria	Tropics	Female *Anopheles* mosquitoes	Coma, obtundation, personality changes, movement disorders, cerebellar ataxia, focal findings (cerebrospinal fluid usually unremarkable)
Entamoeba histolytica	Worldwide	Fecal-oral	Brain abscess
PAM and GAE			
Naegleria fowleri	Worldwide	Freshwater lakes (nasal, via cribriform plate)	Fulminant and rapidly fatal
Acanthamoeba spp.	Worldwide	Brackish warm water (respiratory, eyes, skin)	Chronic granulomatous necrotizing encephalitis in immunocompromised hosts
Balamuthia mandrillaris	Peru, Venezuela, Mexico	?River	Meningoencephalitis
Helminthic			
Neurocysticercosis (*Taenia solium*)	Worldwide	Fecal-oral (ova) (pork meat tapeworm only)	Seizures, hydrocephalic meningitis, cord lesions
Echinococcosis (hydatid disease)			
E. granulosus	South-central Europe, Middle East, South America, Africa, Australia, New Zealand	Fecal-oral from dogs, foxes, etc.	Fewer, larger cysts
E. multilocularis	North America		
E. vogeli	South and Central America		Invasive polycystic disease (extramedullary > brain)
Trichinellosis	Worldwide	Rare pork, bear, horse meat	Focal infections, inflammation, infarction, or hemorrhage
Strongyloides stercoralis	Worldwide	Skin, autoinfection	Immunosuppression causes hematogenous spread of larvae causing brain abscesses, microinfarcts, granuloma formation, or meningitis
Schistosoma japonicum	Orient, Southeast Asia	Swimming in freshwater containing infected snails	Encephalitis, seizures, focal findings
S. haematobium	Africa, South America		Myelopathy, seizures
S. mansoni	Asia, Africa, Latin America		Rare cord compression, spinal artery occlusion, myelitis
Paragonimus westermani	Asia	Eating raw freshwater crustaceans	"Soap-bubble" central nervous system (CNS) calcifications with cavitary lung lesions, occasional seizures, meningitis, focal findings
Paragonimus mexicanus	Costa Rica	Crustaceans	Focal CNS hemorrhage
Helminthic Causes of Eosinophilic Meningitis:			
Angiostrongylus cantonensis	Southeast Asia	Freshwater crustaceans (infected from domestic rat)	Usually self-limited meningitis
Gnathostoma spinigerum	Southeast Asia	Freshwater fish, frogs, snakes, and paratenic poultry, ducks	Meningitis with residual neurologic deficits (45%)
Toxocara canis	Worldwide	Pica, puppy feces	Rare meningoencephalitis
Baylisascaris procyonis	Worldwide	Tree bark contaminated by raccoon feces	Rare meningoencephalitis

GAE, granulomatous amebic encephalitis; PAM, primary amebic meningoencephalitis.

Meningitides

The various forms of meningitis usually present with fever, headache, photophobia, mental confusion, or seizures. The classical triad of fever, neck stiffness, and altered consciousness is found in fewer than 50% of adult patients, though most have at least two of these three features.[8] For infants and very young children, signs of meningeal irritation may not be obvious, and it may present with either seizures in the setting of fever, mildly impaired consciousness or drowsiness, and occasionally a bulging anterior fontanelle. Acute bacterial meningitis generally has a rapid onset and progression. In the tropics, meningococcal meningitis usually occurs in epidemics, affecting mainly children and young adults living within arid geographic regions such as sub-Saharan Africa.[9]

Pneumococcal meningitis can present with markedly raised intracranial pressure and coma. It usually occurs in adults and is particularly common in patients with sickle cell hemoglobinopathy, HIV infection, and functional or anatomic asplenia. *Haemophilus influenzae* meningitis occurs in unvaccinated children or older adults and is associated commonly with seizures linked with fever in children. Complications of bacterial meningitis include cranial nerve palsies, deafness, and subdural effusion in children. The presentations of viral meningitis are typically less severe and without altered consciousness; the infection is commonly due to enteroviruses, such as echovirus. In recent years, there have been large outbreaks of human enterovirus 71 causing aseptic meningitis, and other CNS complications, in the Asia Pacific area.[10]

Subacute and chronic meningitis due to CNS tuberculosis, fungi, or late chronic neurosyphilis have a less fulminant onset and a slow disease progression.[11] However, aseptic meningitis in secondary syphilis mimics acute viral disease and additionally may cause cranial nerve palsies, particularly in HIV-infected patients. In the early phase of tuberculous meningitis, symptoms may be vague with complaints of headache, insomnia, and body pains. Unless there is a high level of suspicion, the diagnosis could be missed at an early stage of the disease, particularly in adults. Later stages are associated with cranial nerve palsies due to basilar meningitis, though presentations with dementia are not unknown. Characteristically, chronic inflammation occurring at the base of the brain also entraps cerebral blood vessels and may lead to vascular compromise and stroke. Hemiplegia is a potential outcome. Focal tuberculous infections (tuberculomas) present as mass lesions and may be mistaken for brain tumors.[12]

Parasitic disease such as acute amebic meningoencephalitis usually presents with features similar to acute bacterial meningitis but with an associated characteristic olfactory involvement based on presumed entry of the organism through the cribriform plate.[13] Seizures and coma rapidly progress in this disease, even in previously healthy persons. *Naegleria fowleri*, the causative organism, is found in warm, freshwater streams and pools, and obtaining a history of such exposure is highly relevant. Motile flagellated amebic trophozoites may be identified during microscopic examination of a wet CSF preparation. *Acanthamoeba* species are more commonly identified as causative organisms in debilitated, immunosuppressed persons, usually producing a subacute or chronic encephalitis. Angiostrongyliasis and gnathostomiasis may cause eosinophilic meningitis, as well as multiple brain abscesses with focal neurologic signs. Strongyloidiasis occurs in specific populations of immunosuppressed persons such as patients given corticosteroids, transplant recipients, or those infected with human T-cell lymphotropic virus type 1 (HTLV-1). Paragonimiasis may involve the CNS in young children with severe consequences of chronic meningoencephalitis. Trichinosis occasionally involves the CNS, causing seizures, meningoencephalitis, or hemorrhagic infarction from larval invasion of the microvasculature. Cerebral edema and death from brainstem herniation may occur.[4]

Encephalopathies

Encephalopathy means a reduction in consciousness level, and when this is due to inflammation of the brain substance, the term encephalitis is used. Encephalitis is most often caused by viruses, though parasites, such as trypanosomiasis, and some bacteria, are also important causes. The term "meningoencephalitis" is often used to reflect the fact that many pathogens cause features of meningitis and encephalitis, and there is overlap of the clinical syndromes. The signs and symptoms of encephalitis include headache, lethargy, stupor, delirium, seizures, hyperreflexia, and spasticity, sometimes with a positive Babinski sign. Coma and signs of raised intracranial pressure may be present. There may be clinical clues to the particular virus; for example, tremors, rigidity spasms, and other movement disorders suggest involvement of the basal ganglia, which is often seen in encephalitis caused by flaviviruses such as Japanese encephalitis virus and West Nile virus.[14] Alphaviruses such as eastern equine encephalitis can cause a similar syndrome. In herpes simplex type 1 encephalitis, a focal neurologic disorder of the temporal lobe is almost always documented on brain imaging, and characteristic periodic complexes are often observed in the EEG. In African trypanosomiasis, somnolence alternating with insomnia is characteristic, and these patients have a course that evolves to manifestations of abnormal movement and gait, total indifference, and eventually stupor.[15] Cerebral malaria is a complication of severe *Plasmodium falciparum* infection and causes encephalopathy, with little or no inflammation, rather than encephalitis; it is particularly common in children and pregnant women living in endemic areas.[16] Cerebral malaria often rapidly progresses to seizures and coma in febrile patients who go undiagnosed.[17] Prevention is of particular importance for nonimmune adult visitors, who are at even greater risk for this complication of severe malaria. They must receive prophylaxis or presumptive therapy that covers potentially resistant strains of *P. falciparum*. Severe malaria may also cause hypoglycemia and mimic the early symptoms of cerebral malaria. Quinine administration can accentuate this problem by enhancing insulin release from the pancreas and contributing to hypoglycemia. Artemether, and related drugs, based on the Chinese herb qinghaosu, do not have this problem, but as for all other antimalarials, drug resistance is a continuing problem.[18]

Postimmunization and Postinfectious Encephalitides

Postimmunization encephalitis has occurred following immunization against yellow fever or rabies, especially in the past when earlier vaccines were utilized.[19] Newer vaccines produced from cell culture are less likely to cause such complications. Postviral encephalitis is well described following measles vaccination in older children. It is characterized by a reduced level of consciousness and multifocal neurologic signs, including hemiparesis and paraparesis.

Brain Abscess and Other Intracranial Mass Lesions

Brain abscess presents with features of raised intracranial pressure, seizure disorders, and focal neurologic deficits but not necessarily with fevers. Brain abscesses are often caused by mixed anaerobic bacteria, but Gram-negative organisms are commonly isolated after middle ear or sinus infections and trauma. Hematogenous dissemination of bacteria such as *Staphylococcus aureus* to the CNS may also result in staphylococcal brain abscess formation. Subdural empyema may present with headache, fever, altered mental status, seizures, nuchal rigidity, and focal neurologic deficits. Most subdural empyemas occur as a consequence of contiguous spread from sinusitis, otitis media, or mastoiditis. Increasing injected drug abuse, chronic immunosuppression, such as HIV and sickle cell disease, and surgery are all important risk factors.[20] Rupture of a CNS tuberculoma to produce meningitis is particularly common in the tropics, and there may be coexistent reactivation of pulmonary tuberculosis.

Neurocysticercosis may produce cystic parenchymal lesions and also causes chronic inflammation of the subarachnoid space with resultant hydrocephalus. Amebic brain abscess from *Entamoeba histolytica* occurs generally in a setting of disseminated disease with concomitant liver abscess. Paragonimiasis can produce mass lesions, chronic meningitis, cerebral infarction, and hemorrhage. Hydatid cyst disease causes local inflammation as well as mechanical obstruction of CSF flow with resulting hydrocephalus.

It is useful to characterize some of the more common clinical scenarios associated with parasitic infections of the CNS, since these syndromes often generate requests for tropical medicine consultation from other practitioners. It is relatively easy to produce a rather long list of diagnostic possibilities when a patient comes in with what appears to be a possible mass lesion of the CNS, but discerning one entity from another on a clinical basis in order to direct the remainder of the diagnostic workup is a challenging task for any consultant. The following clinical paradigms can be considered in sorting out just such cases when they present for evaluation. The reader is referred to other sections for detailed diagnostic workup and treatment.

Neurocysticercosis (see also Chapter 119)

Neurocysticercosis often presents with a new seizure disorder.[21] In the developing world, cysticercosis is one of the most common causes of seizures. In the tropics, patients are often children, who suffer concomitant injuries, such as burns, when seizures occur near open fires.

Pork ingestion is not necessary for the development of cysticercosis. Human ingestion of the ova produced by pork tapeworms poses the threat of neurocysticercosis. Most commonly, the disease is acquired by ingestion of ova that contaminate foodstuffs grown in soil. Rarely, the source of these ova can be the patients themselves, who may have previously acquired pork tapeworm infection by eating undercooked pork containing the larvae of *Taenia solium*. The ova passed in their stools are produced by adult tapeworms and are potentially infectious to both themselves (autoinfection) and others in the immediate household environment. Within communities of the developed world, where food may be prepared by *T. solium*-infected persons who have recently migrated from endemic areas, employers and families are at risk of acquiring this disease.

Larvae-containing cysticerci infecting the CNS do not result in any single disease pattern. The clinical presentation depends on the intensity of infection; the number, size, and localization of cysts; and the intensity of the immunologic responses to their presence. The cysts expand slowly, and larvae within these cysts eventually die. Inflammation follows, sometimes associated with seizures. The lesions ultimately calcify. If an intraventricular cyst suddenly blocks the flow of CSF, causing obstructive hydrocephalus, rapid deterioration or death may occur. Ocular infections (which may occur in about 20% of cases) should be ruled out before the institution of any antiparasitic therapy to prevent further irreparable ocular damage from additional inflammatory responses. If evidence of ocular infection is present, corticosteroids should be administered prior to the antiparasitic agent.

In the diagnostic workup of patients with suspected neurocysticercosis, CT and MRI have enhanced our ability to diagnose these disorders and have delineated different patterns of disease in adults and children. Adults from an endemic area are more likely to have older calcified lesions, which show very little contrast enhancement on CT scanning. These patients generally will *not* have demonstrable *Taenia* ova in their stools. In contrast, children are more likely to have acute lesions with contrast enhancement secondary to host inflammatory responses. These reactions represent immune responses to degeneration of the parasites themselves and account for the acute presentations with seizures. The therapeutic decisions surrounding the use of antiparasitic agents, and the potential use of corticosteroids during treatment of acute lesions, are based on these differences.

Echinococcosis (Hydatid Disease; see also Chapter 120)

Although echinococcosis is also characterized by cystic lesions of the CNS, which can be difficult to distinguish from those of cysticercosis, the epidemiology of human infections and clinical presentations differ considerably from those of neurocysticercosis. Echinococcal cysts tend to be larger and fewer in number, and unlike cysticercosis, echinococcal cysts are not usually found in cerebral parenchyma. They are more likely to infect and destroy vertebral bone, resulting in spinal cord compression from their continuous expansion. Hydatid disease of the CNS only occurs in 1–2% of human echinococcosis cases, and CNS infections are more common in children. Compression of the spinal cord is the most common CNS manifestation of this disease.

When children or adults with CNS echinococcosis also have a history of contact with dogs or sheep in areas endemic for this disease, the diagnosis of hydatid disease should be considered. The sequence of infection first involves one of several species of cestodes of the genus *Echinococcus* infecting carnivores, such as dogs. Within the canine gastrointestinal tract, the parasites grow into adult tapeworms, and humans become infected by accidental ingestion of ova excreted by the infected dog, as in the case of the most common species of parasite infecting humans, *Echinococcus granulosus*.

CT scanning or MRI is useful for demonstrating typical extramedullary cord compression and vertebral involvement. Enzyme-linked immunosorbent assays are replacing the haemagglutination inhibition assay as the screening test of choice, with specific confirmation by immunoblot.[22] As serologic diagnosis becomes more sensitive and specific, a positive antibody titer in conjunction with a typical appearance of cysts on CT scanning or MRI, or vertebral radiographs demonstrating osseous lesions and the appearance of moth-eaten vertebrae, with a supportive epidemiologic history, should suggest the diagnosis once spinal cord and vertebral involvement by large cystic lesions is confirmed.

Cerebral Paragonimiasis (see also Chapter 123)

The pulmonary presentation of infections with the lung fluke *Paragonimus westermani* is easily mistaken for tuberculosis. The appearance of multiple cavitary lesions in a young patient with chronic hemoptysis and CNS symptoms mimics the spread of pulmonary tuberculosis to the CNS associated with tuberculous meningitis. This picture can be even more confusing when the disease occurs in a population that has a high incidence of positive tuberculin skin test reactivity.

However, when a patient is from an endemic area for paragonimiasis, such as Southeast Asia, where crustaceans or their juices are commonly eaten raw, there is the potential for the complex life cycle of this parasite to involve the human host. Children are particularly susceptible to ectopic cerebral infections with these migrating flukes, particularly if infected early in life, since most cerebral infections occur before 10 years of age. The most common neurologic symptoms include seizure disorders, headache, and visual disturbances; the majority of patients in various clinical series of cerebral paragonimiasis have abnormal eye findings. They include impaired visual acuity, homonymous hemianopsia, optic atrophy, papilledema, nystagmus, and pupillary abnormalities.

A clue to the presence of cerebral paragonimiasis may often be found in plain skull films obtained on patients who have cerebral infection with the adult lung flukes. As the ectopic adult flukes degenerate, skull films may show punctate or nodular calcifications, or even advanced lesions with a "soap-bubble" appearance. *Paragonimus* ova can be found in sputum, feces, pleural and peritoneal fluid, or biopsy tissue.

Hence, any clinical presentation that suggests chronic cavitary pulmonary tuberculosis in a young patient with apparent CNS infection, and particularly ocular involvement, might lead to further questioning to obtain the appropriate epidemiologic data indicating that the patient had been at risk for paragonimiasis. Radiologic evaluation with skull films or CT scanning, observation of typical ova, and confirmatory serologic testing aid in diagnosis.

Other Potential Parasitic CNS Infections

Several patterns of parasitic infections of the CNS lead to rapid consideration of other potential parasitic causes of CNS infections. Patients with intestinal *amebiasis* caused by *E. histolytica* generally do *not* develop a brain abscess unless there is a generalized and disseminated amebic infection. It is extremely unusual to have an amebic brain abscess develop without an antecedent liver abscess in patients with amebiasis. Even in the presence of an amebic liver abscess, the incidence of brain abscess is usually less than 10%.

Prior to the current acquired immunodeficiency syndrome (AIDS) pandemic, abscess formation due to *Toxoplasma gondii* infection was rare. It was most likely to occur as reactivation of a latent *Toxoplasma* infection in a compromised host receiving chemotherapy for a disease such as lymphoma, which compromised cell-mediated immunity. However, with the emergence of AIDS, toxoplasmosis became the most common opportunistic CNS infection early in the epidemic, and it has been documented in at least 25% of patients. Because the organisms are sensitive to folic acid antagonists, which are now the drugs of choice for prophylaxis against *Pneumocystis jirovecii* pulmonary infections, the incidence of *Toxoplasma* reactivation has diminished considerably. Previously infected but asymptomatic patients not receiving prophylaxis, whose HIV infections are not under intensive therapy and who present with multiple ring-enhancing lesions on CT scanning or MRI, are likely to have reactivated this infection.

Many anticipated that the AIDS pandemic would result in large numbers of patients chronically infected with *Strongyloides stercoralis* succumbing to disseminated infections. Filariform larvae reach the CNS via hematogenous spread and would occlude small vessels, resulting in microinfarcts, abscesses, or bacterial meningitis (from carriage of bacteria within the larvae). In some cases, the larvae traverse the perivascular spaces to cause granuloma formation in the meninges or parenchyma, as they have in immunocompromised patients such as transplant recipients. To date, this has not been a major problem, with only about 20 such instances described. However, clinicians should be aware of the increasing recognition of disseminated *Strongyloides* infections that occur together with HTLV-1 infections and their associated lymphomas. The presence of disseminated strongyloidiasis in a patient with HIV infections should lead to a consideration of potential coinfection with HTLV-1.

Infections Involving the Brainstem and Spinal Cord

These infections cause paraparesis, paraplegia, or tetraparesis and occasionally cranial nerve dysfunction. In acute transverse myelitis associated with viral infections, fever, backache, leg weakness, sensory disturbances, and sphincter dysfunction may occur. During the acute phase of illness, flaccid paralysis, with absent or reduced tendon reflexes, is observed. Spasticity and hyperactive tendon reflexes may occur later in the course of the disease. A sensory level is usually identified at the involved level of the cord. Transverse myelitis may be a nonspecific complication following a number of viral infections. However, some viruses specifically attack the anterior horn cells of the spinal cord to confer an acute flaccid paralysis in which there may be few sensory symptoms and signs, and no upper motor neuron features. Poliovirus is the classic cause of this syndrome, but other enteroviruses (e.g., human enterovirus 71) and flaviviruses (e.g., Japanese encephalitis and West Nile virus) can also cause a polio-like syndrome.[23] Rabies virus can also present as a painful flaccid paralysis, which ascends to ultimately give a fatal encephalitis.

Cord compression from an epidural abscess produces similar symptoms and signs as transverse myelitis, but MRI or myelography demonstrates evidence of the cord compression. Most patients with a spinal epidural abscess present with focal spinal back pain, aching or tenderness at the level of infection, followed by nerve root pain radiating from the spinal level of involvement. Subsequently, paraparesis with bladder involvement may progress to complete paraplegia.

In spinal tuberculosis, granulomatous arachnoiditis may arise at any level and subsequently cause radiculomyelopathy. Patients present with a combination of nerve root and cord compression. Tuberculous granulomatous masses or abscess formation may be confined to the epidural space and produce cord compression. However, involvement of vertebral bodies, i.e., tuberculous spondylitis, may lead to vertebral collapse with spinal cord compression. *Schistosoma mansoni* and *Schistosoma haematobium* may also cause true granulomatous inflammation of the spinal cord associated with spastic paraplegia and anesthetic sensory levels.[24]

Tropical spastic paraplegia is common in some parts of the tropics, such as Jamaica or southern Japan, where HTLV-1 infections are more common, and can evolve into a chronic inflammatory disease of the spinal cord. This is a slowly progressive paraparesis with both increased tendon reflexes and Babinski signs, sphincter dysfunction, and sensory impairment. Paraparesis has been reported in varicella-zoster infections, in herpes simplex myelitis, and in vacuolar myelopathy seen in advanced HIV infection.

Infections Affecting Peripheral Nerves and Muscles

Acute Paralysis

Acute inflammatory polyneuropathy (Guillain–Barré syndrome) occurs in children and adults following a wide variety of microbial infections; examples include Epstein–Barr virus, other herpesviruses, and bacteria-causing enteritis, such as *Campylobacter jejuni*. It can also follow vaccines, most notably that used against swine flu in 1976.[25] Symmetric weakness of the lower limbs progresses rapidly to involve the upper limbs and later the trunk and the intercostal, cervical, and cranial nerves. Weakness progresses to paralysis and absent tendon reflexes. Disturbances of autonomic functions may occur. In botulism, the clostridial toxins interfere with release of acetylcholine at the neuromuscular junction and cause acute paralysis.[26] Botulism frequently, but not always, produces diplopia and failure of pupillary constriction, which are rarely seen in the Guillain–Barré syndrome. Diphtheria presents as an acute flaccid paralysis weeks to months after a patient has recovered from the acute illness.[27] It is more common in those whose acute illness was severe, with myocarditis, but can occur in patients whose initial illness was so mild they did not seek medical attention; such cases will be diagnosed only by taking a careful history about a preceding sore throat.

Chronic Neuropathy

Gradually evolving neuropathy in tropical countries is often due to leprosy, a result of direct invasion of nerves by *Mycobacterium leprae*. In tuberculoid leprosy, where few organisms are present in nerves, patches of superficial sensory loss and granulomatous enlargement of subcutaneous nerves, such as the ulnar, median, peroneal, posterior auricular, and facial nerves, occur in association with sensory or motor deficits. In lepromatous leprosy, lack of resistance to intracellular bacterial growth causes widespread mycobacterial invasion of cutaneous sensory nerves and a symmetrical pattern of pain and temperature loss with anesthesia involving most of the cutaneous surfaces. Since small sensory fibers are predominantly involved, tendon reflexes are usually preserved, but anesthesia leads to widespread tissue injuries and trophic changes that result from loss of innervation.

Myositis and Other Muscle Diseases

In tetanus, persistent spasms of the skeletal muscles occur owing to the effects of tetanus toxin on the normally inhibitory spinal neurons (e.g., Renshaw cells) which usually function to inhibit the activity of motor neurons.[28] Reflex muscle spasm occurs in response to various visual, tactile, or auditory stimuli. Spontaneous muscle spasms occur in severe cases, and death from respiratory arrest or laryngeal spasm may occur. In trichinosis parasitic muscle invasion causes deposition of larvae in muscle with considerable muscle pain, periorbital edema, and eosinophilia. Staphylococci and streptococci can directly invade muscle to cause bacterial myositis, often a disease of patients with diabetes mellitus but which is now being seen more frequently in association with HIV infection.

THERAPEUTIC APPROACHES

Initial Approach

The initial approaches to emergent problems are outlined in ***Table 136.2***.

Specific Conditions

In *meningitis*, appropriate treatment with antibiotics should be started immediately to minimize neurologic complications and should not be delayed to await imaging studies. The choice of empirical antibiotics depends on the age of the patient, the clinical features, the CSF Gram stain, and current local epidemiologic factors. The most commonly

Table 136.2 Initial Approaches to Emergent Problems in Patients with Neurologic Dysfunction

Problem	Approach
Suspected bacterial meningitides	Location- and age-specific appropriate empirical antibiotic therapy
Increased intracranial pressure	Mannitol 0.25 g/kg; hyperventilation to $PaCO_2$ near 30 mmHg; corticosteroids (e.g., dexamethasone 10 mg)
Shock	Intravenous fluid support (e.g., saline) and vasopressor support (e.g., norepinephrine, phenylephrine, epinephrine)
Seizures or status epilepticus	If acute treatment required, begin with an intravenous benzodiazepine (e.g., lorazepam or clonazepam), followed by intravenous phenytoin 20 mg/kg
Acute paraplegia or quadriplegia	Consider high-dose methylprednisolone 30 mg/kg
Acute respiratory failure	Endotracheal intubation and mechanical ventilation; if elevated ICP is suspected, premedicate with either intravenous lidocaine 1.0–1.5 mg/kg or thiopental 3–5 mg/kg

ICP, intracranial pressure; $PaCO_2$, arterial carbon dioxide tension.

utilized antibiotic agents include penicillins and second- or third-generation cephalosporins. The use of corticosteroids remains controversial. Although dexamethasone significantly reduced death and neurologic sequelae in European adults, results in the tropical setting have been less clear. In two trials in children (one in Malawi, one in Latin America), and one trial in adults (in Malawi), dexamethasone failed to make a difference[29–31]; however in a trial in adults in Vietnam, dexamethasone did reduce mortality and disability in those with microbiologically proven bacterial meningitis.[32]

In *tuberculous meningitis*, corticosteroids are used to minimize complications arising from chronic inflammation and arachnoiditis, particularly at the base of the brain, and have recently been shown to reduce the risk of death.[33] In an accessible *brain abscess*, CT- or MRI-guided aspiration and antibiotics are the treatment of choice. Anaerobic coverage is usually indicated, since mixed anaerobic infections are often the cause of such abscesses and may not be recovered from the abscess for technical reasons. Surgical drainage and excision of the abscess cavity may be necessary when aspiration is not feasible or is contraindicated. Long-term therapy with antibiotics is usual and in rare cases may be the only treatment required.

In *cerebral malaria*, intravenous antimalarials, such as quinine or quinidine, are often used, though drugs such as artemether, based on the Chinese herb qinghaosu, are being used increasingly.[34] Concomitant glucose infusions are important in preventing drug-induced hypoglycemia, which could easily be confused with cerebral malaria. In *cerebral neurocysticercosis*, both oral praziquantel and albendazole treatment are effective in reducing the number and size of brain cysts. Adjunctive treatment is largely symptomatic; *epilepsy* is treated with anticonvulsants, *hydrocephalus* by ventricular shunting, and *cerebral edema* with dexamethasone. *Postinfection* or *postimmunization encephalomyelitis* usually responds incompletely to corticosteroids. Acute cerebellar ataxia following malaria usually responds completely to treatment with corticosteroids. *Acute paraplegia* resulting from transverse myelitis due to viral infections or specifically, HTLV-1, may respond to treatment with corticosteroids, but paraplegia resulting from vacuolar myelopathy from advanced HIV infection is not treated with corticosteroids but may respond to successful antiretroviral treatment. *Tuberculous radiculomyelitis* responds to antituberculous chemotherapy, but *psoas abscess* or *vertebral collapse* may also require drainage, laminectomy, and decompression of the spinal cord. *Tetanus* is treated with tetanus immunoglobulin to neutralize the toxin, metronidazole, wound treatment to kill the causative bacteria, and large doses of intravenous benzodiazepines to relax the involved muscles; magnesium sulfate may reduce the need for benzodiazepines, but has no impact on outcome.[35] In severe cases, tracheostomy, neuromuscular junction blockade, and mechanical ventilation may be necessary.

Whatever the cause of CNS infection, in addition to treating the specific condition attention should be paid to the nonspecific complications and sequelae. In particular, secondary pneumonias are common in patients with reduced consciousness; bedsores, spasticity, and contractures are problems in patients bed-bound for any length of time. Good nursing care and physiotherapy can make an enormous difference to the eventual outcome.

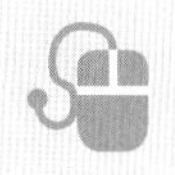

Access the complete reference list online at
http://www.expertconsult.com

CHAPTER 137

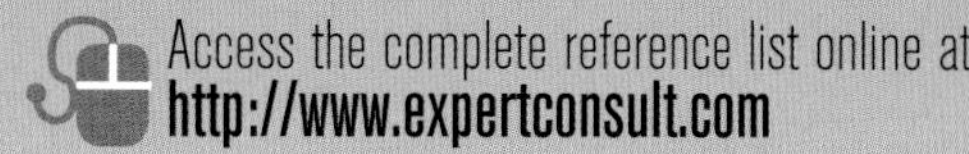
Access the complete reference list online at
http://www.expertconsult.com

Approach to the Patient in the Tropics with Anemia

Saad H. Abdalla • Geoffrey Pasvol

INTRODUCTION

Anemia is a major problem in tropical areas because of a high prevalence of infections and infestations, the presence of dietary deficiencies, and inherited red blood cell (RBC) disorders causing anemia. Limited resources compel the physician to rely on observational and clinical skills rather than complex laboratory tests. This chapter outlines a rational approach to management of anemia in these challenging and diverse settings.

DEFINITION

Anemia can be defined as a hemoglobin (Hb) value below the reference range for age, sex, and ethnic origin. In tropical countries, reference ranges are difficult to define. Ideally, a reference range should be established by measuring Hb in healthy volunteers. The definition of a healthy volunteer is difficult in this setting, especially under conditions in which groups with asymptomatic parasitic or inherited disease constitute a large proportion of the population.

The World Health Organization (WHO) Definition of Anemia[1]

In Children

- 6 months to 2 years: Hb less than 11 g/dL
- 2–12 years: Hb less than 12 g/dL

In Adults

- 13 g/dL for males
- 12 g/dL for nonpregnant females
- 11 g/dL for pregnant females

A definition of anemia with a more practical approach for use in a tropical setting is shown in ***Table 137.1***. In addition, consideration needs to be given as to whether anemia develops acutely or over a more prolonged period (chronic). Acute anemia may demand intervention, such as blood transfusion, whereas compensatory mechanisms may render these interventions unnecessary in the chronic anemias.

PATHOPHYSIOLOGY

Anemia leads to a reduction in oxygen-carrying capacity and in work performance with important economic consequences for the individual and society. Examples of these have been well demonstrated in various settings involving, e.g., sugar cutters in Guatemala,[2] latex tappers in Indonesia,[3] and tea pickers in Sri Lanka.[4] In all three, the reduction in work capacity was reversed by correction of anemia. When more severe, anemia can lead to morbidity and sometimes death.

Interactions between anemia and infection are complex and subject to controversy. A full description cannot be provided here, but three major arguments emerge[5]:

1. Anemia increases the risk of infection shown in iron-deficient individuals and in subjects with megaloblastic anemia, but it can be argued that infected subjects utilize or lose folate more rapidly and the association is that of increased need rather than increased susceptibility. Several studies demonstrated reduction in cell-mediated immunity in iron and folate deficiency.[5]
2. Correction of anemia may have a deleterious effect on infection. This concept has been proposed as a possible cause of exacerbation of malaria in refed malnourished patients. Other factors, such as the increased incidence of malaria and bacterial infections in refugees, may be due to exposure to pathogens to which they have no immunity. The subject is complex: see Abdalla.[6]
3. Anemia may be a nonspecific protective response to infection or perhaps a byproduct of that response. This view has been proposed in the context of the anemia of chronic disease (ACD). The inflammatory response to infection is important as a nonspecific protective mechanism but also results in ACD.[7]

MECHANISM AND CLASSIFICATION OF ANEMIA

Anemias can be classified in various ways. Three major etiologic factors are: (1) infections; (2) dietary deficiency; and (3) inherited disorders (***Box 137.1***). Pathogenesis may be multifactorial. A laboratory-oriented method is to classify anemias as to the Hb content (hypochromic or normochromic) and red cell size (microcytic, normocytic, or macrocytic).

CLINICAL APPROACH

Recognition of severe anemia is often easy clinically. Iron deficiency, often due to hookworm infestation,[8] and malaria are the two most common causes of anemia. Points in the history and clinical examination may help to narrow the diagnosis. Preschool children and women of child-bearing age, especially during pregnancy, are two susceptible groups; multiple factors may contribute.

HISTORY

Geographic locality is pertinent to malaria, hookworm infestation, tuberculosis, human immunodeficiency virus (HIV) infection, and other less frequent causes such as leishmaniasis and trypanosomiasis. Dietary practices are important:

- Hematinic, protein, and vitamin content of common staple local foods, seasonal variation and availability

Table 137.1 Practical Definition of Anemia Severity

Degree	Possible Consequences	Hemoglobin Level (g/dL)
Mild anemia	Minimal or no work or exercise intolerance	>10
Moderate anemia	Some impairment but still able to function	7–10
Severe anemia	Marked impairment of function but not at rest	4–7
Life-endangering anemia	Impending cardiac decompensation, dyspnea at rest	<4

Box 137.1 Major Causes of Anemia in the Tropics

Infection

Bacteria
- Severe acute or chronic bacterial sepsis
- Tuberculosis

Viruses
- Human immunodeficiency virus infection
- Parvovirus (in the presence of hemolytic anemia)

Protozoa
- Malaria
- Amebiasis
- Leishmaniasis
- Trypanosomiasis

Helminths
- Hookworm
- Schistosomiasis
- Trichuriasis

Dietary Deficiency
- Iron deficiency
- Folate deficiency
- Vitamin B_{12} deficiency
- Protein/calorie malnutrition

Inherited Disorders

Hemoglobinopathies
- Hemoglobin (Hb) variants: Hb S, C, D, E, etc.
- α- and β-thalassemia

Red blood cell enzyme deficiency
- Glucose-6-phosphate dehydrogenase deficiency

Red blood cell membrane defects (minor decrease in Hb only)
- Elliptocytosis, spherocytosis
- Southeast Asian (band III) ovalocytosis

- Local restrictive diets, such as vegetarianism
- Feeding practices for infants and young children (e.g., age at weaning and weaning foods)

The clinician needs to be aware of the local prevalence of Hb and other genetic RBC disorders, such as sickle cell anemia (SCA), thalassemia, glucose-6-phosphate dehydrogenase (G6PD) deficiency, and RBC membrane defects. Knowledge of the local epidemiology of malaria as well as drug resistance patterns are important, as is whether anemia has been present from birth, suggesting an inherited disorder, or is of recent onset. A detailed gastrointestinal history, particularly with regard to diet, abdominal pain, and the color and frequency of stool, is important. A history of fevers may suggest malaria, common in primigravidas and children aged less than 5 years. Mild jaundice may be present in hemolytic conditions. It is important to determine whether the jaundice is intermittent and whether precipitating factors are present, as occurs in G6PD-deficient patients. A family history may be relevant. Bone and joint pains suggest sickling disorders. In women of child-bearing age, parity and previous menstrual history are important. People with HIV infection are susceptible to anemia, which may be exacerbated by drugs such as antifolates.[9]

PHYSICAL EXAMINATION

Examination often yields little apart from pallor. A high-grade fever is suggestive of malaria. Koilonychia (spoon-shaped nails) and, less commonly, esophageal and pharyngeal webs suggests iron-deficiency anemia. Angular or atrophic stomatitis is seen in vitamin B_{12} or folate deficiency, but is not specific. Atrophic glossitis with jaundice occurs in megaloblastic anemias. Pallor and mild or moderate jaundice may point to a hemolytic anemia. Signs of peripheral neuropathy suggest vitamin B_{12} deficiency.

Splenomegaly is suggestive of malaria or typhoid fever but also visceral leishmaniasis, hyperreactive malarial splenomegaly, hemoglobinopathies, thalassemia, and lymphomas. In HIV disease cachexia, oral candidiasis, generalized lymphadenopathy, and thrombocytopenia may be suggestive.

Basic laboratory requirements for the diagnosis of anemia in the primary health care setting should include the following relatively simple tests:

1. Hb estimation will confirm and quantitate the degree of severity according to the criteria described previously (see *Table 137.1*), and facilitate the monitoring of treatment.
2. Blood film examination is one of the most useful single tests but requires investment of two types: a microscope of reasonable quality with an adequate light source and a person with appropriate training. Examination of blood smears (including a thick film) remains the gold standard in the diagnosis of the species and parasitemia in malaria. Occasionally, trypanosomes, microfilariae, or spirochetes may be seen on the film. The thin blood film provides a starting point in the diagnostic algorithm because it can be used to divide anemia into useful categories:
   a. Microcytic hypochromic anemia: the RBCs are small or there is an increase in the normal area of central pallor in the cells (normal, up to one-third of the cell diameter). Microcytic hypochromic anemia is most commonly seen in iron deficiency (*Fig. 137.1*), thalassemia (*Fig. 137.2*), and, in some cases of ACD.
   b. Normocytic, normochromic anemia is often found in ACD, which in a tropical setting is most often due to infection, but also in acute blood loss, hypersplenism, certain hemolytic anemias, and anemias due to the underproduction of RBCs (e.g., aplastic anemia and bone marrow infiltration).

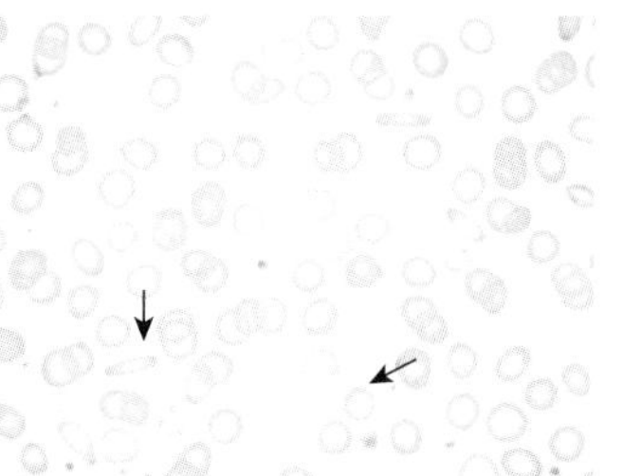

Figure 137.1 Severe iron-deficiency anemia. Peripheral blood film. Note the hypochromia and elongated red blood cell, sometimes referred to as a "pencil cell," typical of iron deficiency.

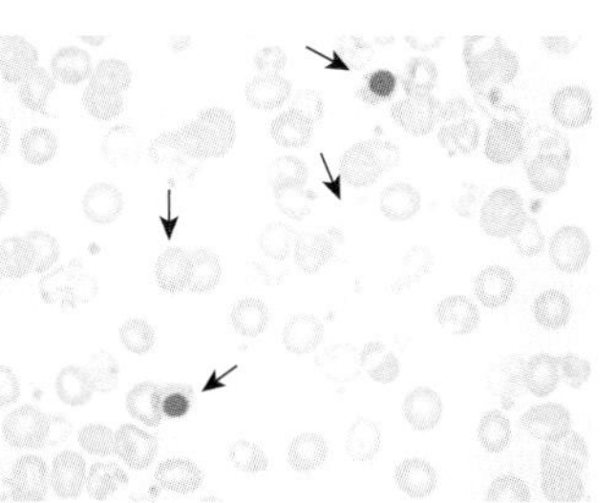

Figure 137.2 Thalassemia major. Blood film from an inadequately transfused patient with numerous nucleated red blood cells. There are a small number of poorly hemoglobinized red blood cells and some target cells, but the majority of red blood cells are normal ones from the transfusion.

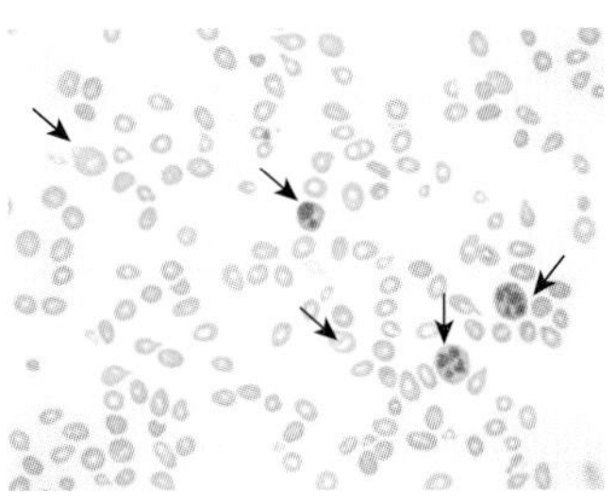

Figure 137.3 Severe megaloblastic anemia. Peripheral blood film showing poikilocytosis and an oval macrocyte. The two neutrophils are hypersegmented. There is also an abnormal megaloblast (thick arrow).

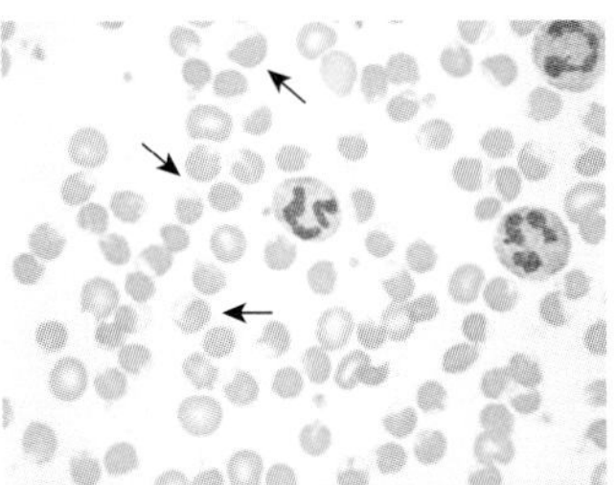

Figure 137.4 Blood film from a patient with infection and glucose-6-phosphate dehydrogenase deficiency showing numerous irregularly contracted red blood cells. These appearances are caused by oxidant damage to hemoglobin with retraction from the red cell membrane. The cells are called "hemighosts" or sometimes "blister cells."

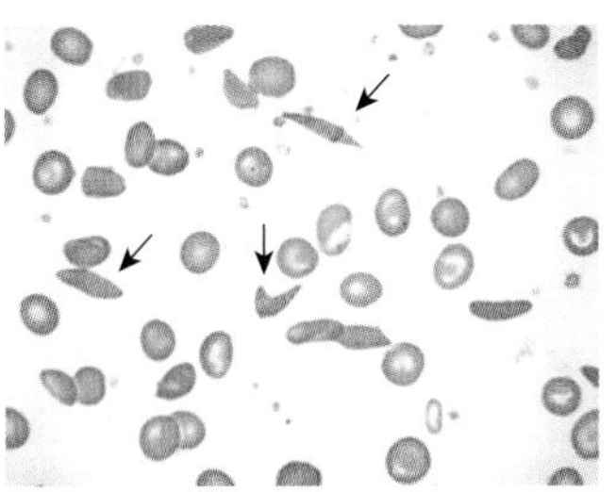

Figure 137.5 Sickle cell anemia. Peripheral blood film showing elongated red blood cells that have pointed ends and no central pallor. Not all cells have the classic curved sickle shape.

c. Macrocytic anemias may be of two types. Oval macrocytes and hypersegmented neutrophils (neutrophils with more than five lobes or 5% with five lobes) are suggestive of a megaloblastic anemia, such as vitamin B_{12} or folate deficiency, whereas round macrocytes without hypersegmented neutrophils occur in the nonmegaloblastic macrocytic anemias seen in excess alcohol consumption, liver disease, hypothyroidism, and other disorders (***Fig. 137.3***).

The blood film may also demonstrate:

a. Polychromasia: (diffuse bluish RBC discoloration) which correlates with the presence of reticulocytes. Polychromasia suggests an adequate response to anemia in hemorrhage, hemolysis, and hematinic replacement. The absence of polychromasia in the face of anemia suggests dietary deficiency or marrow suppression due to some other cause.
b. Abnormal RBC shape: irregularly contracted RBCs suggest oxidant damage as in acute hemolysis (***Fig. 137.4***); sickle cells in SCA (***Fig. 137.5***), RBC fragments in microangiopathic hemolyic anemias (***Fig. 137.6***). Spherocytes in hereditary spherocytosis (***Fig. 137.7***) or other abnormal cells include elliptocytes (in hereditary elliptocytosis), pencil cells (in iron

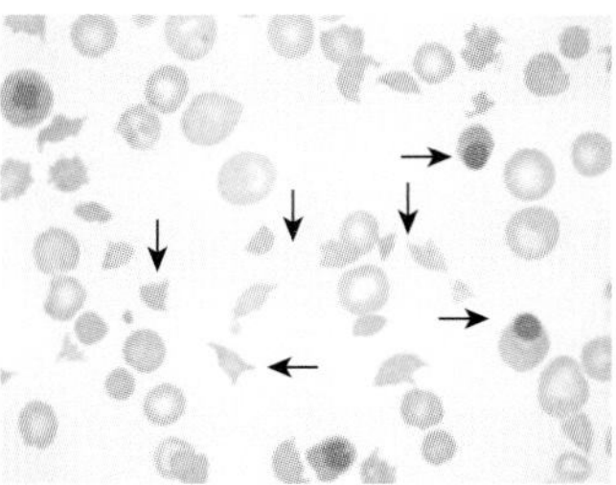

Figure 137.6 Microangiopathic hemolytic anemia (MAHA) showing numerous red cell fragments due to mechanical hemolysis and also numerous nucleated red cells and polychromasia in response to the hemolysis. MAHA can be accompanied by a coagulopathy as in hemolytic–uremic syndrome, or platelet consumption without coagulopathy, as in thrombotic thrombocytopenic purpura.

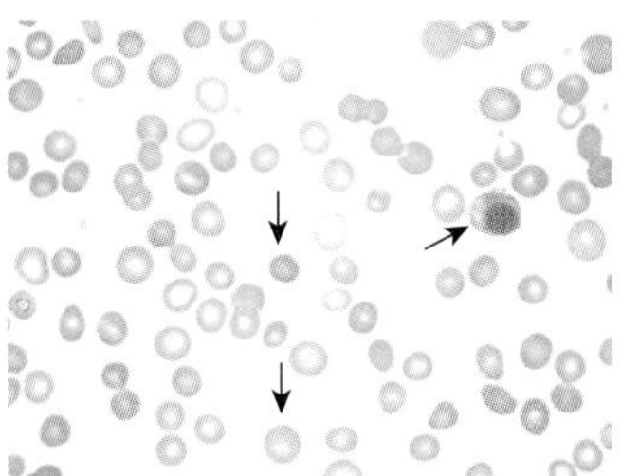

Figure 137.7 Hereditary spherocytosis. Blood film showing spherocytes, round cells with lack of central pallor, and polychromasia and nucleated red cells due to accelerated red cell turnover.

deficiency; ***Fig. 137.1***), and teardrop cells (in thalassemias and marrow infiltration, e.g., myelofibrosis or bone marrow secondaries).

3. Microscopic examination of the stool for cysts and ova of parasites.
4. Tests for fecal occult blood to exclude gastrointestinal hemorrhage.
5. A therapeutic trial: where resources are limited, it may be cost-effective or necessary to embark on a therapeutic trial to treat anemia. Such a trial may involve an antimalarial, iron, or both.

FURTHER INVESTIGATIONS

Undiagnosed or unresponsive cases of anemia or those requiring special treatment, such as blood transfusion, may be referred to a center with additional facilities, such as:

1. Electronic cell count: this will provide RBC indices: mean corpuscular volume (MCV), RBC count, mean corpuscular Hb (MCH), mean corpuscular Hb concentration (MCHC), a white blood cell count (with or without a differential), and platelet count. The RBC indices will confirm whether the anemia is microcytic, hypochromic; normocytic, or normochromic, or macrocytic.
2. Bone marrow examination: this needs to be interpreted by someone with special training. The information obtained is not always diagnostic, but will assist in defining marrow cellularity and provide an estimate of body iron stores. The marrow will indicate whether erythropoiesis is normoblastic, micronormoblastic, megaloblastic, or dysplastic. Marrow infiltrations, e.g., by malignancy or infection can be detected. Marrow examination will also help define the maturation of the myeloid and megakaryocytic series. Findings in some common conditions are as follows:
   a. Microcytic hypochromic anemias
      - Iron deficiency demonstrates micronormoblasts (***Fig. 137.8***), with absent iron stores on Perls' staining (an iron-specific reagent) and no hemosiderin granules in erythroblasts.

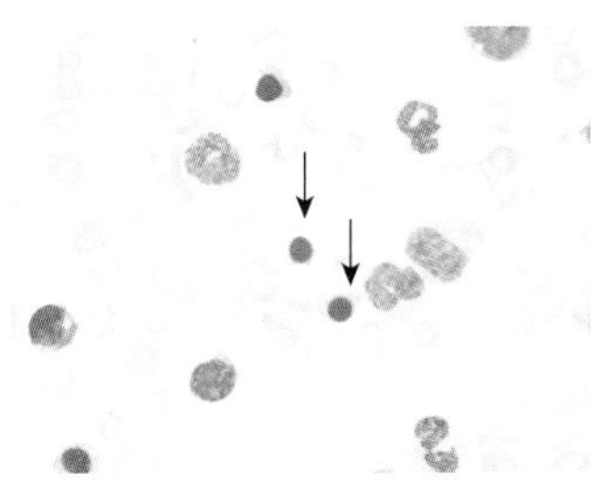

Figure 137.8 Severe iron-deficiency anemia. Bone marrow film showing micronormoblastic erythropoiesis (arrows). The changes are seen in intermediate and late erythroblasts and consist of cells that are smaller than normal with poor irregular cytoplasmic hemoglobinization.

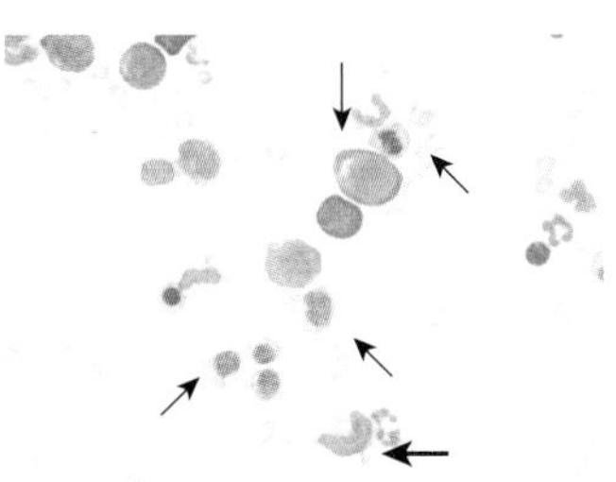

Figure 137.9 Severe megaloblastic anemia. Bone marrow film showing megaloblastic changes of the erythroid series consisting of erythroblasts that are larger than normal, asynchrony of maturation in which the cytoplasm is more mature than the nucleus, and a rather grainy erythroblast nucleus. In addition, there is a giant metamyelocyte (thick arrow) that is twice the size of a normal metamyelocyte and has a contorted nucleus.

- In the thalassemias, the erythroblasts show poor hemoglobinization with hemosiderin granules present in erythroblasts.
- ACD may be hypochromic with increased iron stores but an absence of hemosiderin granules in erythroblasts – the so-called "iron utilization block."
- Sideroblastic anemias show increased iron stores with characteristic "ring sideroblasts."

b. Macrocytic anemias can be classified into:
- Megaloblastic anemia, with megaloblastic changes in the erythroblasts and giant metamyelocytes due to vitamin B_{12} or folate deficiency (*Fig. 137.9*).
- Normoblastic hemopoiesis, as occurs in liver and thyroid disease, and alcoholism.

c. Normocytic anemias, to establish cellularity:
- A hypocellular bone marrow is characteristic of aplastic anemia consequent to drugs such as chloramphenicol or industrial pollutants or toxins.
- A selective reduction in erythropoiesis but with normal myelopoiesis is found in parvovirus infection and other more rare causes, e.g., selective RBC aplasia.
- A normocellular bone marrow is found in a variety of anemias.
- A hypercellular bone marrow is found in hemolytic anemias, leukemias, megaloblastic anemias, and dyserythropoietic anemias, congenital or acquired.

3. Investigation of hemoglobinopathies: important in geographic areas where Hb disorders are common. Tests include:
   a. The sickle solubility test (using sodium metabisulfite) is based on the insolubility of HbS. Hb electrophoresis should be carried out in cases with a positive solubility test to distinguish between patients with sickle cell trait (AS), SCA, or other compound heterozygotes such as S-β-thalassemia and SC. The sickle solubility test does not detect sickle Hb at low levels (<20%) and is therefore of no use in screening infants up to 6 months of age.
   b. Hb electrophoresis will confirm the presence of Hb S and other major Hb variants, such as HbC, D, and E, and also distinguish between hetero- and homozygotes. Hb electrophoresis will also detect fetal Hb (HbF) levels higher than approximately 2%.
   c. Quantitation of HbF using an alkali denaturation method is important in the diagnosis of β-thalassemia major and intermedia.
   d. Quantitation of HbA_2 using a column elution method is important to diagnose β-thalassemia trait – higher than 3.5% in carriers. Accurate diagnosis is relevant where genetic counseling is important in preventing β-thalassemia major.
4. A low serum ferritin or a low serum iron with a raised transferrin suggests iron-deficiency anemia, whereas a low serum iron and low transferrin suggest secondary anemia (e.g., to infections or inflammation).
5. Vitamin B_{12} and RBC folate assays: serum vitamin B_{12} levels are usually low in megaloblastic anemias due to vitamin B_{12} deficiency, but can be low without anemia in vegans. RBC folate is a more stable measure of storage folate than labile serum folate and shows a moderate to severe reduction in folate deficiency. Care must be taken in interpreting the results because folate can also be reduced in vitamin B_{12} deficiency.
6. HIV testing is crucial: a positive test has considerable management implications.

IMPORTANT ANEMIAS IN THE TROPICS

Anemia of Malaria

In areas of high endemicity, severe and sometimes fatal anemia associated with malaria occurs in children up to 5 years of age.[10,11] Severe anemia most commonly occurs in a younger age group (often <2 years) than in those suffering from cerebral malaria. In contrast, in areas where malaria is epidemic rather than endemic, the age distribution of malarial anemia is less well defined and may also occur in adult semi-immune individuals, especially in primigravidas. The importance of anemia as a cause of death in malaria may well be underestimated because of the difficulty in diagnosis.[12] Attributing malaria as the cause of anemia in a tropical setting is often difficult. Some sources have included a minimal arbitrary Hb and parasitemia (<5 g/dL in the presence of parasitemia >10 000/μL) to define severe malarial anemia.

The pathogenesis of the anemia of malaria is both complex and multifactorial but is largely due to hemolysis of both infected and uninfected RBCs – the decline in Hb is often far in excess of what can be accounted for by the loss of infected RBCs alone.[13] The anemia of malaria is usually normochromic, normocytic.

Two clinical patterns predominate: severe acute malaria, in which anemia supervenes,[14] and anemia that has developed usually over a prolonged period of time.[10] In the first, patients suffering a severe acute attack of malaria, and seen early after the onset of clinical symptoms, are initially not anemic and without splenomegaly. However, anemia may develop rapidly during the course of infection, which has been associated with a shortened survival of uninfected RBCs, sometimes well after parasites have disappeared from the blood film.[15] The cause of anemia in these acute episodes is probably multifactorial and may include, in addition to hemolysis, inhibition of erythropoietin secretion, which is low and associated with an initial poor reticulocyte response.[16]

The second pattern of malarial anemia occurs particularly in endemic areas.[10] These patients, usually children, become gradually anemic, often without a clear history of repeated attacks of malaria.[17] The history may be one of intermittent fevers and general symptoms of ill health occurring insidiously over weeks rather than days. Splenomegaly of varying degree

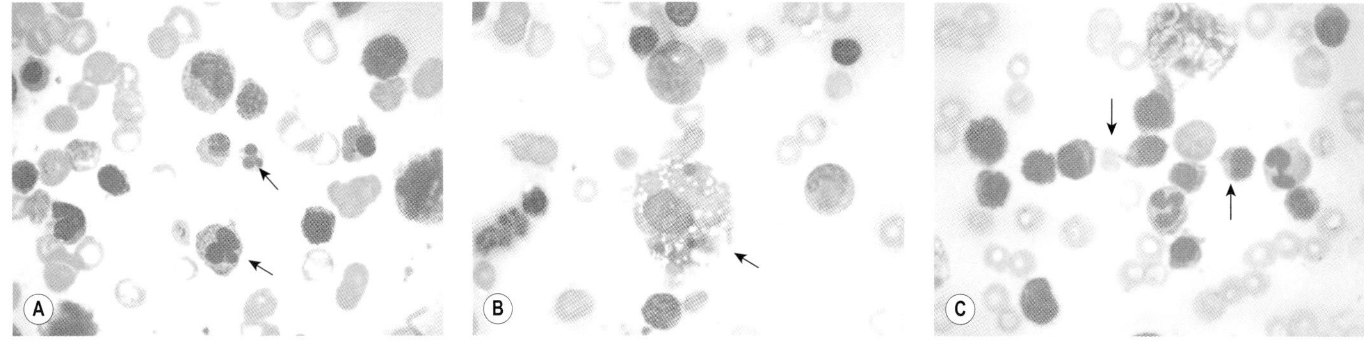

Figure 137.10 Bone marrow of a child with chronic malaria. **(A)** Severe dyserythropoiesis with irregular nuclear lobulation of erythroblasts (karyorrhexis). **(B)** Macrophage showing phagocytosis. **(C)** There is an increase in the proportion of erythroblasts showing intracytoplasmic bridges.

may be present and the peripheral blood film may show minimal parasitemia with only the presence of gametocytes and malarial pigment within phagocytic cells. The bone marrow often shows the picture of dyserythropoiesis,[10] with multinuclearity of erythroid precursors, mitotic figures, and intercytoplasmic bridging between dividing cells (*Fig. 137.10*). In functional terms, these appearances are associated with ineffective erythropoiesis (i.e., the marrow is active but not producing RBCs). Unlike the acute situation, erythropoietin levels are increased.[18]

Great difficulty remains in attributing the relative roles of each mechanism to the anemia of malaria, such as intravascular hemolysis, extravascular clearance of RBCs, and marrow dysfunction. The major mechanisms are RBC destruction and decreased RBC production. The former includes loss of infected cells by rupture or phagocytosis, removal of uninfected cells due to antibody sensitization or other physicochemical membrane changes, and increased reticuloendothelial activity, particularly in the spleen and bone marrow.[10,11] Shortened RBC survival may persist well after parasite clearance[15] and may be related to reduced RBC deformability.[19] Decreased production tends to predominate in acute infections and dyserythropoiesis in more prolonged infections.[20]

Eradication of the malarial parasite is paramount in management. Malaria on its own does not result in iron or folate deficiency, although there is evidence that children given iron but not folate at the time of an acute attack have higher mean Hb levels at follow-up.[21] Blood transfusion may be required in selected severe cases, although most patients have a brisk increase in Hb levels with antimalarial treatment.[22] There is insufficient evidence concerning whether giving blood routinely to children with severe anemia reduces mortality.[23] A suggested guideline for transfusion in severe malarial anemia, based on Hb level, a safe blood supply, and the presence of severe complications (notably respiratory distress), has been proposed.[24] Insecticide-treated bed nets may have a role to play in prevention.[25,26]

Anemia of Human Immunodeficiency Virus Infection

Anemia is common in HIV infection and present in almost all with acquired immunodeficiency syndrome (AIDS).[9,27] The prevalence of anemia in HIV infection is said to vary greatly, from 1.3% to 95%, depending on definition and other factors such as age, sex, pregnancy, and stage of the disease.[28] The anemia is more serious in women, children, and injecting drug users, and with more advanced disease. Anemia and its severity are predictors of mortality and risk of progression to AIDS in adults and children.[29] The anemia is often normochromic and normocytic, with low reticulocyte counts and erythropoietin levels but normal or increased iron stores and serum ferritin levels. The cause is multifactorial and complex. The anemia is more severe in the presence of mycobacterial (*Mycobacterium tuberculosis* and *M. avium* complex), fungal (e.g., cryptococcal) and parvoviral B19 infection, lymphoma, and some drugs. Important drugs are the antiviral drug zidovudine, but also other anti-infective agents, such as dapsone, sulfonamides, primaquine, isoniazid, rifampicin, pyrimethamine, and trimethoprim. Blood loss occurs in gastrointestinal Kaposi's sarcoma, cytomegalovirus, or lymphoma.

Anemia responds to effective antiretroviral therapy. Zidovudine should be avoided. There is evidence that administration of recombinant erythropoietin may improve Hb levels and reduce transfusion requirements.[30] It is important to exclude other causes of anemia, such as malaria and iron deficiency.

Box 137.2 Causes of Iron Deficiency in the Tropics

Reduced Intake	Other Causes Found Worldwide
Late weaning	Hiatal hernia
Poor diet	Peptic ulcer
Increased Demand	Aspirin
Growth	Hemorrhoids
Childhood	Malignancy
Adolescence	**Reduced Absorption**
Pregnancy	Malabsorption
Blood loss	Tuberculosis
Menstruation	Lymphoma
Gastrointestinal	Giardiasis
Hookworm	Bacterial overgrowth
Schistosomiasis	Celiac disease (uncommon)
Helicobacter pylori infection	
Trichuriasis	

Nutritional Anemias

Nutritional anemias result from discrepancy between the supply of and demand for specific nutritional elements.

Iron-deficiency anemia is the most common cause of anemia worldwide[31]; the major causes are shown in ***Box 137.2***. This deficiency predominates because of the extremely tight regulation of iron absorption by the intestinal mucosa and because of the generally poor bioavailability of iron from most diets in tropical areas. Local factors may contribute to negative iron balance, such as hookworm, schistosomiasis, and other gut infestations. Iron status and iron deficiency may be evaluated using a number of indicators (see ***Box 137.2***).

The differential diagnosis of a hypochromic anemia may require additional investigations, such as HbA_2 estimation (to exclude β-thalassemia trait) or HbF estimation (supportive of a diagnosis of β-thalassemia major or intermedia), or by bone marrow examination (***Table 137.2***). The true incidence of iron deficiency may be overestimated or underestimated depending on definition. A single indicator is often unreliable and extensive studies may be difficult to carry out. Often, a therapeutic trial is the only practical management strategy.

Table 137.2 Differential Diagnosis of Hypochromic Anemia in the Tropics

Indices	IDA	ACD	Thalassemia Trait (α or β)
Degree of anemia	Any	Rarely <9 g/dL	Mild
MCV	Reduced (<76 fL or μm^3)	Normal or reduced	Very reduced
MCH, MCHC	Reduced	Reduced	Reduced
RBC count	Normal or reduced	Normal or reduced	Increased
RDW	Increased	Normal or increased	Normal or increased
Blood film	Microcytic, hypochromic	Microcytic, hypochromic; may be normochromic, normocytic	Microcytic, hypochromic; teardrop cells, basophilic stippling, target cells
Serum iron	Reduced	Normal or reduced	Normal
Serum transferrin	Increased	Reduced	Normal
Iron-binding saturation (%)	Very low	Low	Normal
Serum ferritin	Reduced	Normal or increased	Normal
Bone marrow	Mildly hypocellular	Normocellular or hypocellular	Mildly hypercellular
	Micronormoblastic erythropoiesis	Hypercellular when neutrophil leukocytosis is present	Some dyserythropoiesis
	Absent marrow iron	Marrow iron present	Present
Serum transferrin receptor	Increased levels specific for iron deficiency	Normal	Normal
Response to therapeutic trial of iron replacement	Good	None except when IDA and ACD coexist	Potential iron overload
Other		Raised ESR	

IDA, iron-deficiency anemia; ACD, anemia of chronic disease; MCV, mean corpuscular volume; MCH, mean corpuscular hemoglobin; MCHC, mean corpuscular hemoglobin concentration; RBC, red blood cell; RDW, red blood cell distribution width (index); ESR, erythrocyte sedimentation rate.

Folate Deficiency

Folate is found in most foodstuffs, especially liver, meat, green vegetables, and some fruits, and is destroyed by prolonged boiling. Absorption occurs throughout the small intestine.[2] Folate deficiency is rarely due to dietary deficiency and may be due to increased utilization, e.g., in pregnancy, lactation, and malabsorption states. Folate is essential for methyl group transfer and nucleic acid synthesis. Deficiency manifests as megaloblastic anemia and also leads to mucosal atrophy.

Serum folate is labile and reflects a transit pool of folate that may be depressed to very low levels rapidly on a deficient diet. RBC folate, on the other hand, represents a storage pool formed during erythropoiesis and changes more slowly after deprivation. Stores last 4 or 5 months, after which deficiency occurs. The diagnosis of anemia due to folate deficiency is based on a macrocytic anemia with oval macrocytes and hypersegmented neutrophils on blood film and a megaloblastic bone marrow together with a low RBC folate.

Folate deficiency may arise acutely during pregnancy, during acute alcohol intake with a poor diet, and in patients in intensive care. This picture may also be seen when patients with borderline folate stores are given antifolate drugs such as sulfonamides and antimalarials, e.g., pyrimethamine and proguanil. Folate deficiency is treated with 5 mg/day folic acid. This pharmacologic dose is well absorbed. Prophylactic folate should be given in pregnancy and to patients with chronic hemolytic anemias such as SCA.

Vitamin B_{12} Deficiency

Vitamin B_{12} deficiency is not a major problem in the tropics; there are some situations in which its recognition is important. These include areas where veganism is common for religious or other reasons. Vitamin B_{12} deficiency may also occur in abdominal tuberculosis when the terminal ileum is involved. Pernicious anemia is said to be rare in tropical countries, although there are no studies of pernicious anemia in Africa other than case reports that suggest that the condition may occur at a much earlier age than in northern Europe.[32]

Deficiency of vitamin B_{12} can lead to megaloblastic anemia, symmetrical polyneuropathy, and, less frequently, gonadal dysfunction and glossitis. Subacute degeneration of the cord may ensue.

Anemia of Chronic Disease

ACD describes a normocytic or sometimes a microcytic, hypochromic anemia that occurs in patients with infectious, inflammatory, or neoplastic disease.[7,33–35] Important causes include infections such as pneumonia or septicemia, chronic infections such as tuberculosis and HIV infection, renal impairment and only rarely autoimmune disorders such as rheumatoid arthritis and systemic lupus erythematosus.

Pathogenesis

ACD is characterized by underproduction of RBCs; the reticulocyte count is usually low. The bone marrow is normocellular or hypocellular, but occasionally hypercellular due to increased granulocytic activity (see *Table 137.2*). The pathogenesis of ACD is complex, but the cause is an immune-driven process with release of proinflammatory cytokines and activation of cells of the immune system. There is dysregulation of iron homeostasis, erythropoietin production, erythroid cell proliferation, and a reduction in red cell life span.[36] Dysregulation of iron metabolism is seen with an increase of serum ferritin and a reduction in serum iron levels. At the cellular level there is a block in the incorporation of iron into erythroblasts with an increase in macrophage iron.

More recently the molecular basis of this block has been elucidated.[36] The macrophage plays an important role in the regulation of iron in erythropoiesis. Macrophages obtain iron either by erythrophagocytosis of senescent cells, through transferrin–transferrin receptors, induced by interleukin-10 (IL-10), or through a transmembrane protein the divalent metal transporter (DMT), induced by interferon-γ. Increased production of these cytokines leads to increase in macrophage iron as erythrophagocytosis, and iron transport into macrophages through transferrin receptor route via the DMT-1 route is also increased. Release of iron from macrophages is controlled by another transmembrane protein, ferroportin 1. A soluble acute-phase protein hepcidin, produced by hepatocytes, has a negative effect on ferroportin and also on intestinal absorption of iron. In addition to the above, IL-1, interferon-γ and tumor necrosis factor-α lead to an inhibition of erythropoiesis.[36]

ACD can lead to diagnostic difficulties, especially when iron deficiency coexists. The ferritin can be in the normal range and diagnosis requires measurement of serum iron and transferrin to elucidate further.

Management

ACD resolves after treatment of the underlying condition. In untreatable conditions or where there is limited response or in the initial phases, other approaches can be used, such as blood transfusion. Despite low serum iron, administration of iron is of limited or no benefit. ACD responds to recombinant erythropoietin,[36] but this treatment is often restricted by limited resources.

INHERITED RED BLOOD CELL DISORDERS

There is a high prevalence of RBC genetic disorders in tropical areas where malaria is or has been endemic. Carriers of these disorders are relatively protected against malaria. The "malaria hypothesis" proposes that the protective benefit of the carrier state leads to a better survival advantage than either the normal or affected homozygote.

The majority of these disorders lead to hemolytic anemia, e.g., sickling disorders, the thalassemia syndromes, and G6PD deficiency.

Sickling Disorders

Sickle cell anemia (SCA) is a major cause of morbidity and mortality in children in rural Africa.[37–39] A single DNA base substitution leads to an amino acid substitution from valine to glutamic acid in position 6 of the β globin chain. This causes a major change in the solubility of HbS under hypoxic conditions, leading to the formation of "tactoids" – elongated crystalline structures that can lead to irreversible RBC sickling. SCA occurs in homozygotes for the sickle gene. The precipitating factors for sickling include infections, hypoxia, and dehydration, but there may not be an obvious precipitating cause.

Other milder sickling disorders include the coinheritance of HbS with β^+- or β^0-thalassemia (i.e., HbS β-thalassemia) or HbC trait (Hb SC) or HbD (Hb SD). There is thus major variability due to the interaction of a variety of genotypes, the level of HbF, interaction with α-thalassemia, unknown genetic factors, and environmental factors (e.g., altitude).

The first manifestation of the disease usually occurs after 6 months of life, most commonly a dactylitis (***Box 137.3***). As the child grows, other manifestations include painful crises due to vascular occlusion in bone and sometimes other organs, such as the brain, gastrointestinal tract, and lung. The typical crisis is due to multiple painful microinfarcts in bone. More serious complications include sequestration crises in the lungs, spleen, or, less commonly, the brain, ranging from minor strokes to repeated infarcts and major cerebral infarcts. Children frequently die at an early age from SCA, often with sepsis. Patients with SCA are especially susceptible to infection with *Streptococcus pneumoniae* and *Salmonella* spp. Heterozygotes with sickle cell trait are not anemic and rarely symptomatic, except with travel in unpressurized aircraft and during anesthesia.

Box 137.3 Clinical Manifestations of Sickle Cell Anemia

Bone Marrow and Bone

Expansion of hematopoiesis leading to:
- Dactylitis (hand and foot syndrome), especially at 4–6 months of age
- Prognathism
- Bossing of the skull
- Chronic hemolytic anemia
- Painful crises due to microinfarction of bone
- Osteomyelitis, often due to *Salmonella* spp.

Lungs

- Acute chest syndrome with breathlessness, reduced oxygen saturation (<70%), and radiographic changes
- Lung infections often complicated; if hypoxia results, this may precipitate a crisis
- Ultimately may lead to pulmonary fibrosis and cor pulmonale

Heart

- Cardiomegaly due to chronic anemia
- Congestive cardiac failure in later life

Spleen

- Hypoactivity leading to susceptibility to infection, including encapsulated organisms and malaria
- Acute sequestration crisis with rapid enlargement and anemia, especially in infancy, and which tends to recur
- Chronic splenic enlargement with hypersplenism (anemia, leukopenia, and thrombocytopenia)

Liver and Gallbladder

- Acute liver sequestration
- Gallstones

Kidneys

- Renal tubular defect leads to inability to concentrate urine, leading to enuresis
- Dehydration, which may precipitate crises
- Tubular necrosis
- Intermittent hematuria
- Chronic renal failure

Brain

- Recurrent cerebral infarction (may be silent)
- Stroke

Skin

- Chronic leg ulcers (seen especially in Jamaica)

Management

Treatment of acute crises in SCA involves adequate hydration, oxygenation, and analgesia; vigorous treatment of the underlying infection; keeping patients warm in cold weather; and reversal of acidosis. More severe complications, such as acute anemia due to splenic sequestration, increased hemolysis, parvovirus infection, or lung sequestration, are treated with transfusion when the Hb falls below 5 g/dL. Where the Hb is higher and in the presence of certain complications, such as chest syndrome, priapism, and severe abdominal sickling, exchange transfusions are advocated to reduce the HbS percentage to less than 20% and to continue with monthly transfusion.

Pain management is important; pain is often severe and may require opiate analgesia. The particular opiate used (e.g., diamorphine or morphine) is dependent on local preference. Opiates have the disadvantage of a depressive effect on respiratory drive, which may worsen hypoxia, and potential addiction when used for repeated attacks. A study in Jamaica showed that even in the steady state a considerable degree of hypoxia may be found in patients with sickling disorders.[40] Nonsteroidal anti-inflammatory drugs may be useful for bone pain provided there are no contraindications to their use.

Prevention of Complications

Prevention of complications depends on the recognition and avoidance of precipitating factors of acute attacks, such as exposure to cold (e.g., swimming), dehydration, infections, altitude, travel in nonpressurized aircraft, anesthesia, and extremes of physical activity. Parents and patients should be taught to recognize the manifestations of disease, such as dactylitis or splenic sequestration early. Because these patients are effectively autosplenectomized, they should receive pneumococcal, *Haemophilus influenzae* type b and meningococcal vaccinations as well as prophylactic antimalarials, sleep under impregnated bed nets, and receive early malaria treatment. Hepatitis B vaccination should be considered, especially when patients require transfusion and donors are not screened. Folate 5 mg/day should also be given because of high RBC turnover.

Hydroxycarbamide (previously known as hydroxyurea) reduces the frequency of painful crisis, chest syndrome, and transfusion requirements in both adults and children with severe sickle cell disease. Hydroxycarbamide also appears to improve growth and possibly prevent hyposplenism in children. It has not been proven to prevent stroke or avascular necrosis in joints, and is the subject of ongoing trials in Europe and North America.[37] Caution is advised, however, because its long-term profile is unknown. For guidelines on the use of hydroxycarbamide in SCA, see ***Box 137.4***.

Box 137.4 Hydroxycarbamide (Hydroxyurea) in Sickle Cell Disease

Patient Exclusion Criteria

Regular transfusion regimen

Abnormal liver function tests (aspartate aminotransferase or alanine aminotransferase >2 × upper limit of normal)

Inability to attend clinic regularly for follow-up

Patient Eligibility

Patients (Hb SS or Sβ^0-thalassemia, not Hb SC) with a severe clinical course may be offered hydroxylcarbamide, i.e., with

- Three admissions with painful crisis within 1 year, or
- Frequent days of pain at home, leading to a lot of time off work, or
- Recurrent acute chest syndrome

The following predict a more severe clinical course and are additional reasons to consider offering hydroxylcarbamide:

- Steady-State Values
  - Hb <7 g/dL
  - White blood cell count >15 × 10^9/L
  - HbF < 6%
- Renal insufficiency due to sickle cell disease

Dose and Monitoring

Start at 15 mg/kg/day (to the nearest 500 mg/day). If no or poor response, increase dose by increments of 5 mg/kg/day every 4 weeks (max. 30 mg/kg/day)

Monitor full blood count, Hb F %, and reticulocytes every 1 or 2 weeks initially, then every 4 weeks when on a stable dose

Monitor biochemistry profile (hydroxyurea has renal excretion and hepatic toxicity)

Thalassemia Syndromes

The thalassemias are a group of disorders in which there is reduced production of one of the two main globin chains, α or β, leading to α- or β-thalassemia, respectively. Thalassemias are widely distributed throughout Africa, the Mediterranean, the Middle East, the Indian subcontinent, and Southeast Asia. β-Thalassemia is especially common in areas such as northern Thailand, Laos, and Vietnam. In these areas, there are complex interactions between these disorders and Hb E, a β-chain variant that is also underexpressed, leading to a thalassemia-like phenotype. In Africa, β-thalassemia occurs in the northern areas of West African countries such as Ghana and Liberia.

The underlying molecular genetic abnormalities of these disorders are complex. Each normal individual has four functioning α genes and two β genes. In α-thalassemia, one, two, or three of the α globin genes may be nonfunctional. Deletion of a single gene in one chromosome is labeled α^+-thalassemia and of two on the same chromosome as α^0. Homozygotes for α^0 (deletion of all four genes) lead to intrauterine or neonatal death from hydrops fetalis. In Hb H disease, α^0/α^+ double heterozygotes, three of the α globin genes are nonfunctional. In β-thalassemia, output from each β globin allele may be reduced (β^+) or absent (β^0). The underproduction of Hb leads to microcytic, hypochromic RBCs.

Globin chain imbalance results in the formation of tetramers of β chain (Hb H) in α-thalassemia or γ chain (Bart's Hb) in the fetus and neonate. In addition to microcytosis, anemia is made worse by ineffective erythropoiesis because of globin chain imbalance in β-thalassemia and by hemolysis in HbH disease since HbH is unstable.

Underexpression of α chains in α-thalassemia may sometimes also be caused by deletions involving gene expression control regions. In contrast, the majority of β chain defects are caused by single-base pair mutations, usually resulting in reduced or absent gene expression (β^+- or β^0-thalassemia) from the single β gene on each chromosome 11. Whatever the cause, underproduction of adult Hb leads to the formation of hypochromic, microcytic RBCs with reduced MCH. The other main thalassemic indices include an elevated RBC count, a low MCV and MCH, and a relatively less reduced MCHC.

Clinically, the thalassemias are grouped into three entities: minor, intermedia, and major:

1. In thalassemia minor, there is only a minor degree of hypochromic anemia (Hb 9–11 g/dL). Some patients may develop clinically significant anemia in certain circumstances, such as pregnancy. Subjects generally appear clinically normal. Examples are α^+ hetero- and homozygotes, α^- heterozygotes, β-thalassemia trait, and the Hb $A^{\text{Constant spring}}$ heterozygote. Diagnosis is made on routine RBC count, most commonly because of the low MCV, which may be confused with iron deficiency (see *Table 137.2*).
2. In thalassemia intermedia, there is a moderate hypochromic, microcytic anemia but the patient is not normally transfusion-dependent. Patients may become transfusion-dependent when exposed to stress. Examples of thalassemia intermedia include HbH disease and interaction between β^0-thalassemia and HbE trait and between β^0- and β^+-thalassemia. Splenomegaly is a common feature in thalassemia intermedia and hypersplenism may occur. Patients may have cardiomegaly and cardiac failure. Even in the absence of transfusion, iron overload results from increased dietary iron absorption due to increased erythropoiesis.
3. In thalassemia major (β^0 homozygotes) there is little or no production of HbA, and there is progressive anemia from a few months of age, leading to an Hb of less than 4 g/dL. In untreated or inadequately treated patients, increased erythropoiesis causes expansion of medullary bone, leading to features such as prognathism and bossing of the skull and hepatosplenomegaly. There is severe growth retardation and pathologic fractures. In untreated cases, death may occur in the first few years of life. Transfused patients may survive longer but develop iron overload with hypogonadism and secondary deposition of iron in the myocardium, pancreas, and liver, leading to death due to cardiac failure, diabetes mellitus, or liver failure.

Management

The cornerstones of management are:

1. Counseling and advice: in thalassemia trait the main problems are to differentiate from iron deficiency to avoid unnecessary and potentially harmful iron therapy and to provide counseling regarding prevention of pregnancy with a thalassemia major child.
2. Transfusion: in HbH disease, a chronic hemolytic state, episodes of acute hemolysis may occur, necessitating transfusion. In the case of thalassemia intermedia, monitoring is required perhaps at 6-month intervals in childhood and annually in adult life,[41] and transfusion may be needed during periods of stress. In thalassemia major, regular transfusions to maintain an Hb higher than 10 g/dL are needed to maintain normal growth and prevent bony deformities. Repeated transfusion carries the risk of iron overload, sensitization to white blood cells causing febrile reactions, and the possibility of transmission of infections such as hepatitis B and C and HIV.
3. Iron chelation with subcutaneous desferrioxamine infusion together with vitamin C: continuous iron chelation is also needed to prevent cardiac, hepatic, and endocrine organ deposition of iron, leading to dysfunction of these organs and ultimately death. This treatment regimen is often unaffordable.
4. Splenectomy: some patients with thalassemia intermedia or major develop hypersplenism with splenic enlargement and increasing anemia, leukopenia, and thrombocytopenia. These patients may require splenectomy. Indications for splenectomy include transfusion dependence, clinically significant thrombocytopenia, and the mechanical effects of the large spleen.
5. Some patients may develop cardiomegaly with compromised myocardial function leading to cardiac failure. Monitoring with chest radiography in the first instance and echocardiography, if available, may be helpful.

Glucose-6-Phosphate Dehydrogenase Deficiency

All cells contain G6PD, an enzyme catalyzing the conversion of glucose-6-phosphate to 6-phosphogluconate, producing reduced NADPH and leading to the five-carbon sugar ribose necessary for nucleotide synthesis. Reduced NADPH is essential to maintaining several intracellular protein and membrane sulfhydryl groups in their reduced state (e.g., glutathione). RBCs are particularly susceptible to oxidant stress because of their function in oxygen carriage.[41]

The G6PD gene is carried on the X chromosome. The enzyme consists of 515 amino acids with a molecular weight of 59 kDa. There are many variants of G6PD; the majority are the result of a single base mutation causing a single amino acid substitution. In some cases such substitutions may have no or minor effects on enzyme function. Using previously agreed World Health Organization methodology, including electrophoretic mobility, kinetics, and other properties, at least 299 variants of G6PD have been described but only a few are encountered frequently in clinical practice (***Table 137.3***). Using more specific DNA characterization, 60 variants have been identified. Deficiency of G6PD is mostly seen in hemizygous males and less frequently in homozygous females. The gene frequency of G6PD mutations is particularly high in Kurdish Jews (0.70) and black Americans (~0.10), black Africans, and some Asians.

Clinical Picture

G6PD deficiency may present with a wide spectrum of clinical manifestations. The generally accepted classification is as follows: (1) class 1, the most severe, is characterized by a chronic nonspherocytic hemolytic anemia; (2) class 2 includes G6PD Mediterranean (Gd Med), in which there is significant hemolysis with exposure to oxidants; and (3) class 3 includes only mild to moderate deficiency, such as Gd A^- found in Africa. Class 1 variants are rare and usually not found as a polymorphism in areas where malaria is endemic. In contrast, class 2 and 3 variants are common in malaria-endemic areas. The most common manifestations of G6PD deficiency are:

- Infection-induced hemolysis: this is the most common manifestations of G6PD deficiency observed in conditions such as viral hepatitis, typhoid, malaria, pneumonia, and severe sepsis. Patients with G6PD deficiency are more likely to develop intravascular hemolysis mimicking blackwater fever with falciparum malaria.
- Drug-induced hemolysis: the range of drugs causing hemolysis in the tropics in G6PD-deficient people may be more limited because of the milder forms of deficiency present in these areas:[41] antimalarials are important. The schizonticidal drugs, chloroquine and quinine, are considered safe in normal therapeutic doses. Combination drugs containing sulfonamide, dapsone, or pyrimethamine should be avoided; dapsone may cause hemolysis even in non-G6PD-deficient subjects. Primaquine is the major drug that should be avoided. The manufacturers of the aminoquinoline drugs, such as ciprofloxacin and ofloxacin, advise caution in G6PD deficiency.
- Neonatal jaundice is a common and potentially serious complication of G6PD deficiency in Asia, Greece, and Africa, leading to kernicterus. Anemia is not always present but the jaundice may be due to hepatocyte, rather than RBC, deficiency of the enzyme. A history of neonatal jaundice may suggest G6PD deficiency in later life.
- Food-induced jaundice: the best known foods inducing jaundice are fava beans and a food coloring in Nigeria called suya.

Table 137.3 Examples of the Most Common Glucose-6-Phosphate Dehydrogenase (G6PD) Variants

Type	Characteristics	G6PD Activity (%)	Distribution
B	Slower electrophoretic mobility than A	100	Common wild type Worldwide
A	Faster electrophoretic mobility than B	70–90	Africa
Deficient variants			
A^-	Drug- and infection-induced; hemolysis self-limited	15–20	Africa
Mediterranean	Severe, sometimes fatal hemolysis	<10	Mediterranean
Mahidol	Severe hemolysis	<10	Thailand, Southeast Asia
Canton	Severe hemolysis	<10	Orientals

Diagnosis

The blood film is normal in patients with G6PD deficiency in the steady state. During a hemolytic crisis changes may be seen, including irregularly contracted RBCs called "hemighosts" (***Fig. 137.4***). In overwhelming hemolysis or in patients who are hyposplenic, a supravital stain will reveal Heinz bodies, which are denatured Hb or globin precipitates associated with red cell membrane.

There are several assays available commercially for the detection of G6PD deficiency: all utilize the reduction of NADP to NADPH in the presence of excess G6PD and red cell lysate. Reduced NADPH is then detected either by fluorescence under ultraviolet light or by an electron transfer reaction involving tetrazolium compounds that are reduced by NADPH to insoluble forms.

G6PD deficiency of all types can be detected easily in male hemizygotes in the steady state and in homozygotes with the more severe class of enzyme deficiencies (e.g., Gd Med). Difficulties may arise in less severe types (class 3, especially GdA^-), in which reticulocytes and young RBCs, relatively rich in enzymes, tend to restore levels to the normal range. This relatively normal G6PD level in otherwise deficient people explains why these milder deficiencies cause self-limited hemolysis. Diagnosis of heterozygotes is more problematic. An intermediate range in the enzyme assay may be diagnostic of heterozygosity in females, but a considerable number will fall within the normal range. Genetic studies using DNA analysis are being increasingly used to diagnose G6PD deficiency and the carrier state, but they are not routinely available in the tropics.

Management

Acute management during a hemolytic crisis includes adequate hydration, maintenance of urinary output, withdrawal of the offending drug or agent responsible for the hemolysis, and transfusion if necessary. In neonatal jaundice, phototherapy or exchange transfusions may be required according to bilirubin levels.

Deficient patients should be counseled to: (1) avoid agents that are potentially hemolytic; (2) report early for treatment in case of infections; and (3) report the onset of jaundice or pallor early.

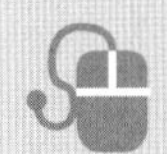

Access the complete reference list online at
http://www.expertconsult.com

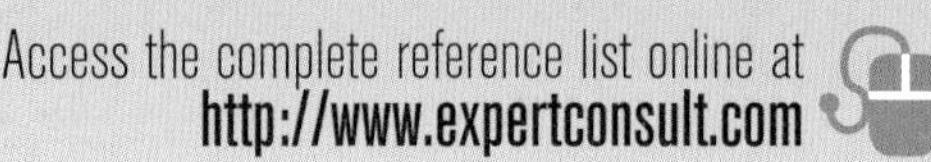
Access the complete reference list online at
http://www.expertconsult.com

CHAPTER 138

Sexually Transmitted and Urinary Tract Infections

Arlene C. Seña • Allan R. Ronald • Kimberley K. Fox • Myron S. Cohen

INTRODUCTION

Sexually transmitted infections (STIs) can lead to serious and sometimes fatal complications, and facilitate the transmission of the human immunodeficiency virus (HIV). In the developing world, STIs, excluding acquired immunodeficiency syndrome (AIDS), are the second leading cause of healthy life lost among women between 15 and 44 years of age.[1] Approximately 340 million new cases of the five curable STIs – gonorrhea, chlamydia, syphilis, chancroid, and trichomoniasis – have been estimated worldwide.[2] In 2003, herpes simplex virus type 2 (HSV-2) infection was newly diagnosed among an estimated 23.6 million persons aged 15–49 years worldwide.[3] The serological prevalence of HSV-2 has increased in sub-Saharan Africa to over 50% among adults in Kenya and Cameroon.[4]

Ecological factors contributing to the high rate of STIs in the tropics include changes in population density (e.g., urbanization); stages of demographic transition (e.g., a high proportion of young people at risk); migration and travel (e.g., increased mobility); and the accessibility, quality, and use of STI health services (e.g., inadequate health facilities). Behavioral factors which vary widely among societies include male circumcision traditions, condom use, spermicide and other contraception practices, and patterns of alcohol or illicit drug use that influence sexual behaviors.[5] Contact with sex workers is an important risk factor for STI acquisition.[6,7] Other STI risk factors include young age, residence in an urban area, multiple sexual partners, and a history of prior STIs.[8]

STI-related syndromes are caused by a multitude of viruses and bacteria (***Table 138.1***). Complications of STIs such as pelvic inflammatory disease (PID), ectopic pregnancy, infertility, epididymitis, urethral strictures, neonatal conjunctivitis, and congenital syphilis occur frequently in tropical settings, in part due to the lack of laboratory resources. Complications may be especially common in patients coinfected with HIV/AIDS.

Laboratory diagnosis of STIs may not be possible in many settings in the developing world. The expanded availability of rapid point-of-care tests may subsequently increase STI diagnosis in resource-poor areas. In the absence of testing, the World Health Organization (WHO) recommends the use of algorithms (also called flowcharts) for STI management based on clinical signs and symptoms.[9] The advantages of syndromic management are the immediate treatment of patients and avoidance of laboratory costs which must be balanced against the disadvantages, including failure to detect subclinical infections and the costs from treatment of uninfected persons. Flowcharts for the management of STI syndromes in men and genital ulcers have proven diagnostic validity in various clinical settings; however, flowcharts for the management of vaginal discharge have poor performance in diagnosing cervical infections.[10–13] These algorithms can be slightly improved with a risk profile approach whereby selected symptoms and signs, as well as demographic and behavioral characteristics, are chosen for their likelihood of association with the STI under consideration.[14]

Urinary tract infections (UTIs) can have similar clinical presentations to STIs. The global incidence of UTIs exceeds 150 million annually and these infections are common everywhere. The epidemiology of UTI in developing countries has not been well studied, and extrapolation from studies in industrialized societies is required to estimate the extent and burden of illness. UTIs are categorized as either "uncomplicated," when they occur in a normal urinary tract with no structural, functional, or underlying host illness to account for the infection, or "complicated," when an underlying abnormality is believed to have enabled the infection to occur.

GENITAL ULCERS

Genital ulcer disease (GUD) occurs frequently in tropical countries, accounting for 10–30% of STI clinic visits in Asia and Africa compared with 2–5% in western Europe and North America.[15] The STIs resulting in GUD include genital herpes, chancroid, syphilis, granuloma inguinale or donovanosis, and lymphogranuloma venereum (LGV). The male-to-female ratio for GUD in tropical areas is at least 4 : 1,[16] which may be partly due to commercial sex, resulting in a higher number of cases in men. *Haemophilus ducreyi* has traditionally been the most common cause of GUD in the tropics; however, there has been a recent decline in the proportion of GUD attributable to chancroid, from 50–60% to 5–11%.[17–20] The increasing prevalence of HSV-2 has now made genital herpes the most common cause of GUD worldwide.[21,22] In Tanzania, HSV-2 accounted for 83% of all identified pathogens in a study of GUD.[20] The prevalence of positive syphilis serology has been reported to be approximately 10% in women attending antenatal and family planning clinics, but considerably higher in groups such as sex workers and men with urethritis (24–42%) in South Africa.[23] Granuloma inguinale occurs most frequently in western Papua New Guinea, India, the Caribbean, and among Australian aborigines. LGV is endemic in parts of Africa, India, Asia, South America, and the Caribbean, but has emerged as a cause of significant morbidity among HIV-positive men who have sex with men in developed countries like the Netherlands and Australia.[24,25]

GUD usually begins as a papule or pustule on the skin or mucous membranes, followed by ulceration and development of inguinal and/or femoral lymphadenopathy. *Treponema pallidum* penetrates through abraded skin or intact mucous membranes within hours to days after exposure, subsequently enters the bloodstream, and disseminates.[26] HSV enters the epidermis and dermis, followed by replication in nerve ganglia and migration via peripheral sensory nerves, potentially leading to development of lesions distant from the primary site of exposure.[27] The other bacterial STIs that cause GUD typically result in localized disease; disseminated disease is rare but has been reported with donovanosis.

Table 138.1 Common Sexually Transmitted Infection-Related Syndromes and Etiologic Agents

Syndrome	Major Etiologic Agents
Genital ulcer disease	
Chancroid	*Haemophilus ducreyi*
Syphilis	*Treponema pallidum*
Genital herpes	Herpes simplex virus
Granuloma inguinale	*Calymmatobacterium granulomatosis*
Lymphogranuloma venereum	*Chlamydia trachomatis* (L serovars)
Nonulcerative genital lesions	
Genital warts	Human papillomavirus
Molluscum contagiosum	Molluscum virus
Scabies	*Sarcoptes scabiei*
Pediculosis[a]	*Phthirus pubis*
Vaginal discharge	
Vaginitis	*Trichomonas vaginalis, Candida albicans*
Bacterial vaginosis	*Gardnerella vaginalis, Mycoplasma hominis*, peptostreptococci, *Bacteroides* species, *Mobiluncus* species
Endocervicitis	*Neisseria gonorrhoeae, C. trachomatis*, herpes simplex virus, *Mycoplasma genitalium*
Ectocervicitis	*T. vaginalis, Herpes simplex* virus
Urethritis (women)	*N. gonorrhoeae, C. trachomatis, Herpes simplex virus*
Urethritis (men)	*N. gonorrhoeae, C. trachomatis, Ureaplasma urealyticum, Mycoplasma genitalium, T. vaginalis, Herpes simplex* virus
Pelvic inflammatory disease	*N. gonorrhoeae, C. trachomatis, M. hominis, M. genitalium*, anaerobic bacteria
Epididymitis	*N. gonorrhoeae, C. trachomatis*
Proctitis	*N. gonorrhoeae, C. trachomatis, T. pallidum*, herpes simplex virus
Pharyngitis	*N. gonorrhoeae, C. trachomatis*
Conjunctivitis	*N. gonorrhoeae, C. trachomatis* (including L serovars)
Hepatitis	Hepatitis A virus, hepatitis B virus, hepatitis C virus, cytomegalovirus

[a]Pediculosis (pubic lice infestation) may be mistaken for genital lesions.

Table 138.2 Typical Clinical Features in the Differential Diagnosis of Genital Ulcer Disease Caused by Sexually Transmitted Infections

Feature	Chancroid	Primary Syphilis	Genital Herpes	Granuloma Inguinale	Lymphogranuloma Venereum
Incubation period	3–7 days	2–4 weeks	2–7 days	1–4 weeks	10–14 days
Number of lesions	Usually 1–3	Usually 1	Multiple	Single or multiple	Usually 1
Genital lesion					
Appearance	Deep, defined, or irregular ulcer	Defined ulcer	Superficial, grouped vesicles or ulcerations	Defined or irregular ulcer; hypertrophic or verrucous	Papule, pustule, vesicle, or ulcer (transient)
Base	Yellow-gray, rough	Red, smooth, shiny	Red, smooth	Red, beefy, rough, usually friable	Variable
Induration	Soft	Firm	None	Firm	None
Pain	Common	None	Common[a]	Rare	Variable
Inguinal lymphadenopathy	Unilateral or bilateral; tender; may suppurate	Unilateral or bilateral; nontender; no suppuration	Bilateral; tender[a]	None; inguinal swelling	Unilateral or bilateral; tender, may suppurate
Constitutional symptoms	Rare	Rare	Common	Rare	Frequent

[a]Occurs more commonly in primary episodes of genital herpes than in recurrences.

CLINICAL MANIFESTATIONS

The manifestations of STIs associated with GUD are outlined in ***Table 138.2***. The clinical features may help differentiate GUD etiology. Chancroid is the most likely disease in a patient presenting with one or more painful genital ulcers accompanied by an inguinal bubo (a group of tender, matted lymph nodes). The ulcers have ragged, undermined borders, a purulent base, and no induration; they may coalesce to form giant lesions. Painful inguinal lymphadenopathy occurs in over half of men with chancroid; it occurs less commonly in women. The lymphadenitis of chancroid is usually unilateral; the bubo can become fluctuant and rupture, resulting in a draining abscess.

In comparison, a patient presenting with a painless solitary ulcer accompanied by nontender unilateral or bilateral inguinal lymphadenopathy most likely has primary syphilis. The ulcer is typically indurated with a defined, raised border and a clear, granular base. Although a solitary painless chancre is the hallmark of primary syphilis, almost half of patients have more than one lesion.[28] Syphilitic chancres are most frequently located on the inner or outer side of the foreskin or coronal sulcus in men, and the labia in women. Approximately one-third of homosexual men with primary syphilis will present with an anorectal lesion.

Table 138.3 Diagnostic Tests and Treatment for the Most Common Causes of Genital Ulcer Disease

	Definitive Diagnosis	Probable Diagnosis	Recommended Treatment Regimes
Chancroid	Culture	Clinical presentation	Azithromycin 1.0 g PO × 1; or ciprofloxacin 500 mg PO bid × 3 days; or erythromycin 500 mg PO tid or qid × 7 days (alternative: ceftriaxone 250 mg IM × 1) (pregnancy: erythromycin or ceftriaxone as above)
Primary syphilis	Dark-field examination; direct immunofluorescence	Clinical presentation; serology	Benzathine penicillin G 2.4 million units IM × 1 (alternatives: procaine penicillin 1.2 million units IM × 10 days; or doxycycline 100 mg PO bid; or tetracycline 500 mg PO qid × 14 days) (pregnancy: penicillin as above)
Genital herpes	Viral culture	Clinical presentation; antigen detection by immunofluorescence or enzyme immunoassay; serology	Acyclovir 200 mg PO 5 × 1 day; or acyclovir 400 mg PO tid; or famciclovir 250 mg PO tid; or valaciclovir 1.0 g PO bid × 7 days[a] (pregnancy: oral acyclovir as above)
Granuloma inguinale	"Donovan bodies" in tissue smear or biopsy specimens	Clinical presentation	Azithromycin 1.0 g × 1, then 500 mg PO every day; or doxycycline 100 mg PO bid for a minimum of 21 days (alternatives: erythromycin 500 mg PO qid, or tetracycline 500 mg PO qid, or trimethoprim (80 mg)–sulfamethoxazole (400 mg) 2 tablets PO bid for a minimum of 21 days) (pregnancy: erythromycin as above)
Lymphogranuloma venereum	Isolation in cell culture	Clinical presentation; serology	Doxycycline 100 mg PO bid × 21 days; or erythromycin 500 mg PO qid × 21 days (alternative: tetracycline 500 mg PO qid × 21 days) (pregnancy: erythromycin as above)

[a]Recommended for the primary episode of genital herpes. For recurrent genital herpes, the recommended regimens include acyclovir 400 mg PO bid × 5 days, acyclovir 800 mg PO bid × 5 days, famciclovir 125 mg PO bid × 5 days, valacyclovir 500 mg PO bid or 1.0 g PO daily × 5 days.

A patient with grouped vesicles or genital ulcers on an erythematous base, especially with a history of similar episodes, has a high likelihood of having herpes. Symptoms of low-grade fever, tender bilateral lymphadenopathy, and severe pain or paresthesias are associated with a primary first episode of genital herpes (i.e., there is no preexisting antibody to HSV-1 or HSV-2).

A prodrome of paresthesias around the outbreak site usually precedes the appearance of lesions by 12–48 hours. Vesicles can last 10–12 days before forming painful shallow ulcers and crusting, which can persist for another 1–2 weeks. Symptoms tend to be milder during the nonprimary first episode of HSV infection, when there are preexisting antibodies to the heterologous HSV type. Homosexual men may have lesions in the anorectal area, which may be accompanied with symptoms of proctitis.

A patient with one or more nonpainful genital ulcers with inguinal swelling (pseudobubo) may have granuloma inguinale, also called donovanosis. This infection is caused by *Calymmatobacterium granulomatis*, a Gram-negative bacillus. Granuloma inguinale may take many forms, including an ulcerative or ulcerogranulomatous lesion (a nontender, beefy-red ulcer with a granulated base); a hypertrophic or verrucous lesion with profuse granulation and friability; a necrotic, painful lesion with a foul-smelling exudate; or a sclerotic bandlike lesion with fibrous tissue formation.

A patient with tender inguinal lymphadenopathy or a suppurating bubo without a visible genital ulcer may have LGV. This syndrome is caused by infection with the serovars L1, L2, and L3 of *Chlamydia trachomatis*. The lesion is transient and frequently goes unnoticed; it precedes the development of unilateral or bilateral lymphadenitis by 7–30 days. The most easily recognized clinical feature of LGV in men is the "groove sign," or the enlargement of nodes above and below the inguinal ligament. The inguinal buboes of LGV may become fluctuant and rupture, or form a hard inguinal mass with suppuration. Women may present with enlarged pelvic nodes and associated pelvic pain, or with symptoms of proctitis due to lymphatic spread to the rectal mucosa.

DIAGNOSIS

The medical history should determine the time of exposure, the nature and duration of the lesions, the presence of pain, and the presence of constitutional symptoms. The physical examination should include the skin, oral cavity, external genitalia, the inguinal or femoral lymph nodes, and the anorectal area. In women, a pelvic examination should be performed whenever possible.

The diagnosis of GUD can be problematic without laboratory testing, since several studies have demonstrated the unreliability of clinical etiologic diagnosis.[29,30] Ideally, the diagnostic workup should include examination for *T. pallidum*, culture for *H. ducreyi*, culture or antigen tests for HSV, and serologic tests for syphilis (***Table 138.3***). Nontreponemal blood tests for syphilis, such as the rapid plasma reagin test or the Venereal Disease Research Laboratory (VDRL) tests, are positive in approximately 80% of primary syphilis cases.[31] False-positive results may occur with the nontreponemal tests due to pregnancy, infections, and autoimmune conditions; therefore confirmation with a specific treponemal test (the *T. pallidum* passive agglutination assay or TPPA; or the *T. pallidum* haemagglutination assay or TPHA) is necessary. The fluorescent treponemal antibody-absorption (FTA ABS) test has the highest sensitivity among the treponemal tests (86–100% for primary syphilis).[31] Rapid treponemal syphilis tests have been extensively evaluated by the WHO, with sensitivities ranging from 85% to 98% and specificities ranging from 93% to 98% compared to the TPPA or TPHA.[32] Rapid treponemal tests may be useful as screening tests in areas of low disease prevalence to identify patients for presumptive treatment. In areas of high disease prevalence, however, the utility of these tests is unclear since they cannot distinguish current from previously treated infections.

Other tests in the laboratory diagnosis of GUD have important limitations. Culture for chancroid is considered to be the definitive test, but has an estimated sensitivity of 75% compared to nucleic acid amplification detection from genital ulcer swabs.[15] If a diagnosis of genital herpes is not certain from the clinical presentation, a culture can provide the most sensitive and specific test when available. The sensitivity of herpes culture approaches 100% for vesicular lesions, but decreases to 33% during the ulcer stage.[33] If the culture for HSV is not available, the Tzanck smear to visualize multinucleated giant cells can provide a probable diagnosis of HSV; its sensitivity is approximately 67% for genital herpes in the vesicular stage and 50% in the ulcer stage.[34] The gold standards for HSV-2 serology are now based on detection of type-specific epitopes on the HSV glycoproteins G and C using Western blot or immunoblot enzyme assays.[35] Rapid tests for the detection of HSV-2 are available but expensive.[36] When granuloma inguinale is suspected, a Giemsa stain or Wright stain of crushed tissue smears or biopsy specimens looking for Donovan bodies (bacillary organisms within histiocytes) should be performed. Donovan bodies can be demonstrated in only 60–80% of cases from either direct smears or biopsy specimens. The isolation of *C. trachomatis* in cell culture provides definitive diagnosis of LGV, but the recovery rate from lymph node aspirates or ulcers is only 50%.[37] Serologic testing with complement fixation (CF) or microimmunofluorescence (MIF) can assist the diagnosis when performed in the appropriate clinical setting, but does not distinguish among infections with other *Chlamydia* serovars and species. Positive titers greater than 1 : 256 with CF or greater than 1 : 128 with MIF are strongly indicative of LGV, although invasive genital infections with the *C. trachomatis* serovars D–K can also give rise to high serum titers.[38] Nucleic acid amplification involving polymerase chain reaction for *T. pallidum, H. ducreyi*, and HSV may be available from some research laboratories as a more sensitive detection method than traditional tests for the diagnosis of genital lesions.[39,40] Coinfection with more than one pathogen has been reported in 5–10% of all GUD cases.[41]

Other causes of genital ulceration to consider in the differential include abrasions and trauma, contact dermatitis, fixed drug eruptions, Reiter's syndrome, Behçet's syndrome, and carcinoma. Atypical presentations of GUD associated with STIs must always be considered and are often seen in the tropics as a result of coinfections, coexistent HIV/AIDS, ineffective self-treatment, use of traditional remedies, superinfections, and other complications due to long-standing disease.

MANAGEMENT

Algorithms for the management of genital ulcers depend on the local prevalence of causal agents. One example of an algorithm for the syndromic management of genital ulcers is the WHO flowchart provided in ***Figure 138.1***, which recommends treatment for chancroid, syphilis, as well as HSV-2 (when the prevalence is >30%) when sores or genital ulcers are present. Otherwise, treatment regimens should be directed towards the most likely diagnosis determined from the clinical presentation and available laboratory studies (see ***Table 138.3***).

In selecting therapy for chancroid, it should be noted that there is widespread resistance of *H. ducreyi* to penicillins (PCNs) and tetracyclines in all geographic areas.[42,43] Azithromycin, ciprofloxacin, erythromycin, and ceftriaxone should be used for chancroid treatment, as noted in ***Table 138.3***. HIV-positive patients may fail single-dose therapy for chancroid,[44] requiring the longer 7-day regimen of erythromycin, and may have increased likelihood of coinfections with syphilis or genital herpes.

Whereas actual resistance of *T. pallidum* to PCN is not known to occur, a significant proportion of patients in the early stages of syphilis fail to demonstrate serologic cure after standard therapy.[45] Serologic cure for syphilis is defined by a fourfold decrease (two or more dilutions) in nontreponemal titers within 6 months after treatment.[46] Serologic treatment failure for primary syphilis has been reported in 5% of HIV-negative patients and 22% of HIV-infected patients at 6 months after standard

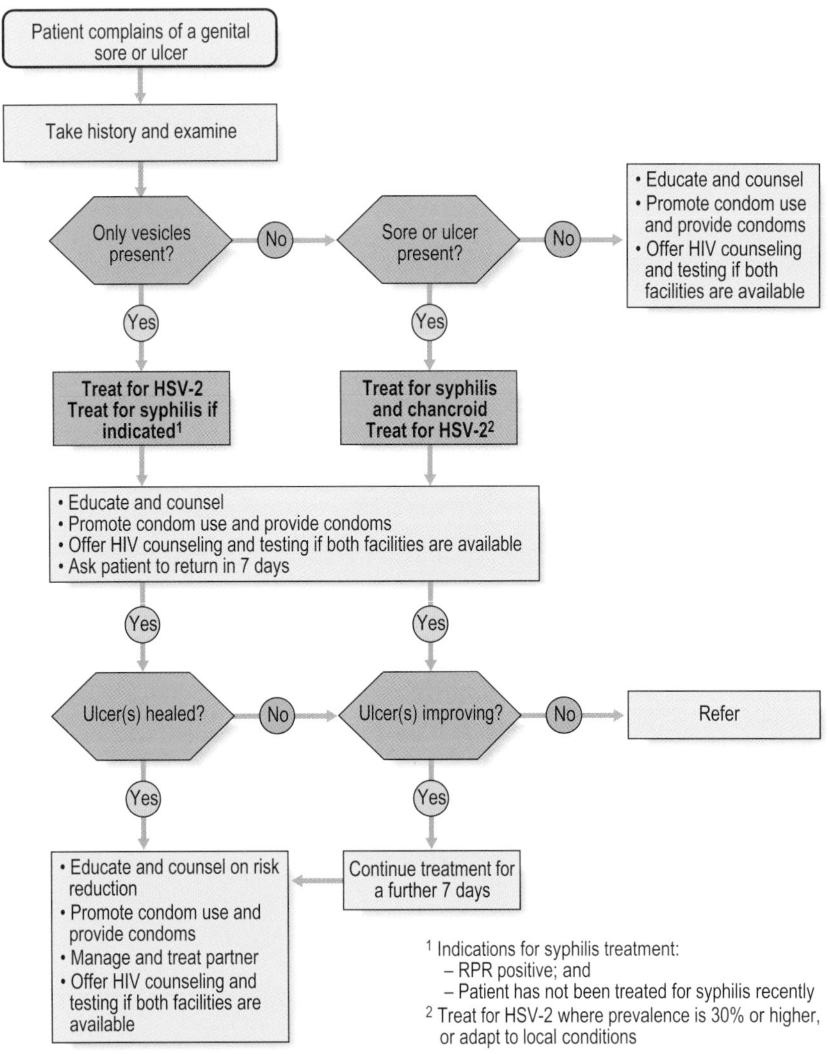

Figure 138.1 World Health Organization flowchart for the syndromic management of patients with a genital sore or ulcer. RPR, rapid plasma reagin. (Redrawn from Guidelines for the Management of Sexually Transmitted Infections. Geneva: World Health Organization; 2003.)

therapy.[45] Primary syphilis unresponsive to a single dose of PCN should be retreated with benzathine PCN 2.4 million units intramuscularly (IM), administered weekly for 3 weeks. Alternative regimens for PCN-allergic patients with early syphilis are doxycycline 100 mg orally twice a day or tetracycline 500 mg orally four times a day for 14 days. Oral therapy with azithromycin at 2.0 g orally in a single dose has been demonstrated to have comparable treatment efficacy as PCN for treatment of early syphilis.[47,48] However, there have been reports of azithromycin resistance from the United States, Ireland, and China, underscoring the importance of determining the local prevalence of azithromycin-resistant *T. pallidum* and providing follow-up of patients treated with azithromycin.[49,50] Pregnant women with syphilis who are allergic to PCN should be desensitized, as alternative therapies are inadequate in preventing congenital syphilis. Treatment regimens for HIV-infected persons with early syphilis are the same as for non-HIV-infected persons. However, examination of cerebrospinal fluid should be considered in HIV-positive patients regardless of their stage of syphilis due to their increased risk for early neurosyphilis. Persons with early syphilis should be re-evaluated clinically and serologically using a nontreponemal test after 6 and 12 months to assess response to therapy. Retreatment should be considered for persons with recurrent clinical signs or symptoms of active syphilis, or persons with a confirmed fourfold (two dilution) increase in the nontreponemal test titers.

There is no cure for genital herpes, but treatment with acyclovir or its analogues initiated promptly after the onset of symptoms reduces the development of new lesions, the duration of pain, and viral shedding (see ***Table 138.3***). Patients with recurrent genital herpes (e.g., six or more recurrences per year) are candidates for daily suppressive therapy with acyclovir 400 mg orally twice a day, famciclovir 250 mg orally twice a day, or valaciclovir 500 mg or 1.0 g orally once daily for 6–12 months,[51] followed by reassessment for continued therapy. The safety and efficacy of suppressive therapy with acyclovir have been assessed up to 5 years; more than 20% of patients on therapy were reported to be recurrence-free during this period.[52] HIV-infected patients with genital herpes can benefit from chronic suppressive therapy, but may develop thymidine-kinase-deficient virus, resulting in difficulties with long-term management.

Patients with granuloma inguinale should be given azithromycin or doxycycline, with the addition of gentamicin at 1.0 mg/kg intravenously every 8 hours in difficult cases involving HIV-infected persons. Other drugs which have been reported to be efficacious for this disease include erythromycin, tetracycline, ciprofloxacin, and streptomycin.[41] LGV should be treated with doxycycline or erythromycin for 21 days. However, some patients with advanced disease may require a longer duration of treatment, and surgery may be required for sequelae such as strictures and/or fistula.

Medical management of sexual contacts of patients with GUD should include an examination for lesions and empirical treatment because of the high likelihood of infection. Sexual contacts of patients with genital herpes are an exception, since the infection is not curable and therapy is provided primarily for palliation of symptoms. In addition, education and counseling are critical.

NONULCERATIVE GENITAL LESIONS

Several STIs may appear as nonulcerative lesions in the genital area (see ***Table 138.1***). Human papillomavirus (HPV) resulting in genital warts is frequently encountered in the tropics. A study of 520 women at an STI clinic in Kenya found that 6% had genital warts.[53] HPV types 6, 11, and other low-risk HPV types cause benign exophytic warts that can occasionally be transmitted to the newborn respiratory tract, but "high-risk" HPV types have been increasingly recognized (especially types 16, 18, 31, 33, and 35) due to their association with cervical and penile carcinoma.[54,55] High-risk HPV types may lead to invasive cervical cancer at a younger age in HIV-infected women compared to HIV-negative women.[56] The pathogenesis of HPV infection involves the squamous epithelium, in which there is viral entry and replication associated with increased proliferation of all the epidermal layers except the basal layer. Molluscum contagiosum is caused by a large DNA virus of the *Poxviridae* family resulting in a superficial cutaneous infection of children and young adults. Molluscum is usually a benign condition which may be transmitted through sexual or other close contact, but can occur as an opportunistic infection in patients with AIDS. Scabies should be included in the differential diagnosis of papular lesions in the genital area, as a condition that can also be transmitted through sexual or other close contact.

CLINICAL MANIFESTATIONS

Genital warts are typically multiple, but may be solitary and can appear as rough, slightly pigmented papules, flat keratotic plaques, or as soft, fleshy, exophytic lesions called condylomata acuminata. Cervical HPV lesions may occasionally present as classic condylomata acuminata, but are more likely to be subclinical. Intra-anal warts are common among men and women who practice receptive anal intercourse.[57] Men with genital warts may complain of penile pruritus or bloody ejaculate due to the presence of intraurethral condylomas.

Molluscum contagiosum presents as small (2–5 mm), dome-shaped papules with characteristic central umbilication. These lesions are usually pearly white, but can be flesh-colored or yellow. They are typically multiple and may be noted in the inguinal area or inner thighs or in extragenital sites such as the palms, soles, eyelids, and conjunctivae. There may be extensive involvement of the face and torso in AIDS patients.

A patient presenting with highly pruritic polymorphic papules should arouse suspicion of scabies. In early lesions, a tiny dot representing the buried mite may be seen at one end of the papule. The lesions can become excoriated, eczematous, and secondarily infected. When sexually transmitted, the lesions are typically found over the lower abdomen, buttocks, inner thighs, and genitalia. Lesions due to scabies can also appear on the finger webs, ventral wrist fold, and underneath the breasts in women.

DIAGNOSIS

The diagnosis of genital warts is made primarily on clinical grounds. Physical examination assisted by bright light and magnification is the recommended approach to primary diagnosis.[58] Histopathology of suspicious lesions should be performed in some cases to rule out malignancies. The differential diagnosis of atypical lesions includes genital herpes, molluscum contagiosum, lichen planus, benign neoplasms, genital squamous cell cancer, and Bowen's disease.

Molluscum contagiosum is also diagnosed based on the clinical appearance of the papules. If confirmation is needed, smears of the caseous material expressed from the lesions or a histologic specimen can be examined for characteristic intracytoplasmic inclusions. The differential diagnosis of these lesions is similar to that for genital warts.

The diagnosis of scabies can be made by identifying the typical elongated burrows within the papules, which may be more visible after application of ink. Scrapings of the lesions can be visualized microscopically for the presence of adult mites, larvae, eggs, or fecal pellets. Scabies may be confused with secondary syphilis, atopic or contact dermatitis, drug eruption, and impetigo.

MANAGEMENT

No therapy will eradicate HPV once acquired. However, external genital warts can be removed if the patient desires with excisional curettage, electrosurgery, or weekly cryotherapy with liquid nitrogen. Podophyllin in a 10–25% solution or trichloroacetic acid in an 80–90% solution can be administered to lesions weekly for up to 6 weeks. Podofilox (a compound purified from podophyllin) in a 0.5% solution may be applied by the patient twice daily for 3 days, followed by 4 days of no treatment, for up to 4 weeks. Imiquimod can be used as patient-administered immunotherapy for external genital and perianal warts in a 5% cream applied three times a week for as long as 16 weeks. During pregnancy, the removal of visible warts is advocated because they tend to proliferate and become friable; however, podophyllin, podofilox, and imiquimod are not recommended as treatment options in pregnancy.[46] Exophytic cervical warts should be evaluated for dysplasia before initiation of therapy. Although HIV-infected persons may have genital warts that may respond poorly to therapy and have more frequent recurrences than immunocompetent individuals,[59] there are no special treatment recommendations for this population.

Molluscum contagiosum rarely requires treatment, but for minor symptoms, excisional curettage or cryotherapy is usually effective. Scabies may be treated with 5% permethrin cream or 1% lindane lotion applied to the body for 8 hours and repeated in 1 week. Pregnant women should not be treated with lindane. Bedding and clothing of affected persons should be decontaminated in hot water or a clothes dryer.

Treatment of sexual contacts is not necessary for genital warts or molluscum contagiosum. However, sexual partners to persons with genital warts should be counseled regarding their exposure and risk for disease. Sexual and other close contacts of patients with scabies should be examined and treated appropriately.

VAGINAL DISCHARGE

Three general syndromes result in a vaginal discharge with specific etiologic agents: (1) vaginitis or vaginosis; (2) endocervicitis; and (3) ectocervicitis (***Table 138.1***). The type of epithelium present and other factors such as the pH in the microenvironment determine the susceptibility of each site to specific pathogens. Trichomoniasis is the most common non-viral STI worldwide, with infection rates as high as 29–34% among women in cities in South Africa with high HIV prevalence.[60] One study conducted from antenatal clinics in Nigeria demonstrated a prevalence of 54% among women aged 16–25 years based on wet mount examination and cultures.[61] Bacterial vaginosis (BV) is also widely prevalent; in parts of Africa, up to 60% of women presenting with a vaginal discharge have been reported to have BV.[62,63] BV is a clinical syndrome resulting from a disequilibrium of the normal vaginal flora, in which there is a massive overgrowth of *Gardnerella vaginalis, Mobiluncus* species, and other anaerobes. The role of sexual transmission in BV is controversial;[64] sexual activity may increase the risk for BV through mechanisms such as alteration of vaginal pH. Factors associated with vulvovaginal candidiasis (VVC) include pregnancy, oral contraceptives, uncontrolled diabetes mellitus, young age, and recent antimicrobial therapy.[63,65] Trichomoniasis and BV have been implicated as causes of obstetric complications (e.g., premature rupture of membranes, low birth weight) and PID.[66–68] However, gonorrhea and chlamydial infection have been strongly associated with upper genital tract disease and complications including adverse obstetric and neonatal outcomes. Subclinical PID, defined by the presence of histologic endometritis, has been reported among 26% of women infected with *Neisseria gonorrhoeae* and 27% of women infected with *C. trachomatis* in the lower genital tract.[69] The population-based prevalence estimate of *Chlamydia* is highest among women aged 15–24 years (4.5%); in contrast, the prevalence of gonorrhea is similar across age groups, at 0.3%.[70] Pregnant women in Botswana were found to have a prevalence of 8% for *Chlamydia* compared to 3% for gonorrhea using highly sensitive nucleic acid amplification tests (NAATs).[13] Among symptomatic women, the prevalence of gonorrhea has been reported as high as 17.1% in Malawi.[71] *N. gonorrhoeae* primarily affects the mucous epithelium of the lower genital tract, resulting in a vigorous neutrophilic response, development of submucosal microabscesses, and exudation of pus. Gonorrhea can also affect the rectum, oropharynx, and conjunctivae; it is discussed in further detail in Chapter 25. The trachoma biovar of *C. trachomatis* primarily affects the squamocolumnar epithelial cells of the endocervix, urethra, rectum, and conjunctiva.[72] Marked inflammation in the upper genital tract of infected women leading to ectopic pregnancy and infertility may be associated with the presence of serum antibodies reactive with the *C. trachomatis* heat-shock protein.[73]

Coinfection with both gonorrhea and *Chlamydia* occurs frequently and should be a consideration in the management of patients with cervicitis. Mucopurulent cervicitis is an STI syndrome that is a diagnosis of exclusion. It has been defined as cervical inflammation that is not secondary to *N. gonorrhoeae*;[74] it may be associated with *C. trachomatis* or less frequently with HSV, but in most cases no pathogen is found by routine testing. *Mycoplasma genitalium* has recently been identified with cervicitis, and has been found to be highly prevalent (26.3%) among female sex workers in sub-Saharan Africa.[75,76]

CLINICAL MANIFESTATIONS

Symptoms of vaginitis may include discharge, odor, external dysuria, and itching of the vulva and perivaginal mucosa. Patients may also complain of vaginal soreness, irritation, discomfort, and dyspareunia. Unfortunately, the symptoms of vaginitis are nonspecific and differentiation of syndromes cannot be based on these findings alone (***Table 138.4***). A patient with BV may present with a "fishy" white, homogeneous vaginal discharge in the absence of irritative symptoms. A patient with trichomoniasis may also have a malodorous discharge, but usually there are accompanying signs of vulvovaginal irritation such as pruritus and dysuria. A patient presenting with a curdlike vaginal discharge and pruritus of the vulva and perivaginal mucosa is more likely to have VVC.

Both gonococcal and chlamydial cervicitis produce few, if any, symptoms. When symptoms do occur, they include vaginal discharge, dysuria, and occasionally minor bleeding. Pelvic examination may reveal a purulent, mucopurulent, or bloody cervical discharge, with edema, erythema, or friability of the cervical os. An obvious endocervical discharge or a purulent vaginal discharge originating from the cervix is present in only 10–20% of women with gonorrhea.[77] Mucopuruluent cervicitis is characterized by the presence of a yellow-green endocervical exudate when viewed on a white cotton swab, or easily induced cervical bleeding when the swab is placed in the endocervix. The presence of mucopurulent discharge along with ulcerations and erythema of the ectocervix should arouse suspicion for HSV.

Table 138.4 Differential Diagnosis of Vaginitis or Vaginosis

Feature	Trichomoniasis	Bacterial Vaginosis	Vulvovaginal Candidiasis
Discharge	Thin; gray to yellow-green frothy; mild to fishy odor	Thin; gray to white homogeneous; fishy odor	Thick; white; often curdlike; minimal odor
Vaginal examination	Vulvovaginal erythema	Minimal or no vulvovaginal erythema	Vulvovaginal erythema; mucosal swelling
Cervical examination	Ectocervical erythema; rare punctate hemorrhages ("strawberry cervix")	Normal	Occasional ectocervical erythema
Wet mount	Trichomonads; increased PMNs	Clue cells; few PMNs	Budding yeast; pseudohyphae; few PMNs
KOH slide	Positive "whiff" test[a] in some cases	Positive "whiff" test[a]	Allows clearer view of yeast
pH of discharge	pH >4.5	pH >4.5	pH normal (4.0–4.5)

PMN, polymorphonuclear leukocytes; KOH, potassium hydroxide.
[a]Intensification of foul fishy odor upon addition of KOH to a sample of vaginal discharge.

DIAGNOSIS

The medical history should include the nature and duration of symptoms, the sexual history (including recent new sex partners), history of prior STIs, past therapy, and response to therapy. The physical examination should include inspection and palpation of the inguinal lymph nodes, vulva, vaginal vestibule, and anorectal area. The color, consistency, volume, and odor of the vaginal secretions should be noted. A speculum examination should be performed to evaluate the vaginal mucosa and cervix for erythema, petechiae, ulceration, edema, atrophy, and adherent discharge.

The differential diagnosis of vaginitis is presented in ***Table 138.4***. A clinical examination should be accompanied by a wet mount, potassium hydroxide (KOH) preparation, and pH determination of the vaginal discharge. The wet mount, performed by mixing vaginal fluid with normal saline on a slide, is examined for polymorphonuclear neutrophils (PMNs), motile trichomonads, and clue cells (exfoliated vaginal squamous epithelial cells covered with bacteria). Increased numbers of PMNs (ratio greater than 1 : 1 relative to epithelial cells) are seen in trichomoniasis, as well as in gonorrhea, *Chlamydia*, and HSV infection. The absence of trichomonads on a wet mount does not exclude the diagnosis since the sensitivity is only 60–70% compared with culture, which detects 95% of *T. vaginalis* infections.[78] A wet mount has a sensitivity of 40–60% for VVC.[62] The sensitivity can be improved by adding a few drops of 10% KOH to vaginal fluid on a slide to dissolve cellular matter, making yeast forms more visible. The finding of pseudohyphae or budding yeast supports the diagnosis of yeast vaginitis in the setting of appropriate symptoms; however, budding yeast may be part of the normal flora if present in small numbers.

Diagnosis of BV requires three of the following four criteria: (1) a homogeneous, white noninflammatory discharge that adheres to the vaginal walls; (2) the presence of clue cells on microscopic examination; (3) vaginal fluid pH greater than 4.5; and (4) a positive whiff test (a fishy odor before or after addition of 10% KOH to a sample of vaginal discharge).[46] A scoring system based on Gram stain of the vaginal discharge (Nugent criteria) can provide a standardized method for the diagnosis of BV, with a sensitivity of 89%.[79] In this scoring system, the absence of lactobacilli, along with the presence of small and curved Gram-variable rods (representing *G. vaginalis, Bacteroides* species, and *Mobiluncus* species), is most predictive of BV.

Patients suspected of or likely to have cervical infection should be tested for *N. gonorrhoeae* and *C. trachomatis*. The most widely available test for gonorrhea is culture on selective media, which has a reported sensitivity of 86–96%.[80] Older detection methods for *C. trachomatis* include enzyme immunoassay (EIA) and direct fluorescent antibody (DFA) tests, with reported sensitivities ranging from 73% to 95% for EIA of cervical specimens,[81,82] and 50–81% for DFA.[83,84] A DNA probe test is also available for the detection of *N. gonorrhoeae* and *C. trachomatis*. The detection of *N. gonorrhoeae* with this test is comparable to culture, and the test has the advantage of requiring only one specimen for identifying both organisms.[85–87] NAATs for *N. gonorrhoeae* and *C. trachomatis* using endocervical and urethral specimens provide greater sensitivity and specificity than traditional tests, and are being increasingly utilized as single or combination assays in areas with laboratory capabilities for these high-complexity methods.[88,89]

Self-inserted vaginal swabs are also an acceptable specimen collection method for NAATs.[90] Urine-based NAATs for *Chlamydia* have the advantage of being noninvasive and have sensitivities equivalent to polymerase chain reaction from endocervical and urethral specimens, but some urine NAATs for gonorrhea have lower sensitivities than swabs from the female genital tract. The cost and the infrastructure required to perform NAATs may limit their utility in tropical settings. Therefore, rapid point-of-care tests have recently been developed as antigen-detection tests for gonorrhea and chlamydia, but require additional field evaluation prior to use. A Gram stain of the cervical discharge with increased PMNs may be correlated with gonococcal or chlamydial infection, but should be interpreted with caution. The presence of intracellular Gram-negative diplococci is 50–60% sensitive and highly specific for gonorrhea, while extracellular diplococci may represent normal genital flora. However, the absence of diplococci on an endocervical smear does not exclude gonococcal infection.

In patients with a vaginal discharge but no obvious infectious cause, the differential diagnosis should include chemical or allergic vulvovaginitis, which can result from contact with deodorants, douches, or spermicides, or the presence of a foreign body in the vagina. Cervical, vaginal, and vulvar neoplasias can also present with discharge.

MANAGEMENT

For settings in which a speculum and bimanual examination cannot be performed, the WHO recommends an algorithm based on the presence of an abnormal discharge, lower abdominal tenderness, and a risk assessment adapted to the local social, behavioral, and epidemiological situation. When the patient has an abnormal discharge and a positive risk assessment, this algorithm recommends empiric treatment for gonococcal, chlamydial and trichomonal infections, and BV (***Fig. 138.2***).[9] However, there are increasing concerns regarding the use of the syndromic approach for vaginal discharge in populations such as pregnant women due to high rates of asymptomatic infections and its poor predictive performance for cervical infections.[13,91] Recommended therapies for vaginitis and cervicitis are provided in ***Table 138.5***. The single oral dose of 2 g metronidazole for trichomoniasis has a cure rate of 82–88%.[91] Due to the occurrence of *T. vaginalis* with resistance to metronidazole, infections that do not respond to the single-dose regimen should be retreated with metronidazole 500 mg twice a day for 7 days. If treatment failure recurs, the patient should be treated with metronidazole 2 g orally once daily for 3–5 days.[46] Women with symptomatic BV should be treated with metronidazole 500 mg orally twice a day for 7 days; the 2-g dose has low efficacy and is not recommended. Pregnant women who have symptomatic BV can be treated with the same dose of metronidazole as nonpregnant women or with 250 mg orally three times a day for 7 days. There are several topical antimycotic agents for VVC with similar clinical efficacies. Oral therapy for VVC with fluconazole 150 mg as a one-time dose is superior to these topical therapies. Recurrent VVC, usually defined as three or more episodes per year, occurs in a minority of patients with risk factors such as immunosuppression or corticosteroid use. The frequency of episodes can be reduced with a regimen of ketoconazole 100 mg orally once daily or fluconazole 100 mg orally once weekly for 6 months.[92] Chronic suppressive therapy may be required for patients with HIV/AIDS who may have severe episodes of VVC and frequent relapses.

Treatment regimens for gonorrhea and chlamydial infection require several considerations, including antimicrobial resistance of *N. gonorrhoeae*, concurrent infection, and involvement of the upper genital tract. Single-dose oral cefixime or intramuscular ceftriaxone, or spectinomycin for cephalosporin-allergic patients, is recommended as therapy for *N. gonorrhoeae*; however, spectinomycin resistance has been reported sporadically, especially in the context of widespread spectinomycin use,[93] and there have been a few reports of resistance to ceftriaxone.[94] Alternative parenteral single-dose regimens for urogenital and anorectal gonorrhea do not offer any advantage over ceftriaxone. Fluoroquinolone resistance has been common in much of Southeast Asia and has been increasing worldwide.[95,96] Therefore, quinolones can no longer be generally recommended for treatment of gonorrhea.

Because of the high likelihood of coinfection, persons treated for gonorrhea should also receive treatment that is effective against *C. trachomatis*. Azithromycin is administered as a single-dose regimen and may be more cost-effective since successful therapy with doxycycline requires compliance with a 7-day course. Empirical treatment of both gonorrhea and chlamydial infection should be considered for patients with mucopurulent cervicitis, especially in populations with a high prevalence of these infections. HIV-infected women with BV, trichomoniasis, vulvovaginal candidiasis, gonorrhea, or *Chlamydia* should receive the same treatment regimens as HIV-negative women.

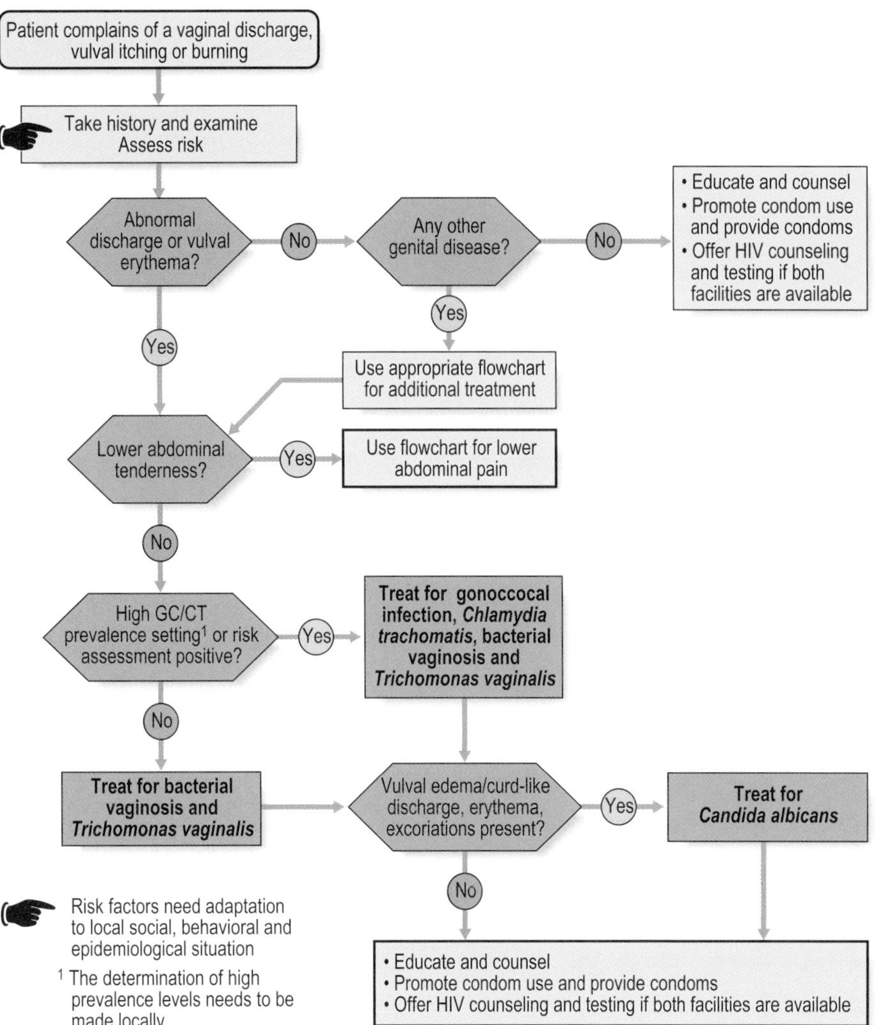

Figure 138.2 World Health Organization flowchart for the syndromic management of patients with a vaginal urethral discharge. GC/CT, gonococcal infection/chlamydia trachomatis infection. (Redrawn from Guidelines for the Management of Sexually Transmitted Infections. Geneva: World Health Organization; 2003.)

Table 138.5 Recommended Treatment Regimens for Vaginitis, Cervicitis, and Urethritis

Trichomonas vaginitis/urethritis	Metronidazole 2 g PO × 1 dose; or tinidazole 2 g PO × 1 dose (alternatives: metronidazole 500 mg PO bid × 7 days; or tinidazole 500 mg PO bid ×5 days) (pregnancy: metronidazole 2 g dose as above)
Bacterial vaginosis	Metronidazole 500 mg PO bid × 7 days (alternatives: metronidazole gel 0.75% 5 g intravaginally bid × 5 days; or clindamycin 300 mg PO bid × 7 days; clindamycin cream 2% 5 g intravaginally at bedtime × 7 days) (pregnancy: oral metronidazole doses as above or 250 mg PO tid × 7 days, oral clindamycin as above)
Candida vaginitis	Miconazole or clotrimazole 200 mg intravaginally every day × 3 days; or clotrimazole 500 mg PO intravaginally × 1 dose; or fluconazole 150 mg PO × 1 dose (alternative: nystatin 100 000 IU intravaginally every day ×14 days) (pregnancy: any 7-day topical treatment)
Gonococcal cervicitis/urethritis[a]	Cefixime 400 mg PO × 1 dose;[c] or ceftriaxone 125 mg IM × 1 dose;[b–d] or spectinomycin 2 g IM × 1 dose[b,d]; *plus* treatment for *C. trachomatis* (pregnancy: cefixime, ceftriaxone, or spectinomycin as above)
Chlamydial cervicitis/ urethritis[a]	Doxycycline 100 mg PO bid × 7 days; or azithromycin 1 g PO × 1 dose (alternatives: amoxicillin 500 mg PO tid × 7 days; erythromycin base 500 mg PO qid × 7 days; ofloxacin 300 mg PO bid × 7 days; tetracycline 500 mg PO qid × 7 days) (pregnancy: azithromycin, amoxicillin, or erythromycin as above)
Nongonococcal urethritis	Doxycycline 100 mg PO bid × 7 days; or azithromycin 1 g PO × 1 dose; or erythromycin base 500 mg PO qid × 7 days

[a]Regimen is for uncomplicated cervicitis or urethritis only.
[b]Regimens recommended for anorectal infections.
[c]Regimens recommended for treatment of gonococcal pharyngitis.
[d]Regimens recommended for treatment of adult gonococcal conjunctivitis.

Treatment and counseling should be provided for sex partners of patients with trichomoniasis, gonococcal, or chlamydial infection. There is an increased cure rate of trichomoniasis in women following treatment of their male sexual partners.[97] In the absence of definitive laboratory diagnosis in women with mucopurulent cervicitis, patients should be told that an infection with an STI is possible but not proven, requiring treatment of the patient and all sex partners. Treatment of sex partners is not required for BV or VVC.

URETHRAL SYNDROMES AND URINARY TRACT INFECTIONS IN WOMEN

Urethral syndromes in women may present as urethritis caused by STIs or cystitis caused by urinary tract pathogens. The causative organisms associated with urethritis in women include *N. gonorrhoeae*, *C. trachomatis*, and HSV infection. The microbiology of UTIs is similar worldwide. Most uncomplicated infections, usually over 80%, are due to *Escherichia coli*. Between 5% and 10% of infections, particularly in females, are due to *Staphylococcus saprophyticus* and the remainder are due to a variety of aerobic organisms. Complicated UTIs are also most commonly due to *E. coli*, but the strains are often more resistant to antimicrobial agents and occur following selection within an institutional environment or secondary to the effects of repeated courses of antibacterial therapy. *Klebsiella* spp., *Proteus* spp., *Pseudomonas aeruginosa*, *Enterococcus* spp., and *Candida* spp. occur much more frequently in patients with underlying structural or functional abnormalities and in patients who have acquired infection nosocomially. Anaerobes and more fastidious organisms are rarely responsible for UTIs and are found in fewer than 3% of patients.

In tropical countries, *Salmonella* spp., particularly *S. typhimurium*, are common causes of UTI. In Egypt, *Salmonella* may account for 10–20% of the complicated urinary infections.[101] *Salmonella* spp. are also very common in patients who have concomitant infection with *Schistosoma haematobium*.[98] These patients may have bladder calculi, so management can be complex. *Mycobacterium tuberculosis* urinary infection is common in tropical countries and must be considered in all patients who present with symptoms of UTI with pyuria and otherwise "sterile" urine cultures. *Brucella* spp. can cause chronic urinary infection with granulomatous pyelonephritis or cystitis.

CLINICAL MANIFESTATIONS

Women with urethritis secondary to STIs may present with dysuria, urinary frequency, and lower abdominal pain, and concomitant symptoms associated with cervicitis or vaginitis. Urethritis should be differentiated from acute cystitis, which may also present with dysuria, frequency, and lower abdominal pain, and be accompanied by urinary urgency and/or gross hematuria.

Additional symptoms of fever, chills, flank pain, and systemic complaints should raise suspicion for pyelonephritis. In about one-fourth of women with pyelonephritis, subsequent bacteremia can lead to the "sepsis syndrome," and require urgent wide-spectrum antimicrobial treatment to prevent serious complications. Asymptomatic bacteriuria occurs commonly with a prevalence of 3–10% in otherwise healthy adult women. Pregnant women with asymptomatic bacteriuria are predisposed to developing invasive pyelonephritis, particularly during the third trimester; therefore, all women should be screened for bacteriuria in early pregnancy.

DIAGNOSIS

Women with urethral symptoms should have a urinalysis, a urine culture, a sexual risk assessment, and a pelvic examination whenever possible to differentiate urinary infection from the various STI syndromes.

The laboratory diagnosis of gonococcal, chlamydial, and HSV infections is discussed in previous sections. Laboratory diagnosis of UTI requires demonstration of pyuria and bacteriuria. A clean-catch midstream urine specimen with 10 or more leukocytes per high-power field (HPF) supports the diagnosis of infection if no other cause of pyuria is present. Leukocyte esterase and nitrite strips can be used to screen urine for evidence of infection, but the sensitivity is usually less than 90% and specificity about 80%.[99] A presumptive diagnosis of UTI may be achieved with a microscopic examination revealing 5–10 organisms per oil immersion field on Gram stain. Quantitative urine cultures should be requested on clean-voided midstream urine and quickly transported to the laboratory. However, if an immediate culture is not feasible, storage for 24 hours at 4°C in a refrigerator maintains bacterial viability and stable bacterial counts. Urine cultures are of no value if specimens have been improperly collected and stored, as bacteria grow readily in urine and urine cultures will be falsely positive. Urine is cultured on blood agar and selective media (such as MacConkey's agar) with a quantitative loop that enables an estimation of the bacterial count (colony-forming units, CFU). Determination of the antimicrobial susceptibilities of the bacterial isolates may be important in patients with complicated infections. Pyuria is almost invariably present in patients with symptomatic urinary infections. Of note, between 10% and 50% of patients with acute symptoms will have bacterial counts of less than 10^8 CFU/L or less than 10^5 CFU/mL.[100] "Low-count" bacteriuria is a real entity; in both males and females with symptoms, it usually portends infection. On the other hand, asymptomatic bacteriuria in females should usually be diagnosed only if at least two urine cultures have counts of greater than 10^8 CFU/L (10^5 CFU/mL). For women who are prone to UTIs and have had multiple recurrences, symptomatic episodes should be managed with as little investigation as possible. A urinalysis may be all that is required for diagnosis.

MANAGEMENT

Management of women with suspected STIs has been discussed previously. Treatment of acute cystitis has been standardized to a 3-day oral regimen with trimethoprim 160 mg and sulfamethoxazole 800 mg (TMP-SMX) twice daily or a fluoroquinolone once daily. Most *E. coli* strains that cause acute uncomplicated cystitis are now resistant to amoxicillin. Women who present with presumed acute pyelonephritis require urgent attention. Alternative diagnoses, particularly surgical conditions, acute PID, ectopic pregnancy, and other illnesses, need to be excluded. About one-third of patients initially diagnosed as having acute pyelonephritis are found to have other illnesses. Women should have urine and blood cultures and be treated immediately with an effective regimen. Ampicillin and gentamicin or a third-generation cephalosporin are appropriate for initial parenteral therapy; oral regimens may then be prescribed for 2 weeks. The fluoroquinolones are satisfactory oral choices for patients with acute pyelonephritis if the infecting pathogen is susceptible.

Recurrence of infection should be anticipated in women with UTIs. Recurrent symptomatic cystitis may be managed by continuous low-dose prophylaxis or with intermittent prophylaxis taken after sexual intercourse.[101] TMP-SMX or a fluoroquinolone is the most effective prophylactic agent. Women with recurrent UTIs may be given medication to initiate self-treatment when their symptoms recur. Postmenopausal women may respond to local vaginal estrogens with reduction in the number of recurring episodes of cystitis.[102] Recurring renal infection mandates studies to exclude abnormalities in the upper tract. Some women will require continuous suppression to prevent recurring symptoms.

All pregnant women should be screened for infection with a urinalysis and a urine culture. Asymptomatic bacteriuria should be treated; this will prevent over 80% of acute episodes of pyelonephritis in pregnancy and will also prevent 10–20% of premature deliveries. All pregnant women who have a urinary infection should be followed with frequent urinalysis throughout their pregnancy. Asymptomatic infections are usually treated in children but not in adults or in individuals with indwelling catheters unless there is evidence of invasive renal disease.

URETHRAL SYNDROMES AND URINARY TRACT INFECTIONS IN MEN

Urethral syndromes in men are classified as urethritis, epididymitis, prostatitis, cystitis, and pyelonephritis. In sexually active men, *N. gonorrhoeae* and *C. trachomatis* are the most common causes of urethritis and epididymitis. The prevalence of gonorrhea among males presenting with a urethral discharge varies from 50% to 60% in Africa.[103,104] In comparison, the prevalence of chlamydial infection among males presenting with a urethral discharge varies from 12.3% in parts of Africa to 53.4% in Jamaica.[71,105] Approximately one-half to three-fourths of cases of nongonococcal urethritis (NGU) are caused by other pathogens, including *Ureaplasma urealyticum, Mycoplasma genitalium, T. vaginalis*, or HSV. *M. genitalium* has gained increased recognition as a causative agent of acute and chronic NGU, and has been detected in 14.4% of male patients with symptomatic urethritis in South Africa.[106] *T. vaginalis* can be a particularly important cause of urethritis in some tropical areas such as Africa, where 19% of males presenting with urethral discharge were diagnosed with *T. vaginalis*.[107,108]

E. coli and other urinary tract pathogens can also present as urethritis, epididymitis, and prostatitis; an initial empirical treatment regimen should include all of these organisms in its spectrum. UTIs occur with an incidence of about 1 per 100 during the first year of life in boys. These infections are often associated with underlying congenital anomalies. The presence of a foreskin increases the incidence of UTIs in boys and in adult men by two- to threefold.[109] During adult life, the annual incidence is approximately 3 per 1000, which increases dramatically during the seventh decade with the onset of prostatic disease.

CLINICAL MANIFESTATIONS

A patient with urethritis may present with urethral discharge, dysuria, or itching at the meatus. Gonorrhea typically develops 2–6 days after exposure, whereas NGU may take 1–5 weeks from exposure to the onset of symptoms. A profuse, yellow-green discharge with an acute onset is suggestive of gonococcal origin, while a mucopurulent or mucoid discharge noted only after urethral stripping or in the morning before voiding is likely to be nongonococcal in etiology. Dysuria is present in both conditions, but the presence of dysuria without a urethral discharge is a very good predictor of NGU. A profuse mucoid discharge with severe dysuria suggests HSV, especially if accompanied by regional lymphadenopathy and external genital lesions.

Urinary frequency, urgency, and hematuria are not generally part of the urethritis syndrome in men, and suggest the presence of prostatitis, cystitis, or other disorders. Asymptomatic bacteriuria is less common in men than women, usually occurring with the onset of prostatic hypertrophy or cancer leading to urinary tract obstruction. Prostatitis usually presents with perineal and lower abdominal pain, fever, burning, frequency, and occasionally with a sepsis-like syndrome.

DIAGNOSIS

A Gram stain should be performed on the urethral discharge and examined for the presence of greater than 4 PMNs per HPF as objective evidence of urethritis. The finding of Gram-negative intracellular diplococci is highly specific for gonococcal urethritis (95% sensitivity, 98% specificity), but a negative smear does not exclude gonorrhea, particularly in cases where self-medication is suspected. If PMNs are present but no intracellular organisms are seen, a tentative diagnosis of NGU should be made. First-void urine can also be centrifuged and analyzed for ≥10 PMNs per HPF, which is indicative of urethritis.[46] Additional tests should be obtained for *N. gonorhoeae* and *C. trachomatis* using urethral or urine-based NAATs whenever possible. In areas with limited laboratory resources, the leukocyte esterase test can be performed on the first-voided portion of urine from symptomatic men with urethritis; this dipstick measurement has a reported sensitivity of 76% and specificity of 80% for the presence of gonorrhea or *Chlamydia* in one study involving STD clinic patients.[110] Trichomonads may occasionally be found on Gram stain or on a wet mount of urethral discharge, but detection of *T. vaginalis* in men is best achieved through cultures or NAATs which are not available in most clinical settings, even in developed countries. Testing for *M. genitalium* using NAATs has only been applied in research studies and detection of *U. urealyticum* is seldom clinically useful since the organism frequently colonizes the urethra.

Males with UTI are often investigated to exclude congenital or acquired abnormalities.[111] An intravenous pyelogram or an ultrasound examination should be combined with a cystoscopic study. Since the majority of adult men will not have an underlying anatomic abnormality as a predisposing factor for their UTIs, the recurrence of infection is an excellent indicator for men who require further investigation. Men with chronic prostatitis should have a culture performed on expressed prostatic secretions to identify the bacterial etiology.

MANAGEMENT

The WHO flowchart (***Fig. 138.3***) illustrates the syndromic management of patients presenting with a urethral discharge, and ***Table 138.5*** provides the recommended therapies for urethritis. In areas with a high prevalence of gonococcal and chlamydial infection, or where tests are not available, empirical treatment aimed at both *N. gonorrhoeae* and *C. trachomatis* for all patients with urethritis can be a cost-effective option. The addition of metronidazole for the initial syndromic treatment of NGU may need consideration in some settings due to the high prevalance of *Trichomonas* in men.[106,112] Because of the high cost of some medications, alternative therapies such as gentamicin and kanamycin for gonorrhea may be reasonable options in some settings depending on local antimicrobial susceptibilities.[113] Men with persistent or recurrent urethritis despite appropriate therapy should be given metronidazole 2 g orally once for trichomoniasis and erythromycin 500 mg orally four times a day for 14 days as treatment for presumptive tetracycline-resistant *U. urealyticum*. Recurrence of NGU days to weeks after therapy may be due to a prostatic focus of infection and may be treated with a 3–6-week course of doxycycline, erythromycin, or azithromycin. Men with gonococcccal urethritis or NGU and HIV infection should receive the same treatment regimen as HIV-negative men. Sex partners of patients with trichomoniasis, gonorrhea, chlamydial infection, or NGU require presumptive treatment and counseling.

Males of all ages with lower-tract infection should be treated with a 14-day course of an effective antibacterial regimen. Trimethoprim–sulfamethoxazole is an acceptable initial regimen. Patients with symptoms of prostatitis and patients who have recurrence after an initial 14-day course of treatment should be given TMP-SMX for at least 6 weeks. Long courses are necessary to eradicate infection in some men. Men with acute pyelonephritis should be treated initially with parenteral regimens; continuing treatment for 14 days should be prescribed with an oral regimen such as TMP-SMX or a fluoroquinolone. These drugs achieve satisfactory levels within prostatic tissue and are more likely to eradicate the organism from this site. For men with relapsing chronic prostatitis, continuous therapy may be necessary to prevent recurrences.

LOWER ABDOMINAL PAIN

Sexually active women presenting with lower abdominal pain should be evaluated for PID, an ascending infection of the uterus, fallopian tubes, and adjacent pelvic structures resulting in endometritis, salpingitis, pelvic peritonitis, or tubo-ovarian abscess. The long-term sequelae of undetected disease include infertility, ectopic pregnancy, and chronic pelvic pain. In sub-Saharan Africa, the majority of cases (85%) of infertility are due to bilateral tubal occlusion resulting from PID.[114] PID is frequently encountered in tropical countries, where the annual incidence in urban women aged 15–35 years has been estimated to be 1–3%.[115] Most cases of PID are caused by *N. gonorrhoeae, C. trachomatis*, and anaerobic flora of

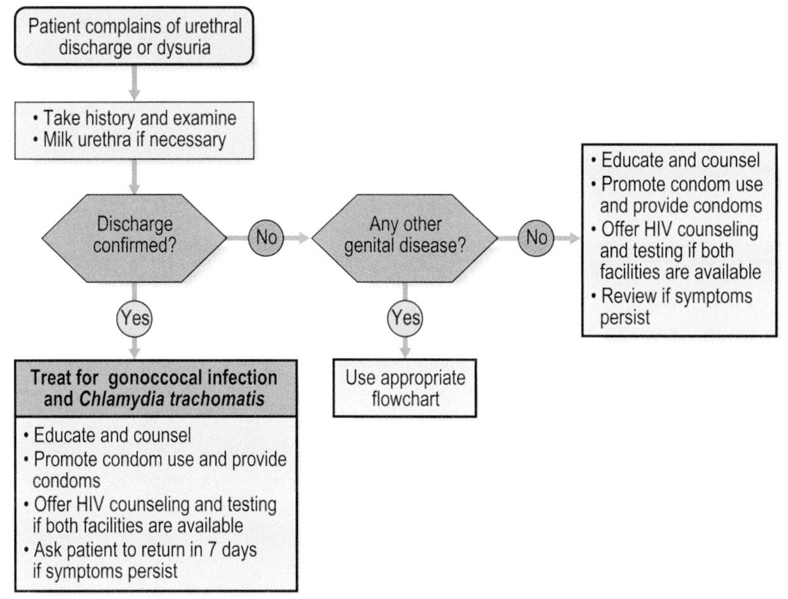

Figure 138.3 World Health Organization flowchart for the syndromic management of patients with a urethral discharge. (Redrawn from Guidelines for the Management of Sexually Transmitted Infections. Geneva: World Health Organization; 2003.)

Table 138.6 Recommended Treatment Regimens for Pelvic Inflammatory Disease

Inpatient regimens	Cefoxitin 2 g IV every 6 hours; or cefotetan 2 g IV every 12 hours; or ceftriaxone 250 mg IM × 1 q day[a] *plus* doxycycline 100 mg IV or PO every 12 hours × 14 days *plus* metronidazole 500 mg IV or PO bid × 14 days Clindamycin 900 mg IV every 8 hours *plus* gentamicin 1.5 mg/kg IV every 8 hours[a,b]
Outpatient regimens	Ceftriaxone 250 mg IM × 1 dose, or cefoxitin 2 g IM with probenecid 1 g PO × 1 dose *plus* doxycycline 100 mg PO bid or tetracycline 500 mg PO qid × 14 days *plus* metronidazole 500 mg PO bid × 14 days Ofloxacin 400 mg PO bid × 14 days; or levofloxacin 500 mg PO once daily × 14 days[c] *plus* metronidazole 500 mg PO bid × 14 days

[a]These regimens should be continued for at least 48 hours after clinical improvement and then followed by an oral regimen to complete 14 days of therapy.
[b]After discontinuation, this regimen should be followed by either doxycycline 100 mg PO bid or tetracycline 500 mg PO qid to complete 14 total days of therapy.
[c]Use of fluoroquinolones as alternative therapy may be considered if the community prevalence and patient's risk for gonorrhea is low. Testing to rule out gonococcal infection is recommended prior to use of this regimen.

the gastrointestinal and genital tracts (e.g., *Bacteroides* spp.). Approximately 30–40% of cases are associated with mixed infections of both aerobic and anaerobic organisms.[116–118] Organisms associated with bacterial vaginosis contribute to some cases of PID,[119] while in 20% of cases no cause has been found.[119] *Mycoplasma genitalium* has been recently associated with PID.[120,121] Predisposing factors for PID include young age, multiple sex partners, use of intrauterine devices, douching, and prior history of PID.[122,123]

CLINICAL MANIFESTATIONS

A patient presenting with lower abdominal pain accompanied by an abnormal vaginal discharge should be suspected of having PID. Other symptoms suggestive of PID include abnormal uterine bleeding, dysuria, dyspareunia, menometrorrhagia, pain associated with menses, nausea, vomiting, and fever. Physical examination may reveal a purulent cervical discharge, cervical motion, and adnexal tenderness. A patient presenting with symptoms of PID and pleuritic upper abdominal pain should raise suspicion for perihepatitis and peritonitis due to extension of the infection to the subphrenic and subdiaphragmatic space, a condition known as the Fitz-Hugh–Curtis syndrome.

DIAGNOSIS

The diagnosis of PID is usually based on the minimum clinical criteria of lower abdominal pain together with cervical motion and adnexal tenderness. Laparoscopic visualization has been considered the gold standard but is usually not warranted. The minimum criteria for PID have a reported sensitivity of 83% compared to endometrial sampling, in comparison with a 95% sensitivity for adnexal tenderness.[124] Additional criteria which may increase the specificity of diagnosis include fever, abnormal discharge, and laboratory documentation of cervical infection. A pelvic examination should be performed to determine the presence of any cervical discharge, uterine, adnexal, or cervical motion tenderness, or masses. Endocervical specimens should be obtained and tested for *N. gonorrhoeae* and *C. trachomatis*. The differential diagnosis of acute lower abdominal pain in women includes pregnancy, appendicitis, ovarian cyst, diverticular disease, urinary tract infections, and enteric illnesses.

MANAGEMENT

Empirical therapy for PID should be instituted in the presence of the minimum clinical criteria and in the absence of another established cause of the patient's symptoms. Because of the difficulty in determining the exact infectious cause of PID, treatment should be directed at all potential pathogens and should be broad-spectrum in nature. Effective inpatient and outpatient regimens for PID are presented in ***Table 138.6***. Antibiotic therapy should be continued for a 10–14-day course; the clinical efficacy of these regimens ranges from 81% to 94%.[125,126] Hospitalization is generally recommended when the diagnosis is uncertain, the possibility of a surgical emergency cannot be excluded, a pelvic abscess is suspected, the patient is pregnant or immunocompromised, severe illness precludes outpatient management, the patient cannot tolerate an outpatient regimen, or the patient has failed to respond to outpatient therapy. Reassessment of the patient after 72 hours is recommended to evaluate the response to outpatient treatment. Because of the risk of reinfection, sex partners of women with PID should be evaluated and empirically treated with regimens that are effective against both *N. gonorrhoeae* and *C. trachomatis*. Bed rest, avoidance of sexual intercourse during therapy, and evaluation of the male sexual partner are integral components of PID management. The woman and her partner(s) should be counseled appropriately; when a definite laboratory diagnosis is not possible, patients should be told that an STI is suspected, requiring treatment of the woman and all partners.

SCROTAL SWELLING

Men presenting with scrotal swelling should be evaluated for epididymitis, an acute inflammation of the epididymis which is usually a complication of gonococcal or chlamydial urethritis in men less than 35 years of age. Extension of the infection to involve the adjacent testicle results in epididymo-orchitis. In older men, epididymitis is more commonly associated with enteric organisms (e.g., *E. coli, Klebsiella* spp.). Other organisms that should be considered as a cause of epididymitis include *Mycobacterium tuberculosis, Brucella* spp., and blastomycosis, which is usually accompanied by orchitis or disease elsewhere such as in the lungs or bones.

CLINICAL MANIFESTATIONS

The presence of acute scrotal swelling with scrotal and inguinal pain suggests the possibility of epididymitis. Testicular torsion can manifest with similar symptoms and must be differentiated because it is a surgical emergency. Symptoms of epididymitis usually begin unilaterally, but may progress to a bilateral epididymo-orchitis. Physical examination may reveal a swollen, tender epididymis and vas deferens, and a red, edematous scrotum. Symptoms of urethritis may also be present. Approximately half of patients presenting with epididymitis of gonococcal origin have a urethral discharge.

DIAGNOSIS

Simple laboratory tests can help with the diagnosis of epididymitis. A urethral smear revealing greater than 4 PMNs per HPF provides objective evidence of urethritis, and supports the diagnosis of epididymitis in a man with scrotal pain. A urethral swab or urine specimen should be obtained and tested for *N. gonorrhoeae* and *C. trachomatis*. Urinalysis and urine culture can determine the presence of an associated urinary tract infection. The differential diagnosis of scrotal swelling includes testicular torsion, orchitis secondary to nonsexually transmitted pathogens, hydrocele, spermatocele, and testicular carcinoma.

MANAGEMENT

Empirical therapy of epididymitis is recommended while awaiting test results. Patients suspected of having an STI should be treated for both *N. gonorrhoeae* and *C. trachomatis*, using ceftriaxone 250 mg IM in a single dose plus doxycycline for 10 days. Ofloxacin 300 mg orally twice a day for 10 days is an alternative regimen that may be considered for treatment of epididymitis negative by gonococcal testing or most likely caused by enteric organisms. Bed rest with scrotal elevation and application of ice packs may assist in decreasing local inflammation and swelling. Sex partners of men with epididymitis thought to be of gonococcal or chlamydial etiology should be evaluated and treated.

OTHER CLINICAL PRESENTATIONS OF SEXUALLY TRANSMITTED INFECTIONS

STIs can present less commonly as other clinical syndromes including proctitis, pharyngitis, conjunctivitis, and hepatitis, depending on the site of exposure or the propensity of the organism to affect certain organ systems (see ***Table 138.1***). Patients with proctitis may present with a rectal discharge, anorectal pain, or tenesmus. In sexually active individuals, especially MSM who engage in receptive anal intercourse, empiric treatment with ceftriaxone 125 mg IM and doxycycline for 7 days should be considered when an anorectal exudate or PMNs on a Gram stain of the anorectal secretions is found on examination. Patients with a history of oral sexual activity, especially fellatio, may present with a sore throat, acute pharyngitis, or tonsillitis secondary to gonorrhea. Chlamydial infection of the pharynx is unusual; however, empiric therapy should be directed towards both pathogens when gonococcal pharyngitis is suspected since coinfections can occur. Conjunctivitis in adults secondary to STIs may result from oculogenital contact, as well as direct or indirect contact from digits or fomites from infected persons. Patients with conjunctivitis secondary to gonorrhea may present with an acute mucopurulent discharge of the conjunctiva, redness, or swelling. The presentation and management of viral hepatitis are presented in greater detail in Chapter 64. Sexual activity is a significant risk factor for acquisition of hepatitis A, hepatitis B, and cytomegalovirus infections; sexual exposure can also result in transmission of hepatitis C.

SEXUALLY TRANSMITTED INFECTIONS–HUMAN IMMUNODEFICIENCY VIRUS INTERACTIONS

The well-established epidemiologic and biologic associations between STIs and HIV infection underscore the importance of integrating STI/HIV management in clinical settings. Many STIs serve as cofactors facilitating HIV transmission, while HIV infection itself appears to alter the natural history and therapeutic response of some STIs. Biological studies have shown that persons with STIs have increased susceptibility to HIV by the presence of increased inflammatory cells and disruptions in their genital mucosa, and that the presence of other STIs in HIV-infected persons facilitates shedding of the virus in their genital tracts, thereby promoting HIV infectiousness.[127–129]

Among the STIs, GUD has been found to have the strongest association with HIV.[130] Studies have also shown associations between HIV infection and gonorrhea,[131,132] chlamydial infection,[133] trichomoniasis,[131] bacterial vaginosis,[134] and genital warts,[135] independent of other risk factors for HIV infection, including sexual behavior. The higher prevalence of nonulcerative STIs makes them equally important as GUD as cofactors for HIV transmission. Therefore, prompt and appropriate treatment of all STIs is important in limiting the spread of HIV infection. HIV voluntary testing and counseling should be offered to patients presenting with STIs, and HIV-infected patients should be screened at baseline and on a regular basis for STIs given their shared risk factors and the high STI prevalence evident among various HIV-infected populations.[136–139] HIV-positive persons may have rapid progression or severe manifestations of STIs such as syphilis, HSV, or HPV. Patients with HIV infection may be less responsive to standard antibiotic therapy for chancroid,[140] syphilis,[45,141] genital HSV,[142] and HPV.[143]

CONTROL OF SEXUALLY TRANSMITTED INFECTIONS

Effective STI control cannot be achieved solely on the basis of correct diagnosis and prompt treatment of symptomatic patients. Primary prevention programs, including culturally appropriate sex education through schools and religious institutions, encouragement of delay in sexual debut among adolescents, programs to encourage gender respect and equity, including educational opportunities for girls, supportive sex worker interventions, marriage support initiatives, prenatal screening programs, and condom access programs, are all important to provide a foundation on which to build secondary control programs. Behavioral change plays a crucial part in the control of STIs and should be addressed through individual counseling or comprehensive health education programs emphasizing safe sex practices and condom use. In developing countries, public health interventions targeting groups with the highest rates of sex partner change (e.g., commercial sex workers) may improve the cost-effectiveness of HIV and other STI prevention efforts. In addition to strategies on the individual level, community-oriented approaches to STI prevention and control may be helpful in settings where STIs are highly prevalent.[144–146] HPV vaccines to prevent genital warts and cervical cancer have been available worldwide since 2006 (Chapter 80), and should be promoted along with hepatitis B vaccination among susceptible populations.

Partner notification and screening among at-risk individuals are integral components of secondary STI control programs due to the fact that a significant proportion of persons infected with STIs, especially women, have no symptoms. Partners of patients with STIs should be contacted for evaluation and treatment to decrease the reservoir of potentially infectious persons.

STI screening should be considered in areas of high prevalence or among high-risk groups, depending on available laboratory techniques and resources. Screening of pregnant women for STIs, especially syphilis, is important and should be performed at the first prenatal visit and again in the third trimester for individuals at high risk for exposure. The promotion of condom use and other barrier methods is imperative and can decrease the rate of transmission of STIs and HIV. Though nonoxynol-9 was not found to reduce male-to-female transmission of STIs,[147,148] efforts are continuing to develop safe and acceptable topical microbicides that could inactivate STIs, including HIV.[149]

Access the complete reference list online at
http://www.expertconsult.com

CHAPTER 139

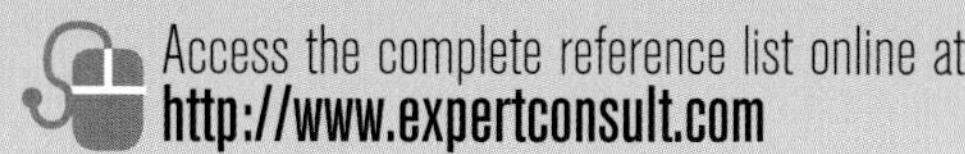
Access the complete reference list online at
http://www.expertconsult.com

Approach to the Patient with HIV and Coinfecting Tropical Infectious Diseases

Christopher L. Karp • Siddhartha Mahanty

All … fall into one of two categories: infected with HIV or at risk for HIV infection (Mary E. Wilson[1])

INTRODUCTION

The morbidity, mortality, and social disruption due to the acquired immunodeficiency syndrome (AIDS) pandemic weigh disproportionately upon resource-poor areas of the tropics.[2] Consequently, the potential for interactions between human immunodeficiency virus (HIV) infection and other tropical infectious diseases is great.

Such interactions are marked by epidemiologic complexity. The AIDS pandemic is best described as the sum of discontinuous and overlapping epidemics of disease among populations of variable and varying risk (see Chapter 81). The predominant modes of transmission of HIV (perinatal, sexual, and parenteral) result in a bimodal distribution of disease, with peaks among young children and young adults. The risk of infection or disease due to tropical pathogens varies widely with differences in ecological, political, and socioeconomic conditions (including access to medical care); related specific host factors such as age of exposure, pregnancy, behavior, and nutrition; and host genetics. Disease due to a coinfecting pathogen may be due to primary infection, recurrent infection, or the reactivation of latent infection. For some pathogens, the risk factor responsible for the acquisition of HIV may also be the risk factor responsible for the acquisition of the coinfecting pathogen. As a consequence of this epidemiologic complexity, both the prevalence and the expression of coinfection are variable across ecological, economic, political, behavioral, and cultural divides.

EFFECTS OF HIV ON TROPICAL COINFECTIONS

Infection with HIV can influence the natural history of infection with other pathogens through: (1) facilitating infection; (2) altering the incidence of disease by increasing the ratio of disease to infection; (3) changing the presentation of disease; or (4) exacerbating the course of disease.[3] Such effects are primarily the result of the immunosuppression associated with HIV infection.

Abnormalities of immune function are found in essentially every cellular and functional compartment of the immune system in AIDS, although profound defects in cell-mediated immunity (CMI) appear to be of greatest clinical importance.[4] *In vitro* correlates include functional abnormalities of:

- $CD4^+$ T cells, with progressive failure of proliferation, interleukin (IL)-2 and interferon-γ (IFN-γ) production,[5,6] dysregulated expression of molecules essential for T-cell/antigen presenting cell interactions;[6] abnormal activation-induced apoptosis,[7,8] preferential loss of Th17-polarized $CD4^+$ T cells in the gastrointestinal (GI) tract;[9,10] and expansion of regulatory T cells that are potent inhibitors of immune responses both to self and to pathogens.[11,12]
- Monocyte/macrophages, with decreased chemotaxis and intracellular microbicidal activity and abnormal cytokine production.[4]
- Dendritic cells, with reduced ability to present antigen and activate T cells (along with efficient transfer of HIV infection to $CD4^+$ T cells)[13] and with depletion of plasmacytoid dendritic cell populations.[14,15]
- $CD8^+$ T cells, with decreased cytotoxic T-lymphocyte (CTL) function[4] and abnormal activation-induced apoptosis.[8]
- Natural killer (NK) cells, with decreased proliferation and IFN-γ production.[16]

Dysregulation of humoral immunity, marked by polyclonal B-cell activation, is also seen.[4] Functionally, abnormalities of $CD4^+$ T-cell, macrophage, and dendritic cell function have been thought to be paramount to the suppression of CMI and the opportunistic infections (OIs) seen in patients with AIDS. In addition to direct effects of HIV infection, the immune system of HIV-infected people may also be compromised in clinically significant ways by profound nutritional and metabolic derangements (e.g., wasting or "slim disease"), therapeutic interventions (e.g., corticosteroids used for the treatment of *Pneumocystis* pneumonia), and immune abnormalities associated with secondary infections (e.g., suppression of CMI seen in visceral leishmaniasis (VL)).

The list of infectious diseases that are exacerbated by HIV coinfection[17] includes many that can be predicted from data demonstrating the important role of CMI in protection from the etiologic agent. Several pathogens for which immunity has been presumed to depend on CMI do not appear to be exacerbated by HIV coinfection, however. The HIV "experiment of nature" has caused a reexamination of the immunology of such "missing infections" in AIDS.[18]

HIV infection can also influence the therapeutic responses of patients with varied tropical infections. The ability to diagnose and monitor coinfection may be compromised by aberrant serologic responses, including false positives due to polyclonal B-cell activation, false negatives due to blunted antigen-specific antibody responses to newly acquired pathogens, and false serologic reversion after treatment in late HIV disease.[4] Diagnosis may also be hindered by unusual presentations of disease with coinfecting pathogens. Finally, a plethora of intercurrent pathologic conditions may lead to a dulling of Ockham's razor during disease evaluation in AIDS patients. A single pathogen, multiple pathogens, HIV infection, side effects of therapeutic drugs, or a combination of these may be responsible for the presenting complaints. Given the suboptimal response to the chemotherapy of many infections in the presence of profound immunosuppression, drugs may need to be given in greater numbers or for a longer duration. With many pathogens, in the absence of immune reconstitution resulting from highly active antiretroviral therapy (HAART), lifelong suppressive therapy is necessary. Drug therapy in the

HIV-infected patient may be complicated further by increased rates of drug allergy as well as by untoward drug interactions in the setting of polypharmacy.[19] Prophylaxis against coinfections may be compromised by substandard vaccination responses. Finally, the presence of HIV coinfection can complicate the public health consequences of tropical diseases. AIDS may increase the transmissibility of secondary infections and provide fertile soil for the development of drug resistance. Public health resources devoted to the AIDS pandemic may divert resources away from the control and prevention of other infectious diseases.

The presence of HIV coinfection can lead to disease of markedly greater incidence or severity (the standard definition of an OI)[17] with some tropical infectious diseases, such as leishmaniasis and American trypanosomiasis. Coinfection has also been demonstrated to have subtle effects on the course of disease with other tropical agents, such as *Schistosoma mansoni*. No robust alteration has been found in the natural history of many tropical infections, including most nematodes. With organisms in the latter groups, the current absence of evidence of significant effects of HIV on the expression of disease or the response to treatment should not be construed as strong evidence for the absence of such effects. Most research resources have been spent on understanding the clinical and epidemiologic manifestations of the HIV pandemic in industrialized countries, where tropical infectious diseases are underrepresented. Where coinfections with HIV and endemic tropical diseases are marked by low prevalence, subtlety of interaction, diagnostic difficulty, or low research priority, the presence and significance of any interaction are likely to be missed. For example, despite the research priority among tropical infections accorded to malaria, the first significant interaction appreciated with HIV infection – the lack of a benefit of increasing parity in the control of malaria in pregnant women – was only discovered 15 years after the AIDS epidemic was recognized.[20] With less heavily studied pathogens, comparatively subtle interactions will likely emerge over time as research resources are appropriately directed.

Focusing on OIs may help to highlight some of the clearest data on the clinical expression of AIDS in the tropics. Of the more than 100 agents known to cause OIs in AIDS patients, several are classic tropical pathogens. These are mostly found among the intracellular protozoans, bacteria, and endemic fungi; there is a marked absence of metazoans. Overall, the clinical expression of AIDS in many resource-poor areas of the tropics appears to involve a different spectrum of OIs than those common in North America and Europe. In place of the high incidences of *Pneumocystis* pneumonia, disseminated *Mycobacterium avium*, and cytomegalovirus (CMV) found in the resource-rich north, the clinical expression of AIDS in much of the tropics has been marked by frequent tuberculosis (the most common serious AIDS OI in the world), chronic diarrhea, wasting, chronic fever without an obvious localizing source, and pulmonary disease.[21]

The contribution of predominantly tropical pathogens to these latter common syndromes is unclear, which illuminates the problems with much of the available data on HIV disease in the tropics. Understanding the spectrum of AIDS-associated OIs in any given area depends on the presence of adequate surveillance systems, which are often lacking in resource-poor regions of the tropics. In the presence of inadequate infrastructures, limited financial resources, and difficult access to medical care on the part of the socially disadvantaged, surveillance is likely to be sporadic and to involve mainly the sampling of subgroups of AIDS patients at late stages of disease.[20] Where resources are limited, diagnostic reporting is likely to be biased in favor of OIs that are inexpensive to diagnose (or misdiagnose).[20] Even the common impression that the progression of AIDS is more rapid in sub-Saharan Africa than in industrialized countries[22–25] rests on data that are less than robust.[26] A more rapid observed course (presumed due to a higher frequency and virulence of coinfection and problems of nutrition and access to medical care) may represent in large part a systematic bias in favor of later initial diagnosis of HIV infection and AIDS.[20,27] Conversely, it has been suggested that the burden of illness and mortality in early HIV disease (often unrecognized as such) due to high-grade pathogens, such as *Streptococcus pneumoniae*, *Mycobacterium tuberculosis*, and the salmonellae, may rival that due to the OIs of late-stage AIDS in the tropics.[27,28]

HIV has shed light on many previously obscure human pathogens. Some, such as the enteric microsporidians, were unknown as agents of human disease prior to the AIDS epidemic. Others, such as *Cryptosporidium parvum*, were underappreciated as causes of disease in normal hosts until their prevalence in AIDS patients led to systematic study in normal hosts.

EFFECTS OF TROPICAL INFECTIONS ON HIV COINFECTION

There are theoretical and experimental reasons to believe that coinfection can significantly alter the course of HIV pathogenesis. The central role of ongoing viral replication in HIV pathogenesis is firmly established, and the set point concentration of plasma viremia correlates well with long-term clinical outcome.[29] It is presumed that any increases in viral replication have the potential for accelerating the course of disease. Efficient replication of HIV in CD4$^+$ T cells is dependent on cellular activation. Similarly, activation of macrophages and dendritic cells can stimulate HIV replication by increasing transcription factor binding to the HIV long terminal repeat region, enhancing transcription. Coinfecting pathogens can stimulate such immune cell activation either directly (e.g., stimulating signaling through Toll-like receptors[30] or upregulating transcription factor transactivation in coinfected immune cells) or indirectly (e.g., promoting the generation of proinflammatory cytokines or activating CD4$^+$T cells as part of the adaptive immune response). Immune activation can also lead to upregulation of the expression of HIV coreceptors,[31] thereby facilitating the infection of fresh cells.

Immunologic responses to pathogens, as well as to purified vaccine antigens, clearly have the potential for enhancing the dynamic burden of HIV replication. *In vitro* studies with diverse pathogens have provided mechanistic support for this idea.[32–34] Experimental evidence has also suggested that immune activation-driven augmentation of the HIV viral burden can occur *in vivo*.[35–42] There is also circumstantial evidence that such immune activation may enhance HIV pathogenesis.[43,44] Both points remain somewhat controversial, however.[45] Whether immune activation-related increases in viral loads actually accelerate the pathogenesis of HIV may depend on whether the changes are transient (as with immunization or with treated acute infection) or chronic (as with untreated infection, or through a resetting of the set point of plasma viremia by a particular coinfection).[46]

Direct equation of immune activation with upregulation of HIV replication is simplistic, however. With CD4$^+$ T cells, the mechanism of activation appears to be critical to whether viral replication is induced or suppressed.[47–49] Furthermore, activation of proinflammatory cytokine production with positive effects on HIV replication goes hand in hand with activation of anti-inflammatory cytokine production, which can inhibit HIV replication. More generally, immune responses reliably induce counterregulatory responses that may well suppress HIV replication.[50,51] It thus should not be surprising that *in vitro* studies have provided mechanistic support for the ability of coinfecting pathogens to suppress HIV replication.[52–55] Indeed, whereas infection with some tropical pathogens (e.g., *Plasmodium falciparum*) has been shown to increase plasma HIV load, the overall effect of acute coinfection with some pathogens, including measles virus, dengue virus, and *Orientia tsutsugamushi*, may be a decrease in HIV viral load.[56–58] That said, measures of persistent immune activation, broadly taken, have been shown to correlate, independently of plasma viral load, with a steeper slope of CD4$^+$ T-cell depletion, disease progression, and mortality risk.[59,60] While the responsible mechanisms remain underdefined, coinfection may thus favor the progression HIV disease independently of effects on viral dynamics. In this context, the provocative finding that HIV infection leads to sustained systemic exposure to microbial products from the gut[61] (something that may well be abetted by tropical gut luminal and tissue pathogens) is potentially of special importance.

In addition to the viral sequelae of generalized immunologic activation, induction of specific alterations in the immunoregulatory environment of the host by ubiquitous tropical pathogens has been postulated to accelerate the course of HIV. Cross-regulating subsets of $CD4^+$ T cells have been distinguished by their cytokine profiles and functional activities: Th1 cells (producing IFN-γ, among other cytokines) are important in classical macrophage activation, the development of CMI, and the generation of humoral responses involving complement-fixing antibody isotypes; Th2 cells (producing IL-4, IL-5, and IL-13, among other cytokines) are important in alternative macrophage activation, the generation of immunoglobulin E (IgE) responses, eosinophilia, mast cell responses, and atopy. The immunologic response to most helminthic parasites is dominated by Th2 cytokine production. Mouse models have shown that helminth-driven Th2 polarization can shift the immunologic response to heterologous antigens and pathogens from a Th1- to a Th2-dominant pattern, as well as significantly suppress $CD8^+$ T-cell-mediated viral clearance.[62,63] Such responses have also been found to impair antigen-specific Th1 immune responses in both mice and humans.[62,64]

Chronic helminthic infections are widespread in the tropics. The resultant Th2 "priming" of the immune system may favor progression of HIV disease.[65] Several mechanisms have been postulated. First, a Th2-polarized immune system may directly suppress $CD8^+$ T-cell-mediated anti-HIV responses.[63] Second, HIV appears to replicate preferentially in Th2 cells,[66] something that may well be due to increased expression of APOBEC3G, a cytidine deaminase with anti-HIV activity, in Th1 cells.[40,41] Third, T cells from HIV-seropositive people undergo abnormal activation-induced apoptosis,[7,8] which is thought to play a role in the depletion of both $CD4^+$ and $CD8^+$ T cells over time.[41] Th2 cytokines can amplify such activation-induced apoptosis.[67] Fourth, Th2 cytokines can upregulate HIV coreceptor expression by $CD4^+$ T cells and monocyte/macrophages.[68] Of note, it has been demonstrated that peripheral blood cells from patients with intestinal helminth infection are more susceptible to *in vitro* infection with HIV than are cells from helminth-uninfected patients.[69,70] Fifth, diverse chronic helminth infections are associated with the development of strong immune counterregulatory responses, which may blunt heterologous anti-HIV immune responses.[43] Finally, both tissue trematodes (e.g., schistosomes) and luminal nematodes (e.g., geohelminths) are likely to have effects on gut mucosal permeability, something that may drive immune activation and disease progression by increasing systemic exposure to gut-derived microbial products.

There is thus clear biological plausibility for the hypothesis that endemic helminth coinfection can lead to acceleration of HIV disease course in the tropics. The hypothesis has been difficult to clearly address experimentally. An initial study in Ethiopia indicated that HIV viral load was significantly higher in individuals with various helminthic infections than in individuals without helminths, correlating positively with the parasite load as well as decreasing after elimination of the worms by antiparasitic treatment.[71] Subsequently, several similar studies from southern Africa failed to replicate these findings,[72,73] one study even reporting significant, transient increases in viral load after therapy for schistosomiasis.[45] A Cochrane Review[49] analyzed the only three randomized, controlled trials published to date on the effects of anthelminthic therapy on HIV disease progression in antiretroviral naïve patients: (1) a randomized trial of praziquantel for schistosomiasis, which found a significant benefit of treatment on plasma HIV-1 RNA load (a lack of an increase with treatment, compared with an increase in viral load in the absence of treatment), with a nonsignificant trend towards a beneficial effect on $CD4^+$ counts in HIV-infected individuals;[50] (2) a randomized, double-blind, placebo-controlled, cross-over trial of diethylcarbamazine for bancroftian filariasis, which reported a decrease in plasma HIV-1 RNA load (and a nonsignificant trend towards a beneficial effect on $CD4^+$ counts) with treatment;[51] and (3) a randomized, double-blind, placebo-controlled trial of albendazole for infection with diverse geohelminths (including hookworms, *Ascaris,* and *Trichuris*), which found a nonsignificant trend towards a beneficial effect of treatment on plasma HIV-1 RNA load, but a significant benefit of treatment on $CD4^+$ T-cell counts, specifically in the subset of patients with *Ascaris* infection.[52] Pooling of data from these three trials – a procedure that seems biologically tenuous – suggested significant (at least short-term) benefit of deworming on plasma HIV-1 mRNA load and $CD4^+$ T-cell counts.[49] The overall hypothesis thus remains compelling. However, given the short-term follow-up, the variable biology and epidemiology of these different organisms, and the different interventions used in these trials, the clearest conclusions to be made are that more data on the subject are needed – something underscored by a recent alarming report that maternal helminth coinfection is associated with a significantly increased risk for mother-to-child transmission of HIV infection.[53]

Other effects of coinfection are perhaps more concrete. Tropical diseases may lead directly to an increased risk of infection with HIV. Treatment of the severe anemia induced by malaria has led to the HIV infection of countless children by transfusion.[74] Genital schistosomiasis, like other genital inflammatory conditions, appears to increase the efficiency of HIV transmission.[75]

CLINICAL SUSPICION OF COINFECTION

The basic biology of HIV; the progression, diagnosis, and treatment of HIV disease; and the epidemiology of HIV/AIDS in the tropics are discussed in Chapter 81. This chapter focuses on tropical infectious diseases that may be OIs in the HIV-infected patient. OIs that are common in the industrialized world are not discussed in depth unless there are compelling clinical or epidemiologic reasons for doing so. Multiple references are available that discuss these cosmopolitan OIs.[17,77–79] Further information on the specific organisms discussed here can be found in the cited pathogen-specific chapters.

The diagnostic, prophylactic, and therapeutic recommendations discussed here describe an approach to the HIV patient that is not limited by scarce medical resources. As such, like many strategies for dealing with HIV disease that have evolved in affluent industrialized countries (including high-technology diagnostics, and multidrug chemoprophylaxis), many of these recommendations may not easily be translated to resource-poor areas of the tropics.

PATHOGENS

Protozoan Infections

Malaria

Malaria (see Chapter 96) remains one of the most important infectious diseases in the world today.[55] Evidence from mouse and human studies suggests an important role for $CD4^+$ T cells in protective immunity to blood-stage malaria. With large areas of shared endemicity, a medically significant interaction between HIV and malaria was thus expected and feared.[79] Initial studies were negative; falciparum malaria did not appear be an OI or to accelerate the progression of HIV disease.[80–84] However, follow-up studies have revealed complex bidirectional interactions between *P. falciparum* and HIV. (There remains little information about the interaction of HIV with *P. vivax*, *P. malariae*, *P. ovale,* or *P. knowlesi*.)

The epidemiology and immunobiology of *P. falciparum* are integral to this complexity. Severe disease and death due to *P. falciparum* occur in those lacking specific acquired immunity, something that only develops in the face of high rates of transmission and over time. With stable, heavy transmission, the greatest burden of disease occurs in young children, travelers, and pregnant women (the latter, for reasons discussed below); nonpregnant adults tend to be parasitemic in the absence of symptoms. With unstable or low transmission rates, the relationship between parasitemia and disease tends to be more direct, and the burden of disease falls more equally.[85] As might be expected, interactions between *P. falciparum* and HIV vary with malaria transmission dynamics.[86]

The first significant clinical effect of HIV on malaria was found in the setting of pregnancy in areas of high malarial endemicity. Despite age-dependent induction of immunity to severe disease in such areas, pregnant women have heightened vulnerablility to both asymptomatic and symptomatic parasitemia;[87] the placental vasculature shields parasitized erythrocytes from the systemic immune response, allowing localized parasite replication. Placental parasitemia has been associated with low birth weight and increased infant mortality. Uteroplacental immune responses do restrict parasite replication, however, and the effectiveness of these responses increases in subsequent pregnancies under pressure of recurrent malarial exposure. Parity-acquired immunity to *P. falciparum* is delayed or impaired in the presence of HIV infection.[88,89] In turn, the beneficial effects (maternal, placental, and neonatal) of parity in the control of parasitemia during pregnancy are markedly attenuated in the face of HIV coinfection.[90–100] HIV infection is associated with increased rates and levels of peripheral and placental parasitemia, clinical malaria, and maternal anemia in pregnant women; and coinfection is associated with a higher risk of low birth weight, preterm birth, intrauterine growth retardation, and postnatal infant mortality. Although placental parasitemia is associated with increased placental HIV viral loads in coinfected patients,[90] it remains unclear as to whether this increases the risk of mother-to-child transmission of HIV. Conflicting results (enhancement, protection, and no effect) have all been published.[96,97,100] A World Health Organization (WHO) technical consultation has recommended that HIV-infected pregnant women at risk for malaria should use insecticide-treated bednets, along with (according to HIV stage) either intermittent preventive treatment with sulfadoxine/pyrimethamine (at higher doses than is recommended for nonpregnant populations) or daily trimethoprim–sulfamethoxazole (TMP-SMX) prophylaxis.[101,102]

In areas with unstable transmission of *P. falciparum*, HIV coinfection is a risk factor for severe malaria in both adults and young children.[101,103,104] In areas of heavy transmission, HIV infection is thought also to be a risk factor for severe malaria in children, although clear data are lacking.[105] In contrast, the presence of HIV coinfection seems to have only a modest impact on risk of parasitemia and clinical malaria in semi-immune adults in such areas. The risk does increase with decreasing $CD4^+$ T-cell numbers, but the correlation is less strong than with other HIV-related OIs.[106–108]

As acquired immunity is important for therapeutic clearance of drug-resistant parasites, one might predict that HIV infection hinders the response to antimalarial therapy, particularly when suboptimal, in adults in areas of heavy transmission. Recent data support this.[109,110] HIV coinfection has also been found to be associated with an increased risk for reinfection after successful treatment for malaria.[111,112] Whether this is due to immunosuppression-associated compromise of immune responses to liver-stage parasites, or to an increased frequency of biting by *Anopheles* mosquitos in the presence of HIV-associated febrile diseases, is unclear.

Daily prophylaxis with TMP-SMX, recommended by WHO for all children and adults in sub-Saharan Africa with $CD4^+$ T-cell counts <500/mm^3, led to a 95% decrease in febrile malaria episode frequency in a study in Uganda.[113] The fact that the addition of antiretroviral therapy was associated with a further >60% decrease in such episodes provides biological support for the link between HIV infection and vulnerability to disease with *P. falciparum*. The use of insecticide-treated bednets lowered the risk further.

HIV replication in peripheral blood cells is enhanced by exposure to *P. falciparum* antigens *in vitro*, in part through induction of TNF-α.[114] HIV-uninfected peripheral blood mononuclear cells challenged with malarial (sporozoite) extracts exhibit increased susceptiblity to HIV infection, and peripheral blood mononuclear cells from HIV-infected individuals exhibit higher levels of HIV replication after exposure to parasite antigens.[115] Increased HIV replication in dendritic cells has also been seen after *in vivo* infection with *P. chabaudi* of mice transgenic for the HIV genome.[116] As might therefore be expected, *P. falciparum* infection has been shown to be associated with increased HIV viral burden in peripheral as well as placental blood.[90,117] Malaria treatment has been associated with reductions in plasma HIV viral load, although the viral burden remained elevated compared to controls for the 4-week duration of the study.[117] Whether or not malaria-mediated increases in HIV replication accelerate the course of HIV disease remains to be determined.[118]

Pharmacological interactions between antiretrovirals and antimalarials have been recognized and studied *in vitro*.[119–121] A number of protease inhibitors (PIs) as well as the nonnucleoside reverse transcriptase inhibitors delaviradine and efavirenz inhibit hepatic cytochrome P450 enzymes. Principal effects are on the CYP3A4 isoform (with ritonavir being the most potent inhibitor), although the CYP2D6 isoform may also be affected.[122,123] Nevirapine and efavirenz cause secondary induction of CYP3A4, an effect of ritonavir and nelfinavir as well.[122] Most antimalarial agents are largely metabolized via P450 enzymes. Mefloquine appears to be no exception, although details remain poorly understood.[124] Proguanil and chloroquine metabolism appears to be largely by the CYP2C19 and CYP2D6 isoforms, respectively.[125–128] Chloroquine also undergoes appreciable renal excretion, whereas doxycycline largely avoids these pathways. However, it should be noted that these interactions are *in vitro* observations, and it is unknown whether these theoretical considerations have practical consequences *in vivo*. Published pharmacokinetic data suggest that: (1) there are no significant drug–drug interactions between nelfinavir or indinavir and mefloquine;[129] (2) ritonavir has minimal effects on mefloquine pharmacokinetics, whereas mefloquine suppresses ritonavir plasma levels;[130] and (3) atovaquone increases serum zidovudine (AZT) levels by approximately 30%, although AZT has no effect on the pharmacokinetics of atovaquone.[131] In summary, the actual pharmacokinetics are not easily predictable from theoretical considerations, and there is a paucity of data. Based on the current data, mefloquine, doxycycline, chloroquine, and malarone (atovaquone + proguanil) are likely to be safe and to retain efficacy for prophylaxis of sensitive strains of malaria.

Among other malaria treatment options, quinidine, quinine, and β-artemether (and possibly other artemesinin compounds) are all predominantly metabolized through CYP3A4 isoforms.[122] Large (more than threefold) increases in the area under the curve for quinidine are expected for ritonavir.[132] As a result, quinidine has been considered to be contraindicated for those on ritonavir,[132] and this likely applies to quinine as well. There are no actual clinical data, however. Whether there are clinically relevant effects of these PIs on the metabolism of artemisinin compounds (dependent at least in part on CYP3A4) remains unknown. Uncomplicated malaria can probably be safely treated with mefloquine (in regions of susceptible strains), or atovaquone/proguanil or artemesinins plus doxycyline. Use of quinine, quinidine, or artemisinin compounds remains essential for the parenteral therapy of severe chloroquine-resistant malaria. For those on ritonavir (and/or other PIs, delaviridine, or efavirenz), the normal loading dose of quinine or quinidine should probably be given, along with some reduction of the maintenance infusion dose. Obviously, careful monitoring needs to be done for the potentially fatal arrhythmic consequences of quinine/quinidine overdosage in this setting. Given the lack of data, however, underdosing may also be a potential problem. The "washout" period for the metabolic effects of ritonavir is thought to be 24–48 hours.

Recent WHO guidelines for malaria treatment recommend artemesinin-based combination therapy containing artemether and lumefantrine or artesunate and amodiaquine, mefloquine or sulfadoxine–pyrimethamine as first-line treatment for uncomplicated malaria.[133] In malaria-endemic regions, first-line treatment for HIV infection includes antiretroviral therapy containing efavirenz,[134] which has been found to elevate amodiaquine levels and half-life.[135–138] These findings raise concerns about the safety of the combination treatments in question. In addition, the rare occurrence of amodiaquine-related hepatotoxicity, along with reports of neutropenia in HIV-infected children treated with artesunate plus amodiaquine, are causes for concern.[139–141]

A higher incidence of allergic responses to sulfonamides makes pyrimethamine–sulfadoxine less attractive as a malaria therapy in HIV-seropositive patients, at least in North American populations.[142] Furthermore, Stevens–Johnson syndrome and related adverse mucocutaneous reactions to the long-acting sulfa compound, sulfadoxine, have contraindicated its use in malaria prophylaxis in developed countries.[143]

The presence of HIV infection alters the predictive value of fever in the empirical diagnosis of malaria. In areas with a high prevalence of both HIV and malaria, the common practice of empirically treating febrile adults for malaria leads to gross overestimation and overtreatment of malaria.[108] Finally, treatment of severe anemia due to malaria is one of the most common reasons for blood transfusion in sub-Saharan Africa. Malaria thus provides an indirect but very important risk factor for the acquisition of HIV infection by children where the blood supply is not well screened for HIV.[144,145]

Babesiosis

A significant clinical interaction with HIV infection has been suggested for *Babesia microti* (see Chapter 97), raising the possibility that infection with other tropical babesial species may be a risk for AIDS patients. There are a handful of reported cases of *B. microti* infection in HIV-infected people.[135,136,146,147] Two occurred in splenectomized patients; in one, chronic low-level hemolysis due to *Babesia* prior to splenectomy was likely. Patients with intact spleens have presented with fevers of unknown origin in the face of CD4 counts less than 200/μL. Quinine plus clindamycin or atovaquone plus azithromycin both appear to have therapeutic efficacy in acute disease. In the face of HIV infection, chronic suppressive therapy appears to be indicated.[146] As with all vector-borne diseases, vector avoidance is the most efficient way to prevent disease. Significant interactions with HIV infection remain to be described for European bovine *Babesia* species (*B. bovis* and *B. divergens*) and the emerging agents of human babesiosis (WA1, CA1, MO1) in North America.

Leishmaniasis

With the exception of *Toxoplasma gondii*, *Leishmania* species (see Chapter 100) are the most common tissue protozoa causing OI in patients with AIDS. This is not surprising because CMI (in particular, Th1-mediated immune responses) is critical for protection from *Leishmania*, and competence of the Th1 axis of cellular response becomes increasingly compromised during the progression of HIV-related immunosuppression. *In vivo*, the overall loss of immunological control of parasite infection is reflected by often-aberrant manifestations of VL in AIDS, including peripheral parasitemia (found in more than 50%) and parasite dissemination to unusual body compartments.[148] An AIDS-related OI occurring at low $CD4^+$ T-cell counts, leishmaniasis may be due either to primary infection or to the reactivation of clinically latent infection.[149,150] Although published data on the interaction of HIV and *Leishmania* focus largely on the effects of HIV on leishmanial infection and disease, there is also both *in vitro* and *in vivo* evidence that *Leishmania* can augment HIV replication.[151–153]

Leishmania normally require an arthropod vector, the sandfly, to move from its zoonotic cycle to human hosts. With certain species of *Leishmania* (*L. tropica* and *L. donovani*) and in some locations (e.g., Syria and India, respectively), an anthroponotic human-to-human cycle via the sandfly can exist. In situations in which intravenous drug use is practiced, transmission is simplified even further by direct person-to-person transfer via contaminated needles and syringes. Generally, however, leishmaniasis is a rural or periurban zoonosis.

The experience with VL complicating HIV/AIDS in Mediterranean countries indicates that many, perhaps most, of the leishmanial infections are acquired with HIV or after HIV infection has already occurred. The transmission of both agents that occurs by sharing of needles and syringes by intravenous drug users could theoretically be reduced by an aggressive program of education and provision of clean needles and syringes. An effective program of sandfly vector control will interrupt transmission from heavily infected human reservoirs to other humans as well as the more usual cycle of infected dogs to humans. Vector control is also the only way to prevent coinfection with *Leishmania* in those who acquire HIV sexually.

From the relatively high prevalence of latent leishmanial infection, it would appear that reactivation of latent infection could account for the increasing numbers of HIV–*Leishmania* coinfections; however, this concept is not always supported by epidemiologic evidence. A greater variability in zymodemes (enzyme markers) has been found in parasite isolates from HIV-infected than uninfected patients. In one series, five isolates were recovered from HIV-infected patients that had previously not been encountered in immunocompetent people with either VL or cutaneous leishmaniasis (CL).[154] The finding that certain strains of *Leishmania* typically causing cutaneous disease are being recovered from the bone marrow of coinfected patients could support either the primary or the reactivation hypothesis.[155] Normally, the age distribution of VL caused by *L. donovani* includes adults as well as children. In contrast, VL due to *L. infantum* affects children predominantly, often age 5 years or younger. In Spain, where intravenous drug use accounts for the majority of HIV–*Leishmania* coinfections, the age distribution of VL has been reversed, with most cases occurring in young adult males.[156] The fact that half of patients have demonstrable organisms in peripheral blood smears[157] and the fact that sandflies can readily be infected by feeding on coinfected patients[158] provide evidence for an additional anthroponotic cycle of transmission in this setting.[155] In summary, although reactivation of latent leishmanial infection is difficult to exclude, increasing evidence – in southern Europe, at least – favors primary infection by certain strains of *Leishmania* as the main mechanism for coinfection with HIV/AIDS.

With the spread of the HIV pandemic, there is increasing epidemiological overlap of areas in which HIV and leishmaniasis occur. Cases have been reported from approximately 40 countries, although the bulk of cases have been reported from southern Europe.[148–150,155,159,160] Of note, relatively few cases of American mucocutaneous leishmaniasis have been recognized in HIV-infected subjects.[161,162] The propensity for disseminated disease in the presence of HIV appears to be limited to certain species of *Leishmania*. The bulk of the information on VL complicating HIV infection involves *L. infantum* in the Mediterranean region. Presumably, the ability to visceralize under the influence of HIV also applies to *L. donovani* in southern Asia and Africa and to *L. chagasi* in Latin America; however, documentation for this is still somewhat meager, one of the possible reasons being the poor overlap between geographic distribution of leishmaniasis caused by these species and the distribution, as well as prevalence, of HIV infection. The species of *Leishmania* that cause CL have been implicated only rarely as OIs in HIV/AIDS. In one instance, *L. braziliensis* was recovered from the bone marrow of a patient with a $CD4^+$ T-cell count of less than 10/μL,[163] but the main clinical picture in this case, as well as in others,[164–166] including a patient infected with *L. major*,[167] has been one of multiple cutaneous lesions resembling diffuse CL. Diffuse CL has also been reported as part of the immune reconstitution inflammatory syndrome (IRIS).[168,169]

A febrile illness of longer than 2 weeks' duration in an HIV-infected person with a lifetime history of travel to *Leishmania*-endemic regions of the world should raise suspicion of leishmaniasis complicating HIV infection. If the patient is an intravenous drug user, travel to southern Europe, especially Spain, France, and Italy, would be particularly pertinent. Clinical diagnosis of VL in *Leishmania*–HIV coinfected people may be difficult. Only 75% of HIV-infected patients, as opposed to 95% of non-HIV-infected patients, exhibit the characteristic clinical pattern, namely fever, splenomegaly, and hepatomegaly.[149,150,155,160,170] With increasing immunosuppression, clinically evident ectopic localization of parasites becomes common.[171] Gastrointestinal, laryngeal, pulmonary, and peritoneal involvement has been reported.[171–178] Single and multiple cutaneous forms and/or mucosal and mucocutaneous lesions have also been described in AIDS patients worldwide.[166,173,179]

In immunocompetent people, serological tests have been very useful in the diagnosis of VL because B-cell activation is prominent, with large amounts of both specific and nonspecific antibody being produced. In contrast, approximately 50% of coinfected patients lack detectable antibody levels.[142,149,150,170] The situation may be different in instances in which leishmanial infection precedes HIV infection and the impaired immune responses that ensue. Gradoni and associates[180] suggested that this type of serologic data could be used as an indicator of the sequence of acquisition of the two infections. Support for this concept is provided by a report from Ethiopia of seven cases of VL with HIV coinfection, all with highly elevated antileishmanial antibody titers.[181] All patients had lived for many years in a leishmaniasis-endemic area of Ethiopia.[181] The recombinant antigen rK-39 appears to be highly sensitive and specific for immunodiagnosis of VL due to *L. donovani* and *L. chagasi* in patients without complicating HIV infection; however, the sensitivity of rK-39 for immunodiagnosis of cutaneous cases from Turkey was greatly reduced compared with most cases of VL.[182] The utility of rK-39-based diagnostics is not clear in HIV-seropositive people. The peripheral parasitemia displayed by many HIV-coinfected individuals allows the detection of parasites from the blood in approximately 50% of cases. Cultures and polymerase chain reaction (PCR) of buffy-coat preparations are positive in 70% and up to 100%, respectively.[149,150,183]

There is abundant evidence that successful treatment of leishmanial disease, regardless of the drugs used, ultimately requires intact CMI. The coinfected patient is the victim of a double insult to the immune system. VL is associated with antigen-specific T-cell unresponsiveness[184] and dysfunctional cytokine responses.[185] This situation is further compounded by the immunologic abnormalities associated with HIV infection.

Therapy for VL in the face of HIV coinfection remains controversial, largely due to a lack of firm data. The same drugs used for treatment of VL in normal hosts (including pentavalent antimonials and amphotericin B preparations) have utility in the treatment of coinfected patients, albeit with significantly less efficacy.[170] Amphotericin B is a conventional drug for all forms of leishmaniasis, including visceral disease. Liposomally encapsulated amphotericin has the theoretical advantage of being targeted to macrophages, host cells for leishmanial parasites. Between 40% and 65% of coinfected patients have initial parasitological cure after treatment with pentavalent antimonials, amphotericin B deoxycholate, or amphotericin B lipid complex.[170,186,187] Among these options, treatment with lipid formulations of amphotericin B appears to have similar efficacy, but less severe toxicity, than the other drugs. However, the experience with lipid formulations of amphotericin B in coinfected patients is limited. These lipid formulations are also quite expensive. Miltefosine, an oral agent that is safe and effective for the treatment of Indian patients with VL,[188] has shown promise in early compassionate-use treatments of VL in HIV-infected subjects.[189]

Even with initial cure, relapse is predictable, occurring in up to 80% of coinfected individuals within 1 year.[169,170,186,190,191] The optimal drug for secondary prophylaxis remains unclear. Pentamidine given once every 3 or 4 weeks[192] and liposome-encapsulated amphotericin every 2 weeks[193] or 3 weeks[191] have been used.

The fact that significant reductions in the incidence of AIDS-related VL were seen in southern Europe after the advent of HAART,[194,195] along with the fact that HAART-related immune reconstitution has allowed secondary prophylaxis for other OIs to be stopped, has raised hope that HAART will allow for safe discontinuance of secondary prophylaxis for VL.[196–198]

American Trypanosomiasis (Chagas Disease)

American trypanosomiasis (see Chapter 99), is a well-recognized OI in AIDS.[199] The causative organism, *Trypanosoma cruzi*, and its triatomine vector are widely distributed from the United States to Chile and Argentina. Because the cases of HIV-related Chagas disease reported to date largely represent reactivation of chronic infection during the course of HIV-induced immunosuppression and not primary infection in the face of AIDS (not surprising given the differing patterns of epidemiological risk for these infections: largely rural for *T. cruzi* and largely urban for HIV), this OI can be expected to appear outside these geographic bounds. It should be noted that activation of latent *T. cruzi* infection, as well as exacerbated primary infection (transmitted by blood transfusion), is also well described in the face of the iatrogenic immunosuppression used for solid-organ transplantation and therapy for hematological malignancies.

Clinical *T. cruzi* reactivation in the face of HIV coinfection appears to occur largely in those with $CD4^+$ T-cell counts less than 200/μL. Clinically, such reactivation most commonly involves the central nervous system (CNS).[199,200] *T. cruzi* was probably late in being recognized as an opportunistic pathogen in this setting because the most prominent features of disease are similar to those of toxoplasmic meningoencephalitis. Enlargement of hemorrhagic foci can produce mass effects simulating brain tumors. Lesions are often multiple, with computed tomographic (CT) scans and magnetic resonance imaging (MRI) showing ring enhancement and preferential involvement of the white matter. Toxoplasmic encephalitis may coexist in the same patient.[201] The cerebrospinal fluid (CSF) findings include a slight pleocytosis, increased protein, slightly decreased glucose in some patients, and the presence of trypanosomes. Histologically, the brain lesions show necrotic foci with hemorrhage and infiltration of inflammatory cells. Amastigote forms of the parasite are abundant in glial cells and macrophages and only occasionally in neuronal cells. Myocarditis is a common autopsy finding in those dying of AIDS-related *T. cruzi* meningoencephalitis.[198] Such myocarditis is often clinically silent. Clinical manifestations, when present, involve arrhythmias and congestive heart failure.[199,202,203] Diagnosis of reactivated *T. cruzi* infection depends, first, on considering the possibility based on the geographic origin of the patient, and on an appreciation of the clinical picture. If neurologic signs are present, performing a CT scan or MRI is key.[204] The imaging pattern of CNS *T. cruzi* infection is indistinguishable from that of toxoplasmic encephalitis. Direct microscopic examination of centrifuged sediment of CSF will often show motile trypanosomes. If fever and other systemic signs are present, direct examination of the buffy coat from the microhematocrit tube may also show motile trypanosomes. Since serum antibodies to *T. cruzi* indicate previous infection with the parasite, this test is only useful for ruling out reactivated infection if it is negative. If other tests are inconclusive, biopsy of a brain lesion to demonstrate characteristic organisms can be done. PCR on blood or CSF requires research laboratory facilities.

Clinically, differentiating HIV-related reactivation of Chagas disease from chronic chagasic disease may be difficult. HIV-related reactivation is associated with high parasitemia, however, whereas the parasitemia of chronic disease is very low.[205] Indeed, even in the absence of overt, clinical reactivation, chronic Chagas disease is associated with a higher percentage and level of parasitemia in those coinfected with HIV (independent of CD4 count) than in HIV seronegatives.[206] The effects of coinfection appear to be bidirectional. HIV viral load has been documented to increase simultaneously with an asymptomatic increase in *T. cruzi* parasitemia, returning to baseline in the face of successful antiparasitic treatment.[207] Nifurtimox and benznidazole, both of which have moderate antitrypanosomal activity, are the standard drugs recommended for treatment of Chagas disease. However, there is not enough experience to evaluate the effectiveness of these drugs in the treatment of *T. cruzi* infections complicating HIV/AIDS, especially in cases with meningoencephalitis. No information is available on the penetration of nifurtimox and benznidazole into the CNS, and the survival time of reported cases of coinfection has been short. A patient reported by Nishioka and coworkers[208] survived for 92 days, with disappearance of trypanosomes from the blood and CSF as well as clearance of a brain lesion while being treated with benznidazole at a dose of 8 mg/kg/day for 80 days. Clinical improvement and reduction in size of a brain lesion were attributed to treatment with benznidazole plus, later, itraconazole and fluconazole in another patient with coinfection who survived for at least 6 months.[209] Itraconazole and ketaconazole have been used and are reported to have reduced parasitemia in one case each,[210] but both cases succumbed to HIV infection. Although there is no other reported experience with the use of itraconazole or fluconazole in the treatment of American trypanosomiasis in humans, itraconazole was reported to be very effective in experimental infections.[211] It has been recommended that treatment of *T. cruzi* infection in the setting of HIV be started early in the reactivation process, when parasitemia is detectable, but before irreversible end-organ damage has occurred.[207] Such a strategy would hinge on serological identification of those at risk, something indicated in all HIV-infected individuals with appreciable risk of *T. cruzi* infection. Although data are lacking, it should be noted that immunological reconstitution through HAART therapy is likely to provide considerable prophylactic and therapeutic benefit in this disease.

African Trypanosomiasis

No significant interactions between the agents of African trypanosomiasis (see Chapter 98) and HIV have been delineated. Although T-cell and macrophage responses are not thought to be important in the protective host response to trypanosomiasis, trypanosomiasis can suppress cellular immune responses, so a biologic interaction between the two is plausible. No significant epidemiologic association between *Trypansoma brucei gambiense* and HIV has been found.[212–215] Whether HIV alters the clinical course of either West or East African trypanosomiasis is unclear.[214] There is anecdotal evidence that HIV may complicate the therapy of West African trypanosomiasis, however. Of 18 patients treated with melarsoprol in a rural hospital in the Congo, all 14 HIV-negative patients recovered, whereas 3 of 4 HIV-positive patients died during treatment (likely due to treatment-related encephalopathy) and the fourth failed to respond to therapy.[216]

Other Trypanosomatids

In addition to the two genera, *Leishmania* and *Trypanosoma*, known to cause disease in humans, the Trypanosomatidae family includes other genera that parasitize other vertebrates, insects, and plants. There have been three reports of HIV-infected individuals presenting with symptoms typical of VL in which ultrastructural, isoenzyme, and/or kinetoplast DNA analyses of the isolated lesional parasites have indicated that the responsible organism actually belongs to one of these latter genera.[217] The strong implication is that HIV-related immunosuppression can render humans vulnerable to normally nonpathogenic lower trypanosomatids.

Toxoplasmosis

Toxoplasma gondii is a ubiquitous parasite of mammals throughout the world (see Chapter 103). Latent infection lasts for the lifetime of the host. Maintenance of latency is dependent on CMI responses. Reactivation of latent infection is common with increasing immunosuppression in AIDS. The principal manifestation of such reactivation, toxoplasmic encephalitis, is thus a common OI in AIDS patients throughout the world. The incidence of toxoplasmic encephalitis is proportional to the prevalence of latent infection in the population at risk of or with AIDS.[218] In the United States, the rate of latent infection varies between 10% and 40%; in Paris, the rate is 90%.[218] Acquisition of *Toxoplasma* infection is age-dependent, but there is wide variation in infection rates even over narrow geographic areas.[219,220] Prevalence rates in the tropics vary from 0% to 90%, with most measured communities falling in a broad middle range.[221–227]

In the United States, prior to the advent of HAART, one-third of *Toxoplasma*-seropositive AIDS patients developed toxoplasmic encephalitis in the absence of prophylaxis,[228] 90% of such cases were in patients with less than 200 $CD4^+$T cells/μL, and 70% in those with less than 100 CD4 T cells/μL.[229] The prevalence of toxoplasmic encephalitis in AIDS patients in the tropics is unclear, but the burden is thought to be immense and underdiagnosed. Autopsy series that have included examination of the brain have suggested disease prevalence rates in late-stage AIDS patients of 15% in Abidjan, Côte d'Ivoire,[230] 25% in Mexico City,[231] and 36% in Kampala, Uganda.[232]

The presumptive diagnosis of toxoplasmic encephalitis is based on clinical presentation, positive *Toxoplasma* serologies, and characteristic neuroradiologic features.[233] A final clinical diagnosis is made based on the clinical and radiographic response to specific chemotherapy. Less common manifestations of toxoplasmosis in AIDS include pneumonia, retinochoroiditis, myocarditis, orchitis, and gastrointestinal involvement. Excellent reviews on *Toxoplasma* in AIDS provide information on the clinical management of this cosmopolitan OI.[17,76,78,234]

Five percent of toxoplasmic encephalitis occurs not as reactivation but as an acute infection.[228] Preventing the transmission of *T. gondii* to *Toxoplasma*-seronegative, HIV-infected people has two facets: (1) avoiding the ingestion of tissue cysts of other intermediate mammalian hosts (i.e., cooking meat well); and (2) avoiding the oocysts of the definitive host, the cat. Avoiding cat feces in and around dwellings is probably not sufficient because the oocysts are viable for up to 18 months in moist soil. Contamination of fresh vegetables may be a common method of human infection, and such foodstuffs should probably be washed well or cooked or both.

Primary prophylaxis (TMP-SMX is preferred)[235] should be taken by all *Toxoplasma*-seropositive HIV patients with a $CD4^+$T-cell count less than 100/μL. It is safe to discontinue both primary and secondary prophylaxis after HAART-related immune reconstitution (sustained $CD4^+$ T-cell counts >200/μL).[76–78]

Free-Living Amebae

Free-living amebae of the *Acanthamoeba* and *Balamuthia* genera (see Chapter 101) are rare causes of opportunistic encephalitis and cutaneous disease in late-stage AIDS. Most case reports have been from the United States, but the worldwide environmental distribution of these ubiquitous protozoans and the fact that diagnosis is often postmortem suggest that underdiagnosis is widespread in the tropics and elsewhere. *Acanthamoeba* and *Balamuthia* have been isolated from soil, water (including tap water, bottled water, chlorinated pools, and natural sources of fresh and seawater), and air throughout the world.[236] The isolation of *Acanthamoeba* from the nasopharynx of healthy adults indicates that these organisms may be common constituents of normal flora.[237] Cellular immunity, along with antibody and complement, appears to be critical for protective immunity.[238] Invasive disease occurs in the immunocompromised and debilitated.[239] Occasionally, encephalitis with *Balamuthia mandrillaris* has occurred in apparently normal hosts.[240–242]

Granulomatous amebic encephalitis (GAE), a subacute to chronic disease of compromised hosts caused by multiple species of *Acanthamoeba* as well as *B. mandrillaris*, generally causes death in weeks to months. Clinical and pathologic data, along with animal models, suggest that the pathogenesis involves hematogenous dissemination to the brain from initial respiratory (or perhaps cutaneous) sites of infection.[239] Pathologic changes, in the form of necrotizing granulomatous inflammation, are found predominantly in the posterior neuraxis.

More than 20 cases of GAE, due to a variety of species, have been reported in AIDS patients.[239,243–253] Disseminated cutaneous disease (subacute granulomatous dermatitis) has been a feature of many of these cases and has preceded clinical cerebral involvement by weeks or months in some. Subacute granulomatous dermatitis has been the sole manifestation of invasive disease in some patients.[254–258] $CD4^+$ T-cell counts in HIV-infected individuals with GAE have been reported to be less than 250/μL (median, 24/μL) at the time of presentation. Where CD4 counts have not been reported, the histories reveal clinical evidence of late-stage AIDS.[236,239]

In AIDS patients, GAE is marked by a more rapid course (with death in 3–40 days)[239] and a paucity of well-formed granulomas in comparison to other hosts with the disease.[239,257] Symptomatic involvement of the nasopharynx, paranasal sinuses, or the skin prior to development of GAE is common in AIDS patients.[239,259] Cutaneous lesions are usually nodular, with subsequent enlargement, ulceration, and metastatic spread. Such lesions can be quite pleomorphic (pustules, plaques, eschars, and cellulitis), however, and have been confused with cat-scratch disease, cryptococcosis, sporotrichosis, bacillary angiomatosis, mycobacterial infections, and vasculitis.[239] The most common presentation of cerebral disease is that of fever and headache.[239,256] Focal neurologic deficits and profound changes in mental status are also frequent. Neuroradiologic findings mimic those of toxoplasmic encephalitis, with multiple enhancing mass lesions and surrounding edema. CSF findings are quite variable.[239,256]

A high index of suspicion and tissue or microbiologic diagnosis are key to the antemortem identification of GAE. Wet mounts of CSF are occasionally useful (perhaps less useful in *Balamuthia* infection).[259] CSF examination generally reveals lymphocytic pleocytosis with mild to severe elevation (≥1000 mg/dL) of protein and normal or low glucose. Both trophozoites and cysts can be found in tissue biopsies. Cysts have been mistaken for the sporangia of *Rhinosporium* or *Prototheca* or for cryptococci; trophozoites have been mistaken for macrophages.[259] *Acanthamoeba* can be isolated by culture on *Escherichia coli*-seeded nonnutrient agar or in tissue culture medium.[239,256] Identification of species (and even differentiation of *Acanthamoeba* from *Balamuthia*) is not possible morphologically. Immunofluorescence techniques can differentiate *Acanthamoeba* to the group level in tissue section or with cultured organisms.

Treatment of disseminated disease due to these organisms is difficult in any host. No chemotherapeutic regimen is clearly efficacious. Miltefosine showed some efficacy in a recently reported case.[260] Other agents with possible clinical utility in combination therapy include pentamidine, 5-fluorocytosine, sulfamethazine, sulfadiazine, fluconazole, itraconazole, ketoconazole, macrolides, phenothiazines, and rifampin.[239,252,254,255,261] There may be value in testing clinical isolates for drug sensitivities. With isolated cerebral lesions, there may be a role for surgical excision.[253]

A case of primary amebic meningoencephalitis due to an apparently newly recognized ameba and not associated with thermally polluted water was reported in a patient with late-stage AIDS in Spain.[262,263]

Enteric Coccidiosis (*Isospora, Cryptosporidium*, and *Cyclospora*)

A trio of coccidian protozoa – *Isospora belli*, *Cryptosporidium* spp., and *Cyclospora* (*Eimeria*) *cayetanensis* – are all prominent causes of self-limited, small-bowel diarrhea in immunologically normal hosts as well as causes of chronic, severe disease in the face of HIV coinfection. All are cosmopolitan infections. Infection with a fourth organism, *Sarcocystis hominis*, responsible for both enteric and disseminated coccidioisis in humans, has been reported as a coinfecting organism in only a handful of cases with HIV infections.[264]

Cryptosporidium spp. (see Chapter 94)

In addition to the most common human pathogen within this genus, *C. hominis*, a variety of zoonotic species also infect humans, including *C. parvum*, *C. canis*, *C. felis*, *C. meleagridis*, and *C. muris*.[265–267] Zoonotic species may cause more severe human disease and may occur more commonly in immunocompromised people. Because of the high prevalence of disease and the lack of effective specific treatment, cryptosporidiosis is a particularly common and severe problem as an OI throughout the world. Chronic infection and disease are most frequent with $CD4^+$ T-cell counts less than 180/μL[268] and are associated with increased mortality.[269–271] The use of HAART therapy has led to a decreasing prevalence of cryptosporidial disease in HIV-infected individuals; however, rates of diarrhea in HIV-infected individuals associated with *Cryoptosporidium* spp. in developing countries remain high, up to 83% in symptomatic and 57% in asymptomatic individuals.[272–274]

Four clinical syndromes of cryptosporidial diarrheal disease in patients with AIDS have been limned: (1) chronic diarrhea (36%); (2) cholera-like disease (33%); (3) transient diarrhea (15%); and (4) relapsing illness (15%). The severe end of the spectrum is seen largely in those with $CD4^+$ T-cell counts less than 180/μL.[275,276] Less commonly, extraintestinal sites are secondarily involved, including biliary tract, stomach, pancreas, lung, paranasal sinuses, and middle ear.[275–278] Of these, biliary tract involvement (presenting with right upper-quadrant pain, nausea, vomiting, and fever) represents the most common, clinically important site, being found in up to one-fourth of patients with AIDS-related intestinal disease prior to the use of HAART.[279] Individuals with $CD4^+$ T-cell counts less than 50/μL are at a particular risk for development of symptomatic biliary disease.[279] No antimicrobial agent has demonstrable, consistent efficacy in HIV-related cryptosporidiosis. Immune reconstitution with HAART should be pursued,[280–283] along with supportive treatment with fluids, nutrition, and antimotility agents.[76–78]

Isospora belli (see Chapter 95)

Disease due to *Isospora* is less cosmopolitan than that due to *Cryptosporidium*, being most common in tropical and subtropical areas.[284] In some regions, it has been reported to be one of the most common parasitic etiologic agents of diarrhea in HIV-infected individuals, rivaling rates for *Cryptosporidium*.[285–287] Rates of infection have fallen dramatically with the introduction of HAART.[288] Isosporiasis usually presents with chronic watery diarrhea and weight loss, with or without vomiting, abdominal pain, and fever.[288] Invasion of gallbladder tissue, similar to that described with *Cryptosporidium*, has been described, along with disseminated involvement of mesenteric and tracheobronchial lymph nodes, in the setting of HIV coinfection.[289,290] Prominent tissue eosinophilia of the involved lamina propria is often present.[284] TMP-SMX provides effective therapy.[291] Pyrimethamine (with leucovorin) provides a second option.[292] Clinical response is usually rapid, but relapses are common. In the absence of immune reconstitution, suppressive therapy is indicated.[76–78]

Cyclospora cayetanensis (see Chapter 95)

The clinical picture of enteric infection with *C. cayetanensis* in AIDS appears to be similar to that due to other coccidia.[293] Biliary tract involvement – manifested as right upper-quadrant pain, elevated alkaline phosphatase, and thickened gallbladder by ultrasound – has also been described in *Cyclospora* infection.[294] Thus, all three human enteric coccidia are capable of invading the gallbladder. As with isosporiasis, cyclosporiasis in AIDS is treatable with TMP-SMX.[293] Follow-up suppressive therapy is indicated.[76–78]

Microsporidiosis

Microsporidia are intracellular protozoans that, due to HIV and AIDS, have emerged from their relative obscurity as pathogens of insects, fish, and laboratory animals to occupy a new role as important OIs of humans.[295] These cosmopolitan emerging pathogens of the immunosuppressed (including *Enterocytozoon bienusi*, *E.* (*Septata*) *intestinalis*, *E. cuniculi*, *E. hellem*, as well as pathogens from several other genera) are considered in Chapter 102.

Other Protozoa

Entamoeba histolytica

This intestinal parasite (see Chapter 92) was initially associated with HIV because of its high prevalence in men who have sex with men (MSM), and seroprevalance studies continue to indicate a high exposure rate in MSM, although the significance of this observation remains unclear.[296–299] Despite considerable evidence that immunity in amebiasis requires the participation of CMI, there is no evidence that patients with HIV infection or AIDS are more likely to develop invasive disease.[297]

Giardia lamblia

As with *E. histolytica*, a high prevalence of infection with *G. lamblia* (see Chapter 93) was found in the 1980s among MSM.[300] A study of MSM performed at that time revealed no increase in prevalence or severity of giardiasis in patients with AIDS.[301] Since then, no evidence has been found of a significant effect of HIV coinfection.[298] Although some studies have indicated a higher prevalence of giardiasis in HIV seropositives, this has not been a consistent finding.[302] Therapy of giardiasis in people with AIDS is usually successful. Some patients, immunocompromised as well as immunocompetent, are refractory to standard therapeutic regimens for giardiasis. It may well be that such refractoriness to standard therapy is found more commonly in the face of HIV coinfection.[303]

Blastocystis hominis

Controversy continues to exist as to the role of this organism as a cause of diarrheal disease in either immunocompetent patients or HIV-infected people.[302,304]

Balantidium coli

No information is available as to whether this organism can serve as an OI in HIV-infected people.

Helminthic Infections

Trematodes

There is no evidence that any trematode infection is more severe or difficult to treat in the face of HIV coinfection. More subtle interactions have been explored in schistosomiasis (see Chapter 122). A study of car washers working on the shores of Lake Victoria in Kenya, a population with a high intensity of exposure to *Schistosoma mansoni* and an HIV seroprevalence of approximately 30%, has provided insights into the bidirectional effects of coinfection.[305] The CD4$^+$ T-cell-dependent granulomatous response to schistosome eggs has been shown to be important in egg migration from venules to the lumen of the intestine in mouse models of disease.[306] As might thereby be expected, a significant suppression of egg excretion efficiency, controlled for the degree of infection, was found in *S. mansoni*-infected patients in the presence of HIV coinfection and low CD4$^+$ T-cell counts.[307] Although successful therapy of *S. mansoni* infection with praziquantel may depend on the host antibody response, praziquantel was efficacious in treating schistosomiasis in this HIV-infected cohort.[308] Given that schistosome infection likely preceded HIV infection in these individuals, whether praziquantel will have equal efficacy in individuals infected first with HIV remains an open question. In this context, a study from Kenya reported that treatment with a standard regimen of praziquantel in coinfected individuals resulted in normal kinetics of reduction in egg excretion, but a slower decline in serum levels of an adult worm antigen – interpreted to indicate less efficient killing of adult worms.[309] Notably, despite similar responses to therapy, individuals with HIV coinfection and low CD4$^+$ T-cell counts showed increased susceptibility to reinfection after therapy,[310] something that appeared to correlate with blunted immunological responses to successful drug therapy (and the resultant release of parasite antigens) in such individuals.[311] A study of HIV/*S. haematobium* coinfection in Zambia mirrored these findings: (1) coinfected individuals had lower egg excretion; and (2) praziquantel retained efficacy in the face of coinfection.[312] No alteration in resistance to reinfection with *S. haematobium* was seen in the face of HIV infection, but CD4$^+$ T-cell counts were not performed in this cohort that lacked clinically evident HIV disease. It thus remains possible that, as with *S. mansoni* infection, resistance to reinfection with *S. haematobium* is decreased with progression of HIV/AIDS.

As for the effects of schistosomiasis on HIV, both female and male urogenital schistosomiasis, like other inflammatory genital diseases, are thought to increase the risk for HIV transmission.[309,313–317] Schistosomiasis is also a prime example of a chronic tropical infection that has been postulated to enhance the pathogenesis of HIV. Schistosome infections act as powerful inducers of Th2 polarization and immune counterregulatory responses in both mice and humans.[309,318–320] Such infections are also likely to alter gut mucosal permeability and systemic exposure to gut-derived microbial products. As noted above, following on the heels of negative studies, a recent randomized trial of praziquantel for schistosomiasis found a significant benefit of treatment on plasma HIV-1 RNA load, along with a nonsignificant trend towards a beneficial effect on CD4$^+$ counts in HIV-infected individuals.[321]

The literature appears to be silent as to whether there are any significant interactions between pulmonary, hepatic, or intestinal trematodes and HIV.

Cestodes

A few unusual manifestations of cestode infection have been reported in AIDS patients. A rapidly expanding, invasive, and ultimately lethal abdominal mass in a patient with a CD4$^+$ T-cell count less than 100/μL was found, by ribosomal DNA amplification and sequencing, to be due to *Hymenolepis nana*.[322,323] Whether this represents merely the fortuitous concurrence of an unusual pathologic finding with dramatic improvements in diagnostic technology (previous rare cases in normal hosts having occurred in the absence of diagnosis) or the recognition of a new disease because its expression is facilitated or dependent on immunosuppression (AIDS patients serving as "sentinel chickens" for the population at large) is unclear. The latter interpretation is favored by a previous similar case report of presumably disseminated cestode infection in the face of immunosuppression due to Hodgkin's disease and its therapy.[324]

Four cases of exuberant subcutaneous disease due to the larval form of *Taenia crassiceps* have been reported in AIDS patients.[325–328] Thus, HIV infection may be a risk for disease with this cestode. A case of hepatic alveolar echinococcal disease in a 6-year-old child with AIDS has been described.[329] Uncommon features of this case include the remarkably young age and hence short incubation period for disease and the complete lack of demonstrable parasite-specific humoral or cellular immune responses. The paucity of reported cases of hydatid disease in HIV-infected patients does not permit any conclusions about the biology or clinical course of coinfection.

Finally, several cases of neurocysticercosis have been reported in HIV-infected patients.[330] Most cases of coinfection have presented with multiple parenchymal lesions.[330] The frequency of giant cysts and racemose forms of disease is elevated in reported cases,[331] again perhaps a reflection of the role of CD4$^+$ T cells in tissue immunity to *T. solium*. Further clinical data on the interaction between HIV and cestode infections are awaited.

Nematodes

Strongyloides stercoralis

Strongyloides stercoralis (see Chapter 117) appeared to qualify as a potential OI because it is one of the two nematodes (apart from *Capillaria philippinensis*; coinfection not yet reported) capable of multiplying in human hosts, especially in immunocompromised subjects.

One way in which immunosuppression enhances *Strongyloides* infection is by permitting or stimulating an increased degree of the normal process of autoinfection.[332] In this process, first-stage rhabditiform larvae (L1) produced by the adult female worm in the upper small bowel are transformed into infective filariform larvae (L3) that can reinvade the colonic intestinal wall or the perianal or perineal areas. Massive upregulation of the autoinfective process results in the hyperinfection syndrome, with the development of many more adult worms, and the production of large numbers of larvae that disseminate to all organs. The clinical picture is dominated by Gram-negative bacterial sepsis, meningitis, and/or pneumonia. Hyperinfection is usually associated with immunosuppression, particularly the administration of corticosteroids.

Strongyloidiasis was initially designated as an AIDS OI based on the past record of *S. stercoralis* in causing hyperinfection in the immunosuppressed.[333] Five years later, when it became apparent that hyperinfection syndrome was not being encountered frequently in patients with AIDS, it was removed from the list of AIDS-defining OIs.[334] Given the low but appreciable rate (3.9%) of strongyloidiasis among men attending sexually transmitted disease clinics in New York City in 1981,[335] the AIDS epidemic in the United States should have provided some clinical evidence of any predisposition of AIDS patients to hyperinfection. This did not occur. The available evidence makes it extremely unlikely that misdiagnosis or underreporting are the relevant factors here; severe strongyloidiasis or hyperinfection syndrome has prominent clinical features and is often fatal if untreated, and it is not likely that the association would escape notice. Few cases of hyperinfection syndrome have been reported in the English-language literature.[336–345] Even among these cases, the presence of hyperinfection is poorly documented in many; and, all too frequently, there is confusion between severe GI disease and hyperinfection.[346]

Diagnosis (as opposed to suspicion) of hyperinfection syndrome depends on the demonstration of markedly increased numbers of filariform larvae in the stool or multiple such larvae in the sputum. The mere presence of filariform larvae in the sputum only indicates the existence of autoinfection. (It should also be noted that the presence of rhabditiform larvae in the sputum points to neither autoinfection nor hyperinfection but to the presence of adult female worms in the lung.)

It is possible that the frequency of severe strongyloidiasis complicating HIV infection is much higher in certain areas of the tropics where both infections are prevalent and medical facilities are lacking; however, an absence of such an association has been noted from just such areas.[18] Petithory and Derouin[347] pointed out that clinical studies of AIDS patients in central Africa, where the prevalence of strongyloidiasis varies from 26% to 48%, did not mention extraintestinal strongyloidiasis. Similarly, a report from Brazil estimated a 1–2% prevalence of *Strongyloides* infection in the population of São Paulo, finding the parasite in 10% of 100 AIDS patients, who showed no evidence of systemic strongyloidiasis.[348] Similar results have been found in Zambia.[349,350] A survey of urban adults in Kinshasa detected *S. stercoralis* in 20% by intensive fecal examinations of single specimens, and estimated a 50% infection rate in the same population on the basis of positive serologies. There were no significant differences in infection rates in those seropositive or seronegative for HIV (F. Neva, unpublished observations).

Taken together, these data suggest that the presence and severity of clinical disease due to *S. stercoralis* are not significantly increased in patients with HIV infection or AIDS alone. A recent study has shed light on the subject.[351] Careful quantitation of the numbers and proportions of free-living adult worms and directly developing L3 larvae in stool cultures revealed a surprising negative correlation between CD4$^+$ T-cell count and the development of infectious larvae in the gut, the latter process being necessary for autoinfection.[352]

More subtle interactions, such as an increased mean GI parasite burden or slower response to therapy, may have been missed. Also, some conditions that cosegregate with HIV/AIDS are known to predispose to the hyperinfection syndrome, including the use of steroids (given for *Pneumocystis* pneumonia and lymphoma in AIDS), inanition (seen in patients with chronic diarrhea, untreated oropharyngeal or esophageal candidiasis, and slim disease), and coinfection with human T-cell lymphotropic virus type I (HTLV-I; see Chapter 81). Strongyloidiasis is an important OI in individuals infected with HTLV-I, and *Strongyloides* infection has been suspected to be a cofactor in the development of acute T-cell leukemia and tropical spastic paraparesis in asymptomatic carriers of HTLV-I.[353,354] Notably, intravenous drug use is a risk factor for infection with both HTLV-I and HIV.

Other Geohelminths

Approximately one-third to one-half of the world's population is thought to be infected with a soil-transmitted geohelminth.[355,356] Apart from *S. stercoralis*, the heaviest public health burdens are posed by *Ascaris lumbricoides*, hookworm species, and *Trichuris trichuria*.[355] There are no published data indicating that infection or disease with any of these latter organisms is excerbated by HIV infection. Indeed, in the case of hookworm, while anemia is an independent risk factor for early death in HIV[357,358] and while hookworm infection can lead to anemia, the actual literature on hookworm infection in HIV has not revealed anything striking apart from the puzzling findings: (1) of a negative association between hookworm infection and HIV infection;[359] (2) of significantly higher CD4$^+$ T cells counts in HIV-infected individuals with hookworm infection than those without hookworm infection;[360] and (3) of a significantly lower prevalence of, and mean intensity of, hookworm infection in those with pulmonary tuberculosis and HIV, than those with pulmonary tuberculosis without HIV.[361] What, if any, significance these observations have remains unclear.

On the other hand, for reasons discussed above, chronic/recurrent geohelminth infection has been suspect as a cofactor for HIV progression. Again, following the publication of conflicting studies, a recent randomized, double-blind, placebo-controlled trial of albendazole for infection with diverse geohelminths (including hookworm, *Ascaris*, and *Trichuris*) found a significant benefit of treatment on CD4$^+$ T-cell counts – specifically in the face of *Ascaris* infection, not in those with the considerably more prevalent hookworm infection.[362] A nonsignificant trend towards a beneficial effect of treatment on plasma HIV-1 RNA load was also seen.[362] More data are needed on the subject.

Filariasis

Among the tissue-infecting filaria, the effect of HIV coinfection has been studied in a large cohort of patients with *Onchocerca volvulus* infection (see Chapter 106). No significant epidemiological association was found between the two infections, nor was there any difference in the efficacy of ivermectin treatment in HIV-infected compared with uninfected patients.[363] Onchocercal skin disease may be worse in the face of HIV infection[364] and HIV-coinfected individuals have lower levels of antibodies to *O. volvulus*.[365]

In contrast, two studies have suggested a significant epidemiological association of lymphatic filariasis (see Chapter 104) with HIV infection.[366] The increased infectability of Th2-polarized CD4$^+$ T cells may underlie this surprising finding – although a similarly increased risk for HIV infection has not been observed with infection with other helminths. As for the effect of lymphatic filariasis on HIV progression, a randomized, double-blind, placebo-controlled, cross-over trial of diethylcarbamazine for *Wuchereria bancrofti* infection reported a significant treatment-associated decrease in plasma HIV-1 RNA load, along with a nonsignificant trend towards a beneficial effect on CD4$^+$ counts.[360]

Arthropods

Sarcoptes scabiei var. *hominis* stands alone among the arthropod and crustacean infestations of humans (see Chapter 124) as a cause of exacerbated disease in the presence of HIV. In normal hosts, scabies is usually manifest as a markedly pruritic, papular, and vesicular dermatitis, with pathognomonic burrows harboring gravid females. Excoriations, nodules, and eczematous or impetiginized plaques may also be found. Relatively few adult mites are normally present. Crusted scabies is seen in neurologically impaired or immunosuppressed patients. Pruritus is often absent or mild. Lesions consist of widespread hyperkeratotic, crusted, scaling, fissured plaques. The nails are frequently involved. Patients tend to be heavily infested, with thousands of adult mites (see Chapter 124). Crusted scabies has been reported as a complication of HIV infection. CD4$^+$ T-cell counts in reported cases have been less than 500/μL.[367–369] Both typical and atypical presentations are seen, the latter including the "pruritus of AIDS," crusting with pruritus, pruritic papular dermatitis, and mimics of Darier's disease and psoriasis.[368] Secondary sepsis and death have been reported.[370] In the face of this clinical variability, the diagnosis of crusted scabies in HIV-seropositive people rests on appropriate clinical suspicion and the demonstration of heavy infestation by microscopic examination of skin scrapings. With such extraordinary mite loads, these patients are remarkably contagious.[371,372] Combination therapy with ivermectin 200 μg/kg and topical benzyl benzoate (or perhaps permethrin) appears to be the treatment of choice.[369,373] Single-dose ivermectin is also effective at preventing transmission in close contacts.

There is no evidence of transmission of HIV by arthropod vectors. Pruritic papular eruptions associated with HIV infection are common in sub-Saharan Africa. The etiology of these intensely pruritic lesions has been attributed to exaggerated immune responses to arthropod bites in HIV-infected individuals.

Fungal Infections

Penicillium marneffei

Disseminated infection with *P. marneffei*, a dimorphic fungus endemic to Southeast Asia and southern China (see Chapter 87), has emerged as an important OI in AIDS patients. It is the third most common OI in HIV disease in northern Thailand, after extrapulmonary tuberculosis and cryptococcal meningitis.[374–376] Infection with *P. marneffei* was a rare event before the arrival of the AIDS pandemic.[376] Since then, thousands of cases have been diagnosed, primarily in southern China, northern Thailand, Hong Kong, Taiwan, Malaysia, Vietnam, Singapore, Indonesia, and Myanmar.[376–380] The overwhelming majority of cases have been in AIDS patients, although normal hosts are also known to develop systemic disease with this fungus.[376,378,381] There is a pronounced intracountry variation in infection rates. In northern Thailand, up to one-fourth of AIDS patients suffer disease with it, whereas in southern Thailand the prevalence is 10-fold less.[380] It remains unresolved whether the human disease, penicilliosis, results from zoonotic or sapronotic transmission. The ecological reservoirs remain unknown despite more than a decade of research. The organism has been isolated from the organs, feces, and burrows of three species of bamboo rats.[374] The geographic range of these rodents overlaps the previously mentioned known areas of endemicity for disease with *P. marneffei*[377–379] and suggests the likelihood that this fungus is also endemic in Laos, Cambodia, and Malaysia.[376] Whether bamboo rats are important reservoirs for human infection or just another natural host is unclear. There is no evidence of transmission between rats and humans. The seasonal distribution of the diagnosis of disseminated disease in AIDS patients suggests expansion of the reservoir during the rainy season.[377] Exposure to soil appears to be a key factor.[382]

The pathogenesis of penicilliosis is presumed, by analogy with other endemic systemic mycoses, to involve transmission by inhalation, with secondary systemic dissemination. Like *Histoplasma capsulatum*, *P. marneffei* is an intracellular parasite of macrophages.[378] Mouse models indicate that T cells play a central role in controlling infection.[383,384] In coinfected patients, disseminated disease is associated with $CD4^+$ T-cell counts less than 100/μL.[376,385]

The largest clinical series of disseminated *P. marneffei* infection reported to date provided detailed information on 80 patients.[376] Symptom onset was generally sudden and intense. The most common presenting symptoms and signs were fever (92%), anemia (77%), weight loss (76%), and skin lesions (71%). Similar patterns of clinical symptoms have also been reported from other endemic regions.[386] Other frequent signs and symptoms included cough (49%), generalized lymphadenopathy (58%), hepatomegaly (51%), and diarrhea (31%). The most common cutaneous manifestation (87%) was a generalized papular rash with central umbilication that resembled the lesions of molluscum contagiosum. These were predominantly found on the face, scalp, and upper extremities but occurred throughout the body, including the palate. Other cutaneous lesions included papules without umbilication, a maculopapular rash, subcutaneous nodules, acne-like lesions, and folliculitis. Chest films were frequently abnormal, with diffuse reticulonodular or localized alveolar infiltrates the most common. The mean duration of illness prior to presentation in this study was 4 weeks.

The incubation period for disseminated disease is unclear, as is the percentage of patients whose disease is a result of reactivation of latent infection, as opposed to new infection or reinfection. The fact that reactivation with increasing immunosuppression occurs is supported by the several cases of disseminated disease reported from nonendemic areas in patients who had a distant history of travel to endemic areas.[385,387,388] Many such patients had spent little time in endemic areas, indicating that infection with *P. marneffei* can occur rapidly. The development of clinically active disease within weeks of exposure in endemic areas[389] and the reports of children with vertically transmitted HIV infection developing disease in the first months and years of life[390] demonstrate that primary infection can quickly lead to disseminated disease. Finally, the pronounced seasonal variation in disease incidence implies an important role for exogenous reinfection in the expression of disease in endemic areas.[377]

The mortality rate of patients with disseminated *P. marneffei* infection is very high in the absence of prompt treatment. Diagnosis depends on a high index of suspicion, including a careful history to assess residence or travel in an endemic area. The differential diagnosis includes tuberculosis, other endemic fungi, and cryptococcosis. Cutaneous lesions may mimic those of AIDS-related molluscum contagiosum, *H. capsulatum* and *Cryptococcus neoformans*. An absence of cutaneous lesions may retard diagnosis. In this regard, a characteristic syndrome of hepatic disease in the absence of skin lesions (fever, hepatomegaly, and markedly elevated serum alkaline phosphatase levels) should be noted.[391] A presumptive diagnosis can be made by the examination of a Wright's-stained bone marrow aspirate, lymph node aspirate, or touch preparations of skin biopsy specimens.[376,378,392] Intracellular and extracellular basophilic elliptic yeast-like organisms with central septation (as opposed to the budding of *H. capsulatum*) are characteristic. *P. marneffei* has characteristic cross-wall formations within macrophages, appearing as transverse cell walls separating individual conidia, which help in distinguishing it from other conidioform fungi. Indirect fluorescent antibody reagents have been developed that may prove useful for differentiating *P. marneffei* from *H. capsulatum* and *C. neoformans* in tissue.[393] Characteristic intracellular organisms have been detected on routine blood smears.[394] In the series discussed above, definitive diagnosis was performed by culture of *P. marneffei* from blood (76%, even in the absence of routine lysis-centrifugation culture), skin biopsy (90%), bone marrow (100%), and sputum (34%). Diagnostic antigenemia tests that may prove valuable for rapid diagnosis have been developed.[395,396] Quantitation of urinary antigen by enzyme immunoassay is especially promising. High sensitivity and specificity were demonstrated in an area of high endemnicity.[397] Of note, *P. marneffei* infection is a known cause of false-positive reactions in the *H. capsulatum* polysaccharide antigen immunoassay, and also crossreacts with antisera raised against *Aspergillus* galactomannan.[374,398] Current serologic assays are unlikely to be helpful in the diagnosis of AIDS patients but, with improved sensitivity, may provide a useful index of infection.[393,399]

Amphotericin B, 0.6 mg/kg/day for 2 weeks, followed by itraconazole, 200 mg twice a day for 10 weeks, is safe and effective.[400] In mild to moderately ill patients, primary therapy with itraconazole may be reasonable. Voriconazole has also shown success in treatment of *P. marneffei* infections in HIV-infected travelers from nonendemic regions.[401] Secondary prophylaxis is mandatory, given relapse rates of 50% within 6 months in its absence.[402] A placebo-controlled, double-blind randomized trial showed that secondary prophylaxis with itraconazole (200 mg once daily) is safe and effective.[78,403] With immune reconstitution as a result of a successful response to HAART, discontinuation of secondary prophylaxis is probably safe.[404] A controlled, double-blind trial of primary prophylaxis with itraconazole (200 mg once daily) in Thai patients with AIDS and $CD4^+$ T-cell counts less than 200/μL showed that the regimen was well tolerated and effective at preventing both cryptococcosis and penicilliosis.[405] No survival benefit was found, but the study was not powered to detect a survival advantage.[405]

Paracoccidioides brasiliensis

The dimorphic fungus, *P. brasiliensis,* is the cause of the most common systemic mycosis in Latin America (see Chapter 86). Two clinical forms are distinguished in normal hosts: an acute or subacute "juvenile" form and a chronic "adult" form. Acute, juvenile disease, occurring in children and young adults and accounting for a small minority of cases (3–5%), is marked by a rapid course, disseminated involvement of macrophages and lymphoid tissue, and severe suppression of CMI. Chronic, adult disease, accounting for the vast majority of cases, is a slowly progressive disease, predominantly of older men. In most patients, the primary clinical and pathologic manifestations are pulmonary, with nodular, infiltrative, or cavitary lesions progressing to fibrosis. Other frequent manifestations of adult disease include infiltrative and ulcerative mucosal lesions of the oro- and nasopharynx, polymorphic cutaneous lesions, lymphadenopathy, and adrenal infiltration. Most infections are subclinical. Long latency has clearly been demonstrated, with a mean of 15 years between leaving an endemic area and presentation.[406]

It is thought that CMI responses are critical to the host defense from disease with *P. brasiliensis*.[406,407] Clinical and experimental evidence indicates that paracoccidioidomycosis is associated with marked abnormalities of immune function, with suppression of CMI responses, polyclonal B-cell activation, and elevation of plasma IgE levels.[406–408] These immunologic perturbations are more common and severe in juvenile disease and are reversed with successful therapy.[406]

Given the immunology of paracoccidioidomycosis, one might expect it to be a prominent OI in South America and among HIV patients with a history of travel there. In fact, fewer than 100 cases have been reported, despite the presumed wide prevalence of infection or coinfection in areas such as urban Brazil.[409–414] Possible reasons for the low number of cases in HIV-seropositive patients include: (1) prophylaxis with TMP-SMX, which has activity against *P. brasiliensis*; (2) the use of ketoconazole for oropharyngeal candidiasis; (3) misdiagnosis as *Pneumocystis carinii* pneumonia, with a therapeutic response to TMP-SMX; (4) lack of diagnosis; and (5) the presence of a particularly subtle interaction between HIV and *Paracoccidioides brasiliensis*.[409,412]

Paracoccidioidomycosis in HIV-seropositive people has been primarily of the "acute" form; however, pulmonary and oral mucosal involvement, more typical of the "chronic" form, often coexists.[410] Although published reports have suggested that this disseminated disease may occur across a broad range of HIV-associated immunosuppression, CD4$^+$ T-cell counts less than 200/μL have been the reported norm.[410,411] More than one-third of patients with paracoccidioidomycosis have presented with another opportunistic coinfection, most frequently oral/esophageal candidiasis or tuberculosis.[410] Reported clinical presentations span a wide spectrum, from relatively indolent to rapidly progressive disease. Clinical manifestations have included prolonged fever, weight loss, cough, dyspnea, generalized lymphadenopathy, hepatosplenomegaly, skin lesions (localized or disseminated maculopapular, nodular, or ulcerative), oral lesions (ulcerative and/or nodular), osteoarticular lesions, and meningitis.[409,410]

Diagnosis in these patients was made by direct examination or culture of clinical specimens, including skin biopsies, lymph node aspirates or biopsies, bone marrow aspirates, CSF, or blood.[409,410] Sputum should also be examined using potassium hydroxide preparations, calcofluor stains, or immunofluorescence. The "pilot wheel" cell, consisting of numerous small buds surrounding the mother cell, is characteristic. Serologies have not been diagnostically helpful. PCR using primers for ITS1 region of the ribosomal gene has been found to be a highly sensitive and specific test that may prove to be useful as a diagnostic tool in the near future.[414]

Mortality in the reported cases of disease in HIV-seropositive people was 30%.[409] No randomized clinical trials have been performed with any of the drugs commonly used for the treatment of *P. brasiliensis* infection (sulfonamides, amphotericin B, ketoconazole, and itraconazole), even in normal hosts. Treatment recommendations are based on data from case series and comparison with historical controls.[412] However, the data are fairly compelling that itraconazole (100 mg/day) is the drug of choice in normal hosts.[406] Published reports of itraconazole treatment in the face of HIV coinfection are scant.[410,411] Although amphotericin B and itraconazole may both have therapeutic roles to play, amphotericin B should probably be used for initial treatment in HIV-coinfected patients. Trials with liposomal formulatins of amphotericin are awaited.[415] Lifelong suppressive therapy is necessary; itraconazole seems to be a reasonable choice.[415]

Histoplasma capsulatum var. *duboisii*

The endemic dimorphic fungus *H. capsulatum* var. *duboisii* is localized to western and central Africa and Madagascar (see Chapter 85). In normal hosts, it tends to cause chronic necrotizing cutaneous and skeletal infections. Disseminated disease is unusual. It may be an emerging OI in AIDS patients. A large retrospective case series, reporting on cases of HIV coinfected with *H. capsulatum* var. *duboisii* presenting to three referral centers in French Guiana, identified *H. capsulatum* infection as an AIDS-defining condition in 200 individuals, with 37% having coinfections with other AIDS-defining infections.[416] However, no increases in the incidence of African histoplasmosis were reported in a study from the People's Republic of the Congo (now Congo Republic) in the 1980s, despite a rapid increase in the AIDS-related incidence of cryptococcal disease.[417] Disease manifestations reported in reported coinfections suggest that AIDS patients are at risk of more severe, disseminated disease.[418–424] Diagnosis is typically by direct examination of clinical specimens and culture. Serodiagnostic tests are cross-reactive with *Aspergillus* and *Penicillium*.[425] The yeast form is larger and has a thicker wall than *H. capsulatum* var. *capsulatum*. Amphotericin B and itraconazole have therapeutic efficacy.[424] With the advent of HAART, there is increasing concern about emergence of *Histoplasma* and other invasive fungi as causes of IRIS.[424]

Sporothrix schenckii

The dimorphic fungus *S. schenckii* has a worldwide distribution, although most reports have been from tropical and subtropical areas of the Americas (see Chapter 90). The highest incidence of disease is thought to be in the highlands of Mexico and in southern Brazil. Recent reports from South Asia suggest high prevalence rates there as well.[426] Cutaneous and lymphocutaneous disease is most common. Extracutaneous involvement, including osteoarticular disease, pneumonia, and meningitis, has been described in both normal and immunosuppressed hosts. A handful of cases of severe, disseminated sporotrichosis in late-stage AIDS have been described.[427–430] Diffuse cutaneous involvement is the norm. Some patients have also presented with CNS, ocular, osteoarticular, splenic, bone marrow, and/or mucosal involvement. It appears likely that disseminated *Sporothrix* will become a more prominent OI in heavily endemic areas. The response to therapy (with amphotericin B, potassium iodide, itraconazole, ketoconazole, and 5-fluorocytosine) has been variable and problematic. Amphotericin B should probably be used for initial treatment, followed by lifelong suppressive therapy with itraconazole.[431]

Other Endemic, Systemic Mycoses

H. capsulatum, *Blastomyces dermatitidis*, and *Coccidioides immitis* are systemic mycoses endemic to the United States that cause AIDS-related OI. As such, they are not distinctly tropical diseases and have been covered in depth elsewhere.[76–78,432–434] The tropical extent of their respective areas of endemicity deserves brief mention, however.

H. capsulatum var. *capsulatum* (see Chapter 85) is found in distinct river basin systems worldwide between 45°N and 30°S of the equator.[432] Progressive disseminated histoplasmosis is common in AIDS patients in endemic areas.[432] In addition to the most prominent worldwide focus (the Ohio and Mississippi river valleys of the United States), cases have been reported from Central and South America, the Caribbean, Africa, Southeast Asia, and Europe.[435,436]

Disease caused by *B. dermatitidis* was originally named North American blastomycosis. It is now clear, however, that the distribution of this fungus is far more cosmopolitan (see Chapter 85). Blastomycosis has been reported in all the major regions of Africa, with a concentration in southern Africa. It is likely underreported.[437] Occasional cases have been reported from Central and South America, the Middle East, and India.[438] African strains of *B. dermatitidis* appear to be antigenically distinct from North American strains. The clinical spectrum likewise appears to be different in African cases, with prominent involvement of bone and chronic draining sinuses. Disseminated blastomycosis is an uncommon, late, frequently fatal OI in patients with AIDS in the United States.[439,440] Cases in Africa are to be expected in the future.

C. immitis is endemic to lower Sonoran life zones in the United States, Mexico, Guatemala, Honduras, Colombia, Venezuela, Bolivia, Paraguay, and Argentina (see Chapter 85). Coccidioidomycosis is a severe, often fatal disease in patients with AIDS and low CD4$^+$ T-cell counts.[434,441,442] Most have presented with diffuse or focal pulmonary disease; extrapulmonary dissemination is not uncommon. In some endemic areas, it is the third most common OI in AIDS patients.[434,441,442]

Cryptococcus neoformans

Cryptococcosis (see Chapter 85) is a common life-threatening fungal infection in AIDS patients.[443] Although *C. neoformans* can disseminate to any organ system in the face of HIV infection, meningitis is the most frequent manifestation. Other relatively common manifestations include pneumonia and cutaneous lesions. Occurring most commonly when CD4 counts fall well below 200/μL, cryptococcosis is a frequent presenting diagnosis in AIDS.[443] Excellent reviews on cryptococcosis in AIDS are available for detailed information on the clinical approach to this ubiquitous OI.[76–78,444,445]

C. neoformans is distributed globally. The distribution of cryptococcus as an OI in AIDS is global as well. Regional differences exist in the prevalence of disease as defined by clinical or autopsy series. The prevalence of cryptococcosis in AIDS patients in the United States was estimated to be 7–8% in the 1980s.[446] In Thailand, it is the second most common OI (after tuberculosis), with a prevalence of 13–44% in different clinical series.[20,447,448] In Africa, the case series prevalence has been variable, from 1% in Soweto, South Africa,[449] to 6–13% in Kinshasa (the former Zaire).[450–452] The prevalence in autopsy series has similarly varied from

3% in Abidjan (Côte d'Ivoire)[230] to 29% in Uganda.[232] Overall, the rates of disease in Africa appear to be higher than those in North America or Europe. Interestingly, a large retrospective case study in London found a significantly higher rate of extrapulmonary cryptococcal disease in Africans attending an HIV clinic than in non-Africans attending the same clinic.[453] Data from case series estimated the prevalence of cryptococcosis in Mexico to be 8–12%[454] and in Haiti 13%.[455] In Brazil, from 1980 to 2002, 6% of patients had cryptococcus as an AIDS-defining diagnosis.[456] Cryptococcal infections have been estimated to contribute to 10–30% of AID-related deaths in developing countries.[457]

C. neoformans exists in two varieties: *C. neoformans* var. *neoformans* and *C. neoformans* var. *gatti*. They inhabit different ecological niches, with *C. neoformans* var. *neoformans* being associated with soil contaminated with bird excrement and *C. neoformans* var. *gatti* having a unique, if poorly understood, association with the tree *Eucalyptus camaldulensis*.[458,459] With the completion of the genomic sequence of *C. neoformans*, enough differences have been found in the sequences of these two fungal subspecies for a proposal to raise *C. neoformans gatti* to its own species, *C. gatti*.[460] Whereas *C. gatti* has a predominantly tropical and subtropical distribution, *C. neoformans* occurs worldwide.[458,459] Of note, although cryptococcosis due to *C. gatti* occurs with some regularity in normal hosts in regions where this variety is endemic, cases of cryptococcosis in AIDS patients have been almost exclusively due to *C. neoformans*.[459,461]

Pneumocystis jirovecii

Throughout the world, there is almost universal serologic evidence of exposure by the age of 2 years to *P. jirovecii*[462] (see Chapter 91). The prevalence of antibodies to specific *P. jirovecii* antigens varies, however, suggesting exposure to antigenically different strains in different areas of the world,[463] which is mirrored by genetic studies revealing strain differences in this organism.[464] Prior to HAART, PCP (*Pneumocystis carinii* pneumonia, based on the prior terminology) occurred in 40–50% of patients in the United States and Europe with a CD4 count less than 100/μL per year, and in 60–80% of patients overall, in the absence of prophylaxis. PCP prevalence appears to be high among AIDS patients in Central and South America and in Asia.[465] Interestingly, however, the incidence of PCP in adult AIDS patients in Africa may be far lower than was seen in the pre-HAART era in industrialized countries.[465] Adult clinical series in Africa have shown prevalence rates of 0–22%.[449,455,466–469] Studies including bronchoscopy for diagnosis have described rates of 0–39% (the highest figures being obtained as a percentage of acid-fast bacillus-negative pneumonias).[455,466,470–472] Autopsy series have had rates of 0–11%.[231,468,473] The reasons for these lower rates are unclear. Possible explanations include less environmental exposure, exposure to differing strains, differences in host susceptibility, earlier deaths in tropical patients with AIDS due to exposure to more virulent organisms, diagnostic difficulties, and host-specific differences in susceptibility.[455,474] The existence of genetically and antigenically distinct human strains is likely; however, pediatric PCP rates in AIDS patients in Africa are quite similar to those in the industrial north.[465,475] Indeed, approximately one-third of HIV-infected infants in Africa die during the first year of life, and PCP is thought to be responsible for 30–50% of such deaths.[476,477] Demise from more virulent pathogens prior to clinical PCP may well occur in adults (and PCP does tend to occur early in the course of HIV disease in North American infants,[478] perhaps with initial exposure).[78] The high prevalence of cryptococcal disease in these same series, which is thought to occur at similar levels of immunosuppression, suggests that this is not the complete answer.[455] More recent studies from Africa, using bronchoscopy and improved microbiological identification, have yielded higher rates of PCP, so it is possible that lower rates in earlier studies may have represented reporting bias introduced by the use of suboptimal diagnostic techniques.[479,480]

The clinical presentation of PCP in the tropics appears to be similar to that in the industrial north.[472] Frequent coinfection with tuberculosis may obscure the diagnosis. Multiple reviews of the clinical approach to PCP in AIDS are available.[481–484]

Other Fungi

Other predominantly tropical fungi, such as the agents of maduromycosis, lobomycosis, rhinosporidiosis, and subcutaneous zygomycosis, may prove to cause OI in AIDS patients but do not appear to have been reported as such. Isolated case reports of infection due to a variety of unusual fungi in AIDS patients have been published (reviewed in references 485 and 486). Some may indeed prove to be OIs, even predominantly tropical OIs, but firm data are lacking. The common occurrence of superficial and invasive infections with *Candida* and the growing problem of *Aspergillus* infection in neutropenic long-term survivors of late-stage AIDS are beyond the scope of this chapter.

BACTERIAL INFECTIONS

Mycobacterial Infections

Mycobacterium tuberculosis

Approximately one-third of those living with HIV worldwide are coinfected with *M. tuberculosis* (see Chapter 35). In developing countries, 50% of patients with HIV infection will develop active TB; in contrast, in the United States, only 4% of patients with AIDS have had TB.[2,487] In some countries in sub-Saharan Africa, more than 70% of TB patients are HIV-seropositive. TB is the leading cause of death among people with HIV infection, accounting for one-third of AIDS deaths worldwide.[488] The introduction of HAART has decreased death and OIs such as TB by 60–90% among people living with HIV worldwide in affluent countries;[489] in developing countries, however, HAART still remains available only to a minority of those who need it.

Mycobacterium avium

The *M. avium* complex (MAC) (see Chapter 35) consists of multiple serovars of two *Mycobacterium* species, *M. avium* and *M. intracellulare*. MAC bacteria are ubiquitous, with organisms commonly being isolated from soil, natural sources of water, tap water, and domestic and wild animals worldwide.[490,491] Most MAC isolates from AIDS patients are *M. avium*; more than 90% are of serovars 1, 4, and 8.[492,493] Disseminated disease due to *M. avium* is the most common systemic bacterial infection in AIDS patients in the industrial north, occurring in up to 43% of AIDS patients in the United States.[494,495] Disease occurs almost exclusively in those with $CD4^+$ T-cell counts less than 100/μL, most frequently in those with $CD4^+$ T-cell counts less than 50/μL.[495] The pathogenesis of disseminated *M. avium* infection in AIDS is thought to involve primary infection (or reinfection) as opposed to reactivation, with initial colonization of the respiratory or GI tracts followed by widespread dissemination.[496–498] Systemic disease is marked by high-grade mycobacteremia (almost exclusively in monocytes) and impressive tissue burdens of bacteria.[499]

The remarkable feature of *M. avium* in the tropics is the apparent virtual absence of disseminated disease in AIDS patients in many areas, predominantly in sub-Saharan Africa. None of 95 blood cultures from severely ill patients with advanced AIDS in Uganda were positive for *M. avium*, nor were any of 165 mycobacterial sputum cultures from HIV-seropositive and seronegative patients at the same hospital found to be positive for *M. avium*.[500,501] None of 202 blood cultures from HIV-positive adult inpatients in Côte d'Ivoire grew *M. avium* (whereas 4% grew *M. tuberculosis*).[502] None of more than 200 diagnostic lymph node biopsies in HIV-seropositive African patients had histology characteristic of disseminated *M. avium* infection.[232] Intestinal biopsies from 98 Ugandan, Zairian, and Zambian patients with chronic HIV-related enteropathy yielded histology suggestive of *M. avium* infection in only 1 patient.[349,503,504] Autopsies on 78 HIV-seropositive children in Côte d'Ivoire revealed no evidence of *M. avium* infection, whereas autopsies on 247 adult HIV patients in Côte d'Ivoire revealed a 3% prevalence of pathologic changes "indicative of atypical mycobacteriosis."[230] In contrast, 3 of 48 (6%) patients hospitalized in Kenya with late-stage HIV disease had *M. avium* bacteremia.[505] Clinical and autopsy series from Mexico have revealed a prevalence of disseminated disease due to *M. avium* of 4–6%,[231,506] whereas 18% of 125 hospitalized patients with AIDS in Brazil had *M. avium* cultured from bone marrow.[507] Few data are available from India and Southeast Asia. One study from East Asia showed patterns of MAC infection similar to those seen in the west, with ~55% of mycobacteremias being identified as due to MAC.[508]

The reasons for the apparent absence of disseminated disease due to *M. avium* in areas of the tropics are unclear. As with the decreased prevalence of PCP, many explanations have been proposed, including less exposure, exposure to less pathogenic variants, differences in host susceptibility, greater acquired immunity to mycobacteria, earlier death by more virulent pathogens, and diagnostic difficulties. Overall exposure to MAC organisms is likely to be similar. Environmental isolation of MAC occurs with similar or greater frequency in Congo and Uganda than in the United States[491,501] and skin test surveys suggest a similar frequency of exposure to MAC in economically developed and developing countries.[509] Piped water systems in the United States and Europe have a higher frequency of MAC isolation, however, and economic conditions may lead to greater exposure to MAC-containing droplets via showerheads in economically developed countries;[490,491,510] such differences, however, are unlikely to lead to an essentially total absence of disease in countries such as Uganda. Exposure to different *M. avium* serovars or strains may well be important. Data on serotyping of African clinical strains are scarce. Preliminary data suggest that African clinical isolates are distinguishable from European and American isolates by restriction fragment length polymorphism analysis.[511] The possibility of underlying genetic differences in host susceptibility is belied by the similar rates of disseminated *M. avium* infection as a presenting diagnosis in African and non-African AIDS patients in a London clinic.[453] Greater acquired immunity to mycobacterial disease through bacille Calmette–Guérin (BCG) vaccination[512] or prior infection with *M. tuberculosis* may exist, but the reported BCG coverage (50%) and purified protein derivative (PPD) reactivity (82%) in Uganda seem unlikely to explain the lack of any disseminated MAC disease.[501] Earlier death due to a greater environmental presence of, or greater latent infection with, more virulent pathogens may occur. This is unlikely to be the entire explanation because patients in many of the previously mentioned studies had clinical late-stage AIDS. Finally, the design of several of the previous studies makes the assertion that the central problem is one of a lack of diagnostic sophistication untenable. Further data from Africa are needed to this puzzling pattern of infections with MAC.

Mycobacterium leprae

The causative agent of leprosy (see Chapter 37) is an incredibly slow-growing parasite of macrophages. For comparative purposes, it may be useful to recall that *Leishmania*, which infects similar cells, is a prominent opportunistic pathogen for patients with HIV infection. The importance of CMI in leprosy and leishmaniasis was emphasized by Turk and Bryceson[513] in their detailed comparison of skin lesions and histopathology of both diseases. Moreover, the immunopathology of both infections is very similar. In view of the widespread prevalence of leprosy in the tropics and subtropics, the immunosuppressive effects of HIV/AIDS on leprosy would be expected to become readily apparent, but there is little or no evidence of this interaction. In fact, in a comprehensive analysis of the possible interaction between HIV/AIDS and leprosy, Lucas concluded that leprosy appears to be another "missing infection in AIDS."[18]

Several studies have examined positive serology for HIV in newly diagnosed leprosy cases. One report from a rural hospital in Zambia found a higher prevalence of reactors compared with blood donors and surgical patients (6 of 18 versus 9 of 105), but the numbers were small and the controls were not adequately matched.[514] A larger study of HIV seroprevalence in northwest Tanzania of 93 new leprosy cases compared with more than 4000 controls found that the presence of HIV antibody was significantly associated with multibacillary disease.[515] The fact that this association was based on only 5 HIV-positive cases with multibacillary disease illustrates the complexity of epidemiologic analysis in a disease such as leprosy. Another comparison of seropositivity for HIV was carried out among 189 new cases of leprosy matched for age, sex, and district of residence with 481 controls in Uganda. No significant difference in overall positive rates was found (12% in cases versus 18% in controls), but again, positive HIV reactions were more frequent among multibacillary cases.[516] A different clinical association was noted in Zambia in leprosy patients with active neuritis, which suggested that HIV-positive cases had poorer recovery of nerve function than controls after treatment with steroids.[517]

A factor that should be considered in evaluating reports of HIV/AIDS in leprosy patients is the greater likelihood of false-positive serologic reactions. One or more positive bands to HIV antigens in Western blots were commonly found in several hundred sera from northern India in the absence of positive enzyme-linked immunosorbent assays (ELISAs).[518] Another report claimed that 3 of 75 (4%) sera from Indonesia and 6 of 100 (6%) sera from Somalia gave positive HIV ELISAs but negative Western blots.[519] These were attributed to leprosy.

Published epidemiological data show neither an increased HIV prevalence among leprosy cases nor a higher rate of HIV among individuals infected with *M. leprae*. Further, there appears to be no striking evidence that HIV infection has an adverse effect on the course of leprosy nor any clear alteration in the clinical spectrum of leprosy among coinfected patients;[520] although some suggest that immune-mediated reactions that complicate leprosy occur at a higher frequency in coinfected patients,[521,522] several of the above reports suggest the possibility that multibacillary disease may develop more readily with coinfection. However, there are several features of leprosy that may tend to obscure an interaction with HIV infection. Both infections are chronic and slow in their progression, so it may simply take more time to recognize an influence of one on the other. Leprosy is predominantly a rural infection; HIV/AIDS is more urban. Patients with AIDS in the tropics may not survive long enough to display interactions with leprosy. Finally, patients in the early stages of leprosy have relatively subtle clinical manifestations with which physicians in the urban environment may not be familiar. Therefore, there may be more going on out there than we realize. Leprosy has now been reported presenting as immune reconstitution disease among patients commencing HAART.[523]

Other Nontuberculous *Mycobacteria*

Disease due to *M. genavense* (see Chapter 35) mimics that due to *M. avium*, causing disseminated disease in AIDS patients with very low $CD4^+$ T-cell counts (mean, <50/μL). Pathogenesis appears to involve initial GI colonization followed by dissemination.[524,525] The important environmental reservoirs are unclear, but pet birds can have extensive GI tract involvement. The organism may also be present in tap water.[526] The geographic range of disease is only beginning to be defined. Cases have been reported from North America, Europe, and Australia.[524] The most common presenting symptoms and signs are fever, weight loss, abdominal pain, chronic diarrhea, lymphadenopathy, hepatosplenomegaly, "pseudo-Whipple's disease," and anemia.[524,527,528] Imaging of the spleen may suggest splenic abscesses;[529] diffuse nodular infiltrates may be seen in the lung.[530] Pathologically, involved organs are filled with histiocytes that are packed with acid-fast bacilli. The diagnosis can be established by the isolation of *M. genavense* from normally sterile sites (blood, bone marrow, lymph node, and spleen). Specific diagnosis is confounded by the fastidious growth requirements of the organism. Primary isolation on solid media is difficult, and growth in liquid broth may have only 50% sensitivity. Definitive identification demands PCR techniques.[524] The clear implication is that a significant percentage of cases ascribed to disseminated *M. avium* are likely due to *M. genavense*.[527] Data on treatment are all retrospective, but therapy appears to be associated both with improvement in symptoms and with survival. Multidrug regimens that include clarithromycin appear to be associated with the best clinical responses.[531,532] Like other nontuberculous mycobacteria, *M. genovense* has also been reported to declare itself during IRIS.[533]

Before the AIDS pandemic, *M. kansasii* was known primarily as a cause of chronic pulmonary disease, resembling TB, in lungs with underlying damage. *M. kansasii* is second to MAC among nontuberculous mycobacteria as a cause of disease in HIV-infected patients in the United States.[534] Although *M. kansasii* has been reported as a cause of pulmonary disease in most areas of the world, most case reports of HIV coinfection are from North America and Europe. However, coinfection may be especially prevalent in the gold mines of the Transvaal in South Africa.[535] In HIV-infected individuals, disease due to *M. kansasii* and *M. tuberculosis* has very similar clinical and radiological characteristics.[536,537] A major difference (with epidemiological and prognostic implications) is that *M. kansasii* disease tends to occur later in the course of HIV infection. The mean CD4$^+$ T-cell count at the time of presentation is approximately 50–60/μL;[536–539] 60–90% present with pulmonary disease alone and 20–35% with disseminated disease.[539,540] The incidence in industrialized countries has plummeted in the HAART era.[541] With all nontuberculous mycobacteria, differentiation between colonization, contamination, and disease can be problematic. Mere colonization of the respiratory tract with *M. kansasii* appears to be infrequent in AIDS patients, however. All pulmonary isolates should be taken seriously.[538,540] Despite relative *in vitro* resistance to isoniazid,[541] the recommended therapy is isoniazid, rifampin, and ethambutol. Therapy clearly alters survival in patients with pulmonary disease.[539,540,542] Disseminated disease has a particularly poor prognosis.

M. malmoense is an uncommon cause of pulmonary disease resembling tuberculosis. The environmental reservoir is unknown. Person-to-person transmission has never been documented. Multisystem disease with bacteremia has rarely occurred in the presence of profound immunosuppression, including several patients with AIDS and low CD4$^+$ T-cell counts. Pulmonary and GI disease, along with bacteremia, is usual.[543,544] *In vitro* susceptibility testing does not correlate well with clinical response.[545] The best regimen for pulmonary disease in the nonimmunosuppressed patient appears to be isoniazid, rifampin, and ethambutol.[545] Optimal therapy in AIDS patients is unclear.

M. haemophilum causes localized lymphadenitis in immunologically healthy children and cutaneous, osteoarticular, and, more rarely, pulmonary or disseminated disease in immunocompromised patients. Several cases have been reported in AIDS patients.[546–551] Cutaneous lesions include furuncles, abscesses, papules, vesicles, and deep ulcers. Such lesions are usually diffuse, most often on the extremities. Culture (at 30–32°C) demands supplementation of media with an iron source. *In vitro* susceptibility data and scattered clinical reports suggest that rifampin plus ciprofloxacin is reasonable empirical therapy. Other agents with good activity include amikacin, ciprofloxacin, and clarithromycin.[548] The environmental source and mode of infection are unclear.

Several other mycobacteria have been demonstrated or suspected to cause opportunistic disease in AIDS patients, including *M. fortuitum* (primary pulmonary disease,[552] disseminated disease,[553] cervical lymphadenitis,[553] and meningitis),[554] *M. marinum* (cutaneous and disseminated disease),[555,556] *M. celatum* (pulmonary and disseminated disease),[557,558] *M. xenopi* (disseminated disease, pulmonary disease, and pulmonary colonization),[559–561] *M. gordonae* (pulmonary, cutaneous, and disseminated disease),[562–564] *M. scrofulaceum* (disseminated disease),[565] *M. bovis* (disseminated disease), and *M. simiae* (disseminated disease).[566–568] Although a smattering of case reports have suggested that HIV does not exacerbate disease due to *M. ulcerans*, the causative agent of Buruli ulcer[569] (see Chapter 36), a recent case report has called this into question.[570]

Spirochetal Infections

Along with other genital inflammatory diseases, syphilis (see Chapter 138) has been implicated as a cofactor in HIV transmission. Many case reports have suggested that HIV infection can alter the course of disease with *Treponema pallidum*. In the presence of concurrent HIV infection, syphilis has been thought to: (1) progress more frequently and rapidly to neurosyphilis;[571,572] (2) lead to an increased incidence of meningitic manifestations of neurosyphilis;[573] (3) lead to an increased frequency of "malignant secondary syphilis" with ulcerating lesions and prominent systemic symptoms;[574] and (4) be less amenable to successful therapy with standard regimens as assessed by clinical or serologic measures (including a lack of appropriate nontreponemal titer reduction or a serologic relapse).[575–580] Higher rates of serological failure continue to be reported in the post-HAART era, but it has become clear that effective suppression of HIV viremia clearly increases the rates of serological responses to standard therapy.[581–584] Concerns about effectiveness of standard therapy for syphilis in HIV-positive individuals, based largely on case reports and retrospective studies, were amplified by the disconcerting finding of *T. pallidum* invasion of the CNS in early syphilis in HIV-infected patients. Such early invasion of the CNS occurs equally frequently in HIV-seropositive and seronegative people, however,[585] and the above "atypical" courses of syphilis were well-known in the pre-AIDS era. Knowledge of the actual frequency and relative significance of such events awaited well-designed prospective studies. Three studies now provide evidence that the clinical presentation and clinical and serologic responses to treatment of syphilis may not be appreciably altered by HIV coinfection.[586–588] A major caveat of these studies is that the mean level of immunosuppression in the patients in these studies, as assessed by CD4$^+$ T-cell counts, was not severe. Furthermore, the number of patients involved was relatively small. Thus, the clinical course of syphilis in the face of severe HIV-induced immunosuppression may in fact be exacerbated, and the response to conventional therapy may lead to the infrequent occurrence of serious adverse treatment outcomes.[588] The clinical approach to the HIV patient infected with this cosmopolitan sexually transmitted disease has been thoroughly discussed elsewhere[76–78,589,590] and will likely continue to evolve.

Whether HIV infection has a deleterious effect on the course of the nonvenereal, endemic treponematoses (see Chapter 43) is unknown, but such an effect has been postulated by analogy with syphilis.[591] No effects of HIV on concurrent infection with the *Borrelia* species that cause relapsing fever have been reported (see Chapter 44). Whether Lyme disease follows an unusual course in HIV-infected people is unclear.[592,593] Finally, initial observations suggest that leptospirosis (see Chapter 45) runs a similar course in patients coinfected with HIV.[594,595]

Rickettsial and Ehrlichial Infections

Among the Rickettsiae and related organisms, only infections with *Coxiella burnetii*, the etiologic agent of Q fever (see Chapter 53) and *Ehrlichia* spp. have been reported to be exacerbated by concurrent HIV infection. Notably, these pathogens are obligate intracellular parasites of monocyte/macrophages. *C. burnetii* lives and multiplies in the phagolysosomes of monocyte/macrophages, and host defense appears to depend on specific T-cell activation of the microbicidal effector functions of infected cells.[596,597] Case series have suggested that patients with immunocompromise due to a variety of causes (including leukemia, Hodgkin's disease, bone marrow and renal transplantation, and alcoholism) are more susceptible to both symptomatic acute and relapsing or chronic disease with *C. burnetii*.[598–600] While the rationale for expecting more frequent or serious disease in the HIV-infected patient is clear, supporting data are sparse. A study from southern France demonstrated a threefold higher prevalence of antibodies to *C. burnetii* in HIV-seropositive people.[601] This suggestion of an increased rate of transmission in HIV-infected people has not been found in other seroprevalence studies from Paris, Spain, or the Central African Republic.[602–604] Given the differential prevalence of risk factors for the acquisition of HIV infection between the studies, the contradictory data strongly suggest that *C. burnetii* can be bloodborne and that intravenous drug use is a risk for its transmission. Two studies from southern Europe have further suggested that HIV infection leads to a higher disease-to-infection ratio with *C. burnetii*.[601,605] A retrospective serologic study of 520 patients with acute Q fever from an area of Spain with a high incidence of both HIV and *C. burnetii* infection revealed no overrepresentation of HIV-infected people, however, with endocarditis being a common presentation.[604,606,607] The clinical features of Q fever do not appear to vary between HIV-infected and uninfected hosts.[601,603–605] However, definitive statements await prospective studies in severely immunosuppressed AIDS patients.

Human monocytic ehrlichiosis (HME), caused by the tick-borne agent *Ehrlichia chaffeensis*, is an acute febrile illness associated with leukopenia, thrombocytopenia, and hepatic enzyme abnormalities (see Chapter 52). While most reports of infection with *E. chaffeensis* have been from the United States, a report of infection in Mali supports a much wider distribution of disease, however.[608] HME appears to be an AIDS-related OI.[608–611] Reported hospitalized cases have had a high rate of complications and a mortality of approximately 30%[609] (compared with an estimated case-fatality rate for HME in the absence of HIV of <3%).[612] Patients with fatal disease had $CD4^+$ T-cell counts less than 200/µL; in patients with less than 100/µL, the mortality rate was more than 50%. Of 8 reported cases of disease caused by *E. ewingii*, a related tick-borne agent, 7 occurred in patients with immune deficiencies, including 4 with HIV infection.[609,612] The suspicion is thus strong that *E. ewingii* is an opportunistic pathogen in the setting of HIV infection.[613] No cases of infection with the tick-borne agent of human granulocytic ehrlichiosis[614] in the face of HIV infection appear to have been reported.

There is no evidence implicating any of the spotted fever or typhus group of Rickettsiae as having a clinically significant interaction with HIV. A prospective study on scrub typhus (due to *Orientia* (formerly *Rickettsia*) *tsutsugamush)* revealed no increase in clinical severity at time of presentation in HIV-infected patients with a median $CD4^+$ T-cell count of 70/µL.[615] Interestingly, rickettsemia occurred significantly less often in the HIV-seropositive patients. Neither the relative prevalence of infection nor the response to treatment was addressed in this study. Of interest, acute infection with *O. tsutsugamushi* has been associated with decreased plasma HIV viral load.[56]

Bacterial Infections

Brucella

A cause of systemic disease worldwide, *Brucella* species are facultative intracellular parasites that infect and multiply in macrophages (see Chapter 40). CMI responses, particularly the activation of monocyte/macrophages by antigen-specific T cells, are important in host resistance. Despite this, the meager published data on coinfection do not support a significant effect of HIV on infection with *Brucella* and, in fact, prior to the AIDS pandemic, only 2 cases of brucellosis in immunocompromised hosts (hairy cell leukemia and IgM deficiency) had been reported.[616,617] A retrospective seroprevalence study found no significant association between *Brucella* serology and HIV serology in a cohort of female sex workers in Kenya.[618] The clinical course of brucellosis in the 18 reported cases with concurrent HIV infection was not outside the spectrum of disease seen in normal hosts.[618–622]

Burkholderia pseudomallei

Melioidosis (see Chapter 33) does not appear to behave as an AIDS-related OI. The disease is endemic in Southeast Asia, particularly in northern Thailand, where the prevalence of AIDS is high. However, only one case of fatal, recrudescent, bacteremic disease in an HIV-seropositive person has been reported, and another study in the same region failed to note any difference in severity of illness in 8 HIV infected individuals compared to HIV-uninfected subjects.[66,623] Clinical series from Thailand are silent with regard to the presence of melioidosis in AIDS patients,[447,448,624,625,626] and a 10-year study of bloodstream infections in a hospital in northern Thailand reported a similar proportion of *B. pseudomallei* isolates in HIV-infected and uninfected patients.[627]

Enteric Bacteria

Several enteric bacterial infections have been reported to cause disease of greater severity, invasiveness, chronicity, or recurrence in the presence of HIV coinfection.[628–630] Enterotoxigenic *Escherichia coli* has not been described as causing more severe disease in HIV-seropositive patients, but *Shigella* species, *Salmonella*, *Campylobacter*, and *Listeria monocytogenes* have all been implicated as causes of more severe or relapsing disease in the presence of HIV. Data from the tropics on enteric bacterial pathogens are scant. Studies of slim disease (enteropathic AIDS) have not revealed an enteric bacterial cause in most cases.[349,503,504] The prevalence of certain enteric pathogens such as *Campylobacter*, *Vibrio*, and enteropathogenic *E. coli* in the tropics has not been accurately assessed because their detection requires the use of special media and experienced laboratory personnel. In the case of less fastidious organisms that are easier to detect, such as *Salmonella* spp., the phenomenon of bacteremia with nontyphoid organisms has been noted in tropical Africa.[27,249,628] Since bacteremia with *Shigella* spp. probably occurs more commonly in patients with HIV disease,[631] this association may be expected to occur in the tropics as well. There is no reported evidence to suggest that cholera is altered in the presence of HIV, although the gastric secretory failure that occurs commonly in AIDS may lead to a greater susceptibility to infection with *Vibrio cholerae*.[632,633] It should be noted that, although the live oral cholera vaccine is considered to be contraindicated in people with HIV infection by the US Public Health Service (USPHS)–Infectious Diseases Society of America (IDSA) working group,[235] it has been shown to be safe and immunogenic in HIV-infected adults in Mali.[634]

Other Bacteria

Although data on HIV infection and epidemic meningococcal meningitis have not provided evidence for a significant interaction,[635] studies suggest that HIV infection may be a risk factor for sporadic meningococcal disease.[636,637] Interactions between HIV and *Bacillus anthracis* or *Yersinia pestis* have not been reported. The globally endemic *Bartonella* species, *B. henselae* and *B. quintana* (see Chapter 39), cause acute and persistent bacteremia as well as localized tissue infection (including bacillary angiomatosis, bacillary peliosis, microscopic abscess formation, and lymphadenitis), primarily in AIDS patients and other immunocompromised people.[55,638–641] The closely related species *B. bacilliformis*, which is geographically restricted to Andean river valleys, causes a similar spectrum of disease (including acute and persistent bacteremia and hemangiomatous nodules resembling those seen in bacillary angiomatosis) in immunologically normal hosts (see Chapter 39). Cases of coinfection with HIV and *B. bacilliformis* do not appear to have been reported.

Viral Infections

Hemorrhagic Fever Viruses, Arboviruses, and Others

No significant interactions have been well documented between HIV and bunyaviruses, hantaviruses, phleboviruses, arenaviruses, alphaviruses, or filoviruses. In part, of course, this may be a function of a lack of sufficient experience with coinfection with these agents. Among the flaviviruses, two uncontrolled series of patients with St Louis encephalitis in Texas have suggested the possibility that the ratio of disease to infection, but not the course of symptomatic disease, is worsened in the presence of HIV infection.[642,643] There are insufficient data to determine whether HIV alters the course of yellow fever (no case reports; 20–50% mortality in the absence of coinfection),[644] West Nile virus infection (a handful of case reports; interestingly, genetic data implicate CCR5, the HIV coreceptor, in resistance to symptomatic West Nile virus infection),[645] or dengue infection (a handful of case reports;[646] interestingly, one report suggests that dengue fever, like acute measles and scrub typhus, may lead to a reversible suppression of HIV replication).[647]

Should the live-attenuated yellow fever vaccine be given to those infected with HIV? There are theoretical risks of vaccine-induced encephalitis and/or hepatic damage due to prolonged viremia in the immunodeficient.[644] A handful of cases of postvaccinial encephalitis or multiple-organ failure (yellow fever vaccine-associated viscerotropic disease) have been reported in presumably immunocompetent patients (against a denominator of approximately 400 million people vaccinated).[644] Of note, 4 of 23 vaccinees who developed yellow fever vaccine-associated viscerotropic disease had undergone thymectomy for thymomas, raising the concern that T-cell deficiency may be a risk factor.[648]

A single case has also been reported of fatal myeloencephalitis after vaccination in a Thai man with asymptomatic HIV infection, albeit a low CD4$^+$ T-cell count and a high viral load.[649] Approximately 100 asymptomatic HIV-seropositive US military personnel received yellow fever vaccination prior to the introduction of routine HIV screening; no adverse effects were detected (R. Redfield, personal communication, 1997). Small published series of travelers have suggested safety and variable efficacy of the 17D yellow fever vaccine in HIV seropositives without severe immunosuppression,[650–652] a concept bolstered by retrospective analysis of 102 patients in the Swiss HIV Cohort Study who received yellow fever vaccine.[653] As might be expected, the latter study noted reduced vaccine immunogenicity and a more rapid decline in titers of neutralizing antibody in those with HIV infection. The immunogenicity of yellow fever vaccination has also been noted to be severely reduced, again in the absence of significant adverse events, in HIV-infected children in Côte d'Ivoire.[654] WHO recommendations are to use yellow fever vaccine in HIV-seropositive patients who are asymptomatic; it remains a part of the WHO EPI.[655] Pending further studies, yellow fever vaccine is not recommended for symptomatic HIV-infected patients by WHO.[655] The ACIP recommends that HIV-infected people without AIDS or other symptomatic manifestations of HIV infection, who have laboratory-established verification of adequate immune function, and who cannot avoid potential exposure to yellow fever be offered the choice of vaccination.[656,657] As genetic evidence has implicated disruption of the CCR5/RANTES axis in a previously healthy, HIV-uninfected vaccinee who developed viscerotropic disease after vaccination,[658] it would be prudent to avoid such vaccination in patients receiving CCR5 antagonists.[659] Given apparent reduced vaccination efficiency, neutralizing antibody titers should probably be measured prior to travel. If travel requirements (as opposed to actual risk of infection) are the only reason for vaccination of an asymptomatic HIV-infected person, a vaccination waiver letter (not accepted at some borders) should be obtained.[657] For all travelers, avoidance of areas of transmission and, if travel to such areas is essential, conscientiously avoiding mosquito exposure is prudent.

Measles Virus

Measles virus (see Chapter 54) causes an annual mortality in the tropics far in excess of that due to the "traditional" tropical disease viruses. In fact, until quite recently[660] the worldwide yearly mortality due to measles was rivaled among single pathogens only by falciparum malaria, TB, and AIDS. This mortality is predominantly in sub-Saharan Africa. Similar to AIDS, infection with measles virus is accompanied by marked abnormalities of CMI that contribute to the increased susceptibility to secondary infections that account for much of the morbidity and mortality of the disease.[661]

Measles is exacerbated in the presence of HIV coinfection.[662] The mortality rate in North American case series and reports of measles in HIV-positive children and adults has been 40%, far higher than the usual 0.1% case fatality rate seen in the United States.[663–673] Although the presentation of disease has been normal in many, up to 40% have had no rash. In these reports, giant cell pneumonitis has been the principal complication and the prime cause of death, although fatal subacute measles encephalitis has also been described. CD4$^+$ T-cell counts have not been reported in many of these cases, but where they have been reported they have generally been less than 500/μL. Such case reports and series are obviously likely to be biased toward the severe end of the spectrum of disease, however.

Four substantial studies have investigated HIV–measles coinfection in sub-Saharan Africa.[662,674–676] A study of children hospitalized with measles in Kinshasa showed similar mortality rates among HIV-seropositive (31.3%) and -seronegative (28%) children.[674] The fact that only severely ill patients, with complications, were hospitalized likely obviated the ability to detect differential mortality in this study. An initial study of children with measles in Lusaka revealed a significantly higher mortality rate in HIV seropositives (28%) than seronegatives (8.3%).[675] A second prospective study in hospitalized children in Lusaka that distinguished between HIV infection and HIV seropositivity found few differences in the clinical presentation, complications, or mortality of HIV-infected compared to -uninfected children with measles.[676] However, enrollment was based on a clinical diagnosis of measles, which would be expected to minimize the ability to detect differences in clinical presentation; there was a bias against enrollment of critically ill children and those dying soon after admission; and there was significantly greater mortality among HIV-infected compared with -uninfected children among those with clinically diagnosed as opposed to confirmed measles.[676] Early death prior to mounting diagnostic measles IgM titers in the face of severe immunosuppression was suspected to be confounding. Indeed, extension of enrollment in this study revealed that HIV coinfection led to a more than two-fold increase in measles mortality.[662] Other positive findings in these studies included a higher proportion of HIV infection among children hospitalized with measles than expected from (maternal) population prevalence rates, a greater proportion of coinfected patients hospitalized with measles younger than the age of 9 months, and a longer duration of illness before hospitalization and longer hospitalization in coinfected children.[676] Follow-up studies have shown that coinfected patients have a higher risk (90.9% vs. 52.8%) for prolonged (30–61 days after rash onset) shedding of measles virus;[677] and that *in vivo* HIV replication is suppressed during acute measles.[678]

No therapies have been rigorously studied. Vitamin A, which has been shown to be protective in severe measles in malnourished children,[679] may be of benefit, especially given the marginal nutritional status of many with HIV infection. Ribavirin has been shown to reduce the severity of measles in normal hosts.[680] Reports of its use in HIV-positive patients with measles pneumonitis have suggested some efficacy, although rigorous data are lacking.[665,666,668,669,672] Intravenous use is probably most effective. Intravenous immunoglobulin (IVIG) may also be of benefit.[666]

Given the severity of measles in HIV patients, prevention is key. Postexposure prophylaxis with intramuscular immunoglobulin attenuates disease in normal hosts. It is recommended by the ACIP[681] in symptomatic HIV patients (and in those with CD4$^+$ T-cell counts <200/μL) regardless of measles serostatus, but it may have limited efficacy in these and other immunosuppressed patients.[669,682] The recommended dose is 0.5 mL/kg (15 mL maximum), given intramuscularly within 6 (or, better, 3) days. Such postexposure prophylaxis is also recommended by the American Academy of Pediatrics (AAP) for all HIV-infected children and adolescents, and for all children of unclear infection status born to HIV-infected women, regardless of measles immunization status or degree of immunosuppression.[683] Preexposure prophylaxis with monthly IVIG has been advocated for HIV-positive children with documented measles vaccine nonresponsiveness during community outbreaks of measles,[669] but this is not likely to be an economically viable option in the resource-poor areas of the tropics where measles is heavily endemic.

Vaccination remains the principal strategy for preventing measles in HIV-infected people. In normal hosts, the protective efficacy of measles vaccination is greater than 95%.[684] Vaccination efficacy data in HIV-seropositive people is lacking, but seroconversion data are available. In adults with HIV infection, there appears to be no waning of measles antibody titers with increasing immunosuppression.[685–687] Unfortunately, there are no clear data on the response to vaccination in those adults who lack antibodies to measles.[688] In children, the situation is different. HIV-infected infants have lower rates of seroconversion after measles vaccination, generate lower titers of antibody on seroconversion, and have a high rate of secondary vaccine failure, with antibody titers that decrease with time and with increasing immunosuppression.[689] In the absence of HAART-related immune reconstitution[690] responses to second doses of vaccine in the face of immune suppression are generally poor.[691]

There is likely benefit to vaccinating early (at 6–9 months of age), both because of lower levels of passively transferred antibodies in infants born to HIV-infected mothers,[692] and because of there being less HIV-related immunosuppression at this early age.[5] While this immunization strategy is clearly immunogenic, a greater percentage of HIV-infected (compared to HIV-uninfected) infants still remain measles-susceptible.[693]

Safety concerns have obviously been of great importance in the use of this live-attenuated vaccine in HIV patients. The use of measles vaccine had appeared to be quite safe in HIV-infected children and adults,[694] although two reports have emphasized the need for some caution. A 20-year-old man with no HIV-related symptoms but a $CD4^+$ T-cell count "too few to enumerate" received a second dose of measles vaccine prior to entry into college. One year after vaccination, he developed progressive, vaccine-associated measles pneumonitis.[695] A study of the effect of HIV on measles mortality in 356 children hospitalized with measles in Lusaka, Zambia, is also troubling.[675] Previous studies have suggested that when prior measles vaccination does not prevent disease, it can reduce the severity of infection.[674] In HIV-seronegative boys hospitalized for measles, prior measles vaccination did lead to a significantly lower case-fatality rate.[675] Although case fatality rates were not significantly lower in vaccinated HIV-seropositive boys or HIV-seronegative girls than in their unvaccinated controls, there was a trend toward a lower case fatality rate in the vaccinees. Surprisingly, however, the case fatality rate was higher in measles-vaccinated than in unvaccinated HIV-seropositive girls. Although this did not reach statistical significance, it is reminiscent of the experience with the high-titered Edmonston–Zagreb (EZ) vaccine. Use of high-titered EZ vaccine at less than 9 months of age was associated with a delayed excess mortality in several study sites.[696–698] This occurred exclusively in female infants for reasons that remain unclear. It is notable that in the Zambian study noted previously, the highest mortality was seen in the youngest, vaccinated HIV-seropositive girls. However, in regions where there is measles transmission, risk–benefit analysis clearly favors measles immunization of all children regardless of HIV status.[691] In regions where measles transmission does not occur and where immune status can be monitored, withholding of measles vaccine from HIV-infected children with severe immune compromise is wise.[691] WHO recommends measles vaccination for all children in developing countries regardless of HIV infection or symptom status because of the high risk and severity of measles in general in such countries.[693,699]

In the United States, the USPHS–IDSA working group and the Advisory Committee on Immunization Practice (ACIP) recommend measles vaccination for HIV-infected people according to the schedule and conditions for normal hosts if they are not severely immunocompromised.[17,56] In addition, the risks and benefits of vaccination or immunoglobulin prophylaxis should be weighed in severely immunocompromised patients who are at increased risk due to travel or outbreaks.[17] AAP recommendations for HIV-infected infants to young adults in the United States include:

- No immunization in the face of severe immunosuppression.
- Use of the measles–mumps–rubella (MMR) vaccine at 12 months of age, with a second dose given as soon as 28 days after the first dose.
- With measles transmission in the community, vaccination of infants as young as 6 months old with MMR or monovalent measles vaccine, and revaccination with MMR at 12 months.
- Vaccination of all measles-susceptible household members of an HIV-infected person.
- Use of immunoglobulin prophylaxis as noted previously.[683]

Few data are available on other paramyxoviruses in AIDS. With respiratory syncytial virus infection, pneumonia may be more common than bronchiolitis with wheezing, and viral carriage may also be prolonged.[700–703] Copathogens may occur more frequently than in normal hosts.[701] As for metapneumovirus infection, emerging data suggest higher rates of hospitalization, bacterial coinfection and mortality in HIV-coinfected infants.[704]

Rabies

Most human rabies (see Chapter 79) occurs in tropical countries where canine rabies is still endemic. The presentation of rabies does not appear to be altered by HIV infection.[705] HIV-infected, immunosuppressed children and adults clearly have substandard responses to rabies vaccination, however.[706–708] WHO recommendations for postexposure prophylaxis in the face of HIV infection include mandatory use of rabies immunoglobulin, use of intramuscular vaccine, and monitoring of neutralizing antibody titers.[709] Revaccination may be necessary. Even multiple-site, double-dose postexposure vaccination has led to poor responses in the face of HIV coinfection in the presence of immunosuppression.[708]

Poliomyelitis

There is no evidence that HIV infection alters the outcome of infection with poliovirus (see Chapter 60). It has been estimated that more than 500 000 HIV-infected children have received live oral polio vaccine (OPV).[691] Only two cases of vaccine-associated paralytic poliomyelitis in HIV-infected children have been reported.[691] If there is greater risk of vaccine-associated disease in the face of HIV infection, the attributable risk is thought to be very low and OPV remains part of the WHO expanded program of immunization for all children.[691] ACIP recommendations have replaced oral polio vaccine with inactivated polio vaccine for all vaccinees in the United States.[710]

Other Enteric Viruses

Chronic diarrhea is a common problem in AIDS patients throughout the world. Although no definite pathogenic role has been ascribed to enteric viruses (small round structured viruses, enteric adenoviruses, and coronaviruses) in AIDS-related diarrhea in either North America or Africa,[711,712] there are some preliminary data suggesting greater disease severity in children coinfected with HIV and astroviruses[712] and an association of picobirnaviruses with diarrhea in HIV-coinfected patients.[713] In noncholera-endemic areas of the tropics, rotavirus is probably the principal cause of diarrheal deaths in HIV-uninfected infants.[714] Rotavirus diarrhea does not appear to be an opportunistic pathogen in children with HIV coinfection. In a large study in Malawi, no differences in the severity of rotavirus gastroenteritis were found between HIV-infected and uninfected children. Interestingly, rotavirus was less frequently detected in HIV-infected children with gastroenteritis. Despite equal resolution of clinical disease, however, the frequency of death after hospital discharge was significantly greater in coinfected children.[715]

Hepatitis Viruses

Infection with hepatitis A virus (HAV) (see Chapter 64) occurs worldwide. In resource-poor countries, especially in the tropics, HAV is hyperendemic, and exposure is essentially universal by the age of 10 years. Virtually all adults are immune. HIV/HAV coinfection appears to be associated with a higher HAV serum viral load, a longer duration of viremia, and lower elevations in serum alanine aminotransferase levels[716] but a similar disease course.[716–718] Vaccination against HAV is safe in HIV-infected patients.[719–721] Efficacy wanes with increasing immunosuppression.[720,721] The CDC, the National Institutes of Health (NIH), and the HIV Medicine Association (HIVMA) of IDSA recommendations are to vaccinate: (1) those with chronic liver disease, MSM, and intravenous drug users; and (2) hepatitis A-susceptible, HIV-infected persons with risk factors for HAV infection.[710]

Infection with hepatitis E virus (HEV) (see Chapter 64) is more localized, with sporadic and epidemic disease being reported in Mexico; North and West Africa; the Middle East; and South, Southeast, and East Asia. Clinical disease occurs in both adults and children. Data are not clear as to whether HEV has a significant interaction with HIV.

With the cosmopolitan hepatitis viruses that are capable of causing chronic disease, however, several potentially important interactions with HIV have been described. The prevalence of coinfection is furthered by the fact that these viruses share routes of transmission with HIV. For hepatitis B virus (HBV) (see Chapter 66), CMI responses are thought to be important both for the resolution of acute disease and for the production of hepatic inflammation in chronic disease. HIV infection has been reported to lead to: (1) at least a threefold increase in risk of the development of a chronic HBV carrier state (with an inverse correlation with the CD4 count), without a significant change in the severity of acute disease; (2) potential reactivation of quiescent HBV infection; (3) increased HBV replication and decreased inflammation in those with[722,723] or without[724] chronic hepatitis; (4) decreased response to HBV vaccination;[725] (5) loss of HBV antibody over time;[725,726] and (6) increased rates of cirrhosis, and liver-related mortality, and increased risk of hepatocellular carcinoma.[727,728]

Vaccination against HBV has reasonable efficacy in HIV-seropositive populations. Interestingly, however, the highest reported rate of development of chronic carrier status in adults (56–80%) occurred in HIV-infected people who were vaccinated at the same time that they developed HBV infection.[729] HBV does not appear to have a significant effect on the clinical course of HIV infection.[730]

Coinfection with hepatitis C virus (HCV) (see Chapter 65) and HIV is associated with reduced likelihood of spontaneous clearance, an increase in HCV viral set point, increased risk of cirrhosis, and reduced likelihood of a successful response to treatment.[731] In the HAART era, HCV-induced liver disease has become a leading cause of mortality in HIV-infected persons. Whether HCV infection has a significant effect on the natural history of HIV infection or the response to HAART remains controversial.[732–736] Maternal HCV infection appears to be associated with an increased risk of HIV vertical transmission.[737]

The data on hepatitis D virus (HDV) are more meager. HDV replication may be prolonged or reactivated in the presence of HIV coinfection.[738,739]

Herpesviruses (see Chapter 56)

As in the industrial world, herpes zoster is quite common in adult AIDS patients in the tropics. A history of shingles is reported by more than 10% of AIDS patients in Africa.[740] In areas of Africa with HIV high seroprevalence, the positive predictive value of a history of shingles for HIV infection is greater than 90%.[740] As elsewhere, zoster tends to develop early in HIV disease; recurrence is common.[740,741]

Chronic genital herpes simplex lesions are common throughout the world in patients with sexually transmitted HIV infection. CMV infection is ubiquitous in most of the tropics.[742] The reported incidence of severe disease due to CMV in AIDS in Africa and Asia (although not Latin America and the Caribbean) has lagged behind that of the industrial north, however, likely because of greater mortality at earlier stages of disease.[743,744] The natural history, diagnosis, and therapy of disease due to coinfection with these cosmopolitan herpesviruses have been discussed elsewhere.[745–747]

Endemic (central Africa), AIDS-related, "classic," and post-transplant Kaposi's sarcoma are all closely associated with human herpesvirus 8 (HHV-8).[748] In the AIDS era, Kaposi's sarcoma has become one of the leading malignancies in areas of sub-Saharan Africa.[749]

Other Viruses

The single case report of severe acute respiratory syndrome coronavirus infection in the face of HIV coinfection was within the described clinical spectrum of this newly emerging virus.[750]

Prevention of Opportunistic Infections

The CDC/NIH/HIVMA/IDSA working group has updated guidelines for preventing OIs in HIV-infected people.[17,78] Several factors were weighed for the generation of these evidence-based recommendations: (1) disease incidence; (2) disease severity in terms of morbidity and mortality; (3) the level of immunosuppression at which disease is most likely to occur; (4) the feasibility, efficacy, and cost of preventive measures; (5) the impact of intervention on quality of life; (6) toxicities, drug interactions, and the potential for drug resistance; and (7) the quality of the evidence supporting each recommendation.[17] The prevention of each OI was evaluated from the standpoint of prevention of exposure, prevention of the first episode of disease (primary prophylaxis), prevention of disease recurrence (secondary prophylaxis), and discontinuance of prophylaxis in those whose $CD4^+$ T-cell counts have risen in response to HAART.[17] These guidelines address specific recommendations for 29 pathogens that interact with HIV, including five pathogens in the tropics, including malaria, penicilliosis, leishmaniasis, Chagas disease, and isosporiasis.[17]

Specific recommendations for prevention of exposure were made for several agents, including *Toxoplasma gondii*, *Cryptosporidium parvum*, *Mycobacterium tuberculosis*, bacterial enteric agents, *Bartonella*, herpes simplex virus (HSV), varicella-zoster virus (VZV), CMV, HHV-8, human papillomavirus, and HCV.[17,78] For adults and adolescents, primary prophylaxis is strongly recommended as a standard of care for *Pneumocystis jirovecii* (daily TMP-SMX (160/800 mg) or thrice-weekly TMP-SMX (320/1600 mg)), *M. tuberculosis* (with tuberculin skin test reactivity, a positive IFN-γ release assay test or contact with a case of active tuberculosis isoniazid daily or twice weekly for 9 months, with pyridoxine to prevent peripheral neuropathy), *T. gondii* (daily or three times weekly TMP-SMX (320/1600 mg); recommended alternative is dapsone–pyrimethamine plus leucovorin), MAC (azithromycin or clarithromycin), and VZV (live attenuated varicella vaccine with exposure to chickenpox or shingles in patients without a history of such, or with negative serologies for VZV and CD4 count ≥200). Primary prophylaxis (vaccination) against HBV, HAV, influenza virus, and *Streptococcus pneumoniae* was generally recommended. Although evidence exists for efficacy, it was not considered sufficiently robust to recommend primary prophylaxis routinely against *Cryptococcus neoformans*, *H. capsulatum*, *Coccidioides immitis*, CMV, or bacterial infection (in the face of neutropenia). For two of these agents (*P. jirovecii* and *M. avium*), primary prophylaxis has been shown to confer a survival benefit.[751–753]

Secondary prophylaxis was strongly recommended as the standard of care for *P. jirovecii*, *T. gondii*, MAC, CMV, *Cryptococcus neoformans*, *H. capsulatum*, *Coccidioides immitis*, and nontyphi *Salmonella* species. Such prophylaxis was recommended for HSV and *Candida* only if subsequent episodes are frequent or severe.[17] With respect to OIs in tropical regions, secondary prophylaxis was recommended for malaria (with drug regimens tailored to specific regions, depending on rates of resistance to commonly used antimalarials), *Penicillium marneffei* (itraconazole), visceral leishmaniasis (amphotericin B lipid complex), Chagas disease (benznidazole for latent disease) and *Isospora belli* (TMP-SMX).[17]

For children and adolescents[78] primary prophylaxis was strongly recommended as a standard of care for *Pneumocystis jirovecii* (TMP-SMX), malaria (mefloquine or atovaquone–proguanil), *M. tuberculosis* (isoniazid or rifampin), MAC (clarithromycin or azithromycin), and VZV (VZIG); generally recommended for *T. gondii* (TMP-SMX), VZV (immunization in the absence of immunosuppression), and influenza virus; and recommended only in unusual circumstances for invasive bacterial infection (hypogammaglobulinemia), *Cryptococcus neoformans* (severe immunosuppression), *H. capsulatum* (severe immunosuppression, endemic geographic area), and CMV (CMV antibody positivity and severe immunosuppression).[78] Primary prophylaxis was also addressed through review of the recommendations for routine immunization schedules in HIV-infected children. In addition to standard schedules for immunization against HBV, HAV, polio, *H. influenzae* type b, diphtheria, tetanus, and pertussis, altered schedules for vaccination against *Streptococcus pneumoniae* (heptavalent pneumococcal conjugate vaccine beginning at 2 months, followed by 23-valent pneumococcal polysaccharide vaccine at 2 years), influenza (yearly), measles–mumps–rubella (no administration to severely immunosuppressed children), and VZV (administration only to asymptomatic, nonimmunosuppressed children) were reviewed.

Recommendations for secondary prophylaxis in children were similar to recommendations for adults.[17,78] The list of pathogens included *P. jirovecii* (TMP-SMX), *T. gondii* (sulfadiazine plus pyrimethamine plus leucovorin), MAC (clarithromycin plus ethambutol ± rifabutin), *Coccidioides* spp. and *Cryptococcus neoformans* (fluconazole), *Histoplasma capsulatum* (itraconazole), *Microsporidia* spp. (albendazole), CMV (ganciclovir), *Bartonella* spp. (doxycycline), *Candida* (fluconazole), and HSV (acyclovir), with the addition of a recommendation for use of TMP-SMX or IVIG to prevent invasive bacterial infection in the presence of more than two such infections in a 1-year period.[78]

These recommendations are likely to find broad applicability in the industrial world, where the OI spectrum, health care priorities, and available prevention options are similar. The applicability to much of the tropics is less clear, however, given differing spectra of OIs, differences in antibiotic resistance patterns, and differences in sociocultural acceptability or feasibility of preventive measures. Limits in the availability of health care resources (including not just an inability to support the cost of many prevention regimens but also an inability to diagnose HIV disease early enough for preventive measures to be effective, to stage the degree of HIV-associated immunosuppression reliably, and to diagnose OIs definitively) also directly influence the range of prevention options and priorities. It should also be noted that, compared with HAART (or prevention of HIV infection), the benefit of OI prevention in reducing HIV-related morbidity and mortality may be somewhat modest.[754] Adequate global provision of HAART represents an ongoing, immense challenge, however, and wide implementation of simple, cheap, effective OI prevention strategies provides an opportunity to reduce morbidity and mortality rapidly and widely.[744]

In 1996, Kaplan and colleagues argued that effective research on OI prevention strategies in the tropics will require an integrated approach, including the area-specific determination of OI spectra, determination of environmental reservoirs of opportunistic pathogens and feasible ways to reduce exposure, assessment of immuno- and chemoprophylaxis against such pathogens, and improvement in the ability to identify and inexpensively stage HIV infection.[20] Since then, data on the efficacy of some OI prevention strategies in resource-poor countries of the tropics have accrued.

First, as noted previously, primary preventive therapy against TB with isoniazid has been shown be effective in HIV-infected individuals, regardless of tuberculin status.[744,755,756] WHO and UNAIDS recommendations are for primary preventive therapy to be given to PPD-positive, HIV-infected individuals who do not have active tuberculosis.[757] In settings where it may not be feasible to do PPD testing, primary preventive therapy should be considered for those living in populations with an estimated prevalence of infection >30%, health care workers, household contacts of TB patients, prisoners, miners, and other groups at high risk of acquisition or transmission of TB.[758]

Second, TMP-SMX – a cheap, widely available antibiotic with activity against a plethora of OIs (including PCP, nontyphoid salmonellosis, pneumococcal disease, and toxoplasmosis) and malaria – has been shown to reduce morbidity and mortality in HIV-infected adults[759–763] and children.[475,764–766] WHO/UNAIDS recommendations are that TMP-SMX be used for prophylaxis in adults and children living with HIV/AIDS in Africa as a minimum package of care.[766] WHO/UNAIDS/UNICEF recommends that such prophylaxis should be offered to adults (defined as those >13 years old) with symptomatic HIV disease, those who are asymptomatic with a CD4 count of 500/μL or less (or total lymphocyte equivalent), and pregnant women after the first trimester.[766] All HIV-exposed children (born to HIV-infected mothers) should get TMP-SMX from the age of 4–6 weeks, as should any child identified as HIV-infected with any clinical signs or symptoms suggestive of HIV, regardless of age or $CD4^+$ T-cell count.[766] It is further recommended that TMP-SMX be discontinued: (1) in HIV-exposed children only once HIV infection has confidently been excluded (and the mother is no longer breastfeeding); (2) in HIV-infected children on antiretroviral therapy when evidence of immune restoration has occurred; and (3) in those with severe cutaneous, renal, hepatic, or hematological toxicity.[767] It has been noted that such mass prophylaxis strategies entail some yet-to-be quantified risks, principally of increasing rates of drug-resistant bacteria and malaria.[768] Studies in Kenya have reported a modest increase in rates of drug-resistant enteric bacteria, without a significant increase in rates of drug-resistant malaria in these settings.[763,769]

Third, a large, randomized, double-blind, placebo-controlled trial of the 23-valent pneumococcal polysaccharide vaccine in HIV-infected Ugandan adults showed no protective effect (with invasive pneumococcal disease as the primary endpoint).[770] Surprisingly, increased rates of pneumococcal disease were seen in vaccine recipients. The potential mechanism remains unclear; not surprisingly, the study remains controversial. The Strategic Advisory Group of Experts of the WHO has recommended that the licensed 7-serotype conjugate vaccine (PCV-7), already used in developed countries, be introduced in countries where HIV is a significant cause of mortality and in populations with a high prevalence of other underlying conditions that increase the risk of pneumococcal disease, such as sickle cell disease.[771] The PCV-7 vaccine can be easily integrated into routine vaccination schedules, with the possibility of being administered at the same time as other vaccines in infant immunization programs.[771]

Fourth, among the specifically tropical OIs, a controlled, double-blind trial of primary prophylaxis with itraconazole in Thailand showed efficacy in preventing penicilliosis (and cryptococcosis), a second study demonstrating efficacy in secondary prophylaxis.[772,773] As a result, daily itraconazole is recommended for secondary prophylaxis by the CDC/IDSA.[17] Recent studies of secondary prophylaxis in visceral leishmaniasis have found that treatment with antileishmanial drugs, including liposomal amphotericin and stibogluconate, reduced relapse rates by 30–40%.[774–777] However, in the absence of head-to-head comparison of drugs, no particular regimen can be recommended.[17] There are little or no data available on the prophylaxis of other tropical OIs, such as American trypanosomiasis, although the utility of avoiding exposures to the vectors of the agents of these diseases should be clear.

More generally, certain options for preventing or reducing exposure to opportunistic pathogens are likely to be broadly useful, including avoiding unboiled water, raw or undercooked foods and unpasteurized milk to prevent enteric bacterial and protozoan infections as well as *T. gondii* exposure, and avoiding contact with patients with TB, for example, in patient care settings. Avoiding exposure to the opportunistic agents of disseminated fungal disease is likely to be impractical in most settings.

Issues pertinent to the HIV-infected traveler are considered in Chapter 126.

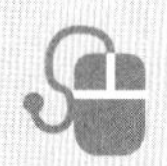

Access the complete reference list online at
http://www.expertconsult.com

CHAPTER 140

Access the complete reference list online at http://www.expertconsult.com

Delusional Parasitosis

Kathryn N. Suh • Jay S. Keystone

Delusional parasitosis (DP) is a rare disorder in which affected individuals have the mistaken but unshakeable belief (delusion) that they are infected by "bugs": parasites, worms, bacteria, mites, or other living organisms. As with all delusions, this belief is unfounded and irrational, but cannot be corrected by reasoning, persuasion, or logical argument. In reality the spectrum of symptoms leading to consideration of the diagnosis of DP can be broad and may encompass a range of symptoms and beliefs. Some individuals are quite functional and merely have the feeling that they are infested; others may experience the sensation of crawling or moving insects in their skin (formication); and yet others may have true delusions of parasitic infection that may interfere with their usual activities to varying degrees.[1]

DP is known by many names, including Ekbom's syndrome, delusory parasitosis, psychogenic parasitosis, delusional infestation, delusional ectoparasitosis, formication, chronic tactile hallucinosis, dermatophobia, parasitophobia, and cocaine bugs.

HISTORICAL PERSPECTIVES

The first reported case of DP is credited to George Thibierge, who coined the term "acaraphobia" in his 1894 description of patients who were convinced they were infected with mites.[2] In 1938, Karl Ekbom described a similar clinical picture that he called "praeseniler Dermatozoenwahn" (presenile dermatozoic delusion),[3] subsequently referred to as Ekbom's syndrome. He postulated that abnormal sensations experienced by patients subsequently led to delusions that parasites were present. This theory was supported over 30 years later by Berrios, who also suggested that the initial sensation *as if* something is crawling on the patient's skin leads to the conviction that something really *is* crawling on the skin.[4]

In 1946, Wilson and Miller[5] described a total of 45 previously reported cases in addition to 6 cases of their own, and introduced the term "delusional parasitosis." Bers and Conrad[6] proposed the term "chronic tactile hallucinosis" in 1954, because of the similarities they observed with alcohol-induced hallucinosis. Munro[7] suggested that DP was a form of monosymptomatic hypochondriasis or monosymptomatic hypochondriacal psychosis (MHP), a fixed, single hypochondriacal belief that exists when no other disorder of thought is present. By 1995, in an extensive review of the topic, Trabert[8] had identified a total of 1223 cases reported in the literature. Many additional case reports and case series have since been reported.

PSYCHIATRIC PERSPECTIVES

The interaction between psychiatric symptoms and dermatologic conditions has been well described. An estimated 30–40% of patients seen in dermatology clinics have some psychiatric symptoms.[9] This is not to suggest, however, that psychiatric illness is the *cause* of dermatologic symptoms in all such patients. Koo[10] described three forms of psychodermatologic conditions in which disorders of skin and mind may be intermingled: psychophysiologic disorders, in which the patient's mental state can directly affect the condition of an underlying skin disease (e.g., eczema worsened by stress); primary psychiatric disorders such as DP, in which cutaneous symptoms or findings can be directly attributed to an underlying psychiatric disease; and secondary psychiatric disorders, such as anxiety or depression, that may result from an intractable disfiguring skin condition (e.g., alopecia; ichthyosis).

In its truest form, DP is a delusional disorder of the somatic type: "delusions that the person has some physical defect of general medical condition."[11] Nonexistent disease or alteration of the body forms the basis of a somatic (or somatoform) delusional disorder. Delusions of parasitosis are classified as one of the MHPs and are the most common form of this disorder.

The etiology of somatic disorders such as DP and mechanisms of its persistence in affected individuals are unknown. One proposed theory is that, for some individuals, distressing symptoms become amplified and are then perpetuated following the result of newly acquired knowledge or awareness of a disease, new or renewed public health interest, or intense media coverage, for example.[12] Fleeting pruritus following an encounter with an individual with scabies may not be uncommon, but for some the pruritus might worsen as they learn more about scabies. The reasons for this degree of symptom amplification are unclear. Some individuals may truly believe that they are sick, others may behave this way because they think that is how they are expected to behave, and others may be seeking secondary gains.[12,13] Regardless, symptoms are continuously intensified with the resulting perception that the individual is now suffering from a serious disease. Patients may also develop a heightened awareness of and misinterpret new sensations or symptoms that they were previously oblivious to, reaffirming their beliefs that they must be sick, and perpetuating the cycle. As with dermatologic disease, stress can also exacerbate other somatic complaints, and the stress induced by the severity of the perceived illness may also act to augment it further.

It has also been proposed that DP may be related to an excess of extracellular dopamine within the striatum of the brain, due to reduced function of the dopamine transporter.[14] Response of many patients to the dopamine antagonist pimozide lends some support to this theory.

CLASSIFICATION OF DELUSIONAL PARASITOSIS

No definite classification of DP exists.[15] However, in broad terms, three different forms can be described based on published accounts of the disease.[16] Primary DP exists when the delusions of parasitic infection are the only manifestation of disease; that is, no other psychiatric or psychological disorder is present. Secondary DP may occur in two settings: (1) in the presence of underlying psychiatric disease, such as schizophrenia or depression, or (2) as a feature of underlying medical condition,

Box 140.1 Diagnostic Criteria for Delusional Disorder

Non-bizarre delusions involving situations that occur in real life, lasting >1 month	Mood episodes, if concurrent, are of brief duration compared with duration of delusions
Does not meet all criteria for diagnosis of schizophrenia (see text)	Substance abuse, medication side effects, and general medical conditions must be ruled out
Function is otherwise not markedly impaired	

(Adapted from American Psychiatric Association. DSM-IV-TR. Diagnostic and Statistical Manual of Mental Disorders: 4th ed. Text Revision. Washington, DC: American Psychiatric Association, 2000:323–329.)

intoxication or substance abuse (e.g., cocaine), or as an adverse effect of some prescription medications.

Primary Delusional Parasitosis

As noted above, primary DP refers to a somatic delusional disorder. By definition, patients with delusional disorders do not meet all of the criteria required for the diagnosis of schizophrenia.[11] Specifically, hallucinations, disorganized speech, schizophrenic behavior, and other "negative" symptoms should be absent, although hallucinations clearly related to the delusional theme (i.e., tactile hallucinations) may be present. Sufferers of DP and other forms of MHP generally have intact mental function, lack other manifestations of psychiatric disease, and have otherwise normal behavior. Their delusions are limited in scope and generally do not encroach on personal and professional aspects of their lives; however, in some cases, severe behavioral abnormalities may occur. Criteria for the diagnosis of delusional disorders are shown in ***Box 140.1***.

Strictly speaking, DP differs from hypochondriasis in that hypochondriacal individuals recognize that fear of illness or disease is unfounded, and differs from phobias in that patients with DP do not have a fear of becoming ill – they believe they *are* ill. Underlying psychiatric disorders, including schizophrenia and mood disorders, and preexisting medical conditions (including true parasitic infections!), substance abuse, and drug side effects must be ruled out prior to establishing the diagnosis of primary DP. Other mood disorders (e.g., anxiety, depression) may be present with primary DP, but they must clearly be secondary to the delusional disorder in order to classify the DP as primary.

Secondary Delusional Parasitosis Associated with Underlying Psychiatric Disease

Delusions of parasitosis may occur in conjunction with other psychiatric symptoms. Some patients with DP are clearly schizophrenic. Others have varying degrees of psychiatric illness including anxiety, depression, obsessive compulsive disorder, schizophreniform disorder, bipolar disorder, or a family history of psychiatric illness.[13,17,18] One case was described in the setting of post-traumatic stress disorder.[19] Delusions of parasitosis in the setting of underlying psychiatric disease must be distinguished from primary DP, as the management differs; however, differentiating these conditions may be challenging, particularly for the family physician or dermatologist who is most likely to encounter such patients. Phobias and hypochondriasis may present with apparent delusions of parasitosis and may be considered as secondary DP by some.[17]

Secondary Delusional Parasitosis Associated with Underlying Medical Conditions

Up to 25% of cases of DP have been attributed to underlying medical diseases.[8,20] Establishing whether or not delusions are related to a concomitant medical disorder, drugs, or toxins is critical, since treatment of the condition (or withdrawal of the offending agent) may lead to resolution of delusional symptoms.

Central nervous system (CNS) disorders appear to be the most common underlying medical conditions associated with DP. Delusions have been described in the setting of dementia of various etiologies,[20,21] head injury,[20] cerebrovascular accidents,[22,23] multiple sclerosis,[22] multiple system atrophy,[24] CNS infections including encephalitis, meningitis, and neurosyphilis,[20] and as a postoperative complication of a neurosurgical procedure.[25]

There is increasing evidence that at least in some patients, DP is associated with structural abnormalities of the brain. A very small, unmatched case series that included five patients with DP secondary to underlying medical conditions reported structural abnormalities in the striatum of the basal ganglia, in particular the putamen and caudate nucleus, in four of these patients using magnetic resonance imaging.[26] Most of these patients responded favorably to dopamine antagonists, again supporting the dopamine transporter theory. Two case reports have described relative regional cerebral hypoperfusion in patients with DP. Successful treatment using risperidone[27] or paroxetine[28] was accompanied in both cases by increased regional blood flow, demonstrated using single photon emission computed tomography. Such findings must be interpreted with caution, however, given the small number of patients studied and the lack of comparison with age-matched controls without DP.

DP has been also associated with diseases of most other organ systems including the hematopoietic,[22] pulmonary,[22] cardiac,[5,29] renal,[22] gastrointestinal,[22] and endocrine systems.[21,22,30] Vitamin B_{12}[22,31] and folate[20,22] deficiencies and pellagra[22,32,33] have also been reported as causes of DP, with resolution of delusional symptoms after nutritional replacement. Delusions of parasitosis may also be associated with malignancy[20,30,34] or systemic infections such as human immunodeficiency virus infection,[35] tuberculosis,[5] and leprosy.[21]

Substance abuse should be considered particularly when DP presents in younger age groups.[18,22] In such instances, delusions are usually transient and of inadequate duration to meet the criteria for delusional disorder. Cocaine, alcohol, and amphetamines (e.g., Ritalin) are common precipitants,[36] and heroin withdrawal has been implicated.[37] Rarely, prescription drugs may induce delusions of parasitosis; DP has been reported with the use of phenelzine,[38,39] pargyline,[39] ketoconazole,[40] corticosteroids,[20] amantadine,[41] ciprofloxacin,[42] pegylated interferon-α,[43] and topiramate.[44] Drug-induced DP generally resolves once the offending drug is discontinued.

A more thorough list of medical conditions and drugs/toxins associated with DP is shown in ***Table 140.1***.

EPIDEMIOLOGY

Delusional disorders in general are rare.[45] Incidence and prevalence of delusional disorders have been estimated to be 0.7–3.0 and 24–30 cases per 100 000 population (upper limits of 0.003% and 0.03%) respectively,[46] although these rates were not determined using currently accepted diagnostic criteria. Delusional disorders are slightly more frequent in women.

Rates of DP are even more difficult to determine. A retrospective study of almost 10 500 psychiatric outpatients in China identified 86 (0.83%) with delusional disorders, 2 of whom had unspecified somatic delusions.[47] In a Norwegian study of over 3000 psychiatric admissions to hospital, 0.4% of patients with paranoid psychoses had hypochondriacal delusions.[48] However, because patients with DP insist that their symptoms do not have a psychiatric basis and hence refuse to seek psychiatric help, the true incidence and prevalence of this disorder may be greatly underestimated in the psychiatric literature. Trabert[49] estimated the incidence of DP to be 16.6 per million population per year, and the prevalence 83.2 cases per million population, in southwest Germany. Although the number of reported cases of DP in the literature continues to increase, it remains an extremely uncommon disorder. Based on Lyell's

Table 140.1 Medical Conditions Associated with Delusions of Parasitosis

Neurologic disorders	Dementia – Alzheimer's – Multi-infarct – Huntington's disease Head trauma Infarction Infection – Meningitis, encephalitis – Human immunodeficiency virus – Neurosyphilis Multiple sclerosis Pernicious anemia Postoperative complication (neurosurgery) Posttraumatic stress disorder Tumors of the central nervous system
Endocrine disorders	Diabetes mellitus Hyperthyroidism
Hematologic disorders	Severe anemia Leukemia Polycythemia vera
Cardiopulmonary disease	Congestive heart failure Hypertension Asthma
Infectious diseases	Human immunodeficiency virus infection Leprosy Tuberculosis Prior infestation
Malignancy	Lymphoma Solid organ: breast, colon, lung
Nutritional deficiency	B_{12}, folate, thiamine deficiency Pellagra
Other miscellaneous disorders	Arthritis Hepatitis Stasis dermatitis Vitiligo
Drugs or toxins	Alcohol Amphetamines including methylphenidate Cocaine Heroin
Prescription medications	Amantadine Ciprofloxacin Corticosteroids Ketoconazole Pargyline Pegylated interferon-α Phenelzine Topiramate

(Adapted from Slaughter JR, Zanol K, Rezvani H, et al. Psychogenic parasitosis: A case series and literature review. Psychosomatics. 1998; 39:491–500; and Johnson GC, Anton RF. Delusions of parasitosis: differential diagnosis and treatment. South Med J. 1985;78:914–918.)

retrospective survey,[22] it is estimated that a practicing dermatologist could expect to see one patient with DP for every 7 years in practice.[1] Most cases have been reported from centers in North America and Europe, and more recently from Asia.

CLINICAL FEATURES AND PRESENTATION

General characteristics of patients with DP are fairly consistent in data reported in two physician surveys[22,29] and several case series.[8,18,20,21,50] DP can affect patients of all ages, but is much more common in older age groups (>50 years).[8,29] The mean age of onset in 802 patients for whom this was recorded in Trabert's review was 57 years;[8] 84% of patients were over age 50. The age of onset does not differ significantly between men and women, although men tend to present at a slightly younger age.[8] Overall, women outnumber men by roughly a 2–3 : 1 ratio.[8,21,22] Although the sex distribution is almost equal in early adulthood, the preponderance of women in older age groups is striking, with the female : male ratio exceeding 3 : 1 in individuals over 50 years of age.[8,22] Younger patients are more likely to have an underlying cause of their delusions, notably head injuries, substance abuse, and schizophrenia, and are more likely to be involved in shared delusions.[18,22]

Patients with primary DP are usually otherwise functional individuals who do not have an antecedent history of psychiatric illness. Apart from their firm belief that they suffer from a parasitic infection, the behavior of affected patients is usually unremarkable. For some patients, delusions may be triggered by an event in which possible exposure to parasites may have occurred – for example, sleeping in unclean bed sheets or borrowing someone else's clothing.[1] Travel to and receipt of gifts from exotic destinations have also precipitated DP.[51,52] Documented parasitic infections predate the development of DP in only 2% of all cases.[22] Patients may be from any socioeconomic background. Many affected individuals are highly functional and highly educated; in Lyell's survey,[22] several of the 282 patients described were professionals, including physicians and psychologists. Despite this they are, by definition, unable to appreciate their delusional state although in some cases of primary DP the unfounded basis of the patient's delusions became apparent to the individual during pharmacologic treatment.[36]

Many patients, but not all, are single and have been categorized as "loners".[7,53] In Trabert's series, only 21% of the 67 patients for whom social interactions were described were considered to have "good and stable social contacts"; 54% were considered "socially isolated."[8] Social isolation appears to be a premorbid state, rather than a consequence of illness. A higher than expected prevalence of personality traits and disorders has also been observed in some case series.[20,22]

Patients with DP often have a long history of dermatologic complaints including rashes, pruritus, and sensations of stinging, biting, and formication. The onset is usually insidious, and most patients have symptoms for at least 6 months and often many years before diagnosis is made.[8,21] In Trabert's review, the average duration of symptoms was 3 years and the median duration 1 year.[8] Typically, patients have sought the help of multiple physicians (most commonly primary care physicians and dermatologists, sometimes infectious diseases physicians, and rarely if ever psychiatrists) or entomologists, usually with little satisfaction. Those who attribute their illness to household pets may have visited veterinarians repeatedly, seeking treatment for their pets. Many patients have received repeated courses of dermatologic and antiparasitic therapies, despite the lack of an objective diagnosis. They often bring in specimens for examination which they have picked from their skin – the "matchbox sign,"[54] or more recently the "Ziploc bag sign."[17] Occasionally these will contain parts of nonpathogenic insects, but most often they will harbor normal skin flakes or dust, hair, or other "flotsam of normal life."[13]

Patients may provide bizarre and unlikely stories concerning their infestation, including exhaustive descriptions and diagrams of the parasites' appearance, habitat, entry and egress to and from various body cavities, and reproductive cycles. Patients often enumerate the parasites and provide details of their activities. Many have repeatedly had exterminators into their homes, consulted pest-control services, and sprayed themselves and their homes with potentially toxic pesticides and other chemicals to eradicate the bugs. Those driven to extremes may move, or rid themselves of some or all of their belongings in the hopes of ending the problem. The fear of contagion and transmission of disease to others may or may not be present.

Other persons may occasionally be drawn into the patient's delusional system; 8–25% of delusions of parasitosis may be shared.[20,22,55,56] Delusions are most often shared with one other person (folie à deux), usually a partner or spouse, or less commonly with offspring,[22] and are usually induced by a woman.[56] On occasion trios (folie à trois), or even larger groups such as entire families or groups of occupational colleagues, have developed shared delusions.

Physical examination is unrevealing apart from ulcers, excoriations and scars that result from attempts to remove the organisms from the skin by using fingernails, knives, pins, or other objects. On exposed skin, lesions may be asymmetric, reflecting the increased range of the patient's dominant hand; this may be particularly evident over the shoulders and scapulae.[22] Lesions are often absent in the upper back where the patient cannot reach. Contact or irritant dermatitis resulting from excessive cleaning or the use of abrasive soaps or chemicals may also be present.

APPROACH TO THE PATIENT WITH DELUSIONAL PARASITOSIS

DP should be suspected when an individual presents with an irrational, fixed belief that he or she is infected with internal or external parasites in spite of reassurance and ample evidence to the contrary. Clearly, it is important to determine the following: (1) is the belief founded in reality? (i.e., is the patient really infected?); (2) if infection can be reliably excluded, is the patient truly delusional, or is the belief "shakeable"? (is the patient merely hypochondriacal; i.e., can the patient possibly be convinced that he or she may not be infected?); and (3) if the patient is delusional, which form of DP is present? (i.e., primary DP, or secondary DP associated with underlying psychiatric disease, medical illness, or medications/toxins). Depending on the answers to these three questions, therapy will differ markedly. Treatment of a previously untreated parasitic infection or medical condition, or cessation of medications that may be triggers, is obviously indicated if possible. If the patient is truly delusional and an organic cause can be ruled out, the major challenge is then to determine whether the patient is suffering from a primary delusional disorder (i.e., MHP) or has an underlying psychiatric illness (i.e., secondary delusions of parasitosis). A psychiatric opinion is invaluable in such instances, but it is often never obtained since patients with DP usually refuse a psychiatric assessment.

One key to the management of patients with DP is the development of a strong, therapeutic relationship with the patient. A significant proportion of these patients, if not the majority, express dissatisfaction with previous physicians, many of whom they believe are incompetent and uncaring. As a result, patients often fail to attend follow-up appointments and receive inadequate or no therapy, whereas many could benefit from readily available and effective therapy if only they would take it. A sympathetic ear, a nonjudgmental approach, acknowledgment that the patient's symptoms are real, and empathetic exploration into the effects their symptoms have had on their daily lives can instill a sense of trust into the relationship.[57] It has been debated whether or not the physician should overtly agree or disagree with the patient's beliefs,[13] but many suggest that a conservative and nonconfrontational approach be employed.[1,13,58,59] Use of phrases such as "I cannot see any parasites today" rather than "there are no parasites,"[22] and acknowledgment that their problem *may* have resulted from a previous infection[17] (perhaps even stating that their persistent symptoms are due to a residual "chemical imbalance") may accomplish this while at the same time further gaining the patient's trust. It is important not to dismiss patients' complaints as trivial, even when it is obvious that they are delusional, but equally important not to overtly support their beliefs and feed into their delusional system. Reassurance that they can be helped is also valuable.

Initial assessment(s) should focus on the patient's primary complaints, attempting to rule out true infection and organic cause(s) of their symptoms. A thorough history, including use of prescription and illicit drugs and travel or geographic exposures, and review of systems should be obtained. Listening carefully to the patient's answers can sometimes provide clues to underlying psychiatric or medical illness. A complete physical examination is warranted, paying particular attention to the skin since most patients have cutaneous symptoms. Careful assessment of any skin lesions is essential; in a small number of cases, patients have a true parasitic infection. Evaluation by a dermatologist, if not already performed, can be beneficial and may provide reassurance to the patient that his/her symptoms are being taken seriously. If the patient has brought his/her own specimens with him/her, reassure the patient that they will be sent to a proper laboratory and/or entomologist for examination. To avoid the argument that the "parasites" have been or will be missed because of improper preservation, the patient should be provided with specimen bottles containing preservative in which he/she may place subsequent samples. Skin biopsies may be indicated in some instances, although rarely; skin scrapings or other cutaneous specimens may be more appropriate and can be readily obtained during an office visit. Negative results, especially from repeated examinations of submitted specimens, can eliminate the possibility of a real parasitic infection.

Possible organic causes of DP may be evident from the history or physical examination (e.g., hyperthyroidism, neurologic disease). Blood tests should be obtained to complete the assessment. Appropriate initial investigations include a complete blood count and differential, electrolytes, urea, creatinine, liver enzymes, fasting blood sugar, thyroid-stimulating hormone level, and B_{12} and folate levels, as well as a chest radiograph. Based on the individual's risk factors, additional tests such as serology for human immunodeficiency virus infection and syphilis, tuberculosis skin testing, or other radiologic imaging (e.g., computed tomography or magnetic resonance imaging of the brain), may be indicated. Those with organic diseases may be better managed by referral to an appropriate specialist (e.g., internist, neurologist) for further management. By means of a thorough history and physical examination and some basic investigations, true infestation and the more commonly reported medical conditions associated with DP can be eliminated.

Over the course of several visits, serial examination of skin lesions can be performed and additional specimens (or other investigations) obtained as required. In addition, follow-up visits provide the opportunity for the patient to develop more trust in the physician. Trust in the physician is crucial if a psychiatric consultation will be requested. Repeated assessments of the patient are helpful in determining whether the patient has a shakeable belief (hypochondriasis) rather than true delusions; he or she may eventually question whether or not the problem may be imaginary or "in his head," or ask the physician's opinion of the problem.[17] Such shakeable beliefs are often associated with anxiety or depression;[17] supportive therapy and anxiolytic or antidepressant therapy is required in these patients. In contrast, antipsychotic therapy is usually indicated for patients with primary DP.

MANAGEMENT

Psychiatric Assessment

Once organic disease has been excluded, a psychiatric referral may be warranted. Effective therapies are available for both primary and secondary DP, but differ. DP associated with underlying psychiatric disorders such as schizophrenia or depression is probably best managed by a psychiatrist and will not be discussed further. While delusions in some patients with organic causes of DP may improve or resolve with treatment of the underlying condition, these individuals may also benefit from psychiatric care. Gould and Gragg[60] have suggested that psychiatric evaluation is appropriate only for selected patients with DP (such as those with schizophrenia), but that many could be adequately managed by primary care physicians, dermatologists, or infectious disease consultants for fear of losing them to medical care altogether by suggesting they see a psychiatrist. However, others suggest that a psychiatrist be at least consulted at some point in the patient's care.[17,18,36] Regardless of the approach used, the treating physician's credibility often dissipates at the mention of the need for psychiatric consultation or therapy.

A thorough psychiatric assessment can provide confirmation of (or establish) the diagnosis; this is perhaps the most important reason for referral, and allows determination of the most appropriate form of therapy. Furthermore, many health care practitioners are not trained or prepared to provide the psychotherapy and/or pharmacotherapy that can benefit both the hypochondriacal patient and the patient with primary or secondary DP. While many hypochondriacal patients will agree to a psychiatric assessment, most patients with DP will not; therefore, some tact and careful strategy may be required to accomplish this.

Convincing patients with DP of the need for and importance of a psychiatric referral is extremely difficult. Gradual introduction of the topic over the course of several office visits, placing emphasis on the need for expert guidance to manage the effects that DP has had on the patient's life (such as stress or depression), may result in greater success. Acceptance of psychiatric referral is also likely to be higher if an on-site psychiatrist is present to perform an immediate assessment, such as in a dermatology–psychiatry liaison clinic, rather than relying on the patient to attend a separate appointment in a different place,[17,36,60] but a significant proportion of patients will still refuse even in this setting.[36] Furthermore, this arrangement is often not practical for physicians practicing outside of academic centers. At a minimum, if a psychiatric evaluation cannot be obtained (the rule rather than the exception), the case should be discussed with a psychiatrist prior to commencing any therapy.

Treatment of Primary Delusions of Parasitosis

Psychotherapy, psychosurgery, and electroconvulsive therapy have had relatively little success in the treatment of DP.[34] Psychotherapy has been successful in only 10% of cases, similar to the rate of resolution in untreated patients.[13] Antidepressant and anxiolytic medications have little or no role in the treatment of primary DP. Secondary mood disorders (i.e., those that are a consequence of the delusional state) may be improved, but delusions will persist. Prior to the introduction of effective neuroleptic therapy, DP was considered to be a progressive disorder with a low rate of spontaneous remission.

Treatment of primary DP has been revolutionized with the use of antipsychotic medications. However, it is important to realize that there is limited evidence of their effectiveness for treatment of DP[61]; few clinical trials, and no substantial randomized controlled trials, have examined the efficacy of neuroleptic medications for the treatment of primary DP. Nonetheless, based on case series and case reports, if the diagnosis has been established with certainty, antipsychotics are now the mainstay of therapy.

Convincing patients to take these medications presents another significant obstacle. Even if patients do agree to start medication, adherence may be an issue. Occasionally bargaining with patients might work; the physician may agree to a patient's request (e.g., treatment with an antiparasitic agent) on condition that the patient also try taking antipsychotic medication.[17] Patients often refuse to try such drugs as risperidone or pimozide if they discover that they are antipsychotic agents. This may be averted by warning the patient that the agent is a commonly used drug for schizophrenia and indicating that "of course, you are not schizophrenic!" Patients are much more likely to agree to take medication for treatment of a "chemical imbalance" than for a psychiatric problem. One additional important strategy is to provide examples of other medications that have multiple indications for their use, such as aspirin for pyrexia and coronary artery disease, or amitriptyline for depression and neuritis. Some, particularly those insistent on knowing if medication will cure their problem, may be persuaded if they are told that patients with a similar condition have experienced great relief in their symptoms with an improvement in their well-being.

Until the introduction of the atypical (second-generation) antipsychotics, pimozide was frequently used as first-line therapy for DP. Today, many psychiatrists would choose the newer antipsychotics over pimozide because of their better safety profile and more specific actions. Publication bias, the paucity of controlled trials, the inclusion of patients with both primary and secondary DP in many studies, and the lack of standardized criteria for assessing response to therapy make efficacy comparisons among different agents challenging.

First-Generation Antipsychotic Agents

Pimozide has been the most extensively used drug and has had the greatest reported success rate for treatment of DP. In the late 1970s, the first case series of DP patients successfully treated with pimozide were published,[7,62] with later case series reporting response rates of up to 87% (33–52% complete, 28–35% partial).[21,63] In retrospective physician surveys, pimozide was reported to effect a clinical response in 73–81% of treated patients,[8,22,29] with a full remission in 50%,[8,22] although like other retrospective studies these data are prone to inherent bias. One placebo-controlled double-blind trial with 10 patients[64] and another double-blind crossover trial with 11 patients[65] both demonstrated efficacy of greater than 90%.

Pimozide is an oral diphenylbutylpiperidine antipsychotic agent, structurally related to butyrophenones, of which haloperidol is the best known. Pimozide selectively blocks dopamine type 2 receptors; it has minimal effect on other CNS neurotransmitters, although its antagonistic effects on opiate receptors may contribute to reducing the sensations of pruritus and formication.[64] Other pharmacologic effects include a mild anticholinergic effect, blockage of calcium channels and of some adrenergic receptors, and induction of prolactin secretion. The most common adverse effects when used at therapeutic doses are extrapyramidal reactions (tremor, bradykinesia, shuffling gait), which occur in up to 15% of patients.[18] Prolongation of the QT interval with the possibility of fatal arrhythmias may occur particularly with higher doses of the drug; a baseline electrocardiogram is recommended prior to starting pimozide and periodically during therapy to monitor the QT interval duration. Increase of the QT interval by 25% or more from baseline, or a QT interval of greater than 520 milliseconds, warrants temporary cessation of the drug and a subsequent dose reduction. Acute dystonic reactions, akathisia, anticholinergic effects, orthostatic hypotension, and galactorrhea are other side effects.

Doses between 1 and 12 mg daily are usually effective for treatment of DP. Pimozide should be instituted at a low dose (0.5–1 mg daily) and increased gradually (e.g., by 1 mg weekly) either until the desired clinical effect has been achieved or to the maximum recommended dose of 20 mg daily. The lowest effective dose should be used, ideally using no more than 10 mg daily. Once a satisfactory response has been obtained, which may require several weeks of therapy, the patient should be maintained on the same dose for at least one and preferably several months.[18,66] The dose should then be tapered gradually (by 1 mg every 1–2 weeks) until it is discontinued, observing carefully for relapses.[18,66] If relapses occur, they often respond to reinstitution of the drug; some patients will require prolonged therapy in order to control their symptoms.

Other first-generation antipsychotics that have been used with success include chlorpromazine, haloperidol, perphenazine, sulpiride, thioridazine, and trifluoperazine.

Second-Generation Antipsychotic (SGA) Agents

Given the side effect profile of pimozide, other neuroleptic agents may be preferable, particularly in elderly patients or those with known cardiac disease. In a recent retrospective case series of patients with both primary and secondary DP treated with various SGAs, partial or full remission was effected in 75% of 63 cases, and overall SGAs were felt to be as effective as traditional first-generation drugs in the treatment of DP, although the rate of complete remission may be lower.[50]

Risperidone has been most widely used SGA, and is considered by some to be the first-line therapy for DP.[67] Risperidone has been effective for some patients who have failed trials of haloperidol and pimozide.[50,68] Serotonin is felt to play a significant role in psychosis;[69] risperidone is one of several atypical antipsychotics that preferentially blocks serotonin receptors while still maintaining some activity against dopamine receptors. Between 0.25 and 8 mg daily, administered in one or two doses, has been required for clinical response.[50] Adverse effects including extrapyramidal reactions can occur, but overall risperidone appears to be a safer and better-tolerated agent than pimozide.[67] Recently there has been suggestion of an increased risk of cerebrovascular accidents in dementia patients receiving risperidone;[70] the evidence is conflicting, and no such association has been reported in patients with delusional disorders.

Olanzipine at doses of 2.5–20 mg daily appears to as effective as risperidone[50] but has been used less frequently. Successful treatment has also been reported with use of amisulpiride, aripiprazole, escitalopram, quetiapine, sertindole, and ziprasidone. Paliperidone (9-hydroxyrisperidone), the active metabolite of risperidone, has also been used with success.[71]

OUTCOME AND PROGNOSIS

DP was previously considered a progressive disorder with little chance of spontaneous improvement; only 10–30% of cases would remit spontaneously prior to the use of neuroleptics.[8,13]

Factors that have been noted to affect the response to therapy include the type of DP (primary versus secondary), duration of illness prior to therapy, and the duration of therapy. In patients treated with SGAs,[50] the time to onset of any effect and to maximal effect was shorter, and response rates higher (80% versus 68%), in secondary DP compared with primary DP, but this difference was not statistically significant. Overall, maximum effects of therapy were noted by 10 weeks in those patients who did respond, suggesting that a lack of response by this time should prompt a change in treatment. The duration of symptoms may also affect outcome. In Trabert's study,[8] the likelihood of a full remission was inversely correlated with the duration of symptoms, but this was not observed in patients treated with SGAs.[50] Regardless, pharmacotherapy has improved the prognosis for patients with DP. In Trabert's series,[8] 52% of patients who were followed after 1960 (after the introduction of neuroleptics for treatment) had a sustained remission during follow-up, compared with 33% who were diagnosed before 1960. Other case series have demonstrated high rates of full recovery using pimozide, with 50–90% of patients achieving a sustained remission.[63,72] An additional one-third of patients may respond well but without achieving full remission.[21,63] In one case series,[50] full remission was achieved in 37% and partial remission in 38% of those treated with SGAs. Relapse rates are difficult to determine, but relapses appear to be common;[22] however, they tend to respond well to reinstitution of therapy, regardless of the neuroleptic agent used.[17,22,30] Sustained therapy of at least 8 weeks' duration and treatment supervision by a psychiatrist may also be associated with improved response rates.[50]

SUMMARY

DP is a rare but treatable disorder. Dermatologists and primary care physicians in particular, being the first physicians who encounter these patients, should consider the diagnosis when patients present with a fixed belief of infestation. True infestation and underlying causes should be ruled out by careful history, physical examination and laboratory investigations. Psychiatric involvement is usually invaluable in these cases, but may be difficult to obtain. Establishing the correct diagnosis is essential in order to offer patients optimal therapy, however. With appropriate treatment, clinical improvement and long-term remission are possible.

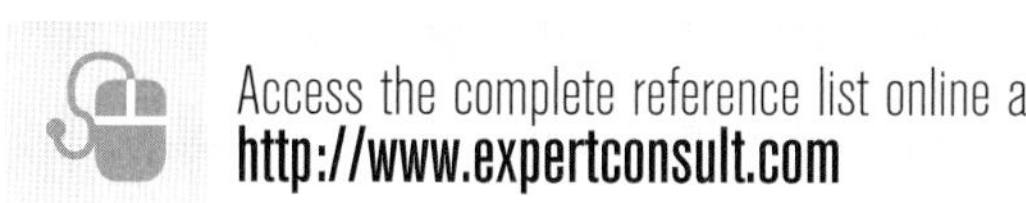
Access the complete reference list online at
http://www.expertconsult.com

CHAPTER 141

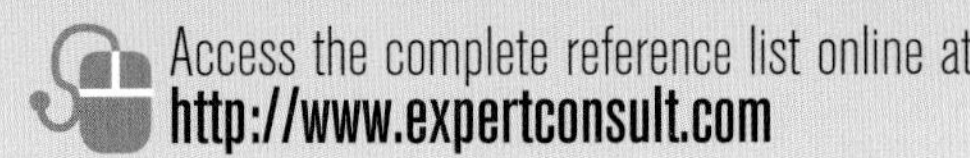
Access the complete reference list online at
http://www.expertconsult.com

Tropical Infectious Disease Concerns in Pregnancy

Raul E. Isturiz • Eduardo Gotuzzo

INTRODUCTION

Tropical infectious diseases that occur during pregnancy, an otherwise healthy, life-affirming state, pose special risks to the mother and fetus. Furthermore, many diagnostic, therapeutic, and preventive measures often must be modified during pregnancy because of their potential for serious side effects. This chapter discusses tropical infectious diseases that, during pregnancy, are especially important to mother or fetus, or that are more common or severe when associated with gestation. The reader must bear in mind that every diagnostic, therapeutic, or preventive strategy applied to a pregnant woman must be individually weighted against the possible side effects both to her and to her developing infant once instituted.

Worldwide, approximately eight million women suffer complications related to their pregnancies every year, and over half a million maternal deaths result. Maternal and neonatal morbidity and mortality show a stark divide between developing and developed countries. In some tropical areas, such as sub-Saharan Africa and central South Asia, one woman in 16 may die of pregnancy-related complications. This compares unfavorably with an average of 1 in 2800 in developed countries. These figures may be an underestimation since the World Health Organization (WHO) estimates that maternal deaths are underreported by as much as 50%. Tragically, motherless children are 10 times more likely to die in childhood than children whose mothers survive. Although maternal infectious diseases in the tropics have an important contributing effect on maternal and childhood morbidity and mortality, their actual impact is unknown.

Based on anecdotal clinical observations and perhaps rooted in a need to explain maternal tolerance of intrauterine fetal tissues, physicians have perceived that the maternal immune response must to some extent be suppressed during gestation. Other than diminished T- and NK-cell function, no measurable suppression has been found in maternal immunity. Neutrophil numbers and function, B-cell counts and subsets, immunoglobulin G (IgG), IgM, and IgA concentrations, antibody-dependent cellular cytotoxicity (ADCC), and complement have been found within the normal limits. Nevertheless, the mild immunosuppression that may accompany pregnancy but that does not last postpartum may play an as yet undefined role in maternal infectious morbidity and mortality by the diseases described in this chapter. The importance of direct or indirect exposure of pregnant women to microorganisms derived from poor tropical areas cannot be overemphasized.

Furthermore, the potential risks of anti-infective drugs in pregnancy also complicate the management of important tropical infectious diseases in pregnant and newborn individuals. The US Food and Drug Administration (FDA) risk category definitions and assignments for selected antimicrobial agents are shown in ***Tables 141.1 and 141.2***.

BRUCELLOSIS (See Chapter 40)

Although teratogenicity has not been described, *Brucella* has been isolated from placental, fetal, and newborn tissues, demonstrating vertical transmission.[1–3] Epidemiologic evidence suggests that *Brucella* species, and *B. melitensis* in particular, can produce preterm and intrauterine fetal death followed by spontaneous abortions in humans, probably more frequently than do other bacterial infections.[4] An increased incidence of fetal loss among infected pregnant women with brucellosis has been repeatedly described.[4–6] In their review of 92 pregnant women with brucellosis in endemic Saudi Arabia, Khan and colleagues note that "although comparative data are limited, the incidence of abortion from 10% to 42% in patients with active brucellosis exceeds that observed in patients infected with other organisms, such as *Campylobacter* species and *Salmonella* species, and suggests that *Brucella* species may indeed produce human abortions more frequently than do other bacterial pathogens." They also recommend prompt antimicrobial therapy in pregnant women with brucellosis.[4]

The absence of erythritol in the human placenta, and anti-*Brucella* activity in human amniotic fluid, may explain why brucellosis causes fewer spontaneous abortions in humans than in farm animals, especially bovine species.[7] *Brucella* has also been isolated from human breast milk and from vaginal swabs from nonpregnant females, but the relevance of these findings remains uncertain.[8–12]

The clinical presentation of brucellosis during pregnancy has prognostic implications for fetal survival. In the Saudi study, during the first and second trimesters, vaginal bleeding with or without febrile illness was associated with spontaneous abortion in all cases of brucellosis, but patients who were treated because they presented with a predominantly febrile illness had no spontaneous abortions.[4] Among 11 patients who were treated because of febrile brucellosis presenting preterm during the third trimester, one spontaneous abortion was observed. Also one spontaneous abortion was documented out of 14 patients that presented with febrile brucellosis at term. The presence of bacteremia or high brucella agglutinin antibody titers did not correlate with the incidence of abortion. In this series, antibiotics used for treatment were trimethoprim-sulfamethoxazole (TMP-SMX) and rifampin.

In a series of studies in Peru, 97 pregnant women with brucellosis have been treated in Lima over a 25-year period.[13,14] Several presented with jaundice, one patient died of hepatic failure in her third trimester, and 7 had spontaneous abortions. Of 22 patients that were admitted to the hospital with threatened abortion, 6 had premature deliveries and 16 eventually delivered a term infant. In this series, rifampin was given for 6 weeks plus an aminoglycoside for the first 2 weeks. Treated patients had no abortions.

Combination treatment of brucellosis is effective,[15–17] but tetracycline is contraindicated in pregnancy. Antepartum treatment with active

Agent	Pregnancy Category[a]
Atovaquone-proguanil	C
Artemisinin	N/A
Azithromycin	B
Aztreonam	B
Chloroquine	N/A (C?)
Chloramphenicol	N/A (C?)
Clarithromycin	C
Cefoperazone	B
Cefotaxime	B
Ceftriaxone	B
Cycloserine	N/A (C)
Clindamycin	B
Dapsone	C
Doxycycline	D
Erythromycin	B
Ethambutol	C
Ethionamide	C
Halofantrine	N/A
Isoniazid	C
Mefloquine	C
Pyrazinamide	C
Quinine	N/A
Rifabutin	B
Rifampicin	C
Rifapentine	C
Spiramycin	N/A
Streptomycin	D
Sulfadoxine	N/A

Table 141.1 Risk Categories of Selected Antimicrobial Agents in Pregnant Women

[a]See Table 141.2.
N/A, not available.

Table 141.2 US FDA Use-in-Pregnancy Ratings

Category	Interpretation	Comments
A	Controlled studies show no risk	No demonstration of risk to the fetus in any trimester
B	No evidence of risk in humans	The chance of fetal harm is remote, but remains a possibility
C	Risk cannot be ruled out	There is a chance of fetal harm, but the potential benefits may outweigh the potential risk
D	Positive evidence of risk	Fetal risk demonstrated; potential benefits may outweigh the risk
X	Contraindicated in pregnancy	Positive evidence of fetal abnormalities or risk that clearly outweighs any possible benefit

antibiotics prevents spontaneous abortion and current information seems enough to recommend treatment of all cases. During pregnancy, combination therapy with rifampin plus TMP-SMX provides the best therapeutic balance to cure the disease, prevent relapses, and protect the developing infant.

CHOLERA (See Chapter 20)

In endemic areas, but especially during epidemics and pandemics, adult individuals including pregnant women can and do acquire cholera.[18–20]

Among pregnant women, cholera is associated with diarrhea and dehydration of such severity that intrauterine suffering and death may occur. In 1892, 57% of pregnant women with cholera died and the abortion rate was estimated around 54%. Conversely, during a 1979–1980 cholera outbreak in Ile-Ife (Nigeria), where 61 pregnant patients were identified, cholera appeared to be less severe and to have a lower mortality in pregnant than in nonpregnant women.[19]

Cholera, a toxin-mediated disease without hematogenous spread or placental invasion, is not transmitted vertically, but intrafamilial transmission from adults with diarrhea is possible in the neonatal period. In Peru, among 626 children with cholera, isolation of *Vibrio cholerae* O1 was possible in 310 (49%), more commonly in children older than 24 months of age.

In a retrospective review of the records of 32 pregnant women treated for cholera of less than 24-hour duration, dehydration was moderate in 62.5% and severe in 37.5%.[21] Two fetal deaths occurred among the patients with severe dehydration, one on arrival and one within 8 hours of emergency room care. This series underscored the immediate favorable outcome for mother and fetus of prompt and vigorous hydration. This was accomplished initially intravenously and after 4 hours orally using the WHO oral rehydration solution (ORS). In another Peruvian series from a university hospital, of 8690 patients with cholera treated, 84 (0.96%) were pregnant women.[22] Eighty-one were treated using a standard rehydration protocol, 20 required hospitalization because of the clinical severity of dehydration, and 64 were treated and discharged from the emergency ward to complete treatment as outpatients. In this series, fetal deaths occurred in 7.7% of first trimester pregnancies, 6.9% in second trimester pregnancies, and 3.6% during the third trimester. Younger pregnant women (<20 years) were more frequently hospitalized (50%) than older mothers and had a higher rate of fetal death associated with the disease. Remarkably, there were no maternal deaths; three patients suffered transitory renal failure that recovered without dialysis.[22]

Treatment for pregnant patients with cholera consists of the rapid and adequate replacement of fluids, electrolytes, and base. There is conclusive evidence that solutions may be given orally and that the WHO ORS is safe and effective for pregnant women.

The rationale for the use of antibiotics for the treatment of cholera is that the duration and volume of fluid loss can be diminished and that clearance of *V. cholerae* from the stools can be hastened. Tetracycline, doxycycline, and quinolones have many more weaknesses than strengths in pregnancy and are not recommended. Ampicillin, TMP-SMX, and erythromycin are safer and can be substituted, provided susceptibility is assured.

Oral cholera vaccines have been available outside of the United States (see Chapter 20), but there are no data on the use of any cholera vaccine during pregnancy. Intrafamilial spread occurs but does not appear to play a major role in transmission to pregnant women.

DENGUE FEVER AND DENGUE HEMORRHAGIC FEVER (See Chapter 75)

Intrauterine transmission of dengue viruses appears to be confirmed by several case reports and small series, but the exact mechanisms of transmission and the fetal pathogenesis have not been elucidated.[23–27] No significant increase in prevalence or in severity of the disease has been noted associated with pregnancy. The review of many small studies of women with clinical diagnosis of dengue fever during pregnancy strongly suggests that the risks of premature birth and fetal death are increased as a consequence of the disease, as are the risks of thrombocytopenia and hemorrhage for both mother and newborn.[23,25,28–30]

Fever is the most common presenting symptom in the mother, and when it occurs near term, the likelihood of hemorrhage is higher.[23] Neonates appear healthy at birth but develop symptoms after 3–7 days.[31,32] They should be thoroughly observed for the development of a sepsis-like illness,[33] even if the mothers are clinically doing well. Maternal monitoring and treatment are as described for nonpregnant individuals. When cesarean section is indicated, platelet transfusions may be necessary.

VIRAL HEPATITIS (See Chapters 64-66)

Infection by the hepatotropic viruses designated A, B, C, D, E, and G constitutes the most common cause of jaundice during pregnancy.[34] Hepatitis A and B viruses are responsible for most of the cases in developing and developed countries, and documentation of infection is most common during the third trimester. The severity and prognosis of maternal acute hepatitis A, B, C, and D does not seem to be affected by pregnancy. Prematurity and perinatal death may be slightly increased, but no increase in congenital malformations, abortion, low birth weight (LBW), or intellectual disabilities has been noted. Maternal management is not altered in any major way by the coexistence of pregnancy.

Hepatitis A

In utero transmission of hepatitis A is not recognized, and transmission by fecal contamination during delivery is rare. Infection during pregnancy or delivery does not appear to result in increased complications in the mother or increased clinical disease in the newborn.[35] Acute hepatitis A in the pregnant woman requires supportive care and recovery is expected; fulminant hepatitis has been observed in less than 1% of the cases. For newborn infants of infected mothers, immunoglobulin (Ig) is given as prophylaxis in postexposure situations.[35] Pregnant women may wish to avoid travel to endemic areas, and when nonimmune to hepatitis A, can receive immunization or Ig prophylaxis when needed.

Hepatitis B

Hepatitis B infection is highly prevalent in the tropics, where large segments of the population are not exposed to universal vaccination programs. Areas such as sub-Saharan Africa, the Amazon basin, most Pacific islands and some Caribbean islands, parts of the Middle East, and China have the highest prevalence of hepatitis B virus (HBV) infection. High prevalence can be expected in these areas during reproductive years.

Acute hepatitis B occurs in approximately 1–2 per 1000 pregnancies,[34] and it does not seem to pose special risks to the mother when compared to background rates for the general population. However, perinatal exposure poses great risk for acquisition of HBV by the infants born to hepatitis B surface antigen (HBsAg)-seropositive mothers. The frequency of chronic hepatitis B in pregnancy is higher (approximately 5–15 per 1000) and also constitutes a risk for vertical transmission. Data from the Centers for Disease Control and Prevention (CDC) analyzed in 1996 estimated that 22 000 children are born to HBV-positive mothers every year in the United States alone. In highly endemic areas, the risk to the neonate to become perinatally infected and to develop chronic infection is very high.[36,37] Therefore, all pregnant women should be screened for HBsAg during prenatal visits. Transmission rates are higher if the mother is also hepatitis B e antigen (HBeAg)-positive.[35] Intrauterine infection occurs as evidenced by the fact that 2.5% of infants born to infected mothers have hepatitis B antigenemia during the neonatal period, but in most cases antigenemia appears later, suggesting transmission at delivery. Maternal blood, amniotic fluid, or feces may contain HBV, but cesarean section delivery and avoidance of breastfeeding do not prevent transmission. Most vertically infected infants carry HBsAg by 2–5 months of age, but in some detection may take longer. Up to 20% of infants born to HBsAg-positive mothers may become infected, and up to 90% of infants infected by their HBeAg-positive mothers may become chronically infected if untreated. Gestational age, birth weight, and viral subtype do not appear to predict the likelihood of the baby becoming a chronic carrier. Although HBsAg has been found in breast milk, breastfeeding does not appear to be a major risk factor for transmission. Most cases of HBV infection during pregnancy are asymptomatic, and when symptomatic the illness is similar to that of the general nonpregnant population. Fulminant hepatitis B[38] has been described at a rate of approximately 1%.

The diagnosis and management of hepatitis B during pregnancy is similar to that of nonpregnant patients. Hepatitis B vaccination is not contraindicated during pregnancy or lactation. Women of unknown HBsAg status who present in labor or after delivery should be considered potentially infected. Infants born to HBsAg-positive mothers or mothers with unknown HBsAg status must receive monovalent hepatitis B vaccine along with 0.5 mL of hepatitis B immunoglobulin (HBIg) at a different anatomical site within 12 hours of birth, and complete a total of four or five doses regardless of gestational age.[39] The series can be completed using combination vaccines. Adoptees should be tested for HBsAg. All children must be vaccinated. Postvaccination testing and revaccination are beyond the scope of this chapter but have been recently investigated.[40]

The management of hepatitis D coinfection during pregnancy does not differ from the management of hepatitis B. Perinatal transmission has been reported. Neonatal prophylaxis as described for HBV may prevent transmission of HDV.

Hepatitis C

A major problem worldwide, infection with the hepatitis C virus (HCV) has not been shown to affect fertility or increase rates of abortion, prematurity, LBW, or obstetric interventions compared to control subjects. There is, however, a risk of transmission from mother to infant of approximately 5%. Although the risk of perinatal transmission and the severity of the maternal disease must be considered, there is no contraindication for pregnancy in HCV-infected females. Vertical transmission *in utero* and during birth canal passage occurs, especially when high maternal viral loads are present[41] and when the expectant mother is an intravenous drug user and/or is coinfected with HIV.[42] Nonviremic mothers (gravidas) rarely transmit HCV, but viremia at delivery reaches 55–75% rates. Current treatment options for hepatitis C such as pegylated interferon plus ribavirin are not used during pregnancy because of the unknown efficacy for treatment and prevention, and the risk of potential side effects for mother and fetus. Delivery by cesarean section and avoidance of breastfeeding may decrease transmission, but data are inconclusive[43] and no formal evidence-based recommendation can be given at this time. Routine screening of all pregnant women is not recommended. Testing can be recommended for high-risk women and their offspring and for potential adoptees. Anti-HCV antibodies are usually present by age 1 year and the polymerase chain reaction (PCR) can detect HCV earlier.

Hepatitis E

There are data that suggest that infection with the hepatitis E virus (HEV), found most commonly in endemic areas of the Indian subcontinent, the Middle East, Southeast Asia, and Latin America, can be associated with higher mortality from fulminant disease during pregnancy,[44] especially when acute disease develops in the third trimester. Intrauterine death has been associated with severe disease and hypoglycemia. Perinatal transmission may occur more commonly than initially estimated[45] and may cause infant mortality as well. Immunoglobulin pooled from patients in endemic areas may prove beneficial.

Hepatitis G

In HIV-1-infected women, hepatitis G virus (HGV) coinfection is common,[46] and HGV can be transmitted sexually. Children born to HGV RNA-positive women coinfected with HIV are also likely to be HGV infected. Transmission appears to occur antenatally. Children remain infected and asymptomatic for long periods.

HUMAN IMMUNODEFICIENCY VIRUS AND ACQUIRED IMMUNODEFICIENCY SYNDROME (See Chapters 81 and 139)

Globally, women represent approximately 60% of the total population of human immunodeficiency virus (HIV)-infected individuals, and the more efficient heterosexual, male-to-female transmission constitutes their greatest exposure risk. Younger women have the highest risk of infection. In areas of sub-Saharan Africa, HIV infection rates in pregnant women may exceed a staggering 25%. The disparity in the delivery of interventions to halt the deleterious effects of HIV and acquired immunodeficiency syndrome (AIDS) between developed and developing countries is very large and growing.

HIV infection is transmitted from an infected mother to her fetus during pregnancy, during delivery, and by breastfeeding. The timing of infection has been estimated and is schematically represented and simplified in ***Table 141.3***. Determinants of transmission efficiency include social factors, concurrent sexually transmitted diseases (STDs), CD4 count and viral load, antiretroviral therapy (ART), as well as obstetric factors and feeding choices. Currently, with the vanishing exception of a few surviving children infected by blood products decades ago, virtually all HIV infections in children less than 13 years of age have been transmitted vertically from their infected mothers. In the United States alone, approximately 7000 HIV-positive women give birth each year. Worldwide, the number of HIV-infected mothers delivering infants is increasing dramatically, mainly in developing areas, while a major decrease has been noted in industrial countries.

Given no comorbidities, and accepting imperfections in the published studies, HIV infection appears to have little if any effect on pregnancy and pregnancy has little if any effect on HIV disease progression. Anemia, LBW, and prolonged labor are more frequently reported from areas where women have more advanced or untreated disease, malnutrition, and coinfections, but pregnancy does not adversely influence survival except in women with very advanced disease.[47,48]

Recurrent vaginal candidiasis is a common presenting complaint during pregnancy in HIV-infected women. With the exception of Kaposi's sarcoma, more common in men, the rates and patterns of symptoms, opportunistic infections, and malignancies are similar in nonpregnant and pregnant women. A somewhat greater predisposition to suffer esophageal candidiasis and bacterial pneumonia has been suggested in the literature. The diagnosis of HIV infection during pregnancy is made in the same manner as in nonpregnant females. Shortcomings of the use of enzyme-linked immunosorbent assay (ELISA) and Western blot tests in pregnant women must be kept in mind. Once diagnosed, a number of interventions to prevent or minimize mother-to-child transmission of HIV become vitally important. In the United States, aiming at the maintenance of the health of the patient and at interventions that sharply reduce vertical transmission, published guidelines recommend voluntary counseling and HIV testing to all pregnant women as early in pregnancy as possible.[49] Counseling must be based on testing that provides definitive information.

Table 141.3 Timing of HIV Transmission from Mother to Infant ($n = 100$)

Gestational Age (in Weeks)	Number Infected
≤14	1
14–36	4
36–labor	12
Intrapartum	8
Breastfeeding	Variable
Total developed countries	14–32%
Total developing countries	25–48%

(Modified from Kourtis AP, Bulterys M, Nesheim SR, et al. Understanding the timing of HIV infection from mother to infant. JAMA. 2001;285:709–712, and several other authors.)

In the developing world, in many areas of Africa, Asia, India, Latin America, and the Caribbean, very large numbers of pregnant women do not recognize the need for prenatal care, have difficulties accessing health facilities and personnel, and receive no or suboptimal diagnostic, prophylactic, and therapeutic interventions. This situation must change. Expert monitoring for health maintenance during pregnancy and for HIV-related issues must be assured. HIV-related monitoring must include timely testing, the prevention and treatment of opportunistic infections including tuberculosis, the use of pregnancy-specific individualized combination ART,[50] the timely election (or not) of the cesarean section, and discouraging (or not) of breastfeeding. These are all desirable, but not always or seldom possible in poor regions.

Current criteria for recommendation of combination ART in females in general apply to pregnant women. During pregnancy, individualization becomes more important and decisions about the initiation, continuation, and choice of treatment include fetal factors. Combination ART offers greater protection against perinatal transmission and should be considered even if the mother does not fulfill criteria for initiation of ART. Zidovudine (ZDV) should be included when possible. A single dose of nevirapine to mothers with HIV, when added to oral ZDV, has recently been proven highly efficacious in reducing vertical transmission of HIV,[51] but resistance mutations may appear in mother and baby.[52] In pregnant HIV-positive women, reverse transcription inhibitors (RTIs) may be responsible for more frequent and pronounced lactic acidosis and even hepatic steatosis. Protease inhibitors (PIs) may worsen insulin resistance and hyperglycemia. Hemolysis, elevated liver function tests, and low platelets, the so-called HELLP syndrome described in late pregnancy in otherwise healthy HIV-infected women, may also be more common with use of RTIs and PIs. Efavirenz is contraindicated in pregnancy because of simian embryopathy. Stavudine and dideoxyinosine (ddI) in combination with either PIs or nevirapine must be avoided or discontinued in pregnancy. An Antiretroviral Pregnancy Registry (www.apregistry.com) has been designed to better understand the strengths and weaknesses of the use of ART during pregnancy and may become an important international tool.

Elective cesarean section reduces the risk of perinatal transmission of HIV even in women who are taking antiretroviral drugs and even at low maternal viral loads,[53] but maternal morbidity is a consideration. With undetectable maternal viral loads, no evidence exists to guide a recommendation at this time.[54] Breastfeeding is discouraged in areas where infant formula is available, but extremely controversial in poor parts of the world where over 95% of HIV-infected women reside[55] who for social, economic, and other reasons will continue to lactate.

To control HIV infection and AIDS in women, pregnant women, and children, major global efforts will be required that close the growing standard of care gap between rich and poor and to ensure that the huge medical advances of the last decades reach as many people as possible.

HUMAN T-LYMPHOTROPIC VIRUS TYPE 1 (See Chapters 81 and 139)

Human T-lymphotropic virus type 1 (HTLV-1) infection, a frequently ignored but important disease, is hyperendemic in the south of Japan and endemic in Africa, the Caribbean, and Latin America. Based on small studies, the clinical course of pregnancy does not seem to be altered by the presence of infection by HTLV-1 and babies appear normal at birth. Vertical transmission does occur in 6–35% of newborns, usually postpartum via breast milk.[56] There is a threefold increased risk of transmission with breastfeeding for more than 6 months; from less than 10% to almost 35%. When breastfeeding was continued for more than one year, the proportion of infected children rose to almost 40% (E. Gotuzzo, unpublished data, 2005). Mothers with strongyloidiasis seem to transmit HTLV-1 with enhanced efficiency, in contrast to asymptomatic mothers or those suffering tropical spastic paraparesis. Intrauterine and intrapartum transmissions also occur, but together they account for approximately 5% of vertical transmission. Perinatally transmitted

HTLV-1 infection poses a risk for the development of adult T-cell leukemia/lymphoma.[57]

Routine combination HTLV-1/2 antibody testing of blood products is a strategy implemented in the United States since 1997, and in countries where the prevalence of infection in pregnant women exceeds 2–4%, screening of all pregnant mothers and formula feeding of infants of infected mothers is a logical strategy that is in use in Japan.[58] It may reduce childhood infection rates by nearly 90% and is a strategy that requires further study in less developed tropical countries. There is no therapy or vaccine available.

LEPTOSPIROSIS (See Chapter 45)

Leptospira survives well in tropical nonsaline waters and leptospirosis is common in several tropical settings.[59,60] In certain endemic areas, up to 5–10% of patients who present to academic or research institutions may have leptospirosis. Data about leptospirosis occurring during gestation are scarce and come from small case series and reviews, case reports, and anecdotal information.[61–66] Little is known about the mutual effects of pregnancy and leptospirosis when they coincide in the same woman. Transplacental transmission is thought to occur and leptospirae have been found in infected organs of mother and fetus. In a series of 11 cases diagnosed by culture or serology in French Guyana, fetal death occurred in over 50% of the cases.[65] In another report of 1 case from Israel and a review of 15 previous cases, 8 pregnancies terminated in abortions, 4 newborns had neonatal leptospirosis, and 4 were uninfected and appeared normal at birth.[62] Stillbirth is recognized as a consequence of infection.[67] During the early months of pregnancy, leptospirosis is more likely to result in spontaneous abortion, and during the last trimesters, more premature deliveries and neonatal disease result. Leptospirosis may present with jaundice and pulmonary abnormalities in a higher percentage of pregnant than nonpregnant women but these observations have not been confirmed.[61] Although mortality occurs,[68] overall maternal mortality seems not affected compared to the background of nonpregnant women. Early diagnosis and antibiotic treatment of leptospirosis during pregnancy is essential. High-dose penicillin or ceftriaxone is associated with faster maternal recovery and improved fetal prognosis. Doxycycline is contraindicated during pregnancy. The Jarisch–Herxheimer reaction occurs rarely.[69]

LISTERIOSIS

Pregnancy is a risk factor for infection with *Listeria monocytogenes*.[70] Listeriosis among pregnant patients mainly affects women who have no comorbidities; cell-mediated immunity depression attributed to pregnancy itself has been cited as a predisposing factor. The incidence of listeriosis is estimated to increase from approximately 0.7 per 100 000 in the general population to approximately 12 per 100 000 in pregnant women, and intrauterine infection has been clearly associated with placental colonization, chorioamnionitis, spontaneous abortion, stillbirth, preterm labor, prematurity, and neonatal infection (including granulomatosis infantisepticum) and significant mortality.[70,71] In humans, there are no convincing data to link the past history of listeriosis with repeated spontaneous abortions. An increasing rate of listeriosis has been reported in Europe.[72]

Maternal infection, which can occur at any gestational age, presents clinically as a mild to moderate febrile illness, but a flulike syndrome is also a common presentation.[70] Maternal infection can occasionally be severe and meningitis and heart block[73] have been reported. A high index of suspicion is essential to obtain specimens for microbiological confirmation of diagnosis. Specimens that are useful for culture of the organisms include maternal blood, placenta, amniotic fluid, cervical secretions, stool, and urine. Blood cultures should be performed to evaluate fever and/or flulike symptoms in pregnant women because they can detect the organism in some 35% of the cases. Gram stains of the placenta, as well as frozen sections when available, can produce a rapid presumptive diagnosis.

Early gestational listeriosis may result in bacteremia and seeding of the uterine contents. Fetal prognosis, worse in early pregnancy, is guarded throughout. Treatment of the disease at early stages is associated with better pregnancy outcomes. Approximately 20% of pregnancies complicated with listeriosis result in fetal death, and approximately two-thirds of the surviving infants develop neonatal disease. Early-onset neonatal listeriosis (<5 days) is predominantly septic and with correct treatment carries a high (approximately 30%) mortality rate; late onset (>5 days) is predominantly meningitic and mortality is lower (approximately 10%) with therapy.[74] A common differential diagnosis is with group B streptococcal sepsis. Disseminated neonatal disease is extremely serious and, if associated with prematurity, has a mortality rate that may approach 90%. Neurologic sequelae have been reported in survivors of neonatal disease. Furthermore, even neonates who do not develop clinically apparent listeriosis but who are born to mothers who suffered listeriosis during their pregnancy may have prolonged hospital stays.

During pregnancy, high-dose ampicillin, considered superior to penicillin for this indication, is felt to be the treatment of choice; adding gentamicin is synergistic and its use must be evaluated in special situations in light of the potential side effects to the fetus. Cephalosporins and clindamycin are not effective. No risk-free alternative exists during pregnancy and when penicillin hypersensitivity is suspected or reported, allergy testing and/or desensitization should be considered. TMP-SMX, active against listeriosis but avoided during pregnancy, may – as is the case with brucellosis – offer benefits that exceed risks in certain cases. Prevention of listeriosis during pregnancy relies on the same principles that prevent listeriosis in general. They should be stressed as most important for women of reproductive capacity and risk factors during pregnancy.[75]

MALARIA (See Chapter 96)

Malaria, the most significant parasitic disease worldwide, remains a major cause of maternal morbidity and mortality.[76] Globally, the pathological effects of infection during gestation and the negative implications for fetal development and survival are underscored by the fact that about 40% of the world's pregnant women (approximately 1 billion) are exposed to the risks of malaria while pregnant. LBW, a common consequence of gestational malaria, is an important risk factor for infant and childhood mortality.[77] In Africa alone, malaria-induced LBW may kill nearly 400 000 infants each year. Recent studies have demonstrated that the frequency and severity of placental malaria and consequential newborn disease and LBW are greater in pregnant women with concomitant HIV infection.

The negative impact of plasmodial infection during pregnancy varies predictably according to maternal immunity, a consequence of the intensity of transmission, and the parasite species. In areas of unstable transmission, where malaria is uncommon except during epidemics and immunity is rare, pregnant women suffer high-level parasitemia with more severe, acute complications including anemia, hypoglycemia, pulmonary edema, the acute respiratory distress syndrome, cerebral malaria, and death. Fetal distress, premature labor, stillbirth, or LBW result.[78] Fetal and perinatal losses have been estimated to be as high as 60–70% in nonimmune pregnant woman. This situation is similar in pregnant women from nonendemic areas or travelers to malarious zones. In contrast, adults who are long-term residents of areas of moderate or high malaria transmission exhibit high-level immunity and infection is usually asymptomatic or mild. But during gestation, this immunity is altered. Infection is still frequently oligo- or asymptomatic and severe disease is uncommon,[78] but it is associated with accumulation of parasitized erythrocytes in the placental microcirculation. In these areas, up to three doses of presumptive intermittent treatment during the duration of gestation has been shown to decrease the risk of severe maternal anemia. Sequestration of *Plasmodium falciparum*-infected red blood cells in the placenta is due to parasite adhesion molecules expressed on the surface of erythrocytes binding to host receptors such as chondroitin sulfate A (CSA). Parasite ligands also mediate placental adhesion. Thus, by invading the placenta,[79] malaria parasites cause more severe maternal anemia and LBW babies. These complications tend to be more common in primi- and secundigravida women with *P. falciparum* infection (weight reduction, approximately 170 g) and in multigravida women with *P. vivax* infection (weight reduction, approximately 100 g). Placental histology is a good indicator of malaria infection at delivery.[80]

Congenital malaria is acquired from the infected, usually nonimmune mother pre- or perinatally in less than 5% of newborns. The transmission efficacy and the clinical severity are functions of the parasite species (more commonly observed with *P. vivax* and *P. malariae* but possible with all human plasmodia) and their density in maternal blood and placenta. In fact, placental malaria is significantly associated with stillbirth regardless of parity. A serious problem in tropical areas, it is rarely reported in the United States. Congenital infection is an important cause of intrauterine growth retardation, premature birth, abortion, miscarriage, stillbirth, and neonatal and infant death. The clinical manifestations can be apparent from the first day after birth to about 1 month later (commonly 10–30 days). They include fever, restlessness, pallor, obtundation, poor feeding, diarrhea, and vomiting. Signs include jaundice, cyanosis, and hepatosplenomegaly. Hypoglycemia is associated with increased mortality and neurologic sequelae.

The clinical features of malaria in obstetric patients, including laboratory and image findings, can be quantitatively more severe and qualitatively unique, but are essentially the same as described in detail for nonpregnant individuals.[81] Features indicating a poor prognosis must always be investigated. Special attention to physical examination, including level of consciousness, blood pressure, urine output, hemoglobinuria, hemoglobin and hematocrit, leukocytes, coagulation tests, arterial blood gases and blood glucose and lactate levels, creatinine, aminotransferases, bilirubin, muscle enzymes, and urate levels as well as chest radiography, is warranted. In serious cases, this is best done in intensive care unit (ICU) settings until clinical stability/improvement. An HIV test is commonly indicated.

Early diagnosis of malaria in pregnancy is extremely important because successful specific treatment can impact mother and child. The diagnosis rests, as in nonpregnant individuals, on the demonstration of asexual plasmodial forms in thick and thin stained smears of peripheral blood. Fluorescence microscopy, rapid detection tests, and PCR are described in Chapter 96. Parasitemias can be very high. Serology has mainly epidemiological uses.

Malaria during pregnancy must be treated with antiparasitic agents, but optimal therapy is difficult to select because there are no reliable clinical data for most oral or parenteral antimalarial drugs to be declared safe for use in pregnant women. The agent or agents of choice and the route of administration also depend on the suspected or demonstrated infecting species and the likelihood of drug resistance. The geographic distribution of drug-resistant malaria parasites can be found elsewhere in this book. Antimalarials with special importance during pregnancy are briefly described here and their administration schedules are found in Chapter 96; drug doses may need to be altered depending on the stage of pregnancy. In pregnancy, the persistence of *P. falciparum* in the placenta after apparently effective treatment has been described.[82]

Chloroquine is generally well tolerated and considered safe in pregnancy[83] and continues to be the drug of choice for all *P. ovale* and *P. malariae* infections and for susceptible *P. falciparum* and *P. vivax* infections.

With the exception of the possibility of stillbirth and LBW, mefloquine, used for treatment and prophylaxis, appears safer for the fetus during any trimester of pregnancy than many other drugs and has been used extensively.[84] In the expectant mother, the drug may produce neuropsychiatric side effects and possibly cardiotoxicity. Combination with halofantrine, not available in the United States, produces prolongation of QTc interval. Tetracyclines and doxycycline are contraindicated during pregnancy; clindamycin (see later discussion) is an alternative. Dapsone in combination with other drugs might provide an alternative to treatment of resistant *P. falciparum* malaria, as suggested by a recent review of 924 pregnancies,[85] but there is no information on hemolytic effects to mother or fetus with or without glucose-6-phosphate dehydrogenase (G6PD) deficiency.

The combination of atovaquone (250 mg) and proguanil (100 mg) is highly effective against chloroquine- and mefloquine-resistant *P. falciparum* malaria, but data in pregnancy are scarce. Combined with artesunate, the combination has been useful and well tolerated in Thailand[86] as rescue treatment of multidrug-resistant *P. falciparum* malaria in pregnant women without recorded maternal or fetal toxicity.

Quinine and quinidine have been given in therapeutic doses to pregnant women throughout gestation;[83] continuous monitoring of vital signs, blood glucose, and electrocardiogram are recommended. Quinine is preferred but availability accounts for greater use of quinidine in North America. Quinine at the intravenous doses used to treat malaria does not induce oxytocic effects. There are concerns about maternal cardiac side effects and tolerance, especially gastrointestinal.

Pyrimethamine-sulfadoxine and clindamycin have also been used in pregnancy with consistent good results; fears of development of kernicterus with the former and colitis with the latter have not materialized. Lower plasma concentrations of both pyrimethamine and sulfadoxine may decrease efficacy.[87] Another problem is the emergence of resistance to drugs used for intermittent preventive treatment of malaria in pregnancy (IPTp).[88] Clindamycin has been used routinely in combination with quinine to treat pregnant patients with multidrug-resistant *P. falciparum* in Brazil for two decades; other than vomiting, no significant side effects have been observed in mothers or fetuses. Quinine should not be used alone because of its slow antimalarial activity.

Artemisinin-derived antimalarials and combinations have considerably faster parasitic clearance rates and shorter half-lives and may be as effective as quinine in treating severe malaria. They can be used orally, intravenously, and rectally. Small studies suggest good tolerance during pregnancy and no evidence of adverse fetal effects.[86] Birth outcomes are similar to community rates for abortion, stillbirth, and congenital anomalies or mean gestation age at delivery. There is a risk of potential teratogenicity if used in the first trimester. Artemether-lumefantrine is now widely used, but altered pharmacokinetics during pregnancy may contribute to high failure rates especially in late pregnancy.[89] A revised dosage in this situation is needed.

The use of intravenous antimalarials in combination with exchange transfusions with careful monitoring should be considered in selected cases of severe complicated malaria in pregnant women.

We recommend hospitalization for pregnant women with suspected malaria at lower levels of severity than for nonpregnant counterparts. This is true for ward and ICU admission. When *P. falciparum* is suspected or demonstrated, or when disease is moderate to severe, hospitalization is always strongly recommended. *P. falciparum* treatment is administered when the organism is demonstrated or suspected (even if not demonstrated) for all infections where one suspects infection with more than one organism, and for severely ill patients.

Chloroquine alone, or with proguanil, remains the preferred drug for chemoprophylaxis for pregnant women in malarial areas where it is still effective. In chloroquine-resistant areas, mefloquine may be used instead. Doxycycline, atovaquone-proguanil, and primaquine are not used for prophylaxis. IPTp with pyrimethamine-sulfadoxine in areas of parasite susceptibility is a common option, but adherence has been poor in some areas.[90] Recently, the use of a double dose was associated with a decrease of maternal parasitemia and newborns with malaria, among nulliparous and primiparous pregnant women in Mozambique. The safety of other prophylactic agents has not been established. Pregnant women from nonmalarial areas should not visit malarial zones, but when unavoidable, antivector strategies cannot be overemphasized.

Women become resistant to pregnancy-associated malaria over successive pregnancies as they acquire antibodies that recognize placental parasites, suggesting that protection by a vaccine during pregnancy is feasible. Insecticide-treated mosquito nets are effective prevention, and systems that facilitate delivery may contribute to household ownership and use.[91]

TETANUS (See Chapter 42)

Maternal tetanus is an extremely serious disease with high morbidity and mortality. It is not communicable, but may be acquired by ways unrelated to pregnancy, such as dirty wounds, or pregnancy-related, such as contaminated delivery or abortion. Tetanus neonatorum, the most common form of tetanus in developing tropical countries, is caused by contamination of the umbilical stump with spores, typically from application of animal dung to the umbilical stump. Virtually all affected are not properly immunized. Symptoms develop after 3–14 days. Even with specific treatment, maternal and neonatal tetanus have high mortality rates.

The clinical picture in mother and infant is secondary to the potent tetanospasmin exotoxin produced during anaerobic growth of *Clostridium tetani* at the site of injury and has been described elsewhere. The diagnosis is clinical, and aggressive treatment, performed in intensive care settings, includes life-sustaining methods, sedation, passive and active immunization, and antibiotics. Tetanus is preventable with the use of one of the safest available immunization products. Immunization of the susceptible pregnant woman should be routine[92,93] and include at least two doses of tetanus toxoid, 4–8 weeks apart, at least 2 weeks before delivery. In pregnancy, Td or Tdap are given in the second and third trimesters and Tdap immediately postpartum. A booster is indicated for pregnant women immunized more than 10 years previously. Partially immunized women should complete a three-dose series. Clean practices for caring for the umbilical stump are clearly to be enforced.

TOXOPLASMOSIS (See Chapter 103)

The incidence of toxoplasmosis during pregnancy is estimated to be similar to that of nonpregnant women of the same age group, and most infections are asymptomatic. In women who are pregnant or of childbearing age, prevalence is high in Latin America, some areas of Eastern and Central Europe including France, the Middle East and parts of Southeast Asia and Africa.[94] A minority of infected patients, calculated at around 20%, develop clinical signs and symptoms of a usually self-limited and rarely prolonged disease.[95] The diagnosis may be made at consultation with symptoms or when specific serological tests are performed after conception.

When infection by *Toxoplasma gondii* is acquired by a woman near the time of conception or during gestation,[96] the organism may be transmitted to the fetus through the placenta. This happens in about one-third of the cases. The incidence of congenital toxoplasmosis in the United States is estimated as 1/1000 to 1/8000 live births or 400–4000 infants per year.

The parasite reaches the placenta after hematogenous spread of tachyzoites released from ingested cysts or oocysts after release of bradyzoites or sporozoites that have invaded the maternal intestinal epithelium. In placental tissue, tachyzoites (demonstrated by Wright, Giemsa, and immunoperoxidase) replicate and cause tissue damage evidenced by chronic inflammation and cysts. From the placenta, hematogenous spread and establishment of a persistent infection with potential for lifelong reactivation and further disease occurs in the fetus.

Before conception, the likelihood of vertical transmission increases from about 6 months to the establishment of pregnancy. Once established, the age of gestation at the time of infection is a critical factor in transmission and fetal outcome. Infections occurring during the first trimester have the lowest vertical transmission (approximately 15%), but the resulting neonatal disease is more severe. The presence of HLA-DQ3 can worsen the prognosis of the fetus when infected in this period. During the third trimester, transmission is greatest (approximately 65%), but clinically apparent neonatal disease is less common or severe. The differences may be explained by placental or immunologic factors.

In severe prenatal infections, intrauterine fetal death may be the consequence of fetal multiorgan failure secondary to parasitic invasion. Acute congenital toxoplasmosis is characterized by intrauterine growth retardation and prematurity, anemia thrombocytopenia and jaundice, hepatosplenomegaly, hydrocephalus, microcephaly, and intracranial calcifications. Surviving congenitally infected babies, including untreated asymptomatic neonates, most often exhibit neurologic sequelae such as chorioretinitis (and visual impairment), seizures, and learning disabilities later in childhood and by adolescence.[95,97–99] Clinical manifestations are often similar in monozygotic twins and different in dizygotic twins. In the latter instance, diagnosis of severe toxoplasmosis in one twin can suggest subclinical disease in the other. Early and appropriate treatment may allow for clinical cure and normal development and is of critical importance.

When clinical manifestations of toxoplasmosis in the pregnant woman become apparent, they do not differ from those described for immunocompetent nonpregnant individuals. Single or multiple, usually nontender cervical lymphadenopathy[100]; nonspecific flulike symptoms such as headache, malaise, fatigue, fever, sore throat, abdominal discomfort, and pain, a maculopapular rash, and meningoencephalitis have been well described. More rarely, lung, pericardium and myocardium, brain, and striated muscles can be affected.

The efficient diagnosis of toxoplasmosis during pregnancy can be extremely challenging. In practice, serologic tests are the most commonly used, but they require experience to be interpreted correctly.[95] Newer tests have become available[101] but their role in the diagnosis of toxoplasmosis in pregnancy has not been fully established. Acute *Toxoplasma* infection can be diagnosed by the isolation of the parasite in blood or body fluid cultures from the mother and any fluid or tissue from the fetus or neonate. Immediate intraperitoneal inoculation of processed blood, body fluids, or tissues into mice, and periodic examination of mouse peritoneal fluid looking for tachyzoites, takes several days; examination of surviving inoculated mice with detectable antibody for brain cysts takes about 6 weeks. Reinoculation of mouse tissues into other mice is even more cumbersome and time-consuming. Thus, cultures are difficult and expensive and, in pregnancy, may not provide a useful window of diagnostic opportunity.

In a pregnant woman with lymphadenopathy, characteristic histological features can support a clinical diagnosis of acute toxoplasmosis.[100] Histologic and histochemical examination of biopsy specimens, bone marrow aspirates, cerebrospinal fluid (CSF), amniotic fluid, and other specimens is rarely performed during pregnancy but can demonstrate tachyzoites. More than one staining method (including immunoperoxidase) is necessary. In the mother, tissue cysts are diagnostic, but the duration of infection cannot be ascertained. Cysts in the placenta or fetal/newborn tissues represent congenital infection.

In broad terms, recent *Toxoplasma* infection can be diagnosed by the presence of *Toxoplasma*-specific IgM antibody, by the simultaneous presence of specific IgM and IgG antibodies, or by demonstration of seroconversion of repeated IgG antibody titers. The presence of IgA antibodies suggests recent infection. A wide range of serologic tests is available commercially, and experience with their utilization varies among laboratories and societies. Systematic serologic screening of all women preconception, during pregnancy, and intrapartum is strongly advised, but in tropical countries this is seldom performed.

IgM-based diagnosis is based on the rapid – few days – rise and fall – weeks to months – of antibodies. It includes the utilization of the IgM indirect fluorescent antibody (IgM-IFA) test, the double-sandwich ELISA, and the immunosorbent agglutination assay (ISAGA). All tests are sensitive and specific. The ELISA is more sensitive and specific than the IgM-IFA test, circumvents the false positive results from rheumatoid factor in the mother and the false negative results from transferred maternal IgG in the newborn, and has been used to detect infection in pregnant women. The ISAGA also avoids false positive results from the presence of rheumatoid factor and antinuclear antibodies. ISAGA IgM is detected earlier, with higher sensitivity, and for a longer time than with the ELISA test. An IgA ELISA is even more sensitive for detection of acute infection in some pregnant women and congenital infection in newborns, but may remain elevated for months to years. A simple, accurate, and inexpensive French agglutination test is available in Europe. Avidity assays[102] are helpful in immunocompetent women. Chemiluminescence screening is fast and commercially available but less sensitive than conventional serology.[103]

IgG titers can be detected in low levels as early as 1–2 weeks after infection, peak with high titers (≥1 : 1000) after 6–8 weeks, and decline to a new individual low level (1 : 4–1 : 64) to persist for life. The Sabin–Feldman dye test, the IgG-IFA, and the ELISA are sensitive and specific and have been in sustained clinical use.

Other serology-based diagnostics include the differential agglutination (HS/SC) test, which may be especially useful to exclude remote infection in pregnant women, the avidity test, and the indirect hemagglutination test (IHA). The IHA should not be relied upon for diagnosis of acute infection during pregnancy because it may remain negative for a prolonged period after infection.

During the acute phase of toxoplasmosis during pregnancy, antigen present in serum samples can be detected by PCR. PCR performed in amniotic fluid is the diagnostic test of choice for congenital fetal infection.[104,105] Timing at 18 weeks of pregnancy is preferred because of optimal sensitivity. A reference laboratory should confirm the diagnosis of acute toxoplasmosis during pregnancy.

Ultrasonography is also useful for fetal diagnosis. Combined with amniocentesis for PCR, a sensitivity of 97% and specificity of 100% for fetal infection is reached.

Appropriate treatment of a woman who acquires *Toxoplasma* infection during pregnancy[96] has been shown to reduce placental invasion and prevent congenital infection of the fetus carried in that pregnancy. Spiramycin (1 g taken every 8 hours by mouth on an empty stomach) is started as soon as possible[99] to prevent fetal infection, because it decreases vertical transmission (from approximately 60% to approximately 20%). When fetal infection seems highly probable or severe and when diagnosis of fetal infection is certain, combination therapy with pyrimethamine (50 mg by mouth once daily) and sulfadoxine (2 g by mouth twice daily) is given with folinic acid (10 mg by mouth once daily). During the first trimester, when pyrimethamine can be teratogenic, spiramycin is substituted and no folinic acid is needed.

No treatment is needed in subsequent pregnancies or for infections acquired over 6 months before any conception provides maternal immunocompetence, but previously infected immunosuppressed women should be given spiramycin for the duration of each pregnancy. In pregnant HIV-infected women, as a reasonable, albeit theoretical approach, spiramycin can be used for the first 17 weeks of gestation followed by pyrimethamine (at a higher dose of 75 mg by mouth once daily), sulfadoxine, and folinic acid until delivery. Clindamycin (1.2 g intravenously every 6 hours) can be used instead of sulfadoxine.

There is no *Toxoplasma* vaccine. Women who do not exhibit specific antibodies against *T. gondii* must be counseled. Avoiding raw meats and contact with cat excreta have proven preventive efficacy. All women not previously tested should have serologic screening at the first prenatal visit and during delivery.

TUBERCULOSIS AND MULTIDRUG-RESISTANT TUBERCULOSIS (See Chapter 35)

The increasing burden of tuberculosis (TB) during pregnancy affects the health of large numbers of mothers and infants.[106] Diagnostic, therapeutic, and prophylactic constraints during gestation include the dangers of X-rays and the intrinsic difficulties in testing anti-TB drugs.

Untreated pulmonary and particularly extrapulmonary TB (other than lymphadenitis) in pregnant women increase the risk for prematurity, fetal growth retardation, LBW, and perinatal mortality.[107,108] The most common mechanism of infection in the newborn is airborne transmission from an adult with pulmonary TB. Congenital TB is rare. It is more likely to be transmitted vertically after primary infection than after reactivation of previous infection. It may occur from a placental lesion through the umbilical vein, from which bacilli reach the fetal liver where a primary focus may be established for hematogenous spread to several organs. In the lungs, oxygenation and pulmonary circulation after birth increase and activate dormant bacilli. A less frequent mechanism is aspiration of infected amniotic fluid. Newborns show signs of TB after the second postnatal week; these are nonspecific and resemble other forms of neonatal sepsis. Fever, respiratory distress, irritability, ear discharge, abdominal symptoms, pulmonary infiltrates, and hilar or generalized lymphadenopathy are common. Up to 50% of infants develop meningitis. Frequently, the mother's disease is discovered as a consequence of the diagnosis in the newborn. The infant's purified protein derivative (PPD) becomes positive after 1–3 months. *M. tuberculosis* can be isolated from middle ear drainage, bone marrow, tracheal aspirate, and liver biopsy, rarely from CSF. Mortality is higher with delayed diagnosis.

Because untreated TB is harmful to both the mother and the fetus, because it represents a great danger to the infant after delivery, and because the disease can be transmitted to others, TB in pregnant women always should be treated without delay. Consensus treatment guidelines have been produced by the American Thoracic Society (ATS), the Infectious Diseases Society of America (IDSA), the CDC,[109] WHO,[110] and the International Union against Tuberculosis and Lung Diseases (IUATLD).[111] The following discussion on anti-TB drug use by pregnant women will closely follow the guidelines. Dosages are individualized during pregnancy and a general discussion can be found in Chapter 35.

The initial regimen, provided no multidrug resistance (MDR) is suspected, consists of isoniazid (INH), rifampin (RIF), and ethambutol (EMB) for a minimum duration of 9 months and with pyridoxine. INH, RIF, and EMB cross the placental barrier but have elicited no teratogenicity.[112] Streptomycin should not be substituted for EMB because it interferes with the development of the ear and hearing loss or vestibular defects may affect the developing fetus (approximately 1–3 per 6 live births) at any period throughout gestation.[113] Presumably, other aminoglycosides such as kanamycin, amikacin, and capreomycin share the ototoxicity potential. The safety of pyrazinamide in pregnancy has not been established and the drug is not recommended for routine use in the United States. Pyrazinamide is listed among the recommendations of the WHO[110] and the IUATLD[111] and has been used without reported adverse events by some public health jurisdictions in the United States. Para-aminosalicylic acid (PAS) was frequently used in combination with INH; no indication of teratogenicity was encountered in children of women who used them during pregnancy. The safety of cycloserine and ethionamide is untested; one report suggested human teratogenicity from ethionamide,[114] a drug that causes birth defects and spontaneous abortion when used in high doses in animals. The fluoroquinolones are avoided in pregnancy because of animal teratogenicity, but may need to be used during pregnancy for treatment of MDR TB infections unresponsive to other drugs.[112] Levofloxacin has been used more often than moxifloxacin for treatment of adults and children, and switching from levofloxacin to moxifloxacin, which may be more active against *M. tuberculosis*, after delivery seems an appropriate option. When anti-TB drugs are to be used during pregnancy, the expectant mother should be counseled concerning the known and unknown risks to the developing fetus of all treatment offered.

High-risk or symptomatic pregnant mothers should be tested with a tuberculin skin test. The PPD or "Mantoux" (5TU) tuberculin test is the most specific and sensitive standardized screening skin test for TB and is preferred. Pregnancy does not measurably affect the response of PPD and there has been no observed evidence of adverse events on women or their children from skin testing. All pregnant women not known previously to be skin reactors and many women of reproductive capacity and high risk (symptomatic, exposed, HIV, diabetes, high prevalence, caretaker, etc.) should ideally be tested.[115] Subsequent investigation of skin reactors facilitates the identification of infected individuals and the treatment of tuberculosis.

Although INH is not teratogenic, the treatment of latent TB infection (LTBI) is often deferred until after delivery, when there may be an increased risk of disease, because of concerns of isoniazid-associated hepatitis, which could be more frequent and/or severe during pregnancy. There might be an exception for pregnant women who have been infected recently; INH in that situation could be started after the first trimester.

Mothers with LTBI do not need to be separated from their infants after delivery and the child needs no special evaluation or treatment provided he or she remains asymptomatic. No treatment is recommended for women with inactive TB if they received adequate treatment in the past.

The diagnosis of maternal TB at delivery requires rapid and thorough evaluation of mother and child. If chest radiography and positive sputum smear confirm the diagnosis, additional steps, such as INH, skin testing follow-up, and rarely separation from the mother are necessary to protect the infant. An HIV test is also indicated.[116]

Because the concentrations of first-line antituberculosis drugs in human breast milk are low, breastfeeding should not be discouraged in nursing mothers treated with them.[117] The risk of toxicity can be minimized if the mother takes her medication after breastfeeding and substitutes saved milk or a bottle for the next feeding. The small concentrations that a baby receives during feeding are not effective as treatment for LTBI or active infection.

TYPHOID FEVER (See Chapter 16)

Studies from the early 1900s, when typhoid fever (TF) was extremely prevalent around the world, suggested an increased severity of TF when it affected pregnant women. In the preantibiotic era, two-thirds of pregnancies complicated by TF resulted in abortion.[118] In one series from the Philippines,[119] mortality rates were 32% and 25% as infection occurred while pregnancy progressed from the first to the third trimester, compared to an accepted general mortality rate of less than 15–20% for the general untreated population. Additionally, fetal prognosis was found to be quite poor, with rates around 60% for fetal demise and 35% for premature labor. Since then, small series, literature reviews, and case reports have produced contradictory reports of more severe versus equally severe clinical manifestations of TF in pregnant women when compared to nonpregnant females. Some of the largest case series of 100 cases from Chile,[120] 81 cases from Mexico,[121] and 129 cases from Peru,[122] though incomplete, are consistent with the notion of increased severity of TF during pregnancy and unequivocal in showing improvement of maternal and fetal prognosis with early antibiotic treatment. They also underscore the continuous presence in tropical and subtropical areas of a disease that has been all but eradicated in societies that have achieved adequate sanitation.

Salmonella enterica serovar Typhi causes sepsis of intestinal origin and colonization of reticuloendothelial tissues such as liver, spleen, lymph nodes, and bone marrow and crosses the placental barrier causing chorioamnionitis and villitis. In autopsy specimens, microscopy has revealed numerous colonies of Gram-negative bacilli within the fibrin between the placental villi. Vertical transmission can also occur in late pregnancy and the perinatal period. Interestingly, cases of chorioamnionitis and transplacental and perinatal infection of a fetus by nontyphoidal *Salmonella* strains have also been described. The neonatal disease begins after an asymptomatic period of 1–3 days after birth. Vomiting, diarrhea, abdominal distension, and fever are common. Seizures may occur. Anorexia and weight loss, hepatomegaly, and jaundice may be severe. Prompt treatment is effective. Maternal long-term asymptomatic carriers may pose a risk for disease in the newborn, and elimination of such state with treatment (15 of 99 in a Japanese study) may prevent infection in the newborn, but no controlled studies exist. The treatment of the carrier state in pregnancy is not known.

In the mother, prolonged fever and gastrointestinal or abdominal symptoms, at times following a nonspecific flulike prodrome, is characteristic but nonspecific for pregnancy. Rose spots, hepatosplenomegaly, and relative bradycardia are very useful when present. Gastrointestinal perforation and hemorrhage are late complications that acutely risk the lives of mother and fetus. Sustained bacteremia without endocarditis is a characteristic of typhoid fever that has three major deleterious consequences: (1) a severe activation and hyperplasia of reticuloendothelial organs, typically the intestinal and mesenteric lymph nodes, the liver, and the spleen; (2) metastatic seeding; and (3) immune complex disease. All have been described in pregnant women. Relapses and long-term carriers have also been seen in pregnancy.

Salmonella Typhi can be found in breast milk (5 of 26 in Chile and 3 of 23 in Peru), but treatment with amoxicillin has been effective in eradicating the organism in 1–3 days. Other drugs have no proof of efficacy and resistance makes this information difficult to interpret.

Whether or not TF is more severe during pregnancy, the disease must be treated to avoid morbidity and mortality in mother and fetus and to decrease transmission.[120–122] Currently, due to the appearance of resistance,[123–125] two drugs, ciprofloxacin and ceftriaxone,[126] are considered first-line and one, azithromycin, is considered alternative. Ciprofloxacin use in pregnancy is controversial and at present not advisable, particularly if there are alternatives, but ceftriaxone has demonstrated safety and efficacy in a series of 25 pregnant patients from French Guiana.[127] Provided susceptibility is assured and in spite of cost considerations, it is the drug of choice during all trimesters. Cefotaxime and cefoperazone are reasonable alternatives, but first- and second-generation cephalosporins, aminoglycosides, and aztreonam are not. Azithromycin use in pregnancy is permitted, but efficacy for treatment of TF is unknown.

Chloramphenicol is not recommended in pregnancy because of *Salmonella* resistance, the fetal risk of gray syndrome, and potential bone marrow toxicity for mother and fetus. Nevertheless, the emergence of quinolone and ceftriaxone resistance,[125] the possible reemergence of susceptibility to chloramphenicol, and the absence of hematologic side effects or gray syndrome in some series, suggest a need to reevaluate the issue.

No trials of corticosteroids in pregnancy have been performed, but their use may be justified in severe cases.

There are no data reported on the use of typhoid vaccines among pregnant women. The CDC advises to avoid vaccinating during pregnancy, but vaccination should be considered in some women (e.g., those allergic to cephalosporins traveling to an endemic area) if actual risk of disease and probable benefits of effective nonlive vaccine (such as the Vi vaccine) outweigh theoretical risks (especially the effect of live bacteria) to the fetus.

Screening with stool cultures of pregnant women seems unjustified in areas of low prevalence. In a large UK study of 30471 mothers over 9 years, only 60 (0.2%) yielded *Salmonella*[128] and 43 (72%) were asymptomatic. Seven of the 60 neonates (12%) excreted *Salmonella* with similar characteristics as their mothers, but no individual suffered invasive disease. However, in other areas like Tuscany (where 7431 pregnant women were studied), stool cultures may be cost effective in late summer and fall.[129] In developing tropical countries, the question is unanswered. The reader is referred to Chapter 16 on TF for detailed discussions of antibiotic dosage and prevention measures.

YELLOW FEVER (See Chapter 74)

The course and severity of yellow fever do not seem affected by pregnancy, but no studies exist to confirm this assessment. Yellow fever is a very severe disease with high mortality and no specific treatment; therefore, in the general population emphasis has been placed on prevention with an easy-to-use, economical, available, safe, and very effective vaccine.

The safety of yellow fever vaccination, a live virus vaccine, has not been established during pregnancy. Studies of infants who were born to mothers that had been vaccinated with the YF17D immunogen during their pregnancies have been analyzed.[130–133] Infection of the fetus with the vaccine strain was documented in one newborn and no congenital abnormalities were observed.[117] In women vaccinated with YF17D early in pregnancy, the relative risk for spontaneous abortion was 2.3, but the difference with unvaccinated cases was not statistically significant. Seventy-four prospectively enrolled cases were analyzed; pregnancies ended in 46 births, five voluntary and seven spontaneous abortions; three newborns had minor defects and two major defects.[130] Although the samples are small, and the follow-up incomplete, these data, plus limited clinical trials in Africa and Europe, suggest that the risk of vaccination of pregnant women who are likely to be exposed to infection with the yellow fever flavivirus in endemic areas is less than the risk of contracting yellow fever. There is a theoretical but unproven risk of transmission of the YF17D strain in human milk during breastfeeding. Small studies from Brazil[131] and Trinidad[132] stress the need for caution. Therefore, pregnant and lactating women who must travel to endemic areas can be offered the vaccine with clear explanations of the risk/benefit ratio as understood at the time of consultation, if the risk of contracting yellow fever is high. Pregnant women who have been inadvertently vaccinated should be reassured. Seroconversion rates during pregnancy can be lower,[133] and immunity should probably be verified.

OTHER INTRAUTERINE INFECTIONS

Cytomegalovirus (See Chapter 56)

Primary cytomegalovirus (CMV) infection during pregnancy may be transmitted to the fetus in 25–75% of cases. Reinfection with a different strain may have lower potential for transmission. Since the use of highly active antiretroviral therapy for prevention of perinatal HIV transmission, the prevalence of congenital CMV infection has decreased in children born to HIV-infected mothers.[134] CMV can persist in a latent stage after primary infection, and reactivate during pregnancy to be transmitted to the fetus. Deleterious developmental outcomes have been observed in infants.[135] There are differences in the sensitivity of commercially available tests for CMV antibodies.[136] A highly sensitive IgM test followed by further serological or virological methods can improve detection of early infection. Treatment with ganciclovir has not been evaluated in pregnancy and is being studied for symptomatic congenital infection.[137]

Herpes Simplex Virus 1 and 2 (See Chapter 56)

Herpes simplex infection is common worldwide.[138] Genital infection by either herpes simplex virus 1 or 2 is rarely transmitted *in utero* to the fetus, but it is more commonly transmitted intrapartum to the newborn. It can also be transmitted later unrelated to pregnancy. Transmission occurs even in asymptomatic women, more efficiently in primary than in reactivated infections. Data on the safety of acyclovir, valacyclovir, and famciclovir are not complete but many specialists recommend their use during pregnancy in several situations.[139] Neonatal disease is very serious, potentially lethal, and has a high risk of severe sequelae and early treatment with intravenous acyclovir reduces but does not eliminate morbidity and mortality.[139] Delivery by cesarean section is advocated to prevent neonatal herpes, but this does not totally eliminate the risk. No effective vaccine is available.

Rubella

Rubella remains prevalent in some areas of the developing world where vaccination programs have not reached the population. The rubella virus interferes with critical steps in fetal organ development during early pregnancy and causes the congenital rubella syndrome (CRS), a disease of poor prognosis and severe sequelae. Global immunization programs and individual vaccination of women before their first pregnancy can prevent CRS.[140]

Syphilis (See Chapter 43)

The risk of syphilis during pregnancy parallels the rates of syphilis in women of childbearing age in a given population. All pregnant women should have a syphilis detection test at the first prenatal visit, and in many instances the test should be repeated one or more times to the time of delivery.[141] All seropositivity should be considered infection unless appropriate treatment can be documented and antibody concentrations decline. Since treatment in pregnancy both prevents and treats fetal infection, it is recommended without delay and consists of the penicillin regimen appropriate for the stage of syphilis diagnosed. Safe and effective alternatives to penicillin are not documented.[142]

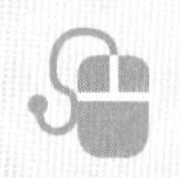

Access the complete reference list online at
http://www.expertconsult.com

INDEX

Note: Page numbers followed by *f* indicate figures, by *t* indicate tables and by *b* indicate boxes. Page numbers preceded by e indicate pages to be found in on-line material only.

A

Abacavir, 103t
  HIV, 553
ABATE larvicide, 761
Abdominal angiostrongyliasis, 776
Abdominal mass, 917t, 921
Abdominal pain, 917t, 920–921
  A. costaricensis infection, 776
  eosinophilia, 945–946, 946b
  giardiasis, 627t
  malaria, 661
  pelvic inflammatory disease *see* Pelvic inflammatory disease treatment, 1043t
Abortion, 271, 273, 1072–1074, 1076–1080
  C. psittaci, 316t
Abscess
  brain, 1020–1022
    amebic, 618
  epidural, 1022
  liver
    amebic, 617–618, 617f, 617t, 976t–977t, 979, 979t
    pyogenic, 976t–977t, 978–979, 978f
  phaeohyphomycosis, 571
  pharyngeal, 263
  psoas, 1023
  staphylococcal, 208–209
Absidia spp., 597
Absidia corymbifera, 601
Acanthamoeba spp., 159, 707–709
  antibodies, 710
  cultivation, 707
  epidemiology, 709
  eradication, 86t–87t
  granulomatous amebic encephalitis *see* Granulomatous amebic encephalitis
  HIV coinfection, 1052
  keratitis, 86t–87t, 707, 710–711, 711f
    diagnosis, 712
    prevention and control, 713
    treatment and prognosis, 713
  life cycle, 707, 708f
  neurologic involvement, 1019t
  taxonomy and classification, 709
Acanthamoeba castellanii, 707, 708f
Acanthamoeba culbertsoni, 707
Acanthamoeba healyi, 707
Acanthamoeba lenticulata, 707
Acanthamoeba polyphaga, 707
Acanthamoeba rhysodes, 707
Acanthocheilonema perstans, 739
Acanthosis, 535
Acaraphobia, 1066
Acaricides, 681
Acarina, 872–873, 873f
Access to care, 19
Accessory cholera enterotoxin, 154
Acetazolamide, altitude sickness, 900–901
Acetylspiramycin, sarcocystosis, 644
Achatina fulica, 774, 776
Achlorhydria, 168
Acinectobacter spp., 184
Acinetobacter calcoaceticus-Acinetobacter baumannii complex, 915
Acquired immunity, genetic variation, 33
Acquired immunodeficiency syndrome *see* HIV/AIDS
Acrodermatitis enteropathica, 25–26, 28
Actin motor, 139–140, 141f
Actinomadura madurae, 565, 567f
Actinomadura pelletieri, 565
Actinomycetoma, 565–566, 566f
Actinomycosis, 917t
  abdominal, 921
  ocular disease, 1001
  oropharyngeal, 919
Active chronic gastritis, 167, 169
Acute disseminated encephalomyelitis (ADEM), 529
Acute flaccid paralysis, 400–401
Acute retinal necrosis, 995
Acyclovir, 102t
  genital herpes, 1035t
  herpesviruses, 356
    cytomegalovirus, 362
    Epstein-Barr virus, 364
    HHV-8, 368
    HSV, 104t, 359
    varicella zoster virus, 104t, 361
  orthopoxviruses, 376
Adaptive immunity, 3, 6t, 56–61
  antigen presentation to T-cells, 58–60, 59f
  attributes of, 53t
  cell types, 57
  cross-presentation, 60
  lymphocyte development/activation, 57–58
  lymphoid organs, 57
  malnutrition effects, 28–30
  maturation of response, 60–61
  MHC *see* Major histocompatibility complex
  protein energy malnutrition, 28–30
  responses, 60
  zinc effects, 30
Adefovir dipivoxil, 102t
  hepatitis B, 436
Adenine arabinoside, human adenovirus, 390
Adenolymphangitis, acute, 731–732
Adenoviruses, 378, 379t–380t, 389–390, 417, 417t
  agent, 389
  capsids, 389
  clinical features, 389
    ocular disease, 991, 992f
  diagnosis, 390
  enteric, 417–418, 417t
  epidemiology, 389
  military cases, 910
  pathogenesis and immunity, 390
  prevention and control, 390
  serotype 14, 910
  treatment, 390
  vaccine, 380t
  see also individual viruses
Adenylate cyclase toxin, 212–213
Adhesins, 4, 114t–115t, 323
  afimbrial, 4, 118
  fimbrial, 118
Adult inclusion conjunctivitis, 997–998
Adult T-cell leukemia, 545
Aedes spp., 49, 442t–443t, 521–522
Aedes aegypti, 40, 47, 51, 442t–443t
  chikungunya virus, 876t
  dengue fever, 504–505, 876t
  distribution in Americas, 506f
  lymphatic filariasis, 730–731
  yellow fever, 494, 876t
Aedes africanus, 493–494
Aedes albopictus, 51, 504, 513
  chikungunya virus, 876t
  dengue fever, 876t
Aedes bromeliae, 493–494
Aedes camptorhynchus, 522
Aedes furcifer, 493–494
Aedes luteocephalus, 493–494
Aedes mcintoshii, 462–463
Aedes (Ochlerotatus) sollicitans, eastern equine encephalitis, 876t
Aedes (Ochlerotatus) triseriatus, La Crosse encephalitis, 876t
Aedes polynesiensis, 522
Aedes vigilax, 522
Aedes vittatus, 493–494
Aeromonas spp., 113, 917t
  toxin, 113
  travelers' diarrhea, 924
Aeromonas hydrophila, toxin, 114t–115t
Aerosol transmission, 910–911
Affected sib pair analysis, 33
Afimbrial adhesins, 4
Africa
  blastomycosis, 576
  causes of fever, 926f
  chromoblastomycosis, 569
  cryptosporidiosis, 636t
  hemorrhagic fevers, 932t
  histoplasmosis, 573–574
  HIV/AIDS, 549–550
  loaiasis, 735
  malaria, 652, 896f
    drug-resistant *P. falciparum*, 654t
    transmission intensity, 652–653
  onchocerciasis, 741–742, 743f
  plague, 278
African green monkey immunodeficiency virus, 542f
African tick bite fever, 323, 875t
  clinical features, 326
    eschar, 955t
African trypanosomiasis *see* Trypanosomiasis, African
Aggregative adherence fimbriae, 117–118
Agrobacterium tumefaciens, 271
Ague *see* Malaria
AIDS *see* HIV/AIDS
'Airport' malaria, 463
Ajellomyces capsulatus, 573
Akodon spp., 276
Alanine aminotransferase, 975
  Crimean-Congo hemorrhagic fever, 467
  hepatitis A, 422
  hepatitis B, 434–435
  hepatitis C, 430
  yellow fever, 496
Alarmins, 53–54
Alastrim, 370
Albendazole
  A. caninum, 77t–79t
  A. cantonensis, 776
  adverse effects, 82b, 629t, 734, 821
  African trypanosomiasis, 687, 688t
  ascariasis, 77t–79t, 797, 918t
  capillariasis, 77t–79t
  cutaneous larva migrans, 77t–79t, 767

cysticercosis, 821
E. granulosus, 80t
echinococcosis
alveolar, 836
cystic, 831
polycystic, 838
Echinostoma spp., 867
embryotoxicity, 76
enterobiasis, 790
fascioliasis, 861
giardiasis, 628t
gnathostomiasis, 77t–79t, 785
gongylonemiasis, 77t–79t
hookworm, 76, 77t–79t, 803
loaiasis, 738
lymphatic filariasis, 734
M. perstans, 77t–79t
microsporidiosis, 86t–89t, 720t, 721
mode of action, 76
neurocysticercosis, 821
subarachnoid, 821–822
Oesophagostomum spp., 781
opisthorchiasis/clonorchiasis, 858
P. philippinensis, 787
perstans filiariasis, 739
strongyloidiasis, 77t–79t, 811, 918t
T. solium, 80t
toxocariasis, 77t–79t, 766
trichinellosis, 77t–79t, 772–773
Trichostrongylus spp., 77t–79t
trichuriasis, 77t–79t, 793
Alcohol, and cancer, 72
Aldolase, trichinellosis, 772
Aleppo evil, 699
Alkhurma virus, 442t–443t, 515, 516f
clinical features, 444t
diagnosis, 447t
Allergens, 61
Allopurinol
adverse reactions, eosinophilia, 947t
cutaneous leishmaniasis, 705
Allpahuayo virus, 450f
Allylamines, dermatophytosis, 563
Alopecia, monkeypox, 371
Alpha level, 12
Alphacoronavirus, 388
Alphaviruses, 519–524, 520t
as bioterrorism agents, 880t, 882
characteristics, 519–521, 520f
clinical features, 523–524
diagnosis, 524, 886
epidemiology, 521–522, 521f
pathogenesis and immunity, 521
prevention and control, 524
skin lesions, 956t, 972t
treatment and prognosis, 524
see also individual viruses
Alternaria alternata, 571
Altitude sickness, 900–901
Alveolar echinococcosis, 824, 833–837
agent *see Echinococcus multilocularis*
clinical features, 834–835, 834f–835f
diagnosis, 835–836, 836f
pathogenesis and immunity, 835
prevention and control, 836–837
sylvatic life cycles, 836
synanthropic cycles, 836–837
transmission, epidemiology and geographic distribution, 833
treatment, 836
Alysiella spp., 184
Amantadine, 102t
influenza, 380t, 382
Amapari virus, 450f, 450t
Amblyomma spp., 329
Amblyomma americanum, 339, 874–875, 875t
Amblyomma aureolatum, 323–326
Amblyomma cajennense, 323–326, 874–875
Amblyomma hebraeum, 324, 875t
Amblyomma maculatum, 875t
Amblyomma triste, 875t
Amblyomma variegatum, 324
Amebae, 1–2
Amebic disease, 614–622
asymptomatic colonization, 616, 616b
colitis, 616–617, 617f, 617t
diagnosis, 620–621, 620t
antigen detection, 620, 620f
colonoscopy, 620
imaging procedures, 620–621, 621f
microscopy, 620
polymerase chain reaction, 620
serology, 620
diarrhea, 616
dysentery and colitis, 616–617, 617f, 617t
epidemiology, 615–616
fever, 926t–927t
granulomatous amebic encephalitis *see* Granulomatous amebic encephalitis
HIV coinfection, 1052–1053
immunity, 619–620, 619f
meningoencephalitis, 711
diagnosis, 712
neurologic involvement, 1019t
prevention and control, 713
treatment and prognosis, 713
metastatic, 618
metastatic amebiasis, 618
ocular involvement, 1011
pathogenesis, 618–619, 618f
pleural effusion, 988t
pruritus, 959t–961t
skin lesions, 962t–968t
treatment and prognosis, 88t–89t, 621–622
vaccines, 621
Amebic liver abscess, 617–618, 617f, 617t, 976t–977t, 979, 979t
incubation period, 929b
Ameboma, 921
American babesiosis, 875t
American boutonneuse fever, 874, 875t
see also Mediterranean spotted fever
American Committee for Immunization Practices, 904
American trypanosomiasis *see* Chagas' disease
Americas
hemorrhagic fevers, 932t
see also Central America; North America; South America
Amikacin, 96t–98t, 100t
actinomycetoma, 568, 568f
MAC, 246
Salmonella resistance, 130t
tuberculosis, 243
Aminoglycosides, 96t–98t, 99
Campylobacter spp., 148
Aminopenicillins, 96t–98t
p-Aminosalicylic acid, tuberculosis, 243
Aminosidine, cryptosporidiosis, 104t
Aminotransferase, trichinellosis, 772
Ammospermophilus spp., 276
Amodiaquine, malaria, 664, 667t, 668
Amoxicillin, 96t–98t
anthrax, 264
H. pylori, 172t, 173b, 918t
Lyme disease, 301
pneumococcal pneumonia, 202
salmonellosis, 135
typhoid/paratyphoid, 125, 125t
Amoxicillin-clavulanate, 96t–98t
melioidosis, 222
Salmonella resistance, 130t
Amphimerus pseudofelineus, 855
Amphotericin B, 93, 100t–101t
blastomycosis, 577
candidemia, 595–596
candidiasis, 590
cardiac, 593
endophthalmitis, 594–595
esophageal, 592
meningitis, 594
oropharyngeal, 592
urinary tract infection, 594
coccidioidomycosis, 579
cryptococcosis, 104t, 580–581
histoplasmosis, 575
leishmaniasis, 91t–92t
mucosal, 705
mucormycosis, 600
Naegleria spp., 86t–87t
P. marneffei infection, 587–588
paracoccidioidomycosis, 584
phaeohyphomycosis, 572
primary amebic meningoencephalitis, 713
sporotrichosis, 604t, 606–607
toxicity, 101t
visceral leishmaniasis, 704
Ampicillin, 96t–98t
adverse reactions, eosinophilia, 947t
Campylobacter spp., 148
cholera, 155–156, 155t
E. coli infection, 119
pneumococcal meningitis, 201
pneumococcal pneumonia, 202
Salmonella spp.
bacteremia, 135
drug-resistant, 129, 130f, 130t
shigellosis, 143f, 143t
Ampicillin-sulbactam, 98f
Amprenavir, HIV, 553–554
Amur virus, 471t, 472
Anajatuba virus, 471t
Anaphylatoxins, 52–53
Anaphylaxis, 55–56
Anaplasma spp., 7, 339
Anaplasma marginale, 339
Anaplasma phagocytophilum, 4, 339, 342–343, 874
babesiosis coinfection, 679
life cycle, 340f
pathogenesis and immunity, 342–343
Anaplasmataceae, 339
Anaplasmosis, 342–343
agent, 342
diagnosis, 343, 343f
disease, 342
epidemiology, 342
granulocytic, 874, 875t
pathogenesis and immunity, 342–343
prevention and control, 343
treatment, 343
Ancylostoma spp., 779–780
proteins secreted by, 803
Ancylostoma braziliense, 799, 800t
cutaneous larva migrans, 766, 800–801
epidemiology, 801
Ancylostoma caninum, 799, 800t
cutaneous larva migrans, 766, 800–801
epidemiology, 801
eradication, 77t–79t
pulmonary disease, 984t
Ancylostoma ceylanicum, 799, 800t
epidemiology, 801
human infection, 800–801
Ancylostoma duodenale, 799–800, 800f, 800t
disease, 802
epidemiology, 801, 802f
larval hypobiosis, 799–800
properties, 800t
pulmonary disease, 984t
skin lesions, 957t
see also Hookworm
Ancylostomiasis, 801
Andes virus, 442t–443t, 471t, 473
animal models, 477
hantavirus pulmonary syndrome, 473, 476
Androctonus australis, 871
Anemia, 1024–1032, e12t–e13t
causes, 1025b
of chronic disease, 1029–1030
management, 1030
pathogenesis, 1029

clinical approach, 1024
definition, 1024, 1025t
WHO, 1024
diseases associated with
African trypanosomiasis, 685
Brucella spp., 273
diphyllobothriasis, 843
HIV/AIDS, 1028
hookworm, 802
malaria, 654–657, 655b, 660, 1027–1028, 1028f
folate deficiency, 1027, 1029
history, 1024–1025
hypochromic microcytic, e12t–e13t
of infection, 26t
inherited red blood cell disorders, 1030–1032
G6PD deficiency, 32, 1025, 1026f, 1032
sickle cell anemia, 1025, 1026f, 1030, 1030b
thalassemia *see* Thalassemia
investigations, 1026–1027
iron deficiency, 26t, 31, 1025f, 1027f
koilonychia, 1025
pencil cells, 1025f, 1026
macrocytic, 1026
mechanism and classification, 1024
megaloblastic, 1025, 1026f–1027f, 1027
microangiopathic hemolytic, 1026f
microcytic hypochromic, 1025
differential diagnosis, 1029t
normocytic normochromic, 1025, 1027
nutritional, 1028
pathophysiology, 1024
physical examination, 1025–1026
vitamin B12 deficiency, 1027, 1029
Anergy, 60
Angiomatosis, bacillary, 266t, 956f
Angiostrongyliasis, 774–777
abdominal, 776
incubation period, 929b
ocular involvement, 1014, 1014f
Angiostrongylus spp., 779–780
Angiostrongylus cantonensis, 77t–79t, 774–776
characteristics, 774, 775f
diagnosis, 775–776
disease, 774–775
eosinophilia, 942t–943t
epidemiology, 774
life cycle, 775f
paratenic hosts, 774
pathogenesis and immunity, 775
prevention and control, 776
treatment and prognosis, 776
Angiostrongylus costaricensis, 77t–79t, 774, 776–777, 917t
abdominal pain, 921
characteristics, 776
diagnosis, 777
disease, 776
eosinophilia, 942t
epidemiology, 776
life cycle, 775f
paratenic hosts, 776
pathogenesis and immunity, 776–777
prevention and control, 777
treatment and prognosis, 777
Anguillula intestinalis, 805
Anguillula stercoralis, 805
Angular cheilitis, 590–592
Angular stomatitis, 28
Anidulafungin, 100t–101t
candidemia, 596
toxicity, 101t
Animal models
arenaviruses, 457
Guanarito virus, 457
hantavirus pulmonary syndrome, 477–478
Junin virus, 457
lymphocytic choriomeningitis, 457
Machupo virus, 457
Anisakiasis, 776–777, 781–783
agent *see Anisakis* spp.
eosinophilia, 942t
eradication, 77t–79t
Anisakis spp., 781–783, 782f, 917t
Anisakis brevispiculata, 781–782
Anisakis pagiae, 781–782
Anisakis pegreffii, 781–782
Anisakis physeteris, 781–782
Anisakis simplex, 781–782
Anisakis typica, 781–782
Anisakis zyphydarum, 781–782
Anncaliia spp., 714
Anncaliia algerae, 714, 715t
clinical manifestations, 718
Anncaliia connori, 715t
Anncaliia vesicularum, 715t
clinical manifestations, 718
treatment, 720t
Anogenital malignancies, 533–534
Anopheles spp., 49, 646, 652
filariasis, 730–731, 876t
malaria, 652, 876t
Anopheles albimanus, 47
Anopheles culicifascies, 47
Anopheles darlingi, 652
Anopheles dirus, 652
Anopheles funestus, 51, 522
Anopheles gambiae, 51, 522, 652
host location, 46
Anopheles stephensi, 650f
Anoplura *see* Lice
Anorectal involvement, lymphogranuloma venereum, 317
Anorexia, giardiasis, 627t
ANOVA, 13
Ansamycins, *H. pylori* infection, 172t
Anthelminthics
adverse effects, 82b
see also individual drugs
Anthracyclines, Kaposi's sarcoma, 368
Anthrax, 261–264
agent *see Bacillus anthracis*
clinical features, 261–263, 262f, 881
cutaneous, 261–262, 954f, 957t, 967t–968t, 972t
eschar, 955t
gastrointestinal, 263, 917t
inhalational, 263, 881
meningitis, 263
ocular involvement, 1002
oropharyngeal, 263, 919
sepsis, 263
diagnosis, 263–264
epidemiology, 261, 262f
global distribution, 262f
incubation period, 929b
pathogenesis and immunity, 263
prevention and control, 264
transmission, 261
treatment and prognosis, 264
Anthrax edema factor, 5
Anthropomorphic indicators of disease effects, 25t
Anti-epileptic drugs
adverse reactions, eosinophilia, 947t
in cysticercosis, 820
Antibiotics *see* Antimicrobials
Antibodies
B. pseudomallei, 221–222
IgM, 54t
protein energy malnutrition, 29
Antibody production, 61
protein energy malnutrition, 29
Antifolates, malaria, 664
Antifungal drugs, 99, 100t–101t, 590
Antigen detection tests
amebiasis, 620, 620f
B. pseudomallei, 221
colonization factor, 113
cysticercosis, 820
Duffy blood group, 4–5
hantavirus, 479
Lewis X, 168
malaria, 662
Salmonella spp., 121
Salmonella typhi, 124
streptococcal superantigen, 208
typhoid/paratyphoid, 124
Antigen presentation, 58–60, 59f
Antigen probes, *C. trachomatis*, 312
Antigen-presenting cells, 33, 56–57
activation of, 55f
Antigenic drift, 6–7
Antigenic variation, 653, 682–683
Antimalarials, 664, 895–898, 897t
active metabolites, 664
adverse effects, 82b
antifolates, 664
artemisinins, 654–655
drug interactions, 664–665
elimination, 664, 665f
pharmacokinetics, 664–665, 665t
quinoline-related or quinoline-like compounds, 664
resistance to, 673–674, 895, 896f
see also individual drugs
Antimicrobial resistance
C. pneumoniae, 95
group A streptococcus
erythromycin, 208
sulfonamide, 208
L. monocytogenes, 95
L. pneumoniae, 95
M. pneumoniae, 95
N. gonorrhoea, 188–189
S. pneumoniae, 95, 201, 201f
Salmonella spp., 129–131, 130f–131f, 130t
Antimicrobials, 95–99, 96t–98t
with antimalarial activity, 668
cholera, 155–156, 155t
E. coli infection, 119
gastrointestinal disease, 918t
gonorrhoea, 189
meningococcal disease, 181–182
mode of action, 98f
in pregnancy, 1073t
trachoma, 312–313
typhoid/paratyphoid, 125–126, 125t
see also individual antimicrobials
Antimony compounds *see* Meglumine antimonate; Sodium stibogluconate
Antimotility agents, *E. coli* infection, 119–120
Antimycobacterial drugs, 99, 100t
see also individual drugs
Antiparasitic drugs, 76–94
Chagas' disease, 694–695
see also individual drugs
Antipsychotic agents, delusional parasitosis, 1070–1071
Antiretroviral therapy, 18, 553–554
adherence to, 20
costs of, 20
drug resistance, 554, 557
efficacy of, 556, 556f
HAART therapy, 553–554
in pregnancy, 1075
recommendations, 554, 557t
see also individual drugs
Antistreptolysin, 207
Antitoxic immunity, 658
Antivirals, 101, 102t–104t
influenza, 380t
chemoprophylaxis, 383
SARS, 397
smallpox, 376–377
see also individual drugs
Apicomplexa, 641
Apodemus spp., 678
Apodemus agrarius, 470, 471t
Apodemus flavicollis, 471t

Apodemus peninsulae, 471t
Apoi virus, 516f
Apophysomyces elegans, 597, 599
Appendicitis, 920
  E. vermicularis, 789–790, 790f
Arabinogalactan, 253
Arachnoiditis, and toxocariasis, 765
Araraquara virus, 471t
Araucária virus, 471t
Arboviruses
  HIV coinfection, 1061–1062
  see also individual viruses
Archaea, evolution, 1
Arcobacter butzleri, 145, 146t
Arcobacter cryaerophila, 145, 146t
Arenaviruses, 442t–443t, 449–461
  agents, 449–452, 450f, 450t
  antigenic and genetic relationships, 451–452, 452f
  clinical features, 444t–445t, 455–457
  diagnosis, 447t, 459–460
    laboratory diagnosis, 459–460
  differential diagnosis
  epidemiology, 452–455
    geography, 450f, 453
    maintenance in rodent host populations, 455
    transmission cycle, 452–453, 452f
    transmission to humans, 453–455
  genomic organization, 449
  pathogenesis and immunity, 458–459
  pathology, 446t, 457–458
    animal models, 457
    human, 457–458
  persistence and defective interfering virus, 451
  prevention and control, 448t, 460–461
    containment of patients, 460
    rodent control, 460–461
  replication, 449–451
  treatment and prognosis, 448t, 460
    supportive, 460
    virus-specific therapy, 460
  vaccines, 461
  virion morphology/structure, 449, 451f
  virology, 451
  see also individual viruses and diseases
Argasidae, 51, 295, 874–875
Argentine hemorrhagic fever, 442t–443t, 450t
  agent *see* Junin virus
  clinical features, 455–456
  epidemiology, 455
  pathogenesis and immunity, 458–459
  pathologic features, 446t
  prevalence, 453f
  transmission, 453–454
  treatment and prevention, 448t, 460
Arginine, 24
Armadillos, leprosy in, 254
Armillifer spp., pulmonary disease, 984t
Armillifer armillatus, 877, 877f
Arms, lymphatic filariasis, 732, 732f
Arteether, malaria prophylaxis, 84–85
Artemether
  C. sinensis, 867
  lung flukes, 867
  malaria, 664
    prophylaxis, 84–85
    severe, 670, 670b
  O. viverrini, 867
  opisthorchiasis/clonorchiasis, 858
  pharmacokinetics, 665t
Artemether-lumefantrine, 83
  adverse effects, 82b, 897t
  malaria, 666–668, 667t, 897t
    dose, 897t
Artemisinins, 654–655
  lung flukes, 867
  malaria, 664
    combination therapies, 17, 20–21
    pregnancy, 671b
  opisthorchiasis/clonorchiasis, 858
  in pregnancy, 1073t
  resistance, 651f
Artemotil
  malaria, 664
    severe, 670
Arteritis, salmonellosis, 132t–133t
Artesunate
  adverse effects, 82b
  C. sinensis, 867
  lung flukes, 867
  malaria, 664, 667t
    combination treatment, 665f
    prophylaxis, 84–85
    severe, 670, 670b
  O. viverrini, 867
  opisthorchiasis/clonorchiasis, 858
  pharmacokinetics, 665t
Artesunate-amodiaquine, malaria, 667
Artesunate-mefloquine, malaria, 666, 667t
Artesunate-sulfadoxine-pyrimethamine, malaria, 667
Arthritis
  Brucella, 272–273, 272t
  candidal, 594
  gonococcal, 187
  loiaisis, 737
  reactive, *C. trachomatis*, 316t, 317
  smallpox, 371
  strongyloidiasis, 810
Arthroconidia, 559
Arthroderma spp., 559
Arthropods, 868
  biting, 871–873, 871f
  as disease vectors, 45, 873–877, 874f
    HIV coinfection, 1055
    military cases, 911–913
  parasitic, 868–870
  stinging, 870–871, 870f
  see also different types
Artibeus spp., 450f
Arvicanthis spp., 276–277, 450f
Arvicolinae, 470
Asbestosis, 987t
Ascariasis, 5, 794–798
  agent *see Ascaris lumbricoides*
  clinical features, 795–796
    eosinophilia, 942t–943t
    hepatobiliary and pancreatic, 796, 976t–977t, 980, 980f
    intestinal, 796, 796f
    ocular involvement, 1013–1014
    pleural effusion, 796, 988t
    skin lesions, 946t
  diagnosis, 797
  epidemiology, 794–795
  eradication, 76, 77t–79t
  pathogenesis and immunity, 796–797
  treatment and prognosis, 797, 918t
    prevention and control, 797–798
  vitamin A malabsorption, 27–28
Ascaridina, 781–784
  Anisakis, 781–783
  Baylisascaris, 783
  Lagochilascaris, 783–784
  Pseudoterranova, 781–783
Ascaris spp., pulmonary disease, 984t
Ascaris lumbricoides, 763, 791, 794, 795f, 917t
  life cycle, 795f
  ova, 795f
  see also Ascariasis
Asia
  causes of fever, 926f
  cryptosporidiosis, 636t
  gnathostomiasis, 784
  hemorrhagic fevers, 932t
  HIV/AIDS, 550–551
  malaria, 652, 652f, 896f
    drug-resistant *P. falciparum*, 654t
  Penicillium marneffei, 586
  plague, 278
  trichinellosis, 770t
Aspartate aminotransferase, 975
  Crimean-Congo hemorrhagic fever, 467
  Hantaan virus, 474–475
  hepatitis A, 422
  yellow fever, 496
Aspergillus spp.
  ocular involvement, 1006
  tuberculosis, 231
Aspirin-induced eosinophilia, 947t
Asplenia, and susceptibility to babesiosis, 678
Association studies, 33–34
  clinical relevance, 39
  infectious diseases, 34–39, 35t–36t
  inherited conditions, 34, 34t–35t
Astroviruses, 416–417, 417t
  characteristics, 416
  diagnosis, 417
  epidemiology, 416
  gastroenteritis, 416–417
  treatment, prognosis and prevention, 417
Atazanavir, 103t
  HIV, 553–554
Atovaquone
  adverse effects, 82b, 85b, 897t
  babesiosis, 680
  malaria, 661, 664, 667t, 897t
    dose, 887–891
    prophylaxis, 84
  pharmacokinetics, 665t
  Pneumocystis jirovecii, 86t–87t
  pneumocystis pneumonia, 104t
  pneumocystosis, 612
  toxoplasmosis, 727
Atovaquone-proguanil
  adverse effects, 897t
  malaria, 83, 666, 668, 897t, 898
    dose, 897t
    prophylaxis, 84, 669t
  in pregnancy, 1073t
Attack rate, 11
  secondary, 11
Attributable risk percent, 14
Aura virus, 520t
Australia
  cryptosporidiosis, 636t
  hemorrhagic fevers, 932t
Autoimmunity, 61
Automeris io, 871
Autonomous Pathogen Detection System, 880
Autumn fever, 303
Azalides, trachoma, 312–313
Azithromycin, 96t–98t, 99, 100t
  babesiosis, 680
  Campylobacter spp., 148
  cat-scratch disease, 269
  cellulitis, 210–211
  cervicitis/urethritis, 1040t
  chancroid, 1035t
  cholera, 155–156, 155t
  cryptosporidiosis, 639
  donovanosis, 197
  E. coli infection, 119
  gonorrhoea, 189
  granuloma inguinale, 1035t
  granulomatous amebic encephalitis, 712
  legionellosis, 218
  lymphogranuloma venereum, 318
  M. avium complex, 104t
  MAC
    in HIV, 246–247
    pulmonary disease, 246
  melioidosis, 222
  meningococcal prophylaxis, 182
  Oroya fever, 269
  pertussis, 214
  in pregnancy, 1073t
  scrub typhus, 338
  shigellosis, 143t
  spotted fever rickettsioses, 328
  syphilis, 292

toxoplasmosis, 727
trachoma, 313
travelers' diarrhea, 894t
typhoid/paratyphoid, 125–126, 125t, 918t
Vibrio spp., 161
Azoles, 590
paracoccidioidomycosis, 584
resistance, 590
see also individual drugs
Aztreonam, 96t–98t
in pregnancy, 1073t

B

B-1 cells, 56
B-cells
development, 57
effector, 57
costimulation, 57
memory, 57
receptors, 57
in zinc deficiency, 30
Babesia spp., 4, 45, 633, 676
see also Babesiosis
Babesia bigemina, life cycle, 676, 677f
Babesia bovis, 48, 676
Babesia capreoli, 676
Babesia divergens, 676
diagnosis, 680f
seasonality and ecology, 677
Babesia duncani, 677–678
clinical manifestations, 678
diagnosis, 680f
Babesia equi, 676
Babesia gibsoni, 677
Babesia microti, 676–677
A. phagocytophilum coinfection, 679
B. burgdorferi coinfection, 679
clinical manifestations, 678–679, 679f
E. chaffeensis coinfection, 679
ecology, 677–678, 678f
Babesia rodhaini, 676
Babesiidae, 676
Babesiosis, 676–681
agent, 646–651
American, 875t
clinical features, 678–679
diagnosis, 679–680, 679f–680f
divergens, 676
epidemiology and distribution, 676–678
HIV coinfection, 678, 1050
pathogenesis and immunity, 678
prevention and control, 681
seasonality and ecology, 677–678
treatment and prognosis, 85, 85b, 86t–87t, 680
Bacillary angiomatosis, 266t, 956f
ocular involvement, 1002
Bacille-Calmette-Guérin *see* BCG
Bacillus anthracis, 4, 261, 262f, 917–918, 955t
agent, 261
as bioterrorism agent, 879, 881
diagnosis, 884–885
see also Anthrax
Bacillus cereus, 917t
food poisoning, 923
Bacitracin
giardiasis, 629
impetigo, 204
Baclofen, tetanus, 287–288
BACTEC 460 system, 239
Bacteremia
plague, 281
Salmonella spp., 131
treatment, 135
without sepsis, 177
Bacterial evolution, 1
Bacterial infection
HIV coinfection, 1058–1065
malaria, 662
ocular disease, 996–1006
see also individual infections and bacteria
Bacterial vaginosis, 1034t
differential diagnosis, 1038t
treatment, 1040t
Bacteriophages, 2
Bacteroides fragilis, 208
Baghdad boil, 699
Bairnsdale ulcer *see Mycobacterium ulcerans*
Balamuthia spp.
epidemiology, 709
HIV coinfection, 1052
taxonomy and classification, 709
Balamuthia mandrillaris, 707–709, 933
cultivation, 708
eradication, 86t–87t
granulomatous amebic encephalitis, 709–710
life cycle, 707–708, 708f
neurologic involvement, 1019t
Balanitis, candidal, 593
Balantidiasis, 1–2
agent *see Balantidium coli*
eradication, 88t–89t
treatment, 628t, 918t
Balantidium coli, 623, 630, 630f, 917t
HIV coinfection, 1053
inflammatory diarrhea, 923
see also Balantidiasis
Bamako Initiative, 19
Bandicota bengalensis, 277
Bandicota indica, 277
Bang's disease, 271
Banzi virus, 492
Barbeiros see Kissing bugs
Barbus barbus, 855
Barking pig syndrome *see* Nipah virus
Barmah Forest virus, 520t
Barriers to care, 17
Bartholinitis, *C. trachomatis*, 317
Bartonella spp., 4, 49, 265, 266t, 552
endocarditis, 266t, 267–268
vectors, 266t
Bartonella alsatica, 265, 266t
endocarditis, 267
Bartonella bacilliformis, 265, 266t
global distribution, 267f
host, 265–267
life cycle, 266f
skin lesions, 957t
see also Oroya fever
Bartonella elizabethae, 265, 266t
endocarditis, 267
Bartonella grahamii, 265, 266t
neuroretinitis, 267
Bartonella henselae, 265, 266t, 271
endocarditis, 267
life cycle, 266f
Bartonella koehlerae, 265, 266t
endocarditis, 267
Bartonella quintana, 265, 266t
endocarditis, 267
life cycle, 266f
Bartonella rochalimae, 265, 266t
bacteremia, 267
Bartonella vinsonii, 265, 266t
endocarditis, 267
Bartonellosis, 265–270
agent, 265
diagnosis, 268–269
disease, 267–268
epidemiology, 265–267
pathogenesis and immunity, 268
prevention and control, 269–270
skin lesions, 962t–966t
treatment and prognosis, 269
see also various Bartonella *spp.*
Basic reproductive number, 11
Basic reproductive rate, 48
Basidiobolomycosis, 603
treatment, 604t
Basidiobolus spp., 603
Basidiobolus baptosporus, 969t–970t
Basidiobolus ranarum, 603
Basilar cisterns, cysticercosis of, 818, 818f
Basophils, 55–56
Bats
as disease vectors, 9
SARS, 392–394
Lagos bat virus, 526t
Baylisascaris spp., 783, 783f
Baylisascaris columnaris, 783
Baylisascaris devosi, 783
Baylisascaris laevis, 783
Baylisascaris procyonis, 776, 783, 1013
Bayou virus, 442t–443t, 471t
BCG vaccine, 64t–65t, 243–244
and tuberculin skin test reaction, 230
Bear Canyon virus, 450f
Beau's lines, 563
Bebaru virus, 520t
Bedbugs, 45, 50–51, 871, 871f
pruritus caused by, 959t–961t
Beef tapeworm *see Taenia saginata*
Beilong virus, 352
Bejel *see* Pinta
Belostomatidae, 248
Bentonite flocculation, trichinellosis, 772
Benzathine penicillin, syphilis, 292, 1035t
Benzimidazoles
adverse effects, 803
contraindication in pregnancy, 831
echinococcosis
alveolar, 836
cystic, 831
hookworm, 803
nematode infections, 76–79
resistance to, 793
trichuriasis, 793
see also individual drugs
Benznidazole, 90
adverse effects, 90b
Chagas' disease, 91t–92t, 694
Trypanosoma cruzi, 91t–92t
Benzodiazepines, tetanus, 287–288
Beriberi, e12t–e13t
Bermejo virus, 471t
Bertiella spp., 813
β-lactam antibiotics, 96t–98t
Borrelia infections, 300
β-lactamase, 261
inhibitors, 96t–98t
Betacoronavirus, 388
Betaherpesviruses, 355–356
Bicarbonate, cholera stools, 153t
Bilharziella spp., 849–850
Biliary tract
ascariasis, 796
fascioliasis, 860
salmonellosis, 132t–133t
see also hepatobiliary disease
Bilirubin, 975
malaria, 655b
Biofilms, 118
Biological Aerosol Sentry and Information System, 880
Biologics license application, 68
Biomphalaria spp., 848
Biosocial model of disease, 17–22
Biosurveillance, 880–881
Bioterrorism, 879–886
Brucella, 274–275
category A agents
bacterial, 881–882
diagnosis, 884–885
toxins, 882
viral, 881–882
category B agents, 882–883
bacterial, 882–883
diagnosis, 885–886
food- and waterborne pathogens, 883

toxins, 883
viral, 882
diagnosis of attack, 883–884, 884t
molecular diagnosis, 884, 884t
epidemiology of attack, 879–881
incubation periods, 880f
laboratory response network, 884t
microorganisms and toxins, 879–886
multiplex detection systems, 886
potential agents, 880t
smallpox, 376
see also individual agents
BioWatch, 880
Bipolaris specifera, 571
Birds, *C. psittaci* transmission, 320
Birnaviruses, 417t, 418
Bismuth subcitrate, *H. pylori*, 172t
Bismuth subsalicylate
E. coli, 119
H. pylori, 172t, 173b, 918t
norovirus, 414
travelers' diarrhea, 893, 894t
Bithionol
fascioliasis, 861
paragonimiasis, 81t, 865
Bithynia fuchsiana, 855
Bithynia siamensis, 855
Biting arthropods, 871–873, 871f, 899–900
spiders, 872, 872f, 967t–968t
Biting insects, 899–900
mosquitoes, 876f
Bitot's spots, 24–25, e12t–e13t
Black Creek Canal virus, 442t–443t, 471t
hantavirus pulmonary syndrome, 476
Black Death, 276, 281
see also Plague
Black flies *see Simulium* spp.
Black widow spider, 872, 872f
Black-dot ringworm, 561, 561f
Blackwater fever, 656, 660–661
Blastocystis hominis, 614, 622
eradication, 88t–89t
HIV coinfection, 1053
Blastomyces dermatiditis, 574–575, 576f
HIV coinfection, 1057
Blastomycosis, 575–577
agent, 574–575, 576f
American *see* Paracoccidioidomycosis
clinical features, 576, 576f
ocular involvement, 1008
skin lesions, 969t–970t
diagnosis, 576
epidemiology, 575–576
keloidal *see* Lobomycosis
pathogenesis and immunity, 576
pregnancy, 577
prevention and control, 577
treatment and prognosis, 577
Blindness, 1016
loaiasis, 737
phythisis bulbi, 1016, 1016f
see also Ocular disease
Blister beetles, 873
Blister cells, 1026f
Bloating, giardiasis, 627t
Blood cell count, 1026
Blood films
anemia, 1025–1026
malaria, 647–649, 662, 662f–663f
gametocytes in, 664
and prognosis, 663–664
Blood group O, malaria protection, 36t
Blood transfusion, malaria transmission, 657
Bloodstream infections, candidal, 595–596
Blow flies, 869
Bluetongue virus, 8–9
Bocaviruses, 378, 379t–380t, 390–391, 416
agent, 390
clinical features, 390
diagnosis, 391
epidemiology, 390
pathogenesis and immunity, 390–391
treatment, prevention and control, 391
Body lice *see Pediculus humanus*
Bolivian hemorrhagic fever, 442t–443t, 450t
agent *see* Machupo virus
clinical features, 456
epidemiology, 453
pathologic features, 446t
transmission, 454
treatment and prevention, 448t
Bolomys lasiurus, 471t
Bolomys obscurus, 450f
Bone involvement, salmonellosis, 132t–133t
Bone marrow examination, 1026–1027
Bordetella avium, 212
Bordetella bronchiseptica, 212
Bordetella hinzii, 212
Bordetella holmesii, 212
Bordetella parapertussis, 212
Bordetella pertussis, 212
adherence factors, 212–213
adhesins, 4
transmission and immunity, 213f
see also Pertussis
Bordetella trematum, 212
Boric acid, vulvovaginal candidiasis, 593
Bornholm disease *see* Pleurodynia
Borrelia spp., 295–302
pathogenesis, 298–299, 299f
reservoirs, 296f
skin lesions, 956t
see also Lyme disease; Relapsing fever
Borrelia afzelii, 295, 296t
Borrelia burgdorferi, 7, 46, 49, 295, 296t
babesiosis coinfection, 679
immunity, 299
skin lesions, 957t
Borrelia crocidurae, 296t
Borrelia duttonii, 296–297, 296t
Borrelia garinii, 295, 296t
Borrelia hermsii, 296t
Borrelia hispanica, 296t
Borrelia latyschewii, 296t
Borrelia lonestari, 295
Borrelia mazzottii, 296t
Borrelia miyamotoi, 295
Borrelia parkeri, 296t
Borrelia persica, 296t
Borrelia recurrentis, 6–7, 295–297, 296t, 499
skin lesions, 957t
Borrelia theileri, 295
Borrelia turicatae, 296t
Borrelia venezuelensis, 296t
Borreliosis *see* Lyme disease; Relapsing fever
Bot fly *see Dermatobia hominis*
Botulinum toxin, 882, 886
Botulism
agent *see Clostridium botulinum*
clinical features, 165
ocular involvement, 1003
diagnosis, 165
epidemiology, 165
immunity, 165
pathogenesis, 165
treatment and prevention, 165–166
Bouboui virus, 492
Bouton d'Alep, 699
Bouton de Briska, 699
Bouton de Crète, 699
Bouton d'Orient, 699
Boutonneuse fever *see* Mediterranean spotted fever
Bovine immunodeficiency virus, 542f
Bovine leukemia virus, 543
Bowenoid papillomatosis, 534
Bowen's disease, 534
Brachiola spp., 714
Brachiola algerae, 714
Brachiola vesicularum, eradication, 86t–87t
Brain abscess, 1020–1022
amebic, 618
Brain drain, 18–19
Brainerd diarrhea, 924
Brainstem infections, 1022
Brazilian hemorrhagic fever, 442t–443t
Brazilian purpuric fever, 1003
Breast, lymphatic filariasis, 732
Breast milk, *M. leprae* transmission, 254
Breastfeeding
HIV/AIDS, 1075t
isoniazid therapy, 242
tuberculosis, 242
Brighton Collaboration, 67
Bromocriptine, pleural effusion, 988t
Bronchiolitis, HPIVs, 385
Bronchitis, *C. pneumoniae*, 316t
Bronchoalveolar lavage
mucormycosis, 599
pneumocystosis, 610
Bronchoscopy, tuberculosis, 239
Brown recluse spider bite, 872, 872f, 967t–968t
eschar, 955t
Bruce, Sir David, 271
Brucella spp., 4, 271
as bioterrorism agent, 274–275, 880t, 883
diagnosis, 886
HIV coinfection, 1061
life cycle, 272f
pathogenesis and immunity, 274
vaccine, 275
see also Brucellosis
Brucella abortus, 271, 883
characteristics, 272t
see also Brucellosis
Brucella canis, 883
Brucella ceti, 271
Brucella melitensis, 271, 883
characteristics, 272t
see also Brucellosis
Brucella microti, 271
Brucella neotomae, 271
Brucella ovis, 271
Brucella pinnipedialis, 271
Brucella suis, 271, 883
Brucellosis, 271–275, 883
acute, 271
agent, 271
chronic, 272
clinical features
arthritis, 272–273, 272t
gastrointestinal, 917, 917t
genitourinary, 273
hematologic involvement, 273
hepatitis, 273
neurologic involvement, 273
ocular involvement, 273, 1002
skin lesions, 957t, 972t
diagnosis, 274–275, 274f
epidemiology, 271
immunocompromised patients, 273–274
incubation period, 929b
pathogenesis and immunity, 274
pediatric, 273
in pregnancy, 273
pregnancy, 273, 1072–1073
prevention and control, 275
relapsing/undulant, 272
treatment and prognosis, 275, 918t
Brudzinski's sign, 401, 711, 1017
Brugia spp., 339, 750, 751t
clinical features, 754f
diagnosis, 755–756, 756f
Brugia beaveri, 755
Brugia buckleyi, 755
Brugia ceylonensis, 751t, 755
Brugia guyanensis, 755
Brugia leporis, 750–752, 755

INDEX

Brugia malayi, 7, 77t–79t, 729, 737
  life cycle, 730f
  lymphatic filariasis, 729
  pulmonary disease, 984t
  skin lesions, 946t
Brugia pahangi, 755
Brugia patei, 755
Brugia timori, 77t–79t, 729
  life cycle, 730f
  lymphatic filariasis, 729
  skin lesions, 946t
Buboes
  lymphogranuloma venereum, 308, 317
  plague, 279–280, 279f
Bubonic plague, 3, 279–280
  symptoms, 279–280, 279f
Buffalopox, 372
Bulbar poliomyelitis, 401
Bulinus spp., 848
Bumble bee, 870f
Bundibugyo ebolavirus, 483, 485t
Bung-eye, 757, 757f
Bunostomum phlebotomum, 957
Bunyaviruses, 9, 442t–443t, 481
  clinical features, 444t, 446t
  Crimean-Congo hemorrhagic fever, 466
  diagnosis, 447t
  hantavirus, 470
  pathologic features, 446t
  Rift Valley fever, 462
  treatment and prevention, 448t
Burkholderia spp., 709
Burkholderia mallei, as bioterrorism agent, 880t
Burkholderia pseudomallei, 219
  as bioterrorism agent, 880t
  fever, 928
  host defense, 221
  skin lesions, 956t
  virulence factors, 221
  see also Melioidosis
Burkitt's lymphoma, 362–363, 363f
  diagnosis, 364
  malaria, 657
  pathogenesis and immunity, 363–364
  treatment and prognosis, 364
  see also Epstein-Barr virus
Burnet, Frank Macfarlane, 344
Buruli ulcer, 248–252, 953f
  agent, 248
  clinical features, 248–250, 249f
  diagnosis, 251
  disseminated disease, 250
    edematous form, 250
    metastatic disease, 250f
    plaque, 250
  epidemiology, 248
  geographic distribution, 249f
  localized disease, 249–250
    nodules, 249, 249f
    nodulo-ulcerative forms, 249–250, 249f–250f
  pathogenesis and immunity, 250–251
  prevention and control, 252
  treatment and prognosis, 251–252, 251f
Burulin, 250–251
Buschke-Löwenstein tumors, 534
Bush yaws, 699
Bwanba virus, 482

C

C proteins, 352–353
C-reactive protein, malaria, 657
C1q, 53
C3, 52–53
C3a, 52–53
C3b, 52–53, 57
C3dg, 53
C3Ig, 55
C4, 53
C4a, 53
C4b, 53
C5, 52–53
  deficiency, 52–53
C5a, 53
C5a peptidase, 208
C5b, 52–53
C5b-9 complex, 52–53
C6, 52–53
  deficiency, 52–53
C7, 52–53
  deficiency, 52–53
C8, 52–53
  deficiency, 52–53
C9, 52–53
  deficiency, 52–53
Cabassou virus, 520t
Caenorhabditis elegans, 808
CagA, 168, 170
Calabar swellings, 735–736, 736f, 962f
  differential diagnosis, 737–738
Calcified parenchymal neurocysticercosis, 817, 817f
  treatment, 821
Caliciviruses, 411–416
  characteristics, 411, 412f–413f
  phylogeny, 413f
  see also Norovirus
Calliphoridae, 869
Callitrichid hepatitis, 457
Calodium hepaticum, 786, 786f
Calomys callosus, 442t–443t, 450f, 454
Calomys hildebrandii, 453, 455
Calomys laucha, 471t
Calomys musculinus, 442t–443t, 450f, 455
Calymmatobacterium granulomatis, 196, 1035
Cambaroides spp., 862
Camelpox, 369
Campylobacter spp., 145–149, 917t
  characterization, 145
  clinical features, 147, 917t
    inflammatory diarrhea
  diagnosis, 148
  epidemiology, 145–147, 146t
  incubation period, 929b
  life cycle, 146f
  military cases, 913
  pathogenesis and immunity, 147–148
  prevention and control, 148–149
  toxin, 113, 114t–115t
  travelers' diarrhea, 892, 924
  treatment and prognosis, 148, 918t
Campylobacter coli, 145, 146t
Campylobacter concisus, 145
Campylobacter curvus, 145
Campylobacter fetus, 145, 146t
Campylobacter hyointestinalis, 145, 146t
Campylobacter insulaenigrae, 145, 146t
Campylobacter jejuni, 4, 145
  and cancer, 73t
  subsp. *doylei*, 145, 146t
Campylobacter lari, 145, 146t
Campylobacter rectus, 145
Campylobacter sputorum, 145, 146t
Campylobacter upsaliensis, 145, 146t
Canada, Global Public Health Intelligence Network, 106
Cancer, 71–75
  infection-related, 71–74, 73t, 74f
    prevention, 74–75
  mortality, 72f
  and paracoccidioidomycosis, 583
Candida spp.
  macronodules, 955t
  vaginitis, 3–4
  see also Candidiasis
Candida albicans, 589–590
Candida dubliniensis, 589, 591
Candida glabrata, 574, 589–590
Candida guilliermondii, 589–590
Candida krusei, 589–590
Candida lusitaniae, 589–590
Candida parapsilosis, 589–590
  candidemia, 595
Candida tropicalis, 589–590
Candidiasis, 589–596
  agents, 589
  balanitis, 593
  bloodstream infections, 595–596
  cardiac involvement, 593
  chronic disseminated, 595
  esophageal, 589, 592
  hepatobiliary disease, 976t–977t
  joint and bone infection, 594
  meningitis and meningoencephalitis, 594
  mucocutaneous, 589, 591
  mucosal, 104t, 589–590, 917t
  ocular involvement, 1006–1007, 1007f
    endophthalmitis, 594–595
  oropharyngeal, 589, 591–592
  pathogenesis and immunity, 589–590
  peritonitis, 595
  pseudomembranous, 591–592
  respiratory tract infections, 593
  skin and nails, 590–591
    angular cheilitis, 590–591
    congenital, 591
    diaper dermatitis, 590–591
    miliaria, 590–591
    paronychia, 591
  systemic, 590
  urinary tract infection, 593–594
  vulvovaginal, 589, 592–593
    diagnosis, 1038t
    treatment, 1040t
Candiduria, 593–594
Cannomys badius, 586
Capillaria hepatica, 942t
Capillaria philippinensis, 917t
  diarrheal disease, 924
  eosinophilia, 942t
  eradication, 77t–79t
Capreomycin, 100t
  tuberculosis, 243
Caprine arthritis and encephalitis virus, 542f
Carbapenems, 96t–98t, 98
Carbenicillin, *E. coli* infection, 119
Carbohydrate metabolism, in infection, 27
Carbon dioxide laser, genital warts, 537
Carboxypenicillins, 96t–98t
Carbuncles, staphylococcal, 208–209
Carcinoembryonic antigen cell adhesion molecules *see* CEACAMs
Cardiac arrhythmias, strongyloidiasis, 810
Cardiopathy, Chagas' disease, 692
Caribbean
  drug-resistant *P. falciparum*, 654t
  measles, 350f
Carios spp., 295
Carp, as intermediate hoses of *C. sinensis*, 855
Carrión's disease, 266f, 267
  ocular involvement, 1002
Case-control studies, 12, 14
Caspofungin, 100t–101t
  candidemia, 596
  candidiasis, 592
  toxicity, 101t
Castelo dos Sonhos virus, 471t
Castleman's disease, 367
Cat-scratch disease, 265, 266f, 266t
  diagnosis, 269
  ocular involvement, 1002
  skin lesions, 962t–966t
  treatment and prognosis, 269
Catarrhal enteritis, 808
Categorical data, 13
Caterpillars
  stinging, 870–871
  urticating, 871
Cathelicidins, 54t

Catostomus commersoni, 855
Cavia spp., 276
CCR3, 5
CCR5, HIV infection, 545
CD1, cross-presentation, 60
CD3, 55
CD4, 5
  abnormalities in HIV/AIDS, 545, 1046
CD8, abnormalities in HIV/AIDS, 1046
CD11b/CD18, 55
CD16, 54–55
CD19, 57
CD21, 53, 57
CD21/CD19, 57
CD28, 57–58
CD32
  malaria protection, 37t
  malaria susceptibility, 37t
CD35, 53, 55
CD36, 658–659
  malaria protection, 37t
CD40, 53–54, 57–58
  malaria protection, 37t
CD44, 207
CD80, 53–54
CD86, 53–54
CD94, 54–55
CD206, 55
CEACAMs, 180, 186
Cefazolin, cellulitis, 210–211
Cefepime, 96t–98t
Cefixime
  cervicitis/urethritis, 1040t
  gonorrhoea, 189
    disseminated, 189
  typhoid/paratyphoid, 125, 125t, 918t
Cefoperazone
  in pregnancy, 1073t
  salmonellosis, 135
Cefoperazone-sulbactam, melioidosis, 222
Cefotaxime, 96t–98t
  H. influenzae, 194
  leptospirosis, 307
  melioidosis, 222
  pneumococcal meningitis, 201
  in pregnancy, 1073t
  typhoid/paratyphoid, 125t
  Vibrio spp., 161
Cefotetan, pelvic inflammatory disease, 190t, 1043t
Cefoxitin
  pelvic inflammatory disease, 190t, 1043t
  Salmonella resistance, 130t
Cefpodoxime
  cellulitis, 210–211
  gonorrhoea, 189
    disseminated, 189
Ceftazidime, 96t–98t
  melioidosis, 222
Ceftriaxone, 96t–98t
  cellulitis, 210–211
  cervicitis/urethritis, 1040t
  chancroid, 1035t
  donovanosis, 197
  gonorrhoea, 189
    disseminated, 189
  H. influenzae, 194
  Lyme disease, 301
  meningococcal disease, 181–182
  meningococcal prophylaxis, 182
  pelvic inflammatory disease, 190t, 1043t
  pneumococcal meningitis, 201
  in pregnancy, 1073t
  Salmonella spp.
    bacteremia, 135
    drug resistance, 130t
  shigellosis, 143t
  typhoid/paratyphoid, 125t, 918t
Cefuroxime, 96t–98t
  cellulitis, 210–211
Cefuroxime axetil
  cellulitis, 210–211
  Lyme disease, 301
Cell-associated virions, 370–372
Cell-mediated immunity, 57, 61
  typhoid/paratyphoid, 124
Cellulitis, 261–262
  H. influenzae, 194t
  S. pyogenes, 204
  staphylococcal, 210–211
Centers for Disease Control and Prevention, 105
  Division of Global Migration and Quarantine, 904
  Global Disease Detection Program, 107, 907
Centipedes, 872, 873f
Central America
  causes of fever, 926f
  malaria, 896f
    drug-resistant, 654t
Central nervous system *see* Neurologic disease
Central Plata virus, 471t
Centruroides exilicauda, 871
Cephalic tetanus, 285–286
Cephalosporins, 95, 96t–98t
  adverse reactions, eosinophilia, 947t
  see also individual drugs
Cephalothin, 96t–98t
  cellulitis, 210–211
  drug-resistant *Salmonella* spp., 130t
  E. coli infection, 119
Cercarial dermatitis, 849–850
  pruritus, 959t–961t
Cercopithecine virus-1, 355, 356t
Cerebral malaria, 655b, 655f–656f
  coma, 660
  immuno-mediated damage, 659–660
Cerebral paragonimiasis, 863–864
Cerebrospinal fluid *see* CSF
Cervical cancer, 71–72, 73t
  C. trachomatis, 317
  HPV, 533–534, 533t
  prevention, 74f
Cervical intraepithelial neoplasia
  HPV, 533t, 534
  visual diagnosis, 536
Cervicitis
  C. trachomatis, 316, 316t
  gonococcal, 186–187
  treatment, 1040t
Cestoda, 813, 824
Cestodaria, 813
Cestodes, 1–2
  chemotherapy, 80–82, 80t
  HIV coinfection, 1054
Chagas' disease, 17, 21, 50, 689–695
  agent, 689
  clinical features, 691–693
    acute disease, 691–692
    cardiopathy, 692
    chronic disease, 692–693
    dysphagia, 919–920
    gastrointestinal, 692–693, 692f
    meningoencephalitis, 691–692
    myocarditis, 691–692, 692f
    Romaña's sign, 691f, 1010, 1010f
    skin lesions, 962t–966t
  diagnosis, 693–694
    acute disease, 693
    chronic disease, 693–694
  epidemiology, 689–691
    Latin America, 689–690
    USA, 691
  geographic distribution, 690f
  HIV coinfection, 693, 899, 1051
  immunosuppressed patients, 693
  incubation period, 929b
  prevention and control, 695
  treatment and prognosis, 90–94, 694–695
    antiparasitic drugs, 694–695
    clinical disease, 695
Chagoma, 691
Chancre, syphilitic, 290
Chancroid, 952t, 967t–968t, 1034t
  agent *see Haemophilus ducreyi*
  clinical features, 1034t
  diagnosis, 1035t
  ocular involvement, 1003
Chapare virus, 442t–443t, 450f, 450t
  maintenance in rodent hosts, 455
  transmission, 454
Charcot-Leyden crystals, 643
  pleuropulmonary paragonimiasis, 863
Cheilosis, 28
Cheilostomatitis, e12t–e13t
Chemokines, disease associations, 36t
Chemoprophylaxis
  cholera, 156
  HIV/AIDS, 554–555
  influenza, 383
  malaria, 895
  meningococcal disease, 182
  travelers' diarrhea, 893–894
Chemotaxis, inhibition of, 7
Chest X-ray
  paracoccidioidomycosis, 583f
  reactivation tuberculosis, 231, 231f
  SARS, 395
Chi-square test, 13
Chickenpox *see* Varicella
Chiclero ulcer, 698t, 699
Chiggers *see* Trombiculid mites
Chikungunya virus, 519, 520t, 876t
  clinical features, 523
    ocular disease, 996
    skin lesions, 956t
  diagnosis, 524
  epidemiology, 522, 523f
  prevention and control, 524
  vectors *see Aedes aegypti*; *Aedis albopictus*
Children
  anemia, 1024
  brucellosis, 273
  gastrointestinal disease, 916
  immunization for travel, 891
  Lassa fever, 456
    swollen baby syndrome, 456
  malaria, 657, 1027, 1028f
    immunity, 653
  mortality
    causes of, 379f
    rate, 25t
  mycobacterial lymphadenitis, 245
  pneumonia
    etiology, 983b
    incidence, 985f
    mortality, 983f, 985f
  toxocariasis, 764–765
  tuberculosis, 232, 242
Chilomastix mesnili, 623, 631–632, 631f
Chimpanzee immunodeficiency virus, 542f
Chincha see Kissing bugs
Chironomus spp., 159
Chlamydia spp., 5
  biology, 314
  classification, 314
  developmental cycle, 315f
  elementary body, 314
  genetics, 314
  human diseases, 316t
Chlamydia abortus, 314, 320
Chlamydia caviae, 314, 320
Chlamydia felis, 314, 320
Chlamydia muridarum, 314, 320
Chlamydia pecorum, 314, 320
Chlamydia pneumoniae, 308, 314, 320
  drug resistance, 95, 308
Chlamydia psittaci, 308, 314, 320
  ocular involvement, 998
  pathogenesis and immunity, 321–322
  see also Psittacosis
Chlamydia suis, 314, 320

Chlamydia trachomatis, 308–309, 314
 antigenic composition and diversity, 309
 biologic characteristics, 308–309
 biovars, 308, 314
 eye infection
  nontrachoma, 997–998
  trachoma *see* Trachoma
 genital infection *see* Lymphogranuloma venereum
 isolation, 311–312
 molecular epidemiology, 315
 neonatal infections, 317
 pathogenesis and immunity, 315–316
 in pregnancy, 317
 serovars, 314
 vaccine, 315
Chlamydia-associated reactive arthritis syndrome, 998
Chlamydial heat shock protein, 316
Chlamydial proteasome-like activity factor, 315
Chlamydophila see Chlamydia
Chloramphenicol, 96t–98t, 99
 Borrelia spp., 300
 cat-scratch disease, 269
 E. coli infection, 119
 melioidosis, 222
 meningococcal disease, 181–182
 Oroya fever, 269
 plague, 282
 in pregnancy, 1073t
 Salmonella spp.
  bacteremia, 135
  drug resistance, 129, 130f, 130t
 scrub typhus, 338
 spotted fever rickettsioses, 328
 typhoid/paratyphoid, 125, 125t, 918t
 typhus, 332–333
Chlorcycloguanil, malaria, 664
Chlorhexidine gluconate
 Acanthamoeba keratitis, 713
 granulomatous amebic encephalitis, 712
Chloride, cholera stools, 153t
Chlorocebus aethiops, 490
Chloroplasts, 1
Chloroquine
 adverse effects, 82b, 897t
 fascioliasis, 861
 malaria, 664, 666, 667t, 895–896, 897t
  dose, 897t
  pregnancy, 671b
  prophylaxis, 83, 669t
 pharmacokinetics, 665t
 in pregnancy, 1073t
Chlorosis, hookworm, 802
Chlorproguanil-dapsone, malaria, 667
Choclo virus, 471t
 animal models, 477–478
 hantavirus pulmonary syndrome, 473
Cholangiocarcinoma, 856–857
Cholangitis, recurrent ascending, 856
Cholera, 150–156
 agent *see Vibrio cholerae*
 complications, 153
 diagnosis, 154
 epidemiology, 151–153
 host risk factors, 153
 incidence and geographic distribution, 151, 151f
 incubation period, 153
 infective agent, 150–151
 international surveillance and disease notification, 153
 modes of transmission, 152–153, 152f
 ocular involvement, 1003, 1004f
 pregnancy, 1073
 prevention and control, 156
  chemoprophylaxis, 156
  safe water and food, 156
  travelers, 156
 reservoirs, 151–152
 seasonality, 151
 stools, 153, 153t
 treatment, 154–156
  antimicrobial therapy, 155–156, 155t, 917t
  fluid therapy, 154
  intravenous rehydration, 154–155
  oral rehydration, 155
 vaccine, 64t–65t, 156, 888t–890t, 891
 see also Vibrio cholerae
Cholera enterotoxin, 150, 154
Cholesterol-dependent cytolysins, 207
Cholestyramine, hepatitis A, 422
Chondroitin sulfate A, 658–659
Chordopoxvirinae, 369
Chromoblastomycosis, 569–570
 agent, 569
 clinical features, 569–570, 570f, 969t–970t
 diagnosis, 570, 570f
 prevention and control, 570
 treatment and prognosis, 570
Chromomycosis *see* Chromoblastomycosis
Chronic granulomatous disease, 34t
Chrysomyia bezziana, 870, 870f, 1016
Chrysops spp., 735, 736f
Chrysops dimidiata, 735
Chrysops silacea, 735
Chvostek's sign, 286
Chyluria, 732
CI-1033, orthopoxviruses, 376–377
Cidofovir, 102t
 cytomegalovirus, 104t
 herpesviruses, 356
  HHV-6, 362
  HHV-7, 366
  HSV, 359
 human adenovirus, 380t, 390
 orthopoxviruses, 376
Ciliates, 1–2
Cimex hemipterus, 50–51, 871
Cimex lectularius see Bedbugs
Cinchona bark, 646
Ciprofloxacin, 96t–98t, 100t
 anthrax, 264
 Campylobacter spp., 148
 chancroid, 1035t
 cholera, 155–156, 155t
 cyclosporiasis, 642–643
 donovanosis, 197
 drug resistant *Salmonella* spp., 130t
 E. coli infection, 119
 gonorrhoea, 189
 H. ducreyi, 191
 H. pylori, 172t
 meningococcal prophylaxis, 182
 mycobacterial infections, 247
 Oroya fever, 269
 plague, 282
 shigellosis, 143f, 143t, 918t
 spotted fever rickettsioses, 328
 travelers' diarrhea, 894t
 typhoid/paratyphoid, 125, 125t, 918t
 Vibrio spp., 161
Circumcision, HPV prevention, 538
Cirrhosis, 917t
 chronic, 976t–977t, 978
Citellophilus spp., 277
Citrobacter spp., 113
Citrobacter freundii, toxin, 114t–115t
Citrobacter rodentium, toxin, 114t–115t
Civil conflict, 20
Cladophialophora bantiana, 571
Cladophialophora carrionii, 569
Clarithromycin, 96t–98t, 99, 100t
 anthrax, 264
 Campylobacter spp., 148
 cat-scratch disease, 269
 cellulitis, 210–211
 granulomatous amebic encephalitis, 712
 H. pylori, 172t, 173b, 918t
 leprosy, 259
 MAC, 246
  in HIV, 246–247
 Mycobacterium avium complex, 104t
 pertussis, 214
 in pregnancy, 1073t
 scrub typhus, 338
 spotted fever rickettsioses, 328
 toxoplasmosis, 727
Climate, 8
Clindamycin, 96t–98t, 99
 anthrax, 264
 babesiosis, 680
 bacterial vaginosis, 1040t
 cellulitis, 210–211
 malaria, 667t
 P. jirovecii, 86t–87t, 104t
 pelvic inflammatory disease, 190t, 1043t
 pneumocystosis, 612
 in pregnancy, 1073t
 staphylococcal toxic shock syndrome, 210
 toxoplasmosis, 727
Clinical studies
 data expression and analysis, 13–14
 design, 11–12
 hypothesis testing, 12–14
Clinical trials, 12
 cohort studies, 12
 equivalence studies, 12
 placebo-controlled, 12
Clobazam, cysticercosis, 820
Clofazimine, 100t
 leprosy, 259
Clonidine, tetanus, 287–288
Clonorchiasis, 854–858
 agent *see Clonorchis sinensis*
 clinical features, 855–857
  acute, 855
  cholangiocarcinoma, 856–857, 976t–977t, 981
  chronic, 855–856
  eosinophilia, 942t–943t
  recurrent ascending cholangitis/pancreatitis, 856
 diagnosis, 857–858
 epidemiology, 854–855
 immunodiagnosis, 858
 pathogenesis and immunity, 857
 treatment, 858
Clonorchis sinensis, 854
 and cancer, 71–72, 73t, 856–857
 diagnosis, 867
 epidemiology, 854
 eradication, 81t
 fish hosts, 855
 geographic distribution, 857f
 life cycle, 856f
 morphology, 854, 857f
 snail vectors, 855
 see also Clonorchiasis
Clostridium spp., 162–166
 characteristics, 162
Clostridium botulinum, 162, 165–166
 as bioterrorism agent, 880t, 882
  diagnosis, 886
 toxin, 882
Clostridium difficile, 3–4, 162–164
 animal infection, 163
 diagnosis, 163–164, 164f
 disease, 163
 environmental sources, 163
 epidemiology, 162–163
 exotoxin, 5
 fulminant colitis, 164
 human carriage, 163
 pathogenesis and immunity, 163
 prevention and control, 164
 recurrent disease, 164
 risk factors, 163
 treatment and prognosis, 164
Clostridium perfringens, 7, 162, 164–165
 agent, 164–165
 diagnosis, 165

disease, 164–165
epidemiology, 164
immunity, 164–165
pathogenesis, 164–165
treatment and prevention, 165
Clostridium septicum, 166
Clostridium tetani, 284, 285f
pathogenesis and immunity, 286
toxin, 2
see also Tetanus
Clotrimazole
candidiasis, 592
dermatophytosis, 563
vulvovaginal candidiasis, 1040t
Cloxacillin, 96t–98t
Clutton's joints, 291
Co-trimoxazole
actinomycetoma, 568
B. hominis, 622
brucellosis, 273, 275
donovanosis, 197
isosporiasis, 644
melioidosis, 222
Q fever, 346
Coagulation defects
malaria, 660
yellow fever, 497–498
Coccidia, 641
Coccidiasina, 633
Coccidiida, 646
Coccidioides immitis, 577, 577f, 605
HIV coinfection, 1057
skin lesions, 957t
Coccidioidomycosis, 577–579
agent *see Coccidioides immitis*
clinical features, 578, 578f
ocular involvement, 1008
pleural effusion, 988t
skin lesions, 969t–970t
diagnosis, 578–579
endemic range, 577f
epidemiology, 577–578
incubation period, 929b
military cases, 914
pathogenesis and immunity, 578
prevention and control, 579
treatment and prognosis, 579
Coccidiosis, HIV coinfection, 1053
Cochliomyia hominivorax, 870, 870f
Cod worm disease *see Pseudoterranova* spp.
Codiella inflata, 855
Codiella leachi, 855
Codiella troscheli, 855
Coenuriasis, 822–823
agent, 822
clinical features, 822
eosinophilia, 942t
ocular involvement, 1015
skin lesions, 962t–966t
diagnosis, 822f, 823
epidemiology, 822
prevention and control, 823
Cohort studies, 12
Cold sores *see* Herpes labialis
Coleoptera, 873
Colitis, amebic, 616–617, 617f, 617t
Collagenases, 4
Colonization, 3–4
Colonization factor antigens, 113
Colorado tick fever, 4, 875t
skin lesions, 956t
Colposcopy, HPV, 536
Commensalism, 1
Common cold, 398
see also Human rhinovirus
Complement fixation test, arenaviruses, 451
Complement system, 33, 52–53
costimulation, 57
inherited disorders, 34t
see also individual proteins
Condoms, HPV prevention, 538
Condylomata acuminata *see* Genital warts
Confidence intervals, 14
Confounding, 12
Congenital disease
candidiasis, 591
cytomegalovirus, 725–726
herpes simplex virus, 725–726
rubella syndrome, 349, 351, 725–726
syphilis, 291
toxoplasmosis, 723f, 724, 725f
varicella syndrome, 360
see also inherited conditions
Congenital rubella syndrome, 349, 351, 725–726
Conidiobolomycosis, 603
treatment, 604t
Conidiobolus spp., 603
Conidiobolus coronatus, 603
Conidiobolus incongruus, 603
Conjunctival papillomas/carcinomas, 533t
Conjunctivitis, 1004, 1005f, 1034t
acute hemorrhagic, 991, 992f
adult inclusion, 997–998
C. trachomatis, 316t, 317
causes, 992b, 1004b
enterovirus, 398, 402
influenza, 991
see also Trachoma
Constipation
brucellosis, 271
giardiasis, 627t
Constitutional symptoms, 27
Continuous ambulatory peritoneal dialysis, candidal peritonitis, 595
Continuous data, 13
Copper, requirements, e12t–e13t
Coquillettidia perturbans, eastern equine encephalitis, 876t
Cordylobia anthropophaga, 870, 1016
Corneal microsporidiosis, *M. africanus*, 718
Corneal opacity, trachoma, 311b
Corneal ulcers, smallpox, 371
Coronavirus-like particles, 418
Coronaviruses, 378, 380t, 388–389, 417t, 418–419
agent, 388
clinical features, 388
diagnosis, 389
epidemiology, 388
pathogenesis and immunity, 388–389
treatment and prevention, 389
Corticosteroids
cysticercosis, 821
extrapulmonary tuberculosis, 242
pneumocystosis, 612
retinochoroiditis, 727
typhoid/paratyphoid, 126
Corynebacterium diphtheriae, 207, 223
life cycle, 224f
see also Diphtheria
Corynebacterium minutissimum, 973t
Corynebacterium pseudotuberculosis, 223
Corynebacterium ulcerans, 223
Cosavirus, 398
Côte d'Ivoire ebolavirus, 483, 485t
Cough, 986
differential diagnosis, 986b
Coumermycins, *Borrelia* spp., 300
Councilman bodies, 458, 499
Cowpox, 369, 371
Cox, Herald Rae, 344
Coxiella spp., 5
Coxiella burnetii, 344, 345f
antibodies to, 344
as bioterrorism agent, 880t, 883
diagnosis, 886
life cycle, 345f
pathogenesis and immunity, 346
skin lesions, 957t
see also Q fever
Coxsackievirus-adenovirus receptor, 403
Coxsackieviruses, 398, 399t
selenium deficiency, 26–27
CR1, 53, 54t, 55–56
malaria protection, 37t
CR2, 54t, 56
CR3, 54t
CR4, 56
Crab lice *see Phthirus pubis*
Cranial neuropathy, syphilitic, 290
Crayfish, spread of *P. westermani*, 862
Creatine phosphokinase
Crimean-Congo hemorrhagic fever, 467
trichinellosis, 772
Creatinine, malaria, 655b
Creeping eruption *see* Cutaneous larva migrans
Cricetidae, 470
Crimean-Congo hemorrhagic fever, 442t–443t, 466–469, 467f
agent, 466
as bioterrorism agent, 880t
clinical features, 444t–445t, 467
diagnosis, 447t, 467
epidemiology, 466, 468f
global distribution, 467f
pathogenesis and immunity, 467
pathologic features, 446t
prevention and control, 448t, 467–469
skin lesions, 956t
transmission, 875t, 932t
treatment and prognosis, 448t, 467–469
CRM197, 226
Cross-presentation, 60
Crotamiton
adverse effects, 94b
scabies, 93t, 868–869
Croup, HPIVs, 385
Cryopyrin, 53, 54t
Cryotherapy
cutaneous leishmaniasis, 705
genital warts, 537
Cryptococcoma, 581
Cryptococcosis, 579–581
agent, 574, 579
clinical features, 580, 580f
ocular involvement, 1007
pleural effusion, 987t
skin lesions, 969t–970t
diagnosis, 580
drug therapy, 104t
epidemiology, 579–580
HIV coinfection, 1057–1058
meningitis, 580
pathogenesis and immunity, 580
prevention and control, 581
treatment and prognosis, 580–581
Cryptococcus gattii, 579–580
Cryptococcus neoformans, 574, 579
Cryptosporidiosis, 633–640
clinical features, 636–637
diarrheal disease, 635, 636f, 922
complications, 637
diagnosis, 638, 639f
epidemiology, 633–636
pathogenesis and immunity, 637–638
pathology, 637
prevention and control, 640
treatment and prognosis, 88t–89t, 104t, 638–640, 918t
Cryptosporidium spp., 1–2, 7, 552, 625, 633
as bioterrorism agent, 880t, 883
diagnosis, 886
history, 633
HIV coinfection, 636, 638, 639f, 1053
life cycle, 633, 635f
oocysts, 634
taxonomy, 633, 634f
travelers' diarrhea, 924
see also Cryptosporidiosis
Cryptosporidium andersoni, 634f
Cryptosporidium baileyi, 634f

Cryptosporidium canis, 634f
Cryptosporidium felis, 634f, 883
Cryptosporidium gaffi, 634f
Cryptosporidium hominis, 627, 634f, 883
Cryptosporidium meleagridis, 634f, 883
Cryptosporidium moinari, 634f
Cryptosporidium muris, 634f, 883
Cryptosporidium nasoris, 634f
Cryptosporidium parvum, 634f, 917t
  diarrheal disease, 922
  life cycle, 635f
Cryptosporidium saurophilium, 634f
Cryptosporidium serpentis, 634f
Cryptosporidium wrairi, 634f
CSF
  A. cantonensis infection, 775–776
  African trypanosomiasis, 685–686
  eosinophilia, 775–776, 947, 947b
  tuberculous meningitis, 235
Ctenocephalides felis, 266t, 267, 330, 876
Ctenoiphthalmus nobilis nobilis, 266t
Ctenopharyngodon idellus, 855
Culex spp., 49, 462–463, 521–522
  filariasis, 730–731, 876t
  West Nile encephalitis, 876t
Culex annulirostris, 522
Culex nigripalpus, St Louis encephalitis, 876t
Culex pipiens, 49
Culex pipiens quinquefasciatus, 51
  St Louis encephalitis, 876t
Culex tarsalis
  St Louis encephalitis, 876t
  western equine encephalitis, 876t
Culex tritaeniorhynchus, 511
  Japanese encephalitis, 876t
Culicoides spp., 8–9, 739
  zoonotic filariasis, 750
Culicoides austeni, 739
Culicoides fulvithorax, 739
Culicoides furens, 739, 740
Culicoides grahamii, 738, 739
Culicoides imicola, 8–9
Culicoides kingi, 739
Culicoides milnei, 739
Culicoides obsoletus, 8–9
Culicoides paraensis, 482
Culicoides pulicaris, 8–9
Culture filtrate protein-10, 230
Cuniculus paca, 837
Cunninghamella bertholletiae, 597
Cupixi virus, 450f
Curvularia lunata, 571
Cutaneous anergy, 23
Cutaneous larva migrans, 766–767, 767f, 800–801, 946t, 950, 958t, 961f
  clinical features
    eosinophilia, 942t
    pruritus, 959t–961t
  eradication, 76, 77t–79t
  fascioliasis, 860
Cutaneous lesions *see* Skin lesions
CXCR4, 5
  HIV infection, 545
Cycloguanil, malaria, 664
Cyclophyllidea, 813
  rostellum, 813, 814f
Cyclops, 759
Cyclops spp., 842–843, 845
Cycloserine, 100t
  in pregnancy, 1073t
  tuberculosis, 243
Cyclospora spp., 552, 634f, 641–643, 642f
Cyclospora cayetanensis, 627, 641, 916, 917t
  characteristics and epidemiology, 641–642
  diarrheal disease, 922–923
  HIV coinfection, 641–642, 1053
  life cycle, 641
  seasonality of infections, 641
  treatment, 918t
  see also Cyclosporiasis
Cyclospora cercopitheci, 641
Cyclospora colobi, 641
Cyclospora papionis, 641
Cyclosporiasis, 641
  children, 641–642
  clinical features, 642
  diagnosis, 642
  prevention and control, 643
  prophylaxis, 643
  treatment and prognosis, 88t–89t, 642–643
  see also Cyclospora cayetanensis
Cynomys gunnisoni, 276
Cynomys ludovicianus, 276
Cyprinus carpio, 855
Cystic echinococcosis, 824–832
  agent *see Echinococcus granulosus*
  clinical features, 826–828, 829f
  diagnosis, 829–831, 830f
  pathogenesis and immunity, 828–829
  prevention and control, 832
  transmission, epidemiology and geographic distribution, 825–826
  treatment and prognosis, 831–832
    chemotherapy, 831
    monitoring of results, 832
    PAIR, 831–832
    surgery, 831
Cystic fibrosis, 33
Cystic fibrosis transmembrane conductance regulator gene, 33
Cystic neurocysticercosis, 817, 817f
  treatment, 821
Cysticercosis, 814–823
  agent *see Taenia solium*
  clinical features, 815–818
    eosinophilia, 939
    extraparenchymal neurocysticercosis, 817–818
    muscular involvement, 818
    ocular involvement, 818, 818f, 1015, 1015f
    parenchymal neurocysticercosis, 817
    skin lesions, 946t, 962t–966t
  diagnosis, 819–820, 820b
  epidemiology, 815
  imaging, 819
  paragonimiasis, 776
  pathogenesis and immunity, 818–819
  prevention, 822
  treatment and prognosis, 820–822
    antiparasitic drugs, 821
    calcified parenchymal neurocysticercosis, 821
    corticosteroids, 821
    parenchymal neurocysticercosis with cystic lesions, 821
    subarachnoid neurocysticercosis and giant cysticerci, 821–822
    symptomatic therapy, 820
    ventricular neurocysticercosis, 821
Cystoisospora belli see Cystoisosporiasis
Cysts, 966
Cytoadherence, 658
Cytokines, 56
  disease associations, 36t
  genetic variation, 33
  leishmaniasis, 702–703
  malaria, 657–658
Cytolysins, cholesterol-dependent, 207
Cytomegalovirus, 4, 355, 356t, 361–362
  agent, 361
  clinical features, 361, 362f, 917t
    ocular disease, 994–995, 994f
    skin lesions, 956t
  congenital, 725–726
  diagnosis, 362
  epidemiology, 361
  incubation period, 929b
  pathogenesis and immunity, 361–362
  pregnancy, 1081
  prevention and control, 362
  treatment and prognosis, 362
    drug therapy, 104t
Cytotoxic T cells, 58

D

Dacryoadenitis, mumps, 993
Dafachronic acid, 808
DALYs, 7, 24
  E. coli infection, 110
DAMPs, 53–54
Dane particles, 433
Dantrolene
  adverse reactions
    eosinophilia, 947t
    pleural effusion, 988t
Dapaong tumor, 781
Dapsone
  actinomycetoma, 568
  adverse effects, 85b
  leprosy, 259
  Pneumocystis jirovecii, 86t–87t
  pneumocystis pneumonia, 104t
  pneumocystosis, 612–613
  in pregnancy, 1073t
  rhinosporidiosis, 605
  toxoplasmosis, 727
Daptomycin, 96t–98t, 98–99
  MRSA, 211
Darmbrand, 165
Darunivir, 103t
  HIV, 553–554
Dasyprocta spp., 837
Data expression, 13–14
DDT, 40
  malaria control, 646
  typhus control, 333
Deafness
  hemorrhagic fevers, 445t
  Lassa fever, 457
Dectin-1, 55
Deep-vein thrombosis, 901
Deer flies, 50, 871–872
Deer tick virus, 516f
DEET, 510, 524, 681, 705
  biting midges, 872
  mosquitoes, 895
Defensins, 52–53, 54t
Deferasirox, mucormycosis, 601
Dehydration
  cholera, 154–155
  dengue shock syndrome, 510
  diarrheal disease, 921–924, 922t
  E. coli infection, 119
  travelers' diarrhea, 894
Dehydroemetine, fascioliasis, 861
Delavirdine, 103t
  HIV, 553–554
Delayed type hypersensitivity, 61
Delhi boil, 699
Deltavirus, 435
Delusional parasitosis, 1066–1071
  approach to, 1069
  classification, 1066–1067
  clinical features and presentation, 1068–1069
  diagnosis, 1067b
  epidemiology, 1067–1068
  history, 1066
  management, 1069–1071
    antipsychotic agents, 1070–1071
    psychiatric assessment, 1069–1070
    treatment, 1070–1071
  outcome and prognosis, 1071
  primary, 1067
  psychiatric manifestations, 1066
  secondary
    underlying medical conditions, 1067, 1068t
    underlying psychiatric disease, 1067
Dementia, e12t–e13t

Demodex brevis, 869
Demodex folliculorum, 869
Dendritic cells, 55–56
abnormalities in AIDS, 1046
follicular, 56
HRSV infection, 384
plasmacytoid, 56
subsets of, 56
Dengue fever, 7, 17, 21, 416, 442t–443t, 504–510, 516f, 876t
agent *see Aedes aegypti*
changing disease patterns, 505–507
classification, 507f
clinical features, 444t–445t, 507–509
fever, 926t–927t
skin lesions, 954f, 956t–957t
diagnosis, 447t, 509–510
epidemiology, 505–507
global distribution, 505f
Americas, 506f
increased incidence, 507
incubation period, 929b
military cases, 912
natural history, 505
pathogenesis and immunity, 509
pathologic features, 446t
pregnancy, 1073–1074
prevention and control, 448t, 510
transmission, 932t
treatment and prognosis, 448t, 510
vectors, 51
with/without warning signs, 507
Dengue hemorrhagic fever, 508–509, 508t
Dengue shock syndrome, 442t–443t, 508–509
clinical features, 444t–445t
diagnosis, 447t
genetic protection, 35t
genetic susceptibility, 35t
pathologic features, 446t
Depurinase, 5
Dermacentor spp., 515
Dermacentor andersoni, 324, 875t
Dermacentor cajennense, 324
Dermacentor marginatus, 875t
Dermacentor nuttalli, 875t
Dermacentor occidentalis, and *A. phagocytophilum*, 342
Dermacentor reticulatus, 515
Dermacentor silvarum, 875t
Dermacentor variabilis, 324, 875, 875t
and *A. phagocytophilum*, 342
Dermanyssus gallinae, 872–873
Dermatitis
cercarial, 849–850, 959t–961t
diaper, 590–591
onchocerciasis, 742–744, 744f
onchodermatitis, 742–744, 744f
plant, 972t
see also Skin lesions
Dermatobia hominis, 869, 869f, 1016
larva, 870f
Dermatolymphangioadenitis, lymphatic filariasis, 731–732
Dermatophytosis, 559–564
agents, 559, 560t
diagnosis, 563
diseases, 559–562
epidemiology, 559
geographic distribution, 560t
in HIV/AIDS, 562
pathogenesis and immunity, 562–563
prevention and control, 564
treatment and prognosis, 563
Dermatosis, 28
Desferrioxamine, 1031
Desmodillus spp., 276–277
Dexamethasone
African trypanosomiasis, 688t
altitude sickness, 900–901
H. influenzae, 194
meningococcal disease, 182
Oroya fever, 269
pneumococcal meningitis, 201
typhoid/paratyphoid, 126
Dhaka Solution, 154–155
Diabetes mellitus, mucormycosis infection, 597–598
Diamanus montanus, 276
Diaper dermatitis, 590–591
Diaptomus spp., 842–843
Diarrheal disease, 17, 23, 28, 917t, 921–924
acute inflammatory diarrhea, 923
acute watery diarrhea, 921–923
amebic, 616
Brainerd diarrhea, 924
C. cayetanensis, 922–923
C. parvum, 922
calicivirus, 412, 414t
Campylobacter see Campylobacter spp.
cholera *see* Cholera
cryptosporidiosis, 635, 636f, 922
dehydration, 922t
E. coli see Escherichia coli
effect on anthropometric indicators, 25t
enteric adenovirus, 418
enterovirus, 402
eosinophilia, 945–946, 946b
and fever, 933–934
gastroenteritis, 923
giardiasis, 627t
military cases, 913
and nutritional status, 27–28
persistent/chronic diarrhea, 923–924
rotavirus, 407f, 408
Salmonella see Salmonellosis
travelers', 887, 892–894, 924
chemoprophylaxis, 893–894
food and water precautions, 892–893
HIV/AIDS infection, 899
self-treatment, 894, 894t
trichinellosis, 770
Vibrio, 160
zinc supplements, 26
see also individual diseases
Diarrhée de la Cochinchine, 805
Diazepam, tetanus, 287–288
Dichotomous data, 13
Diclazuril, isosporiasis, 644
Dicloxacillin, 96t–98t
cellulitis, 210–211
Dicrocoeliasis, 942t
Didanosine, 103t
HIV, 553
Didelphis aurita, 323–324
Dientamoeba fragilis, 622–623, 622t, 631, 631f
treatment, 88t–89t, 628t
Diethylcarbamazine, 79
adverse effects, 82b, 734, 738
filariasis, 77t–79t, 79
lymphatic, 734
loaiasis, 77t–79t, 79, 738
prophylaxis, 900
onchocerciasis, 748
streptocerciasis, 77t–79t, 79, 739
toxocariasis, 766
tropical pulmonary eosinophilia, 77t–79t
Diffuse toxic erythema, 955t
Diffusely adherent *E. coli*, 111t, 118
clinical features, 112t
Difimicin, *C. difficile*, 164
Dihydroartemisinin, 664
pharmacokinetics, 665t
Dihydroartemisinin-piperaquine, malaria, 667–668, 667t
Diloxanide furoate, 89
adverse effects, 85b
amebiasis, 88t–89t, 621
Dimycolate, 236–237
Dinopsyllus spp., 276–277
Dipetalonema spp., 750
Dipetalonema perstans, 739
Dipetalonema semiclarum, 751t, 757
Dipetalonema streptocerca, 738
Dipetalonema-like organisms
diagosis, 756
ocular involvement, 751t
Diphenoxylate
cryptosporidiosis, 638
norovirus, 414
Diphtheria, 223–227, 263
agent, 223
clinical features, 224–226
bull-necked appearance, 224
ocular involvement, 1002–1003
pseudomembrane, 224, 225f
complications, 224–225
myocarditis, 224–225
neuropathy, 225
cutaneous, 225, 967t–968t
diagnosis, 226
epidemiology, 223–224
incidence, 224f
incubation period, 929b
prevention and control, 226–227
treatment and prognosis, 226
vaccine, 64t–65t, 226–227
Diphtheria antitoxin, 226
Diphtheria toxin, 5, 223, 225–226
cross-reacting material, 226
structure, 225f
Diphtheria/tetanus/pertussis vaccine, 888t–890t
requirements for immigrants, 908t
Diphtheria/tetanus/polio vaccine, 64t–65t
Diphyllobothriasis, 841–843
agent *see Diphyllobothrium* spp.
clinical features, 843
diagnosis, 843
epidemiology, 843
prevention and control, 843
treatment and prognosis, 843
Diphyllobothrium spp., 813, 841–843
life cycle, 841–842, 842f
ova, 813–814
Diphyllobothrium cordatum, 843
Diphyllobothrium dalliae, 843
Diphyllobothrium dendriticum, 843
Diphyllobothrium klebaanovskii, 843
Diphyllobothrium latum, 24, 813
epidemiology, 843
eradication, 80t
ova, 842f
proglottids, 842f
scolex, 842f
Diphyllobothrium nihonkaiense, 843
Diphyllobothrium pacificum, 813
epidemiology, 843
life cycle, 840f
Diphyllobothrium ursi, 843
Diplococcus intracellularis meningitidis, 174
Diplogonoporus grandis, 843
Diploscapter coronata, 778–779
Diptera, 45, 49
Dipylidiasis, 845
agent *see Dipylidium caninum*
clinical features, 845, 846f
epidemiology, 845
treatment and prevention, 845
Dipylidium spp., 813
Dipylidium caninum, 845
egg pockets, 846f
eradication, 80t
flea host, 876
life cycle, 846f
proglottids, 846f
scolex, 846f
Direct immunofluorescence
C. trachomatis, 318
Q fever, 346
Directly observed therapy *see* DOT
Dirifolaria repens, 737–738
Dirithromycin, 99
Dirofilaria spp., diagnosis, 755, 755f–756f

Dirofilaria conjunctivae, 750
Dirofilaria immitis, 750, 751t, 808
clinical features, 753f
diagnosis, 755f
pulmonary disease, 984t
Dirofilaria repens, 750, 751t
clinical features, 752f
diagnosis, 755f–756f
Dirofilaria striata, 751t
Dirofilaria tenuis, 750, 751t
clinical features, 752f–753f
diagnosis, 755f
Dirofilaria ursi, 751t
Dirofilariasis, 942t
ocular involvement, 1013, 1013f
skin lesions, 962t–966t
Disability-adjusted life years *see* DALYs
Disease eradication/control, 40–44
barriers to, 17–22
access to care, 19
brain drain, 18–19
civil conflict and natural disaster, 20
economic austerity, 19
economic costs and adherence to HIV therapy, 20
stigma, 20
structural, 18–20
structural adjustment, 19
user fees, 19–20
candidate infectious agents, 40–41, 41f
biological and epidemiological characteristics, 40–41, 41b
feasibility, 41–44, 42t
public health terms describing, 41, 41b, 42t
see also individual diseases
Disease frequency measures, 11
Disease transmission vectors *see* Vector-borne disease transmission
Dispersin, 114t–115t, 118
Disseminated intravascular coagulation, 464, 467
malaria, 655b
Disseminated mucormycosis, 600
DNA gyrase inhibitors, 96t–98t, 99
DNases, 203
group A streptococcus, 207
Dobrava-Belgrade virus, 470–472, 471t
hemorrhagic fever with renal syndrome, 475
n-Docosanol, herpesviruses, HSV, 359
Dog tapeworm *see Dipylidum caninum*
Donovan bodies, 196
Donovanosis, 196–198
characteristics, 196
clinical features, 196–197, 197f
cutaneous lesions, 952t
granuloma inguinale *see* Granuloma inguinale
diagnosis, 197, 197f
epidemiology, 196
HIV coinfection, 196–197
prevention and control, 198
treatment and prognosis, 197–198
Doripenem, 96t–98t, 98
DOT
HIV, 18
tuberculosis, 241
Double-blind randomized trials, 12
Doxycycline
adverse effects, 897t
adverse reactions, 897–898
anthrax, 264
babesiosis, 680
Borrelia infections, 300
brucellosis, 275, 918t
cat-scratch disease, 269
cervicitis/urethritis, 1040t
cholera, 155, 155t, 918t
donovanosis, 197
ehrlichial, anaplasmal and neorickettsial infections, 343
granuloma inguinale, 1035t
legionellosis, 218
leptospirosis, 307
Lyme disease, 301
lymphatic filariasis, 734
lymphogranuloma venereum, 318, 1035t
M. ozzardi, 740
malaria, 667t, 897–898, 897t
dose, 897t
prophylaxis, 84, 669t
melioidosis, 222
mycobacterial infections, 247
onchocerciasis, 748
pelvic inflammatory disease, 190t, 1043t
perstans filiariasis, 739
plague, 281–282
in pregnancy, 1073t
psittacosis, 322
Q fever, 346
scrub typhus, 338
spotted fever rickettsioses, 328
syphilis, 292, 1035t
typhus, 332–333
Dracunculiasis, 759–762
agent *see Dracunculus medinensis*
clinical features, 759, 761f
eosinophilia, 942t
ocular involvement, 1014
pleural effusion, 988t
pruritus, 959t–961t
skin lesions, 946t, 958t, 962t–966t
diagnosis, 759–760
epidemiology, 759, 760f
global distribution, 760f
pathogenesis and immunity, 759–760
prevention and control, 761–762, 761f
treatment and prognosis, 760
Dracunculiasis Eradication Program, 761
Dracunculus medinensis, 41, 759
eradication, 43, 77t–79t
comparison with poliovirus, 43
feasibility, 42t
life cycle, 760f
see also Dracunculiasis
Droplet transmission, 910–911
Drug abuse, overseas medical screening, 904t
Drug interactions, antimalarials, 664–665
Drug resistance
surveillance projects, 108
tuberculosis, 237–238
see also individual organisms
Drug-associated reactions
delusional parasitosis, 1068t
pleural effusion, 988t
skin lesions, 971–973, 974t
Duffy blood group antigen, 4–5, 650
lack of in malaria protection, 36t, 653
Duffy-binding protein, 650
Duncan's disease, 363
Duodenal ulcer, *H. pylori*, 169, 169f
Dust-borne pathogens, military cases, 914–915
Duvenhage virus, 526t
Dwarf tapeworm *see Hymenolepsis nana*
Dysarthria, hemorrhagic fevers, 445t
Dysentery
amebic, 616–617, 617f, 617t
ocular involvement, 1004
protein losses, 27
Shigella spp., 141, 141f
Dyserythropoiesis, malaria, 660
Dyskeratosis, 535
Dysphagia, 592, 917t, 919–920
cephalic tetanus, 285–286
Chagas' disease, 919–920
Dyspnea, trichinellosis, 770

E

E-cadherin, 139–140
E-selectin, 658–659
Early induced response, 6t
Early secreted antigen-6, 230
EAST-1, 118
Eastern equine encephalitis, 520t, 876t
Ebola virus, 7, 442t–443t
as bioterrorism agent, 880f
clinical features, 444t–445t
diagnosis, 447t
incubation period, 929b
pathologic features, 446t
skin lesions, 956t
transmission, 932t
treatment and prevention, 448t
Ebolaviruses, 483
outbreaks, 486f
Ecdysteroids, 807–808
Echinocandins, 100t–101t, 590
candidemia, 595–596
candidiasis, 592
cardiac, 593
chromoblastomycosis, 570
mucormycosis, 601
Echinococcosis, 824–838
alveolar, 824, 833–837
agent *see Echinococcus multilocularis*
clinical features, 834–835, 834f, 988t
diagnosis, 835–836, 836f
pathogenesis and immunity, 835
prevention and control, 836–837
transmission, epidemiology and geographic distribution, 833
treatment, 836
cystic, 824–832
agent *see Echinococcus granulosus*
clinical features, 826–828, 829f
diagnosis, 829–831, 830f
pathogenesis and immunity, 828–829
prevention and control, 832
transmission, epidemiology and geographic distribution, 825–826
treatment and prognosis, 831–832
eosinophilia, 942t
neurologic involvement, 1019t, 1021
ocular involvement, 1015
polycystic, 824, 837–838
agent *see Echinococcus oligarthrus*; *Echinococcus vogeli*
clinical features, 837–838
diagnosis, 838, 838f
prevention and control, 838
transmission, epidemiology and geographic distribution, 837
treatment, 838
skin lesions, 946t, 962t–966t
Echinococcus spp., 813, 824
life cycle, 829f
Echinococcus granulosus, 813, 824–825
eradication, 80t
geographic distribution, 827f
life cycle, 827f, 829f
morphology, 825f
pulmonary disease, 984t
species and strains, 824–825, 826t
Echinococcus multilocularis, 824, 833
eradication, 80t
geographic distribution, 833, 834f
life cycle, 829f, 833f
morphology, 825f
species and strains, 826t
Echinococcus oligarthrus, 824, 826t, 837
life cycle, 829f, 837f
morphology, 825f
Echinococcus shiquicus, 824, 826t
Echinococcus vogeli, 824, 826t, 837
life cycle, 829f, 837f
morphology, 825f
Echinostoma spp., 865–866
characteristics, 866
diagnosis, 867
disease, 866
epidemiology, 866

Echinostoma ilocanum, 866
Echinostoma malayanum, 866
Echinostoma revolutum, 866
Echinostomatidae, 866
Echinostomiasis, 942t
Echoviruses, 398, 399t, 419
Ecthyma gangrenosum, 591, 955t
Ectocervicitis, 1034t
Ectoparasites, treatment, 93t, 94b
Eczema vaccinatum, 375
Edema
  Buruli ulcer, 250
  lymphatic filariasis, 732, 732f
  pulmonary, malaria, 660
  trichinellosis, 770
Edema factor, 263
Edematous enteritis, 808
Edge Hill virus, 492
Efavirenz, 103t
  HIV, 553–554
  TB-HIV, 242–243
Effect, measures of, 11
Effective reproductive number, 11
Eflornithine, 92
  adverse effects, 90b
  African trypanosomiasis, 91t–92t, 686–687, 688t
Ehrlich, Paul, 300
Ehrlichia spp., 7, 339
Ehrlichia canis, 339
Ehrlichia chaffeensis, 339, 874, 933
  B. microti coinfection, 679
  life cycle, 340f
  pathogenesis and immunity, 340–341
Ehrlichia ewingii, 4, 341–342
  life cycle, 340f
Ehrlichia ruminantium, 339
Ehrlichioses, 339–343
  agents, 339
  E. chaffeensis, 339–342
    agent, 339
    diagnosis, 341, 342f
    disease, 340, 341t
    epidemiology, 339–340
    human monocytic, 874, 875t
    pathogenesis and immunity, 340–341
  E. ewingii, 341–342
  HIV coinfection, 1060–1061
  incubation period, 929b
  military cases, 912
  prevention and control, 343
  treatment, 343
Eikenella spp., 184
Eimeria spp., 634f, 641
Eimeriorina, 633
Ekbom's syndrome, 1066
El Moro Canyon virus, 472
Elastase, 5
Electrolytes, cholera stools, 153, 153t
Electromyography, trichinellosis, 771
Electronic disease notification system, 906
Electrosurgery, genital warts, 537
Elephantiasis
  lymphatic filariasis, 729
  streptocerciasis, 738
  treatment, 734
Eliocharis tuberossa, 865
ELISA
  arenaviruses, 451
  Brugia spp., 754
  C. trachomatis, 318
  Chagas' disease, 693
  Crimean-Congo hemorrhagic fever, 467
  cystic echinococcosis, 830
  fascioliasis, 861
  HHV-6, 365
  HSV antigen, 359
  leishmaniasis, 703
  lymphatic filariasis, 733
  lymphogranuloma venereum, 318
  measles, 348
  opisthorchiasis/clonorchiasis, 858
  orthopoxviruses, 373
  paragonimiasis, 865
  rotavirus, 409
  scrub typhus, 337
  strongyloidiasis, 811
  toxocariasis, 766
  toxoplasmosis, 726
  trichinellosis, 772
Elliptocytosis, 1026
Emerging Infections Program, 105
Emerging infectious diseases, 7, 937–938
  global surveillance, 105–109
Emetine
  B. hominis, 622
  fascioliasis, 861
Empyema
  staphylococcal, 209
  tuberculous, 234
Emtricitabine, 103t
  HIV, 553–554
En Niño-Southern Oscillation, 8
Encephalitis, 932–933
  eastern equine, 520t, 876t
  enterovirus, 398, 401–402
  granulomatous amebic, 707, 709–710, 1019t
    prevention and control, 713
    treatment and prognosis, 712
  Japanese, 352, 511–512, 516f, 876t
    clinical features, 512
    diagnosis, 513
    pathogenesis and immunity, 512
    pathology, 512
    prevention and control, 513–514
    treatment and prognosis, 513
    vaccine, 64t–65t, 513, 888t–890t
  La Crosse, 876t
  loaiasis, 737
  measles, 347
  monkeypox, 371
  multifocal necrotizing, 725, 725f–726f
  Murray Valley, 511, 514, 516f
  Nipah virus, 933
  ocular involvement, 996
  postimmunization, 1020
  postinfectious, 1020
  Q fever, 346
  rabies, 933
  St Louis, 516f, 876t
  sandfly fever, 933
  smallpox, 371
  tick-borne, 515–518, 875t
    agent, 515
    clinical features, 516–517, 517t
    diagnosis, 518
    epidemiology, 515, 517f
    pathogenesis and immunity, 517–518
    Siberian subtype, 517, 517t
    treatment and prognosis, 518
    vaccine, 888t–890t
  varicella, 360
  Venezuelan equine, 519, 520t, 876t
  West Nile, 105, 876t
  western equine, 520t, 876t
Encephalitozoon spp., 714
Encephalitozoon bieneusi
  eradication, 86t–87t
  treatment, 720t
Encephalitozoon cuniculi, 634f, 714, 715t
  clinical manifestations, 717
  epidemiology, 716–717
  eradication, 86t–87t
Encephalitozoon hellem, 634f, 715t, 716f
  clinical manifestations, 717
  eradication, 86t–87t
  histology, 719f
  treatment, 720t
Encephalitozoon intestinalis, 715t
  clinical manifestations, 717
  epidemiology, 716–717
  eradication, 76, 86t–87t
  histology, 719f
  treatment, 720t
Encephalomyelitis
  acute disseminated (ADEM), 529
  postvaccinial, 375
Encephalopathy, 1020
  hemorrhagic fevers, 445t
  postvaccinial, 375
  toxocariasis, 765
  yellow fever, 498
Endemic, 11
Endocardial mucormycosis, 599
Endocarditis
  Bartonella, 266t, 267–268
  Brucella spp., 273
  C. psittaci, 316t
  fungal, 593
  prosthetic valve, 593
  Q fever, 346
  S. aureus, 178b, 209
  Salmonella spp., 132t–133t
Endocervicitis, 1034t
Endolimax nana, 614, 621, 622f
Endometritis, *C. trachomatis*, 316–317
Endomyocardial fibrosis, loiasis, 737
Endophthalmitis, 1004–1006, 1006f
  candidal, 594–595
  larva migrans, 765
Endothelium, filovirus infection, 490
Endotoxins, 6
  immune response, 39
Energy parasites, 308
Enfuvirtide, 103t
  HIV, 553–554
Enhanced Refugee Health Program Initiative, 906–908
Enoplida capillarids, 785–787
  C. hepaticum, 786
  P. philippinensis, 786–787
Entamoeba coli, 614, 621, 622f
Entamoeba dispar, 614–615, 615b
  clinical features, 616
Entamoeba gingivalis, 614, 621, 622f
Entamoeba hartmanni, 614, 622f
Entamoeba histolytica, 1–2, 141, 614, 622f, 707, 709, 917t
  cell biology and biochemistry, 614, 615b
  eradication, 85, 88t–89t
  gene structure and organization, 614, 616f
  HIV coinfection, 1053
  inflammatory diarrhea, 923
  life cycle, 614, 615f–616f
  neurological involvement, 1019t
  phagocytic killing, 7
  pulmonary disease, 984t
  taxonomy, 614, 615b
  treatment, 918t
  see also Amebic disease
Entamoeba moshkovskii, 614–615, 615b
  clinical features, 616
Entamoeba polecki, 614, 621, 622f
Entecavir, hepatitis B, 436
Enteric adenovirus, 417–418, 417t
  diagnosis, 418
  diarrheal disease, 418
  epidemiology, 417–418
  fastidious, 417
  treatment, prognosis and prevention, 418
Enteric fever, 916–919, 917t, 926t–927t
  brucellosis *see* Brucellosis
  treatment, 918t
  typhoid/paratyphoid *see* Typhoid/paratyphoid
Enteric viral hepatitis *see* Hepatitis A; Hepatitis E
Enteritis
  Salmonella, 132
  strongyloidiasis, 808
Enteroaggregative *E. coli*, 111t, 117–118
  clinical features, 112t
Enterobacter spp., 113
  toxin, 113, 114t–115t

Enterobiasis, 788–790
agent *see Enterobius vermicularis*
clinical features, 789–790, 790f
eosinophilia, 942t
diagnosis, 790, 790f
epidemiology, 788
pregnancy, 790
prevention and control, 790
treatment and control, 790
Enterobiinae, 788
Enterobius gregorii, 788
Enterobius vermicularis, 777, 788, 789f
eradication, 76, 77t–79t
life cycle, 788, 789f
pruritus, 959t–961t
Enterococcus spp., skin lesions, 956t
Enterocytozoon spp., 714
Enterocytozoon bieneusii, 634f, 714, 715t
epidemiology, 716–717
histology, 719f
Enterohemorrhagic *E. coli*, 111t, 117, 117f
clinical features, 112t
Enteroinvasive *E. coli*, 111t, 118
clinical features, 112t
Enteromonas hominis, 623, 632f
Enteropathogenic *E. coli*, 111t, 113–115, 116f–117f
clinical features, 112t
Enterotoxigenic *E. coli*, 111t, 113
clinical features, 112t
Enterotoxins, 113, 114t–115t
cholera, 150
heat-stable, 116f
staphylococcal, 210
Enteroviruses, 387, 398–405
characteristics, 398
classification, 398, 399t
clinical manifestations, 400–402
conjunctivitis, 398, 402, 991, 992f
diarrhea, 402
encephalitis, 398, 401–402
hand, foot and mouth disease, 398, 401–402
herpangina, 398, 402
meningitis, 398, 400–401
myocarditis, 398, 402
neonatal, 402
pericarditis, 402
pleurodynia, 402
poliomyelitis *see* Poliomyelitis
short fever with maculopapular rash, 402
skin lesions, 956t, 972t
coxsackieviruses, 398, 399t
diagnosis, 404
echoviruses, 398, 399t
epidemiology, 398–400
EV70, 401
EV71, 401
pathogenesis and immunity, 403–404
poliovirus *see* Poliovirus
prevalence, 399
prevention and control, 404–405
immunization, 404–405
polio eradication, 405
shedding, 399
transmission, 399
treatment and prognosis, 404
Entomologic inoculation rate, 652
Entomophthorales, 597
Entomophthoramycosis, 603–604
clinical features, 603
ocular involvement, 1009, 1009f
skin lesions, 969t–970t
diagnosis, 603–604
epidemiology, 603
pathogenesis and immunity, 603
treatment and prognosis, 604, 604t
Entomopoxvirinae, 369
Entrapment neuropathy, loaiasis, 737
Entropion, trachoma, 311b
Env, 543, 545
Environmental changes, 8
Environmentally induced pulmonary disease, 989–990
Enzootic, 11
Enzyme immunoassay *see* ELISA
Enzyme-linked immunoabsorbent assay *see* ELISA
Enzyme-linked immunotransfer blot assay, cysticercosis, 820
Eosinopenia, visceral leishmaniasis, 701
Eosinophils, 55–56
Eosinophil cationic protein, 55–56
Eosinophil peroxidase, 55–56
Eosinophilia, 939–949, 940b
abdominal pain, 945–946, 946b
ascariasis, 796
aspergillosis, 940b
basidiobolomycosis, 940b
coccidioidomycosis, 940b
CSF, 775–776, 947, 947b
D. fragilis, 940b
diarrheal disease, 945–946, 946b
drug-associated reactions, 947t
epidemiology, 941–943
fever, 947, 947b
filariasis, 942t, 944
hepatobiliary disease, 946–947, 947b
HIV, 940b, 944
hookworm, 803
host factors affecting, 941, 941b
I. belli, 940b
immunobiology, 940–941
loaiasis, 736–737
M. ozzardi, 740
myiasis, 940b
noninfectious diseases, 947–948, 947t
paracoccidioidomycosis, 940b
parasitic infections, 940b, 943t
pathogenesis, 939–940
patient evaluation, 947–948, 948b
patterns of, 941, 942t
persistent, 943b
pleural effusion, 945b
psittacosis, 321
pulmonary disease, 944, 944b, 987
response to treatment, 948, 949b
scabies, 940b
schistosomiasis, 944
skin diseases, 946, 946t
strongyloidiasis, 943–944
taeniasis, 839
trichinellosis, 771, 771f
tropical pulmonary, 945
eradication, 77t–79t
lymphatic filariasis, 733
visceral larva migrans, 765
Eosinophilic meningitis, 774
EphrinB2, 353
Epidemics, 3, 11
control of, 21–22
and social conditions, 17
Epidemiology, 11–16
Epidermophyton spp., 559
Epidermophyton floccosum, 560t
onychomycosis, 562
tinea corporis, 561
tinea cruris, 561
Epididymitis, 1034t, 1044
C. trachomatis, 316, 316t
clinical features, 1044
diagnosis, 1044
gonococcal, 185, 316
management, 1044
Epidural abscess, 1022
Epiglottitis
candidal, 593
H. influenzae, 194t
Epizootic, 11
Epstein-Barr virus, 355, 356t, 362–364, 416
agent, 362–363
Burkitt's lymphoma *see* Burkitt's lymphoma
and cancer, 71–72, 73t
clinical features, 363
ocular disease, 995
skin lesions, 957t
diagnosis, 364
epidemiology, 363
malaria, 657
pathogenesis and immunity, 363–364
prevention and control, 364
Equine infectious anemia virus, 542f
Equine morbillivirus, 352
Equivalence studies, 12
Erb's paralysis, syphilitic, 290
Ergosterol, 590
Eriocheir spp., 862
Erisipela de la costa, 744, 744f
Eristalis tenax, 869
Ertapenem, 98
Erysipelas, 204, 261–262
Erythema migrans, relapsing fever, 298
Erythema multiforme, 951, 951f
causes, 951b
Erythema nodosum, 951, 951f
differential diagnosis, 951b
Erythrasma, 973t
Erythroblastosis fetalis, 725–726
Erythrocyte sedimentation rate, malaria, 657
Erythrocytes
aggregation, 659
deformability, 659
rosetting, 659
Erythromycin, 96t–98t, 99
Borrelia spp., 300
Campylobacter spp., 148, 918t
cat-scratch disease, 269
cellulitis, 210–211
cervicitis/urethritis, 1040t
chancroid, 1035t
cholera, 155–156, 155t
diphtheria, 226
granuloma inguinale, 1035t
group A streptococcus resistance, 208
H. ducreyi, 191
legionellosis, 218
lymphogranuloma venereum, 318, 1035t
Oroya fever, 269
pertussis, 214
in pregnancy, 1073t
psittacosis, 322
staphylococcal toxic shock syndrome, 210
trachoma, 312–313
Erythroplasia of Queyrat, 534
Eschar, 955t
scrub typhus, 337
spotted fever rickettsioses, 327
see also skin lesions
Escherichia coli, 3, 5, 709
as bioterrorism agent, 880t
diagnosis, 886
diagnosis, 118–119
diffusely adherent, 111t–112t, 118
disease, 112–113, 112t
enteroaggregative, 111t–112t, 117–118
enterohemorrhagic, 111t–112t, 117, 117f
enteroinvasive, 111t, 118
enteropathogenic, 111t–112t, 113–115, 116f–117f
enterotoxigenic, 111t–112t, 113
epidemiology, 110–112, 111f
GroEL protein, 316
pathogenesis and immunity, 113–118, 114t–115t, 116f
prevention and control, 120
properties, 110
serogroups, 111t
travelers' diarrhea, 892
treatment and prognosis, 119–120
antimicrobial therapy, 119
antimotility agents, 119–120
bismuth subsalicylate, 119
probiotics, 120
rehydration, 119

Esmolol, tetanus, 287–288
Esomeprazole, *H. pylori*, 172t, 173b
Esophageal candidiasis, 589, 592
Esophageal varices, 917t
Espundia *see* Leishmaniasis, mucosal
Esthiomene, 318
Ethambutol, 100t
adverse effects, 240
M. avium complex, 104t
MAC, 246
in pregnancy, 1073t
resistance, 237–238
tuberculosis, 239t, 240
tuberculous meningitis, 236
Ethionamide, 100t
leprosy, 259
in pregnancy, 1073t
tuberculous meningitis, 236
Etravirine, 103t, 553–554
Eucalyptus camaldulensis, 579–580
Eucoccidiorida, 633, 641
Eukaryotes, evolution, 1
Eukhornia crassipes, 865
Eumolpianus eumolpi, 276
Eumycetoma, 565–566, 566f
Euproctis chrysorrhoea, 871
Europe
cryptosporidiosis, 636t
E. multilocularis, 834f
hemorrhagic fevers, 932t
trichinellosis, 770t
European bat lyssavirus, 526t
Evans's syndrome, 273
Everglades virus, 520t
Exanthem, febrile, 398
Exanthem subitum, 358f, 364–365
diagnosis, 365
Exchange transfusion, babesiosis, 680
Exfoliatin, 5
Exophiala jeanselmei, 571
Exophiala moniliae, 571, 572f
Exophiala spinifera, 571
Exotoxins, 5
streptococcal pyrogenic, 203, 205
Exserohilum rostratum, 571
Extracellular enveloped virions, 370–372
Extracorporeal membrane oxygenation, 384–385
Extrapolation, 14
Extrapulmonary tuberculosis, 233–236
meningeal, 231, 233
miliary, 231, 233
tuberculous pleurisy, 233–234
Eye worm, 736, 736f, 1012–1013, 1012f
oriental, 785
see also Loa loa
Eyelid, ulcerative lesions, 1005b

F

F proteins, 353
Face washing, 313
Factor H, 34t, 39, 52–53
Factor I, 34t
Faget's sign, 496
False negatives, 14–15
False positives, 14–15
Famciclovir, 102t
genital herpes, 1035t
herpesviruses, 356
HSV, 359
varicella zoster virus, 361
Famine fever, 297
Fannia scalaris, 869
Fasciola spp., 783
Fasciola gigantica, 854, 858
geographic distribution, 860f
life cycle, 859f
Fasciola hepatica, 80, 854, 858
eradication, 81t
life cycle, 859f
morphology, 854, 858f
ova, 858f
Fascioliasis, 858–862
agent *see Fasciola hepatica*
clinical features, 859–860
acute hepatic (invasive) stage, 859–860
chronic biliary (obstructive) stage, 860
eosinophilia, 942t–943t
hepatobiliary disease, 976t–977t, 980–981
skin lesions, 946t, 958t
diagnosis, 861
epidemiology, 859
geographic distribution, 860f
incubation period, 929b
pathogenesis and immunity, 860–861
treatment and vaccination, 861–862
Fasciolidae, 854, 866
Fasciolopsiasis, 942t
eosinophilia, 943t
Fasciolopsis buski, 865
characteristics, 865
diagnosis, 867
disease, 865
epidemiology, 865
eradication, 81t
morphology, 854
Favus, 560–561, 560f
Fc receptors, 56–57
Fc-δ receptor IIa *see* CD32
Febendazole, toxocariasis prophylaxis, 767
Feline immunodeficiency virus, 542f
Fever blisters *see* Herpes labialis
Fevers, 925–938
approach to, 928–931
exposure, 930t
history, 928–931, 930b
host factors, 931
timing, 928, 929b, 929t
associated symptoms/clinical findings, 932–937
CNS findings, 932–933
diarrhea, 933–934
hemorrhage, 932
hepatitis, 934
lymphadenopathy, 935
rash, 934–935
respiratory symptoms, 933
causes, 926f, 931–932
duration and pattern, 931
clinical manifestations, undifferentiated, 931–932
emerging diseases and difficulties, 937–938
eosinophilia, 947, 947b
epidemiology, 925–928
evaluation, 926b
giardiasis, 627t
HIV-infected, immunocompromised and pregnant patients, 937
malaria, 925
non-infection-related, 936–937
pathogenesis, 925
patient evaluation, 937, 937b
persistent, 935–936, 936b
relapsing *see* Relapsing fever
remote residence in tropical areas, 936
returning travelers, 926t–927t
viral hemorrhagic see Viral hemorrhagic fevers
see also individual fevers
Fibrinolysis, 4
Ficolins, 52–53
Filamentous hemagglutinin, 212–213
Filaria conjunctivae, 750
Filaria dance sign, 733
Filaria lacrimalis see Loa loa
Filaria loa see Loa loa
Filaria oculi humani see Loa loa
Filaria subconjunctivalis see Loa loa
Filariasis, 17, 21, 876t
clinical features
eosinophilia, 942t, 944
pleural effusion, 988t
skin lesions, 946t, 962t–966t
eradication, 43, 77t–79t
genetic associations
protection, 35t
susceptibility, 35t
HIV coinfection, 1055
incubation period, 929b
lymphatic, 729–734, 950–951
agent, 729–730, 730f
clinical features, 731–733, 732f, 1013
diagnosis, 733–734
epidemiology, 730–731, 731f
pathogenesis and immunity, 733
prevention and control, 734
treatment and prognosis, 734
perstans, 738
agent, 739
clinical features, 739
diagnosis, 739
epidemiology, 739
pathogenesis and immunity, 739
prevention and control, 740
treatment and prognosis, 739
Wolbachia-related complications, 343
zoonotic, 750–758
agent, 750, 751t
clinical features, 752–754
diagnosis, 754–757
epidemiology, 750–752, 751f
prevention and control, 758
treatment and prognosis, 758
Filobasidiella bacillispora, 579
Filobasidiella neoformans, 579
Filoviruses, 442t–443t, 483–491
characteristics, 483–484
genome organization and replication, 483
taxonomy, 483
virion structure, 483
virus proteins, 483–484
clinical features, 444t–445t, 488
diagnosis, 447t, 490
ecology, 484
epidemiology, 484, 485t–486t, 486f
pathologic features, 446t
pathology, 488–489, 489f
prevention, 448t
prevention and control, 491
role of endothelium, 490
sequence of infection, 489
transmission, 484–488, 487f
treatment and prognosis, 448t, 490–491
virus spreading, 490
see also individual viruses
Fimbriae, 212–213
aggregative adherence, 117–118
Fimbrial adhesins, 4
Fine needle aspiration cytology, mycetoma, 567
First-aid kit for travelers, 901, 901b
Fish hosts
C. sinensis, 855
O. felineus, 855
Fish tapeworm *see Diphyllobothrium* spp.
Fite-Faraco stain, *M. leprae*, 253
Fitz-Hugh-Curtis syndrome, 187, 1043
C. trachomatis, 316–317, 316t
Flagellates, 1–2
Flagellin, 118, 221
Flatulence, giardiasis, 627t
Flaviviruses, 427, 442t–443t
clinical features, 444t–445t
dengue, 505
diagnosis, 447t
Japanese encephalitis *see* Japanese encephalitis
pathologic features, 446t
tick-borne encephalitis, 517–518
treatment and prevention, 448t
West Nile virus *see* West Nile virus
yellow fever *see* Yellow fever
Flea-borne spotted fever, 323

- Fleas, 50, 876
  - pruritus caused by, 959t–961t
  - *see also individual species*
- Fleroxacin, travelers' diarrhea, 893
- Flesh flies, 869
- Flexal virus, 450f, 450t
- Flinders Island spotted fever, 323
- Flour mites, 872–873
- Flucloxacillin, 96t–98t
- Fluconazole, 94, 100t–101t
  - blastomycosis, 577
  - candidemia, 596
  - candidiasis, 590
    - balanitis, 593
    - cardiac, 593
    - endophthalmitis, 594–595
    - esophageal, 592
    - oropharyngeal, 592
    - urinary tract infection, 594
    - vulvovaginal, 593
  - coccidioidomycosis, 579
  - cryptococcosis, 580–581
    - prophylaxis, 581
  - dermatophytosis, 563
  - granulomatous amebic encephalitis, 712
  - histoplasmosis, 575
  - leishmaniasis, cutaneous, 705
  - mucosal candidiasis, 104t
  - onychomycosis, 563
  - *P. marneffei*, 587–588
  - paracoccidioidomycosis, 584
  - phaeohyphomycosis, 572
  - resistance, 581
  - toxicity, 101t
  - vulvovaginal candidiasis, 1040t
- Flucytosine, 590
  - candiduria, 594
  - cryptococcosis, 580–581
  - granulomatous amebic encephalitis, 712
  - *P. marneffei*, 587–588
  - phaeohyphomycosis, 572
  - toxicity, 101t
- Fluid therapy *see* Rehydration therapy
- Flukes *see* Trematodes
- Fluoroquinolones, 96t–98t
  - ehrlichial, anaplasmal and neorickettsial infections, 343
  - melioidosis, 222
  - *N. gonorrhoea* resistance, 189
  - Q fever, 346
  - *Salmonella* bacteremia
  - salmonellosis, 135
  - staphylococcal toxic shock syndrome, 210
  - urinary tract infection, 1041
  - *see also individual drugs*
- 5-Fluorouracil, HPV, 537
- Fluoxetine, pleural effusion, 988t
- Fly larvae, parasitic, 869–870, 869f
- Focal epithelial hyperplasia of Heck, 533t
- Folate
  - deficiency, 1027, 1029
  - requirements, e12t–e13t
- Follicle mites, 869
- Folliculitis
  - barbae, 208–209
  - staphylococcal, 208–209
- Fomiversen, 102t
- *Fonsecaea compacta*, 569
- *Fonsecaea monophora*, 569
- *Fonsecaea pedrosoi*, 569, 570f
  - micromorphology, 570f
- Food, precautions, 892–893
- Food poisoning
  - *B. cereus*, 923
  - *C. difficile*, 164–165
  - staphylococcal, 923
- Food-borne pathogens, 883
- Forest yaws, 698t
- Fort Morgan virus, 520t
- Fosamprenavir, 103t
- Foscarnet, 102t
  - cytomegalovirus, 104t
  - herpes simplex virus, 104t
  - herpesviruses, 356
    - Epstein-Barr virus, 364
    - HHV-6, 362
    - HHV-7, 366
    - HHV-8, 368
    - HSV, 359
    - varicella-zoster virus, 104t
- Frambesioma, 293f
- *Francisella tularensis*, 709
  - as bioterrorism agent, 880t, 881
    - diagnosis, 885
- FTI-277, hepatitis D, 440
- FTI-2153, hepatitis D, 440
- Fumagillin, microsporidiosis, 86t–89t, 720–721, 720t
- *Funambulus* spp., 277
- Fungal balls, 593
- Fungal infections
  - *Aspergillus* spp., 231
  - dermatophytosis *see* Dermatophytosis
  - endocarditis, 593
  - HIV coinfection, 1055–1058
  - keratitis, 1006
  - neurologic involvement, 599
  - ocular involvement *see* ocular disease, fungal infection
  - sinusitis, 1009
  - skin lesions, 969t–970t
  - treatment, 99, 100t–101t, 590
  - *see also individual infections*
- Furazolidone
  - adverse effects, 629t
  - *B. hominis*, 622
  - cholera, 155–156, 155t
  - giardiasis, 88t–89t, 628t
  - *H. pylori*, 172t, 173b
- Furin, 263
- Furious rabies, 527–528, 527t, 528f
- Furuncle, 261–262
- *Fusarium* spp., 563
- Fusion inhibitors, 103t, 553–554
- *Fusobacterium necrophorum*, 919

G

- G6PD *see* Glucose-6-phosphate dehydrogenase deficiency
- Gadgets Gully virus, 516f
- *Gag*, 543, 545
- *Galago crassicaudatus*, 495
- *Galea* spp., 276
- Gallbladder, typhoid bacilli in, 124
- Gammaherpesviruses, 355–356, 363
- Ganciclovir, 102t
  - cytomegalovirus, 104t
  - herpesviruses, 356
    - cytomegalovirus, 362
    - HHV-6, 362
    - HHV-7, 366
    - HHV-8, 368
- Gangrene
  - gas, 166
  - peripheral, 955t
  - streptococcal *see* Necrotizing fasciitis
- Gas gangrene, *C. septicum*, 166
- Gasterophilidae, 1016
- Gastric cancer, *H. pylori*, 170
- Gastric ulcer, *H. pylori*, 169, 169f
- Gastritis, active chronic, 167, 169
- *Gastrodiscoides hominis*, 866
- Gastroenteritis, 923
  - astrovirus, 416–417
  - food poisoning, 923
  - norovirus, 411–412, 414t, 923
  - rotavirus, 923
  - *Salmonella*, 131
    - treatment, 135
  - *Vibrio*, 160
- Gastrografin, ascariasis, 797
- Gastrointestinal bleeding, 917t, 920
- Gastrointestinal involvement, 916–924
  - anthrax, 263, 917t
  - antimicrobial therapy, 918t
  - brucellosis, 917
  - Chagas' disease, 692–693, 692f
  - enteric fever, 916–919
  - hookworm, 802, 917t
  - leprosy, 917t
  - malaria, 661
  - mucormycosis, 599
  - and nutritional status, 27–28
  - paracoccidioidomycosis, 917t
  - patient history, 917b
  - *Salmonella* spp., 130f, 132
  - strongyloidiasis, 809
  - symptoms and syndromes, 916–924, 917t–918t
  - syphilis, 917t
  - tuberculosis, 917t, 920
  - *see also individual diseases*
- Gatifloxacin, 96t–98t, 100t
  - tuberculosis, 242
  - typhoid/paratyphoid, 125t
- Genetic dissection, 33–34
  - association studies *see* Association studies
- Genetic immunodeficiency syndromes, 35t
- Genetic markers, 32–33
- Genetics, 32–39
  - immune system, 33
- Genital herpes, 1034t
  - clinical features, 1034t
  - diagnosis, 1035t
  - HIV coinfection, 1064
- Genital lymphedema, 732
- Genital salmonellosis, 132t–133t
- Genital ulcer disease, 1033–1037, 1034t
  - clinical features, 1034–1035, 1034t
  - diagnosis, 1035–1036, 1035t
  - management, 1036–1037, 1036f
- Genital warts, 533t, 534, 1034t
  - clinical features, 1037
  - diagnosis, 1037
  - histological features, 535f
  - pregnant women, 538
  - treatment, 536–537
  - visual diagnosis, 536
  - *see also* Human papillomavirus
- Genome-based surveillance, 880
- Genome-wide association studies, 33–34
- Genomics, 3
- Gentamicin, 96t–98t
  - brucellosis, 275, 918t
  - cat-scratch disease, 269
  - donovanosis, 197
  - *E. coli* infection, 119
  - gonorrhoea, 189
  - pelvic inflammatory disease, 190t, 1043t
  - plague, 281–282
  - *Salmonella* spp.
    - bacteremia, 135
    - drug resistance, 130t
- Gentian violet, candidiasis, 592
- Geometric mean, 13
- Geophagia, 764, 767, 791
- Getah virus, 520t
- Ghon complex, 230, 230f
- *Giardia agilis*, 624t
- *Giardia ardae*, 624t
- *Giardia duodenalis see* Giardiasis
- *Giardia lamblia*, 1–2, 623–630, 917t
  - categorization, 623f
  - characteristics, 623–625
  - eradication, 85
  - HIV coinfection, 1053
  - life cycle, 624f
  - morphologic forms, 623
    - cyst, 623f, 625f
    - trophozoite, 623f–625f
  - travelers' diarrhea, 924
- *Giardia microti*, 624t

Giardia muris, 624t
Giardia psittaci, 624t
Giardiasis
agent *see Giardia lamblia*
clinical features, 627, 627t
chronic diarrhea, 923–924
fever, 926t–927t
ocular involvement, 1011
pruritus, 959t–961t
vitamin A malabsorption, 27–28
diagnosis, 627–628
epidemiology, 625–626
pathogenesis and immunity, 626–627
prevention and control, 629–630
transmission, 625
treatment and prognosis, 88t–89t, 628–629, 628t
adverse events, 629t
antimicrobials, 918t
Glanders, 219, 261–262
skin lesions, 962t–968t
Glaucomys volans, 329
Gleevec, orthopoxviruses, 376–377
Gliclazide, pleural effusion, 988t
Global AIDS Program, 907
Global Alliance for Vaccines and Immunization, 64–66
Global Disease Detection Program, 107
Global Foodborne Infections Network, 107
Global Immunization Vision and Strategy, 66
Global Influenza Surveillance Network, 107, 107f
Global Laboratory Network for Poliomyelitis Eradication, 107
Global Outbreak Alert and Response Network, 106–108
Global Programme to Eliminate Lymphatic Filariasis, 734
Global Project on Anti-Tuberculosis Drug Resistance Surveillance, 108
Global surveillance, 105–109
communication, 108
role of laboratory, 108
surveillance and response networks, 107–108
Global warming, 8
Glomerulonephritis, poststreptococcal, 206
Glossina spp., 683, 877
Glossina fuscipes, 683, 877
Glossina morsitans, 683, 877
Glossina pallidipes, 683, 877
Glossina palpalis, 683, 877
Glossina swynnertoni, 683, 877
Glossina tachinoides, 683, 877
Glossitis, median rhomboid, 591–592
Glucan receptors, 55
Gluconeogenesis, 27
Glucose-6-phosphate dehydrogenase deficiency, 32, 1025, 1026f, 1032
clinical features, 1032, 1032t
diagnosis, 1026f, 1032
hemighosts, 1026f, 1032
and malaria resistance, 36t, 653, 668
management, 1032
Glufanide disodium, Kaposi's sarcoma, 368
Glutamine, 24, 28
Glycomes, 52
Glycophorin B deficiency, malaria protection, 36t
Gnathostoma spp., 783–785, 785f
Gnathostoma binucleatum, 784
Gnathostoma doloresi, 784
Gnathostoma hispidum, 784
Gnathostoma malaysiae, 784
Gnathostoma nipponicum, 784
Gnathostoma spinigerum, 776, 784, 957
pulmonary disease, 984t
see also Gnathostomiasis
Gnathostomiasis, 776
clinical features
eosinophilia, 942t–943t
ocular involvement, 785, 1014–1015, 1014f
pruritus, 959t–961t
skin lesions, 946t, 958t, 962t–966t
eradication, 77t–79t
Goiter, e12t–e13t
Gongylonema pulchrum, 785, 785f
Gongylonemiasis, 785, 785f
eradication, 77t–79t
Gonococcal infections, 184–190
see also Neisseria
Gonococcal Isolate Surveillance Project, 105
Gonorrhea, 184–190
antimicrobial therapy, 189
clinical features, 184–185
cutaneous lesions, 952t
fever, 926t–927t
in men, 184–185
in women, 185–187
diagnosis, 186–188
disseminated disease, 187
drug resistance, 188–189
epidemiology, 184
pathogenesis and immunity, 185–186
pharyngeal, 187
in pregnancy, 189
prevention and control, 190
transmission, 184
treatment and prognosis, 188–189
see also Neisseria gonorrhoeae
Gowers, Sir William, 284
Grain mites, 872–873, 873f
Gram staining, *N. gonorrhoea*, 188
Granulocyte transfusion, 601
Granulocyte-macrophage colony-stimulating factor, 601
Granuloma
doughnut, 345
tick, 959t–966t
Granuloma inguinale, 952t, 953f, 962t–968t, 1034t
clinical features, 1034t
diagnosis, 1035t
Granulomatous amebic encephalitis, 707, 709–710
clinical features, 709f–710f
neurologic involvement, 1019t
diagnosis, 712
neuroimaging, 712
in HIV/AIDS, 707, 709f, 1052–1053
pathogenesis and immunity, 710–711
prevention and control, 713
treatment and prognosis, 712
Greek goat encephalitis virus, 516f
Grimontia hollisae, 157, 158t, 161
Griseofulvin, tinea capitis, 563
Groove sign, 317
Ground itch, 802, 950, 959t–961t, 961f
Group A streptococcus
acquisition of, 205
antimicrobial resistance
erythromycin, 208
sulfonamide, 208
bacterial cell structure, 207–208
capsule, 207
cell wall, 207
cytoplasmic membrane, 207
C5a peptidase, 208
clinical isolates, 205
diphtheria, 224
DNases, 207
hyaluronidase, 207
interleukin-8 cleaving enzyme, 208
M proteins, 206–207
protein F, 208
streptococcal pyrogenic exotoxins, 203, 205
streptolysin O, 203, 206–207
treatment and prognosis, 208
see also S. pyogenes
Group C virus, 482
Guana virus, 482
Guanarito virus, 442t–443t, 450f, 450t
animal models, 457
incubation period, 929b
maintenance in rodent hosts, 455
see also Venezuelan hemorrhagic fever
Guarnieri bodies, 373, 373f, 885
Guillain-Barré syndrome, 147, 401, 526–527, 531, 1022
and *Cyclospora cayetanensis* infection, 642
Guinea worm *see Dracunculus medinensis*
Gumma, syphilitic, 290–291
Gyraulus spp., 865

H

HAART therapy, 553–554
Haemagogus spp., 493, 495, 522
Haemaphysalis spp., 514
Haemaphysalis longicornis, 342
Haemophilus aegyptius, skin lesions, 956t
Haemophilus ducreyi, 191–192
characteristics, 191
diagnosis, 191
disease, 191
epidemiology, 191
pathogenesis and immunity, 191
treatment and prognosis, 191
prevention and control, 191–192
Haemophilus influenzae, 3, 177–178, 178b, 193–195, 308–309
characteristics, 193
diagnosis, 194
disease spectrum, 193, 194t
meningitis, 193, 194t
sepsis, 178
epidemiology, 193
pathogenesis and immunity, 193–194
prevention and control, 194
skin lesions, 956t
treatment and prognosis, 194
type b, 193–194
vaccine, 64t–65t, 194, 195f
Haemosporidiidea, 646
Halicephalobus spp., 778, 779f
Halofantrine
malaria, 661, 664, 668
prophylaxis, 84
pharmacokinetics, 665t
in pregnancy, 1073t
Hand, foot and mouth disease, 398, 401–402
Hanging groin, 744f, 745
Hansen's disease *see* Leprosy
Hantaan virus, 471t, 472
hemorrhagic fever with renal syndrome, 471f, 473–475
Hantavirus cardiopulmonary syndrome, 476
Hantavirus pulmonary syndrome, 442t–443t, 475–476
Andes virus, 473, 476
animal models, 477–478
Choclo virus, 473
clinical course, 475f
clinical features, 444t–445t
diagnosis, 447t
differential diagnosis, 478
geographic range, 473
global distribution, 471f
incubation period, 929b
pathologic features, 446t
prevention, 448t
prognosis, 479
Sin Nombre virus, 473, 475–476
transmission, 932t
treatment, 448t, 479
Hantaviruses, 8, 442t–443t, 470–480
agent, 470–473, 471f, 471t
as bioterrorism agent, 880t
diagnosis, 478–479
epidemiology, 473
laboratory diagnosis, 478–479
antigen detection, 479
nucleic acid detection, 479
serology, 478–479
virus, 479
natural host relationships and ecology, 470–473
pathogenesis and immunity, 476–478, 476t

prevention and control, 480
skin lesions, 956t
transmission cycle, 472f
treatment and prognosis, 479
vaccines, 480
see also individual viruses
Haptoglobin
disease associations, 36t
malaria susceptibility, 37t
Hartmannella spp., 709
Hartmannella vermiformis, 217
Harvest mites *see* Trombiculid mites
HAV *see* Hepatitis A
Hb C, malaria protection, 36t
Hb E, malaria resistance, 36t, 653
Hb F, malaria resistance, 36t, 653
Hb S, malaria resistance, 36t
HCV *see* Hepatitis C
Head lice *see Pediculus humanus*
Headache
malaria, 654–655
neurocysticercosis, 818
trichinellosis, 770
Health care workers
burn-out, 19
loss of, 18–19
Heart transplantation, Chagas' disease, 695
Heat acclimatization, 900
Heat therapy
chromoblastomycosis, 570
phaeohyphomycosis, 572
Heat-labile toxin, 116f
Heat-resistant agglutinin 1, 117–118
Heatstroke, 178b
Heck's disease, 534
Helicobacter cinaedi, 145, 146t
Helicobacter fennilliae, 145, 146t
Helicobacter pullorum, 146t
Helicobacter pylori, 2, 5, 167–173, 627, 917t
abdominal pain, 920
active chronic gastritis, 169
adhesins, 4
asymptomatic infection, 169
and cancer, 71–72, 73t
characteristics, 167, 168f
culture, 167
diagnosis, 170–171, 170t
culture, 171
histology, 171
non-invasive tests, 171, 172f
urease test, 171
diagnostic criteria, 170t, 171
duodenal and gastric ulcer, 169, 169f
epidemiology, 167–168
gastric cancer, 170
adenocarcinoma, 170
lymphoma, 170
ulcer-cancer controversy, 170
identification, 167
natural history, 171f
pathogenesis and immunity, 168–169
acute infection, 168
attachment, 168
cytotoxins, 168–169, 168f
pitfalls, 167
prevalence, 168f
prevention and control, 173
selective media, 167
treatment and prognosis, 171–173, 172t, 173b, 917t
Helicobacter rappini, 146t
Helminthic infections
eosinophilia, 942t
genetic associations, 38
neurologic involvement *see* neurologic disease, helminthic infection
ocular involvement *see* ocular disease, helminthic infection
treatment *see* Anthelminthics
see also individual infections
Helminths, 1–2, 5
adaptive mechanisms, 7
hematogenous seeding, 945
pulmonary parenchymal invasion, 945
Hemagglutination test, trichinellosis, 772
Hemagglutinin neuraminidase, 353
Hematogenous spread of microorganisms, 4
Hematologic involvement
brucellosis, 273
yellow fever, 497–498
Hematological malignancy, mucormycosis infection, 598
Hematopoietic stem cell transplantation, mucormycosis infection, 598
Hematuria, Q fever, 346
Hemighosts, 1026f, 1032
Hemileuca maia, 871
Hemimetabolous insects, 45, 46f
Hemin, 193
Hemiptera *see* Bedbugs; Kissing bugs
Hemoglobin
electrophoresis, 1027
estimation of, 1025
see also Hb
Hemoglobin H disease, 1031
Hemoglobinopathy, 1027
Hemoglobinuria, malaria, 656, 660–661
Hemolysins, 160–161, 221
Hemolytic-uremic syndrome, 178b
E. coli infection, 113
Hemoptysis, 986, 987b
tuberculosis, 231
Hemorrhagic fever with renal syndrome, 442t–443t, 473–475
clinical features, 444t–445t, 474–475, 474f
diagnosis, 447t
differential diagnosis, 478
Hantaan virus, 471f, 473–475
incubation period, 929b
military cases, 913–914
pathologic features, 446t
prevention, 448t
prognosis, 479
Puumala virus, 471f, 475
Seoul virus, 473, 475
transmission, 932t
treatment, 448t, 479
Hemorrhagic fevers, 932, 932t
viral *see* viral hemorrhagic fevers
see also individual diseases
Hemozoin, 664
Hendra virus, 9, 352–354
agent, 352–353
clinical features, 353–354
epidemiology, 353
gene function, 352
genome structure, 352
membrane glycoproteins, 353
P, C, V and L proteins, 352–353
prevention and control, 354
treatment and prognosis, 354
Henipavirus, 9, 352
HEPA filters, 602
Hepacivirus, 427
Hepadnaviridae, 433
Hepatic calodiasis, 786
Hepatic hydatid disease, 976t–977t, 979–980, 979f
Hepatitis, 1034t
acute sporadic, 975, 976t–977t
Brucella, 273
callitrichid, 457
chronic, 976t–977t, 978
enteric, 420–426
epidemic, 975–978, 976t–977t
and fever, 934
HIV coinfection, 1063–1064
ocular involvement, 996
Q fever, 345
see also different types
Hepatitis A, 420–423
characteristics, 420, 421f
clinical features, 422f
fever, 926t–927t
diagnosis, 422
disease, 421–422
epidemiology, 420–421
genome, 421f
geographic distribution, 421f
incubation period, 929b
pathogenesis and immunity, 422
pregnancy, 1074
prevention and control, 423
treatment and prognosis, 422
vaccine, 64t–65t, 69t, 423, 888t–890t, 891
requirements for immigrants, 908t
Hepatitis B, 433–440
and cancer, 71–72, 73t, 433
characteristics, 433
clinical features, 434–435
acute, 434
chronic, 433–435
pruritus, 959t–961t
diagnosis, 435–436
epidemiology, 433, 434t
genetic associations, 38–39
protection, 35t
genetic drift, 435f
pathogenesis and immunity, 435
pregnancy, 1074
prevalence, 433, 434f
prevention and control, 437
treatment and prognosis, 436–437
clinical and surrogate endpoints, 436
drug treatment strategies, 437
interferon-alfa, 436
nucleos(t)ide analogs, 436–437
vaccine, 64t–65t, 69t, 437, 888t–890t, 891–892
requirements for immigrants, 908t
Hepatitis C, 427–432
antibody, 429f–430f
testing for, 431, 431t
and cancer, 71–72, 73t
characteristics, 427–428, 428f
diagnosis, 431, 431t
disease, 430–431
chronic, 430
epidemiology, 428–430, 428f
genetic diversity, 427
genetic protection, 35t
genome, 428f
pathogenesis and immunity, 431
pregnancy, 1074
prevalence, 428f
age-specific, 429f
prevention and control, 432
replicons, 428
transmission, 429f
occupational, 429–430
perinatal, 430
sexual activity, 430
treatment and prognosis, 431–432
Hepatitis D, 437–440, 934
characteristics, 437–438
diagnosis, 439
epidemiology, 438–439, 438f
genotypes, 438
natural history, 438–439, 439f, 439t
pathogenesis and immunity, 439
prevalence, 438f
replication, 438
transmission, 438
treatment and prognosis, 439–440
Hepatitis E, 423–426, 934
characteristics, 423–424
clinical course, 425f
diagnosis, 425
disease, 424–425, 425f
epidemiology, 424
genome, 423f

incubation period, 929b
pathogenesis and immunity, 425
pregnancy, 1074
prevention and control, 425–426
treatment and prognosis, 425
vaccine, 426
Hepatitis G, pregnancy, 1074
Hepatobiliary disease, 975–981, 976t–977t
amebic liver abscess, 617–618, 617f, 617t, 976t–977t, 979, 979t
ascariasis, 796, 976t–977t, 980, 980f
candidiasis, 976t–977t
chronic hepatitis/cirrhosis, 976t–977t, 978
clonorchiasis, 976t–977t, 981
diagnosis, 975
eosinophilia, 946–947, 947b
fascioliasis, 976t–977t, 980–981
hepatic hydatid disease, 976t–977t, 979–980, 979f
hepatitis viruses, 975–978, 976t–977t
HIV cholangiopathy, 976t–977t, 981
hyperinfection syndrome, 976t–977t
leptospirosis hepatitis, 305, 305f, 976t–977t
liver failure, 976t–977t, 978
malaria-related, 976t–977t
opisthorchiasis, 976t–977t, 981
pyogenic liver abscess, 976t–977t, 978–979, 978f
salmonellosis, 132t–133t
schistosomiasis, 976t–977t, 980, 980f
tropical splenomegaly syndrome, 976t–977t
tuberculosis, 976t–977t, 981
typhoid hepatitis, 976t–977t
Hepatomegaly
fascioliasis, 859–860
polycystic echinococcosis, 838
Q fever, 346
with rash, 955b
visceral larva migrans, 765
Hepatotoxicity
anti-tuberculosis drugs, 241
see also individual drugs
Hepatovirus, 398
Hepeviridae, 423
Hepevirus, 423
Herbert's peripheral pits, 310, 310f
Herpangina, enterovirus, 398, 402
Herpes genitalis, 357, 358f
Herpes gladiatorum, 357
Herpes labialis, 357, 358f, 359
treatment, 359
Herpes simplex virus, 356–359
agent, 356–357
clinical features, 357–358, 917t
ocular infection, 993, 993t
skin lesions, 952t, 967t–968t, 972t
congenital, 725–726
diagnosis, 359
epidemiology, 357
genital *see* Genital herpes
HSV-1, 355–357, 356t, 357f
clinical features, 357
drug therapy, 104t
latent, 357
HSV-2, 355–357, 356t
clinical features, 357
latency-associated transcript, 358–359
neonatal, 357–358
pathogenesis and immunity, 358–359
pregnancy, 1081
prevention and control, 359
treatment and prognosis, 359
Herpes zoster virus, 358f, 360
clinical features, 358f
HIV coinfection, 1064
Herpesviruses *see* Herpes simplex virus; Herpes zoster virus; Human herpesviruses
Herring worm disease *see* Anisakiasis
Heterophyes heterophyes, 865–866
diagnosis, 867
eradication, 81t
Heterophyes nocens, 866
Heterophyiasis, 942t
Heterophyidae, 865–866
Heterophyids, 866
disease, 866
epidemiology, 866
see also individual types
HEV *see* Hepatitis E
Hexamidine, *Acanthamoeba* keratitis, 713
HHV *see* Human herpesvirus
Highlands J virus, 520t
Hippeutis spp., 865
Hippletes spp., 310
Hirudin, 877–878
Hirudinea, 877–878
Hirudo medicinalis, 878
Histoplasma capsulatum, 573, 574f
Histoplasmosis, 573–581
African, 573–574
agent, 573
clinical features, 573–574, 574f, 917t
abdominal mass, 921
chronic diarrhea, 924
ocular involvement, 1007–1008, 1008f
pleural effusion, 988t
skin lesions, 969t–970t
diagnosis, 574–575
epidemiology, 573, 574f
HIV coinfection, 573–574, 574f, 1057
incubation period, 929b
pathogenesis and immunity, 574
prevention and control, 575
treatment and prognosis, 575
HIV antibody assays, 552–553
HIV wasting syndrome, 552
HIV-1, 2, 5, 541–542
and cancer, 73t
cell entry, 5
genetic organization, 545
origins of, 543
HIV-2, 2, 542
and cancer, 73t
genetic organization, 545
HIV/AIDS, 3, 8, 17, 21, 541–558, 1046–1065
attachment, penetration and uncoating, 543–544
barriers to control, 18–20
case history, 17–18, 18f
CD4 abnormalities, 545, 1046
CD8 abnormalities, 1046
cell tropism, 545
clinical manifestations, 552, 552b
anemia, 1028
cholangiopathy, 976t–977t, 981
cutaneous lesions, 952t
eosinophilia, 940b, 944
fevers, 937
Kaposi's sarcoma *see* Kaposi's sarcoma
oropharyngeal candidiasis, 591
pulmonary disease, 989
clinical manifestations ocular disease, 995, 995f
coinfection, 1046–1047
African trypanosomiasis, 1052
amebiasis, 1052–1053
arboviruses, 1061–1062
arthropod-borne diseases, 1055
babesiosis, 678–679, 1050
bacillary angiomatosis, 266t, 956f
brucellosis, 1061
C. cayetanensis, 641–642, 1053
Campylobacter spp., 147
cestodes, 1054
Chagas' disease, 693, 899, 1051
clinical suspicion, 1048
coccidiosis, 1053
Cryptosporidium spp., 636, 638, 639f, 1053
donovanosis, 196–197
effects of tropical infections on, 1047–1048
ehrlichioses, 1060–1061
filariasis, 1055
hemorrhagic fever viruses, 1061–1062
hepatitis, 1063–1064
herpesviruses, 1064
histoplasmosis, 573–574, 574f, 1057
HPV, 533, 555
leishmaniasis, 701, 899, 1050–1051
leprosy, 260, 1059
M. avium-intracellulare complex, 246–247, 1058–1059
malaria, 654, 899, 1048–1050
measles, 1062–1063
melioidosis, 1061
microsporidiosis, 717–718, 717f, 1053
onchocerciasis, 745
paracoccidioidomycosis, 552, 584, 1056–1057
pneumococcal disease, 200–201
pneumocystosis, 608–613, 1058
poliomyelitis, 1063
protozoa, 1053
rabies, 1063
rickettsioses, 1060–1061
S. pneumoniae, 555
salmonellosis, 131–132, 134
strongyloidiasis, 552, 810, 1054–1055
syphilis, 1060
tinea, 562–563
toxoplasmosis, 725–727, 725f, 1052
trematodes, 1054
trichinellosis, 771
tuberculosis, 229–230, 232–233, 232f, 242–243, 552, 1058
see also individual diseases and organisms
counselling of patients and families, 555
defining conditions, 552b
dendritic cell abnormalities, 1046
diagnosis and prognosis, 552–553
HIV antibody assays, 552–553
HIV nucleic acids, 553
immunologic assessment, 553
disseminated MAC disease, 246–247
DNA synthesis, nuclear transport and integration, 544
economic cost, 20
future challenges, 557
gene expression, 544–545
particle assembly and budding, 544–545
genetic associations, 37
protection, 35t
susceptibility, 35t
global funding, 556–557
global molecular epidemiology, 548–551
global statistics and projections, 548–549
granulomatous amebic encephalitis, 707, 709f, 1052–1053
history, 541–542
immigrants, 903–904
identification of infection, 905, 905t
immunity, 551–552
incubation period, 929b
IRIS, 260
life cycle, 543, 544f
mechanism of immune dysfunction, 551
natural killer cells in, 1046
opportunistic infections
prevention, 1064–1065
treatment, 547–548
origins of, 543, 543f
pathogenesis and natural history, 551
pregnancy, 1075, 1075t
prevalence, 546, 546f–547f
prevention and control, 555–557
behavioral prevention in at-risk populations, 555–556
HIV testing, 555
recurrent *Salmonella* bacteremia, 135
regional epidemics, 549–551
Asia, 550–551
North Africa and Middle East, 550
sub-Saharan Africa, 549–550
STD interactions, 548, 1044–1045
stigma, 20
taxonomy, 542

transmission, 546–548
biologic factors affecting, 548
parenteral, 547–548
perinatal, 547, 547f
sexual, 546–547
travelers, 899
diarrheal disease, 899
immunizations, 899
treatment, 553–555
adherence to, 20
antiretroviral therapies *see* Antiretroviral therapy
chemoprophylaxis, 554–555
DOT, 18
drug resistance, 554
economic costs, 20
vaccines, 556
vertical transmission, 1075t
viral genome organization, 543
WHO classification system, 558b
yellow fever vaccination, 503
Hobo spider, 872
Holometabolous insects, 45, 46f
Hookworm, 5, 779–781, 799–804, 800t
clinical features, 802
abdominal pain, 920
anemia, 802
eosinophilia, 942t–943t
gastrointestinal, 802, 917t
ground itch, 802, 950, 959t–961t, 961f
ocular involvement, 1014
pulmonary disease, 802, 984t
skin lesions, 946t, 958t, 972t
diagnosis, 803
epidemiology, 801–802
eradication, 40, 76, 77t–79t
life cycle, 799, 800f
military cases, 914
pathogenesis and immunity, 803
prevention and control, 804
treatment and prognosis, 803–804
see also individual species
Hoplopsyllus anomalus, 276
Horder's spots, 321
Horse flies, 46, 50, 871–872, 871f
Host defences, 3–6, 3f
epithelial barrier, 3–4
normal flora, 3–4
Host response, *Salmonella*, 134
Host specificity, 46
Host-parasite interactions, 1–7
immune evasion, 6–7, 6t
microbial factors, 1–3
House dust mites, 873
House flies, 869
HPIVs *see* Human parainfluenza virus
HPV *see* Human papillomavirus
HRSV *see* Human respiratory syncytial viruses
Hsp60, 316
HSV *see* Herpes simplex virus
HTLV, 543
prevalence, 545–546
HTLV-1, 2, 7, 541, 545–546
cancer, 71–72, 73t
ocular disease, 995–996
pregnancy, 1075–1076
strongyloidiasis, 810
HTLV-2, 545–546
HTLV-3, 541
HTLV-associated myelopathy, 545
Hu39694 virus, 471t
Human granulocytotropic anaplasmosis *see* Anaplasmosis
Human herpesviruses, 355–368, 356t
agent, 355–356
see also individual viruses
Human herpesvirus-6, 355, 356t, 364–365
agent, 364–365
clinical features, 365
diagnosis, 365
epidemiology, 365
exanthem subitum, 358f, 364–365
genome, 365
prevention and control, 365
treatment and prognosis, 365
Human herpesvirus-7, 355, 356t, 365–366
agent, 365
clinical features, 366
diagnosis, 366
epidemiology, 366
prevention and control, 366
treatment and prognosis, 366
Human herpesvirus-8, 355, 356t, 366–368
agent, 366
and cancer, 73t
Castleman's disease, 367
diagnosis, 368
epidemiology, 366
Kaposi's sarcoma, 358f, 366–367
multiple myeloma, 367
pathogenesis and immunity, 367–368
prevention and control, 368
primary effusion lymphoma, 367
treatment and prognosis, 368
Human Hookworm Vaccine Initiative, 804
Human immunodeficiency virus *see* HIV/AIDS
Human metapneumovirus, 7, 378, 379t–380t, 386–387
agent, 386
clinical features, 386
diagnosis, 386–387
epidemiology, 386
pathogenesis and immunity, 386
treatment, prevention and control, 387
vaccine, 380t
Human papillomavirus, 532–540, 533t
agent, 532
and cancer, 71–72, 73t
clinical features, 534
anogenital malignancies, 533–534
genital warts, 533t, 534, 535f
mucosal, 534
penile, vulvar, vaginal and cervical cancers, 533t, 534
recurrent respiratory papillomatosis, 533t, 534
diagnosis, 536
colposcopy, 536
cytology, 536
histology, 536
nucleic acid detection tests, 536
visual examination, 536
epidemiology, 532–533
HIV coinfection, 533, 555
incidence and prevalence, 532–533
natural history, 75f
pathogenesis and immunity, 534–536
prevention and control, 538–540
circumcision and condoms, 538
environmental precautions, 538
screening, 539–540
transmission, 533–534
treatment and prognosis, 536–538
treatment approaches, 538
treatment methods, 536–537
vaccine, 64t–65t, 538–539, 539t
Human parainfluenza virus, 379t–380t, 385–386
agent, 385
clinical features, 385
diagnosis, 386
epidemiology, 385
pathogenesis and immunity, 385–386
prevention and control, 385–386
treatment, 386
vaccine, 380t
Human parechoviruses, 419
Human respiratory syncytial viruses, 378, 379t, 383–385
agent, 383
clinical features, 384
diagnosis, 384
epidemiology, 383–384
pathogenesis and immunity, 384
treatment and prognosis, 384–385
vaccine, 380t, 385
Human rhinovirus, 378, 379t–380t, 387–388
agent, 387
clinical features, 387
diagnosis, 388
epidemiology, 387
pathogenesis and immunity, 387–388
prevention and control, 388
serotypes, 387
treatment, 388
Human T-lymphotropic virus *see* HTLV
Humoral response, 57
Hutchinson's incisors, 291
Hyalomma spp., 442t–443t, 466, 515
Hyalomma anatolicum, 875t
Hyalomma marginatum, 875t
Hyaluronic acid, 658–659
Hyaluronidase, 4, 200
group A streptococcus, 203, 207
Leptospira, 305
Hybrid vigor, 32
Hydatid disease
liver, 827–828, 830f, 976t–977t, 979–980, 979f
lung, 828
treatment
PAIR, 831–832
surgical removal, 831
see also Cystic echinococcosis
Hydrobiidae, 862
Hydrocele
loaiasis, 737
lymphatic filariasis, 729, 732, 732f
Hydrocephalus
congenital toxoplasmosis, 725f
cysticercosis, 820
tuberculous meningitis, 236
ventricular neurocysticercosis, 821
Hydrocortisone, paracoccidioidomycosis, 584
Hydrogen peroxide, 200
Hydrophobia, 527
Hydroxycarbamide, sickle cell anemia, 1030, 1031b
Hydroxychloroquine
adverse effects, 897t
malaria, 897t
dose, 897t
prophylaxis, 669t
Q fever, 346
Hylomyscus simus, 473
Hymenolepiasis, 843–845
agent *see Hymenolepsis* spp.
clinical features, 845
eosinophilia, 942t
diagnosis, 845
epidemiology, 845
prevention and control, 845
treatment and prognosis, 845
Hymenolepsis spp., 813, 843–845
Hymenolepsis diminuta, 813–814, 844–845
Hymenolepsis nana
cysticercoid stage, 844f
eradication, 80t
life cycle, 844f
ova, 813–814, 843–845, 844f
proglottids, 844f
scolex, 844f
Hyper-IgM syndrome, 34t
Hyperalaninemia, malaria, 661
Hyperamylasemia, leptospirosis, 304
Hyperbaric oxygen
adverse effects, 601
mucormycosis, 601
Hypergammaglobulinemia
loaiasis, 737
malaria, 657
toxocariasis, 766
Hyperglycaemia, correction of, 601
Hyperinfection syndrome, 976t–977t

Hyperinsulinemia, 27
  malaria, 661
Hyperkeratosis, 535
Hyperlactatemia, malaria, 655b, 661
Hyperreactive malaria splenomegaly, 657
Hypersensitivity
  delayed type, 61
  immediate, 61
Hypocalcemia, cholera, 153
Hypochloremia, malaria, 660
Hypochlorhydria, 170
Hypochromic microcytic anemia, e12t–e13t
Hypoglycemia
  cholera, 153
  malaria, 655b, 656, 661
Hypokalemia, cholera, 153
Hyponatremia
  cholera, 153
  malaria, 660
  shigellosis, 141–144
Hypotension, yellow fever, 498
Hypothesis testing, 12–14
  alpha level, 12
  null hypothesis, 12
  P value, 12
  power, 12
  type I errors, 12
  type II errors, 12
Hypothyroidism, e12t–e13t
Hypovolemic shock, cholera, 153
Hystricognath rodents, 837

I

IC3b, 53
ICAM-1, 5, 56
  cytoadherence, 658–659
  enterovirus infection, 403
  malaria protection, 37t
Icterus, hemorrhagic fevers, 445t
Idoxuridine, herpesviruses, HSV, 359
IgA
  H. pylori infection, 171
  properties of, 58t
  trichuriasis, 793
IgA protease, 186
IgD, properties of, 58t
IgE
  ascariasis, 796
  loaiasis, 737
  onchocerciasis, 747
  properties of, 58t
  toxocariasis, 765
  trichinellosis, 772
IgG
  properties of, 58t
  protein energy malnutrition, 29
  tick-borne virus-specific, 448t
IgG antibodies, 348
  B. mandrillaris, 712
  HEV, 424
  orthopoxviruses, 373
  T. cruzi, 693
  toxoplasmosis, 726
  trichuriasis, 793
IgM
  H. pylori infection, 171
  HSV-specific, 359
  properties of, 58t
  trichuriasis, 793
IgM antibodies, 54t
  B. mandrillaris, 712
  HAV, 422
  measles, 348
IgM-ELISA, toxoplasmosis, 726
IgM-ISAGA, toxoplasmosis, 726
Ilesha virus, 482
Ilheus virus, 511, 514
Imidazoles, dermatophytosis, 563
Imipenem, 96t–98t, 98
  melioidosis, 222
  mycobacterial infections, 247
Imiquimod, HPV, 537
Immediate hypersensitivity, 61
Immigrants, 902–909
  admission to USA, 903f
  classification of medical conditions, 904
  electronic disease notification system, 906
  health screening, 902–903
    conditions identified, 905t
    required medical examinations, 903–905, 904f–905f, 904t
  vaccination requirements, 908t
Immune evasion, 6–7, 6t
Immune reconstitution inflammatory syndrome *see* IRIS
Immune system, 3
  genetic variation, 33
  malnutrition effects, 24b
Immunity, *Salmonella*, 134
Immunization
  overseas medical screening, 904t
    requirements for immigrants, 908t
  private-public partnerships, 64–67
    advance market commitments, 66
    Global Alliance for Vaccines and Immunization, 64–66
    Global Immunization Vision and Strategy, 66
    Program for Appropriate Technology in Health, 66
    United Nations Prequalified Vaccines, 66–67
    World Health Organization, 66, 66b
  routine, 63, 64t–65t
  travelers, 894t
    altered immunocompetence, 890–891
    HIV-infected, 899
    hypersensitivity to vaccine components, 890
    immunoglobulins, 887–890
    infants, 891
    interrupted multidose schedules, 887
    pregnancy, 891
    recommended, 887, 888t–890t, 891–892
    required, 887, 888t–890t, 891
    routine, 887, 888t–890t, 891
    simultaneous administration of vaccines, 887
  see also Vaccines
Immunocompromised patients, 62
  brucellosis, 273–274
  Chagas' disease, 693
  fevers in, 937
  immunization for travel, 890–891
  microsporidiosis, 717–718, 717f
  Q fever, 346
  strongyloidiasis, 810
  tuberculosis, 232
  see also HIV/AIDS
Immunofluorescence assay, orthopoxviruses, 373
Immunoglobulinopathy, strongyloidiasis, 810
Immunoglobulins
  antirabies, 530
  HRSV, 380t
  human metapneumovirus, 380t
  properties of, 58t
  staphylococcal toxic shock syndrome, 210
  travelers, 887–890, 888t–890t
  see also Ig
Immunology, 52–62
  adaptive immunity *see* Adaptive immunity
  immunodeficiency, 62
  innate immunity *see* Innate immunity
  vaccines *see* Vaccines
Immunomodulators, SARS, 397
Immunopathology, 61–62
  autoimmunity, 61
Immunoproteosomes, 58
Immunoreceptor tyrosine-based activation motif *see* ITAM
Immunoreceptor tyrosine-based inhibitory motif *see* ITIM
Immunostimulators, Rift Valley fever, 465
Immunotherapy, rotavirus, 409
Impetigo, 261–262, 972t
  staphylococcal, 209
Impetigo contagiosa, 204
Incidence, 11
Incubation period, 11
India
  drug-resistant *P. falciparum*, 654t
  leishmaniasis, 697–698
Indinavir, 103t
  herpesviruses, HHV-8, 368
  HIV, 553–554
Indirect immunofluorescent antibody test, arenaviruses, 451
Inducible nitric oxide synthase promoter, malaria susceptibility, 37t
Inermicapsifer spp., 813
Infants *see* Children
Infection
  and cancer, 71–74, 73t, 74f
    prevention, 74–75
  causes
    individuals, 2
    populations, 3
  gastrointestinal, 27–28
  mycobacterial, 245–247, 245t
  and nutritional status, 27, 27b
    carbohydrate metabolism, 27
    constitutional symptoms, 27
    mineral metabolism, 27
    protein metabolism, 27
  susceptibility to, 32–39
Infectious agents, 1
Infectious diseases
  genetic influence of, 34–39, 35t
  inherited conditions predisposing to, 34, 34t
Inflammasomes, 53–54
Inflammation, 61
Infliximab, complications, tuberculosis, 233
Influenza, 7, 378–383, 379t, 419
  A strain, 379–380
  agent, 378–380, 380f
  B strain, 379–380
  C strain, 379–380
  clinical features, 381
    conjunctivitis, 991
  diagnosis, 382
  epidemiology, 380–381
  incubation period, 929b
  military cases, 910
  N1N1 strain, 106f
  pathogenesis and immunity, 381–382
  prevention and control, 383
  transmission, 381
  treatment and prognosis, 382–383
  vaccine, 64t–65t, 380t, 383, 888t–890t
    requirements for immigrants, 908t
Inhalational anthrax, 263
Inherited conditions
  association studies, 34, 34t–35t
  complement system, 34t
  polygenic inheritance, 32
  predisposition to infectious disease, 34, 34t
  red blood cell disorders, 1030–1032
    G6PD deficiency, 32, 1025, 1026f, 1032
    sickle cell anemia, 1025, 1026f, 1030, 1030b
    thalassemia see Thalassemia
  see also congenital disease
Innate immunity, 3, 6t, 52–56
  attributes of, 53t
  cellular constituents, 54–56
  components of, 53t
  epithelial barrier surfaces, 3–4
  genetic variation, 33
  malnutrition effects
    phagocytic cells, 28
    physical barriers, 28
  pattern recognition molecules, 52–54
  synthesis, 56

Insect vectors, 45
hemimetabolous, 45, 46f
holometabolous, 45, 46f
see also individual insect species
Insecticide-treated bednets, 17, 20–21, 646, 654, 673, 673f, 895
free distribution, 21
willingness to pay, 21
Insecticides
DDT *see* DDT
DEET, 510, 524, 681, 705
lindane, 333, 868–869
Insulin resistance, 27
Insulin-like growth factor-1, trichuriasis, 793
Integrase inhibitors, 103t, 553–554
α/β-Integrin, 658–659
Interferons, 56
hepatitis D, 439
pegylated, hepatitis D, 439
Rift Valley fever, 465
Interferon-alfa, 102t
hepatitis B, 436
Kaposi's sarcoma, 368
pegylated
hepatitis B, 436
hepatitis C, 431
Interferon-γ
cysticercosis, 819
disease associations, 36t
malaria, 657–658
Interferon-γ release assays, 230
Intergovernmental Panel on Climate Change, 8
Interleukin-1, 27
cysticercosis, 819
disease associations, 36t
malaria, 657–658
Interleukin-2, cysticercosis, 819
Interleukin-4, toxocariasis, 765
Interleukin-5
alveolar echinococcosis, 835
loiaisis, 737
toxocariasis, 765
Interleukin-6
cysticercosis, 819
malaria, 657–658
Interleukin-8
disease associations, 36t
malaria, 657–658
Interleukin-8 cleaving enzyme, 208
Interleukin-10
alveolar echinococcosis, 835
disease associations, 36t
leishmaniasis, 702
malaria, 657–658
Interleukin-12
cysticercosis, 819
malaria, 657–658
Interleukin-12 receptor, disease associations, 36t
Interleukin-18, malaria, 657–658
International Health Regulations, 106
International System for Total Early Disease Detection (InStedd), 880
Intestinal ascariasis, 796, 796f
Intestinal flukes, 865
diagnosis, 867
prevention and control, 867
treatment and prognosis, 867
Intestinal obstruction, 921
Intestinal protozoa, 621–622, 622f
see also Amebic disease
Intimin, 114t–115t
Intracellular adhesion molecule-1 *see* ICAM-1
Intracellular enveloped virion, 370–372
Intracranial pressure, raised, tuberculous meningitis, 236
Iodamoeba butschlii, 614, 621–622, 622f
Iodine, requirements, e12t–e13t
Iododeoxyuridine, human adenovirus, 390
Iodoquinol, 90
adverse effects, 85b
amebiasis, 88t–89t, 621
balantidiasis, 88t–89t, 628t, 630
D. fragilis, 88t–89t, 628t
E. histolytica, 918t
Ipaf, 53, 54t
Ipomoea aquatic, 865
Ippy virus, 450f
IRIS
HIV, 260
tuberculosis, 234–236
Iron, 24, 26
requirements, e12t–e13t
Iron deficiency, 26, 26t, 1028b
immune effects, 24b
Iron deficiency anemia, 26t, 31, 1025f, 1027f
koilonychia, 1025
pencil cells, 1025f, 1026
Iron supplements, 26
Iron utilization block, 1027
ISD sensor, 54t
Isoniazid, 100t
adverse reactions, 240
peripheral neuropathy, 240
breastfeeding, 242
chemoprophylaxis, 555
in pregnancy, 242, 1073t
resistance, 237–238
tuberculosis, 239t, 240
prophylactic, 244–245
tuberculous meningitis, 236
tuberculous pleurisy, 234
Isospora spp., 634f
Isospora belli, 627, 641, 643–644, 917t
characteristics and epidemiology, 643
HIV coinfection, 1053
see also Isosporiasis
Isosporiasis, 643
agent *see Isospora belli*
clinical features, 643
chronic diarrhea, 924
diagnosis, 643–644
prophylaxis, 643
treatment and prognosis, 88t–89t, 644, 918t
Isotretinoin, pleural effusion, 988t
ITAM, 54–55
ITIM, 54–55
Itraconazole, 94, 100t–101t
basidiobolomycosis, 604t
blastomycosis, 577
candidiasis, 590–591
esophageal, 592
oropharyngeal, 592
vulvovaginal, 593
chromoblastomycosis, 570
coccidioidomycosis, 579
conidiobolomycosis, 604t
cryptococcosis, 580–581
dermatophytosis, 563
entomophthoramycosis, 604t
granulomatous amebic encephalitis, 712
histoplasmosis, 575
leishmaniasis
cutaneous, 705
visceral, 704
microsporidiosis, 720t
mucosal candidiasis, 104t
onychomycosis, 563
P. marneffei, 587–588
paracoccidioidomycosis, 584
phaeohyphomycosis, 572
sporotrichosis, 604t, 606–607
tinea capitis, 563
toxicity, 101t
Ivermectin, 79
adverse effects, 82b, 734
African trypanosomiasis, 687, 688t
ascariasis, 77t–79t
cutaneous larva migrans, 77t–79t, 767
enterobiasis, 790
gnathostomiasis, 77t–79t, 785
loaiasis, 738
louse eradication, 93t
lymphatic filariasis, 734
M. ozzardi, 740
nematode infections, 77t–79t
onchocerciasis, 77t–79t, 79, 747–748, 748f
prophylaxis, 749
perstans filariasis, 739
scabies, 93t, 868–869
streptocerciasis, 77t–79t, 739
strongyloidiasis, 76, 77t–79t, 811, 918t
toxocariasis, 766
prophylaxis, 767
trichuriasis, 77t–79t, 793
Ixodes spp., 515
Lyme disease, 297
Ixodes dammini, 875
babesiosis, 677, 678f
Ixodes dentatus
A. phagocytophilum, 342
B. divergens, 677
Ixodes granulatus
babesiosis, 677f
ecology, 678
Ixodes holocyclus, 324–326, 875t
Ixodes ovatus
babesiosis, 677f
ecology, 678
Ixodes pacificus, 296t, 342
Ixodes persulcatus, 296t, 297, 342, 515, 677
and *A. phagocytophilum*, 342
Ixodes ricinus, 296t, 875t
babesiosis, 676–677
ehrlichiosis, 342
Lyme disease, 297, 676
tick-borne encephalitis, 515
Ixodes scapularis, 46, 49, 296t, 297, 342, 875, 875t
and *A. phagocytophilum*, 342
babesiosis, 677f
Ixodes trianguliceps, and *A. phagocytophilum*, 342
Ixodidae, 45, 51, 874–875

J

J virus, 352
James' dots, 647–649
Janeway lesions, 950, 955t
Japanese encephalitis, 352, 511–512, 516f, 876t
clinical features, 512
diagnosis, 513
incubation period, 929b
military cases, 912
pathogenesis and immunity, 512
pathology, 512
prevention and control, 513–514
treatment and prognosis, 513
vaccine, 64t–65t, 513, 888t–890t, 892
Japanese spotted fever, 323
Jarisch-Herxheimer reaction
leptospirosis, 307
Q fever, 346
relapsing fever, 301
syphilis, 292
Jaundice
leptospirosis, 304f, 305
malaria, 654–656, 655b, 661
returning travelers, 973b
Jet lag, 900
Joint involvement, salmonellosis, 132t–133t
Josamycin
H. pylori infection, 172t
spotted fever rickettsioses, 328
Jugra virus, 492
Junin virus, 442t–443t, 450f, 450t
animal models, 457
as bioterrorism agent, 880t
incubation period, 929b
skin lesions, 956t
transmission, 932t
rodent hosts, 455

vaccine, 461
see also Argentine hemorrhagic fever
Juquitiba virus, 471t
hantavirus pulmonary syndrome, 476

K

Kadam virus, 516f
Kala-azar *see* Leishmaniasis, visceral
Kanamycin, 100t
gonorrhoea, 189
tuberculosis, 243
Kaposi's sarcoma, 72, 358f, 366–367, 1064
geographic distribution, 367f
histopathology, 367f
Kaposi's varicelliform eruption, 357
Karshi virus, 516f
Katayama fever, 701, 849, 918
incubation period, 929b
Kato template technique, 852
Kelly's medium, 300
Keratitis, 1004, 1004f–1005f
Acanthamoeba, 86t–87t, 707, 710–711, 711f, 1011, 1011f
diagnosis, 712
prevention and control, 713
treatment and prognosis, 713
causes, 1005b
fungal, 1006
measles, 992–993, 992f–993f
onchocerciasis, 1012f
rubella, 993
smallpox, 371
Keratoconjunctivitis
adenovirus, 389, 992f
HSV-1, 357
Keratomalacia, 992f
Kernig's sign, 1017
Keshan's disease, 26–27, e12t–e13t
Ketoacidosis, malaria, 661
Ketoconazole, 94, 100t–101t
basidiobolomycosis, 604t
candidiasis, 592
vulvovaginal, 593
conidiobolomycosis, 604t
dermatophytosis, 563
entomophthoramycosis, 604t
eumycetoma, 568
histoplasmosis, 575
leishmaniasis
cutaneous, 705
visceral, 704
P. marneffei infection, 587–588
paracoccidioidomycosis, 584
phaeohyphomycosis, 572
toxicity, 101t
Kexin, 609
Kidney *see* Renal involvement
Killer inhibitory receptors, 54–55, 54t
Kinetoplastids, 682, 696
adverse effects, 90b
treatment, 90–94, 91t–92t
Kingella spp., 184
Kinjin virus, 516f
Kinyoun stain, *M. tuberculosis*, 238
Kissing bugs, 45, 50, 874, 874f
pruritus caused by, 959t–961t
Klebsiella spp., 113
toxin, 113, 114t–115t
Klebsiella granulomatis, 196
see also Donovanosis
Klebsiella rhinoscleromatis, 196, 962t–966t
Kobuvirus, 398
Koch, Robert, 150
Koilocytes, HPV infection, 536
Koilonychia
hookworm, 802
iron deficiency anemia, 1025
Koplik's spots, 348
Kruskal-Wallis test, 13
Kumusi ulcer *see Mycobacterium ulcerans*
Kwashiorkor, 23
skin lesions, 28
Kyasanur Forest disease, 442t–443t, 511, 514–515, 516f
clinical features, 444t–445t
skin lesions, 956t
diagnosis, 447t
pathologic features, 446t
transmission, 932t

L

L proteins, 352–353
La Crosse encephalitis, 876t
Labetalol, tetanus, 287–288
Laboratory tests, 14–16, 14f
false negatives, 14–15
false positives, 14–15
sensitivity, 14
specificity, 14
Lacazia loboi, 604
Lacaziosis *see* Lobomycosis
Lactase deficiency, rotavirus-induced, 409
Lactate dehydrogenase
Crimean-Congo hemorrhagic fever, 467
trichinellosis, 772
Lactic acidosis, malaria, 661
Lactobacillus spp., rotavirus, 409
Lactobacillus GG, *E. coli* infection, 120
Lagochilascaris spp., 783–784
Lagochilascaris minor, 783–784, 784f
Lagos bat virus, 526t
Lagovirus, 411
Laguna Negra virus, 471t
hantavirus pulmonary syndrome, 476
Lake Victoria marburgvirus, 483
Laminin-2, 254
Lamivudine, 102t–103t, 553
hepatitis B, 436
HIV, 553
Langat virus, 516f
Langerhans cells, 56
Lansoprazole, *H. pylori* infection, 172t
Large-loop excision of transformation zone (LLETZ), 537
Larva currens, 810, 961f
Larva migrans, 763
cutaneous, 766–767, 767f, 800–801
eradication, 76, 77t–79t
fascioliasis, 860
ocular, 763, 764t, 765, 765f
trematode, 864
visceral, 763, 764t, 765
see also Toxocariasis
Laryngitis, candidal, 593
Laryngotracheobronchitis *see* Croup
Lasègue's sign, 272
Lassa fever, 7, 442t–443t, 450f, 450t
as bioterrorism agent, 880t
children, 456
swollen baby syndrome, 456
clinical features, 444t–445t, 456–457
liver infection, 458f
skin lesions, 956t–957t
diagnosis, 447t
epidemiology, 453
incubation period, 929b
maintenance in rodent hosts, 455
pathologic features, 446t
transmission, 454–455, 932t
treatment and prevention, 448t, 460
Latency, 11
Latex agglutination, trichinellosis, 772
Latin America
candidemia, 595
Chagas' disease *see* Chagas' disease
chromoblastomycosis, 569
coccidioidomycosis, 578
cryptosporidiosis, 636t
histoplasmosis, 573
measles, 350f
Latino virus, 450f
Latrodectus mactans, 872, 872f
Lechiguanas virus, 471t
hantavirus pulmonary syndrome, 476
Lecithinase, 221
Lecithodendridae, 866
Lectin pathway, 52–53
Leeches, 877–878
Legionella spp., 5, 709
Legionella pneumophila, 215
developmental cycle, 217f
drug resistance, 95
see also Legionellosis
Legionellosis, 215–218
agent, 215
diagnosis, 218
disease, 216–217, 216t, 217f
epidemiology, 215–216, 216f
incubation period, 929b
pathogenesis and immunity, 217–218, 217f
prevention and control, 218
treatment and prognosis, 218
Legionnaire's disease *see* Legionellosis
Legs, lymphatic filariasis, 732, 732f
Leishmania spp., 5, 45, 48–49, 574, 696, 698t
amastigotes, 696, 697f
life cycle, 697f
transmission, 696
Leishmania aethiopica, 697
clinical syndrome and geographic distribution, 698t, 699f
Leishmania amazonensis, 697
clinical syndrome and geographic distribution, 698t
Leishmania braziliensis, 696–697
clinical syndrome and geographic distribution, 698t, 699f
Leishmania chagasi, 49
geographic distribution, 699f
Leishmania colombiensis, clinical syndrome and geographic distribution, 698t
Leishmania donovani, 552, 697
clinical syndrome and geographic distribution, 698t, 699f
pulmonary disease, 984t
Leishmania garnhami, clinical syndrome and geographic distribution, 698t
Leishmania guyanensis, 697
clinical syndrome and geographic distribution, 698t
Leishmania infantum, 696
clinical syndrome and geographic distribution, 698t, 699f
Leishmania infantum chagasi, 697–698
clinical syndrome and geographic distribution, 698t
vectors, 697
Leishmania major, 49, 696
clinical syndrome and geographic distribution, 698t, 699f
Leishmania mexicana, 697
clinical syndrome and geographic distribution, 698t, 699f
Leishmania panamensis, 697
clinical syndrome and geographic distribution, 698t
Leishmania peruviana, 697
clinical syndrome and geographic distribution, 698t
vectors, 697
Leishmania pifanoi, clinical syndrome and geographic distribution, 698t
Leishmania tropica, 697
clinical syndrome and geographic distribution, 698t, 699f
Leishmania venezuelensis, clinical syndrome and geographic distribution, 698t
Leishmania viannia braziliensis, 919

Leishmaniasis, 17, 21, 261–262, 696–706, 697f
agent, 696, 698t
American mucocutaneous, 698t
clinical features, 698–701
ocular involvement, 1010–1011
cutaneous, 696
clinical features, 699–700, 700f, 957f, 957t, 962t–968t, 972t
differential diagnosis, 700
diffuse, 698t, 700
New World, 697, 698t
Old World, 697, 698t
treatment and prognosis, 704–705
diagnosis, 703
parasite identification, 703
serology, 703
skin test, 703
epidemiology, 696–698
genetic protection, 35t
geographic distribution, 696
HIV coinfection, 899, 1050–1051
immunology, 701–703
cellular and cytokine responses, 702–703
Leishmania-macrophage interactions, 702
incubation period, 929b
military cases, 912–913
mucosal, 697
clinical features, 700–701, 700f, 917t
differential diagnosis, 701
treatment and prognosis, 705
post-kala-azar dermal, 701
prevention and control, 705–706
treatment and prognosis, 90–94, 91t–92t, 700
visceral (kala-azar), 696–698, 698t
clinical features, 701, 962t–966t
differential diagnosis, 701
distribution, 699f
pigmentation changes, 973t
treatment and prognosis, 704
viscerotropic, 701
Lentiviruses
cell tropism, 545
genetic organization, 545
life cycle, 543, 544f
phylogeny, 542f
see also HIV/AIDS
Leopard skin, 744f
Lepromin, 253
Leprosy, 253–260
agent, 253
clinical features
gastrointestinal symptoms, 917t
Mitsuda reaction, 254–255
ocular involvement, 998–999, 998f
oropharyngeal lesions, 919
pigmentation changes, 973t
skin lesions, 962t–968t
diagnosis, 258–259
histopathology, 258–259
laboratory findings, 258
physical examination, 258
differential diagnosis, 259
epidemiology, 253–254, 254f
genetic, 254
eradication, 43
erythema nodosum leprosum, 258f
treatment, 259
genetic associations, 38
susceptibility, 35t
geographic distribution, 254f
history, 253
HIV coinfection, 260, 1059
Lucio, 257
overseas medical screening, 904t
pathogenesis and immunity, 254–258
clinical leprosy, 255–257
immunopathogenesis, 254–255, 255t
prevention and control, 260
reversal reaction, 258, 258f
treatment, 259
Ridley-Jopling classification, 254–255, 255t
borderline, 255t, 256–257, 257f
borderline-lepromatous, 255t, 257f
borderline-tuberculoid, 255t, 256–257
indeterminate, 255t, 256f
lepromatous, 255t, 257, 257f
tuberculoid, 255t, 256, 256f
transmission, 254
treatment and prognosis, 259–260
multibacillary regimen, 259, 259t
paucibacillary regimen, 259
reactions, 259–260
single lesion regimen, 259
Leptospira spp., 303
skin lesions, 957t
Leptospira borgpeterseni, 303
Leptospira inadai, 303
Leptospira interrogans, 303, 307
skin lesions, 956t
Leptospira kirschneri, 303
Leptospira noguchii, 303
Leptospira santarosai, 303
Leptospira weillii, 303
Leptospirosis, 303–307
agent, 303
clinical features, 303–305
jaundice, 304f, 305
kidney, 305f
liver, 305, 305f, 976t–977t
ocular involvement, 1001
pulmonary hemorrhage, 304f–305f
skin lesions, 962t–966t
uveitis, 304f
diagnosis, 305–307, 306f
epidemiology, 303, 304f
geographic distribution, 304f
icteric, 303
incubation period, 929b
military cases, 914
pathogenesis and immunity, 305, 305f–306f
pregnancy, 1076
prevention and control, 307
treatment and prognosis, 307
Leptotrombidium akamushi, 334
Leptotrombidium arenicola, 334
Leptotrombidium chiangraiensis, 334
Leptotrombidium deliense, 334
Leptotrombidium imphalum, 334
Leptotrombidium pallidum, 334
Leptotrombidium pavlovsky, 334
Leptotrombidium scutellare, 334
Lethal factor, 263
Leucovorin, pneumocystosis, 613
Leukemia, strongyloidiasis, 810
Leukocyte count, hemorrhagic fevers, 445t
Leukonychia, 563
Leukopenia
Brucella, 273
dengue hemorrhagic fever, 509
visceral leishmaniasis, 701
yellow fever, 498
Leukoplakia, candidal, 591–592
Leukovorin, toxoplasmosis, 727
Levamisole
ascariasis, 797
trichuriasis, 793
Levofloxacin, 96t–98t
H. pylori infection, 172t, 173b
legionellosis, 218
pelvic inflammatory disease, 1043t
travelers' diarrhea, 894t
tuberculosis, 242–243
Lewis X antigen, 168
Lice, 50, 868
pruritus caused by, 959t–961t
treatment, 93t
see also Louse
Lichenified onchodermatitis, 743, 744f
Lictheimia spp., 597
Limestone Canyon virus, 472
Limnatis nilotica, 878
Lindane
scabies, 868–869
typhus control, 333
Linezolid, 96t–98t, 98–99
MRSA, 211
Linguatula serrata, 877f
life cycle, 877
pulmonary disease, 984t
Lipase, 221
Lipoarabinomannan, 236–237
Lipooligosaccharide, 185
Lipophosphoglycan, 702
Lipoteichoic acid, 207
Listeria spp., 5, 7, 725–726
Listeria monocytogenes, 4
Listeriolysins, 5
Listeriosis
agent *see Listeria monocytogenes*
drug resistance, 95
pregnancy, 1076
Liver abscess
amebic, 617–618, 617f, 617t, 976t–977t
pyogenic, 976t–977t
Liver biopsy
hepatitis B, 436
hepatitis C, 431
Liver failure
acute, 976t–977t, 978
acute on chronic, 976t–977t
subacute, 976t–977t, 978
Liver flukes, 854
life cycle, 856f
see also Clonorchiasis; Fascioliasis; Opisthorchiasis
Liver involvement
cirrhosis, 917t
doughnut granuloma, 345
hydatid cysts, 827–828, 830f
leptospirosis, 305, 305f
malaria, 661
schistosomiasis, 851
Swiss cheese, 220f
yellow fever, 497
see also Hepatobiliary disease
Loa loa, 735
life cycle, 736f
microfilaria, 735f
pulmonary disease, 984t
vectors of, 50
see also Loiasis
Loaina spp., 751t
Loboa loboi, 604
Lobomycosis, 604–605
clinical features, 604
skin lesions, 969t–970t
diagnosis, 604–605
epidemiology, 604
pathogenesis and immunity, 604
treatment and prognosis, 604t, 605
Lobo's disease *see* Lobomycosis
Lockjaw, 284–285
see also Tetanus
Löffler's syndrome, 6, 944–945
Loiasis, 735–738
agent, 735
clinical features, 736–737
Calabar swellings, 735–738, 736f, 962f
eosinophilia, 943t
ocular involvement, 736, 736f, 1012–1013, 1012f
pleural effusion, 988t
pruritus, 959t–961t
skin lesions, 946t, 958t, 962t–966t
complications, 737
diagnosis, 737–738
epidemiology, 735–736
eradication, 77t–79t
pathogenesis and immunity, 737
pigmentation changes, 973t
prevention and control, 738
treatment and prognosis, 738

- Lone Star tick *see Amblyomma americanum*
- Loop electrosurgical excisional procedure (LEEP), 537
- Loop-mediated isothermal amplification, 221
- Loperamide
  - cryptosporidiosis, 638
  - *E. coli*, 119–120
  - norovirus, 414
- Lopinavir
  - HIV, 553–554
  - SARS, 397
- Lorazepam, tetanus, 287–288
- Louping ill virus, 515, 516f
- Louse-borne relapsing fever, 295–302
  - clinical/laboratory features, 297t
  - ecology and epidemiology, 296–297, 297f
  - life cycle, 297f
  - prevention, 301
- Louse-borne typhus, 329, 330f
  - skin lesions, 331f
- Low birth weight, malaria, 656–657
- Löwenstein-Jensen medium, 238
- *Loxosceles reclusa*, 872, 872f, 955t
- *Lucilia sericata*, 869
- Ludwig's angina, 263
- Lues maligna, 290
- Lujo virus, 442t–443t, 450f, 450t
  - clinical features, 457
  - transmission, 455
- Lumefantrine
  - malaria, 661, 664
  - pharmacokinetics, 665t
- Lung flukes, 862–865, 984t
  - *see also individual types*
- Lung infections *see* Pulmonary disease
- *Lutzomyia* spp., 49, 697
  - leishmaniasis, 696
- *Lutzomyia columbiana*, 265–267
- *Lutzomyia longipalpis*, 49
- *Lutzomyia verrucarum*, 265–267, 266f, 266t
- Lyme disease, 45, 295
  - agent, 295, 296t
  - clinical/laboratory features, 297–298, 297t
  - diagnosis, 299–300, 300f
  - ecology and epidemiology, 297, 297f
  - genetic susceptibility, 35t
  - immunity, 299
  - pathogenesis, 298–299, 299f
  - pathology, 299
  - prevention and control, 302
  - prognosis, 301
  - transmission, 874, 875t
  - treatment and prognosis, 300–301
  - *see also* Relapsing fever
- Lymphadenitis, 266t
  - loaiasis, 737
  - mycobacterial, 245
- Lymphadenopathy
  - African trypanosomiasis, 685
  - cutaneous leishmaniasis, 700f
  - differential diagnosis, 954b
  - and fever, 935
  - monkeypox, 371
  - onchocerciasis, 745
  - paracoccidioidomycosis, 583f
  - tick-borne, 326–327
  - *see also* Skin lesions
- Lymphangitis, 204
- Lymphatic filariasis, 729–734
  - agent, 729–730, 730f
  - clinical features, 731–733, 732f
    - acute adenolymphangitis, 731–732
    - arms, legs and breasts, 732, 732f
    - chyluria, 732
    - genitourinary system, 732, 732f
    - subclinical patent infection, 731
    - tropical pulmonary eosinophilia, 733
  - diagnosis, 733–734
  - epidemiology, 730–731, 731f
  - expatriates and travelers, 733
  - global distribution, 731f
  - pathogenesis and immunity, 733
  - prevention and control, 734
  - treatment and prognosis, 734
    - chemotherapeutic agents, 734
    - pathology based therapy, 734
  - zoonotic, 753–754, 754f
- Lymphatic spread of infection, 4
- *Lymphcryptovirus*, 362–363
- Lymphedema therapy, 734
- Lymphocytes
  - development and activation, 57–58
  - *see also* B-lymphocytes; T-lymphocytes
- Lymphocytic choriomeningitis, 450f, 450t
  - animal models, 457
  - clinical features, 457
  - epidemiology, 453
  - maintenance in rodent hosts, 455
  - ocular involvement, 996
  - transmission, 454
- Lymphogranuloma venereum, 308, 314–319, 1034t
  - clinical features, 316–318, 1034t
    - anorectal involvement, 317
    - buboes, 308, 317
    - cutaneous lesions, 952t
    - esthiomene, 318
    - extragenital infection, 317
    - groove sign, 317
    - inguinal form, 317
    - men, 316
    - ocular, 998
    - skin lesions, 952t, 962t–966t
    - women, 316–317
  - diagnosis, 318, 1035t
    - culture, 318
    - direct immunofluorescence, 318
    - ELISA, 318
    - nucleic acid amplification tests, 318
    - point of care tests, 318
    - serologic tests, 318
  - epidemiology, 315
  - incidence, 315
  - molecular epidemiology, 315
  - pathogenesis and immunity, 315–316
  - prevention and control, 319
  - primary stage, 317
  - secondary stage, 317
  - sex ratio, 315
  - tertiary stage, 318
  - treatment and prognosis, 318
  - *see also Chlamydia trachomatis*
- Lymphoid organs, 57
- Lymphoma
  - gastric, *H. pylori*, 170
  - primary effusion, 367
- Lymphopenia, *Brucella*, 273
- Lyssaviruses, 526t, 530t

M

- M proteins, 206–207
- MAC *see Mycobacterium avium-intracellulare* complex
- *Macaca fascicularis*, 477
- Machupo virus, 442t–443t, 450f–451f, 450t
  - animal models, 457
  - as bioterrorism agent, 880t
  - incubation period, 929b
  - skin lesions, 956t
  - transmission, 932t
    - rodent hosts, 455
  - *see also* Bolivian hemorrhagic fever
- Macrocytic anemia, 1026
- Macrolides, 96t–98t, 99
  - *Borrelia* spp., 300
  - *Campylobacter* spp., 148
  - *H. pylori*, 172t
  - lymphogranuloma venereum, 318
  - pertussis, 214
  - trachoma, 312–313
  - *see also individual drugs*
- Macronodules, 955t
- Macrophages, 55
  - effects of malnutrition, 28
  - *Leishmania* interactions, 702
  - microorganisms in, 5
  - *Salmonella* interactions, 134
  - trachoma, 311
- Macular retinopathy, loaiasis, 737
- Macular skin lesions, 956–957, 956f, 957t
  - differential diagnosis, 957t
- Madarosis, 998, 1000
- *Madurella grisea*, 565, 567
- *Madurella mycetomatis*, 565, 567
- Magnesium sulfate, tetanus, 287–288
- Majocchi's granuloma, 561
- Major basic protein, 55–56
- Major histocompatibility complex, 54–55, 58–60
  - associations with infectious disease, 35t
  - diversity, 60
  - MHCI, 58, 59f
  - MHCII, 60
- Major outer membrane protein, 309, 314
- Mal morado, 744
- Malabsorption
  - ascariasis, 27–28
  - giardiasis, 27–28
  - strongyloidiasis, 809
  - vitamin A, 27–28
- Malaria, 17, 21, 646–675, 876t
  - adaptive immunity, 653
    - late infancy through childhood, 653
    - neonatal period and early infancy, 653
  - Africa, 652
    - transmission intensity, 652–653
  - agent, 646–651
  - 'airport', 463
  - Asia, 652, 652f
  - bacterial infection, 662
  - blood films, 647–649, 662, 662f–663f
    - gametocytes in, 664
    - and prognosis, 663–664
  - Burkitt's lymphoma, 657
  - cerebral, 655b, 655f–656f, 659–660, 1019t, 1023
  - children, 657
  - clinical features, 646, 654–657
    - anemia, 654–657, 655b, 660, 1027–1028, 1028f
    - coagulopathy, 660
    - fever, 926t–927t
    - headache, 654–655
    - hepatitis, 976t–977t
    - jaundice, 654–656, 655b, 661
    - liver dysfunction, 661
    - myalgia, 654–655
    - ocular involvement, 1010, 1010f
    - pulmonary edema, 660
    - renal failure, 656, 660
    - seizures, 649f, 655, 655b
    - splenomegaly, 654–655, 657, 661
  - cost of, 20–21
  - diagnosis, 662–664
    - rapid diagnostic tests, 663
  - effect on anthropometric indicators, 25t
  - endemicity, 647b
    - holoendemic, 647b
    - hyperendemic, 647b
    - hypoendemic, 647b
    - mesoendemic, 647b
  - epidemiology, 651–654, 651f–652f
  - Epstein-Barr virus, 657
  - eradication and control, 40, 654, 672–675
    - artemisinin-based combination therapies, 17, 20–21
    - case management, 673
    - control and prevention tools, 673
    - drug resistance and new drug development, 673–674
    - drug safety and contraindications, 672
    - indoor residual spraying, 673
    - insecticide-treated bednets, 17, 20–21, 646, 654, 673, 673f, 895

intermittent preventive treatment, 673
program goals, 673
residents of malaria-endemic areas, 672
visitors to malaria-endemic areas, 652f, 672
falciparum, 2, 655–656
genetic protection, 35t
fluid space and electrolyte changes, 660
gastrointestinal dysfunction, 661
genetic resistance, 34–37, 35t–37t
sickle cell trait, 32
thalassemia, 34
global distribution, 647f
health impact of, 646
hemoglobinuria, 656, 660–661
HIV coinfection, 654, 899, 1048–1050
human behavior and environment, 653–654
hyperalaninemia, 661
hyperinsulinemia, 661
hyperlactatemia, 655b, 661
hypochloremia, 660
hypoglycemia, 655b, 656, 661
hyponatremia, 660
immunologic processes, 659–662
incubation period, 647–649, 647b, 929b
innate immunity, 653
G6PD deficiency, 36t, 653
Hb E, 36t, 653
Hb F, 36t, 653
Hb S, 36t
lack of Duffy antigen, 36t, 653
sickle cell trait, 32, 653
thalassemia, 34, 36t, 653
iron supplements, 26
laboratory findings, 657
lactic acidosis, 661
metabolic acidosis, 655b, 656–657
military cases, 911
parasite density, 655b, 662–663
and prognosis, 663
parasite genomics, 650–651
pathogenesis, 657–659
erythrocyte deformability, 659
rosetting and aggregation, 659
sequestration and cytoadherence, 656f, 658
toxicity and role of cytokines, 657–658
vascular endothelial ligands, 658–659
pigment (hemozoin), 664
pregnancy, 654, 656–657, 1076–1077
placental dysfunction, 662
treatment, 671–672, 671b
prepatent period, 647–649, 647b
prognosis
antiparasite antibodies, 664
blood films, 663–664
gametocytes in blood films, 664
mature parasites, 655b, 664
parasite density, 663
pigment in polymorphonuclear leukocytes, 664
prophylaxis, 83
quartan, 650
nephropathy, 657
recurrence, 647b
Roll Back Malaria campaign, 20–21, 646
severe, 668–672
follow-up treatment, 672
treatment, 670–671, 670b
South America, 652
tertian, 650
thrombocytopenia, 656, 660
transfusion, 657
transmission intensity, 652–653
entomologic inoculation rate, 652
reproductive rate, 652
travelers, 887, 894–898, 895b
antimalarial drugs, 895–898, 897t
chemoprophylaxis, 895
malaria-endemic countries, 896f
personal protection measures, 895
recommended regimens, 897t, 898
self-treatment, 898
treatment
adjuvant, 671
antimalarials *see* Antimalarials
classification of patients for, 665
drug regimens, 666–668, 667t
P. vivax, *P. ovale* or *P. malariae* malaria, 668
in pregnancy, 671–672
pregnancy, 671–672, 671b
severe malaria, 668–672, 670b
supportive care, 671
uncomplicated *P. falciparum* malaria, 665–668
vaccines, 674–675, 674f
zinc supplements, 26
see also Plasmodium falciparum; Plasmodium malariae; Plasmodium ovale; Plasmodium vivax
Malassezia furfur, 969t–970t
Malathion
adverse effects, 94b
louse eradication, 93t
Malignant disease *see* Cancer
Malleobactin, 221
Malnutrition
clinical pointers, 30–31
immune effects, 24b, 28–30
and infection, 24–27, 25t
lymphoid atrophy, 30–31
protein energy, 23–24
Malta fever, 271–272, 883
Mammomogamus spp., 779–780, 780f
Mammomogamus laryngeus, 780f
Mammtrifluridine, herpesviruses, 356
Mandril immunodeficiency virus, 542f
Mann-Whitney *U*-test, 13
Mannan, 563
Mannan-binding lectin, 52–53, 54t
disease associations, 36t
Mannose receptor, 55
Mannose-binding lectin, 33, 34t
Mannose-binding receptors, 54t
Mansonella interstitium, 756
Mansonella ozzardi, 740
characteristics, 740
clinical features, 740
diagnosis, 740
epidemiology, 740
eradication, 77t–79t
pathogenesis and immunity, 740
prevention and control, 740
treatment and prognosis, 740
Mansonella perstans, 737, 739
eradication, 77t–79t
ocular involvement, 757f, 1013
see also Perstans filariasis
Mansonella rhodhaini, 750, 751t, 757
Mansonella streptocerca, 738, 757
eradication, 77t–79t
see also Streptocerciasis
Mansonellosis, 943t
Mansonia spp., filariasis, 730–731, 876t
Maporal virus, 477
Maraviroc, 103t
HIV, 553–554
Marboran, smallpox, 376
Marburg virus, 442t–443t, 487t
as bioterrorism agent, 880f
clinical features, 444t–445t
diagnosis, 447t
incubation period, 929b
pathologic features, 446t
skin lesions, 956t–957t
transmission, 932t
treatment and prevention, 448t
Marburgviruses, 483
outbreaks, 486f
Maribavir, herpesviruses, cytomegalovirus, 362
Marmota spp., 277
Mast cells, 55–56
Mastadenovirus, 389, 417
Mastocytosis, ascariasis, 796
Mastomys spp., 276–277, 442t–443t, 450f
Mastomys natalensis, 453
Matrix metalloproteinase 9, *C. trachomatis* infection, 316
Mauer's clefts, 647–649
Mayaro virus, 519, 520t
clinical features, 523
epidemiology, 522
Mazzotti reaction, 745–747, 746f
MDA5, 54t
Meaban virus, 516f
Mean, 13
geometric, 13
Measles, 3–4, 23, 347–351
agent, 347
Americas, 350f
clinical course, 348f
clinical features, 347
cough, 347
febrile convulsions, 347
keratitis, 992–993, 992f–993f
Koplik's spots, 348
pneumonia, 347
rash, 347, 348f, 972t
control of outbreaks, 350–351
diagnosis, 348
differential diagnosis, 348
effect on anthropometric indicators, 25t
elimination, 350
epidemiology, 347
HIV coinfection, 1062–1063
incubation time, 347
Latin America and Caribbean, 350f
malnourished children, 347
mortality, 347
pathogenesis and immunity, 351
skin lesions, 347, 348f, 956t
treatment and prognosis, 348
vaccine, 64t–65t, 348–351, 888t–890t
contraindications, 348
live vaccine, 348
maintenance of status, 350
Moraten strain, 348
Pan American Health Organization campaign, 349
and vitamin A deficiency, 25
Mebendazole
A. caninum, 77t–79t
A. cantonensis infection, 776
adverse effects, 82b
ascariasis, 77t–79t, 797, 918t
capillariasis, 77t–79t
E. vermicularis, 77t–79t
echinococcosis
alveolar, 836
cystic, 831
enterobiasis, 790
fascioliasis, 861
hookworm, 76, 77t–79t, 803
loaiasis, 738
M. perstans infection, 77t–79t
P. philippinensis infection, 787
perstans filariasis, 739
toxocariasis, 77t–79t, 766
trichinellosis, 77t–79t, 772–773
Trichostrongylus spp., 77t–79t
trichuriasis, 77t–79t, 793
Mecillinam, shigellosis, 143f
Mectizan Donation Program, 749
Median, 13
Mediterranean spotted fever, 875t
clinical features, 326
eschar, 955t
fever, 926t–927t
Mefloquine
adverse effects, 82b, 84, 897t
malaria, 664, 666, 667t, 668, 896–897, 897t
dose, 897t
pregnancy, 671b
prophylaxis, 84, 669t
pharmacokinetics, 665t

in pregnancy, 1073t
resistance, 83, 652f
Megacolon
Chagas' disease, 692f
treatment, 695
Megaesophagus
Chagas' disease, 692f
treatment, 695
Megaloblastic anemia, 1025, 1026f–1027f, 1027
vitamin B12 deficiency, 1027
Megalopyge opercularis, 871
Meglumine antimonate, 93
adverse effects, 90b
leishmaniasis, 91t–92t
cutaneous, 704–705
visceral, 704
Melanesian ovalocytosis, malaria protection, 36t
Melanoconion spp., 482
Melanoides tuberculatus, 855
Melarsoprol, 92
adverse effects, 90b
African trypanosomiasis, 91t–92t, 686–687, 688t
Melioidosis, 219–222
agent *see Burkholderia pseudomallei*
clinical features, 219–221
skin lesions, 967t–968t
diagnosis, 221–222
antibodies, 221–222
antigens and nucleic acids, 221
microscopy and culture, 221
epidemiology, 219
descriptive, 219
geographic distribution, 219
HIV coinfection, 1061
incubation period, 929b
latent infections, 220
localized, 220–221, 220f
mild and subclinical infections, 220
military cases, 914
outcome and follow-up, 222
pathogenesis and immunity, 221
pathology, 221
prevention and control, 222
reservoirs and transmission, 219
septicemic, 220, 220f
treatment and prognosis, 222
specific, 222
supportive, 222
Mellardia meltada, 277
Meloidae, 873
Membrane attack complex, 52–53
Men
Chlamydia prostatis, 316
epididymitis *see* Epididymitis
gonococcal infection, 184–185
gonorrhea, 184–185
lymphogranuloma venereum, 316
scrotal swelling, 1044
urethral syndromes, 1042
urinary tract infection, 1042
Meningeal plague, 280
Meningitis, 1019–1020
anthrax, 263
bacterial
H. influenzae, 193, 194t
symptoms and signs, 177t
with or without meningococcemia, 177
candidal, 594
cryptococcosis, 580
enterovirus, 398, 400–401
eosinophilic, 774–775
paragonimiasis, 863–864
pneumococcal, 201
Q fever, 346
Toscana virus, 481
toxocariasis, 765
tuberculous, 231, 233–236, 235f
CSF findings, 235
diagnosis, 236
symptoms, 235
treatment, 236, 1023
vaccine, 64t–65t, 183
viral, 178b
Meningitis belt, 175f
Meningococcal disease, 174–183
agent, 174–175
characteristics, 177–179
diagnosis, 181, 181f
differential diagnosis, 178b
epidemiology, 175–177
genetic associations, 39
history, 174
incidence, 177f
incubation period, 929b
military cases, 911
myocardial dysfunction, 179
pathogenesis and immunity, 179–181
pericarditis, 178
peritonitis, 179
prevention and control, 182–183
chemoprophylaxis, 182
immunoprophylaxis, 182–183
respiratory tract infections, 179
risk factors, 180
transmission and carriage, 175
treatment and prognosis, 181–182
antimicrobial and adjunctive therapies, 181–182
supportive care, 182
vaccines, 183, 888t–890t, 891–892
requirements for immigrants, 908t
Meningococcal sepsis, 178
Meningococcemia
chronic, 179
complement deficiency, 179
incubation period, 929b
without meningitis, 177
Meningococci, 174–175
virulence factors, 180b
Meningoencephalitis, 177
candidal, 594
Chagas' disease, 691–692
Halicephalobus, 778
paracoccidioidomycosis, 584
primary amebic, 707, 711
diagnosis, 712
neurologic involvement, 1019t
prevention and control, 713
treatment and prognosis, 713
toxocariasis, 765
Meningonema peruzzii, 750, 754, 757
Menkes' disease, e12t–e13t
Meriones spp., 277
Meropenem, 96t–98t, 98
melioidosis, 222
Mesalamine, pleural effusion, 988t
Mesocestoides spp., 813
Mesocricestus auratus, 454, 477
Metabolic acidosis
cholera, 153
malaria, 655b, 656–657
Metagonimiasis, 942t
Metagonimus yokogawai, 855f, 865–866
diagnosis, 867
eradication, 81t
Metapneumovirus, 386
Methicillin-resistant *Staphylococcus aureus see* MRSA
Methotrexate, cysticercosis, 821
Methylbenzethonium, leishmaniasis, cutaneous, 705
Methylprednisolone, histoplasmosis, 575
Metorchis conjunctus, 854–855
eradication, 81t
morphology, 855f
Metrifonate, schistosomiasis, 853
Metronidazole, 85–89, 96t–98t
adverse effects, 85b, 629t
amebiasis, 88t–89t, 621
amebic liver abscess, 979
B. hominis, 622
bacterial vaginosis, 1040t
balantidiasis, 88t–89t, 628t, 630, 918t
C. difficile, 164
Campylobacter spp., 148
D. fragilis, 88t–89t, 628t
E. histolytica, 918t
giardiasis, 88t–89t, 628t, 918t
H. pylori, 172t, 173b, 918t
pelvic inflammatory disease, 190t, 1043t
T. vaginalis, 88t–89t
tetanus, 287–288
trichomoniasis, 1040t
urinary tract infection, 1042
MGUS, 367
MHC *see* Major histocompatibility complex
Micafungin, 100t–101t
candidemia, 596
toxicity, 101t
Miconazole
candidiasis, 591
dermatophytosis, 563
P. marneffei infection, 587–588
primary amebic meningoencephalitis, 713
vulvovaginal candidiasis, 1040t
Microangiopathic hemolytic anemia, 1026f
Microarrays, orthopoxviruses, 373
Microcytic hypochromic anemia, 1025
differential diagnosis, 1029t
Microfilaria bolivarensis, 750, 751t, 757
Microfilaria diurna, 735
Microfilaria semiclarum, 750
Microfilarial infections, 754
Microimmunofluorescence test
C. psittaci, 322
C. trachomatis, 312, 315
Micronema deletrix, 778
Micronutrients, 24, e12t–e13t
requirements, e12t–e13t
Microorganisms
classification, 1–2
epithelial adhesion, 4
evolution, 1–2
host interactions, 3–6, 3f
localization in host, 4–5
extracellular, 5
intracellular, 4–5
normal flora, 3–4
penetration of epithelial barrier, 4
spread of, 4
tissue damage, 5–6
host cell function, 5–6
indirect, 6
virulence, 2
alteration of, 2
Microphallidae, 866
Microscopic agglutination test, leptospirosis, 306
Microsporidia, 7, 552, 714–716, 715t
characteristics, 714, 715f–716f
global distribution, 715f
life cycle, 714–716, 716f
Microsporidiosis, 714–721
diagnosis, 718–720
coprodiagnosis, 718–719
cytology, 719, 719f
electron microscopy, 719
histology, 719, 719f
immunofluorescence, 720
molecular diagnosis, 720
epidemiology, 716–717
HIV coinfection, 717–718, 717f, 1053
immunocompetent hosts, 718
immunosuppressed hosts, 717–718, 717f
intestinal, treatment, 88t–89t
ocular involvement, 1009, 1009f
pathogenesis and immunity, 718
prevention and control, 721
treatment and prognosis, 86t–87t, 720–721, 720t
Microsporidium spp., 634f, 714
Microsporidium africanus, 715t
corneal microsporidiosis, 718

Microsporidium ceylonesis, 715t
clinical manifestations, 718
Microsporum spp., 559
Microsporum audouinii, 560t
tinea capitis, 560
Microsporum canis, 560t
tinea capitis, 560
Microsporum ferrugineum, 560t
Microsporum gypseum, 560, 560t
tinea capitis, 560
Microtus spp., 276
Midazolam, tetanus, 287–288
Middelburg virus, 520t
Middle East
malaria, 896f
trichinellosis, 770t
Midges, 872
Migrants, 902–909
health screening, USA, 902–903
Migratory rash, 957, 958t, 961f
Miliaria rubra, 957
Miliary tuberculosis, 231, 233–234, 234f, 235t
Military forces, infectious diseases in, 910–915
arthropod-transmitted diseases, 911–913
droplet/aerosol transmission, 910–911
fecal-oral transmission, 913
multidrug-resistant war wound infections, 915
soil and dust transmission, 914–915
zoonotic diseases, 913–914
Milker's nodule, 261–262, 962t–966t
Miller Fisher syndrome, 346
Millipedes, 873, 873f
Miltefosine, 92–93
adverse effects, 90b
leishmaniasis, 91t–92t
cutaneous, 705
mucosal, 705
visceral, 704
Mimiviruses, 709
Mineral metabolism, in infection, 27
Minocycline
cat scratch disease, 269
leprosy, 259
meningococcal prophylaxis, 182
toxoplasmosis, 727
Vibrio spp., 161
Mites, 868–869
biting, 872–873, 873f
flour, 872–873
follicle, 869
grain, 872–873, 873f
house dust, 873
trombiculid *see* Trombiculid mites
Mitogenic factor, 208
Mitsuda reaction, 254–255
MMR vaccine, requirements for immigrants, 908t
Mobala virus, 450f, 450t
Modoc virus, 516f
Mokola virus, 526t
Molluscum contagiosum, 1034t
clinical features, 1037
diagnosis, 1037
Moniliformis moniliformis, eradication, 77t–79t
Monkeypox, 105, 369, 371–372
clinical features, 370, 370f
skin lesions, 972t
Monoclonal gammopathy of undetermined significance *see* MGUS
Monocytes, 55
Mononegavirales, 352–353, 483
Mononucleosis *see* Epstein-Barr virus
Montana myotis leukoencephalitis, 516f
Montenegro skin test, 703
Mopeia virus, 450f, 450t
Moraxella spp., 184
Morbillivirus, 347
Morera's disease, 776
Morganella spp., toxin, 113
Morphine sulfate, tetanus, 287–288
Mortality
children, odds ratio, 25t
travelers, 887, 899
Mosquito-borne diseases, 876t
see also chikungunya virus; dengue fever; malaria; and other diseases
Mosquitoes, 46, 49, 875–876
bites, 876f
feeding, 876f
life cycle, 45
pruritus caused by, 959t–961t
see also Aedes spp.; *Anopheles* spp.; *Culex* spp.; *Plasmodium* spp.
Mosso das Pedras virus, 520t
Motavizumab, HRSV, 385
Motor vehicle accidents/injuries, 899
Mousepox, 372
Moxidectin, onchocerciasis, 748
Moxifloxacin, 96t–98t, 100t
leprosy, 259
tuberculosis, 242
MRSA, 211
Mucambo virus, 520t
Mucorales, 597
Mucormycosis, 597–602
clinical features, 598–600
cutaneous mucormycosis, 599
gastrointestinal, 599
ocular involvement, 1008–1009
pulmonary, 599
sinuses, 598–599
diagnosis, 600
direct examination, 600
disseminated, 600
epidemiology, 598
histopathology, 600
microbiology, 597
pathogenesis and host-pathogen interactions, 597–598
prevention and control, 602
treatment and prognosis, 600–602
amphotericin B, 600
deferasirox, 601
echinocandins, 601
hyperbaric oxygen, 601
posaconazole, 600–601
reversal of host impairment, 601
surgical debridement, 601–602
Mucosal atrophy, 28
Mulberry stomatitis, paracoccidioidomycosis, 583f
Multifocal necrotizing encephalitis, 725, 725f–726f
Multilocus sequence typing, 175
C. trachomatis, 315
Multiple myeloma, HHV-8, 367
Mumps
dacryoadenitis, 993
skin lesions, 972t
vaccine, 64t–65t, 888t–890t
Mupirocin, impetigo, 204
Muridae spp., 442t–443t, 470
Murine typhus, 329–330
clinical features, 331
Murray Valley encephalitis, 511, 514, 516f
Mus musculus, 450f, 453, 477
Musca domestica, 869
Musca sorbens, 310
Musca vetustissima, 310
Muscidae, 869
Muscle involvement
cysticercosis, 818
salmonellosis, 132t–133t
trichinellosis, 770
Mutualism, 1
Myalgia, malaria, 654–655
Mycetoma, 231, 565–568
actinomycetoma, 565–566, 566f
treatment, 568, 568f
agents, 565
clinical features, 565–566
skin lesions, 962t–966t, 969t–970t
culture, 567
diagnosis, 566–567
histologic, 567
molecular, 567
differential diagnosis, 566
epidemiology, 565
eumycetoma, 565–566, 566f
treatment, 568, 568f
fine needle aspiration cytology, 567
imaging, 566–567, 566f
ultrasonic, 567, 567f
management, 567
pathogenesis and immunity, 566
serodiagnosis, 567
site of, 566, 566f
surgery, 568
Mycobacterial infections, 245–247, 245t
chronic pulmonary disease, 246
HIV coinfection, 1058–1060
see also individual infections
lymphadenitis, 245
skin and soft tissue, 245–246
treatment, 247
see also Leprosy; Tuberculosis; and *Mycobacterium* spp.
Mycobacterium spp., 5, 709
atypical, 245–247, 245t
classification, 245
Mycobacterium abscessus, 245t
Mycobacterium africanum, 228
see also Tuberculosis
Mycobacterium avium-intracellulare complex, 245t, 246–247, 552, 606
chronic pulmonary disease, 246
drug therapy, 104t
HIV coinfection, 246–247, 1058–1059
Mycobacterium bovis, 228
see also Tuberculosis
Mycobacterium chelonae, 245–246, 245t, 606
Mycobacterium fortuitum complex, 245–246, 245t, 606
treatment, 247
Mycobacterium genavense, 245t
Mycobacterium haemophilum, 245–246, 245t
Mycobacterium kansasii, 245–247, 245t, 606
treatment, 247
Mycobacterium leprae, 4, 7, 253
cell wall, 253
pathogenesis and immunity, 254–258
see also Leprosy
Mycobacterium malmoense, 245t, 246
Mycobacterium marinum, 245–246, 245t, 248, 606
skin lesions, 962t–966t, 971f
treatment, 247
Mycobacterium scrofulaceum, 245t
treatment, 247
Mycobacterium simiae, 245t
Mycobacterium szulgai, 245t
Mycobacterium terrae, 245t
Mycobacterium tuberculosis, 7, 228, 253, 267
as bioterrorism agent, 880t
pathogenesis and immunity, 236–238
sequencing of, 228
single nucleotide polymorphisms, 228
skin lesions, 972t
see also Tuberculosis
Mycobacterium ulcerans, 245–246, 245t, 248–252
and cancer, 73–74, 73t
pathogenesis and immunity, 250–251
skin lesions, 962t–966t
see also Buruli ulcer
Mycobacterium xenopi, 245t, 246
Mycocladus spp., 597
Mycocladus circeneloides, 597
Mycolactone, 248
Mycolates, 253
Mycoplasma spp.
ocular disease, 1001
skin lesions, 972t
Mycoplasma genitalium, 3
Mycoplasma hominis, ocular disease, 1001

Mycoplasma pneumoniae, 6
drug resistance, 95
military cases, 910
ocular disease, 1001
Myelitis, toxocariasis, 765
Myiasis, 869–870, 869f, 953f
clinical features
ocular involvement, 1016, 1016f
pleural effusion, 988t
pruritus, 959t–961t
skin lesions, 953f, 958t, 962t–966t
facultative, 869
obligate, 869–870
Mymphaea lotus, 865
Myocardial dysfunction, meningococcal disease, 179
Myocarditis
candidal, 593
Chagas' disease, 691–692, 692f
diphtheria, 224–225
enterovirus, 398, 402
relapsing fever, 298
toxoplasmic, 725
trichinellosis, 770–771
yellow fever, 406, 497
Myodes glareolus, 471t, 472–473
Myonecrosis, *S. pyogenes*, 204–205
Myopericarditis, postvaccinial, 375–376
Myositis, 1022
S. pyogenes, 204–205

N

Naegleria spp.
eradication, 86t–87t
taxonomy and classification, 709
Naegleria fowleri, 707–709, 933
cultivation, 708
epidemiology, 709
life cycle, 708, 708f
neurologic involvement, 1019t
primary amebic meningoencephalitis, 711, 711f
Nafcillin, 96t–98t
cellulitis, 210–211
staphylococcal toxic shock syndrome, 210
Nail infections
candidiasis, 590–591
onychomycosis, 559, 562, 562f, 591
paronychia, 591
Nairoviruses
Crimean-Congo hemorrhagic fever, 466
Rift Valley fever, 462
Nalidixic acid
Salmonella resistance, 130t
shigellosis, 143f
NALP3, 54t
Nanjianyin virus, 515
Nanophyetus salmincola, 855f, 866
eradication, 81t
Nasturtium officinale, 865
National Molecular Subtyping Network for Foodborne Disease Surveillance *see* PulseNet International
National Regulatory Authorities, 68
Natural disasters, 20
Natural killer cells, 54–55
abnormalities in AIDS, 1046
activation, 619
Natural killer T cells, 619
Naucoris spp., 248
Nausea, giardiasis, 627t
Ndumu virus, 520t
Neacomys guianae, 450f
Nebovirus, 411
Necator spp., 779–780
Necator americanus, 799, 800f, 800t
disease, 802
epidemiology, 801, 801f
properties, 800t
pulmonary disease, 984t
skin lesions, 957t
see also Hookworm
Necator brasiliense, pulmonary disease, 984t
Necrotizing enteritis, *C. difficile*, 165
Necrotizing fasciitis, 204
Nef, 543
Negative predictive value, 15
Neglected diseases, 17
Negri bodies, 525–526
Neisseria spp., 174
Neisseria gonorrhoeae, 5, 184
adhesins, 4
antimicrobial resistance, 188–189
complement deficiency predisposing to, 52–53
identification
culture, 187–188
Gram staining, 188
nucleic acid amplification tests, 188
ocular involvement, 1003
pathogenesis and immunity, 185–186
IgA protease, 186
lipooligosaccharide, 185
opacity proteins, 186
porin, 186
reduction modifiable protein, 186
type IV pilus, 185
skin lesions, 955t–956t
see also Gonorrhea
Neisseria lactamica, 180, 184
Neisseria meningitidis, 2, 60, 174, 184
atypical sites, 179
complement deficiency predisposing to, 52–53
ocular involvement, 1003
serogroups, 177t
A, 175–176, 175f–176f
B, 176, 176f
C, 176–177, 177f
W-135, 177
Y, 177
skin lesions, 955t–956t
see also Meningococcal disease
Nelfinavir, 103t
HIV, 553–554
Nematode infections, 1–2, 778–787
chemotherapy, 76–79, 77t–79t
HIV coinfection, 1054–1055
see also individual infections
Neonatal intensive care units, candidal infections, 595
Neonates
C. trachomatis infection, 317
enterovirus disease, 402
herpes virus, 357–358
malaria immunity, 653
tetanus, 284, 286
treatment, 288
see also Children
Neorickettsia helminthoeca, 866
Neorickettsia sennetsu, 339, 343
prevention and control, 343
treatment, 343
Neotestudina rosatii, 565
Neotoma spp., 276
Neotoma albigula, 450f
Neotominae, 470
Nephropathia epidemica, 473
Nephropathy, quartan malarial, 657
Neuraminidase, 154, 200
Neuraminidase inhibitors, influenza, 382
Neurobrucellosis, 273
Neurocysticercosis, 815, 1019t, 1020–1021
cerebral, treatment, 1023
epidemiology, 815, 816f
eradication, 76
extraparenchymal, 817–818
spinal, 818
subarachnoid, 817–818, 818f
ventricular, 817, 818f
parenchymal, 817
calcifications, 817, 817f
cystic and enhancing lesions, 817, 817f
treatment, 821
Neurologic disease, 1017–1023, 1018b
brain abscess, 1020–1022
brainstem and spinal cord, 1022
brucellosis, 273
encephalopathy *see* Encephalopathy
examination, 1017
fever *see* Encephalitis
fungal infection, mucormycosis, 599
Guillain-Barré syndrome, 147, 401, 526–527, 531, 1022
helminthic infection, 1019t
echinococcosis, 1019t, 1021
sparganosis, 846–847, 847f
history, 1017
investigations, 1017–1018
meningitis *see* Meningitis
parasitic infection, 1019t
malaria, 655b, 655f–656f, 659–660, 1019t, 1023
paragonimiasis, 1019t, 1021
schistosomiasis, 852
strongyloidiasis, 809, 810f
primary amebic meningoencephalitis, 1019t
protozoa, 1019t
Q fever, 346
salmonellosis, 132t–133t
syndrome-based diagnosis, 1018b, 1019t
treatment, 1022–1023, 1023t
tropical spastic paraparesis, 545, 1022
yellow fever vaccine-associated, 502–503
Neuropathy, 1022, e12t–e13t
isoniazid-induced, 240
Neuroretinitis, 266t
Neurotrichinosis, 771
Neutralization assay, arenaviruses, 451
Neutralizing antibodies
filoviruses, 490
Rift Valley fever, 465
Neutropenia, yellow fever, 498
Neutrophils, 55
effects of malnutrition, 28
hypersegmented, 1026f
Nevirapine, 103t
HIV, 553–554
New York virus, 470, 471t, 472–473
Niacin, requirements, e12t–e13t
Niclosamide, 81–82
adverse effects, 82
diphyllobothriasis, 80t, 843
dipylidiasis, 845
F. buski, 867
H. heterophyes, 867
hymenolepiasis, 845
T. saginata, 80t
T. solium, 80t
taeniasis, 840–841
Nifedipine, altitude sickness, 900–901
Nifurtimox, 90
adverse effects, 90b
African trypanosomiasis, 687
Chagas' disease, 91t–92t, 694
T. cruzi, 91t–92t
Night blindness *see* Xerophthalmia
Nikolsky's sign, 972f
Nipah virus, 7–10, 352
agent, 352–353
as bioterrorism agent, 880t
clinical features, 353–354
epidemiology, 353
gene function, 352
genome structure, 352
membrane glycoproteins, 353
mortality, 354
P, C, V and L proteins, 352–353
prevention and control, 354
treatment and prognosis, 354

Nitazoxamide
adverse effects, 629t
hymenolepiasis, 845
taeniasis, 840–841
Nitazoxanide, 90
adverse effects, 85b
ascariasis, 798
balantidiasis, 88t–89t
C. difficile, 164
cryptosporidiosis, 104t, 639, 918t
giardiasis, 88t–89t, 628t
H. nana, 80t
Nitric oxide, 619
Nitric oxide resistance, 134
Nitric oxide synthase, malaria protection, 37t
Nitrofurans
Campylobacter spp., 148
H. pylori, 172t
Nitrofurantoin, pleural effusion, 988t
Nitroimidazoles, *H. pylori* infection, 172t
NMSO3, human metapneumovirus, 380t
Nocardia spp., ocular disease, 1001–1002
Nocardia brasiliensis, 565, 606
Nocardia otitidiscaviarum, 565
Nocardia transvalensis, 565
Nod-like receptors, 53
Nod1, 54t
Nod2, 54t
Nodular skin lesions, 962, 962f, 962t–966t
differential diagnosis, 962t–966t
fungal, 969t–970t
Noma, 917t
Non-nucleoside reverse transcriptase inhibitors, 553–554
Nonoxynol-9, 190
Norfloxacin
donovanosis, 197
shigellosis, 918t
travelers' diarrhea, 894t
Normal distribution, 13, 13f
Normocytic normochromic anemia, 1025
Norovirus, 411
diagnosis, 414
diarrheal disease, 412, 414t
epidemiology, 411–412
gastroenteritis, 411–412, 414t
military cases, 913
pathogenesis and immunity, 412–414
prevention and control, 414–415
outbreaks, 414–415
sporadic disease, 415
treatment and prognosis, 414
vaccine development, 415
North America
babesiosis, 677
blastomycosis, 575, 576f
cryptosporidiosis, 636t
trichinellosis, 770t
see also USA
North Asian tick typhus, 955t
Norwalk virus, 411, 412f
Norwegian scabies, 868–869
Nose, in mucosal leishmaniasis, 700–701, 700f
Nosema spp., 634f
Nosema algerae, 714
Nosema apis, 720–721
Nosema corneum, 714
Nosema ocularum, 715t
Nosopsyllus spp., 277, 844–845
NSAIDs
adverse reactions, eosinophilia, 947t
histoplasmosis, 575
Nucleic acid amplification tests
B. anthracis, 884–885
C. trachomatis, 311, 318
N. gonorrhoea, 188
Nucleic acid detection tests
HIV, 553
HPV, 536
Nucleic acid probes, *C. trachomatis*, 312
Nucleic acids, 1
Nucleoside analog reverse transcriptase inhibitors, 553
Nucleos(t)ide analogs, hepatitis B, 436–437
Null hypothesis, 12
Nutrition, 23–31
Nutrition-infection interactions, 23, 24f
Nutritional anemia, 1028
Nutritional status
effects of infection, 27, 27b
and gastrointestinal infection, 27–28
Nystagmus, e12t–e13t
Nystatin
candidiasis
mucosal, 104t, 591
oral, 592
vulvovaginal, 593, 1040t

O

Occupational pulmonary disease, 989–990
Ochonta spp., 833
Ochotona curzoniae, 824
Octreotide, cryptosporidiosis, 640
Ocular disease, 991–1016
bacterial infection, 996–1006
actinomyces, 1001–1002
adult inclusion conjunctivitis, 997–998
anthrax, 1002
B. ceylonensis, 751t, 752–753
bacillary dysentery, 1004
Bartonella spp., 1002
botulism, 1003
Brazilian purpuric fever, 1003
brucellosis, 273, 1002
C. psittaci, 998
chancroid, 1003
Chlamydia-associated reactive arthritis syndrome, 998
cholera, 1003, 1004f
diphtheria, 1002–1003
lymphogranuloma venereum, 998
melioidosis, 1004
mycobacteria, 998–999
Mycoplasma spp., 1001
Neisseria spp., 1003
ophthalmia neonatorum, 997
orbital cellulitis, 1006
Q fever, 1002
Rickettsia spp., 1001
spirochetes, 1000–1001
tetanus, 1003
trachoma *see* Trachoma
tularemia, 1002
typhoid, 1003
conjunctivitis *see* Conjunctivitis
Dipetalonema-like organisms, 751t
ectoparasites, 1015–1016
myiasis, 1016, 1016f
pentastomiasis, 1015
endophthalmitis *see* Endophthalmitis
fungal infection, 1006–1009
aspergillosis, 1006
blastomycosis, 1008
candidiasis, 1006–1007, 1007f
coccidioidomycosis, 1008
cryptococcosis, 1007, 1007f
entomophthoramycosis, 1009, 1009f
histoplasmosis, 1007–1008, 1008f
mucormycosis, 1008–1009
mycotic infection and fungal sinusitis, 1009
paracoccidioidomycosis, 1008
rhinosporidiosis, 1009, 1009f
sporotrichosis, 1008
helminthic infection, 1011–1015, 1011b
angiostrongyliasis, 1014, 1014f
ascariasis, 1013–1014
baylisascariasis, 783, 1013
coenuriasis, 1015
cysticercosis, 818, 818f, 1015, 1015f
dirofilariasis, 751t, 1013, 1013f
dracunculiasis, 1014
echinococcosis, 1015
filariasis, 752–753, 752f–753f, 1013
gnathostomiasis, 785, 1014–1015, 1014f
hookworm, 1014
Loaina spp., 751t
loiasis, 736, 736f, 1012–1013, 1012f
M. perstans, 757f, 1013
onchocerciasis, 745, 751t, 1011–1012, 1012f
paragonimiasis, 1015
schistosomiasis, 1015
sparganosis, 847, 1015
thelaziasis, 1014
toxocariasis, 763, 764t, 765, 765f, 1013, 1013f
trichinellosis, 1015
W. bancrofti, 752–753
keratitis *see* Keratitis
keratoconjunctivitis *see* Keratoconjunctivitis
parasitic infection, 1009–1016
African trypanosomiasis, 1010
amebiasis, 1011
Chagas' disease, 691f, 1010, 1010f
giardiasis, 1011
leishmaniasis, 1010–1011
malaria, 1010, 1010f
microsporidiosis, 717f, 1009, 1009f
toxoplasmosis, 724–725, 1009–1010, 1010f
Parinaud's ocular glandular syndrome, 1001–1002, 1005b
uveitis *see* Uveitis
viral infection, 991–996
acute retinal necrosis, 995
adenovirus, 991, 992f
chikungunya virus, 996
cytomegalovirus, 994–995, 994f
encephalitis, 996
enteroviruses, 991, 992f
Epstein-Barr virus, 995
hepatitis viruses, 996
herpes simplex virus, 993, 993f
HIV, 995, 995f
HTLV-1, 995–996
influenza, 991
lymphocytic choriomeningitis virus, 996
mumps, 993
rabies, 996
rubella, 993
varicella zoster, 994, 994f
viral hemorrhagic fevers, 996
Ocular toxicity, ethambutol, 240
Oculogyric crisis, 286
Odocoileus virginianus, 339
Odynophagia, 592, 920
Oecomys spp., 450f
Oesophagostomum spp., 779–781, 781f
Oesophagostomum aculeatum, 780
Oesophagostomum apiostomum, 780
Oesophagostomum bifurcum, 780
eradication, 77t–79t
Oesophagostomum stephanostomum, 780
Oestrus ovi, 1016
Ofloxacin, 96t–98t, 100t
cervicitis/urethritis, 1040t
gonorrhoea, 189
H. pylori infection, 172t
leprosy, 259
lymphogranuloma venereum, 318
meningococcal prophylaxis, 182
pelvic inflammatory disease, 190t, 1043t
travelers' diarrhea, 894t
tuberculosis, 243
typhoid/paratyphoid, 125, 125t
Oka vaccine, 361
Olanzipine, delusional parasitosis, 1071
Oligochaetes, 813
Oligoryzomys chacoensis, 471t
Oligoryzomys flavescens, 471t
Oligoryzomys fornesi, 471t
Oligoryzomys fulvescens, 471t

Oligoryzomys longicaudatus, 471t
Oligoryzomys nigripes, 471t
Oliveros virus, 450f
Omeprazole, *H. pylori*, 172t, 173b, 918t
OmpA, 323
OmpB, 323, 327
Omsk hemorrhagic fever, 442t–443t, 515–518, 516f
agent, 515
clinical features, 444t–445t, 516–517, 517t
diagnosis, 447t, 518
epidemiology, 515, 517f
pathogenesis and immunity, 517–518
pathologic features, 446t
skin lesions, 956t
transmission, 932t
treatment and prevention, 518
Onchocerca spp., 339, 750, 751t
diagnosis, 756, 756f–757f
Onchocerca cervicalis, 741
Onchocerca gibsoni, 741
Onchocerca lienalis, 741
Onchocerca ochengi, 741
Onchocerca stilesi, 757f
Onchocerca volvulus, 737, 741
history, 741
life cycle, 741, 742f
vectors, 741, 877
see also Onchocerciasis
Onchocerciasis, 7, 17, 21, 739, 741–749
agent *see Onchocerca volvulus*
clinical features, 742–745
dermatitis *see* Onchodermatitis
eosinophilia, 943t
eye, 745
lymphadenopathy, 745
ocular involvement, 1011–1012, 1012f
pigmentation changes, 973t
pruritus, 959t–961t
skin lesions, 946t, 957t, 962t–966t
subcutaneous nodules, 742, 743f
diagnosis, 746–747
clinical examination, 746
problems of, 747
epidemiology, 741–742, 743f
eradication, 43, 77t–79t
genetic protection, 35t
HIV coinfection, 745
laboratory diagnosis, 746–747
blood examination, 747
demonstration of adult parasite, 747
DNA diagnosis, 747
eosinophil count, 747
IgE levels, 747
Mazzotti reaction, 745–747, 746f
serologic tests, 747
skin snips, 746–747
ultrasound, 747
urine and other fluids, 747
pathogenesis and immunity, 745–746
local immune responses, 745
protective immune responses, 745
systemic immune responses, 745
Wolbachia endosymbionts, 745–746, 746f
prevention and control, 749
mass ivermectin distribution, 749
prophylaxis, 749
vector control, 749
socioeconomic consequences, 742
treatment and prognosis, 747–749
diethylcarbamazine, 748
doxycycline, 748
ivermectin, 77t–79t, 79, 747–748, 748f
moxidectin, 748
nodulectomy, 749
suramin, 749
see also Streptocerciasis
Onchocerciasis Control Program, 749
Onchodermatitis, 742–744, 744f, 962f
acute papular, 743, 744f
atrophy, 743–744
chronic papular, 743, 744f
depigmentation, 744, 744f
lichenified, 743, 744f
sowda, 742, 744f
Oncomelania spp., 848
Ondansetron, rotavirus, 409
One Health Initiative, 105
Onychomycosis, 559, 562, 562f
Candida, 591
O'nyong-nyong virus, 519, 520t
clinical features, 524
epidemiology, 522
skin lesions, 972t
Opacity proteins, 186
Open reading frames, 433
Ophthalmia neonatorum, 997
Ophthalmomyiasis, 1016, 1016f
Ophthalmoplegia, e12t–e13t
Opisocrostis spp., 276
Opisthorchiasis, 854–858
agent *see Opisthorchis* spp.
clinical features, 855–857
acute, 855
cholangiocarcinoma, 856–857, 976t–977t, 981
chronic, 855–856
eosinophilia, 942t–943t
recurrent ascending cholangitis/pancreatitis, 856
diagnosis, 857–858
epidemiology, 854–855
immunodiagnosis, 858
pathogenesis and immunity, 857
treatment, 858
Opisthorchiidae, 854
geographic distribution, 857f
Opisthorchis felineus, 854
epidemiology, 854–855
fish hosts, 855
geographic distribution, 857f
life cycle, 856f
snail vectors, 855
Opisthorchis guayaquilensis, 854–855
Opisthorchis viverrini, 854
and cancer, 71–72, 73t, 856–857
diagnosis, 867
epidemiology, 854–855
eradication, 81t
geographic distribution, 857f
life cycle, 856f
snail vectors, 855
Opsonization, 53
Oral hairy leukoplakia, 363
Oral lesions, 917t
Oral rehydration solution, 155
enteric adenovirus, 418
norovirus, 414
rotavirus, 409
Orán virus, 471t
Orbital cellulitis, 1006
Orchiepididymitis, *Brucella*, 273
Orchitis
SARS, 395
smallpox, 371
Orchopeas spp., 276
Ordinal data, 13
Orf, 261–262, 962t–966t, 972t
Organ transplantation, malaria transmission, 657
Oriental eye worm, 785
Oriental sore, 699
Orientia tsutsugamushi, 51, 334–336
antigenic heterogeneity, 336
genome, 336
membrane proteins, 334–336
pathogenesis and immunity, 336–337
target cells, 337
see also Scrub typhus
Ornithodoros spp., 295, 301–302, 875t
feeding, 295
Ornithodoros coriaceus, 51
Ornithodoros erraticus, 296t
Ornithodoros hermsi, 296t
Ornithodoros marocanus, 296t
Ornithodoros moubata, 296t
Ornithodoros parkeri, 296t
Ornithodoros rudis, 296t
Ornithodoros talaje, 296t
Ornithodoros tartakovskyi, 296t
Ornithodoros tholozani, 296t
Ornithodoros turicata, 295f, 296t
Oropharyngeal lesions, 919
actinomycosis, 919
anthrax, 263, 919
candidiasis, 589, 591–592
F. necrophorum, 919
leprosy, 919
paracoccidioidomycosis, 919
syphilis, 919
tuberculosis, 919
Oropouche fever, 482
Oropsylla spp., 277
Oropsylla idahoensis, 276
Oropsylla montana, 276
Oroya fever, 265, 266f, 266t
diagnosis, 268–269, 269f
pathogenesis and immunity, 268
treatment and prognosis, 269
Orthobunyaviruses, 466
Orthomyxoviridae, 378–379
Orthopoxviruses, 369
B-type inclusions, 369–370
classification, 369
diseases, 370–372
cowpox, 369, 371
monkeypox, 105, 369, 371
smallpox *see* Smallpox
immunodiagnosis, 373
laboratory diagnosis, 373
morphology, 369
nucleic acid diagnosis, 373–374
phenotypic diagnosis, 373, 373f
phylogeny, 369
replication, 369–370
Oryzomus palustris, 471t
Oryzomys spp., 276, 450f
Oryzomys albigularis, 450f
Oryzomys bicolor, 450f
Oryzomys buccinatus, 450f
Oseltamivir, 102t
influenza, 380t, 382
resistance, 382–383
Osler's nodes, 950, 955t
Osteomyelitis
candidal, 594
H. influenzae, 194, 194t
smallpox, 371
Osteoperiostitis, yaws, 293f
Otitis media
adenovirus, 389
C. trachomatis, 317
pneumococcal, 202
Otomys spp., 276–277
Outbreaks, 11
Outer membrane proteins *see* Omp
Ovalocytosis, 653
Overseas medical screening, 903–905, 904f–905f, 904t
drug abuse, 904t
health conditions identified through, 905–906, 905t
immunization, 904t
leprosy, 904t
psychiatric disorders, 904t
STDs, 904t
tuberculosis, 904t, 905f
Oxacillin, 96t–98t
Oxamniquine, 82
adverse effects, 82b
schistosomiasis, 81t, 853
Oxygen, hyperbaric, mucormycosis, 601
Oysters, *Vibrio* spp. in, 159

P

P proteins, 352–353
P value, 12
P-selectin, 658–659
PA-824, tuberculosis, 242
Pachyonychia congenita, 563
Paclitaxel, Kaposi's sarcoma, 368
Palivizumab, HRSV, 380t, 385
PAMPs, 52, 54t
Pancreatic ascariasis, 796, 976t–977t, 980, 980f
Pancreatitis, recurrent ascending, 856
Pancuronium bromide, tetanus, 287–288
Pancytopenia, *Brucella*, 273
Panstrongylus spp., 50
Panstrongylus megistus, 689, 874
Panton-Valentine leukotoxin, 210–211
Pantoprazole, *H. pylori* infection, 172t
Pantothenic acid, 24
Papanicolaou stain, 536
Papilledema, *A. cantonensis* infection, 774–775
Papillomatosis, 535, 535f
Papillomaviruses, 532
Papular skin lesions, 956–957, 956f, 957t
  differential diagnosis, 957t
Para-aminosalicylic acid, 100t
Paracapillaria philippinensis, 786–787, 787f
Parachlamydia spp., 709
Paracoccidioides brasiliensis, 582
Paracoccidioides loboi, 604
Paracoccidioides lutzii, 582
Paracoccidioidomycosis, 582–585
  agent, 582, 583f
  clinical features, 582–583, 583f, 953f
    chronic diarrhea, 924
    gastrointestinal, 917t
    lymphadenopathy, 583f
    mulberry stomatitis, 583f
    ocular involvement, 1008
    oropharyngeal lesions, 919
    skin lesions, 969t–970t
  diagnosis, 584
  epidemiology, 582, 583f
  HIV coinfection, 552, 584, 1056–1057
  pathogenesis and immunity, 583–584
  prevention and control, 585
  treatment and prognosis, 584
  and tuberculosis, 584
Parafossarulus manchouricus, 855
Paragonimiasis
  agent *see Paragonimus* spp.
  clinical features, 862–864
    cerebral paragonimiasis, 863–864
    cutaneous paragonimiasis, 864
    eosinophilia, 942t–943t
    extrapulmonary, 863
    neurologic involvement, 1019t, 1021
    ocular involvement, 1015
    pleuropulmonary, 863, 988t
    skin lesions, 864, 946t, 958t, 962t–966t
  diagnosis, 865
  epidemiology, 862
  geographic distribution, 863f
  immunodiagnosis, 865
  pathogenesis and immunity, 864–865
  treatment and prognosis, 865
Paragonimus spp., 783, 862
  geographic distribution, 863f
Paragonimus africanus, 862
  epidemiology, 862
  pulmonary disease, 984t
Paragonimus caliensis, pulmonary disease, 984t
Paragonimus heterotremus, 862
  epidemiology, 862
Paragonimus hueitungensis, 862
  epidemiology, 862
Paragonimus kellicotti, 862
Paragonimus mexicanus, 862
  epidemiology, 862
Paragonimus miyazakii, 862
  epidemiology, 862
Paragonimus skrjabini, 862
  epidemiology, 862
Paragonimus uterobilateralis, 862
  epidemiology, 862
Paragonimus westermani, 854, 862
  epidemiology, 862
  eradication, 81t
  life cycle, 864f
  morphology, 862f
  ova, 862f
  pulmonary disease, 984t
  snail vectors, 862
Parainfluenza virus, 378
Parakeratosis, 535
Paralytic rabies, 527t, 528
Paramyxoviruses, 9, 347, 352, 383, 385
  attachment proteins, 353
  F proteins, 353
Paraná virus, 450f
Parapharyngeal abscess, 263
Parapneumoic effusion, 988t
Parasitic cirrhosis, 786
Parasitic infections
  chemotherapy, 76–94
  eosinophilia, 940b, 943t
  neurologic involvement *see* neurologic disease, parasitic infection
  ocular involvement *see* ocular disease, parasitic infection
  vaccines, 69t
  see also individual diseases
Parasitism, 1
Parastrongylus cantonensis, 785
Paratenic hosts
  A. cantonensis, 774
  A. costaricensis, 776
  Gnathostoma spp., 784
  T. canis, 763
Paratrachoma, *C. trachomatis*, 317
Paratyphoid *see* Typhoid/paratyphoid
Parechoviruses, 398, 416
Paresthesia
  A. cantonensis infection, 774–775
  Q fever, 346
Parinaud's ocular glandular syndrome, 1001–1002
  causes, 1005b
Paromomycin, 89
  adverse effects, 85b, 629t
  amebiasis, 88t–89t, 621
  balantidiasis, 918t
  cryptosporidiosis, 638–639, 918t
  D. fragilis, 88t–89t, 628t
  E. histolytica, 918t
  giardiasis, 88t–89t, 628t
  leishmaniasis, 91t–92t
    cutaneous, 705
    visceral, 704
Paronychia, 591
Parotitis, suppurative, 220f
Parrot beak sign, 272–273
Partial thromboplastin time, malaria, 657
Parvoviruses, 390, 419
Pasteurization, 275
Pathogen-associated molecular patterns *see* PAMPs
Pattern recognition molecules, 52–54
  cell-associated, 53–54, 54t, 55f
  host fluid phase, 52–53, 54t
Peau d'orange appearance, genital lymphedema, 732
Pebrine, 714
PECAM, 658–659
Pediatric *see* Children
Pediculus humanus, 50, 266t, 267, 296t, 329, 868
  body louse, 869f
  head louse, 869f
  nits, 868
  relapsing fever, 296–297
  treatment, 93t
Pefloxacin, leprosy, 259
Pegylated interferons
  hepatitis B, 436
  hepatitis C, 431
  hepatitis D, 439
Pellagra, 28, e12t–e13t
Pelodera strongyloides, 778, 779f
Pelvic inflammatory disease, 190t, 1034t, 1042–1044
  C. trachomatis, 316–317, 316t
  clinical features, 1043
  diagnosis, 1043
  management, 1043–1044, 1043t
Penciclovir, 102t
  herpesviruses, 356
    HSV, 359
Pencil cells, 1025f, 1026
Penicillins, 95–98, 96t–98t
  adverse reactions, eosinophilia, 947t
  diphtheria, 226
  group A streptococcus, 208
  leptospirosis, 307
  penicillinase-resistant, 96t–98t
  pneumococcal meningitis, 201
  pneumococcal pneumonia, 202
  Salmonella bacteremia, 135
  syphilis, 104t
Penicillin G
  anthrax, 264
  Borrelia infections, 300
  diphtheria prophylaxis, 226
  Lyme disease, 301
Penicillin V, anthrax, 264
Penicilliosis
  pleural effusion, 988t
  skin lesions, 969t–970t
Penicillium marneffei, 552, 586–588
  clinical features, 586, 587f
  diagnosis, 586–587, 587f
  epidemiology, 586, 587f
  HIV coinfection, 1055–1056
  pathogenesis and immunity, 586
  prevention and control, 588
  treatment and prognosis, 587–588
Penile cancer, 534
Penis, ram horn, 732
Pentamidine, 90–92
  adverse effects, 90b
  African trypanosomiasis, 91t–92t, 686, 688t
    prophylaxis, 683
  B. hominis, 622
  granulomatous amebic encephalitis, 712
  leishmaniasis, visceral, 704
  P. jirovecii, 86t–87t
  pneumocystis pneumonia, 104t
  pneumocystosis, 612–613
Pentastomiasis, 877
  ocular involvement, 1015
Pentastomida, 877
Pentatrichomonas hominis, 623, 631–632, 631f
Pentoxifylline, leishmaniasis, mucosal, 705
Peptidoglycan, 206–207, 253
Peramivir, influenza, 382–383
Pericarditis
  enterovirus, 402
  meningococcal, 178
Peritonitis, 921
  candidal, 595
  meningococcal, 179
  tuberculous, 920
  see also Abdominal pain
Permethrin
  adverse effects, 94b
  louse eradication, 93t
  mosquitoes, 895
  scabies, 93t, 868–869
  typhus control, 333
Peromyscus californicus, 450f
Peromyscus leucopus, 471t, 472–473
Peromyscus maniculatus, 276, 470, 471t, 472–473

Perstans filariasis, 738
agent, 739
clinical features, 739
diagnosis, 739
epidemiology, 739
pathogenesis and immunity, 739
prevention and control, 740
treatment and prognosis, 739
Pertactin, 212–213
Pertussis, 212–214
agent *see Bordetella pertussis*
characteristics, 212
diagnosis, 213–214
epidemiology, 212, 213f
pathogenesis and immunity, 212–213
prevention and control, 214
treatment, 214
Pertussis toxin, 5, 213
Pestiviruses, 427
Pet, 118
Petechiae, 955–956, 955t–956t
differential diagnosis, 956t
PfEMP1, 651
antibodies, 653
cytoadherence, 658
Phaeoacremonium parasiticum, 571
Phaeohyphomycosis, 571–572
agent, 571
clinical features, 571, 571f
diagnosis, 571–572, 572f
prevention and control, 572
treatment and prognosis, 572
Phaeoid fungi, 569
Phagocytes, 33
Phagocytic cells, 55
Phagocytic killing, 7
Phagolysosomes, 55
Phagosomes, 55
Pharyngeal gonorrhoea, 187
Pharyngeal plague, 280
Pharyngitis, 1034t
adenovirus, 389
HPIVs, 385
streptococcal, 263
Phenylalanine, 27
Phenytoin
adverse reactions, eosinophilia, 947t
cysticercosis, 820
Phialemonium obovatum, 571
Phialophora repens, 571
Phialophora verrucosa, 569
Phlebotomus fever *see* Sandfly fever
Phlebotomus spp., 49
leishmaniasis, 696
Phlebotomus papatasi, 481
Phlebotomus perfiliewi, 481
Phlebotomus perniciosus, 481
Phleboviruses, 9, 462, 466
PhoP/PhoQ regulon, 134
Phormia regina, 869
Phosphoenolpyruvate carboxykinase, 27
Phosphorodiamidate morpholino oligomers, 490
Phthiraptera, 868
Phthirus pubis, 868, 869f, 1034t
treatment, 93t
Phylogeny, 1
Physiotherapy, decongestive, 734
Phythisis bulbi, 1016, 1016f
Pian bois, 699
Pic, 118
Pica, 764, 767
Picaridin, biting midges, 872
Pichindé virus, 450f, 450t
pathogenesis and immunity, 459
Picobirnavirus, 417t, 418–419
Picornaviruses
enteroviruses *see* Enteroviruses
hepatitis A, 420
rhinoviruses, 387
Saffold virus, 378
Pigbel, 165
Pigmentation changes, 971, 973t
Pigs, Nipah virus in, 353–354
Pila spp., 774
PilC proteins, 185
Pimozide, delusional parasitosis, 1070
Pinta, 289, 292–294
clinical features, 293
pigmentation changes, 973t
pruritus, 959t–961t
transmission, 290f
Pintids, 293
Pinworm *see Enterobius vermicularis*
Piperacillin-tazobactam, 96t–98t
Piperaquine
malaria, 664
pharmacokinetics, 665t
Piperazine, 76
enterobiasis, 790
Piperonyl butoxide, adverse effects, 94b
Pirital virus, 450f, 450t
see also Venezuelan hemorrhagic fever
Pirodavir, human rhinovirus, 380t
Piroplasmidora, 676
Pityriasis versicolor, 969t–970t, 973t
Pivamdinocillin, shigellosis, 143t
Pixuna virus, 520t
Placebo-controlled clinical trials, 12
Placental dysfunction, malaria, 662
Plagiorchiidae, 866
Plague, 261–262, 276–283
agent *see Yersinia pestis*
bubonic, 3, 279–280, 279f
diagnosis, 281
drug resistance, 282
epidemiology, 277–279, 277f, 278b
foci
African, 278
Asian, 278
North American, 278
South American, 278
global distribution, 277f
historical aspects, 276
incubation period, 929b
meningeal, 280
pandemics, 276
pathogenesis and immunity, 280–281
pharyngeal, 280
pneumonic, 276, 280–281
incubation period, 881
prevention and control, 282–283
prophylaxis, 282
pruritus, 959t–961t
septicemic, 280
skin lesions, 956t–957t, 967t–968t
transmission cycles, 279f
treatment and prognosis, 281–282
vaccines, 282–283
Plant dermatitis, 972t
Plaque reduction neutralization tests, Crimean-Congo hemorrhagic fever, 467
Plasma viscosity, malaria, 657
Plasmid, 2
Plasmodiidae, 646
Plasmodium spp., 4, 45, 48–49, 633, 646, 652–654
genomics, 650–651
life cycle, 649f
metabolism and transport in, 651
pulmonary disease, 989
Plasmodium falciparum, 646, 652
and babesiosis, 679
characteristics, 648t
drug resistance, 651f
distribution of, 654t
mefloquine, 652f
genomics, 650–651
incubation period, 647–649
life cycle, 647–650, 648t, 650f, 674f
gametocytes, 650f, 657, 664
hypnozoites, 649–650
merozoites, 647–649, 650f
sporozoites, 647, 650f
metabolism and transport in, 651
morphology in blood films, 647–649, 663f
onset time, 929t
prophylaxis, 83
pulmonary disease, 984t
skin lesions, 956t
Plasmodium knowlesi, 646
characteristics, 648t
epidemiology, 652
incubation period, 647–649
life cycle, 648t, 650
morphology in blood films, 647–649
prophylaxis, 83
Plasmodium malariae, 646, 652
characteristics, 648t
incubation period, 647–649
life cycle, 647–649
morphology in blood films, 647–649
onset time, 929t
prophylaxis, 83
treatment, 668
Plasmodium ovale, 646, 652
characteristics, 648t
incubation period, 647–649
life cycle, 649–650
morphology in blood films, 647–649
onset time, 929t
prophylaxis, 83
treatment, 668
Plasmodium vivax, 4–5, 646, 652
adaptive immunity, 653
characteristics, 648t
genomics, 650
incubation period, 647–649
life cycle, 649–650
merozoites, 650
military cases, 911
morphology in blood films, 647–649, 663f
onset time, 929t
prophylaxis, 83
treatment, 668
Platelet count, malaria, 657
Platelet-activating factor, 199
Platyhelminthes, 813
Pleconaril, human rhinovirus, 380t
Pleisiomonas shigelloides, 138
Pleistophora spp., 634f, 714, 715t
eradication, 86t–87t
Pleistophora ronneafiei, 715t
clinical manifestations, 718
Pleochaetis spp., 276
Plesiomonas spp., 113
toxin, 113
Plesiomonas shigelloides, 917t
toxin, 114t–115t
travelers' diarrhea, 924
Pleural effusion, 987–988, 987t–988t
eosinophilic, 945b, 988t
loaiasis, 737
Pleurisy, tuberculous, 233–234
Pleurocercidae, 862
Pleurodynia, 398
enterovirus, 402
Pleuropulmonary paragonimiasis, 863
Pneumococcal disease, 199–202
diagnosis, 201
HIV coinfection, 200–201
prevention and control, 202
treatment and prognosis, 201–202
vaccine, 64t–65t, 202, 888t–890t
requirements for immigrants, 908t
see also S. pneumoniae; and individual diseases
Pneumocystis spp., 608
life cycle, 609f
Pneumocystis carinii, 608
Pneumocystis jirovecii, 552, 574, 608, 610f, 725, 984t
eradication, 86t–87t
HIV coinfection, 1058

INDEX

Pneumocystis murina, 608
Pneumocystis octolagii, 608
Pneumocystis pneumonia
  clinical features, 608, 609f–610f
  treatment, 85, 85b, 86t–87t, 104t
Pneumocystis wakefieldiae, 608
Pneumocystosis, 608–613
  agent, 608, 609f
  clinical features, 608–609, 609f–610f
  diagnosis, 610–611, 610f–611f
  epidemiology, 608
  pathogenesis and immunity, 609–610
  prevention and control, 613
  treatment and prognosis, 611–613, 611f
Pneumolysin, 200
Pneumonia, 982–986
  Ascaris spp., 796
  C. psittaci, 316t
  children
    etiology, 983b
    incidence, 985f
    mortality, 983f, 985f
  community-acquired, *C. pneumoniae*, 316t
  effect on anthropometric indicators, 25t
  H. influenzae, 193, 194t
  HPIVs, 385
  measles, 347
  neonatal, *C. trachomatis*, 316t
  pneumococcal, 202
    military cases, 910
  Pneumocystis, 552, 574, 608, 609f–610f, 725, 984t
    eradication, 86t–87t
    HIV coinfection, 1058
    treatment, 85, 85b, 86t–87t, 104t
  Q fever, 345, 345f
Pneumonic plague, 276, 280–281
Pneumonitis, hookworm, 802
Pneumovirinae, 386
PNU-100480, tuberculosis, 242
Podophyllin, HPV, 536–537
Podophyllotoxin, 536–537
Podophyllum emodi, 536–537
Podophyllum peltatum, 536–537
Poikilocytosis, 1026f
Point of care tests, *C. trachomatis*, 318
Pol, 543, 545
Poliomyelitis, 398, 400–401
  acute flaccid paralysis, 398, 400
  bulbar, 401
  eradication, 405
  HIV coinfection, 1063
  incubation period, 929b
  post-polio syndrome, 401
  provocation, 403
  see also Poliovirus
Poliovirus, 4, 398, 399t
  circulating vaccine-derived, 405
  epidemiology, 399
  eradication, 42–43
    comparison with dracunculiasis, 43
    feasibility, 42t
  global distribution, 400f
  neurovirulence, 403
  ocular disease, 991
  vaccines, 42–43, 64t–65t, 399, 404–405, 888t–890t
    requirements for immigrants, 908t
Polychromasia, 1026
Polycystic echinococcosis, 824, 837–838
  agent *see Echinococcus oligarthrus*; *Echinococcus vogeli*
  clinical features, 837–838
  diagnosis, 838, 838f
  prevention and control, 838
  transmission, epidemiology and geographic distribution, 837
  treatment, 838
Polyenes, 590
Polygenic inheritance, 32
Polygenis spp., 276
Polyhexamethylene biguanide, *Acanthamoeba* keratitis, 713
Polymerase chain reaction
  amebiasis, 620
  B. pertussis, 213
  brucellosis, 274
  C. burnetii, 346
  C. cayetanensis, 642
  Chagas' disease, 694
  donovanosis, 197
  enteroviruses, 404
  leptospirosis, 306
  loiasis, 737
  lymphatic filariasis, 733
  M. ulcerans, 248
  malaria, 662
  microsporidiosis, 720
  orthopoxviruses, 373
Polymorphonuclear leukocytes, malaria pigment, 664
Polyparasitism, 3
Polyradiculoneuritis, Q fever, 346
Pomacea caniculata, 774, 776
Pontiac fever, 215
PorB, 186
Porin, 186
Pork, preparation for cooking, 773
Pork tapeworm *see Taenia solium*
Posaconazole, 100t–101t
  candidiasis, esophageal, 592
  chromoblastomycosis, 570
  cryptococcosis, 581
  mucormycosis, 600–601
  toxicity, 101t
Positive predictive value, 15
Post-kala-azar dermal leishmaniasis, 701
Post-polio syndrome, 401
Post-tussive rales, 231
Postherpetic neuralgia, 360
  treatment, 361
Potamon spp., 862
Potassium, cholera stools, 153t
Potassium iodide, sporotrichosis, 606–607
Potiskum virus, 492
Poverty, and disease, 17
Powassan virus, 515, 516f
Poxviruses, 369–370
Praomys spp., 450f
Praziquantel
  A. cantonensis infection, 776
  adverse effects, 81
  cystic echinococcosis, 831
  cysticercosis, 821
  D. caninum, 80t
  D. latum, 80t
  diphyllobothriasis, 843
  dipylidiasis, 845
  F. buski, 81t
  H. heterophyes, 81t
  H. nana, 80, 80t
  hymenolepiasis, 845
  intestinal flukes, 867
  M. conjunctus, 81t
  M. yokogawai, 81t
  N. salmincola, 81t
  O. viverrini, 81t
  opisthorchiasis/clonorchiasis, 858
  paragonimiasis, 81t, 865
  schistosomiasis, 81t, 852–853
  T. saginata, 80t
  T. solium, 80t
  taeniasis, 840–841, 841f
Prednisolone
  A. cantonensis infection, 776
  African trypanosomiasis, 687, 688t
  cysticercosis, 821
  trichinellosis, 772–773
Prednisone
  cysticercosis, 821
  histoplasmosis, 575
  pneumocystis pneumonia, 104t
  toxocariasis, 766
Pregnancy, 1072–1081
  blastomycosis, 577
  brucellosis, 273, 1072–1073
  C. trachomatis in, 317
  cholera, 1073
  cytomegalovirus, 1081
  dengue fever/dengue hemorrhagic fever, 1073–1074
  enterobiasis, 790
  fevers in, 937
  genital warts, 538
  gonococcal infection, 189
  hepatitis A, 1074
  hepatitis B, 1074
  hepatitis C, 1074
  hepatitis E, 1074
  hepatitis G, 1074
  herpes simplex virus, 1081
  HIV/AIDS, 1075, 1075t
  hookworm, 802
  HTLV-1, 1075–1076
  immunization for travel, 891
  leptospirosis, 1076
  listeriosis, 1076
  malaria, 654, 656–657, 1076–1077
    placental dysfunction, 662
    treatment, 671–672, 671b
  psittacosis, 321
  Q fever, 346
  risks of antimicrobial therapy, 1073t
  rubella, 1081
  syphilis, 292, 1081
  tetanus, 1078
  toxoplasmosis, 727, 1078–1079
  tuberculosis, 242, 1079–1080
  typhoid/paratyphoid, 1080
  yellow fever, 1080–1081
Prenylation inhibitors, hepatitis D, 440
Prevalence, 11
Prickle cell layer, 534
Prickly heat, 957
Primaquine
  adverse effects, 82b, 897t, 898
  malaria, 664, 898
    dose, 897t
    prophylaxis, 669t, 897t
  P. jirovecii, 86t–87t
  pharmacokinetics, 665t
  pneumocystosis, 612
  prophylaxis, 83
Primary amebic meningoencephalitis, 707, 711, 711f
  diagnosis, 712
  neurologic involvement, 1019t
  pathogenesis and immunity, 711–712
  prevention and control, 713
  treatment and prognosis, 713
Primary effusion lymphoma, 367
Priority diseases, 68–70, 69b, 69t
Probenecid, pelvic inflammatory disease, 1043t
Probiotics
  C. difficile, 164
  E. coli infection, 120
Proctitis, 1034t
  C. trachomatis, 316, 316t
  gonococcal, 187
Proctocolitis, *C. trachomatis*, 316t
Procyclin, 682
Procyon lotor, 750
Proechimys spp., 837
Program for Appropriate Technology in Health, 66
Program for Monitoring Emerging Diseases, 106
Proguanil
  adverse effects, 82b
  malaria, 897t, 898
    prophylaxis, 84
  pharmacokinctics, 665t
Prokaryotes, phylogeny, 1
Propamidine gluconate, *Acanthamoeba* keratitis, 713

Proptosis, causes, 1005b
Prosecutor's wart, 228
Prospect Hill virus, 470
Prostatitis, *C. trachomatis*, 316
Prostigmata, 869, 873
Protease inhibitors, 103t
Protective immunity, 6t
Protein energy malnutrition, 23–24
and adaptive immunity, 28–30
antibody production, 29
Protein F, 208
Protein metabolism, in infection, 27
Proteolysis, 27
Prothionamide, leprosy, 259
Prothrombin time, malaria, 657
Proton pump inhibitors, *H. pylori* infection, 172t
Protozoa, 1–2
Pruritus, 957, 959t–961t, 962f
giardiasis, 627t
hookworm, 802, 950, 959t–961t, 961f
prickly heat, 957
swimmer's itch, 849–850, 950
Pseudocowpox, 261–262, 962t–966t
Pseudomembranous candidiasis, 591–592
Pseudomonas spp., exotoxin, 5
Pseudomonas aeruginosa
exotoxin, 5
skin lesions, 956t
Pseudophyllidea, 813
bothria, 813
Pseudoraspora parva, 855
Pseudorubella, 364–365
Pseudoterranova spp., 781–783
Pseudoterranova decipiens, 782
Pseudotetanus, 286
Psittacosis, 320–322
agent, 320
clinical features, 321
Horder's spots, 321
diagnosis, 322
distribution, 321f
epidemiology, 320
pathogenesis and immunity, 321–322
pregnancy, 321
prevention and control, 322
treatment and prognosis, 322
see also Chlamydia psittaci
Psoas abscess, 1023
Psorophora spp., 521–522
Psorophora columbiae, Venezuelan equine encephalitis, 876t
Psychiatric disorders
delusional parasitosis, 1066–1071
overseas medical screening, 904t
Psychiatric manifestations
Brucella, 273
neurocysticercosis, 818
Pteropus spp., 352
Pteropus alacto, 353
Pteropus conspicillatus, 353
Pteropus giganteus, 352–353
Pteropus hypomelanus, 353
Pteropus poliocephalus, 353
Pteropus rufus, 353
Pteropus scapulatus, 353
Pteropus vampyrus, 353
Pubic lice *see Phthirus pubis*
Public Health Emergency of International Concern, 106
Public health surveillance, 105–106
Pulex irritans, 276
Pulex simulans, 266t
Pulmonary disease, 982–990, 983t
D. immitis, 751t
and fever, 933
hantavirus pulmonary syndrome, 442t–443t, 473, 475–476
hemorrhagic fevers, 445t
HIV-associated, 989
M. avium-intracellulare complex, 246
mucormycosis, 599
mycobacterial, 246
occupational/environmental, 989–990
P. jirovecii see Pneumocystis jirovecii
parasite-associated, 984t
ascariasis, 796
hookworm, 802, 984t
hydatid disease, 828
paragonimiasis, 863
Plasmodium spp., 989
pneumonia *see* Pneumonia
respiratory tract infections
acute, 982–986
candidiasis, 593
meningococcal, 179
viral *see* Respiratory viral infections
rheumatic heart disease, 989
salmonellosis, 132t–133t
strongyloidiasis, 809, 809f
symptoms
cough, 986, 986b
eosinophilia, 944, 944b, 987
hemoptysis, 986, 987b
pulmonary effusion *see* Pulmonary effusion
tobacco-associated, 989
tuberculosis *see* Tuberculosis
zoonotic filariasis, 753, 753f
Pulmonary edema, malaria, 660
Pulmonary embolism, 988t
Pulmonary eosinophilia, 944, 944b
tropical *see* Tropical pulmonary eosinophilia
Pulmonary hemorrhage, leptospirosis, 304f–305f
PulseNet International, 105, 107
Punctate epithelial keratopathy, *E. hellem*, 717f
Purpura, 955t
differential diagnosis, 956t
Purpura fulminans, 591
meningococcal, 178f
Puumala virus, 442t–443t, 470, 471t
hemorrhagic fever with renal syndrome, 471f, 475
nephropathia epidemica, 473
Pyemotes tritici, 872–873
Pyoderma, streptococcal, 204
Pyogenic liver abscess, 976t–977t, 978–979, 978f
Pyomyositis, *S. aureus*, 208–209
Pyrantel pamoate
A. caninum, 77t–79t
adverse effects, 82b
ascariasis, 797, 918t
E. vermicularis, 77t–79t, 79
hookworm, 76, 77t–79t
M. moniliformis, 77t–79t
Oesophagostomum spp., 781
Ternidens infection, 781
trichinellosis, 772–773
Trichostrongylus spp., 77t–79t
trichuriasis, 793
Pyrazinamide, 100t
adverse effects, 240
in pregnancy, 1073t
tuberculosis, 239t, 240
tuberculous meningitis, 236
tuberculous pleurisy, 234
Pyrenochaeta mackinnonii, 565
Pyrenochaeta romeroi, 565, 567
Pyrethrins
adverse effects, 94b
louse eradication, 93t
Pyrexia *see* Fever
Pyridoxal kinase, malaria protection, 36t
Pyridoxine, requirements, e12t–e13t
Pyridoxine deficiency, 28
Pyrimethamine
adverse effects, 85b
isosporiasis, 644
malaria, 664, 667t
prophylaxis, 84
pharmacokinetics, 665t
pneumocystosis, 613
toxoplasmosis, 104t, 727
Pyrimidine analogs, 590
Pyronaridine
malaria, 664
pharmacokinetics, 665t
Pyrvinium pamoate, enterobiasis, 790

Q

Q fever, 344–346, 883
agent *see Coxiella burnetii*
clinical features, 344–346, 345f
acute, 345–346
chronic, 346
hepatitis, 345
neurologic manifestations, 346
ocular involvement, 1002
pneumonia, 345, 345f
self-limited illness, 345
diagnosis, 346
epidemiology, 344
immunocompromised patients, 346
incubation period, 345, 929b
Jarisch-Herxheimer reaction, 346
military cases, 913
pathogenesis and immunity, 346
pregnancy, 346
prevention and control, 346
transmission, 344–345
treatment and prognosis, 346
Quartan malaria, 650
nephropathy, 657
Queensland coastal fever, 955t
Quinacrine
adverse effects, 629t
B. hominis, 622
giardiasis, 88t–89t, 628t, 918t
Quinidine
malaria, 664
prophylaxis, 84
severe, 670b
pharmacokinetics, 665t
Quinine, 646
adverse effects, 82b, 897t
babesiosis, 680
malaria, 664, 666, 667t, 897t
dose, 897t
pregnancy, 671b
prophylaxis, 83
severe, 670–671, 670b
pharmacokinetics, 665t
in pregnancy, 1073t
Quinolones
Campylobacter spp., 148
H. pylori infection, 172t
legionellosis, 218
meningococcal prophylaxis, 182
travelers' diarrhea, 893
Quinupristin/dalfopristin, 96t–98t

R

Rabbitpox, 372
Rabeprazole, *H. pylori* infection, 172t, 173b
Rabies, 525–531, 526t
agent, 525
animal, 528
epidemiology, 526
susceptibility, 527t
diagnosis, 529
differential diagnosis, 529
disease, 527–528
epidemiology, 525–526
established disease, 527–528
furious, 527–528, 527t, 528f
HIV coinfection, 1063
hydrophobia, 527
incubation period, 527, 527t, 929b
mortality, 526t

non-neurologic findings, 528
ocular involvement, 996
paralytic, 527t, 528
pathogenesis, 528–529
immune response, 528–529
pathology, 526–527
postexposure prophylaxis, 530, 530t
postexposure treatment, 530–531
prevention and control, 529–531
prodrome, 527
transmission, 527, 527t
treatment and prognosis, 529
vaccine, 64t–65t, 529–531, 531f, 888t–890t, 892
Racecadotril, rotavirus, 409
Radiculomyelitis, gnathostomiasis, 784–785
Radiculomyeloencephalitis, gnathostomiasis, 784–785
Radioimmunoassay, orthopoxviruses, 373
Raillietina spp., 813
Raltegravir, 103t
Ram horn penis, 732
Ramoplanin, *C. difficile*, 164
Ramsay Hunt syndrome, 360
Randomized clinical trials, 12
double-blind, 12
Range, 13
Ranitidine, adverse reactions, eosinophilia, 947t
Ranke complex, 230, 230f
RANTES, disease associations, 36t
Rapid fluorescent focus inhibition test, 529
Rashes *see* Skin lesions
Rasmussen's aneurysm, 231
Rat bite fever, 959t–961t
Rat lungworm *see Angiostrongylus cantonensis*
Rattus spp., 276–277, 678
Rattus exulans, 277
Rattus norvegicus, 277, 471t
Rattus rattus, 277
Reactive arthritis
C. trachomatis, 316t, 317
Shigella spp., 142
Recall bias, 12
Receptors, disease associations, 36t
Recovirus, 411
Rectal prolapse, shigellosis, 141f
Recurrent respiratory papillomatosis, 533t, 534
see also Human papillomavirus
Red blood cell disorders, inherited, 1030–1032
G6PD deficiency, 32, 1025, 1026f, 1032
sickle cell anemia, 1025, 1026f, 1030, 1030b
thalassemia, 1025, 1029t, 1031
intermedia, 1031
major, 1025f, 1031
and malaria resistance, 34, 36t, 653
management, 1031
minor, 1031
Red-man syndrome, 98
Reduction modifiable protein, 186
Refugees, 902–909
diseases of concern, 907f
electronic disease notification system, 906
enhanced health program initiative, 906–908
health screening, conditions identified, 905t
USA, 903f
Regulatory T cells *see* Tregs
Rehydration therapy, 922, 922t
cholera, 154
intravenous, 154–155
oral, 155
dengue shock syndrome, 510
E. coli infection, 119
travelers' diarrhea, 894
Reiter's syndrome, 317
and *C. cayetanensis* infection, 642
Shigella, 142
Relapsing fever, 295–302, 935–936, 936b
agent, 295, 296t
diagnosis, 299–300, 300f
immunity, 299
incubation period, 929b
louse-borne
clinical/laboratory features, 297–298, 297t
ecology and epidemiology, 296–297, 297f
life cycle, 297f
ocular involvement, 1001
pathogenesis, 298–299, 299f
pathology, 299
prevention and control, 301–302
prognosis, 301
pruritus, 959t–961t
tick-borne
clinical/laboratory features, 297–298, 297t
ecology and epidemiology, 295–296, 295f
life cycle, 296f
temperature curves, 298f
treatment and prognosis, 300–301
Jarisch-Herxheimer reaction, 301
see also Lyme disease
Relative risk, 13–14
Renal involvement
hemorrhagic fever with renal syndrome *see* Hemorrhagic fever with renal syndrome
hemorrhagic fevers, 445t
leptospirosis, 305f
loaiasis, 737
malaria, 656, 660
quartan malarial nephropathy, 657
schistosomiasis, 851–852
yellow fever, 496–497
Renal mucormycosis, 599
Reoviridae, 8–9, 406
Respiratory tract infections
candidiasis, 593
meningococcal, 179
viral *see* Respiratory viral infections
Respiratory viral infections, 378–391, 379f, 379t
detection of
community-based studies, 379t
hospital-based studies, 379t
HPIVs, 379t–380t, 385–386
HRSV, 378, 379t, 383–385
human adenovirus, 379t–380t, 389–390
human bocavirus, 378, 379t–380t, 390–391
human coronavirus, 378, 380t, 388–389
human metapneumovirus, 7, 378, 379t–380t, 386–387
human rhinovirus, 378, 379t–380t, 387–388
influenza viruses, 378–383
Respiroviruses, 385
hemagglutinin neuraminidase, 353
Reston ebolavirus, 483, 486t
Restriction fragment-length polymorphism, orthopoxviruses, 373
Retinal artery occlusion, loaiasis, 737
Retinal hemorrhage, malaria, 655b, 655f
Retinal lesions, hemorrhagic fevers, 445t
Retinitis, cytomegalovirus, 362f
Retinochoroiditis, toxoplasmosis, 724–725, 725f
Retinoic acid, Kaposi's sarcoma, 368
Retinoic acid-inducible gene 1-like receptor *see* RIG-1
Retortamonas intestinalis, 623, 632f
Retrobulbar neuritis, ethambutol-induced, 240
Retroviruses, 2, 541–558
endogenous, 545
HIV *see* HIV
HTLV *see* HTLV
transposable elements, 545
Rev, 543
Reverse transcriptase inhibitors, 103t
Reverse transcription-polymerase chain reaction
hepatitis A, 422
influenza virus, 382
rabies, 529
viral hemorrhagic fevers, 441
Reversed halo sign, 599
Reye's syndrome, 381, 383
Rhabditida, 778–779, 805
Diploscapter, 778–779
Halicephalobus, 778
Pelodera, 778
Rhabditis, 778
Turbatrix, 778–779
Rhabditis spp., 778
Rhabditis axei, 778
Rhabdoviridae, 525
Rhadinopsylla spp., 277
Rheumatic fever, 203, 205–206
Rheumatic heart disease, 989
Rhinitis, HPIVs, 385
Rhinocladiella cerophilum, 569
Rhinoscleroma, 962t–966t
Rhinosporidiosis, 605
clinical features, 605
ocular involvement, 1009, 1009f
skin lesions, 969t–970t
diagnosis, 605
epidemiology, 605
pathogenesis and immunity, 605
treatment and prognosis, 604t, 605
Rhinosporidium seeberi, 605, 969t–970t
Rhipicephalus appendiculatus, 875t
Rhipicephalus microplus, 48
Rhipicephalus sanguineus, 324–326, 875t
Rhizomys pruinosus, 586
Rhizomys sinensis, 586
Rhizomys sumatranensis, 586
Rhizopus microsporus, 597, 601
Rhizopus oryzae, 597, 601
Rhizopus rhizopodiformis, 597
Rho GA, 132
Rhodnius spp., 50
Rhodnius prolixus, 689, 690f, 874
Rhodococcus spp., 552
Rhomboid protein, 618
Ribavirin, 102t
Bolivian hemorrhagic fever, 448t
Crimean-Congo hemorrhagic fever, 448t, 469
hemorrhagic fever with renal syndrome, 448t, 479
hepatitis C, 431
HRSV, 380t, 385
human metapneumovirus, 380t, 387
human parainfluenza virus, 380t
Lassa fever, 448t, 460
Nipah virus, 354
Rift Valley fever, 448t, 465
SARS, 397
South American hemorrhagic fevers, 460
yellow fever, 499
Riboflavin, 24
requirements, e12t–e13t
Rice harvest jaundice, 303
Ricin, 880t, 883
detection of, 886
Ricinis communis, 883
Rickets, e12t–e13t
Ricketts, Howard, 323
Rickettsia spp., 5, 7, 323
eschar, 955t
ocular disease, 1001
Rickettsia aeschlimannii, 323, 324t
Rickettsia africae, 323, 324t, 955t
Rickettsia akari, 323, 324t, 955t
Rickettsia amblyommii, 324t
Rickettsia australis, 323, 324t, 955t
Rickettsia conorii, 323, 324t, 955t
Rickettsia felis, 323, 324t
Rickettsia heilongjiangiensis, 323, 324t
Rickettsia helvetica, 323, 324t
Rickettsia honei, 323, 324t
Rickettsia japonica, 323, 324t
Rickettsia massiliae, 323, 324t
Rickettsia monacensis, 323, 324t
Rickettsia parkeri, 323, 324t
Rickettsia prowazekii, 5, 329
as bioterrorism agent, 880t, 882–883
diagnosis, 885–886
life cycle, 330f
skin lesions, 956t–957t
see also Typhus
Rickettsia quintana, skin lesions, 957t

Rickettsia rickettsii, 323, 324t
as bioterrorism agent, 882–883
diagnosis, 885–886
petechiae/purpura, 955t
skin lesions, 956t
Rickettsia sibirica, 323, 324t, 955t
Rickettsia slovaca, 323
Rickettsia tsutsugamushi, 955t
Rickettsia typhi, 329
life cycle, 330f
prevalence, 331f
skin lesions, 956t–957t
Rickettsialpox, 955t, 972t
Rickettsioses, 178b
HIV coinfection, 1060–1061
spotted fever *see* Spotted fever rickettsioses
typhus group, 329–333
see also individual Rickettsia *spp.*
Rifabutin, 100t
H. pylori infection, 172t
MAC in HIV, 246–247
Mycobacterium avium complex, 104t
in pregnancy, 1073t
toxoplasmosis, 727
Rifampicin, 100t
actinomycetoma, 568
adverse effects, 240
anthrax, 264
brucellosis, 273, 275, 918t
Buruli ulcer, 251–252
cat-scratch disease, 269
ehrlichial, anaplasmal and neorickettsial infections, 343
interactions, 240
legionellosis, 218
leprosy, 259
MAC, 246
meningococcal prophylaxis, 182
in pregnancy, 1073t
pregnancy and lactation, 242
primary amebic meningoencephalitis, 713
Q fever, 346
resistance, 237–238
scrub typhus, 338
staphylococcal toxic shock syndrome, 210
TB-HIV, 242–243
trachoma, 312–313
tuberculosis, 231, 239t
tuberculous meningitis, 236
tuberculous pleurisy, 234
Rifampin *see* Rifampicin
Rifapentine
in pregnancy, 1073t
tuberculosis, 242
Rifaximin
C. difficile, 164
E. coli infection, 119
travelers' diarrhea, 893, 894t
Rifins, 651
Rift Valley fever, 8–9, 442t–443t, 462–465
agent, 462, 463f
as bioterrorism agent, 880t
clinical features, 444t–445t, 464
diagnosis, 447t, 465
laboratory, 465
differential diagnosis, 465
epidemiology, 462–464
geography, 463
transmission cycle, 462–463, 463f, 464t
transmission to humans, 463–464
incubation period, 929b
military cases, 912
pathogenesis and immunity, 464–465
pathologic features, 446t
prevention and control, 465
skin lesions, 956t
transmission, 932t
treatment and prevention, 448t
treatment and prognosis, 465
vaccines, 465
RIG-1, 53, 54t
Rimantadine, influenza, 380t, 382
RING finger motif, 449
Ring sideroblasts, 1027
Ringer's lactate, 154–155
Ringworm *see* Tinea corporis
Rio Bravo virus, 516f
Rio Negro virus, 520t
Risk factors, 13–14
Risperidone, delusional parasitosis, 1070
Risus sardonicus, 285f
Ritonavir, 103t
HIV, 553–554
SARS, 397
River blindness *see* Onchocerciasis
RNA replicase, 427
RNA silencers, hepatitis D, 440
Rocky Mountain spotted fever, 323, 882–883
clinical features, 326
cutaneous lesions, 954f
military cases, 912
transmission, 875t
Rodent control, 460–461
Rodent vectors
arenaviruses, 455
Chapare virus, 455
Guanarito virus, 455
hystricognath rodents, 837
Junin virus, 455
Lassa fever, 455
lymphocytic choriomeningitis, 455
Machupo virus, 455
see also individual rodent species
Roll Back Malaria campaign, 20–21, 646
Romaña's sign, 691f, 1010f
Rose spots, 950, 955t
Roseola infantum *see* Exanthem subitum
Rosetting, 659
Ross River virus, 519, 520t
clinical features, 523
skin lesions, 972t
epidemiology, 522
military cases, 912
Rotavirus, 406–410, 407b
characteristics, 406
complications, 409
diagnosis, 409
diarrheal disease, 407f, 408
epidemiology, 406–408
mortality, 406–407
pathogenesis and immunity, 408–409
prevention and control, 409–410
recurrent infection, 408–409
transmission, 407–408
treatment and prognosis, 409–410
vaccine, 64t–65t, 409
requirements for immigrants, 908t
virulence, 408
Roundworm *see* Ascariasis
Rousettus aegyptiacus, 484
Roxithromycin
isosporiasis, 644
scrub typhus, 338
toxoplasmosis, 727
Rubella, 348–349
congenital rubella syndrome, 349, 351, 725–726
elimination of, 350, 350f
keratitis, 993
pregnancy, 1081
vaccine, 64t, 66b, 888t–890t
Rubulavirus, 385

S

Saaremaa virus, 471t, 472–473
hemorrhagic fever with renal syndrome, 475
Sabaeus monkey immunodeficiency virus, 542f
Saber shins, 291
Sabethes albiprivus, 493
Sabethes chloropterus, 493
Sabiá virus, 442t–443t, 450f, 450t
clinical features, 456
incubation period, 929b
transmission, 932t
Sabin-Feldman dye test, 726
Saboya virus, 492
Saccharomyces boulardii, 621
E. coli infection, 120
Saccharomyces cerevisiae, 651, 714
Sacroiliitis, *Brucella* spp., 272
Saffold virus, 378
St Louis encephalitis, 516f, 876t
Saliva, in parasite transmission, 49
Salmonella spp., 5, 60, 128, 917t
antimicrobial resistance, 129–131, 130f–131f, 130t
as bioterrorism agent, 880t, 883
diagnosis, 886
chronic carrier state, 132
drug resistance, 121
enteritis, 132
flagellar antigens, 121
gastrointestinal effects, 130f, 132
nontyphoidal *see* Salmonellosis
pathogenesis and immunity, 132–134
gastrointestinal tract and enteritis, 132
host response and immunity, 134
macrophage interactions, 134
systemic infection, 134
polymorphous lesions, 955t
rose spots, 955t
taxonomy, 121
toxin, 113, 114t–115t
travelers' diarrhea, 892, 924
type III secretion system, 132
Salmonella bongori, 121, 128
Salmonella choleraesuis, 128
bacteremia, 131
Salmonella dublin, bacteremia, 131
Salmonella enterica, 121, 138–139
Salmonella isangi, antimicrobial resistance, 129
Salmonella paratyphi, 121
bacteriology, 124
genomics, 122
pathogenesis, 123
Salmonella typhi, 4, 121
bacteriology, 124
in bile, 124
and cancer, 73t
genomics, 122
host factors, 124
intestinal perforation, 124f
skin lesions, 957t
Salmonella typhimurium, 4
antimicrobial resistance, 129
Salmonellosis, 128–136, 917t
clinical features, 131–132
bacteremia, 131
gastroenteritis, 131
HIV infection, 131–132
diagnosis, 134–135
isolation and identification, 134
molecular typing, 134–135
epidemiology, 128–131
extraintestinal complications, 132t–133t
incidence, 128, 129f–130f
incubation period, 929b
international spread of, 131
localized infections, 132, 132t–133t
prevention and control, 135–136
reservoirs, 128
transmission to humans, 128
treatment and prognosis, 135, 918t
AIDS patients, 135
bacteremia, 135
chronic carrier state, 135
gastroenteritis, 135
see also Salmonella spp.

Sandflies, 49, 876–877, 876f
see also Lutzomyia spp.; *Phlebotomus* spp.
Sandfly fever, 481
Sapovirus, 411, 412f
Sappinia spp., 707
epidemiology, 709
taxonomy and classification, 709
Sappinia diploidea, 708, 709f
eradication, 86t–87t
Sappinia pedata, 708, 709f
Saquinavir, 103t
HIV, 553–554
Saransinula plebeia, 776
Sarcocystis spp., 634f, 641, 644
characteristics, 644, 645f
Sarcocystis bovihominis, 644
Sarcocystis hirsuta, 644
Sarcocystis hominis, life cycle, 645f
Sarcocystis suihominis, 644
Sarcocystosis
clinical features, 644
diagnosis and treatment, 644
epidemiology, 644, 645f
prevention and control, 644
see also Sarcocystis spp.
Sarcophagidae, 869
Sarcoptes scabiei, 803, 868, 869f
see also Scabies
Sargramostim, candidiasis, 592
SARS, 392–397
agent, 392–394
animal reservoir, 392–394
chest X-ray findings, 395
diagnosis, 396–397
serologic diagnosis, 397
virus detection, 396–397
epidemiological parameters, 394
epidemiology, 394
extrapulmonary involvement, 395
incidence, 393f
incubation period, 394, 929b
laboratory findings, 395–396
life cycle, 393f
pathogenesis and immunity, 396
genetic predisposition, 396
viral load and mortality, 396
presentation, 394, 394t
prevention and control, 397
progression and clinical spectrum, 394–395
transmission routes, 394, 395f
treatment and prognosis, 397
antiviral agents, 397
clinical prognostic indicators, 397
immunomodulators, 397
long-term prognosis, 397
supportive care, 397
SARS-CoV, 7–8, 392–394
genetic evolution, 394
Saumarez reef virus, 516f
Sca1, 323
Sca2, 323
Scabies, 952t, 962t–966t, 1034t
agent *see Sarcoptes scabiei*
diagnosis, 868–869, 1037
dog, 869
HIV coinfection, 1055
horse, 869
Norwegian, 868–869
pruritus, 959t–961t
treatment, 93t, 868–869
Scarlet fever, 203–204, 950
septic, 205–206
Schistosoma haematobium, 132, 848
and cancer, 71–72, 73t
eradication, 81t
geographic distribution, 849f
life cycle, 851f
ova, 848, 850f
pulmonary disease, 984t
snail vector, 848
Schistosoma intercalatum, 848
ova, 850f
pulmonary disease, 984t
Schistosoma japonicum, 848
and cancer, 73t
eradication, 81t
geographic distribution, 850f
life cycle, 851f
ova, 848, 850f
pulmonary disease, 984t
snail vector, 848
Schistosoma mansoni, 848
eradication, 81t
genetic associations, 38
geographic distribution, 849f
life cycle, 851f
ova, 848, 850f
pulmonary disease, 984t
snail vector, 848
Schistosoma mekongi, 848
eradication, 81t
ova, 850f
Schistosomiasis, 17, 21, 776, 848–853
agent *see Schistosoma* spp.
clinical features, 849–852, 851f
acute, 850–851
cercarial dermatitis, 849–850
chronic, 851
chronic diarrhea, 924
eosinophilia, 942t–943t, 944
hepatobiliary disease, 976t–977t, 980, 980f
intestinal, 851, 917t, 920
Katayama fever, 701, 849
neurologic involvement, 1019t
ocular involvement, 1015
pruritus, 959t–961t
skin lesions, 946t, 962t–966t
diagnosis, 852
epidemiology, 848–849
genetic susceptibility, 35t
incubation period, 929b
pathogenesis and immunity, 852
prevention and control, 853, 900
treatment and prognosis, 852–853
Schizosaccharomyces pombe, 650–651
Schuffner's dots, 647–649
Sciurus niger, 276
Scopulariopsis spp., 563
Scorpions, 871, 871f, 900
Screening, HPV, 539–540
Screwworm fly *see Chrysomyia bezziana*
Scrotal swelling, 1044
Scrub typhus, 334–338
agent, 334–336
clinical features, eschar, 955t
diagnosis, 337
disease, 336
epidemiology, 334
geographic distribution, 335f
incubation period, 929b
military cases, 912
pathogenesis and immunity, 336–337
prevention and control, 338
treatment and prognosis, 338
Scrumpox, 357
Scurvy, 28, e12t–e13t
Scutula, 560–561, 560f
Scytalidium spp., 563
SDF-1, disease associations, 36t
Searles' ulcer *see Mycobacterium ulcerans*
Secernentea, 805
Segmentina spp., 865
Seizures
malaria, 655, 655b
neurocysticercosis, 817
toxocariasis, 765
Selamectin, toxocariasis prophylaxis, 767
Selenium, 26–27
requirements, e12t–e13t
Semliki virus, 520t
Seoul virus, 442t–443t, 470, 471t, 472
hemorrhagic fever with renal syndrome, 473, 475
Sepik virus, 492
Sepsis
anthrax, 263
meningococcal, 178
Septata spp., 714
Septata intestinalis, 634f
Septic shock, 178b
meningococcal, 178f
Septicemia
H. influenzae, 194t
melioidosis, 220, 220f
Vibrio spp., 160
Septicemic plague, 280
Sequestration, 656f, 658
Séreny test, 118–119
Serodiagnosis
C. trachomatis, 318
typhoid/paratyphoid, 125
Serologic tests
amebiasis, 620
echinococcosis
cystic, 830
polycystic, 838
hantaviruses, 478–479
leishmaniasis, 703
loaiasis, 737
lymphogranuloma venereum, 318
onchocerciasis, 747
SARS, 397
schistosomiasis, 852
toxoplasmosis, 726
trachoma, 312
Severe acute respiratory syndrome *see* SARS
Severe combined immunodeficiency syndrome, 34t
Sexually acquired reactive arthritis, 316t, 317
Sexually transmitted diseases, 1033–1045, 1034t
clinical presentations, 1044
control of, 1044–1045
genital ulcers *see* Genital ulcer disease
HIV interactions, 548, 1044–1045
non-ulcerative genital lesions, 1034t, 1037–1038
clinical features, 1037
diagnosis, 1037
management, 1037–1038
see also individual lesions
overseas medical screening, 904t
skin lesions, 952, 952t
travelers, 898–899
vaccines, 69t
vaginal discharge, 1034t, 1038–1041
see also individual diseases
Sheep bot fly *see Oestrus ovi*
Sheep maggot fly *see Wohlfahrtia magnifica*
Shiga spp., exotoxin, 5
Shiga toxin, 140–141
Shiga-like toxins, 117f
Shigella spp., 5, 137, 917t
antimicrobial sensitivity, 143f
as bioterrorism agent, 880t
life cycle, 138f
lipopolysaccharide, 139
travelers' diarrhea, 892, 924
see also Shigellosis
Shigella boydii, 138, 139f
Shigella dysenteriae, 117, 137–138, 139f
as bioterrorism agent, 883
diagnosis, 886
toxin, 114t–115t
Shigella flexneri, 60, 118, 137–138, 139f
pathogenesis, 140f
Shigella sonnei, 137–138, 139f
Shigellosis, 137–144
agent, 137
clinical manifestations and complications, 141–142
dysentery, 141, 141f
rectal prolapse, 141f
toxic megacolon, 141f
diagnosis, 142, 142f

epidemiology, 137–138
incidence, 138
incubation period, 929b
pathogenesis and immunity, 138–141, 140f–141f
prevention and control, 144
treatment and prognosis, 142–144, 143f, 143t, 918t
Shingles *see* Herpes zoster
Shock, yellow fever, 498
Sialic acids, 52–53
Siberian tick typhus, 875t
Sibine stimulea, 871
Sick euthyroid syndrome, 661
Sickle cell anemia, 1025, 1026f, 1030
clinical features, 1030b
management, 1030
hydroxycarbamide, 1030, 1031b
prevention of complications, 1030
Sickle cell trait, malaria resistance, 32, 653
Sickle solubility test, 1027
Sigmodon spp., 276, 462
Sigmodon alstoni, 450f, 454
Sigmodon hispidus, 450f, 471t, 776
Sigmodontinae, 470
Signal 1, 57–58
Signal 2, 57–58
Silicosis, 989
Simian immunodeficiency virus, 542f, 543
Simisulcospica libertina, 855
Simon's foci, 230, 230f
Simonsiella spp., 184
Simulium spp., 50, 741, 742f, 877f
zoonotic filariasis, 750
Simulium amazonicum, 740
Simulium damnosum, 741, 742f
Simulium leonense, 741
Simulium neavei, 50
Simulium ochraceum, 741
Simulium sanctipauli, 741
Simulium sirbanum, 741
Simulium squamosum, 741
Simulium yahense, 741
Sin Nombre virus, 7, 442t–443t, 470, 471t, 472–473, 472f
hantavirus pulmonary syndrome, 473, 475–476
host, 470, 471t
pulmonary syndrome, 471f
Sindbis viruses, 519, 520t
skin lesions, 972t
Single nucleotide polymorphisms, 33–34
SARS, 396
Sinton and Mulligan's stippling, 647–649
Sinus mucormycosis, 598–599
Sinusitis, fungal, 1009
SipA, 132
SipC, 132
Siphonaptera *see* Fleas
Skin, eye or mouth disease, 357–358
Skin lesions, 950–974
alphaviruses, 956t, 972t
amebiasis, 962t–968t
anthrax, 261–262, 954f, 957t, 967t–968t, 972t
approach to, 951–952
ascariasis, 946t
B. bacilliformis, 957t
B. burgdorferi, 957t
B. malayi, 946t
B. pseudomallei, 956t
B. recurrentis, 957t
B. timori, 946t
bartonellosis, 962t–966t
blastomycosis, 969t–970t
blister beetles, 873
Borrelia spp., 956t
brucellosis, 957t, 972t
Buruli ulcer, 248–252, 953f
C. burnetii, 957t
C. immitis, 957t
candidiasis, 590–591, 955t
cat-scratch disease, 962t–966t
characterization of, 955
chromomycosis, 969t–970t
coccidioidomycosis, 969t–970t
coenurisis, 962t–966t
Colorado tick fever, 956t
Crimean-Congo hemorrhagic fever, 956t
cryptococcosis, 969t–970t
cysticercosis, 946t, 962t–966t
cysts, 966
cytomegalovirus, 956t
dengue fever, 954f, 956t–957t
dermatitis *see* Dermatitis
differential diagnosis, 954b
diffuse toxic erythema, 955t
diphtheria, 225, 967t–968t
Dirofilaria spp., 751t
dirofilariasis, 962t–966t
donovanosis, 952t
dracunculiasis, 946t, 958t, 962t–966t
drug-related, 971–973, 972t, 974t
Ebola virus, 956t
echinococcosis, 946t, 962t–966t
ecthyma gangrenosum, 591, 955t
Enterococcus spp., 956t
enteroviruses, 402, 956t, 972t
entomophthoramycosis, 969t–970t
with eosinophilia, 946, 946t
Epstein-Barr virus, 957t
eschar *see* Eschar
etiology, 952b
fascioliasis, 946t, 958t
and fever, 934–935
filariasis, 946t, 962t–966t
gangrene, 955t
glanders, 962t–968t
gnathostomiasis, 946t, 958t, 962t–966t
H. aegyptius, 956t
H. influenzae, 956t
hantaviruses, 956t
hemorrhagic, 955–956, 955t–956t
hemorrhagic fevers, 445t
with hepatomegaly, 955b
herpes simplex virus, 952t, 967t–968t, 972t
histoplasmosis, 969t–970t
history, 952–953, 952b
HIV/AIDS, 952t
hookworm, 946t, 957t–958t, 972t
impetigo, 972t
Janeway lesions, 950, 955t
Junin virus, 956t
kwashiorkor, 28
Kyasanur Forest disease, 956t
L. interrogans, 956t
larva migrans *see* Cutaneous larva migrans
Lassa fever, 956t–957t
leishmaniasis
cutaneous *see* Leishmaniasis, cutaneous
visceral, 962t–966t
leopard skin, 744f
leprosy, 962t–968t
Leptospira spp., 957t
leptospirosis, 962t–966t
lobomycosis, 969t–970t
loiasis, 946t, 958t
louse-borne typhus, 331f
M. marinum, 962t–966t, 971f
M. rhodhaini, 751t
M. tuberculosis, 972t
M. ulcerans, 962t–966t
Machupo virus, 956t
macronodules, 955t
macules and papules, 956–957, 956f, 957t
Marburg virus, 956t–957t
measles, 347, 348f, 956t, 972t
melioidosis, 967t–968t
migratory rash, 957, 958t, 961f
monkeypox, 972t
mucormycosis, 599
mumps, 972t
mycetoma, 962t–966t, 969t–970t
mycobacterial infections, 245–246
Mycoplasma spp., 972t
myiasis, 953f, 958t, 962t–966t
N. meningitidis, 955t–956t
nodules and ulcers, 962, 962f, 962t–968t
Omsk hemorrhagic fever, 956t
Onchocerca spp., 751t
onchocerciasis, 946t, 957t, 962t–966t
orf, 261–262, 962t–966t, 972t
Osler's nodes, 950, 955t
P. aeruginosa, 956t
P. falciparum, 956t
paracoccidioidomycosis, 969t–970t
paragonimiasis, 864, 946t, 958t, 962t–966t
pathogenesis, 950–951
penicilliosis, 969t–970t
petechiae and purpura, 955–956, 955t
differential diagnosis, 956t
physical examination, 953–971, 954b
pigmentation changes, 971, 973t
pityriasis versicolor, 969t–970t
plague, 956t–957t, 967t–968t
pruritic *see* Pruritus
pseudocowpox, 261–262, 962t–966t
R. prowazekii, 956t–957t
R. quintana, 957t
R. rickettsii, 956t
R. typhi, 956t–957t
rhinoscleroma, 962t–966t
rhinosporidiosis, 969t–970t
rickettsialpox, 955t, 972t
Rift Valley fever, 956t
Rocky Mountain spotted fever, 954f
rose spots, 950, 955t
S. minus, 957t
S. moniliformis, 956t–957t
S. typhi, 957t
scabies *see* Scabies
schistosomiasis, 946t, 962t–966t
sparganosis, 946t, 958t, 962t–966t
with splenomegaly, 955b
sporotrichosis, 969t–970t, 971f
staphylococcal scalded skin syndrome, 209b, 950
STDs, 952, 952t
chancroid, 952t, 967t–968t
gonorrhea, 952t
granuloma inguinale, 952t, 953f, 962t–968t
lymphogranuloma venereum, 952t, 962t–966t
syphilis, 952t, 962t–968t
strongyloidiasis, 810, 946t, 957t
T. gondii, 956t–957t
T. pallidum, 956t–957t
T. spiralis, 956t
tanapox, 972t
tick granuloma, 959t–966t
tinea imbricata, 561, 561f, 969t–970t
toxic epidermal necrolysis, 972f, 972t
trichinellosis, 946t
tropical ulcer, 967t–968t
trypanosomiasis
African, 959t–966t
American, 962t–966t
tuberculosis, 967t–968t
tularemia, 967t–968t
tungiasis, 959t–966t
V. vulnificus, 956t, 972t
vaccinia, 972t
varicella, 358f, 360, 972t
variola, 972t
verruga peruana, 267f
vesicles, 966–971, 972t
visceral larva migrans, 946t, 962t–966t
W. bancrofti, 946t
West Nile virus, 957t
yaws, 952t, 962t–966t
yellow fever, 956t
see also Lymphadenopathy

Skin tests
leishmaniasis, 703
Montenegro, 703
tuberculosis, 228–230
false positives, 229
SLC11A1, disease associations, 36t
Sleeping sickness *see* Trypanosomiasis, African
Smallpox, 3, 369–377
bacterial superinfection, 371
as bioterrorism agent, 376, 880t, 881–882
diagnosis, 885
clinical diagnosis, 372
clinical features, 41, 370, 882
flat-type, 370–371
rash, 370f
disease burden, 41, 41f
environmental persistence, 41
eradication, 40–41
Guarnieri bodies, 373, 373f, 885
laboratory diagnosis, 373
long-term effectiveness of interventions, 41
mortality, 41f
pathogenesis and immunity, 372, 372f
prevention and control, 374–376
inoculation, 374
variolation, 374
susceptibility to reinfection, 41
transmission potential, 41
treatment and prognosis, 376–377
antiviral drugs, 376–377
passive immunization, 376
vaccination, 374–375
adverse events, 375–376
contraindications, 375
outcome, 375
see also Orthopoxviruses
Smoking, and cancer, 72
Snail fever *see* Katayama fever
Snail vectors
A. cantonensis by, 774
clonorchiasis/opisthorchiasis, 855
control of, 853
F. buski, 865
P. westermani, 862
Schistosoma spp. by, 848
see also individual species
Snow, John, 150
Social inequality, 21–22
Sodium, cholera stools, 153t
Sodium stibogluconate
adverse effects, 90b
leishmaniasis, 91t–92t
cutaneous, 704–705
visceral, 704
Soft tissue infections
mycobacterial, 245–246
salmonellosis, 132t–133t
Soilborne pathogens, 900
military cases, 914–915
Solid organ transplantation, mucormycosis infection, 598
Sooty mangabey immunodeficiency virus, 542f
Soricomorpha, 470
Source-sink model, 2
South America
causes of fever, 926f
Chagas' disease *see* Chagas' disease
coccidioidomycosis, 578
malaria, 652, 896f
drug-resistant, 654t
paracoccidioidomycosis, 582, 583f
trichinellosis, 770t
South American blastomycosis *see* Paracoccidioidomycosis
South American hemorrhagic fever
clinical features, 444t–445t
diagnosis, 447t
Sowda, 742, 744f
Spanish sheep encephalitis virus, 516f
Sparganosis, 813, 845–847
agent *see Spirometra* spp.
clinical features, 846–847, 847f
eosinophilia, 942t
ocular involvement, 847, 1015
skin lesions, 946t, 958t, 962t–966t
diagnosis, 847, 847f
epidemiology, 845
treatment and prevention, 847
Sparganum spp., 783
Sparganum proliferum, 847
Spectinomycin
cervicitis/urethritis, 1040t
gonorrhoea, 189
disseminated, 189
Spermophilus spp., 276–277
Spherocytosis, 1026f
Spiders, 872
Spinal cord infections, 1022
Spinal neurocysticercosis, 818
treatment, 822
Spiramycin
adverse effects, 85b
cryptosporidiosis, 639
in pregnancy, 1073t
toxoplasmosis, 727
Spirillum minus, 957t
Spirometra spp., 813, 845
see also Sparganosis
Spirometra mansonoides, 814
Spirurida, 784–785
Gnathostoma, 784–785
Gongylonema, 785
Thelazia, 785
Spleen, pitting, 661
Splendore-Hoeppli phenomenon, 603–604, 606
Splenectomy, 1031
Splenic salmonellosis, 132t–133t
Splenomegaly, 1025
African trypanosomiasis, 685
malaria, 654–655, 657, 661
Q fever, 346
with rash, 955b
tropical splenomegaly syndrome, 976t–977t
Spondylitis
Brucella spp., 272–273, 273t
parrot beak sign, 272–273
differential diagnosis, 273t
tuberculous, 234, 235f, 273t
Sporothrix schenckii, 605
HIV coinfection, 1057
Sporotrichosis, 605–607
agent, 605
clinical features, 606
ocular involvement, 1008
skin lesions, 969t–970t, 973t
diagnosis, 606
epidemiology, 606
pathogenesis and immunity, 606
prevention and control, 607
treatment and prognosis, 604t, 606–607
Sporozoa, 1–2
Sporozoasida, 633
Spotted fever rickettsioses, 323–328
agent, 323
clinical features, 326–327
diagnosis, 327
epidemiology, 323–326, 324t, 325f
incubation period, 929b
pathogenesis and immunity, 327
prevention and control, 328
treatment and prognosis, 328
see also individual fevers
Sputum specimens, tuberculosis, 238–239
SpvB, 134
SQ-109 (ethylenediamine), tuberculosis, 242
ST-246, orthopoxviruses, 376
Standard deviation, 13
Standard error of mean, 13
Staphylinidae, 873
Staphylococcal enterotoxins, 210
Staphylococcal scalded skin syndrome, 209b, 950
Staphylococcal toxic shock syndrome, 209–210
clinical presentation, 210
epidemiology, 209
pathogenesis and immunity, 210
treatment and prognosis, 210–211
Staphylococcus spp., 208–211
characteristics, 208
disease spectrum, 208–210, 209b
cellulitis, 210–211
empyema, 209
endocarditis, 209
folliculitis, carbuncles and abscesses, 208–209
impetigo, 209
pyomyositis, 209
epidemiology, 208
prevention and control, 211
Staphylococcus aureus, 208, 917t
diffuse toxic erythema, 955t
disease spectrum
endocarditis, 178b, 209
impetigo, 209
pyomyositis, 208–209
sepsis, 178
exotoxin, 5
Janeway lesions, 955t
methicillin-resistant *see* MRSA
Osler's nodes, 955t
superinfection, 360
Staphylococcus aureus Enterotoxin B, 880t, 883
detection, 886
Staphylococcus epidermidis, 208
Staphylococcus intermedius, 208
Staphylococcus saprophyticus, 208
Statistical significance, 12
Statistical tests
ANOVA, 13
chi-square test, 13
Kruskal-Wallis test, 13
Mann-Whitney *U*-test, 13
Wilcoxon matched rank test, 13
Stavudine, 103t
HIV, 553
STDs *see* Sexually transmitted diseases
Stegomyia spp., 504
Stevens-Johnson syndrome, 99, 951
STEVORs, 651
Stibogluconate, 93
Stigma, 20
Stinging arthropods, 899–900
caterpillars, 870–871
insects, 868, 870f
Stivalius cognatus, 277
Stratum acanthosum, 534
Stratum corneum, 534
Stratum granulosum, 534
Streptobacillus moniliformis, skin lesions, 956t–957t
Streptocerciasis, 738–739
agent *see Mansonella streptocerca*
clinical features, 738
diagnosis, 739
epidemiology, 738
pathogenesis and immunity, 738
prevention and control, 739
treatment and prognosis, 739
Streptococcal infections *see S. pyogenes*
Streptococcal M protein, 203
Streptococcal pyoderma, 204
Streptococcal pyrogenic exotoxins, 206–208
Streptococcal superantigen, 208
Streptococcal toxic shock syndrome, 203, 205
bacteriologic cultures, 205
clinical course, 205
group A streptococcus acquisition, 205
laboratory test results, 205
physical findings, 205
predisposing factors, 205
symptoms, 205
Streptococcus spp., Janeway lesions, 955t

Streptococcus pneumoniae, 53, 60, 178b, 199, 200f
antimicrobial resistance, 95, 201, 201f
characteristics, 199
drug resistance, 95
epidemiology, 200–201
HIV patients, 555
military cases, 910
pathogenesis and immunity, 199–200, 200f
host targeting, 199–200
inflammation in response to cell wall, 200
inflammation in response to toxins, 200
pneumococcal clearance, 200
sepsis, 178
see also Pneumococcal infections
Streptococcus pyogenes, 203
asymptomatic carriers, 203
characteristics, 203
diffuse toxic erythema, 955t
disease spectrum, 204b
cellulitis, 204
erysipelas, 204
lymphangitis, 204
myositis and myonecrosis, 204–205
necrotizing fasciitis, 204
pharyngitis, 203
scarlet fever, 203–204
streptococcal pyoderma, 204
streptococcal toxic shock syndrome *see* Streptococcal toxic shock syndrome
epidemiology, 203
military cases, 910
pathogenesis and immunity, 206–208
phagocytic killing, 7
postinfectious sequelae, 205–206
glomerulonephritis, 206
rheumatic fever, 205–206
superinfection, 360
Streptolysin O, 203, 206–207
Streptolysins, 5
Streptomyces avermitilis, 811
Streptomyces somaliensis, 565
Streptomycin, 96t–98t, 100t
actinomycetoma, 568
brucellosis, 275, 918t
Buruli ulcer, 251–252
MAC, 246
plague, 281
in pregnancy, 1073t
resistance, 237–238
Salmonella resistance, 130t
toxicity, 281
tuberculosis, 239–240, 239t
Strongylida, 779–781
Mammomonogamus, 780
Oesophagostomum, 780–781
Ternidens, 781
Trichostrongylus, 780
Strongyloides fuelleborni, 805
Strongyloides myopotami, 957
Strongyloides papillosus, 805
Strongyloides ransomi, 805
Strongyloides ratti, 805
Strongyloides stercoralis, 767, 805, 917t
hyperinfection syndrome, 976t–977t
life cycle and morphology, 805, 806f–807f
pulmonary disease, 984t
see also Strongyloidiasis
Strongyloides venezuelensis, 805
Strongyloides westeri, 805
Strongyloidiasis, 776, 805–812
agent *see Strongyloides stercoralis*
autoinfection, 805–807
clinical features, 808–810
chronic diarrhea, 924
eosinophilia, 942t, 943–944
gastrointestinal, 809
intestinal obstruction, 921
neurologic, 809, 810f, 1019t
pruritus, 959t–961t
pulmonary, 809, 809f, 988t
skin lesions, 810, 946t, 957t
diagnosis, 810–811
disseminated, 806–807, 809
epidemiology, 805–806, 807f
eradication, 76, 77t–79t
HIV coinfection, 552, 810, 1054–1055
HTLV-1 and leukemia, 810
military cases, 914
pathogenesis and immunity, 806–808
pathology, 808, 808f–809f
prevention and control, 811–812
treatment and prognosis, 811, 918t
albendazole, 77t–79t, 811
ivermectin, 811
thiabendazole, 811
Strongyloididae, 805
Structural adjustment programs, 19
Strychnine poisoning, comparison with tetanus, 286
Study design, 11–12
Subacute sclerosing panencephalitis, measles, 347
Subarachnoid hemorrhage, gnathostomiasis, 784–785
Subarachnoid neurocysticercosis, 817–819, 818f
treatment, 821–822
Subcutaneous infections, filarial, 752, 752f
Sudan ebolavirus, 483, 485t
Sudan Guinea Worm Eradication Program, 762
Sulfadiazine
granulomatous amebic encephalitis, 712
sarcocystosis, 644
toxoplasmosis, 727
Sulfadoxine-pyrimethamine
malaria, 666, 667t
pregnancy, 671b
in pregnancy, 1073t
resistance, 651f
Sulfamethoxazole
cholera, 155–156
Salmonella resistance, 130t
Sulfonamides, 96t–98t, 99
group A streptococcus resistance, 208
paracoccidioidomycosis, 584
toxoplasmosis, 727
trachoma, 312–313
Suncus murinus, 277
Sundathelphusa spp., 862
Superoxide dismutase, 346
Suramin, 90
adverse effects, 90b
African trypanosomiasis, 91t–92t, 687, 688t
onchocerciasis, 749
Surfactant protein A, 54t
Surfactant protein D, 54t
Surgical treatment
cystic echinococcosis, 831
mucormycosis, 601–602
mycetoma, 568
trachoma, 312
see also individual procedures
Surveillance studies, 11–12
Swimmer's itch, 849–850, 950
Swiss cheese liver, 220f
Swollen baby syndrome, 456
Sykes' monkey immunodeficiency virus, 542f
Sylvilagus floridianus, 837
Symbiosis, 1
Syndecans, 534–535
Syndrome of inappropriate antidiuretic hormone secretion, malaria, 660
Syndromic surveillance, 880
Syngamus spp., 780
Syphilis, 289, 1034t
clinical features, 290–291, 1034t
chancre, 290
CNS symptoms, 290
gastrointestinal, 917t
gumma, 290–291
lues maligna, 290
ocular involvement, 1000, 1000f
pigmentation changes, 973t
pruritus, 959t–961t
skin lesions, 952t, 962t–968t
congenital, 291
cutaneous lesions, 952t
diagnosis, 291–292, 291f, 1035t
drug therapy, 104t
endemic, 289, 292–294
epidemiology, 289–290, 290f, 290t
global burden, 290t
history, 289
HIV coinfection, 1060
overseas medical screening, 904t
in pregnancy, 292
pregnancy, 292, 1081
prevention and control, 292
tertiary, 290–291
transmission, 290f
treatment and prognosis, 292
Jarisch-Herxheimer reaction, 292
see also Treponema pallidum
Syphilitic chancre, 261–262
Syringes, reuse of, spread of HCV infection, 429

T

T-cells
anergy, 250–251
antigen presentation, 58–60
cytotoxic *see* Cytotoxic T cells
development, 57
effector, 57
costimulation, 57–58
maturation defects, 28–29
memory, 57
regulatory *see* Tregs
response to infectious agents, 59f
in zinc deficiency, 30
T-helper cells, 57–58
antigen presentation, 60
immune regulation, 60
Th1, 61
Th2, 61
Th17, 61
Tacaribe virus, 450f
Taenia spp., 813
ovum, 840f
Taenia asiatica, 839–840
Taenia crassiceps, 841, 841f
Taenia multiceps, 814, 822, 822f
see also Coenuriasis
Taenia saginata, 813, 839, 840f
cysticercus, 814–815, 839
eradication, 80t
life cycle, 840f
ova, 813–814
proglottid, 841f
scolex, 840f
Taenia serialis, 822
Taenia solium, 785, 814f, 815, 839, 840f
cysticercosis *see* Cysticercosis
cysticercus, 814, 839
eradication, 80t
global distribution, 816f
life cycle, 815, 816f
proglottid, 839, 840f
scolex, 840f–841f
Taeniasis, 839–841
agent *see Taenia saginata*; *Taenia solium*
clinical features, 839, 841f
diagnosis, 839–840, 841f
epidemiology, 839
prevention and control, 841
treatment and prognosis, 840–841, 841f
Taeniidae, 824
Tafenoquine, malaria, 664
Tamiami virus, 450f
Tamias spp., 276
Tanabids *see* Deer flies; Horse flies
Tanapox, 972t

Tapeworms, 813–814, 839–847
characteristics, 813
ova, 813–814, 840f
proglottids, 839, 841f
scolex, 813, 840f
taeniasis, 839–841
vaccines, 814
see also Diphyllobothrium spp.; *Dipylidium* spp.; *Hymenolepsis* spp.; *Spirometra* spp.; *Taenia* spp.
Tat, 543
Tataguine virus, 482
Tatera spp., 276–277
Tatera indica, 277
Taterapox, 369
TB 7.7, 230
TcdA, 163
TcdB, 163
Teicoplanin, cellulitis, 210–211
Telbivudine, hepatitis B, 436
Telithromycin, scrub typhus, 338
Tenebrio spp., 844–845
Tenofovir, 103t
hepatitis B, 436
HIV, 553–554
Terbinafine
candidiasis, 592
chromoblastomycosis, 570
dermatophytosis, 563
onychomycosis, 563
phaeohyphomycosis, 572
sporotrichosis, 604t, 606–607
Ternidens spp., 779–780
Ternidens deminutus, 781
Tertian malaria, 650
Tetanic spasms, 285
Tetanolysin, 286
Tetanospasmin, 285–286
Tetanus, 284–288
agent, 284
cephalic tetanus, 285–286
clinical features, 284–286
ocular involvement, 1003
diagnosis, 286
differential diagnosis, 286
epidemiology, 284
generalized tetanus, 284–285
risus sardonicus, 285f
trismus, 284–286
global incidence, 285f
historical aspects, 284
localized tetanus, 285
neonatal, 284, 286, 288
pathogenesis and immunity, 286
pregnancy, 1078
prevention and control, 288, 288t
treatment, 287–288, 287b
Tetanus antitoxin, 288
Tetanus immunoglobulin, 287–288
Tetanus/diphtheria vaccine, 888t–890t
requirements for immigrants, 908t
Tetracyclines, 96t–98t, 99
adverse reactions, eosinophilia, 947t
balantidiasis, 88t–89t, 628t, 630, 918t
Borrelia spp., 300
brucellosis, 275
Campylobacter spp., 148
cat-scratch disease, 269
cervicitis/urethritis, 1040t
cholera, 155, 155t, 918t
D. fragilis, 88t–89t, 628t
E. coli infection, 119
ehrlichial, anaplasmal and neorickettsial infections, 343
granuloma inguinale, 1035t
H. pylori infection, 172t, 173b
lymphogranuloma venereum, 318, 1035t
melioidosis, 222
plague, 282
psittacosis, 322
Q fever, 346
Salmonella resistance, 130t
scrub typhus, 338
spotted fever rickettsioses, 328
syphilis, 292, 1035t
trachoma, 312–313
typhus, 332–333
Vibrio spp., 161
Tetrapetalonema perstans, 739
Tetrapetalonema streptocerca, 738
Thalassemia, 1025, 1031
intermedia, 1025
major, 1025f, 1031
and malaria resistance, 34, 36t, 653
management, 1031
minor, 1025
Thalidomide
erythema nodosum leprosum, 259–260
Kaposi's sarcoma, 368
Theileria spp., 45, 676
Thelazia californiensis, 737–738, 785, 1014
Thelazia callipaeda, 785, 1014
Thiabendazole
C. hepaticum, 786
cutaneous larva migrans, 767
P. strongyloides infection, 778
strongyloidiasis, 76–79, 77t–79t, 811, 918t
Ternidens spp., 781
toxocariasis, 766
trichinellosis, 772–773
Thiacetazone, tuberculosis, 241
Thiamine, 24
requirements, e12t–e13t
Thiaridae, 862
Thrassis spp., 276
Thrombocytopenia
Brucella spp., 273
Crimean-Congo hemorrhagic fever, 467
hemorrhagic fevers, 445t
malaria, 656, 660
shigellosis, 142
Sin Nombre virus, 475–476
Thrombospondin, 658–659
Thrombospondin-related anonymous protein (TRAP), 647
Thrombotic thrombocytopenic purpura, 178b
Thrush, 591–592
Thymosin, 29
Thymulin, 29
inhibition by zinc deficiency, 30
Ticarcillin-clavulanate, 96t–98t
Ticks, 45, 51, 873f
as disease vectors, 874
hard (Ixodidae), 51, 874–875
life cycle, 45
lifespan, 48
removal of, 875, 875f
soft (Argasidae), 51, 295, 874–875
see also individual species
Tick granuloma, 959t–966t
Tick paralysis, 875t
Tick-borne diseases, 875t
military cases, 912
see also individual diseases
Tick-borne encephalitis, 515–518, 875t
agent, 515
clinical features, 516–517, 517t
diagnosis, 518
epidemiology, 515, 517f
incubation period, 929b
military cases, 912
pathogenesis and immunity, 517–518
Siberian subtype, 517, 517t
treatment and prognosis, 518
vaccine, 888t–890t
Tick-borne lymphadenopathy, 326–327
Tick-borne relapsing fever, 295–302, 875t
clinical/laboratory features, 297t
ecology and epidemiology, 295–296, 295f
life cycle, 296f
prevention, 301
temperature curves, 298f
Tigecycline, 96t–98t
MRSA, 211
TIGER, 886
Tinca tinca, 855
Tinea, HIV coinfection, 562–563
Tinea capitis, 559–561
endothrix, 560–561, 561f
favus, 560–561, 560f
Tinea corporis, 559, 560f, 561
Tinea cruris, 559, 561
Tinea imbricata, 561, 561f, 969t–970t
Tinea pedis, 559, 561–562, 562f
moccasin foot, 563
Tinea unguium, 559, 562, 562f
Tinga penetrans, 876
Tinidazole, 89
adverse effects, 85b, 629t
amebiasis, 88t–89t, 621
E. histolytica, 918t
giardiasis, 88t–89t, 628t, 918t
H. pylori, 172t
sarcocystosis, 644
Trichomonas vaginalis, 88t–89t
trichomoniasis, 1040t
Tipranivir, 103t
HIV, 553–554
Tissue damage, 5–6
host cell function, 5–6
TLR1, 54t
TLR2, 54t
TLR3, 54t
TLR4, 54t
TLR5, 54t
TLR6, 54t
TLR7, 54t
TLR8, 54t
TLR9, 54t
TMC-207 (diarylquinoline), tuberculosis, 242
TNF inhibitors, complications, tuberculosis, 233
Tobacco-associated pulmonary disease, 989
Tobramycin, 96t–98t
Tolerance, 60
Tolevamer, *C. difficile*, 164
Toll-like receptors, 33, 53
disease associations, 36t
leishmaniasis, 702
M. tuberculosis infection, 236–237
P. brasiliensis infection, 583–584
salmonellosis, 134
TLR-4, 39
Tonate virus, 520t
Tongue worms, 877, 877f
Tonsillar size estimation, 30–31
Tonsillitis, 263
Toroviruses, 417t, 419
Torticollis, 286
Toscana virus, 481
Tospoviruses, 466
Toxic epidermal necrolysis, 972f, 972t
Toxic megacolon, 163
shigellosis, 141f
Toxic shock syndrome, 950
staphylococcal *see* Staphylococcal toxic shock syndrome
streptococcal *see* Streptococcal toxic shock syndrome
Toxin coregulated pili, 154
Toxins, 2
category A, 880–881
category B, 883
Toxocara spp., 763
Toxocara canis, 763–764
life cycle, 763, 764f
paratenic hosts, 763
pulmonary disease, 984t
Toxocara cati, 763–764
life cycle, 763
pulmonary disease, 984t

Toxocara leonina, 763
Toxocariasis, 763–767
clinical features, 763, 764t, 765
ocular larva migrans, 763, 764t, 765, 765f, 1013, 1013f
pleural effusion, 988t
visceral larva migrans, 763, 764t, 765
covert, 764t, 765
diagnosis, 766
epidemiology, 764–765
eradication, 77t–79t
pathogenesis and immunity, 765–766, 766f
prevention and control, 767
treatment and prognosis, 766
Toxoplasma spp., 4
Toxoplasma gondii, 634f, 644, 722
bradyzoites, 723f
history and taxonomy, 722
life cycle, 722, 723f
pulmonary disease, 984t
skin lesions, 956t–957t
tachyzoites, 723f
see also Toxoplasmosis
Toxoplasmosis, 5, 7, 722–728
agent *see Toxoplasma gondii*
clinical features
neurologic involvement, 1019t
ocular involvement, 724–725, 725f, 1009–1010, 1010f
congenital, 723f, 724, 725f
diagnosis, 725–726
detection/isolation of parasites, 726
serologic tests, 726
specific symptoms, 726
differential diagnosis, 725–726
ecology, epidemiology and distribution, 722–724
HIV coinfection, 725–727, 725f, 1052
diagnosis, 726
treatment, 727
incubation period, 929b
multifocal necrotizing encephalitis, 725, 725f–726f
pathogenesis, pathology and clinical features, 724–725
pregnancy, 727, 1078–1079
prevention and control, 727–728
primary, 724
treatment and prognosis, 85, 85b, 86t–87t, 104t, 727
immunocompromised patients, 727
indications and treatment regimens, 727
ToxR, 154
Tracheal cytotoxin, 212–213
Trachipleistophora spp., 714
eradication, 86t–87t
Trachipleistophora anthropopthera, 715t
Trachipleistophora hominis, 715t
clinical manifestations, 718
treatment, 720t
Trachoma, 308–313, 316t, 996–997
agent, 308–309
blinding, 309–310
classification, 997b, 997f
clinical features, 310–311, 311b, 997f
entropion, 997f
Herbert's peripheral pits, 310, 310f
papillary hypertrophy, 310f
scarring, 310f
trichiasis, 310f, 997f
diagnosis, 311–312
antigen and nucleic acid probes, 312
isolation, 311–312
serology and immunology, 312
elimination, 313
epidemiology, 309–310
global distribution, 309f
pathogenesis and immunity, 311
post-trachomatous degeneration, 311
treatment and control, 312–313
antibiotics, 312–313
environment, 313
face washing and hygiene, 313
surgery, 312
Transforming growth factor-β, leishmaniasis, 702
Transfusion malaria, 657
Transovarial transmission, 48
Transposons, 2
Trapa bicornis, 865
Trapa natans, 865
Travelers
advice for, 887–901
altitude sickness, 900–901
bloodborne pathogens, 898–899
cholera prevention, 156
cutaneous larva migrans, 767
deep-vein thrombosis, 901
diarrheal disease, 887, 892–894, 924
chemoprophylaxis, 893–894, 924
food and water precautions, 892–893
HIV/AIDS infection, 899
self-treatment, 894, 894t, 924
fever in, 926t–927t
first-aid kit, 901, 901b
health considerations, 899–901
adaptation to environment, 900–901
bites and stings, 899–900
mortality, 887, 899
motor vehicle accidents/injuries, 899
soil/water-transmitted diseases, 900
health problems, 887, 888t–890t
heat acclimatization, 900
HIV-infected, 899
immunization, 888t–890t
altered immunocompetence, 890–891
hypersensitivity to vaccine components, 890
immunoglobulins, 887–890
infants, 891
interrupted multidose schedules, 887
pregnancy, 891
recommended, 887, 891–892
required, 887, 891
routine, 887, 891
simultaneous administration of vaccines, 887
see also Vaccines
infections and fatal accidents, 888f
jaundice, 973b
jet lag, 900
loaiasis, 735, 738
lymphatic filiariasis, 733
malaria, 887, 894–898, 895b
antimalarial drugs, 895–898, 897t
chemoprophylaxis, 895
malaria-endemic countries, 896f
personal protection measures, 895
recommended regimens, 897t, 898
self-treatment, 898
pre-existing health problems, 887
STDs, 898–899
trichinellosis, 769
tuberculosis, 892
typhoid fever, 887
vaccines, 63
Tregs, 61
leishmaniasis, 703
Trehalose, 236–237
Trematode larva migrans, 864
Trematodes, 1–2, 854–867
eradication, 80–82, 81t
HIV coinfection, 1054
intestinal, 865
liver, 854
lung, 862–865
morphology, 855f
see also individual species
Tremor, hemorrhagic fevers, 445t
Trench fever, 266f, 266t
agent *see Bartonella quintana*
characteristics, 268
ocular involvement, 1002
skin lesions, 957t
Treponema carateum, 289
Treponema pallidum, 7, 289
skin lesions, 956t–957t
subsp. *endemicum*, 289
subsp. *pallidum*, 289
subsp. *pertenue*, 289
Treponemal infections, 289–294
endemic, 292–294
geographic distribution, 293f
ocular involvement, 1000–1001
history, 289
ocular involvement, 1000, 1000f
pinta *see* Pinta
syphilis *see* Syphilis
yaws see Yaws
see also Treponema carateum; Treponema pallidum
Triatoma spp., 50
Triatoma dimidiata, 50, 874
Triatoma infestans, 689, 874
Triazoles, dermatophytosis, 563
Tribendimidine
ascariasis, 798
C. sinensis, 867
lung flukes, 867
O. viverrini, 867
opisthorchiasis/clonorchiasis, 858
Tricarboxylic acid cycle, 651
Trichiasis, 310f, 311b, 997f
Trichinella spp., 768, 769t
Trichinella britovi, 769t
life cycle, 769f
Trichinella murrelli, 769t
life cycle, 769f
Trichinella nativa, 769t
life cycle, 769f
Trichinella nelsoni, 769t
life cycle, 769f
Trichinella papuae, 768, 769t
life cycle, 769f
Trichinella pseudospiralis, 768, 769t
life cycle, 769f
Trichinella spiralis, 768, 769t, 791
life cycle, 769f
pulmonary disease, 984t
skin lesions, 956t
see also Trichinellosis
Trichinella zimbabwensis, 768, 769t
life cycle, 769f
Trichinellosis, 768–773
agent, 768
clinical features, 769–771
eosinophilia, 942t–943t
neurologic involvement, 1019t
ocular involvement, 1015
pruritus, 959t–961t
skin lesions, 946t
diagnosis, 771–772, 772t
epidemiology, 768–769, 770t
eradication, 76, 77t–79t
incubation period, 929b
pathogenesis and immunity, 771
prevention and control, 773
treatment and prognosis, 772–773
Trichinellotic syndrome, 769–770
Trichiniasis *see* Trichinellosis
Trichinosis *see* Trichinellosis
Trichloroacetic acid, HPV, 537
Trichobilharzia spp., 849–850
Trichocephalus spp., 791
Trichomonas spp., 1–2
Trichomonas hominis, 623
Trichomonas tenax, 631–632
Trichomonas vaginalis, eradication, 85, 88t–89t
Trichomoniasis
diagnosis, 1038t
treatment, 1040t
Trichophyton spp., 559

Trichophyton concentricum, 560t
tinea imbricata, 561, 561f
Trichophyton gourvilii, 560t
Trichophyton megninii, 560t
Trichophyton mentagrophytes, 560t, 561
onychomycosis, 562
tinea capitis, 560
tinea corporis, 561
tinea cruris, 561
tinea pedis, 562
Trichophyton rubrum, 560t
onychomycosis, 562
tinea corporis, 561
tinea cruris, 561
tinea pedis, 562
Trichophyton schoenleinii, 560t
tinea capitis, 560–561
Trichophyton soudanenese, 560t
Trichophyton tonsurans, 560t
onychomycosis, 562
tinea capitis, 561, 561f
Trichophyton verrucosum, 560t, 561
tinea capitis, 560
Trichophyton violaceum, 560t
tinea capitis, 561
Trichophyton yaoundei, 560t
Trichostrongyliasis, 942t
Trichostrongylus spp., 779–780, 780f
eradication, 77t–79t
Trichostrongylus axei, 780
Trichostrongylus capricola, 780
Trichostrongylus colubriformis, 780
Trichostrongylus orientalis, 780
Trichostrongylus probolurus, 780
Trichostrongylus skrjabini, 780
Trichostrongylus vitrinus, 780
Trichuriasis, 5, 791–793
clinical features, 791
diagnosis, 793
epidemiology, 791
eradication, 76, 77t–79t
pathogenesis and immunity, 791–793
prevalence, 792f
prevention and control, 793
treatment and prognosis, 793
Trichuris spp., 791
Trichuris muris, 793
Trichuris suis, 793
Trichuris trichiura, 791
diarrheal disease, 924
life cycle, 792f
see also Trichuriasis
Trichuroidea, 791
Triclabendazole
Fasciola hepatica, 80
fascioliasis, 861
intestinal flukes, 867
paragonimiasis, 865
Trifluridine, 102t
herpesviruses, HSV, 359
Trimethoprim
E. coli infection, 119
malaria, 664
Salmonella resistance, 130t
Trimethoprim-sulfamethoxazole, 90, 96t–98t, 99
adverse reactions, 611–612
basidiobolomycosis, 604
Campylobacter spp., 148
chemoprophylaxis, 555
cholera, 155–156, 155t
cyclosporiasis, 88t–89t, 642–643, 918t
cystoisosporiasis, 88t–89t
E. coli infection, 119
granuloma inguinale, 1035t
granulomatous amebic encephalitis, 712
histoplasmosis, 575
isosporiasis, 643–644, 918t
melioidosis, 222
mycobacterial infections, 247
P. jirovecii, 86t–87t
paracoccidioidomycosis, 584
pertussis, 214
plague, 282
pneumocystis pneumonia, 104t
pneumocystosis, 611–613
retinochoroiditis, 727
S. pneumoniae resistance, 201
Salmonella spp.
bacteremia, 135
drug resistance, 129, 130f
salmonellosis, 135
shigellosis, 143f, 143t
typhoid/paratyphoid, 125t
urinary tract infection, 1041–1042
Trismus, 284–285
Trocara virus, 520t
Trombiculid mites, 51, 873
life cycle, 334, 335f
scrub typhus transmission, 334, 873
Tropheryma whipplei, 1002
Trophozoites, 614
Tropical enteropathy, 924
Tropical infectious diseases, 7
Tropical phagedenic ulcer, 953f
Tropical pulmonary eosinophilia, 945
eradication, 77t–79t
lymphatic filariasis, 733
Tropical spastic paraparesis, 545, 1022
Tropical splenomegaly syndrome, 976t–977t
Tropical sprue, 924
Tropical ulcer, 967t–968t
Trousseau's sign, 286
Trovofloxacin, donovanosis, 197
Trypanosoma spp., 48–49, 682, 683f
life cycle, 682, 684f
variant surface glycoprotein, 682–683, 685
Trypanosoma brucei brucei, 682
Trypanosoma brucei gambiense, 6–7, 90, 682
animal infection, 684
treatment regimen, 688t
vector, 683, 877
see also Trypanosomiasis, African
Trypanosoma brucei rhodesiense, 90, 682, 683f
treatment regimen, 688t
vector, 683, 877
see also Trypanosomiasis, African
Trypanosoma cruzi, 7, 45, 90, 552, 689, 725–726
distribution, 689–691
epizootiology, 689
geographic distribution, 690f
life cycle, 690f
trypomastigotes, 691f
vectors, 50, 689, 690f–691f
see also Chagas' disease
Trypanosoma rangeli, 689
Trypanosomatidae, 696
Trypanosomiasis
African, 17, 21, 682–688
agent, 682–683
clinical features, 685, 917t, 959t–966t, 1010
diagnosis, 686
differential diagnosis, 686
distribution, 684f
epidemiology, 683–684
HIV coinfection, 1052
pathogenesis and immunity, 685–686
prevention and control, 687–688
case-finding, 688
treatment and prognosis, 90–94, 91t–92t, 686–687, 688t
Winterbottom's sign, 1017
American *see* Chagas' disease
Tsetse flies, 46, 50, 682–683, 877, 877f
TSST-1, 210
Tsutsugamushi disease *see* Scrub typhus
Tuberculin skin test, 228–230
false positives, 229
Tuberculoma, 234
Tuberculosis, 3, 17, 21, 228–247, 988–989
agent, 228
barriers to control, 18–20
case history, 17–18, 18f
as complication of TNF inhibitor treatment, 233
control, 243–244
BCG vaccine, 64t–65t, 243–244
diagnosis, 238–239
drug resistance, 237–238
acquired, 238, 238b
multidrug resistance, 237–238
primary, 238
treatment options, 243
epidemiology, 228–230
effect of immigration, 902, 904t
USA, 903f
extrapulmonary, 233–236
cutaneous, 967t–968t
gastrointestinal bleeding, 920
hepatobiliary, 976t–977t, 981
meningeal, 231, 233–236, 235f
miliary, 231, 233–234, 234f, 235t
ocular involvement, 999, 999f
oropharyngeal lesions, 919
treatment, 242
tuberculous pleurisy, 233–234
gastrointestinal symptoms, 917t
genetic associations, 37–38
protection, 35t
susceptibility, 35t
HIV coinfection, 229, 232–233, 232f, 552, 1058
paradoxical reactions, 242
treatment, 242–243
immunocompromised patients, 232
incubation period, 929b
infection risk, 228
IRIS, 234–236
latent infection, 229
treatment, 244–245, 244b
military cases, 910–911
overseas medical screening, 904t, 905f
and paracoccidioidomycosis, 583
pathogenesis and immunity, 236–238
pediatric, 232, 242
pregnancy and lactation, 242, 1079–1080
primary, 230
Ghon complex, 230, 230f
Ranke complex, 230, 230f
Simon's foci, 230, 230f
progressive primary, 231
reactivation (postprimary), 231–232
chest X-ray, 231, 231f
symptoms, 231
remote arrested, 230f
risk factors for progression to active disease, 230
spread of, 228
symptoms
cough, 986
pleural effusion, 988t
travelers, 892
treatment, 239–243, 239t
DOT, 241
drug resistance, 243
first-line drugs, 239–240
initial regimens, 241–242, 241b
latent infection, 244–245, 244b
patient compliance, 241
second-line drugs, 240
see also individual drugs
Tuberculous meningitis, 231, 233–236, 235f
CSF findings, 235
diagnosis, 236
symptoms, 235
treatment, 236, 1023
Tuberculous peritonitis, 920
Tuberculous radiculomyelitis, 1023
Tuberculous spondylitis, 234, 235f, 273t
TUBEX test, 125
Tula virus, 470

Tularemia
agent *see Francisella tularensis*
incubation period, 929b
ocular involvement, 1002
skin lesions, 967t–968t
transmission, 875t
ulceroglandular, 261–262
Tumbu fly, 870
Tumor necrosis factor-α, 27, 56
cysticercosis, 819
disease associations, 36t
malaria, 37t, 657–658
Tumors *see* Cancer
Tunga penetrans, 959t–961t
Tungiasis, 959t–966t
Turbatrix aceti, 778–779
Turkish sheep encephalitis virus, 516f
TyphiDot test, 125
Typhoid/paratyphoid, 121–127, 916
agent, 121–122
chronic carriers, 123
clinical features, 123, 917t
bacteremia, 124
hepatitis, 976t–977t
ileal perforation, 921
ocular involvement, 1003
complications, 123
intestinal perforation and hemorrhage, 123, 124f
diagnosis, 124–125
antigen detection, 124
clinical bacteriology, 124
nucleic acid-based detection, 124
serodiagnosis, 125
epidemiology, 122
gastrointestinal bleeding, 920
genetic protection, 35t
genetic susceptibility, 35t
geographic distribution, 122
host factors, 124
immune response, 124
incidence, 122
incubation period, 929b
modes of transmission, 122
molecular epidemiology, 122
pathogenesis, 123–124
pregnancy, 1080
prevention and control, 126–127
safe water/food, 126
relapse, 123
reservoirs of infection, 122
seasonality, 122
treatment and prognosis, 125–126
antimicrobials, 125–126, 125t, 918t
corticosteroids, 126
vaccines, 64t–65t, 126–127, 127t, 888t–890t, 892
Typhus, 3, 329–333
agent, 329
bioterrorism, 333
clinical features, 330–331
pruritus, 959t–961t
rash, 331f
diagnosis, 332
epidemic, 882–883
epidemiology, 329–330, 330f
louse-borne, 329, 330f–331f
murine, 329–331
clinical features, 331
pathogenesis and immunity, 331–332
prevention and control, 333
scrub, 334–338
agent, 334–336
diagnosis, 337
disease, 336
epidemiology, 334
pathogenesis and immunity, 336–337
prevention and control, 338
treatment and prognosis, 338
treatment and prognosis, 332–333
vaccine, 333
Typhus group rickettsioses, 329–333
incubation period, 929b
Tyuleniy virus, 516f
Tzanck test, 359

U

Uganda S virus, 492
Ulcerative enteritis, 808
Ulcerative skin conditions, 962, 962f, 962t–966t
Buruli ulcer, 248–252, 953f
differential diagnosis, 967t–968t
fungal, 969t–970t
tropical phagedenic ulcer, 953f
tropical ulcer, 967t–968t
Ulcers
chiclero, 698t, 699
duodenal, 169, 169f
gastric, 169, 169f
genital *see* Genital ulcer disease
Ultrasound, onchocerciasis, 747
Una virus, 520t
Uncinaria stenocephala, 800t, 957
Uncinariasis, 801
Undulant fever, 883
UNICEF, Bamako Initiative, 19
United Nations, Prequalified Vaccines, 66–67
Urea breath test, 172f
Ureaplasma urealyticum, ocular disease, 1001
Urease test, 171
Ureidopenicillins, 96t–98t
Urethral syndromes
men, 1042
women, 1041
Urethritis
C. trachomatis, 316t
men, 316
women, 316
gonococcal, 184–185
men, 1034t
treatment, 1040t
women, 1034t
Urinary salmonellosis, 132t–133t
Urinary tract infection, 1033
candidal, 593–594
men, 1042
clinical features, 1042
diagnosis, 1042
management, 1042, 1043f
women, 1041
clinical features, 1041
diagnosis, 1041
management, 1041
see also Sexually transmitted diseases
Urticaria *see* Pruritus
US-Mexico Border Infectious Disease Surveillance, 105–106
USA
Centers for Disease Control and Prevention, 105
Division of Global Migration and Quarantine, 904
Global Disease Detection Program, 107, 907
Chagas' disease, 691
coccidioidomycosis, 577
electronic disease notification system, 906
Enhanced Refugee Health Program Initiative, 906–908, 907f
immigration
classification of medical conditions, 904
health screening, 902–903
number admitted, 903f
overseas medical screening, 903–905, 904f–905f, 904t
health conditions identified through, 905–906, 905t
refugee arrivals, 903f
trichinellosis, 770t
tuberculosis, 903f
User fees, 19–20
Uta, 698t, 699
Uukuniemi virus, 462
Uveitis, 1005b
leptospirosis, 304f
loaiasis, 737

V

V proteins, 352–353
VacA, 168–169
Vaccination *see* Immunization; Vaccines
Vaccines, 17, 62–70
amebiasis, 621
anthrax, 264
arenaviruses, 461
bacterial diseases, 69t
BCG, 64t–65t, 243–244
Brucella, 275
cancer-related diseases, 69t
Chlamydia trachomatis, 315
cholera, 64t–65t, 156, 888t–890t, 891
development, 67–68
basic science/discovery, 67
clinical research, 68
economics of, 63–64
preclinical, 67–68
priority diseases, 68–70, 69b, 69t
diphtheria, 64t–65t, 226–227
diphtheria/tetanus/pertussis, 888t–890t
diphtheria/tetanus/polio, 64t–65t
enteric diseases, 69t
fascioliasis, 861–862
H. influenzae, 64t–65t, 194, 195f
hantaviruses, 480
hepatitis, 69t
hepatitis A, 64t–65t, 69t, 423, 888t–890t, 891
hepatitis A/hepatitis B, 888t–890t
hepatitis B, 64t–65t, 69t, 437, 888t–890t, 891–892
hepatitis E, 426
herpesviruses
cytomegalovirus, 362
varicella zoster virus, 361
HIV, 556
HPV, 65t, 538–539, 539t
HRSV, 380t, 385
human adenovirus, 380t
human metapneumovirus, 380t
human parainfluenza virus, 380t
hypersensitivity to components of, 890
influenza, 64t–65t, 380t, 383, 888t–890t
Japanese encephalitis, 64t–65t, 513, 888t–890t, 892
leprosy, 260
malaria, 674–675, 674f
measles, 64t–65t, 348–351, 888t–890t
contraindications, 348
live vaccine, 348
maintenance of status, 350
Moraten strain, 348
Pan American Health Organization campaign, 349
meningitis, 64t–65t, 183
meningococcal disease, 183, 888t–890t, 891–892
mumps, 64t–65t, 888t–890t
National Regulatory Authorities, 68
Nipah virus, 354
parasitic diseases, 69t
pertussis, 214
plague, 282–283
pneumococcal disease, 202, 888t–890t
poliovirus, 42–43, 64t–65t, 399, 404–405, 888t–890t
Q fever, 346
rabies, 64t–65t, 529–531, 531f, 888t–890t, 892
respiratory diseases, 69t
Rift Valley fever, 465
rotavirus, 64t–65t, 409
rubella, 64t, 66b, 888t–890t

safety, 67
simultaneous administration, 887
smallpox, 374–375
STDs, 69t
tapeworms, 814
tetanus, 288
tetanus/diphtheria, 888t–890t
tick-borne encephalitis, 888t–890t
travelers, 63
typhoid/paratyphoid, 64t–65t, 126–127, 127t, 888t–890t, 892
new generation vaccines, 126–127
Ty21a live oral vaccine, 126
Vi polysaccharide parenteral vaccine, 126
typhus, 333
varicella zoster virus, 361, 888t–890t
vector-borne viral diseases, 69t
West Nile virus, 514
yellow fever, 64t–65t, 499–500, 888t–890t, 891
adventitious viruses, 500
adverse events, 501
dose, route of administration and preparations, 500
efficacy, 501
failure of, 501
genetic stability, 500
HIV patients, 503
immune response, 500
prior flavivirus immunity, 500–501
revaccination, 500
safety, 501
viremia after, 500
zoonotic diseases, 69t
see also Immunization; and individual diseases
Vaccinia, 369, 375–376
skin lesions, 972t
Vaccinia immune globulin, 375–376
Vagabond fever, 297
Vaginal discharge, 1034t, 1038–1041
clinical features, 1038, 1038t
diagnosis, 1039
management, 1039–1041, 1040f, 1040t
Vaginal microbicidal agents, 190
Vaginal neoplasia, 534
Vaginitis, 1034t
differential diagnosis, 1038t
treatment, 1040t
Vaginosis *see* Bacterial vaginosis
Vaginulus plebeius, 776
Vahlkampfia spp., 709
Valaciclovir, 102t
genital herpes, 1035t
herpesviruses, 356
HSV, 359
varicella zoster virus, 361
Valganciclovir, 102t
herpesviruses, cytomegalovirus, 362
Vancomycin, 96t–98t, 98
anthrax, 264
Borrelia infections, 300
cellulitis, 210–211
Clostridium difficile, 164
MRSA, 211
pneumococcal meningitis, 201
red-man syndrome, 98
staphylococcal toxic shock syndrome, 210
Vannella spp., 709
Variable membrane proteins, 298
Varicella, 23, 358f, 359–360
clinical features, 358f, 360
ocular disease, 994
congenital varicella syndrome, 360
Varicella zoster virus, 355, 356t, 359–361
agent, 359
clinical features, 358f, 360
ocular disease, 994, 994f
skin lesions, 972t
diagnosis, 361
drug therapy, 104t
epidemiology, 360
pathogenesis and immunity, 360
prevention and control, 361
superinfection, 360
treatment and prognosis, 361
vaccine, 361, 888t–890t
requirements for immigrants, 908t
Variola, 369–370
clinical features, 370–371, 972t
major, 369–370
major *see* Smallpox
minor, 369–370
Rao classification, 370–371
sine eruptione, 370–371
Variolation, 374
Varivax vaccine, 356
Vascular endothelial ligands, 658–659
Vasculitis, 178b
VCAM, 658–659
Vector competence, 46–47
Vector longevity, 48
Vector potential, 46–47
Vector-borne disease transmission, 45–51
arthropods, 45
basic reproductive rate, 48
control, 51
defecation, 48–49
extrinsic incubation period, 45
host location, 46
host specificity, 46
life cycle, 45
life span, reproductive capacity and abundance, 45–46
saliva, 49
transovarial transmission, 48
see also individual vectors
Vectorial capacity, 47–48, 47f
Vecuronium, tetanus, 287–288
Venereal syphilis, 289
Venereal warts *see* Genital warts
Venezuelan equine encephalitis, 519, 520t, 876t
as bioterrorism agent, 882
clinical features, 523
diagnosis, 524
epidemiology, 521–522, 521f
prevention and control, 524
treatment and prognosis, 524
Venezuelan hemorrhagic fever, 442t–443t, 450t
agent *see* Guanarito virus
clinical features, 456
epidemiology, 453
pathologic features, 446t
transmission, 454, 932t
Ventricular neurocysticercosis, 817, 818f
treatment, 821
Verruca vulgaris, 534
Verruga peruana, 265, 266f, 266t
pathogenesis and immunity, 268
skin lesions, 267f
Vesicular skin lesions, 966–971, 972t
differential diagnosis, 972t
Vesiculovirus, 525
Vesivirus, 411
Viannia spp., 696
Vibrio spp., noncholera, 157–161
carriage, 157–158
diagnosis, 161
disease, 160
ecology, distribution and seasonality, 159
encapsulation, 161
endemic areas, 158f
epidemiology, 157–160
host factors, 160
incidence, 157
pathogenesis and immunity, 160–161
prevention and control, 161
prognosis, 161
transmission, 158–159, 159f
treatment, 161
Vibrio alginolyticus, 157, 158t
Vibrio carchariae, 26, 157, 158t
Vibrio cholerae, 5, 138–139, 150, 158t, 917t
as bioterrorism agent, 880t
classical, 150
El Tor, 150–151
immune response, 154
Inaba, 150
life cycle, 152f
molecular epidemiology, 153
nonepidemic, 157–158, 158t
encapsulation, 161
Ogawa, 150
pathogenesis, 153–154
serotypes, 150
toxin, 113, 114t–115t
see also Cholera
Vibrio cincinnatiensis, 26, 157, 158t
Vibrio damsela, 157, 158t
Vibrio fluvialis, 157–158, 158t
Vibrio furnissii, 157, 158t
Vibrio metschnikovii, 26, 157, 158t
Vibrio mimicus, 157–158, 158t
Vibrio parahaemolyticus, 157–158, 158t
dissemination, 159f
distribution, 159
human illness, 159
pathogenicity, 160
Vibrio vulnificus, 26, 157–158, 158t
distribution, 159
encapsulation, 161
host factors, 160
human illness, 159
skin lesions, 956t, 972t
Vidarabine, 102t
herpesviruses, 356
Epstein-Barr virus, 364
HSV, 359
varicella zoster virus, 361
Vif, 543
Vinblastine, Kaposi's sarcoma, 368
Vincent's angina, 263
Vinchuca see Kissing bugs
Vincristine, Kaposi's sarcoma, 368
Vinegar eelworm, 778–779
Violin spider, 872
Viral encephalitides, 882
Viral hemorrhagic fevers, 441–448
agent, 441, 442t–445t
as bioterrorism agents, 879, 880t, 882
diagnosis, 885
clinical features, 444t
ocular involvement, 996
petechiae/purpura, 955t
diagnosis, 441–447, 447t
HIV coinfection, 1061–1062
pathogenesis and immunity, 441, 446t
treatment and prevention, 447, 448t
see also individual diseases and viruses
Viral infections, 1
in bioterrorism, 881–882
HIV coinfection, 1061–1064
meningitis, 178b
ocular involvement *see* Ocular disease, viral infection
respiratory tract *see* Respiratory viral infections
treatment see antivirals
see also individual viruses
Viroids, 1
Virulence, 2
alteration of, 2
source-sink model, 2
Virusoids, 1
Visceral larva migrans, 763, 764t, 765
eosinophilia, 942t–943t
skin lesions, 946t, 962t–966t
Vitamin A, 24–25
deficiency, 23, 28
immune effects, 24b, 30
measles, 25, 348, 992f
prevalence, 31

malabsorption, 27–28
mortality, 348
requirements, e12t–e13t
supplements, 23, 25
Vitamin B_1 *see* Thiamine
Vitamin B_2 *see* Riboflavin
Vitamin B6 *see* Pyridoxine
Vitamin B_{12}
deficiency, 1027, 1029
requirements, e12t–e13t
Vitamin C, requirements, e12t–e13t
Vitamin D_3, requirements, e12t–e13t
Vitamin E, requirements, e12t–e13t
Vitamin K, requirements, e12t–e13t
Vittaforma corneae, 714, 715t
eradication, 86t–87t
Vomiting
giardiasis, 627t
trichinellosis, 770
Voriconazole, 100t–101t
blastomycosis, 577
candidemia, 596
candidiasis, esophageal, 592
chromoblastomycosis, 570
cryptococcosis, 581
histoplasmosis, 575
phaeohyphomycosis, 572
toxicity, 101t
Vpr, 543
Vpu, 543, 545
Vulpes ferrilata, 824
Vulvar intraepithelial neoplasia, 534
treatment, 538
Vulvovaginal candidiasis, 589, 592–593
diagnosis, 1038t
treatment, 1040t

W

Wakana disease, 802
Wangiella dermatitidis, 569, 571, 571f
Warfarin, pleural effusion, 988t
Wasting, severe, 30
Water, precautions, 892–893
Water fleas, 759
Waterborne pathogens, 883, 900
WEEV virus, 520t
Weight loss, giardiasis, 627t
Weil-Felix test, 337
Weil's disease, 303, 307
Wernicke-Korsakoff dementia, e12t–e13t
Wesselsbron virus, 492
West Nile encephalitis, 105, 876t
West Nile virus, 7, 511–512, 516f
clinical features, 512
diagnosis, 513
incubation period, 929b
pathogenesis and immunity, 512
pathology, 512
prevention and control, 514
skin lesions, 957t
treatment and prognosis, 513
Western equine encephalitis, 520t, 876t
Whataroa virus, 520t
Whipple's disease, ocular involvement, 1002
Whipworm *see* Trichuriasis
Whitewater Arroyo virus, 450f
WHO
Bamako Initiative, 19
definition of anemia, 1024
Global Foodborne Infections Network, 107
Global Outbreak Alert and Response Network, 106–107, 880
HIV/AIDS classification system, 558b
Poliovirus Laboratory Network, 399–400
recommendations
antiretroviral therapy, 557t
rabies postexposure prophylaxis, 530t
Roll Back Malaria campaign, 20–21
Safe Injection Global Network (SIGN), 432
vaccine programs, 66, 66b
Working Together for Health, 19
Whooping cough *see* Pertussis
Widal test, 125, 918–919
Widow spider, 872, 872f
Wilcoxon matched rank test, 13
Winterbottom's sign, 1017
Wiskott-Aldrich syndrome, 34t
Wohlfahrtia magnifica, 870, 1016
Wolbachia spp., 339
complications of filariasis, 343
endosymbionts, 745–746, 746f
Wolbachia pipientis, 339
Women
genital warts, 538
gonococcal infection, 185–187
gonorrhea, 187
lymphogranuloma venereum, 316–317
pelvic inflammatory disease, 190t, 1034t, 1042–1044
C. trachomatis, 316–317, 316t
urethral syndromes, 1041
urethritis, 316, 1034t
urinary tract infection, 1041
see also Pregnancy
Woolsorter's disease, 263
World Health Organization *see* WHO
Wound infections, multidrug-resistant, 915
Wuchereria spp., 48–49
Wuchereria bancrofti, 77t–79t, 729, 737
life cycle, 730f
lymphatic filariasis, 729
ocular involvement, 752–753
pulmonary disease, 984t
skin lesions, 946t

X

X-linked agammaglobulinemia, 34t
X-linked immunodeficiency syndromes, 34t
Xenopsylla spp., 276–277, 844–845
Xenopsylla cheopis, 330, 876
Xerophthalmia, 23–25, 31, 993f, e12t–e13t
vitamin A deficiency, 992–993, 992f

Y

Yaws, 289, 292–294
clinical features, 293f
pigmentation changes, 973t
skin lesions, 952t, 962t–966t
eradication, 40
transmission, 290f
Yellow fever, 5, 303, 442t–443t, 492–503, 516f, 876t
agent, 492–493
genetic variation, 492–493
replication, 492
viral structure, 492, 493t
clinical features, 444t–445t, 495–497, 496f
coagulation defects, 497–498
encephalopathy, 498
hepatic failure, 497
hypotension and shock, 498
myocarditis, 406, 497
renal failure, 497
triphasic disease, 496–497
diagnosis, 447t, 499
epidemiology, 493–495
disease susceptibility, 495
geographic distribution and incidence, 495
geography, 493, 493f
mosquito vectors, 494
seasonality, 495
transmission patterns and ecology, 493–494, 494f
vertebrate hosts, 495
eradication, 40
immune response
adaptive, 498–499
innate, 498
incubation period, 929b
mortality, 497
pathogenesis and pathophysiology, 497
pathologic features, 446t
pregnancy, 1080–1081
prevention, 448t
prevention and control, 499–503
personal protection, 499
prognosis, 499
risk factors for illness, 497
skin lesions, 956t
transmission, 932t
treatment, 448t, 499
vaccine, 64t–65t, 499–500, 888t–890t, 891
adventitious viruses, 500
adverse events, 501
dose, route of administration and preparations, 500
efficacy, 501
failure of, 501
genetic stability, 500
HIV patients, 503
immune response, 500
prior flavivirus immunity, 500–501
revaccination, 500
safety, 501
viremia after, 500
Yellow fever vaccine-associated neurologic disease, 502–503
risk assessment, 503
risk factors, 503
thymus and autoimmune disease, 503
Yellow fever vaccine-associated viscerotropic disease, 501–502
risk assessment, 503
risk factors, 503
thymus and autoimmune disease, 503
Yellow jacket, 870f
Yersinia spp., 113
vectors, 50
Yersinia enterocolitica, 4, 917
toxin, 114t–115t
Yersinia pestis, 3–4, 276–277, 277f
agent, 276–277
as bioterrorism agent, 880t, 881
diagnosis, 885
biotypes, 277
life cycle, 279f
pathogenesis and immunity, 280–281
see also Plague
Yersinia pseudotuberculosis, 4, 277
toxin, 114t–115t
Yersiniosis, 917t
Yokose virus, 516f

Z

Zaire ebolavirus, 483, 485t
Zalcitabine, 103t
HIV, 553
Zanamivir, 102t
influenza, 380t, 382
Zidovudine, 103t
avoidance in anemia, 1028
HIV, 553
Salmonella bacteremia, 135
Ziehl-Neelsen stain
M. leprae, 253
M. tuberculosis, 238
M. ulcerans, 255, 256f
Zika virus, 511, 514
Zinc
deficiency, 23, 25–26
immune effects, 24b, 30
requirements, e12t–e13t

supplements
acute diarrhea, 26
malaria, 26
Zinc protease, 5
Zizania aquatic, 865
Zonula occludens toxin, 154
Zoonotic filariasis, 750–758
agent, 750, 751t
clinical features, 752–754
eye infections, 752–753, 752f–753f
lung infections, 753, 753f
lymphatic infections, 753–754, 754f
microfilarial infections, 754
subcutaneous infections, 752, 752f
diagnosis, 754–757
Brugia, 755–756, 756f
Dipetalonema-like species, 756
Dirofilaria, 755, 755f–756f
Onchocerca, 756, 756f–757f
species of uncertain origin, 757, 757f
epidemiology, 750–752, 751f
life cycle, 751f
prevention and control, 758
treatment and prognosis, 758
Zostavax vaccine, 356, 361
Zoster *see* Varicella-zoster virus
Zygodontomys spp., 276
Zygodontomys brevicauda, 442t–443t, 450f, 453–454
Zygomycetes, 597
Zygomycosis, 597